Bailey's
Head and Neck Surgery—
OTOLARYNGOLOGY

FIFTH EDITION

SECTION EDITORS

Basic Science/General Medicine
Shawn D. Newlands
Karen T. Pitman

Rhinology and Allergy
Berrylin J. Ferguson
Matthew W. Ryan

General Otolaryngology
David E. Eibling
Shawn D. Newlands

Laryngology
Milan R. Amin
Michael M. Johns III

Trauma
Grant S. Gillman
Jonathan M. Sykes
Stephen S. Park

Pediatric Otolaryngology
Margaretha L. Casselbrant
Charles M. Myer III

Head and Neck Surgery
Christine G. Gourin
Anna M. Pou

Sleep Medicine
Ryan J. Soose
Edward M. Weaver

Otology
Barry E. Hirsch
Robert K. Jackler

Facial Plastic and Reconstructive Surgery
Grant S. Gillman
Jonathan M. Sykes
Stephen S. Park

Contemporary Issues in Medical Practice
Shawn D. Newlands
Karen T. Pitman

Radiology
Barton F. Branstetter

VOLUME TWO

Bailey's
Head and Neck Surgery—
OTOLARYNGOLOGY

FIFTH EDITION

■ **JONAS T. JOHNSON, MD**

Professor and Chairman, Department of Otolaryngology
The Dr. Eugene N. Myers Professor and Chairman of Otolaryngology
Professor, Department of Radiation Oncology, University of Pittsburgh School
  of Medicine
Professor, Department of Oral and Maxillofacial Surgery, University of Pittsburgh
  School of Dental Medicine
Pittsburgh Pennsylvania

■ **CLARK A. ROSEN, MD**

Professor, Department of Otolaryngology
University of Pittsburgh Medical Center
Director, University of Pittsburgh Voice Center
Professor, Department of Communication Sciences Disorders
University of Pittsburgh
Pittsburgh, Pennsylvania

380 Contributors

Illustrations by Victoria J. Forber, Anthony Pazos
  and Christine Gralapp

🔹 Wolters Kluwer | Lippincott Williams & Wilkins
Health

Philadelphia · Baltimore · New York · London
Buenos Aires · Hong Kong · Sydney · Tokyo

Acquisitions Editor: Ryan Shaw
Product Manager: Dave Murphy
Production Project Manager: David Saltzberg
Marketing Manager: Lisa Lawrence
Manufacturing Manager: Beth Welsh
Design Manager: Steven Druding
Production Services: SPi Global

Fifth Edition

Copyright © 2014 Lippincott Williams & Wilkins, a Wolters Kluwer business.

Fourth Edition © 2006 Lippincott Williams & Wilkins
Third Edition © 2001 Lippincott Williams & Wilkins
Second Edition ©1998 Lippincott- Raven Publishers

351 West Camden Street
Baltimore, MD 21201

Two Commerce Square
2001 Market Street
Philadelphia, PA 19103

Printed in China

Library of Congress Cataloging-in-Publication Data
Bailey's head and neck surgery—otolaryngology / [edited by] Jonas T. Johnson, Clark A. Rosen. — 5th ed.
        p. ; cm.
    Head and neck surgery—otolaryngology
    Otolaryngology
    Rev. ed. of: Head & neck surgery—otolaryngology / [edited by] Byron J. Bailey. 4th ed. c2006.
    Includes bibliographical references and index.
    ISBN 978-1-60913-602-4
    I. Johnson, Jonas T. II. Rosen, Clark A. III. Bailey, Byron J., 1934– IV. Head & neck surgery—otolaryngology. V. Title: Head and neck surgery—otolaryngology. VI. Title: Otolaryngology.
    [DNLM: 1. Otorhinolaryngologic Diseases—surgery. 2. Head—surgery. 3. Neck—surgery. WV 168]
    RF51
    617.5'1059—dc23

2013011054

DISCLAIMER
Care has been taken to confirm the accuracy of the information present and to describe generally accepted practices. However, the authors, editors, and publisher are not responsible for errors or omissions or for any consequences from application of the infor-mation in this book and make no warranty, expressed or implied, with respect to the currency, completeness, or accuracy of the contents of the publication. Application of this information in a particular situation remains the professional responsibility of the practitioner; the clinical treatments described and recommended may not be considered absolute and universal recommendations.

The authors, editors, and publisher have exerted every effort to ensure that drug selection and dosage set forth in this text are in accordance with the current recommendations and practice at the time of publication. However, in view of ongoing research, changes in government regulations, and the constant flow of information relating to drug therapy and drug reactions, the reader is urged to check the package insert for each drug for any change in indications and dosage and for added warnings and precau-tions. This is particularly important when the recommended agent is a new or infrequently employed drug.

Some drugs and medical devices presented in this publication have Food and Drug Administration (FDA) clearance for lim-ited use in restricted research settings. It is the responsibility of the health care provider to ascertain the FDA status of each drug or device planned for use in their clinical practice.

To purchase additional copies of this book, call our customer service department at **(800) 638-3030** or fax orders to **(301) 223-2320**. International customers should call (301) 223-2300.

Visit Lippincott Williams & Wilkins on the Internet: http://www.lww.com. Lippincott Williams & Wilkins customer service repre-sentatives are available from 8:30 am to 6:00 pm, EST.

CCS0513

9 8 7 6 5 4 3 2 1

CONTENTS

Contributing Authors xiii
Foreword xxix
Preface xxxi

VOLUME ONE

SECTION I: BASIC SCIENCE/GENERAL MEDICINE 1

1   Surgical Anatomy of the Head and Neck 3
Michael D. Maves

2   Basic Surgical Principles 18
A. Bradley Boland and Emily Rogers

3   Perioperative Management Issues 26
David M. Barrs

4   Operative Technologies 49
Paul G. van der Sloot and Runhua Hou

5   Critical Care 55
Jon D. Simmons and Kimberly A. Donnellan

6   Dynamic Wound Healing 75
Gina D. Jefferson

7   Understanding Data and Interpreting the Literature 86
Richard M. Rosenfeld

8   Outcomes Research and Evidence-Based Medicine 102
Michael G. Stewart

9   Introduction to Otolaryngic Genetics 111
Selena E. Heman-Ackah and Anil K. Lalwani

10   Microbiology, Infections, and Antibiotic Therapy 131
Thuy-Anh N. Melvin and Murugappan Ramanathan Jr.

11   Head and Neck Imaging 141
Tanya J. Rath

12   Surgical Pathology in Otolaryngologic Practice 178
Matthew C. Miller and Christa L. Whitney-Miller

13   Neurology in Otolaryngology 199
Rachel E. Roditi and Benjamin T. Crane

14   Ophthalmology 217
Jean Edwards Holt and G. Richard Holt

15   Anesthesiology 235
Stewart J. Lustik and Shawn D. Newlands

16   Endocrinology 250
Paul G. van der Sloot and Runhua Hou

17   Rheumatologic, Granulomatous, and Other Systemic Diseases Affecting the Head and Neck 267
Valentin D. Marian, Anurag Gandhi, and Shawn D. Newlands

18   Geriatric Otolaryngology 298
David E. Eibling and Sarah H. Kagan

19   Headache and Facial Pain 305
Chase H. Miller and Alfredo S. Archilla

20   Complementary and Alternative Medicine 316
Li-Xing Man and Nicholas C. Sorrel

21   Tobacco Cessation: How-to Guidance and Resources for Practitioners 329
Henry R. Diggelmann and Grant S. Hamilton III

22   Palliative Care and Pain Management 340
Robert M. Taylor and Amit Agrawal

SECTION II: RHINOLOGY AND ALLERGY 357

23   Sinonasal Anatomy and Physiology 359
Randy M. Leung, William E. Walsh, and Robert C. Kern

24   Olfaction 371
Eric H. Holbrook and Donald A. Leopold

25   Immunology and Allergy 379
Mohamad Raafat Chaaban and Robert M. Naclerio

26   Allergy Testing 412
James W. Mims

27   Diagnostic Imaging 422
Jenny K. Hoang and Adam M. Becker

28   Diagnostic Tools for Sinonasal Disease and Role of Office Imaging 446
Luke Rudmik and Timothy L. Smith

29   Allergic Rhinitis 460
James T. O'Neil and James W. Mims

30 Nonallergic Rhinitis 469
    Teresa V. Chan

31 Systemic Diseases that Affect the Nose
    and Sinuses 489
    David A. Zopf and Mark A. Zacharek

32 Epistaxis 501
    Benjamin S. Bleier and Rodney J. Schlosser

33 Acute Rhinosinusitis 509
    Elizabeth K. Hoddeson and Sarah K. Wise

34 Chronic Rhinosinusitis with Nasal Polyposis 525
    Matthew W. Ryan

35 Nonpolypoid Rhinosinusitis: Pathogenesis,
    Diagnosis, Staging, and Treatment 535
    Zara M. Patel and Peter H. Hwang

36 The Unified Airway 550
    Jeb M. Justice and Richard R. Orlandi

37 Fungal Rhinosinusitis 557
    Robert T. Adelson, Bradley F. Marple, and
    Matthew W. Ryan

38 Complications of Rhinosinusitis 573
    Carla M. Giannoni

39 Medical Management of Chronic Sinusitis 586
    Jeffrey D. Suh and Alexander G. Chiu

40 Endoscopic Sinus Surgery for Chronic
    Rhinosinusitis 595
    Barry M. Schaitkin and Kenneth D. Rodriguez

41 External Approaches in Sinus Surgery 604
    Carlos D. Pinheiro-Neto and Carl H. Snyderman

42 Septoplasty, Turbinate Reduction, and Correction
    of Nasal Obstruction 612
    Neal C. Gehani and Steven M. Houser

43 Endoscopic Orbital and Lacrimal Surgery 622
    Erik Kent Weitzel and Raymond I. Cho

44 Complications of Sinus Surgery 638
    James A. Stankiewicz and Kevin C. Welch

45 Endoscopic Evaluation and Treatment of CSF
    Leaks 662
    Pete S. Batra

46 Frontal Sinus Surgery 675
    Yuresh S. Naidoo and Peter-John Wormald

SECTION III: GENERAL OTOLARYNGOLOGY 689

47 Anatomy and Physiology of the Salivary
    Glands 691
    Rohan R. Walvekar, Bridget C. Loehn, and
    Meghan N. Wilson

48 Nonneoplastic Diseases of the Salivary
    Glands 702
    Rohan R. Walvekar and Matthew A. Bowen

49 Outcomes, Effectiveness, and Quality of Life:
    Measuring Clinical Effectiveness 717
    Maureen Hannley

50 Taste 729
    Natasha Mirza

51 Stomatitis 736
    Richard O. Wein and Miriam O'Leary

52 Pharyngitis 757
    Stephen R. Hoff and Kay W. Chang

53 Odontogenic Infections 770
    Timothy D. Doerr

54 Management of Temporomandibular Joint Pain
    and Dysfunction 782
    Joseph J. Fantuzzo and Sveta Karelsky

55 Deep Neck Infections 794
    Behrad B. Aynehchi and Gady Har-El

SECTION IV: LARYNGOLOGY 815

56 Upper Digestive Tract Anatomy and Physiology 817
    Libby J. Smith and Roxann Diez Gross

57 Functional Assessment of Swallowing 825
    Maggie A. Kuhn and Peter C. Belafsky

58 Nonsurgical Management of Swallowing
    Disorders 838
    Shaum S. Sridharan, Cathy L. Lazarus,
    and Milan R. Amin

59 Esophageal Disorders 852
    Catherine Rees Lintzenich

60 Management of Intractable Aspiration 859
    David E. Eibling

61 Upper Airway Anatomy and Function 868
    Gayle E. Woodson

62 Upper Airway Stenosis: Evaluation
    and Management 879
    Philip A. Weissbrod and Albert L. Merati

63 Complex Upper Airway Problems 896
    Jay B. Tuchman and Deepak K. Mehta

64 Advanced Airway Management—Intubation
    and Tracheotomy 908
    Karen M. Kost

65 Voice: Anatomy, Physiology, and Clinical
    Evaluation 945
    Lucian Sulica

66 Laryngopharyngeal Reflux 958
    Joel H. Blumin and Nikki Johnston

67 Infection, Infiltration, and Benign Neoplasms
    of the Larynx 978
    Craig R. Villari and Melissa M. Statham

68 Benign Vocal Fold Lesions and
    Phonomicrosurgery 989
    John W. Ingle and Clark A. Rosen

69 Treatment of Vocal Fold Paralysis 1004
    VyVy N. Young and C. Blake Simpson

70 Neurologic Disorders of the Larynx 1026
    John P. Ney and Tanya K. Meyer

71 Voice Therapy for the Treatment of Voice
    Disorders 1048
    Jackie Gartner-Schmidt

72 Care of the Professional Voice 1059
    Julina Ongkasuwan and Mark S. Courey

73 Office-Based Procedures in Laryngology 1078
    Manish D. Shah and Michael M. Johns III

SECTION V: TRAUMA 1091

74 Principles of Trauma 1093
    Peter J. Koltai and James Chan

75 Management of Soft Tissue Injuries
    of the Face 1108
    Scott Shadfar and William W. Shockley

76 Penetrating Face and Neck Trauma 1131
    Michael G. Stewart

77 Laryngeal Trauma 1141
    J. Randall Jordan, Byron K. Norris,
    and Scott P. Stringer

78 Principles in Rigid Fixation of the Facial
    Skeleton 1153
    Robert M. Kellman and Sherard A. Tatum

79 Surgical Approaches to the Craniofacial
    Skeleton 1171
    John F. Hoffmann

80 Mandibular Fractures 1195
    Brett A. Miles and Jesse E. Smith

81 Midface Fractures 1209
    Brendan C. Stack Jr., and Francis P. Ruggiero

82 Orbital Fractures 1225
    Clinton D. Humphrey and J. David Kriet

83 Nasal Fractures 1241
    Grant S. Gillman and Carlos M. Rivera-Serrano

84 Frontal Sinus Fractures 1255
    E. Bradley Strong

85 Pediatric Facial Fractures 1272
    Peter C. Revenaugh and Paul Krakovitz

SECTION VI: PEDIATRIC OTOLARYNGOLOGY 1285

86 Pediatric Otolaryngology 1287
    Stephen C. Maturo and Michael Cunningham

87 Congenital Aerodigestive Tract
    Anomalies 1306
    Christopher T. Wootten and Charles M. Myer III

88 Neonatal Respiratory Distress 1328
    Mark Boston

89 Stridor, Aspiration, and Cough 1338
    Joseph E. Dohar and Samantha Anne

90 Laryngeal Stenosis 1356
    Michael J. Rutter, Aliza P. Cohen, and Alessandro de
    Alarcón

91 Pediatric Voice 1372
    Susan Baker Brehm, Melissa M. Statham, and
    Alessandro de Alarcón

92 Pediatric Tracheotomy 1382
    Jeffrey P. Simons

93 Ingestion Injuries and Foreign Bodies in the
    Aerodigestive Tract 1399
    Warren K. Yunker and Ellen M. Friedman

94 Recurrent Respiratory Papillomatosis 1409
    Craig S. Derkay and Cristina M. Baldassari

95 Adenotonsillar Disease in Children 1430
    Anita Jeyakumar, Sean Miller, and Ron B. Mitchell

96 Congenital Anomalies of the Nose 1445
    John P. Bent and David E. Conrad

97 Pediatric Rhinosinusitis 1455
    Rodney P. Lusk

98 Salivary Gland Disease in Children 1467
    Matthew K. Whitley and Karen B. Zur

99 Otitis Media in the Age of Antimicrobial
    Resistance 1479
    Margaretha L. Casselbrant and Ellen M. Mandel

100 Pediatric Audiology and Implantable Hearing
    Devices 1507
    David H. Chi and Diane L. Sabo

101 Nongenetic Hearing Loss 1523
    Margaret A. Kenna

102 Genetic Hearing Loss 1541
     John Greinwald and Catherine Hart

103 Comprehensive Cleft Care 1556
     *Alexander J. Davit III, Todd Otteson,
     and Joseph E. Losee*

104 Congenital Vascular Lesions 1574
     Ravindhra G. Elluru

105 Head and Neck Masses in Children 1589
     Cuneyt M. Alper and Jacob G. Robison

106 Congenital Cysts and Sinuses of the Head
     and Neck 1607
     Robert F. Yellon

107 The Syndromal Child 1617
     Ted L. Tewfik

VOLUME TWO

SECTION VII: HEAD AND NECK SURGERY 1643

108 Head and Neck Tumor Biology 1645
     Alec Vaezi and Jennifer R. Grandis

109 Principles of Patient Care 1672
     *Rohan R. Walvekar, Marcie C. Tauzin, and Neelima
     Tammareddi*

110 Principles of Radiation Oncology 1682
     Umamaheswar Duvvuri and Gregory J. Kubicek

111 Chemoradiation 1692
     Christine G. Gourin and Arlene A. Forastiere

112 Therapeutic Options for Patients Who Fail
     Primary Chemoradiation 1708
     Steven B. Cannady and Mark K. Wax

113 Cutaneous Malignancy 1723
     Cherie-Ann O. Nathan and Timothy S. Lian

114 Malignant Melanoma of the Head and
     Neck Region 1739
     *Aaron J. Berger, Jeffrey N. Myers, Andrew J. Nemechek,
     and Mike Yao*

115 Salivary Gland Neoplasms 1760
     *Young S. Oh, Matthew S. Russell, and David
     W. Eisele*

116 Lip Cancer 1788
     *Liana Puscas, Michael A. Fritz, and Ramon M.
     Esclamado*

117 Neck Dissection 1807
     Jesus E. Medina and Nilesh R. Vasan

118 Controversies in Management of the N0 Neck
     in Squamous Cell Carcinoma of the Upper
     Aerodigestive Tract 1839
     Ryan Case and Karen T. Pitman

119 Oral Cavity Cancer 1849
     Daniel G. Deschler and Audrey B. Erman

120 Nasopharyngeal Carcinoma 1875
     William Ignace Wei and Daniel T. T. Chua

121 Oropharyngeal Cancer 1898
     Anna M. Pou and Jonas T. Johnson

122 Hypopharyngeal and Cervical Esophageal
     Carcinoma 1917
     Mihir Kiran Bhayani and Randal S. Weber

123 Early Laryngeal Cancer 1940
     *Parul Sinha, Oluwafunmilola Okuyemi, and Bruce H.
     Haughey*

124 Advanced Laryngeal Cancer 1961
     *Bridget C. Loehn, Melda Kunduk, and Andrew J.
     McWhorter*

125 Voice Rehabilitation Following Laryngectomy 1978
     Anna M. Pou

126 Tracheal Tumors 1990
     Kevin L. Potts and Jeffrey M. Bumpous

127 Vascular Tumors of the Head and Neck 1999
     Mark Persky and Spiros Manolidis

128 Lymphomas of the Head and Neck 2032
     *Raymond L. Chai, Andrew B. Tassler, and
     Seungwon Kim*

129 Neoplasms of the Nose and Paranasal Sinuses 2044
     Lee A. Zimmer and Ricardo L. Carrau

130 Orbital Tumors 2063
     *Neda Esmaili, Michael E. Stadler, and Adam M.
     Zanation*

131 Cranial Base Surgery 2081
     *Carlos D. Pinheiro-Neto, Carl H. Snyderman, and Paul
     A. Gardner*

132 Odontogenic Cysts, Tumors, and Related Jaw
     Lesions 2097
     *William L. Chung, Kurt F. Summersgill, and
     Mark W. Ochs*

133 Treatment of Thyroid Neoplasms 2115
     *Irene Zhang, Samantha DeMauro-Jablonski, and
     Robert L. Ferris*

134 Hyperparathyroidism: Evaluation
     and Surgery 2131
     Maisie L. Shindo

SECTION VIII: SLEEP MEDICINE 2147

135 Sleep Medicine for the Otolaryngologist 2149
     Pell Ann Wardrop and Kathleen L. Yaremchuk

136 Medical Therapy for Obstructive Sleep
     Apnea 2174
     Ryan J. Soose and Patrick J. Strollo

137 Nasal and Palatal Surgery for OSA 2191
     Peter D. O'Connor and Tucker Woodson

138 Hypopharyngeal and Skeletal Surgery
     for OSA 2206
     Eric James Kezirian and Edward M. Weaver

139 Pediatric Sleep-Disordered Breathing 2220
     Stacey L. Ishman, David F. Smith, and Sally R. Shott

SECTION IX: OTOLOGY 2237

140 Development of the Ear 2239
     *Michael John Wareing, Anil K. Lalwani, Abbas A.
     Anwar, and Robert K. Jackler*

141 Anatomy and Physiology of Hearing 2253
     Peter C. Weber and Samir Khariwala

142 Assessment of Peripheral and Central Auditory
     Function 2274
     James W. Hall III and Patrick J. Antonelli

143 Vestibular Function and Anatomy 2291
     J. Christopher Holt and Shawn D. Newlands

144 Vestibular and Balance Laboratory
     Studies 2302
     *Neil T. Shepard, Kristen L. Janky, and Jaynee A.
     Handelsman*

145 Neurophysiologic Intraoperative
     Monitoring 2314
     *Brannon D. Mangus, Betty S. Tsai, and David S.
     Haynes*

146 Diseases of the External Ear 2333
     Christopher J. Linstrom and Frank E. Lucente

147 Neoplasms of the Ear and Lateral
     Skull Base 2358
     Bradley P. Pickett and Brianna K. Crawley

148 Congenital Malformation of the Ear 2384
     Paul R. Lambert

149 Intratemporal and Intracranial Complications
     of Otitis Media 2399
     H. Alexander Arts and Meredith E. Adams

150 Middle Ear and Temporal Bone Trauma 2410
     Rodney C. Diaz, Sally M. Kamal, and Hilary A. Brodie

151 Cholesteatoma 2433
     *Ted A. Meyer, Chester L. Strunk Jr., and
     Paul R. Lambert*

152 Surgery of the Mastoid and Petrosa 2447
     *Richard A. Chole, Hilary A. Brodie, and
     Abraham Jacob*

153 Reconstruction of the Tympanic Membrane
     and Ossicular Chain 2465
     John L. Dornhoffer and Michael B. Gluth

154 Otosclerosis 2487
     *Brandon Isaacson, Joe Walter Kutz Jr., and Peter S.
     Roland*

155 Acute Paralysis of the Facial Nerve 2503
     Jeffrey T. Vrabec and Jerry W. Lin

156 Otologic Manifestations of Systemic Disease:
     Includes Autoimmune Inner Ear Disease 2519
     Arnaud F. Bewley and Michael J. Ruckenstein

157 Noise-Induced Hearing Loss 2530
     Robert A. Dobie

158 Ototoxicity 2542
     Kay W. Chang

159 Cerebellopontine Angle Tumors 2556
     Matthew L. Bush and D. Bradley Welling

160 Sudden Sensory Hearing Loss 2589
     Eric R. Oliver and George T. Hashisaki

161 Tinnitus and Hyperacusis 2597
     Maura K. Cosetti and Pamela C. Roehm

162 Aging and the Auditory and Vestibular
     System 2615
     *Joe Walter Kutz Jr., Brandon Isaacson, and
     Peter S. Roland*

163 Cochlear Implants and Other Implantable
     Auditory Prostheses 2624
     Oliver F. Adunka and Craig A. Buchman

164 Hearing Aids and Assistive Listening
     Devices 2654
     Catherine V. Palmer and Barry E. Hirsch

165 Clinical Evaluation of the Patient with
     Vertigo 2673
     Courtney C. J. Voelker and Joel A. Goebel

166 Peripheral Vestibular Disorders 2701
     Yuri Agrawal, Lloyd B. Minor, and John P. Carey

167 Central Vestibular Disorders 2717
     Gail Ishiyama and Akira Ishiyama

168 Vestibular Rehabilitation 2733
     Susan L. Whitney and Yael Raz

169 Regenerative Strategies for Overcoming
     Deafness 2747
     Alan G. Cheng and Stefan Heller

SECTION X: FACIAL PLASTIC AND RECONSTRUCTIVE SURGERY 2755

170 Preoperative Evaluation and Facial Analysis in
     Facial Plastic Surgery 2757
     Andrew Winkler and Justin M. Wudel

171 Pictorial Documentation: Digital Imaging and
     Traditional Photography 2772
     Andrew K. Patel, Amir M. Karam, and Samuel M. Lam

172 Grafts and Implants in Facial, Head, and Neck
     Surgery 2784
     G. Richard Holt and Christian L. Stallworth

173 Local Cutaneous Flaps and Grafts 2797
     Brian Jewett

174 Reconstructive Microsurgery of the Head
     and Neck 2824
     Douglas B. Chepeha

175 Tissue Expanders 2849
     Jonathan Liang and Jonathan M. Sykes

176 Scar Camouflage 2859
     Shawn M. Stevens and Krishna G. Patel

177 Nasal Reconstruction 2871
     Stephen S. Park

178 Facial Reanimation 2905
     Tessa A. Hadlock

179 Surgical Anatomy of the Nose: A Foundation
     for Rhinoplasty 2919
     David W. Kim and Ted Mau

180 Rhinoplasty: Incisions, Approaches
     and Analysis 2941
     Grant S. Gillman

181 The Nasal Dorsum: Management of the Upper
     Two-Thirds of the Nose 2952
     Randolph B. Capone and Ira D. Papel

182 Nasal Tip Surgery 2964
     Tatiana K. Dixon and Dean M. Toriumi

183 Management of the Crooked Nose 2977
     Craig S. Murakami and Richard A. Zoumalan

184 Revision Rhinoplasty 2989
     Richard E. Davis

185 The Aging Forehead 3053
     Kian Karimi and Peter A. Adamson

186 Upper Eyelid Blepharoplasty 3074
     Jonathan M. Sykes and Christina K. Magill

187 Lower Eyelid Blepharoplasty 3085
     Stephen W. Perkins and Jess Prischmann

188 Rhytidectomy (Face-Lift) 3103
     Russell W. H. Kridel and Zahi Abou Chacra

189 The Aging Neck 3131
     Edwin Francis Williams and Henry Haipei Chen

190 Otoplasty: Anatomy, Embryology, and
     Technique 3142
     Steven Ross Mobley and Nathan Todd Nelson Schreiber

191 Congenital Auricular Malformation 3161
     Eugenio A. Aguilar III and Anthony Echo

192 Chin Augmentation 3176
     Jonathan M. Sykes and Christina K. Magill

193 Redefining Skin Resurfacing: The Hetter Chemical
     Peel 3189
     Devinder S. Mangat

194 Lasers in Facial Plastic Surgery 3200
     William Russell Ries and Joseph E. Hall

195 Management of Benign Facial Lesions 3212
     Karen J. Sundby, and John A. Zitelli

196 Management of Alopecia 3229
     Raymond J. Konior and Steven Gabel

197 Cosmetic Uses of Neurotoxins and Injectable
     Fillers 3239
     Grant S. Gillman

SECTION XI: CONTEMPORARY ISSUES IN MEDICAL PRACTICE 3253

198 Patient Safety 3255
     David E. Eibling

199 Business Law and the Practice of
     Otolaryngology 3270
     *Robert S. Iwrey, Stephanie P. Ottenwess, Jessica L.
     Gustafson, Kathryn Hickner-Cruz, David M. Ottenwess,
     and Reginald Baugh*

200 Compliant Documentation, Coding, and Billing
     in the Practice of Otolaryngology—Head and Neck
     Surgery 3303
     Stephen R. Levinson

201 Clinic Management 3332
     Dana E. Habers and Scott P. Stringer

202 Comparative Medical Systems 3341
     William Anthony Wood

203   **Effective Education in Medical Practice** 3349
      John M. Schweinfurth

204   **Medical Informatics and Databases** 3354
      John C. Sok and Richard K. McHugh

205   **Telemedicine for Otolaryngology** 3361
      John Kokesh, Chris Patricoski, and A. Stewart Ferguson

206   **Quality Improvement in Otolaryngology** 3372
      Rahul K. Shah, Jean Brereton, and David W. Roberson

207   **Conflict of Interest** 3380
      Andrew H. Murr and Susan J. Murr

Subject Index I-1

CONTRIBUTING AUTHORS

MEREDITH E. ADAMS, MD   Assistant Professor, Departments of Otolaryngology–Head and Neck Surgery and Neurosurgery, University of Minnesota; Attending Surgeon, Departments of Otolaryngology–Head and Neck Surgery and Neurosurgery, University of Minnesota Medical Center, Fairview, Minneapolis, Minnesota

PETER A. ADAMSON, BSc, MD, FRCSC, FACS   Professor, Head, Division of Facial Plastic and Reconstructive Surgery, Department of Otolaryngology–Head and Neck Surgery, University of Toronto, Toronto, Ontario, Canada

ROBERT T. ADELSON, MD   Chief, Division of Facial Plastic and Reconstructive Surgery, Assistant Professor, Department of Otolaryngology, University of Florida College of Medicine, Gainesville, Florida

OLIVER F. ADUNKA, MD   Associate Professor, Department of Otolaryngology–Head and Neck Surgery, University of North Carolina at Chapel Hill; Attending Physician, Department of Otolaryngology–Head and Neck Surgery, UNC Health Care, Chapel Hill, North Carolina

AMIT AGRAWAL, MD   Associate Professor, Department of Otolaryngology–Head and Neck Surgery, The Ohio State University; Attending Surgeon, Department of Otolaryngology–Head and Neck Surgery, Arthur G. James Cancer Hospital and Richard J. Solove Research Institute, The Ohio State University Wexner Medical Center, Columbus, Ohio

YURI AGRAWAL, MD   Assistant Professor, Division of Otology, Neurotology and Skull Base Surgery, Department of Otolaryngology–Head and Neck Surgery, The Johns Hopkins University School of Medicine, Baltimore, Maryland

EUGENIO A. AGUILAR III, MD   Professor, Division of Plastic Surgery, Department of Surgery, Baylor College of Medicine, Houston, Texas

CUNEYT M. ALPER, MD   Professor, Departments of Otolaryngology, University of Pittsburgh School of Medicine; Pediatric Otolaryngologist, Department of Pediatric Otolaryngology, Children's Hospital of Pittsburgh of UPMC, Pittsburgh, Pennsylvania

H. ALEXANDER ARTS, MD   Professor, Department of Otolaryngology and Neurosurgery, University of Michigan, Ann Arbor, Michigan

MILAN R. AMIN, MD   Associate Professor, Department of Otolaryngology–Head and Neck Surgery, New York University School of Medicine; Associate Professor, Department of Otolaryngology–Head and Neck Surgery, NYU Langone Medical Center, New York, New York

SAMANTHA ANNE, MD, MS   Assistant Professor of Surgery, Head and Neck Institute, Cleveland Clinic Foundation, Cleveland, Ohio

PATRICK J. ANTONELLI, MD, MS   Professor and Chair, Department of Otolaryngology, University of Florida; Chair, Department of Otolaryngology, Shands at the University of Florida, Gainesville, Florida

ABBAS A. ANWAR, MD   Resident Physician, PGY-1, Department of Otolaryngology–Head and Neck Surgery, New York University Langone Medical Center, New York, New York

ALFREDO S. ARCHILLA, MD   Director, Center for Advanced Sinus and Nasal Care, Otolaryngology Consultants, PA, Boynton Beach, Florida

BEHRAD B. AYNEHCHI, MD   Assistant Clinical Instructor, Department of Otolaryngology–Head and Neck Surgery, SUNY Downstate Medical Center, Brooklyn, New York

ALESSANDRO DE ALARCÓN, MD, MPH   Assistant Professor, Department of Otolaryngology, University of Cincinnati College of Medicine; Assistant Professor, Department of Otolaryngology, Cincinnati Children's Hospital Medical Center, Cincinnati, Ohio

CRISTINA M. BALDASSARI, MD, FAAP   Assistant Professor, Department of Pediatric Otolaryngology, Eastern Virginia Medical School; Assistant Professor, Department of Pediatric Otolaryngology, Children's Hospital of the King's Daughters, Norfolk, Virginia

DAVID M. BARRS, MD   Consultant, Department of Otolaryngology, Mayo Clinic Arizona, Phoenix, Arizona

PETE S. BATRA, MD, FACS   Associate Professor, Department of Otolaryngology–Head and Neck Surgery, University of Texas Southwestern Medical Center; Co-Director, Comprehensive Skull Base Program, University Hospitals, Dallas, Texas

REGINALD BAUGH, MD   Professor, Department of Surgery, The University of Toledo; Chief, Division of Otolaryngology–Head and Neck Surgery, University of Toledo Medical Center, Toledo, Ohio

ADAM M. BECKER, MD   Assistant Professor of Surgery, Division of Otolaryngology, Department of Surgery, Duke University Medical Center, Durham, North Carolina

PETER C. BELAFSKY, MD, MPD, PhD   Professor, Department of Otolaryngology–Head and Neck Surgery, University of California, Davis Medical Center, Sacramento, California

JOHN P. BENT, MD Associate Professor, Department of Otolaryngology–Head and Neck Surgery, Albert Einstein College of Medicine; Director, Division of Pediatric Otolaryngology, Children's Hospital at Montefiore, Bronx, New York

AARON J. BERGER, MD, PhD Chief Resident, Division of Plastic Surgery, Department of Surgery, Stanford Hospital and Clinics, Palo Alto, California; Chief Resident, Division of Plastic Surgery, Department of Surgery, Stanford Hospital and Clinics, Stanford, California

ARNAUD F. BEWLEY, MD Head and Neck/Microvascular Fellow, Department of Otolaryngology–Head and Neck Surgery, Medical University of South Carolina, Charleston, South Carolina

MIHIR KIRAN BHAYANI, MD Clinical Assistant Professor, Department of Surgery, Pritzker School of Medicine, University of Chicago, Chicago, Illinois; Otolaryngologist, Department of Surgery, Kellogg Cancer Center, North Shore University Health System, Evanston, Illinois

BENJAMIN S. BLEIER, MD Assistant Professor, Department of Otology and Laryngology, Harvard Medical School, Boston, Massachusetts

JOEL H. BLUMIN, MD, FACS Associate Professor and Chief, Division of Laryngology and Professional Voice, Department of Otolaryngology and Communication Sciences, Medical College of Wisconsin, Milwaukee, Wisconsin

A. BRADLEY BOLAND, MD Professor, Department of Surgery, University of Mississippi Medical Center, Jackson, Mississippi

MARK BOSTON, MD Pediatric Otolaryngologist, San Antonio Military Medical Health System, San Antonio, Texas

MATTHEW A. BOWEN, MD Resident Physician, Department of Otolaryngology–Head and Neck Surgery, Louisiana State University Health Sciences Center, New Orleans, Louisiana

SUSAN BAKER BREHM, PhD Associate Professor, Department of Speech Pathology and Audiology, Miami University, Oxford, Ohio; Research Associate, Department of Speech Language Pathology, Cincinnati Children's Hospital Medical Center, Cincinnati, Ohio

D. BRADLEY WELLING, MD, PhD, FACS Professor and Chair, Department of Otolaryngology–Head and Neck Surgery, The Ohio State University; Professor, Department of Otolaryngology–Head and Neck Surgery, The Ohio State University Wexner Medical Center, Columbus, Ohio

BARTON F. BRANSTETTER, MD Professor of Radiology, Otolaryngology, and Biomedical Informatics, Department of Radiology, University of Pittsburgh Medical Center, Pittsburgh, Pennsylvania

JEAN BRERETON, MBA Senior Director, Research and Quality, American Academy of Otolaryngology–Head and Neck Surgery, Alexandria, Virginia

HILARY A. BRODIE, MD, PhD Professor and Chairman, Division of Otology and neurotology, Department of Otolaryngology, UC Davis Health System, Sacramento, California

CRAIG A. BUCHMAN, MD, FACS Harold C. Pillsbury Distinguished Professor, Department of Otolaryngology and Head and Neck Surgery, University of North Carolina at Chapel Hill; Physician Service Leader, Department of Otolaryngology–Head and Neck Surgery, UNC Health Care, Chapel Hill, North Carolina

JEFFREY M. BUMPOUS, MD Professor and Chief, Division of Otolaryngology–Head and Neck Surgery, School of Medicine, University of Louisville, Louisville, Kentucky

MATTHEW L. BUSH, MD Assistant Professor, Department of Otolaryngology–Head and Neck Surgery, University of Kentucky; Chief of Otolaryngology, Department of Surgery, Veterans Affairs Medical Center, Lexington, Kentucky

STEVEN B. CANNADY, MD Assistant Professor, Department of Otolaryngology, SUNY Downstate Medical Center; Chief, Head and Neck Surgery at University Hospital Brooklyn, Department of Otolaryngology, SUNY Downstate Medical Center, Brooklyn, New York

RANDOLPH B. CAPONE, MD Director, Baltimore Center for Facial Plastic Surgery, Baltimore, Maryland

JOHN P. CAREY, MD Professor, Chief, Division of Otology, Neurotology, and Skull Base Surgery, Department of Otolaryngology–Head and Neck Surgery, Johns Hopkins Hospital, Baltimore, Maryland

RICARDO L. CARRAU, MD Professor, Department of Otolaryngology, The Ohio State University College of Medicine; Director of the Comprehensive Skull Base Surgery Program, Department of Otolaryngology, The Ohio State University Wexner Medical Center, Columbus, Ohio

RYAN CASE, MD Resident, Department of Otolaryngology and Communicative Sciences, University of Mississippi Medical Center, Jackson, Mississippi

MARGARETHA L. CASSELBRANT, MD, PhD Eberly Professor of Pediatric Otolaryngology, Department of Otolaryngology, University of Pittsburgh School of Medicine; Director, Department of Pediatric Otolaryngology, Children's Hospital of Pittsburgh of UPMC, Pittsburgh, Pennsylvania

MOHAMAD RAAFAT CHAABAN, MD Rhinology Fellow/Instructor, Division of Otolaryngology–Head and Neck Surgery, Department of Surgery, University of Alabama at Birmingham, Birmingham, Alabama; Director, Lanier Nasal & Sinus Institute, Valley, Alabama

ZAHI ABOU CHACRA, MD Surgeon, Department of Otolaryngology, Westmount Square Medical Center, Westmount, Quebec, Canada

RAYMOND L. CHAI, MD Resident, Department of Otolaryngology, University of Pittsburgh Medical Center, Pittsburgh, Pennsylvania

JAMES CHAN, MD Department of Otolaryngology–Head and Neck Surgery, Providence Medical Center, Portland, Oregon

TERESA V. CHAN, MD Assistant Professor, Department of Otolaryngology–Head and Neck Surgery, University of Texas Southwestern Medical Center; Chief, Department of Otolaryngology–Head and Neck Surgery, Parkland Health and Hospital System, Dallas, Texas

KAY W. CHANG, MD Associate Professor, Department of Otolaryngology, Stanford University, Stanford, California

HENRY HAIPEI CHEN, MD, MBA Attending Physician, Department of Otolaryngology–Head and Neck Surgery, Cedars-Sinai Medical Center, Los Angeles, California

ALAN G. CHENG, MD Assistant Professor, Department of Otolaryngology–Head and Neck Surgery, Stanford University School of Medicine, Stanford, California

DOUGLAS B. CHEPEHA, MD, MSPH, FRCSC Professor and Director of Microvascular, Reconstructive Surgery, Department of Otolaryngology–Head and Neck Surgery, University of Michigan, Ann Arbor, Michigan

DAVID H. CHI, MD Assistant Professor, Department of Otolaryngology, University of Pittsburgh School of Medicine; Pediatric Otolaryngologist, Department of Pediatric Otolaryngology, Children's Hospital of Pittsburgh of UPMC, Pittsburgh, Pennsylvania

ALEXANDER G. CHIU, MD Professor and Chief, Division of Otolaryngology–Head and Neck Surgery, Arizona Health Science Center, University of Arizona, Tucson, Arizona

RAYMOND I. CHO, MD, FACS Assistant Professor, Department of Surgery, Uniformed Services University of the Health Sciences; Director, Oculoplastic and Orbital Surgery, Department of Ophthalmology, Walter Reed National Military Medical Center, Bethesda, Maryland

RICHARD A. CHOLE, MD, PhD Lindburg Professor and Head, Department of Otolaryngology, Washington University School of Medicine; Chief, Department of Otolaryngology, Barnes-Jewish Hospital, St Louis, Missouri

DANIEL T. T. CHUA, MBChB, MD, FRCR, FHKCR, FHKAM Associate Director, Comprehensive Oncology Centre, Associate Director, Department of Radiotherapy, Department of Medicine, Department of Radiotherapy, Hong Kong Sanatorium and Hospital, Hong Kong SAR

WILLIAM L. CHUNG, DDS, MD Associate Professor, Department of Oral and Maxillofacial Surgery, School of Dental Medicine, University of Pittsburgh; Associate Professor, Department of Oral and Maxillofacial Surgery, University of Pittsburgh Medical Center, Pittsburgh, Pennsylvania

ALIZA P. COHEN, MA Medical Writer, Division of Pediatric Otolaryngology–Head and Neck Surgery, Cincinnati Children's Hospital Medical Center, Cincinnati, Ohio

DAVID E. CONRAD, MD Resident, Department of Otorhinolaryngology–Head and Neck Surgery, Albert Einstein College of Medicine–Montefiore Medical Center, Bronx, New York

MAURA K. COSETTI, MD Assistant Professor, Departments of Otolaryngology–Head and Neck Surgery and Neurosurgery, Shreveport, Louisiana

MARK S. COUREY, MD Professor, Department of Otolaryngology–Head and Neck Surgery, University of California, San Francisco; Director, Division of Laryngology, University of California, San Francisco, San Francisco, California

BENJAMIN T. CRANE, MD, PhD Assistant Professor, Department of Otolaryngology, Bioengineering, Neurobiology and Anatomy, University of Rochester; Assistant Professor, Department of Otolaryngology, Strong Memorial Hospital, Rochester, New York

BRIANNA K. CRAWLEY, MD Chief Resident, Department of Surgery, University of New Mexico; Department of Surgery, University of New Mexico Health Sciences Center, Albuquerque, New Mexico

MICHAEL CUNNINGHAM, MD Professor, Department of Otology and Laryngology, Harvard Medical School; Otolaryngologist in Chief, Department of Otolaryngology and Communication Enhancement, Boston Children's Hospital, Boston, Massachusetts

J. DAVID KRIET, MD, FACS WS and EC Jones Chair in Craniofacial Reconstruction, Associate Professor, Director, Division of Facial Plastic and Reconstructive Surgery, Department of Otolaryngology–Head and Neck Surgery, University of Kansas School of Medicine, Kansas City, Kansas

RICHARD E. DAVIS, MD Voluntary Professor of Otolaryngology, Department of Otolaryngology, University of Miami, Miller School of Medicine, Miami, Florida

ALEXANDER J. DAVIT III, MD Assistant Professor, Department of Plastic Surgery, University of Pittsburgh School of Medicine; Attending, Department of Plastic Surgery, Children's Hospital of Pittsburgh of UPMC, Pittsburgh, Pennsylvania

SAMANTHA DeMAURO-JABLONSKI, MD Clinical Assistant Professor, Internal Medicine, University of Pittsburgh; Clinical Assistant Professor, Internal Medicine, University of Pittsburgh Medical Center, Pittsburgh, Pennsylvania

CRAIG S. DERKAY, MD, FACS Professor, Department of Otolaryngology–Head and Neck Surgery, Eastern Virginia Medical School; Director, Department of Pediatric Otolaryngology, Children's Hospital of the King's Daughters, Norfolk, Virginia

DANIEL G. DESCHLER, MD, FACS Professor, Department of Otology and Laryngology, Harvard Medical School; Director, Division of Head and Neck Surgery, Department of Otolaryngology–Head and Neck Surgery, Massachusetts Eye and Ear Infirmary/Massachusetts General Hospital, Boston, Massachusetts

RODNEY C. DIAZ, MD Assistant Professor, Department of Otolaryngology, UC Davis Health System, Sacramento, California

HENRY R. DIGGELMANN, MD Chief Resident, Department of Otolaryngology–Head and Neck Surgery, University of Iowa Hospitals and Clinics, Iowa City, Iowa

TATIANA K. DIXON, MD Fellow, Division of Facial Plastic and Reconstructive Surgery, Department of Otolaryngology–Head and Neck Surgery, University of Illinois at Chicago, Chicago, Illinois

ROBERT A. DOBIE, MD Clinical Professor, Department of Otolaryngology, University of Texas Health Science Center at San Antonio, San Antonio, Texas

TIMOTHY D. DOERR, MD, FACS Associate Professor and Program Director, Department of Otolaryngology–

Head and Neck Surgery, University of Rochester School of Medicine; Director of Facial Plastic Surgery, Department of Otolaryngology, University of Rochester Medical Center, Rochester, New York

JOSEPH E. DOHAR, MD, MS Professor, Department of Otolaryngology, University of Pittsburg School of Medicine; Professor, Staff Otolaryngologist, Department of Pediatric Otolaryngology, Children's Hospital of Pittsburgh of UPMC, Pittsburgh, Pennsylvania

KIMBERLY A. DONNELLAN, MD Adjunct Professor, Department of Surgery, University of South Alabama School of Medicine; Adjunct Professor, IMC Otolaryngology and Facial Plastic Surgery, Mobile Infirmary Medical Center, Mobile, Alabama

JOHN L. DORNHOFFER, MD, FACS Professor and Vice-Chair of Adult Services, Department of Otolaryngology, University of Arkansas for Medical Sciences; Professor and Vice-Chair of Adult Services, Department of Otolaryngology, University Hospital, Little Rock, Arkansas

UMAMAHESWAR DUVVURI, MD, PHD Assistant Professor, Department of Otolaryngology, University of Pittsburgh School of Medicine; Director of Head and Neck Robotic Surgery, Eye and Ear Institute, Pittsburgh, Pennsylvania

ANTHONY ECHO, MD Staff Physician, Division of Plastic Surgery, Department of Surgery, Methodist Institute for Reconstructive Surgery, Houston, Texas

DAVID E. EIBLING, MD, FACS Professor, Department of Otolaryngology–Head and Neck Surgery, University of Pittsburgh School of Medicine; Assistant Chief of Surgery, Surgery Service Line, VA Pittsburgh Healthcare System, University Drive C SSSL, Pittsburgh, Pennsylvania

DAVID W. EISELE, MD, FACS Andelot Professor and Director, Department of Otolaryngology–Head and Neck Surgery, Johns Hopkins University School of Medicine; Department of Otolaryngologist–Head and Neck Surgeon in Chief, The Johns Hopkins Hospital, Baltimore, Maryland

RAVINDHRA G. ELLURU, MD, PHD Associate Professor, Department of Otolaryngology–Head and Neck Surgery, University of Cincinnati College of Medicine; Associate Professor, Department of Pediatric Otolaryngology, Cincinnati Children's Hospital, Cincinnati, Ohio

AUDREY B. ERMAN, MD Assistant Professor, Co-director, Head and Neck Oncology Program, Division of Otolaryngology–Head and Neck Section, University of Arizona College of Medicine, Tucson, Arizona

RAMON M. ESCLAMADO, MD Richard H. Chaney Sr., Professor and Chief, Division of Otolaryngology–Head and Neck Surgery, Department of Surgery, Duke University, Durham, North Carolina

NEDA ESMAILI, MD Clinical Instructor, Section of Oculofacial and Orbital Surgery, Department of Ophthalmology, Medical College of Wisconsin, Milwaukee, Wisconsin

JOSEPH JOHN J. FANTUZZO, DDS, MD Associate Professor, Department of Oral and Maxillofacial Surgery, University of Rochester; Chair and Program Director, Department of Oral and Maxillofacial Surgery, University of Rochester Medical Center, Strong Memorial Hospital, Rochester, New York

A. STEWART FERGUSON, PhD Chief Information Officer (CIO), Health Information Technology, Alaska Native Tribal Health Consortium, Anchorage, Alaska

BERRYLIN J. FERGUSON, MD Professor of Otolaryngology, Director, Division of Sino-Nasal Disorders and Allergy; Assistant Professor, Department of Otolaryngology, University of Pittsburgh School of Medicine, UPMC Mercy, Pittsburgh, Pennsylvania

ROBERT L. FERRIS, MD, PhD, FACS UPMC Endowed Professor, Department of Medicine, Immunology, University of Pittsburgh School of Medicine; Chief, Head and Neck Surgery, Department of Otolaryngology, University of Pittsburgh Medical Center, Pittsburgh, Pennsylvania

ARLENE A. FORASTIERE, MD Professor, Department of Oncology, Johns Hopkins University; Active Staff, The Johns Hopkins Hospital, Baltimore, Maryland

ELLEN M. FRIEDMAN, MD Otolaryngology Center Staff Physician, Texas Children's Hospital, Bobby Alford Chair in Pediatric Otolaryngology; Professor and Chief of Service, Baylor College of Medicine, Houston, Texas

MICHAEL A. FRITZ, MD Staff Member, Department of Otolaryngology, Cleveland Clinic, Cleveland, Ohio

STEVEN GABEL, MD, FACS Gabel Hair Restoration Center, Hillsboro, Oregon

ANURAG GANDHI, MD Fellow, Infectious Disease Division, University of Rochester Medical Center, Rochester, New York; Physician, Infectious Disease, Gadsden Regional Medical Center, Gadsden, Alabama

PAUL A. GARDNER, MD Assistant Professor, Department of Neurology Surgery, University of Pittsburgh School of Medicine; Co-Director, Center for Cranial Base Surgery, University of Pittsburgh Medical Center, Pittsburgh, Pennsylvania

JACKIE GARTNER-SCHMIDT, PHD Associate Professor, Department of Otolaryngology, University of Pittsburgh; Associate Director/Speech Language Pathologist, UPMC Voice Center, UPMC Mercy, Pittsburgh, Pennsylvania

NEAL C. GEHANI, MD Staff Physician, Department of Otolaryngology, Milford Regional Medical Center, Milford, Massachusetts

CARLA M. GIANNONI, MD Associate Professor, Department of Otolaryngology, Baylor College of Medicine; Associate Professor, Department of Pediatric Otolaryngology, Texas Children's Hospital, Houston, Texas

GRANT S. GILLMAN, MD, FRCS Associate Professor, Director, Division of Facial Plastic Surgery, Department of Otolaryngology–Head and Neck Surgery, University of Pittsburgh School of Medicine, Pittsburgh, Pennsylvania

MICHAEL B. GLUTH, MD Assistant Professor, Division of Otolaryngology–Head and Neck Surgery, Department of Surgery, Pritzker School of Medicine University of Chicago; Director, University of Chicago Listening Center, Division of Otolaryngology–Head and Neck Surgery, University of Chicago Medical Center, Chicago, Illinois

JOEL A. GOEBEL, MD, FACS, FRCS Professor and Vice Chairman, Department of Otolaryngology–Head and Neck

Surgery, Washington University School of Medicine; Attending Surgeon, Barnes-Jewish Hospital, St Louis, Missouri

CHRISTINE G. GOURIN, MD, MPH, FACS Associate Professor, Department of Otolaryngology–Head and Neck Surgery, Johns Hopkins University; Active Staff, The Johns Hopkins Hospital, Baltimore, Maryland

JENNIFER R. GRANDIS, MD, FACS Fulltime Faculty, Department of Otolaryngology and Pharmacology, University of Pittsburgh; Fulltime Faculty, Department of Otolaryngology and Pharmacology, University of Pittsburgh School of Medicine, Pittsburgh, Pennsylvania

JOHN GREINWALD, MD, FAAP Professor, Department of Otolaryngology and Pediatrics, University of Cincinnati College of Medicine; Professor, Department of Otolaryngology–Head and Neck Surgery, Auditory Genetics Lab (Director), Cincinnati Children's Hospital Medical Center, Cincinnati, Ohio

ROXANN DIEZ GROSS, PhD Director of Research, The Children's Institute, Pittsburgh, Pennsylvania

JESSICA L. GUSTAFSON, Esq Partner, The Health Law Partners, PC, Southfield, Michigan

DANA E. HABERS, MPH Chief Operating Officer, USC Care Faculty Practice Plan, Keck Medical Center of USC, Los Angeles, California

TESSA A. HADLOCK, MD Director, Facial Nerve Center, Department of Otolaryngology, Massachusetts Eye and Ear Infirmary, Boston, Massachusetts

JOSEPH E. HALL, MD Resident, Department of Otolaryngology, Vanderbilt University Medical Center, Nashville, Tennessee

JAMES W. HALL III, PhD Extraordinary Professor, Department of Communication Pathology, University of Pretoria, Pretoria, South Africa

GRANT S. HAMILTON III, MD Assistant Professor, Department of Otorhinolaryngology, Mayo Clinic; Senior Associate Consultant, Department of Otorhinolaryngology, Mayo Clinic, Rochester, Minnesota

JAYNEE A. HANDELSMAN, PhD Clinical Assistant Professor, Department of Otolaryngology–Head and Neck Surgery, University of Michigan Medical School; Director, Pediatric Audiology, Department of Otolaryngology–Head and Neck Surgery, University of Michigan C.S. Mott Children's Hospital, Ann Arbor, Michigan

MAUREEN HANNLEY, PhD Clinical Associate Professor, Department of Otolaryngology–Head and Neck Surgery, University of Arizona Medical Center, Tucson, Arizona

GADY HAR-EL, MD, FACS Professor, Department of Otolaryngology and Neurosurgery, SUNY Downstate Medical Center, Brooklyn, New York; Chairman, Department of Otolaryngology–Head and Neck Surgery, Lenox Hill Hospital, New York, New York

CATHERINE HART, MD Assistant Professor, Department of Pediatric Otolaryngology, University of Cincinnati College of Medicine; Assistant Professor, Department of Pediatric Otolaryngology–Head and Neck Surgery, Cincinnati Children's Hospital Medical Center, Cincinnati, Ohio

GEORGE T. HASHISAKI, MD Associate Professor, Department of Otolaryngology–Head and Neck Surgery, University of Virginia Health System, Charlottesville, Virginia

BRUCE H. HAUGHEY, MBChB, FACS, FRACS Kimbrough Professor and Director, Head and Neck Surgical Oncology, Department of Otolaryngology–Head and Neck Surgery, Washington University School of Medicine; Kimbrough Professor and Director, Head and Neck Surgical Oncology, Department of Otolaryngology–Head and Neck Surgery, Barnes-Jewish Hospital, St. Louis, Missouri

DAVID S. HAYNES, MD, FACS Professor of Otolaryngology, Neurosurgery and Hearing and Speech Sciences, Neurotology Division/Fellowship Program/Cochlear Implant Program Director, Department of Otolaryngology, Vanderbilt University Medical Center, The Otology Group of Vanderbilt; Vanderbilt University Hospital, Vanderbilt University Medical Center, Nashville, Tennessee

STEFAN HELLER, PhD Professor, Department of Otolaryngology–Head and Neck Surgery, Stanford University School of Medicine, Stanford, California

SELENA E. HEMAN-ACKAH, MD, MBA Clinical Instructor, Division of Otolaryngology, Department of Surgery, Beth Israel Deaconess Medical Center, Boston, Massachusetts

KATHRYN HICKNER-CRUZ, Esq Partner, The Health Law Partners, PC, Southfield, Michigan

BARRY E. HIRSCH, MD Professor, Department of Otolaryngology, Neurological Surgery, and Communication Science and Disorders, University of Pittsburgh, Eye and Ear Institute; Director, Division of Otology/Neurotology, Department of Otolaryngology, Neurological Surgery, and Communication Science and Disorders, University of Pittsburgh Medical Center, Pittsburgh, Pennsylvania

JENNY K. HOANG, MD Assistant Professor of Radiology and Radiation Oncology, Department of Radiology, Duke University, Durham, North Carolina

ELIZABETH K. HODDESON, MD Resident Physician, Department of Otolaryngology–Head and Neck Surgery, Emory University; Resident Physician, Department of Otolaryngology–Head and Neck Surgery, Emory University Hospital, Atlanta, Georgia

STEPHEN R. HOFF, MD Assistant Professor, Department of Otolaryngology–Head and Neck Surgery, Northwestern University, Feinberg School of Medicine, Chicago, Illinois

JOHN F. HOFFMANN, MD, FACS Spokane Center for Facial Plastic Surgery, Spokane, Washington

ERIC H. HOLBROOK, MD Assistant Professor, Department of Otology and Laryngology, Harvard Medical School; Surgeon; Co-Director of the Sinus Center, Department of Otolaryngology–Head and Neck Surgery, Massachusetts Eye and Ear Infirmary, Boston, Massachusetts

G. RICHARD HOLT, MD, D Bioethics Professor Emeritus, Department of Otorhinolaryngology–Head and Neck Surgery, University of Texas Health Science Center at San Antonio, San Antonio, Texas

J. CHRISTOPHER HOLT, PhD Assistant Professor, Department of Otolaryngology and Neurobiology and Anatomy, University of Rochester Medical Center, Rochester, New York

JEAN EDWARDS HOLT, MD, MPH Clinical Professor, Department of Ophthalmology, University of Texas Health Science Center at San Antonio, San Antonio, Texas

RUNHUA HOU, MD Assistant Professor, Division of Endocrinology and Metabolism, Department of Medicine, University of Rochester Medical Center, Rochester, New York

STEVEN M. HOUSER, MD, FAAOA Associate Professor of Otolaryngology, Department of Otolaryngology, Case Western Reserve University School of Medicine; Director of Rhinology, Allergy, and Sinus, Department of Otolaryngology, MetroHealth Medical Center, Cleveland, Ohio

CLINTON D. HUMPHREY, MD, FACS Assistant Professor, Division of Facial Plastic and Reconstructive Surgery, Department of Otolaryngology–Head and Neck Surgery, University of Kansas School of Medicine, Kansas City, Kansas

PETER H. HWANG, MD Professor, Department of Otolaryngology–Head and Neck Surgery, Stanford University School of Medicine; Chief, Division of Rhinology and Endoscopic Skull Base Surgery, Department of Otolaryngology–Head and Neck Surgery, Stanford University School of Medicine, Stanford, California

JOHN W. INGLE, MD Clinical Instructor, Department of Otolaryngology, University of Pittsburgh; Laryngologist/Surgeon, UPMC Voice Center, UPMC Mercy, Pittsburgh, Pennsylvania

BRANDON ISAACSON, MD Associate Professor, Department of Otolaryngology–Head and Neck Surgery, University of Texas Southwestern Medical Center, Dallas, Texas

AKIRA ISHIYAMA, MD Professor, Department of Head and Neck Surgery, UCLA, David Geffen School of Medicine; Surgeon, Department of Head & Neck Surgery, Ronald Reagan UCLA Medical Center, Los Angeles, California

GAIL ISHIYAMA, MD Associate Professor in Residence, Department of Neurology, UCLA, David Geffen School of Medicine; Attending Neurologist, Department of Neurology, Ronald Reagan UCLA Medical Center, Los Angeles, California

STACEY L. ISHMAN, MD, MPH Associate Professor, Department of Otolaryngology–Head and Neck Surgery, Pediatrics, Internal Medicine–Division of Pulmonary and Critical Care, Anesthesia and Critical Care Medicine, Johns Hopkins School of Medicine, Baltimore, Maryland

ROBERT S. IWREY, Esq Partner, The Health Law Partners, PC, Southfield, Michigan

ROBERT K. JACKLER, MD Sewall Professor and Chair, Department of Otolaryngology–Head and Neck Surgery, Stanford University School of Medicine, Stanford, California

ABRAHAM JACOB, MD Associate Professor of surgery and Director of the UA Ear Institute, Division of Otolaryngology, Department of Surgery, The University of Arizona, Tucson, Arizona

KRISTEN L. JANKY, PhD Coordinator, Vestibular Services; Director, Vestibular Lab, Department of Audiology, Boys Town National Research Hospital, Omaha, Nebraska

GINA D. JEFFERSON, MD, MS Assistant Professor, Department of Otolaryngology and Communicative Sciences, University of Mississippi Medical Center, Jackson, Mississippi

BRIAN JEWETT, MD Assistant Professor, Department of Otolaryngology, University of Miami Health Systems, Miami, Florida

ANITA JEYAKUMAR, MD Assistant Professor, Department of Otorhinolaryngology, Louisiana State University Health Science Center; Faculty, Department of Otorhinolaryngology, Children's Hospital New Orleans, New Orleans, Louisiana

MICHAEL M. JOHNS III, MD Associate Professor-Otolaryngology, Director–Emory Voice Center, Emory University, Atlanta, Georgia

KAREN J. JOHNSON, MD Associate Clinical Professor, Department of Dermatology, University of Colorado Health Sciences Center, Denver, Colorado

JONAS T. JOHNSON, MD Professor and Chairman, Department of Otolaryngology; The Dr. Eugene N. Myers Professor and Chairman of Otolaryngology; Professor, Department of Radiation Oncology, University of Pittsburgh School of Medicine; Professor, Department of Oral and Maxillofacial Surgery, University of Pittsburgh School of Dental Medicine, Pittsburgh, Pennsylvania

NIKKI JOHNSTON, PhD Assistant Professor, Director of Airway, Digestive and Voice Research, Division of Research, Department of Otolaryngology and Communication Sciences, Medical College of Wisconsin, Milwaukee, Wisconsin

J. RANDALL JORDAN, MD, FACS Professor and Vice Chair, Department of Otolaryngology Head and Neck Surgery and Communicative Sciences, University of Mississippi Medical Center, Jackson, Mississippi

JEB M. JUSTICE, MD Assistant Professor, Department of Otolaryngology, University of Florida, Gainesville, Florida

SARAH H. KAGAN, PhD, RN Professor-Clinician Educator, University of Pennsylvania School of Nursing; Clinical Nurse Specialist, Abramson Cancer Center at the University of Pennsylvania, Philadelphia, Pennsylvania

SALLY M. KAMAL, MD Resident Physician, Department of Otolaryngology, UC Davis Health System, Sacramento, California

AMIR M. KARAM, MD Director, Carmel Valley Facial Plastic Surgery, San Diego, California

SVETA KARELSKY, MD Assistant Professor, Department of Otolaryngology–Head and Neck Surgery, University of Rochester Medical Center, Rochester, New York

KIAN KARIMI, MD Cosmetic and Reconstructive Facial Plastic Surgeon, Pacific Eye and Ear Specialists, Los Angeles, California

ROBERT M. KELLMAN, MD Professor and Chair, Department of Otolaryngology, SUNY Upstate Medical University, Syracuse, New York

MARGARET A. KENNA, MD, MPH Professor, Department of Otology and Laryngology, Harvard Medical School; Director of Clinical Research, Department of Otolaryngology and Communication Enhancement, Boston Children's Hospital, Boston, Massachusetts

ROBERT C. KERN, MD Professor and Chairman, Department of Otolaryngology–Head and Neck Surgery, Northwestern University; Chairman, Department of Otolaryngology–Head and Neck Surgery, Northwestern Memorial Hospital, Chicago, Illinois

ERIC JAMES KEZIRIAN, MD, MPH Associate Professor in Residence, Department of Otolaryngology–Head and Neck Surgery, University of California, San Francisco, San Francisco, California

SAMIR KHARIWALA, MD Assistant Professor, Department of Otolaryngology, University of Minnesota Medical Center, Minneapolis, Minnesota

SEUNGWON KIM, MD Assistant Professor, Department of Otolaryngology–Head and Neck Surgery, University of Pittsburgh, Pittsburgh, Pennsylvania

DAVID W. KIM, MD, FACS Associate Clinical Professor, Facial Plastic and Reconstructive Surgery, Department of Otolaryngology–Head and Neck Surgery, University of California, San Francisco, San Francisco, California

JOHN KOKESH, MD Chief, Department of Otolaryngology, Alaska Native Medical Center, Anchorage, Alaska

PETER J. KOLTAI, MD, FACS Professor of Otolaryngology and Pediatrics, Department of Otolaryngology–Head and Neck Surgery and Pediatrics, Stanford University School of Medicine, Stanford, California; Chief, Department of Pediatric Otolaryngology, Lucile Packard Children's Hospital, Palo Alto, California

RAYMOND J. KONIOR, MD Clinical Professor, Department of Otolaryngology–Head and Neck Surgery, Loyola University Medical Center, Maywood, Illinois

KAREN M. KOST, MD Assistant Professor, Department of Otolaryngology, McGill University Health Center, Montreal, Quebec, Canada

PAUL KRAKOVITZ, MD, Section Head, Head and Neck Institute, Department of Otolaryngology, Cleveland Clinic, Cleveland, Ohio

RUSSELL W. H. KRIDEL, MD, FACS Clinical Professor and Chief of Division of Facial Plastic Surgery, Department of Otolaryngology–Head and Neck Surgery, University of Texas–Health Science Center at Houston; Facial Plastic Surgeon, Facial Plastic Surgery Associates, Houston, Texas

GREGORY J. KUBICEK, MD Assistant Professor, Department of Radiation Oncology, University of Pittsburgh Medical Center, Pittsburgh, Pennsylvania

MAGGIE A. KUHN, MD Fellow, Laryngology and Broncho-esophagology, Department of Otolaryngology, University of California, Davis Medical Center, Sacramento, California

MELDA KUNDUK, PhD, CCC-SLP Associate Professor, Department of Communication Science and Disorder, Louisiana State University, Baton Rouge, Louisiana

JOE WALTER KUTZ JR, MD Assistant Professor, Department of Otolaryngology–Head and Neck Surgery, University of Texas Southwestern Medical Center, Dallas, Texas

ANIL K. LALWANI, MD Professor and Vice Chairman, Department of Otolaryngology–Head and Neck Surgery, Columbia University College of Physicians and Surgeons; Chief, Division of Otology, Neurotology, and Skull Base Surgery, Director, Columbia Cochlear Implant Program, Department of Otolaryngology–Head and Neck Surgery, New York-Presbyterian Hospital, New York, New York

SAMUEL M. LAM, MD, FACS Director, Willow Bend Wellness Center, Plano, Texas

PAUL R. LAMBERT, MD Professor and Chair, Department of Otolaryngology–Head and Neck Surgery, Medical University of South Carolina, Charleston, South Carolina

CATHY L. LAZARUS, PhD Associate Professor, Department of Otorhinolaryngology–Head and Neck Surgery, Albert Einstein College of Medicine, Bronx, New York; Research Director, THANC Foundation Research Center, Department of Otolaryngology–Head and Neck Surgery, Beth Israel Medical Center, New York, New York

DONALD A. LEOPOLD, MD Professor, Department of Surgery, Division of Otorhinolaryngology–Head and Neck Surgery, University of Vermont; Surgery, Fletcher Allen Health Care, Burlington, Vermont

RANDY M. LEUNG, MD, FRCSC Clinical Lecturer, Department of Otolaryngology–Head and Neck Surgery, University of Toronto; Rhinologist, Department of Otolaryngology–Head and Neck Surgery, Royal Victoria Hospital, Barrie, Ontario, Canada

STEPHEN R. LEVINSON, MD ASA, LLC, Easton, Connecticut

TIMOTHY S. LIAN, MD, FACS Associate Professor, Department of Otolaryngology–Head and Neck Surgery, Louisiana State University-Health, Shreveport; Vice-Chairman, Department of Otolaryngology–Head and Neck Surgery, Louisiana State University-Health, Shreveport, Shreveport, Louisiana

JONATHAN LIANG, MD Resident Physician, Department of Otolaryngology, UC Davis Health System, Sacramento, California

JERRY W. LIN, MD, PhD Otolaryngology Associates, PC, Fairfax, Virginia

CHRISTOPHER J. LINSTROM, MD, CM Professor, Department of Otolaryngology–Head and Neck Surgery, New York Medical College, Valhalla, New York; Surgeon Director, Department of Otolaryngology–Head and Neck Surgery, New York Eye and Ear Infirmary, New York, New York

CATHERINE REES LINTZENICH, MD Associate Professor, Department of Otolaryngology, Wake Forest School of Medicine, Medical Center Boulevard, Winston Salem, North Carolina

BRIDGET C. LOEHN, MD Resident, Department of Otolaryngology, Louisiana State University Health Sciences Center, New Orleans, Louisiana

JOSEPH E. LOSEE, MD, FACS, FAAP Professor and Vice Chair, Department of Plastic Surgery, University of Pittsburgh

Medical Center; Chief, Division of Plastic Surgery, Children's Hospital of Pittsburgh, Pittsburgh, Pennsylvania

FRANK E. LUCENTE, MD   Professor and Former Chairman, Department of Otolaryngology, SUNY Downstate Medical Center, Brooklyn, New York

RODNEY P. LUSK, MD   Director: ENT Institute, Boys Town National Research Center, ENT, Boys Town National Research Center; Boys Town National Research Hospital, ENT, Boys Town National Research Center, Omaha, Missouri

STEWART J. LUSTIK, MD, MBA   Professor, Department of Anesthesiology, University of Rochester Medical Center; Department of Anesthesiology, Strong Memorial Hospital, Rochester, New York

CHRISTINA KENNEY MAGILL, MD   Surgeon, Department of Otolaryngology, Alyeska Facial Plastic Surgery ENT, Anchorage, Alaska

LI-XING MAN, MSc, MD, MPA   Assistant Professor, Department of Otolaryngology–Head and Neck Surgery, University of Rochester–School of Medicine and Dentistry; Attending Physician, Department of Otolaryngology–Head and Neck Surgery, University of Rochester Medical Center, Rochester, New York

ELLEN M. MANDEL, MD   Associate Professor, Department of Otolaryngology, University of Pittsburgh School of Medicine; Research Pediatrician, Department of Pediatric Otolaryngology, Children's Hospital of Pittsburgh of UPMC, Pittsburgh, Pennsylvania

DEVINDER S. MANGAT, MD   Mangat-Kuy-Holzapfel Plastic Surgery, Edgewood, Kentucky

BRANNON D. MANGUS, MD   Resident Physician, Department of Otolaryngology–Head and Neck Surgery, Vanderbilt University Medical Center, Nashville, Tennessee

SPIROS MANOLIDIS, MD   Associate Professor, Department of Otolaryngology, Albert Einstein School of Medicine; Faculty, Department of Otolaryngology, Beth Israel Hospital, New York, New York

VALENTIN D. MARIAN, MD   Administrator Department of Rheumatology, Department of Medicine, Jersey City Medical Center, Jersey City, New Jersey

BRADLEY F. MARPLE, MD   Professor, Vice Chairman, Department of Otolaryngology–Head and Neck Surgery, University of Texas Southwestern Medical Center, Dallas, Texas

STEPHEN C. MATURO, MAJ, USAF, MC, FS   Assistant Professor, Department of Surgery, Uniformed Services University of the Health Sciences, Bethesda, Maryland; Pediatric Otolaryngologist, Department of Otolaryngology, San Antonio Military Medical Center, Fort Sam Houston, Texas

TED MAU, MD   Assistant Professor, Department of Otolaryngology–Head and Neck Surgery, University of Texas Southwestern Medical Center, Dallas, Texas

MICHAEL D. MAVES, MD   Executive Vice President and Chief Executive Officer, American Medical Association, Chicago, Illinois

JESUS E. MEDINA, MD   Paul and Ruth Jonas Professor, Department of Otorhinolaryngology, University of Oklahoma Health Sciences Center, Oklahoma City, Oklahoma

DEEPAK K. MEHTA, MD   Assistant Professor, Department of Otolaryngology, University of Pittsburgh School of Medicine; Assistant Professor, Staff Otolaryngologist, Department of Pediatric Otolaryngology, Children's Hospital of Pittsburgh of UPMC, Pittsburgh, Pennsylvania

THUY-ANH N. MELVIN, MD   Instructor, Department of Otolaryngology–Head and Neck Surgery, Johns Hopkins University School of Medicine; Department of Otolaryngology–Head and Neck Surgery, The Johns Hopkins Hospital, Baltimore, Maryland

ALBERT L. MERATI, MD, FACS   Professor and Chief, Division of Laryngology, Department of Otolaryngology–Head and Neck Surgery, University of Washington School of Medicine; Chief, Laryngology Service, Department of Otolaryngology–Head and Neck Surgery Center, University of Washington Medical Center, Seattle, Washington

TED A. MEYER, MD   Assistant Professor, Director, Cochlear Implant Center, Department of Otolaryngology–Head and Neck Surgery, Medical University of South Carolina, Charleston, South Carolina

TANYA K. MEYER, MD   Assistant Professor, Department of Otolaryngology–Head and Neck Surgery, University of Washington; Attending Surgeon, Department of Otolaryngology–Head and Neck Surgery, University of Washington Medical Center, Seattle, Washington

BRETT A. MILES, DDS, MD   Assistant Professor, Department of Otolaryngology–Head and Neck Surgery, Mount Sinai School of Medicine, New York, New York

CHASE H. MILLER, MD   Associate Professor of Clinical Otolaryngology, Department of Otolaryngology, University of Rochester; Attending, Department of Otolaryngology, Strong Memorial Hospital, Rochester, New York

MATTHEW C. MILLER, MD   Assistant Professor, Department of Otolaryngology–Head and Neck Surgery and Neurosurgery, University of Rochester; Attending Surgeon, Department of Otolaryngology–Head and Neck Surgery and Neurosurgery, University of Rochester Medical Center, Rochester, New York

SEAN MILLER, MD   Resident, Department of Otolaryngology, Saint Louis University, St Louis, Missouri

JAMES W. MIMS, MD   Associate Professor, Department of Otolaryngology, Wake Forest School of Medicine, Medical Center Boulevard; Medical Staff Member, Department of Otolaryngology, Wake Forest Baptist Health, Medical Center Boulevard, Winston Salem, North Carolina

LLOYD B. MINOR, MD   Professor of Otolaryngology–Head and Neck Surgery, Andelot Professor and Director, Department of Otolaryngology–Head and Neck Surgery, Johns Hopkins Outpatient Center, Baltimore, Maryland

NATASHA MIRZA, MD   Professor, Department of Otolaryngology, University of Pennsylvania; Department of Otolaryngology, Hospital of the University of Pennsylvania, Philadelphia, Pennsylvania

RON B. MITCHELL, MD   Professor, Departments of Otolaryngology–Head and Neck Surgery and Pediatrics, William Beckner Distinguished Chair in Otolaryngology,

University of Texas Southwestern Medical Center; Chief, Department of Pediatric Otolaryngology, Children's Medical Center Dallas, Dallas, Texas

STEVEN ROSS MOBLEY, MD Associate Professor, Division of Otolaryngology–Head and Neck Surgery, University of Utah; Attending Physician, Division of Otolaryngology–Head and Neck Surgery, University of Utah Hospitals and Clinics, Salt Lake City, Utah

CRAIG S. MURAKAMI, MD Clinical Associate Professor, Department of Facial Plastic Surgery and Otolaryngology, University of Washington, Virginia Mason Medical Center, Seattle, Washington

ANDREW H. MURR, MD, FACS Professor and Interim Chairman, Roger Boles, M.D. Endowed Chair in Otolaryngology Education, Department of Otolaryngology–Head and Neck Surgery, University of California, San Francisco School of Medicine; Chief of Service, Department of Otolaryngology–Head and Neck Surgery, San Francisco General Hospital, San Francisco, California

SUSAN J. MURR, JD Vice President, Commercial Assurance and Privacy, Becton Dickinson and Company, Franklin Lakes, New Jersey

CHARLES M. MYER III, MD Professor-Vice-Chairman, Department of Otolaryngology–Head and Neck Surgery, University of Cincinnati–Academic Health Center; Residency Program Director, Department of Otolaryngology–Head and Neck Surgery, Cincinnati Children's Hospital Medical Center, Cincinnati, Ohio

JEFFREY N. MYERS, MD, PhD, FACS Hubert L. and Olive Stringer Distinguished Professor in Cancer Research Professor and Director of Research Deputy Chair for Academic Programs, Department of Head and Neck Surgery, University of Texas M.D. Anderson Cancer Center, Houston, Texas

RICHARD K. McHUGH, MD, PhD Assistant Professor, Division of Otolaryngology–Head and Neck Surgery, Department of Surgery, University of Alabama at Birmingham; Assistant Professor of Surgery, Division of Otolaryngology–Head and Neck Surgery, Department of Surgery, UAB Hospital, Birmingham, Alabama

ANDREW J. McWHORTER, MD Associate Professor, Director OLOL/LSU Voice Center, Department of Otolaryngology–Head and Neck Surgery, Louisiana State University Health Sciences Center, New Orleans, Louisiana

ROBERT M. NACLERIO, MD, FACS Professor and Chief, Department of Otolaryngology–Head and Neck Surgery, Surgery, University of Chicago, Chicago, Illinois

YURESH S. NAIDOO, BE, MBBS, FRACS Rhinology and Skull Base Surgeon, Department of Otorhinolaryngology Head and Neck Surgery, Australian School of Advanced Medicine, Macquarie University, Sydney, Australia

CHERIE-ANN O. NATHAN, MD, FACS Professor, Department of Otolaryngology–Head and Neck Surgery, Louisiana State University-Health, Shreveport; Chairman, Department of Otolaryngology–Head and Neck Surgery, Louisiana State University-Health, Shreveport, Shreveport, Louisiana

ANDREW J. NEMECHEK, MD, FACS Assistant Clinical Professor, Otolaryngology–Head and Neck Surgery, Department of Family Medicine, University of Colorado School of Medicine, Aurora, Colorado; Medical Director, Multidisciplinary, Head and Neck Tumor Program, Porter Adventist Hospital, Denver, Colorado

SHAWN D. NEWLANDS, MD, PhD, MBA, FACS Professor and Chair, Department of Otolaryngology, University of Rochester Medical Center; Chief, Department of Otolaryngology, Strong Memorial Hospital, Rochester, New York

JOHN P. NEY, MD, MPH Acting Instructor, Department of Neurology, University of Washington; Attending Neurologist, Department of Neurology, Puget Sound, VAMC, Seattle, Washington

BYRON K. NORRIS, MD ENT of Athens, Academic Institution, Athens, Georgia

MARK W. OCHS, DMD, MD Professor and Chair, Department of Oral and Maxillofacial Surgery, School of Dental Medicine, University of Pittsburgh; Associate Dean for Hospital Affairs, Department of Oral and Maxillofacial Surgery, University of Pittsburgh Medical Center, Pittsburgh, Pennsylvania

PETER D. O'CONNOR, MD, OD Assistant Professor of Surgery, Department of Surgery, Uniformed Services University of the Health Sciences, Bethesda, Maryland; Chief, Sleep Surgery Division, Department of Surgery/ENT Service, San Antonio Military Medical Center, San Antonio, Texas

YOUNG S. OH, MD, FACS Assistant Clinical Professor, Department of Otolaryngology–Head and Neck Surgery, University of California, Irvine School of Medicine; Staff Surgeon, Department of Head and Neck Surgery, Southern California Permanente Medical Group, Kaiser Foundation Hospital–Orange County (CA), Irvine, California

OLUWAFUNMILOLA OKUYEMI, MD Post-Doctoral Research Scholar, Department of Otolaryngology, Washington University School of Medicine; Resident Physician, Department of Otolaryngology–Head and Neck Surgery, Barnes-Jewish Hospital, St Louis, Missouri

MIRIAM O'LEARY, MD Assistant Professor, Department of Otolaryngology–Head and Neck Surgery, Tufts University School of Medicine; Assistant Professor, Department of Otolaryngology–Head and Neck Surgery, Tufts Medical Center, Boston, Massachusetts

ERIC R. OLIVER, MD Assistant Professor, Department of Otolaryngology–Head and Neck Surgery, Wake Forest School of Medicine, Medical Center Boulevard; Assistant Professor, Division of Surgical Science, Wake Forest Baptist Health, Medical Center Boulevard, Winston Salem, North Carolina

JAMES T. O'NEIL, MD Chief Resident, Department of Otolaryngology, Wake Forest School of Medicine; Chief Resident, Department of Otolaryngology, Wake Forest Baptist Hospital, Winston-Salem, North Carolina

JULINA ONGKASUWAN, MD Assistant Professor, Department of Otolaryngology–Head and Neck Surgery, Baylor College of Medicine; Assistant Professor, Department of Otolaryngology–Head and Neck Surgery–Pediatric Otolaryngology, Baylor College of Medicine/Texas Children's Hospital, Houston, Texas

RICHARD R. ORLANDI, MD, FACS Professor, Department of Otolaryngology–Head and Neck Surgery, University of Utah; Professor, Department of Otolaryngology–Head and Neck Surgery, University of Utah Hospital and Clinics, Salt Lake City, Utah

DAVID M. OTTENWESS, Esq Managing Partner, Ottenwess, Allman & Taweel, PLC, Detroit, Michigan

STEPHANIE P. OTTENWESS, Esq Partner, Ottenwess, Allman & Taweel, PLC, Detroit, Michigan

TODD OTTESON, MD, MPH Associate Professor, Department of Otolaryngology, University of Pittsburgh School of Medicine; Pediatric Otolaryngologist, Division of Pediatric Otolaryngology, Children's Hospital of Pittsburgh of UPMC, Pittsburgh, Pennsylvania

CATHERINE V. PALMER, PhD Associate Professor, Communication Science and Disorder, Department of Otolaryngology, University of Pittsburgh; Director, Audiology, Department of Otolaryngology, University of Pittsburgh Medical center, Pittsburgh, Pennsylvania

IRA D. PAPEL, MD Associate Professor, Department of Otolaryngology–Head and Neck Surgery, Johns Hopkins University, Baltimore, Maryland

STEPHEN S. PARK, MD Director, Division of Facial Plastic and Reconstructive Surgery, Department of Otolaryngology–Head and Neck Surgery, University of Virginia, Charlottesville, Virginia

ANDREW K. PATEL, MD Fellow, Department of Otolaryngology, Mayo Clinic Hospital, Phoenix, Arizona

KRISHNA G. PATEL, MD Director of Facial Plastic and Reconstructive Surgery, Medical University of South Carolina, Charleston, South Carolina

ZARA M. PATEL, MD Assistant Professor, Department of Otolaryngology–Head and Neck Surgery, Emory Health Care, Atlanta, Georgia

CHRIS PATRICOSKI, MD, FAAFP Clinical Director of Telemedicine, Health Information Technology, Alaska Native Tribal Health Consortium (ANTHC), Primary Care Physician, Anchorage, Alaska

STEPHEN W. PERKINS, MD, FACS Clinical Associate Professor, Department of Otolaryngology–Head and Neck Surgery, Indiana University School of Medicine; Private Practice, Meridian Plastic Surgery Center, Indianapolis, Indiana

MARK PERSKY, MD Professor of Clinical Otolaryngology, Departments of Otolaryngology, Albert Einstein College of Medicine, Bronx, New York; Chairman, Departments of Otolaryngology–Head and Neck Surgery, Beth Israel Medical Center, New York, New York

BRADLEY P. PICKETT, MD Assistant Professor, Department of Surgery, University of New Mexico; Division of Otology/Neurotology, Department of Surgery, University of New Mexico Health Sciences Center, Albuquerque, New Mexico

CARLOS D. PINHEIRO-NETO, MD, PhD Assistant Professor, Department of Otolaryngology and Neurology Surgery, Albany Medical College; Skull Base and Cranio-Maxillofacial Surgeon, Department of Otolaryngology, Albany Medical Center, Albany, New York

KAREN T. PITMAN, MD, FACS Professor, Department of Otolaryngology and Communicative Sciences, University of Mississippi Medical Center, Jackson, Mississippi

KEVIN L. POTTS, MD, FACS Assistant Professor, Division of Otolaryngology, Department of Surgery, University of Louisville; Department of Surgery, University of Louisville, Louisville, Kentucky

ANNA M. POU, MD, FACS Professor, Department of Otolaryngology–Head and Neck Surgery, Louisiana State University Health Sciences Center–New Orleans, New Orleans, Louisiana; Program Director, Department of Head and Neck Surgery, Our Lady of the Lake Regional Medical Center, Baton Rouge, Louisiana

JESS PRISCHMANN, MD Private Practice, Prischmann Facial Plastic Surgery, Edina, Minnesota

LIANA PUSCAS, MD, MHS Assistant Professor, Department of Surgery, Division of Otolaryngology–Head and Neck Surgery, Duke University; Attending Physician, Department of Surgery, Division of Otolaryngology–Head and Neck Surgery, Duke University Hospital, Durham, North Carolina

MURUGAPPAN RAMANATHAN JR., MD Assistant Professor, Department of Otolaryngology–Head and Neck Surgery, Johns Hopkins University School of Medicine; Department of Otolaryngology–Head and Neck Surgery, The Johns Hopkins Hospital, Baltimore, Maryland

TANYA J. RATH, MD Assistant Professor, Director of Head and Neck Imaging, Department of Radiology, University of Pittsburgh School of Medicine; Assistant Professor, Department of Radiology, University of Pittsburgh Medical Center, Pittsburgh, Pennsylvania

YAEL RAZ, MD Assistant Professor, Department of Otolaryngology, University of Pittsburgh, Eye and Ear Institute, Pittsburgh, Pennsylvania

PETER C. REVENAUGH, MD Head and Neck Institute, Cleveland Clinic, Cleveland, Ohio

WILLIAM RUSSELL RIES, MD Professor, Carol and John S. Odess Chair in Facial and Plastic Reconstructive Surgery, Department of Otolaryngology, Vanderbilt University Medical Center, Nashville, Tennessee

CARLOS M. RIVERA-SERRANO, MD Resident, Department of Otolaryngology–Head and Neck Surgery, University of Pittsburgh School of Medicine, Pittsburgh, Pennsylvania

DAVID W. ROBERSON, MD Associate Professor in Otolaryngology, Harvard Medical School; Associate in Otolaryngology, Boston Children's Hospital, Boston, Massachusetts

JACOB G. ROBISON, MD, PhD Fellow, Departments of Otolaryngology, University of Pittsburgh, Eye and Ear Institute; Fellow, Department of Pediatric Otolaryngology, Children's Hospital of Pittsburgh, Pittsburgh, Pennsylvania

RACHEL E. RODITI, MD   Resident, Otolaryngology, Department of Otolaryngology–Head and Neck Surgery, University of Rochester–School of Medicine and Dentistry; Resident, Otolaryngology, Department of Otolaryngology–Head and Neck Surgery, Strong Memorial Hospital, Rochester, New York

KENNETH D. RODRIGUEZ, MD   Chief Resident, Department of Otolaryngology, University of Pittsburgh, Pittsburgh, Pennsylvania

PAMELA C. ROEHM, MD, PhD   Assistant Professor, Department of Otolaryngology, New York University School of Medicine, New York, New York

HENRY H. ROENIGK JR, MD, FACP   Professor Emeritus, Department of Dermatology, Northwestern University Medical School, Chicago, Illinois

EMILY ROGERS, MD   Resident, Department of Surgery, University of Mississippi Medical Center, Jackson, Mississippi

PETER S. ROLAND, MD   Professor and Chairman, Department of Otolaryngology–Head and Neck Surgery, University of Texas Southwestern Medical Center, Dallas, Texas

CLARK A. ROSEN, MD   Professor, Department of Otolaryngology, University of Pittsburgh Medical Center; Director, University of Pittsburgh Voice Center; Professor, Department of Communication Sciences Disorders, University of Pittsburgh, Pittsburgh, Pennsylvania

RICHARD M. ROSENFELD, MD, MPH   Professor and Chairman, Department of Otolaryngology, SUNY Downstate Medical Center; Chairman, Department of Otolaryngology, University Hospital of Brooklyn at LICH, Brooklyn, New York

MICHAEL J. RUCKENSTEIN, MD, FSc, FACS   Professor, Vice Chairman, Department of Otorhinolaryngology–Head and Neck Surgery, University of Pennsylvania Health System, Philadelphia, Pennsylvania

LUKE RUDMIK, MD, FRCSC   Clinical Assistant Professor, Department of Otolaryngology–Head and Neck Surgery, University of Calgary; Clinical Assistant Professor, Department of Otolaryngology–Head and Neck Surgery, Foothills Medical Centre, Calgary, Alberta, Canada

FRANCIS P. RUGGIERO, MD   ENT–Head and Neck Surgery of Lancaster, Lancaster, Pennsylvania

MATTHEW S. RUSSELL, MD   Assistant Professor, Department of Otolaryngology–Head and Neck Surgery, University of California, San Francisco; Otolaryngology Hospitalist, Department of Otolaryngology–Head and Neck Surgery, University of California, San Francisco Medical Center, San Francisco, California

MICHAEL J. RUTTER, MD   Professor, Department of Otolaryngology–Head and Neck Surgery, University of Cincinnati; Attending/Faculty, Department of Otolaryngology–Head and Neck Surgery, Cincinnati Children's Hospital Medical Center, Cincinnati, Ohio

MATTHEW W. RYAN, MD   Assistant Professor, Department of Otolaryngology, University of Texas Southwestern Medical Center, Dallas, Texas

DIANE L. SABO, PhD   Associate Professor, Department of Communication Science and Disorders, University of Pittsburgh; Director, Department of Audiology and Speech-Language Pathology, Children's Hospital of Pittsburgh, Pittsburgh, Pennsylvania

BARRY M. SCHAITKIN, MD   Professor, Department of Otolaryngology–Head and Neck Surgery, University of Pittsburgh; Chief, Division of Otolaryngology, UPMC Shadyside Hospital, Pittsburgh, Pennsylvania

RODNEY J. SCHLOSSER, MD   Professor and Director of Rhinology, Department of Otolaryngology–Head and Neck Surgery, Medical University of South Carolina; Staff Surgeon, Department of Surgery (Otolaryngology), Ralph H. Johnson VA Medical Center, Charleston, South Carolina

NATHAN TODD NELSON SCHREIBER, MD   Staff Physician, Department of Otolaryngology, Sequoia Hospital, San Mateo, California

JOHN M. SCHWEINFURTH, MD   Professor, Department of Otolaryngology, University of Mississippi; Professor, Department of Otolaryngology, University of Mississippi Medical Center, Jackson, Mississippi

SCOTT SHADFAR, MD   Chief Resident, Department of Otolaryngology–Head and Neck Surgery, University of North Carolina, Chapel Hill, North Carolina

MANISH D. SHAH, MD, MPhil, FRCS(C)   Assistant Professor, Department of Otolaryngology–Head and Neck Surgery, University of Toronto; Attending Physician, Department of Otolaryngology–Head and Neck Surgery, North York General Hospital, Toronto, Ontario, Canada

RAHUL K. SHAH, MD, FACS, FAAP   Associate Professor, Department of Otolaryngology and Pediatrics, The George Washington University School of Medicine and Health Sciences; Associate Surgeon-in-Chief, Joseph E. Robert Jr. Center for Surgical Care, Children's National Medical Center, Washington, District of Columbia

FRED F. SHAHAN, MD   Staff Physician, Department of Dermatology, Alvarado Hospital Medical Center, San Diego, California

NEIL T. SHEPARD, PhD   Professor of Audiology, Department of Otolaryngology, Mayo Medical School; Chair of Audiology, Mayo Clinic, Rochester, Minnesota

MAISIE L. SHINDO, MD, FACS   Professor of Otolaryngology, Director of Thyroid and Parathyroid Center, Department of Otolaryngology, Oregon Health and Science University, Portland, Oregon

WILLIAM W. SHOCKLEY, MD, FACS   W. Paul Biggers Distinguished Professor of Otolaryngology/Head and Neck Surgery, Chief, Division of Facial Plastic and Reconstructive Surgery, Department of Otolaryngology–Head and Neck Surgery, University of North Carolina, Chapel Hill, North Carolina

SALLY R. SHOTT, MD   Professor, Department of Otolaryngology–Head and Neck Surgery, University of Cincinnati; Professor, Department of Pediatric Otolaryngology, Cincinnati Children's Hospital Medical Center, Cincinnati, Ohio

JON D. SIMMONS, MD   Assistant Professor, Department of Surgery, University of South Alabama School of Medicine; Assistant Professor, Department of Surgery, University of South Alabama Medical Center, Mobile, Alabama

JEFFREY P. SIMONS, MD Assistant Professor, Department of Otolaryngology, University of Pittsburgh School of Medicine; Assistant Professor, Staff Otolaryngologist, Department of Pediatric Otolaryngology, Children's Hospital of Pittsburgh of UPMC, Pittsburgh, Pennsylvania

C. BLAKE SIMPSON, MD Professor, Department of Otolaryngology–Head and Neck Surgery, University of Texas Health Science Centre at San Antonio, San Antonio, Texas

PARUL SINHA, MBBS, MS Research Fellow, Department of Otolaryngology–Head and Neck Surgery, Washington University School of Medicine, St Louis, Missouri

DAVID F. SMITH, MD, PhD House Staff, Department of Otolaryngology–Head and Neck Surgery, Johns Hopkins University School of Medicine, Baltimore, Maryland

JESSE E. SMITH, MD Assistant Clinical Professor, Department of Otolaryngology, University of Texas Southwestern Medical Center, Dallas, Texas; Facial Plastic Reconstructive Surgeon, Department of Surgery, John Peter Smith Hospital, Fort Worth, Texas

LIBBY J. SMITH, DO, FAOCO Associate Professor, Department of Otolaryngology, University of Pittsburgh; Laryngologist/Surgeon, UPMC Voice Center, UPMC Mercy Academic Institution, Pittsburgh, Pennsylvania

TIMOTHY L. SMITH, MD, MPH, FACS Professor, Department of Otolaryngology–Head and Neck Surgery, Oregon Health and Science University; Director, Oregon Sinus Center, Department of Otolaryngology–Head and Neck Surgery, Oregon Health and Science University, Portland, Oregon

JOHN C. SOK, MD, PhD Assistant Professor, Department of Otolaryngology–Head and Neck Surgery, Loma Linda University School of Medicine; Director, Loma Linda University Voice and Swallow Center, Department of Otolaryngology–Head and Neck Surgery, Loma Linda University Medical Center, Loma Linda, California

RYAN J. SOOSE, MD Assistant Professor, Department of Otolaryngology, University of Pittsburgh School of Medicine; Director, Division of Sleep Surgery, Department of Otolaryngology, University of Pittsburgh Medical Center, Pittsburgh, Pennsylvania

NICHOLAS C. SORREL, MD Physician in Training, Department of Otorhinolaryngology and Head and Neck Surgery, University of Texas at Houston; Physician in Training, Department of Otorhinolaryngology and Head and Neck Surgery, Memorial Herman Hospital, Houston, Texas

SHAUM S. SRIDHARAN, MD Resident, Department of Otolaryngology–Head and Neck Surgery, New York University; Chief Resident, Department of Otolaryngology–Head and Neck Surgery, New York University, New York, New York

BRENDAN C. STACK JR, MD, FACS, FACE Professor, Department of Otolaryngology–Head and Neck Surgery, University of Arkansas; Professor, Department of Otolaryngology–Head and Neck Surgery, University Hospital of Arkansas, Little Rock, Arkansas

MICHAEL E. STADLER, MD Assistant Professor, Division of Head and Neck Surgical Oncology and Reconstructive Surgery, Department of Otolaryngology and Communication Sciences, Medical College of Wisconsin, Milwaukee, Wisconsin

CHRISTIAN L. STALLWORTH, MD Assistant Professor, Department of Otolaryngology–Head and Neck Surgery, University of Texas Health Science Center at San Antonio; Staff Otolaryngology, Department of Otolaryngology–Head and Neck Surgery, University Hospital System, San Antonio, Texas

JAMES A. STANKIEWICZ, MD Professor, Department of Otolaryngology–Head and Neck Surgery, Loyola University School of Medicine; Chairman, Department of Otolaryngology–Head and Neck Surgery, Loyola University/Trinity Health Care Center, Maywood, Illinois

MELISSA M. STATHAM, MD Assistant Professor, Department of Otolaryngology–Head and Neck Surgery, Emory University School of Medicine; Assistant Professor, Department of Otolaryngology–Head and Neck Surgery, Emory Voice Center, Emory University Hospital–Midtown, Atlanta, Georgia

SHAWN M. STEVENS, MD Resident Physician, Department of Otolaryngology, Medical University of South Carolina, Charleston, South Carolina

MICHAEL G. STEWART, MD Professor and Chairman, Department of Otolaryngology–Head and Neck Surgery, Vice Dean of the Medical College, Weill Cornell Medical College; Chief of Service, Department of Otolaryngology–Head and Neck Surgery, New York–Presbyterian Hospital/Weill Cornell Medical Center, New York, New York

SCOTT P. STRINGER, MD, MS Professor and Chairman, Department of Otolaryngology and Communicative Sciences, University of Mississippi Medical Center, Jackson, Mississippi

PATRICK J. STROLLO JR, MD, FCCP, FAASM Professor of Medicine and Clinical and Translational Science, Department of Medicine, University of Pittsburgh School of Medicine, UPMC Montefiore; Medical Director, UPMC Sleep Medicine Center, Montefiore University Hospital, University of Pittsburgh Medical Center, Pittsburgh, Pennsylvania

E. BRADLEY STRONG, MD Professor, Department of Otolaryngology, University of California, Davis; Vice Chairman, Department of Otolaryngology, University of California, Davis, School of Medicine, Sacramento, California

CHESTER L. STRUNK JR, MD Clinical Assistant Professor, Department of Otolaryngology, The University of Texas Medical Branch at Galveston, Galveston, Texas; Bay Area Ear, Nose and Throat Specialists, Pearland, Texas

JEFFREY D. SUH, MD Assistant Professor, Department of Head and Neck Surgery, University of California, Los Angeles, Los Angeles, California

LUCIAN SULICA, MD Associate Professor and Director, Laryngology/Voice Disorders, Department of Otolaryngology–Head and Neck Surgery, Weill Cornell Medical College; Attending Otolaryngologist, Department of Otolaryngology–Head and Neck Surgery, New York-Presbyterian Hospital, New York, New York

KURT F. SUMMERSGILL, DDS, PhD Associate Professor, Diagnostic Sciences, University of Pittsburgh–School of Dental

Medicine; Consultant, Department of Oral and Maxillofacial Surgery, University of Pittsburgh Medical Center, Pittsburgh, Pennsylvania

JONATHAN M. SYKES, MD, FACS Professor of Otolaryngology, Director, Facial Plastic and Reconstructive Surgery, Department of Otolaryngology–Head and Neck Surgery, University of California, Davis Medical Center, Sacramento, California

CARL H. SNYDERMAN, MD, MBA, FACS Professor, Department of Otolaryngology and Neurology Surgery, University of Pittsburgh School of Medicine; Co-Director, Center for Cranial Base Surgery, University of Pittsburgh Medical Center, Pittsburgh, Pennsylvania

NEELIMA TAMMAREDDI, MD Resident, Department of Otolaryngology, Louisiana State University Health Sciences Center–New Orleans, New Orleans, Louisiana

ANDREW B. TASSLER, MD Assistant Professor, Department of Otorhinolaryngology–Head and Neck Surgery, Albert Einstein College of Medicine; Assistant Professor, Department of Otorhinolaryngology–Head and Neck Surgery, Montefiore Medical Center, Bronx, New York

SHERARD A. TATUM, MD Professor, Department of Otolaryngology, SUNY Upstate Medical University, Syracuse, New York

MARCIE C. TAUZIN, MD Attending Staff, Touro Infirmary, New Orleans, Louisiana

ROBERT M. TAYLOR, MD Associate Professor, Departments of Neurology and Internal Medicine, The Ohio State University College of Medicine; Associate Professor, Division of Palliative Medicine, Department of Internal Medicine, The Ohio State University Wexner Medical Center, Columbus, Ohio

TED L. TEWFIK, MD Professor and Director of CME, Department of Otolaryngology–Head and Neck Surgery; Professor of Pediatric Surgery, McGill University, Montreal, QC, Canada

DEAN M. TORIUMI, MD Professor, Head of Division of Facial Plastic and Reconstructive Surgery, Department of Otolaryngology–Head and Neck Surgery, University of Illinois at Chicago, Chicago, Illinois

BETTY S. TSAI, MD Assistant Professor, Department of Otorhinolaryngology, The University of Oklahoma Health Sciences Center; Attending Physician, Department of Otorhinolaryngology, OU Physicians, Oklahoma City, Oklahoma

JAY B. TUCHMAN, MD, FAAP Assistant Professor, Department of Anesthesiology, University of Pittsburgh School of Medicine; Assistant Professor, Department of Pediatric Anesthesiology, Children's Hospital of Pittsburgh, Pittsburgh, Pennsylvania

ALEC VAEZI, MD Assistant Professor, Department of Otolaryngology, University of Massachusetts Medical School, Department of Otolaryngology, University of Massachusetts Memorial Medical Center, Worcester, Massachusetts

PAUL G. VAN DER SLOOT, MD, MS Assistant Professor, Otolaryngology–Head and Neck Surgery, University of Rochester Medical Center, Rochester, New York

NILESH R. VASAN, MD, FRACS Assistant Professor, Department of Otorhinolaryngology, University of Oklahoma Health Sciences Center, Oklahoma City, Oklahoma

CRAIG R. VILLARI, MD Resident Physician, PGY-4, Department of Otolaryngology–Head and Neck Surgery, Emory University School of Medicine, Atlanta, Georgia

COURTNEY C. J. VOELKER, MD, PhD Clinical Fellow, House Ear Clinic; Clinical Fellow, St. Vincent's Medical Center, Los Angeles, California

JEFFREY T. VRABEC, MD Associate Professor, Bobby R Alford Department of Otolaryngology–Head and Neck Surgery, Baylor College of Medicine, Houston, Texas

WILLIAM E. WALSH, MD Assistant Professor, Facial Plastic and Reconstructive Surgeon, Otolaryngologist, Department of Otolaryngology–Head and Neck Surgery, University of Minnesota Medical Center, Fairview, Minneapolis, Minnesota

ROHAN R. WALVEKAR, MD Associate Professor, Department of Otolaryngology–Head and Neck Surgery, Louisiana State University Health Sciences Center, New Orleans, Louisiana

PELL ANN WARDROP, MD Assistant Professor, Department of Otolaryngology, University of Kentucky; Medical Director, Sleep Disorder Center, St Joseph Hospital, Lexington, Kentucky

MICHAEL JOHN WAREING, BSc, MBBS, FRCS (ORL-HNS) Lead Clinician, Department of Otolaryngology–Head and Neck Surgery, Barts and The London NHS Trust; Consultant Surgeon, ENT, The London Clinic, London, United Kingdom

MARK K. WAX, MD FACS FRCS(C) Professor Otolaryngology–Head and Neck Surgery, Professor Oral Maxillo Facial Surgery; Program Director, Chief Microvascular and Reconstructive Surgery, Department of Otolaryngology–Head and Neck Surgery, Oregon Health and Sciences University, Portland, Oregon

EDWARD M. WEAVER, MD, MPH Professor, Chief of Sleep Surgery, Department of Department of Otolaryngology–Head and Neck Surgery, University of Washington; Co-Director, UW Medicine Sleep Center, Harborview Medical Center, Seattle, Washington

PETER C. WEBER, MD, MBA Professor, Department of Otolaryngology, Rocky Mountain Ear Institute/Swedish Hospital, Englewood, Colorado

RANDAL S. WEBER, MD Professor and Chairman, Department of Head and Neck Surgery, University of Texas, MD Anderson Cancer Center, Houston, Texas

WILLIAM IGNACE WEI, MD Honorary Clinical Professor, Department of Surgery, The University of Hong Kong; Director of Li Shu Pui ENT Head and Neck Surgery Centre, Head, Department of Surgery, Department of Surgery, Hong Kong Sanatorium and Hospital, Hong Kong SAR

RICHARD O. WEIN, MD, FACS Associate Professor, Tufts University School of Medicine, Associate Professor, Department of Otolaryngology–Head and Neck Surgery, Tufts Medical Center, Boston, Massachusetts

PHILIP A. WEISSBROD, MD Assistant Professor, Division of Otolaryngology–Head and Neck Surgery, University of

California, San Diego, San Diego, California; Director, Center for Voice and Swallowing, Division of Otolaryngology–Head and Neck Surgery, UC San Diego Health System, La Jolla, California

ERIK KENT WEITZEL, MD Assistant Professor, Department of Otolaryngology–Head and Neck Surgery, SAUSHEC Joint Base San Antonio; Chief of Rhinology, Department of Otolaryngology–Head and Neck Surgery, San Antonio Military Medical Center, San Antonio, Texas

KEVIN C. WELCH, MD Assistant Professor, Department of Otolaryngology–Head and Neck Surgery, Loyola University School of Medicine, Maywood, Illinois

MATTHEW K. WHITLEY, MD Attending Physician, Department of Otolaryngology–Head and Neck Surgery, Pediatric Ear Nose and Throat of Atlanta, Atlanta, Georgia

SUSAN L. WHITNEY, PT, DPT, PhD, NCS, ATC, FAPTA Professor, Department of Physical Therapy and Otolaryngology, University of Pittsburgh; Program Director, Centers for Rehab Services, University of Pittsburgh Medical Center, Pittsburgh, Pennsylvania

CHRISTA L. WHITNEY-MILLER, MD Assistant Professor, Department of Pathology and Laboratory Medicine, University of Rochester–School of Medicine and Dentistry; Staff Surgical Pathologist, Department of Pathology and Laboratory Medicine, Strong Memorial Hospital, Rochester, New York

EDWIN FRANCIS WILLIAMS, MD Medical Director, Williams Center Plastic Surgery Specialists, Latham, New York

MEGHAN N. WILSON, MD Resident, Department of Otolaryngology, Louisiana State University Health Sciences Center–New Orleans; Resident, Department of Otolaryngology, Louisiana State University Health Sciences Center–New Orleans, New Orleans, Louisiana

ANDREW WINKLER, MD Assistant Professor, Department of Otolaryngology, University of Colorado Denver; Director-Facial Plastic and Reconstructive Surgery, Department of Otolaryngology, University of Colorado Hospital, Aurora, Colorado

SARAH K. WISE, MD, MSCR Assistant Professor, Department of Otolaryngology–Head and Neck Surgery, Emory University; Staff Physician, Department of Otolaryngology–Head and Neck Surgery, Emory University Hospital, Atlanta, Georgia

WILLIAM ANTHONY WOOD, MD, FACS, FAAOA Staff Otolaryngologist, Brattleboro Memorial Hospital, Brattleboro, Vermont

GAYLE E. WOODSON, MD Professor and Chair, Division of Otolaryngology, Head and Neck Surgery, Department of Surgery, SIU School of Medicine; Otolaryngology, Head and Neck Surgery, St. John's Hospital, Springfield, Illinois

TUCKER WOODSON, MD Professor and Chief Division Sleep Medicine, Department of Otolaryngology, Medical College of Wisconsin; Staff, Department of Otolaryngology, Froedtert Hospital, Milwaukee, Wisconsin

CHRISTOPHER T. WOOTTEN, MD, FACS Assistant Professor, Department of Otolaryngology, Vanderbilt University; Surgical Director, Complex Aerodigestive Evaluation Team,

Department of Pediatric Otolaryngology, Monroe Carell Jr. Children's Hospital at Vanderbilt, Nashville, Tennessee

PETER-JOHN WORMALD, MD, FRACS, FCS(SA), FRCS(ED), MBChB Professor and Chairman, Department of Otolaryngology–Head and Neck Surgery, The University of Adelaide; Chairman, Department of Otolaryngology–Head and Neck Surgery, The Queen Elizabeth Hospital, Woodville South, South Australia, Australia

JUSTIN M. WUDEL, MD Resident, Department of Otolaryngology–Head and Neck Surgery, University of Colorado School of Medicine; Resident, Department of Otolaryngology–Head and Neck Surgery, University of Colorado Hospital, Aurora, Colorado

MIKE YAO, MD Clinical Associate Professor, Department of Otolaryngology, New York Medical College, Valhalla, New York

KATHLEEN L. YAREMCHUK, MD, MSA Chair, Department of Otolaryngology–Head and Neck Surgery, Henry Ford Hospital, Detroit, Michigan

ROBERT F. YELLON, MD Professor, Department of Otolaryngology, University of Pittsburgh School of Medicine; Co-Director, Department of Pediatric Otolaryngology, Children's Hospital of Pittsburgh of UPMC, Pittsburgh, Pennsylvania

VyVy N. YOUNG, MD Assistant Professor, Department of Otolaryngology, University of Pittsburgh; Assistant Professor, Department of Otolaryngology, University of Pittsburgh Medical Center, UPMC Mercy, Pittsburgh, Pennsylvania

WARREN K. YUNKER, BSc, MD, PhD, FRCS(C) Assistant Professor, Department of Surgery, Foothills Medical Centre, University of Calgary; Assistant Professor, Department of Surgery, Alberta Children's Hospital, Calgary, Alberta, Canada

MARK A. ZACHAREK, MD, FACS, FAAOA Clinical Associate Professor, Department of Otolaryngology–Head and Neck Surgery, University of Michigan Health System, Associate Professor and Associate Program Director; Director Michigan Sinus Center, Department of Otorhinolaryngology, University of Michigan Health Systems, Ann Arbor, Michigan

ADAM M. ZANATION, MD Assistant Professor, Department of Otolaryngology–Head and Neck Surgery, University of North Carolina at Chapel Hill; Physician, Department of Otolaryngology–Head and Neck Surgery, University of North Carolina at Chapel Hill, Chapel Hill, North Carolina

IRENE ZHANG, MD Fellow, Head and Neck Surgery, Department of Otolaryngology, University of Pittsburgh Medical Center; Fellow, Head and Neck Surgery, Department of Otolaryngology, Eye and Ear Institute, University of Pittsburgh Medical Center, Pittsburgh, Pennsylvania

LEE A. ZIMMER, MD, PhD Associate Professor, Department of Otolaryngology–Head and Neck Surgery, University of Cincinnati; Associate Professor, Department of Otolaryngology–Head and Neck Surgery, UC Health, Cincinnati, Ohio

JOHN A. ZITELLI, MD, PC Clinical Associate Professor, Department of Dermatology and Otolaryngology, University of Pittsburgh Medical Center; Staff Doctor, Zitelli & Brodland, PC, Skin Cancer Center, Mohs Surgery and Surgical Dermatology, Pittsburgh, Pennsylvania

DAVID A. ZOPF, MD Resident Surgeon, Department of Otolaryngology–Head and Neck Surgery, University of Michigan, Ann Arbor, Michigan

RICHARD A. ZOUMALAN, MD Clinical Professor, Department of Otolaryngology–Head and Neck Surgery, University of California, Los Angeles; Attending Surgeon, Department of Otolaryngology–Head and Neck Surgery, Cedars Sinai Medical Center, Beverly Hills, California

KAREN B. ZUR, MD Assistant Professor, Department of Otolaryngology–Head and Neck Surgery, Perelman School of Medicine, University of Pennsylvania; Director, Pediatric Voice Program; Associate Director, The Center for Pediatric Airway Disorders, Department of Otolaryngology–Head and Neck Surgery, The Children's Hospital of Philadelphia, Philadelphia, Pennsylvania

FOREWORD

The editorial team of this fifth edition of *Head and Neck Surgery—Otolaryngology* is pleased to present you with the newest and most up-to-date version of the foremost textbook in *Head and Neck Surgery—Otolaryngology*. The fifth edition features a revised and more comprehensive table of contents authored by the thought leaders in our field focusing upon the modern practice of medicine.

This text is intended for use by students and practitioners at every level. The pace of the development of new material and information in the world of biomedical science has made information management a contemporary challenge. There is an increasing demand for the practice of evidence-based medicine. Clinical proficiency and mastery of the information are presented in a concise and clear manner in this text and will serve the practitioner in his/her preparation for the future.

The editorial team remains grateful for this opportunity to continue their pioneering efforts of Byron J. Bailey, MD, and the many section editors and authors who have contributed so much to making this the preeminent text of our field. Special thanks also goes to Jackie Lynch for her editorial assistance and a special acknowledgment of the detailed, meticulous artwork of Anthony Pazo.

Clark A. Rosen, MD
Jonas T. Johnson, MD

"More than a textbook—it's a learning system." That has been our challenging goal since the first edition of "*Head and Neck Surgery—Otolaryngology*" went to the printer 20 years ago. Once again, we began the planning of this fifth edition with the recruiting of experienced and expert authors capable of providing our readers with the most current and useful evidence-based information available for residents and practicing physicians intent on mastering the practice of our specialty.

Comprehensive, concise, and practical content that is presented in the format designed to increase the understanding, retention, and application of knowledge is the end result of the efforts of our outstanding team of Section Editors led by Jonas Johnson and Clark Rosen. Useful illustrations, helpful summary tables, and supplemental video segments enhance the effort of the learner to retain and apply the information contained in these volumes. A new and valuable study guide companion, *Bailey's Head and Neck Surgery: Otolaryngology Review*, will be published separately to assist with benchmarks of the progress that the reader has made.

And now, with sincere thanks to the authors and editors who have made this learning system possible, we have arrived once again at the point where vision becomes reality.

Many months of hard work have been transformed into a product with the potential to move clinical care to a higher level, and that is always the foundation of our striving.

We welcome our new readers and we applaud your decision to join us in this quest for greater understanding for ourselves and improved care for our patients.

Byron J. Bailey, MD, FACS
Chairman Emeritus, Department of Otolaryngology
The University of Texas Medical Branch
Galveston, Texas

VII

Head and Neck Surgery

Christine G. Gourin   Anna M. Pou

Head and Neck Tumor Biology 108

Alec Vaezi *Jennifer R. Grandis*

The treatment of head and neck squamous cell carcinoma (HNSCC) evolved slowly over most of the 20th century, with important breakthroughs including the description of the radical neck dissection by George Crile (1) in 1906 with an improvement of 3-year survival from 19% to 75%, the report of modified radical neck dissection by Suarez et al. (2) in 1963, the introduction of postoperative adjuvant external beam radiotherapy in the 1970s, and the use of adjuvant chemotherapy in the late 1980s. However, the last 20 years have brought considerable advances in the understanding of head and neck cancer tumor biology. Molecular techniques helped epidemiologists identify and characterize human papillomavirus (HPV)-associated HNSCC, which is currently responsible for an epidemic of oropharyngeal HNSCC extending throughout North America and, to a lesser extent, Europe. In addition, with better understanding of the genetic and molecular changes that characterize HNSCC, novel therapeutic agents have been designed and used with success in the treatment of HNSCC, such as the EGFR-blocking antibody cetuximab (Erbitux). Furthermore, novel prognostic and predictive biomarkers are being evaluated in the clinical setting to inform personalized cancer treatments in which the treatment is tailored to the biology of an individual tumor. HNSCC vaccine trials are currently accruing patients, and the role of cancer stem cells (CSCs), angiogenesis, and microRNAs is under study. Very recently, the HNSCC cancer genome has been outlined by sequencing the genomes or exomes of nearly 75 tumors (3). In sum, these times are exciting not only for head and neck tumor biologists but also for clinicians and patients who are already seeing the benefit of scientific discoveries in the clinical setting.

As basic science increasingly merges with clinical medicine, it is important for the clinician to be familiar with the different molecular pathways contributing to HNSCC development. A working knowledge of this biology has become essential for understanding treatment options for HNSCC in the 21st century. This chapter reviews selected major molecular pathways contributing to HNSCC. These include the mitogen signaling cascade, the cell cycle and its regulation, the major DNA repair pathways, and protection against apoptosis. The concept of solid tumor stem cells and angiogenesis is also discussed. For each section, a current model for the pathway is described, highlighting how deregulation of this pathway participates in tumor development. Examples illustrate how each pathway is involved in HNSCC tumor biology, and its clinical relevance. However, it is important to remember that basic science is in constant evolution. What appears meaningful today may be obsolete tomorrow. Every effort has been made to provide models backed by strong evidence that are likely to withstand the test of time.

DIFFERENT SUBTYPES OF HNSCC IDENTIFIED BASED ON RISK FACTORS AND GENETICS

Head and neck cancer is an important cause of death and morbidity worldwide. It is the eighth most frequent type of cancer in the USA with nearly 50,000 new cases diagnosed every year accounting for 11,000 deaths (4). Similar to other cancer types, HNSCC is proportionally even more deadly worldwide, where 510,000 new cases of HNSCC will be diagnosed yearly and more than half of these patients will succumb to their disease (5). Each of these cancers is the result of a multistep accumulation of genetic mutations in a progenitor cancer cell (6–8). Subsequent proliferation of mutated progenitor cells results in clonal expansion. With further accumulation of mutations, the clonal outgrowth becomes unregulated and irreversible. The nascent tumor progressively acquires new phenotypes including the capacity for invasiveness and metastasis. It was previously thought that head and neck cancers resulted from 6 to 10 independent significant genetic mutations acquired over a period of 20 years (9). However, recent data from head and neck cancer genome sequencing suggest that many more mutations accumulate, although most of these may be of little consequence (i.e., passenger mutations) (3). In HNSCC, on average, 1 to 15 base pairs are mutated for each megabase of exome (3), which suggests there may be at least 6,000 to 90,000 mutations for the 6.4 billion base pairs in the human diploid genome.

Over the past 15 years, it has been increasingly evident that all tumors labeled as HNSCC may not represent the same clinical entity (10). For instance, HNSCC tumors have different prognosis depending on the affected site. A tonsil cancer from a middle-age smoker–drinker behaves differently than a lateral tongue cancer from an elderly woman who never smoked or drank, or a tonsil cancer from a young nonsmoker. Epidemiologic and clinical studies suggest that even HNSCCs with a similar histologic appearance may represent different types of tumors based on molecular heterogeneity, pathogenesis, risk factors, and clinical outcomes.

Exposure to carcinogens present in tobacco or betel quid is a major factor for head and neck cancer that has been recognized for years. Tobacco derivates contain a potent carcinogen, which damage the DNA and mutate the genome of progenitor cancer cell; tobacco smoke contains more than 4,000 toxic compounds including 81 carcinogens (11), and smokeless tobacco contains mutagenic nitrosamines (11). Interestingly, *in vitro*, one of the most potent carcinogens found in cigarette smoke, named benzo[a]pyrene diol epoxide, preferentially mutates p53 at hot spots found in lung cancer (12). It is therefore perhaps not surprising that p53 is the most frequently mutated gene in HNSCC, since tobacco consumption and synergistically excessive alcohol intake are the two major risk factors for HNSCC in the USA; "heavy" tobacco consumption increases the cancer risk by 5.8 times, "heavy" drinking by 7.4 times, and combination of the 2 increases the risk by 38 times in male and 100 times in females (13). In eastern countries, areca nut chewing in betel quid has been identified as a risk factor for HNSCC. The areca nut does not contain a single organic chemical responsible for the cancer formation, but rather a combination of chemicals that affect distinct steps of carcinogenesis. Areca alkaloids have genotoxic effects and participate in tumor initiation, and arecaidine contributes to tumor promotion (14).

After HPV was identified in oropharyngeal cancers (15–19), it became evident that a subset of oropharyngeal HNSCC is not associated with smoking and drinking but rather with promiscuous oral sex behavior and to seropositivity of sexually transmitted HPV16 (18,20). HPV-positive HNSCC found in nonsmokers has a better prognosis than traditional HNSCC found in smoker/drinkers (21,22). That these tumors represent two groups of HNSCC with distinct tumor biology is also evident at a genetic level: considerably fewer mutations are found in HPV-positive tumors from nonsmoker patients (3). Interestingly, retrospective analyses of archived tumors suggest that oropharyngeal HPV-positive tumors represent a relatively recent entity; also, to date, this epidemic has spread more extensively in the USA than in Europe. HPV-positive HNSCC in nonsmokers is now widely recognized as a distinct group of HNSCC (21). With further progress in the genetic and molecular understanding of HNSCC tumor biology, novel groups of HNSCC are likely to be characterized.

Other subtypes of HNSCC may originate on particular genetic backgrounds. Humans are not identical due to a certain genetic variability, or polymorphism, observed within the human population. In certain instances, the polymorphism has a profound effect on the function of a cancer susceptibility gene and induces a cancer-prone syndrome, sometimes an HNSCC-prone syndrome. For instance, patients with a congenital deficiency in one of the multiple genes coding for the Fanconi anemia DNA repair pathway proteins are 500 to 700 times more prone to HNSCC compared to other patients. Fanconi anemia patients, recognized at birth by finger aplasia, abnormal facies, and short stature, develop childhood aplastic anemia due to apoptosis of hematopoietic cells, and myelodysplastic syndrome in adolescence, with an 800-fold increased chance of myeloid leukemia (23). These patients are exquisitely sensitive to genotoxic stress by cross-linking agents (such as mitomycin C) because they cannot efficiently repair mutagenic DNA *inter*strand cross-links; as a consequence, their cells rapidly accumulate mutations when exposed to carcinogens (23). In a similar vein, it has been proposed that polymorphisms in DNA repair genes that mildly affect DNA repair capacity may lead to increased susceptibility to HNSCC due to hypersensitivity to environmental DNA-damaging agents. However, increased HNSCC susceptibility due to polymorphisms in DNA repair genes remains largely unproven (24).

PATHOGENESIS AND FIELD CANCERIZATION

Most of our knowledge about HNSCC pathogenesis comes from oral cancer. Precursor lesions of oral SCC are *oral leukoplakia* and *erythroplakia*. Clinically evident premalignant lesions are prevalent in less than 0.5% of the population where the rate of progression to cancer is estimated to be 1% to 2% per year (25). The leukoplakia is an exclusion diagnosis. It is a clinical term referring to a patch of white mucosa that does not disappear by rubbing. More specifically, a workshop coordinated by the World Health Organization defines leukoplakia as "white plaques of questionable risk having excluded (other) known diseases or disorders that carry no increased risk for cancer" (26). The erythroplakia is a clinical term reserved as an exclusion diagnosis for a red velvety mucosal lesion that cannot be classified otherwise. These are clinical terms based on the macroscopic appearance, the lesion, and not pathologic diagnoses, and inference on the histopathology of the lesion should not be made. Histologically, most leukoplakia are the consequence of a hyperkeratotic response to an irritant, and only 20% shows evidence of dysplasia or carcinoma on histology (27,28), while 90% of erythroplakia demonstrate changes consistent with premalignancy or early malignancy (29). However, it is now evident that the macroscopically normal mucosa that surrounds the excision site of HNSCC may also represent mucosa in an inconspicuous state of premalignancy, and may be the source of recurrence (10). As early as the 1950s, the concept of field cancerization that the mucosa is diffusely diseased and at higher risk of developing tumor was proposed (30). Scientific advances over the past 20 years have begun to describe the pathogenesis of HNSCC at a molecular and genetic level.

Experimental animal models of tumor formation have identified chemical tumorigenesis as a two-step process. First, a mutagen, such as dimethylbenzanthracene (DMBA) or 4NQO, is applied to the epithelium (31). During this step, called *tumor induction*, genotoxic stress induces DNA damage, which, if not repaired, leads to mutation of the genome of a precursor cancer cell. In this model, mutations are not sufficient to induce cancer. The mutated precursor cancer cell needs to be stimulated to proliferate to progress to cancer. In skin carcinogenesis, application of croton's oil stimulates the protein kinase C (PKC) signaling cascade (see below) and induces epithelial and precursor cancer cell proliferation; this step is called *tumor promotion* (32). With further mutations, clonal outgrowth becomes irreversible and unregulated.

The critical mutations leading to cancer development occur in two major gene categories: *proto-oncogenes* and *tumor suppressors*. Proto-oncogenes are genes involved in normal cellular functions such as cell proliferation or cell death (33). Ras and epidermal growth factor receptor (EGFR) are proto-oncogenes. A proto-oncogene with a mutation that renders it capable of transforming a cell

is called an *oncogene*. Since oncogenic mutations represent genetic gain of function, mutation in only one of the two gene copies (alleles) is sufficient to confer a growth advantage. For example, only one mutated copy of an activated EGFR is sufficient to drive proliferation. In contrast, tumor suppressors are genes that prevent carcinogenesis. Mutations of both alleles are required to remove a normal cellular block to cancer development (33). Often one copy is inactivated by mutation, and the other is lost secondary to loss of heterozygosity (LOH). For instance, p53 is a tumor suppressor, as it prevents cell proliferation and induces apoptosis. With a mutation that inactivates only one copy of p53, the cell can still efficiently regulate the cell cycle via the remaining non-mutated copy. If copies are lost or inactivated, the cell cycle block is removed. Ironically, p53 was initially identified in a screen designed to identify oncogenes (34–36). The mutant copy of p53 that was thought to be an oncogene was later recognized to be a dominant negative form, in which the mutated p53 prevented the function of the normal allele (37,38). When this was understood, p53 was recognized to be a tumor suppressor (39,40). A list of putative and confirmed oncogenes and tumor suppressors in HNSCC and their respective chromosomal locations is provided (Table 108.1).

A multistep model of HNSCC progression proposes that mutations may be acquired in a progenitor cancer cell in a successive manner, ultimately leading to carcinoma formation (Fig. 108.1) (7,8,33,41). This model resulted from the analysis of cancers and cancer precursors in which histology was linked to genetic analysis (42). LOH of chromosome 3p and 9p, which contains the tumor suppressor p16, is frequently found in dysplasias, and is thought to be involved early during carcinogenesis (6,8). Loss of 17p, the part of the genome that contains p53, occurs at the transition from a noninvasive to an invasive lesion (6). In contrast, alteration of chromosomes 4q, 11q, and 8 is found

TABLE 108.1	**TUMOR SUPPRESSORS AND ONCOGENES IN HNSCC**		
Tumor Suppressor	Location	Oncogenes	Location
p16 (CDKN2A)	**3p21**	**Cyclin D1(CCND1)**	**11q13**
p53 (TP53)	**17p13**	**EGFR**	**7p11**
PTEN	**10q23**	**PI3KCA**	**3q26**
SMAD4	**18q21**	**MET**	**7q31**
PTPRD	**9p23**	Cyclin L1 (CCNL1)	3q25
CSMD1	**8p23**	PARP1	3q25
RASSF1A	**3p21**	TP63	3q26
FHIT	**3p14**	Dcun1D1	3q26
		Myc	8q24
		PTK2	8q24
		Cortactin	11q13
		FADD	11q13

Bold indicates established tumor suppressor or oncogenes.
Derived from Leemans CR, Braakhuis BJ, Brakenhoff RH. The molecular biology of head and neck cancer. *Nat Rev Cancer* 2011;11:9–22.

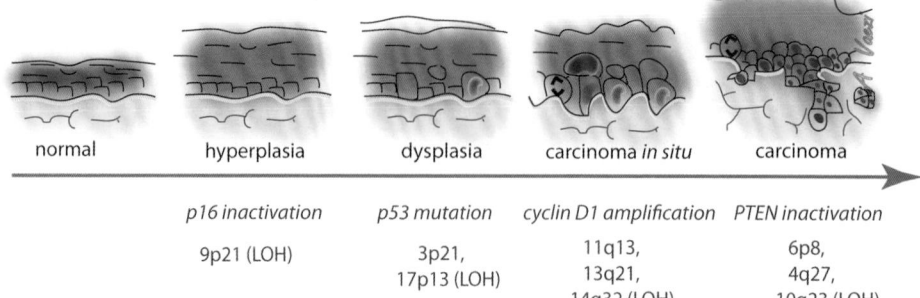

Figure 108.1 Tumor progression in HNSCC. Timeline representing the correlation between histopathology and cytogenetics in HNSCC and its precursor lesions. Histology is represented on the top, cytogenetic abnormalities on the bottom.

preferentially in carcinomas and is thought to represent late events in the carcinogenic process (6,7). 11q amplification corresponds to cyclin D1 overexpression.

In LOH and chromosomal amplification, a group of genes located in one region of a chromosome are all lost or amplified at once. Genetic mapping of the lost/amplified portion of the chromosome helps delineate genes potentially involved in tumor formation. In addition, cells with common genetic alterations can be identified on histology and mark clonal expansion of cancer progenitors. By labeling cells bearing these chromosomal markers together with p53 mutations on histologic slides, it was found that in 35% of oral carcinomas the macroscopically normal mucosa surrounding the tumor contained genetic alteration (43). Eradication of the mucosa bearing genetic alterations at the time of surgery is critical to reduce local recurrences (44). These data support the field cancerization theory put forward in the 1950s.

With the principles of carcinogenesis in mind, we can probe into the major molecular pathways that are dysregulated in cancer precursor cells and are instrumental in driving cancer progression. The clonal growth of a cancer precursor cell can be viewed as the product of a steady state equation in which the rate of proliferation is greater than the rate of cell death, leading to a net overgrowth of the clone. At the core of proliferation lies the cell cycle and its tight regulation. Before elaborating on this, it is important to review the major autocrine and paracrine signals that drive the cell cycle.

UPSTREAM OF THE CELL CYCLE: EPIDERMAL GROWTH FACTOR RECEPTOR AND TGFβ

Epidermal Growth Factor

Under physiologic conditions, epithelial cells proliferate in response to mitogens of the epidermal growth factor (EGF) family of ligands that are secreted in autocrine or paracrine fashion, or presented via cell–cell contact and activate the EGF receptor (EGFR) (Fig. 108.2A). For instance, cells are stimulated to proliferate via EGF during wound healing. The signal is initiated by 1 of 11 members of the EGF family. All EGF family ligands exist in pro-form as transmembrane

precursor proteins. They are converted to an active diffusible form by extracellular cleavage of the membrane protein. Six members of the EGF family are expressed in most SCC cell lines and activate the EGFR: EGF, transforming growth factor alpha (TGFα), HB-EGF, amphiregulin, betacellulin, and heregulin (45). HB-EGF is particularly interesting. The proform may either be cleaved to generate a diffusible factor by matrix metalloproteases (MMPs) that degrade extracellular matrix during cell migration (46), or it may activate EGFR as a transmembrane protein via cell-cell interaction, acting in a juxtacrine fashion. The effects on the target cell are different depending on whether HB-EGF is soluble or membrane bound. (Singh AB, Harris R. Autocrine, paracrine and juxtacrine signaling by EGFR ligands. *Cell Signal* 2005;10:1183–1193.)

Growth factors present in the interstitial space can also act on other receptors of the EGFR family (also called the ErbB family) that include ErbB1 (EGFR), ErbB2 (HER2/c-neu), ErbB3 (Her3), and ErbB4 (Her4) (45). In absence of ligand, most ErbB-family receptors are present at the cell surface of epithelial cells in the form of monomeric inactive transmembrane tyrosine kinase receptors. Binding of bivalent extracellular ligand triggers receptor dimerization, which brings catalytic cytoplasmic tails into close proximity, allowing trans-autophosphorylation of the cytoplasmic tails on tyrosine, serine, and threonine residues (47,48). ErbB receptors present at the cell surface are not a static pool of proteins. The receptors constantly cycle between an endosomal reservoir and the cell surface, where they become exposed to the ligands (49). After being activated, the receptor is endocytosed and either degraded or recycled (47,49).

Upon activation and transphosphorylation, active EGFR triggers three major signaling pathways. First, it activates the Ras–Map kinase pathway. Autophosphorylation sites on the cytoplasmic tail become docking sites for the adaptor protein SHC, which in turn recruits Grb2, which recruits Sos. Sos is a guanosine exchange factor for Ras, a small GTPase bound to the inner leaflet of the plasma membrane where it cycles between GDP and GTP bound forms (50,51). Ras acts as a molecular switch which is turned "on" when bound to GTP (52). The Sos activates Ras by mediating the exchange of GDP for GTP. Active Ras recruits the scaffolding protein Raf to the membrane (53). This leads to activation of the map kinase cascade, ultimately leading to ERK

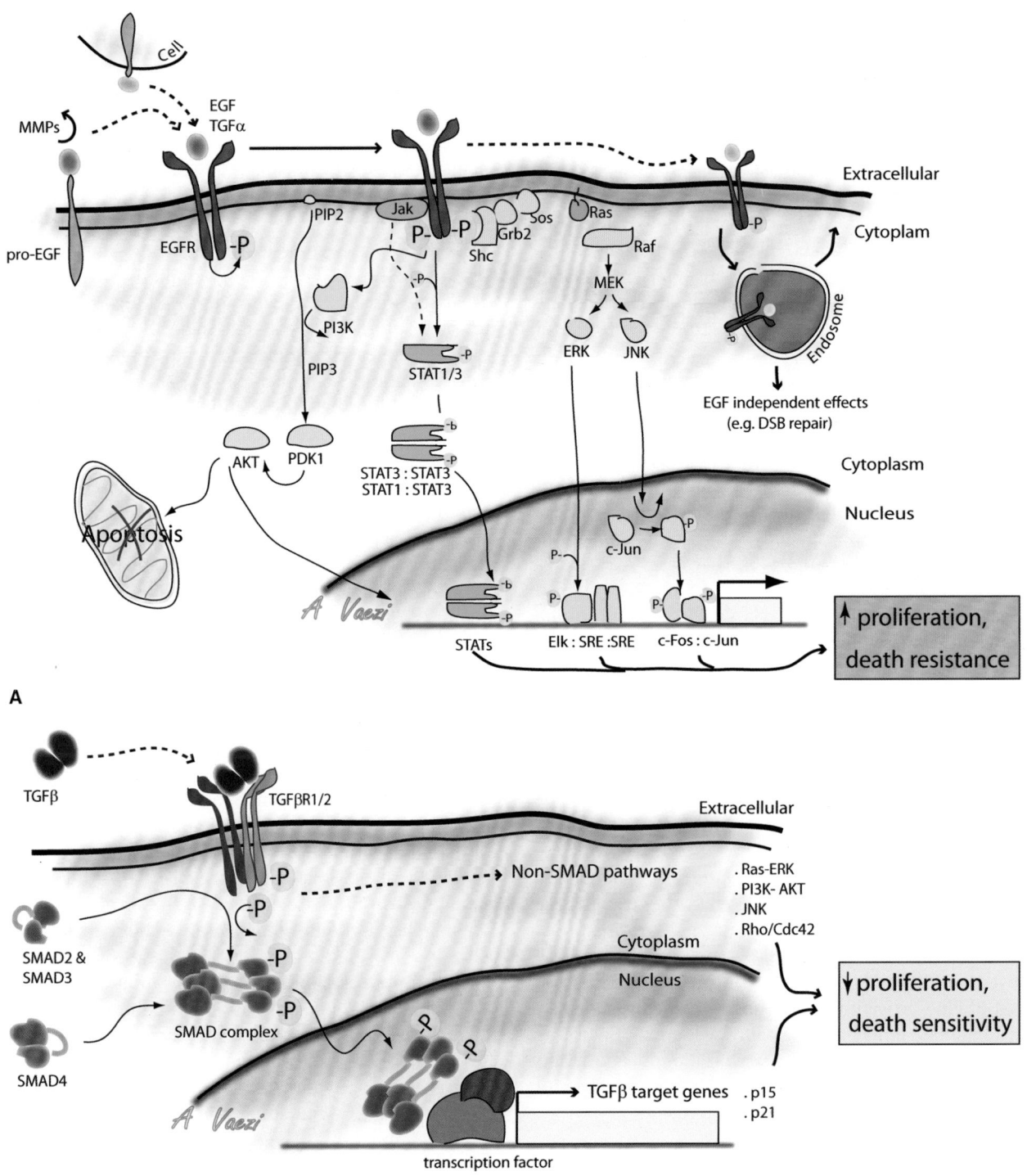

Figure 108.2 Signaling upstream of the cell cycle. Model for EGFR **(A)** and TGF-β **(B)** signaling pathways are represented. See text for details.

and Jun kinase (JNK) phosphorylation and activation (54). JNK is a serine/threonine kinase, which phosphorylates the c-Jun transcription factor. Phosphorylated c-Jun forms a heterodimer with phosphorylated c-fos, which together constitutes the AP-1 early response transcription factor that drives cell proliferation (55). ERK can also phosphorylate and activate transcription factors responsible for cell proliferation and cell migration.

The second signaling pathway activated by EGFR is the Jak/STAT pathway. Inactive STAT (signal transducer and activator of transcription) proteins are located in the cytoplasm. Activated EGFR recruits and activates the transcription factor STAT3 via two mechanisms: via Janus kinase (Jak) or via direct interaction with STAT3. Jak is a tyrosine kinase that binds to the juxtamembrane intracellular portion of activated receptors. Active Jak then phosphorylates and activates STAT1 or STAT3 proteins (56). An alternate mode of activation of STAT3 is via direct interaction with EGFR (57). STAT3 is recruited to active EGFR, where it binds to specific phosphotyrosine residues of the receptor via its Src homology domain (SH2). STAT3 is then directly phosphorylated by the receptor on critical tyrosine and serine residues. Phosphorylation of STAT3, either via Jak or via EGFR, leads to its dimerization, either as STAT3 homodimers or as STAT3:STAT1 heterodimers (58). Activated STAT transcription factor dimers translocate either to mitochondria where they regulate metabolism characteristic of cancer cells (59,60) or to the nucleus where they regulate growth factor/cytokine-directed gene expression (56) and increase cell motility (61,62).

Finally, EGFR also activates the PI3 kinase/Akt pathway that promotes cell survival by suppressing apoptosis. Activated EGFR recruits and activates phospholipase-Cγ, which directs the hydrolysis of the phosphatidylinositol biphosphate (PIP2) at the plasma membrane. This hydrolysis generates an insoluble diacyl glycerol, which activates PKC, and a soluble phosphatidyl (1,4,5) triphosphate in the cytosol (32). There, IP3 (1,4,5) releases Ca^{2+} stores from the endoplasmic reticulum. Activated EGFR can also recruit and activate PI3 kinase, via the SH2 domain of the kinase. PI3 kinase then phosphorylates PIP2 to generate phosphatidylinositol-(3,4,5) triphosphate (PIP3) that remains membrane bound (63). Proteins with a pleckstrin homology (PH) domain such as Akt and PDK migrate to and associate with PIP3 located at the plasma membrane (63). Close proximity of Akt and PDK leads to Akt phosphorylation and activation. Akt renders the cell more resistant to apoptosis and increases proliferation. In addition, Akt also induces a motile and invasive cell phenotype. PTEN, an important tumor suppressor that is frequently mutated in cancers, counteracts Akt effects (64,65). PTEN's sequence resembles serine, threonine, and tyrosine phosphatases, but it acts principally as a lipid phosphatase converting PIP3 into PIP2 (64). Thus, PTEN tempers the effect of PI3K activation by limiting PIP3-mediated signaling. PI3 kinase lipid signaling pathway is a major pathway linking EGFR activation to increased cell proliferation and motility and decreased cell death, and is often involved in carcinogenesis.

Clinical Implications of EGF Pathway in HNSCC

EGFR is frequently upregulated in HNSCC (66–68), and in general EGFR upregulation correlates with a worse prognosis (68–70), including more rapid disease progression and the presence of lymphatic metastasis, through its effect on proliferation, motility, and angiogenesis (71). The mechanisms leading to EGFR overexpression in HNSCC are still unclear. Genome sequencing suggests that EGFR is not mutated in HNSCC, in contrast to other tumor types (3). It is rarely amplified (less head than 10% of HNSCC). However,

a peculiarity of HNSCC is the common overexpression of a truncated mutant of the receptor (EGFRvIII) in 40% of HNSCC (72). EGFRvIII, which is constitutively active and has degradation prolonged half-life, is found exclusively in tumors, making it a prime target for anticancer therapy with specific monoclonal antibodies. Because of the high frequency of EGFR upregulation HNSCC, EGFR-targeting strategies have been extensively investigated. Both small molecule EGFR tyrosine kinase inhibitors and monoclonal antibodies have been tested for activity against HNSCC. Cetuximab, an EGFR-blocking antibody, demonstrated activity against HNSCC, with improved locoregional control and survival compared to radiotherapy alone (73) and with improved response rate and survival when used in combination chemotherapy (74). Cetuximab (Erbitux) is now used routinely to potentiate radiotherapy. To date, while tyrosine kinase inhibitors targeting EGFR (such as gefitinib and erlotinib) have activity in HNSCC, they have not demonstrated prolonged survival in Phase III clinical studies (75). This discrepancy suggests that EGFR-blocking antibody has effects other than inhibition of the signaling pathway; the antibody could have an effect on immunity (76,77), or on EGF-independent effects such as DNA repair (78,79).

In addition to targeting EGFR itself, considerable effort has been invested in inhibiting downstream targets. STAT3 homodimers, which have oncogenic properties, are overexpressed in HNSCC and are the target of anticancer therapies (80). Specifically, STAT3 inhibitory strategies using dimerization-disrupting agents or competitive inhibitors of the DNA-binding domain of STAT3 have been proposed to combat HNSCC (80–82); the latter was used in a clinical trial with promising results. HNSCC genome sequencing found that 5% of tumors display H-Ras mutations, leading to constitutive activation of the small GTPase (3). Whether Ras is mutated or simply subject to sustained activation by EGFR, it is a seductive therapeutic target. Ras may be inhibited via blocking farnesylation of the protein (63), an essential posttranslational modification required for its targeting to the plasma membrane where it mediates its effects. In addition, the PIP3 lipid pathway is also relatively frequently mutated in HNSCC. PTEN is mutated in 7% of HNSCC with some cancers bearing both H-Ras and PTEN mutations (3,83). The inactivation of PTEN promotes PIP3 accumulation and activation of downstream targets such as Akt. PI3KCA, a catalytic subunit of PI3 kinase, is also mutated in HNSCC (3,84). These mutations underscore how frequently the inositol lipid pathway is the target of carcinogenic mutations. While the contribution of these mutations to protein function or prognosis is yet unknown, they will likely be the subject of exciting HNSCC tumor biology discoveries in the near future. To date, therapeutic strategies targeting the PI3K/Akt pathway in HNSCC remain mostly limited to the preclinical setting (63). Pharmacologic inhibitors being developed include a water-soluble form of wortmannin, an inhibitor of PI3K.

Importantly, mTOR, a downstream target of Akt, can be inhibited with rapamycin, the RAD001(Everolimus), and CCI-779 (Temsirolimus) compounds and is the focus of innovative anti-HNSCC therapeutic strategies that are already being tested in Phase I and II clinical trials (85).

Transforming Growth Factor Beta

The transforming growth factor beta (TGF-β) superfamily of ligands regulates both embryologic processes and adult tissue homeostasis. These ligands act as tumor suppressors by inhibiting proliferation of epithelial cells, and by sensitizing cells to apoptosis; in that respect, TGF-β effects are opposite to those of EGFR. It is therefore not surprising that TGF-β signaling is also the target of carcinogenic mutations.

The TGF-β superfamily includes TGF-βs (TGF-β 1, 2, and 3), bone morphogenic protein, growth and differentiation factors, nodal, activin (involved in embryogenesis and bone formation), and anti-mullerian hormone (86,87). TGF-β is secreted as inactive precursors that are proteolytically activated by extracellular proteinases (86,88). The biologically active cytokine is present in the interstitial compartment; the signal is triggered when TGF-β binds a dimeric *Type II* TGFβ receptor. TGF-β receptors are single-span transmembrane receptors with serine/threonine kinase activity (Fig. 108.2B). Upon activation, dimeric type II receptors recruit and associate with dimeric *Type I* receptors, another transmembrane serine/threonine kinase receptor, to form a tetrameric receptor complex (86–88). Both receptors are then in close proximity, leading to the phosphorylation and activation of the Type I receptor by the Type II receptor. In turn, activated Type I receptor recruits an adaptor protein named SARA (Smad anchor for receptor activation) that mediates transient binding between the Type I receptor and SMADs, a family of transcription factors present in the cytoplasm. The SMAD family of proteins has eight members, SMAD 1–8, which come in three types: receptor-activated SMADS (R-SMADS), co-SMADS, and inhibitory SMADS (I-SMADS) (89). R-SMADS involved in TGF-β signaling are SMAD2 and SMAD3. SARA brings SMAD 2 and 3 in close proximity to the catalytic site of the Type I receptor, which then phosphorylates the R-SMAD C-terminus (87,88). This posttranslational modification induces a conformational change that allows interaction with a co-SMAD (SMAD4). The newly assembled SMAD:co-SMAD complex translocates to the nucleus where it interacts with other transcription regulators, to control expression of genes involved in apoptosis, and cell cycle repressors including p15 and p21(87). However, TGF-β signaling does not necessarily involve SMADs, and SMADs are not necessarily activated by Type I receptors. Recently, important cross talk between the MAP kinase pathway and SMADs has been revealed: ERK has been shown to phosphorylate SMADS (90). Reciprocally, TGF receptors can regulate important targets in a SMAD-independent manner, including the Map kinase pathway (90) and the Rho family of small GTPases (91), which are "molecular switches" similar to Ras, but are involved in the regulation of actin dynamics, cell migration, and metastasis (51). This represents one way in which TGF-β regulates cell morphology and migration.

The TGF-β pathway is negatively regulated at three levels. First, at the level of the extracellular matrix, the small proteoglycan decorin inhibits TGF-β receptor signaling (92). Decorin has antitumoral activity *in vitro*. Second, intracellular I-SMADs prevent binding of R-SMADs to the activated Type I receptor, and thus negatively impact SMAD signaling. Third, both the receptor and SMADs can be targeted for proteasome-mediated degradation, regulated by E3 ubiquitin ligases SMURF1 and SMURF2 (93,94). Interestingly, SMURF1 not only downregulates the TGF-β signaling pathway but also enhances cancer cell migration and invasion by targeting the GTPase Rho A for degradation, thereby reducing stress fibers and enhancing cell protrusions and motility (91). In summary, TGF-β signaling is at the crossroads of cell proliferation, cell death, and migration, and it is involved in many aspects of carcinogenesis.

Clinical Implications of TGF-β Pathway in HNSCC

The role of TGF-β signaling in tumorigenesis is multifaceted. While TGF-β has tumor suppressive effects, cancer cells can circumvent the suppressive component of the pathway and use TGF-β stimulation to their advantage to promote invasion and secretion of mitogens and pro-metastatic cytokines. This explains why TGF-β signaling is inhibited in certain cancers and upregulated in others. HNSCC is no exception. For instance, TGF-β receptor and SMADS are often downregulated in HNSCC (95). The downregulation may occur via loss of heterozygosity of chromosome q18, which contains TGFβRI and SMAD genes, or via DNA methylation-mediated gene repression (88). In addition, inactivating mutations in TGFβRI or II and SMADs have been reported in HNSCC, and may be present in up to 20% of neck metastasis (TGFβRI) (96–98). However, exosome sequencing of 80 HNSCC primary tumors found no mutations in TGF-β pathway, indicating that inactivating mutations are probably not a frequent event (3). An elegant demonstration that the downregulation of TGF-β signaling participates in HNSCC formation comes from a genetic mouse model in which the loss of TGFβRII, in the presence of an activating Ras mutation, induces head and neck tumors that closely resemble human HNSCC.

As above, TGF-β1 is actually frequently overexpressed in HNSCC, by about five times the normal levels in 40% of HNSCC (99). TGF-β1 is not only upregulated in the tumor but also in the surrounding normal-appearing tissue, suggesting that the tumor microenvironment contributes to tumorigenesis. This hypothesis was confirmed in a transgenic animal model where the induction of TGF-β1 overexpression in oral mucosa led to mucosal hyperproliferation and angiogenesis (99). This suggests that TGF-βR ligand stimulation may be upregulated in HNSCC and have a profound effect on tumorigenesis and tumor biology. In addition, modulation of TGF-β signaling mediators downstream of the receptor also contributes to HNSCC tumorigenesis. For instance, SMAD2 and 4, but not SMAD3, are frequently downregulated in HNSCC, correlating with a worse prognosis (100,101). Here again, a genetic animal model in which SMAD4 is deleted demonstrates that loss of SMAD4 interferes with DNA repair pathways and results in the spontaneous development of invasive head and neck tumors (101). In a similar vein, TGF-β inhibitors interfering with SMAD signaling also contribute to tumorigenesis. The overexpression of SMURF2, which enhances cell migration and invasion *in vitro*, is a marker of bad prognosis in esophageal SCC (102); whether SMURFs have prognostic value in HSNCC has not yet been tested.

THE CELL CYCLE ORCHESTRATES CELL PROLIFERATION

Multiple extracellular mitogenic signals such as EGF, the sensing of neighboring cells via cell–cell interactions, or tissue oxygenation are integrated via distinct signaling pathways that converge to regulate the cell cycle. The integration of these signals informs the cell of the decision to proliferate. The cell cycle-regulating machinery is a prime target for oncogenic mutations, since cancer is a disease of unregulated cell proliferation.

In the resting state, the cell is quiescent, termed the G0 phase of the cell cycle. In this dormant stage, the pocket family proteins (Rb, p107, and p130) act as transcriptional cofactors that inhibit expression of proliferation-related genes (103). Among other effects, Rb inhibits the transcription factor E2F that drives the expression of proliferation genes (33,103). However, in the presence of growth factors, the Ras/Raf/ERK pathway becomes activated, leading to the phosphorylation and activation of transcription factors driving expression of proliferation genes, including cyclin D (Fig. 108.3) (104). Cyclin proteins are expressed for a limited period during the cell cycle and are rapidly degraded via ubiquitin-mediated protein degradation, leading to oscillating concentration during the cell cycle (105). There are several members of the cyclin family, each specific for a phase of the cell cycle. Cyclins have no intrinsic enzymatic activity, but associate with and partially activate cyclin-dependent kinases (Cdk), whose expression levels remain constant during the cell cycle. A second posttranslational modification, such as phosphorylation of the cyclin:Cdk complex by a Cdk-activating kinase (CAK or cylinH:Cdk7) at a specific threonine site (Thr 160) (106) or dephosphorylation of an active site by cdc25 (107), is also required for full activity of the complex.

Early in the G1 phase, cyclin D is synthesized as a consequence of ERK activation (104). Cyclin D accumulates as long as the growth factor is present, but in the absence of growth stimuli, the protein is quickly degraded, and progression through the cell cycle stops. Cyclin D associates with Cdk4/6, the effector kinases of the G1 phase of the cell cycle. Active cyclinD:Cdk4/6 complex acts in a positive feedback loop during the G1 phase to promote cyclin D expression. The active kinase complex mediates the inhibitory phosphorylation of pocket proteins, which repress E2F. As a result, E2F-dependent transcription is derepressed, and cyclin D synthesis increases (104). The same mechanism is responsible for the accumulation of cyclin E later in G1.

As cyclin E levels increase in somatic cells, it associates with Cdk2 to form an active complex that governs the G1/S transition. This cyclin:Cdk complex has distinct functions to prepare cell for DNA synthesis and mitosis. First, it induces duplication of the centrosome (108), a membraneless organelle responsible for microtubule network and mitotic spindle assembly. Second, it renders the cell competent for DNA synthesis, but does not start DNA synthesis (109). Third, it phosphorylates and inactivates a cell cycle inhibitor named p27 (110). The transcription of cyclin A thus far inhibited by p27 is now induced. Cyclin E is present at high levels only at the G1/S transition in somatic cells and is targeted for ubiquitin-mediated degradation in early S phase. As cyclin E levels decrease, the free pool of Cdk2 instead associates with the increasingly abundant cyclin A. The active cyclin A:Cdk2 then stimulates DNA replication by activating the replication complex, completing the transition from G1 to S phase (104,109).

After completion of DNA replication, cyclin A changes kinase partner, now associating with Cdk1, which drives the G2 and M phases. G2 is a phase of preparation for mitosis that is incompletely understood. G2 is not an absolute requirement for division, as cancer cells may skip this stage and directly progress to mitosis. In early G2, cyclin B accumulates. As the cell progresses through G2, cyclin A is targeted for ubiquitin-mediated degradation, increasing the pool of free Cdk1 available for association with cyclin B. With rising cyclin B:Cdk1 activity by the end of G2, nuclear breakdown occurs, chromosomes condense, and the cell enters mitosis (111).

Mitosis is a highly orchestrated phenomenon. During this phase, 46 duplicated chromosomes need to be distributed equally between two future daughter cells. Faulty distribution results in aneuploidy, which is most often incompatible with cell survival, at least under physiologic conditions (112). The central regulator of proper cell division, ensuring correct distribution of genetic material between daughter cells, is an ubiquitin ligase complex called the anaphase-promoting complex (APC). APC targets mitosis regulatory proteins for degradation. The specificity of APC for its targets is dependent on Cdc20; if Cdc20 is inhibited, APC cannot degrade regulators essential for progression through mitosis, and the cell cycle is stalled before anaphase (105).

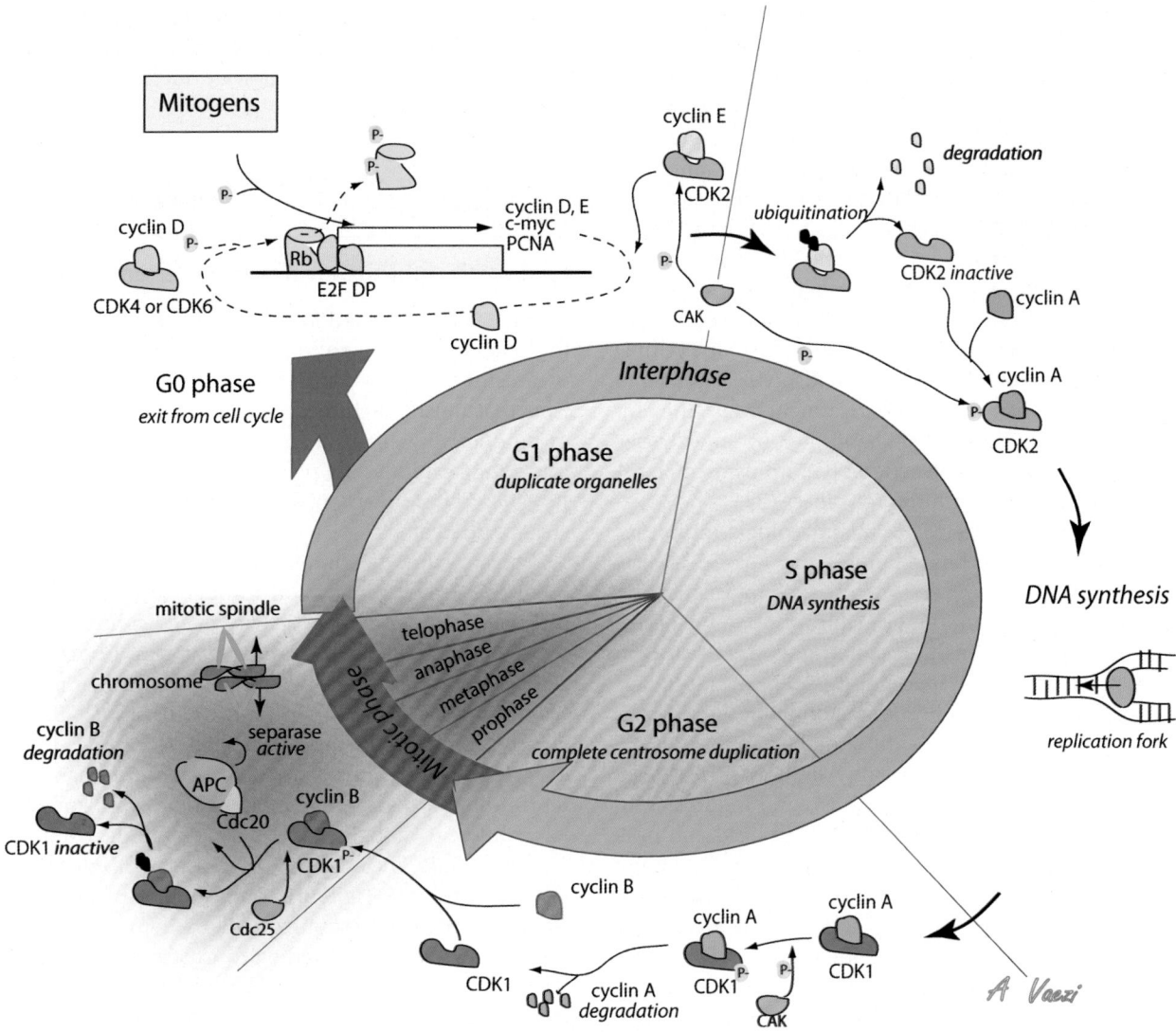

Figure 108.3 Cell cycle proteins regulate cell replication. Cyclin:Cdk complexes orchestrate progression through the cell cycle. Mitogen signals triggering proliferation are represented on the top left; regulation of cyclin:Cdk complexes is represented on the rest of the figure. See text for details.

During mitosis, chromosomes condense, the nuclear envelope breaks down, a bipolar mitotic spindle forms, and each chromosome attaches to the mitotic spindle at the chromosome center, or kinetochore. To ensure symmetry, the "mitotic checkpoint" ensures that no cell division starts before each and every chromosome is attached to both mitotic spindles (113). The molecular mechanism responsible for preventing premature division is only partially understood. Uncaptured kinetochores bind to protein complexes formed by Bub and Mad proteins (114,115). These complexes generate, through an unknown mechanism, an inhibitory signal that represses Cdc20. Thus, only when all kinetochores are captured by the spindle, and therefore the division is expected to unfold symmetrically, does the inhibitory signal stop. Cdc20 can then direct APC to target mitotic regulators for degradation (105). APC instructs the degradation of securin, which is essential to prevent the premature separation of sister chromosomes.

Securin binds to and inhibits separase, a protease that cleaves cohesin, the "glue" that holds the two sister chromatids together. When securin is degraded, active separase cleaves cohesin, freeing the sister chromatids from each other and allowing the chromosomes to be freely pulled in opposite directions by each mitotic spindle (116). By this elegant mechanism, symmetrical segregation of genetic material is ensured. APC:Cdc20 also targets cyclin B for degradation, which inactivates Cdk1; this constitutes a major signal to start anaphase and complete cell division.

Clinical Implications of Cyclins and Cdks for HNSCC

Since cyclins and Cdks drive the cell cycle, they are obvious targets for oncogenic mutations. In HNSCC, cyclin D gene or protein expression level was identified as a prognostic factor in HSNCC in most but not all studies (117–122) and has been proposed to be an early event in tumor progression. Interestingly, cyclin D is part of an amplicon present in 30% of tumors, which may explain why HNSCC overexpresses this cyclin (123–125). Conceptually, the presence of the amplicon may be of no consequence if the amplified chromosome does not translate to elevated levels of protein expression. In some but not all studies, the presence of the amplicon correlated with increased cyclin D expression, establishing a possible link between the genetic abnormality and elevated protein expression (126–128). In addition, a particular genetic polymorphism in cyclin D that increases the protein half-life predisposes its carrier to HNSCC and predicts response to treatment (129); the cancer predisposition results were confirmed by an extensive meta-analysis analyzing genetic polymorphisms in DNA repair genes associate with risk for cancer (24).

Cdks are being targeted by pharmacologic inhibitors, such as seliciclib. Preclinical studies and Phase I clinical trials point to promising effects in nasopharyngeal cancer (130). However, the antitumoral efficacy of a nonspecific modulator of G1 cyclins/Cdk (small molecule E7070) in a Phase II trial was disappointing (131). The drug was effective in reducing Rb phosphorylation, but the trial was aborted early due to lack of antitumoral effect.

Spindle checkpoint abnormality induces mis-segregation of genetic material during mitosis and induces chromosomal instability in animal models. In head and neck cancer, the level of expression of a mitotic checkpoint protein named BubR1, which is involved in pairing kinetochores with spindles, has been identified as a potential biomarker for HNSCC clinical outcome (132,133). Low expression, which may mark a defective spindle checkpoint, correlated with worse outcome. This may suggest that in the presence of an abnormal checkpoint, the segregation of chromosomes is not maintained, leading to chromosomal instability, a hallmark of aggressive cancers. Most

importantly, taxanes are microtubule stabilizing drugs that interfere with the normal function of the mitotic spindle and prevent anaphase. Taxanes are increasingly used in HNSCC treatment.

CELL CYCLE REGULATORS: A CHECK ON PROLIFERATION

Cell Cycle Inhibitors: INKs, KIPs, and Wee1

Unregulated proliferation has disastrous consequences for living organisms, not only for a complex multicellular organisms at risk for cancer but also for unicellular organisms that must match their growth rate to the availability of nutrients present in their environment. There is therefore strong evolutionary pressure to regulate the cell cycle. In cancer, these mechanisms are almost invariably deficient or altered.

Active cyclin:Cdk complexes are the terminal signaling event that drives progression through the cell cycle. Cell cycle regulators modulate activity of the cyclin:Cdk complexes using different molecular strategies. Conceptually, cell cycle inhibitors can be categorized in three families: the inhibitors of cyclin-dependent kinases (INKs), the kinase inhibitor proteins (KIPs), and Wee1 (Fig. 108.4A) (134,135). Each family has a different mechanism of repression, blocks different phases of the cycle, and inhibits a different range of cyclins or cyclin:Cdk complexes. The INK family includes p15 (INK4b), p16 (INK4a), p18 (INK4c), and p19 (INK4b). These inhibitors are specific for the G1 phase and suppress Cdk4 activity (Fig. 108.4A). INKs act by physically binding to Cdk to prevent interaction with cyclin D. When cellular levels of p16 are persistently elevated, cells permanently withdraw from the cell cycle, a process known as cellular senescence. p16 is an important tumor suppressor; it is frequently the target of repression in cancer via microRNA or gene methylation,

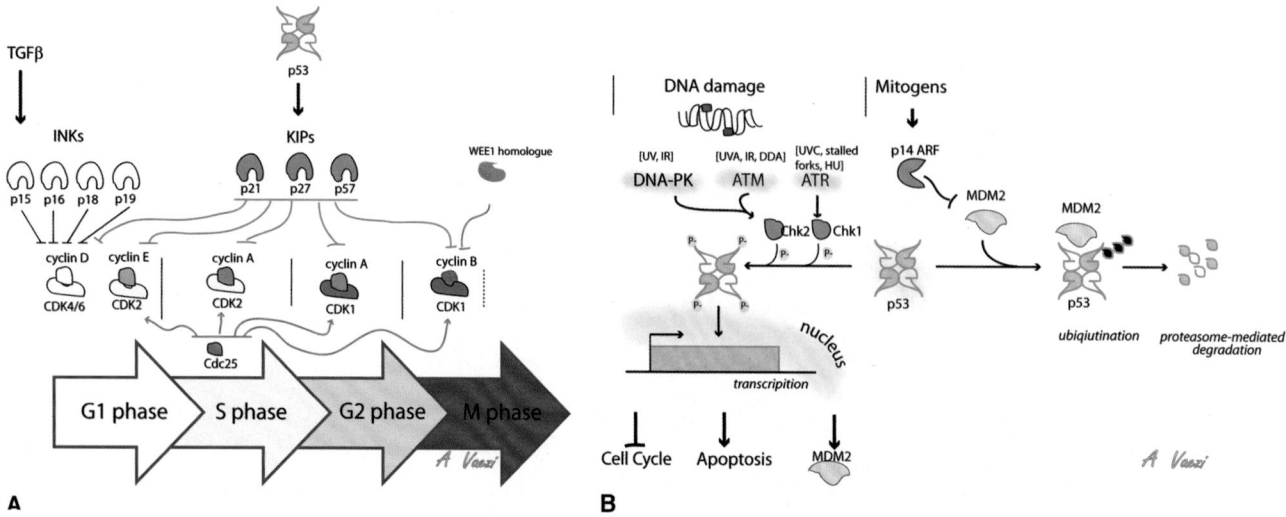

A   **B**

Figure 108.4 Activators and repressors of the cell cycle. **A**: INKs, CIP/KIP, and Wee1 repress cyclin:Cdk complexes and the cell cycle, while CDC25 activates them. **B**: p53 stabilization in response to cellular stress represses the cell cycle and stimulates apoptosis. See text for details.

and overexpression of p16 in mice confers a protective effect against cancer development (136).

KIPs have a wider scope of action. The KIP family consists of p21, p27, and p57. In contrast to INKs, these proteins counteract active cyclin:Cdk complexes after cyclins are already loaded on the kinase. KIPs also principally inhibit G1 phase Cdks, but are not restricted to this phase of the cell cycle, as KIPs also inhibit both cyclin:Cdk2 and cyclin:Cdk1 complexes involved at the G2/M transition (135). p27 represses cyclin A expression in G1, and inactivation of p27 by phosphorylation mediated by cyclinE:Cdk2 permits cyclin A synthesis. However, the actions of KIPs are more complex as in addition to their negative effect on cyclin E-, A-, and Cdk complexes. They act as positive regulators of cyclinD:Cdk4/6 and can also affect apoptosis, transcription, and cell motility (137).

The Wee1 family of proteins prevent cells from entering mitosis by inactivating cyclinB:Cdk1. Wee1 phosphorylates Cdk1 on critical threonine residues located in the ATP-binding loop necessary for Cdk function, keeping the kinase in check (138). Wee1 action is opposed by Cdc25 phosphatases, which permit entry into mitosis. Cdc25 activates Cdks throughout the cell cycle, including G1 and S phase. It is therefore not surprising that Cdc25 is overexpressed in many cancers (107). Overexpression of Cdc25 in animal model induces tissue proliferation, suggesting a tumor promoter effect, but mutagens are required to induce cancer.

P53, A Master Regulator of Cell Proliferation

The tumor suppressor p53 plays a major role in preventing progress through the cell cycle under conditions in which mitosis might be deleterious for the cell, such as DNA damage or sustained proliferation stimuli. p53 blocks proliferations and induces apoptosis. p53, a transcription factor that exists mainly as a homotetramer, has a high turnover rate, constantly being synthesized and degraded (Fig. 108.4B). p53 activity is regulated at two levels: (a) by inactivation through degradation and (b) by stabilization through phosphorylation (139). At steady state, the murine double-minute protein (MDM2) oncogene, an E3 ubiquitin ligase, binds to and ubiquitinates p53, targeting it for proteasome-mediated degradation (139). When p53 levels are low, the cell cycle can progress. However, in the setting of potentially hazardous events for the cell such as constant mitogen stimulation or DNA damage, degradation of p53 is blocked, and the transcription factor accumulates in the cytoplasm. p53 then shuttles to the nucleus where it increases transcription of KIPs to block the cell cycle, and of proapoptotic factors that trigger cell death. This selectively activates transcription of down targets depending on the level and type of posttranslational modifications such as phosphorylation, acetylation, neddylation, or sumoylation (139). Specifically, during persistent proliferation signals caused by sustained exposure to mitogens or by oncogenic stimulation, constant Ras or myc activation induces the expression of p14ARF, which is coded by a single gene locus with alternate reading frames responsible for expression of two INKs (p15 and p16) and p14ARF (136). p14ARF inhibits MDM2, which prevents ubiquitin-mediated degradation of p53, thus stabilizing p53. Through this pathway, p53 level rises and the cell is protected from sustained mitogenic activation.

DNA damage is sensed through different mechanisms depending on the type of damage encountered, but severe DNA damage also leads to p53 stabilization. For instance, irradiation generates severe oxidative stress that provokes DNA lesions. DNA double-strand breaks (DSBs) are particularly toxic as they may lead to genetic rearrangement events. DSB leads to activation of the gigantic ataxia telangectasia mutated (ATM) kinase (350 kD) (140). Upon activation, ATM induces a rapid and robust phosphorylation of proteins (141). On the one hand, it phosphorylates proteins involved in DNA repair pathways as explained in detail below. On the other hand, it activates the effector kinase Chk2, which in turn phosphorylates p53 (142). The addition of the phosphate group prevents association between p53 and MDM2. p53 then ceases to be degraded and accumulates, leading to cell cycle arrest or apoptosis if the damage is severe (141). Other types of DNA damage, such as when alkylating chemicals covalently modify DNA, prevent the replication fork from processing. A stalled replication fork is an unstable and dangerous event for the cell since it may result in DNA DSBs that are very toxic. Stalled replication forks are recognized by and activate another kinase named ATM- and Rad3-related (ATR) protein kinase. ATR is believed to stabilize p53 via activation of Chk1 protein kinase, which like Chk2 prevents association of p53 and MDM2, leading to accumulation of p53 (141,142). The ATM and ATR pathways leading to p53 accumulation and cell cycle arrest constitute the major DNA damage checkpoints of the cell cycle: cell proliferation is prevented until the DNA is repaired, ensuring conservation of genetic information. Since cancer escapes the DNA damage checkpoints, and proliferates despite persistent mitogenic stimuli, it is not surprising that p53 mutations have been found in most cancers.

Clinical Implications of Regulators of the Cell Cycle for HNSCC

The p16 INK is frequently lost early in SCC carcinogenesis, whether secondary to promoter methylation of genetic rearrangements (143). LOH in 9p is found in dysplastic mucosa (144), and in 20% to 75% of HNSCC (143–146). Loss of p16 locus is a biomarker of poor prognosis in some but not all studies, underscoring the importance of p16 in preventing head and neck cancers (124,143,147). Furthermore, p16 positivity, which occurs more frequently in HPV-related tumors, is a marker of better prognosis (21,148–153). p16-positive tumors in nonsmokers have a far better prognosis than p16-negative tumors when treated with chemoradiation therapy (21). At this juncture, it is not possible to determine whether p16 positivity simply correlates with outcome or whether p16 is directly responsible for a biologic activity that generates a favorable prognosis.

Cdc25A and B, the phosphatases that activate cyclins/Cdk complexes and promote progression through the cell cycle, are upregulated in 96% (Cdc25A) and 57% (Cdc25B) of laryngeal tumors (154). The proportion of overexpressing tumors increases with progression. However, overexpression does not correlate with clinical prognosis and upregulation of this phosphatase does not necessarily translate to increased phosphatase activity. The meaning of this upregulation needs to be determined (107).

p53 is heavily mutated upon exposure to tobacco smoke, and 50% of HNSCC tumors harbor mutations in p53 (3,155). Because of a high prevalence p53 mutations that negatively impact protein expression level, p53 expression is low in HNSCC, which in turn correlates with poor prognosis in large studies (155). The multistep HNSCC carcinogenesis model proposes that LOH in p53 may represent a genetic event that marks the transition from a noninvasive to an invasive cancer (6). In fact, p53 mutations may occur earlier, in normal-appearing mucosa; loss of p53 is now accepted as an early genetic event in HNSCC tumorigenesis (156,157). Using an elegant technique to detect mutations in p53, it has been shown that p53 mutations exist in normal-appearing mucosa present near tumor margins (44). This is an important finding as excision of these mutated cancer progenitors is essential to prevent locoregional recurrence. p53 is thus a prime candidate for cancer screening methods in HNSCC.

The elevated rate of p53 mutations observed in HNSCC opens therapeutic opportunities for preferential pharmacologic targeting of cells lacking this tumor suppressor. Despite the strong rationale, clinical success has been limited. Exposure of tumors (by intra-tumoral injection or mouthwashes) to Onyx virus, which supposedly replicates in and preferentially kills cells lacking p53, showed efficacy (158,159). For instance, virus mouthwashes transiently reduce precancerous lesions (160). However, the specificity of the virus for p53 mutated cancers has been questioned, stopping progression to Phase III trials, except in China.

p53 downregulation is intimately linked with HPV infection. While the mechanism by which HPV 16 causes tumors is not completely elucidated, HPV produces early genes E6 and E7. E6 protein associates with a cellular ubiquitin ligase that targets p53 for proteosomal degradation, but it also interferes with p53 acetylation required for some of its function (161). In addition, E7 not only competes with Rb for binding to E2F transcription regulatory sequence but also neutralizes p21 and p27. As a result, Rb is displaced and E2F is derepressed, triggering synthesis of proliferation genes such as c-myc and cyclin D and E (161). In the presence of both E7 and E6, the cell receives a constant proliferative stimulus, but has lost the protection conferred by p53. Proliferation continues contributing to carcinogenesis. Interestingly, cancer exome sequencing confirmed that nonsmokers with HPV-positive tumors have fewer p53 mutations, underscoring the interrelation between HPV and p53 in HNSCC (3).

DNA REPAIR PATHWAYS MAINTAIN GENOME INTEGRITY

p53 stabilization is a major event inducing cell cycle arrest in response to DNA damage. The delay in cell cycle progression provides time for DNA repair to occur. Failure to repair damaged DNA leads to mutations, a change in genetic sequence, which propagate in progeny of each additional cell division. Appearance of mutations occurs because the damaged DNA cannot be replicated properly during DNA synthesis. The replication machinery may, for instance, incorporate a mismatched base opposite to the damage. The replication fork may also be stalled when the damage is encountered, leading to its collapse and creation of secondary chromosome breaks and rearrangements (162). The resulting mutations are not detected as being abnormal by the cell and will be replicated and propagated as normal genome with each cell division.

DNA repair pathways are multiple and complex, and common components are often shared between pathways, adding a level of complexity. A comprehensive description of all the pathways involved in DNA repair is beyond the scope of this chapter; selected repair pathways are discussed. An essential concept in DNA repair is that the type of DNA repair is specific to the type of DNA damage encountered. For example, a DSB is repaired by a different pathway than a single-strand break (SSB) or a bulky DNA adduct that distorts the double helix. Often the repair pathway is able to correct the damage and restore the original DNA sequence, but not always (163). Certain types of damage are repaired without preservation of the genome fidelity, via "error-prone" repair mechanisms. Why cells adopt error-prone repair is not completely understood, but it is believed that the introduction of a mutation may be preferable for the cell or the organism, rather than maintaining a hazardous DNA lesion that is incompatible with cell survival.

Nucleotide Excision Repair and Interstrand Cross-Link Repair

Bulky chemical DNA adducts such as those caused by cisplatin result in intrastrand cross-links and distortion of the double helix (164,165). Such lesions are recognized and repaired via nucleotide excision repair (NER) (Fig. 108.5). This efficient mechanism is faithful; genome sequence is conserved at the end of the repair. In NER, the distortion of the DNA double helix is detected by XPC-hHR23B complex, in some cases with the assistance of XPE–DDB. Xeroderma pigmentosum (XP) proteins (e.g., XPE, XPF, XPG, XPD) were found to be congenitally mutated in patients diagnosed with XP, a syndrome characterized by a high propensity for skin cancer and exquisite sensitivity

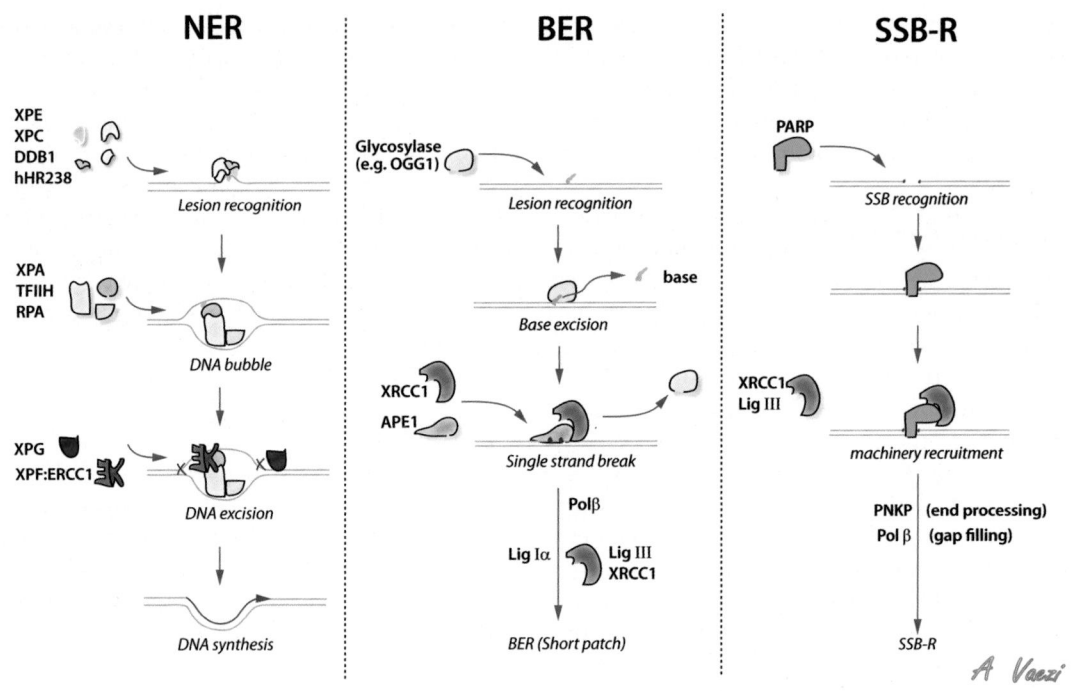

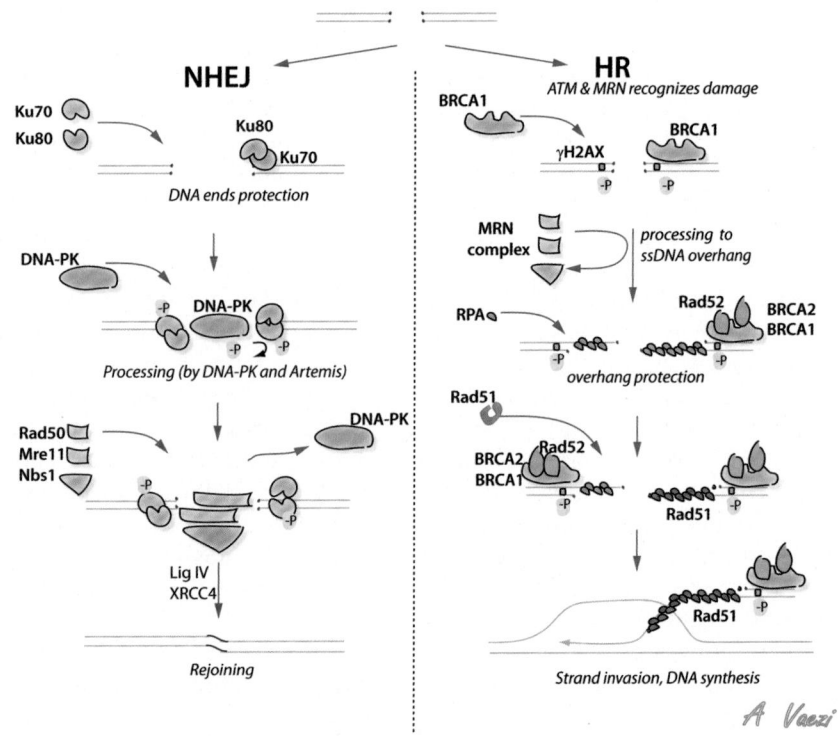

Figure 108.5 DNA repair pathways. Model of selected DNA repair pathways. From top right to bottom left, nucleotide excision repair (NER), base excision repair (BER), single strand break repair (SSB-R), and double-strand break repair (DSB-R) with non-homologous end joining (NHEJ) and homologous recombination (HR) are represented.

to DNA-damaging agents. The XPE:DDB protein complex signals the damage by binding to the damaged DNA. The complex recruits TFIIH, which unwinds the DNA around the adduct, creating a single-stranded DNA bubble

centered on the damage. XPA and RPA, which bind ssDNA, stabilize the open complex and recruit the ERCC1:XPF endonuclease. XPF:ERCC1 is a bipartite endonuclease that cuts the damaged strand 5′ to the adduct. TFIIH recruits a second endonuclease, XPG, which cuts 3′ of the lesion. The damaged base is removed as part of a single-stranded oligonucleotide. The replication machinery uses the 3′-OH created by ERCC1-XPF incision to prime DNA synthesis to fill the gap. After ligation, the integrity of the DNA is fully restored (166,167).

In addition to intrastrand cross-link and bulky DNA adducts, cisplatin also creates interstrand cross-link (ICLs), in which both strands are covalently linked by the chemical. The consequence of this lesion is catastrophic for the cell, as it prevents transcription and constitutes an absolute block for DNA replication machinery at the replication fork. The stalled replication fork collapses and creates DSB. The fork cannot progress until the DNA is repaired. ERCC1-XPF cuts near the ICL to release it from one strand, allowing bypass of the adduct by a trans-lesion polymerase such as REV1/Polζ (164,165). This type of repair is error-prone. An error-free repair has also been documented, which involves the formation of a DSB followed by homologous recombination (HR) (see below). The importance of intact NER and ICL repair to prevent cancer is illustrated by the genetic disorder XP, and alteration in these pathways could be an important carcinogenic event.

Base Excision Repair

Physiologic metabolism generates oxidative reactive species, which cause an estimated 1,000 to 1,000,000 DNA lesions per day. Oxidative stress, like alkylating agents or ionizing radiation, generates small genotoxic oxidative base lesions, which do not distort the DNA double helix, and are principally repaired through the base excision repair (BER) pathway. In BER, damaged bases are recognized and excised by glycosylases, such as OGG1, which removes the abundant oxidative lesion 8-oxodeoxyguanosine. Excision of the damaged base leaves an abasic (AP) site, while leaving the DNA backbone intact. The backbone adjacent to the AP site is then incised by APE1 endonuclease to create an SSB. XRCC1, a platform protein with no enzymatic activity that is critical for the scaffolding of proteins involved in BER is recruited to the site of damage. The recruitment is mediated either by the glycosylase/AP1 complex or by PARP1, which recognizes and binds SSBs. DNA polymerase β (Polβ) then fills the gap. XRCC1 subsequently forms a complex with ligase 3 (LIG3). The ligase seals the SSB created during the repair process to complete BER in an error-free fashion (165,168).

Single-Strand Break Repair

Energy release by free radicals generated by ionizing radiation disrupts phosphodiester bonds in the DNA backbone and can cause either SSB or DSB, the latter being very toxic. SSB is repaired by the single-strand break repair (SSB-R) pathway which shares many components with BER; this is not surprising since the BER mechanism creates an SSB

intermediate product. In SSB-R, the severed DNA strand is detected by PARP that binds to the lesion to protect the ends against processing. It then recruits the scaffolding protein XRCC1. The XRCC1:PARP complex recruits PNKP, a bifunctional polynucleotide kinase/phosphatase, which processes the ends of the broken DNA. Once the gap has been tailored, it is filled by Polβ, using the intact complementary DNA strand as template. The newly completed DNA strand is then ligated to complete SSB-R. DNA integrity is restored with maintenance of the genetic sequence via an error-free repair mechanism (162,169,170).

Double-Strand Break Repair

Ionizing radiation or stalled replication forks are very hazardous for a cell. Both create double-strand DNA breaks that can lead to genome rearrangement if left unrepaired. Here we discuss two mechanisms directed to the repair of double-stand breaks: nonhomologous end-joining (NHEJ) and HR repair. These pathways are different in multiple aspects. NHEJ occurs at all stages of the cell cycle, but during the repair, the broken ends have been processed before being rejoined, which leads to loss of DNA. On the other hand, HR is faithful as the processed broken DNA ends are copied from intact DNA from a sister chromatid, but the repair is restricted to S phase and G2.

In NHEJ, the site where both strands of the double helix are severed is recognized by two proteins of the Ku family (Ku70 and 80). Ku70/80 dimers rapidly bind to the free end of the broken DNA to prevent processing of the ends. These protein foci located at DSB recruit the large protein DNA-dependent serine/threonine protein kinase (DNA-PK). The kinase autophosphorylates itself and also phosphorylates the Ku proteins. As a consequence, the Ku proteins translocate slightly away from the broken DNA end, giving space for DNA-PK and a protein named Artemis to process the free ends of the broken DNA double helix; Artemis resolves DNA hairpins formed due to sequence homology in the broken DNA. After this first step of end processing, a complex of three proteins (Mre11, Rad50, and Nbs1) named MRN is recruited at the DSB foci. MRN catalyzes further the ends processing and produce single-stranded ends. XRCC4 is then recruited to the site of damage, and in tight association with ligase IV, it reseals the broken ends together. During end processing, DNA is lost: This repair is error-prone (162,171). However, the pathway as described here is simplified and does not account for all the observations. For instance, cells are able to undergo NHEJ in the absence of Ku/DNA-PK, demonstrating the presence of an alternative pathway, which may be error-free and involve the protein breast cancer 1 (BRCA1) (172).

An alternate way to repair DSB involves HR with intact DNA borrowed from sister chromatids or homologous chromosomes. This type of repair happens preferentially when the DNA has been duplicated in S or G2 phase. Initially, the DSB is detected by ATM and the MRN complex. ATM rapidly phosphorylates the Chk2 kinases involved in stabilizing p53 to activate the DNA damage checkpoint as described above. ATM also phosphorylates histone H2A at the site of damage, on a serine (Ser139); the phosphorylated histone is called γH2AX. Within 1 hour of damage, BRCA1, which was identified as being mutated in familial breast cancers, is recruited to sites of DSB containing γH2AX. The MRN complex also localizes early at the site of DSB, where it processes the broken DNA ends to form single-stranded overhangs on each side of the lesion. The single-stranded DNA ends are rapidly covered by replication protein A (RPA), which forms a filament and prevents the formation of secondary DNA structures. RPA also activates ATR, leading to p53-mediated DNA damage checkpoint. At this stage, BRCA1 recruits two other proteins, BRCA2 and Rad52, which load the recombinase Rad51 onto the single-stranded overhang. RPA is dislodged by Rad51 polymer, which forms a filament composed of protein and DNA named the presynaptic filament. Rad51 then searches for homologous sequences via strand invasion of the sister chromatid or the homologous chromosome. The DNA is copied from the undamaged DNA and results, after resolution of complex DNA intermediate structures, in HR and in faithful repair of DNA (162,171–173).

Clinical Implications of DNA Repair Pathways for HNSCC

HNSCC are generally treated with DNA-damaging agents such as ionizing radiation and platinum-based chemotherapy, either in a primary or adjuvant setting. Tumors with an altered capacity to repair DNA respond differently to these treatments. During treatment with DNA-damaging agents, genotoxic lesions accumulate both in normal tissue and in cancer cell DNA. In this context, cancer cells with a low level of DNA repair machinery accumulate damage and mutations more rapidly, and are thus more sensitive to DNA-damaging agents. Hence, therapeutic compounds that inhibit DNA repair pathways are relatively cytotoxic for tumors and may sensitize cancers to DNA-damaging agents. For instance, a novel class of antitumor drugs, PARP inhibitors, showed promising results in preclinical studies and are currently being tested in Phase I and Phase II clinical trial in breast and other cancers (174). Other compounds showing promising results in the preclinical setting include the Chk1/2 inhibitors (175), DNA-PK (175), ATM kinase (175), RPA (176), and MGMT (177) inhibitors, although results of MGMT inhibition in clinical trials were disappointing (177,178). It is with great hope that we follow the evolution of these new therapies as they are tested in clinical settings in HNSCC.

Abnormalities in DNA repair pathways of a given tumor may predict sensitivity to DNA-damaging agents and inform the head and neck oncologist on the most appropriate treatment to administer for a given tumor. In the growing field of personalized oncology, there is great interest in estimating the DNA repair capacity of HNSCC

prospectively. The tumor expression level of ERCC1 and XPF generally correlates with survival in HNSCC treated with DNA-damaging agents, although the results are not uniform (165,179–183). Platinum-based compounds such as cisplatin and carboplatin are the most commonly used chemotherapeutic agents for HNSCC. These genotoxic drugs form bulky chemical adducts and cause intrastrand and interstrand cross-links, which are repaired via NER and ICL repair. The bipartite endonuclease ERCC1:XPF is the only DNA repair protein involved in the repair of all DNA damage generated by cisplatin, and cells deficient in ERCC1:XPF are exquisitely sensitive to DNA-damaging agents such as cisplatin. This explains why a low level of ERCC1:XPF correlates with enhanced sensitivity to cisplatin and ionizing radiation, and predicts clinical outcome in HNSCC. Surprisingly, when the level of expression of more than 30 genes involved in DNA repair was evaluated in HNSCC, Ku80, which is involved in NHEJ, was the only gene studied associated with prognosis (184). Another DNA repair protein identified as potential biomarker is XRCC1 (BER pathway), for which the expression level associates with clinical outcome in HNSCC (185). With further validation through independent prospective clinical trials, these biomarkers will instruct the personalized treatment of HNSCC to maximize survival and minimize unnecessary toxicity.

It has also been proposed that polymorphisms in DNA repair genes may correlate with altered capacity for repairing DNA, and therefore may indicate risk for HNSCC. Single nucleotide polymorphisms (SNPs) are defined as single-base changes that occur in more than 1% of the population. Depending on the location of the SNP, it may alter protein expression level or activity. A meta-analysis of HNSCC cancer risk in relation to SNPs in DNA repair genes revealed that XRCC1 codon 194 is associated with cancer risk (24). Mutation in DNA repair genes, such as the numerous genes in involved in Fanconi anemia, causes a high risk of HNSCC. It is therefore possible that genetic variants in the same or other DNA repair genes may have a more subtle clinical phenotype to increase HNSCC risk, response to treatment, or treatment toxicity.

APOPTOSIS COUNTERBALANCES PROLIFERATION

Proliferating tissues such as skin and the mucosa of the gastrointestinal, respiratory, and aerodigestive tracts are in constant turnover. Some cells proliferate, while others die, often through programmed cell death, but under physiologic conditions, the overall number of cells within the tissue remains constant. In cancer, this balance is lost and net gain of cells occurs; this results from both unregulated proliferation and impaired programmed cell death. The molecular pathways leading to programmed cell death, or apoptosis, can be divided in two categories: the extrinsic pathway, which is triggered by the activation of death receptors at the cell surface, and the intrinsic pathway, which is activated by radiation, cytotoxic drugs, cellular stress, or growth factor withdrawal (186). Both pathways are mediated through activation of a cascade of intracellular proteases called caspases that cleave multiple intracellular targets (187). The hallmarks of apoptosis are DNA fragmentation as a result of DNA cleavage between nucleosomes and nuclear disintegration into small vesicles, which leads to the characteristic appearance of apoptotic cells. Caspases are zymogens that are activated by cleavage and can be grouped in two categories: *initiator* or apical caspases, which transduce the apoptotic signal, and *effector* caspases, which break down the cell and execute apoptosis (187).

In the extrinsic apoptotic pathway (Fig. 108.6), caspases are activated by a protein platform called death-inducing signaling complex (DISC), which forms at the plasma membrane. Death receptors of the TNF receptor superfamily, which include the FAS receptors and the CR4 and CR5 receptors, are used by neutral killer cell to kill cancer cells. FAS ligand binding to FAS receptor or Apo2L/TRAIL binding to CR4/CR5 initiates clustering of the receptors and DISC formation (186). The transmembrane receptors homo-trimerize and recruit an adaptor protein (FADD) to form an active DISC. The protein platform then recruits and activates procaspase 8 or procaspase 10 (187). The active caspase is released from the DISC and remains in the cytosol where it cleaves and activates effector caspases, in particular caspase 6, 7, and 3, which execute cell autodestruction. The extrinsic pathway is also connected to the intrinsic pathway as described below.

The mitochondria play a central role in mediating apoptosis via the intrinsic pathway. In the intrinsic pathway, proapototic proteins located in the mitochondrial membrane trigger the release of cytochrome C from the mitochondrion. The cytochrome C is located in the space between the mitochondrial inner and outer membranes and is sequestered from the cytoplasm in the absence of a death signal. Cytoplasmic release of cytochrome C, instrumental in activating caspases and apoptosis in the intrinsic pathway (188,189), is regulated by proteins of the BCL-2 family. The BCL-2 family contains 21 proteins, which can be divided into 3 classes: multidomain anti-apoptotic (including BCL-2, BCL-XL, MCL-1), multidomain proapototic (including BAX and BAK), and single-domain proapoptotic activators (including BID, BIN) or sensitizers (including BAD, NOXA, PUMA); the single domain of the activators/sensitizers resembles a portion of BLC-2 and is termed Bcl-2 homology 3 (BH3) domain that is important in drug development (190). Under physiologic conditions, in the absence of death signals, the multidomain anti-apoptotic BCL-2 and proapoptotic protein BAX are constitutively inserted in the outer leaflet of the mitochondrial outer membrane (MOM), where they neutralize each other. Upon activation by death signals, apoptotic activators such as BIN disrupt this interaction, via their BH3 domains. The freed pool of BAX then oligomerizes into channels that permeabilize the MOM, leading to leakage of cytochrome C. BAK, on the other hand, is mainly

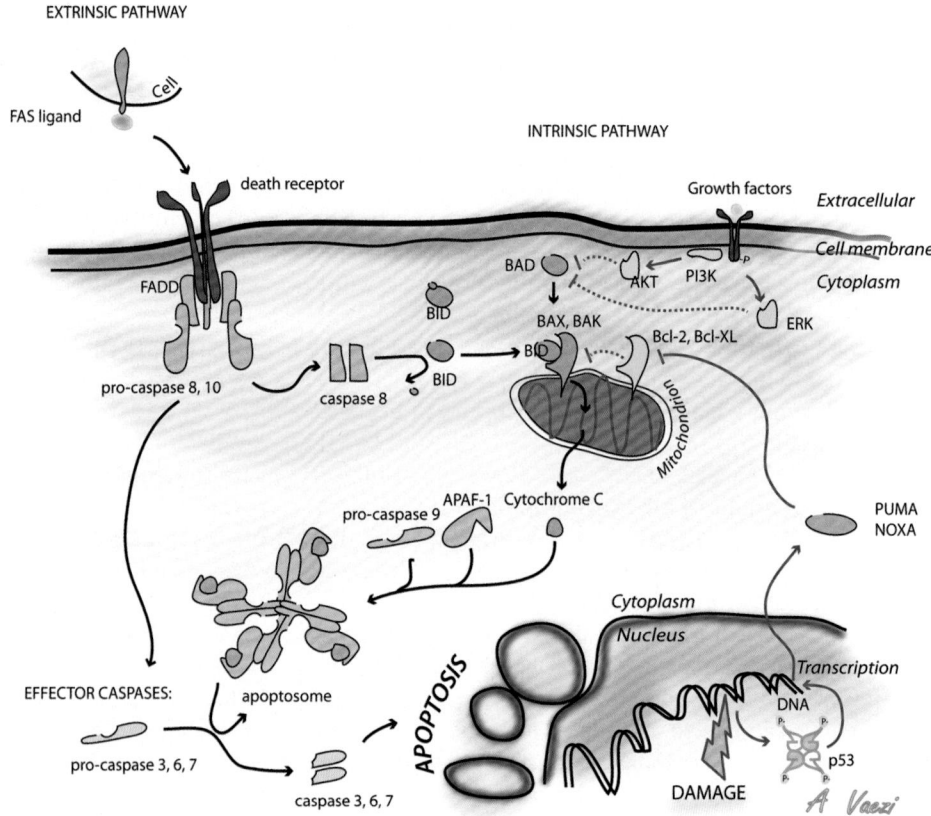

Figure 108.6 Pathways to apoptosis. Model of the extrinsic (**left**) and intrinsic (**right**) apoptosis pathways and their cross talk is represented. See text for details.

cytoplasmic; activation by apoptotic signals induces a conformational change in the protein that leads to its insertion into the MOM. Upon binding and activation by the cytosolic proapoptotic activator or sensitizer, BAK forms pores and releases cytochrome C from the mitochondrion, like BAX (190). Once in the cytoplasm, cytochrome C permits the formation of a large multiprotein platform called the apoptosome. This propeller-like structure is composed of APAF1, procaspase 9 dimers, and cytochrome C (190). It acts as an effector caspase activator platform, where procaspase 9 is activated and cleaves the *effector* caspases 6, 7, and 3 (187).

The extrinsic pathway and the intrinsic pathway interact. In the cytoplasm, the initiator caspase of the extrinsic pathway, caspase 8, cleaves the self-inhibitory portion of the single-domain proapoptotic activator BID (187). BID then translocates to the mitochondrial membrane where it binds BAX and BAK, triggering the intrinsic pathway and the release of cytochrome C. Of interest, mitogenic pathways also have cross talk with the intrinsic pathway. Growth factors enjoy both positive effects on cell proliferation and pro-survival effects by inhibiting apoptosis. Growth factor receptors, such as EGFR, activate PI3 kinase. The formation of PI3P (3,4,5) in inner leaflet of the plasma membrane creates docking and activation sites for PH domain proteins, in particular Akt (63). Activated Akt phosphorylates BAD, a single-domain proapoptotic protein (191,192). Phosphorylated BAD is unable to activate BAX or BAK, rendering the cell increasingly resistant to apoptosis. EGFR signaling also counteracts apoptotic signals via the MAP kinase ERK, which activates RSK kinase, which, similar to Akt, inhibits BAD (193). Finally, p53 activates apoptotic pathways in response to DNA damage. Phosphorylated p53 increases transcription of PUMA (194) and NOXA (195), two apoptotic sensitizers. PUMA is the more potent apoptosis activator, inhibiting all multidomain anti-apoptotic proteins including Bcl-2, Bcl-X_L (194), and MCL-1, while NOXA inhibits only Bcl-X_L and MCL-1.

Defective apoptotic pathways, for instance when Bcl-2 is overexpressed, are beneficial for a cancer cell, because they are resistant to death signals from TNF or FAS ligand induced by contact with a cell responsible for immune surveillance. In addition, it will also be more protected against apoptotic signals triggered by oncogenic activation of Ras or Myc. In this case, the cancer cell may progress through the cell cycle despite DNA damage, leading to accumulation of further mutations. This also renders apoptosis-deficient cells resistant to chemotherapy by DNA-damaging agents. Escape from apoptosis clearly favors carcinogenesis.

Clinical Implications of Apoptosis for Prognosis and Treatment of HNSCC

Cancer results from a disequilibrium between cell proliferation and cell death, and HNSCC is not an exception. The apoptotic pathways are frequently impaired in HNSCC, with repercussions on tumor behavior and resistance to

treatment. For instance, the anti-apoptotic proteins Bcl-2 and Bcl-X_L of the intrinsic pathway are often overexpressed in HNSCC (196). Overexpression of Bcl-2 or Bcl-X_L conferred resistance to apoptosis and associated with a worse clinical prognosis in some but not all retrospective analysis (149,196,197). Curiously, Bcl-2 overexpression had opposite effects in two studies, where it associated with better clinical response to hyperfractionated radiotherapy and laryngeal preservation strategies (196,198). Probably higher level of clinical evidence via prospective analysis or meta-analysis is needed to clarify the role of Bcl-2 family of protein as biomarkers in HNSCC. In addition, the apical caspase of the extrinsic pathway, caspase 8, is mutated in 8% of HNSCC, as identified by HNSCC exome sequencing (3). The majority of the mutations identified are nonsense mutations, coding for a premature stop codon. Interestingly, caspase 8 appears to be the only apoptotic gene mutated in the 80 tumors sequenced; the reason for this peculiarity remains to be understood. Taken together, these results underscore how frequently the intrinsic and the extrinsic apoptosis pathway are altered in HNSCC, suggesting an important role of apoptosis suppression in HNSCC carcinogenesis.

The frequent resistance to apoptosis in HNSCC, conferred in part by Bcl-2 overexpression, renders HNSCC an attractive target for new generation Bcl-2 inhibitors (199,200). While four Bcl-2 family targeting agents are currently being studied in a preclinical setting, four are already being used in Phase I, II, or III clinical trials, although for cancers other than HNSCC (200). An important compound being tested in Phase III trial is oblimersen sodium, an antisense oligonucleotide that interferes with Bcl-2 mRNA. Oblimersen shows survival benefit in melanoma (201) and to a certain degree in chronic lymphocytic leukemia (CLL) (202); however, the positive effect may be only partially related to Bcl-2 inhibition, as oblimersen appears to stimulate local immunity independently of its effect on Bcl-2 (200). Another class of agents that deserves attention is BH3 mimetic compounds. BH3 mimetics bind to and sequester Bcl-2, thereby facilitating oligomerization of Bax and Bak and related cell death induction. Gossypol (AT-101), a toxin isolated from cotton seed half a century ago, is under clinical investigation, but is toxic for the GI tract limiting its use (200). A novel BH3 mimetic ABT-737 recently showed promising effects in a clinical trial as a radiosensitizer or chemosensitizer in hematogenous malignancies and solid non-HNSCC tumors (200); ABT-737 oral counterpart ABT-263 is under current investigation (203,204). Therefore, the overexpression of Bcl-2 family proteins or mutations in caspase 8 observed in HNSCC may serve to identify tumors that are most likely to benefit from Bcl-2 targeting therapies.

Triggering the extrinsic apoptotic pathway is another angle to attack cancer. Two approaches are employed. On the one hand, soluble human recombinant death receptor ligands are administered systemically. Interaction between ligand and CR4 and CR5 receptors triggers receptor clustering and leads to activation of the extrinsic pathway. Phase

II clinical trials are under way in non-small cell lung cancer using soluble recombinant human Apo2L/TRAIL (186). An alternative approach consists of monoclonal antibodies directed against death receptors. Antibodies such as mapatumumab, lexatumumab, and apomab induce DISC formation and cell death (186). Phase II trials are under way for cancers other than HNSCC.

CANCER STEM CELLS CONTRIBUTE TO TUMOR HETEROGENEITY

The dysfunction of the signaling pathways described above explains how a single cell may grow in an unregulated manner, resulting in clonal expansion of the diseased cell. The expected product of the clonal expansion of a single cell is a homogenous mass of cells. However, tumors are extraordinarily heterogeneous, and multiple theories attempt to reconcile this paradox. The stochastic genetic mutation theory proposes that mutations occur randomly in the initial clone, leading to the generation of subclone populations. However, another concept, now widely accepted in hematopoietic malignancies, may also be true for solid tumors. The hierarchical CSC theory proposes that only a small pool of self-renewing cancer cells have the exclusive ability to maintain the tumor. It is still unclear whether CSCs originate from mutated tissue stem cells or whether CSC come from more differentiated cells which acquire stem cell properties via a dedifferentiation process. In any case, by definition, the CSC must (a) have an unlimited self-renewal capacity to maintain the pool of CSC and (b) divide asymmetrically to provide a differentiated progeny that accounts for heterogeneity and the bulk of the tumor (205,206). For instance, in hematopoietic malignancies, a progenitor may acquire transforming mutations responsible for clonal expansion of itself while maintaining the ability to produce partially or completely differentiated cell progeny. On a blood smear, the abundant differentiated progeny will account for the vast majority of cancer cells seen; however, only a few cells, the cancer progenitors, sustain continuous proliferation and are responsible for maintaining the tumor (205). All the other tumor cells, despite their abundance, are incapable of recreating a hematopoietic malignancy when transplanted into immunodeficient animals, the gold standard test of isolation of CSC (207). Thus, novel CSC therapies are aimed at eradicating the CSC responsible of tumor maintenance and recurrences, irrespective of whether the tumor bulk is affected initially. The goal is to kill the cancer at its roots (Fig. 108.7).

In 2003, Clarke et al. applied the concept of CSC to solid tumors and isolated the first solid tumor CSCs in breast cancer (208). CSCs have now been isolated from brain, colon, prostate, pancreas, melanoma, and HNSCC tumors (206). Interestingly, there is, to date, not a single marker common for all CSCs. Often, however, solid tumor CSCs express a molecular signature of gene products involved in epithelial–mesenchymal transition (EMT) (209,210).

EMT denotes a change in cell phenotype seen during gastrulation in which epithelial cells acquire a mesenchymal phenotype. Cell–cell adhesions are lost, the cytoskeleton is remodeled with adoption of a spindle cell morphology, and cells acquire an invasive phenotype. Specifically, the cell–cell adhesion molecule E-cadherin is downregulated, while mesenchymal markers such as α-smooth muscle actin and MMPs are upregulated; TGF-β via SMAD3 and 2 and tyrosine kinase receptors induce EMT (211).

The concept of EMT may be reversible in CSC, leading to the theory of migratory CSC.

This model proposes that CSC could be divided into stationary (sCSC) and migratory CSC (mCSC) (212). The sCSCs would be entrenched to the core of the tumor, while mCSC are located at the periphery and represent CSCs that underwent EMT. mCSCs are responsible of locoregional and distant metastasis. Since EMT appears reversible in cancer, it has been proposed that the mCSC cells undergo EMT reversal, or mesenchymal–epithelial transition, at the site of metastasis (212). The exciting field of CSC is in rapid evolution, and the future will tell what proportion of this theory will prove correct.

Like tissue stem cells, CSCs live in stem cell niches poor in oxygen content, where they are protected from oxidative stress. While this has advantages for genome protection, radiation therapy, which is more effective in well-oxygenated tissues, is less effective against CSC. This may account for radioresistance and locoregional failure. Not only are CSCs relatively protected from free radicals by their location in the tissue, but they also overexpress free radical scavengers such as the glutathione reductase system (213). In addition to being resistant to oxidative stress, CSCs are also resistant to chemotherapy agents. They express drug evacuation channels such as multidrug resistance gene 1 (MDR1), which is an ATP-binding cassette transporter which lowers the intracellular concentration of chemicals and chemotherapeutic agents including taxol (214).

However, there are also differences between tissue stem cells and CSCs. Tissue stem cells are rare, but CSCs may be abundant. While the CSC population in leukemia represents a rare portion (<1%) of cancer cells (205), in HNSCC, they may represent between less than 1% and 45% of the tumors (215). It is therefore conceptually important to understand that in some tumors up to half of the cells have tumor-maintaining capacity. Another level of complexity is the tumoral environment. The gold standard test used to define CSC populations, the xenograft model, has limitations: Tumor stroma and associated cells including supporting cells, endothelial cells, and immune cells are missing. It is therefore possible that cells that act as stem cells in the native tumoral environment may lose tumor-forming ability when deprived of their native environment (205). Thus, the concept of CSC continues to evolve, but it opens new perspective for treatment.

The models of CSC, stochastic mutations, and field cancerization in HNSCC may coexist (Fig. 108.7A).

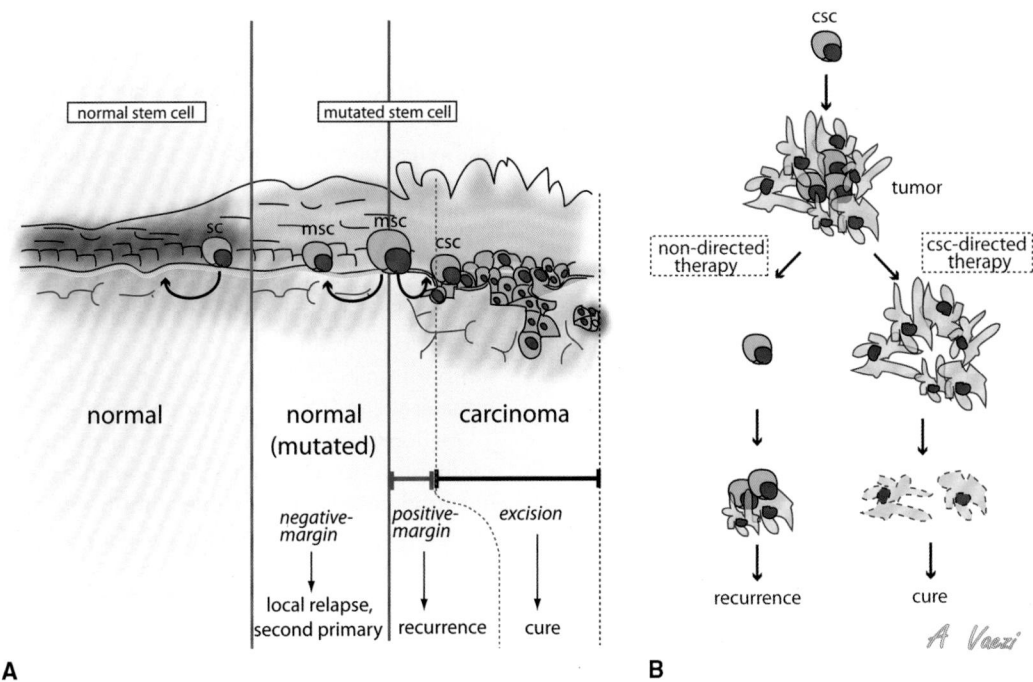

Figure 108.7 Cancer stem cells. **A:** Model integrating the concept of CSC and field cancerization, with emphasis on consequences for surgical margins. (Inspired from Leemans CR, Braakhuis BJ, Brakenhoff RH. The molecular biology of head and neck cancer. *Nat Rev Cancer* 2011;11:9–22.) **B:** Model of CSC-targeted therapies.

Transforming mutations due to alcohol and tobacco consumption in aerodigestive tract progenitors may lead to clonal expansion of CSC progenitors. It has also been proposed that transforming mutations occur in a more differentiated cell that undergoes dedifferentiation as a result of the mutation, thereby acquiring stem cell features (212). Both alternatives are possible and could lead to expansion of CSC precursors, which could lead to progressive replacement of large portions of the normal mucosa by the cancer progenitor and its differentiated progeny: the fields of cancerization. With further mutations acquired by a stochastic mutation model, CSCs arise in a cancer progenitor cell. The tumor may be the consequence of both (a) differentiation of the CSC and (b) novel mutations acquired stochastically within the clone. CSCs become mCSCs at the tumor periphery, detaching from the primary tumor to form metastatic seeds. Metastatic cells may be detected in the lymph and the circulation, but will not necessarily cause metastasis. When mCSCs home to a favorable distant site, they may grow into a metastasis (212). Resection of the primary tumor may leave either CSC or CSC progenitors at microscopically negative and possibly normal-appearing margins (10). Failure to resect these progenitors may increase the chance of recurrence.

Clinical Implications of Cancer Stem Cells in HNSCC

Little is known about HNSCC stem cells, but knowledge is increasing rapidly. In 2007, Prince et al. (215) reported CSC isolation in HNSCC for the first time. The population was initially isolated by FACS sorting with two markers; CSCs were enriched in the CD44$^+$CD24$^-$ cell population. The CSCs were found to express an oncogene BMI-1 (215), a polycomb family protein involved in chromatin remodeling and gene regulation, including p16. However, CD44 was found to be widely expressed in HNSCC; other markers have now been identified. For instance, aldehyde dehydrogenase 1 (Aldh1) expression can be used to narrow the CSC population (216). In laryngeal cancer, CD133 was identified as a sorting marker for CSCs (217,218). In addition, a less specific marker of CSC is exclusion of nuclear dye by cells with stem cell proprieties; the efflux of dye is mediated via a membrane channel of the same family as multidrug resistance gene 1 (MDR1), which also evacuates chemotherapy drugs (219). This test can be used to detect a cell population enriched in stem cells, which, as predicted, is resistant to chemotherapy.

CSCs are functionally different, and more radioresistant, than non-CSCs. CSCs are relatively resistant to chemotherapy and ionizing radiation. This explains why, while ionizing radiation is effective at reducing the global volume of head and neck tumors in xenograft models, it resulted in a relative enrichment in CSCs (213); radiation therapy and chemotherapy may select for and enrich CSCs that are resistant to treatment. As a corollary, the HNSCC CSC marker high CD44+ predicts response to treatment and is associated with increased local recurrence after radiotherapy in laryngeal cancer (220).

Novel treatment strategies target CSCs specifically. The primary goal of treatment is to attack the cancer at its regenerating roots, rather than simply reducing the tumor bulk (Fig. 108.7B). However, these strategies have not yet been translated to HNSCC clinical trials. Specific attempts to target CSCs in HNSCC include immunotherapeutic strategies targeted to CSC markers, either using anti-CD133 antibodies (221) or tumor vaccines targeting Aldh1+ cells. To date, however, no antibody specific for HNSCC CSC has been found. Another therapeutic approach is the downregulation of BMI-1, the transcription factor essential in maintenance of the self-renewal proprieties of CSCs, via siRNA strategies (217). Much hope is being invested in CSC-targeting therapies.

ANGIOGENESIS AND VASCULOGENESIS FEED TUMOR GROWTH

Tumor cells are dependent on their microenvironment and their supporting cells. For instance, independent of the existence of CSC, the tumor cannot grow without blood vessels to bring oxygen and nutrients vital for survival of the cell, and evacuation of catabolic products toxic for the cell. In absence of blood vessels, tumors cannot grow more than 1 to 2 mm in diameter (222). New blood supply is provided either through the formation of new blood vessels arising from preexisting vessels in a process termed *angiogenesis* or via the recruitment of bone marrow-derived cells and *de novo* formation of blood vessels through the process of *vasculogenesis* (223).

Angiogenesis occurs in orchestrated steps, in which a preexisting capillary sprouts new endothelial tubes which appear as finger projections of proliferating endothelial cells. Initially, endothelial cells differentiate into a motile "tip cells" that lead a trail of proliferating endothelial cells and the "stalk cells," constituting the core of the finger projection, through the hypoxic tissue (224). The endothelial tube then encounters and fuses with other capillaries, forming a complex vascular network. The immature newly formed endothelial vessels are stabilized after association with pericytes originating either from the preexisting capillaries or from the bone marrow (225). In cancer, the mature capillaries are different than normal capillaries, being more tortuous and leaky.

The molecular mechanisms involved in angiogenesis are partially understood. Capillary endothelial cells are sensitive to tissue hypoxia. In response to the lack of O_2, hypoxia-inducible factor 1α (HIF-1α) accumulates in the endothelial cell (222). HIF-1α is a transcription factor that is continuously degraded via ubiquitin-mediated degradation dependent on oxygen. Hypoxia blocks the degradation of HIF-1α, leading to its accumulation (226). HIF-1α partners with HIF-1β to induce expression of hypoxia genes including the vascular endothelial growth factor A (VEGF-A) and the VEGF receptor 2 (VEGFR2) (222). VEGF-A is a potent endothelial mitogenic factor that acts on tyrosine kinase receptors of the VEGF family. A VEGF-A gradient induces differentiation of a pioneering "tip cell," which acquires a proteolytic phenotype and degrades laminin in the basement membrane. With erosion of the basement membrane, interstitial collagen is exposed, leading to a change in cell morphology with appearance of cell protrusions and finger-like cell projections known as filopodia, which sense the VEGF gradient in the hypoxic tissue and direct the growth of the endothelial chords (222). VEGF also induces expression of the receptor notch and its ligand delta present on "stalk cells," which counteract the proliferation and migration of the endothelial chord (222). Later, association with the pericytes induces the production of metallo-protease inhibitors in both pericytes and endothelial cells, which terminates the proteolytic phenotype of the endothelial cells.

Angiogenesis is a particularly attractive target for anticancer therapy, because the cells responsible for the formation of blood vessels vital for the tumor are not transformed. They have fewer mechanisms in place to evade radio- or chemotherapy.

Vasculogenesis occurs during embryogenesis and in tumors. It involves the migration of endothelial progenitor cells (EPC) originating from bone marrow into hypoxic tissue, where EPC contribute to new vessel formation. EPC are characterized by surface markers including CD34, endothelial surface makers, and CD11, a cell substratum adhesion molecule (223). In response to tumor hypoxia, EPC home in the tumor bed in a process involving HIF-1α. HIF-1α induces secretion of stromal cell-derived factor 1 (SDF-1) in the hypoxic tissue, which activates CXCR4, a cytokine receptor present on the EPC cell surface. SDF-CXCR4 constitutes the recruiting signal for EPC into hypoxic tissue (227). Experimental evidence supporting the presence of EPC in cancer comes from animal models where EPC are genetically labeled with a color marker. In xenograft experiments, EPC contributed to 25% of the tumor vasculature within a week of tumor implantation, but the number decreased to 1% by 1 month (228). Whether or not EPC is an artifact seen in animal models is debatable, but in one study of patients who received gender mismatched bone marrow transplants showed that EPC do contribute to tumor vasculature in patients. EPC contributed to 1% to 12% of the tumor vasculature depending of the tumor type (229). The role played by EPC in tumor regrowth after irradiation was elegantly demonstrated in animal model. Blocking EPC migration through HIF-1α, or SDF-CXRCC4 inhibitors, prevented homing of EPC at the site of tumor xenograft and blocked regrowth of tumors after radiation (227).

Clinical Implication of Hypoxia, Angiogenesis, and Vasculogenesis in HNSCC

Tumoral hypoxia has long been recognized as a resistance factor for radiation therapy, and tumor tissue with oxygen tension under 0.5 mm Hg is considered resistant to radiation. Tumor hypoxia measured in pretreatment tissue specimens is an independent prognostic factor for survival, but measurements are not done routinely in clinic. HIF-1 was proposed to be a predictive biomarker for clinical outcome (230–234), but clinical results for this marker are equivocal (235–237). Another hypoxia biomarker is carbonic anhydrase IX (CA-IX), a target of HIF-1 that regulates local pH, is elevated in hypoxic regions of HNSCC, and is a confirmed marker of tumor hypoxia (231,232). Unfortunately, the prognostic value of CA-IX is disappointing. In a large retrospective analysis of a prospective study of HSNCC treated with radiotherapy with or without the hypoxia sensitizer nimorazole, CA-IX had no prognostic value, even for tumors treated with nimorazole (238). In contrast, tumoral VEGF expression as a biomarker is promising. VEGF, also a HIF-1 target, correlated with worse prognosis in several studies, and the results were confirmed in a meta-analysis (239).

Therapeutic strategies have been used to target the hypoxic regions of HNSCC. For instance, tirapazamine becomes activated in a cytotoxic radical only in hypoxic cells and was proposed as a radiosensitizer of choice to target hypoxic-resistant cells. Unfortunately, after a promising Phase II trial, the drug showed no benefit over standard cisplatin plus radiation therapy in a Phase III, multiinstitutional trial (240). Another therapeutic angle is to neutralize tumor angiogenesis. Anti-VEGF therapies are used clinically to combat HNSCC. The compound SU5416 (semaxanib), a pharmacologic inhibitor of VEGF receptor 2, was tested in HNSCC with limited efficacy (241). In contrast, some Phase III HNSCC clinical trials using bevacizumab (Avastin), a monoclonal anti-VEGF antibody, have been completed, and other Phase II trials are under way in combination with other drugs. In a double-blind, placebo-controlled, randomized trial of non-small cell lung cancer salvage therapy with erlotinib with or without bevacizumab, the addition of the VEGF-blocking agent did not improve overall survival, despite an encouraging but nonsignificant improvement in disease-free survival (242). However, in HNSCC, Phase I/II showed encouraging results (243), and promising Phase II trials testing the activity of bevacizumab and the antimetabolite pemetrexed in HNSCC are actively accruing patients. It is conceivable that only tumors expressing high levels of VEGF are sensitive to bevacizumab, and tumoral VEGF expression could be used as predictive biomarker to select patients who would benefit from antiangiogenic therapy. Novel therapeutic agents are in the preclinical study pipeline, such as PG545, which is a heparan sulfate mimetic that sequesters tumor angiogenic factors in the interstitium (244). This is another example where the understanding of the biology of angiogenesis led to the development of innovative therapies.

CONCLUSION

The information on biology of head and neck cancers is vast. In this chapter, we have focused on a description of basic concepts with an emphasis on the clinical implications of each pathway. It is crucial for the clinician to understand the molecular pathways contributing to tumorigenesis of HNSCC in order to understand and participate actively in the development of novel anticancer therapies.

The pathways described herein are interconnected. The mitogenic signal starts with growth factors of the EGF family, which lead to activation of the Map kinase, PI3K, and STAT signaling pathways leading to cell proliferation and promotion of cell survival, as well as increased motility. In contrast, TGF-β counterbalances EGF effects by restraining the cell cycle and enhancing cell death. However, TGF-β has dual effects; it also appears important in EMT and possibly metastasis. These two essential pathways appear to be essential for HNSCC carcinogenesis.

The cell cycle, activated by mitogenic signals, is ultimately orchestrated by the oscillating expression of cyclins, and activation of Cdks, the effector kinases responsible of signaling progression through the cell cycle. Multiple checkpoints must be passed in order for the cell to proliferate, and multiple inhibitors including INKs, KIPs, and Wee1 proteins stall the cell cycle to ensure appropriate proliferation. Malfunction(s) in the series of molecular events linking mitogens to cell division is an opportunity for uncontrolled cell proliferation and cancer formation.

However, tumor biology is more complex than an imbalance between proliferation and cell death leading to the clonal expansion of one cell. The tumor, like an organ, depends on supporting cells, blood vessels, and subject to an immune surveillance. Cancer cells are not homogenous within the tumor. This may be explained by the presence of solid CSCs, which may self-renew, may maintain the cancer, and may differentiate into other subpopulation of cancer cells found in the tumor. However, CSC is a model that is not mutually exclusive. The traditional stochastic mutation model with development of subclone population probably also contributes to the tumor heterogeneity. Furthermore, the HNSCC should be viewed as an abnormal organ in which cancer cells of epithelial origin interact with the stroma and blood vessels, essential for its growth.

Any of the molecular mechanisms leading to or supporting the tumor growth are potential anticancer treatment targets. Understanding the basic concepts of tumor biology is crucial to the development of rationale therapies.

HIGHLIGHTS

- Tumors labeled as HNSCC are not homogenous, but represent different clinical entities based on their pathogenesis, such as smoker–drinker, HPV infection, or genetic defects in DNA repair genes.
- HPV16 is a sexually transmitted disease causing oropharyngeal HNSCC; these cancers are p16 positive and have a favorable clinical outcome in non-smokers when treated with chemoradiation therapy.

- EGFR, tyrosine kinase transmembrane receptors of the ErbB family that drive proliferation, resistance to apoptosis, and migration, is upregulated in HNSCC. EGFR acts via Ras/Raf/MapKinase as well as PI3K/Akt and STAT pathways. Agents targeting the EGFR pathway have clinical utility against HNSCC (cetuxumab, erlotinib).

- TGF-β signaling is frequently deregulated in HNSCC. Cancer cells can circumvent tumor suppressor components of this pathway and use TGF-β stimulation to promote invasion, EMT, secretion of mitogens, and pro-metastatic cytokines.

- Cell cycle progression is regulated by cyclin proteins. Cyclin family members, each specific for a phase of the cell cycle, have no intrinsic enzymatic activity, but associate with and activate Cdk. CCND1, the gene coding for cyclin D1 that regulates progression through G1 phase, is frequently amplified in HNSCC.

- Cyclin:Cdk complexes are inhibited by INKs, CIP/KIPs, and Wee1 homologues and are activated by CDC25 phosphatases. CIP/KIPs are upregulated in response to cellular stresses, via p53. p53, the gatekeeper of the human genome that mediates cell cycle arrest in response to DNA damage, is inactivated in 50% of HNSCC.

- DNA repair processes are important to prevent conversion from damage to mutation. Impaired DNA repair predisposes to HNSCC cancer (e.g., Fanconi anemia) but also renders tumors more sensitive to DNA-damaging agents such as ionizing radiation and cisplatin. Reduced levels of DNA damage proteins are emerging as predictive biomarkers in HNSCC.

- Apoptosis, or programmed cell death, is mediated via the extrinsic pathway involving TNF superfamily death receptors, or via the intrinsic pathway involving release of cytochrome C by the mitochondrion. Caspases are proteases that are the machinery of apoptosis. Proapoptotic drugs are part of the new armamentarium of oncologists.

- The concept of CSC is gaining traction in solid tumors including HNSCC. CSCs have unlimited self-renewal capacity and divide asymmetrically to provide differentiated progeny that make up the bulk of the tumor. CSC are the target of novel anticancer therapeutic strategies.

- Blood supply is critical to tumor growth. New blood vessels form from preexisting capillaries (angiogenesis) or via the formation of new blood vessels from bone marrow-derived cells (vasculogenesis). Hypoxic tumor cells are resistant to radiation, and are therefore the target of anti-hypoxic adjuvant therapeutic agents.

REFERENCES

1. Crile W. Excision of cancer of the head and neck. With special reference to the plan of dissection based on one hundred and thrity-two operations. *JAMA* 1906;47:1780–1786.
2. Suarez A. El problema de las metastasis linfaticas y alejadas del cancer de laringe e hipofaringe. *Rev Otorrinolaryngol* 1963;23:83–99.
3. Stransky N, Egloff A-M, Tward A, et al. The mutational landscape of head and neck squamous cell carcinoma. *Science* 2011;333:1157–1160.
4. Jemal A, Siegel R, Ward E, et al. Cancer statistics, 2009. *CA Cancer J Clin* 2009;59:225–249.
5. Boyle P, Levin B, International Agency for Research on Cancer., World Health Organization. World cancer report 2008. Lyon, France: International Agency for Research on Cancer; Distributed by WHO Press, 2008.
6. Forastiere A, Koch W, Trotti A, et al. Head and neck cancer. *N Engl J Med* 2001;345:1890–1900.
7. Argiris A, Karamouzis MV, Raben D, et al. Head and neck cancer. *Lancet* 2008;371:1695–1709.
8. Haddad RI, Shin DM. Recent advances in head and neck cancer. *N Engl J Med* 2008;359:1143–1154.
9. Renan MJ. How many mutations are required for tumorigenesis? Implications from human cancer data. *Mol Carcinog* 1993;7:139–146.
10. Leemans CR, Braakhuis BJ, Brakenhoff RH. The molecular biology of head and neck cancer. *Nat Rev Cancer* 2011;11:9–22.
11. Brunnemann KD, Scott JC, Hoffmann D. N-nitrosomorpholine and other volatile N-nitrosamines in snuff tobacco. *Carcinogenesis* 1982;3:693–696.
12. Denissenko MF, Pao A, Tang M, et al. Preferential formation of benzo[a]pyrene adducts at lung cancer mutational hotspots in P53. *Science* 1996;274:430–432.
13. Franceschi S, Talamini R, Barra S, et al. Smoking and drinking in relation to cancers of the oral cavity, pharynx, larynx, and esophagus in northern Italy. *Cancer Res* 1990;50:6502–6507.
14. Jeng JH, Chang MC, Hahn LJ. Role of areca nut in betel quid-associated chemical carcinogenesis: current awareness and future perspectives. *Oral Oncol* 2001;37:477–492.
15. Mork J, Lie AK, Glattre E, et al. Human papillomavirus infection as a risk factor for squamous-cell carcinoma of the head and neck. *N Engl J Med* 2001;344:1125–1131.
16. Maden C, Beckmann AM, Thomas DB, et al. Human papillomaviruses, herpes simplex viruses, and the risk of oral cancer in men. *Am J Epidemiol* 1992;135:1093–1102.
17. Smith EM, Hoffman HT, Summersgill KS, et al. Human papillomavirus and risk of oral cancer. *Laryngoscope* 1998;108:1098–1103.
18. Schwartz SM, Daling JR, Doody DR, et al. Oral cancer risk in relation to sexual history and evidence of human papillomavirus infection. *J Natl Cancer Inst* 1998;90:1626–1636.
19. Snijders PJ, Cromme FV, van den Brule AJ, et al. Prevalence and expression of human papillomavirus in tonsillar carcinomas, indicating a possible viral etiology. *Int J Cancer* 1992;51:845–850.
20. D'Souza G, Kreimer AR, Viscidi R, et al. Case-control study of human papillomavirus and oropharyngeal cancer. *N Engl J Med* 2007;356:1944–1956.
21. Ang KK, Harris J, Wheeler R, et al. Human papillomavirus and survival of patients with oropharyngeal cancer. *N Engl J Med* 2010;363:24–35.
22. Gillison ML, Koch WM, Capone RB, et al. Evidence for a causal association between human papillomavirus and a subset of head and neck cancers. *J Natl Cancer Inst* 2000;92:709–720.
23. Niedernhofer LJ, Lalai AS, Hoeijmakers JH. Fanconi anemia (cross)linked to DNA repair. *Cell* 2005;123:1191–1198.
24. Vineis P, Manuguerra M, Kavvoura FK, et al. A field synopsis on low-penetrance variants in DNA repair genes and cancer susceptibility. *J Natl Cancer Inst* 2009;101:24–36.
25. Silverman S, Jr, Gorsky M, Lozada F. Oral leukoplakia and malignant transformation. A follow-up study of 257 patients. *Cancer* 1984;53:563–568.

26. Warnakulasuriya S, Johnson NW, van der Waal I. Nomenclature and classification of potentially malignant disorders of the oral mucosa. *J Oral Pathol Med* 2007;36:575–580.

27. Haya-Fernandez MC, Bagan JV, Murillo-Cortes J, et al. The prevalence of oral leukoplakia in 138 patients with oral squamous cell carcinoma. *Oral Dis* 2004;10:346–348.

28. Axell T, Pindborg JJ, Smith CJ, et al. Oral white lesions with special reference to precancerous and tobacco- related lesions: conclusions of an international symposium held in Uppsala, Sweden, May 18–21 1994. International Collaborative Group on Oral White Lesions. *J Oral Pathol Med* 1996;25:49–54.

29. Shafer WG, Waldron CA. Erythroplakia of the oral cavity. *Cancer* 1975;36:1021–1028.

30. Slaughter DP, Southwick HW, Smejkal W. Field cancerization in oral stratified squamous epithelium; clinical implications of multicentric origin. *Cancer* 1953;6:963–968.

31. Tanaka T, Ishigamori R. Understanding carcinogenesis for fighting oral cancer. *J Oncol* 2011: 2011;603–740.

32. Griner EM, Kazanietz MG. Protein kinase C and other diacylglycerol effectors in cancer. *Nat Rev Cancer* 2007;7:281–294.

33. Vogelstein B, Kinzler KW. Cancer genes and the pathways they control. *Nat Med* 2004;10:789–799.

34. Parada LF, Land H, Weinberg RA, et al. Cooperation between gene encoding p53 tumour antigen and ras in cellular transformation. *Nature* 1984;312:649–651.

35. Eliyahu D, Raz A, Gruss P, et al. Participation of p53 cellular tumour antigen in transformation of normal embryonic cells. *Nature* 1984;312:646–649.

36. Jenkins JR, Rudge K, Currie GA. Cellular immortalization by a cDNA clone encoding the transformation-associated phosphoprotein p53. *Nature* 1984;312:651–654.

37. Herskowitz I. Functional inactivation of genes by dominant negative mutations. *Nature* 1987;329:219–222.

38. Lane DP. Cancer. p53, guardian of the genome. *Nature* 1992;358:15–16.

39. Finlay CA, Hinds PW, Levine AJ. The p53 proto-oncogene can act as a suppressor of transformation. *Cell* 1989;57:1083–1093.

40. Lane DP, Benchimol S. p53: oncogene or anti-oncogene? *Genes Dev* 1990;4:1–8.

41. Perez-Ordonez B, Beauchemin M, Jordan RC. Molecular biology of squamous cell carcinoma of the head and neck. *J Clin Pathol* 2006;59:445–453.

42. Califano J, van der Riet P, Westra W, et al. Genetic progression model for head and neck cancer: implications for field cancerization. *Cancer Res* 1996;56:2488–2492.

43. Tabor MP, Brakenhoff RH, van Houten VM, et al. Persistence of genetically altered fields in head and neck cancer patients: biological and clinical implications. *Clin Cancer Res* 2001;7:1523–1532.

44. Brennan JA, Mao L, Hruban RH, et al. Molecular assessment of histopathological staging in squamous-cell carcinoma of the head and neck. *N Engl J Med* 1995;332:429–435.

45. Morgan S, Grandis JR. ErbB receptors in the biology and pathology of the aerodigestive tract. *Exp Cell Res* 2009;315:572–582.

46. Nanba D, Higashiyama S. Dual intracellular signaling by proteolytic cleavage of membrane-anchored heparin-binding EGF-like growth factor. *Cytokine Growth Factor Rev* 2004;15:13–19.

47. Lemmon MA, Schlessinger J. Cell signaling by receptor tyrosine kinases. *Cell* 2010;141:1117–1134.

48. Hynes NE, Lane HA. ERBB receptors and cancer: the complexity of targeted inhibitors. *Nat Rev Cancer* 2005;5:341–354.

49. von Zastrow M, Sorkin A. Signaling on the endocytic pathway. *Curr Opin Cell Biol* 2007;19:436–445.

50. Choy E, Chiu VK, Silletti J, et al. Endomembrane trafficking of ras: the CAAX motif targets proteins to the ER and Golgi. *Cell* 1999;98:69–80.

51. Bar-Sagi D, Hall A. Ras and Rho GTPases: a family reunion. *Cell* 2000;103:227–238.

52. Vigil D, Cherfils J, Rossman KL, et al. Ras superfamily GEFs and GAPs: validated and tractable targets for cancer therapy? *Nat Rev Cancer* 2010;10:842–857.

53. Stokoe D, Macdonald SG, Cadwallader K, et al. Activation of Raf as a result of recruitment to the plasma membrane. *Science* 1994;264:1463–1467.

54. Johnson GL, Lapadat R. Mitogen-activated protein kinase pathways mediated by ERK, JNK, and p38 protein kinases. *Science* 2002;298:1911–1912.

55. Davis RJ. Signal transduction by the JNK group of MAP kinases. *Cell* 2000;103:239–252.

56. O'Shea JJ, Gadina M, Schreiber RD. Cytokine signaling in 2002: new surprises in the Jak/Stat pathway. *Cell* 2002;109(Suppl): S121–S131.

57. David M, Wong L, Flavell R, et al. STAT activation by epidermal growth factor (EGF) and amphiregulin. Requirement for the EGF receptor kinase but not for tyrosine phosphorylation sites or JAK1. *J Biol Chem* 1996;271:9185–9188.

58. Quesnelle KM, Boehm AL, Grandis JR. STAT-mediated EGFR signaling in cancer. *J Cell Biochem* 2007;102:311–319.

59. Wegrzyn J, Potla R, Chwae YJ, et al. Function of mitochondrial Stat3 in cellular respiration. *Science* 2009;323:793–797.

60. Gough DJ, Corlett A, Schlessinger K, et al. Mitochondrial STAT3 supports Ras-dependent oncogenic transformation. *Science* 2009;324:1713–1716.

61. Andl CD, Mizushima T, Oyama K, et al. EGFR-induced cell migration is mediated predominantly by the JAK-STAT pathway in primary esophageal keratinocytes. *Am J Physiol Gastrointest Liver Physiol* 2004;287:G1227–G1237.

62. Hou SX, Zheng Z, Chen X, et al. The Jak/STAT pathway in model organisms: emerging roles in cell movement. *Dev Cell* 2002;3:765–778.

63. Fresno Vara JA, Casado E, de Castro J, et al. PI3K/Akt signalling pathway and cancer. *Cancer Treat Rev* 2004;30:193–204.

64. Salmena L, Carracedo A, Pandolfi PP. Tenets of PTEN tumor suppression. *Cell* 2008;133:403–414.

65. Zhang S, Yu D. PI(3)king apart PTEN's role in cancer. *Clin Cancer Res* 2010;16:4325–4330.

66. Grandis JR, Tweardy DJ. TGF-alpha and EGFR in head and neck cancer. *J Cell Biochem Suppl* 1993;17F:188–191.

67. Ozanne B, Richards CS, Hendler F, et al. Over-expression of the EGF receptor is a hallmark of squamous cell carcinomas. *J Pathol* 1986;149:9–14.

68. Dassonville O, Formento JL, Francoual M, et al. Expression of epidermal growth factor receptor and survival in upper aerodigestive tract cancer. *J Clin Oncol* 1993;11:1873–1878.

69. Rubin Grandis J, Melhem MF, Gooding WE, et al. Levels of TGF-alpha and EGFR protein in head and neck squamous cell carcinoma and patient survival. *J Natl Cancer Inst* 1998;90:824–832.

70. Burtness B, Goldwasser MA, Flood W, et al. Phase III randomized trial of cisplatin plus placebo compared with cisplatin plus cetuximab in metastatic/recurrent head and neck cancer: an Eastern Cooperative Oncology Group study. *J Clin Oncol* 2005;23: 8646–8654.

71. Ang KK, Berkey BA, Tu X, et al. Impact of epidermal growth factor receptor expression on survival and pattern of relapse in patients with advanced head and neck carcinoma. *Cancer Res* 2002;62:7350–7356.

72. Sok JC, Coppelli FM, Thomas SM, et al. Mutant epidermal growth factor receptor (EGFRvIII) contributes to head and neck cancer growth and resistance to EGFR targeting. *Clin Cancer Res* 2006;12:5064–5073.

73. Bonner JA, Harari PM, Giralt J, et al. Radiotherapy plus cetuximab for squamous-cell carcinoma of the head and neck. *N Engl J Med* 2006;354:567–578.

74. Vermorken JB, Mesia R, Rivera F, et al. Platinum-based chemotherapy plus cetuximab in head and neck cancer. *N Engl J Med* 2008;359:1116–1127.

75. Stewart JS, Cohen EE, Licitra L, et al. Phase III study of gefitinib compared with intravenous methotrexate for recurrent squamous cell carcinoma of the head and neck [corrected]. *J Clin Oncol* 2009;27:1864–1871.

76. Lee SC, Srivastava RM, Lopez-Albaitero A, et al. Natural killer (NK):dendritic cell (DC) cross talk induced by therapeutic monoclonal antibody triggers tumor antigen-specific T cell immunity. *Immunol Res* 2011;50:248–254.

77. Ferris RL, Jaffee EM, Ferrone S. Tumor antigen-targeted, monoclonal antibody-based immunotherapy: clinical response, cellular immunity, and immunoescape. *J Clin Oncol* 2010;28: 4390–4399.

78. Huang SM, Harari PM. Modulation of radiation response after epidermal growth factor receptor blockade in squamous cell carcinomas: inhibition of damage repair, cell cycle kinetics, and tumor angiogenesis. *Clin Cancer Res* 2000;6:2166–2174.

79. Dittmann K, Mayer C, Rodemann HP. Inhibition of radiation-induced EGFR nuclear import by C225 (Cetuximab) suppresses DNA-PK activity. *Radiother Oncol* 2005;76:157–161.

80. Johnston PA, Grandis JR. STAT3 signaling: anticancer strategies and challenges. *Mol Interv* 2011;11:18–26.

81. Song JI, Grandis JR. STAT signaling in head and neck cancer. *Oncogene* 2000;19:2489–2495.

82. Xi S, Gooding WE, Grandis JR. In vivo antitumor efficacy of STAT3 blockade using a transcription factor decoy approach: implications for cancer therapy. *Oncogene* 2005;24:970–979.

83. Okami K, Wu L, Riggins G, et al. Analysis of PTEN/MMAC1 alterations in aerodigestive tract tumors. *Cancer Res* 1998;58:509–511.

84. Qiu W, Schonleben F, Li X, et al. PIK3CA mutations in head and neck squamous cell carcinoma. *Clin Cancer Res* 2006;12: 1441–1446.

85. Hennessy BT, Smith DL, Ram PT, et al. Exploiting the PI3K/AKT pathway for cancer drug discovery. *Nat Rev Drug Discov* 2005;4:988–1004.

86. Massague J. TGFbeta in cancer. *Cell* 2008;134:215–230.

87. Massague J, Blain SW, Lo RS. TGFbeta signaling in growth control, cancer, and heritable disorders. *Cell* 2000;103:295–309.

88. Malkoski S, Lighthall JGW, Wang XJ. *Oral cancer metastasis*, 1st ed. New York, NY: Springer, 2010.

89. Liu F. *Transforming growth factor-β in cancer therapy*. New York, NY: Humana Press, 2008.

90. Kretzschmar M, Doody J, Massague J. Opposing BMP and EGF signalling pathways converge on the TGF-beta family mediator Smad1. *Nature* 1997;389:618–622.

91. Ozdamar B, Bose R, Barrios-Rodiles M, et al. Regulation of the polarity protein Par6 by TGFbeta receptors controls epithelial cell plasticity. *Science* 2005;307:1603–1609.

92. Yamaguchi Y, Mann DM, Ruoslahti E. Negative regulation of transforming growth factor-beta by the proteoglycan decorin. *Nature* 1990;346:281–284.

93. Lo RS, Massague J. Ubiquitin-dependent degradation of TGF-beta-activated smad2. *Nat Cell Biol* 1999;1:472–478.

94. Zhu H, Kavsak P, Abdollah S, et al. A SMAD ubiquitin ligase targets the BMP pathway and affects embryonic pattern formation. *Nature* 1999;400:687–693.

95. Lu SL, Herrington H, Reh D, et al. Loss of transforming growth factor-beta type II receptor promotes metastatic head-and-neck squamous cell carcinoma. *Genes Dev* 2006;20:1331–1342.

96. Qiu W, Schonleben F, Li X, et al. Disruption of transforming growth factor beta-Smad signaling pathway in head and neck squamous cell carcinoma as evidenced by mutations of SMAD2 and SMAD4. *Cancer Lett* 2007;245:163–170.

97. Chen T, Yan W, Wells RG, et al. Novel inactivating mutations of transforming growth factor-beta type I receptor gene in head-and-neck cancer metastases. *Int J Cancer* 2001;93:653–661.

98. Wang D, Song H, Evans JA, et al. Mutation and downregulation of the transforming growth factor beta type II receptor gene in primary squamous cell carcinomas of the head and neck. *Carcinogenesis* 1997;18:2285–2290.

99. Lu SL, Reh D, Li AG, et al. Overexpression of transforming growth factor beta1 in head and neck epithelia results in inflammation, angiogenesis, and epithelial hyperproliferation. *Cancer Res* 2004;64:4405–4410.

100. Mangone FR, Walder F, Maistro S, et al. Smad2 and Smad6 as predictors of overall survival in oral squamous cell carcinoma patients. Mol Cancer 2010;9:106.

101. Bornstein S, White R, Malkoski S, et al. Smad4 loss in mice causes spontaneous head and neck cancer with increased genomic instability and inflammation. *J Clin Invest* 2009;119: 3408–3419.

102. Fukuchi M, Fukai Y, Masuda N, et al. High-level expression of the Smad ubiquitin ligase Smurf2 correlates with poor prognosis in patients with esophageal squamous cell carcinoma. *Cancer Res* 2002;62:7162–7165.

103. Burkhart DL, Sage J. Cellular mechanisms of tumour suppression by the retinoblastoma gene. *Nat Rev Cancer* 2008;8:671–682.

104. Massague J. G1 cell-cycle control and cancer. *Nature* 2004;432: 298–306.

105. Murray AW. Recycling the cell cycle: cyclins revisited. *Cell* 2004;116:221–234.

106. Fisher RP, Morgan DO. A novel cyclin associates with MO15/CDK7 to form the CDK-activating kinase. *Cell* 1994;78:713–724.

107. Boutros R, Lobjois V, Ducommun B. CDC25 phosphatases in cancer cells: key players? Good targets? *Nat Rev Cancer* 2007;7: 495–507.

108. Hinchcliffe EH, Li C, Thompson EA, et al. Requirement of Cdk2-cyclin E activity for repeated centrosome reproduction in Xenopus egg extracts. *Science* 1999;283:851–854.

109. Sherr CJ, Roberts JM. Living with or without cyclins and cyclin-dependent kinases. *Genes Dev* 2004;18:2699–2711.

110. Vlach J, Hennecke S, Amati B. Phosphorylation-dependent degradation of the cyclin-dependent kinase inhibitor p27. *EMBO J* 1997;16:5334–5344.

111. Gavet O, Pines J. Activation of cyclin B1-Cdk1 synchronizes events in the nucleus and the cytoplasm at mitosis. *J Cell Biol* 2010;189:247–259.

112. Holland AJ, Cleveland DW. Boveri revisited: chromosomal instability, aneuploidy and tumorigenesis. *Nat Rev Mol Cell Biol* 2009;10:478–487.

113. Rieder CL, Schultz A, Cole R, et al. Anaphase onset in vertebrate somatic cells is controlled by a checkpoint that monitors sister kinetochore attachment to the spindle. *J Cell Biol* 1994;127:1301–1310.

114. Chen RH, Waters JC, Salmon ED, et al. Association of spindle assembly checkpoint component XMAD2 with unattached kinetochores. *Science* 1996;274:242–246.

115. Chan GK, Jablonski SA, Sudakin V, et al. Human BUBR1 is a mitotic checkpoint kinase that monitors CENP-E functions at kinetochores and binds the cyclosome/APC. *J Cell Biol* 1999;146:941–954.

116. Nasmyth K. How do so few control so many? *Cell* 2005;120: 739–746.

117. Fortin A, Guerry M, Guerry R, et al. Chromosome 11q13 gene amplifications in oral and oropharyngeal carcinomas: no correlation with subclinical lymph node invasion and disease recurrence. *Clin Cancer Res* 1997;3:1609–1614.

118. Michalides R, van Veelen N, Hart A, et al. Overexpression of cyclin D1 correlates with recurrence in a group of forty-seven operable squamous cell carcinomas of the head and neck. *Cancer Res* 1995;55:975–978.

119. Michalides RJ, van Veelen NM, Kristel PM, et al. Overexpression of cyclin D1 indicates a poor prognosis in squamous cell carcinoma of the head and neck. *Arch Otolaryngol Head Neck Surg* 1997;123:497–502.

120. Mineta H, Miura K, Takebayashi S, et al. Cyclin D1 overexpression correlates with poor prognosis in patients with tongue squamous cell carcinoma. *Oral Oncol* 2000;36:194–198.

121. Vielba R, Bilbao J, Ispizua A, et al. p53 and cyclin D1 as prognostic factors in squamous cell carcinoma of the larynx. *Laryngoscope* 2003;113:167–172.

122. Akervall J, Bockmuhl U, Petersen I, et al. The gene ratios c-MYC:cyclin-dependent kinase (CDK)N2A and CCND1:CDKN2A correlate with poor prognosis in squamous cell carcinoma of the head and neck. *Clin Cancer Res* 2003;9:1750–1755.

123. Jares P, Fernandez PL, Campo E, et al. PRAD-1/cyclin D1 gene amplification correlates with messenger RNA overexpression and tumor progression in human laryngeal carcinomas. *Cancer Res* 1994;54:4813–4817.

124. Namazie A, Alavi S, Olopade OI, et al. Cyclin D1 amplification and p16(MTS1/CDK4I) deletion correlate with poor prognosis in head and neck tumors. *Laryngoscope* 2002;112:472–481.

125. Callender T, el-Naggar AK, Lee MS, et al. PRAD-1 (CCND1)/cyclin D1 oncogene amplification in primary head and neck squamous cell carcinoma. *Cancer* 1994;74:152–158.

126. Akervall J, Borg A, Dictor M, et al. Chromosomal translocations involving 11q13 contribute to cyclin D1 overexpression in squamous cell carcinoma of the head and neck. *Int J Oncol* 2002;20:45–52.

127. Akervall JA, Michalides RJ, Mineta H, et al. Amplification of cyclin D1 in squamous cell carcinoma of the head and neck and

the prognostic value of chromosomal abnormalities and cyclin D1 overexpression. *Cancer* 1997;79:380–389.

128. Greer RO, Jr, Said S, Shroyer KR, et al. Overexpression of cyclin D1 and cortactin is primarily independent of gene amplification in salivary gland adenoid cystic carcinoma. *Oral Oncol* 2007;43:735–741.

129. Matthias C, Branigan K, Jahnke V, et al. Polymorphism within the cyclin D1 gene is associated with prognosis in patients with squamous cell carcinoma of the head and neck. *Clin Cancer Res* 1998;4:2411–2418.

130. Hsieh WS, Soo R, Peh BK, et al. Pharmacodynamic effects of seliciclib, an orally administered cell cycle modulator, in undifferentiated nasopharyngeal cancer. *Clin Cancer Res* 2009;15:1435–1442.

131. Haddad RI, Weinstein LJ, Wieczorek TJ, et al. A phase II clinical and pharmacodynamic study of E7070 in patients with metastatic, recurrent, or refractory squamous cell carcinoma of the head and neck: modulation of retinoblastoma protein phosphorylation by a novel chloroindolyl sulfonamide cell cycle inhibitor. *Clin Cancer Res* 2004;10:4680–4687.

132. Rizzardi C, Torelli L, Barresi E, et al. BUBR1 expression in oral squamous cell carcinoma and its relationship to tumor stage and survival. *Head Neck* 2011;33:727–733.

133. Hannisdal K, Burum-Auensen E, Schjolberg A, et al. Correlation between reduced expression of the spindle checkpoint protein BubR1 and bad prognosis in tonsillar carcinomas. *Head Neck* 2010;32:1354–1362.

134. Vermeulen K, Van Bockstaele DR, Berneman ZN. The cell cycle: a review of regulation, deregulation and therapeutic targets in cancer. *Cell Prolif* 2003;36:131–149.

135. Sherr CJ, Roberts JM. CDK inhibitors: positive and negative regulators of G1-phase progression. *Genes Dev* 1999;13:1501–1512.

136. Kim WY, Sharpless NE. The regulation of INK4/ARF in cancer and aging. *Cell* 2006;127:265–275.

137. Besson A, Dowdy SF, Roberts JM. CDK inhibitors: cell cycle regulators and beyond. *Dev Cell* 2008;14:159–169.

138. Parker LL, Atherton-Fessler S, Piwnica-Worms H. p107wee1 is a dual-specificity kinase that phosphorylates p34cdc2 on tyrosine 15. *Proc Natl Acad Sci U S A* 1992;89:2917–2921.

139. Kruse JP, Gu W. Modes of p53 regulation. *Cell* 2009;137:609–622.

140. Niida H, Nakanishi M. DNA damage checkpoints in mammals. *Mutagenesis* 2006;21:3–9.

141. Yang J, Yu Y, Hamrick HE, et al., ATR and DNA-PK: initiators of the cellular genotoxic stress responses. *Carcinogenesis* 2003;24:1571–1580.

142. Smith J, Tho LM, Xu N, et al. The ATM-Chk2 and ATR-Chk1 pathways in DNA damage signaling and cancer. *Adv Cancer Res* 2010;108:73–112.

143. Koscielny S, Dahse R, Ernst G, et al. The prognostic relevance of p16 inactivation in head and neck cancer. *ORL J Otorhinolaryngol Relat Spec* 2007;69:30–36.

144. van der Riet P, Nawroz H, Hruban RH, et al. Frequent loss of chromosome 9p21-22 early in head and neck cancer progression. *Cancer Res* 1994;54:1156–1158.

145. Gonzalez MV, Pello MF, Lopez-Larrea C, et al. Deletion and methylation of the tumour suppressor gene p16/CDKN2 in primary head and neck squamous cell carcinoma. *J Clin Pathol* 1997;50:509–512.

146. Jares P, Nadal A, Fernandez PL, et al. Disregulation of p16MTS1/CDK4I protein and mRNA expression is associated with gene alterations in squamous-cell carcinoma of the larynx. *Int J Cancer* 1999;81:705–711.

147. Lydiatt WM, Davidson BJ, Schantz SP, et al., Chaganti RS. 9p21 deletion correlates with recurrence in head and neck cancer. *Head Neck* 1998;20:113–118.

148. Fakhry C, Westra WH, Li S, et al. Improved survival of patients with human papillomavirus-positive head and neck squamous cell carcinoma in a prospective clinical trial. *J Natl Cancer Inst* 2008;100:261–269.

149. Kumar B, Cordell KG, Lee JS, et al. EGFR, p16, HPV Titer, Bcl-xL and p53, sex, and smoking as indicators of response to therapy and survival in oropharyngeal cancer. *J Clin Oncol* 2008;26:3128–3137.

150. Lassen P, Eriksen JG, Hamilton-Dutoit S, et al. HPV-associated p16-expression and response to hypoxic modification of radiotherapy in head and neck cancer. *Radiother Oncol* 2010;94:30–35.

151. Rischin D, Young RJ, Fisher R, et al. Prognostic significance of p16INK4A and human papillomavirus in patients with oropharyngeal cancer treated on TROG 02.02 phase III trial. *J Clin Oncol* 2010;28:4142–4148.

152. Reimers N, Kasper HU, Weissenborn SJ, et al. Combined analysis of HPV-DNA, p16 and EGFR expression to predict prognosis in oropharyngeal cancer. *Int J Cancer* 2007;120:1731–1738.

153. Weinberger PM, Yu Z, Haffty BG, et al. Molecular classification identifies a subset of human papillomavirus-associated oropharyngeal cancers with favorable prognosis. *J Clin Oncol* 2006;24:736–747.

154. Gasparotto D, Maestro R, Piccinin S, et al. Overexpression of CDC25A and CDC25B in head and neck cancers. *Cancer Res* 1997;57:2366–2368.

155. Poeta ML, Manola J, Goldwasser MA, et al. TP53 mutations and survival in squamous-cell carcinoma of the head and neck. *N Engl J Med* 2007;357:2552–2561.

156. Nees M, Homann N, Discher H, et al. Expression of mutated p53 occurs in tumor-distant epithelia of head and neck cancer patients: a possible molecular basis for the development of multiple tumors. *Cancer Res* 1993;53:4189–4196.

157. Waridel F, Estreicher A, Bron L, et al. Field cancerisation and polyclonal p53 mutation in the upper aero-digestive tract. *Oncogene* 1997;14:163–169.

158. Nemunaitis J, Ganly I, Khuri F, et al. Selective replication and oncolysis in p53 mutant tumors with ONYX-015, an E1B-55kD gene-deleted adenovirus, in patients with advanced head and neck cancer: a phase II trial. *Cancer Res* 2000;60:6359–6366.

159. Khuri FR, Nemunaitis J, Ganly I, et al. a controlled trial of intratumoral ONYX-015, a selectively-replicating adenovirus, in combination with cisplatin and 5-fluorouracil in patients with recurrent head and neck cancer. *Nat Med* 2000;6:879–885.

160. Rudin CM, Cohen EE, Papadimitrakopoulou VA, et al. An attenuated adenovirus, ONYX-015, as mouthwash therapy for premalignant oral dysplasia. *J Clin Oncol* 2003;21:4546–4552.

161. Moody CA, Laimins LA. Human papillomavirus oncoproteins: pathways to transformation. *Nat Rev Cancer* 2010;10:550–560.

162. Friedberg EC, Walker GC, Wolfram S, et al. DNA repair and mutagenesis, 2nd ed. Hoboken, NJ: Wiley, 2006.

163. Hoeijmakers JH. DNA damage, aging, and cancer. *N Engl J Med* 2009;361:1475–1485.

164. McHugh PJ, Spanswick VJ, Hartley JA. Repair of DNA interstrand crosslinks: molecular mechanisms and clinical relevance. *Lancet Oncol* 2001;2:483–490.

165. McCabe KM, Olson SB, Moses RE. DNA interstrand crosslink repair in mammalian cells. *J Cell Physiol* 2009;220:569–573.

166. Vaezi A, Feldmand CH, Niedernhofer LJ. ERCC1 and XRCC1 as biomarkers for liung and head and neck cancer. *Pharacogenomics Pers Med* 2011;4:47–63.

167. Friedberg EC. How nucleotide excision repair protects against cancer. *Nat Rev Cancer* 2001;1:22–33.

168. Jacobs DE, Kelly T, Sobolewski J. Linking public health, housing, and indoor environmental policy: successes and challenges at local and federal agencies in the United States. *Environ Health Perspect* 2007;115:976–982.

169. Caldecott KW. Mammalian single-strand break repair: mechanisms and links with chromatin. *DNA Repair (Amst)* 2007;6:443–453.

170. Caldecott KW. Single-strand break repair and genetic disease. *Nat Rev Genet* 2008;9:619–631.

171. O'Driscoll M, Jeggo PA. The role of double-strand break repair—insights from human genetics. *Nat Rev Genet* 2006;7:45–54.

172. Zhang J, Powell SN. The role of the BRCA1 tumor suppressor in DNA double-strand break repair. *Mol Cancer Res* 2005;3:531–539.

173. Helleday T, Lo J, van Gent DC, et al. DNA double-strand break repair: from mechanistic understanding to cancer treatment. *DNA Repair (Amst)* 2007;6:923–935.

174. Helleday T, Petermann E, Lundin C, et al. DNA repair pathways as targets for cancer therapy. *Nat Rev Cancer* 2008;8:193–204.

175. Peng G, Lin SY. Exploiting the homologous recombination DNA repair network for targeted cancer therapy. *World J Clin Oncol* 2011;2:73–79.

176. Shuck SC, Turchi JJ. Targeted inhibition of replication protein A reveals cytotoxic activity, synergy with chemotherapeutic DNA-damaging agents, and insight into cellular function. *Cancer Res* 2010;70:3189–3198.

177. Ranson M, Middleton MR, Bridgewater J, et al. Lomeguatrib, a potent inhibitor of O_6-alkylguanine-DNA-alkyltransferase: phase I safety, pharmacodynamic, and pharmacokinetic trial and evaluation in combination with temozolomide in patients with advanced solid tumors. *Clin Cancer Res* 2006;12:1577–1584.

178. Rosell R, Robinet G, Szczesna A, et al. Randomized phase II study of cetuximab plus cisplatin/vinorelbine compared with cisplatin/vinorelbine alone as first-line therapy in EGFR-expressing advanced non-small-cell lung cancer. *Ann Oncol* 2008;19:362–369.

179. Fountzilas G, Kalogera-Fountzila A, Lambaki S, et al. MMP9 but Not EGFR, MET, ERCC1, P16, and P-53 is associated with response to concomitant radiotherapy, cetuximab, and weekly cisplatin in patients with locally advanced head and neck cancer. *J Oncol* 2009:2009;305–908.

180. Vaezi A, Wang X, Buch SC, et al. XPF expression correlates with clinical outcome in squamous cell carcinoma of the head and neck. *Clin Cancer Res* 2011.

181. Handra-Luca A, Hernandez J, Mountzios G, et al. Excision repair cross complementation group 1 immunohistochemical expression predicts objective response and cancer-specific survival in patients treated by Cisplatin-based induction chemotherapy for locally advanced head and neck squamous cell carcinoma. *Clin Cancer Res* 2007;13:3855–3859.

182. Jun HJ, Ahn MJ, Kim HS, et al. ERCC1 expression as a predictive marker of squamous cell carcinoma of the head and neck treated with cisplatin-based concurrent chemoradiation. *Br J Cancer* 2008;99:167–172.

183. Koh Y, Kim TM, Jeon YK, et al. Class III beta-tubulin, but not ERCC1, is a strong predictive and prognostic marker in locally advanced head and neck squamous cell carcinoma. *Ann Oncol* 2009;20:1414–1419.

184. Moeller BJ, Yordy JS, Williams MD, et al. DNA repair biomarker profiling of head and neck cancer: Ku80 expression predicts locoregional failure and death following radiotherapy. *Clin Cancer Res* 2011;17:2035–2043.

185. Nix P, Greenman J, Stafford N, L. C. Expression of XRCC1 and ERCC1 proteins in radioresistant and radiosensitive laryngeal cancer. *Cancer Therapy* 2004;47–53.

186. Ashkenazi A. Directing cancer cells to self-destruct with pro-apoptotic receptor agonists. *Nat Rev Drug Discov* 2008;7:1001–1012.

187. Kurokawa M, Kornbluth S. Caspases and kinases in a death grip. *Cell* 2009;138:838–854.

188. Li P, Nijhawan D, Budihardjo I, et al. Cytochrome c and dATP-dependent formation of Apaf-1/caspase-9 complex initiates an apoptotic protease cascade. *Cell* 1997;91:479–489.

189. Zou H, Henzel WJ, Liu X, et al. Apaf-1, a human protein homologous to C. elegans CED-4, participates in cytochrome c-dependent activation of caspase-3. *Cell* 1997;90:405–413.

190. Danial NN. BCL-2 family proteins: critical checkpoints of apoptotic cell death. *Clin Cancer Res* 2007;13:7254–7263.

191. del Peso L, Gonzalez-Garcia M, Page C, et al. Interleukin-3-induced phosphorylation of BAD through the protein kinase Akt. *Science* 1997;278:687–689.

192. Datta SR, Dudek H, Tao X, et al. Akt phosphorylation of BAD couples survival signals to the cell-intrinsic death machinery. *Cell* 1997;91:231–241.

193. Bonni A, Brunet A, West AE, et al. Cell survival promoted by the Ras-MAPK signaling pathway by transcription-dependent and -independent mechanisms. *Science* 1999;286:1358–1362.

194. Yu J, Zhang L, Hwang PM, et al. PUMA induces the rapid apoptosis of colorectal cancer cells. *Mol Cell* 2001;7:673–682.

195. Oda E, Ohki R, Murasawa H, et al. Noxa, a BH3-only member of the Bcl-2 family and candidate mediator of p53-induced apoptosis. *Science* 2000;288:1053–1058.

196. Trask DK, Wolf GT, Bradford CR, et al. Expression of Bcl-2 family proteins in advanced laryngeal squamous cell carcinoma: correlation with response to chemotherapy and organ preservation. *Laryngoscope* 2002;112:638–644.

197. Kumar B, Cordell KG, D'Silva N, et al. Expression of p53 and Bcl-xL as predictive markers for larynx preservation in advanced laryngeal cancer. *Arch Otolaryngol Head Neck Surg* 2008;134:363–369.

198. Buffa FM, Bentzen SM, Daley FM, et al. Molecular marker profiles predict locoregional control of head and neck squamous cell carcinoma in a randomized trial of continuous hyperfractionated accelerated radiotherapy. *Clin Cancer Res* 2004;10:3745–3754.

199. Lessene G, Czabotar PE, Colman PM. BCL-2 family antagonists for cancer therapy. *Nat Rev Drug Discov* 2008;7:989–1000.

200. Kang MH, Reynolds CP. Bcl-2 inhibitors: targeting mitochondrial apoptotic pathways in cancer therapy. *Clin Cancer Res* 2009;15:1126–1132.

201. Bedikian AY, Millward M, Pehamberger H, et al. Bcl-2 antisense (oblimersen sodium) plus dacarbazine in patients with advanced melanoma: the Oblimersen Melanoma Study Group. *J Clin Oncol* 2006;24:4738–4745.

202. O'Brien S, Moore JO, Boyd TE, et al. 5-year survival in patients with relapsed or refractory chronic lymphocytic leukemia in a randomized, phase III trial of fludarabine plus cyclophosphamide with or without oblimersen. *J Clin Oncol* 2009;27:5208–5212.

203. Tse C, Shoemaker AR, Adickes J, et al. ABT-263: a potent and orally bioavailable Bcl-2 family inhibitor. *Cancer Res* 2008;68:3421–3428.

204. Ackler S, Mitten MJ, Foster K, et al. The Bcl-2 inhibitor ABT-263 enhances the response of multiple chemotherapeutic regimens in hematologic tumors in vivo. *Cancer Chemother Pharmacol* 2010;66:869–880.

205. Rosen JM, Jordan CT. The increasing complexity of the cancer stem cell paradigm. *Science* 2009;324:1670–1673.

206. Ailles LE, Weissman IL. Cancer stem cells in solid tumors. *Curr Opin Biotechnol* 2007;18:460–466.

207. Clarke MF, Dick JE, Dirks PB, et al. Cancer stem cells—perspectives on current status and future directions: AACR Workshop on cancer stem cells. *Cancer Res* 2006;66:9339–9344.

208. Al-Hajj M, Wicha MS, Benito-Hernandez A, et al. Prospective identification of tumorigenic breast cancer cells. *Proc Natl Acad Sci U S A* 2003;100:3983–3988.

209. Shipitsin M, Campbell LL, Argani P, et al. Molecular definition of breast tumor heterogeneity. *Cancer Cell* 2007;11:259–273.

210. Mani SA, Guo W, Liao MJ, et al. The epithelial-mesenchymal transition generates cells with properties of stem cells. *Cell* 2008;133:704–715.

211. Thiery JP, Acloque H, Huang RY, et al. Epithelial-mesenchymal transitions in development and disease. *Cell* 2009;139:871–890.

212. Chen ZG. The cancer stem cell concept in progression of head and neck cancer. *J Oncol* 2009: 2009;894–1064.

213. Diehn M, Cho RW, Lobo NA, et al. Association of reactive oxygen species levels and radioresistance in cancer stem cells. *Nature* 2009;458:780–783.

214. Maugeri-Sacca M, Vigneri P, De Maria R. Cancer Stem Cells and Chemosensitivity. *Clin Cancer Res* 2011;17:4942–4947.

215. Prince ME, Sivanandan R, Kaczorowski A, et al. Identification of a subpopulation of cells with cancer stem cell properties in head and neck squamous cell carcinoma. *Proc Natl Acad Sci U S A* 2007;104:973–978.

216. Chen YC, Chen YW, Hsu HS, et al. Aldehyde dehydrogenase 1 is a putative marker for cancer stem cells in head and neck squamous cancer. *Biochem Biophys Res Commun* 2009;385:307–313.

217. Chen H, Zhou L, Dou T, et al. BMI1'S maintenance of the proliferative capacity of laryngeal cancer stem cells. *Head Neck* 2010.

218. Okamoto A, Chikamatsu K, Sakakura K, et al. Expansion and characterization of cancer stem-like cells in squamous cell carcinoma of the head and neck. *Oral Oncol* 2009;45:633–639.

219. Tabor MH, Clay MR, Owen JH, et al. Head and neck cancer stem cells: the side population. *Laryngoscope* 2011;121:527–533.

220. de Jong MC, Pramana J, van der Wal JE, et al. CD44 expression predicts local recurrence after radiotherapy in larynx cancer. *Clin Cancer Res* 2010;16:5329–5338.

221. Damek-Poprawa M, Volgina A, Korostoff J, et al. Targeted inhibition of CD133+ cells in oral cancer cell lines. *J Dent Res* 2011;90:638–645.

222. Chung AS, Lee J, Ferrara N. Targeting the tumour vasculature: insights from physiological angiogenesis. *Nat Rev Cancer* 2010;10:505–514.

223. Ahn GO, Brown JM. Role of endothelial progenitors and other bone marrow-derived cells in the development of the tumor vasculature. *Angiogenesis* 2009;12:159–164.

224. Carmeliet P, De Smet F, Loges S, et al. Branching morphogenesis and antiangiogenesis candidates: tip cells lead the way. *Nat Rev Clin Oncol* 2009;6:315–326.

225. Folkman J, D'Amore PA. Blood vessel formation: what is its molecular basis? *Cell* 1996;87:1153–1155.

226. Schofield CJ, Ratcliffe PJ. Oxygen sensing by HIF hydroxylases. *Nat Rev Mol Cell Biol* 2004;5:343–354.

227. Kioi M, Vogel H, Schultz G, et al. Inhibition of vasculogenesis, but not angiogenesis, prevents the recurrence of glioblastoma after irradiation in mice. *J Clin Invest* 2010;120:694–705.

228. Nolan DJ, Ciarrocchi A, Mellick AS, et al. Bone marrow-derived endothelial progenitor cells are a major determinant of nascent tumor neovascularization. *Genes Dev* 2007;21:1546–1558.

229. Peters BA, Diaz LA, Polyak K, et al. Contribution of bone marrow-derived endothelial cells to human tumor vasculature. *Nat Med* 2005;11:261–262.

230. Winter SC, Shah KA, Han C, et al. The relation between hypoxia-inducible factor (HIF)-1alpha and HIF-2alpha expression with anemia and outcome in surgically treated head and neck cancer. *Cancer* 2006;107:757–766.

231. Hoogsteen IJ, Marres HA, Bussink J, et al. Tumor microenvironment in head and neck squamous cell carcinomas: predictive value and clinical relevance of hypoxic markers. A review. *Head Neck* 2007;29:591–604.

232. Schrijvers ML, van der Laan BF, de Bock GH, et al. Overexpression of intrinsic hypoxia markers HIF1alpha and CA-IX predict for local recurrence in stage T1-T2 glottic laryngeal carcinoma treated with radiotherapy. *Int J Radiat Oncol Biol Phys* 2008;72:161–169.

233. Koukourakis MI, Giatromanolaki A, Danielidis V, et al. Hypoxia inducible factor (HIf1alpha and HIF2alpha) and carbonic anhydrase 9 (CA9) expression and response of head-neck cancer to hypofractionated and accelerated radiotherapy. *Int J Radiat Biol* 2008;84:47–52.

234. Koukourakis MI, Bentzen SM, Giatromanolaki A, et al. Endogenous markers of two separate hypoxia response pathways (hypoxia inducible factor 2 alpha and carbonic anhydrase 9) are associated with radiotherapy failure in head and neck cancer patients recruited in the CHART randomized trial. *J Clin Oncol* 2006;24:727–735.

235. van den Broek GB, Wildeman M, Rasch CR, et al. Molecular markers predict outcome in squamous cell carcinoma of the head and neck after concomitant cisplatin-based chemoradiation. *Int J Cancer* 2009;124:2643–2650.

236. Kappler M, Taubert H, Holzhausen HJ, et al. Immunohistochemical detection of HIF-1alpha and CAIX in advanced head-and-neck cancer. Prognostic role and correlation with tumor markers and tumor oxygenation parameters. *Strahlenther Onkol* 2008;184: 393–399.

237. Roh JL, Cho KJ, Kwon GY, et al. The prognostic value of hypoxia markers in T2-staged oral tongue cancer. *Oral Oncol* 2009;45: 63–68.

238. Eriksen JG, Overgaard J. Lack of prognostic and predictive value of CA IX in radiotherapy of squamous cell carcinoma of the head and neck with known modifiable hypoxia: an evaluation of the DAHANCA 5 study. *Radiother Oncol* 2007;83:383–388.

239. Kyzas PA, Cunha IW, Ioannidis JP. Prognostic significance of vascular endothelial growth factor immunohistochemical expression in head and neck squamous cell carcinoma: a meta-analysis. *Clin Cancer Res* 2005;11:1434–1440.

240. Rischin D, Peters LJ, O'Sullivan B, et al. Tirapazamine, cisplatin, and radiation versus cisplatin and radiation for advanced squamous cell carcinoma of the head and neck (TROG 02.02, HeadSTART): a phase III trial of the Trans-Tasman Radiation Oncology Group. *J Clin Oncol* 2010;28:2989–2995.

241. Fury MG, Zahalsky A, Wong R, et al. A Phase II study of SU5416 in patients with advanced or recurrent head and neck cancers. *Invest New Drugs* 2007;25:165–172.

242. Herbst RS, Ansari R, Bustin F, et al. Efficacy of bevacizumab plus erlotinib versus erlotinib alone in advanced non-small-cell lung cancer after failure of standard first-line chemotherapy (BeTa): a double-blind, placebo-controlled, phase 3 trial. *Lancet* 2011;377:1846–1854.

243. Cohen EE, Davis DW, Karrison TG, et al. Erlotinib and bevacizumab in patients with recurrent or metastatic squamous-cell carcinoma of the head and neck: a phase I/II study. *Lancet Oncol* 2009;10:247–257.

244. Dredge K, Hammond E, Handley P, et al. PG545, a dual heparanase and angiogenesis inhibitor, induces potent anti-tumour and anti-metastatic efficacy in preclinical models. *Br J Cancer* 2011;104:635–642.

109 Principles of Patient Care

Rohan R. Walvekar   *Marcie C. Tauzin*   *Neelima Tammareddi*

Principles of care for the head and neck patient can be defined by understanding of the concepts of quality health care and the methods and processes necessary to secure it. An appropriate definition of quality care must be agreed upon in order to implement it. There are several mechanisms that have been introduced in current medicine as ways to measure, implement, and audit quality health care and ensure an equitable and ethical practice of medicine. *Clinical guidelines* and *critical pathways* are used to direct medical decision making. The appropriate evaluation of clinical outcomes through evidence-based research provides a reasonable justification for everyday clinical decision making. Multidisciplinary team (MDT) approaches ensure complete and efficient care for the patient. In addition, safety, standardization of care, and associated costs can be examined to allocate health care resources in an equitable fashion.

PURPOSE

The aim of this chapter is to highlight the importance of quality care, particularly with regard to the head and neck cancer patient. We define the different components of quality care and describe the various tools used to improve it. Reviews of current literature are used to support the importance of this topic and offer examples of implementation. The goal is to emphasize the need for high-quality medical care and to provide a resource that explains how it can be incorporated into the care of a head and neck cancer patient.

QUALITY OF CARE

Historical Background

Beginning in the 1990s and rising over the last two decades, there has been an increasing focus on the quality of medical care in the United States. It has prompted the development of several organizations to assess and improve health care, including the Agency for Healthcare Research and Quality (AHRQ), which oversees the National Guideline Clearinghouse (NGC), the Patient-Centered Outcomes Research Institute, and the National Quality Forum (NQF). In addition, there was rapid growth of existing programs such as the Institute of Medicine (IOM), which is the health arm under the National Academy of Sciences, dating back to the 1860s. Some of these initiatives are government-based, some are nonprofit, and others are professionally associated. The Clinical Guidelines Task Force established by the American Academy of Otolaryngology (AAO) and the Quality of Care Committee created by the American Head and Neck Society (AHNS) are organizations specific to otolaryngology. The emphasis on quality improvement also coincided with a new shift toward the use of evidence-based medicine (EBM). It has become increasingly important in all aspects of health care, especially those that affect the quality of health care delivery.

Defining Quality Care

In 2001, the IOM published a report entitled "Crossing the Quality Chasm: A New Health System for the 21st Century," which highlighted the disparity between optimal care based on the best evidence and the quality of care that is delivered. In this report the IOM proposed six critical goals to redefine health care: improved safety, effectiveness, timeliness, efficiency, individualization, and equality of delivery of health care. It defined quality as "the degree to which health services for individuals and populations increase the likelihood of desired heath outcomes and are consistent with current professional knowledge" (1). The AHRQ simplified this definition as "doing the right thing, at the right time, in the right way, for the right person—and having the best possible results" (2,3).

The three general aspects studied in assessing quality of care are structure, process, and outcomes. *Structure* refers to health system characteristics. *Process* refers to the role of the health care provider. *Outcome* refers to what happens to the patient (3,4). These three concepts are intertwined and must all be addressed for effective quality improvement. This involves analysis of how organizations and systems fail and the practice of devising, testing, and evaluating tools and techniques to address those deficiencies.

Organizations For Improved Quality

The national initiatives dedicated to the improvement of quality health care all work together but also focus on different aspects of the same goal. The AHRQ focuses on research that promotes improvement of health care quality, safety, efficiency, and effectiveness. The IOM identifies key health care areas that need to be addressed more urgently. The Patient-Centered Outcomes Research Institute commissions research focused on evidence-based information as well as specific values and interests of patients. The NQF was formed in 1999 to identify and enforce performance measures and disseminate quality measures. Currently, there are 55 of these performance quality measures pertaining to oncology; however, none that explicitly pertain to head and neck cancer.

The Clinical Guidelines Task Force of the AAO was formed for the development of rigorous evidence-based guidelines in head and neck surgery. There are several published treatment guidelines available such as those for hoarseness (5), otitis externa (6), and acute sinusitis (7). These focus on improving quality of care and standardizing clinical protocols and algorithms for patients with specific otolaryngologic diagnoses based on best current evidence. They describe accurate diagnosis, treatment options, and prevention measures.

The Quality of Care Committee, formed in 2007 by the AHNS, works to establish consensus quality measures in head and neck cancer care and to promote compliance with these standards as a framework for measuring quality of care in head and neck surgery. Currently, there are quality measures for the two most common head and neck cancers: oral cavity and laryngeal cancer, approved by the AHNS in 2007 and 2009, respectively. Pretreatment measures include histopathologic confirmation of diagnosis, appropriate Tumor Node Metastasis (TNM) staging (8), and tobacco cessation counseling. Treatment-related measures involve referrals to radiation oncology, medical oncology, and speech pathology when necessary. Appropriate follow-up for symptom management and cancer surveillance encompasses the posttreatment measures (4).

Outcomes of Care

Another important aspect of quality health care is assessing the outcomes of care received. The IOM defines three general categories of outcomes: clinical status, functional status, and patient satisfaction. *Clinical status* is defined as the biologic outcome of disease, for example, 30-day mortality rates. *Functional status* is the patient's physical, emotional, and cognitive activity levels as the disease affects them, for example, Karnofsky score (4). Quality of life has become an important goal for head and neck oncology outcomes, in addition to cancer control and overall survival. Attempts to measure health-related quality of life have led to an increase in production of formal assessments to evaluate physical, mental, and social function for a variety of clinical topics. A frequently used example of such a tool is the University of Washington Quality of Life Revised Version 4 (9). Finally, *patient satisfaction* is a measure of patients' opinions about the care they receive, for example, Likert scale (10). It should be noted that patient satisfaction and high-quality care have not been shown to be correlative, and thus, it may not be the best means of measuring quality of care (4). Quality of care can be improved by considering these three aspects of clinical outcomes.

CLINICAL GUIDELINES

Clinical practice guidelines present systematically and precisely developed evidence-based recommendations for diagnostic procedures and medical treatment options that are used for standard patients (11). They use EBM to help set national standards and aid in decisions regarding appropriate health care for specific clinical circumstances. While there is increasing integration of evidence-based practice into clinical decision making, most clinical practice is still not based on the best available evidence. Guidelines are tools used to ensure that this evidence is put into current practice. They serve not only as references for clinical decision making and best practices but also as criteria for performance evaluation (12).

The general goals of developing clinical guidelines are to improve the quality of clinical care by helping physicians and patients in decision making and to support the delivery of cost-effective care by reducing unwarranted variations in clinical practice (13). In addition to promoting improved decision making, they can be used to initiate improvement strategies, prioritize research goals, and support reimbursement for particular services.

However, physicians must be careful in the use of guidelines. A flawed guideline can impair the whole health care system through the same pathways that an effective one makes improvements. There is a potential threat to individualized patient care if guidelines are used without proper evaluation. Every clinician must remember that in medicine every patient and every situation is slightly different. Guidelines must be developed in a very strict fashion to prevent inappropriate use (12,14).

Many review articles, consensus statements, practice parameters, and policy recommendations are labeled as "guidelines," without possessing the diligent methodology to merit such a designation (12). A variety of tools such as the Conference on Guideline Standardization (COGS) checklist, the Grading of Recommendations Assessment, Development and Evaluation (GRADE) approach (11), and the Appraisal of Guidelines Research and Evaluation (AGREE) instrument exist to measure the quality of guidelines. The AGREE instrument is a widely used generic measure of guideline quality characterized by the attributes outlined in Table 109.1 (15).

Clinical guidelines for a variety of otolaryngologic issues can be found through several different databases. The NGC database, an initiative of the AHRQ, is a repository that includes national guidelines that meet specific criteria. As of the publication date, the NGC database contains a total of 151 published guidelines with the search term "head and neck" and 71 with the search term "otolaryngology." A few resources for finding guidelines are listed in Table 109.2.

TABLE 109.1	AGREE INSTRUMENT PRINCIPLES

1. Scope and purpose
   a. Overall objective(s) of the guideline described
   b. Clinical questions detailed
   c. Intended target patient population identified
2. Stakeholder involvement
   a. Guideline development group of individuals from all relevant professional groups
   b. Incorporation of patients' views and preferences
   c. Clear definition of target users
   d. Pilot testing of guideline for further validation
3. Rigor of development
   a. Systematic methods used to search for evidence
   b. Criteria for evidence selection described
   c. Methods used to formulate of recommendations described
   d. Recommendations account for health benefits, side effects, and risks
   e. Explicit link between recommendations and supporting evidence
   f. External review of guideline
   g. Process for updating guideline provided
4. Clarity of presentation
   a. Specific and unambiguous recommendations
   b. Different options of management presented
   c. Key recommendations easily identifiable
   d. Supported with tools for application
5. Applicability
   a. Potential organizational barriers in applying recommendations discussed
   b. Potential cost of applying recommendations considered
   c. Key review criteria for monitoring or audit purposes
6. Editorial independence
   a. Editorially independent from funding body
   b. Conflicts of interests acknowledged

From Rosenfeld RM, Shiffman RN. Clinical practice guideline development manual: a quality-driven approach for translating evidence into action. *Otolaryngol Head Neck Surg* 2009;140 (6 Suppl 1):S1–S43; *Appraisal of Guidelines for Research and Evaluation (AGREE) Instrument 2001*, AGREE Collaboration: London, September 2011.

TABLE 109.2	RESOURCES FOR CLINICAL PRACTICE GUIDELINES

- National Guidelines Clearinghouse, http:www.guidelines.gov
- Guidelines International Network, http:www.g-i-n.net
- American Academy of Otolaryngology, http:www.entnet.org/Practice/clinicalPracticeguidelines.cfm
- National Comprehensive Cancer Network Treatment Guidelines, http:www.nccn.org
- Centers for Disease Control Morbidity and Mortality Weekly Report, http:*www.cdc.gov/mmwr*
- MD Consult, http:www.mdconsult.com/das/guidelines/268935093-2/1/toc?tab=topic

CLINICAL PATHWAYS

Clinical pathways are manifestations of guidelines, typically set up by a single institution, to specify care through protocols and to provide action plans with the appropriate support systems in place. Also known as critical pathways, they are developed by MDTs and establish the optimum timing of essential care in the management of patients who have specific conditions or undergo specific procedures. The development of these pathways through critical analysis has become a way to further streamline the clinical workup, treatment, and follow-up of head and neck cancer patients (16). By utilizing evidence-based interventions and reducing variations in care, the development of pathways can benefit patients by reducing complications, providing better quality of life, improving survival, and allowing more cost-effectiveness (17).

Several institutions have described experiences with critical pathways in head and neck oncology, reporting on associations between the implementation of a pathway and lengths of stay (LOS) in the hospital. Some studies compare observational cohorts of critical pathway patients to prepathway historical cohorts for the same or similar procedure. Others controlled for changes in medical care over time by comparing pathway cohorts with nonpathway counterparts during the same time frame. Pathway implementation does appear to decrease LOS, but the effect is confounded by temporal trends such as increased utilization review, more cost-conscious care, and better-educated medical providers regarding the importance of minimizing hospitals stays (17).

Chen et al. examined the implementation of a clinical pathway for unilateral neck dissection. Pathway patients were compared with historical controls and with a nonpathway contemporaneous cohort. Significantly decreased LOS and median costs were seen in pathway patients. Interestingly, LOS and median cost of care for the nonpathway contemporaneous control group was in between that of the pathway patients and historical controls. This suggests that care was made more efficient and cost-effective through both changes over time as well as through the clinical pathway (18).

Gendron et al. examined the effect of a clinical pathway for head and neck cancer patients on health care efficiency. Several aspects of hospital courses were reviewed for 3 years. Intensive care LOS, incidence of postoperative pneumonia, 30-day readmission rates, and median total costs decreased across the 3 years with implementation of the pathway. Median total LOS and nonintensive care LOS decreased over the first year but remained stable through year three (3,19).

Yueh et al. critically evaluated the impact of critical pathways on LOS after laryngectomy. This study compared a hospital that implemented a critical pathway for laryngectomy and a contemporary control group that did not utilize a critical pathway at a separate institution. After controlling for temporal trends and clinical variables, the direct impact of a clinical pathway on LOS in relatively low-volume procedures such as laryngectomy was noted to be limited. However, the simple process of thinking about and developing a pathway can help patients, whether they are managed using it or not, by encouraging those involved to more critically evaluate the care that is provided (17).

Clinical pathways ideally function to maximize quality of care in a resource-effective manner and may serve as a working model to readily implement clinical guidelines.

An example of a pathway for the care of a patient with an unknown primary associated with squamous cell carcinoma of the neck is illustrated in Figure 109.1. In general, the aforementioned findings suggest that successful clinical pathway implementation confers, either directly or indirectly, sustained efficacy and continual potential for improvement of health care quality (3).

MULTIDISCIPLINARY TEAM APPROACH

Even with medical advances, the 5-year survival rate of head and neck cancer patients has not substantially improved during the last 30 years. There has been a movement toward centralized multidisciplinary clinics and tumor conferences and cancer treatment programs in an effort to provide high-quality individualized patient care, which encompasses medical, surgical, social, emotional, and rehabilitative needs of the head and neck cancer patient. In addition, the goals of these centralized services are to improve and standardize treatment outcome, improve access to clinical trials, and improve survival outcomes (20). The variability of head and neck cancer presentation along with the complexity of cancer care warrants multidisciplinary coordination and centralization of care to optimize treatment.

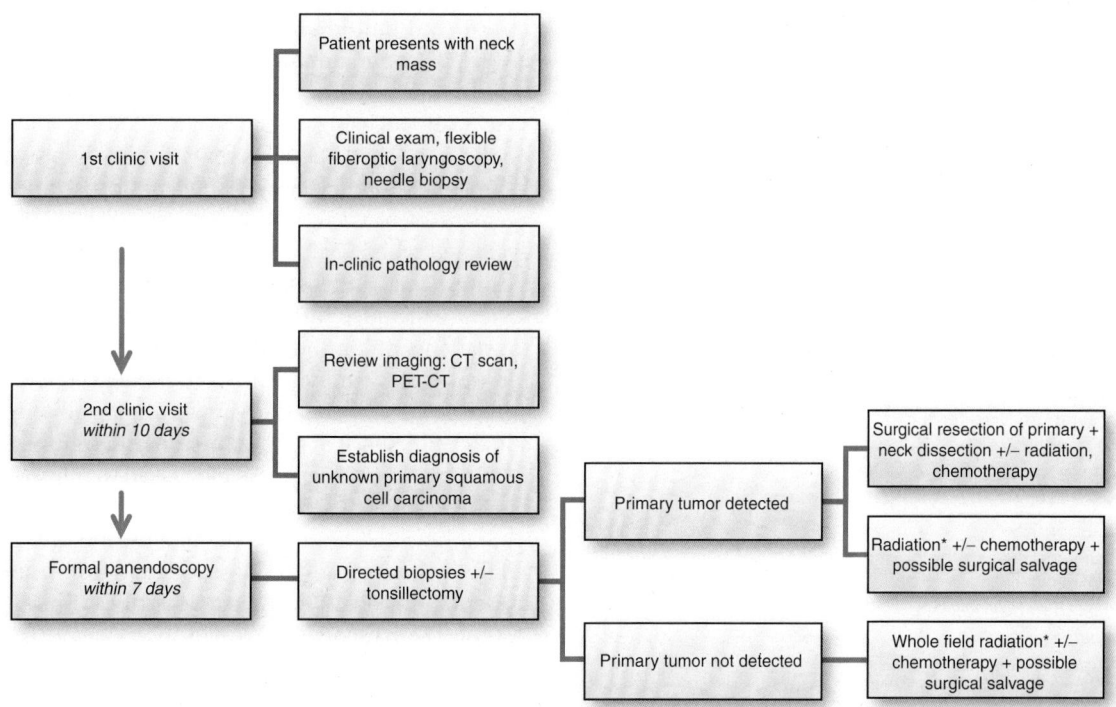

* Radiation therapy can be tailored to inclusion of the primary tumor and nodal basins most likely to be involved if Primary tumor is detected. When no primary tumor is detected, the radiation field should include all potential epicenters of cancer from the skull base to the clavicles and include all nodal basins.

Figure 109.1 Clinical pathway example for neck mass with unknown primary tumor.

The purpose of a MDT meeting is to ensure the quality of the health care provided to patients with head and neck cancer. The team includes physicians such as otolaryngologists and radiation oncologists, as well as allied health professionals who provide adjunctive care to head and neck cancer patients. Table 109.3 lists the essential components of this team.

The main goals of a MDT meeting are to define the true anatomical extension of the tumor, assign accurate TNM staging, and offer appropriate treatment recommendations. Proposed benefits of MDTs include more standardized care, better coordinated continuity of care, cost-effective care, improved communication among health professionals, improved clinical outcomes, and increased recruitment into clinical trials (16).

Multidisciplinary Team Presentations

Every patient with a newly diagnosed head and neck cancer, all patients who have undergone initial surgery, and all patients with newly identified recurrent or metastatic disease

TABLE 109.3	MULTIDISCIPLINARY HEAD AND NECK ONCOLOGY TEAM

Physicians
- Otolaryngologist/head and neck surgeon
- Subspecialty surgical consultants
  - General surgeon
  - Plastic and reconstructive surgeon
  - Oral maxillofacial surgeon
- Radiologist—interventional and diagnostic
- Radiation oncologist
- Medical oncologist
- Internal medicine physician
- Anesthesiologist
- Pathologist

Nurses
- Head and neck surgery clinic
- Operating room
- Postanesthesia care unit
- Intensive care unit
- Postsurgical unit
- Rehabilitation, long-term care, or nursing home
- Home health care

Allied health members
- Dentist
- Prosthodontist
- Speech–language pathologist
- Audiologist
- Physical therapist
- Occupational therapist
- Nutritionist or dietician

Other core members
- Social worker
- Religious or spiritual counselor
- Mental health specialists

From Chalian AA, Kagan SH. Guidelines for patient care. In: Johnson JT, Bailey BJ, Newlands SD, eds. *Head & neck surgery—otolaryngology*, Lippincott Williams & Wilkins, 2006:1419–1426.

should be presented to a MDT meeting. Adequate preparation and complete workup of the patient prior to meeting are essential to the working process of establishing a multidisciplinary accurate diagnostic TNM stage and treatment plan.

To ensure accurate TNM staging, satisfactory documentation of head and neck tumors should include a verbal description, precise measurement, illustrative representation, photographic recording, and appropriate radiographic imaging techniques such as computerized tomography (CT), magnetic resonance imaging, positron emission tomography (PET), and finally pathology reports and demonstrative histologic slides (21). Simo et al. presented their experience utilizing concise integrated multimedia Microsoft PowerPoint presentations including all of the aforementioned data, which could later be integrated into a centralized database. Figure 109.2 shows a good example of effective and complete MDT presentation using the format from Simo et al. as a guideline. The highlighted advantages include comprehensive and complete information available for each member to give expert opinion, educational benefit to medical and nonmedical team members, comparative baseline multimedia presentation in cases of recurrence, and a valuable adjunct to long-term clinical monitoring (21).

Efficacy of Multidisciplinary Teams

Despite more than 30 years of experience with MDTs in several countries, such as Sweden, the evolution to centralization and multidisciplinary care is supported mostly by lower power and anecdotal evidence with an obvious lack of fully high-quality evidence (16). There are few studies specifically focusing on the quality, efficacy, and efficiency of MDTs for head and neck that warrant discussion.

In a literature review, Westin et al. focused on the management of head and neck cancers using MDT meetings, evaluated whether this entity is beneficial to patients and treating staff, and determined if it is cost-effective. The review concluded that MDTs provide quality assurance for patients on an individual basis. They provide a forum for up-to-date individualized treatment plans, facilitate coordinated and timely treatment, and enhance the personal competence of clinical members. Additionally, MDTs within cancer care networks likely lead to improved patient outcomes and cost-effectiveness (16).

Stalfors et al. evaluated the quality and effectiveness of MDTs by collecting data prospectively from tumor board presentations on 329 consecutive patients. They found that 236 of 324 patients (73%) had their diagnosis and treatment plans established at the first meeting and were thus regarded as successes. However, 27% of patients were presented before all the necessary data were available, and the need to have more complete routine workup of patients prior to the MDT was emphasized. After presentation at the MDT, the TNM classification was only changed in 1.4% of patients. This attests to the high quality of decisions

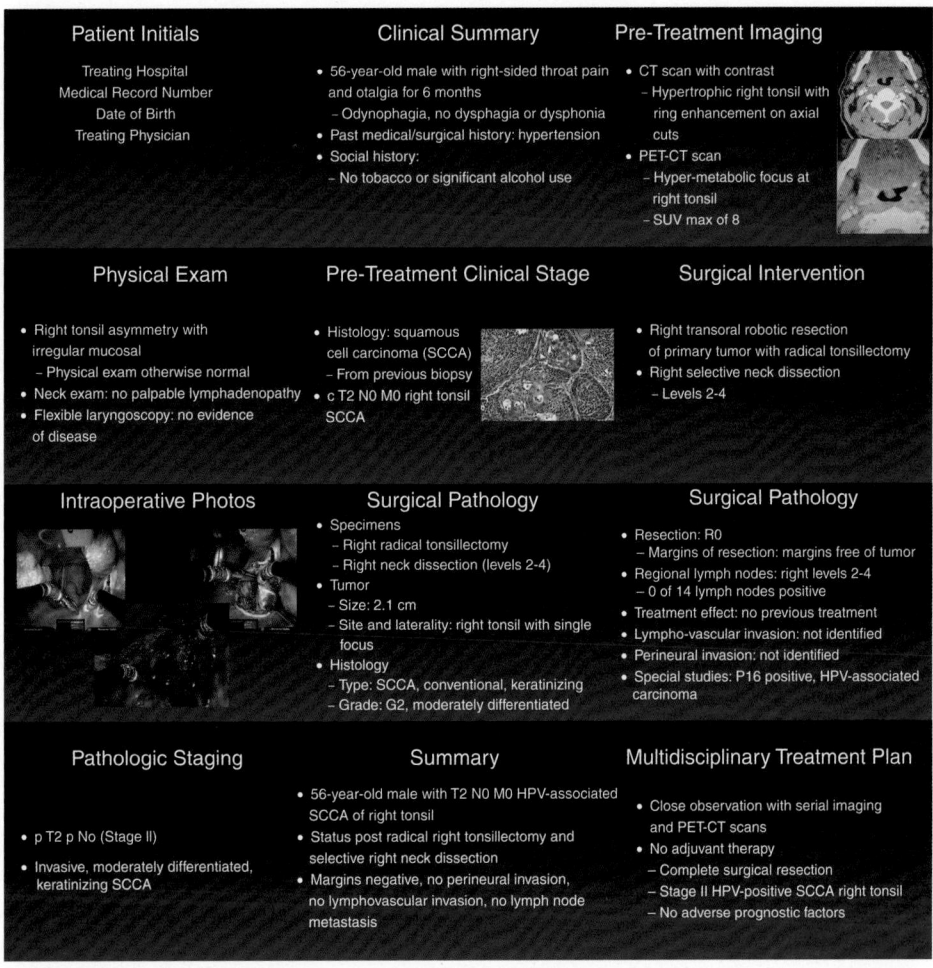

Figure 109.2 Integrated media presentation for MDT. (From Simo R, et al. Integrated media presentation in multidisciplinary head and neck oncology meetings. *Eur Arch Otorhinolaryngol* 2009;266:261–265.)

made at the MDT meeting and indicates that waiting time recorded in this study (median 38 days) does not appear to jeopardize the medical safety of patients. The study concluded that while the quality of decisions made at MDT meetings is good, there is a need to improve the quality of premeeting workup (20). Likewise focusing on efficiency, Nouraei et al performed a systematic analysis of the MDT to identify factors delaying treatment planning and implemented a system-wide Internet-based database. After the database was employed, significant improvements were made in cross-specialty coordination resulting in statistically significantly fewer delays in treatment due to unavailability of adjunctive investigations. Overall efficiency of the MDT was improved by 60% (22).

In a prospective study, Wheless et al. concentrated on the efficacy of the MDT in altering diagnosis, stage, and treatment plan in patients with head and neck cancers. The study population consisted of 120 patients, and 27% overall had some change in tumor diagnosis, stage, or treatment plan after MDT presentation. Change in treatment plan occurred in one out of every five patients (18.3%).

Treatment changes were significantly more common in cases of malignant tumors (24% vs. 6% benign tumors) and typically involved escalation in management by adding multimodality care (23).

As the management of head and neck tumors has become increasingly complex with multiple treatment modalities, the multidisciplinary tumor approach has become critical in optimizing treatment planning and patient outcomes. The available data show that tumor board meetings significantly affect diagnosis, treatment decisions, and delays in appropriate care. Many argue that multidisciplinary tumor boards are essential to managing head and neck cancer patients and represent a new standard of care (23).

MEDICAL ERRORS AND PATIENT SAFETY

Patient safety is a serious public health issue and is fundamental to achieving quality health care. In recent years, the importance of improving patient safety has been a priority both nationally and globally. It is also one of the core goals defined by the IOM. Compared to health care, industries with a perceived higher risk such as aviation have much better safety records. There is a one in 1,000,000 chance of an aircraft traveler being harmed during a flight. In comparison, there is a one in 300 chance of a patient being harmed while receiving health care. The economic benefits of improving patient safety are compelling. Studies show that additional hospitalization, litigation costs, infections acquired in hospitals, lost income, disability, and medical expenses have cost some countries between US$ 6 billion and US$ 29 billion a year (24).

Medical Errors

Estimates show that as many as 1 in 10 patients is harmed on some level while receiving hospital care in developed countries. A range of errors or adverse events may lead to the injury. The American health care system, one of the most advanced and costly in the world, still has an unacceptably high number of medical errors. Estimates indicate that nearly 100,000 patients die each year from medical errors in the United States. In addition, patient safety measures have worsened by nearly 1% each year for the past decade (24).

In an effort to develop a classification system for errors in otolaryngology, Shah et al. conducted a retrospective anonymous survey to members of the AAO. The survey asked participants to disclose any errors that occurred in their practice in the last 6 months and to describe the error, its consequences, and the corrective measures taken. There was an 18.6% (488/2,500) survey response rate with 216 errors reported by otolaryngologists, including 78 cases of major morbidity and 9 deaths. From these data, errors were classified into several categories: history and physical, differential or final diagnosis, testing, surgical planning, wrong site surgery, anesthesia-related, wrong drug/dilution on the surgical field, technical, retained foreign body, equipment-related, postoperative care, medical management, nursing/ancillary, administrative, communication, and miscellaneous. The most common errors were technical errors (19.3%) and medication errors (13.7%). From these data, the authors proposed a "Top Ten Safety Recommendations" list for otolaryngologists. It cautions against dependence on image guidance for sinus surgery and intraoperative nerve monitoring, emphasizes the importance of adequate preparation before surgeries with testing of necessary equipment and examination of all tests and consults, and highlights the effectiveness using the "time-out" at the beginning of each procedure (25).

Patient Safety

Patient safety research is an emerging field important to improve these statistics. The World Health Organization (WHO) has developed a set of patient safety research core competencies and describes a cycle of five key areas of patient safety research. These include measuring harm through quantification of morbidities and mortalities,

understanding the causes of adverse events, developing the solutions to reduce patient harm, evaluating the impact of solutions, and translating these improvements into policy and practice (26).

Surgery is one of the most complex health interventions to deliver. More than 100 million people require surgical treatment every year for different medical reasons. Problems associated with surgical safety in developed countries account for half of the avoidable adverse events that result in death or disability (24). A current example of a tool developed to improve surgical safety and reduce surgical adverse events is the WHO's Surgical Safety Checklist. Figure 109.3 shows an adapted version of this checklist. According to the WHO 2007–2008 pilot study for this checklist, the incidence of surgery-related deaths and complications can be reduced by one-third during major operations (9). These results have been reproducible in recent studies (27). The use of checklists significantly reduces surgical morbidity and mortality.

Helmio et al. detailed the feasibility of implementing of the WHO surgical checklist into the process of otorhinolaryngology–head and neck surgery and investigated whether it would have an impact on the awareness of safety-related issues. A structured questionnaire was given to the operating room team 1 month prior to and 1 month after surgical checklist implementation. Statistically significant findings after checklist implementation included improved verification of the patient's identity and awareness of the patient's medical history, medications, and allergies. Otolaryngologists and anesthesiologists more frequently discussed potential critical events. The authors concluded that the incorporation of the WHO surgical safety checklist into otolaryngology–head and neck surgery improved the sharing of patient-related medical information between team members (28).

DISPARITIES IN HEALTH CARE

One of the critical goals of the IOM's "Crossing the Quality Chasm" focused on establishing equitable care, both on the individual and population levels (29). Health care providers are to treat all individuals fairly and deliver high-quality care regardless of personal characteristics such as age, gender, race, ethnicity, education, disability, sexual orientation, income, or location of residence. More broadly, the health care system's goal is to improve health status and reduce disparities among subgroups. Multiple studies have examined these disparities among patients with head and neck cancer based on demographic factors such as race, socioeconomic status, and education.

Goodwin et al. performed a retrospective analysis evaluating racial disparities in the incidence and survival of head and neck cancer. Data showed that African American males have higher age-adjusted incidences and mortality rates for laryngeal and oral cavity/oropharyngeal cancers than black females, white males, and white females. Similarly, age-adjusted mortality rates were higher in black males for these subsites. Additionally, African American males have

Before induction of anesthesia	Before skin incision	Before patient leaves operating room
Nurse and anesthetist	*Nurse, anesthetist, and surgeon*	*Nurse, anesthetist, and surgeon*
◎ Confirm identity, site, procedure and consent with patient	◎ Introduce all team members by name and role	◎ Verbal confirmation of procedure and complete instrument counts
◎ Surgical site marked	◎ Confirm patients' name, procedure and site of incision	◎ Read specimen lables aloud
◎ Yes	◎ Antibiotic prophylaxis within 60 min of incision	◎ Address any equipment problems
◎ Not applicable—midline or bilateral sites	◎ Yes	◎ Discuss key concerns for recovery and management
◎ Check anesthesia machine and medications	◎ Not applicable	
◎ Pulse oximeter in place and functioning	◎ Display any essential imaging	
◎ Identify any patient allergies	*Anticipated critical events*	
◎ Difficult airway or aspiration risk	Surgeon:	
◎ No	◎ Identify critical or non-routine steps	
◎ Yes → Ensure appropriate precautions	◎ Estimated operating time	
	◎ Anticipated blood loss	
◎ Risk of >500 mL blood loss	Anesthetist:	
◎ No	◎ Recognize any patient-specific concerns	
◎ Yes → Prepare for fluid/blood replacement as necessary	Nurses:	
	◎ Confirm sterility	
	◎ Check for any equipment issues	

Figure 109.3 Surgical safety checklist. (From Haynes AB, Weiser T, Berry WR, et al. A surgical safety checklist to reduce morbidity and mortality in a global population. *N Engl J Med* 2009;360:491–499.)

a lower overall survival for these cancers when controlling for stage of presentation (29,30).

Beitler et al. examined health literacy as a factor in access to quality health care, specifically for head and neck cancer patients who have undergone total laryngectomy. The National Institutes of Health defines health literacy as the "degree to which individuals have the capacity to obtain, process, and understand basic health information and services needed to make appropriate health care decisions" (31). The patients in this study had dismal results with more than half being unable to interpret an appointment card or determine the correct time to take a medication (32). Such deficiencies may have severe consequences on the degree and quality of care these patients receive. This can be further translated to highlight the potentially serious implications poor health literacy has on access to care and overall quality of care.

Recent head and neck oncology literature emphasizes variations in patient care, specifically regarding high-volume versus low-volume centers and socioeconomic status. Two papers have reported that treatment for head and neck cancer is more likely to be concordant with guidelines when it is performed at tertiary care centers (4). Additionally, treatment at low-volume facilities has been associated with higher risk for death in patients with early-stage laryngeal cancer (29). Investigators have also reported that care for advanced laryngeal cancer in centers other than academic medical centers is associated with higher risk for death.

COST OF CARE

With the rising price of health care in America, it has become increasingly important to practice cost-conscious medicine. Utilization reviews use cost analysis and other measures to justify appropriate allocation of resources and delivery of care. Inefficient care causes costs to increase unnecessarily and can negatively affect access to health care. Thus, appropriate quality care must be evaluated through clinical research to identify what the actual cost of care is and where improvements can be made. Yet, few studies address this topic, specifically regarding the cost of care for patients with head and neck cancer.

The economics of medicine is not like that of other industries; cost can never be fully separated from medical decision making. In a review published in 1989, Eisenberg explained that the economic medicine does not imply that less money can or should be spent on health care but rather that efficient utilization of resources is essential. The review goes on to break down clinical economics into three dimensions of care: types of analysis, points of view, and types of cost. There are three types of analysis. *Cost identification*, most frequently used in clinical research, answers the question "what is the cost." It compares the lowest cost of different available diagnostic or treatment regimens, assuming that the outcomes of each are equal. *Cost-effectiveness* determines the net cost of a service and incorporates different outcomes through "cost per unit outcomes" measures. *Cost-benefit* analysis evaluates if the cost is truly worth the benefit by describing both aspects in equal units, typically currency. The patient, the payer, the provider, and society are the four perspectives to be considered. Finally, the types of cost are direct medical costs, direct nonmedical costs, indirect morbidity and mortality costs, and intangible costs. These dimensions of clinical economics are the tools used to further evaluate medical costs (33).

Westin et al. performed a comparative cost-identification analysis of total laryngectomy with postoperative radiotherapy versus preservation treatment for the larynx with chemotherapy/radiotherapy. The same survival was demonstrated with each treatment plan, but direct medical costs were nearly US$ 3,000 less for the surgical arm. This shows cost efficiency, but it has to be weighed against the loss of the larynx and its effect on quality of life of the patient (16).

Dedhia et al. also performed a cost-identification analysis of 119 patients undergoing total laryngectomy with bilateral neck dissections. The study revealed that mean total hospital cost for this relatively standardized procedure was $29,563 with a range from $10,915 to $120,345. Length of hospital stay was noted to correlate with cost. Most of the hospital costs were incurred on the day of admission (postoperative day 0), primarily attributed to operating room costs, which averaged 24% of total hospital costs (34).

Rabalais et al. evaluated the utility of PET–CT imaging for surveillance of neck disease and need for surgical intervention versus upfront neck dissection for patients who were treated with chemotherapy and radiation for cancers of the oropharynx with N2 neck disease. The study found that in patients who had a complete response to treatment at the primary site and neck, upfront neck dissection strategies had a 0.6% advantage in preventing neck recurrences as compared to the PET–CT strategies. The incremental cost-effectiveness ratio, that is, the additional cost if upfront neck dissection strategies were utilized as compared to PET–CT surveillance per patient cured, was calculated to be $3,854,397. This difference was so large because of the minimal difference in effectiveness of the strategies (35).

Further research evaluating the cost and outcomes of care will allow the health care system to better allocate needed resources and enable the provider to be a better-informed patient advocate.

CONCLUSION

In order to provide quality health care to the head and neck cancer patient, providers and members of the health care system must be educated on the benefits of utilizing clinical guidelines and pathways. In addition, development and utilization must be fostered. Centralized care through MDTs can help by facilitating better communication among treating physicians and improving access to efficient multidisciplinary evaluations for patients. Adverse events and patient safety must be carefully examined to reduce medical errors and to continually assess where improvements can be made. Measures should also be taken to address the disparities that exist in health care delivery and find ways to decrease them. Finally, appropriate cost analysis of treatment regimens is needed to ensure that limited health care resources are allocated appropriately.

Quality health care involves system-wide evaluations and improvements and is important from the perspective of the individual caregiver. The described principles of patient care stem from the basic medical ethics that guide each provider in conscientious medical decision making. Incorporating these components into everyday care will make for better providers and also aid in system-wide changes and improvements to provide the optimal care for patients.

HIGHLIGHTS

- Clinical guidelines and pathways incorporate EBM to provide individualized care for the head and neck cancer patient.
- MDTs incorporate clinical experience with EBM and provide the opportunity for the creation of individualized treatment protocols for diverse head and neck cancer patients.
- Multidisciplinary approaches incorporating clinical, functional, social, emotional, and rehabilitative aspects of patient care permit a comprehensive, effective, and efficient mechanism for management of the complex care of head and neck cancer patients.
- Cost-effective medicine is a crucial component to ensuring the appropriate utilization and allocation of limited health care resources.
- Providers of head and neck cancer care should be aware of the disparities in health care and address them through improved patient education.
- Few disease-specific guidelines exist for head and neck cancer care, and there is a significant need for development of clinical guidelines and incorporation of clinical pathways dedicated to various aspects of care of the head and neck cancer patient.

REFERENCES

1. Crossing the Quality Chasm: A New Health System for the 21st Century. Institute of Medicine, 2001.
2. *National Healthcare Quality Report* 2010. Available from *http://www.ahrq.gov/qual/qrdr09htm*. Accessed July 2011.
3. Lewis C, Weber R, Hanna E. Quality of care in head and neck cancer. *Curr Oncol Rep* 2011;13(2):120–125.
4. Chen A. Quality initiatives in head and neck cancer. *Curr Oncol Rep* 2010;12(2):109–114.
5. Schwartz SR, et al. Clinical practice guideline: hoarseness (dysphonia). *Otolaryngol Head Neck Surg* 2009;141(3 Suppl 2):S1–S31.
6. Rosenfeld RM, et al. Clinical practice guideline: acute otitis externa. *Otolaryngol Head Neck Surg* 2006;134(4 Suppl):S4–S23.
7. Rosenfeld RM, et al. Clinical practice guideline: adult sinusitis. *Otolaryngol Head Neck Surg* 2007;137(3 Suppl):S1–S31.
8. *What is Cancer Staging?* May 5, 2010. Available from *http://www.cancerstaging.org/mission/whatis.html*. Accessed August 2011.
9. Haynes AB, Weiser T, Berry WR, et al. A surgical safety checklist to reduce morbidity and mortality in a global population. *N Engl J Med* 2009;360:491–499.
10. Trochim WM. *Likert Scaling*. Research Methods Knowledge Base. October 20, 2006. Available from *http://www.socialresearchmethods.net/kb/scallik.php*. Accessed August 2011.
11. Brozek JL, et al. Grading quality of evidence and strength of recommendations in clinical practice guidelines: Part 1 of 3. An overview of the GRADE approach and grading quality of evidence about interventions. *Allergy* 2009;64:669–677.
12. Rosenfeld RM, Shiffman RN. Clinical practice guideline development manual: a quality-driven approach for translating evidence into action. *Otolaryngol Head Neck Surg* 2009;140(6 Suppl 1):S1–S43.
13. Medina J. *Clinical practice guidelines for the diagnosis and management of cancer of the head and neck*. 1995. Available from *http://www.ahns.info/clinicalresources/guidelines.php*. Accessed July 2011.
14. Chalian AA, Kagan SH. Guidelines for patient care. In: Johnson JT, Bailey BJ, Newlands SD, eds. *Head & neck surgery—otolaryngology*, Philadelphia, PA: Lippincott Williams & Wilkins, 2006:1419–1426.
15. *Appraisal of Guidelines for Research and Evaluation (AGREE) Instrument* 2001. AGREE Collaboration: London, September 2011.
16. Westin T, Stalfors J. Tumour boards/multidisciplinary head and neck cancer meetings: are they of value to patients, treating staff or a political additional drain on healthcare resources? *Curr Opin Otolaryngol Head Neck Surg* 2008;16(2):103–107. Doi:10.1097/MOO.0b013e3282f6a4c4.
17. Yueh Bevan, et al. A critical evaluation of critical pathways in head and neck cancer. *Arch Otolaryngol Head Neck Surg* 2003;129:89–95.
18. Chen AY, et al. The impact of clinical pathways on the practice of head and neck oncologic surgery: the University of Texas M. D. Anderson Cancer Center Experience. *Arch Otolaryngol Head Neck Surg* 2000;126:322–326.
19. Gendron K, et al. Clinical care pathway for head and neck cancer: a valuable tool for decreasing resource utilization. *Arch Otolaryngol Head Neck Surg* 2002;128:258–262.
20. Stalfors J, Lundberg C, Westinn T. Quality assessment of a multidisciplinary tumour meeting for patients with head and neck cancer. *Acta Otolaryngol* 2007;127(1):82–87.
21. Simo R, et al. Integrated Media Presentation in Multidisciplinary Head and Neck Oncology Meetings. *Eur Arch Otorhinolaryngol* 2009;266:261–265.
22. Nouraei SA, et al. Reducing referral-to-treatment waiting times in cancer patients using a multidisciplinary database. *Ann R Coll Surg Engl* 2007;89(2):113–117.
23. Wheless SA, McKinney KA, Zanation AM. A prospective study of the clinical impact of a multidisciplinary head and neck tumor board. *Otolaryngol Head Neck Surg* 2010;143(5):650–654.
24. *10 Facts on Patient Safety*. 2011. Available from *http://www.who.int/features/factfiles/patient_safety/en/index.html*. Accessed July 2011.
25. Shah RK, et al. Classification and consequences of errors in otolaryngology. *Laryngoscope* 2004;114(8):1322–1335.
26. *Cases on Patient Safety Research*. 2011. Available from *http://www.who.int/patientsafety/research/strengthening_capacity/classics/en/index.html*. Accessed August 2011.
27. de Vries EN, Prins HA, Crolla RM, et al. Effect of a comprehensive surgical safety system on patient outcomes. *N Engl J Med* 2010;363:1928–1937.
28. Helmiö P, et al. Towards better patient safety: WHO Surgical Safety Checklist in otorhinolaryngology. *Clin Otolaryngol* 2011;36(3):242–247.
29. Chen AY, Halpern M. Factors predictive of survival in advanced laryngeal cancer. *Arch Otolaryngol Head Neck Surg* 2007;133:1270–1276.
30. Goodwin WJ, Thomas GR, Parker DF, et al. Unequal burden of head and neck cancer in the United States. *Head Neck* 2008;30(3):358–371.
31. Parker RM, Ratzan SC, Lurie N. Health literacy: a policy challenge for advancing high-quality health care. *Health Aff* 2003;22:147–153.
32. Beitler JJ, et al. Health literacy and health care in an inner-city, total laryngectomy population. *Am J Otolaryngol* 2010;31(1):29–31.
33. Eisenberg JM. Clinical economics: a guide to the economic analysis of clinical practices. *JAMA* 1989;262(20):2879–2886.
34. Dedhia RC, et al. Cost-identification analysis of total laryngectomy: an itemized approach to hospital costs. *Otolaryngol Head Neck Surg* 2011;144(2):220–224.
35. Rabalais A, Walvekar RR, Johnson JT, et al. A cost-effective analysis of positron emission tomography-computed tomography surveillance versus upfront neck dissection for management of the neck for N2 disease after chemoradiotherapy. *Laryngoscope* 2012;122(2):311–314.

110 Principles of Radiation Oncology

Umamaheswar Duvvuri   *Gregory J. Kubicek*

Radiation oncology plays an important role in the treatment of head and neck cancers, both in the adjuvant and the definitive setting. Radiation is an important modality and has a large influence in terms of both survival and toxicity for patients. The field of radiation oncology is rapidly evolving, and head and neck oncologists should be aware of some of the important and changing features of this field to ensure that the patients they refer are treated appropriately. The goals of this chapter are to review the fundamental basis of radiation oncology (radiobiology), to describe some of the everyday aspects of radiation therapy delivery and toxicity, and finally to describe some of the new innovations in the field of radiation oncology.

RADIOBIOLOGY

Radiobiology describes the effects of ionizing radiation on the cellular level. Ionizing radiation induces cell death via DNA damage. DNA damage occurs when radiation interacts directly with the DNA strand or, more commonly, when the radiation interacts with a water molecule with secondary DNA damage. When ionizing radiation hits a water molecule, it forms free radicals; these free radicals are very unstable and, if formed in the vicinity of the DNA strand, are able to inflict damage.

DNA damage does not always lead to cell death; the cell has the capability of repairing radiation-induced damage to DNA. The rate and capability for repair are different for different types of cells. In general, more rapidly growing cells are more susceptible to damage from radiation (the process of cell division makes the DNA more susceptible to damage and also DNA damage is declared during DNA division). This is why the mucosa of the oral cavity (which is always dividing and being replaced) is very sensitive to the effects of radiation. In general, normal tissues have greater capacity for DNA repair than cancer tissues; one

of the rationales for fractionation of radiation is to allow repair of normal tissues during fractions.

The more radiation damage that is inflicted upon a population of cells, the more cell death; the initial radiation dose causes damage to the cell population but does not necessarily cause cell death. As the radiation damage accumulates, cell death starts to occur. A simplistic way to view this is to imagine that both strands of the DNA must be damaged before the cell is irreversibly killed; the initial dose of radiation is most likely to damage a number of single strands and occasionally both strands in a single cell. As radiation dose continues, it becomes more likely that double-strand damage occurs in more cells and thus causes cell death. During the initial (single strand) DNA damage, there is potential for the cell to repair the single-strand break and undo the radiation damage. The differential ability for DNA repair has led to the terms "radiosensitive" and "radioresistant." Although the exact terms are very subjective, the basic principle is that some types of cells and tumors have very little repair ability and die rapidly from even low doses of radiation. On the other side are "radioresistant" tumors; such tumors have ability to repair DNA, which makes them less likely to undergo cell death from radiation damage. Some typical radiosensitive tumors include lymphomas, while radioresistant tumors include sarcomas and melanomas. In Figure 110.1 we have three cell populations; cell population A would be radiosensitive (note the lack of a shoulder region and the immediate linear decline in surviving cells; such a curve is seen in blood cells that lack any repair mechanisms). Population C has a wide shoulder representing a radioresistant cell population; the initial portion of the curve is where cell repair is occurring preventing death from the radiation.

In addition to the capacity for DNA repair, another component that affects radiation sensitivity (and the slope of the cell death curve) is oxygenation. Under hypoxic conditions, it is thought that the free radicals, which are

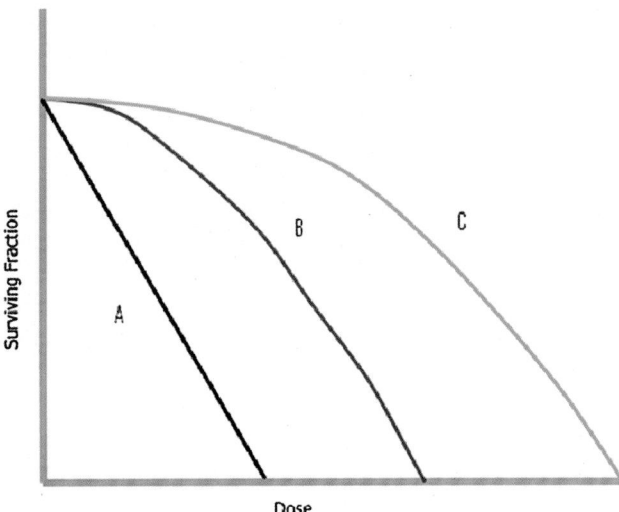

Figure 110.1 Three cell populations showing different levels of sensitivity to radiation. Cell population *A* would be radiosensitive (note the lack of a shoulder region and the immediate linear decline in surviving cells, such a curve is seen in blood cells that lack any repair mechanisms). Population *C* has a wide shoulder representing a radioresistant cell population; the initial portion of the curve is where cell repair is occurring preventing death from the radiation.

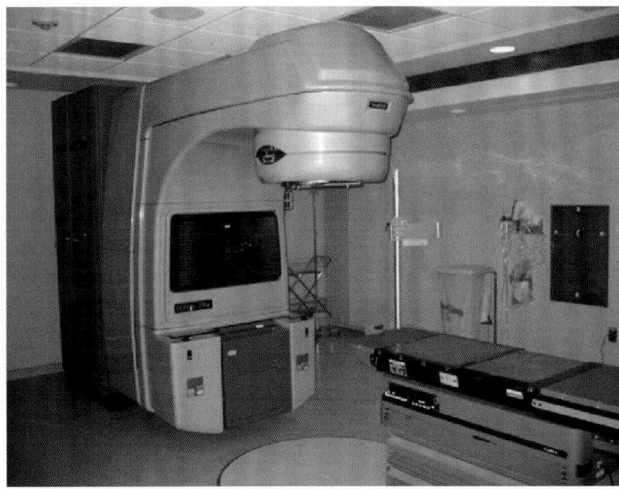

Figure 110.2 Linear accelerator.

responsible for DNA damage, can be scavenged by the hypoxia-induced acidic environment and that oxygen itself may play a role in continuing the cascade of the free radical formation. Large tumors tend to grow faster than their blood supply, leading to hypoxic areas in the center of large tumors. This phenomenon is thought to contribute to the relatively poor control rates for large head and neck cancers treated with ionizing radiation.

DOSE AND DELIVERY

The most commonly used form of radiation is photons, but other particles can also be used, including electrons, protons, neutrons, and carbon ions. Electrons are widely available but not as commonly used as photons. Electrons have a short depth of penetration; this allows for good dose to the surface and minimal dose to deeper levels (e.g., 6 MV electrons will deposit 90% of their energy 2 cm into tissue). Because of the dose distribution, electrons are a very good treatment option for the treatment of skin cancers. Protons and carbon ions are other forms of radiation and are less frequently used. Protons, neutrons, and carbon ions (referred to as heavy particle radiation) are not produced by normal radiation oncology linear accelerators and require special (and very expensive) accelerators to produce this type of radiation (see below for a more detailed description of proton radiation oncology).

It should be noted that all types of radiation work via the same basic mechanisms although some of the logistics of delivery are different. For photon radiation (usually just described as radiation), the radiation is produced by a

linear accelerator (Fig. 110.2). The patient lies on the treatment table, and the linear accelerator rotates around the patient to deliver the radiation. In order to ensure that the patient is not moving while the radiation is being delivered, an immobilization device is used; for HNC this typically consists of the thermoplastic head mask (Fig. 110.3).

Radiation is described in terms of dose; the common convention for dose is the gray (Gy). The definition of a Gy is the amount of energy dose absorbed per unit mass (1 Gy = 1 J/kg). Less often used is rads, 1 rad is equal to 0.01 Gy. The typical total dose for treatment of HNC is 60 to 66 Gy for adjuvant radiation and 70 to 74 Gy for definitive radiation. By comparison, doses for lymphoma would be 30 to 40 Gy, and the dose for a computed tomography (CT) scan is 0.1 to 0.2 Gy.

The total dose of radiation is divided into smaller doses called fractions. The dose for a fraction of radiation is usually between 1.8 and 2.0 Gy, although there can be a wide range (e.g., the dose for radiosurgery in the treatment of

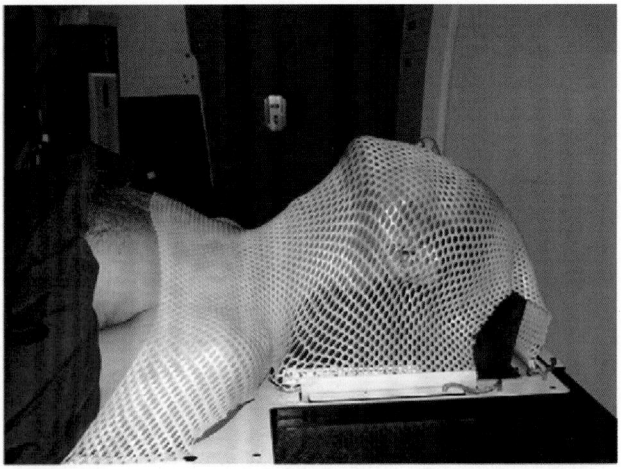

Figure 110.3 Thermoplastic head mask used for immobilization.

trigeminal neuralgia can be as high as 80 Gy in a single fraction). The purpose of delivering the total dose of radiation as a number of smaller fractions is to take advantage of normal tissue repair of DNA damage. For the most part, normal tissues have a much greater ability for DNA repair than do cancer cells. Thus, if damage is incurred to both normal tissues and cancer cells, the normal tissues will repair themselves while the cancer cells will die (this is not completely accurate as there is still a lot of normal tissue damage as discussed later).

The interplay between dose and fraction is sometimes referred to as "radiobiologically equivalent dose." Several mathematical models exist to convert from one dose and fractionation to another dose at a different fractionation (e.g., in terms of spinal cord tolerance, at 3 Gy per fraction, the maximum dose is 30 Gy, whereas at 2.0 Gy per fraction, the maximum dose is 45 Gy). The differential in repair between normal and cancer cells is magnified as radiation is delivered over a long period of time. This allows for improvement of the toxicity profile and minimizes toxicity to normal tissues.

FRACTIONATION AND TREATMENT TIME

The most common fractionation pattern is to deliver the radiation every day (Monday through Friday) and is referred to as "conventional" or standard fractionation. Hypofractionation is delivering less than one fraction per day (typically done in radiosurgery where the fraction is given every other day). Hyperfractionation is delivering more than one fraction per day. While there is repair of normal tissue DNA between radiation fractions, there is also (hopefully to a lesser extent) repair of cancer DNA and potential growth of the cancer itself. In order to decrease this risk, there have been several studies that have investigated the potential advantages of hyperfractionation.

The most well-known study is RTOG 90-03 (1). In this study, patients with stage III and IV HNC where randomized to conventional radiation (standard arm), hyperfractionation with twice daily treatments, hyperfractionation with twice daily treatments with a planned 2-week break during the radiation, and accelerated hyperfractionation or concomitant boost (which consists of daily radiation until the final 12 treatments at which time radiation is given twice daily). The results of this study showed an improvement in local control in the hyperfractionation and accelerated hyperfractionation arms (survival had a trend toward improvement, but did not reach statistical significance). Several other studies have shown similar results including DHANCA where patients were randomized to five versus six treatments per week, and local control was found to be improved with the six fraction regimen (5 year local control 70% vs. 60%) (2).

It should be noted that while tumor control appears to be improved with a reduction in treatment time, there is also an increase in acute toxicity (the normal tissues now have less ability to repair). However, the studies have not found a significant increase in late toxicity.

While hyperfractionation appears to be one method to improve outcome, chemotherapy is another. Chemotherapy has been shown to improve outcome versus radiation alone in both the definitive and the adjuvant setting. Brizel et al. (3) found that concomitant chemotherapy delivered with hyperfractionation provided better locoregional control than hyperfractionated radiation alone (70% vs. 44%). Brizel et al. (4) performed a mathematical analysis of the data obtained from RTOG 90-03 to determine what the impact of chemotherapy was on the radiobiologically equivalent dose. They determined that a 1% increase in radiobiologically equivalent dose lead to a 1.1% increase in locoregional control. Similarly, the addition of chemotherapy effectively increased the total radiobiologically equivalent dose by about 10 Gy. The authors concluded that this increase in effective radiation dose could not be safely achieved by simply increasing the amount of radiation delivered to the patient.

RTOG 0129 (5) set out to examine if chemotherapy (cisplatin 100 mg/m^2 every 3 weeks) plus hyperfractionated radiation (concomitant boost) was better than the same chemotherapy plus standard (once daily) radiation. The study did not find a difference between the two arms, and given the increase in acute toxicity and logistical difficulties with hyperfractionation, most institutions use once daily treatments for locally advanced HNC treated with chemoradiotherapy.

In summary, based on the known benefits of chemotherapy and the negative RTOG 0129 study, hyperfractionation is typically only used for patients who cannot get chemotherapy and have to be treated with radiation alone.

The overriding principle for the benefits of hyperfractionation is that a reduction in overall treatment time corresponds to an improvement in tumor control. The opposite is also true; when the overall treatment time is extended, tumor control decreases (6–9). RTOG (6) looked at the importance of treatment time in HNC radiation and found that local failure increased when the total treatment time (from surgery to completion of radiation) exceeded 11 weeks. This is why treatment breaks should be avoided unless absolutely necessary.

RADIATION ONCOLOGY PLANNING

The first step in radiation oncology planning is consultation with a radiation oncologist to examine the patient and discuss the risks and benefits of therapy. After this, a radiation planning CT scan is performed. This is similar to a diagnostic CT scan except that the CT scan is performed with the patient in the same position as they will be when receiving the daily radiation treatments. In order to reduce setup error between and during treatments, patients will have a plastic mask made that conforms to their facial anatomy (Fig. 110.3). Because of the special positioning (including the mask), a diagnostic CT scan cannot be used as a substitute for a radiation planning scan (although the information from a diagnostic CT scan can certainly be used to help in planning). Sometimes a positron emission tomography (PET) scan can be done at the same time as radiation planning (see section on PET scans).

After the radiation planning scan has been performed, the radiation oncologist will begin planning the radiation beams. This process has evolved over time (see below) but in all cases involves distinguishing normal structures from areas that are targeted for radiation. Several terms are commonly used to describe this process (Table 110.1). Gross tumor volume (GTV) represents the areas of actual tumor; this can be defined either radiographically (CT, PET, MRI) or clinically. In patients who have had surgery, there should not be a GTV since there is no longer any gross disease. Clinical tumor volume (CTV) defines areas that are at risk for harboring microscopic disease (such as lymph node basins); there can be discrepancy between different physicians in deciding the CTV volumes (e.g., does the contralateral neck need to be covered in a patient with tonsil cancer). Planning tumor volume (PTV) is a small expansion on the CTV or GTV to account for errors in daily setup. A typical PTV expansion is 0.3 to 1.0 cm. At our institution, we use daily imaging verification to reduce random setup error and are able to use a smaller PTV margin (3 to 5 mm). Organ at risk (OAR) is defined as normal tissue that is not involved with cancer and needs to be protected from radiation (examples include the spinal cord, parotid glands, mandible, etc.). Depending on the degree of risk, different areas will receive different doses of radiation. For example, the gross disease (GTV) will typically receive 70 to 74 Gy; areas of low risk (uninvolved lymph node basins) are treated to 50 to 54 Gy, while intermediate risk regions receive 60 to 66 Gy (Table 110.2).

TABLE 110.1	ORADIATION TERMS	
Term	**Definition**	
Hyperfractionation	Delivery of more than one fraction of radiation a day	
Hypofractionation	Delivery of less than one fraction of radiation a day	
Gross tumor volume	Gross disease as defined by radiology and physical exam	
Clinical tumor volume	Areas at high risk for microscopic tumor involvement	
Planning tumor volume	Treatment field, which includes margin for setup error and other uncertainty	
Organ at risk	Normal structure (such as spinal cord) that must be protected to some extent from radiation	

TABLE 110.2	TARGET DOSES	
Target	**Dose Range**	**Description**
High risk	70–74	Gross disease plus small margin
Intermediate risk	60–66	In adjuvant setting, tumor bed and resected but involved lymph node basins. In adjuvant or definitive setting, lymph node basins at high risk for failure
Low risk	50–54	In adjuvant and definitive setting, uninvolved lymph node basins at low risk for failure

After the radiation oncologist has distinguished the different target volumes, there is some time required for the radiation planning (mapping out the number and direction of the radiation beams) done by a dosimetrist and physicist. This can take anywhere between 10 minutes and 3 days depending on the complexity of the plan. When the radiation plan has been completed, the radiation oncologist will evaluate the plan to make sure that the target volumes (GTV, CTV, PTV, etc.) are adequately covered by radiation dose while simultaneously sparing the normal structures (OARs). There are general guidelines for how much radiation dose a normal structure can tolerate (Table 110.3). In order to evaluate a radiation plan and determine if it is safe for normal structures (OARs), a dose volume histogram (DVH) is constructed. A DVH plots percent volume of a structure versus the radiation dose. Oftentimes in order to cover the tumor, it is necessary to deliver radiation doses beyond tolerance to some normal tissue; this can lead to some of the long-term toxicities of radiation (discussed later). In the DVH shown in Figure 110.4 (patient with left base of tongue cancer), we see that the right parotid is being spared, because of the location of the tumor; the left parotid, being too close to the tumor, will receive dose that will likely make the

TABLE 110.3	NORMAL STRUCTURE DOSE TOLERANCE	
Structure	**Dose Limit**	**Toxicity**
Spinal cord	45 Gy (point dose)	Paralysis
Mandible	70 Gy	Osteoradionecrosis
Parotids	25 Gy (50% of gland)	Xerostomia
Pharyngeal constrictor muscles	55 Gy (50%)	Swallowing difficulties
Optic chiasm	54 Gy	Blindness
Lens	10 Gy	Cataracts

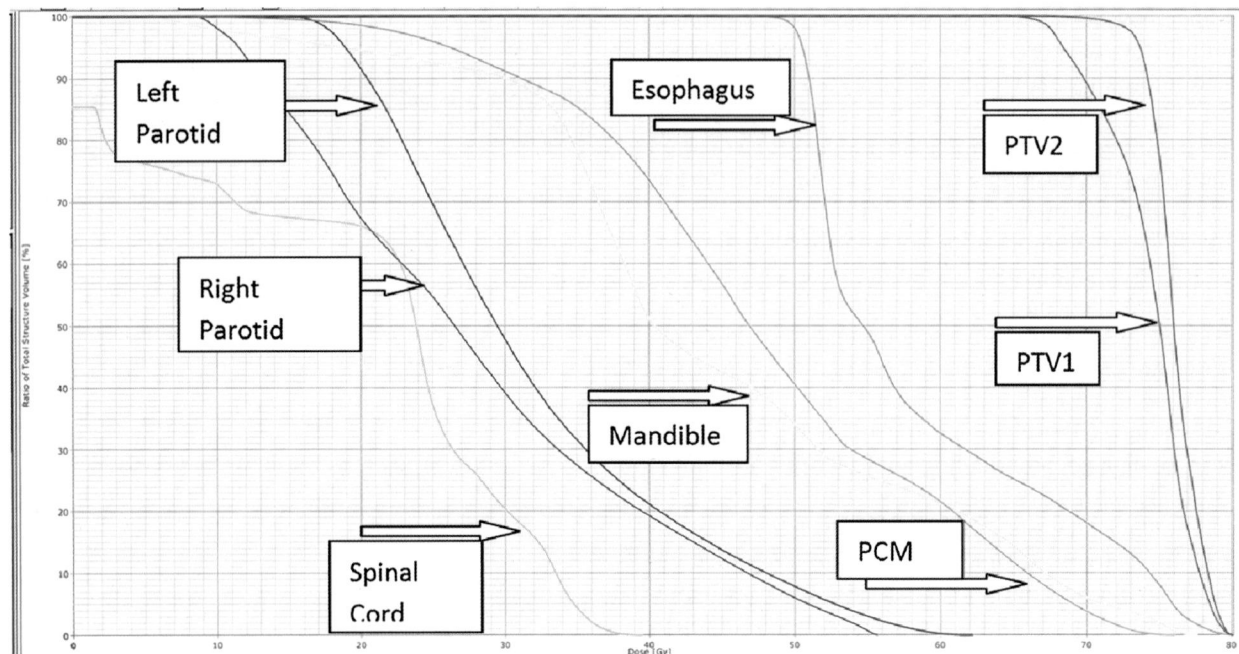

Figure 110.4 Dose volume histogram. This plots the percent volume of a structure (*y*-axis) versus the radiation dose (*x*-axis). In this DVH we see that the right parotid is receiving less radiation than the left parotid.

parotid nonfunctional (as seen in Table 110.3, the dose limit for parotid glands is 25 Gy at 50% of the organ; in Figure 110.4 we see that right parotid is getting about 25 Gy to 50% of the organ whereas the left parotid is getting 25 Gy to greater than 70% of the organ).

A typical time from consult to the start of radiation is a week to 2 weeks; this can be longer if a dental extraction is required or if patients are not compliant with appointments. As discussed above, overall treatment time is a very important metric in HNC outcomes; this is why it is valuable to have the consultation with the radiation oncologist within the first week of surgery for patients who may need adjuvant radiation. This allows everything to be set up and ready to start without undue delay.

The radiation therapy is typically delivered once daily (see above for discussion on fractionation). A typical treatment time is 5 to 10 minutes, and the entire session will be completed in about half an hour (time from in the door to out the door). The radiation oncologist will see the patient at a minimum of once per week; oftentimes there will also be weekly appointments with nursing and dietary staff as well. A typical course of radiation is 7 weeks for a definitive case and 6 weeks for adjuvant.

More details on the indications for adjuvant radiation are available in individual chapters, but in general, radiation is recommended in the adjuvant setting for positive lymph nodes, large tumor size (T3 or T4), perineural invasion (PNI), and positive surgical margins. Chemotherapy is added to radiation in the setting of positive margins and extracapsular extension (ECE) of a lymph node (see Table 110.4).

RADIATION DELIVERY

As computer technology continues to improve so does the delivery of radiation. Radiation delivery has evolved over time and continues to improve. The most basic system for radiation delivery is 2D (two dimensional) and involves planning the radiation from plain x-ray films. For 2D radiation delivery, a radiation planning CT scan would not be used. In 3D (three-dimensional) radiation delivery, an extra dimension is added to 2D planning; this incorporates imaging data from the CT scan used for radiation planning. 3D planning has the advantage of being able to accurately calculate doses to normal structures. The next step in radiation oncology evolution is intensity-modulated radiation therapy (IMRT). IMRT improves upon 3D radiation planning

TABLE 110.4	INDICATIONS FOR RADIATION AND CHEMORADIATION

Recommendations for adjuvant radiation
+ margins
+ lymph nodes (N+)
Large tumor size (T3, T4)
Perineural invasion

Recommendations for adjuvant chemoradiation
Extracapsular extension
+ margins

by using multiple radiation beams (referred to as beamlets) from different directions, all of which can potentially have different intensities of radiation. IMRT allows the radiation dose to "bend" around normal structures. In Figure 110.5 is a patient who had both a 3D and an IMRT plan. In the 3D plan, there is a beam from the right and a second beam from the left; everything in the radiation field gets a fairly high dose of radiation. In the IMRT plan, the dose is able to be shaped and bent; this allows less the radiation dose to the parotid glands to be drastically reduced. The consequence of this is an increase in the low-dose region with the IMRT plan as compared to the 3D plan (bottom row of Fig. 110.5). IMRT involves a large amount of planning. While a 3D plan can be generated within an hour, an IMRT plan can take up to a week to plan. The main catalyst for the evolution from 3D to IMRT is the multileaf collimator (MLC), an attachment to the head of the linear accelerator that allows the radiation beams to be modulated. MLCs are

relatively cheap and easy to implement. As a result, IMRT is available essentially everywhere that radiation is available (at least in the United States).

There are obvious advantages to IMRT; with reduction in dose to normal structures, there is a reduction in the likelihood of late radiation-induced toxicity. As shown in Figure 110.5, the radiation dose delivered to the parotid glands is reduced; this will hopefully result in a reduction of xerostomia. However, IMRT also has some significant (and perhaps underappreciated) disadvantages. First of all, IMRT takes significantly longer to plan and is much more expensive than 3D. For patients with rapidly growing or bleeding tumors, it often makes sense to start with a 3D plan, which can begin rapidly and then convert to an IMRT plan to complete the radiation. Another disadvantage is the distribution of low-dose radiation. While Figure 110.5 shows a clear reduction in the areas of high radiation dose, we also see an increase in the low dose

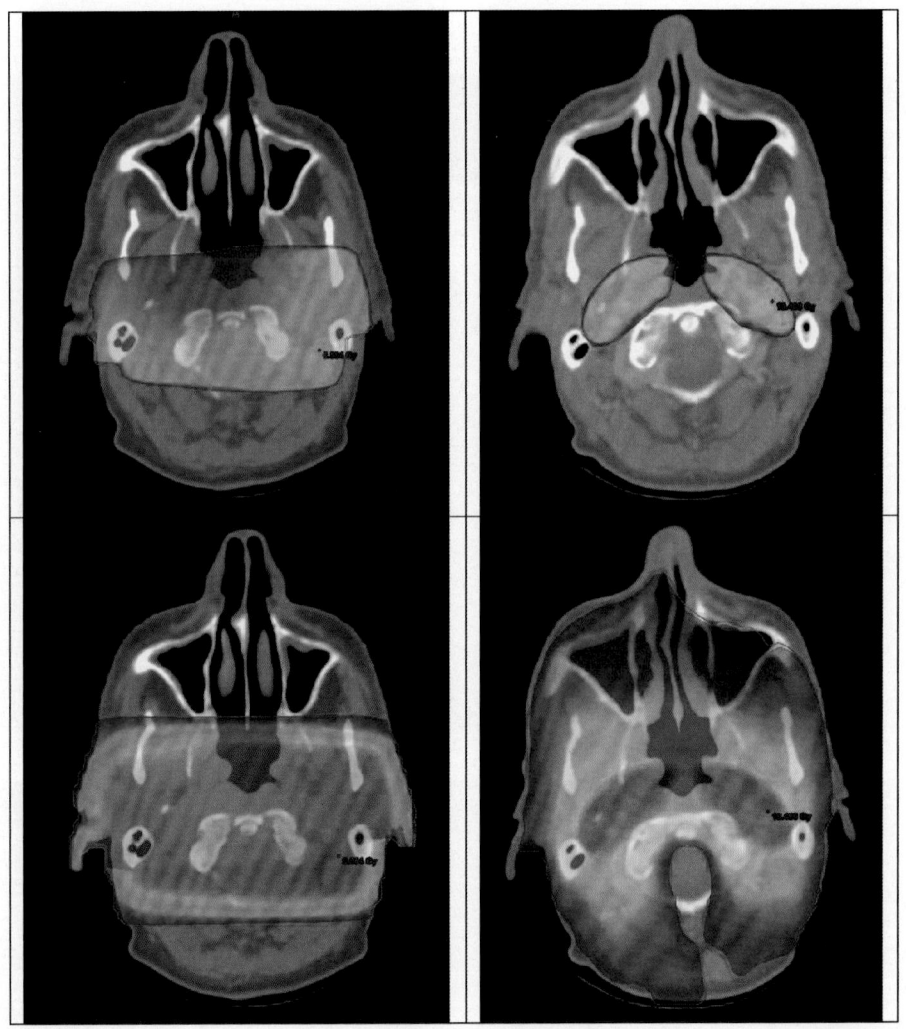

Figure 110.5 IMRT versus 3D plan The left hand column is a 3D plan (two opposed lateral beams). The right hand is the same patient with an IMRT plan. Notice that the top row is the high-dose region and it is much more conformal in the IMRT plan. The bottom row is the low-dose region and is much larger in the IMRT plan.

of radiation. In IMRT there is a significantly higher volume of tissues getting a low dose of radiation. The volume of low-dose radiation has some repercussions. There are toxicities that are seen in IMRT that were not seen in 3D planning; one of these side effects is nausea from radiation beams going through the brainstem. If the radiation oncologist does not mark an area as an OAR, the computer will not see it as being at risk, and this area will receive higher doses of radiation in the computer's attempt to spare areas that were marked as OARs. Another concern of the low-dose volume in IMRT is that this might confer a higher chance of a radiation-induced cancer. This risk is mainly theoretical, although it should be noted that IMRT has only been used in high volume recently and the average time to develop a radiation-induced cancer is 10 to 20 years. Figure 110.6 represents a typical IMRT plan for a base of tongue cancer.

Most of the date describing IMRT outcomes is retrospective, but there are some limited phase III data. The published level I evidence consists of two randomized prospective trials treating nasopharyngeal cancer (NPC). Similar in design, each trial randomized locally advanced NPC patients between conventional radiation and IMRT along with concurrent chemotherapy. The results showed that salivary gland (parotid) function was significantly and dramatically improved in the IMRT arms in both studies. Kam et al. (10) found a reduction in observer-rated xerostomia from 82.1% with conventional radiotherapy to 39.3% with IMRT and also measured improvements in measured parotid flow rates. Similarly, Pow et al. (11) found an improvement in stimulated saliva flow with IMRT and also found that patients treated with IMRT had an improvement in patient-reported quality of life scores. The primary end point for both studies was parotid function; neither trial was powered or intended to examine the role of IMRT in disease control or overall survival. Retrospective data in both nasopharyngeal (12–15) and nonnasopharyngeal HNC (16–21) compare very favorably to historical norms. It should be noted that the essentially all of the phase III HNC data acquired thus far

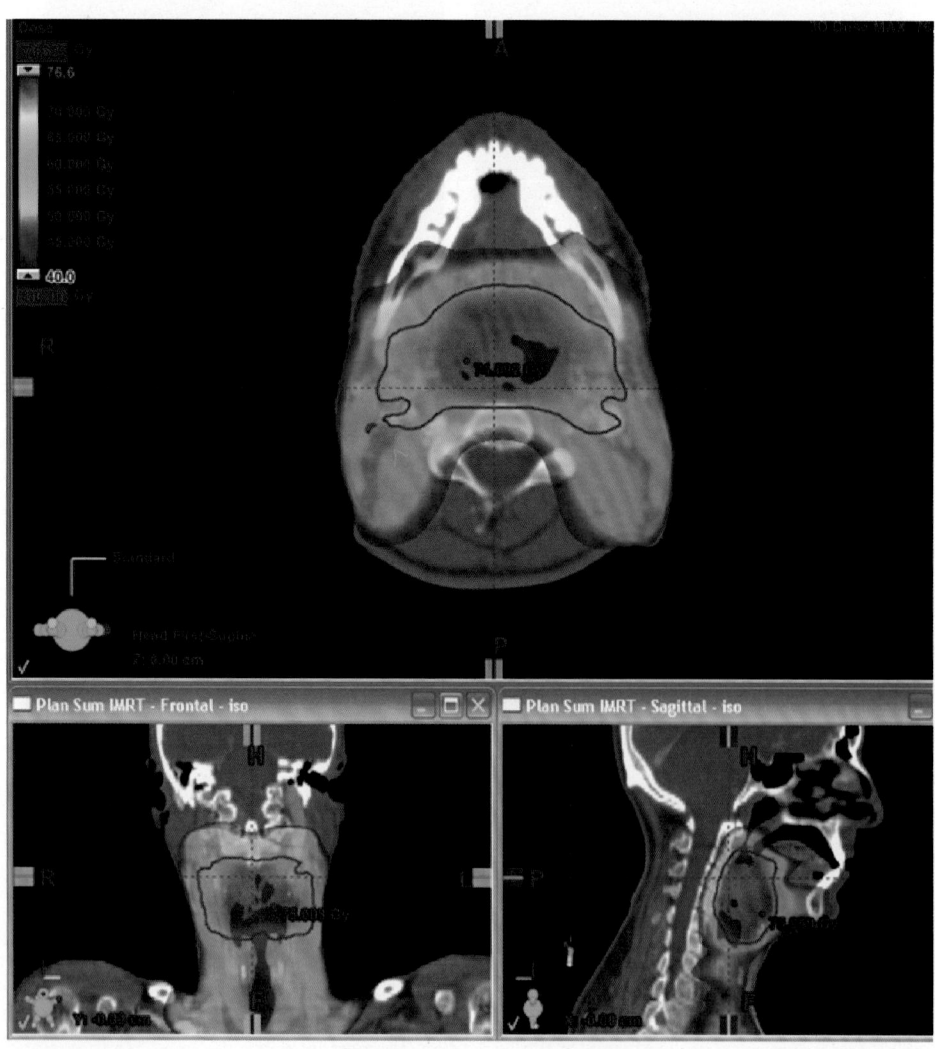

Figure 110.6 Base of tongue IMRT plan.

are from 2D or 3D radiation planning but that the general acceptance of IMRT technology has led to its inclusion in RTOG trials; RTOG 0234 and 0522 are the first major US cooperative group studies incorporating IMRT into radiotherapy planning.

RADIATION TOXICITY

Radiation has multiple side effects and toxicities, some of which occur during treatment (acute) and others that occur months to years after therapy (late). If chemotherapy is added to the radiation, there is a significant increase in the rate of acute toxicities, although late toxicities appear to be similar. There is a significant amount of variation between patients and how the radiation is tolerated, but some general remarks can be made. During radiation, the first 2 weeks typically proceed without much difficulty unless the first round of chemotherapy causes toxicity such as nausea and vomiting or dehydration. After the second week, the acute radiation steadily escalates; toxicities include pain (sore mouth and sore throat) from mucositis, taste changes, loss of facial hair (in treatment field) and skin irritation, thick mucus, and dry mouth. These toxicities will typically escalate until they plateau around week 5 to 6 and remain constant through the remainder of the therapy. The majority of patients state that pain is the most difficult of the side effects and often requires narcotic medications.

After the completion of radiation, the side effects slowly subside. The first-week postradiation remains a difficult time with modest improvement in pain and other side effects; around the 2-week mark, patients begin to feel some noticeable improvement in toxicity, and this continues for the next several weeks. Skin breakdown typically heals in about 2 weeks, thick mucus resolves around week 3 to 4, and the pain improves but is often still present until 8 to 12 weeks after radiation. Fatigue and ability to return to work are dependent on a number of factors, but in general most patients are able to return to work around 8 weeks after radiation.

In addition to the acute toxicities, there are a number of late radiation associated side effects. One of the most common side effects is xerostomia (dry mouth) from damage to the salivary glands; this sometimes responds to pilocarpine (Salagen), but oftentimes patient will need to carry a bottle of water around and may have difficulty swallowing dry meats and breads. Taste changes typically resolve by 3 months after radiation although patients may have some food items that never regain taste and develop intolerance to spicy foods (which taste too spicy). Some late side effects that develop months and even years after the radiation include hypothyroidism, neck fibrosis, carotid artery stenosis, osteoradionecrosis (the incidence of which can be increased by dental work after radiation), and dysphagia with concomitant aspiration. As seen in Table 110.3, there are general dose guidelines for how much radiation certain tissues can tolerate. Radiation tolerance doses are put together by a combination of retrospective studies and animal studies and while this data are tentative for obvious reasons cannot be easily expanded upon.

In general, toxicity rates are poorly documented and recorded; hence, a wide range of toxicity rates are reported in the literature. Machtay reported on the toxicity with chemotherapy and non-IMRT radiation in several RTOG studies; 43% of patients had severe late toxicity, mostly consisting of pharyngeal and laryngeal dysfunction (22). Eisbruch and coworkers recently published their prospective data using IMRT to treat oropharyngeal tumors (23). Swallowing function was assessed by two methods, videofluoroscopy and subjective symptom score assessment. Videofluoroscopy demonstrated that on average, mild pretreatment dysphagia progressed to moderate dysphagia after chemoradiotherapy. While many patients experienced recovery of swallowing function, some patients never had full recovery.

INNOVATIONS IN RADIATION PLANNING

In addition to IMRT, there have been several other innovations in radiation therapy, which have promise to improve outcomes in HNC. Some of the recent innovations in HNC radiation oncology have included incorporation of imaging such as PET scans, proton therapy, and radiosurgery.

One major innovation to the treatment of HNC has been PET scans. While the imaging aspect of PET scans is described elsewhere, there is also an important role for PET scans in radiation treatment planning. Geets et al. (24) reported that the use of pretreatment FDG–PET in combination with pretreatment CT or MRI improves target definition in oropharyngeal cancer and results in more normal tissue sparing. The same group also examined the role of PET contouring in larynx cancer, by comparing standard imaging techniques and PET findings with the pathologic specimens (25). They reported significantly smaller target volumes when targets were drawn on FDG-PET as opposed to CT scan. PET-based tumor volumes also showed better correlation with pathologic findings compared with CT, both for the primary tumor and the locoregional lymph nodes (26). Long-term clinical data are emerging; favorable 3-year overall state and disease-free survival rates have been shown in IMRT patients who all had PET-based contouring (27).

Proton therapy represents another possible evolution in radiation oncology. Protons are fundamentally different than photon radiation and are attractive because of its theoretical dose distribution in normal tissue. Photons lose energy slowly as they travel through tissue; energy is deposited in the tumor but is also in the normal tissue both in front and in back of the tumor. Protons on the other hand have very low energy loss until they reach a certain depth at which point all of the proton's energy is released at once. Tissue distal to this point has almost no radiation dose. This sudden peak in dose is known as the "Bragg peak" and can allow the proton beam to be targeted on the tumor and has very little dose to normal structures on the other side (very little exit dose). Theoretic plans have been created testing conventional IMRT versus intensity-modulated proton therapy, showing a significant advantage in tumor coverage and normal tissue sparing with the intensity-modulated proton therapy plans (28,29). It should be emphasized that these were theoretic plans and not actual treatments. Currently, most proton treatments are given with conventional (3D; anteroposterior–posteroanterior, lateral) proton beams.

Protons are currently only available in a limited number of centers, and experience and published results are very limited, especially in the treatment of head and neck cancer. The majority of reported results of proton therapy in head and neck cancer involve rare and difficult to treat tumors, such as chordomas and other skull-base tumors (30). A small series from Loma Linda looked at 29 oropharyngeal HNC patients treated with a proton boost (66% of the radiation was delivered via photons); the study showed good local control and toxicity (31) but larger and more heterogeneous series are certainly needed.

Another radiation oncology innovation is radiosurgery. Radiosurgery is similar to IMRT in the delivery of the photon radiation; the only difference between conventional radiation and radiosurgery is in patient immobilization and image verification techniques. Radiosurgery requires very stringent immobilization and alignment techniques; this allows for high doses of radiation to be delivered in a highly conformal manner. There are multiple platforms that can be used for delivery of radiosurgery; some of the common devices include CyberKnife, Gamma Knife, Trilogy, and TrueBeam. Although some of the details differ, the basic performance for all of the machines capable of radiosurgery is similar. Because of the precise nature of radiosurgery, much higher doses per fraction can be used, which allows for fewer overall fractions. For example, in the treatment of early-stage lung cancer, 3 fractions of 20 Gy per fraction is a common radiosurgery schedule as compared to 35 fractions of 2 Gy per fraction for nonradiosurgery HNC. Most of the radiosurgery data in radiation oncology are in the treatment of central nervous system (CNS) disease (such as brain metastatic lesions) and in early-stage lung cancer. However, there are growing data in the use of radiosurgery in the treatment of head and neck cancer (32). Radiosurgery in the HNC setting is most often in recurrent HNC; the current approach at our institution is to use radiosurgery (40 to 44 Gy in five fractions) for patients with recurrent HNC that is not amenable to surgical salvage. This is a growing field and will certainly continue to evolve.

HIGHLIGHTS

- Conventional fractionated irradiation therapy is undertaken to allow normal tissue repair of DNA damage between fractions while cancer cells die.
- Hyperfractionation (more than one fraction per day) appears to improve outcome in patients treated with radiation alone. However, it is also associated with increased acute toxicity, and the benefit appears to be lost in patients treated with both radiation and chemotherapy.
- Common indications for radiation include T3–T4 tumors, positive lymph nodes, and positive or close margins, PNI.
- Tumor control decreases when total treatment time exceeds 11 weeks.
- Use of IMRT allows for the sparing of normal tissues such as parotids, mandible, and pharyngeal constrictor muscles.

REFERENCES

1. Fu KK, Pajak, TF, Trotti A. A radiation therapy oncology group (RTOG) phase III randomized study to compart hyperfraction-ation and two variants of accelerated fractionation to standard fractionation radiotherapy for head and neck squamous cell carcinomas: first report of RTOG 9003. *Int J Radiat Oncol Biol Phys* 2000;48(1):7–16.
2. Overgaard J, Hansen HS, Specht L, et al. Five compared with six fractions per week of conventional radiotherapy of squamous-cell carcinoma of head and neck: DAHANCA 6 and 7 randomised controlled trial. *Lancet* 2003;362(9388):933–940.
3. Brizel DM, Albers ME, Fisher SR. Hyperfractionated irradiation with or without concurrent chemotherapy for locally advanced head and neck cancer. *N Engl J Med* 1998;338(25):1798–1804.
4. Kasibhatla M, Kirkpatrick JP, Brizel DM. How much radiation is the chemotherapy worth in advanced head and neck cancer? *Int J Radiat Oncol Biol Phys* 2007;68(5):1491–1495.
5. Ang KK, Harris J, Wheeler R. Human papillomavirus and survival of patients with oropharyngeal cancer. *N Engl J Med* 2010;363(1):24–35.
6. Ang KK, Trotti A, Brown BW, et al. Randomized trial addressing risk features and time factors of surgery plus radiotherapy in advanced head-and-neck cancer. *Int J Radiat Oncol Biol Phys* 2001;51(3):571–578. PMID: 11597795.
7. Rosenthal DI, Liu L, Lee JH, et al. Importance of the treatment package time in surgery and postoperative radiation therapy for squamous carcinoma of the head and neck. *Head Neck* 2002;24(2):115–126.
8. Parsons JT, Mendenhall WM, Stringer SP, et al. An analysis of factors influencing the outcome of postoperative irradiation for squamous cell carcinoma of the oral cavity. *Int J Radiat Oncol Biol Phys* 1997;39(1):137–148. PMID: 9300748.
9. Muriel VP, Tejada MR, de Dios Luna del Castillo J. Time-dose-response relationships in postoperatively irradiated patients with head and neck squamous cell carcinomas. *Radiother Oncol* 2001;60(2):137–145.
10. Kam MK, Leung SF, Zee B, et al. Prospective randomized study of intensity modulated radiotherapy on salivary gland function in early stage nasopharyngeal carcinoma patients. *J Clin Oncol* 2007;25(31):4873–4879.

11. Pow EH, Kwong DL, McMillian AS, et al. Xerostomia and quality of life after intensity modulated radiotherapy vs. conventional radiotherapy for early-stage nasopharyngeal carcinoma: initial report on a randomized controlled clinical trial. *Int J Radiat Oncol Biol Phys* 2006;66:981–991.

12. Wolden SL, Chen WC, Pfister DG, et al. Intensity-modulated radiation therapy (IMRT) for nasopharyngeal cancer: update of the memorial Sloan-Kettering experience. *Int J Radiat Oncol Biol Phys* 2006;64:57–62.

13. Kam MK, Teo PM, Chau RM, et al. Treatment of nasopharyngeal carcinoma with intensity-modulated radiotherapy: the Hong Kong experience. *Int J Radiat Oncol Biol Phys* 2004;60:1440–1450.

14. Lee N, Xia P, Quivey JM, et al. Intensity-modulated radiotherapy in the treatment of nasopharyngeal carcinoma: an update of the UCSF experience. *Int J Radiat Oncol Biol Phys* 2002;53:12–22.

15. Bucci M, Xia P, Lee N, et al. Intensity modulated radiation therapy for carcinoma of the nasopharynx: an update of the UCSF experience. *Int J Radiat Oncol Biol Phys* 2004;60:S317–S318.

16. Chao KS, Low DA, Perez CA, et al. Intensity-modulated radiation therapy in head and neck cancers: the Mallinckrodt experience. *Int J Cancer* 2000;90:92–103.

17. Garden AS, Morrison W, Rosenthal D, et al. Intensity modulated radiation therapy (IMRT) for metastatic cervical adenopathy from oropharynx carcinoma. *Int J Radiat Oncol Biol Phys* 2004;60:S318.

18. Huang K, Lee N, Xia P. Intensity-modulated radiotherapy in the treatment of oropharyngeal carcinoma: a single institutional experience. *Int J Radiat Oncol Biol Phys* 2003;57:S302.

19. de Arruda FF, Puri DR, Zhung J, et-al. Intensity-modulated radiation therapy for the treatment of oropharyngeal carcinoma: the memorial Sloan-Kettering cancer center experience. *Int J Radiat Oncol Biol Phys* 2006;64(2):363–373.

20. Yao M, Dornfield KJ, Buatti JM, et al. Intensity-modulated radiation treatment for head-and-neck squamous cell carcinoma: the University of Iowa experience. *Int J Radiat Oncol Biol Phys* 2005;63:410–421.

21. Dawson LA, Anzai Y, Marsh L, et al. Patterns of local-regional recurrence following parotid-sparing conformal and segmental intensity-modulated radiation therapy for head and neck cancer. *Int J Radiat Oncol Biol Phys* 2000;46:1117–1126.

22. Machtay M, Moughan J, Trotti A, et al. Factors associated with severe late toxicity after concurrent chemoradiation for locally advanced head and neck cancer: an RTOG analysis. *J Clin Oncol* 2008;26(21):3582–3589.

23. Feng FY, Kim HM, Lyden TH. Intensity-modulated chemoradiotherapy aiming to reduce dysphagia in patients with oropharyngeal cancer: clinical and functional results. *J Clin Oncol* 2010;28(16):2732–2738.

24. Geets X, Daisne JF, Tomsej M, et al. Impact of the type of imaging modality on target volumes delineation and dose distribution in pharyngolaryngeal squamous cell carcinoma: comparison between pre and per-treatment studies. *Radiother Oncol* 2006;78:291–297.

25. Daisne JF, Duprez T, Weynand B, et al. Tumor volume in pharyngolaryngeal squamous cell carcinoma: comparison at CT, MR imaging, and FDG PET and validation with surgical specimen. *Radiology* 2004;233:93–100.

26. Burri RJ, Rangaswamy B, Kostakoglu L, et al. Correlation of positron emission tomography standard uptake value and pathologic specimen size in cancer of the head and neck. *Int J Radiat Oncol Biol Phys* 2008;71:682–628.

27. Vernon MR, Maheshwari M, Schultz CJ, et al. Clinical outcomes of patients receiving integrated PET/CT-guided radiotherapy for head and neck carcinoma. *Int J Radiat Oncol Biol Phys* 2008;70:678–684.

28. Steneker M, Lomax A, Schneider U. Intensity modulated photon and proton treatment of head and neck tumors. *Radiother Oncol* 2006;80(2): 263–267.

29. Taheri-Kadkhoda Z, Björk-Eriksson T, Nill S. Intensity-modulated radiotherapy of nasopharyngeal carcinoma: a comparative treatment planning study of photons and protons. *Radiat Oncol* 2008;3:4.

30. Ares C, Hug EG, Lomax AJ, et al. Effectiveness and safety of spot scanning proton radiation therapy for chordomas and chondrosarcomas of the skull base: first long-term report. *Int J Radiat Oncol Biol Phys* 2009;75:1111–1118.

31. Slater JD, Yonemoto LT, Mantik DW, et al. Proton radiation for treatment of cancer of the oropharynx: early experience at Loma Linda University Medical Center using a concomitant boost technique. *Int J Radiat Oncol Biol Phys* 2005;62:494–500.

32. Heron DE, Ferris RL, Karamouzis M. Stereotactic body radiotherapy for recurrent squamous cell carcinoma of the head and neck: results of a phase I dose-escalation trial. *Int J Radiat Oncol Biol Phys* 2009;75(5):1493–1500.

Chemoradiation

Christine G. Gourin   *Arlene A. Forastiere*

OVERVIEW

The addition of chemotherapy to radiation treatment, often referred to as chemoradiation, has been increasingly used since initial clinical trials in the 1990s showed that chemoradiation achieved comparable survival outcomes to surgery with postoperative radiation for patients with stage III advanced laryngeal cancer. Such patients formerly were only offered surgery with postoperative radiation; radiation alone was less effective than when combined with surgery to treat advanced head and neck cancer. The findings of these studies, and numerous phase II and III studies performed since then, have ushered in a new era for patients with head and neck cancer, many of whom can be treated with intent to cure using chemoradiation.

Chemotherapy refers to drugs that are cytotoxic—that is, they cause cell death. There are different types of chemotherapy drugs, all with different mechanisms of action that result in cell death. Chemotherapy may enhance the effects of radiation therapy, but chemotherapy by itself is not a curative modality. Though these drugs can result in impressive initial tumor shrinkage, the drugs may not reach cells in the center of the tumor. In addition, tumor cells vary in their response to chemotherapy—the less "normal" a cancer cell is, the less likely it is that the cells use normal cell growth patterns to divide and grow, and therefore, chemotherapy may not be effective. Head and neck cancer cells can also demonstrate resistance, both innate and acquired, to chemotherapy.

Chemotherapy has been shown to increase the effect of radiation on tumor cells when used with radiation therapy. Chemotherapy acts as a radiosensitizer, making cancer cells more sensitive to the effects of radiation and when used with radiation, utilizes the radiosensitizing effects of chemotherapy as well as the systemic cytotoxic properties of chemotherapy. It is indicated for patients with advanced stage head and neck cancers, who are at high risk for distant metastases. It is not indicated for patients with previously untreated stage I, II, or low-volume stage III disease (a small primary tumor with or without a single ipsilateral node measuring 3 cm or less in diameter). Initial studies of chemoradiation employed induction chemotherapy, where three courses of chemotherapy were administered several weeks apart: patients with a response to induction chemotherapy subsequently received definitive radiotherapy, while patients who didn't respond were treated with surgery and postoperative radiation. Induction chemotherapy regimens are still in use, but have been largely supplanted by concurrent or concomitant chemoradiation, where chemotherapy is given concurrently with radiation therapy, either as weekly treatments or for a total of three treatments during the 6- to 8-week course of radiation therapy, based on studies showing improved tumor response rates with this approach. The use of chemotherapy alone is reserved for palliation of patients with metastatic disease.

The radiosensitizing effect of chemotherapy on radiation means that the side effects of chemoradiation are greater than for radiation alone. All of the side effects associated with radiation occur; however, the mucositis of the tissues lining the mouth and throat are more severe with the addition of chemotherapy to radiation, and swallowing difficulties both during and after treatment may be more severe in intensity and duration.

CHEMOTHERAPY DRUGS USED TO TREAT HEAD AND NECK CANCER

The most commonly used cytotoxic drugs to treat recurrent or metastatic squamous cell cancers of the head and neck are cisplatin, carboplatin, docetaxel, paclitaxel, 5-fluorouracil (5-FU), and methotrexate. Activity also has been demonstrated for more recent biologic agents that target the epidermal growth factor receptor (EGFR) such as cetuximab.

Platinum-Based Agents

Platinum analogs represent a class of drugs that are platinum complexes, with biologic and chemical similarities to alkylating agents. The two platinum analogs used for head and neck cancer are cisplatin (*cis*-diamminedichloroplatinum II) and carboplatin (*cis*-diammine [1,1 cyclobutanedicarboxylate] platinum II). The major cytotoxic action of cisplatin results from the formation of covalent adducts with DNA that are capable of blocking DNA replication and transcription (1). Cytotoxicity of non-target tissues is common. Cisplatin is associated with renal toxicity, gastrointestinal toxicity largely resulting from mucositis with nausea and vomiting, myelosuppression, ototoxicity and neurotoxicity including peripheral neuropathy, visual impairment, and rarely, seizures. The effects of neurotoxicity and nephrotoxicity are cumulative with repeated administration of the drug; while nephrotoxicity may be prevented by aggressive hydration and diuresis, there are no methods for preventing or treating neurotoxicity or ototoxicity. Cisplatin-induced hearing loss results in loss of outer hair cells in the cochlea through generation of reactive-oxygen species, which deplete the cochlear antioxidant system (2). Hearing loss is usually bilateral and irreversible, and may occur in more than 75% of patients treated with cisplatin.

Carboplatin, in contrast, is associated with lower rates of nephrotoxicity and neurotoxicity, with less nausea and emesis reported; however, it is somewhat less active than cisplatin. Resistance to platinum-based agents may occur and can be either intrinsic or acquired.

5-Fluorouracil

5-FU is a fluorinated pyrimidine that was synthesized to specifically take advantage of the observation that carcinoma cells utilize uracil to a greater degree than normal cells. The cytotoxic effects of 5-FU result from its conversion via multiple alternate biochemical pathways to several different active cytotoxic forms that inhibit DNA synthesis by binding with thymidylate synthase with subsequent depletion of precursor proteins for DNA synthesis, and through incorporation into nuclear and cytoplasmic RNA and DNA (3,4). 5-FU is specific for cells in the S phase of the cell cycle. Resistance has been correlated with reduced levels of enzymes required for 5-FU activation and mutations in thymidylate synthase that decrease binding affinity. Side effects are primarily related to bone marrow suppression and gastrointestinal mucositis, but dermatologic manifestations including hyperpigmentation, dermatitis, and alopecia have been described. Ocular toxicity can occur resulting from an acute inflammatory response causing conjunctivitis, blepharitis, and epiphora.

5-FU has synergistic effects with other chemotherapeutic agents and with radiotherapy and is used in combination with other drugs to exploit this effect.

Taxanes

Taxanes represent a class of drugs that specifically target mitosis by binding to microtubules, stabilizing them and disrupting microtubule dynamics thus inhibiting spindle function. Docetaxel and paclitaxel are the most commonly used taxanes in head and neck cancer (5). Taxanes induce mitotic arrest, which is typically followed by the induction of apoptosis (6). Because microtubules are required for protein transport as well as cell division, the cytotoxicity of taxanes may also result from microtubule dysfunction causing dysregulation of motility and transport.

The toxicity of taxanes is primarily myelosuppression with neutropenia, which may be dose limiting, and hair loss. Docetaxel is associated with fluid retention and paclitaxel has been associated with peripheral neuropathy and arthralgia (6). Neurotoxicity is more common when taxanes are given in combination with platinum-based agents.

Methotrexate

Methotrexate is an antifolate antimetabolite that inhibits dihydrofolate reductase, a key enzyme in intracellular folate metabolism. This effect is thought to be the main mechanism by which methotrexate produces cytotoxicity (7). Inhibition of dihydrofolate reductase prevents normal thymidylate and purine nucleotide synthesis, which results in single- and double-stranded DNA breaks, and leads to the accumulation of dihydrofolate polyglutamates, which are potent inhibitors of folate-dependent enzymes. Additional cytotoxicity may result from transformation of methotrexate to polyglutamate forms, which are preferentially retained within cells. Methotrexate is most active against rapidly proliferating cells and active during the S phase of the cell cycle.

The primary toxicities of methotrexate are myelosuppression and gastrointestinal mucositis, although nephrotoxicity, hepatotoxicity, and neurotoxicity can also occur. Gastrointestinal symptoms and myelosuppression occur in a dose-dependent fashion, although myelosuppression can occur with even small doses in patients with compromised renal function. Acute and chronic hepatic dysfunction has been associated with methotrexate use and is dose and schedule dependent. Rarely, cirrhosis of the liver has been reported. High doses of methotrexate have been associated with encephalopathy and dementia. Polymorphisms in folate metabolizing enzymes and blood–brain barrier transporter genes may increase susceptibility to central nervous system toxicity (8).

Biologic Modifiers

Various biologic agents that target the EGFR pathway are under study in combination with chemotherapy, as single agents, and as multiple targeted agents. EGFR is highly expressed in virtually all squamous cell cancers of the head and neck, and expression is inversely associated with prognosis. EGFR is a transmembrane receptor belonging to a family of ErbB receptors, which contain an extracellular ligand binding region and a cytoplasmic tyrosine kinase-containing domain. Ligand binding signals receptor auto-phosphorylation through intracellular tyrosine kinase activity, which triggers a series of intracellular pathways leading to cell proliferation, inhibition of apoptosis, activation of invasion and metastasis, and neovascularization (9). Monoclonal antibodies to the EGFR such as cetuximab and panitumumab and small molecule tyrosine kinase inhibitors such as gefitinib and erlotinib ultimately target tyrosine kinase activity with downregulation of pathways including the PI3K-Akt, MAPK, Src, and STAT pathways and block the proliferation of tumor cells. A major response is seen in approximately 10% of patients who are platinum refractory.

Cetuximab is the only biologic agent in its class approved for use in head and neck cancer, although clinical trials are in progress to test the efficacy of newer agents. Compared to conventional chemotherapy agents, cetuximab is associated with less systemic toxicity, but is associated with the development of an acneiform rash in 84% of patients during treatment, which resolves after discontinuation of drug (10).

ADMINISTRATION SCHEDULES

There are different ways to administer chemotherapy when used in conjunction with radiation therapy. Induction chemotherapy, sometimes referred to as neoadjuvant chemotherapy, refers to the use of chemotherapy before definitive treatment. Concurrent or concomitant chemotherapy is given simultaneously with radiotherapy.

Sequential therapy describes the use of induction chemotherapy followed by concurrent chemoradiation. Adjuvant chemotherapy refers to the use of chemotherapy after surgery. Treatment recommendations for chemotherapy administration vary by primary tumor site, extent of disease, and evidence-based data used to support the use of a particular chemotherapeutic approach generated by clinical trials.

CLINICAL TRIALS

Chemotherapeutic agents used in the treatment of head and neck cancer are initially offered in the setting of a clinical trial. Clinical trials test the efficacy and safety of new agents before they are introduced into clinical practice. Clinical trials are performed in phases, with each phase designed to answer a different research question.

Phase I Trials

Phase I trials are designed to test tolerance and safety in drugs that have already passed through phase 0 trials, which involve animal testing. These trials have a study endpoint of determining the maximal tolerated dose and toxicity usually through dose escalation; while the clinical intent of the eventual use of the drug is efficacy, phase I trials are largely safety trials and generally are limited to a small number of patients who may have a variety of tumor types. The maximal tolerated dose determined by phase I trials is then further studied in phase II trials.

Phase II Trials

Phase II trials are designed to determine the response of the tumor to treatment in order to provide an estimate of drug activity. The study endpoint is response of tumor to treatment, usually measured by a reduction in tumor size. Responses may be complete (no measurable disease) or partial (a 50% or greater reduction in disease), and must last a minimum of 28 days to be considered clinically significant. Disease that does not demonstrate a response is graded as stable (no change in size) or progressive (an increase in tumor burden). If 20% or more of study participants demonstrate a response of any kind to treatment, the treatment is considered to be successful. A secondary endpoint is usually toxicity as well. A larger number of patients are required for a phase II trial than for a phase I trial. Such trials are used to determine if a drug warrants further testing in a phase III trial.

Phase III Trials

Phase III trials are designed to compare the response of the new treatment to a treatment that is already in clinical use. This type of study requires large numbers of patients to participate in order to detect meaningful differences in survival, and usually has strict inclusion criteria limited to a particular tumor site or stage. Patients are usually randomized to treatment arm, which is the gold standard for a phase III trial, and the study endpoint is usually survival, although toxicity and symptom palliation may be study endpoints depending on the clinical research question. Phase III trials represent level I evidence, which is the best evidence to support treatment approaches to head and neck cancer (11) (Table 111.1).

USE OF CHEMOTHERAPY IN HEAD AND NECK CANCER

Chemotherapy is used in the management of advanced head and neck cancers as initial treatment when administered with radiotherapy for organ preservation or for locally advanced, unresectable disease; in the postoperative setting concurrent with radiotherapy for high-risk disease; and for palliation of recurrent, inoperable disease.

TABLE 111.1	OXFORD CENTRE FOR EVIDENCE-BASED MEDICINE—LEVELS OF EVIDENCE	
Level	**Therapy/Prevention or Etiology/ Harm Study**	**Prognosis Study**
1a	SR[a] of randomized controlled trials	SR of prospective cohort studies
1b	Individual randomized controlled trial	Individual prospective cohort study
2a	SR of cohort studies	SR of retrospective cohort studies
2b	Individual cohort study[b]	Individual retrospective cohort study
2c	Outcomes research[c]	Outcomes research
3a	SR of case–control studies	
3b	Individual case–control study	
4	Case series	Case series
5	Expert opinion	Expert opinion

[a]SR, systematic review of published studies, for example, a meta-analysis.
[b]Cohort study, longitudinal multivariable epidemiologic study.
[c]Outcomes research, observational study with defined variables and validated outcome assessment.
From Oxford Centre for Evidence Based Medicine—Levels of Evidence (March 2009). Available at: http://www.cebm.net/. Accessed April 5, 2009.

CHEMORADIATION FOR ORGAN PRESERVATION

The first prospective randomized controlled clinical trial that integrated chemotherapy into the curative treatment of patients with advanced head and neck cancer was the Head and Neck Contracts Program, a multi-institutional collaboration of surgeons, medical oncologists, and radiation oncologists (12). This trial randomized 462 patients into a control group of surgery and postoperative radiotherapy, an experimental arm of one cycle of induction chemotherapy with cisplatin and bleomycin followed by surgery and postoperative radiotherapy or a second experimental arm of induction chemotherapy with cisplatin and bleomycin followed by surgery and postoperative radiotherapy, followed by six cycles of adjuvant cisplatin. Study results were reported in 1987 and demonstrated that the group that received adjuvant cisplatin after definitive therapy had a lower rate of distant metastases; however, the addition of chemotherapy in both experimental arms did not impact survival (13). However, some laryngectomy specimens in patients with an apparent complete response to induction chemotherapy were found to be histologically free of tumor after resection. These findings drove subsequent studies of the feasibility of larynx preservation with induction chemotherapy followed by radiotherapy, with surgery reserved for patients without a response to induction chemotherapy or for salvage of patients with persistent or recurrent disease following radiotherapy.

Larynx Cancer

The current era of chemoradiation was ushered in by the Veterans Affairs (VA) Laryngeal Cancer Study Group, who performed a landmark randomized controlled clinical trial to determine if induction chemotherapy followed by definitive radiation, with laryngectomy reserved for salvage, was a viable option to the gold standard of total laryngectomy with postoperative radiotherapy for patients with advanced stage laryngeal cancer (14). Patients with stage III or IV laryngeal cancer who would have required total laryngectomy for cure were randomized to receive either three cycles of induction chemotherapy with cisplatin and 5-FU followed by radiotherapy, or surgery and postoperative radiotherapy. Clinical tumor response was assessed after two cycles of chemotherapy, and patients with a response to induction received a third cycle followed by definitive radiation therapy. Patients without a tumor response or patients with progressive disease, including nodal disease, underwent immediate surgical resection followed by postoperative radiotherapy; patients with recurrent disease following chemotherapy and radiation underwent salvage laryngectomy.

The VA study results were published in 1991 and showed that organ preservation could be attempted in patients with advanced laryngeal cancer with chemoradiation without reducing survival in patients who would otherwise have undergone total laryngectomy, with laryngeal preservation in 64% of patients. Patterns of failure did differ between treatment groups, with significantly more patients in the induction chemotherapy group failing locally and significantly fewer patients failing at distant sites, in comparison with the surgical control group. Rates of second primary cancers were significantly higher in the surgery group. This study demonstrated that for some patients with advanced laryngeal cancer, laryngeal preservation with chemoradiation was feasible. Significant predictors of the need for salvage surgery were T4 and stage IV disease. Salvage laryngectomy was required in 56% of T4 lesions compared with 29% of smaller primary tumors, and in 44% of patients with stage IV disease compared with 29% for stage III disease. Patients with T4 lesions comprised 26% of participants in the VA study, with T4N0 disease present in 12% of patients. The subset of patients with T4N0 disease had significantly reduced survival in the nonoperative treatment arm compared to the surgical arm (15), suggesting that the encouraging results of organ preservation do not apply to this subgroup.

Advanced stage nodal disease is a known adverse prognostic factor and was related to the poorer survival of stage IV disease in the VA study, which includes N2 and N3 nodal disease by definition. When organ preservation therapy is used in patients with advanced neck disease, the response in the neck may be independent of the response at the primary site. A follow-up study of patients in the VA study showed poorer survival in patients with N2 or N3 disease and a partial response in the neck following induction chemotherapy, who subsequently required salvage neck dissection because of inability to control disease in the neck, compared to those with a complete response to induction therapy (16). The incorporation of early, planned posttreatment neck dissection after induction but prior to radiotherapy in such patients resulted in improved regional control and no difference in survival between patients with a partial response compared to complete responders (17).

A follow-up phase III study designed by the Radiation Therapy Oncology Group (RTOG) was designed to determine the contribution of chemotherapy and radiotherapy to larynx preservation to investigate three radiation-based treatments: induction cisplatin and 5-FU followed by radiotherapy in responders, similar to the induction arm of the VA study; chemotherapy with cisplatin administered concurrently with radiotherapy; and radiotherapy alone (18). Unlike the VA study, there was no primary surgical arm. The concurrent treatment arm was designed to test observations of the enhancement of radiation effects on tumor by concurrent treatment with cisplatin. Patients with stage III or IV laryngeal cancer, excluding T1 disease, were included. As a result of the poorer outcomes for patients with T4 disease in the VA study, patients with large volume T4 disease, defined as extension through cartilage or greater than 1 cm of base of tongue involvement, were excluded from the RTOG 91-11 trial. Patients with low volume T4 disease were incorporated into RTOG 91-11 and represented 10% or less of patients in each arm.

The RTOG 91-11 study demonstrated that overall survival rates were similar in all three treatment groups; however, locoregional control rates were significantly better in the concurrent chemoradiation arm (78%) compared with induction (61%) and radiation alone (56%) and 2-year laryngeal preservation rates were higher for concurrent therapy (88%) compared with induction (75%) or radiation alone (70%). Induction chemotherapy had the same rate of acute toxicity as concurrent chemotherapy; however,

acute mucosal toxicity was twice as frequent in the concurrent chemotherapy arm as in the induction or radiotherapy alone arms and was associated with delayed recovery of swallowing function at 1-year assessment.

These data established concurrent chemoradiation with cisplatin as the standard of care for organ preservation in advanced laryngeal cancer, excluding T4 tumors with tongue base or cartilage invasion. A follow-up of RTOG 91-11 evaluating the subset of patients who required salvage laryngectomy confirmed that salvage laryngectomy was required significantly less often following concurrent chemoradiation (16%), compared with the induction (28%) and radiotherapy alone (31%) arms (19). However, among patients surviving at least 1 year, overall survival was significantly worse for patients who required salvage laryngectomy compared to those who did not, by approximately 10%. There was no statistically significant difference in survival among patients undergoing salvage total laryngectomy as a function of initial nonoperative treatment.

Severe late toxicity after concurrent chemoradiation causing dysphagia secondary to dysfunction of the larynx and/or pharynx is progressive over time and in an RTOG analysis of several RTOG studies, including 91-11, was present in as many as 43% of patients at 3 years, after excluding patients with pretreatment severe laryngopharyngeal dysfunction (20). On multivariate analysis, older age, advanced primary tumor stage and laryngeal or hypopharyngeal primary site disease were significant predictors of late toxicity, emphasizing the importance of careful patient selection for aggressive organ-sparing treatment and swallowing exercises.

Taken together, these landmark randomized controlled clinical trials established concurrent chemoradiation as the standard of care for laryngeal preservation in advanced laryngeal cancer, with the caveat that patient selection should consider whether survival *and* function with an organ-sparing approach can be anticipated to be equivalent to the standard of laryngectomy with postoperative radiotherapy. Patients with T4 disease have poorer survival with chemoradiation and should undergo primary laryngectomy. Patients with pretreatment organ dysfunction are inappropriate for organ preservation because of predicted laryngopharyngeal dysfunction and feeding tube dependence resulting from severe late toxicities associated with chemoradiation. The cohort of patients with advanced primary stage disease and evidence of pretreatment organ dysfunction are better served with primary surgery and reconstruction rather than attempting to preserve a dysfunctional organ. Finally, patients should be aware that salvage laryngectomy is associated with a decrease in survival.

Hypopharyngeal Cancer

Organ preservation strategies for hypopharyngeal cancer are associated with a lower laryngeal preservation rate than those reported for advanced laryngeal cancer. The only randomized, prospective trial to date comparing chemoradiation to surgery with postoperative radiotherapy in hypopharyngeal cancer was conducted by the European Organization for Research and Treatment of Cancer (EORTC) Head and Neck Cancer Cooperative group (21). Modeled after the VA laryngeal cancer study, patients with T2–T4 lesions who required total laryngectomy as part of definitive surgical treatment were randomized to receive either induction chemotherapy with cisplatin and 5-FU followed by definitive radiotherapy, or surgery with postoperative radiotherapy. Patients with T4 lesions comprised 6% of participants. This trial found no significant difference between the induction chemotherapy arm and the surgery arm in local (12% and 17%, respectively) or regional (19% and 23%) recurrence rates and 5-year disease-free survival (25% and 27%).Overall survival was less than 30% and did not differ between treatment groups. Successful organ preservation was far less likely when compared with laryngeal cancer, with only 17% of patients treated with induction chemotherapy followed by radiation alive and laryngectomy-free at 5 years.

A subsequent phase III study, also conducted by the EORTC, directly compared induction cisplatin and 5-FU followed by radiotherapy in patients with a complete response at the primary site with a regimen of alternating cisplatin and 5-FU and radiotherapy (22). No significant difference in laryngeal preservation or survival rates was demonstrated, and at the present time, induction chemotherapy followed by radiotherapy is the evidence-based standard of care for laryngeal preservation in hypopharyngeal cancers, in the absence of site-specific trials evaluating concurrent chemoradiation.

A third trial was conducted by the European Groupe Oncologie Radiothérapie Tête et Cou (GORTEC) study group for organ preservation in patients with advanced cancer of the larynx or hypopharynx who, similar to the EORTC study, would be candidates for total laryngectomy for cure (23). A total of 220 patients were randomly assigned, and of those, just more than one-half had a hypopharynx primary tumor. The majority of patients had T3 primary tumors. The two treatment arms consisted of standard cisplatin and 5-FU for three cycles (control group) or combination docetaxel, cisplatin, and 5-FU for three cycles. Following induction of both therapies, responding patients received 70 Gy of standard radiation; patients without a response to induction chemotherapy underwent surgery. The three-drug therapy was shown to be statistically superior for the endpoints of response to the induction regimen (80% vs. 59%) and preservation of a functional larynx at 3 years (70% vs. 58%). Based on these data, induction therapy with the triple-drug combination of docetaxel, cisplatin, and 5-FU is superior to cisplatin and 5-FU for organ preservation in advanced hypopharyngeal cancer.

While subsite analysis was not described in the EORTC report, others have shown in retrospective studies that survival is better with surgery and postoperative radiotherapy compared with chemoradiation, and in such series the volume of disease and laryngeal involvement were factors that adversely impacted survival (24–26). As for advanced laryngeal cancer, patients with severe pretreatment organ dysfunction are inappropriate for chemoradiation because permanent laryngeal dysfunction and gastrostomy tube dependence are expected sequelae of nonoperative treatment. Hypopharyngeal cancer is a significant predictor of pharyngoesophageal stricture, with rates of gastrostomy tube dependence following chemoradiation twice as high as for laryngeal primary tumors (27). The hypopharynx is particularly predisposed to stricture formation because the dose to the pharyngeal constrictors cannot be reduced as the structures related to swallowing dysfunction are the primary target. Taken together, these data suggest that organ preservation in hypopharyngeal cancer should be reserved for those patients with stage III disease with low volume primary tumors. As for laryngeal cancer, patients with T4 disease have poorer survival with chemoradiation and should undergo primary laryngectomy (28).

Oropharyngeal Cancer

Concurrent chemoradiation has increasingly replaced surgery in the initial treatment of advanced stage oropharyngeal cancer, despite a lack of trials directly comparing surgery with postoperative radiation to concurrent chemoradiation. In contrast to the data for larynx and hypopharyngeal cancer, there are no clinical trial data that compare control rates and survival for patients with advanced oropharyngeal cancer treated with surgery with postoperative radiation versus chemoradiation, and therefore equivalence cannot be shown. Surgery with postoperative radiation therapy results in superior survival compared with radiation therapy alone, and has been the standard of care for patients with advanced stage oropharyngeal cancer. There has been one randomized controlled trial limited to patients with oropharyngeal cancer (29–31) and several nonrandomized or mixed primary site trials (31–36) that demonstrate improved locoregional control and survival rates with concurrent chemoradiation (cisplatin and 5-FU) of approximately 20% compared to radiation alone for advanced stage disease, which are comparable to the historical results of surgery and postoperative radiation (34,37–42) with organ preservation rates of 77% to 84%. No difference was observed between chemoradiation and radiation alone in the distant metastatic rate. Mucositis, related weight loss and need for a feeding tube, and hematologic toxicity occurred more frequently in the chemoradiotherapy group.

Despite the absence of level I evidence comparing concurrent chemoradiation to primary surgery, most oncologists consider these data sufficient evidence to offer organ preservation using concurrent cisplatin and 5-FU to patients with oropharyngeal cancer. Exceptions are stage I or II disease, which is treated with either surgery or radiotherapy, and a subset of stage III oropharyngeal cancers with T1 or T2 lesions and N1 disease, who do not appear to receive significant benefit from the addition of chemotherapy and may be treated with primary radiation therapy alone (43). A major topic of debate is the influence of human papillomavirus (HPV) associated tumors on clinical trial results, which primarily involves males under age 65, and is increasing in incidence in the United States and Europe (44). The favorable response of oropharyngeal cancer to chemoradiation may be due to a subset of patients with HPV-associated disease, who have improved response rates to chemoradiation primarily due to improved disease-free survival (45). HPV-positive tumors have been shown to have improved survival and disease control rates compared to HPV-negative tumors, and this survival benefit is independent of treatment modality (46–50). Patients with HPV-positive tumors are more likely to present with smaller primary site disease and more advanced nodal disease (51,52). Advanced nodal stage is a poor prognostic factor for HPV-negative tumors, but does not carry the same adverse prognosis in HPV-positive disease that it does for HPV-negative tumors (52–54). The improved survival in HPV-positive disease has been attributed to increased radiosensitivity, but has been shown to be independent of treatment modality (46,47,49). Other factors such as a lower risk of distant disease and second primary cancers and an inverse correlation with adverse tumor biomarkers such as EGFR, p53 mutations, and survivin are equally plausible (46). Advanced primary site stage has been shown to be an independent risk factor for recurrence and survival after controlling for HPV status (54).

HPV-positive lesions appear to have increased sensitivity to radiotherapy and may not require intensive concurrent chemoradiation regimens for treatment with the attendant effects on swallowing function without further improvements in survival. This premise is the focus of current clinical trials and it will be several years before data are available. Current research is focused on delineating differences in patients with oropharyngeal cancer based on HPV status. The presence of a high proportion of HPV-positive patients confounds the interpretation of efficacy in novel regimens investigating both chemoradiation and surgical treatment. The favorable impact of HPV on oropharyngeal squamous cell cancer outcomes is a relatively recent discovery, and to date the majority of studies regarding oropharyngeal cancer outcomes does not include HPV status in outcome analysis. Patients with HPV-positive tumors appear to have a different disease, with improved locoregional control and survival despite a preponderance of advanced stage disease. This difference may be due to smaller primary site disease at presentation, or to differences in tumor

biology conferred by HPV infection, including p53 and EGFR expression.

It is important to recognize that although initial disease control rates following chemoradiation are higher for oropharyngeal cancer than they are for larynx or hypopharynx tumors, successful salvage of oropharyngeal primary site recurrence is far less likely (55). Fewer than 20% of patients with recurrent disease are candidates for salvage surgery, which is associated with increased complication rates and the median survival of patients with recurrence in less than 1 year (31,36,55–57). The majority of patients with recurrence develop a second recurrence in less than 12 months (56,58). Patients with the greatest likelihood of salvage following chemoradiation failure are those with early stage primary tumors and no recurrent nodal disease (56,58). These data emphasize that successful locoregional control with initial therapy is a critical determinant of long-term survival. Patients with initial early stage disease who receive chemoradiation have been shown to have an increased risk of second recurrences after salvage surgery (56), and chemoradiation failure is associated with poorer survival even after controlling for other variables (55). These data suggest that chemotherapy may select for more aggressive tumor biology in a subset of patients. Because nonoperative therapy appears less likely to be successful in HPV-negative disease and the results of surgical salvage are poor, risk stratification of patients by biomarker status including HPV infection is an area of active investigation to optimize treatment selection and outcomes and may result in tailored therapeutic recommendations in the future.

Patients with T4 disease invading the mandible have been excluded from chemoradiation trials because of the high incidence of osteoradionecrosis resulting from chemoradiation, and such patients should undergo primary surgery with reconstruction and postoperative radiation therapy.

Nasopharyngeal Cancer

Nonoperative treatment is standard of care for the initial treatment of nasopharyngeal cancer in light of the close proximity of the nasopharynx to critical skull base structures, which makes surgical extirpation with adequate margins challenging, and the unique radiosensitivity of nasopharyngeal tumors. The clinical behavior of nasopharyngeal cancer varies by histologic subtype. World Health Organization (WHO) type I (squamous cell cancer) is more common in the United States than in endemic areas, with local–regional behavior that is similar to that of other head and neck cancers. WHO types II (nonkeratinizing cancer) and III (undifferentiated cancer) predominate in endemic areas, such as southern China and northern Africa, and have a higher propensity for distant metastases. WHO types II and III are more responsive to radiotherapy and chemotherapy than those with differentiated squamous histology, and more than 90% of WHO type II and III cases are associated with the Epstein-Barr virus.

Radiation has historically been the mainstay of treatment for disease above the clavicles. The management of locally advanced nasopharyngeal cancer dramatically changed a decade ago after publication of the results of the Intergroup 0099 study, which was designed to test concurrent chemoradiation in nasopharyngeal cancer in an effort to improve locoregional control and to decrease the distant metastatic rate by the addition of adjuvant chemotherapy (59). In this trial, patients with stage III or IV nasopharyngeal cancer were randomly assigned to either radiation alone or radiation with three cycles of concomitant cisplatin administered every 21 days, followed by three cycles of adjuvant cisplatin and 5-FU. Most patients (91%) had stage IV disease, and WHO type I histology was more common compared with published series from endemic areas. Overall survival at 5 years was significantly improved for patients who received combined-modality therapy (67% vs. 37%, $P < 0.001$), as was progression-free survival (58% vs. 29%, $P < 0.001$). The survival advantage of combined therapy was significant even though only 63% of patients received all three planned cycles of cisplatin during radiation and only 55% received all three cycles of adjuvant cisplatin and 5-FU.

One criticism of the Intergroup 0099 study is that the relative contributions of concurrent and adjuvant therapy could not be determined, and clinical trial results may be less applicable to endemic areas where WHO type I histologic subtypes are infrequent. However, subsequent randomized trials (60–62) in endemic areas and two meta-analyses (63,64) have confirmed a significant survival advantage for concurrent platinum-based chemoradiation over radiation alone. In contrast, randomized trials of induction chemotherapy followed by radiation compared with radiation alone have shown no significant improvement in overall survival (65–68), although some reported improved disease-free survival. Two meta-analyses of clinical trials that compared any sequence of chemotherapy and radiotherapy with radiotherapy alone have been published. A meta-analysis of the published results of six randomized trials comprising 1,500 patients (63) reported that at 4 years, chemotherapy improved progression-free survival by 34% and overall survival by 20%. The second meta-analysis used updated individual patient data from eight randomized trials (1,753 patients) with locally advanced disease, covering 1966 to 2003 (64). The effect of adding chemotherapy to radiotherapy on overall survival resulted in an absolute survival benefit of 6% (56% to 62%) at 5 years (hazard ratio [HR] of death = 0.82; $P = 0.006$). The effect on event-free survival was an absolute benefit of 10% (42% to 52%) at 5 years (HR of tumor failure [local, regional, or distant] or death = 0.76; $P < 0.0001$). There was a significant interaction between the timing of chemotherapy and radiotherapy and overall survival, with the highest benefit resulting from concomitant administration of chemotherapy and radiotherapy ($P = 0.005$).

Based on these data, concurrent cisplatin-based chemotherapy and radiation provides a clear survival benefit and is the accepted standard of care within and outside of the United States. The benefit of adjuvant chemotherapy, which theoretically will suppress distant metastases common in nasopharyngeal cancer, is less widely accepted. In the United States, the standard of care for treatment of patients with nasopharyngeal cancer stages IIB, III, IVA (T4, N0 to N2, M0), and IVB (any T, N3, M0) is radiotherapy with concurrent high-dose cisplatin on days 1, 22, and 43, followed by three courses of adjuvant cisplatin and infusional 5-FU dosing as administered in the Intergroup 0099 trial (59). Radiotherapy alone is indicated for stages I and IIA (N0 disease with no parapharyngeal space involvement).

Current areas of investigation in the management of nasopharyngeal cancer include the potential benefit of changing the sequencing of the three cycles of chemotherapy from adjuvant (after chemoradiation) to sequential (prior to chemoradiation) and the exploration of alternative cytotoxic regimens. The high incidence of distant metastases coupled with the limited ability to successfully deliver all three cycles of adjuvant chemotherapy in only 55% of patients in the Intergroup 0099 trial has motivated the investigation of sequential chemotherapy followed by chemoradiation. However, there is concern that this sequence of treatment might compromise the delivery of chemoradiation, the critical curative component of the treatment. The early results from several single-institution trials of sequential therapy have shown feasibility and encouraging response and survival data, and multicenter trials are under consideration. Circulating Epstein-Barr viral DNA can be quantitated by real-time polymerase chain reaction (PCR) in 96% of patients and predicts tumor load and risk of recurrence; this biomarker may have a role in stratifying patients by risk for additional systemic therapy (69). Pretreatment levels appear predictive of distant failure in patients with stage I or II disease, while posttreatment levels correlate with disease-free survival (70,71), and a validation trial is now in progress.

Oral Cavity Cancer

Cancer of the oral cavity should be distinguished from other sites as biologically distinct, and is managed surgically. Data from patients with advanced oral cavity treated with concurrent chemoradiation in phase I or II trials show equivalent survival compared to historic control patients treated with primary surgery, but a high rate of osteoradionecrosis (72–74). There are no level I data to suggest that nonoperative treatment effectively controls advanced oral cavity tumors, which is reflected in the 2011 National Comprehensive Cancer Network (NCCN) guidelines that recommend surgery as the preferred modality of treatment for advanced oral cavity cancer (28).

CHEMORADIATION FOR LOCALLY ADVANCED UNRESECTABLE DISEASE

Inoperable disease is defined as tumor that invades the base of the skull, prevertebral fascia, pterygoid musculature, or encases the carotid artery. Historically patients with inoperable disease were managed with radiotherapy alone, with a median survival time of 12 months and only 20% of patients alive at 2 years. The radiosensitizing properties of chemotherapy were explored in this population in several randomized controlled clinical trials that showed the potential for improved survival. The focus of these studies has been on drugs that show activity against both the disease and radiation-enhancement properties (e.g., cisplatin and 5-FU). The three general strategies that can be employed are (1) concomitant single-agent or combination chemotherapy with continuous-course radiation; (2) combination chemotherapy with planned split-course radiation; and (3) rapidly alternating chemotherapy and radiation. More recently, altered-fractionation radiation approaches have become an additional radiotherapy option. Currently, the best evidence supports concurrent chemoradiotherapy with a platinum-based agent as the standard of care for locally advanced head and neck cancer, but recommendations may change as new data become available.

Concurrent Chemoradiation

The first study to investigate concomitant chemoradiotherapy for the treatment of unresectable advanced head and neck cancer was reported in 1992 (75). The investigators randomly assigned 157 patients with unresectable squamous cell cancer of the head and neck were randomly assigned to radiation alone (70 Gy, conventional fractionation) or to a cisplatin and 5-FU combination alternating with radiation (60 Gy). Compared to patients treated with radiation alone, the group treated with chemotherapy showed significantly better complete response rates (43% vs. 22%) and survival (41% vs. 23%; $P = 0.01$).

A subsequent trial randomized 295 patients with unresectable squamous cell cancer of the head and neck to one of three treatment groups: radiation alone, radiation with concurrent cisplatin on days 1, 22, and 43; or split-course radiation with three cycles of concurrent bolus cisplatin and infusional 5-FU. Surgical resection was offered for patients in all three groups if feasible after the completion of treatment; patients in the third arm had an option for surgical resection after the second cycle of chemotherapy, if feasible (76). This study demonstrated a significant survival advantage at 3 years for patients treated with concurrent cisplatin and radiation (37%) compared with radiation alone (23%; $P = 0.014$). The split-course

concurrent regimen offered no survival advantage (27%) over radiation alone. Grade 3 toxicity or higher was significantly more common with concurrent therapy (89%) compared with radiation alone (52%; $P < 0.0001$). This study established radiation with concurrent high-dose cisplatin as the standard of care for locally advanced unresectable head and neck cancer.

A meta-analysis by Pignon et al. (77), the Meta-Analysis of Chemotherapy in Head and Neck Cancer (MACH-NC), highlighted the favorable results seen with a concurrent approach. Despite significant heterogeneity in study trial designs, overall concurrent chemoradiotherapy regimens were associated with an 8% absolute benefit in survival at 5 years compared with radiation alone (HR = 0.81; $P < 0.0001$). An updated analysis of 87 trials and more than 16,000 patients showed the same absolute benefit for survival with concomitant treatment (HR = 0.81; $P < 0.0001$) (78).

A meta-analysis of randomized concurrent chemoradiotherapy studies for patients with locally advanced squamous cell cancer of the head and neck was performed to develop clinical recommendations (79). Subgroup analysis of data from 1,514 patients in nine trials demonstrated that platinum-based concurrent programs offered the greatest survival advantage compared with radiation alone (odds ratio [OR] = 0.57; $P < 0.00001$). The meta-analysis suggested that platinum-based regimens for concurrent chemoradiation that were associated with a positive trial and a more favorable side-effect profile should be used. Overall, cisplatin-based chemoradiotherapy provided the most significant benefit in terms of survival and local–regional control (80).

In summary, concurrent chemoradiotherapy leads to improved disease control compared with radiation alone for patients with unresectable squamous cell cancer of the head and neck and represents standard treatment for patients who are able to tolerate the additional treatment-related toxicity of chemotherapy. The data showing improvement are best established for platinum-based concurrent regimens; an advantage for the use of chemotherapy persists even when newer altered-fractionation radiotherapy approaches are employed.

Induction Chemotherapy Using Cisplatin and 5-Fu with a Taxane

Three randomized controlled trials have directly compared induction chemotherapy using a combination of docetaxel, cisplatin, and 5-FU to standard cisplatin plus 5-FU in unresectable head and neck cancer (81,82). The TAX 323 trial enrolled more than 300 patients with locally advanced unresectable disease. The control arm consisted of four cycles of the two-drug combination followed by radiotherapy, and the experimental arm consisted of four cycles of the three-drug combination (docetaxel, cisplatin, 5-FU) followed by radiotherapy (81). The response rate to induction with the three-drug regimen was significantly higher compared with that of the two-drug regimen (68% vs. 54%, $P = 0.006$) as was overall survival (HR = 0.73; $P = 0.016$). Less toxicity was observed with the three-drug combination than with the two-drug combination.

Similarly, the TAX 324 trial randomly assigned 501 patients with unresectable or resectable disease (all sites) to three cycles of standard cisplatin and 5-FU or to combination docetaxel, cisplatin, and 5-FU (docetaxel, cisplatin, 5-FU) (82). Definitive local therapy in both arms consisted of standard radiotherapy plus weekly carboplatin. Overall survival was significantly improved for patients who received the three-drug therapy (HR = 0.70; $P = 0.0058$).

A third phase III trial compared induction combination paclitaxel, cisplatin, and 5-FU to induction cisplatin and 5-FU in a heterogeneous population of patients with both resectable and unresectable cancer (83). Chemoradiation was planned following induction chemotherapy but the actual treatment was not uniform. The taxane-containing treatment group had a higher overall response rate (80% vs. 68%); however, the difference in overall survival was not significant.

These trials demonstrate that the combination of docetaxel, cisplatin, and 5-FU followed by radiotherapy alone or radiotherapy and concurrent carboplatin is superior to cisplatin and 5-FU followed by the same definitive local therapy. The three-drug regimen administered in the TAX 323 trial seems to have an acceptable toxicity profile with lower rates of severe and life-threatening myelosuppression than observed with the two-drug regimen (81). These trials indicate that treatment with a taxane plus cisplatin and 5-FU is more effective than cisplatin and 5-FU alone when using response rate as the outcome measure. They do not indicate that induction combination docetaxel, cisplatin, and 5-FU is the standard of care, but provide support for a prospective, randomized controlled trial that compares induction chemotherapy followed by chemoradiation (termed sequential treatment) against the standard of care of chemoradiation for nonsurgical management of resectable disease or for management of unresectable disease. Several such trial designs are in progress in the United States. Combination docetaxel, cisplatin, and 5-FU should replace cisplatin and 5-FU as a new standard regimen for induction chemotherapy and is being used in ongoing trials. A second approach for patients with unresectable disease focuses on the addition of biologic agents to chemoradiation and trials by both ECOG and the RTOG testing the addition of cetuximab to concurrent chemoradiation are in progress. The results of these trials may redefine the standard of care for unresectable disease.

POSTOPERATIVE CHEMORADIATION FOR HIGH-RISK DISEASE

Two randomized controlled trials have investigated the role of chemoradiation in the postoperative adjuvant setting when compared with radiotherapy alone. A study conducted by EORTC (22931) (84) and a trial conducted by the RTOG (9501) (85) were designed to address the issue of whether the addition of cisplatin to standard postoperative radiotherapy based on adverse pathologic criteria would improve disease control and survival. The experimental arms of both studies consisted of standard fractionation radiation with concurrent cisplatin on days 1, 22, and 43. At 5 years, the EORTC study demonstrated significant improvement in disease-free survival (47% vs. 36% for radiation alone, $P = 0.04$), and overall survival (53% vs. 40% for radiation alone, $P = 0.02$) for the arm treated with concurrent cisplatin and radiation. The RTOG study demonstrated a significant advantage with combined-modality adjuvant therapy for disease-free survival, but not for overall survival. In both studies, concurrent chemoradiotherapy was associated with greater toxicity.

While the experimental treatment arms were similar for both studies, the definition of high-risk pathologic features differed between studies. The RTOG study defined high-risk pathologic features as the presence of multiple positive nodes, extracapsular extension of nodal disease, or a positive surgical resection margin. In contrast, the EORTC trial defined high-risk pathologic features as a positive surgical resection margin, extracapsular extension of nodal disease, vascular embolisms, or perineural disease; for oral cavity or oropharynx primary sites, high-risk pathologic features included positive nodes in level IV or V. These differences may in part explain the variable outcome of the two trials. In an attempt to reconcile the differing results of these two trials, a pooled analysis was performed which showed that the subset of patients in both trials who received a significant benefit from the addition of cisplatin to postoperative radiotherapy had either microscopically involved margins or extracapsular extension of disease in neck nodes (86). The presence of either or both of these risk factors is therefore now considered a definite indication for adjuvant chemoradiation. Patients who were enrolled only because of tumor present in multiple positive lymph nodes did not benefit from the addition of chemotherapy to postoperative radiation.

Since these analyses were performed, the RTOG trial data have been reanalyzed with longer follow-up times and now demonstrate a significant advantage for chemoradiation in local–regional control, with locoregional failure in 21% of patients receiving adjuvant chemoradiation compared with 33% of patients treated with radiation alone (87,88). The difference in disease-free survival was marginally significant (18% vs. 12%; $P = 0.05$). These results do not change current treatment recommendations, which are adjuvant chemoradiation in patients with extracapsular spread or a positive surgical margin on final pathology.

BIOLOGIC THERAPY

EGFR is highly expressed in head and neck squamous cell cancer, and the expression of EGFR has an inverse relationship with prognosis. Inhibitors of the EGFR have been the focus of targeted therapy trials in head and neck cancer. Cetuximab is a chimeric immunoglobulin G antibody that binds to EGFR with high affinity. In preclinical studies, cetuximab demonstrated at least additive effects when combined with radiotherapy or with cisplatin, paclitaxel, and other cytotoxics. Cetuximab was approved by the FDA for use in combination with radiotherapy in patients with advanced head and neck cancer based on a multicenter trial phase III trial published by Bonner et al. (89). This trial randomly assigned patients with locally advanced squamous cell cancers of the oropharynx, larynx, and hypopharynx to treatment with radiotherapy alone (using either standard or altered fractionation schedules) or to radiotherapy with concurrent weekly cetuximab. The addition of cetuximab significantly improved local–regional failure-free survival and overall survival rates: median local–regional failure-free survival was 24.4 months with cetuximab and 14.9 months with RT alone ($P = 0.005$), and 5-year overall survival rates were 45% with cetuximab and 36% with radiotherapy alone ($P = 0.018$) (10). Cetuximab had no effect on distant metastases. Cetuximab is associated with the development of an acneiform rash in 84% of patients during treatment, which is prominent in 73% of patients. Of the patients who received cetuximab, those who developed a prominent cetuximab-induced acneiform rash had longer overall survival (69 months) compared to those with mild rash (26 months), which was significant ($P = 0.002$). There was no association between the cumulative dose of cetuximab and rash.

A limitation to this study is extrapolation of the results to the larger head and neck cancer population: cetuximab was only studied in combination with radiotherapy, using radiation alone as the control group. In addition, the study population was heterogeneous with respect to resectability, primary site, and radiation schedule. Whether the combination of radiotherapy and cetuximab is as effective as the standard of chemoradiation is unknown. At the present time, the only indication for cetuximab with radiotherapy is in the treatment of patients whose age, performance status, or comorbidity precludes treatment with platinum-based chemoradiation. Cetuximab with radiotherapy provides a 9% absolute survival advantage at 5 years over radiotherapy alone. Numerous trials are currently testing the addition of cetuximab or small-molecule tyrosine kinase inhibitors to chemoradiation in various disease settings. One such trial, RTOG 0522, directly compared concurrent cisplatin and radiation with or without cetuximab: preliminary data presented at the American Society of Clinical Oncology annual meeting in 2011 showed no survival benefit with the addition of cetuximab (90).

INCURABLE RECURRENT OR DISTANT METASTATIC DISEASE

Inoperable disease that has been previously irradiated or disease that involves distant organs is considered incurable. Commonly used chemotherapeutic agents to treat recurrent or metastatic squamous cell cancers of the head and neck are cisplatin, carboplatin, docetaxel, paclitaxel, 5-FU, and methotrexate. Less commonly used drugs that also show some activity against head and neck tumors are bleomycin, irinotecan, gemcitabine, capecitabine, oxaliplatin, cyclophosphamide, ifosfamide, pemetrexed, and biologic agents such as cetuximab. Randomized trials comparing combination chemotherapy and single-agent therapy show an approximate doubling of the response rate with platinum-based combinations of chemotherapy, but the duration of response is brief (2 to 4 months) and does not significantly impact overall survival (91–93).

Combination chemotherapy is associated with greater toxicity. In a meta-analysis of all studies in which cisplatin and 5-FU, the gold-standard combination drug regimen, was compared with single-agent therapy, a significant improvement in response (OR = 0.43) was documented, which translated into only a 2-week difference in the median survival (94). Toxicity was greater for patients who received combination therapy. While numerous single agents have activity against head and neck cancers and can be used, weekly methotrexate is the historical gold standard because of its ease of administration, lower toxicity profile, and relative lower costs (95). Combination chemotherapy should be limited to patients who have a good performance status (ECOG performance status of 0 to 1) and as a result are better able to tolerate the added toxicity: in such patients the higher response rate may translate into better palliation, although no objective quality of life data exist to support this concept. A poor response to palliative chemotherapy can be predicted for patients with poor performance status, the presence of comorbidities, bulky local–regional disease or high tumor volume, and prior treatment for recurrence.

Despite the favorable results of the use of taxanes in induction chemotherapy protocols, no improvement in survival with the use of taxanes has been documented for patients with recurrent disease. A study comparing two different weekly schedules of paclitaxel in patients with recurrent disease offered no advantage compared with weekly single-agent methotrexate (96). The addition of paclitaxel to cisplatin did not significantly impact outcomes when compared to the use of standard cisplatin plus 5-FU with respect to median survival times (9 vs. 8 months) and the 1-year survival rates (30% vs. 41%), although the paclitaxel regimen was better tolerated (97).

Cetuximab is the only biologic agent to be approved for use in head and neck cancer, but as previously mentioned, its only approved indication is in patients who are resistant to or cannot receive platinum-based agents. In phase II trials of cetuximab alone or combined with cisplatin in patients who had either stable or progressive disease, the best response rates are in the range of 10% to 13% (98–100). In a randomized trial of 123 patients comparing the combination of cisplatin and placebo with cisplatin and cetuximab, no significant difference was found in median progression-free survival (2.7 months compared with 4.2 months, respectively; P = 0.27), although the rate of a major complete or partial response was significantly higher for patients who received cisplatin and cetuximab (10% compared with 26%, respectively; P = 0.03) (101).

Another phase III trial randomized 442 patients to receive either cisplatin–5FU–cetuximab or cisplatin–5FU as first-line treatment in patients with recurrent or metastatic squamous-cell carcinoma of the head and neck (102). The addition of cetuximab to cisplatin/5-FU prolonged the median overall survival from 7.4 to 10.1 months (HR for death, 0.80; P = 0.04), prolonged the median progression-free survival time from 3.3 to 5.6 months (HR for progression, 0.54; P < 0.001) and increased the response rate from 20% to 36% (P < 0.001). This was the first trial to show any improvement in overall survival by the addition of cetuximab when compared with the standard regimen of cisplatin/5-FU, although gains were modest.

Interest has been generated in the use of the small molecule tyrosine kinase inhibitors gefitinib and erlotinib, which have modest activity in the setting of recurrent disease, including responses in patients who have received prior chemotherapy. In a phase II trial of 52 patients, the administration of 500 mg/d of gefitinib resulted in an 11% major response rate (103). In a phase II trial in 115 patients, the administration of 150 mg/d of erlotinib resulted in a 4% major response rate (104). Stable disease was demonstrated in 50% of patients. Combination trials using other agents directed at EGFR pathway downstream targets, such as the vascular endothelial growth factor (VEGF) inhibitor, are in progress (105). In a phase II trial, the combination of erlotinib and bevacizumab resulted in a 17% response rate, with median survival of 7.5 months in patients previously treated for recurrent disease (106).

CONCLUSIONS

In summary, concurrent chemoradiotherapy leads to improved disease control compared with radiation alone for patients with unresectable squamous cell cancer of the head and neck and represents standard treatment for patients who are able to tolerate the anticipated added treatment-related toxicity. There also is a role for this approach in the organ-preservation and larynx-preservation setting and for advanced local–regional nasopharyngeal cancer. The data showing improvement are best established for platinum-based concurrent regimens; an advantage persists even when newer altered-fractionation approaches are employed. Induction chemotherapy results in superior rates of laryngeal preservation in advanced hypopharyngeal cancer. Adjuvant chemoradiation is indicated for patients with high-risk pathologic features of extracapsular spread or positive margins. The use of biologic therapy with radiation provides a survival benefit in patients with advanced head and neck cancer who would otherwise only be candidates for radiation alone because of contraindications to the use of chemotherapy. Current evidence-based indications for standard of care use of chemoradiation are listed in Table 111.2. Clinical trials testing the addition of cetuximab to concurrent chemoradiation, and induction chemotherapy with the addition of a taxane are in progress. The results of these trials may redefine the standard of care for both resectable and unresectable disease.

TABLE 111.2	CURRENT EVIDENCE-BASED INDICATIONS FOR CHEMOTHERAPY IN THE MANAGEMENT OF ADVANCED HEAD AND NECK CANCER	
Primary Site	**Regimen**	**References**
Organ preservation, larynx (resectable stage III and IV disease, excluding T1 disease)	XRT 70 Gy + high-dose cisplatin	(18,19)
Organ preservation, hypopharynx (resectable stage III and IV disease, excluding T1 disease)	Cisplatin (100 mg/m²) + 5-FU (1,000 mg/m²/d × 4) × 3 cycles followed by XRT 70 Gy	(21,23)
Oropharynx, resectable T3–T4 or N2–N3	XRT 70 Gy + cisplatin or carboplatin (70 mg/m²/d × 4) + 5-FU (600 mg/m²/d × 4) × 3 cycles	(29–31)
Nasopharynx, stages IIB, III, IVA, IVB	XRT 70 Gy + high-dose cisplatin, adjuvant cisplatin (80 mg/m²) + 5-FU (1,000 mg/m²/d × 4) × 3 cycles	(59)
Unresectable, all sites	XRT 70 Gy + high-dose cisplatin	(76)
Postoperative adjuvant high-risk factors: extracapsular spread or margin positive	XRT 70 Gy + high-dose cisplatin	(84–88)
Contraindications to systemic chemotherapy, stage III or IV disease	Cetuximab (400 mg/m²) followed by XRT 70 Gy + cetuximab (250 mg/m²/wk)	(10,89)

High-dose cisplatin = 100 mg/m² days 1, 22, and 43. XRT = external beam radiation therapy.

- In patients with unresectable squamous cell cancer of the head and neck, concomitant cisplatin and radiotherapy significantly improves survival, compared with radiotherapy alone, and is the standard of care.

- Concomitant cisplatin and radiotherapy is the standard of care for postoperative adjuvant treatment for patients with positive resection margins or extracapsular extension of nodal disease.

- To preserve the larynx of patients with locally advanced, resectable laryngeal cancer, concomitant cisplatin and radiotherapy is the standard of care. T4 disease is associated with poorer outcomes and survival following chemoradiation, and should be treated with primary laryngectomy.

- To preserve the oropharyngeal functions of speech and swallowing in patients with locally advanced, respectable oropharyngeal cancer, concomitant chemotherapy and radiotherapy is the standard of care for T3 to T4 or N2 to N3 disease.

- To preserve the larynx of patients with locally advanced, resectable cancer of the hypopharynx, induction chemotherapy and radiotherapy is the standard of care based on randomized controlled trials.

- The standard of care for treatment of nasopharyngeal cancer is radiotherapy alone for early stage disease (stages I and IIa), and concurrent cisplatin and radiotherapy followed by three cycles of adjuvant cisplatin and 5-FU for advanced stage disease (stages IIb, III, IVA, and IVB).

- Cetuximab when added to radiotherapy for definitive treatment of locally advanced cancer showed significantly improved survival compared with radiotherapy alone. However, no indications for using cetuximab plus radiotherapy in place of standard platinum-based chemotherapy plus radiotherapy have been established.

- Induction chemotherapy using a taxane with cisplatin plus 5-FU regimen followed by concomitant chemoradiation (sequential therapy) shows promise in improving disease-control and survival, but this is not at present standard of care. Trials comparing chemoradiation with or without induction chemotherapy in high-risk populations are in progress.

- Combination chemotherapy in the palliative setting leads to increased response rates as well as increased toxicity over single-agent chemotherapy, but does not significantly improve survival compared with single-agent methotrexate, a platinum-based agent, or 5-FU.

- Various biologic agents that target the EGFR pathway are under study in combination with chemotherapy, as single agents, and as multiple targeted agents. Antibodies to the EGFR and small molecule tyrosine kinase inhibitors cause major response in approximately 10% of patients who do not respond to platinum agents. Cetuximab is the only biologic agent approved for use in head and neck cancer.

REFERENCES

1. Pasheva EA, Ugrinova I, Spassovska NC, et al. The binding affinity of HMG1 protein to DNA modified by cis-platin and its analogs correlates with their antitumor activity. *Int J Biochem Cell Biol* 2002;34:87–92.
2. Mukherjea D, Rybak LP. Pharmacogenomics of cisplatin-induced ototoxicity. *Pharmacogenomics* 2011;12:1039–1050.
3. Walko CM, Lindley C. Capecitabine: a review. *Clin Ther* 2005;27:23–44.
4. Patel PA. Evolution of 5-fluorouracil-based chemoradiation in the management of rectal cancer. *Anticancer Drugs* 2011;22:311–316.
5. Huszar D, Theoclitou ME, Skolnik J, et al. Kinesin motor proteins as targets for cancer therapy. *Cancer Metastasis Rev* 2009;28:197–208.
6. Bernier J, Vrieling C. Docetaxel in the management of patients with head and neck squamous cell carcinoma. *Expert Rev Anticancer Ther* 2008;8:1023–1032.
7. McGuire JJ. Anticancer antifolates: current status and future directions. *Curr Pharm Des* 2003;9:2593–2613.
8. Froklage FE, Reijneveld JC, Heimans JJ. Central neurotoxicity in cancer chemotherapy: pharmacogenetic insights. *Pharmacogenomics* 2011;12:379–395.
9. Burgos-Tiburcio A, Santos ES, Arango BA, et al. Development of targeted therapy for squamous cell carcinomas of the head and neck. *Expert Rev Anticancer Ther* 2011;11:373–386.
10. Bonner JA, Harari PM, Giralt J, et al. Radiotherapy plus cetuximab for locoregionally advanced head and neck cancer: 5-year survival data from a phase 3 randomised trial, and relation between cetuximab-induced rash and survival. *Lancet Oncol* 2010;11:21–28.
11. Oxford Centre for Evidence Based Medicine—Levels of Evidence (March 2009). Available at: http://www.cebm.net/. Accessed April 5, 2009.
12. Head and Neck Contracts Program. Adjuvant chemotherapy for advanced head and neck squamous carcinoma: Final report of the Head and Neck Contracts Program. *Cancer* 1987;60:301–311.
13. Jacobs C, Makuch R. Efficacy of adjuvant chemotherapy for patients with resectable head and neck cancer: a subset analysis of the Head and Neck Contracts Program. *J Clin Oncol* 1990;8:838–847.
14. The Department of Veterans Affairs Laryngeal Cancer Study Group. Induction chemotherapy plus radiation compared with surgery plus radiation in patients with advanced laryngeal cancer. *N Eng J Med* 1991;324:1685–1690.
15. Wolf GT. Routine computed tomography scanning for tumor staging in advanced laryngeal cancer: implications for treatment selection. *J Clin Oncol* 2010;29:2315–2317.
16. Wolf GT, Fisher SG. Effectiveness of salvage neck dissection for advanced regional metastases when induction chemotherapy and radiation are used for organ preservation. *Laryngoscope* 1992;102:934–939.
17. Thomas GR, Greenberg J, Wu KT, et al. Planned early neck dissection before radiation for persistent neck nodes after induction chemotherapy. *Laryngoscope* 1997;107:1129–1137.

18. Forastiere A, Goepfert H, Maor M, et al. Concurrent chemotherapy and radiotherapy for organ preservation in advanced laryngeal cancer. *N Eng J Med* 2003;349:2091–2098.

19. Weber RS, Berkey BA, Forastiere A, et al. Outcome of salvage total laryngectomy following organ preservation therapy: the Radiation Therapy Oncology Group Trial 91-11. *Arch Otolaryngol Head Neck Surg* 2003;129:44–49.

20. Machtay M, Moughan J, Trotti A, et al. Factors associated with severe late toxicity after concurrent chemoradiation for locally advanced head and neck cancer: an RTOG analysis. *J Clin Oncol* 2008;26:3582–3589.

21. Lefebvre JL, Chevalier D, Luboinski B, et al. Larynx preservation in piriform sinus cancer: preliminary results of a European Organization for Research and Treatment of Cancer phase III trial. *J Natl Cancer Inst* 1996;88:890–899.

22. Lefebvre JL, Horiot J, Rolland F, et al. Phase III study on larynx preservation comparing induction chemotherapy and radiotherapy versus alternating chemoradiotherapy in resectable hypopharynx and larynx cancers. EORTC protocol 24954–22950. *Proc Am Soc Clin Oncol* 2007;25.

23. Pointreau Y, Garaud P, Chapet S, et al. Randomized trial of induction chemotherapy with cisplatin and 5-5-FU with or without docetaxel for larynx preservation. *J Natl Cancer Inst* 2009;101:498–506.

24. Kraus DH, Zelefsky MJ, Brock HA, et al. Combined surgery and radiation therapy for squamous cell carcinoma of the hypopharynx. *Otolaryngol Head Neck Surg* 1997;116:637–641.

25. Tsou YA, Lin MH, Hua CH, et al. Survival outcome by early chemoradiation therapy salvage or early surgical salvage for the treatment of hypopharyngeal cancer. *Otolaryngol Head Neck Surg* 2007;137:711–716.

26. Zelefsky MJ, Kraus DH, Pfister DG, et al. Combined chemotherapy and radiotherapy versus surgery and postoperative radiotherapy for advanced hypopharyngeal cancer. *Head Neck* 1996;18:405–411.

27. Lee NY, O'Meara W, Chan K, et al. Concurrent chemotherapy and intensity-modulated radiotherapy for locoregionally advanced laryngeal and hypopharyngeal cancers. *Int J Radiat Oncol Biol Phys* 2007;69:459–468.

28. The NCCN Clinical Practice Guidelines in Oncology™ Head and Neck Cancers (Version 2.2011). © 2011 National Comprehensive Cancer Network, Inc. Available at: http: NCCN.org. Accessed July 1, 2011.

29. Calais G, Alfonsi M, Bardet E, et al. Randomized trial of radiation therapy versus concomitant chemotherapy and radiation therapy for advanced stage oropharynx carcinoma. *J Natl Cancer Inst* 1999;91:2081–2086.

30. Denis F, Garaud P, Bardet E, et al. Late toxicity results of the GORTEC 94-01 randomized trial comparing radiotherapy with concomitant radiochemotherapy for advanced-stage oropharynx carcinoma: comparison of LENT/SOMA, RTOG/EORTC, and NCI-CTC scoring systems. *Int J Radiat Oncol Biol Phys* 2003;55:93–98.

31. Denis F, Garaud P, Bardet E, et al. Final results of the 94-01 French Head and Neck Oncology and Radiotherapy Group randomized trial comparing radiotherapy alone with concomitant radiochemotherapy in advanced-stage oropharynx carcinoma. *J Clin Oncol* 2004;22:69–76.

32. Adelstein DJ, Lavertu P, Saxton JP, et al. Mature results of a phase III randomized trial comparing concurrent chemoradiotherapy with radiation therapy alone in patients with stage III and IV squamous cell carcinoma of the head and neck. *Cancer* 2000;88:876–883.

33. Adelstein DJ, Saxton JP, Rybicki LA, et al. Multiagent concurrent chemoradiotherapy for locoregionally advanced squamous cell head and neck cancer: mature results from a single institution. *J Clin Oncol* 2006;24:1064–1071.

34. Machtay M, Rosenthal DI, Hershock D, et al. Organ preservation therapy using induction plus concurrent chemoradiation for advanced resectable oropharyngeal carcinoma: a University of Pennsylvania Phase II Trial. *J Clin Oncol* 2002;20:3964–3971.

35. Vokes EE, Stenson K, Rosen FR, et al. Weekly carboplatin and paclitaxel followed by concomitant paclitaxel, fluorouracil, and hydroxyurea chemoradiotherapy: curative and organ-preserving therapy for advanced head and neck cancer. *J Clin Oncol* 2003;21: 320–326.

36. Fallai C, Bolner A, Signor M, et al. Long-term results of conventional radiotherapy versus accelerated hyperfractionated radiotherapy versus concomitant radiotherapy and chemotherapy in locoregionally advanced carcinoma of the oropharynx. *Tumori* 2006;92:41–54.

37. Skoner JM, Andersen PE, Cohen JI, et al. Swallowing function and tracheotomy dependence after combined-modality treatment including free tissue transfer for advanced-stage oropharyngeal cancer. *Laryngoscope* 2003;113:1294–1298.

38. Shiley SG, Hargunani CA, Skoner JM, et al. Swallowing function after chemoradiation for advanced stage oropharyngeal cancer. *Otolaryngol Head Neck Surg* 2006;134:455–459.

39. Gourin CG, Johnson JT. Surgical treatment of squamous cell carcinoma of the base of tongue. *Head Neck* 2001;23:653–660.

40. Udoff RA, Elam JC, Gourin CG. Primary surgery for oropharyngeal cancer. *Otolaryngolo Head Neck Surg* 2010;143:644–649.

41. Malone JP, Stephens JA, Grecula JC, et al. Disease control, survival, and functional outcome after multimodal treatment fo,r advanced-stage tongue base cancer. *Head Neck* 2004;26:561–572.

42. Denittis AS, Machtay M, Rosenthal DI, et al. Advanced oropharyngeal carcinoma treated with surgery and radiotherapy: oncologic outcome and functional assessment. *Am J Otolaryngol* 2001;22:329–335.

43. Garden AS, Asper JA, Morrison WH, et al. Is concurrent chemodiation the treatment of choice for all patients with Stage III or IV head and neck carcinoma? *Cancer* 2004;100:1171–1178.

44. Marur S, D'Souza G, Westra WH, et al. HPV-associated head and neck cancer: a virus-related cancer epidemic. *Lancet Oncol* 2010;11:781–789.

45. Ang KK, Harris J, Wheeler R, et al. Human papillomavirus and survival of patients with oropharyngeal cancer. *N Engl J Med* 2010;363:24–35.

46. Adelstein DJ, Ridge HA, Gillison ML, et al. Head and neck squamous cell cancer and the human papillomavirus: summary of a National Cancer Institute State of the Science meeting, November 9–10, 2008, Washington, DC. *Head Neck* 2009;31(11): 1393–1422.

47. Fischer CA, Zlobec I, Green E, et al. Is the improved prognosis of p16 positive oropharyngeal squamous cell carcinoma dependent of the treatment modality? *Int J Cancer* 2009;126:1256–1262.

48. Fakhry C, Westra WH, Li S, et al. Improved survival of patients with human papillomavirus-positive head and neck squamous cell carcinoma in a prospective clinical trial. *J Natl Cancer Inst* 2008;100:261–269.

49. Licitra L, Perrone F, Bossi P, et al. High-risk human papillomavirus affects prognosis in patients with surgically treated oropharyngeal squamous cell carcinoma. *J Clin Oncol* 2006;24:5630–5636.

50. Ragin CC, Taioli E. Survival of squamous cell carcinoma of the head and neck in relation to human papillomavirus infection: review and meta-analysis. *Int J Cancer* 2007;121:1813–1820.

51. Hafkamp HC, Manni JJ, Haesevoets A, et al. Marked differences in survival rate between smokers and nonsmokers with HPV 16-associated tonsillar carcinomas. *Int J Cancer* 2008;122: 2656–2664.

52. Straetmans JM, Olthof N, Mooren JJ, et al. Human papillomavirus reduces the prognostic value of nodal involvement in tonsillar squamous cell carcinomas. *Laryngoscope* 2009;119:1951–1957.

53. Rischin D. Oropharyngeal cancer, human papillomavirus, and clinical trials. *J Clin Oncol* 2010;28:1–3.

54. Sedaghat AR, Zhang Z, Begum S, et al. Prognostic significance of human papillomavirus in oropharyngeal squamous cell carcinomas. *Laryngoscope* 2009;119:1542–1549.

55. Goodwin WJ Jr. Salvage surgery for patients with recurrent squamous cell carcinoma of the upper aerodigestive tract: when do the ends justify the means? *Laryngoscope,* 2000;110(Suppl 93): 1–18.

56. Zafereo ME, Hanasono MM, Rosenthal DI, et al. The role of salvage surgery in patients with recurrent squamous cell carcinoma of the oropharynx. *Cancer* 2009;115:5723–5733.

57. Cmelak AJ, Li S, Goldwasser MA, et al. Phase II trial of chemoradiation for organ preservation in resectable stage III or IV squamous cell carcinomas of the larynx or oropharynx: results of Eastern Cooperative Oncology Group Study E2399. *J Clin Oncol* 2007;25:3971–3977.

58. Kostrzewa JP, Lancaster WP, Iseli TA, et al. Outcomes of salvage surgery with free flap reconstruction for recurrent oral and oropharyngeal cancer. *Laryngoscope* 2010;120:267–272.

59. Al-Sarraf M, LeBlanc M, Giri PG, et al. Chemoradiotherapy versus radiotherapy in patients with advanced nasopharyngeal cancer: Phase III randomized Intergroup study 0099. *J Clin Oncol* 1998;16:1310–1317.

60. Chan AT, Teo PM, Nga, RK, et al. Concurrent chemotherapy-radiotherapy compared with radiotherapy alone in locoregionally advanced nasopharyngeal carcinoma: progression-free survival analysis of a phase III randomized trial. *J Clin Oncol* 2002;20:2038–2044.

61. Chan AT, Leung SF, Ngan RK, et al. Overall survival after concurrent cisplatin-radiotherapy compared with radiotherapy alone in locoregionally advanced nasopharyngeal carcinoma. *J Natl Cancer Inst* 2005;97:536–539.

62. Lin JC, Jan JS, Hsu CY, et al. Phase III study of concurrent chemoradiotherapy versus radiotherapy alone for advanced nasopharyngeal carcinoma: positive effect on overall and progression-free survival. *J Clin Oncol* 2004;21:631–637.

63. Huncharek M, Kupelnick B. Combined chemoradiation versus radiation therapy alone in locally advanced nasopharyngeal carcinoma: results of a meta-analysis of 1,528 patients from six randomized trials. *Am J Clin Oncol* 2002;25:219–223.

64. Baujat B, Audry H, Bourhis J, et al. Chemotherapy in locally advanced nasopharyngeal carcinoma: an individual patient data meta-analysis of eight randomized trials and 1753 patients. *Int J Radiat Oncol Biol Phys* 2006;64:47–56.

65. Chua DT, Ma J, Sham JS, et al. Long-term survival after cisplatin-based induction chemotherapy and radiotherapy for nasopharyngeal carcinoma: a pooled data analysis of two phase III trials. *J Clin Oncol* 2005;23:1118–1124.

66. Chan AT, Teo PM, Leung TW, et al. A prospective randomized study of chemotherapy adjunctive to definitive radiotherapy in advanced nasopharyngeal carcinoma. *Int J Radiat Oncol Biol Phys* 1995;33:569–577.

67. Roussy IG. Preliminary results of a randomized trial comparing neoadjuvant chemotherapy (cisplatin, epirubicin, bleomycin) plus radiotherapy vs. radiotherapy alone in stage IV (>or=N2, M0) undifferentiated nasopharyngeal carcinoma: a positive effect on progression-free survival. International Nasopharynx Cancer Study Group. VUMCA I trial. *Int J Radiat Oncol Biol Phys* 1996;35:463–469.

68. Ma J, Mai HQ, Hong MH, et al. Results of a prospective randomized trial comparing neoadjuvant chemotherapy plus radiotherapy with radiotherapy alone in patients with locoregionally advanced nasopharyngeal carcinoma. *J Clin Oncol* 2001;19:1350–1357.

69. Leung SF, Tam JS, Chan AT, et al. Improved accuracy of detection of nasopharyngeal carcinoma by combined application of circulating Epstein-Barr virus DNA and anti-Epstein-Barr viral capsid antigen IgA antibody. *Clin Chem* 2004;50:339–345.

70. Leung SF, Chan AT, Zee B, et al. Pretherapy quantitative measurement of circulating Epstein-Barr virus DNA is predictive of post-therapy distant failure in patients with early-stage nasopharyngeal carcinoma of undifferentiated type. *Cancer* 2003;98:288–291.

71. Chan AT, Lo YM, Zee B, et al. Plasma Epstein-Barr virus DNA and residual disease after radiotherapy for undifferentiated nasopharyngeal carcinoma. *J Natl Cancer Inst* 2002;94:1614–1619.

72. Stenson KM, Kunnavakkam R, Cohen EE, et al. Chemoradiation for patients with advanced oral cavity cancer. *Laryngoscope* 2010;120(1):93–99.

73. Pederson AW, Salama JK, Witt ME, et al. Concurrent chemotherapy and intensity-modulated radiotherapy for organ preservation of locoregionally advanced oral cavity cancer. *Am J Clin Oncol* 2011;34:356–361.

74. Cohen EE, Baru J, Huo D, et al. Efficacy and safety of treating T4 oral cavity tumors with primary chemoradiotherapy. *Head Neck* 2009;31:1013–1021.

75. Merlano M, Benasso M, Corvo R, et al. Five-year update of a randomized trial of alternating radiotherapy and chemotherapy compared with radiotherapy alone in treatment of unresectable squamous cell carcinoma of the head and neck. *J Natl Cancer Inst* 1996;88:583–589.

76. Adelstein DJ, Li Y, Adams GL, et al. An intergroup phase III comparison of standard radiation therapy and two schedules of concurrent chemoradiotherapy in patients with unresectable squamous cell head and neck cancer. *J Clin Oncol* 2003;21:92–98.

77. Pignon JP, Bourhis J, Domenge C, et al. Chemotherapy added to locoregional treatment for head and neck squamous-cell carcinoma: three meta-analyses of updated individual data. MACH-NC Collaborative Group. Meta-Analysis of Chemotherapy on Head and Neck Cancer. *Lancet* 2000;355:949–955.

78. Bourhis J, Armand C, Pignon JP. Update of MACH-NC database focused on concomitant chemoradiotherapy. *Proc Am Soc Clin Oncol* 2004;22:488.

79. Browman GP, Hodson DI, Mackenzie RJ, et al. Choosing a concomitant chemotherapy and radiotherapy regimen for squamous cell head and neck cancer: a systematic review of the published literature with subgroup analysis. *Head Neck* 2001;23:579–589.

80. Bourhis J, Le Maitre A, Baujat B, et al. Individual patients' data meta-analyses in head and neck cancer. *Curr Opin Oncol* 2007;19:188–194.

81. Vermorken JB, Trigo J, Hitt R, et al. Cisplatin and 5-FU alone or with docetaxel in head and neck cancer. *N Engl J Med* 2007;357:1705–1715.

82. Posner MR, Hershock DM, Blajman CR, et al. Cisplatin and fluorouracil alone or with docetaxel in head and neck cancer. *N Engl J Med* 2007;357:1705–1715.

83. Hitt R, Lopez-Pousa A, Martinez-Trufero J, et al. Phase III study comparing cisplatin plus fluorouracil to paclitaxel, cisplatin, and fluorouracil induction chemotherapy followed by chemoradiotherapy in locally advanced head and neck cancer. *J Clin Oncol* 2005;23:8636–8645.

84. Bernier J, Domenge C, Ozsahin M, et al. European Organization for Research and Treatment of Cancer Trial 22931: postoperative irradiation with or without concomitant chemotherapy for locally advanced head and neck cancer. *N Engl J Med* 2004;350:1945–1952.

85. Cooper JS, Pajak TF, Forastiere AA, et al. Postoperative concurrent radiotherapy and chemotherapy for high-risk squamous-cell carcinoma of the head and neck. *N Engl J Med* 2004;350:1937–1944.

86. Bernier J, Coope, JS, Pajak TF, et al. Defining risk levels in locally advanced head and neck cancers: a comparative analysis of concurrent postoperative radiation plus chemotherapy trials of the EORTC (#22931) and RTOG (# 9501). *Head Neck* 2005;27:843–850.

87. Cooper JS, Pajak TF, Forastiere A, et al. Long-term survival results of a phase III intergroup trial (RTOG 95-01) of surgery followed by radiotherapy vs. radiochemotherapy for resectable high risk squamous cell carcinoma of the Head and Neck. *Int J Radiat Oncol Biol Phys* 2006;66:S14.

88. Cooper JS, Zhang Q, Pajak TF, et al. Long-term follow-up of the RTOG 9501/Intergroup phase III trial: postoperative concurrent radiation therapy and chemotherapy in high-risk squamous cell carcinoma of the head and neck. *Int J Radiat Oncol Biol Phys* 2012. In press.

89. Bonner JA, Harari PM, Giralt J, et al. Radiotherapy plus cetuximab for squamous-cell carcinoma of the head and neck. *N Engl J Med* 2006;354:567–578.

90. Radiation Therapy Oncology Group News. Available at: http://www.rtog.org/News/tabid/72/articleType/ArticleView/articleId/15/RTOG-0522-Initial-Results-Reported-at-ASCO.aspx. Accessed June 7, 2011.

91. Forastiere AA, Metch B, Schuller DE, et al. Randomized comparison of cisplatin plus fluorouracil and carboplatin plus fluorouracil versus methotrexate in advanced squamous-cell carcinoma of the head and neck: a Southwest Oncology Group study. *J Clin Oncol* 1992;10:1245–1251.

92. Jacobs C, Lyman G, Velez-Garcia E, et al. A phase III randomized study comparing cisplatin and fluorouracil as single agents and in combination for advanced squamous cell carcinoma of the head and neck. *J Clin Oncol* 1992;10:257–263.

93. Clavel M, Vermorken JB, Cognetti F, et al. Randomized comparison of cisplatin, methotrexate, bleomycin and vincristine (CABO) versus cisplatin and 5-fluorouracil (CF) versus cisplatin (C) in recurrent or metastatic squamous cell carcinoma of the head and neck. A phase III study of the EORTC Head and Neck Cancer Cooperative Group. *Ann Oncol* 1994;5:521–526.

94. Browman GP, Cronin L. Standard chemotherapy in squamous cell head and neck cancer: what we have learned from randomized trials. *Semin Oncol* 1994;21:311–319.

95. Colevas AD. Chemotherapy options for patients with metastatic or recurrent squamous cell carcinoma of the head and neck. *J Clin Oncol* 2006;24:2644–2652.

96. Vermorken JB, Catimel G, Mulder PD, et al. Randomized phase II trial of weekly methotrexate (MTX) versus two schedules of triweekly paclitaxel (Taxol) in patients with metastatic or recurrent squamous cell carcinoma of the head and neck (SCCHN). *Proc Am Soc Clin Oncol* 1999;18:395.

97. Gibson MK, Li, Y, Murphy B, et al. Randomized phase III evaluation of cisplatin plus fluorouracil versus cisplatin plus paclitaxel in advanced head and neck cancer (E1395): an intergroup trial of the Eastern Cooperative Oncology Group. *J Clin Oncol* 2005;23:3562–3567.

98. Vermorken JB, Trigo J, Hitt R, et al. Open-label, uncontrolled, multicenter phase II study to evaluate the efficacy and toxicity of cetuximab as a single agent in patients with recurrent and/or metastatic squamous cell carcinoma of the head and neck who failed to respond to platinum-based therapy. *J Clin Oncol* 2007;25:2171–2177.

99. Herbst RS, Arquette M, Shin DM, et al. Phase II multicenter study of the epidermal growth factor receptor antibody cetuximab and cisplatin for recurrent and refractory squamous cell carcinoma of the head and neck. *J Clin Oncol* 2005;23:5578–5587.

100. Baselg, J, Trigo JM, Bourhis J, et al. Phase II multicenter study of the antiepidermal growth factor receptor monoclonal antibody cetuximab in combination with platinum-based chemotherapy in patients with platinum-refractory metastatic and/or recurrent squamous cell carcinoma of the head and neck. *J Clin Oncol* 2005;23:5568–5577.

101. Burtness B, Goldwasser MA, Flood W, et al. Phase III randomized trial of cisplatin plus placebo compared with cisplatin plus cetuximab in metastatic/recurrent head and neck cancer: an Eastern Cooperative Oncology Group study. *J Clin Oncol* 2005;23:8646–8654.

102. Vermorken JB, Mesia R, Rivera F, et al. Platinum-based chemotherapy plus cetuximab in head and neck cancer. *N Engl J Med* 2008;359:1116–1127.

103. Cohen EE, Rosen F, Stadler WM, et al. Phase II trial of ZD1839 in recurrent or metastatic squamous cell carcinoma of the head and neck. *J Clin Oncol* 2003;21:1980–1987.

104. Cohen EE. Role of epidermal growth factor receptor pathway-targeted therapy in patients with recurrent and/or metastatic squamous cell carcinoma of the head and neck. *J Clin Oncol* 2006;24:2659–2665.

105. Seiwert TY, Haraf DJ, Cohen EE, et al. A phase I study of bevacizumab (B) with fluorouracil (F) and hydroxyurea (H) with concomitant radiotherapy (X) (B-FHX) for poor prognosis head and neck cancer (HNC). *Proc Am Soc Clin Oncol* 2006;24.

106. Vokes EE, Cohen EE, Mauer AM, et al. A phase I study of erlotinib and bevacizumab for recurrent or metastatic squamous cell carcinoma of the head and neck (HNC). *Proc Am Soc Clin Oncol* 2005;23.

112 Therapeutic Options for Patients Who Fail Primary Chemoradiation

Steven B. Cannady *Mark K. Wax*

Single institution reports, randomized controlled trials, and meta-analyses have established that chemoradiotherapy protocols improve locoregional control and reduce distant metastases in patients with head and neck squamous cell carcinoma (HNSCC) (1–9). These protocols have been collectively termed "organ preservation strategies" as they inherently maintain the anatomic structure being treated. Increased usage of organ preservation strategies has led to scenarios in which surgical salvage for recurrent or persistent disease requires removal of an organ from a significantly treated soft tissue and vascular bed. Studies have confirmed that operating in the previously treated field leads to a greater risk of complications resulting in added morbidity after surgery (10,11). In patients with advanced recurrent HNSCC, long-term survival is rare, and the quality of life (QOL) cost to such added morbidity and decreased function may outweigh the benefit of surgery unless adequate reconstruction is feasible (12,13). The advent of microvascular free tissue transfer has reduced the risk of complication and increased the possibility of regaining function in the posttreatment patient, rendering salvage more appealing even for short-term control of disease, amelioration of pain, or improvement of function (14–24).

Free tissue transfer has revolutionized the management of posttreatment sequelae encountered following nonsurgical upfront treatment of HNSCC. The functional consequences of high dose radiation therapy with concomitant chemotherapy can now be surgically addressed in the cured patient to improve QOL (14), swallowing, and deglutition (25). Microvascular techniques also allow for preservation of normal tissue outside the body during chemotherapy and radiotherapy (CRT) with reimplantation afterward as in the case of submandibular gland preservation techniques.

Within this chapter, treatment options following failed chemoradiation are discussed. The applications of microvascular free tissue transfer in the treatment of recurrent HNSCC following previous nonsurgical treatment are reviewed. The relative merits of free tissue transfer in the treatment of each subsite of HNSCC are assessed. The use of free tissue transfer in the reconstruction of treatment-related complications is also discussed.

Surgical salvage after failed chemoradiation is by far the most common treatment option available for these patients. Other options that that have been described include chemotherapy, reirradiation (external beam and brachytherapy), and hospice care. Each of these is briefly described.

(CHEMO) RADIOTHERAPY EFFECTS ON TISSUES OF THE HEAD AND NECK

Before we can discuss the possible treatment options for patients that have failed chemoradiation, we must understand the underlying tissue consequences of the initial treatment.

The role of chemotherapy in the treatment of head and neck oncology is well discussed in a previous chapter in this textbook. There are many agents available for treatment in the primary setting. Investigational agents have been used in Phase I and Phase II trials, and there is some question about whether, in Phase III trials, chemotherapy as a single modality treatment may be efficacious. Chemotherapy in the majority of head and neck tumors is combined with radiation therapy in a protocol known as chemoradiation. Here, the chemotherapy may be used as a sensitizing agent or as a direct combination therapy with the radiation to kill the tumor cells. Consequently, the majority of patients who present for salvage treatment, who have had chemotherapy, will have had this as a combined modality treatment with radiation therapy.

Chemotherapy has been demonstrated to not only enhance the tumor kill effectiveness of the radiation therapy but also to increase the postoperative complications in patients who require salvage surgery. The effects of radiation therapy on the tissues have been described both from a short- and long-term toxicity perspective. Chemotherapy will adversely affect patients in the short term as well as in the long term. Patients who recur and who require salvage treatment in the close term will oftentimes be debilitated, have lost significant amounts of body weight, and still be suffering from some of the acute toxicity, such as mucositis and soft tissue necrosis. These patients will have underlying metabolic disorders and will be in a high catabolic state. Their ability to heal their wounds will be less than patients who have not undergone this treatment. Consideration of these issues should be undertaken with nutritional supplementation, and g-tube placement will need to be considered in these patients.

The effects on soft tissue of chemotherapy and chemoradiation will be greater than that of just radiation alone. The soft tissue fibrosis and long-term scarring will be more extensive. Combined with the patient's inability to heal well, the patients who undergo salvage surgery following chemoradiation are more prone to develop local morbidities and complications from poor tissue and wound healing. Not only must the primary closure site of the ablated defect be considered, but the prophylactic reconstruction of the soft tissues that have been affected by the previous treatments must also be considered if one is to rehabilitate these patients and allow them to heal the arterial response to radiation that occurs most severely within the capillary endothelium and is the mechanism of late tissue manifestations of radiation therapy (XRT). The results of histologic changes to the capillaries lead to tissue anoxia and dilation of remaining capillaries (26,27). Larger arteries have different responses to XRT based on their sizes; small (less than 100 μm) to medium (100 to 500 μm) vessels suffer adventitial fibrosis, medial hyalinization, and intimal foam cell accumulation, whereas large arteries (greater than 500 μm) tend to be more resistant to these changes (28–30). Large arteries can suffer complications associated with neointimal proliferation, atheromatosis, thrombosis, and rupture, whereas the effect of chronic radiation on medium to large vessels is caused by injury to the vasa vasorum owing to a greater incidence of atherosclerosis within these vessels—a major concern in the use of microvascular free flaps (Fig. 112.1). This phenomenon is well documented in studies of irradiated carotid arteries, to which most head and neck reconstructive free flaps are anastamosed (31). Finally, the vascular physiology itself is altered by radiation therapy such that less blood flow occurs due to increased smooth muscle vasoconstriction and increased pressure in the capillary system secondary to tissue fibrosis of surrounding tissues (32).

Additional tissue-specific treatment effects of particular interest to oncologic surgeons include late toxicity to the skin, mucosa, salivary tissue, mandible, and laryngotracheal cartilages. It is well established that when exposed to radiation therapy, mucocutaneous tissue changes that

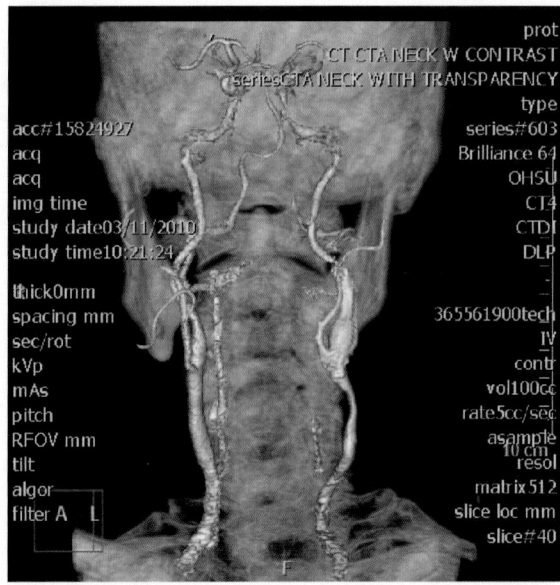

Figure 112.1 This CT angio of the carotids demonstrates severe disease of the left carotid system. There is a stent present, but the common carotid below the stent has severe atherosclerotic changes.

include increases in vascular permeability, fibrin deposition, collagen formation, and ultimately, tissue fibrosis occur (33). Salivary tissue is exquisitely sensitive to XRT causing marked degeneration and loss of saliva. In a series of studies on XRT-related damage to the mandible, Marx (34) demonstrated that the triad of hypoxia, hypocellularity, and hypovascularity in posttreatment bone leads to tissue breakdown and chronic nonhealing wounds associated with osteoradionecrosis (ORN) of the jaw. It is thought that this process occurs in up to 56% of patients that undergo XRT to the head and neck, but it is unclear how many will manifest clinical symptoms; however, as many as half of those that become clinically apparent will require surgical interventions (35) (Fig. 112.2). A similar process is plausible in the cartilaginous structures of the

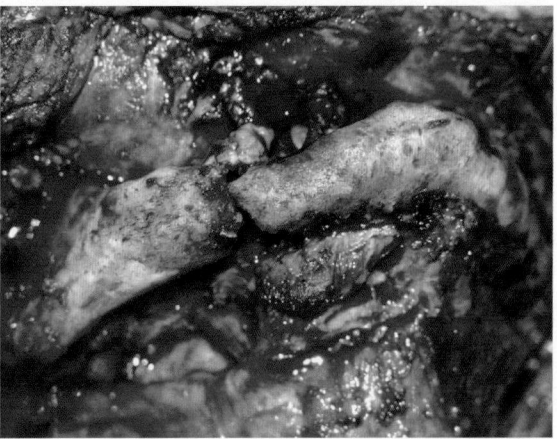

Figure 112.2 This intraoperative photograph demonstrates ORN with a fracture. The bone around the fracture site is dead.

upper aerodigestive tract leading to chondroradionecrosis (CRN) with less frequency than mandible necrosis—5% to 12% of radiated laryngeal cancers (36). These latter two tissue effects can mimic cancer recurrence and thus often require a thorough workup for recurrence. In addition, the effects on bone and cartilage may be severe enough to warrant ablative surgery of the structure in question with reconstruction, even in the absence of recurrent disease, to improve pain and function.

RECURRENT HNSCC: EFFICACY OF TREATMENT

Surgery remains the standard of care and occasionally is the only available treatment for recurrent HNSCC that is deemed resectable by multidisciplinary care teams (37). In a large meta-analysis, Goodwin established the survival, complications, operative mortality, and treatment effect of salvage surgery for patients with recurrent HNSCC (13). In addition, his concomitant observational study collected QOL data, performance status, and financial considerations to assess the overall effectiveness of salvage on these parameters.

It was established within Goodwin's meta-analysis that the 5-year overall average survival after salvage surgery is 39%, but a large separation was noted between early (Stage I or II) larynx recurrence (83%) versus late (Stage III or IV) larynx (37%), oral cavity (43%), and pharynx (26%) recurrences. Disease-free survival was similarly stratified denoting a clear difference in outcome for patients with early laryngeal recurrence. Surgical complications and mortality were also assessed in this analysis with a 5.2% risk of death from surgical salvage or its complications. Although the definition of major and minor complication is variable within the literature, a consistent risk in the range of 30% to 40% for salvage surgery of the primary is cited in the literature (10,11), with better outcomes in patients requiring only planned neck dissections or dissections for persistent disease (38).

In the prospective arm of Goodwin's study, survival for 109 patients was 21.5 months. Recurrent stage was again a significant survival predictor, with decreasing survival as stage advanced, but original cancer stage was not a predictive factor. Interestingly, patients that had received prior chemotherapy had worse survival than those that did not, but no survival effect was noted for prior radiation or surgical treatments. QOL was assessed by the Functional Living Index-Cancer Questionnaire before and after surgery and demonstrated a decline with increasing stage of recurrent disease; the percentage of patients showing improvement was 64%, 65%, 41%, and 39% for Stage I, II, III, and IV, respectively. No significant difference in QOL existed for site of recurrent disease. Performance status was also assessed via the Performance Status Scale for Head and Neck Cancer Patients. Normalcy of diet varied considerably by site of recurrence and declined with advancing stage of recurrence and showed that only 47% of patients had a

successful outcome after surgery. Forty-one percent (41%) had a successful outcome with respect to understandability of speech following surgery. Public eating behavior was improved in 50% of patients following surgery and again varied with recurrent stage. Operative mortality was slightly less (1.8%) in this series than in the retrospective review as were complications (20.2%). Average length of stay in the hospital following salvage was 11.5 days with an average cost of $5,700 per day in the year 2000.

This study was paramount to the understanding of outcomes for patients undergoing surgical salvage of recurrent HNSCC; however, many of these patients had undergone radiotherapy as the sole modality of treatment, and there was no analysis of free-flap surgery's contributions to complications, QOL, or performance status. Recent studies have suggested that QOL may be maintained at a stable level (despite some performance impairments) with the use of free-flap reconstruction after head and neck ablative surgery (14). Bozec et al. employed the European Organization for Research and Treatment of Cancer's Core Quality of Life Questionnaire (EORTC-QLQ-C30) before surgery and at 6 and 12 months in 13 patients with recurrent tumors to determine that no drop in global QOL occurred.

In addition, Kim et al. (22) studied the outcomes of patients undergoing salvage surgery with free-flap reconstruction for recurrent HNSCC. One hundred and six patients treated at the University of California at Los Angeles were reviewed. Sixty-nine patients were radiation alone failures, 14 were chemoradiation failures, and the remaining patients failed after either surgery alone or combined therapy. Major perioperative complications occurred in 34% of patients and were comprised mostly of skin necrosis (7.5%) or fistula (3.8%). Many of these patients re-recurred (74%) at an average time interval of nine months, an occurrence that was predicted by recurrent T class and persistent smoking. These results are disappointing with respect to tumor control, but remain consistent with Goodwin's review and reflect similar rates of survival and complications to reirradiation protocols (37,39–42). No functional or QOL data are available from this study; however, based on the previously mentioned QOL study by Bozec, one can extrapolate that patients may die before reaching maximal QOL; average time to death was 9 months in the 74% of patients that re-recurred, but QOL is not maximized until between 6 and 12 months following surgery. This creates a significant treatment dilemma that requires sound clinical judgment and open communication with patients to make appropriate decisions on an individual basis.

Although some evidence exists suggesting that primary closure is superior to flap reconstruction for swallowing outcomes following ablative head and neck surgery, previous treatment limits the availability of healthy tissue for primary closure (43). As evidenced by Khariwala et al. (25), four out of five patients undergoing ablation followed by free-flap reconstruction will resume oral intake, which compares favorably to historical data using pedicled or local tissue reconstructions. In this study, nearly half of patients had been previously irradiated, and nearly 20% had previous surgery, further adding to the impressiveness of their swallowing results. They also determined that preoperative irradiation, total glossectomy, hypopharyngeal defect, base of tongue surgery, and oropharyngeal surgery were risk factors for poor swallowing (g-tube dependence) following reconstruction. The authors recognized that in addition to subsite importance, the size of defect and reconstruction was important to include in the swallowing prognosis when counseling a patient.

Taken as a whole, these studies suggest that salvage surgery offers a viable, albeit low likelihood, chance for long-term survival with acceptable QOL and swallowing rates. Therefore, in properly selected patients that are motivated to attempt salvage, ablation with free tissue reconstruction should be considered after in-depth counseling.

FREE TISSUE TRANSFER TO A PREVIOUSLY TREATED FIELD

Free tissue transfer is now accepted as the standard of care in the reconstruction of many head and neck defects, with high probability success rates (95%) (44). However, transferring free tissue to a previously treated head and neck site poses several challenges. Whether the initial treatment was surgery, radiation, chemoradiation, or a combination thereof, clear tissue effects may limit local reconstructive options as well as the ability to transfer free tissue (45).

Multiple studies document that decreased vascularity of skin results in relatively high rates of local skin flap necrosis for salvage surgery following XRT or CRT (Fig. 112.3) (10,11,22). The reconstructive surgeon must be prepared to deal with local wound complications resulting from skin changes and should counsel patients preoperatively of the potential for a protracted wound healing course. Some authors advocate the use of concomitant regional

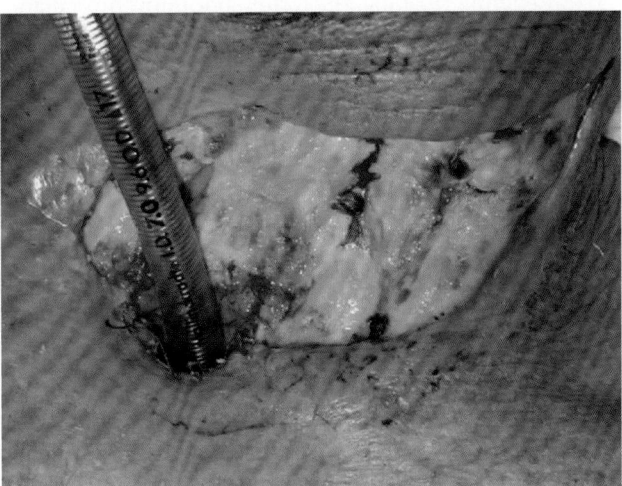

Figure 112.3 Representative example of skin flap necrosis—a common wound complication encountered in salvage surgery.

flaps for superficial coverage of important structures due to the expectation of some degree of skin loss in the heavily treated neck, particularly when single free-flap procedures will not be adequate to provide the volume of tissue necessary to reconstitute the internal defect and bolster marginal skin (19). Surgical planning is paramount to limiting skin flap loss, as prior incisions must be coordinated with planned salvage incisions in a way that limits devascularization of tenuous skin. Proper planning can limit minor skin flap loss as well as potentially lethal exposures of deeper neck structures such as the carotid arteries.

Nonetheless, free tissue transfer has proven feasible in the previously treated patient with similar rates of flap failure (15–17,19,22–24,46). In a study by Choi et al. (16) which compared patient cohorts that had no XRT to those undergoing preoperative or postoperative XRT, no difference in rate or severity of local postoperative complications was noted, but high complication rates were cited in all groups (46% to 65%). Additionally, Cohn et al. (17) examined the use of free tissue reconstruction after twice previous chemoradiation and found that wound complication was common (66%), but flap loss was not (6%). However, of the 24 patients undergoing free-flap reconstruction, four required additional free flaps for wound healing issues, and eight required additional regional flaps for the same.

In contrast, other authors have noted increased free-flap loss in addition to expected delays in wound healing and increased infections in second flap procedures (21). The largest such cohort examined results with 50 second flaps and 12 third flaps and reported 88% and 75% success, respectively, compared with 94% in primary flap surgery (45). Whether the lower success rates are related to vessel selection, flap choice, patient physiology, or other reasons remains speculative.

The emerging sentiment from these studies seems to be that even though free-flap success rates are high, the surgeon should expect some degree of minor wound complication with the potential for more severe healing problems that require second flaps. The small cohort of patients reported by Dubsky et al. (19) lends promise to the concept of double flap reconstruction; they utilized jejunum-free tissue with pectoralis major rotational flaps in the reconstruction of recurrent hypopharyngeal tumors and suffered no flap losses or wound complications requiring further surgical therapy.

The selection of recipient vessels remains a challenge in the previously treated patient; some authors report a 50% rate of contralateral vessel use when previous neck surgery had been performed, necessitating long vascular pedicles in reconstruction (47). In addition, the surgeon must be prepared to utilize out of field recipient vessels if the health of in-field vessels is suboptimal. Particularly in the previously irradiated and surgically treated neck, the internal mammary artery and transverse cervical arteries and veins should be held in reserve, and saphenous vein grafts may be necessary (17) (Fig. 112.4).

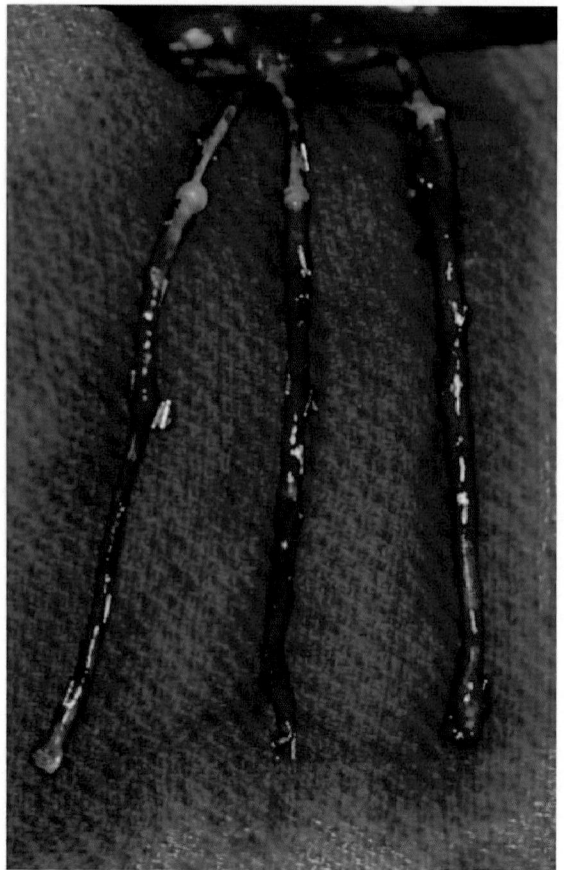

Figure 112.4 A RFFF is demonstrated here. The vascular pedicle has been lengthened by the addition of saphenous vein grafts to the radial artery and the two venae comitantes.

Few papers exist specifically addressing the use of free flaps in the salvage setting. Below is a summary of pertinent literature on the use of free flaps in previously treated patients. Some reference is made to larger series that include treated and treatment naïve patients in the interest of completeness.

Nasopharynx/Skull Base/Paranasal Sinuses

Intergroup Study 0099, a phase III randomized controlled study comparing chemoradiotherapy to XRT alone for nasopharyngeal carcinoma (NPC), established chemoradiation as the primary treatment of NPC (48). Recurrent nasopharyngeal HNSCC occurs in approximately 30% of patients; treatment options include reirradiation with either external beam or brachytherapy or nasopharyngectomy (49). Survival following reirradiation ranges between 16% and 45% with 5-year local control of 50% to 60%. Reirradiation of locally recurrent NPC has been well described in the literature. The inaccessibility and the reluctance of many centers to undertake nasopharyngectomy have led to a large experience in the management of local failure. The patients with local recurrence do well with nasopharyngeal retreatment. Mortality rates are less than 5%. Patients who have limited volume or current disease may be treated with break therapy and also have excellent local control rates.

While local control rates with reirradiation can be achieved, the patient population often is preselected. Patients will have significant morbidity secondary to the tumor as well as from the treatment. The definitive answer to the role of reirradiation awaits being answered by a multiinstitutional controlled study. Nasopharyngectomy results in survival between 4% and 67% with local control from 43% to 67% (50). QOL studies indicates that nasopharyngectomy using the anterolateral or maxillary swing approach results in acceptable outcomes (51,52).

When larger resections of the nasopharynx, skull base, or paranasal sinuses are necessary, a free flap may be required to reconstitute nasal–cranial separation or to cover vital structures. As nasopharyngectomy must remove the nasopharynx, pterygoid musculature, Eustachian tubes, and pre-/post-styloid tissues, it is often performed via an anterolateral approach which also provides access for reconstruction (53). In 2005, Bridger et al. (53) studied 11 patients who underwent nasopharyngectomy for recurrence, seven of which were reconstructed with radial forearm free flaps (RFFF). The facial vessels were used as recipient artery and vein, and there were no instances of flap loss. The authors felt that the inset of free flaps was feasible when anterolateral approaches were used, but recognized the potential for bone loss with this approach with later need for bone replacement. Following extensive nasopharyngectomy, it is important to reline both the skull base and parapharyngeal space to avoid carotid and brain exposure whenever possible.

Skull base tumor resections require extensive reconstruction particularly when performed in the setting of previous surgery or radiation as regional tissue may not be suitable for use (54). A large series of patients who underwent craniofacial resection with free-flap reconstruction was reported by Chiu et al. in 2008 (54). In this series from Memorial Sloan-Kettering Hospital, the rectus abdominis myocutaneous flap was used in 68 patients, a radial forearm in one, and latissimus flap in one; all 70 free flaps survived. It is difficult to separate complications that are directly related to free-flap surgery; however, early and late complication rates were similar to reports that did not use free-flap reconstruction (54). Speech, oral intake, globe position and vision, and aesthetics were all assessed postoperatively with acceptable results. Cerebrospinal fluid (CSF) leak was avoided in 93% percent of patients. Weber et al. reported on the Oregon Health and Sciences University Hospital experience and reported similar results with the use primarily of radial forearm (25), rectus abdominis (12), latissimus (4), and one each of anterolateral thigh (ALT), scapula, serratus anterior, and ulnar flaps for post-surgical or post-traumatic defects. In their study, seven patients (18.4%) required second flaps for flap death (3), partial necrosis (2), pneumocephalus (1), or tumor recurrence (1) (55).

Although these groups did not specifically address results in recurrent disease, it is known that complication rates are higher in this setting; the University of Michigan has published results with the use of free flaps in recurrent skull base resections (15). Chepeha et al. performed free-flap reconstructions on 20 patients following recurrent tumor surgery. All patients underwent radial forearm flap surgery, six with bony components for orbital rim reconstruction. Local complications were common (35%), but major complications were rare (15%), with only one instance of CSF leak. Complications attributed to reconstruction were CSF leak (5%) and venous compromise (5%)—both were resolved with single reoperation. Given the usually high rate of major complication with skull base surgery (27% to 75%), and even higher incidence in patients with previous treatment, the use of free tissue seems to improve results (15).

Review of these studies suggests that free flaps may reduce complication rate and severity in surgery for recurrent nasopharyngeal and skull base. When the degree of resection dictates reconstruction, free tissue should be considered safe and potentially useful in wound healing.

Oral Cavity

The oral cavity encompasses the following subsites of the head and neck: lip, buccal mucosa, lower alveolar ridge, retromolar trigone, upper alveolar ridge and hard palate, and floor of mouth and anterior tongue. Because the oral cavity is essential in the handling of food boluses, taste, and speech, microsurgical reconstruction of the oral cavity has emerged as a well-established and effective technique for rehabilitation following primary ablative procedures in these areas (56). The 5-year survival for oral cavity cancer is 46% to 59%, but is significantly related to site and stage, Stage I—53% to 90%, Stage II—54% to 100%, Stage III—37% to 71%, and Stage IV—15% to 50% (57). Primary surgery is common for tumors of the oral cavity, and postoperative XRT is employed frequently; therefore, recurrences occur in an irradiated, previously operated field.

Local recurrences generally require more aggressive ablative procedures, and locoregional tissues are less available due to prior surgery and/or radiation. Thus, microvascular free-flap reconstruction is frequently employed to reconstruct re-resected structures. Often, initial surgery will have resulted in a prior reconstruction with a free flap. However, second flap surgery has been shown feasible with acceptable results for both soft tissue and bone reconstruction (56,58). In the largest study of second free flaps for recurrent cancer, Demirkan et al. (56) studied 35 patients who underwent a total of 75 free tissue transfers for their first and second reconstructions. Second resections were reconstructed with more bone flaps since the second resection more frequently required segmental mandibulectomy. Flap survival rate was 94.6% in salvage surgery with a re-exploration rate of 13.5% (56). The same group also demonstrated that a third flap after a third resection is feasible (59). In contrast, Ross et al. (45) recently showed that free-flap success rates decline for second flaps (88%) and third flaps (75%) compared with primary flaps (95%) in their series of patients.

Evidence suggests that free-flap reconstruction in the oral cavity allows the patient better opportunity for functional rehabilitation than local flap closure (25). Swallowing data from the Khariwala et al. study showed that free-flap reconstruction of the buccal mucosa, or mandible, resulted in no significant impact on swallowing. These patients tended to have normal or soft solid diets. In addition, few patients with ventral tongue or hemiglossectomy defects were unable to swallow after microvascular reconstruction (19% to 22%). Total glossectomy defects had much worse swallowing results and will be addressed as part of the oropharynx subsite. A large number of these patients underwent prior treatment, so this study gives the best estimate available of swallowing outcomes after salvage surgery with free-flap reconstruction in the oral cavity. In addition, decannulation rates are in the 85% to 100% range and are superior to pedicled flaps in this regard (60).

Optimal free-flap choice for oral reconstruction is debatable. Some authors suggest ALT flaps are superior to RFFF because they do not sacrifice a major blood vessel and are usually primarily closed (61). However, flap selection should consider the donor site defect as well as the optimal reconstruction on an individual defect basis. The majority of oral cavity defects may be reconstructed with ALT or RFFF. More extensive defects may required musculocutaneous free tissue transfer as in the case of through and through resections involving buccal mucosa and cheek skin. A special consideration is that of bony defect in oral cavity reconstruction. Bony reconstitution is best for long-term function and can be accomplished with fibula free flaps, osteocutaneous RFFF, iliac crest free flaps, or scapula free flaps (Fig. 112.5). Each has relative merits and should all be considered part of the armamentarium of reconstructive flaps available to the surgeon—these are further explored in a section on ORN reconstruction later in this chapter. Regardless of flap choice, successful rehabilitation of speech and swallowing requires mobile tongue and ability to use it in the transit of a food bolus through the oral cavity.

Oropharynx

Chemoradiation protocols are well established as upfront organ-sparing treatments for Stage III and IV tumors of the oropharynx and N2–N3 neck disease (62). No trials exist that have compared surgery and reconstruction to organ-sparing treatment as an upfront treatment; however, when compared with historical data, chemoradiation affords increased overall survival, disease-free survival, and locoregional control over radiation alone or surgery. With a reported 66% rate of locoregional control, roughly a third of patients will go on to require surgery in a heavily treated bed. Thus, salvage surgery, when viable, should be coupled with reconstruction

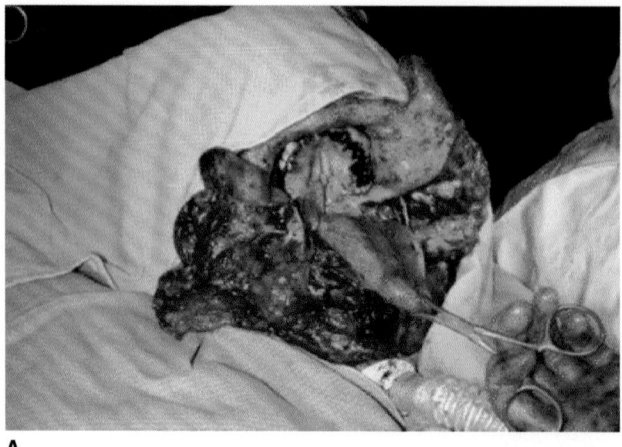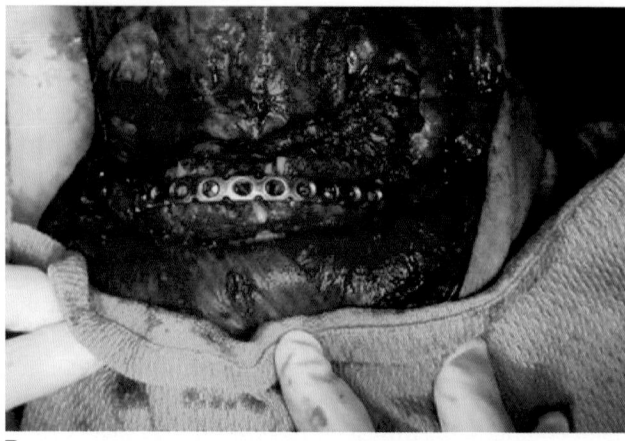

A   **B**

Figure 112.5 This patient presented with recurrent oral cavity tumor that required surgical resection. **A:** Oral cavity resection including the floor of mouth and angle-to-angle mandibulectomy. **B:** A fibula free flap was used to reconstruct the soft tissue defect and the bone.

to employ vascularized tissue in the form of rotational or free flaps. More recently, several retrospective reviews have begun to investigate the role for upfront surgery in the form of transoral robotic surgery, transoral laser surgery, or traditional open surgery for oropharyngeal cancers (63–66). However, many patients still undergo postoperative radiation or chemoradiation protocols, and salvage surgery will still occur in the radiated field for these patients.

Literature exists to suggest primary closure of oropharyngeal defects in the untreated patient affords improved swallowing of liquids, less pharyngeal residue, and shorter pharyngeal delay times on videofluoroscopic studies compared with patients undergoing myocutaneous rotational flaps or free flaps (43). In the previously treated patient, especially when chemoradiation has been employed, there is little disagreement among experts that local tissue is not often a viable option for large defects. In smaller resections for T1 recurrent disease, primary closure or local flaps are still an option. Examples of local options include primary closure, buccal flaps, facial artery myocutaneous flaps, tongue flaps, palatal island flaps, and submental island flaps. Compromised vascularity, fibrosis, and limited viable tissue make local reconstructions difficult in previously treated beds. Rotational flaps should be considered in the reconstructive ladder when assessing the oropharyngeal defect. However, recent data suggest that function is improved with free-flap reconstruction over rotational flaps (25). The authors prefer reconstruction of most oropharyngeal salvage defects with free-flap reconstruction. Information on free-flap success for oropharyngeal salvage is sparse; however, most of the patients in Kim et al. series were oropharyngeal reconstructions, and a high rate of success was encountered (no free-flap failures) (22).

Shiley et al. examined 30 patients treated by chemoradiation for advanced-stage oropharyngeal cancer. They reported that 82% of patients required g-tubes at some point in their treatment. After 1 year of follow-up, patients

without recurrence required g-tubes 31% of the time to maintain their weight. In contrast, a study from the same institution that reviewed patients treated by surgery involving free-flap reconstruction reported that 50% of patients were g-tube dependent. While the number was small, the patients that are salvageable can be expected to achieve relative good swallow function when considered in the context of their prior treatment status.

Depending on which subsites (tongue base, tonsil, pharyngeal walls, soft palate) of the oropharynx and adjacent structures (mandible) are involved in a resection, the optimal free flap used in reconstruction may vary considerably (44). As previously mentioned, operations in the previously chemoradiated field are associated with increased rate of complications, some of which can be catastrophic. Therefore, the goal of reconstruction is to reconstitute the deficient tissue in a functional way, circumvent complications such as fistula, and avoid compromise of the adjacent normal tissue and its functions. The tongue base requires bulky reconstruction to allow for its function in propelling food boluses posterior by abutting the oropharynx. When adjacent oropharynx is involved with a resection, a more complex three-dimensional reconstruction is important to preserve function and swallowing. As expected, when multiple subsites of the oropharynx are involved in a resection, swallowing tends to be poorer with a 59 times greater likelihood of poor swallowing outcomes (25). RFFF allows for resurfacing of large area of defect without adding excess bulk that might impede breathing or swallowing while affording a long vascular pedicle that can reach second or third choice donor vessels often employed for salvage surgery. The radial forearm flap may also be transferred as a sensate flap to aid in swallowing. Alternatives include the lateral arm flap, or ALT, both of which tend to be of thicker caliber, with shorter pedicle length; however, they may be useful in reconstruction of the tongue base where bulk is desirable (44).

Important QOL outcomes following oropharyngeal reconstruction with free flaps have been evaluated and indicate excellent results. The vast majority of patients achieve tracheotomy decannulation (44). Khariwala et al. found that over 70% of reconstructed patients achieve the ability to swallow after oropharynx resection and free flap. However, the total glossectomy defect is unique in that no patients were able to resume oral intake (25). Total glossectomy defects combine oral cavity and oropharyngeal resections and have poorer swallowing results than for either site alone. A bulkier flap can be effective at providing tissue to oppose the pharynx and soft palate in attempts to swallow; however, it is infrequently sufficient alone to rehabilitate swallowing. In addition, an increased risk of aspiration is associated with this defect and reconstruction, therefore resulting in fewer decannulations (44).

Larynx

Level I evidence now exists to establish concomitant chemoradiotherapy as an accepted method for definitive organ preservation treatment in advanced laryngeal cancer based on multiple important studies starting with The Department of Veterans Affairs Larynx Trial as well as Radiation Therapy Oncology Group Trial 91-11 (RTOG 91-11) (1,8). In a follow-up study to RTOG 91-11, Weber et al. examined a cohort of 129 patients from the trial that required total laryngectomy (TL) after an attempt at upfront organ preservation strategy (67). The incidence of TL was 5% for aspiration of chondronecrosis with the remaining TL for recurrence or persistence. The incidence of complications was 52% to 59%, with fistula formation in 15% to 30%. The concomitant chemoradiotherapy group experienced minor complication rates of 41% and major complication rate of 5%. Locoregional control was 74% to 90% depending on upfront treatment. Thus, data support an upfront nonsurgical management strategy for organ preservation with excellent salvage rates for persistent or recurrent disease. Hence, the heavily treated salvage bed scenario is frequently encountered in salvage laryngeal surgery.

Free tissue transfer is a useful adjunct in salvage TL surgery that has been shown to reduce the risk of leak and complication. Fung et al. reported results from the University of Michigan in which patients undergoing salvage laryngectomy after failed radiotherapy or concurrent chemoradiotherapy received free-flap reconstruction to reinforce the pharyngeal flap closure (patients that required skin paddle for closure were excluded). These patients were compared with a historical control of 27 patients from RTOG 91-11 with the same eligibility criteria but did not undergo free tissue reinforcement. The fistula rate was comparable between groups, but the rate of major wound complication was reduced from 14.8% without a flap to 0% in the flap group (20). Further, Winthrow et al. demonstrated that even when sufficient mucosa is present to close the defect primarily, free-flap reconstruction results in a lower rate of fistula (18%), stricture (18%), and feeding tube dependence (23%) than primary closure (50%, 25%, and 45%, respectively) (24). In their series, the free flap was used as a patch to supplement the anterior post laryngectomy defect and take it off tension; 16 were RFFF, and one was a rectus.

The RFFF is well suited for reconstruction of the post laryngectomy defect (Fig. 112.6). It is thin and has adequate pedicle length to reach multiple donor vessel choices. Thicker fasciocutaneous flaps are less desirable due to the relative fibrosis of posttreatment skin and inability to close it well primarily with added bulk. Both the Michigan series and Winthrow et al. relied primarily on forearm flaps with good success. The authors advocate for the use of this flap given its success. Based upon the two studies described, swallowing results are good overall following laryngectomy with free-flap closure and represent an improvement over primary closure alone. When the laryngectomy is extended to include partial or total pharyngeal defects, the reconstructive options change as described in the hypopharynx section below. Others studies have confirmed that pectoralis muscle flaps either to provide coverage of the pharyngeal repair or as a patch graft also if effective means of preventing leaks (68–70).

Partial laryngeal surgery appears oncologically safe in some sets of circumstances in recurrent laryngeal cancer (71–74). No data exist to support the use of free flaps in this setting; however, as more conservation surgery is employed, these data will likely follow. Currently, free fasciocutaneous tissue is used at our institution on a case-by-case basis with data forthcoming on its relative benefits.

Hypopharynx

Recurrent tumors involving the hypopharynx presumably extend the tissue deficit after resection and the need for free tissue to reconstitute the swallowing tract. Multiple small series demonstrate the feasibility of total laryngopharyngectomy with free-flap reconstruction with acceptable functional and wound outcomes (19,75,76). Disease-specific survival at 5 years is low in recurrent hypopharyngeal carcinoma (20%) (13,77). When resection is possible, free tissue has provided a tool to decrease severe complications, shorten hospital stay, and speed time to resumption of oral intake as compared with pedicled (78).

QOL studies confirm that the use of free jejunal tissue transfer in the reconstruction of total laryngopharyngectomy (TLP) defects results in acceptable QOL with mildly perceived clinical dysphagia; however, radiologic assessment often showed disturbed bolus transport through the jejunal segment. The radiologic and clinical findings did not seem to correlate suggesting that the flap functions well even when radiographic tests suggest abnormal swallowing (75).

Most series that directly investigate post-CRT or XRT-free tissue reconstruction of TLP are too small to remark

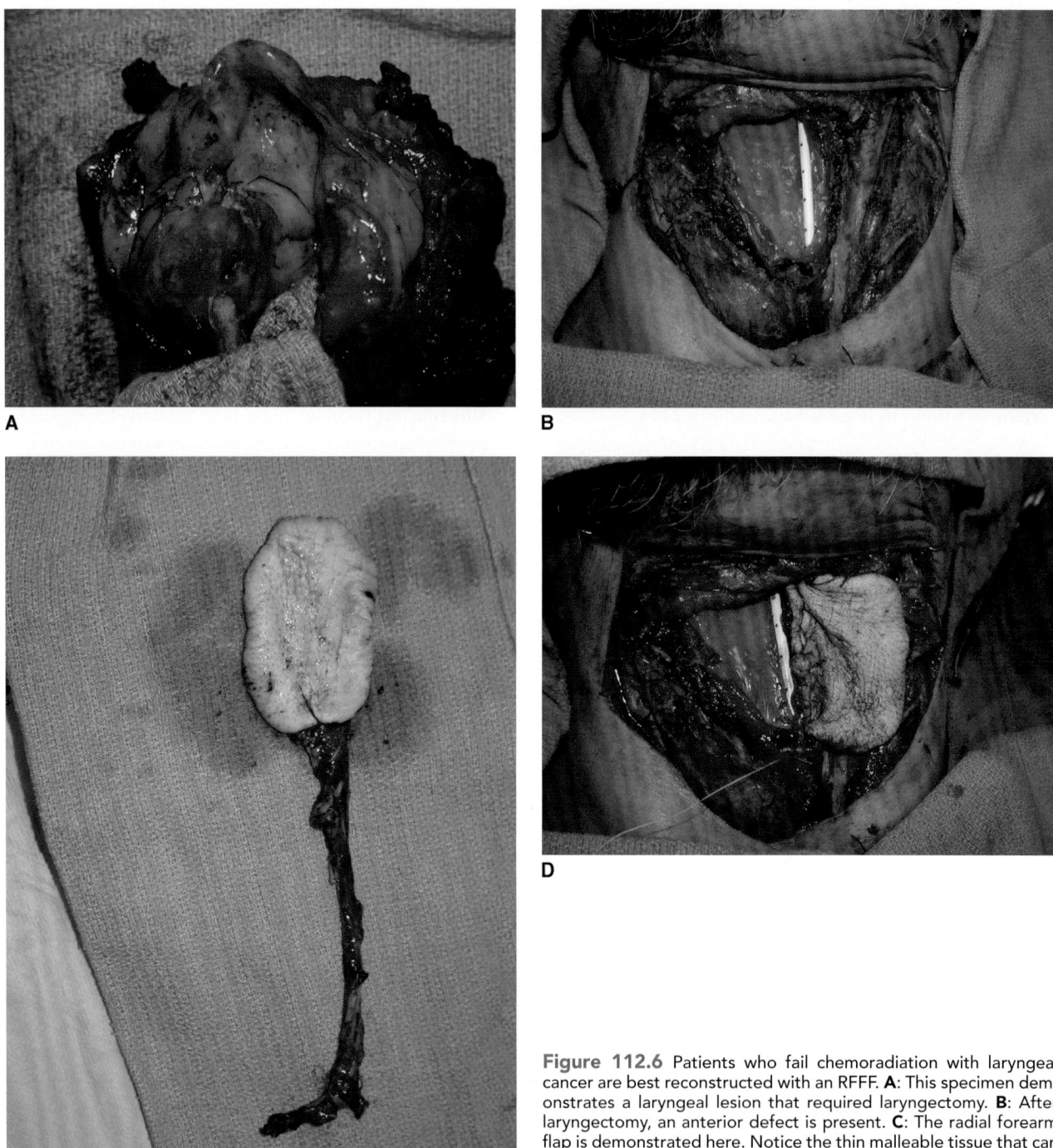

A

B

C

D

Figure 112.6 Patients who fail chemoradiation with laryngeal cancer are best reconstructed with an RFFF. **A:** This specimen demonstrates a laryngeal lesion that required laryngectomy. **B:** After laryngectomy, an anterior defect is present. **C:** The radial forearm flap is demonstrated here. Notice the thin malleable tissue that can be used to reconstruct the anterior defect. **D:** The radial forearm is being sewn in to reconstruct the pharynx.

on complication rates; however, the series' sited state that the perioperative courses were unremarkable—no significant complications occurred after jejunal free tissue was transferred. The possibility of soft tissue breakdown led Dubsky et al. to provide additional coverage with a pectoralis major rotational flap when they performed TLP with jejunal free flap with no complications. However, it is unclear whether this is necessary without direct comparison to cases in which no regional flap was used. In another study, the use of a second jejunal free flap after failed first surgery was proven feasible—an important consideration

in surgery for recurrent disease in which a first flap may have already been utilized (79).

The jejunal free flap is well suited for large segment reconstructions of the TLP defect with extension to the cervical esophagus (Fig. 112.7). The flap can be harvested in a two-team approach, and bowel complications are rare following the harvest. The flap is easily transferred to the head and neck on large-caliber vessels that usually result in one draining vein and one feeding artery. Additional flap choices have been described and include tubed radial forearm or ALT free flap. The disadvantage of tubed skin flaps

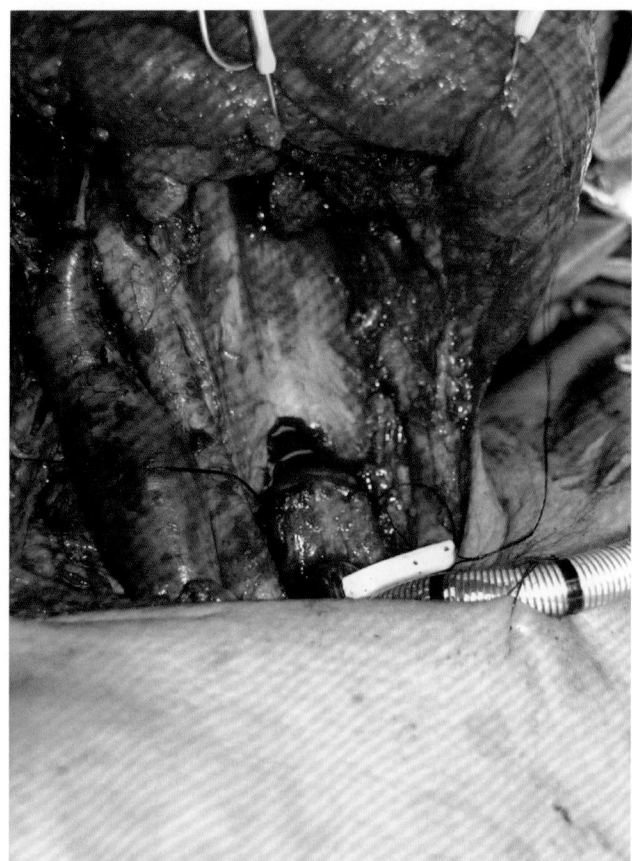

A

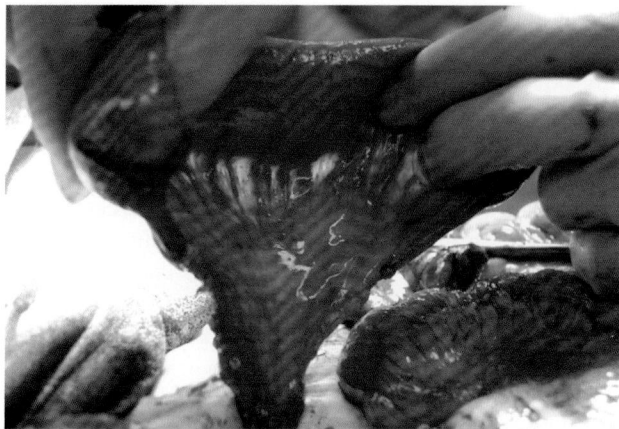

B

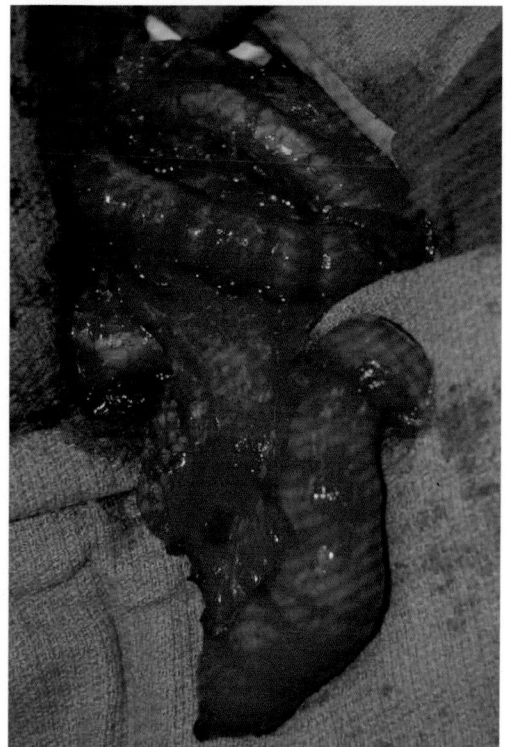

C

Figure 112.7 Patients with recurrent hypopharyngeal cancer or extensive laryngeal lesions may require total laryngopharyngectomy. **A:** This photograph demonstrates a defect after total laryngopharyngectomy. **B:** The jejunum is harvested based on a single vascular pedicle. **C:** Enough jejunum is used to reconstruct the pharyngeal defect and to provide for an external monitor.

is in their lack of mucous-secreting glands and peristalsis that comes along with jejunum. Therefore, at our institution, the jejunum is preferred when possible. However, Genden reported good success with the tubed ALT without any stenoses in 12 patients, compared with 3 stenoses out of 11 radial forearm flaps (80). The low complication rates associated with fasciocutaneous flaps and elimination of abdominal complications have led some authors to suggest that these flaps are preferred. As more functional data emerge, the question of what flap to use will be clarified, but it remains clear that single stage reconstruction is best for patients to regain function and QOL fast.

A significant local complication is that of an anastomotic leak. Leaks are difficult to treat as they often result in a local infection in a poorly vascularized bed. Neck wraps

are not useful as the vascular pedicle may be compressed. Therefore, local wound care with fistula packing, antibiotics, and observation is preferred. Some patients will require second operations to address the leak with salivary diversion or bypass followed by delayed reconstruction. This scenario seems to be rare in the reported literature, but anecdotal reports of frequent local wound problems are found.

UNRESECTABLE

There exists a subset of patients who are not candidates for surgical resection, having failed primary chemoradiation. This may be on the basis of a technically unresectable disease, being medically unfit due to a significant comorbid condition, or patient refusal to undergo significant, long-term debility because of the sacrifice of multiple structures. In this select group of patients, reradiation may be the only potentially curative treatment. Two Phase II studies using chemotherapy and reirradiation have been performed by the RTOG. Survival rates of between 8.5 and 12 months, with a 2-year survival rates of 15% to 25%, were obtained. Of significance was the acute toxicity that developed in all patients. Death was seen in 5% of patients undergoing these secondary treatments. Grade III and IV toxicity occurred in more than half of the patients. No QOL information was available from these studies or in the literature. Certainly in selected cases, reirradiation may be indicated. Chemotherapy as a single modality of treatment in the salvage patient has not been shown to be efficacious in prolonging life. Short-term local response is possible but not maintained.

USES OF MICROVASCULAR SURGERY IN THE MANAGEMENT OF CRT COMPLICATIONS

Osteoradionecrosis

Chemoradiotherapy modalities may result in long-term tissue fibrosis and ORN. When conservative measures are unsuccessful at resolving pain, tissue loss, or pathologic fractures, a more aggressive approach is warranted. Previous studies have established antibiotic treatment and hyperbaric oxygen treatment as a first-line treatment in management of early ORN (34,81–83). However, the degree of necrosis observed following concurrent chemo radiotherapy (CCRT) may exceed the ability of conservative therapy to cure, in which case surgical treatments may be required. Mandibular reconstruction for nonhealing ORN has grown in favor owing to its ability to remove necrotic tissue and restore dental function (84). The fibula, scapula, and iliac crest free flap have been shown to be useful in the reconstruction of the mandible and can serve to reconstitute the entire mandible including the temporomandibular joint (85).

The pathogenesis of ORN of the mandible has been alluded to previously; it occurs as the result of a complex interplay between impaired bone healing ability, load bearing stress on the mandible, and the frequent need for post-XRT dental extractions that result in chronic infection and fracture (35). In recent years, there has been a downward trend in occurrence likely due to increased awareness of the implications of ORN and management by multidisciplinary teams accustomed to dealing with post-CCRT-type patients.

Causes of ORN include dental extractions, spontaneous, surgery related, and from prosthetics in descending order of frequency (86). Diagnosis of ORN is both clinically and radiographically based. However, a universal staging system is lacking in the literature (87). Diagnosis requires the absence of recurrent disease as a prerequisite (which may occur in 10% to 21% of ORN cases), the observation

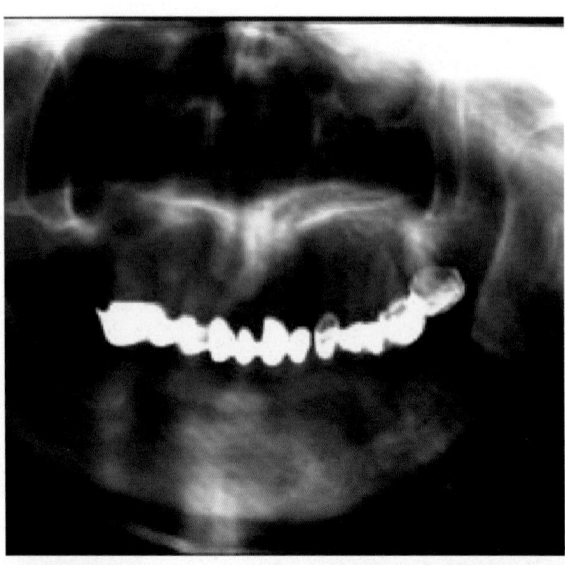

Figure 112.8 This panorex demonstrates the classic findings of a destructive lesion of the mandible secondary to ORN. Tumor has been ruled out.

of exposed bone and/or deficient mucosal covering, and lytic x-ray changes on panorex or maxillofacial computed tomography (CT) (88). Often, biopsy is performed of the questionable area as it can be difficult to differentiate recurrence from necrosis (84) (Fig. 112.8).

Treatment for ORN begins with prevention. Superior oral care is paramount to maintain the health of existing teeth and prevent progressive deterioration of those that are beginning to decay. Care of xerostomia, oral rinses, gum care, and prosthetic care should be adhered to carefully. Marx' protocols appear to be capable of managing early ORN with acceptable cure rates (83). However, one recent review and meta-analysis by Wahl indicated that prophylactic hyperbaric oxygen is not of clear benefit in ORN prevention (86). Once ORN segments occur, local treatment can be viewed as a stepwise effort starting with minor surgical intervention such as sequestrectomy and ending with major reconstruction and segmental resection +/– soft tissue resection and reconstruction. Microvascular reconstructive options have expanded the ability to restore bone and remove bone in the process of necrosis in order to speed the recovery and rehabilitation of suffering patients.

The ability to use free tissue in reconstruction is not impeded by use of prior hyperbaric oxygen, and therefore, conservative therapies should not be bypassed (89). However, if a reconstruction is performed, it is best to resect all questionable bone segments to avoid the need for later surgery when marginal bone necroses. QOL studies indicate that mandibular reconstruction afforded by free flaps results in significant improvements in cosmesis and swallowing function (14).

Reconstructive options following ORN resections include osteocutaneous free tissue or fasciocutaneous free tissue without bony reconstitution of the mandible. The osteocutaneous free flap serves as an excellent tool in the surgical management of mandibular ORN as it is best served to restore long segments of resected bone. Among the options, radial forearm, fibular, scapular, and iliac crest flaps are best described. Osteocutaneous forearm flaps are extensively utilized by the group at University of Kansas in the management of segmental mandibulectomy defects and have therefore been studied in the setting of ORN reconstruction (90). In a pair of publications, Militsakh et al. showed that osteocutaneous radial forearm flaps for mandibular reconstruction result in low rates of complications, good restoration of mandibular continuity, and resumed PO diet intake. In addition, they found that the forearm osteocutaneous flap afforded comparable morbidity at the primary and donor site and functional outcomes to that of patients reconstructed with fibular or scapular free flaps (91). Critics of radial forearm reconstruction cite the risk of pathologic radius fracture and inability to place dental implants as the major deterrents to routine use of this flap for ORN.

The workhorse of oromandibular reconstruction is the fibular free flap (Fig. 112.9). It provides a long segment (up to 20 cm) of solid bone stock capable of angle-to-angle reconstructions and large soft tissue paddles for orocutaneous fistula separation (89). The Chang Gung Memorial Hospital experience with 780 fibula flaps for segmental resections of the mandible effectively established the merits of a lengthy bicortical bone with long, large-caliber pedicles, minimal donor site morbidity, and the ability to sculpt the donor tissue to suit the defect (92). Success of this flap in the setting of ORN is well established, although, so is a high rate of wound complication (21% to 43%) and resultant protracted healing (89, 93). With a rate of flap loss that is higher than that of other free tissue defect reconstruction, it is wise to counsel patients of the potential need for second free flaps and comparable morbidity with the first flap (58). Studies exist that suggest removing the temporomandibular joint and reconstructing with free fibular bone with or without an Alloderm covering may be functionally better than attempting to achieve bone–bone union with a small segment of condyle (85, 94).

Scapular or iliac crest free flaps are also established means of mandibular reconstruction. The scapula flap can provide sufficient bone for unilateral body defects, but must be harvested in the prone position after resection has occurred. It also affords the advantage of multiple skin paddles, should both intraoral and external skin be required to replace badly damaged, or chronically fistulized tissue. Similarly, the iliac crest provides adequate bone for hemimandible defects and additional muscle and cutaneous tissue for soft tissue reconstruction (95).

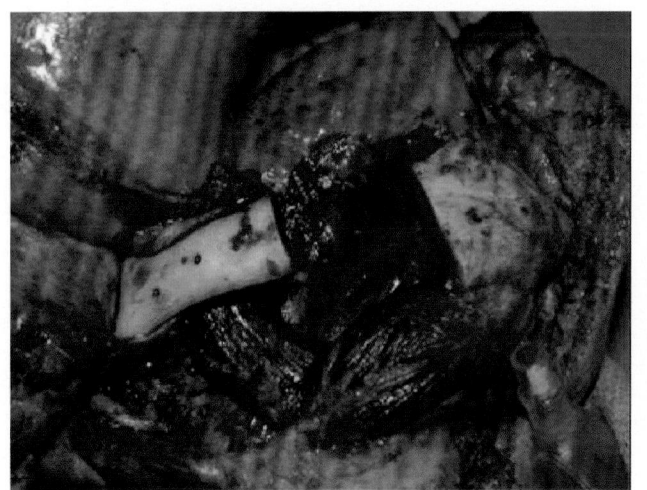

A

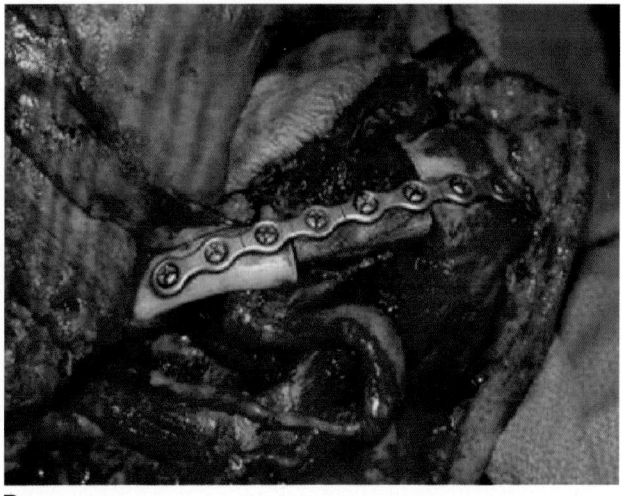

B

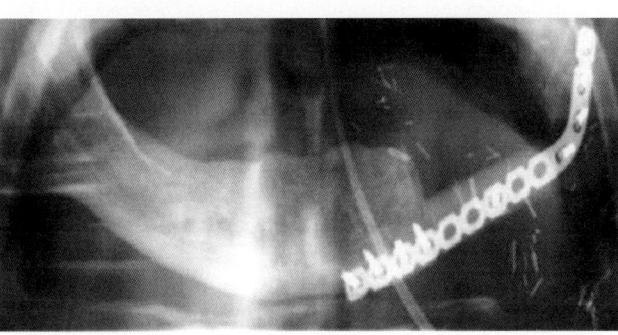

C

Figure 112.9 This patient had ORN that required surgical resection. **A:** The dead bone has been resected back to living healthy bone. **B:** A radial forearm osteocutaneous free flap has been used to reconstruct the bony defect. **C:** A postoperative panorex shows good bony union.

The psychological impact of surviving one's cancer only to be handicapped by treatment sequelae cannot be ignored, and free tissue affords surgeon's the ability to restore what is lost to an extent. However, it seems clear that ORN surgery comes with a significant risk of complication (21% to 43%) and flap loss (0% to 14%), and thus, should not be offered without restraint or until deemed absolutely necessary (84,89).

Chondroradionecrosis

The application of free tissue transfer in the management of CRN is less well established. The Chandler classification, established in 1979, is still widely accepted as the standard grading system for CRN ranging from I to IV depending on symptoms and signs present. Previously, Grades III and IV frequently resulted in TL, but recent advances in conservative therapy, including antibiotic treatment and hyperbaric oxygen (HBO), have limited this practice (35). When necessary, TL with free-flap reconstruction can rehabilitate patients suffering from debilitating pain and swallowing handicaps. Some emerging evidence suggests that partial laryngeal surgery is oncologically sound for laryngeal cancer recurrence with acceptable wound complications, and therefore, these techniques may be employed for CRN in similar fashion. Adjunctive fasciocutaneous free flaps should decrease fistula rates in partial laryngeal surgery in the post-XRT setting similarly to their role in TL (71–74). This finding suggests that revascularization of cartilage may occur through the free tissue and may represent a viable method to reverse CRN short of requiring laryngectomy, but no literature has yet been published to support this use.

CONCLUSIONS

Microvascular free tissue transfer has revolutionized the field of head and neck surgery and added greatly to the ability to treat recurrent disease that would otherwise have left patients with debilitating tissue loss. Free tissue may be applied in an organized fashion to allow for reconstruction of most head and neck subsites, and the review above indicates that this approach remains viable even in the previously treated patient. With the greater use of nonsurgical upfront treatment for HNSCC, recurrences increasingly occur in settings where native tissue is not sufficient for reconstruction after ablation. Therefore, regional, and now free flap, reconstructions have become the standard of care for bringing healthy tissue into the treated bed. High success rates and improving functional results underscore the impact of free tissue on ablative surgery for recurrence. Although recurrent HNSCC carries a poor prognosis, when surgery is an option for cure or treatment sequelae, free tissue remains a strong ally in the overall care of these patients.

HIGHLIGHTS

- Chemoradiation affects all the tissue of the head and neck adversely and will lead to a greater incidence of operative wound complications.
- Oftentimes the only option for salvage of a failed chemoradiation protocol is surgery.
- Reconstruction of the salvage patient is best accomplished with free tissue transfer.
- Surgical ablation will yield a complex composite defect that can be reconstructed with composite tissue to achieve adequate functional and cosmetic outcomes.
- Reconstruction of patients with complications from primary treatment for head and neck cancer is efficacious but complex.

REFERENCES

1. Induction chemotherapy plus radiation compared with surgery plus radiation in patients with advanced laryngeal cancer. The Department of Veterans Affairs Laryngeal Cancer Study Group. *N Engl J Med* 1991;324:1685–1690.
2. Adelstein DJ, Li Y, Adams GL, et al. An intergroup phase III comparison of standard radiation therapy and two schedules of concurrent chemoradiotherapy in patients with unresectable squamous cell head and neck cancer. *J Clin Oncol* 2003;21:92–98.
3. Adelstein DJ, Saxton JP, Lavertu P, et al. A phase III randomized trial comparing concurrent chemotherapy and radiotherapy with radiotherapy alone in resectable stage III and IV squamous cell head and neck cancer: preliminary results. *Head Neck* 1997;19:567–575.
4. Adelstein DJ, Saxton JP, Rybicki LA, et al. Multiagent concurrent chemoradiotherapy for locoregionally advanced squamous cell head and neck cancer: mature results from a single institution. *J Clin Oncol* 2006;24:1064–1071.
5. Bernier J, Domenge C, Ozsahin M, et al. Postoperative irradiation with or without concomitant chemotherapy for locally advanced head and neck cancer. *N Engl J Med* 2004;350:1945–1952.
6. Cooper JS, Pajak TF, Forastiere AA, et al. Postoperative concurrent radiotherapy and chemotherapy for high-risk squamous-cell carcinoma of the head and neck. *N Engl J Med* 2004;350:1937–1944.
7. Denis F, Garaud P, Bardet E, et al. Final results of the 94-01 French Head and Neck Oncology and Radiotherapy Group randomized trial comparing radiotherapy alone with concomitant radiochemotherapy in advanced-stage oropharynx carcinoma. *J Clin Oncol* 2004;22:69–76.
8. Forastiere AA, Goepfert H, Maor M, et al. Concurrent chemotherapy and radiotherapy for organ preservation in advanced laryngeal cancer. *N Engl J Med* 2003;349:2091–2098.
9. Pignon JP, Bourhis J, Domenge C, et al. Chemotherapy added to locoregional treatment for head and neck squamous-cell carcinoma: three meta-analyses of updated individual data. MACH-NC Collaborative Group. Meta-Analysis of Chemotherapy on Head and Neck Cancer. *Lancet* 2000;355:949–955.
10. Lavertu P, Bonafede JP, Adelstein DJ, et al. Comparison of surgical complications after organ-preservation therapy in patients with stage III or IV squamous cell head and neck cancer. *Arch Otolaryngol Head Neck Surg* 1998;124:401–406.
11. Sassler AM, Esclamado RM, Wolf GT. Surgery after organ preservation therapy. Analysis of wound complications. *Arch Otolaryngol Head Neck Surg* 1995;121:162–165.
12. Arnold DJ, Goodwin WJ, Weed DT, et al. Treatment of recurrent and advanced stage squamous cell carcinoma of the head and neck. *Semin Radiat Oncol* 2004;14:190–195.

13. Goodwin WJ Jr. Salvage surgery for patients with recurrent squamous cell carcinoma of the upper aerodigestive tract: when do the ends justify the means? *Laryngoscope* 2000;110:1–18.

14. Bozec A, Poissonnet G, Chamorey E, et al. Free-flap head and neck reconstruction and quality of life: a 2-year prospective study. *Laryngoscope* 2008;118:874–880.

15. Chepeha DB, Wang SJ, Marentette LJ, et al. Radial forearm free tissue transfer reduces complications in salvage skull base surgery. *Otolaryngol Head Neck Surg* 2004;131:958–963.

16. Choi S, Schwartz DL, Farwell DG, et al. Radiation therapy does not impact local complication rates after free-flap reconstruction for head and neck cancer. *Arch Otolaryngol Head Neck Surg* 2004;130:1308–1312.

17. Cohn AB, Lang PO, Agarwal JP, et al. Free-flap reconstruction in the doubly irradiated patient population. *Plast Reconstr Surg* 2008;122:125–132.

18. Deutsch M, Kroll SS, Ainsle N, et al. Influence of radiation on late complications in patients with free fibular flaps for mandibular reconstruction. *Ann Plast Surg* 1999;42:662–664.

19. Dubsky PC, Stift A, Rath T, et al. Salvage surgery for recurrent carcinoma of the hypopharynx and reconstruction using jejunal free tissue transfer and pectoralis major muscle pedicled flap. *Arch Otolaryngol Head Neck Surg* 2007;133:551–555.

20. Fung K, Teknos TN, Vandenberg CD, et al. Prevention of wound complications following salvage laryngectomy using free vascularized tissue. *Head Neck* 2007;29:425–430.

21. Halle M, Bodin I, Tornvall P, et al. Timing of radiotherapy in head and neck free flap reconstruction - a study of postoperative complications. *J Plast Reconstr Aesthet Surg* 2009;62:889–895.

22. Kim AJ, Suh JD, Sercarz JA, et al. Salvage surgery with free flap reconstruction: factors affecting outcome after treatment of recurrent head and neck squamous carcinoma. *Laryngoscope* 2007;117:1019–1023.

23. Klug C, Berzaczy D, Reinbacher H, et al. Influence of previous radiotherapy on free tissue transfer in the head and neck region: evaluation of 455 cases. *Laryngoscope* 2006;116:1162–1167.

24. Withrow KP, Rosenthal EL, Gourin CG, et al. Free tissue transfer to manage salvage laryngectomy defects after organ preservation failure. *Laryngoscope* 2007;117:781–784.

25. Khariwala SS, Vivek PP, Lorenz RR, et al. Swallowing outcomes after microvascular head and neck reconstruction: a prospective review of 191 cases. *Laryngoscope* 2007;117:1359–1363.

26. Reinhold HS, Keyeux A, Dunjic A, et al. The influence of radiation on blood vessels and circulation. XII. Discussion and conclusions. *Curr Top Radiat Res Q* 1974;10:185–198.

27. Dimitrievich GS, Fischer-Dzoga K, Griem ML. Radiosensitivity of vascular tissue. I. Differential radiosensitivity of capillaries: a quantitative in vivo study. *Radiat Res* 1984;99:511–535.

28. Fajardo LF. Morphologic patterns of radiation injury. *Front Radiat Ther Oncol* 1989;23:75–84.

29. Fajardo LF. The pathology of ionizing radiation as defined by morphologic patterns. *Acta Oncol* 2005;44:13–22.

30. Fajardo LF, Berthrong M. Vascular lesions following radiation. *Pathol Annu* 1988;23(Pt 1):297–330.

31. Murros KE, Toole JF. The effect of radiation on carotid arteries. A review article. *Arch Neurol* 1989;46:449–455.

32. O'Connor MM, Mayberg MR. Effects of radiation on cerebral vasculature: a review. *Neurosurgery* 2000;46:138–149;discussion 150–151.

33. Cooper JS, Fu K, Marks J, et al. Late effects of radiation therapy in the head and neck region. *Int J Radiat Oncol Biol Phys* 1995;31:1141–1164.

34. Marx RE. Osteoradionecrosis: a new concept of its pathophysiology. *J Oral Maxillofac Surg* 1983;41:283–288.

35. Hunter SE, Scher RL. Clinical implications of radionecrosis to the head and neck surgeon. *Curr Opin Otolaryngol Head Neck Surg* 2003;11:103–106.

36. Fitzgerald PJ, Koch RJ. Delayed radionecrosis of the larynx. *Am J Otolaryngol* 1999;20:245–249.

37. Langendijk JA, Bourhis J. Reirradiation in squamous cell head and neck cancer: recent developments and future directions. *Curr Opin Oncol* 2007;19:202–209.

38. Morgan JE, Breau RL, Suen JY, et al. Surgical wound complications after intensive chemoradiotherapy for advanced squamous cell carcinoma of the head and neck. *Arch Otolaryngol Head Neck Surg* 2007;133:10–14.

39. Kasperts N, Slotman B, Leemans CR, et al. A review on re-irradiation for recurrent and second primary head and neck cancer. *Oral Oncol* 2005;41:225–243.

40. Langer CJ, Harris J, Horwitz EM, et al. Phase II study of low-dose paclitaxel and cisplatin in combination with split-course concomitant twice-daily reirradiation in recurrent squamous cell carcinoma of the head and neck: results of Radiation Therapy Oncology Group Protocol 9911. *J Clin Oncol* 2007;25:4800–4805.

41. Nagar YS, Singh S, Datta NR: Chemo-reirradiation in persistent/recurrent head and neck cancers. *Jpn J Clin Oncol* 2004;34:61–68.

42. Pomp J, Levendag PC, van Putten WL. Reirradiation of recurrent tumors in the head and neck. *Am J Clin Oncol* 1988;11:543–549.

43. McConnel FM, Pauloski BR, Logemann JA, et al. Functional results of primary closure vs flaps in oropharyngeal reconstruction: a prospective study of speech and swallowing. *Arch Otolaryngol Head Neck Surg* 1998;124:625–630.

44. Smith RB, Sniezek JC, Weed DT, et al. Utilization of free tissue transfer in head and neck surgery. *Otolaryngol Head Neck Surg* 2007;137:182–191.

45. Ross GL, Ang SWE, Lannon D, et al. A ten-year experience of multiple flaps in head and neck surgery: how successful are they? *J Reconstr Microsurg* 2008;24:183–187.

46. Teknos TN, Myers LL, Bradford CR, et al. Free tissue reconstruction of the hypopharynx after organ preservation therapy: analysis of wound complications. *Laryngoscope* 2001;111:1192–1196.

47. Head C, Sercarz JA, Abemayor E, et al. Microvascular reconstruction after previous neck dissection. *Arch Otolaryngol Head Neck Surg* 2002;128:328–331.

48. Al-Sarraf M, LeBlanc M, Giri PG, et al. Chemoradiotherapy versus radiotherapy in patients with advanced nasopharyngeal cancer: phase III randomized Intergroup study 0099. *J Clin Oncol* 1998;16:1310–1317.

49. Wei WI. Cancer of the nasopharynx: functional surgical salvage. *World J Surg* 2003;27:844–848.

50. Fee WE Jr, Moir MS, Choi EC, et al. Nasopharyngectomy for recurrent nasopharyngeal cancer: a 2- to 17-year follow-up. *Arch Otolaryngol Head Neck Surg* 2002;128:280–284.

51. Ng RW, Wei WI. Quality of life of patients with recurrent nasopharyngeal carcinoma treated with nasopharyngectomy using the maxillary swing approach. *Arch Otolaryngol Head Neck Surg* 2006;132:309–316.

52. Hao SP, Tsang NM, Chang KP, et al. Nasopharyngectomy for recurrent nasopharyngeal carcinoma: a review of 53 patients and prognostic factors. *Acta Otolaryngol* 2008;128:473–481.

53. Bridger GP, Smee R, Baldwin MA, et al. Salvage nasopharyngectomy for radiation recurrences. *ANZ J Surg* 2005;75:1065–1069.

54. Chiu ES, Kraus D, Bui DT, et al. Anterior and middle cranial fossa skull base reconstruction using microvascular free tissue techniques: surgical complications and functional outcomes. *Ann Plast Surg* 2008;60:514–520.

55. Weber SM, Kim JH, Wax MK. Role of free tissue transfer in skull base reconstruction. *Otolaryngol Head Neck Surg* 2007;136:914–919.

56. Demirkan F, Wei FC, Chen HC, et al. Microsurgical reconstruction in recurrent oral cancer: use of a second free flap in the same patient. *Plast Reconstr Surg* 1999;103:829–838.

57. Campana JP, Meyers AD. The surgical management of oral cancer. *Otolaryngol Clin North Am* 2006;39:331–348.

58. Ghaheri BA, Kim JH, Wax MK. Second osteocutaneous fibular free flaps for head and neck defects. *Laryngoscope* 2005;115:983–986.

59. Demirkan F, Wei FC, Chen HC, et al. Oromandibular reconstruction using a third free flap in sequence in recurrent carcinoma. *Br J Plast Surg* 1999;52:429–433.

60. Haughey BH, Taylor SM, Fuller D. Fasciocutaneous flap reconstruction of the tongue and floor of mouth: outcomes and techniques. *Arch Otolaryngol Head Neck Surg* 2002;128:1388–1395.

61. Wei FC, Jain V, Celik N, et al. Have we found an ideal soft-tissue flap? An experience with 672 anterolateral thigh flaps. *Plast Reconstr Surg* 2002;109:2219–2226;discussion 2227–2230.

62. Calais G, Alfonsi M, Bardet E, et al. Randomized trial of radiation therapy versus concomitant chemotherapy and radiation therapy for advanced-stage oropharynx carcinoma. *J Natl Cancer Inst* 1999;91:2081–2086.

63. Moncrieff M, Sandilla J, Clark J, et al. Outcomes of primary surgical treatment of T1 and T2 carcinomas of the oropharynx. *Laryngoscope* 2009;119:307–311.

64. Jaber JJ, Moreira J, Canar WJ, et al. A 25-year analysis of veterans treated for tonsillar squamous cell carcinoma. *Arch Otolaryngol Head Neck Surg* 2009;135:1147–1153.

65. Moore EJ, Olsen KD, Kasperbauer JL. Transoral robotic surgery for oropharyngeal squamous cell carcinoma: a prospective study of feasibility and functional outcomes. *Laryngoscope* 2009;119:2156–2164.

66. Poulsen M, Porceddu SV, Kingsley PA, et al. Locally advanced tonsillar squamous cell carcinoma: Treatment approach revisited. *Laryngoscope* 2007;117:45–50.

67. Weber RS, Berkey BA, Forastiere A, et al. Outcome of salvage total laryngectomy following organ preservation therapy: the Radiation Therapy Oncology Group trial 91–11. *Arch Otolaryngol Head Neck Surg* 2003;129:44–49.

68. Gil Z, Gupta A, Kummer B, et al. The role of pectoralis major muscle flap in salvage total laryngectomy. *Arch Otolaryngol Head Neck Surg* 2009;135:1019–1023.

69. Mebeed AH, Hussein HA, Saber T, et al. Role of pectoralis major myocutaneuos flap in salvage laryngeal surgery for prophylaxis of pharyngocutaneous fistula and reconstruction of skin defect. *J Egypt Natl Canc Inst* 2009;21:23–32.

70. Patel UA, Keni SP. Pectoralis myofascial flap during salvage laryngectomy prevents pharyngocutaneous fistula. *Otolaryngol Head Neck Surg* 2009;141:190–195.

71. Deganello A, Gallo O, De Cesare JM, et al. Supracricoid partial laryngectomy as salvage surgery for radiation therapy failure. *Head Neck* 2008;30:1064–1071.

72. Holsinger FC, Funk E, Roberts DB, et al. Conservation laryngeal surgery versus total laryngectomy for radiation failure in laryngeal cancer. *Head Neck* 2006;28:779–784.

73. Pellini R, Pichi B, Ruscito P, et al. Supracricoid partial laryngectomies after radiation failure: a multi-institutional series. *Head Neck* 2008;30:372–379.

74. Piazza C, Peretti G, Cattaneo A, et al. Salvage surgery after radiotherapy for laryngeal cancer: from endoscopic resections to open-neck partial and total laryngectomies. *Arch Otolaryngol Head Neck Surg* 2007;133:1037–1043.

75. Bergquist H, Andersson M, Ejnell H, et al. Functional and radiological evaluation of free jejunal transplant reconstructions after radical resection of hypopharyngeal or proximal esophageal cancer. *World J Surg* 2007;31:1988–1995.

76. Bergquist H, Ejnell H, Fogdestam I, et al. Functional long-term outcome of a free jejunal transplant reconstruction following chemoradiotherapy and radical resection for hypopharyngeal and proximal oesophageal carcinoma. *Dig Surg* 2004;21:426–431; discussion 432–433.

77. Stoeckli SJ, Pawlik AB, Lipp M, et al. Salvage surgery after failure of nonsurgical therapy for carcinoma of the larynx and hypopharynx. *Arch Otolaryngol Head Neck Surg* 2000;126:1473–1477.

78. Benazzo M, Bertino G, Occhini A, et al. Functional outcomes in patients reconstructed with flaps following surgery for hypopharyngeal cancer. *Acta Otorhinolaryngol Ital* 2006;26:127–132.

79. Bertino G, Benazzo M, Occhini A, et al. Reconstruction of the hypopharynx after free jejunum flap failure: is a second free jejunum transfer feasible? *Oral Oncol* 2008;44:61–64.

80. Genden EM, Jacobson AS. The role of the anterolateral thigh flap for pharyngoesophageal reconstruction. *Arch Otolaryngol Head Neck Surg* 2005;131:796–799.

81. Marx RE. A new concept in the treatment of osteoradionecrosis. *J Oral Maxillofac Surg* 1983;41:351–357.

82. Marx RE, Johnson RP. Studies in the radiobiology of osteoradionecrosis and their clinical significance. *Oral Surg Oral Med Oral Pathol* 1987;64:379–390.

83. Marx RE, Johnson RP, Kline SN. Prevention of osteoradionecrosis: a randomized prospective clinical trial of hyperbaric oxygen versus penicillin. *J Am Dent Assoc* 1985;111:49–54.

84. Chang DW, Oh HK, Robb GL, et al. Management of advanced mandibular osteoradionecrosis with free flap reconstruction. *Head Neck* 2001;23:830–835.

85. Wax MK, Winslow CP, Hansen J, et al. A retrospective analysis of temporomandibular joint reconstruction with free fibula microvascular flap. *Laryngoscope* 2000;110:977–981.

86. Wahl MJ. Osteoradionecrosis prevention myths. *Int J Radiat Oncol Biol Phys* 2006;64:661–669.

87. Schwartz HC, Kagan AR. Osteoradionecrosis of the mandible: scientific basis for clinical staging. *Am J Clin Oncol* 2002;25:168–171.

88. Hao SP, Chen HC, Wei FC, et al. Systematic management of osteoradionecrosis in the head and neck. *Laryngoscope* 1999;109:1324–1327;discussion 1327–1328.

89. Gal TJ, Yueh B, Futran ND. Influence of prior hyperbaric oxygen therapy in complications following microvascular reconstruction for advanced osteoradionecrosis. *Arch Otolaryngol Head Neck Surg* 2003;129:72–76.

90. Militsakh ON, Wallace DI, Kriet JD, et al. The role of the osteocutaneous radial forearm free flap in the treatment of mandibular osteoradionecrosis. *Otolaryngol Head Neck Surg* 2005;133:80–83.

91. Militsakh ON, Werle A, Mohyuddin N, et al. Comparison of radial forearm with fibula and scapula osteocutaneous free flaps for oromandibular reconstruction. *Arch Otolaryngol Head Neck Surg* 2005;131:571–575.

92. Schrag C, Chang YM, Tsai CY, et al. Complete rehabilitation of the mandible following segmental resection. *J Surg Oncol* 2006;94:538–545.

93. Cannady SB, Dean N, Kroeker A, et al. Free flap reconstruction for osteoradionecrosis of the jaws—outcomes and predictive factors for success. *Head Neck* 2011;33:424–428.

94. Khariwala SS, Chan J, Blackwell KE, et al. Temporomandibular joint reconstruction using a vascularized bone graft with Alloderm. *J Reconstr Microsurg* 2007;23:25–30.

95. Ang E, Black C, Irish J, et al. Reconstructive options in the treatment of osteoradionecrosis of the craniomaxillofacial skeleton. *Br J Plast Surg* 2003;56:92–99.

Cutaneous Malignancy 113

Cherie-Ann O. Nathan   Timothy S. Lian

Skin cancer is the most common human malignancy, with an estimated 3,500,000 nonmelanoma skin cancers cases in the United States annually (1). Most tumors arise on the sun-exposed regions of the head and neck. Basal cell carcinoma is the predominant histologic type and accounts for about 90% of all cutaneous neoplasms in the head and neck region. Second in incidence is squamous cell carcinoma. Less common is melanoma, which accounts for approximately 8,700 deaths each year in the United States. There are 3,000 additional deaths related to other forms of cutaneous cancer (2). Cutaneous malignancies are classically divided into epidermal, dermal, adnexal, and melanocytic. Malignant melanoma has a distinct biologic behavior and is addressed separately in Chapter 114. Other rare skin malignancies of the dermis and adnexa are not discussed specifically, but principles of evaluation and treatment of cutaneous cancers are applicable. This chapter is dedicated to a discussion of nonmelanoma cutaneous malignancy, specifically basal cell carcinoma, squamous cell carcinoma, Merkel cell carcinoma (MCC), their precursors, and associated epidermal neoplasms.

RISK FACTORS

Risk factors for basal and squamous cell carcinomas are strikingly similar. These lesions, although seen in younger age groups, are most often encountered in patients 60 years of age or older.

The mechanism by which ultraviolet (UV) light causes sun-damaged skin has been extensively studied. Laboratory experiments indicate that the wavelengths with the most potential for carcinogenesis are those in the range of 280 to 320 nm, the UVB band. This UVB is responsible for the common sunburn. The transition from normal to actinic (i.e., sun damaged) to cancerous skin is usually a progressive process that occurs over several decades. With the current environmental changes occurring with the earth's protective ozone layer, the concern for skin cancer becomes much more significant. A dramatic ozone depletion above the Antarctic continent has been detected (3). For each 1% reduction in atmospheric ozone concentration, there is a concomitant 2% increase in UVB penetration (4). Approximately 90% of nonmelanoma skin cancers are estimated to be associated with exposure to UV radiation from the sun (5).

The carcinogenesis of epidermal tumors parallels the multistep development of other neoplasms. As with other neoplasms, certain characteristics render the host more susceptible to the development of cancer. Traits that are associated with an increased incidence of skin cancer include fair complexion, light hair, blue or green eyes, inability to tan, propensity to sunburn, history of multiple or severe sunburns, and Celtic ancestry (6). Other factors implicated include age, occupation, habits (tanning booths), and residential geography, which are considered indirect causes of increased sun exposure.

The bulbs used in tanning booths are almost exclusively UVA wavelength and are promoted as providing a safe suntan. However, recent evidence indicates that UVA (320 to 400 nm) synergistically augments UVB responses and is independently capable of producing deleterious skin alterations and neoplasias (7).

Other etiologic factors are associated with the development of cutaneous carcinoma (6). Chronic exposure to chemical agents, such as arsenic in patients treated with Fowlers solution, has been associated with the development of multiple squamous and basal cell tumors. Patients with chronic radiodermatitis, resulting from superficial radiation therapy, demonstrate a propensity to develop multiple and aggressive lesions. Trauma in the form of burns, ulcers, and scars is also associated with the development of skin cancer (i.e., Marjolin ulcer). Immunosuppression, common in transplant patients and patients with leukemia or lymphoma, can be complicated by an increased incidence or aggressiveness of skin malignancies (8).

Studies of human papillomavirus offer additional support for the importance of immune dysfunction in the development of skin squamous cell carcinoma. One study showed human papillomavirus presence in 60% of cutaneous squamous cell carcinoma lesions found in renal autograft recipients. Moreover, human papillomavirus presence was significantly higher than that found in matched transplant recipients without cutaneous malignancy (9). Furthermore, there is evidence to suggest that human papillomavirus may be related to the development of some nonmelanoma cutaneous malignancies not necessarily associated with immune suppression.

Genetic syndromes, such as xeroderma pigmentosum (autosomal recessive) and nevoid basal cell carcinoma syndrome (autosomal dominant), are associated with a predilection for developing multiple basal cell carcinomas, often at an early age.

BASAL CELL CARCINOMA

There are several clinical types of basal cell carcinoma. Smith (10) outlined five clinical forms: nodular or noduloulcerative, morphea-like or sclerosing, superficial multicentric, pigmented, and fibroepithelioma. Although other less common types exist, subclassification is not clinically useful. The most common type is the nodular or noduloulcerative lesion. This lesion typically presents as a discrete, raised, circular lesion that appears pink and waxy with a capillary network that is easily visible. There is often an area of central ulceration and the border of the lesion is rolled. This is the type of basal cell carcinoma that is easiest to recognize and treat. A variant of this lesion is cystic basal cell carcinoma, which is also waxy and well demarcated but is more cystic in appearance.

The superficial basal cell carcinoma lesion shows evidence of scarring and atrophy, with a thread-like waxy border. This lesion may consist of one or several red scaling patches. These crusted lesions have irregular borders and gradually increase in size by peripheral extension. They are relatively uncommon in the head and neck and more frequently occur on the trunk or extremities.

The most aggressive clinical form of basal cell carcinoma is the morphea type, also called sclerosing or fibrosing basal cell carcinoma. This variety is typified by its macular, whitish, or yellowish plaque. Some physicians have noticed an increased incidence among women. The margins may be quite indistinct, and the lesion may go unnoticed for years in some patients. Complete excision is difficult because of ill-defined margins. The lesion may look like a scar, may develop telangiectasia, or may ulcerate.

A less common basal cell carcinoma variant is pigmented basal cell carcinoma, which is characterized by its brown pigmentation and may resemble a pigmented nevus or a melanoma. The appearance and behavior of this lesion seems to parallel that of nodular basal cell carcinoma. Pigmented basal cell carcinoma differs from the noduloulcerative type only by the brown pigmentation

of the lesion. This type of lesion may also be mistaken for seborrheic keratosis, melanoma, or dermatofibroma.

Fibroepitheliomas, another variant, present as firm pedunculated lesions that resemble fibromas. It was first described in 1953 by Pinkus (11). These lesions commonly occur on the back.

The nevoid basal cell carcinoma syndrome is an autosomal dominant disease. During childhood, small cutaneous nodules appear, often numbering in the hundreds. These lesions initially have a rather indolent course during the nevoid phase, but as the patient ages, a neoplastic phase may occur in which the lesions show a marked change in aggressiveness. The lesions become invasive, destructive, and mutilating. Abnormalities associated with nevoid basal cell carcinoma syndrome include jaw cysts, bifid ribs, scoliosis, mental retardation, and frontal bossing.

The characteristic cell in basal cell carcinoma has a large, oval, or elongated nucleus with relatively little cytoplasm. These cells may resemble the basal cells of the epidermis, but the neoplastic forms lack intercellular bridges. The nuclei are rather uniform in size and configuration. A connective tissue stroma proliferates with the tumor and is oriented in parallel bundles around the tumor masses, causing peripheral palisading of the cells and stromal retraction. This is commonly referred to as peritumoral lacunae. The stroma is often mucinous. Because mucin shrinks with dehydration and fixation of the specimen, the stroma may show retraction from the tumor islands. This detachment of tumor islands from the stroma is known as clefting and is a helpful diagnostic sign.

Lever (12) divided basal cell carcinoma into four basic histologic patterns: solid, keratotic, cystic, and adenoid. In the solid pattern, the cells show no differentiation. This type generally displays tumor masses of various sizes and shapes embedded in the dermis (Fig. 113.1). The peripheral cell layer may show a palisading of the nuclei. Basal cell carcinomas that differentiate toward hair structures are referred to as keratotic. This lesion is typified by undifferentiated cells in combination with parakeratotic cells and horn cysts (Fig. 113.2). Cystic tumors show differentiation toward sebaceous glands. Histologically, there may be one or several cystic spaces within the tumor lobules. In the adenoid variety of basal cell carcinoma, the tumors display a tubular or glandular formation. The strands of epithelial cells commonly form a lace-like pattern (Fig. 113.3).

Keratotic basal cell carcinoma, also known as basosquamous cell carcinoma or metatypical carcinoma, has been the subject of much controversy. The confusion arises because histologically there are coexistent features of both basal cell and squamous cell carcinomas in the same lesion, frustrating accurate assessment of prognosis and behavior. Most dermatopathologists currently believe that basosquamous tumor is a variant basal cell carcinoma, referred to by many as keratotic basal cell carcinoma (12). Although there is limited potential for metastasis, keratotic basal cell carcinoma is thought to be more biologically aggressive than many of the other types of basal cell carcinomas.

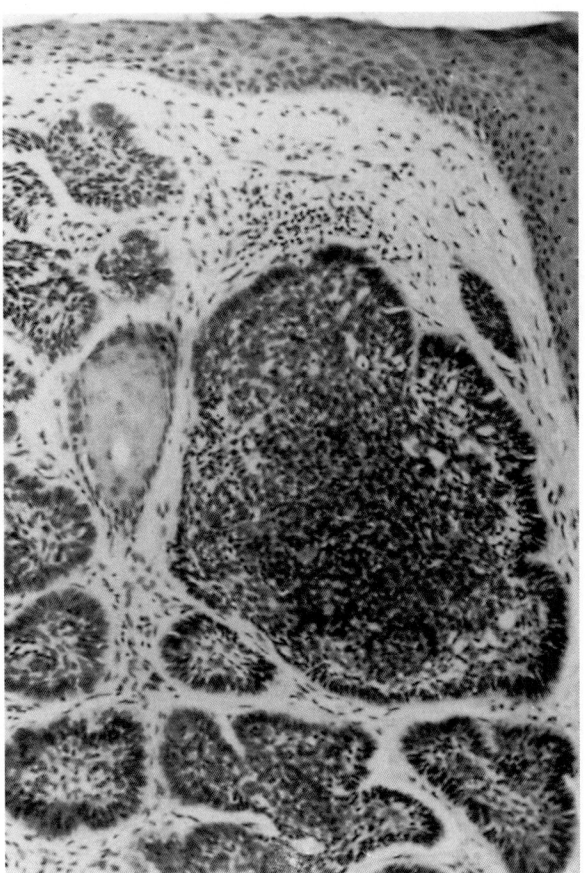

Figure 113.1 Basal cell tumor masses (solid type).

SQUAMOUS CELL CARCINOMA

Far less common than basal cell carcinoma, squamous cell carcinoma accounts for approximately 10% of skin malignancies. As with its counterpart, basal cell carcinoma, squamous cell carcinoma is related to chronic (i.e., 10 to 20 years) sun exposure. As the equator is approached, the relative incidence of squamous cell carcinoma increases compared with basal cell carcinoma. Cutaneous squamous cell carcinoma, like basal cell carcinoma, is more common in men.

Squamous cell carcinoma of the skin usually presents as an erythematous, ulcerated, crusting lesion. The tumor often demonstrates a granular base that may be friable and tends to bleed with minimal trauma. There is usually an elevated area of induration at the lesion edge and there may be an inflammatory response in the adjacent tissues.

These lesions present in different patterns. Squamous cell carcinoma can present as a thickened hyperkeratotic patch or an area of crusting. Under this crust is an ulcerated base with a rolled margin. Other lesions may be recognized as areas of persistent ulceration, possibly in the site of previous trauma, burns, or an old scar (i.e., Marjolin ulcer). Neoplastic change in a chronic ulcer may result in basal cell or squamous cell carcinoma and is associated with a poorer prognosis and higher rates of metastasis. Superficial multifocal lesions can arise in actinic skin. These lesions are usually accompanied by a scaling patch that bleeds with minimal trauma. Diagnosis and determination of the extent of the lesion can be difficult, and multiple biopsies may be necessary. Squamous cell carcinoma occasionally presents as a nodular exophytic lesion. Initially cystic, it later tends to become ulcerative and progressively enlarges. These lesions may also demonstrate a sudden growth spurt.

Several histologic characteristics are important in analyzing squamous cell carcinoma. The usual histologic picture of squamous cell carcinoma of the skin is that of irregular masses of epidermal cells that proliferate downward and invade the dermis. The tumor masses may be well differentiated or may show atypical or anaplastic cells. The differentiated tumors tend to be associated with evidence of keratinization, such as keratin pearls.

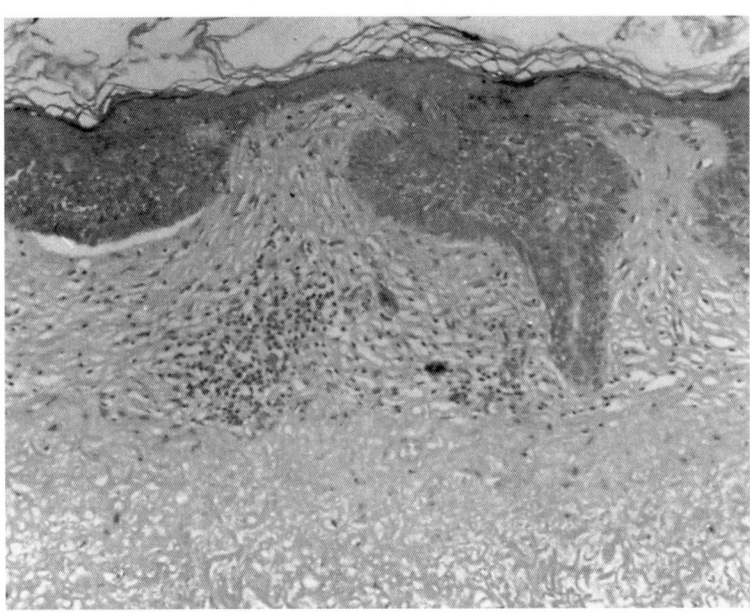

Figure 113.2 Undifferentiated cells with parakeratotic and horn cysts (keratotic type).

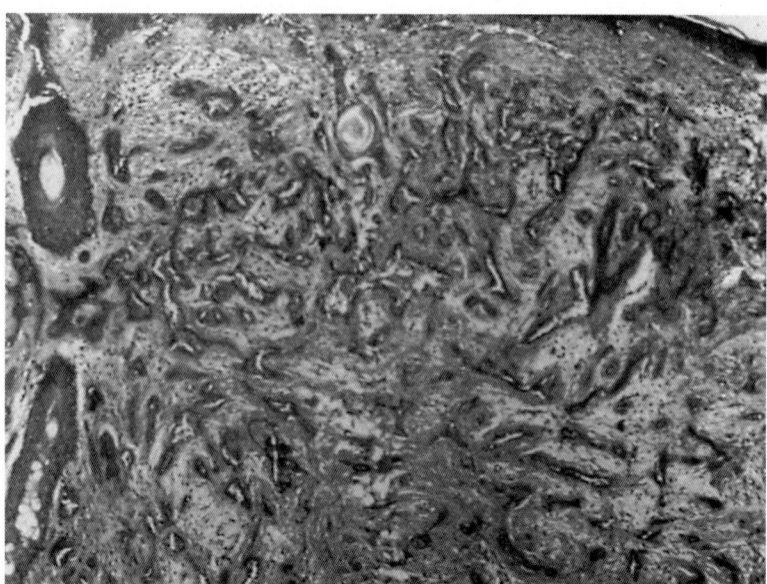

Figure 113.3 Lace-like patterns of epithelial cells (adenoid type).

Some squamous cell carcinomas are actinically induced, and some arise *de novo*. Lesions arising in sun-exposed areas appear to follow a more benign course with a low incidence of metastasis. The *de novo* lesions are more aggressive in their behavior and exhibit greater potential for metastasis. It has been estimated that up to 54% of patients with *de novo* lesions develop regional or distant metastases (13). It is often possible to differentiate clinically between the two types of squamous cell carcinoma. Histologically, a determination can usually be made by looking for actinic changes in the skin adjacent to the squamous cell carcinoma.

Squamous cell carcinoma has metastatic potential, and regional metastatic spread is correlated with depth of invasion. Squamous cell carcinoma lesions that penetrate to Clark level IV or V are associated with a 20% regional metastatic rate.

Histologic variations of squamous cell carcinoma are numerous and include adenoid, bowenoid, verrucous, and spindle–pleomorphic types (14). The generic type is characterized by actinic changes. In the adenoid type, there is a pseudoglandular arrangement. These tubular or alveolar formations result from dyskeratosis and subsequent acantholysis. The lumina are lined with one or several layers of epithelium and are filled with desquamated acantholytic cells. The bowenoid type of squamous cell carcinoma is characterized by evidence of invasion coexistent with the findings of Bowen disease.

Verrucous carcinoma is seldom seen as a skin neoplasm on the head and neck, but it is well known as a tumor of the oral cavity and larynx. It presents as a white cauliflower-like lesion. The tumor is well differentiated, demonstrating hyperkeratosis, parakeratosis, and acanthosis. Clinical and pathologic correlations are needed to confirm the diagnosis.

In the spindle–pleomorphic type of squamous cell carcinoma, there is little evidence of differentiation. These tumors are anaplastic, show little or no keratinization, and are usually considered to be a Broders grade 4 tumor. The spindle cells are intermingled with collagen, may be arranged in whorls, and can be associated with pleomorphic giant cells.

PREMALIGNANT LESIONS

Several skin lesions are considered premalignant. This group includes a low-grade malignancy that can be treated as if it was a premalignant lesion. The most common of these are actinic keratosis, Bowen disease, and keratoacanthoma.

Actinic Keratoses

Actinic keratoses (i.e., solar keratoses or senile keratoses) is the most common premalignant lesion of the head and neck and is seen almost exclusively in sun-exposed areas of the skin. The lesions are generally less than 1 cm in diameter and are commonly located on the face, scalp, hands, and forearms (Fig. 113.4). They are considered precancerous. The chance of progression to epidermal cutaneous carcinoma has been estimated to be as great as 20% (12). They usually present as an erythematous patch, often covered by an adherent scale. Clinically, they show little or no sign of inflammation. Occasionally, there is a marked hyperkeratosis, giving the appearance of a cutaneous horn. A sandpaper-like scale is the most distinctive feature on clinical examination. Because these lesions have malignant transformation potential, most physicians believe they should be treated. Depending on the clinical setting, superficial shave excision, cryosurgery, topical treatment

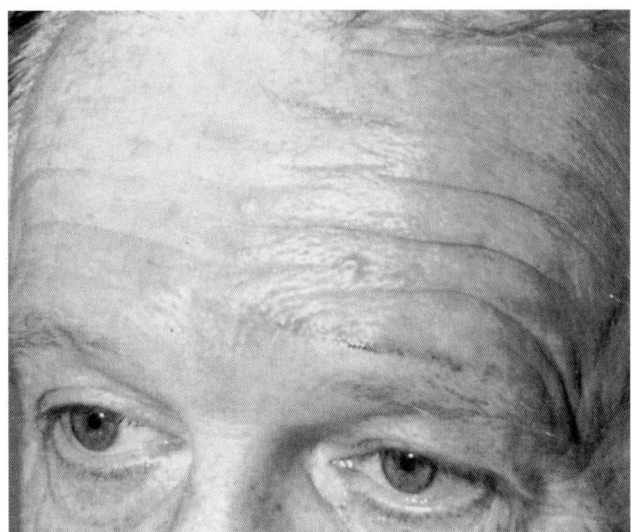

Figure 113.4 Actinic keratosis on forehead.

with 5-fluorouracil, or trichloroacetic acid peel may provide effective treatment. The differential diagnosis includes seborrheic keratosis, benign lentigo, squamous cell carcinoma, and basal cell carcinoma.

Bowen Disease

Bowen disease is considered a preinvasive form of squamous cell carcinoma. It can be considered synonymous with carcinoma *in situ* of the skin. Histologically, there is full-thickness dysplasia of the epidermis without evidence of invasion. Clinically, the lesion presents as a well-circumscribed, erythematous, scaly patch or plaque with an irregular border. As with squamous cell carcinoma, these lesions generally occur in sun-exposed areas. They are particularly common in patients with a history of chronic arsenic ingestion in whom lesions often occur on nonexposed skin. The lesion may resemble a superficial basal cell carcinoma, but it lacks the fine pearly border.

Keratoacanthoma

Keratoacanthoma is a benign usually self-limited epithelial tumor that is easily confused clinically and histopathologically with squamous cell carcinoma. It is more common in males and typically presents in older patients. There is a history of rapid growth, usually over 2 to 6 months. The lesion begins as a smooth rounded nodule, but with further enlargement, the center becomes ulcerated and filled with keratinous material, taking on a volcano-like appearance. The hallmark of keratoacanthoma is rapid growth over weeks or months.

The most common site affected is the nose. Although histologically the lesion resembles a squamous cell carcinoma (Fig. 113.5), it may involute spontaneously, leaving only a depressed scar. Because of the lack of predictability, surgical excision is recommended.

TUMOR BEHAVIOR

Staging for cutaneous basal cell carcinoma and squamous cell carcinoma has been defined by the American Joint Committee on Cancer using the TNM classification as shown in Table 113.1 (15). Tumor histology, local extent or infiltration, tumor size, anatomic site, associated risk factors (e.g., age, prior irradiation, genetic syndromes), and previous treatment must be considered in determining the risk of recurrence for a given lesion. High-risk features include depth and extent of invasion, anatomic location, and histologic differentiation (Table 113.2).

The clinical and histologic types are significant prognostic variables. The morphea type of basal cell carcinoma is well known for its subversive attitude. This lesion generally spreads centrifugally by way of finger-like projections

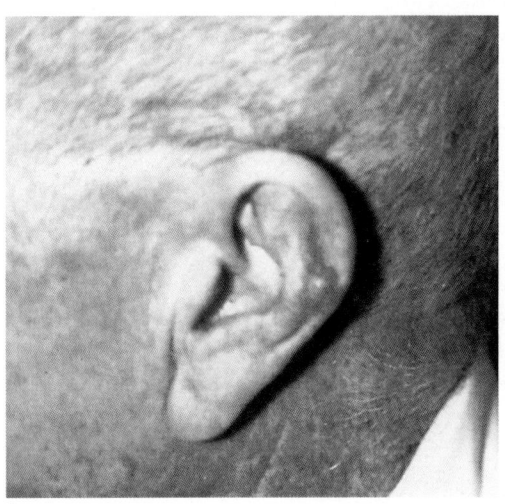

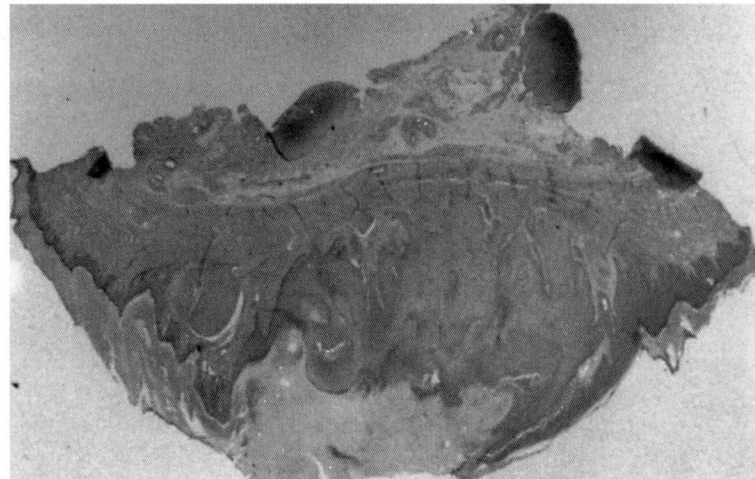

A   B

Figure 113.5 **A:** Keratoacanthoma of the auricle. **B:** Histologic volcano-appearance.

TABLE 113.1	AJCC CLASSIFICATION FOR CUTANEOUS SQUAMOUS CELL CARCINOMA AND OTHER CUTANEOUS CARCINOMAS (EXCLUDING THE EYELID)

Primary tumor (T)

TX: Primary tumor cannot be assessed.

T0: No evidence of primary tumor

Tis: Carcinoma *in situ*

T1: Tumor 2 cm or less in greatest dimension with less than two risk features

T2: Tumor >2 cm or tumor of any size with two or more high-risk features

T3: Tumor with invasion of the maxilla, mandible, orbit, or temporal bone

T4: Tumor with invasion of the skeleton (axial or appendicular) or perineural invasion of the skull base

Regional lymph nodes (N)

NX: Regional lymph nodes cannot be assessed.

N0: No regional lymph node metastasis

N1: Metastasis in a single ipsilateral lymph node, 3 cm or less

N2a: Metastasis in a single ipsilateral lymph node, more than 3 cm but not more than 6 cm

N2b: Metastasis in multiple ipsilateral lymph nodes with none more than 6 cm

N2c: Metastasis in bilateral or contralateral lymph nodes with none more than 6 cm

N3: Metastasis in a lymph node more than 6 cm

Distant metastasis (M)

M0: No distant metastasis

M1: Distant metastasis

of tumor. It is deceptive in its behavior and can be difficult to evaluate and control. Keratotic (i.e., basosquamous), recurrent basal cell, and spindle cell variants of squamous cell carcinomas are also associated with worse prognoses. Poorly differentiated or undifferentiated tumors are considered high-risk features for staging purposes.

Squamous cell lesions can be virulent. They have the potential to metastasize to regional nodes and are sometimes associated with distant metastases. Locally, these tumors are more likely to grow in a vertical fashion and less likely to respect the barriers of cartilage and bone than basal cell carcinoma. It is prudent to evaluate the regional lymphatic drainage when dealing with squamous cell carcinoma. Tumor thickness greater or equal to 2 mm, Clark level IV or greater, and perineural invasion are high-risk features with regard to staging.

The anatomic location influences the prognosis because various regions of the head and neck have a propensity for tumor recurrence. Lesions on the nose and ear have higher rates of recurrence, which is probably associated with embryonic fusion planes (16). These embryologic sites of fusion afford greater access for tumors, which use the planes as avenues for spread. The most prominent sites are the preauricular and postauricular regions, the floor of the nose and columella, and the nose–cheek crease. The periorbital region is also at risk for tumors tracking along the bone or periosteum, particularly in the medial canthal region. Mohs (17) speculated that basal cell tumor cells migrate along the periosteum or perichondrium of the nose and the medial canthi because of the close apposition of the skin to the bone and cartilage in these locations.

Swanson (18) determined that the high-risk sites fall within an "H" zone on the face (Fig. 113.6). In highlighting the specific regions at risk, he cited the junction of the ala with the nasolabial fold, the nasal septum, the nasal ala, the inner canthi and lower eyelids of the periorbital region, the periauricular region extending to the temple, and certain scalp lesions. Primary tumor site of the ear or non–hair-bearing lip are considered high-risk features for staging purposes (Table 113.2).

TABLE 113.2	HIGH-RISK FEATURES OF CUTANEOUS SQUAMOUS CELL CARCINOMA AND OTHER CUTANEOUS MALIGNANCIES

Depth/invasion	More than 2 mm of thickness
	Clark level IV or greater
	Perineural invasion
Location	Ear
	Non–hair-bearing lip
Differentiation	Poorly differentiated or undifferentiated

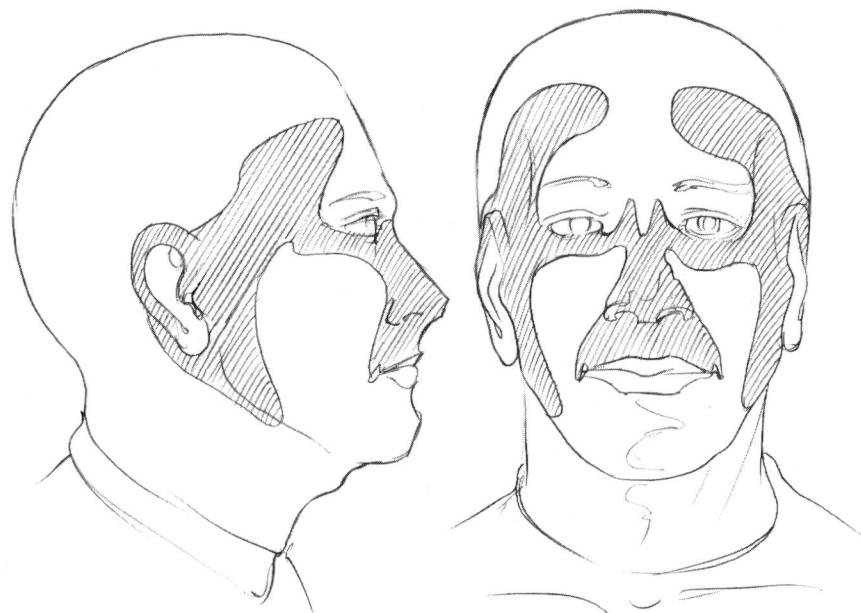

Figure 113.6 H zone: high-risk areas of aggressive cutaneous malignancies. (Adapted from Swanson NA. Mohs surgery: technique, indications, applications, and the future. *Arch Dermatol* 1983;119:761.)

RECURRENT CUTANEOUS LESIONS

A recurrent carcinoma of the skin presents a much more challenging problem than the primary lesion. Recurrent cancer indicates inadequate initial therapy or a persistence of disease in the tissue adjacent to the original lesion. Levine and Bailin (18) evaluated 496 cases of recurrent basal cell carcinoma in an attempt to identify significant risk factors. They found the midface region was involved in 57.6% of the cases and the auricular and preauricular areas accounted for 13.4% of the recurrences. The nose is the most common location of recurrence (25.5% to 41%).

The relative risk for recurrence was calculated in one study for different locations (19). In order of decreasing magnitude of risk, the locations are the nose (2.38), the ears (1.43), the periorbital areas (1.17), the remainder of the face (1.04), and the neck and scalp (0.55). The distribution of these recurrent tumors is shown in Figure 113.7. It is suggested that treatment of positive margins in the immediate postoperative period may decrease the recurrence rate and thus avoid a more extensive treatment if the cancer were to recur (20).

Jackson and Adams (21) described 33 cases of extensive basal cell carcinoma. These lesions were large (greater than

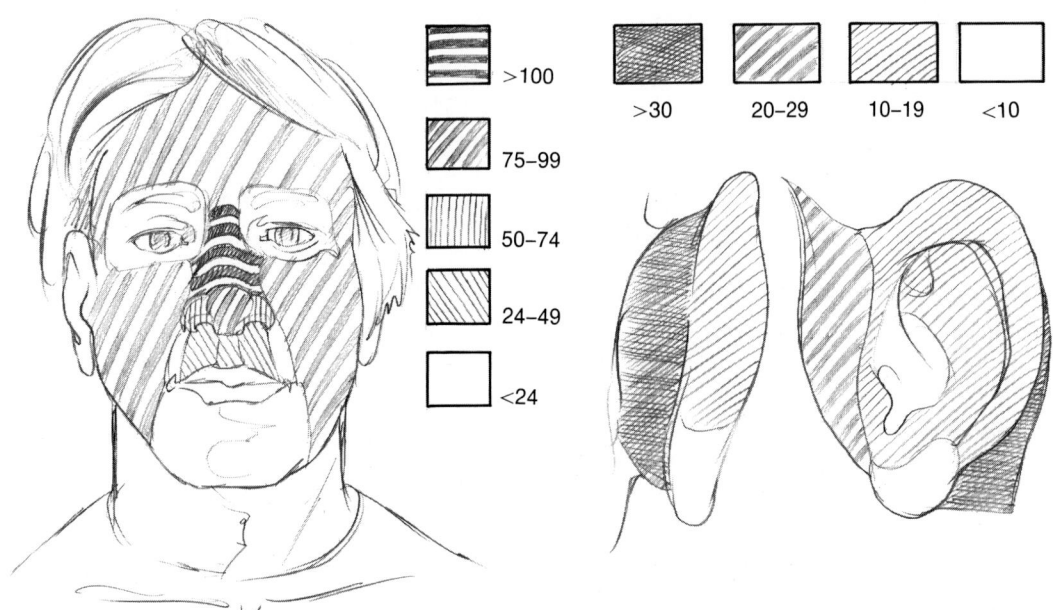

>100

75–99

50–74

24–49

<24

>30   20–29   10–19   <10

Figure 113.7 Distribution of recurrent cutaneous malignancies.

3 cm), destructive, locally uncontrollable, or metastatic. In defining the predominant characteristic of each lesion, they found that 18 were large, 6 destructive, 5 locally uncontrollable, and 4 metastatic. They concluded that these neglected tumors usually had an onset before age 40 and recurred more than twice despite adequate treatment and that each recurrence appeared sooner and became larger than the preceding tumor. In many patients, underlying conditions predisposed them to cutaneous basal cell carcinoma, including arsenic ingestion, nevoid basal cell syndrome, preexisting burns, and radiodermatitis.

Levine (22) studied the pathogenesis and treatment of large recurrent cutaneous neoplasms. The advanced lesions, called massive or previously uncontrolled, met one or more of the following criteria: diameter greater than 3 cm, involvement deeper than skin and subcutaneous fat, four or more previous treatments without control, or proven metastatic disease.

MANAGEMENT OF CUTANEOUS SQUAMOUS CELL AND BASAL CELL CARCINOMA

An advantage of nonsurgical management of primary skin malignancies is cure rates reported in excess of 95% for selected skin malignancies. These nonsurgical modalities use field therapy for their mechanism of treatment. Skin cancers grow both radially and vertically in a predictable and proportional manner. Field therapy uses these growth characteristics to treat a defined area containing both tumor and a surrounding layer of normal tissue.

Curettage With Electrodesiccation

One of the most common treatments for basal cell carcinoma is curettage excision combined with electrodesiccation, also known as electrosurgery or electrodesiccation with curettage. It is used primarily by dermatologists, who manage most of these lesions, and is quite successful when used appropriately, yielding cure rates of 81% to 97% (23).

The rationale for using this modality is that basal cell and squamous cell tumors have a soft feel that can be detected as a lesion is curetted. In experienced hands, this allows the removal of all palpable tumors with different sizes of curettes. After normal-feeling tissue is encountered over the entire base of the excision, electrodesiccation or fulguration of the wound is performed. This process is completed from two to six times, and the wound is treated topically and allowed to heal by second intention.

The advantages of electrosurgery include maximal sparing of normal tissue, ease of performance, and expediency. The disadvantages include care of an open wound, depressed or hypertrophic scarring, and delayed bleeding. Electrosurgery should be used only in selected lesions, usually basal cell lesions less than 2 cm in diameter. Contraindications for this treatment modality include

lesions with deep invasion, morphea-like and sclerotic basal cell carcinomas, and recurrent tumors. If squamous cell tumors are treated by this modality, they should be carefully selected.

Cryosurgery

Cryosurgery is another treatment option that may be appropriate for some basal cell lesions. As with electrosurgery, the skill and experience of the treating physician are critical. The most common cryogen used is liquid nitrogen. A temperature of at least 30°C is considered to be lethal to cutaneous malignant tissue, although some surgeons consider –50°C to be more appropriate. The tumor and an area of surrounding tissue are frozen to ensure the adequacy of the ablation. A thermocouple inserted at the margin of the treatment area ensures that the proper temperature for cell killing is reached. The tissue is allowed to thaw, and after an appropriate period, the freeze–thaw cycle is repeated.

Proponents of this technique cite as advantages its high cure rate, tissue-sparing capabilities, and expedience (24). It is thought to be useful in tumors overlying cartilage that can be frozen without undergoing necrosis. It may be particularly useful in patients with multiple lesions. The disadvantages include a prolonged healing phase and wound care. Hypopigmentation and unsatisfactory scarring can occur. Its use should be limited to lesions with well-defined borders and should not be used for morphea-like tumors or recurrent skin cancers.

Radiation Therapy

Radiation therapy has the capability of effectively treating skin cancers successfully and has been used extensively in the past (25). As more expedient and less radical methods of treatment have become popular, its use in recent years has waned. The advantages of irradiation include the ability to treat a wide field of tumor and avoidance of surgery. The disadvantages include the protracted treatment course, expense, adjacent tissue effects, limited effectiveness if tumors involve cartilage or bone, and the possibility of radiodermatitis and delayed carcinogenesis. Radiation therapy is currently used in the treatment of poor operative candidates, as an adjuvant to surgery, or for palliation in advanced lesions. It can be curative, but careful selection of lesions and patients is crucial.

Photodynamic Therapy for Cutaneous Malignancy of the Head and Neck

Photodynamic therapy (PDT) is a therapeutic modality using a photosensitizing drug that selectively localizes in tumors and that, on being activated by exposure to light, causes preferential tumor necrosis. Despite its initial promise, PDT remains an investigational modality at the present time. The two components needed for this therapy are a photosensitizer drug and a laser to activate the drug. The most widely used drug in head and neck has been porphyrin. Some of the other drugs that have been used as photosensitizers are tetracyclines, fluorescein, rhodamine, and more recently sulfonated metallophthatlocyanines. The light source consists of a laser either delivered down a fiber for surface illumination (which is the technique of choice for superficial cancer) or implanted into the substance of the tumor (used for bulky tumors). The argon ion dye pumped laser is most commonly used in North America.

Review of the literature reveals that initially this treatment was used predominantly for palliation of advanced skin cancer. Most series reveal a dramatic initial response in many patients, but long-term follow-up was rarely possible because of the advanced nature of these cancers (26). The response was variable and unpredictable, and severe pain and skin necrosis were common. A major problem in evaluating the literature is the tremendous variability in technique, drug, and light dosage in the reported series.

The advantages of PDT are that multiple lesions can be treated at the same time, it has good cosmetic results, and no anesthesia is required. The disadvantages include lack of predictable response in more advanced lesions and occasional photosensitivity. Once the technique has been further refined, it has great potential in the management of skin cancers.

Interferon-Alpha

Interferon-alpha (IFN-α) has been demonstrated to be useful for the treatment of select primary skin cancer. Studies demonstrated that basal cell carcinoma of the nodular and superficial types shows excellent responses (27,28). Treatment is typically initiated with low-dose intralesional IFN-α three times a week. Local reactions include pain and persistent erythema. The most common side effect is a flu-like illness, the symptoms of which respond to acetaminophen. Hematologic side effects include leukocytopenia and thrombocytopenia.

The mechanism is believed to be due to the antiproliferative and immunomodulating properties of interferon. Through a nonspecific stimulating effect on macrophages and natural killer cells, localized administration of IFN-α focally increases the host response to the neoplastic tissue.

Excisional Surgery

Surgical excision for cutaneous neoplasms is the modality with which most head and neck surgeons have the most experience. The success rate for this method of treatment is 86% to 97% (29). The major advantages of excisional surgery include the ability to obtain tissue for diagnosis and to assess the completeness of excision. By use of frozen sections, the surgeon can evaluate the margins of excision histologically. Another benefit is the excellent

cosmesis, particularly if defects are amenable to primary closure. The disadvantages are that excisional surgery can be more time consuming, inconvenient, and expensive for the patient than other treatments. Most surgeons believe that the histologic confirmation of the adequacy of excision outweighs these relatively minor disadvantages. The carbon dioxide (CO_2) laser can also be used for excision of cutaneous carcinomas.

Mohs Surgery

Mohs pioneered a new technique for removal of cutaneous neoplasms while he was a medical student in the 1930s. His first results were published in 1941, and the new modality was dubbed chemosurgery technique (30). With this method, zinc chloride paste (a chemical fixative) was applied to the cancer, fixing it *in situ* and permitting careful serial excisions with examination of the entire specimen histologically. This permitted him to map extensions of residual tumor, so that reexcision of these pockets of cancer was possible. The cure rates associated with the technique range from 96% to 99% (30,31). Tromovitch and Stegman (32) revised the original technique and used a fresh-tissue technique that adhered to the same tenets of serial excisions and mapping of residual tumor deposits. The nomenclature for the techniques has now evolved to the point that Mohs chemosurgery implies a fixed tissue technique and Mohs micrographic surgery indicates use of the fresh-tissue technique. Most dermatologic surgeons now use the fresh-tissue technique, commonly called Mohs surgery. Details of the technique are published in numerous sources (30,31). A schematic of this process is shown in Figure 113.8.

The advantages of Mohs surgery lie in its ability to examine the resection margins in their entirety, unlike routine or frozen-section margins that evaluate a random sampling of margins. Microscopic foci of tumor can be identified, mapped, and reexcised with this technique. It also allows removal of the neoplasm with maximal preservation of surrounding normal tissue. Another benefit of the Mohs fresh-tissue technique is the ability to immediately reconstruct the defects that have been created. The major advantage is that this technique has the highest cure rate in the management of advanced, high-risk, or recurrent lesions. Mohs surgery is most useful in the high-risk lesions. The disadvantages of the Mohs technique are the special expertise, time, and expense involved. Someone with this special training may not be available in all communities. These drawbacks are compensated for by achieving a disease-free status.

Carbon Dioxide Laser

Laser excision is appropriate in the management of some skin malignancies. It is indicated instead of standard excision for patients whose cardiac status or other medical

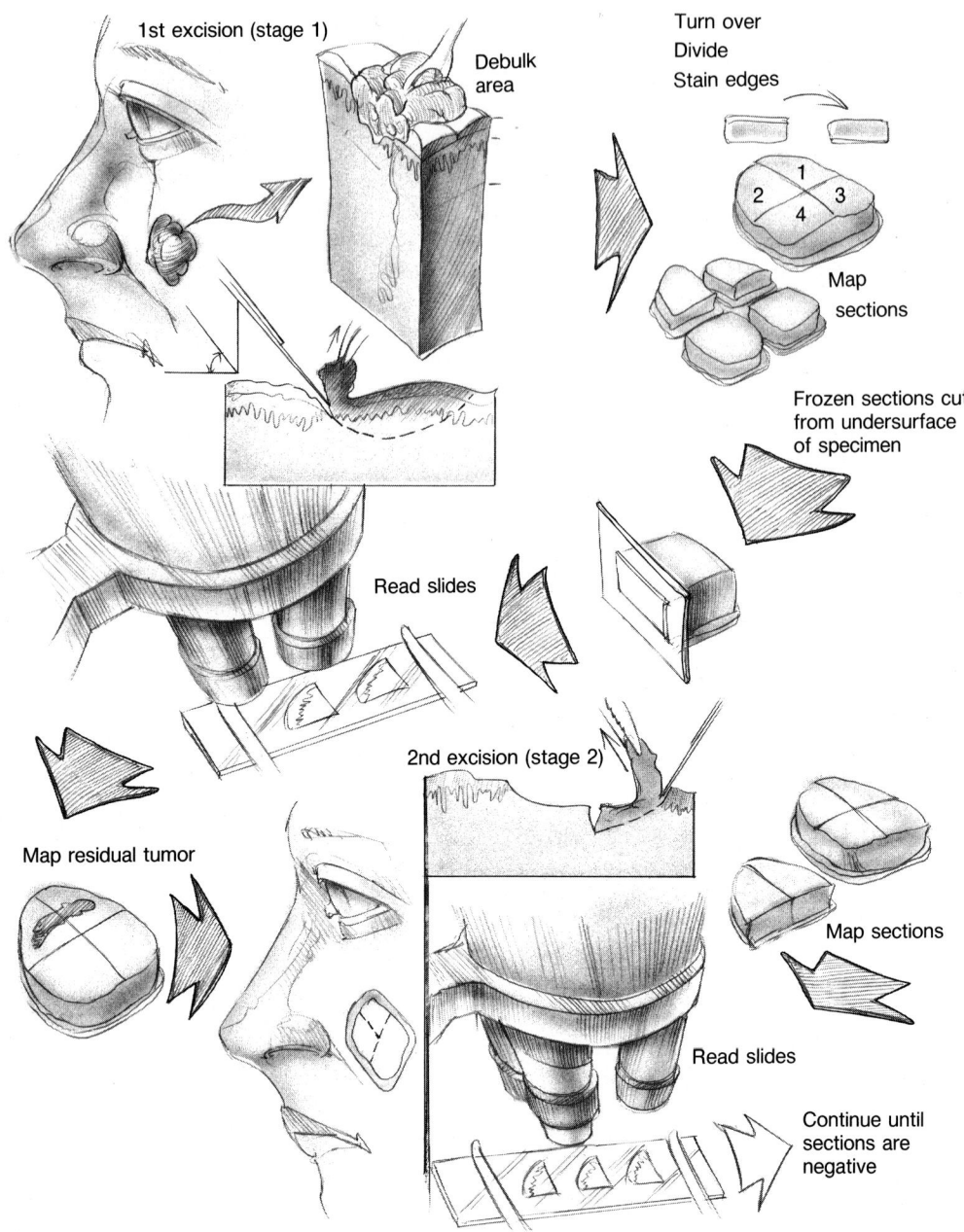

1st excision (stage 1)

Debulk area

Turn over
Divide
Stain edges

Map sections

Frozen sections cut from undersurface of specimen

Read slides

Map residual tumor

2nd excision (stage 2)

Map sections

Read slides

Continue until sections are negative

Figure 113.8 Schema used by micrographic cutaneous tumor excision. (Modified from Mohs FE. Microcontrolled surgery for skin cancer. In: Epstein E, Epstein E, eds. *Skin surgery*. Philadelphia, PA: W.B. Saunders, 1987, with permission.)

conditions render it unwise to use epinephrine in the local anesthesia. Lidocaine without the addition of a vasoconstrictor has a duration of approximately 15 minutes, more than adequate time for the few minutes required to resect most facial lesions in a bloodless fashion with the CO_2 laser. If margins are positive, more anesthesia is infiltrated where required and more tissue removed as needed. After margins are determined to be free of tumor, the area of the local flap is infiltrated and the reconstruction carried out. We have also found laser excision to be of benefit in patients with bleeding disorders.

Another indication for use of the CO_2 laser is the resection or vaporization of small multiple lesions that then require no reconstruction. Lesions as large as 7 to 8 mm can be resected bloodlessly and are left with a physiologic dressing that heals completely within 10 days, resulting in excellent cosmesis. This method is particularly effective in managing multiple premalignant or potentially malignant lesions in patients with skin cancer.

Palliation of the neglected lesion in the very elderly or debilitated patient whose skin cancer is of less concern than more major health considerations is carried out with alacrity using the CO_2 laser. These patients often reside in limited-care facilities, and palliation can be directed toward improved nursing care, better patient comfort, and convenience. These goals prompt some type of treatment,

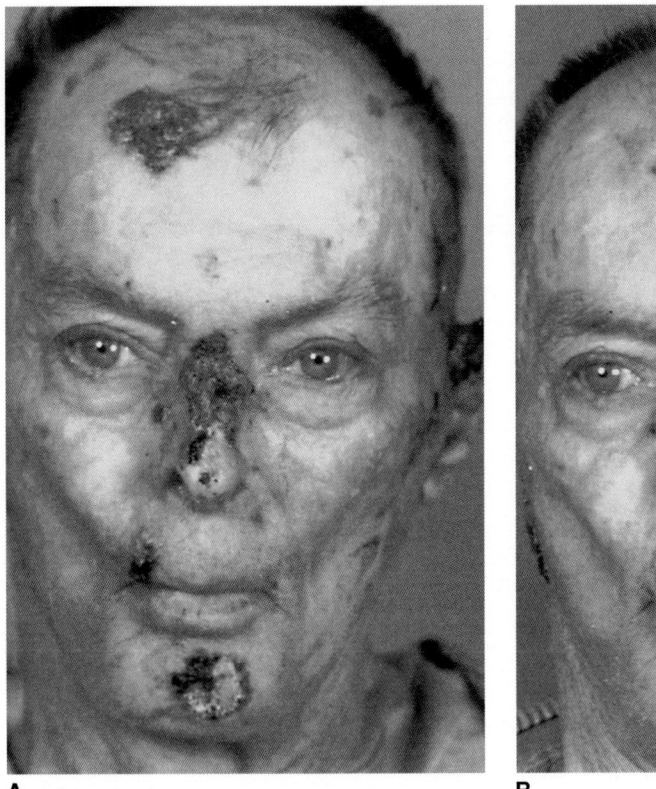

A   B

Figure 113.9 **A:** Multiple basal cell cancers palliated with laser. **B:** Six weeks after laser ablation.

although cure may not be realistic or possible (Fig. 113.9). Success rates for the various treatment modalities of basal cell carcinoma are outlined in Table 113.3. Our approach to management techniques is summarized in Table 113.4.

Surgical Reconstruction

There are three fundamental methods of managing the defects created by excisional surgery for skin cancer: no reconstruction, immediate repair, or delayed reconstruction. The first alternative is used if the wound is allowed to heal by second intention or is covered by a graft and the subsequent defect not reconstructed. This may be appropriate for patients who are palliated or who for other reasons are not candidates for reconstruction. Other patients may be candidates or better served with a prosthesis. The

surgeon's choice is influenced by many factors, such as the general health of the patient and his or her life expectancy. The location and extent of the lesion and the social situation of the patient may play a role in the decisions concerning reconstruction. Large defects are of little concern to some people, but a minimal defect can be devastating to others.

Functional restoration takes precedence over cosmesis if this choice must be made (e.g., reconstruction of the upper lip to ensure a competent oral sphincter before embarking on a nasal reconstruction). Early reconstruction of nasal ala and eyelid defects is of paramount concern because reconstruction after contracture has occurred is rarely satisfactory.

In addition to functional restoration, anatomic, pathologic, and cosmetic considerations influence the surgeon's choice of reconstructive method. Basic to any flap reconstruction is the secondary tissue deficit that, when closed, results in increased tension on the surrounding local tissue. Scar contraction has the potential to distort and create a greater deformity. The use of a skin graft decreases this likelihood by harvesting tissue where there is an abundance, usually some distance from the defect, and substituting this tissue for the resected tumor.

Anatomic considerations control surgical options by imposing constraints such as symmetry, facial landmarks and structures, and the lack of availability of adequate local or adjacent tissue. All flaps create a secondary defect that must be attended to in some manner. This is most often

TABLE 113.3	R̲x TREATMENT BASAL CELL CARCINOMA

Treatment Method	Success Rate (%)
Electrosurgery	81–97
Excisional surgery	86–97
Cryosurgery	83–96
Radiation surgery	90–93
Mohs surgery	97–99

TABLE 113.4	℞ TREATMENT CUTANEOUS MALIGNANCIES

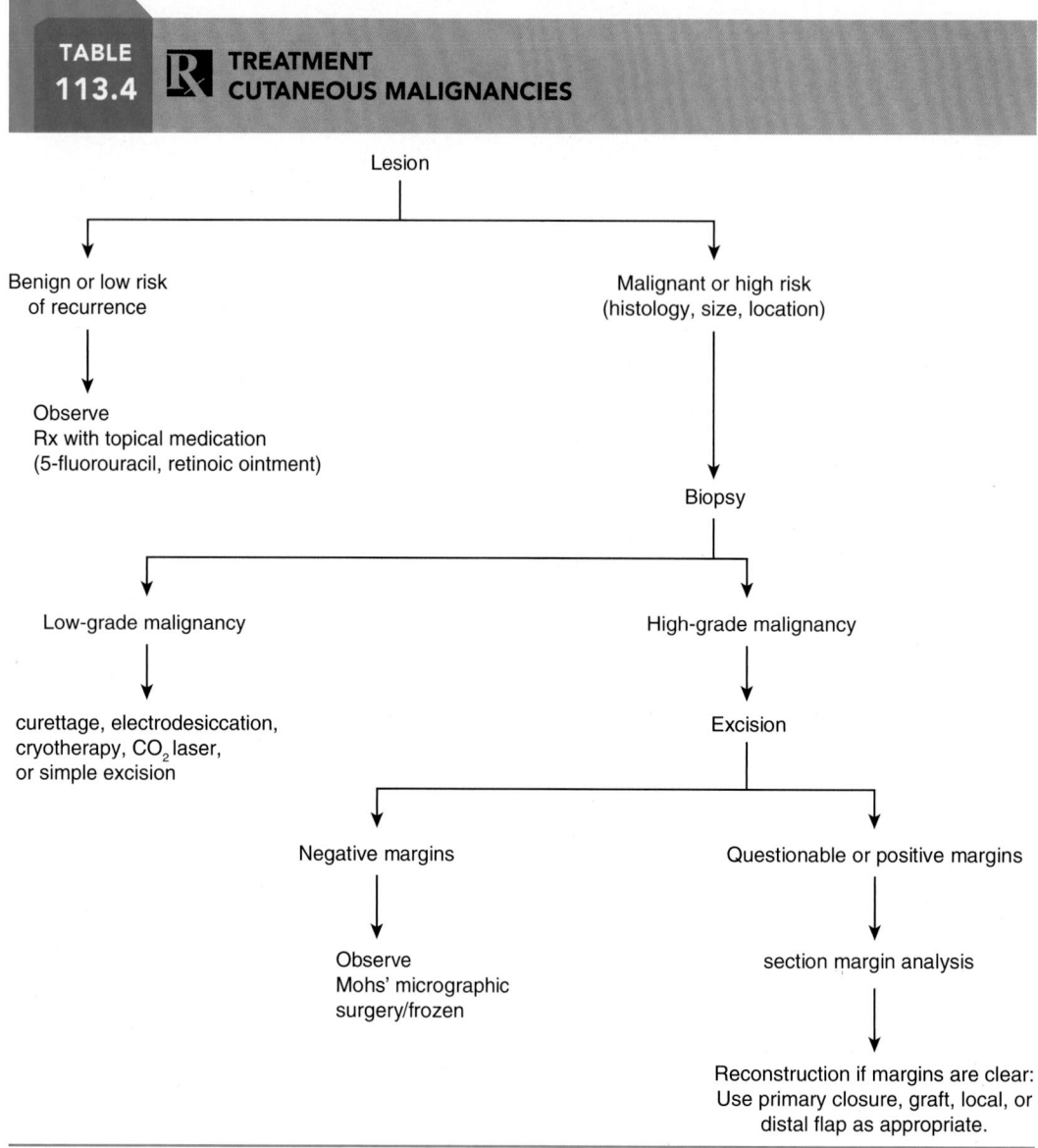

Lesion

Benign or low risk of recurrence

Malignant or high risk (histology, size, location)

Observe
Rx with topical medication
(5-fluorouracil, retinoic ointment)

Biopsy

Low-grade malignancy

High-grade malignancy

curettage, electrodesiccation, cryotherapy, CO$_2$ laser, or simple excision

Excision

Negative margins

Questionable or positive margins

Observe
Mohs' micrographic surgery/frozen

section margin analysis

Reconstruction if margins are clear:
Use primary closure, graft, local, or distal flap as appropriate.

done by primary closure, but the surgeon can use another flap or a graft.

Pathologic considerations influence reconstructive choices. The defects related to certain histologic tumor types might best be covered with a skin graft rather than have potential tumor hidden by a thick flap. Questionable margins are another factor that might prompt a more conservative choice. Tumors located in areas known clinically to be more virulent (e.g., medial canthus, nasal spine, external ear canal) might best not be reconstructed with a thick flap. Squamous cell carcinomas of the skin are usually more aggressive and infiltrative than basal cell carcinomas, and this affects their management. An exception to this is the morphea type of basal cell carcinoma, which is infiltrative. Its iceberg-like subdermal extension may make elaborate reconstructive efforts futile and perhaps devastating for the patient. It is wise to defer immediate reconstruction and allow healing by second intention or cover the defect with

a skin graft. When the recipient bed has a marginal blood supply, delayed skin grafting is recommended. The wound area is allowed to granulate for 21 days. Then a 1- to 2-mm circumferential strip is removed, followed by cross-hatching of the area. A thick (0.45- to 0.5-mm) split-thickness skin graft is placed. If further reconstruction is needed, it can be undertaken when the patient is confirmed to be tumor free, usually after a period of observation of 1 to 2 years.

Planning Reconstruction

In designing local flap reconstruction, the surgeon must first consider the effects on adjacent tissues and structures. It is essential that the tissue to be moved into the defect is lax and abundant enough to close the surgical void. The donor site must also be closed, usually primarily, without unacceptable consequences to adjacent tissues or structures. Utmost in the surgeon's mind must be the placement of incisions. Closure lines should be in skin creases, facial structural demarcations, or relaxed skin tension lines. The tension and direction of maximal pull must not distort, create asymmetry, or result in an unacceptable scar. The ultimate contracture of the resulting scars should not create a deformity.

A review of our surgical cases indicates that the most common management after resection is advancement and primary closure. Obviously, this technique is propitious for most small lesions. For those requiring a more sophisticated form of reconstruction, there are several reliable reconstructive options. Reconstruction options and techniques are discussed in Chapters 162, 166, and 169.

Additional Considerations

In dealing with facial cutaneous malignancies, the temptation to avoid disfigurement is great. Unfortunately, this often results in an inadequate excision, dooming the patient to recurrence and quite possibly a much worse prognosis. Perhaps the most important lesson that the Mohs technique has taught us is the insidious behavior of some cutaneous malignancies. Therefore, margins must always be checked and histology confirmed. Questionable margins should not be reconstructed primarily but instead reconstructed at a later date once margin status has been confirmed on permanent histopathologic analysis.

What may originally be considered a simple excision is occasionally complicated by positive margins. The surgeon must be flexible. If the patient is under local anesthesia, general anesthesia may be needed. If the patient was not aware of the extent of the resection and subsequent repair, the surgeon should stage the surgery and discuss with the patient what may be involved. In considering reconstruction, function is always more important than cosmesis. The surgeon should avoid designing flaps that adversely affect function (i.e., cheek flap producing ectropion).

Regional nodal metastasis from cutaneous basal cell carcinoma is rare, occurring in up to 0.5% of patients (33). Nodal metastasis from cutaneous squamous cell carcinoma occurs in up to 12.5% of patients (34). Thus, in dealing with squamous cell carcinoma, regional lymph nodes must be carefully evaluated. Regional nodal metastasis from cutaneous malignancies in the head and neck most frequently involve the parotid nodes followed by upper cervical nodes. For cutaneous lesions larger than 3 cm, neck dissections or adjuvant therapy should be considered. It is mandatory to follow all patients with cutaneous malignancies, and biopsies should be performed for suspicious areas. Follow-up of patients with basal cell carcinoma should be every 6 months for 5 years as just over one-third of patients will develop a second primary basal cell carcinoma within 5 years. In many patients with skin cancers, constant vigilance is the key to a successful outcome. Potential problems and complications that can occur when managing these cutaneous malignancies are outlined in Table 113.5.

MERKEL CELL CARCINOMA

MCC is a rare but aggressive cutaneous malignancy with a mortality rate more than twice that of melanoma. The incidence of MCC is low relative to other cutaneous malignancies; however, the incidence has tripled from 1986 to 2001 representing an annual increase of 8% (35). MCC appears most frequently in those patients who are white with 95% of newly diagnosed MCC occurring in people over 50 years of age. Currently, approximately 1,500 cases of MCC are diagnosed per year (36).

TABLE 113.5	SUMMARY OF THE DIAGNOSIS, MANAGEMENT, AND COMPLICATIONS ASSOCIATED WITH CUTANEOUS MALIGNANCIES			
Lesion	Diagnosis	Treatment	Closure	Problems or Complications
Superficial basal cell carcinoma	History of sun exposure, red scaly patches, occasionally central ulceration, rolled border	Small: electrodissection and curettage, cryosurgery, excisional biopsy	Primary if excised	Lesion recurs; large excision with frozen section or Mohs surgery
Morpheaform basal cell carcinoma	Macular rough patch, skip lesions, extension down natural fascial planes	Resection often to bone, including periosteum, frozen sections of deep layers	Delay reconstruction if margins are uncertain	Recurrence common; primary excision is aggressive, possible role for adjuvant therapy
Squamous cell carcinoma	Erythematous and patchy, usually history of actinic keratosis, friable	Evaluate regional nodes, neck dissection and postoperative radiation if indicated	Local flap, graft, or distant flap	Recurrent and large lesions; requires large en bloc resection; failure to identify lymph node involvement

Merkel cells, described by Friedrich Merkel in 1875, are large pale cells found in the basal layer of the epidermis that resemble cells of the diffuse neuroendocrine system and function as mechanoreceptors. Indeed it has been demonstrated that Merkel cells are neural crest in origin. Ultrastructurally Merkel cells are characterized by having projections and cytoplasmic dense core granules facing nerve terminals. Merkel cells are highly specific for cytokeratins to include CK-20 as is MCC; thus, MCC is thought to arise from Merkel cells.

MCC most commonly presents in the head and neck as well as the extremities. Indeed 70% to 90% of case of MCC present in these areas. MCC has a propensity to metastasize to regional lymph node basins with regional disease found in 52% to 59% of patients (37). In the clinically N0 necks, 32% have been found to have microscopic evidence of metastasis (38). Distant metastasis is found in 32% to 34% of cases to include, in order of highest frequency, distant skin, lung, central nervous system, bone, and liver (37). Risk factors implicated in the development of MCC include age greater than 50 years, white skin, suppressed immune system, and overexposure to sunlight/UV radiation to include UVB radiation. Merkel cell Polyomarvirus has been identified in some cases of MCC; however, its precise role in MCC remains to be determined.

MCC characteristically presents in an elderly white individual of either sex. The clinical presentation of the lesion itself can be rather nonspecific; however, a common presentation involves the presentations of a rapidly enlarging, nonulcerative, violaceous, nodular cutaneous, or subcutaneous lesion. Indeed on clinical presentation, MCC is rarely suspected and the diagnosis is only made after biopsy. Light microscopy reveals a small blue cell tumor, and the diagnosis is confirmed with immunohistochemistry using

CK-20 (Fig. 113.10). In the head and neck, the periorbital/cheek areas have been reported as the most common sites of involvement. On presentation, 25% of patients have palpable regional adenopathy, and 5% have distant metastatic disease.

With the diagnosis of MCC established via histopathologic analysis of biopsy specimens, workup includes a complete evaluation of the skin and regional lymph nodes. Imaging consists of CT scan, MRI, and PET scanning where appropriate. Primary treatment depends on the staging of MCC as defined by the AJCC (Table 113.6). For lesions where pretreatment staging does not indicate regional or distant metastasis, wide local excision and lymph node assessment is appropriate. Margins ranging from 1 to 2 cm have been advised as well as the use of intraoperative margin analysis to ensure negative resection margins. It has been reported that in the N0 neck, elective lymph node dissection decreased regional recurrence rates and improved survival (39). Pathologic nodal staging is associated with improved survival and a decrease in nodal recurrence. Typically, sentinel node biopsy is performed, and if positive, neck dissection is then performed to optimize the treatment. Postoperative radiation to the primary tumor bed and lymphatics is appropriate to minimize postoperative recurrence. Chemotherapy is typically reserved for those patients with distant metastatic disease.

Despite the method of treatment, the overall recurrence rate ranges from 40% to 75% with over 90% of recurrences occurring within 2 years of the initial diagnosis of MCC. The overall 5-year survival is 30% to 64%; however, those who have developed distant metastasis have an 11% 2-year survival rate (40). Median survival for patients with regional nodal metastatic disease is reported as 11 months.

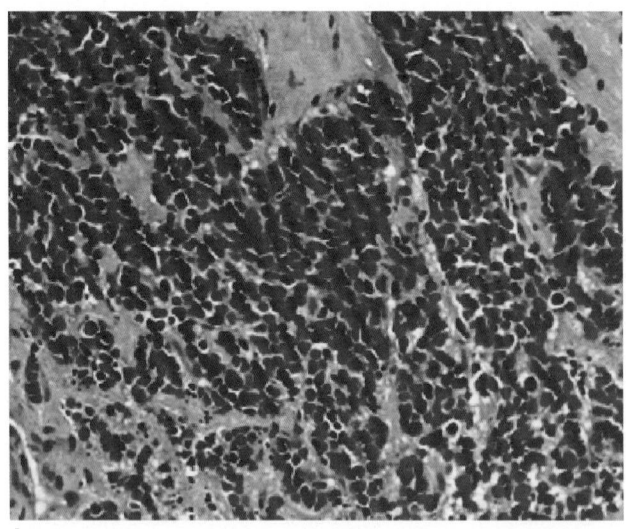

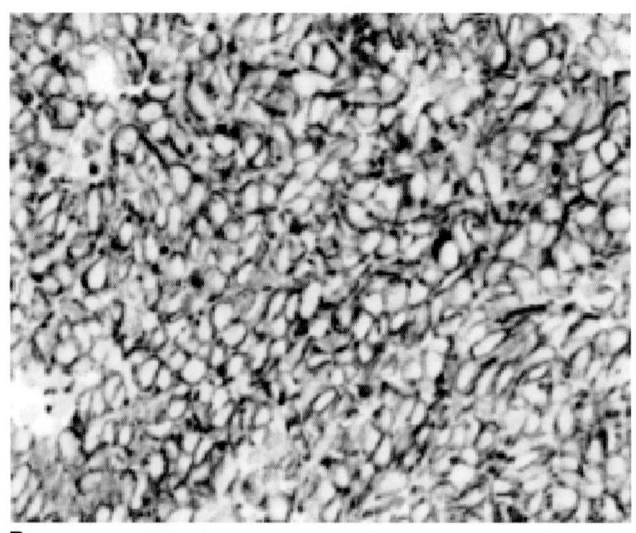

Figure 113.10 A: H & E staining of MCC demonstrating diffuse atypical blue cells with minimal cytoplasm and many mitoses. **B**: MCC positive demonstrating a paranuclear dot staining pattern with CK-20.

TABLE 113.6	AJCC CLASSIFICATION FOR MCC

Primary tumor (T)

TX: Primary tumor cannot be assessed.

T0: No evidence of primary tumor

Tis: Carcinoma *in situ*

T1: Tumor 2 cm or less in greatest dimension

T2: Tumor >2 cm but not more than 5 cm in greatest dimension

T3: Tumor >5 cm in greatest dimension

T4: Tumor invades bone, muscle, fascia, or cartilage

Regional lymph nodes (N)

NX: Nodes cannot be assessed.

N0: No regional lymph node metastasis

cN0: Nodes negative by clinical exam

pN0: Nodes negative by pathologic exam

N1: Regional lymph node metastasis

N1a: Micrometastasis as seen on sentinel node biopsy or elective neck dissection

N1b: Macrometastasis as seen on clinical exam and confirmed by pathologic exam

N2: In transit metastasis

Distant metastasis (M)

M0: No distant metastasis

M1: Distant metastasis beyond regional nodal basin

M1a: Metastasis to skin, subcutaneous tissues, or distant lymph nodes

M1b: Lung metastasis

M1c: Metastasis to other visceral sites

HIGHLIGHTS

- Sun exposure is associated with all forms of skin cancer.
- Unlike other forms of basal cell cancer, the morphea type is particularly difficult to excise because of indistinct margins, skip lesions, and a propensity for deep invasion.
- *De novo* squamous cell cancer tends to be far more aggressive locally and metastatically than cancer that develops after actinic changes.
- High-risk features of cutaneous carcinoma include thickness more than 2 mm, perineural invasion, ear or non–hair-bearing lip involvement, and poorly differentiated or undifferentiated pathology.
- Premalignant and low-grade lesions can be managed by topical chemotherapy (i.e., 5-fluorouracil), electrodesiccation and curettage, or CO_2 laser. All other lesions should be excised with clear margins to maximize success.
- Consider excising additional tissue to incorporate a complete facial unit if more than one-third is involved. This produces a more cosmetic and symmetric repair.

- If confronted with indistinct deep margins or a high probability of recurrence, consider skin grafting and observation for 6 to 12 months.
- Planned reconstruction should never limit oncologic resection.
- If possible, place incisions in a facial crease, hair-bearing areas, junctions of facial units, and parallel to relaxed skin tension lines.
- If using a local facial flap, consider the donor site defect and its effect on functional structures (e.g., eyelid, mouth).
- For MCC, sentinel node biopsy is appropriate if adenopathy is not clinically present.

REFERENCES

1. Rogers, HW, Weinstock, MA, Harris AR, et al. Incidence estimate of nonmelanoma skin cancer in the United States, 2006. *Arch Dermatol* 2010;146(3):283–287.
2. American Cancer Society. *Cancer facts and figures 2010.* Available at: www.cancer.org. Accessed May 2011.
3. Farman J, Gardiner B, Shanklin J. Large losses of total ozone in Antarctica reveal seasonal Clx/NOx interaction. *Nature* 1985;315:207.
4. Cutchis P. Stratospheric ozone depletion and solar ultraviolet radiation on earth. *Science* 1974;184:13.
5. Pleasance ED, Cheetham RK, Stephens PJ, et al. A comprehensive catalogue of somatic mutations from a human cancer genome. *Nature* 2009;463:191–196.
6. Wagner RF, Casciato DA. Skin cancers. In: Casciato DA, Lowitz BB, eds. *Manual of clinical oncology,* 4th ed. Philadelphia, PA: Lippincott Williams & Wilkins, 2000:336–373.
7. Karagas MR, Stannard VA, Mott LA, et al. Use of tanning devices and risk of basal cell and squamous cell skin cancers. *J Natl Cancer Inst* 2002;94:224–226.
8. Bavinck JN, Feltkamp M, Struijk L, et al. Human papillomavirus infection and skin cancer risk in organ transplant recipients. *J Investig Dermatol Sym Proc* 2001;6:207–211.
9. Karagas MR, et al. Genus β human papillomaviruses and incidence of basal cell and squamous cell carcinomas of skin: population based case-control study. *BMJ* 2010;341:c2986.
10. Smith JL. Pathology of skin tumors of the head and neck. In: Thawley SE, Panje WR, eds. *Comprehensive management of head and neck tumors.* Philadelphia, PA: W.B. Saunders, 1985:1173.
11. Pinkus H. Premalignant fibroepithelial tumors of the skin. *Arch Dermatol Syph* 1953;67:598–615.
12. Lever WF. *Histopathology of the skin,* 10th ed. Philadelphia, PA: Lippincott Williams & Watkins, 2009:823–835.
13. Sabin SR, Goldstein G, Rosenthal HG, et al. Aggressive squamous cell carcinoma originating as a Marjolin's ulcer. *Dermatol Surg* 2004;30(2, Part 1):229–230.
14. Yanofsky VR. Histopathological variants of cutaneous squamous cell carcinoma: a review. *J Skin Cancer* 2011;210:813.
15. American Joint Committee on Cancer. Carcinoma of the skin (excluding eyelid, vulva, and penis). In: *American Joint Committee on Cancer: Staging Manual,* 7th ed. New York: Springer, 2010:359–376.
16. Gurudutt VV, Genden EM. Cutaneous squamous cell carcinoma of the head and neck. *J Skin Cancer* February 21, 2011;Article ID 502723.
17. Mohs FE. Chemosurgery for the microscopically controlled excision of skin cancer. *J Surg Oncol* 1971;3:257–267.
18. Swanson NA. Mohs surgery: technique, indications, applications, and the future. *Arch Dermatol* 1983;119:761.
19. Levine HL, Bailin PL. Basal cell carcinoma of the head and neck: identification of the high risk patient. *Laryngoscope* 1980;90:955.

20. Robinson JK, Fisher SG. Recurrent basal cell carcinoma after incomplete resection. *Arch Dermatol* 2000;136(11):1318–1324.

21. Jackson R, Adams RH. Horrifying basal cell carcinoma: a study of 33 cases and a comparison with 435 non-horror cases and a report of four metastatic cases. *J Surg Oncol* 1973;5:431.

22. Levine H. Cutaneous carcinoma of the head and neck: management of massive and previously uncontrolled lesions. *Laryngoscope* 1983;93:87.

23. Ceilley RI, Del Rosso JQ. Current modalities and new advances in the treatment of basal cell carcinoma. *Int J Dermatol* 2006;45(5):489–498.

24. Thissen MR, Nieman FH, Ideler AH, et al. Cosmetic results of cryosurgery versus surgical excision for primary uncomplicated basal cell carcinomas of the head and neck. *Dermatol Surg* 2000;26:759–764.

25. Hernández-Machin B, Borrego L, Gil-García M, et al. Office-based radiation therapy for cutaneous carcinoma: evaluation of 710 treatments. *Int J Dermatol* 2007;46(5):453–459.

26. Carruth JAS, McKenzie AL. Preliminary report of a pilot study of photoradiation therapy for the treatment of superficial malignancies of the skin, head and neck. *Eur J Surg Oncol* 1985;11:47–50.

27. Greenway HT, Cornell RC, Tanner DJ, et al. Treatment of BCC with intralesional interferon. *J Am Acad Dermatol* 1986;15:437–443.

28. Kim KH, Yavel RM, Gross VL, et al. Intralesional interferon alpha-2b in the treatment of basal cell carcinoma and squamous cell carcinoma: revisited. *Dermatol Surg* 2004;30:1116–1120.

29. Nagore E, Grau C, Molinero J, et al. Positive margins in basal cell carcinoma: relationship to clinical features and recurrence risk. A retrospective study of 248 patients. *J Eur Acad Dermatol Venereol* 2003;17:167–170.

30. Mohs FE. Chemosurgery: a microscopically uncontrolled method of cancer excision. *Arch Surg* 1941;42:279.

31. Mohs FE. Microcontrolled surgery for skin cancer. In: Epstein E, Epstein E, eds. *Skin surgery*. Philadelphia, PA: W.B. Saunders, 1987.

32. Tromovitch TA, Stegman SJ. Microscopically controlled excision of skin tumors. Chemosurgery (Mohs): fresh tissue technique. *Arch Dermatol* 1974;110:231.

33. Malone JP. Basal cell carcinoma metastatic to the parotid: report of a new case and review of the literature. *ENT* 2000;79:511.

34. Cherpelis BS, Marcusen C, Lang PG. Prognostic factors for metastasis in squamous cell carcinoma of the skin. *Dermatol Surg* 2002;28:268–273.

35. Hodgson NC. Merkel cell carcinoma: changing incidence trends. *J Surg Oncol* 2005;89:1–4.

36. Lemos B, Nghiem P. Merkel cell carcinoma: more deaths but still no pathway to blame. *J Investig Dermatol* 2007;127:2100–2103.

37. Medina-Franco H, Urist MM, Fiveash J, et al. Multimodality treatment of Merkel cell carcinoma: case series and literature review of 1024 cases. *Ann Surg Oncol* 2001;8:204–208.

38. Gupta SG, Wang LC, Gellenthin M, et al. Sentinel lymph node biopsy for evaluation and treatment of patients with Merkel cell carcinoma: the Dana-Farber experience and meta-analysis of the literature. *Arch Dermatol* 2006;142(6):685–690.

39. Lawenda BD, Thiringer JK, Foss RD, et al. Merkel cell carcinoma arising in the head and neck: optimizing therapy. *Am J Clin Oncol* 2001;24:35–42.

40. Allen PJ, Bowne WB, Jaques DP, et al. Merkel cell carcinoma: prognosis and treatment of patients from a single institution. *J Clin Oncol* 2005;23:2300–2309.

Malignant Melanoma of the Head and Neck Region

Aaron J. Berger   **Jeffrey N. Myers**   **Andrew J. Nemechek**
Mike Yao

The incidence of cutaneous malignant melanoma (CMM) continues to increase at a remarkable rate, and mortality from this disease also continues to rise. Despite our best attempts to understand the molecular basis of CMM, only recently have some of the critical molecular determinants of this disease been uncovered and used as a basis for new medical treatments. Thus, successful treatment of this disease relies heavily upon the surgeon. In this chapter, we will review some of the recent developments in the staging, evaluation, and treatment of CMM and present guidelines for treatment and management of melanoma of the head and neck.

EPIDEMIOLOGY

Despite an overall modest decrease in cancer incidence and cancer-related deaths over the past 20 years (largely related to lung, colon, breast, and prostate cancers), melanoma incidence rates and deaths continue to rise yearly. In the United States alone for 2013, it is estimated that 76,690 new melanoma cases will be diagnosed, and 9,480 deaths will be attributed to melanoma (1). While melanoma accounts for roughly 4% of all skin cancers, it is responsible for more than 77% of skin cancer deaths.

The major risk factors for development of cutaneous melanoma include fair complexion, tendency to sunburn easily, large congenital nevi (greater than 20 cm), presence of atypical/dysplastic nevi (2,3), a personal history of skin cancer (melanoma or otherwise) (4–7), genetic predisposition (8), and immunosuppression (9). Head and neck melanomas occur more commonly in men (2:1), with a median age at diagnosis of 55 years, and a range of 12 to 92 years (10).

Epidemiologic studies demonstrate higher rates of melanoma in those living in geographic areas that are exposed to intense sunlight (i.e., Australia). This finding and investigations in the laboratory demonstrate that exposure to ultraviolet light plays a major role in the pathogenesis of melanoma, and UV-A and UV-B radiation have both been implicated. This is further supported by the lower rates of melanoma reported in people whose skin natively has more pigmentation, and the incidence of melanoma is approximately 10 times higher in whites than in blacks in the same geographic region (11).

Although the combined head and neck region accounts for only 9% of body surface area, 15% to 30% of all melanomas arise within the head and neck (12,13). Multiple factors may contribute to this anatomic predilection for the skin of the head and neck, including higher levels of sun exposure and melanocyte content of the skin that is two- to threefold higher than other regions (14). Of note, melanomas arising on the face and scalp are associated with higher rates of local recurrence and regional lymph node disease than melanomas arising in other parts of the body.

CLINICAL PRESENTATION AND DIAGNOSIS

The classic hallmark finding that raises suspicion for malignant melanoma is the presence of a pigmented lesion that changes over a period of weeks to months. Lesions that change substantially in size or color over time should prompt medical attention. Other features of pigmented lesions, which should alert one to the possibility of a malignant process, include changes in diameter or height, variations in border, color, ulceration, itching, pain, and bleeding (15). Melanomas also may show signs of regression with involution of a primary lesion, which is often manifested by a "halo" lesion with a central area of decreased pigmentation. However, the clinical diagnosis of this disease may not always be straightforward; not all melanomas are pigmented. As many as 10% of melanomas may lack melanin, some may resemble other cutaneous lesions such as basal cell carcinoma, and some tumors may not have a surface component. Patients also may be seen initially with metastasis to cervical lymph nodes with no identifiable primary tumor.

Once a suspicion of melanoma exists, relevant historic factors associated with increased risk of developing this disease should be ascertained. These factors include a history of childhood sun exposure with episodes of severe sunburns and a family history of cutaneous malignancies, including melanomas. Other types of pigmented lesions are important to note as well. These include junctional or acquired nevi that are found in the skin of most adults and are generally smaller than 5 mm. Dysplastic nevi tend to be larger and have irregular borders with variation in color. The identification of a dysplastic nevus should prompt dermatologic evaluation and excision because of an increased risk of developing a malignant melanoma within these lesions.

When a patient's skin lesion is suggestive of malignant melanoma by both history and physical examination, biopsy is performed. The clinician should document clearly the presence or absence of ulceration before biopsy, as this plays a role in staging. The technique for obtaining tissue for pathologic analysis has been the subject of considerable debate. A properly performed biopsy not only establishes a diagnosis but also provides critical prognostic data and assists in formulating a specific treatment plan. The type of biopsy is dictated by factors such as the size of the lesion and its anatomic location in relation to vital structures in the head, face, and neck. The site of origin of a primary melanoma in the head and neck also can be of prognostic significance, because lesions of the scalp and neck are associated with a worse prognosis than are melanomas of the face. Excisional biopsies are the favored technique to obtain tissue for diagnosis, and several studies have demonstrated an association between decreased survival and incisional or manipulative biopsies (16). Excision is performed with a narrow margin of normal-appearing tissue and should include subcutaneous fat for complete evaluation of the depth.

After excisional biopsy, the specimen is oriented and discussed with the pathologist. If the lesion's size or other anatomic or cosmetic constraints preclude excision, incisional or punch biopsy techniques are acceptable alternatives. Shave biopsies are acceptable, but should only be performed by experienced practitioners to ensure that the biopsy fully assesses the thickness of the lesion, or in cases with low suspicion. All biopsy techniques should sample the most representative portion of the lesion. Punch biopsy may include sampling the most raised area of the lesion or an area with the most pigmentation. Lesions with variable heights, colors, and borders may require biopsies of multiple areas to be performed for accurate and proper diagnosis. Traditional stains such as hematoxylin–eosin are used. The immunohistochemical stains S-100, HMB-45, and melan-A have helped standardize pathologic evaluation of cutaneous lesions (Fig. 114.2).

Fine-needle aspiration and curettage techniques have no role in evaluation of suspected invasive cutaneous melanoma, as they are inadequate in providing precise information regarding the depth of invasion. It should also be clearly stated that the initial excisional biopsy with negative margins is not considered adequate therapy for invasive melanoma but does allow re-excision with the opportunity to perform lymphatic mapping and sentinel lymph node biopsy (SLNB) at the time of re-excision.

MELANOMA SUBTYPES

Melanoma is divided into four distinct clinicopathologic subtypes: lentigo maligna melanoma (LMM), superficial spreading, nodular, and acral lentiginous melanoma. These lesions demonstrate either a radial (intraepithelial) or vertical (intradermal) growth phase or a combination of the two. Radial growth is circumferential in nature and confined to the dermal–epidermal junction. The vertical growth phase (intradermal) demonstrates invasion through the dermal–epidermal junction. The radial growth phase may indicate a lesion's capacity for growth and invasion into the papillary dermis. These lesions may lack metastatic potential. Conversely, cells in the vertical growth phase may represent a clonal change in cells with a growth advantage over neighboring cells, resulting in the clone's ability to invade and metastasize.

Cutaneous melanomas may mimic a host of other pathologic cutaneous lesions.

Differential diagnosis includes seborrheic keratosis, benign nevi (including junctional, compound, and dermal), hemangioma, blue nevi, pyogenic granuloma, and pigmented basal cell carcinoma.

Lentigo maligna (LM), also known as melanoma *in situ*, is a premalignant pigmented lesion that frequently develops in the head and neck region of elderly patients (Fig. 114.1A). Known historically as Hutchinson melanotic freckle, these lesions are associated with solar skin damage and feature atypical melanocytes, which spread radially along the dermal–epidermal junction, exhibit focal nesting, and occasionally extend along skin appendages into the dermis. Up to 5% of LMs or melanomas in situ progress to invasive LMM. LMM lesions should be excised with 0.5- to 1.0-cm margins, although prediction of tumor margins can prove difficult. This is the least common type of cutaneous melanoma and accounts for between 6% and 10% of melanoma lesions. Its growth is characterized by a slow radial phase that may take up to 10 years to progress. At first, they are quite slow to invade deeply, and affected patients have a better prognosis when compared with those with other forms of melanoma.

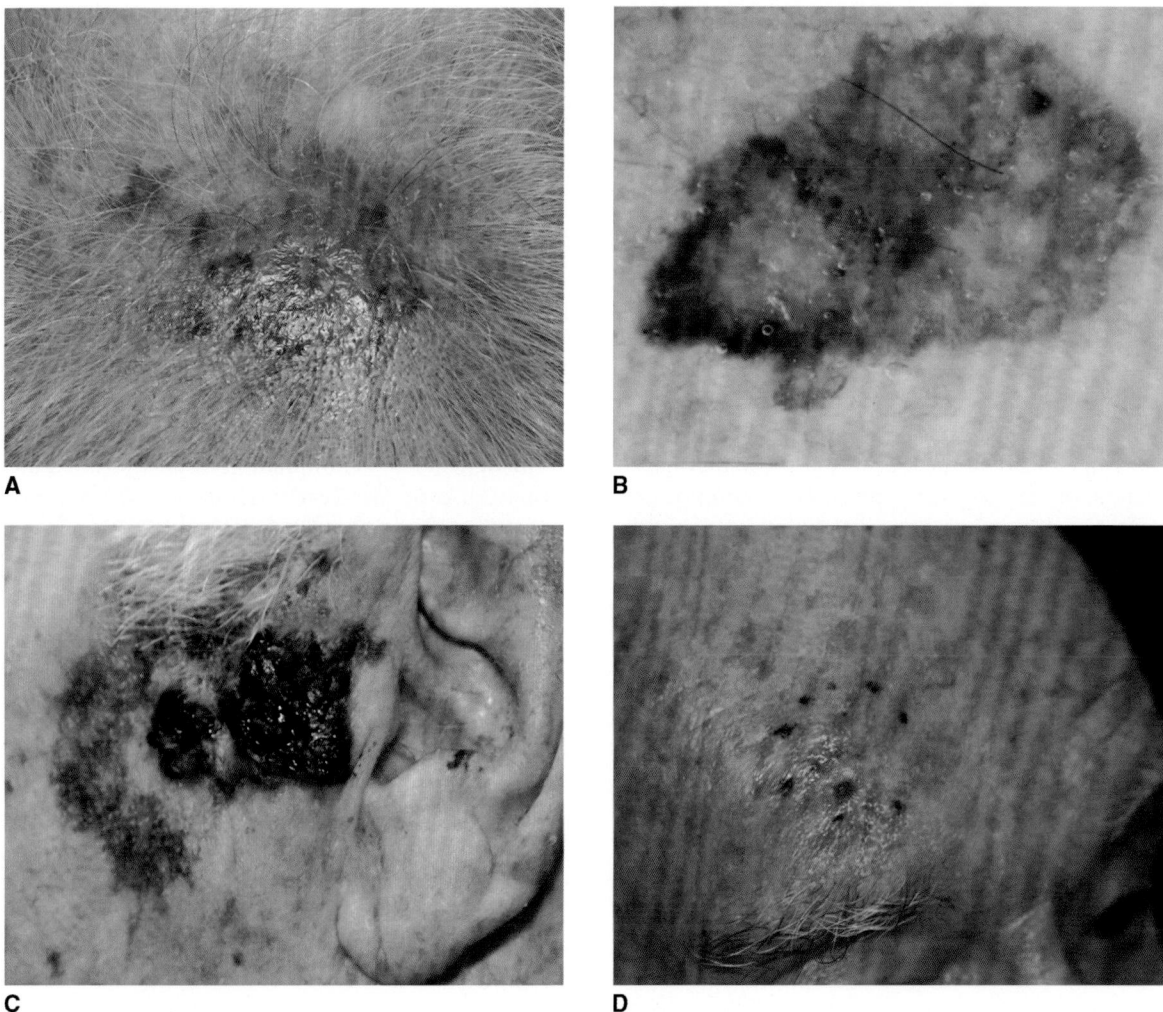

Figure 114.1 Photographs of the different subtypes of melanoma. **A:** Lentigo maligna invasive melanoma, Breslow depth 1.35 mm, Clark's level IV, no ulceration, mitotic index of 4, sentinel lymph nodes negative. **B:** Superficial spreading melanoma, Breslow depth 1.36 mm, Clark's level III, no ulceration, mitotic index of 5, sentinel lymph nodes negative. **C:** Nodular melanoma, Breslow depth of at least 3.9 mm, no ulceration, mitotic index of 4, sentinel lymph node negative. Case confounded by concurrent chronic lymphocytic leukemia. **D:** Desmoplastic melanoma, Breslow depth of 9 mm, Clark's level V, ulcerated, mitotic index of 5, sentinel lymph nodes negative. An SLNB was performed because the initial biopsy showed a spindle cell melanoma that was not thought to be a desmoplastic melanoma.

Superficial spreading melanoma represents the most common type of melanoma and comprises between 65% and 75% of cases (Fig. 114.1B). These lesions may demonstrate a wide variety of colors, including pink, blue–gray, brown, tan, and black. They also may demonstrate radial growth for 5 to 7 years and then become invasive, an event frequently heralded by ulceration and bleeding. High cure rates have been reported when these lesions are clinically detected in the radial growth phase. Spontaneous regression of superficial spreading melanomas also has been reported.

Acral lentiginous is the most common type of melanoma seen in the African American population. Because these lesions commonly occur on the soles of the feet, surfaces of the hand, and oral/anogenital mucosa, head and neck surgeons less commonly encounter them.

Nodular melanoma comprises between 10% and 15% of all melanomas and may affect areas of both exposed and non–sun-exposed areas of the skin (Fig. 114.1C). They tend to develop in patients older than 50 years. Nodular melanoma is considered to be the most invasive of the cutaneous melanomas, and affected patients have the poorest prognosis.

Desmoplastic melanoma is a histologic variant of melanoma that accounts for fewer than 1% of melanoma cases overall (Fig. 114.1D). However, as many as 75% of these tumors occur in the head and neck region. Clinically, desmoplastic melanomas may be amelanotic, a feature that impedes early recognition and often leads to significant delays in diagnosis and treatment. Another important characteristic feature of these lesions is their neurotropism.

This predisposes them to perineural invasion and spread that often accounts for local recurrence despite histologically "negative margins" with recurrence rates reported between 23% and 48% (17–22). Therefore, it is suggested that wider resection margins be taken around a desmoplastic tumor and that adjuvant radiation is often recommended after definitive excision. Multiple studies have demonstrated a lower rate of regional nodal spread in patients with desmoplastic melanoma as compared to other histologic subtypes of melanoma (23–27). The lower rate of positive sentinel lymph nodes has made the role of SLNB in this population less widely recommended (25). However, a distinction needs to be made between those lesions which are purely desmoplastic and are associated with a low rate of nodal metastasis and those that have a combination of desmoplastic and a more conventional melanoma histology which spread to lymph nodes at the higher frequency associated with the nondesmoplastic histology (25,26). Therefore, SLNB can be recommended in the combined desmoplastic cases, which meet other criteria for performing the biopsy such as depth of invasion, number of mitoses, and/or ulceration.

MUCOSAL MELANOMA

A relatively rare entity, mucosal melanoma deserves special mention. Primary melanoma may arise in the mucosa of the respiratory, alimentary, and genitourinary tracts, as they all contain melanocytes. Mucosal melanoma accounts for 1% to 2% of all melanomas, with the majority being found in the head and neck region (28). More than 50% of reported cases arise within the nasal cavity. Other affected areas include the paranasal sinuses, nasopharynx, oral cavity, and oropharynx. Esophageal mucosa can also be affected. Nasal obstruction is the most common presenting symptom for sinonasal lesions. However, a significant number of mucosal melanomas may be asymptomatic until they have progressed to an advanced stage, which contributes to the poor prognosis of patients with this diagnosis. Stern and colleagues (29) at the M.D. Anderson Cancer Center found an average of 9 months between the first onset of symptoms and physician intervention. In addition to delay in diagnosis, the poorer prognosis associated with mucosal melanomas may also be related to an inherently more aggressive behavior of mucosal melanomas, or earlier dissemination, because of the rich lymphatic and vascular supply of the mucosa.

The differential diagnosis includes vascular lesions, angiomas, and dental amalgam tattoos. It is not uncommon for the characteristic melanosis to be absent in mucosal melanoma lesions. Biopsy is usually confirmatory, and immunohistochemistry may be used to assist in diagnosis. Desmoplastic variants of mucosal melanoma have been described in the head and neck (30). No studies have conclusively demonstrated that depth of invasion is of prognostic importance in mucosal melanoma.

The majority of these patients have a poor prognosis. These tumors have a high rate of local recurrence, which is typically a harbinger of disseminated disease, and most of these patients die from complications related to distant metastases.

Anatomic constraints frequently preclude the use of excisional biopsy techniques in most patients with mucosal melanoma. Although wide local excision is the mainstay of therapy, radiation therapy has been used as a primary modality and postoperative adjuvant therapy with unclear benefit (31–33). It should especially be considered in situations when adequate resection margin is not possible, where it may help prevent local recurrence (34).

Patients may experience multiple local recurrences and ultimately die of a combination of uncontrolled local and distant disease. Five-year survival rates for mucosal melanoma range between 10% and 45% (35–39).

MELANOMA STAGING SYSTEM

The staging of malignant melanoma has evolved over the past half century in efforts to more reliably determine prognosis and to identify the most appropriate treatment schemes. Clark and Breslow made significant contributions to the microscopic grading of primary cutaneous melanoma. Clark (40) described five levels of anatomic invasion through the layers of the skin. In the Breslow system (41), the maximum thickness of melanomas is used as a prognostic indicator.

The current staging system for melanoma developed by the American Joint Committee on Cancer (AJCC) and adopted by the International Union for Cancer Control, relies upon assessment of the primary tumor (T), regional lymph nodes (N), and distant metastatic sites (M). The seventh, and most recent, edition of this staging system is based upon long-term analysis of over 38,900 patients with cutaneous melanoma (42) (Table 114.1).

Primary Tumor

Tumor thickness, presence or absence of ulceration, and mitotic rate are the histopathologic details factored into staging, as they have been demonstrated to correlate closely with prognosis. Clark level has clinical utility in the evaluation and treatment of patients with thin melanomas, and thus, is only included in the staging of melanomas less than or equal to 1 mm in thickness.

Regional Nodal Staging

Regional nodal status is the most powerful predictor of survival for patients with melanoma (43) and has led to the widespread adoption of SLNB in the evaluation of patients with primary cutaneous melanomas. For patients with clinically detectable lymph nodes on presentation, regional imaging (CT or MRI) as well as fine-needle aspiration

TABLE 114.1	CUTANEOUS MELANOMA TNM STAGING

Melanoma TNM Classification

T Classification	Thickness	Ulceration Status
T_{is}	Not applicable	Not applicable
T1	≤1.0 mm	A: w/o ulceration and mitosis <1/mm^2
		B: with ulceration or mitosis ≥1/mm^2
T2	1.01–2.0 mm	A: w/o ulceration
		B: with ulceration
T3	2.01–4.0 mm	A: w/o ulceration
		B: with ulceration
T4	>4.0 mm	A: w/o ulceration
		B: with ulceration

N Classification	Number of Metastatic Nodes	Nodal Metastatic Mass
N1	One node	A: micrometastasis[a]
		B: macrometastasis[b]
N2	—Two to three nodes	A: micrometastasis[a]
		B: macrometastasis[b]
		C: in-transit met(s)/satellite(s) *without* metastatic nodes
N3	Four or more metastatic nodes, or matted nodes, or in-transit met(s)/ satellite(s) *with* metastatic node(s)	

M Classification	Site	Serum LDH
M1a	Distant skin, subcutaneous, or nodal metastases	Normal
M1b	Lung metastases	Normal
M1c	All other visceral metastases	Normal
	Any distant metastasis	Elevated

[a]Micrometastases are diagnosed after sentinel or elective lymphadenectomy.
[b]Macrometastases are defined as clinically detectable nodal metastases confirmed by therapeutic lymphadenectomy or when nodal metastasis exhibits gross extracapsular extension.
Used with the permission of the American Joint Committee on Cancer (AJCC), Chicago, Illinois. The original and primary source for this information is the AJCC Cancer Staging Manual, Seventh Edition (2010) published by Springer Science and Business Media LLC (SBM).

may be performed to confirm the presence of melanoma; if found, therapeutic lymph node dissection and systemic staging are recommended (Fig. 114.2). The extent of dissection remains controversial and will be addressed later in this chapter.

The decision to perform SLNB is typically based upon characteristics of the primary tumor, as the risk of regional metastasis is known to correlate with tumor thickness and ulceration (44–48); high mitotic rate and younger patient age have also been associated with SLN positivity rates (49–51). With respect to SLN status, patients with T1 lesions have a 3% to 5% risk of SLN positivity; T2, 8% to 12%; T3, 23% to 27%; and T4, 24% to 44% (46,50,52).

When reporting the pathologic nodal status after SLNB or a more comprehensive lymphadenectomy, it is important to include the number of nodes involved (53), micro- versus macrometastases (53), and the presence or absence of in-transit metastases. In-transit metastases are a unique manifestation of intralymphatic tumor dissemination, characterized by the presence of melanoma in either cutaneous or subcutaneous tissue situated between the primary tumor and the draining regional lymph node basin (54). In

early stage disease, these develop in 2% to 13% of patients (55,56), and based on poor patient outcomes associated with their presence, they are considered equivalent to the presence of significant nodal disease (Table 114.1).

The prognosis for patients with microscopic metastases found at the time of SLNB (67% 5-year survival) is better than for patients with macroscopic metastases detected clinically (43% 5-year survival) (57). For patients with microscopic metastases, the number of tumor containing nodes is the most important prognostic indicator followed by the mitotic rate (57). For patients with macroscopic metastases, the number of nodes, primary ulceration, and patient age are the most important prognostic factors (57). Buzaid et al. (58) showed that the number of lymph nodes involved with regional metastases is more predictive of treatment outcomes than is the size of lymph nodes harboring metastatic disease.

In the head and neck, lateralized tumors may drain into the primary echelon nodal basins, including preauricular, parotid, postauricular, suboccipital, posterior cervical, anterior cervical (external or internal jugular), and supraclavicular nodal groups. Nodal drainage basins in the

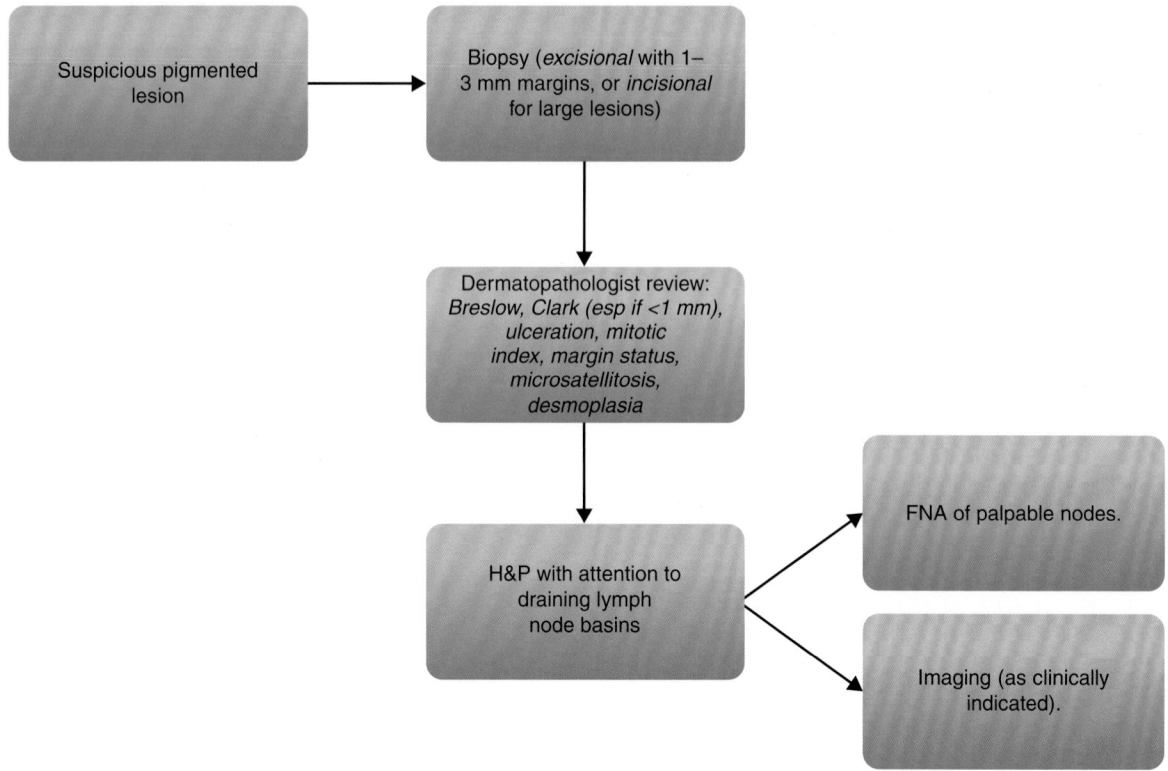

Figure 114.2 Initial management of cutaneous melanoma (Adapted from NCCN). H&P, History and Physical Examination; FNA, Fine-needle aspiration.

head and neck are less predictable when compared with trunk and extremity sites. Although some areas on the scalp, face, and ears may have predictable lymphatic drainage, bilateral or contralateral metastases are not uncommon, and ambiguous drainage patterns can be seen in up to 55% of patients (59). Preoperative and intraoperative lymphoscintigraphy helps to precisely define an individual's pattern of lymphatic drainage in primary melanomas of the head and neck region (60).

Metastatic Workup

The National Comprehensive Cancer Network (NCCN) guidelines for melanoma do not recommend routine use of imaging studies such as CT, MRI, or PET scans for the systemic staging of patients with thin melanomas (stage I and II) since the risk of distant metastasis is exceedingly low in this group of patients (61). For patients with thin melanomas with adverse features such as positive deep margins, lymphovascular invasion, or mitotic rate greater than 1 per mm^2, imaging is recommended only to investigate specific signs or symptoms that may be attributable to a metastatic lesion.

For patients with stage III melanomas (metastatic disease in a lymph node, satellite, or in-transit metastases), the NCCN guidelines do not make specific recommendations and leave the workup to the discretion of the treating physician. Without any signs or symptoms, the likelihood

of finding an occult metastatic lesion with screening CT or PET scan is low.

For stage IV (distant metastases), the NCCN guidelines recommend an LDH level plus chest x-ray and/or chest CT (Fig. 114.3). A brain MRI or CT scan with contrast should be performed if the patients have even minimal suggestions of symptoms or physical findings of brain involvement or if the results would affect treatment decisions. LDH levels have been shown to correlate with melanoma-specific survival (62). Nevertheless, in our practices, in order to help select and prioritize treatments for patients with Stage III or IV disease, we will often perform systemic imaging to include and brain MRI and either a PET/CT or CT of the head and neck, chest, abdomen, and pelvis. As an example, a patient presenting with regional nodal metastatic disease found to have distant metastatic disease on systemic imaging might be offered systemic treatment rather than surgery and radiation as initial treatment. Thus, we find imaging quite helpful in these instances to make informed treatment decisions.

DETECTION OF OCCULT LYMPH NODE DISEASE

As stated previously, the most powerful predictor of survival is lymph node status. In patients with lesions less than 0.75 mm in depth, lymph node observation is appropriate. Patients with lesions between 0.76–1.0 mm in depth, without ulceration and less than 1 mitosis per mm^2

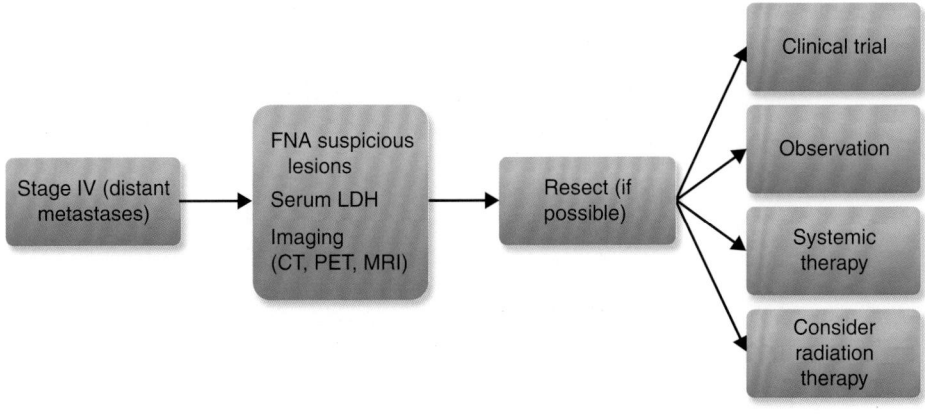

Figure 114.3 Management of metastatic melanoma (Adapted from NCCN).

should consider lymph node evaluation. Patients with lesions between 0.76–1.0 mm in depth with ulceration or ≥1 mitosis per mm^2 or with lesions >1 mm with any characteristic should be offered lymph node evaluation. Of the two main ways of evaluating for occult lymph node metastases, SLNB has supplanted elective lymph node dissection (ELND) as the preferred method.

The rationale for determination of nodal status is to appropriately stage patients and to identify patients who may benefit from regional therapy with surgery, radiation, or both to improve locoregional control. The goal is to also identify patients at greater risk for systemic recurrence who could potentially benefit from systemic adjuvant therapy.

Elective Lymph Node Dissection

The utility of ELND in the initial management of patients with CMM of intermediate-thickness or thicker lesions is questionable in the current era of SLNB. In terms of using ELND to attempt surgical cure, four prospective randomized clinical trials failed to show a benefit from ELND in melanoma (63–66). However, data from the World Health Organization (WHO) Melanoma group Trial 14 and the Intergroup Melanoma Surgical Trial suggest that certain subgroups of patients may benefit from ELND (44,67,68). In particular, patients in the WHO study with truncal melanoma greater than 1.5 mm thick and microscopic regional nodal disease had improved survival compared to those patients in whom lymph node dissection was delayed until they developed palpable lymphadenopathy (5-year survival 48.2% vs. 26.9%, $P = 0.04$). In the intergroup study, patients younger than 60, with nonulcerated primary lesions 1 to 2 mm thick, had a survival benefit from ELND. While these studies demonstrate survival benefits in select groups of melanoma patients with clinically undetectable disease, the majority of patients (80% to 85%) will not have occult metastases.

The development of SLNB has enhanced the sensitivity and specificity of lymph node biopsy, and it has replaced ELND, a procedure with greater potential morbidity and disability, in the *initial* assessment of regional metastatic disease in patients with CMM of the head and neck region.

Sentinel Lymph Node Identification and Biopsy

Seminal work by Dr. Donald Morton (14) and others has supported the hypothesis that, within each nodal basin, an orderly progression of lymphatic drainage is found from a first-echelon or sentinel node to nodes of lower echelons. This implies that if one can identify the sentinel lymph node in a basin at risk for spread from a melanoma and find it to be free of metastasis, then the remainder of nodes in that basin should also be free of metastatic tumor. This concept has been subsequently supported in a number of trials for non–head and neck CMM. Universal adoption of SLNB for CMM of the head and neck was somewhat delayed secondary to the belief that nodal drainage patterns in the head and neck region might be too complex to make SLNB feasible. Eicher et al. were among the first to dispel this notion (69), demonstrating SLNs in 98% of patients in whom SLNB was performed in the context of a regional lymphadenectomy in patients with intermediate-thickness cutaneous melanomas in the head and neck region. No patients were found to have a positive non-SLN when the SLN was negative. Overall, studies reflect that the predictive value of a negative SLN approaches 99% and that the SLNB procedure has a low false-negative rate (less than 4%) (70,71); however, this rate may be slightly higher in head and neck melanomas as compared to the trunk or extremities (72). Studies of SLNB for patients with head and neck primary melanomas report a range of regional recurrence from 2% to 8% in patients who had negative SLN (67,70,72).

Patients with melanomas ≤0.75 mm in depth with or without adverse characteristics are not offered sentinel lymph node biopsy. Patients with melanomas 0.76–1.0 mm in depth without ulceration and <1 mitosis per mm^2 should consider SLNB. Patients with melanomas 0.76–1.0 mm in depth with ulceration or ≥1 mitosis per mm^2, or >1 mm in depth with any characteristic should be offered SLNB (61) (Fig. 114.4).

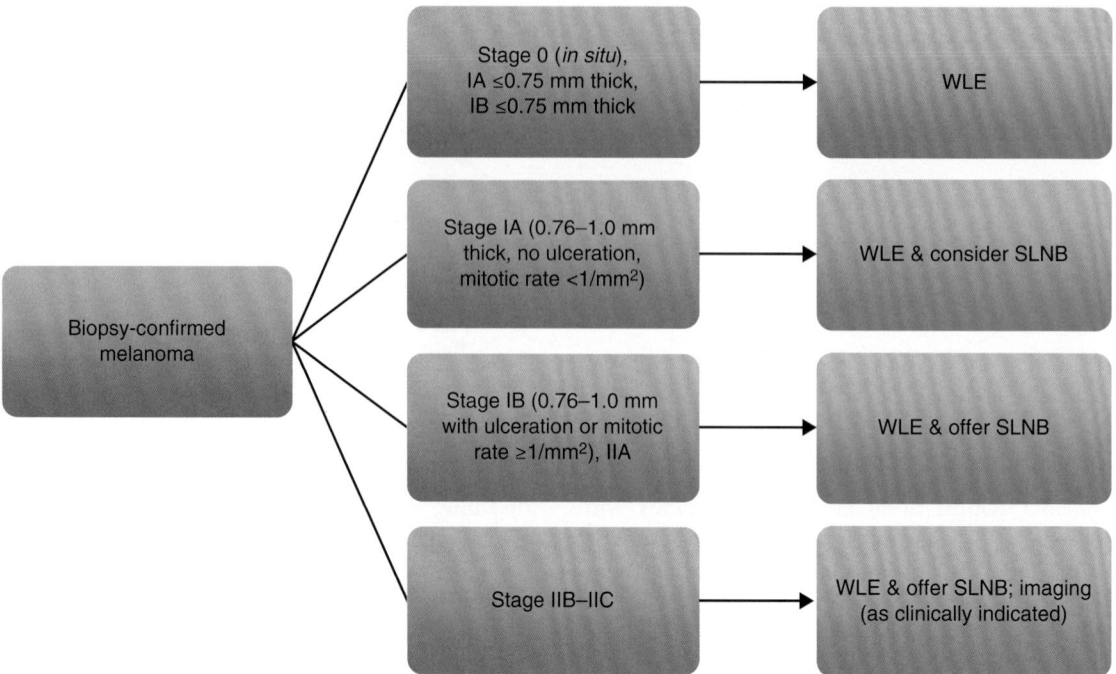

Figure 114.4 Surgical management of cutaneous melanoma (Adapted from NCCN). WLE, wide local excision (see Primary Resection section for suggested margin of resection); SLNB, sentinel lymph node biopsy; imaging modalities to consider: Chest x-ray, CT ± PET, MRI.

Technical Considerations

Localization and mapping of sentinel lymph nodes typically involves preoperative cutaneous lymphoscintigraphy as well as intraoperative localization of lymph nodes with vital blue dye and handheld gamma probe detection of lymph nodes harboring technetium-99m (^{99}Tc)-labeled sulfur colloid. SLNB is usually performed at the time of wide excision of the primary tumor. Preoperative lymphoscintigraphy involves intradermal (not subcutaneous) injection of ^{99}Tc-labeled sulfur colloid divided into four quadrants around the melanoma. SPECT imaging (single photon emission computed tomography) of the draining radioactive colloid identifies the regional nodal basins at risk, and, in some cases, the number and location of SLNs within the basin. Intraoperative injection of blue dye and ^{99}Tc-labeled sulfur colloid intradermally around the intact tumor/biopsy site is taken up by the lymphatic system, and the afferent lymphatic channels and SLNs are identified by the uptake of blue dye and radioactive signal (using handheld gamma probe). The addition of radiocolloid to blue dye increases the surgeon's ability to identify the SLN from 84% to 85% accuracy with blue dye alone to 96% to 99% (45). By performing the lymphoscintigraphy the morning of surgery, the radioactivity from the lymphoscintigraphy can be used for intraoperative localization, and a second injection of the radioactive colloid is not needed. If the delay between lymphoscintigraphy and SLNB is more than a few hours, a second injection of the radiolabelled sulfur colloid is performed (73–75).

Lymphazurin (1% isosulfan blue, US Surgical Corp, Norwalk, CT) was the first blue dye to be approved by the FDA for lymphangiography and is considered the gold standard dye for SLNB (76). However, due to shortages and anaphylactic reactions to the isosulfan blue, other blue dyes such as methylene blue have been successfully used (77).

In the head and neck, lymphatic basins can overlap with the primary tumor site making identification of the SLN difficult. Rasgon (78) advocated the use of lower levels of radioactivity (0.1 to 0.6 mCi) for lymphoscintigraphy and SLNB. We have had similar problems with radioactivity from ear, cheek, or neck melanomas obscuring evaluation of the underlying lymph nodes. As a result, in these areas, we have lowered the injected level of radioactivity from 1 to 0.4 mCi. Another effective strategy for dealing with this "shine-through" from the primary injection obscuring the sentinel lymph nodes nearby is to remove the primary tumor prior to sentinel node identification.

More recently, SPECT–CT has been used to aid in identification of sentinel lymph nodes in the head and neck, providing higher sensitivity for SLN detection and detailed anatomic localization (79,80) (Fig. 114.5). This technique has proven particularly useful in determining the extent of parotid gland LN involvement, assisting the surgeon in determining the necessary extent of parotid dissection (81). Another area in which this imaging adjunct has been useful is discerning whether high cervical lymph nodes are in the external or internal jugular chains, facilitating preoperative counseling about incisions and potential risk to vital structures such as the spinal accessory nerve.

For the SLNB to be accurate, all true SLNs, regardless of location, must be identified and harvested, since the

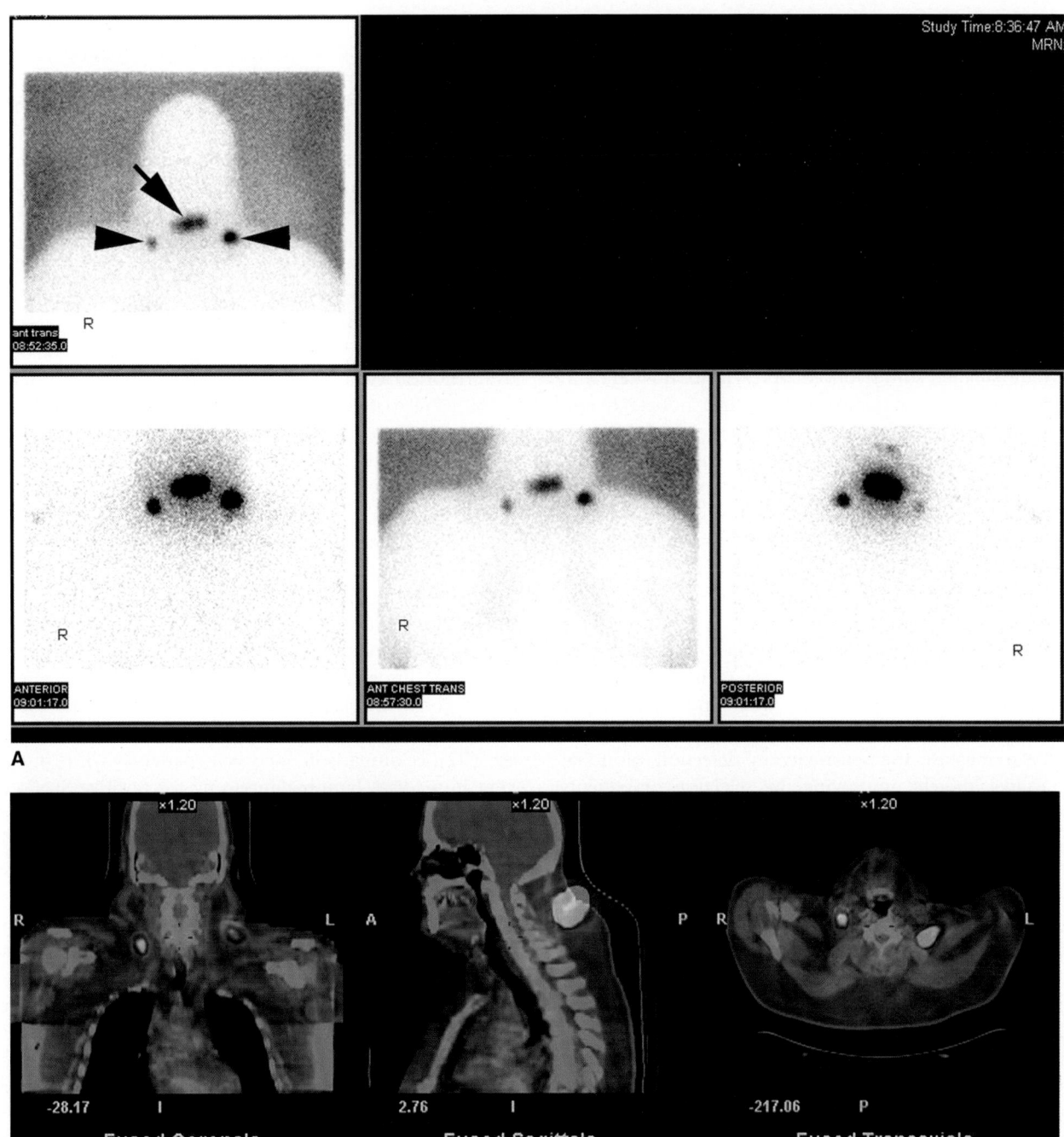

Figure 114.5 Patient with superficial spreading type melanoma of the posterior neck. **A:** Lymphoscintigraphy showing the injection site (*large arrow*). The sentinel lymph nodes are seen laterally in the neck bilaterally (*arrowhead*). **B:** SPECT/CT showing much improved anatomic detail of the radioactive lymph nodes in the supraclavicular fossa bilaterally. SLNB successfully identified three sentinel lymph nodes. Two sentinel lymph nodes on the left and one on the right all harbored metastatic disease. Subsequent bilateral neck dissections did not reveal any metastatic disease in the nonsentinel lymph nodes.

histologic status of one draining basin does not predict the status of other basins in patients with melanomas that drain to multiple regional basins. Eicher et al. (69) found that head and neck primary melanomas drain to an average of 2.2 nodal basins per patient, with drainage to nonadjacent nodal basins in 42% of patients. Reynolds et al.

(82) performed an extensive review of lymphoscintigraphy results from 929 patients with head and neck melanoma, demonstrating that the lymphatic drainage patterns in the head and neck are not always predictable. O'Brien et al. (59), at the Sydney Melanoma Unit, performed lymphatic mapping in the treatment of head and neck

melanoma in 97 patients. The authors found a high rate (34%) of disagreement between clinically predicted lymphatic drainage pathways in the head and neck region and those demonstrated on lymphoscintigraphy. Their analysis also revealed a large number of SLNs for each patient: 13 patients had a single SLN, 33 patients had two SLNs, 3 had three SLNs, 15 had four SLNs, and 6 had five SLNs, indicating some of the complexity of lymphatic mapping in the head and neck region.

We recommend removing lymph nodes identified with the handheld gamma probe until all lymph nodes with counts per minute greater than 10% of the counts per minute found in the lymph node with the highest uptake of the radiolabelled sulfur colloid (83,84). Abou-Nukta and Ariyan reported that removing the three hottest lymph nodes and all of the blue lymph nodes detected 100% of the positive SLNs. In addition, 98% of the positive SLNs in their study had radioactivity counts greater than 30% of the hottest lymph node. They have suggested that the removal of lymph nodes with radioactivity less than 30% of the hottest lymph node is unnecessary (85).

Pathologic Analysis of SLNs

An additional benefit of SLNB is that it can focus a more extensive evaluation of lymph nodes at risk for subclinical metastases. Workers at the M.D. Anderson Cancer Center have shown that analysis of serial sections of an SLN can increase the sensitivity in detection of nodal metastases, thereby improving the selection of patients who receive regional and systemic treatment (86). The use of frozen sections for evaluation of an SLN is not recommended because false negatives have been reported, secondary to inferior quality relative to permanent sections. Immunohistochemistry for S-100, HMB-45, MART-1/ melan-A, or, more recently, the reverse transcriptase polymerase chain reaction (RT-PCR) is required since hematoxylin and eosin alone will miss up to 12% of positive nodes (87). It is important to note that in the new AJCC staging system, immunohistochemically detected SLN metastases are formally considered evidence of node-positive disease (88). With respect to RT-PCR analysis of SLN, it remains investigational and should not be used outside of a clinical trial to direct further therapy (89).

The role of SLNB continues to be refined in the management of CMM of the head and neck region. The complexity of lymphatic drainage patterns and the frequent need to remove SLNs from the parotid gland, placing the facial nerve at risk, initially made head and neck surgical oncologists somewhat slow to adapt this method. Multiple centers have reviewed their experience with lymphatic mapping by using preoperative lymphoscintigraphy and intraoperative blue-dye localization and a handheld gamma probe (75,86). The University of Michigan group reported no facial nerve injuries in 19 patients with SLNs removed from the parotid gland (90), and this technique of removing parotid nodes without performing a complete parotidectomy has become widely adopted. The low false-negative rate of lymphatic mapping lends further support for the use of this method for staging the regional lymphatics (91). Data from these studies suggest that lymphatic mapping by using the combination of blue dye and a handheld gamma probe is an effective method for ruling out regional metastases in patients with melanoma and identifying patients who might benefit from further lymph node dissection, radiation, and/or systemic adjuvant therapy.

Potential Therapeutic Benefit from SLNB

In an effort to determine the impact of SLNB on survival, Morton et al. (92) performed a prospective analysis of 1,269 patients with intermediate stage melanoma (1.2- to 3.5-mm depth) and no lymphadenopathy. The patients were randomly assigned to receive wide excision and postoperative observation of regional lymph nodes, or wide excision and SLNB with immediate lymphadenectomy if nodal micrometastases were detected. Five-year melanoma-specific survival was not significantly different between the two groups (87.1% vs. 86.6%; $P = 0.58$). However, the group performed several subgroup analyses and clearly demonstrated that SLNB provides important prognostic information, identifying patients with microscopic nodal metastases, a median of 16 months earlier than presentation of clinically evident nodal metastases (92). Comparison between patients who underwent immediate lymphadenectomy for positive SLN and patients who underwent delayed lymphadenectomy for clinically detected nodal relapse, 5-year melanoma-specific survival, was significantly better in the SLN group (72.3% vs. 52.4%; $P = 0.004$) (92).

The value of SLNB lies in its ability to improve staging accuracy and, in turn, the ability to obtain regional disease control early, as melanoma-specific survival is better when lymphadenectomy is performed in patients with *microscopic* nodal burden than in patients with multiple nodal metastases (53,93–95). The presumption is that once nodal disease becomes clinically evident (palpable), metastatic deposits may already be present at distant sites.

While primarily advocated for patients with intermediate-thickness melanomas, SLNB should not be omitted from the workup of patients with thick (greater than 4 mm) melanomas, as it remains a prognostically powerful tool in this patient cohort (96–100).

TREATMENT: PRIMARY RESECTION

After an appropriate preoperative workup, therapeutic options are discussed with the patient. Surgical resection has been the mainstay of therapy in the treatment of primary cutaneous melanoma in the head and neck. Treatment includes resection of the primary melanoma or previous biopsy site with a rim of normal-appearing tissue surrounding it.

The minimal resection margin necessary for adequate resection has been the topic of debate. Historically, 5-cm excision margins were suggested, based on the propensity of melanomas to recur in areas adjacent to the primary site, although no survival advantage could be demonstrated. Based on subsequent retrospective analyses, it was suggested that narrower resection margins might be appropriate for thin or intermediate-thickness lesions (101). Recent randomized trials concluded that local and regional control rates and survival were not different when excisions with large (5-cm) margins, and those using more conservative (2-cm) margins were compared (102).

In a collaborative review, investigators at the University of Texas M.D. Anderson Cancer Center and the Moffitt Cancer Center found no increase in local recurrence rates or worse survival rates in patients when thick primary melanomas (larger than 4 mm) were excised with a margin of 10 mm or less (103). Of note, a recent Cochrane review of surgical excision margins for primary cutaneous melanoma (including five randomized controlled trials) was unable to demonstrate a statistically significant difference in overall survival between narrow and wide excision margins (104).

According to the NCCN, current guidelines for adequate resection margins of cutaneous melanoma are the following (which may be modified to accommodate individual anatomic or functional considerations) (61):

In Situ (T_{is})	0.5 cm
≤1 mm (T1)	1 cm
1.01–2.0 mm (T2)	1–2 cm
2.01–4.0 mm (T3)	2 cm
>4 mm (T4)	2 cm

Frequently, in the head and neck, proximity of structures such as the eyes, nose, ears, and circumoral anatomy effectively limits the borders for excision. Excisions are carried out in a full-thickness fashion down to underlying fascia such that all margins, including those that are deeply invaded, may be effectively evaluated.

Significant controversy exists regarding the use of frozen section for evaluation and diagnosis. Zitelli et al. (105) and other Mohs surgeons have reported that frozen sections of analysis for surgical margins of melanoma had sensitivity and specificity of 100% and 90%, respectively. However, many dermatopathologists believe that the use of frozen sections is inadequate to distinguish the margins of pigmented lesions. Therefore, we recommend control of margins by permanent-section pathologic analysis and often delay reconstruction until margin analysis has been completed. However, Mohs' surgery may be useful for extensive contiguous disease such as large, clinically ill-defined in situ melanoma of the lentigo maligna type. Alternatively, for some of these lesions, with positive surgical margins showing in situ disease, topical imiquimod or radiotherapy may be considered (61).

Methods of reconstruction after resection for melanoma are beyond the scope of this chapter. However, most lesions can be closed either primarily with the use of local advancement flaps or with the use of skin-grafting techniques. Skin grafting may allow closer surveillance for earlier detection of recurrent disease, and may also serve as a bridge to later definitive flap reconstruction.

Though more rare than cutaneous melanoma, mucosal melanoma deserves some mention in this section. While early detection is unlikely because of the occult anatomic locations, diagnosis must be established through full-thickness biopsy if possible. If the size or location of the lesion precludes excisional biopsy, incisional biopsy should include a representative sample from the border of the lesion, to assist the pathologist in differentiating a primary mucosal melanoma from mucosal melanoma metastasis. The primary approach to treatment of mucosal melanoma is wide surgical resection, for which the 5-year overall survival is only 13% to 22% (106,107). As a result of these poor outcomes and concern regarding adequate resection, radiotherapy and chemotherapy are often pursued as adjuvant therapies in the treatment of mucosal melanoma.

LYMPHADENECTOMY: THERAPEUTIC NECK DISSECTION AND PAROTIDECTOMY

For patients with clinically positive lymph nodes, neck dissection is indicated (Fig. 114.6). However, the extent of neck dissection remains an area of controversy but ranges from removal of gross disease by selective lymphadenectomy to radical neck dissection and its modifications.

Studies from Memorial Sloan-Kettering Cancer Center, the Melanoma Unit in Sydney, Australia, and Duke University have investigated the effect of neck dissection on outcome for patients with melanoma (108,109). Shah and colleagues (110) concluded that in the presence of clinically positive lymph nodes, a comprehensive neck dissection should be carried out. The type of neck dissection was tailored to the site of the primary tumor. For instance, in patients with melanomas of the face, ear, and anterior scalp, dissection of the parotid gland and lymph node levels I through IV was carried out. Patients with lesions in the postauricular and posterior scalp and neck required dissections of levels II through V. A complete discussion as to type and technique of neck dissection can be found elsewhere in this chapter.

For patients with positive SLNs, treatment options include observation, completion lymphadenectomy, and/or radiation therapy. In approximately 20% of SLN-positive patients, completion lymphadenectomy reveals additional melanoma-containing lymph nodes (111). Thus, completion lymphadenectomy is highly recommended for patients with positive SLN to ensure regional control. However, the multicenter selective lymphadenectomy trial (MSLT–II), which is currently in progress, is

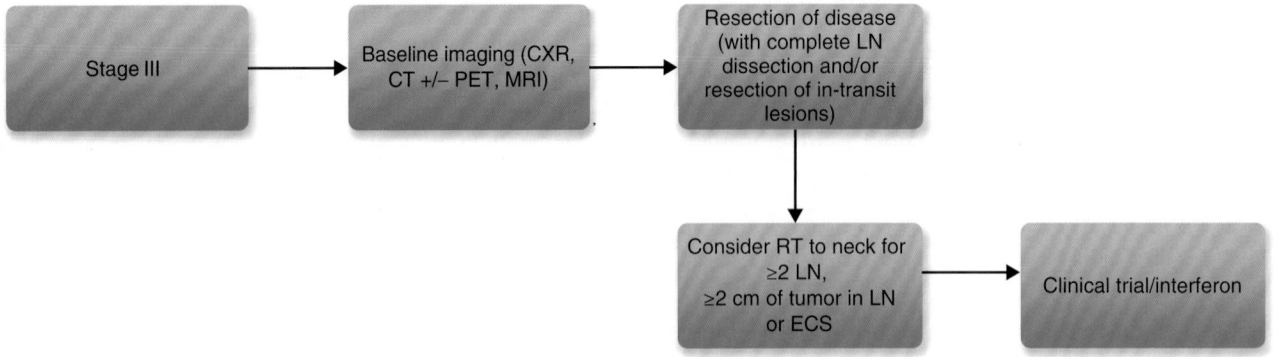

Figure 114.6 Management of node-positive melanoma (Adapted from NCCN). LN, lymph node; ECS, extra ≥2 cm tumor within lymph node capsular spread.

investigating the use of serial nodal ultrasound to identify those SLN-positive patients who will need completion lymphadenectomy, sparing up to 80% of patients a potentially unnecessary operation (112). The use of radiation therapy for SLN-positive patients will be addressed later in this chapter.

RADIOTHERAPY

Like many issues important to the treatment of malignant melanoma, radiotherapy, both as the primary modality of therapy and in the adjuvant setting, has sparked much controversy in the past century. Conflicting reports as to its efficacy included investigators unabashedly stating that malignant melanoma cells were radioresistant. However, groundbreaking work by Barranco et al. (113) found that cultured malignant melanoma cells differ from other types of tumor cells in their radiosensitivity. The observed radio resistance of melanoma could be overcome by increasing the individual dose fraction. These studies have helped form the basis for clinical practice, and subsequent studies helped to determine the ideal fraction size and total therapeutic dose that effectively treats melanoma.

Radiotherapy is not generally recommended for the primary treatment of CMM. However, in some exceptional circumstances, its use is advocated. In patients who are poor candidates for surgical resection, radiotherapy may offer an acceptable alternative.

For those patients with extensive facial LM melanoma that precludes adequate surgical resection based on functional or cosmetic considerations, radiotherapy has been used and has provided excellent outcomes (114). However, more recently, advances in topical therapies such as imiquimod are supplanting radiation therapy in the nonsurgical treatment of LMM.

In prospective nonrandomized clinical trials carried out at The University of Texas M.D. Anderson Cancer, three subgroups of patients were studied (115). The first group had primary lesions thicker than 1.5 mm or had lesions extending to Clark level IV or V and received elective

radiation after a wide local resection. The second group had palpable lymphadenopathy and received radiation in the adjuvant setting after excision of primary lesions coupled with a therapeutic neck dissection (selective or modified radical). The last group of patients underwent radiation after therapeutic neck dissection for regionally recurrent melanoma. Hypofractionated radiotherapy was delivered in five fractions of 6 Gy, twice weekly, to a total dose of 30 Gy. Theoretically, the large radiation fractions were used to overcome the melanoma radioresistance. Only 6 of 174 patients developed recurrence above the clavicles, but 58 patients developed distant metastases. The 5-year survival rate was 47%, and the local–regional control rate was 88% for all patients. The 5-year survival rates compared favorably with historical controls, and the radiation side effects were tolerable. These studies formed the basis for the use of hypofractionated radiation in melanoma.

Later studies from this group evaluated the outcome of patients with clinically apparent cervical lymph node metastases from malignant melanoma managed with surgical resection and adjuvant radiation (116). After 10-year follow-up, the group demonstrated a 94% regional control rate. Radiation-related complications for the patients were rare and manageable (116). The same group evaluated the utility of radiation therapy alone in the treatment of 36 patients with positive SLNB (*in lieu* of completion lymphadenectomy) and demonstrated 93% regional control over 5 years (117).

The Trans Tasman Radiation Oncology Group and Australia and New Zealand Melanoma Trials Group reported on a prospective study of radiation versus observation after lymphadenectomy on patients from 16 different centers (118). Inclusion criteria included greater than or equal to one parotid, greater than or equal to two cervical or axillary, or greater than or equal to three groin-positive nodes; extra nodal spread of tumor; or minimum metastatic node diameter of 3 cm (neck or axilla) or 4 cm (groin). Radiation was given as 2.4 Gy in 20 fractions over 4 weeks. There was a statistically significant improvement in lymph node field control with radiotherapy: 20 of 109 radiation and 34 of 108 observation patients relapsed regionally ($P = 0.04$). Despite improved local regional control, the overall survival was better in the observation group (47 months median survival) versus the radiation group (31 months median survival) although this was not statistically significant ($P = 0.14$). These data have raised concerns about possible deleterious effects of radiation as a contributor to the development of distant metastases. This question remains to be answered.

The NCCN recommends adjuvant radiation for patients with desmoplastic melanoma with narrow margins, recurrent disease, extensive neurotropism, gross nodal extracapsular extension, ≥2 lymph nodes, ≥2 cm of tumor in a lymph node, or unresectable nodal, satellite or in-transit disease (Fig. 114.6). Additionally, radiotherapy should be considered after excision of mucosal melanomas, which may or may not be amenable to complete excision (32,120).

SYSTEMIC THERAPY

Two major indications exist for systemic therapy in the management of patients with CMM. The first indication is the *adjuvant* treatment of patients who have completed locoregional therapy and have no evidence of local, regional, or systemic disease but who are thought to be at high risk for systemic relapse. The second indication for systemic treatment is the presence of distant metastases. A number of systemic therapy options are available to treat patients with either of these indications, including single-agent or multiple-agent chemotherapy, biochemotherapy, or strategies using immune modulation.

A number of clinical studies have been designed to evaluate the role of systemic adjuvant therapies for patients who have completed local–regional treatment and who are believed to be at high risk for the development of distant metastatic disease. Although no universal definition exists for the high-risk patient, a number of studies have accrued patients with primary lesions that are ulcerated, more than 4 mm in depth or Clark level IV, or those patients with satellitosis, in-transit disease, or nodal metastases. It is well established that the prognosis of patients with metastatic melanoma is poor; those with liver, brain, or bone metastasis have a median survival of only 3 to 4 months.

Interferon

Interferon alfa is one of the most well-studied agents for the systemic adjuvant therapy of CMM arising from all sites (121,122). However, it has yet to be shown unequivocally to improve overall survival for these patients. The interferons are a family of proteins that have both immunostimulatory and antiangiogenic activity and have excellent preclinical antitumor activity in a number of systems. Interferons enhance phagocytosis and free radical production in macrophages and increase activity of natural killer cells.

A prospective, randomized, clinical trial of high-dose interferon alfa-2b in the treatment of patients with high-risk melanoma was conducted by the Eastern Cooperative Oncology Group (122). High risk was defined as thick melanomas greater than 4 mm in Breslow depth and lymph node involvement by melanoma. High-risk patients were given high-dose interferon alfa-2b, 20 MU/m^2/d intravenously for 4 weeks. This was followed by 10 MU/m^2/d, administered subcutaneously, 3 days weekly for the remainder of the year. An increase in survival of 2.8 to 3.8 years was observed, and the recurrence-free survival ranged from 1 month to 1.7 years. The survival advantages were statistically significant in patients with regional lymph node metastasis. Most patients experienced significant toxicity that included chills, fevers, myalgias, and other constitutional symptoms including fatigue and anorexia. A follow-up trial of high- and low-dose interferon alfa-2b in high-risk melanoma, E1690, was reported by the intergroup (121). This study did not confirm the earlier improvement in overall survival but did demonstrate a dose-dependent improvement in 5-year recurrence-free survival rates from 35% to 44%. This is the 9% improvement in survival that many practitioners quote when discussing this treatment with patients.

The EORTC protocol 18,991 randomized 1,256 patients with stage III melanoma that had been completely resected to either observation or treatment with pegylated interferon alfa for an intended duration of 5 years. Four-year relapse-free survival was significantly better in the interferon group compared to the observation group (45.6% vs. 38.9%), but there was no significant effect of pegylated interferon on overall survival (123). Of note, a recent study (124) demonstrated that the appearance of autoantibodies or clinical manifestations of autoimmunity (i.e., vitiligo) during treatment with interferon alfa-2b is associated with statistically significant improvements in relapse-free survival and overall survival, though this has been disputed by others (125).

Low-dose and intermediate-dose trials of interferon alfa (EORTC 18952 and AIM HIGH Study) did not show improvement in progression-free or overall survival (126,127). Currently, when interferon is recommended as adjuvant therapy, only the high-dose regimens are recommended.

Recently, the Hellenic Cooperative Oncology Group reported on a prospective randomized study of 4 weeks of high-dose induction interferon (15 MU/m^2/d) versus the same induction regimen followed by 11 months of lower dose interferon (10 MU/m^2/d three times a week) (128). They found no difference in relapse-free survival (24.1 vs. 27.9 months [$P = 0.9$]) and median overall survival (64.4 vs. 65.3 months [$P = 0.49$]) (128). There were more side effects in the group with prolonged therapy. These findings were encouraging that a shorter treatment might be equally efficacious; however, subsequently, the Eastern Cooperative Oncology Group (ECOG) trial 1697: Phase III

Randomized Study of Four Weeks High Dose IFN-A2B in Stage T2B NO, T3A-B NO, T4A-B NO, and T1-4, N1A, 2A (microscopic) melanoma compared 1 month of high-dose interferon to observation. This study was halted in October of 2010 after the third interim analysis because there was no evidence of benefit in the interferon treatment group and no meaningful possibility that the study would show a benefit. These results have not been published yet, but based on the limited information that is publicly available, only treating with 1 month of interferon is not advisable.

The NCCN guidelines recommend consideration of the use of high-dose interferon alfa for treatment of patients with stage IIB (2.01 to 4 mm thick with ulceration or greater than 4 mm thick without ulceration), IIC (greater than 4.0 mm thick with ulceration), III (lymph node, in-transit, or satellite metastases), or IV (distant metastatic) disease.

Tumor Vaccines

Tumor vaccines are another widely studied strategy for systemic adjuvant therapy of the high-risk melanoma patient, and a variety of different immunization approaches have been used. These studies are predicated on several clinical observations and lines of basic investigation that indicate that the immune system can eradicate melanoma cells and that immune stimulation can overcome immune tolerance to tumor antigens to enhance the immune surveillance of tumor cells. Although a comprehensive review of available vaccine strategies is beyond the scope of this chapter, some of the more encouraging studies are discussed.

Ganglioside GM2, an antigen overexpressed by many melanoma cells, given in combination with Bacille Calmette-Guérin (BCG) or other immune adjuvants, was developed by Dr. Alan Haughton and colleagues at Memorial Sloan-Kettering Cancer Center. Initial clinical trials suggested promising results (129); however, further studies failed to show clinical benefit of this adjuvant treatment. Kirkwood et al. (130) reported their experience comparing high-dose interferon alfa-2b and GM-2 ganglioside vaccine for patients with resected melanoma, demonstrating superior performance of interferon. Additionally, a randomized Phase III trial (EORTC 18961) of adjuvant GM2-KLH21 in 1,314 patients with stage II melanoma was closed early by the data monitoring committee because of inferior survival in the vaccine arm (131).

Investigators at the John Wayne Cancer Center developed a polyvalent melanoma cell vaccine capable of inducing humoral- and cell-mediated immune responses to melanoma-specific antigens (132,133). Dr. Steven Rosenberg and coinvestigators at the surgery branch of the National Cancer Institute have identified other cancer vaccines by using specific peptide antigens recognized by autologous tumor-specific T-cell clone reactivity (134). These peptide vaccines are most often administered with cytokine or cellular immune adjuvants such as dendritic cells. DiFronzo et al. (135) demonstrated that enhanced humoral responses in patients treated with polyvalent vaccines resulted in limited but improved disease-free survival. Schwartzentruber et al. (136)

showed increased survival of 17.8 months compared to 11.1 months in treatment with a vaccine (gp100:209-217(210M)) and interleukin-2 (IL-2) as compared to IL-2 alone. It is difficult to advocate any of the current vaccine strategies over another. Therefore, we recommend that patients with high-risk melanoma be enrolled into prospective trials to test these adjuvant therapeutic strategies.

Interleukin-2

Interleukin-2 (IL-2) was approved by the Food and Drug administration (FDA) for treatment of metastatic melanoma in 1998. High-dose intravenous bolus IL-2 treatment resulted in overall objective response rates of about 17% (137). In a highly selected patient population ($n = 270$), IL-2 was able to induce durable complete responses (median response duration over 59 months) in approximately 6% of patients and partial responses in 10% of patients with metastatic melanoma, albeit with high levels of toxicity (138,139). A recent study demonstrated increased response rate in metastatic melanoma when IL-2 was given with the 210M peptide vaccine (22%) compared to IL-2 (13%) alone (140).

Ipilimumab

Despite many preclinical and clinical studies evaluating multiple cytokines, vaccines, antibodies, and other types of immune modulation, alone or in combination with chemotherapy, only *IL-2* for metastatic disease and *interferon alfa* for surgical adjuvant treatment have demonstrated sufficient success to warrant approval by regulatory authorities (138,141). Nevertheless, there has been continued optimism that immune modulation can become an effective treatment for patients with melanoma driven largely by key advances in tumor immunobiology, including the potential to manipulate and disrupt immune activation checkpoints and tumor defense mechanisms; newer approaches to antigen presentation for immune activation; refinements to procedures for antigen-specific T-cell expansion; gene transfer to alter lymphocyte specificity and function; and the potential for discovery of improved predictive biomarkers to select patients for individual treatments (142).

Along these lines, Hodi et al. induced antitumor immunity in patients with metastatic melanoma using ipilimumab, an antibody directed against the cytotoxic T-lymphocyte-associated antigen CTLA-4 (143). CTLA-4 is an immune checkpoint molecule that downregulates T-cell activation, and blocking this molecule is known to promote antitumor immunity (143). In their multicenter clinical trial, patients with metastatic melanoma were randomly assigned to receive either an anti–CTLA-4 agent (ipilimumab), a vaccine based on a melanoma antigen, or a combination of the anti–CTLA-4 agent and the vaccine. An improvement in overall survival, as well as an improvement in progression-free survival and best overall response rate, was seen in the patients who received anti–CTLA-4 therapy, as compared with the patients who received the vaccine only (143). Of note, the side effect profile of ipilimumab deserves mention, as 60% of patients suffered adverse events, mostly immune related. However, this randomized, controlled trial showed that there was a significant improvement in overall survival among melanoma patients treated with ipilimumab. Robert et al. (144) showed improved survival of 20.8% from 12.2% at 3 years for patients treated with ipilimumab plus dacarbazine versus dacarbazine alone. Based on these trials, ipilimumab is a preferred therapy option for advanced or metastatic melanoma in the NCCN guidelines.

Chemotherapeutic Agents

Chemotherapy regimens using single-agent dacarbazine (DTIC) or combinations such as bis(2-chloroethyl)nitrosourea (BCNU), cisplatin, lomustine, and hydroxyurea have been reported. The trials comparing DTIC alone or in combination with other agents have shown a significant though brief improvement in survival (145). Unfortunately, there is little consensus regarding a standardized chemotherapeutic regimen for metastatic melanoma. According to the NCCN, dacarbazine remains a standard of care in community practice and has been used as a standard for comparing the efficacy of new regimens (61,146). Dacarbazine and temozolomide have been shown to have similar response rates (~10% to 20%) and survival (147); median response duration with these drugs is 3 to 4 months (145,147). Temozolomide can cross the "blood–brain barrier," making it an attractive agent for treating melanoma, which has a propensity for metastasis to the brain.

Combination chemotherapy regimens such as CVD (dacarbazine plus cisplatin and vinblastine) or the Dartmouth regimen (dacarbazine, carmustine, cisplatin, and tamoxifen) initially reported higher response rates (148,149), but subsequent clinical trials have not replicated these high response rates (150). Paclitaxel alone or in combination with carboplatin may provide clinical benefit to some patients with metastatic melanoma; however, the duration of clinical benefit is short (2 to 7 months) (151,152).

Molecularly Targeted Therapy of Melanoma

Recent groundbreaking work has been reported on molecularly targeted chemotherapy in melanoma. In 2002, it was demonstrated that approximately 50% of human melanomas harbor an activating mutation in BRAF, in which glutamic acid is substituted for valine (the V600E mutation) (153). BRAF is an upstream component of the growth-promoting mitogen-activated protein (MAP) kinase pathway. It has been established that melanoma cells containing mutant BRAF are dependent on MAP kinase signaling for their growth and survival (154). These findings suggested the possibility that melanoma may be amenable to targeted therapy. Initial studies performed with sorafenib, a multikinase anti-BRAF agent, were disappointing showing no difference between standard chemotherapy and the addition of sorafenib (155,156). However, vemurafenib (PLX4032

Plexxikon; RG7204, Roche Pharmaceuticals), a potent inhibitor of BRAF with the V600E mutation, has been shown to be remarkably successful therapeutic option in properly selected patients (157). Eighty-one percent of patients with metastatic melanomas harboring the activating mutation in BRAF (V600E) had a response—complete or partial tumor regression—to treatment with vemurafenib in a multicenter, phase 1 and 2, dose escalation trial. Responses were observed at all sites of disease, including bone, liver, and small bowel.

A phase 3 randomized clinical trial comparing vemurafenib with dacarbazine in 675 patients with previously untreated, metastatic melanoma with the BRAF V600E mutation showed improved 6 month survival of 84% versus 64% in the vemurafenib versus the dacarbazine group (158). Response rates were 48% for vemurafenib and 5% for dacarbazine (158). Endpoints for improved survival with vemurafenib were met at the interim analysis and patients were recommended to crossover from dacarbazine to vemurafenib.

It seems clear that melanomas can be categorized by specific molecular changes that drive their proliferation (159); targeting the activated pathways in individual tumors may lead to tumor regression and possible cure. This type of personalized cancer therapy will likely play a prominent role in the care of patients with melanoma and other cancers in the coming decade.

Biochemotherapy

Another approach to systemic treatment of melanoma includes the use of biochemotherapy in which conventional chemotherapeutic drugs are combined with the biologically active agents interferon alfa and IL-2. In single institutional phase II trials, biochemotherapy (cisplatin, vinblastine, dacarbazine, interferon alfa, and IL-2) produced an overall response rate of 27% to 64% and a complete response rate of 15% to 21% in patients with metastatic melanoma (160–162). A report of a small phase III randomized trial comparing sequential biochemotherapy (dacarbazine, cisplatin, vinblastine with IL-2, and interferon alfa administered on a distinct schedule) with combined cisplatin, vinblastine, and dacarbazine (CVD) showed response rates of 48% for the biochemotherapy regimen compared to 25% for CVD alone; median survival for patients treated with biochemotherapy was 11.9 versus 9.2 months for CVD (163). In a phase III randomized intergroup trial (E3695), biochemotherapy (cisplatin, vinblastine, dacarbazine, IL-2, and interferon alfa-2b) produced a slightly higher response rate and progression-free survival than CVD alone, but it was not associated with either improved quality of response or overall survival in patients with metastatic melanoma (164). Biochemotherapy was substantially more toxic than CVD. Additional attempts to decrease toxicity of biochemotherapy by administering subcutaneous outpatient IL-2 did not show a substantial benefit of biochemotherapy versus chemotherapy alone (165–167). Notably, a recent meta-analysis demonstrated that although biochemotherapy seemed to improve overall response rates, there was no survival benefit for patients with metastatic melanoma (168). Some current studies are focused on the use of IL-2 given with melanoma peptide antigens or melanoma-specific in vitro expanded autologous tumor-infiltrating lymphocytes. A combination of systemic therapies such as interferon alfa, IL-2, cisplatin, dacarbazine, and tamoxifen also has been reported to have activity in patients with metastatic disease (169).

Nevertheless, given the overall poor performance of agents in this cohort of patients, continued basic and translational research is warranted to identify active agents for these unfortunate patients. Preemptive strategies are also being developed. Because a majority of patients with CMM have some identifiable risk factor (i.e., sun exposure), chemoprevention using carotenoids and inhibitors of cyclooxygenase-2 (COX-2), vascular endothelial growth factor (VEGF) receptor, and cytochrome P-450 is actively being investigated (170). Outcomes of this work are much anticipated.

SURVEILLANCE

With the rapidly increasing rate of melanoma worldwide, the importance of surveillance of even benign-appearing lesions is understood. The importance of dermatologic evaluation, photo documentation, and close follow-up cannot be overstated. In patients with a diagnosed malignant melanoma, between 55% and 70% of recurrences appear within the first 2 years of therapy, and up to 80% of recurrences will be diagnosed in the first 3 years after treatment. Those with regional metastasis at presentation may have clinically evident tumor recurrences within 24 months. The time to recurrence also correlates with primary tumor thickness, ulceration, and increasing patient age. Screening

is typically by physical examination, liver-function serology, and chest x-ray, which will detect most of these recurrences; therefore, routine screening with CT of the head, chest, and abdomen is not recommended. In general, the use of chest x-rays and liver serology is known to have an extremely low yield (171). The utility of PET or PET–CT imaging for the surveillance of affected patients is still under investigation. Additionally, the prospect of using specific serum screening tools such as tyrosinase mRNA detected by RT-PCR is both clinically exciting and ethically challenging (172).

The National Cancer Institute reported a consensus statement on the follow-up evaluation of patients with early melanoma. Most patients without a family history and no atypical nevi should have follow-up evaluations every 6 months for the first 2 years.

Thereafter, yearly follow-up is appropriate. Those with a family history or atypical nevi are followed up every 3 months. The recommended surveillance for patients without any evidence of disease after treatment for CMM is shown in Figure 114.7 (173).

CONCLUSION

The incidence and mortality rate of CMM are rapidly increasing worldwide. Features of the history and physical examination that are suggestive of malignant melanoma include changes in size or color, sensation of the lesion, and variations in color and margin, and thickness. The presence of ulceration also is quite important. When a suggestive lesion is encountered, excisional biopsy is recommended, and should include subcutaneous fat for complete evaluation of lesion depth. Biopsy techniques that do not evaluate depth, such as fine-needle aspiration and

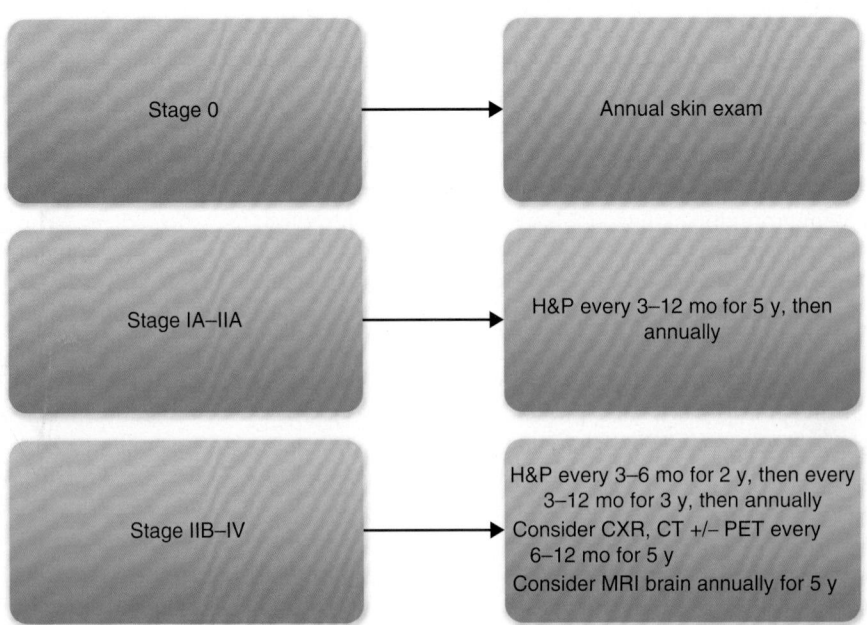

Figure 114.7 Surveillance recommendations (Adapted from NCCN).

curettage, have no role in evaluation in suspected melanoma. Once invasive melanoma is diagnosed, histologic type is assessed, and lesion thickness is established. Tumor thickness (Breslow), level of invasion (Clark), presence of ulceration and microscopic satellitosis, and number of mitoses are prognostically important and aid the clinician in the decision to perform SLNB. Staging in relation to the presence of regional and distant metastasis is established by physical examination, liver function serology, and chest radiograph in stage I and II disease. Additionally, imaging of the brain, head, neck, chest, and abdomen is recommended for patients with stage III and IV disease.

Lymphoscintigraphy with SLNB provides an adjunctive method of identifying SLNs and defining routes of lymphatic spread, especially in patients with primary tumors located in the midline that have predicted drainage basins that are ambiguous or include both parotid glands. After staging, a treatment strategy is formulated. For melanomas less than 0.75 mm in thickness and with no evidence of regional metastasis, surgical excision is carried out with close surveillance thereafter. Current recommendations for adequate resection margins, dependent on anatomic constraints, range from 0.5 to 2 cm, depending on the thickness of the primary lesion. For patients with lesions more than 0.75 mm thick without regional metastasis, excision is offered, along with SLNB. Once SLNB is performed, serial sectioning of the lymph node(s) with immunohistochemical evaluation is carried out on histologically negative SLNs to increase the sensitivity of pathologic identification of metastases.

In patients with regional lymph nodes that are found to be pathologically positive, therapeutic lymphadenectomy and/or radiotherapy is offered.

Patients with clinically positive lymph nodes should undergo excision of the primary lesion and a therapeutic neck dissection that may be modified to preserve neurovascular structures. Parotidectomy is performed if parotid lymph nodes are included in nodal drainage basins. These patients also should be evaluated for systemic therapy, as should those who have or develop distant metastasis. The use of systemic therapy includes chemotherapy, bioimmunotherapy, vaccination, and more recently, molecularly targeted therapy, all of which can be used to treat metastatic disease or in the adjuvant setting for patients without evidence of disease who are at high risk for systemic failure. The importance of treating these patients within the confines of thoughtfully designed, prospective clinical trials cannot be overemphasized.

The number of patients affected with melanoma is increasing. However, survival rates are improving because of early-detection programs and heightened awareness of the general population. It is hoped that this heightened awareness, coupled with progress made in improved pathologic description and staging and the use of systemic therapies, including immune modulation and molecularly targeted therapy, will result in continued improvement in our ability to cure patients with this disease.

HIGHLIGHTS

- Melanoma is divided into four distinct clinicopathologic subtypes: LMM, superficial spreading, nodular, and acral lentiginous melanoma. Desmoplastic melanomas are a fifth, less common subtype of melanoma that are characterized by perineural invasion, high local recurrence rates, and low rates of lymph node metastases.
- Histologic evaluation must include the following: Breslow depth/thickness, presence or absence of ulceration, and mitotic rate. Clark level may have clinical utility in the evaluation and treatment of patients with thin melanomas.
- Staging of melanoma includes the presence of satellite lesions, in-transit disease, the number (rather than the size of) involved lymph nodes, and distant metastases.
- Recommended excision margins for melanoma are dictated by Breslow depth. *In situ* melanoma requires a 0.5-cm margin of normal skin, lesions less than or equal to 1 mm in depth require a 1-cm margin, lesions 1.01 to 2.0 mm in depth require a 1- to 2-cm margin depending upon surrounding structures, and lesions greater than 2.01 mm in depth require a 2-cm margin.
- SLNB is considered or offered to patients with melanomas greater than 0.75 mm in thickness. The likelihood of a positive sentinel lymph node increases with the depth of the primary melanoma: T1 lesions have a 3% to 5% risk of SLN positivity; T2, 8% to 12%; T3, 23% to 27%; and T4, 24% to 44%.
- For patients with thin, nonulcerated primary tumors without evidence of regional or distant spread on physical examination (stages I and II), chest radiograph and liver function tests compose the recommended workup. For patients with regional or systemic metastases or both, a comprehensive staging workup should include MRI of the brain and contrast-enhanced CT of the neck, chest, abdomen, and pelvis. PET imaging has been used to aid in detecting regional and distant metastasis.
- Adjuvant radiation therapy should be considered for patients with desmoplastic melanoma with narrow margins, recurrent disease, extensive neurotropism, gross nodal extracapsular extension, ≥2 lymph nodes, ≥2 cm of tumor in a lymph node, or unresectable nodal, satellite or in-transit disease.
- Patients with high-risk primary tumors, regional metastasis, or distant metastases should be evaluated for systemic adjuvant therapies. Interferon alfa, ipilimumab, vemurafenib and high-dose IL-2 are effective in this setting.

REFERENCES

1. Siegel R, et al. Cancer statistics, 2013. *CA Cancer J Clin* 2013;63:11–30.
2. Olsen CM, Carroll HJ, Whiteman DC. Estimating the attributable fraction for cancer: a meta-analysis of nevi and melanoma. *Cancer Prev Res (Phila)* 2010;3(2):233–245.
3. Kang S, et al. Melanoma risk in individuals with clinically atypical nevi. *Arch Dermatol* 1994;130(8):999–1001.
4. Bradford PT, et al. Increased risk of second primary cancers after a diagnosis of melanoma. *Arch Dermatol* 2010;146(3):265–272.
5. Kahn HS, et al. Increased cancer mortality following a history of nonmelanoma skin cancer. *JAMA* 1998;280(10):910–912.
6. Marghoob AA, et al. Basal cell and squamous cell carcinomas are important risk factors for cutaneous malignant melanoma. Screening implications. *Cancer* 1995;75(2 Suppl):707–714.
7. Goggins WB, Tsao H. A population-based analysis of risk factors for a second primary cutaneous melanoma among melanoma survivors. *Cancer* 2003;97(3):639–643.
8. Goldstein AM, et al. Linkage of cutaneous malignant melanoma/dysplastic nevi to chromosome 9p, and evidence for genetic heterogeneity. *Am J Hum Genet* 1994;54(3):489–496.
9. Penn I. Malignant melanoma in organ allograft recipients. *Transplantation* 1996;61(2):274–278.
10. O'Brien CJ, et al. Experience with 998 cutaneous melanomas of the head and neck over 30 years. *Am J Surg* 1991;162(4):310–314.
11. Weinstock MA. Epidemiology of melanoma. *Cancer Treat Res* 1993;65:29–56.
12. Gibbs P, et al. Management of primary cutaneous melanoma of the head and neck: the University of Colorado experience and a review of the literature. *J Surg Oncol* 2001;77(3):179–185, discussion 186–187.
13. Golger A, et al. Epidemiological features and prognostic factors of cutaneous head and neck melanoma: a population-based study. *Arch Otolaryngol Head Neck Surg* 2007;133(5):442–447.
14. Lentsch EJ, Myers JN. Melanoma of the head and neck: current concepts in diagnosis and management. *Laryngoscope* 2001;111(7):1209–1222.
15. Abbasi NR, et al. Early diagnosis of cutaneous melanoma: revisiting the ABCD criteria. *JAMA* 2004;292(22):2771–2776.
16. Austin JR, et al. Influence of biopsy on the prognosis of cutaneous melanoma of the head and neck. *Head Neck* 1996;18(2):107–117.
17. Egbert B, Kempson S, Sagebiel R. Desmoplastic malignant melanoma. A clinicohistopathologic study of 25 cases. *Cancer* 1988;62(9):2033–2041.
18. Beenken S, et al. Desmoplastic melanoma. Histologic correlation with behavior and treatment. *Arch Otolaryngol Head Neck Surg* 1989;115(3):374–379.
19. Smithers BM, McLeod GR, Little JH. Desmoplastic melanoma: patterns of recurrence. *World J Surg* 1992;16(2):186–190.
20. Carlson JA, et al. Desmoplastic neurotropic melanoma. A clinicopathologic analysis of 28 cases. *Cancer* 1995;75(2):478–494.
21. Quinn MJ, et al. Desmoplastic and desmoplastic neurotropic melanoma: experience with 280 patients. *Cancer* 1998;83(6):1128–1135.
22. Payne WG, et al. Desmoplastic melanoma. *Am Surg* 2001;67(10):1004–1006.
23. Murali R, et al. Prognostic factors in cutaneous desmoplastic melanoma: a study of 252 patients. *Cancer* 2010;116(17):4130–4138.
24. Gyorki DE, et al. Sentinel lymph node biopsy for patients with cutaneous desmoplastic melanoma. *Ann Surg Oncol* 2003;10(4):403–407.
25. Pawlik TM, et al. Assessment of the role of sentinel lymph node biopsy for primary cutaneous desmoplastic melanoma. *Cancer* 2006;106(4):900–906.
26. Sassen S, et al. The complex relationships between sentinel node positivity, patient age, and primary tumor desmoplasia: analysis of 2303 melanoma patients treated at a single center. *Ann Surg Oncol* 2008;15(2):630–637.
27. George E, et al. Subclassification of desmoplastic melanoma: pure and mixed variants have significantly different capacities for lymph node metastasis. *J Cutan Pathol* 2009;36(4):425–432.
28. Chang AE, Karnell LH, Menck HR. The National Cancer Data Base report on cutaneous and noncutaneous melanoma: a summary of 84,836 cases from the past decade. The American College of Surgeons Commission on Cancer and the American Cancer Society. *Cancer* 1998;83(8):1664–1678.
29. Stern SJ, Guillamondegui OM. Mucosal melanoma of the head and neck. *Head Neck* 1991;13(1):22–27.
30. Prasad ML, Patel SG, Busam KJ. Primary mucosal desmoplastic melanoma of the head and neck. *Head Neck* 2004;26(4):373–377.
31. Douglas CM, et al. Mucosal melanoma of the head and neck: radiotherapy or surgery? *J Otolaryngol Head Neck Surg* 2010;39(4):385–392.
32. Temam S, et al. Postoperative radiotherapy for primary mucosal melanoma of the head and neck. *Cancer* 2005;103(2):313–319.
33. Owens JM, Roberts DB, Myers JN. The role of postoperative adjuvant radiation therapy in the treatment of mucosal melanomas of the head and neck region. *Arch Otolaryngol Head Neck Surg* 2003;129(8):864–868.
34. Krengli M, et al. Radiotherapy in the treatment of mucosal melanoma of the upper aerodigestive tract: analysis of 74 cases. A Rare Cancer Network study. *Int J Radiat Oncol Biol Phys* 2006;65(3):751–759.
35. Dauer EH. et al. Sinonasal melanoma: a clinicopathologic review of 61 cases. *Otolaryngol Head Neck Surg* 2008;138(3):347–352.
36. Bachar G, et al. Mucosal melanomas of the head and neck: experience of the Princess Margaret Hospital. *Head Neck* 2008;30(10):1325–1331.
37. Meleti M, et al. Head and neck mucosal melanoma: experience with 42 patients, with emphasis on the role of postoperative radiotherapy. *Head Neck* 2008;30(12):1543–1551.
38. Yii NW, et al. Mucosal malignant melanoma of the head and neck: the Marsden experience over half a century. *Clin Oncol (R Coll Radiol)* 2003;15(4):199–204.
39. Patel SG, et al. Primary mucosal malignant melanoma of the head and neck. *Head Neck* 2002;24(3):247–257.
40. Clark WH Jr, et al. The histogenesis and biologic behavior of primary human malignant melanomas of the skin. *Cancer Res* 1969;29(3):705–727.
41. Breslow A. Thickness, cross-sectional areas and depth of invasion in the prognosis of cutaneous melanoma. *Ann Surg* 1970;172(5):902–908.
42. Balch CM, et al. Final version of 2009 AJCC melanoma staging and classification. *J Clin Oncol* 2009;27(36):6199–6206.
43. Gershenwald JE, et al. Multi-institutional melanoma lymphatic mapping experience: the prognostic value of sentinel lymph node status in 612 stage I or II melanoma patients. *J Clin Oncol* 1999;17(3):976–983.
44. Balch CM, et al. Long-term results of a multi-institutional randomized trial comparing prognostic factors and surgical results for intermediate thickness melanomas (1.0 to 4.0 mm). Intergroup Melanoma Surgical Trial. *Ann Surg Oncol* 2000;7(2):87–97.
45. Gershenwald JE, et al. Improved sentinel lymph node localization in patients with primary melanoma with the use of radiolabeled colloid. *Surgery* 1998;124(2):203–210.
46. Wagner JD, et al. Predicting sentinel and residual lymph node basin disease after sentinel lymph node biopsy for melanoma. *Cancer* 2000;89(2):453–462.
47. Rousseau DL Jr, et al. Revised American Joint Committee on Cancer staging criteria accurately predict sentinel lymph node positivity in clinically node-negative melanoma patients. *Ann Surg Oncol* 2003;10(5):569–574.
48. McMasters KM, et al. Factors that predict the presence of sentinel lymph node metastasis in patients with melanoma. *Surgery* 2001;130(2):151–156.
49. Sondak VK, et al. Mitotic rate and younger age are predictors of sentinel lymph node positivity: lessons learned from the generation of a probabilistic model. *Ann Surg Oncol* 2004;11(3):247–258.
50. Kruper LL, et al. Predicting sentinel node status in AJCC stage I/II primary cutaneous melanoma. *Cancer* 2006;107(10):2436–2445.
51. Paek SC, et al. The impact of factors beyond Breslow depth on predicting sentinel lymph node positivity in melanoma. *Cancer* 2007;109(1):100–108.
52. Ellis MC, et al. Sentinel lymph node staging of cutaneous melanoma: predictors and outcomes. *Am J Surg* 2010;199(5):663–668.

53. Balch CM, et al. Prognostic factors analysis of 17,600 melanoma patients: validation of the American Joint Committee on Cancer melanoma staging system. *J Clin Oncol* 2001;19(16): 3622–3634.

54. Pawlik TM, et al. The risk of in-transit melanoma metastasis depends on tumor biology and not the surgical approach to regional lymph nodes. *J Clin Oncol* 2005;23(21):4588–4590.

55. Cascinelli N, et al. Regional non-nodal metastases of cutaneous melanoma. *Eur J Surg Oncol* 1986;12(2):175–180.

56. Borgstein PJ, Meijer S, van Diest PJ. Are locoregional cutaneous metastases in melanoma predictable? *Ann Surg Oncol* 1999;6(3):315–321.

57. Balch CM, et al. Multivariate analysis of prognostic factors among 2,313 patients with stage III melanoma: comparison of nodal micrometastases versus macrometastases. *J Clin Oncol* 2010;28(14):2452–2459.

58. Buzaid AC, et al. Prognostic value of size of lymph node metastases in patients with cutaneous melanoma. *J Clin Oncol* 1995;13(9):2361–2368.

59. O'Brien CJ, et al. Prediction of potential metastatic sites in cutaneous head and neck melanoma using lymphoscintigraphy. *Am J Surg* 1995;170(5):461–466.

60. Cochran AJ, Huang R, Guo J. Current management issues in malignant melanoma. *ASCO* 2003:189–194.

61. NCCN Clinical Practice Guidelines in oncology: melanoma. 2012 (cited 2013 January 20); Version 2.2013. Available from: http://www.nccn.org/professionals/physician_gls/PDF/melanoma.pdf

62. Neuman HB, et al. A single-institution validation of the AJCC staging system for stage IV melanoma. *Ann Surg Oncol* 2008;15(7):2034–2041.

63. Balch CM, et al. A comparison of prognostic factors and surgical results in 1,786 patients with localized (stage I) melanoma treated in Alabama, USA, and New South Wales, Australia. *Ann Surg* 1982;196(6):677–684.

64. Reintgen DS, et al. Efficacy of elective lymph node dissection in patients with intermediate thickness primary melanoma. *Ann Surg* 1983;198(3):379–385.

65. Sim FH, et al. Lymphadenectomy in the management of stage I malignant melanoma: a prospective randomized study. *Mayo Clin Proc* 1986;61(9):697–705.

66. Veronesi U, et al. Inefficacy of immediate node dissection in stage 1 melanoma of the limbs. *N Engl J Med* 1977;297(12):627–630.

67. Balch CM, et al. Efficacy of an elective regional lymph node dissection of 1 to 4 mm thick melanomas for patients 60 years of age and younger. *Ann Surg* 1996;224(3):255–263, discussion 263–266.

68. Caraceni A, et al. Neurotoxicity of interferon-alpha in melanoma therapy: results from a randomized controlled trial. *Cancer* 1998;83(3):482–489.

69. Eicher SA, et al. A prospective study of intraoperative lymphatic mapping for head and neck cutaneous melanoma. *Arch Otolaryngol Head Neck Surg* 2002;128(3):241–246.

70. Morton DL, et al. Validation of the accuracy of intraoperative lymphatic mapping and sentinel lymphadenectomy for early-stage melanoma: a multicenter trial. Multicenter Selective Lymphadenectomy Trial Group. *Ann Surg* 1999;230(4):453–463, discussion 463–465.

71. Karim RZ, et al. False negative sentinel lymph node biopsies in melanoma may result from deficiencies in nuclear medicine, surgery, or pathology. *Ann Surg* 2008;247(6):1003–1010.

72. Carlson GW, et al. Regional recurrence after negative sentinel lymph node biopsy for melanoma. *Ann Surg* 2008;248(3):378–386.

73. Gennari R, et al. Sentinel node localization in primary melanoma: preoperative dynamic lymphoscintigraphy, intraoperative gamma probe, and vital dye guidance. *Surgery* 2000;127(1):19–25.

74. Bostick P, et al. Comparison of blue dye and probe-assisted intraoperative lymphatic mapping in melanoma to identify sentinel nodes in 100 lymphatic basins. *Arch Surg* 1999;134(1):43–49.

75. Patel SG, et al. Sentinel lymph node biopsy for cutaneous head and neck melanomas. *Arch Otolaryngol Head Neck Surg* 2002;128(3):285–291.

76. Morton DL, et al. Technical details of intraoperative lymphatic mapping for early stage melanoma. *Arch Surg* 1992;127(4): 392–399.

77. Liu Y, Truini C, Ariyan S. A randomized study comparing the effectiveness of methylene blue dye with lymphazurin blue dye in sentinel lymph node biopsy for the treatment of cutaneous melanoma. *Ann Surg Oncol* 2008;15(9):2412–2417.

78. Rasgon BM. Use of low-dose technetium Tc 99 m sulfur colloid to locate sentinel lymph nodes in melanoma of the head and neck: preliminary study. *Laryngoscope* 2001;111(8):1366–1372.

79. Uren RF. SPECT/CT Lymphoscintigraphy to locate the sentinel lymph node in patients with melanoma. *Ann Surg Oncol* 2009;16(6):1459–1460.

80. Vermeeren L, et al. SPECT/CT for sentinel lymph node mapping in head and neck melanoma. *Head Neck* 2011;33(1):1–6.

81. Yang AD, et al. *Comparison of SPECT/CT to planar lymphoscintigraphy for sentinel lymph node biopsy of melanoma draining to the head and neck.* Houston, TX: The University of Texas MD Anderson Cancer Center, 2011.

82. Reynolds HM, et al. Three-dimensional visualization of skin lymphatic drainage patterns of the head and neck. *Head Neck* 2009;31(10):1316–1325.

83. Emery RE, et al. Sentinel node staging of primary melanoma by the "10% rule": pathology and clinical outcomes. *Am J Surg* 2007;193(5):618–622, discussion 622.

84. McMasters KM, et al. Sentinel lymph node biopsy for melanoma: how many radioactive nodes should be removed? *Ann Surg Oncol* 2001;8(3):192–197.

85. Abou-Nukta F, Ariyan S. Sentinel lymph node biopsies in melanoma: how many nodes do we really need? *Ann Plast Surg* 2008;60(4):416–419.

86. Gershenwald JE, et al. Patterns of recurrence following a negative sentinel lymph node biopsy in 243 patients with stage I or II melanoma. *J Clin Oncol* 1998;16(6):2253–2260.

87. Yu LL, et al. Detection of microscopic melanoma metastases in sentinel lymph nodes. *Cancer* 1999;86(4):617–627.

88. Balch CM. Melanoma of the skin. In: Edge SB, et al., eds. *AJCC cancer staging manual.* New York: Springer-Verlag, 2010.

89. Chapman PB. Detection of melanoma cells in sentinel lymph nodes by PCR is not yet ready for prime time. *Pigment Cell Res* 2007;20(5):343–344.

90. Schmalbach CE, et al. Reliability of sentinel lymph node mapping with biopsy for head and neck cutaneous melanoma. *Arch Otolaryngol Head Neck Surg* 2003;129(1):61–65.

91. Chao C, et al. Sentinel lymph node biopsy for head and neck melanomas. *Ann Surg Oncol* 2003;10(1):21–26.

92. Morton DL, et al. Sentinel-node biopsy or nodal observation in melanoma. *N Engl J Med* 2006;355(13):1307–1317.

93. Balch CM, Cascinelli N. Sentinel-node biopsy in melanoma. *N Engl J Med* 2006:355(13):1370–1371.

94. Morton DL, et al. Improved long-term survival after lymphadenectomy of melanoma metastatic to regional nodes. Analysis of prognostic factors in 1134 patients from the John Wayne Cancer Clinic. *Ann Surg* 1991;214(4):491–499; discussion 499–501.

95. Cascinelli N, et al. Immediate or delayed dissection of regional nodes in patients with melanoma of the trunk: a randomised trial. WHO Melanoma Programme. *Lancet* 1998:351(9105): 793–796.

96. Scoggins CR, et al. Prognostic information from sentinel lymph node biopsy in patients with thick melanoma. *Arch Surg* 2010;145(7):622–627.

97. Gajdos C, et al. Is there a benefit to sentinel lymph node biopsy in patients with T4 melanoma? *Cancer* 2009;115(24): 5752–5760.

98. Cecchi R, et al. Sentinel lymph node biopsy in patients with thick (= 4 mm) melanoma: a single-centre experience. *J Eur Acad Dermatol Venereol* 2007;21(6):758–61.

99. Gutzmer R, et al. Sentinel lymph node status is the most important prognostic factor for thick (> or = 4 mm) melanomas. *J Dtsch Dermatol Ges* 2008;6(3):198–203.

100. Vermeeren L, et al. Thick melanoma: prognostic value of positive sentinel nodes. *World J Surg* 2009;33(11):2464–2468.

101. O'Rourke MG, Altmann CR. Melanoma recurrence after excision. Is a wide margin justified? *Ann Surg* 1993;217(1):2–5.

102. Karakousis CP, et al. Local recurrence in malignant melanoma: long-term results of the multiinstitutional randomized surgical trial. *Ann Surg Oncol* 1996;3(5):446–452.

103. Heaton KM, et al. Surgical margins and prognostic factors in patients with thick (>4 mm) primary melanoma. *Ann Surg Oncol* 1998;5(4):322–328.

104. Sladden MJ, et al. Surgical excision margins for primary cutaneous melanoma. *Cochrane Database Syst Rev* 2009;(4):CD004835.

105. Zitelli JA, Moy RL, Abell E. The reliability of frozen sections in the evaluation of surgical margins for melanoma. *J Am Acad Dermatol* 1991;24(1):102–106.

106. Gorsky M, Epstein JB. Melanoma arising from the mucosal surfaces of the head and neck. *Oral Surg Oral Med Oral Pathol Oral Radiol Endod* 1998;86(6):715–719.

107. Loree TR, et al. Head and neck mucosal melanoma: a 32-year review. *Ear Nose Throat J* 1999;78(5):372–375.

108. O'Brien CJ, et al. Radical, modified, and selective neck dissection for cutaneous malignant melanoma. *Head Neck* 1995;17(3):232–241.

109. Fisher SR. Elective, therapeutic, and delayed lymph node dissection for malignant melanoma of the head and neck: analysis of 1444 patients from 1970 to 1998. *Laryngoscope* 2002;112(1):99–110.

110. Shah JP, et al. Patterns of regional lymph node metastases from cutaneous melanomas of the head and neck. *Am J Surg* 1991;162(4):320–323.

111. Lee JH, et al. Factors predictive of tumor-positive nonsentinel lymph nodes after tumor-positive sentinel lymph node dissection for melanoma. *J Clin Oncol* 2004;22(18):3677–3684.

112. Morton DL, et al. Sentinel node biopsy for early-stage melanoma: accuracy and morbidity in MSLT-I, an international multicenter trial. *Ann Surg* 2005;242(3):302–311; discussion 311–313.

113. Barranco SC, Romsdahl MM, Humphrey RM. The radiation response of human malignant melanoma cells grown in vitro. *Cancer Res* 1971;31(6):830–833.

114. Farshad A, et al. A retrospective study of 150 patients with lentigo maligna and lentigo maligna melanoma and the efficacy of radiotherapy using Grenz or soft X-rays. *Br J Dermatol* 2002;146(6):1042–1046.

115. Ang KK, et al. Postoperative radiotherapy for cutaneous melanoma of the head and neck region. *Int J Radiat Oncol Biol Phys* 1994;30(4):795–798.

116. Ballo MT, et al. Adjuvant irradiation for cervical lymph node metastases from melanoma. *Cancer* 2003;97(7):1789–1796.

117. Ballo MT, et al. Melanoma metastatic to cervical lymph nodes: can radiotherapy replace formal dissection after local excision of nodal disease? *Head Neck* 2005;27(8):718–721.

118. Burmeister B, Thompson HMJ, Fisher R, et al. Adjuvant radiotherapy improves regional (lymph node field) control in melanoma patients after lymphadenectomy: results of an intergroup randomized trial (TROG 02.01/ANZMTG 01.02). I. *J Radiat Oncol* 2009;75(3 Suppl 2009):S2.

119. Chen JY, et al. Desmoplastic neurotropic melanoma: a clinicopathologic analysis of 128 cases. *Cancer* 2008;113(10):2770–2778.

120. Krengli M, et al. What is the role of radiotherapy in the treatment of mucosal melanoma of the head and neck? *Crit Rev Oncol Hematol* 2008;65(2):121–128.

121. Kirkwood JM, et al. High- and low-dose interferon alfa-2b in high-risk melanoma: first analysis of intergroup trial E1690/S9111/C9190. *J Clin Oncol* 2000;18(12):2444–2458.

122. Kirkwood JM, et al. Interferon alfa-2b adjuvant therapy of high-risk resected cutaneous melanoma: the Eastern Cooperative Oncology Group Trial EST 1684. *J Clin Oncol* 1996;14(1):7–17.

123. Eggermont AM, et al. Adjuvant therapy with pegylated interferon alfa-2b versus observation alone in resected stage III melanoma: final results of EORTC 18991, a randomised phase III trial. *Lancet* 2008;372(9633):117–126.

124. Gogas H, et al. Prognostic significance of autoimmunity during treatment of melanoma with interferon. *N Engl J Med* 2006;354(7):709–718.

125. Bouwhuis MG, et al. Autoimmune antibodies and recurrence-free interval in melanoma patients treated with adjuvant interferon. *J Natl Cancer Inst* 2009;101(12):869–877.

126. Hancock BW, et al. Adjuvant interferon in high-risk melanoma: the AIM HIGH Study—United Kingdom Coordinating Committee on Cancer Research study of adjuvant low-dose extended-duration interferon Alfa-2a in high-risk resected malignant melanoma. *J Clin Oncol* 2004;22(1):53–61.

127. Eggermont AM, et al. Post-surgery adjuvant therapy with intermediate doses of interferon alfa 2b versus observation in patients with stage IIb/III melanoma (EORTC 18952): randomised controlled trial. *Lancet* 2005;366(9492):1189–1196.

128. Pectasides D, et al. Randomized phase III study of 1 month versus 1 year of adjuvant high-dose interferon alfa-2b in patients with resected high-risk melanoma. *J Clin Oncol* 2009;27(6):939–944.

129. Saleh MN, et al. Phase I trial of the murine monoclonal anti-GD2 antibody 14G2a in metastatic melanoma. *Cancer Res* 1992;52(16):4342–4347.

130. Kirkwood JM, et al. High-dose interferon alfa-2b significantly prolongs relapse-free and overall survival compared with the GM2-KLH/QS-21 vaccine in patients with resected stage IIB–III melanoma: results of intergroup trial E1694/S9512/C509801. *J Clin Oncol* 2001;19(9):2370–2380.

131. Eggermont AM, et al. EORTC 18961: post-operative adjuvant ganglioside GM2-KLH21 vaccination treatment vs observation in stage II (T3-T4N0M0) melanoma: 2nd interim analysis led to an early disclosure of the results. *J Clin Oncol (Meeting Abstracts)* 2008;26(15 Suppl):9004.

132. Chung MH, et al. Humoral immune response to a therapeutic polyvalent cancer vaccine after complete resection of thick primary melanoma and sentinel lymphadenectomy. *J Clin Oncol* 2003;21(2):313–319.

133. Hsueh EC, Morton DL. Antigen-based immunotherapy of melanoma: Canvaxin therapeutic polyvalent cancer vaccine. *Semin Cancer Biol* 2003;13(6):401–407.

134. Rosenberg SA, Yang JC, Restifo NP. Cancer immunotherapy: moving beyond current vaccines. *Nat Med* 2004;10(9):909–915.

135. DiFronzo LA, et al. Enhanced humoral immune response correlates with improved disease-free and overall survival in American Joint Committee on Cancer stage II melanoma patients receiving adjuvant polyvalent vaccine. *J Clin Oncol* 2002;20(15):3242–3248.

136. Schwartzentruber DJ, Lawson DH, Richards JM, et al. gp100 peptide vaccine and interleukin-2 in patients with advanced melanoma. *N Engl J Med* 2011;364(22):2119–2127.

137. Rosenberg SA, et al. Treatment of 283 consecutive patients with metastatic melanoma or renal cell cancer using high-dose bolus interleukin 2. *JAMA* 1994;271(12):907–913.

138. Atkins MB, et al. High-dose recombinant interleukin 2 therapy for patients with metastatic melanoma: analysis of 270 patients treated between 1985 and 1993. *J Clin Oncol* 1999;17(7):2105–2116.

139. Atkins MB, et al. High-dose recombinant interleukin-2 therapy in patients with metastatic melanoma: long-term survival update. *Cancer J Sci Am* 2000;6(Suppl 1):S11–S14.

140. Smith FO, et al. Treatment of metastatic melanoma using interleukin-2 alone or in conjunction with vaccines. *Clin Cancer Res* 2008;14(17):5610–5618.

141. Kirkwood JM, et al. A pooled analysis of eastern cooperative oncology group and intergroup trials of adjuvant high-dose interferon for melanoma. *Clin Cancer Res* 2004;10(5):1670–1677.

142. Sznol M. Betting on immunotherapy for melanoma. *Curr Oncol Rep* 2009;11(5):397–404.

143. Hodi FS, et al. Improved survival with ipilimumab in patients with metastatic melanoma. *N Engl J Med* 363(8):711–723.

144. Robert C, Thomas L, Bondarenko I, et al. Ipilimumab plus dacarbazine for previously untreated metastatic melanoma. *N Engl J Med* 2011;364(26):2517–2526.

145. Atallah E, Flaherty L. Treatment of metastatic malignant melanoma. *Curr Treat Options Oncol* 2005;6(3):185–193.

146. Serrone L, et al. Dacarbazine-based chemotherapy for metastatic melanoma: thirty-year experience overview. *J Exp Clin Cancer Res* 2000;19(1):21–34.

147. Middleton MR, et al. Randomized phase III study of temozolomide versus dacarbazine in the treatment of patients with advanced metastatic malignant melanoma. *J Clin Oncol* 2000;18(1):158–166.

148. Legha SS, et al. A prospective evaluation of a triple-drug regimen containing cisplatin, vinblastine, and dacarbazine (CVD) for metastatic melanoma. *Cancer* 1989;64(10):2024–2029.

149. McClay EF, et al. Combination chemotherapy and hormonal therapy in the treatment of malignant melanoma. *Cancer Treat Rep* 1987;71(5):465–469.

150. Chapman PB, et al. Phase III multicenter randomized trial of the Dartmouth regimen versus dacarbazine in patients with metastatic melanoma. *J Clin Oncol* 1999;17(9):2745–2751.

151. Agarwala SS, et al. Randomized phase III study of paclitaxel plus carboplatin with or without sorafenib as second-line treatment in patients with advanced melanoma. *J Clin Oncol (Meeting Abstracts)* 2007;25(18 Suppl):8510.

152. Rao RD, et al. Combination of paclitaxel and carboplatin as second-line therapy for patients with metastatic melanoma. *Cancer* 2006;106(2):375–382.

153. Davies H, et al. Mutations of the BRAF gene in human cancer. *Nature* 2002;417(6892):949–954.

154. Wellbrock C, Karasarides M, Marais R. The RAF proteins take centre stage. *Nat Rev Mol Cell Biol* 2004;5(11):875–885.

155. Hauschild A, et al. Results of a phase III, randomized, placebo-controlled study of sorafenib in combination with carboplatin and paclitaxel as second-line treatment in patients with unresectable stage III or stage IV melanoma. *J Clin Oncol* 2009;27(17):2823–2830.

156. Flaherty KT, et al. Final results of E2603: A double-blind, randomized phase III trial comparing carboplatin (C)/paclitaxel (P) with or without sorafenib (S) in metastatic melanoma. *J Clin Oncol (Meeting Abstracts)* 2010;28(15 Suppl):8511.

157. Flaherty KT, et al. Inhibition of mutated, activated BRAF in metastatic melanoma. *N Engl J Med* 2010;363(9):809–819.

158. Chapman et al. Improved survival with vemurafenib in melanoma with BRAF V600E mutation. *N Engl J Med* 2011;364(26):2507–2516.

159. Curtin JA, et al. Distinct sets of genetic alterations in melanoma. *N Engl J Med* 2005;353(20):2135–2147.

160. Legha SS, et al. Treatment of metastatic melanoma with combined chemotherapy containing cisplatin, vinblastine and dacarbazine (CVD) and biotherapy using interleukin-2 and interferon-alpha. *Ann Oncol* 1996;7(8):827–835.

161. Legha SS, et al. Development of a biochemotherapy regimen with concurrent administration of cisplatin, vinblastine, dacarbazine, interferon alfa, and interleukin-2 for patients with metastatic melanoma. *J Clin Oncol* 1998;16(5):1752–1759.

162. O'Day SJ, et al. Maintenance biotherapy for metastatic melanoma with interleukin-2 and granulocyte macrophage-colony stimulating factor improves survival for patients responding to induction concurrent biochemotherapy. *Clin Cancer Res* 2002;8(9):2775–2781.

163. Eton O, et al. Sequential biochemotherapy versus chemotherapy for metastatic melanoma: results from a phase III randomized trial. *J Clin Oncol* 2002;20(8):2045–2052.

164. Atkins MB, et al. Phase III trial comparing concurrent biochemotherapy with cisplatin, vinblastine, dacarbazine, interleukin-2, and interferon alfa-2b with cisplatin, vinblastine, and dacarbazine alone in patients with metastatic malignant melanoma (E3695): a trial coordinated by the Eastern Cooperative Oncology Group. *J Clin Oncol* 2008;26(35):5748–5754.

165. Ridolfi R, et al. Cisplatin, dacarbazine with or without subcutaneous interleukin-2, and interferon alpha-2b in advanced melanoma outpatients: results from an Italian multicenter phase III randomized clinical trial. *J Clin Oncol* 2002;20(6):1600–1607.

166. Keilholz U, et al. Dacarbazine, cisplatin, and interferon-alfa-2b with or without interleukin-2 in metastatic melanoma: a randomized phase III trial (18951) of the European Organisation for Research and Treatment of Cancer Melanoma Group. *J Clin Oncol* 2005;23(27):6747–6755.

167. Bajetta E, et al. Multicenter phase III randomized trial of polychemotherapy (CVD regimen) versus the same chemotherapy (CT) plus subcutaneous interleukin-2 and interferon-alpha2b in metastatic melanoma. *Ann Oncol* 2006;17(4):571–577.

168. Ives NJ, et al. Chemotherapy compared with biochemotherapy for the treatment of metastatic melanoma: a meta-analysis of 18 trials involving 2,621 patients. *J Clin Oncol* 2007;25(34):5426–5434.

169. Rosenberg SA, et al. Prospective randomized trial of the treatment of patients with metastatic melanoma using chemotherapy with cisplatin, dacarbazine, and tamoxifen alone or in combination with interleukin-2 and interferon alfa-2b. *J Clin Oncol* 1999;17(3):968–975.

170. Demierre MF, Nathanson L. Chemoprevention of melanoma: an unexplored strategy. *J Clin Oncol* 2003;21(1):158–165.

171. Weiss M, et al. Utility of follow-up tests for detecting recurrent disease in patients with malignant melanomas. *JAMA* 1995;274(21):1703–1705.

172. Mellado B, et al. Tyrosinase mRNA in blood of patients with melanoma treated with adjuvant interferon. *J Clin Oncol* 2002;20(19):4032–4039.

173. Poo-Hwu WJ, et al. Follow-up recommendations for patients with American Joint Committee on Cancer Stages I–III malignant melanoma. *Cancer* 1999;86(11):2252–2258.

115 Salivary Gland Neoplasms

Young S. Oh   *Matthew S. Russell*   *David W. Eisele*

Neoplasms of the salivary glands represent a diverse group of benign and malignant tumors with varying degrees of behavior. Accurate pathologic diagnosis is key to the management of these lesions because of their varied clinical behaviors. The otolaryngologist-head and neck surgeon must understand the behavior of each tumor type to develop an appropriate treatment plan for a given patient.

ANATOMY AND PHYSIOLOGY

Salivary glands are divided into major and minor glands. The major salivary glands consist of the paired parotid, submandibular, and sublingual glands. The minor salivary glands consist of 600 to 1,000 glands distributed throughout the upper aerodigestive tract. The World Health Organization histologic classification scheme for salivary gland tumors is presented in Table 115.1.

The incidence rate for salivary gland neoplasms is near 1/100,000 with little variance over the last several decades. Approximately 70% of salivary gland tumors originate in the parotid gland. Of parotid gland tumors, approximately 75% to 80% are benign. About 10% of salivary gland tumors arise from the submandibular gland with the distribution of benign and malignant tumors being similar to the parotid gland. Finally, approximately 20% arise from the minor salivary glands, and a higher proportion (50% to 75%) of these neoplasms are malignant (1).

In adults, the vast majority of salivary gland tumors are benign. Malignancies make up 5% of all head and neck cancers and less than 0.5% of all cancers (2). The most common benign tumor for all salivary glands is the pleomorphic adenoma. Tables 115.2 to 115.4 list series in the literature detailing the distribution of neoplasms of the parotid, submandibular, and minor salivary glands, respectively (3–5).

Salivary gland tumors are far less common in the pediatric population. Only about 5% of all epithelial salivary gland tumors will occur in children and adolescents. Unlike adults, benign vascular and lymphatic tumors are the most common pediatric salivary gland masses (6). Infectious, inflammatory, and congenital conditions should also be considered in the differential diagnosis of pediatric salivary gland lesions. The majority of epithelial neoplasms in children are malignant (Tables 115.5 and 115.6) (7).

BENIGN NEOPLASMS

Pleomorphic Adenoma

Pleomorphic adenoma (benign mixed tumor) accounts for approximately 65% of all salivary gland tumors. These tumors are most often found in the parotid gland, followed by the submandibular gland, and the minor salivary glands. They also represent the most common tumor of each type of salivary gland.

Benign mixed tumor describes the mesenchymal and epithelial components of the tumor. The gross appearance is smooth and lobular with a well-defined capsule. Microscopically, the tumor consists of epithelial and mesenchymal elements. The epithelial component forms a trabecular pattern with a mesenchymal stroma (Fig. 115.1). The mesenchymal portion may be myxoid, chondroid, fibroid, or osteoid. The stroma varies from tumor to tumor and may have a combination of any of these tissue types within it. Histologically, encapsulation may be incomplete with pseudopod extensions of the tumor (8).

Historically, unacceptably high recurrence rates of 20% to 45% have been observed with simple tumor enucleation. Thus, complete surgical resection with an adequate margin of normal tissue is advocated. In the past, for the parotid gland, this constituted a complete superficial parotidectomy. Although this technique is highly effective, there can be some unwanted sequelae such as temporary or permanent facial nerve injury, cosmetic soft tissue defects, or Frey syndrome. Presently, tumor resection by partial parotidectomy

TABLE 115.1	THE WORLD HEALTH ORGANIZATION HISTOLOGIC CLASSIFICATION OF TUMORS OF THE SALIVARY GLANDS

Malignant epithelial tumors	*Benign epithelial tumors*
Acinic cell carcinoma	Pleomorphic adenoma
Mucoepidermoid carcinoma	Myoepithelioma
Adenoid cystic carcinoma	Basal cell adenoma
PLGA	Warthin tumor
Epithelial-Myoepithelial carcinoma	Oncocytoma
Clear cell carcinoma, NOS	Canalicular adenoma
Basal cell adenocarcinoma	Sebaceous adenoma
Sebaceous carcinoma	Lymphadenoma
Cystadenocarcinoma	Sebaceous
Low-grade cribriform cystadenocarcinoma	Nonsebaceous
Mucinous adenocarcinoma	Ductal Papillomas
Oncocytic carcinoma	Inverted ductal papilloma
Salivary duct carcinoma	Intraductal papilloma
Adenocarcinoma NOS	Sialadenoma papilliferum
Myoepithelial carcinoma	Cystadenoma
Carcinoma ex pleomorphic adenoma	*Soft tissue tumors*
Carcinosarcoma	Hemangioma
Metastasizing pleomorphic adenoma	*Hematolymphoid tumors*
Squamous cell carcinoma	Hodgkin lymphoma
Small cell carcinoma	Diffuse large B-cell lymphoma
Large cell carcinoma	Extranodal marginal zone B-cell lymphoma
LEC	*Secondary tumors*
Sialoblastoma	

LEC, Lymphoepithelial carcinoma; NOS, Not otherwise specified.
From Barnes L, Eveson JW, Reichart P, et al., eds. *World Health Organization Classification of Tumors. Pathology and Genetics of Head and Neck Tumours.* Lyon, France: IARC Press, 2005, with permission.

with facial nerve preservation is advocated. This procedure is defined as any parotidectomy in which less than the entire lobe or less than all the branches of the facial nerve are dissected. Lower rates of facial nerve weakness and Frey syndrome are observed with this approach (9).

Rarely, pleomorphic adenoma can metastasize and yet remain benign appearing histologically. Reported sites of metastases include bone, head and neck regions, lungs, and skin. When feasible, surgical resection of the metastatic site is the optimal treatment. Incomplete excision or

TABLE 115.2	DISTRIBUTION OF PAROTID GLAND NEOPLASMS

Histologic Type	Parotid Gland N (%)
Pleomorphic adenoma	256 (66.8)
Warthin tumor	87 (22.8)
Other	40 (10.4)
Total benign	**383 (100)**
Mucoepidermoid carcinoma	41 (32.5)
Adenoid cystic carcinoma	20 (15.9)
Ca ex pleomorphic adenoma	17 (13.5)
Acinic cell carcinoma	13 (10.3)
Adenocarcinoma NOS	6 (4.7)
Basal cell adenocarcinoma	5 (3.9)
Clear cell adenocarcinoma	4 (3.2)
Myoepithelial carcinoma	3 (2.4)
Salivary duct carcinoma	3 (2.4)
Other malignant	14 (11.2)
Total malignant	**126 (100)**

From Luksic I, Virag M, Manojlovic S, et al. Salivary gland tumors: 25 years of experience from a single institution in Croatia. *J Craniomaxillofac Surg* 2011; 40(3):e75–e81. doi:10.1016/j.jcms.2011.05.002.

TABLE 115.3	DISTRIBUTION OF SUBMANDIBULAR GLAND NEOPLASMS

Histologic Type	Submandibular Gland N (%)
Pleomorphic adenoma	479 (97.8)
Other	11 (2.2)
Total benign	**490 (100)**
Adenoid cystic carcinoma	74 (43)
Mucoepidermoid carcinoma	28 (16)
Ca ex pleomorphic adenoma	27 (16)
Acinic cell carcinoma	7 (4)
Adenocarcinoma NOS	6 (3.5)
LEC	12 (7)
Myoepithelial carcinoma	6 (3.5)
Other malignant	12 (7)
Total malignant	**172 (100)**

From Zian T, Li L, Wang L, et al. Salivary gland neoplasms in oral and maxillofacial regions: a 23-year retrospective study of 6982 cases in an eastern Chinese population. *Int J Oral Maxillofac Surg* 2010;39:235–242.

TABLE 115.4	INCIDENCE OF MINOR SALIVARY GLAND NEOPLASMS BY TUMOR TYPE	
Tumor Type		**Incidence (%)**
Pleomorphic adenoma		22.16
Basal cell adenoma		1.08
Cystadenoma		0.54
Myoepithelioma		0.54
Oncocytoma		0.54
Other benign		0.54
Total benign		**25.4**
Mucoepidermoid carcinoma		34.05
Adenoid cystic carcinoma		14.59
PLGA		9.73
Adenocarcinoma not specified		7.57
Basal cell adenocarcinoma		4.86
Clear cell carcinoma		1.08
Salivary duct carcinoma		1.08
Carcinoma ex pleomorphic adenoma		0.54
Mucinous adenocarcinoma		0.54
Sebaceous carcinoma		0.54
Total malignant		**74.6**

PLGA, Polymorphous low-grade adenocarcinoma.
From Vani NV, Ponniah I. The frequency and distribution pattern of minor salivary gland tumors in a government dental teaching hospital, Chennai, India. *Oral Surg Oral Med Oral Pathol Oral Radiol Endod* 2011;111:e33.

rupture of the primary is thought to be a risk factor for the development of distant metastases (10,11).

Warthin Tumor

Warthin tumor (papillary cystadenoma lymphomatosum) is the second most common benign salivary gland neoplasm constituting 5% to 6% of all benign tumors. The majority of Warthin tumors occur in the parotid gland. However, extraparotid sites can be involved as

TABLE 115.5	BENIGN SALIVARY GLAND TUMORS IN CHILDREN	
Tumor Type		**Number of Patients**
Hemangioma		191
Pleomorphic adenoma		182
Lymphangioma		48
Neurogenic		11
Embryoma		5
Lymphoepithelial lesion		3
Cystadenoma		3
Warthin tumor		3
Other		9
Total patients		**668**
Total benign		**68%**

From Luna MA, Batsakis JG, El-Naggar AK. Salivary gland tumors in children. *Ann Otol Rhinol Laryngol* 1991;100:869–871, with permission.

TABLE 115.6	MALIGNANT SALIVARY GLAND TUMORS IN CHILDREN	
Histologic Type		**N (%)**
Mucoepidermoid carcinoma		47 (42)
Acinic cell carcinoma		38 (34)
Rhabdomyosarcoma		8 (7)
Lymphoma/Hodgkin's		9 (8)
Adenocarcinoma		4 (4)
Adenoid cystic carcinoma		2 (2)
Other malignant		5 (4)
Total malignant		**113 (100)**

From Shapiro N, Bhattacharyya N. Clinical characteristics and survival for major salivary gland malignancies in children. *Otolaryngol Head Neck Surg* 2006;134:631–634.

well, typically in the cervical lymph nodes (12). Smoking is a clear etiologic factor for this tumor. Classically, this is a tumor that occurs more commonly in men, but the incidence has increased in women. This is thought to be due to the increased relative rate of smoking in women. Rates of multicentricity for this tumor has been reported from 12% to 50% depending on the series (Fig. 115.2). Bilateral tumor can be seen in up to 12% of patients (13,14).

The gross appearance of the tumor is smooth with a well-defined capsule. Cut sections reveal multiple cystic spaces that can be filled with a thick, mucinous exudate. Microscopically, Warthin tumor has a characteristic appearance with a papillary epithelium with a lymphoid stroma projecting into cystic spaces (Fig. 115.3). The epithelium is a double layer of oxyphilic granular cells, with cells of the inner layer having the nuclei oriented toward the basement membrane. The cells in the outer layer have nuclei toward the cystic space.

Complete surgical excision is recommended. Tumor "recurrences" are thought to result from unrecognized multicentric tumors (13).

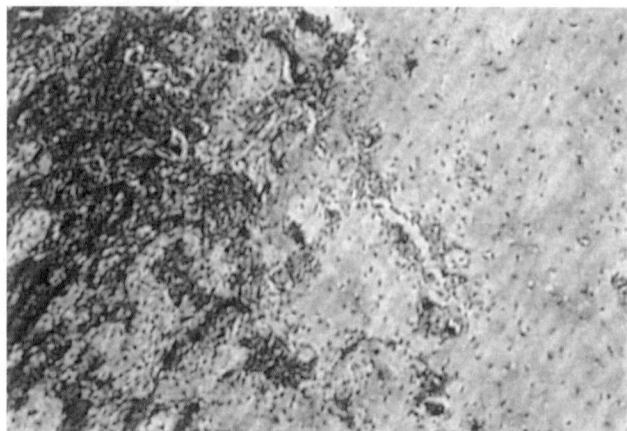

Figure 115.1 Pleomorphic adenoma. The histologic appearance shows characteristic epithelial and mesenchymal elements.

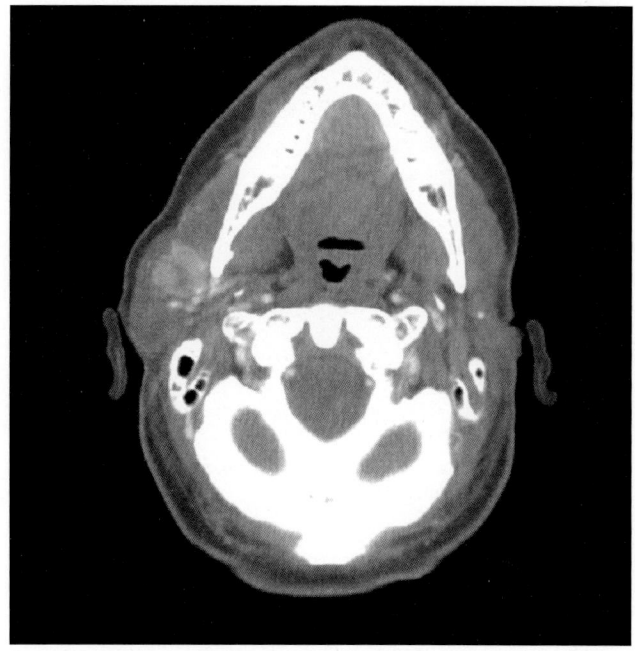
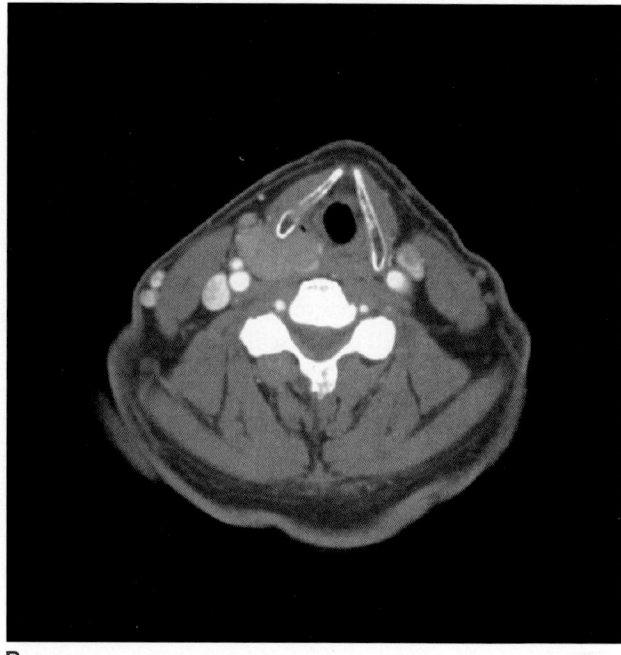

A   B

Figure 115.2 A: Axial contrast-enhanced CT shows a sharply marginated, heterogeneous attenuation lesion in the superficial lobe of the right parotid gland. **B:** Axial contrast-enhanced CT demonstrates a well-circumscribed enhancing mass, medial to the sternocleidomastoid muscle, which displaces the right thyroid cartilage anteriorly and laterally. This lesion proved to be an additional focus of Warthin tumor.

Oncocytoma

Oncocytoma is an uncommon salivary gland tumor that accounts for about 1% of all salivary gland neoplasms (15). It occurs almost exclusively in the parotid gland. This tumor occurs most frequently in the fifth and sixth decades of life and with equal distribution between men and women (16). Oncocytoma usually presents as a painless mass in the superficial lobe of the parotid gland.

These tumors are noncystic, firm, and rubbery. Microscopically, these neoplasms are composed of brown, plump, granular eosinophilic cells with small indented nuclei (Fig. 115.4). A mitochondria-filled cystoplasm is a characteristic finding on electron microscopy. Malignant degeneration is rare. A possible explanation for these tumors is an acquired genetic defect leading to mitochondrial dysfunction; however, an exact molecular mechanism has not been established (17). Immunohistochemical studies have found that oncocytoma demonstrated positive reactivity to CK5/6, CK8/18, CK19, and EMA. It was negative to S100 and SMA (16).

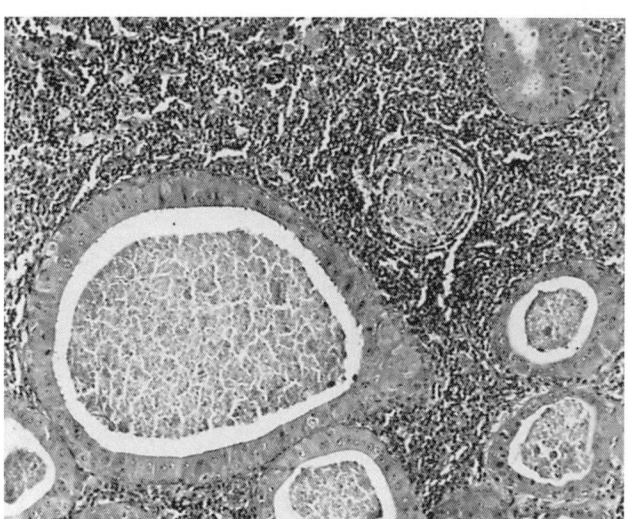

Figure 115.3 Warthin tumor. Lymphoid stroma and double-layered epithelium surround the cystic spaces.

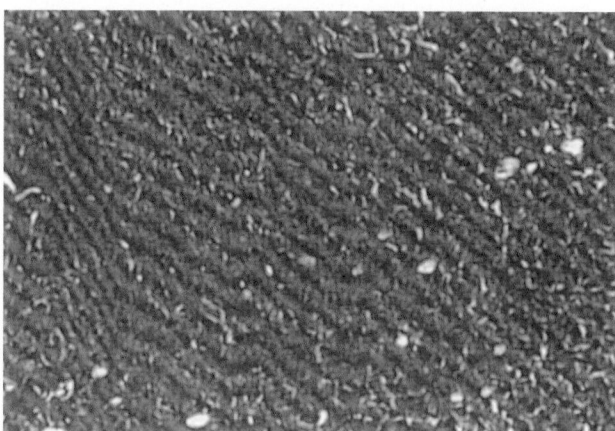

Figure 115.4 Oncocytoma. The histologic appearance is that of typical plump, granular eosinophilic cells.

Complete tumor resection is the treatment of choice for oncocytoma.

Basal Cell Adenoma

Basal cell adenoma represents about 2% to 3% of all salivary gland tumors. It usually occurs in the sixth to seventh decades of life, and it occurs most often in the parotid gland. The remainder are divided between the submandibular and the minor salivary glands. It affects more women than men (18).

These tumors are well circumscribed and encapsulated. The membranous histologic variant can be multinodular. Microscopically, it can demonstrate four different histologic patterns. The solid pattern consists of sheets of basaloid cells. The tubular pattern consists of small ductules linked by the basaloid cells. The trabecular pattern has plexiform bands of the tumor cells. Finally, the membranous pattern consists of differing sizes of islands of basaloid cells. The membranous pattern can show multicentric tumor patterns and has a higher rate of recurrence after surgery (18).

Basal cell adenoma is considered a benign, nonaggressive tumor. Treatment consists of complete surgical resection with a margin of normal tissue.

MALIGNANT NEOPLASMS

Mucoepidermoid Carcinoma

Mucoepidermoid carcinoma is the most common malignant neoplasm of the salivary glands. It presents most frequently in the parotid gland, for which it is the most common malignant tumor. It is the second most common malignant tumor of the submandibular gland. Mucoepidermoid carcinoma constitutes approximately 30% to 35% of all malignant tumors of the salivary glands (19,20). This is a cancer that usually occurs between the third and sixth decades of life with a slight predominance in women.

Mucoepidermoid carcinomas are usually classified as low-grade or high-grade tumors. However, some pathologists also include an intermediate grade. Low-grade tumors have a higher proportion of mucous cells to epidermoid cells. These lesions behave more like benign neoplasms but in rare cases are capable of local invasion and metastasis. High-grade tumors have a higher proportion of epidermoid cells and may be difficult to differentiate from squamous cell carcinoma. High-grade lesions are aggressive tumors with a high propensity for metastasis. Intermediate-grade lesions have been found to behave like high-grade tumors. Thus, the grade and stage of these neoplasms are important prognostic variables (21).

Low-grade tumors are usually small and partially encapsulated. High-grade neoplasms are usually larger and locally invasive. On cut sections, low-grade mucoepidermoid carcinoma may contain mucinous fluid, whereas high-grade tumors are typically solid. Microscopically, low-grade mucoepidermoid carcinoma demonstrates aggregates of

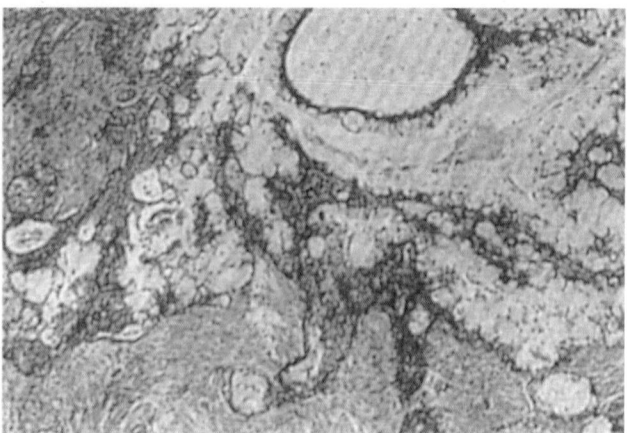

Figure 115.5 Low-grade mucoepidermoid carcinoma. Note the epithelial and glandular elements.

mucoid cells separated by strands of epidermal cells (Fig. 115.5). High-grade tumors have few mucoid elements, and the epidermoid cells predominate (Fig. 115.6).

The treatment of this cancer depends on the grade and stage of the tumor. For small, low-grade cancers, complete surgical resection is recommended. Elective treatment of the neck is not recommended for in the clinically N0 neck because of the incidence of occult nodal involvement is very low (21). If the surgical margins are clear and there are no adverse pathologic features, adjuvant radiation therapy is not recommended. Prognosis for this cancer is excellent with locoregional recurrence rates of 10% and 5-year overall survival of 97% (22).

For high-grade tumors, the treatment is tailored to the extent of the disease. As in low-grade disease, complete surgical resection of the primary site is recommended. If the tumor involves the parotid gland, the facial nerve is spared, if possible. Cervical nodal metastases are managed by a comprehensive neck dissection at the time of the resection of the primary. Occult metastases rates have been shown to be approximately 21%; therefore, an elective neck dissection can be considered in a patient with a clinically N0

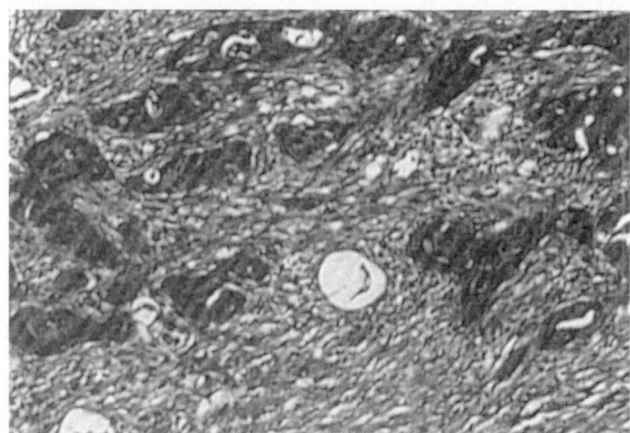

Figure 115.6 High-grade mucoepidermoid carcinoma. Note the relative lack of glandular elements.

neck (22). In most cases of high-grade mucoepidermoid carcinoma, adjuvant radiation therapy is recommended to improve locoregional control (23). High-grade mucoepidermoid carcinoma is an aggressive tumor with a poorer prognosis than the low-grade variant. Locoregional recurrence has been shown to occur 43.5% of the time with 3-year disease-free survival reported to be 55% and 5-year disease-free survival at 30% (21,24).

Adenoid Cystic Carcinoma

Adenoid cystic carcinoma accounts for approximately 10% of all salivary gland neoplasms. It is the second most common malignancy of the parotid gland but is the most common malignancy of the submandibular and minor salivary glands (25). Adenoid cystic carcinoma occurs with equal frequency in men and women, usually in the fifth decade of life. Facial paralysis and pain occur as initial symptoms in a small proportion of patients.

Adenoid cystic carcinoma has a contradictory clinical course. The tumor is slow growing, but its clinical course is relentless. Multiple local recurrences can occur despite adequate surgical intervention, and although regional metastatic spread is uncommon, distant spread, especially to the lungs, is common.

Grossly, the tumor is usually monolobular and either nonencapsulated or partially encapsulated. The mass often demonstrates infiltration of surrounding normal tissue. Microscopically, adenoid cystic carcinoma has a basaloid epithelium arranged in cylindric formations in an eosinophilic hyaline stroma (Fig. 115.7). Different histologic patterns have been identified including cribriform, solid, and tubular. The solid histologic pattern appears to have a worse prognosis in terms of distant metastases and long-term survival (26).

Perineural invasion is a typical feature of adenoid cystic carcinoma. This explains the difficulty in tumor eradication despite the appearance of complete tumor removal. Complete surgical excision and postoperative radiation therapy is recommended for the management of this tumor (27). For select small tumors that are completely excised, however, postoperative radiation therapy may not be needed (28).

There is evidence that fast neutron radiotherapy may be more effective than conventional photon radiation therapy as primary therapy for select adenoid cystic carcinomas that are not amenable to surgery (29,30).

Long-term follow-up is mandatory for these patients because of the slow, relentless disease progression. Recurrences have been shown to occur at an average of 63 months from the time of initial treatment (31). Thus, 5-year survival is not adequate to detail the outcomes of this malignancy. Ten-year overall survival has been reported to be from 55% to 64%. Recurrence rates can be broken down as 42% with distant metastases only, 39% with locoregional recurrences only, and 19% with both locoregional and distant disease (27,31).

Because of the low incidence of occult metastases, elective neck dissection for the N0 neck is not usually performed. However, the presence of nodal metastases at the time of diagnosis is an important prognostic factor because overall survival is significantly lowered when metastases are present (31).

Acinic Cell Carcinoma

Acinic cell carcinoma constitutes approximately 17% of all salivary gland cancers. Up to 98% of these occur in the parotid gland. It affects women more often than men and occurs in the fourth to sixth decade of life. The tumor can be multicentric in 2% to 5% of cases, and it can involve both parotid glands (32,33).

Grossly, this well-circumscribed tumor often has a fibrous capsule. There are two populations of cells: those resembling serous acinar cells of the salivary gland and those with a clear cytoplasm. Tumors occur in several configurations, including cystic, papillary, vacuolated, or follicular. There is often a lymphoid infiltrate, and cells are characteristically positive on periodic acid–Schiff staining (Fig. 115.8).

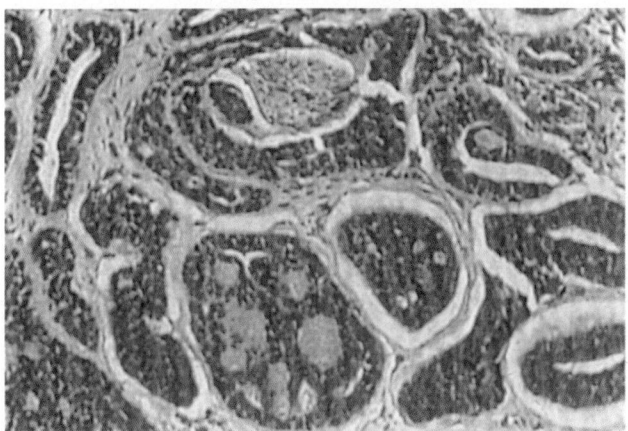

Figure 115.7 Adenoid cystic carcinoma, showing the characteristic histologic appearance with eosinophilic hyaline stroma and perineural invasion.

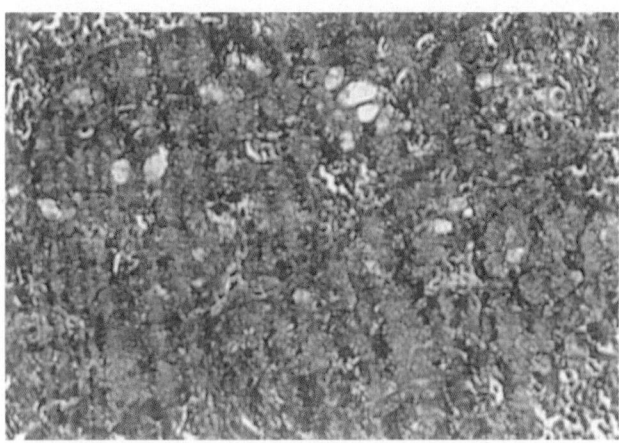

Figure 115.8 Acinic cell carcinoma. Note cells similar to serous acinar cells and cells with clear cytoplasm.

Treatment consists of complete surgical resection with adjuvant radiotherapy reserved for indicators of a poor prognosis (e.g., facial nerve involvement, neck metastases, and skin involvement). Elective treatment of the neck is indicated for high-grade cases of acinic cell carcinoma (32). Although acinic cell carcinoma is typically categorized as an indolent, slow-growing tumor, the average rate of recurrence has been found to be about 35% (32,33). Long term follow-up is mandatory because late local recurrences have been shown to occur many years after initial treatment. For low-grade lesions, 5- and 10-year disease-free survivals have been reported to be approximately 91% and 88%, respectively (34). Five-year overall survival for high-grade acinic cell carcinoma is much poorer at 33% (33).

Adenocarcinoma

Adenocarcinoma most commonly occurs in the minor salivary glands followed by the parotid gland. This neoplasm represents approximately 12% of malignant parotid neoplasms (35). Adenocarcinomas occur equally in both sexes and usually present as a palpable mass. They behave aggressively with a strong propensity to recur and metastasize.

Grossly, adenocarcinoma is firm or hard and attached to the surrounding tissue. Microscopically, the cylindric cells of variable height form papillae, acini, or solid masses. Most neoplasms produce mucus, which can be detected by mucicarmine stain. Adenocarcinoma can be differentiated from mucoepidermoid carcinoma by the lack of keratin staining. The degree of glandular formation has been used as a means of grading these tumors.

Complete surgical resection with postoperative radiation therapy is the recommended treatment for this high-grade malignancy. Five- and ten-year overall survivals are 52% and 36%, respectively (36).

Polymorphous Low-Grade Adenocarcinoma

Polymorphous low-grade adenocarcinoma (PLGA) occurs almost exclusively in the minor salivary glands. The neoplasm most commonly occurs in the palate, buccal mucosa, and the upper lip. Women are affected more commonly than men, and most of these neoplasms occur in the sixth decade of life. The typical presentation of this tumor is of a long-standing, asymptomatic mass on the palate (37).

Histologically, PLGA demonstrates a variable tumor cell differentiation and organization. Mitotic figures and necrosis are unusual features. Tumors typically have an infiltrative growth pattern with frequent perineural invasion. Typical histologic patterns include solid, trabecular, glandular, cribriform, fascicular, cord-like, and papillary. Because of this, careful pathologic diagnosis is mandatory as this neoplasm can be mistaken for pleomorphic adenoma or adenoid cystic carcinoma. Immunohistochemical staining has not been helpful in differentiating adenoid cystic carcinoma from polymorphous low-grade adenocarcinoma (38).

Treatment is wide local surgical excision. Cervical metastases are very uncommon, so a neck dissection is performed only for clinically positive nodes. In a recent review of the three largest series on PLGA, it was found that local recurrences occur anywhere from 10% to 33% of the time. These recurrences can occur up to 15 years after treatment. Even with recurrences, death from tumor progression is rare (39). In general, adjuvant radiotherapy is not recommended for this cancer (40).

Carcinoma Ex Pleomorphic Adenoma

Carcinoma ex pleomorphic adenoma represents a malignant tumor that has risen from a preexisting or recurrent pleomorphic adenoma. The malignant component and metastases from this tumor are purely epithelial in origin. This malignancy represents 2% to 5% of all salivary gland tumors. Rarely, the malignancy can take the form in which the tumor contains both mesenchymal and epithelial components.

Grossly, the tumors are firm with minimal encapsulation. The lesion is widely infiltrative with regions of necrosis and hemorrhage. Microscopically, the malignant neoplasm arises in a background that is characteristic of a benign mixed tumor (Fig. 115.9). Neurovascular invasion and necrosis are frequent findings. The malignant portion of the tumor can take the form of an adenocarcinoma, salivary duct carcinoma, adenosquamous carcinoma, undifferentiated carcinoma, or other malignancy (41). The tumor can also be classified as noninvasive (*in situ*), minimally invasive (less than 1.5 mm), or invasive (greater than 1.5 mm). The majority of these neoplasms are invasive (41,42).

The diagnosis may be confusing because of the differing proportions of benign and malignant elements of the

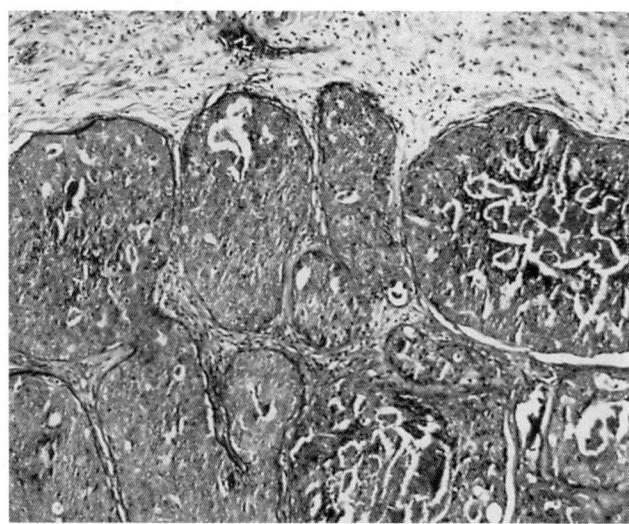

Figure 115.9 Carcinoma ex pleomorphic adenoma is seen in a preexisting pleomorphic adenoma.

tumor. Most cases, however, will have predominantly the malignant component (41,42).

Local and distant metastases are common with this tumor when compared to other salivary gland malignancies. Elective treatment of the neck is recommended because rates of occult metastases have been shown to be about 20%. The recurrence rate is 32% with most occurring in the first year following treatment. Overall survival is 48% at 5 years.

Nodal status is a major determinant of overall survival. In one study, patients who were N+ had 5-year survival at 16% compared to 67% of patients who were N0 (43). Other prognostic factors include pathologic stage, tumor size, grade, proportion of cancer, and extent of invasion (41). Complete surgical resection with postoperative radiation therapy is the recommended treatment for this high-grade malignancy (43).

Primary Squamous Cell Carcinoma

Primary squamous cell carcinoma of the salivary glands represents a rare neoplasm that constitutes less than 1% of all salivary gland cancers (44). This malignancy occurs more often in the submandibular gland than the parotid gland. Rarely, this tumor can also occur in the minor salivary glands (45). Proper diagnosis of squamous cell carcinoma requires exclusion of contiguous spread of a squamous cell carcinoma into the gland, metastases to the gland, high-grade mucoepidermoid carcinoma, and metastatic squamous cell carcinoma from a cutaneous primary.

These tumors usually present as firm indurated masses and occur more commonly in men, usually in the seventh decade of life. Histologically, these tumors reveal intracellular keratinization, intercellular bridges, and keratin pearl formation. However, they do not produce mucus (45). There is a high incidence of regional and distant metastases. Therapy consists of complete surgical resection and postoperative radiation therapy. The prognosis for squamous cell carcinoma of the salivary gland is fair with 5-year disease-free survival at 33% (44).

Undifferentiated Carcinoma

Undifferentiated carcinoma is a rare salivary gland malignancy. These tumors can be further subtyped as small cell undifferentiated carcinoma (SCUC), large cell undifferentiated carcinoma (LCUC), and lymphoepithelial carcinoma (LEC). The vast majority of these tumors occur in the parotid gland.

There is a high incidence of these tumors in Southeast China and among the Inuit Eskimos of North America where the presence of the Epstein-Barr virus (EBV) is more widespread. Studies have shown that the LEC subtype is strongly associated with EBV whereas the LCUC and the SCUC are not. However, even in these endemic geographic areas, the incidence of this malignancy is still very

uncommon. A recent study from Taiwan reported 16 cases of LEC and 12 cases of large cell over nearly 30 years (46).

Overall survival is excellent for LEC with 5-year survival being 85%. However, survival is worse in LCUC with overall 2-year survival being 36%.

Salivary Duct Carcinoma

Salivary duct carcinoma is a rare but aggressive malignancy of the salivary glands. It affects primarily men in the seventh decade of life. The majority occur in the parotid gland (78%), followed by the submandibular gland, and then the minor salivary glands (47).

The tumor is poorly circumscribed and unencapsulated. Cut sections are white-tan and solid, often with cystic areas and necrosis. Microscopically, salivary duct carcinoma resembles high-grade breast carcinoma. Classic examples show Roman bridge structures. Comedonecrosis is often seen. The constituent cells have eosinophilic cytoplasm and exhibit moderate to marked nuclear pleomorphism (Fig. 115.10).

In a recent series, cervical metastases were present in 56% of patients at the time of initial diagnosis. Local recurrence occurred in 48% of patients with an average time to recurrence being 17.4 months. Distant metastases occurred also in 48% of patients with an average time of onset being 29 months after initial treatment. The average time of survival was found to be about 56 months (47).

Immunohistochemical studies reveal a similarity of this cancer and infiltrating ductal carcinoma. Approximately 20% of these tumors are strongly positive for HER2/neu. Having HER2/neu positivity is associated with a poorer prognosis with 5-year survival of 0% for strongly positive tumors compared to 11% for weakly positive cancers (47). Recommended treatment is wide surgical resection with ipsilateral neck dissection followed by adjuvant radiotherapy. Preliminary findings on the use of trastuzumab as a

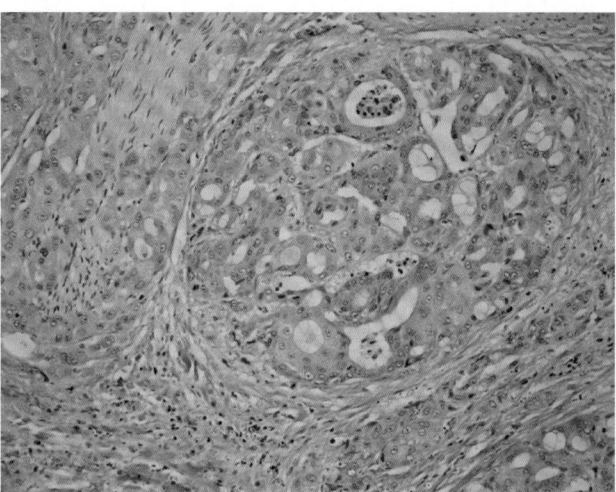

Figure 115.10 Salivary duct carcinoma. The tumor has cribriform architecture with mucin in small glandular spaces. Upper left hand portion of the image shows tumor wrapping around a nerve.

palliative chemotherapeutic agent has been reported in the case of recurrent salivary duct carcinoma (48).

Sarcoma

Sarcomas arising in the parotid gland are rare (49). These aggressive malignancies occur more commonly in men than in women and usually present as an enlarging, yet painless mass. Rhabdomyosarcoma and fibrosarcoma are the most common histopathologic subtypes. Diagnosis of a primary sarcoma requires the exclusion of metastatic spread of the sarcoma to the gland or glandular invasion from local soft tissues. Primary sarcomas behave like other soft tissue sarcomas, and the prognosis correlates with tumor size, type, and degree of histopathologic differentiation (49).

Lymphoma

Primary lymphoma occurs uncommonly in the salivary glands. When present, it usually affects the parotid gland more commonly than the other glands. Lymphoma occurs frequently in patients who have chronic autoimmune diseases such as Sjogren syndrome. Mucosa-associated lymphoid tissue lymphomas are the most common form of primary lymphoma (50). Primary lymphoma usually runs an indolent course with a favorable prognosis (51).

ASSESSMENT AND DIAGNOSIS

Etiologic Factors

Etiologic factors for salivary gland neoplasms are not well understood. Tobacco use has been clearly associated with the risk of developing Warthin tumor. There is no increased risk of developing other salivary gland neoplasms from tobacco use (52). Also, alcohol consumption has not been shown to increase the risk of developing salivary gland tumors (53).

Studies have examined viruses such as the EBV as etiologic factors and, except for LEC, there has not been a demonstrated role for viral infection as a factor in the pathogenesis of salivary gland neoplasms (54).

Low-dose radiation is considered a risk factor for the development of salivary gland neoplasms. A wide range in the dosage of radiation and age of exposure has been seen. This suggests that exposure at any age and any dose may predispose one to the development of a salivary gland tumor (55). The most common malignant radiation-related tumors are mucoepidermoid carcinoma and adenocarcinoma (56).

History

Patients with salivary gland neoplasms usually present with asymptomatic masses. Benign parotid gland neoplasms typically occur in the region of the tail of the gland. Pain is unusual with benign neoplasms but can occur due to associated infection, hemorrhage, or cystic enlargement.

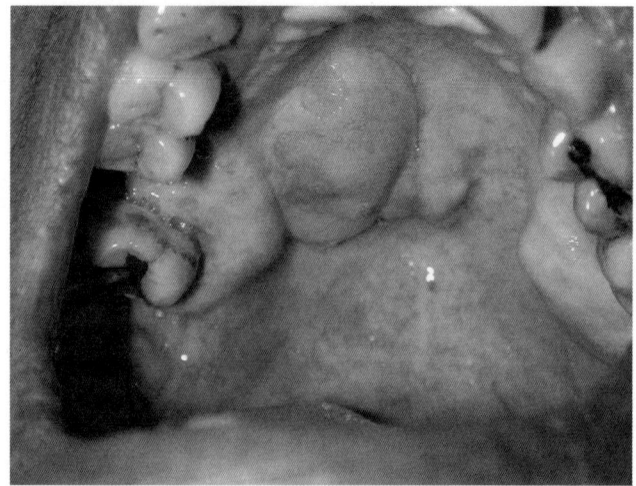

Figure 115.11 Low-grade polymorphous adenocarcinoma presenting as a smooth painless mass of the hard palate.

In malignant neoplasms, pain is usually indicative of neural invasion by the tumor and portends a worse prognosis than a malignant tumor that is not painful. However, pain is not a reliable indicator for malignancy.

Submandibular gland neoplasms present in a similar manner as parotid tumors. Minor salivary gland tumors usually present as nonulcerated, painless submucosal masses involving the oral cavity, typically the hard or soft palate (Fig. 115.11).

Patients with nasal and paranasal sinus neoplasms usually present with advanced symptoms such as nasal obstruction or epistaxis. In the upper aerodigestive tract, minor salivary gland tumors can cause hoarseness, respiratory complaints, or dysphagia, depending on the location. Sublingual gland tumors usually present as masses in the floor of the mouth and may have associated discomfort.

Tumors located in the parapharyngeal space (PPS) are usually asymptomatic and may be noted on routine oropharyngeal examination (Fig. 115.12) or as a neck mass. As

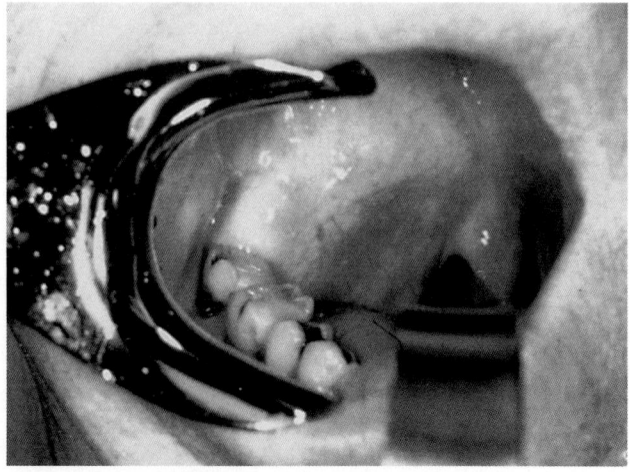

Figure 115.12 Pleomorphic adenoma of the PPS. Note the uvular deviation to the opposite site.

| TABLE 115.7 | ACCURACY OF FNA TECHNIQUE IN DISTINGUISHING MALIGNANT FROM BENIGN AND NONNEOPLASTIC LESIONS | | | |

Histology	Cytology			
	Malignant	Benign	Nonneoplastic	Total
Malignant	387 (93.25%)	55 (4.31%)	42 (19%)	484
Benign	22 (5.3%)	1,219 (95.46%)	34 (15.38%)	1,275
Nonneoplastic or normal tissue	6 (1.45%)	3 (0.23%)	145 (65.61%)	154
Total	415	1,277	221	1,913

From Colella G, Cannavale R, Flamminio F, et al. Fine-needle aspiration cytology of salivary gland lesions: a systemic review. *J Oral Maxillofac Surg* 2010;68:2146–2153, with permission.

the tumor enlarges, alterations in speech and swallowing function may occur.

Physical Examination

In a patient with a salivary gland neoplasm, a thorough head and neck examination is indicated. Attention should be directed to the size, location, and mobility of the tumor. The presence or absence of tenderness to the mass should be noted. Facial nerve function should also be assessed. The presence of facial nerve paralysis should raise the suspicion of malignancy, although rarely, a benign tumor can cause facial nerve paralysis.

Fine Needle Aspiration Biopsy

Fine needle aspiration (FNA) biopsy of a salivary gland tumor is a simple and accurate aid for the diagnosis of salivary gland neoplasms. Its primary value is to establish the need for surgery, not to establish a definitive diagnosis. As such, it is helpful to avoid surgery in select patients with a reactive lymph node, lymphoma, or nonneoplastic disorders.

Adequate tissue sampling is necessary, and clinicopathologic correlation is important. Image guidance with ultrasound or computed tomography (CT) scan is sometimes helpful. FNA offers several advantages including the ability to obtain a definitive diagnosis of a neoplasm and to aid in preoperative patient counseling regarding extent of surgery, timing of surgery, and use of imaging studies (Table 115.7) (57).

Imaging

Head and neck imaging is discussed in detail in Chapter 11. Imaging of salivary gland tumors is important to help in the evaluation of malignant or recurrent tumors, suspected PPS involvement, or suspected involvement in structures that would indicate tumor unresectability. The primary modalities used are CT and magnetic resonance imaging (MRI).

MRI is the imaging modality of choice in evaluating salivary gland tumors. MRI is superior to CT in its soft tissue differentiation. Also, MRI can also provide valuable information on deep tissue invasion, bone marrow infiltration, and perineural spread of tumor (58). The superiority of its soft tissue definition allows MRI to be a useful tool in assessing the PPS. The periparotid fat strip separating the deep lobe of the parotid gland from the PPS is an important anatomic landmark and allows for the differentiation of deep lobe parotid tumors extending into the PPS from tumors that arise from ectopic salivary gland tissue.

CT is helpful in identifying bony erosion or invasion. In cases of minor salivary gland tumors or tumors arising in the paranasal sinuses, CT and MRI frequently provide complimentary information to assess the extent of invasion of the malignancy (Figs. 115.13 and 115.14).

Recently, ultrasound has been more utilized for the assessment of major salivary gland masses. Since the lateral

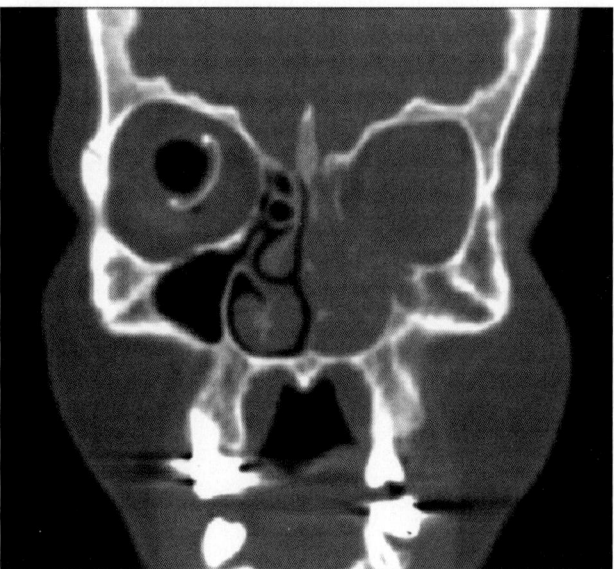

Figure 115.13 Coronal CT with bone windows demonstrates a large neoplasm in the left maxillary sinus with extension into the nasal cavity and orbit. Bone destruction is evident in the inferior orbital wall and a portion of the lateral wall of the left maxillary sinus.

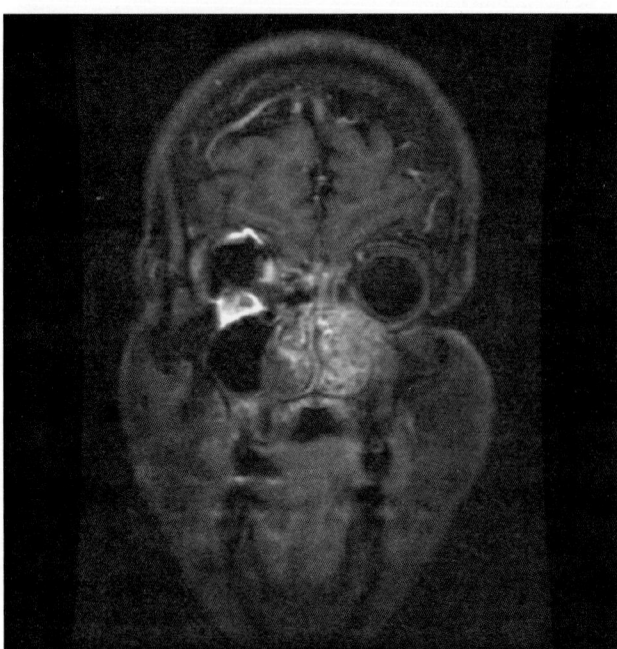

Figure 115.14 Coronal T1 fat-saturation MR image shows avid enhancement of the large neoplasm of the left maxillary sinus with extension in the orbit.

lobe of the parotid gland is a superficial structure, tumors of this lobe can be readily visualized with ultrasound. Advantages of ultrasound include relative low cost, ease of use, and the avoidance of ionizing radiation. A disadvantage of ultrasound, however, is that deep lobe tumors may not be accurately assessed. In some areas, ultrasound has replaced MRI and CT in preoperative imaging of benign parotid tumors (59). Accuracy in FNA has also been increased by using ultrasound to guide biopsy (60).

Fluorine-18 fluorodeoxyglucose positron emission tomography (PET) is uncommonly utilized to assess salivary gland neoplasms because many benign tumors and inflammatory conditions can be reported as falsely positive (61). It may provide additional information regarding the extent of disease for select malignant salivary gland neoplasms. A recent review reported a sensitivity of 74.4%, specificity of 100%, positive predictive value of 100%, and negative predictive value of 61.5% for combined PET/CT (62).

Diagnostic Surgery

Surgical biopsy of a parotid gland tumor should be avoided if possible. Excisional biopsy or tumor enucleation is associated with high rates of recurrence, particularly for pleomorphic adenoma. The standard surgical approach for parotid neoplasms is to perform complete surgical resection by parotidectomy with identification and preservation of the facial nerve. This ensures an adequate margin of tissue surrounding the tumor. This approach is diagnostic and curative in most cases. The facial nerve is identified to

allow tumor excision and to avoid facial nerve injury. This technique has excellent rates of tumor control. However, risks of facial nerve paralysis (permanent vs. transient), cosmetic defects, and Frey syndrome still exist (63).

Some surgeons manage select parotid pleomorphic adenomas by careful extracapsular dissection. This surgical method is not the same as simple tumor enucleation. In this technique, the tumor is dissected with a thin cuff of normal parotid tissue around it (2 to 3 mm). Recent reports of this approach demonstrate low rates of tumor recurrence, facial nerve injury rates similar to standard parotid techniques, and low rate of Frey syndrome (64,65).

Staging

The AJCC staging system (2010) for major salivary gland malignancies is described in Table 115.8.

Differential Diagnosis

Normal anatomic structures can often be confused with salivary gland tumors. The masseter muscle, transverse process of the C1 vertebral body, and mandibular processes can mimic parotid lesions (Fig. 115.15). Inflammatory diseases, nutritional deficiencies, and infections can cause diffuse parotid enlargement. Parotid cysts are uncommon but may mimic tumor. Cystic lymphoepithelial lesions observed in patients who are positive for the human immunodeficiency virus or have Sjogren syndrome may be confused with tumor as well (Fig. 115.16).

Cutaneous malignancies can metastasize to the intraparotid lymph nodes. Melanoma and squamous cell carcinoma account for the majority of these metastatic tumors. Infraclavicular tumors such as lung, kidney, breast, and colorectal cancers can spread to the salivary glands.

Necrotizing sialometaplasia is a benign lesion of salivary tissue that may be confused with a minor salivary gland tumor. Other lesions of the palate that may be mistaken for a minor salivary gland tumor include mucus retention cyst, epidermoid cyst, fibroma, and a palatine torus.

MANAGEMENT

Surgery

The treatment of choice for most salivary gland neoplasms is complete surgical excision. Because most parotid tumors occur in the region of the tail of the gland and are superficial to the facial nerve, parotidectomy with identification and preservation of the facial nerve is diagnostic and curative in most cases. The tumor should be removed with an adequate margin of normal tissue to ensure complete tumor excision and, in the case of pleomorphic adenoma, to avoid tumor rupture and spillage.

(Text continued on page 1775)

TABLE 115.8	STAGING SYSTEM FOR MAJOR SALIVARY GLAND MALIGNANCY, AMERICAN JOINT COMMITTEE ON CANCER, 2010

MAJOR SALIVARY GLANDS STAGING FORM

CLINICAL *Extent of disease before any treatment*	STAGE CATEGORY DEFINITIONS		PATHOLOGIC *Extent of disease through completion of definitive surgery*
☐ y clinical – staging completed after neoadjuvant therapy but before subsequent surgery	**TUMOR SIZE:** _____	**LATERALITY:** ☐ left ☐ right ☐ bilateral	☐ y pathologic – staging completed after neoadjuvant therapy AND subsequent surgery
	PRIMARY TUMOR (T)		
☐ TX	Primary tumor cannot be assessed		☐ TX
☐ T0	No evidence of primary tumor		☐ T0
☐ T1	Tumor 2 cm or less in greatest dimension without extraparenchymal extension*		☐ T1
☐ T2			☐ T2
☐ T3	Tumor more than 2 cm but not more than 4 cm in greatest dimension without extraparenchymal extension*		☐ T3
☐ T4a	Tumor more than 4 cm and/or tumor having extraparenchymal extension*		☐ T4a
☐ T4b	Moderately advanced disease 　Tumor invades skin, mandible, ear canal, and/or facial nerve Very advanced disease 　Tumor invades skull base and/or pterygoid plates and/or encases carotid artery *Note:* Extraparenchymal extension is clinical or macroscopic evidence of invasion of soft tissues. Microscopic evidence alone does not constitute extraparenchymal extension for classification purposes.		☐ T4b
	REGIONAL LYMPH NODES (N)		
☐ NX	Regional lymph nodes cannot be assessed		☐ NX
☐ N0	No regional lymph node metastasis		☐ N0
☐ N1	Metastasis in a single ipsilateral lymph node, 3 cm or less in greatest dimension		☐ N1
☐ N2	Metastasis in a single ipsilateral lymph node, more than 3 cm but not more than 6 cm in greatest dimension, or in multiple ipsilateral lymph nodes, none more than 6 cm in greatest dimension, or in bilateral or contralateral lymph nodes, none more than 6 cm in greatest dimension		☐ N2
☐ N2a	Metastasis in a single ipsilateral lymph node, more than 3 cm but not more than 6 cm in greatest dimension		☐ N2a
☐ N2b	Metastasis in multiple ipsilateral lymph nodes, none more than 6 cm in greatest dimension		☐ N2b
☐ N2c	Metastasis in bilateral or contralateral lymph nodes, none more than 6 cm in greatest dimension		☐ N2c
☐ N3	Metastasis in a lymph node, more than 6 cm in greatest dimension		☐ N3
	DISTANT METASTASIS (M)		
☐ M0	No distant metastasis (no pathologic M0; use clinical M to complete stage group)		
☐ M1	Distant metastasis		☐ M1

HOSPITAL NAME/ADDRESS	PATIENT NAME/INFORMATION

MAJOR SALIVARY GLANDS STAGING FORM

ANATOMIC STAGE • PROGNOSTIC GROUPS

	CLINICAL					**PATHOLOGIC**		
GROUP	**T**	**N**	**M**		**GROUP**	**T**	**N**	**M**
☐ I	T1	N0	M0		☐ I	T1	N0	M0
☐ II	T2	N0	M0		☐ II	T2	N0	M0
☐ III	T3	N0	M0		☐ III	T3	N0	M0
	T1	N1	M0			T1	N1	M0
	T2	N1	M0			T2	N1	M0
	T3	N1	M0			T3	N1	M0
☐ IVA	T4a	N0	M0		☐ IVA	T4a	N0	M0
	T4a	N1	M0			T4a	N1	M0
	T1	N2	M0			T1	N2	M0
	T2	N2	M0			T2	N2	M0
	T3	N2	M0			T3	N2	M0
	T4a	N2	M0			T4a	N2	M0
☐ IVB	T4b	Any N	M0		☐ IVB	T4b	Any N	M0
	Any T	N3	M0			Any T	N3	M0
☐ IVC	Any T	Any N	M1		☐ IVC	Any T	Any N	M1

☐ Stage unknown   ☐ Stage unknown

PROGNOSTIC FACTORS (SITE-SPECIFIC FACTORS)

REQUIRED FOR STAGING : None

CLINICALLY SIGNIFICANT:

Size of Lymph Nodes _____

Extracapsular Extension from Lymph Nodes for Head & Neck _____

Head & Neck Lymph Nodes Levels I-III _____

Head & Neck Lymph Nodes Levels IV-V _____

Head & Neck Lymph Nodes Levels VI-VII _____

Other Lymph Nodes Group _____

Clinical Location of cervical nodes _____

Extracapsular spread (ECS) Clinical _____

Extracapsular spread (ECS) Pathologic _____

Histologic Grade (G) (also known as overall grade)

Grading system	*Grade*
☐ 2 grade system	☐ Grade I or 1
☐ 3 grade system	☐ Grade II or 2
☐ 4 grade system	☐ Grade III or 3
☐ No 2, 3, or 4 grade system is available	☐ Grade IV or 4

General Notes:

For identification of special cases of TNM or pTNM classifications, the "m" suffix and "y," "r," and "a" prefixes are used. Although they do not affect the stage grouping, they indicate cases needing separate analysis.

m suffix indicates the presence of multiple primary tumors in a single site and is recorded in parentheses: pT(m)NM.

y prefix indicates those cases in which classification is performed during or following initial multimodality therapy. The cTNM or pTNM category is identified by a "y" prefix. The ycTNM or ypTNM categorizes the extent of tumor actually present at the time of that examination. The "y" categorization is not an estimate of tumor prior to multimodality therapy.

r prefix indicates a recurrent tumor when staged after a disease-free interval and is identified by the "r" prefix: rTNM.

a prefix designates the stage determined at autopsy: aTNM.

HOSPITAL NAME/ADDRESS	PATIENT NAME/INFORMATION

(Continued)

MAJOR SALIVARY GLANDS STAGING FORM

ADDITIONAL DESCRIPTORS

Lymphatic Vessel Invasion (L) and Venous Invasion (V) have been combined into Lymph-Vascular Invasion (LVI) for collection by cancer registrars. The College of American Pathologist (CAP) Checklist should be used as the primary source. Other sources may be used in the absence of a Checklist. Priority is given to positive results.

❑ Lymph-vascular Invasion Not Present (absent)/Not Identified
❑ Lymph-vascular Invasion Present/Identified
❑ Not Applicable
❑ Unknown/Indeterminate

Residual Tumor (R)

The absence or presence of residual tumor after treatment. In some cases treated with surgery and/or with neoadjuvant therapy there will be residual tumor at the primary site after treatment because of incomplete resection or local and regional disease that extends beyond the limit of ability of resection.

❑ RX Presence of residual tumor cannot be assessed
❑ R0 No residual tumor
❑ R1 Microscopic residual tumor
❑ R2 Macroscopic residual tumor

General Notes (continued):

surgical margins is data field recorded by registrars describing the surgical margins of the resected primary site specimen as determined only by the pathology report.

neoadjuvant treatment is radiation therapy or systemic therapy (consisting of chemotherapy, hormone therapy, or immunotherapy) administered prior to a definitive surgical procedure. If the surgical procedure is not performed, the administered therapy no longer meets the definition of neoadjuvant therapy.

❑ Clinical stage was used in treatment planning (describe): _____

❑ National guidelines were used in treatment planning ❑ NCCN ❑ Other (describe): _____

_____

_____

Physician signature   Date/Time

HOSPITAL NAME/ADDRESS	PATIENT NAME/INFORMATION

MAJOR SALIVARY GLANDS STAGING FORM

Illustration

Indicate on diagram primary
tumor and regional nodes
involved.

1.

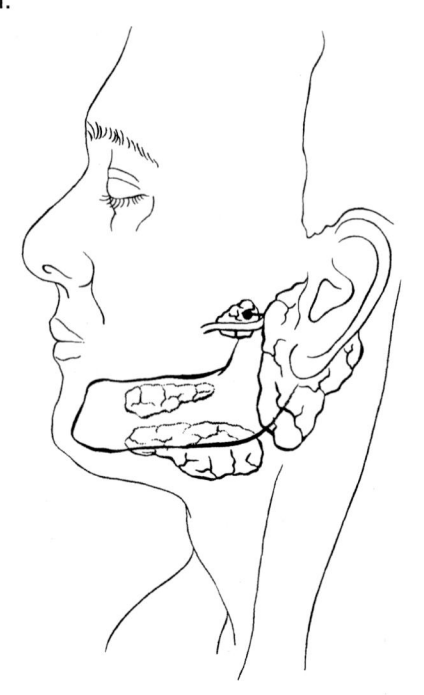

2.

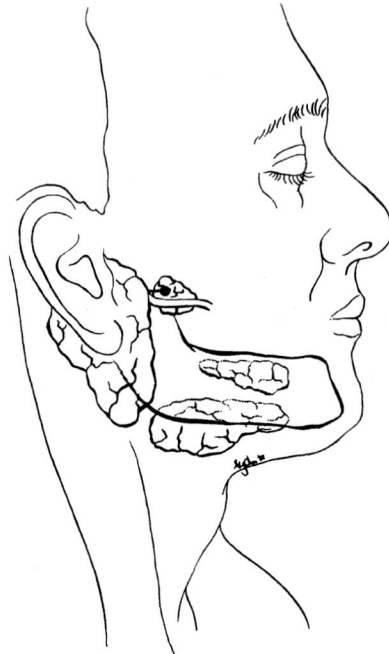

3.

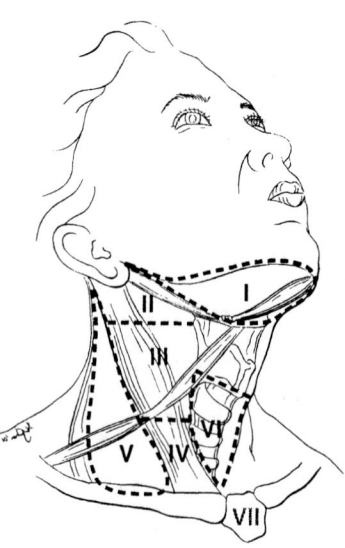

4.

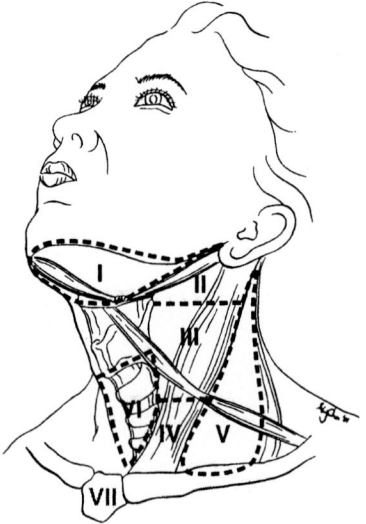

HOSPITAL NAME/ADDRESS	PATIENT NAME/INFORMATION

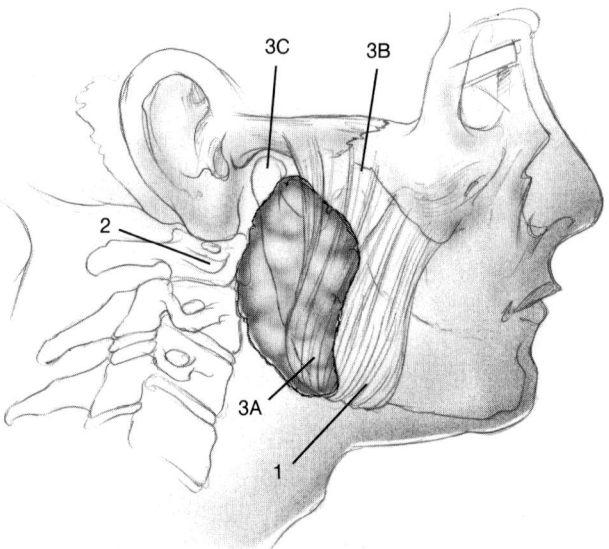

Figure 115.15 Normal anatomic structures are sometimes mistaken for parotid neoplasms. *1*, masseter; *2*, transverse process of C1; *3*, mandibular processes: *A*, angle; *B*, coronoid; *C*, condyle.

Complete excision by parotidectomy (Fig. 115.17) is considered adequate therapy for superficial low-grade malignancies (e.g., low-grade mucoepidermoid carcinoma and acinic cell carcinoma).

Complete surgical resection by parotidectomy is recommended for high-grade malignancies. The facial nerve is to be preserved if it functions normally and is not invaded by tumor. Facial nerve involvement by tumor requires facial nerve resection. Frozen sections are used to ensure negative

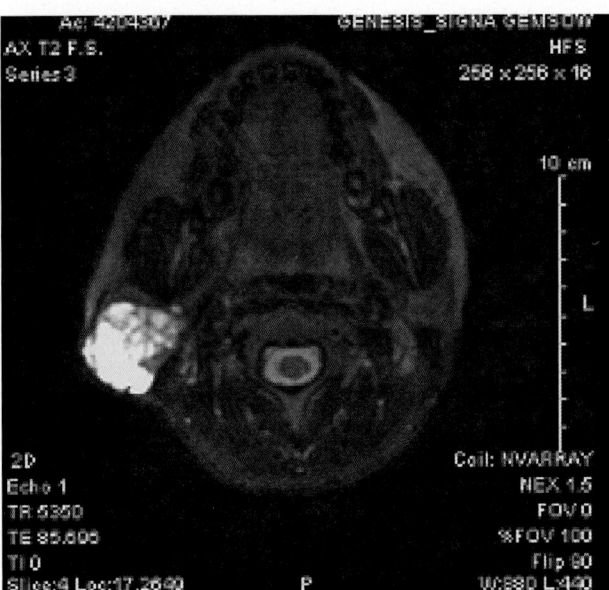

Figure 115.16 Fat-saturation T2-weighted magnetic resonance image demonstrates multiple cysts within the right parotid gland. This lesion is hyperintense on T2-weighted images.

nerve margins both proximally and distally. Immediate facial nerve grafting should be considered.

During parotidectomy for malignancy, the neck is addressed with a comprehensive neck dissection for any known positive nodal disease. For the N0 neck, the role of elective neck dissection is controversial.

In general, high-grade tumors are more frequently associated with occult metastasis than low-grade tumors. Thus, malignancies such as high-grade mucoepidermoid or carcinoma ex pleomorphic adenoma have relatively high rates of occult disease. Other high-risk tumors include adenocarcinoma, primary squamous cell carcinoma, and salivary duct carcinoma. Low-risk tumors include low-grade mucoepidermoid carcinoma and acinic cell carcinoma. Although adenoid cystic carcinoma is considered a high-grade malignancy, it is associated with a low rate of occult metastases, and thus, elective neck dissection is not recommended for this cancer.

Some advocate that all salivary gland malignancies be managed with elective neck dissection of levels I, II, and III. A rationale is that in less than half the cases, the exact grade and histologic type of tumor is indeterminate prior to definitive resection (66).

There are also some who do not advocate elective neck dissection at all. Some suggest sampling the nodal tissue in levels I and II and making a decision based on frozen section whether or not to perform a neck dissection (67). A recent review on the management of the neck in salivary gland cancer summarizes the reasonable considerations for elective neck dissection as high-grade tumor, large tumor size, facial paralysis, extraglandular spread, age greater than 54, and perilymphatic invasion (68).

Parotidectomy Technique

The face and neck are prepared and draped with a transparent adhesive drape to allow for visualization of the face during the procedure. A preauricular incision is made extending inferiorly along the line of attachment of the ear lobule and curving into an upper neck crease. Alternatively, a modified face-lift incision can be used for selected patients. An anterior skin flap is elevated superficial to the parotid fascia. The flap is raised to the posterior border of the masseter muscle. The tail of the parotid is then dissected from the sternocleidomastoid muscle and the posterior branch of the greater auricular nerve is preserved if possible.

The digastric muscle is then exposed as the tail of the parotid is elevated. This serves as an important landmark in identifying the facial nerve. The second plane of dissection is then developed in the pretragal region. This space is opened with blunt dissection parallel to the course of the facial nerve. This exposes the tragal pointer and opens a plane from the zygoma superiorly to just above the styloid process inferiorly. With the tail and the pretragal portions of the parotid mobilized, the remaining parotid fascial attachments to the mastoid are divided. The facial nerve is then identified using the exposed anatomic landmarks (Table 115.9).

If the main trunk of the facial nerve cannot be identified, then peripheral facial nerve branches can be dissected in a retrograde fashion. Alternatively, when there is significant scarring or distortion of the normal anatomy, a mastoidectomy can be performed and the facial nerve identified within the temporal bone.

After the main branch of the facial nerve is identified, individual facial nerve branches are followed peripherally and the gland is dissected off the nerve branches. After tumor removal, hemostasis is ensured and the wound closed over a closed-suction drain.

Total parotidectomy involves removal of parotid gland tissue both superficial and deep to the facial nerve. For deep lobe tumors, the facial nerve is exposed by removing the superficial lobe of the parotid gland. The deep lobe is then removed by first carefully mobilizing the branches of the facial nerve and removing the tissue deep to the nerve.

For parotid malignancies, the extent of the resection is determined by the extent of the disease. Frozen sections may guide the need for removal of any tissues that are invaded beyond the gland.

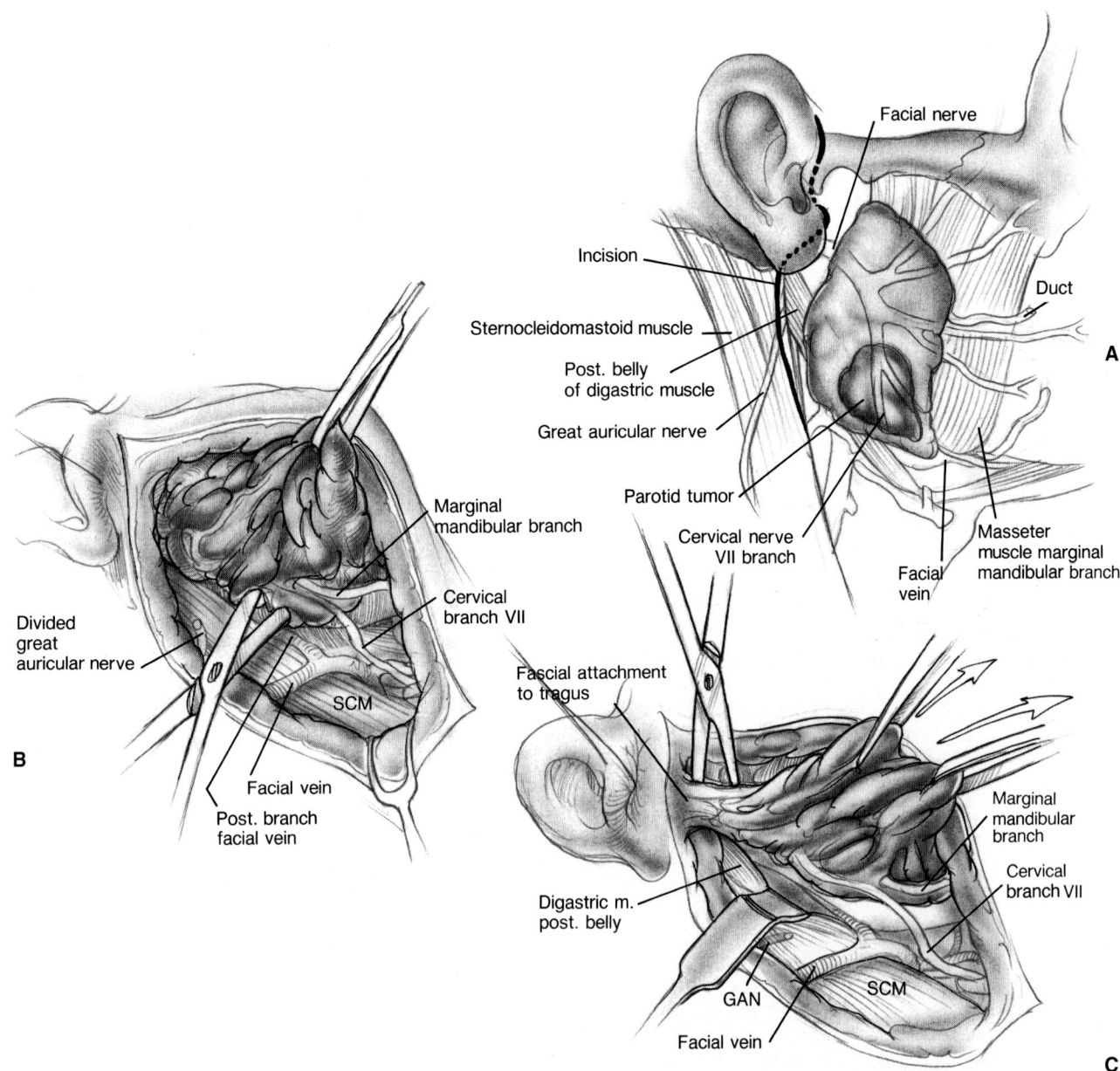

Figure 115.17 Techniques of parotidectomy. **A:** Anatomy of parotid area. **B:** Dissection of the inferior pole of the gland takes place before dissection of the facial nerve and its branches. **C:** Anterior retraction and blunt dissection above the main trunk of the facial nerve follows the mobilization of the inferior pole of the gland.

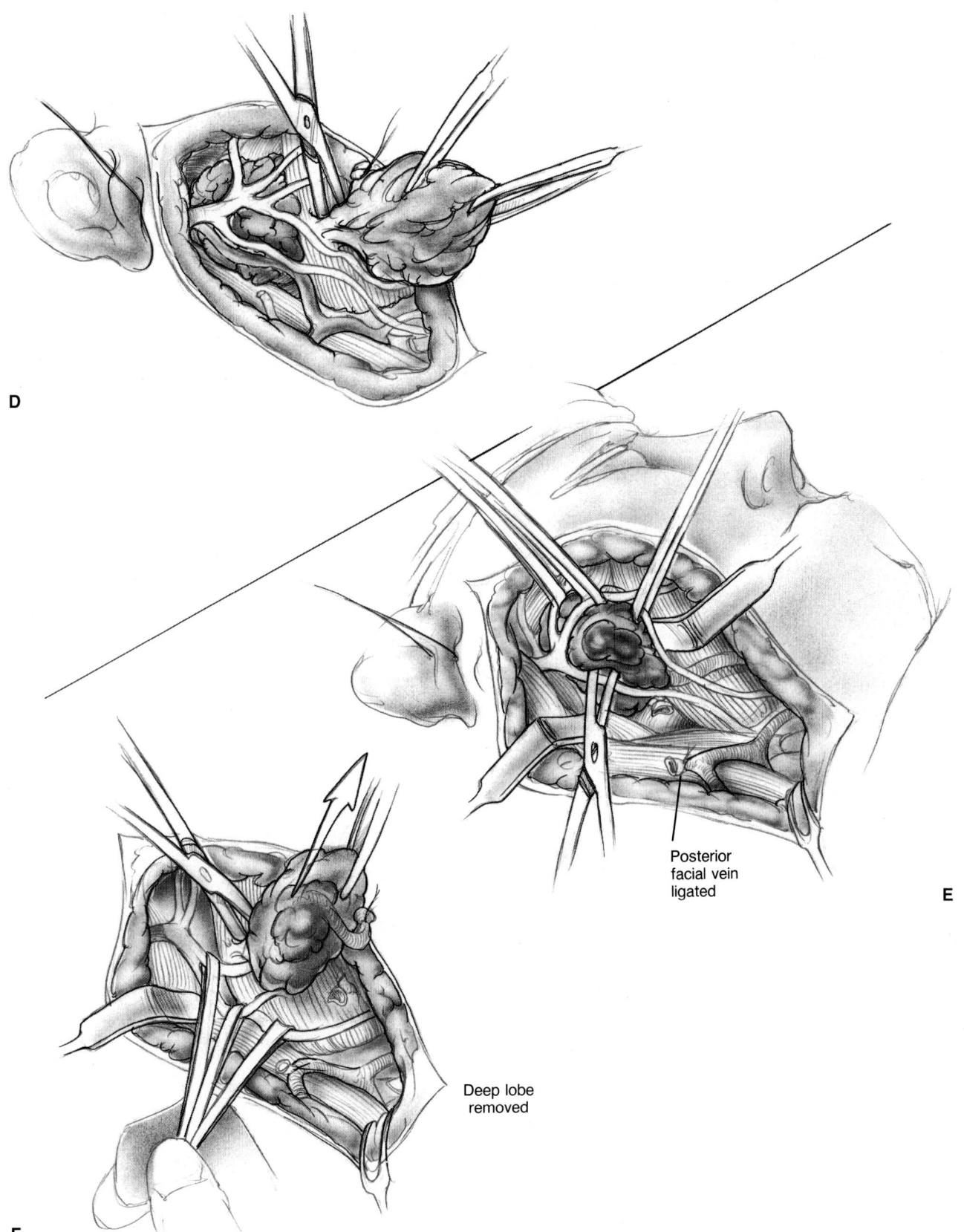

D

Posterior
facial vein
ligated

E

Deep lobe
removed

F

Figure 115.17 *(Continued)* **D:** All nerve branches are successively dissected and identified. Then the gland is removed in a single block. **E:** Deep lobe parotidectomy. Facial nerve is visualized, and dissection is continued deep to it. **F:** The deep lobe is removed. GAN, greater auricular nerve; SCM, sternocleido-mastoid muscle.

TABLE 115.9	ANATOMIC LANDMARKS FOR FACIAL NERVE IDENTIFICATION DURING PAROTIDECTOMY

Tragal pointer
Tympanomastoid suture line
Digastric muscle attachment to digastric groove
Retrograde dissection from distal nerve branch
Nerve within the temporal bone

Surgical Treatment of Parapharyngeal Space Tumors

The PPS is located lateral to the pharynx and is shaped as an inverted pyramid with its base at the skull base and its apex at the hyoid bone. It is bounded posteriorly by the prevertebral fascia, medially by the pharyngeal constrictor muscles, and laterally by the mandibular ramus and the deep lobe of the parotid.

Parotid neoplasms may involve the PPS by two routes. Round tumors extend posterior to the stylomandibular ligament. Dumbbell tumors have waist-like constrictions that form as they penetrate between the mandible and the stylomandibular ligament (Figs. 115.18 and 115.19).

Most tumors of the PPS can be removed through a transcervical approach. The submandibular gland is then mobilized, which allows access to the anterior compartment of the PPS. Most PPS tumors can be bluntly dissected from the surrounding structures. This dissection must be done gently to avoid tumor rupture and seeding of the PPS.

If exposure needs to be increased, techniques such as division of the stylomandibular ligament and division of the stylohyoid and digastric muscles can enhance exposure (69). If additional exposure is required, a mandibulotomy may be needed. The mandibular osteotomies should be made in manner to preserve the inferior alveolar nerve.

For select benign tumors, a transoral approach to the PPS can be considered. Preoperative imaging is important in patient selection for this approach (70). Transoral biopsy of PPS tumors should be avoided. This carries risks of injury to the carotid artery, tumor spillage, seeding the tumor into the oropharyngeal tissues, and formation of adhesions. A transoral or image-guided FNA biopsy usually provides diagnostic information without these risks (71).

Surgical Treatment of Submandibular Gland Neoplasms

Tumors involving the submandibular gland are usually limited to the gland. For benign tumors, submandibular gland excision is therapeutic. Malignant tumors require complete surgical resection. Malignant tumors are usually confined to the gland, and thus, surgical resection is usually confined to the contents of the submandibular triangle. All nerves are preserved unless there is evidence of tumor involvement. For malignant tumors invading the surrounding tissue, the surgical resection is extended to

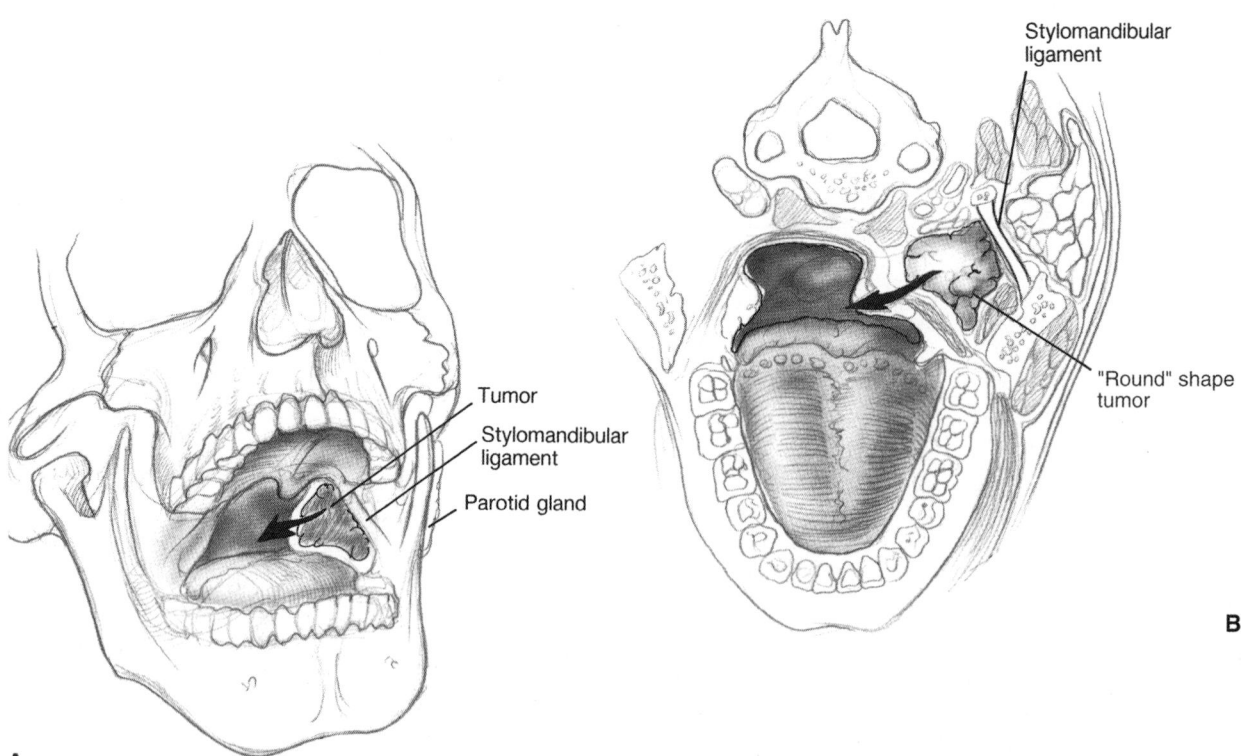

Figure 115.18 Round tumor involving the PPS. **A:** Three-fourths view. **B:** Axial view.

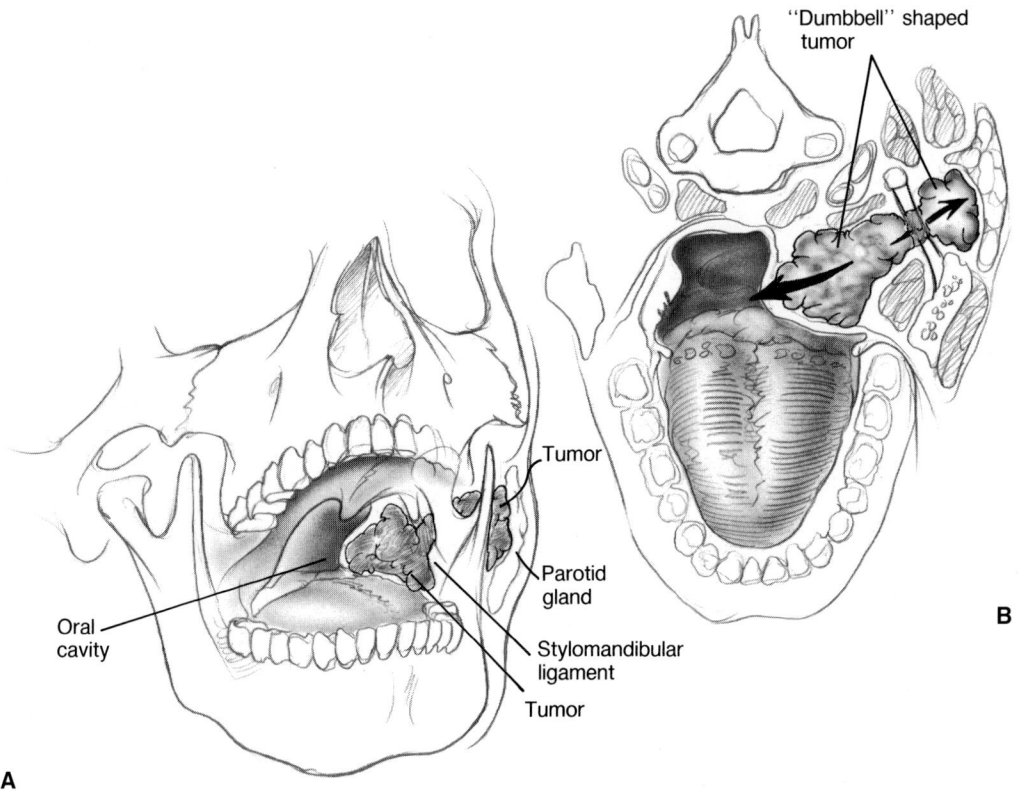

Figure 115.19 Dumbbell tumor involving the PPS. **A:** Three-fourths view. **B:** Axial view.

include the involved structures with an appropriate tumor-free margin. The involved structures may include the marginal mandibular branch of the facial nerve, the hypoglossal nerve, the lingual nerve, the mandible, the tongue, the floor of mouth, and the skin. The extent of surgical resection depends on the extent of the disease.

Submandibular Gland Excision Technique

The neck is prepared and draped in a sterile fashion. The incision is made below the inferior border of the mandible in a skin crease (Fig. 115.20). The incision is carried through the platysma muscle, and subplatysmal flaps are elevated with care to avoid injury to the marginal mandibular nerve. The Hayes Martin maneuver can be used to protect the marginal mandibular nerve at this point. The fascia overlying the submandibular gland is then incised and raised, exposing the gland itself. However, if enlarged facial nodes are present, the marginal mandibular nerve may need to be completely dissected and mobilized superiorly to ensure complete nodal removal. The dissection is then performed superiorly, and the facial artery is divided and ligated. The mylohyoid muscle is retracted anteriorly, and the gland is retracted posteroinferiorly, exposing the lingual nerve and Wharton duct. The submandibular ganglion is divided, freeing the lingual nerve. Wharton duct is then divided and ligated. The hypoglossal nerve runs superficial to the hyoglossus muscle. The hypoglossal nerve is preserved as the inferior border of the

gland is dissected free. The facial artery is encountered again, and it is divided and ligated. After ensuring hemostasis, the wound is closed in layers over a drain.

Surgical Treatment of Minor Salivary Gland Neoplasms

Surgical therapy depends on the location and extent of disease. Complete surgical excision is therapeutic for benign tumors. Adenoid cystic carcinoma most commonly involves the oral cavity, nasal cavity, and paranasal sinuses. Adenocarcinomas most commonly involve the paranasal sinuses and nasal cavities. Malignant minor salivary gland tumors involving the larynx are usually adenoid cystic carcinoma or adenocarcinoma. The surgery for malignant minor salivary gland tumors may be extensive and may require maxillectomy, craniofacial resection, mandibulectomy, laryngectomy, or tracheal resection.

Radiation Therapy

Adjuvant radiation therapy has improved the locoregional control and survival for patients with carcinoma of the salivary glands (72). Indications for adjuvant radiotherapy include lymph node metastasis, high tumor grade, positive surgical margins and T3-T4 tumor stage (73). Although surgery remains the mainstay in the treatment of salivary gland malignancies, radiation therapy alone may be an

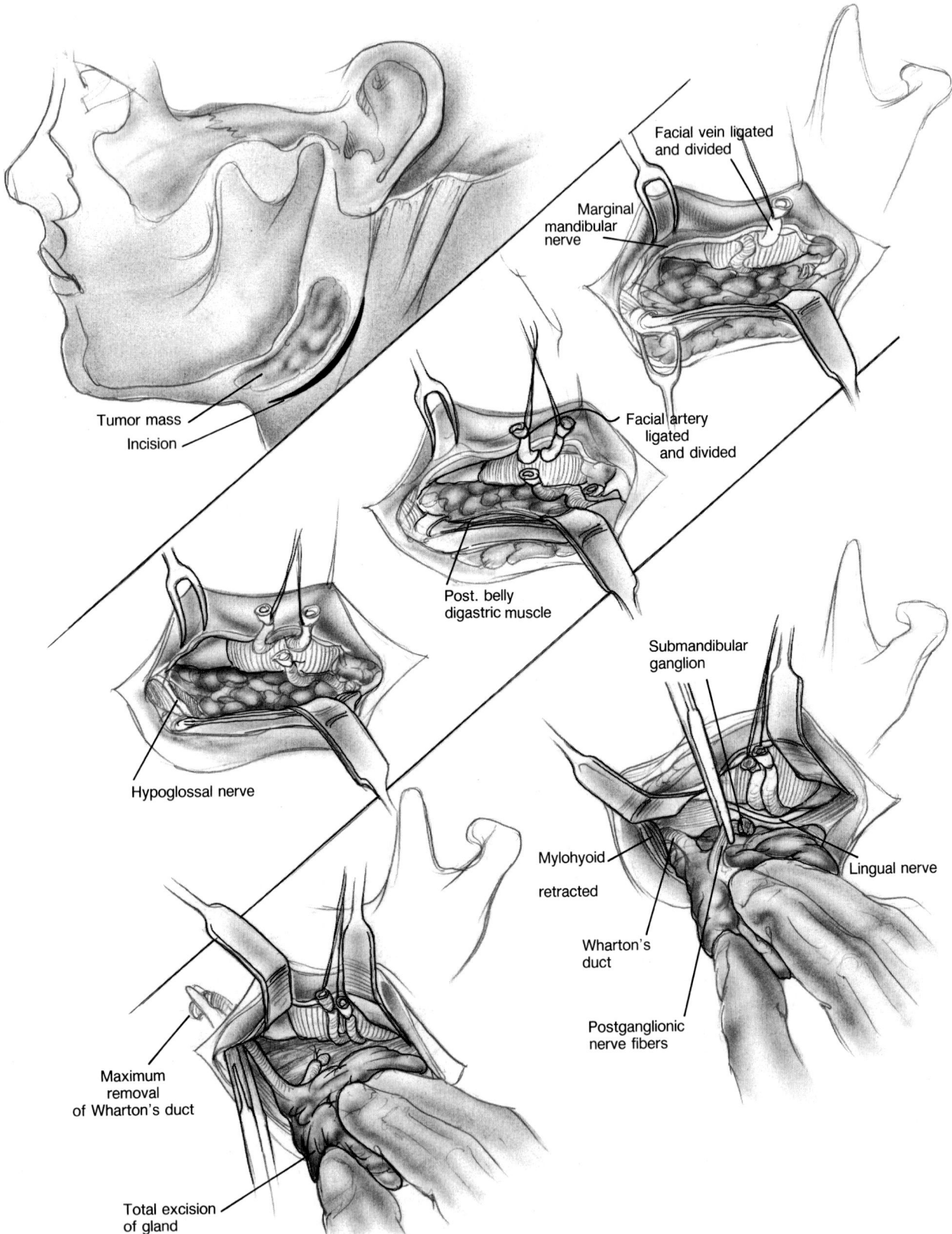

Tumor mass

Incision

Facial vein ligated and divided

Marginal mandibular nerve

Facial artery ligated and divided

Post. belly digastric muscle

Hypoglossal nerve

Submandibular ganglion

Mylohyoid retracted

Lingual nerve

Wharton's duct

Postganglionic nerve fibers

Maximum removal of Wharton's duct

Total excision of gland

Figure 115.20 Technique for submandibular gland excision. See text for discussion.

TABLE 115.10	PHASE II TRIALS OF TARGETED THERAPY FOR SALIVARY GLAND CANCER					
	ACC No.	Non-ACC No.	Target(s)	Drug	Response Rate (%)	Stable Disease (%) (>6 mo)
Haddad et al.	2	12	HER2	Trastuzumab	8	Not reported
Glisson et al.	19	9	EGFR	Gefitinib	0	67% (0%)
Hottle et al.	16	0	c-kit	Imatinib	0	60% (13%)
Pfeiffer et al.	10	0	c-kit	Imatinib	0	20% (20%)
Agulnik et al.	19	17	HER2/EGFR	Lapatinib	0	59% (47%)
Locati et al.	23	7	EGFR	Cetuximab	0	80% (50%)

ACC, Adenoid cystic carcinoma; EGFR, Epidermal growth factor receptor; HER2 - Human epidermal growth factor receptor 2.
From Adelstein DJ, Rodriguez CP. What is new in the management of salivary gland cancers? *Curr Opin Oncol* 2011;23:249–253, with permission.

option in cases where surgery is not possible or would result in unacceptable morbidity (74).

Adjuvant radiotherapy has been shown to be beneficial following resection of recurrent pleomorphic adenoma of the parotid, thus making it an option in selected cases (75). Fast neutron radiotherapy also shows promise as another modality for the treatment of recurrent pleomorphic adenoma (76).

Because of the proximity of important structures, it is difficult to deliver curative doses of radiation using conventional photons for tumors of the skull base or paranasal sinuses. Because of the radiobiologic properties of heavy particles, a larger dose of radiation can be delivered to the tumor while sparing the surrounding tissue. As mentioned earlier in this chapter, fast neutron radiotherapy may be more effective than conventional photon radiotherapy as the primary treatment modality in select cases of unresectable adenoid cystic carcinoma (29,30). In addition, conformal proton radiotherapy has shown promise in the treatment of adenoid cystic carcinoma of the skull base in cases of partial or incomplete resection of tumor (77).

Chemotherapy

Historically, the primary role for chemotherapy has been for palliation in the setting of symptomatic, unresectable disease. The role for chemotherapy continues to be investigated. At this point, there are very limited data for the role of chemotherapy in salivary gland cancer. It should be noted, however, that adenoid cystic carcinoma constitutes a large number of patients in these trials, thus making extrapolation of the outcomes to other malignancies difficult (1).

Single agent paclitaxel has been studied by the Eastern Cooperative Oncology Group. In their Phase II trial, they found a partial response rate in 26% of patients with mucoepidermoid carcinoma or adenocarcinoma but zero responders in those with adenoid cystic carcinoma. Median survival was 12.5 months (78). Gemcitabine combined with either cisplatin or carboplatin has also demonstrated modest response rates (79).

Small retrospective studies have demonstrated a potential benefit in adjuvant chemoradiation with platinum

compounds (80). Currently, prospective studies are under way to determine its utility.

Development of therapeutic agents directed against specific molecular targets has also found its way in salivary gland cancers. No study thus far, however, has demonstrated meaningful responses, despite the overexpression of various markers in some neoplasms (Table 115.10).

COMPLICATIONS

Parotidectomy

There are both early and late complications of parotidectomy (Table 115.11). Partial or complete paralysis involving some or all branches of the facial nerve can occur as an early complication. Temporary facial nerve paralysis involving one or all branches of the nerve occurs in 10% to 30% of parotidectomies. Permanent facial nerve paralysis occurs in fewer than 3% of parotidectomies. The incidence of facial nerve paralysis is higher with total parotidectomy than with superficial parotidectomy. Facial nerve injury is also more common during reoperation for recurrent tumors. The nerve at most risk for injury during parotidectomy is the marginal mandibular branch. Temporary paresis usually resolves from weeks to months postoperatively. Complete nerve transection can occur during surgery and should be identified and immediately repaired.

TABLE 115.11	COMPLICATIONS OF PAROTIDECTOMY	
Early		**Late**
Facial nerve paralysis		Frey syndrome
Bleeding		Recurrent tumor
Infection		Poor cosmesis
Skin flap necrosis		Soft tissue deficit
Trismus		Hypertrophic scar or keloid
Sialocele		
Seroma		

There are many factors that influence the risk of facial nerve injury. These include tumor size, location, type, extent of surgery, and reoperation. Mechanisms of injury include nerve transection, stretch, compression, thermal/electrical injury, and ischemia.

Continuous facial nerve monitoring has been gaining in popularity in recent years (81). In this technique, facial muscle electromyographic (EMG) activity is monitored. Commercially available, multichannel systems can track facial muscle activity and have a built-in pulse generator for nerve stimulation at varying strengths. Data for these systems are easy to interpret and do not require the presence of a neurophysiologic nerve monitoring team. Intraoperatively, the surgeon must be able to differentiate true EMG events from artifacts that are usually caused by contact of metal instruments on the operative field. Wave form analysis and the context in which the artifactual alert occurs can aid in differentiating these from true events.

The literature suggests a reduction in the rate of temporary facial nerve paresis and possible decreased operating time with facial nerve monitoring during parotidectomy. Studies to date, however, preclude conclusions regarding a benefit for permanent facial paralysis reduction due to lack of sufficient power (82,83). There are benefits to the use of the facial nerve monitor including minimizing trauma to the nerve during its dissection, improved ability to differentiate the facial nerve from nonnerve tissue, and alert to the surgeon regarding facial nerve proximity (84). The use of monitoring technology, however, should not replace the identification of the facial nerve using known anatomic landmarks.

Corticosteroids have been used by some surgeons in the hopes of avoiding postoperative paresis of the facial nerve by reducing edema and inflammation of the nerve. Studies, however, have failed to demonstrate a benefit of perioperative corticosteroids on facial nerve paresis rates (85).

Hemorrhage or hematoma is an uncommon complication and is usually related to incomplete hemostasis at the end of the procedure. Treatment consists of evacuation of the hematoma and surgical control of the bleeding vessels.

Infection is rare after parotidectomy and is avoided by the use of aseptic technique and careful handling of tissues. The rarity of infection is probably related to the rich vascular supply to this anatomic region. Treatment of infection consists of surgical drainage, if necessary, and antibiotics.

Skin-flap necrosis most commonly occurs in the distal tip of the postauricular skin flap. Care must be taken in designing this portion of the skin flap in avoiding this complication. Smoking, prior radiation therapy, and diabetes mellitus are risk factors for this complication.

Trismus may occur related to inflammation and fibrosis of the masseter muscle. This complication is usually mild and self-limited with jaw range of motion exercises.

Salivary fistula or sialocele is a relatively common complication after parotidectomy. This usually results from the cut edges of the remaining salivary gland leaking saliva and then collecting beneath the flap. This complication is usually self-limited when treated with needle aspirations. A chronic salivary fistula is rare.

Frey syndrome or gustatory sweating is a relatively common long-term complication of parotidectomy (Fig. 115.21). This is thought to occur as a result of aberrant

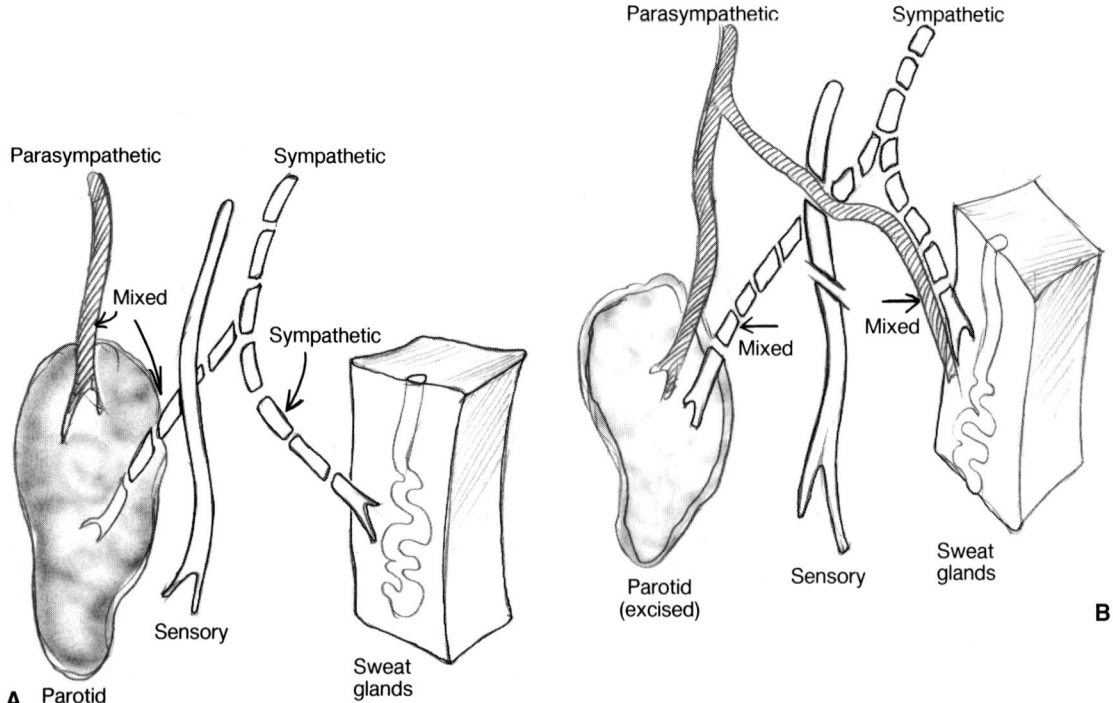

Figure 115.21 A: Normal innervation of parotid and sweat glands. **B:** Proposed mechanism of Frey syndrome.

regeneration of nerve fibers from the postganglionic secretomotor parasympathetic innervation of the parotid gland to the severed postganglionic sympathetic fibers that supply the sweat glands of the skin of the face. As a result, sweating or dermal flush occurs during salivary stimulation. Frey syndrome has been reported for 30% to 60% of patients undergoing parotidectomy. Only about 10% of patients, however, have symptomatic Frey syndrome.

Most patients with Frey syndrome do not seek therapy. Medical treatment of symptomatic Frey syndrome has included topical application of antiperspirant, topical anticholinergics, and injections of botulinum toxin, which provides excellent control for prolonged periods. Surgical techniques during parotidectomy that can reduce the risk of Frey syndrome include elevation of a thick skin flap and performance of partial parotidectomy (86). In addition, interpositional barriers such as fat, acellular dermal grafts, and muscle flaps have been used with success in the prevention of Frey syndrome (87–89). These surgical methods are uncommonly utilized presently due to the effectiveness of botulinum toxin therapy.

First bite syndrome can occur following deep lobe parotid and PPS neoplasms and manifests with recurrent severe pain with initial oral intake that subsides with successive bites. This problem is thought to result from interruption of the sympathetic innervation of the parotid gland with denervation supersensitivity of myoepithelial cell receptors. The severity of this condition usually diminishes over time. Severe cases may benefit from botulinum toxin injection of residual gland tissue.

Malignant and even benign tumors can recur. High-grade malignancies can have a high rate of recurrence despite combined therapy. Benign tumors such as pleomorphic adenoma, however, recur in less than 1% of patients who have proper surgery. Most recurrences occur after incomplete tumor resection or tumor spillage from tumor capsule rupture.

Recurrent pleomorphic adenoma is difficult to treat because they tend to be larger than suspected, lie at a deeper level than expected, and are multicentric (90). The treatment of recurrent pleomorphic adenoma consists of comprehensive resection of recurrent tumor nodules by revision parotidectomy with facial nerve preservation. A decrease in the rate of surgical control occurs with subsequent recurrences. Thus, postoperative radiation therapy may be recommended in certain cases to reduce the likelihood of recurrence following revision surgery. En bloc resection with immediate nerve grafting is necessary for recurrences encasing the facial nerve.

Submandibular Gland Excision

The complications of submandibular gland excision are listed in Table 115.12. Injury to the marginal mandibular

TABLE 115.12	COMPLICATIONS OF SUBMANDIBULAR GLAND EXCISION

Hemorrhage
Infection
Marginal mandibular branch of facial nerve injury
Hypoglossal nerve injury
Lingual nerve injury
Poor scar formation

branch of the facial nerve results in loss of lip depressor function. Temporary paresis of this nerve can occur from nerve stretch injury during retraction. Other nerves at risk include the hypoglossal nerve and lingual nerve resulting in ipsilateral tongue paralysis and anesthesia of the anterior two-thirds of the tongue, respectively.

Hemorrhage, particularly from the facial artery, results in vigorous bleeding and can contribute to airway compromise. Wound re-exploration and control of hemorrhage is necessary. Infection is uncommon after submandibular gland excision.

PROGNOSTIC FACTORS

Histopathology

Many studies over the years have demonstrated that tumor histopathology is a strong prognostic factor in predicting the behavior of a malignancy. In general, low-grade tumors such as low-grade mucoepidermoid carcinoma or acinic cell carcinoma are usually well controlled with single-modality therapy. Whereas high-grade lesions such as high-grade mucoepidermoid carcinoma or salivary duct carcinoma require aggressive surgical treatment with adjuvant radiotherapy because they have a greater likelihood of metastasis and locoregional failure. An epidemiologic study was performed looking at data in the Swedish Cancer Society to look at the relative survival of different cancer types in the parotid and submandibular glands (Tables 115.13 and 115.14) (36). A classification scheme dividing tumors into low-risk and high-risk cancers is presented in Table 115.15 (91).

Tumor Size

Tumor size has been considered a major prognostic indicator for salivary gland malignancies with increased size resulting in poor prognosis and decreased survival (92,93). Increased tumor size also correlates with high rates of regional and distant metastases and increased rates of recurrence (95).

TABLE 115.13	RELATIVE SURVIVAL RATES FOR CANCER OF THE PAROTID	
Tumor Type	**5-y Survival (95% CI)**	**10-y Survival (95% CI)**
Carcinoma ex pleomorphic	76 (69–82)	73 (65–81)
Adenoid cystic carcinoma	85 (79–90)	74 (66–82)
Acinic cell carcinoma	93 (88–98)	88 (80–95)
Mucoepidermoid carcinoma	82 (77–87)	80 (73–87)
Adenocarcinoma	63 (57–70)	55 (48–75)
Undifferentiated carcinoma	48 (40–56)	40 (25–61)

Adapted from Wahlberg P, Anderson H, Bjorklund A, et al. Carcinoma of the parotid and submandibular glands: a study of survival in 2465 patients. *Oral Oncol* 2002;38:706–713.

Facial Nerve Paralysis

Facial nerve paralysis associated with malignant tumors indicates a poor prognosis. Facial nerve paralysis is also associated with higher incidences of regional and distant metastases (95).

Regional Lymphatic Metastases

Regional lymph node metastases are associated with a poorer prognosis than for nonmetastatic disease (67,94). Factors associated with a higher risk of metastases have already been discussed earlier in the chapter. Other factors include tumor size, facial nerve paralysis, age of patient, histologic type, and grade of tumor.

Distant Metastases

Distant metastases indicate a poor prognosis. Distant metastases occur in approximately 20% of parotid malignancies, and they occur most frequently in adenoid cystic carcinoma and undifferentiated carcinoma. The most common sites for distant metastases are lung, bone, and brain. The length of survival after distant failure varies according to the tumor type. Some patients with adenoid cystic carcinoma may survive for many years due to slow tumor progression. The most important factors for predicting the development of distant metastases are the size of the tumor, presence or absence of regional metastases, and histologic type of tumor (93).

Location

There appears to be no difference in survival based on the location of a malignancy within the parotid gland, but PPS involvement by a malignancy is associated with a poor prognosis. In general, parotid malignancies have a better prognosis than salivary carcinomas arising in other locations.

For adenoid cystic carcinoma, tumors in the major salivary glands are associated with a better prognosis than those in the minor salivary glands.

TABLE 115.14	RELATIVE SURVIVAL RATES FOR CANCER OF THE SUBMANDIBULAR GLAND	
Tumor Type	**5-y Survival (95% CI)**	**10-y Survival (95% CI)**
Carcinoma ex-pleomorphic	71 (54–86)	62 (43–82)
Adenoid cystic carcinoma	84 (76–90)	73 (63–82)
Acinic cell carcinoma	83 (50–100)	86 (46–100)
Mucoepidermoid carcinoma	55 (42–69)	53 (37–71)
Adenocarcinoma	43 (29–61)	42 (25–65)
Undifferentiated carcinoma	50 (32–70)	53 (32–81)

Adapted from Wahlberg P, Anderson H, Bjorklund A, et al. Carcinoma of the parotid and submandibular glands: a study of survival in 2465 patients. *Oral Oncol* 2002;38:706–713.

TABLE 115.15	RISK STRATIFICATION OF SALIVARY GLAND CANCERS

Low Risk	High Risk
Acinic cell carcinoma	Sebaceous carcinoma and lymphadeno carcinoma
Low-grade mucoepidermoid carcinoma	High-grade mucoepidermoid carcinoma
Epithelial–myoepithelial carcinoma	Adenoid cystic carcinoma
Polymorphous low-grade adenocarcinoma	Mucinous adenocarcinoma
Clear cell carcinoma	Squamous cell carcinoma
Basal cell adenocarcinoma	Small cell carcinoma
Low-grade salivary duct carcinoma (low-grade cribriform cystadenocarcinoma)	Large cell carcinoma
Myoepithelial carcinoma	LEC
Oncocytic carcinoma	Metastasizing pleomorphic adenoma
Carcinoma ex pleomorphic adenoma (intracapsular/minimally invasive or with low-grade histology)	Carcinoma ex pleomorphic adenoma (widely invasive or high-grade histology)
Sialoblastoma	Carcinosarcoma
Adenocarcinoma NOS and cystadenocarcinoma, low grade	Adenocarcinoma and cystadenocarcinoma, NOS, high grade

From Seethala RR. An update on grading of salivary gland carcinomas. *Head Neck Pathol* 2009;3:69–77, with permission.

HIGHLIGHTS

- Salivary gland neoplasms represent a diverse group of benign and malignant tumors.
- In the parotid gland, 75% to 80% of tumors are benign and 25% malignant.
- In the submandibular gland, a higher proportion of neoplasms are malignant compared to the parotid gland.
- In the minor salivary glands, most neoplasms are malignant.
- An accurate diagnosis is important for guiding proper therapy.
- Most salivary gland tumors develop in the parotid gland.
- Low-dose radiation exposure has been implicated as an etiologic factor for salivary gland neoplasms.
- A mass in the region of the parotid gland should be considered a salivary gland neoplasm until proven otherwise.
- FNA biopsy is an accurate method to confirm the diagnosis of a salivary gland neoplasm.
- Parotidectomy with identification and preservation of the facial nerve is diagnostic and curative for most parotid gland neoplasms.
- In select cases, extracapsular dissection of pleomorphic adenoma of the parotid gland yields low rates of recurrence and complications.
- Combined surgery and radiation therapy has improved locoregional control and survival in patients with carcinoma of the major salivary glands.
- Tumor grade, stage, and histologic type are important prognostic variables for salivary gland malignancies.

REFERENCES

1. Adelstein DJ, Rodriguez CP. What is new in the management of salivary gland cancers? *Curr Opin Oncol* 2011;23:249–253.
2. Kokemueller H, Brueggeman N, Swennen G, et al. Mucoepidermoid carcinoma of the salivary glands: clinical review of 42 cases. *Oral Oncol* 2005;41:3–10.
3. Luksic I, Virag M, Manojlovic S, et al. Salivary gland tumors: 25 years of experience from a single institution in Croatia. *J Craniomaxillofac Surg* 2011;40(3):e75–e81. doi:10.1016/j.jcms.2011.05.002.
4. Zian T, Li L, Wang L, et al. Salivary gland neoplasms in oral and maxillofacial regions: a 23-year retrospective study of 6982 cases in an eastern chinese population. *Int J Oral Maxillofac Surg* 2010;39:235–242.
5. Vani NV, Ponniah I. The frequency and distribution pattern of minor salivary gland tumors in a government dental teaching hospital, Chennai, India. *Oral Surg Oral Med Oral Pathol Oral Radiol Endod* 2011;111:e33.
6. Luna MA, Batsakis JG, El-Naggar AK. Salivary gland tumors in children. *Ann Otol Rhinol Laryngol* 1991;100:869–871.
7. Shapiro N, Bhattacharyya N. Clinical characteristics and survival for major salivary gland malignancies in children. *Otolaryngol Head Neck Surg* 2006;134:631–634.
8. Stennert E, Guntinas-Lichius O, Klussmann JP, et al. Histopathology of pleomorphic adenoma in the parotid gland: a prospective unselected series of 100 cases. *Laryngoscope* 2001;111:2195–2200.
9. Upton DC, McNamar JP, Connor NP, et al. Parotidectomy: ten-year review of 237 cases at a single institution. *Otolaryngol Head Neck Surg* 2007;136:788–792.
10. Bae CH, Kim YD, Song SY. Benign pleomorphic adenoma of the soft palate metastasizing to the sphenoid sinus. *Clin Exp Otorhinolaryngol* 2010;3172–3175.
11. Nouraei SAR, Ferguson MS, Clarke PM, et al. Metastasizing pleomorphic salivary adenoma. *Arch Otolaryngol Head Neck Surg* 2006;132:788–793.
12. Shah N, Tighe JV, Barrett AW, et al. Bilateral intraparotid and extraparotid Warthin's tumours. *Br J Oral Maxillofac Surg* 2007;45:238–239.
13. Ethunandan M, Pratt CA, Higgins B, et al. Factors influencing the occurrence of multicentric and 'recurrent' Warthin's tumour: a cross sectional study. *Int J Oral Maxillofac Surg* 2008;37:831–834.
14. Teymoorthash A, Krasnewicz Y, Werner JA. Clinical features of cystadenolymphoma (Warthin's tumor) of the parotid gland: a retrospective comparative study of 96 cases. *Oral Oncol* 2006;42:569–573.

15. Huvos AG. Oncocytoma. In: Barnes L, Eveson JW, Reichart P, et al. eds., *World Health Organization classification of tumours: pathology and genetics, head and neck tumours*. Lyon, France: IARC Press, 2005:242–243.

16. Zhou CX, Gao Y. Oncocytoma of the salivary glands: a clinicopathologic and immunohistochemical study. *Oral Oncol* 2009;45:232–238.

17. Capone RB, Ha PK, Westra WH, et al. Oncocytic neoplasms of the parotid gland: a 16 year institutional review. *Otolaryngol Head Neck Surg* 2002;126:657–662.

18. Torske KR. Basal cell adenoma. In: Thompson LDR, Wenig BM, Nelson BL, et al., eds. *Diagnostic pathology head and neck*. Manitoba, Canada: Amirsys, 2011:5.39.

19. Boahene KO, Olsen KD, Lewis JE, et al. Mucoepidermoid carcinoma of the parotid gland: the Mayo Clinic experience. *Arch Otolaryngol Head Neck Surg* 2004;130:849–856.

20. Spight PM, Barrett AW. Salivary gland tumors. *Oral Dis* 2002;8:229–240.

21. Aro K, Leivo I, Makitie AA. Management and outcome of patients with mucoepidermoid carcinoma of major salivary gland origin: a single institution's 30-year experience. *Laryngoscope* 2008;118:258–262.

22. Laskar-Ghosh S, Murthy V, Wadasadawala T, et al. Mucoepidermoid carcinoma of the parotid gland: factors affecting outcome. *Head Neck* 2011;22:497–503.

23. Mendenhall WM, Morris CG, Amdur RJ, et al. Radiotherapy alone or combined with surgery for salivary gland carcinoma. *Cancer* 2005;45:52–55.

24. Emerick KS, Fabian RL, Deschler DG. Clinical presentation, management, and outcome of high-grade mucoepidermoid carcinoma of the parotid gland. *Otolaryngol Head Neck Surg* 2007;136:783–787.

25. Bradley PJ. Adenoid cystic carcinoma of the head and neck: a review. *Curr Opin Otolaryngol Head Neck Surg* 2004;12: 127–132.

26. Bianchi B, Copelli C, Cocchi R, et al. Adenoid cystic carcinoma of the intraoral minor salivary glands. *Oral Oncol* 2008;44: 1026–1031.

27. Chen AM, Bucci MK, Weinberg V, et al. Adenoid cystic carcinoma of the head and neck treated by surgery with or without postoperative radiation therapy: prognostic features of recurrence. *Int J Radiat Oncol Biol Phys* 2006;66:152–159.

28. Silverman DA, Carlson DL, Khuntia D, et al. Role of postoperative radiation therapy in adenoid cystic carcinoma of the head and neck. *Laryngoscope* 2004;114:1194–1199.

29. Huber PE, Debus J, Latz D, et al. Radiotherapy for advanced adenoid cystic carcinoma: neutrons, photons, or mixed beam? *Radiother Oncol* 2001;59:161–167.

30. Douglas JG, Koh WJ, Austin-Seymour M, et al. Treatment of salivary gland neoplasms with fast neutron radiotherapy. *Arch Otolaryngol Head Neck Surg* 2003;129:944–948.

31. Oplatek A, Ozer E, Agrawal A, et al. Patterns of recurrence and survival of head and neck adenoid cystic carcinoma after definitive resection. *Laryngoscope* 2010;120:65–70.

32. Hoffman HT, Karnel LH, Robinson R, et al. National Cancer Database report on cancer of the head and neck: acinic cell carcinoma. *Head Neck* 1999;21:297–309.

33. Federspil PA, Constantinidis J, Karapantzos I, et al. Acinic cell carcinomas of the parotid gland. A retrospective analysis. *HNO* 2001;49:825–830.

34. Al-Zaher N, Obeid A, Al-Salam S, et al. Acinic cell carcinoma of the salivary glands: a literature review. *Hematol Oncol Stem Cell Ther* 2009;2:259–264.

35. Bjorndal K, Krogdahl A, Therkildsen MH, et al. Salivary gland carcinoma in Denmark 1990–2005: a national study of incidence, site and histology. Results of the Danish Head and Neck Cancer Group (DAHANCA). *Oral Oncol* 2011;47:677–682.

36. Wahlberg P, Anderson H, Bjorklund A, et al. Carcinoma of the parotid and submandibular glands—a study of survival in 2465 patients. *Oral Oncol* 2002;38:706–713.

37. El-Naaj IA, Leiser Y, Wolff A, et al. Polymorphous low grade adenocarcinoma: case series and review of surgical management. *J Oral Maxillofac Surg* 2011;69(7):1967–1972. Epub Ahead of Print.

38. McHugh JB, Visscher DW, Barnes EL. Update on selected salivary gland neoplasms. *Arch Pathol Lab Med* 2009;133:1763–1774.

39. Pogodzinski MS, Sabri AN, Lewis JE, et al. Retrospective study and review of polymorphous low-grade adenocarcioma. *Laryngoscope* 2006;116:2145–2149.

40. Paleri V, Robinson M, Bradley P. Polymorphous low-grade adenocarcinoma of the head and neck. *Curr Opin Otolaryngol Head Neck Surg* 2008;16:163–169.

41. Olsen KD, Lewis JE. Carcinoma ex-pleomorphic adenoma: a clinicopathologic review. *Head Neck* 2001;23:705–712.

42. Zbaren P, Zbaren SY, Caversaccio MD, et al. Carcinoma ex pleomorphic adenoma: diagnostic difficulty and outcome. *Otolaryngol Head Neck Surg* 2008;138:601–605.

43. Chen AM, Garcia J, Bucci MK, et al. The role of postoperative radiation therapy in carcinoma ex-pleomorphic adenoma of the parotid gland. *Int J Radiat Oncol Biol Phys* 2007;67:138–143.

44. Lee S, Kim GE, Park CS, et al. Primary squamous cell carcinoma of the parotid gland. *Am J Otolaryngol* 2001;22:400–406.

45. Brennand-Rober MJ, Pring M, Hughes CW, et al. Minor salivary gland squamous cell carcinoma of the lower lip demonstrating striking perineural invasion. *Oral Surg Oral Med Oral Pathol Oral Radiol Endod* 2010;110:e28–e32.

46. Wang CP, Chang YL, Ko JY, et al. Lymphoepithelial carcinoma versus large cell undifferentiated carcinoma of the major salivary glands. *Cancer* 2004;101:2020–2027.

47. Jaehne M, Roeser K, Jaekel T, et al. Clinical and immunohistologic typing of salivary duct carcinoma: a report of 50 cases. *Cancer* 2005;103:2526–2533.

48. Nabili V, Tan JW, Bhuta S, et al. Salivary duct carcinoma; a clinical and histologic review with implications for trastuzumab therapy. *Head Neck* 2007;29(10):907–912.

49. Luna MA, Tortoledo ME, Ordonez NG, et al. Primary sarcomas of the major salivary glands. *Arch Otolaryngol Head Neck Surg* 1991;117:302–306.

50. Dunn P, Kuo TT, Shih LY, et al. Primary salivary gland lymphoma: a clinicopathologic study of 23 cases in Taiwan. *Acta Haematol* 2004;112:203–208.

51. Roh JY, Huh JR, Suh CW. Primary non-Hodgkin's lymphomas of the major salivary glands. *J Surg Oncol* 2008;97:35–39.

52. Sadetzki S, Oberman B, Mandelzweig L, et al. Smoking and risk of parotid gland tumors: a nationwide case-control study. *Cancer* 2008;112:1974–1982.

53. Forrest J, Campbell P, Kreiger N, et al. Salivary gland cancer: an exploratory analysis of dietary factors. *Nutr Cancer* 2008;60: 469–473.

54. Laane CJ, Murr AH, Mattre AN, et al. Role of Epstein-Barr virus and cytomegalovirus in the etiology of benign parotid tumors. *Head Neck* 2002;24:443–450.

55. Beal KP, Sing B, Kraus D, et al. Radiation induced salivary gland tumors: a report of 18 cases and a review of the literature. *Cancer J* 2003;9:467–471.

56. Boukheris H, Ron E, Dores GM, et al. Risk of radiation-related salivary gland carcinomas among survivors of Hodgkin lymphoma: a population-based analysis. *Cancer* 2008;113:3153–3159.

57. Alphs HH, Eisele DW, Westra WH. The role of fine needle aspiration in the evaluation of parotid masses. *Curr Opin Otolaryngol Head Neck Surg* 2006;14:62–66.

58. Lee YY, Wong KT, King AD, et al. Imaging of salivary gland tumors. *Eur J Radiol* 2008;66:419–436.

59. Brennan PA, Herd MK, Howlett DC, et al. Is ultrasound alone sufficient for imaging superficial lobe benign parotid tumours before surgery? *Br J Oral Maxillofac Surg* 2012;50(4):333–337. doi:10.1016/j.bjoms.2011.01.018.

60. Sharma G, Jung AS, Maceri DR, et al. US-guided fine-needle aspiration of major salivary gland masses and adjacent lymph nodes: accuracy and impact on clinical decision making. *Radiology* 2011;259:471–478.

61. Lee SK, Rho BH, Won KS. Parotid incidentaloma identified by combined 18-F-fluorodeoxyglucose whole-body positron emission tomography and computed tomography: findings at grayscale and power Doppler ultrasonography and ultrasound-guided fine-needle aspiration biopsy or core-needle biopsy. *Eur Radiol* 2009;19:2268–2274.

62. Razfar A, Heron DE, Branstetter BF, et al. Positron emission tomography-computed tomography adds to the management of salivary gland malignancies. *Laryngoscope* 2010;120:734–738.

63. Johnson JT, Ferlito A, Fagan JJ, et al. Role of limited parotidectomy in management of pleomorphic adenoma. *J Laryngol Otol* 2010;121:1126–1128.

64. Klintworth N, Zenk J, Koch M, et al. Postoperative complications after extracapsular dissection of benign parotid lesions with particular reference to facial nerve function. *Laryngoscope* 2010;120:484–490.

65. Shehata EA. Extra-capsular dissection for benign parotid tumors. *Int J Oral Maxillofac Surg* 2010;39:140–144.

66. Zbaren P, Schupbach J, Nuyens M, et al. Elective neck dissection versus observation in primary parotid carcinoma. *Otolaryngol Head Neck Surg* 2005;132:387–391.

67. Korkmaz H, Yoo GH, Du W, et al. Predictors of nodal metastasis in salivary gland cancer. *J Surg Oncol* 2002;80:186–189.

68. Gold DR, Annino DJ. Management of the neck in salivary gland carcinoma. *Otolaryngol Clin N Am* 2005;38:99–105.

69. Cohen SM, Burkey BB, Netterville JL. Surgical management of parapharyngeal space masses. *Head Neck* 2005;27:669–675.

70. Ducic Y, Oxford L, Pontius AT. Transoral approach to the superomedial parapharyngeal space. *Otolaryngol Head Neck Surg* 2006;134:466–470.

71. Oliai BR, Sheth S, Burroughs FH, et al. Parapharyngeal space tumors: a cytopathological study of 24 cases on fine-needle aspiration. *Diagn Cytopathol* 2005;32:11–15.

72. Schoenfeld JD, Sher DJ, Norris CM, et al. Salivary gland tumors treated with adjuvant intensity-modulated radiotherapy with or without concurrent chemotherapy. *Int J Radiat Oncol Biol Phys* 2010. doi:10.1016/j.ijrobp.2010.09.042.

73. Chen AM, Granchi PJ, Garcia J, et al. Local-regional recurrence after surgery without postoperative irradiation for carcinomas of the major salivary glands: implications for adjuvant therapy. *Int J Radiat Oncol Biol Phys* 2007;67:982–987.

74. Chen AM, Bucci MK, Quivey JM, et al. Long-term outcome of patients treated by radiation therapy alone for salivary gland carcinomas. *Int J Radiat Oncol Biol Phys* 2006;66:1044–1050.

75. Chen AM, Garcia J, Bucci MK, et al. Recurrent pleomorphic adenoma of the parotid gland: long-term outcome of patients treated with radiation therapy. *Int J Radiat Oncol Biol Phys* 2006;66:1031–1035.

76. Douglas JG, Einck J, Austin-Seymour M, et al. Neutron radiotherapy for recurrent pleomorphic adenomas of major salivary glands. *Head Neck* 2001;23:1037–1042.

77. Pommier P, Liebsch NJ, Deschler DG, et al. Proton beam radiation therapy for skull base adenoid cystic carcinoma. *Arch Otolaryngol Head Neck Surg* 2006;132:1242–1249.

78. Gilbert J, Li Y, Pinto HA, et al. Phase II trial of Taxol in salivary gland malignancies (E1394): a trial of the eastern cooperative oncology group. *Head Neck* 2006;28:197–204.

79. Laurie SA, Siu LL, Winquist E, et al. A phase 2 study of platinum and gemcitabine in patients with advanced salivary gland cancer: a trial of the NCIC Clinical Trials Group. *Cancer* 2010;116:362–368.

80. Tanvetyanon T, Quin D, Padhya T, et al. Outcomes of postoperative concurrent chemoradiotherapy for locally advanced major salivary gland carcinoma. *Arch Otolaryngol Head Neck Surg* 2009;135:687–692.

81. Lowry TR, Gal TJ, Brennan JA. Patterns of use of facial nerve monitoring during parotid gland surgery. *Otolaryngol Head Neck Surg* 2005;133:313–318.

82. Lopez M, Quer M, Leon X, et al. Usefulness of facial nerve monitoring during parotidectomy. *Acta Otorrinolaringol Esp* 2001;52:418–421.

83. Grosheva M, Klussmann JP, Grimminger C, et al. Electromyographic facial nerve monitoring during parotidectomy for benign lesions does not improve the outcome of postoperative facial nerve function: a prospective two-center trial. *Laryngoscope* 2009;119:2299–2305.

84. Eisele DW, Wang SJ, Orloff LA. Electrophysiologic facial nerve monitoring during parotidectomy. *Head Neck* 2010;32:399–405.

85. Lee KJ, Fee WF, Terris DJ. The efficacy of corticosteroids in post-parotidectomy facial nerve paresis. *Laryngoscope* 2001;112:1958–1963.

86. De Bree R, van der Wall I, Leemans CR. Management of Frey syndrome. *Head Neck* 2007;29:773–778.

87. Sinha UK, Saadat D, Doherty CM, et al. Use of AlloDerm implant to prevent Frey syndrome after parotidectomy. *Arch Facial Plast Surg* 2003;5:109–112.

88. Kim JT, Naidu S, Kim YH. The buccal fat: a convenient and effective autologous option to prevent Frey syndrome and for facial contouring following parotidectomy. *Plast Reconstr Surg* 2010;125:1706–1709.

89. Sanabria A, Kowalski LP, Bradley PJ, et al. Sternocleidomastoid muscle flap in preventing Frey's syndrome after parotidectomy: a systematic review. *Head Neck* 2012;34(4):589–598. Doi: 10.1002/hed.21722.

90. Leonetti JP, Marzo SJ, Petruzzelli GJ, et al. Recurrent pleomorphic adenoma of the parotid gland. *Otolaryngol Head Neck Surg* 2005;133:319–322.

91. Seethala RR. An update on grading of salivary gland carcinomas. *Head Neck Pathol* 2009;3:69–77.

92. Kokemueller H, Swennen G, Brueggemann N, et al. Epithelial malignancies of the salivary glands: clinical experience of a single institution—a review. *Int J Oral Maxillofac Surg* 2004;22:423–432.

93. Terhaard CHJ, Lubsen H, Van der Tweel I, et al. Salivary gland carcinoma: independent prognostic factors for locoregional control, distant metastases, and overall survival: results of the Dutch Head and Neck Oncology Cooperative Group. *Head Neck* 2004;26:681–693.

94. Hocwald E, Korkmaz H, Yoo GH, et al. Prognostic factors in major salivary gland cancer. *Laryngoscope* 2001;111:1434–1439.

116 Lip Cancer

Liana Puscas   *Michael A. Fritz*   *Ramon M. Esclamado*

Lip cancer is one of the most common malignant tumors of the head and neck. The typical patient is a white male smoker with a fair complexion in his sixth to seventh decade of life who presents with a squamous cell carcinoma (SCCA) involving the lower lip. As the lips are in a prominent position on the face, appropriate management of this malignancy should have as its goals maximizing survival while minimizing the functional and cosmetic morbidity associated with treatment. This requires a thorough understanding of the functional anatomy of the lips, the biologic behavior of the disease, treatment options, and reconstructive considerations.

FUNCTIONAL ANATOMY

The lips form the anterior boundary of the oral cavity and function as a mobile oral sphincter that prevents dribbling of fluids and assists in mastication, deglutition, and articulation. The lips are also important aesthetically, contributing to appearance and facial expression. The anatomic extent of the lips includes only the vermilion, or that portion of the lip mucosa that contacts the opposing lip. Anteriorly, the lip ends at the vermilion border, which is the junction of the vermilion with the skin. The lower lip vermilion in repose is more everted than the upper lip. The transverse length of the upper lip is slightly longer: about 8.0 cm compared with 7.5 cm for the lower lip.

The orbicularis oris muscle is the sphincter that lies within the lip and encircles the oral aperture. Superiorly, it extends almost to the columella and attaches to the anterior nasal spine. Inferiorly, it interdigitates with the mentalis muscles to form the mental crease. Numerous paired muscles of facial expression insert on its lateral deep surface and contribute to oral competence and the diversity of lip movement (Fig. 116.1). The deep surface of the orbicularis oris is covered by loosely attached mucous membranes containing numerous minor salivary glands. Superficially, it is loosely attached to overlying skin.

The sensory and motor innervations of the lips are separate. The infraorbital branch of the maxillary division of the trigeminal nerve (V2) provides the major sensory supply to the skin and mucous membrane of the upper lip. The oral commissure area is supplied by the buccal branch of the mandibular division of the trigeminal nerve (V3), whereas sensation of the lower lip skin and mucosa is derived from the mental branch of the mandibular division. The seventh cranial nerve (facial nerve) provides the motor innervation of the lip. The upper lip musculature is supplied by the buccal branch of the facial nerve, whereas the marginal mandibular branch innervates the lower lip musculature.

The main blood supply to the lips consists of the superior and inferior labial arteries, which travel between the submucosa of the lip and the orbicularis at the level of the vermilion cutaneous junction. The vessels branch from the facial artery just lateral to the oral commissure. These paired vessels create a circumoral vascular arcade that provides the anatomic basis for the classic lip-switch procedures and other local myocutaneous flaps. Efforts should therefore be made to preserve the facial vessels when performing concomitant neck dissections. The arteries have accompanying veins that drain to the anterior facial veins.

The lymphatics of the lips (Fig. 116.2) begin as a fine capillary network in the vermilion border and combine to form collecting trunks. The trunks from the upper lip and commissure drain first to the ipsilateral preauricular, infraparotid, submandibular, and submental lymph nodes. No contralateral drainage occurs because the embryonic fusion plane of the central frontonasal process separates the lateral maxillary processes and their associated neurovascular and lymphatic connections. The lower lip lymphatics drain first to the submental and submandibular nodes. Because the mandibular processes fuse in

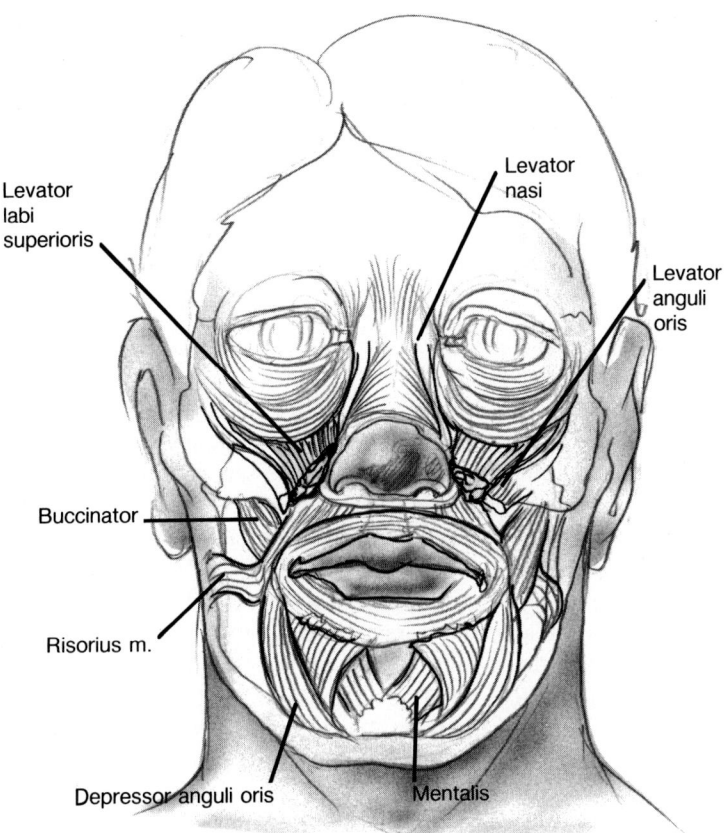

Figure 116.1 Musculature of the lips. The orbicularis oris muscle is the sphincter lying within the lip and encircles the oral aperture. Numerous paired muscles of facial expression insert on its lateral deep surface to contribute to oral competence and the diversity of lip movement.

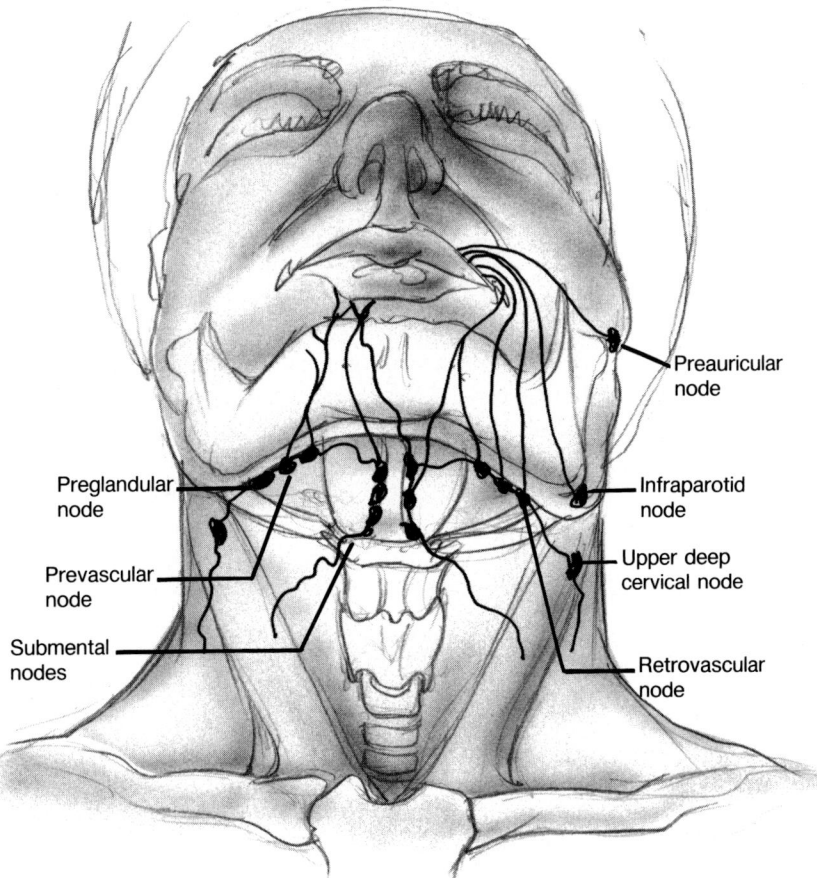

Figure 116.2 Lymphatic drainage of the lips. Lymphatic channels of the upper lip and commissure drain to the ipsilateral preauricular, infraparotid, submandibular, and submental lymph nodes. The lower lip lymphatics drain to both ipsilateral and contralateral submental and submandibular lymph nodes. The second nodal station for both lips is the upper deep jugular nodes and occasionally the middle deep jugular nodes.

the midline, numerous anastomoses cross the midline to drain bilaterally. Lower lip lymphatics also enter the mental foramen in 22% of patients. The second nodal station for both upper and lower lips is the upper deep jugular nodes (level II) or occasionally the middle deep jugular nodes (level III).

BIOLOGIC BEHAVIOR

The age-standardized rate (ASR) of lip cancer varies according to gender, race, and geography. Around the world, lip cancer rates are highest in white males (1). In the United States, the ASR for white males is 2.5/100,000 per year compared to 0.3/100,000 per year for white females (2). South Australia has the highest ASR of lip cancer in the world: over 15/100,000 per year in men and 4/100,000 per year in women (3). Lip cancer is rare in Asia and in blacks (1,4,5). In the United States, for example, the ASR for both black males and females is 0.1/100,000 per year (2). The most common type of lip cancer is SCCA that is usually found on the lower lip in men. Basal cell carcinoma (BCCA) is the second most common malignancy and is found most frequently on the upper lip in women (6,7). Most cancers are found in individuals in their sixth to seventh decade of life (6–8).

The etiology is multifactorial and includes prolonged exposure to ultraviolet radiation, use of tobacco, consumption of alcohol, poor dental hygiene, and low socioeconomic status (6–9). Actinic cheilitis, or actinic keratosis of the lip, is considered to be a premalignant condition that doubles the risk of lip SCCA (10,11). Immunosuppression also significantly increases the risk of lip cancer as evidenced by higher rates in organ transplant patients. Unfortunately, both SCCA and BCCA arising in this setting are more aggressive in their behavior. Interestingly, failure of a transplanted kidney with its attendant cessation of immunosuppression decreases the risk of lip cancer to baseline (12).

Lip cancer is one of the most readily curable malignancies of the head and neck. When diagnosed at an early stage, 10-year cause-specific survival is as high as 98%, with a recurrence-free survival of 92.5% (13). The prominent location of the lips typically allows for early detection and treatment of this lesion. Characteristically, a history of crusting that bleeds on removal and a nonhealing blister for several months to years has been noted. When left untreated, the tumor progresses to involve skin of the mentum and alveolar mucosa. In advanced cases, mandibular bone, floor of the mouth, and tongue can be involved, which renders the patient an oral cripple. Metastasis to cervical nodes develops with advanced lesions, and ultimately distant metastasis occurs. In a retrospective study of 1,036 patients with lip cancer (14), multivariate analysis yielded several prognostic factors predictive for significantly decreased determinate survival: patients with primary tumors larger than 3 cm, presence of cervical metastasis,

poorly differentiated or undifferentiated histology, and involved surgical margins. The risk of cervical metastases is increased in large primary tumors (greater than 3 cm), particularly if the oral commissure is involved; locally recurrent tumors; tumors thicker than 5 mm; poorly differentiated histology; or if perineural invasion is present (15–18).

CLINICAL EVALUATION

Lip carcinoma should be readily recognized and diagnosed (see Table 116.2). Its early stages can be indolent and protracted. As previously mentioned, the patient may present with a history of lower lip crusting that bleeds on removal or a nonhealing blister present for several months to years. Physical examination typically reveals an area of crusting with surrounding induration in an area of leukoplakia of the lower lip. In more advanced stages, a large bleeding mass may be present that can involve chin skin, the oral commissure, the upper lip, or the mandible. The integrity of the mental nerve must be evaluated even in early lesions, because tumor may track along the mental nerve and involve the mandible by direct extension, perineural invasion, or lymphatic spread into the mental foramen.

The diagnosis is established by incisional biopsy, which should include part of the deep or lateral tumor margin. This allows the pathologist to determine the pattern of invasion and the presence of perineural invasion. Prophylactic antibiotics are not necessary for simple biopsies (19). Ancillary radiographic studies such as a Panorex, computerized tomography (CT), and magnetic resonance imaging (MRI) are indicated when tumor is attached to the mandible or extends over the gingiva into a tooth root, when dentition is loose, or when hypesthesia of the mental nerve is present. Positron emission tomography (PET) resolution is too imprecise to correctly define the extent of the tumor compared to CT or MRI. Ipsilateral enlargement of the mental nerve foramen is a sign of mandibular invasion via the mental nerve, and obliteration of fat in the masticator space, in the pterygopalatine fossa, or along the mandibular canal must be regarded as suspicious for tumor spread, even in the absence of gross osteolytic changes (20). An aggressive metastatic workup is not indicated in previously untreated lip carcinomas, because fewer than 2% of patients have distant metastases at the time of initial evaluation (21). The staging of SCCA of the lip, as defined by the American Joint Committee on Cancer, is outlined in Table 116.1.

Although 90% of lower lip malignancies are SCCA (22), it is important to keep in mind the differential diagnosis of other nonhealing or ulcerative lesions of the lips, particularly when the clinical presentation is atypical for squamous cell cancer. BCCA is the second most common malignancy of the perioral region. Cancers of the upper lip are nearly always BCCA (6,14). It rarely arises on lip mucosa; rather, it involves the lip by direct extension of

TABLE 116.1	STAGING OF SCCA OF THE LIP: PRIMARY TUMOR (T)

TX	Primary tumor cannot be assessed.
T0	No evidence of primary tumor
Tis	Carcinoma *in situ*
T1	Tumor ≤2 cm in greatest dimension
T2	Tumor >2 cm but ≤4 cm in greatest dimension
T3	Tumor >4 cm in greatest dimension
T4a	Moderately advanced local disease: Tumor invades through cortical bone, inferior alveolar nerve, floor of mouth, or skin of face (e.g., chin or nose).
T4b	Very advanced local disease: Tumor invades masticator space, pterygoid plates, or skull base and/or encases internal carotid artery.

a perioral skin lesion. This is most commonly seen with sclerosing BCCAs. These tumors usually have a distinct clinical appearance of a pearly white nodule with central dimpling, although larger tumors may appear similar to squamous cell tumors. They grow very slowly, rarely metastasize to cervical lymph nodes, and when located near embryonic fusion planes tend to track deeply into the soft tissues along these planes.

Overall, minor salivary gland tumors (MSGT) comprise less than 3% of all head and neck neoplasms, but the lips are the second most common site after the hard palate for the occurrence of MSGT (23). A neoplasm arising from the minor salivary glands typically presents as a smooth, firm, nonulcerated mass, very often involving the upper lip. However, when a MSGT presents on the lower lip, it is far more likely to be malignant. Overall, MSGT have about a 25/75 distribution between benign and malignant, but on the lip, they are more likely to be benign due to the great preponderance of pleomorphic adenomas. The most common malignant MSGT are mucoepidermoid and adenoid cystic carcinoma (23,24). Other rare malignant lesions of the lips include melanoma, microcystic adnexal carcinoma, Merkel cell carcinoma, malignant fibrous histiocytoma, and malignant granular cell tumors. Keratoacanthoma is a benign self-limiting epithelial neoplasm that can mimic SCCA. It is commonly seen in patients aged 60 to 80 years. It has an initial rapid growth phase (over several weeks) to 1 to 2 cm in diameter and then stabilizes and spontaneously regresses after several weeks to months. It occurs on the lips in 8.1% of cases, appearing as an ulcerated circumscribed lesion with elevated or rolled margins, a keratinized central region, and an indurated base. It is firm in consistency, and the central keratin core can desquamate, leaving an ulcer. Diagnosis is established by incisional biopsy, which is reported to accelerate its involution (25) (Table 116.2). Excisional biopsy, sparing as much normal tissue as possible, is indicated for persistent or enlarging lesions over several months, when SCCA cannot be excluded after previous incisional biopsies.

Again, a high index of suspicion for tumor should prompt a biopsy in the face of an abnormal physical exam of the lip. Common signs and symptoms of actinic cheilitis include dryness, atrophy, scaliness, swelling, erythema, ulceration, loss of distinction of the vermilion border, and the formation of transverse fissures (11). When any of these changes or leukoplakia or hyperkeratosis is seen, either as an isolated lesion or if the lesion progresses in size, biopsy is indicated. Other ulcerative inflammatory lesions involving the lips, including viral stomatitis and the primary chancre of syphilis, can mimic lip carcinoma but are acute in onset, and the lip lesion heals spontaneously.

MANAGEMENT

The most efficacious treatment modality for lip carcinoma is one that allows adequate treatment of the primary tumor, appropriate management of cervical lymph nodes,

TABLE 116.2	Ⓓ DIAGNOSIS LIP CANCER

Diagnosis	Symptoms and Signs	Tests
Squamous cell cancer	Nonhealing blister or recurrent crusting, lip induration, ulcer or mass for months to years, mental nerve numbness	Panorex CT/MRI Biopsy
BCCA	Pearly nodule with central dimpling, upper lip, or perioral skin	Biopsy
Minor salivary gland tumor	Submucosal mass, usually upper lip	Biopsy
Keratoacanthoma	Rapid growth then spontaneous regression, may mimic SCCA in appearance	Incisional biopsy

CT, computed tomography; MRI, magnetic resonance imaging.
From Baker SR, Krause CJ. Pedicled flaps in reconstruction of the lip. *Facial Plast Surg* 1983;1:68–69, with permission.

and successful reconstruction. The treatment plan should have the following goals:

1. Extirpate all tissue involved with cancer, both at the primary site and regional lymph nodes
2. Maintain oral competence in terms of speech, mastication, and retention of saliva
3. Maintain satisfactory lip cosmesis
4. Permit early rehabilitation and return to daily activities

Surgery and radiation therapy are equally effective in controlling T1, T2, and T3 lesions, while T4 lesions require combined modality treatment (26–28). In a series of 323 patients, of which 91% were T1 or Tcis treated primarily by surgery, cause-specific survival at 10 years was 98% (29). In a series of 158 stage I and II patients, 108 (68%) of whom were treated with surgery, and 50 (32%) of whom were treated with XRT; determinate survival rates were 95% for stage I and 90% for stage II without any difference between the treatment received (30). Another group reported on their 228 patients of whom 197 (86%) were treated only with surgery and 205 (90%) of whom were stage I and II. Their actuarial disease-specific survival for all stages was 92% at 5 years (22). A study of 256 stage I patients treated either with surgery (*n* = 90) or XRT (*n* = 166) found no difference between the two groups in local control or overall survival rates; however, disease-free survival rates were higher for those treated with surgery (31). A very large European study of 1,870 patients looking at the effectiveness of brachytherapy showed 5-year local control rates of 98% for T1, 97% for T2, and 90% for T3 lesions (27). In another set of 85 N0 patients treated primarily with XRT, the actuarial 5-year survival rate was 97% with a locoregional control rate of 93% in patients who had T1–T3 disease (26).

Patients with higher overall stages, and especially those with higher nodal stages, have a worse prognosis. In the series mentioned earlier with 5-year determinate survival rates of 95% for stage I and 90% for stage II, patients with stage III and IV lip cancers had a 37% 5-year determinate survival rate (30). In one series of 118 patients treated with surgery and post-op XRT as indicated, determinate 5-year survival rates were 100% for stage I, 94% for stage II, 67% for stage III, and 49% for stage IV. Not surprisingly, patients in stage IV also had the highest rate of recurrence (32).

Radiation therapy is a low-risk noninvasive technique that avoids the potential complications associated with general anesthesia and surgical morbidity (Table 116.3). However, the treatment time is prolonged (as much as 5 to 6 weeks for external beam XRT, 1 week for brachytherapy), a whistle deformity may result from tissue loss and wound contracture with very large tumors, osteoradionecrosis of the mandible may develop, and future reconstructive options may be limited. It is contraindicated as primary therapy in patients with definite bony involvement. Studies looking at the sequelae of XRT have

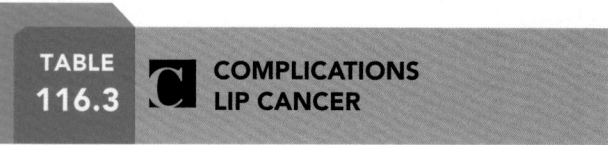

TABLE 116.3	**C**	**COMPLICATIONS LIP CANCER**

Surgical
  Wound infection and dehiscence
  Incompetent oral sphincter
  Microstomia
  Poor cosmetic result
Radiation
  Whistle deformity
  Osteoradionecrosis

found that the majority of patients have good aesthetic and functional outcomes, especially with smaller or intermediate tumors (26,27), but the great difficulty with XRT as primary therapy (especially for larger tumors) is that when complications occur, surgical reconstruction becomes more difficult. Primary radiation therapy may be most useful in the treatment of commissure lesions due to aesthetic and reconstructive considerations in this setting (27).

In the United States, surgical management is recommended for most patients. The oncologic, functional, and cosmetic outcome is usually excellent in early T stage disease, and the oncologic outcome is poor with primary radiation of advanced tumors, particularly when it is close to or involves the mandible. We prefer a combination of surgery and postoperative radiotherapy for stage III disease with high-risk features, stage IV disease, and for recurrent disease after primary surgical treatment.

Vermilionectomy is indicated in Tcis, superficial carcinoma limited to mucosa, or multicentric or premalignant lesions such as actinic cheilitis (10). The standard approach to surgical resection of the primary lip lesion is full-thickness excision and careful intraoperative frozen-section evaluation of the surgical margins. The appropriate margin around a T1 primary lip tumor is controversial. A study of 72 stage I and II patients reported a 2.8% local recurrence rate when a 3-mm margin of normal tissue was obtained and frozen-section margins were negative (33). When tumor margins were 2 mm or less, local recurrence was seen in 13% of patients, half of whom had received postoperative radiation therapy (34). Even with 5 to 10 mm of seemingly normal tissue as a margin, 17 of 131 (13%) T1–T3 patients had positive margins on frozen sections, and 9 of 131 (7%) had a "close" margin in which the tumor was within 5 mm on permanent histologic examination. Sixteen of the seventeen patients had T1 tumors (35). In T2 tumors, we advocate a 5- to 8-mm margin of normal tissue because tendency to underestimate margins is more common and reported local recurrence rates have been higher than anticipated.

The primary goal of therapy is eradication of all tumor tissue, without limitation of extirpation for reconstructive considerations. More advanced tumors may require resection of chin skin, mandibular bone, or oral cavity soft tissues to allow a 1- to 2-cm margin. Skin incisions should be planned so as to minimize the secondary deformity and to facilitate reconstruction but not at the expense of compromising tumor margins. BCCA should also be treated with margins of at least 4 mm to improve control rates (36). The importance of frozen section margin control and the achievement of negative margins in the treatment of cancer cannot be overemphasized as it is well known that positive margins decrease locoregional control rates and may require the addition of another treatment modality (e.g., XRT).

Mohs micrographic surgery is an accepted treatment for cutaneous carcinomas and is recommended as first-line therapy in the following settings due to superior cure rates: BCCA greater than 2 cm, SCCA greater than 1 cm, tumors at high risk for recurrence (tumors in the H-zone or embryonic fusion planes, tumors in immunocompromised patients, tumors with aggressive histologic features), tumors with indistinct clinical margins (e.g., morpheaform BCCA), and especially recurrent tumors (37). Looking specifically at the performance of Mohs in the setting of lip carcinoma, two different studies with 5 years of follow-up have shown a recurrence rate of 3% for BCCA and 8% for SCCA (38,39). A metaanalysis of cutaneous, lip, and ear SCCA showed a 5-year local recurrence rate of 10.5% in 7,022 patients treated with non-Mohs modalities versus 2.3% in 952 patients undergoing Mohs micrographic surgery (40). However, in this study, electrodesiccation and curettage were also included in the non-Mohs modalities, and not every series included in the metaanalysis may have used frozen section control of the margins. In a study of 599 facial BCCA lesions (lips *n* = 29) with 5-year follow-up comparing surgical excision with 3-mm margins and frozen section control against Mohs, there was not a significant difference between the two regarding recurrence of primary BCCA, but Mohs did show a statistically significant lower rate of recurrence in the treatment of recurrent BCCA (41).

The management of regional lymph nodes in patients with lip carcinoma is controversial and requires a thorough understanding of the risk of nodal metastasis and the patterns of nodal spread. In contrast to other SCCAs of the oral cavity, lip carcinoma uncommonly metastasizes to regional lymph nodes. However, when nodal metastasis occurs, 5-year determinate survival is significantly decreased as discussed earlier. In fact, nodal disease is the single most important prognostic factor of survival in lip cancer (15). Regional nodal metastasis is present at the time of initial diagnosis in up to 15% of patients, and up to another 15% of patients will develop delayed nodal metastasis (15,30). Therefore, appropriate management of the neck in lip cancer requires separate decision making for clinically palpable disease versus occult metastatic nodal disease in the newly diagnosed, untreated patient. For patients with recurrent disease, the cervical lymph nodes must be addressed.

In patients with clinically palpable, suspicious lymph nodes, the rate of pathologically positive nodes ranges from 44% to 97% (15,17,42). If the primary tumor was on the lateral one-third of the lip, the ipsilateral nodes were involved 84% of the time and were limited to levels I to III (42). Bilateral or contralateral metastasis was seen 3% to 14% of patients and was usually associated with larger tumors that crossed the midline of the lower lip (15,17,42). Neck dissection of the ipsilateral side alone is recommended if radiation therapy is planned postoperatively and includes the contralateral, undissected, clinically N0 neck. Indications for postoperative radiation therapy include a T3 or T4 primary tumor, a recurrent tumor, extracapsular spread, metastasis in multiple levels or more than two nodes, or perineural invasion. A modified radical or radical neck dissection is performed for bulky (greater than 3 cm) nodal disease in levels II/III, but a selective neck dissection of levels I to III is oncologically sound if the nodes are freely mobile, and postoperative radiation therapy is used for extracapsular spread, more than two pathologically positive nodes, or multiple levels are involved (15,30,43,44).

Decision making for treating clinically N0 necks is more complex. Sentinel node biopsy for lip cancer is slowly growing in usage, and it holds promise as in other oral cavity sites (45,46). Current studies will help to determine its place in the treatment algorithm. T1 lesions rarely need the neck addressed, because the risk of nodal metastasis is approximately 3% (29). The risk for occult metastases increases with increased primary tumor size as evidenced in a large study of 617 patients: only 4% of T1/T2 patients had occult metastasis versus 23% of T3/T4 patients ($P < 0.001$) (17). The likely location of possible occult metastases is determined by the lymph node drainage basin of the primary lesion as described earlier.

Our treatment philosophy is to perform ipsilateral selective neck dissection, levels I to III and contralateral level I in N0 necks when a significant risk (20%) of occult metastasis is present and radiation therapy is not planned. As previously mentioned, there is a higher risk of cervical metastasis in primary tumors greater than 3 cm, particularly if the oral commissure is involved; locally recurrent tumors; tumors thicker than 5 mm; poorly differentiated histology; or if perineural invasion is present (15–17,30). We also perform ipsilateral selective neck dissection, levels I to III and contralateral level I when ipsilateral N1 disease is present, the contralateral neck is N0, and postoperative radiation therapy is not planned, or when reconstruction requires revascularized tissue transfer. Bilateral I to III SND can be performed for primary lesions greater than 3 cm crossing the midline, but neck dissection is unnecessary if postoperative radiation will be used to treat the primary site, because the neck can be included in the treatment fields.

LIP RECONSTRUCTION

Lip reconstruction must be carefully considered when managing lip carcinomas and requires meticulous planning to achieve optimal functional and cosmetic results. The ideal reconstructive procedure should result in a lip that is sensate; has sphincter or muscle function that maintains a watertight continent seal; allows sufficient opening for food, dentures, and oral hygiene; and is aesthetically acceptable. It is not possible to satisfy all these criteria in every instance; therefore, reconstructive goals must be prioritized. The most critical component of successful reconstruction is oral continence, which is a function of sensation and two sphincteric mechanisms oriented at right angles. The deep orbicularis and buccinator muscle interplay to create an axial force that seals the lips against the teeth, and the superficial orbicularis functions as a coronal sphincter, pursing and sealing the opposing lips (47). This complex relationship is best preserved when circumferential continuity of the orbicularis is maintained; however, larger defects often mandate alternative solutions to avoid compromising oral aperture size.

Multiple preoperative factors will influence reconstructive plans including defect size, tissue laxity, and patient factors such as dentures. In addition, planned adjunctive surgery, which may affect vascular supply (e.g., neck dissection), previous radiation therapy, or surgery, may compromise vascularity and affect design or preclude pedicled flaps. To optimize reconstructive and oncologic results, it is best to employ a flexible game plan of lip repair, with multiple options in mind, choosing the technique that best fits the final oncologic defect and the patient's specific tissue characteristics. It is important to keep in mind priorities of structure, function, and form (in that order), realizing that satisfaction of all goals often requires more than one stage, particularly with regard to large or complex defects. If possible, incisions should be placed within the circumoral relaxed skin tension lines (oriented radially), at borders of lip subunits or at boundaries such as the melolabial crease and labiomental sulcus. Tattooing the white scroll at the vermilion border with a fine needle and methylene blue dye ensures accurate postoperative realignment of this aesthetically critical boundary.

Partial-Thickness Defects

Partial-thickness or mucosal loss at the vermilion only is most commonly encountered when vermilionectomy or lip shave is performed for diffuse premalignant or superficial malignant disease or preventatively in conjunction with primary tumor resection when actinic cheilitis is present in remaining lip tissue. The most commonly used method of reconstitution of lining involves submucosal dissection and advancement of labial buccal mucosa. Undermining is performed deep to minor salivary glands and superficial to the orbicularis oris muscle and labial artery, and it can be extended to the apex of the buccal

sulcus to ensure tension-free redraping. Problems with this technique include thinning of lip, persistent deep red color of advanced mucosa (more of a problem for males), and potential inversion of hairs at the vermillion border with irritation. These drawbacks can be avoided with carbon dioxide laser lip shaves and mucosalization by secondary intention, although healing time requires 2 to 3 weeks. Other less commonly used two-stage techniques for vermillion mucosa replacement include bipedicle visor-type flaps from the undersurface of the opposing lip, ventral tongue flaps, and cross-lip mucosal flaps (48). Small vermilion deficiencies can be managed with V-Y advancement flaps.

Small partial-thickness defects involving the lips are managed following basic principles of cutaneous surgery. Optimal reconstructive results are often achieved when the defect can be converted to a wedge or pentagonal defect oriented within relaxed skin tension lines. M-plasty is used when possible to avoid scars that cross the boundaries of the lip subunits. Extending resections through uninvolved vermilion and orbicularis often achieves better cosmetic results than A-to-T methods that create horizontal scars parallel to the mucocutaneous junction (48,49).

Larger partial-thickness defects mandate consideration of lip subunits. Upper lip subunits include a central segment composed of the philtrum and philtral ridges and two trapezoid-shaped lateral segments (50). The lower lip consists of a single subunit. Similar to principles of nasal reconstruction, absence of the majority of a subunit is often best repaired after excision of the remaining portion. Medial advancement of lateral upper lip skin is aided greatly by the excision of perialar crescents of skin and anchoring dermis to pyriform periosteum deep to the ala. Partial-thickness defects of the central segment are amenable to full-thickness skin grafting or healing by secondary intention—with the intention of narrowing the philtrum as little as possible. Patients with flat, less distinct philtral columns may be an exception to this rule (47). Large cutaneous lateral defects are optimally resurfaced with V to Y island flaps or with inferiorly or superiorly based melolabial transposition flaps (Fig. 116.3).

Full-Thickness Defects

Isolated full-thickness defects of vermilion only (mucosa and orbicularis) are uncommon, but full-thickness deficiencies along the length of the vermilion are almost always present after extensive reconstructions with local or distant flaps. Several techniques have therefore been designed to address this issue. Small complete vermilion defects can be addressed with a full-thickness horizontal releasing incision at the vermilion–cutaneous junction of the longer portion of the remaining lip (48). Vermilion is then advanced laterally into the defect. Another option is to convert the defect to a full-thickness wedge through the cutaneous lip.

When extensive vermilion substance has been lost, a muscle-mucosal flap from the ventral surface of the tongue may be used. This flap is based posteriorly with the free

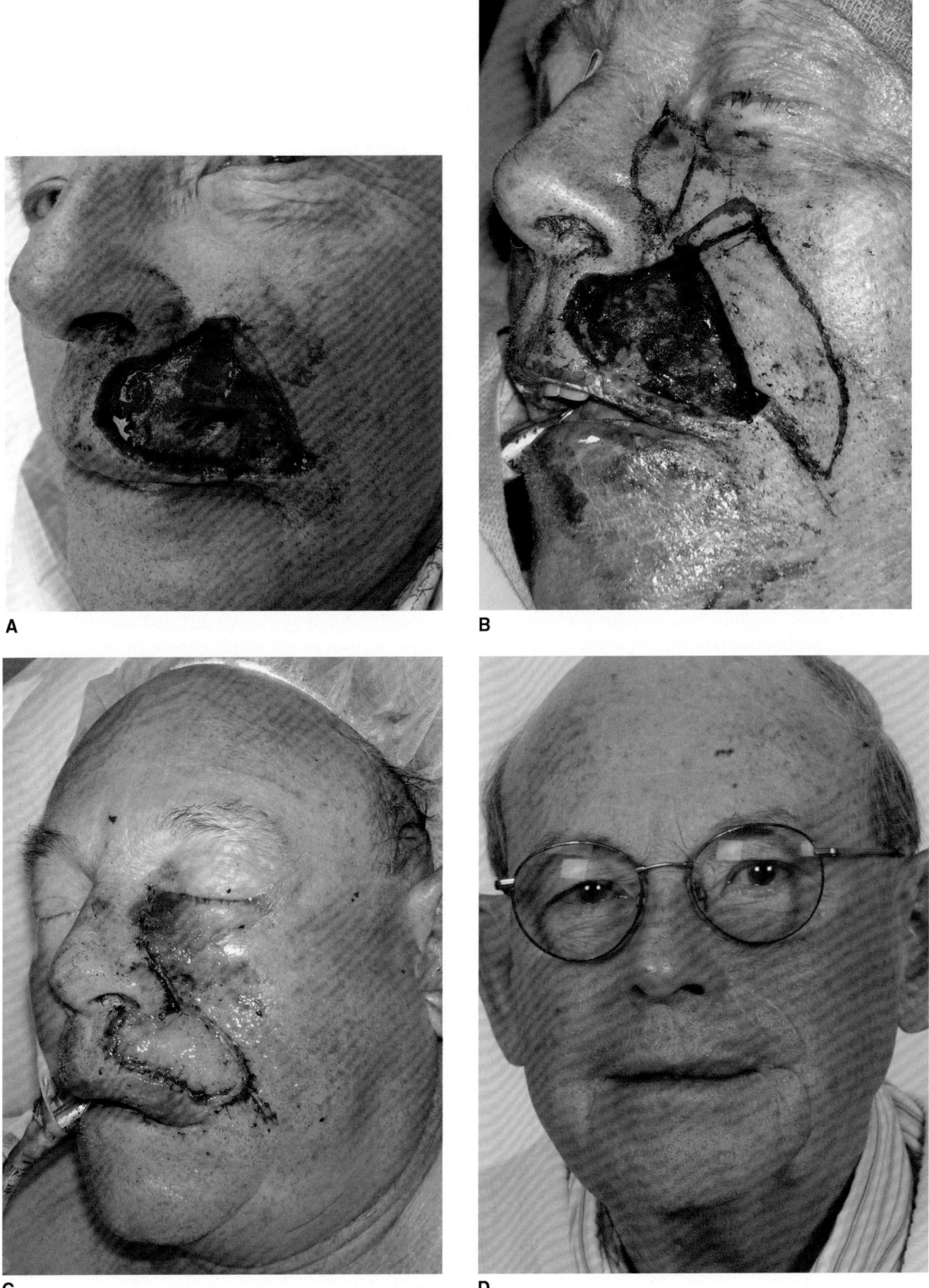

Figure 116.3 A: Large upper lip and cheek defect after Mohs resection of basal cell carcinoma. **B:** Design of V to Y island flap from nasolabial fold and cheek advancement. **C:** Appearance following flap inset. **D:** Result at 1 year following nasolabial fold revision.

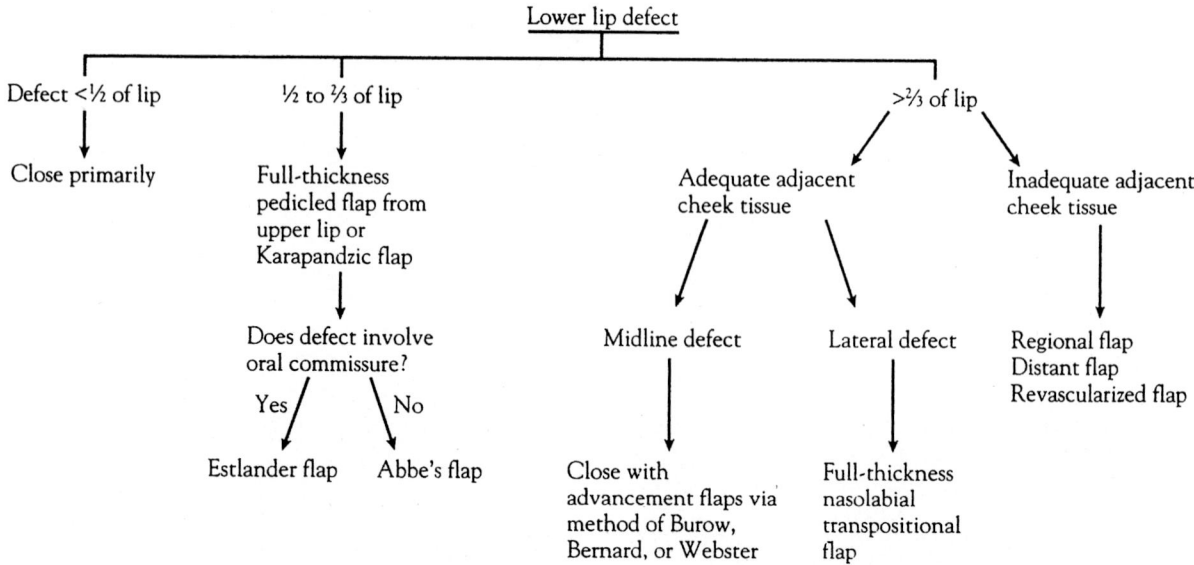

Figure 116.4 Lower lip reconstruction. From Baker SR, Krause CJ. Pedicled flaps in reconstruction of the lip. *Facial Plast Surg* 1983;1:68–69, with permission.

edge of the flap attached to the mucocutaneous border. Two to three weeks later, the pedicle is transected at the junction of the lateral and ventral tongue, retaining muscle for bulk and mucosa for vermilion reconstruction. This technique does not limit tongue mobility; however, the newly created vermillion has a pebbled surface (51). A better alternative for more extensive defects may be the facial artery musculomucosal (FAMM) flap (52). This axial flap containing buccal mucosa, submucosa, and a small amount of buccinator muscle is based on the facial artery as it courses through the cheek lateral to the buccinator muscle and medial to other muscles of facial expression. Inferiorly based FAMM flaps incorporate the facial artery as it enters the face at

the anterior edge of the masseter muscle, whereas superiorly based FAMM flaps are perfused retrograde through the angular artery. Both designs allow for a long thin flap to be harvested without compromise of viability—this both minimizes donor site morbidity and enables single-stage reconstructions of the entire vermillion. Bilateral and unilateral FAMM flaps have been used with particular success as adjuncts in total lip reconstruction for color and contour-appropriate replacement of vermilion deficiencies.

The algorithms in Figures 116.4 and 116.5 outline an excellent general approach to upper and lower lip reconstruction (51). The relative proportion of total lip length that can be excised and closed directly without distortion

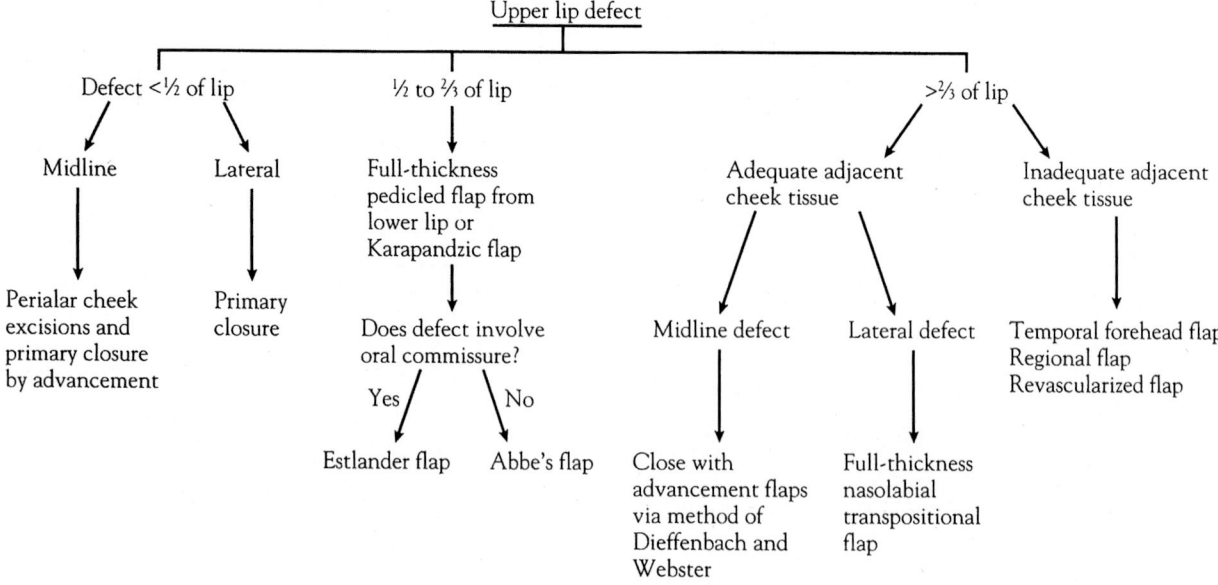

Figure 116.5 Upper lip reconstruction. From Baker SR, Krause CJ. Pedicled flaps in reconstruction of the lip. *Facial Plast Surg* 1983;1:68–69, with permission.

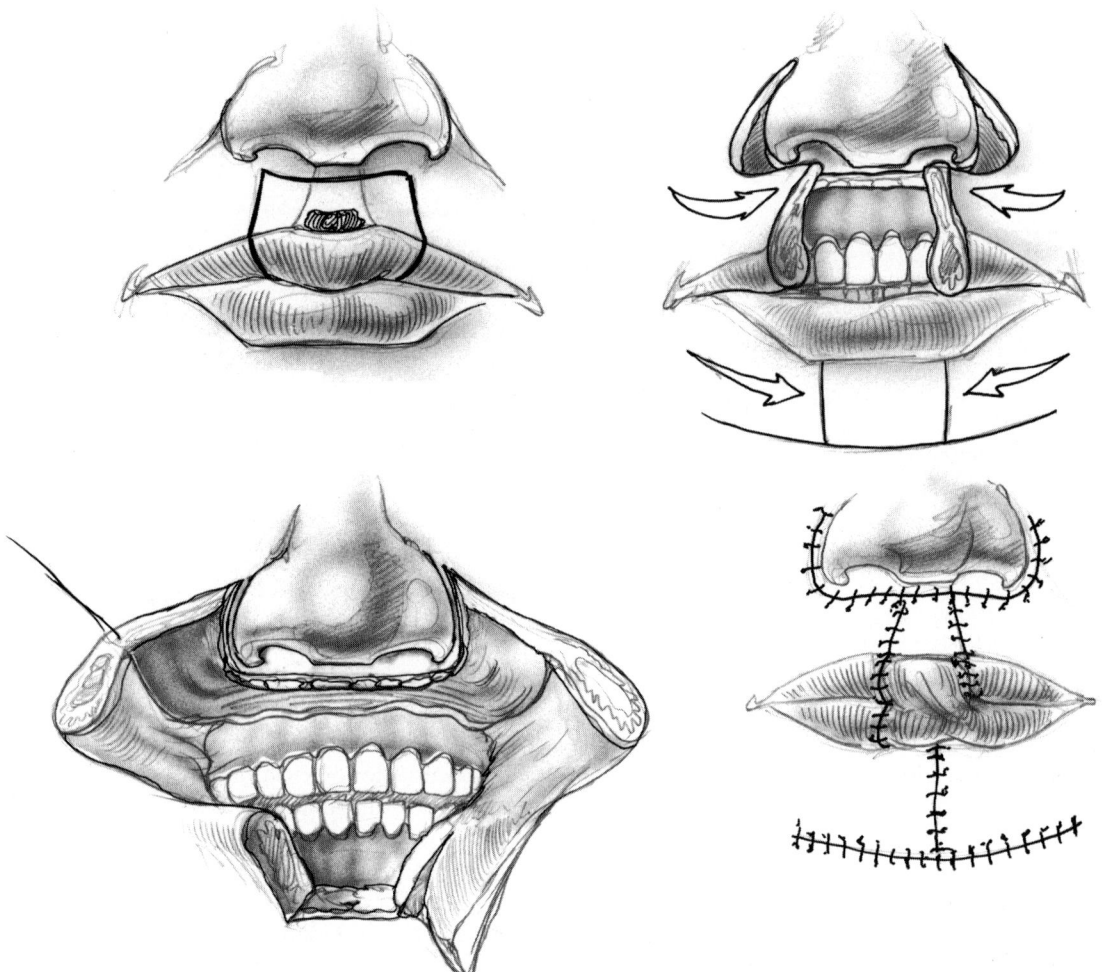

Figure 116.6 Primary closure of defects in the midline of the upper lip can be facilitated by excising crescents of cheek skin in the perialar regions. An Abbe flap can be added in the midline if the wound closure is under excessive tension.

varies between individuals and depends on overall lip length and tissue laxity. In general, one-fourth to one-third of the upper lip may be closed directly with larger lateral resections sometimes amenable to direct closure. Lower lip defects of one-third to one-half lip length may be closed primarily. Shield or V excision is usually adequate with closure in three layers (mucosa, muscle, skin) and meticulous reapproximation of the orbicularis and white scroll at the vermilion border on either side of the defect.

In the lower lips, lateral advancement with incisions placed in the mental crease may be required when the defect base is broad. Every attempt should be made not to extend incisions beyond the mental crease to avoid a pointed chin deformity. Just as in partial-thickness defects, full-thickness advancement in the mesial upper lip is facilitated by excising a crescent of cheek skin in the perialar region and anchoring the lateral flap to periosteum (53) (Fig. 116.6). This method is similar to that described by Diffenbach and Webster and lessens tension on remaining lip segments after primary closure (48). An Abbe flap may

be used in the midline to replace the central subunit and prevent excessive tension on the wound closure.

Defects of One-Third to Two-Thirds of the Lip

The majority of these defects are amenable to closure using rotated or pedicled tissue from the opposing lip. Three procedures constitute the majority of reconstructions in this group: the Karapandzic labioplasty, the Abbe cross-lip flap, and the Estlander cross-lip flap. Each method has advantages and disadvantages and individual surgeons favor different techniques (48,54).

The Karapandzic labioplasty, described in 1974, modified older circumoral advancement techniques to preserve vascularity, sensation, and motor innervation to the lips. This single-stage reconstructive procedure has gained popularity to become the favored reconstructive method of many surgeons for moderate-sized defects (48). This technique (Fig. 116.7) is more commonly used for lower lip defects but can be applied to upper defects as well. Circumoral

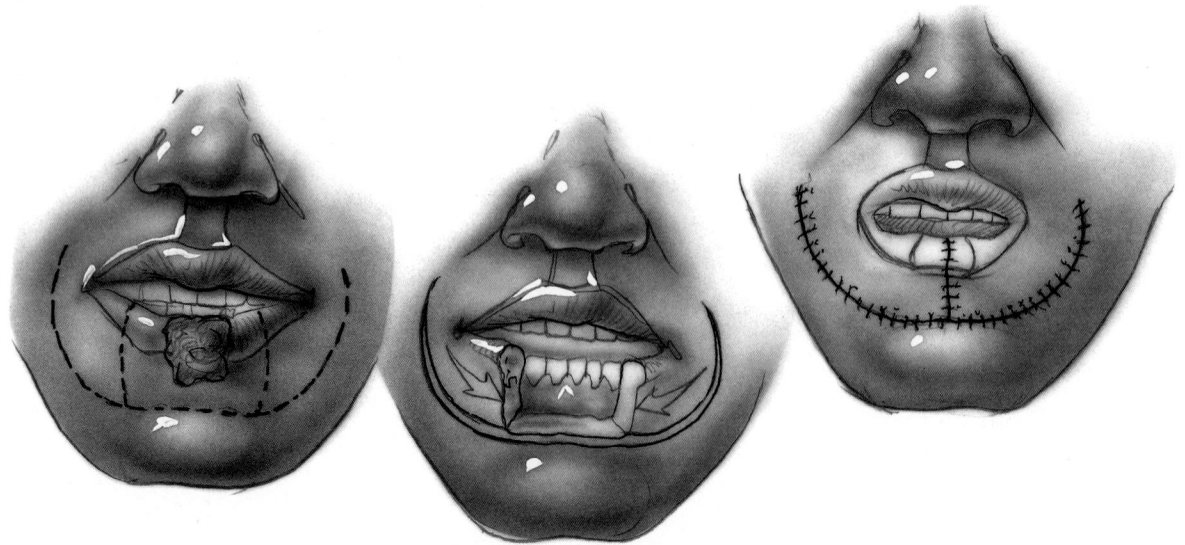

Figure 116.7 The Karapandzic labioplasty. Circumoral skin incisions are made within the naso-labial and mental creases. The orbicularis oris muscle is bluntly dissected from supporting perioral muscles, taking care to preserve the neuromuscular pedicles, which enter from the periphery. The oral mucosa usually does not require transection.

incisions are begun in the mental crease and carried around the oral commissures into the melolabial sulci. An important technical point is to maintain appropriate flap width in the area of the oral commissure. Flap width in this area must approximate the height of the lip portion, which it will replace after rotation. Incisions, therefore, cannot remain within the melolabial sulcus where it runs very close to the commissures. After incisions are carried through skin and subcutaneous tissue, the lateral border of the orbicularis oris muscle is mobilized from the other supporting perioral muscles to allow rotation of segments and tension-free closure. Blunt dissection of the muscle allows identification and preservation of the superior and inferior labial arteries and the neurovascular pedicles that enter the orbicularis muscle from its periphery. The underlying oral mucosa usually does not require transection for mobilization. Flaps are rotated and advanced into their new positions and divided perioral muscles and reattached at appropriate positions along the repositioned lip.

The advantages of the Karapandzic flap are its ease of design and the preservation of oral competence. Disadvantages include blunting of the commissures; circumoral scars, which can be unsightly; and the potential for microstomia, which may preclude the use of dentures. One potential solution to microstomia is to initially reconstruct with this technique, accept temporary microstomia, and allow tissues to stretch with time and use, then perform a cross-lip procedure to improve oral opening (54,55).

Abbe and Estlander flaps transfer full-thickness tissue between opposing lips pedicled on the labial artery. These techniques allow precise flap design, typically result in less microstomia than rotation flap reconstruction, and avoid circumoral incisions (54). Abbe flaps preserve the aesthetically important oral commissure but require a second stage for flap division. Additional disadvantages include denervation of tissue with variable reinnervation over time and the potential for pincushioning or trapdoor deformity in a lip segment surrounded by scars on three sides (56). The Abbe flap was originally designed to close medial defects, and it can be based either medially or laterally, depending on the location of the defect and blood supply. There are several important points for consideration in Abbe flap design (Fig. 116.8). Flap height should equal the height of the defect. Flap width is classically designed to be one-half the width of the defect, but more modern approaches advocate reconstruction of upper lip subunit defects with like-size flaps from the lower lip when possible (50,56). Creation of the flap involves full-thickness incisions through all portions except the region of the pedicle, which consistently is found at the level of the vermilion border on the posterior surface of the orbicularis muscle just deep to the labial submucosa (57). The pedicle should be narrow to facilitate rotation, and extension of anterior incisions into the vermilion allows for more accurate alignment of vermilion borders. Because the pedicle does not contain an associated major venous structure, it is important to leave a fairly wide mucosal bridge posteriorly to allow venous return. The donor site defect and flap reconstruction should be closed in three layers, with careful alignment of both orbicularis muscle and vermilion. When an Abbe flap is designed from the upper lip, lateral lip tissue should be used with medial incisions placed on the philtral ridges to camouflage donor site closure (54). This closure is facilitated by advancement of the lateral upper lip segment and excision of perialar crescents as described earlier. In general, cross-lip pedicles may be divided in 3 weeks.

The Estlander flap uses the same techniques as the Abbe flap to create a flap based a narrow labial artery pedicle

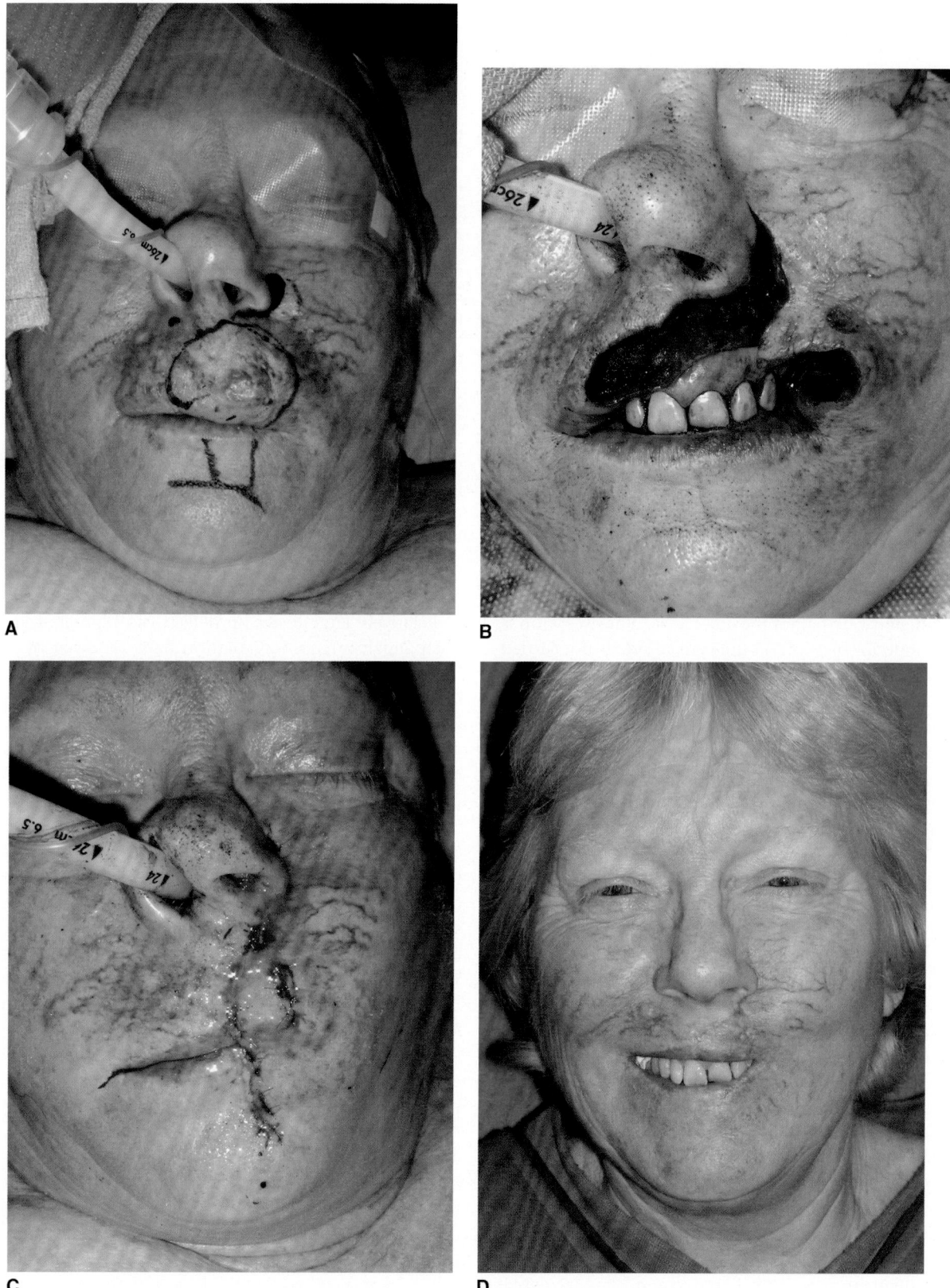

Figure 116.8 A: Large recurrent upper lip arteriovenous malformation following previous lip wedge resections. Anticipated resection with planned Abbe flap design. **B:** Defect involving two-third of upper lip following lesion removal. **C:** Closure with Abbe flap and cheek advancement with peri-alar crescent removal. **D:** Appearance following Abbe flap division.

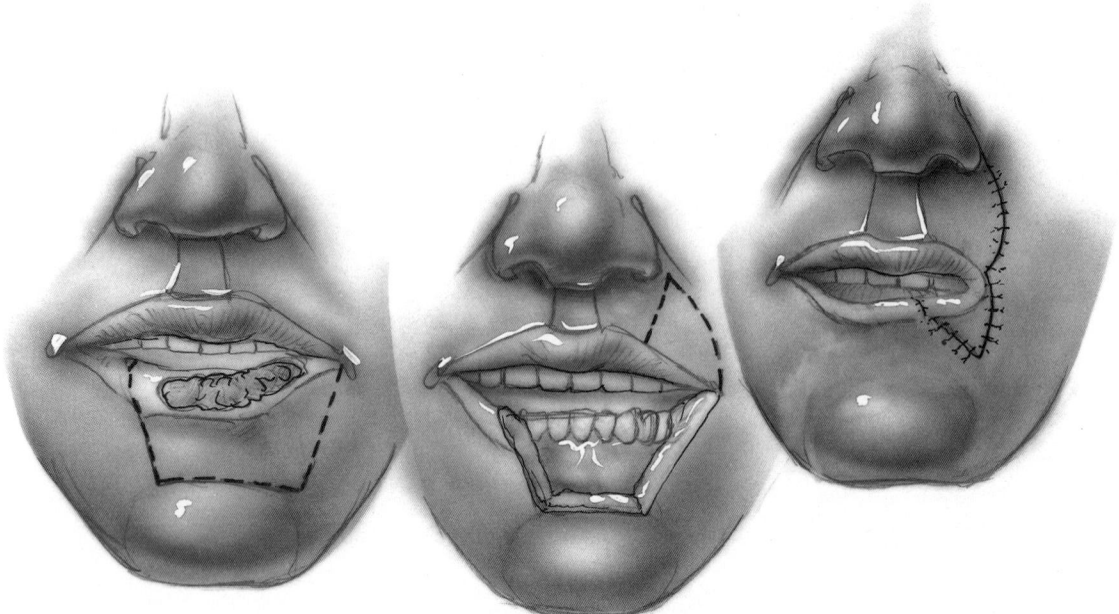

Figure 116.9 The superiorly based Estlander flap may be modified from its original description by designing the flap so that it lies within the nasolabial fold.

approximately one-half of the defect size. One exception is that the anterior incision on the pedicle side is not carried into the vermilion. Superiorly based Estlander flaps should be modified to incorporate scars within the nasolabial fold (Fig. 116.9). Donor tissue is rotated around the oral commissure to the opposing lip, and therefore, this single-stage procedure is only applied to defects involving the commissure. This technique results in blunting of the oral commissure that, unlike the symmetric blunting of circum-oral advancement, is starkly contrasted by the unviolated opposing commissure. As a result, secondary commissuro-plasty is often performed to minimize this disparity.

Defects Greater Than Two-Thirds of the Lip

Lip reconstruction with locoregional tissue is favored if possible, particularly techniques that allow for salvage of dynamic muscle function and color-matched skin. Cross-lip flaps may be combined with lateral advancement flaps for larger central upper lip defects (Fig. 116.6), but this technique is not sufficient for total upper lip reconstruction. Modified cheek flaps that preserve neurovascular structures and the original position of the oral commis-sures have been used with success in reconstruction of near total and total upper lip defects (58). The main disadvantage of this technique is large transverse scars that cross the cheeks. Bilateral superiorly based composite nasolabial flaps have also provided reasonable aesthetic and functional results (59). Free temporal scalp flaps based on the superficial temporal vessels have been used with some success to import hair-bearing tissue to restore male beard patterns and provide camouflage (60). A major disadvantage of this technique is the lack of innervated tissue.

Relatively large lower lip defects can be managed with Karapandzic circumoral rotation flaps followed by cross-lip flaps as previously described. Extended Karapandzic flaps and bilateral Karapandzic flaps have also been used with success for total and subtotal lower lip defects, provided tissue inferior and lateral to the oral commissures has been spared (61). Buccal advancement flaps allow for mucosal restoration.

Midline lower lip defects may be corrected by using any of several modifications of the Bernard repair, which essentially uses full-thickness advancement flaps of adjacent cheek tissue. These techniques have the advantage of single-stage reconstruction with innervated flaps but frequently result in a tight lower lip with poor function (48,54,62). The Webster modification of the Bernard cheiloplasty employs Burow triangles whose medial vertical limbs lie within the melolabial fold (Fig. 116.10). The width of the base of the triangles is calculated so that the distance from the oral commissure to the lateral portion of the base equals one-half the width of lip tissue excised. Skin and subcutaneous tissue only are excised from the triangles, and incisions are deepened along its base, identifying and preserving the neurovascular supply to the orbicularis oris and buccina-tor muscles. A mucosal flap based on the superior margin of the cheek flap is elevated to create a new vermilion or a tongue flap may be employed. Usually, incisions through skin and muscle are required around the mental crease, with Burow triangles strategically placed in the submental area to allow sufficient advancement of the cheek flaps.

Full-thickness inferiorly based nasolabial flaps have been used to reconstruct subtotal lower lip defects (54). The disadvantage of this technique is that the flaps are not innervated, and in raising the flaps, the upper lip is

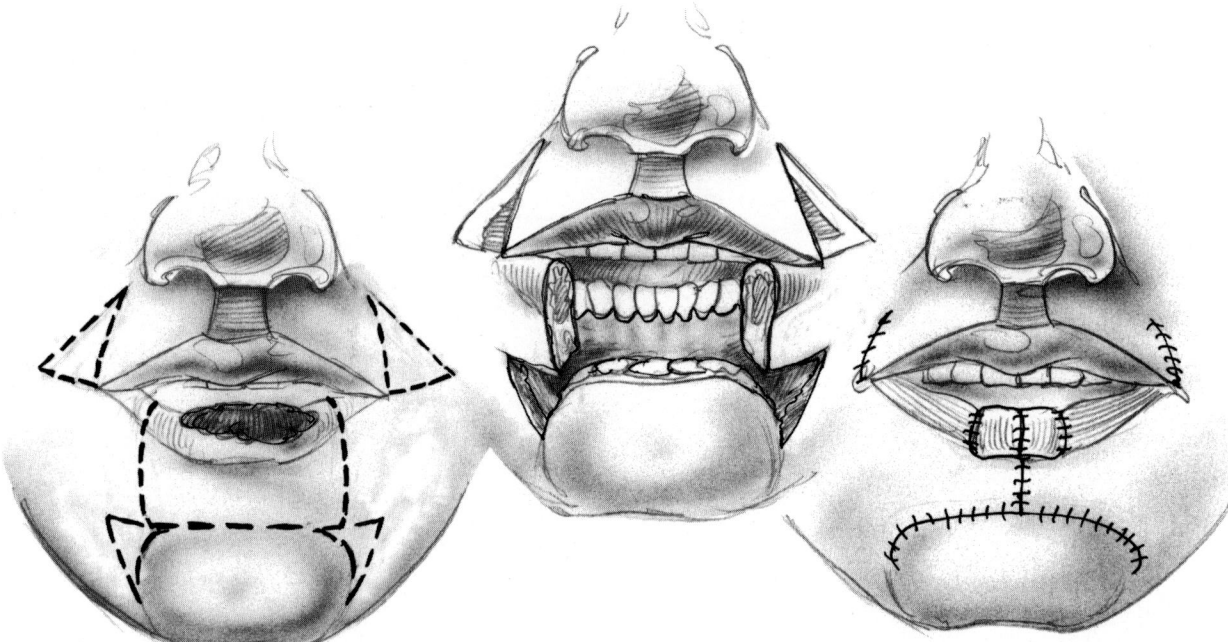

Figure 116.10 Webster modification of Bernard cheiloplasty. *Cross-hatched area* denotes mucosal flap used to create new vermilion (see text).

usually denervated. To avoid this complication, total lower lip reconstruction with skin only nasolabial flaps has been described with good aesthetic results and preservation of oral competence (63). Consistent functional reconstruction of total and subtotal defects has also been described using musculocutaneous island flaps based on the facial artery and innervated depressor anguli oris (DAO) muscle (62). Similarly, an unequal double Z-plasty transferring the DAO and platysma has been utilized with success, achieving sensation, sphincter function, and acceptable cosmesis (64).

Defects involving the entire lower lip and adjacent soft tissue of the cheek or chin require reconstruction with distant flaps. A variety of axial or myocutaneous flaps, particularly the pectoralis myocutaneous flap, have been utilized for extensive reconstructions, but variable flap bulk, inferior tension, and the lack of sensory reinnervation resulted in less consistent outcomes than those provided by free tissue transfer.

The composite radial forearm free flap with palmaris longus tendon has yielded reliable reconstructive results and remains the most commonly employed method (65–67). The skin paddle is folded over the palmaris longus tendon (or harvested fascia lata when palmaris is absent) to provide internal and external lip lining. The tendon ends are suspended superiorly to attain lip support and function. Various tendon inset methods described include fixation to orbicularis muscle at the modiolus, circumferential tunneling within the remaining lip, and attachment into medial upper lip orbicularis or tendon suspension to zygomatic arch periosteum (68). Although all described methods reportedly yield competence, long-term dynamic function is

difficult to achieve and often elusive in the face of postoperative radiation (which is often required) (67). One promising alternative is to attach palmaris longus or fascia lata suspensions to bilateral orthodromic temporalis tendon transfers (TTTs), providing long-term support and dynamic voluntary closure. Experience using TTT in facial reanimation including bilateral facial paralysis has demonstrated long-term support and dynamic control of the lower lip (Fig. 116.11).

To facilitate sensory recovery, the lateral antebrachial cutaneous nerve can be neurotized to the stump of the mental or inferior alveolar nerve (69). The vermilion can be established on a deepithelialized segment of the forearm flap using a facial artery myomucosal flap as described earlier or with mucosal flaps from the tongue, upper lip, or cheek (52,65,66). Medical tattooing has also been used with acceptable results.

Anterolateral thigh flaps and free innervated gracilis flaps have also been utilized with success in lower lip reconstruction. While the former has become a dominant reconstructive flap at many centers due to its minimal harvest site morbidity and abundant available tissue, variable thickness, less favorable color match, and perforators less tolerant of aggressive suspension have maintained radial forearm dominance in this subsite. Innervated gracilis flaps have shown significant promise with advantages of true dynamic function mediated by facial nerve branches and better color match when external full-thickness skin grafts are employed (70,71). Despite reported successes, experience with this technique has been limited, and performance in the face of extensive mucosal defects and postoperative radiation has not been established.

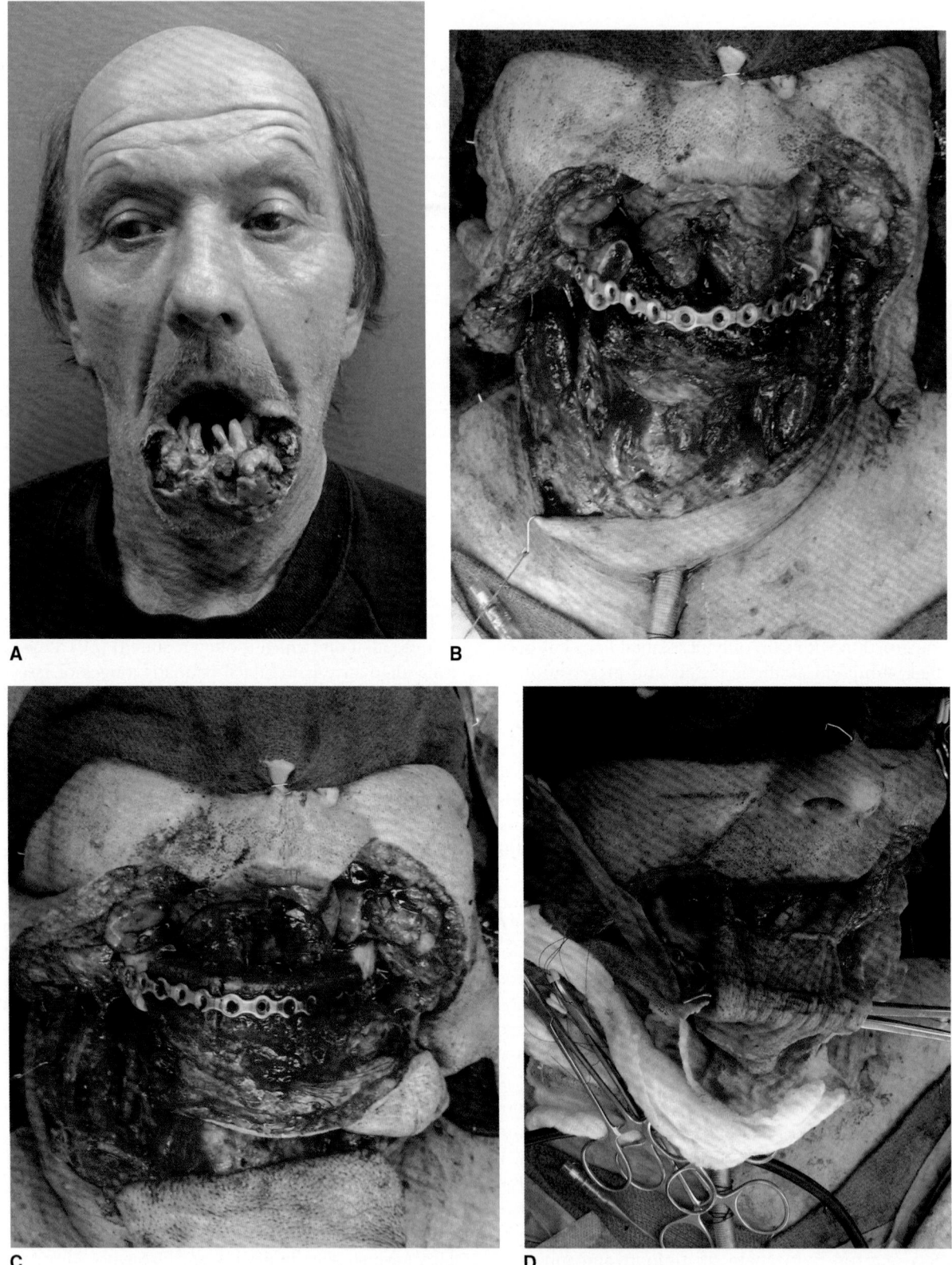

Figure 116.11 A: Advanced lower lip squamous cell carcinoma with mandibular invasion. **B:** Composite defect following resection and margin clearance involving total lower lip and one-third upper lip, commissures and medial cheek, anterior mandible, floor of mouth chin, and central neck. **C:** Mandibular reconstruction with fibula segments. **D:** Radial forearm free flap secured to intraoral fibula paddle and suspended with tunnelled fascia lata graft secured to bilteral orthodromic temporalis tendon transfers (prolene sutures).

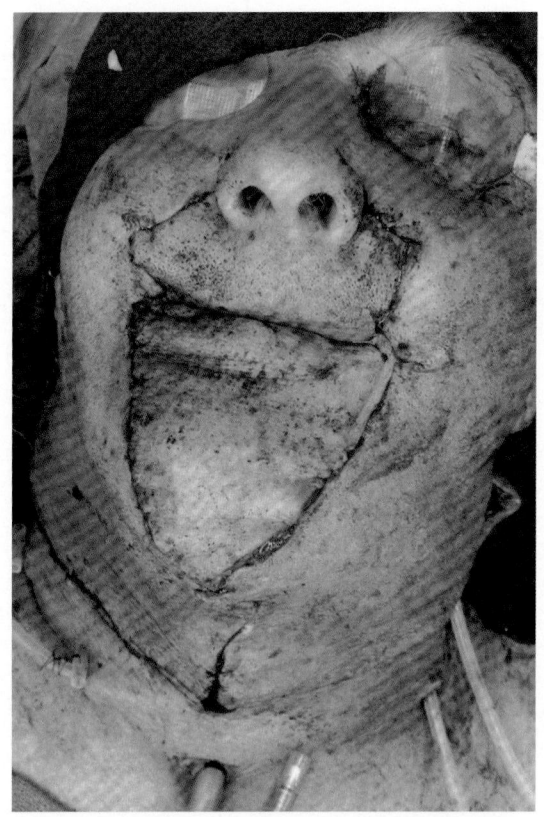

E

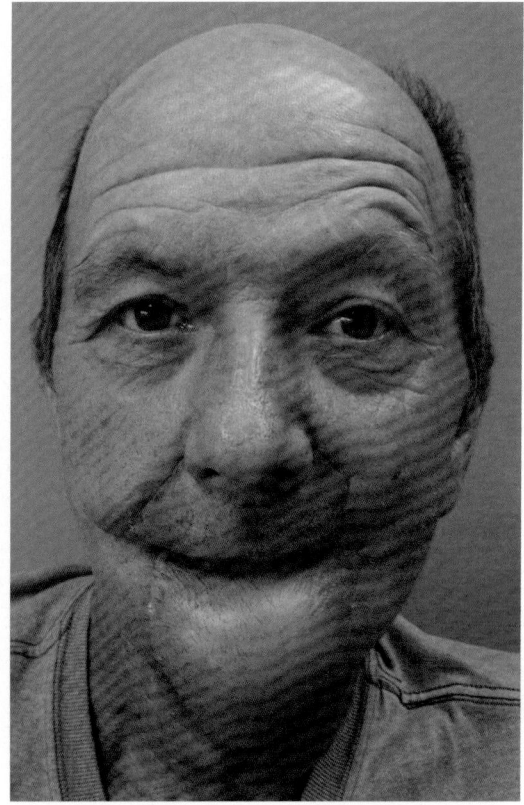

F

G

Figure 116.11 *(Continued)* **E:** Defect closed after cheek and neck advancement, fibula and radial forearm free flaps. **F,G:** Oral competence and dynamic closure 9 months after completion of postoperative radiation therapy.

When the anterior mandibular arch has been resected along with the lower lip, vascularized osteomyocutaneous flaps allow for immediate single-stage reconstruction with cosmetically and functionally acceptable results. The flap selected is dependent on bone and soft tissue requirements. For anterior mandible and lip alone, an osteocutaneous radial forearm or fibular flap is an option, whereas larger defects may require use of scapular flap or more commonly two separate free flaps (e.g., fibula and radial forearm). In the latter case, the fibula flap provides internal lining (e.g., buccal, floor of mouth, tongue), while the forearm is utilized for lip and additional external coverage (Fig. 116.11). Anterolateral thigh flaps have the advantage of providing greater coverage and may be superior for massive external defects.

COMPLICATIONS

Complications of radiation therapy, as discussed previously, include a prolonged treatment time, with delayed rehabilitation; a whistle deformity from tissue loss and scar contracture with large tumors, which may require secondary reconstruction; osteoradionecrosis of the mandible; and limitation of future reconstructive options. Surgical complications include those associated with general anesthesia, neck dissection, and wound infection and dehiscence. In regard to lip reconstruction, complications include fistula, an incompetent oral sphincter, microstomia, or poor cosmetic result. To avoid these complications, the surgeon must thoroughly understand the biologic behavior of lip carcinoma and its management principles and must carefully plan and meticulously execute the reconstructive option chosen.

EMERGENCIES

There are very few situations in which patients with lip carcinoma require emergent intervention (Table 116.4). As previously mentioned, lip carcinoma is usually a slow-growing lesion and is usually diagnosed relatively early. Large tumors involving the tongue and the floor of the mouth may cause airway problems when general anesthesia is required; this is readily managed by initial tracheotomy under local anesthesia. Patients with large tumors may be malnourished, in part due to oral incompetence; adequate preoperative nutritional assessment is important when major resection and reconstructive procedures are contemplated.

TABLE 116.4	⚕ EMERGENCIES LIP CANCER

Airway compromise with large tumors

HIGHLIGHTS

- The lips are important functionally in maintaining oral competence and aesthetically by contributing to appearance and facial expression. The lips are characterized by the vermilion, or that lip mucosa that contacts the opposite lip mucosa.
- The orbicularis oris muscle serves as the oral sphincter and is innervated by branches of the facial nerve. The blood supply is from the labial branches of the facial artery. Sensation is provided by the paired mental nerves.
- Lymphatic drainage from the lower lip is to the submental and submandibular nodes bilaterally; the upper lip drains to the ipsilateral parotid and submandibular nodes.
- Lip carcinoma is the most common malignancy of the oral cavity. As a rule of thumb, 90% are SCCA, 90% occur on the lower lip, and the overall 5-year determinate survival rate is 90%. Sunlight is thought to be the principal etiologic factor in its development.
- The diagnosis is established by biopsy but is suggested by a history of recurrent crusting or a nonhealing area of lip induration noted over several months. With a high index of suspicion, lip carcinoma is easily diagnosed and successfully managed if treated in its early stages.
- Surgery and radiation therapy are equally efficacious for lesions less than 3 cm. Surgery is preferred, because it offers the advantages of tumor margin assessment, rapid rehabilitation through immediate reconstruction, and avoidance of radiation complications. For advanced lesions, surgery combined with postoperative radiation therapy is indicated.
- Indicators predictive of poor outcome are large primary tumors, mandibular involvement, mental nerve involvement, cervical node metastases, recurrent disease, and undifferentiated histology.
- The goal of lip reconstruction is to provide the patient with a sensate innervated lip that functions as a competent oral sphincter of adequate size while remaining aesthetically acceptable. Successful reconstruction requires careful preoperative planning and meticulous execution of the appropriate technique.
- Defects of less than one-third of the upper lip and one-half of the lower lip can be closed primarily. Defects of one-third to two-thirds of the lip can be closed with an Abbe-Estlander flap or Karapandzic labioplasty. Both techniques require an intact labial artery.
- When the entire lip or surrounding soft tissue or mandibular bone is resected, reconstruction requires a distant flap. The ideal technique uses revascularized fasciocutaneous or osteomyocutaneous composite flaps, which can be done in a single stage for immediate reconstruction.

REFERENCES

1. Yako-Suketomo H, Marugame T. Comparison of time trends in lip cancer incidence (1973–1997) in East Asia, Europe and USA, from Cancer Incidence in Five Continents, Vols IV-VIII. *Jpn J Clin Oncol* 2008;38(6):456–457.

2. Canto MT, Devesa SS. Oral cavity and pharynx cancer incidence rates in the United States, 1975–1998. *Oral Oncol* 2002;38(6):610–617.

3. Moore SR, Allister J, Roder D, et al. Lip cancer in South Australia, 1977–1996. *Pathology* 2001;33(2):167–171.

4. Chidzonga MM, Mahomva L. SCCA of the oral cavity, maxillary antrum and lip in a Zimbabwean population: a descriptive epidemiological study. *Oral Oncol* 2006;42(2):184–189.

5. Effiom OA, Adeyemo WL, Omitola OG, et al. Oral squamous cell carcinoma: a clinicopathologic review of 233 cases in Lagos, Nigeria. *J Oral Maxillofac Surg* 2008;66:1595–1599.

6. Czerninski R, Zini A, Sgan-Cohen HD. Lip cancer: incidence, trends, histology and survival: 1970-2006. *Br J Dermatol* 2010;162:1103–1109.

7. Abreu L, Kruger E, Tennant M. Lip cancer in Western Australia, 1982–2006: a 25-year retrospective epidemiological study. *Aus Dent J* 2009;54:130–135.

8. Perea-Milla Lopez E, Minarro-del Moral RM, Martinez-Garcia C, et al. Lifestyles, environmental and phenotypic factors associated with lip cancer: a case-control study in southern Spain. *Br J Cancer* 2003;88:1702–1707.

9. Pukkala E, Martinsen JI, Lynge E, et al. Occupation and cancer—follow up of 15 million people in five Nordic countries. *Acta Oncol* 2009;48(5):646–790.

10. Shah AY, Doherty SD, Rosen T. Actinic cheilitis: a treatment review. *Int J Dermatol* 2010;49:1225–1234.

11. Cavalcante ASR, Anbinder AL, Carvalho YR. Actinic cheilitis: clinical and histologic features. *J Oral Maxillofacial Surg* 2008;66:498–503.

12. van Leeuwen MT, Grulich AE, McDonald SP, et al. Immunosuppression and other risk factors for lip cancer after kidney transplantation. *Cancer Epidemiol Biomarkers Prev* 2009;18(2):561–569.

13. McCombe D, MacGill K, Ainslie J, et al. Squamous cell carcinoma of the lip: a retrospective review of the Peter MacCallum Cancer Institute experience 1979–88. *Aust N Z J Surg* 2000;70:358–361.

14. Zitsch RP, Park CW, Renner GJ, Rea JL. Outcome analysis for lip carcinoma. *Otolaryngol Head Neck Surg* 1995;113:589–596.

15. Gooris PJJ, Vermey A, de Visscher JGAM, et al. Supraomohyoid neck dissection in the management of cervical lymph node metastases of squamous cell carcinoma of the lower lip. *Head Neck* 2002;24:679–683.

16. Onerci M, Yilmaz T, Gedikoglu G. Tumor thickness as a predictor of cervical lymph node metastasis in squamous cell carcinoma of the lower lip. *Otolaryngol Head Neck Surg* 2000;122:139–142.

17. Vartanian JG, Carvalho AL, Filho M, et al. Predictive factors and distribution of lymph node metastasis in lip cancer patients and their implications on the treatment of the neck. *Oral Oncol* 2004;40:223–227.

18. Fernandez-Angel I, Rodriguez-Archilla A, Aneiros Cachaza J, et al. Markers of metastasis in lip cancer. *Eur J Dermatol* 2003;13:276–279.

19. Dixon AJ, Dixon MP, Askew DA, Wilkinson D. Prospective study of wound infections in dermatologic surgery in the absence of prophylactic antibiotics. *Dermatol Surg* 2006;32(6):819–826.

20. Matzko J, Becker DG, Phillips CD. Obliteration of fat planes by perineural spread of squamous cell carcinoma along the inferior alveolar nerve. *Am J Neuroradiol* 1994;15:1843–1845.

21. Betka J. Distant metastases from lip and oral cavity cancer. *J Otorhinolaryngol Relat Spec* 2001;63(4):217–221.

22. Casal D, Carmo L, Melancia T, et al. Lip cancer: a 5-year review in a tertiary referral centre. *J Plast Recon Aesthetic Surg* 2010;63: 2040–2045.

23. Wang D, Li Y, He H, et al. Intraoral minor salivary gland tumors in a Chinese population: a retrospective study on 737 cases. *Oral Surg Oral Med Oral Pathol Oral Radio Endod* 2007;104:94–100.

24. Yih WY, Kratochvil FJ, Stewart JCB. Intraoral Minor Salivary Gland Neoplasms: review of 213 cases. *J Oral Maxillofacial Surg* 2005;63:805–810.

25. Ramos LMA, Cardoso SV, Loyola AM, et al. Keratoacanthoma of the inferior lip: review and report of case with spontaneous regression. *J Appl Oral Sci* 2009;17(3):262–265.

26. Gooris PJJ, Maat B, Vermey A, et al. Radiotherapy for cancer of the lip. *Oral Surg Oral Med Oral Pathol Oral Radiol Endod* 1998;86:325–330.

27. Casino AR, Toledano IP, Jorge JF, et al. Brachytherapy in lip cancer. *Med Oral Pathol Oral Cir Bucal* 2006;11:E223–E229.

28. Guinot JL, Arribas L, Chust ML, et al. Lip cancer treatment with high dose rate brachytherapy. *Radiother Oncol* 2003;69:113–115.

29. McCombe D, MacGill K, Ainslie J, et al. Squamous cell carcinoma of the lip: a retrospective review of the Peter MacCallum Cancer Institute experience 1979–88. *Aust N Z J Surg* 2000;70: 358–361.

30. Kornevs E, Skagers A, Tars J, et al. 5 year experience with lower lip cancer. *Stomatologija, Baltic Dent Maxillofacial J* 2005;7(3): 95–98.

31. de Visscher JGAM, Botke G, Schakenraad JACM, et al. A comparison of results after radiotherapy and surgery for stage 1 squamous cell carcinoma of the lower lip. *Head Neck* 1999;21:526–530.

32. Bilkay U, Kerem H, Ozek C, et al. Management of lower lip cancer: a retrospective analysis of 118 patients and review of the literature. *Ann Plast Surg* 2003;50:43–50.

33. de Visscher JG, Gooris PJ, Verney A, Roodenburg JL. Surgical margins for resection of squamous cell carcinoma of the lower lip. *Int J Oral Maxillofacial Surg* 2002;31:154–157.

34. Babington S, Veness MJ, Cakir B, et al. Squamous cell carcinoma of the lip: is there a role for adjuvant radiotherapy in improving local control following incomplete or inadequate excision? *ANZ J Surg* 2003;73:621–625.

35. Gooris PJJ, Vermey B, de Visscher JGAM, Roodenburg JLN. Frozen section examination of the margins for resection of squamous cell carcinoma of the lower lip. *J Oral Maxillofac Surg* 2003;61:890–894.

36. Kimyai-Asadi A, Alam M, Goldberg LH, et al. Efficacy of narrow-margin excision of well-demarcated primary facial basal cell carcinomas. *J Am Acad Dermatol* 2005;53:464–468.

37. Minton TJ. Contemporary Mohs surgery applications. *Curr Opin Otolaryngol Head Neck Surg* 2008;16:376–380.

38. Leibovitch I, Huilgol SC, Selva D, et al. Cutaneous lip tumors treated with Mohs micrographic surgery: clinical features and surgical outcome. *Br J Dermatol* 2005;153:1147–1152.

39. Holmkvist KA, Roenigk RK. Squamous cell carcinoma of the lip treated with Mohs micrographic surgery: outcome at 5 years. *J Am Acad Dermatol* 1998;38:960–966.

40. Rowe DE, Carroll RJ, Day CL. Prognostic factors for local recurrence, metastasis, and survival rates in squamous cell carcinoma of the skin, ear and lip. *J Am Acad Dermatol* 1992;26:976–990.

41. Mosterd K, Krekels GAM, Nieman FHM, et al. Surgical excision versus Mohs micrographic surgery for primary and recurrent basal cell carcinoma of the face: a prospective randomized controlled trial with 5 years' follow-up. *Lancet Oncol* 2008;9: 1149–1156.

42. Zitsch RP III, Lee BW, Smith RB. Cervical lymph node metastases and squamous cell carcinoma of the lip. *Head Neck* 1999;21: 447–453.

43. Chepeha D, Hoff P, Taylor R, et al. Selective neck dissection for the treatment of neck metastasis from squamous cell carcinoma of the head and neck. *Laryngoscope* 2002;112:434–438.

44. Anderson PE, Warren F, Spiro J, et al. Results of selective neck dissection in management of the node-positive neck. *Arch Otolaryngol Head Neck Surg* 2002;128:1180–1184.

45. Altinyollar H, Berberoglu U, Celen O. Lymphatic mapping and sentinel lymph node biopsy in squamous cell carcinoma of the lower lip. *Eur J Surg Oncol* 2002;28:72–74.

46. Khalil HH, Elaffandi AH Afifi A, et al. Sentinel lymph node biopsy (SLNB) in management of N0T1-T2 lip cancer as a "same day" procedure. *Oral Oncol* 2008;44(6):608–612.

47. Dupin C, Metzinger S, Rizzuto R. Lip reconstruction after ablation for skin malignancies. *Clin Plast Surg* 2004;31:69–85.

48. Renner GJ. Reconstruction of the lip. In: Baker SR, ed. *Local flaps in facial reconstruction.* St. Louis, MO: Mosby, 1995:345–396.
49. Godek CP, Weinzweig J, Bartlett SP. Lip reconstruction following Mohs' surgery, the role for composite resection and primary closure. *Plast Reconstr Surg* 2000;106:798–804.
50. Burget GC, Menick FJ. Aesthetic restoration of one-half of the upper lip. *Plast Reconstr Surg* 1986;78:583–593.
51. Baker SR, Krause CJ. Pedicled flaps in reconstruction of the lip. *Facial Plast Surg* 1983;1:68–69.
52. Pribaz JJ, Meara JG, Wright S, et al. Lip and vermillion reconstruction with the facial artery musculomucosal flap. *Plast Reconstr Surg* 2000;105:864–872.
53. Webster JP. Crescentic peri-alar cheek excision for upper lip flap advancement with a short history of upper lip repair. *Plast Reconstr Surg* 1955;16:434–464.
54. Luce EA. Reconstruction of the lower lip. *Clin Plastic Surg* 1995;22:109–120.
55. Kroll SS. Staged sequential flap reconstruction for large lower lip defects. *Plast Reconstr Surg* 1991;88:620–625.
56. Galyon SW, Frodel JL. Lip and perioral defects. *Otolaryngol Clin North Am* 2001;34:647–664.
57. Kroll SS. Lip reconstruction. In: Kroll SS, ed. *Reconstructive plastic surgery for cancer.* St. Louis, MO: Mosby, 1996:201–209.
58. Chowchuen B, Surakunprapha P. Modified bilateral neurovascular cheek flaps: a new technique for reconstruction of extensive upper lip defects. *Ann Plast Surg* 2001;47:64–69.
59. Sarifakioglu N, Aslan G, Terzloglu A, Ates L. New technique of one-stage reconstruction of a large full-thickness defect in the upper lip: bilateral reverse composite nasolabial flap. *Ann Plast Surg* 2002;49:207–210.
60. Chang KP, Lai CS, Tsai CC, et al. Total upper lip reconstruction with a free temporal scalp flap: long-term follow-up. *Head Neck* 2003;25:602–605.
61. Hanasono MM, Langstein HN. Extended Karapandzic flaps for near-total and total lower lip defects. *Plast Reconst Surg* 2011;127:1199–1205.
62. Yotsuyanagi T, Nihei Y, Yokoi K, Sawada Y. Functional reconstruction using a depressor anguli oris musculocutaneous flap for large lower lip defects, especially for elderly patients. *Plast Reconstr Surg* 1999;103:850–855.
63. Rudkin GH, Carlsen BT, Miller TA. Nasolabial flap reconstruction of large defects of the lower lip. *Plast Reconstr Surg* 2003;111: 810–817.
64. Mutaf M, Bulut O, Sunay M, Can A. Bilateral musculocutaneous unequal-Z procedure, a new technique for reconstruction of total lower-lip defects. *Ann Plast Surg* 2008;60:162–168.
65. Jeng SF, Kuo YR, Wei FC, et al. Total lower lip reconstruction with a composite radial forearm-palmaris longus tendon flap: a clinical series. *Plast Reconstr Surg* 2004;113:19–23.
66. Daya M, Nair V. Free radial forearm flap lip reconstruction, a clinical series and case reports of technical refinements. *Ann Plast Surg* 2009;62:361–367.
67. Wax MK, Kim J, Ducik Y. Update on major reconstruction of the head and neck. *Arch Facial Plast Surg* 2007;9:392–399.
68. Rudkin GH, Carlsen BT, Miller TA. Nasolabial flap reconstruction of large defects of the lower lip. *Plast Reconstr Surg* 2003;111: 810–817.
69. Serletti JM, Tavin ET, Moran SL, Coniglio JU. Total lower lip reconstruction with a sensate composite radial forearm-palmaris longus free flap and a tongue flap. *Plast Reconstr Surg* 1997;99:559–561.
70. Ninkovic M, Spanio di Spilimbergo S, Ninkovic M. Lower lip reconstruction: introduction of a new procedure using a functioning gracilis muscle free flap. *Plast Reconstr Surg* 2007;119:1472–1480.
71. Cordova A, D'Arpa S, Moschella F. Gracilis free muscle transfer for morpho-functional reconstruction of the lower lip. *Head Neck* 2008;30:684–689.

Neck Dissection

117

Jesus E. Medina   Nilesh R. Vasan

ANATOMY

Any student of neck dissection must understand the vascular supply of the skin of the neck and the anatomic characteristics and relationships of certain structures that are encountered within the course of performing a neck dissection.

Vascular Supply to the Skin of the Neck

To avoid complications such as wound breakdown, skin flap necrosis, and exposure of the carotid artery after neck dissection, the incisions must be placed correctly.

The skin of the anterior lateral aspect of the neck is supplied by descending branches of the facial, submental, and occipital arteries and by ascending branches of the transverse cervical and suprascapular artery (Fig. 117.1). These arterial branches anastomose, forming a superficial network of vessels that runs predominantly in a vertical direction. Although some or all the main arteries or their perforating branches may be ligated or divided during a neck dissection, the superficial, predominantly vertical, vascular plexus must remain intact to ensure adequate blood supply to the skin flaps. Thus, the incisions in the neck that are more likely to safeguard the blood supply to the skin flaps are the single transverse incision in the mid portion of the neck, the superiorly based apron-like incision from mastoid to mentum for combined neck dissection with intraoral procedures (Fig. 117.2A), and the apron-like incision used when a neck dissection is performed in conjunction with a laryngectomy (Fig. 117.2B).

The Y incision and the double-Y incision jeopardize the blood supply to the inferior and middle skin flaps, respectively, and suffer from placing a trifurcate incision over the carotid artery (Fig. 117.2C and D). The modification of the Schobinger incision creates a long anterior medial flap, the tip of which may necrose as a result of the limited ascending blood supply (Fig. 117.2E). The MacFee double transverse incision transects the ascending and descending blood supply to the central portion of the flap (Fig. 117.2F). This flap, however, usually fares well even in the previously irradiated patient.

Platysma Muscle

Located in the anterolateral aspect of the neck, the platysma is a wide, quadrangular, sheet-like muscle that extends obliquely from the upper chest to the lower face. This muscle, a remnant of the *panniculus carnosus*, is located immediately deep to the subcutaneous tissue and thus provides an easily identifiable plane to raise skin flaps during neck surgery. In most neck dissections, flaps are elevated by dissecting in a plane immediately deep to the platysma; however, when the extent of the disease is such that the platysma must be left attached to the specimen, flaps can be elevated easily in a plane immediately superficial to this muscle. The beginning head and neck surgeon must remember that, because of its oblique direction, the platysma does not cover an inferiorly based triangle in the anterior aspect of the neck and most of the posterolateral aspect of the neck. Here, flaps must be elevated in a subcutaneous plane created by the surgeon. While making the incisions for a neck dissection and elevating the skin flaps, it is helpful to remember that the posterior border of the platysma is either over or slightly anterior to the external jugular vein and the greater auricular nerve.

Marginal Mandibular Branch of the Facial Nerve

Identifying the marginal mandibular branch is essential to perform an adequate excision of the lymph nodes in the submandibular triangle. The practice of ligating the anterior facial vein low in the submandibular triangle and

1807

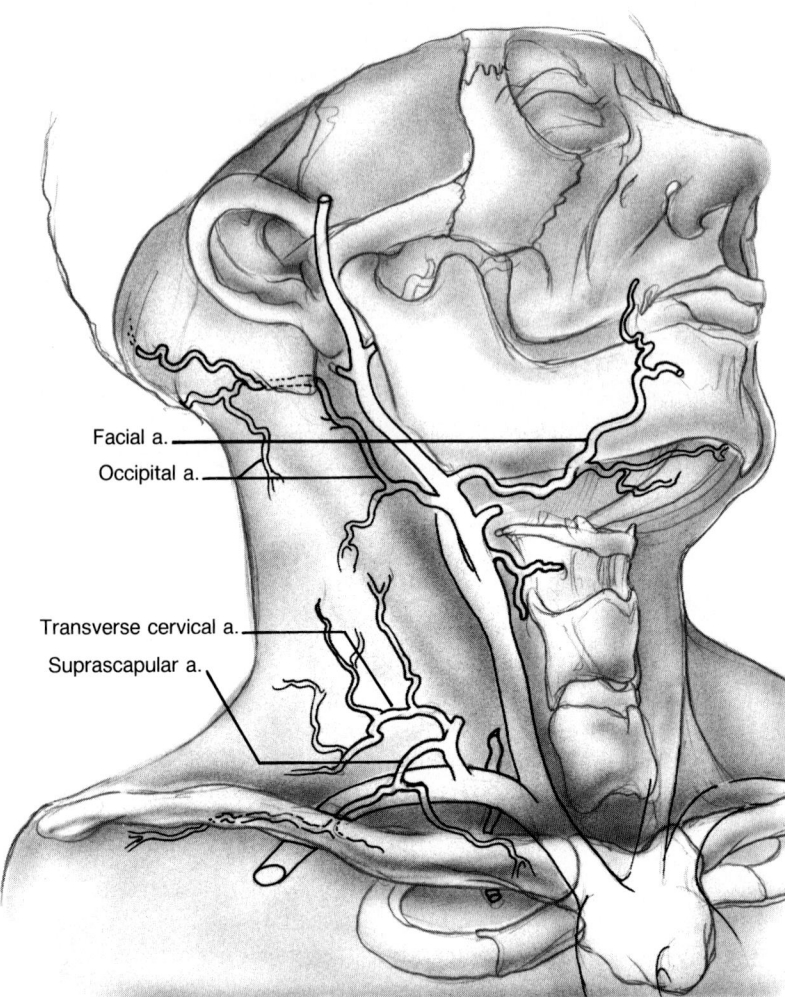

Facial a.

Occipital a.

Transverse cervical a.

Suprascapular a.

Figure 117.1 Vascular supply of the neck skin. (Adapted from Freelend AP, Rogers JH. The vascular supply of the cervical skin with reference to incision planning. *Laryngoscope* 1975;85:714, with permission.)

retracting it superiorly to "protect the marginal branch" can also result in elevation of the prevascular and retrovascular lymph nodes, thus precluding their appropriate removal. When indicated, it is preferable to identify the nerve and thoroughly remove these lymph nodes.

The nerve can be identified about 1 cm in front of and below the angle of the mandible by incising the superficial layer of the deep cervical fascia that envelops the submandibular gland, immediately above the gland, in a direction parallel to the direction of the nerve. The incised fascia then is gently pushed superiorly, exposing the nerve that lies deep to it but superficial to the adventitia of the anterior facial vein. The submandibular retrovascular lymph nodes are usually near the nerve and must be carefully dissected away from it. As this is done, the facial vessels are exposed and can be divided.

Spinal Accessory Nerve

Below the jugular foramen, the external branch of the spinal accessory nerve is located medial to the digastric and stylohyoid muscles and lateral or immediately posterior to

the internal jugular vein (IJV). Occasionally, the uppermost portion of the nerve is posteriomedial to the vein. From here, the nerve runs obliquely downward and backward to reach the medial surface of the sternocleidomastoid muscle (SCM) near the junction of its superior and middle thirds (two to three finger breadths below the tip of the mastoid). Although the nerve can continue its downward course entirely medial to the muscle (18%), more commonly, it traverses and appears in the posterior border of it (82%) (1). Here, the nerve is always located above the point where the greater auricular nerve turns around the posterior border of the SCM, also known as Erb point (2). The mean distance between Erb point and the spinal accessory nerve is 10.7 mm, SD ± 6.3. It then runs through the posterior triangle of the neck and crosses the anterior border of the trapezius muscle. The mean distance between this point and the clavicle is 51.3 mm, SD ± 17 (2). Two anatomic characteristics of this portion of the nerve are relevant to avoid injuring it in the course of a neck dissection. First, the spinal accessory nerve is located rather superficially as it courses through the middle and low posterior triangle of the neck, and it can be easily injured while elevating the

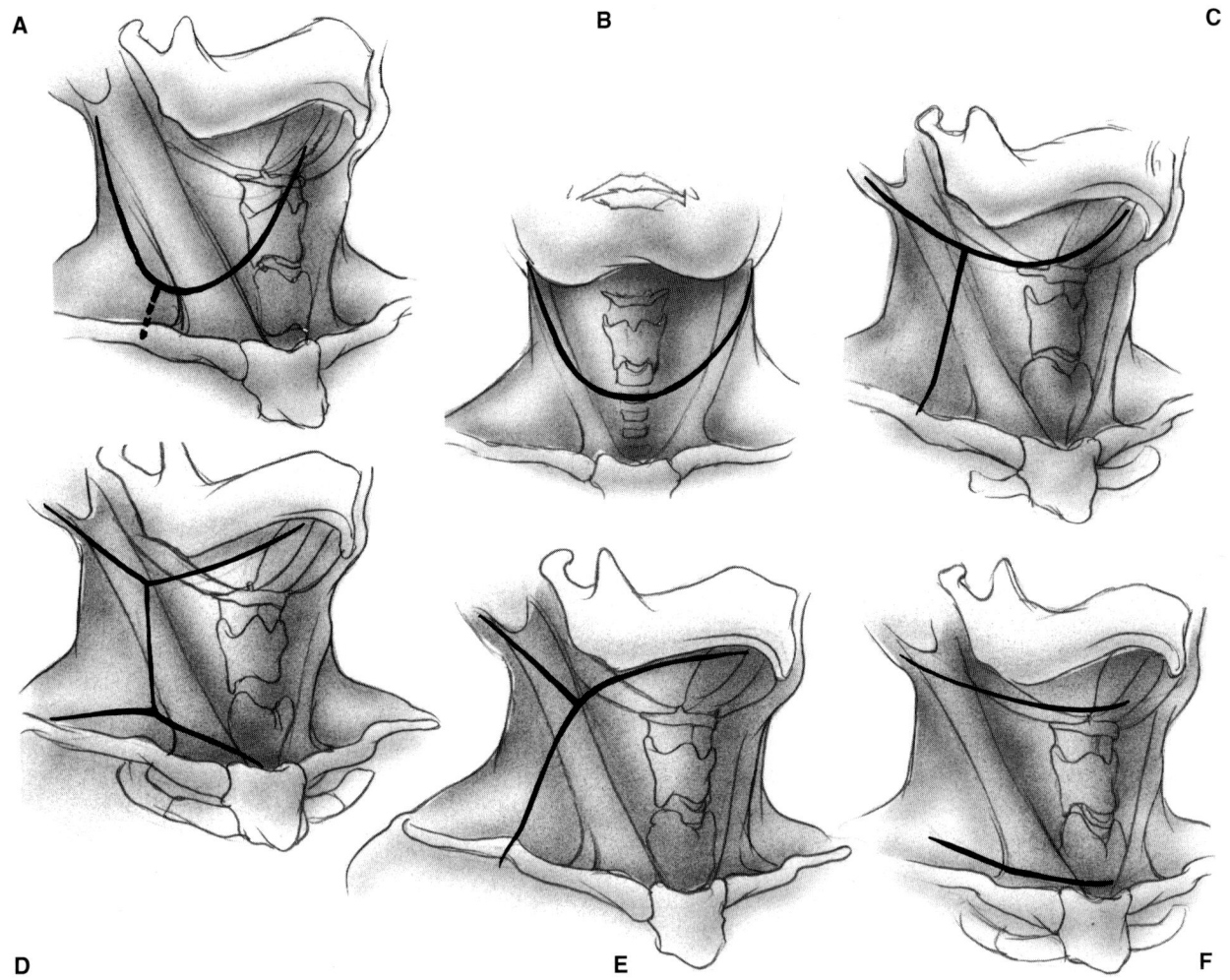

Figure 117.2 Neck dissection incisions. **A:** Latyschevsky and Freund. **B:** Freund. **C:** Crile. **D:** Martin. **E:** Babcock and Conley. **F:** MacFee.

posterior skin flaps. Second, the nerve does not enter the trapezius muscle at the anterior border of it but courses along the deep surface of the muscle in close relationship with the transverse cervical vessels. Therefore, isolating the nerve to the level of the anterior border of the trapezius does not ensure its preservation during surgical dissection below this point, particularly in a bloody operative field.

Nerve to the Levator Scapulae Muscle

The levator scapulae is a triangular muscle located deep in the lateral aspect of the neck, anterior and medial to the splenius capitis muscle. It extends from the transverse process of the atlas and the next three cervical vertebrae to the superior angle and the spine of the scapula. The action of levator scapulae is to raise the medial angle of the scapula and incline the neck to the corresponding side with rotation of the neck in the same direction. With the trapezius muscle, the levator scapulae makes a shrug possible.

The nerves to the levator scapulae, which vary in number from 1 to 3, branch off the fourth and fifth cervical nerves

and travel posteriorly and inferiorly. They cross the anterior border of the levator scapulae and remain on the surface of the muscle for a short distance. The nerves to levator scapulae are under the fascia of this muscle; thus, in the course of any neck dissection, but especially in a radical neck dissection (RND) or a modified radical neck dissection (MRND), it is crucial to keep the plane of dissection superficial to the fascia of the levator in order to preserve these nerves. The dorsal scapular nerve is inconsistent in its anatomic relations in the posterior triangle of the neck and contributes to the innervation of the levator scapulae in a minority of cases (3).

Because one of the functions of the levator is to draw the scapula and the shoulder upward and medially, inadvertent or unnecessary resection of the nerves to it during an RND may add to the resulting deformity and functional disability of the shoulder.

Thoracic Duct

At the base of the neck, the thoracic duct is located medial to and behind the left common carotid artery and the vagus nerve. From here, it arches upward, forward, and laterally, passing behind the IJV and in front of the anterior scalene muscle and the phrenic nerve. It then opens into the IJV, the subclavian vein, or the angle formed by the junction of these two vessels. The duct is anterior and medial to the thyrocervical trunk and the transverse cervical artery. Precise knowledge of these anatomic relationships is important to avoid injuring the duct during a neck dissection. It is even more important when the surgeon is called on to search for and repair a chyle leak during or after a neck dissection. To prevent a chyle leak, the surgeon also must remember that the thoracic duct may be multiple in its upper end and that at the base of the neck it usually receives a jugular, a subclavian, and usually other minor lymphatic trunks, which must be ligated or clipped individually.

Fascial Compartments of the Neck

The deep cervical fascia of the neck is divided into three layers: superficial, middle, and deep (Fig. 117.3). The superficial or investing layer surrounds the entire neck. It arises from the vertebral spinous processes and the ligamentum nuchae and encircles the entire neck to attach itself again to the spinous processes on the opposite side. This fascia divides to enclose the trapezius muscle. At the anterior border of this muscle, the two layers fuse into a single layer that crosses the posterior triangle of the neck. It divides again to surround the inferior belly of the omohyoid muscle and the sternomastoid muscle. At the lateral border of the strap muscles, it sends fibers between them before fusing in front of them as it extends onto the other side of the neck. This fascia also envelops the submandibular and parotid glands.

The middle layer of the deep cervical fascia, also called the visceral fascia, surrounds the visceral structures of the anterior portion of the neck. The deep layer of the deep cervical fascia or prevertebral fascia surrounds the deep muscles of the neck. Among them, it covers the splenius capitis, the levator scapulae, and the scalene muscles. It extends onto the other side of the neck, covering the prevertebral muscles.

The carotid sheath encircling the jugular vein, common carotid artery, and vagus nerve is formed by all layers of the deep cervical fascia. The carotid sheath originates superiorly at the jugular foramen, where it attaches to the skull base. It then follows the course of the vessels, traversing the anterior cervical triangle and extending inferiorly into the thoracic inlet.

Lymphatics of the Neck

The lymph node regions of the neck are shown in Figure 117.4. The six levels currently used encompass the complete topographic anatomy of the neck. The concept of sublevels has been introduced into the classification since certain zones have been identified within the six levels, which may have clinical significance.

Level I is divided in two sublevels: sublevel IA (submental), which includes the lymph nodes within the triangle bound by the anterior bellies of the digastric muscles and the mylohoid muscle, and sublevel IIB (submandibular), which includes the lymph nodes with the boundaries of the triangle formed by the anterior and posterior bellies of the digastrics and body of the mandible.

Level II (upper jugular) includes the lymph nodes located around the upper third of the IJV and adjacent spinal accessory nerve extending from the level of the

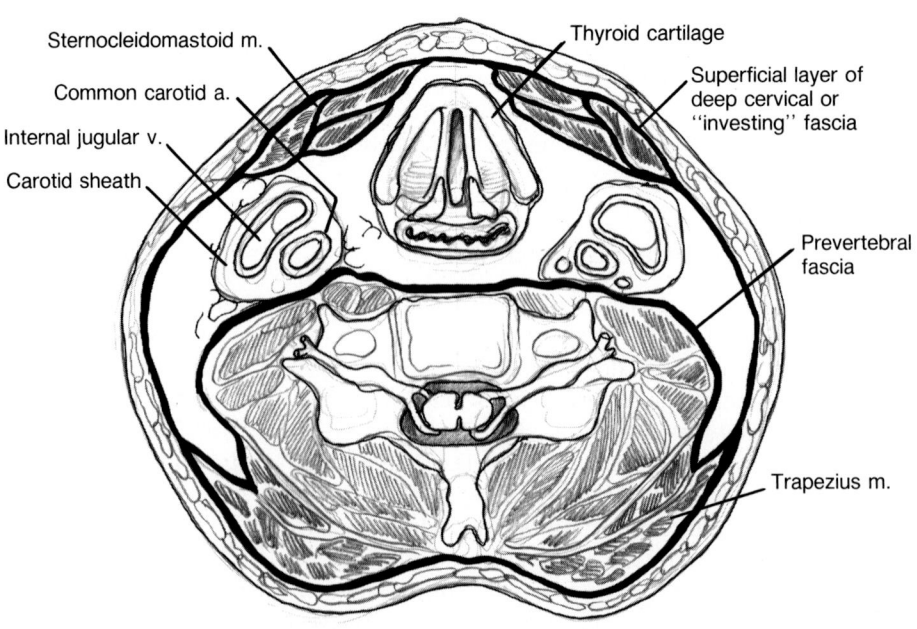

Sternocleidomastoid m.

Common carotid a.

Internal jugular v.

Carotid sheath

Thyroid cartilage

Superficial layer of deep cervical or "investing" fascia

Prevertebral fascia

Trapezius m.

Figure 117.3 Layers of the cervical fascia.

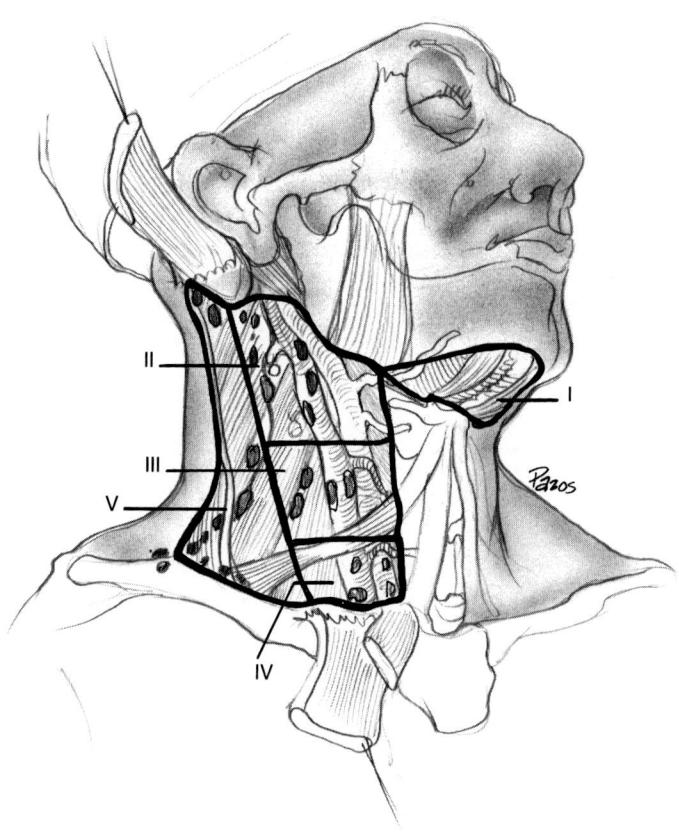

Figure 117.4 Lymph node regions of the neck.

skull base to the level of the inferior border of the hyoid. The anterior/medial boundary is the stylohyoid muscle (the radiologic correlate is the vertical plane defined by the posterior surface of the submandibular gland), and the posterior (lateral) boundary is the posterior border of the SCM. Two sublevels are recognized in level II: sublevel IIA contains nodes in the region anterior to the spinal accessory nerve (SAN) and sublevel IIB contains nodes posterior to the SAN.

Level III (midjugular) includes the lymph nodes located around the middle third of the IJV extending from the inferior border of the hyoid bone to the inferior border of cricoid cartilage. The anterior/medial boundary is the lateral border of the sternohyoid muscle, and the posterior/lateral boundary is the posterior border of the SCM.

Level IV (lower jugular) encompasses the lymph nodes located around the lower third of the IJV extending from the inferior border of the cricoid cartilage to the clavicle.

The anatomic boundary that separates the medial border of levels III and IV from the lateral border of level VI has traditionally been the lateral border of the sternohyoid muscle, a landmark that cannot be easily discerned on imaging studies. Therefore, the medial aspect of the common carotid artery has been suggested as an alternate boundary to separate these levels in an axial plane in imaging studies (4).

Level V (posterior triangle) comprises predominantly of the lymph nodes located along the lower half of the spinal accessory nerve and the transverse cervical artery. The supraclavicular nodes are also included in posterior triangle group. The superior boundary is the apex formed by convergence of the sternocleidomastoid and trapezius muscles, the inferior boundary is the clavicle, the anterior boundary is the posterior border of the SCM, and the posterior boundary is the anterior border of the trapezius muscle. A horizontal plane marking the inferior border of the anterior cricoid arch separates two sublevels. Sublevel VA, above this plane, includes the spinal accessory nodes. Sublevel VB, below this plane, includes the nodes that follow the transverse cervical vessels and the supraclavicular nodes with the exception of Virchow node, which is located in level IV.

Level VI (anterior compartment): Lymph nodes in this compartment include the pre- and paratracheal nodes, precricoid (delphian) node, and the perithyroidal nodes including the lymph nodes along the recurrent laryngeal nerves. The superior boundary is the hyoid bone, the inferior boundary is the suprasternal notch, and the lateral boundaries are the common carotid arteries.

Other lymph node groups: Lymph nodes involving regions not located within these levels should be referred to by the name of their specific nodal group; examples of these are the superior mediastinum, the retropharyngeal, the periparotid, the buccinator, the postauricular, and the suboccipital lymph nodes.

TABLE 117.1	PERCENTAGE OF METASTATIC LYMPH NODES INVOLVED IN ELECTIVE AND THERAPEUTIC RNDs							
	Primary Site							
Level of Metastatic Lymph Nodes	**Oral Cavity**		**Oropharynx**		**Hypopharynx**		**Larynx**	
	Elective	Therapeutic	Elective	Therapeutic	Elective	Therapeutic	Elective	Therapeutic
I	58	61	7	17	0	10	14	8
II	51	57	80	85	75	78	52	68
III	26	44	60	50	75	75	55	70
IV	9	20	27	33	0	47	24	35
V	2	4	7	11	0	11	7	5

Modified from Shah JP. Patterns of cervical lymph node metastasis from squamous carcinomas of the upper aerodigestive tract. *Am J Surg* 1990;160(4):405–409.

Patterns of Lymph Node Metastases

Lindberg first described the clinical pattern of cervical metastases for various primary sites in 1972 (5). Shah (6), in 1990, examined the distribution of nodal metastases in 1,119 RNDs performed both electively and therapeutically for squamous cell carcinoma (SCCA) of the oral cavity, oropharynx, hypopharynx, and larynx. He found a consistent distribution of cervical metastases (Table 117.1). The majority of metastases from cancer of the oral cavity were found in lymph nodes in levels I, II, and III. On the other hand, most metastases from carcinomas of the oropharynx, hypopharynx, and larynx were found in levels II, III, and IV. The lymph nodes in level V were not involved in the absence of metastases at other levels.

The significance of other lymphatic groups, such as the retropharyngeal lymph nodes (RPLNs) and paratracheal nodes, has also been characterized (7). Metastases to the RPLNs can occur with SCCA of the hypopharynx, tonsil, soft palate, posterior and lateral oropharynx, nasopharynx, and supraglottis.

Metastases from cancers of the larynx can occur to the paratracheal lymph nodes (PTLNs). In a study of 91 selected patients with carcinoma of the larynx who underwent PTLN dissection, Weber et al. (8) found that metastases to these lymph nodes occurred primarily in patients with subglottic and transglottic tumors, but they also occurred in patients with glottic tumors. In a prospective study of 45 patients with advanced glottic cancers, who underwent bilateral paratracheal node dissection as part of their treatment, Shenoy et al. (9) found metastases in the ipsilateral paratracheal nodes in 4% of the cases and contralateral metastases in 2%. Failure to address the paratracheal nodes for laryngeal cancer is a known cause of stomal recurrence.

PHYSIOLOGY

The trapezius is a fan-shaped muscle composed of upper, middle, and lower segments, each of which functions in a different but complementary manner. The trapezius and the

other muscles that insert on the scapula stabilize and control the shoulder girdle during arm movement. The levator scapulae acts synergistically with the upper division of the trapezius to elevate the scapula; the rhomboid assists the middle part of the trapezius in retracting and stabilizing the scapula against the posterior thoracic cage. The simultaneous action of the upper and lower divisions of the trapezius muscle results in a unique rotatory action of the scapula. The upward rotation of the scapula, in combination with abduction of the arm at the glenohumeral joint, permits elevation of the arm beyond 90 degrees at the shoulder level.

As is discussed in detail later in this chapter, paralysis of the trapezius muscle causes a syndrome characterized by weakness and deformity of the shoulder girdle, usually accompanied by pain.

DIAGNOSTIC EVALUATION

Clinical Examination

Clinical examination of the neck by palpation is not uniformly reliable in the detection of cervical lymph node metastases, particularly of lymph nodes minimally involved by the tumor. The reported error rate in assessing the presence or absence of cervical lymph node metastases by palpation ranges from 20% to 50%. The factors responsible for this variation are not only the ability and experience of the examiner but also the patient's habitus and previous treatment to the neck with surgery or radiation therapy. With the advent of modern imaging techniques, it was hoped that the clinician would not have to rely solely on clinical examination to make decisions in the treatment of the neck.

Imaging Studies

Using the histologic demonstration of metastasis in a lymph node as the gold standard, several studies have shown that ultrasonography (US), computed tomography (CT), and magnetic resonance imaging (MRI) have a higher sensitivity and specificity than clinical examination in the detection of metastases in lymph nodes. In a prospective study of 48 patients who were to undergo neck dissection, Haberal et al. (10) found that the sensitivity and specificity of palpation for the detection of metastases in the lymph nodes were 64% and 85%, respectively, while the corresponding values were 72% and 96% for US and 81% and 96% for CT. Adams et al. (11) reported similar results for US and CT; in addition, they reported a sensitivity of 80% and a specificity of 79% for MRI. What these observations indicate is that a "negative" US, CT, or MRI of the neck cannot be relied to withhold elective treatment of the cervical lymph nodes, since they cannot detect metastases in 19% to 28% of the patients staged clinically N0. Obviously the imaging criteria used to diagnose metastasis in a lymph node are not absolutely reliable. The imaging criterion used most often to consider a cervical node suspicious for metastasis is size larger than 1.5 cm in maximum diameter for nodes located in levels I and II and larger than 1 cm for nodes in other regions of the neck (12). Although a correlation exists between the size of a lymph node and the presence of histologic metastasis (Table 117.2), it is clear that not all enlarged lymph nodes contain metastatic deposits and that nodes smaller than 1 or 1.5 cm can indeed contain metastases. Thirty-three percent of all metastases from SCCAs of the head and neck are found in lymph nodes smaller than 1 cm, 10% of tumor-positive neck dissection specimens contain only metastases less than 3 mm in diameter, and, more importantly, 25% of all clinically occult lymph node metastases are too small to be detected by any of the currently available imaging techniques (13). DiNardo (14) demonstrated that 88% of metastases from the carcinomas of the floor of the mouth were found in nodes that were 1 cm or less in diameter.

The presence of a central area of lucency within a node shown on CT was at one time considered equivalent to the presence of necrotic tumor within a node; however, such a finding can be caused by an artery with plaque formation or a fatty inclusion in a lymph node. Another imaging criterion used to "diagnose" metastasis in a lymph node is the shape of the node, as determined by the ratio of its long (l) and short (s) axis diameters. In a study by Steinkamp et al. (15), 730 enlarged cervical lymph nodes in 285 patients were examined using ultrasound, and the l/s ratio was calculated. Histologic examination after neck dissection revealed that 95% of the enlarged cervical nodes, shown on ultrasound to have a l/s ratio of more than 2, were correctly diagnosed as benign. Nodes presenting with a more circular shape and a l/s ratio of less than 2 were diagnosed correctly as metastases with 95% accuracy.

Ultrasound Guided Fine-Needle Aspiration Biopsy

In an attempt to overcome the lack of sensitivity of morphologic imaging criteria, US was combined with fine needle aspiration biopsy (US-FNAB). This technique appeared more promising for the preoperative evaluation of the N0 neck as it enables sampling of lymph nodes as small as 3 mm in diameter and adds the advantages of cytologic evaluation (16). However, the usefulness of this technique is strongly dependent on the skill and time of the ultrasonographer and on the experience of the cytopathologist. Furthermore, the outcomes of a wait-and-see policy after negative US-FNAB have been disappointing. In a study of 92 patients with tumors of the oral cavity, staged T1 and T2, who were observed after a negative US-fine-needle aspiration (US-FNA), metastases in neck nodes became apparent subsequently in 19 (21%) (17). In a more recent study, Wensing et al. (18) found that palpation and US with or without US-FNAB missed occult lymph node metastases in 22% of the patients with oral cavity SCCA. These figures are troubling because the incidence of lymph node metastases in patients with such tumors, who are observed without any intervention to the neck, is about 25%.

TABLE 117.2	NODAL SIZE AND PRESENCE OF HISTOLOGIC METASTASES		
	Histologic Status (%)		
Node Size (cm)	**Negative**	**Positive**	**Positive with Extranodal Extension**
1	67	33	14
2	38	62	26
3	19	81	49
4	12	88	71
5	0	100	76

From Hamakawa H, Fukizumi M, Bao Y, et al. Genetic diagnosis of micrometastasis based on SCCA antigen mRNA in cervical lymph nodes of head and neck cancer. *Clin Exp Metastasis* 1999;17(7):593–599, with permission.

Positron Emission Tomography

Prospective studies using 18-fluorodeoxyglucose (FDG) positron emission tomography (PET) to assess lymph node metastases from SCCAs of the oral cavity have shown a sensitivity and specificity higher than MRI, CT, and US. However, current FDG-PET techniques are also limited in the detection of tumor foci smaller than 1 cm (19,20). Kyzas et al. (21) performed a meta-analysis of 32 studies that assessed the diagnostic performance of PET scans in patients with SCCA of the head and neck. In patients staged clinically N0, the sensitivity of 18 PET scan was only 50% (95% CI: 37% to 63%), whereas specificity was 87% (95% CI: 76% to 93%). These authors also compared the performance of PET scan with that of "conventional diagnostic methods," that is, CT, MRI, and ultrasound with fine-needle aspiration (FNA) by analyzing studies that had also used these diagnostic methods on the same patients. The sensitivity and specificity of PET scans were 80% and 86%, respectively, and of "conventional diagnostic tests" were 75% and 79%. Thus, at the present time, the role for PET scan in the evaluation of the N0 neck is limited as it will not detect metastases in 20% to 50% of the cases.

In another effort to overcome the limitations of current imaging techniques, particularly their inability to differentiate a tumor-infiltrated lymph node from a normal or a reactive one, de Bree et al. (22) have experimented with radioimmunoscintigraphy (RIS). With this technique, SCCA specific monoclonal antibodies labeled with ^{99}mTc were given intravenously to patients with SCCA who underwent neck dissection. Unfortunately, RIS was not superior to CT and MRI for the detection of lymph node metastases.

CT and MRI are valuable in the evaluation of lymph nodes that are not easily accessible to the hands of the examiner, such as the retropharyngeal, upper mediastinal, and, in some patients, the PTLNs. They are also valuable in the assessment of resectability of large metastatic deposits in the neck, because in most instances they can define the relationship of a metastatic tumor with critical structures, such as the common and the internal carotid artery, the cervical spine, the vertebral artery, and the brachial plexus. If tumor involvement of the common or the internal carotid artery is suspected, a systematic preoperative evaluation should include four-vessel cerebral angiography to determine the status of the contralateral carotid and to assess collateral intracerebral circulation. In addition, an attempt should be made during the angiography to measure carotid back pressure and to assess dynamically the collateral circulation by using balloon occlusion techniques while monitoring the patient for evidence of neurologic deficits under normotensive and hypotensive conditions.

Fine-Needle Aspiration

FNA has become a valuable diagnostic tool in patients with a mass in the neck in whom metastatic carcinoma is suspected.

According to numerous recent reports, the specificity of FNA ranges from 94% to 100% and the sensitivity ranges from 92% to 98%. The interobserver variability between cytopathologists in one series has been reported as 8%. FNA has been found to be most accurate in the diagnosis of epithelial malignancies, achieving nearly 100% accuracy.

FNA is indicated in the patient with a solid mass in the neck after a thorough examination of the mucosal surfaces and skin of the head and neck region fails to reveal a primary tumor. If the mass is located in the supraclavicular area, FNA is essential in the initial evaluation of the patient. The cytopathology findings then can guide the clinician's search for a primary tumor below the clavicles.

Sentinel Node Biopsy

Sentinel lymph node biopsy (SLNB) is feasible and useful as a staging procedure in patients with early carcinomas of the oral cavity and in particular for patients with cancers of the oral tongue. Proponents of this technique point out that it allows accurate histopathologic staging of the neck by examining the sentinel lymph node (SLN) with serial sectioning and immunohistochemistry, and it avoids unnecessary neck dissection and its possible complications.

The SLNB is based on the belief that cancers metastasize via lymphatics to regional lymph nodes in an orderly fashion, that this process is embolic in nature, and that the lymph node that first receives lymphatic drainage from the primary site can be identified and excised for histologic analysis (23).

Early studies in patients with SCCAs of the mucosal surfaces of the head and neck investigated the methodology and feasibility of SLNB (23–26). In general, the primary cancer should be accessible to infiltration with a radioisotope-labeled colloid to perform a lymphoscintigraphy and a blue dye to aid in intraoperative localization of the sentinel node. These localizing methods have been shown to be complementary. Ross et al. (26) in a multicenter study investigated SLNB in 134 patients with SCCA of the oral cavity and oropharynx, staged T1/T2 N0. Lymphoscintigraphy was performed preoperatively; blue dye and a gamma probe were used intraoperatively to aid in the identification of sentinel nodes. Sentinel nodes were identified in 93% of the cases. The number of sentinel nodes varies, but in a series of 48 patients studied by Ross et al. (24), the mean number of sentinel nodes harvested was 2.4.

Subsequent studies have examined the utility of SLNB in patients with oral cavity or oropharyngeal cancers staged T1/T2 N0. The sensitivity of the procedure is 90% when the histopathology of the sentinel node is compared with that of the neck dissection specimen (27). It results in histopathologic upstaging of the clinically N0 neck in 36% of the patients when the nodes are examined with routine hematoxylin–eosin staining; serial sectioning and immunohistochemistry upstage an additional 8% of the cases (24). The detection of micrometastases can be further enhanced by using highly specific tumor markers and molecular methods (28,29).

Recently, Civantos et al. (30) reported the results of a North American Multi-Institutional Prospective Study that evaluated the utility of SLNB in T1/T2 oral SCCAs. The study included 140 patients (68% oral tongue, 19% the floor of the mouth) from 25 institutions who underwent SLNB and selective neck dissection (SND) (levels I–IV). The negative predictive value (NPV) was 94% when the SLNs were examined with hematoxylin–eosin stains and 96% when they were examined with serial sectioning and immunocytochemistry (30). The NPV among experienced surgeons was 100% versus 95% for less experienced ones. The SLN was the only positive node in 51% of the cases with a positive SLN. The false-negative rate was 9.8% overall. Interestingly, however, the false-negative rate was 10% in patients with cancers of the oral tongue but was 25% in patients with cancers of the floor of the mouth. In the experience of the University of Miami (31), the NPV of SLNB was 88.5% in patients with cancers of the floor of mouth (FOM) and 95.8% when these patients were excluded. Similarly, Ross et al. (26) have reported that the identification of SLNB in patients with FOM cancers was lower (86%) than in patients with tumors in other locations (97%); the sensitivity of SLNB in FOM cancers was also lower (80%), compared with other tumor locations (100%). It appears that lymphoscintigraphy in cancers of the FOM is not as helpful in identifying the SLN due to the shine-through effect of the radioactivity at the primary site; it obscures the lymph nodes in level I, which are one of the primary echelons of lymphatic drainage for the FOM and lower gum. Obviously, this limits the utility of SLNB in patients with tumors in these locations.

STAGING

At completion of the clinical evaluation of a patient with SCCA of the head and neck region, the disease should be classified according to stage. The staging for the lymph nodes proposed by the American Joint Committee on Cancer in 2009 (32) is outlined below:

NX: Regional lymph nodes cannot be assessed.
N0: No regional lymph node metastasis.
N1: Metastasis in a single ipsilateral lymph node, 3 cm or less in greatest dimension.
N2: Metastasis in a single ipsilateral lymph node, more than 3 cm but not more than 6 cm in greatest dimension; or in multiple ipsilateral lymph nodes, none more than 6 cm in greatest dimension; or in bilateral or contralateral lymph nodes, none more than 6 cm in greatest dimension.
N2a: Metastasis in a single ipsilateral lymph node more than 3 cm but not more than 6 cm in greatest dimension.
N2b: Metastasis in multiple ipsilateral lymph nodes, none more than 6 cm in greatest dimension.
N2c: Metastasis in bilateral or contralateral nodes no more than 6 cm in greatest dimension.
N3: Metastasis in a lymph node more than 6 cm in greatest dimension.

Staging of the neck in nasopharyngeal carcinoma patients is different because the distribution and the prognostic impact of regional lymph node spread from nasopharynx cancer, particularly of the undifferentiated type, are different from those of other head and neck mucosal cancers and justify the use of the following scheme:

NX: Regional lymph nodes cannot be assessed.
N0: No regional lymph node metastasis.
N1: Unilateral metastasis in lymph node(s), 6 cm or less in greatest dimension, above the supraclavicular fossa.
N2: Bilateral metastasis in lymph node(s), 6 cm or less in greatest dimension, above the supraclavicular fossa.
N3: Metastasis in a lymph node(s) greater than 6 cm and/or to supraclavicular fossa.
N3a: Greater than 6 cm in dimension.
N3b: Extension to the supraclavicular fossa.

CLASSIFICATION OF NECK DISSECTIONS

Several cervical lymph node dissections are currently used for the surgical treatment of the neck in patients with cancer of the head and neck region. To standardize the nomenclature used to refer to these operations, it is essential to adopt a common nomenclature for the lymph node groups of the neck, such as the one outlined earlier in this chapter. The current classification of neck dissections recommended by the American Academy of Otolaryngology-Head and Neck Surgery (Table 117.3) takes into account the lymph node groups of the neck that are removed and secondarily the anatomic structures that may be preserved, such as the spinal accessory nerve and the IJV. Analyzing neck dissections from these two points of view, there are essentially four anatomic types of neck dissections: radical, modified radical, selective, and extended. Recently, clinicians from around the world have proposed a nomenclature for neck dissection that, if recognized internationally, would be "logical, unambiguous, precise, and easy to remember" (33).

In this classification, the following three descriptors are used to label a neck dissection:

1. "ND" to represent neck dissection that is prefaced by either "L" or "R" for side. If bilateral, both sides must be classified independently.
2. The levels and sublevels of lymph nodes removed designated by Roman numerals I through VII in ascending order. For levels that contain sublevels (I, II, and V), listing of the level without a sublevel indicates that the entire level (both A and B) was excised.
3. The nonlymphatic structures removed designated by their internationally recognized initials, that is, SCM for sternocleidomastoid muscle, IJV for internal jugular vein.

It is hoped that this new classification system will convey precisely the extent of lymphatic and nonlymphatic structures removed in a neck dissection that will then allow better comparison of results between studies.

TABLE 117.3 CLASSIFICATION OF NECK DISSECTIONS	
2001 Classification	**2010 Proposed Classification**
1. Radical neck dissection	1. ND (I–V, SCM, IJV, CNXI)
2. Modified radical neck dissection	2. ND (I–V, SCM, IJV), ND (I–V, IJV, CNXI), ND (I–V)
3. Selective neck dissection (SND):	3.
SND (I–III/IV)	ND (I, II, II/IV)
SND (II–IV)	ND (II–IV)
SND (II–V, postauricular, suboccipital)	ND (II–V, postauricular, suboccipital)
SND (level VI)	ND (VI)
4. Extended neck dissection	4. ND (levels removed, nodes or structures removed)

Lastly, the surgeon must orient the surgical specimen for the pathologist and identify the different lymph node groups it contains. Only then can the pathologist be expected to generate a clinically and prognostically meaningful report that describes the location and number of lymph nodes examined, the number of nodes that contain the tumor, and the presence or absence of extranodal extension of the tumor.

ND (I–V, SCM, IJV, CN XI)

Radical Neck Dissection

This operation is defined as the en bloc removal of the lymph node–bearing tissues of one side of the neck, from the inferior border of the mandible to the clavicle and from the lateral border of the strap muscles to the anterior border of the trapezius. Included in the resected specimen are the spinal accessory nerve, the IJV, and the SCM (Fig. 117.5). A comprehensive description of the surgical technique of this operation was recently provided by McCammon and Shah (34).

Rationale

The first description of the systematic en bloc removal of the lymphatics of the neck was published by Crile in 1906. The operation he described came to be known as the RND. Although Crile believed that removing the IJV was essential because of the intimate relation of this structure with the lymph nodes of the neck, it is interesting to note that the drawings that illustrate his publication indicate that the spinal accessory nerve and the ansa hypoglossi were preserved. It was Martin et al. in the 1950s who championed the concept that a cervical lymphadenectomy for cancer was inadequate unless all the lymph node–bearing tissues of one side of the neck were removed and that this was impossible unless the spinal accessory nerve, the IJV, and the SCM were included in the resection. In fact, they categorically stated, "any technique that is designed to preserve the spinal accessory nerve should be condemned unequivocally."

In describing the RND, Crile contended that an en bloc removal of the primary tumor and the lymphatic system of the neck should be carried out in a manner similar to the Halstead operation for breast cancer. He believed that

normal lymph flow is interrupted by metastasis in a lymph node, causing further tumor dissemination to occur in any direction, and that a less radical "incomplete" operation would disseminate and stimulate the growth of the tumor. Like Crile, Martin et al. believed that it was impossible to remove the lymphatics of the neck completely without resecting the SCM and IJV because of the close association of the lymphatics in this area with the vein walls.

Removing the SCM unquestionably facilitates access to the jugular vein and the removal of the lymph node–bearing tissues of the neck. In some instances, the muscle must be removed because it is involved by the tumor. However, removal of this muscle is no longer justified for ease or exposure alone.

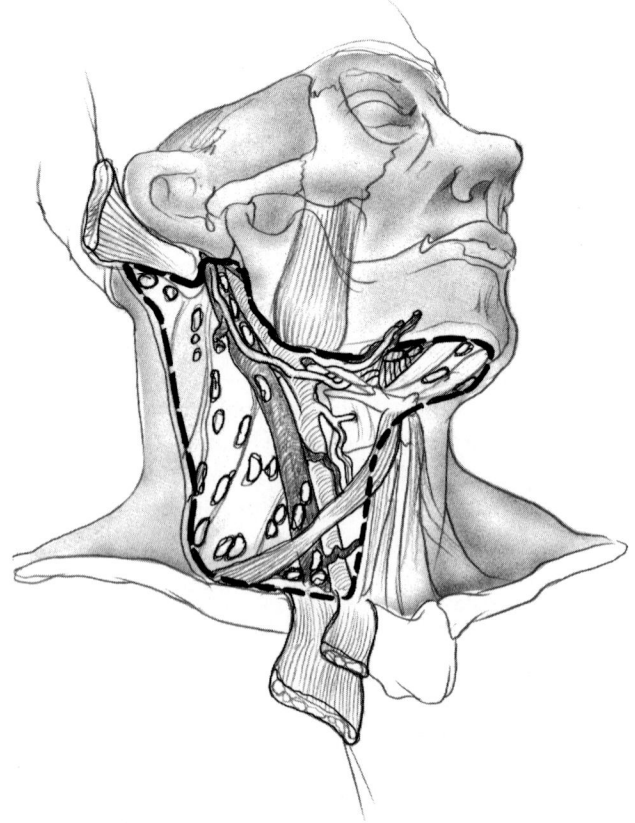

Figure 117.5 Radical neck dissection.

An RND is not indicated in the absence of palpable cervical metastases (i.e., in the treatment of the N0 neck). Currently, RNDs represent less than 20% of all neck dissection done at many institutions (35), as familiarity with the other types of neck dissection has increased.

Indications

An RND is indicated when there are multiple clinically obvious cervical lymph node metastases, particularly when they involve the lymph nodes of the posterior triangle of the neck and are found to involve or to be tightly related to the spinal accessory nerve. An RND is also indicated when there is a large metastatic tumor mass or when multiple matted nodes are present in the upper part of the neck. In such instances, it is unwise to preserve the sternocleidomastoid or the internal jugular or to dissect the spinal accessory nerve and risk entering the tumor. A similar situation can be created by the inflammation, hematoma, or ecchymosis that follows ill-advised excisional biopsies of neck metastases. An RND may be the safest option in such patients.

ND (I–V, SCM, IJV, CN XI)

Modified Radical Neck Dissection (MRND)

This category includes modifications of the RNDs developed with the intention of reducing the morbidity of the operation by preserving one or more of these structures: the spinal accessory nerve, the IJV, or the SCM.

The three neck dissections that can be included in this category are outlined in Table 117.3. They differ from each other only in the number of neural, vascular, and muscular structures that are preserved. Therefore, they can be subclassified as follows:

- ND (I–V, SCM, IJV) (MRND type I) with preservation of the spinal accessory nerve
- ND (I–V, SCM) (MRND type II) with preservation of the spinal accessory nerve and the IJV
- ND (I–V) (MRND type III) with preservation of the spinal accessory nerve, the IJV, and the SCM. This corresponds to the operation often called "functional neck dissection."

ND (I–V, SCM, IJV)

Modified Radical Neck Dissection with Preservation of the Spinal Accessory Nerve

This operation is defined as the en bloc removal of the lymph node–bearing tissues of one side of the neck, from the inferior border of the mandible to the clavicle and from the lateral border of the strap muscles to the anterior border of the trapezius, preserving the spinal accessory nerve. The IJV and the SCM are included in the resected specimen (Fig. 117.6). The surgical technique is essentially the same as that of the RND.

Rationale

The following observations have compelled surgeons, for several decades, to explore and develop alternatives to the RND:

- The morbidity associated with the RND, especially the shoulder disability that results from the resection of the spinal accessory nerve and, to a lesser extent, the cosmetic deformity that results from this operation, particularly when it is done on both sides of the neck

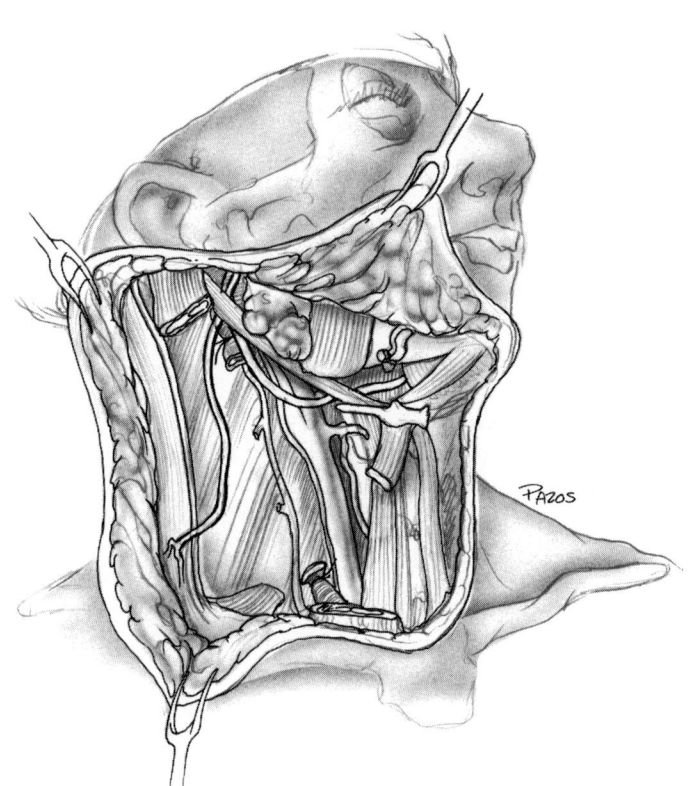

Figure 117.6 MRND (type I) with preservation of the spinal accessory nerve.

■ The realization that in many instances the spinal accessory nerve is not in close proximity to the nodes grossly involved by the tumor and that its preservation does not compromise the oncologic soundness of the operation

Indications

This type of neck dissection is used in the surgical treatment of the neck of patients with clinically obvious lymph node metastases when the spinal accessory nerve is not directly involved by the tumor, regardless of the number, size, and location of the involved lymph nodes. The decision to preserve the spinal accessory nerve is, therefore, a delicate intraoperative judgment call. Much like the philosophy about preservation of the facial nerve during surgery for parotid tumors, the spinal accessory nerve can be preserved whenever there is a clearly identifiable, not an artificially created, plane of dissection between the tumor and the nerve. The reported rate of recurrence in the neck when used for the treatment of the N+ neck in combination with postoperative radiation is 8.1% (36).

ND (I–V, SCM)

Modified Radical Neck Dissection with Preservation of the Spinal Accessory Nerve and the Internal Jugular Vein

In this type of dissection, the lymph node–bearing tissues of one side of the neck are removed en bloc, preserving the spinal accessory nerve and the IJV. This operation is seldom planned. It is done occasionally when in the course of a neck dissection the metastatic tumor in the neck is noted to be adherent to the SCM but away from the accessory nerve and the jugular vein. This situation occurs occasionally in patients with hypopharyngeal or laryngeal tumors with metastases under the middle third of the SCM.

ND (I–V, SCM, IJV, CN XI)

Modified Radical Neck Dissection with Preservation of the Spinal Accessory Nerve, the Internal Jugular Vein, and the Sternocleidomastoid Muscle

This operation consists of the en bloc removal of the lymph node–bearing tissues of one side of the neck, including lymph nodes in levels I through V, preserving the spinal accessory nerve, the IJV, and the SCM. The submandibular gland may or may not be removed (Fig. 117.7). A description of the operative technique of this operation, as it is currently advocated by most European surgeons, can be found in a publication by Gavilan et al. (37).

Rationale

The muscular and vascular aponeurosis of the neck demarcate compartments filled with fibroadipose tissue that contains lymph nodes. In the early 1960s, Suárez observed that the lymph nodes of the neck are not located within the muscular aponeurosis of the SCM and do not form part of the adventitia of nearby blood vessels, particularly veins. He then showed that it was technically feasible and

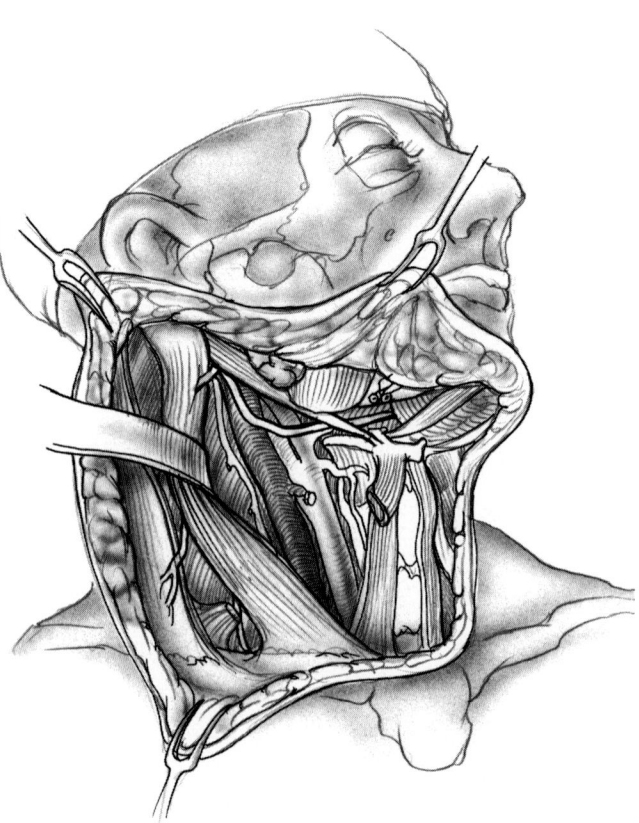

Figure 117.7 MRND (type III) with preservation of the spinal accessory nerve, the internal jugular vein, and the SCM.

oncologically sound to perform a comprehensive removal of the lymph node–bearing tissues of one or both sides of the neck without removing the SCM, the submandibular gland, and the IJV (38). It should be pointed out that the nerves of the neck do not follow the aponeurotic compartment distribution, except for the vagus nerve that is contained within the carotid sheath. The phrenic nerve and the brachial plexus are partially within a compartment; the hypoglossal and the spinal accessory nerves run across several compartments. Unless these nerves are directly involved by the tumor, they can be dissected free and preserved.

Indications

This operation was widely used, particularly in Europe, as the neck dissection of choice for the treatment of the N0 neck in patients with SCCA of the upper aerodigestive tract, especially when the primary tumor was in the larynx or hypopharynx. It is now considered an unnecessarily extensive procedure for the treatment of the clinically negative neck in patients with head and neck cancers. A multi-institutional prospective randomized study comparing MRND to ND (levels II–IV)) in patients with laryngeal cancer was performed by the Brazilian Head and Neck Cancer Study Group (39). All patients had previously untreated T2–T4 N0M0 supraglottic and transglottic squamous carcinoma. Pathologically positive nodes were found in 26% of the patients, and most positive nodes were located at levels II and III. There were six ipsilateral neck recurrences (four in the MRND group and two in the lateral neck dissection ND II–IV group). Five-year actuarial survival calculated by the Kaplan-Meier method was 72.3% in the MRND group and 62.4% in the ND (II–III) (log-rank test $P = 0.312$). Another prospective study and a recent retrospective study also support the practice of not dissecting level V in patients with clinically N0 laryngeal and hypopharyngeal cancers (40,41).

According to some surgeons, this operation is indicated for the treatment of the N1 neck, when the metastatic nodes are mobile and no greater than 2.5 to 3 cm. The reported rates of recurrence in the neck with this type of neck dissection range between 0% and 16.6% for the clinically N0 neck and between 3.7% and 25% for the N+ neck (42–47).

This type of MRND remains the operation of choice for most patients with differentiated carcinoma of the thyroid who have palpable lymph node metastases in the lateral compartment of the neck.

Selective Neck Dissections

The SNDs consist of the removal of only the lymph node groups at highest risk of containing metastases according to the location of the primary tumor, preserving the spinal accessory nerve, the IJV, and the SCM. There are four main types of SNDs:

- SND of levels I–III or ND (I–III) (commonly referred to as "supraomohyoid" neck dissection) (Fig. 117.8) and SND of levels I–IV or ND (I–IV) (also referred to as

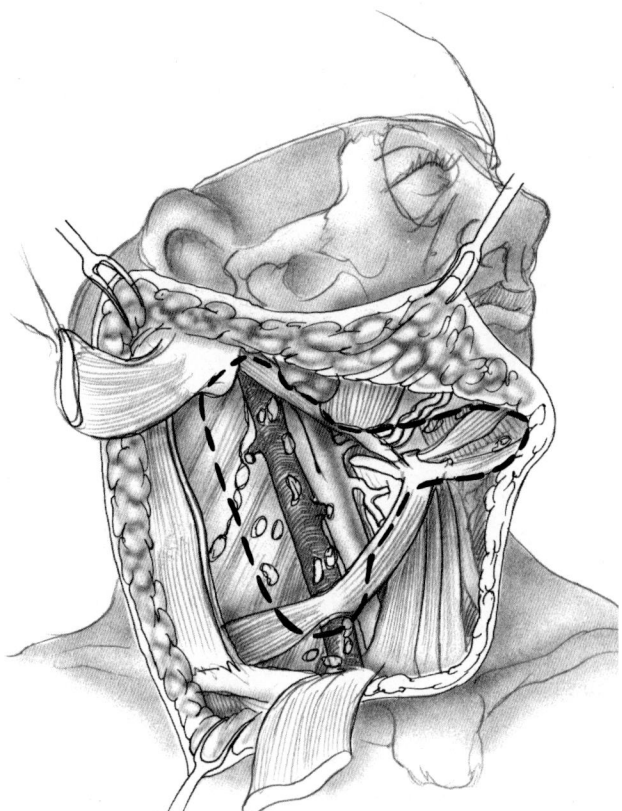

Figure 117.8 Supraomohyoid neck dissection.

"extended supraomohyoid" neck dissection). These are the neck dissections commonly used in the treatment of patients with SCCA of the oral cavity. The lymph nodes removed are those contained in the submental and submandibular triangles (level I), the upper jugular region (level II), and the midjugular region (level III). The posterior limit of the dissection is marked by the cutaneous branches of the cervical plexus and the posterior border of the SCM. The inferior limit is the omohyoid muscle as it crosses the IJV. Some surgeons prefer to perform an SND of level I–IV in cases with cancer of the oral tongue (48). For cancers of the oral cavity that are close to or involve the midline, either type of SND is done bilaterally, since the lymph nodes in both sides of the neck are at risk. These operations have been described in detail by Medina and Byers (49).

- SND of levels II–IV or ND (II–IV) (Fig. 117.9). This neck dissection, commonly referred to as the "lateral" neck dissection, is used in the treatment of patients with SCCA of the larynx, oropharynx, and hypopharynx. It consists of the removal of the upper (level II), middle (level III), and lower (level IV) jugular lymph nodes. The superior limit of the dissection is the digastric muscle and the mastoid tip. The inferior limit is the clavicle. The anteriomedial limit is the lateral border of the sternohyoid muscle. The posterior limit of the dissection is marked by the cutaneous branches of the cervical plexus and the posterior border of the SCM. For tumors of the supraglottic

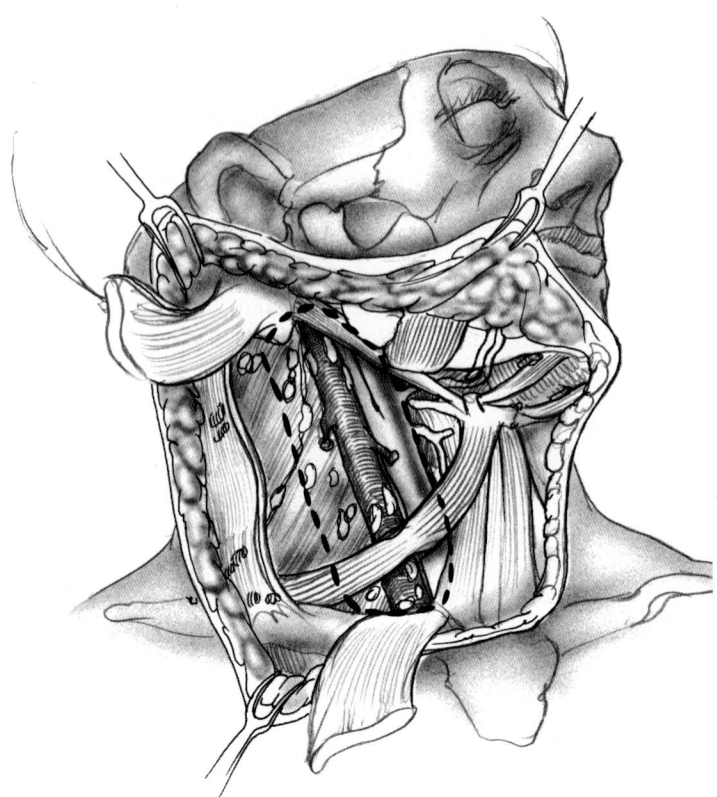

Figure 117.9 Lateral neck dissection.

larynx and posterior pharyngeal walls, the dissection is often bilateral. A recent description of the technique of this operation has been provided by Khafif (50).

- SND of level VI or ND (VI). This operation is also called "anterior" neck dissection or "central compartment" dissection. It is used in the treatment of patients with cancer of the midline structures of the anterior inferior aspect of the neck and thoracic inlet, such as the thyroid, the glottic and subglottic regions of the larynx, the pyriform sinus, and the cervical esophagus and trachea. It consists of the removal of the prelaryngeal, pretracheal lymph nodes, as well as the PTLNs on both sides. However, using a single denomination (i.e., SND of level VI) to refer to any dissection of the lymph nodes in this region is confusing. For instance, if the surgeon elects to remove the prelaryngeal, pretracheal, and the right PTLNs, the operation would have the same designation as one in which only the left paratracheal nodes are removed. Therefore, until consensus is reached about grouping of the lymph nodes in this area (i.e., level VIA and VIB), it is best to describe the operation in terms of the specific lymph nodes removed (e.g., left thyroid lobectomy with dissection of level VI that included the pretracheal and left paratracheal nodes) (51). These operations have been described recently by Weber and Holsinger (52).

- SND for cutaneous malignancies of the head and neck. The extent of the regional node dissection in patients with cutaneous malignancies depends on the location

of the primary lesion and the lymph node groups that are likely to harbor metastases. For skin cancers originating from the posterior scalp and the upper-lateral aspect of the neck, the operation most commonly done is an ND (levels II–V, retroauricular, suboccipital), which is also known as the "posterolateral" neck dissection (Fig. 117.10). The superior limit of this dissection is the posterior belly of the digastric muscle and the mastoid tip anterior laterally and the nuchal line/ridge posteriorly. The inferior limit is the clavicle. The anteriomedial limit is the lateral border of the sterno-hyoid muscle. The posteriolateral limit of the dissection is marked by the anterior border of the trapezius muscle inferiorly and the posterior midline of the neck superiorly (53). The regional node dissection often performed for cutaneous malignancies originating from the periauricular skin, anterior scalp, and temporal region is an SND (parotid, facial and external jugular nodes, levels II, III, VA).

Rationale

In the 1960s, surgeons at The University of Texas MD Anderson Cancer Center modified the concept of the RND by selectively removing only those lymph node groups that, based on the location of the primary tumor, were at highest risk of containing metastases" (54). These operations were eventually called "SNDs" (55) and their current use is based on the following observations:

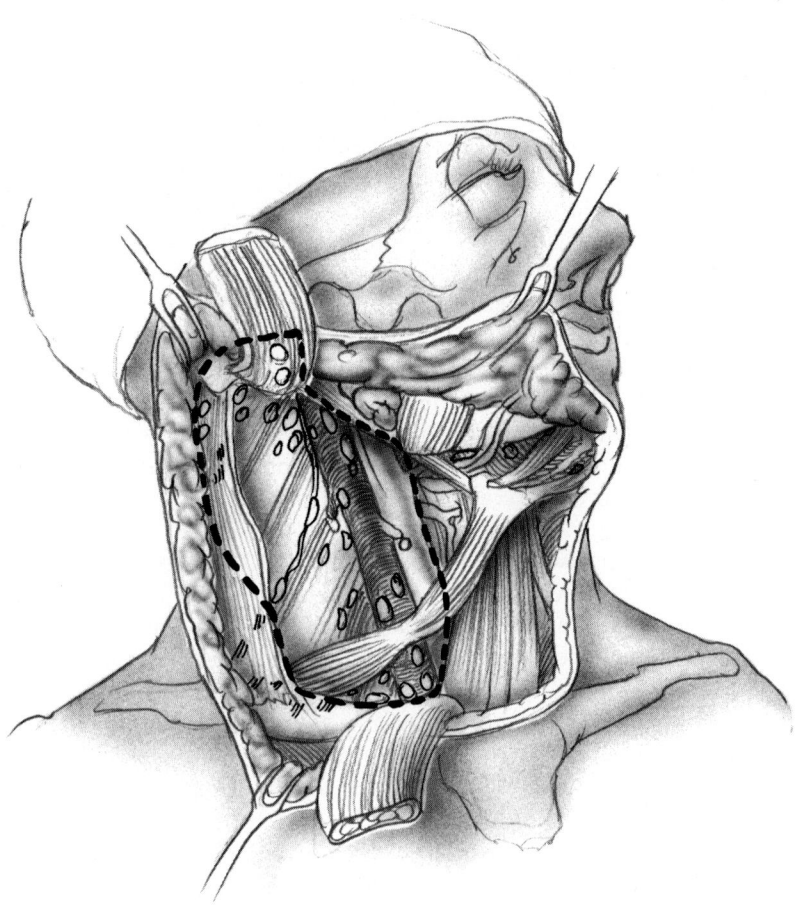

Figure 117.10 Posterolateral neck dissection.

1. Anatomic, pathologic, and clinical investigations (5,6,48,56–64) and recent prospective studies (39,40) have demonstrated that cervical lymph node metastases occur in predictable patterns in patients with SCCA of the head and neck.

The lymph node groups most frequently involved in patients with carcinomas of the oral cavity are the nodes in levels II and III. In addition, the nodes in level I are frequently involved in patients with carcinoma of the floor of the mouth, anterior oral tongue, and buccal mucosa. These tumors frequently metastasize to both sides of the neck, and they can skip levels I and II, metastasizing first to the nodes in level III. In a retrospective study of 1,119 RNDs, Shah (6) found that tumors of the oral cavity metastasized most frequently to the neck nodes in levels I, II, and III, whereas carcinomas of the oropharynx, hypopharynx, and larynx involved mainly the nodes in levels II, III, and IV.

It has been demonstrated that in the absence of metastases to the first-echelon nodes, tumors of the oral cavity and oropharynx rarely involve the nodes in level IV and level V. The nodes in level V are not commonly involved, regardless of the site of the primary tumor and the presence or absence of metastases in the jugular nodes (41), conceivably because there is no

retrograde flow from the jugular nodes into the spinal accessory nodes.

The predictability of lymphatic spread applies to both occult (N0 neck) and clinically evident (N+ neck) lymph node metastases. In an analysis of the distribution of lymph node metastasis in a cohort of 164 patients with oral cancer, who had a single clinically positive node (N1 or N2a), Kowalski and Carvalho (60) found that there were no isolated lymph node metastases in levels IV or V. These findings suggest that an SND of levels I–III could encompass the tumor in the neck in these patients. In other reports, the prevalence of metastases in level IV in clinically N+ cases is 17%, suggesting that it is a safer practice to include level IV whenever an SND is done for an N+ neck in patients with cancer of the oral cavity. The prevalence of nodal metastases in level V, on the other hand, is so low (0.5% in cN0 and 3% in cN+) that dissection of this region of the neck is rarely necessary (6). Similarly, in a prospective analysis of the prevalence and distribution of histologic lymph node metastases in 100 consecutive neck dissections done as part of the initial treatment of laryngeal and hypopharyngeal cancer, Buckley and MacLennan (40) found that all metastases in N0 and N1 cases were confined to levels II, III, IV, and VI. Metastases to levels I and V were infrequent, even in N+ disease, and occurred only in cases with N2c and N3 disease. These results support the use of dissection of nodes in levels II–IV for N0 and selected N+ cases with laryngeal and hypopharyngeal cancer.

2. SNDs provide the surgeon with the same staging information as the more extensive radical and MRNDs. There is substantial evidence that, at this time, micrometastases cannot be detected consistently by noninvasive methods (6). To detect such metastatic deposits, it is necessary to remove the regional lymph nodes, guided either by lymphoscintigraphy or by the anticipated pattern of metastases, and scrutinize them histopathologically. Thus, an SND serves as a staging procedure and can be used for decision making regarding the need for adjuvant postoperative radiation therapy. The concept of disease staging in the neck is important in patients whose primary tumors are amenable to treatment with surgery alone but who are highly likely to produce metastases to the cervical lymph nodes. Patients who have T2N0 and T3N0 SCCAs of the oral cavity and faucial arch region are excellent examples of this situation. Because the probability of lymph node metastasis is high in most of these patients, the neck dissection may only have the value of a staging procedure, the results of which determine whether or not postoperative radiation therapy is necessary. If the lymph nodes are histologically negative, no further therapy is indicated and the patient is treated with surgery alone. However, to make this decision with confidence, all the lymph nodes at risk of containing metastases must be evaluated. This evaluation requires dissecting both sides of the neck in patients with lesions of the anterior tongue and floor of the mouth, with the attendant morbidity of a bilateral RND. On the other hand, if the nodal metastases are multiple or the tumor extends beyond the capsule of a lymph node, the neck dissection alone is associated with a high incidence of recurrence in the neck (6,65,66). In these situations, the addition of postoperative radiation therapy results in better regional control of the disease (67).

3. When SND is utilized for the elective treatment of the regional lymphatics, regional control and survival rates are similar to those of more extensive neck dissections (39,40,68–78).

4. SNDs result in less postoperative morbidity. The dysfunction of the trapezius muscle produced by SNDs is minimal and, unlike that produced by the RND, is usually temporary and reversible (79–84).

Indications

Elective SND: N0 Neck

ND I–III/IV (Supraomohyoid Neck Dissection and Extended Supraomohyoid Neck Dissection). This SND is indicated in the surgical management of patients with SCCA of the oral cavity staged T2–T4 N0. The procedure is performed on both sides of the neck in patients with cancers of the anterior tongue and floor of the mouth. This type of dissection is performed when an elective neck dissection is indicated in the management of patients who have SCCA of the lip or skin of the midportion of the face and when these lesions are associated with clinically discrete, single metastases to the submental or submandibular nodes. A bilateral dissection is performed when the lesion is located at or near the midline.

The need to remove routinely the nodes in level IV in patients with cancer of the oral tongue is controversial. Byers et al. (48) reported finding "skip metastases" in 15.8% of patients with oral tongue cancer. In these cases, metastases to either level IV or level III were the only manifestation of the disease in the neck. In a similar more recent review of 119 neck dissections in patients with cancer of the oral cavity, De Zinis et al. (85) found metastases in level IV nodes in 15% of the patients and 28% of them were skip metastases. In another study of 49 patients with cancer of the oral cavity, staged N0, undergoing "extended supraomohyoid" neck dissection, occult metastases in level IV were found in 10% of the cases (86). These and other authors contend that the supraomohyoid neck dissection is inadequate for a complete pathologic evaluation of all the nodes at risk, and they recommend dissecting the nodes in level IV when performing an elective neck dissection in patients with cancer of the oral tongue.

The opposing point of view has been advanced by Khafif et al. (87) whose practice has been to dissect level IV only when a suspicious node is found at level III or there are multiple obviously involved lymph nodes. They reported their findings in a cohort of 58 patients with SCCA of the oral tongue (stage T1–T2 N0). The node dissections performed included levels I through III in 42 patients (69%), levels I through IV in 16 patients (26%), and levels I through V in 1 patient (5%). A positive node was found in level IV in only one instance (1/54, 1.8%), and no recurrences were observed in level IV. Ambrosch et al. (68) reported similar observations in a study of 167 patients with cancer of the oral cavity and oropharynx of whom 82 had a clinically staged N0 neck. They dissected level IV only when multiple metastases were suspected during the neck dissection. At a median follow-up of 34 months, the rate of regional recurrence in that series was 5.4%. Shah et al. (62) studied RND specimens performed as elective treatment for oral cavity tumors and found metastatic involvement of level IV in 3% of the patients. Li et al. (88) studied 153 patients who had an RND for oral cavity cancer (60 therapeutic and 93 elective) and found metastases to level IV in 3.2% of the patients. Wang et al. (89) studied 116 patients with oral tongue cancer, staged N0, who underwent comprehensive neck dissections and 5 patients who had SND. Metastases in level IV or level V were found in only one patient each. Interestingly, there were five cases with level III involvement as a first echelon of metastasis.

These studies and others (90) have shown that the risk of metastases to level IV in patients with cancer of the oral tongue with clinically negative neck is low, thus the controversy about the routine inclusion of this level in such patients.

ND II–IV (Lateral Neck Dissection). This type of SND is indicated in patients with tumors of the larynx, oropharynx, and hypopharynx staged T2–T4 N0. Because the lymphatic drainage of these regions is such that metastases are frequently bilateral, the operation is often done on both sides of the neck.

The need to dissect the lymph nodes of sublevel IIB and level IV in every patient undergoing elective SND for laryngeal cancer has recently been questioned. In 2006, Rinaldo et al. (91) collected data from five prospective, multi-institutional studies of neck dissection specimens using pathologic and molecular analysis. These studies included 211 patients with laryngeal cancer and clinically N0 neck. Only three patients (1.4%) were found to have positive lymph nodes at sublevel IIB (one patient had also lymph node metastases to sublevel IIA and level III; the other two patients had also a positive lymph node at sublevel IIA). In a more recent prospective multi-institutional study, metastases in sublevel IIB nodes were found in only 2% of 92 neck dissections done for laryngeal cancer (92). This and other recent studies have shown that the incidence of sublevel IIB metastases in patients undergoing elective neck dissection for hypopharyngeal and oropharyngeal cancers is also low, ranging between 5% and 9% for hypopharyngeal cancer and between 0% and 6% for oropharyngeal cancer (92–94). These observations strongly suggest that dissection of sublevel IIB is not necessary in patients with larynx, oropharynx, and hypopharynx cancer and clinically N0 neck. Since dissection of this region requires, in most patients, a more extensive manipulation of the spinal accessory nerve, avoiding it can decrease operative time and the risk of postoperative dysfunction of this nerve, as it has been suggested by a recent study using electromyography (95). The need to electively dissect level IV in patients with laryngeal cancer has also been questioned recently. In a review of 43 patients with laryngeal SCCA who underwent elective ND of levels II–IV, Khafif et al. (96) found that only one patient (2.3%) had metastases in level IV nodes and that patient also had metastases in level II nodes. Others have reported similar observations indicating that the prevalence of positive nodes found in level IV in the absence of palpable metastases elsewhere in the neck varies from 0% to 2.3% (73,97). Furthermore, a recent analysis of the data from three prospective multi-institutional studies of neck dissection specimens, including 175 patients with laryngeal cancer and clinically N0 necks, revealed only 6 patients (3.4%) with positive lymph nodes at level IV (98,99). Based on a thorough review of prospective multi-institutional studies published to date, Ferlito et al. (100) concluded that dissection of sublevel IIa

and level III appears to be adequate for the elective surgical treatment of the neck in supraglottic and glottic carcinomas. Appropriate outcome studies are now needed to ascertain that not dissecting these areas of the neck will not have a negative effect on regional control of the disease.

There appears to be a role for elective SND in patients previously treated with primary radiation therapy or chemoradiation for SCCA of the head and neck, who had recurrence or persistent disease at the primary site or develop a second primary tumor. In a retrospective study of 69 such patients who underwent SND as part of their treatment, Solares et al. (101) found metastases evident histologically in 23% of the SND specimens. There were no cases of recurrence in the neck when the primary site remained controlled. All patients who had more than two positive nodes had recurrence either at the primary site or distant metastasis. The authors concluded that SND is oncologically safe in the management of the N0 previously irradiated neck and that the finding of more than two positive nodes is associated with a poor outcome.

SND of Level VI. The role of elective dissection of the lymph nodes in level VI, also referred to as the central compartment dissection, is the main controversy in the surgical management of differentiated carcinoma of the thyroid today (102). The most recent guidelines published by the American Thyroid Association state that "prophylactic central-compartment neck dissection (ipsilateral or bilateral) may be performed in patients with papillary thyroid carcinoma with clinically uninvolved central neck lymph nodes, especially for advanced primary tumors (T3 or T4)" (103).

SND is now the preferred type of neck dissection for the elective surgical management of the cervical lymph nodes in patients with malignant tumors of the head and neck. The effectiveness of the ND (I–III/"supraomohyoid") and the ND (II–IV/"lateral") in the treatment of the N0 and N1 neck in patients with SCCA of the upper aerodigestive tract has been evaluated in a prospective analysis of our practice in which the indications for the operations, the surgical technique, and the indications for postoperative radiation were standardized. The overall recurrence rates observed in the dissected side of the neck at 2 years, with the primary tumor under control, was 3.4% when the lymph nodes removed were histologically negative and 12.5% when multiple positive nodes or extracapsular invasion were found. These results are typical of what has been reported in the literature during the past two decades regarding the effectiveness of SND in the management of the N0 neck (39,40,68–78,104).

Therapeutic SND: N+ Neck. SND is being used with increasing frequency in the management of selected patients with clinically obvious lymph node metastases (N+). In order to determine the feasibility of doing a supraomohyoid neck dissection in patients with oral cavity carcinoma who have a single clinically metastatic lymph node smaller than 6 cm (N1 and N2a), Kowalski and Carvalho (60) studied 164 oral cavity cancer patients with clinically N1 or N2a stage cancer submitted to RND. Interestingly, metastases were found in level IV lymph nodes in only one patient (0.6%), and metastases were not found in level V nodes. The authors concluded that in patients with clinical N1 stage in whom the metastasis is at level I, a supraomohyoid neck dissection (extended or not to level IV) is feasible instead of an RND. Andersen et al. (105) recently reported a 10-year multi-institutional retrospective review of pooled data from 106 previously untreated clinically and pathologically node-positive patients undergoing 129 SNDs and followed for a minimum of 2 years or until death. The neck was clinically staged N1 in 58 patients (57.7%), N2a in 5 (4.7%), N2b in 28 (26.4%), N2c in 14 (13.2%), and N3 in 1 (0.9%). Extracapsular extension of the tumor was present pathologically in 36 patients (34.0%), and postoperative radiation therapy was administered to 76 patients (71.7%). Overall, nine patients had recurrence in the neck. Six of these recurrences were in the areas of the neck that had been dissected during the SND, for a regional recurrence rate of 5.7%. The recurrence rates reported by others using SND in the N+ neck range from 5.5% to 11.1% (mean recurrence rate of 8.3%) (106,107). These rates are comparable to those reported after MRND or RND (36,42,43,54, 108–110) although absolute comparison is difficult because the SND patients represented a more selected sample (67). Nonetheless, these observations support the use of SND in selected patients with clinically positive nodal metastasis from SCCA of the upper aerodigestive tract.

Extended Neck Dissections

Any of the neck dissections described herein can be "extended" to include either lymph node groups that are not routinely removed (i.e., retropharyngeal, paratracheal, upper mediastinal) or other structures that are not routinely removed (i.e., skin of the neck, carotid artery, levator scapulae, vagus or hypoglossal nerve).

Skin, Muscles, Nerves
In a review of 106 cases of extended neck dissections, the largest review on record in the literature, involvement of the skin occurred in 18% of cases (111). Involvement of the skin did not have a significant prognostic implication.

Involvement of muscles requiring extension of the neck dissection may affect superficial, prevertebral, and paraspinal muscles. The superficial group is composed of the strap muscles (sternohyoid, sternothyroid, and omohyoid), the mylohyoid, and the digastric/stylohyoid muscle complex. Removal of one or more of these muscles was the reason for extending neck dissections in as many as 62% of the cases studied by Carew and Spiro (111), the digastric muscle being among the structures sacrificed in 51% of cases. The functional deficit resulting from removal of

these muscles is of little consequence and their removal usually does not require reconstruction. The dissection was extended to include the prevertebral muscles in only 3% of the cases. The muscles deep to the sternocleidomastoid that may be involved by a tumor are the splenius capitis, the levator scapulae, and the semispinalis capitis muscles. Involvement of these muscles occurs most commonly just lateral to the carotid artery. It was the reason to extend a neck dissection in 14% to 18% of cases.

Tumors may be adherent to or involve several important nerves in the neck. Since the lymph nodes in level II are the most common site of metastases, it stands to reason that the nerve most commonly involved is the hypoglossal nerve (41%). This is followed distantly by the sympathetic chain (8%), the lingual nerve (7%), the vagus nerve (4%), the superior laryngeal nerve (3%), the phrenic nerve (3%), and the glossopharyngeal nerve (2%) (111). When a nerve is resected, it is advisable to obtain an intraoperative frozen section of the margin of resection even if the appearance of the nerve is normal; perineural tumor spread is initially axial and may not result in thickening of the nerve until late (112).

Retropharyngeal Lymph Node Dissection
The RPLNs lie within a fat pad located behind the posterior wall of the pharynx and anterior to the prevertebral fascia and the cervical sympathetic trunk and ganglion. This fat pad extends from about the level of the carotid bifurcation to just below the skull base. The RPLNs are divided into medial and lateral groups; the medial group of nodes lies behind the pharyngeal midline at a level between the first and fourth cervical vertebrae. The lateral group of nodes, better known as the nodes of Rouviere, are the nodes removed in an RPLN dissection. They are contained within a sliver of fatty tissue located immediately medial to the internal carotid artery. The RPLNs receive lymphatic drainage from the nasopharynx, tonsillar fossa, oropharyngeal and hypopharyngeal walls, and the posterior ethmoidal sinuses.

Clinically, involvement of the retropharyngeal nodes by the tumor may be signaled by pain and stiffness in the neck. More ominous and characteristic is an ipsilateral occipitoparietal headache described by the patient as pain located behind the eye. Also ominous is the presence of a Horner syndrome that results from tumor involvement of the cervical sympathetic trunk.

The highest incidence of RPLN metastases is associated with advanced cancers of the oropharynx and hypopharynx in patients who present with neck metastases. Therefore, elective RPLN dissection is indicated when these patients are treated surgically. An RPLN dissection should also be performed in patients in whom imaging studies suggest the presence of metastases in the RPLN. An RPLN dissection should also be considered in patients with advanced cancer of the oropharynx and hypopharynx who are treated with organ preservation protocols, have an incomplete response of the tumor in the neck, and require a neck dissection. An RPLN dissection in these situations is likely to afford the patient perhaps a last opportunity to prevent recurrence in the RPLN.

Dissection of the retropharyngeal nodes can be performed separately or in continuity with the resection of the primary tumor. When it is done electively, this operation is relatively simple and it takes only a few minutes. On the other hand, when the RPLNs are grossly involved by the tumor, the operation may be difficult and sometimes not feasible. The proximity of the nodes to the internal carotid artery and prevertebral structures is such that these structures may be involved as soon as tumor extends beyond the capsule of the lymph nodes. The technique of retropharyngeal node dissection has been described in detail by Vasan and Medina (7).

In a retrospective study designed to assess the frequency of RPLN metastases in 774 patients with SCCA of the nasopharynx, oropharynx, hypopharynx, and supraglottis, using enlargement of the RPLN on CT scans as an indicator of the presence of metastases, McLaughlin et al. (113) found an overall incidence of radiologically "positive" RPLN of 9% in the patients. The highest incidence was seen in patients with cancer of the nasopharynx (74%) and the pharyngeal walls (19%). They also noted that in patients with advanced cancer of the oropharyngeal walls and hypopharynx, the incidence of radiologically positive RPLN was higher in patients with cervical metastases (N+ necks) than in those with an N0 neck (pharyngeal wall: N+ 21%, N0 16%; hypopharynx: N+ 9%, N0 0%) (113).

Amatsu et al. (114) studied 82 patients who had RPLN dissection for SCCA of the hypopharynx and cervical esophagus. They reported finding metastases in the RPLN in 16 patients (20%) (114). Fourteen of these patients had hypopharyngeal cancer, and the posterior pharyngeal wall was involved in 57% of them. In keeping with the studies mentioned previously, the majority of patients with RPLN metastases also had metastases in other neck nodes. However, in 15% of the patients with RPLN metastases, the neck was staged N0 (114).

In these studies, the presence of RPLN metastases did not appear to influence survival (115,116). Recently, Gross et al. (117) found no statistically significant difference in the rate of local/regional recurrence, survival, or distant metastases between patients with RPLN metastases and those without them. These authors attribute this finding to more aggressive, multimodality treatment of these patients, and they advocate performing RPLN in patients with advanced tumors of the oropharynx, hypopharynx, and supraglottic larynx (117).

Paratracheal and Upper Mediastinal Lymph Node Dissection

The paratracheal nodes are a common site of metastases for laryngeal carcinomas that involve the subglottic region and for carcinomas of the cervical esophagus.

In a study that included 91 patients with carcinoma of the larynx who underwent PTLN dissection, Weber et al. found that metastases to these lymph nodes occurred more often in patients with subglottic tumors (40%) and transglottic tumors (21.4%), but they also occurred in patients with glottic (13%) and supraglottic tumors (15.7%). The presence of PTLN metastases had a significant negative impact on survival. While the survival at 48 months for the entire group of 141 patients was 60%, none of the 29 patients with PTLN metastases survived beyond 42 months ($P > 0.001$) (8). In 2005, Plaat et al. performed a retrospective study of 85 patients who underwent total laryngectomy and PTLN dissection for laryngeal and hypopharyngeal carcinomas. The prevalence of PTLN metastases was 30%, 12%, and 67% in patients with supraglottic, glottic, and subglottic carcinomas, respectively. Among all laryngeal carcinomas with subglottic extension, PTLN metastases were found in 27% of the cases (118).

Based on the anatomy of the lymphatic drainage of the different laryngeal sites and on the pertinent clinical observations described in the literature, dissection or treatment with radiation of the lymph nodes in level VI is indicated in the following situations (51):

1. Primary subglottic carcinomas. Treatment/dissection in these cases should include the pretracheal and the paratracheal nodes on both sides.
2. Advanced (T3–T4) glottic carcinomas particularly those with involvement of the anterior commissure and with subglottic extension. In tumors confined to one side of the larynx, treatment/dissection should include the prelaryngeal, pretracheal, and the ipsilateral paratracheal nodes. In tumors involving both sides of the larynx, treatment should include the paratracheal nodes on both sides.
3. Advanced (T3–T4) supraglottic carcinomas, particularly those with involvement of the ventricle/ paraglottic space, those with the anterior commissure, and those with clinically apparent lymph node metastases in the lateral compartment of the neck. In tumors confined to one side of the larynx, treatment/dissection should include the prelaryngeal, pretracheal, and the ipsilateral paratracheal nodes. In tumors involving both sides of the larynx, treatment should include the paratracheal nodes on both sides.

In these situations, a neck dissection may need to be extended to include the paratracheal and pretracheal lymph nodes; failure to do so may predispose to the development of peristomal recurrence. It should also be emphasized that the presence of metastases in PTLN has been found to be associated with increased tumor recurrence (51).

In addition, lymph node metastases from thyroid carcinomas tend to occur first in the paratracheal nodes regardless of the location of the primary within the thyroid gland (119).

Resection of the Carotid Artery

Controversy still exists about the advisability of extending a neck dissection to resect the common or the internal carotid artery. Initial reports on carotid artery resection showed very poor results, with approximately 50% of patients suffering either a severe stroke or death. Recent reports have shown a decrease in these events to approximately 25%, with modest improvement in survival compared to those who did not undergo resection. This is epitomized by the recent report by Freeman et al. (120) of their experience with 58 patients with neck metastasis adherent to the internal or common carotid artery. Angiography was used in patients who demonstrated fixation of the tumor to the carotid artery on examination or imaging, followed by balloon test occlusion and single photon emission computer tomography (SPECT) brain scanning. In most patients (70%), the carotid was reconstructed with a vein graft, especially if there was insufficient collateral cerebral circulation. In addition, these patients were given 15 to 20 Gy of intraoperative radiation. In their more recent cases, the carotid was permanently occluded preoperatively when possible. Unfortunately, in spite of such aggressive treatment preceded by a systematic, "state of the art" preoperative assessment, the median disease-specific survival was 12 months and 11 patients (19%) suffered a stroke (120). The mean 1-year disease-free survival rates reported in the literature after resection and reconstruction of the carotid vary between 0% and 44% (121).

When considering resection of the carotid the surgeon must make critical preoperative, intraoperative, and postoperative decisions. Preoperative evaluation of these patients requires a clear understanding of the methods available for assessment of the cerebral circulation. Several tests are available that involve occlusion of the carotid artery with either digital pressure (Matas test) or using a balloon during arteriography. The objective of each method is to determine a "critical point" that indicates when reconstruction of the artery is necessary. With the transcranial color Doppler method, the "critical point" is reverse flow from the external carotid artery to the internal carotid. Technetium-99m hexamethylpropyleneamine oxime brain SPECT measures cerebral perfusion. A 19% to 29% reduction in radioactivity is considered the "critical point." Unlike some of the other methods, this is not a real-time measurement but requires delayed imaging. Another method uses Xenon in an aerosolized mixture that is inhaled by the patient, and then cerebral perfusion is measured by CT scan. Xenon is concentrated in areas of the brain that are well perfused, correlating with blood flow. Two CT scans are obtained to assess cerebral blood flow: the first one during balloon occlusion and the second after the balloon is released. The "critical point" is a 25% reduction in the degree of enhancement on the first occlusion scan compared to the open study. Electroencephalography has a distinct disadvantage

compared to other methods. It does not evaluate blood flow volume to the brain directly. However, it has the advantage that it can be used intraoperatively. The "critical point" is a 50% attenuation of the somatosensory-evoked cortical potential in relation to the preoperative exam. Finally, stump pressure measurements can be taken during angiography to determine the pressure on the distal side of the balloon when it is occluded. The critical point is a measurement of less than 50 mm Hg. There is significant individual variability with this measurement, as it is affected by systemic blood pressure.

Intraoperatively, patients with frank involvement of the carotid wall whose preoperative evaluation indicates intolerance to carotid ligation should have the carotid reconstructed. Saphenous vein grafts are preferred over prosthetic grafts for reconstruction, and if the skin has been heavily radiated or a portion of skin over the carotid is resected, an appropriate flap should be used to cover the graft. There is still considerable debate regarding the routine use of intraoperative shunts, and to date, there has not been a prospective study to prove their usefulness. However, shunting is clearly indicated when there is angiographic evidence of inadequate flow through the circle of Willis.

Postoperatively, delayed strokes can occur in as many as 25% of patients who have undergone carotid artery resection without reconstruction, even if they "passed" the balloon occlusion test (122). Flow from the contralateral side through the circle of Willis prevents a stroke initially. However, the resection creates an arterial stump that begins at the takeoff of the middle cerebral artery and continues down to the level of the resection. This can be a site for thrombus formation, which can then propagate up into the circle of Willis. Alternatively, the thrombus may produce emboli that can travel into the distribution of the middle cerebral artery. While these mechanisms have not been conclusively proven, many surgeons advocate the use of heparin postoperatively to prevent delayed strokes following resection of the internal carotid artery. Recommended doses range from 5,000 units subcutaneously twice a day to full therapeutic anticoagulation (123). The benefit of anticoagulation has not been shown in a prospective controlled study.

"CONTRAINDICATIONS" TO NECK DISSECTION

It is not advisable to attempt a neck dissection when the diagnostic evaluation of the patient reveals any of the following circumstances: (a) frank involvement of the carotid wall in patients whose preoperative evaluation indicates intolerance to carotid ligation, and the location and extent of the tumor in the neck is near the skull base, precluding reconstruction of the carotid artery and (b) involvement of the base of the skull, paraspinal muscles, and transverse processes of the cervical vertebrae and the brachial plexus.

ADJUVANT THERAPY FOLLOWING NECK DISSECTION

Numerous studies in the 1980s showed that the rate of tumor recurrence in the neck is decreased by the addition of postoperative radiation, when multiple nodes are involved at multiple levels of the neck, and when extracapsular spread (ECS) of the tumor is found (124–126). Since then, it has also been accepted that timing of the initiation of radiotherapy is important; delays beyond 6 weeks may compromise tumor control (125). The seminal study of Peters et al. in the early 1990s established the dose of postoperative radiation therapy that is essential to achieve optimal results. Daily fractions of 1.8 Gy to a total dose of 57.6 Gy to the entire operative bed is currently recommended. Sites of increased risk for recurrence, such as areas of the neck where ECS of the tumor was found, should be boosted to 63 Gy (127). A prospective, randomized clinical study published in 2004 showed that the concurrent postoperative administration of chemotherapy (cisplatin 100 mg/m² on days 1, 22, and 43) and radiotherapy (60 to 66 Gy in 30 to 33 fractions over 6 to 6.6 weeks) significantly improved the rates of local and regional control and disease-free survival in patients with high-risk resected head and neck cancers (128). The high-risk criteria included any or all of the following: histologic evidence of metastases in two or more lymph nodes, ECS, and microscopically involved margins of resection. Although the study subjects were stratified according to the presence or absence of microscopically positive margins, the published results did not include an analysis of outcomes with and without concomitant chemotherapy in the cohort of patients with microscopically negative margins, which would have elucidated whether or not the addition of chemotherapy was beneficial to patients with high-risk neck disease. A similar study by the European Organization for Research and Treatment of Cancer (EORTC), published at the same time, included patients with various clinical (primary tumor and nodal volume and nodal site) and pathologic (involved margins of resection, ECS, perineural involvement, and vascular embolism) high-risk factors related to neck metastases (129). It also showed that concomitant postoperative chemoradiation was significantly more efficacious than radiation alone in these high-risk patients. However, resection margins were positive in 30% of the patients included in the study and the design did not include an analysis focused on the neck disease factors. Nonetheless, both of these studies suggest that the addition of chemotherapy may be beneficial to patients with resectable head and neck cancers who have advanced neck metastases, N2–N3, and to patients with N0 or N1 disease who are found to have multiple histologically positive nodes or ECS of the tumor.

In a subsequent analysis of both the EORTC and Radiation Therapy Oncology Group (RTOG) studies, Bernier et al. (130) found that chemoradiation improved overall survival in patients with ECS and/or positive margins in both studies (EORTC $P = 0.0019$; RTOG $P = 0.0.63$). Thus, in regard to adjuvant treatment of neck metastases following neck dissection, the presence of ECS of the tumor is currently considered an indication for postoperative concurrent chemoradiation.

CURRENT CONTROVERSIES

Pertinent controversies regarding neck dissection concern the need for postoperative radiation in patients with pathologically proven metastasis in a single cervical lymph node (pN1) and the need for and the extent of "planned" neck dissection in patients with SCCA of the upper aerodigestive tract who have clinically obvious neck node metastases (N+ neck) and are treated with radiation alone or in combinations with chemotherapy.

IS Postoperative Radiation Beneficial in the Pathologically N_1 (pN$_1$) Neck?

When a single metastasis is found (pN$_1$) in a neck dissection specimen, surgery alone has been considered adequate treatment. Recently, however, regional recurrence rates from 16% to 25% have been reported with surgery alone, and it has been suggested that postoperative radiation may be beneficial (73,131).

In a retrospective analysis of 517 SNDs performed in 363 patients, Byers et al. found 51 (17.6%) patients who had metastases in only one lymph node (pathologically N1) with or without ECS. A regional failure occurred in 2 of 36 (5.6%) of these patients who received postoperative radiation and in 5 of 14 patients (35.7%) who did not. All recurrences were within the dissected area of the neck (73). More recently, Chen et al. (132) analyzed 59 patients with T1–T2/N0–N1 SCCA of the oral cavity to determine the effect of postoperative radiation. Of the patients staged pathologically N1, 28 received postoperative radiation and 31 did not. With a mean follow-up period of 46 months (12–109), locoregional recurrences occurred in 14% of the patients who received postoperative radiation and in 39% of the patients who did not. As in the Byers' study, all regional recurrences occurred within the dissected neck. To characterize further the impact of the N1 status and radiation, the authors excluded from the analysis patients with ECS, positive margins, lymphovascular invasion, and perineural invasion and compared those who had received post-op XRT with those who did not. The 5-year disease-free survival rate and overall survival were 95% and 92.3%, respectively, for the group that received postoperative radiation and 54.7% and 54.9%, respectively, for the group that did not. On the other hand, radiation was not found to be beneficial in an unpublished retrospective review we conducted of 58 patients with T1/T2 SCCA of the oral tongue treated with surgery, which included an ipsilateral SND, who were found to have metastasis in a single lymph node. These patients were treated at seven institutions and were followed for a minimum of 2 years. Twenty-two (38%) patients were treated with surgery alone, while 36 (62%) received postoperative radiation. In the group treated with surgery alone, two patients had recurrence at the primary site and in the neck. Of the remaining 20 patients, 6 patients (30%) had recurrences in the neck (5 contralateral and 1 simultaneous ipsilateral and contralateral). In the surgery plus radiation group, four (11%) tumors recurred in the neck, all within the operative field. The difference in the rate of recurrence in the neck for the two groups was not statistically significant.

Thus, it appears that a prospective randomized study is necessary to determine in a controlled manner whether or not postoperative radiation is beneficial in patients whose neck is pathologically staged N1.

"Planned" Neck Dissection After "Organ Preservation" for Squamous Cell Carcinoma of the Head and Neck

The treatment of advanced carcinomas of the larynx and pharynx has evolved from surgery and postoperative radiation to "organ preservation" strategies with hyperfractionated radiation and more recently with various combinations of radiation and chemotherapy. This has brought up several dilemmas in the management of patients with clinically obvious lymph node metastases, particularly those with advanced neck disease (N2–N3).

The first dilemma is whether or not a planned neck dissection should be performed, irrespective of the response of the tumor in the neck to the treatment with radiation or chemoradiation. Some clinicians argue that a neck dissection should be carried out as part of the treatment plan, irrespective of the response of the tumor in the neck, because the clinical and pathologic responses of the tumor in the neck correlate poorly with each other. In a study by Brizel et al. (133), a planned neck appeared to confer a disease-free survival and overall-survival advantage in patients with N2–N3 disease undergoing chemoradiation, with acceptably low morbidity. This was a retrospective study of a cohort of 108 patients with advanced squamous carcinoma of the head and neck, who presented with nodal disease and were treated with hyperfractionated radiotherapy and concurrent cisplatinum and 5-fluorouracil. A "modified neck dissection" was performed in 65 patients, while 29 patients did not undergo neck dissection because of "the physician and/or patient preference." The 4-year disease-free survival was 70% for patients with N1 disease, irrespective of the clinical response or whether a neck dissection was performed. For patients with N2–N3 disease who had a complete clinical response to chemoradiation, the 4-year disease-free survival rate was 75% for those who had a neck dissection and 53% for those who did not. This difference was not statistically significant ($P = 0.08$). However, the 4-year overall survival rate was significantly better (77% vs. 50%) for the group treated with

neck dissection ($P = 0.04$). These authors and others have suggested that a planned neck dissection be considered for all patients with N2 and N3 disease (133,134).

On the other hand, some clinicians argue that it is not necessary to perform a "planned" neck dissection when the tumor in the neck undergoes a complete response to the treatment (135,136). This position is based on the observation that less than a third of patients with clinically positive nodes before therapy have histologic evidence of metastases at neck dissection (137), even when there is residual clinical or radiologic "adenopathy" in the neck after completion of (chemo)radiation (138,139). Furthermore, when the tumor in the neck undergoes a complete response to the treatment, the probability of an isolated recurrence in the neck is low (0% to 11%) if the patients are simply observed (135–141).

The controversy over whether or not a planned neck dissection (PND) is needed is in good part due to the inability to determine, preoperatively, when a complete clinical response is associated with the presence or absence of viable tumor cells. PET scanning may be useful in identifying the subset of patients who need a neck dissection, since this imaging modality has been shown to be more accurate than others in the evaluation of patients following treatment (142). However, the timing of posttreatment PET imaging appears to be important. In a series of 12 patients studied prospectively by Rogers et al. (143) a positive PET 1 month after radiation therapy accurately indicated the presence of residual disease in all cases; however, a negative PET indicated absence of disease in only 14% of the cases. Other studies have also shown that PET scan obtained 1 month after completion of treatment with radiation was inaccurate in predicting the presence of residual cancer (144). In contrast, a PET scan done 12 weeks after completion of treatment with radiation or chemoradiation may be more useful (145). Porceddu et al. (146) evaluated the utility of PET imaging in 39 N+ patients who achieved a complete response at the primary site but had a residual mass in the neck, 8 weeks or more after definitive (chemo)radiotherapy. The PET scan was performed at a median of 12 weeks (range, 8 to 32 weeks) after treatment. Interestingly, the PET scan showed no metabolic activity in the residual mass in 32 patients. Five of these patients had a neck dissection and the neck dissections were all pathologically negative. The remaining 27 patients were observed for a median of 34 months (range 16 to 86 months), and only one of them had a locoregional recurrence. Thus, the NPV of PET for viable disease in a residual anatomic abnormality in the neck was 97%. These authors concluded that a neck dissection is not necessary in patients who have achieved a complete response at the primary site but have a residual abnormality in the neck that is PET negative approximately 12 weeks after treatment and that these patients can be observed safely. Others have reported similar results. Rabalais et al. (147) in a retrospective analysis of 52 patients treated with chemoradiation therapy (CRT) found that 10 (19.2%) had a positive PET scan on an average 11.8 weeks after completion of treatment. Three of the ten underwent neck dissection of which two partial responders had residual disease and the one complete responder did not. The remaining 7 (70%) patients were observed only. One of these patients was shown to have residual tumor on FNA but was not a surgical candidate for neck dissection and another had disease in the neck in addition to persistent disease at the primary site. Of the five remaining patients with positive PET-CT results who did not undergo PND, all five showed gradual resolution of the disease on serial PET-CT scans with no failures in the neck. Of the 42 (81%) who had a negative posttreatment PET finding, 2 underwent neck dissection for palpable lymphadenopathy and 3 had neck dissections as a component of salvage surgery for the primary tumor. None of the five neck dissection specimens revealed residual tumor. There were no isolated neck recurrences in the remaining 37 patients (average follow-up of 60.4 weeks). Recently, Corry et al. (148) reviewed their experience with N2/N3 disease following CRT in 102 patients. Of the 28 patients in whom there was a complete response within the primary and a partial response in the neck, 11 patients demonstrated resolution of their adenopathy with continued observation, 1 was diagnosed with metastatic disease prior to any further therapy, and 16 patients had a neck dissection of which 9/16 (65%) were pathologically negative. In another study, patients with a clinically complete response to chemoradiation who were observed rather than having a neck dissection demonstrated a regional failure rate of 3% to 8%, and if negative PET imaging was included as part of the definition of a complete response, the regional failure rate decreased to 0% to 3% (149). Thus, it appears from this information that observation with a PET-CT obtained at least 12 weeks after completion of chemoradiation is a reasonable alternative to a "routine" planned neck dissection (149).

The second dilemma regarding "planned" neck dissections is the extent of the operation. Traditionally, surgeons performed comprehensive neck dissections (levels I–V) with or without preservation of nonlymphatic structures (150). Recently, however, surgeons have reported performing SNDs with reasonable results (151). Robbins et al. (140,151) performed 33 SNDs in patients treated with targeted intra-arterial high-dose cisplatin infusions combined with radiation therapy (RADPLAT). There was only one recurrence in the neck. Stenson et al. (152) reported the results in 69 patients who had planned neck dissections after various concomitant chemoradiation protocols. The majority of them (56/69) underwent an SND and only one patient had a recurrence in the neck. These studies suggest that SND may be an appropriate option for some patients with an N+ neck who are treated with organ preservation regimens.

Robbins et al. (153) in 2005 reported the results of 106 neck dissections performed in 84 patients with advanced N stage disease (N2–N3) that were treated with the RADPLAT protocol. Fourteen neck dissections were radical or modified radical, eighty-one were selective, and eleven were dissections of levels II and III and were labeled as "super selective neck dissections" (SSNDs). Interestingly, there were no recurrences in the neck in the group that underwent SSND. The authors outlined the indications for the different types of neck dissection as follows: In general, an RND or MRND was performed in patients in whom the residual lymphadenopathy involved multiple levels, an SND was performed when the residual disease was confined to two levels involving the lymph node groups at greatest risk, and an SSND was performed when the residual lymphadenopathy was confined to one level.

Vasan et al., at our institution, investigated the feasibility of performing a "single-level dissection." To that end, they studied a cohort of 51 patients, treated between January 1999 and March 2005, who underwent a total of 55 "planned" neck dissections for clinically or radiologically apparent residual disease in the neck, after definitive treatment of the primary tumor and neck with radiation therapy alone or with chemotherapy (138). The primary tumor was in the tonsil in 20 (39%) patients, base of the tongue in 12 (23%), supraglottic larynx in 10 (20%), hypopharynx in 4 (8%), faucial arch in 3 (6%), and "unknown" in 2 (4%). The neck was staged N1 in 19 (38%) patients, N2A in 8 (16%), N2B in 10 (20%), N2C in 6 (12%), and N3 in 7 (14%). All patients were treated with radiation therapy with curative intent. The mean radiation dose was 7,077 cGy and 5,814 cGy to the primary and neck, respectively. Twelve patients also received chemotherapy. The neck dissections performed included lymph node levels II–IV in 32 (58%) of the cases, II–III in 16 (29%), I–IV in 4 (7.1%), and one each of I–IV, II–V, and II only. In 19 dissections (34%), nonlymphatic structures were removed, including the IJV (19/34%), a portion or all of the SCM (14/25%), the digastric (5/9%), and the cranial nerve XI (4/7%). Interestingly, Robbins et al. (140,151) also reported the need to remove one or more of these nonlymphatic structures in 24% of "planned" SNDs. The pathologists found histologically "viable looking" tumor in one or more lymph nodes in 15 of the 55 neck dissection specimens; thus, the yield of histologically positive nodes was 27.2%. In the analysis of the distribution of the positive nodes, five patients had clinical or radiologic evidence of metastases of one or more nodes in level II only; in all of them (5/5), histologically positive nodes were found only in level II. Eight patients had clinical/radiologic evidence of metastases in one or more nodes in levels II and III (one patient also had a node in level V); histologically positive nodes were found in level II in one instance, in level III in four, and in levels II, III, and IV in three. Two patients had clinically/radiologically positive nodes in levels I and II; histologically positive nodes were found in levels I and II in one of them and in levels I and III in the other. Over a mean follow-up time of 25.9 months, there were only two recurrences in the neck (4%).

These findings confirm the effectiveness of SND in the management of residual disease in the neck. In addition, they suggest that it may be feasible to perform a single-level dissection in patients whose disease is confined to level II nodes, before, during, and after treatment with radiation with or without chemotherapy. Boyd et al. (154) noted a predictable pattern of residual metastases following irradiation and suggested that a lateral (II–IV) neck dissection may be appropriate in the majority of patients. In this study, of nine positive specimens, six revealed malignant cells in a single nodal echelon. Obviously such an approach must be investigated further in prospective studies.

More recently, investigators have used CT scans of the neck following chemoradiation to determine the extent of neck dissection. Goguen et al. (155) and Yeung et al. (156) noted that the NPV for CT for the posttreatment neck was 95%. They noted that an SND or SSND guided by posttreatment CT would have captured all disease in 95% and 93% of the cases, respectively.

SEQUELAE OF NECK DISSECTION

The most notable sequelae observed in patients who have undergone an RND are related to removal of the spinal accessory nerve. The resulting denervation of the trapezius muscle, one of the most important shoulder abductors, causes destabilization of the scapula with progressive flaring at the vertebral border, drooping, and lateral and anterior rotation. The loss of trapezius function decreases the patient's ability to abduct the shoulder above 90 degrees. These physical changes result in the recognized shoulder syndrome of pain, weakness, and deformity of the shoulder girdle commonly associated with the RND. It should also be noted that preserving the cervical plexus contributions to the spinal accessory nerve may not decrease shoulder morbidity significantly (157). Furthermore, shoulder disability after neck dissection results not only from the spinal accessory nerve dysfunction but also from secondary glenohumeral stiffness caused by weakness of the scapulohumeral girdle muscles and postoperative immobility.

A number of studies have demonstrated that when compared with the RND, neck dissections that preserve the spinal accessory nerve are associated with less shoulder pain (158), better shoulder function, and overall quality of life (79–83,159). However, these studies also provide evidence that even procedures that involve minimal dissection of the spinal accessory nerve can result in shoulder dysfunction. Although this dysfunction is often reversible, it behooves the surgeon to make every effort to avoid undue trauma to the nerve, particularly stretching, during any neck dissection in which the nerve is preserved. In addition, every patient who undergoes neck dissection must be questioned about the function of the shoulder and must be evaluated by a physical therapist early in the postoperative period. If any deficit is detected, the patient should be properly counseled and coached to ensure proper rehabilitation of the shoulder. Physical therapy aimed to early recovery of passive motion and to avoid the occurrence of joint fibrosis has been shown to be beneficial (160). It has also been suggested that progressive resistance exercise training may be a useful adjunct to standard physical therapy (161). It should be kept in mind, as mentioned earlier, that shoulder pain after neck dissection may not be the result of dysfunction of the spinal accessory nerve. Consequently, if a patient experiences shoulder pain after neck dissection, the trapezius muscle and active bilateral abduction of the shoulder should be examined to determine if the spinal accessory nerve is involved (162).

COMPLICATIONS OF NECK DISSECTION

In addition to the medical complications that can occur after any surgical procedure in the head and neck region, several surgical complications can be related solely or in part to neck dissection.

Infection

Following clean neck dissections, those in which the upper aerodigestive tract is not entered, wound infections are not common. Interestingly, however, a recent prospective study, designed to evaluate the effects of a prophylactic antibiotic regimen (ampicillin–sulbactam for 24 hours) on the incidence of infection after clean neck dissection, showed that the infection rate in patients who were treated with the antibiotic was 1.7% compared to a significantly higher rate (13.3%) among patients who did not receive an antibiotic ($P = 0.02$) (163).

Air Leaks

Circulation of air through a wound drain is a common complication that usually is encountered during the first postoperative day. The point of entrance of air may be located somewhere along the skin incision. If the drains are connected to suction in the operating room near the completion of the wound closure, however, such an air leak usually becomes apparent then and can be corrected. Other points of entrance may not become apparent until after surgery, when the position of the neck changes or the patient begins to move. The typical example of this situation is the improperly secured suction wound drain that gets displaced, exposing one or more of the drain vents. A similar situation can occur when a skin graft to reconstruct a cutaneous defect is created in conjunction with the neck dissection. Movement of the neck can produce an air leak even after meticulous suturing of the skin graft. This can be prevented by applying an adhesive vinyl drape over the graft and surrounding skin to seal any possible air leak instead of or in addition to the bolster of gauze traditionally used to immobilize a skin graft.

Air leaks with potentially more serious consequences are those that occur through a communication of the neck wound with the tracheostomy site or through a mucosal suture line. In addition to air, contaminated secretions may be circulated through the wound. Thus, early identification of the site of leakage is desirable but may not be a simple task, and correcting it may require revision of the wound closure in the operating room.

Bleeding

Postoperative hemorrhage usually occurs immediately after surgery. External bleeding through the incision, without distortion of the skin flaps, often originates in a subcutaneous blood vessel. In most instances, this bleeding can be controlled readily by ligation or infiltration of the surrounding tissues with an anesthetic solution containing epinephrine. On the other hand, pronounced swelling or ballooning of the skin flaps in the immediate postoperative period, with or without external bleeding, must be attributed to a hematoma in the wound. If detected early, milking the drains occasionally may result in evacuation of the accumulated blood and resolve the problem. If this is not accomplished immediately or if blood reaccumulates quickly, however, it is best to return the patient to the operating room and to explore the wound under sterile conditions, evacuate the hematoma, and control the bleeding. Attempting to do this in the recovery room or at the bedside may be ill-advised, because lighting may be inadequate, surgical equipment improvised, and sterile conditions precarious. Failure to recognize or to manage properly a postoperative hematoma may predispose the patient to the development of a wound infection. Although bulky pressure dressings may be useful in curtailing postoperative edema, they do not prevent hematomas and may in fact delay their recognition.

Chylous Fistula

The reported incidence of chyle fistula following neck dissection varies between 1% and 2.5%. In most patients who develop a postoperative chylous fistula, a chylous leakage is identified and apparently controlled intraoperatively (164). These observations behoove the surgeon to avoid injury to the thoracic duct proper and also to ligate or clip any visualized or potential lymphatic tributaries in the area of the thoracic duct, which may be accomplished with relative ease if the operative field is kept bloodless when dissecting in this area of the neck. Furthermore, as soon as the dissection of this area is completed and again before closing the wound, the area is observed for 20 or 30 seconds while the anesthesiologist increases the intrathoracic pressure.

Even the smallest leak of chylous material must be pursued seriously until it is arrested. Direct clamping and ligating may be difficult and sometimes counterproductive as a result of the fragility of the lymphatic vessels and the surrounding fatty tissue. Hemoclips are ideal to control a source of leakage that is clearly visualized. Otherwise, it is preferable to use suture ligatures with pliable material, such as 5 to 0 silk, that are tied over a piece of hemostatic sponge to avoid tearing. In the immediate postoperative period, serum and drainage levels of triglycerides and cholesterol obtained on the first postoperative day may be useful parameters to predict early the occurrence of a chyle fistula (165).

Management of a chyle leak noted postoperatively depends on the time of onset of the leak, the amount of chyle drainage in a 24-hour period, and the presence or absence of accumulation of chyle under the skin flaps (164,166). When the daily output of chyle exceeds 600 mL in a day or 200 to 300 mL/day for 3 days, especially when the chyle fistula becomes apparent immediately after surgery, conservative closed wound management is unlikely to succeed (167). In such cases, it is preferable to explore the wound early, before the tissues exposed to the chyle become markedly inflamed and before the fibrinous material that coats these tissues becomes adherent, obscuring and jeopardizing important structures such as the phrenic and the vagus nerves. Surgical exploration is also warranted when chyle accumulates under the skin flaps either because of inadequate drain size or because of the volume or consistency of the chyle causes partial or compete obstruction of the drains.

On the other hand, chylous fistulae that become apparent later in the postoperative period, after enteral feedings are resumed, or those that drain less than 200 to 300 mL of chyle per day are initially managed conservatively with closed wound drainage, pressure dressings (which are cumbersome to secure in this area of the neck), repeated aspirations, and diet modifications aimed at decreasing chyle drainage while maintaining nutritional support. Usually, nutrition can be provided enterally using elemental diets supplemented with medium-chain triglycerides, which are absorbed directly into the portal circulation bypassing the lymphatic system. In some patients, parenteral nutrition may be necessary (168). If these measures fail, the neck is surgically explored and the leak is identified and dealt with appropriately. Sometimes, this intervention is unsuccessful and the leak persists. The use of fibrin glue and a clavicular periosteal flap may be useful to control the leak in such cases (169). Percutaneous lymphangiography guided cannulation and embolization of the thoracic duct is an effective minimally invasive alternative to open surgical intervention (170). Success with this technique has been reported in as many as 45% to 70% of the cases (167). In a recent report, Nyquist et al. described a case in which a chylous fistula stopped draining 24 hours after the administration of octreotide (100 micrograms given subcutaneously three times a day). These authors postulate that the effect of octreotide on chylous fistulae may be due to its ability to reduce gastrointestinal and pancreatic secretions, decrease hepatic venous pressure, and reduce splanchnic blood flow, which may decrease thoracic duct flow and relative concentration of triglycerides (171).

Ipsilateral chylothorax can occur following neck dissection. Bilateral chylothorax as a complication of neck dissection is extremely rare, but it is potentially serious and sometimes fatal (172,173).

Facial or Cerebral Edema

Synchronous bilateral RNDs, in which both IJVs are ligated, can result in the development of facial edema, cerebral edema, or both. The facial edema sometimes can be dramatically severe. It appears to be a mechanical problem of venous drainage, which resolves to a variable extent with time as collateral circulation is established. It appears to be more common and more severe in patients who had previous radiation to the head and neck and in those patients in whom the resection includes large segments of the lateral and posterior pharyngeal walls. We have been able to prevent massive facial edema by preserving at least one external jugular vein whenever a bilateral RND is anticipated. The external jugular usually is separated from the tumor in the neck by the SCM and can be dissected free between the tail of the parotid and the subclavian vein. Others have reconstructed one internal jugular using various techniques including vein with saphenous vein grafts or by using a segment of one of the resected jugular veins, distal to the site of tumor involvement (174,175). The development of cerebral edema may be at the root of the impaired neurologic function and even coma that can occur after bilateral RND. Following neck dissection, a syndrome of inappropriate secretion of antidiuretic hormone (SIADH) occurs in 8% to 30% of patients. This is a disorder in which release of antidiuretic hormone is independent of plasma osmolarity, resulting in fluid retention and development of dilutional hyponatremia. It occurs significantly more often in patients who have a history of smoking and it has been noted to resolve within 72 hours (176). It is commonly believed that synchronous, bilateral RND causes the SIADH, presumably as a result of increased intracranial pressure. This belief is based mainly on the results of an experimental study published in 1978 in which occlusion of the superior vena cava in dogs resulted in increased intracranial pressure and SIADH. Using an animal model that more closely resembles the clinical condition of bilateral RND, Khafif and Medina (177) found that bilateral synchronous IJV ligation and bilateral RNDs did not result in SIADH in dogs. As these results contradict a commonly held belief in clinical practice, a prospective evaluation of the physiologic changes after bilateral RNDs is warranted. Nevertheless, it is possible that an expansion of extracellular fluids and dilutional hyponatremia that occurs in some patients after neck dissection could aggravate cerebral edema, creating a vicious cycle. In practice, this behooves the surgeon and the anesthesiologist to curtail the administration of fluids during and after bilateral RNDs. Furthermore, perioperative management of fluid and electrolytes in these cases should not be guided solely by the patient's urine output, but also

by monitoring central venous pressure, cardiac output, and serum and urine osmolarity.

Blindness

Blindness after bilateral RND is a rare but catastrophic complication (178). The pathogenesis of it remains unclear. In one of the few cases reported in the literature, histologic examination revealed intraorbital optic nerve infarction, suggesting intraoperative hypotension and severe venous distention as possible etiologic factors. In another case, bilateral occipital lobe infarcts were demonstrated on CT scan (179).

Apnea

Some patients may become apneic as a result of loss of their hypoxic ventilatory responses due to carotid body denervation after bilateral neck dissection.

Jugular Vein Thrombosis

Preservation of the IJV during neck dissection does not ensure its patency after surgery, particularly when radiation therapy is also used. Cotter et al. (180) used preoperative and postoperative CT or MRI on 69 patients undergoing 79 vein-sparing neck dissections. Sixty-eight veins (86%) were patent postoperatively. Interestingly, radiation therapy appears to influence patency of the IJV. Cappiello et al. studied the patency of the IJV following selective lateral neck dissection in a cohort of 34 patients. A preoperative baseline study of vein patency and flow by US was obtained followed by postoperative evaluations at 1 week, 1 month, and 3 months. At 1 week postoperatively, 50% of the IJVs did not present any alteration in patency, 46% had reduced flow, and 4% showed absent flow. However, at 3 months, none of the patients showed evidence of IJV occlusion. Postoperative radiotherapy did not have a statistically significant impact on IJV patency ($P = 0.09$) (181).

A recent report describes the rate of complications after planned posttreatment neck dissections in patients enrolled in organ preservation protocols. The authors conclude that the rate is similar to that previously for neck dissections (37%) and that the rate increases when higher preoperative radiation therapy doses are used (182).

EMERGENCIES

Carotid Artery Rupture

The most feared and most commonly lethal complication after neck surgery is exposure and rupture of the carotid artery, the carotid blowout syndrome (CBS). Therefore, every effort must be made to prevent it. If the skin incisions have been designed properly, the carotid seldom becomes exposed in the absence of a salivary fistula. Fistula formation and flap breakdown are more likely to occur in the presence of malnutrition, diabetes, and prior radiation therapy, which impair healing capacity and compromise vascular supply. Faced with any of these risk factors, the surgeon must use flawless surgical technique in closing oral and pharyngeal defects. Use of perioperative antibiotics and, more importantly, use of free and pedicled vascularized flaps (which provide skin for closure of mucosal defects and variably bulky muscle that can protect the carotid) have rendered nearly obsolete the use of "protective" measures such as dermal grafts, levator scapulae muscle flaps, and controlled pharyngostomies.

Fortunately, CBS has become less frequent; however, its frequency may increase again as more salvage procedures are done in patients whose tumors fail to respond to chemoradiation regimens. Therefore, it is essential for all head and neck surgeons to be familiar with the current management of CBS. In a retrospective review of all HNC patients with a diagnosis of CBS seen at our tertiary cancer hospital from 1994 to 2009, we found eight patients who developed CBS. Powitzky et al. (183) recently published an analysis of these cases and a review of 21 studies published in the English-language literature within the past 15 years. They summarized the presentation, treatment, and outcomes of a total of 132 patients. Patients with CBS typically have a history of radiotherapy (89%), nodal metastasis (69%), and neck dissection (63%). Rupture of the carotid usually occurs proximal to the carotid bifurcation and is commonly associated with soft tissue necrosis in the neck (55%) and mucocutaneous fistulas (40%). Half of CBS patients present with sentinel bleeding, but 60% of patients will develop a life-threatening hemorrhage requiring emergent intervention. Over 90% of the cases reported with initial and recurrent CBS were treated with endovascular embolization (56%) or stenting (36%). Ligation was used in only 7% for primary management of CBS. Those clinicians who used endovascular stenting did so because it provides constructive repair and allows preservation or revascularization of the cerebral blood flow. Overall, however, stent placement was associated with a higher risk of CBS recurrence (44%) than embolization (10%) or surgical ligation (25%). Cerebrovascular accidents occurred in 12 patients and were the most common cause of death next to tumor progression. The mortality rate of patients with CBS was high (63%). Only 23% of the patients have survived without evidence of disease (average follow-up of 17 months).

CBS has a spectrum of presentations that range from exposure of the carotid artery to hemorrhage from the carotid artery system. Three types of CBS can be recognized. Type I or threatened CBS, when exposure of the carotid artery is found on clinical examination or imaging studies (i.e., air surrounding the vessel, adjacent abscess, or tumor associated with a fistula or areas of arterial wall disruption found on vascular imaging studies). Type II or impending blowout, when bleeding episodes occur that resolve temporarily with pressure and wound packing. In many cases, these are self-limiting, single incidents that may cause little suspicion to those unaware of the patient's history and risk factors for CBS. Sentinel bleeding can occur moments to months before hemorrhage. High-risk head and neck cancer (HNC) patients should be educated to report any occurrences of soft tissue breakdown or bleeding so that they may be properly evaluated for potential CBS and associated risk factors. Management of the exposed carotid depends on the likelihood of rupture, based on the length of the exposed segment, the condition of the surrounding tissues, and the size of the oropharyngocutaneous fistula. Large cutaneous defects or large high-output fistulae in previously irradiated patients are not likely to heal by secondary intention in a timely manner. The likelihood of rupture of the carotid in these conditions is extremely high. Therefore, an attempt should be made to repair the defect and to cover the carotid using well-vascularized tissue early, before the vessel has been irreversibly damaged. Whenever the carotid is exposed, it is advisable to take the following carotid rupture precautions:

- Warn and instruct nursing personnel and house staff about the possibility of a carotid rupture, the site of potential rupture, and the steps to be taken in the event of bleeding.
- Have compatible blood available.
- Keep appropriate surgical instruments at the bedside.

Type III or hemorrhage from the carotid system is usually rapidly fatal especially when it occurs outside the hospital setting. Bleeding can occur externally through a neck wound or "internally" into the pharynx/mouth (less common). In the latter cases, the possibility exists for airway compromise. Identification of the early stages and prevention of type III CBS are crucial, as patients with CBS who undergo therapy before the development of hemorrhage have been shown to have a lower complication rate than do those who wait until hemorrhage develops. CT and MRI are helpful in finding type I situations, such as an exposed carotid vessel within a fistula tract or recurrent tumor with carotid space invasion. Computed tomographic angiography, magnetic resonance angiography, and arteriography can also be helpful in evaluating patents at risk for CBS. Findings include endoluminal and vessel wall irregularities and pseudoaneurysm formation and extravasation. Angiography is the gold standard for diagnosing arterial disorders and is preferred because of its therapeutic capabilities; however, it is important to be aware of the 8.5% complication rate associated with this procedure.

When a carotid rupture occurs, it is usually possible to stop the bleeding with manual pressure while blood and fluids are given to restore and maintain the patient's blood pressure. Often, in emergency situations, medical staff place multiple dressings over the wound, which will not apply focused pressure over the bleeding site, and the patient may continue to exsanguinate around them. It is more effective to place a gloved finger for pressure to temporarily control the bleeding until definitive treatment is undertaken. Blood pressure must be addressed aggressively with proper resuscitation. Only then is the patient taken to surgery, since the risk of morbidity with ligation increases significantly in the setting of hypotension, which is the greatest predictor of a poor outcome in the acute treatment of CBS. Attempts to repair the area of rupture are futile. Introducing Fogarty catheters through the area of rupture helps control the bleeding temporarily while the artery is exposed and ligated proximally and distally to the area of rupture.

Endovascular embolization—whether it be with balloons, coils, or other materials—is more precise than ligation, as it targets the exact location of the arterial defect. It also decreases the hospital stay and causes less of the collateral morbidity that is sometimes associated with emergent open ligation procedures, such as injury of cranial nerves or ligation of the incorrect trunk or branch of the carotid system. Endovascular embolization also has the ability to help predict cerebrovascular complications with temporary balloon occlusion and collateral cerebral blood flow analysis. Carotid artery embolization is associated with 15% to 20% long-term neurologic morbidity rate and a much lower incidence of associated mortality.

More recently, constructive endovascular management of CBS became available for patients who have risk factors for neurologic sequelae after embolization. Constructive methods utilize intravascular stents to control vascular wall instability while allowing adequate cerebral perfusion. Some indications used for arterial stenting include an incomplete circle of Willis, significant contralateral carotid artery atherosclerosis or narrowing, inability to perform balloon occlusion tests (proximal atherosclerotic stenosis or unstable clinical scenario), and failure to tolerate balloon test occlusion on either clinical or cerebral blood flow criteria (decrease of cerebral blood flow of more than 20%).

Regardless of the treatment used, anticoagulation therapy may be required to prevent thrombosis distal to the ligation or endovascular occlusion site or to prevent stent thrombosis. Patients with an exposed carotid artery require wound management with flap placement to cover and protect these vessels.

Although endovascular treatment within the carotid system can have a significant risk of mortality and neurologic morbidity, it has become the treatment of choice for CBS.

Jugular Vein "Blowout"

This complication is seen more often because the IJV is preserved more frequently during neck dissection. Jugular vein rupture should be considered in patients undergoing primary tumor excision with MRND complicated by a pharyngocutaneous fistula. In a recent study of six patients who experienced rupture of the IJV, Cleland-Zamudio et al. (184) found that patients who have a complete circumferential dissection of the IJV low in the neck and go on to have fistulas develop may be more prone to this complication. Typically, bleeding is venous and occurs repeatedly. Treatment consists of surgical exploration and ligation of the jugular vein above and below the level of rupture.

HIGHLIGHTS

- A comprehensive knowledge of anatomy and physiology is necessary to understand the nuances of surgical planning and technique as well as the prevention and management of the sequelae and complications of neck dissection.
- At the present time, the role of imaging studies including PET/CT in the evaluation of the N0 neck is limited as it will not detect subclinical metastases in 20% to 50% of the cases.
- SLNB is feasible and useful as a staging procedure in patients with early carcinomas of the oral cavity, particularly for patients with cancers of the oral tongue.
- There is finally consensus about a classification of neck dissections that conveys more precisely the extent of lymphatic and nonlymphatic structures removed in a neck dissection.
- There is now a better understanding of the indications and limitations of the different neck dissections.
- The rate of tumor recurrence in the neck is decreased by the addition of postoperative radiation, when multiple nodes are involved at multiple levels of the neck, and when ECS of the tumor is found.
- The presence of ECS of the tumor is currently considered an indication for postoperative concurrent chemoradiation.
- The most common sequelae following any type of neck dissection is related to weakness or paralysis of the trapezius muscle. Early recognition and rehabilitation are paramount in the management of such patients.

REFERENCES

1. Guo CB, Zhang Y, Zhang L, et al. [Surgical anatomy and preservation of the accessory nerve in radical functional neck dissection]. [Chinese]. [*Chung-Hua Kou Chiang i Hsueh Tsa Chih*] *Chin J Stomatol* 2003;38(1):12–15.
2. Hone SW, Ridha H, Rowley H, et al. Surgical landmarks of the spinal accessory nerve in modified radical neck dissection. *Clin Otolaryngol Allied Sci* 2001;26(1):16–18.

3. Frank DK, Wenk E, Stern JC, et al. A cadaveric study of the motor nerves to the levator scapulae muscle. *Otolaryngol Head Neck Surg* 1997;117(6):671–680.

4. Robbins KTM, Shaha ARM, Medina JEM, et al. Consensus statement on the classification and terminology of neck dissection. *Arch Otolaryngol Head Neck Surg* 2008;134(5):536–538.

5. Lindberg R. Distribution of cervical lymph node metastases from squamous cell carcinoma of the upper respiratory and digestive tracts. *Cancer* 1972;29(6):1446–1449.

6. Shah JP. Patterns of cervical lymph node metastasis from squamous carcinomas of the upper aerodigestive tract. *Am J Surg* 1990;160(4):405–409.

7. Vasan NR, Medina JE. Retropharyngeal node dissection. *Oper Tech Otolaryngol Head Neck Surg* 2004;15(3):180–183.

8. Weber RS, Marvel J, Smith P, et al. Paratracheal lymph node dissection for carcinoma of the larynx, hypopharynx, and cervical esophagus. *Otolaryngol Head Neck Surg* 1993;108(1):11–17.

9. Shenoy AM, Nanjundappa A, Kumar P, et al. Interjugular neck dissection and post-operative irradiation for neck control in advanced glottic cancers—are we justified? *J Laryngol Otol* 1994;108(1):26–29.

10. Haberal I, Celik H, Gocmen H, et al. Which is important in the evaluation of metastatic lymph nodes in head and neck cancer: palpation, ultrasonography, or computed tomography? *Otolaryngol Head Neck Surg* 2004;130(2):197–201.

11. Adams S, Baum RP, Stuckensen T, et al. Prospective comparison of F-FDG PET with conventional imaging modalities (CT, MRI, US) in lymph node staging of head and neck cancer. *Eur J Nucl Med* 1998;25(9):1255–1260.

12. Sakai O, Curtin HD, Romo LV, et al. Lymph node pathology. Benign proliferative, lymphoma, and metastatic disease. [Review] [57 refs]. *Radiol Clin North Am* 2000;38(5):979–998.

13. van den Brekel MWM, van der Waal I, Meijer CJLM, et al. The incidence of micrometastases in neck dissection specimens obtained from elective neck dissections. *Laryngoscope* 1996;106(8):987–991.

14. DiNardo LJ. Lymphatics of the submandibular space. *Laryngoscope* 1998;108(2):206–214.

15. Steinkamp HJ, Cornehl M, Hosten N, et al. Cervical lymphadenopathy: ratio of long- to short-axis diameter as a predictor of malignancy. *Br J Radiol* 1995;68(807):266–270.

16. van den Brekel MW, Castelijns JA, Stel HV, et al. Modern imaging techniques and ultrasound-guided aspiration cytology for the assessment of neck node metastases: a prospective comparative study. *Eur Arch Otorhinolaryngol* 1993;250(1):11–17.

17. Nieuwenhuis E, Castelijns J, Pijpers R, et al. Wait-and-see policy for the N0 neck in early-stage oral and oropharyngeal squamous cell carcinoma using ultrasonography-guided cytology: is there a role for identification of the sentinel node? *Head Neck* 2002;24(3):282–289.

18. Wensing BM, Merkx MA, De Wilde PC, et al. Assessment of preoperative ultrasonography of the neck and elective neck dissection in patients with oral squamous cell carcinoma. *Oral Oncol* 2010;46(2):87–91.

19. Braams JW, Pruim J, Freling NJ, et al. Detection of lymph node metastases of squamous-cell cancer of the head and neck with FDG-PET and MRI. *J Nucl Med* 1995;36(2):211–216.

20. Stokkel MP, ten Broek FW, Hordijk GJ, et al. Preoperative evaluation of patients with primary head and neck cancer using dual-head 18-fluorodeoxyglucose positron emission tomography. *Ann Surg* 2000;231(2):229–234.

21. Kyzas PA, Evangelou E, Denaxa-Kyza D, et al. 18F-fluorodeoxyglucose positron emission tomography to evaluate cervical node metastases in patients with head and neck squamous cell carcinoma: a meta-analysis. [Article]. *J Natl Cancer Inst* 2008;100(10):712–720.

22. de Bree R, Roos JC, Verel I, et al. Radio immunodiagnosis of lymph node metastases in head and neck cancer. *Oral Dis* 2003;9(5):241–248.

23. Shoaib T, Soutar DS. Sentinel node biopsy in head and neck cancer. [Miscellaneous Article]. *Curr Opin Otolaryngol Head Neck Surg* 2001;9(2):79–84.

24. Ross GL, Soutar DS, MacDonald DG, et al. Improved staging of cervical metastases in clinically node-negative patients with head

and neck squamous cell carcinoma. *Ann Surg Oncol* 2004;11(2):213–218.

25. Mozzillo N, Chiesa F, Botti G, et al. Sentinel node biopsy in head and neck cancer. *Ann Surg Oncol* 2001;8(Suppl 9):S105.

26. Ross GL, Soutar DS, Gordon MD, et al. Sentinel node biopsy in head and neck cancer: preliminary results of a multicenter trial. *Ann Surg Oncol* 2004;11(7):690–696.

27. Ross GL, Shoaib T, Soutar DS, et al. The First International Conference on sentinel node biopsy in mucosal head and neck cancer and adoption of a multicenter trial protocol. *Ann Surg Oncol* 2002;9(4):406–410.

28. Hamakawa H, Fukizumi M, Bao Y, et al. Genetic diagnosis of micrometastasis based on SCC antigen mRNA in cervical lymph nodes of head and neck cancer. *Clin Exp Metastasis* 1999;17(7):593–599.

29. Shores CG, Yin X, Funkhouser W, et al. Clinical evaluation of a new molecular method for detection of micrometastases in head and neck squamous cell carcinoma. *Arch Otolaryngol Head Neck Surg* 2004;130(8):937–942.

30. Civantos FJ, Zitsch RP, Schuller DE, et al. Sentinel lymph node biopsy accurately stages the regional lymph nodes for T1-T2 oral squamous cell carcinomas: results of a prospective multi-institutional trial. *J Clin Oncol* 2010;28(8):1395–1400.

31. Civantos F, Zitsch R, Bared A. Sentinel node biopsy in oral squamous cell carcinoma. *J Surg Oncol* 2007;96(4):330–336.

32. Edge SB, Byrd DR, Compton CC, et al. *AJCC cancer staging manual*, 7th ed., New York: Springer, 2009.

33. Ferlito A, Robbins KT, Shah JP, et al. Proposal for a rational classification of neck dissections. *Head Neck* 2011;33(3):445–450.

34. McCammon S, Shah J. Radical neck dissection. *Oper Tech Otolaryngol Head Neck Surg* 2004;15(3):152–159.

35. Pinsolle J, Pinsolle V, Majoufre C, et al. Prognostic value of histologic findings in neck dissections for squamous cell carcinoma. *Arch Otolaryngol Head Neck Surg* 1997;123:145–148.

36. Andersen P, Shah J, Cambronero E, et al. The role of comprehensive neck dissection with preservation of the spinal accessory nerve in the clinically positive neck. *Am J Surg* 1994;168(5):499–502.

37. Gavilan J, Herranz J, Martin L. Functional neck dissection: the Latin approach. *Oper Tech Otolaryngol Head Neck Surg* 2004;15(3):168–175.

38. Ferlito A, Rinaldo A, Osvaldo Suarez. Often-forgotten father of functional neck dissection (in the non-Spanish-speaking literature). [Article]. *Laryngoscope* 2004;114(7):1177–1178.

39. Brazilian Head and Neck Cancer Study Group. End results of a prospective trial on elective lateral neck dissection vs type III modified radical neck dissection in the management of supraglottic and transglottic carcinomas. *Head Neck* 1999;21(8):694–702.

40. Buckley JG, MacLennan K. Cervical node metastases in laryngeal and hypopharyngeal cancer: a prospective analysis of prevalence and distribution. *Head Neck* 2000;22(4):380–385.

41. Naiboglu B, Karapinar U, Agrawal A, et al. When to manage level V in head and neck carcinoma? *Laryngoscope* 2011;121(3):545–547.

42. Lingeman R, Stephens R, Helmus C, et al. Neck dissection: radical or conservative. *Ann Otol* 1977;86:737.

43. Molinari R, Chiesa F, Cantu G, et al. Retrospective comparison of conservative and radical neck dissection in laryngeal cancer. *Ann Otol* 1980;89:578.

44. Joseph C, Gregor R, Davidge-Pitts K. The role of functional neck dissection in the management of advanced tumors of the upper aerodigestive tract. *S Afr J Surg* 1985;23:83.

45. Gavilan C, Gavilan J. Five-year results of functional neck dissection for cancer of the larynx. *Arch Otolaryngol Head Neck Surg* 1989;115:1193.

46. Bocca E, Pignataro O, Oldini C. Functional neck dissection: an evaluation and review of 843 cases. *Laryngoscope* 1984;94:942.

47. Calearo C, Teatini G. Functional neck dissection: anatomical grounds, surgical technique, clinical observations. *Ann Otol Rhinol Laryngol* 1983;92:215.

48. Byers R, Weber R, Anderws T, et al. Frequency and therapeutic implications of "skip metastases" in the neck from squamous carcinoma of the oral tongue. *Head Neck* 1997;19:14–19.

49. Medina J, Byers R. Supraomohyoid neck dissection: rationale, indications and surgical technique. *Head Neck Surg* 1989;11:111.

50. Khafif A. Lateral neck dissection. *Oper Tech Otolaryngol Head Neck Surg* 2004;15(3):160–167.

51. Medina JE, Ferlito A, Robbins KT, et al. Central compartment dissection in laryngeal cancer. *Head Neck* 2011;33(5):746–752.

52. Weber R, Holsinger F. Central compartment dissection (of levels VI and VII for carcinoma of the larynx, hypopharynx, cervical esophagus, and thyroid). *Oper Tech Otolaryngol Head Neck Surg* 2004;15(3):190–195.

53. Medina J. Posterolateral neck dissection. *Oper Tech Otolaryngol Head Neck Surg* 2004;15(3):176–179.

54. Jesse RH, Ballantyne AJ, Larson D. Radical or modified neck dissection: a therapeutic dilemma. *Am J Surg* 1978;136(4):516–519.

55. Medina JE. A rational classification of neck dissections. *Otolaryngol Head Neck Surg* 1989;100(3):169–176.

56. Byers R, Wolf P, Ballantyne A. Rationale for elective modified neck dissection. *Head Neck* 1988;10:160–167.

57. Candela F, Kothari K, Shah J. Patterns of cervical node metastases from squamous cell carcinoma of the oropharynx and hypopharynx. *Head Neck* 1990;12:197–203.

58. Candela F, Shah J, Jaques D, et al. Patterns of cervical node metastases from squamous cell carcinoma of the larynx. *Arch Otolaryngol Head Neck Surg* 1990;116:432–435.

59. Fisch U, Sigel M. Cervical lymphatic system as visualized by lymphography. *Ann Otol Rhinol Laryngol* 1964;73:869.

60. Kowalski L, Carvalho A. Feasibility of supraomohyoid neck dissection in N1 and N2a oral cancer patients. *Head Neck* 2002;24:921–924.

61. Mukherji S, Armao D, Joshi V. Cervical nodal metastases in squamous cell carcinoma of the head and neck: what to expect. *Head Neck* 2001;23:995–1005.

62. Shah J, Candela F, Poddar A. The patterns of cervical lymph node metastases from squamous cell carcinoma of the oral cavity. *Cancer* 1990;66:109–113.

63. Skolnik E. The posterior triangle in radical neck surgery. *Arch Otolaryngol* 1976;102:1.

64. Wong R, Rinaldo A, Ferlito A, et al. Occult cervical metastasis in head and neck cancer and its impact on therapy. *Acta Otolaryngol* 2002;122:107–114.

65. Ferlito A, Rinaldo A, Devaney K, et al. Prognostic significance of microscopic and macroscopic extracapsular spread from metastatic tumor in the cervical lymph nodes. *Oral Oncol* 2002;38:747–751.

66. Woolgar J, Rogers S, Lowe D, et al. Cervical lymph node metastasis in oral cancer: the importance of even microscopic extracapsular spread. *Oral Oncol* 2003;39:130–137.

67. Ferlito A, Buckley J, Shaha A, et al. Rationale for selective neck dissection in tumors of the upper aerodigestive tract. *Acta Otolaryngol* 2001;121:548–555.

68. Ambrosch P, Freudenberg L, Kron M, et al. Selective neck dissection in the management of squamous cell carcinoma of the upper digestive tract. *Eur Arch Otorhinolaryngol* 1996;253:329–335.

69. Zhang B, Xu Z, Tang P. Lateral neck dissection vs radical neck dissection in the management of supraglottic carcinoma with pathologically negative nodes. *Chin J Otorhinolaryngol* 2003;38(6):426–429.

70. Leon X, Quer M, Orus C, et al. Selective dissection of levels II-III with intraoperative control of the upper and middle jugular nodes: a therapeutic option for the N0 neck. *Head Neck* 2001;23:441–446.

71. Pitman K, Johnson J, Myers E. Effectiveness of selective neck dissection for management of the clinically negative neck. *Arch Otolaryngol Head Neck Surg* 1997;123:917–922.

72. Spiro R, Gallo O, Shah J. Selective jugular node dissection in patients with squamous carcinoma of the larynx or pharynx. *Am J Surg* 1993;166:399–402.

73. Byers R, Clayman G, McGill D, et al. Selective neck dissections for squamous carcinoma of the upper aerodigestive tract: patterns of regional failure. *Head Neck* 1999;21:499–505.

74. Myers E, Fagan J. Management of the neck in cancer of the larynx. *Ann Otol Rhinol Laryngol* 1999;108:828–832.

75. Davidson J, Khan Y, Gilbert R, et al. Is selective neck dissection sufficient treatment for the N0/Np+ neck? *J Otolaryngol* 1997;26:229–231.

76. Clayman G, Frank D. Selective neck dissection of anatomically appropriate levels is as efficacious as modified radical neck dissection for elective treatment of the clinically negative neck in patients with squamous cell carcinoma of the upper respiratory and digestive tracts. *Arch Otolaryngol Head Neck Surg* 1998;124:348–352.

77. Houck J, Medina J. Management of cervical lymph nodes in squamous carcinomas of the head and neck. *Semin Surg Oncol* 1995;11:228–239.

78. Pellitteri P, Robbins K, Neuman T. Expanded application of selective neck dissection with regard to nodal status. *Head Neck* 1997;19:260–265.

79. van Wilgen C, Dijkstra P, van der Laan BF, et al. Shoulder complaints after nerve sparing neck dissections. *Int J Oral Maxillofac Surg* 2004;33(3):253–257.

80. Caversaccio M, Negri S, Nolte L, et al. Neck dissection shoulder syndrome: quantification and three-dimensional evaluation with an optoelectronic tracking system. *Ann Otol Rhinol Laryngol* 2003;112(11):939–946.

81. Zhang B, Tang P, Xu Z, et al. Functional evaluation of the selective neck dissection in patients with carcinoma of the head and neck. *Chin J Otorhinolaryngol* 2004;39:28–31.

82. Laverick S, Lowe D, Brown J, et al. The impact of neck dissection on health-related quality of life *Arch Otol Head Neck Surg* 2004;130:149–154.

83. van Wilgen C, Dijkstra P, Nauta J, et al. Shoulder pain and disability in daily life, following supraomohyoid neck dissection: a pilot study. *J Craniomaxillofac Surg* 2003;31:183–186.

84. Cheng P, Hao S, Lin Y, et al. Objective comparison of shoulder dysfunction after three neck dissection techniques. *Ann Otol Rhinol Laryngol* 2000;109:761–766.

85. De Zinis LO, Bolzoni A, Piazza C, et al. Prevalence and localization of nodal metastases in squamous cell carcinoma of the oral cavity: role and extension of neck dissection. *Eur Arch Otorhinolaryngol* 2006;263(12):1131–1135.

86. Crean SJ, Hoffman A, Potts J, et al. Reduction of occult metastatic disease by extension of the supraomohyoid neck dissection to include level IV. *Head Neck* 2003;25(9):758–762.

87. Khafif A, Lopez-Garza JR, Medina JE. Is dissection of level IV necessary in patients with T1-T3 N0 tongue cancer? *Laryngoscope* 2001;111(6):1088–1090.

88. Li XM, Wei WI, Guo XF, et al. Cervical lymph node metastatic patterns of squamous carcinomas in the upper aerodigestive tract. *J Laryngol Otol* 1996;110(10):937–941.

89. Wang X, Tu G, Tang P. The treatment of tongue squamous cell with N0. [Chinese]. [*Zhonghua Kou Qiang Yi Xue Za Zhi*] *Chin J Stomatol* 2000;35(1):12–14.

90. Akhtar S, Ikram M, Ghaffar S. Neck involvement in early carcinoma of tongue. Is elective neck dissection warranted? *J Pak Med Assoc* 2007;57(6):305–307.

91. Rinaldo A, Elsheikh MN, Ferlito A, et al. Prospective studies of neck dissection specimens support preservation of sublevel IIB for laryngeal squamous carcinoma with clinically negative neck. [Review]. *J Am Coll Surg* 2006;202(6):967–970.

92. Villaret AB, Piazza C, Peretti G, et al. Multicentric prospective study on the prevalence of sublevel IIB metastases in head and neck cancer. [Article]. *Arch Otolaryngol Head Neck Surg* 2007;133(9):897–903.

93. Kim YHM, Koo BSM, Lim YCM, et al. Lymphatic metastases to level IIb in hypopharyngeal squamous cell carcinoma. [Article]. *Arch Otolaryngol Head Neck Surg* 2006;132(10):1060–1064.

94. Lee SY, Lim YC, Song MH, et al. Level IIb lymph node metastasis in elective neck dissection of oropharyngeal squamous cell carcinoma. *Oral Oncol* 2006;42(10):1017–1021.

95. Köybasioglu A, Bora Tokçaer A, Inal E, et al. Accessory nerve function in lateral selective neck dissection with undissected level IIB. *ORL* 2006;68(2):88–92.

96. Khafif A, Fliss DM, Gil Z, et al. Routine inclusion of level IV in neck dissection for squamous cell carcinoma of the larynx: is it justified? *Head Neck* 2004;26(4):309–312.

97. Hua H, Liu Q, Han Z, et al. [The study on the occult metastases to cervical lymph node in squamous cell carcinoma of the larynx and hypopharynx]. [Chinese]. [*Lin Chuang Erh Pi Yen Hou Ko Tsa Chih*] *J Clin Otorhinolaryngol* 2001;15(9):391–392.

98. Elsheikh MN, Ferlito A, Rinaldo A, et al. Do pathologic and molecular analyses of neck dissection specimens justify the preservation of level IV for laryngeal squamous carcinoma with clinically negative neck? *J Am Coll Surg* 2006;202(2):320–323.

99. Ferlito A, Silver CE, Suarez C, et al. Preliminary multi-institutional prospective pathologic and molecular studies support preservation of sublevel IIB and level IV for laryngeal squamous carcinoma with clinically negative neck. [Review] [22 refs]. *Eur Arch Otorhinolaryngol* 2007;264(2):111–114.

100. Ferlito A, Silver CE, Rinaldo A. Selective neck dissection (IIA, III): a rational replacement for complete functional neck dissection in patients with n0 supraglottic and glottic squamous carcinoma. *Laryngoscope* 2008;118(4):676–679.

101. Solares CA, Fritz MA, Esclamado RM. Oncologic effectiveness of selective neck dissection in the N0 irradiated neck. *Head Neck* 2005;27(5):415–420.

102. Mazzaferri EL, oherty GM, Steward DL. The pros and cons of prophylactic central compartment lymph node dissection for papillary thyroid carcinoma. *Thyroid* 2009;19(7):683–689.

103. Cooper DS, Doherty GM, Haugen BR, et al. Revised American Thyroid Association Management Guidelines for patients with thyroid nodules and differentiated thyroid cancer. *Thyroid* 2009;19(11):1167–1214.

104. Ambrosch P, Kron M, Pradier O, et al. A review of 503 cases of elective and therapeutic treatment of the neck in squamous cell carcinoma of the upper aerodigestive tract. *Otolaryngol Head Neck Surg* 2001;124:180–187.

105. Andersen P, Warren F, Spiro J, et al. Results of selective neck dissection in management of the node-positive neck. *Arch Otol Head Neck Surg* 2002;128:1180–1184.

106. Robbins K, Clayman G, Levine P, et al. Neck dissection classification update. Revision proposed by the American Head and Neck Society and the American Academy of Otolaryngology-Head and Neck Surgery. *Arch Otol Head Neck Surg* 2002;128:751–758.

107. Buckley J, Feber T. Surgical treatment of cervical node metastases from squamous carcinoma of the upper aerodigestive tract: evaluation of the evidence for modifications of neck dissection. *Head Neck* 2001;23:907–915.

108. Brandenburg J, Lee C. The XI nerve in radical neck surgery. *Laryngoscope* 1981;91:1851.

109. Deutsch E, Skolnik E, Friedman M, et al. The conservation neck dissection. *Laryngoscope* 1985;95:561–565.

110. Mann W, Wolfensberger M, Fuller U, et al. Radical versus modified neck dissection. Cancer-related and functional viewpoints. *Laryngorhinootologie* 1991;70:32–35.

111. Carew J, Spiro R. Extended neck dissection. *Am J Surg* 1997;174(5):485–489.

112. Osguthorpe J, Abel C, Lang P. Neurotropic cutaneous tumors of the head and neck. *Arch Otolaryngol* 1997;123:871–876.

113. McLaughlin M, Mendenhall W, Mancuso A, et al. Retropharyngeal adenopathy as a predictor of outcome in squamous cell carcinoma of the head and neck. *Head Neck* 1995;17:190–198.

114. Amatsu M, Mohri M, Kinishi M. Significance of retropharyngeal node dissection at radical surgery for carcinoma of the hypopharynx and cervical esophagus. *Laryngoscope* 2001;111:1099–1103.

115. Ballantyne A. Significance of retropharyngeal nodes in cancer of the head and neck. *Am J Surg* 1964;108:500.

116. Hasegawa Y, Matsuura H. Retropharyngeal node dissection in cancer of the oropharynx and hypopharynx. *Head Neck* 1994;16:173–180.

117. Gross N, Ellington T, Wax M, et al. Impact of retropharyngeal lymph node metastases in head and neck squamous cell carcinoma. *Arch Otolaryngol Head Neck Surg* 2004;130:169–173.

118. Plaat RE, de BR, Kuik DJ, et al. Prognostic importance of paratracheal lymph node metastases. *Laryngoscope* 2005;115(5):894–898.

119. Khafif A, Medina J. Management of the neck in differentiated thyroid carcinoma. In: Randolph G, ed. *Surgery of the thyroid and parathyroid glands*. Saunders, Elsevier Science, 2003:409–418.

120. Freeman SB, Hamaker RC, Borrowdale RB, et al. Management of neck metastasis with carotid artery involvement. *Laryngoscope* 2004;114(1):20–24.

121. Nemeth Z, Domotor G, Talos M, et al. Resection and replacement of the carotid artery in metastatic head and neck cancer: literature review and case report. *Int J Oral Maxillofac Surg* 2003;32(6):645–650.

122. de Vries E, Sekhar L, Horton J, et al. A new method to predict safe resection of the internal carotid artery. *Laryngoscope* 1990;100(1):85–88.

123. Wright J, Nicholson R, Schuller D, et al. Resection of the internal carotid artery and replacement with greater saphenous vein: a safe procedure for en bloc cancer resections with carotid involvement. *J Vasc Surg* 1996;23(5):775–780.

124. Johnson J, Myers E, Bedetti C, et al. Cervical lymph node metastases. *Arch Otolaryngol Head Neck Surg* 1985;111:534–537.

125. Vikram B, Strong E, Shah J, et al. Failure in the neck following multimodality treatment for advanced head and neck cancer. *Head Neck Surg* 1984;6:724.

126. O'Brien C, Smith J, Soong S, et al. Neck dissection with and without radiotherapy: prognostic factors, patterns of recurrence, and survival. *Am J Surg* 1986;152:456–463.

127. Peters L, Goepfert H, Kiang A, et al. Evaluation of the dose for postoperative radiation therapy of head and neck cancer: first report of a prospective randomized trial. *Int J Rad Oncol Biol Phys* 1993;26:3–11.

128. Cooper J, Pajak T, Forastiere A, et al. Postoperative concurrent radiotherapy and chemotherapy for high-risk squamous cell carcinoma of the head and neck. *N Engl J Med* 2004;350:1937–1944.

129. Bernier J, Domenge C, Ozsahin M, et al. Postoperative irradiation with or without concomitant chemotherapy for locally advanced head and neck cancer. *N Engl J Med* 2004;350:1945–1952.

130. Bernier J, Cooper JS, Pajak TF, et al. Defining risk levels in locally advanced head and neck cancers: a comparative analysis of concurrent postoperative radiation plus chemotherapy trials of the EORTC (#22931) and RTOG (# 9501). *Head Neck* 2005;27(10):843–850.

131. Yuen A, Lam K, Chan A, et al. Clinicopathological analysis of elective neck dissection for N0 neck of early oral tongue carcinoma. *Am J Surg* 1999;177(1):90–92.

132. Chen TC, Wang CT, Ko JY, et al. Postoperative radiotherapy for primary early oral tongue cancer with pathologic N1 neck. *Head Neck* 2010;32(5):555–561.

133. Brizel DM, Prosnitz RG, Hunter S, et al. Necessity for adjuvant neck dissection in setting of concurrent chemoradiation for advanced head-and-neck cancer. *Int J Rad Oncol Biol Phys* 2004;58(5):1418–1423.

134. McHam SA, Adelstein DJ, Rybicki LA, et al. Who merits a neck dissection after definitive chemoradiotherapy for N2-N3 squamous cell head and neck cancer? *Head Neck* 2003;25(10):791–798.

135. Corry J, Smith J, Peters L. The concept of a planned neck dissection is obsolete. *Cancer J* 2001;7:472–474.

136. Mendenhall W, Villaret D, Amdur R, et al. Planned neck dissection after definitive radiotherapy for squamous cell carcinoma of the head and neck. *Head Neck* 2002;24:1012–1018.

137. Wanebo H, Chougule P, Ready N, et al. Surgical resection is necessary to maximize tumor control in function-preserving, aggressive chemoradiation protocols for advanced squamous cancer of the head and neck (stage III and IV). *Ann Surg Oncol* 2001;8(8):644–650.

138. Medina JE, Vaasan NR, Krempl GA. Management of the neck after treatment with radiation with or without chemotherapy. *Current Treat Options Oncol* 2007;8(3):261–264.

139. Yao M, Graham SM, Hoffman H, et al. The role of post-radiation FDG pet in prediction of necessity for post-radiation therapy neck dissection in locally Advanced head and neck squamous cell carcinoma. *Int J Rad Oncol Biol Phys* 2004 15;59(4):1001–1010.

140. Robbins KT, Wong F, Kumar P, et al. Efficacy of targeted chemoradiation and planned selective neck dissection to control bulky nodal disease in advanced head and neck cancer. *Arch Otolaryngol Head Neck Surg* 1999;125:670–675.

141. Chan AW, Ancukiewicz M, Carballo N, et al. The role of postradiotherapy neck dissection in supraglottic carcinoma. *Int J Rad Oncol Biol Phys* 2001;50:367–375.

142. Ware RE, MathewsJP, Hicks RJ. Usefulness of fluorine-18 fluorodeoxyglucose positron emission tomography in patients with a residual structural abnormality after definitive treatment for squamous cell carcinoma of the head and neck. *Head Neck* 2007;26:1008–1017.

143. Rogers J, Greven K, NcGuirt W, et al. Can post-RT neck dissection be omitted for patients with head and neck cancer who have a negative PET scan after definitive radiation therapy? *Int J Rad oncol Biol Phys* 2004;58:694–697.

144. Greven KM, Williams DW, McGuirt WF, et al. Serial positron emission tomography scans following radiation therapy of patients with head and neck cancer. *Head Neck* 2001;23(11):942–946.

145. Ware RE, Matthews JP, Hicks RJ, et al. Usefulness of fluorine-18 fluorodeoxyglucose positron emission tomography in patients with a residual structural abnormality after definitive treatment for squamous cell carcinoma of the head and neck. *Head Neck* 2004;26(12):1008–1017.

146. Porceddu SV, Jarmolowski E, Hicks R, et al. Utility of positron omission tomography for the detection of disease in residual neck nodes after (chemo) radiotherapy in head and neck cancer. *Head Neck* 2005;27:175–181.

147. Rabalais AG, Walvekar R, Nuss D, et al. Positron emission tomography -computed tomography surveillance for the node-positive neck after chemoradiotherapy. *Laryngoscope* 2009;119(6):1120–1124.

148. Corry J, Peters L, Fisher R, et al. N2-N3 neck nodal control without planned neck dissection for clinical/radiologic complete responders: results of Trans Tasman Radiation Oncology Group Study 98.02. *Head Neck* 2008;30(6):737–742.

149. Gourin CG, Boyce BJ, Williams HT, et al. Revisiting the role of positron-emission tomography/computed tomography in determining the need for planned neck dissection following chemoradiation for advanced head and neck cancer. *Laryngoscope* 2009;119(11):2150–2155.

150. Lavertu P, Adelstein DJ, Saxton JP, et al. Management of the neck in a randomized trial comparing concurrent chemotherapy and radiotherapy with radiotherapy alone in resectable stage III and IV squamous cell head and neck cancer. *Head Neck* 1919;7:559–566.

151. Robbins KT, Ferlito A, Suarez C, et al. Is there a role for selective neck dissection after chemoradiation for head and neck cancer? *J Am Coll Surg* 2004;199(6):913–916.

152. Stenson K, Haraf DJ, Pelzer H, et al. The role of cervical lymphadenectomy after aggressive concomitant chemoradiotherapy: the feasibility of selective neck dissection. *Arch Otolaryngol Head Neck Surg* 2000;126:950–956.

153. Robbins K, Doweck I, Samant S, et al. Effectiveness of superselective and selective neck dissection for advanced nodal metastases after chemoradiation. *Arch Otolaryngol Head Neck Surg* 2005;131(11):965–969.

154. Boyd TS, Harari PM, Tannehill SP, et al. Planned postradiotherapy neck dissection in patients with advanced head and neck cancer. *Head Neck* 1998;20(2):132–137.

155. Goguen LA, Chapuy CI, Sher DJ, et al. Utilizing computed tomography as a road map for designing selective and superselective neck dissection after chemoradiotherapy. *Otolaryngol Head Neck Surg* 2010;143(3):367–374.

156. Yeung AR, Liauw SL, Amdur RJ, et al. Lymph node-positive head and neck cancer treated with definitive radiotherapy. *Cancer* 2008;112(5):1076–1082.

157. El Ghani F, van den Brekel M, De Goede C, et al. Shoulder function and patient well-being after various types of neck dissections. *Clin Otolaryngol Allied Sci* 2002;27:403–408.

158. Terrell J, Welsh D, Bradford C, et al. Pain, quality of life, and spinal accessory nerve status after neck dissection. *Laryngoscope* 2000;110:620–626.

159. Kuntz A, Weymuller EJ. Impact of neck dissection on quality of life. *Laryngoscope* 1999;109:1334–1338.

160. Salerno G, Cavaliere M, Foglia A, et al. The 11th nerve syndrome in functional neck dissection. *Laryngoscope* 2002;112:1299–1307.

161. McNeely M, Parliament M, Courneya K, et al. A pilot study of a randomized controlled trial to evaluate the effects of progressive resistance exercise training on shoulder dysfunction caused by spinal accessory neurapraxia/neurectomy in head and neck cancer survivors. *Head Neck* 2004;26:518–530.

162. van Wilgen C, Dijkstra P, van der Laan BF, et al. Shoulder complaints after neck dissection; is the spinal accessory nerve involved? *Bri J Oral Maxillofacial Surg* 2003;41:7–11.

163. Seven H, Sayin I, Turgut S. Antibiotic prophylaxis in clean neck dissections. *J Laryngol Otol* 2004;118(3):213–216.

164. Nussenbaum B, Liu J, Sinard R. Systematic management of chyle fistula: the Southwestern experience and review of the literature. *Otolaryngol Head Neck Surg* 2000;122:31–38.

165. Erisen L, Coskun H, Basut O. Objective and early diagnosis of chylous fistula in the postoperative period. *Otolaryngol Head Neck Surg* 2002;126:172–175.

166. Kannan R, Mahajan V, Ayyappan S. Management of chyle fistulae following surgery in the neck. *Indian J Cancer* 2001;38:117–120.

167. Scorza LB, Goldstein BJ, Mahraj RP. Modern management of chylous leak following head and neck surgery: a discussion of percutaneous lymphangiography-guided cannulation and embolization of the thoracic duct. *Otolaryngol Clin North Am* 2011;41:1231–1240.

168. Morris S, Taylor S. Peripheral parenteral nutrition in a case of chyle leak following neck dissection. *J Hum Nutr Diet* 2004;17:153–155.

169. Yoshimura Y, Kondoh T. Treatment of chylous fistula with fibrin glue and clavicular periosteal flap. *Br J Oral Maxillofac Surg* 2002;40:138–139.

170. Repko BM, Scorza LB, Mahraj RP. Recurrent chylothorax after neck surgery: percutaneous thoracic duct embolization as primary treatment. *Otolaryngol Head Neck Surg* 2009;141(3):426–427.

171. Nyquist G, Hagr A, Sobol S, et al. Octreotide in the medical management of chyle fistula. *Otolaryngol Head Neck Surg* 2003;128:910–911.

172. Jortay A, Bisschop P. Bilateral chylothorax after left radical neck dissection. *Acta Otorhinolaryngol* 2001;55:285–289.

173. Kamasaki N, Ikeda H, Wang Z, et al. Bilateral chylothorax following radical neck dissection. *Int J Oral Maxillofac Surg* 2003;32(1):91–93.

174. Padilla Parrado M, Galan Morales J, Abril Garcia A, et al. Bilateral neck dissection and venous reconstruction with internal saphenous vein in cancer of the larynx. *Ann Otol* 2002;29:367–376.

175. Katsuno S, Ishiyama T, Nezu K, et al. Three types of internal jugular vein reconstruction in bilateral radical neck dissection. *Laryngoscope* 2000;110:1578–1580.

176. Zacay G, Bedrin L, Horowitz Z, et al. Syndrome of inappropriate antidiuretic hormone or arginine vasopressin secretion in patients following neck dissection. *Laryngoscope* 2002;112(11):2020–2024.

177. Khafif A, Medina J. The syndrome of inappropriate antidiuretic hormone secretion after bilateral radical neck dissections. *Acta Otolaryngol* 2002;122:907–909.

178. Worrell L, Rowe M, Petti G. Amaurosis: a complication of bilateral radical neck dissection. *Am J Otolaryngol* 2002;23:56–59.

179. Raj P, Moore P, Henderson J, et al. Bilateral cortical blindness: an unusual complication following unilateral neck dissection. *J Laryngol Otol* 2002;116:227–229.

180. Cotter C, Stringer S, Landau S, et al. Patency of the internal jugular vein following modified radical neck dissection. *Laryngoscope* 1994;104:841–845.

181. Cappiello J, Piazza C, Berlucchi M. Internal jugular vein patency after lateral neck dissection: a prospective study. *Arch Otorhinolaryngol* 2002;259:409–412.

182. Davidson B, Newkirk K, Harter W, et al. Complications from planned, posttreatment neck dissections. *Arch Otol Head Neck Surg* 1999;125:401–405.

183. Powitzky R, Vasan N, Krempl G, et al. Carotid blowout in patients with head and neck cancer. *Ann Otol Rhinol Laryngol* 2010;119(7):476–484.

184. Cleland-Zamudio S, Wax M, Smith J, et al. Ruptured internal jugular vein: a postoperative complication of modified/selected neck dissection. *Head Neck* 2003;25:357–360.

Controversies in Management of the N0 Neck in Squamous Cell Carcinoma of the Upper Aerodigestive Tract

118

Ryan Case   Karen T. Pitman

Cervical lymph node metastasis is the single most adverse prognostic factor in patients with head and neck squamous cell carcinoma (HNSCC) without distant metastases. The clinically negative neck (cN0) is defined by the absence of palpable or radiographically suspicious lymphadenopathy. Patients who are cN0 can harbor lymphatic metastases that are too small to be detected by imaging or palpation. A discordance between the clinical and pathologic nodal (pN) stage results when subclinical or occult metastases not appreciated on imaging are detected on pathologic examination of the lymph nodes (LNs) following neck dissection.

Management of the cN0 neck is controversial, the decision being to treat or observe the neck. Advocates of observation (OBS), or watchful waiting, will examine the neck during follow-up visits and reserve neck dissection for patients who develop regional metastases. Elective neck dissection (END) or elective neck irradiation (ENI) are management options when the decision is to treat the neck. These management options have been long discussed among head and neck surgeons and the controversy persists despite significant advances in imaging and surgical techniques. The extent of controversy is illustrated by two studies that examined the variability in management strategies of the cN0 neck among otolaryngologists (1,2). A survey of 763 otolaryngologists in the United States showed 13% of the responders would observe the neck in all cN0 patients, 66% would perform END and 19% would recommend ENI. There was also little agreement about the extent of neck dissection among surgeons who operate on the cN0 neck. Similarly, the most recent National Comprehensive Cancer Network (NCCN) treatment guidelines leave the decision of END for early stage (T1 and T2) oral cavity, oropharynx, and supraglottic cancers largely to the discretion of the surgeon (3). NCCN treatment guidelines are based on the consensus of a multidisciplinary panel of experts who have reviewed the best available evidence.

The controversy over management of the N0 neck arises for several reasons. Proponents of OBS argue that the risk of isolated regional recurrence is small and does not warrant the morbidity of END in the majority of patients. Another presumption of OBS is that patients who do recur can be detected early enough for salvage treatment to be effective. Advocates of END argue that pathologic staging provides objective data that guide decisions about adjuvant treatment, as well as accurate prognostic information. All are factors that contribute to the decision about how the cN0 neck is managed.

This chapter explores the controversies that surround management of the cN0 neck. As a starting point, consider the following questions as related to the management options. (a) What is the incidence of occult metastases in the cN0 neck? (b) Do occult metastases impact patient outcome? (c) Can radiographic imaging detect occult metastases with acceptable accuracy?

INCIDENCE OF OCCULT METASTASES

Tumor site, its stage, and in some sites tumor thickness are important determinants of the occult metastases. Estimates of the occult metastatic rate can be obtained by studying the regional recurrence rate in patients who are followed clinically, or by looking at the pN+ rate after END. Using the first method, studies that report on patients who develop isolated regional metastases during OBS are assumed to have had occult neck disease at the time of diagnosis. Data from four studies on the regional recurrence rate of early stage oral tongue and floor of mouth squamous cell carcinoma (SCC) during OBS suggest that the occult metastatic rate approaches 40% (4–7). Reports on the pathologic N stage following END are also available

TABLE 118.1	OCCULT METASTATIC RATE: PATHOLOGIC N STAGE

Primary Site	pN+ (%)		
	Pitman et al.	Byers et al.	Shah
Oral cavity	41	45	34
Oropharynx	36	39	31
Hypopharynx	36	56	17
Larynx (supraglottic/ advanced glottic)	30	26	37

and data from three studies reporting on the pN stage in oral cavity, oropharynx, larynx and hypopharynx SCC, and with the exception of the hypopharynx, showed an occult metastatic rate of greater than 30% for all sites, as shown in Table 118.1 (8–10).

IMPACT OF OCCULT METASTASES

Several studies have sought to correlate patient outcome with the presence or absence of occult metastases. A highly significant survival difference is reported in pN0 versus pN+ patients who are cN0 prior to neck dissection (11,12). Extracapsular spread (ECS) in occult metastases further downgrades disease-related survival, and some reports suggest that ECS in occult nodes has the same impact as it does in palpable nodes (11–14). The number of pathologically positive occult LNs also correlates with survival. Patients with two or more positive nodes have significantly worse survival compared to those with less than two positive nodes (15). Additionally, the impact of nodal ratio (positive:total LNs in the neck dissection specimen) on survival has been evaluated for HNSCC, with increasing nodal ratio negatively impacting survival (16). These data are strong evidence that occult metastases do impact the disease-specific survival. pN staging provides very accurate information about the risk of disease recurrence and is used to select those patients who will benefit from adjuvant radiation with or without chemotherapy.

RADIOGRAPHIC IMAGING

Clinical nodal staging is a multidisciplinary diagnostic problem that starts with palpation of the neck. It is estimated that 1.0 cm is the lower size limit that LNs can be appreciated by palpation, with accuracy of between 59% and 84%. Imaging studies provide an assessment of LN size and shape, as well as information about architecture. Suspicious LNs are spherical and greater than 1.0 to 1.5 cm. LNs that demonstrate central necrosis, surrounding soft tissue invasion, irregular borders, or groups of greater than 2 LNs also heighten suspicion for metastases. Imaging is also helpful in patients when palpation is less accurate, especially patients with a thick or previously treated neck or those who are at risk for metastases to the retropharyngeal and parapharyngeal space LNs. Today, computed tomography (CT), magnetic resonance imaging (MRI), ultrasound (US), and positron emission tomography (PET) scan are utilized to evaluate the N0 neck. Contemporary high-resolution imaging detects a certain percentage of suspicious LNs that are not appreciated on palpation and provides a slight to moderate increase in the detection rate. If imaging can reduce the risk of undetected occult metastases to less than 15%, head and neck surgeons may opt to observe cN0 patients. The question is whether imaging can achieve this aim.

COMPUTED TOMOGRAPHY AND MAGNETIC RESONANCE IMAGING

Studies that corroborate radiographic and pathologic staging provide meaningful information about the accuracy of radiographic staging. Curtin et al. (17) performed one of the most rigorous studies reporting on 213 cN0 patients with SCC of the oral cavity, oropharynx, hypopharynx, and larynx. All patients who had pretreatment CT and MRI of the neck and the imaging results were compared with pN staging. The results were used to calculate the negative and positive predictive value (NPV and PPV) for node sizes from 5.0 to 15.0 mm in 1.0-mm increments. The authors showed that a 5.0-mm node had a PPV of 44% and a NPV of 90%. When a 10-mm threshold was utilized, the PPV and NPV were 50% and 84%, respectively. Accordingly, for every increase in LN size the false-positive rate decreases, but so too does the ability to detect patients that are truly diseased. The accuracy of CT and MRI was approximately equal in this study. Dr. Curtin concluded, "It is unlikely that any imaging study will distinguish normal from metastatic lymph nodes in the 5 to 10 mm range, because nodes less than 5 to 10 mm rarely show internal abnormalities that are used to distinguish suspiciouslymph nodes."

Size measurements of metastatic LNs in END specimens reflect the difficulty with their clinical detection. Approximately two-thirds of occult metastases were less than 10 mm, and of these, up to 50% are less than 3 mm. Importantly, ECS was found in 33% to 36% of occult positive nodes (11).

More recent studies substantiate Curtin's findings. Yuen et al. (18) found that occult metastases were present in 34% of T1/T2 oral tongue SCC patients who were cN0 based on imaging. Another study demonstrated the differences between pathologic and clinical staging with CT and US were highly significant ($P = 0.0001$) (19).

Imaging can also show false positives when corroborated with pN stage. For example, Walvekar et al. (20) showed that 21% of patients were downstaged from cN+ to pN0 when CT findings and pathology were compared. In addition to downstaging, 26% patients who were cN0 by imaging were upstaged to pN+ following neck dissection. Overall, this study reported a discrepancy between pathologic and clinical nodal stage in 47% of patients with T1/T2 oropharyngeal cancer. The authors of these studies, all performed more recently than Curtin's original study, suggest that radiographic imaging is not accurate enough to take the place of pathologic staging for at-risk patients.

ULTRASOUND-GUIDED FINE NEEDLE ASPIRATION

Ultrasound-guided fine-needle aspiration (USGFNA) of suspicious LNs is another method to evaluate patients who are N0 by palpation. US examination of the neck and biopsy is typically performed by the head and neck surgeon familiar in lymphatic drainage patterns and risk factors for occult metastases. US criteria for suspicious nodes are similar to those used for CT and MRI and according to published protocols at least one suspicious node per patient is sampled by fine-needle biopsy under US guidance. US measurements of LNs are highly accurate making it an excellent method to detect serial changes in LNs during follow-up. When fine-needle aspiration (FNA) results are positive, the neck is treated. FNA negative patients are staged N0 and followed clinically with frequent US examination of the neck. The low cost of examinations, accurate measurements of LN size, the lack of exposure to ionizing radiation, and the ability to needle biopsy suspicious nodes during the examination highlight the appeal of this technique. Isolated regional recurrences detected with follow-up US examinations are reported by three groups studying early stage tongue cancer, ranging from 18% to 31% (21–23).

van den Brekel et al. (21) studied 77 patients with oral cavity lesions staged cN0 by USGFNA. Tumors were resected transorally and the neck was followed with US at 2- to 3-month intervals. The regional recurrence rate during follow-up was 18%. Six recurrences were detected on US, eight patients presented with palpable nodes, and the salvage rate was 71.4%. In two similar studies, patients with T1 and T2 oral tongue tumors who were cN0 by US were followed. The incidence of isolated regional recurrences was 28.5% and 31%, with salvage rates of 46% and 100% (22,23). The authors of these three studies advocate the use of USGFNA nodal staging. Close clinical follow-up and strict patient compliance are required for early detection of recurrences and meaningful salvage. Notably, the 100% salvage rate was reported by for patients enrolled in a prospective trial (23).

POSITRON EMISSION TOMOGRAPHY

PET is a functional imaging modality that provides information about the metabolic activity of tissues. Because the metabolic rate of SCC is higher than surrounding normal tissue, Fluorodeoxyglucose—the radioactively glucose analog used for imaging, accumulates in cancer cells at increased rates resulting in higher standard uptake values. Combined PET/CT scanners are now available and provide the anatomic detail of CT and the whole body sensitivity of PET. Three studies using PET for the cN0 neck showed NPVs of 88% to 92% (24–26) and found that false positives were possible in conditions that increased glucose metabolism including inflammation, sarcoidosis, and normal salivary tissue. False negatives occurred with necrotic LNs and when metastatic LNs were less than 5.0 mm, suggesting that a minimum tumor volume must be present to detect a difference in glucose utilization above background. Two studies have demonstrated that at least 5-mm tumor must be present to be detected and suggest PET does not achieve the diagnostic accuracy of END (26,27).

More recent studies using higher resolution fused PET/CT scanners show a significant false-positive rate of 16% to 27%. The authors of these studies conclude PET is a valuable test for detection of unknown and second primary tumors as well as distant metastases, but does not currently have the accuracy to replace END or guide therapeutic decisions in the N0 neck (27–30).

In 2011, Stoeckli et al. (31) compared CT, PET/CT, US, and USGFNA for neck staging in a prospective study of 76 patients. The study protocol included imaging with all four radiographic modalities prior to surgery that included neck dissection. Results showed that USGFNA overstaged the fewest, with only 7% false positive (7% to 16%). Understaging was equivalent for all modalities with false-negative rates of 21% to 25%. Despite significant improvements in imaging technology over the past decade, even recent data suggest no imaging study can assess N stage with 100% accuracy. Size and changes in LN architecture or metabolic activity determine if a study is positive or negative. Since a significant percentage of occult nodes fall outside of these radiographic parameters, both the false-positive and false-negative rates are significant. Further prospective studies that correlate the pN stage with combined PET/CT findings are required to determine if it can reduce the risk of undetected metastases to an acceptable level.

MANAGEMENT STRATEGY FOR THE N0 NECK

Patient and tumor-related factors impact the decision to electively treat the neck. Many clinicians cite unreliable patient follow-up as justification for elective treatment of the neck. ENI is used when radiation is used to treat the primary tumor so the patient is treated with a single modality. If the neck will be entered for resection of the tumor or reconstruction, most surgeons advocate END. Accordingly, END becomes a question when treatment of the primary does not involve access to the neck. Examples include transoral resection of oral cavity and oropharyngeal tumors and transoral laser or robotic excision of laryngeal or pharyngeal tumors.

Surgeons typically use a 15% to 20% or greater risk of occult metastases as the threshold to perform END. Table 118.2 shows estimates of the likelihood of occult metastases based on the site and stage of the primary tumor. The threshold of 20% is based on a decision analysis performed by Weiss et al. published in 1994 (32) that compared survival outcomes for patients managed by END versus OBS. The method for a decision analysis concerning management of the N0 neck involves the use of decision trees using the alternative management options and probabilities based on published data. It is used to guide management decisions when no clear consensus emerges from the available data. Weiss et al. (32) reviewed outcome data for END versus OBS published in the 1980s, and some authors believe older results no longer be relevant given advances in technology and surgical technique. Using more recent data, the decision analysis by Okura et al. (33) suggested that a threshold of 44% could be utilized because detection of occult metastases, salvage rates, and the morbidity of END had all improved. In contrast, Song et al. (34) suggested that an 18% risk of occult metastases would provide benefit for END in patients with early stage tongue cancer. Their model showed that OBS would be an acceptable strategy only if the occult metastatic rate is less than 18% and salvage rates for regional recurrences is 73% or greater. These three decision analyses use theoretical models based on published data from the literature reporting on the risk of occult metastases and salvage rates.

Elective Neck Dissection

The procedural details of END have evolved from the use of radical neck dissection (RND) over 100 years ago, to more targeted, selective operations that are widely used today. Based on OBSs that regional recurrence rates were lower in some cN0 patients whose necks were dissected electively, Crile (35) introduced the concept of END in 1905. Hayes Martin popularized the concept of RND and described it as en bloc resection of levels I to V that included the sternocleidomastoid muscle, CN XI, and internal jugular vein and this became the standard for END in the United States (36,37). Martin's precepts were not challenged until the 1960s when Bocca proposed a conservation technique that preserved major structures (38). The rationale for preserving structures was based on OBSs that the lymphatic system of the neck is contained within the adipose tissue and does not extend beyond the fascial sheaths. By removing the fascia surrounding the sternocleidomastoid muscle, internal jugular vein, and CN XI, the cervical LNs in level I to V are completely excised. Subsequent studies have shown that modified radical neck dissection (MRND) is as effective as RND for both elective and therapeutic neck dissection when the preserved structures are not involved by tumor. Aside from the obvious functional and cosmetic advantages, MRND made simultaneous bilateral neck dissections a safe alternative when operating on both necks. The concept of selective neck dissections (SNDs) emerged as clinical studies suggested that metastases travel from the primary site to predictable first echelon nodal groups and then on to adjacent nodal basins. Retrospectively analyzing the location of occult metastases following elective MRND, Shah and Byers independently reported on the patterns of occult metastases from primary sites of the head and neck (8,9,39). SNDs were defined as a dissection that removes only the cervical levels that are at greatest risk for metastases. Today most surgeons remove levels I to III or I to IV for oral cavity primaries and levels II to IV for laryngeal, hypopharyngeal, and oropharyngeal primaries, and may include level VI in select laryngeal and hypopharyngeal sites. Treatment of the contralateral neck is given consideration for supraglottic, base of tongue, palate, and primary tumors that approach or cross the midline (3). Advantages of selective procedures are the reduction in surgical morbidity and cosmetic impact compared to RND and MRND. During the 1980s and 1990s surgeons at most centers in the United States adopted SNDs as the preferred procedure for END.

TABLE 118.2	RISK OF OCCULT METASTASES BY SITE AND STAGE OF PRIMARY TUMOR	
	Stage	Site
<15%–20%	T1	Glottis (T1/T2), retromolar trigone, gingiva, hard palate, buccal mucosa
>20%–30%	T1	Oral tongue, soft palate, pharyngeal wall, supraglottic larynx, tonsil
	T2	Floor of mouth, oral tongue, retromolar trigone, gingiva, hard palate, buccal mucosa
		T1–4 nasopharynx, piriform sinus, base of tongue
	T2–4	Soft palate, pharyngeal wall, supraglottic larynx, tonsil
	T3–4	Floor of mouth, oral tongue, retromolar trigone, gingiva, hard palate, buccal mucosa

Modified from Mendenhall et al. (42).

Regional recurrences following END occur at a rate of 3% to 6% regardless of the procedure utilized (RND, MRND, or SND) (10). Regional recurrences can be thought of as either an error in surgical technique or in the pathologic sampling technique. If the surgeon does not completely dissect the levels at risk, or the tumor has metastasized to levels not predicted by the primary tumor recurrences are possible. The accuracy of pathologic staging also depends on how carefully the pathologist examines the neck specimen. The detection rate is higher when cervical nodes are serially sectioned with thin cuts versus bisecting LNs; and a small percent of occult metastases are likely beyond the resolution of light microscopy. Immunohistochemical (IHC) analysis for several tumor markers in electively dissected neck specimens showed that 20% to 30% of the nodes that were pN0 on light microscopy had evidence micrometastases of on IHC analysis (40,41).

Elective Neck Irradiation

The factors that influence the decision to irradiate the cN0 neck are similar to those for END. ENI is the treatment of choice when the primary tumor is irradiated and the risk of occult metastases is greater than 15% to 20%. It is also an option for patients who are poor surgical candidates. Patients' compliance with follow-up and the morbidity of ENI are also considered. Patients who are cN0 receive substantially lower radiation doses to the neck than cN+ patients and have an associated reduction in the treatment-related morbidity. The availability of conformational and intensity modulated radiation therapy has minimized the volume of normal tissue that is included in the treatment portals further reducing the morbidity of ENI. Mendenhall et al. (42) have reported regional recurrences in less than 5% of patients following ENI. One advantage of ENI is the ability to address groups of nodes that are not typically included in END. These include the retropharyngeal and parapharyngeal space LNs that are at risk of harboring occult metastases in tumors of the oropharynx, hypopharynx, nasopharynx, and nasal cavity.

A significant shortcoming of ENI is that the prognostic information from pathologic staging is not known. It is also more difficult to detect recurrences following ENI and the use of reirradiation can be limited.

END Controversies

Central to the debate surrounding the value of END is whether removing occult neck disease affords a survival advantage when compared to a policy of clinical OBS. There are four prospective randomized reports comparing END to OBS for oral cavity cancers treated with transoral excision or irradiation. They span 30 years and report a wide range of salvage rates. Disease-free survival rates for the OBS groups range from 49% to 87% in these studies. Only one study showed a statistically significant advantage for END (43), and another showed an advantage but state

their study group was too small to achieve statistical significance (6). One study randomized patients after receiving interstitial radiation to tumors of the oral tongue (44). The most recent study followed patients in the OBS group with monthly neck US examination and reported a 100% salvage rate for isolated regional recurrences in the OBS group (23). The results of this prospective study are in marked contrast to a retrospective study published 10 years earlier by the same group. Their earlier study reported a 50% salvage rate and a statistically significant improvement in disease-free survival for END (45). The authors attribute disparate results to the rigorous schedule of follow-up with monthly US for patients enrolled in the prospective clinical trial. All four studies showed that END markedly improved the regional control rate with regional recurrences in 6% to 30% of the END group versus 37% to 58% in the OBS group. Fansula et al. (46) performed a meta-analysis of these four studies. By combining outcomes for the 283 patients from these reports, they showed that END significantly reduced the disease-specific mortality and acknowledged the advantage for END in early tongue cancer. Meta-analysis was used in this case to increase the sample size, hence the statistical power, to provide a more accurate estimate of the true effect of END.

Retrospective studies also show mixed results. Smith et al. (47) reported on the outcome of 150 patients with T1 to T4 N0 oral cavity and oropharyngeal tumors. There were 75 patients in the END group based on a greater than 20% risk of occult metastases or if the neck was entered for the tumor resection or microvascular reconstruction. The other 75 patients were managed with OBS based on less than 20% risk of occult disease. Despite a statistically significant difference in the regional recurrence rate, 5% for the END group and 20% for the OBS group, the difference in the 5-year survival rate between the two groups was not significant. The authors did show highly significant differences in 5-year survival rates based on the number of pathologically positive nodes ($P < 0.001$).

Duvvuri et al. (48) compared the outcome of 359 patients with T1 to T4 N0 oral cavity and oropharyngeal tumors managed with END versus OBS. The treatment groups were based on time period they were treated, for example, before or after 1990 when the management strategy changed END was performed routinely in N0 patients. The 5-year overall survival between END and OBS groups was not different, but the difference in the regional recurrence rate, 15% versus 27% for the END and OBS groups, respectively, was highly significant ($P < 0.0001$). In both studies, more patients in the END group received adjuvant radiation, a direct result of the pathologic staging information.

A similar study (49) analyzed 54 patients with T1 to T3 N0 oral cavity tumors managed with END versus OBS. There was no difference in the overall survival between treatment groups. But when stratified by T stage, for T1 tumors there was no difference between the treatment groups for the regional recurrence rate or overall survival. But for patients with T2 and T3 tumors, the regional recurrence rate and the associated mortality were significantly higher in the patients in the OBS group and the authors advocated END.

Other retrospective studies have shown a significant survival advantage for patients who receive END. Yuen et al. (45) performed a retrospective review of 63 patients with T1 and T2 oral tongue tumors. For the 33 patients in the END group, both regional recurrences and 5-year overall survival rate were significantly improved compared to the 30 patients who were observed ($P = 0.0008$ and $P = 0.01$, respectively). Despite surgical salvage of 50% of the regional recurrences in the OBS group, the regional recurrence-related mortality in this group was 23% compared to 3% in the END group and this benefit translated to a significant improvement in 5-year overall survival. In another study that examined 153 patients with T1/T2 oral SCC with thickness 4 mm or more showed a statistically significant ($P = 0.001$) improvement in regional recurrence-related survival for END compared to OBS (50).

In a detailed analysis of patients with T1 and T2 N0 oral tongue tumors, Haddadin et al. (51) compared the outcome of 64 patients who were observed to that of 37 who received END. The institutional policy was to observe the neck in all patients with T1 or T2 oral tongue tumors unless the neck was entered to resect the primary or perform reconstruction. The authors did show a trend toward improved 5-year overall survival for the END cohort. Subset analysis of the T2 tumors demonstrated a highly significant survival advantage for END ($P = 0.0007$). The authors also showed that the incidence of greater than 2 LNs and/or ECS was significantly higher in the patients who required therapeutic neck dissection than in patients who received END ($P = 0.001$ and $P < 0.0001$). The impact of this finding is illustrated by comparing the 5-year survival of patients who were pN+ after END versus therapeutic dissections, which was 69% versus 35%, respectively ($P = 0.04$). Another retrospective report showed no significant difference in survival outcomes for patients treated with END versus observation for oral cavity, larynx and pharynx (52).

These seven retrospective studies all show significant improvements in the regional recurrence rate for patients managed with END. The benefit in disease-related survival is less clear and retrospective studies will probably never conclusively answer the question. Rodrigo et al. (53) performed a meta-analysis of 21 prospective and retrospective studies comparing END to OBS in N0 patients with early stage oral, oropharyngeal, and supraglottic cancers. Their conclusion was that based on the best available evidence, END does not appear to provide a survival advantage over OBS, but the studies analyzed are not of sufficient quality to provide definitive recommendations for management of the cN0 neck. These patient cohorts are difficult to analyze because of differences in institutional treatment plans, time period, and the significant number of patients

who succumb to local and distant recurrences or medical comorbidities, ultimately leaving the number of patients who develop isolated regional recurrences and can be analyzed relatively small. While END may not show benefit when the entire cohort is analyzed, scrutinizing the outcome of pN+ patients may demonstrate a benefit.

Other Considerations

END is a consideration for patients with unilateral N+ disease and contralateral N0 disease in a malignancy for sites that bilateral END is not usually recommended, such as tonsil, oral tongue, and piriform sinus cancers. This was addressed for tonsil cancer by Lim et al. (54), who found that in patients with tonsillar cancer who were ipsilateral N+, there was a 21% rate of contralateral neck disease which portended a poorer survival. Contralateral neck disease was also influenced by T stage, and the authors concluded that the contralateral neck should be addressed in patients with ipsilateral neck metastasis or advanced T stage (T3 to T4). Koo et al. (55) examined patients with piriform sinus SCC and found that ipsilateral neck disease and extension of the primary across midline was associated with occult disease in the contralateral neck and therefore recommended bilateral neck treatment in the aforementioned situations. In the oral cavity, END of the contralateral N0 neck has not shown to improved survival in patients with early stage SCC of the oral tongue (56).

Salvage surgery for recurrent head and neck tumors that were treated with primary radiation and remain N0, with isolated primary recurrences is another area of discussion. If the necks received ENI, the dilemma in patients who remain N0 is whether to perform END at the time of salvage surgery. Bohannon et al. (57) compared 38 patients who underwent END with salvage laryngectomy with 33 whose necks were not dissected. Their results were mixed with higher fistula and complication rates in patients undergoing END, but lower rate of regional failure (7.9% vs. 15%). There was no statistically significant survival difference between the two groups. A similar study examined 57 patients with recurrent oropharyngeal, hypopharyngeal, and laryngeal cancers treated with primary radiation and were N0 at recurrence. Dagan et al. (58) concluded that adding END to the salvage surgery increased morbidity while there was no benefit in survival or locoregional control when initial treatment included ENI.

FUTURE DIRECTIONS

More accurate, less invasive methods to evaluate the cN0 neck are active areas of investigation. Sentinel lymph node biopsy (SLNB) and pathologic predictors of occult metastases are two techniques that demonstrate potential for routine clinical use in the future. The concept of the sentinel lymph node (SLN) is described as the first echelon lymph node that is most likely to contain metastases if they are present. Morton et al. at the John Wayne Cancer Center are credited with the development of the technique for selective identification and biopsy of the SLN in patients with intermediate thickness cutaneous melanoma (CM). SLNB is based on the premise that metastases travel sequentially from the primary tumor, to the SLN and then on to the remaining regional LNs. Therefore, the histopathologic status of the SLN accurately reflects the pathologic status of the remaining regional lymphatics and patients with pathologically negative SLNs can be spared the morbidity of regional lymphadenectomy. Since Morton's original description of the SLNB technique, investigators worldwide have contributed to the evolution and refinement of the technique that is currently used. Multiple studies show highly acceptable sensitivity and false-negative rates for SLNB (59) and today SLNB is considered the standard of care for patients with intermediate thickness CM (60).

Preoperative lymphoscintigraphy performed by nuclear medicine uses peritumoral injection of a radiotracer, directing the surgeon to the lymphatic regions at risk (Fig. 118.1). In the operating room, the surgeon uses a gamma probe to identify radioactive SLNs and may use blue dye injections around the tumor for visual identification.

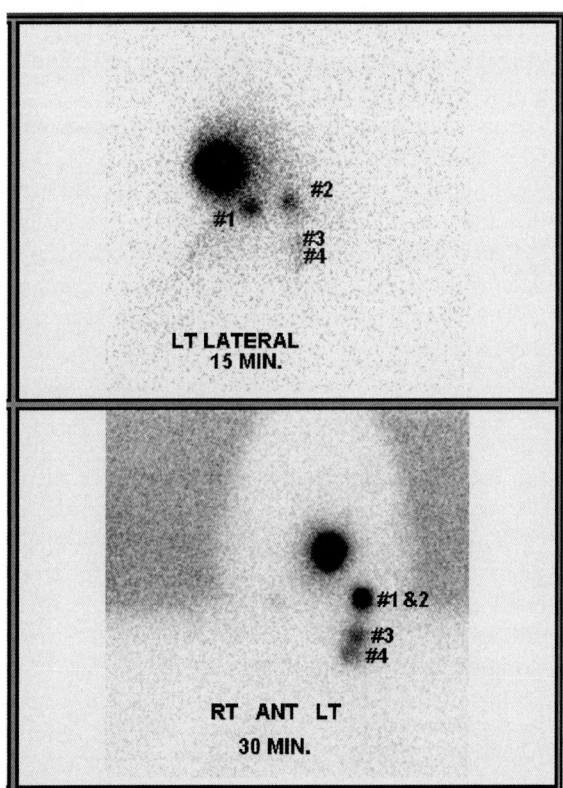

Figure 118.1 Lateral and anterior-posterior lymphoscintigraphy images at 15 and 30 minutes postinjection of Technetium–sulfa colloid. The patient is a 42-year-old man with a cT1N0M0 SCC of the left lateral tongue. Surgical pathology was SCC, 1.2 cm in greatest diameter, with maximum depth of invasion 4.1 mm. SLNB results: SLN 1 was a 7 × 5 × 2 mm LN with a 1-mm focus of SCC. SLN 2–4 showed no evidence of carcinoma on H&E or cytokeratin immunohistochemical staining.

The SLN is exposed through a small skin incision and is identified by the presence of blue staining and/or radiotracer uptake detected by the gamma probe. The SLN(s) are removed and sent to the pathologist for histologic and IHC analysis. Therapeutic node dissection is performed only in patients whose SLN is positive.

SLNB has been studied in head and neck cancer patients who are cN0. Guidelines published in 2010 describe the indications as well as the radiologic, surgical, and pathologic techniques for localizing, obtaining, and processing SLNB in patients with oral/oropharyngeal SCC (61). The preliminary experience in HNSCC was summarized by Ross et al. (62) and included data from 22 centers. Analysis of 316 cN0 necks showed that the SLN was identified in 95% with an overall accuracy of 90%. When the results from centers that performed less than 10 cases were excluded, the sensitivity of SLNB was 94% relative to simultaneous END. The ACOSOG multi-institutional study compared the accuracy of SLNB versus END in patients with T1/T2 N0 oral cavity SCC. SLNB compared favorably to END, with a 96% NPV for SLNB (63). SLNB for oral cavity tumors appears to offer patients a reduction in the overall morbidity and cost compared to a blanket policy of END (64).

Advantages of SLNB specific to head and neck tumors include the ability of preoperative lymphoscintigraphy to map the patient's unique lymphatic drainage pattern and direct the surgeon to cervical levels that may not have been predicted by the site and stage of the primary tumor. Results of preoperative lymphoscintigraphy show a significant rate of aberrant lymphatic draining for the head and neck. Three independent studies have shown that 15% to 20% of ENDs for HNSCC, and over 30% for head and neck CM would have been misdirected had they been based solely on classical anatomic studies (59,65,66). Another advantage is that SLNB is a cost-effective method for pathologic examination of select LNs. Rather than examining all of the nodes in a neck dissection specimen, SLNB identifies an average of two or three nodes per patient. This facilitates the routine use of more costly and time-consuming serial sectioning and IHC required to accurately diagnose occult metastases. Using SLNB and IHC, several investigators have shown significant improvements in the accuracy of staging the cN0 neck (61,67,68). A recent review of the literature of SLNB for the cN0 head and neck patients confirms the conclusions of preliminary reports: that SLNB is safe and efficacious, although a learning curve does exist with high volume centers better equipped to achieve consistent results (69).

Ferris et al. (70) have designed a rapid, quantitative PCR assay that accurately identifies positive SLNs in the operating room. Further study and validation at other institutions will rectify one of the major drawbacks of SLNB, namely that for patients whose SLNs are positive, neck dissection is deferred to a separate procedure due to the time required for accurate step sectioning on permanent section.

PATHOLOGIC PREDICTORS OF METASTASES

The site and stage of the primary tumor are important considerations in assessing the risk of occult metastases. While there is a direct correlation between tumor stage and the occult metastatic rate for some sites, for example, in glottic SCC, tumor thickness has been shown to be a predictor of occult metastases for some sites including the oral tongue, floor of mouth, and oropharynx (71). Tumor thickness has been most intensively studied for oral tongue tumors (72,73). Yuen et al. (74) examined several histopathologic characteristics of 72 patients with T1 and T2 oral tongue tumors that were correlated with occult metastases. On multivariate analysis, tumor thickness was the only factor that correlated with occult metastases and 5-year survival. The pN+ rate for tumor thickness 3 mm or less was 8%. Metastases occurred in 44% of tumors between 3 and 9 mm, and in 53% of those tumors with thickness greater than 9 mm. The 5-year survival by thickness grouping was 100%, 77%, and 66%, respectively. Other studies have examined other histomorphologic features including perineural, lymphovascular, and the mode of invasion and grade of differentiation as risk factors for occult metastases and shown correlations (75–78).

Pathologic findings highlight one of the shortcomings of the current tumor nodal metastasis staging system. For instance, oral cavity tumor stage is defined primarily by tumor size and these studies suggest that some early stage tumors may have very aggressive characteristics. Investigators seeking to improve the prognostic capabilities of tumor staging have focused on characteristics of the primary tumor that are correlated with nodal metastases. Pathologic predictors of occult metastases that can be characterized with light microscopy, IHC (79), DNA analysis (80), and expression profiling (81) are currently under investigation. Many studies suggest that the specific correlates of metastases may be different for different anatomic sites. Additionally, combinations of parameters may more accurately predict the risk of metastases because it is unlikely that a single characteristic of the tumor will have a distinct cut off point in differentiating metastatic from nonmetastatic disease. A histologic malignancy score for oral cavity tumors based on a several histologic findings such as the keratinization, frequency of mitotic figures, pattern of invasion, perineural and perivascular invasion has been proposed (75,77). When these were applied prospectively to newly diagnosed patients, metastases were accurately predicted in these reports. Takes et al. (82) used a combination of histologic and IHC findings and showed that LN metastases from laryngeal tumors were accurately predicted ($P = 0.002$).

Once the characteristics of primary tumors that correlate with occult metastases are accurately identified, biologic tumor staging will be possible. One of the goals of these studies is to integrate the biologic correlates of metastases into the tumor staging system so clinicians can make management decisions about head neck based on the results of the pretreatment biopsy.

CONCLUSION

Management of the cN0 neck is controversial. The aim of the pretreatment evaluation of cN0 patients is to accurately identify patients with occult metastases who will benefit from treatment of the neck. Review of the methods that are currently in use for evaluation of the cN0 neck shows that radiographic imaging, and even PET/CT does not distinguish patients with microscopic cervical metastases from N0 patients with acceptable sensitivity and specificity. Biologic tumor staging and SLNB are promising techniques that have the potential to accurately stage the cN0 neck patients before treatment is initiated. Until these investigational staging methods are refined and validated in prospective trials, pathologic examination of the neck contents remains the most accurate method to assess cervical LNs, accurately estimate disease-free survival, and guide the administration of adjuvant therapies.

HIGHLIGHTS

- The incidence of occult cervical metastases is greater than 20% for most head and neck mucosal sites. The exceptions are T1 tumors of the retromolar trigone, buccal mucosal, gingiva, hard palate, and T1 and T2 glottic tumors (Table 118.1).
- The pN status of cN0 patients is strongly correlated with the disease-related outcome.
- Radiographic imaging provides anatomic information that identifies lymph nodes that are suspicious for metastases. It does not have the accuracy to determine whether the N0 neck requires treatment.
- END is currently the most accurate method to stage the cN0 neck. END is a staging procedure that is used to guide subsequent treatment. Its therapeutic value has not been conclusively documented.
- Elective versus therapeutic neck dissection describes the indication for neck dissection. A neck dissection is performed *electively* when there is no clinical evidence of metastases. *Therapeutic* neck dissection refers to procedures that are performed for suspicious adenopathy that is palpable or detected on radiographic imaging.
- Comprehensive versus SND describes what cervical levels are removed. *Comprehensive* neck dissection removes levels I to V. RNDs and all three types of MRNDs are comprehensive procedures. SND removes less than five levels and are named according to the levels removed, for example, SND I to III. Both selective and comprehensive procedures can be used for END.
- Techniques that are less invasive than END and more accurate than radiographic imaging for staging the cN0 neck are under active investigation and hold promise for routine clinical use in the future.

REFERENCES

1. Werning J, Heard D, Pagano C, et al. Elective management of the clinically negative neck by otolaryngologists in patients with oral tongue cancer. *Arch Otolaryngol Head Neck Surg* 2003;129:83–88.

2. Dunne AA, Folz BJ, Kuropkat C, et al. Extent of surgical intervention in case of N0 neck in head and neck cancer patients: an analysis of data collection of 39 hospitals. *Eur Arch Otorhinolaryngol* 2004;261:295–303.

3. NCCN Guidelines Head and Neck Cancers Version 2.2011. NCCN.org

4. Yuen AP, Wei WI, Wong Y, et al. Elective neck dissection versus observation in the treatment of early oral tongue carcinoma. *Head Neck* 1997;19:583–588.

5. McGuirt WF, Johnson JT, Myers EN, et al. Floor of mouth carcinoma. The management of the clinically negative neck. *Arch Otolaryngol Head Neck Surg* 1995;121:278–282.

6. Fakih AR, Rao RS, Borges AM, Patel AR. Elective versus therapeutic neck dissection in early carcinoma of the oral tongue. *Am J Surg* 1989;158:309–313.

7. Vandenbrouck C, Sancho-Garnier H, Chassagne D, et al. Elective versus therapeutic radical neck dissection in epidermoid carcinoma of the oral cavity: results of a randomized clinical trial. *Cancer* 1980;15:386–390.

8. Shah JP. Patterns of cervical lymph node metastasis from squamous carcinomas of the upper aerodigestive tract. *Am J Surg* 1990;160:405–409.

9. Byers RM, Wolf PF, Ballentyne AJ. Rationale for elective modified neck dissection. *Head Neck Surg* 1988;10:160–167.

10. Pitman KT, Johnson JT, Myers EN. Effectiveness of selective neck dissection for management of the clinically negative neck. *Arch Otolaryngol Head Neck Surg* 1997;123:917–922.

11. Jose J, Coatesworth AP, MacLennan K. Cervical metastases in upper aerodigestive tract squamous cell carcinoma: the significance of extracapsular spread and soft tissue deposits in the neck. *Head Neck* 2003;25:194–197.

12. Gourin CG, Conger BT, Porubsky ES, et al. The effect of occult nodal metastases on survival and regional control in patients with head and neck squamous cell carcinoma. *Laryngoscope* 2008;118:1191–1194.

13. Dias F, Lima R, Manfro G. Management of the N0 neck in moderately advanced squamous carcinoma of the larynx. *Otolaryngol Head Neck Surg* 2009;141:59–65.

14. Shaw RJ, Lowe D, Woolgar JA, et al. Extracapsular spread in oral squamous cell carcinoma. *Head Neck* 2010;32:714–722.

15. Colnot DR, Nieuwenhuis EJ, Kuik DJ, et al. Clinical significance of micrometastatic cells detected by E48 (Ly-6D) reverse transcription-polymerase chain reaction in bone marrow of head and neck cancer patients. *Clin Cancer Res* 2004;10:7827–7833.

16. Ebrahimi A, Clark JR, Zhang WJ, et al. Lymph node ratio as an independent prognostic factor in oral squamous cell carcinoma. *Head Neck* 2010;33:1–8.

17. Curtin H, Ishwaran H, Mancuso A, et al. Comparison of CT and MR imaging in staging of neck metastases. *Radiology* 1998;207:123–130.

18. Yuen AP, Lam KY, Chan AC, et al. Clinicopathological analysis of elective neck dissection for N0 neck of early oral tongue carcinoma. *Am J Surg* 1999;177:90–92.

19. Haberal I, Celik H, Gocmen H, et al. Which is important in the evaluation of metastatic lymph nodes in head and neck cancer: Palpation, ultrasonography, or computed tomography? *Otolaryngol Head Neck Surg* 2004;130:197–201.

20. Walvekar RR, Li RJ, Gooding WE, et al. Role of surgery in limited (T1–2, N0–1) cancers of the oropharynx. *Laryngoscope* 2008;118:2129–2134.

21. van den Brekel M, Castelijns J, Leemans C, et al. Outcome of observing the N0 neck using ultrasonographic-guided cytology for follow-up. *Arch Otolaryngol Head Neck Surg* 1999;125:153–156.

22. Tsang RK, Chung JC, To VS, et al. Efficacy of salvage neck dissection for isolated nodal recurrences in early carcinoma of oral tongue with watchful waiting management of initial N0 neck. *Head Neck* 2011;33(10):1482–1485.

23. Yuen AP, Chow TL, Cheung WY, et al. Prospective randomized study of selective neck dissection versus observation for N0 neck of early tongue carcinoma. *Head Neck* 2009;31:765–772.

24. Myers L, Wax M, Nabi H. Positron emission tomography in the evaluation of the N0 neck. *Laryngoscope* 1998;108:232–236.

25. Wensing B, Vogel WV, Marres HA, et al. FDG-PET in the clinically negative neck in oral squamous cell carcinoma. *Laryngoscope* 2006;119:809–813.

26. Hansono MM, Kunda LD, Segal GM, et al. Uses and limitations of FDG positron emission tomography in patients with head and neck cancer. *Laryngoscope* 1999;109:880–885.

27. Fleming AJ Jr, Smith SP Jr, Paul CM, Hall NC. Impact of [18F]-2-fluorodeoxyglucose-positron emission tomography/computed tomography on previously untreated head and neck cancer patients. *Laryngoscope* 2007;117(7):1173–1179.

28. Richard C, Prevot N, Timoshenko AP, et al. Preoperative combined 18-fluorodeoxyglucose positron emission tomography and computed tomography imaging in head and neck cancer: does it really improve initial N staging? *Acta Otolaryngol* 2010;130(12):1421–1424.

29. Gordin A, Golz A, Keidar Z, et al. The role of FDG-PET/CT imaging in head and neck malignant conditions: Impact on diagnostic accuracy and patient care. *Otolaryngol Head Neck Surg* 2007;137:130–137.

30. Iyer NG, Clark JR, Singham S, Zhu J. 3 Role of pretreatment ^{18}FDG-PET/CT in surgical decision-making for head and neck cancers. *Head Neck* 2010;32:1202–1208.

31. Stoeckli SJ, Haerle SK, Strobel K, et al. Initial staging of the neck in head and neck squamous cell carcinoma: a comparison of CT, PET/CT, and ultrasound-guided fine-needle aspiration cytology. *Head Neck* 2012;34(4):469–476.

32. Weiss MH, Harrison LB, Isaacs RS, et al. Use of decision analysis in planning a management strategy for the stage N0 neck. *Arch Otolaryngol Head Neck Surg* 1994;120:699–702.

33. Okura M, Aikawa T, Sawai NY, et al. Decision analysis and treatment threshold in a management for the N0 neck of the oral cavity carcinoma. *Oral Oncol* 2009;45:908–911.

34. Song T, Bi N, Gui L, Peng Z. Elective neck dissection or "watchful waiting": optimal management strategy for early stage N0 tongue carcinoma using decision analysis techniques. *Chin Med J* 2008;121:1646–1650.

35. Crile G. Landmark article Dec 1, 1906: Excision of cancer of the head and neck with special reference to the plan of dissection based on 132 operations. By George Crile. *JAMA* 1987;258:3286–3293.

36. Martin H, Del Valle B, Ehrlich HE, Cahan WG. Neck dissection. *Cancer* 1951;4:441–499.

37. Martin H. Radical neck dissection. *Clin Symp* 1961;13:103–120.

38. Bocca E, Pignataro O. A conservation technique in radical neck dissection. *Ann Otol Rhinol Laryngol* 1967;76:975–987.

39. Byers RM. Modified neck dissection. A study of 967 cases from 1070–1980. *Am J Surg* 1985;150:414–421.

40. Ferlito A, Rinaldo A, Devaney KO, et al. Detection of lymph node micrometastasis in patients with squamous cell carcinoma of the head and neck. *Eur Arch Otorhinolaryngol* 2008;265:1147–1153.

41. Barrera JE, Miller ME, Said S, et al. Detection of occult cervical micrometastases in patients with head and neck squamous cell cancer. *Laryngoscope* 2003;113:892–896.

42. Mendenhall WM, Million RR. Elective irradiation for squamous cell carcinoma of the head and neck: analysis of dose related factors and causes of failure. *Int J Radiant Oncol Biol Phys* 1986;12:741–746.

43. Kligerman J, Lima RA, Soares JR, et al. Supraomohyoid neck dissection in the treatment of T1/T2 squamous cell carcinoma of the oral cavity. *Am J Surg* 1994;168:391–394.

44. Vandenbrouck C, Sancho-Garnier H, Chassagne D, et al. Elective versus therapeutic radical neck dissection in epidermoid carcinoma of the oral cavity: results of a randomized clinical trial. *Cancer* 1980;15:386–390.

45. Yuen AP, Wei WI, Wong YM, Tang KC. Elective neck dissection versus observation in the treatment of early oral tongue carcinoma. *Head Neck* 1997;19:583–588.

46. Fansula AJ, Greene BH, Timmesfeld N, et al. A meta-analysis of the randomized controlled trials on elective neck dissection versus therapeutic neck dissection in early oral cavity cancers with clinically node negative neck. *Oral Oncol* 2011;5:320–324.

47. Smith GI, O'Brien CJ, Clark J, et al. Management of the neck in patients with T1 and T2 cancer in the mouth. *Br J Oral Maxillofacial Surg* 2004;42:494–500.

48. Duvvuri U, Simental AA, D'Angelo G, et al. Elective neck dissection and survival in patients with squamous cell carcinoma of the oral cavity and oropharynx. *Laryngoscope* 2004;114:2228–2234.

49. Persky M, Lagmay V. Treatment of the clinically negative neck in oral squamous cell carcinoma. *Laryngoscope* 1999;109: 1160–1164.

50. Ebrahimi A, Ashford BG, Clark JR. Improved survival with elective neck dissection in thick early stage oral squamous cell carcinoma. *Head Neck* 2012;34(5):709–716.

51. Haddadin K, Soutar D, Oliver R, et al. Improved survival for patients with clinically T1/T2, N0 tongue tumors undergoing prophylactic neck dissection. *Head Neck* 1999;21:517–525.

52. Layland M, Sessions D, Lenox J. The influence of lymph nodes metastasis in the treatment of squamous cell carcinoma of the oral cavity, oropharynx, larynx, and hypopharynx: N0 versus N+. *Laryngoscope* 2005;115:629–639.

53. Rodrigo JP, Shah JP, Silver CE. Management of the clinically negative neck in early-stage head and neck cancers after transoral resection. *Head Neck* 2011;33:1210–1219.

54. Lim YC, Lee SY, Lim JY, et al. Management of the contralateral neck in tonsillar squamous cell carcinoma. *Laryngoscope* 2005;115:1672–1675.

55. Koo BS, Lim YC, Lee JS, et al. Management of the contralateral N0 neck in pyriform sinus carcinoma. *Laryngoscope* 2006;116: 1268–1272.

56. Lim YC, Lee JS, Koo BS, et al. Treatment of contralateral N0 neck in early squamous cell carcinoma of the oral tongue: elective neck dissection versus observation. *Laryngoscope* 2006;116:461–465.

57. Bohannon IA, Desmond RA, Clemons L, et al. Management of the N0 neck in recurrent laryngeal squamous cell carcinoma. *Laryngoscope* 2010;120:58–61.

58. Dagan R, Morris CG, Kirwan JM, et al. Elective neck dissection during salvage surgery for locally recurrent head and neck squamous cell carcinoma after radiotherapy with elective nodal irradiation. *Laryngoscope* 2010;120:945–952.

59. Morton DL, Wen DR, Foshag LJ, et al. Intraoperative lymphatic mapping and selective cervical lymphadenectomy for early stage melanomas of the head and neck. *J Clin Oncol* 1993;11: 1751–1756.

60. Balch CM, Buzaid AC, Soong SJ, et al. Final version of the American Joint Committee on Cancer staging system for cutaneous melanoma. *J Clin Oncol* 2001;15:3635–3648.

61. Alkureishi LW, Burak Z, Alvarez JA, et al. Joint practice guidelines for radionuclide lymphoscintigraphy for sentinel node localization in oral/oropharyngeal squamous cell carcinoma. *Ann Surg Oncol* 2009;16:3190–3210.

62. Ross GL, Soutar DS, MacDonald GD, et al. Sentinel node biopsy in head and neck cancer: Preliminary results of a multicenter trial. *Ann Surg Oncol* 2004;11:690–696.

63. Civantos F, Zitsch RP, Schuller DE. Sentinel lymph node biopsy accurately stages the regional lymph nodes for T1-T2 oral squamous cell carcinomas: results of a prospective multi-institutional trial. *J Clin Oncol* 2010;28:1395–1400.

64. Murer K, Huber GF, Halle SR, Stoeckli SJ. Comparison of morbidity between sentinel node biopsy and elective neck dissection for treatment of the N0 neck in patients with oral squamous cell carcinoma. *Head Neck* 2011;33(9):1260–1264.

65. Pitman KT, Johnson JT, Brown ML, et al. Sentinel lymph node biopsy in head and neck squamous cell carcinoma. *Laryngoscope* 2002;112:2101–2113.

66. Hyde NC, Prvulovich E, Newman L, et al. A new approach to pretreatment assessment of the N0 neck in oral squamous cell carcinoma: the role of sentinel lymph node biopsy and positron emission tomography. *Oral Oncol* 2003;39:350–260.

67. Burcia V, Costes V, Faillie JL. Neck restaging with sentinel node biopsy in T1-T2N0 oral and oropharyngeal cancer: Why and how?. *Otolaryngol Head Neck Surg* 2010;142:592–597.

68. Civantos FJ, Moffat FL, Goodwin WJ. Lymphatic mapping and sentinel lymphadenectomy for 106 head and neck lesions: contrasts between oral cavity and cutaneous malignancy. *Laryngoscope* 2006;116(Suppl 109):1–15.

69. Alkureishi LW, Ross GL, Shoaib T, Soutar DS. Sentinel node biopsy in head and neck squamous cell cancer: 5-year follow-up of a European multicenter trial. *Ann Surg Oncol* 2010;17: 2459–2464.

70. Ferris RL, Xi L, Seethala RR, et al. Intraoperative qRT-PCR for deection of lymph node metastasis in head and neck cancer. *Clin Cancer Res* 2011;17:1858–1866.

71. O'Brien CJ, Traynor SJ, McNeil E, et al. The use of clinical predictors alone in the management of the clinically negative neck among patients with squamous cell carcinoma of the oral cavity and oropharynx. *Arch Otolaryngol Head Neck Surg* 2000;126: 360–365.

72. Lim YC, Choi EC. Unilateral, clinically T2N0, squamous cell carcinoma of the tongue: surgical outcome analysis. *Int J Oral Maxillofac Surg* 2007;36:610–614.

73. Veness MJ, Morgan GJ, Sathiyaseelan Y, Gebski V. Anterior tongue cancer and the incidence of cervical lymph node metastases with increasing tumour thickness: Should elective treatment to the neck be standard practice in all patients? *ANZ J Surg* 2005;75:101–105.

74. Yuen AP, Lam KY, Lam LK, et al. Prognostic factors of clinically Stage I and II oral tongue carcinoma-A comparative study of stage, thickness, shape, growth pattern, invasive front malignancy grading, Martinez-Gimeno score, and pathologic features. *Head Neck* 2002;24:513–520.

75. Goerkem M, Braun J, Stoeckli SJ. Evaluation of clincal and histomorphological parameters as potential predictors of occult metastases in sentinel lymph nodes of early squamous cell carcinoma of the oral cavity. *Ann Surg Oncol* 2010;17:527–535.

76. Sparano A, Weinstein G, Chalian A, et al. Multivariate predictors of occult neck metastases in early tongue cancer. *Otolaryngol Head Neck Surg* 2004;131:472–476.

77. Kurokawa H, Zhang M, Matsumoto S, et al. The high prognostic value of histologic grade at the deep invasive front of tongue squamous cell carcinoma. *J Oral Pathol Med* 2005;34:329–333.

78. Brandwein-Gensler M, Lewis C, Lee B, et al. Oral squamous cell carcinoma: histologic risk assessment, but not margin status, is strongly predictive of local disease free and overall survival. *Am J Surg Pathol* 2005;20:167–178.

79. Rinaldo A, Devaney KO, Ferlito A. Immunohistochemical studies in the identification of lymph node micrometastases in patients with squamous cell carcinoma of the head and neck. *ORL J Otorhinolaryngol Relat Spec* 2004;66:38–41.

80. Roepman P, Wessels LF, Kemmeren P, et al. An expression profile for diagnosis of lymph node metastases from primary head and neck carcinomas. *Nat Genet* 2005;37:182–186.

81. Roepman P, Wessels LF, Kettelariji N, et al. An expression profile for diagnosis of lymph node metastases from primary head and neck squamous cell carcinomas. *Nat Genet* 2005;37:182–186.

82. Takes RP, Batenburg RJ, Schuuring E, et al. Markers for assessment of nodal metastases in laryngeal carcinoma. *Arch Otolaryngol Head Neck Surg* 1997;123:412–418.

Oral Cavity Cancer

119

Daniel G. Deschler   *Audrey B. Erman*

ANATOMY

The oral cavity represents one of the most anatomically diverse regions within the head and neck. Within this relatively confined space operate highly specialized and important physiologic activities, beginning with the ability to communicate through facial animation and articulation. Deglutition originates with the maintenance of oral competence at the anterior oral cavity and then relies on subsequent lubrication, mastication, bolus formation, and then bolus transfer to the oropharynx. Similarly, within the oral cavity, sensory innervation for touch, pressure, temperature, and taste function is notable for its high degree of cortical representation. In order to achieve these critical functions, numerous tissue types are represented within the oral cavity including the mucosal lining, muscle, bone as well as unique tissues including teeth, salivary glands, and epithelium for taste. These tissues are supported by the region's vast and redundant blood supply and innervation (Figs. 119.1 to 119.3).

The oral cavity itself has a strict anatomic demarcation as a head and neck subsite. The boundaries of the oral cavity begin with the lips anteriorly and extend posteriorly to the vertical plane beginning at the junction of the hard and soft palate, continuing inferiorly through the circumvallate papillae at the sulcus terminalis and ending at the hyoid bone. The oral cavity is further divided into subareas including the *"lips, alveolar ridge, floor of mouth, oral tongue, hard palate, retromolar trigone, and the lateral buccal mucosa"* (Fig. 119.4). Each of these subareas has distinct anatomic features and lymphatic drainage pathways, the knowledge of which is imperative in the management of neoplasms of the oral cavity (Table 119.1).

At the most anterior boundary of the oral cavity are the specialized myomucosal element of the *"lips."* Anatomically the region of the lip begins anteriorly with the vermilion border and extends posteriorly along the red

lip into the mucosal elements at the labial sulcus. The lateral demarcations of the lip are the bilateral commissures. The philtrum, or Cupid's bow, occupies the midline superiorly and directly opposes the labial tubercle in the midline of the lower lip. The lip has a dense sensory innervation provided by the third branch of the trigeminal nerve and consists of its epithelial lining, muscle, and minor salivary glands. The blood supply is provided bilaterally by the labial arteries, which originate from the facial arterial system. The lymphatic drainage of the lower lip is primarily to the submental and submandibular triangles with subsequent drainage to the upper jugular chain. The lower lip demonstrates propensity for contralateral drainage and therefore bilateral metastasis. The upper lip does not demonstrate significant lymphatic crossover, and lesions of this region will usually metastasize to ipsilateral lymph nodes in level IB, periparotid lymph nodes, and level II jugulodigastric lymph nodes.

The *"lower alveolar ridge"* begins immediately behind the lower lip and its labial sulcus, and is composed of the specialized tooth-bearing bone of the mandible. The oral cavity components of the mandible include the symphysis, perisymphysis, and the bilateral mandibular bodies extending toward the ramus. The visible component of the alveolar ridge has a tightly adherent mucosal and gingival coverage that surrounds dentition where it is present. The bone of the alveolus, or the tooth-bearing component of the mandible, is characterized by thin bone surrounding the tooth with the tooth roots extending deeply into the cortical bone of the mandible. This becomes important as this thin bone can be susceptible to bone erosion by tumors, while the tooth root allows access to the deeper components of the mandible including the marrow space. The inferior aspect of the mandible is composed of dense cortical bone, which provides sufficient support, and this is the supporting bone that remains when teeth are lost and there is regression of the alveolus.

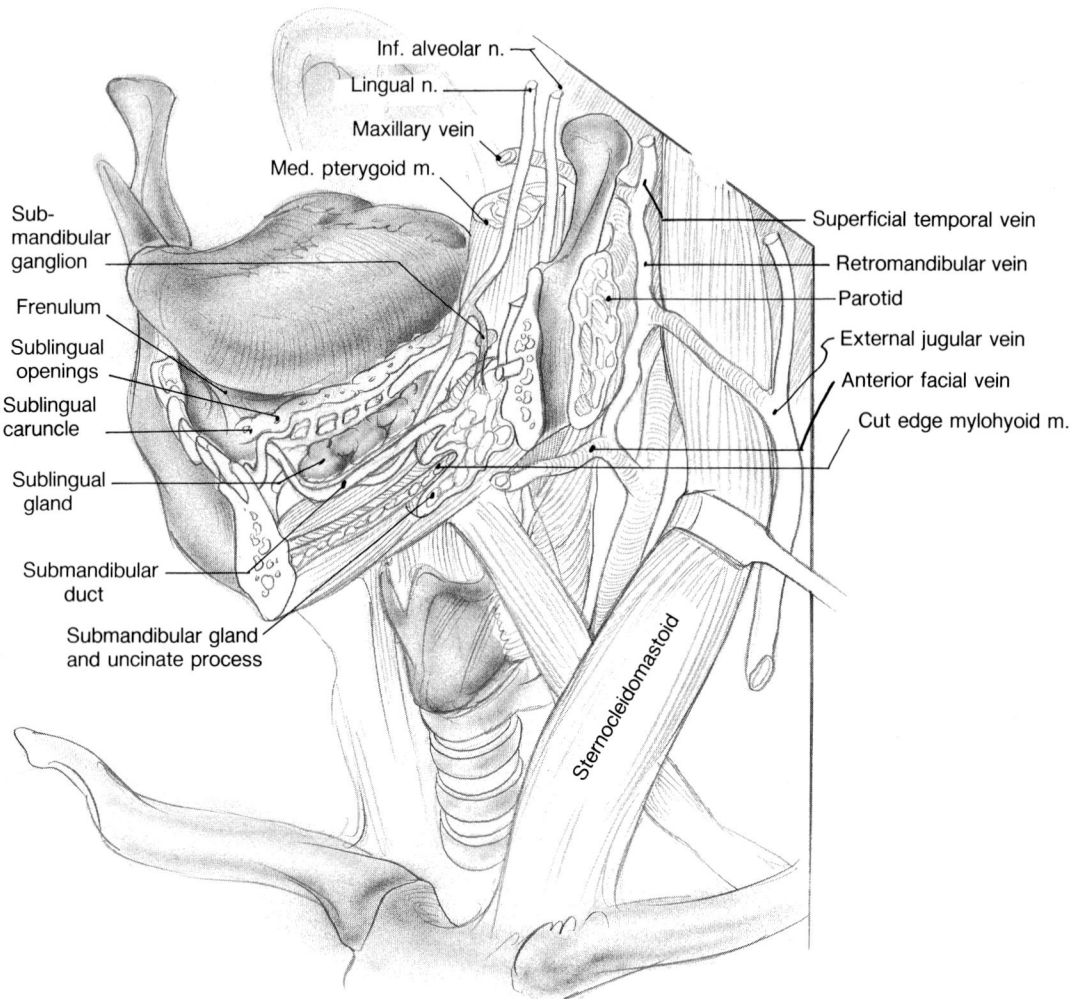

Figure 119.1 Superficial anatomic landmarks and structure of the oral cavity.

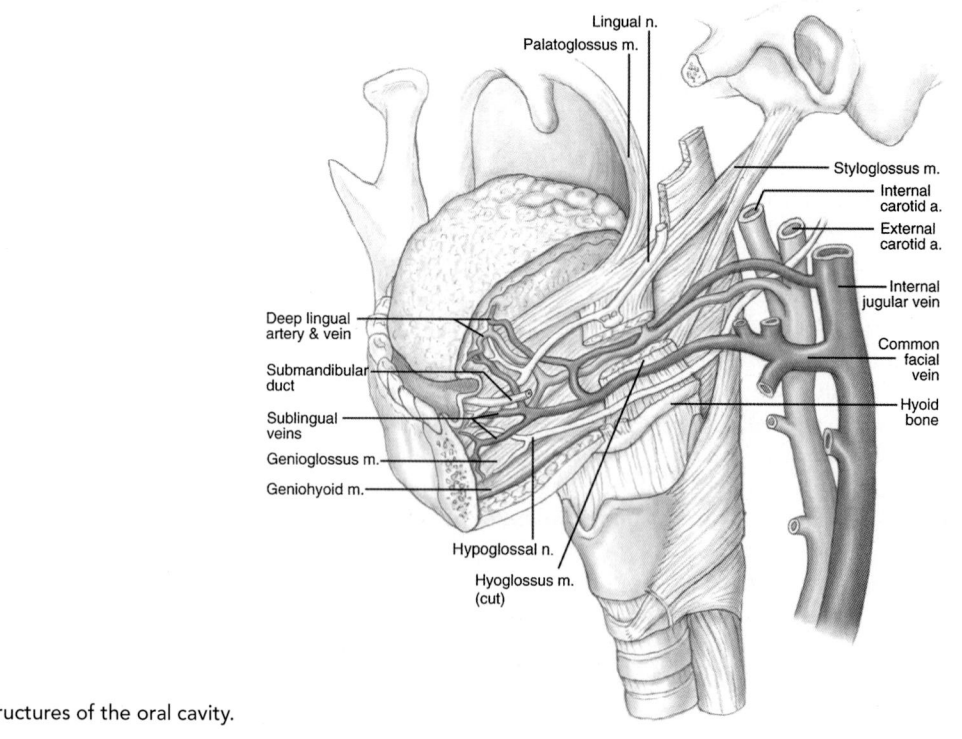

Figure 119.2 Deep anatomic structures of the oral cavity.

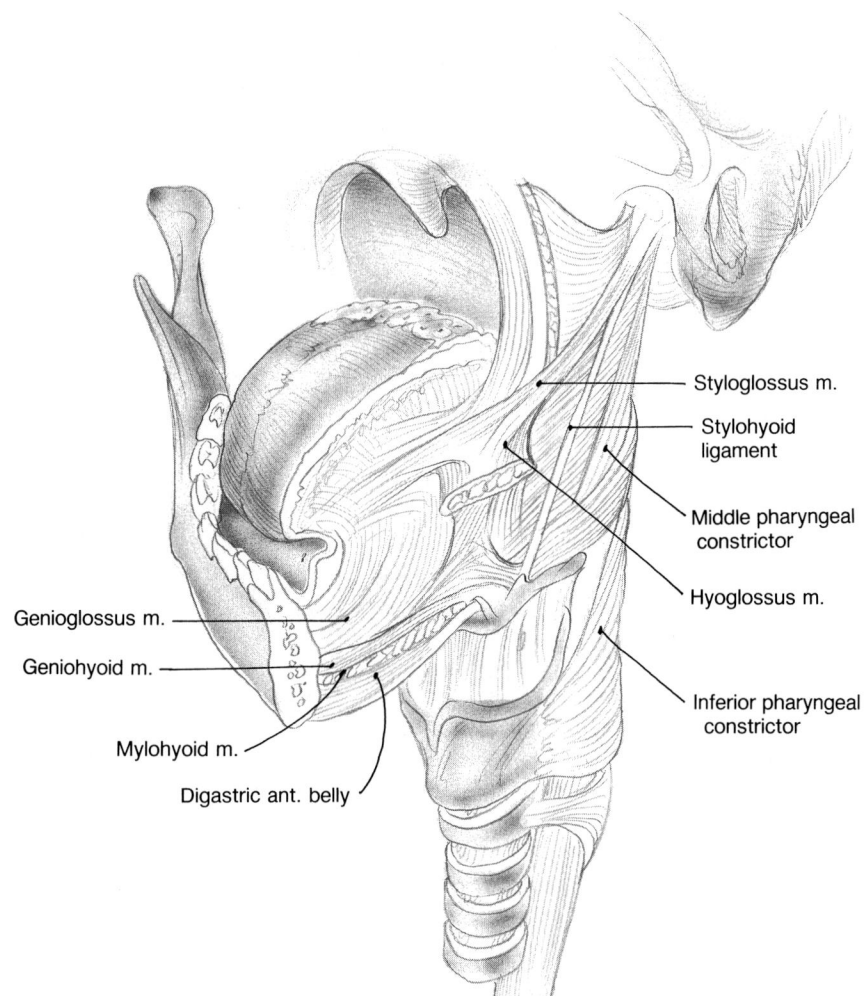

Styloglossus m.

Stylohyoid
ligament

Middle pharyngeal
constrictor

Hyoglossus m.

Inferior pharyngeal
constrictor

Genioglossus m.

Geniohyoid m.

Mylohyoid m.

Digastric ant. belly

Figure 119.3 Musculature of the oral cavity.

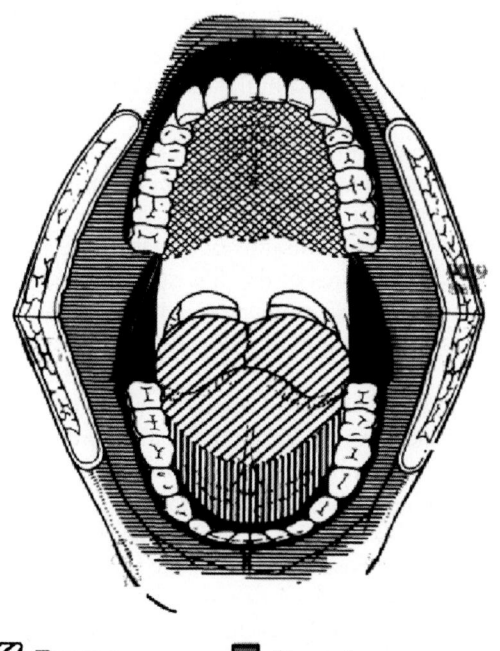

▨ Tongue   ▤ Buccal mucosa
▥ Floor of mouth ■ Retromolar trigone
■ Gingiva   ▨ Hard palate

Figure 119.4 Labeled diagram from AJCC Staging Manual.

TABLE 119.1	PATTERNS OF LYMPHATIC DRAINAGE BY SUBSITE OF ORAL CAVITY

Subsite	Common Level of Regional Lymph Node Metastasis
Upper lip	Ipsilateral level IB, perifacial, periparotid, level II
Lower lip	Bilateral levels IA and IB, perifacial, level II
Upper alveolar ridge	Ipsilateral levels IB and II If midline—bilateral
Lower alveolar ridge	Ipsilateral levels IA, IB and II If midline—bilateral
Floor of mouth	Ipsilateral levels IA, IB and II If midline—bilateral
RMT	Ipsilateral levels IIA, IIB and III
Hard palate	Bilateral levels IB and II, retropharyngeal and perifacial
Buccal mucosa	Ipsilateral levels IB, level II

Medially, the mucosal surface of the alveolar ridge extends down the mandibular surface to the mylohyoid muscle and becomes one with the floor of mouth. Laterally, this region will extend to the gingival buccal sulcus and the insertion of the buccinator muscle. The notable tissues within the alveolar ridge include the mucosal and gingival lining as well as bone, muscle, marrow, minor salivary glands, and the teeth. The blood supply to the lower alveolar ridge is comprised of both an endosteal and a periosteal blood supply. Primary innervation is via the inferior alveolar nerve from V3, which enters the mandible at the mandibular canal within the medial ramus and exits at the mental foramen, as the mental nerve. The drainage of the alveolar ridge is dependent upon its location. Anterior lesions drain to level I and have bilateral drainage to level IB. Lateral lesions will drain to level IB as well as level II.

Directly within the lower alveolar ridge lies the crescent-shaped region known as the *"floor of mouth"* (Fig. 119.5). The floor of mouth extends from the attached gingiva of the medial alveolar ridge to the muscular tongue. Anteriorly, the region begins just posterior to the incisors and extends bilaterally to the anterior tonsillar pillars. The mucosal covering here is a very thin layer with a high degree of mobility. Within the floor of mouth are numerous salivary glands including minor salivary glands, the sublingual glands, as well as the ductal apparatus of the paired submandibular glands. All of these salivary glands have a drainage pathway within the floor of mouth, with the submandibular glands draining through Wharton duct and emptying anteriorly into the oral cavity on either side of the midline frenulum. The primary vascular supply to the floor of mouth is from the lingual artery and elements of the facial system with the primary neural supply being from the third branch of the trigeminal nerve via the lingual nerve. Anatomic injection studies demonstrate both a superficial and deep lymphatic drainage system for the oral cavity (1). This superficial system can demonstrate bilateral drainage, whereas the deep system will drain primarily

to the ipsilateral level I and upper jugular chain. Anterior floor of mouth lesions will have propensity to drain to the levels of IA and IB.

The *"oral tongue"* consists of that portion of the tongue that extends from the tip to the region of the circumvallate papillae and constitutes two-thirds of the entire tongue. The oral tongue has four distinct anatomic regions: the tip, the lateral borders, the dorsum, and the ventral surface. The oral tongue is a highly specialized muscular unit with a similarly specialized mucosal lining having a dense innervation for touch and specialized epithelium for taste. The muscular component of the oral tongue is composed of six paired muscles (Fig. 119.6). The three extrinsic muscle groups include the paired genioglossus, hyoglossus, and styloglossus muscles that achieve the gross movements of the body of the tongue. The intrinsic musculature of the tongue includes the lingual muscles and the vertical and transverse muscular units that provide most of the tongue's bulk. These muscles have intricate mobility and interaction critical for the functions of speech and deglutition. The motor innervation of the tongue is provided by the twelfth cranial nerve with sensory innervation from the lingual nerve via V3. Taste sensation is delivered from thousands of gustatory receptors located within the taste buds of the oral cavity through the chorda tympani and the glossopharyngeal nerve. Lesions on the tip of the tongue and midline dorsum can have a propensity for bilateral lymphatic spread as well as spread to level IA. Lateral tongue lesions will primarily spread to the ipsilateral level IB and level II. Additionally, there are anatomic and clinical series alerting practitioners to the potential of spread to levels III and IV of the neck from tongue carcinomas even in the absence of spreads to level I or level II.

Proceeding posteriorly from the upper lip, begins the "upper alveolar ridge." In parallel to the lower alveolar ridge, this region is characterized by dense tooth-bearing bone and has similarly specialized tissues. Most anteriorly in the upper alveolar ridge is the triangular-shaped premaxilla. This portion of the maxillary alveolar ridge

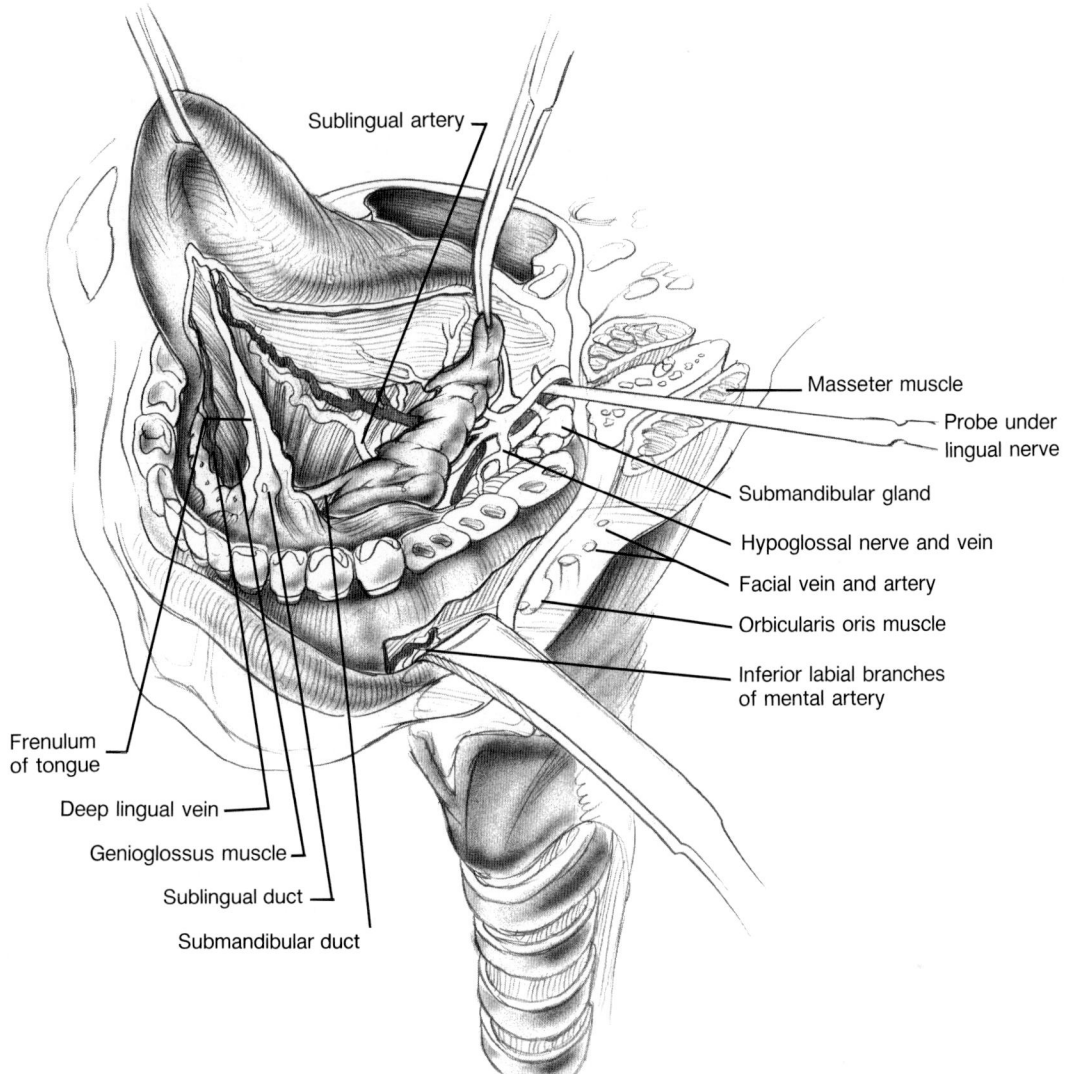

Sublingual artery

Masseter muscle

Probe under
lingual nerve

Submandibular gland

Hypoglossal nerve and vein

Facial vein and artery

Orbicularis oris muscle

Inferior labial branches
of mental artery

Frenulum
of tongue

Deep lingual vein

Genioglossus muscle

Sublingual duct

Submandibular duct

Figure 119.5 Floor of the mouth.

contains the incisors and has its apex at the incisive foramen. Posteriorly, the upper alveolar ridge extends to the maxillary tuberosities bilaterally. Similar to the lower alveolar ridge, the mucosa and gingiva are firmly adherent to the underlying bone, conferring the same propensity for cortical erosion, and spread down tooth roots, which exit in the lower alveolar ridge. In contrast to the lower alveolar ridge, the deep bone of the upper alveolar ridge lacks the same dense cortical characteristics of the mandible and instead thins as the maxillary sinuses begin. The thin bone at this interface is less resistant and readily allows tumor spread into the sinuses. The upper alveolar ridge is innervated by the second branch of the trigeminal nerve and has a considerable blood supply from the facial artery as well as branches of the internal maxillary artery including the sphenopalatine artery. Lymphatic drainage is to level IB, periparotid lymph nodes, and level II.

Within the bony borders of the upper alveolar ridge rests the anatomic unit of the "hard palate." The hard palate is primarily thin bone with a very tight mucosal layer overlying it on both the oral and nasal surfaces. The paired palatine processes of the maxilla extend to the level of the second posterior molar and form the bulk of the hard palate. At the most posterior edges are the paired horizontal processes of the palatine bone through which the greater palatine nerve and vessels exit via the greater palatine foramen. Although the periosteum overlying the hard palate is very dense and resistant to tumor invasion, there are important areas of potential tumor spread related to the foramen of the hard palate including the greater palatine, the lesser palatine, and the incisive foramen. In addition to its mucosal covering, there are numerous minor salivary glands throughout the hard palate region. Primary lymphatic drainage is to levels I and II.

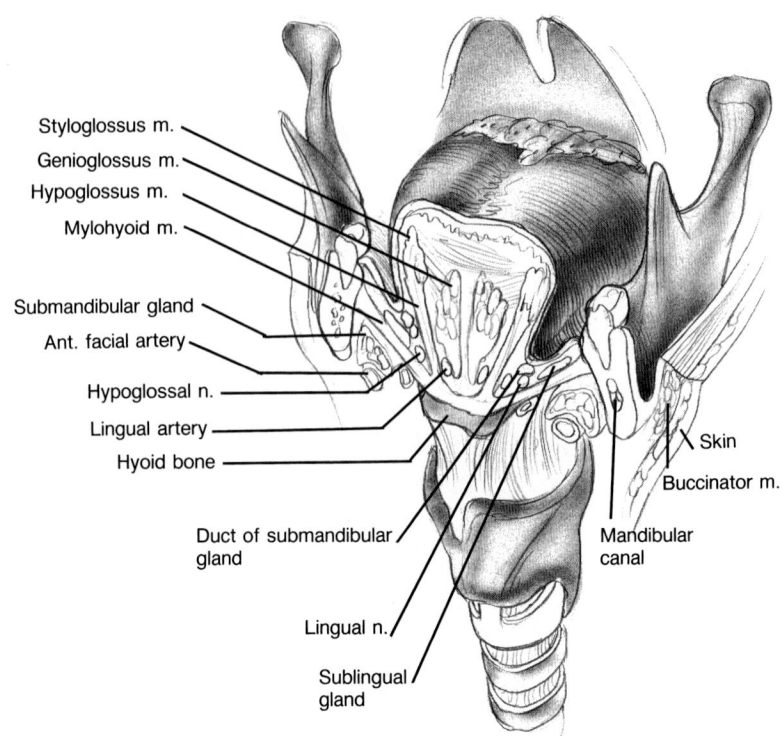

Styloglossus m.
Genioglossus m.
Hypoglossus m.
Mylohyoid m.

Submandibular gland
Ant. facial artery

Hypoglossal n.
Lingual artery
Hyoid bone

Skin
Buccinator m.

Duct of submandibular
gland

Mandibular
canal

Lingual n.

Sublingual
gland

Figure 119.6 Intrinsic muscles of the tongue.

At the most posterior margin of the oral cavity is the *"retromolar trigone or RMT."* This region consists of a mucosally covered triangular area that overlies the ascending ramus of the mandible. The base of this triangle rests at the last lower molar of the lower alveolar ridge and the posterior body of the mandible. The apex of the RMT is the maxillary tuberosity. The medial border is the anterior tonsillar pillar, and the lateral border is the buccal mucosa. The mucosa of the RMT is very tightly adherent to the underlying mandible and is an area prone to mandibular invasion even with small lesions. The lymphatic drainage of this area is to levels I and II, but because of its proximity to the oropharynx, a special consideration must be given to both levels IIA and IIB with RMT lesions.

The last and most lateral component of the oral cavity is represented by the *"buccal mucosa."* This region extends from the RMT and the pterygomandibular raphae posteriorly to the oral commissure and lips bilaterally. The region has a mucosal lining surface that extends from the upper alveolar ridge superiorly to the inferior alveolar ridge inferiorly. Deep to the mucosal lining is the pharyngobuccal fascia and the buccinator muscle. The parotid duct pierces the buccinator and the pharyngobuccal fascia to exit at the Stensen duct lateral to the upper second molar. Tumors penetrating these anatomic layers can readily involve the laterally placed buccal fat pad and the subcutaneous as well as cutaneous structures of the cheek. Sensation to this region is provided by nerves from the second and third branch of the trigeminal system, whereas the buccinator muscle is innervated by the seventh cranial nerve. The lymphatic

drainage to the buccal mucosa is quite dense and primarily drains to levels I and II but may extend to the periparotid lymph nodes as well.

EPIDEMIOLOGY

Assessment of statistics related to oral cavity cancer must done with care as often cancers of the oropharynx, a distinct subsite of the head and neck with a unique epidemiology, are included under the term "oral cancers." True oral cavity malignancies are the 10th most common cancer worldwide in men with over 170,000 new cases per year and a mortality rate approaching 50% and the 15th most common in women with over 83,000 cases and a similar mortality rate (2). Globally, the incidence of oral cavity cancer is 1.5 times higher in men than women (3), whereas in the US the male:female ratio is 2:1 (4). Certain geographic regions have a very high incidence such as Micronesia with 24 cases per 100,000 in men compared to 6.7 per 100,000 men in Western Europe (5).

In the US, head and neck cancer—inclusive of all subsites—is the sixth most commonly occurring cancer. Review of the Surveillance, Epidemiology and End Results (SEER) data base indicates that 38% of these occur in the oral cavity, making it the most common subsite. Thirty-two percent will occur in the oral tongue and 20% in the floor of mouth, making these the most commonly affected sub areas within the oral cavity (6). In 2011, the American Cancer Society estimated that 25,820 new cases of oral cavity cancer would occur in the US of which nearly 12,000 would originate in the tongue (7). Five to six thousand oral cavity cancer–related deaths occur per year (7). Yet, the incidence and mortality rates of oral cavity cancer have been declining, albeit in small increments, over the past few decades. From 1975 to 2008, the incidence of oral cavity in the United States decreased by 1%, and the mortality declined by 1.3% (8). This likely reflects decreases in tobacco consumption within the population. Racial disparities also exist. Although the incidence of oral cavity and oropharynx cancers is essentially equal among African American and White US males, death rate of African American males is nearly twice that of Whites (9). Although the average age of occurrence of an oral cavity cancer is approximately 60 years and nearly 95% of patients will be over 40 years old at the time of presentation, there is concern that the incidence of tongue cancer in younger patients has been steadily increasing over the same time period (10,11).

The overwhelming majority, nearly 95%, of oral cavity cancers will be squamous cell carcinomas (SCCA) arising from the squamous epithelium lining the oral cavity. The next most common histology is tumors of salivary gland origin. Because of the diverse tissues within the oral cavity, a wide variety of tumors may occur in this region. Sarcomas of bone (osteosarcoma), muscle (rhabdomyosarcomas), and other soft tissues (fibrosarcomas and liposarcomas) may occur. Similarly, lymphomas, mucosal melanomas, and nerve sheath tumors may also present in the oral cavity. Tumors of dental origin, both benign and malignant, complete the differential of primary lesions within the oral cavity. Metastatic lesions, albeit rare, can also occur (Table 119.2).

TABLE 119.2	TUMORS OF THE ORAL CAVITY

SCCA
Salivary gland masses
  Malignant
    Mucoepidermoid carcinoma
    Adenoid cystic carcinoma
    Acinic cell carcinoma
    Salivary ductal carcinoma
    Carcinoma ex pleomorphic adenoma
  Benign
    Pleomorphic adenoma
    Oncocytic lesions (Warthin tumors)
    Mucoceles
  Sarcomas
    Osteosarcoma
    Rhabdomyosarcoma
    Fibrosarcoma
    Liposarcoma
Lymphomas
Mucosal melanomas
Nerve sheath tumors
Metastatic lesions

ETIOLOGY

Use of tobacco and related products, as well as alcohol consumption, are the greatest risk factors for developing the most common carcinoma of the oral cavity—SCCA. Approximately 75% of oral cavity carcinomas will be related to tobacco and alcohol use (12). The risk of developing oral cavity cancer is correlated with tobacco use in a dose-dependent fashion. Oral cavity cancer risk increases 1.5-fold in light smokers (less than 10 cigarettes per day) and increases to a fourfold greater risk in smokers of greater than 30 cigarettes per day (13). The risk markedly increases with a smoking history of longer than 20 years and greater than 20 cigarettes daily (13). In Europe and South America, non–alcohol users who smoked had a threefold greater incidence of oral cavity SCCA than nonsmoking non-drinkers. In former smokers, the risk of developing cancer declines with time. After 9 years of cessation, patients had a 50% reduction of risk of cancer (14), and patients have only a 1.5-fold increase in cancer rates after 20 years of cessation in comparison to nonsmokers (14). In patients cured of a primary oral cancer malignancy, 40% recurred or developed a secondary head and neck primary, whereas only 6% of patients recurred after smoking cessation (15).

Tobacco use in any form has been associated with oral cancer. Although not as strongly and directly correlated with oral cavity SCCA, smokeless tobacco (snuff) may confer as great as a fourfold increase in oral cavity carcinoma (16). A cohort study of women in India revealed a greater than ninefold increase in the incidence of oral cavity cancer in women who used chewing tobacco greater than 10 times per day and was also related to duration of use (17). Pipe smoking has been associated with cancers of the oral cavity, pharynx, and esophagus, with heavy drinking increasing the risk multiplicatively (18). Pipe smoking associated with cancer of the lip is due to both the temperature and permeability of the pipe stem (19). The lateral tongue and floor of mouth also warrant close consideration.

Similar to tobacco for the stimulant and carcinogenic effects, the areca nut is the seed of the Areca palm and when wrapped in the betel leaf is referred to as "betel nut." In India and Southeast Asia, the betel nut is chewed with a mixture of other flavorings, cured tobacco, and lime and called "quid." Betel nut quid has been shown to be highly carcinogenic (20). Buccal mucosa cancers are nearly eight times more prevalent in betel nut users and in high-use regions such as India, Southeast Asia and northeast Brazil, where oral cavity cancers can account for between 25% and 50% of all cancers (21). In a cohort study of over 10,000 participants in Taiwan, users of tobacco, alcohol, and betel nut quid had a greater than 46-fold increase in oral cavity cancers (22). Other alternative uses of tobacco and like products also increase the risk of oral cancers. The practice of reverse smoking—placing the lit end of the cigarette in the mouth during inhalation—is associated with a 47-fold increase in rates of hard palate carcinoma among women in India (23).

The synergistic effect of tobacco and alcohol consumption has long been recognized in the development of head and neck cancer. An estimated 75% of all head and neck cancers are caused by tobacco and alcohol combined, and those who smoke two packs per day and drink four units of alcohol per day are 35 times more likely to develop cancer compared with healthy controls (12). Significant overlap in the consumption of tobacco and alcohol can confound epidemiologic attempts at risk stratification. Yet, studies indicate an independent role for alcohol in inducing malignancy of the oral cavity, in a dose-dependent fashion (24,25). Dose–response curves demonstrate a doubling in relative risk for light users of alcohol (30 g/day) compared to a nearly 10-fold increase in relative risk for heavy users of alcohol (130 g/day) (26). The effect is consistent across types of alcoholic beverages including beer, wine, and hard alcohol (27). No clear trend is identifiable for duration of alcohol use. Decreased risk of head and neck cancer can be achieved with alcohol cessation but requires years of abstinence, and the return to the risk level of nonalcohol users does not standardly occur until 20 years after cessation (27).

The human papilloma virus (HPV) infects epithelial cells and has been implicated as an early carcinogenic event in head and neck cancer with the HPV-16 subtype being the most common. There has been a significant increase in HPV+ oropharyngeal cancers, which demonstrate an overall favorable prognosis when compared to traditional oropharyngeal squamous cell cancers (28). However, HPV+ oropharyngeal SCCA is a distinct clinical entity highly selective to the oropharyngeal subsites. HPV DNA has been variably isolated from a wide range of oral cavity cancer specimens (29). Review often indicates significant overlaps with the oropharyngeal subsites and not true oral cavity origin. The same increase in cure rates of oral cavity cancers has not yet been observed, and therefore, current treatment methods for oral cavity squamous cell cancers should not be altered. Efforts to test oral cavity cancers for HPV and related markers may be helpful in future treatment algorithms, but a clear trend needs to be established prior to altering management.

Nonsmokers and nondrinkers may also present with oral cavity cancers, and fortunately, many of these present with early-stage disease affording a favorable prognosis. A greater proportion of these patients are female, and the common sites include the lateral tongue, maxillary alveolar ridge, and buccal regions. There is also an observed trend for an increased incidence in patients under 40 years of age (6).

Lichen planus is a chronic, inflammatory process affecting the oral cavity with a predilection for the buccal regions. Reports describe squamous cell cancers arising within areas of lichen planus, but the true malignant transformation rate is demonstrated to be less than 2% (30). Lichen planus has an unclear etiology and often responses to topical steroids. Patients with lichen planus should be observed closely for the formation of dominant and rapidly progressive lesions more consistent with carcinoma. Such observation and the use of judicious biopsy will prevent concerning lesions from proliferating under the supposition of a benign process.

Another small but important subgroup of patients warranting close observation are those who have undergone allogenic bone marrow transplantation. A chronic inflammatory process accompanies graft versus host disease (GVHD) in these patients, and although the most common second cancers noted after transplantation are hematologic, squamous cell cancer is the most common solid tumor seen in GVHD patients (31). All regions of the oral cavity are susceptible to GVHD and therefore warrant close observation.

PRESENTATION

Oral cavity neoplasms present in a variety of forms (Fig. 119.7A–F). Growths will usually present as an atypical area affecting the lining of one of the specific subsites of the oral cavity. This may be as simple as a small rough

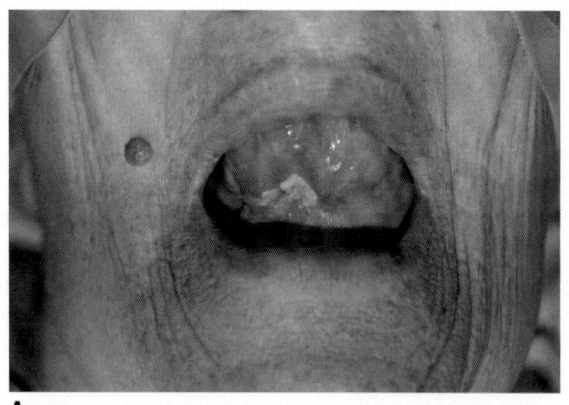

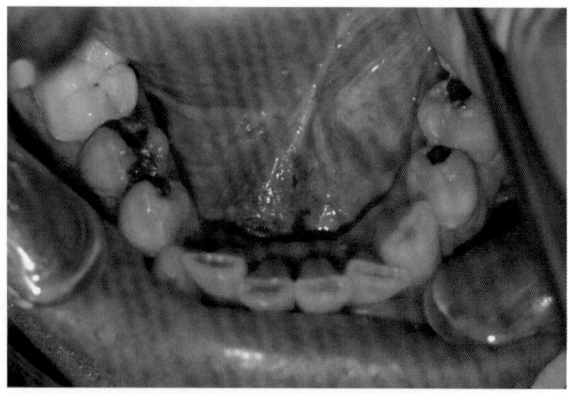

A   **B**

Figure 119.7 A: Leukoplakia at the junction of the floor of mouth and tongue. **B:** Erythroplakic lesion of the floor of mouth positive for SCCA.

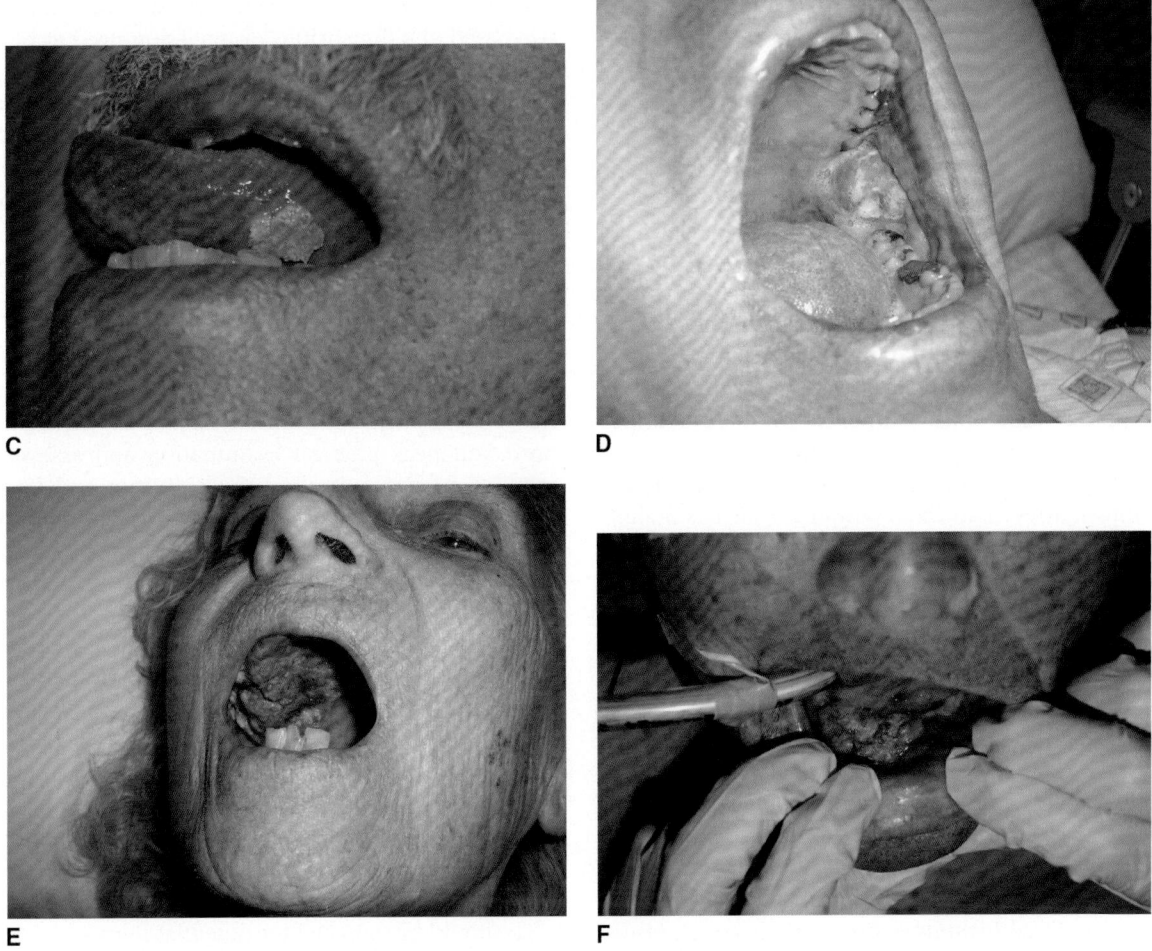

Figure 119.7 *(Continued)* **C:** Exophytic and pedunculated lesion of the lateral oral tongue positive for SCCA. **D:** SCCA at the junction of the RMT and the posterior buccal mucosa. **E:** SCCA of the right upper alveolar ridge. **F:** SCCA of the lower alveolar ridge invasion into cortical bone.

area or may be quite extensive involving multiple subsites. Leukoplakia is a commonly used term to describe a discrete persistent white patch in the oral cavity. These areas cannot be wiped off and are usually the result of chronic irritation. The malignant potential of leukoplakia is rather small, but it is generally felt that between 5% and 15% of these lesions can harbor malignancy (32). A baseline biopsy is not an unreasonable initial approach to the management of the leukoplakic lesion. Erythroplakia, a red plaque, is a more concerning entity. Erythroplakic lesions are felt to have a much greater potential for malignant transformation that can be five to seven times that of leukoplakia. All erythroplakic lesions warrant a biopsy for full evaluation and close follow-up if found to be nonmalignant.

Oral cavity lesions may also present as an ulcerative lesion within one of the subsites. This can be a shallow area without deep infiltration but also can manifest a significant infiltrative pattern into involved regions such as the tongue, floor of mouth, or alveolar ridges. Often,

these deeply infiltrative ulcerative lesions are quite painful. At the other extreme, some lesions may be highly exophytic and present with a small base of true invasion. Likewise, an exophytic lesion can have a broad base with deep infiltration. These lesions also can present with pain.

Other manifestations of oral cavity neoplasms include bleeding without any predisposing trauma. As noted, persistent pain of the oral cavity lasting longer than 3 weeks is concerning for a neoplasm. Patients may also complain of new loose teeth in either the upper or lower alveolar ridges without any significant predisposing trauma, dental issues, or lack of hygiene. Another less common presentation is that of bad breath secondary to necrotic tumor. Oral cavity neoplasms can also present as a painless submucosal masses that can be quite extensive. Neoplasms such as this should raise concern for an etiology other than that from the squamous mucosal lining of the oral cavity. Salivary gland neoplasms would be the most common such lesions, especially in the floor of mouth or a buccal region. Tumors originating from the mandible or maxilla, as well as from the teeth, also warrant consideration.

DIAGNOSIS AND EVALUATION

Although lesions of the oral cavity are usually quite visible compared to other head and neck subsites such as the oropharynx, larynx, hypopharynx, and sinonasal tract, a large proportion will present at an advanced local stage. A complete history will elucidate the clinical course. The timing of presentation and relative growth of the primary lesion will alert to rapidly progressive tumors that require urgent intervention before nutritional and airway issues become critical. Similarly, the presence and growth pattern of any clinical neck disease will be informative. Associated symptoms such as otalgia can portend more advanced disease than may be initially noted. Trismus also carries significant implications as it can be a harbinger of deep infiltration into the pterygoid musculature. Oral pain and odynophagia are often early symptoms but indicate advanced disease. Functional issues such as dysphagia and dysarthria may be related to tumor-associated pain or the physical presence of tumor in the oral cavity. Tumors may also involve cranial nerves, V, VII, IX, X, and XII. Weight loss, halitosis, or loose teeth can indicate advanced disease. Dysarthria may be secondary to pain or signal involvement of the hypoglossal nerve. A thorough past medical history should be obtained including current medications (anticoagulants), previous interventions (biopsies, lesion excisions, or aerodigestive malignancy treatments), and medical comorbidities that will be of critical importance for surgical planning (coronary artery disease, chronic obstructive pulmonary disease).

A history of salient risk factors is mandatory not only for assessment of causation but also to begin treatment planning. Smokers should be advised to stop and cessation counseling undertaken. Numerous studies indicate that patients who smoke tobacco during head and neck cancer treatment have significantly worse treatment courses and overall survival compared to those who stop smoking (33). Continued alcohol use and abuse may also have significant negative impact. Alcohol use comorbidities, including cirrhosis and encephalopathy, can seriously affect treatment planning and long-term care. Furthermore, the abrupt cessation of alcohol use, which normally accompanies impatient surgical care, may place patients at significant risk for alcohol withdrawal syndrome and its sequalae (34,35).

Cancers involving the oral cavity are readily assessed by physical examination in the clinic. The overall quality of the tumor should be described: exophytic, ulcerative, pedunculated, etc. A clear demarcation of the specific subsite of the oral cavity affected by the neoplasm is essential: tongue, floor of mouth, etc. As tumor staging in the oral cavity is size based, the dimensions of the lesion need to be clearly defined with particular attention to the demarcation points of 2 and 4 cm. If a lesion extends from one head and neck subsite to another, this too must be noted such as a tongue cancer extending into the floor of mouth. Palpation is essential to determine factors such as depth, degree of infiltration, immobility, and adherence to bone—all of which portend more serious disease. Likewise, palpation of the base of tongue, although unpleasant for the patient, offers critical information.

As the primary risk factors for oral cavity malignancies are also prime risk factors for other upper aerodigestive tract subsites, such as oropharynx and larynx, a complete head and neck physical examination and assessment is required of not only the primary tumor and its associated anatomical extension, but a thorough appraisal of the upper aerodigestive tract to evaluate for second primary tumors. The process of field cancerization—"*the development of premalignant clones of cells throughout the aerodigestive tract because of repeated exposure of the tissue to carcinogens in tobacco products*" (36)—accounts for the significant rates of second primary tumors in head and neck cancer patients with primary tumors of subsites separate from the second lesion. Mirror exam or fiberoptic examination of all visible upper aerodigestive tract mucosal surfaces should be undertaken as part of the initial clinical evaluation.

Assessment of regional spread is required. The entire neck should be palpated for potential metastatic spread of disease with particular attention paid to the assessment of the lymphatic levels at greatest risk for each specific region of the oral cavity (Table 119.1). Bimanual palpation, with one gloved finger in the mouth and the other palpating the external neck, is beneficial for assessment of the submental and submandibular triangles. Mobility of suspicious nodes should be noted. Fixed adenopathy is a poor prognostic feature and can indicate carotid encasement as well as deep muscle infiltration, factors ultimately affecting resectability.

The appropriate use of imaging for the evaluation of the primary tumor, regional lymph node basins, and chest imaging further augments the comprehensive assessment of oral cavity neoplasms and should be addressed at the earliest clinical time point. If possible, imaging is usually recommended prior to tissue acquisition by biopsy or fine needle aspiration (FNA) to limit any effect these interventions may have on radiologic findings. Plain films currently have little utility in evaluation of oral cavity cancers. With recent technologic advances such as reformatting, image acquisition speed, and low-dose scanning, much greater detail can be obtained with computed tomography (CT) imaging in a similar amount of time with minimal increase in radiation dosage. CT imaging provides excellent bony definition, which is critical in many oral cavity subsites. When combined with contrast utilization, CT imaging can also provide excellent soft tissue definition. The rapid acquisition time of CT scans is also an important consideration as some patients with advanced oral cavity cancers may not be able to tolerate the positioning and necessity of prolonged immobility required for other imaging techniques.

Magnetic resonance imaging (MRI), with contrast enhancement and use of differential weighting, can provide truly outstanding soft tissue definition and demarcation of tumor involvement. Similarly, evidence of perineural spread and cranial nerve involvement may be obtained with MRI. MRI evaluates mandibular invasion with greater sensitivity than CT, though with less specificity (37). Although delivering no ionizing radiation, MRI does have disadvantages of increased cost, geographic inaccessibility, and longer acquisition times.

As both CT and MRI have specific advantages and disadvantages, choice of imaging modality will be determined by the primary site of the lesion and the specific clinical information desired in the evaluation of the primary site and the regional lymphatics (Figs. 119.8 to 119.11). Assessment of bone involvement is best evaluated with CT scan and is critical in alveolar ridge, RMT, and hard palate sites. The RMT can be particularly challenging to assess, and studies demonstrate that bone invasion may not be notable on preoperative CT imaging in one-quarter of patients evaluated (38). Bone involvement by tumors originating in soft tissue sites such as tongue and floor of mouth has significant impact on

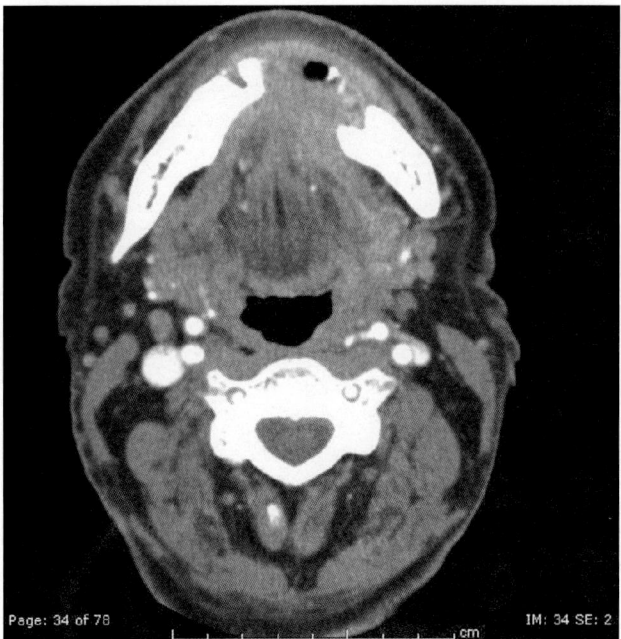

Figure 119.9 Contrast axial CT demonstrating floor of mouth oral cavity cancer eroding the anterior mandible.

treatment planning. Specifically, the evaluation of mandibular involvement is important in primary tumor staging and surgical planning. Again, high-resolution CT scanning is the current imaging modality of choice, although recent studies indicate the increasing utility of MRI, especially for marrow and nerve involvement. The

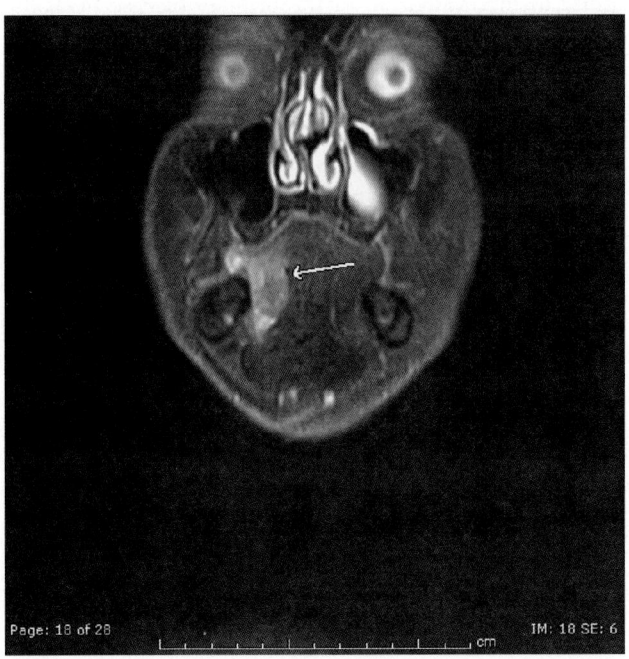

Figure 119.8 T2-weighted coronal MRI demonstrating infiltrating lateral tongue cancer, abutting the lingual artery (*arrow*).

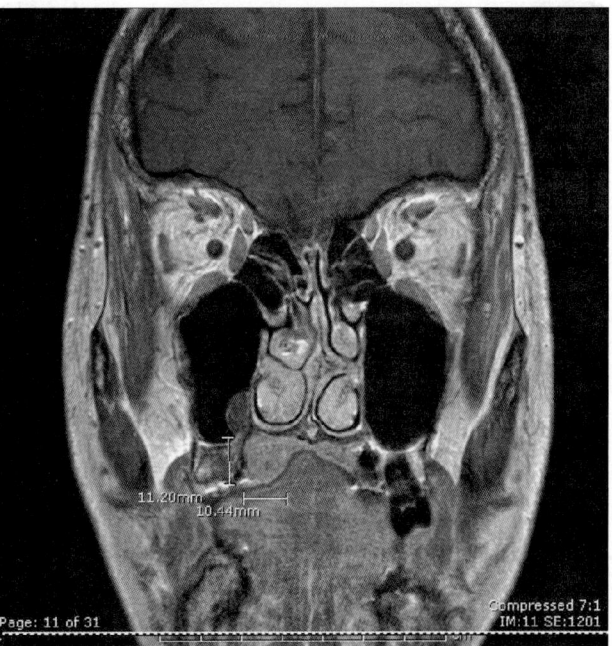

Figure 119.10 Postcontrast T1-weighted coronal MRI demonstrating low-grade polymorphous adenocarcinoma of the hard palate.

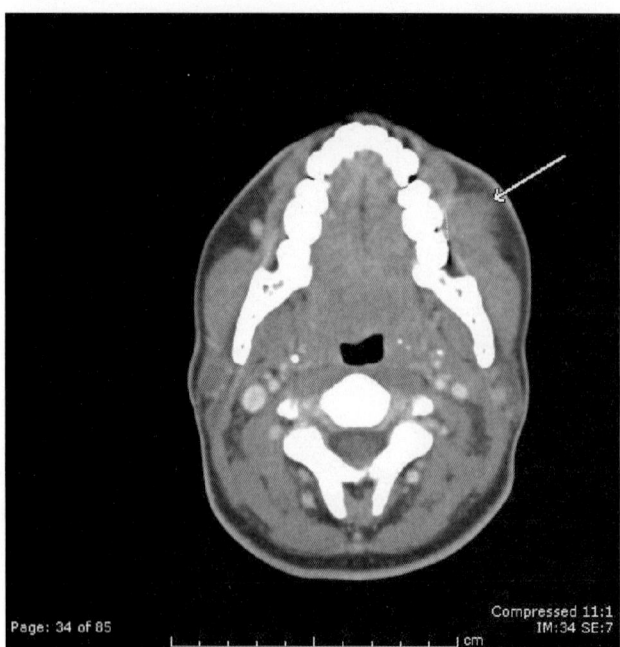

Page: 34 of 85   Compressed 11:1
                                  IM:34 SE:7

Figure 119.11 Contrast axial CT demonstrating extension of buccal carcinoma into the subcutaneous tissues of the cheek.

use of CT scanning has been shown to be helpful in clinical evaluation of the primary tongue tumors (39). Due to the well-established fascial planes surrounding the lingual artery and hypoglossal nerve, a CT scan will aid in the surgical evaluation for a partial glossectomy, as the surgeon evaluates the ability to save the neurovascular bundle on one side of the tongue. This has been greatly aided by high-quality reformatting allowing assessment of the coronal, sagittal, and axial planes. Yet, MRI provides superior definition of tumor extent and involvement in soft tissue areas such as the tongue, floor of mouth, and buccal region and should be considered for these lesions. Patients with clinical evidence of neural involvement and with tumors predisposed to perineural involvement, such as floor of mouth adenoid cystic carcinomas or palatal or alveolar ridge carcinomas, can also benefit from MRI to assess potential proximal neural involvement.

In the United States, CT and MRI are the most commonly used imaging modalities to evaluate for regional metastasis, though with somewhat limited accuracy (40). Definition of clinical evident adenopathy is straightforward with attention focused on overall size, multifocality, evidence of extracapsular spread, deep muscle involvement, carotid involvement, and skull base involvement. The clinically negative neck provides a greater challenge. Criteria for positivity can vary but often include size greater than 10 mm, evidence of central necrosis, loss of ovoid shape, loss of fatty hilum, and the presence of extracapsular extension (41). Though not widely used in the United States, ultrasound has been

shown to be more accurate in the assessment of metastatic lymph nodes, specifically in assessing the integrity of the hilar architecture and blood flow in benign appearing lymph nodes (42). In the evaluation of the combination of selective ultrasound-guided FNA biopsy, several European studies indicate the usefulness of these techniques for assessment of the occult metastatic neck disease (43–45).

The role of positron emission tomography (PET) scans in the staging of oral cavity cancer has not yet been defined. The combination of the PET imaging with CT scanning to provide PET/CT modality has increased the applicability of this imaging technique, yet limitations remain. The CT images obtained with combined PET/CT are often not of the detail and quality obtained with dedicated high-resolution, contrast-enhanced CT scans and therefore should not be considered a replacement. PET imaging offers little added information over standard imaging for assessment of primary lesions. In the assessment of regional disease, PET is often confirmatory, not enlightening. PET also demonstrates limitations in the assessment of the clinical negative neck especially for nodes less than 1 cm. Despite equivocal evidence, PET/CT scans are often obtained in the preoperative setting. Although PET/CT may be of limited use in management of the primary disease, it can aid in the detection of distant metastatic disease (46). Therefore, patients at high risk for metastatic disease such as those with recurrent disease, large primary site tumors, extensive and low neck adenopathy, as well as patients requiring surgical intervention with significant potential morbidity should be considered for evaluation of potential distant metastatic disease with PET/CT. Thus, although of limited utility in the evaluation of the primary disease (47), the more significant role of PET/CT imaging may be in post-treatment assessment in distinguishing posttreatment effect from neoplasm in cases of recurrence or persistent tumors (48).

Pulmonary metastasis is the most common site of distant disease spread in oral cavity, and formal evaluation of the chest is mandatory. Furthermore, widespread tobacco use by patients with oral cavity cancer predisposes this risk group to increased rates of synchronous primary lung cancers. For patients at low risk for distant spread or primary lung cancer, chest x-ray (CXR) is sufficient for evaluation of the chest. If there is greater concern for pulmonary metastasis because of risk factors noted above, excessive tobacco use, or suspicious chest plain film, then chest CT is indicated. When clinical circumstances warrant it, PET/CT imaging may be alternatively employed.

Comprehensive staging of the oral cavity tumors performed in the clinic setting requires tissue for diagnosis. As the oral cavity subsites are quite accessible in the office exam, a biopsy of the primary site can readily be obtained with minimal issue under local anesthesia. This can be completed with an incisional technique or cup forceps.

Care must be taken to obtain adequate and analyzable tissue with biopsy. A specimen of adequate depth, to assess invasion, and viability should be the goal. Biopsies of frankly necrotic tumor or superficial biopsies can be of limited usefulness. The use of a 3- to 4-mm dermatologic punch is an excellent means of obtaining an adequate tissue specimen with minimal morbidity. Acquiring a tissue sample will have minimal effect on subsequent treatment. An exception is the mobile submucosal mass in the floor of mouth or buccal region without evidence of mucosal involvement. Because salivary gland neoplasms can present in this fashion, a mucosa-disrupting biopsy should be avoided, and tissue diagnosis can be achieved with transoral FNA. Finally, if lymphoma is a serious consideration at the time of biopsy, the specimen should be sent fresh in saline to allow assessment by flow cytometry.

Palpable and suspicious lymphadenopathy can be further assessed with outpatient FNA. In experienced centers, FNA is highly accurate in diagnosing metastatic SCCA (49). Again, adequate specimen acquisition and fixation are critical (50,51). Although confirmatory, an FNA of clinically evident lymphadenopathy in the setting of a biopsy-confirmed, primary oral cavity cancer is not mandatory.

Upon completion of the outpatient evaluation, patients with oral cavity malignancies should undergo formal evaluation under anesthesia (EUA). This should include direct laryngoscopy and pharyngoscopy, with consideration of flexible bronchoscopy and esophagoscopy if warranted. During the EUA, complete assessment of the primary site can be achieved without the limitations of patient discomfort and compliance. Thorough palpation for size and extent of involvement can be undertaken. The remaining subsites in the upper aerodigestive tract can also be thoroughly evaluated to rule out second primary disease. Finally, initial or additional tissue sampling can be obtained (Table 119.3).

TABLE 119.3	DIAGNOSIS AND EVALUATION

Complete history and physical examination
  (1) History
      (a) Length, severity, and quality of symptoms, with specific attention to dysphagia, odynophagia, otalgia, and dyspnea
      (b) Previous treatments relating to oral lesion
      (c) Social history including drug and alcohol exposure
      (d) Comorbid factors important in surgical planning
  (2) Physical
      (a) Assess overall characteristics of tumor including subsite, invasion of local structures; assess for reconstructive options
      (b) Assess for multiple primary sites and regional spread
      (c) Stage tumor using AJCC staging TNM guidelines
  (3) Biopsies
      (a) Biopsy of the primary tumor in the office if possible and appropriate
      (b) FNA of regional neck metastatic disease if present

Imaging
  (1) CT and/or MRI of the primary tumor and regional lymph node basins
  (2) CXR or CT of the chest
  (3) PET/CT if concerns for metastases
  (4) May consider panorex or barium swallow

Laboratory tests
  (1) Complete blood count, electrolytes, and liver function panel based on preoperative assessment and anesthetic considerations
  (2) Electrocardiogram and further cardiac evaluation based on patient's medical history

Consultations
  (1) Dental evaluation
  (2) Radiation oncology evaluation
  (3) Medical oncology evaluation
  (4) Pretreatment medical evaluation
  (5) Appropriate subspecialty consultations
  (6) May also consider speech pathology, internal medicine, and anesthesiology

Examination under anesthesia
  (1) Direct laryngoscopy and pharyngoscopy
  (2) Esophagoscopy if physical examination warrants further evaluation
  (3) Bronchoscopy if physical examination warrants further evaluation
  (4) Palpation of oral cavity and oropharynx

STAGING AND PROGNOSIS

The staging for oral cavity carcinoma follows the American Joint Committee on Cancer (AJCC) staging format, most recently updated in 2010. Staging criteria may be found in Table 119.4. The standard TNM classification system is utilized to arrive at a stage rated from I to IV. The T status is determined by the size of the tumor for T1, T2, and T3 and the degree of associated involvement for T4 lesions. Tumors achieve a T4a status with invasion: through cortical bone, into deep, extrinsic muscles of the tongue, into the maxillary sinus and skin of the face. T4b tumors invade one or more of the following structures—Masticator space, pterygoid plates, the skull base, and carotid artery—and

may therefore be unresectable. The N status is determined by size, location, and number of lymph nodes involved ranging from N0 to N3. The presence of metastatic disease is denoted by the M status.

Though the current AJCC staging criteria are based on clinical and radiologic diagnoses, multiple histologic characteristics of the primary tumor have been shown to impact prognosis. These are discussed under the "Management of the N0 Neck" but include depth of invasion of the primary tumor, perineural spread, perivascular spread, perilymphatic spread, poorly differentiated tumors, and infiltrative tumors. Tumors of the oral tongue and floor of mouth with invasion less than 2 mm have a 13% metastatic rate to the regional lymph node basin and

---

TABLE 119.4   CLINICAL CLASSIFICATION OF SQUAMOUS CELL CARCINOMA OF THE ORAL CAVITY

Primary Tumor (T)

Tx	Unassessable
T0	No evidence of primary tumor
Tis	Carcinoma *in situ*
T1	Tumor 2 cm or less in greatest dimension
T2	Tumor 2 cm but not >4 cm in greatest dimension
T3	Tumor >4 cm in greatest dimension
T4a	Moderately advanced disease (resectable)
Lip	Tumor invades through the cortical bone, inferior alveolar, floor of mouth, or skin of face (chin, nose, etc.)[a]
Oral cavity sites	Tumor invades through adjacent structures only such as cortical bone (mandible or maxilla), into deep extrinsic muscles of tongue (genioglossus, hyoglossus, palatoglossus, styloglossus), into maxillary sinus or skin of face[a]
T4b	Very advanced disease (unresectable) Tumor invades masticator space, pterygoid plates, or skull base and/or encases internal carotid artery

Regional Lymph Nodes (N)

NX	Unassessable
N0	No regional lymph node metastasis
N1	Single ipsilateral lymph node, 3 cm or less in greatest dimension
N2a	Single ipsilateral lymph node >3 cm but not >6 cm in greatest dimension
N2b	Multiple ipsilateral lymph nodes, none >6 cm in greatest dimension.
N2c	Bilateral or contralateral lymph nodes, none >6 cm in greatest dimension.
N3	Any lymph node >6 cm

Distant Metastasis (M)

MX	Unassessable
M0	No distant metastasis (no pathologic M0; use clinical M to complete stage group)
M1	Distant metastasis

Stage Grouping

M0	T1	T2	T3	T4a	T4b
N0	I	II	III	IVA	IVB
N1	III	III	III	IVA	IVB
N2	IVA	IVA	IVA	IVA	IVB
N3	IVB	IVB	IVB	IVB	IVB

All M1	IVC

[a]Superficial erosion alone of bone/tooth socket by gingival primary is not sufficient to classify a tumor as T4.

a 95% disease-specific survival, while tumors 2.1 to 9 mm in depth have a metastatic rate of 46% and survival drops to 85% (52). Patients with tumors exhibiting perineural invasion have both decreased locoregional control of their disease and decreased disease-specific survival. The border of the tumor with the native tissue as well as the type of invasion also affect prognosis. Tumors with well-defined or "pushing" borders confer a better prognosis than those with less well-defined borders and deep infiltration (53).

The single most important factor in overall survival is the presence of positive cervical lymph nodes, and is reflected in the current AJCC staging guidelines. Extracapsular extension, as evaluated in the excised specimen, has been shown to be an independent predictor of development of regional recurrence and distant metastatic disease (54). In one single-institution study, the "lymph node density," or ratio of metastatic to benign lymph nodes in the surgical specimen, was found to have important prognostic implications. Patients with a higher lymph node density had decreased overall and disease-specific 5-year survival rates, though replication of these results may be hindered by institutional variation in both surgical neck dissection technique and pathologic examination (55).

Overall survival rates based on stage alone are detailed in Figure 119.12. Statistics for each individual patient, however, remain difficult to predict, as many important prognostic features are not included in the current staging system. Recently, a nomogram including various other patient and tumor characteristics has been developed and externally validated, which may aid in the assessment of each individual's locoregional recurrence-free survival

(56). This study validated the negative poor prognostic influence of advanced T stage, advanced N status, and close or positive margins.

TREATMENT

Treatment options for oral cavity carcinoma include surgery, radiation, chemotherapy, or some combination of the above. For early-stage tumors, both primary surgery and radiation have been shown to be equally effective. Therefore, treatment decisions are based on anatomical subsite and the associated morbidity of surgery or of radiation to that region, the patient's comorbidities, and physician and patient preference. Chemotherapy has no role as a single-modality curative therapy, but recent experience has demonstrated usefulness in the adjuvant setting. For later-stage tumors, or tumors with other poor prognostic features, patients benefit from multimodality treatment with the proper sequence of surgery and radiation with or without chemotherapy.

Radiation

Early-stage tumors may be treated with primary radiation therapy. The standard dosing regimen for external beam radiation is 1.8 to 2 gray (Gy) daily for a total dose of 62 to 70 Gy. For locally advanced head and neck cancer, hyperfractionated radiation dosing with concomitant boost protocols provides better locoregional control than standard daily dosing, although no significant differences were seen in overall survival. Furthermore, patients

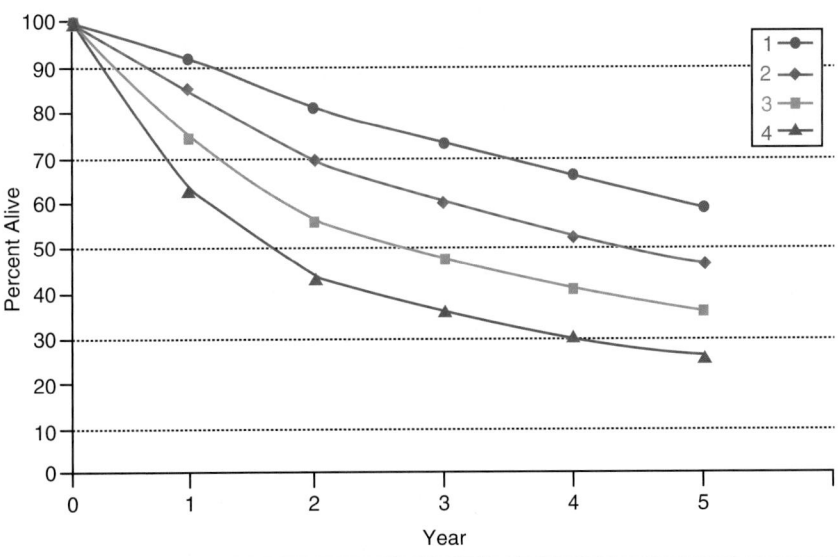

Observed Survival	1	2	3	4	5	95% Cls	Cases
1	92.4	81.3	73.6	66.4	59.2	57.5–60.8	4660
2	85.8	69.8	60.2	52.8	46.9	45.0–48.9	3315
3	74.9	56.4	47.9	41.1	36.3	34.1–38.6	2239
4	63.6	43.7	35.8	30.7	26.5	25.2–27.8	5431

Figure 119.12 AJCC graph of survival by stage.

receiving hyperfractionated dosing experienced more severe acute side effects including radiation burns to the skin, mucositis, and xerostomia (57). Indications for postoperative radiation therapy to the primary site include positive or close surgical margins (less than 5 mm), perineural or perivascular invasion, or T_3 or T_4 tumors (58). Patients with multiple positive nodes or lymph nodes with extracapsular extension in the neck also benefit from postoperative radiation therapy. In any treatment protocol, every effort should be made to reduce the total treatment time (from surgery to the completion of radiation therapy) to less than 100 days, as decreased treatment time increases locoregional control and overall survival (59). Curative unimodality radiation therapy can be limited by several technical challenges in delivering consistent dosage to the target area. These challenges include mobility of the target tissue such as the tongue and the presence of dense materials such as bone and dental restorations in the field. These factors can often be overcome with the use of interstitial implant and brachytherapy. The most common use of radiation therapy for oral cavity cancer is in the adjuvant setting with planned surgery. Adjuvant radiation is usually done in the postoperative setting as no survival benefit exists when radiation is given preoperatively (60).

Radiation toxicities to the oral cavity include xerostomia, dysgeusia, dysphagia, dental decay, and osteoradionecrosis of the mandible. The duration of treatment is also significant with treatment courses averaging 6 to 7 weeks. Due to the extensive side effect profile, primary surgical resection is favored over radiation for early-stage oral cavity carcinoma. The use of intensity-modulated radiation therapy (IMRT) for advanced-stage oral cavity carcinoma has improved side effect profiles, in which dosing is maximized to tumor volume but minimized to surrounding normal structures. The use of IMRT decreases the incidence and severity of late xerostomia (61). Though sparing of the submandibular and parotid glands when possible may minimize xerostomia, this technique is more feasible for sites outside of the oral cavity (62,63).

Chemotherapy

Chemotherapy, as a single treatment modality, has no role in the primary treatment of oral cavity carcinoma but has a well-established role in the adjuvant setting for advanced-stage disease. Randomized studies by both the European Organization Research and Treatment of Cancer and the Radiation Therapy Oncology Group show that adding concomitant cisplatin to postoperative radiation improves both locoregional control and disease-free survival in patients with advanced-stage disease (64,65). Side effect profiles, however, remain poor, and the addition of chemotherapy adds significant adverse toxicity to therapy (64). Retrospective subgroup analysis of these studies demonstrated that only patients exhibiting either

extracapsular extension or positive margin status were found to have significant survival benefits from the addition of chemotherapy. Though there was a trend toward increased survival with advanced-stage (III and IV) tumors, these results were not statistically significant. Interestingly, the presence of multiple positive lymph nodes without ECS was not shown to have benefited from the addition of chemotherapy (66).

The use of primary chemoradiation therapy for surgically resectable advanced-stage oral cavity cancer is currently under investigation in several centers. Various treatment protocols have been proposed using neoadjuvant, concurrent, and sequential treatment algorithms, with potentially encouraging results in selected patient groups. Further investigation is necessary before widespread adoption is advocated.

Surgery (By Subsite)

Cancers of the oral cavity are best managed by primary surgery. Many early T-stage tumors may be managed by transoral resection. For larger intraoral tumors, or tumors extending posteriorly towards the base of tongue, transoral approaches may not be sufficient for access. Adequate access and visualization are maximized by various surgical approaches. For buccal lesions, the addition of a lip-split incision may be required. This can be expanded to include mandibulotomy to afford the surgeon excellent posterior visualization for resection, and wide access for reconstructive options. This approach does, however, place the patient at risk for postoperative nonunion of the mandible, especially in patients who will be receiving postoperative irradiation. Furthermore, patients are left with a midline lip-split scar, and numbness in the distribution of the inferior alveolar nerve. In lieu of a mandibulotomy approach, most tumors without mandibular involvement may be approached through a visor flap and some form of lingual release. Liberal transcervical access allows for adequate visualization for ablation and access for reconstructive efforts. No significant difference in locoregional control or margin status has been found between the two approaches (67,68).

Surgical decision making must also take into consideration the management of the neck as well as the primary site. For clinically, radiographically, or pathologically positive regional neck disease, formal neck dissection is recommended. Historically, the use of the modified radical neck dissection for node positive disease was advocated. Currently, thorough selective neck dissections of involved lymph node levels and levels at risk for specific subsites are reported as equally effective in controlling neck disease. Advanced neck disease with sternocleidomastoid involvement, jugular vein involvement, and accessory nerve encasement warrants treatment with classic radical neck dissections and consideration of accessory nerve reconstruction.

Management of the N0 Neck

The management of patients with oral cavity malignancies and N0 neck stage deserves specific consideration. The N0 status must be strictly demonstrated by both physical exam and radiologic criteria. Regardless of negative assessment on both these factors, between 20% and 40% of patients with oral cavity cancer and N0 neck will demonstrate regional metastasis (69–71). The salvage rates for subsequent neck recurrence are poor, approximately 25%, and underscore the importance of adequate up-front treatment of the N0 neck (72).

Therefore, judicious surgical and pathologic assessment of the lymphatic basins at risk with specific oral cavity subsites is warranted. Such intervention not only provides a therapeutic benefit of removing any potentially occult metastatic disease within the neck but also provides more thorough pathologic staging information. Pathologic information from the surgical specimen can guide the appropriate decision making for adjuvant therapy such as radiation therapy or a combination of chemoradiation therapy. Factors taken into account include multifocality of the metastatic disease, evidence of extracapsular spread, and further assessment of potentially important biologic markers.

Classic evaluation of the N0 neck was defined using the modified radical neck dissection and clearance of levels one through five. Experience over the last two decades has demonstrated that the selective neck dissection of levels I, II and III, *the supraomohyoid neck dissection*, is as efficacious as the modified radical neck dissection (72,73) with less morbidity (74,75). The selective neck dissection demonstrates similarly low recurrence rates of less than 5% when compared to the modified radical neck dissection.

Specific consideration should be given to thorough dissection of level 1A for all anterior tongue and anterior floor of mouth lesions. Similarly, potential dissection of bilateral necks should be considered for such anterior lesions. Studies have indicated that level IIB is a rare site for occult metastasis from most oral cavity malignancies (76). This has significant importance as the dissection of only level IIA carries significantly lower risk of 11th cranial nerve dysfunction secondary to surgical issues related to direct trauma, tissue retraction, and decreased vascularity involved with circumferential neural dissection. Eleventh nerve dysfunction along with praxis of the lower seventh nerve branches and resultant smile dysfunction as well as contour deformity are the main postoperative issues associated with selective neck dissection and deserve specific consideration in discussing such intervention with patients (74,75). A consideration for level IIB dissection can be undertaken with RMT carcinomas and lesions with a more posterior location that abut or potentially cross into the oropharyngeal subsite.

Advanced oral cavity lesions, T3–T4 tumors, have a significantly higher degree of occult metastasis in the N0 neck and should be addressed with a selective neck dissection. This issue is less controversial as surgical exploration of the neck is usually required as a component of the ablative approach to the resection of such tumors. Similarly, necessary reconstructive efforts such as regional and free tissue flap reconstructions may require intervention in the neck.

The more challenging question is the management of the early-stage oral cavity cancer, T1–T2 tumors, with the N0 neck. Currently, between 15% and 20% of such early-stage malignancies will demonstrate occult metastasis on formal surgical evaluation of the neck. This risk of occult metastasis increases with certain factors, most notably, size of the tumor with T2 lesions having a greater metastatic potential than smaller T1 lesions. Depth of invasion has been evaluated in numerous studies and found to be significantly correlated with occult metastatic disease (52). Varying cutoff points between 2 and 4 mm have been evaluated to demonstrate an appropriate threshold for proceeding with surgical treatment and evaluation of the selective neck dissection (77). Studies support the cutoff of 4 mm or greater depth of invasion as an indication to proceed with selective neck dissection. Although not as strongly correlated with occult metastasis as depth of invasion, other factors such as poorly differentiated tumors, tumors demonstrating lymphovascular invasion, and tumors with an infiltrative growth pattern can confer and increased risk (78). Neck dissection should also be recommended in such cases.

For early-stage tumors, one clinical approach is to proceed with the surgical management of the early-stage primary tumor and allow the presence of poor pathologic features on final pathology to determine the need for adjuvant treatment of the neck with radiation therapy. Yet, even in tumors with poor prognostic features, this would lead to significant overtreatment with radiation therapy and its associated short- and long-term side effects. Similarly, after surgical treatment of the primary cancer and the identification of poor prognostic pathologic features, a recommendation could also be made to then formally proceed with surgical management of the neck with neck dissection. Results of this intervention can guide potential adjuvant treatment. This approach has the drawback of requiring two distinct anesthetic procedures.

The most thorough and streamlined approach in patients with T1/T2 primary site cancers and the N0 neck is to proceed with selective neck dissection at the same time as the primary surgical therapy. Results of the primary site pathologic assessment as well as the pathologic assessment of surgical basins at risk will then form the basis of adjuvant treatment planning.

As a corollary to the positive experience with sentinel lymph node biopsy techniques in the management of malignant melanoma, the use of radionucleotide-guided sentinel lymph node biopsy for T1 and T2 oral cavity carcinomas with an N0 neck is currently under evaluation. Prospective studies have indicated a negative predictive value in the 90% range utilizing radionucle-otide-guided sentinel lymph node biopsy techniques (79). These studies also indicate that the optimal utilization of the sentinel lymph node biopsying technique requires experienced operators to increase the negative predictive value. More intensive pathologic analysis is required including immunohistochemistry techniques not standardly utilized in the pathologic assessment of standard neck dissection specimens. Also of note, a greater accuracy has been shown when focusing on the oral tongue subsite as compared to other subsites within the oral cavity (80). Other accurate, but effort-intense means of assessing the N0 neck include the use of ultrasound-guided FNA, which has demonstrated a favorable experience in numerous European studies (43–45,81). Although ultrasound-guided FNA and a radionucleotide-guided sentinel lymph node biopsy demonstrate potential benefit in selected cases, utilization of the selective neck dissection in T1 and T2 N0 carcinomas of the oral cavity is recommended.

Mandibular Involvement

As discussed earlier in regards to preoperative imaging, tumors of the oral cavity should be assessed for mandibular involvement both clinically and radiographically. The mandible may be either abutted or completely invaded by tumor, and anticipating mandibular involvement will help in both ablative and reconstructive planning. Two forms of mandibular resection are available. The *marginal mandibulectomy* removes a portion of the mandibular cortex but does not interrupt the continuity of the mandible nor significantly alter its function. The *segmental mandibulectomy* involves the removal of an entire segment of the mandible—through the entire cortex—and, by definition, interrupts the continuity of the mandible significantly affecting function. Reconstruction of marginal mandibulectomy defects primarily involves soft tissue coverage, whereas reconstruction of the segmental defect usually requires the restoration of mandibular continuity. Marginal mandibulectomy is considered for tumors abutting the periosteum or superficially involving the alveolar mandible, whereas segmental resection is reserved for patients with clear bone involvement with significant cortical bone erosion and potential marrow involvement. The mandibular periosteum is thought to act as a barrier to tumor spread, and patients with microscopic disease may undergo marginal mandibulectomy of either cortex with preservation of at least 1 cm of alveolar height. Patients with invasion of the periosteum or superficial invasion of either cortex may also undergo marginal mandibulectomy without limitation in oncologic control. In these cases, multiple studies have demonstrated no changes in locoregional control or disease-specific survival with marginal mandibulectomy over segmental mandibulectomy (82,83). Segmental

mandibulectomy is reserved for patients with extensive mandibular destruction or bone marrow involvement. Intraoperative frozen sections of bone marrow or the inferior alveolar nerve may help intraoperative decision making. Suspicion of significant bone involvement should expand preoperative planning—raising the consideration of necessary reconstructive options (84).

Lip

Cancers of the lip present more often on the lower lip than on the upper lip, most likely secondary to the increased sun exposure of the lower lip. The majority of lip lesions are SCCA, while basal cell carcinomas can also occur. The majority of patients present with early-stage primary tumors without cervical metastases, and surgery is the preferred method of primary treatment (85).

Reconstructive principles of the lip include cosmesis as well as maintaining oral competence. Reconstruction is based on the percentage and site of lip resection. In general terms, for defects less than 33%, a wedge excision and primary closure provide excellent results. For lesions involving a greater percentage of the lip length, a procedure mobilizing the available remaining lip is preferred. Options include the Abbe, Estlander, and Karapandzic flaps. Distinct advantages of the Karapandzic flap include the maintenance of lip sensation, mobility, and oral competence. Resultant microstomia needs to be carefully considered. Larger defects require utilization of nonlip tissue such as modified Webster flaps and the radial forearm free flap. The lower lip drains bilaterally, most commonly affecting the perifacial, submandibular, and submental lymph nodes. Cancers of the upper lip and oral commissures are often more aggressive and confer a worse prognosis. Drainage patterns remain ipsilateral for upper lip carcinoma, and the cervical metastatic rate is slightly higher than for lower lip though the overall rate remains low. The 5-year survival for stage I and II lesions is 90%, and survival drops to 50% with the involvement of cervical lymph nodes (86). Further discussions of lip cancer and its management are provided in Chapter 116.

Alveolar Ridge

The majority of primary alveolar ridge carcinomas occur in the mandible with the posterior body being most common. Although SCCA are by far the most common, consideration to tumors of dental origin, osteosarcomas, and salivary gland cancers must be given. The prognosis of early-stage disease remains relatively favorable with 70% to 80% survival, while prognosis significantly worsens with advancing stage based on size, bone invasion, and nodal metastases. Unimodality treatment for early-stage disease is primarily surgical with the consideration of adjuvant radiation therapy for advanced-stage disease.

The surgical approach to resection of both upper and lower alveolar ridge carcinoma follows the same basic principles as outlined above in the section on mandibular involvement. Tumors with minimal bone disruption at the dental interface can be addressed with marginal resections and acceptable oncologic control. Potential contraindications to marginal mandibulectomy include previous loss of alveolar height, radiographic evidence of marrow involvement, intraoperative evidence of deep bone erosion, and previous radiation therapy. Intraoperative assessment is critical in the treatment of these lesions, and evidence of disease that is more advanced than previously appreciated needs to be addressed with appropriate expansion of the ablative procedure. For lesions with significant erosion and bone involvement, *en bloc* removal of the affected segment with maxillectomy for upper alveolar ridge lesions and segmental mandibulectomy for mandibular lesions is recommended.

Reconstruction will be dictated by the specifics for the surgical defects. Limited upper and lower alveolar ridge resection can be allowed to heal secondarily or augmented with intraoral local flaps. Larger upper alveolar ridge lesion will result in connection to the sinonasal tract and are most often addressed with obturating prostheses. Soft tissue and bone containing free flaps are effective and necessary for large upper alveolar ridge defects.

The marginal mandibular defect will often require intraoral soft tissue coverage, and skin flaps such as the submental and radial forearm free flap are effective in achieving coverage without compromising oral function. Segmental mandibular defects provide a greater challenge. Reconstructive options are many and are determined by the location of the bone deficit and the associated soft tissue defect. The lateral defect can be addressed with a large soft tissue flap, such as the pectoralis major flap, without restoring mandibular continuity. This will result in malocclusion and mandibular shift but can be appropriate in select cases. Attempts to restore continuity of the mandible are the standard. This can be achieved with an appropriately sized reconstruction plate and soft tissue coverage that can include regional flap and free tissue transfer. Risks include potential plate fracture and plate exposure. The restoration of mandibular continuity with vascularized bone is the gold standard for segmental mandible reconstruction (87). Although optional in the lateral defect, vascularized bone is mandatory for the anterior defect as synthetic prostheses will uniformly erode secondary to tissue contracture. The fibula osseocutaneous flap in the most commonly used free flap for mandibular reconstruction secondary to numerous favorable qualities. Other options include the scapular osseocutaneous flap, the iliac crest osseomyocutaneous flap, and the radial forearm osseocutaneous flap.

Floor of Mouth

More than one-third of patients with floor of mouth cancer present with advanced T-stage disease, and nearly 40% of patients have clinically positive regional metastases (88,89). For T_1 tumors, the rate of occult metastasis is 21%, and it is 62% for T_2 tumors (89). Early in the disease process, cancer of the floor of mouth is often asymptomatic, with pain, bleeding, and submandibular duct obstruction more common as tumor size progresses. The floor of mouth musculature, specifically the mylohyoid muscle, as well as the mandibular periosteum may act as barriers to tumor spread, though when involved by tumor require comprehensive clearance. Many patients require either marginal or segmental mandibulectomy for small, but invasive lesions. Involvement of the ventral aspect of the tongue may require partial glossectomy. Such tumors can also readily involve the root of the tongue necessitating significant resection into the tongue base, which can place the neurovascular pedicles of the tongue at risk. Invasion through the submandibular duct is best treated with resection of the submandibular gland and sublingual glands with the primary specimen.

Mucosal lesions sparing the mandible are optimally managed with transoral surgical resection. Anterior defects larger than 2 cm have the potential to tether the ventral aspect of the tongue, and formal reconstruction should be considered. For smaller mucosal lesions, a split-thickness skin graft may be used with the application of a bolster dressing. For larger lesions, tissue flap reconstruction may be required. Multiple pedicled flap options are available including the submental flap, the nasolabial flap, and the platysma flap. The myocutaneous pectoralis flap may be used, although it can be somewhat bulky. For larger defects requiring vascularized tissue reconstructions, microvascular free flaps are the superior choice with the radial forearm free flap offering the greatest coverage and flexibility for large mucosal defects, although the perforator anterior lateral thigh flap is another excellent option.

As discussed above, partial mandibulectomy does not compromise oncologic control. Required marginal mandibulectomy may involve the lingual cortex or the alveolar ridge, as dictated by the disease location. Care must be taken to leave the outer cortex or 1 cm of inferior cortex respectively for such marginal bone resections. Segmental mandibulectomy is reserved for patients with gross destruction of the mandible seen on clinical or radiographic examination (82,83). Mucosal defects with a marginal mandibulectomy may be reconstructed with appropriate tissue flaps as discussed above. Segmental mandibulectomy defects may be left unreconstructed if lateral, but usually an effort is made to restore continuity. Lateral defects can be reconstructed with a reconstruction bar and soft tissue flap, but do benefit from the use of vascularized osseocutaneous flaps such from the fibula, radius, scapular and iliac crest. Microvascular free flap reconstruction is mandatory for anterior defects as alloplastic techniques will break down and extrude.

The floor of mouth drains directly to the submental and submandibular lymph node basins, with the submandibular lymph nodes the most frequently involved. Bilateral neck disease should be addressed at the time of primary resection, as cervical metastatic disease confers a grim prognosis with poor rates of surgical salvage. The 5-year survival rates for floor of mouth carcinoma are 90%, 80%, 65%, and 30% for stages I to IV disease respectively (88,90).

Oral Tongue

Though early T-stage tumors of the oral tongue have equivalent survival rates when treated with surgery or radiation, surgical treatment is preferred to avoid the acute and late side effects of radiation (91,92). Another drawback of radiation is the prolonged treatment course and recovery period. The majority of tongue cancers will present on the lateral border of the tongue, and patients have minimal symptoms. Dorsal tongue cancer is rare, representing 3% to 5% of oral tongue cancers, but can have significant delay in diagnosis because of the unusual location (93). Recent reviews of the SEER database revealed that early-stage oral tongue carcinoma confers a poorer prognosis than carcinoma of other sites of the oral cavity. Five-year overall survival rates from the dataset for oral tongue cancers revealed 67% and 51% for stage I and stage II tumors, respectively (94), whereas other oral cavity subsites reviewed in the same series noted disease-specific 5-year survival rates at 94% and 85% for stage I and stage II disease, respectively. Yet, other studies reveal a less dramatic difference while reiterating the negative effect of advanced disease stage on the survival statistics for oral tongue cancer, with overall 5-year survival of 75% for stage I or II tumors, and 40% for stage III or IV tumors (95,96).

Standard surgical management of oral cavity cancers includes a partial glossectomy with at least 1-cm margins. As both specimen shrinkage and muscle distortion after resection may alter incised planes, margin status at the mucosal level and along the deep tongue musculature must be assessed with caution. Intraoperative frozen sections can be utilized to confirm clear margins around the tumor, and are best taken from the patient along the resected mucosal and muscular borders. Means of resection can affect margin assessment. Animal studies demonstrate that the use of scalpel will give the most representative tissue margin and the other techniques, such as electrocautery and ultrasonic device will have varying degrees of tissue disruption affecting margin assessment (97). Due to the difficult nature of assessing muscle margins, postoperative radiation may be considered in patients with initial positive surgical margins, despite further resection to clear margins (98).

Once complete surgical resection of the tumor has been achieved, attention can be focused on appropriate reconstructive efforts. The primary goal of tongue reconstruction is to limit tongue tethering and any other restraints on mobility that would significantly affect speech and swallow function. Partial glossectomy defects including less than one-third of the tongue may heal by secondary intention, or a split-thickness skin graft may be used for limited extension along the floor of mouth to decrease tongue tethering. For larger defects of the tongue or floor of mouth, multiple reconstructive options may be explored. In addition to maximizing mobility, reconstructive efforts should include augmenting tongue volume as needed. Increasing tongue volume, while maintaining mobility in reconstructing the tongue defect, helps in secretion management, transfer of the food bolus posteriorly, and articulation. Maintaining premaxillary contact and palatal contact aids in speech production, while having full excursion past the alveolar ridge aids in the clearing of secretions (99). Fasciocutaneous free flaps such as the radial forearm or anterolateral thigh flap offer adequate tissue for larger partial glossectomy reconstruction, with or without a floor of mouth component. A comparative study of the submental flap and the radial forearm flap used to reconstruct partial glossectomy defects demonstrated equivalent speech and swallow results, while patients receiving a submental flap had decreased operative time and hospitalization (100).

For advanced disease, multimodality treatment is required. Surgery followed by either radiation or chemoradiation has better disease control than either surgery or radiation alone (95,101). Postoperative radiation therapy has been shown to increase locoregional control rates, with a positive surgical margin the only factor predictive of recurrence, though the majority of patients in this study recurred within 2 years (95).

Hard Palate

SCCA makes up the vast majority of oral cavity cancers, but the hard palate has equal incidence of minor salivary gland tumors. In one series, SCCA represented only 50% of cancers originating in the hard palate (102). Other tumors include adenoid cystic carcinoma, polymorphous low-grade adenocarcinoma, adenocarcinoma, and mucoepidermoid carcinoma (103). Early lesions of any pathology of the hard palate most often involve the underlying bone, and are therefore best treated with primary surgical therapy (104).

Transoral resection of the tumor may include an alveolectomy or inferior maxillectomy in addition to palatectomy (105). Because of the dense innervation of the hard palate and the foramina through which the nerves run, consideration must be given to perineural spread of disease and direct extension via the foramina. Adequate margin assessment of these regions is required.

Reconstruction of oroantral fistulae may be accomplished by intraoperative placement of palatal prosthesis after packing the remaining maxillary sinus. The prosthesis and packing is removed in clinic, and a more long-term prosthesis fitted. For larger defects, or defects involving the premaxilla, free tissue transfer is indicated and offers the benefit of providing stable projection in this region. Reconstruction of the premaxilla maintains facial contour and prevents erosion of the prosthesis through the upper lip. Often, a combination of a free flap with a prosthesis offers the best cosmetic and functional result for hard palate defects (106).

The hard palate drains to level I and level II lymph nodes but also may involve retropharyngeal and perifacial nodes. Historically, the rate of occult cervical metastatic disease has been considered low, and routine elective neck dissections have not been recommended (102,107). More recently, however, studies have indicated higher occult rates than previously thought, from 27% to 30%, with variable rates of surgical salvage for regionally recurrent disease (108,109). Regional failure was associated with increasing T classification, which also was an independent predictor of recurrence-free survival on multivariable analysis (109). Elective treatment of the neck with either surgery or radiation is therefore recommended (108,109).

Retromolar Trigone

Cancer of the RMT is often diagnosed at a later stage than other oral cavity tumors, due to both a difficult clinical examination of the site and its close proximity to the mandible. Again SCCA is the most common pathology, but salivary gland malignancies require consideration. The mucosa of the RMT directly abuts the periosteum of the mandible, and mandibular invasion occurs in up to 50% of tumors on initial diagnosis (59). Because of the critical anatomic location, this can occur even with small tumors. Trismus indicates involvement of the pterygoid musculature, and extension to the tonsillar pillars, soft palate, and base of tongue is common.

A transoral surgical approach is appropriate for many tumors of the RMT if adequate visualization and access for instrumentation is available. In cases where this is not achievable, the combined use of a transcervical visor flap or cheek flap will be helpful and may be required if there is significant extension to multiple subsites or with large tumors. Patients requiring segmental mandibulectomy will require a transcervical approach for extirpative and reconstructive access. Small defects may be closed primarily, left to heal by secondary intention, or reconstructed with a pedicled buccal fat graft. Larger mucosal defects or defects including a marginal mandibulectomy benefit from free tissue transfer technique providing adequate, pliable lining such as the radial forearm free flap. Defects including a segmental mandibulectomy benefit from restoration of mandibular continuity by reconstruction with osseocutaneous free flaps.

The RMT drains to lymph nodes in levels II and III. As RMT tumors usually present with advanced stage, elective neck dissection should be performed in any patient undergoing transcervical approach for primary tumor resection, regardless of clinical nodal stage. Patients with clinically positive disease should be managed with a therapeutic neck dissection followed by radiation therapy. Overall survival decreases with N stage, with a 69% 5-year survival in patients with N_0 disease, 56% for N_1, and a 26% survival rate for those with N_2 disease (60).

Buccal Mucosa

SCCA of the buccal mucosa represents 5% to 10% of oral cavity cancers in the United States (110), though in India it accounts for over 40% due to betel nut use (20). Buccal cancer often presents as advanced-stage disease, as there is no lateral anatomic barrier to spread. The buccal fat pad and musculature are easily invaded by carcinoma, and facial paralysis, skin invasion, and trismus are not unusual in primary presentation.

Surgery is the treatment of choice for buccal cancer, most often through transoral excision (111). Larger lesions may require a combined oral and transcervical approach. The addition of a lip splitting incision can add critical access to visualization and surgical resection of this region. For smaller lesions, primary closure or skin grafting may be considered. For larger lesions, soft tissue reconstruction with pedicled regional flaps such the submental flap or temporoparietal fascial flap or fasciocutaneous free flaps may be required to avoid contracture and trismus. The risk of cervical metastatic disease is related to both T stage and the depth of invasion of the primary tumor. Advanced T stage III and IV and invasion greater than 5 mm has been associated with increased risk of cervical metastatic spread, and elective neck dissection for those with clinically negative lymph node basins should be considered (112).

Buccal carcinoma can bestow a grave prognosis, with some evidence that it is worse than other sites of the oral cavity (111). For patients with unresectable disease, primary chemoradiation therapy may be considered, though patients treated with radiation alone have high recurrence rates and decreased overall survival (113,114).

COMPLICATIONS

Complications from treatment of oral cavity neoplasms depend on not only the type of treatment but the extent and location of the original lesion. Acute complications due to treatment effects are usually managed without treatment breaks, but complications may continue to arise many years after treatment has finished.

Radiation to the oral cavity has close proximity to the salivary tissues and the mandible, and thus treatment is wrought with acute and long-term complications.

Universally, patients develop superficial burns to the skin and the mucous membranes during treatment, which may persist for weeks after treatment has completed. Mucositis is very painful and may become suprainfected with bacteria or fungus (115). Mouthwash with a mixture of lidocaine and an antifungal may provide some relief, and many patients benefit from enteral nutrition via nasogastric or gastric tube. After treatment, many patients are permanently left with xerostomia and dysgeusia (116). While not painful, the decreased saliva production and altered taste leaves eating difficult and less enjoyable. Tooth decay results from decreased saliva production, and impeccable dental hygiene is essential (117). Though the introduction of IMRT and salivary-sparing techniques have relieved the severity of xerostomia (118), the problem still exists, especially for those with tumors located in the floor of mouth with close proximity to the submandibular glands. Mastication can also be significantly affected, especially when combined with surgery (119). Other late complications of radiation include soft tissue radionecrosis and osteoradionecrosis of the mandible. Soft tissue necrosis presents as a nonhealing ulcer, and biopsies must be taken to exclude the possibility of recurrent cancer. Osteoradionecrosis presents as bone loss and mandibular exposure, either intraorally or externally through the skin. This is often precipitated by dental trauma, underscoring the need for extensive pretreatment evaluation by a dentist. Exposed mandible often becomes infected and results in an orocutaneous fistula. Treatment with antibiotics, conservative sequestrectomy, and hyperbaric oxygen may help early lesions (120). Pathologic fractures due to radiation damage, or osteoradionecrosis not helped by other measures, benefit from free tissue transfer of bone. Microvascular reconstruction replaces necrotic tissue and reestablishes blood flow to the hypoxic bed.

Surgical complications are varied and depend on the extent of the tumor resection and reconstruction (Table 119.5). Due to the causative effects of oral cavity cancer, most patients present with numerous comorbid states, placing them at increased surgical risk. Patients with head and neck cancer are at increased risk for postoperative pulmonary embolism, cardiac complications, delirium tremens, and aspiration pneumonia (121,122). Careful preoperative optimization of other medical problems helps minimize intra- and postoperative medical complications.

Airway management must remain a priority. The most drastic and emergent complication of oral cavity cancer and its treatment is acute airway obstruction. This may evolve from increasing mass or edema from the tumor itself obstructing the oral cavity. Less commonly, primary radiation may result in tissue edema causing acute airway obstruction before treatment. Postoperatively, tissue swelling or hematoma formation may occlude the airway, and patients undergoing extensive surgical resection and reconstruction may require a tracheotomy or

TABLE 119.5	SURGICAL COMPLICATIONS RELATED THE TREATMENT OF ORAL CAVITY CANCER AND MANAGEMENT

Airway obstruction: prophylactic or emergent tracheotomy
Postoperative hemorrhage: secure airway, cardiopulmonary stabilization, operative or interventional radiology control
Postoperative fistula: local wound care with salivary diversion from vascular structures
   Prevent great vessel compromise with appropriate vascularized flap coverage if warranted
   Secondary wound closure with appropriate flap reconstruction
Graft compromise or loss
   Split thickness skin flap: debride and allow secondary intention
   Pedicled or free flap compromise
      Explore and assess pedicle integrity, if hematoma or seroma—drain, if vessel compromise—revise
      If partial loss—debride, if complete loss—remove and revise with second flap
Final margins return positive: Re-resect is possible, consider adjuvant treatment

prolonged intubation to avoid airway difficulty. Though rare, this devastating complication may be prevented. Thorough evaluation of the patient's airway at the time of presentation and at every subsequent interaction either in clinic appointments or in the pre- or postoperative setting will alert the clinician to impending airway obstruction. Signs such as tachypnea, drooling, inability to lie flat, stridor, anxiety or the sense of impending doom all may indicate an airway problem. Desaturation seen on pulse oximetry is a late finding necessitating immediate intervention. For prevention and treatment of all airway obstruction, tracheostomy is the treatment of choice.

Immediate postoperative surgical complications such as bleeding or hematoma formation warrant immediate intervention in the operating room. Further postoperative complications include many related to wound healing problems, especially for patients with poor nutritive status, or those who have been previously treated with radiation. Wound breakdown may occur along the reconstructed areas or neck flaps. Salivary contamination, wound infections, and fistulae can occur with varying frequency and may be managed conservatively with meticulous wound dressings and antibiotics. Optimization of thyroid function, nutrition status, and blood glucose levels provides significant benefit. Neck wounds with potential great vessel exposure require tissue coverage with either a local or a free flap, and surgical diversion of salivary contaminants to aid in healing and to prevent carotid rupture.

Late surgical complications may involve both the soft tissue and the bone involved in the resection and reconstruction. Soft tissue loss due to graft loss or inadequate graft volume may result in tethering of the tongue or oral commissure. Recent studies indicate significant decrease in mastication function after treatment of oral cavity cancer. In addition to osteoradionecrosis discussed above, surgical complications of the bone may also occur. In patients who have undergone marginal mandibulectomy, at least 1 cm of height should be left to prevent pathologic fracture (123). Despite these guidelines, some patients go on to develop fractures, especially in the setting of previous radiation treatment. A midline mandibulectomy for access will predispose the patient to nonunion, causing infection, pain, and possibly an orocutaneous fistula.

FUTURE DIRECTIONS

Despite decades of research on head and neck cancer, the overall mortality for oral cavity cancer remains high, without significant improvement. Patients with clinically similar disease may have variable response to treatment, and specific outcomes can be difficult to assess. The current staging system based on clinically obtainable data may not be predictive of outcome for all patients, as oral cavity cancer proves itself a heterogeneous disease.

Surgery remains the mainstay of treatment for oral cavity cancer, and there have been many additions to the extirpative arsenal in the hopes to make surgical ablation faster, more accurate, and with less blood loss. Most surgeons prefer electrocautery over cold techniques for ablation, though this may affect the examination of surgical margins. The addition of the ultrasound scalpel in tongue ablations may help minimize surgical distortion while maintaining hemostasis (97). Some surgeons use the laser or the surgical robot to help ablative visualization, though this may be more useful in oropharyngeal primaries with less surgical access than the oral cavity. Though industry will no doubt provide further technology with which to ablate, it is unclear whether these tools will provide drastic improvement over the scalpel.

Over the past 30 years, the single most important surgical advancement in the treatment of oral cavity cancer has been the addition of free tissue transfer. For large ablative defects, a free flap affords the patient increased speech and swallow function and without the donor site morbidity of a pectoralis major flap. Further advances in technique and critical examination of function will likely elucidate additional surgical measures important in maintaining oral function.

Quite possibly, however, the greatest advancements in overall cancer survival may come from greater precision in selecting patients who will benefit from adjuvant postoperative treatment. As we continue to learn about individual tumor biology, it is becoming clear that biomarkers will play an increasingly important role in prognosis and treatment of oral cavity cancer. Multiple prognostic biomarkers have been identified to date: some predicting overall survival, others predicting lymph node or distant metastatic disease (124). Further research will hopefully illuminate biomarker profiles indicating not only prognostic information but also specific sensitivity to various treatments (125). As an early example, some centers use epidermal growth factor receptor expression as a contributing factor in the decision to add adjuvant treatment. As we gain more information of biomarkers and their importance, we hope to individualize treatment, with the molecular profile of any specific tumor dictating treatment decision trees.

Fortunately, the rates of oral cavity cancer are relatively rare in comparison to other solid tumors. This does, however, make large clinical studies difficult. The vast majority of current oral cavity cancer research comes from single-institution, retrospective studies. While useful, these studies do not provide the level-1 evidence needed for sweeping changes in clinical practice, and result in inter- and even intrainstitutional variation in treatment. Powering large prospective studies to answer clinically relevant questions will require standardization of protocols and multicenter involvement.

HIGHLIGHTS

- In the United States, oral cancer is the most common of the head and neck sites involved by cancer.
- Tobacco and alcohol use remain the carcinogens most commonly linked to oral cancer.
- Cervical metastases are frequently associated with oral cancer.
- PET/CT may be indicated to complete staging for patients with advanced tumors.
- Surgery remains the mainstay of therapy for early cancer.
- Adjuvant chemoradiotherapy is indicated for advanced cancer after resection.

REFERENCES

1. Ossoff RH, Bytell DE, Mast MH, et al. Lymphatics of the floor of mouth and periosteum: anatomic studies with possible clinical correlations. *Otolaryngol Head Neck Surg* 1980;88:652–660.
2. http://globocan.iarc.fr/factsheets/populations/factsheet.asp?uino=900
3. Warnakulasuriya S. Living with oral cancer: epidemiology with particular reference to prevalence and life-style changes that influence survival. *Oral Oncol* 2010;26:407–410.
4. Funk GF, Karnell LH, Robinson RA, et al. Presentation, treatment, and outcome of oral cavity cancer: a National Cancer Data Base Report. *Head Neck* 2002;24:165–180.
5. Jemal A, Bray F, Center MM, et al. Global cancer statistics. *CA Cancer J Clin* 2011;61(2):69–90.
6. http://seer.cancer.gov/csr/1975_2008/index.html.
7. http://www.cancer.org/acs/groups/content/@epidemiologysurveilance/documents/document/acspc-029771.pdf.
8. Howlader N, Noone AM, Krapcho M, eds. SEER Cancer Statistics Review, 1975–2008, National Cancer Institute.

9. http://www.cancer.org/acs/groups/content/@epidemiologysurveilance/documents/document/acspc-027765.pdf.

10. Patel SC, Carpenter WR, Tyree S, et al. Increasing incidence of oral tongue squamous cell carcinoma in young white women, age 18 to 44 years. *J Clin Oncol* 2011;29(11):1488–1494.

11. Myers JN, Elkins T, Roberts D, et al. Squamous cell carcinoma of the tongue in young adults: increasing incidence and factors that predict treatment outcomes. *Otolaryngol Head Neck Surg* 2000;122:44–51.

12. Blot WJ, McLaughlin JK, Winn DM, et al. Smoking and drinking in relation to oral and pharyngeal cancer. *Cancer Res* 1988;48:3282–3287.

13. Hashibe M, Brennan P, Benhamou S, et al. Alcohol drinking in never users of tobacco, cigarette smoking in never drinkers, and the risk of head and neck cancer: pooled analysis in the International Head and Neck Cancer Epidemiology Consortium. *J Natl Cancer Inst* 2007;99(10):777–789.

14. Macfarlane GJ, Zheng T, Marshall JR, et al. Alcohol, tobacco, diet and the risk of oral cancer: a pooled analysis of three case-control studies. *Eur J Cancer B Oral Oncol* 1995;31B:181–187.

15. Schlecht NF, Franco EL, Pintos J, et al. Effect of smoking cessation and tobacco type on the risk of cancers of the upper aerodigestive tract in Brazil. *Epidemiology* 1999;10:412–418.

16. Winn DM, Blot WJ, Shy CM, et al. Snuff dipping and oral cancer among women in the southern United States. *N Engl J Med* 1981;304:745–749.

17. Jayalekshmi PA, Gangadharan P, Akiba S, et al. Tobacco chewing and female oral cavity cancer risk in Karunagappally cohort, India. *Br J Cancer* 2009;100(5):848–852.

18. Randi G, Scotti L, Bosetti C, et al. Pipe smoking and cancers of the upper digestive tract. *Int J Cancer* 2007;121:2049–2051.

19. Franceschi S, Talamini R, Barra S, et al. Smoking and drinking in relation to cancers of the oral cavity, pharynx, larynx, and esophagus in northern Italy. *Cancer Res* 1990;50:6502–6507.

20. Jussawalla DJ, Deshpande VA. Evaluation of cancer risk in tobacco chewers and smokers: an epidemiologic assessment. *Cancer* 1971;28:244–252.

21. http://www.who.int/oral_health/publications/oral_cancer_brochure.pdf.

22. Lin WJ, Jiang RS, Wu SH, et al. Smoking, alcohol, and betel quid and oral cancer: a prospective cohort study. *J Oncol* 2011;2011:525976.

23. Baden E. Prevention of cancer of the oral cavity and pharynx. *CA Cancer J Clin* 1987;37:49–62.

24. Znaor A, Brennan P, Gajalakshmi V, et al. Independent and combined effects of tobacco smoking, chewing and alcohol drinking on the risk of oral, pharyngeal and esophageal cancers in Indian men. *Int J Cancer* 2003;105:681–686.

25. Ng SK, Kabat GC, Wynder EL. Oral cavity cancer in non-users of tobacco. *J Natl Cancer Inst* 1993;85:743–745.

26. Turati F, Garavello W, Tramacere I, et al. A meta-analysis of alcohol drinking and oral and pharyngeal cancers: part 2: results by subsites. *Oral Oncol* 2010;46:720–726.

27. Goldstein NY, Chang S, Hashibe M, et al. Alcohol consumption and cancer of the oral cavity and pharynx from 1988–2009: an update. *Eur J Cancer Prev* 2010;19:431–465.

28. Ang KK, Harris J, Wheeler R, et al. Human papillomavirus and survival of patients with oropharyngeal cancer. *N Engl J Med* 2010;363(1):24–35.

29. http://www.cdc.gov/cancer/hpv/statistics/cases.htm

30. Lodi G, Scully C, Carrozzo M, et al. Current controversies in oral lichen planus: part 2: clinical manifestations and malignant transformation. *Oral Surg Oral Med Oral Pathol Oral Radiol Endod* 2005;100:164–178.

31. Demarosi F, Siligo D, Lodi G, et al. Squamous cell carcinoma of the oral cavity associated withgraft versus host disease: report of a case and review of the literature. *Oral Surg Oral Med Oral Pathol Oral Radiol Endod* 2005;100:63–69.

32. Amagasa T, Yamashiro M, Uzawa N. Oral premalignant lesions: from a clinical perspective. *Int J Clin Oncol* 2011;16(1):5–14.

33. Chen AM, Chen LM, Vaughan A, et al. Tobacco smoking during radiation therapy for head-and-neck cancer is associated with unfavorable outcome. *Int J Radiat Oncol Biol Phys* 2011;79(2):414–419.

34. Lansford CD, Guerriero CH, Kocan MJ, et al. Improved outcomes in patients with head and neck cancer using a standardized care protocol for postoperative alcohol withdrawal. *Arch Otolaryngol Head Neck Surg* 2008;134(8):865–872.

35. Neyman KM, Gourin CG, Terris DJ. Alcohol withdrawal prophylaxis in patients undergoing surgical treatment of head and neck squamous cell carcinoma. *Laryngoscope* 2005;115(5):786–790.

36. Slaughter DP, Southwick HW, Smejkal W. "Field cancerization" is stratified squamous epithelium. *Cancer* 1953;6:963–968.

37. van den Brekel MW, Runne RW, Smeele LE, et al. Assessment of tumour invasion into the mandible: the value of different imaging techniques. *Eur Radiol* 1998;8:1552–1557.

38. Lane AP, Buckmire RA, Mukherji SK, et al. Use of computed tomography in the assessment of mandibular invasion in carcinoma of the retromolar trigone. *Otolaryngol Head Neck Surg* 2000;122:673–677.

39. Muraki AS, Mancuso AA, Harnsberger HR, et al. CT of the oropharynx, tongue base, and floor of the mouth: normal anatomy and range of variations, and applications in staging carcinoma. *Radiology* 1983;148:725–731.

40. Curtin HD, Ishwaran H, Mancuso AA, et al. Comparison of CT and MR imaging in staging of neck metastases. *Radiology* 1998;207:123–130.

41. van den Brekel MW. Lymph node metastases: CT and MRI. *Eur J Radiol* 2000;33:230–238.

42. Sumi M, Ohki M, Nakamura T. Comparison of sonography and CT for differentiating benign from malignant cervical lymph nodes in patients with squamous cell carcinoma of the head and neck. *AJR Am J Roentgenol* 2001;176:1019–1024.

43. van den Brekel MW, Castelijns JA, Stel HV, et al. Occult metastatic neck disease: detection with US and US-guided fine-needle aspiration cytology. *Radiology* 1991;180(2):457–461.

44. Snow GB, Patel P, Leemans CR, et al. Management of cervical lymph nodes in patients with head and neck cancer. *Eur Arch Otorhinolaryngol* 1992;249(4):187–194.

45. Knappe M, Louw M, Gregor RT. Ultrasonography-guided fine-needle aspiration for the assessment of cervical metastases. *Arch Otolaryngol Head Neck Surg* 2000;126(9):1091–1096.

46. Teknos TN, Rosenthal EL, Lee D, et al. Positron emission tomography in the evaluation of stage III and IV head and neck cancer. *Head Neck* 2001;23:1056–1060.

47. Dammann F, Horger M, Mueller-Berg M, et al. Rational diagnosis of squamous cell arcinoma of the head and neck region: comparative evaluation of CT, MRI, and 18FDG PET. *AJR Am J Roentgenol* 2005;184:1326–1331.

48. Farber LA, Benard F, Machtay M, et al. Detection of recurrent head and neck squamous cell carcinomas after radiation therapy with 2-18F-fluoro-2-deoxy-D-glucose positron emission tomography. *Laryngoscope* 1999;109:970–975.

49. Layfield LJ. Fine-needle aspiration of the head and neck. *Pathology (Phila)* 1996;4(2):409–438.

50. Layfield LJ. Fine-needle aspiration in the diagnosis of head and neck lesions: a review and discussion of problems in differential diagnosis. *Diagn Cytopathol* 2007;35(12):798–805.

51. Tatomirovic Z, Skuletic V, Bokun R, et al. Fine needle aspiration cytology in the diagnosis of head and neck masses: accuracy and diagnostic problems. *J BUON* 2009;14(4):653–659.

52. Spiro RH, Huvos AG, Wong GY, et al. Predictive value of tumor thickness in squamous carcinoma confined to the tongue and floor of the mouth. *Am J Surg* 1986;152:345–350.

53. Bundgaard T, Rossen K, Henriksen SD, et al. Histopathologic parameters in the evaluation of T1 squamous cell carcinomas of the oral cavity. *Head Neck* 2002;24:656–660.

54. Myers JN, Greenberg JS, Mo V, et al. Extracapsular spread. A significant predictor of treatment failure in patients with squamous cell carcinoma of the tongue. *Cancer* 2001;92:3030–3036.

55. Gil Z, Carlson DL, Boyle JO, et al. Lymph node density is a significant predictor of outcome in patients with oral cancer. *Cancer* 2009;115:5700–5710.

56. Gross ND, Patel SG, Carvalho AL, et al. Nomogram for deciding adjuvant treatment after surgery for oral cavity squamous cell carcinoma. *Head Neck* 2008;30:1352–1360.

57. Fu KK, Pajak TF, Trotti A, et al. A Radiation Therapy Oncology Group (RTOG) phase III randomized study to compare

hyperfractionation and two variants of accelerated fractionation to standard fractionation radiotherapy for head and neck squamous cell carcinomas: first report of RTOG 9003. *Int J Radiat Oncol Biol Phys* 2000;48:7–16.

58. Hinerman RW, Mendenhall WM, Morris CG, et al. Postoperative irradiation for squamous cell carcinoma of the oral cavity: 35-year experience. *Head Neck* 2004;26:984–994.
59. Rosenthal DI, Liu L, Lee JH, et al. Importance of the treatment package time in surgery and postoperative radiation therapy for squamous carcinoma of the head and neck. *Head Neck* 2002;24:115–126.
60. Snow JB, Guber RD, Kramer S, et al. Randomized preoperative and postoperative radiation therapy for patients with carcinoma of the head and neck: preliminary report. *Laryngosocpe* 1980;90:930–945.
61. Gomez DR, Zhung JE, Gomez J, et al. Intensity-modulated radiotherapy in postoperative treatment of oral cavity cancers. *Int J Radiat Oncol Biol Phys* 2009;73:1096–1103.
62. Deasy JO, Moiseenko V, Marks L, et al. Radiotherapy dose-volume effects on salivary gland function. *Int J Radiat Oncol Biol Phys* 2010;76:S58–S63.
63. Eisbruch A, Ship JA, Dawson LA, et al. Salivary gland sparing and improved target irradiation by conformal and intensity modulated irradiation of head and neck cancer. *World J Surg* 2003;27:832–837.
64. Cooper JS, Pajak TF, Forastiere AA, et al. Postoperative concurrent radiotherapy and chemotherapy for high-risk squamous-cell carcinoma of the head and neck. *N Engl J Med* 2004;350:1937–1944.
65. Bernier J, Domenge C, Ozsahin M, et al. Postoperative irradiation with or without concomitant chemotherapy for locally advanced head and neck cancer. *N Engl J Med* 2004;350:1945–1952.
66. Bernier J, Cooper JS, Pajak TF, et al. Defining risk levels in locally advanced head and neck cancers: a comparative analysis of concurrent postoperative radiation plus chemotherapy trials of the EORTC (#22931) and RTOG (#9501). *Head Neck* 2005;27:843–850.
67. Cilento BW, Izzard M, Weymuller EA, et al. Comparison of approaches for oral cavity cancer resection: lip-split versus visor flap. *Otolaryngol Head Neck Surg* 2007;137:428–432.
68. Devine JC, Rogers SN, McNally D, et al. A comparison of aesthetic, functional and patient subjective outcomes following lip-split mandibulotomy and mandibular lingual releasing access procedures. *Int J Oral Maxillofac Surg* 2001;30(3):199–204.
69. Pillsbury HC, Clark M. A rationale for therapy of the N0 neck. *Laryngoscope* 1997;107:1294–1315.
70. Alvi A, Johnson JT. Extracapsular spread in the clinically negative neck (N0): implications and outcomes. *Otolaryngol Head Neck Surg* 1996;114:65–70.
71. Rassekh CH, Johnson JT, Myers EN. Accuracy of intraoperative staging of the N0 neck in squamous cell carcinoma. *Laryngoscope* 1995;105:1334–1336.
72. Kligerman J, Lima RA, Soares JR, et al. Supraomohyoid neck dissection in the treatment of T1/T2 squamous cell carcinoma of oral tongue. *Am J Surg* 1994;168:391–394.
73. Clayman GL, Frank DK. Selective neck dissection of anatomically appropriate levels is as efficacious as modified radical neck dissection for elective treatment of the clinically negative neck in patients with squamous cell carcinoma of the upper aerodigestive tract. *Arch Otolaryngo Head Neck Surg* 1998;124:348–352.
74. Chepea DB, Taylor RJ, Chepea JC, et al. Functional assessment using constant's shoulder scale after modified and selective neck dissection. *Head Neck* 2002;24:432–436.
75. Kuntz AL, Weymuller EA. Impact of neck dissection on quality of life. *Laryngoscope* 1999;109:1334–1338.
76. Lea J, Bachar G, Sawka AM, et al. Metastases to level IIb in squamous cell carcinoma of the oral cavity: a systematic review and meta-analysis. *Head Neck* 2010;32(2):184–190.
77. Lin MJ, Guiney A, Iseli CE, et al. Prophylactic neck dissection in early oral tongue squamous cell carcinoma 2.1 to 4.0 mm depth. *Otolaryngol Head Neck Surg* 2011;144(4):542–548.
78. Martinez-Gimeno C, Rodriguez EM, Vila CN, et al. Squamous cell carcinoma of the oral cavity: a clinocopathological scoring system for evaluating risk of cervical lymph node metastasis. *Laryngoscope* 1995;105:728–733.

79. Civantos FJ, Zitsch RP, Schuller DE, et al. Sentinel lymph node biopsy accurately stages the regional lymph nodes of T1-2 oral squamous cell carcinomas: results of a prospective multi-institutional trial. *J Clin Oncol* 2010;28:1395–1400.
80. Civantos FJ, Stoeckli SJ, Takes RP, et al. What is the role of sentinel lymph nodes biopsy in the management of oral cancer in 2010? *Eur Arch Otorhinolaryngol* 2010;267:839–844.
81. De Bondt RB, Nelemans PJ, Hoffman PA, et al. Detection of lymph node metastasis in head and neck cancer: a meta-analysis comparing US, USgFNAC, CT and MRI. *Eur J Radiol* 2007;64(2):266–272.
82. Patel RS, Dirven R, Clark JR, et al. The prognostic impact of extent of bone invasion and extent of bone resection in oral carcinoma. *Laryngoscope* 2008;118:780–785.
83. Chen YL, Kuo SW, Fang KH, et al. Prognostic impact of marginal mandibulectomy in the presence of superficial bone invasion and the nononcologic outcome. *Head Neck* 2011;33:708–713.
84. Varvares M. Frozen section assessment of marrow margins during mandibulectomy. *AHNS Poster Presentation*. 2011.
85. Baker SR, Krause CJ. Carcinoma of the lip. *Laryngoscope* 1980;90:19–27.
86. Baker SR. Current management of cancer of the lip. *Oncology (Williston Park)* 1990;4:107–120; discussion 122–124.
87. Mehta RP, Deschler DG. Mandibular reconstruction in 2004: an analysis of different techniques. *Curr Opin Otolaryngol Head Neck Surg* 2004;12(4):288–293.
88. Shaha AR, Spiro RH, Shah JP, et al. Squamous carcinoma of the floor of the mouth. *Am J Surg* 1984;148:455–459.
89. Hicks WL Jr, Loree TR, Garcia RI, et al. Squamous cell carcinoma of the floor of mouth: a 20-year review. *Head Neck* 1997;19:400–405.
90. Rodgers LW Jr, Stringer SP, Mendenhall WM, et al. Management of squamous cell carcinoma of the floor of mouth. *Head Neck* 1993;15:16–19.
91. Wendt CD, Peters LJ, Delclos L, et al. Primary radiotherapy in the treatment of stage I and II oral tongue cancers: importance of the proportion of therapy delivered with interstitial therapy. *Int J Radiat Oncol Biol Phys* 1990;18:1287–1292.
92. Fujita M, Hirokawa Y, Kashiwado K, et al. An analysis of mandibular bone complications in radiotherapy for T1 and T2 carcinoma of the oral tongue. *Int J Radiat Oncol Biol Phys* 1996;34:333–339.
93. Goldenberg D, Ardekian L, Rachmiel A, et al. Carcinoma of the dorsum of the tongue. *Head Neck* 2000;22:190–194.
94. Rusthoven K, Ballonoff A, Raben D, et al. Poor prognosis in patients with stage I and II oral tongue squamous cell carcinoma. *Cancer* 2008;112:345–351.
95. Franceschi D, Gupta R, Spiro RH, et al. Improved survival in the treatment of squamous carcinoma of the oral tongue. *Am J Surg* 1993;166:360–365.
96. Lydiatt DD, Robbins KT, Byers RM, et al. Treatment of stage I and II oral tongue cancer. *Head Neck* 1993;15:308–312.
97. Kakarala K, Faquin WC, Deschler DG. Effect of glossectomy technique on histopathologic assessment in a rat model. *Head Neck* 2011;33:1576–1580.
98. Scholl P, Byers RM, Batsakis JG, et al. Microscopic cut-through of cancer in the surgical treatment of squamous carcinoma of the tongue. Prognostic and therapeutic implications. *Am J Surg* 1986;152:354–360.
99. Chepeha DB, Teknos TN, Shargorodsky J, et al. Rectangle tongue template for reconstruction of the hemiglossectomy defect. *Arch Otolaryngol Head Neck Surg* 2008;134:993–998.
100. Paydarfar JA, Patel UA. Submental island pedicled flap vs radial forearm free flap for oral reconstruction: comparison of outcomes. *Arch Otolaryngol Head Neck Surg* 2011;137:82–87.
101. Fein DA, Mendenhall WM, Parsons JT, et al. Carcinoma of the oral tongue: a comparison of results and complications of treatment with radiotherapy and/or surgery. *Head Neck* 1994;16:358–365.
102. Petruzzelli GJ, Myers EN. Malignant neoplasms of the hard palate and upper alveolar ridge. *Oncology (Williston Park)* 1994;8:43–48; discussion 50, 53.
103. Beckhardt RN, Weber RS, Zane R, et al. Minor salivary gland tumors of the palate: clinical and pathologic correlates of outcome. *Laryngoscope* 1995;105:1155–1160.

104. Yorozu A, Sykes AJ, Slevin NJ. Carcinoma of the hard palate treated with radiotherapy: a retrospective review of 31 cases. *Oral Oncol* 2001;37:493–497.
105. Truitt TO, Gleich LL, Huntress GP, et al. Surgical management of hard palate malignancies. *Otolaryngol Head Neck Surg* 1999;121:548–552.
106. Futran ND, Mendez E. Developments in reconstruction of midface and maxilla. *Lancet Oncol* 2006;7:249–258.
107. Evans JF, Shah JP. Epidermoid carcinoma of the palate. *Am J Surg* 1981;142:451–455.
108. Simental AA Jr, Johnson JT, Myers EN. Cervical metastasis from squamous cell carcinoma of the maxillary alveolus and hard palate. *Laryngoscope* 2006;116:1682–1684.
109. Morris LG, Patel SG, Shah JP, et al. High rates of regional failure in squamous cell carcinoma of the hard palate and maxillary alveolus. *Head Neck* 2011;33(6):824–830.
110. Holmstrup P, Thorn JJ, Rindum J, et al. Malignant development of lichen planus-affected oral mucosa. *J Oral Pathol* 1988;17:219–225.
111. Diaz EM Jr, Holsinger FC, Zuniga ER, et al. Squamous cell carcinoma of the buccal mucosa: one institution's experience with 119 previously untreated patients. *Head Neck* 2003;25:267–273.
112. Jing J, Li L, He W, et al. Prognostic predictors of squamous cell carcinoma of the buccal mucosa with negative surgical margins. *J Oral Maxillofac Surg* 2006;64:896–901.
113. Coppen C, de Wilde PC, Pop LA, et al. Treatment results of patients with a squamous cell carcinoma of the buccal mucosa. *Oral Oncol* 2006;42:795–799.
114. Pop LA, Eijkenboom WM, de Boer MF, et al. Evaluation of treatment results of squamous cell carcinoma of the buccal mucosa. *Int J Radiat Oncol Biol Phys* 1989;16:483–437.
115. Sonis ST. Mucositis: the impact, biology and therapeutic opportunities of oral mucositis. *Oral Oncol* 2009;45:1015–1020.
116. Porter SR, Fedele S, Habba KM. Taste dysfunction in head and neck malignancy. *Oral Oncol* 2010;46:457–459.
117. Jham BC, Reis PM, Miranda EL, et al. Oral health status of 207 head and neck cancer patients before, during and after radiotherapy. *Clin Oral Investig* 2008;12:19–24.
118. Eisbruch A. Radiotherapy: IMRT reduces xerostomia and potentially improves QoL. *Nat Rev Clin Oncol* 2009;6:567–568.
119. Speksnijder CM, van der Bilt A, Abbink JH, et al. Mastication in patients treated for malignacies in the tongue and/or floor of mouth: 1 year prospective study. *Head Neck* 2011;33:1013–1020.
120. Chrcanovic BR, Reher P, Sousa AA, et al. Osteoradionecrosis of the jaws–a current overview—part 2: dental management and therapeutic options for treatment. *Oral Maxillofac Surg* 2010;14:81–95.
121. Lansford CD, Guerriero CH, Kocan MJ, et al. Improved outcomes in patients with head and neck cancer using a standardized care protocol for postoperative alcohol withdrawal. *Arch Otolaryngol Head Neck Surg* 2008;134:865–872.
122. Spires JR, Byers RM, Sanchez ED. Pulmonary thromboembolism after head and neck surgery. *South Med J* 1989;82:1111–1115.
123. Barttelbort SW, Ariyan S. Mandible preservation with oral cavity carcinoma: rim mandibulectomy versus sagittal mandibulectomy. *Am J Surg* 1993;166:411–415.
124. Chang SS, Califano J. Current status of biomarkers in head and neck cancer. *J Surg Oncol* 2008;97:640–643.
125. Wolf GT. Integrating surgery into treatment paradigms for organ preservation: tailoring treatment to biology improves outcomes. *Int J Radiat Oncol Biol Phys* 2007;69:S4–S7.

Nasopharyngeal Carcinoma

120

William Ignace Wei   *Daniel T. T. Chua*

Anatomically, the nasopharynx is situated behind the posterior choanae and is continuous with the posterior aspect of the nasal cavities. Inferiorly, it is separated from the oropharynx by the soft palate and it is the air passage during breathing. Because of its bony framework, it remains patent under normal circumstances. Nasopharyngeal carcinoma (NPC) is a squamous cell carcinoma (SCC) arising from the epithelial lining of the nasopharynx. This neoplasm may arise from any site in the nasopharynx and is more frequently seen at the lateral wall, from the fossa of Rosenmüller, the recess located medial to the medial crura of the opening of the auditory tympanic tube or the Eustachian tube.

A group of 14 patients suffering from this malignancy was first reported in the English literature in 1901 (1). The first comprehensive series reporting clinicopathologic features of 114 patients suffering from NPC in Hong Kong was published in 1941 (2).

NPC is a relatively uncommon malignant disease in most countries with its age-adjusted incidence being less than 1 per 100,000 (3). It constitutes 0.7% of all cancers, and is rated the 23rd common new cancer in the world (4). It occurs frequently in the Inuits of Alaska (5) and ethnic Chinese in Southern part of China, especially from the province of Guangdong. The recent reported incidence of NPC among men and women in Hong Kong, in the southern part of the Guangdong province, was 17.8 per 100,000 and 6.7 per 100,000, respectively (3). A range of intermediate rates are observed in populations of North Africa (6) and the Middle East (7). The incidence of NPC remains high among those Chinese who have immigrated to Southeast Asia countries or North America, but is low among those Chinese born in North America (8,9). This suggests that genetic, ethnic, and environmental factors may play a role in the etiology of the disease.

One of the etiologic factors of NPC frequently referred to is the consumption of salted fish. This may be related to the carcinogenic compound, nitrosamine, detected on the salted fish (10). A case–control study has shown that weekly consumption of salted fish before 10 years of age is associated with a threefold increased risk of developing NPC (11). The consumption of salted fish at childhood rather than adulthood contributes to the increased incidence (12). The Epstein-Barr virus (EBV) has also been considered to play an oncogenic role in this tumor, as the EBV genome is frequently detected in the biopsy specimens of NPC (13). Additionally, patients suffering from NPC also have higher EBV antibody titers than controls, especially the IgA antibodies to viral capsid antigen (VCA) and early antigen (EA) (14,15).

In view of the ubiquitous presence of this virus in the human population, it is unlikely that EBV is the only causative agent of NPC. In the first-degree relatives of patients suffering from NPC, their incidence of developing this malignancy is 4 to 10 times higher than controls (16). This suggests that genetic factor might have an important role in the etiology of NPC. Comparative genomic hybridization studies have demonstrated several genomic spots where chromosomal losses and gains were identified in NPC (17). These losses on chromosomes 3p, 9p, 11q, 13q, and 14q suggested that tumor suppressor genes at these loci might be involved in NPC development (18,19).

HISTOPATHOLOGY

The malignant epithelial cells of NPC are large polygonal cells with a syncytial character. Their nuclei are round or oval with scanty chromatin and distinct nucleoli. The cells are frequently intermingled with lymphoid cells in the nasopharynx, giving rise to the term lymphoepithelioma (20). Electron microscopy studies have confirmed the squamous origin of these cells including those undifferentiated carcinoma that are a form of epidermoid SCC with minimal differentiation (21).

The histologic classification of NPC proposed by the World Health Organization (WHO) (22) in 1978 categorized tumors into three groups:

1. Type I included those typical keratinizing SCCs with intercellular bridges, similar to those found in the rest of the upper aerodigestive tract (Fig. 120.1).
2. Type II included nonkeratinizing epidermoid carcinomas. They showed evidence of maturation but without definite squamous differentiation (Fig. 120.2).
3. Type III included undifferentiated carcinomas or poorly differentiated carcinoma. These cells have indistinct cell margins with hyperchromatic nuclei (Fig. 120.3).

In North America, around 25% of patients have tumor with Type I histology, 12% with Type II, and 63% with Type III. The corresponding histologic distribution in southern Chinese patients is 3%, 2%, and 95%, respectively (23).

An alternative classification divided tumors into two histologic types, namely, SCCs and undifferentiated carcinomas of the nasopharyngeal type (UCNTs) (24). This second classification took into consideration the correlation of the tumor with EBV serology. Patients with SCCs have a lower EBV titer, while those with UCNTs have elevated titers.

On clinical grounds, biopsies obtained from patients suffering from NPC sometimes show a mixed histologic pattern. The recent WHO classification has taken this mixed pattern into account as well as the association of the EBV with Type II and III tumors. The histologic types of NPC are classified into two groups; the first group comprises the SCCs or nonkeratinizing carcinomas, and the second group is subdivided into differentiated and

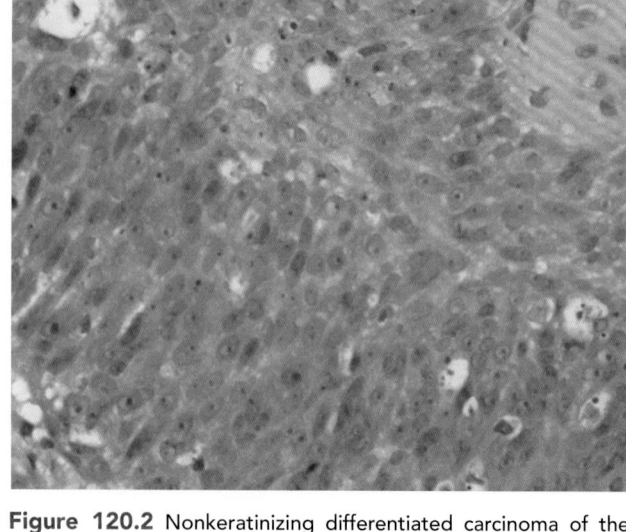

Figure 120.2 Nonkeratinizing differentiated carcinoma of the nasopharynx. The tumor cells have a papillary configuration and the cells appear more hyperchromatic than the undifferentiated carcinoma. The nuclei at the periphery show palisading (hematoxylin and eosin ×400).

undifferentiated carcinomas (25). This new classification has also been shown to have a prognostic bearing; the undifferentiated carcinomas have a higher local tumor control rate with radiotherapy (RT) and a higher incidence of distant metastasis (26,27).

CLINICAL PRESENTATIONS

Comparing with other head and neck cancers, NPC affects relatively younger age group of patients (28). Patients suffering from NPC may present with one or more of the four groups of symptoms. These groups of symptoms are

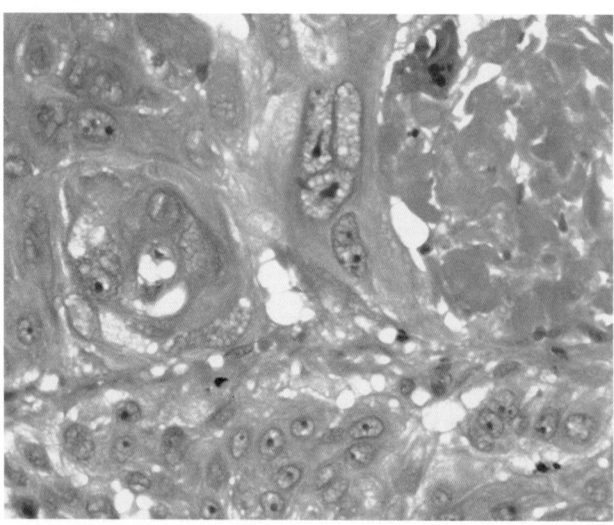

Figure 120.1 SCC of the nasopharynx. The tumor cells are large with eosinophilic cytoplasm and show features of keratinization (hematoxylin and eosin ×400).

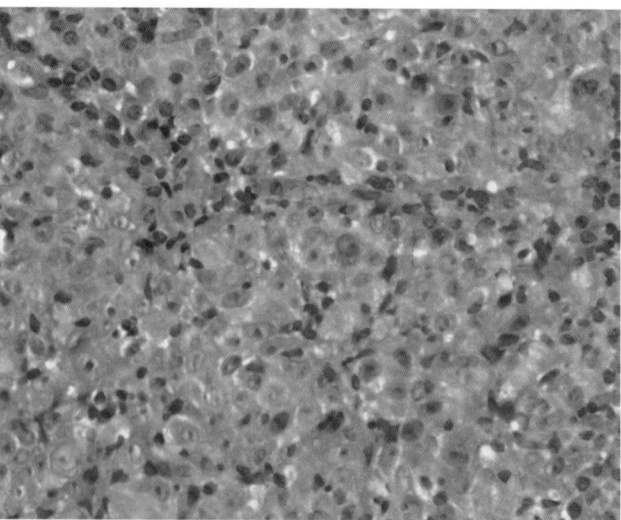

Figure 120.3 Undifferentiated carcinoma of the nasopharynx. Tumor cells are typically composed of nests or islands of pleomorphic polygonal cells with large vesicular nuclei and prominent nucleoli. The tumor nests are often surrounded by a lymphoid stroma, which is part of the nasopharyngeal stroma (hematoxylin and eosin ×400).

related to the location of the primary tumor, infiltration of structures in the vicinity of the nasopharynx, or metastasis to cervical lymph nodes.

The presence of tumor mass in the nasopharynx may lead to the symptoms of nasal obstruction and discharge. With a small tumor, the obstruction is unilateral and with tumor growth the symptoms may become bilateral. When the tumor ulcerates, the patient may present with epistaxis. The amount of bleeding is usually trivial and the frequent presentation is the presence of altered blood in the postnasal drip, especially in the morning.

The tumor bulk in the nasopharynx with or without posterolateral extension into the paranasopharyngeal space is frequently associated with dysfunction of the Eustachian tube. This may lead to the collection of fluid in the middle ear and the patients may experience unilateral deafness that is conductive in nature and other otologic symptoms such as otalgia and tinnitus. When a Chinese adult patient presents with serous otitis media, the otolaryngologist should consider the possibility of NPC (29).

When the primary tumor grows superiorly to infiltrate the skull base, the patient experiences headache. When the

upward extension of tumor affects the cavernous sinus and its lateral wall, cranial nerves III, IV, and VI may be affected and the patient will present with diplopia (Fig. 120.4). When the tumor extends to involve the foramen ovale, the cranial nerve V may be affected (30) and there may be facial pain and numbness. Cranial nerve involvement in patients suffering from NPC is in the region of 13% (31) to 30% (32) depending on the stage of the disease.

In view of the high propensity of NPC to metastasize to cervical lymph nodes, the most frequent presenting symptom is painless neck masses, frequently appearing in the upper neck (Figs. 120.5 and 120.6). As the nasopharynx is a midline structure, it is not uncommon to see patients presenting with bilateral cervical lymph nodes.

Patients presenting with symptoms related to distant metastasis are relatively uncommon in NPC. Common distant metastatic sites are the vertebra, liver and lung.

Unfortunately, because of the nonspecific nature of the nasal and aural symptoms and the inconspicuous nature of the painless cervical lymph node, the majority of NPC patients are only diagnosed when their tumor have reached advanced stages. A retrospective analysis of 4,768 patients showed that the symptoms at presentation were neck mass

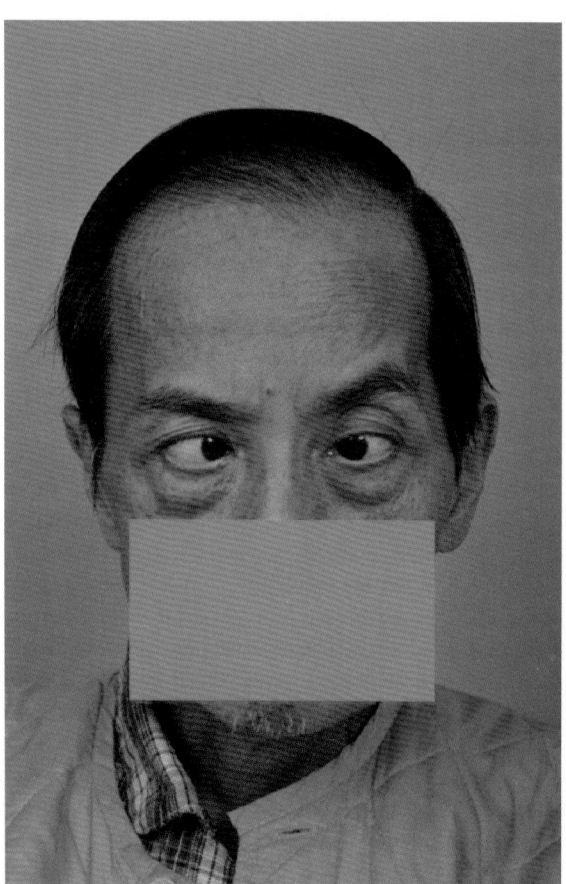

Figure 120.4 Clinical photograph showing a patient with paralyzed right eye lateral rectus muscle due to involvement of the right abducent nerve by NPC.

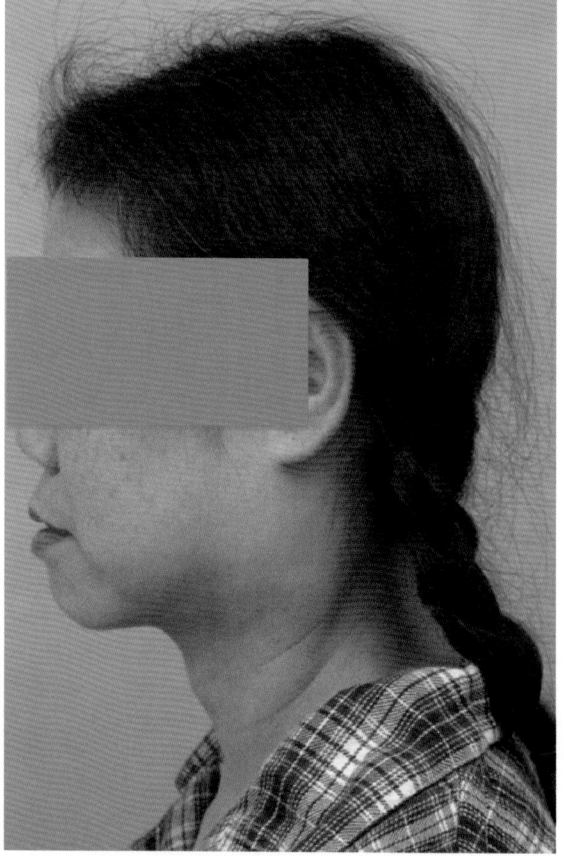

Figure 120.5 Clinical photograph showing a patient with an enlarged upper cervical lymph node (lateral view).

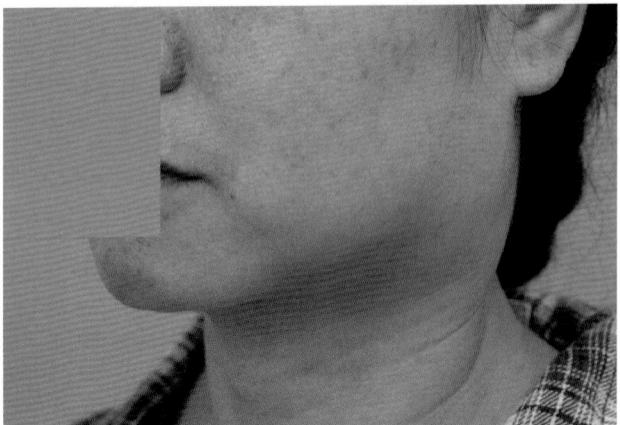

Figure 120.6 Clinical photograph of the same patient showing enlarged upper cervical lymph node (anterolateral view).

in 76%, nasal symptoms in 73%, aural symptoms in 62%, and cranial nerve palsy in 20% of patients (33). In most reports, the male-to-female ratio was 3:1, and the median age was 50 years.

DIAGNOSIS

When patients present with symptoms of NPC, they should be evaluated clinically for physical signs of NPC such as the presence of lymph nodes in the neck, fluid in the middle ear, and cranial nerve involvement. Indirect examination of the postnasal space should be carried out with a mirror although, in some patients, the anatomical variation of the nasopharynx precludes an adequate evaluation of the region. Other investigations toward the diagnosis of NPC are the estimation of antibody levels against EBV, imaging studies and endoscopic examination of the nasopharynx, and biopsy.

SEROLOGY

EBV affects human in various forms. It may cause infectious mononucleosis and has also been found to be associated with Burkitt lymphoma and NPC. EBV belongs to the herpes virus family, and the EBV-specific antigens can be grouped into early replicative antigens, latent-phase antigens, and late antigens. In patients suffering from NPC, their antibody, immunoglobulin A (IgA), response to the EA of the first group, and the VCA of the third group have been shown to be of diagnostic value (34). When a spectrum of antibodies against one of the latent-phase antigens, the EBV-associated nuclear antigen (EBNA), was evaluated, both the specificity and sensitivity of the test exceed 92% (35).

Most of the studies on the EBV serology for early diagnosis of NPC were carried out in the 1980s. In a recent meta-analysis on 20 these types of studies showed that IgA anti-VCA when elevated has a sensitivity of 91% and

specificity of 92% in the diagnosis of NPC (36). A recent report from Taiwan studied 9,699 men, who had a one-off blood sample for their EBV serology, and this was subsequently correlated with the cancer registry and death registry over a 15-year period. Those with elevated anti-EBV titers have a 30 times more chance of developing NPC (15). The level of IgA anti-VCA in monitoring tumor response to treatment and in the detection of recurrence has not been established.

In recent years, cell-free DNA of the EBV in NPC patients was detected by real-time quantitative PCR, and it has been evaluated as a tumor marker (37). Increased copies of EBV DNA were found in the blood during the initial phase of RT as the viral DNA was released into the circulation after cell death (38). This has been shown to be more sensitive than the antibody titers against the various EBV antigens in the diagnosis of NPC (39). The quantity of free plasma EBV DNA has been shown relating to the stage of disease (40), and it is reliable in detecting distant metastases (41). The quantities of EBV DNA copies detected before and after treatment were significantly related to the rates of overall and disease-free survival (42). It has also been used to monitor recurrent disease following treatment (43); however, elevated levels of EBV DNA were only detected in 67% of patients with small locoregional recurrence (44).

IMAGING STUDIES

Clinical examination together with endoscopic examination can provide valuable information on tumor extension on the mucosal surface in nasopharynx. This procedure cannot determine the third dimension of tumor growth, that is, its deep extension and this includes skull base erosion and intracranial spread. This information is provided by cross-sectional imaging studies (45). These investigations are essential to document the extent of disease in the nasopharynx and its involvement of surrounding tissue. They are mandatory for the planning of RT.

Computed tomography (CT) can demonstrate the soft tissue extension in the nasopharynx and laterally into the paranasopharyngeal space (Fig. 120.7). It is sensitive in detecting bone erosion especially that of the skull base (46) (Fig. 120.7). Intracranial tumor extension through the foramen ovale with perineural spread can also be detected and this provides evidence of cavernous sinus involvement without skull base erosion (47). The information provided through CT is important for staging and also the choice of therapeutic measures for some patients (48). CT is capable of showing bone regeneration after therapy and this indicates complete eradication of tumor (49). CT, however, in general has poor tumor enhancement and in contrast magnetic resonance imaging (MRI) has better soft tissue specificity. Besides its ability to provide multiplanar imaging abilities (Fig. 120.8),

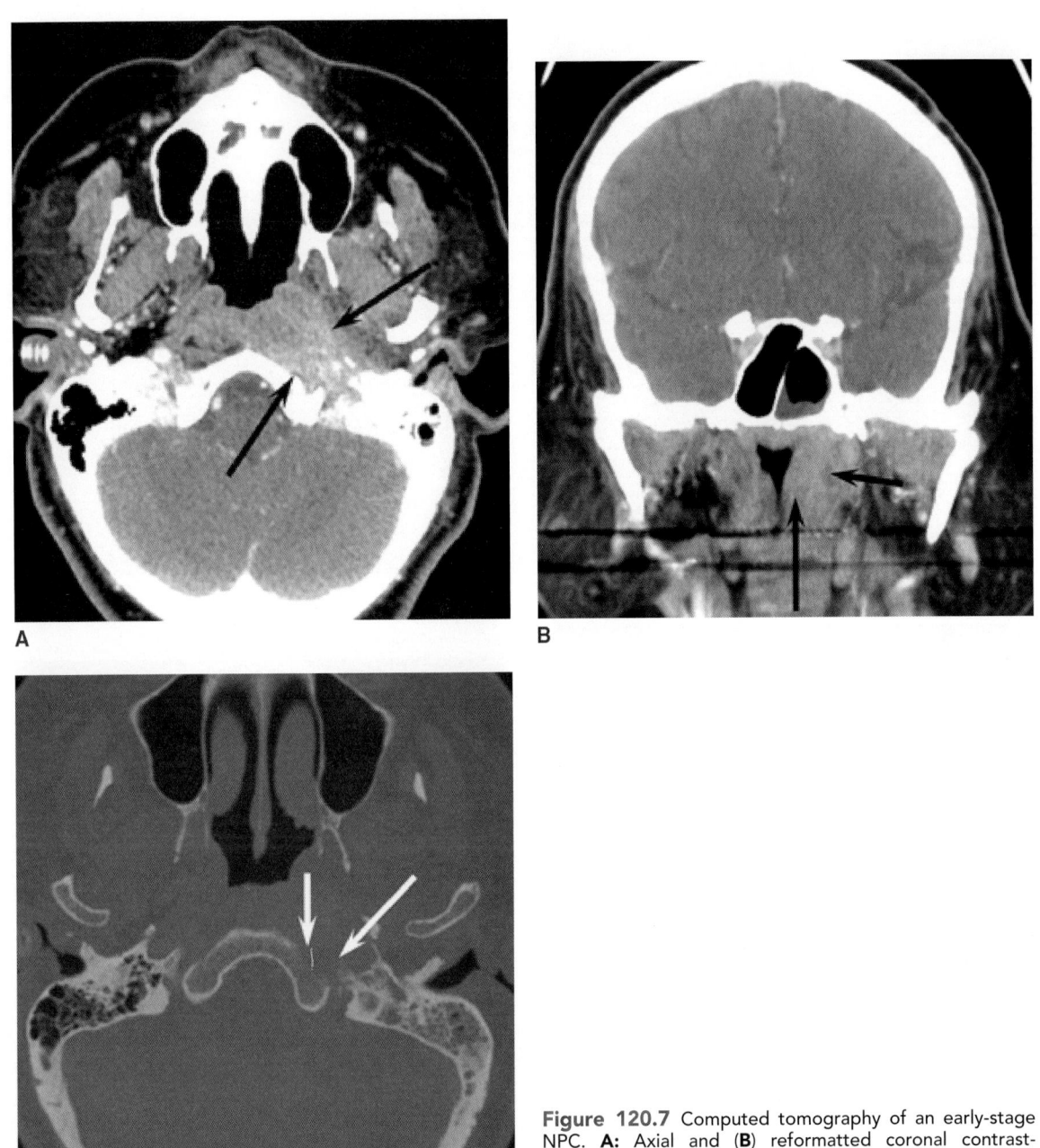

Figure 120.7 Computed tomography of an early-stage NPC. **A:** Axial and (**B**) reformatted coronal contrast-enhanced CT images show a left-sided NPC (*black arrows*). Enhancing soft tissue infiltrates the normal anatomy of the soft tissues near the skull base, obliterating the normal fat planes that can still be seen on the right. **C:** Erosion of the clivus (*white arrows*) is best seen on bone window CT.

MRI is better than CT in the differentiation of tumor from soft tissue inflammation, especially in the paranasal sinuses (Fig. 120.9). MRI is also more sensitive at evaluating retropharyngeal and deep cervical nodal metastases (Figs. 120.10 and 120.11). MRI is able to detect bone marrow infiltration by tumors (50), while CT can only detect this kind of infiltration when there is associated bony erosion. MRI, however, is unable to evaluate details of bone erosion.

Another contribution of cross-sectional imaging in NPC is the therapeutic aspects. As CT or MRI determines the primary tumor extent with precision (Figs. 120.12 to 120.14), it enables RT treatment to be designed and administered accurately and effectively, resulting in an improved outcome (51). This is particularly applicable with the intensity modulated radiotherapy (IMRT), which makes use of composite CT-MRI targets (52), enabling radiation energy to be targeted even more accurately to

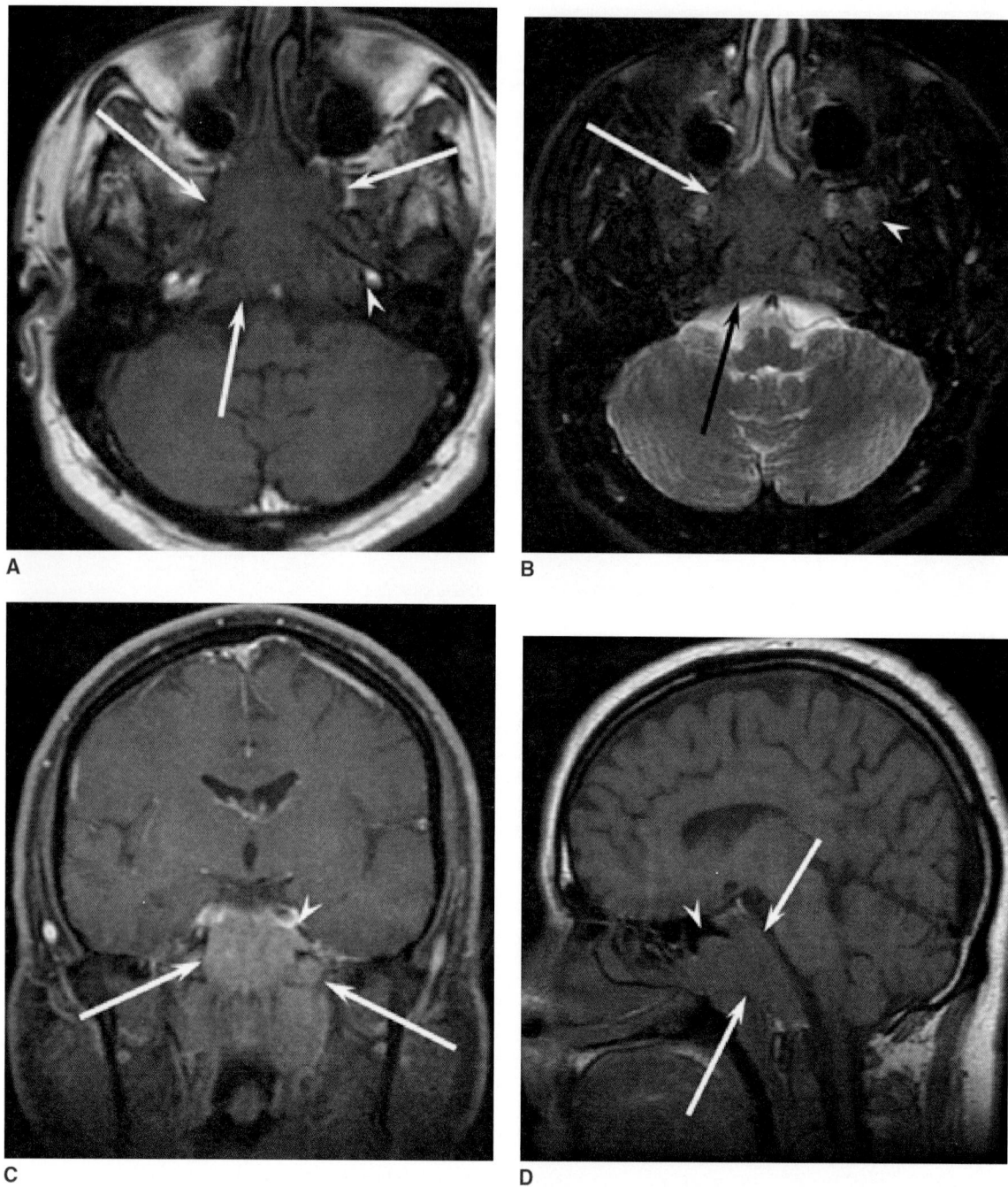

Figure 120.8 MRI of an advanced NPC. **A**: Axial unenhanced T1-weighted, (**B**) axial fat-suppressed T2-weighted, (**C**) coronal postcontrast fat-suppressed T1-weighted, and (**D**) sagittal unenhanced T1-weighted images of the nasopharynx demonstrate a large tumor (*arrows*) that has destroyed most of the central skull base. The tumor is isodense to brain (**A**), but dark on T2 (**B**) because of its high nuclear-to-cytoplasmic ratio. This tumor enhances uniformly (**C**), although many large NPCs have central necrosis resulting in heterogeneous enhancement. There is extensive involvement of surrounding structures such as the petrous carotid (*arrowhead* in **A**), the pterygopalatine and infra-temporal fossae (*arrowhead* in **B**), the cavernous sinus (*arrowhead* in **C**), the clivus (*arrows* in **D**), and the sphenoid sinus (*arrowhead* in **D**).

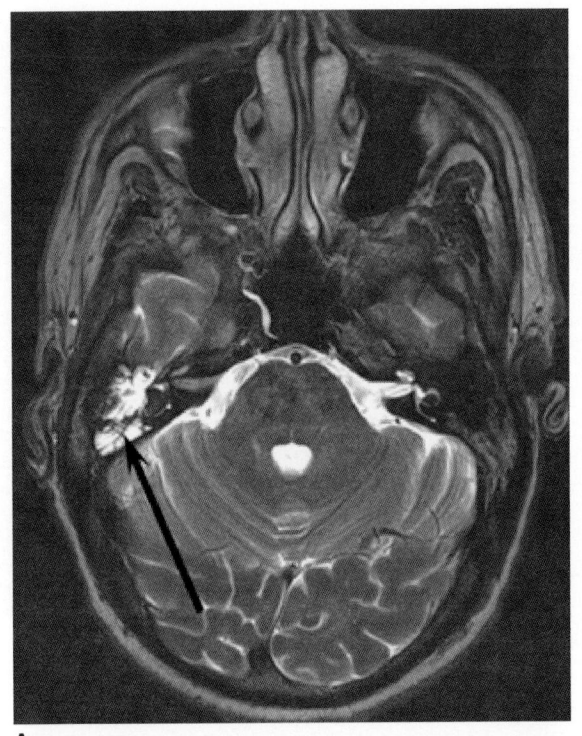

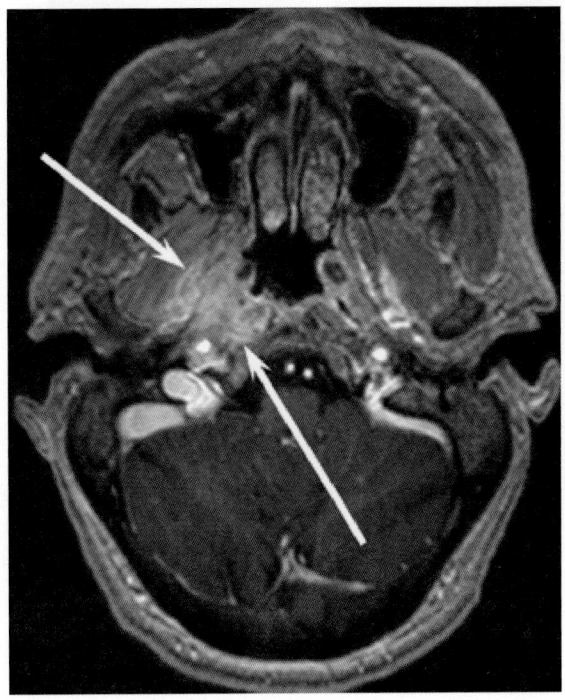

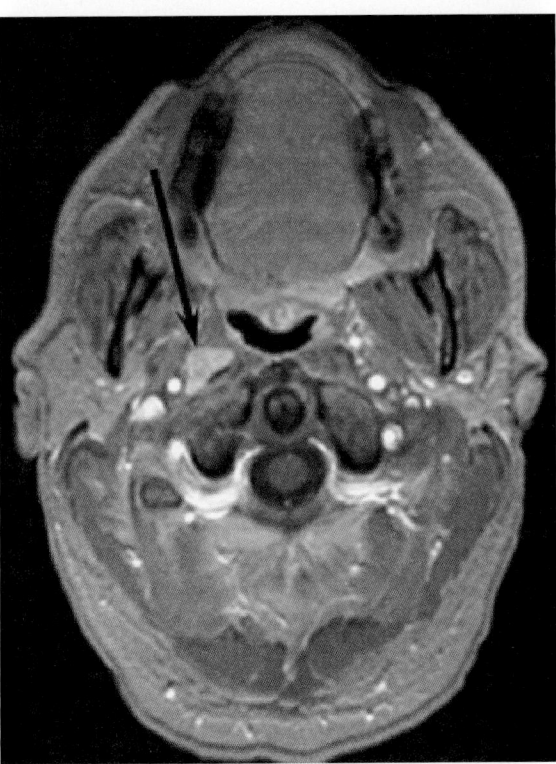

Figure 120.9 A patient presenting with hearing loss undergoes MRI, including (**A**) axial T2-weighted and (**B**) axial fat-suppressed enhanced T1-weighted (**C**) images of the skull base, as well as enhanced T1-weighted images of the neck. There is a right-sided mastoid effusion (*arrow* in **A**), which should always prompt an evaluation of the nasopharynx for Eustachian tube dysfunction. There is an enhancing, infiltrative mass (*arrows* in **B**) that obscures and destroys the normal right-sided nasopharyngeal anatomy and extends into the carotid sheath. Although NPC often spreads to Level II lymph nodes, it is famed for spread to retropharyngeal nodes (*arrow* in **C**), which are critical to identify radiographically because they are not palpable.

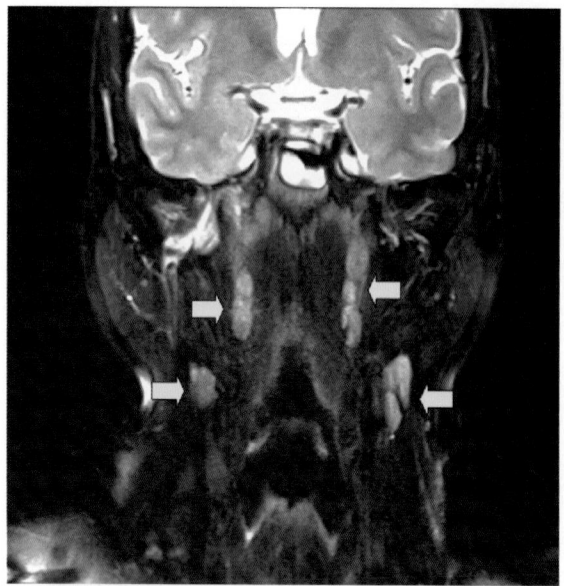

Figure 120.10 Coronal T2-weighted MRI demonstrates multiple bilateral pathologically enlarged cervical lymph nodes (*arrows*), representing metastatic NPC.

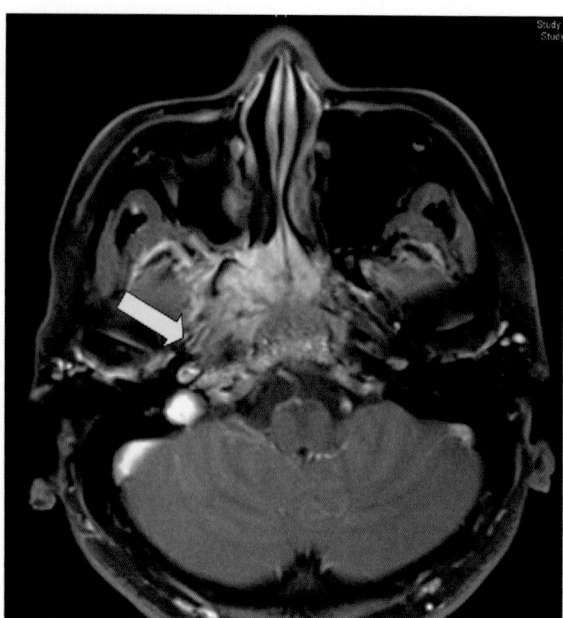

Figure 120.12 Axial fat-suppressed enhanced T1-weighted MRI shows NPC invading the greater sphenoid wing (*arrow*).

tumor while at the same time sparing adjacent normal tissues.

Positron emission tomography (PET) is useful to show the primary NPC with the metastatic lymph nodes (Figs. 120.15 and 120.16). For locally advanced NPC, the fluor-18-fluorodeoxyglucose (^{18}F-FDG) uptake as measured by standard uptake value (SUV_{max}) has been shown to have prognostic significance (53); those patients with SUV_{max} of higher than five have poor outcome (54). The hypermetabolic site locates the presence of tumor (Fig. 120.17).

The detection of distant metastases at diagnosis is difficult. Conventional studies such as bone scans, liver scintigraphy (55), and marrow biopsy (56) are of little value. They should only be carried out for those patients with high risk of distant spread such as those with N3 disease (57).

The role of PET in the detection of distant metastases in NPC and other malignancies was first noted in 2003 (58) (Fig. 120.18). In newly diagnosed NPC, PET is not more sensitive than MRI in the detection of distant metastasis (59). PET, however, has also been reported to

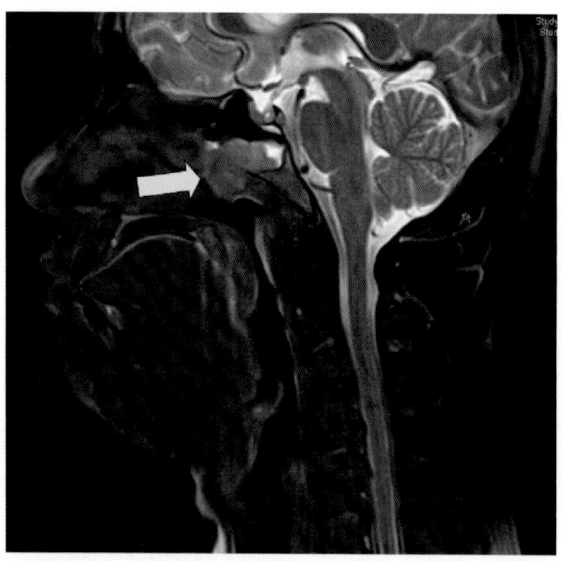

Figure 120.11 Sagittal T2-weighted MRI demonstrates NPC invading the sphenoid sinus (*arrow*).

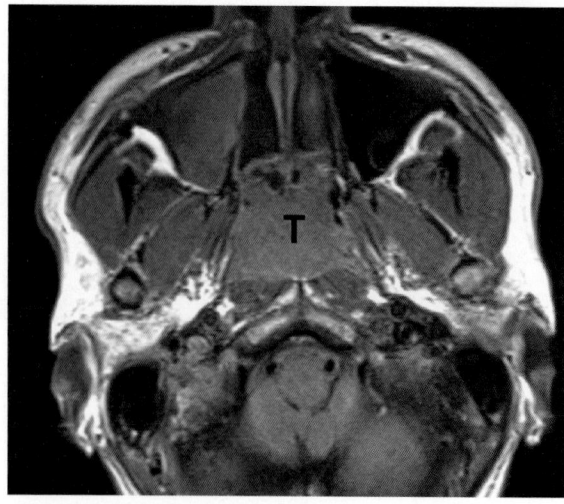

Figure 120.13 Axial unenhanced T1-weighted image shows a bulky tumor (T) filling the nasopharynx and extending into the nasal cavity bilaterally.

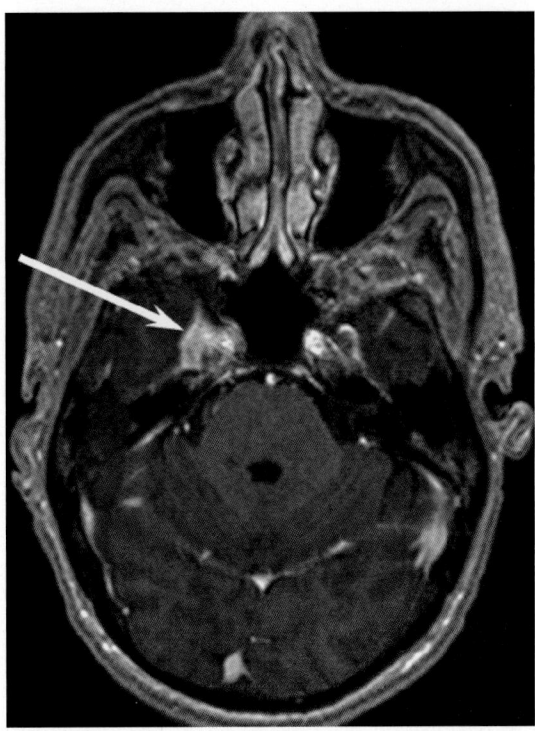

Figure 120.14 Axial T1-weighted MRI shows an enhancing mass (*arrow*) in the cavernous sinus and right middle cranial fossa, representing direct spread of NPC.

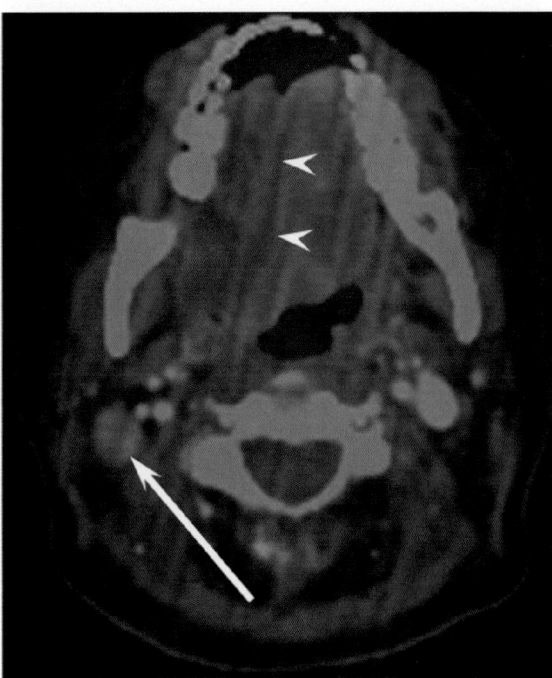

Figure 120.16 Combined PET-CT axial image shows an enlarged, FDG-avid Level II lymph node (*arrow*) representing metastatic NPC. The *arrowheads* show denervation atrophy of the tongue reflecting involvement of the hypoglossal nerve.

be more sensitive than cross-sectional imaging studies in detecting persistent and recurrent NPC (60), both at the primary site and in the neck. A recent systemic review showed that PET was better with dual-section and multi-section helical CT (61).

In summary, MRI is the preferred modality for local staging and detection of local recurrence. In patients with advanced disease, a PET/CT from the skull base to mid-thigh is useful to ascertain the extent of disease in the body.

ENDOSCOPIC EXAMINATION

The confirmation of the diagnosis of NPC requires a positive biopsy taken from the tumor in the nasopharynx. The nasopharynx can be adequately examined under topical anesthesia with endoscopes (Fig. 120.19). The rigid Hopkins telescopes, both 0° and 30°, give an excellent view of the nasopharynx on the side of insertion (Figs. 120.20 and 120.21). A 70° endoscope inserted behind the soft palate allows visualization of the roof of nasopharynx and both Eustachian tube openings (Fig. 120.22). These 3- or 4-mm-diameter rigid endoscopes do not have a suction or biopsy channel. Blood and mucus covering the tumor have to be removed by a separate suction catheter for a clear view of the pathology. Biopsy forceps should also be inserted alongside the endoscope for taking a biopsy of the tumor under direct vision.

The flexible endoscope allows thorough examination of the entire nasopharynx even when it is inserted through one nasal cavity. Its tip can be maneuvered behind the nasal septum to the opposite side. It has a suction channel and a biopsy forceps can be inserted through it to take a biopsy of the tumor under direct vision (Figs. 120.23

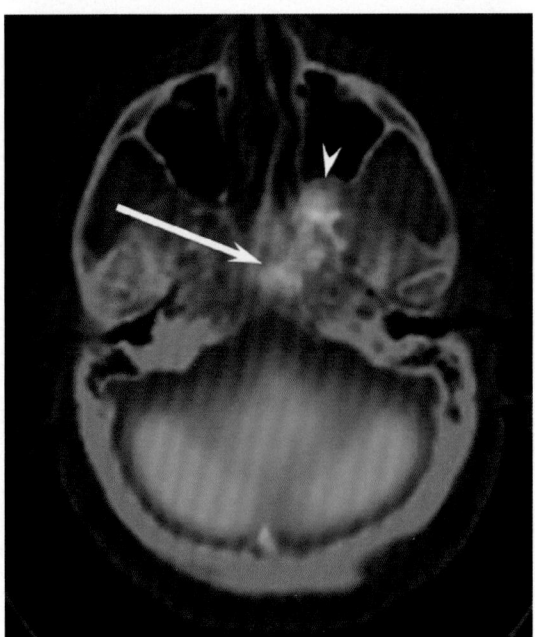

Figure 120.15 Combined PET-CT axial image shows increased activity in the middle skull base (*arrow*) and in the pterygopalatine fossa (*arrowhead*), demonstrating direct spread of primary NPC.

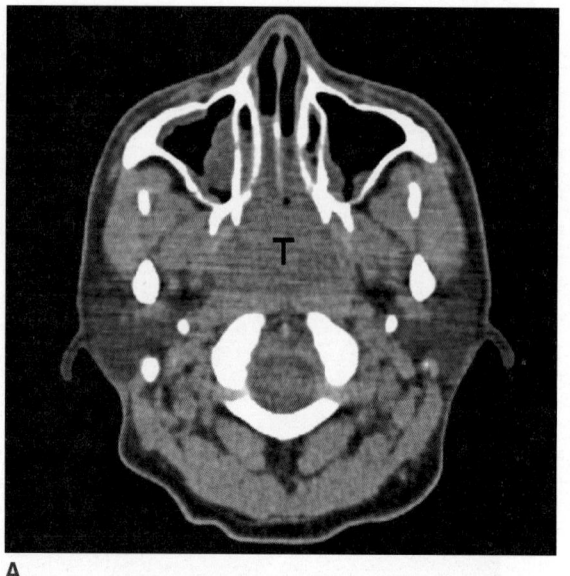
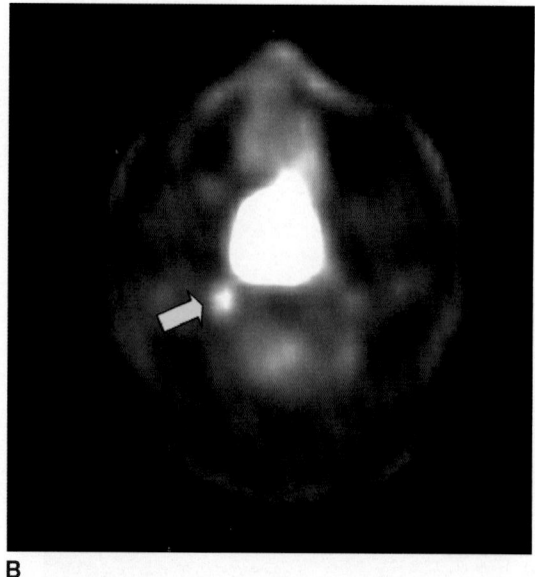

A **B**

Figure 120.17 Axial CT (**A**) shows a large tumor in the nasopharynx, but the soft tissue in the nasal cavity and sinuses is equivocal for tumor. Corresponding PET image (**B**) shows the tumor is confined to the nasopharynx, and also identifies an unseen retropharyngeal node (*arrow*).

and 120.24). Despite all these advantages, the visual image gathered with the flexible endoscope is inferior to that of the rigid endoscope. The size of the biopsy forceps is also small thus the amount of tissue obtained might not be enough. Sometimes a larger biopsy forceps might

have to be inserted by the side of the flexible endoscope to obtain more substantial amount of tissue for histologic examination.

STAGING

A clinical staging system for NPC is essential for treatment planning and evaluation of therapeutic outcome. Over the years, a few staging systems were used for NPC; the Union International Contre le Cancer (UICC) system and the American Joint Committee on Cancer Staging (AJCC) system are preferred in Europe and America, respectively, while Ho system (62) is frequently used in Asia.

Both the UICC and the AJCC systems assess tumor extent in the nasopharynx by considering the number of tumor-affected sites within the nasopharynx while the

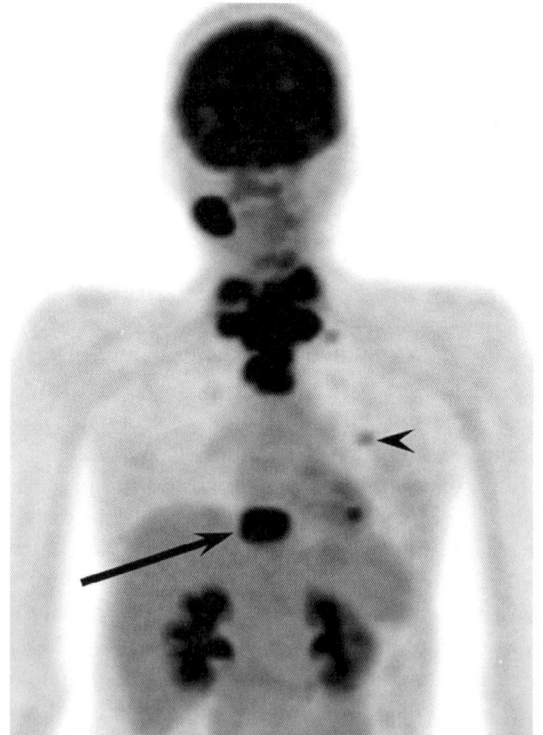

Figure 120.18 Frontal-projection MIP of a PET scan shows extensive NPC metastases in the neck and upper mediastinum, as well as unsuspected metastasis in the lower mediastinum (*arrow*) and the lung (*arrowhead*).

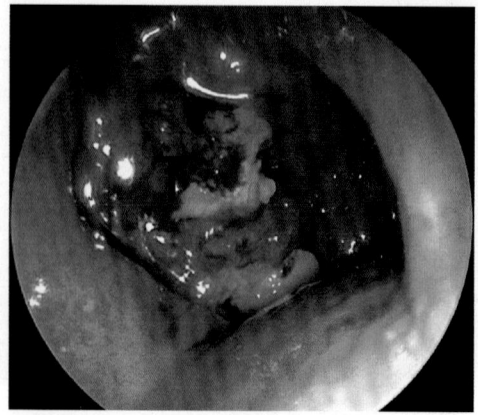

Figure 120.19 Rigid endoscope (0°) inserted through the right nasal cavity showing a fleshy tumor in the nasopharynx (T).

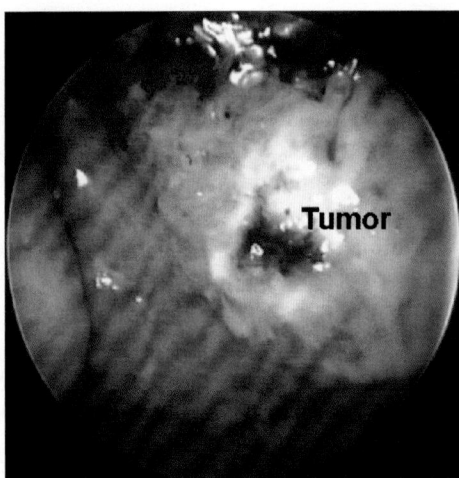

Figure 120.20 Rigid endoscope (0°) inserted through the right nasal cavity and tumor in the nasopharynx is identified (Tumor).

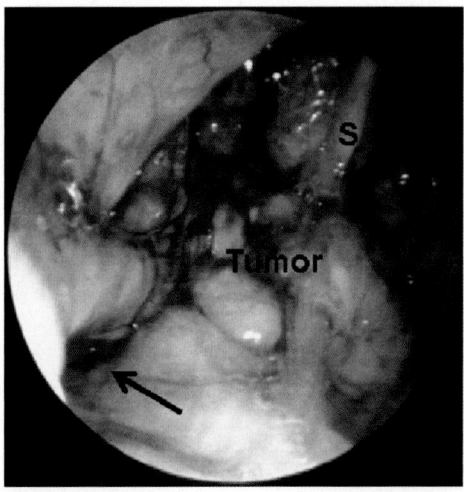

Figure 120.22 Rigid endoscope (70°) inserted through the oral cavity, inspecting the nasopharynx from below. Posterior edge of the nasal septum (S). Right Eustachian tube orifice (*arrow*) and nasopharyngeal tumor can be seen extending from the right lateral wall onto the roof of the nasopharynx (Tumor).

Ho system classifies all tumors confined to the nasopharynx as T1 disease. UICC and AJCC systems have unified since 1992. In the recent staging system of 2009, T1 stage included all tumors that confine to the nasopharynx or extend locally such as inferiorly to the oropharynx or anteriorly to the nasal cavity (63,64) (Table 120.1). On the other hand, lateral tumor extension to the paranasopharyngeal space indicates more advanced disease. T2 stage includes tumor that has extended to the paranasopharyngeal space. The T3 disease covers tumors that have involved the skull base or the paranasal sinuses. T4 tumors are those that have extended to the infratemporal fossa, orbit, hypopharynx, and cranium, or have affected the cranial nerves.

The UICC/AJCC staging systems recognize the size of the cervical lymph node as an important factor. For other head and neck cancers, N1 is less than 3 cm in size and N2 is greater than 3 cm. The difference between N2 and

N3 is a nodal size of 6 cm. The retropharyngeal nodes, which are the first-echelon nodes, are not taken into account by all staging systems. CT or MRI now detects these nodes (65).

These factors are all addressed in the nodal staging section of the recent UICC/AJCC for nasopharyngeal cancer staging system (Table 120.1). The measurement of 6 cm is the only factor for size. Laterality and site of involvement such as the retropharyngeal region and the supraclavicular fossa are other important factors in determining the N staging. Under the current system, N1 referred to unilateral nodal involvement less than 6 cm in diameter and not reaching the supraclavicular fossa. Bilateral retropharyngeal nodes as long as they are less than 6 cm are still N1. Bilateral cervical nodal disease that has not reached

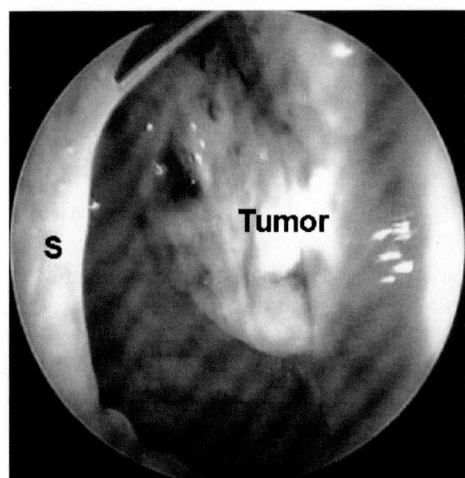

Figure 120.21 Rigid endoscope (30°) inserted through the left nasal cavity of the same patient and tumor in the nasopharynx identified (Tumor). The posterior edge of the septum is visible (S).

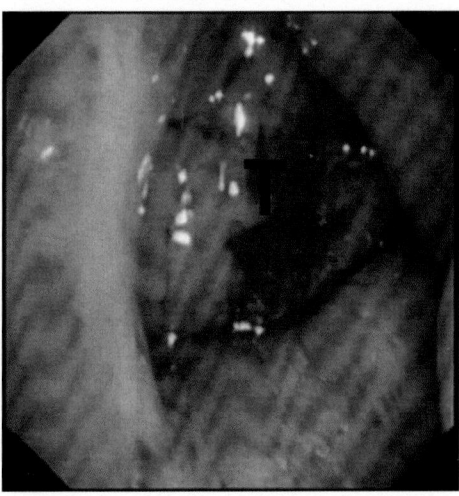

Figure 120.23 Flexible endoscope (videoendoscope) inserted through the left nasal cavity showing the tumor (T) on the right side.

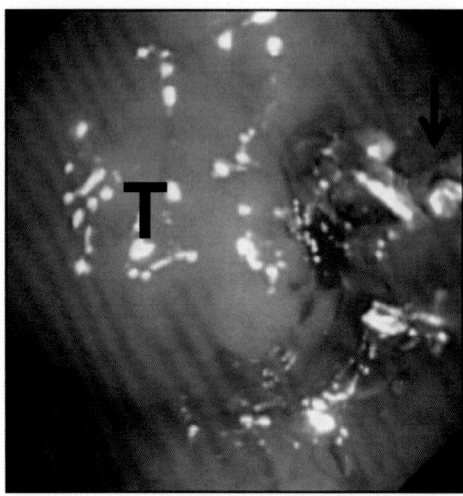

Figure 120.24 Flexible endoscope (videoendoscope) inserted through the left nasal cavity a biopsy forceps (*arrow*) is inserted through the biopsy channel and guided to the tumor (T).

N3 designation, irrespective of size, number, and location is classified N2. Stage N3 disease referred to lymph nodes larger than 6 cm (N3a), or nodes that had extended to the supraclavicular fossa (N3b). For M-staging, M1 represents distant metastases, including any lymph node involvement below the level of the clavicle. The current unified staging system has enabled patients to be staged more precisely and simply; it is also considered as a better predictor of prognosis (66–68).

TREATMENT

Radiotherapy

In view of the location of the nasopharynx, lying in close proximity to important structures and the infiltrative nature of NPC, surgical resection of the primary tumor is challenging. NPC, however, is radiosensitive and thus RT has been the primary treatment modality for decades. RT though effective may also produce undesirable complications as the radiation might affect the structures around the nasopharynx. These structures include the brain stem, spinal cord, pituitary–hypothalamic axis, temporal lobes, eyes, middle and inner ears, and parotid glands. These structures limit the amount of radiation that can be delivered to the tumor. As NPCs tend to infiltrate and spread toward these dose-limiting organs, it is difficult to shield these structures without compromising the dose delivered to the primary tumor with conventional RT using two-dimensional treatment planning and custom block for shielding. Because of the high incidence of occult neck node involvement, the neck is usually included in the radiation field electively (69). A good locoregional control could be achieved and once there is a locoregional relapse there is an increased risk of developing distant metastases (70).

During the two-dimensional RT era, RT for NPC usually starts with large lateral opposing faciocervical fields that cover the primary tumor and the upper neck lymphatics in one volume, with matching lower anterior cervical field for lower neck lymphatics (71). In general, the radiation dose given to the primary tumor is in the range of 65 to 75 Gy and that to the involved neck nodes 65 to 70 Gy. For elective radiation of node-negative neck, the dose given is 50 to 60 Gy. This treatment has successfully controlled T1 and T2 tumors in between 75% to 90% of cases, and T3 and T4 tumors in 50% to 75% of cases (72,73). Nodal control is achieved in 90% of patients with N0 and N1 diseases, but the regional control rate drops to 70% for N2 and N3 cases (58).

Sometimes for T1 and T2 tumors, employing a booster dose using intracavitary brachytherapy has shown to improve tumor control by 16% (74). Although stereotactic radiosurgery has also been used for delivery of the booster dose (75), the hypofractionated treatment is associated with undesirable side effects and is probably better reserved for the treatment of persistent and recurrent disease (76).

The major limitations of two-dimensional planning for NPC can now be eliminated with three-dimensional conformal RT and IMRT (77,78). When the tumor extension was close to the dose-limiting organs, IMRT is distinctly useful as it further improves the dose differential between the tumor and the dose-limiting organs (79,80). IMRT is a complicated technique that allows the delivery of highly conformed dose distribution to the target and critical structures through optimization of intensity of multiple beams, that is, the beams are shaped so that high dose can be conformed to match the target while selective avoidance of dose to critical structures can be achieved at the same time. The advantages of IMRT include the ability to deliver highly conformal RT to irregular target, in particularly when the target volume wraps around critical structures such as brain stem and spinal cord. It also has the ability to treat primary and regional lymphatic in one volume thus eliminating the dose uncertainty problem at the junction between the primary tumor and neck lymphatic target volumes.

IMRT is ideal for treatment of NPC and has already achieved excellent local control rates for newly diagnosed NPC, with reported local control rate of 92% to 97% at 3 to 4 years (81,82). Apart from improvement of tumor control, IMRT also reduces the risk of late complications such as xerostomia in early stage disease. A prospective study has confirmed the recovery of salivary functions within 2 years (83). Satisfactory results were also achieved with IMRT for recurrent NPC, and the degree of short-term control was encouraging (84). The limitation of IMRT remains to be the precision of determining the junction of tumor and the adjacent normal structures and the accurate determination of this safety margin is crucial for an optimal treatment outcome.

TABLE 120.1	THE AMERICAN JOINT COMMITTEE ON CANCER STAGING

Primary tumor in nasopharynx (T)

T1—Tumor confined to the nasopharynx, or tumor extends to oropharynx and/or nasal cavity without parapharyngeal extension

T2—Tumor with parapharyngeal extension

T3—Tumor involves bony structures of skull base and/or paranasal sinuses

T4—Tumor with intracranial extension and/or involvement of cranial nerves, hypopharynx, orbit, or with extension to the infratemporal fossa/masticator space

Regional lymph nodes (N)

The distribution and the prognostic impact of regional lymph node spread from nasopharynx cancer, particularly of the undifferentiated type, are different from those of other head and neck mucosal cancers and justify the use of a different N classification scheme.

NX—Regional lymph nodes cannot be assessed

N0—No regional lymph node metastasis

N1—Unilateral metastasis in lymph node(s), 6 cm or less in greatest dimension, above the supraclavicular fossa, and/or unilateral or bilateral, retropharyngeal lymph nodes, 6 cm or less, in greatest dimension

N2—Bilateral metastasis in lymph node(s), 6 cm or less in greatest dimension, above the supraclavicular fossa

N3—Metastasis in a lymph node(s) >6 cm and/or to supraclavicular fossa

    N3a—>6 cm in dimension

    N3b—extension to the supraclavicular fossa

Distant metastasis (M)

M0—No distant metastasis

M1—Distant metastasis

Stage groups

Stage 0	T1s	N0	M0
Stage I	T1	N0	M0
Stage II	T1	N1	M0
	T2	N0	M0
	T2	N1	M0
Stage III	T1	N2	M0
	T2	N2	M0
	T3	N0	M0
	T3	N1	M0
	T3	N2	M0
Stage IVA	T4	N0	M0
	T4	N1	M0
	T4	N2	M0
Stage IVB	Any T	N3	M0
Stage IVC	Any T	Any N	M1

Edge SB, Byrd DR, Compton CC, et al. *AJCC cancer staging hand book*, 7th ed. New York, NY: Springer, 2010:63–79.

Other attempts to enhance the results of RT included accelerated fractionation (85), accelerated hyperfractionation (86), combination of one or other of these treatments with chemotherapy (87,88).

Chemotherapy

For the management of NPC patients especially those with advanced locoregional disease, chemotherapy has been applied in combination with RT. The chemotherapy can be given before, during, or after radiation, and are named as neoadjuvant, concurrent, and adjuvant chemotherapy, respectively.

The Intergroup 1997 study first showed that employing chemotherapy together with radiation improved overall survival when compared to using RT alone (89). The Intergroup trial employed both concurrent and adjuvant chemotherapy in the study arm and reported an absolute improvement of survival of 31% at 3 years. This study included many patients with well-differentiated carcinoma and there were initially doubts whether it was applicable to NPC in the endemic areas. Subsequent randomized trials conducted in endemic regions have confirmed the benefits of concurrent chemoradiotherapy for locoregionally advanced NPC, although different regimens and schedule were being employed in these studies (90–93).

Four randomized phase III studies comparing neoadjuvant chemotherapy followed by RT versus RT alone in NPC have been reported (94–97). All these studies failed to demonstrate any survival benefits with addition of chemotherapy prior to RT. Two of these studies were recently updated and the data pooled for analysis, and although significant improvement in disease-free survival in the chemotherapy arm was observed, overall survival was not improved (98). Two adjuvant chemotherapy phase III studies have been reported, and both showed no survival benefits (99,100). Both adjuvant chemotherapy trials had limitations since nonplatinum chemotherapy was used in one study and chemotherapy compliance was rather poor in the other study. These studies showed that induction chemotherapy alone has limited role in NPC, whereas the role of adjuvant chemotherapy remains undefined.

Another new approach being investigated currently is the combination of neoadjuvant chemotherapy and concurrent chemoradiotherapy for locoregional advanced NPC, since it may be easier to administer chemotherapy before than after concurrent chemotherapy with the added benefit of rapid tumor shrinkage prior to RT, and preliminary reports showed that excellent control can be achieved using this approach in advanced T stage tumors (101). Another study on neoadjuvant chemotherapy followed by concomitant chemoradiotherapy also reported excellent overall survival with acceptable toxicity (102). In view of the ototoxicity of cisplatin, other chemotherapeutic agents have been used. A study using cisplatin concurrently with RT, followed by adjuvant ifosfamide, 5-fluorouracil, and leucovorin in patients with stage IVb NPC has been reported. Although these patients have more advanced disease, the outcome of the treatment was comparable to other platinum-based adjuvant chemotherapy studies and the compliance rate was acceptable (103). Another study employed oxaliplatin instead of cisplatin as concurrent chemotherapy during RT, with favorable toxicity profile and superior outcome than RT alone (104).

In summary, current evidence indicates that concurrent chemoradiotherapy has a major role in advanced stage NPC. A recent meta-analysis that included eight trials with 1,753 patients showed an absolute survival benefit of 6% at 5 years from the addition of chemotherapy (from 56% to 62%) to RT in NPC, and the benefit was essentially observed when chemotherapy was administered concomitantly with RT (105). Based on current evidence, concurrent chemoradiotherapy should be given to all patients with nodal disease and/or T3-4 disease, whereas RT alone should be reserved for those with T1-2 N0 disease.

MANAGEMENT OF PERSISTENT OR RECURRENT DISEASE

Although concurrent chemoradiation is effective in the management of NPC, local or regional failure presenting as persistent or recurrent tumor still occurs. The incidence of local failure was around 8.3% (106) and they may present as residual or recurrent tumor, and the incidence

of isolated failure in the neck in recent years was around 1.6% (107). To attain a high successful salvage rate, early detection and administration of the appropriate therapy is essential. Imaging studies such as CT and MRI at one time cannot give a definite diagnosis but on sequential imaging a progressive enlarging mass would suggest the presence of disease. PET scan has been reported to be superior to conventional imaging studies to provide the diagnosis of persistent or recurrent disease (108). The presence of malignancy can usually be confirmed with biopsy through endoscopic examination. Persistent or recurrent tumor in the neck node after chemoradiotherapy, however, is notoriously difficult to confirm, as in some lymph nodes only clusters of tumor cells were present. Fine needle aspiration cytology was diagnostic only in 50% of the time and frequently surgery has to be carried out for progressive enlarging cervical lymph node, either clinically or on sequential imaging.

Aggressive treatment for locally recurrent NPC is warranted as although survival after retreatment for extensive disease remains poor, it is still higher than that of those managed with supportive treatment only. Even when there were synchronous locoregional failures, aggressive treatment should be considered for selected patients (109).

Persistent or Recurrent Tumor in Neck Lymph Nodes

When the persistent or recurrent neck nodes are managed with another course of external RT, the reported overall 5-year survival rate was only 19.7% (110). Radical neck dissection performed as surgical salvage has reported to achieve a 5-year tumor control rate of 66% in the neck (111) and a 5-year disease progression free 44% (112). Pathologic studies have shown that for those persistent or recurrent tumors in the neck nodes, the disease involvement of the local tissue was extensive. Many lymph nodes appeared free of tumor macroscopically were identified to harbor malignant cells on histologic examination. Malignant cells could be seen to extend outside the capsule of the lymph nodes and lying close to the accessory nerve and internal jugular vein. Tumor clusters were also seen in the stern mastoid muscle and among other tissues in the neck (113). A radical neck dissection was considered essential for salvage treatment for the cervical nodal metastasis after RT in patients with NPC. A recent study showed that as the neck nodes in level I was infrequently involved, level I should be preserved in the neck dissection (114).

When tumor in the neck node extends beyond the confines of the lymph node, such as infiltrating the floor of the neck or the overlying skin, then brachytherapy should be applied to the tumor bed in addition to radical neck dissection (Figs. 120.25 and 120.26). With this adjuvant therapy, the 3-year actuarial control rate of neck disease

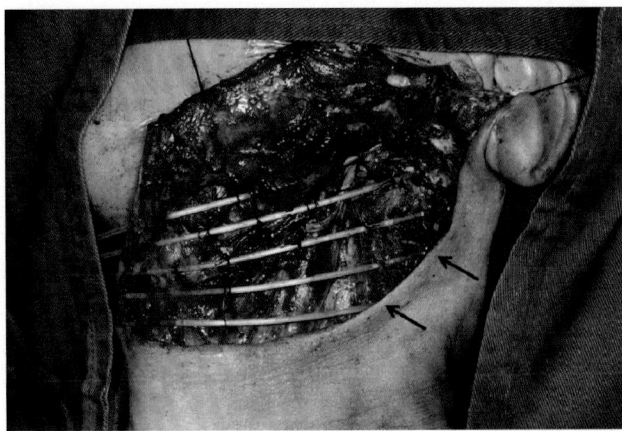

Figure 120.25 Following radical neck dissection for the extensive neck node, the overlying neck skin was also removed. Hollow nylon tubes (*arrows*) were placed in the tumor bed for postoperative brachytherapy.

was reported to be around 60% (115). This became similar to the local disease control rate when a radical neck dissection was carried out for less extensive neck disease.

Persistent or Recurrent Tumor in the Nasopharynx

Persistent or recurrent disease in the nasopharynx after the initial radical dose of radiation can still be managed with a second course of external RT with a larger radiation dose. The complications arising from the second dose of external RT affect significantly the quality of life of these patients. However, with the development of precision RT, such as IMRT, a second course of external RT could be given with sufficient efficacy and acceptable side effects. A salvage rate of 32% has been reported although the cumulative incidence of late post-reirradiation sequelae was 24%, with a treatment mortality of 1.8% (116). To alleviate the complications of reirradiation, alternative salvage measures have been introduced. These include stereotactic

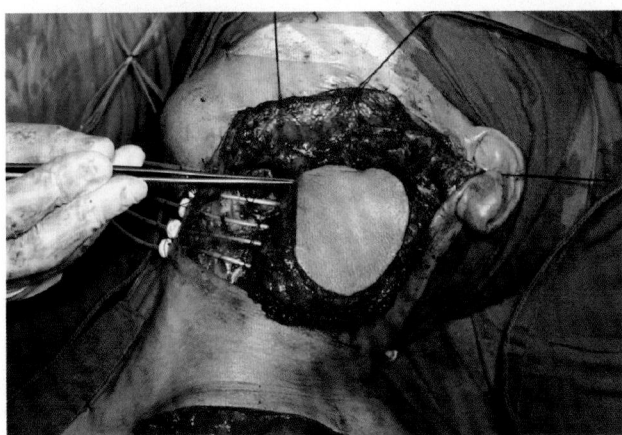

Figure 120.26 The neck skin defect was covered with a pectoralis major myocutaneous flap.

RT, brachytherapy, and surgical resection. These treatment options are applicable when the persistent or recurrent tumor is small and localized in the nasopharynx.

Stereotactic Radiotherapy

The local tumor control rate achieved with stereotactic RT for management of persistent or recurrent tumor was 72% at 2 years and 86% at 3 years (117). A recent study with 90 patients treated employing this approach for locally persistent and recurrent disease reported a 3-year local control rate of 83% (118). For small volume disease, using stereotactic RT with single fraction treatment achieved excellent result that appears to be comparable to gold grain implantation (119) and fractionated dose of stereotactic RT (120).

Brachytherapy

With brachytherapy, the radiation source is placed directly into the tumor. Thus, the radiation dose is highest at the source in the tumor, and this declines with increasing distance from the tumor. This allows the delivery of a high therapeutic radiation dose to the persistent or recurrent tumor in the nasopharynx while the surrounding tissue is irradiated with a much smaller dose. The brachytherapy radiation source also delivers radiation at a continuous rate, and this gives radiobiologic advantage over fractionated external radiation. Intracavitary brachytherapy has been used for NPCs both as a boost of the primary treatment and for persistent or recurrent disease (121). The radiation source was placed either in a tube or a mould and then inserted into the nasopharynx. Good local control has been reported with intracavitary brachytherapy (122). However, in view of the irregular contour of the primary tumor within the nasopharynx, it is difficult to apply the radiation source accurately to each part of the tumor to produce a tumoricidal effect. To circumvent this problem, radioactive interstitial implants have been used to treat small and localized persistent or recurrent tumor in the nasopharynx (123). The frequently used interstitial implant is radioactive gold grains (^{198}Au). They are implanted either transnasally or using the split-palate approach (124). The split-palate approach gives the surgeon a direct view of the tumor and enables the implantation of the desired number of gold grains permanently into the tumor with precision (Figs. 120.27 and 120.28). The surgical procedure is simple with limited morbidity (125). When gold grain implants were used to treat persistent and recurrent tumors after RT, the reported 5-year local tumor control rates were 87% and 63%, respectively, and the corresponding 5-year disease-free survival rates were 68% and 60%, respectively (126).

Nasopharyngectomy

When the persistent or recurrent tumor in the nasopharynx has extended to the paranasopharyngeal space or is too bulky for brachytherapy to be successful, then the

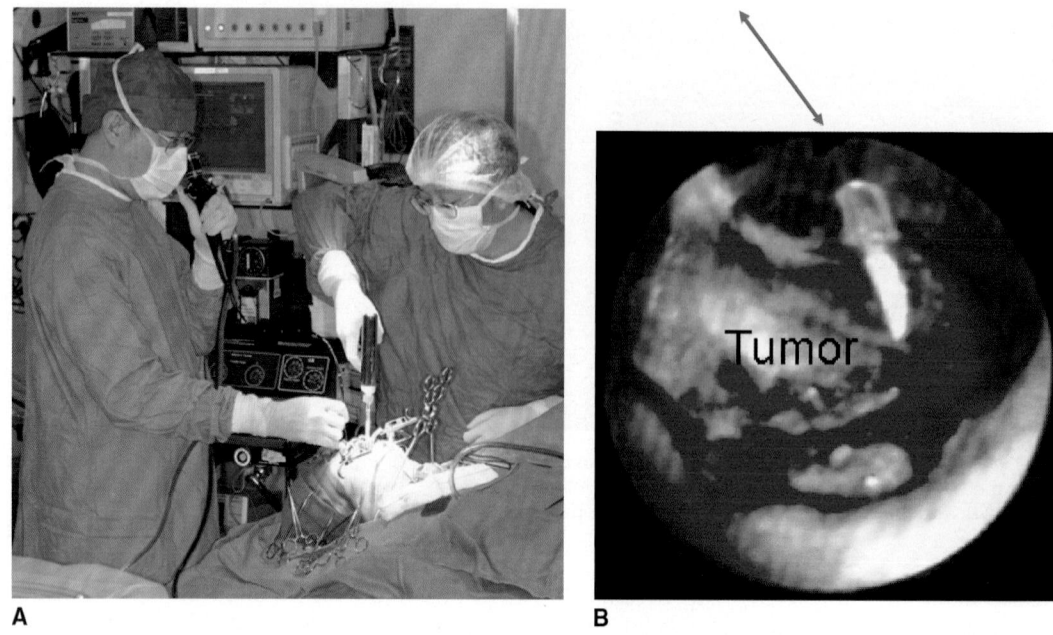

A   B

Figure 120.27 A: The surgeon (**left**), after splitting the palate, holds a flexible endoscope placed in the nasopharynx to provide illumination and guidance. The oncologist (**right**) uses the gold grain applicator to insert the radioactive grains directly into the tumor. **B:** endoscopic view showing the tip of the gold grain applicator (*arrow*) before inserting into the tumor (Tumor).

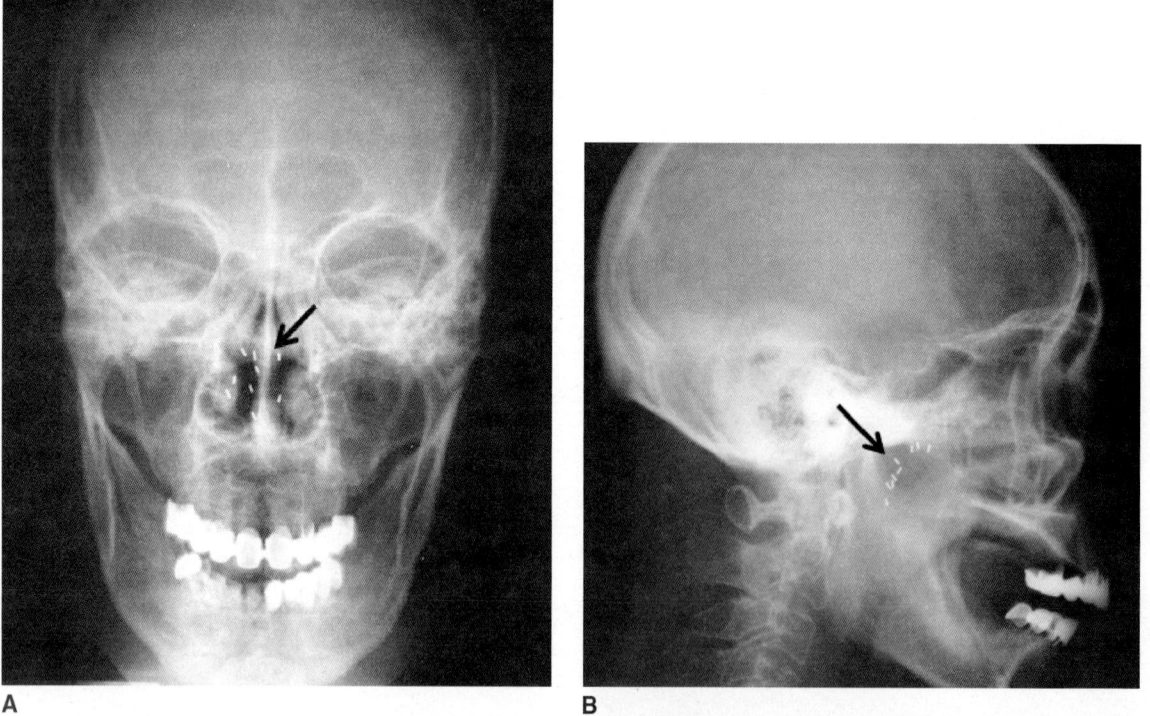

A   B

Figure 120.28 A: Frontal and (**B**) lateral conventional radiographs demonstrate gold grains (*arrows*) embedded in the nasopharynx.

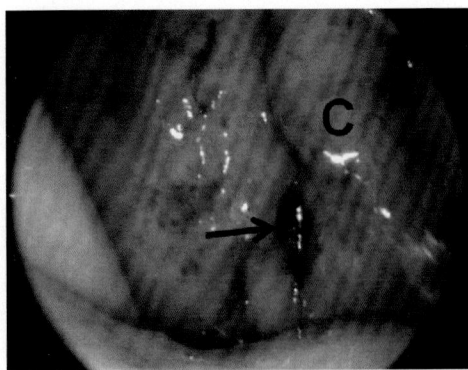

Figure 120.29 Endoscopic view showing a small recurrent tumor (*arrow*) situated medial to the medial crura of the left Eustachian tube (C).

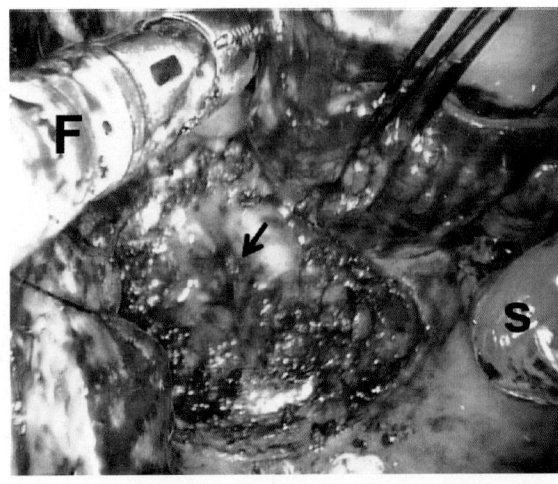

Figure 120.31 Through a split-palate approach, the endowrists of the da Vinci robot is employed to remove the tumor (*arrow*) under direct vision. Endowrist with grasping jaw (F) is shown on the left and the scissors with diathermy capabilities (S) on the right.

next salvage option is surgery. Nasopharyngectomy is effective in the eradication of localized disease in selected patients.

Adequate resection of small but thick tumor located in the posterior wall of the nasopharynx could be achieved with endoscope inserted through the nasal and oral cavities (127–129) (Figs. 120.29 and 120.30). Microwave coagulation therapy has also been reported with success when applied transnasally (130). The rigid endoscopic instruments, however, limit the removal of tumor located over the lateral wall of the nasopharynx. These localized tumors not involving the paranasopharyngeal space, however, might be resected employing the versatile endowrists of the da Vinci Robot. The robotic arms and the three-dimensional camera could be inserted to the nasopharynx through a split-palate approach (131) (Fig. 120.31).

For more extensive disease in the nasopharynx, open approach resection is necessary. A successful surgical salvage depends on adequate tumor removal with a negative resection margin (132) and thus wide exposure of the tumor and its vicinity is essential. The anatomical location of the nasopharynx is in the central part of the head. It is difficult to expose the region adequately to carry out an oncologic resection. The brain and the spinal cord render

superior and posterior approaches not practical. The transantral and midfacial deglove procedures to reach the nasopharynx from the front do not provide adequate exposure of the whole nasopharynx. These anterior approaches, even with the down-fracture of the hard palate, only expose the posterior wall of the nasopharynx and not the lateral walls adequately. Despite these, satisfactory results of surgical salvage of recurrent tumor in the nasopharynx have been reported (133–136). The nasopharynx can be approached through the infratemporal fossa from the lateral aspect (137). It is applicable for lesions localized to the lateral wall. Recently, there was a report on 11 patients salvaged with this approach, resulting a 2-year disease-free survival rate of 72% (138). With this approach, however, it is difficult to remove adequately those tumors that have crossed the midline.

To remove tumor in nasopharynx from the inferior aspect, employing the transpalatal, transmaxillary, and transcervical approach is possible (139,140). It is useful for tumors located in central nasopharynx and not extending too far laterally.

To approach the nasopharynx anterolaterally with the maxillary antrum swung laterally provides adequate exposure of the tumor in nasopharynx and the paranasopharyngeal region (141). Following appropriate osteotomies, the maxilla bone attached to the anterior cheek flap can be swung laterally as one osteocutaneous complex (Fig. 120.32). This exposes the entire nasopharynx and the paranasopharyngeal space so that an oncologic surgical procedure can be carried out. The operative procedure is simple and similar to a maxillectomy (Figs. 120.33 to 120.35). It also provides good control of the internal carotid artery. The procedure has limited morbidity (142,143) and is the appropriate surgical salvage procedure for most residual or recurrent tumors in the nasopharynx (144). As all these patients had previously undergone

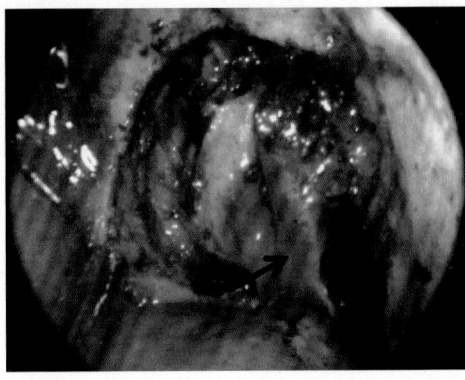

Figure 120.30 The tumor is resected with margin (*arrow*) employing diathermy under direct vision of the endoscope.

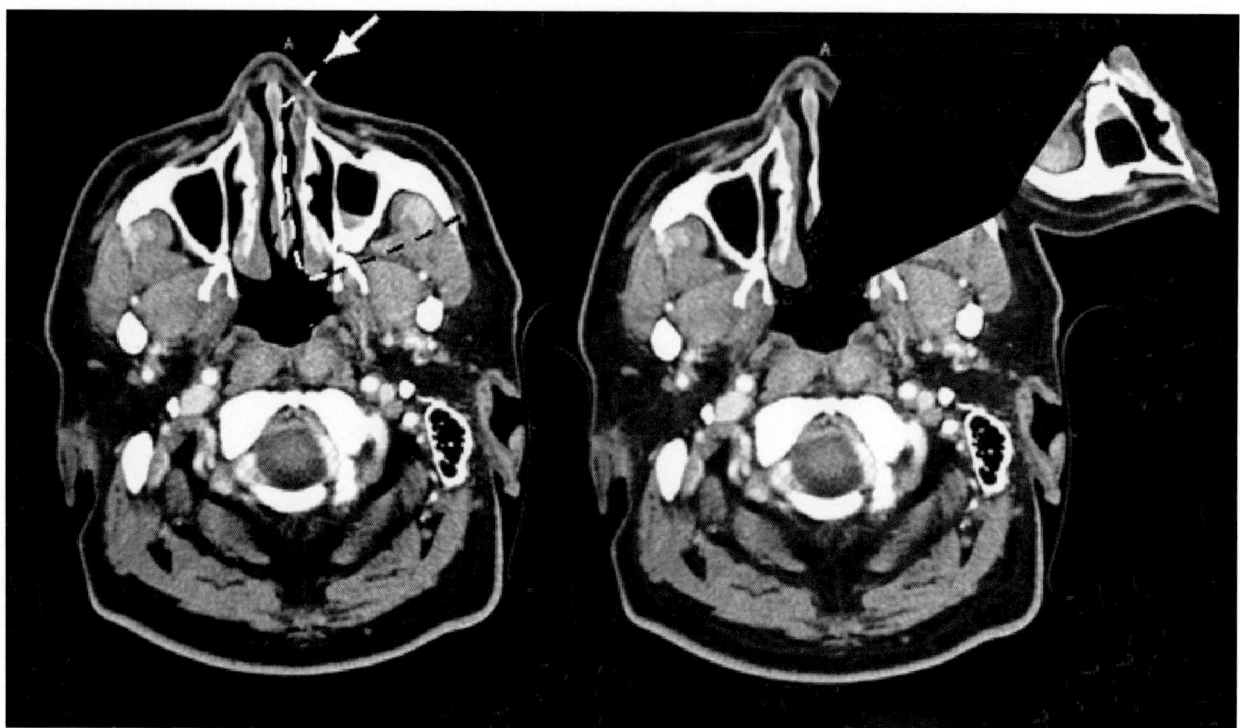

Figure 120.32 Schematic computed tomography. **Left:** Planned osteotomies of the maxilla and the posterior part of the nasal septum (*arrow* and *broken line*). **Right:** The maxilla is swung laterally while still attached to the cheek flap.

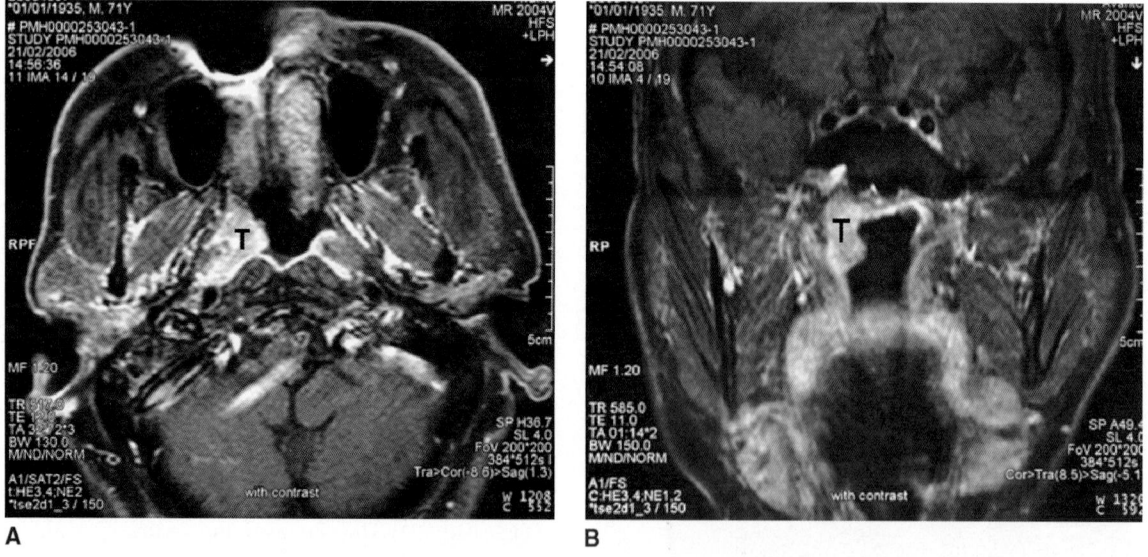

A   B

Figure 120.33 Recurrent NPC. **A:** Axial and (**B**) coronal fat-suppressed enhanced T1-weighted MR images show a bulky enhancing tumor (T) in the right nasopharynx. Bulky enhancement indicates recurrence, whereas infiltrative or linear enhancement may be related to treatment.

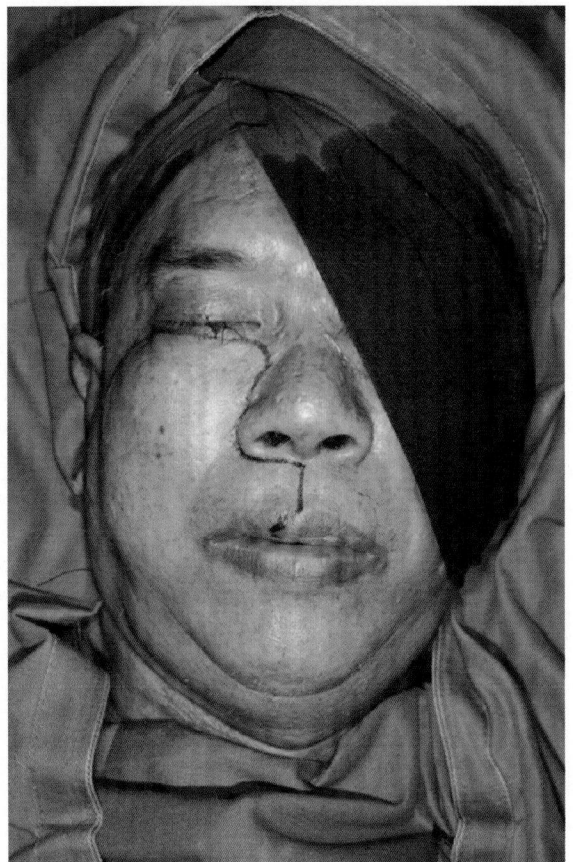

Figure 120.34 Facial incision marked on the patient with the MRI in Figure 120.33 for right maxillary swing approach to expose the nasopharynx for resection of recurrent NPC.

radical RT, complete wound healing might take some time and around 25% of patients developed trismus. In general, as long as the persistent or recurrent tumor can be resected with a clear margin, the long-term results have been satisfactory. Salvage nasopharyngectomy with this approach

carried out for 246 selected patients showed a 5-year local control of disease of 74% and the 5-year disease-free survival was 56% (145).

External Radiotherapy, Chemotherapy, and Targeted Therapy

Reirradiation with external beam is the only option when the recurrence involves skull base. For these extensive recurrences, conformal RT such as IMRT is applicable. For 29 patients who had reirradiation with and without brachytherapy boost, the 5-year local control rate of 52% has been reported (146). In another study, for 31 patients, the 1-year locoregional control was 56% employing IMRT for reirradiation (147). With a shorter follow-up of 9 months, 100% local control has been reported following reirradiation with IMRT (148).

Induction chemotherapy has been employed to reduce the tumor bulk before reirradiation (149), or it was administered concurrent with reirradiation (150). Cisplatin-based agents combined with other agents give an overall response rate of 50% to 70%. Other drugs such as capecitabine (151,152), taxane (153,154), and gemcitabine (155,156) can be used either as a single agent or in combination with cisplatin. Oxaliplatin is also active in NPC and can be used in place of cisplatin (157).

There are only limited studies on the use of molecular targeted therapy in NPC. One study showed that addition of cetuximab to carboplatin in platinum-refractory disease resulted in a modest response rate of 11.7% and the median survival was 233 days (158). Studies using small molecular inhibitors such as gefitinib (159,160) and sunitinib (161) in recurrent and metastatic NPC failed to show any benefits. Currently there is no established role of molecular targeted therapy in the management of NPC, and treatment using such approach should not be routinely given outside the context of clinical trial.

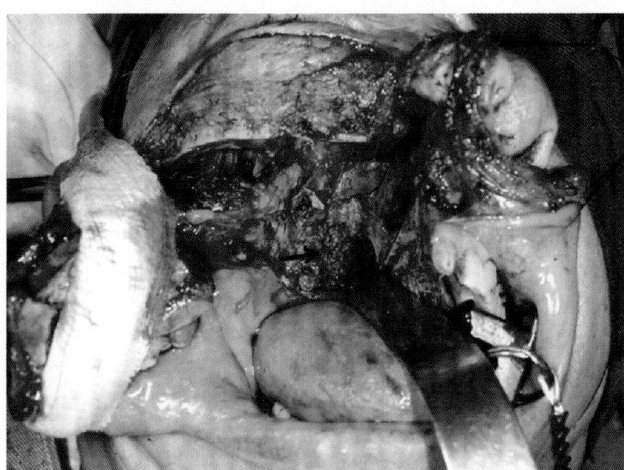
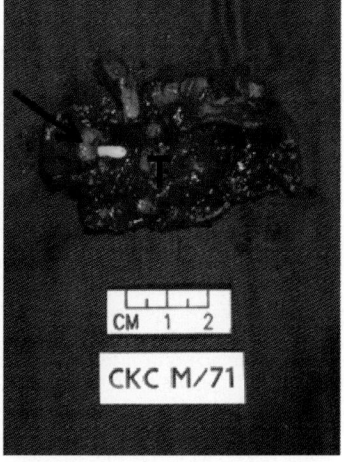

Figure 120.35 The same patient as in Figure 120.34, the right maxilla is swung laterally to expose the nasopharynx with recurrent tumor (*arrow*). Inset: Nasopharyngectomy specimen showing tumor (T). The Eustachian tube opening is marked with a yellow tube (*arrow*).

HIGHLIGHTS

- NPC is common among southern Chinese, and a combination of genetic, viral, and environmental factors contributes to the etiology.
- The diagnosis of NPC depends on the clinical features, serologic tests, and imaging features. The confirmation of the disease is through endoscopic examination and biopsy.
- The extent of the disease is determined by clinical examination, imaging studies, and endoscopic findings.
- The treatment of early stage NPC is by radiation alone while for advanced stage disease, concurrent chemoradiation gives the best outcome.
- The incidence of local/regional residual of recurrent disease after radiation/chemoradiation is around 10% and the outcome of salvage with further radiation, brachytherapy, and surgery depends on the extent of the disease.
- For salvage of localized lymph nodes confined to the neck, surgery with neck dissection gives satisfactory results.
- The choice of surgical approach for resection of recurrent NPC in the nasopharynx depends on the size, location, extent of disease, and condition of the patient. In general, the 5-year local tumor control rate following surgical salvage is around 74% and the 5-year disease-free survival rate is 56%.

REFERENCES

1. Jackson C. Primary carcinoma of the nasopharynx. A table of cases. *JAMA* 1901;37:371–377.
2. Digby KH, Fook WL, Che YT. Nasopharyngeal carcinoma. *Br J Surg* 1941;28:517–537.
3. Curado MP, Edwards B, Shin HR, et al., eds. *Cancer incidence in five continents*, Vol. IX. Lyon, France: IARC Scientific Publications, 2007:141–143.
4. Parkin DM, Bray F, Ferlay J, et al. Global cancer statistics 2002. *CA Cancer J Clin* 2005;55(2):74–108.
5. Nielsen NH, Mikkelsen F, Hansen JP. Nasopharyngeal cancer in Greenland. The incidence in an Arctic Eskimo population. *Acta Pathol Microbiol Scand [A]* 1977;85:850–858.
6. Zanetti R, Tazi MA, Rosso S. New data tells us more about cancer incidence in North Africa. *Eur J Cancer* 2010;46(3):462–466.
7. Al-Rajhi N, El-Sebaie M, Khafaga Y, et al. Nasopharyngeal carcinoma in Saudi Arabia: clinical presentation and diagnostic delay. *East Mediterr Health J* 2009;15(5):1301–1307.
8. Dickson RI, Flores AD. Nasopharyngeal carcinoma: an evaluation of 134 patients treated between 1971–1980. *Laryngoscope* 1985;95:276–283.
9. Buell P. The effect of migration on the risk of nasopharyngeal cancer among Chinese. *Cancer Res* 1974;34:1189–1191.
10. Zou XN, Lu SH, Liu B. Volatile N-nitrosamines and their precursors in Chinese salted fish-a possible etiological factor for NPC in china. *Int J Cancer* 1994;59(2):155–158.
11. Yu MC, Ho JH, Lai SH, et al. Cantonese-style salted fish as a cause of nasopharyngeal carcinoma: report of a case-control study in Hong Kong. *Cancer Res* 1986;46(2):956–961.
12. Gallicchio L, Matanoski G, Tao XG, et al. Adulthood consumption of preserved and nonpreserved vegetables and the risk of nasopharyngeal carcinoma: a systematic review. *Int J Cancer* 2006;119(5):1125–1135.
13. zur Hausen H, Schulte-Holthausen H, Klein G, et al. EBV DNA in biopsies of Burkitt tumours and anaplastic carcinomas of the nasopharynx. *Nature* 1970;228:1056–1058.
14. Lin TM, Yang CS, Chiou JF, et al. Antibodies to Epstein-Barr virus capsid antigen and early antigen in nasopharyngeal carcinoma and comparison groups. *Am J Epidemiol* 1977;106(4):336–339.
15. Chien YC, Chen JY, Liu MY, et al. Serologic markers of Epstein-Barr virus infection and nasopharyngeal carcinoma in Taiwanese men. *N Engl J Med* 2001;345(26):1877–1882.
16. Complex segregation analysis of nasopharyngeal carcinoma in Guangdong, China: evidence for a multifactorial mode of inheritance (complex segregation analysis of NPC in China). *Eur J Hum Genet* 2005;13(2):248–252.
17. Li X, Wang E, Zhao YD, et al. Chromosomal imbalances in nasopharyngeal carcinoma: a meta-analysis of comparative genomic hybridization results. *J Transl Med* 2006;4:4.
18. Hu LF, Eiriksdottir G, Lebedeva T, et al. Loss of heterozygosity on chromosome arm 3p in nasopharyngeal carcinoma. *Genes Chromosomes Cancer* 1996;17(2):118–126.
19. Chien G, Yuen PW, Kwong J, et al. Comparative genomic hybridization analysis of nasopharyngeal carcinoma: consistent patterns of genetic aberrations and clinicopathological correlations. *Cancer Genet Cytogenet* 2001;126(1):63–67.
20. Godtfredsen E. On the histopathology of malignant nasopharyngeal tumors. *Acta Pathol Microbiol Scand* 1944;55(suppl):308–319.
21. Prasad U. Cells of origin of nasopharyngeal carcinoma: an electron microscopical study. *J Laryngol Otol* 1974;88:1087.
22. Shanmugaratnam K, Sobin LH. Histological typing of upper respiratory tract tumors. In: Shanmugaratnam K, Sobin LH, eds. *International histological classification of tumours: No 19*. Geneva, Switzerland: World Health Organization, 1978:32–33.
23. Nicholls JM. Nasopharyngeal carcinoma: classification and histological appearances. *Adv Anat Path* 1997;4:71–84.
24. Michaeu C, Rilke F, Pilotti S. Proposal for a new histopathological classification of the carcinomas of the nasopharynx. *Tumori* 1978;64:513–518.
25. Shanmugaratnam K, Sobin LH. Histological typing of tumors of upper respiratory tract and ear. In: Shanmugaratnam K, Sobin LH, eds. *International histological classification of tumours*, 2nd ed. Geneva, Switzerland: World Health Organization, 1991:32–33.
26. Reddy SP, Raslan WF, Gooneratne S, et al. Prognostic significance of keratinization in nasopharygeal carcinoma. *Am J Otolaryngol* 1995;16:103–108.
27. Marks JE, Philips JL, Menck HR. The National Cancer Data Base report on the relationship of race and national origin to the histology of nasopharyngeal carcinoma. *Cancer* 1998;83:582–588.
28. Lee AW, Foo W, Mang O, et al. Changing epidemiology of nasopharyngeal carcinoma in Hong Kong over a 20-year period (1980–99): an encouraging reduction in both incidence and mortality. *Int J Cancer* 2003;103(5):680–685.
29. Ho KY, Lee KW, Chai CY, et al. Early recognition of nasopharyngeal cancer in adults with only otitis media with effusion. *J Otolaryngol Head Neck Surg* 2008;37(3):362–365.
30. Cui C, Liu L, Ma J, et al. Trigeminal nerve palsy in nasopharyngeal carcinoma: correlation between clinical findings and magnetic resonance imaging. *Head Neck* 2009;31(6):822–828.
31. Sham JS, Cheung YK, Choy D, et al. Cranial nerve involvement and base of the skull erosion in nasopharyngeal carcinoma. *Cancer* 1991;68(2):422–426.
32. Turgut M, Erturk O, Saygi S, et al. Importance of cranial nerve involvement in nasopharyngeal carcinoma. A clinical study comprising 124 cases with special reference to clinical presentation and prognosis. *Neurosurg Rev* 1998;21:243–248.
33. Lee AW, Foo W, Law SC, et al. Nasopharyngeal carcinoma: presenting symptoms and duration before diagnosis. *Hong Kong Med J* 1997;3:355–361.
34. Ho HC, Ng MH, Kwan HC, et al. Epstein-Barr-virus-specific IgA and IgG serum antibodies in nasopharyngeal carcinoma. *Br J Cancer* 1976;34:655–660.

35. Cheng WM, Chan KH, Chen HL, et al. Assessing the risk of naso-pharyngeal carcinoma on the basis of EBV antibody spectrum. *Int J Cancer* 2002;97:489–492.

36. Li S, Deng Y, Li X, et al. Diagnostic value of Epstein-Barr virus capsid antigen-IgA in nasopharyngeal carcinoma: a meta-analysis. *Chin Med J (Engl)* 2010;123(9):1201–1205.

37. Mutirangura A, Pornthanakasem W, Theamboonlers A, et al. Epstein-Barr viral DNA in serum of patients with nasopharyngeal carcinoma. *Clin Cancer Res* 1998;4(3):665–669.

38. Lo YM, Leung SF, Chan LY, et al. Kinetics of plasma Epstein-Barr virus DNA during radiation therapy for nasopharyngeal carcinoma. *Cancer Res* 2000;60(9):2351–2355.

39. Shao JY, Li YH, Gao HY, et al. Comparison of plasma Epstein-Barr virus (EBV) DNA levels and serum EBV immunoglobulin A/virus capsid antigen antibody titers in patients with nasopharyngeal carcinoma. *Cancer* 2004;100(6):1162–1170.

40. Lo YM, Leung SF, Chan LY, et al. Plasma cell-free Epstein-Barr virus DNA quantitation in patients with nasopharyngeal carcinoma: correlation with clinical staging. *Ann N Y Acad Sci* 2000;906:99–101.

41. Hong RL, Lin CY, Ting LL, et al. Comparison of clinical and molecular surveillance in patients with advanced nasopharyngeal carcinoma after primary therapy: the potential role of quantitative analysis of circulating Epstein-Barr virus DNA. *Cancer* 2004;100(7):1429–1437.

42. Lin JC, Wang WY, Chen KY, et al. Quantification of plasma Epstein-Barr virus DNA in patients with advanced nasopharyngeal carcinoma. *N Engl J Med* 2004;350(24):2461–2470.

43. Lo YM, Chan LY, Chan AT, et al. Quantitative and temporal correlation between circulating cell-free Epstein-Barr virus DNA and tumor recurrence in nasopharyngeal carcinoma. *Cancer Res* 1999;59(21):5452–5455.

44. Wei WI, Yuen AP, Ng RW, et al. Quantitative analysis of plasma cell-free epstein-barr virus DNA in nasopharyngeal carcinoma after salvage nasopharyngectomy. a prospective study. *Head Neck* 2004;26(10):878–883.

45. Goh J, Lim K. Imaging of nasopharyngeal carcinoma. *Ann Acad Med Singapore* 2009;38(9):809–816.

46. Roh JL, Sung MW, Kim KH, et al. Nasopharyngeal carcinoma with skull base invasion: a necessity of staging subdivision. *Am J Otolaryngol* 2004;25(1):26–32.

47. Chong VF, Ong CK. Nasopharyngeal carcinoma. *Eur J Radiol* 2008;66(3):437–447.

48. Hu YC, Chang CH, Chen CH, et al. Impact of intracranial extension on survival in stage IV nasopharyngeal carcinoma: identification of a subset of patients with better prognosis. *Jpn J Clin Oncol* 2011;41(1):95–102.

49. Fang FM, Leung SW, Wang CJ, et al. Computed tomography findings of bony regeneration after radiotherapy for nasopharyngeal carcinoma with skull base destruction: implications for local control. *Int J Radiat Oncol Biol Phys* 1999;44:305–309.

50. Glastonbury CM. Nasopharyngeal carcinoma: the role of magnetic resonance imaging in diagnosis, staging, treatment, and follow-up. *Top Magn Reson Imaging* 2007;18(4):225–235.

51. Cellai E, Olmi P, Chiavacci A, et al. Computed tomography in nasopharyngeal carcinoma: Part II: Impact on survival. *Int J Radiat Oncol Biol Phys* 1990;19:1177–1182.

52. Emami B, Sethi A, Petruzzelli GJ. Influence of MRI on target volume delineation and IMRT planning in nasopharyngeal carcinoma. *Int J Radiat Oncol Biol Phys* 2003;57:481–488.

53. Xie P, Yue JB, Fu Z, et al. Prognostic value of 18F-FDG PET/CT before and after radiotherapy for locally advanced nasopharyngeal carcinoma. *Ann Oncol* 2010;21(5):1078–1082.

54. Liu WS, Wu MF, Tseng HC, et al. The role of pretreatment FDG-PET in nasopharyngeal carcinoma treated with intensity-modulated radiotherapy. *Int J Radiat Oncol Biol Phys* 2012;82:561–566.

55. Kraiphibul P, Atichartakarn V, Clongsusuek P, et al. Nasopharyngeal carcinoma: value of bone and liver scintigraphy in the pre-treatment and follow-up period. *J Med Assoc Thai* 1991;74:276–279.

56. Sham JS, Chan LC, Loke SL, et al. Nasopharyngeal carcinoma: role of marrow biopsy at diagnosis. *Oncology* 1991;48:480–482.

57. Kumar MB, Lu JJ, Loh KS, et al. Tailoring distant metastatic imaging for patients with clinically localized undifferentiated nasopharyngeal carcinoma. *Int J Radiat Oncol Biol Phys* 2004;58:688–693.

58. Nakamoto Y, Osman M, Wahl RL. Prevalence and patterns of bone metastases detected with positron emission tomography using F-18. FDG. *Clin Nucl Med* 2003;28(4):302–307.

59. Ng SH, Chan SC, Yen TC, et al. Pretreatment evaluation of distant-site status in patients with nasopharyngeal carcinoma: accuracy of whole-body MRI at 3-Tesla and FDG-PET-CT. *Eur Radiol* 2009;19:2965–2976.

60. Yen RF, Hung RL, Pan MH, et al. 18-fluoro-2-deoxyglucose positron emission tomography in detecting residual/recurrent nasopharyngeal carcinomas and comparison with magnetic resonance imaging. *Cancer* 2003;98:283–287.

61. Liu T, Xu W, Yan WL, et al. FDG-PET, CT, MRI for diagnosis of local residual or recurrent nasopharyngeal carcinoma, which one is the best? A systematic review. *Radiother Oncol* 2007;85(3):327–335.

62. Ho JH. Stage Classification of nasopharyngeal carcinoma: a review. *IARC Sci Publ* 1978;(20):99–113.

63. Sobin LH, Gospodarowicz MK, Wittekind CH, eds. *TNM classification of malignant tumours*, 7th ed. New York, NY: Wiley-Blackwell, 2009:30–38.

64. Edge SB, Byrd DR, Compton CC, et al. *AJCC cancer staging handbook*, 7th ed. New York, NY: Springer, 2010:63–79.

65. Chua DT, Sham JS, Kwong DL, et al. Retropharyngeal lymphadenopathy in patients with nasopharyngeal carcinoma: a computed tomography-based study. *Cancer* 1997;79(5):869–877.

66. Lee AW, Foo W, Law SC, et al. Staging of nasopharyngeal carcinoma: from Ho's to the new UICC system. *Int J Cancer* 1999;84(2):179–187.

67. Özyar E, Yildiz F, Akyol FH, et al. Comparison of AJCC 1988 and 1997 classifications for nasopharyngeal carcinoma. *Int J Radiat Oncol Biol Phys* 1999;44(5):1079–1087.

68. Chua DT, Sham JS, Wei WI, et al. The predictive value of the 1997 American Joint Committee on Cancer stage classification in determining failure patterns in nasopharyngeal carcinoma. *Cancer* 2001;92(11):2845–2855.

69. Lee AW, Sham JS, Poon YF, et al. Treatment of stage I nasopharyngeal carcinoma: analysis of the patterns of relapse and the results of withholding elective neck irradiation. *Int J Radiat Oncol Biol Phys* 1989;17:1183–1190.

70. Kwong D, Sham J, Choy D. The effect of loco-regional control on distant metastatic dissemination in carcinoma of the nasopharynx: an analysis of 1301 patients. *Int J Radiat Oncol Biol Phys* 1994;30:1029–1036.

71. Mesic JB, Fletcher GH, Goepfert H. Megavoltage irradiation of epithelial tumors of the nasopharynx. *Int J Radiat Oncol Biol Phys* 1981;7:447–453.

72. Chua DT, Sham JS, Wei WI, et al. The predictive value of the 1997 American Joint Committee on Cancer stage classification in determining failure patterns in nasopharyngeal carcinoma. *Cancer* 2001;92:2845–2855.

73. Lee AW, Poon YF, Foo W, et al. Retrospective analysis of 5037 patients with nasopharyngeal carcinoma treated during 1976–1985: overall survival and patterns of failure. *Int J Radiat Oncol Biol Phys* 1992;23:261–270.

74. Levendag PC, Lagerwaard FJ, de Pan C, et al. High-dose, high-precision treatment options for boosting cancer of the nasopharynx. *Radiother Oncol* 2002;63:67–74.

75. Le QT, Tate D, Koong A, et al. Improved local control with stereotactic radiosurgical boost in patients with nasopharyngeal carcinoma. *Int J Radiat Oncol Biol Phys* 2003;56:1046–1054.

76. Chua DT, Sham JS, Kwong PW, et al. Linear accelerator-based stereotactic radiosurgery for limited, locally persistent, and recurrent nasopharyngeal carcinoma: efficacy and complications. *Int J Radiat Oncol Biol Phys* 2003;56:177–183.

77. Waldron J, Tin MM, Keller A, et al. Limitation of conventional two dimensional radiation therapy planning in nasopharyngeal carcinoma. *Radiother Oncol* 2003;68:153–161.

78. Cheng JC, Chao KS, Low D. Comparison of intensity modulated radiation therapy (IMRT) treatment techniques for nasopharyngeal carcinoma. *Int J Cancer* 2001;96:126–131.

79. Wu VW, Kwong DL, Sham JS. Target dose conformity in 3-dimensional conformal radiotherapy and intensity modulated radiotherapy. *Radiother Oncol* 2004;71:201–206.

80. Hsiung CY, Yorke ED, Chui CS, et al. Intensity-modulated radiotherapy versus conventional three-dimensional conformal radiotherapy for boost or salvage treatment of nasopharyngeal carcinoma. *Int J Radiat Oncol Biol Phys* 2002;53:638–647.

81. Lee N, Xia P, Quivey JM, et al. Intensity-modulated radiotherapy in the treatment of nasopharyngeal carcinoma: an update of the UCSF experience. *Int J Radiat Oncol Biol Phys* 2002;53:12–22.

82. Kam MK, Teo PM, Chau RM, et al. Treatment of nasopharyngeal carcinoma with intensity-modulated radiotherapy: the Hong Kong experience. *Int J Radiat Oncol Biol Phys* 2004;60:1440–1450.

83. Kwong DL, Pow EH, Sham JS, et al. Intensity-modulated radiotherapy for early-stage nasopharyngeal carcinoma: a prospective study on disease control and preservation of salivary function. *Cancer* 2004;101:1584–1593.

84. Lu TX, Mai WY, Teh BS, et al. Initial experience using intensity-modulated radiotherapy for recurrent nasopharyngeal carcinoma. *Int J Radiat Oncol Biol Phys* 2004;58:682–687.

85. Lee AW, Sze WM, Yau TK, et al. Retrospective analysis on treating nasopharyngeal carcinoma with accelerated fractionation (6 fractions per week) in comparison with conventional fractionation (5 fractions per week): report on 3-year tumor control and normal tissue toxicity. *Radiother Oncol* 2001;58:121–130.

86. Franchin G, Vaccher E, Talamini R, et al. Nasopharyngeal cancer WHO type II-III: monoinstitutional retrospective analysis with standard and accelerated hyperfractionated radiation therapy. *Oral Oncol* 2002;38:137–144.

87. Wolden SL, Zelefsky MJ, Kraus DH, et al. Accelerated concomitant boost radiotherapy and chemotherapy for advanced nasopharyngeal carcinoma. *J Clin Oncol* 2001;19:1105–1110.

88. Jian JJ, Cheng SH, Tsai SY, et al. Improvement of local control of T3 and T4 nasopharyngeal carcinoma by hyperfractionated radiotherapy and concomitant chemotherapy. *Int J Radiat Oncol Biol Phys* 2002;53:344–352.

89. Al-Sarraf M, Leblanc M, Giri PG, et al. Chemoradiotherapy versus radiotherapy in patients with advanced nasopharyngeal cancer: phase III randomized Intergroup Study 0099. *J Clin Oncol* 1998;16:1310–1317.

90. Lin JC, Jan JS, Hsu CY, et al. Phase III study of concurrent chemoradiotherapy versus radiotherapy alone for advanced nasopharyngeal carcinoma: Positive effect on overall and progression-free survival. *J Clin Oncol* 2003;21:631–637.

91. Chan AT, Leung SF, Ngan RK, et al. Overall survival after concurrent cisplatin-radiotherapy compared with radiotherapy alone in locoregionally advanced nasopharyngeal carcinoma. *J Natl Cancer Inst* 2005;97:536–539.

92. Wee J, Tan EH, Tai BC, et al. Randomized trial of radiotherapy versus concurrent chemoradiotherapy followed by adjuvant chemotherapy in patients with American Joint Committee on Cancer/International Union Against Cancer Stage III and IV nasopharyngeal cancer of the endemic variety. *J Clin Oncol* 2005;23:6730–6738.

93. Kwong DL, Sham JS, Au GK, et al. Concurrent and adjuvant chemotherapy for nasopharyngeal carcinoma: a factorial study. *J Clin Oncol* 2004;22:2643–2653.

94. International Nasopharynx Cancer Study Group: VUMCA I Trial: Preliminary results of a randomized trial comparing neoadjuvant chemotherapy (cisplatin, epirubicin, bleomycin) plus radiotherapy vs. radiotherapy alone in stage IV (≥N2, M0) undifferentiated nasopharyngeal carcinoma: A positive effect on progression-free survival. *Int J Radiat Oncol Biol Phys* 1996;35:463–469.

95. Chua DTT, Sham JST, Choy D, et al. Preliminary report of the Asian-Oceanian Clinical Oncology Association randomized trial comparing cisplatin and epirubicin followed by radiotherapy versus radiotherapy alone in the treatment of patients with locoregionally advanced nasopharyngeal carcinoma. *Cancer* 1998;83:2270–2283.

96. Ma J, Mai H, Hong M, et al. Results of a prospective randomized trial comparing neoadjuvant chemotherapy plus radiotherapy with radiotherapy alone in patients with locoregionally advanced nasopharyngeal carcinoma. *J Clin Oncol* 2001;19:1350–1357.

97. Hareyama M, Sakata K, Shirato H, et al. A prospective, randomized trial comparing neoadjuvant chemotherapy with radiotherapy alone in patients with advanced nasopharyngeal carcinoma. *Cancer* 2002;94:2217–2223.

98. Chua DT, Ma J, Sham JS. Long-term survival after cisplatin-based induction chemotherapy and radiotherapy for nasopharyngeal carcinoma: a pooled data analysis of two phase III trials. *J Clin Oncol* 2005;23:1118–1124.

99. Rossi A, Molinari R, Boracchi P, et al. Adjuvant chemotherapy with vincristine, cyclophosphamoide, and doxorubicin after radiotherapy in local-regional nasopharyngeal cancer: results of a 4-year multicenter randomized study. *J Clin Oncol* 1988;6:1401–1410.

100. Chi KH, Chang YC, Guo WY, et al. A phase III study of adjuvant chemotherapy in advanced nasopharyngeal carcinoma patients. *Int J Radiat Oncol Biol Phys* 2002;52:1238–1244.

101. Rischin D, Corry J, Smith J, et al. Excellent disease control and survival in patients with advanced nasopharyngeal cancer treated with chemoradiation. *J Clin Oncol* 2002;20:1845–1852.

102. Oh JL, Vokes EE, Kies MS, et al. Induction chemotherapy followed by concomitant chemoradiotherapy in the treatment of locoregionally advanced nasopharyngeal cancer. *Ann Oncol* 2003;14:564–569.

103. Chua DT, Sham JS, Au GK. A concurrent chemoirradiation with cisplatin followed by adjuvant chemotherapy with ifosfamide, 5-fluorouracil, and leucovorin for stage IV nasopharyngeal carcinoma. *Head Neck* 2004;26:118–126.

104. Zhang L, Zhao C, Peng PJ, et al. Phase III study comparing standard radiotherapy with or without weekly oxaliplatin in treatment of locoregionally advanced nasopharyngeal carcinoma: preliminary results. *J Clin Oncol* 2005;23:8461–8468.

105. Baujat B, Audry H, Bourhis J, et al. Chemotherapy in locally advanced nasopharyngeal carcinoma: an individual patient data meta-analysis of eight randomized trials and 1753 patients. *Int J Radiat Oncol Biol Phys* 2006;64(1):47–56.

106. Ng WT, Lee MC, Hung WM, et al. Clinical outcomes and patterns of failure after intensity-modulated radiotherapy for nasopharyngeal carcinoma. *Int J Radiat Oncol Biol Phys* 2011;79(2):420–428.

107. Lee AW, Sze WM, Au JS, et al. Treatment results for nasopharyngeal carcinoma in the modern era: the Hong Kong experience. *Int J Radiat Oncol Biol Phys* 2005;61(4):1107–1116.

108. Kao CH, Tsai SC, Wang JJ, et al. Comparing 18-fluoro-2-deoxy-glucose positron emission tomography with a combination of technetium 99m tetrofosmin single photon emission computed tomography and computed tomography to detect recurrent or persistent nasopharyngeal carcinomas after radiotherapy. *Cancer* 2001;92(2):434–439.

109. Chua DT, Wei WI, Sham JS, et al. Treatment outcome for synchronous locoregional failures of nasopharyngeal carcinoma. *Head Neck* 2003;25:585–594.

110. Sham JS, Choy D. Nasopharyngeal carcinoma: treatment of neck node recurrence by radiotherapy. *Australas Radiol* 1991;35:370–373.

111. Wei WI, Lam KH, Ho CM, et al. Efficacy of radical neck dissection for the control of cervical metastasis after radiotherapy for nasopharyngeal carcinoma. *Am J Surg* 1990;160:439–442.

112. Tsang RK, Chung JC, Ng YW, et al. Efficacy of neck dissection for locoregional failures versus isolated nodal failures in nasopharyngeal carcinoma. *Head Neck* 2012;34:638–642.

113. Wei WI, Ho CM, Wong MP, et al. Pathological basis of surgery in the management of postradiotherapy cervical metastasis in nasopharyngeal carcinoma. *Arch Otolaryngol Head Neck Surg* 1992;118:923–929.

114. Khafif A, Felito A, Takes RP, et al. Is it necessary to perform radical neck dissection as a salvage procedure for persistent or recurrent neck disease after chemoradiotherapy in patients with nasopharyngeal carcinoma? *Euro Arch Otorhinolaryngol* 2010;267(7):997–999.

115. Wei WI, Ho WK, Cheng AC, et al. Management of extensive cervical nodal metastasis in nasopharyngeal carcinoma after radiotherapy: a clinicopathological study. *Arch Otolaryngol Head Neck Surg* 2001;127(12):1457–1462.

116. Lee AW, Law SC, Foo W, et al. Retrospective analysis of patients with nasopharyngeal carcinoma treated during 1976–1985: survival after local recurrence. *Int J Radiat Oncol Biol Phys* 1993;26:773–782.

117. Yau TK, Sze WM, Lee WM, et al. Effectiveness of brachytherapy and fractionated stereotactic radiotherapy boost for persistent nasopharyngeal carcinoma. *Head Neck* 2004;26:1024–1030.

118. Wu SX, Chua DT, Deng ML, et al. Outcome of fractionated stereotactic radiotherapy for 90 patients with locally persistent and recurrent nasopharyngeal carcinoma. *Int J Radiat Oncol Biol Phys* 2007;69:761–769.

119. Chua DT, Wei WI, Sham JS, et al. Stereotactic radiosurgery versus gold grain implantation in salvaging local failures of nasopharyngeal carcinoma. *Int J Radiat Oncol Biol Phys* 2007;69:469–474.

120. Chua DT, Wu SX, Lee V, et al. Comparison of single versus fractionated dose of stereotactic radiotherapy for salvaging local failures of nasopharyngeal carcinoma: a matched-cohort analysis. *Head Neck Oncol* 2009;1:13.

121. Wang CC, Busse J, Gitterman M. A simple afterloading applicator for intracavitary irradiation of carcinoma of the nasopharynx. *Radiology* 1975;115:737–738.

122. Law SC, Lam WK, Ng MF, et al. Reirradiation of nasopharyngeal carcinoma with intracavitary mold brachytherapy: an effective means of local salvage. *Int J Radiat Oncol Biol Phys* 2002;54:1095–1113.

123. Harrison LB, Weissberg JB. A technique for interstitial nasopharyngeal brachytherapy. *Int J Radiat Oncol Biol Phys* 1987;13:451–453.

124. Wei WI, Sham JS, Choy D, et al. Split-palate approach for gold grain implantation in nasopharyngeal carcinoma. *Arch Otolaryngol Head Neck Surg* 1990;116:578–582.

125. Choy D, Sham JS, Wei WI, et al. Transpalatal insertion of radioactive gold grain for the treatment of persistent and recurrent nasopharyngeal carcinoma. *Int J Radiat Oncol Biol Phys* 1993;25:505–512.

126. Kwong DL, Wei WI, Cheng AC, et al. Long term results of radioactive gold grain implantation for the treatment of persistent and recurrent nasopharyngeal carcinoma. *Cancer* 2001;91:1105–1113.

127. Wen YH, Wen WP, Chen HX, et al. Endoscopic nasopharyngectomy for salvage in nasopharyngeal carcinoma: a novel anatomic orientation. *Laryngoscope* 2010;120:1298–1302.

128. Chen MK, Lai JC, Chang CC, et al. Minimally invasive endoscopic nasopharyngectomy in the treatment of recurrent T1–2a nasopharyngeal carcinoma. *Laryngoscope* 2007;117:894–896.

129. Chen MY, Wen WP, Guo X, et al. Endoscopic nasopharyngectomy for locally recurrent nasopharyngeal carcinoma. *Laryngoscope* 2009;119:516–522.

130. Mai HQ, Mo HY, Deng JF, et al. Endoscopic microwave coagulation therapy for early recurrent T1 nasopharyngeal carcinoma. *Eur J Cancer* 2009;45:1107–1110.

131. Wei WI, Ho WK. Transoral robotic resection of recurrent nasopharyngeal carcinoma *Laryngoscope* 2010;120:2011–2014.

132. Vlantis AC, Tsang RK, Yu BK, et al. Nasopharyngectomy and surgical margin status: a survival analysis. *Arch Otolaryngol Head Neck Surg* 2007;133:1296–1301.

133. Shu CH, Cheng H, Lirng JF, et al. Salvage surgery for recurrent nasopharyngeal carcinoma. *Laryngoscope* 2000;110:1483–1488.

134. To EW, Lai EC, Cheng JH, et al. Nasopharyngectomy for recurrent nasopharyngeal carcinoma: a review of 31 patients and prognostic factors. *Laryngoscope* 2002;112:1877–1882.

135. Wei WI. Cancer of the nasopharynx: functional salvage. *World J Surg* 2003;27:844–848.

136. Hao SP, Tsang NM, Chang KP, et al. Nasopharyngectomy for recurrent nasopharyngeal carcinoma: a review of 53 patients and prognostic factors. *Acta Otolaryngol* 2008;128:473–481.

137. Fisch U. The infratemporal fossa approach for nasopharyngeal tumors. *Laryngoscope* 1983;93:36–44.

138. Danesi G, Zanoletti E, Mazzoni A. Salvage surgery for recurrent nasopharyngeal carcinoma. *Skull Base* 2007;17:173–180.

139. Fee WE Jr, Roberson JB Jr, Goffinet DR. Long-term survival after surgical resection for recurrent nasopharyngeal cancer after radiotherapy failure. *Arch Otolaryngol Head Neck Surg* 1991;117:1233–1236.

140. Morton RP, Liavaag PG, McLean M, et al. Transcervico-mandibulo-palatal approach for surgical salvage of recurrent nasopharyngeal cancer. *Head Neck* 1996;18:352–358.

141. Wei WI, Lam KH, Sham JS. New approach to the nasopharynx: the maxillary swing approach. *Head Neck* 1991;13:200–207.

142. Ng RW, Wei WI. Elimination of palatal fistula after the maxillary swing procedure. *Head Neck* 2005;27:608–612.

143. Ng RW, Wei WI. Quality of life of patients with recurrent nasopharyngeal carcinoma treated with nasopharyngectomy using the maxillary swing approach. *Arch Otolaryngol Head Neck Surg* 2006;132:309–316.

144. Vlantis AC, Yu BK, Kam MK, et al. Nasopharyngectomy: does the approach to the nasopharynx influence survival? *Otolaryngol Head Neck Surg* 2008;139:40–46.

145. Wei WI, Chan JYW, Ng RW, et al. Surgical salvage of persistent or recurrent nasopharyngeal carcinoma with maxillary swing approach–critical appraisal after 2 decades. *Head Neck* 2011;33:969–975.

146. Koutcher L, Lee N, Zelefsky M, et al. Re-irradiation of locally recurrent nasopharynx cancer with external beam radiotherapy with or without brachytherapy. *Int J Radiat Oncol Biol Phys* 2010;76:130–137.

147. Chua DT, Sham JS, Leung LH, et al. Reirradiation of nasopharyngeal carcinoma with intensity-modulated radiotherapy. *Radiother Oncol* 2005;77:290–294.

148. Lu TX, Mai WY, Teh BS, et al. Initial experience using intensity-modulated radiotherapy for recurrent nasopharyngeal carcinoma. *Int J Radiat Oncol Biol Phys* 2004;58:682–687.

149. Chua DT, Sham JS, Au GK. Induction chemotherapy with cisplatin and gemcitabine followed by reirradiation for locally recurrent nasopharyngeal carcinoma. *Am J Clin Oncol* 2005;28:464–471.

150. Nakamura T, Kodaira T, Tachibana H, et al. Chemoradiotherapy for locally recurrent nasopharyngeal carcinoma: treatment outcome and prognostic factors. *Jpn J Clin Oncol* 2008;38:803–809.

151. Chua D, Wei WI, Sham JS, et al. Capecitabine monotherapy for recurrent and metastatic nasopharyngeal carcinoma. *Jpn J Clin Oncol* 2008;38:244–249.

152. Li YH, Wang FH, Jiang WQ, et al. Phase II study of capecitabine and cisplatin combination as first line chemotherapy in Chinese patients with metastatic nasopharyngeal carcinoma. *Cancer Chemother Pharmacol* 2008;62:539–544.

153. Chua DT, Sham JS, Au GK. A phase II study of docetaxel and cisplatin as first-line chemotherapy in patients with metastatic nasopharyngeal carcinoma. *Oral Oncol* 2005;41:589–595.

154. Yeo W, Leung TW, Chan AT, et al. A phase II study of combination paclitaxel and carboplatin in advanced nasopharyngeal carcinoma. *Eur J Cancer* 1998;34:2027–2031.

155. Ngan RK, Yiu HH, Lau WH, et al. Combination gemcitabine and cisplatin chemotherapy for metastatic or recurrent nasopharyngeal carcinoma: report of a phase II study. *Ann Oncol* 2002;13:1252–1258.

156. Foo KF, Tan EH, Leong SS, et al. Gemcitabine in metastatic nasopharyngeal carcinoma of the undifferentiated type. *Ann Oncol* 2002;13:150–156.

157. Ma BB, Hui EP, Wong SC, et al. Multicenter phase II study of gemcitabine and oxaliplatin in advanced nasopharyngeal carcinoma–correlation with excision repair cross-complementing-1 polymorphisms. *Ann Oncol* 2009;20:1854–1859.

158. Chan AT, Hsu MM, Goh BC, et al. Multicenter, phase II study of cetuximab in combination with carboplatin in patients with recurrent or metastatic nasopharyngeal carcinoma. *J Clin Oncol* 2005;23:3568–3576.

159. Chua DT, Wei WI, Wong MP, et al. Phase II study of gefitinib for the treatment of recurrent and metastatic nasopharyngeal carcinoma. *Head Neck* 2008;30:863–867.

160. Ma B, Hui EP, King A, et al. A Phase II study of patients with metastatic or locoregionally recurrent nasopharyngeal carcinoma and evaluation of plasma Epstein-Barr virus DNA as a biomarker of efficacy. *Cancer Chemother Pharmacol* 2008;62:59–64.

161. Hui EP, Ma BB, King AD, et al. Hemorrhagic complications in a phase II study of sunitinib in patients of nasopharyngeal carcinoma who has previously received high dose radiation. *Ann Oncol* 2011;22:1280–1287.

121 Oropharyngeal Cancer

Anna M. Pou   *Jonas T. Johnson*

Cancer of the oropharynx is relatively uncommon, accounting for fewer than 1% of all new cancers. Cancer data reported combine oral cavity sites with oropharyngeal sites. It has been estimated that over 39,000 cases of oral cavity and pharyngeal cancer will be diagnosed in the United States in 2010 (1). Approximately one-third of these will be expected to arise in the oropharynx. Its peak incidence is between the sixth and seventh decades of life; however, cases in the fifth and fourth decades of life are not uncommon. The disease has a distinct male predominance, but recent data show an increased incidence among women. Squamous cell carcinoma (SCC) and its variants account for more than 90% of malignant oropharyngeal lesions. Historically, the most important etiologic factor was the exposure to tobacco and alcohol; however, the majority of cases seen today are HPV associated (2). Treatment of this disease is complex, and a team including a head and neck surgeon, reconstructive surgeon, radiation oncologist, medical oncologist, prosthodontist, and speech and language pathologist offers the patient the best opportunity for disease control with management of treatment-related toxicities.

ANATOMY

The oropharynx is the midportion of the pharynx that connects the nasopharynx superiorly to the oral cavity anteriorly and to the hypopharynx inferiorly. It extends from an imaginary horizontal plane through the hard palate to another through the hyoid bone (Fig. 121.1). As it opens into the oral cavity, it is bounded by the circumvallate papillae, anterior tonsillar pillars, and the junction of the hard and soft palates. The posterior limit of the oropharynx is the posterior pharyngeal wall, which lies anterior to the prevertebral fascia. The lateral boundary includes the tonsillar fossae and pillars and the lateral pharyngeal walls. The superior limit is contiguous with the inferior boundary of the nasopharynx. Clinically, the oropharynx is divided into four subsites: base of tongue, soft palate, the palatine tonsillar fossa and pillars, and pharyngeal walls.

The pharyngeal walls are made of multiple layers, which include from surface to deep the mucosa, submucosa, pharyngobasilar fascia, constrictor muscles (superior and upper fibers of middle), and buccopharyngeal fascia. The superficial anatomy of the lateral walls includes the anterior tonsillar pillars (palatoglossus muscle); the palatine tonsillar tissue, which lies in the tonsillar fossae; posterior tonsillar pillars (palatopharyngeal muscle); and a small portion of lateral pharyngeal walls. The palatine tonsils, when present, often have an irregular surface filled with crypts, which are blind tubules of epithelium that invaginate deep within the lymphoid tissue of the tonsil.

The soft palate is a fibromuscular structure that projects posteriorly and downward into the oropharynx. It is composed of the palatine aponeurosis, which forms the skeleton and includes the tensor veli palatini, levator veli palatini, uvular, palatoglossus, and palatopharyngeal muscles.

The base of the tongue is the anterior wall of the oropharynx and extends from the circumvallate papillae back to the pharyngoepiglottic ligament and glossoepiglottic folds. The lingual tonsils lie superficial and lateral on either side and cause its mucosal surfaces to be irregular. The paired valleculae mark the transition of the base of the tongue into the epiglottis. This relationship explains why the submucosal spread of tumor from the base of the tongue may involve the supraglottic larynx or, conversely, laryngeal tumors may grow into the base of the tongue.

Most of the oropharynx is supplied with sensory and motor innervation through the glossopharyngeal (cranial nerve IX) and vagus (cranial nerve X) nerves. The hypoglossal nerve (cranial nerve XII) supplies motor innervation to the base of the tongue. The motor and most of the sensory innervation of the soft palate comes from the trigeminal nerve.

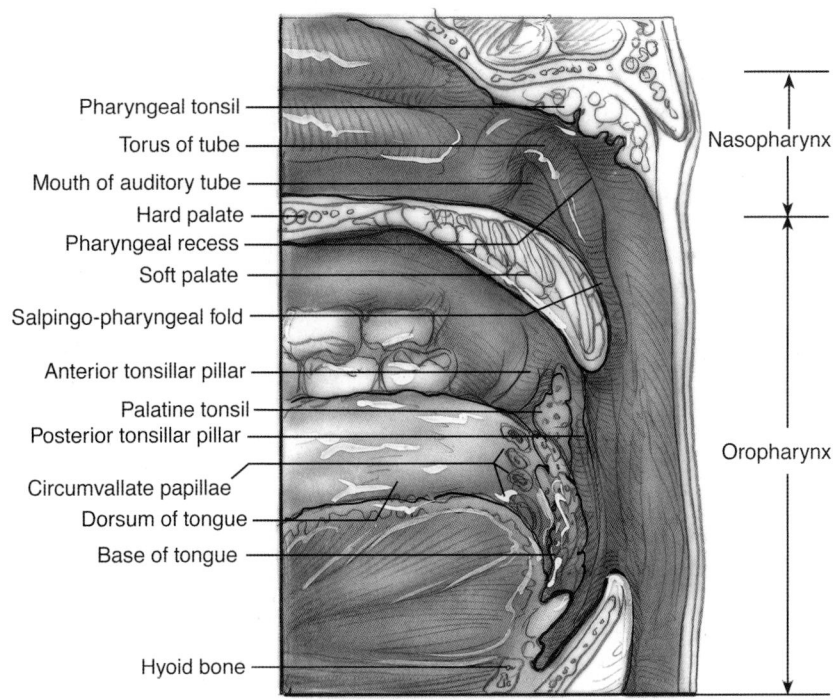

Pharyngeal tonsil
Torus of tube
Mouth of auditory tube
Hard palate
Pharyngeal recess
Soft palate
Salpingo-pharyngeal fold
Anterior tonsillar pillar
Palatine tonsil
Posterior tonsillar pillar
Circumvallate papillae
Dorsum of tongue
Base of tongue
Hyoid bone

Nasopharynx

Oropharynx

Figure 121.1 Surface anatomy of the oropharynx.

The oropharynx is abundantly supplied with blood from most branches of the external carotid artery, particularly the ascending pharyngeal. The lymphatic drainage is primarily to levels II and III, with midline structures such as the tongue base, soft palate, and posterior pharyngeal wall draining to both sides of the neck. The posterior pharyngeal wall, soft palate, and tonsillar region also drain to the retropharyngeal nodes, which in turn drain to the upper level II nodes.

The oropharynx is surrounded on three sides by potential fascial spaces. The retropharyngeal space is an area of loose connective tissue lying behind the pharynx between the buccopharyngeal fascia of the pharynx and the alar layer of the prevertebral fascia. The retropharyngeal space extends from the skull base to the superior mediastinum and communicates with the parapharyngeal space laterally. The parapharyngeal space is defined by fascial planes extending from the skull base to the greater cornu of the hyoid bone and lying lateral to the pharyngeal walls. It has the shape of an inverted pyramid, and its boundaries include the skull superiorly, pterygomandibular raphe anteriorly, prevertebral fascia posteriorly, and the pharynx medially. The lateral boundary is the most complex and is formed by the fascia overlying the medial pterygoid muscle, a portion of the mandible, deep lobe of the parotid, and the posterior belly of the digastric muscle. This fascia extends superiorly, incorporating the stylomandibular ligament, and fuses with the strong interpterygoid fascia to attach to the skull base in a line passing medial to the foramen ovale and spinosum. It also separates the parapharyngeal space from the infratemporal fossa and masticator space and places the trigeminal nerve within the latter (3). The parapharyngeal space can be further divided by a layer

of fascia running from the tensor veli palatini muscle to the styloid and its related structures into two compartments. The prestyloid compartment contains fat, variable portions of the deep lobe of the parotid, and a small branch of the trigeminal nerve to the tensor veli palatini. The poststyloid compartment contains the carotid artery, jugular vein, cranial nerves IX to XII, sympathetic chain, and lymph nodes.

There are multiple aspects of oropharyngeal anatomy that are clinically important. The irregular surfaces of the tongue base and the tonsils make it difficult to identify small tumors. The vagus and glossopharyngeal nerves have tympanic and auricular branches (Jacobson and Arnold nerves), which cause the referred otalgia associated with tumors of this area. The retropharyngeal and parapharyngeal spaces also serve as potential routes for cancer spread. Surgical margins may be difficult to achieve in some patients because oropharyngeal structures lack natural boundaries. Tumors that involve the palate or tonsillar pillar may invade or encase bone of the mandible or maxilla. Involvement of the muscles of mastication results in pain and trismus. Base of tongue tumors may spread in all directions to involve larynx, palatine tonsil, or oral tongue.

PHYSIOLOGY

The oropharynx is essential for normal speech production, respiration, and deglutition. These highly coordinated functions require intact sensory and motor input and intact structures. A detailed understanding of these coordinated events is crucial. All treatment modalities may result in dysfunction.

Deglutition is the most complex of these functions and can be divided into four phases: (a) oral preparatory, (b) oral, (c) pharyngeal, and (d) esophageal. The oropharynx plays an important role in the first three phases. The soft palate is pulled forward while the tongue base is slightly elevated during both oral phases to prevent food from spilling prematurely into the pharynx. The food bolus at the end of the oral phase is propelled between the tongue and palate, past the tongue base and faucial arches, triggering the pharyngeal phase. This phase culminates with the propulsion of the food bolus into the esophagus through the following events: (a) velopharyngeal closure, (b) elevation and closure of the larynx, (c) contraction of the pharyngeal muscles and retraction of the tongue base, and (d) opening of the cricopharyngeal region. The major driving force of the bolus through the pharyngeal phase is the pressure developed by the tongue base; pharyngeal contraction and peristalsis serve mostly to clear the residual material present at the end (4).

Extirpative surgery of the oropharynx may result in poor speech production, dysphagia, and aspiration. This may be a result of velopharyngeal incompetence, pharyngeal stenosis, inappropriate functioning of the tongue base tethering or volume reduction, decreased pharyngeal contraction, sensory denervation, and delayed triggering of the pharyngeal swallow because of decreased sensation. Avoidance of these undesirable sequelae may be mitigated with proper patient selection for surgery, appropriate reconstruction, and vigorous rehabilitation. Use of tissue sparing such as intensity-modulated radiation therapy (IMRT) radiation techniques and less toxic regimens may be appropriate in some cases. Evaluation of speech and swallowing should occur before, during, and after treatment to allow for the best outcomes and quality of life (5).

ETIOLOGY

SCC of the head and neck is known to arise from the accumulation of multiple genetic alterations to genes important to the regulation of cellular growth and death. These alterations, which may be inherited but are more often acquired from exposure to environmental agents, provide the cell with a selective growth advantage. The cells then undergo further selection, which eventually results in a clone that overcomes the normal growth controls and host defenses to establish the tumor (6).

Multiple environmental factors are associated with SCC of the oropharynx. Historically the most important was exposure to tobacco and alcohol. Heavy tobacco users have a 5- to 25-fold higher risk of developing head and neck cancer than nonsmokers (7). The effect of these agents is dose related, and concurrent exposure is synergistic, resulting in a risk that is greater than the sums of the risks of either one alone (8). The relative risk of developing cancer increases from 2.7 in those who smoke up to 10 cigarettes per day to 9 in those who smoke 1 pack per day. The relative risk also increases with an increase in alcohol consumption; the relative risk rises to 8.8 in those who consume 30 or more drinks per week compared to 1.2 in

those who consume 1 to 4 drinks per week. The combination of smoking and drinking has a greater than additive effect as mentioned earlier; a person who has greater than a 40-pack-year history of smoking who consumes 5 alcoholic drinks per day has a relative risk of 40 (9,10).

Viruses have been shown to be a probable etiologic agent in development of SCC. The most extensively studied virus is the human papillomavirus (HPV) (11). In a study by Kerimer et al., a systematic review of 5,046 head and neck SCC specimens from 60 studies worldwide was performed to determine the worldwide prevalence and types of HPV in head and neck cancer (11). The overall prevalence of HPV was 25.9%: 35.6% in oropharyngeal SCC, 23.5% in oral cavity SCC, and 24.0% in laryngeal SCC. HPV 16 was the most common type detected: It accounted for 30.9% of oropharyngeal SCC, 16% of oral cavity SCC, and 16.6% of laryngeal SCC. HPV-positive tumors are more likely to originate in the oropharynx, to be poorly differentiated, have basaloid features, and present with a lower T stage than HPV-negative tumors. Prognosis and response to treatment are strongly associated with HPV status, and those who are positive appear to be more responsive to treatment and thus have a survival advantage (12).

Individuals with HPV-positive tumors have different risk factors than those who are HPV negative. HPV-positive SCC's were independently associated with sexual behavior and marijuana use but not with tobacco or alcohol use or poor oral hygiene. On the other hand, those tumors that were HPV negative were associated with heavy alcohol and tobacco use and poor oral hygiene, but not sexual behavior or marijuana use (13). D'Souza et al. (14) found that oral HPV infection is strongly associated with oropharyngeal SCC among those with or without established risk factors of alcohol and tobacco use. In addition, Mork et al. (15) found a 14-fold increase in risk of developing oropharyngeal SCC in those who are seropositive for PGY 16. Oropharyngeal tumors should be tested for HPV 16 status.

Dietary factors such as vitamin deficiency (Vitamin A, iron deficiency of Plummer-Vinson syndrome), poor nutrition, poor oral hygiene, syphilis, occupational exposure, and previous irradiation also have been implicated as etiologic agents; however, evidence is limited overshadowed by the evidence supporting the carcinogenic effects of tobacco and alcohol.

Immunosuppression due to heredity, transplantation, or human immunodeficiency virus (16,17) may accelerate the development of SCC, lymphoma, and other tumors of the oropharynx by impairing normal immune surveillance mechanisms.

HISTOPATHOLOGY

The oropharynx consists of different types of epithelium pending on the subsite. The oropharyngeal epithelium arises from stratified squamous epithelium and transitions where the soft palate contacts the posterior pharyngeal wall (Passavant ridge) into ciliated respiratory epithelium of the nasopharynx.

Minor salivary glands can be found in the soft palate, tonsillar pillars, and lingual tonsils, and therefore, tumors of minor salivary gland origin can be found in these places. Lymphoepithelium can be found in the subsites that form Waldeyer ring (nasopharynx, palliative tonsils, and tongue base).

Premalignant lesions occur in the oropharynx; however, they are rarely recognized. Lesions are seen most commonly on the soft palate and anterior tonsillar pillars and include leukoplakia (white plaque lesion), erythroplakia (sharply demarcated red lesion), and lichen planus (white, lacy lesion). Diagnosis requires biopsy.

SCC (keratinizing and nonkeratinizing) and its variants account for more than 90% of malignant oropharyngeal lesions. The spindle cell variant is clinically and biologically similar to SCC, whereas others behave differently. Basaloid appearance of SCC may be an indication of HPV-positive status (12).

Verrucous carcinoma is a fungating, slow-growing tumor with well-differentiated keratinizing epithelium and rare cellular atypia or mitosis on histology. These tumors have "pushing" margins. They rarely metastasize and are considered a low-grade malignancy. Lymphoepitheliomas arise from Waldeyer ring. This tumor is nonkeratinizing and is similar in behavior to the undifferentiated type of nasopharyngeal carcinoma. These lesions usually occur in the tonsillar region of young adults that do not have typical risk factors. Lymphoma may occur in Waldeyer ring (usually non-Hodgkin lymphoma). Minor salivary gland tumors, mucosal melanomas, and sarcomas are other malignant lesions found in the oropharynx.

Minor salivary gland malignancies are relatively rare. The most common types include adenoid cystic carcinoma, mucoepidermoid carcinoma, and adenosquamous carcinoma. These tumors are treated with primary surgical excision and postoperative radiotherapy depending on high-risk features (perineural invasion, close or positive margins, nodal metastases, high-grade disease).

Some benign lesions, such as minor salivary gland tumors, pseudoepitheliomatous hyperplasia, necrotizing sialometaplasias, Crohn disease, papillomas, pyogenic granulomas, and median rhomboid glossitis, may clinically mimic malignant lesions. Biopsy is usually required to distinguish among these entities.

NATURAL HISTORY

Prolonged exposure of the upper aerodigestive surfaces to carcinogens results in molecular changes throughout the mucosa. With time, certain areas may undergo further change, giving rise to premalignant and malignant lesions. This concept of "field cancerization" or "condemned mucosa" applies to all mucosal head and neck cancers and results in the high rates of second primaries in patients with oropharyngeal cancer (18) (Table 121.1).

SCC usually starts on the surface. Invasion of vessels and thick fascia such as the prevertebral fascia or periosteum is uncommon until late stages, but perineural invasion may occur at any time. Bone involvement is also rare, occurring in only 17% of the lesions (19). Invasion into the parapharyngeal and retropharyngeal spaces allows easy spread to the skull base and neck with possible involvement of the internal carotid artery, cranial nerves IX through XII, and the sympathetic chain. Invasion of the masticator and infratemporal spaces results in trismus.

Lymphatic metastases at presentation are common because the oropharynx is richly supplied with lymphatics and the tumors are generally advanced (20) (Table 121.1). Tumors of the oropharynx may be remarkably asymptomatic. Symptoms of sore throat, otalgia, and dysphagia are commonly misinterpreted or overlooked. For many patients, the first acknowledged observation is the presence of a cervical metastasis.

Oropharyngeal cancer tends to metastasize early. The first echelon nodes are level II, III, or retropharyngeal. Metastasis may be altered by obstruction of the lymphatic channels caused by inflammation, previous surgery, radiation, or large metastatic deposits. Oropharyngeal cancers have a tendency to metastasize to both necks, especially if

TABLE 121.1	THE INCIDENCE OF NODAL DISEASE AT PRESENTATION, SECOND PRIMARIES, AND DISTANT METASTASIS		
Site	Palpable Nodes at Presentation (%)	Second Primary (%)[a]	Distant Metastasis[b] (%)
Base of tongue	72	19	18
Tonsillar region	58	25	15
Soft palate	45	26	7.5
Posterior wall	52	29	11

[a]Incidence of synchronous and metachronous second primaries.
[b]Incidence of distant metastasis with control above the clavicles.

the lesion is midline. The rate of occult neck metastases in the clinically negative neck is estimated at greater than 20% for all lesions larger than T1.

Distant metastases are rare at presentation, occurring in 2% to 5% of patients, but with control of the disease above the clavicles, the incidence of overt distant metastasis increases (18,21) (Table 121.1). The most common sites affected by distant metastases are lung, liver, and bones.

DIAGNOSIS

History

A complete history, including a review of systems and past medical, social, and family history, is essential in planning the proper therapy. Patients with oropharyngeal cancer often have very subtle symptoms such as nonspecific sore throat or unilateral otalgia. Hemoptysis may occur but is relatively uncommon. Frequently the first time a patient presents is because of a neck mass. A history of tobacco use *is not* required to be suspicious. The prevalence of HPV-related cancer in patients who are younger nonsmokers has dramatically modified the profile. The physician must be alert to the asymptomatic patient who demonstrates a cervical cyst, which may be found to be a cystic metastasis (22).

Physical Examination

A complete physical and a thorough head and neck examination should be routinely performed on all patients. Systematic visualization of all the mucosal surfaces of the upper aerodigestive tract is essential due to the field cancerization phenomenon. This examination is greatly facilitated by the use of a fiberoptic nasopharyngolaryngoscope, especially in patients with trismus. The mandibular opening and cranial nerve function are also examined, with cranial nerve deficits indicating extension into the mandible, parapharyngeal, or masticator spaces. Palpation of the primary tumor is always performed in order to judge the extent of submucosal spread. All nodal levels of the neck are systematically evaluated, and size, location, and mobility of these nodes are documented. Dentition is also assessed because restoration or extraction may be required before initiation of treatment. The remainder of the physical exam is performed with emphasis on the cardiopulmonary and nutritional status of the patient.

Further Evaluation

The extent of the tumor, neck metastasis, distant metastasis, and the medical condition of the patient should be assessed completely before a treatment plan is devised or implemented (Table 121.2). In patients with biopsy-proven cancer, positron emission tomography (PET)/computed tomography (CT) has largely replaced other modalities in offering whole body evaluation, which can alert the treatment team to metastasis and synchronous cancers. In

TABLE 121.2	**DIAGNOSIS OROPHARYNGEAL CANCER**

1. History
   Alcohol and tobacco abuse
   Pain and dysphagia
2. Physical
   Nodal enlargement
   Trismus
   Cranial nerve deficits
3. Biopsy of the primary lesion and fine-needle aspiration of enlarged nodes
4. Imaging studies
   PET/CT—for Stages III and IV
   Chest radiograph—if not evaluated by CT or PET/CT
   CT scan/MRI—to evaluate bone and deep invasion
5. Laboratory studies
   Complete blood count and chemistry
   Liver function tests
   ECG
6. Examination under anesthesia
   Look for second primaries
   Assessment of submucosal spread, mandibular invasion, and tumor fixation

patients with cystic neck metastasis, PET scan can be helpful in detecting the occult primary tumor, which is usually found in the tonsils or base of tongue. Most oncologists employ PET/CT to evaluate patients with stage III/IV disease.

CT with iodine contrast and/or magnetic resonance imaging (MRI) with gadolinium may be employed during the diagnostic workup before a histologic diagnosis is established. A fine-cut CT may be needed for evaluating bony structures such as mandibular invasion. MRI is best at evaluating soft tissue involvement, such as the tongue base, parapharyngeal space, or prevertebral fascia. Special tests:

a. Barium swallow is performed on patients with dysphagia. The barium study may alert the treatment team to a synchronous primary in the esophagus. Also, the movement of the posterior wall on the cervical spine observed during fluoroscopy is an indication that the prevertebral fascia is not involved by tumors of the posterior pharyngeal wall.

b. Angiography with the balloon test occlusion and cerebral blood flow evaluation should be considered if the tumor involves the carotid and resection is contemplated.

c. Speech and swallowing evaluation including a modified barium swallow. Patients should be evaluated before, during, and after treatment in order to achieve the best functional results (5,23).

d. Laboratory evaluation of oropharyngeal cancer patients includes a complete blood count, blood chemistry, liver function tests, and an electrocardiogram. Thyroid function and nutritional evaluation may be included in this.

Tissue diagnosis is obtained with fine-needle aspiration (FNA) of enlarged nodes and/or biopsy of the oropharyngeal lesion. This can usually be performed in the office or clinic, but biopsy under general anesthesia should be reserved for patients with trismus, tenuous airway, or lesions that are not accessible transorally. FNA may need to be performed with ultrasound guidance especially in patients with cystic masses in order to obtain sufficient epithelial cells to make a diagnosis (22).

Staging Endoscopy

Patients with epithelial primary tumors should undergo examination under anesthesia irrespective of the size of the tumor or the adequacy of the initial assessment. Complete visualization and palpation of the tumor greatly facilitate the assessment of submucosal spread and invasion of surrounding structures such as the prevertebral fascia and mandible, especially in patients with trismus. A thorough search for a synchronous second primary tumor, which occurs in approximately 8% of patients (15), is conducted via systematic examination of the upper aerodigestive tract and esophagus. Bronchoscopy is optional in patients with normal chest radiographs (16), but we usually perform a tracheobronchoscopy in patients who have not undergone a PET scan, because small lesions in the trachea or hilum are not readily seen on routine radiographs. Biopsies are performed at the end of the endoscopy to allow the examination to proceed unhindered by bleeding from the biopsy site. If lymphoma is suspected, the pathologist should be notified in advance, and an adequate sample of tissue is submitted fresh to allow for receptor typing. The teeth are evaluated and restored or extracted as needed at the end of the procedure. The findings of endoscopy and tumor mapping are then recorded and the patient is staged. Table 121.2 shows the tumor staging for the oropharynx. Many patients with oropharyngeal cancer present initially with an unknown primary with a cervical metastasis. Panendoscopy is crucial in these patients, and bilateral tonsillectomy and bilateral biopsies of the base of the tongue and nasopharynx are recommended if the primary tumor is not found. Recently authors have demonstrated the potential value of transoral tongue base resection in patients with occult HPV cervical metastasis (24). The neck staging and stage groupings are the same as other sites of the head and neck (Table 121.3).

TREATMENT

The treatment of oropharyngeal cancers, especially for patients with advanced tumors and those involving the base of the tongue, has evolved dramatically in the past decade. The initial shift away from primary surgery to "organ preservation" strategies employing CRT was reflective of the success of CRT in avoidance of laryngectomy in patients with laryngeal cancer. The community of head and neck oncologists seemed anxious to avoid the significant functional

TABLE 121.3	TUMOR (T) STAGING FOR THE OROPHARYNX
Stage	**Description**
Tx	Carcinoma *in situ*
T1	Tumor 2 cm or less in greatest dimension
T2	2–4 cm in greatest dimension
T3	>4 cm in greatest dimension
T4a	Tumor invades the larynx, deep/extrinsic muscles of the tongue, medial pterygoid, hard palate, or mandible
T4b	Tumor invades lateral pterygoid muscle, pterygoid plates, lateral nasopharynx, or skull base, or encases carotid artery

Greene FL, Page DL, Fleming ID, et al. *AJCC cancer staging manual*, 6th ed. New York: Springer, 2010.

morbidity of open surgical approaches to the oropharynx. Unfortunately, the initial enthusiasm for nonoperative primary therapy has been tempered by the high rate of treatment related toxicity associated with CRT (25). These dilemmas are not resolved at the time of this writing. Recent advances in minimally invasive transoral surgery of the oropharynx offer the potential for enhanced functional results.

The treatment of oropharyngeal cancer is complex and requires a multidisciplinary team approach, which offers the patient the best opportunity for a comprehensive treatment plan. This team includes a head and neck surgeon, reconstructive surgeon, radiation oncologist, medical oncologist, dental oncologist, prosthodontist, and speech and language pathologist. The surgeon must consider an array of factors when deciding on the optimal treatment regimen for the individual patient. These include the type of treatment needed for the primary tumor and the neck, the modality best suited for functional preservation or restoration, the general medical condition of the patient, and, most importantly, the patient's preferences. The availability of facilities, expertise, and social support also play a role (Table 121.4). All patients should be counseled and aided in cessation of smoking and alcohol consumption at the time of diagnosis. While the relationship of HPV with these tumors is generally accepted, little is known about the potential of transmission at the time of diagnosis.

Squamous Cell Carcinoma

Surgery and radiation therapy, alone or combined, have been the mainstays of treatment for squamous cell oropharyngeal cancer, but the treatment paradigm regarding advanced disease has changed over the past several years. Early-stage oropharyngeal cancer can be successfully treated with radiotherapy (26), and concurrent chemoradiation is the standard of care for advanced cancers, both resectable and nonresectable (27). Further details of nonsurgical treatment are discussed in Chapters 110 and 111.

TABLE 121.4	R TREATMENT OROPHARYNGEAL CANCER

1. Team approach
2. Primary tumor treatment
   a. T1 and T2: single modality surgery or radiation
   b. T3 and T4: combined modality (chemoradiation or surgery and postoperative radiation)
3. Neck treatment
   a. N0 and N1: surgery or radiation
   b. N2 and N3: combined modality (surgery and postoperative chemoradiation or chemoradiation)
   c. Both sides of neck are treated with midline lesions
   d. Retropharyngeal nodes are always treated when cervical nodes are treated

TABLE 121.5	INDICATIONS FOR POSTOPERATIVE RADIATION (± CHEMO)

Tumor factors
1. Close or involved resection margins
2. Perineural or vascular invasion
3. T3
4. T4

Neck factors
1. Clinically N0 or N1 neck
   a. Two or more histologically positive nodes
   b. Histologically positive nodes at multiple sites
   c. Perineural or vascular invasion
   d. Extracapsular nodal spread
2. N2
3. N3

Those patients with HPV-negative tumors and direct mandibular invasion may be better served with primary surgery. Similarly the availability of minimally invasive transoral resection techniques, either laser or robotic, offers the potential to cure patients with small tumors with surgery alone (28). Surgical resection also may afford the treatment team an opportunity to deintensify chemoradiation and further limit treatment related toxicity. The potential merits of this approach are being evaluated in many centers, but Level I evidence is not available at the time of this writing.

PET–CT is widely advocated at 12 weeks post-CRT to assess for residual disease. Intraoperative assessment with biopsies and/or neck dissection are performed if residual tumor persists.

Primary Tumor

Surgery and radiation alone are similar in controlling T1 and T2 oropharyngeal cancers. The high incidence of occult clinical metastatic deposits mandates the neck be treated electively with either modality in all patients except those with very small primary tumors. In patients who undergo primary surgery, the indications for postoperative radiotherapy (± chemotherapy) are listed in Table 121.5 (29,30). The decision to treat even the smallest oropharyngeal primary with surgery alone must be based upon favorable histologic findings. Stage T3 and T4 tumors can be controlled with surgery and postoperative radiation, but concurrent chemoradiation or hyperfractionated radiotherapy is now considered standard of care especially for patients who are HPV positive and for those in whom the morbidity from surgery is deemed too high to tolerate or in whom the regain of function is unlikely.

Neck

Almost all patients with oropharyngeal SCC require some treatment of the neck because of the high rate of clinically positive nodes and occult nodal metastasis at presentation. The choice of initial treatment modality (surgery or radiation) for the neck and retropharyngeal nodes is usually dictated by that used for the primary tumor. Stage N0 and N1 neck disease are effectively controlled with a single modality. Neck dissection has the added benefit of providing pathologic staging and may allow single modality surgery to be used for small primaries. The use of selective neck dissection in ruling out regional spread following transoral excision of the primary is not as reliable in oropharyngeal cancer as in oral cancer. This is due to the less predictable lymphatic pathways and the increased difficulty accessing the retropharyngeal nodes. For this reason, radiotherapy is often used even when the primary is treated surgically. Following combined chemoradiation surgery results in better regional control in stage N2 and N3 neck disease (31). Both necks should be treated when there is clinical disease in one side of the neck, and the lesion is midline or crosses the midline. The retropharyngeal lymph nodes (RPLNs) must always be considered in the neck treatment plan.

A recent study evaluated the pattern of cervical lymph node metastasis including RPLN metastasis in 76 patients presenting with SCC of the tonsil. 81.6% were stages III and IV. Sixteen patients were treated with surgery only. Seventy-one therapeutic and twenty-seven elective neck dissections were performed. Thirty-four patients underwent RPLN dissection. The rate of contralateral occult metastasis was 28.6%, and the rate of RPLN metastasis was 26.5%. The predictors of contralateral metastasis were stages T3–T4 disease, lesions close to the midline, and ipsilateral multilevel involvement. The predictors of RPLN metastasis were positive preoperative imaging, posterior pharyngeal wall invasion, more than N2 stage, contralateral nodal metastasis, or ipsilateral multilevel involvement. The authors recommend that an elective RPLN dissection be considered in patients with advanced T and N stage, particularly for tumors with posterior pharyngeal wall involvement (32). Although these authors did not discuss function, severe dysphagia can result due to disruption of the pharyngeal plexus when dissecting RPLN's. In a previous study, Tauzin et al. (33) also found that RPLN metastasis was associated with advanced T and N stage. Tonsil was the primary site (82%) of those with RPLN metastasis. This is probably primarily reflective of the fact that tonsil cancers are far more common than posterior wall tumor. They also concluded that pretreatment PET/CT can be used as a single tool to aid in planning treatment of the neck in oropharyngeal tumors as their results were consistent with those reported in the literature. They suggest that pretreatment PET/CT may identify a subset of patients who can be treated with surgery only, negating the need for radiation therapy for treatment of the RPLN's in early-stage disease.

Nonsurgical Management

Nonsurgical management consists of radiotherapy with or without concurrent chemotherapy. Most chemotherapy regimens are based on platinum agents. The radiation course usually consists of delivering a dose of 60 to 70 Gy through an external-beam shrinking field to the primary lesion and necks over a 6- to 7-week period. Other strategies, such as brachytherapy, hyperfractionation, and electron boost to the neck, are used in some centers to enhance the effectiveness of radiation therapy in more advanced lesions. Radiation is typically delivered using IMRT (34,35). Patients treated nonsurgically should be evaluated using a posttreatment PET/CT to determine response at 8 to 12 weeks after completion of therapy. Patients who presented with N2 and N3 disease should undergo a neck dissection (36) if PET/CT-positive disease persists. If a complete clinical response is obtained, there are data to support a watchful waiting approach as this usually predicts a complete tumor control (37).

Surgery

Primary Tumor

Most oropharyngeal tumors are amenable to surgical excision; however, the best evidence suggests that CRT offers similar tumor control when compared to surgery and radiation. This is especially true for patients with advanced tumors because of poor disease control and the severe functional impairment associated with resection of these large tumors. This is true when tumor involves more than 1/2 of the tongue base extends to the oral tongue, or extends to the larynx. Extension into the parapharyngeal space, prevertebral fascia, or involvement of the carotid artery makes tumor control unlikely. Successful extirpation of oropharyngeal cancers hinges on good exposure and wide resection margins (1 to 2 cm), because these tumors have the propensity for submucosal spread; frozen-section clearance obtained of all the margins is needed. Patients with microscopically positive margins that are found intraoperatively or postoperatively after the permanent sections are examined should undergo 1-cm resection of the involved

margin if possible and adjuvant radiation therapy. The use of robotics and transoral laser microsurgical resection is currently under investigation. The potential that minimally invasive resection can offer some patients single modality tumor control and de-intensification of adjuvant CRT, better functional recovery may result. This is the topic of ongoing clinical trials.

Surgical Approaches

Transoral

The transoral approach to the oropharynx involves resection of the tumor through the open mouth with no external incisions. Caution should be exercised before recommending this approach because it provides limited exposure. It may be indicated for small (T1), superficial, or exophytic cancers of the upper or anterior sites of the oropharynx, such as lesions of the soft palate, anterior tonsillar pillar, tonsil, and posterior wall. The surgeon must ensure that there is good visualization of not only the entire tumor but a 1- to 2-cm resection perimeter surrounding it on all sides, including the deep margin. Trismus, height of the mandible, and presence of teeth may further hinder visualization, making adequate resection almost impossible. Resections through this approach are quick and have minimal morbidity, but visualization of the posterior and deep resection margins tends to be very poor.

For tumors that are difficult to access, transoral microsurgical approaches using the CO_2 laser can be a valuable tool. Although tumors of the soft palate and tonsil may be removed with cautery, the laser is more precise. The CO_2 laser and microscope may be used to resect tumors that are otherwise difficult to access transorally including such as those involving the lateral and posterior pharyngeal walls, posterior tongue base, and vallecula. Good local control rates and functional results have been obtained. Steiner et al. (38) reported the use of transoral laser microsurgery for resection of tongue base tumors ($n = 48$) with 94% belonging to stages III and IVa. Forty-three patients underwent selective neck dissections and twenty-three patients underwent postoperative radiotherapy with or without chemotherapy. There was no local recurrence rate for T1 and T2 lesions but a 20% local recurrence rate for T3 and T4 tumors, with a 5-year disease-free survival rate of 73%. Function was preserved in the majority of patients. Laccourreye and colleagues reported a 5-year local control rate of 82% in patients with tonsillar cancer undergoing transoral laser microsurgery. The 5-year local control rate was 89% for T1 and T2 tumors and 63% with T3 lesions (39).

Transoral Robotic Surgery

The use of the robot has allowed the surgeon to manipulate the instruments and endoscopes simultaneously with improved dexterity by allowing more degrees of freedom (40). The advantages of transoral robotic surgery (TORS) include improved optics, three-dimensional tumor visualization, and tremor filtration. Due to these advantages TORS is gaining popularity. In order to determine if the patient's anatomy is accessible to the use of any transoral approach, access should be evaluated and include evaluation of teeth/mandible, trismus, tori, tongue, size, and flexibility of the neck and tumor extent (28).

TORS has been used successfully for the resection of tongue base and tonsillar tumors (41,42). In a study by O'Malley et al., three patients with T1/T2 base of tongue tumors underwent successful TORS with clear margins and post-TORS neck dissection. One patient experienced a postoperative bleed, which was controlled with surgical intervention. All three patients were treated with adjuvant therapy. In another study, 27 patients with T1–3, N0–2 tumors were resected using TORS and underwent post-TORS neck dissection. Seventy-five percent of these tumors were T1–2. Thirty percent (8/27) required an additional unplanned operation and functional outcomes were good. TORS has also been shown to be a safe alternative to open salvage resection for selected tumors (43).

The oncologic benefit for TORS is still unclear. Many patients in the studies mentioned above required postoperative radiation therapy or chemoradiation therapy. Considering the fact that many patients with oropharyngeal tumors are treated successfully with primary radiation with or without chemotherapy, the additional benefit of surgery is unknown. Transoral approaches may be best suited for treatment of small primary tumors. For instance, patients with T1–2 N0–1 tumor may be considered for surgical

therapy employed as a single modality. The potential to deintensify adjuvant therapies in advanced cancer may serve as a motive for surgical resection. Additional follow-up regarding oncologic and functional outcomes is needed to determine the utility of these novel approaches.

Open Procedures

The major open procedures were developed during a time when surgery was the primary mode of therapy for most patients. These procedures have been largely obsoleted as primary therapy because of the success of CRT and minimally invasive transoral surgical approaches. Open approaches may still be required in patients who are HPV negative and in very advanced cancer with bone involvement. Open approaches may be needed for salvage of CRT failures.

Mandibular Lingual Release

The mandibular lingual release or pull-through approach to the oropharynx is indicated for lesions confined mostly to the base of the tongue. The technique involves a standard apron flap elevated in the subplatysmal plane to the lower border of the mandible. Neck dissections are performed as needed. An incision is made through the lingual mucoperiosteum and the periosteum at the lower edge of the mandible (Fig. 121.2A). The anterior mandibular muscles are released with the periosteum from the inner mandibular table, delivering the tongue and floor of mouth into the neck. The lesion can then be resected with excellent direct visualization (Fig. 121.2B). This approach does not require

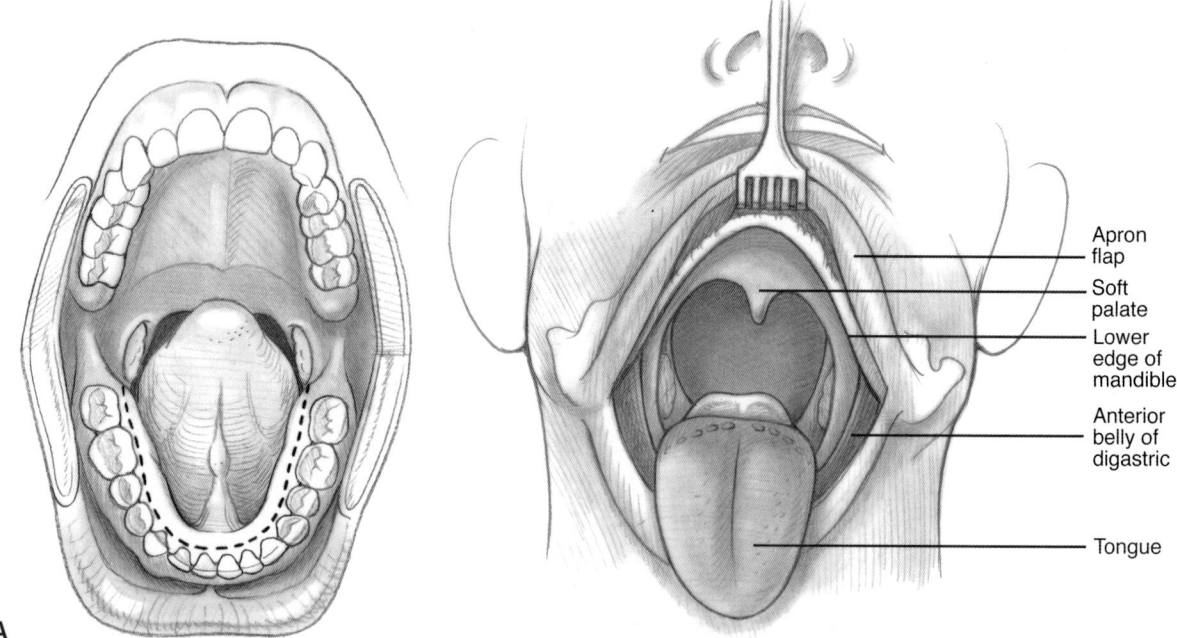

A   B

Apron flap
Soft palate
Lower edge of mandible
Anterior belly of digastric
Tongue

Figure 121.2 Mandibular lingual release. **A:** An incision is made through the lingual mucoperiosteum and the periosteum at the lower edge of the mandible. **B:** The anterior mandibular muscles are released with the periosteum from the inner mandibular table, delivering the tongue and floor of mouth into the neck.

mandibulotomy or a lower lip split, but it offers less access to the lateral pharynx and parapharyngeal spaces than the transmandibular approaches. The lingual arteries, lingual nerves, and hypoglossal nerves are also at risk for damage.

Transpharyngeal Approaches

Suprahyoid Pharyngotomy

The suprahyoid approach is useful for small tumors of the base of the tongue and pharyngeal walls. The pharynx is entered through the vallecula, and the resection is performed from the neck with preservation of the lingual arteries and the hypoglossal nerves (Fig. 121.3). The pharyngotomy also can be extended laterally and inferiorly along the thyroid ala to widen the exposure. This approach results in an excellent functional and cosmetic outcome, but the visualization of the superior margin in larger tumors is inadequate, and there is a risk of cutting into cancer if there is extensive involvement of the tongue base or vallecula. Following resection, the remaining base of tongue is sutured to the valleculae. The remainder of the pharyngotomy defect is then closed. This open technique places the lingual arteries, hypoglossal, and superior laryngeal nerves at risk.

Lateral Pharyngotomy

The lateral pharyngotomy may be used for small lesions of the base of the tongue and pharyngeal walls. The pharynx is entered posterior to the thyroid ala on the least affected side. The hypoglossal and superior laryngeal nerves are dissected and retracted superiorly and inferiorly. Once the pharynx has been entered, the larynx is retracted to the opposite side, providing a good view of the entire posterior pharyngeal wall, opposite lateral wall, and base of the tongue

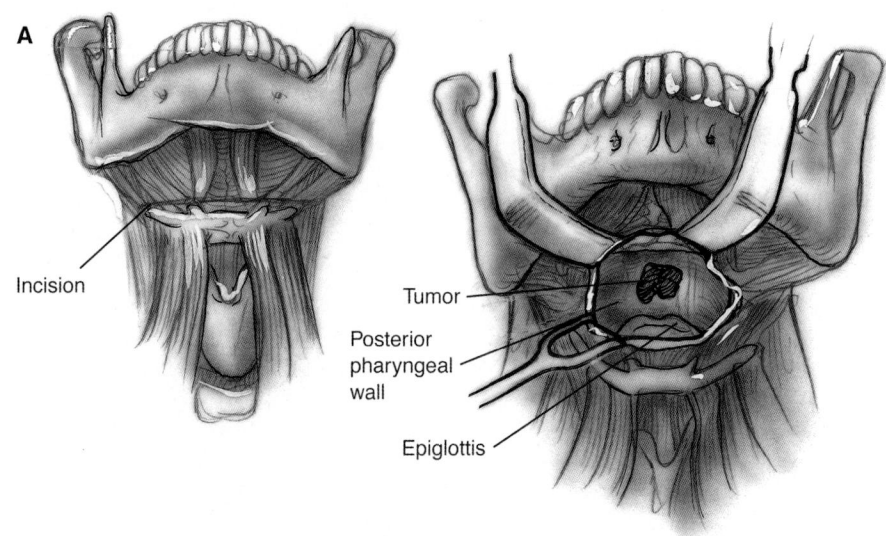

A

Incision

Tumor

Posterior
pharyngeal
wall

Epiglottis

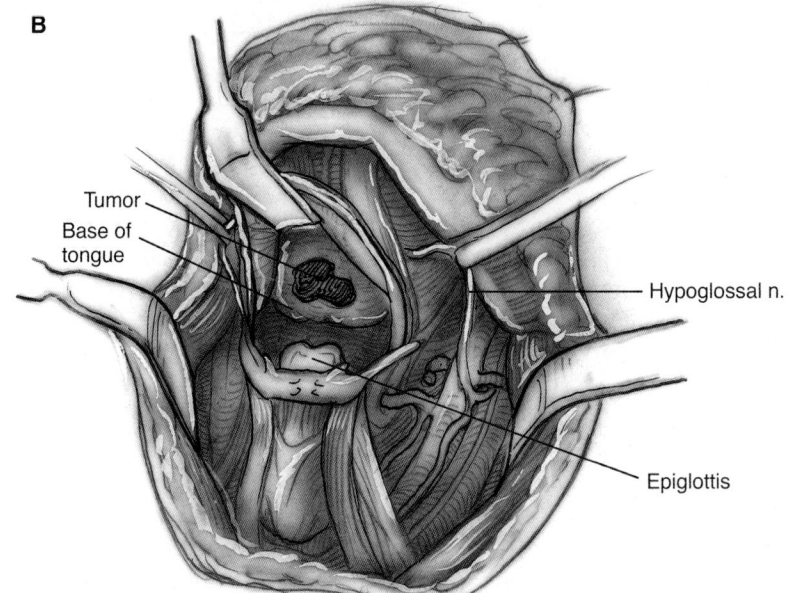

B

Tumor

Base of
tongue

Hypoglossal n.

Epiglottis

Figure 121.3 Suprahyoid pharyngotomy. **A:** Incision above the hyoid through the vallecula with exposure of the posterior pharyngeal wall. **B:** Exposure of the tongue base.

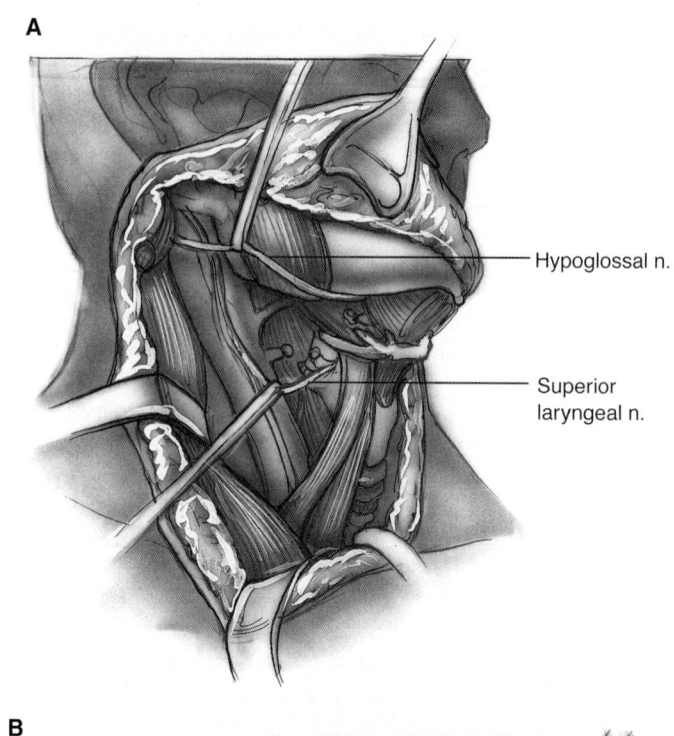

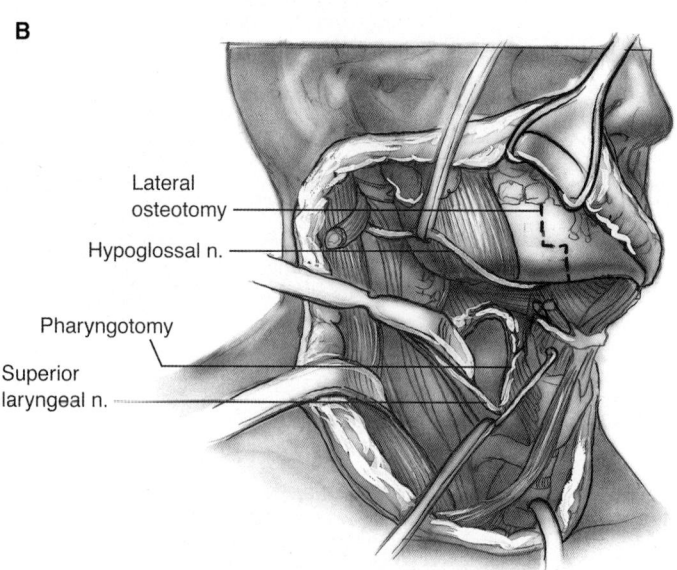

Figure 121.4 Lateral pharyngotomy. **A**: Retraction of the hypoglossal and superior laryngeal nerves. **B**: Exposure of the lower oropharynx and the hypopharynx. Further superior exposure is obtained with lateral mandibulotomy.

(Fig. 121.4A). Further superior exposure can be achieved by extending the pharyngotomy across the vallecula or by combining this approach with a lateral mandibulotomy (Fig. 121.4B). The disadvantages of this approach are the limited superior visualization and the risk of damage to the hypoglossal and superior laryngeal nerves. The lateral mandibulotomy also results in transection of the inferior alveolar nerve resulting in ipsilateral lower lip anesthesia.

Transmandibular

Midline Labiomandibular Glossotomy
The midline labiomandibular glossotomy is rarely used today. The approach involves splitting of the lip (44), gingiva, mandible, and anterior tongue in the midline. The incision can be carried through the base of the tongue down to the hyoid bone if wide exposure of the posterior wall is required (Fig. 121.5). Bleeding and neurologic deficits are minimal because the hypoglossal nerves and lingual arteries are usually not disrupted. However, the approach does not provide access to the parapharyngeal space or lateral oropharyngeal sites.

Mandibular Swing Approach
The mandibular swing approach provides wide exposure to the entire oropharynx and allows an en bloc resection of the cancer and the draining nodes. It can be used for resecting a variety of oropharyngeal cancers that do not involve the mandible, especially those that include multiple sites and the parapharyngeal space. The technique involves a

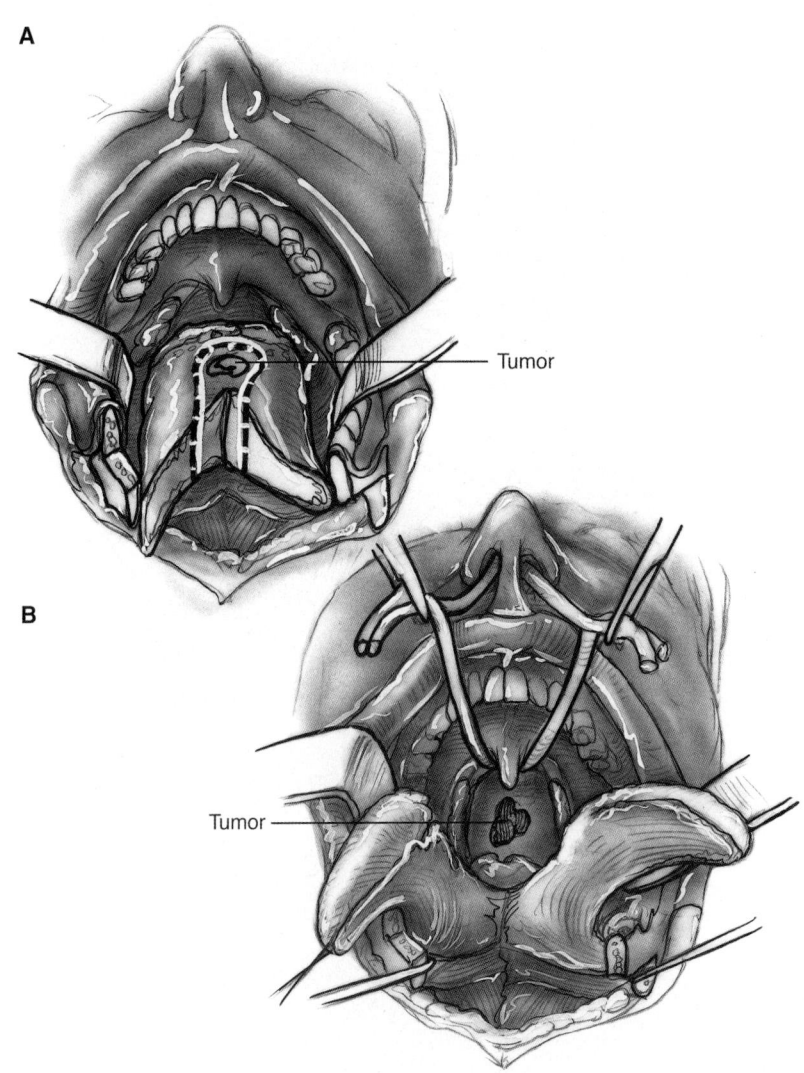

A

Tumor

B

Tumor

Figure 121.5 Midline labiomandibular glossotomy. **A**: The lip, mandible, and tongue are split in midline for a base of tongue lesion. **B**: Exposure of the posterior pharyngeal wall after division of the tongue base.

standard apron flap elevated in the subplatysmal plane to the lower border of the mandible. Neck dissections are performed as needed, identifying the carotid sheath structures and lingual and hypoglossal nerves in the process. The lip then is split. Visor flaps to preserve the continuity of the lip can be used but require division of both mental nerves and result in suboptimal posterior exposure. The osteotomy is performed anterior to the mental nerve on the ipsilateral side through the site of a missing or extracted tooth. Lateral osteotomies that are posterior to the mental foramen are not recommended because they result in the division of the inferior alveolar nerve and have more limited exposure. Prior to the mandibulotomy, compression plates are bent and screwed into place on either side of the planned cut. A full-thickness soft tissue cut then is made through the floor of the mouth and continued posteriorly to the anterior margin of resection, transecting the lingual nerve if needed. The mandibular segments and tongue are distracted, exposing the tumor and parapharyngeal space (Fig. 121.6). Closure of the soft tissue defect usually requires a flap, and the mandible is reapproximated using

the previously bent compression plates. These plates are flashed prior to replacing them in the "clean" wound. The main disadvantage of using this approach is the potential sacrifice of the whole hemimandible if unsuspected mandibular involvement that is not amenable to a marginal resection is found after the mandibulotomy. This problem can be avoided in most cases by careful evaluation at endoscopy and review of the imaging modalities.

Mandibulectomy

Oropharyngeal composite resection with mandibulectomy is used in advanced cancers in which there is overt bony invasion or in situations in which mandibular invasion cannot be ruled out. Usually, the resection is preceded by a neck dissection, leaving the specimen attached to the inferior border of the angle of the mandible. The lip is divided and a cheek flap is developed by performing a full-thickness incision through the buccogingival sulcus. The uninvolved outer periosteum of the mandible may be left on the cheek flap. The anterior mandibular cut is performed well clear of the tumor (1 to 2 cm), preserving as much of the

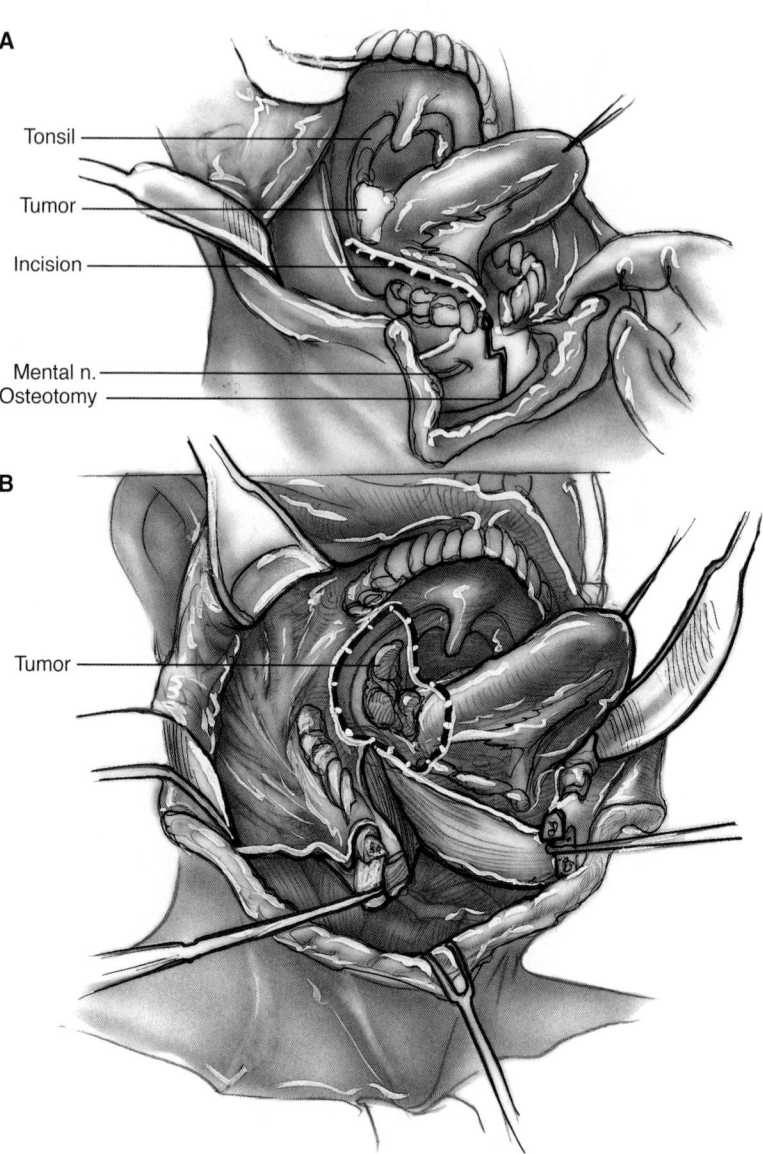

Tonsil

Tumor

Incision

Mental n.
Osteotomy

Tumor

Figure 121.6 Mandibular swing approach. **A:** Osteotomy is placed anterior to the mental foramen. **B:** The full thickness of the floor of the mouth is incised. The mandibular segments are then retracted laterally, allowing good access to the oropharyngeal structures and parapharyngeal space.

mandibular body as possible, and frozen sections of the inferior alveolar nerve are obtained. However, the entire mental canal must be resected, placing the mandibular body osteotomy anterior to the mental foramen, if there is overt mandibular canal invasion or hypesthesia in the inferior alveolar distribution, or if the nerve is positive on frozen section, because there is no reliable method of assessing bony tumor extension intraoperatively. The cranial mandibular cuts are placed along the ramus, but resection of the coronoid process and the condyle may be required with extensive tumors. The mandible then is retracted laterally, and the remaining tumor cuts are performed (Fig. 121.7). The main disadvantage of this approach is the resultant functional and cosmetic deficits, especially if the defect is closed primarily. Reconstruction using free tissue transfer (osteocutaneous flap) is ideal. However, reconstruction of the soft tissue defect takes precedence over reconstruction of the lateral mandibular defect if both soft tissue and bone cannot be reconstructed. However, in order to rehabilitate

mastication, bony reconstruction with dental implants is necessary. Mandibulectomy and mandibulotomy approaches compare favorably (45) for tumor control.

RECONSTRUCTION

The reconstruction of oropharyngeal cancer defects has been revolutionized in the past two decades by the development of pedicled regional myocutaneous flaps and free tissue transfer. The objective of modern reconstruction is to restore the integrity of the oropharynx and its essential functions of deglutition, respiration, and speech production.

Successful reconstruction requires the surgeon to have a detailed knowledge of the various reconstructive techniques and an understanding of their limitations. A variety of techniques have been described over the years, but none has achieved the ideal reconstruction of replacing the resected structure with tissue that matches its form and function. The reconstructive capabilities at present are limited to

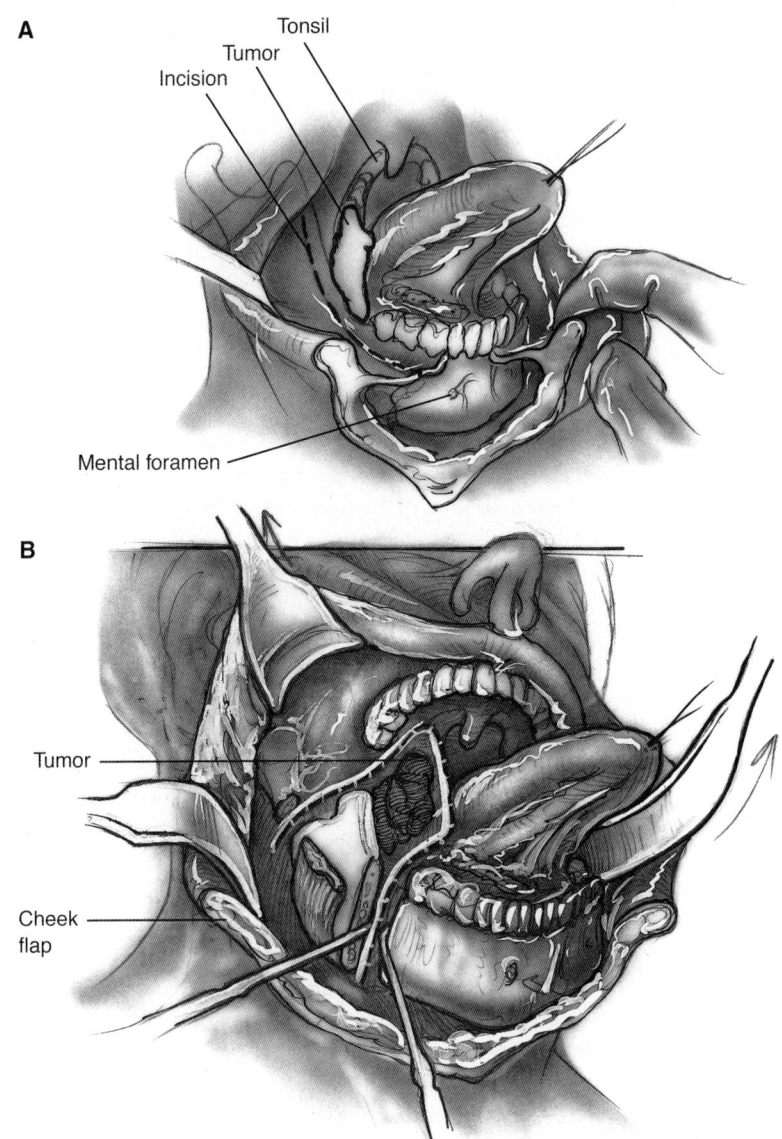

A

Tonsil
Tumor
Incision

Mental foramen

B

Tumor

Cheek
flap

Figure 121.7 Mandibulectomy. **A:** A cheek flap is developed through a full-thickness incision of the gingivobuccal sulcus, exposing the mandible. **B:** The mandibular cuts are made well clear of the tumor and anterior to the mental foramen if the mandibular canal or inferior alveolar nerve is involved with tumor. The mandible is then retracted laterally and the soft tissue cuts are performed.

restoration of integrity, bulk, and sensation, but the complex motor functions of the oropharynx cannot be duplicated.

The use of local flaps has decreased significantly in the past two decades as a result of the limited amount of tissue they provide and their inferior functional results when compared with regional flaps and free tissue transfer. The regional flaps reliably provide abundant well-vascularized tissue that can be used for single-stage reconstruction, they are easy to harvest, and they do not require microvascular expertise. Their disadvantages include the limited superior reach, bulk, and the significant rate of marginal necrosis of the distal skin, especially with pectoralis major flaps. They also can rarely be tailored to reconstruct a defect that involves multiple sites. The free microvascular flaps overcome most deficiencies of the regional flaps and have the added advantage of sensory or motor reinnervation. The use of free tissue transfer along with conservative approaches to the mandible significantly decreases morbidity and length of hospitalization and results in improved

function at a cost comparable with regional myocutaneous flaps (46–48). The main disadvantages of free microvascular flaps that have prevented them from wide acceptance by head and neck surgeons are the prolongation of operative time and the need for special expertise. A free skin graft is also often a very viable method (48).

The other component essential for successful reconstruction is an intimate understanding of the ablated tissue's functional and cosmetic capacities. The tongue base is the structure most important to the function of the oropharynx, because it is responsible for pharyngeal closure during the oral phase and is the main driving force of the bolus through the pharyngeal phase (5). Optimal functional restoration requires the presence of at least one intact hypoglossal nerve and lingual artery to allow for mobility and survival of the remaining tongue. The reconstruction must restore some of the bulk, the glossopharyngeal fold, and ensure continued mobility of this organ (49,50). The pharyngeal walls help generate the pressure needed for appropriate movement of the food bolus and clear material remaining in the pharynx after a swallow. The remaining pharynx and the tongue can easily compensate for these functions after partial resection (51); therefore, a reconstruction that maintains the integrity of the pharynx and function of the base of the tongue is required. The soft palate is the most important component of the velopharyngeal mechanism, which also includes the lateral and posterior pharyngeal walls. Restoration of the soft palate's complex dynamic fibromuscular structure is not possible, but good velopharyngeal function is obtained if the reconstruction allows for the closure of the naso-pharynx with swallowing and an opening of no more than 20 mm² during speech (52). Defects that involve multiple sites provide a considerable challenge, and elaborate tech-niques often are required to achieve the reconstructive objectives because of the different requirements of each site. Patients with extensive defects involving most of the oropharyngeal walls or tongue base may require laryn-geal manipulation (suturing the thyroid ala anteriorly and superiorly to the mandible) to prevent chronic aspiration. Despite reconstruction, function may be suboptimal.

Soft Tissue Reconstruction

Choosing the appropriate reconstruction requires an indi-vidualized treatment plan based on careful consideration of all pertinent tumor-, defect-, and patient-related factors. Generally, the least complex method that restores function and form is selected. Sensory reinnervation of the flaps is pre-ferred whenever feasible, because pharyngeal function may benefit from such a reconstruction. Small defects of the pha-ryngeal walls up to 3 cm in largest dimension and those less than one-third the volume of the tongue base can be closed primarily, reconstructed using a split-thickness skin graft, or left to granulate if the defect does not communicate with the

neck. There are minimal functional deficits with these small defects. Larger lesions require some form of reconstruction, because primary closure results in poor function due to tongue tethering or pharyngeal stenosis. Free fasciocutane-ous flaps are well suited for these reconstructions, especially when the defect involves multiple sites, such as the pharyn-geal wall, soft palate, and tongue base. The thin and pliable nature of these flaps is ideal for pharyngeal wall reconstruc-tion, and bulk for the tongue base may be obtained by deep-ithelializing and burying part of the flap (50) (Fig. 121.8). Adequate reconstruction with myocutaneous regional flaps is achieved when the defect is mostly base of tongue, but these flaps tend to be too bulky for pharyngeal wall or soft pal-ate reconstruction, especially when mandibular continuity is maintained. In these situations, regional myofascial flaps are better suited because of the decreased bulk. It is important to remember, however, that only vascularized fat maintains its bulk, and following atrophy of these myofascial flaps, there may be insufficient bulk to sustain good results.

Small tumors of the soft palate that can be removed with partial-thickness resection and preservation of the poste-rior mucosa may be left to granulate with excellent func-tional results. Full-thickness defects are best reconstructed with fasciocutaneous flaps that are folded onto themselves and sutured to the remaining nasal and oral aspects of the soft palate (Fig. 121.8). Surgical adhesions are fashioned between the neopalate and the posterior pharyngeal wall to narrow the adynamic reconstructed segment of the velopha-ryngeal complex when the defect involves more than half the soft palate. Alternatively, a combination of fasciocuta-neous flaps and pharyngeal flaps also can be used (53,54). These reconstructions result in immediate and excellent function in most cases and may be further augmented with a prosthesis if needed after the radiation mucositis resolves. The use of prosthetics only is also an option, with good

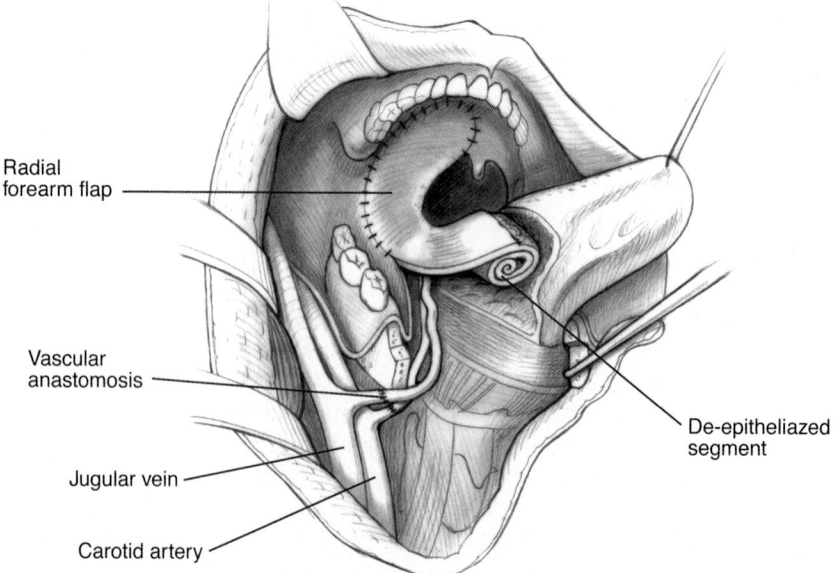

Figure 121.8 Reconstruction of the pha-ryngeal wall and tongue base with radial fore-arm fasciocutaneous flap. The distal flap is deepithelialized and rolled on itself to replace tongue base volume. The proximal flap is folded onto itself and sutured to the remain-ing nasal and oral aspects of the soft palate.

Radial forearm flap

Vascular anastomosis

Jugular vein

Carotid artery

De-epitheliazed segment

results obtained when the defect involves the total palate, movement of the residual velopharyngeal complex exists, and the patient has good supporting tissue to anchor the palatal device properly (49). The main disadvantage of prosthetics is the potential delay in function because definitive obturation cannot be performed until postoperative healing is complete and the acute radiation changes resolve. Also, foods can become trapped on the nasal side of the prosthesis with foul-smelling debris in the mouth.

Mandibular Reconstruction

Oropharyngeal cancers rarely invade the mandible, and with the use of mandibular preservation techniques, segmental resections are infrequent. Controversy exists regarding reconstruction of the lateral mandible; however, to achieve the best aesthetic and functional results, this defect should be reconstructed. Lateral mandibular defects can be reconstructed with bone containing free flaps, but newer generation reconstruction plates with soft tissue reconstruction have been shown to be an alternative for some patients (55).

COMPLICATIONS

Complications related to the management of oropharyngeal cancer patients are the same as those of any head and neck cancer patient and are listed in Table 121.6. Surgical

TABLE 121.6	COMPLICATIONS OROPHARYNGEAL CANCER TREATMENT

1. Radiation
   Mucositis
   Xerostomia
   Taste dysfunction
   Dysphagia
   Fibrosis
   Ulceration and tissue necrosis
   Osteoradionecrosis of the mandible
   Hypoglossal palsy
2. Surgical
   A. Approach related
      Damage to teeth
      Damage to nerves
      Cerebral embolism and carotid artery thrombosis
   B. Resection and reconstruction related
      Hemorrhage
      Wound infection and dehiscence
      Positive resection margin
      Pharyngocutaneous fistula
      Aspiration
      Dysphagia
      Poor speech
      Velopharyngeal incompetence
      Eustachian tube dysfunction
      Nonunion and osteomyelitis of the mandible
      Malocclusion and TMJ dysfunction

TABLE 121.7	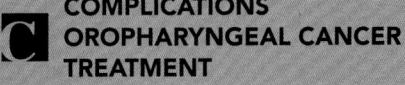 EMERGENCY CARE

1. Airway obstruction
2. Bleeding
3. Free tissue transfer vascular compromise

complications are more likely in patients previously treated with radiotherapy or chemoradiation. Radiotherapy complications can be reduced by using IMRT, but caution is advised as altered patterns of local recurrence have been reported in patients treated with IMRT (56).

EMERGENCIES

The most urgent problems that arise in oropharyngeal cancer patients are airway obstruction, bleeding, and free flap vascular compromise after reconstruction (Table 121.7). Airway obstruction is usually due to large exophytic tumors or edema from treatment. Imminent obstruction should be managed with a tracheotomy in the operating room with an anesthesiologist experienced in fiberoptic intubation. Bleeding from the tumor is usually controlled with selective cautery or embolization, but surgery with ligation of the carotid artery or its branches may be required in extreme situations. Bleeding from the carotid artery system itself (due to fistula or other wound complications) is life threatening, and hemorrhage can be controlled with embolization, endovascular stenting, or, as a last resort, carotid artery ligation. When free tissue transfer is used to reconstruct the surgical defect, any signs of arterial or venous compromise require immediate exploration of the vessels in an attempt to salvage the failing flap.

FOLLOW-UP

Oropharyngeal cancer patients require close observation initially to detect recurrences and lifelong follow-up after to identify second primaries. A general follow-up schedule after completion of treatment is provided in Table 121.8 (25). Chest radiographs, liver enzymes,

TABLE 121.8	FOLLOW-UP SCHEDULE AFTER COMPLETION OF TREATMENT

Years Posttreatment	Follow-Up
1st	1–3 mo
2nd	2–4 mo
3rd	3–6 mo
4th and 5th	4–6 mo
After 5th	Every 12 mo

and thyroid-stimulating hormone levels are obtained as indicated. Many centers now use a schema of serial PET/CT evaluation beginning 2 to 3 months after completion of therapy. Concurrent use of chest x-ray and CT seems wasteful. Recurrence after a normal post treatment PET/CT is unusual.

PROGNOSIS

Table 121.9 shows the expected actuarial 5-year survival of patients with oropharyngeal cancers (57). As previously mentioned, for selected groups, better results have been reported. Patients with early-stage cancer die of unrelated diseases or second primary tumors, because they are usually cured of their index tumor, whereas patients who have advanced disease often die of locoregional recurrence or distant metastasis. Patients with advanced disease treated with surgery and postoperative radiotherapy can be expected to have approximately a 50% 3-year survival and greater than 70% local control rate (58). The results are very similar with concurrent chemoradiation (59). HPV-positive cancers are more effectively controlled. HPV-positive patients with tobacco exposure represent an intermediate risk population. Clinical trials are seeking to optimize results while reducing toxicities.

NEW AND DEVELOPING TREATMENTS

The continued discovery of more active chemotherapeutic and biologic agents such as the monoclonal antibody inhibitor and tyrosine kinase inhibitors offers hope for the future. Refinement of diagnostic and reconstructive techniques offers improved cure rates and better function for oropharyngeal cancer patients. PET/CT scan has allowed detection of occult metastatic disease and persistent disease following nonsurgical therapy and may help in the future to guide the extent of surgery and the role of adjuvant therapy (59). Lymphoscintigraphy and sentinel node mapping and biopsy for oral cancer are now being studied in a multicenter cooperative group trial in the United States. Preliminary experience also suggests that it may be feasible in oropharyngeal carcinomas (60). Properly conducted quality of life studies with larger patient numbers will help predict functional outcomes for different treatments and

help determine which patients would be better served with a nonsurgical approach (49,54,61).

HIGHLIGHTS

- Cancer of the oropharynx is relatively uncommon; however, the incidence is rising primarily attributable to HPV-related tumor.
- SCC and its variants account for 90% of primary malignant oropharyngeal lesions, whereas lymphomas, minor salivary gland tumors, melanomas, and sarcomas make up the rest.
- The concept of "field cancerization" or "condemned mucosa" applies to all mucosal head and neck cancers and is the reason for the high rate of second primaries in oropharyngeal cancer patients.
- The complete visualization and palpation of the tumor under general anesthesia greatly facilitate the assessment of submucosal spread, invasion of surrounding structures such as the prevertebral fascia and mandible, and identification of second primary tumors.
- Almost all patients with oropharyngeal squamous cell cancers require some treatment of the neck because of the high rate of clinically positive nodes and occult nodal metastasis at presentation.
- N0 and N1 are usually adequately treated with a single modality, whereas a combined modality results in better regional control in N2 and N3 neck disease. Treatment often includes both necks and retropharyngeal nodes. Sentinel node mapping remains investigational.
- Successful extirpation of oropharyngeal cancers hinges on good exposure and wide resection margins because these tumors have the propensity for submucosal spread. Mandibular sparing procedures are used whenever possible.
- The appropriate reconstruction requires an individualized treatment plan based on careful consideration of all pertinent tumor-, defect-, and patient-related factors. Generally, the least complex method that restores function and form is selected. If good function cannot be maintained with surgery, a nonsurgical approach should be considered.
- Oropharyngeal cancer patients require close observation initially to detect recurrences and lifelong follow-up afterward to identify second primary tumors. Patients with early-stage cancer die of unrelated diseases or second primary tumors, whereas those with advanced disease die of locoregional recurrence or distal metastasis.
- HPV 16 is an independent risk factor for oropharyngeal carcinoma. HPV-positive tumors respond better to treatment and appear to have a survival benefit.

TABLE 121.9	THE 5-YEAR SURVIVAL OF OROPHARYNGEAL CANCER PATIENTS BY STAGE

Stage	5-Year Survival (%)
1	67
2	46
3	31
4	32

REFERENCES

1. Siegel R, Ward, E, Brawley O, et al. Cancer statistics, 2011. *CA Cancer J Clin* 2011;61:212–236.
2. Chaturvedi, AK, Engels EA, Anderson WF, et al. Incidence trends for human papillomavirus-related and -unrelated oral squamous cell carcinomas in the United States. *J Clin Oncol* 2008;26:612–619.
3. Jemal A, Tiwari RC, Murray T, et al.; American Cancer Society. Cancer statistics, 2004. *CA Cancer J Clin* 2004;54:829.
4. Curtin HD. Separation of the masticator space from the parapharyngeal space. *Radiology* 1987;163(1):195–204.
5. Rosenthal KI, Lewin JS, Eisbruch A. Prevention and treatment of dysphagia and aspiration after chemoradiation for head and neck cancer. *J Clin Oncol* 2006;24:2636–2643.
6. Myers JN. Molecular pathogenesis of squamous cell carcinoma of the head and neck. In: Myers EN, Suen JY, eds. *Cancer of the head and neck.* Philadelphia, PA: WB Saunders, 1996:5–16.
7. Marur S, Forastiere AA. Head and neck cancer: changing epidemiology, diagnosis and treatment. *Mayo Clin Proc* 2008;83:489–501.
8. Mashberg A, Boffetta P, Winkelman R, et al. Tobacco smoking, alcohol drinking and cancer of the oral cavity and oropharynx among US veterans. *Cancer* 1993;72:1369–1375.
9. Gassner HG, Sabri AN, Olsen KD. Oropharyngeal malignancy. In: Cummings CW, ed. *Cummings's otolaryngology-head and neck surgery.* St. Louis, MO: Mosby, 2005.
10. Goldenberg D, Lee J, Koch WM, et al. Habitual risk factors for head and neck cancer. *Otolaryngol Head Neck Surg* 2004;131(6):986–993.
11. Kreimer AR, Clifford GM, Boyle P, et al. Human papillomavirus types in head and neck squamous cell carcinomas worldwide: a systematic review. *Cancer Epidemiol Biomarkers Prev* 2005;14(2):467–475.
12. Fakhry C, Westra WH, Li S, et al. Improved survival of patients with human papillomavirus-positive head (Fakhry and neck squamous cell carcinoma in a prospective clinical trial. *J Natl Cancer Inst* 2008;100:261–269.
13. Gillison ML, D'Souza G, Westra W, et al. Distinct risk factor profiles for human papillomavirus type 16-positive and human papillomavirus type 16-negaive head and neck cancers. *J Natl Cancer Inst* 2008;100:407–420.
14. D'Souza G, Kerimer AR, Viscidi R, et al. Case-control study of human papillomavirus and oropharyngeal cancer. *N Engl J Med* 2007;356:1944–1956.
15. Mork J, Lie AK, Glattre E, et al. Human papillomavirus infection as a risk factor for squamous-cell carcinoma of the head and neck. *N Engl J Med* 2001;244:1125–1131.
16. Singh B, Balwally AN, Shaha AR, et al. Upper aerodigestive tract squamous cell carcinoma. The human immunodeficiency virus connection. *Arch Otolaryngol Head Neck* 1996;122:639–643.
17. Chandler SW, Rassekh CH, Rodman SM, et al. Immunohistochemical localization of interleukin-10 in human oral and pharyngeal carcinomas. *Laryngoscope* 2002;112:808–815.
18. Zelefsky MJ, Harrison LB, Armstrong JG. Long-term treatment results of postoperative radiation therapy for advanced stage oropharyngeal carcinoma. *Cancer* 1992;70:2388–2395.
19. Tsue TT, McCulloch TM, Girod DA, et al. Predictors of carcinomatous invasion of the mandible. *Head Neck* 1994;16:116–126.
20. Jesse RH, Fletcher GH. Metastasis in cervical lymph node from oropharyngeal carcinoma treatment and results. *AJR Am J Roentgenol* 1963;90:990–996.
21. Chung TS, Stefani S. Distant metastases of carcinoma of tonsillar region: a study of 475 patients. *J Surg Oncol* 1980;14:5–9.
22. Gourin CG, Johnson JT. Incidence of unsuspected metastases in lateral cervical cysts. *Laryngoscope* 2000;110:1637–1641
23. Carroll WR, Locher JL, Canon CL, et al. Pretreatment swallowing exercises improve swallow function after chemoradiation. *Laryngoscope* 2008;118:39–43.
24. Karni RJ, Rich JT, Sinha P, et al. Transoral laser microsurgery: a new approach for unknown primaries of the head and neck. *Laryngoscope* 2011;121:1194–1201.
25. Machtay M, Rosenthal DI, Hershock D, et al. Organ preservation therapy using induction plus concurrent chemoradiation for advanced resectable oropharyngeal carcinoma: University of Pennsylvania Phase II trial. *J Clin Oncol* 2002;20:3964–3971.
26. Selek U, Garden AS, Morrison MF, et al. Radiotherapy for early-stage carcinoma of the oropharynx. *Int J Radiat Oncol Biol Phys* 2004;59:743–751.
27. Fu KK, Pajak TF, Trotti A, et al. Radiotherapy Oncology Group (RTOG) phase III randomized study to compare hyperfractionation and two variants of accelerated fractionation to standard fractionation radiotherapy for head and neck squamous cell carcinomas: fist report of RTOG 9003. *Int J Radiat Oncol Biol Phys* 2000;48:7–16.
28. Rich JT, Milov S, Lewis JS, Thorstad WL, et al. Transoral laser microsurgery (TLM) ± adjuvant therapy for advanced stage oropharyngeal cancer. *Laryngoscope* 2009;119:1709–1719.
29. Houck JR, Shaha A. Oropharynx. In: Medina JE, Chairman, eds. *Clinical practice guidelines for the diagnosis and management of cancer of the head and neck. Presented at the meeting of the American Society for Head and Neck Surgery and the Society of Head and Neck Surgeons.* Los Angeles, CA: The American Society for Head and Neck Surgery, 1996:25–29.
30. Galati LT, Myers EN, Johnson JT. Primary surgery as a treatment for early squamous cell carcinoma of the tonsil. *Head Neck* 2000;22:294–296.
31. Cooper JS, Pajak TF, Forastiere AA, et al. Radiation Therapy Oncology Group 9501/Intergroup. Postoperative concurrent radiotherapy and chemotherapy for high-risk squamous-cell carcinoma of the head and neck. *N Engl J Med* 2004;350:1937–1944.
32. Chung EJ, Oh JI, Choi KY, et al. Pattern of cervical lymph node metastasis in tonsil cancer: predictive factor analysis of contralateral and retropharyngeal lymph node metastasis. *Oral Oncol* 2011;47(8):758–762.
33. Tauzin M, Rabalais A, Hagan JL, et al. PET-CT staging of the neck in cancers of the oropharynx: patterns of regional and retropharyngeal nodal metastasis. *World J Surg Oncol* 2010;8:70–74.
34. Chen KS, Majhail N, Huang CJ, et al. Intensity-modulated radiation therapy reduces late salivary toxicity without compromising tumor control in patients with oropharyngeal carcinoma: a comparison with conventional techniques. *Radiother Oncol* 2001;61:275–280.
35. Smith RV, Goldman SY, Beitler JJ, et al. Decreased short-and-long-term swallowing problems with altered radiotherapy dosing used in an organ-sparing protocol for advanced pharyngeal carcinoma. *Arch Otolaryngol Head Neck Surg* 2004;130:831–836.
36. Brizel DM, Prosnitz RG, Hunter S, et al. Necessity for adjuvant neck dissection in setting of concurrent chemoradiation for advanced head-and-neck cancer. *Int J Radiat Oncol Biol Phys* 2004;58:1418–1423.
37. Nayak JV, Walvekar RR, Andrade RS, et al. Deferring planned neck dissection following chemoradiation for stage IV head and neck cancer. The utility of PET-CT. *Laryngoscope* 2007;117:2129–2134.
38. Steiner W, Fierek O, Ambrosch P, et al. Transoral laser microsurgery for squamous cell carcinoma of the base of the tongue. *Arch Otolaryngol Head Neck Surg* 2003;129:36–43.
39. Laccourreye O, Hans S, Menard M, et al. Transoral lateral oropharyngectomy for squamous cell carcinoma of the tonsillar region: II. An analysis of the incidence, related variable, and consequences of local recurrence. *Arch Otolaryngol Head Neck Surg* 2005;131:592–599.
40. Hockstein NG, O'Malley BW Jr, Weinstein GS. Assessment of intraoperative safety in transoral robotic surgery. *Laryngoscope* 2006;116:165–168.
41. O'Malley BW Jr, Weinstein GS, Snyder W, et al. Transoral robotic surgery (TORS) for base of tongue neoplasms. *Laryngoscope* 2006;116:1465–1472.
42. Weinstein GS, O'Malley BW Jr, Snyder W, et al. Transoral robotic surgery: radical tonsillectomy. *Arch Otolaryngol Head Neck Surg* 2007;133:1220–1226.
43. Dean NR, Rosenthal EL, Carroll WR, et al. Robotic-assisted surgery for primary or recurrent oropharyngeal carcinoma. *Arch Otolaryngol Head Neck Surg* 2010;136(4):380–384.
44. Rassekh CH, Janecka IP, Calhoun KH. Lower lip splitting incisions: anatomic considerations. *Laryngoscope* 1995;105(8 Pt 1):880–883.
45. Christopoulos E, Canan R, Segas T, et al. Transmandibular approaches to the oral cavity and oropharynx—a functional assessment. *Arch Otolaryngol Head Neck Surg* 1992;118:1164–1167.

46. O'Brien CJ, Nettle W, Lee KK. Changing trends in the management of carcinoma of the oral cavity and oropharynx. *Aust N Z J Surg* 1993;63:270–274.

47. Tsue TT, Desyatnikova SS, Deleyiannis FW, et al. Comparison of cost and function in reconstruction of posterior oral cavity and oropharynx. Free vs pedicled soft tissue transfer. *Arch Otolaryngol Head Neck Surg* 1997;123:731–737.

48. Sabri A. Oropharyngeal reconstruction: current state of the art. *Curr Opin Otolaryngol Head Neck Surg* 2003;11:251–254.

49. Friedlander P, Caruana S, Singh B, et al. Functional status after primary surgical therapy for squamous cell carcinoma of the base of the tongue. *Head Neck* 2002;24:111–114.

50. Salibian AH, Allison GR, Krugman ME, et al. Reconstruction of the base of tongue with the microvascular ulnar forearm flap: a functional assessment. *Plast Reconstruct Surg* 1995;96:1081–1089.

51. Walther EK. Dysphagia after pharyngolaryngeal cancer surgery. Part 1: pathophysiology of postsurgical deglutition. *Dysphagia* 1995;10:275–278.

52. Curtis TA, Beumer J III. Speech, velopharyngeal function, and restoration of soft palate defects. In: Curtis TA, Beumer J III, Marunick MT, eds. *Maxillofacial rehabilitation prosthodontic and surgical consideration*. St. Louis, MO: Ishiyaku EuroAmerica, 1996:285–329.

53. Brown JS, Zuydam AC, Jones DC, et al. Functional outcome in soft palate reconstruction using a radial forearm free flap in conjunction with a superiorly based pharyngeal flap. *Head Neck* 1997;19:524–534.

54. Seikaly H, Rieger J, Wolfaardt J, et al. Functional outcomes after primary oropharyngeal cancer resection and reconstruction with the radial forearm free flap. *Laryngoscope* 2003;113:897–904.

55. Blackwell KE, Lacombe V. The bridging lateral mandibular reconstruction plate revisited. *Arch Otolaryngol Head Neck Surg* 1999;125:988–993.

56. Eisbruch A, Marsh LH, Dawson LA, et al. Recurrence near base of skull after IMRT for head-and-neck cancer: implications for target delineation in high neck and for parotid gland sparing. *Int J Radiat Oncol Biol Phys* 2004;59:28–42.

57. Pugliano FA, Piccirillo JF, Zequeira MR, et al. Clinical severity staging system for oropharyngeal cancer: five-year survival rates. *Arch Otolaryngol Head Neck Surg* 1997;123:1118–1124.

58. Denittis AS, Machtay M, Rosenthal DJ, et al. Advanced oropharyngeal carcinoma treated with surgery and radiotherapy: oncologic outcome and functional assessment. *Am J Otolaryngol* 2001;22:329–335.

59. Mantz CA, Vokes EE, Stenson K, et al. Induction chemotherapy followed by concomitant chemoradiotherapy in the treatment of locoregionally advanced oropharyngeal carcinoma. *Cancer J* 2001;7:140–148.

60. Ross G, Shoaib T, Soutar DS, et al. The use of sentinel node biopsy to upstage the clinically N0 neck in head and cancer. *Arch Otolaryngol Head Neck Surg* 2002;128:1287–1291.

61. Gillespie MB, Brodsky MB, Day TA, et al. Swallowing-related quality of life after head and neck cancer treatment. *Laryngoscope* 2004;114:1362–1367.

Hypopharyngeal and Cervical Esophageal Carcinoma

122

Mihir Kiran Bhayani   *Randal S. Weber*

Hypopharyngeal and cervical esophageal malignancies are rare upper aerodigestive tract cancers that create a treatment challenge for head and neck surgeons. Although the hypopharynx and cervical esophagus are two separate subsites, the management of carcinoma in this area is, for the most part, similar. These tumors are characterized by multicentricity, submucosal spread, and early lymphatic metastasis. Patients typically present with advanced-stage disease and severe malnutrition that requires a multidisciplinary approach to their care. This multidisciplinary team must consist of the head and neck surgeon, radiation oncologist, medical oncologist, plastic surgeon, speech pathologist, and nutritionist to help guide the treatment to not only remove the disease but to maintain as much of the patient's baseline function from before the tumor arose.

Despite these efforts from multiple fronts, the overall prognosis of patients with these tumors is poor. Advancements in surgical technique have been expanded to transoral techniques that may minimize the morbidity from major resections. Sequential chemotherapy and innovations with radiation techniques as part of clinical trials have resulted in larynx preservation without compromising survival (1–3). Together, these improvements result in improved function without compromising disease-free intervals. Enhanced microsurgical techniques with a diverse range of reconstructive flaps have created many options for surgical approaches in the primary and salvage setting. Thus, the development of a sound approach to patients with these tumors must include a thorough understanding of the anatomy, pathology, and clinical signs when preparing the most appropriate treatment.

ANATOMY

The hypopharynx begins at the level of the hyoid bone where it borders the oropharynx superiorly and funnels inferiorly to the cervical esophagus at the level of the inferior cricoid cartilage (Fig. 122.1). Three subsites make up the hypopharynx: the pyriform sinuses laterally, the postcricoid area anteriorly, and the pharyngeal wall posteriorly (Fig. 122.2). The paired pyriform sinuses lie in the form of inverted pyramids that begin at the pharyngoepiglottic folds superiorly and the apex blending into the cervical esophagus at its inferior extent. The postcricoid area represents the mucosa overlying the posterior portion of the cricoid ring. It extends from the arytenoid cartilage to the inferior border of the cricoid cartilage. The proximity of the pyriform sinuses and the postcricoid area to the larynx can lead to direct invasion of tumors of these regions into the paraglottic space and laryngeal skeleton. The posterior pharyngeal wall is the portion of the hypopharynx overlying the vertebrae. Tumors of this area can directly invade the potential retropharyngeal space, paraspinous muscles, and prevertebral fascia, making complete resection extremely difficult.

The lining of the hypopharynx is stratified squamous epithelium that overlies a submucosal loose areolar tissue layer, followed by a muscular layer made up of the posterior cricoarytenoid muscles anteriorly and the middle/inferior pharyngeal constrictors posteriorly and laterally. These structures are enclosed by the buccopharyngeal fascia. The muscular layer is notable because tumor extension from the posterior cricoid mucosa can invade into the posterior cricoarytenoid muscles causing vocal cord fixation, and the inferior constrictor muscles blend into the cricopharyngeus muscle inferiorly where the potential area weakness, Killian triangle, is located. Although this region is noted for the site of pharyngeal diverticula, tumor extension to the prevertebral space is also possible.

The vascular supply of the hypopharynx comes from the external carotid system and includes branches of the superior thyroid artery and ascending pharyngeal and lingual arteries. Venous drainage mirrors the arterial system in addition to the prevertebral venous plexus.

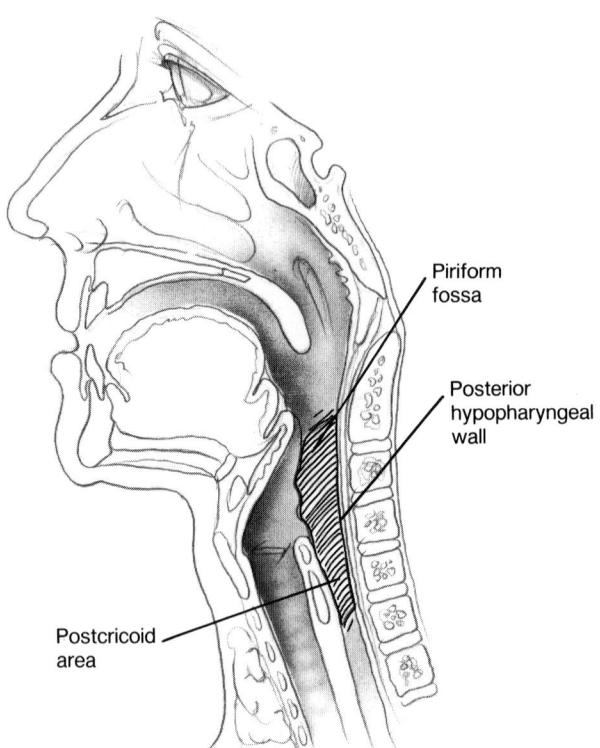

Figure 122.1 The hypopharyngeal region extends from a point at the superior edge of the body of the hyoid bone down to the inferior aspect of the cricoid cartilage; it is composed of the piriform fossa, the posterior hypopharyngeal wall, and the postcricoid area.

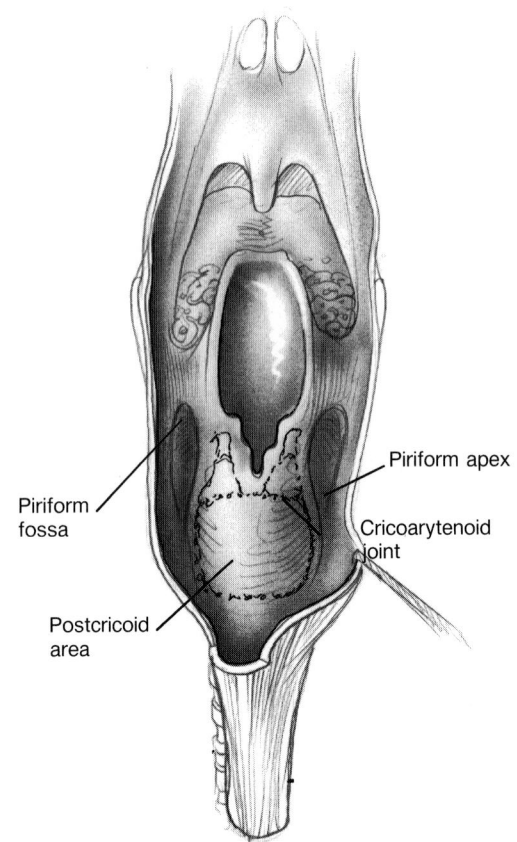

Figure 122.2 The piriform apex is at the junction between the inferior aspect of the piriform fossa and the postcricoid region. It marks the location of the cricoarytenoid joint.

Sensory innervation to the hypopharynx is derived from branches of the glossopharyngeal and vagus nerves via the pharyngeal plexus and the internal branch of the superior laryngeal nerve. The latter nerve pierces the thyrohyoid membrane and joins with the vagus nerve where fibers coalesce with branches of Arnold nerve to the external auditory canal. This connection can result in the referred otalgia seen in many patients with hypopharyngeal pathology. Motor innervation to the pharyngeal constrictors comes from the pharyngeal plexus, while the posterior cricoarytenoid muscles are innervated by the recurrent laryngeal nerve.

The hypopharynx has an extensive network of lymphatics. Drainage can occur laterally to the jugulodigastric nodes (Fig. 122.3). The second drainage pathway is posterior to the retropharyngeal nodes and can extend as high as the skull base in the nodes of Rouviere. Inferiorly, nodal metastases can occur in the paratracheal and paraesophageal nodes (4). Bilateral drainage is common, especially for lesions located in the medial pyriform and posterior pharyngeal wall.

The cervical esophagus begins at the inferior extent of the hypopharynx and extends to the thoracic inlet. It can vary in length depending on the length and angle of the neck. The lining of the cervical esophagus is stratified squamous epithelium that covers a submucosal layer that is rich in lymphatic vessels. The muscular layer contains the bilayered esophageal muscles, with an internal circular layer and external longitudinal layer. The serosa is a continuation of the buccopharyngeal fascia. Arterial supply to this region comes from the inferior thyroid circulation off the thyrocervical trunk, and venous drainage occurs via the inferior thyroid veins. Innervation is derived from the recurrent laryngeal nerve and sympathetic chain. Lymphatic drainage occurs in the paraesophageal and paratracheal nodes, which can then spread to the superior mediastinum or lateral cervical nodes.

EPIDEMIOLOGY

In the United States and Canada, two large studies of national cancer registries have shed light on the presence of hypopharynx carcinoma in the population. In a review of the National Cancer Data Base (NCDB), a hospital-based cancer registry that covers the entire United States, hypopharyngeal carcinomas account for approximately 3% to 4% of all head and neck cancers, which account for approximately 3% of all cancers (5,6). Of note, this report also showed that the percentage of hypopharyngeal carcinoma cases decreased nearly 30% from 2000 to 2004 compared to the 1990 to 1994 (5). This number has been attributed to the decrease in cigarette smoking among

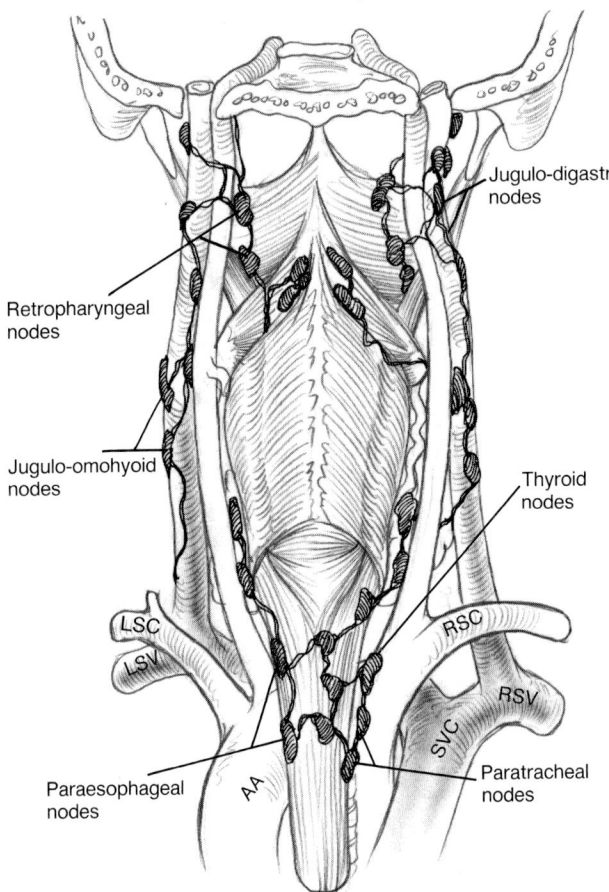

Figure 122.3 The primary lymph node drainage of the hypopharynx. Cancers of the superior hypopharynx metastasize to the jugulodigastric and retropharyngeal nodes, whereas those of the inferior hypopharynx, including the piriform apex, metastasize to the jugulo-omohyoid, paraesophageal, paratracheal, and thyroid lymph nodes. AA, aortic arch; LSC, left subclavian artery; LSV, left subclavian vein; RSC, right subclavian artery; RSV, right subclavian vein; SVC, superior vena cava.

Americans (7). A previous review of the NCDB revealed that 77% of patients with hypopharynx carcinoma present with stage III or IV disease (8). Of note, the survival in the most recent update of the NCDB showed hypopharynx carcinoma to have the worst survival of any primary head and neck mucosal surface malignancy, with a 5-year overall survival around 35% (5).

A review of the data pooled from multiple Canadian cancer registries from 1990 to 1999 revealed that hypopharynx cancer is 5% of all head and neck cancers (9). In Canada, this represents an incidence of approximately 0.8 new cases per 100,000 persons/year. Peak incidence was seen in the sixth and seventh decades of life with 80% of cases being male. Similar to the NCDB data, 74% of patients presented with advanced-stage disease, and survival was 35% at 5 years.

Cervical esophageal carcinoma is difficult to assess, as they are very rare and many times mislabeled as thoracic esophageal carcinoma or hypopharyngeal carcinoma as

the tumors grow. They have been reported to account for between 2% and 10% of all esophageal carcinomas (10). In 2010, esophageal carcinoma represented 5% of all digestive system cancers, estimated at 16,640 new cases with 14,500 deaths, thus explaining the paucity of data with cervical esophageal carcinoma (6).

ETIOLOGY

Tobacco smoking and alcohol are well-established risk factors for upper aerodigestive tract tumors. In a recent study reviewing smoking in Europeans, the association with active tobacco smoking was strongest for cancer risk of hypopharynx compared to the oral cavity, oropharynx, and esophagus (11). Alcohol intake appears to be more common in patients with hypopharyngeal cancer when compared with laryngeal cancer and is considered an independent risk factor in the development of hypopharyngeal carcinoma when controlled for smoking (12). Daily consumption of alcohol has been found to increase the risk of hypopharyngeal carcinoma by 2.2 (13). The mechanism of carcinogenesis by alcohol is unclear. Many believe it has a direct carcinogenic effect on the hypopharyngeal mucosa, potentiates tobacco, or is related to the poor nutritional status in alcoholics that contributes to the development of hypopharyngeal carcinoma (14). The use of smokeless tobacco products has also been implicated as a cause of hypopharynx cancer increasing the risk by 4.6 in a study from India (13).

Another causative factor for hypopharyngeal carcinoma that is specifically associated with the postcricoid mucosa is Plummer-Vinson syndrome. This syndrome is characterized by dysphagia, iron deficiency anemia, and hypopharyngeal webs. Chronic irritation of the webs is thought to be the causative factor in the progression to carcinoma.

DIAGNOSIS

Patient Evaluation

Most patients with hypopharyngeal and cervical esophageal carcinoma present at an advanced stage with a multitude of presenting symptoms. A review of the Canadian Cancer Registry found that the most common symptoms in patients presenting with hypopharyngeal carcinoma were dysphagia (53%), hoarseness (39%), neck mass (37%), weight loss (36%), sore throat (34%), and otalgia (30%) (9). Airway distress and voice changes can be seen in advanced tumors by direct invasion into the larynx. Progressive dysphagia for liquids and solids points to larger primary tumors. Chronic throat clearing and globus sensation may initially be diagnosed as reflux disease, but in cases that are refractory to medical therapy, hypopharyngeal or esophageal carcinoma should be ruled out. Unilateral otalgia with a normal otologic exam should lead to full evaluation of the upper aerodigestive tract.

After evaluation of presenting symptoms, a comprehensive medical history includes information regarding smoking and alcohol use. A prior history of iron deficiency anemia in middle-aged women points to Plummer-Vinson syndrome. Pulmonary and cardiac history is assessed in planning for future treatment. A review of systems can elicit significant weight loss and malnutrition (Table 122.1)

Physical Exam

The general status of the patient is the initial observation during the physical examination of patients with hypopharyngeal or cervical esophageal carcinoma. With chronic alcoholism, patients typically have nutritional deficiencies and weight loss. Patients may appear thin and dehydrated and have poor hygiene.

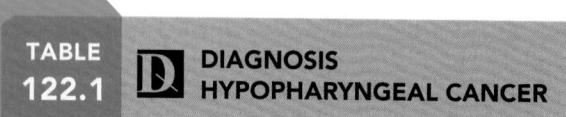

| TABLE 122.1 | **D** DIAGNOSIS HYPOPHARYNGEAL CANCER |

History
Treated for pharyngitis
Tobacco and ethanol abuse
Weight loss
Dehydration
Odynophagia
Dysphagia
Hoarseness
Dyspnea
Otalgia
Neck mass
Airway obstruction
Support group status

Physical
Weight loss or cachexia
Decreased skin turgor
Hyporesonant voice
Hoarseness
Stridor
Status of dentition
Indirect examination with mirror
Flexible fiberoptic laryngoscopy
Full neck examination

Radiology
Chest radiograph
Barium swallow
CT or MRI of the neck

Laboratory
Complete chemistries
Staging endoscopy and biopsy
Control of airway
Complete paralysis
Gross characteristics of tumor
Three-dimensional relationships of tumor
Biopsy
Determination of inferior border
Esophagoscopy
Bronchoscopy, if warranted

CT, computed tomography; MRI, magnetic resonance imaging.

The head and neck examination begins with evaluation of the facial skin, which can have decreased turgor and increased pallor. Examination of the oral cavity includes a dental evaluation since most patients will require radiation therapy. Poor dentition is also an indicator of malnutrition and hypovitaminosis. The oral cavity and oropharynx also needs to be evaluated for second primary malignancies.

Evaluation of the hypopharynx and larynx can be done using indirect mirror exam, if possible. If secretions or patient comfort does not allow full mirror exam, then endoscopic evaluation is performed. Appearance of the larynx must rule out obstructing mass, direct tumor invasion, or vocal cord paralysis. Evaluation of the hypopharynx should include assessment of any ulceration or mass lesion present in the pyriform fossae, pharyngeal wall, or postcricoid area. The pyriform fossae are best seen when the patient performs a puffed cheek maneuver. Evaluation of the cervical esophagus is limited in the office setting and should be reserved for a flexible or rigid evaluation under sedation.

Palpation of the neck to evaluate for clinically apparent nodes is a necessity. Hypopharyngeal and cervical esophageal carcinomas have a high rate of cervical metastasis; therefore, a thorough evaluation of the neck is mandatory.

Imaging

The goal of imaging in patients with hypopharyngeal and cervical esophageal carcinoma is to evaluate the extent of the primary disease and presence of regional or distant metastasis. Since hypopharyngeal and cervical esophageal carcinoma are characterized by submucosal spread of disease, the ideal imaging modality should facilitate identification of the full extent to the primary. Computed tomography (CT) of the neck with IV contrast is the imaging modality of choice to assess the primary disease by most practitioners. Magnetic resonance imaging (MRI) is an alternative to CT and can provide greater soft tissue delineation; however, the patient with an obstructing hypopharyngeal and cervical esophageal carcinoma may find it difficult to lay supine for extended period due to aspiration risk. CT has been historically used to detect cartilage invasion, but multiple studies have found MRI to be equivalent compared to CT in detecting neoplastic cartilage invasion (15). A study from Switzerland investigated the accuracy of MRI and CT in a cohort of 44 patients undergoing surgical resection of their hypopharyngeal cancer. The authors found that MRI was more sensitive than CT in detecting neoplastic invasion of the laryngeal cartilage, but CT was more specific. Overall accuracy of both modalities was equivalent (MRI, 78% and CT, 75%) (16). Due to practical reasons and patient comfort, though, CT is the preferred modality for many practitioners.

In evaluating for regional disease, contrast-enhanced CT has been the imaging modality of choice since the primary site is also covered. Distant disease can be evaluated using multiple imaging modalities. Many patients with early-stage disease may have a chest radiograph as the only screening radiograph. With higher nodal stage, the risk of distant metastasis increases. Therefore, chest CT is the preferred imaging modality (17,18). A study from Toronto found that higher stage hypopharynx primary disease (T3–4/N2–3) has five times the increased risk of having either synchronous second primary or distant metastasis, and they recommend chest CT in all patients with advanced-stage hypopharynx primary tumors (19). Another imaging modality used to investigate distant metastasis or synchronous second primary tumor is 18-fluorodeoxyglucose positron-emission tomography (FDG-PET). PET scans can be fused with CT scans for improved evaluation of the anatomic location of FDG avid lesions. It has been found superior to chest radiograph and chest CT in many studies (20–22). The advantage of PET–CT is whole body scanning for distant metastasis at the time of diagnosis. However, further studies need to be performed to evaluate the cost-effectiveness of PET–CT over traditional chest CT and bone scanning for screening of distant metastasis in patients with hypopharynx and cervical esophageal cancer.

Nutritional Evaluation

Standard laboratory evaluation should be performed on all patients who present with hypopharyngeal and cervical esophageal cancer at the initial visit. Blood counts, electrolytes, thyroid stimulating hormone, vitamin, iron, prealbumin, transferrin, and albumin levels are appropriate initial tests that are completed. In severely malnourished patients, a referral to a dietician and placement of a feeding tube are appropriate. Prior to placement of feeding tube, one must consider the reconstructive method to be carried out since location of the tube in either the stomach or jejunum can affect reconstructive options.

PATHOLOGY

Squamous cell carcinoma is the most common histology seen in the hypopharyngeal and cervical esophageal cancer, representing over 95% of cases (9). Three variants are commonly seen in the hypopharynx. The first is basaloid squamous cell carcinoma, which has a more aggressive course. Lymphoepithelial carcinomas are similar in nature to nasopharyngeal carcinoma. Adenosquamous carcinoma is the third variant with a similar aggressive course to basaloid squamous cell carcinoma. The remaining 5% of histologies consist of adenocarcinomas, thought to arise from ectopic gastric mucosa, lymphomas, and sarcomas (8).

Patterns of Spread

A distinguishing feature of hypopharyngeal and cervical esophageal carcinomas is submucosal extension of the tumors. An understanding of the patterns of spread of tumors begins with the site of origin. Most hypopharynx

		Stage			
TABLE 122.2	**HYPOPHARYNGEAL CANCER: STAGING (EASTERN VIRGINIA MEDICAL SCHOOL EXPERIENCE)**				
Location	No. (%)	I	II	III	IV
Piriform fossa	63 (64)	11	10	24	18
Posterior wall	30 (30)	5	15	8	2
Postcricoid	4 (4)	—	—	3	1

Eastern Virginia Medical School experience of 97 previously untreated patients, 1972 to 1985.

cancers are located in the pyriform sinuses, followed by the posterior pharyngeal wall, and then the postcricoid mucosa (Table 122.2) (23). Submucosal extension is more common in the inferior hypopharynx and cervical esophagus, thought to be caused by the rich submucosal lymphatic network seen at the pharyngoesophageal junction. Satellite lesions are also a characteristic of these tumors; however, it is difficult to determine if these tumors are separate primary tumors or metastatic lesions. The presence of submucosal extension, especially in the inferior hypopharynx and cervical esophagus, must be taken into account when assessing margins during surgical resection. It has generally been recommended that 3-cm margins be taken in the cervical esophagus and inferior hypopharynx, 2 cm laterally and 1.5 cm along the superior margin.

Tumors of the pyriform fossae can spread laterally to the thyroid cartilage and soft tissues of the neck. Medial extension of these tumors will involve the larynx and the paraglottic space (Fig. 122.4). Postcricoid tumors tend to grow circumferentially. Inferior extension via submucosal spread involves the cervical esophagus. Anterior extension spreads to the cricoarytenoid joint and posterior cricoarytenoid muscles causing vocal cord immobility (Fig. 122.5). Advanced cases of hypopharyngeal carcinoma can present with direct invasion into the thyroid gland (24).

Lymph node metastases are common in hypopharyngeal carcinoma with 64% to 90% of patients presenting with nodal disease and bilateral disease seen in 8% to 16% of cases (9,25,26). Regional metastasis occurs in levels II to IV, with rare involvement of levels I and V (25,27). Invasion of the pyriform apex (20%), postcricoid mucosa (57%), and subglottis is associated with metastasis in the paratracheal and paraesophageal nodes (4,28,29). Mediastinal nodal involvement is noted in 73% to 80% of T4 hypopharynx cancers and 33% to 62% of cervical esophageal carcinomas of all stages (30,31). Forty-three percent of cervical esophageal carcinomas are noted to have paratracheal and paraesophageal nodal disease (29). Retropharyngeal nodal disease is seen in 20% to 50% of patients with hypopharyngeal and cervical esophageal cancers (32–34). The significant percentage of nodal metastasis in hypopharyngeal and cervical esophageal percentage

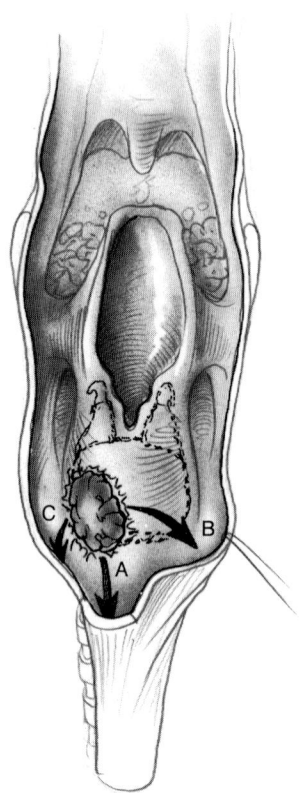

Figure 122.4 Lymph node and submucosal spread of piriform fossa cancer. Submucosal spread inferiorly (*A*) can involve the piriform apex and then metastases to the paratracheal, paraesophageal, thyroid, and jugulo-omohyoid nodes (*B*). Medial extension (*C*) involves the arytenoid and perilaryngeal compartments.

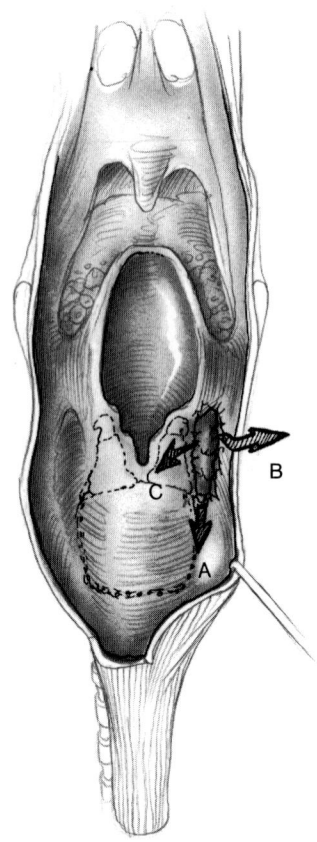

Figure 122.5 Lymph node and submucosal spread of postcricoid cancer. Submucosal spread inferiorly (*A*) can be extensive, and these lesions frequently metastasize to the paratracheal, thyroid, and paraesophageal nodes (*B,C*).

requires treatment of the nodal basins that are specific to each subsite of these regions.

Staging

The seventh edition of the American Joint Committee on Cancer Staging Manual has similar TNM staging compared to the sixth edition manual. This staging system facilitates the study of prognostic variables as related to the volume of local, regional, and distant disease. T4 tumors are divided into T4a (resectable; advanced local disease) and T4b (low likelihood of resection free margins; very advanced local disease). This has led to stratification of stage IV disease into IVA (moderately advanced local/regional disease), IVB (very advanced local/regional disease), and IVC (distant metastatic disease). The TNM staging for the hypopharynx is as follows:

TX: Primary tumor cannot be assessed.

T0: No evidence of primary tumor

Tis: Carcinoma *in situ*

T1: Tumor limited to one subsite and ≤2 cm in greatest dimension

T2: Tumor invades more than one subsite of the hypopharynx or adjacent site, or measures greater than

2 cm but not ≤4 cm in greatest dimension without larynx fixation.

T3: Tumor greater than 4 cm in greatest dimension or with fixation of the hemilarynx

T4a: Tumor invades thyroid/cricoids cartilage, hyoid bone, thyroid gland, esophagus, or central compartment soft tissue.

T4b: Tumor invades prevertebral fascia, encases carotid artery, or involves mediastinal structure.

NX: Regional lymph nodes cannot be assessed.

N0: No regional lymph node metastasis

N1: Metastasis in a single ipsilateral lymph node less than 3 cm in greatest dimension

N2a: Metastasis in a single ipsilateral lymph node ≥3 cm but less than 6 cm in greatest dimension

N2b: Metastasis in multiple ipsilateral lymph nodes, all less than 6 cm in greatest dimension

N2c: Metastasis in bilateral lymph nodes, all less than 6 cm in greatest dimension

N3: Metastasis in lymph node is ≥6 cm in greatest dimension

MX: Distant metastasis cannot be assessed.

M0: No distant metastasis

M1: Distant metastasis

The TNM staging system for the cervical esophagus is different from the hypopharynx. T stage is based on tumor depth of invasion, and N stage is based on the number of nodes present. The staging system has been updated since the sixth edition and is as follows:

TX: Primary tumor cannot be assessed.

T0: No evidence of primary tumor

Tis: Carcinoma *in situ*

T1: Tumor invades lamina propria or submucosa.

T2: Tumor invades muscularis propria.

T3: Tumor invades adventitia.

T4: Tumor invades adjacent structures (hypopharynx, thyroid gland, carotid sheath).

    T4a: Resectable disease

    T4b: Unresectable disease

NX: Regional lymph nodes cannot be assessed.

N0: No regional nodal metastasis

N1: Regional lymph node metastasis 1 to 2 nodes

N2: Regional lymph node metastasis in 3 to 6

N3: Regional lymph node metastasis in greater than 7 nodes

MX: Distant metastasis cannot be assessed

M0: No distant metastasis

M1: Distant metastasis

Molecular Staging

Hypopharyngeal and cervical esophageal cancers have distinct clinical behavior compared to other head and neck cancers; however, no specific molecular markers have paralleled this behavior. One study found an association between the stem cell markers, Oct4 and Sox2, and hypopharyngeal cancer progression, but the authors in this study did not compare their results to other head and neck sites (35). The recent interest in human papillomavirus (HPV) in head and neck carcinoma has not translated to hypopharyngeal carcinoma. A study from M.D. Anderson Cancer Center revealed the presence of HPV correlated with poor prognosis in hypopharyngeal carcinoma (36). Another study from Belgium identified no difference in survival between HPV-positive and HPV-negative hypopharyngeal carcinomas despite the presence of HPV in 74% of patients (37). This may represent the molecular heterogeneity within hypopharyngeal carcinoma that makes HPV status irrelevant, but future study is warranted.

PROGNOSIS

Overall survival for patients with hypopharyngeal cancer who receive no treatment is dismal, with a 1-year survival of 10%. Conversely, those who seek treatment have 1-year overall survival of 48% (9). Five-year overall survival for advanced-stage cancer ranges from 18% to 47%, while early-stage cancers have much improved survival ranging from 64% to 78% (Table 122.3) (23,38). The improvements in treatment protocols are reflected in the change in 5-year disease-specific survival rates for hypopharyngeal cancer patients. Between 1980 and 1985, 5-year disease-specific survival was 4.2%, and between 1990 and 1999, the 5-year disease-specific survival increased to 35% (8,9).

Lymph node status affects survival in hypopharyngeal carcinoma (Table 122.4) (23). A review of 132 patients treated with surgery and radiation revealed patients with N0 or N1 disease had 5-year survival of 54%, which drops to 20% in those with N2 or greater disease (39).

Prognostic information for cervical esophageal carcinoma is limited because most analyses are combined with all esophageal carcinomas. A large study from Hong Kong outlined the treatment of 124 patients with cervical esophageal carcinoma. They found that the primary surgery group had 2-year overall survival of 38% with median survival of 20 months and the chemoradiation-treated group had 2-year overall survival of 48% with median survival of 24 months, although the differences were not statistically significant (40). Five-year survival was noted to be 33% in a Japanese series of 84 patients with cervical esophageal

TABLE 122.3	HYPOPHARYNGEAL CANCER: 5-YEAR SURVIVAL BY STAGE[a]				
	Stage				
Location No.	**I**	**II**	**III**	**IV**	**Overall**
Piriform fossa (63)	6/11 54%	5/10 50%	7/24 29%	1/18 5%	19/63 30%
Posterior wall (30)	5/5 100%	11/15 75%	1/8 12%	0/2 0%	17/30 56%
Postcricoid (4)			1/3 33%	0/1 0%	1/4 25%
Totals	11/16 68%	16/25 64%	9/35 25%	1/21 4%	37/97 38%

[a]Eastern Virginia Medical School, 1972 to 1985; 97 patients.

TABLE 122.4	HYPOPHARYNGEAL CANCER:5-YEAR SURVIVAL BY LYMPH NODE STATUS (EASTERN VIRGINIA MEDICAL SCHOOL EXPERIENCE)[a]		
Node Location (n)	Negative (n)	Positive (n)	5-Year Survival (%)
Piriform fossa (63)	14	49	8/14 (57) 11/49 (22)
Posterior wall (30)	7	23	5/7 (71) 12/23 (52)
Postcricoid (4)	1	3	1/1 (100) 0/3 (0)
Totals	22	75[b]	14/22 (63) 23/75 (30)

[a]Eastern Virginia Medical School 1972 to 1985; 97 patients.
[b]Bilateral nodes in 10 of 97 (10%) of entire group or 10 of 75 (13%) of those with positive nodes. Only 1 of 10 (10%) survived 5 years.

carcinoma treated with surgery and radiation (41). Another review of 32 patients with cervical esophageal carcinoma treated with primary surgery found a 5-year disease-free survival of 33% in higher stage tumors and 47% in early-stage tumors (10).

MANAGEMENT

Since the majority of patients present with advanced-stage disease, multimodality therapy is required, which would consist of surgery, radiation, and chemotherapy. Presentation at a multidisciplinary conference is a necessity to reach a consensus opinion on the management of patients; however, patients should be treated according to evidence-based guidelines or entered into an institutional review board approved protocol (42). In lieu of a therapeutic trial, treatment should comply with treatment guidelines put forth by the National Comprehensive Cancer Network (43). Functional rehabilitation, facilitated by speech pathology and dental and nutrition services in addition to the treating oncologists, is required as part of the recovery process. Typically, early-stage tumors are treated with surgery or definitive radiation. Advanced-stage disease requires combination therapy with two to three modalities. The following sections outline surgical (open and minimally invasive) and nonsurgical treatments for hypopharyngeal and cervical esophageal carcinoma. When considering treatment options, it is vital for the practitioner not to compromise oncologic outcome for preservation of organ function or application of unproven technology.

Surgery of the Hypopharynx

Preoperative Considerations

Patients who present with hypopharyngeal carcinoma typically are malnourished and have multiple comorbidities. These issues must be addressed and managed as much as possible prior to undertaking surgical resection to ensure optimal outcomes. Nutritional deficits can be identified with preoperative evaluation of weight loss and laboratory testing to assess the degree of malnutrition (e.g., anemia, low serum prealbumin and transferrin). A dietician can assist with improving diet, or recommendation can be made for temporary feeding tube. Respiratory status must also be optimized, especially if the patient is undergoing partial laryngeal resection.

Early-Stage Pyriform Sinus Cancer

Surgical approaches to early-stage pyriform sinus cancers can result in preservation of the larynx that involves the medial or lateral walls of the pyriform sinus that does not extend to the pyriform sinus apex or postcricoid mucosa. Selection for patients with early-stage tumor resections must also take into account the predilection for submucosal extension in hypopharyngeal tumors.

One approach to resection of these early-stage tumors in the superior pyriform fossae is a partial laryngopharyngectomy (Figs. 122.6 to 122.8). This procedure involves resection of the involved pyriform sinus with a partial laryngectomy. Tumor visualization is via a transhyoid or lateral pharyngotomy. Entry into the pharynx is through the contralateral side. With the tumor in full view, a mucosal incision is carried along the posterior pharyngeal wall to the involved side maintaining an adequate 1- to 1.5-cm margin. The contralateral aryepiglottic fold is incised and extended inferiorly into the laryngeal ventricle and anteriorly to the anterior commissure (Fig. 122.9).

Next, attention is directed to interarytenoid space with a vertical incision carried to the superior border of the cricoid cartilage. This incision is then directed laterally to the ipsilateral cricoarytenoid joint, orienting the incision superiorly and anteriorly across the vocal process. The cut is then directed anteriorly across the ipsilateral ventricle to the anterior commissure, joining it with the contralateral cuts. The specimen is now centered on the tumor,

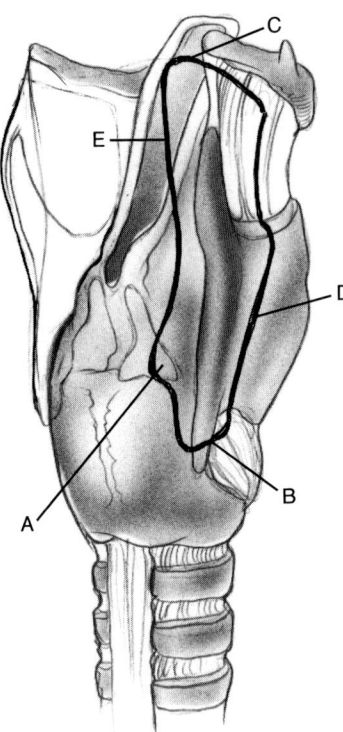

Figure 122.6 External surgical anatomic projections of the piriform fossa. The piriform apex (A) is just above the cricothyroid articulation at the inferior cornu (B). The superior border is at the inferior margin of the hyoid bone (C). The anterior border is at the junction of the anterior and posterior halves of the thyroid cartilage (D). The posterior edge of the thyroid cartilage marks the posterior border of the piriform fossa (E).

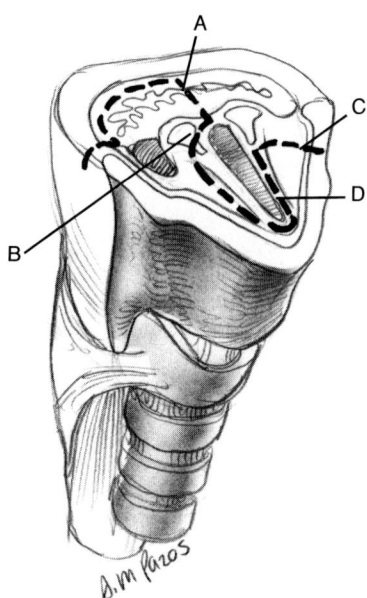

Figure 122.7 Partial laryngopharyngectomy (PLP) for cancer of the superior piriform fossa. The key elements of the PLP involve an interarytenoid incision (A) that extends across the vocal process (B) on the ipsilateral side and an incision in the aryepiglottic fold (C) and ventricle (D), similar to that used for supraglottic laryngectomy on the contralateral side.

which is resected with adequate margins. Frozen sections should be used to evaluate mucosal and soft tissue margins. Reconstruction of the laryngopharyngeal defect is accomplished by suturing of the vocal cord remnant to the posterior–superior cricoid cartilage, and the tongue base is sutured to the thyroid cartilage perichondrium. Reinforcement of the pharyngeal closure can be accomplished with the remaining strap muscles or a sternocleidomastoid flap (Figs. 122.10 and 122.11). A cricopharyngeal myotomy is performed, and either a nasogastric feeding tube or gastrostomy tube is placed. The airway is secured temporarily with a tracheostomy.

This procedure was studied by Makeieff et al. (44) in 87 patients with early-stage tumors. He found a 5-year overall survival of 60% in his cohort of T1 and T2 tumors with a local recurrence rate of 19.9%. Ninety-three percent of patients resumed normal oral diet after a median duration of nasogastric tube alimentation for 20 days. Another recent series reviewing 48 patients with selected T1 and T2 tumors of the pyriform fossae found a 5-year local control rate of 98% and 5-year actuarial survival of 47% (45). All patients in this series returned to normal diet after 1 month. In both of these series, postoperative radiotherapy was used in 90% of the patients.

Another approach to larger tumors of the pyriform fossae is the supracricoid hemilaryngectomy. Invasion of the pyriform apex, postcricoid mucosa, and posterior pharyngeal wall and vocal cord immobility are relative contraindications to this procedure. The efficacy of this procedure was studied in France with a cohort of 147 patients who received induction chemotherapy followed by surgery (46). Half of the patients went on to receive adjuvant radiotherapy. He found a 5-year local control rate of 90%, including 63% for T4a tumors. Lesions invading the pyriform sinus apex and posterior pharyngeal wall were associated with increased rate of recurrence. Normal deglutition was observed in 64.6% after 1 month and 92% after 1 year. Only 1.5% of the patients in the cohort required completion laryngectomy. In the United States, this procedure has gained little acceptance.

Currently, most of these early-stage tumors are treated with definitive radiotherapy with or without chemotherapy. In addition, endoscopic laser or transoral robotic techniques have replaced these open partial laryngeal procedures. These points will be discussed in other sections.

Advanced-Stage Pyriform Sinus Cancer
In T3 and T4 tumors of the pyriform sinus, treatment centers on surgery and adjuvant radiation. Conservation surgery may be possible, but local control is poor (47). Therefore, surgical resection involves total laryngectomy with partial or total pharyngectomy. The surgeon must take into account the propensity for submucosal spread when addressing margins. Varying amounts of cervical esophagus or thoracic esophagus must be resected based on size of the primary tumor. In one study from Australia, 180

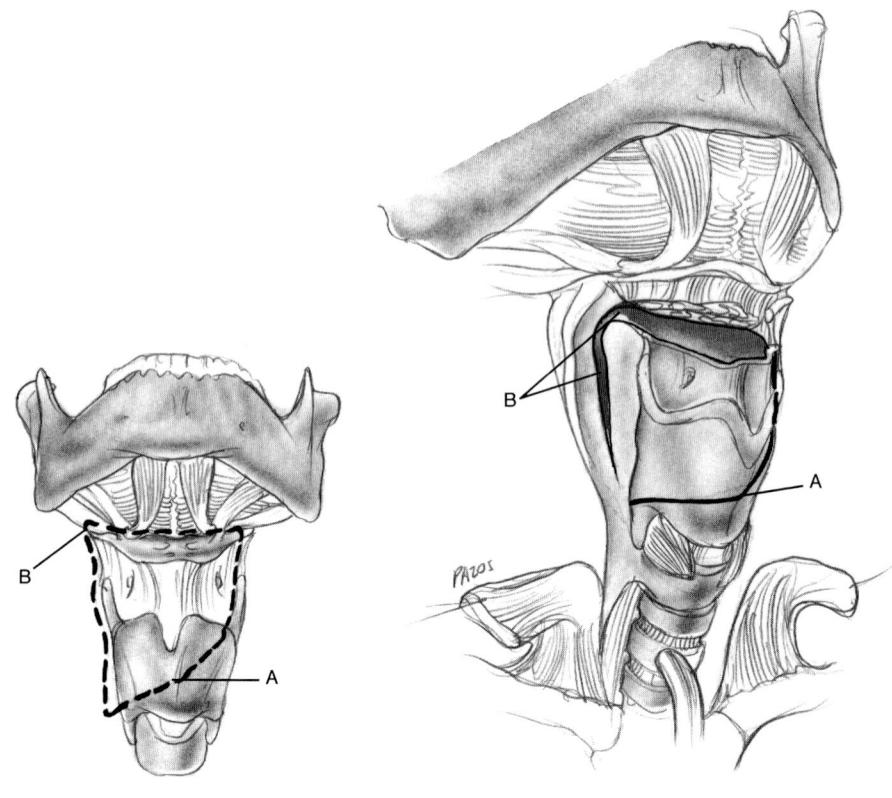

Figure 122.8 Partial laryngopharyngectomy for cancer of the superior piriform fossa. The cartilage cuts begin at a point above the anterior commissure (*A*) and extend laterally and inferiorly on the ipsilateral side and laterally and superiorly on the contralateral side. The pharynx is entered through a combination of suprahyoid and lateral pharyngotomy incisions (*B*).

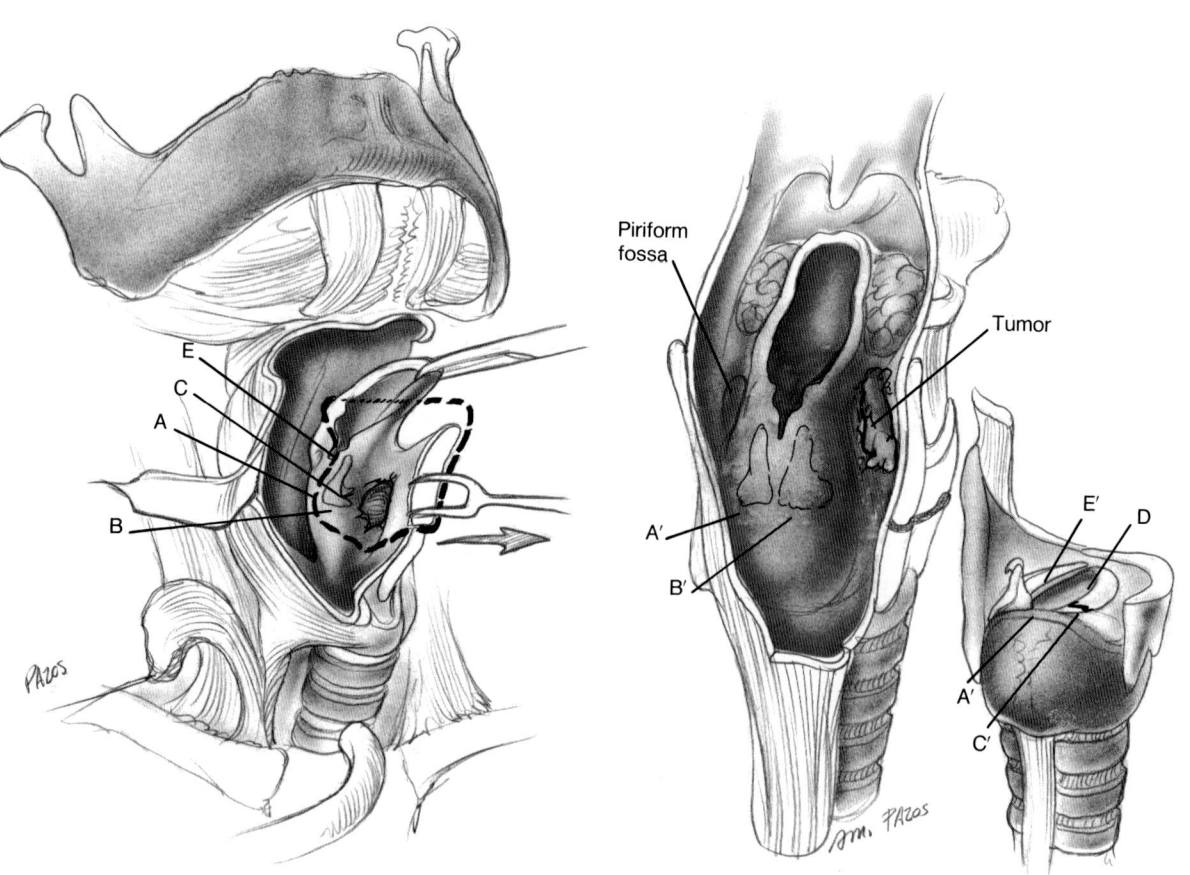

Figure 122.9 Partial laryngopharyngectomy for cancer of the superior piriform fossa. The interarytenoid incision (*A*) is carried down to the cricoid cartilage through the cricoarytenoid joint (*B*), across the vocal process (*C*), and anteriorly through the ventricle (*D*). The contralateral aryepiglottic fold and ventricular incisions (*E*) also extend forward to the anterior commissure.

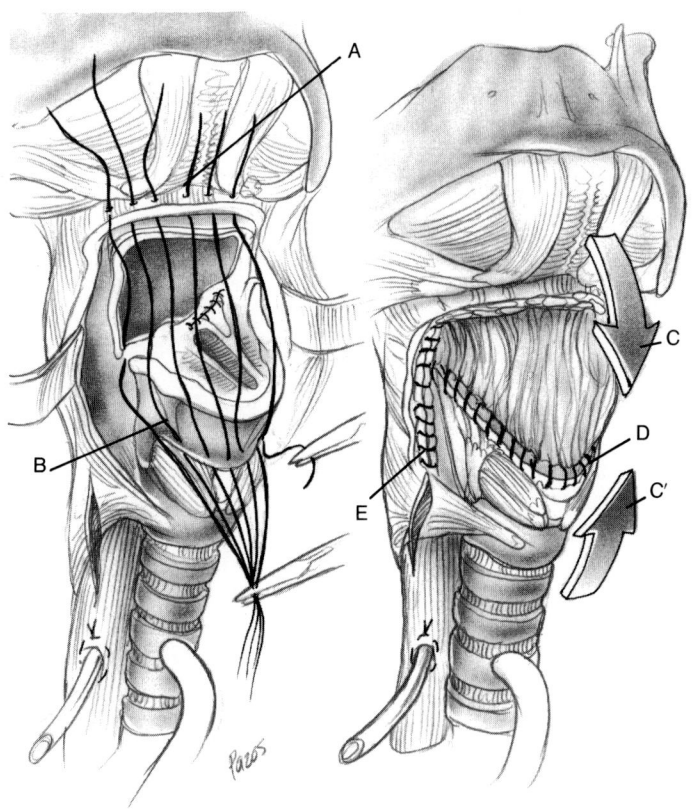

Figure 122.10 Partial laryngopharyngectomy for cancer of the superior piriform fossa. A watertight closure of the pharyngotomy is accomplished with a combination of sutures from the tongue base (*A*) to the thyroid perichondrium (*B*). Head flexion allows tongue base and laryngeal relaxation (*C*) with closure of the horizontal segment of the pharyngotomy (*D*). The lateral pharyngotomy is sutured vertically (*E*).

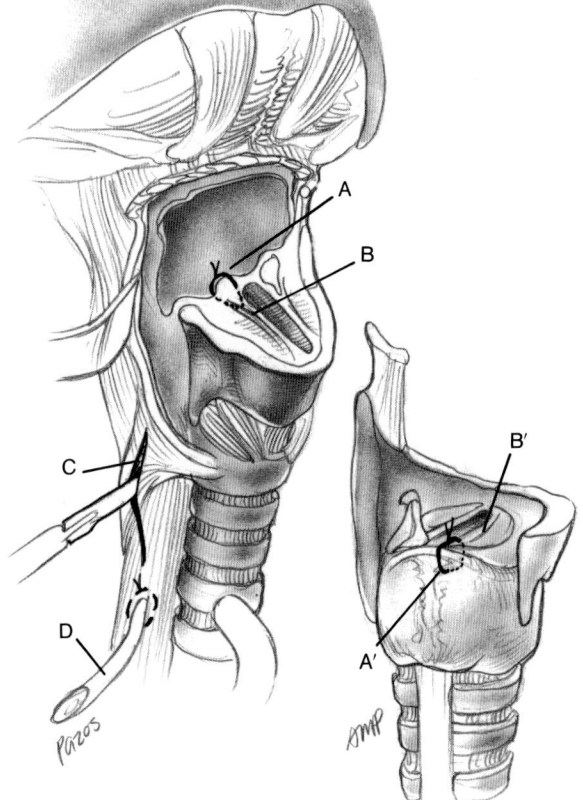

Figure 122.11 Partial laryngopharyngectomy for cancer of the superior piriform fossa. The vocal cord retention suture (*A*) is placed through the lateral aspect of the vocal process remnant, through the cricoid cartilage, and then tied down to bring the cord (*B*) to the midline. A cricopharyngeal myotomy (*C*) is performed, and a feeding esophagostomy tube (*D*) placed.

patients had total laryngopharyngectomy followed by postoperative radiation treatment (48). Local/regional control rate was 82% with 5-year survival of 52%. These results illustrate the aggressive nature of these tumors. Organ preservation protocols are a valid alternative to total laryngopharyngectomy and will be discussed subsequently.

Posterior Hypopharyngeal Wall Cancer

These lesions are typically localized and exophytic, allowing for wide excision and reconstruction. Advanced-stage tumors are typically fixed to the prevertebral fascia and not amenable to surgery. The approach requires either a lateral pharyngotomy or transhyoid pharyngotomy (Fig. 122.12). Once the vallecula has been entered, the incision is extended along the hyoid bone on either side ensuring the superior laryngeal neurovascular bundles are hypoglossal nerves that are protected. The hyoid and larynx can be retracted inferiorly to provide excellent exposure of the pharyngeal wall (Fig. 122.13). Resection of the tumor should involve the prevertebral musculature if the prevertebral fascia is involved. In this setting, local control is poor with surgery alone. Retropharyngeal node dissection should be performed as well. If these nodes are not dissected, then adjuvant radiotherapy must cover the retropharyngeal nodal basin. One problem with surgery is the denervation of the pharyngeal plexus, which can result in significant dysphagia and aspiration in larger tumor resections.

Reconstruction of a small posterior pharyngeal wall defect can be achieved with a split-thickness skin graft

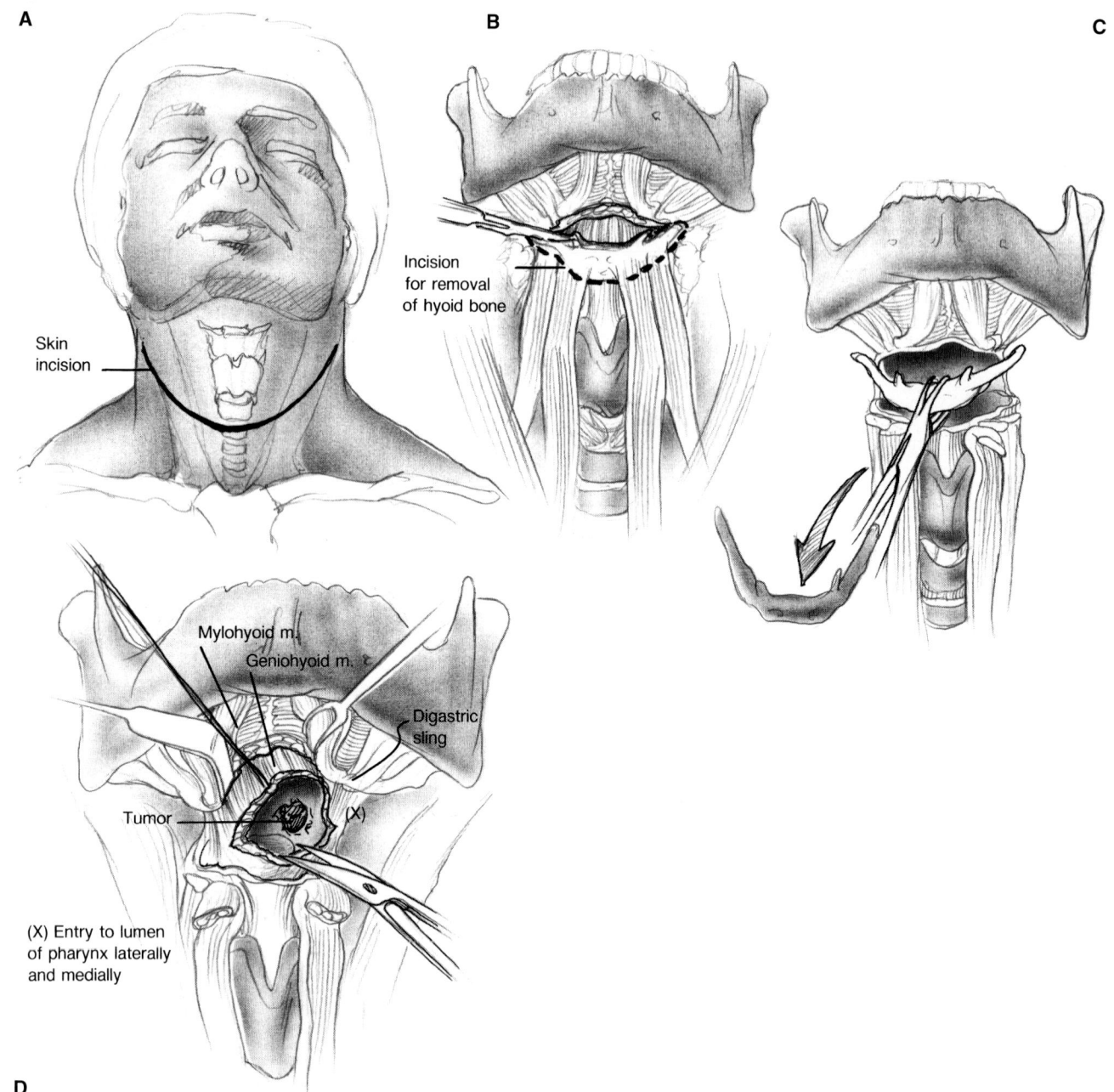

A

Skin incision

B

Incision for removal of hyoid bone

C

D

Mylohyoid m.
Geniohyoid m.
Digastric sling
Tumor
(X)

(X) Entry to lumen of pharynx laterally and medially

Figure 122.12 Suprahyoid pharyngotomy for posterior hypopharyngeal cancer. The initial incision (**A** and **B**) extends along the superior border of the hyoid for its entire length. The hyoid then is removed (**C**) to facilitate completion of the pharyngotomy (**D**).

(Fig. 122.14). A bolster is placed over the graft and can be removed transorally in 5 days. If the resection involves removal of the lateral wall of the pyriform sinus, the defect size will not support a skin graft alone (Figs. 122.15 and 122.16). In this situation, a pectoral myocutaneous flap, platysma myocutaneous flap, or free fasciocutaneous flap (e.g., radial forearm or anterolateral thigh) can repair this defect. A local alternative can be achieved with bilateral advancement of the prevertebral muscles with a skin graft (Figs. 122.17 and 122.18). Reconstruction of posterior hypopharyngeal wall defects is fraught with significant morbidity (49,50). For

example, a series from Memorial Sloan-Kettering reported a 67% complication rate after surgery, and only 33% of the patients in the series resumed a full oral diet (49).

If surgery is considered for posterior pharyngeal wall tumors, the surgeon must understand that resection will likely involve the pharyngeal plexus and patients may experience significant swallowing dysfunction as well as the high complication rate associated with the reconstruction. Definitive radiation is an alternative therapy to achieve good local control with adequate function posttreatment, and the retropharyngeal lymph nodes will be treated.

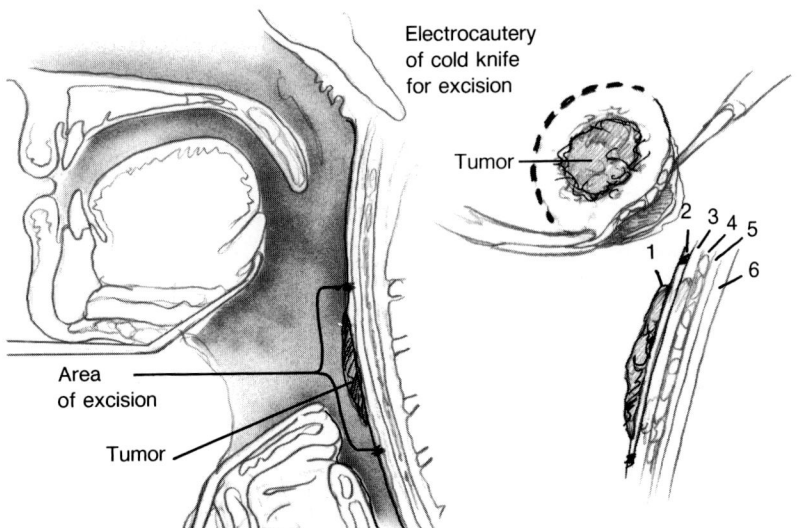

Figure 122.13 Suprahyoid pharyngotomy for posterior hypopharyngeal cancer. After the hyoid is removed and the pharyngotomy completed, superior and inferior retraction provides excellent exposure for wide excision of the cancer. *1*, tumor; *2*, mucosa; *3*, constrictor; *4*, longus colli; *5*, retropharyngeal space; *6*, prevertebral fascia.

Postcricoid Cancer

Tumors of the postcricoid region typically do not present until reaching an advanced stage. The lesions have invaded the cricoid cartilage and posterior cricoarytenoid muscles. Inferior extension into the cervical esophagus is common. Therefore, surgery should involve total laryngopharyngectomy and cervical esophagectomy with postoperative radiation therapy. Again, organ preservation approaches can be presented to patients who do not desire total laryngectomy.

Minimally Invasive Approaches

Transoral laser surgery was initially developed for laryngeal carcinoma in head and neck cancers, but its use has been translated to the hypopharynx. Multiple case series have been published detailing the personal experiences of individual surgeons. All stages have been evaluated for transoral laser surgery. Local control rates have been reported between 90% and 95% in early-stage tumors and 47% and 69% in advanced-stage tumors (51–53). The purported advantages of transoral laser surgery compared to open functional surgery are avoidance of tracheotomy in most cases, a feeding tube is not required in many cases, and the hospital stay is shorter. Moreover, endoscopic laser surgery, in contrast to open surgery, better spares the pharyngeal sensory innervation, thus improving the capability of protecting the airway during swallowing (52).

Transoral robotic surgery is a new technique that is gaining popularity in some centers. Its application in oropharyngeal carcinoma has been well documented (54). However, only small series have included hypopharyngeal cancers, with the largest personal series being 10 patients with T1 or T2 tumors (55,56). Feasibility of surgery has been limited to the posterior pharyngeal wall and lateral pyriform sinus due to restricted space that safely allows the robotic arms to perform the resection.

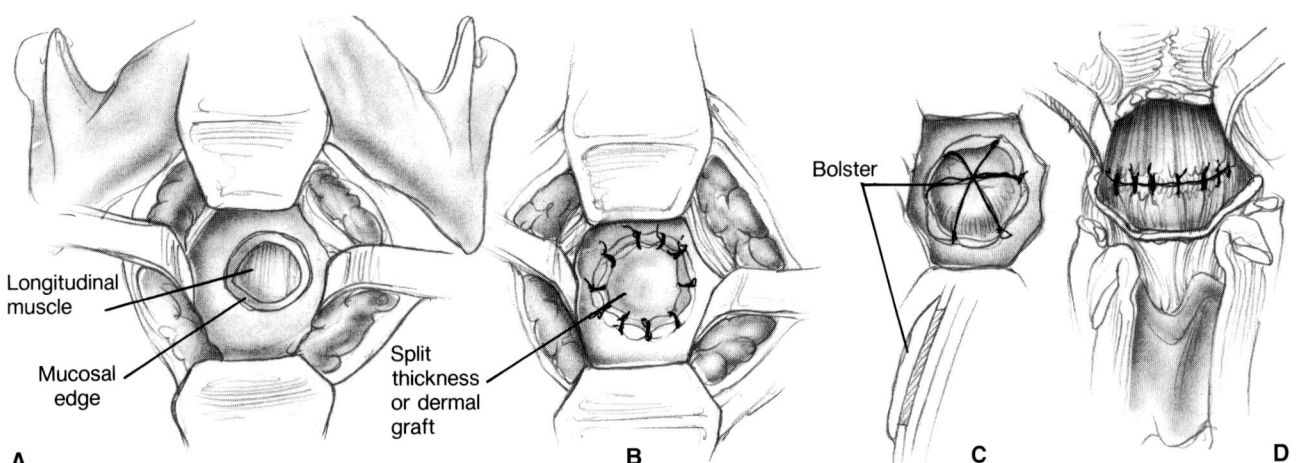

Figure 122.14 Suprahyoid pharyngotomy for posterior hypopharyngeal cancer. The incision is usually carried down to the prevertebral fascia (**A**), which acts as the surgical plane for excision. The defect then is covered with a split-thickness or dermal skin graft (**B**). This is held in place with a bolster (**C**) of nylon sheeting stuffed with cotton balls. The pharyngotomy is closed in layers, avoiding suture ligation of the hypoglossal and superior laryngeal nerves (**D**).

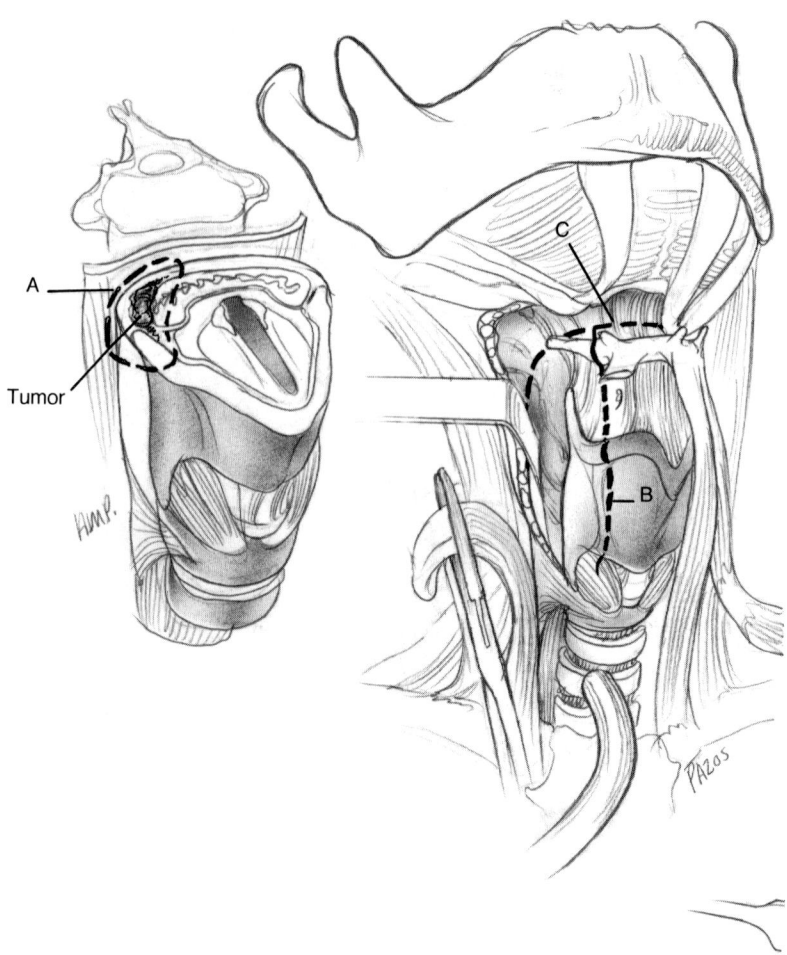

Figure 122.15 Combined suprahyoid and lateral pharyngotomy for posterolateral hypopharyngeal cancer. These cancers (*A*) are approached by excising the posterior third of the thyroid cartilage and combining the anterolateral pharyngotomy incision (*B*) with the suprahyoid incision (*C*).

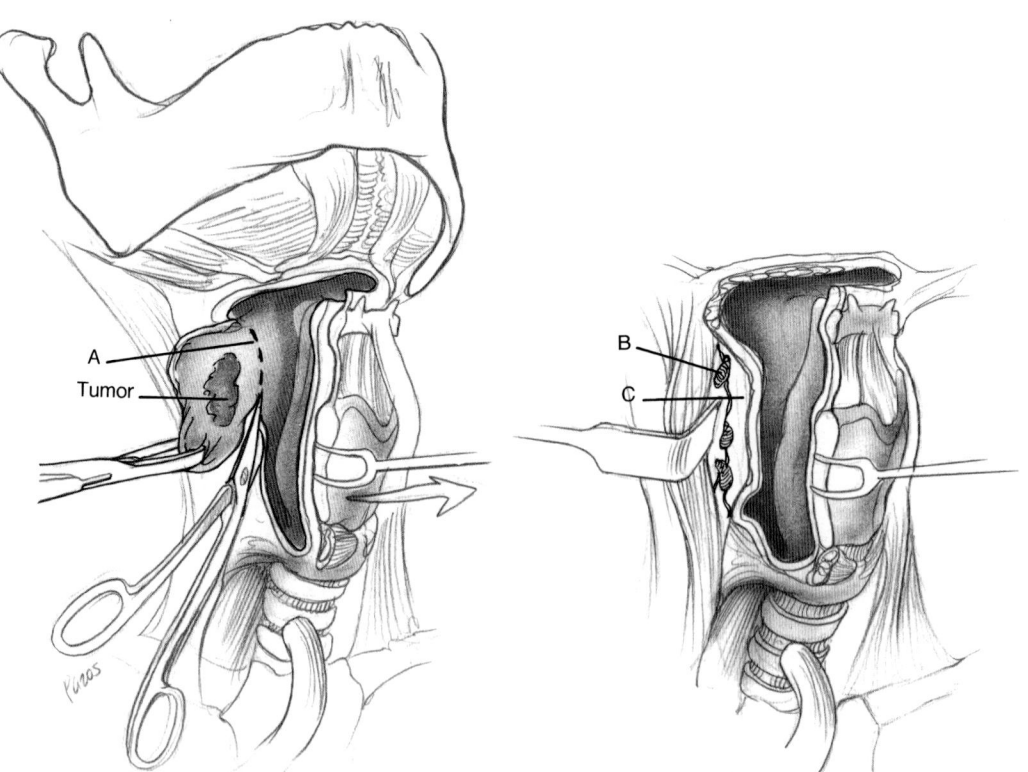

Figure 122.16 Combined suprahyoid and lateral pharyngotomy for posterolateral hypopharyngeal cancer. The final incision (*A*) is made under direct vision. The cervical sympathetic ganglion (*B*) should be preserved if it is not involved with the cancer. Reconstruction can be accomplished by using a portion of the prevertebral muscle (*C*) as a backing for a skin graft.

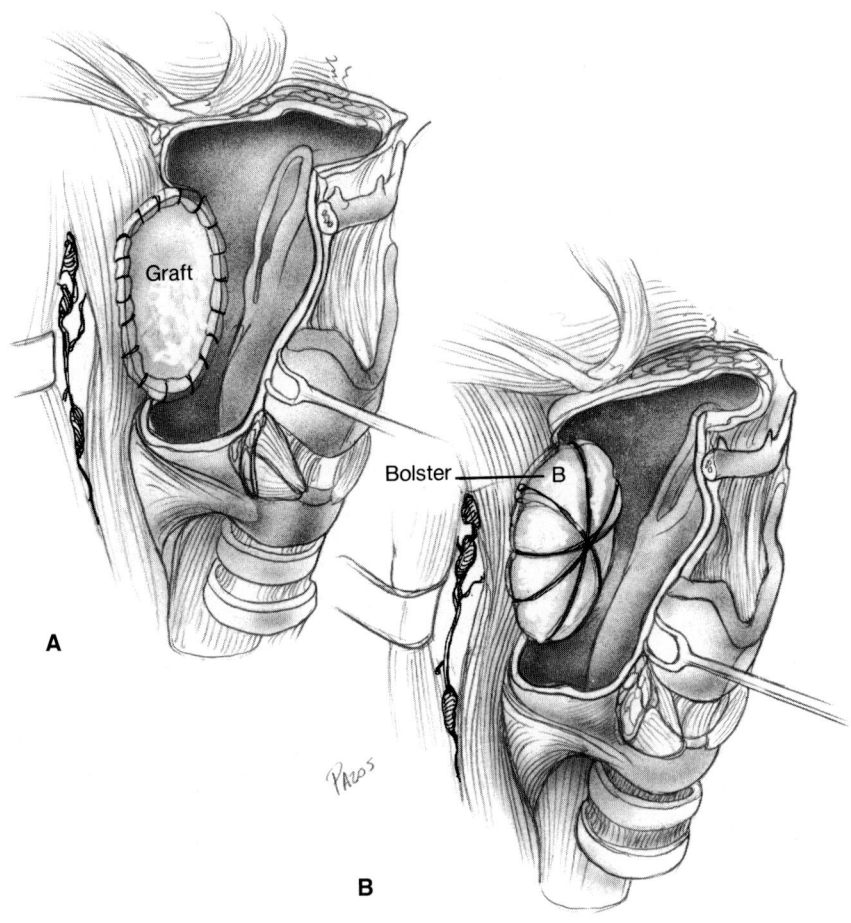

Figure 122.17 Combined suprahyoid and lateral pharyngotomy for posterolateral hypopharyngeal cancer. The split-thickness or dermal skin graft is sutured to the prevertebral muscle (A) and held in place with a nylon mesh and cotton-ball bolster (B).

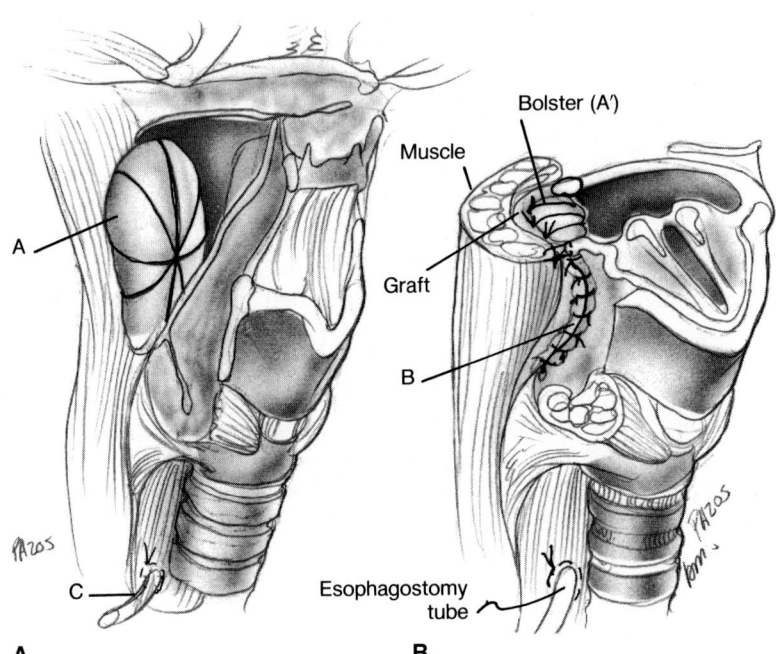

Figure 122.18 Combined suprahyoid and lateral pharyngotomy for posterolateral hypopharyngeal cancer. After the steps illustrated in Figures 122.15 and 122.16 the prevertebral muscle is mobilized as a bipedicled flap for medial rotation of the skin graft–bolster combination (A). The bolster is sutured in place with long sutures from the graft. A water-tight closure of the pharyngotomy (B) is then accomplished, and a feeding esophagostomy is placed.

SURGERY OF THE CERVICAL ESOPHAGUS

Tumors of the cervical esophagus typically present at an advanced stage; therefore, a limited local surgery is rare. Because the proximal cervical esophagus is adjacent to the larynx, total laryngopharyngectomy with cervical esophagectomy is often the indicated procedure, both to obtain an adequate upper surgical margin and to avoid postoperative aspiration. In instances where the tumor extends inferiorly into the thoracic esophagus, total esophagectomy is required. Tumors that do not invade into the hypopharynx or larynx may be amenable to larynx-preserving cervical esophagectomy with adequate functional and oncologic outcomes (10).

MANAGEMENT OF THE NECK

Nodal metastasis is common in hypopharyngeal and cervical esophageal carcinoma. Therefore, nodal basins must be addressed by either surgery or radiation. Lymph node metastases are common in hypopharyngeal carcinoma with 64% to 90% of patients presenting with nodal disease and bilateral disease seen in 8% to 16% of cases (9,25,26). Ipsilateral neck dissection is adequate for early-stage tumors of the lateral pyriform sinus. However, tumors approaching the midline require bilateral dissection. For the hypopharynx, nodal dissection should involve the levels II, III, and IV. Elective dissection of the paratracheal and paraesophageal nodes is unclear at this time. A high rate of paratracheal nodal metastasis is seen in advanced-stage disease and tumors involving the postcricoid mucosa (57%) (28,31,57); therefore, paratracheal dissection is indicated in advanced hypopharyngeal carcinoma. Bilateral paratracheal dissection and total thyroidectomy are indicated in midline lesions or lesions involving the cervical esophagus (57). Mediastinal dissection is advocated in T4 hypopharynx tumors because of nodal metastasis rate that approaches up to 40% (30,31).

The cervical esophagus has a propensity to metastasize to bilateral paratracheal and paraesophageal basins (29). Therefore, elective bilateral central compartment dissection is advocated in cervical esophageal carcinoma. Mediastinal dissection is also recommended due to high rate of mediastinal nodal metastasis (30,31).

Retropharyngeal nodal disease is seen in 20% to 50% of patients with hypopharyngeal and cervical esophageal cancers (32–34). These data suggest the importance of treating the retropharyngeal nodes with surgery or radiation. Gross retropharyngeal nodal disease that is noted with preoperative imaging should be removed at the time of surgery. Radiation can be used in the adjuvant setting or in the elective setting when there is no apparent retropharyngeal nodal disease.

RECONSTRUCTION

Small defects of the hypopharynx are amenable to reconstruction via a split-thickness and local advancement flaps. It is best to avoid primary closure of a mucosal remnant less than 2 cm because of concerns for stricture. These larger defects are better suited for reconstruction with pedicled myocutaneous flaps, such as the pectoral myocutaneous or deltopectoral flap. The pedicled flaps are reliable with minimal complications (58). Free tissue transfer with a radial forearm flap or anterolateral thigh (ALT) flap is another option in the reconstruction of these defects with acceptable functional results (59). Bulky flaps should be avoided in cases of laryngeal preservation, as this may interfere with swallowing and cause intractable aspiration.

Total pharyngeal defects are best reconstructed with free tissue flaps. Tubed fasciocutaneous flaps from the radial forearm and ALT or free enteral grafts are the common choices by the reconstructive surgeons. The ALT flap has good versatility with only a 5% stricture rate reported in one study (60). Another review from Korea found 92% of patients undergoing reconstruction with a tubed free fasciocutaneous flap returned to normal oral diet, and only 6% experienced stricture (61). Enteric flaps have the advantages of tissue pliability, tubed shape, ease of contouring, intrinsic peristalsis, and the ability to secrete mucus. However, it has been observed that many patients have inferior vocal quality that is described as "wet" due to the increased mucus secretion (62). In addition, jejunal grafts can be harvested with laparoscopic techniques, thus, avoiding a laparotomy incision (63).

Surgery of the cervical esophagus many times requires resection of the entire esophagus posing a challenge in the reconstruction. Tubed fasciocutaneous flaps are not an option in these cases due to length of the defect. Colon interposition is an option in the reconstruction of the esophagus because it does not involve microvascular anastomosis (Fig. 122.19). However, postoperative infection is common with devastating consequences; therefore, this technique is only used when other options are not available.

Gastric transposition has several advantages in the reconstruction with a robust blood supply and creation of a single pharyngeal anastomosis. Blunt dissection from the abdomen and posterior mediastinum can mobilize the stomach. In addition, mobilization of the duodenum allows the stomach to be pulled up to the level of the nasopharynx (Fig. 122.20). Complications of this procedure commonly involve fluid collections within the pleural space causing pneumo/hemothorax. This complication can be resolved with a thoracostomy tube. Mortality of this procedure is approximately 5% to 15% (64,65).

The jejunal graft is an excellent option in reconstruction of the cervical esophagus as described above. In cases where total esophagectomy is required, additional length can be obtained by "supercharging" the jejunum with a distal pedicle supplying the enteric anastomotic end (66). The stomach

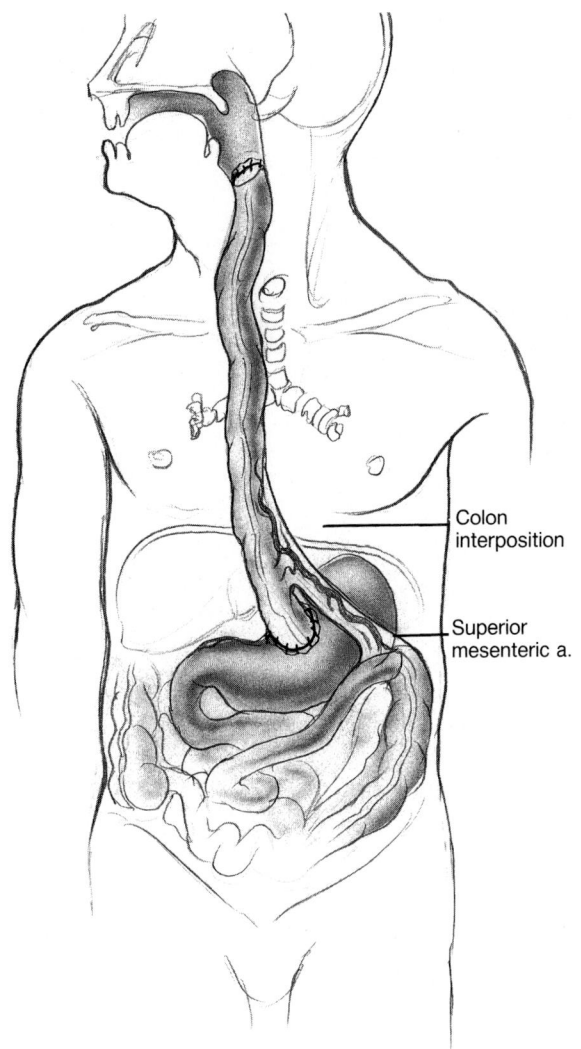

Figure 122.19 Colon interposition allows one-stage reconstruction or bypass of the entire esophagus. A high incidence of septic complications is associated with this procedure.

remains *in situ* and serves as a reservoir, thus avoiding reflux seen in the gastric pull-up. Another advantage of this surgery is it requires one microvascular anastomosis in the neck with acceptable operative morbidity. In fact, 90% of the patients are able to return to normal oral diet.

Many reconstructive options exist for the closure of hypopharyngeal and cervical esophageal defects. It is imperative that the reconstructive surgeon plays a role in the multidisciplinary team. However, oncologic safety must not be compromised for a specific reconstructive method.

NONSURGICAL THERAPIES FOR HYPOPHARYNGEAL AND CERVICAL ESOPHAGEAL CARCINOMA

Primary radiation is the treatment of choice in many early-stage hypopharyngeal carcinomas. Disease-specific survival and local control rates are similar to published surgical series of similar stage cases with acceptable morbidity (67,68). Advanced-stage tumors typically are treated with surgery followed by postoperative radiation. Local control rates in this situation range between 76% and 79% (69).

Although chemotherapy is not used as a definitive treatment in hypopharyngeal carcinoma, its use in the neoadjuvant or concomitant role has proven beneficial in many patients. A meta-analysis of over 87 trials using chemotherapy in head and neck cancers between 1965 and 2000 revealed an absolute survival benefit of 4.5% (70). The use of concurrent chemotherapy had a more pronounced survival benefit at 6.5%. Therefore, the addition of chemotherapy to protocols in the treatment of hypopharyngeal carcinoma may improve survival. Although induction chemotherapy did not show a survival benefit in these studies, more recent studies have shown the addition of taxanes (docetaxel) to the previous platinum-based regimen (cisplatin and 5-fluorouracil) provides a significant survival benefit over the platinum-based regimen alone (1).

The addition of chemotherapy in the postoperative radiation setting has been studied by two cooperative trials, RTOG 95-01 and EORTC 22391 (71,72). These two trials compared the addition of chemotherapy to postoperative radiation to conventional postoperative radiation alone in patients with high-risk head and neck cancer (defined as extranodal spread, multiple positive nodes, and positive surgical margins). Hypopharynx carcinomas constituted 20% of the European Organization for Research and Treatment of Cancer (EORTC) group, 12% of the Radiation Therapy Oncology Group (RTOG) radiation arm, and 7% of the RTOG concurrent chemoradiation arm. Both trials showed improved local and regional control in the chemotherapy arms with an increase in control rate of 10% and 11% in RTOG and EORTC trials, respectively. Only the EORTC found a significant survival benefit in the chemotherapy arm (13% difference at 2 years). Therefore, the conclusions of these two studies are addition of chemotherapy in high-risk head and neck cancer will improve local and regional control and survival.

The results of the Veterans Affairs Laryngeal Cancer Study and the RTOG have encouraged treatment regimens using chemotherapy and radiation therapy to preserve the larynx (73,74). The use of chemotherapy as part of induction or concurrent treatment has resulted in improved local/regional control rates and decreased distant metastasis. These results have not compromised survival rates when compared to surgery and adjuvant radiation. However, these studies looked at patients with larynx cancers alone without any hypopharyngeal carcinomas.

The promising results of the VA trial led to consideration for organ preservation protocols in the treatment of hypopharyngeal carcinoma. The first such study was a retrospective review from M.D. Anderson Cancer Center comparing induction chemotherapy and radiation therapy to surgery in patients with laryngeal and hypopharyngeal

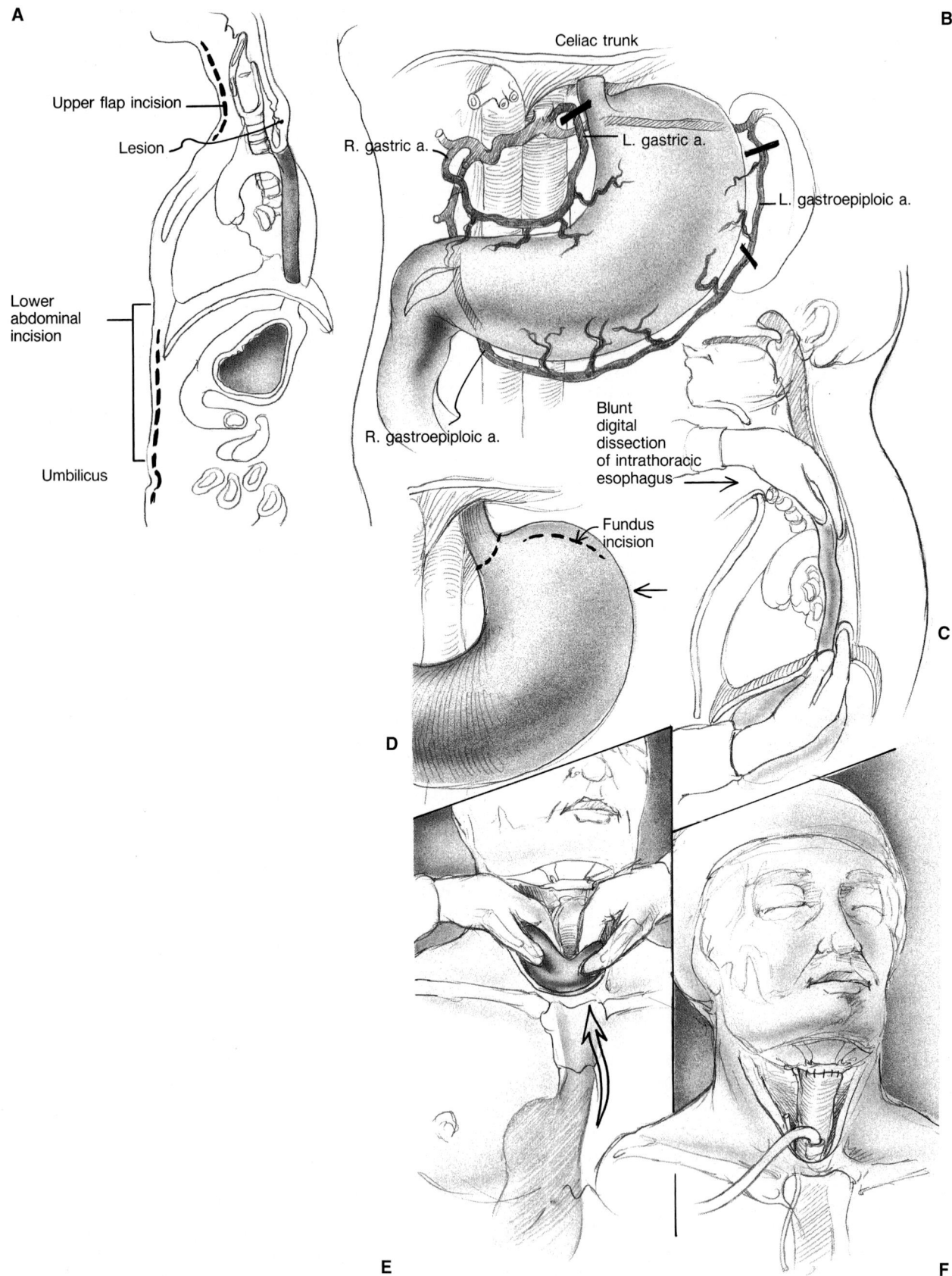

Figure 122.20 A: Gastric pull-up with pharyngogastric anastomosis is commonly used to reconstruct total esophageal defects. **B:** The intraabdominal procedure includes vagotomy with pyloroplasty. The duodenum is mobilized with the Kocher maneuver. **C:** The esophagus is removed without thoracotomy, using bimanual transabdominal and transcervical dissection. The stomach is brought up through the chest into the neck in the posterior mediastinum. **D:** The fundus is opened to provide the greatest length for anastomosis. **E:** Fundus in neck. **F:** Fundus surgery.

carcinomas (75). They reported a response rate of 78% in all hypopharyngeal patients and complete response rate of 83% in patients who had a response to induction chemotherapy. The larynx was preserved in 69% of the patients. Most importantly, there was not a significant survival difference between the nonsurgical group and the surgical group. These results were followed by a prospective evaluation of larynx preservation in hypopharynx cancer developed by the EORTC. It was a phase III, randomized controlled trial comparing induction cisplatin and 5-fluorouracil (FU) followed by radiation therapy and conventional surgery with adjuvant radiation therapy (2). No difference was found in local/regional control rates and disease-free survival at 5 years. Functional laryngeal preservation was 35% at 5 years. This study concluded that functional larynx preservation is possible without compromising survival in hypopharyngeal carcinoma.

The EORTC reported on a second larynx preservation for hypopharyngeal comparing induction chemotherapy to concurrent chemoradiation, similar to RTOG 91-11. This trial had 51% of patients with hypopharyngeal carcinoma (3). Patients were staged T2-4/N0-2 at the hypopharynx for entry into the trial and assigned to receive induction chemotherapy followed by radiotherapy or an alternating chemoradiation regimen. Local control rates were similar in each group at 32% at 5 years. Survival was not significantly different, with median survival 4.4 years (5-year overall survival estimate 48.5%) in the induction arm and 5.1 years (5-year overall survival estimate 51.9%) in the chemoradiation arm. The main weakness of this study is the alternating fractionation of the radiation, with the treatment regimen lasting greater than 7 weeks, and total dose delivered was reduced to 60 Gy. Due to these differences in treatment regimen, it is difficult to compare this result to conventional concurrent chemoradiation protocols. In contrast, the results of the RTOG 91-11 have shown that concurrent chemoradiotherapy had a greater loco/regional control compared to the sequential arm and radiation alone (74). This trial did not include hypopharynx carcinoma patients, but it does demonstrate that concurrent treatment similar to current regimens can result in improved locoregional control.

Chemotherapy and radiation have also been studied in the treatment of cervical esophageal carcinoma. Results of these studies combined all esophageal carcinomas. One study from M.D. Anderson Cancer Center retrospectively reviewed 132 patients who received concurrent chemoradiation (76). Sixty patients underwent esophagectomy after treatment and compared to the remaining 72 patients who had no surgery. Significant findings were noted in the surgical arm for local control (67% vs. 22%) and 5-year overall survival (52.6% vs. 6.5%). The addition of induction chemotherapy was found to be superior to concurrent chemoradiation and surgery alone in a subsequent study (77). The 5-year overall survival in the induction arm followed by concurrent chemoradiation and surgery was 71% compared to 22% in the concurrent chemoradiation and surgery arm. Additional investigation is required to validate the findings in these studies, but multimodality therapy in the treatment of esophageal carcinoma is noted to have significant survival benefit.

SALVAGE SURGERY

Salvage surgery for persistent or recurrent disease of the hypopharynx or cervical esophagus following the completion of chemoradiation therapy may be particularly challenging but can prolong disease-free interval (78). Uneven tumor regression, ill-defined tumor borders, radiation-induced soft tissue fibrosis, and poor wound healing make salvage surgery a challenging endeavor (79). However, median survival in patients with recurrent head and neck cancer without any additional therapy is 3.8 months (80). With salvage surgery, median survival increases to 14 months after treatment of recurrent disease in the pharynx (78). From these two observations, salvage surgery is a viable option to prolong survival.

A follow-up study to the RTOG 91-11 trial revealed that 24.9% of all the patients required salvage laryngectomy (81). No significant survival difference was observed in any of the treatment arms (range 69% to 76%), which makes the point that surgical salvage is independent of prior therapy. Another study with promising result in salvage pharyngectomy for recurrent hypopharyngeal carcinoma comes from Toronto (82). They reviewed 72 patients with recurrent hypopharyngeal carcinoma who presented for surgical salvage. Their results demonstrated a 5-year overall survival of 31% with 5-year local and regional control rate of 70% and 71%. The presence of extracapsular extension, positive surgical margins, lymphovascular invasion, and nodal status was a negative predictor of local and regional control. These data are comparable to results from M.D. Anderson Cancer Center, where the authors reviewed their experience with induction chemotherapy and radiation for patients with hypopharyngeal carcinoma (75). They found 2-year survival after salvage laryngopharyngectomy was 75%. Another report from Germany presented results that are more dismal after salvage laryngopharyngectomy (83). They reviewed 28 patients with recurrent/persistent hypopharyngeal carcinoma, out of 134 patients who originally had organ preserving therapy, for surgical salvage. They found that only 2 of the 20 patients who had histologically proven recurrence were actually tumor free and alive after a mean observation time of 43.9 months. The authors concluded that patients must be informed of high morbidity and poor oncologic outcome after salvage surgery.

An important point to address from these studies is the high morbidity in salvage surgery. The Toronto group reported a 75% pharyngocutaneous fistula, and the

German study reported 73% fistula rate (83,84). The high perioperative morbidity in the setting of marginal oncologic control points to careful patient selection when performing salvage surgery for the hypopharynx.

FUNCTIONAL OUTCOMES

The hypopharynx and cervical esophagus represent the region of tightest control of bolus passage in the upper aerodigestive tract. Therefore, patients can feel a significant impact in their ability to maintain oral intake after treatment for their cancer. In surgical series of laryngopharyngectomy patients, despite good local control, the permanent gastrostomy rate still approaches 16% (38). In a review of the reconstruction of 153 postlaryngopharyngectomy patients, a stricture rate of 15% was also observed (82).

Organ preservation protocols also have significant dysphagia during and after treatment (85). Stricture rates have been reported as high as 20% postradiotherapy, with the hypopharynx primary being the most significant predictive factor (86). The introduction of intensity-modulated radiation therapy presents a recent advancement in the treatment of head and neck carcinoma with the advantage of a more accurate delineation of target volumes to spare the pharyngeal constrictors. However, this benefit may not be relevant in hypopharyngeal and cervical esophageal carcinoma (87,88). A recent series at M.D. Anderson Cancer demonstrated a 7% gastrostomy tube rate 2 years after organ preservation treatment for hypopharyngeal primary (Bhayani, et al. 2012, unpublished data). The authors found that patients who performed therapeutic exercises under the guidance of a speech pathologist and maintained some oral intake through radiation were less likely to have long-term gastrostomy tube dependence. Therefore, the incorporation of the speech pathologist in the multidisciplinary team is critical to the functional preservation of swallowing in patients with hypopharyngeal and cervical esophageal carcinoma.

Restoration of speech following total laryngopharyngectomy is accomplished with a tracheoesophageal puncture (TEP) and voice prosthesis. Because the presence of a bulky flap and variable position of the esophagus and neopharynx may interfere with TEP success, placement of the TEP is preferred as secondary procedure (89,90). Vocal intelligibility was between 72% and 81% in these case series, which is similar to another series from Australia (91). Primary TEP in the surgical series by Yu and colleagues found speech intelligibility of 41%, owing the poor result to perioperative complications and poor patient selection; therefore, the authors recommended secondary TEP for voice rehabilitation in complex pharyngoesophageal reconstruction.

Functional rehabilitation of speech and swallowing is possible with any curative therapy. The presence of speech pathology service dedicated to head and neck rehabilitation is a necessity to ensure optimal functional results.

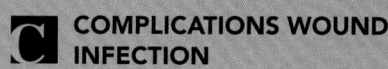

TABLE 122.5	COMPLICATIONS WOUND INFECTION

Hemorrhage
Fistula
Aspiration
Stricture

COMPLICATIONS

Complications encountered in surgery of the hypopharynx and cervical esophagus are similar to other major head and neck tumor resections (Tables 122.5 and 122.6). Poor wound healing and its sequelae, such as pharyngeal fistula, are the most common complications seen in the postoperative period. Patient comorbidities, such as malnutrition, prior radiation therapy, hypothyroidism, and hypovitaminosis, are critical factors in contributing to these complications. Technical details, such as suture type, tension at mucosal anastomosis, tumor at the pharyngeal margin, and reconstructive flap choice, also contribute to fistula formation.

Maintenance of a patent stoma is also a critical aspect in avoiding acute complications. Mucus plugging is a common occurrence postlaryngectomy. Diligent nursing care and frequent suctioning can avoid significant airway obstruction. This aspect also applies to patients who are tracheostomy dependent following partial laryngeal surgery.

Common delayed complications of surgery are stenosis and aspiration. Speech pathology consultation can provide therapeutic exercises to improve swallowing and reduce the risk of these issues. Regular dilation by either the head and neck surgeon or gastroenterologist, in conjunction with therapeutic exercises from the speech pathologist, can improve stenosis (92).

TABLE 122.6	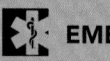 EMERGENCY CARE

Obstruction
Airway
Tracheotomy
Laser debulking
Esophagus
Feeding tube
Fluid resuscitation
Disimpaction
Hemorrhage
Isolate source
Angiography
Embolization
Surgical ligation

HIGHLIGHTS

- Patients with hypopharyngeal and cervical esophageal carcinoma are typically malnourished, causing multiple medical problems.
- Submucosal extension with satellite lesions and ill-defined margins is a hallmark of these tumors.
- Hypopharyngeal carcinoma patients have a 60% to 80% rate of lymphatic metastasis at presentation. Most common site of lymphatic metastasis is located in the jugulodigastric nodes. Paratracheal and paraesophageal nodal metastases are common in advanced-stage tumors.
- Cervical esophageal carcinoma patients have nodal spread to the paratracheal, paraesophageal, and upper mediastinal nodes.
- Retropharyngeal nodal involvement is common in tumors that extend into the retropharyngeal space. Surgical dissection of the space or radiation to these nodal levels is required as part of the treatment.
- Multidisciplinary evaluation by the head and neck surgeons, medical oncologists, radiation oncologists, plastic surgeon, radiologist, dentist, nutritionist, and speech pathologist is required prior to initiating treatment.
- Definitive radiation is an appropriate treatment for early-stage tumors of the hypopharynx. Surgery for these lesions may disrupt the pharyngeal plexus, which can create significant swallowing dysfunction.
- Advanced-stage tumors are best managed with total laryngopharyngectomy ± esophagectomy with free tissue reconstruction. Oncologic resection should not be compromised by reconstructive method.
- Organ preservation using chemotherapy and radiation therapy provides good local and regional control rates with acceptable morbidity. Surgical salvage is possible in the appropriately selected patient.
- Successful rehabilitation of speech and swallowing is feasible no matter the treatment modality in the motivated patient with a well-trained speech pathologist.

REFERENCES

1. Posner MR, et al. Sequential therapy for the locally advanced larynx and hypopharynx cancer subgroup in TAX 324: survival, surgery, and organ preservation. Ann Oncol 2009;20(5):921–927.
2. Lefebvre JL, et al. Larynx preservation in pyriform sinus cancer: preliminary results of a European Organization for Research and Treatment of Cancer phase III trial. EORTC Head and Neck Cancer Cooperative Group. J Natl Cancer Inst 1996;88(13):890–899.
3. Lefebvre JL, et al. Phase 3 randomized trial on larynx preservation comparing sequential vs. alternating chemotherapy and radiotherapy. J Natl Cancer Inst 2009;101(3):142–152.
4. de Bree R, et al. Paratracheal lymph node dissection in cancer of the larynx, hypopharynx, and cervical esophagus: the need for guidelines. Head Neck 2011;33(6):912–916.
5. Cooper JS, et al. National Cancer Database report on cancer of the head and neck: 10-year update. Head Neck 2009;31(6):748–758.
6. Jemal A, et al. Cancer statistics, 2010. CA Cancer J Clin 2010;60(5):277–300.
7. Sturgis EM, Cinciripini PM. Trends in head and neck cancer incidence in relation to smoking prevalence: an emerging epidemic of human papillomavirus-associated cancers? Cancer 2007;110(7):1429–1435.
8. Hoffman HT, et al. The National Cancer Database report on cancer of the head and neck. Arch Otolaryngol Head Neck Surg 1998;124(9):951–962.
9. Hall SF, et al. The natural history of patients with squamous cell carcinoma of the hypopharynx. Laryngoscope 2008;118(8):1362–1371.
10. Kadota H, et al. Larynx-preserving esophagectomy and jejunal transfer for cervical esophageal carcinoma. Laryngoscope 2009;119(7):1274–1280.
11. Lee YC, et al. Active and involuntary tobacco smoking and upper aerodigestive tract cancer risks in a multicenter case-control study. Cancer Epidemiol Biomarkers Prev 2009;18(12):3353–3361.
12. Menvielle G, et al. Smoking, alcohol drinking and cancer risk for various sites of the larynx and hypopharynx. A case-control study in France. Eur J Cancer Prev 2004;13(3):165–172.
13. Sapkota A, et al. Smokeless tobacco and increased risk of hypopharyngeal and laryngeal cancers: a multicentric case-control study from India. Int J Cancer 2007;121(8):1793–1798.
14. Franceschi S, et al. Alcohol and cancers of the upper aerodigestive tract in men and women. Cancer Epidemiol Biomarkers Prev 1994;3(4):299–304.
15. Becker M, et al. Imaging of the larynx and hypopharynx. Eur J Radiol 2008;66(3):460–479.
16. Zbaren P, Becker M, Lang H. Pretherapeutic staging of hypopharyngeal carcinoma. Clinical findings, computed tomography, and magnetic resonance imaging compared with histopathologic evaluation. Arch Otolaryngol Head Neck Surg 1997;123(9):908–913.
17. Hsu YB, et al. Role of chest computed tomography in head and neck cancer. Arch Otolaryngol Head Neck Surg 2008;134(10):1050–1054.
18. Houghton DJ, et al. Role of chest CT scanning in the management of patients presenting with head and neck cancer. Head Neck 1998;20(7):614–618.
19. Loh KS, et al. A rational approach to pulmonary screening in newly diagnosed head and neck cancer. Head Neck 2005;27(11):990–994.
20. Gourin CG, et al. Identification of distant metastases with positron-emission tomography-computed tomography in patients with previously untreated head and neck cancer. Laryngoscope 2008;118(4):671–675.
21. Krabbe CA, et al. FDG-PET and detection of distant metastases and simultaneous tumors in head and neck squamous cell carcinoma: a comparison with chest radiography and chest CT. Oral Oncol 2009;45(3):234–240.
22. Wax MK, et al. Positron emission tomography in the evaluation of synchronous lung lesions in patients with untreated head and neck cancer. Arch Otolaryngol Head Neck Surg 2002;128(6):703–707.
23. Marks JE, et al. The need for elective irradiation of occult lymphatic metastases from cancers of the larynx and pyriform sinus. Head Neck Surg 1985;8(1):3–8.
24. Ceylan A, et al. Thyroid gland invasion in advanced laryngeal and hypopharyngeal carcinoma. Kulak Burun Bogaz Ihtis Derg 2004;13(1–2):9–14.
25. Buckley JG, MacLennan K. Cervical node metastases in laryngeal and hypopharyngeal cancer: a prospective analysis of prevalence and distribution. Head Neck 2000;22(4):380–385.
26. Koo BS, et al. Management of contralateral N0 neck in pyriform sinus carcinoma. Laryngoscope 2006;116(7):1268–1272.
27. Mercante G, et al. Involvement of level I neck lymph nodes and submandibular gland in laryngeal and/or hypopharyngeal squamous cell carcinoma. J Otolaryngol 2006;35(2):108–111.
28. Joo YH, et al. The impact of paratracheal lymph node metastasis in squamous cell carcinoma of the hypopharynx. Eur Arch Otorhinolaryngol 2010;267(6):945–950.

29. Timon CV, Toner M, Conlon BJ. Paratracheal lymph node involvement in advanced cancer of the larynx, hypopharynx, and cervical esophagus. *Laryngoscope* 2003;113(9):1595–1599.

30. Hirano S, et al. Upper mediastinal node dissection for hypopharyngeal and cervical esophageal carcinomas. *Ann Otol Rhinol Laryngol* 2007;116(4):290–296.

31. Martins AS. Neck and mediastinal node dissection in pharyngolaryngoesophageal tumors. *Head Neck* 2001;23(9):772–779.

32. Amatsu M, Mohri M, Kinishi M. Significance of retropharyngeal node dissection at radical surgery for carcinoma of the hypopharynx and cervical esophagus. *Laryngoscope* 2001;111(6):1099–1103.

33. Coskun HH, et al. Retropharyngeal lymph node metastases in head and neck malignancies. *Head Neck* 2011;33(10):1520–1529.

34. Gross ND, et al. Impact of retropharyngeal lymph node metastasis in head and neck squamous cell carcinoma. *Arch Otolaryngol Head Neck Surg* 2004;130(2):169–173.

35. Ge N, et al. Prognostic significance of Oct4 and Sox2 expression in hypopharyngeal squamous cell carcinoma. *J Transl Med* 2010;8:94.

36. Clayman GL, et al. Human papillomavirus in laryngeal and hypopharyngeal carcinomas. Relationship to survival. *Arch Otolaryngol Head Neck Surg* 1994;120(7):743–748.

37. Ernoux-Neufcoeur P, et al. Combined analysis of HPV DNA, p16, p21 and p53 to predict prognosis in patients with stage IV hypopharyngeal carcinoma. *J Cancer Res Clin Oncol* 2011;137(1):173–181.

38. Takes RP, et al. Current trends in initial management of hypopharyngeal cancer: the declining use of open surgery. *Head Neck* 2012;34(2):270–281.

39. Kraus DH, et al. Combined surgery and radiation therapy for squamous cell carcinoma of the hypopharynx. *Otolaryngol Head Neck Surg* 1997;116(6 Pt 1):637–641.

40. Tong DK, et al. Current management of cervical esophageal cancer. *World J Surg* 2011;35(3):600–607.

41. Daiko H, et al. Surgical management of carcinoma of the cervical esophagus. *J Surg Oncol* 2007;96(2):166–172.

42. Wheless SA, McKinney KA, Zanation AM. A prospective study of the clinical impact of a multidisciplinary head and neck tumor board. *Otolaryngol Head Neck Surg* 2010;143(5):650–654.

43. Lewis CM, et al. Prereferral head and neck cancer treatment: compliance with National Comprehensive Cancer Network treatment guidelines. *Arch Otolaryngol Head Neck Surg* 2010;136(12):1205–1211.

44. Makeieff M, et al. Supraglottic hemipharyngolaryngectomy for the treatment of T1 and T2 carcinomas of laryngeal margin and piriform sinus. *Head Neck* 2004;26(8):701–705.

45. Chevalier D, et al. Supraglottic hemilaryngopharyngectomy plus radiation for the treatment of early lateral margin and pyriform sinus carcinoma. *Head Neck* 1997;19(1):1–5.

46. Laccourreye O, et al. Supracricoid hemilaryngopharyngectomy in patients with invasive squamous cell carcinoma of the pyriform sinus. Part I: technique, complications, and long-term functional outcome. *Ann Otol Rhinol Laryngol* 2005;114(1 Pt 1):25–34.

47. Kania R, et al. Supracricoid hemilaryngopharyngectomy in patients with invasive squamous cell carcinoma of the pyriform sinus. Part II: incidence and consequences of local recurrence. *Ann Otol Rhinol Laryngol* 2005;114(2):95–104.

48. Bova R, et al. Total pharyngolaryngectomy for squamous cell carcinoma of the hypopharynx: a review. *Laryngoscope* 2005;115(5):864–869.

49. Lydiatt WM, et al. Posterior pharyngeal carcinoma resection with larynx preservation and radial forearm free flap reconstruction: a preliminary report. *Head Neck* 1996;18(6):501–505.

50. Jol JK, et al. Larynx preservation surgery for advanced posterior pharyngeal wall carcinoma with free flap reconstruction: a critical appraisal. *Oral Oncol* 2003;39(6):552–558.

51. Steiner W, et al. Organ preservation by transoral laser microsurgery in piriform sinus carcinoma. *Otolaryngol Head Neck Surg* 2001;124(1):58–67.

52. Kutter J, et al. Transoral laser surgery for pharyngeal and pharyngolaryngeal carcinomas. *Arch Otolaryngol Head Neck Surg* 2007;133(2):139–144.

53. Martin A, et al. Organ preserving transoral laser microsurgery for cancer of the hypopharynx. *Laryngoscope* 2008;118(3):398–402.

54. Bhayani MK, Holsinger FC, Lai SY. A shifting paradigm for patients with head and neck cancer: transoral robotic surgery (TORS). *Oncology (Williston Park)* 2010;24(11):1010–1015.

55. Boudreaux BA, et al. Robot-assisted surgery for upper aerodigestive tract neoplasms. *Arch Otolaryngol Head Neck Surg* 2009;135(4):397–401.

56. Park YM, et al. Feasibility of transoral robotic hypopharyngectomy for early-stage hypopharyngeal carcinoma. *Oral Oncol* 2010;46(8):597–602.

57. Weber PC, Johnson JT, Myers EN. Impact of bilateral neck dissection on recovery following supraglottic laryngectomy. *Arch Otolaryngol Head Neck Surg* 1993;119(1):61–64.

58. Spriano G, Pellini R, Roselli R. Pectoralis major myocutaneous flap for hypopharyngeal reconstruction. *Plast Reconstr Surg* 2002;110(6):1408–1413; discussion 1414–1416.

59. Hong JW, et al. Hypopharyngeal reconstruction using remnant narrow pharyngeal wall as omega-shaped radial forearm free flap. *J Craniofac Surg* 2009;20(5):1334–1340.

60. Spyropoulou GA, et al. Reconstruction of the hypopharynx with the anterolateral thigh flap: defect classification, method, tips, and outcomes. *Plast Reconstr Surg* 2011;127(1):161–172.

61. Joo YH, et al. Fasciocutaneous free flap reconstruction for squamous cell carcinoma of the hypopharynx. *Eur Arch Otorhinolaryngol* 2011;268(2):289–294.

62. Clark JR, et al. Morbidity after flap reconstruction of hypopharyngeal defects. *Laryngoscope* 2006;116(2):173–181.

63. Wadsworth JT, Futran N, Eubanks TR. Laparoscopic harvest of the jejunal free flap for reconstruction of hypopharyngeal and cervical esophageal defects. *Arch Otolaryngol Head Neck Surg* 2002;128(12):1384–1387.

64. Ferahkose Z, et al. Comparison of free jejunal graft with gastric pull-up reconstruction after resection of hypopharyngeal and cervical esophageal carcinoma. *Dis Esophagus* 2008;21(4):340–345.

65. Richmon JD, Brumund KT. Reconstruction of the hypopharynx: current trends. *Curr Opin Otolaryngol Head Neck Surg* 2007;15(4):208–212.

66. Poh M, et al. Technical challenges of total esophageal reconstruction using a supercharged jejunal flap. *Ann Surg* 2011;253(6):1122–1129.

67. Foote RL. Radiotherapy alone for early-stage squamous cell carcinoma of the larynx and hypopharynx. *Int J Radiat Oncol Biol Phys* 2007;69(2 Suppl):S31–S36.

68. Yoshimura R, et al. Outcomes in patients with early-stage hypopharyngeal cancer treated with radiotherapy. *Int J Radiat Oncol Biol Phys* 2010;77(4):1017–1023.

69. Hinerman RW, et al. Surgery and postoperative radiotherapy for squamous cell carcinoma of the larynx and pharynx. *Am J Clin Oncol* 2006;29(6):613–621.

70. Pignon JP, et al. Meta-analysis of chemotherapy in head and neck cancer (MACH-NC): an update on 93 randomised trials and 17,346 patients. *Radiother Oncol* 2009;92(1):4–14.

71. Cooper JS, et al. Postoperative concurrent radiotherapy and chemotherapy for high-risk squamous-cell carcinoma of the head and neck. *N Engl J Med* 2004;350(19):1937–1944.

72. Bernier J, et al. Postoperative irradiation with or without concomitant chemotherapy for locally advanced head and neck cancer. *N Engl J Med* 2004;350(19):1945–1952.

73. The Department of Veterans Affairs Laryngeal Cancer Study Group. Induction chemotherapy plus radiation compared with surgery plus radiation in patients with advanced laryngeal cancer. *N Engl J Med* 1991;324(24):1685–1690.

74. Forastiere AA, et al. Concurrent chemotherapy and radiotherapy for organ preservation in advanced laryngeal cancer. *N Engl J Med* 2003;349(22):2091–2098.

75. Clayman GL, et al. Laryngeal preservation for advanced laryngeal and hypopharyngeal cancers. *Arch Otolaryngol Head Neck Surg* 1995;121(2):219–223.

76. Liao Z, et al. Esophagectomy after concurrent chemoradiotherapy improves locoregional control in clinical stage II or III esophageal cancer patients. *Int J Radiat Oncol Biol Phys* 2004;60(5):1484–1493.

77. Jin J, et al. Induction chemotherapy improved outcomes of patients with resectable esophageal cancer who received chemoradiotherapy

followed by surgery. *Int J Radiat Oncol Biol Phys* 2004;60(2): 427–436.

78. Goodwin WJ Jr. Salvage surgery for patients with recurrent squamous cell carcinoma of the upper aerodigestive tract: when do the ends justify the means? *Laryngoscope* 2000;110(3 Pt 2, Suppl 93):1–18.

79. Wong RJ, Shah JP. The role of the head and neck surgeon in contemporary multidisciplinary treatment programs for advanced head and neck cancer. *Curr Opin Otolaryngol Head Neck Surg* 2010;18(2):79–82.

80. Kowalski LP, Carvalho AL. Natural history of untreated head and neck cancer. *Eur J Cancer* 2000;36(8):1032–1037.

81. Weber RS, et al. Outcome of salvage total laryngectomy following organ preservation therapy: the Radiation Therapy Oncology Group trial 91–11. *Arch Otolaryngol Head Neck Surg* 2003;129(1):44–49.

82. Clark JR, et al. Primary and salvage (hypo)pharyngectomy: analysis and outcome. *Head Neck* 2006;28(8):671–677.

83. Relic A, et al. Salvage surgery after induction chemotherapy with paclitaxel/cisplatin and primary radiotherapy for advanced laryngeal and hypopharyngeal carcinomas. *Eur Arch Otorhinolaryngol* 2009;266(11):1799–1805.

84. Dirven R, et al. The assessment of pharyngocutaneous fistula rate in patients treated primarily with definitive radiotherapy followed by salvage surgery of the larynx and hypopharynx. *Laryngoscope* 2009;119(9):1691–1695.

85. Rosenthal DI, Lewin JS, Eisbruch A. Prevention and treatment of dysphagia and aspiration after chemoradiation for head and neck cancer. *J Clin Oncol* 2006;24(17):2636–2643.

86. Lee WT, et al. Risk factors for hypopharyngeal/upper esophageal stricture formation after concurrent chemoradiation. *Head Neck* 2006;28(9):808–812.

87. Caudell JJ, et al. Factors associated with long-term dysphagia after definitive radiotherapy for locally advanced head-and-neck cancer. *Int J Radiat Oncol Biol Phys* 2009;73(2):410–415.

88. Eisbruch A, et al. Dysphagia and aspiration after chemoradiotherapy for head-and-neck cancer: which anatomic structures are affected and can they be spared by IMRT? *Int J Radiat Oncol Biol Phys* 2004;60(5):1425–1439.

89. LeBert B, et al. Secondary tracheoesophageal puncture with in-office transnasal esophagoscopy. *Arch Otolaryngol Head Neck Surg* 2009;135(12):1190–1194.

90. Yu P, et al. Pharyngoesophageal reconstruction with the anterolateral thigh flap after total laryngopharyngectomy. *Cancer* 2010; 116(7):1718–1724.

91. Sharp DA, et al. Long-term functional speech and swallowing outcomes following pharyngolaryngectomy with free jejunal flap reconstruction. *Ann Plast Surg* 2010;64(6):743–746.

92. Ahlawat SK, Al-Kawas FH. Endoscopic management of upper esophageal strictures after treatment of head and neck malignancy. *Gastrointest Endosc* 2008;68(1):19–24.

123 Early Laryngeal Cancer

Parul Sinha   *Oluwafunmilola Okuyemi*   *Bruce H. Haughey*

The term *"early laryngeal cancer"* refers to a mucosally derived neoplastic lesion that may invade deeply into soft tissue, but not into the underlying cartilage. The majority of literature reports include carcinoma *in situ* (CIS), T1 and T2 lesions in the spectrum of early laryngeal cancer. At the glottic level, early cancer implies a local lesion limited to single or multiple sites in the glottis or adjacent laryngeal subsites that might impair the cord mobility but does not cause cord fixation. Overall, these lesions display pathologic invasiveness and a potential to metastasize, which exceeds that of CIS but is less than deeply infiltrating carcinoma (1). By contrast, early supraglottic cancer may not be confined to the primary site because of its regional metastatic behavior. Pathologic invasion of the epiglottic cartilaginous foramina, short of entering the preepiglottic space (PES), is included.

EPIDEMIOLOGY

Laryngeal cancer is the second most common type of head and neck cancer worldwide, with an estimated incidence of 151,000 cases resulting in about 82,000 deaths annually (2). With a male-to-female ratio of 6:1, laryngeal cancer is also the 13th most common cancer in men worldwide (2). Geographic variations in the incidence and mortality of laryngeal cancer suggest that a larger proportion of the cases occur in South-Central Asia, Eastern Asia, Central Europe, and Eastern Europe (2): incidence in the United States has declined, associated with reduced smoking (3).

In the United States, laryngeal cancer accounts for about one-fourth of the annual cases of head and neck cancer with an estimated incidence of 12,720 cases (4). Overall, about 60% of laryngeal cancer cases are diagnosed as *"early laryngeal cancer"* and encompass the Tis, T1N0M0, or T2N0M0 categories (5). These commonly arise from the glottis and are mostly squamous cell carcinoma (6). Variation in site predominance, however, has been reported across ethnic groups; for example, glottic cancers appear to be the most common in Caucasians, while in African Americans, the incidence of glottic and supraglottic cancers appear to be equal (7).

RISK FACTORS

Smoking and alcohol consumption are well-established etiologic factors for laryngeal cancers. Their combined use has been associated with a multiplicative effect for the risk of developing laryngeal cancer (8,9). A recent study by Hashibe et al. (10) showed that the incidence of cancers attributable to tobacco and alcohol exposure was the highest in larynx of all head and neck cancer sites at 89%. About 5% of laryngeal cancers occur in nonsmokers and nondrinkers, suggesting that other factors such as diet, gastroesophageal reflux, previous radiation, and viral infection may also contribute (11). Human papillomavirus types 16 and 18 have been detected in frequencies ranging from 5% to 32% of analyzed samples in laryngeal cancer (11). Occupational exposures to wood dust, polycyclic hydrocarbons, and asbestos have also been associated with increased risk for developing laryngeal cancer (12).

TUMOR BIOLOGY

Genetics

Genetic alterations have been shown to underlie the development of precancerous lesions and their progression to invasive laryngeal carcinoma (13–15). Loss of heterozygosity and microsatellite instability at certain genetic loci has been identified in the progression to invasive laryngeal cancer (13).

1. Mutations in *p16*, a tumor suppressor gene located at chromosome 9p21, occur in over half of laryngeal squamous cell carcinomas and are believed to occur early in the progression to invasive squamous cell carcinoma (SCC) of the larynx (16).
2. Overexpression of *cyclin D1*, a key cell-cycle regulatory protein, results in increased cellular proliferation and tumorigenesis (17). It has also been shown to correlate with poor prognosis, recurrence, and lymph node metastasis (18).
3. Alterations in *p53*, a tumor suppressor gene that maps to the 17p13 locus, result in destabilization of genomic repair processes leading to tumorigenesis (17).

Pathology

Laryngeal cancer is thought to arise from precancerous lesions. These precancerous lesions are characterized by atypical cellular changes with malignant features (loss of cell maturation, nuclear atypia, increased mitotic activity) that occur in response to carcinogenic exposures especially tobacco smoke and alcohol. The precancerous lesions include *dysplasia* (graded from "mild" to "severe" depending on the extent of epithelial involvement) and CIS (involvement of the whole thickness of the epithelium). These preinvasive lesions are, by definition, confined to the epithelium of the larynx with an intact basement membrane. Progression to microinvasive and invasive carcinoma is characterized by infiltration of basement membrane and the underlying tissue.

Histologically, squamous cell carcinomas account for over 95% of primary laryngeal cancers and arise from the stratified squamous epithelium lining the larynx (8). Other less-commonly encountered histologic types of primary laryngeal cancer include verrucous squamous cell carcinoma (a highly differentiated variant with low incidence for metastases), adenocarcinoma, spindle cell carcinoma, fibrosarcoma, and chondrosarcoma. Neuroendocrine tumors, though rare, are the most common nonsquamous tumors encountered and have a predilection for the supraglottic larynx.

ANATOMY OF THE LARYNX

The laryngeal skeleton is composed of cartilages—thyroid, cricoid, arytenoids, epiglottis, cuneiform, and corniculate—interconnected with ligaments and membranes and moved by groups of intrinsic and extrinsic laryngeal muscles (see Fig. 124.2).

Anatomical subsites: The larynx is divided into three regions: supraglottis, glottis, and subglottis. The *supraglottis* extends from the epiglottis to the ventricular apices, encompassing the false cords, aryepiglottic folds, the arytenoids, and the laryngeal surface of the epiglottis. The *glottis* contains the true vocal cords, the anterior commissure, the interarytenoid region, and the floor of the ventricles. It extends inferiorly to 1 cm below the plane of the apex of the ventricles.

The true vocal cords thicken at the anterior commissure and form the *macula flava*, anterior to which the ligaments merge into the Broyle tendon. The Broyle tendon, also known as anterior commissure tendon, gets inserted into the thyroid cartilage. The *subglottis* extends from 1 cm below the apex of ventricles to the lower border of the cricoid cartilage.

Laryngeal membranes: The *conus elasticus* or the cricovocal membrane arises from the inner surface of the cricoid arch and extends superiorly to attach anteriorly to the inner surface of the thyroid cartilage and posteriorly to the tip of the vocal process of arytenoids. Its free upper border thickens to form the vocal ligament. The *quadrangular membrane* extends between the arytenoids and epiglottis. Its upper border forms the aryepiglottic fold, while the free lower border constitutes the false cord. The *thyrohyoid membrane* is another fibroelastic membrane that attaches inferiorly to the upper border of the thyroid cartilage and superiorly to the posterior surface of hyoid bone.

Laryngeal spaces: Knowledge of laryngeal spaces is important to the understanding of the spread of laryngeal cancer and, therefore, planning of conservation surgical procedures. The *preepiglottic* space or the *space of Boyer* lies anterior to the infrahyoid epiglottis. It is bounded superiorly by the hyoepiglottic ligament, inferiorly by the attachment of epiglottis to the thyroid and anteriorly by the thyrohyoid membrane and upper part of the thyroid cartilage. It contains fibrofatty tissue and numerous lymphatic channels. Laterally, it merges with the paraglottic space. The *paraglottic space* surrounds the laryngeal ventricle and is bounded anterolaterally by the thyroid cartilage, posterolaterally by pyriform sinus mucosa, superomedially by quadrangular membrane, and inferomedially by conus elasticus. The paraglottic space provides an important route to extralaryngeal spread of cancer.

Lymphatic pathways: The supraglottis has a rich lymphatic network. The lymphatics drain primarily to the upper jugular (level II) chain of lymph nodes. It can extend to the middle (level III) and lower jugular groups (level IV), and depending on the site of tumor, cross-drainage may occur to the contralateral nodes. Lymphatic drainage from the glottis is essentially nonexistent although the cords themselves have a network of superficial mucosal lymphatics. The paratracheal (level VI) group of lymph nodes is the primary echelon of lymphatic drainage from the subglottis that may further spread to the delphian node and upper mediastinal (level VII) or the level IV nodes.

Blood supply: The arterial blood supply to the supraglottic larynx is derived from the superior laryngeal artery, a branch of the superior thyroid artery; the lower half of the larynx is supplied by the inferior laryngeal branch of the inferior thyroid artery.

Nerve supply: Sensation above the vocal fold is supplied by the internal branch of the superior laryngeal nerve, whereas the external branch provides motor supply to the cricothyroid muscles. Both sensory and motor innervations below the vocal fold are provided by the recurrent laryngeal nerve.

EARLY SUPRAGLOTTIC CANCER

Supraglottic squamous cell cancers comprise 30% to 40% of laryngeal cancers in the United States (5,19). The lesions are often silent in their early stages and may present with non–site-specific symptoms such as a sore throat or referred otalgia. Persistent dysphagia or aspiration does not usually manifest until the primary tumor attains significant bulk. Due to abundant lymphatic outflow, an enlarged metastatic neck node is another mode of presentation for early supraglottic tumors. The incidence of cervical metastasis at presentation, however, depends upon the T stage, location, and differentiation of the primary tumor and is reported to vary from zero to approximately 33% in T1–T2 tumors (20).

Surgical Pathology

Whole-organ laryngeal section studies (21,22) and numerous clinical observations (23–25) have postulated the supraglottic larynx as a distinct anatomic laryngeal subunit, above the true vocal cords. This compartmentalization is partly attributed to separate embryologic derivations, with the supraglottic structures emanating from branchial arches III and IV (buccopharyngeal anlage) and the glottic–subglottic structures from branchial arch VI (tracheopulmonary anlage). However, no specific anatomical structure has been identified that might act as a barrier between the supraglottic and glottic regions (23).

Early tumors spread within the confines of the supraglottic unit. This concept combined with an understanding of the key avenues of extension, makes supraglottic laryngectomy (SGL), endoscopic or open, a highly effective option for treatment of early-stage cancers. Infrequently, invasion of the glottis can occur when the tumor of the epiglottic petiole extends inferiorly or when extension from the undersurface of the false cord reaches the ventricle.

A certain subset of tumors arises in the (infrahyoid) angle between the epiglottis and the anterior false cord. Dubbed "engelkarzinom" by our German colleagues, this presentation may have considerable deep extension toward or into the PES.

The epiglottic perichondrium and the thyroepiglottic ligament limit anterior extension, but the tumor spreads into the fatty areolar tissue of the PES via infiltration through the epiglottic cartilage fenestrations. Involvement of PES implies a T3 stage, but insidious extension in this direction can occur in early supraglottic lesions, particularly if the tumor originates in the infrahyoid epiglottis. In the PES, there is a transition of the tumor edge from "infiltrating" to broad, "pushing" type with a pseudocapsule, probably arising from the expanded epiglottic perichondrium (21). A tumor-free space usually exists between the hyoid bone and the advancing front of the tumor, a feature that makes preservation of the hyoid in SGL oncologically safe and functionally superior. In late tumors, extralaryngeal spread occurs when extension is observed anteriorly from the PES, breaching the thyrohyoid membrane, sometimes reaching the strap muscles. Another late route of extralaryngeal spread is through the hyoepiglottic ligament to the vallecula and tongue base superiorly. Deep lateral extension of the supraglottic tumor to the thyroid cartilage is rare; ossified cartilage has higher susceptibility to invasion. Lesions of the aryepiglottic fold may spread laterally to involve the medial wall of pyriform sinus.

Staging and Treatment Planning

A complete workup to assess the patient, the subsite and stage of primary tumor, and the presence of cervical lymphadenopathy is indicated (Table 123.1). This includes a thorough history and physical examination, including neck palpation and fiberoptic laryngoscopy. This affords direct visualization of the tumor extent, arytenoid involvement, and cord mobility. Cord hypomobility implies paraglottic space invasion, and cord fixation upstages the primary tumor to T3.

Assessment of comorbidity, particularly, pulmonary diseases, is a crucial component of preoperative planning for conservation surgery. Patients with poor pulmonary reserve, as determined by forced expiratory volume in one second (FEV1) of greater than 75% or FEV1/FVC (functional vital capacity) ratio of less than 65%, are at greater risk of troublesome aspiration.

For T2 lesions, radiologic evaluation with computed tomography (CT) or magnetic resonance imaging (MRI) is performed to determine the extent of the primary and to rule out involvement of the PES, the paraglottic space, or the inner thyroid cortex, factors that escalate the T stage. CT, MRI, and especially gray-scale ultrasonography can reliably assess cervical lymphadenopathy, supplemented by ultrasound-guided fine-needle aspiration (FNA), if indicated. The latter is particularly useful in decision making for or against treating the contralateral neck (see "Management of the Neck"). Chest radiography, CT, or positron emission tomography (PET) is used to evaluate distant metastasis or second primary tumors in smokers.

Operative direct laryngoscopy should be performed along with photodocumentation to accurately assess the primary tumor and obtain biopsies for diagnosis and/or mapping in postradiation, recurrent cases. It also provides the opportunity to determine the suitability for a conservation procedure and decide the ideal approach—transoral or open. Occasionally, exophytic bulk conceals the accurate determination of the inferior tumor extent, whereupon rigid telescopes may be helpful. To detect synchronous primaries, a complete examination of the upper aerodigestive tract (UADT) mucosa is performed.

Treatment

Single-modality therapy with primary surgery or definitive radiotherapy (RT) are the two alternative treatment approaches for early supraglottic tumors. RT alone,

TABLE 123.1	DIAGNOSTIC APPROACH TO EARLY SUPRAGLOTTIC AND GLOTTIC CANCERS

Supraglottis	Glottis

• History and physical examination, office-based fiberoptic laryngoscopy
• Imaging: Office neck ultrasonography, CT/MRI for assessment of primary tumor and neck, chest CT or PET
• Pulmonary function test
• Direct laryngoscopy under anesthesia for biopsy and assessment of
  – Site, size, and extent of primary tumor
  – Tumor extension to vallecula, tongue base, pharyngeal wall, medial wall of piriform sinus, arytenoid/ventricle
  – Cord mobility
  – Palpation of neck nodes
  – Adequacy of transoral exposure
  – UADT examination for second primaries
	• History and physical examination, office-based fiberoptic laryngoscopy and videostroboscopy
	• Imaging: Limited role, evaluation of invasion in bulky lesions
	• Pulmonary function test
	• Direct laryngoscopy under anesthesia for biopsy and assessment of
	  – Site, size, surface, and extent of primary tumor
	  – Tumor extension to subglottis, arytenoid, supraglottis, anterior commissure, petiole of epiglottis
	  – Cord mobility
	  – Adequacy of transoral exposure, especially anterior commissure
	  – UADT examination for second primaries

UADT, upper aerodigestive tract.

however, is less effective for local control (26), and high laryngectomy rates (14% to 31%) for recurrent tumors (27,28) have made this option less acceptable than primary surgery. T1 and T2 primaries are amenable to curative treatment by conservation surgery with an optimum oncologic control and minimal functional morbidity. Total laryngectomy was the only procedure commonly used for treatment of supraglottic cancer until 1946 when Alonso (29) first described the procedure of SGL. The SGL technique was later refined by Joseph Ogura in 1958 (30) and Max Som in 1959 (24). The modern paradigm of conservation surgery for supraglottic tumors, however, is minimally invasive, endoscopic transoral laser microsurgery (TLM), first introduced by Vaughan et al. in 1978 (31) and further popularized by Davis et al. (32) and Steiner (33–36). Numerous publications within the last two decades on TLM for supraglottic tumors demonstrate evidence of both comparable (or superior) survival rates and functional preservation rates compared to open surgical procedures. This makes TLM a widely preferred surgical tool in the armamentarium of organ preservation treatment for supraglottic cancer (37,38). Limited reports of technical feasibility also now exist for use of the da Vinci robotic surgical system (39).

SURGERY

Endoscopic Procedures

Transoral Laser Microsurgery

The concept of endoscopic management of supraglottic cancer dates back to 1939 when Jackson and Jackson (40) first described the use of the laryngoscope for resection of cancer of the suprahyoid epiglottis (Figs. 123.1A, 123.2,

and 123.3). Coupling of the carbon dioxide (CO_2) laser to the operating microscope in 1969 by Strong and Jako (41) heralded the advent of TLM. The basic technique of *transtumoral* cuts to assess the depth of disease and *multibloc* transoral laser resection is distinct from the time-honored principle of *en bloc* tumor resection, espoused in open techniques, where exposure of large surface areas of dissected tissue occurs. The transoral approach, however, makes it possible to resect the primary tumor with optimally cleared histologic margins and, at the same time, preserve the anatomical and functional integrity of the noninvolved, surrounding tissue. The resection can be tailored according to tumor location and extension. A classification of different types of endoscopic SGL has been described by the European Laryngological Society (ELS) (Table 123.2) (42). The fundamental requirements for TLM include careful training in technique, knowledge of site-specific "inside out" anatomy, good endoscopic access, and strict enforcement of laser-specific precautions in the operating room.

Contraindications: The major contraindication to TLM for early supraglottic cancers is inadequate transoral access to the entire tumor. We have proposed 8 'T's (45) as limitations of endoscopic access: teeth (prominent), trismus, transverse dimensions (narrow mandibular arch), tori (mandibular), tongue (bulk), tilt (atlanto-occipital extension), treatment (prior radio- or chemoradiotherapy), and tumor (site and size). Once adequate exposure is obtained, there are few technical constraints in terms of curative resection with TLM, even in the presence of intraoperative upgrade of T2 tumors to T3, secondary to spread into the preepiglottic or paraglottic space, glottis, arytenoid, or thyroid cartilage. A further contraindication is disease that requires bilateral arytenoid resection, which causes a high

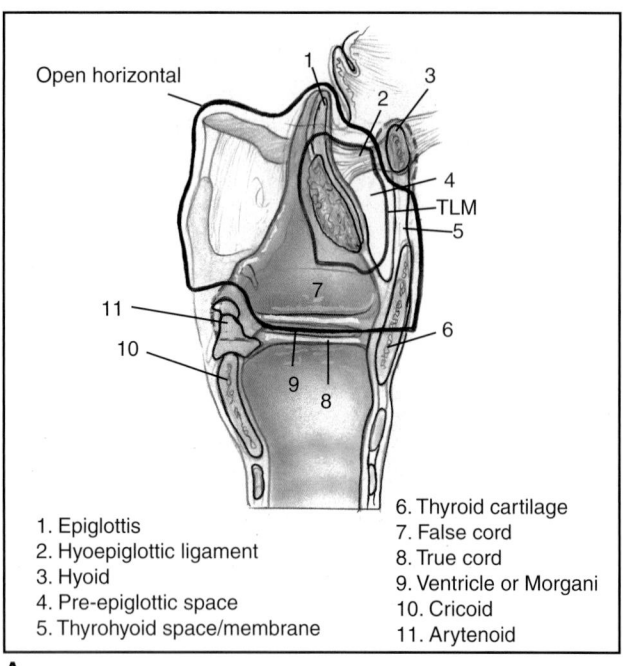

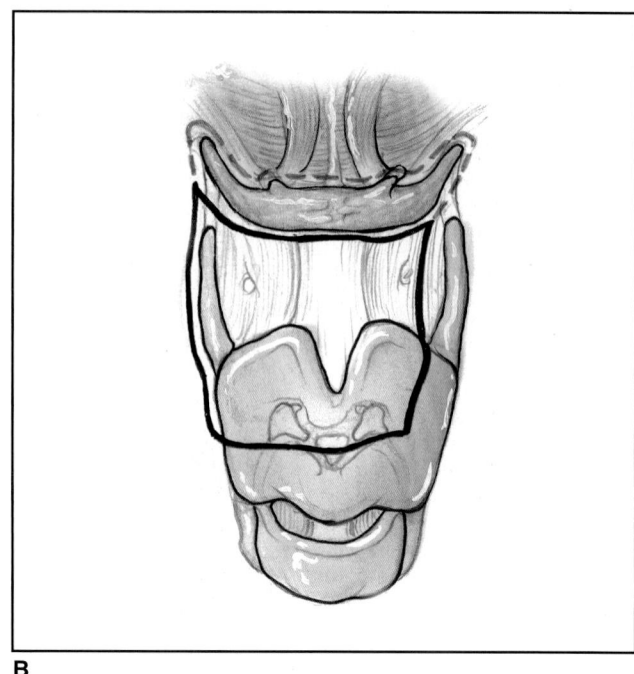

Open horizontal

TLM

1. Epiglottis
2. Hyoepiglottic ligament
3. Hyoid
4. Pre-epiglottic space
5. Thyrohyoid space/membrane
6. Thyroid cartilage
7. False cord
8. True cord
9. Ventricle or Morgani
10. Cricoid
11. Arytenoid

A   **B**

Figure 123.1 Supraglottic Laryngectomy. **A:** Incisions for TLM *(red)* and open horizontal *(black)* procedures, *sagittal view.* **B:** External incisions for open horizontal procedure. Note less resection of normal structures in TLM. Extensions *(dotted line)* in either technique may include hyoid and/or arytenoid.

potential for defunctionalization of safe swallowing, especially in context of poor pulmonary reserve, other major comorbidities, or compromised performance status.

Surgical technique: After induction of anesthesia and intubation with a 5-mm inner diameter (preferable) laser endotracheal tube, the usual safety precautions are observed for protection of eyes and face of the patient.

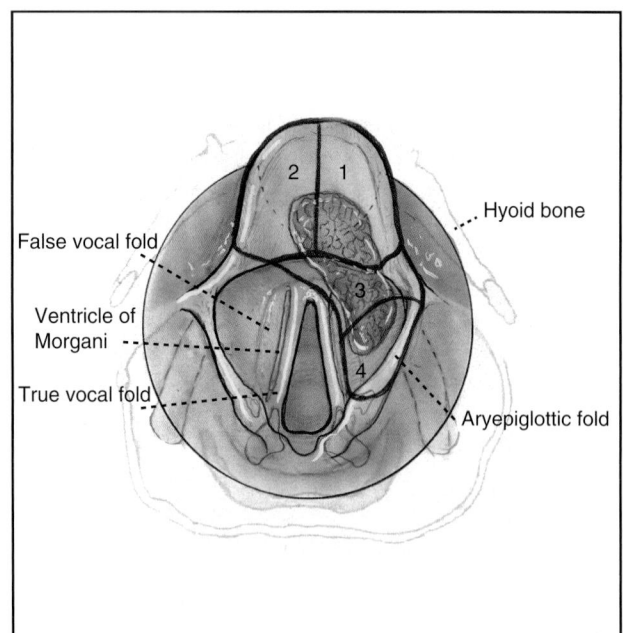

False vocal fold

Ventricle of Morgani

True vocal fold

Hyoid bone

Aryepiglottic fold

Figure 123.2 Incisions for multibloc TLM resection of supraglottic tumor. Blocs *1–4* are removed in numerical order.

An Aquaplast mouth guard is fashioned to protect the patient's teeth and upper gingiva. Optimum visualization of the operative site is obtained with introduction of laryngoscopes, standard tubed or bivalved, for example, Steiner, Weerda, Kleinsasser. The laryngoscopes may need to be changed or repositioned during the procedure for a satisfactory exposure. Transoral resection is performed with a CO_2 laser beam delivered either via micromanipulator or a handheld device, although rapid debulking may initially be performed with electrocautery. For margin management, the high-precision and relatively bloodless cutting characteristics of laser, under high magnification, facilitate clear intraoperative distinction between tumor and normal tissue. Surgical techniques specific to tumor size and subsite are described below.

Suprahyoid epiglottis: Small and well-circumscribed primaries may be resected *en bloc* for efficiency of margin evaluation. For larger lesions, the epiglottis is divided sagittally from superior to inferior, followed by lateral cuts across the vallecula, lateral pharyngoepiglottic fold, and the epiglottis, bilaterally if necessary, to complete resection of the tumor. Wide resection margins can be obtained at this site without swallowing morbidity.

Infrahyoid epiglottis: Early primaries of the infrahyoid epiglottis need to be addressed with caution because of close proximity to the PES. However, some tumors may be "keyholed" out of the epiglottis by excising a disc of mucosa and epiglottic cartilage containing the disease, with perichondrium, using the preepiglottic fat as the deep margin. When the disease is more extensive across the laryngeal surface of the epiglottis, the suprahyoid epiglottis may

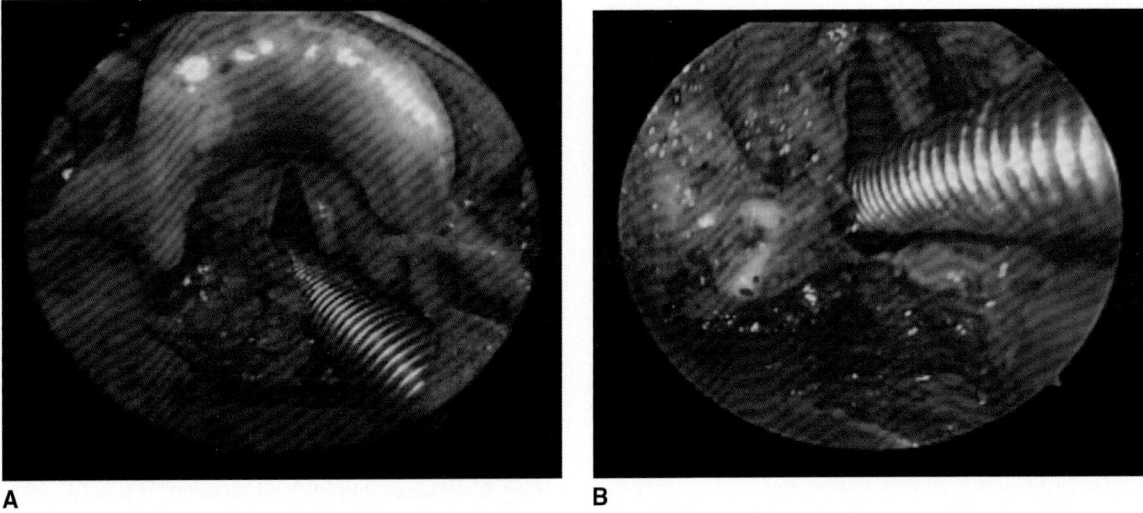

Figure 123.3 Endoscopic image of T2 supraglottic tumor, **(A)** pre- and **(B)** post-TLM resection.

be split sagittally (Fig. 123.2) and an ipsilateral hemiepiglottectomy performed. A second, medial to lateral cut is made in the nadir of vallecula to incise around the epiglottis with adequate margins of at least 5 mm. As this incision progresses to transect the lateral pharyngoepiglottic fold, identification of the superior laryngeal artery and/or its branches may be necessary. When identified, they should be clipped before division, failing which they may retract into the lateral soft tissues. Incisions are further made laterally, until the hyoid is reached, to detach the specimen and also partially excise the fatty areolar tissue in the PES. This is facilitated by application of neck pressure applied

externally on the larynx to bring the hyoid into laryngoscopic view.

Should there be PES involvement, this tissue is completely excised by advancing the dissection caudal to the hyoid and peeling tissue off the inner thyrohyoid membrane until the superior border of the thyroid cartilage is identified. The dissection is continued further anteroinferiorly, along the thyroid inner perichondrium, past the midline thyroid notch to reach the level of the petiole immediately above the anterior commissure.

To facilitate removal of inferior tumor or remaining epiglottis, a mucosal incision is made across the aryepiglottic

TABLE 123.2	ELS CLASSIFICATION OF ENDOSCOPIC SURGERIES FOR EARLY SUPRAGLOTTIS AND GLOTTIS CANCER

Endoscopic SGL (42)	Endoscopic Cordectomy (43,44)
Type I, limited excision of small size, superficial lesions in any part of the supraglottis	Type I, subepithelial cordectomy

Type II, medial SGL without resection of the PES
  Type IIa, superior hemiepiglottectomy
  Type IIb, total epiglottectomy
	Type II, subligamental cordectomy

Type III, medial SGL with resection of the PES
  Type IIIa, without extension to the ventricular fold
  Type IIIb, with extension to the ventricular fold
	Type III, transmuscular cordectomy

Type IV, lateral SGL
 	
  Type IVa, includes ventricular fold
  Type IVb, includes arytenoid
	Type IV, total cordectomy

	Type V, extended cordectomy
	  Type Va, encompassing the contralateral vocal fold and the anterior commissure
	  Type Vb, encompassing the arytenoid
	  Type Vc, encompassing the ventricle
	  Type Vd, encompassing subglottis (1 cm)

	Type VI cordectomy for cancers of the anterior commissure Extension to one or both of the vocal folds, without infiltration of the thyroid cartilage

fold and extended inferiorly to cross the false cord, then proceeding anteriorly in the ventricle toward the midline, allowing removal of the remaining epiglottis. These incisions are made uni- or bilaterally according to tumor distribution.

False cord: Tumors at these sites can be completely resected using similar TLM techniques. The depth of excision is determined by a transverse cut through the tumor's epicenter, and the surface extent of tumor determines the design of the mucosal incisions; inferiorly, the dissection is usually carried to the level of the ventricle or the superior vocal cord. A safe lateral oncologic margin of 5 mm can be obtained for lesions confined to the false cord without any significant functional impairment. However, the inferior deep margin may be closer (1 to 2 mm) and histologic negativity is confirmed with frozen section.

Aryepiglottic fold: Small and superficial lesions can be excised *en bloc*. The resection is tailored depending on the tumor extent and any extension to arytenoids or medial hypopharyngeal wall is carefully assessed and addressed. The general principle is to split transversely through the tumor and the fold until sufficient deep tissue margin (2 to 5 mm) is established, followed by appropriately oriented perimeter cuts for mucosal clearance. When necessary, the arytenoid may be shaved away serially from anterior to posterior, leaving the posterior body undisturbed.

Hemostasis: Meticulous hemostasis should be ensured during and at completion of all TLM procedures for supraglottic tumors. Bipolar cautery using the 22-cm Stryker Silverglide bipolar forceps design, directly down the endoscope, is especially useful for mucosal bleeding, common along epiglottic and base of the tongue incisions. Because of proximity to or exposure of the superior laryngeal artery or its branches, hemostasis is critical when the procedure involves transection of lateral pharyngoepiglottic fold or dissection of lateral supraglottic mucosa. This vessel should be doubly or triply clipped at identification during TLM. It is also prudent to clip the superior laryngeal and/or superior thyroid artery during any neck dissection, to further obviate the risk of delayed primary or secondary hemorrhage. Before extubation, the laryngoscope is desuspended to allow for reduction of any temporary hemostatic tamponade, and Valsalva maneuvers are used to stimulate dormant bleeders. A tracheostomy, of course, provides optimal protection against major, unexpected late hemorrhage into the airway.

Frozen section analysis: Meticulous orientation of the specimen by marker (e.g., suture or clip) is recommended before removal from the patient, following which the surgical margin is inked carefully for pathologic analysis. It is incumbent on the surgeon to inform the pathologist that part of the specimen intentionally contains a nonmargin area of tumor cut through. Mono- or multibloc resection is performed until histologically negative margins are secured on frozen section. A minor discrepancy of about 2% (46) has been reported to occur between frozen section

and permanent section results, but this can be adequately addressed with margin re-resection using repeat TLM. Heat or crush artifact may sometimes make adequate pathologic determination of the resection margin difficult and the surgeon's discretion becomes important in such situations to judge the adequacy of the actual extent of margin resection.

Postoperative care: A 3-week course of broad-spectrum antibiotics and antireflux measures is instituted in the postoperative period. Resection for early supraglottic cancer seldom requires prolonged intubation or tracheostomy. Nasogastric feeding is usually avoided for small resections but may be prudent in the initial postoperative period. Rehabilitation measures to improve swallowing with postural modifications and a supraglottic diet are commenced at an early stage. Functional recovery is usually rapid, with return to normal swallowing function within a relatively short period, facilitated by good pain control.

Complications: TLM procedures pose a risk of airway laser fire and methods of prevention include reduction of the inspiratory oxygen concentration to less than 30% (47), use of a laser endotracheal tube, or placement of laserproof covering over nonlaser tubes. There is a risk of secondary hemorrhage following TLM during postoperative day 0 to day 21. This can be obviated by taking adequate precautions during the procedure as discussed above (48). Postresection edema of the remaining supraglottic mucosa, especially on the arytenoids, may compromise the airway in the postoperative period. This often resolves with administration of steroids in limited resection. Tracheostomy is seldom required. Airway obstruction may be more persistent after TLM for radiation-recurrent tumors, sometimes necessitating a tracheostomy or transoral laser resection of edematous supraglottic mucosa. Severe aspiration can result in pulmonary complications but is infrequently seen for early supraglottic tumor resection. Resection of the arytenoid, aryepiglottic fold, or tongue base will increase the risk of aspiration. Extensive defects may result in supraglottic stenosis. Complications due to laryngoscope pressure such as dental and mandibular trauma, pharyngeal tears, tongue swelling, laceration, and numbness or loss of taste may also occur.

Transoral Robotic Surgery

Transoral surgery using the da Vinci robotic surgical system was recently reported to be suitable for performing SGL in humans (38). The three-armed robotic system is said to confer improved, three-dimensional optics and tissue manipulating/cutting maneuverability. However, some optical resolution is lost over a high-quality operating microscope. The "endowrist" design allows for flexibility in movement at the *end* of the robotic instruments. However, the arms carrying such flexible working tips are straight, are rigid, and cannot be maneuvered down a laryngoscope, necessitating spatulate retraction of the tongue. In reality, laryngoscopic exposure may be required to obtain optimum exposure and the rigid robotic arms cannot be used inside laryngoscopes, needing approximately 30 degrees of axial offset angle to work through the mouth and pharynx. Furthermore, with a 12-mm diameter endoscope for viewing plus two 8-mm (or 5-mm) surgical arms and a suction device, there is significant instrument crowding that currently limits this instrument's application in supraglottic tumors.

As a fledgling transoral approach, the setup time, expense, and compatibility issues of transoral robotic surgery (TORS) with the routine operating requirements, such as neck dissection, confine its niche to select treatment centers. Currently, the robot appears to offer no advantage over endoscopic laser resection although its application in supraglottic tumors may increase with future refinements.

Open Conservation Procedures

Horizontal Supraglottic Laryngectomy (see Fig. 123.1A,B)

"Open" SGL entails resection of the epiglottis, false cord, aryepiglottic folds, hyoid, and upper half of the thyroid cartilage. It includes complete resection of PES. This procedure spares the true cords, at least one arytenoid, and the tongue base, structures that are vital to phonation, respiration, and deglutition, and also avoids the need of a permanent tracheostomy. In early-stage tumors, the basic SGL can be modified to preserve the hyoid bone. "Extended" SGL may be performed for lesions extending to vallecula, tongue base, ipsilateral arytenoid, and medial wall of pyriform sinus. A tracheostomy is always required at the time of resection.

Contraindications: Paraglottic space involvement, cord fixation, thyroid cartilage invasion, bilateral arytenoid or interarytenoid space involvement, tumor extension to the pyriform sinus apex, and extensive tongue base involvement are contraindications for open SGL. The procedure is also contraindicated in patients with poor motivation and respiratory insufficiency.

Surgical technique: A preoperative laryngoscopy is performed to reassess the extent of primary tumor and a preliminary tracheostomy is secured. An apron incision is made and subplatysmal flaps are raised. The hyoid bone is skeletonized and infrahyoid muscles are detached from the body and greater cornua of the hyoid, in preparation for the superior pharyngotomy. The greater cornu should be skeletonized with care because of proximity to the hypoglossal nerve.

The superior thyroid neurovascular pedicle is divided and ligated on the side of the tumor and the constrictors are separated from the posterior edge of the ipsilateral thyroid ala. An incision is made through the perichondrium along the superior border of the thyroid cartilage and a perichondrial flap is reflected inferiorly below the level of the true cord, thus exposing the upper two-thirds of the thyroid cartilage. The thyroid cartilage is transected horizontally just

above the midpoint between the thyroid notch and lower border including the superior cornu on the tumor side. The incision is extended horizontally across to the other side or obliquely to preserve the contralateral superior cornua of the thyroid cartilage.

The pharynx is entered superiorly infrahyoid, through the vallecula if the tumor is confined to the supraglottic larynx. For tumors with extension to the vallecula, a suprahyoid or lateral pharyngotomy approach through the contralateral pyriform sinus is utilized. The epiglottis is delivered outward through the pharyngotomy and retracted to visualize the laryngeal introitus. Connecting mucosal incisions are made through the aryepiglottic folds on both sides, anterior to the arytenoids. The cuts are extended through the posterior part of the false cords into the ventricle and connected to the thyroid cartilage incisions to complete resection. An inferior margin of about 2 to 3 mm normal mucosa has been found to be adequate to prevent recurrence at the glottic level (49). Resection of all supraglottic mucosa including uninvolved false cord is recommended to prevent postoperative edema. The role of cricopharyngeal myotomy in SGL for better swallowing outcomes lacks consensus.

After securing complete hemostasis, the defect is reconstructed by suturing the thyroid perichondrial flap to the deep musculature of the tongue base with 3-0 Vicryl. A second reinforcing layer is created by suturing the suprahyoid muscles to the cut edges of infrahyoid musculature. The neck incision is closed after placement of a closed suction drain. The tracheostomy tube is reinserted through a separate incision in the lower skin flap and care is taken to isolate the stoma from the major resection wound in order to prevent contamination of the neck.

Postoperative care: Routine care of wound, tracheostomy, and neck drain is instituted. Feeding is initiated through a nasogastric tube. As the postoperative edema resolves, the tracheostomy cuff is deflated, and depending upon the patient's tolerance and absence of signs of aspiration, a decannulation trial is commenced. Intensive swallow rehabilitation is initiated under supervision, with a "supraglottic" diet initially followed by a normal diet as judged by the patient's ability to swallow without difficulty or aspiration.

Complications: Severe aspiration after SGL can lead to recurrent aspiration pneumonia. Intractable life-threatening aspiration, particularly in patients undergoing extended SGL for tongue base or arytenoid involvement, may require a functional total laryngectomy. Hemorrhage, infection, accidental decannulation, and subcutaneous emphysema are other possible complications.

Supracricoid Laryngectomy

Supracricoid laryngectomy (SCL) was first introduced by Majer and Reider in 1959 as a conservation procedure for laryngeal cancer with later refinements in the procedure proposed by Labayle, Bismuth and Piquet (50). It entails *en bloc* resection of the PES, paraglottic space, and thyroid cartilage, yielding outcomes comparable to total laryngectomy in selected cases but preserving functions of phonation and deglutition without a permanent tracheostoma. The indications of SCL in T2 supraglottic cancers are lesions that are not ideal candidates for SGL by the virtue of their extension to the ventricle, the anterior commissure, or the glottis with or without impaired cord mobility.

Contraindications: Invasion of the cricoid cartilage, bilateral arytenoid involvement, extension into the base of the tongue, vallecula or hypopharynx, and fixation of arytenoids are contraindications for SCL.

Surgical technique: A direct laryngoscopy is recommended at the onset for reevaluation of the tumor and its suitability for resection with SCL. After adequately skeletonizing the larynx, the inferior constrictors are incised along the lateral border of the thyroid cartilage followed by release of the pyriform sinuses from the inner thyroid cartilage. The external thyroid perichondrium is preserved bilaterally. During division of the superior laryngeal vascular pedicle, care is taken to preserve the internal branch of the superior laryngeal nerve. The cricoarytenoid joints are disarticulated with care bilaterally to preserve both recurrent laryngeal nerves, which lie just medial and posterior to this joint. A cricothyrotomy is performed just immediately above the cricoid following which ventilation continues through this new opening.

The pharyngotomy is performed by entering the vallecula on the uninvolved side, grasping and retracting the epiglottis through the vallecular incision. Sharp dissection is continued alongside the epiglottis to the aryepiglottic fold and in front of the arytenoid bilaterally, down to the cricoid cartilage and the cricothyrotomy incision, thus releasing the specimen. On the side of the tumor, incisions are made ensuring safe resection margins. If one of the arytenoids needs to be included in the surgical specimen, the incision down the aryepiglottic fold is made posterior to, instead of anterior to, arytenoid on the ipsilateral side.

Before closure, hemostasis is secured and the mucosa is approximated over the arytenoid in a manner that does not limit its movement. To prevent posterior prolapse of arytenoid, a single 3-0 Vicryl suspension suture is passed through the arytenoid, anchoring it forward to the cricoid cartilage. Neck extension is removed to perform laryngoplasty by approximating the cricoid and hyoid using interrupted, nonabsorbable 1-0 Vicryl sutures passed submucosally, one in the midline and one 1 cm on either side of the midline. Tightening of these cricohyoidopexy (CHP) sutures brings the arytenoids(s) closer to the tongue base. This facilitates vibration of the mucosa over arytenoids(s) against the tongue base, a mechanism that is responsible for phonation in these patients.

Once the trachea has been stretched up by the CHP, tracheostomy is performed at an appropriate site that allows the tube to exit skin through the neck incisions. The inferior and superior margins of strap muscle flaps are approximated to reinforce the CHP area. Neck incisions are closed after placement of suction drains.

Postoperative care: Routine care of wound, tracheostomy, and neck drain is instituted in the postoperative period. The patient is nursed in a position that ensures that the head is flexed toward the chest. Feeding is initiated through a nasogastric tube or a gastrostomy in the immediate postoperative period followed by swallow rehabilitation exercises. A decannulation trial is commenced after 6 weeks provided there are no symptoms of aspiration and good airway is maintained. Voice therapy is initiated after completion of wound healing.

Complications: Aspiration occurs commonly after SCL resulting in morbid pulmonary complications such as atelectasis and pneumonia (51). Older patients (greater than 60 years), chronic airway disease, smoking status, extent of arytenoid resection, and CHP are some of the factors associated with a greater risk of postoperative pulmonary complications. More frequent rates of aspiration have been observed in CHP versus cricohyoidoepiglottopexy (CHEP), possibly because of the absence of epiglottis and inadequate neoglottic closure in the former. Precautions recommended for prevention of aspiration are preservation of the superior laryngeal nerves, anterosuperior suturing and positioning of the cricoarytenoid unit, early decannulation, and early onset of swallowing rehabilitation (52). Hemorrhage, infection, wound dehiscence, accidental decannulation, subcutaneous emphysema, and pharyngocutaneous fistula are other possible complications.

Management of the Neck

Clinically or radiologically positive neck disease requires the patient to undergo neck dissection. Ipsilateral N+ necks require ipsilateral dissection, and bilateral or contralateral N+ necks require bilateral neck dissection. Neck dissection is performed at the same operative session as primary tumor resection, although a staged contralateral neck dissection may be carried out later if the ipsilateral neck was pathologically positive. Selective, lateral dissection of levels II, III, and IV is an effective and adequate procedure for management of the neck in early supraglottic cancer. For T1–T2 cancer of the infrahyoid epiglottis or lesions crossing midline, our preferred approach is to carefully assess the neck for ipsilateral and contralateral cervical metastasis by office ultrasound ± ultrasound-guided FNA.

Presence of multinodal or multilevel neck disease with extracapsular spread is an indication for postoperative RT or chemoradiotherapy. However, such adjuvant treatments should be used with caution since the potential is high for airway compromise due to stenosis or arytenoid edema.

The standard of care in early supraglottic tumors with an N0 neck is controversial. An occult metastatic rate ranging from 4% to 35% (20), combined with a high risk of contralateral metastasis, is cited as a rationale for performing a routine bilateral neck dissection. However, early cancer confined to the suprahyoid epiglottis and well-lateralized primaries not crossing the midline are exceptions. Moreover, less than 10% of the early T1–T2 lesions are reported at risk of contralateral spread, which is infrequent in the absence of ipsilateral neck disease (53,54). Evidence from some studies indicates that bilateral dissection of the clinically N0 neck in T1 to T2 supraglottic cancer may not always be necessary (54,55) and its routine practice leads to overtreatment in 70% to 80% of cases with unnecessary increase in treatment-related morbidity (20,56).

Although surgery is preferred in neck management, RT alone to one or both necks can be used to control N0 or N1 necks. However, unwanted radiation to the larynx will occur, even with intensity-modulated radiation therapy, adding to the risk of prolonged airway edema and obstruction from arytenoid swelling.

OUTCOMES

Surgical therapy alone achieves oncologic outcomes equivalent to combined therapy in early supraglottic cancer. Postoperative RT is known to adversely affect the functional results of conservation surgery by increasing edema (especially arytenoid mucosa), which in turn compromises airway patency and voice, and may cause strictures. The decision for administering adjuvant RT should be judicious and based on high-risk neck indications. Lymph node metastasis is the most important prognostic factor in supraglottic cancer. In one of the most recent reviews of laryngeal cancer cases recorded in National Cancer Data Base (1985 to 2002), a decline in survival was observed among the early-stage supraglottic cancers, T1N0M0 and T2N0M0 (5). At this stage, no definitive links can be identified between outcomes and patterns of surgical treatment.

Oncologic: Excellent oncologic outcomes have been reported for TLM in early supraglottic cancer. A 5-year recurrence-free survival of 83% for early tumors, a 5-year local control rate of 100% for T1 and 89% to 97% for T2 tumors, and a 5-year laryngeal preservation rate of 86% to 100% are observed from the various studies reporting outcomes for laser resection (37,57). Few comparative studies found a higher 5-year disease-free survival (80% vs. 72%), 5-year laryngeal preservation rate (86% vs. 80%), and a 5-year disease-specific survival (89% vs. 80%) in the endoscopic laser group compared to open SGL group (57,58).

Functional: The functional results of transoral laser resection for early supraglottic cancers are superior to open conservation procedures by virtue of shorter hospital stays, lower tracheostomy rate, and better swallowing outcomes. The resection of critical barriers to aspiration in open surgery for SGL cancers combined with a sensory deficit from superior laryngeal nerve section results in interference with food bolus recognition and also weakening of the "glottic closure" reflex (59). Aspiration-related

secondary laryngectomy rates for open conservative surgery have been reported to range between 3.5% and 12.5% (59). Preservation of normal structures including the cartilaginous framework and avoidance of damage to superior laryngeal nerve make rapid restoration of swallowing function feasible in endoscopic laser surgery. In spite of pulmonary status being a better predictor of aspiration pneumonia than a particular surgical approach, a lower incidence of aspiration pneumonia has been observed in patients undergoing TLM (11.5%) compared to open surgery (40%) for supraglottic cancer (60,61). Avoidance of wound dehiscence and pharyngocutaneous fistula are other advantages of endoscopic versus open resection for supraglottic cancers.

RADIOTHERAPY

Definitive RT is another treatment modality reported to be effective for management of early supraglottic cancers. The local control rates observed from review of large RT series (61,62) range from 75% to 100% for T1 tumors and 71% to 83% for T2 tumors, with a laryngeal preservation rate of about 80% (62). The success of RT is often correlated with the tumor volume; better results are reported for superficial and small-volume tumors (62). In the era of endoscopic approaches to early supraglottic tumors, RT is indicated for treatment of patients who are not physiologically suitable for conservation surgery because of cardiac or pulmonary insufficiency.

Recurrences after primary RT for early supraglottic cancer have been reported to be as high as 29% (63). Surgical salvage with conservation procedures or total laryngectomy is associated with a greater risk of complications, especially pharyngocutaneous fistula, tissue necrosis, wound breakdown, and carotid artery rupture. The rate of complications has been related to the dose of radiation therapy (64).

EARLY GLOTTIC CANCER

Glottic cancer accounts for about 50% to 60% of all laryngeal cancer cases. A change in voice with varying severity of hoarseness is almost universally associated with glottic tumors resulting in diagnosis at an early stage (5). These lesions do not cause airway obstruction or swallowing difficulty unless they progress to higher T stages. Lymphatic spread of early glottic cancer is extremely rare.

Surgical Pathology

Glottic cancer mostly arises on the mucosa of anterior true cords, a region with paucity of lymphatics. Tumor extension occurs along the cord in the submucosal space. The chief barriers to spread of glottic cancer are the vocal ligament, conus elasticus, and the thyroid perichondrium and cartilage. Spread may occur across the anterior commissure to the opposite cord. The Broyle ligament offers a tough barrier to superior and anterior spread of the tumor. However, the site of insertion of the Broyle ligament at the anterior commissure is devoid of inner thyroid perichondrium, and once involved, it serves as a portal of entry of the tumor into the thyroid cartilage from where it can spread to involve the ossified portions of the cartilage or further to the extralaryngeal structures. Posteriorly, the lesions can spread to involve the thyroarytenoid muscle. This may result in impaired mobility, which should be carefully assessed during preoperative planning to differentiate from cord fixation. Further posterior spread may occur to involve the arytenoid cartilage or the posterior commissure.

Inferior extension can occur to the subglottis; spread of more than 1 cm below the free edge of the true cord can invade the cricoid cartilage. With superior extension, the tumor can spread along the floor of the ventricle and invade the glottic musculature. Extension to the false cords, filling the ventricle, makes the lesion transglottic. This is one of the mechanisms for involvement of paraglottic space from where the tumor can breach the cricothyroid membrane and involve the cricoid cartilage or extralaryngeal soft tissues and thyroid gland. Paraglottic space can also be involved following spread across the conus elasticus or lateral spread of the tumor along the superior surface of the true cord.

Staging and Pretreatment Planning

A detailed history of presenting symptoms, smoking, and reflux along with office flexible laryngoscopic evaluation of the upper aerodigestive tract mucosa is the initial step in management of patients presenting with hoarseness (Table 123.1). The site, size, appearance, and extent of the lesion are noted along with the cord mobility. Evaluation of fine cord mobility, amplitude of vibration, and mucosal wave by videostroboscopy facilitates assessment of the superficial extent as well as the infiltrative depth of early lesions (65). Imaging has a limited role in pretreatment planning of early glottic cancers and is usually not recommended except in bulky T2 lesions, for a better assessment of supraglottic or subglottic extensions and involvement of the thyroid cartilage.

A direct laryngoscopy and biopsy under anesthesia with additional telescope examination allows for accurate assessment and photodocumentation of the site, size, surface, and extent of the primary tumor. The procedure also facilitates evaluation of cord mobility, detection of second primaries, and adequacy of transoral exposure.

Treatment

The fundamental goals of treatment for early glottic cancer are disease cure, voice preservation, airway protection, and maintenance of function-preserving options for

management of recurrences. Primary transoral laser microsurgical cordectomy (Table 123.2), open surgery (cordectomy, hemilaryngectomy), or RT are the three effective treatment modalities. All these have been reported to have excellent patient survival outcomes; thus, the decision for treatment of choice in a particular individual is guided by other variables. These include patient preference, age, and expectations for quality of voice; tumor stage, site, for example, extension to anterior commissure; the physician's expertise and skills; and treatment-related factors such as morbidity, cost-effectiveness, and availability of function-preserving salvage options.

Carcinoma In situ

CIS can exist alone, involving limited or extensive areas of true cords, or it can coexist with foci of invasive squamous cancer. Management plans described in literature include "watchful waiting" (66), cord stripping, excisional biopsy, transoral laser excision, or RT. A watch-and-wait approach, however, is not practical since 66% of the patients in a study reporting this policy progressed to squamous cell carcinoma (66). Modest local control rates from 56% to 72% and worsening of voice have been reported for vocal cord stripping as a surgical intervention for CIS (67–69). Cord stripping and excisional biopsy with cold instruments such as small cup forceps may not include truly representative samples for pathologists to rule out basement membrane involvement (70,71). In comparison, excisional biopsy with TLM not only improves the diagnostic yield for CIS by better estimation of the depth but also offers option of complete removal of all macroscopic disease in the same setting (72). A safety margin of normal tissue is taken around the superficial lesion. Recent publications by experienced practitioners (73–75) favor at least ELS type 2 resections (Table 123.2), that is, removal of the entire cord and ligament. A review of literature for TLM in glottic CIS reveals high local control rates ranging from 75% to 100% (67).

Definitive treatment with RT is preferred at a few centers for the treatment of CIS (70), but the long-term complications and increased treatment time and costs for comparable local control rates make this option less desirable than excision biopsy by TLM alone (76). It also exhausts the option of subsequent radiation for recurrent or second primary tumor.

Approximately 29% of the laryngeal CIS lesions have a potential to progress to SCC, transformation rates being higher (33% to 92%) in untreated cases (72,77). This forms a basis for recommendation of close follow-up in patients with CIS irrespective of the treatment modality used. Presence of CIS at the anterior commissure has a greater risk of conversion to invasive squamous cancer than CIS at the membranous cord, 92% versus 17%, respectively. This has been reported in one of the studies analyzing predictive factors for progression of CIS to SCC (72).

Invasive Squamous Cell Carcinoma
Surgery

Endoscopic Procedures. The concept of endoscopic excision of early glottic cancer was pioneered by Lynch in 1920 using suspension laryngoscopy (71). Excellent outcomes were reported by New and Dorton in 1941 with transoral diathermy excision of glottic cancers, followed by De Santo in 1973 (71). The results for transoral CO_2 laser excision of glottic cancer were first published by Strong in 1975 (78) and popularized later by Steiner in 1980s (33). Since then, the use of laser with its hemostatic properties has evolved to become the optimal tool of endoscopic excision, although cold steel is still used. Glottic tumors are difficult to access through the currently available robotic arms and exposure devices. Robotic laryngeal surgery was found technically feasible for cordectomy in a canine model (79) and a human pilot study of four patients with glottic cancer (80), although access is severely limited once the narrow restrictions of the larynx are reached, given the angle of approach needed for the da Vinci robotic arms.

Transoral Laser Microsurgery. Surgical technique: Adequate laryngoscopic exposure of glottis is the basic technical requirement for TLM (Figs. 123.4 and 123.5). For procedures restricted to true cord, the laser is usually kept at continuous super pulse mode and low power settings ranging from 1 to 3 W. Modern CO_2 lasers allow tumor dissection in bloodless field with minimal char formation; thus, the use of electrocautery for hemostasis is almost eliminated in glottic lesions, which translates to lesser tissue injury and better functional results.

T1a (Unilateral) and T1b (Bilateral) Glottic Tumor. Small superficial lesions can be excised *en bloc*. Resection of larger microinvasive tumors, as judged intraoperatively, is performed in two or more pieces with the first incision passing through the middle of the tumor for depth assessment. Prior resection, partial or complete, of the ipsilateral false cord may be required. Resection is commenced by this first incision through the center followed by a further incision in normal tissue, lateral and posterior to the tumor. The first specimen is obtained by continuing the dissection posteriorly, forward to backward direction, to excise the posterior half of the tumor. Next, the anterior resection is completed by making an incision in the normal tissue lateral to the tumor and advancing the dissection anteriorly to resect the anterior half of the tumor. A deep margin of 1 to 3 mm and mucosal margin of 1 to 2 mm are recommended. If the tumor reaches the vocal process, mucosa is resected in close approximation, anterior to the arytenoid cartilage, and depending upon the extent of involvement, the vocal process may need to be included in the resection specimen. Bilateral tumors can be removed transorally in two sessions to prevent web formation.

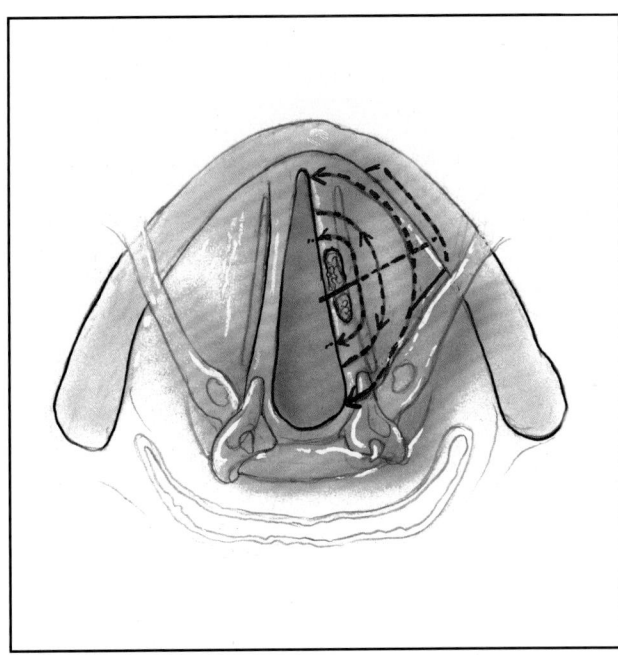

Figure 123.4 Transoral laser cordectomy for glottic tumors. *Dotted lines* indicate extended resections for lesions of increasing depth.

T2 Glottic Tumor (Supraglottis and/or Subglottis Extension, and/or Impaired Vocal Cord Mobility). T2 glottic cancers are amenable to complete excision with TLM irrespective of tumor extension into supraglottis, subglottis, or anterior commissure. The surgical principles applied are similar to laser surgery for other subsites. Again, false cord resection may be necessary for access to the ventricle and the paraglottic space. Tumor debulking is done for larger lesions followed by an incision through the tumor and further resection as necessary.

For tumors extending to supraglottic larynx across the arytenoid cartilage or interarytenoid mucosa, it is usually possible to preserve the arytenoid by peeling the tumor off the cartilage, if superficial. The exposed cartilage gets epithelialized after 3 to 4 weeks (36). Every attempt is made to preserve the posterior uninvolved mucosal cover of arytenoid for prevention of aspiration.

For tumors with suspected inferior extension, the subglottis is carefully evaluated, a procedure that often needs repositioning of the endotracheal tube and transoral access through smaller-caliber laryngoscopes for optimum exposure. The tumor is followed along the subglottic extensions if any, securing an adequate inferior margin.

Early Glottic Tumor with Anterior Commissure Involvement. In T1a tumors extending to the anterior commissure, a small tumor-free margin of the anterior part of contralateral cord should be included in the resection. This is sometimes associated with web formation at the anterior commissure. In T1b tumors, the bilateral cord lesion is usually resected together with the anterior commissure. The dissection is

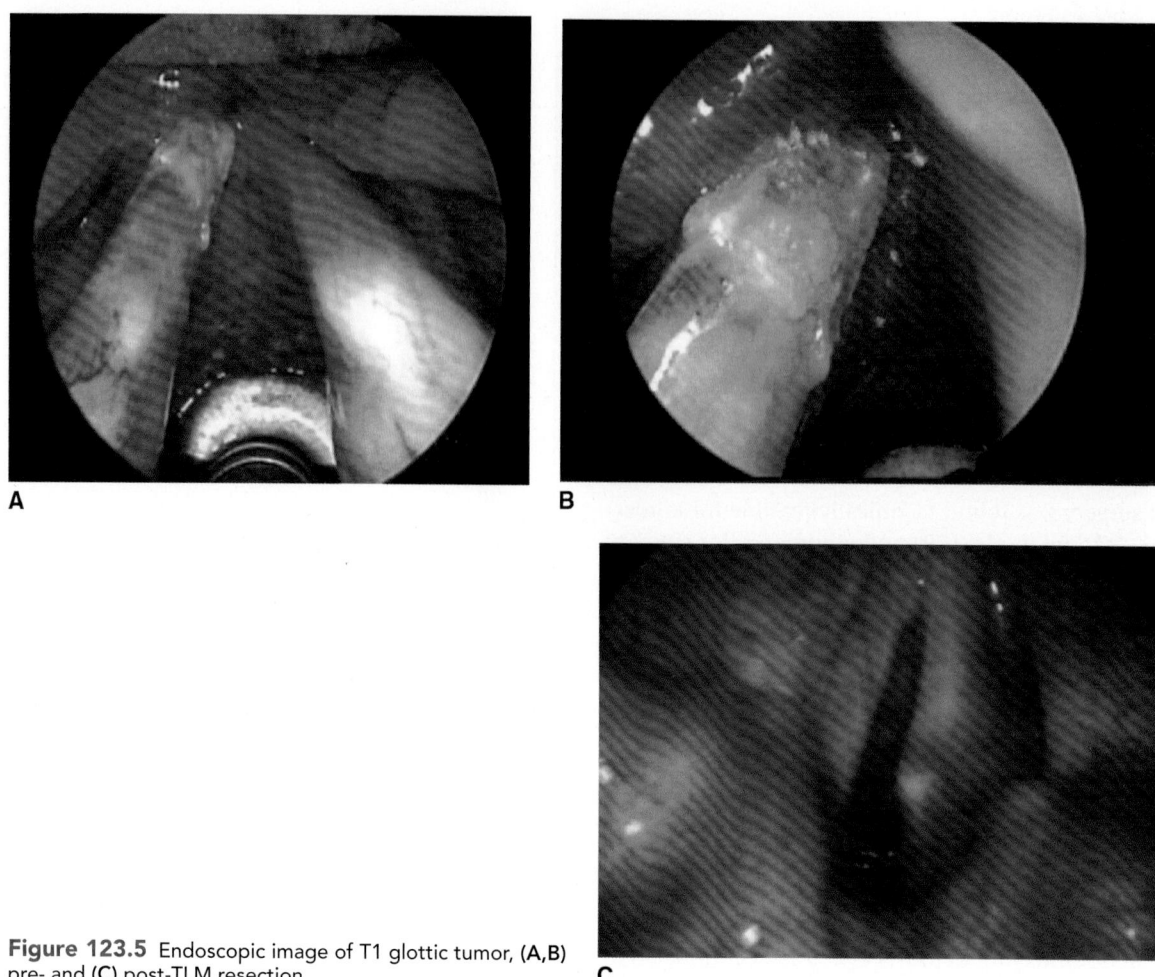

Figure 123.5 Endoscopic image of T1 glottic tumor, (A,B) pre- and (C) post-TLM resection.

also continued anteriorly along the thyroid cartilage, and with the help of frozen sections, it is ensured that the perichondrium toward the inside of the thyroid cartilage is free from the tumor.

Application of fibrin at the site of tumor resection at anterior commissure has been shown to reduce the incidence of web formation. If necessary, a silicone stent may be placed endoscopically as a prophylactic measure, which is removed after 6 weeks.

Postoperative care: Follow-up is recommended after 2 weeks. Strategies for cessation of smoking and alcohol consumption form an important component of postoperative counseling. Adequate gastroesophageal reflux preventive measures are initiated in all patients as reflux may impair wound healing, promote granulation tissue formation, and prolong edema. Wound healing is usually complete in 4 to 6 weeks following which voice rehabilitation therapy is scheduled. A small number of patients with persistent granulation or granuloma formation may require a second-look laryngoscopy.

Complications: Secondary hemorrhage is rare following resection of glottic tumors and can be managed conservatively if minor or with cautery at microlaryngoscopy.

Postoperative laryngeal or tongue edema can occur particularly after resection of bulky T2 tumors with supraglottic spread to arytenoids. The airway obstruction may necessitate tracheostomy but is frequently managed by administration of intravenous corticosteroids and aerosolized topical vasoconstrictors. In certain patients, wound healing elicits a strong inflammatory response and formation of exuberant granulation tissue. If the granulation persists for more than 6 to 12 weeks or is a source of compromised voice quality, surgical removal may be required. Laryngeal stenosis occurs as a rare, late complication if tumor resection involved extensive subglottic, interarytenoid, or near circumferential resections. This phenomenon is more likely to occur in patients undergoing TLM for radiation failures. Poor voice quality is universally observed prior to epithelialization. Thereafter, quality of voice recovery is related to volume of tissue loss and recruitment of supraglottic vibratory structures.

Phonosurgical Management After Endoscopic Partial Laryngectomy. Endoscopic laser excision for early glottic tumors does not usually require any reconstruction of the glottic defect as in open conservation surgery. However, in cordectomies requiring vocal muscle excision, poorer voice quality may result due to an aerodynamic glottic insufficiency caused by the concavity of the neocord (81). In such cases, phonosurgical techniques to augment the paraglottic space by microlaryngoscopic lipoinjection or cord medialization with Gore-Tex have been applied to optimize the voice restoration (81,82).

Open Conservation Procedures

Laryngofissure and Cordectomy. Laryngofissure and cordectomy are indicated for T1 lesions of vocal cord limited to the membranous cord when transoral resection is not possible. An endoscopy is performed prior to the surgery to reevaluate the suitability of the tumor for the procedure. A transverse skin incision is made at the level of midportion of the thyroid cartilage. Superior and inferior flaps are raised, strap muscles are retracted, and the thyroid cartilage is exposed in the midline. A midline vertical thyrotomy is performed and the larynx is entered through a short incision in the cricothyroid membrane. The thyroid ala is retracted laterally and the anterior ends of vocal folds are separated in the midline at the anterior commissure. The resection can include the true and false cords anterior to the vocal process of arytenoid, underlying thyroarytenoid muscle, internal thyroid perichondrium, and anterior commissure. The anterior commissure is reconstructed by anchoring the anterior end of the uninvolved cord to the thyroid lamina. The perichondrium and strap muscles are approximated and the incision is closed (Fig. 123.6).

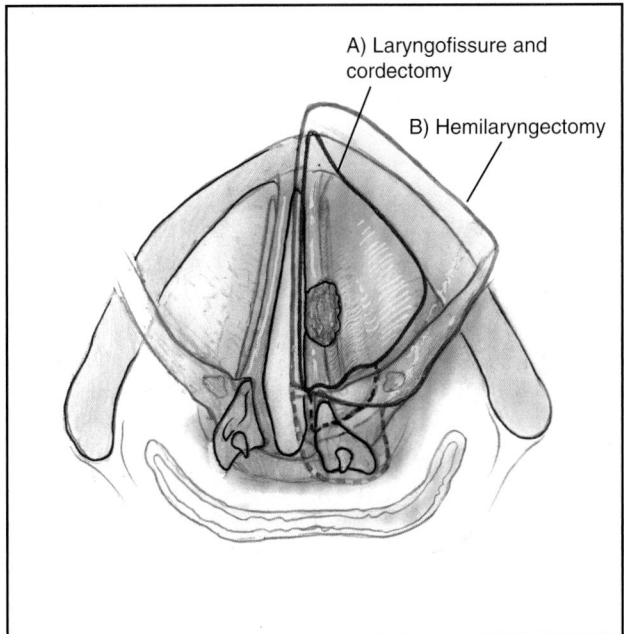

A) Laryngofissure and cordectomy

B) Hemilaryngectomy

Figure 123.6 Extent of resection in laryngofissure and cordectomy (**A**) and hemilaryngectomy (**B**). Extensions (*dotted line*) in either procedures may include the vocal process of the arytenoids, if required.

Postoperative care and complications: Tracheostomy is generally not required in cordectomy due to enlargement of the laryngeal inlet by cord resection; exceptions are patients with unfavorable body habitus. Feeding can be successfully initiated on the day following the surgery. Subcutaneous emphysema has been reported as one of the complications and can be prevented by pressure dressing and a wound drain.

Vertical Partial Laryngectomy. Hemilaryngectomy: This procedure involves resection of the ipsilateral thyroid cartilage, arytenoid, true cord and false cord, underlying muscle, and mucosa from the aryepiglottic fold to the upper border of the cricoid cartilage from the posterior to anterior midline. For early glottic tumors, its indications include T1 lesions with suspicion of deeply infiltrating tumor or T2 lesions of vocal cords with extension to arytenoids (Fig. 123.6).

Frontolateral vertical hemilaryngectomy: The procedure is indicated for T1 cord lesions approaching or extending to the anterior commissure and not more than 1 to 2 mm of the contralateral cord. The thyrotomy incisions are made bilaterally on either side of the midline and the larynx is entered through the cricothyroid membrane, on the side of lesser involvement. The resection includes true and false cords and ventricle on the ipsilateral side, arytenoid when necessary, anterior commissure, and anterior contralateral cord. The contralateral mucosa is sutured to the external perichondrium in order to resurface the larynx.

Anterior commissure technique/anterior frontal vertical partial laryngectomy: The procedure is indicated for T1 and T2 cord lesions with significant "horseshoe" involvement of the opposite vocal cord. The vertical midline portion of the thyroid cartilage, inner perichondrium, true cord, false cord, and ventricle up to the vocal process, bilaterally, are included in the resection. Reconstruction is performed by silastic or keel insertion to allow epithelialization on either side without web formation. The keel is usually removed after 6 to 8 weeks.

Reconstruction after partial laryngectomy: The glottic defect from open partial laryngectomy procedures may result in unsatisfactory voice outcomes. Resurfacing and reconstruction of the glottic defect enable better functional restoration. Several techniques are described of which more commonly applied are strap muscle flaps. Mucosal flaps, external thyroid perichondrium flap, a muscle-based cartilage flap, or imbrication laryngoplasty are alternatives.

Postoperative care: Care of the tracheostomy tube to maintain a patent airway is important in patients undergoing vertical hemilaryngectomy. Decannulation is deferred until the patient's swallowing improves and wound healing is complete. Voice usually tends to be breathy following hemilaryngectomy and speech therapy is initiated after decannulation. This procedure may temporarily require feeding through nasogastric tube or a gastrostomy but improves with swallowing rehabilitation.

Complications: Airway obstruction after vertical hemi-laryngectomy from prolapse of supraglottic tissue or formation of excessive granulation tissue is managed by maintenance of the tracheostomy. Progression to glottic stenosis is a possible complication in postradiation cases, which may need to be addressed by surgical intervention. Dysphagia and aspiration may occur in immediate postoperative period, particularly in patients with arytenoid resection. In a study of 438 patients comparing outcomes for different surgical approaches, a lower complication rate of 1.2% including stenosis, dyspnea, bleeding, fistula, and aspiration has been noted for TLM compared to 17.6% in open cordectomy, 9.4% in vertical partial laryngectomy, and 13.6% in frontolateral laryngectomy (83).

Supracricoid Laryngectomy. SCL may be an effective procedure to conserve the larynx for T2 glottic cancers that involve the anterior commissure, ventricle, and bilateral vocal cords. The surgical details have been discussed earlier. Reconstruction in these cases may include a CHEP.

OUTCOMES

Early glottic tumors have a good prognosis and failure occurs mainly at the primary site. T stage, anterior commissure involvement, and epidermal growth factor receptor expression are correlated with poorer local control in early glottic cancer (84). In addition, overall treatment time greater than 50 days and total dose less than or equal to 65 Gy, especially for T2 tumors, have been found to be significant for reduced local control in studies of early glottic cancers treated by definitive RT (84).

Oncologic: A review of studies reporting on TLM for T1 glottic cancers from various centers reveals a 5-year local control rate ranging from 88% to 94% and laryngeal preservation in more than 94% of cases (34,85–91). Sjögren et al. (92) compared results of TLM versus RT in T1 glottic cancer and found a local control rate of 89% versus 75% and a laryngeal preservation rate of 100% versus 83%. In a similar study by Schrijvers et al. (93), local control rates between the two groups were similar but laryngeal preservation was 95% for TLM versus 77% for RT. Also, in patients with T2 neoplasms, good local control ranging from 75% to 85% for local control has been observed in patients with T2 neoplasms (87,94–97).

A comparison of outcomes for external versus endoscopic approach for patients with early glottic tumors revealed similar oncologic results. The group treated by laser surgery, however, was found to have a shorter clinical course, lower complications, and the best possibility of salvage therapy in the case of local recurrence (83,98,99). Depending upon the stage and site of recurrence following TLM, options for treatment include laser resection,

partial laryngectomy, RT, or total laryngectomy. In a study investigating prognostic factors for local recurrence, the anterior commissure was the site of recurrent tumor in 54% of the cases, vocal muscle infiltration and subglottic involvement correlated with poor disease-free survival, and 91% of the recurrent cases could be retreated successfully (100).

Outcome for lesions involving anterior commissure: Involvement of the anterior commissure is considered to be a poor prognosticator for local control in early glottic cancer irrespective of the treatment modality. With exception of a few (101), most authors report lower responses to RT, possibly due to underdosage. The observed rates for local control in T1 carcinoma with anterior commissure extension vary from 57% to 89% (102–107). The organ preservation rates for tumors treated with RT range from 80% to 85% (103,106). Open procedures have been shown to offer higher organ preservation rates. These are correlated with good local control from 80% to 90% after frontolateral partial laryngectomy (108,109) and SCL (110,111) in early glottic cancers involving the anterior commissure.

TLM has been found to be effective for treatment of early glottic lesions with anterior commissure involvement, but the local tumor control rate has been found to be affected by the T stage as in other treatment modalities (104,112). In a study by Steiner et al., the 5-year local control rate varied from 84% for T1a to 73% for T1b and 79% for T2 lesions. The organ preservation rate in this study was high ranging from 93% for T1a to 88% in T1b and 93% in T2 lesions (112). The oncologic outcomes for open surgery were found to be comparable with TLM but functionally less favorable in terms of speech, swallowing, and a provisional tracheostomy (83). Measures cited to improve local control rates for TLM resections include adequate exposure, surgical experience and skill, resection of the thyroid cartilage, and careful attention to subglottic extension (36,113).

Functional: TLM is associated with minimal functional impairment. Tracheotomy is avoided in most patients undergoing TLM for early laryngeal cancer. Unlike open procedures, there is no disruption of structural integrity including the cartilaginous framework or the strap muscles. This results in better protection of the airway and swallowing that facilitate faster functional recovery. Furthermore, avoidance of RT preserves salivation and pharyngeal lubrication that assists in speech (104). The quality of voice is affected by the extent of cordectomy (114) and unsatisfactory outcome can be improved using phonomicrosurgical techniques. Whereas some authors advocate better voice outcomes with radiation than laser surgery (115), others have observed dysphonia due to RT-induced scarring and dryness of normal mucosa (116). Most of the comparative analyses show a reduced impact on patients' perception of voice quality after treatment with RT compared to TLM, but no significant difference could be detected by objective measurements (117–119).

RADIOTHERAPY

RT is employed as a treatment of choice for early glottic cancers at a number of centers. The cure rates for T1 lesions range from 71% to 95% (63,106,120–122). For treatment with RT, an endoscopic staging biopsy, usually under general anesthesia, is required to establish a histologic diagnosis followed by 5 to 6 weeks of treatment. Excision biopsy using transoral laser alone has been observed to yield a 92% recurrence-free survival at 3 years for T1 glottic cancers (71). Compared to this, definitive RT for CIS or T1 lesions is a radical treatment. The local control rates in studies advocating RT sometimes include surgical salvage of recurrences (106). Moreover, biopsy for making the histologic diagnosis is quite likely to remove the entire tumor in early localized lesions even before the initiation of radiation treatment (123). For T2 glottic cancer, the local control rates with RT vary from 50% to 80% (84,120). Successful local control and laryngeal preservation with RT have been shown to be affected by several factors including high tumor volume/bulk (102), anterior commissure involvement (124), and subglottic extension (125). Hyperfractionated RT has been associated with improved local control rates in patients with T2N0 glottic cancer compared to conventional RT (126).

Recent studies have employed chemotherapeutic agents such as carboplatin, tegafur-uracil, and fluoropyrimidine to improve results with RT in T2 glottic cancer (127–129). In a retrospective study of 30 patients, better 3-year local control rate could be achieved only when chemoradiotherapy was combined with transoral debulking microsurgery (95%) versus chemoradiotherapy alone (61%) (127).

Suitable candidates for radiation in early glottic cancer may include elderly patients with poor general health who are at greater risk of surgery-related complications, tumor extending to both cords, or when the physician lacks surgical expertise. Avoidance of RT is recommended in the younger populations for prevention of morbidity from both acute and late RT-related complications. In a prospective study of T1 glottic cancers treated with definitive RT (N = 180), a high rate of acute complications such as patchy or diffuse mucosal coating (65%) and chronic complications such as persistent arytenoid edema/polypoid lesions (8%) was observed (122). Other complications include xerostomia, persistent laryngeal edema, cervical fibrosis, glottic stenosis, hypothyroidism, chondronecrosis, and radiation-induced malignancy.

Management of Radiation Recurrences

Recurrences after failed radiation are often advanced at the time of diagnosis. A minority of radiation-recurrent glottic carcinomas can be salvaged by conservation surgery, but persistent aspiration, pharyngocutaneous fistula, delayed decannulation, and laryngeal stenosis can make such procedures particularly challenging with many tumors. Salvage partial surgery for localized T1 and T2 recurrences has shown acceptable survival rates and laryngeal preservation (130,131);

however, total laryngectomy may be commonly required for radiation failures (113,132,133).

TLM has been identified as one of the effective salvage procedures in selected cases involving glottic post-RT recurrences. Radiation-recurrent tumors are also, frequently, submucosal and discontinuous in nature. Magnification with TLM helps in identification of atypical-appearing mucosa though with greater difficulty compared to primary tumors. Using TLM, Steiner et al. (132) reported a successful salvage in 71%, with laryngectomy needed in 21% cases only. Another study by Ansarin et al. (134) reported TLM as an effective salvage for early RT recurrent tumors with laryngeal preservation rate of 70%. The outcomes for TLM as surgical salvage therapy, however, may depend on the individual surgeon's skill and experience. The results may also be affected by tumor extension to the anterior commissure or the arytenoids (133,135).

PHOTODYNAMIC THERAPY

Photodynamic therapy (PDT) utilizes the activation of tumor-selective photosensitizing agents with light to induce tumor necrosis (136) by increased production of oxygen radicals and decreased vascular supply. The photosensitizer is delivered intravenously, topically, or orally followed by subsequent treatment with a pulsed dye laser. PDT is usually performed as an outpatient procedure and the known complications of the procedure include glottic edema, pain, necrosis, and sun-induced photosensitivity (136). PDT is U.S. Food and Drug Administration approved for clinical treatment of early glottic cancers; however, its application as a single-modality, minimally invasive treatment modality is still limited.

EARLY SUBGLOTTIC CANCER

Primary lesions originating in the subglottis are rare and account for about 1% to 5% of all laryngeal cancers (137,138). More common are secondary extensions of carcinoma from the glottis. About 68% of patients were reported to present with early subglottic cancer in a series of 39 patients (137); however, most of the other published studies have observed 60% to 80% of the tumors presenting at late stages with dyspnea and stridor that may necessitate tracheostomy (138,139). Hoarseness can also occur as an initial presenting symptom (140). The incidence of nodal metastases at presentation varies widely from 4% to 33% depending on the disease stage (138–140).

Surgical Pathology and Treatment Planning

Subglottic cancers are known to have a typical circumferential and inferior pattern of intraluminal spread. Tumor extension is contained in the early stages by the conus elasticus; invasion through this barrier can involve the vocal musculature resulting in impaired mobility or fixation of the true cord. Vertical spread can occur toward the trachea caudally or the paraglottic space superiorly. Anterior spread through the cricothyroid membrane to involve the thyroid cartilage and the thyroid gland is a common mode of extralaryngeal spread.

CT and MRI with contrast are important for better delineation of the inferior extent of the tumors, invasion of the cricoid or thyroid cartilage, and the presence of cervical lymphadenopathy. Definitive diagnosis requires direct laryngoscopy with biopsy under general anesthesia.

TREATMENT

The rarity of subglottic tumors and variation in presenting stage preclude adoption of a uniform treatment paradigm. While surgery is recommended either as a part of combined modality or as definitive treatment for all stages of subglottic cancer in certain studies (137,141), some centers advocate definitive RT to the primary site, lower neck, and upper mediastinum with surgery reserved for salvage as an appropriate treatment for T1 and T2 cancers (139,140). Santoro et al. (142) reported that the 5-year disease-free survival rate for subglottic cancer was 0% with RT alone and 47% with surgery.

Using long, small-caliber laryngoscopes, resection with TLM combined with level VI neck dissection, if indicated, can be effectively employed to treat early lesions. Small, superficial-appearing tumors with deep infiltration can be dissected off the inside of the cricoid cartilage provided an adequate exposure is obtained (37). Infravestibular horizontal partial laryngectomy has been described for treatment of small series of patients with early subglottic lesions (142). Conservation of the upper half of the thyroid cartilage followed by adequate laryngeal reconstruction allowed restoration of natural phonation and respiration without requiring a tracheostomy in 75% of treated patients (143); however, application of this surgical procedure has not been widely reported.

Local recurrence of tumor is relatively common and is the primary cause of mortality in subglottic cancer (137,142). The most common site of recurrence is at the peristomal level, mostly attributed to nodal metastasis to the paratracheal lymph nodes (142,144). This emphasizes the need to address level VI nodes as an essential part of management for subglottic cancers (144). Distant metastasis is reported to occur in 12% to 50% patients with subglottic cancer (137,140,142). In a series reporting 15% of distant metastasis, three-fourths occurred in patients with early-stage disease at presentation (137), all of whom succumbed to the metastatic disease.

SUMMARY

TLM is an effective single-modality treatment for early laryngeal cancer and has supplanted the open conservation surgery with optimum oncologic outcomes, low morbidity, reduced hospital stay, reduced treatment time, and reduced cost (104,145–147). It has been established, by consensus

of ABEA, as an oncologically safe procedure for laryngeal cancer when applied judiciously and by a skilled surgeon (147). The main advantage lies in the possibility of offering individualized treatment by tailoring the surgical resection to precise extent of the tumor, thereby preserving the uninvolved healthy tissues. Moreover, TLM does not preclude further treatment options in the form of functional salvage surgery or RT for recurrent or second primary tumors. Its repeatability has been observed to result in lower laryngectomy rate compared with the published series on RT (148). Though no randomized trial has been conducted to compare the outcomes for TLM versus open conservation procedures or RT, a sufficient quantum of evidence from various centers establishes TLM as a minimally invasive, tumor-targeted therapeutic procedure. Comparative meta-analyses have shown no differences in oncologic outcome between TLM and RT (119,149) with no significant difference in objective voice analyses. TLM was also found to be superior to RT from a cost-utility point of view (149).

Patient selection for TLM, however, remains paramount and open conservation surgery can be a valuable approach to treat patients not suitable for a transoral laser excision. Open partial laryngectomy is a salvage option in selected radiation-recurrent tumors though it is associated with higher rates of failure as well as complications in the form of aspiration and tracheostomy dependence that may culminate in total laryngectomy.

HIGHLIGHTS

- Larynx cancer incidence is on the decline in the United States: Early glottic tumor incidence is greater than supraglottic, due to symptom development.
- Supraglottic tumors spread early to the preepiglottic space (PES) via the epiglottic foramina.
- For glottic tumors, deep lateral spread is from the cord to the paraglottic space.
- The fundamental goals of treatment are cure with no ultimate compromise in voice and swallowing.
- TLM is an effective and efficient minimally invasive option.
- For TLM, endoscopic access is paramount for patient selection.
- *"en bloc"* resection is performed for small tumors, and transtumoral, multibloc for larger tumors.
- Open partial procedures confer excellent and equivalent levels of local control.
- RT, while offering local control, may impair laryngeal physiology and reduce options for function-preserving salvage.
- Level II, III, and IV dissection is adequate for surgical management of neck metastasis in supraglottic cancer.

REFERENCES

1. Ferlito A. The natural history of early vocal cord cancer. *Acta Otolaryngol* 1995;115:345–347.

2. Ferlay J, Shin H, Bray F, et al. GLOBOCAN 2008, Cancer Incidence and Mortality Worldwide. *IARC CancerBase No 10 [internet]* 2010; Available at: URL: http://globocan.iarc.fr. Accessed June 1, 2011.

3. Sturgis EM, Cinciripini PM. Trends in head and neck cancer incidence in relation to smoking prevalence: an emerging epidemic of human papillomavirus-associated cancers. *Cancer* 2007;110:1429–1435.

4. Jemal A, Siegel R, Xu J, et al. Cancer statistics, 2010. *CA Cancer J Clin* 2010;60:277–300.

5. Hoffman HT, Porter K, Karnell LH, et al. Laryngeal cancer in the United States: changes in demographics, patterns of care, and survival. *Laryngoscope* 2006;116:1–13.

6. Back G, Sood S. The management of early laryngeal cancer: options for patients and therapists. *Curr Opin Otolaryngol Head Neck Surg* 2005;13:85–91.

7. Rafferty MA, Fenton JE, Jones AS. The history, aetiology and epidemiology of laryngeal carcinoma. *Clin Otolaryngol Allied Sci* 2001;26:442–446.

8. Marioni G, Marchese-Ragona R, Cartei G, et al. Current opinion in diagnosis and treatment of laryngeal carcinoma. *Cancer Treat Rev* 2006;32:504–515.

9. Talamini R, Bosetti C, La VC, et al. Combined effect of tobacco and alcohol on laryngeal cancer risk: a case-control study. *Cancer Causes Control* 2002;13:957–964.

10. Hashibe M, Brennan P, Chuang SC, et al. Interaction between tobacco and alcohol use and the risk of head and neck cancer: pooled analysis in the International Head and Neck Cancer Epidemiology Consortium. *Cancer Epidemiol Biomarkers Prev* 2009;18:541–550.

11. Baumann JL, Cohen S, Evjen AN, et al. Human papillomavirus in early laryngeal carcinoma. *Laryngoscope* 2009;119:1531–1537.

12. Purdue MP, Jarvholm B, Bergdahl IA, et al. Occupational exposures and head and neck cancers among Swedish construction workers. *Scand J Work Environ Health* 2006;32:270–275.

13. Califano J, van der RP, Westra W, et al. Genetic progression model for head and neck cancer: implications for field cancerization. *Cancer Res* 1996;56:2488–2492.

14. Veltman JA, van WI, Aubele M, et al. Specific steps in aneuploidization correlate with loss of heterozygosity of 9p21, 17p13 and 18q21 in the progression of pre-malignant laryngeal lesions. *Int J Cancer* 2001;91:193–199.

15. Ha PK, Califano JA III. The molecular biology of laryngeal cancer. *Otolaryngol Clin North Am* 2002;35:993–1012.

16. Nadal A, Cardesa A. Molecular biology of laryngeal squamous cell carcinoma. *Virchows Arch* 2003;442:1–7.

17. Almadori G, Bussu F, Cadoni G, et al. Multistep laryngeal carcinogenesis helps our understanding of the field cancerisation phenomenon: a review. *Eur J Cancer* 2004;40:2383–2388.

18. Rydzanicz M, Golusinski P, Mielcarek-Kuchta D, et al. Cyclin D1 gene (CCND1) polymorphism and the risk of squamous cell carcinoma of the larynx. *Eur Arch Otorhinolaryngol* 2006;263:43–48.

19. Karatzanis AD, Psychogios G, Zenk J, et al. Evaluation of available surgical management options for early supraglottic cancer. *Head Neck* 2010;32:1048–1055.

20. Yüce I, Cağli S, Bayram A, et al. Occult metastases from T1-T2 supraglottic carcinoma: role of primary tumor localization. *Eur Arch Otorhinolaryngol* 2009;266:1301–1304.

21. Kirchner JA, Carter D. Intralaryngeal barriers to the spread of cancer. *Acta Otolaryngol* 1987;103:503–513.

22. Tucker GF Jr, Smith HR Jr. A histological demonstration of the development of laryngeal connective tissue compartments. *Trans Am Acad Ophthalmol Otolaryngol* 1962;66:308–318.

23. Kirchner JA. Glottic-supraglottic barrier: fact or fantasy? *Ann Otol Rhinol Laryngol* 1997;106:700–704.

24. Som ML. Conservation surgery for carcinoma of the supraglottis. *J Laryngol Otol* 1970;84:655–678.

25. Lutz CK, Johnson JT, Wagner RL, et al. Supraglottic carcinoma: patterns of recurrence. *Ann Otol Rhinol Laryngol* 1990;99:12–17.

26. Scola B, Fernández-Vega M, Martínez T, et al. Management of cancer of the supraglottis. *Otolaryngol Head Neck Surg* 2001;124: 195–198.

27. Johansen LV, Overgaard J, Hjelm-Hansen M, et al. Primary radiotherapy of T1 squamous cell carcinoma of the larynx: analysis of 478 patients treated from1963 to 1985. *Int J Radiat Oncol Biol Phys* 1990;18:1307–1313.

28. Mendenhall WM, Parsons JT, Mancuso AA, et al. Radiotherapy for squamous cell carcinoma of the supraglottic larynx: an alternative to surgery. *Head Neck* 1996;18:24–35.

29. Alonso JM. Conservative surgery of cancer of the larynx. *Trans Am Acad Ophthalmol Otolaryngol* 1947;51:633–642.

30. Ogura JH. Selection of patients for conservation surgery of the larynx and pharynx. *Trans Am Acad Ophthalmol Otolaryngol* 1972;76:741–751.

31. Vaughan CW, Strong MS, Jako GJ. Laryngeal carcinoma: transoral treatment utilizing the CO2 laser. *Am J Surg* 1978;136:490–493.

32. Davis RK, Shapsay SM, Strong MS, et al. Transoral partial supraglottic resection using the CO2 laser. *Laryngoscope* 1983;93:429–432.

33. Steiner W. Experience in endoscopic laser surgery of malignant tumours of the upper aero-digestive tract. *Adv Otorhinolaryngol* 1988;39:135–144.

34. Steiner W. Results of curative laser microsurgery of laryngeal carcinomas. *Am J Otolaryngol* 1993;14:116–121.

35. Ambrosch P, Kron M, Steiner W. Carbon dioxide laser microsurgery for early supraglottic carcinoma. *Ann Otol Rhinol Laryngol* 1998;107:680–688.

36. Steiner W, Ambrosch P, Knappe MV. *Endoscopic laser surgery of the upper aerodigestive tract: with special emphasis on cancer surgery.* New York: Thieme Medical Publishers, 2001.

37. Ambrosch P. The role of laser microsurgery in the treatment of laryngeal cancer. *Curr Opin Otolaryngol Head Neck Surg* 2007;15:82–88.

38. Grant DG, Repanos C, Malpas G, et al. Transoral laser microsurgery for early laryngeal cancer. *Expert Rev Anticancer Ther* 2010;10:331–338.

39. Weinstein GS, O'Malley BW Jr, Snyder W, et al. Transoral robotic surgery: supraglottic partial laryngectomy. *Ann Otol Rhinol Laryngol* 2007 J;116:19–23.

40. Jackson C, Jackson CL. *Cancer of the larynx.* Philadelphia, PA: WB Saunders, 1939.

41. Strong MS, Jako G. Laser surgery in the larynx. Early clinical experience with continuous CO2 laser. *Ann Otol Rhinol Laryngol* 1972;81:791–798.

42. Remacle M, Hantzakos A, Eckel H, et al. Endoscopic supraglottic laryngectomy: a proposal for a classification by the working committee on nomenclature, European Laryngological Society. *Eur Arch Otorhinolaryngol* 2009;266:993–998.

43. Remacle M, Eckel HE, Antonelli A, et al. Endoscopic cordectomy. A proposal for a classification by the Working Committee, European Laryngological Society. *Eur Arch Otorhinolaryngol* 2000;257:227–231.

44. Remacle M, Van Haverbeke C, Eckel H, et al. Proposal for revision of the European Laryngological Society classification of endoscopic cordectomies. *Eur Arch Otorhinolaryngol* 2007;264: 499–504.

45. Rich JT, Milov S, Lewis JS Jr, et al. Transoral laser microsurgery (TLM) ± adjuvant therapy for advanced stage oropharyngeal cancer: outcomes and prognostic factors. *Laryngoscope* 2009;119:1709–1719.

46. Cooley ML, Hoffman HT, Robinson RA. Discrepancies in frozen section mucosal margin tissue in laryngeal squamous cell carcinoma. *Head Neck* 2002;24:262–267.

47. Lierz P, Heinatz A, Gustorff B, et al. Management of intratracheal fire during laser surgery. *Anesth Analg* 2002;95:502.

48. Salassa JR, Hinni ML, Grant DG, et al. Postoperative bleeding in transoral laser microsurgery for upper aerodigestive tract tumors. *Otolaryngol Head Neck Surg* 2008;139:453–459.

49. Silver CE. *Surgery for cancer of the larynx and related structures.* New York: Churchill Livingstone, Inc., 1981.

50. Vincentiis M, et al. Supracricoid laryngectomy with cricohyoidopexy in the treatment of laryngeal cancer: a functional and oncological experience. *Laryngoscope* 1996;106:1108–1114.

51. Joo YH, Sun DI, Cho JH, et al. Factors that predict postoperative pulmonary complications after supracricoid partial laryngectomy. *Arch Otolaryngol Head Neck Surg* 2009;135:1154–1157.

52. Yücetürk AV, Tarhan S, Günhan K, et al. Videofluoroscopic evaluation of the swallowing function after supracricoid laryngectomy. *Eur Arch Otorhinolaryngol* 2005;262:198–203.

53. Oztürkcan S, Katilmiş H, Ozdemir I, et al. Occult contralateral nodal metastases in supraglottic laryngeal cancer crossing the midline. *Eur Arch Otorhinolaryngol* 2009;266:117–120.

54. Cağli S, Yüce I, Yiğitbaşi OG, et al. Is routine bilateral neck dissection absolutely necessary in the management of N0 neck in patients with supraglottic carcinoma? *Eur Arch Otorhinolaryngol* 2007;264:1453–1457.

55. Rodrigo JP, Cabanillas R, Franco V, et al. Efficacy of routine bilateral neck dissection in the management of the N0 neck in T1–T2 unilateral supraglottic cancer. *Head Neck* 2006;28:534–539.

56. Ferlito A, Silver CE, Rinaldo A. Selective neck dissection (IIA, III): a rational replacement for complete functional neck dissection in patients with N0 supraglottic and glottic squamous carcinoma. *Laryngoscope* 2008;118:676–679.

57. Suárez C, Rodrigo JP, Silver CE, et al. Laser surgery for early to moderately advanced glottic, supraglottic, and hypopharyngeal cancers. *Head Neck* 2012;34(7):1028–1035.

58. Bussu F, Almadori G, De Corso E, et al. Endoscopic horizontal partial laryngectomy by CO(2) laser in the management of supraglottic squamous cell carcinoma. *Head Neck* 2009;31:1196–1206.

59. Suarez C, Rodrigo JP, Herranz J, et al. Complications of supraglottic laryngectomy for carcinomas of the supraglottis and the base of the tongue. *Clin Otolaryngol Allied Sci* 1996;21:87–90.

60. Köllisch M, Werner JA, Lippert BM, et al. Functional results following partial supraglottic resection. Comparison of conventional surgery vs. transoral laser microsurgery. *Adv Otorhinolaryngol* 1995;49:237–240.

61. Cabanillas R, Rodrigo JP, Llorente JL, et al. Functional outcomes of transoral laser surgery of supraglottic carcinoma compared with a transcervical approach. *Head Neck* 2004;26:653–659.

62. Orus C, Leon X, Vega M, et al. Initial treatment of the early stages (I, II) of supraglottic squamous cell carcinoma: partial laryngectomy versus radiotherapy. *Eur Arch Otorhinolaryngol* 2000; 257:512–516.

63. Hafidh M, Tibbo J, Trites J, et al. Radiotherapy for T1 and T2 laryngeal cancer: the Dalhousie University experience. *J Otolaryngol Head Neck Surg* 2009;38:434–439.

64. McLaughlin MP, Parsons JT, Fein DA, et al. Salvage surgery after radiotherapy failure in T1-T2 squamous cell carcinoma of the glottic larynx. *Head Neck* 1996;18:229–235.

65. Hirano M. Video-stroboscopic advances. In: Smee R, Bridgers GP, eds. *Laryngeal cancer proceedings of the second world congress on laryngeal cancer*. Oxford, UK: Elsevier, 270–272. International Congress Scene No. 1963. 20-24 Feb 1994.

66. Hintz BL, Kagan AR, Nussbaum H, et al. A 'watchful waiting' policy for in situ carcinoma of the vocal cords. *Arch Otolaryngol* 1981;107:746–751.

67. Roedel RM, Christiansen H, Mueller RM, et al. Transoral laser microsurgery for carcinoma in situ of the glottic larynx. A retrospective follow-up study. *ORL J Otorhinolaryngol Relat Spec* 2009;71:45–49.

68. Le QT, Takamiya R, Shu HK, et al. Treatment results of carcinoma in situ of the glottis: an analysis of 82 cases. *Arch Otolaryngol Head Neck Surg* 2000;126:1305–1312.

69. Garcia-Serra A, Hinerman RW, Amdur RJ, et al. Radiotherapy for carcinoma in situ of the true vocal cords. *Head Neck* 2002;24: 390–394.

70. Hinerman RW, Mendenhall WM, Amdur RJ, et al. Early laryngeal cancer. *Curr Treat Options Oncol* 2002;3:3–9.

71. Blakeslee D, Vaughan CW, Shapshay SM, et al. Excisional biopsy in the selective management of T1 glottic cancer: a three-year follow-up study. *Laryngoscope* 1984;94:488–494.

72. Myssiorek D, Vambutas A, Abramson AL. Carcinoma in situ of the glottic larynx. *Laryngoscope* 1994;104:463–467.

73. Peretti G, Nicolai P, Redaelli De Zinis LO, et al. Endoscopic CO2 laser excision for Tis, T1, and T2 glottic carcinomas: cure rate and prognostic factors. *Otolaryngol Head Neck Surg* 2000;123:124–131.

74. Damm M, Sittel C, Streppel M, et al. Transoral CO2 laser for surgical management of glottic carcinoma in situ. *Laryngoscope* 2000;110:1215–1221.

75. Peretti G, Nicolai P, Piazza C, et al. Oncological results of endoscopic resections of Tis and T1 glottic carcinomas by carbon dioxide laser. *Ann Otol Rhinol Laryngol* 2001;110:820–826.

76. Murty GE, Diver JP, Bradley PJ. Carcinoma in situ of the glottis: radiotherapy or excision biopsy? *Ann Otol Rhinol Laryngol* 1993;102(8 Pt 1):592–595.

77. Nguyen C, Naghibzadeh B, Black MJ, et al. Carcinoma in situ of the glottic larynx: excision or irradiation? *Head Neck* 1996;18:225–228.

78. Daly CJ, Strong EW. Carcinoma of the glottic larynx. *Am J Surg* 1975;130:489–492.

79. O'Malley BW Jr, Weinstein GS, Hockstein NG. Transoral robotic surgery (TORS): glottic microsurgery in a canine model. *J Voice* 2006;20:263–268.

80. Park YM, Lee WJ, Lee JG, et al. Transoral robotic surgery (TORS) in laryngeal and hypopharyngeal cancer. *J Laparoendosc Adv Surg Tech A* 2009;19:361–368.

81. Zeitels SM. Optimizing voice after endoscopic partial laryngectomy. *Otolaryngol Clin North Am* 2004;37:627–636.

82. Remacle M, Lawson G, Hedayat A, et al. Medialization framework surgery for voice improvement after endoscopic cordectomy. *Eur Arch Otorhinolaryngol* 2001;258:267–271.

83. Karatzanis AD, Psychogios G, Zenk J, et al. Comparison among different available surgical approaches in T1 glottic cancer. *Laryngoscope* 2009;119:1704–1708.

84. Nur DA, Oguz C, Kemal ET, et al. Prognostic factors in early glottic carcinoma implications for treatment. *Tumori* 2005;91: 182–187.

85. Gallo A, de Vincentiis M, Manciocco V, et al. CO2 laser cordectomy for early-stage glottic carcinoma: a long-term follow-up of 156 cases. *Laryngoscope* 2002;112:370–374.

86. Peretti G, Piazza C, Bolzoni A, et al. Analysis of recurrence in 322 Tis, T1, or T2 glottic carcinomas treated by carbon dioxide laser. *Ann Otol Rhinol Laryngol* 2004;113:853–858.

87. Motta G, Esposito E, Motta S, et al. CO2 laser surgery in the treatment of glottic cancer. *Head Neck* 2005;27:566–574.

88. Sigston E, de Mones E, Babin E, et al. Early-stage glottic cancer: oncological results and margins in laser cordectomy. *Arch Otolaryngol Head Neck Surg* 2006;132:147–152.

89. Ledda GP, Puxeddu R. Carbon dioxide laser microsurgery for early glottis carcinoma. *Otolaryngol Head Neck Surg* 2006;134: 911–915.

90. Hartl DM, de Monès E, Hans S, et al. Treatment of early-stage glottic cancer by transoral laser resection. *Ann Otol Rhinol Laryngol* 2007;116:832–836.

91. Grant DG, Salassa JR, Hinni ML, et al. Transoral laser microsurgery for untreated glottic carcinoma. *Otolaryngol Head Neck Surg* 2007;137:482–486.

92. Sjögren EV, Langeveld TP, Baatenburg de Jong RJ. Clinical outcome of T1 glottic carcinoma since the introduction of endoscopic CO2 laser surgery as treatment option. *Head Neck* 2008;30:1167–1174.

93. Schrijvers ML, van Riel EL, Langendijk JA, et al. Higher laryngeal preservation rate after CO2 laser surgery compared with radiotherapy in T1a glottic laryngeal carcinoma. *Head Neck* 2009;31:759–764.

94. Eckel HE, Thumfart WF, Jungehulsing M, et al. Transoral laser for early glottic carcinoma. *Eur Arch Otorhinolaryngol* 2000;257:221–226.

95. Peretti G, Piazza C, Mensi MC, et al. Endoscopic treatment of cT2 glottic carcinoma: prognostic impact of different pT subcategories. *Ann Otol Rhinol Laryngol* 2005;114:579–586.

96. Davis RK, Hadley K, Smith ME. Endoscopic vertical partial laryngectomy. *Laryngoscope* 2004;114:236–240.

97. Pradhan SA, Pai PS, Neeli SI, et al. Transoral laser surgery for early glottic cancers. *Arch Otolaryngol Head Neck Surg* 2003;129: 623–625.

98. de Campora E, Radici M, de Campora L. External versus endoscopic approach in the surgical treatment of glottic cancer. *Eur Arch Otorhinolaryngol* 2001;258:533–536.

99. Puxeddu R, Argiolas F, Bielamowicz S, et al. Surgical therapy of T1 and selected cases of T2 glottic carcinoma: cordectomy, horizontal glottectomy and CO2 laser endoscopic resection. *Tumori* 2000;86:277–282.

100. Mortuaire G, Francois J, Wiel E, et al. Local recurrence after CO2 laser cordectomy for early glottic carcinoma. *Laryngoscope* 2006;116:101–105.

101. Mendenhall WM, Parsons JT, Million RR, et al. T1-T2 squamous cell carcinoma of the glottic larynx treated with radiation therapy: relationship of dose-fractionation factors to local control and complications. *Int J Radiat Oncol Biol Phys* 1988;15: 1267–1273.

102. Reddy SP, Mohideen N, Marra S, et al. Effect of tumour bulk on local control and survival of patients with T1. *Radiother Oncol* 1998; 47:161–166.

103. Marshak G, Brenner B, Shvero J, et al. Prognostic factors for local control early glottic cancer: the Rabin Medical Center retrospective study on 207 patients. *Int J Radiat Oncol Biol Phys* 1999;43:1009–1013.

104. Pearson BW, Salassa JR. Transoral laser microresection for cancer of the larynx involving the anterior commissure. *Laryngoscope* 2003;113:1104–1112.

105. Gowda RV, Henk JM, Mais KL, et al. Three weeks radiotherapy for T1 glottic cancer: the Christie and Royal Marsden Hospital experience. *Radiother Oncol* 2003;68:105–111.

106. Cellai E, Frata P, Magrini SM, et al. Radical radiotherapy for early glottic cancer: results in a series of 1087 patients from two Italian radiation oncology centers. II. The case of T1N0 disease. *Int J Radiat Oncol Biol Phys* 2005;63:1378–1386.

107. Bradley PJ, Rinaldo A, Suárez C, et al. Primary treatment of the anterior vocal commissure squamous carcinoma. *Eur Arch Otorhinolaryngol* 2006;263:879–888.

108. Rucci L, Gallo O, Fini-Storchi O. Glottic cancer involving anterior commissure: surgery vs radiotherapy. *Head Neck* 1991;13: 403–410.

109. Zohar Y, Rahima M, Shvili Y, et al. The controversial treatment of anterior commissure carcinoma of the larynx. *Laryngoscope* 1992;102:69–72.

110. Chevalier D, Laccourreye O, Brasnu D, et al. Cricohyoidoepiglottopexy for glottic carcinoma with fixation or impaired motion of the true vocal cord: 5-year oncologic results with 112 patients. *Ann Otol Rhinol Laryngol* 1997;106:364–369.

111. Laccourreye O, Muscatello L, Laccourreye L, et al. Supracricoid partial laryngectomy with cricohyoidoepiglottopexy for "early" glottic carcinoma classified as T1-T2N0 invading the anterior commissure. *Am J Otolaryngol* 1997;18:385–390.

112. Steiner W, Ambrosch P, Rodel RMW, et al. Impact of anterior commissure involvement on local control of early glottic carcinoma treated by laser microresection. *Laryngoscope* 2004;114:1485–1491.

113. Silver CE, Beitler JJ, Shaha AR, et al. Current trends in initial management of laryngeal cancer: the declining use of open surgery. *Eur Arch Otorhinolaryngol* 2009;266:1333–1352.

114. Vilaseca I, Huerta P, Blanch JL, et al. Voice quality after CO2 laser cordectomy—what can we really expect? *Head Neck* 2008;30:43–49.

115. Krengli M, Policarpo M, Manfreda I, et al. Voice quality after treatment for T1a glottic carcinoma-radiotherapy versus laser cordectomy. *Acta Oncol* 2004;43:284–289.

116. Lehman JJ, Bless DM, Brandenburg JH. An objective assessment of voice production after radiation therapy for stage I squamous cell carcinoma of the glottis. *Otolaryngol Head Neck Surg* 1988;98:121–129.

117. Sjögren EV, van Rossum MA, Langeveld TP, et al. Voice outcome in T1a midcord glottic carcinoma: laser surgery vs radiotherapy. *Arch Otolaryngol Head Neck Surg* 2008;134:965–972.

118. Núñez Batalla F, Caminero Cueva MJ, Señaris González B, et al. Voice quality after endoscopic laser surgery and radiotherapy for early glottic cancer: objective measurements emphasizing the Voice Handicap Index. *Eur Arch Otorhinolaryngol* 2008;265:543–548.

119. Higgins KM, Shah MD, Ogaick MJ, et al. Treatment of early-stage glottis cancer: meta-analysis comparison of laser excision versus radiotherapy. *J Otolaryngol Head Neck Surg* 2009;38:603–612.

120. Mendenhall WM, Amdur RJ, Morris CG, et al. T1-T2 N0 squamous cell carcinoma of the glottic larynx treated with radiation therapy. *J Clin Oncol* 2001;19:4029–4036.

121. Jones DA, Mendenhall CM, Kirwan J, et al. Radiation therapy for management of T1-T2 glottic cancer at a private practice. *Am J Clin Oncol* 2010;33:587–590.

122. Yamazaki H, Nishiyama K, Tanaka E, et al. Radiotherapy for early glottic carcinoma (T1N0M0): results of prospective randomized study of radiation fraction size and overall treatment time. *Int J Radiat Oncol Biol Phys* 2006;64:77–82.

123. Neel HB III, Devine KD, Desanto LW. Laryngofissure and cordectomy for early cordal carcinoma: outcome in 182 patients. *Otolaryngol Head Neck Surg* 1980;88:79–84.

124. Zouhair A, Azria D, Coucke P, et al. Decreased local control following radiation therapy alone in early-stage glottic carcinoma with anterior commissure extension. *Strahlenther Onkol* 2004;180:84–90.

125. Dagan R, Morris CG, Bennett JA, et al. Prognostic significance of paraglottic space invasion in T2N0 glottic carcinoma. *Am J Clin Oncol* 2007;30:186–190.

126. Haugen H, Johansson KA, Mercke C. Hyperfractionated-accelerated or conventionally fractionated radiotherapy for early glottic cancer. *Int J Radiat Oncol Biol Phys* 2002;52:109–119.

127. Ohguri T, Imada H, Nakano K, et al. Concurrent hyperfractionated radiotherapy and carboplatin with transoral debulking microsurgery for T2N0 glottic cancer. *Head Neck* 2008;30: 1027–1034.

128. Niibe Y, Nakayama M, Matsubayashi T, et al. Effectiveness of concurrent radiation therapy with UFT or TS-1 for T2N0 glottic cancer in Japan. *Anticancer Res* 2007;27:3497–3500.

129. Taguchi T, Tsukuda M, Mikami Y, et al. Concurrent chemoradiotherapy with carboplatin and uracil-ftegafur in patients with stage two (T2 N0 M0) squamous cell carcinoma of the glottic larynx. *J Laryngol Otol* 2006;120:478–481.

130. Shah JP, Loree TR, Kowalski L. Conservation surgery for radiation-failure carcinoma of the glottic larynx. *Head Neck* 1990;12:326–331.

131. Nibu K, Kamata S, Kawabata K, et al. Partial laryngectomy in the treatment of radiation-failure of early glottic carcinoma. *Head Neck* 1997;19:116–120.

132. Steiner W, Vogt P, Ambrosch P, et al. Transoral carbon dioxide laser microsurgery for recurrent glottic carcinoma after radiotherapy. *Head Neck* 2004;26:477–484.

133. Ferlito A, Silver CE, Howard DJ, et al. The role of partial laryngeal resection in current management of laryngeal cancer: a collective review. *Acta Otolaryngol* 2000;120:456–465.

134. Ansarin M, Planicka M, Rotundo S, et al. Endoscopic carbon dioxide laser surgery for glottic cancer recurrence after radiotherapy: oncological results. *Arch Otolaryngol Head Neck Surg* 2007;133:1193–1197.

135. de Gier HH, Knegt PP, de Boer MF, et al. CO2-laser treatment of recurrent glottic carcinoma. *Head Neck* 2001;23:177–180.

136. Biel MA. Photodynamic therapy treatment of early oral and laryngeal cancers. *Photochem Photobiol* 2007;83:1063–1068.

137. Dahm JD, Sessions DG, Paniello RC, et al. Primary subglottic cancer. *Laryngoscope* 1998;108:741–746.

138. Smee RI, Williams JR, Bridger GP. The management dilemmas of invasive subglottic carcinoma. *Clin Oncol (R Coll Radiol)* 2008;20:751–756.

139. Ferlito A, Rinaldo A. The pathology and management of subglottic cancer. *Eur Arch Otorhinolaryngol* 2000;257:168–173.

140. Garas J, McGuirt WF Sr. Squamous cell carcinoma of the subglottis. *Am J Otolaryngol* 2006;27:1–4.

141. Davis LW. Controversy in the management of laryngeal tumors: radiation therapy perspective. In: Thawley S, Panje W, Batsakis J, et al., eds. *Comprehensive management of head and neck tumors*, 2nd ed., Vol. 2. Philadelphia, PA: WB Saunders, 1999: 1081–1089.

142. Santoro R, Turelli M, Polli G. Primary carcinoma of the subglottic larynx. *Eur Arch Otorhinolaryngol* 2000;257:548–551.

143. Bartual J, Roquette J. Infravestibular horizontal partial laryngectomy. A new surgical method. *Arch Otorhinolaryngol* 1978;220: 213–220.

144. Weber RS, Marvel J, Smith P, et al. Paratracheal lymph node dissection for carcinoma of the larynx, hypopharynx, and cervical esophagus. *Otolaryngol Head Neck Surg* 1993;108: 11–17.

145. Brandenburg JH. Laser cordotomy versus radiotherapy: an objective cost analysis. *Ann Otol Rhinol Laryngol* 2001;110: 312–318.

146. Myers EN, Wagner RL, Johnson JT. Microlaryngoscopic surgery for T1 glottic lesions: a cost-effective option. *Ann Otol Rhinol Laryngol* 1994;103:28–30.

147. Burns JA, Har-El G, Shapshay S, et al. Endoscopic laser resection of laryngeal cancer: is it oncologically safe? Position statement from the American Broncho-Esophagological Association. *Ann Otol Rhinol Laryngol* 2009;118:399–404.

148. Kennedy JT, Paddle PM, Cook BJ, et al. Voice outcomes following transoral laser microsurgery for early glottic squamous cell carcinoma. *J Laryngol Otol* 2007;121:1184–1188.

149. Higgins KM. What treatment for early-stage glottic carcinoma among adult patients: CO2 endolaryngeal laser excision versus standard fractionated external beam radiation is superior in terms of cost utility? *Laryngoscope* 2011;121:116–134.

Advanced Laryngeal Cancer

124

Bridget C. Loehn   **Melda Kunduk**   **Andrew J. McWhorter**

Laryngeal cancer affects nearly 12,720 men and women, and approximately 3,600 people will die of laryngeal cancer in the United States per year (1). The overall incidence of developing laryngeal cancer is approximately 0.7% with a mortality of 0% to 0.3% (2). If detected early, it can be effectively treated; however, over 40% of laryngeal cancers present with advanced-stage disease (3). Advanced-stage laryngeal cancer is defined as Stage III or IV disease, which includes not only T3 and T4 tumors but also tumors with regional cervical metastasis (N1 to N3 disease) (4).

The larynx produces one of the most complex motor functions of the body. It provides airway protection for respiration and deglutition as well as phonation. Any malignancy that affects the larynx can alter one or more of these main functions. Effects on this complex mechanism must be taken into account when formulating a treatment plan. The ultimate goal is to cure the patient of disease but with secondary goals to preserve phonation and deglutition and maintain a safe airway. There are many different treatment options for laryngeal cancer, but the clinician must balance quality of life (QOL) issues with the survival advantage of therapy. The treatment of laryngeal cancer should be a multidisciplinary approach to provide the patient with every opportunity available and the best oncologic and functional outcome.

Treatment of laryngeal cancer has evolved as medical advances have created more treatment options. Total and partial laryngectomy surgeries were the initial treatment for laryngeal cancer and were developed in the 19th century. Billroth is credited with the first laryngectomy in 1873 (5). Surgical advances in technique and antisepsis were major accomplishments that standardized surgical treatments and created reliable and safe conservation laryngeal surgery. With advances in radiation and chemotherapy and the use of multicentered prospective randomized trials, organ preservation therapy evolved to replace many of the surgical treatments and became the most common treatment

for advanced laryngeal cancer. This shift in treatment paradigm during the early 1990s, from surgical excision to organ preservation using concurrent chemoradiation therapy, has provided similar survival to the gold standard total laryngectomy with postoperative radiation therapy but with a 73% organ preservation rate (6). Disappointing functional outcomes and new developments in minimally invasive techniques have further changed the treatment of laryngeal cancer with the popularization of endoscopic laser surgical resections in the 21st century.

EPIDEMIOLOGY

The larynx is the second most common site of primary epithelial malignant tumors of the head and neck. Laryngeal cancer accounts for 0.3% of all cancer-related deaths (2). Unfortunately, the 5-year survival for all stages of laryngeal cancer has worsened over the past 30 years despite efforts to improve treatment protocols. In between 1975 and 1977, the 5-year survival was 67%, and between 1999 and 2005, the 5-year survival has statistically decreased to 63% (1,7). There is an ongoing debate as to the etiology of the decrease in survival as to whether using chemoradiation versus total laryngectomy for earlier stage disease is the cause.

Laryngeal malignancies can occur in all three subsites of the larynx. The glottis is the most common site for laryngeal malignancy (51%), followed by the supraglottis (32%) and the subglottis (2%) (8) (Fig. 124.1).

From 2003 to 2007, the median age of diagnosis was 65 years with the highest incidence in the sixth and seventh decades (7). Men are more commonly affected than women with a male to female ratio of 3.6:1. The ratio of male:female has decreased over the years likely secondary to the increased rate of tobacco use in females. There are also differences in the 5-year survival according to race. Caucasians have a higher 5-year survival (67%) than African Americans (53%).

Laryngeal Malignancy

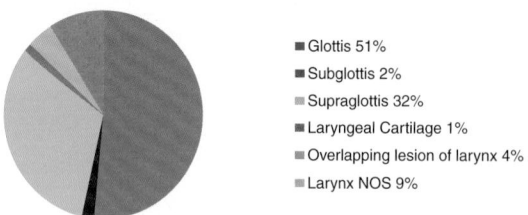

- ■ Glottis 51%
- ■ Subglottis 2%
- ■ Supraglottis 32%
- ■ Laryngeal Cartilage 1%
- ■ Overlapping lesion of larynx 4%
- ■ Larynx NOS 9%

Figure 124.1 Incidence of laryngeal cancer by subsite. Compiled from the National Cancer Database and Hoffman et al. (8). Approval for use obtained.

Over 40% of laryngeal cancers present as advanced stage disease. The 5-year survival also varied according to clinical stage (Table 124.1). Stage III supraglottic and glottic cancer had a 5-year survival of 50% to 60%. Stage IV supraglottic cancer has a 5-year survival of less than 50%, and Stage IV glottic cancer has a 5-year survival of 30% to 57% (3).

ANATOMY

The larynx is found in the anterior neck at the level of the C3 to C5 vertebrae and connects the hypopharynx with the trachea. The larynx functions in airway protection, phonation, and respiration. These functions are made possible by the three valves contained within the larynx. These valves include the true vocal cords, false vocal cords, and epiglottis to the arytenoids. Any dysfunction of these valves can lead to aspiration, airway obstruction, and changes in voice. The larynx is divided anatomically and clinically into the supraglottis, glottis, and subglottis.

The supraglottic larynx is composed of the epiglottis (lingual and laryngeal aspects), aryepiglottic folds, arytenoids, and bilateral false vocal cords. Clinically, the inferior border of the supraglottis, according to the American Joint Committee on Cancer (AJCC), is defined by a horizontal plane passing through the lateral margin of the ventricle at its junction with the superior surface of the vocal cord (4). Anatomically, the inferior border is defined by the arcuate line, which marks the change from respiratory to squamous epithelium and is not reliably located at the apex of the ventricle. For staging purposes, the epiglottis is divided into suprahyoid and infrahyoid portions by a plane at the level of the hyoid bone. Histologically, the supraglottis is lined with ciliated columnar epithelium.

The glottic larynx is comprised of the superior and inferior surfaces of the true vocal cords, including both the anterior and posterior commissures. The inferior border is defined as the line 1 cm below the apex of the ventricle (4). Histologically, the glottis is lined with stratified squamous epithelium. The layers of the true vocal cord from outward to inside are the following: stratified squamous epithelium, lamina propria, and vocalis muscle. The lamina propria is composed of three layers: a superficial layer that is composed of loose fibrous tissue and creates Reinke space an intermediate layer and a deep layer composed of elastic and collagen fibers that create the vocal ligament.

The subglottic larynx is the region below the glottis down to the inferior rim of the cricoid cartilage (4). The subglottis has no subsites. It is rarely the primary site of laryngeal cancer but is commonly involved in the inferior extent of glottic tumors. Histologically, the subglottis is lined with ciliated columnar epithelium (Fig. 124.2).

PATTERNS OF SPREAD

The larynx contains several fibroelastic membranes and ligaments that divide the larynx into compartments, limit the spread of early cancers, and allow for partial resections with adequate margins. Tumors tend to grow in the path of least resistance into preexisting compartments including the preepiglottic space and paraglottic space. The preepiglottic space is bound by the thyroepiglottic ligament inferiorly, the hyoepiglottic ligament superiorly, and the epiglottis posteriorly. At this level, the thyroepiglottic ligament is an ineffective barrier and offers little resistance to tumor spread. Tumor may also spread directly into the

TABLE 124.1	OVERALL 5-YEAR SURVIVAL BY SUBSITE AND STAGE (8,9)		
	Supraglottis	**Glottis**	**Subglottis**
Stage III	50%–60%	50%–60%	43%
Stage IV	28%–53%	22%–52%	25%

A. Supraglottis
B. Glottis
C. Subglottis

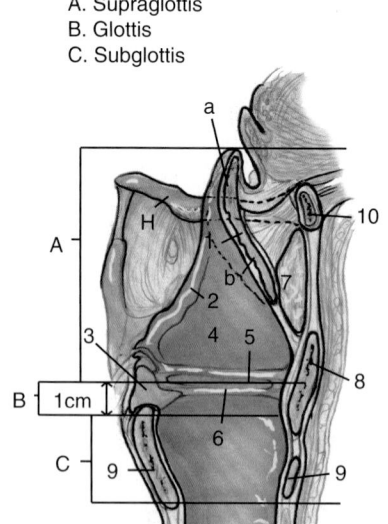

1. Epiglottis
   a. Surahyoid portion
   b. Infrahyoid portion
2. Aryepiglottic fold
3. Arytenoid cartilage
4. False vocal fold
5. Ventricle of Morgani
6. True vocal fold
7. Pre-epiglottic space
8. Thyroid cartilage
9. Cricoid cartilage
10. Hyoid bone

Staging larynx anatomy

Figure 124.2 Midline sagittal section of the larynx demonstrating the supraglottis, glottis and subglottis.

preepiglottic space by traveling through lacunae on the laryngeal surface of the epiglottis into the space. The paraglottic space is another potential space bound laterally by the perichondrium of the thyroid cartilage and cricothyroid membrane and posteriorly by the mucosa of the pyriform sinus. Medially, the paraglottic space is bound by the quadrangular membrane above the ventricle and the conus elasticus below the ventricle. The conus elasticus extends superiorly from the superior border of the cricoid cartilage to merge with the inferomedial border of the vocal ligament. This ligament resists the extralaryngeal spread of early glottic and subglottic tumors. The paraglottic space allows tumors to become transglottic (superior and inferior to the ventricle) tumors and also to impair the movement of the true vocal cord. The preepiglottic space and paraglottic space communicate with each other.

At the level of the glottis, the vocalis tendon attaches to the thyroid cartilage through Broyles ligament, which is an ineffective barrier and will allow tumors to spread into the thyroid cartilage and preepiglottic space. This region where the tendon attaches to the thyroid cartilage has no perichondrium. The perichondrium is considered another barrier to the spread of early cancers. As previously discussed, the true vocal cords contain a lamina propria consisting of three layers. The superficial layer (Reinke's space) contains loose fibrous tissue and is almost void of lymphatics and blood vessels creating a resistance to the spread of early glottic tumors.

Lymphatic spread of the tumor usually occurs in a predictable manor and follows the embryologic origins of the larynx. The supraglottis is derived from the midline buccopharyngeal primordium and branchial arches 3 and 4. The supraglottis has a rich lymphatic supply. The glottis is derived from the tracheobronchial primordium and branchial arches 4, 5, and 6. In contrast to the supraglottis, the glottis has a very low lymphatic supply. These differences account for the high incidence of lymphatic spread for supraglottic carcinomas and the low incidence of lymphatic spread in glottic carcinomas. As a result of the rich lymphatic supply to the supraglottis, there is also a greater incidence of bilateral lymph node metastasis as compared to the unilateral spread in glottic tumors (10).

Since the lymphatic drainage of these sites is predictable, this allows surgeons to limit neck dissections to the lymph node levels most at risk. In 1972, Lindberg mapped out affected lymph nodes based on the primary site of the tumor. This study demonstrated that laryngeal carcinoma has lymphatic drainage to Levels II to V and that supraglottic tumors have a greater incidence of bilateral neck involvement (11) (Fig. 124.3).

STAGING

The current staging system for laryngeal cancer is the Tumor-Node-Metastasis (TNM) staging system of the

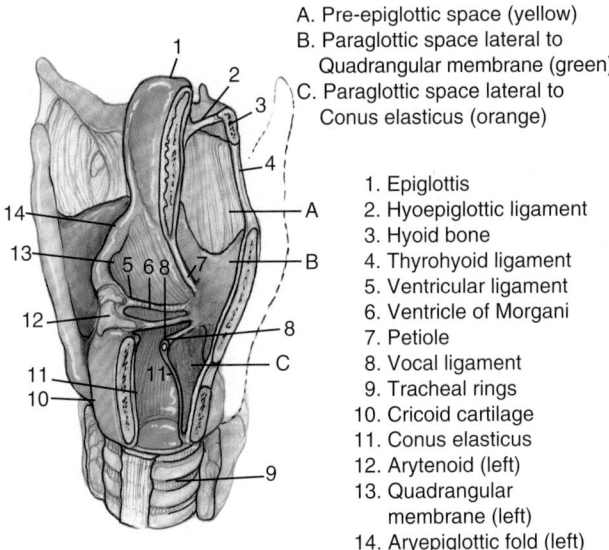

A. Pre-epiglottic space (yellow)
B. Paraglottic space lateral to Quadrangular membrane (green)
C. Paraglottic space lateral to Conus elasticus (orange)

1. Epiglottis
2. Hyoepiglottic ligament
3. Hyoid bone
4. Thyrohyoid ligament
5. Ventricular ligament
6. Ventricle of Morgani
7. Petiole
8. Vocal ligament
9. Tracheal rings
10. Cricoid cartilage
11. Conus elasticus
12. Arytenoid (left)
13. Quadrangular membrane (left)
14. Aryepiglottic fold (left)

Figure 124.3 Parasagittal view of larynx demonstrating laryngeal spaces and cartilages and ligaments that compose them.

AJCC. This system is an anatomical staging system characterized by the extent of invasion of the primary tumor, cervical lymph node involvement, and distant metastasis. This information is obtained through physical examination, imaging, and endoscopic examination and finally confirmed by surgical pathology from the resected tumor. For purposes of this chapter, advanced laryngeal cancer will be defined as Stage III or IV on the AJCC staging system (4) (Table 124.2).

While this system stages tumors based on size and extent of the tumor, other important prognostic factors are not included. There are histologic factors that can indicate a poorer prognosis including perineural invasion, angiolymphatic spread, extracapsular spread of nodal metastasis, and histologic grade of the tumor. There are also studies showing that multiple chromosomal and molecular markers are indicative of a poor prognosis. Some of these markers include overexpression of mutant p53 protein (12), a high Ki67 or proliferating cell nuclear antigen score, and the expression of c-myc oncogene or int-2 gene (13,14). Bradford et al. (12) in 1997 found that high levels of mutant p53 are associated with decreased survival.

Other staging systems have been proposed for laryngeal cancer. Some propose using a high-resolution computed tomography (CT) to assess the volume of tumor. Others suggest that any tumor with any change in vocal cord mobility be considered a T3 or T4. There was also a five-part system devised that used the TNM system but separated it into clinical/diagnostic, surgical, pathologic, retreatment, and autopsy. Other research is including comorbidities into the staging system and is looking at how it relates to the overall outcome (15) (Table 124.2).

TABLE 124.2	STAGING LARYNGEAL CARCINOMA

Primary tumor (T): TX: Primary tumor cannot be assessed T0: No evidence of primary tumor Tis: Carcinoma *in situ*

Supraglottis

T1: Tumor limited to one subsite[a] of supraglottis with normal vocal cord mobility

T2: Tumor invades mucosa of more than one adjacent subsite[a] of supraglottis or glottis or region outside the supraglottis (e.g., mucosa of base of tongue, vallecula, medial wall of pyriform sinus) without fixation of the larynx

T3: Tumor limited to larynx with vocal cord fixation and/or invades any of the following: postcricoid area, preepiglottic tissues, paraglottic space, and/or minor thyroid cartilage erosion (e.g., inner cortex)

T4a: Tumor invades through the thyroid cartilage and/or invades tissues beyond the larynx (e.g., trachea, soft tissues of the neck including deep extrinsic muscle of the tongue, strap muscles, thyroid, or esophagus)

T4b: Tumor invades prevertebral space, encases carotid artery, or invades mediastinal structures

Glottis

T1: Tumor limited to the vocal cord(s) (may involve anterior or posterior commissure) with normal mobility

T1a: Tumor limited to one vocal cord T1b: Tumor involves both vocal cords

T2: Tumor extends to supraglottis and/or subglottis, and/or with impaired vocal cord mobility

T3: Tumor limited to the larynx with vocal cord fixation and/or invades paraglottic space, and/or minor thyroid cartilage erosion (e.g., inner cortex)

T4a: Tumor invades through the outer cortex of the thyroid cartilage and/or invades tissues beyond the larynx (e.g., trachea, soft tissues of neck, including deep extrinsic muscle of the tongue, strap muscles, thyroid, or esophagus)

T4b: Tumor invades prevertebral space, encases carotid artery, or invades mediastinal structures

Subglottis

T1: Tumor limited to the subglottis

T2: Tumor extends to vocal cord(s) with normal or impaired mobility

T3: Tumor limited to larynx with vocal cord fixation

T4a: Tumor invades cricoid or thyroid cartilage and/or invades tissues beyond the larynx (e.g., trachea, soft tissues of neck, including deep extrinsic muscles of the tongue, strap muscles, thyroid, or esophagus)

T4b: Tumor invades prevertebral space, encases carotid artery, or invades mediastinal structures

Regional lymph nodes (N) NX: Regional lymph nodes cannot be assessed

N0: No regional lymph node metastasis

N1: Metastasis in a single ipsilateral lymph node, 3 cm or less in greatest dimension

N2a: Metastasis in a single ipsilateral lymph node more than 3 cm but not more than 6 cm in greatest dimension

N2b: Metastasis in multiple ipsilateral lymph nodes, not more than 6 cm in greatest dimension

N2c: Metastasis in bilateral or contralateral lymph nodes, not more than 6 cm in greatest dimension

N3: Metastasis in a lymph node more than 6 cm in greatest dimension

Distant metastasis (M) MX: Distant metastasis cannot be assessed

M0: No distant metastasis

M1: Distant metastasis

Stage

Stage 0: Tis, N0, M0

Stage I: T1, N0, M0

Stage II: T2, N0, M0

Stage III: T3, N0, M0 or T1, N1, M0 or T2, N1, M0 or T3, N1, M0

Stage IVA: T1, N2, M0 or T2, N2, M0 or T3, N2, M0 or T4a, N2, or less M0

Stage IVB: T4b, any N, M0 or any T, N3, M0

Stage IVC: Any T, any N, M1

[a]Subsites include the following: suprahyoid epiglottis, infrahyoid epiglottis, vestibular folds (false vocal cords), aryepiglottic folds, arytenoids (each fold is one subsite).

Adapted from AJCC. Larynx. In: Edge SB, Byrd DR, Compton CC, et al., eds. *AJCC Cancer Staging Manual*, 7th ed. New York: Springer, 2010:57–62.

EVALUATION AND DIAGNOSIS

History and Physical Examination

The majority of the time, the diagnosis of laryngeal cancer can be made through a complete history and physical examination. Presenting complaints can be site specific. Patients may complain of hoarseness (glottic carcinoma), muffled/ hot potato voice (supraglottic carcinoma), dyspnea, dysphagia, and otalgia (usually supraglottic). Patients may also present with a history of aspiration pneumonia, stridor, hemoptysis, or sore throat. Constitutional symptoms may include weight loss, fevers, chills, and night sweats. Often, the initial complaint is that of a cervical mass. Glottic tumors usually present earlier than supraglottic cancers due to the early change in voice. Supraglottic tumors present with fewer symptoms in the early stage and therefore are usually diagnosed at a later stage. Patients with supraglottic tumors tend to present with pain, dysphagia, and cervical metastasis. Subglottic tumors typically present as advanced stage disease with airway obstruction.

Past medical history is also important in assessing patient comorbidities, history of cancer, and immunologic status. Social history is important in assessing patient risk factors. More than 95% of patients with laryngeal cancer have a significant history of tobacco abuse (3). There is a positive relationship between the quantity of cigarettes consumed and the increased risk of developing laryngeal cancer. There is also a synergistic effect when tobacco is combined with alcohol use leading to even higher rates of malignancy (16). However, alcohol may be a risk factor by itself, but its role is less defined. Treatment of tobacco and alcohol dependency must be considered in the postoperative period. Delirium tremens and tobacco withdrawal can lead to a complicated and prolonged postoperative course and impaired healing.

Other risk factors include human papillomavirus, especially subtypes 16 and 18 (17); gastroesophageal reflux disease; and occupational exposures as seen in patients who are metal workers, construction workers (asbestos), and textile processors.

A complete examination including a complete head and neck exam should be performed on all patients to determine staging, the presence of second primaries, and other findings/comorbidities that may influence recommended treatments. A complete head and neck examination includes examination of the skin, eyes, ears, oral cavity, and pharynx, including palpation of the floor of mouth, base of tongue, and tonsils in addition to the larynx, neck, and cranial nerves. Dentition should be assessed for caries and periodontal disease. A more detailed exam of the larynx and pharynx is performed using flexible fiberoptic laryngoscopy at which time. The extent of the lesion as well as the mobility and position of the vocal cords are assessed. This also allows for assessment of the airway. Videostroboscopy can also be used to detect subtle changes in vocal cord function and mobility but is more helpful in early-stage disease. Palpation of the neck should occur bilaterally noting the location, size, and relationship of the lymph nodes to adjacent structures (18,19) (Fig 124.4).

Imaging

Physical examination is often limited in the evaluation of tumor depth and nodal metastases, and radiographic imaging is helpful in determining the extent of the disease. Imaging can provide information regarding cartilage invasion, extension into the preepiglottic and paraglottic spaces, and extralaryngeal spread of tumor. Imaging studies can also be used to assess cervical nodal disease. Both CT and magnetic resonance imaging are useful tools for

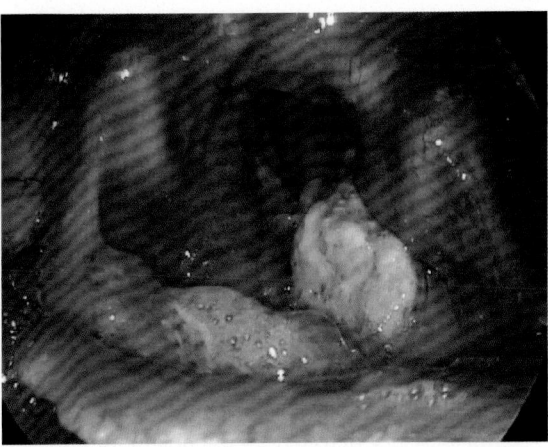

Figure 124.4 Seventy-degree fiberoptic view of T3N0M0 SCCA supraglottis. Tumor extends from epiglottis onto left false fold.

this assessment. The CT scan is more specific for cartilage invasion (20), and in most centers, CT is considered the standard imaging modality for advanced laryngeal cancers (Fig 124.5).

Chest radiograph (CXR) should be obtained on all patients in the preoperative evaluation and staging of laryngeal cancer. This allows for the diagnosis of acute/chronic pulmonary disease as well as a synchronous or metastatic lung mass/tumor. Patients with abnormalities on CXR will usually require additional imaging (chest CT) for further work-up.

Another imaging modality used in the staging of many cancers, including laryngeal cancer, is positron emission tomography (PET). PET is a nuclear medicine technique that produces a three-dimensional image of the functional processes of the body. It utilizes fluorescence-tagged glucose molecules and then measures the uptake within the tissues. The hypermetabolic state of most malignancies will lead to increased uptake (10). PET has evolved to be an essential imaging modality in the assessment of advanced laryngeal cancer. It has limited utility in determining the

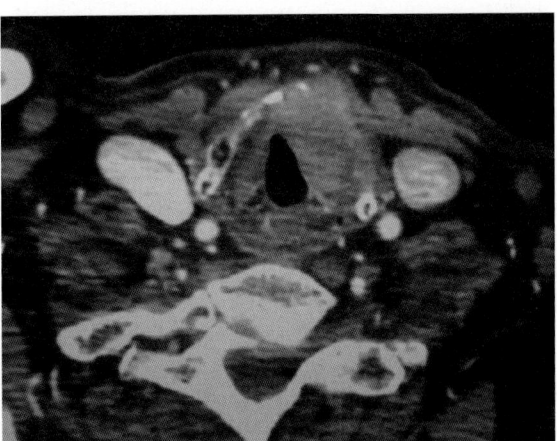

Figure 124.5 Axial contrast CT scan, T4N0M0 transglottic SCCA demonstrating paraglottic space involvement and thyroid cartilage invasion with extralaryngeal spread.

extent of the primary tumor; however, it is becoming the standard in the assessment of regional cervical metastasis as well as distant metastasis (21). The sensitivity and specificity of PET in detecting cervical metastatic disease range from 74% to 94% and from 82% to 100%, respectively, compared with the sensitivity and specificity of CT, which ranged from 67% to 81% and from 47% to 81%, respectively (22–27). Kyzas et al. (28) found that the overall sensitivity of PET in detecting cervical nodal metastasis was 79%; however, in tumors with nodal status as N0, the sensitivity decreased to 50%. Yamazaki et al. (27) found that metastatic nodes measuring greater than 1cm were detected 100% of the time whereas nodes measuring less than 5 mm were not detected. In the posttreatment period, PET has become useful in the identification of residual and recurrent disease (21). In the assessment of distant metastasis, Gourin et al. (29) reported that the sensitivity and specificity of PET–CT detecting distant metastasis were 86% and 84%, respectively.

Ultrasound is another useful imaging tool in the determination of nodal disease. This is most commonly used in Europe but is gaining prevalence in the United States. This tool is noninvasive, low cost, and is a good technique for lymph node assessment.

Laboratory Tests

Laboratory tests are ordered as part of the preoperative and metastatic workup, usually according to patient factors and institutional guidelines. These tests typically include complete blood count, complete metabolic panel, coagulation studies, as well as other tests. If abnormal liver function tests and calcium and alkaline phosphatase levels are noted, abdominal CT, bone scan, or PET can be utilized to further determine the etiology of these abnormalities.

Consultations

A multidisciplinary approach is used in the treatment of advanced laryngeal cancer. Prior to the start of treatment, other specialists, who will assist in the treatment, as well as posttreatment care, should evaluate the patient. The members of the multidisciplinary team usually include radiation oncology, hematology oncology, dental oncology, speech pathology, nutritional services, and spiritual care. The speech pathologist is critical in pretreatment assessment, counseling, education regarding changes in voice and swallowing including alaryngeal speech, and posttreatment rehabilitation.

Surgical Evaluation

Panendoscopy is a term used to describe the endoscopic evaluation of the entire upper aerodigestive tract. This includes direct laryngoscopy, tracheobronchoscopy, and esophagoscopy and is typically done under general anesthesia. With the advent of advanced flexible scopes and the advancements of in-office procedures, panendoscopy has been performed successfully in this setting (30); however, if conservation laryngeal surgery is being considered, it should not replace the operative endoscopy.

Exam under anesthesia allows the surgeon to make an accurate assessment of the boundaries of the primary site (T stage) and determine if the patient is a candidate for conservation laryngeal surgery by allowing superb visualization of the complex endolaryngeal anatomy. This assessment also allows for the evaluation of a second primary tumor. The overall incidence of second primary tumors is 8.9% creating a 5-year disease-specific survival of 35%. Second primary tumors are not statistically related to the primary tumor site, stage, or presence of regional or distant metastases (31).

Evaluation of the upper aerodigestive tract begins with a thorough examination and palpation of the oral cavity; oropharynx, including base of tongue and tonsil; and nasopharynx.

Direct laryngoscopy is then performed to assess the extent of the tumor, carefully mapping its margins. Rigid telescopes (0, 30, and 70 degree) are helpful in examining the ventricles as well as the subglottis and for photodocumentation (Fig. 124.6). The true vocal cords, vocal processes, and arytenoids are palpated to assess cricoarytenoid joint mobility and to differentiate vocal cord immobility from vocal cord fixation. Tumor involvement in the preepiglottic space and base of tongue is assessed through bimanual palpation. Biopsies are taken at the primary site to obtain the pathological diagnosis. Flexible or rigid esophagoscopy is performed to assess esophageal involvement by tumor, skip lesions in the esophagus or second primaries. Tracheobronchoscopy can also be performed; however, the

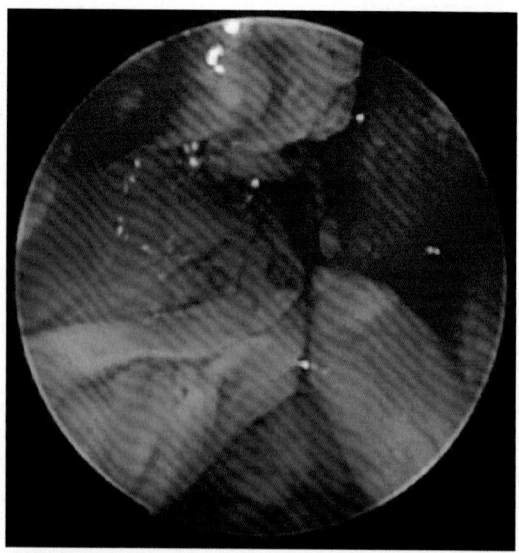

Figure 124.6 Seventy-degree telescope evaluation of left ventricle with SCCA involving left false vocal fold with clear ventricle and true vocal fold.

yield is low in the asymptomatic patient due to the limitation of only visualizing endobronchial lesions. With the patient fully relaxed, a complete neck examination is performed to assess for occult nodal disease that might have been missed on in-office examination.

DIFFERENTIAL DIAGNOSIS

Squamous cell carcinoma (SCCA) comprises 95% to 99% of laryngeal malignancies. SCCA can be represented by a linear continuum from dedifferentiation through invasive carcinoma. There are multiple histologic variants of SCCA. The most common of these is verrucous carcinoma representing 1% to 3% of all laryngeal malignancies. This variant has "pushing borders" with a high propensity for local recurrence but an extremely low rate of distant metastasis. It has the classic appearance of exophytic white-gray fronds. The treatment remains controversial, but as of now, surgery remains the treatment of choice (10,32,33).

Although SCCA accounts for the majority of laryngeal cancers, many granulomatous and neoplastic lesions can mimic its appearance, and therefore, a biopsy must always be obtained. Granulomatous diseases such as tuberculosis, Wegener granulomatosis, sarcoidosis, histoplasmosis, and blastomycosis may present with an exophytic or fungating mass resembling SCCA. Of the neoplastic lesions, the most common are sarcomas, minor salivary gland tumors, and neuroendocrine tumors. Multiple sarcomas have been described in the larynx, with chondrosarcoma being the most common sarcoma in the larynx, usually arising from the cricoid cartilage (Fig. 124.7).

Minor salivary tumors include adenoid cystic carcinoma, mucoepidermoid carcinoma, acinic cell carcinoma, adenocarcinoma, and malignant mixed carcinoma. These tumors are most commonly found in the supraglottis but can also be found in the subglottis (adenoid cystic carcinoma). Neuroendocrine malignancies are comprised of paragangliomas, large cell tumors, and small cell tumors and usually involve the supraglottis. Lymphoproliferative lesions also usually occur in the supraglottis, and the most common type is mucosal-associated lymphoid tissue, a subtype of non-Hodgkin lymphoma. Granular cell tumors usually affect the younger patient population and can be difficult to distinguish from invasive carcinoma.

It is also important to remember that the larynx can be the site of secondary spread through direct extension from neighboring structures such as the thyroid gland. Metastatic lesions can also occur in the larynx. Adenocarcinoma can metastasize most commonly from the breast or colon. However, renal cell carcinoma is the most common laryngeal metastasis (34).

TREATMENT

Through the use of history and physical examination, imaging studies, laboratory data, and diagnostic surgery, the tumor can be accurately staged, and the appropriate treatment plan can be recommended. The treatment is then divided into surgical and nonsurgical pathways. Unlike early-stage laryngeal cancer, advanced laryngeal cancer usually requires multimodality treatment with surgery followed by radiation or radiation and chemotherapy. The goal of treatment for advanced laryngeal cancer is to cure the patient with secondary goals of preserving speech and swallowing function. The patient should be included in all aspects of the decision-making process and be allowed to make an informed decision on which treatment option is best for him or her.

Nonsurgical Treatment

Radiation Therapy

External beam radiation uses ionizing radiation to generate free radicals within cell nuclei creating cellular and DNA damage resulting in cell death. The goal of radiation therapy is to achieve better outcomes with tumor eradication while preserving normal tissue. Intensity-modulated radiation therapy was most recently designed to better achieve the above goals. It allows the radiation beams to be more precisely focused to limit the effects of the radiation on surrounding tissue.

The typical total treatment dose of radiation is 6,000 to 7,000 cGy given 5 days per week over a period of 6 to 7 weeks. Primary radiation therapy is indicated for T1, T2, and small T3 tumors. The necks are included in the field of radiation if there is N+ disease or if there is greater than a 20% to 30% risk of cervical regional metastasis. It is also useful in palliation in unresectable tumors and in patients who are poor surgical candidates. Adjuvant radiation may also be given in the postoperative period. Indications for

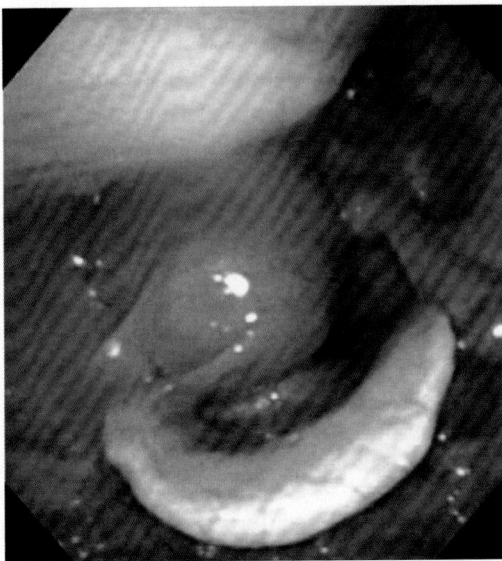

Figure 124.7 Chondrosarcoma with cricoid and right arytenoid cartilage involvement with airway obstruction.

this include advanced stage disease, positive margins, extracapsular spread of tumor in a lymph node, perineural or angiolymphatic spread of tumor, multiple cervical lymph node involvement, and subglottic extension of tumor. Radiation therapy alone for advanced laryngeal cancer has a 5-year disease-specific survival of 56.5% for Stage III laryngeal cancers and 50% for Stage IV laryngeal cancers (35,36).

Complications of radiation therapy are divided into early and late. Early complications include mucositis, odynophagia, dysphagia, skin breakdown, loss of taste, and edema. These side effects can last up to 6 weeks after the completion of radiation. As a result of the dysphagia and edema associated with radiation, the patient may require the placement of a tracheotomy as well as a percutaneous gastrostomy to maintain nutrition. The late complications include fibrosis, xerostomia, edema, loss of taste, hypothyroidism, laryngeal stenosis, esophageal stenosis, chondroradionecrosis, and osteoradionecrosis. Chondroradionecrosis occurs in approximately 5% of patients with laryngeal cancer. The most common cartilage to be affected is the arytenoid cartilage (37). Osteoradionecrosis can be prevented by having a thorough dental exam prior to the start of radiation.

Chemotherapy

Chemotherapy is another modality used in the treatment of laryngeal cancer. It is most often used in conjunction with radiation therapy. The two most common methods of chemotherapy are induction and concomitant. Concomitant chemoradiation therapy has added a new dimension to the treatment of laryngeal cancer. The chemotherapeutic agent is used as a radiosensitizer while also providing a systemic antineoplastic effect.

Cisplatin and 5-fluorouracil are the two most commonly used agents. Chemotherapy may also be used in palliation when radiation therapy is not an option.

Concurrent Chemotherapy and Radiation Therapy

In 2003, a landmark trial (RTOG 91-11) by Forastiere et al. was conducted, which was the first prospective randomized trial specifically addressing the role of concurrent chemoradiotherapy in laryngeal preservation. Five hundred and forty-seven patients with resectable Stage III or IV SCCA of the larynx were randomized to one of three treatment arms. The three treatments included (a) induction chemotherapy followed by chemoradiation or surgery and postoperative radiation, (b) concurrent chemoradiation, and (c) radiation alone. Exclusions to the trial included all T1 tumors, T4 tumors if the tumor penetrated through cartilage or invaded greater than 1 cm into the base of tongue and any patients with distant metastasis. Any patient who presented with N2 or N3 disease had a planned neck dissection 8 weeks after completing radiation. Indications for total laryngectomy were inadequate response after two cycles of induction

chemotherapy, biopsy-proven disease at the primary site at least 8 weeks after radiation therapy, or laryngeal dysfunction with aspiration or laryngeal necrosis. At 2 years, the patients who had an intact larynx after concurrent chemoradiation (88%) differed significantly from the groups given induction chemotherapy followed by radiation (75%) and radiation therapy alone (70%). The locoregional control was also found to be significantly better with concurrent chemoradiation as compared to induction chemotherapy and radiation and radiation alone. Overall 2-year survival was 76% for induction chemotherapy group, 74% for concurrent chemoradiation group, and 75% for radiation alone (38).

In 2006, Forastiere et al. performed a follow-up study to the original RTOG 911-11 trial, which examined this same group of patients 5 years after treatment. The 5-year results differ from the 2-year results by a significant improvement in laryngectomy-free survival for both the induction chemotherapy followed by radiation (44.6%) and concurrent chemoradiation (46.6%) compared to radiation alone (33.9%). The 5-year disease-free survival was better with induction chemotherapy followed by radiation (38.6%) or concurrent chemoradiation (39%) compared to radiation alone (27.3%) which is similar to the 2-year disease-free survival statistics. The overall 5-year survival was similar for the three treatments: induction chemotherapy followed by radiation (59.2%), concurrent chemoradiation (54.6%), and radiation alone (53.5%) (39).

Induction Chemotherapy

Induction chemotherapy has been found to have high response rates. The response to induction chemotherapy predicts the success of subsequent therapy with additional chemotherapy and radiation. In the original RTOG study, the early data on induction chemotherapy suggested a lower survival, but the follow-up study showed an increase in laryngectomy-free survival with induction chemotherapy (38,39). Recent studies have shown that there have been no adverse effects from the delay in surgery or radiation therapy with induction. There has been no difference in survival, but there is a decrease in distant metastasis in patients treated with induction chemotherapy (40,41).

The Veterans Affairs Study Group provided a landmark induction study for laryngeal cancer. Patients in the experimental arm were treated with two cycles of cisplatin and 5-fluorouracil and then reassessed. If there was a partial response, a third round was given followed by radiation. Poor responders after two cycles of chemotherapy were treated with surgery. The experimental arm was compared to the standard therapy of surgery and postoperative radiation. Patients treated with induction chemotherapy followed by radiation had a similar survival to those treated with total laryngectomy and postoperative radiation (68% at 5 years) (40). One of the limitations of this study was that there was no radiation-therapy-alone arm for direct comparison.

The European Organization for Research and Treatment of Cancer performed a study to determine if induction chemotherapy followed by radiation was comparable to surgery and postoperative radiation in patients with T2–T4, N0–N2b SCCA of the pyriform sinus or aryepiglottic fold. Two hundred and two patients were enrolled in the study. The induction chemotherapy patients underwent three cycles of cisplatin and 5-fluorouracil. Partial response and complete response were assessed after each cycle. Only the patients with complete response underwent radiation. The surgical group underwent partial laryngopharyngectomy and postoperative radiation. The results showed for the chemotherapy group a 3-year and 5-year disease-free survival of 43% and 25%, respectively, and the surgical group 32% and 27%, respectively. The overall survival at 3 years was 57% for the chemotherapy group and 43% for the surgical group. There was no difference in survival at 5 years between the two groups. There was also found to be no difference in local regional failure. There were fewer distant metastases and increased time to distant metastases in the chemotherapy arm of the study. A complete response was found in 82% of T2 tumors, 48% of T3, and 0% of T4 (41).

Both of these trials suggest that organ preservation is possible in patients with advanced stage laryngeal or hypopharyngeal cancer. Distant metastases appear to be decreased with chemotherapy. They also suggest that head and neck SCCA is sensitive to cisplatin and 5-fluorouracil.

A new development has been the addition of a taxane (T) (docetaxel) to the traditional doublet cisplatin and 5-fluorouracil (PF) regimen, thus creating a highly active triplet induction regimen, TPF (docetaxel, cisplatin, 5-fluorouracil). Data from randomized trials indicate that TPF sequential therapy may be an effective alternative to concurrent chemoradiation for some patients with locally advanced laryngeal cancer with extensive tumor load or low-neck disease. The TPF is well tolerated but is associated with higher incidence of hematologic events (neutropenia) than traditional PF. These side effects can be managed using prophylactic G-CSF and antibodies (42). In 2007, Posner et al. compared induction chemotherapy with TPF and with PF, both followed by chemoradiation. The 3-year overall survival was 62% in the TPF group compared to 48% in the PF regimen. There was better locoregional control in the TPF group, but the incidence of distant metastasis was not significantly different. The TPF group had higher rates of neutropenia, but there were more treatment delays in the PF group secondary to hematologic events (43).

Surgical Treatment

There are many surgical options for laryngeal cancer. The spectrum ranges from the less invasive microlaryngeal technique to the most invasive, total laryngectomy. The key to the surgical treatment of laryngeal cancer is to determine the correct patient for the correct procedure while accounting for the expertise of the surgeon. Not all patients are amenable to surgical options; however, this can be determined through a complete and thorough preoperative evaluation.

Endoscopic Transoral Laser Microsurgery

Endoscopic resection of laryngeal tumors was first designed for T1 and T2 tumors, but through experience in treating early disease and technical recent advancements, the procedure can be utilized for selected T3 and T4 tumors. The field was born in 1972 when Strong and Jako (44) first introduced the laser through the laryngoscope. The field of endoscopic transoral laser microsurgery was initially slow to develop, but through the work of Wolfgang Steiner and other European experts, it has become more widely accepted and commonly used in the United States in the 21st century. This technique utilizes endoscopes, carbon dioxide laser, and the microscope to excise both glottic and supraglottic tumors by following the pathway of the tumor. It challenged traditional views by transection of the tumor to assess tumor depth and to remove tumors larger than the laryngoscope in a multipiece fashion. This technique is less invasive than traditional open procedures. It does not deconstruct the larynx or its support mechanisms and does not require reconstruction, and major complications are very uncommon. This field is continuing to evolve and is used mainly for early laryngeal cancers, but its development has led to less open conservation laryngeal surgery for advanced laryngeal cancer. The major advantages of this procedure over open procedures are the frequent avoidance of a tracheotomy, swallowing rehabilitation is of shorter duration, and it does not remove the laryngeal support structures. Limitations to this procedure include surgical expertise and special instrumentation (Fig. 124.8).

Hinni et al. in 2007 performed a multicenter study on 117 patients with advanced laryngeal cancer of the glottis or supraglottis treated with transoral laser microsurgery from 1997 to 2004. They examined laryngeal preservation, overall survival, disease-free survival, local control, locoregional control, and distant metastasis. At 2 years, 92% of patients had an intact larynx after treatment. The 5-year Kaplan-Meier estimates were local control 74%, locoregional control 68%, disease-free survival 58%, overall survival 55%, and distant metastasis 14%. They concluded that in patients with advanced laryngeal cancer, transoral laser microsurgery with or without postoperative radiation therapy is a valid treatment option for organ preservation with low mortality and morbidity with good outcomes (44). Vilaseca et al. (45) found that vocal cord fixation and cartilage invasion were found to be negative prognostic factors for transoral laser microsurgery.

Open Conservation Laryngeal Surgery

Conservational laryngeal surgery is any procedure that maintains physiologic speech and swallowing without the need for permanent tracheostoma. The goal is to preserve maximal laryngeal function without compromising cure

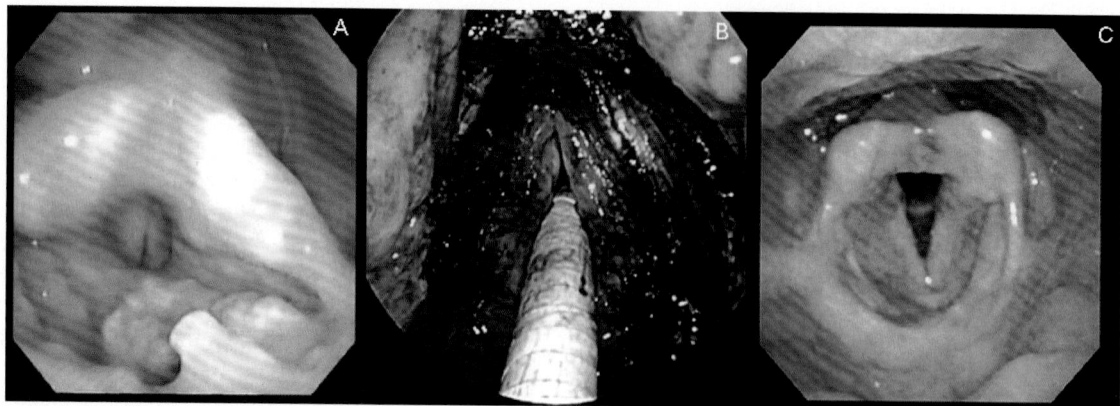

Figure 124.8 T3N0M0 SCCA treated with transoral laser microsurgery. **A:** Pre-op flexible laryngoscopy image demonstrating ulcerative cancer of laryngeal surface of the epiglottis in phonation. **B:** Intraoperative telescopic image in surgical position demonstrating postsurgical defect with hyoid visible superiorly with visible thyroid cartilage status post removal of false folds, epiglottis, and preepiglottic space with laser-shielded endotracheal tube. **C:** Postoperative flexible healed supraglottic laryngectomy defect on inhalation.

rates. Malignant disease is resected while preserving swallowing, respiration, phonation, and airway protection. In conservational laryngeal surgery, proper patient selection is critical. As long as one cricoarytenoid joint is preserved and one laryngeal valve (epiglottis, false vocal cords, or true vocal cords) is maintained, the patient is a potential candidate. The following are the partial surgical procedures and their indications.

Vertical Hemilaryngectomy

The vertical hemilaryngectomy is an organ-sparing procedure used for the treatment of glottic malignancies. This procedure allows for the en bloc removal of the involved vocal cord and a portion of the thyroid cartilage. It also addresses tumors that extend into the paraglottic space. In order for the tumor to be resected by a vertical hemilaryngectomy procedure, the tumor can be up to 5 mm onto the contralateral true vocal fold, up to 15 mm of subglottic extension anteriorly, up to 5 mm of subglottic extension posteriorly, and can extend superiorly up to the free edge of the false vocal fold. Candidates for this procedure include T1, T2, selected T3, and rare T4 glottic tumors. First, endoscopy and tracheotomy are performed. A horizontal skin incision is made separate from the tracheotomy incision. The strap muscles are retracted laterally to expose the larynx. The external perichondrium and musculature are elevated. A midline thyrotomy, cricothyrotomy, and a superior incision across the petiole are made. The lesion and thyroid cartilage are removed en bloc. The raised perichondrium and occasionally the strap muscles are used to reconstruct the neoglottis. Contraindications to this procedure include fixed true vocal fold, posterior commissure/interarytenoid involvement, invasion of bilateral arytenoids, bulky transglottic lesion, thyroid cartilage invasion, preepiglottic space involvement, subglottic extension that involves the cricoid cartilage, and extralaryngeal spread. Survival is similar between radiation and open surgical techniques. Voice outcomes are generally considered inferior to primary radiotherapy.

The extended vertical hemilaryngectomy can be subdivided into frontolateral vertical hemilaryngectomy and the posterolateral vertical hemilaryngectomy. The frontolateral hemilaryngectomy is for glottic lesions involving the anterior commissure and can encompass up to the anterior one-third of the contralateral vocal cord. The posterolateral vertical hemilaryngectomy is for lesions involving the ipsilateral arytenoid without fixation.

Vertical partial laryngectomies are used mainly for T1 and T2 tumors. Brumund et al. in 2005 studied 270 patients with previously untreated SCCA of the true vocal cord (232 T1N0M0, 35 T2N0M0, and 3 T3N0M0). These patients were treated with frontolateral vertical partial laryngectomy. The 5-year Kaplan-Meier survival estimate was 83.1% for T1 tumors and 67.2% for T2 tumors, and the local control estimate was 91% for T1 tumors and 68.7% for T2 tumors. Reduced survival was seen with advanced T stage, local failure, and nodal failure (46).

Supraglottic Laryngectomy

The supraglottic laryngectomy is also known as the horizontal hemilaryngectomy, which is used to remove the supraglottic structures superior to the true vocal cords including the preepiglottic space and leaves a portion of the thyroid cartilage and both arytenoid cartilages behind. The supraglottic laryngectomy does not clear the paraglottic space. This procedure may be indicated in T1, T2, or T3 supraglottic tumors with limited preepiglottic space involvement. Patients undergoing this procedure must have mobile vocal cords, no cartilage involvement, limited base of tongue extension, no pyriform sinus involvement, and good pulmonary reserve. All patients will have a temporary tracheotomy placed for pulmonary toilet. All patients aspirate after supraglottic laryngectomy, which is why the patients must have good cardiopulmonary reserve.

An apron incision is made separate from the tracheotomy incision, and the strap muscles are retracted laterally to expose the larynx. The perichondrium is elevated off of the larynx, and a transverse incision is made in the thyroid cartilage at the junction of the superior one-third and inferior two-thirds. The supraglottic larynx up to the hyoid is removed. The perichondrium is then sutured to the base of tongue. Contraindications include anterior commissure or thyroid cartilage invasion, vocal cord fixation, or involvement of the pyriform apex, postcricoid mucosa base of tongue, bilateral arytenoids, and posterior commissure. The expected functional outcome is for excellent voice results and safe swallowing utilizing a supraglottic swallow.

Chun et al. in 2010 analyzed 68 patients with Stage I–IV laryngeal cancer. Forty-eight patients were initially treated with supraglottic partial laryngectomy (SPL), and 20 patients were treated with radiation therapy. In the patients receiving SPL, if they had positive nodal disease, they received postoperative radiation. The 5-year disease-free survival for patients with Stage I or II disease was 89% for SPL and 100% for radiation. The overall 5-year survival was 87% and 80% for SPL and radiation therapy, respectively. In patients with Stage III or IV disease, the 5-year disease-free survival was 85% for patients receiving SPL and 52% for radiation therapy. The overall 5-year survival was 83% and 61% for SPL and radiation therapy, respectively (47).

Supracricoid Partial Laryngectomy

This technique adds to the previous supraglottic laryngectomy to remove the supraglottis plus the true vocal cords and thyroid cartilage. This procedure not only clears the preepiglottic space but can also clear the paraglottic space. Supracricoid laryngectomy was first described by Majer and Rieder in 1959, as an alternative to total laryngectomy (48), and popularized in the United States through the work of Laccourreye and Weinstein (49,50). One functional arytenoid must be preserved; therefore, careful patient selection is critical. Indications for this procedure include supraglottic cancer with glottic and anterior commissure involvement, ventricle invasion, thyroid cartilage invasion, true vocal cord immobility, paraglottic space invasion, moderate preepiglottic space involvement, and transglottic tumors. The cricoid cartilage, hyoid bone, and at least one arytenoid cartilage are spared. This procedure is indicated for T2, T3, and T4 cancers of the glottis and supraglottis. As with supraglottic laryngectomy, the patient must have good cardiopulmonary reserve. The type of supracricoid laryngectomy is named for its reconstruction. Reconstruction is by cricohyoidopexy or cricohyoidoepiglottopexy depending on the absence or presence of an epiglottic remnant. This also determines whether the tumor that is being treated is supraglottic (cricohyoidopexy) or glottic (cricohyoidoepiglottopexy). This reconstruction helps to restore a symmetric valve, which aids the patient in voicing as well as airway protection. The functional outcome for voice and swallow is good, but like most conservation procedures requires a dedicated period of rehabilitation.

In 1990, Laccourreye et al. examined 36 patients with SCCA of the glottis who underwent partial horizontal supracricoid laryngectomy with cricohyoidoepiglottopexy. All 36 recovered physiologic deglutition and phonation. None required tracheotomy. The 3-year survival rate was 86.5% with a recurrence rate of 5.5% (50). Also in 1990, Laccourreye et al. examined 68 patients with supraglottic carcinoma who underwent supracricoid laryngectomy with cricohyoidopexy. Supraglottic laryngectomy was contraindicated in all patients. 95.4% of the patients recovered physiologic deglutition. The 3-year survival was 71.4%, and no local recurrences were noted (49). This procedure has been found to be a useful alternative for the treatment of selected cases of laryngeal cancer (Fig. 124.9).

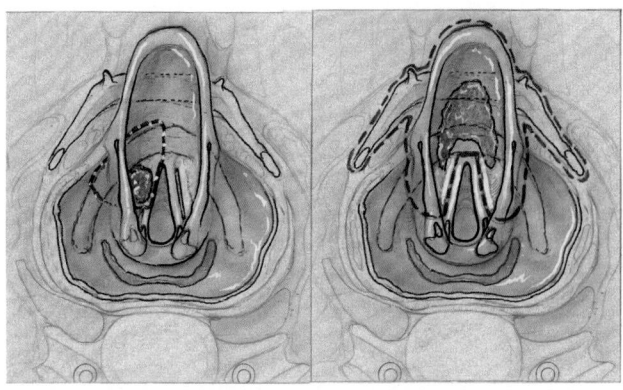

A. Vertical hemilaryngectomy   B. Supraglottic laryngectomy

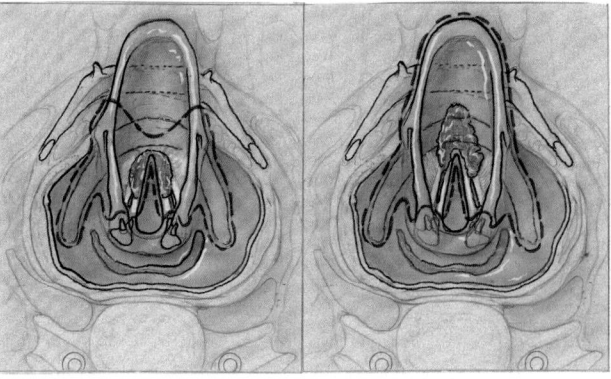

C. Supracricoid partial laryngectomy with CHEP   D. Supracricoid partial laryngectomy with CHP

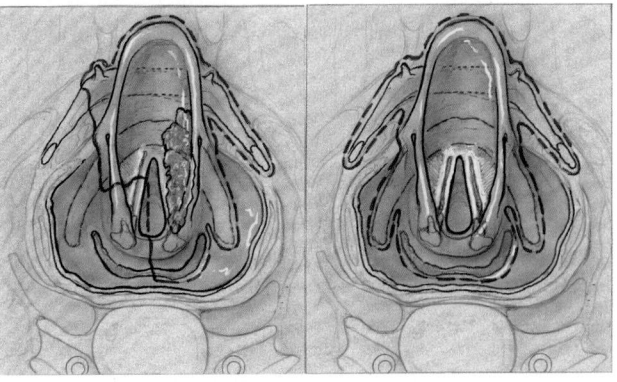

E. Near total laryngectomy   F. Total laryngectomy

Figure 124.9 A–F: Resection outline by conservation procedure.

Near-Total Laryngectomy

Near-total laryngectomy, or the Pearson procedure, is a voice preservation surgery used for large T3 and T4 lesions of the unilateral larynx not amenable to supraglottic or supracricoid laryngectomy. The procedure includes resection of one hemilarynx with the anterior portion of the contralateral cord. It also includes the ipsilateral cricoid and can include a portion of the proximal trachea. A permanent tracheostoma is created for respiration, and voice is produced through a dynamic tracheoesophageal conduit. Contraindications to this procedure include interarytenoid involvement, postcricoid involvement, and the inability to preserve two-thirds of the contralateral cord. Functional outcomes include a permanent tracheostoma, normal swallow, and a speech fistula. This technique is technically challenging.

In 1998, Pearson et al. studied 233 patients who underwent near-total laryngectomy for laryngeal or pharyngeal cancer. They found that the control rates were similar to that expected for total laryngectomy of total laryngopharyngectomy. Conversational voice was achieved in 85% of patients surviving greater than 1 year. There were eight local recurrences (7%). Five of the eight recurrences occurred in patients whose near-total laryngectomy was for surgical salvage or irradiation failure. They concluded that near-total laryngectomy was an alternative to total laryngectomy but that it should not be used for surgical salvage (51).

Total Laryngectomy

Total laryngectomy is the gold standard treatment for laryngeal cancer and has the best oncologic outcome for which all partial laryngectomies should strive to achieve. It was first successfully performed by Billroth in 1873 (5) but has been further refined by Gluck and Sorenson in 1894 (52). It is indicated for T3 and T4 advanced stage laryngeal cancers, chemotherapy and radiation failures, and conservation laryngeal surgery failures. Total laryngectomy provides excellent control rates but with the sacrifice of natural voice. The procedure includes an en bloc resection of the larynx, including the hyoid bone, thyroid cartilage, and cricoid cartilage to the proximal tracheal rings inferiorly. Combined with this procedure may be resection of the pharyngeal wall and base of tongue. The trachea is then sutured to the skin to form a tracheostoma. The pharyngeal wall is closed upon itself to form a digestive path separate from respiration.

The key to success in total laryngectomy is maximizing QOL by maximizing alaryngeal function. Carefully creating an accessible stoma by releasing the sternal heads of the sternocleidomastoid muscle and suspending the trachea to prevent traction that can lead to stomal stenosis are helpful in patients managing their stomas and easing voice restoration with tracheoesophageal speech. In order to improve deglutition and alaryngeal voicing, a complete cricopharyngeal myotomy or pharyngeal plexus neurectomy

should be performed. If not performed adequately, the patient may have difficulty swallowing and require esophageal dilatations or other measures to improve voice and swallowing. Voice restoration is obtained through tracheoesophageal speech, esophageal speech, or an artificial larynx.

Overall 5-year disease-free survival for T3 glottic tumors treated with total laryngectomy varies according to the study but ranges 49% to 80% (53–55). The 5-year overall survival is 54% (35). For T4 tumors of the glottis, the 5-year overall survival after total laryngectomy ranges from 32% to 63% (36,54,55). The overall recurrence rate for Stage III and IV glottic tumors was 37% with 19% recurring at the primary site and 17% recurring in the neck (36).

Advanced laryngeal tumors can involve structures outside of the larynx. Tumors can extend to directly involve the hypopharynx or oropharynx. Hypopharyngeal tumors with the piriform sinuses and postcricoid mucosa making up two of the hypopharyngeal sites are in direct contact with the larynx. Tumors that cross these boundaries frequently require extended surgical resections that can encompass the entire pharynx, namely, a laryngopharyngectomy. Similarly large tumors that involve the subglottis or the hypopharynx often involve the trachea and/or the esophagus necessitating extended excisions that may require an esophagectomy to ensure adequate margins.

Salvage Total Laryngectomy

Patients who fail organ preservation therapy with chemoradiation therapy for their advanced laryngeal cancer require surgical salvage. Once the patient has received chemoradiation therapy, only in highly selected cases are patients still candidates for conservation laryngeal surgery with most requiring salvage total laryngectomy. Many studies looking at overall survival in treatment with chemotherapy and radiation therapy include salvage laryngectomy in their outcome data. Patients requiring surgical salvage whether it is through conservation surgery or with total laryngectomy have a higher surgical complication rate. Salvage total laryngectomy is also frequently required if a patient fails conservation laryngeal surgery. In 2006, Fowler et al. examined the overall survival in patients undergoing salvage total laryngectomy. They found the 5-year and 10-year overall survival after salvage total laryngectomy to be 65.2% and 37.7%, respectively (56).

Postlaryngectomy Recurrence

Laryngeal cancer not only has a risk of regional and distant metastases; it can recur locally as well after total laryngectomy or salvage total laryngectomy. The most common location for the local recurrence is in the tracheal stoma. The incidence of stomal recurrence is 2% to 25% (57). The Sisson classification was developed to identify the location of the recurrence and the appropriate management and outcome (58). Type I is localized to the superior aspect of the stoma without esophageal involvement. Type II is localized to the superior aspect of the stoma with esophageal involvement. Type III originates in the inferior aspect of the stoma with involvement of the superior mediastinum. Type IV has extension laterally beneath the clavicle and into the superior mediastinum. Type I and II stomal recurrences are best treated with salvage therapy. However, Sisson type III and IV are generally considered unresectable, and nonoperative management involving chemoradiation or re-irradiation should be used (59,60).

Subglottic Carcinoma

Subglottic carcinoma usually presents with airway obstruction and hemoptysis. It is rare to find a primary subglottic carcinoma. Since there are so few, there are no studies examining treatment protocols and outcomes. Subglottic carcinomas have no barriers to the spread of disease and usually present with extensive cartilage invasion. The accepted treatment for subglottic carcinoma is total laryngectomy and tracheal resection below the level of the disease.

In 1998, Dahm et al. performed a retrospective review of 39 patients treated for primary subglottic cancer. 32.1% of the patients were diagnosed with advanced stage subglottic cancer. The 5-year overall survival and disease-free survival were 57.7% and 46.2%, respectively. Patients treated with radiotherapy alone, surgery alone, or both had disease-free 5-year survival of 22.2%, 41.7%, and 100%, respectively (9).

Surgery versus Chemoradiation

Over the last two decades, survival from laryngeal cancer has unfortunately decreased. There has been a great interest in determining the etiology associated with the decreased survival. In 2009, Gourin et al. performed a retrospective review of patients diagnosed with laryngeal cancer between 1985 and 2002. They found the 5-year survival rates were 85% for Stage I, 77% for Stage II, 51% for Stage III, and 35% for Stage IV disease. Survival for patients with Stage I–III disease was similar for patients treated operatively and nonoperatively. Patients with Stage III disease had a worse survival when treated with radiation alone as compared to chemoradiation. Patients with Stage IV disease had better survival after surgery (55%) as compared to chemoradiation (25%) or radiation alone (0%) (61).

In 2007, Chen et al. examined factors predictive of survival in advanced laryngeal cancer. During 1995 to 1998, 10,590 patients (7,019 patients included in the study) with Stage III or IV SCCA of the larynx were examined. These patients were treated with total laryngectomy, radiotherapy, or chemoradiation. They found that total laryngectomy, when compared with radiation therapy or chemoradiation, had increased survival. Death rates with radiotherapy alone and chemoradiation were 60% and 30% higher, respectively, than those following total laryngectomy. In Stage IV disease, the death rate was 43% higher with chemoradiation than with total laryngectomy.

In Stage III disease, there is no significant disadvantage for chemoradiation relative to total laryngectomy. However, radiation alone was associated with significantly higher death rates relative to total laryngectomy in stage III as well as stage IV patients. They found that overall survival was decreased in men, African American patients as compared to Caucasians and in patients with Medicare, Medicaid, or uninsured (62).

In 2010, Chen et al. identified 19,326 patients through the National Cancer Database who were diagnosed with advanced laryngeal cancer between 1996 and 2002 and were treated with chemoradiation therapy, total laryngectomy, or radiotherapy. The objective was to determine if patients treated at a high volume teaching facility had a better survival. They found that patients who received treatment at low volume facilities had a poorer survival when compared to those treated at higher volume facilities. It was also found that patients with advanced T4 disease who were treated with total laryngectomy had an increased survival when compared to chemoradiation therapy (63).

Treatment of the Neck

When deciding whether to treat the neck, the likelihood of regional spread into the cervical lymphatics must be taken into account. As previously stated, the supraglottic larynx has a rich lymphatic supply as compared to the glottis, and also tends to spread to bilateral cervical lymph nodes. As a result of the poor lymphatic supply to the glottis, there is unlikely to be cervical spread until the primary tumor is stage T3 or greater. The nodal basins that are of greatest risk are levels II–IV and the central compartment level VI. Generally accepted guidelines suggest that the neck should be treated if there is a 20% to 30% chance of regional metastasis. T3 glottic tumors have a 10% to 20% risk of regional spread, and T4 glottic tumors have a 25% to 40% risk of spread. Whereas T3 supraglottic tumors have a risk of 38% to 65%, T4 supraglottic tumors have a greater than 57% risk of lymphatic spread (64–69) (Table 124.3).

The N0 neck at risk for nodal metastasis and the N1 neck can be treated with radiation or surgery depending on the treatment of the primary tumor. If radiation is the treatment option, the field can be extended to include the nodal basins at risk. If surgery is the best treatment option, a selective neck dissection can be performed with limited morbidity. For N2 and N3 disease, the neck is best treated with multimodality therapy including surgery and radiation therapy. Occasionally, advanced neck disease will require a more extensive neck dissection including levels II–V as a modified radical or radical neck dissection depending on which structures are involved.

Surgical Complications

As with all head and neck surgery, complications arise including hematoma, infection, and skin flap necrosis.

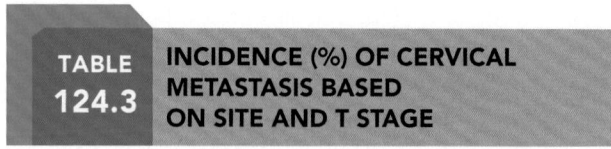

| TABLE 124.3 | INCIDENCE (%) OF CERVICAL METASTASIS BASED ON SITE AND T STAGE |

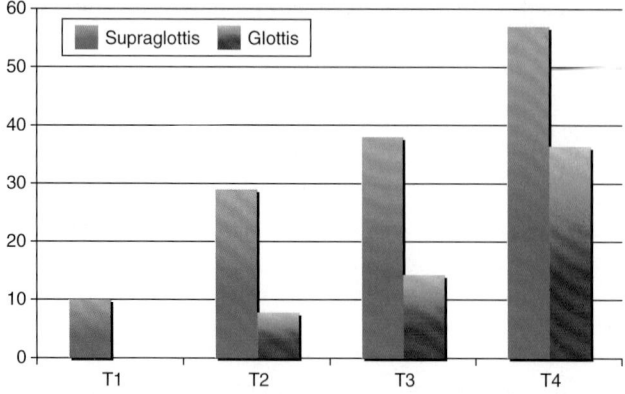

Redaelli de Zinis LO, et al. The distribution of lymph node metastases in supraglottic squamous cell carcinoma: therapeutic implications. *Head Neck* 2002;24(10):913–920; Zhang B, Xu ZG, Tang PZ. Elective lateral neck dissection for laryngeal cancer in the clinically negative neck. *J Surg Oncol* 2006;93(6):464–467.

Head and neck surgery is considered a clean-contaminated procedure, and the risk of postoperative infection is increased. Therefore, prophylactic, perioperative antibiotics are given. There are many other complications that occur specific to laryngeal surgery. One important early complication is pharyngocutaneous fistula. This occurs as a result from failed surgical closure of the pharynx or larynx allowing contents to travel from the pharynx/larynx through the neck to the skin. The risk of fistula formation increases with poor nutritional status, previous radiation therapy, and in patients who received preoperative chemotherapy and radiation therapy. Small fistulas can be treated conservatively with holding of oral feeds and local wound care. Larger fistulas may require additional surgical procedures including debridement, closure of the fistula, regional tissue transfer, or free tissue transfer. Recurrence or residual cancer should be suspected for fistulas that fail to respond to treatment or for late-occurring fistulas. Other early complications include aspiration pneumonia, wound dehiscence, hypocalcemia, and chyle leak/fistula. This can be avoided by meticulous dissection in Level IV to avoid injuring the thoracic duct.

Late complications include pharyngeal/esophageal stricture, which can lead to swallowing dysfunction and failure of esophageal and tracheoesophageal speech. This may require periodic esophageal dilation. Tracheal stoma stenosis is another late complication that can be prevented by avoiding excess tension on the stoma, by releasing the medial heads of the sternocleidomastoid muscle, by beveling the transected trachea when making the tumor cuts, and by "walking" the stoma out to the skin while sewing it during stomal construction. Hypothyroidism can also occur after surgery or radiation. Serial thyroid-stimulating hormone testing should be used to prevent the consequences of hypothyroidism (Fig. 124.10).

POSTTREATMENT QUALITY OF LIFE AND FUNCTIONAL OUTCOMES

The larynx's primary function is airway protection with its vital role in breathing and swallowing. It is equally essential in voice, and all three functions are at risk with laryngeal cancer and its treatment. Surgery, chemotherapy, radiotherapy, and combined modality treatments can have transient or permanent effects on voice, swallowing, and breathing. The resulting deficits have a direct impact on patient's QOL, and pretreatment perceptions of these risks frequently color a patient's choice of therapy. Patients with voice and swallowing difficulties may experience tremendous frustration that can lead to severe depression due to the loss of social, cultural, and personal satisfaction associated with talking, eating, and drinking. Loss of voice can also impact the patient's work and income. Different treatment modalities for advanced laryngeal cancers may offer similar survival but may differ in health-related quality of life (HRQOL). It is very important to consider the potential HRQOL changes and organ function as an outcome of these treatment modalities and a component in helping patients select the optimal treatment modality.

One of the first studies to assess QOL issues in patients with laryngeal cancer was the "Fireman study" by McNeil et al. in 1981. In this study, 37 healthy volunteers (12 firefighters and 25 executives) were asked to choose a treatment option based on perceived changes in QOL after total

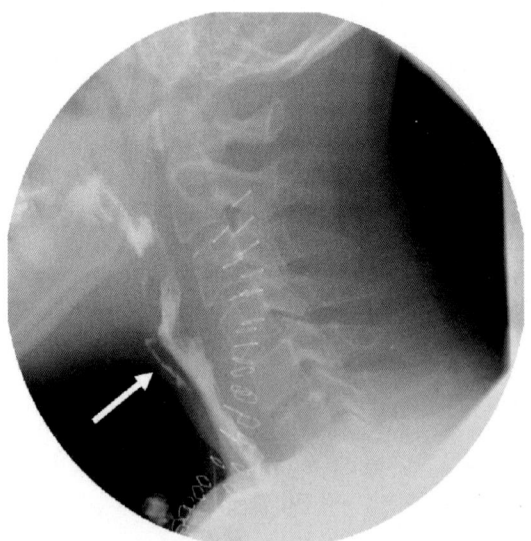

Figure 124.10 Post total laryngectomy pharyngocutaneous fistula on barium esophagram. Lateral cervical x-ray with *arrow* pointing to contrast leaking from pharyngeal closure, staple line visible.

laryngectomy. Patients were also given a questionnaire to determine what impact these changes would have on them. Based on the questionnaires, McNeil et al. found that 10 years of survival with normal speech was equivalent to 7 years survival with artificial speech. They also found that 20% of subjects would choose a treatment to preserve their larynx even if it meant a possible shorter survival, based on the perceived adverse effect to QOL after total laryngectomy (70).

Terrell et al. (71) investigated the long-term QOL in surviving patients with advanced laryngeal cancer that originally participated in the Veterans Affairs Laryngeal Cancer Study (40). They used the University of Michigan Head and Neck Quality of Life (HNQOL) instrument (72) and Medical Outcomes Studies Short Form-36 (SF-36) (73). They found that the chemoradiation group (CT + RT) had better QOL scores than the laryngectomy and radiation group (TL + RT) after 10 or more years following initial grouping. They concluded that this result appeared to be related to more freedom from pain, better emotional well-being, and lower levels of depression rather than preservation of speech function. The authors reported that there were no statistical differences between the two groups in speech and swallowing domains of the HNQOL in the study. The authors also noted that the detectable speech intelligibility scores differences at 24 months between CT + RT and TL + RT groups as initially reported by Hillman et al. study (74) disappeared in their 10-year follow-up study. Fung et al. (75) measured the vocal function using Voice-Related Quality of Life Measure and reported that the chemoradiation group had worse scores compare to normal subjects but better scores than the salvage laryngectomy group. With respect to swallowing function, they further reported that the chemoradiated patients did as well as the laryngectomies but had more dietary restrictions.

Different studies however support different conclusions on functional outcomes. Hanna et al. (76), in a retrospective study, reported treatment-related toxic effects in patients who received intensive CT + RT for their advanced cancer of head and neck. The authors reported dehydration, pneumonia, and malnutrition as some of the most frequent causes for the unscheduled hospitalizations of the subjects, which had significant effect on the overall cost of treatment. In addition, 93% of their subjects required G-tube placement to offset weight loss, poor oral intake, dehydration, and malnutrition and electrolyte imbalance. Weight loss was a considerable problem among their patients despite the PEG-tube placement not only during treatment but even 1 year after treatment. In addition, PEG-tube placement did not substantially reduce the unscheduled hospitalizations in their study. The study also found that 40% of the subjects changed their diet posttreatment due to dysphagia. Other studies, however, (77,78) have reported similar overall QOL scores for patients undergoing total laryngectomy with those that receive chemotherapy and radiation therapy.

Conservation laryngeal surgery techniques such as supraglottic and supracricoid partial laryngectomy can be performed for advanced laryngeal cancers as a first-line organ-sparing procedure or as salvage following radiation failure. The success of these procedures depends not only on tumor characteristics but also on appropriate patient selection. Adequate pulmonary function and commitment to rehabilitation are as important as the remaining larynx being functional enough to ensure prevention of aspiration, while maintaining voice and airway. Almost all patients initially aspirate, and postoperative rehabilitation for voice and swallowing function begins as early as possible to restore swallowing function. The successful rehabilitation of voice and swallowing following conservation laryngeal surgery depends on comprehensive evaluation and teamwork between the surgeon, patient and family, and the rehabilitation team. An optimal protocol should begin with preoperative counseling and functional assessment as well as posttreatment evaluation and rehabilitation of voice and swallowing function.

EMERGENCIES

As with all emergencies, the airway must be established first, and patients with advanced laryngeal cancer can initially present with symptoms of airway distress and impending airway obstruction. Similarly, patients who receive radiation therapy can develop airway edema and airway obstruction. Managing airway distress without a tracheotomy when safe is preferable in untreated laryngeal cancer patients. If possible, the patient should undergo fiberoptic nasotracheal intubation followed by debulking of the tumor. If the patient must undergo tracheotomy, the tracheotomy should be performed high so that the tracheostomy may be removed with the resection. Other emergencies in advanced laryngeal cancer include complications of chondroradionecrosis or pharyngocutaneous fistula putting the great vessels of the neck at risk. It is important to have an awareness of these complications and provide appropriate management to avoid these emergencies.

HIGHLIGHTS

- The larynx produces one of the most complex motor functions in the body. It provides an airway for respiration, deglutition, and phonation. Laryngeal cancer can alter one or more of these functions.
- Five-year overall survival has worsened over the past 30 years (67% to 63%) despite efforts to improve treatment.
- The larynx contains several fibroelastic membranes, ligaments, and spaces that divide the larynx into compartments, limit the spread of early cancers, and allow for partial resections with adequate margins.

- Careful preoperative evaluation includes history and physical, flexible endoscopy, imaging through CT (to assess extent of invasion), and PET (to assess regional and distant metastasis).
- Surgical endoscopy is critical to map out the boundaries of the tumor, to determine cricoarytenoid joint mobility, and to differentiate vocal cord immobility from vocal cord fixation in order to accurately stage the tumor and develop the best treatment plan.
- Ninety-five to ninety-nine percent of laryngeal malignancies are SCCA.
- Treatment for advanced laryngeal cancer is multimodality therapy with surgery followed by radiation or radiation and chemotherapy.
- Endoscopic laser resection is used mainly for early laryngeal cancers, but its use on certain T3 and T4 tumors is becoming more accepted.
- Conservation laryngeal surgery is an option for advanced laryngeal cancer, but the tumor must be accurately staged and boundaries identified in order for these procedures to be performed.
- Total laryngectomy remains the gold standard surgical procedure for advanced laryngeal cancer from which all other surgeries are derived.
- Postoperative radiation improves locoregional control and survival.
- Chemotherapy (induction or concurrent) decreases the risk of distant metastasis.
- Treatment of the neck for nodal metastasis must be considered if the nodal metastases risk is greater than 20% to 30% or if there is palpable nodal disease.
- Postoperative complications increase after prior radiation therapy.

REFERENCES

1. Jemal A, et al. Cancer statistics, 2010. *CA Cancer J Clin* 2010; 60(5):277–300.
2. Jemal A, et al. Global cancer statistics. *CA Cancer J Clin* 2011; 61(2):69–90.
3. Shah JP, et al. Patterns of care for cancer of the larynx in the United States. *Arch Otolaryngol Head Neck Surg* 1997;123(5): 475–483.
4. AJCC. Larynx. In: Edge SB, Byrd DR, Compton CC, et al., eds. *AJCC Cancer Staging Manual*, 7th ed. New York: Springer, 2010: 57–62.
5. Alberti, PW. Panel discussion: the historical development of laryngectomy. II. The evolution of laryngology and laryngectomy in the mid-19th century. *Laryngoscope* 1975;85(2):288–298.
6. Worden FP, et al. Chemoselection as a strategy for organ preservation in patients with T4 laryngeal squamous cell carcinoma with cartilage invasion. *Laryngoscope* 2009;119(8):1510–1517.
7. National cancer Institute. U.N.I.o. Health, Editor. *Surveillance epidemiology and end result—Cancer statistics review laryngeal cancer 1975-2007*.
8. Hoffman HT, et al. Laryngeal cancer in the United States: changes in demographics, patterns of care, and survival. *Laryngoscope* 2006; 116(9 Pt 2 Suppl 111):1–13.
9. Dahm JD, et al. Primary subglottic cancer. *Laryngoscope* 1998; 108(5):741–746.
10. Hunt JP, McWhorter AJ. Malignant neoplasms of the larynx. In: Merati AL, Bielamowicz SA, eds. *Textbook of laryngology*. San Diego, CA: Plural Publishing, 2006.
11. Lindberg R. Distribution of cervical lymph node metastases from squamous cell carcinoma of the upper respiratory and digestive tracts. *Cancer* 1972;29(6):1446–1449.
12. Bradford CR, et al. p53 mutation as a prognostic marker in advanced laryngeal carcinoma. Department of Veterans Affairs Laryngeal Cancer Cooperative Study Group. *Arch Otolaryngol Head Neck Surg* 1997;123(6):605–609.
13. Welkoborsky HJ, et al. Predicting recurrence and survival in patients with laryngeal cancer by means of DNA cytometry, tumor front grading, and proliferation markers. *Ann Otol Rhinol Laryngol* 1995;104(7):503–510.
14. Truelson JM, et al. DNA content and histologic growth pattern correlate with prognosis in patients with advanced squamous cell carcinoma of the larynx. The Department of Veterans Affairs Cooperative Laryngeal Cancer Study Group. *Cancer* 1992;70(1):56–62.
15. Piccirillo JF, et al. New clinical severity staging system for cancer of the larynx. Five-year survival rates. *Ann Otol Rhinol Laryngol* 1994;103(2):83–92.
16. Falk RT, et al. Effect of smoking and alcohol consumption on laryngeal cancer risk in coastal Texas. *Cancer Res* 1989; 49(14):4024–4029.
17. Kiyabu MT, et al. Detection of human papillomavirus in formalin-fixed, invasive squamous carcinomas using the polymerase chain reaction. *Am J Surg Pathol* 1989;13(3):221–224.
18. Practice Guidelines Committee. *American Head and Neck Society Clinical Practice Guidelines. Larynx, Supraglottis.* 1995.
19. Practice Guidelines Committee. *American Head and Neck Society Clinical Practice Guidelines. Larynx, Glottis.* 1995.
20. Zbaren P, Becker M, Lang H. Staging of laryngeal cancer: endoscopy, computed tomography and magnetic resonance versus histopathology. *Eur Arch Otorhinolaryngol* 1997;254(Suppl 1):S117–S122.
21. Chu MM, et al. FDG PET with contrast-enhanced CT: a critical imaging tool for laryngeal carcinoma. *Radiographics* 2010;30(5):1353–1372.
22. Hannah A, et al. Evaluation of 18 F-fluorodeoxyglucose positron emission tomography and computed tomography with histopathologic correlation in the initial staging of head and neck cancer. *Ann Surg* 2002;236(2):208–217.
23. Braams JW, et al. Detection of lymph node metastases of squamous-cell cancer of the head and neck with FDG-PET and MRI. *J Nucl Med* 1995;36(2):211–216.
24. Laubenbacher C, et al. Comparison of fluorine-18-fluorodeoxyglucose PET, MRI and endoscopy for staging head and neck squamous-cell carcinomas. *J Nucl Med* 1995;36(10):1747–1757.
25. McGuirt WF, et al. A comparative diagnostic study of head and neck nodal metastases using positron emission tomography. *Laryngoscope* 1995;105(4 Pt 1):373–375.
26. Kau RJ, et al. Lymph node detection of head and neck squamous cell carcinomas by positron emission tomography with fluorodeoxyglucose F 18 in a routine clinical setting. *Arch Otolaryngol Head Neck Surg* 1999;125(12):1322–1328.
27. Yamazaki Y, et al. Assessment of cervical lymph node metastases using FDG-PET in patients with head and neck cancer. *Ann Nucl Med* 2008;22(3):177–184.
28. Kyzas PA, et al. 18F-fluorodeoxyglucose positron emission tomography to evaluate cervical node metastases in patients with head and neck squamous cell carcinoma: a meta-analysis. *J Natl Cancer Inst* 2008;100(10):712–720.
29. Gourin CG, et al. Identification of distant metastases with PET-CT in patients with suspected recurrent head and neck cancer. *Laryngoscope* 2009;119(4):703–706.
30. Andrus JG, Dolan RW, Anderson TD. Transnasal esophagoscopy: a high-yield diagnostic tool. *Laryngoscope* 2005;115(6):993–996.
31. Spector JG, et al. Delayed regional metastases, distant metastases, and second primary malignancies in squamous cell carcinomas of the larynx and hypopharynx. *Laryngoscope* 2001;111(6): 1079–1087.
32. McCaffrey TV, Witte M, Ferguson MT. Verrucous carcinoma of the larynx. *Ann Otol Rhinol Laryngol* 1998;107(5 Pt 1):391–395.

33. Maurizi M, et al. Verrucous squamous cell carcinoma of the larynx: diagnostic and therapeutic considerations. *Eur Arch Otorhinolaryngol* 1996;253(3):130–135.
34. Batsakis JG, Luna, MA, Byers RM. Metastases to the larynx. *Head Neck* 1985;7(6):458–460.
35. Sessions DG, et al. Management of T3N0M0 glottic carcinoma: therapeutic outcomes. *Laryngoscope* 2002;112(7 Pt 1):1281–1288.
36. Spector GJ, et al. Management of stage IV glottic carcinoma: therapeutic outcomes. *Laryngoscope* 2004;114(8):1438–1446.
37. Zbaren P, et al. Radionecrosis or tumor recurrence after radiation of laryngeal and hypopharyngeal carcinomas. *Otolaryngol Head Neck Surg* 2006;135(6):838–843.
38. Forastiere, AA, et al. Concurrent chemotherapy and radiotherapy for organ preservation in advanced laryngeal cancer. *N Engl J Med* 2003;349(22):2091–2098.
39. Forastiere AA, Maor M, Weber RS, et al. Long-term results of Intergroup RTOG 91–11: a phase III trial to preserve the larynx—induction cisplatin/5-FU and radiation therapy versus concurrent cisplatin and radiation therapy versus radiation therapy, in 2006 ASCO Annual Meeting Proceedings. Part I. *J Clin Oncol* 2006;24(18 Suppl):5517.
40. Induction chemotherapy plus radiation compared with surgery plus radiation in patients with advanced laryngeal cancer. The Department of Veterans Affairs Laryngeal Cancer Study Group. *N Engl J Med* 1991;324(24):1685–1690.
41. Lefebvre JL, et al. Larynx preservation in pyriform sinus cancer: preliminary results of a European Organization for Research and Treatment of Cancer phase III trial. EORTC Head and Neck Cancer Cooperative Group. *J Natl Cancer Inst* 1996;88(13):890–899.
42. Budach V. TPF sequential therapy: when and for whom? *Oncologist* 2010;15(Suppl 3):13–18.
43. Posner MR, et al. Cisplatin and fluorouracil alone or with docetaxel in head and neck cancer. *N Engl J Med* 2007;357(17):1705–1715.
44. Hinni ML, et al. Transoral laser microsurgery for advanced laryngeal cancer. *Arch Otolaryngol Head Neck Surg* 2007;133(12):1198–1204.
45. Vilaseca I, Bernal-Sprekelsen M, Luis Blanch, J. Transoral laser microsurgery for T3 laryngeal tumors: prognostic factors. *Head Neck* 2010;32(7):929–938.
46. Brumund KT, et al. Frontolateral vertical partial laryngectomy without tracheotomy for invasive squamous cell carcinoma of the true vocal cord: a 25-year experience. *Ann Otol Rhinol Laryngol* 2005;114(4):314–322.
47. Chun JY, et al. The oncologic safety and functional preservation of supraglottic partial laryngectomy. *Am J Otolaryngol* 2010; 31(4):246–251.
48. Majer EH, Rieder, W. Technic of laryngectomy permitting the conservation of respiratory permeability (cricohyoidopexy). Annales d'oto-laryngologie et de chirurgie cervico faciale: bulletin de la Societe d'oto-laryngologie des hopitaux de Paris. *Ann Otolaryngol* 1959;76:677–681.
49. Laccourreye H, et al. Supracricoid laryngectomy with cricohyoidopexy: a partial laryngeal procedure for selected supraglottic and transglottic carcinomas. *Laryngoscope* 1990;100(7):735–741.
50. Laccourreye H, et al. Supracricoid laryngectomy with cricohyoidoepiglottopexy: a partial laryngeal procedure for glottic carcinoma. *Ann Otol Rhinol Laryngol* 1990;99(6 Pt 1):421–426.
51. Pearson BW, et al. Results of near-total laryngectomy. *Ann Otol Rhinol Laryngol* 1998;107(10 Pt 1):820–825.
52. Henley J, Souliere C Jr. Tracheoesophageal speech failure in the laryngectomee: the role of constrictor myotomy. *Laryngoscope* 1986;96(9 Pt 1):1016–1020.
53. Skolnik EM, et al. Carcinoma of the laryngeal glottis therapy and end results. *Laryngoscope* 1975;85(9):1453–1466.
54. Vermund H. Role of radiotherapy in cancer of the larynx as related to the TNM system of staging. A review. *Cancer* 1970;25(3):485–504.
55. Yuen A, et al. Management of stage T3 and T4 glottic carcinomas. *Am J Surg* 1984;148(4):467–472.
56. Fowler BZ, et al. Factors influencing long-term survival following salvage total laryngectomy after initial radiotherapy or conservative surgery. *Head Neck* 2006;28(2):99–106.
57. Kowalski LP, et al. Stomal recurrence: pathophysiology, treatment and prevention. *Acta Otolaryngol* 2003;123(3):421–432.
58. Sisson GA, Bytell DE, Becker SP. Mediastinal dissection—1976: indications and newer techniques. *Laryngoscope* 1977;87(5 Pt 1):751–759.
59. Gluckman JL, et al. Surgical salvage for stomal recurrence: a multi-institutional experience. *Laryngoscope* 1987;97(9):1025–1029.
60. Ampil F, et al. Post-laryngectomy stomal cancer recurrences, retreatment decisions and outcomes: case series. *J Craniomaxillofac Surg* 2009;37(6):349–351.
61. Gourin CG, et al. The effect of treatment on survival in patients with advanced laryngeal carcinoma. *Laryngoscope* 2009;119(7):1312–1317.
62. Chen AY, Halpern M. Factors predictive of survival in advanced laryngeal cancer. *Arch Otolaryngol Head Neck Surg* 2007;133(12):1270–1276.
63. Chen AY, et al. Improved survival is associated with treatment at high-volume teaching facilities for patients with advanced stage laryngeal cancer. *Cancer* 2010;116(20):4744–4752.
64. Redaelli de Zinis LO, et al. Incidence and distribution of lymph node metastases in supraglottic squamous cell carcinoma: therapeutic implications. *Acta Otorhinolaryngol Ital* 1994;14(1):19–27.
65. Johnson JT, Myers EN. Cervical lymph node disease in laryngeal cancer. In: Silver CE, ed. *Laryngeal Cancer*. New York: Thieme, 1991.
66. Daly CJ, Strong EW. Carcinoma of the glottic larynx. *Am J Surg* 1975;130(4):489–492.
67. Jesse RH. The evaluation of treatment of patients with extensive squamous cancer of the vocal cords. *Laryngoscope* 1975;85(9):1424–1429.
68. Redaelli de Zinis LO, et al. The distribution of lymph node metastases in supraglottic squamous cell carcinoma: therapeutic implications. *Head Neck* 2002;24(10):913–920.
69. Zhang B, Xu ZG, Tang PZ. Elective lateral neck dissection for laryngeal cancer in the clinically negative neck. *J Surg Oncol* 2006;93(6):464–467.
70. McNeil BJ, Weichselbaum R, Pauker SG. Speech and survival: tradeoffs between quality and quantity of life in laryngeal cancer. *N Engl J Med* 1981;305(17):982–987.
71. Terrell JE, Fisher SG, Wolf GT. Long-term quality of life after treatment of laryngeal cancer. The Veterans Affairs Laryngeal Cancer Study Group. *Arch Otolaryngol Head Neck Surg* 1998;124(9):964–971.
72. Terrell JE, et al. Head and neck cancer-specific quality of life: instrument validation. *Arch Otolaryngol Head Neck Surg* 1997;123(10):1125–1132.
73. Ware JE. *SF 36 Health survey: Manuel and Interpretation Guide*, Boston, MA: T.H. Institute, 1993.
74. Hillman RE, et al. Functional outcomes following treatment for advanced laryngeal cancer. Part I—Voice preservation in advanced laryngeal cancer. Part II—Laryngectomy rehabilitation: the state of the art in the VA System. Research Speech-Language Pathologists. Department of Veterans Affairs Laryngeal Cancer Study Group. *Ann Otol Rhinol Laryngol Suppl* 1998;172:1–27.
75. Fung K, et al. Voice and swallowing outcomes of an organ-preservation trial for advanced laryngeal cancer. *Int J Radiat Oncol Biol Phys* 2005;63(5):1395–1399.
76. Hanna E, et al. Intensive chemoradiotherapy as a primary treatment for organ preservation in patients with advanced cancer of the head and neck: efficacy, toxic effects, and limitations. *Arch Otolaryngol Head Neck Surg* 2004;130(7):861–867.
77. Hanna E, et al. Quality of life for patients following total laryngectomy vs chemoradiation for laryngeal preservation. *Arch Otolaryngol Head Neck Surg* 2004;130(7):875–879.
78. Maclean J, Cotton S, Perry A. Dysphagia following a total laryngectomy: the effect on quality of life, functioning, and psychological well-being. *Dysphagia* 2009;24(3):314–321.

125 Voice Rehabilitation Following Laryngectomy

Anna M. Pou

The larynx is the second most common site for cancer in the upper aerodigestive tract, of which squamous cell carcinoma (SCCA) is the predominant type (95%) (see Chapters 123 and 124). Although organ preservation protocols and conservation laryngeal surgeries are in use today, patients with advanced or recurrent SCCA of the larynx continue to undergo total laryngectomy in the course of their treatment.

The operative procedure of total laryngectomy results in separation of the aerodigestive tract, establishing a permanent tracheostoma at the base of the neck. The pharynx is closed by simply closing the mucosa or, in more complex cases, by placing a flap to preserve an adequate lumen for swallowing. Total laryngectomy profoundly alters speech, lung function, respiration, and sense of smell and taste. It is the loss of voice that is most responsible for the psychosocial and economic consequences following laryngectomy. Effective voice restoration is essential for the rehabilitation of these patients.

Total laryngectomy includes removal of the entire larynx, hyoid bone, portions of the pharynx, the strap muscles, one or more rings of the trachea, and part or all of the thyroid gland. The resection may include neck dissection, upper mediastinal lymph node dissection, and dissection of portions of the tongue base. In order to resect the larynx, entrance into the pharynx away from the epicenter of the tumor is required. The resulting defect, a pharyngotomy, consists of varying amounts of pharyngeal and esophageal mucosa, constrictor muscle remnants, and tongue base. The closure of this defect depends upon the amount of remaining mucosa; it is closed using continuous or interrupted Connell sutures in a vertical or "T" fashion. Flap reconstruction (free fasciocutaneous flap; pectoral major flap) is used when there is insufficient mucosa to close the pharynx.

The usual approach to laryngectomy separates the pharyngeal constrictor muscles at the oblique line of the thyroid cartilage (Fig. 125.1). Specifically this includes the inferior pharyngeal constrictor and cricopharyngeus muscles. The junction of the pharynx and esophagus has been studied by speech pathologists as the sound source for alaryngeal speech and is called the "PE" segment. It is difficult to predict resultant voice or quality because of variations in anatomy, tumor extent, muscle bulk, and operative technique. Pharyngeal closure after laryngectomy is generally concerned with controlling secretions, swallowing, and prevention of fistula formation. In addition, attention has been directed to alaryngeal voice acquisition and the possibilities for maximizing voice results.

There are three methods of alaryngeal speech: electrolarynx speech, esophageal speech, and tracheoesophageal (TE) speech. Historically speaking, esophageal speech was the method of choice by which all others were compared. In this method, air is injected into the cervical esophagus and immediately expelled causing the vibration of the opposing mucosal surfaces of the pharyngoesophagus, which is then articulated into speech by structures of the oral cavity. This method is very difficult to learn, and only about 26% of patients are able to use this method in daily communications (1). Consequently, tracheoesophageal puncture (TEP) has replaced esophageal speech as the gold standard. All methods of alaryngeal speech are taught by a speech pathologist.

The characteristic esophageal voice is low in fundamental frequency (~65 Hz), is of short duration, and requires some effort to produce. The most common method involves trapping air in the mouth or pharynx and then injecting it into the esophagus by the propulsive action of the tongue. With diaphragmatic effort, the air refluxes through the esophagus and crosses the upper esophageal sphincter. The mucosa of this region is vibrated by the released air and produces a characteristic belch-like

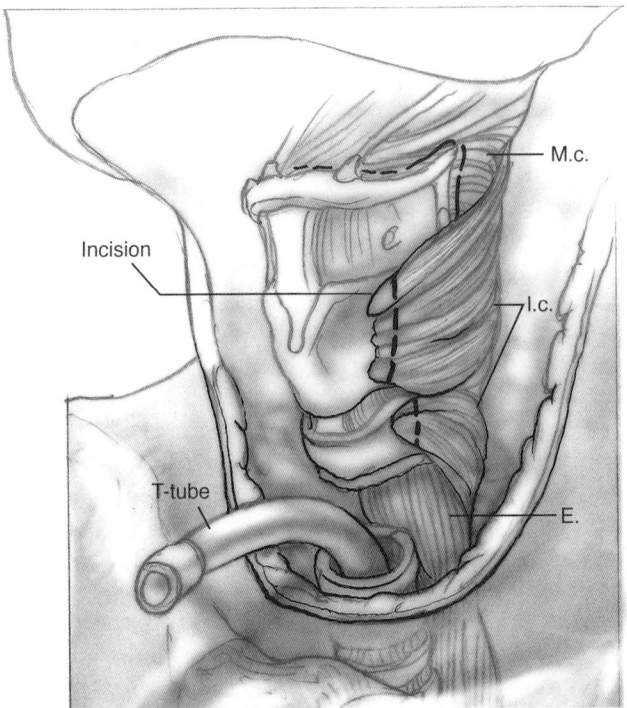

Figure 125.1 Separation of the pharyngeal constrictors from the larynx. E, esophagus; Ic, inferior constrictor; Mc, middle pharyngeal constrictor.

sound. This sound is then articulated into speech using the tongue, lips, and teeth. Rapid repetitive movements of injection and release produce fluent and understandable speech.

The artificial larynx is an instrument that serves as a voicing source. It introduces a mechanical sound into the tissues and air spaces of the vocal tract. This sound, emanating from the mouth, is again articulated into speech by structures in the oral cavity. The most common types of electrolarynx include one that is placed against a supple point on the neck or one that uses a tube adapter to direct the sound to the oral cavity, where it can be articulated with some reduction in intelligibility. The oral adapter is useful for patients whose necks do not transmit the electrical sound or in the immediate postoperative period when the neck is healing. A newer device consists of an electric sound source that is housed in a denture and is activated by a hand control or by the tongue (2).

The artificial larynx is rapidly learned and does not delay or interfere with the acquisition of other forms of alaryngeal speech. It has the advantages of low cost, availability, short learning time, and loudness. Its disadvantages are dependence on batteries (cost often not covered by insurance), mechanical sound, conspicuous appearance, loss of hands-free speech, and hygiene of the intraoral tubes or dental appliance. It also relies on the use of batteries and is often not covered by insurance policies. Nevertheless, many laryngectomized patients use the artificial devices as the primary method for speech communication.

SHUNTS AND VALVES

From the time of the first laryngectomies, it was known that tracheal air during exhalation can be shunted to the pharynx or esophagus through a planned fistula or tract, and this pulmonary-driven insufflation can produce effective speech. The same principles of speech production apply with articulation at the oral cavity and sound produced in the upper esophageal sphincter. The shunts, however, persisted with problems: shunt closure due to stenosis at the level of the trachea or pharynx and leakage of esophageal contents into the trachea through the patent shunt with resultant aspiration. For these reasons, some investigators developed mechanical valves to divert the secretions from the trachea or attempted to devise biologic valves (sphincters) for airway protection, but most of them failed.

The creation of a successful, surgical voice restoration technique did not occur until the introduction of the TEP by Singer and Blom in 1979. It was proposed as a secondary salvage technique for those who failed esophageal speech or those who were displeased with the electrolarynx voice (3). The guidelines used to create this revolutionary method for voice restoration were no oncologic compromise; applicability in an irradiated field; normal swallowing without aspiration; reliable voice; surgical simplicity; rapid recovery; reliability and reproducibility; inclusion of an uncomplicated, cost-effective prosthetic valve to prevent stenosis and aspiration; and limited cost (4). TE voice restoration has gained worldwide acceptance over the past 32 years and is the preferred method of postlaryngectomy speech. TEP is safe, reliable, and reproducible and should be considered in all patients undergoing total laryngectomy and in those who have failed to master other methods of alaryngeal speech.

The TEP pioneered by Singer and Blom (3) is not very different from the self-inflicted TEP made by a laryngectomy patient using an ice pick in 1931. An endoscopic puncture is made through the party wall through which a one-way silicone valve is placed. This tubular prosthesis (silicone) maintains the puncture site, protects the airway from aspiration of saliva and foods, and allows pulmonary air to be directed across the pharyngoesophageal mucosa for voice production. Airflow is only limited by the vital capacity of the lungs. The prosthesis is biologically compatible, removable, and inexpensive. Various modifications and improvements have been made on the prosthesis since 1978 (3). Other prostheses have also been introduced (Provox, Groningen).

SECONDARY TRACHEOESOPHAGEAL PUNCTURE

Patient Selection and Timing

There are a few factors that guide patient selection and they are similar to those listed for primary TEP. The timing of secondary puncture depends upon the extent of resection, the complexity of reconstruction, and the need for postoperative radiation therapy. Secondary voice restoration should be delayed at least 8 weeks following postoperative radiation therapy or until the peristomal skin has recovered from radiation toxicity and at least 6 weeks following recovery from reconstruction of a total laryngopharyngoesophagectomy defect in order to allow healing of the flap to the posterior tracheal wall. Patients undergoing flap reconstruction for pharyngeal defects should also undergo barium swallow to evaluate the reconstructive changes and for the presence of a stricture. The stoma is outlined with a radiopaque marker, and the site for the proposed puncture is determined in relationship to the pharyngoesophageal segment. Pharyngoesophageal dilatation is performed if necessary (5).

Stoma size is critical to successful use of the voice prosthesis. Stoma size under 2 cm is suboptimal; this small size makes it difficult to place the prosthesis and may compromise the airway due to the prosthesis size. If microstomia is present, the stoma can be serially dilated using silicone laryngectomy tubes, or a stomaplasty can be performed at the time of puncture. Patients who have undergone radiation therapy whose tissues appear to be at risk are better managed by the former method. If a laryngectomy tube is used, it can be fenestrated posteriorly and simultaneously worn with the prosthesis in place. When necessary, the stomaplasty is performed prior to the puncture leaving the posterior wall intact. The stoma is enlarged using a Z-plasty technique on each side (5).

In order for fluent TE speech to occur, there must be sufficient relaxation of the pharynx. There was a subset of patients (20% to 40%) identified early on who presented with hypertonic or spastic speech. It was determined that failure to maintain fluent speech was due to spasm of the cricopharyngeus and inferior and middle constrictor muscles when speech was attempted (6,7). A hypopharyngeal bar corresponding to these muscles can be seen using barium swallow. A column of air distends the esophagus proximal to the bar when phonation is attempted. The status of the pharynx can be evaluated prior to puncture using the transnasal esophageal insufflation test (5).

The transnasal esophageal insufflation test is a subjective test that is used to assess the pharyngeal constrictor muscle response to esophageal distention in the laryngectomy patient (8). The test is performed using a disposable kit consisting of a 50-cm-long catheter and tracheostoma tape housing with a removable adaptor. The catheter is placed through the nostril until the 25-cm mark is reached. This should place the catheter in the cervical esophagus adjacent to the proposed TEP. The catheter and the adaptor are taped into place. The patient is then asked to count from 1 to 15 and to sustain an "ah" for at least 8 seconds without interruption. Multiple trials are performed to allow the patient to produce a reliable sample.

One of four responses is obtained following the insufflation test: fluent, sustained voice production with minimal effort indicating relaxed pharyngoesophageal muscles; a breathy, hypotonic voice indicating the absence of pharyngeal constrictor muscle tone; hypertonic voice characterized by intermittent production of effortful speech with gastric distension and posttrial burping; and spasm, which is characterized by no production of voice even with substantial pulmonary airflow. Insufflation testing is also done after flap reconstruction or gastric pull-up to determine the quality of voice (5). The voice quality is usually "wet" following jejunal reconstruction and hollow or breathy following gastric pull-up. Compression of the neck with an elastic band can enhance voice quality in the latter situation.

Examiner error can obscure the results of the test. Common errors include improper placement of the catheter (not inserted 25 cm into the cervical esophagus), too much digital pressure exerted by the patient or examiner on the tracheostoma, and attempting to swallow saliva or inject air from the mouth into the esophagus while simultaneously insufflating the esophagus. The patient errors can be prevented by having the patient self-monitor using a mirror (5).

Surgical Procedure

This procedure was first described by Singer and Blom in 1979 (3) and has been modified over the years. The following procedure is performed in the operating room under general anesthesia. The Blom-Singer tracheostoma puncture kit (InHealth Technologies, Carpinteria, CA) allows the surgeon to perform the secondary puncture in less than 30 minutes. Following esophagoscopy, the esophagoscope (surgeon's choice) is withdrawn to the level of the stoma with the bevel positioned against the posterior wall of the trachea so that the light can be seen and the bevel palpated. The position of the esophagoscope also protects the posterior esophageal wall from penetration. A number 14 sheathed catheter is introduced into the bevel of the esophagoscope about 5 mm below the mucocutaneous junction. The needle is withdrawn leaving the sheath in place (Fig. 125.2). A wire on a tapered catheter is threaded through the sheath and pulled out of the mouth of the esophagoscope. The wire is cut from the end of the catheter, which is then directed down the scope into the esophagus. The catheter is secured into place at the stoma (5). This kit can be replaced by using a curved 18-gauge needle, a 24-gauge wire, red rubber catheter, number 15 scalpel blade, and hemostat. The prosthesis can be placed immediately, but most clinicians wait 48 hours.

This technique has been modified by many clinicians over the years to include the use of local anesthesia, transnasal esophagoscopy (TNE), and the use of the KTP laser, among other methods (9–12). In patients who present with a stricture, fibrosis of the neck tissues following radiation therapy, or cervical spine deformity, it is often impossible to perform a secondary TEP using a rigid esophagoscope.

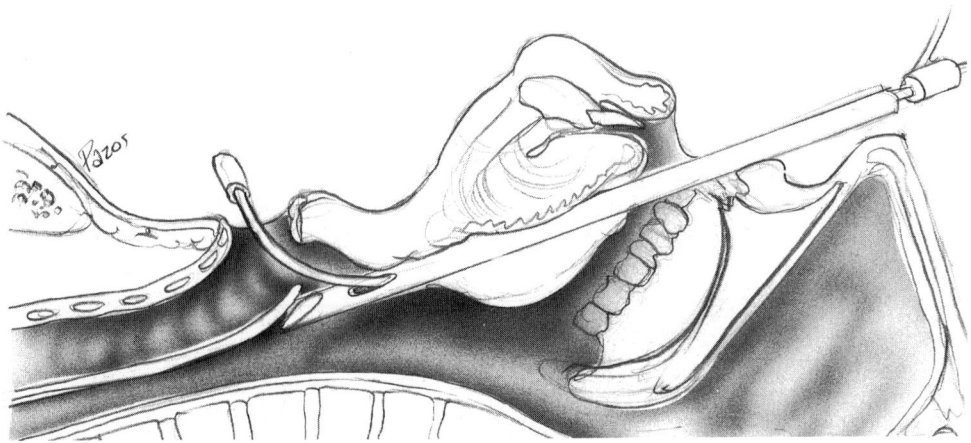

Figure 125.2 Endoscopic voice restoration (TEP).

Many surgeons have developed their own techniques for dealing with this problem, but the most common way to deal with this now is using flexible esophagoscopy in the office under local anesthesia (11,12). In a study performed by LeBert et al. (11), the overall success rate of TNE-assisted TEP was 97%. Only 1/39 patient attempts was unsuccessful. Regarding previous radiation therapy, myotomy, and type of reconstruction, there was no statistically significant difference among patients regarding difficulty with placement of prosthesis, development of complications, use of TEP prosthesis, or speech intelligibility.

The method of TNE-assisted TEP is described below. Pontocaine and Neo-Synephrine are sprayed into the more patent nare. Up to 1.0 mL of 1% lidocaine with 1:100,000 epinephrine is injected into the posterior tracheal wall at the intended TEP site. Pledgets soaked with 4% lidocaine or 2% lidocaine jelly are placed in the nasal cavity. The TNE scope is also coated with 2% lidocaine jelly. The TNE scope is advanced through the nasopharynx and oropharynx into the hypopharynx to reach the upper esophageal inlet. The anatomic subsites are evaluated for abnormal function and masses. The patient is then asked to swallow to assist with advancement of the scope into the esophagus. Flexible esophagoscopy to the limits of the lower esophageal sphincter is then performed under direct visualization, maintaining the view by air insufflation as needed. The exam is visualized using the video monitor. The endoscope is withdrawn until the light at the tip of the scope transilluminates the site of puncture of the anterior esophageal wall. This site is then confirmed by visualization of the indentation of the posterior tracheal wall by ballottement. A number 11 blade is used to incise the posterior tracheal wall. The esophageal wall is entered under direct visualization. A hemostat is used to dilate the puncture site. A dilator is introduced into the new TEP site and then removed. The prosthesis can be immediately placed if desired or the puncture site can be stented open with a 16-French red rubber catheter until the prosthesis is placed. If there

is difficulty transilluminating the TEP site due to a bulky flap or scar tissue, this technique can be modified using the Seldinger guide wire technique (11).

PRIMARY VOICE RESTORATION

Selection Criteria

Maves and Lingeman (13) and Hamaker et al. (14) were the first to introduce TEP as a primary technique at the time of laryngectomy. Primary voice restoration developed from the concepts of secondary voice restoration. The only absolute contraindication to primary voice restoration is separation of the party wall at the puncture site. This occurs if the surgeon inadvertently separates the party wall or when a patient undergoes a total laryngopharyngoesophagectomy with gastric pull-up. If a puncture is performed following separation of the party wall, abscess formation, sloughing of the posterior tracheal wall, and possibly mediastinitis can occur.

Relative contraindications to primary (and secondary) TEP include the complexity of the reconstruction and the patient's inability to use and care for the prosthesis due to impaired mental status or decrease in manual dexterity due to age, arthritis, or neurologic insult/disease. With the introduction of the indwelling prosthesis and the hands-free valve, most of these obstacles have become manageable with the assistance of a care taker. Bilateral severe sensorineural hearing loss and limited pulmonary function are also relative contraindications to primary TEP due to the fact that the patient cannot hear the TE voice and limited pulmonary air restricts the fluency and volume of speech, respectively (15). Preoperative radiation therapy or the need for postoperative radiation therapy is not a contraindication for this procedure (14–16). Studies have shown that there is no difference in complication rates between these groups of patients (15,17). In addition, the rate of pharyngocutaneous fistula, wound breakdown, stomal stenosis, and esophageal stenosis are similar to those reported in patients undergoing total laryngectomy without primary TEP (17).

If a patient is indecisive regarding primary TEP, a puncture can be performed and then allowed to close if the patient does not wish TE speech. This allows the use of the catheter for feeding until the pharyngeal closure is healed. This obviates the need for placement of a nasogastric tube (NGT) through the fresh pharyngeal closure, which may reduce the pharyngocutaneous fistula rate (17). When undecided preoperatively, the patient often commits to this form of alaryngeal speech in the immediate postoperative period after he/she understands stoma care and has had time to psychologically adjust to laryngectomy.

Primary TEP is felt to be safer than secondary TEP in the fact that there is less risk of mediastinal dissection and posterior esophageal perforation and there is elimination of an additional anesthesia (17).

Surgical Technique

The technique for primary voice restoration includes five basic steps, which are to be done in an ordered sequence to provide success without complication. These steps include incision (laryngectomy), followed by tracheostoma construction, TEP, unilateral pharyngeal constrictor myotomy or pharyngeal plexus neurectomy and buttressing the TE party wall (14).

Tracheostoma Construction
Following laryngectomy, the stoma is constructed. The optimal tracheal diameter is 3 cm or greater in order to prevent stenosis. The midline inferior skin flap is sewn to the midline anterior tracheal ring using half vertical mattress sutures, which allow coverage of the cartilage. Interrupted sutures are placed at 5-mm intervals on either side of the midline, pulling the trachea laterally. This creates a straight, horizontal membranous trachea, which is sewn to the superior skin flap. If the trachea is smaller than 3.0 cm, a stomaplasty is performed (14). The trachea is incised bilaterally for a vertical distance of 1 cm (two tracheal rings in length) between the midline and the most posterolateral aspect. An "X" is drawn in the midline of the inferior skin flap at the proposed stoma site. The skin and subcutaneous tissues of the superior and inferior areas of the "X" incision are discarded. The lateral triangles of skin are sewn into the apex of the lateral tracheal ring incisions causing the trachea to enlarge (5).

Tracheoesophageal Puncture
The TEP is then performed using a ruler, right-angled clamp, and a number 15 scalpel blade. The puncture is made 1.0 to 1.5 cm below the posterior cut edge of the stoma. A right-angled hemostat is placed in the esophagus

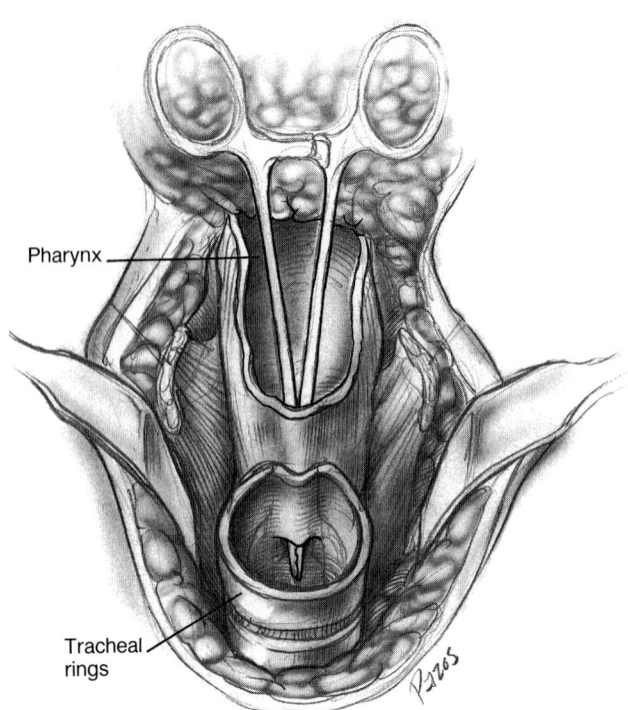

Figure 125.3 Primary placement of the TEP via the pharyngotomy.

through the pharyngotomy and pushed against the posterior tracheal wall. A 4-mm horizontal incision is made over the tip of the hemostat and the hemostat is pushed into the tracheal lumen (Fig. 125.3). The jaws of the hemostat are opened and a number 16-French Silastic Foley catheter is grasped and pulled through the party wall and fed down into the esophagus. Care should be taken at this step to ensure that the catheter is firmly grasped by the hemostat so that it does not slip while it is being pulled through the party wall. The catheter is sewn to the superior skin flap after the skin is closed and can be used to feed the patient in the immediate postoperative period (5,14).

Alternatively, the prosthesis can be primarily placed and the patient fed through a NGT. This is popular in Europe but has not gained wide acceptance in the United States. When using this method, after the red rubber catheter is pulled through the puncture into the esophagus, a prosthesis is attached to the catheter using a silk suture and pulled through the esophagus to the puncture site. The tab and tracheal flange are delivered through the puncture tract to the tracheal side.

The advantages of primary placement include no longer requiring a separate consultation for prosthesis placement; the prosthesis being more stable than the catheter and taking up less space, which allows for easier stoma care and placement of a laryngectomy tube; and the low profile of the prosthesis on the esophageal side that also allows for placement of a Montgomery bypass salivary stent. The only significant disadvantage is the need for an NGT or percutaneous gastrostomy (PEG) for feeding (18).

Pharyngeal Constrictor Myotomy

As mentioned previously, management of the pharyngeal constrictor muscles to prevent pharyngeal spasm is key to successful TE speech. The most reliable method for preventing spasm, if done properly, is a pharyngeal constrictor myotomy. The pharynx is rolled over a tubular structure, most often a finger, and the muscles are incised vertically in the posterior midline of the pharynx from the level of the puncture to the tongue base. The muscles are cut to the level of the submucosa. If bleeding occurs, careful use of bipolar cautery is recommended. If an inadvertent pharyngotomy is made, the mucosa is repaired at this time. If flap reconstruction of the pharynx is performed, the segment of muscle from the puncture site to the inferior flap is myotomized (5,14).

An alternative method that can be performed to prevent pharyngeal spasm is a unilateral pharyngeal plexus neurectomy (Fig. 125.4) (19). After laryngectomy, the pharyngeal muscles lay medially at the level of the superior thyroid artery. The plexus is found within the middle constrictor muscle. A nerve stimulator is used to identify three to five nerve branches by eliciting muscle contraction. The nerve branches are then cut and coagulated. If poor muscle contraction is seen following stimulation, this method is abandoned, and a myotomy is performed. This method is also useful when the pharynx is already closed and a myotomy was inadvertently not performed.

Buttressing of the TE Party Wall

The party wall usually separates about 3 to 5 mm above the site of the puncture. The party wall is buttressed using interrupted sutures of 3-0 chromic or 4-0 Vicryl, which obliterates this space. This prevents the collection of saliva in this area if a fistula develops and helps to maintain the integrity of the posterior stoma. If separation of the party wall extends below the area of the planned puncture, then the puncture is delayed as this can lead to pocket formation with abscess and loss of the posterior tracheal wall (5,14).

The voice prosthesis can be placed at the time of primary TEP as mentioned above until anytime after the patient is taking per oral feeds. Voicing, however, is delayed until 2 weeks postoperatively in order to allow the hypopharyngeal closure to heal. Voicing prior to this time may place too much air pressure on the new closure, disrupting the suture line. If the patient is discharged from the hospital with the Foley catheter in place, the balloon is filled with 2 mL of normal saline to prevent accidental dislodgement of the catheter from the puncture site (15). The patient is also given varying sizes of red rubber catheters and instructed on how to replace the catheter if it becomes dislodged.

Primary TEP results in development of successful TE speech in 50% to 93% of patients depending on patient selection criteria and the use of an indwelling prosthesis (14–,20). During postoperative radiation therapy, voicing may become interrupted due to mucositis or the patient's inability to occlude the stoma due to pain. Although not used, the prosthesis may remain in place during this time (14).

Despite an overall excellent success rate, some clinicians are still hesitant to perform primary TEPs based on lack of experience and fear of complications. Previous radiation therapy and flap reconstruction, as long as the party wall is not separated, are not contraindications to primary TEP; however, these two variables most commonly dissuade surgeons. When not performed primarily, TEP is rarely done as a secondary procedure likely due to patients' bias toward their initial form of speech and their reluctance to undergo another surgical procedure (17).

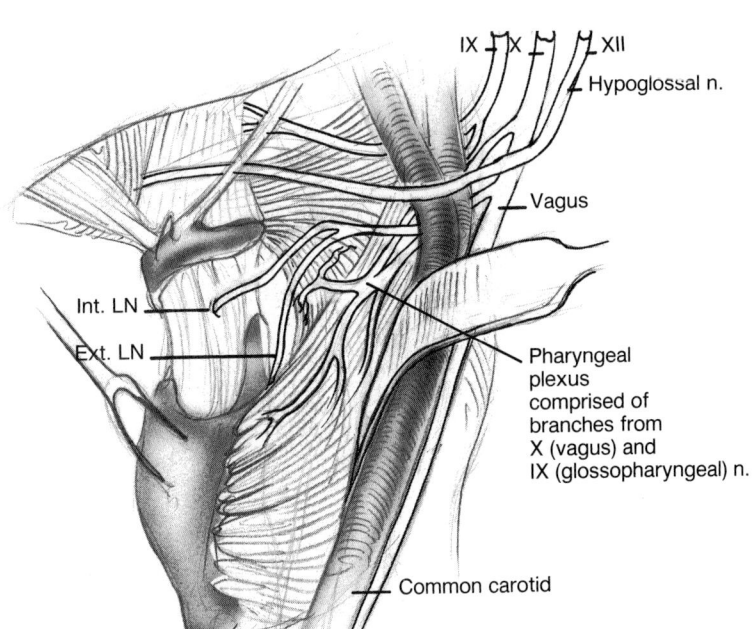

Figure 125.4 Surgical anatomy of the pharyngeal plexus during laryngectomy.

TREATMENT OF PHARYNGEAL CONSTRICTOR SPASM

Hypertonicity or spastic TE speech occurs when the esophagus extends with air on attempted phonation and the PE segment (cricopharyngeus, inferior and middle constrictor muscles) fails to relax to permit airflow for voicing. When the insufflation test reveals hypertonic or spastic speech or the patient fails the "open track" test following primary TEP, this must be addressed to obtain fluent speech. It was thought by some that a nonmuscle closure of the pharynx could prevent spasm, but this did not prove to be true over time (21). Injection of Botox toxin A has been found to be effective in treating spasm. It can be injected under electromyographic guidance or fluoroscopy into the pharyngeal constrictor muscles as chemical denervation of these muscles (22–25). Its effect usually occurs within 72 hours after injection and may require repeated injections approximately every 6 months. Open secondary pharyngeal constrictor myotomy, with its associated complication of fistula, and pharyngeal plexus neurectomy have essentially been replaced with Botox A injections to the PE segment. Recurrent tumor, pharyngeal stenosis, and fibrosis of the tissues should be identified as these patients will not benefit from this procedure.

When pharyngoesophageal spasm is suspected, it can be confirmed by anesthetic block of the pharyngeal plexus. The most effective method for analysis combines radiographic assessment with a plexus block. The patient is evaluated by videofluoroscopy using barium; the lateral view is preferred. An at-rest view is first obtained to rule out stricture, fistula tract, or persistent neoplasm. Several views during voicing are taken. Fluoroscopic visualization reveals a pronounced, transient, posterior pharyngeal muscle mass that protrudes into the lumen and restricts the egress of air. This is seen in the retropharyngeal radiographic plane as a bar (Fig. 125.5) (22).

The study is followed by the pharyngeal plexus block with local anesthesia (150 to 200 mg of 2% lidocaine without epinephrine). The neck skin is entered at the level of C2 to C3 immediately parapharyngeal and medial to the carotid sheath. The lidocaine is injected with a 23-gauge needle placed at the level of the prevertebral fascia. After 3 to 5 minutes, the patient is instructed to attempt voicing. The anesthetic can temporarily inhibit reflex tonicity resulting in fluent speech. The voicing dynamics are now analyzed by fluoroscopy. The typical appearance shows a reduction in the mass of the constrictor muscles, including the axial length, which is documented by radiographic examination. This indicates that the use of botulinum toxin A will most likely be successful in treating pharyngoesophageal spasm. Hamaker and Blom (22) reported a success rate of 79% following one injection of 100 units of Botox A under EMG and fluoroscopic guidance into the posterior pharyngeal "bar" seen with phonation. The patient undergoes preinjection videofluoroscopy to

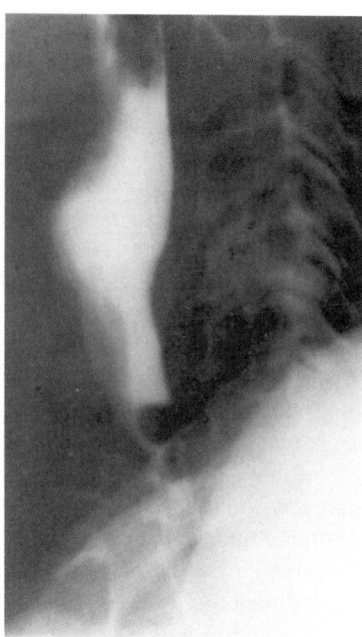

Figure 125.5 Lateral radiograph demonstrating the constrictor mass during esophageal distention. (Reprinted from Singer MI, Blom ED. A selective myotomy for voice restoration after total laryngectomy. *Arch Otolaryngol* 1981;107:670–673, with permission.)

identify the area of spasm. The patient is asked to phonate and the area of spasm is marked. In addition, the area 1 cm above and 1 cm below the level of the spasm is marked in order to include all the muscles. EMG guidance is also used when injecting the Botox (the patient is asked to swallow and/or phonate to confirm the area). Fifty-five percent of these patients had fluent speech for more than 6 months. Following a second and/or third injection with Botox A, 66% of patients required no further treatment without relapse. It has been postulated that the sustained effects of Botox is related to the degree of surgical and/or radiation damage of the neuromuscular junction preventing regeneration. Other studies using slightly different techniques reported 88% and 87% success rates following subsequent injections with Botox, which were sustained (24,25).

COMPLICATIONS

The most common complications encountered following primary and secondary TEP include loss of the puncture site by dislodgment of the catheter placed at the time of puncture or partial or complete extrusion of the prosthesis, migration of the puncture site, formation of granulation tissue, aspiration of the prosthesis, cellulitis, stomal stenosis, and pharyngoesophageal stenosis (15,26–28). Sternoclavicular arthritis and manual pressure necrosis have also been reported (29). Violation of the posterior esophageal wall, passage of the catheter through a false passage, and esophageal perforation are unique to secondary TEP and can result in deep neck space infections, epidural abscess, vertebral osteomyelitis, and mediastinitis (28).

TABLE 125.1	**C**	**COMPLICATIONS**

Epidural abscess or vertebral osteomyelitis secondary to violation of posterior esophageal wall during secondary TEP
Mediastinitis secondary to dissection of party wall
Loss of the puncture site by dislodgment of the catheter placed at the time of puncture
Partial or complete extrusion of the prosthesis
Migration of the puncture site
Formation of granulation tissue
Stomal or pharyngoesophageal stenosis
TEP enlargement
Aspiration of saliva and foods through puncture site

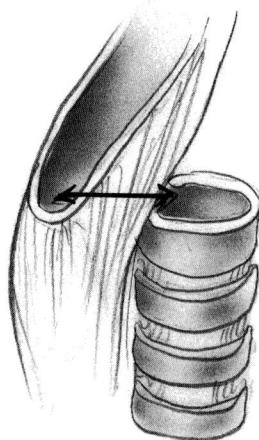

Figure 125.6 Fitting distance from the posterior trachea to the anterior esophagus.

An important local complication is enlargement of the puncture site relative to the size of the prosthesis resulting in leakage around the prosthesis and aspiration of foods and saliva (Table 125.1). The most common causes of enlargement of the puncture site are repeated trauma due to changing the prosthesis or thinning of the party wall. Recurrent tumor should always be considered as a cause. There are many ways in which to manage this problem. One way is to remove the prosthesis and place a red rubber catheter through which the patient can be fed and the fistula can contract around. Other ways include cautery of the edges, surgical closure, local flaps placed between the trachea and esophagus, and more recently the injection of biomaterials (collagen, Cymetra, Bioplastique) around the site to reduce its size and to stop leakage (28,30). Silicone "washers" can be placed behind the prosthesis against the posterior tracheal wall to increase the thickness of the party wall.

Reflux-associated morbidity includes prosthesis erosion, leakage, and granulation tissue formation, but reflux does not appear to effect intelligibility and overall quality of TE speech (31). Previous radiation (32,33), diabetes mellitus, chronic obstructive pulmonary disease, alcoholism, and extended laryngectomy have not been found to be significant risk factors for complications (34).

POSTOPERATIVE REHABILITATION

Postoperative TE voice rehabilitation is usually taught by a speech and language pathologist. There are three basic treatment goals following TEP. The first is to dilate and measure the puncture followed by placement of the prosthesis, the second is to instruct the patient and family in routine care of the prosthesis, and the third is to instruct the patient in finger occlusion of the tracheostoma and to apply and use a tracheostomal valve (35).

Briefly, the puncture must be dilated to the appropriate size to accommodate the prosthesis (e.g., 22 French for a 20-French prosthesis). A measuring device is then placed into the puncture and slowly withdrawn until the retention collar sits against the inner surface of the esophageal wall

and the length of the prosthesis is measured (Fig. 125.6). If the length lies between sizes, the longer size is chosen to prevent underfitting, which can cause the puncture to heal from behind.

The type of prosthesis to be used is chosen. The duckbill and low-pressure prostheses (Figs. 125.7 and 125.8) are removable prostheses, which the patient learns to clean and replace into the puncture. The indwelling low-pressure prosthesis is placed and removed by the physician or speech and language pathologist. The indwelling prosthesis is used in patients who cannot or prefer not to use the removable prosthesis. The life of any prosthesis in

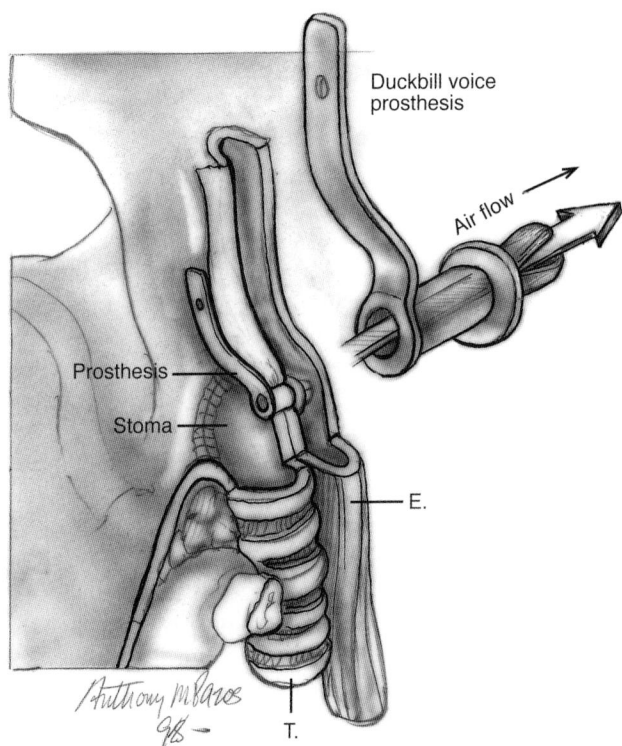

Figure 125.7 Duckbill (slit-valve) voice prosthesis.

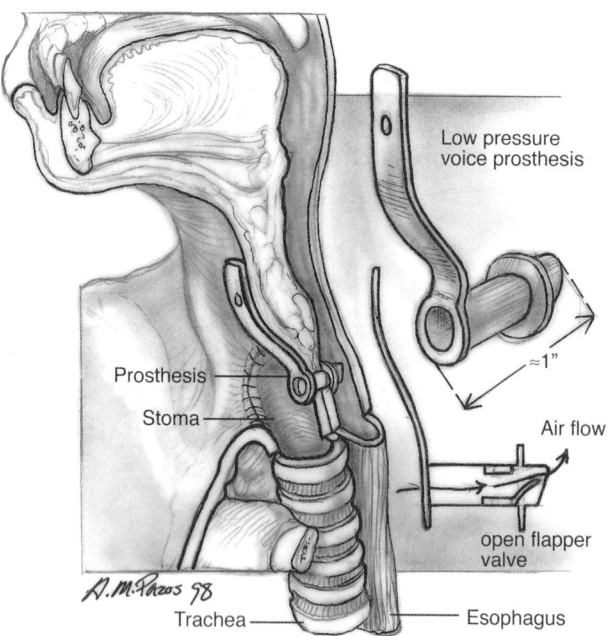

Low pressure
voice prosthesis

Prosthesis

Stoma

≈1"

Air flow

open flapper
valve

A. M. Pazos 98

Trachea ———— Esophagus

Figure 125.8 Voice prosthesis in place in the TEP.

general is about 3 to 6 months. It is the colonization of yeast (more common in indwelling prosthesis) that usually destroys the integrity of the valve, which causes leakage of saliva and foods and decreases the life expectancy of the prosthesis (14,15). A prescription for oral nystatin should be given to all patients for daily use to prevent yeast colonization, or the newly available pretreated prosthesis can be used. Prior to placing the voice prosthesis, an "open tract" test is performed. The patient is asked to voice without prosthesis in place. Poor voicing is either due to pharyngeal constrictor spasm or excessive finger pressure occlusion of the stoma.

The next steps include patient and family education regarding care of the prosthesis and patient instruction regarding finger occlusion of the prosthesis. It is usually necessary to assist the patient with accurate occlusion of the stoma at the initial visit while the patient watches in the mirror. About six sessions are required for the average patient to master removal, cleaning, and reinsertion of the standard voice prosthesis. For those patients who find finger occlusion unacceptable, a hands-free valve can be used.

PREDICTORS OF SUCCESSFUL TRACHEOESOPHAGEAL SPEECH

TE speech is closer to laryngeal speech than esophageal speech because its air supply is pulmonary; voice parameters including fundamental frequency, jitter, shimmer, words per minute, and maximum phonation time are closer to laryngeal speech.

Many variables have been studied by various clinicians in order to predict those patients who will achieve

successful TE speech with primary or secondary puncture (17,33,34,36). The results of these studies have varied, although age, sex, and tumor size/stage appear to have no influence. Ethanol abuse and lack of transportation to follow-up visits correlated well with TE speech failure in some studies, but were not significant in others (17,36). However, many clinicians can anecdotally report alcohol abuse as a contributor to rehabilitation failure. In a study by Cantu et al. (36), 36 patients undergoing either primary or secondary TEP were evaluated for long-term success and predictors of successful TE speech. Nearly two-thirds had successful communication at an average of 4 years postpuncture. For the remaining patients who were judged as unsuccessful, reduced vision, limited hand and arm movement, and history of radiation therapy (but not timing of radiation therapy) were found to be significant. However, there were patients with good vision and hand coordination who did not develop good speech and those with previous radiation therapy who did develop successful speech. In a 16-year retrospective outcomes analysis of primary and secondary TEPs, neither pre- nor postoperative radiotherapy had any effect on voice restoration or complications (33). Therefore, the presence of these factors does not necessarily predict lack of success. The introduction of the indwelling prosthesis has reduced the problems associated with decreased function.

A study by Bozec et al. (37) evaluated patients using prosthetic voice restoration for clinical factors that correlated with functional outcomes. One hundred and three patients who underwent total laryngectomy or pharyngolaryngectomy were evaluated regarding speech and swallowing. Eighty-two percent of patients had successful voice rehabilitation. Hypopharyngeal tumors, circular laryngopharyngectomies, and the use of pectoralis major myocutaneous flaps were associated with the placement of a secondary TEP, and the only factor that correlated with speech failure was a high level of comorbidity (American Association of Anesthesiologist (ASA) score greater than or equal to 3). It is thought that reduced vital lung capacity, neurologic disabilities altering hand coordination, decreased motivation, chronic asthenia, and dyspnea, which are frequent in patients with severe comorbidities, could be the possible causes of unsuccessful vocal rehabilitation. Decreased life of the prosthesis was seen with flap reconstruction, which could be explained by decreased pharyngeal motility with food stasis around the valve resulting in more *Candida* colonization.

The timing of TEP does not appear to appear the influence communication effectiveness and the absence of pharyngeal stricture was the only significant predictor of good to excellent speech results in secondary TEP (34). In another study, it was found that 77.8% of patients undergoing primary TEP achieved excellent voice quality and 78.4% of these patients consistently used TE speech, while only 50% of those undergoing secondary TEP achieved excellent voice quality and only 70.6% consistently used TE speech (33). Primary TEP may be preferable in view of superior voice quality, a shorter period of aphonia, and the fact that there is no need for a second procedure for voice restoration (33). In addition, primary TEP precludes major complications in the visceral compartment. As one can see, there are variable results found in multiple studies, which can make predicting success of TE speech challenging.

VOICE QUALITY

Preoperative and postoperative evaluation by a speech and language pathologist is vital to successful TE speech. The goal of voice restoration is to provide fluent, effortless, and intelligible speech. The patients should understand that voice quality cannot be controlled.

TE speech does generally improve over time and its use does not preclude the use of other methods of alaryngeal speech.

TE voice quality is usually harsh and often loses its sexual characterization (38). However, patients undergoing total laryngectomy already have varying degrees of dysphonia, and voice should be compared to the preoperative voice quality. In a study by Cantu et al. (36), one-third of patients or their significant others judged the success of their TE speech at a lower level than that of the primary investigator. This indicates that the clinician and patient may be using different standards of success; the patient and significant other may be using an "idealized" voice standard that cannot be produced using TEP. The patients should realize that there is a learning curve associated with TE speech and it generally improves over time (27). In addition, a functionally rehabilitated TE prosthesis user may find it easier to switch to esophageal speech (27). Acoustic analysis of TE speech has been compared to laryngeal, esophageal, and electrolarynx speech by many (39–41). The fundamental frequency, intensity, and rate of TE speech approximate that of normal speech. In a study by Robbins et al. (42), esophageal and TE speakers were analyzed for intensity, frequency, and rate of speech production. TE speech was found to be more similar to laryngeal speech than esophageal speech. When compared to esophageal speech, it gives superior voice quality in reference to volume and phrase length and is much easier to learn. Also, the rate of speech is faster and the intelligibility is superior to that acquired using the artificial larynx or esophageal speech (41,43,44). However, in the presence of noise, there is a lower rate of listener intelligibility of TE speech compared to laryngeal speech (40).

The prevention of pharyngeal spasm is paramount to the production of successful TE speech as mentioned previously. Acoustic analysis of TE speech was studied following three different surgical methods used to address the pharynx: pharyngeal plexus neurectomy, pharyngeal constrictor myotomy, and unilateral pharyngeal plexus neurectomy with a drainage myotomy limited to the cricopharyngeus. Patients undergoing pharyngeal plexus neurectomy had the highest fundamental frequency, which may be due to the residual resting tone in the pharyngoesophageal segment (39). Management of the pharynx with neurectomy may be desirable in women undergoing laryngectomy with voice restoration.

TE speech has been rated the most desirable form of alaryngeal speech by both speech pathologist and patients (45) and is the preferred method of alaryngeal speech by naïve listeners (41).

In a study by Gerwin and Culton (46), greater than 80% of laryngectomy patients ($n = 16$) reported a good quality of life satisfaction with TE speech using the University of Washington Quality of Life Scale and Functional Assessment of Cancer Therapy.

EMERGENCIES

Two urgent conditions may result for prosthesis users and should be attended to without delay. For patients who routinely change their prostheses, the inability to insert the tip of the prosthesis and collar into the lumen of the esophagus may occur, which results initially in increased voice resistance and, in some cases, complete loss of voice. The TEP tract will close over time from inside out, and it will be impossible after 24 to 48 hours to reenter the lumen. If this occurs, the TEP can be serially dilated with plastic catheters ranging from 10F to 18F and then stented with a flexible catheter for several hours before the voice prosthesis is replaced. Laryngeal and urethral dilators are also an effective instrument for TEP dilatation. Dilatation must be performed with as little resistance as possible because it is possible to dissect into the TE party wall and enter the anterior mediastinum.

The second urgent condition is aspiration of the voice prosthesis. This condition usually occurs when patients attempt to replace the device in the TEP and a cough is stimulated. The most common location for device impaction is at the level of the upper right mainstem bronchus and carina. This usually is well tolerated, but an uncomfortable dyspnea is present. Furthermore, if the TEP is not stented with a red rubber catheter, tracheal aspiration of saliva may occur. Should aspiration of the prosthesis occur, the patient should first securely stent the puncture and then attempt to bend over as far as possible and cough out the prosthesis. In the event of failure, the patient should go to an emergency medical facility as soon as possible. The size of the prosthesis prevents it from occluding the airway. The most efficient method for prosthesis retrieval is to use topical anesthesia and flexible bronchoscope with grasping forceps. After removing the foreign body, the TEP can be replaced. The patient may require additional training regarding removal and reinsertion of the prosthesis.

HIGHLIGHTS

- Alaryngeal voice restoration can be attained with the use of an electrolarynx speech, esophageal speech, and TE speech.

- TE speech is more acoustically similar to normal laryngeal speech and more intelligible than standard esophageal speech.

- Restoration of the voice after total laryngectomy must not compromise the established principles of surgical oncology.

- TE speech dysfluency may be the result of pharyngeal constrictor tonicity, excessive resistance to airflow by a prosthesis with high-resistance characteristics, or tissue changes related to edema, fibrosis, or recurrent disease.

- There are no absolute contraindications to secondary TEP.

- The only absolute contraindication to primary TEP is separation of the party wall. Separation of the party wall below the puncture site can lead to abscess formation, necrosis of the posterior tracheal wall, and possibly mediastinitis.

- Relative contraindications to primary and secondary TEP include the patient's inability to use and care for the prosthesis due to impaired mental status or decrease in manual dexterity, bilateral severe sensorineural hearing loss (patient cannot hear the TE voice), and limited pulmonary function (restricts the fluency and volume of speech).

- It is imperative that the puncture is through the party wall to prevent mediastinal dissection with the catheter resulting in mediastinitis.

- Radiation therapy is not a contraindication for TEP.

- Botulinum toxin A injections can be used to treat hypertonic or spastic TE speech.

- Secondary voice restoration can be performed using the TNE scope under local anesthesia in the office setting. It is especially useful in patients with esophageal strictures, fibrosis of the neck due to surgery, and radiation and cervical spine deformity causing rigid esophagoscopy to be challenging if not impossible.

- Pharyngeal constrictor myotomy or pharyngeal plexus neurectomy at the time of laryngectomy are paramount to attaining fluent TE speech.

REFERENCES

1. Gates GA, Ryan W, Cooper JC Jr, et al. Current status of laryngectomy rehabilitation: results of therapy. *Am J Otolaryngol* 1982;3:1–7.
2. *Ultra voice.* Malvern, PA: Health Concepts.
3. Singer MI, Blom ED. An endoscopic technique for restoration of voice after laryngectomy. *Ann Otol Rhinol Laryngol* 1980;89:529–533.
4. Blom ED. Current status of voice restoration following total laryngectomy. *Oncology (Williston Park)* 2000;14(6):915–922.
5. Blom ED, Hamaker RC. Tracheoesophageal voice restoration following total laryngectomy. In: Myers EN, Suen JY, eds. *Cancer of the head and neck,* 3rd ed. Philadelphia, PA: WB Saunders, 1996:839–852.
6. Singer MI. The development of successful tracheoesophageal voice restoration. *Otolaryngol Clin North Am* 2004;37:507–517.
7. Kirchner JA, Dey FL, Shedd DP. The pharynx after laryngectomy. *Laryngscope* 1963;73:18–33.
8. Blom ED, Singer MI, Hamaker RC. An improved esophageal insufflation test. *Arch Otolaryngol* 1985;111:211–212.
9. Desyatnikova S, Caro JJ, Cohen JI, et al. Tracheoesophageal puncture in the office setting with local anesthesia. *Ann Otol Rhinol Laryngol* 2001;110:613–616.
10. Bach KK, Postma GN, Koufman JA. In-office tracheoesophageal puncture using transnasal esophagoscopy. *Laryngoscope* 2003;113(1):173–176.
11. LeBert B, McWhorter AW, Kunduk M, et al. Secondary tracheoesophageal puncture with in-office transnasal esophagoscopy. *Arch Otolaryngol Head Neck Surg* 2009;135(12):1190–1194.
12. Doctor VS. In-office unsedated tracheoesophageal puncture. *Curr Opin Otolaryngol Head Neck Surg* 2007;15:405–408.
13. Maves MD, Lingeman RE. Primary vocal rehabilitation using the Blom-Singer and Panje voice prosthesis. *Ann Otol Rhinol Laryngol* 1982;1:458–460.
14. Hamaker RC, Singer MI, Blom ED, et al. Primary voice restoration at laryngectomy. *Arch Otolaryngol* 1985;111:182–186.
15. Silverman AH, Black MJ. Efficacy of primary tracheoesophageal puncture in laryngectomy rehabilitation. *J Otolaryngol* 1994;23(5):370–377.
16. Kao WW, Mohr RM, Kimmel CA, et al. The outcome and techniques of primary and secondary tracheoesophageal puncture. *Arch Otolaryngol Head Neck Surg* 1994;120:310–307.
17. Karlen RG, Maisel RH. Does primary tracheoesophageal puncture reduce complications after total laryngectomy and improve patient communication? *Am J Otolaryngol* 2001;22(5):324–328.
18. Deschler DG, Bunting GW, Lin DT, et al. Evaluation of voice prosthesis placement at the time of primary tracheoesophageal puncture with total laryngectomy. *Laryngoscope* 2009;119(7):1353–1357.
19. Singer MI, Blom ED, Hamaker RC. Pharyngeal plexus neurectomy for alaryngeal speech rehabilitation. *Laryngoscope* 1986;96:50–53.
20. Singer MI, Blom ED, Hamaker RC, et al. Application of the voice prosthesis during laryngectomy. *Ann Otol Rhinol Laryngol* 1989;98:921–925.
21. Clevens RA, Esclamado RM, Hartshorn DO, et al. Voice rehabilitation after total laryngectomy and tracheoesophageal puncture using nonmuscle closure. *Ann Otol Rhinol Laryngol* 1993;102:792–796.
22. Hamaker R, Blom E. Botulinum neurotoxin for pharyngeal constrictor muscle spasm in tracheoesophageal voice restoration. *Laryngoscope* 2003;113(9):1479–1482.
23. Chao SS, Graham SM, Hoffman HT. Management of pharyngoesophageal spasm with Botox. *Otolaryngol Clin North Am* 2004;37:559–556.
24. Lewin JS, Bishop-Leone JK, Forma AD, et al. Further experience with Botox injection for tracheoesophageal speech failure. *Head Neck* 2001;23:456–460.
25. Hoffman HT, McCulloch TM. Botulinum neurotoxin for tracheoesophageal voice failure. In: BLom ED, Singer MI, Hamaker RC, eds. *Tracheoesophageal voice restoration following total laryngectomy.* San Diego, CA, London: Singular Publishing Group, Inc, 1998:83–87.
26. Ramirez MJF, Domenech FG, Durban SB, et al. Surgical voice restoration after total laryngectomy: long-term results. *Eur Arch Otorhinolaryngol* 2001;258:463–466.
27. Hotz MA, Baumann A, Schaller I, et al. Success and predictability of Provox voice rehabilitation. *Arch Otolaryngol Head Neck Surg* 2002;128(6):687–691.
28. Malik T, Bruce L, Cherry J. Surgical complications of tracheoesophageal puncture and speech valves. *Curr Opin Otolaryngol Head Neck Surg* 2007;15(20):117–122.

29. Mehle ME, Lavertu P. Sternoclavicular joint arthritis and manual pressure necrosis: two potential complications of tracheoesophageal puncture. *Otolaryngol Head Neck Surg* 1991;105:130–133.

30. Seshamani M, Ruiz C, Kasper Schwartz S, et al. Cymetra injections to treat leakage around a tracheoesophageal puncture. *ORL J Otorhinolaryngol Relat Spec* 2006;68(3):146–148.

31. Jobe BA, Rosenthal E, Wiesberg TT, et al. Surgical management of gastroesophageal reflux and outcome after laryngectomy in patients using tracheoesophageal speech. *Am J Surg* 2002;183(5):539–543.

32. LaBruna A, Klatsky I, Huo J, et al. Tracheoesophageal puncture in irradiated patients. *Ann Otol Rhinol Laryngol* 1995;104(4 Pt 1): 279–281.

33. Cheng E, Ho M, Ganz C, et al. Outcomes of primary and secondary tracheoesophageal puncture: a 16-year retrospective analysis. *Ear Nose Throat J* 2006;85(4):262–267.

34. Lavertu P, Guay ME, Meeker SS, et al. Secondary tracheoesophageal puncture: factors predictive of voice quality and prosthesis use. *Head Neck* 1996;18(5):393–398.

35. Blom ED. Tracheoesophageal speech. *Semin Speech Lang* 1995;16 (3):191–204.

36. Cantu E, Ryan WJ, Tansey S, et al. Tracheoesophageal speech: predictors of success and social validity ratings. *Am J Otolaryngol* 1998;9(1):12–17.

37. Bozec A, Poissonnete G, Chamorey E, et al. Results of vocal rehabilitation using tracheoesophageal voice prosthesis after total laryngectomy and their predictive factors. *Eur Arch Otorhinolaryngol* 2010;267:751–758.

38. Mendelsohn M, Morris M, Galllagher R. Speaking proficiency after primary tracheoesophageal puncture. *J Otolaryngol* 1993;22(6):435–437.

39. Blom ED, Pauloski BR, Hamaker RC. Functional outcome after surgery for prevention of pharyngospasms in tracheoesophageal speakers. Part I: speech characteristics. *Laryngoscope* 1995;105:1093–1103.

40. McColl D, Fucci D, Petrosino L, et al. Listener ratings of the intelligibility of tracheoesophageal speech in noise. *J Commun Disord* 1998;31(4):279–289.

41. Merwin GE, Goldstein LP, Rothman HB. A comparison of speech using artificial larynx and tracheoesophageal puncture with valve in the same speaker. *Laryngoscope* 1985;95:730–734.

42. Robbins J, Fisher HA, Blom ED, et al. Selected acoustic features of tracheoesophageal, esophageal and laryngeal speech. *Arch Otolaryngol* 1984;110:670–672.

43. Pindzola R, Cain B. Acceptability rating of tracheoesophageal speech. *Laryngoscope* 1988;98:394–397.

44. Williams S, Watson B. Speaking proficiency variation according to method of alaryngeal voicing. *Laryngoscope* 1987;97: 737–739.

45. Culton GL, Gerwin JM. Current trends in laryngectomy rehabilitation: a survey of speech-language pathologists. *Otolaryngol Head Neck Surg* 1998;118:458–463.

46. Gerwin JM, Culton GL. Quality of life in prosthetic voice users. *Otolaryngol Head Neck Surg* 2005;133(5):685–688.

126 Tracheal Tumors

Kevin L. Potts   *Jeffrey M. Bumpous*

Tracheal neoplasms are rare, accounting for only 1% of all malignancies (1), but the impact on the individual is generally severe (2–4). With regard to incidence, these tumors may also be underreported, incompletely diagnosed, and undertreated because of the rarity, lack of mandatory registration, limited surgical experience, and the relative sporadic nature of the lesions (4). The most common tumors are classified as benign, primary malignant and secondary malignant in Table 126.1. Because these tumors occupy the main airway conduit, as they enlarge, the impact and potential fatality increase. Stridor, hemoptysis, and shortness of air are the most common symptoms, and many patients present in need of acute airway management. Injudicious airway management may precipitate airway obstruction and/or potentially interfere with subsequent definitive surgical management (4,5).

CLINICAL PRESENTATION

History

Tracheal tumors tend to cause progressive symptoms over several months to years due to their slow-growing nature often causing accurate diagnosis to be delayed (6). Gaissert et al. (7) reviewed 270 cases of squamous cell and adenoid cystic carcinoma of the trachea and carina, and the mean duration of symptoms was 12.2 months. The duration of symptoms was longer in adenoid cystic carcinoma and in tumors that were deemed to be unresectable (resected adenoid cystic carcinoma 18.3 months, resected squamous cell carcinoma 4.54 months, unresectable adenoid cystic carcinoma 23.7 months, unresectable squamous cell carcinoma 7.58 months, $P < 0.0001$) (6).

Symptoms at presentation depend largely on extent of airway obstruction and tumor type, but not location within the tracheobronchial tree (8). Dyspnea with exertion or phonation is the primary symptom when the tumor has caused significant airway obstruction. If lesions are ulcerative and mucosal irritation is severe, chronic cough and hemoptysis are common. Wheezing, stridor, hoarseness, difficulty clearing secretions, and frequent respiratory infections are also encountered.

Presentation may vary with tumor type with hemoptysis being the main symptom in patients with squamous cell carcinoma, and wheezing and dyspnea predominate in those with adenoid cystic carcinoma (Table 126.2) (9). Wheezing is often misdiagnosed as "asthma" and is refractory to bronchodilator therapy. Prolonged use of systemic corticosteroids is common, and patients may even be secondarily cushingoid at presentation (10).

Imaging

Imaging studies that are most frequently employed are CT scan with contrast and in some instances PET–CT. CT with contrast allows for adequate multiplanar imaging of the airway from hyoid to segmental bronchi. CT can be further exploited to derive three-dimensional images allowing for "virtual endoscopy." It is useful in the identification of involvement of mediastinal soft tissues, esophagus, and vasculature. It is additionally helpful in demonstrating coexisting pulmonary metastatic disease. PET–CT may be useful in distinguishing more aggressive pathology and may be more sensitive in the detection of paratracheal and mediastinal nodal involvement. MRI scanning may be useful in the examination of the cervical trachea, but mediastinal and thoracic structures may be significantly be distorted by motion artifact due to respiratory and circulatory movement (11–13). Figure 126.1A and B represent a demonstration of a high tracheal adenoid cystic carcinoma in both the axial and coronal planes.

TABLE 126.1	PATHOLOGY OF TRACHEAL TUMORS

Primary Tumor	Tumor Type
Epithelial (benign)	Papilloma
	Adenoma
	Myoepithelial tumor
	Pleomorphic adenoma
	Oncocytoma
Epithelial (malignant)	Squamous cell carcinoma
	Adenoid cystic carcinoma
	Adenocarcinoma
	Mucoepidermoid carcinoma
	Large cell undifferentiated carcinoma
	Carcinoma ex-pleomorphic adenoma
	Neuroendocrine tumors:
	Typical and atypical carcinoids
	Large cell neuroendocrine tumor
	Small cell carcinoma
Mesenchymal (benign)	Lipoma
	Neurofibroma
	Fibroma
	Pyogenic granuloma
	Plexiform neurofibroma
	Benign fibrous histiocytoma
	Hemangioma
	Hemangiopericytoma
	Chondroma
	Leiomyoma
	Chondroblastoma
	Granular cell tumor
	Plasmacytoma
	Paraganglioma
	Schwannoma
	Glomus tumor
Mesenchymal (malignant)	Chondrosarcoma
	Malignant melanoma
	Malignant lymphoma
	Leiomyosarcoma
	Spindle cell sarcoma
	Malignant fibrous histiocytoma
	Carcinosarcoma
	Rhabdomyosarcoma
Secondary Tumor	**Tumor Type**
Local invasion	Thyroid carcinoma
	Lung carcinoma
	Esophageal carcinoma
Metastatic	Renal cell carcinoma
	Colon carcinoma
	Breast carcinoma
	Metastatic melanoma

TABLE 126.2	PRESENTING SYMPTOMS IN 270 PATIENTS WITH PRIMARY TRACHEAL CARCINOMA

Symptoms (%)	Adenoid Cystic	Squamous Cell
Dyspnea	65	50
Cough	55	52
Hemoptysis	29	60
Wheeze	44	27
Stridor	21	27
Hoarseness	10	13
Dysphagia	7	7
Fever	7	4
Other	12	14

Gaissert HA, Grillo H, Mathisen D, et al. Long-term survival after resection of primary adenoid cystic and squamous cell carcinoma of the trachea and carina. *Ann Thorac Surg* 2004;78:1889–1897.

INITIAL AIRWAY MANAGEMENT

For tracheal tumors, bronchoscopy is the mainstay of initial airway management and diagnosis. If the airway is stable at presentation, elective bronchoscopy can be arranged. However, in patients with acute airway compromise, urgent bronchoscopy may be needed to stabilize the airway. Bronchoscopy allows accurate estimation of the extent of airway pathology and airway obstruction. The exact tumor location, length of tracheal involvement, and its proximity to key anatomical structures can be determined. Tissue diagnosis is obtained during initial bronchoscopy, and margin mapping can be performed to help with treatment planning. For proximal tracheal tumors, rigid bronchoscopy is preferred over flexible bronchoscopy due to its ability to ventilate during the evaluation. Flexible bronchoscopy can provide additional information concerning the more distal airways.

Patients are sometimes able to tolerate significant obstruction (75% or more), but can decompensate rapidly with increased secretions or inflammation. In the event of an urgent airway, endotracheal intubation may not be feasible and could cause tumor dislodgement with subsequent complete airway obstruction. In this setting, rigid bronchoscopy can help stabilize the airway by dilating the stenotic segment, and tumor debulking can be performed. Flexible bronchoscopy alone can be dangerous, potentially causing edema and bleeding, which can precipitate complete airway obstruction. A rigid bronchoscope has the ability to tamponade bleeding while bypassing the site of obstruction for ventilation.

Emergency intervention via a surgical airway could prove troublesome depending on tumor location. Injudicious tracheotomy may transgress a lesion or make subsequent tracheal resection and reconstruction more difficult. If tracheotomy can be safely accomplished distal to the lesion, it may be warranted if the tumor is unresectable or patient comorbidities preclude definitive surgical management.

Finally, in addition to stabilizing the airway, therapeutic bronchoscopy can prepare and optimize a patient for airway surgery (14). Inflammation adjacent to the lesion may represent malignant submucosal extension or benign reactive changes. By delaying the resection and palliating the airway through repeated bronchoscopic

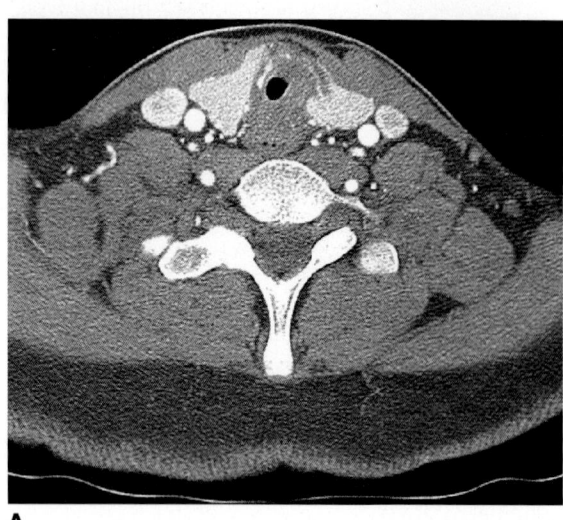
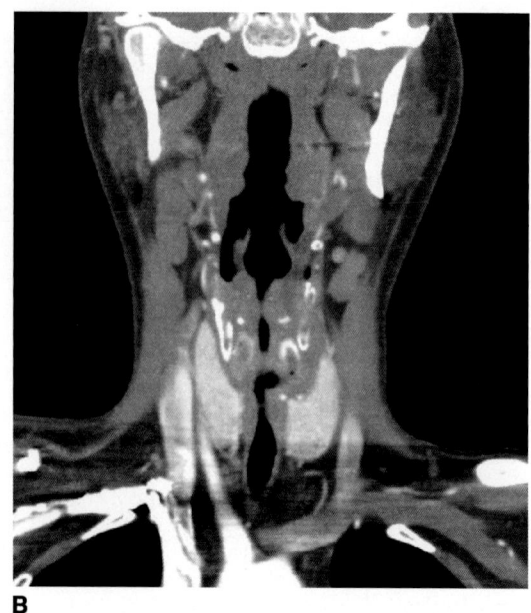

Figure 126.1 A,B: Adenoid cystic carcinoma. Contrast-enhanced axial CT showing a mass involving the lateral and posterior aspect of the proximal trachea. Adenoid cystic carcinoma. Coronal CT shows a submucosal lesion similar in appearance to tracheal stenosis.

intervention, obstructive pneumonia with resulting airway inflammation can be resolved. This allows for better delineation of margins and may decrease perioperative complications such as wound disruption and pneumonia (14).

DEFINITIVE SURGICAL MANAGEMENT

Tracheal Resection

Tracheal resection and primary reanastamosis is the preferred treatment for the majority of both benign and malignant tracheal neoplasms. The ability to perform this preferred management is predicated upon patient-, tumor-, and surgeon-related factors. Patient factors that are important include body habitus, medical comorbidities, and patient preference. Increasing body mass index (BMI) and a thick and short neck may be impediments to the execution of tracheal resection and reanastamosis. In this patient group, the mobilization of the trachea inferiorly and superiorly may be limited, and access to the segment of trachea containing the tumor may not be able to be accomplished solely through a cervical approach. Patients with coexisting chronic obstructive pulmonary disease may require a longer intubation and may be more prone to coughing exacerbations that may place additional strain on the tracheal repair. Furthermore, patients who have diabetes mellitus or are otherwise immunocompromised may have poorer wound healing, especially with longer segment resections that are under tension.

Tumor factors are important in decision making. The length of the proposed segment that would require

resection for adequate margins represents one of the key factors in determination of treatment. Segmental resections of greater than 4 cm or six tracheal rings represent conditions in which the tracheal repair is under increased tension and dehiscence may be more likely. Submucosal, esophageal, mediastinal, and extensive tracheal or bronchial extension may require combined cervicothoracic procedures or nonsurgical treatment. A variety of extended tracheobronchial resections have been described and are best managed in a multidisciplinary approach with otolaryngologist and thoracic surgeon. Premature tracheotomy in the securing of an airway may create additional scar tissue and potential seeding of the soft tissues of the neck and make subsequent surgical resection efforts more difficult. Prior radiation therapy may additionally have an impact on the ability to dissect soft tissues, mobilize the trachea and larynx, identify critical structures, and allow for optimal wound healing.

Surgeon preference and experience may influence approach. Experience with benign tracheal stenosis, laryngectomy, and tracheal resection increases the confidence and ability of the surgeon to manage these lesions. Cooperation between otolaryngologists and thoracic surgeons allows for improved patient selection, procedure selection, and technical execution of these complicated cases (2–5,15). Contraindications for tracheal resection are relative rather than absolute in many cases. Because airway patency represents a fundamental goal in the management of patients with tracheal neoplasms, resection may be offered even in the face of primary tracheal tumors with regional or distant metastatic disease as well as selected metastatic lesions to the trachea. Lesions that are involve greater than 4 cm or are greater than six tracheal rings may not be eligible for resection; factors ultimately affecting this decision include body habitus, ability to adequately mobilize the upper respiratory tract, and experience of the surgical team in both the procedure and management of its complications. Extensive extratracheal disease in the mediastinum involving the esophagus, mediastinal vessels, and prevertebral spaces represents cases in which resection is contraindicated and tracheotomy, endoscopic tumor ablation, and stent placement may be preferred.

Standard resection steps are predicated upon adequate bronchoscopic evaluation of the airway, imaging of the trachea and related neck and mediastinal structures, pathological confirmation, surgical team selection and approach, anesthetic preparation and management plan, and finally execution of the procedure. The steps of the tracheal resection procedure are as follows: transverse cervical incision outlined in cervical crease at midpoint between the sternal notch and the inferior border of the cricoid cartilage that are readily palpable landmarks. In extended cases or in cases in which cervical and extensive mediastinal dissection or proximity to the innominate artery is anticipated, both the neck and chest should be sterilely prepped and draped. The transverse cervical incision can be readily connected to a vertical chest incision for addition of a median sternotomy (total or partial). After preparation and skin incision choices are made, the steps of tracheal resection with primary repair are as follows:

1. Elevation of a subfascial, supramuscular flap above the strap musculature and the sternomastoid muscles sternal heads both superiorly and inferiorly into the suprasternal space of Burns.

2. Separation of the strap muscles from the thyroid cartilage to the sternal and clavicular origins of the muscles. Retraction of the wound may be done with a variety of self-retaining retractors, elastic stays, or sutures.

3. Exposure of the trachea requires the surgeon to anticipate extratracheal extension. For example, thyroidectomy may be required if resection is being performed because of well-differentiated thyroid cancer with focal tracheal invasion. In cases of endoluminal primary tracheal neoplasms, the thyroid isthmus should be divided with careful hemostasis, and the thyroid lobes mobilized laterally.

4. Recurrent (inferior) laryngeal nerve identification is not performed routinely, although identification of the nerve may be required for adjunctive procedures such as thyroidectomy, central lymphadenectomy, or extended cricotracheal procedures. Monitoring of the recurrent nerves may be helpful in maintaining integrity of the nerves and monitoring the condition of the nerve during retraction; there is no current evidence that use of neural monitoring improves recurrent laryngeal nerve outcome in these procedures.

5. Tracheal mobilization. The trachea should be carefully mobilized from the cricoid to two to three rings below the intended inferior margin of resection. Concomitant use and measuring of the lesion with imaging studies and intraoperative bronchoscopy may add accuracy to the determination of the segment requiring resection. Mobilization of the resection segment must be circumferential. Beyond the resection segment inferiorly, care should be taken to perform anterior and posterior mobilization, but careful lateral preservation of soft tissues in order to preserve the blood supply to the distal trachea from the inferior thyroid artery and other thyrocervical trunk arterial tributaries.

6. The majority of mobilization occurs from inferior mobilization for cervical tracheal defects.

7. Superior mobilization may provide from 1 to 2 cm of additional length. This may include either infra- or suprahyoid muscle release, which in effect allows for stretching or elongation of the thyrohyoid membrane.

8. The anesthesiologist and operative room team should be notified to remove any shoulder roll that was placed and to place the head in a neutral to flexed position.

9. Closure of the trachea should be performed with reabsorbable interrupted sutures. I prefer 3-0 dyed polyglactin-coated vicryl sutures. The posterior sutures are placed first. Placing a 0 silk suture through the Murphy Eye of the endotracheal tube allows for it to be withdrawn and retrieved safely without accidental extubation. All of the sutures posteriorly to up to the 3 and 9 o'clock positions of the trachea should be placed prior to tying the sutures. These sutures are then tied sequentially, while the surgical assistant removes tension from the proximal and distal ends of the trachea. The anterior sutures are then placed extraluminally around one tracheal ring inferiorly and one tracheal ring or the cricoid cartilage superiorly. Each of these sutures is interrupted and should be thrown but not tied. Once all anterior sutures are placed, they may then be tied by the surgeon (I prefer hand tying to monitor tension rather than instrument tying); while the surgical assistant removes tension from the proximal and distal tracheal segments.

10. Buttressing extraluminal permanent sutures (i.e., 3-0 Prolene or nylon) may be thrown from tracheal rings or laryngeal cartilages above and below the primary tracheal repair line in order to further remove tension of closure. This is not always feasible, and care must be taken not to tear the trachea or larynx.

11. The wound is then irrigated, and hemostasis is reviewed and insured. The surgeon should ask the anesthesiologist to perform a Valsalva or positive pressure ventilation with the endotracheal cuff inflated to review hemostasis and then with the endotracheal cuff deflated, while the wound is flooded with sterile irrigation in order to determine if the repair is air tight.

12. A drain may or may not be placed and is the preference of the surgeon based on the condition of the wound.
13. The strap muscles are closed.
14. Subcutaneous tissues and skin are closed.
15. A large retention stitch ("Grillo stitch") may be placed from the mandibular skin and periosteum to the sternal skin and periosteum with the patient's head in a flexed position in order to keep the head in this position in the postoperative period in order to reduce tension on the tracheal repair.
16. The patient may then be extubated when awake and able to protect his/her airway. This should be done in the operating room with both anesthesiologist and surgeon present in the untoward event that airway obstruction and subsequent reintubation or surgical management is required.
17. In extended procedures such as cricotracheal resections, a tracheotomy inferior to the repair site may be performed if laryngeal patency is in question.
18. If the procedure has been prolonged or significant edema of the airway is suspected, intubation over 24 hours with subsequent controlled extubation may be performed.

In the postoperative period, several potential problems must be actively monitored for and managed. Minor wound complications such as hematoma, seroma, or wound infection are rare, but they may become major complications if there is wound disruption of the tracheal repair itself. Earlier tracheal disruption may manifest with wound crepitance, extended neck and chest crepitance, and in its most extreme forms, pneumomediastinum and pneumothorax. This may require opening of the wound with placement of a drain, tracheal repair or tracheotomy, and chest tube placement. Late disruption is more likely to occur subsequent to wound infection and may require incision and drainage and possible tracheotomy placement depending on the severity of the wound and the airway condition. The second most serious condition is the development of tracheal granulation tissue. Suture granulation/granuloma occurring at the suture line may require bronchoscopy and removal either mechanically or by laser with possible adjuncts such as dilation, steroid injection, or topical application of substances such as mitomycin-c. In severe cases, stent placement or tracheotomy may be considered. Complication rates in experienced hands range from 17% to approximately 30%. Long-term restenosis is uncommon occurring at 1% to 14% of cases. The management of restenosis may require re-resection of the stenotic segment, endoscopic management with or without stenting, or placement of a tracheotomy (16,17).

Multiple surgical series have demonstrated that the overall survival of these rare tumors is best accomplished with surgical resection (16–18). Adenoid cystic carcinomas fare better than squamous cell carcinomas, which have as a category the worst prognosis. Negative surgical margins at the

	TABLE 126.3	TRACHEA SURVIVAL		
Tumor Type	5-Y Overall Survival (%)	5-Y Disease-Free Survival (%)		Sources
Adenoid cystic	31.6	47.4–77.9		9,10
Squamous	6	29		9
Other	19–90	38–90		7,9
Overall	21	27		9

time of resection predict improved disease-free and overall survival for all malignant tumors (19). Application of adjuvant radiotherapy may improve survival for all squamous cell carcinomas and for other tumors with microscopic residual disease (17–19). Carcinoid tumors, sarcomas, and mucoepidermoid carcinomas demonstrate survival in excess of 78% with complete resection in experienced centers (18). Without surgical resection, long-term survival for malignant tracheal tumors is dismal (16–19). Extension of squamous cell carcinomas of the trachea into the thyroid or the regional lymphatics is a poor prognosticator, diminishing overall survival by more than 50% (20). (See Table 126.3 Survival For Malignant Tracheal Tumors for a summary of survivorship for common tracheal malignancies.)

Cricotracheal Resection

Cricotracheal resections may be appropriate for selected subglottic laryngeal tumors as well as proximal extension of primary tracheal tumors. This is most commonly applied for subglottic tumors that may have tracheal extension, for example, chondrosarcomas arising from the cricoid cartilage (21). Contraindications to cricotracheal resection included involvement of the true vocal cord and/or arytenoid. Tumor extension beyond the airway to involve the mediastinal vasculature or prevertebral fascia represents additional contraindications. The execution of a cricotracheal resection is similar to tracheal resection in terms of exposure and precautions regarding the length of resection. In addition, all or portion of the cricoid may be removed. Removal of the anterior cricoid represents a relatively technically easy exercise. The posterior cricoid is both taller vertically and thicker. Care must be taken in removing the posterior cricoid to avoid resection or damage to the arytenoid cartilages and to avoid inadvertent entry into the esophagus. Closure is accomplished by circumferential tracheal suture with suspension to the fibrous-mucosal cuff posteriorly and to the thyroid cartilage superiorly. If the thyroid cartilage is calcified, drilling holes with a surgical drill facilitates the placement of these suspension sutures (5,20,22). In experienced hands, successful airway patency without tracheotomy may be obtained in over 90% of patients (17).

Distally Extended Resections

Extended resections distally in the trachea may involve resection of segments of trachea greater than 4 cm, resections of the trachea with one mainstem bronchus, carinal resections, or resections combined with pneumonectomy. These extended thoracic procedures may be approached through median sternotomy, thoracotomy, or combinations depending on the extent of resection and if pneumonectomy is included. Some of these extended resections may require cardiopulmonary bypass (23,24). Overall 1-, 2-, and 3-year survivals in these extended tracheobronchial resections for malignancy are approximately 98%, 54%, and 50% (24). The majority of extended resections are reconstructed with tracheobronchoplasties that are tailored to the specific resection (23–25). Other reconstructive methods and tracheal replacement methods have also been described for extended tracheobronchial resections including the use of flaps (pectoralis major flap and engineered radial forearm) and aortic homografts (25–27).

Laryngeal–Tracheal Resections with Permanent Stoma

Some tracheal tumors with extensive laryngeal framework involvement, recurrent laryngeal nerve involvement, and significant laryngeal dysfunction may require laryngectomy, laryngopharyngectomy, or laryngopharyngoesophagectomy; in these cases, mediastinal resections with flap reconstruction, innominate artery mobilization, and management and creation of a mediastinal tracheostoma may be indicated. Overall survival at 3 and 5 years for these types of resections is approximately 57% and 43% (28).

Lymph Node Management

The role of lymphadenectomy in primary tracheal tumors is controversial. Obviously involved, resectable paratracheal and mediastinal nodes should be removed. In the case of the clinically uninvolved neck, the role of elective removal of paratracheal lymph nodes is less well understood. The presence of positive lymph nodes does not appear to adversely affect prognosis; however, over 80% of patients with pathologically positive lymph nodes have also received adjuvant radiation therapy in addition to resection (29).

ENDOSCOPIC AND NONOPERATIVE MANAGEMENT

Debulking and Stents

Tumor debulking is a good initial diagnostic and temporary therapeutic endeavor. Given comorbidities, the management may precede other nonsurgical interventions such as radiation therapy. Debulking can occur by mechanical removal, laser ablation, and cryoablation. These methods can provide in general short-term relief of airway obstruction, but are otherwise palliative rather than definitive treatment (30). Stents may be applied following biopsy or debulking procedures as a temporizing measure preceding definitive resection or as a means of extending palliative relief of airway obstruction. Stents may be placed by means of flexible bronchoscopy for metal-based stents or rigid bronchoscopy for metal or other plastic polymer stents. Additionally, drug-eluting stents have been used in the context of both benign and malignant airway stenosis management (1,30–35). Complications occurring most frequently with airway stent use include mucous plugging, stent displacement, granulation tissue formation, and rarely erosion (30,34). It is important to emphasize that although stents are used in the management of the airway for patients with tracheal tumors, with or without adjuvant therapies such as radiation, when complete tumor resection is feasible, it is the preferred management due to better long-term airway patency and oncologic outcomes (4,5).

Radiation Therapy

Radiation therapy may be utilized as either a primary or adjunctive modality in the treatment of tracheal neoplasms. Radiation may be delivered through external beam or brachytherapy techniques. In large series, upwards of 50% of patients receive radiation in addition to definitive surgical management (34). Indications for adjuvant external beam irradiation therapy include positive surgical margins, high-grade histopathology, lymphatic involvement, perineural invasion, and invasion that extends outside of the airway (18,36). External beam radiation therapy may be delivered to airway neoplasms using a variety of sources, energies, and techniques. Hypofractionated tomotherapy allows for three-dimensional coverage of at-risk areas following surgical resection and may limit dose to the esophagus and surrounding trachea, lung, and mediastinum and therefore lessen the side effects of radiation (37). Primary external beam irradiation therapy may be applied as primary therapy in patients who are not suitable candidates for surgical resection. The radiation therapy may be delivered with electrons or neutrons. Ideal fractionation and dosing has not been established. Fast neutron beam irradiation therapy for adenoid cystic carcinoma in median doses of 19.2 Gy offers actuarial 5-year overall survival of 54% with or without an endobronchial brachytherapy boost with [192]iridium. Neutrons may be superior to electrons in these minor salivary gland cancers (38). Neutron radiation therapy is not as widely available, however, and may not differ significantly with electrons with endobronchial brachytherapy boost. External beam irradiation therapy may also play a role in increasing locoregional control in patients with well-differentiated thyroid cancers that have required shave excisions from the airway (51% with radiation vs. 8% without) (39). However, segmental resection and reanastamosis of the involved airway may provide superior control in well-differentiated thyroid cancers. In general, endoluminal or full-thickness involvement of the airway by well-differentiated thyroid cancers should be managed with segmental resections of the airway or laryngectomy and addition of adjuvant irradiation therapy (40,41). Endobronchial brachytherapy may be administered as a boost to external beam irradiation as discussed above or may be utilized as a largely palliative modality to limit endoluminal tumor growth in tracheal malignancy. Endobronchial brachytherapy requires special expertise, and while it may temporarily enhance tumor control, it may also be complicated by serious hemoptysis due to vascular erosion (30,42,43).

Chemotherapy

The role, either adjunctive or palliative, of chemotherapy in the management of tracheal malignancy is poorly defined. Unlike laryngeal cancer, there are no multicenter clinical trial results that define the role of combined radiation and chemotherapy for organ preservation. In unresectable or certain aggressive neoplasms such as basaloid squamous cancer of the trachea, concomitant chemotherapy and irradiation therapy may represent a possible management strategy (44).

PATHOLOGY

Tracheal tumors are uncommon with an overall incidence of 0.2 per 100,000 persons per year, and 80% of these neoplasms are malignant. Primary tumors originate most frequently from the epithelium or glandular tissues of the trachea. Squamous cell carcinomas and adenoid cystic carcinomas are the most common, occurring in equal proportions. These two carcinomas have been reported to represent between two-thirds and three-fourths of tracheal neoplasms (6,45). There are numerous additional benign and malignant neoplasms that have been described, and this group of heterogeneous lesions comprises the remaining one-fourth to one-third of tracheal tumors (Table 126.1) (6,7,18,29,45). Tracheal tumors occur equally among men and women; however, squamous cell carcinoma affects men at least twice as often as women. Adenoid cystic carcinoma occurs equally between men and women. A history of smoking tobacco is associated with squamous cell carcinoma, but not with adenoid cystic carcinoma. In a retrospective chart review of malignant tracheal neoplasms by Webb et al. (18), 75 patients with malignant tracheal neoplasms were identified, and there was a strong correlation between smoking and squamous cell carcinoma, but not adenoid cystic carcinoma.

Squamous Cell Carcinoma

This very aggressive epithelial malignancy can be ulcerative or exophytic. Arising from the surface respiratory epithelium, squamous cell carcinomas can occur throughout the entire trachea, and have been known to invade surrounding structures in the neck and mediastinum. Squamous cell carcinoma of the trachea is notorious for rapid growth and early regional lymph node metastasis. Synchronous or metachronous lesions are common (30% to 40%) and occur most frequently in the lung, larynx, and oropharynx, regions where smoking-related neoplasms are also common (45).

Adenoid Cystic Carcinoma

Adenoid cystic carcinoma arises from the minor salivary gland epithelium within the trachea, and they are usually indolent in their presentation and course. One study reviewed 208 patients with tracheal tumors and found that those with adenoid cystic carcinoma had symptoms three times as long as patients with squamous cell carcinoma (29). There is low risk for regional lymph node involvement; however, perineural invasion and hematogenous metastasis are encountered frequently. These tumors tend to displace surrounding structures rather than invade them. Hematogenous metastasis occurs in approximately 50% of patients and most commonly involves the lungs (46). Recurrence after definitive primary treatment is common and occurs at an average of 51 months compared to 18 months for other tracheal tumors (29).

Secondary Tracheal Tumors

Tumors from adjacent structures can invade the cervical or thoracic trachea. Cervical trachea invasion can occur from well-differentiated thyroid carcinoma, anaplastic thyroid carcinoma, cervical esophageal cancers, and advanced metastatic cervical lymph node disease. Thoracic trachea involvement can result from lung carcinoma, as well as esophageal and mediastinal lymph node disease similar to the cervical trachea.

Although death from thyroid cancer is the exception rather than the rule, when it does occur, tracheal invasion with airway obstruction and bleeding is the cause over 50% of the time (47). Invasion is often identified at the time of thyroidectomy unless luminal invasion has occurred with resulting airway symptoms. Management of tracheal invasion from thyroid carcinoma depends on the extent of invasion, histology, and patient-related factors. Early invasion can be addressed by shaving the tumor from the trachea with the expectation that adjuvant radiotherapy will be given postoperatively. Although controversial, tracheal resection with primary reanastamosis is also an option especially in advanced cases of invasion with intraluminal involvement and may offer more robust disease control (48). Invasion of the trachea or carina can occur from direct extension of a bronchogenic lung cancer. Resection is recommended if there is no regional lymph node involvement or distant metastasis. Tracheal invasion from esophageal carcinoma or metastatic lymph node disease should be considered unresectable, and nonsurgical therapy and palliation is recommended.

Metastatic Tumors

Metastatic tumors of the trachea have been reported and are most commonly from breast cancer, colon cancer, and cutaneous melanoma. Metastasis from renal cell carcinomas, adrenal gland tumors, and testicular cancers has also been described. As with any metastatic disease, prognosis is poor, and palliative treatment is recommended.

HIGHLIGHTS

- Tracheal neoplasms, either benign or malignant, are rare.
- Early biopsy, careful endoscopic mapping, and endoscopic debulking help establish both the airway and diagnosis.
- Prior to definitive management, imaging with CT, MRI, or PET–CT may be helpful in determining extent of disease, lymph node involvement, or extension of tumor outside of the airway.
- Segmental resection of the airway is preferable to nonsurgical or endoscopic management only.
- Extended resections such as cricotracheal resection, laryngotracheal resections with mediastinal tracheostoma, and tracheocarinal resections may be necessary in advanced tumors.
- Adjuvant radiation therapy is helpful in reducing locoregional recurrence in malignant tracheal tumors that have positive resection margins, high-grade histopathology, lymphatic involvement, and perineural invasion.
- In patients in which tumors are not resectable, endoscopic debulking with laser, radiofrequency ablation, or cryotherapy or by mechanical means and placement of airway stents may be helpful in palliation and airway protection.
- External beam radiation, with either electrons or neutrons, along with endobronchial brachytherapy may be used in the treatment of unresectable malignant tracheal tumors.
- The role of chemotherapy, especially in combination with radiotherapy, is emerging, but is poorly characterized. Squamous cell carcinoma is the predominant histopathology and is aggressive with frequent nodal metastasis.
- Adenoid cystic carcinoma is also relatively common and is less aggressive than squamous cell carcinoma and is more likely to exhibit perineural and hematogenous spread. A myriad group of tumors may present in the trachea, which makes accurate biopsy and diagnosis of paramount importance prior to instituting treatment.

REFERENCES

1. Gaissert HA, Mark EJ. Tracheobronchial gland tumors. *Cancer Control* 2006;13(4):286–294.
2. Hoerbelt R, Padberg W. Primary tracheal tumors of the neck and mediastinum: resection and reconstruction procedures. *Chirurg* 2011;82(2):125–133.
3. Honings J, Gaissert HA, van der Heijden HF, et al. Clinical aspects and treatment of primary tracheal malignancies. *Acta Otolaryngol* 2010;130(7):763–772.
4. Honings J, Gaissert HA, Verhagen AF, et al. Undertreatment of tracheal carcinoma: multidisciplinary audit of epidemiologic data. *Ann Surg Oncol* 2009;16(2):246–253.
5. Zhengjaiang L, Pingzhang T, Dechao Z, et al. Primary tracheal tumours: 21 years of experience at Peking Union Medical College, Beijing, China. *J Laryngol Otol* 2008;122(11):1235–1240.
6. Grillo HC, Mathisen DJ. Primary tracheal tumors: treatment and results. *Ann Thorac Surg* 1990;49:69.
7. Gaissert A, Grillo HC, Shadmehr MC, et al. Uncommon primary tracheal tumors. *Ann Thorac Surg* 2006;82:268.
8. Gaissert HA. Primary tracheal tumours. *Chest Surg Clin North Am* 2003;13:247–256.
9. Gaissert HA, Grillo H, Mathisen DJ, et al. Long-term survival after resection of primary adenoid cystic and squamous cell carcinoma of the trachea and carina. *Ann Thorac Surg* 2004;78:1889–1897.
10. Wood DE. Management of malignant tracheobronchial obstruction. *Surg Clin North Am* 2002;82:621–642.
11. Ferretti GR, Bithigoffer C, Righini CA, et al. Imaging of tumors of the trachea and central bronchi. *Radiol Clin North Am* 2009;47(2):227–241.
12. Koletsis EN, Kalogeropoulou C, Prodromaki E, et al. Tumoral and non-tumoral trachea stenoses: evaluation with three-dimensional CT and virtual bronchoscopy. *J Cardiothorac Surg* 2007;2:18.
13. Park CM, Goo JM, Lee HJ, et al. Tumors in the tracheobronchial tree: CT and FDG PET features. *Radiographics* 2009;29(1):55–71.
14. Wood DE. Bronchoscopic preparation for airway resection. *Chest Surg Clin N Am* 2001;11:735–748.
15. Honings J, van Dijck JA, Verhagen AF, et al. Incidence and treatment of tracheal cancer: a nationwide study in the Netherlands. *Ann Surg Oncol* 2007;14(2):968–976.
16. Gaissert HA, Grillo HC, Shadmehr MB, et al. Uncommon primary tracheal tumors. *Ann Thorac Surg* 2006;82(1):268–272; discussion 272–273.
17. Amorós JM, Ramos R, Villalonga R, et al. Tracheal and cricotracheal resection for laryngotracheal stenosis: experience in 54 consecutive cases. *Eur J Cardiothorac Surg* 2006;29(1):35–39.
18. Webb BD, Walsh GL, Roberts DB, et al. Primary tracheal malignant neoplasms: the University of Texas MD Anderson Cancer Center experience. *J Am Coll Surg* 2006;202(2):237–246.
19. Shadmehr MB, Farzanegan R, Graili P, et al. Primary major airway tumors; management and results. *Eur J Cardiothorac Surg* 2011;39(5):749–754.
20. Honings J, Gaissert HA, Ruangchira-Urai R, et al. Pathologic characteristics of resected squamous cell carcinoma of the trachea: prognostic factors based on an analysis of 59 cases. *Virchows Arch* 2009;455(5):423–429.
21. Obeso S, Llorente JL, Díaz-Molina JP, et al. Surgical treatment of head and neck chondrosarcomas. *Acta Otorrinolaringol Esp* 2010;61(4):262–271.
22. Hong P, Taylor SM, Trites JR, et al. Chondrosarcoma of the head and neck: report of 11 cases and literature review. *J Otolaryngol Head Neck Surg* 2009;38(2):279–285.
23. Parissis H, Young V. Carinal surgery: experience of a single center and review of the current literature. *J Cardiothorac Surg* 2010;5:51.
24. Liu FY, Liu XY, Wang Z, et al. The long-term outcome and prognostic analysis of surgically treated patients with trachea tumors. *Zhonghua Wai Ke Za Zhi* 2009;47(14):1055–1057.
25. He J, Xu X, Chen M, et al. Novel method to repair tracheal defect by pectoralis major myocutaneous flap. *Ann Thorac Surg* 2009;88(1):288–291.
26. Maciejewski A, Szymczyk C, Półtorak S, et al. Tracheal reconstruction with the use of radial forearm free flap combined with biodegradative mesh suspension. *Ann Thorac Surg* 2009;87(2):608–610.

27. Anoosh F, Hodjati H, Dehghani S, et al. Tracheal replacement by autogenous aorta. *J Cardiothorac Surg* 2009;4:23.

28. Conti M, Benhamed L, Mortuaire G, et al. Indications and results of anterior mediastinal tracheostomy for malignancies. *Ann Thorac Surg* 2010;89(5):1588–1595.

29. Regnard JF, Fourquier P, Levasseur P. Results and prognostic factors in resections of primary tracheal tumors: a multicenter retrospective study. The French Society of Cardiovascular Surgery. *J Thorac Cardiovasc Surg* 1996;111(4):808–813, discussion 813–814.

30. Chhajed PN, Somandin S, Baty F, et al. Therapeutic bronchoscopy for malignant airway stenoses: choice of modality and survival. *J Cancer Res Ther* 2010;6(2):204–209.

31. Saueressig MG, Sanches PR, Macedo Neto AV, et al. Novel silicone stent to treat tracheobronchial lesions: results of 35 patients. *Asian Cardiovasc Thorac Ann* 2010;18(6):521–528.

32. Kirsner KM, Sarkiss M, Brydges GJ. Treatment of tracheal and bronchial tumors and tracheal and bronchial stent placement. *AANA J* 2010;78(5):413–419.

33. Kim WK, Shin JH, Kim JH, et al. Management of tracheal obstruction caused by benign or malignant thyroid disease using covered retrievable self-expandable nitinol stents. *Acta Radiol* 2010;51(7):768–774.

34. Lee P, Kupeli E, Mehta AC. Airway stents. *Clin Chest Med* 2010;31(1):141–150.

35. Chin CS, Litle V, Yun J, et al. Airway stents. *Ann Thorac Surg* 2008;85(2):S792–S796.

36. Honings J, Gaissert HA, Weinberg AC, et al. Prognostic value of pathologic characteristics and resection margins in tracheal adenoid cystic carcinoma. *Eur J Cardiothorac Surg* 2010;37(6):1438–1444.

37. Alongi F, Di Muzio N, Motta M, et al. Adenoid cystic carcinoma of trachea treated with adjuvant hypofractionated tomotherapy. Case report and literature review. *Tumori* 2008;94(1):121–125.

38. Bittner N, Koh WJ, Laramore GE, et al. Treatment of locally advanced adenoid cystic carcinoma of the trachea with neutron radiotherapy. *Int J Radiat Oncol Biol Phys* 2008;72(2):410–414.

39. Keum KC, Suh YG, Koom WS, et al. The role of postoperative external-beam radiotherapy in the management of patients with papillary thyroid cancer invading the trachea. *Int J Radiat Oncol Biol Phys* 2006;65(2):474–480.

40. Ark N, Zemo S, Nolen D, et al. Management of locally invasive well-differentiated thyroid cancer. *Surg Oncol Clin N Am* 2008;17(1):145–155, ix.

41. Price DL, Wong RJ, Randolph GW. Invasive thyroid cancer: management of the trachea and esophagus. *Otolaryngol Clin North Am* 2008;41(6):1155–1168, ix–x.

42. Becker HD. Endobronchial treatment of malignant airway obstructions. *Dtsch Med Wochenschr* 2009;134(10):454–460.

43. Matsumoto I, Oda M, Imagawa T, et al. Management of tracheobronchial ulceration induced by high-dose brachytherapy. *Ann Thorac Surg* 2009;87(4):1301–1303.

44. Joshi NP, Haresh KP, Das P, et al. Unresectable basaloid squamous cell carcinoma of the trachea treated with concurrent chemoradiotherapy: a case report with review of literature. *J Cancer Res Ther* 2010;6(3):321–323.

45. Macchiarini P. Primary tracheal tumours. *Lancet Oncol* 2006;7:83–91.

46. Azar T, Abdul-Karim FW, Tucker HM. Adenoid cystic carcinoma of the trachea. *Laryngoscope* 1998;108:1297–1300.

47. Honings J, Stephen AE, Marres HA, et al. The management of thyroid carcinoma invading the larynx or trachea. *Laryngoscope* 2010;120:682.

48. Hammoud ZT, Mathisen DJ. Surgical management of thyroid carcinoma invading the trachea. *Chest Surg Clin N Am* 2003;13:359.

Vascular Tumors of the Head and Neck

127

Mark Persky   **Spiros Manolidis**

Vascular tumors of the head and neck consist of a variety of different entities that are unrelated to each other. This chapter focuses on acquired vascular tumors that present vexing clinical problems. Based on Batsakis classification of vascular tumors, a differentiation can be made: tumors that are congenital and/or arise on behalf of syndromes and those that are acquired (Table 127.1). This chapter focuses on acquired tumors.

PARAGANGLIA AND PARAGANGLIOMAS

Anatomy and Physiology of the Paraganglia

Paraganglia are part of a system of cell clusters that facilitate the baroreceptive and chemoreceptive reflexes of the cardiovascular system. They are diffusely distributed throughout the upper body. They contain cells that are capable of secreting neuropeptides that have the capability to influence vascular reflexes.

These structures are part of the diffuse neuroendocrine system that are derived from neural crest origin cells. Neural crest derivatives, produce the C cell of the thyroid gland, the melanocyte, and the paraganglia. Paraganglia are found in the adrenal medulla or diffusely distributed as the extra-adrenal paraganglia (1,2).

The latter, the diffusely distributed extra-adrenal paraganglia are divided into branchiomeric paraganglia and vagal paraganglia. The branchiomeric paraganglia are distributed along arteries and cranial nerves in the head and neck. The jugulotympanic paraganglia arise from the second branchial arch while the carotid paraganglia arise from the third branchial arch. The intravagal paraganglia do not follow this embryologic pharyngeal pouch distribution and are thus classified separately. Even so, unusual paraganglioma locations have been recorded that do not fit this classification: larynx, orbit, thyroid, nasal cavity, and sinuses as well as intracranial (3) (Fig. 127.1).

The carotid body is a chemoreceptor that senses changes in arterial oxygen pressure, pH, and carbon dioxide. Along with the cardiac and aortic bodies, these are the only chemoreceptors in the paraganglia. The carotid body is a discrete oval structure situated behind the carotid bifurcation and receives its blood supply directly from the carotid bifurcation via the glomic arteries. The afferent reflex is mediated by a branch of the glossopharyngeal nerve (nerve of Hering) (4) (Fig. 127.2).

The jugulotympanic paraganglia are distributed within the temporal bone in close association with the tympanic branch of the glossopharyngeal nerve (Jacobson nerve) and the auricular branch of the vagus nerve (Arnold nerve). The majority of the temporal bone paraganglia are located in the jugular fossa and the rest are located in the bony canal that transmits Jacobson nerve or in the submucosa of the tympanic cavity. There is a marked difference in the clinical behavior of tumors arising from the jugular paraganglia versus the tympanic paraganglia. This has significant therapeutic implications (5) (Fig. 127.3).

The vagal paraganglia are distinctly different from the jugulotympanic paraganglia. They do not form discrete bodies and are incorporated within the vagus nerve underneath the perineurium or interspersed within the vagal nerve fibers in the pars nervosa of the jugular foramen (which transmits the lower cranial nerves IX, X, and XI). The superior vagal ganglion is found at the level of the jugular foramen. The nodose vagal ganglion lies just below the jugular foramen. Both ganglia are in close proximity to cranial nerves IX through XII, the pars venosa of the jugular foramen, as well as the ascending portion of the petrous internal carotid artery (6). Thus vagal paragangliomas have distinct therapeutic implications based on their close association with the superior portion of the vagal nerve and their adjacent neurovascular structures.

The microanatomy of normal paraganglia is that of clusters that contain chief cells (type I cells) surrounded by

TABLE 127.1	CLASSIFICATION OF VASCULAR TUMORS OF THE HEAD AND NECK		
Congenital	Localized		Hemangioma
			Lymphangioma
			Hemangiolymphoma
	Generalized		Angiomatosis
			Cystic hygroma
Inflammatory			Arterio-venous malformation
			Aneurism
			Phlebectasia
Syndromic			Osler-Weber-Rendu
			Sturge-Weber
			Maffucci
			von Hippel-Lindau
Acquired benign	APUD		Paraganglioma
			Carotid
			Vagus
			Larynx
			Jugular
			Tympanic
			Aortic
Acquired malignant			Angiosarcoma
Acquired indeterminate			Hemangiopericytoma

sustentacular cells (type II). These clusters are interspersed by a web of blood vessels. The equivalent structures seen in paragangliomas are termed Zellballen, which retain part of this structural arrangement. The sustentacular cells do not secrete catecholamines and are similar in nature to the Schwann cells enveloping autonomic ganglia. The chief cells have abundant secretory granules, a characteristic of secreting cells. The biochemistry of paraganglia chief cells is characterized by catecholamine production (7). This sequence is characterized by enzymatic conversion of tyrosine to dopamine, norepinephrine, and epinephrine. Extra-adrenal paraganglia lack methyltransferase that is required for the conversion of

norepinephrine to epinephrine. The metabolic breakdown of catecholamines to metanephrine (from epinephrine) and normetanephrine (from norepinephrine) as well as vanillyl-mandelic acid (VMA) can be detected in the urine. Actively secreting paragangliomas can be thus detected with appropriate urine and serum analysis (Fig. 127.4).

Paraganglioma Epidemiology and Pathophysiology

Paragangliomas are neoplasms of the paraganglia. Paragangliomas of the head and neck are rare tumors, comprising about 1 in 10,000 of all tumors in the head and neck area excluding intracranial tumors. The annual incidence of extra-adrenal paragangliomas is estimated at 1 in 300,000 (8). Carotid body tumors and jugulotympanic tumors account for approximately 80% of these, and vagal paragangliomas add another 5%. Significant referral pattern distortions make these numbers less reliable. Multiple paragangliomas are present in up to 22% of all patients with a paraganglioma, and these are frequently hereditary in nature with a family history of such tumors. Approximately 10% of sporadic cases will have a concurrent second paraganglioma. Multiple tumors may be metachronous, and this has implications for surveillance of patients with a paraganglioma. The most common pattern of a synchronous secondary paraganglioma is a second carotid body tumor, which is present in 20% of carotid body tumors. Bilateral carotid body tumors as well as an additional paraganglioma ipsilaterally or contralaterally present significant and challenging treatment problems due to the potential for cranial nerve deficits and loss in baroreceptor function, which results in labile hypertension (9–11).

Other than genetics, the only known predisposition for a paraganglioma is high-altitude living associated with chronic hypoxemia. Several studies show that there is an increased incidence of these tumors with high-

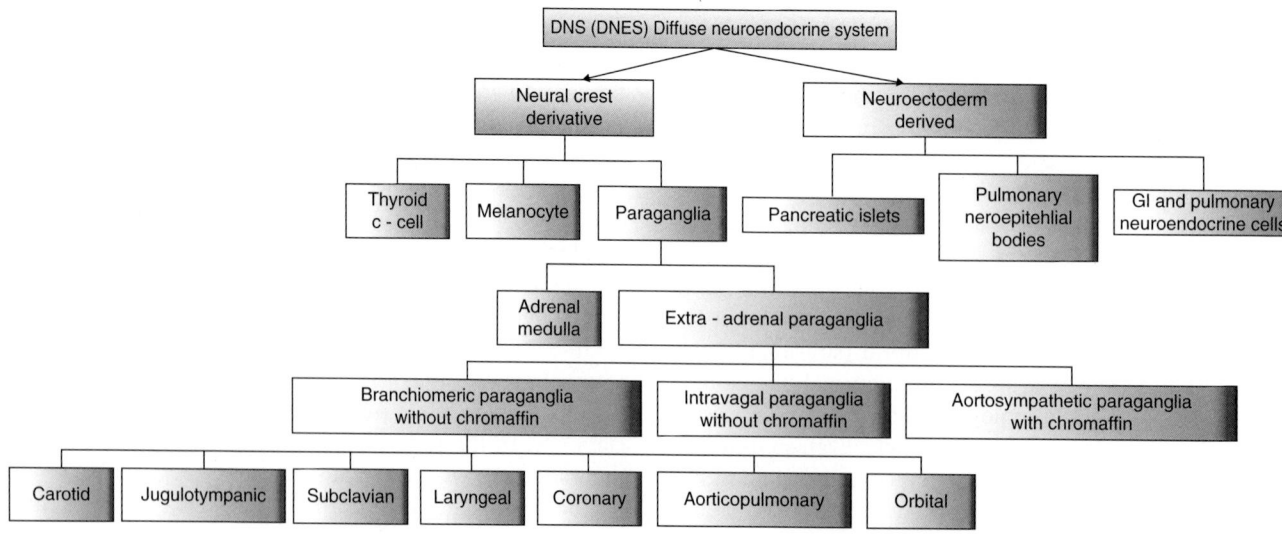

Figure 127.1 Classification of the diffuse neuroendocrine system.

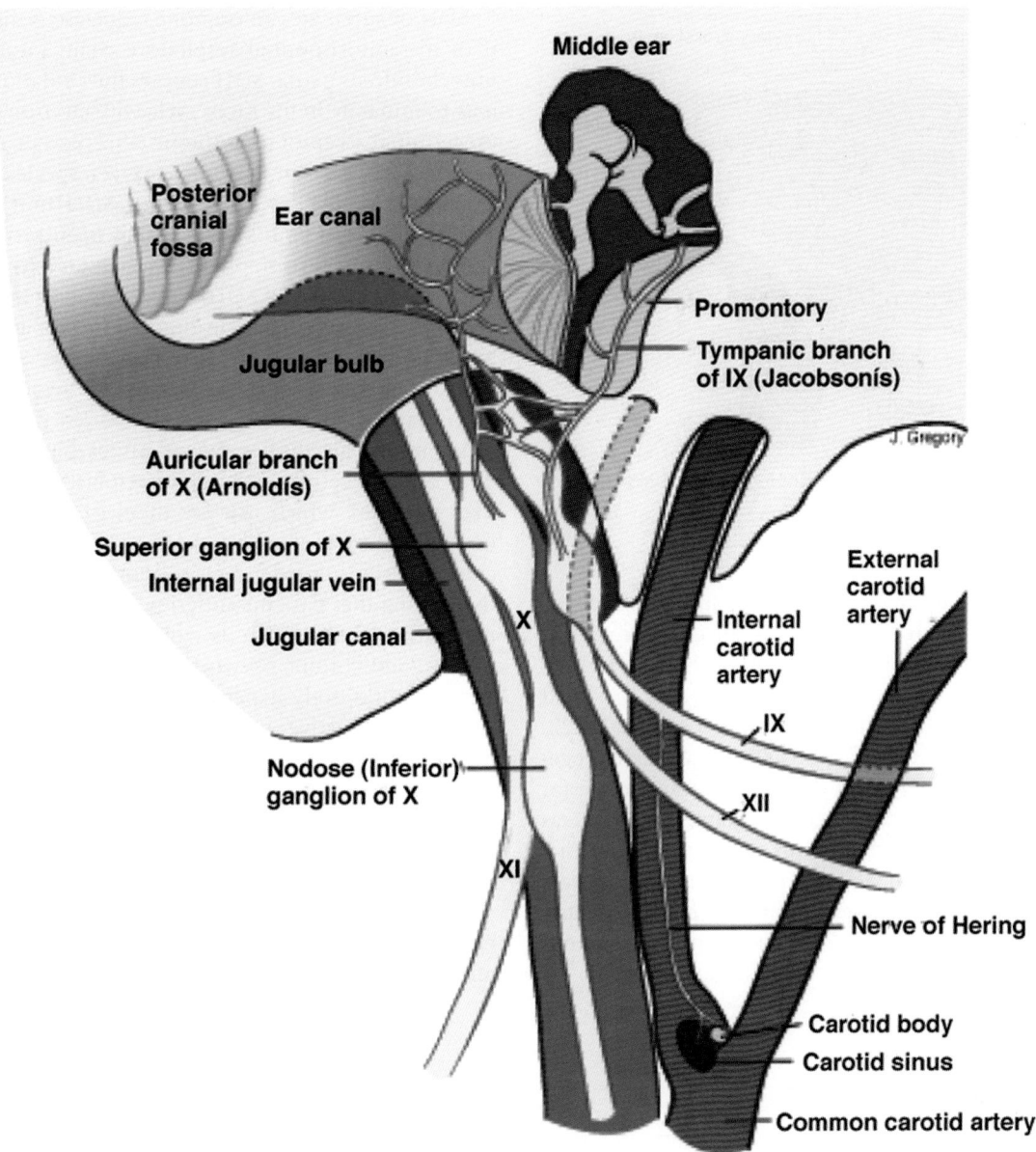

Figure 127.2 Schematic representation of lower cranial nerves at the level of jugular foramen.

altitude living, a ninefold increase for those living between 2 and 3 km and 12-fold increase for those living between 3 and 4.5 km above sea level. Patients forming these tumors at higher altitude show a lower rate of bilaterality and a lesser degree of familial history of paragangliomas (12–14).

Approximately 1% to 3% of paragangliomas secrete catecholamines. A fivefold increase in catecholamines is sufficient to produce symptoms. Secreting paragangliomas account for approximately 2% of all instances of secondary hypertension. Twenty-four–hour urine collection in these patients will show elevated levels of the catecholamine metabolites metanephrine and VMA. Serum catecholamines will show elevated levels of norepinephrine in functioning extra-adrenal paragangliomas. Elevated serum epinephrine is indicative of a concurrent pheochromocytoma (3,15).

Malignant paragangliomas represent a small subset of extra-adrenal paragangliomas that have a propensity for regional lymph nodes and distant metastatic disease, primarily to the lungs, liver, and bones. Sporadic paragangliomas have a higher rate of malignancy than familial-type paragangliomas. PGL4 syndrome is associated with a very high rate of malignancy as high as 54%. The rate of malignancy is site specific. Orbital and laryngeal paragangliomas have the highest rate of malignancy, approximately 25%. Vagal paragangliomas have a malignancy rate of up to 10%, followed by jugulotympanic paragangliomas with a malignancy rate of 5% and carotid body tumors being last at 3% to 6%. There are no histologic criteria by which primary tumor malignancy can be diagnosed. Malignancy is confirmed by tumor present in lymph nodes or distant metastatic sites. The presence of malignancy has profound implications in the treatment of these tumors (16–18).

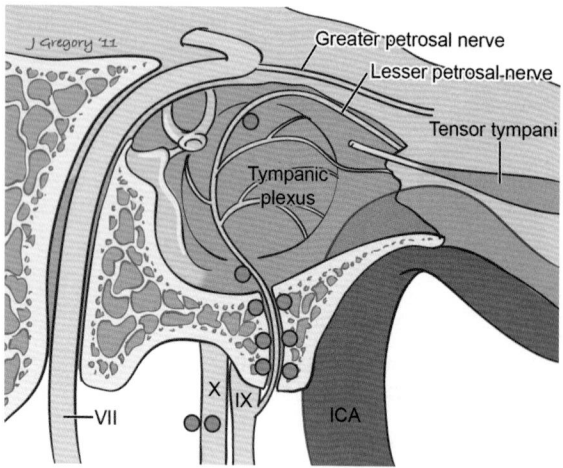

Figure 127.3 Distribution of frequent locations for glomus bodies in the temporal bone.

Genetics

Hereditary susceptibility to paragangliomas, mainly of the head and neck region, was recognized at least two decades ago and led to the identification through linkage analysis of three loci on chromosomes 11 and 1, named PGL1 on 11q23, PGL2 on 11q11.3, and PGL3 on 1q21–23. Following the discovery of SDHD (succinate dehydrogenase [SDH] subunit D gene) as the gene responsible for PGL1 in familial head and neck paragangliomas, it was recognized that two other subunits of this mitochondrial enzyme, SDHC (PGL3) and SDHB (PGL4, 1p36), were associated with heritable pheochromocytoma and/or paraganglioma. To date, the gene for PGL2 has not been identified (12,19–22).

SDH or succinate–ubiquinone reductase is the complex II of the mitochondrial respiratory chain located in the mitochondrial matrix. SDH couples the oxidation of succinate to fumarate in the Krebs cycle with electron transfer to the terminal acceptor ubiquinone. This prevents formation of potentially dangerous reactive oxygen species.

The molecular cascade between SDH mutations and tumor formation is unknown. It has been proposed that SDHD is a critical component of a cellular oxygen-sensing system. Mutations in SDHD may incapacitate the oxygen-sensing mechanism, leading to an apparent or real hypoxic state accompanied by chronic hypoxic stimulation and cell proliferation. Support for hypoxia-induced hyperplasia comes from evidence obtained in high-altitude physiologic studies. Cows, guinea pigs, rabbits, and dogs experience carotid body hyperplasia when living at high altitudes, which exposes them to a hypoxic condition, and this has also been described in humans. Another clinical observation lending support to these theories is the finding that patients suffering from conditions resulting in hypoxemia, such as cystic fibrosis, cyanotic heart disease, and chronic obstructive pulmonary disease experience carotid body hyperplasia and those suffering from chronic obstructive pulmonary disease have a higher rate of carotid body tumors. This relationship between SDHD, SDHC, and SDHB mutations and the oxygen-sensing mechanism, and the cascade of events between these mutations and tumor formation are not completely known (12,13,19–22).

SDH is an enzyme complex composed of four subunits encoded by four nuclear genes (SDHA, SDHB, SDHC, and SDHD). SDHC (cybL, 15 kDa, 169 amino acids) and

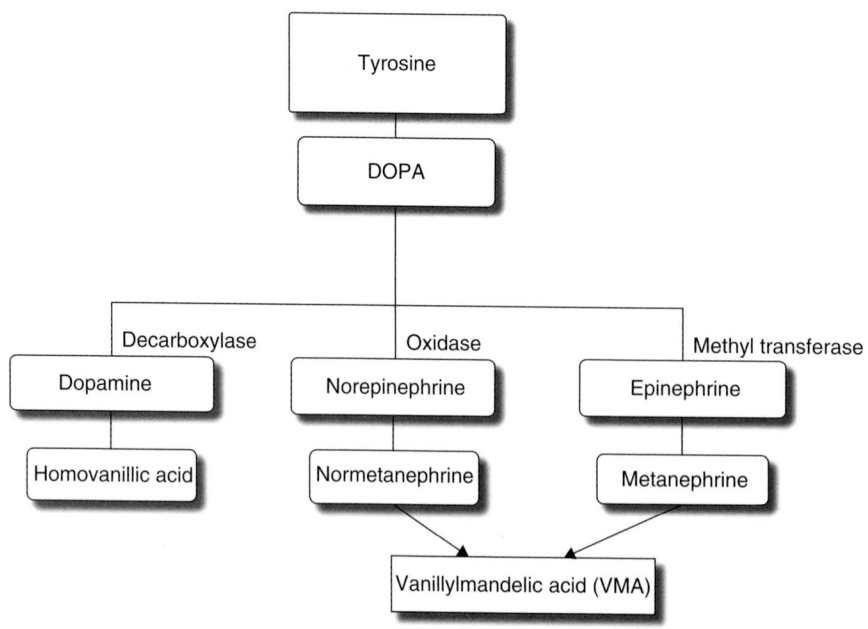

Figure 127.4 Biochemical pathway for catecholamine metabolism.

SDHD (cybS, 12 kDa, 159 amino acids) subunits are hydrophobic and provide membrane anchor and the binding site for ubiquinone. SDHA (flavoprotein, 70 kDa, 664 amino acids) and SDHB (iron–sulfur protein, 27 kDa, 280 amino acids) are hydrophilic with the former involved in substrate binding and oxidation and the latter in electron transfer. Both the SDHB (35.4 kb, 8 exons) and the SDHC (50.3 kb, 6 exons) genes are located on chromosome 1, the short and long arm respectively. The SDHD gene located on 11q23.1 spans 8.9 kb and contains 4 exons while SDHA lies on the short arm of chromosome 5 (5p15) and is composed of 15 exons spread in a genomic region of 38.4 kb. While homozygote germline mutations affecting the SDHA gene cause Leigh syndrome, a subacute necrotizing encephalomyelopathy during infancy, SDHD, SDHB, and SDHC heterozygous mutations cause a genetic predisposition to head and neck paragangliomas and adrenal/extra-adrenal pheochromocytomas (23). This inherited tumorigenic predisposition is transmitted in an autosomal dominant fashion with age-dependent and incomplete penetrance. However, for SDHD located on chromosome 11q, a parent-of-origin effect is apparent as the disease is manifest almost exclusively when the mutation is transmitted from the father. A maternal imprinting has therefore been postulated but despite the pattern of inheritance, SDHD shows bi-allelic expression in normal tissues and neural crest-derived tissues (12,18).

Neurofibromatosis type 1 is also associated with both pheochromocytomas and glomus tumors. Pheochromocytomas are also associated with multiple endocrine neoplasia type II with RET gene mutations, and with von Hippel-Lindau syndrome and mutations in the VHL gene (24).

In cases where successive generations of a family have been harboring the mutations, patients develop tumors at progressively younger ages. This finding is a good example of genetic anticipation, in which the mutation appears to be more severe with succeeding generations.

Familial glomus tumors constitute approximately 20% of affected patients, for which the genetic defects are known. One subgroup (10% of all glomus tumors) appears to be caused by sporadic mutations in SDHB and SDHD. The pathogenesis of the remaining 80% of tumors remains a mystery. Oncology research implicates several processes as important to tumor formation and growth. Two that attract a significant amount of attention are angiogenesis and apoptosis, and these processes have been examined in paragangliomas as well (25).

Angiogenesis is a critical event in the development and sustained growth of several tumor types. Given the vascular nature of paraganglion tissue, questions about the role that angiogenesis plays in the development of paragangliomas.

Vascular endothelial growth factor (VEGF) and platelet-derived endothelial growth factor (PD-ECGF) as well as endothelin-1 have been found in the majority of specimens examined. It has been postulated that this was consistent with a paracrine mechanism for tumor development (26).

Additionally, hypoxia induces expression of hypoxia-inducible factor 1, which participates in the angiogenesis cascade. Pheochromocytomas exhibit ubiquitous hypoxia-inducible factor 1 secondary to mutations resulting in cell hypoxia. This may represent a link between the mutation and tumor development (27).

In summary, the genetic associations in these paraganglioma syndromes are as follows:

- Patients with PGL develop tumors at a younger age than sporadic cases
- Other tumor syndromes: Neurofibromatosis type 1, MEN type 2 and von Hippel-Lindau predispose to paragangliomas
- In PGL 1, 2, and 3, the genetic transmission is autosomal dominant, with highly variable expressivity and reduced penetrance. Genomic imprinting is seen: the paternally transmitted genes lead to tumor development and the maternally transmitted gene gives carrier status without developing tumors
- PGL1 and PGL4 show multicentricity and pheochromocytomas
- PGL4 shows a marked increase in malignant paragangliomas
- PGL3 shows exclusively benign paragangliomas with no multifocality and no association to pheochromocytomas.

Clinical Presentation, Classification

The clinical presentation of paragangliomas is location specific. As these tumors enlarge, they tend to produce cranial neuropathies. Additionally, secreting tumors can produce hypertension, tachycardia, sweating, and nervousness secondary to catecholamine release.

Carotid Body Tumors

Carotid body tumors typically present as a slowly enlarging asymptomatic deep neck mass at the level of the carotid bifurcation. In a small minority of patients, pain is present around the tumor. Because of the association with the carotid artery they are laterally mobile, but rostrocaudally fixed on examination. As the tumor enlarges, a bruit may be auscultated and in addition to a neck mass, a parapharyngeal extension results in the lateral displacement of the soft palate medially and anteriorly. Cranial nerve paralysis symptoms are unusual and present in very large tumors with superior extension toward the jugular foramen. Shamblin classification is commonly used to stage carotid body tumors, and though this is based on intraoperative findings, it can be applied to radiologic findings prior to treatment (Table 127.2, Fig. 127.5).

Jugulotympanic Paragangliomas

Jugular and tympanic paragangliomas occur predominantly in the fifth and sixth decades of life with an overwhelming female predominance. They are slow growing,

TABLE 127.2	SHAMBLIN CLASSIFICATION OF CAROTID BODY TUMORS
Type 1	Relatively small tumor with minimal attachment to the carotid vessels
Type 2	Larger tumor with moderate attachment to carotid vessels but resectable with preservation of the carotid vessels
Type 3	Tumor encases the carotid vessel requiring arterial sacrifice with reconstruction

and their pattern of growth follows the pathways of least resistance in the temporal bone and surrounding skull base structures. In their later stages, both types produce similar symptoms including cranial nerve deficits, while in the early stages tympanic and jugular paragangliomas differ in presentation.

Tympanic paragangliomas present early with pulsatile tinnitus and conductive hearing loss. On otomicroscopic examination, a red–blue middle ear mass that blanches with positive pressure on pneumatic otoscopy is appreciated (Brown sign). With subsequent growth, there is ossicular erosion and filling of the middle ear cleft. Extension through the tympanic membrane will produce an ear canal polypoid mass that may spontaneously cause bloody otorrhea. Extension to the mastoid can occur through a number of pathways. Involvement of the facial nerve, usually in the mastoid, can produce facial paralysis as a presenting symptom. Anterior growth toward the pericarotid air cells can involve the petrous carotid artery and occupy the eustachian tube. Medial growth into the infralabyrinthine air cells can reach the petrous apex and petroclival area as well as cavernous sinus. Intracranial extension is possible through extension through the jugular foramen and/or petrous apex. More infrequently, there is involvement of the otic capsule and the inner ear with attendant sensorineural hearing loss and vertigo at presentation.

Jugular paragangliomas, due to their origin location within the jugular bulb, have the capacity for early and extensive skull base invasion with involvement of cranial nerves 9 through 12. Growth through Jacobson nerve canal and the hypotympanic air cells leads to involvement of the middle ear and mastoid bone leading to conductive hearing loss, tinnitus, and facial paralysis. Intracranial involvement through the jugular foramen is frequent. Erosion of the jugulocarotid spine leads to involvement of the vertical petrous carotid artery, and further anterior extension leads to involvement of the horizontal portion of the petrous carotid artery. More medial extension to the infralabyrinthine air cells lead to involvement of the petrous apex. Further medial extension along this pathway leads to involvement of the clivus and cavernous sinus. Occasionally, jugular paragangliomas will escape the confines of the temporal bone and involve the infratemporal fossa and parapharyngeal space. Lower cranial nerve involvement is frequent and ranges from 38% to 58% (28,29). Multiple cranial nerves are frequently involved with Vernet syndrome (paralysis of cranial nerves 9, 10, and 11) or Collet-Sicard syndrome (paralysis of cranial nerves 9, 10, 11, and 12) in at least 10% of those with jugular paragangliomas (Fig. 127.6). The attendant symptomatology is hoarseness, swallowing difficulty, hemipalatal dysfunction with nasal air escape, shoulder motion restriction, and dysarthria due to tongue hemiparalysis. Two surgical classification systems are in wide use today and can be used preoperatively based on radiographic findings: the Fisch classification system, which makes no distinction between tympanic and jugular paragangliomas and is predicated

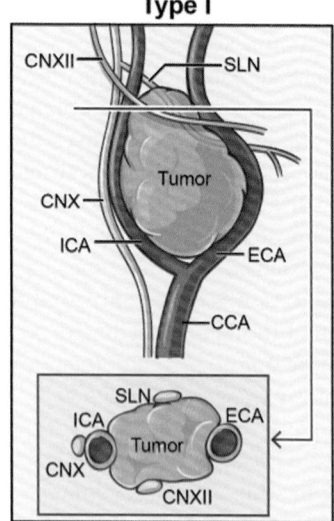
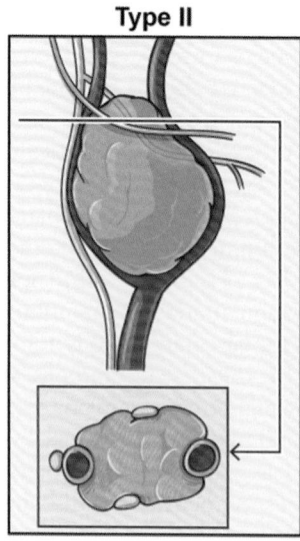
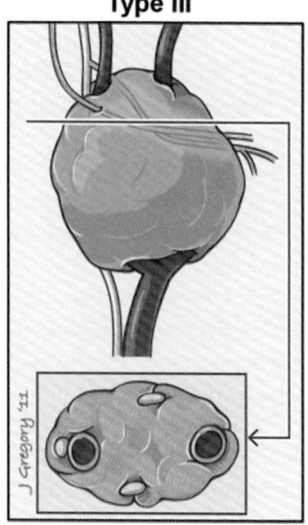

Figure 127.5 Shamblin classification of carotid body tumors.

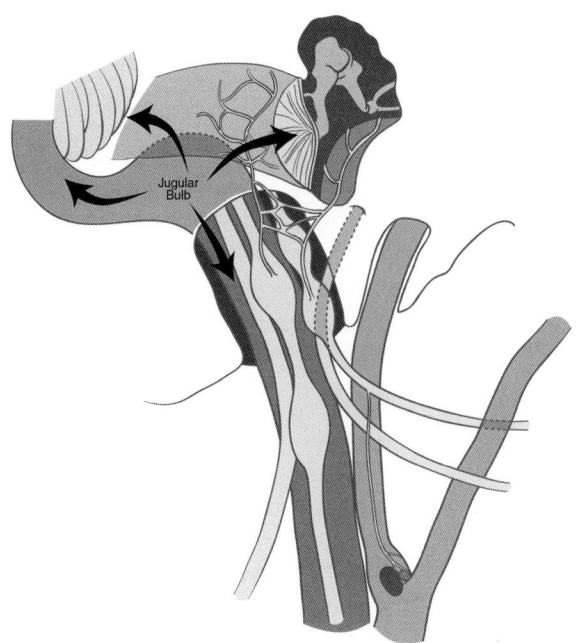

Figure 127.6 Modes of spread for jugular paragangliomas.

on detailed patterns of progressive disease extension, and the Glasscock-Jackson classification system, which treats tympanic and jugular paragangliomas differently (15,28) (Tables 127.3 and 127.4).

Vagal paragangliomas account for 5% of all head and neck paragangliomas and originate in the vagus nerve where the paraganglia are diffusely distributed in the

TABLE 127.3	FISCH CLASSIFICATION OF JUGULOTYMPANIC PARAGANGLIOMAS
Class A	Tumors arising on the tympanic plexus confined to the middle ear
Class B	Tumors arising from the inferior tympanic canal in the hypotympanum with middle ear and/or mastoid invasion, but jugular bulb and carotid canal intact
Class C	Tumors arising in the dome of the jugular bulb and involving the overlying cortical bone
C1	Tumors eroding the carotid canal but not involving the carotid artery
C2	Tumors involving the vertical petrous carotid artery
C3	Tumors involving the horizontal carotid canal but not foramen lacerum
C4	Tumors involving the foramen lacerum and cavernous sinus
Class D	Tumors with intracranial extension
De1	Extradural extension of <2 cm medial dural displacement
De2	Extradural extension of >2 cm medial dural displacement
Di1	Intradural extension of <2 cm
Di2	Intradural extension of >2 cm
Di3	Neurosurgically unresectable tumors

TABLE 127.4	GLASSCOCK-JACKSON CLASSIFICATION OF JUGULOTYMPANIC PARAGANGLIOMAS
Glomus tympanicum	
Type 1	Small mass limited to the promontory
Type 2	Tumor completely filling the middle ear
Type 3	Tumor filling the middle ear and mastoid
Type 4	Tumor completely filling the middle ear, extending into the mastoid or through the external auditory canal. May also extend anteriorly to involve the carotid artery
Glomus jugulare	
Type 1	Small tumor involving the jugular bulb, middle ear, and mastoid
Type 2	Tumor extending under the internal auditory canal. May have intracranial extension
Type 3	Tumor extending to the petrous apex. May have intracranial extension
Type 4	Tumor extending beyond the petrous apex into the clivus or infratemporal fossa. May have intracranial extension.

superior, middle, and inferior vagal ganglia. There is a female preponderance of 3:1. Tumors originating superiorly will often present with a dumbbell appearance with an intracranial component in the posterior cranial fossa. Tumors originating inferiorly will extend into the post-styloid compartment of the parapharyngeal space. Vagal paragangliomas are frequently associated with multiple cranial neuropathies at presentation in up to 50% of patients. The vagus nerve is affected most commonly, followed by the hypoglossal and spinal accessory (30) (Fig. 127.7).

Diagnostic Imaging Studies

Computed Tomography

Computed tomography (CT) with contrast is an excellent imaging choice for the diagnosis and delineation of paragangliomas. Since these tumors are highly vascular, early and intense contrast enhancement is seen. The relation of the tumor to the external and internal carotid arteries, as well as the jugular vein, makes this modality essentially diagnostic (31). The delineation of the pattern of invasion of the temporal bone and skull base is indispensable in treatment and especially preoperative planning for paragangliomas. Carotid body tumors display the characteristic splaying of the internal and external carotid arteries by a well-circumscribed mass occupying the carotid bifurcation. Carotid body tumors displace the internal carotid artery posterolaterally. Vagal paraganliomas typically will displace the internal carotid artery anteriorly and occupy the high parapharyngeal space, with or without involvement of the skull base. Jugulotympanic paragangliomas can be distinguished in their early phases, especially when a tympanic paraganglioma is confined to the tympanic

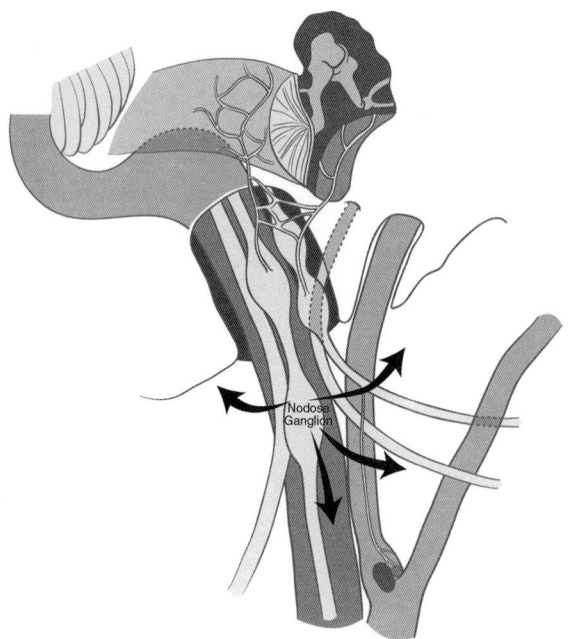

Figure 127.7 Modes of spread for vagal paragangliomas.

cavity. Characteristic patterns of bone destruction occur with jugulotympanic paragangliomas. These include erosion of the jugulotympanic spine, enlargement of the jugular foramen with bone destruction, and involvement of the middle ear and mastoid (31,32). Multiplanar reconstruction of high-resolution CT scans in the axial, sagittal, and coronal planes is of great assistance in the planning of operative management of these tumors. Middle ear and/or eustachian tube involvement will create postobstructive

fluid accumulation in the aerated spaces of the temporal bone, including the mastoid (Fig. 127.8).

Magnetic Resonance Imaging

Magnetic resonance imaging (MRI) is a complementary and equally important imaging modality in the evaluation and treatment of head and neck paragangliomas. MRI with gadolinium contrast serves three purposes: delineation of the tumor in question, surveillance and detection of concurrent paragangliomas of the head and neck, and confirmation of the diagnosis of paraganglioma. The classic, "salt and pepper" appearance of paragangliomas on T2-weighted images is due to the high-flow vascular voids that are essentially pathognomonic. Paragangliomas show intense signal enhancement with gadolinium contrast (33). Fat-suppressed sequences are exceptionally useful in delineating the extent of the tumor. Patterns of carotid artery displacement can be accurately determined distinguishing carotid body tumors from vagal paragangliomas (33). More importantly, in tumors with intracranial extension, intradural versus extradural involvement can be appreciated, and the relationship of the tumor to important intracranial structures can be delineated. Specialized techniques such as MR angiography and contrast time-of-flight three-dimensional angiography increase the sensitivity of the diagnosis of concurrent tumors but do not supplant selective angiography in the preoperative planning setting (34,35) (Figs. 127.9 and 127.10).

Angiography

With the evolution of detailed MRI and CT techniques, angiography plays a much more limited role in the

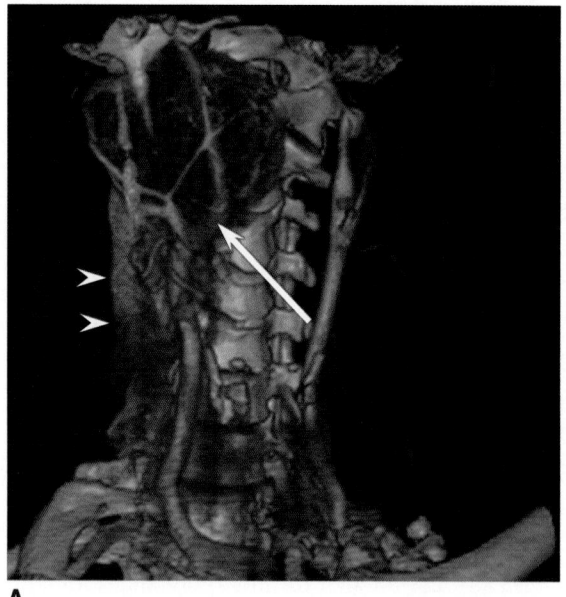

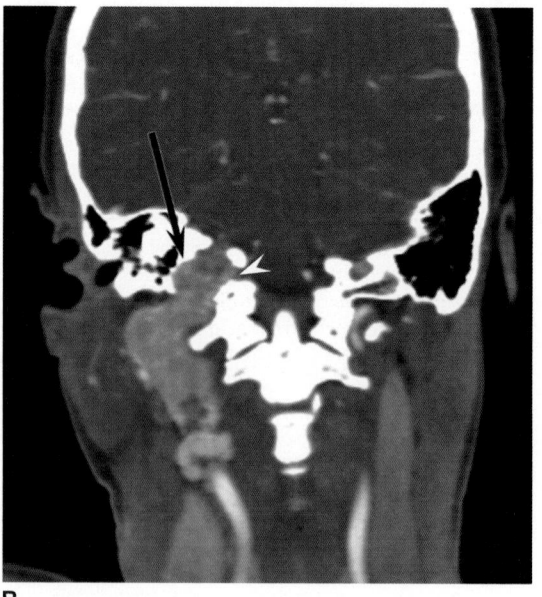

A   **B**

Figure 127.8 CT angiogram of a patient with a large paraganglioma. **A:** Volumetric surface rendering shows anterolateral displacement of the internal carotid artery (*arrow*) and narrowing of its lumen. Note the filling of the internal jugular vein (*arrowheads*) with contrast posterior to the common carotid artery, demonstrating the high flow within this tumor. **B:** Coronal reformat demonstrates involvement of the jugular foramen (*arrow*) as well as the hypoglossal canal (*arrowhead*) by tumor.

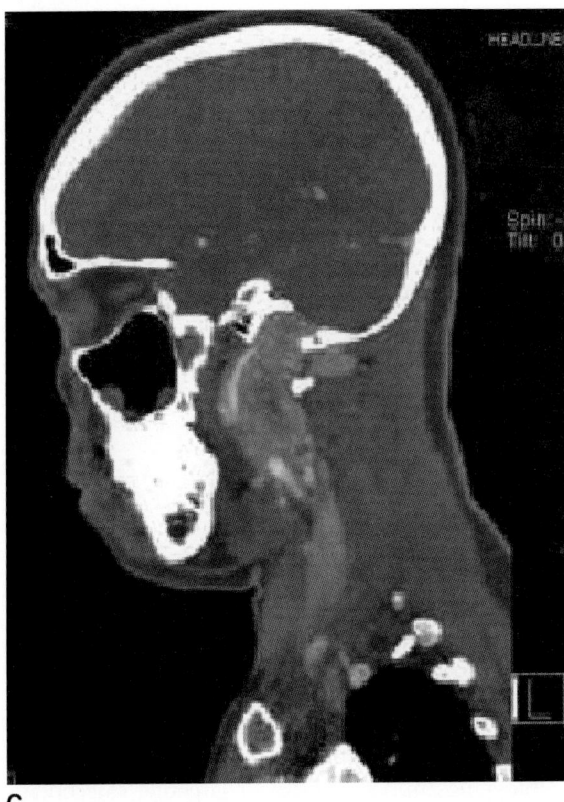

Figure 127.8 *(Continued)* **C:** Sagittal reformat demonstrates circumferential involvement of the internal carotid artery (*arrow*) with anterior displacement, with extensive involvement of the jugular foramen to its intracranial portion.

diagnosis of head and neck paragangliomas but is of paramount importance in preoperative planning for resection of these tumors. Angiography is essential in providing a detailed map of tumor blood supply and venous drainage, demonstrating the tumor flow dynamics and detailing the general vascular anatomy of the head and neck and intracranial space. Four-vessel cerebral angiography allows for qualitative and quantitative blood flow studies of the cerebral circulation. Preoperative preparation through superselective embolization of the feeding arterial supply to the tumor decreases the risk of intraoperative blood loss.

Arterial supply of carotid body tumors takes place directly from the feeding vessels to the carotid body that hypertrophies when a tumor is present (15,28,36). Arterial supply of jugulotympanic tumors is well defined when these tumors are early in their development and involve the ascending pharyngeal artery. As these tumors grow, they recruit additional blood supply that comes from the internal carotid circulation via the caroticotympanic arteries. With invasion of the posterior fossa and medial extension of the tumor toward the cavernous sinus, additional vascular recruitment is possible through the posterior circulation via the vertebral arteries through the clival anastomoses as well as the cavernous sinus microcirculation. This is significant in the preoperative angiographic and embolization management of these tumors. Assessing tolerance to interruption of the internal carotid artery is of paramount importance for extensive paragangliomas that involve the internal carotid artery that can be injured during surgery

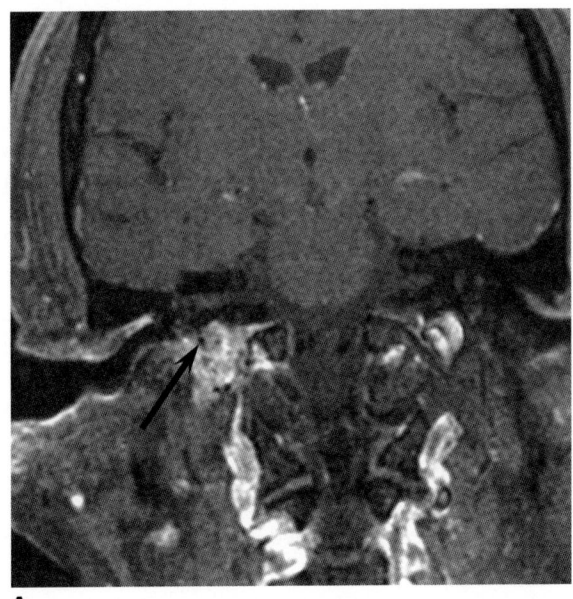

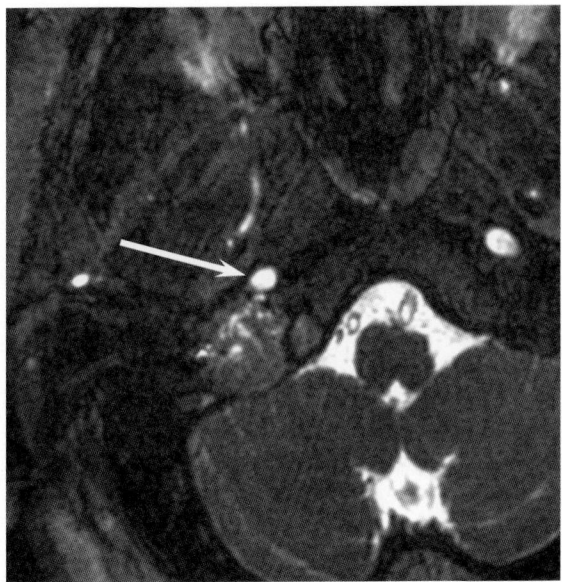

Figure 127.9 Jugular paraganglioma. **A:** Coronal enhanced fat-suppressed T1-weighted image shows avid enhancement with focal round flow voids (*arrow*) indicating large feeding vessels. **B:** Axial fat-suppressed T2-weighted image demonstrates the proximity of the tumor to the vertical portion of the petrous internal carotid artery (*arrow*) as well as the intracranial but extradural component of the tumor in the jugular foramen posteriorly.

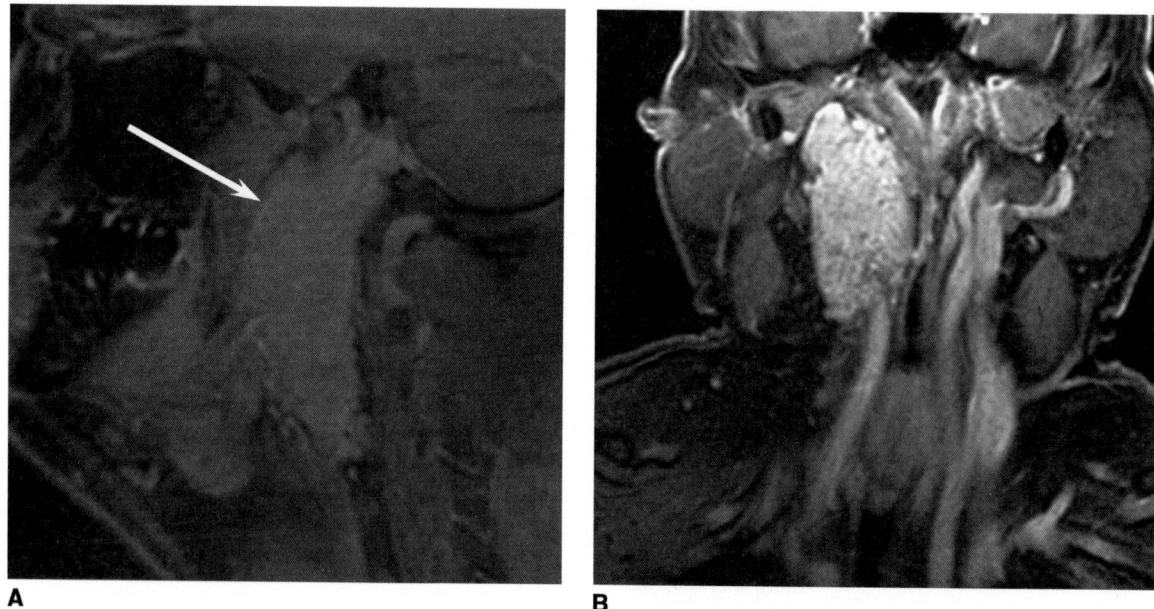

Figure 127.10 Vagal paraganglioma. Sagittal **(A)** and coronal **(B)** enhanced fat-suppressed T1-weighted images demonstrate typical rostrocaudal growth. The internal carotid artery (*arrow*, **A**) is displaced anteriorly.

or where a planned internal carotid resection is contemplated. An angiographic balloon occlusion test involves the threading of a transfemoral catheter to the internal carotid and involves temporarily occluding the internal carotid artery, usually at the carotid siphon within the cavernous sinus to determine whether there will be neurologic deficit (9,11). Several modalities for neurologic monitoring during balloon occlusion testing of the internal carotid artery are available. In order of decreasing sensitivity, they are clinical neurologic examination, electroencephalography (EEG), and quantitative blood flow examination through xenon CT concurrent examination. Xenon CT angiography is a precise quantitative study with the best sensitivity but is cumbersome and rarely available (37,38) (Fig. 127.11).

Radionuclide Imaging

Radionuclide imaging of paragangliomas targets the biochemical pathways of catecholamine synthesis, storage, and secretion by chromaffin tumor cells. A variety of different imaging techniques exist:

[123]I-metaiodobenzylguanidine (MIBG), ^{18}F-3,4 dihydroxyphenylalanine–positron emission tomography (^{18}F-DOPA–PET), ^{18}F-fluorodopamine (^{18}F-FDA–PET), ^{18}F-fluoro-2-deoxyglucose (^{18}F-FDG–PET) and Indium octreotide scanning (^{111}In-octreoscan) (39,40).

Different functional imaging agents target paraganglioma tumor cells through different mechanisms. [123]I- and ^{131}I-labeled MIBG and ^{18}F-FDA are actively transported into neurosecretory granules of catecholamine-producing cells via the vesicular monoamine transporters after uptake into cells by the norepinephrine transporter. In contrast, ^{18}F-DOPA enters the cell via the amino acid transporter based on the capability of PGL and other neuroendocrine

tumors to take up, decarboxylate, and store amino acids and their biogenic amines. Instead of targeting catecholamine pathways, ^{18}F-FDG enters the cell via the glucose transporter, and its accumulation is an index of increased glucose metabolism whereas ^{111}In-octreoscan images indicate somatostatin type 2 receptors that are expressed in paragangliomas (9,10).

[111]In-octreoscan specificity and sensitivity is approximately 90% in head and neck paragangliomas, which makes it a very effective way to screen for secondary tumors and postoperatively screen for recurrent disease when structural studies like CT and MRI may be compromised postoperatively. ^{123}I-MIBG shows similar sensitivities and specificities. Malignant and metastatic paragangliomas are best imaged with ^{18}F-FDG–PET, which shows sensitivities of 74% to 88% (9,10).

It is increasingly understood that there is a link between genotype-specific tumor biology and imaging. For example, ^{18}F-FDG–PET has an excellent sensitivity for paragangliomas due to SDHB-associated mutation. The SDHB gene encodes for subunit B of the mitochondrial SDH complex II that catalyzes the oxidation of succinate to fumarate in the Krebs cycle and feeds electrons to the respiratory chain, which ultimately leads to the generation of ATP (oxidative phosphorylation). SDHB mutations can lead to complete loss of SDH enzymatic activity in malignant paragangliomas, with up-regulation of hypoxic-angiogenetic responsive genes (23). Impairment of mitochondrial function due to loss of SDHB function may cause tumor cells to shift from oxidative phosphorylation to aerobic glycolysis, a phenomenon known as the Warburg effect. Higher glucose requirements for anaerobic metabolism explain the increased ^{18}F-FDG uptake by malignant SDHB-related paragangliomas (40).

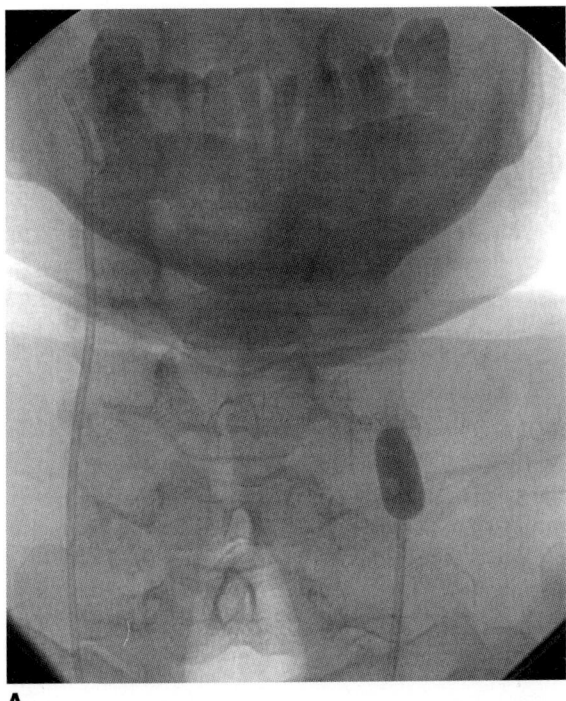

A

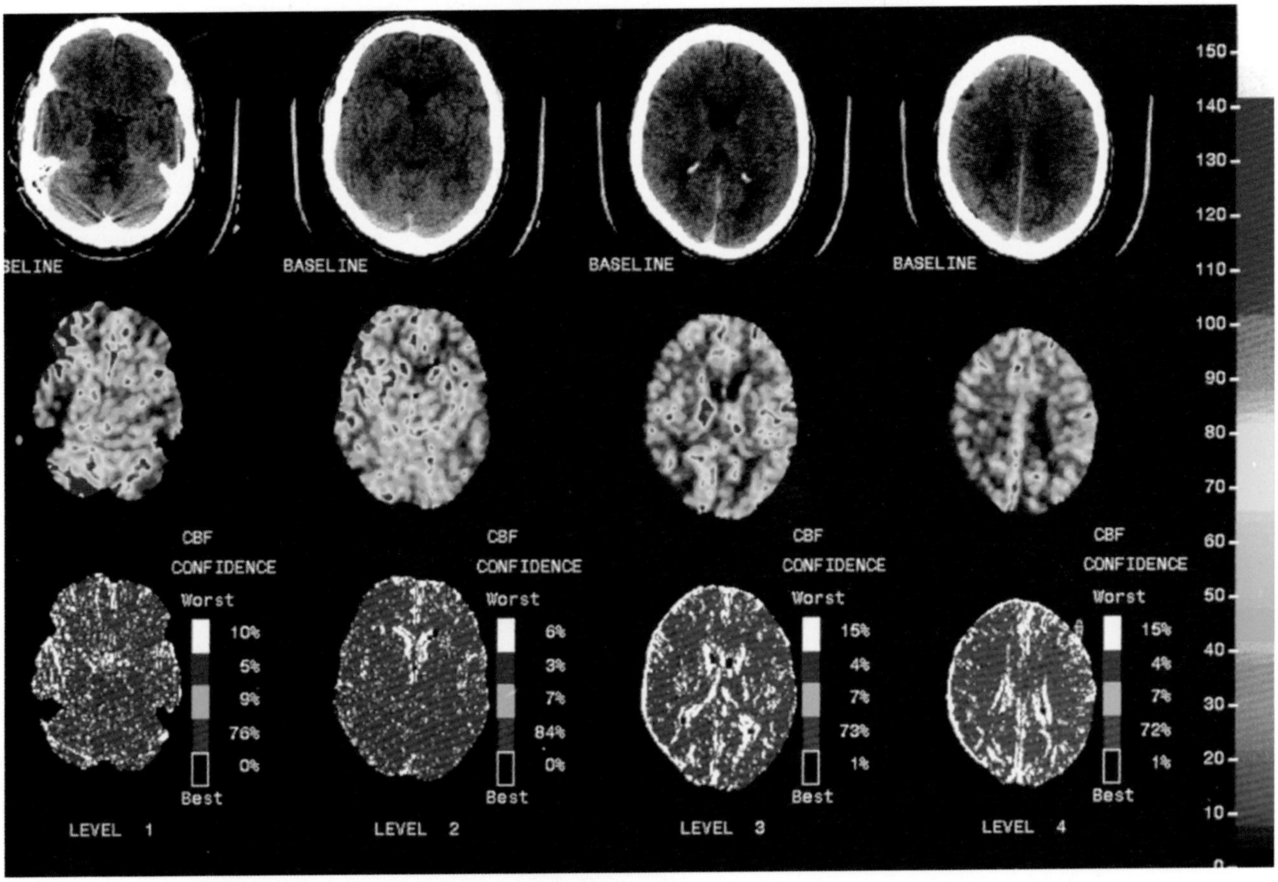

B

Figure 127.11 Balloon occlusion testing. **A:** Frontal angiographic image shows the inflated radiodense balloon in the proximal left internal carotid artery, occluding flow. **B:** Quantitative cerebral blood flow images created by inhaling xenon gas during dynamic CT. The color images reveal reduced flow (blue instead of red) in the left MCA distribution.

Treatment

Surgical resection has been the traditional treatment for paragangliomas of the head and neck. Microsurgical skull base techniques such as the Fisch infratemporal fossa approaches were developed to specifically resect temporal bone paragangliomas (Fig. 127.12). The refinement of these surgical techniques with the assistance of preoperative embolization has significantly reduced morbidity and has minimized mortality associated with surgery. However, when complete tumor extirpation is contemplated, lower cranial nerve resection or inadvertent injury to the lower cranial nerves can result in significant morbidity affecting phonation and deglutition with a risk for aspiration.

Radiation therapy, which was initially used for the treatment of unresectable tumors or for surgical treatment failures, has become an acceptable treatment modality and has been incorporated into the treatment algorithms for head and neck paragangliomas. External beam radiation, intensity-modulated radiation therapy (IMRT), and, more recently, stereotactic radiation have all been used with excellent results.

In deciding what modality of treatment to select, the following factors should be taken into account: the patient's age and medical comorbidities, the type of paraganglioma in question (vagal, tympanic, jugular, carotid body), the presence of concurrent paragangliomas, the extent of the tumor as well as any preoperative cranial nerve deficits, whether partial or complete. When surgery is contemplated, a surgical team with experience in lateral skull base surgery, head and neck surgery and interventional neuroradiology is a requisite.

Surgery

Preparation for surgery requires angiographic evaluation for most paragangliomas. Anesthesia requirements should take into consideration tumors that may be actively secreting catecholamines, which will require alpha and beta adrenergic blockade. Continuous arterial pressure monitoring is required and transfusions may be necessary. Central venous pressure monitoring may be required depending on the underlying comorbidities.

Angiographic Evaluation

Superselective angiography is an invaluable adjunct for planning surgery in paragangliomas by providing an arterial map that identifies the feeding blood vessels as well as providing the flow dynamics to the tumor. This is especially useful in larger tumors where multiple feeding vessels from both the internal and external circulation may be present with anastomoses between the external and internal carotid systems (41). Similarly, the internal carotid artery can be evaluated for structural integrity and areas of constriction or irregularity, which would imply involvement of the vessel and the potential need for sacrifice. The venous phase of angiography is equally important in identifying the draining vessels and, in jugulotympanic paragangliomas, the degree of occlusion of the jugular bulb, sigmoid sinus, and jugular vein.

Equally important is the angiographic evaluation of adequate cerebral circulation in the event of internal carotid artery disruption or sacrifice. There are many methods

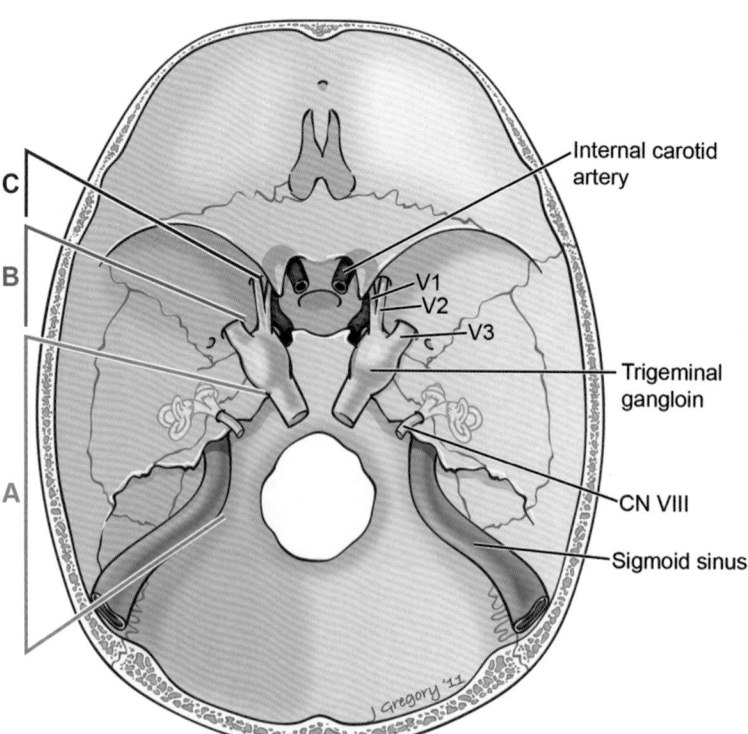

Figure 127.12 Fisch classification of infratemporal fossa approaches. Type A, exposure to the level of the anterior eustachian tube, middle meningeal artery/foramen spinosum. Type B, exposure to the foramen ovale, V3. Type C, exposure to the foramen rotundum, V2.

for assessing adequate contralateral cerebral circulation. Xenon CT scanning with concurrent balloon occlusion is a quantitative analysis of cerebral flow and is the most precise method of cerebral circulation evaluation, though it is cumbersome and not readily available (37,38). Temporary balloon occlusion of the carotid with monitoring of the clinical neurologic examination in the presence of a patent circle of Willis is easier to perform and also very reliable. EEG monitoring can be performed during balloon occlusion as well as hypotensive challenge during the period of balloon occlusion. Approximately 93% of patients can tolerate sacrifice of the carotid artery based on angiographic evaluation. It should be noted that intraoperative conditions may be different in terms of cerebral delivery of oxygen than those in the angiographic suite (11). Tolerance of temporary internal carotid occlusion does not predictably avoid the possibility of a delayed postoperative cerebrovascular ischemic event. The venous outflow of the ipsilateral and contralateral sigmoid and jugular systems should be noted, especially in jugulotympanic paragangliomas. Since there are anatomic variants, a contralateral hypoplastic or absent jugular system would be a contraindication for surgery as this would raise the possibility of a postoperative venous stroke unacceptably (42–44) (Fig. 127.13).

Embolization

Embolization is an exceptionally useful adjunct in the surgery of large paragangliomas. In experienced hands, it carries very low morbidity. The risk of embolization is the escape of embolizing particles into the cerebral circulation thus causing a stroke. This can occur through external–internal carotid circulation anastomoses or flow reversal from the arterial supply of the tumor. The advantages of embolization are tumor shrinkage and decreased blood flow with profound surgical benefits. Less intraoperative bleeding diminishes the requirement of potential transfusions and provides for a much easier dissection with better-defined tissue planes leading to less risk to normal anatomic structures, including cranial nerves. Larger paragangliomas have multiple arterial feeding vessels that need to be individually addressed through superselective angiography. In doing so, with each successive embolization of these vessels, additional compartments of the tumor are devascularized until finally with further injection of contrast in the arterial circulation, there is absence of a tumor "blush." Surgery should be performed within 48 hours of embolization to avoid recruitment of collateral circulation, and administration of steroids is useful in reducing the post-embolization inflammatory response (41,45) (Figs. 127.5 and 127.14).

Surgery
Carotid Body Tumors
Smaller carotid body tumors can be approached through a transverse neck incision, larger ones through an oblique vertical incision along the anterior border of the sternocleidomastoid muscle. Proximal and distal dissection to

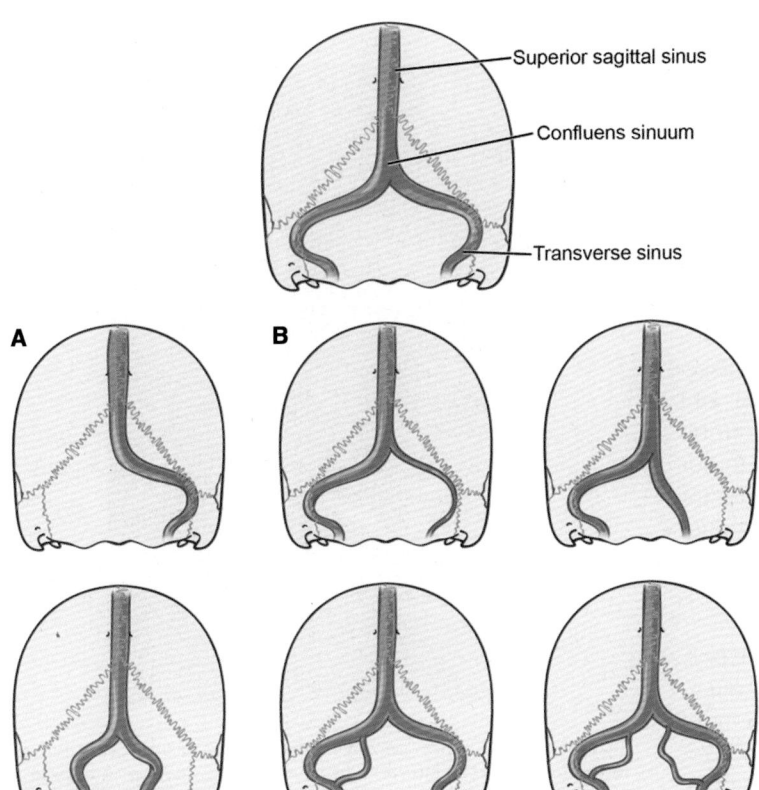

Figure 127.13 Variations of the intracranial posterior venous outflow system at the level of the transverse sinus, sigmoid sinus, and jugular bulb. Variations **A** and **B** would have a high surgical significance if a lesion were to involve the dominant side.

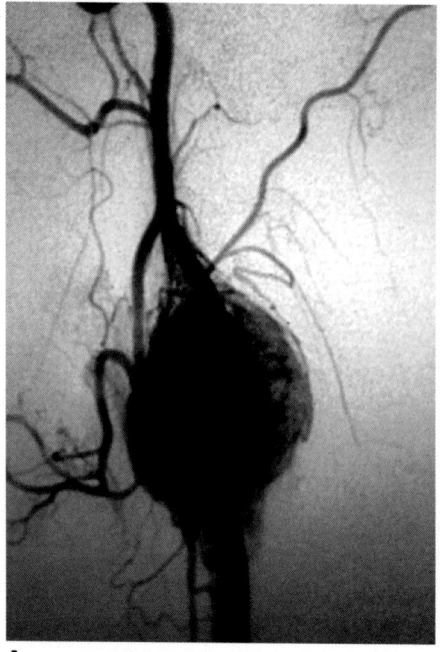

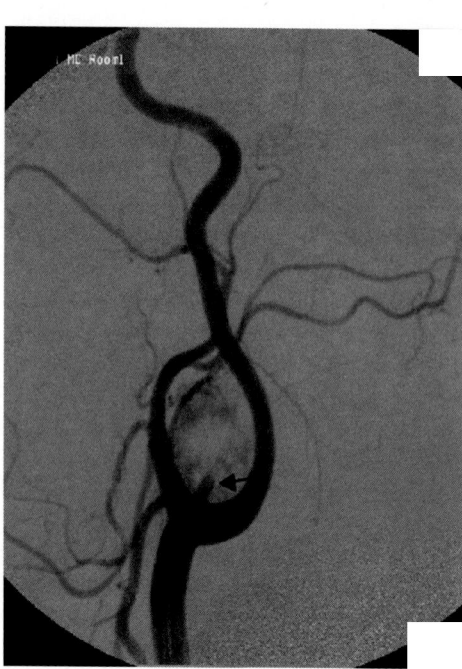

Figure 127.14 Preoperative embolization of a carotid body tumor. **A:** Pre-embolization lateral angiogram shows early, intense blush reflecting high vascular flow with multiple collateral feeding vessels. **B:** Postembolization frontal angiogram shows marked reduction in vascularity. The primary feeding vessel (*arrow*) terminates abruptly.   **A**   **B**

the tumor identifies the common carotid artery, internal and external carotid arteries, and jugular vein. Vessel loop control is applied. Carotid bypass precautions should be available. The entire course of the internal carotid artery is then exposed with the vessel being typically displaced posterolaterally. The dissection of the tumor is in the subadventitial plane and must be done with extreme care. The tumor may have to be split as it encases the internal carotid artery. In a similar fashion, the external carotid artery is then addressed. Encasement and infiltration of the external carotid artery may necessitate its sacrifice, though this should be avoided if possible. The dissection of the tumor at the bifurcation of the carotid is left last since this is the most vulnerable point for breaching the artery as it is intimately associated with the arterial wall where the tumor originates from the carotid body. The surrounding cranial nerves in carotid body tumors show marked hyperemia of their vasa nervosum of the nerve sheath. In larger tumors, these nerves may be intimately involved and their dissection may cause dysfunction of the vagus, hypoglossal, and glossopharyngeal nerves. Ligation of the external carotid artery as a means to control blood flow to the tumor should be avoided as this maneuver does not affect tumor blood flow since collateral circulation may be profuse (Figs. 127.15 and 127.16).

Jugulotympanic Paragangliomas

Small tympanic paragangliomas (Glascock-Jackson type I, Fisch class A) can be approached through a transcanal/inferiorly based tympanomeatal flap. Embolization of these tumors is not required. Bipolar electrocautery microforceps can be used to shrink the tumor and resect it. Larger tympanic paragangliomas confined to the middle

ear and/or mastoid without breaching the bone overlying the jugular bulb or the jugulocarotid spine can be exposed through a combined postauricular/endaural approach with a canal wall up mastoidectomy and extended facial recess approach inferiorly that sacrifices the chorda tympani and removes the vaginal process of the tympanic bone to expose the hypotympanum.

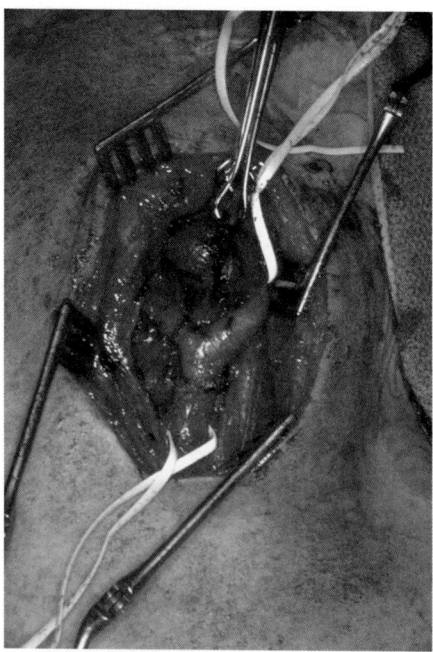

Figure 127.15 Intraoperative picture of a carotid body tumor. Tenaculum is on the lateral tumor surface. Vessel loops are around the common carotid artery (inferiorly) and internal carotid artery (superiorly).

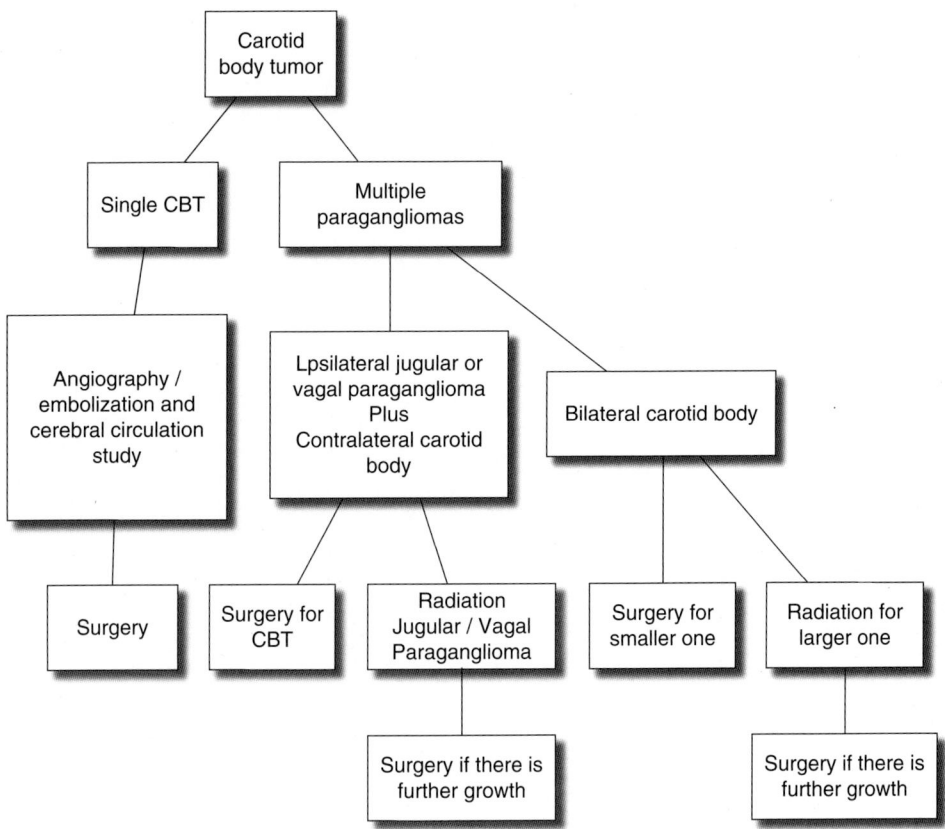

Figure 127.16 Decision analysis tree for the treatment of carotid body tumors.

When the jugular bulb is involved, a combined temporal/cervical approach is required. An extended mastoidectomy and extended facial recess approach is performed with skeletonization of the sigmoid sinus and exposure of the jugular bulb through the retrofacial air cells. The internal carotid artery is dissected superiorly and controlled. Cranial nerves 9, 10, and 11 are identified and traced proximally and distally. The internal jugular vein is then ligated superiorly and dissected toward the jugular bulb in the neck. The sigmoid sinus is occluded and ligated above the tumor extension. Contralateral venous outflow should be verified through preoperative studies. When occlusion of the sigmoid sinus is performed, this should be done in a manner that avoids interfering with the outflow from the anastomotic vein of Labbe that drains the temporoparietal cortex, thereby avoiding the risk of a venous stroke (46). Once the sigmoid sinus is opened and the jugular vein is ligated inferiorly, hemostatic agents can be injected to gently occlude the inferior petrosal veins. Dissection of the tumor should proceed with irrigating bipolar electrocautery. At the level of the jugular bulb, the dissection should proceed with extreme caution since the cranial nerve rootlets of the glossopharyngeal and vagus are at their most vulnerable. In jugulotympanic paragangliomas, these rootlets are displaced medially and are thus in a favorable position. If the tumor does not extend into the pars nervosa/medial jugular bulb compartment, preservation of the cranial nerves is feasible and desirable (47).

More advanced tumors that involve the vertical and/or horizontal petrous carotid artery with possible intracranial extension require a postauricular infratemporal fossa approach. These approaches begin with an extended mastoidectomy, removal of the external auditory canal, tympanic membrane, malleus, and incus. The external canal is permanently oversewn, which commits the patient to ipsilateral conductive hearing loss. The peritubal and pericarotid air cells are removed and the intrapetrous carotid artery is skeletonized proximal to the tumor extent. This may involve sacrifice of the middle meningeal artery and removal of the foramen spinosum as well as the foramen ovale if the tumor has extended toward the cavernous sinus. The tumor is removed from the carotid, middle ear, and sigmoid/jugular bulb/jugular vein (Fig. 127.17). Extension of the tumor to the medial jugular bulb compartment or intracranially places the nerve rootlets of cranial nerves 9, 10, and 11 in an unfavorable position, and more frequently than not these need to be sacrificed. If there is no such extension, an effort is made to gently dissect the tumor away from the nerves. The eustachian tube should be permanently occluded to avoid postoperative cerebrospinal fluid rhinorrhea. Intracranial extension is addressed by opening the dura in the presigmoid area down to the tumor extension at the level of the jugular bulb. Tumor extension

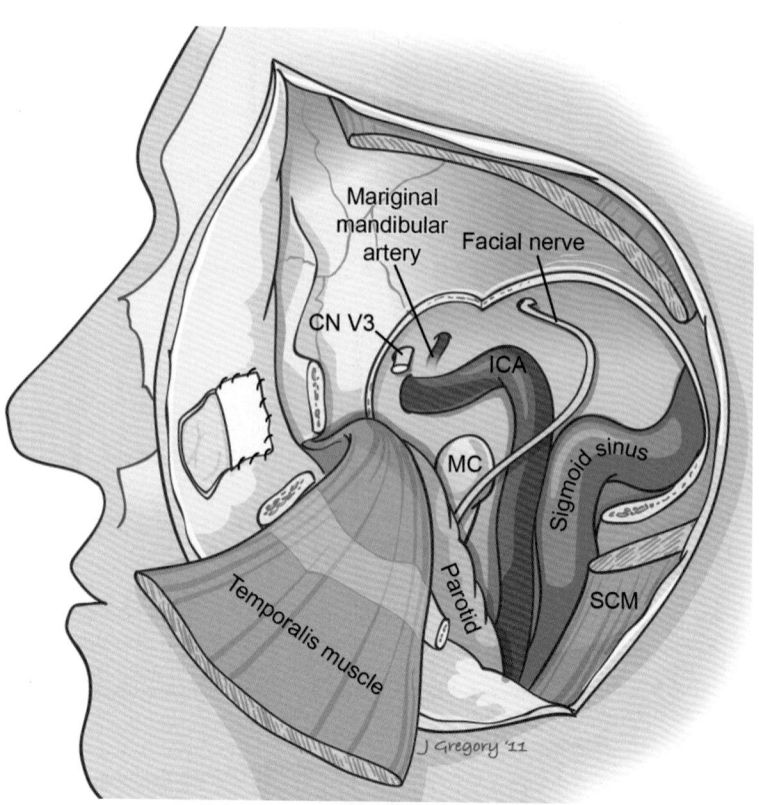

Figure 127.17 Schematic representation of a type B infratemporal fossa approach. Lateral temporal bone has been removed exposing the petrous carotid artery, jugular vein, jugular bulb, and sigmoid sinus. Facial nerve has been mobilized in its horizontal and vertical portions. The third division of the trigeminal nerve (V3) has been divided as well as the middle meningeal artery right behind it. MC, mandibular condyle; SCM, sternocleidomastoid muscle; ICA, internal carotid artery.

toward the petrous apex and clivus may necessitate a translabyrinthine/transcochlear approach. In these approaches, the facial nerve is mobilized out of the fallopian canal in its vertical and horizontal portion to the geniculate ganglion. This will result in temporary facial paralysis due to interruption of the blood supply to the nerve as well as the retraction anterosuperiorly (15,28,48). Incomplete recovery of facial nerve function is a possible outcome. Reconstruction with temporoparietal fascia flap or temporalis muscle is done at the conclusion to assist healing and prevent a cerebrospinal fluid leak. Lumbar drainage for a limited period of time in the immediate postoperative recovery may be indicated for the prevention of a cerebrospinal fluid leak. When cranial nerves have been sacrificed, immediate surgical amelioration with a concurrent vocal cord medialization and a pharyngoplasty with cricoesophageal myotomy at the same sitting have been recommended.

Refinement of these surgical techniques includes the juxtacondylar approach as well as the transjugular craniotomy (47). These modifications have in common the shifting of the surgical angle of approach more posteriorly. The advantages are that they obviate the need for facial nerve transposition and improve the control and preservation of the lower cranial nerves in the jugular foramen. The limitation is that they cannot address tumors that involve the petrous carotid artery.

Vagal Paragangliomas

Most vagal paragangliomas originate in the nodose (inferior) vagal ganglion, which is situated 2 cm below the jugular foramen. Their bidirectional growth along the vagus results in involvement of the jugular bulb superiorly and poststyloid parapharyngeal space inferiorly. The internal carotid artery is displaced anteriorly (30). Vagal paragangliomas originating in the superior and middle ganglia, which are situated within the jugular foramen, cause early skull base invasion with intracranial extension. The surgical techniques to approach these tumors are identical to those for jugulotympanic paragangliomas when the skull base is involved. The inferior extent of vagal paragangliomas require detaching the digastric muscle from its origin and removing the styloid process to access the parapharyngeal space extension. Sacrifice of the vagus nerve in these tumors is inevitable. With involvement of the jugular foramen and skull base, additional cranial nerve deficits are to be expected as these tumors extend medial to the cranial nerve rootlets, within the pars nervosa of the jugular foramen.

Complications

Vascular Injury

Early surgical series for paraganglioma surgery reported a stroke rate of 10% to 20%. More recent series report a stroke rate of 0% to 2%. With more recent diagnostic evaluations, preoperative planning, and microsurgical techniques, the risk of injury or need for internal carotid sacrifice is minimal. For carotid body tumors, the risk of injury and need for vessel sacrifice is size specific, with tumors larger than 5 cm likely requiring carotid reconstruction. In addition, preoperative findings of stenosis and irregularity on angiography and/or circumferential involvement on MRI with loss of the pericarotid advential plane should dictate preoperative preparation for carotid resection and reconstruction (49–52).

Vagal paragangliomas differ from carotid body tumors and jugulotympanic paragangliomas as they are not intimately associated with the carotid artery. In advanced tumors, both vagal and jugulotympanic, the internal carotid artery can be completely encased in its petrous portion. With adequate surgical exposure and microsurgical technique, injury should be infrequent in experienced hands. Internal carotid sacrifice in this location is fraught with problems, and therefore if sacrifice is contemplated, consideration for alternate treatment in these instances is important. If the vessel is at high risk for injury within the petrous carotid portion and the patient has safely passed balloon occlusion testing, permanent preoperative occlusion of the carotid distal to the tumor should be considered.

More recently, a novel approach to the artery at risk is to place a vascular endoprosthesis and then perform the surgery several weeks later. Fibrosis around the self-expanding stent creates a leak-proof artery. This has the advantage of reducing blood flow to the tumor as well as preventing vascular injury (53).

Baroreflex Failure

Surgery for removal of bilateral carotid body tumors results in loss of the baroreceptor reflex with bilateral denervation of the carotid sinus. In the immediate postoperative period, this results in labile refractory hypertension, tachycardia, diaphoresis, and headache, which may be managed with sodium nitroprusside. The long-term treatment is controlled with clonidine (54). Alternative therapy may be considered on one of the tumors to avoid long-term blood pressure lability.

Cranial Nerve Injury

The risk to the lower cranial nerves in surgery for paragangliomas is location specific and tumor size specific. The surgical treatment of the following tumors, in decreasing order, pose risk to the cranial nerves: vagal, jugulotympanic, and lastly carotid body paragangliomas. Size of lesion is especially important in vagal and jugulotympanic paragangliomas. Tumors with extensive skull base involvement, intracranial, and/or infratemporal fossa extension are likely to have extensive involvement of the lower cranial nerves with at least one lower cranial nerve involved and often times multiple cranial nerve deficits preoperatively. Involvement of the facial nerve with preoperative paralysis is a sign of such extensive involvement (15,28,29,55,56).

Postoperative individual cranial nerve deficits most often result in a temporary deglutition, phonation, tongue motion, and/or aspiration problem. Multiple cranial nerve deficits have additive effects and are poorly tolerated. In older patients, recovery is often very difficult and permanent aspiration requiring management with a gastrostomy and tracheostomy is a possibility, especially in high vagal nerve injuries. Bilateral lower cranial nerve paralysis, especially of the vagus nerve as a result of therapy or progression of tumor in bilateral disease is a devastating injury that results in inability to swallow and phonate.

The deficit in vagal nerve injuries is proportionate to the level of the injury. Low vagal nerve injuries distal to the origin of the superior laryngeal nerve will result in vocal cord paralysis that can be mitigated relatively easily. Injury to the vagus at the nodose ganglion or at the level of the jugular foramen results in vocal cord paralysis, anesthesia of the ipsilateral hemilarynx, supraglottic structures, and paralysis of the ipsilateral soft palate. The deficit results in aspiration due to lack of sensory input from the larynx with paralysis of the pharyngeal musculature and the vocal cord. In addition, there is air and food escape into the nasopharynx due to the paralysis of the soft palate. Vagal nerve injuries at the jugular foramen are often associated with glossopharyngeal nerve injuries, which add ipsilateral pharyngeal anesthesia, further compromising swallowing function. Superior vagal injuries require immediate and intensive swallowing therapy with surgical management of the vocal cord paralysis (Fig. 127.18). Most injuries at the level of the jugular foramen are permanent, and immediate surgical management to mitigate deficits is indicated. Vocal cord medialization with a thyroplasty combined with cricopharyngeal myotomy will improve phonation and deglutition as well as minimize the risk of aspiration. An ipsilateral palatal adhesion procedure can mitigate the hypernasality in speech and nasal bolus escape during deglutition. Additional lower cranial nerve injuries are seen in 30% to 50% of patients with a vagal nerve injury significantly complicating recovery (57–60).

Accessory nerve injury results in loss of trapezius and sternocleidomastoid muscle function. Physical therapy is required to avoid should pain secondary to shoulder "drop" and limitation of motion. If the nerve is injured below the jugular foramen it may be amenable to primary repair either directly or through a nerve graft (59).

Injury to the hypoglossal nerve results in ipsilateral tongue paralysis. Hemiatrophy of the tongue is the eventual outcome within a few months. When this is in combination with additional cranial nerve injuries swallowing therapy is of paramount importance in preventing aspiration. Swallowing therapy is directed at teaching the patient to move the bolus to the functioning side (59).

Injury to the sympathetic chain is seen in approximately 25% of patients postoperatively as a result of interruption of the sympathetic ganglia. This results in partial or complete Horner syndrome. The resultant ptosis can be easily rectified through a Müller muscle eyelid-tightening procedure. "First bite syndrome," which is intense pain with the first bite, can develop as a result of denervation hypersensitivity of the myoepithelial cells of the parotid gland. This problem improves gradually and spontaneously in most patients.

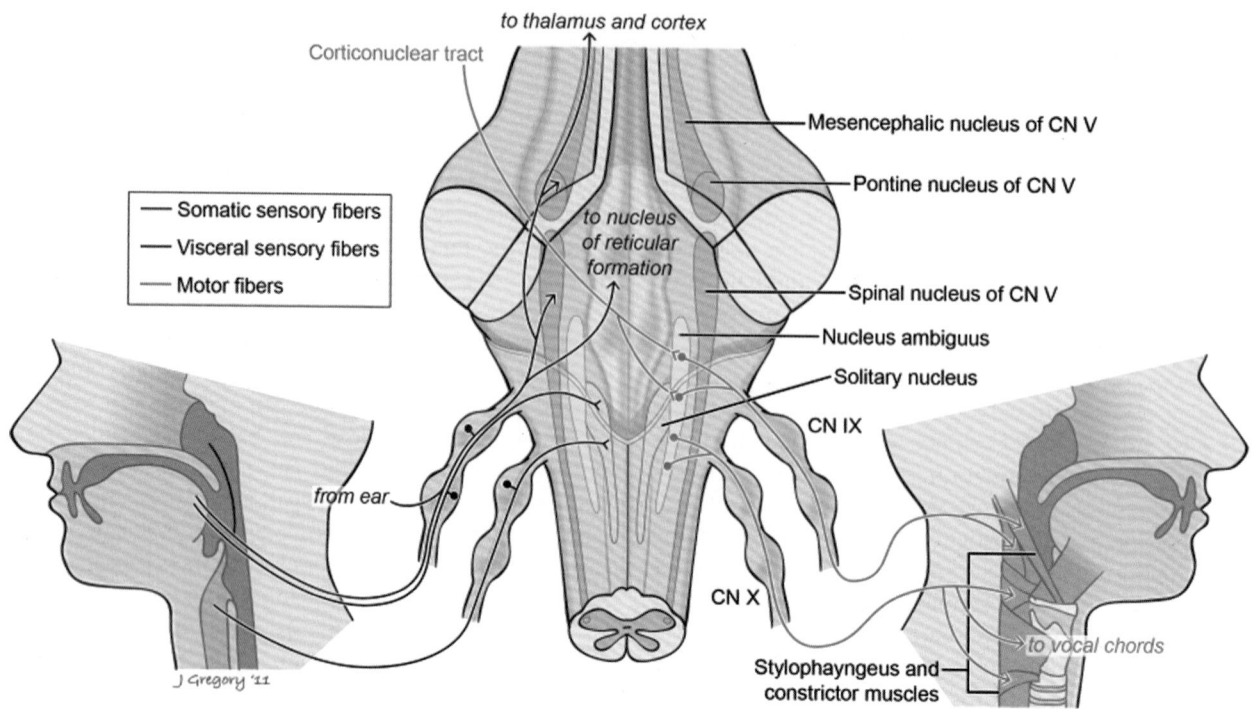

Figure 127.18 Schematic representation of the afferent and efferent swallowing reflex.

Postoperative cranial nerve deficits in carotid body tumor surgery are seen in up to 40% of patients and are associated with large tumor size. The majority of these deficits are transient and related to the manipulation of cranial nerves during dissection. Vagal nerve injury is most common. In jugulotympanic paragangliomas, the most common nerve deficit is also vagal (27%), followed by the glossopharyngeal (18%), the accessory, and hypoglossal (8%) (9–11,29,59).

External Beam Radiation

Paragangliomas are responsive to radiation treatment. On the basis of histologic studies, the primary effect of radiation is obliterative endarteritis at the capillary level, followed by fibrosis within several months. However, chief cells remain viable in the specimens studied following radiation. It is difficult to state whether these cells retain their capacity to proliferate. Traditionally, radiation was relegated for tumors that were deemed unresectable or tumors in elderly and medically infirm patients deemed not able to tolerate surgical resection. The optimal dose appears to be 45 Gy/over 5 weeks.

Local control with radiation therapy is defined as tumor shrinkage or nonprogression. An analysis of 36 series with over 1,000 tumors treated spanning the period of 1964 to 2001 shows an average local control of 90% with a range of 65% to 100%. Other reviews of the radiation therapy literature provide similar control rates of 90% and 91%, respectively. Follow-up in these series is wide, ranging from 1.5 to 30 years. The intriguing aspect of radiation is the minimal additional damage to cranial nerves. New cranial neuropathies range from 1% to 4% with existing cranial neuropathies improving in an average 35%. The incidence of severe complications is 6% with a mortality of 0.6%. These include radiation osteoradionecrosis, temporal bone complications, and brain complications and are associated with older radiation techniques or higher radiation dosages. In addition, there are well recognized and reported cases of secondary malignancy from radiation to the temporal bone (61).

Stereotactic Radiation

The principle of stereotactic radiation is to deliver a one-time high dose of radiation to the target in question, which is highly focused and has a sharp drop off to spare surrounding normal tissue. This can be achieved through the Gamma Knife that utilizes cobalt as a source of radiation or radiation generated in a linear accelerator—LINAC. The advantages are similar to those of external beam therapy with preservation of cranial nerve function and minimal significant complications, in addition to the therapy being delivered in one sitting. This modality cannot be used for tumors larger than 4 cm and cannot be used for carotid body tumors as well as tumors that extend caudal to the skull base as they are out of the stereotactic frame field. Local control rates for stereotactic radiation range from 82% to 100% albeit with limited follow-up ranging from 19 months to 4.2 years (62–66).

Treatment Comparisons

The results of surgery, external beam radiation, and stereotactic radiation show similar efficacy in affecting cure:

approximately 90%. The definition of cure is different for surgery and radiation. Surgical cure is total resection with no evidence of tumor regrowth by serial radiologic imaging. With radiation, a fraction of tumors show some reduction in size and the majority remain stable in size. Two more factors are important in interpreting results: recurrences and disease progression. Tumor growth for paragangliomas is very slow with a mean growth rate of 1 mm/y and an average tumor doubling time of 4.2 years. In comparing external beam radiation to surgery, the recurrence rates are similar at 7% to 8%, respectively. Salvage therapy for recurrent disease is effective in 88% of patients. Disease progression and death from paraganglioma tumor occurs in 2.5% of those treated by surgery and 6% of those treated by radiation (disease specific mortality). In comparing surgery versus stereotactic radiation, the control rate was 86% for surgery with an 88-month average follow-up versus a 95% control rate for stereotactic radiation with a 71-month follow-up. Others have found a control rate of 92% versus 97% for surgery versus stereotactic radiation, albeit with a shorter follow-up period (61).

Treatment Strategies

Patients presenting with signs and symptoms consistent with paraganglioma and patients referred for treatment with a radiographically confirmed paraganglioma should undergo a thorough history and examination. Attention should be focused on signs and symptoms of a secreting tumor, a familial history of paragangliomas, MEN type 2, and von Hippel-Lindau syndromes. Examination should focus on cranial nerve function, and any dysfunction should be documented thoroughly. Genetic testing for PGL gene should be done if there is a positive family history and other members of the family should be screened for paragangliomas. Multiple paragangliomas can be screened by ^{123}I-MIBG or ^{111}In-octreotide scans as well as (18)F-DOPA PET scans. If malignant paraganglioma is suspected, (18)F-FDG PET scan should be the modality of choice. Twenty-four–hour urine as well as serum catecholamine screening for norepinephrine, epinephrine, and their metabolites should be performed to exclude a functioning tumor. Contrast-enhanced CT scans with thin cuts as well as MRI scans should be done for pretreatment evaluation. If surgery is contemplated, angiographic evaluation with superselective embolization in preparation for surgery should be performed for the appropriately selected tumors. Similarly, cerebral angiography for adequacy of collateral blood flow and temporary balloon occlusion studies will be required in selected patients. A fine needle biopsy is not indicated in most instances as the radiographic studies are pathognomonic (9,10,15,61).

Noting that the definition of cure is different for surgery than radiation and assuming that the two are equal concerning "cure," treatment algorithms can be constructed for paragangliomas that maximize the long-term control and minimize the potential morbidities of each modality.

Therefore, for unilateral small- to moderate-sized carotid body tumors as well as tympanic paragangliomas without cranial nerve dysfunction, primary surgery is the first line of choice. In bilateral carotid body tumors, surgery on both sides should be avoided because of labile hypertension. However, this needs to be weighed against radiation risks for accelerated atherosclerosis and radiation-induced malignancy risk especially in young patients. Radiation therapy is a highly effective treatment for jugulotympanic and vagal paragangliomas without cranial nerve dysfunction. For patients with jugulotympanic as well as vagal paragangliomas, surgery should be the primary modality when lower cranial nerve dysfunction is present, especially vagal paralysis. Radiation therapy as a primary modality is best suited for those who have medical comorbidities and those who have no lower cranial deficits at presentation. Elderly patients can either be observed or treated with radiation as the primary treatment. Salvage therapy for recurrent tumors should be offered (Figs. 127.16 and 127.19).

Catecholamine-secreting tumors should be managed by surgery as primary treatment as these tumors continue to secrete after radiation despite radiographic evidence of arrest of growth (61).

Paragangliomas suspected or proved to be malignant, either by fine needle biopsy of suspicious lymph nodes and/or positive PET–FDG scans, should also be managed by surgery as the primary modality, given the unknown response rate to radiation alone as well as the frequent need to perform neck dissection for staging and comprehensive treatment. Additionally, in patients who have been genetically screened and found to have a PGL4 mutation, because of the marked increase in incidence of malignant paragangliomas, surgery should be considered as the first line of treatment.

Finally, despite advances in surgical treatment as well as radiation techniques, these tumors have the potential for significant morbidity. Overriding factors such as the patient's wishes, the patient's lifestyle, and family support structure may alter the treatment choices. Regardless of the modality of treatment, long-term follow-up with serial scanning is indicated.

HEMANGIOPERICYTOMA

Hemangiopericytoma (HPC) is an uncommon tumor that arises from the pericytes of Zimmerman that are found spiraling around capillaries and postcapillary venules. The function of the cell is to control vascular tone in these capillary beds and this tumor can theoretically arise wherever capillary beds are found. HPC was first described by Stout and Murray in 1942. The pathologic diagnosis is vexing and frequently confused with synovial cell sarcoma, epithelioid hemangioendothelioma and solitary fibrous tumor (SFT). The architectural pattern of HPC is similar to that of other mesenchymal neoplasms, for example, sarcomas (67).

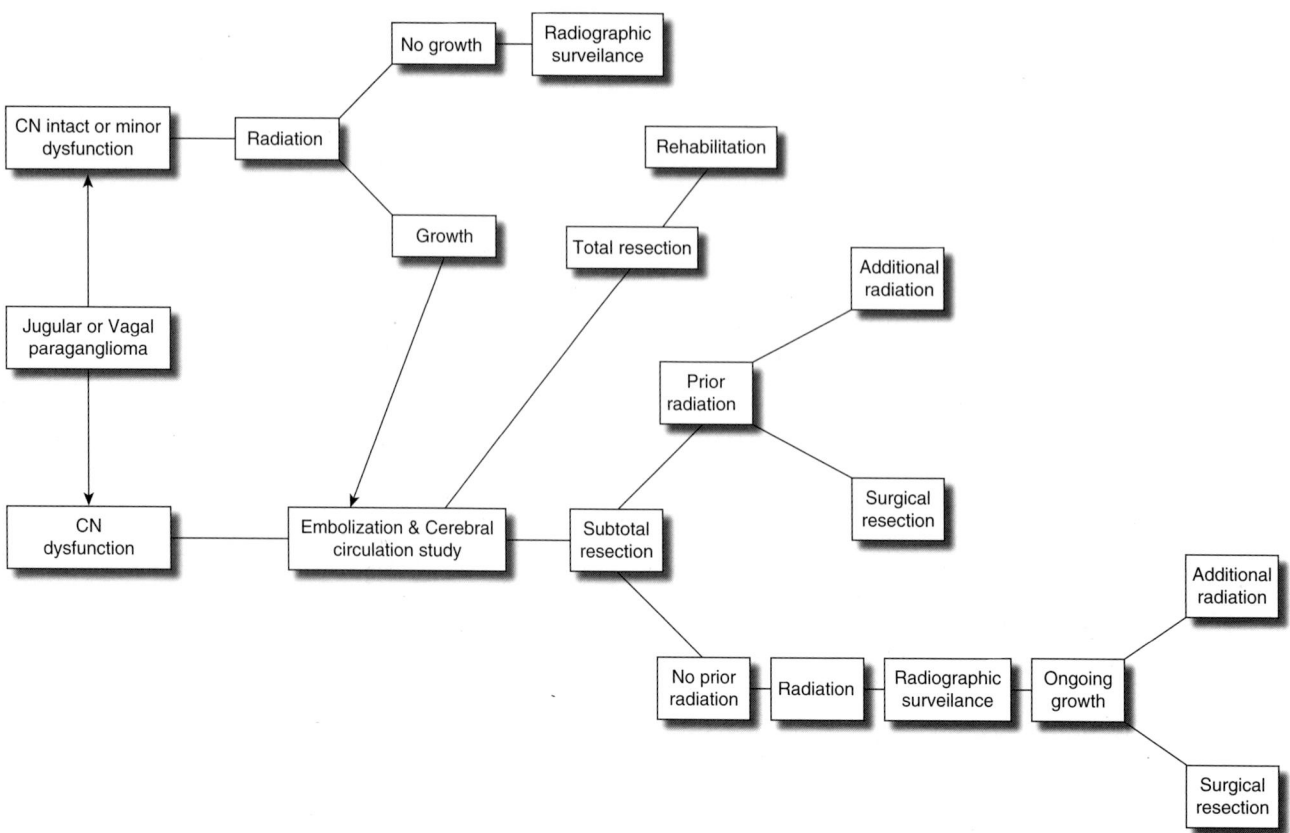

Figure 127.19 Decision analysis tree for the treatment of vagal and/or jugular paragangliomas.

An ongoing debate currently exists among sarcoma experts as to how best to classify HPC and SFT. Because of the large overlap of morphologic and clinical features between HPC and SFT and a lack of clear diagnostic criteria, the two entities have been frequently misdiagnosed for each other. In the most recent WHO classification of soft tissue sarcomas, the concept of HPC as a vascular, pericyte-derived tumor was abandoned in favor of a fibroblastic cell of origin, thus aligning HPC more closely with SFT. SFT in particular displays two different types: a fibrous variant and a cellular variant. The latter is virtually indistinguishable from HPC. The current paradigm tends to view HPC and SFT as a spectrum of a single entity (68).

The diagnosis of HPC is one of exclusion and relies on the presence of characteristic histologic features. Older studies have characterized a low-grade versus a high-grade variant of this tumor based on the presence and number of mitoses, presence of necrosis, and cellular anaplasia. Ten-year survival was markedly different between the two groups: 77% for those with low grade, versus 29% for those with high-grade tumors. More recently, reverse transcriptase polymerase chain reaction has helped distinguish HPC variants such as lipomatous HPC, glomangiopericytoma, and myopericytoma, which have a much more benign course and require much less aggressive therapy than HPC (68).

Of interest is that an infantile or congenital HPC exists that differs substantially clinically and pathologically from the adult form. Congenital HPCs are predominantly subcutaneous head and neck lesions that display an indolent behavior despite worrisome histologic features such as extensive necrosis and hemorrhage, hypercellularity, and increased mitotic figures. These tumors spontaneously regress and behave biologically in a much more benign fashion despite their aggressive histologic features (69). Similarly, sinonasal HPCs behave biologically in a more benign fashion than other head and neck sites (70,71).

Overall, it is difficult to predict biologic behavior of the HPC on conventional histopathologic parameters.

Clinical Behavior

In descending order of frequency, these tumors occur in the extremities, particularly the lower extremity, the pelvis and retroperitoneum, the head and neck as well as the meninges. Fifteen percent to twenty-five percent of these tumors occur in the head and neck. Meningeal HPCs were initially thought to be variants of meningioma (hemangioblastic meningioma) and were reclassified by the WHO in 1993. In the head and neck, they can be mucosal, arising in the sinonasal tract as well as the oral cavity or in the soft tissues of the neck, particularly of the scalp. Orbital HPC tumors have also been described. Sinonasal HPCs behave clinically in a less aggressive fashion with lower rates of metastases (72,73).

Overall, the clinical course of HPC may vary from indolent, with a low rate of local recurrence, to aggressive, with rapid development of metastases.

The tumor presents most frequently as a painless mass, predominantly in the sixth and seventh decades with a median age of 45 at presentation and no sex predilection. Pain is associated with advanced presentation. Satellite nodules around the primary tumor can be frequently seen, though they are not specific for this lesion. The etiology of HPC is unknown, although the presence of HPC has been linked to trauma, prolonged steroid use, and hormonal imbalance.

Treatment

No treatment modality for HPC/SFT has been evaluated prospectively, but several retrospective analyses suggest that complete surgical resection of the tumor, whenever possible, should be the treatment of choice. Earlier studies have demonstrated an overall 10-year survival of 54% to 89% after complete surgical resection. However, it is worth noting that earlier series may include patients who were histologically classified as an HPC when in fact these tumors were sarcomas. The rate of regional metastasis from HPC is low, and most patients fail at a local or distant site. Local recurrence and distant metastases are often noted after a significant disease-free period, which necessitates continuous surveillance. Series have shown that over 80% survival rates have been faulted by limited follow-up, especially for a tumor that has indolent and unpredictable behavior (72,74–76).

In comparison with other soft tissue sarcomas, HPCs fare much better in terms of recurrence and overall survival. Development of distant metastatic disease is a poor predictor of survival.

Management of HPC/SFT patients who develop locally recurrent or metastatic disease has been challenging, for no clearly effective therapy exists. Re-resection and/or metastasectomy can lead to improvement in tumor-free survival and should be considered if technically feasible.

Radiation Therapy

Radiation therapy has been used, both as adjuvant therapy in patients considered at risk for local recurrence and as primary therapy in unresectable cases. The best evidence for effectiveness of external beam radiation is for meningeal HPCs. In one study with long follow-up, adjuvant external beam radiation extended the disease-free interval from 154 months to 254 months, providing patients with an increased recurrence-free interval and overall survival (72).

Chemotherapy

Conventional chemotherapy for HPC is based on anthracycline agents that involve significant toxicity. Limited data are available for the effectiveness of systemic chemotherapy in advanced HPC. Although a few responses have been reported, systemic chemotherapy has not shown significant clinical response, and its effects on disease progression and/or survival advantage are difficult to prove (77,78).

More recently, inhibition of angiogenesis pathways with monoclonal antibodies has provided a target for this tumor with limited but promising data for disease stabilization. In a study of temozolomide and bevacizumab for both HPCs and SFTs considered unresectable, disease stabilization was demonstrated. These agents had a 10% mortality in this cohort of medically compromised patients. Bevacizumab is a recombinant monoclonal antibody that targets VEGF, a key mediator of a signaling pathway that affects many vital cellular processes, including angiogenesis and vascular permeability. Bevacizumab has shown antitumor activity when combined with a number of cytotoxic chemotherapeutic agents. Other specific target agents that have been used are sunitinib, sorafenib, and pazopanib, which target broadly the tyrosine kinase receptors and block multiple pathways of tumorigenesis. The results of these studies are difficult to extrapolate to this specific tumor because of its rarity and the fact that it is included in studies that include multiple soft tumor types (79).

ANGIOSARCOMA

Epidemiology

Angiosarcomas are a subtype of soft tissue sarcoma and are aggressive malignancies arising from the vascular endothelium of blood vessels or lymphatics. Fewer than 5% of all soft tissue sarcomas occur in the head and neck, and approximately 10% of these head and neck soft tissue sarcomas are angiosarcomas (80). Angiosarcomas are the fourth most frequent sarcoma of the skin, after Kaposi sarcoma, dermatofibrosarcoma protuberans, and leiomyosarcoma. The incidence of angiosarcoma has risen over the past 30 years, but whether this is a true increase is unclear. The rise could be related to greater use of radiotherapy and improved diagnosis. Angiosarcomas have a similar distribution between sexes, can develop at any age, and are more common in older patients. Angiosarcoma can arise in any soft tissue structure or viscera, and cutaneous angiosarcomas typically involve the head and neck, particularly the scalp. Cutaneous head and neck angiosarcomas account for 62% of all angiosarcomas, have a male predilection, and 88% occur in the Caucasian population (81).

Treatment Is Challenging and Prognosis Is Poor

Angiosarcomas of the face and scalp are insidious, and their clinical presentation varies widely. In their early stages, they frequently appear clinically innocent and may even show benign capillary hemangioma-like structures histologically. There is a frequent delay in clinical diagnosis. This pattern, however, is deceiving because angiosarcomas usually have an aggressive course. Tumor cells are located mainly in the dermis and may extend into the subcutaneous tissue.

Results of treatment are difficult to interpret due to the rarity of the tumor and paucity of adequate studies. There have been no phase-3 and few phase-2 treatment trials in angiosarcomas. In the past, the prognosis of cutaneous angiosarcoma was considered extremely poor, with an overall 5-year survival rate less than 20%. Age, (less than 50 years), tumor stage (localized), and anatomical site (trunk) confer a favorable prognosis. Locations other than the head and neck (i.e., trunk and extremities) confer a better survival prognosis, which is similar to Merkel cell carcinomas. The tendency of angiosarcoma for early regional and distant metastases, as well as local recurrences after years of apparent remission, is well recognized (81,82).

Etiologic Factors

Most angiosarcomas arise spontaneously, but there are a few reports of malignant transformation within pre-existing benign vascular lesions. Several well-described risk factors exist (Table 127.5).

Chronic lymphoedema of any origin is associated with the development of angiosarcoma, (Stewart-Treves syndrome). Lymphoedema caused by Milroy disease and chronic infections, such as filariasis, have been linked to the development of angiosarcomas.

Radiotherapy is an independent risk factor. Although the association between radiotherapy and subsequent angiosarcoma is best described for breast cancer therapy, it is not exclusive to breast lesions (82). In a review of the Surveillance of Epidemiology and End Results (SEER), data showed an increased risk of soft tissue sarcomas (particularly angiosarcomas) after adjuvant radiotherapy, with a peak incidence 5 to 10 years after treatment. Angiosarcoma of the breast is associated with previous treatment by radiation with subsequent lymphoedema as well as treated breast cancers with mutations in the DNA repair genes, BRCA1 and BRCA2. Other familial syndromes such as Maffucci syndrome and Klippel-Trenaunay have been associated with increased incidences of angiosarcoma (81,82).

Various chemicals are associated with the development of angiosarcomas, particularly within the liver. Occupational exposure to vinyl chloride as well as thorium dioxide is associated with hepatic angiosarcomas. Exposure to arsenic, radium, and anabolic steroids is also associated with angiosarcomas. Reports of angiosarcoma associated with foreign bodies include accidentally retained surgical gauzes as well as surgical prostheses (82).

Pathology

Angiosarcomas are infiltrative and do not have a capsule or a clear border.

Abnormal, pleomorphic, malignant endothelial cells are the hallmark of angiosarcoma and can have an epithelioid appearance. In well-differentiated tumors, abnormal endothelial cells retain vascular structures with functioning vascular channels. With increasing dedifferentiation, the vascular architecture disappears with abnormal cells becoming multilayered and forming papillary-like projections. In poorly differentiated areas, the malignant endothelial cells form continuous sheets with areas of necrosis, which can make differentiation from anaplastic carcinoma or melanoma difficult (82).

Angiosarcomas typically express endothelial markers including von Willebrand factor, CD34, CD31, Ulex europaeus agglutinin 1, and VEGF. Immunohistochemistry is therefore important in confirming the diagnosis. von Willebrand factor, U europaeus agglutinin 1, and CD31 are the most useful markers in poorly differentiated cases. However, progressive tumor dedifferentiation can lead to a loss of these markers. The absence of melanocytic markers (S100), human melanoma black-45, and melanoma antigen can help distinguish angiosarcoma from melanoma. Additionally, epithelioid angiosarcomas can express cytokeratins, leading to confusion with poorly differentiated carcinomas (82,83).

Molecular Studies

Because angiosarcomas are endothelial-cell tumors, there is great interest in the role of angiogenesis and the angiogenic factors associated with their pathogenesis, and how they might be used as targets for treatment. VEGF and its receptors can be overexpressed in angiosarcomas. VEGF-A is the most studied cytokine and is consistently expressed at higher concentrations in angiosarcomas than in benign vascular or normal-tissue controls (82).

All three subtypes of VEGF receptors (VEGFRs) have been detected in angiosarcomas. VEGF-A expression is correlated with VEGFR-1 expression, VEGFR-2 is correlated with prognosis, and the loss of expression of VEGFR-2 is associated with a significantly poorer prognosis (84,85).

TABLE 127.5	RISK FACTORS FOR ANGIOSARCOMA

Chronic Lymphoedema (Stewart-Treves syndrome)
   Postsurgery or radiation therapy
   Milroy syndrome (congenital lower extremity lymphoedema)
   Filariasis (parasitic lymphoedema)
Carcinogens
   Vinyl chloride
   Thorium dioxide
   Arsenic
   Anabolic steroids
   Foreign bodies
Syndromes
   Neurofibromatosis type 1
   Maffucci syndrome
   Klippel-Trenaunay syndrome
   BRCA-1 or BRCA-2 mutations

Activation of the RAS pathway is often tumorigenic. Although immortalized murine endothelial cells form benign hemangiomas *in vivo*, the addition of activated HRAS produces rapidly growing, poorly differentiated angiosarcomas. In clinical cases, KRAS mutations have been reported in liver and cardiac angiosarcomas.

Consistent with the invasive and metastatic potential of angiosarcoma, overexpression of the transcription factor ETS1 results in increased production of metalloproteinases (particularly MMP1, MMP3, and uPA), resulting in increased extracellular proteolysis and decreased amounts of the major basement membrane components. Angiosarcomas recruit inflammatory cells, particularly mast cells, that drive positive feedback loops by causing further release of cytokine growth signals, including basic fibroblast growth factor (bFGF) and VEGF (79,85,86).

Because of the success of KIT–tyrosine-kinase inhibitors in treating some other sarcomas, investigators have studied KIT expression in various forms of angiosarcoma. Results pooled from three separate series showed KIT positivity in 50% of the samples examined. KIT-mutation analysis has been done for a handful of angiosarcomas; however, no unique abnormalities to angiosarcomas have been to date identified. Conversely, although angiosarcomas are tumors of malignant endothelial cells, increased expression of angiogenic cytokines, including VEGF and its receptors, bFGF, platelet-derived growth factor (PDGF), and the angiopoietin system, have been reported in other cancers including soft tissue sarcomas of nonendothelial vascular origin (79,85,86).

Pathologically, the distinction between angiosarcoma and a benign capillary lesion or an HPC or Kaposi sarcoma is difficult and fraught with error on routine light microscopy.

Staging

Soft tissue sarcomas are staged using the International Union Against Cancer and American Joint Committee on Cancer (UICC/AJCC) system. This is based on the TNM (tumor–node–metastasis) staging system (Table 127.6). Angiosarcomas are not graded according to histology as they all are considered high grade. Various authors have tried staging angiosarcomas, and in a review of the SEER data, three stages were identified: local, regional, and distant disease.

Approximately 10% of patients with head and neck angiosarcoma will show regional metastases at presentation. Eighty-two percent of primary tumors are larger than 5 cm at presentation. Satellite lesions are seen in 46% of patients and these are an ominous prognostic sign. Approximately 10% of patients will have distant metastases at presentation. The lungs followed by the liver and bones are the most common sites of distant metastatic disease (81).

Treatment

There are no randomized trials and few prospective studies; most published reports of angiosarcoma treatment are

TABLE 127.6	TNM SARCOMA STAGING	
T stage		
Tx		Primary tumor cannot be assessed
T0		No primary tumor found
T1		Tumor <5 cm diameter
T2		Tumor >5 cm diameter
N stage		
Nx		Cannot be assessed
N0		No regional lymph-node involvement
N1		Regional lymph-node involvement
M stage		
Mx		Cannot be assessed
M0		No distant metastasis
M1		Distant metastasis

retrospective case series. Treatment guidelines for angiosarcoma have been included in guidelines for other soft tissue sarcomas. Such guidelines have been published by the European Society for Medical Oncology and the National Comprehensive Cancer Network.

Radical surgery with complete (R0) resection is the primary treatment of choice. Involved margins (R1 or R2 resection) are common because of the invasive and often multifocal nature of angiosarcomas, which confer a worse prognosis.

Wide margins are recommended but are difficult to achieve in the head and neck and particularly the scalp because of extensive microscopic spread, surrounding function—critical structures, and cosmesis. Compounding this problem is the inability of intraoperative frozen section to evaluate correctly for microscopic margins. In one study, the negative predictive value of frozen section was 33.3% with 79% of patients having residual microscopic disease despite multiple attempts at achieving clear microscopic margins (80). Therefore, what appears to be a clinical T1 stage will be very frequently upstaged to a pathologic T2 stage in angiosarcoma. Because of these limitations, the use of Mohs surgery does not confer an advantage in treatment.

Some have argued that since an R0 resection rarely results in clear margins of resection, the goal should be an R1 or R2 resection with rapid wound closure to expedite adjuvant therapy. However, with the availability of reliable free tissue transfer to close large wound defects, margins need not be compromised for prompt delivery of adjuvant therapy (Figs. 127.20 to 127.22).

Additional surgery in locally recurrent disease to achieve a pathologic complete resection may improve survival. Because of the high risk of local recurrence, adjuvant radiotherapy, with large doses (greater than 50 Gy) and wide treatment fields, is recommended. Radiation treatment alone is generally thought to be inadequate treatment for angiosarcoma and further radiotherapy is usually avoided for radiation-induced angiosarcomas (84).

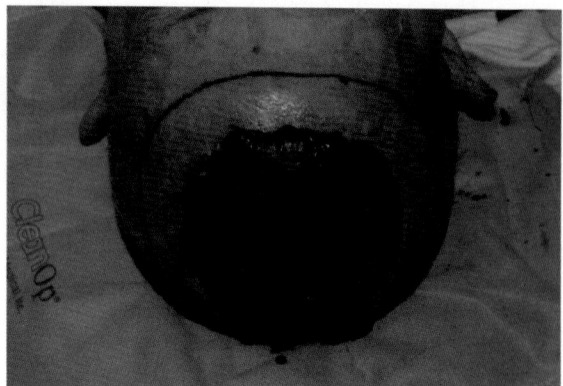

Figure 127.20 Extensive recurrent angiosarcoma of the scalp.

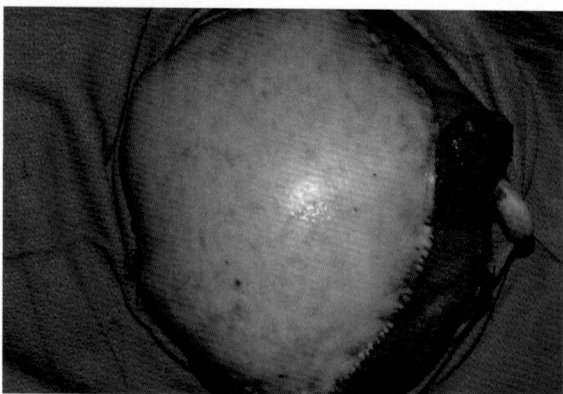

Figure 127.22 Same patient as in Figures 127.20 and 127.21 after reconstruction with a latissimus dorsi free flap.

Chemotherapy has not been shown to improve either overall or disease-specific survival in large series and there is no convincing evidence to support the use of chemotherapy in the neoadjuvant or adjuvant setting after definitive surgery and radiotherapy for angiosarcoma. However, in view of the risk of distant metastasis, in the setting of local failure, a compelling argument can be made for adjuvant chemotherapy.

Chemotherapy is the primary treatment option for metastatic angiosarcoma, although the evidence base for this is limited. Drugs that have been used include: doxorubicin, ifosfamide, and taxanes. Many angiosarcoma patients are elderly, so comorbidities and the risk of treatment-related toxicity can limit the use of chemotherapy.

In soft tissue sarcomas, doxorubicin and ifosfamide as single drugs show response rates of 16% to 36% (87,88). Combination chemotherapy is associated with increased toxicity but not necessarily with better outcomes. The addition of cisplatin, vinorelbine, and gemcitabine to doxorubicin and ifosfamide has shown no proven benefit to the treatment of angiosarcoma. Liposomal doxorubicin has the theoretic advantage of higher vascular tissue accumulation of the drug (89).

Response rates for taxane-based drugs in other soft tissue sarcomas have been disappointing, but taxanes have antiangiogenic activity and are therefore of particular interest in the management of angiosarcomas. The results have been mixed with studies reporting short-lived response rates of 63% to 75% and small gains in progression-free intervals (90). In one study, though the response rate was low at 17%, three patients with otherwise unresectable disease went subsequently to surgery with complete pathologic response (91).

Biologic Molecules

Although the pathogenic pathways underlying angiosarcoma are not fully understood, there is interest in exploring the potential of antiangiogenic molecules in the treatment of angiosarcomas. Encouraging reports on the use of the VEGF-A monoclonal antibody, bevacizumab, include one of two patients with nasal angiosarcomas who achieved pathologic-complete responses to treatment with bevacizumab and radiotherapy (92,93). A phase 1/2 study of bevacizumab, in combination with docetaxel and gemcitabine chemotherapy in advanced and recurrent soft tissue sarcomas, included three angiosarcomas, with complete responses reported in two of them (87).

There is evidence to suggest activity of the targeted treatments, bevacizumab and sorafenib, in angiosarcoma; however, biologic agents are not recommended,

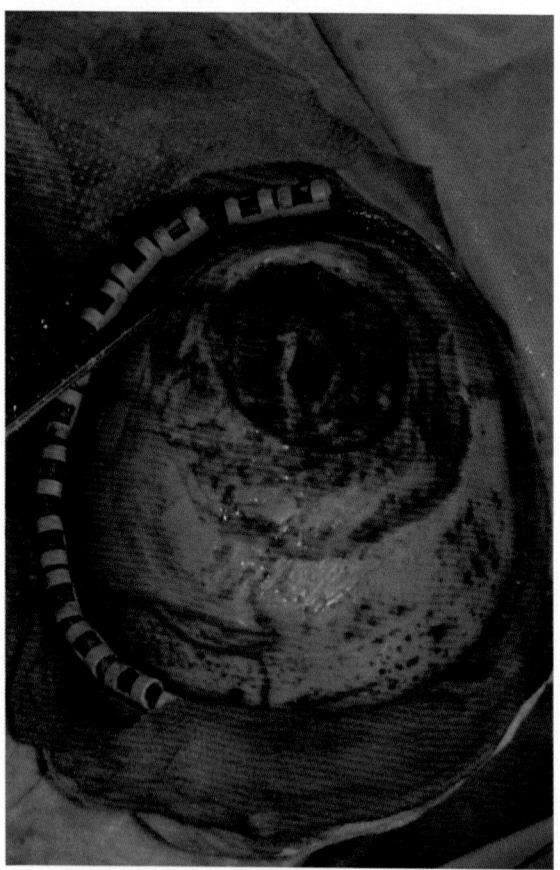

Figure 127.21 Same patient as in Figure 127.20 after resection including sagittal craniectomy.

either as monotherapy or in combination with cytotoxic chemotherapy, outside of clinical trials.

Results

Disease variables that affect survival in angiosarcoma of the head and neck include: anatomic location, size of tumor at presentation, presence of regional or distant metastatic disease, presence of satellite lesions as well as age at presentation.

In the SEER study, head and neck angiosarcomas had a 13.8% 10-year relative survival rate, whereas tumors arising in the trunk resulted in a 75.3% 10-year survival rate. Angiosarcomas of the scalp are particularly problematic. Patients with scalp angiosarcoma show significantly poorer prognosis than patients with angiosarcoma of the face. Size of lesion at presentation shows significant difference in survival and this is more pronounced for the scalp. Patients with T1 lesions have a 71.4% disease survival rate versus those with T2 lesions who show a 9.5% survival rate (81).

Overall patients with angiosarcomas localized to the skin show a 54% 10-year relative survival rate, those with regional metastases a 19% 10-year relative survival rate, and those with distant metastases a 6.1% survival rate (81).

The vast majority (85%) of patients with angiosarcomas of the skin are older than 60 years. The SEER epidemiologic data show that patients younger than 50 years have a 10-year relative survival rate of 71.7%, whereas patients 50 years and older have a 36.8% 10-year survival rate (81).

Disease relapse occurs frequently, and in one large series, 53% developed local recurrence, 36% developed distant metastases, and 21% developed regional metastases. Overall, almost two-thirds of patients experienced local recurrence of their disease, and 36% developed distant metastases. Isolated local recurrence portends a poor prognosis that leads to the development of distant metastases. This highlights the critical role definitive local management plays in controlling this disease. Most local relapses occur in the first 5 years (92%), but local relapses up to 10 years after successful initial treatment have also been reported. Similarly, the interval for distant metastases after successful treatment spans to 10 years (80,82,94,95).

JUVENILE NASOPHARYNGEAL ANGIOFIBROMA

Epidemiology and Pathogenesis

Juvenile nasopharyngeal angiofibromas (JNAs) are rare fibrovascular tumors that account for less than 0.5% of all head and neck tumors. The incidence of JNA is approximately 1:150,000, and it affects adolescent boys and men between the ages of 14 and 25 years. Rare cases have been reported in men over 25 years old and in adolescent girls. Although benign, they are locally invasive with a capacity for extensive bone destruction and remodeling (96,97).

The most widely accepted theory of formation of JNA is that the tumor originates from embryologic chondrocartilage during the development of the cranial bones. The site of origin is the superior margin of the sphenopalatine foramen, which is formed by the junction of the palatine bone, horizontal ala of the vomer, and the root of the pterygoid process (98).

Histologically, JNA shows a biphasic pattern. There is a component of fibrous stroma of spindle cells in a dense collagen matrix and a component of a rich network of vascular channels of varying sizes in clusters. These vascular channels lack the surrounding smooth muscle of normal blood vessels and it has been theorized that this is related to their capacity to profusely bleed when surgically manipulated. JNAs are nonencapsulated and are mucosa covered on their nasal and nasopharyngeal aspect (99,100).

Because of this tumor's sex selectivity and young age at diagnosis, early research focused on steroid hormones. Trials of estrogen treatment showed variable response of JNAs to this therapy and have been largely abandoned. Accelerated tumor growth was described with testosterone treatment that led to studies of flutamide (antiandrogen) treatment preoperatively that showed minimal tumor reduction. More recently, androgen receptors have been identified suggesting that JNA may be androgen dependent (101). Angiogenic and growth factors have also been studied, and bFGF and transforming growth factor-beta 1 have been found in the stromal component of JNAs implicating these growth factors in tumorigenesis. VEGF, as well as VEGFR-2, and PDGF have been found in the vascular component of JNAs (102). Chromosomal studies of JNA show that DNA gains are remarkably more common than DNA losses, with loss of chromosome Y reported in all these studies. The association of JNA with familial adenomatous polyposis has been a focus of studies on the adenomatous polyposis coli tumor suppressor gene (APC) located on chromosome 5q21. The APC gene regulates the level of beta-catenin, which in turn regulates cell–cell adhesion as well as an activator of the Wnt signaling pathway implicated in carcinogenesis (97,103). Beta-catenin products are found in the majority of JNAs in the stromal but not vascular component of the tumor. Furthermore, beta-catenin functions as a coactivator of androgen receptor that may possibly increase tumor androgen sensitivity. Other studies have focused on the oncogenes C-KIT and C-MYC that regulate cell differentiation, cell proliferation, and apoptosis among numerous other functions (100). JNAs are positive for these oncogenes again in the stromal compartment. Though the molecular tumorigenesis of JNAs remains elusive, these studies collectively suggest that the stromal component of the tumor is the neoplastic element of JNAs and that deregulated vessel growth is driven by stromal growth factors. Furthermore, the loss of chromosome Y and the presence of androgen receptors and beta-catenin suggest an androgen-related pathophysiologic response of these tumors (97).

Patterns of Growth

Although histologically benign, the tumor exhibits aggressive local behavior with extensive bone erosion and remodeling and extensive invasion of adjacent structures. The location of origin of JNAs allows these tumors to spread simultaneously toward multiple locations that can involve the nasopharynx, nasal cavity and paranasal sinuses, the infratemporal fossa, and inferior orbital fissure via the pterygomaxillary fissure as well as the skull base and splanchnocranium. However, the early stages are characterized by an indolent growth phase with minimal symptoms. These include unilateral nasal obstruction and epistaxis that tend to be ignored for prolonged periods of time. This is why the majority of patients present with advanced disease. Significant morbidity can occur in the later stages of growth, and even death from hemorrhage and/or intracranial extension (Fig. 127.23).

Medial growth of the tumor fills the nasopharynx and ipsilateral nasal cavity. Anterior growth invades the posterior aspect of the maxillary sinus and more superiorly the ethmoid air cells. With lateral growth, the pterygoid plates are eroded, and the tumor extends into the pterygomaxillary fissure. From here it invades the infratemporal fossa and gains access to the inferior orbital fissure with erosion of the greater wing of sphenoid. The orbit is frequently involved through the inferior orbital fissure as well as through the lamina papyracea from the ethmoid tumor component. When the orbit is involved, additional symptoms of diplopia, visual loss, and proptosis may develop. Proptosis may be due to increased orbital volume from

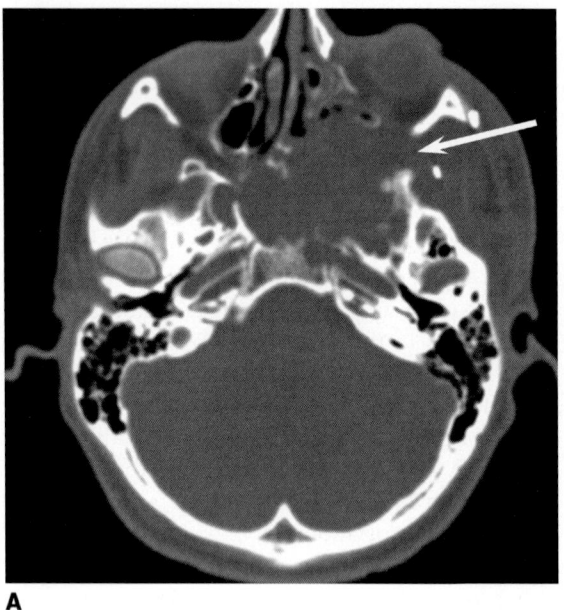

A

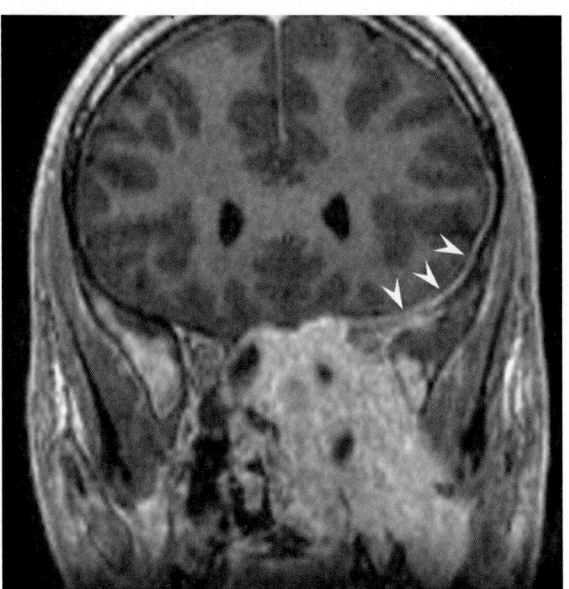

B

Figure 127.23 Recurrent juvenile nasopharyngeal angiofibroma. **A:** Axial bone-window CT demonstrates a widened pterygopalatine fossa (*arrow*) and extensive skull base erosions in the body of the sphenoid. **B:** Coronal enhanced T1-weighted image demonstrates extensive intracranial involvement with abnormal dural enhancement (*arrowheads*). **C:** Coronal T2-weighted image demonstrates invasion of the cavernous sinus (*arrow*) and the infratemporal fossa (*arrowhead*).

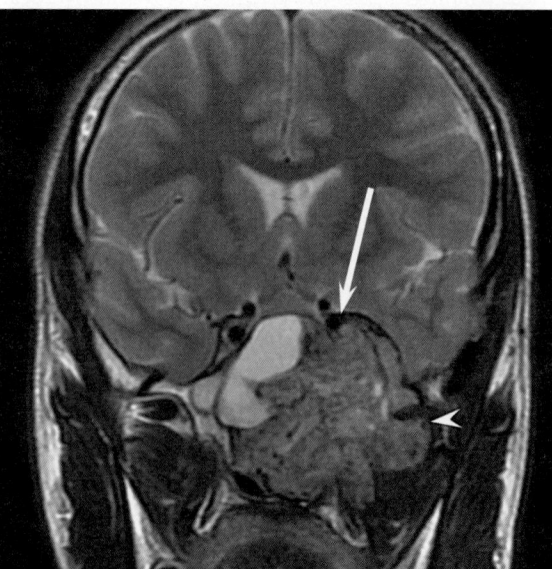

C

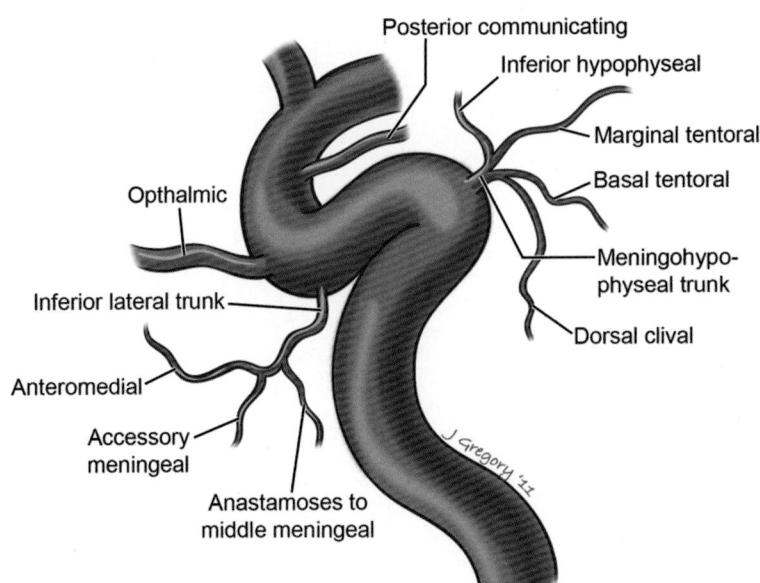

Figure 127.24 Schematic representation of the cavernous carotid artery with hypophyseal and meningeal branches.

tumor growth or increased venous pressure with involvement of the orbital apex.

Superior growth of the tumor involves the base of the pterygoid plates and the body of the sphenoid. Intracranial involvement has been reported to occur in 10% to 36% of all cases in western series. In published data from India, intracranial involvement is as high as 90% (104–106).

Four routes of intracranial invasion have been described: direct extension through the foramen rotundum, ovale, and lacerum; from the infratemporal fossa directly into the middle cranial fossa; from the pterygomaxillary fissure through the inferior and superior orbital fissures into the middle cranial fossa; rarely through the ethmoid lamina and cribriform plate into the anterior cranial fossa with ethmoid air cell involvement; and finally a particularly vexing intracranial extension through the roof of the sphenoid sinus into the sella and medial to the cavernous sinus. With intracranial extension, JNAs recruit blood supply from the internal circulation through the hypophyseal plexus (Fig. 127.24). Invasion of the cavernous sinus and sella will threaten the pituitary, the optic chiasm, optic nerve as well as cranial nerves 3, 4, and 6.

Diagnostic Studies

The diagnosis of a JNA is usually made by nasal endoscopy based on suspected presenting symptomatology. Histopathologic confirmation is not necessary as subsequent radiographic studies are virtually pathognomonic. Biopsy of a suspected JNA prior to imaging may lead to severe epistaxis and blood loss.

Both CT and MRI are essential for the assessment of JNAs. CT is invaluable for providing bony anatomy reference points as well as degree of erosion and remodeling of the sphenopalatine area and the skull base. MRI with gadolinium contrast is essential in determining the difference between tumor and surrounding soft tissues, the delineation between tumor and obstructive sinus disease as well as the interface between tumor and intracranial structures. The determination of dural invasion by MRI is not precise and caution should be exercised when interpreting MRIs for dural invasion. When surgery is planned, specialized CT scanning for intraoperative navigation is essential for tumors that have intracranial invasion (106).

Angiography and embolization should be performed in patients when surgery is contemplated. The vascular anatomy of JNA is important in the planning of surgical resection. Blood supply is determined by the size and extension of the tumor. In the initial stages, there is a consistent vascular supply from the branches of the internal maxillary artery via the sphenopalatine branches. In advanced stage with intracranial extension, blood supply may be through both the internal and external carotid circulation, especially the ophthalmic artery, the ethmoid arteries, and branches of the cavernous carotid. In recurrent or residual JNAs, this vascular supply may become even more complex. Residual tumor blush after angiographic embolization may necessitate further angiographic procedures for control. These should be performed by an experienced interventional neuroradiology team (107,108) (Fig. 127.25).

Balloon occlusion of the internal carotid artery should be done in patients in whom intracranial extension encroaches the cavernous carotid or the horizontal petrous carotid.

Staging

Multiple staging systems have been elaborated for JNAs. The most commonly used system is that of Radkowski

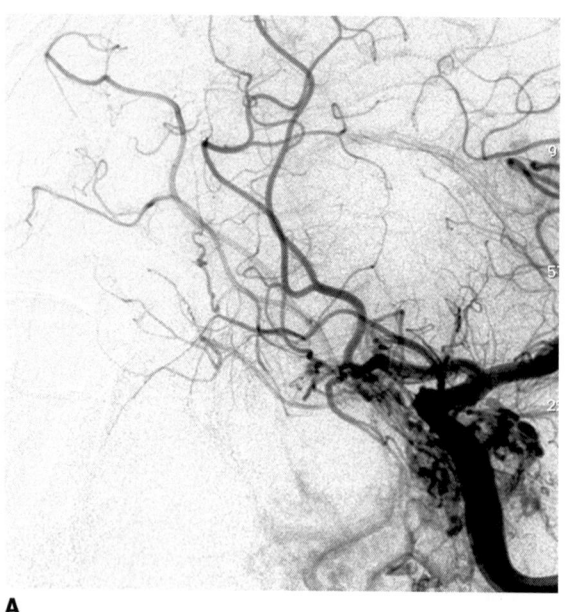

A

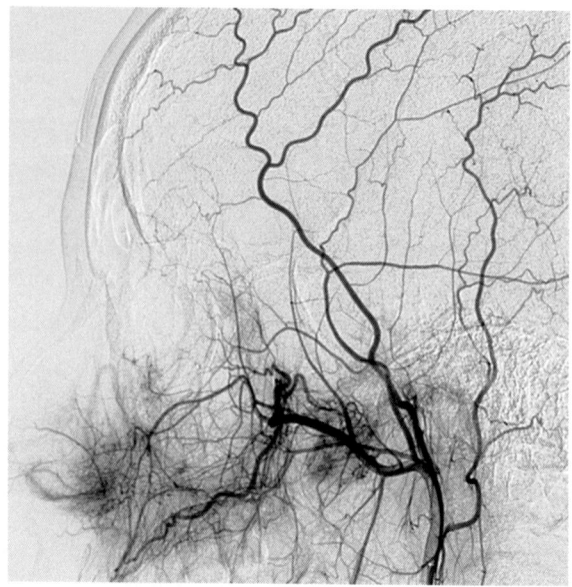

B

Figure 127.25 Collateral vessels feeding a large JNA. **A:** Pre-embolization oblique angiographic image after internal carotid injection shows the extensive blood supply to the tumor from the internal circulation. **B:** Post-embolization lateral angiographic image after external carotid injection shows residual blush through orbital collaterals. **C:** Postembolization frontal angiographic image shows residual flow through meningohypophyseal branches.

C

et al. (109). Variations of these systems have been used recently such as the modified Fisch system and the system proposed by Snyderman for endoscopic resection of tumors (110,111) (Table 127.7).

Treatment Options

The treatment of choice for JNAs is surgical excision. Smaller tumors without intracranial extension can be effectively removed through endoscopic approaches. More extensive tumors are now also amenable to endoscopic approaches due to intraoperative navigation, improved surgical tools, and surgical experience. Extensive intracranial involvement of JNA requires an open approach of which there is a wide variety. However, even extensive JNAs with intracranial involvement can be approached through an extracranial approach. These tumors do not tend to invade or adhere to the adjacent dura. Previous surgery and

radiation limit the utility of extracranial approaches for intracranial invasion (Table 127.8).

Open Surgery

Tumors that infiltrate the infratemporal fossa, the sphenoid sinus, the base of the pterygoids, the cavernous sinus, the foramen lacerum, and the anterior fossa are at higher risk for recurrence. With the refinement of surgical approaches and skull-base techniques, these lesions can routinely undergo total resection.

Choice of Surgical Approach

Combined intracranial and extracranial approaches may be necessary. Surgical approaches can be modified according to the extent of the tumor. The selection of the surgical approach is dictated by the ability to expose the tumor and

| TABLE 127.7 | RADOWSKI CLASSIFICATION OF JNA |

Stage	Tumor Extent
Ia	Limited to the posterior nares and/or nasopharyngeal vault
Ib	Involving the posterior nares and/or nasopharyngeal vault with involvement of at least one paranasal sinus
IIa	Minimal lateral extension to the pterygomaxillary fossa
IIb	Full occupation of the pterygomaxillary fossa with or without erosion of orbital bones
IIc	Extension into the infratemporal fossa or extension posterior to the pterygoid plates
IIIa	Erosion of the base of skull (middle cranial fossa/base of pterygoids)—minimal intracranial extension
IIIb	Extensive intracranial extension with or without extension into the cavernous sinus.

critical structures, control bleeding, avoid growth centers in the craniofacial skeleton of young patients and finally avoid facial scars if possible.

Open Surgery

Open surgical techniques can be classified according to the following scheme (Table 127.8).

These approaches can be classified according to the incision placement and the type of bone work required. Thus, the anterior approaches can be intraoral without external incisions or extraoral anterior with facial incisions

| TABLE 127.8 | OPEN APPROACHES FOR JNA SURGICAL RESECTION |

Open anterior approaches Intraoral	Degloving-Le fort-I osteotomy and downward palatal translocation
	Degloving, transantral approach
	Degloving modified transantral approach with medial maxillectomy and lateral buttress removal
	Degloving, maxillary/zygomatic removal and re–insertion
	Transpalatal and modified transpalatal approach
Open anterior approaches Facial incision	Weber-Ferguson and extended WF incision with facial translocation (removal and reinsertion of zygomatic bone including orbit floor and lateral wall)
Open lateral approaches	Fisch type D transtemporal approach with facial nerve mobilization
	Preauricular infratemporal fossa approach with zygomatic arch displacement and pterional craniectomy extradural approach

or lateral with coronal/hemicoronal incision. In terms of bone work, these can be broadly categorized as those that remove bone and those that displace bone (bone is temporarily translocated and placed back at closure), or a combination of the two.

The choice of approach is largely dependent on tumor extent and the facility of the surgical team.

With the transpalatal approach, the soft palate is mobilized and retracted to the opposite side of the tumor once the greater and lesser palatine vessels and nerves on the ipsilateral side have been sacrificed. The posterior hard palate along with the posterior upper molars may be resected and the corresponding alveolus drilled down along with the hard palate, the pterygoid plates leading to the base of the sphenoid. Once in this location, using as landmarks the dura of middle cranial fossa, V2 and V3 and their bony foramina and the sphenoid sinus, the skull base can be widely exposed and the tumor removed. A facial degloving with Le Fort-I achieves a very similar result in terms of exposure. A facial degloving with a medial maxillectomy and resection of the posterior lateral walls of the maxilla can effectively expose the nasal cavity, nasopharynx, pterygomaxillary space, and infratemporal fossa with excellent tumor exposure and removal. An anterior approach with a Weber-Ferguson facial incision can be combined with the removal of the zygomatic bone (including the orbital floor and lateral wall) possibly with a Le Fort-I osteotomy to provide wide access. This bone is removed, the tumor is removed, and then the bone segment is replaced and fixed with osteosynthesis plates.

With the preauricular infratemporal fossa approach, an extended hemicoronal incision is made, the zygomatic arch is transected and the temporalis muscle is inferiorly displaced from the temporal fossa. Soft tissue elevation exposes the body of the sphenoid and base of pterygoid plates. After a pterional craniectomy, the sphenoid wing and middle cranial fossa floor are removed, which provides contiguous access along the middle cranial fossa up to the cavernous sinus. The limits of this are the superior orbital fissure, optic canal, and horizontal petrous carotid artery. The lateral preauricular approaches are largely reserved for intracranial extension and can be combined in the same sitting as an anterior approach or as a separate procedure.

The postauricular transtemporal approach requires sacrifice of the middle ear structures and mobilization of the facial nerve. This indirect approach is used for more extensive petrous involvement.

The concerns with open approaches, especially those that involve bone displacement or resection in children and adolescents, are that bone growth may be affected with resultant facial symmetry and malocclusion. None of these concerns have been substantiated to date. Facial incisions, which are ideally placed correctly at the border of adjacent facial aesthetic units and closed meticulously, will leave almost imperceptible scarring (112).

Open approaches will achieve approximately 80% complete resection avoiding tumor recurrence even in advanced and salvage cases (96,106,109).

Endoscopic and Endoscopic-Assisted Approaches

There are increasing numbers of endoscopic and endoscopic-assisted approaches for JNA. Few authors have considerable experience with very advanced disease. Previous limitations of endoscopic approaches include extensive intracranial extension, tumor extension lateral to the cavernous sinus or posterior to the pterygoid plates.

Improved technique and intraoperative navigation have extended the successful endoscopic approach for these extensive tumors. Patient selection and the experience of the endoscopic surgeons are of paramount importance (111,113).

Radiotherapy

Radiation therapy is effective at controlling JNA. Rates of control of over 80% have been reported. Conventional radiation therapy of 30 to 35 Gy can achieve these results. IMRT can also be used, and excellent control has been reported. The advantage of IMRT is the precise computer-controlled dosing, which can potentially eliminate significant complications. Stereotactic radiation has also been used, especially in the setting of residual small volume tumor remnants after surgery (114–116).

Complications from radiation have included well-documented secondary malignancies, cataracts, CNS complications as well as panhypopituitarism. The risks of radiation should be carefully weighed against other available modalities especially in these young patients.

Surveillance

Symptoms and physical examination, including serial endoscopic examinations are unreliable for the detection of recurrent JNA, especially in previously treated advanced tumors. Serial radiographic imaging by contrast-enhanced CT and/or MRI is the choice of follow-up. Gadolinium-enhanced MRI is particularly sensitive for residual disease. Findings consistent with residual disease should be followed for at least 2 years before a decision for additional treatment is made.

HIGHLIGHTS

- Paraganglia facilitate the baroreceptive and chemoreceptive reflexes of the vascular system. In the head and neck, the carotid body only facilities the chemoreceptive reflex.
- The carotid body is a separate structure that lies at the carotid bifurcation. The jugulotympanic paraganglia are distributed in the temporal bone along Jacobson nerve while the vagal paraganglia are found within the vagus nerve at the level of the jugular foramen.
- Genetics and hypoxemia, such as high-altitude living, predispose to the paragangliomas.
- Mutations in the gene encoding for the mitochondrial enzyme SDH, a key enzyme in the Krebs cycle, are responsible for the genetic etiology of paraganglioma formation. PGL1 and PGL4 mutations show multicentricity and pheochromocytomas. PGL4 is associated with higher rate of malignant paraganglioma.
- Both radiation and surgery are effective treatments for paragangliomas. Selection of treatment depends on existing cranial nerve deficits, bilateral and/or multicentric tumors as well as age of patient.
- Surgery for paragangliomas requires extensive preparation including serum and urine catecholamine screening for functioning tumors, detailed radiographic investigations as well as superselective angiography with preoperative embolization. Jugulotympanic and vagal paragangliomas require an infratemporal fossa approach tailored to the size and extent of the lesion.
- HPCs are rare tumors. Twenty-five percent of them occur in the head and neck including the meninges. Ten-year survivals of 54% to 89% can be achieved with complete surgical resection, which is the primary mode of treatment.
- Angiosarcomas account of 10% of all head and neck sarcomas; they are much more aggressive than other body sites. They are difficult to distinguish pathologically from other vascular lesions.
- The treatment of angiosarcoma is wide resection with the goal of negative margins, which are difficult to achieve. Adjuvant therapy in the form or radiation and chemotherapy should be considered, but there is little evidence for their efficacy. Ten-year survival is approximately 14%.
- JNAs are highly vascular tumors that occur exclusively in adolescent and young adult males. They express indolent behavior with continued growth, which frequently extends to involve the skull base.
- The management of JNAs is surgical. Endoscopic techniques are indicated for early-stage tumors while a variety of open approaches are applicable to advanced disease.

REFERENCES

1. Pearse AG. The diffuse neuroendocrine system: peptides, amines, placodes and the APUD theory. *Prog Brain Res* 1986;68:25–31.
2. Pearse AG. The diffuse endocrine system and the implications of the APUD concept. *Int Surg* 1979;64:5–7.
3. Schwaber MK, Glasscock ME, Nissen AJ, et al. Diagnosis and management of catecholamine secreting glomus tumors. *Laryngoscope* 1984;94:1008–1015.

4. Fitzgerald RS, Eyzaguirre C, Zapata P. Fifty years of progress in carotid body physiology—invited article. *Adv Exp Med Biol* 2009;648:19–28.

5. Glenner GG, Grimley P. *Tumors of the Extra-Adrenal Paraganglion System (Including Chemoreceptors). Atlas of Tumor Pathology.* Washington, DC: Armed Forces Institute of Pathology, 1974:1–90.

6. Plenat F, Leroux P, Floquet J, et al. Intra and juxtavagal paraganglia: a topographical, histochemical, and ultrastructural study in the human. *Anat Rec* 1988;221:743–753.

7. Shibahara J, Goto A, Niki T, et al. Primary pulmonary paraganglioma: report of a functioning case with immunohistochemical and ultrastructural study. *Am J Surg Pathol* 2004;28: 825–829.

8. Gardner P, Dalsing M, Weisberger E, et al. Carotid body tumors, inheritance, and a high incidence of associated cervical paragangliomas. *Am J Surg* 1996;172:196–199.

9. Hu K, Persky MS. The multidisciplinary management of paragangliomas of the head and neck, part 2. *Oncology (Williston Park)* 2003;17:1143–1153; discussion 1154, 1158, 1161.

10. Hu K, Persky MS. Multidisciplinary management of paragangliomas of the head and neck, part 1. *Oncology (Williston Park)* 2003;17:983–993.

11. Persky MS, Setton A, Niimi Y, et al. Combined endovascular and surgical treatment of head and neck paragangliomas—a team approach. *Head Neck* 2002;24:423–431.

12. Hensen EF, Bayley JP. Recent advances in the genetics of SDH-related paraganglioma and pheochromocytoma. *Fam Cancer* 2011;10:355–363.

13. Cerecer-Gil NY, Figuera LE, Llamas FJ, et al. Mutation of SDHB is a cause of hypoxia-related high-altitude paraganglioma. *Clin Cancer Res* 2010;16:4148–4154.

14. Astrom K, Cohen JE, Willett-Brozick JE, et al. Altitude is a phenotypic modifier in hereditary paraganglioma type 1: evidence for an oxygen-sensing defect. *Hum Genet* 2003;113:228–237.

15. Jackson CG, Glasscock ME III, Nissen AJ, et al. Glomus tumor surgery: the approach, results, and problems. *Otolaryngol Clin North Am* 1982;15:897–916.

16. Müller U. Pathological mechanisms and parent-of-origin effects in hereditary paraganglioma/pheochromocytoma (PGL/PCC). *Neurogenetics* 2011;12:175–181.

17. Timmers HJ, Gimenez-Roqueplo AP, Mannelli M, et al. Clinical aspects of SDHx-related pheochromocytoma and paraganglioma. *Endocr Relat Cancer* 2009;16:391–400.

18. Baysal BE. Genomic imprinting and environment in hereditary paraganglioma. *Am J Med Genet C Semin Med Genet* 2004; 129C:85–90.

19. Pigny P, Cardot-Bauters C. Genetics of pheochromocytoma and paraganglioma: new developments. *Ann Endocrinol (Paris)* 2010; 71:76–82.

20. Cascon A, Pita G, Burnichon N, et al. Genetics of pheochromocytoma and paraganglioma in Spanish patients. *J Clin Endocrinol Metab* 2009;94:1701–1705.

21. Gimenez-Roqueplo AP, Burnichon N, Amar L, et al. Recent advances in the genetics of phaeochromocytoma and functional paraganglioma. *Clin Exp Pharmacol Physiol* 2008;35:376–379.

22. Gimenez-Roqueplo AP. New advances in the genetics of pheochromocytoma and paraganglioma syndromes. *Ann N Y Acad Sci* 2006;1073:112–121.

23. Parfait B, Chretien D, Rotig A, et al. Compound heterozygous mutations in the flavoprotein gene of the respiratory chain complex II in a patient with Leigh syndrome. *Hum Genet* 2000;106:236–243.

24. Moley JF, Wallin GK, Brother MB, et al. GM. Oncogene and growth factor expression in MEN 2 and related tumors. *Henry Ford Hospital Medical Journal* 1992;40(3–4):284–288.

25. Chetty R. Familial paraganglioma syndromes. *J Clin Pathol* 2010;63:488–491.

26. Zhang X, Xu W, Sun J, et al. VEGF mRNA expression in jugulotympanic paraganglioma. *Eur J Cancer Care (Engl)* 2010;19: 816–819.

27. Span PN, Rao JU, Oude Ophuis SB, et al. Overexpression of the natural antisense hypoxia-inducible factor-1{alpha} transcript is associated with malignant pheochromocytoma/paraganglioma. *Endocr Relat Cancer* 2011;18:323–331.

28. Jackson CG, McGrew BM, Forest JA, et al. Lateral skull base surgery for glomus tumors: long-term control. *Otol Neurotol* 2001;22:377–382.

29. Manolidis S, Jackson CG, Von Doersten PG, et al. Lateral skull base surgery: the otology group experience. *Skull Base Surg* 1997;7: 129–137.

30. Netterville JL, Jackson CG, Miller FR, et al. Vagal paraganglioma: a review of 46 patients treated during a 20-year period. *Arch Otolaryngol Head Neck Surg* 1998;124:1133–1140.

31. Rao AB, Koeller KK, Adair CF. From the archives of the AFIP. Paragangliomas of the head and neck: radiologic-pathologic correlation. Armed Forces Institute of Pathology. *Radiographics* 1999;19:1605–1632.

32. Valavanis A, Schubiger O, Oguz M. High-resolution CT investigation of nonchromaffin paragangliomas of the temporal bone. *AJNR Am J Neuroradiol* 1983;4:516–519.

33. Som PM, Braun IF, Shapiro MD, et al. Tumors of the parapharyngeal space and upper neck: MR imaging characteristics. *Radiology* 1987;164:823–829.

34. van den Berg R, Verbist BM, Mertens BJ, et al. Head and neck paragangliomas: improved tumor detection using contrast-enhanced 3D time-of-flight MR angiography as compared with fat-suppressed MR imaging techniques. *AJNR Am J Neuroradiol* 2004;25:863–870.

35. Neves F, Huwart L, Jourdan G, et al. Head and neck paragangliomas: value of contrast-enhanced 3D MR angiography. *AJNR Am J Neuroradiol* 2008;29:883–889.

36. Jackson CG, Cueva RA, Thedinger BA, et al. Cranial nerve preservation in lesions of the jugular fossa. *Otolaryngol Head Neck Surg* 1991;105:687–693.

37. Carlson A, Yonas H. Xenon techniques in predicting patients at risk for stroke after balloon test occlusion. *Neurosurgery* 2009;64:E1206.

38. Barr JD, Lemley TJ, McCann RM. Carotid artery balloon test occlusion: combined clinical evaluation and xenon-enhanced computed tomographic cerebral blood flow evaluation without patient transfer or balloon reinflation: technical note. *Neurosurgery* 1998;43:634–637; discussion 637–638.

39. Chrisoulidou A, Kaltsas G, Ilias I, et al. The diagnosis and management of malignant phaeochromocytoma and paraganglioma. *Endocr Relat Cancer* 2007;14:569–585.

40. Brink I, Hoegerle S, Klisch J, et al. Imaging of pheochromocytoma and paraganglioma. *Fam Cancer* 2005;4:61–68.

41. Young NM, Wiet RJ, Russell EJ, et al. Superselective embolization of glomus jugulare tumors. *Ann Otol Rhinol Laryngol* 1988;97:613–620.

42. Piazza P, Di Lella F, Menozzi R, et al. Absence of the contralateral internal carotid artery: a challenge for management of ipsilateral glomus jugulare and glomus vagale tumors. *Laryngoscope* 2007;117:1333–1337.

43. Forshaw MA, Higgins N, Hardy DG, et al. Rupture of an internal carotid artery aneurysm in the petrous temporal bone. *Br J Neurosurg* 2000;14:479–482.

44. Andrews JC, Valavanis A, Fisch U. Management of the internal carotid artery in surgery of the skull base. *Laryngoscope* 1989;99:1224–1229.

45. Gardner G, Cocke EW Jr, Robertson JH, et al. Skull base surgery for glomus jugulare tumors. *Am J Otol* 1985;(Suppl):126–134.

46. Bigelow DC, Hoffer ME, Schlakman B, et al. Angiographic assessment of the transverse sinus and vein of labbe to avoid complications in skull base surgery. *Skull Base Surg* 1993;3:217–222.

47. Oghalai JS, Leung MK, Jackler RK, et al. Transjugular craniotomy for the management of jugular foramen tumors with intracranial extension. *Otol Neurotol* 2004;25:570–579; discussion 579.

48. Jackson CG, Glasscock ME III, Harris PF. Glomus tumors. Diagnosis, classification, and management of large lesions. *Arch Otolaryngol* 1982;108:401–410.

49. Lim JY, Kim J, Kim SH, et al. Surgical treatment of carotid body paragangliomas: outcomes and complications according to the shamblin classification. *Clin Exp Otorhinolaryngol* 2010;3:91–95.

50. Vogel TR, Mousa AY, Dombrovskiy VY, et al. Carotid body tumor surgery: management and outcomes in the nation. *Vasc Endovascular Surg* 2009;43:457–461.

51. Kotelis D, Rizos T, Geisbusch P, et al. Late outcome after surgical management of carotid body tumors from a 20-year single-center experience. *Langenbecks Arch Surg* 2009;394:339–344.

52. Sajid MS, Hamilton G, Baker DM. A multicenter review of carotid body tumour management. *Eur J Vasc Endovasc Surg* 2007;34:127–130.

53. Sanna M, De Donato G, Piazza P, et al. Revision glomus tumor surgery. *Otolaryngol Clin North Am* 2006;39:763–782, vii.

54. Maturo S, Brennan J. Baroreflex failure: a rare complication of carotid paraganglioma surgery. *Laryngoscope* 2006;116:829–830.

55. Glasscock ME III. The history of glomus tumors: a personal perspective. *Laryngoscope* 1993;103:3–6.

56. Jackson CG, Harris PF, Glasscock ME III, et al. Diagnosis and management of paragangliomas of the skull base. *Am J Surg* 1990;159:389–393.

57. Netterville JL, Vrabec JT. Unilateral palatal adhesion for paralysis after high vagal injury. *Arch Otolaryngol Head Neck Surg* 1994;120:218–221.

58. Netterville JL, Civantos FJ. Defect reconstruction following neurotologic skull base surgery. *Laryngoscope* 1993;103:55–63.

59. Netterville JL, Civantos FJ. Rehabilitation of cranial nerve deficits after neurotologic skull base surgery. *Laryngoscope* 1993;103:45–54.

60. Netterville JL, Jackson CG, Civantos F. Thyroplasty in the functional rehabilitation of neurotologic skull base surgery patients. *Am J Otol* 1993;14:460–464.

61. Mark S, Persky KH. Paragangliomas of the head and neck. In: Louis B. Harrison RBS, Waun Ki Hong, eds. *Head and neck cancer: a multidisciplinary approach.* Philadelphia, PA: Lippincott Williams and Wilkins, 2009:655–687.

62. Wegner RE, Rodriguez KD, Heron DE, et al. Linac-based stereotactic body radiation therapy for treatment of glomus jugulare tumors. *Radiother Oncol* 2010;97:395–398.

63. Lim M, Gibbs IC, Adler JR Jr, et al. Efficacy and safety of stereotactic radiosurgery for glomus jugulare tumors. *Neurosurg Focus* 2004;17:E11.

64. Pollock BE. Stereotactic radiosurgery in patients with glomus jugulare tumors. *Neurosurg Focus* 2004;17:E10.

65. Maarouf M, Voges J, Landwehr P, et al. Stereotactic linear accelerater-based radiosurgery for the treatment of patients with glomus jugulare tumors. *Cancer* 2003;97:1093–1098.

66. Foote RL, Pollock BE, Gorman DA, et al. Glomus jugulare tumor: tumor control and complications after stereotactic radiosurgery. *Head Neck* 2002;24:332–338; discussion 338–339.

67. Billings KR, Fu YS, Calcaterra TC, et al. Hemangiopericytoma of the head and neck. *Am J Otolaryngol* 2000;21:238–243.

68. Park MS, Araujo DM. New insights into the hemangiopericytoma/solitary fibrous tumor spectrum of tumors. *Curr Opin Oncol* 2009;21:327–331.

69. Chen KT, Kassel SH, Medrano VA. Congenital hemangiopericytoma. *J Surg Oncol* 1986;31:127–129.

70. Gillman G, Pavlovich JB. Sinonasal hemangiopericytoma. *Otolaryngol Head Neck Surg* 2004;131:1012–1013.

71. Harrison JM, Fazekas MA, Palacios E. Sinonasal hemangiopericytoma. *Ear Nose Throat J* 2002;81:141.

72. Schiariti M, Goetz P, El-Maghraby H, et al. Hemangiopericytoma: long-term outcome revisited. Clinical article. *J Neurosurg* 2011;114:747–755.

73. Carew JF, Singh B, Kraus DH. Hemangiopericytoma of the head and neck. *Laryngoscope* 1999;109:1409–1411.

74. Spitz FR, Bouvet M, Pisters PW, et al. Hemangiopericytoma: a 20-year single-institution experience. *Ann Surg Oncol* 1998;5:350–355.

75. Thompson LD, Miettinen M, Wenig BM. Sinonasal-type hemangiopericytoma: a clinicopathologic and immunophenotypic analysis of 104 cases showing perivascular myoid differentiation. *Am J Surg Pathol* 2003;27:737–749.

76. Espat NJ, Lewis JJ, Leung D, et al. Conventional hemangiopericytoma: modern analysis of outcome. *Cancer* 2002;95:1746–1751.

77. Chamberlain MC, Glantz MJ. Sequential salvage chemotherapy for recurrent intracranial hemangiopericytoma. *Neurosurgery* 2008;63:720–726; author reply 726–727.

78. Celik I, Bascil N, Yalcin S, et al. Ifosfamide-based chemotherapy for recurrent or metastatic hemangiopericytoma. *Acta Oncol* 1997;36:348.

79. Park MS, Ravi V, Araujo DM. Inhibiting the VEGF-VEGFR pathway in angiosarcoma, epithelioid hemangioendothelioma, and hemangiopericytoma/solitary fibrous tumor. *Curr Opin Oncol* 2010;22:351–355.

80. Pawlik TM, Paulino AF, McGinn CJ, et al. Cutaneous angiosarcoma of the scalp: a multidisciplinary approach. *Cancer* 2003;98:1716–1726.

81. Albores-Saavedra J, Schwartz AM, Henson DE, et al. Cutaneous angiosarcoma. Analysis of 434 cases from the Surveillance, Epidemiology, and End Results Program, 1973-2007. *Ann Diagn Pathol* 2011;15:93–97.

82. Young RJ, Brown NJ, Reed MW, et al. Angiosarcoma. *Lancet Oncol* 2010;11:983–991.

83. Deyrup AT, Miettinen M, North PE, et al. Pediatric cutaneous angiosarcomas: a clinicopathologic study of 10 cases. *Am J Surg Pathol* 2011;35:70–75.

84. Mendenhall WM, Mendenhall CM, Werning JW, et al. Cutaneous angiosarcoma. *Am J Clin Oncol* 2006;29:524–528.

85. Tokuyama W, Mikami T, Masuzawa M, et al. Autocrine and paracrine roles of VEGF/VEGFR-2 and VEGF-C/VEGFR-3 signaling in angiosarcomas of the scalp and face. *Hum Pathol* 2010;41:407–414.

86. Deyrup AT, Miettinen M, North PE, et al. Angiosarcomas arising in the viscera and soft tissue of children and young adults: a clinicopathologic study of 15 cases. *Am J Surg Pathol* 2009;33:264–269.

87. Shkoukani MA, Carron MA, Tulunay O, et al. Angiosarcoma of the scalp with complete response to a biweekly gemcitabine and docetaxel (GEMDOC) chemotherapy regimen. *Ear Nose Throat J* 2011;90:E26–E29.

88. Asmane I, Litique V, Heymann S, et al. Adriamycin, cisplatin, ifosfamide and paclitaxel combination as front-line chemotherapy for locally advanced and metastatic angiosarcoma. Analysis of three case reports and review of the literature. *Anticancer Res* 2008;28:3041–3045.

89. Holloway CL, Turner AR, Dundas GS. Cutaneous angiosarcoma of the scalp: a case report of sustained complete response following liposomal Doxorubicin and radiation therapy. *Sarcoma* 2005;9:29–31.

90. Nagano T, Yamada Y, Ikeda T, et al. Docetaxel: a therapeutic option in the treatment of cutaneous angiosarcoma: report of 9 patients. *Cancer* 2007;110:648–651.

91. Penel N, Bui BN, Bay JO, et al. Phase II trial of weekly paclitaxel for unresectable angiosarcoma: the ANGIOTAX study. *J Clin Oncol* 2008;26:5269–5274.

92. Fuller CK, Charlson JA, Dankle SK, et al. Dramatic improvement of inoperable angiosarcoma with combination paclitaxel and bevacizumab chemotherapy. *J Am Acad Dermatol* 2010;63:e83–e84.

93. Koontz BF, Miles EF, Rubio MA, et al. Preoperative radiotherapy and bevacizumab for angiosarcoma of the head and neck: two case studies. *Head Neck* 2008;30:262–266.

94. Guadagnolo BA, Zagars GK, Araujo D, et al. Outcomes after definitive treatment for cutaneous angiosarcoma of the face and scalp. *Head Neck* 2011;33:661–667.

95. Lydiatt WM, Shaha AR, Shah JP. Angiosarcoma of the head and neck. *Am J Surg* 1994;168:451–454.

96. Bales C, Kotapka M, Loevner LA, et al. Craniofacial resection of advanced juvenile nasopharyngeal angiofibroma. *Arch Otolaryngol Head Neck Surg* 2002;128:1071–1078.

97. Coutinho-Camillo CM, Brentani MM, Nagai MA. Genetic alterations in juvenile nasopharyngeal angiofibromas. *Head Neck* 2008;30:390–400.

98. Howard DJ, Lloyd G, Lund V. Recurrence and its avoidance in juvenile angiofibroma. *Laryngoscope* 2001;111:1509–1511.

99. Schuon R, Brieger J, Heinrich UR, et al. Immunohistochemical analysis of growth mechanisms in juvenile nasopharyngeal angiofibroma. *Eur Arch Otorhinolaryngol* 2007;264:389–394.

100. Renkonen S, Hayry V, Heikkila P, et al. Stem cell-related proteins C-KIT, C-MYC and BMI-1 in juvenile nasopharyngeal angiofibroma—do they have a role? *Virchows Arch* 2011;458:189–195.

101. Thakar A, Gupta G, Bhalla AS, et al. Adjuvant therapy with flutamide for presurgical volume reduction in juvenile nasopharyngeal angiofibroma. *Head Neck* 2011;33:1747–1753.

102. Brieger J, Wierzbicka M, Sokolov M, et al. Vessel density, proliferation, and immunolocalization of vascular endothelial growth factor in juvenile nasopharyngeal angiofibromas. *Arch Otolaryngol Head Neck Surg* 2004;130:727–731.

103. Ponti G, Losi L, Pellacani G, et al. Wnt pathway, angiogenetic and hormonal markers in sporadic and familial adenomatous polyposis-associated juvenile nasopharyngeal angiofibromas (JNA). *Appl Immunohistochem Mol Morphol* 2008;16:173–178.

104. Roche PH, Paris J, Regis J, et al. Management of invasive juvenile nasopharyngeal angiofibromas: the role of a multimodality approach. *Neurosurgery* 2007;61:768–777; discussion 777.

105. Browne JD, Jacob SL. Temporal approach for resection of juvenile nasopharyngeal angiofibromas. *Laryngoscope* 2000;110: 1287–1293.

106. Danesi G, Panizza B, Mazzoni A, et al. Anterior approaches in juvenile nasopharyngeal angiofibromas with intracranial extension. *Otolaryngol Head Neck Surg* 2000;122:277–283.

107. Wu AW, Mowry SE, Vinuela F, et al. Bilateral vascular supply in juvenile nasopharyngeal angiofibromas. *Laryngoscope* 2011;121: 639–643.

108. Wilms G, Peene P, Baert AL, et al. Pre-operative embolization of juvenile nasopharyngeal angiofibromas. *J Belge Radiol* 1989; 72:465–470.

109. Radkowski D, McGill T, Healy GB, et al. Angiofibroma. Changes in staging and treatment. *Arch Otolaryngol Head Neck Surg* 1996; 122:122–129.

110. Zhang M, Garvis W, Linder T, et al. Update on the infratemporal fossa approaches to nasopharyngeal angiofibroma. *Laryngoscope* 1998;108:1717–1723.

111. Carrau RL, Snyderman CH, Kassam AB, et al. Endoscopic and endoscopic-assisted surgery for juvenile angiofibroma. *Laryngoscope* 2001;111:483–487.

112. Enepekides DJ. Recent advances in the treatment of juvenile angiofibroma. *Curr Opin Otolaryngol Head Neck Surg* 2004;12:495–499.

113. Douglas R, Wormald PJ. Endoscopic surgery for juvenile nasopharyngeal angiofibroma: where are the limits? *Curr Opin Otolaryngol Head Neck Surg* 2006;14:1–5.

114. Lee JT, Chen P, Safa A, et al. The role of radiation in the treatment of advanced juvenile angiofibroma. *Laryngoscope* 2002;112: 1213–1220.

115. Reddy KA, Mendenhall WM, Amdur RJ, et al. Long-term results of radiation therapy for juvenile nasopharyngeal angiofibroma. *Am J Otolaryngol* 2001;22:172–175.

116. Cummings BJ, Blend R, Keane T, et al. Primary radiation therapy for juvenile nasopharyngeal angiofibroma. *Laryngoscope* 1984; 94:1599–1605.

128 Lymphomas of the Head and Neck

Raymond L. Chai   *Andrew B. Tassler*   *Seungwon Kim*

Lymphoma, a malignancy of lymphoid tissue characterized by the proliferation of lymphoid cells or their precursors, is the most common nonepithelial malignancy of the head and neck. Because lymphoma typically manifests as a neck mass, otolaryngologists are frequently involved in diagnosis. However, as it is a disease treated primarily by radiation and medical oncologists, the role of the otolaryngologist generally diminishes once a diagnosis is obtained. Nonetheless, as a participant of a multidisciplinary team, it is imperative for the otolaryngologist to be well versed in not only comprehensive management of the disease but also the controversies of classification and treatment. Moreover, the otolaryngologist will often be the diagnosing physician for lymphomas that present in the head and neck, and thus a high index of suspicion must be maintained, especially for lymphomas occurring at extranodal sites.

There are two main types of lymphoma: Hodgkin lymphoma (HL) and non-Hodgkin lymphoma (NHL). HL is typically characterized by the orderly spread of disease through contiguous groups of lymph nodes. In contrast, NHL can manifest in extranodal sites such as Waldeyer ring, salivary glands, and thyroid in addition to occurring in the nodal basins of the head and neck.

EPIDEMIOLOGY

NHL accounts for 86% of all lymphoma cases and is the fifth most common malignancy in the United States, excluding skin cancers (1). It is primarily a disease of adults, with less than 10% of overall cases occurring in children (2). NHL results from chromosomal translocations in B or T/ natural killer (NK) cells that lead to either the inactivation of tumor suppressor genes or activation of oncogenes (3). B-cell lymphomas compromise roughly 90% of all NHLs; the two most common histologic subtypes are follicular lymphoma and the more aggressive diffuse large B-cell lymphoma (DLBCL) (4). Risk factors include male gender,

long-term immunosuppression, exposure to radiation or pesticides, and autoimmune diseases such as systemic lupus erythematous (5). Infections including human immunodeficiency virus (HIV), human T-cell lymphotropic virus 1 (HTLV-1), human herpesvirus-8 (HHV-8), and Epstein-Barr virus (EBV) have also been associated with the development of lymphoma (6).

The less common HL is a highly curable disease with an estimated 5-year relative survival of 86% (2). The incidence of HL has a bimodal distribution, with the disease primarily occurring in young adults and patients 55 years and older (7). Much like in NHL, risk factors for the development of HL include viral exposure, immune suppression, and familial factors (8). Although HL originally had been subdivided into four categories, the most recent World Health Organization (WHO) classification has separated the disease into the more common classical HL and the rare nodular lymphocyte-predominant HL (9). The diagnosis of HL is made with the identification of Reed-Sternberg cells, a binucleated or multinucleated giant cell of germinal center B-cell origin (Fig. 128.1) (10). HL is unique in that malignant cells compromise the minority (estimated at 0.1% to 10%) of the cellular population of the tumor (11). Thus, obtaining ample biopsy specimen is critical for accurate diagnosis of the disease.

In 2010, the American Cancer Society estimates that 74,030 new lymphoma cases will be diagnosed and 21,530 deaths due to lymphoma will occur in the United States (2). An analysis of the National Cancer Data Base (NCDB) revealed that the proportion of lymphoma cases among all head and neck tumors increased from 14.7% between 1985 and 1989 to 15.4% between 1990 and 1994 (12). This increase has been postulated to be attributable to an increase in immunodeficiency secondary to both HIV and patients receiving organ transplants. Interestingly, more recent data from the NCDB suggest both an absolute and proportionate decrease (to 12.4%) in the prevalence of lymphoma from 2000 to 2004, perhaps reflecting the use

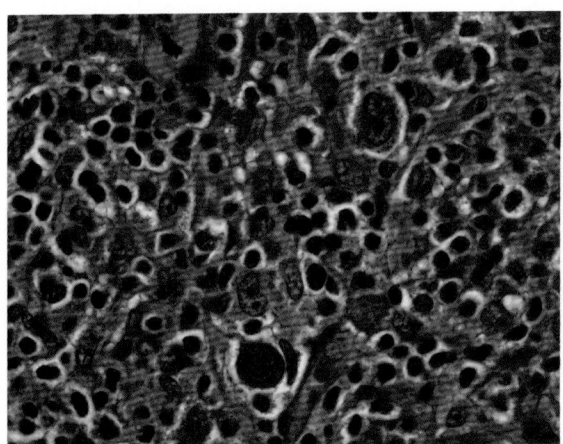

Figure 128.1 Reed-Sternberg cell in a lymph node involved by HL.

of combination antiretroviral therapy for patients with acquired immune deficiency syndrome (AIDS) (13).

CLINICAL DIAGNOSIS AND IMAGING

The majority of lymphoma cases present with nontender lymphadenopathy of greater than 2 weeks duration, usually in the neck or supraclavicular area (14). Systemic symptoms including fever greater than 38°C, drenching night sweats, and unintentional weight loss of greater than 10% of body weight over a period of 6 months or less are known collectively as B symptoms. B symptoms are established negative prognostic factors in both HL and NHL and predict worse treatment response and survival. Recently, B symptoms, a marker of systemic inflammation, have been established as an independent predictor of increased toxicity from chemotherapy in NHL patients (15).

Although HL is primarily a disease confined to lymph nodes, primary extranodal involvement occurs in 25% to 40% of NHL patients at initial diagnosis (16). Roughly a third of all primary extranodal lymphomas occur in Waldeyer ring, a circle of lymphoid tissue in the pharynx formed by the palatine and pharyngeal tonsils as well as the lymphatic follicles at the base of tongue (17). Several European studies have shown an even higher incidence of extranodal disease in Waldeyer ring, likely related to the routine biopsy of this area in all patients with NHL (18,19). Lymphomas in this region compromise greater than half of all primary extranodal lymphomas of the head and neck (20). Less commonly, primary lymphoma in the head and neck can manifest in salivary glands, the sinonasal region, the thyroid, and the larynx.

Diagnosis of lymphoma in the head and neck includes a combination of history and physical, including a full head and neck exam. Either mirror exam or flexible laryngoscopy should be performed to visualize Waldeyer ring, the larynx, and hypopharynx. Routine hematologic and biochemical profiles, renal and liver profiles, as well as imaging should

be obtained as well. Cardiac assessment including clinical examination, electrocardiography (EKG), and echocardiogram should be performed for all patients greater than 65 years of age and when otherwise indicated.

Serum lactate dehydrogenase (LDH) level should be measured in all patients and is an important predictor of survival, with elevated levels indicating tissue damage, lymphoma relapse, or renewed growth. As a component of the International Prognostic Index (IPI), pretreatment LDH is used to stratify patient populations into appropriate treatment regimens (21). β-2 microglobulin testing, which has been shown to predict response rate and duration of remission, is also routinely performed in some centers (22). Bone marrow aspirate and biopsy, typically of the bilateral iliac crests, is also routinely performed to define the extent of disease in initial staging. Marrow involvement is found in 5% to 15% of HL patients at diagnosis and up to 30% of newly diagnosed NHL cases (23,24). Cerebrospinal fluid (CSF) evaluation should be performed in patients with paranasal sinus or nasopharyngeal involvement due to disease proximity to the skull base. CSF analysis should also be considered in patients with large cell lymphoma presenting with an elevated LDH and/or involvement of multiple extranodal sites (25).

Contrast-enhanced computerized tomography (CT) of the head, neck, chest, abdomen, and pelvis is routinely performed for evaluation of both nodal and nonnodal lymphoma involvement. CT of the head and neck is also useful for the assessment of any bony involvement or destruction of the mandible, maxilla, paranasal sinuses, and skull base. Although it is difficult to distinguish HL and NHL by CT alone, lymphoma is suspected when multiple, nonenhancing, large, homogeneous lymph nodes are present, particularly in unusual nodal chains such as the retropharyngeal, occipital, and parotid nodes (Fig. 128.2) (26). Because nodal necrosis is present in the majority of lymph nodes involved with squamous cell carcinoma (SCC) larger than 3 cm, lymphoma is implicated with the presence of large nonnecrotic nodes (27). Pretreatment nodal necrosis, when seen, is usually found in high-grade lymphomas (28).

Fluorine-18-fluorodeoxyglucose positron emission tomography-computed tomography (^{18}F-FDG-PET-CT) superimposes anatomic detail from CT images with functional imaging obtained by PET. ^{18}F-FDG-PET-CT is a good choice as the initial imaging study in patients with FDG avid lymphomas such as HL, B-cell lymphoma, or follicular lymphoma. A pretreatment ^{18}F-FDG-PET-CT is used in most centers for initial staging and allows for subsequent monitoring of response to treatment and assessment of recurrent or residual disease. Because it evaluates metabolic activity, ^{18}F-FDG-PET-CT can also help differentiate malignant and nonmalignant lymph nodes in small lymph nodes that are negative by CT size criteria. Improved accuracy in staging with ^{18}F-FDG-PET-CT may help avoid overtreatment and its associated toxicities.

Recent studies have shown upstaging of disease in up to 20% of cases using PET-CT with improved detection of

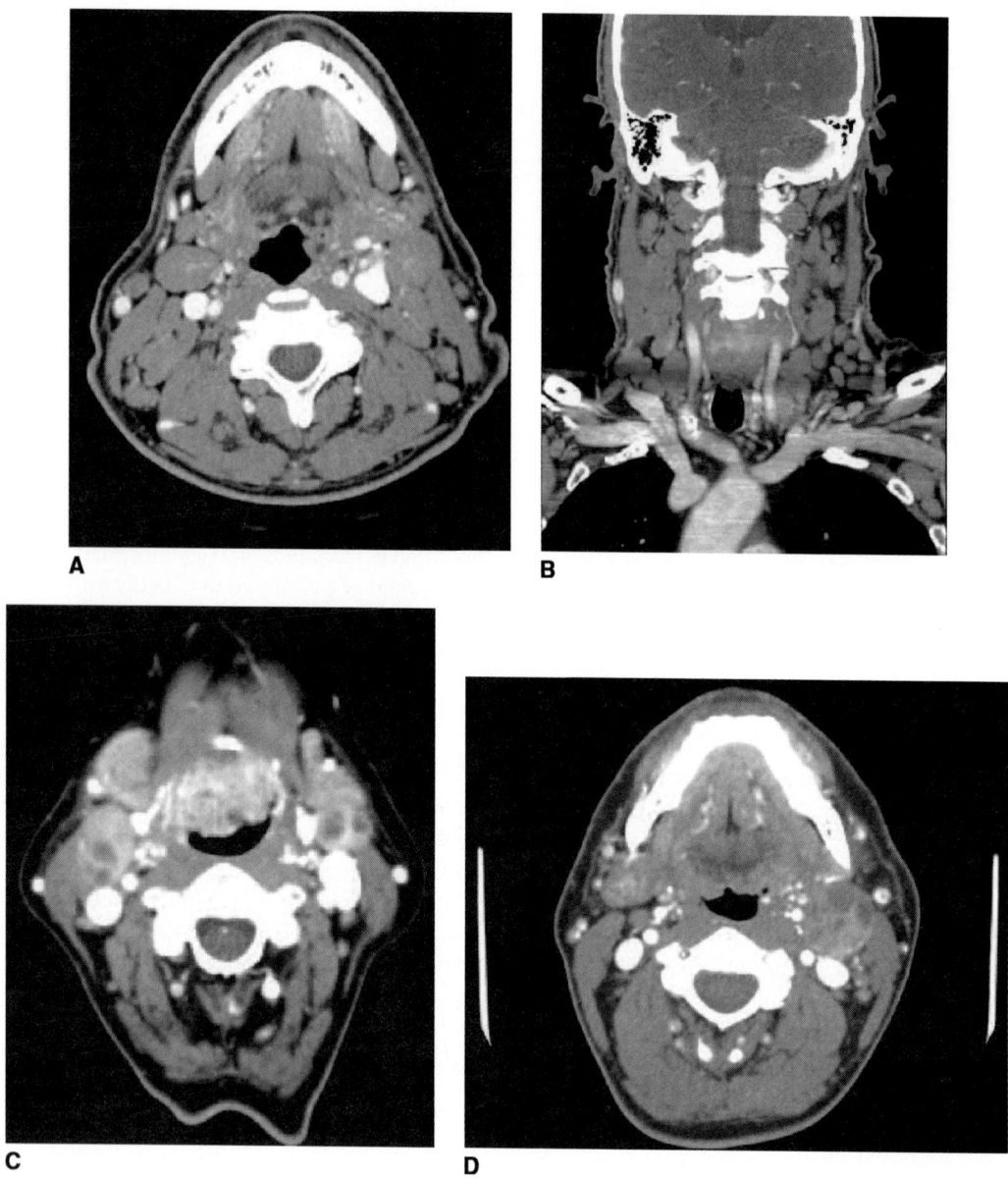

Figure 128.2 Contrast-enhanced (**A**) axial and (**B**) coronal CT images from patient with B-cell lymphoma, demonstrating multiple enlarged lymph nodes with poor contrast enhancement and uniform appearance. In contrast, lymph nodes with metastatic SCC demonstrate (**C**) heterogeneous enhancement as well as (**D**) central necrosis.

occult splenic involvement and exclusion of bone marrow involvement in aggressive B-cell NHL (29). A meta-analysis of 20 studies including seven prospective trials on the effectiveness of PET in lymphoma staging showed an overall change-in-management rate of 30% based on imaging findings (30). ^{18}F-FDG-PET-CT is less useful in low-grade NHL because of low metabolic uptake in malignant nodes (31).

TISSUE DIAGNOSIS

In order to institute appropriate therapy, adequate tissue sampling is needed for both diagnosis and definitive subclassification of lymphoma. As such, the gold standard

for diagnosis of lymphoma in the head and neck is open excisional biopsy. However, with the advent of new classification schemes such as the Revised European-American Lymphoma classification (REAL) in the mid-1990s and more recently the WHO classification, new emphasis has been placed on immunophenotypic and cytogenetic characteristics rather than architectural features in the categorization of tumors. Thus, recent investigations have focused on the utility of both fine needle aspiration (FNA) and core needle biopsy (CNB) as independent diagnostic tools for lymphoma diagnosis.

FNA has become widely used in the head and neck in the evaluation of both lymphadenopathy as well as primary lesions such as parotid and thyroid tumors. In comparison to surgical biopsy, FNA offers advantages in speed, cost, and minimal complications. Needle aspirates can provide material for both cytomorphology and flow cytometry, a technique that selects for specific surface antigens that determine lymphoid and/or myeloid cell lineages. It is possible to diagnose most lymphomas in general terms on the basis of characteristic cytologic morphology. FNA cytology has shown to have a high accuracy rate, ranging from 80% to 90%, in the diagnosis of both HL and NHL (32–36). Flow cytometry alone has also been shown to be an accurate independent ancillary test, with a large series from the University of Iowa demonstrating a sensitivity of 91.8% and a specificity of 95.5% in the diagnosis of B-cell NHL (37). Multiple studies have shown, however, that the malignant Reed-Sternberg cells that characterize HL are almost never detected by flow cytometry (38,39).

The primary limitation of FNA is the relatively small amount of material available for phenotyping. Although helpful in the diagnosis of lymphoma, flow cytometry has been shown to not aid in the subclassification of disease (40). A complete histologic diagnosis using the WHO classification is possible in only a minority of FNA specimens (41). FNA alone is thus clinically insufficient to design appropriate treatment plans for lymphoma patients. However, the utility of FNA has become widely accepted in certain clinical conditions, such as the documentation of recurrent lymphoma and the diagnosis of posttransplant lymphoproliferative disorder (PTLD) (42,43).

CNB is an intermediate step between FNA and open surgical biopsy. By using a larger sized needle (14 to 18 gauge), CNB provides sufficient sample for both immunohistochemistry and conventional histopathology. CNB is now commonly accepted as an initial procedure for patients with deep-seated lymph nodes, particularly in the mediastinum or abdomen (44). Two recent studies investigating ultrasound-guided CNB in cervical lymphadenopathy have shown full subclassification in 89.7% and 92.3% of lymphoma cases, respectively (45,46). Factors such as nodal necrosis or infarct significantly reduce the success of diagnosis, particularly for HL. Although promising, further investigation is needed in evaluating the full utility of this technique.

STAGING

First proposed in 1971 for HL and later adapted for NHL, the Ann Arbor staging system is the most widely used criterion for determining prognosis and treatment (Table 128.1) (47). This system is based on the region and number of affected lymph nodes as well as the presence of extranodal sites and constitutional symptoms. The Ann Arbor staging system that was originally developed for HL is currently used to stage both HL and NHL. In 1989, the Ann Arbor system was refined with the Cotswalds modification, which takes into account the importance of bulky disease as a negative prognostic factor (48).

TABLE 128.1	ANN ARBOR STAGING SYSTEM FOR LYMPHOMA
Stage I	Involvement of a single lymph node region (I) or of a single extralymphatic organ or site (IE)
Stage II	Involvement of two or more lymph node regions or lymphatic structures on the same side of the diaphragm alone (II) or with involvement of limited, contiguous extralymphatic organ or tissue (IIE)
Stage III	Involvement of lymph node regions on both sides of the diaphragm (III) that may include the spleen (IIIS) or limited, contiguous extralymphatic organ or site (IIIE) or both (IIIES)
Stage IV	Diffuse or disseminated foci of involvement of one or more extralymphatic organs or tissues, with or without associated lymphatic involvement

All cases are subclassified to indicate absence (A) or presence (B) or systemic symptoms of significant unexplained fever, night sweats, and unexplained weight loss exceeding 10% of body weight during the 6 mo prior to diagnosis.
The designation "S" refers to the involvement of the spleen.
The designation "E" refers to extranodal contiguous extension.

The Ann Arbor system does not, however, take into account the grade and biologic behavior of a given lymphoma and has been shown to be inadequate as a sole predictor of overall survival for patients with aggressive NHL (49). In 1993, the IPI was proposed. Based on a retrospective series of over 2,000 patients in an international multi-institutional study, this model uses age, Ann Arbor tumor stage, serum LDH, performance status, and number of extranodal disease sites to stratify patients into four risk groups (50). Because younger patients may tolerate more aggressive therapy and thus have different outcomes, an age-adjusted index was proposed in the same study for patients younger than 60. This simplified criteria use only stage, LDH, and performance status to predict outcomes. Similar to the IPI, the Follicular Lymphoma International Prognostic Index (FLIPI) was designed as a prognostic model for patients with indolent lymphoma (51). Factors in this index include age, stage, number of involved lymph node areas, serum hemoglobin level, and serum LDH.

These systems alone are not, however, sufficient for initiating treatment, as outcome is highly variable and dependent on tumor histology and morphology. In 1982, the Working Formulation, a now-obsolete classification of NHL tumors, subdivided lymphomas by morphology alone (52). The REAL and later the WHO classification groups differentiated NHLs by cell lineage and unique phenotypic, molecular, and cytogenetic characteristics. The fourth edition of the WHO classification, which is the most recent update, was introduced in 2008 and classifies NHL as indolent, aggressive, and highly aggressive tumors (9). However, it should be kept in mind that the WHO classification system is not a staging system. The Ann Arbor staging system, despite its shortcomings, remains the best mean of staging lymphomas and has been adopted by the

American Joint Committee on Cancer (AJCC) as well as Union for International Cancer Control (UICC) as the official system for classifying the extent of anatomic involvement and for staging of both HL and NHL.

THERAPY

Radiation therapy and/or combination chemotherapy is the current mainstay of treatment for both NHL and HL of the head and neck. Advances in molecular biology have led to the development of novel therapies for NHL such as monoclonal antibodies and radioimmunoconjugates. Although surgery does play a role in the management of lymphoma, particularly in localized gastrointestinal disease, its utility in the head and neck is typically limited to diagnostic biopsy.

Hodgkin Lymphoma

Initial therapy for early stage HL (I–IIA) may vary depending on the center instituting treatment. Extended-field radiation had been the standard of care for decades. However, with 5-year survival rates for patients with early-stage disease of 90% or higher, long-term complications from radiation therapy are not insignificant (53). Second malignancies such as breast cancer occur roughly 1% a year for at least 30 years after treatment (54). Other long-term side effects include mediastinal fibrosis, myelitis, and hypothyroidism (55). For favorable early-stage disease, short-term chemotherapy with doxorubicin, bleomycin, vinblastine, and dacarbazine (ABVD) alone or combined chemotherapy with involved-field radiation therapy to involved lymph nodes regions only is now recommended (56).

Tumor bulk, high erythrocyte sedimentation rate, multiple sites, age 50 or greater, and massive splenic disease have been identified as factors defining unfavorable disease in HL (57). Although the subject of ongoing debate, the usage of combination chemotherapy plus involved-field radiotherapy rather than extended-field radiation is a generally accepted protocol (58). For the rare nodular lymphocyte-predominant HL, with its improved prognosis, reduced intensity protocols have been advocated for early stage tumors (59).

In patients with advanced stage III to IV HL, the ongoing challenge involves developing regimens that maximize survival rates while limiting the development of long-term toxicities. The first combination chemotherapy used for these patients was the MOPP (mechlorethamine, vincristine, procarbazine, and prednisone) protocol. Developed in 1970 for patients with disease progression after radiotherapy, this regimen markedly improved survival rates (60). In 1975, the ABVD regimen was shown to have similar clinical activity (61). A regimen utilizing alternating cycles of ABVD and MOPP was later shown to have superior overall survival rates (62). More recently, a large multi-institutional trial established ABVD as the standard regimen for treatment of advanced HL, with the hybrid MOPP/ABV regimen associated with greater toxicity (63). Thus, the primary treatment strategy at many centers is ABVD combined with involved-field radiotherapy. Similar regimens are typically used for advanced stage nodular lymphocyte-predominant HL (64).

Indolent Non-Hodgkin Lymphoma

Indolent lymphoma comprises 40% of all NHLs, with follicular lymphomas the most common subtype. The majority of these patients are initially asymptomatic and typically present at advanced stage. Although these tumors have a long median survival, the majority of patients are incurable, with the exception of rare early stage disease (65). The goal of treatment should be complete remission but often is focused toward alleviating localized symptoms and compromised organ function. There is significant controversy in treatment options because despite the wide range of available therapeutic approaches, most patients ultimately relapse. However, despite some data suggesting that overall survival for these patients has not improved in the last several decades, recent studies have shown survival improvements, particularly from the introduction of biologic therapies (66).

Data from large prospective trials have shown no significant difference between observation and the initiation of immediate treatment in advanced indolent lymphoma patients (67). Watchful waiting, particularly in patients older than 70 years of age, is thus an accepted initial option. In symptomatic patients, combination chemotherapy and immunotherapy is considered to be standard therapy. The addition of the anti-CD20 monoclonal antibody rituximab with the standard CHOP (cyclophosphamide, doxorubicin, vincristine, and prednisone) regimen (R-CHOP) has shown significant improvement in outcome without additional major toxicity (68). The addition of rituximab has demonstrated clinical benefit as well for symptomatic elderly patients with relevant comorbidities (69). Rituximab as maintenance therapy is recommended for relapsed or refractory advanced disease (70). Radioimmunotherapy using monoclonal antibodies covalently bound to radionuclides such as Yttrium-90 ibritumomab tiuxetan and iodine-131 tositumomab has shown efficacy in both consolidation therapy and rituximab-refractory tumors, respectively (71,72).

Aggressive Non-Hodgkin Lymphoma

The majority of NHL cases are aggressive lymphomas, with DLBCL as the most common histologic subtype in the head and neck (73). Treatment has evolved over the last 30 years from the primary usage of radiotherapy to combination chemotherapy with immunotherapy. Current National Comprehensive Cancer Network (NCCN) guidelines provide oncologists with the option of utilizing either three cycles of R-CHOP plus involved-field radiation therapy or six to eight cycles of R-CHOP with or without involved-field radiation therapy for both bulky and nonbulky early-stage disease (74). The addition of radiation therapy, however, is controversial, and the majority of oncologists utilize the extended combination chemotherapy protocol alone (75).

For advanced stage DLBCL, R-CHOP is considered to be the standard of care in the United States. Large prospective studies in both France and the United States have found significant improvement in both progression-free and overall survival with R-CHOP compared to CHOP in elderly patients over 60 years of age (76,77) These findings have been confirmed in both younger patients (age less than 60) and in a population-based study in British Columbia (78,79). However, as cure rates with R-CHOP range from 30% to 70%, treatment protocols continue to seek further refinement.

Highly Aggressive Non-Hodgkin Lymphoma

Highly aggressive lymphomas include lymphoblastic lymphoma and Burkitt lymphoma. These diseases are uncommon in adults and encompass roughly 5% of all NHL cases in the United States. Lymphoblastic lymphomas are treated with modified acute lymphoblastic leukemia (ALL)-type regimens including intensive multiagent induction therapy, consolidation, and maintenance therapy (80). Central nervous system (CNS) prophylaxis with intrathecal chemotherapy is widely accepted, as the incidence of CNS relapse in patients not receiving prophylaxis approaches 30% (81). Similar approaches with induction chemotherapy and CNS prophylaxis but without prolonged maintenance therapy are used for Burkitt lymphoma (82).

LYMPHOMA SPECIFIC TO THE HEAD AND NECK

Waldeyer Ring Lymphoma

Roughly half of all Waldeyer ring NHLs arise in the palatine tonsil, 20% of which are bilateral (83). In decreasing order, lymphomas in this region also arise from the pharyngeal tonsil, base of tongue or lingual tonsil, or involve multiple primary sites (84). Symptoms correspond with the location of disease. NHL of the tonsil and base of tongue typically present with unilateral odynophagia and dysphagia while nasopharyngeal NHL can manifest with nasal obstruction, eustachian tube dysfunction, persistent epistaxis, or cranial neuropathy. On physical examination, NHL lesions are mostly submucosal, unlike the ulcerated lesions seen with SCC.

The vast majority of patients present with early stage I or stage II disease, with B symptoms occurring in less than 15% of patients (85). The most common histologic subclassification in this region is by far DLBCL, which is present in up to 85% of cases (86). Although large prospective

series are not available, combined chemoradiotherapy has consistently shown superior disease-free survival compared with chemotherapy or radiotherapy alone (85,87). Out-of-field recurrences are the primary pattern for failure, with up to a third of patients developing relapse in the gastrointestinal tract (88).

CT imaging of Waldeyer ring NHL commonly shows a large homogeneous mass of similar intensity to surrounding lymphoid tissue in either the lingual or palatine tonsil, or the nasopharynx (Fig. 128.3) (89). Unlike in nasopharyngeal carcinoma, skull base erosion from nasopharyngeal lymphoma is rare. Associated lymphadenopathy on the ipsilateral side of the lesion is common and usually nonnecrotic in imaging appearance.

Sinonasal Lymphoma

Sinonasal lymphoma is uncommon and represents less than 1% of overall NHL cases. Similar to Waldeyer ring NHL, DLBCL is the most common subgroup of disease found in this location (90). The vast majority of sinonasal DLBCL tumors involve the paranasal sinuses but not the nasal cavity. The next most common subgroup, NK/T-cell lymphoma, is more prevalent in Asia than in Western countries and is associated with EBV infection (91). Unlike DLBCL, NK/T-cell lymphoma nearly always arises from the nasal cavity. Most patients with sinonasal lymphoma present with early stage disease. In contrast to most large Asian studies, a recent clinicopathologic analysis of tumors from the United States showed that NK/T-cell lymphomas had a favorable prognosis with similar outcomes to patients with DLBCL tumors (92). On magnetic resonance imaging (MRI), sinonasal lymphomas are more homogeneous on T2 sequences and mildly enhance when compared with carcinoma. They may present with bony remodeling and/or erosion and can radiographically mimic destructive nasal lesions such as Wegener granulomatosis.

Low-grade sinonasal lymphomas present with obstructive symptoms while high-grade tumors can manifest with cranial neuropathies, pain, and epistaxis. DLBCL tumors have a propensity for soft tissue or osseous destruction near the orbit and can have ophthalmic symptoms such as proptosis. In contrast, true to their alternative name of lethal midline granuloma, NK/T-cell tumors are associated with nasal septal ulceration and destruction (93). Treatment includes combination chemotherapy, most commonly CHOP, and radiation therapy (94). Though uncommon, lymphoma should remain in the differential diagnosis of many sinonasal lesions; a high index of suspicion often must be maintained to make the diagnosis.

Salivary Gland Lymphoma

Between 2% and 5% of salivary gland neoplasms are primary lymphomas. Patients with this tumor typically present with an asymptomatic mass of their parotid or submandibular gland. Pain and facial nerve paresis are very uncommon. Most of these tumors are early stage, and 70% to 80% of them arise from the parotid gland (95). Lymphoma is rarely suspected preoperatively, and many of these patients undergo invasive procedures such as superficial parotidectomy prior to obtaining a diagnosis of lymphoma. Histologic subtypes in this region include, in decreasing frequency, mucosa-associated lymphoid tissue (MALT) lymphoma, follicular lymphoma, and DLBCL (96). Lymphomas of the salivary glands have a favorable overall survival rate compared to other extranodal sites in the head and neck and are typically treated with primary radiotherapy (97).

There is controversy in the literature over the terms *primary, secondary, nodal,* and *extranodal* with respect to NHL

of the parotid gland. Some investigators distinguish disease arising from the parenchyma and tumors of the periparotid and intraparotid lymph nodes. Other reports differentiate tumors arising in the background of known malignant lymphoma or in patients with established autoimmune disease (98). Compared with normal age-matched cohorts, patients with Sjogren disease have an over 40 times greater relative risk of developing NHL within the affected parotid glands (99). For patients with the Sjogren disease, there is an overall 4% prevalence of NHL (100).

CT imaging of salivary gland lymphomas shows homogeneity and mild enhancement (Fig. 128.3) (101). Aggressive tumors can exhibit infiltration of surrounding tissue with necrotic or cystic changes in the tumor itself (102). Ultrasound, an often used modality in the work-up of parotid

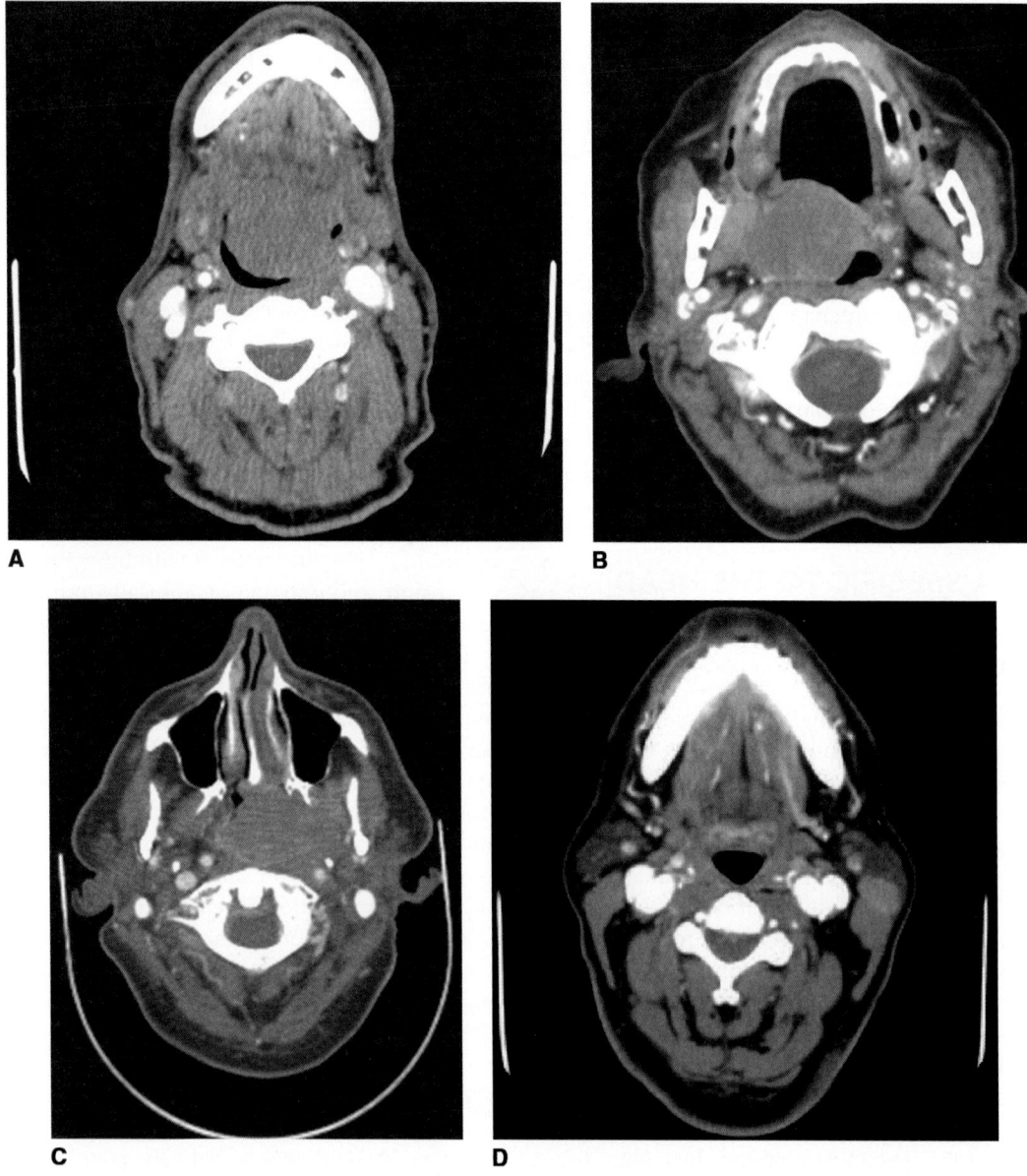

Figure 128.3 Contrast-enhanced axial CT images from patients with lymphoma of the (**A**) base of tongue, (**B**) left tonsil, (**C**) nasopharynx, (**D**) the left parotid gland.

masses, typically shows a well-circumscribed, hypoechoic mass with marked intratumoral vascularization (103).

Thyroid Lymphoma

Primary thyroid lymphoma is uncommon, comprising less than 5% of all thyroid malignancies (104). The most common presentation of disease is a rapidly growing thyroid mass. Patients with primary lymphoma of the thyroid are often younger than those with anaplastic thyroid cancer—the other major disease of concern for those presenting with a rapidly enlarging thyroid mass. Compressive symptoms including hoarseness, dysphagia, and stridor occur in roughly 30% to 50% of patients (105). Although not often on the differential diagnosis of a thyroid mass, prompt diagnosis of primary thyroid lymphoma is critical in that the disease has favorable rates of curability when confined to the thyroid itself. Five-year overall survival for stage I disease is higher than 80% while advanced stage disease (III or IV) has survival rates less than 35% (106). Because of a high relapse rate even for early stage MALT lymphomas, a combination of CHOP and irradiation is used in most centers for all primary thyroid NHLs (107).

The normal thyroid gland does not contain lymphoid tissue. Acquisition of lymphoid tissue in this organ is almost entirely found in patients with autoimmune thyroiditis (108). Chronic lymphocytic thyroiditis (Hashimoto's) has been estimated to confer a 40- to 80-times higher risk for developing thyroid lymphoma in comparison to the general populace (109). It takes an average of 20 to 30 years for lymphoma to develop after the onset of Hashimoto's (110). Most patients are euthyroid.

DLBCL is the most common histologic subtype, occurring in roughly 70% of cases (111). High-grade transformation to DLBCL from MALT lymphoma, the next most common subtype, has been seen on rare occasions (112). Similar to other extranodal lymphomas, most primary thyroid NHLs present in early stage I or stage II disease (113). Although open surgical biopsy has traditionally been required for diagnosis, FNA with modern immunotyping is reasonable for diagnosis in suspicious lesions, particularly for high-grade tumors (114). CNB may provide adequate tissue as well if the diagnosis of thyroid lymphoma is entertained.

Although imaging can be helpful in determining the extent of disease and monitoring treatment efficacy, it is difficult radiographically to distinguish primary thyroid lymphomas from other rapidly enlarging thyroid masses such as anaplastic carcinoma. On ultrasound, most tumors show a well-defined hypoechoic mass with low echogenicity (115). One series reports that nearly all thyroid NHLs have a characteristic asymmetric pseudocystic pattern on ultrasound (116). On CT imaging, a lack of necrosis and calcification in a rapidly growing thyroid mass is suggestive of lymphoma (117). A "donut sign" on CT has been described because of the propensity for the disease to encircle the trachea (118).

Laryngeal Lymphoma

Primary laryngeal lymphoma is an exceedingly rare disease, with less than 100 cases reported in the literature. Common symptoms include dyspnea, hoarseness, and stridor. Most cases manifest as a nonulcerated submucosal mass in the supraglottis, which is the location of organized lymphoid tissue in the larynx (119). Most cases on histology are either MALT lymphomas or DLBCL (120). Although these lesions are noted to be exquisitely radiosensitive, most centers utilize combined chemoradiotherapy for treatment (121). On CT imaging, characteristic features of laryngeal NHL include a uniformly enhancing supraglottic mass without necrosis, calcification, or cervical lymphadenopathy (122).

AIDS-Related Lymphoma

Nearly 500,000 Americans live with AIDS, with 50,000 new HIV infections diagnosed yearly in the United States (123). An estimated 40% of patients with AIDS will develop cancer during their lifetime (124). Cervical carcinoma, Kaposi sarcoma, and NHL constitute the three AIDS-defining malignancies (125). The development of AIDS increases the relative risk of developing lymphoma by 165-fold, with a roughly 4% incidence of NHL amongst those with the diagnosis of AIDS (126). There is evidence, however, to suggest that the overall incidence of AIDS-related NHL has declined since the introduction of modern highly active antiretroviral therapy (HAART) (127). HAART therapy though has not been shown to improve survival time for patients with NHL (128).

HIV-associated B-cell dysregulation secondary to immunodeficiency is considered to be the primary contributing factor to the development of lymphomas. As such, DLBCL is the most common subtype amongst AIDS-related NHL cases (129). Interestingly, although rituximab plus intravenous bolus chemotherapy is the standard of care for immunocompetent patients with aggressive B-cell lymphomas, prospective studies have suggested that R-CHOP has an unacceptable rate of toxicity for patients with AIDS (130). Infusional therapy is now being used in many centers as it has been demonstrated to have similar to greater efficacy while minimizing toxicity (131).

Posttransplant Lymphoproliferative Disorder

Given the increasing number of transplantation procedures being performed, the otolaryngologist must be familiar with the manifestations of PTLD and its manifestations in the head and neck. First described by Starzl in 1968, PTLD involves a spectrum of abnormal lymphoid proliferations that occur after either solid organ transplant or hematopoietic stem cell transplantation (132). PTLDs can be subclassified into four distinct categories: early lesions (plasmacytic hyperplasia), polymorphic disease, monomorphic disease (B- and T-cell neoplasms), and classical HL (133). The majority of PTLD cases (roughly 70%) are associated with EBV infection (134). In patients receiving long-term immunosuppression therapy such as cyclosporine, T-lymphocyte suppression allows for unchecked proliferation of EBV-infected B cells. Thus, the primary risk factors for the development of PTLD include the EBV serostatus of both the donor and recipient as well as intensity of immunosuppression (135). The incidence of PTLD is highest in combined heart-lung transplants and small bowel transplants (roughly 20%) and lowest after kidney transplantation (less than 1%) (136). Extranodal involvement is seen in up to 85% of cases (137).

Head and neck manifestations of PTLD vary depending on the site of involvement. These can include constitutional B symptoms, enlargement of Waldeyer ring, and cervical lymphadenopathy. Most patients presenting with head and neck symptoms within 1 year of transplantation will present with a mononucleosis-like syndrome with rapid swelling of lymphoid tissue (138). Imaging reveals focal masses, particularly in Waldeyer ring, as well as a predilection for submucosal extension through fascial planes (139). Unlike with immunocompetent patients, central lymph node necrosis is commonly seen.

First described over 25 years ago, the initial therapeutic approach for the management of PTLD remains reduction of immunosuppression (RI) (140). The goal of this strategy is to allow the body to recover normal immune surveillance function. Independent prognostic factors associated with a poor response to RI include organ dysfunction, multiorgan involvement, and elevated LDH (141). However, the utility of RI in aggressive PTLDs has been questioned. A recent retrospective analysis of patients with aggressive PTLDs revealed a less than 10% rate of remission from RI alone (136). Another drawback in the usage of RI is the expected risk of organ rejection (142).

Although there is evidence supporting RI alone in the treatment of early stage PTLD, many centers now utilize rituximab-based therapy in patients who either fail or do not tolerate RI (143). In the largest prospective trial of PTLD patients to date, the usage of rituximab monotherapy followed by sequential cycles of R-CHOP demonstrated a complete response rate of roughly 70% (144). For patients receiving CHOP therapy, immunosuppression can continue to be withheld without increased risk for graft failure. It has been suggested that the inherent immunosuppressive activity of chemotherapy can compensate for any negative effects of RI (145).

CONCLUSION

The otolaryngologist is often the first physician to evaluate a patient with lymphoma given the propensity of the disease to present in the head and neck. A high index of suspicion must often be maintained, and recognition of the various manifestations of this diverse group of tumors

is critical for facilitating prompt diagnosis and treatment. Communication with colleagues in the specialties of hematology/oncology, pathology, and, increasingly, infectious disease and transplant surgery is important as well.

With the development of novel diagnostic, staging, and therapeutic regimens, the outcome for individuals diagnosed with lymphoma will continue to improve.

HIGHLIGHTS

- Otolaryngologists will often be called upon to make diagnosis of lymphomas in the head and neck area.
- Lymphoma in the head and neck area presents most commonly as enlarged cervical lymph nodes or hypertrophic lymphoid tissues within the Waldeyer ring.
- Definitive biopsy requires tissue sampling for histologic examination and flow cytometry. Gold standard is excisional biopsy of involved lymph node. CNB may be appropriate also.
- CT with contrast is adequate for the initial evaluation of patients with suspected lymphoma in the head and neck area.
- The Ann Arbor staging system is the most widely used system for classifying the extent of anatomic involvement in lymphomas and for staging of both HL and NHL.
- The most common type of NHL is follicular lymphoma, which is often indolent and does not require active treatment.
- Radiation therapy and/or combination chemotherapy is the current mainstay of treatment for both NHL and HL of the head and neck. Advances in molecular biology have led to the development of novel therapies for NHL such as monoclonal antibodies and radioimmunoconjugates.

REFERENCES

1. Lu P. Staging and classification of lymphoma. *Semin Nucl Med* 2005;35(3):160–164.
2. Jemal A, et al. Cancer statistics, 2010. *CA Cancer J Clin* 2010;60(5):277–300.
3. Chaganti RS, et al. Recurring chromosomal abnormalities in non-Hodgkin's lymphoma: biologic and clinical significance. *Semin Hematol* 2000;37(4):396–411.
4. Good DJ, Gascoyne RD. Classification of non-Hodgkin's lymphoma. *Hematol Oncol Clin North Am* 2008;22(5):781–805, vii.
5. Alexander DD, et al. The non-Hodgkin lymphomas: a review of the epidemiologic literature. *Int J Cancer* 2007;120(Suppl 12):1–39.
6. Harris NL, et al. A revised European-American classification of lymphoid neoplasms: a proposal from the International Lymphoma Study Group. *Blood* 1994;84(5):1361–1392.
7. Glaser SL, Jarrett RF. The epidemiology of Hodgkin's disease. *Bailliere's Clin Haematol* 1996;9(3):401–416.
8. Lynch HT, Marcus JN, Lynch JF. Genetics of Hodgkin's and non-Hodgkin's lymphoma: a review. *Cancer Invest* 1992;10(3):247–256.

9. Jaffe ES. The 2008 WHO classification of lymphomas: implications for clinical practice and translational research. *Hematology Am Soc Hematol Educ Program* 2009:523–531.

10. Marafioti T, et al. Hodgkin and reed-sternberg cells represent an expansion of a single clone originating from a germinal center B-cell with functional immunoglobulin gene rearrangements but defective immunoglobulin transcription. *Blood* 2000;95(4):1443–1450.

11. Pui CH, Campana D. New definition of remission in childhood acute lymphoblastic leukemia. *Leukemia* 2000;14(5):783–785.

12. Hoffman HT, et al. The National Cancer Data Base Report on cancer of the head and neck. *Arch Otolaryngol Head Neck Surg* 1998;124(9):951–962.

13. Cooper JS, et al. National Cancer Database report on cancer of the head and neck: 10-year update. *Head Neck* 2009;31(6): 748–758.

14. Nogova L, Rudiger T, Engert A. Biology, clinical course and management of nodular lymphocyte-predominant hodgkin lymphoma. *Hematology Am Soc Hematol Educ Program* 2006:266–272.

15. Sharma R, et al. Inflammatory (B) symptoms are independent predictors of myelosuppression from chemotherapy in Non-Hodgkin Lymphoma (NHL) patients—analysis of data from a British National Lymphoma Investigation phase III trial comparing CHOP to PMitCEBO. *BMC Cancer* 2009;9(1):153.

16. Krol ADG, et al. Primary extranodal non-Hodgkin's lymphoma (NHL): the impact of alternative definitions tested in the Comprehensive Cancer Centre West population-based NHL registry. *Ann Oncol* 2003;14(1):131–139.

17. Bajetta E, et al. Non-Hodgkin's lymphomas of Waldeyer's ring. *Tumori* 1983;69(2):129–136.

18. Saul SH, Kapadia SB. Primary lymphoma of Waldeyer's ring. Clinicopathologic study of 68 cases. *Cancer* 1985;56(1): 157–166.

19. Albada J, et al. Non-Hodgkin's lymphoma of Waldeyer's ring. *Cancer* 1985;56(12):2911–2913.

20. Jacobs C, Hoppe RT. Non-Hodgkin's lymphomas of head and neck extranodal sites. *Int J Radiat Oncol Biol Phys* 1985;11(2): 357–364.

21. Schneider RJ, et al. Prognostic significance of serum lactate dehydrogenase in malignant lymphoma. *Cancer* 1980;46(1): 139–143.

22. Johnson PW, et al. Beta-2 microglobulin: a prognostic factor in diffuse aggressive non-Hodgkin's lymphomas. *Br J Cancer* 1993;67(4):792–797.

23. Mauch PM, et al. Patterns of presentation of Hodgkin disease. Implications for etiology and pathogenesis. *Cancer* 1993;71(6):2062–2071.

24. Arber DA, George TI. Bone marrow biopsy involvement by non-Hodgkin's lymphoma: frequency of lymphoma types, patterns, blood involvement, and discordance with other sites in 450 specimens. *Am J Surg Pathol* 2005;29(12):1549–1557.

25. van Besien K, et al. Risk factors, treatment, and outcome of central nervous system recurrence in adults with intermediate-grade and immunoblastic lymphoma. *Blood* 1998;91(4):1178–1184.

26. Harnsberger HR, et al. Non-Hodgkin's lymphoma of the head and neck: CT evaluation of nodal and extranodal sites. *AJR Am J Roentgenol* 1987;149(4):785–791.

27. Som PM. Detection of metastasis in cervical lymph nodes: CT and MR criteria and differential diagnosis. *AJR Am J Roentgenol* 1992;158(5):961–969.

28. Fishman EK, Kuhlman JE, Jones RJ. CT of lymphoma: spectrum of disease. Radiographics: a review publication of the Radiological Society of North America, Inc. *Radiographics* 1991;11(4):647–669.

29. Ngeow JY, et al. High SUV uptake on FDG-PET/CT predicts for an aggressive B-cell lymphoma in a prospective study of primary FDG-PET/CT staging in lymphoma. *Ann Oncol* 2009;20(9):1543–1547.

30. Isasi CR, Lu P, Blaufox MD. A metaanalysis of 18F-2-deoxy-2-fluoro-D-glucose positron emission tomography in the staging and restaging of patients with lymphoma. *Cancer* 2005;104(5):1066–1074.

31. Fletcher JW, et al. Recommendations on the use of 18F-FDG PET in oncology. *J Nucl Med* 2008;49(3):480–508.

32. Qizilbash AH, et al. Aspiration biopsy cytology of lymph nodes in malignant lymphoma. *Diagn Cytopathol* 1985;1(1):18–22.

33. Das DK, et al. FNA cytodiagnosis of non-Hodgkin's lymphoma and its subtyping under working formulation of 175 cases. *Diagn Cytopathol* 1991;7(5):487–498.

34. Das DK. Value and limitations of fine-needle aspiration cytology in diagnosis and classification of lymphomas: a review. *Diagn Cytopathol* 1999;21(4):240–249.

35. Das DK, Gupta SK. Fine needle aspiration cytodiagnosis of Hodgkin's disease and its subtypes. II. Subtyping by differential cell counts. *Acta Cytol* 1990;34(3):337–341.

36. Friedman M, et al. Appraisal of aspiration cytology in management of Hodgkin's disease. *Cancer* 1980;45(7):1653–1663.

37. Savage EC, et al. Independent diagnostic accuracy of flow cytometry obtained from fine-needle aspirates: a 10-year experience with 451 cases. *Am J Clin Pathol* 2011;135(2):304–309.

38. Jorgensen JL. State of the Art Symposium: flow cytometry in the diagnosis of lymphoproliferative disorders by fine-needle aspiration. *Cancer* 2005;105(6):443–451.

39. Caraway NP. Strategies to diagnose lymphoproliferative disrders by fine-needle aspiration by using ancillary studies. *Cancer* 2005;105(6):432–442.

40. Amador-Ortiz C, et al. Combined core needle biopsy and fine-needle aspiration with ancillary studies correlate highly with traditional techniques in the diagnosis of nodal-based lymphoma. *Am J Clin Pathol* 2011;135(4):516–524.

41. Hehn ST, Grogan TM, Miller TP. Utility of fine-needle aspiration as a diagnostic technique in lymphoma. *J Clin Oncol* 2004;22(15):3046–3052.

42. Gong JZ, et al. Fine-needle aspiration in non-Hodgkin lymphoma: evaluation of cell size by cytomorphology and flow cytometry. *Am J Clin Pathol* 2002;117(6):880–888.

43. Gattuso P, Manosca F. Fine-needle aspiration of posttransplant lymphoproliferative disorders: a review. *Diagn Cytopathol* 2005;33(4):273–278.

44. Loubeyre P, et al. Diagnostic precision of image-guided multisampling core needle biopsy of suspected lymphomas in a primary care hospital. *Br J Cancer* 2009;100(11):1771–1776.

45. Huang PC, et al. Ultrasound-guided core needle biopsy of cervical lymphadenopathy in patients with lymphoma: the clinical efficacy and factors associated with unsuccessful diagnosis. *Ultrasound Med Biol* 2010;36(9):1431–1436.

46. Pfeiffer J, Kayser G, Ridder GJ. Sonography-assisted cutting needle biopsy in the head and neck for the diagnosis of lymphoma: can it replace lymph node extirpation? *Laryngoscope* 2009;119(4):689–695.

47. Carbone PP, et al. Report of the Committee on Hodgkin's Disease Staging Classification. *Cancer Res* 1971;31(11):1860–1861.

48. Lister TA, et al. Report of a committee convened to discuss the evaluation and staging of patients with Hodgkin's disease: Cotswolds meeting. *J Clin Oncol* 1989;7(11):1630–1636.

49. Rosenberg SA. Validity of the Ann Arbor staging classification for the non-Hodgkin's lymphomas. *Cancer Treat Rep* 1977;61(6):1023–1027.

50. Cleland JGF, et al. A predictive model for aggressive non-hodgkin's lymphoma. *N Engl J Med* 1993;329(14):987–994.

51. Solal-Celigny P, et al. Follicular lymphoma international prognostic index. *Blood* 2004;104(5):1258–1265.

52. Robb-Smith AH. U.S. National Cancer Institute working formulation of non-Hodgkin's lymphomas for clinical use. *Lancet* 1982;2(8295):432–434.

53. Rueda Dominguez A, et al. Treatment of stage I and II Hodgkin's lymphoma with ABVD chemotherapy: results after 7 years of a prospective study. *Ann Oncol* 2004;15(12):1798–1804.

54. Franklin J, et al. Second malignancy risk associated with treatment of Hodgkin's lymphoma: meta-analysis of the randomised trials. *Ann Oncol* 2006;17(12):1749–1760.

55. Brusamolino E, et al. Early-stage Hodgkin's disease: long-term results with radiotherapy alone or combined radiotherapy and chemotherapy. *Ann Oncol* 1994;5(Suppl 2):S101–S106.

56. Bonadonna G, et al. ABVD plus subtotal nodal versus involved-field radiotherapy in early-stage Hodgkin's disease: long-term results. *J Clin Oncol* 2004;22(14):2835–2841.

57. Josting A, et al. Prognostic factors and treatment outcome in primary progressive Hodgkin lymphoma: a report from the German Hodgkin Lymphoma Study Group. *Blood* 2000;96(4):1280–1286.

58. Engert A, et al. Involved-field radiotherapy is equally effective and less toxic compared with extended-field radiotherapy after four cycles of chemotherapy in patients with early-stage unfavorable hodgkin's lymphoma: results of the HD8 Trial of the German Hodgkin's Lymphoma Study Group. *J Clin Oncol* 2003;21(19):3601–3608.

59. Nogova L, Rudiger T, Engert A. Biology, clinical course and management of nodular lymphocyte-predominant Hodgkin lymphoma. *Hematology* 2006:266–272.

60. Longo DL, et al. Twenty years of MOPP therapy for Hodgkin's disease. *J Clin Oncol* 1986;4(9):1295–1306.

61. Bonadonna G, et al. Combination chemotherapy of Hodgkin's disease with adriamycin, bleomycin, vinblastine, and imidazole carboxamide versus MOPP. *Cancer* 1975;36(1):252–259.

62. Bonadonna G, Valagussa P, Santoro A. Alternating non-cross-resistant combination chemotherapy or MOPP in Stage IV Hodgkin's disease. *Ann Intern Med* 1986;104(6):739–746.

63. Duggan DB, et al. Randomized Comparison of ABVD and MOPP/ABV hybrid for the treatment of advanced hodgkin's disease: report of an intergroup trial. *J Clin Oncol* 2003;21(4):607–614.

64. Fuchs M, et al. Nodular lymphocyte-predominant Hodgkin lymphoma. *Curr Hematol Malign Rep* 2008;3(3):126–131.

65. Young GA, Iland HJ. Clinical perspectives in lymphoma. *Intern Med J* 2007;37(7):478–484.

66. Liu Q, et al. Improvement of overall and failure-free survival in stage IV follicular lymphoma: 25 years of treatment experience at The University of Texas M.D. Anderson Cancer Center. *J Clin Oncol* 2006;24(10):1582–1589.

67. Ardeshna KM, et al. Long-term effect of a watch and wait policy versus immediate systemic treatment for asymptomatic advanced-stage non-Hodgkin lymphoma: a randomised controlled trial. *Lancet* 2003;362(9383):516–522.

68. Hiddemann W, et al. Frontline therapy with rituximab added to the combination of cyclophosphamide, doxorubicin, vincristine, and prednisone (CHOP) significantly improves the outcome for patients with advanced-stage follicular lymphoma compared with therapy with CHOP alone: results of a prospective randomized study of the German Low-Grade Lymphoma Study Group. *Blood* 2005;106(12):3725–3732.

69. Griffiths R, et al. Survival in elderly follicular lymphoma patients who receive frontline chemo-immunotherapy. *Am J Hematol* 2010;85(12):963–967.

70. Vidal L, et al. Rituximab maintenance for the treatment of patients with follicular lymphoma: systematic review and meta-analysis of randomized trials. *J Natl Cancer Inst* 2009;101(4):248–255.

71. Morschhauser F, et al. Phase III trial of consolidation therapy with yttrium-90–ibritumomab tiuxetan compared with no additional therapy after first remission in advanced follicular lymphoma. *J Clin Oncol* 2008;26(32):5156–5164.

72. Horning SJ, et al. Efficacy and safety of tositumomab and iodine-131 tositumomab (bexxar) in b-cell lymphoma, progressive after rituximab. *J Clin Oncol* 2005;23(4):712–719.

73. Lee Y, et al. Lymphomas of the head and neck: CT findings at initial presentation. *Am J Roentgenol* 1987;149(3):575–581.

74. Zelenetz AD, et al. Non-Hodgkin's lymphomas. *J Natl Comprehen Cancer Netw* 2010;8(3):288–334.

75. Yahalom J. Radiation therapy after R-CHOP for diffuse large b-cell lymphoma: the gain remains. *J Clin Oncol* 2010;28(27):4105–4107.

76. Coiffier B, et al. CHOP chemotherapy plus rituximab compared with CHOP alone in elderly patients with diffuse large-B-cell lymphoma. *N Engl J Med* 2002;346(4):235–242.

77. Hochster H, et al. Maintenance rituximab after cyclophosphamide, vincristine, and prednisone prolongs progression-free survival in advanced indolent lymphoma: results of the randomized phase III ECOG1496 Study. *J Clin Oncol* 2009;27(10):1607–1614.

78. Pfreundschuh M, et al. Prognostic significance of maximum tumour (bulk) diameter in young patients with good-prognosis diffuse-large-B-cell lymphoma treated with CHOP-like chemotherapy with or without rituximab: an exploratory analysis of the MabThera International Trial Group (MInT) study. *Lancet Oncol* 2008;9(5):435–444.

79. Sehn LH, et al. Introduction of combined CHOP plus rituximab therapy dramatically improved outcome of diffuse large B-cell lymphoma in British Columbia. *J Clin Oncol* 2005;23(22):5027–5033.

80. Thomas DA, et al. Outcome with the hyper-CVAD regimens in lymphoblastic lymphoma. *Blood* 2004;104(6):1624–1630.

81. Coleman CN, et al. Treatment of lymphoblastic lymphoma in adults. *J Clin Oncol* 1986;4(11):1628–1637.

82. Mead GM, et al. An international evaluation of CODOX-M and CODOX-M alternating with IVAC in adult Burkitt's lymphoma: results of United Kingdom Lymphoma Group LY06 study. *Ann Oncol* 2002;13(8):1264–1274.

83. Zucca E, et al. Primary extranodal non-Hodgkin's lymphomas. Part 2: Head and neck, central nervous system and other less common sites. *Ann Oncol* 1999;10(9):1023–1033.

84. Saul SH, Kapadia SB. Primary lymphoma of waldeyer's ring clinicopathologic study of 68 cases. *Cancer* 1985;56(1):157–166.

85. Ezzat AA, et al. Localized non-Hodgkin's lymphoma of Waldeyer's ring: clinical features, management, and prognosis of 130 adult patients. *Head Neck* 2001;23(7):547–558.

86. Nayak LM, Deschler DG. Lymphomas. *Otolaryngol Clin North Am* 2003;36(4):625–646.

87. Chang DT, et al. Long-term outcomes for stage I-II aggressive non-Hodgkin lymphoma of Waldeyer's ring. *Am J Clin Oncol* 2009;32(3):233–237. doi:10.1097/COC.0b013e318187ddbb.

88. Avilés A, et al. Treatment of non-Hodgkin's lymphoma of waldeyer's ring: radiotherapy versus chemotherapy versus combined therapy. *Eur J Cancer* 1996;32(1):19–23.

89. Aiken AH, Glastonbury C. Imaging Hodgkin and non-Hodgkin lymphoma in the head and neck. *Radiol Clin North Am* 2008;46(2):363–378, ix–x.

90. Shohat I, et al. Primary non-Hodgkin's lymphoma of the sinonasal tract. *Oral Surg Oral Med Oral Pathol Oral Radiol Endod* 2004;97(3):328–331.

91. Hongyo T, et al. Specific c-kit mutations in sinonasal natural killer/t-cell lymphoma in China and Japan. *Cancer Res* 2000;60(9):2345–2347.

92. Cuadra-Garcia I, et al. Sinonasal lymphoma: a clinicopathologic analysis of 58 cases from the Massachusetts General Hospital. *Am J Surg Pathol* 1999;23(11):1356.

93. Abbondanzo SL, Wenig BM. Non-Hodgkin's lymphoma of the sinonasal tract. A clinicopathologic and immunophenotypic study of 120 cases. *Cancer* 1995;75(6):1281–1291.

94. Cheung MM, et al. Primary non-Hodgkin's lymphoma of the nose and nasopharynx: clinical features, tumor immunophenotype, and treatment outcome in 113 patients. *J Clin Oncol* 1998;16(1):70–77.

95. Wolvius EB, et al. Primary non-Hodgkin's lymphoma of the salivary glands. An analysis of 22 cases. *J Oral Pathol Med* 1996;25(4):177–181.

96. Kojima M, et al. Primary salivary gland lymphoma among Japanese: a clinicopathological study of 30 cases. *Leukemia Lymphoma* 2007;48(9):1793–1798.

97. Anacak Y, Miller RC, Constantinou N, et al. Primary mucosa-associated lymphoid tissue lymphoma of the salivary glands: a multicenter rare cancer network study. *Int J Radiat Oncol Biol Phys* 2012;82(1):315–320.

98. Barnes L, Myers EN, Prokopakis EP. Primary malignant lymphoma of the parotid gland. *Arch Otolaryngol Head Neck Surg* 1998;124(5):573–577.

99. Kassan SS, et al. Increased risk of lymphoma in sicca syndrome. *Ann Intern Med* 1978;89(6):888–892.

100. Voulgarelis M, Moutsopoulos HM. Mucosa-associated lymphoid tissue lymphoma in Sjogren's syndrome: risks, management, and prognosis. *Rheum Dis Clin North Am* 2008;34(4):921–933, viii.

101. Chua SC, Rozalli FI, O'Connor SR. Imaging features of primary extranodal lymphomas. *Clin Radiol* 2009;64(6):574–588.

102. Hirokawa N, et al. Diagnosis and treatment of malignant lymphoma of the parotid gland. *Jpn J Clin Oncol* 1998;28(4):245–249.

103. Eichhorn KW, Arapakis I, Ridder GJ. Malignant non-Hodgkin's lymphoma mimicking a benign parotid tumor: sonographic findings. *J Clin Ultrasound* 2002;30(1):42–44.

104. Ha CS, et al. Localized non-Hodgkin lymphoma involving the thyroid gland. *Cancer* 2001;91(4):629–635.

105. Hwang YC, et al. Clinical characteristics of primary thyroid lymphoma in Koreans. *Endocr J* 2009;56(3):399–405.

106. Pyke CM, et al. Non-Hodgkin's lymphoma of the thyroid: is more than biopsy necessary? *World J Surg* 1992;16(4):604–609; discussion 609–610.

107. Doria R, Jekel JF, Cooper DL. Thyroid lymphoma. The case for combined modality therapy. *Cancer* 1994;73(1):200–206.

108. Kossev P, Livolsi V. Lymphoid lesions of the thyroid: review in light of the revised European-American lymphoma classification and upcoming World Health Organization classification. *Thyroid* 1999;9(12):1273–1280.

109. Holm LE, Blomgren H, Lowhagen T. Cancer risks in patients with chronic lymphocytic thyroiditis. *N Engl J Med* 1985;312(10):601–604.

110. Pedersen RK, Pedersen NT. Primary non-Hodgkin's lymphoma of the thyroid gland: a population based study. *Histopathology* 1996;28(1):25–32.

111. Widder S, Pasieka JL. Primary thyroid lymphomas. *Curr Treat Opt Oncol* 2004;5(4):307–313.

112. Thieblemont C, et al. Primary thyroid lymphoma is a heterogeneous disease. *J Clin Endocrinol Metab* 2002;87(1):105–111.

113. Ruggiero FP, Frauenhoffer E, Stack BC Jr. Thyroid lymphoma: a single institution's experience. *Otolaryngology* 2005;133(6):888–896.

114. Morgen EK, et al. The role of fine-needle aspiration in the diagnosis of thyroid lymphoma: a retrospective study of nine cases and review of published series. *J Clin Pathol* 2010;63(2):129–133.

115. Kwak JY, et al. Primary thyroid lymphoma: role of ultrasound-guided needle biopsy. *J Ultrasound Med* 2007;26(12):1761–1765.

116. Matsuzuka F, et al. Clinical aspects of primary thyroid lymphoma: diagnosis and treatment based on our experience of 119 cases. *Thyroid* 1993;3(2):93–99.

117. Ishikawa H, et al. Comparison of primary thyroid lymphoma with anaplastic thyroid carcinoma on computed tomographic imaging. *Radiat Med* 2002;20(1):9–15.

118. Kim HC, et al. Primary thyroid lymphoma: CT findings. *Eur J Radiol* 2003;46(3):233–239.

119. Horny HP, Ferlito A, Carbone A. Laryngeal lymphoma derived from mucosa-associated lymphoid tissue. *Ann Otol Rhinol Laryngol* 1996;105(7):577–583.

120. Markou K, et al. Primary laryngeal lymphoma: report of 3 cases and review of the literature. *Head Neck* 2010;32(4):541–549.

121. Ansell SM, et al. Primary laryngeal lymphoma. *Laryngoscope* 1997;107(11 Pt 1):1502–1506.

122. Siddiqui NA, et al. Imaging characteristics of primary laryngeal lymphoma. *AJNR Am J Neuroradiol* 2010;31(7):1261–1265.

123. Hall HI, et al. Estimation of HIV Incidence in the United States. *JAMA* 2008;300(5):520–529.

124. Levine AM. AIDS-related malignancies: the emerging epidemic. *J Natl Cancer Inst* 1993;85(17):1382–1397.

125. Burgi A, et al. Incidence and risk factors for the occurrence of non-AIDS-defining cancers among human immunodeficiency virus-infected individuals. *Cancer* 2005;104(7):1505–1511.

126. Cote TR, et al. Non-Hodgkin's lymphoma among people with AIDS: incidence, presentation and public health burden. AIDS/Cancer Study Group. *Int J Cancer* 1997;73(5):645–650.

127. Diamond C, et al. Changes in acquired immunodeficiency syndrome-related non-Hodgkin lymphoma in the era of highly active antiretroviral therapy: incidence, presentation, treatment, and survival. *Cancer* 2006;106(1):128–135.

128. Pipkin S, et al. The effect of HAART and calendar period on Kaposi's sarcoma and non-Hodgkin lymphoma: results of a match between an AIDS and cancer registry. *AIDS* 2011;25(4):463–471. doi:10.1097/QAD.0b013e32834344e6.

129. Gucalp A, Noy A. Spectrum of HIV lymphoma 2009. *Curr Opin Hematol* 2010;17(4):362–367.

130. Kaplan LD, et al. Rituximab does not improve clinical outcome in a randomized phase 3 trial of CHOP with or without rituximab in patients with HIV-associated non-Hodgkin lymphoma: AIDS-Malignancies Consortium Trial 010. *Blood* 2005;106(5):1538–1543.

131. Sparano JA, et al. Rituximab plus concurrent infusional EPOCH chemotherapy is highly effective in HIV-associated B-cell non-Hodgkin lymphoma. *Blood* 2010;115(15):3008–3016.

132. Murray JE, et al. Five years' experience in renal transplantation with immunosuppressive drugs: survival, function, complications, and the role of lymphocyte depletion by thoracic duct fistula. *Ann Surg* 1968;168(3):416–435.

133. Swerdlow SH. Post-transplant lymphoproliferative disorders: a morphologic, phenotypic and genotypic spectrum of disease. *Histopathology* 1992;20(5):373–385.

134. Paya CV, et al. Epstein-Barr virus-induced posttransplant lymphoproliferative disorders. ASTS/ASTP EBV-PTLD Task Force and The Mayo Clinic Organized International Consensus Development Meeting. *Transplantation* 1999;68(10):1517–1525.

135. Dharnidharka VR, et al. Risk factors for posttransplant lymphoproliferative disorder (PTLD) in pediatric kidney transplantation: a report of the North American Pediatric Renal Transplant Cooperative Study (NAPRTCS). *Transplantation* 2001;71(8):1065–1068.

136. Knight JS, et al. Lymphoma after solid organ transplantation: risk, response to therapy, and survival at a transplantation center. *J Clin Oncol* 2009;27(20):3354–3562.

137. Ghobrial IM, et al. Prognostic analysis for survival in adult solid organ transplant recipients with post-transplantation lymphoproliferative disorders. *J Clin Oncol* 2005;23(30):7574–7582.

138. Vargas H, et al. Posttransplant lymphoproliferative disorder of the nasopharynx. *Am J Rhinol* 2002;16(1):37–42.

139. Loevner LA, et al. Posttransplantation lymphoproliferative disorder of the head and neck: imaging features in seven adults. *Radiology* 2000;216(2):363–369.

140. Starzl TE, et al. Reversibility of lymphomas and lymphoproliferative lesions developing under cyclosporin-steroid therapy. *Lancet* 1984;1(8377):583–587.

141. Tsai DE, et al. Reduction in immunosuppression as initial therapy for posttransplant lymphoproliferative disorder: analysis of prognostic variables and long-term follow-up of 42 adult patients. *Transplantation* 2001;71(8):1076–1088.

142. Reshef R, et al. Reduction of immunosuppression as initial therapy for posttransplantation lymphoproliferative disorder(bigstar). *Am J Transpl* 2011;11(2):336–347.

143. Elstrom RL, et al. Treatment of PTLD with rituximab or chemotherapy. *Am J Transpl* 2006;6(3):569–576.

144. Trappe RU, et al. Risk stratified sequential treatment with rituximab and chop chemotherapy in b-cell PTLD—defining a new standard of care: results from a prospective international multicenter trial: 1322. *Transplantation* 2010;90:257.

145. Trappe R, et al. Treatment of PTLD with rituximab and CHOP reduces the risk of renal graft impairment after reduction of immunosuppression. *Am J Transpl* 2009;9(10):2331–2337.

129

Neoplasms of the Nose and Paranasal Sinuses

Lee A. Zimmer   *Ricardo L. Carrau*

EPIDEMIOLOGY

Malignant tumors of the sinonasal tract constitute about 3% of tumors arising in the upper respiratory tract. They occur most commonly in whites, and the incidence in males is twice the incidence in females (1). Exposure to industrial fumes, wood dust, nickel-refining processes, and leather tanning has been implicated in the carcinogenesis of certain types of sinonasal malignant tumors. Other industrial exposures associated with an increased incidence of sinonasal cancer include mineral oils, chromium and chromium compounds, isopropyl oils, lacquer paint, soldering and welding, and radium dial painting. A recent report demonstrates a higher incidence of nasal cancers in cigarette smokers (1).

EVALUATION

Diagnosis

Tumors of the sinonasal tract commonly present with symptoms similar to those caused by inflammatory sinus disease, such as nasal airway obstruction, epistaxis, headache, facial pain, and nasal discharge, and are frequently asymptomatic in 9% to 12% of patients, contributing to a delay in the diagnosis and advanced stage of disease. Regional and distant metastases are infrequent despite the advanced stage of the primary tumor. The incidence of cervical metastases on initial presentation varies from 1% to 26%, with most series reporting less than 10%. In one large series, the 5-year incidence of neck metastasis is 4.3% for primary ethmoid malignancies and 12.5% for primary maxillary malignancies (2). This number decreases in patients treated with radiation to the neck. The presence of distant metastasis on initial presentation is even less common, with most authors reporting an incidence of less than 7%.

The physical examination should be thorough, with emphasis on the sinonasal region, orbit, cranial nerves, and should include nasal endoscopy. Although not pathognomonic, numbness or hypoesthesia of the infraorbital (V2) or supraorbital (V3) nerve strongly suggests malignant invasion. Other findings such as proptosis, chemosis, extraocular muscle impairment, mass effect in the cheek, gingiva or gingivobuccal sulcus (e.g., ill-fitting dentures), and loose dentition also suggest the presence of a sinonasal tumor. Table 129.1 provides a summary of diagnostic techniques.

Radiologic imaging is essential for staging. Plain films may demonstrate bone destruction; however, a significant number will be interpreted as normal. A screening computed tomography (CT) scan is more accurate than plain films to evaluate the bony framework of the paranasal sinuses and compares favorably with the cost of plain films. High-risk patients with a history of carcinogen exposure, severe persistent pain, cranial neuropathies, exophthalmos, chemosis, and sinonasal disease and those with persistent symptoms after adequate medical treatment should be evaluated with an axial and coronal CT scan with contrast or magnetic resonance imaging (MRI) with contrast. CT scanning is superior for the evaluation of the bony confines of the sinonasal tract and skull base. The use of contrast provides an estimate of the tumor vascularity and its relationship to the carotid artery.

MRI differentiates adjacent tumor from soft tissue, differentiates secretions in an obstructed sinus from a space-occupying lesion, demonstrates perineural spread, suffers less artifact effect with dental fillings, offers the advantage of imaging in the sagittal plane, and does not involve exposure to ionizing radiation. Coronal MRI images are superior for the evaluation of the foramen rotundum, vidian canal, foramen ovale, and optic canal. Sagittal images are most useful to demonstrate the replacement of the normal low-intensity signal of Meckel's cave and the high-intensity signal of fat in the pterygopalatine fossa (PtPF) by tumor signals similar to brain. MRI, however, is more expensive than CT scan, more prone to motion artifact, and less tolerated due to claustrophobia.

TABLE 129.1	DIAGNOSIS PARANASAL TUMORS TECHNIQUE	
History and Physical	**Risk Factors/Cranial Nerve Deficits, Nasal Mass**	
Imaging		
CT scanning	Evaluation of bony boundaries of PNS; not cost-effective	
MRI	Evaluation of soft tissue invasion and perineural spread; differentiate retained secretions from tumor	
PET	Routine evaluation for recurrent disease after primary treatment and distant metastasis; useful for SCCA; cost-effectiveness unknown	
Biopsy		
Sinus lavage/cytology		
Fine needle aspiration		
Transnasal biopsy	Direct or endoscopic. Preferred modality	

Positron emission tomography (PET) is commonly used for malignancies of the head and neck for staging and surveillance. The combined PET/CT scanner adds anatomical detail which aids in surgical planning by defining the extent of tumor. Although many reports have documented the use of PET in head and neck cancer, none have evaluated the use of this modality for malignant tumors of the nose and paranasal sinuses.

Angiography with carotid flow study is reserved for surgical candidates presenting with tumors that surround the carotid artery or when sacrifice of the vessel is anticipated to obtain clear margins. Balloon occlusion tests, used with SPECT, Xenon CT scan, or Transcranial Doppler, offer a reasonable estimate of the risk of ischemic brain infarction if the internal carotid artery is sacrificed. These tests, however, cannot predict ischemia at marginal ("watershed") areas or embolic phenomena.

A CT scan of the chest and abdomen is recommended for patients presenting with tumors that metastasize hematogenously, such as sarcomas, melanoma, and adenoid cystic carcinoma. Metastatic evaluation is important if an extensive resection is considered. A lumbar puncture, brain and spine imaging are recommended for tumors that invade the meninges or brain.

Pathology

The sinonasal tract pathology, with certain important exceptions, reflects the pathology found in other areas of the head and neck (Table 129.2). We provide a brief description of the most common histologic diagnoses.

Benign Epithelial Tumors

Papillomas arise from squamous or schneiderian epithelium. The keratotic papilloma of the vestibule (vestibular wart) behaves like other cutaneous counterparts. It is easily treated by simple excision or cauterization.

TABLE 129.2	TUMORS OF THE SINONASAL TRACT
Epithelial	
Benign	Exophytic papilloma
	Inverted papilloma
	Columnar papilloma
	Adenoma
Malignant	Squamous cell carcinoma
	Transitional cell carcinoma
	Adenocarcinoma
	Adenoid cystic carcinoma
	Melanoma
	Olfactory neuroblastoma
	Undifferentiated carcinoma
Nonepithelial	
Benign	Fibroma
	Chondroma
	Osteoma
	Neurilemmoma
	Neurofibroma
	Hemangioma
Malignant	Soft tissue sarcoma
	Rhabdomyosarcoma
	Leiomyosarcoma
	Fibrosarcoma
	Liposarcoma
	Angiosarcoma
	Myxosarcoma
	Hemangiopericytoma
	Connective tissue sarcoma
	Chondrosarcoma
	Osteosarcoma
Lymphoreticular tumors	
	Lymphoma
	Plasmacytoma
	Giant cell tumor
Metastatic carcinoma	

TABLE 129.3 PAPILLOMAS OF THE SINONASAL TRACT			
	Inverted Papillomas	Fungiform Papilloma	Cylindrical Papilloma
Site of origin	Lateral wall	Septum	Lateral wall
Frequency	47%	50%	3%
Recurrence rate	27%–73%	22%–50%	25%–35%
Associated with malignancy	13%	3%–5%	15%

Adapted from Barnes EL. *Surgical pathology of the head and neck*, Vol. 1. New York: Marcel Dekker, 1985.

Papillomas of the nasal cavity may be classified in three distinct categories (Table 129.3). Fungiform papillomas arise from the nasal septum, while inverted and cylindrical papillomas typically arise from the lateral nasal wall. Although benign in nature, extension beyond their site of origin can destroy bone, recur when not excised completely, and may be associated with malignant tumors (3,4). They are most commonly diagnosed in white males during the fifth to seventh decades (mean 50 years). En bloc resection has been the gold standard for the treatment of these lesions (Table 129.4). MRI, CT scanning, and nasal endoscopy permit an accurate preoperative mapping of these lesions, allowing a more conservative resection through less invasive approaches. During the last decade, various endoscopic, transnasal techniques for the resection of inverting papillomas have been reported (4,5). Transnasal techniques avoid the use of incisions and usually require a shorter hospital stay than external approaches. The endoscopic approach provides superior visualization of the posterior ethmoid cells, especially those that extend lateral to the sphenoid sinus or around the optic nerve (Onodi cells). In expert hands, resection with an endonasal, medial maxillectomy approach has equal recurrence rates as traditional open, en bloc resections (Table 129.5) (5).

Adenomas of the sinonasal tract arise more commonly in the nasal septum. Most are found during the fourth to the seventh decade, occurring with an equal sex distribution. The recurrence rate is low following complete removal (10%).

Malignant Epithelial Tumors

Squamous cell carcinoma (SCCA) is the most common tumor of the sinonasal tract. It is most commonly reported in white males in their fifth to sixth decade. The prognosis is related to the extent of the tumor and the site of origin.

TABLE 129.4 OPEN MEDIAL MAXILLECTOMY RECURRENCE RATES FOR INVERTING PAPILLOMA		
Authors	Lateral Rhinotomy-Medial Maxillectomy	Conservation Resection[a]
Benninger et al. (1991)	0% (0/20)	36% (5/14)
Myers et al. (1990)	5% (1/22)	0% (0/4)
Pelausa and Fortier (1992)	7% (1/14)	77% (37/48)
Outzen et al. (1991)	7% (3/44)	27% (3/11)
Lawson et al. (1989)	9% (7/77)	10% (1/10)
Segal et al. (1986)	10% (1/10)	70% (10/14)
Kristensen et al. (1985)	12% (7/57)	38% (8/21)
Phillips et al. (1990)	13% (9/72)	44% (4/9)
Smith and Gullane (1987)	27% (3/11)	57% (4/7)
Dolgin et al. (1992)	29% (4/14)	44% (4/9)
Weissler et al. (1986)	29% (37/126)	67% (103/153)
Bielamowicz et al. (1993)	30% (60/20)	74% (17/23)
Averages	16% (79/487)	60% (209/350)

[a]Does not include reports of endoscopic resection.
Adapted from Lawson W, Ho BT, Shaari CM, et al. Inverted papillomas: a report of 112 cases. *Laryngoscope* 105:282–288.

TABLE 129.5	ENDOSCOPIC RECURRENCE RATES FOR INVERTING PAPILLOMA

Authors	Recurrence Rates
Sham et al. (2009)	30% (8/26)
Lawson et al. (2009)	6%
Kim (2008)	4% (4/94)
Mackle (2008)	7% (4/55)
Sautter (2007)	22% (11/49)
Holzmann (2007)	4% (2/51)
Minovi (2006)	10% (5/48)
Pasquini (2004)	3% (1/36)
Tomenzoli (2004)	0% (0/47)

Adenocarcinomas make up 4% to 8% of all sinonasal tumors. They originate most commonly in the ethmoid sinuses and nasal cavity and are associated with exposure to hardwood dust. Adenocarcinomas may be divided into low and high grades according to their histologic characteristics and behavior. Low-grade tumors present a uniform glandular architecture and cytologic characteristics, with rare mitoses and seldom perineural invasion or distant metastases. Low-grade adenocarcinomas tend to recur locally. High-grade adenocarcinoma has a solid growth pattern with poorly defined margins, prominent pleomorphism, and large number of mitoses. One-third of patients with high-grade adenocarcinomas will present with distant metastases. Approaches to adenocarcinomas of the paranasal sinuses include anterior craniofacial resection, lateral rhinotomy, and endonasal techniques with or without radiotherapy. The 5-year disease-specific survival for patients with adenocarcinoma of the nose and paranasal sinuses following surgery and radiation therapy is 100% for T1, 93% for T2, 60% for T3, and 0% for T4 lesions (6). Disease extension to the orbit, infratemporal fossa, frontal sinus and dura are poor prognostic indicators.

Adenoid cystic carcinomas of the sinonasal tract comprise 14% to 20% of all the adenoid cystic carcinomas arising in the head and neck. They are characterized by early spread to neurovascular structures, submucosal spread, and advanced stage at the time of diagnosis. Low-grade tumors are defined by histology with less than 30% solid architecture and include the cribriform and tubular patterns. High-grade tumors correspond to those with a histologic pattern with more than 30% solid cellular architecture. The incidence of perineural invasion is similar for both grades, but the incidence of local recurrence and metastases is higher in the solid type. High rates of recurrence (50% to 76%) are likely due to perineural spread and positive microscopic margins not identified at the time of surgery (7,8). The treatment of adenoid cystic carcinoma of the sinonasal tract is primarily surgical, although combined surgery and postoperative radiation therapy appear to yield better local control.

In the MD Anderson experience, among the 105 patients presenting with ACC of the sinonasal tract, most patients presented with locally advanced disease (8). Tumor extended to the skull base in 28% of patients and invaded the skull base and brain in 24%. Margins are difficult to clear even with extensive craniofacial resection due to the proximity to vital structures and the propensity for perineural spread, which in this series was 60% of patients. The survival rate at 2 years was 46% following primary treatment and 15% following salvage surgery. Patients recurred locally (31%), and 38% developed regional or distant recurrence. Overall 5-year survival was 50% for stage I to III and 20% for stage IV.

Melanoma of the sinonasal tract may be primary or metastatic. Although 20% of all melanomas originate in the head and neck, less than 1% arises from the sinonasal tract. They are most commonly found in the nasal cavity, followed by the maxillary sinus, ethmoid sinus, and frontal sinus, in descending order. Most patients present with disease confined to the site of origin but show a tendency toward early vascular and lymphatic invasion with a high incidence of local recurrence after surgical excision. Postoperative radiation therapy may be beneficial, although its impact on survival and local control has not been addressed in scientific trials. The median survival for patients presenting with sinonasal melanoma is 15 months with a 5-year overall survival of 23% (9). The most common cause of failure is local recurrence, whereas the most important factor in predicting survival is metastatic disease (9,10).

Olfactory neuroblastoma is a rare tumor arising in the olfactory epithelium. Patients often present with nasal obstruction and epistaxis. It has a bimodal frequency at 10 to 20 and 50 to 60 years of age, with a similar incidence in males and females. Its prognosis is related to the extent of disease and resectability on initial presentation. Most institutions have adopted combined therapies based on the Kadish staging system (Table 129.6). The UCLA classification (Table 129.7), however, provides better prognostication regarding local recurrences as factors such as intradural and orbital invasion are not considered in the Kadish staging system. The advent of open or endoscopic craniofacial resection with postoperative radiation to the primary site and neck has improved the therapeutic results (11). In a recent meta-analysis, the 5-year disease-free survival for all stages is 78% following combined surgery with radiotherapy and 47% for Kadish stage C (12).

TABLE 129.6	KADISH STAGING SYSTEM FOR OLFACTORY NEUROBLASTOMA

Stage A	Tumor confined to the nasal cavity
Stage B	Tumor in nasal cavity extending to paranasal sinus
Stage C	Tumor extending to orbit, base of skull, cranial cavity or with cervical/distant metastasis

TABLE 129.7	UCLA STAGING SYSTEMS FOR OLFACTORY NEUROBLASTOMA

Stage	Description
T1	Tumor involving the nasal cavity and/or paranasal sinuses (excluding sphenoid), sparing the most superior ethmoidal air cells
T2	Tumor involving the nasal cavity and/or paranasal sinuses (including the sphenoid) with extension to or erosion of the cribriform plate
T3	Tumor extending into the orbit or protruding into the anterior cranial fossa
T4	Tumor involving the brain

Sinonasal undifferentiated carcinomas are usually composed of small and medium-sized cells and must be differentiated from rhabdomyosarcomas, melanoma, olfactory neuroblastoma, lymphoma, and SCCA. The progression of symptoms is very rapid, and they usually present with very advanced stage involving multiple sinuses. Treatment includes trimodal therapy employing chemotherapy (cyclophosphamide, doxorubicin and vincristine), radiation therapy, and, in appropriate cases, surgery. Patients with intracranial disease fared poorly despite aggressive combination therapy.

Benign Nonepithelial Tumors

Fibro-osseous lesions, including osteomas, fibromas, and chordomas, are the most common benign tumors of the sinonasal tract. Their growth is usually slow and self-limited. Simple surgical excision is recommended when a histologic diagnosis is needed or to relieve obstructive symptoms.

Fewer than 4% of benign peripheral nerve sheath tumors of the head and neck arise in the nose and paranasal sinuses. They present as polypoid, slow-growing masses, reaching a very large size and often causing facial deformities and local destruction of adjacent structures. Ninety percent of the nerve sheath tumors show a benign histology. Two-thirds of these tumors are schwannomas and one-third neurofibromas. Unlike other regions, schwannomas of the nose and paranasal sinuses often lack tumor encapsulation, with neoplastic cells undermining adjacent respiratory mucosa (13). Treatment is by complete surgical excision, or partial removal for massive neurofibromas involving vital areas.

Malignant Nonepithelial Tumors

Neurogenic sarcomas are rare in the head and neck and commonly associated with neurofibromatosis. Neurogenic sarcomas are locally aggressive and frequently present with distant metastases. Surgery plays a primary role in their therapy; radiation and chemotherapy are usually reserved

for incomplete removal, inoperable cases, or recurrences (14). The 5-year survival rate is 60% although sarcomas associated with neurofibromatosis behave more aggressively, yielding a 5-year survival rate of 30% (14).

Rhabdomyosarcomas arise in the head and neck in 35% to 45% of cases. In 10% of patients, they originate in the paranasal sinuses (15). These tumors may assume the morphology of any of the developmental stages of striated muscle, hence the classification into embryonal, alveolar, and pleomorphic types. There is a bimodal distribution pattern in childhood, with the embryonal occurring in the first decade and the alveolar type in adolescents. Rhabdomyosarcomas have a less favorable outcome in adults, with a 5-year survival rate of only 35% (16). The head and neck region is less involved in adults, with the viscera and extremities the most common sites of presentation.

Rhabdomyosarcomas of the sinonasal tract are classified as nonorbital parameningeal and behave more aggressively than those arising in other locations. Systemic and regional metastases are common. In 1987, the Intergroup Rhabdomyosarcoma Study I reported the use of intensive radiation and chemotherapy on patients with nonorbital parameningeal rhabdomyosarcoma showing an improvement of the survival rate from 51% to 81%. In 2002, Intergroup Rhabdomyosarcoma Study IV reported further improvements in survival for those patients with cranial parameningeal involvement (17). Patients with cranial parameningeal sarcomas, but without meningeal invasion, require multiagent chemotherapy followed by radiation therapy. High-risk tumors defined as intracranial tumors, tumors that eroded the base of skull or that caused a cranial neuropathy were treated with triple intrathecal chemotherapy, whole brain radiation, and spinal radiation. At 5 years, 73% of patients were alive, compared with 45% in IRS I. Overall survival for patients with paranasal sinus involvement was 76% for the low-risk group and 57% for the high-risk group. Failure-free survival was 57% for the low-risk group and 52% for the high-risk group. Aggressive initial surgical therapy was not warranted. These results, however, have never been confirmed in adults. Adult rhabdomyosarcoma is usually treated by wide surgical excision. Radiation is recommended for positive margins or inoperable or recurrent disease. Chemotherapy has a palliative role that must be weighed against its possible morbidity.

Fibrosarcoma is a tumor arising from fibroblasts, thus, the term encompasses a spectrum of malignancies that ranges from low-grade fibromatosis to high-grade tumors. Misdiagnosis is very common. Radiation and trauma have been implicated as possible etiologic factors. The treatment of choice is wide surgical excision for previously untreated tumors. Radiation is recommended for involved margins or recurrent or inoperable tumors.

Hemangiopericytoma is a very rare, highly vascular tumor arising from the pericapillary pericytes of Zimmerman. Histologic examination reveals oval- and spindle-shaped pericytes. Benign and malignant varieties have been described. Malignant tumors are distinguished by increased mitotic activity, high cell density, and necrotic and hemorrhagic zones. They invade locally and metastasize in 10% to 15% of cases. Hematogenous metastases involve lung, liver, and bone. Sixteen percent are found in the head and neck, with about 50 reported cases arising in the sinonasal tract (18). Their prognosis relates to the size of the lesion, number of mitoses, and metastases. The primary treatment is surgical excision.

Osteogenic sarcoma is the most common primary tumor of bone in the United States, with an estimated incidence of one case per 100,000. Those originating within the jaws constitute 7% to 10% of all osteosarcomas. Etiologic factors include ionizing, radiation, fibrous dysplasia, trauma, Paget disease, and the gene associated with retinoblastoma. The most effective therapy is surgical excision. However, during the past decade, several reports have suggested that adjunctive radiation and chemotherapy may improve survival. A multi-institutional review and meta-analysis demonstrated a 2- and 5-year disease-free survival for maxillary osteosarcomas of 65% and 38%, respectively (19). Adjuvant therapy, including radiation, chemotherapy, or combination therapy, failed to improve outcome. Nonetheless, these authors acknowledge a selection bias and therefore the role of adjuvant therapy remains unresolved.

Chondrosarcomas are slow-growing tumors that usually arise from cartilaginous structures. These tumors have been graded from I to III on the basis of the rate of mitoses, cellularity, and nuclear size. Size of the tumor and grading correlates with the rate of metastasis, local aggressiveness, and ultimate survival. Surgical removal with wide margins is the treatment of choice. Gross total removal with postoperative radiation is recommended for those involving vital structures.

Although the metastatic potential and oncologic outcome of sarcomas arising in the sinonasal tract is variable among the different histologic types, the local behavior of sarcomas is similar. Sarcomas are infiltrative, usually advancing to areas farther than what is appreciated by the naked eye; thus, they are often incompletely resected and therefore recur locally. Wide excision improves the local control, but this is difficult to perform when dealing with the sinonasal tract, which is adjacent to important if not vital structures. Cranial base surgery may improve the local control of sarcomas of the sinonasal tract.

Lymphoma of the sinonasal tract accounts for only 0.17% of all lymphomas. T-cell lymphomas are more common in Asian populations, while B-cell lymphomas are more common in Western populations. The primary sites of occurrence in the sinonasal tract are the maxillary sinus (79%) and nasal cavity (20%) (20). The treatment includes radiation therapy for localized lesions and chemotherapy to prevent systemic recurrence. The biologic behavior is remarkably different in the pediatric and adult populations. Adults suffer frequent relapses, commonly involving the abdomen, and show a 5-year survival rate of

around 45%. Distant metastases are often associated with failure to treat with chemotherapy in the primary setting (20). In children, complete remissions are more common, involvement of the gastrointestinal tract is rare, and the 5-year survival rate is close to 75%.

Eighty to ninety percent of patients with extramedullary plasmacytoma have involvement of the head and neck region, 40% arise in the sinonasal tract. It is more common in the sixth to seventh decades. It tends to spread locally, and can be found in the cervical nodes in less than 25% of the cases. The prognosis is unpredictable, and a variable number of the patients will be diagnosed with multiple myeloma. It is of utmost importance to rule out this diagnosis on the initial presentation. Most of these lesions will respond to radiation therapy in doses of 4,000 to 5,000 cGy administered over 4 to 5 weeks.

Metastatic Tumors

Metastatic tumors to the sinonasal tract produce symptoms similar to those of primary tumors. More than 100 cases have been reported, metastasizing to the maxillary, ethmoid, frontal, and sphenoid sinus in descending order. The most common primary sources are the kidneys, breasts, and lungs. The treatment is palliative, using radiation, surgery, or chemotherapy to relieve obstructive and compressive symptoms or pain.

STAGING

A staging system provides a guide to define the extent and prognosis of a tumor and also serves as a communication tool, allowing different institutions to compare their experience with the use of different therapeutic modalities. The American Joint Committee on Cancer (AJCC) TNM staging system of the nose and paranasal sinuses is provided (Table 129.8). The AJCC recommends a different system for soft tissue sarcomas. This system includes a histologic grading system that differs from the system used for epithelial tumors. Grading is thought to be the most significant prognostic factor in patients with mesenchymal tumors and is based on the number of mitoses, degree of cellularity, amount of stroma, degree of maturation, nuclear pleomorphism, and presence or absence of necrosis.

PRINCIPLES OF TREATMENT

Surgery

Diagnostic (Biopsy)

Tissue sampling may be performed using endoscopic sinus surgery instruments or through open transcutaneous or transoral procedures (e.g., Caldwell-Luc antrostomy, external ethmoidectomy, rhinotomy). The former is preferred since it provides good access and hemostatic control with less morbidity, and does not contaminate other soft tissues.

TABLE 129.8	MAXILLARY SINUS TNM STAGING FOR PRIMARY TUMOR (T)
TX	Primary tumor cannot be assessed
T0	No evidence of primary tumor
Tis	Carcinoma *in situ*
T1	Tumor limited to maxillary sinus mucosa with no erosion or destruction of bone
T2	Tumor causing bone erosion or destruction including extension into the hard palate and/or middle nasal meatus, except extension to posterior wall of maxillary sinus and pterygoid plates
T3	Tumor invades any of the following: bone of the posterior wall of the maxillary sinus, subcutaneous tissues, floor or medial wall of orbit, pterygoid fossa, ethmoid sinuses
T4a	Tumor invades anterior orbital contents, skin of cheek, pterygoid plates, infratemporal fossa, cribriform plate, sphenoid or frontal sinuses
T4b	Tumor invades any of the following: orbital apex, dura, brain, middle cranial fossa, cranial nerves other than maxillary division of trigeminal nerve (V2), nasopharynx, or clivus

American Joint Committee on Cancer. *Manual for staging of cancer*, 6th ed. New York: Springer-Verlag, 2002:61.

Drainage/Debridement

An adequate drainage port (e.g., nasoantral window) should be opened in patients presenting with secondary bacterial sinusitis and in patients who will require radiation therapy as primary treatment.

Resection

Surgical resection is usually recommended with curative intent. Palliative excision may be considered to alleviate intractable pain, to provide rapid decompression of vital structures, or to debulk a massive lesion, thus freeing the patient from social embarrassment. Surgery as a single treatment modality for malignant tumors of the sinonasal tract has yielded 5-year survival rates from 19% to 86%. Figures 129.1 through 129.6 demonstrate the most common surgical approaches and techniques.

With recent advances in preoperative imaging, intraoperative image guidance systems, endoscopic instrumentation, and materials for hemostasis, endonasal techniques for the removal of nasal and paranasal sinus tumors may be a viable alternative to the traditional open techniques. Endoscopic approaches can access and visualize tumors in the nasal cavity, ethmoid, sphenoid, medial frontal, and medial maxillary sinuses. Frozen sections must be utilized as the tumor is often removed in a piecemeal fashion. Improvements in functional recovery and long-term survival, however, are yet to be described. A recent review of 134 patients undergoing endoscopic resection of sinonasal malignancies revealed a 5-year disease-free survival rate 91% and a 59% survival rate for open procedures (21). Unfortunately, the data were not stratified by stage.

Rehabilitation

The main goals of postsurgical rehabilitation are primary wound healing, preservation or reconstruction of the facial contour, and restoration of oronasal separation, thus facilitating speech and swallowing. Functional considerations take precedence over aesthetics. Rehabilitation after surgical resection may be achieved with a dental prosthesis or reconstructive flaps, such as temporalis muscle flaps with and without the inclusion of cranial bone, pedicled or microvascular free myocutaneous flaps (e.g., pectoralis major, latissimus dorsi, trapezius), and cutaneous flaps (e.g., forehead, scalp, deltopectoral). Flaps are recommended to replace resected skin, to provide support for the orbit or brain, or to isolate the cranial cavity from the upper aerodigestive tract.

A total maxillectomy defect should not be obliterated at the initial operation; an open cavity facilitates cleansing and direct visual inspection during the follow-up period. Patients requiring a craniofacial resection, especially those needing an orbital exenteration deserve special consideration, since a recurrence after an adequate craniofacial resection is uniformly lethal. From the functional standpoint, patients require immediate separation of the cranial cavity from the upper aerodigestive tract and support of the brain. A pericranial flap and transfer of a temporalis muscle flap achieves these goals. The temporalis muscle, however, is often devascularized after an infratemporal fossa dissection or its bulk may be inadequate to obliterate the dead space. Under these circumstances, the maxillectomy cavity may be obliterated with a free microvascular flap, offering immediate palliation and oronasal separation without the need for a prosthesis.

Radiation Therapy

The response of sinonasal tract tumors to radiation varies with the stage and histology of the tumor. Radiation may be used as a single modality, as an adjunct to surgery, or as palliative therapy. Recent reports indicate that postoperative radiation improves local control but not cause specific or absolute survival (22). Radiation therapy is the primary treatment for lymphoreticular tumors, for patients who are poor surgical candidates and for those patients who refuse surgery. Preoperative and postoperative radiation therapy seems to produce similar results. We and others favor postoperative radiation since there is a smaller volume of tumor cells to kill, the margins of the nonradiated tumor can be better defined during surgery and the postoperative wound healing is more predictable.

Chemotherapy

The role of chemotherapy for the treatment of tumors of the sinonasal tract is usually palliative, using its cytoreductive effect to relieve pain, obstruction, or to debulk a massive external lesion. Nevertheless, the failure of combination therapy, including surgery and radiation, to achieve local control, the need for deforming procedures,

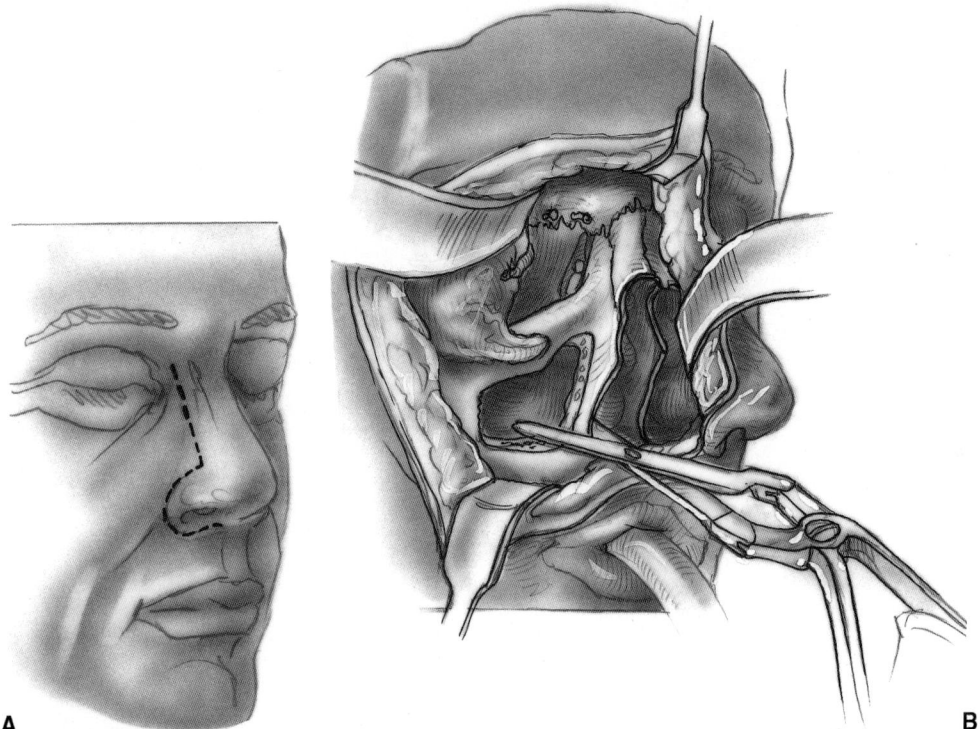

A   **B**

Figure 129.1 Medial maxillectomy. Lateral rhinotomy: **A:** The skin incision begins beneath the medial aspect of the eyebrow and continues 4 to 5 mm anterior to the medial canthus and over the nasal bone along the deepest portion of the nasomaxillary groove and following the alar crease. A lip-splitting extension of the incision is not necessary. To expose the surgical area, the cheek flap is elevated subperiosteally over the maxilla and around the infraorbital nerve. The periorbita is elevated over the lamina papyracea, and the frontoethmoid suture is identified and followed posteriorly until the anterior and posterior ethmoid arteries are identified. The anterior wall of the antrum is penetrated at the canine fossa using a 4-mm chisel. The antrostomy is enlarged with a Kerrison rongeur around the infraorbital nerve and superiorly toward the inferior orbital rim. **B:** Bone is removed across the orbital rim, including the lacrimal fossa. The nasolacrimal duct is divided and the lacrimal sac is opened and marsupialized (**C**). **D:** Osteotomies and removal of the specimen. The first osteotomy involved in the actual removal extends through the piriform aperture at the level of the nasal floor, directed posteriorly until the osteotomy perforates the posterior wall of the antrum. The orbit is retracted laterally, and a second osteotomy is performed at the frontoethmoid suture, extending posteriorly to a point 2 to 3 mm posterior to the posterior ethmoid artery (i.e., anterior to the optic foramen). **E:** The thin bone of the medial floor of the orbit is sawed following a line that joins the lacrimal fossa with the superior osteotomy. The final bone cut involves three steps. First, a 2-mm osteotome is introduced through the anterior antrostomy and directed through the medial posterior antral wall. The osteotome is advanced superiorly to reach the level of the superior osteotome and is then pushed medially. Second, a wide osteotome, introduced through the nose, is impacted into the anterior wall of the sphenoid sinus, and then pushed laterally. Heavy right-angle scissors (e.g., upper-lateral-cartilage scissors) are guided through the inferior osteotomy with one blade in the nose and the other in the antrum to start the posterior cut, behind the turbinates. **F:** Heavy curved scissors are then introduced with one blade in the nasal cavity and the other in the superior osteotomy, directed through or along the posterior attachments of the turbinates. The specimen is removed by anterior and inferior traction. Hemostasis is achieved by direct clamping or cautery. The bony edges are smoothed with a rongeur. Residual ethmoid mucosa is removed with ethmoid forceps, and a wide sphenoidotomy is opened with Kerrison rongeurs. The cavity is covered with Gelfoam for hemostasis. The medial canthal tendon is sutured to the periosteum of the nasal bones. The wound is closed using a meticulous layered closure. AEF, anterior ethmoidal foramen; OF, optic foramen; PEF, posterior ethmoidal foramen.

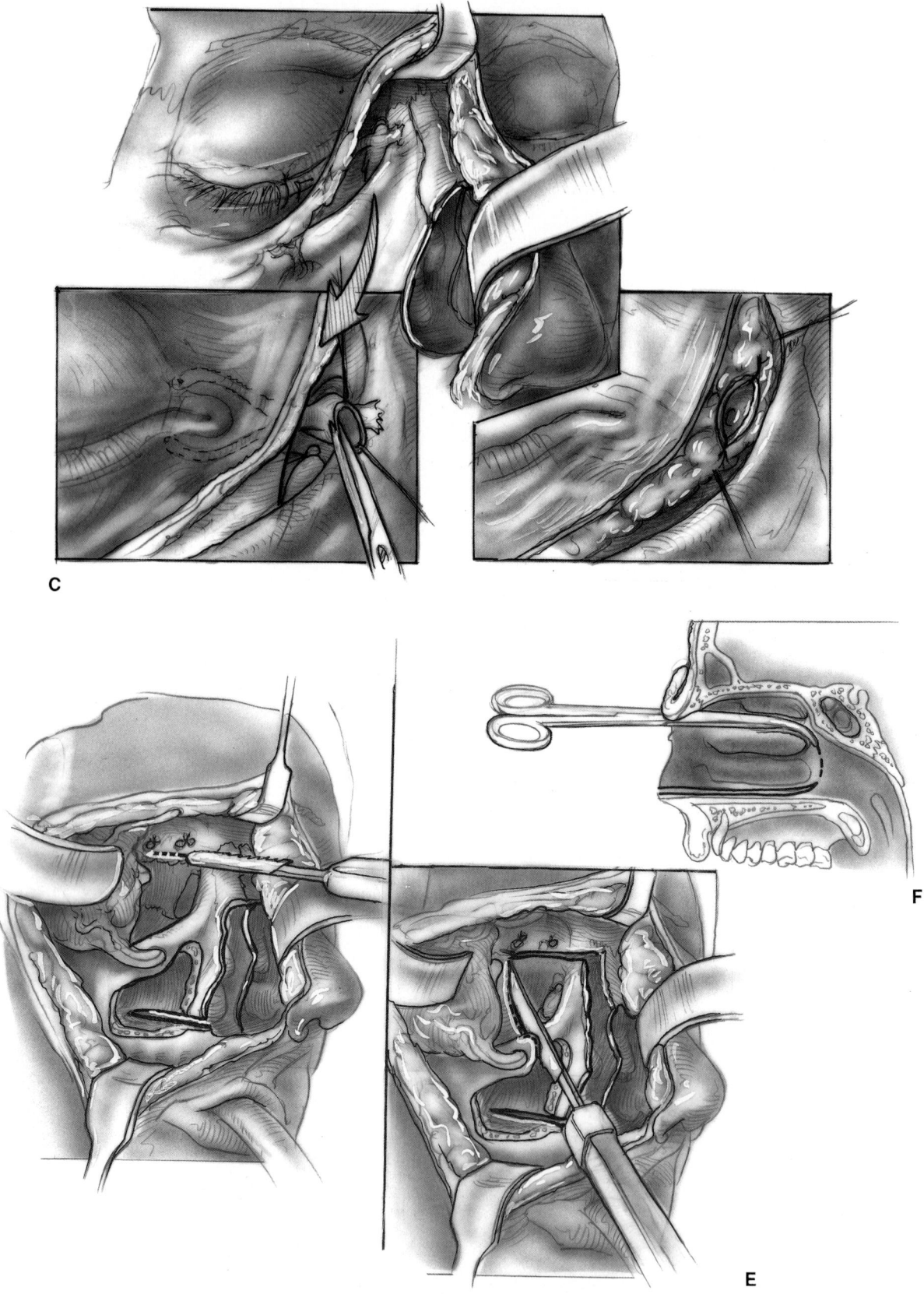

Figure 129.1 *(Continued)*

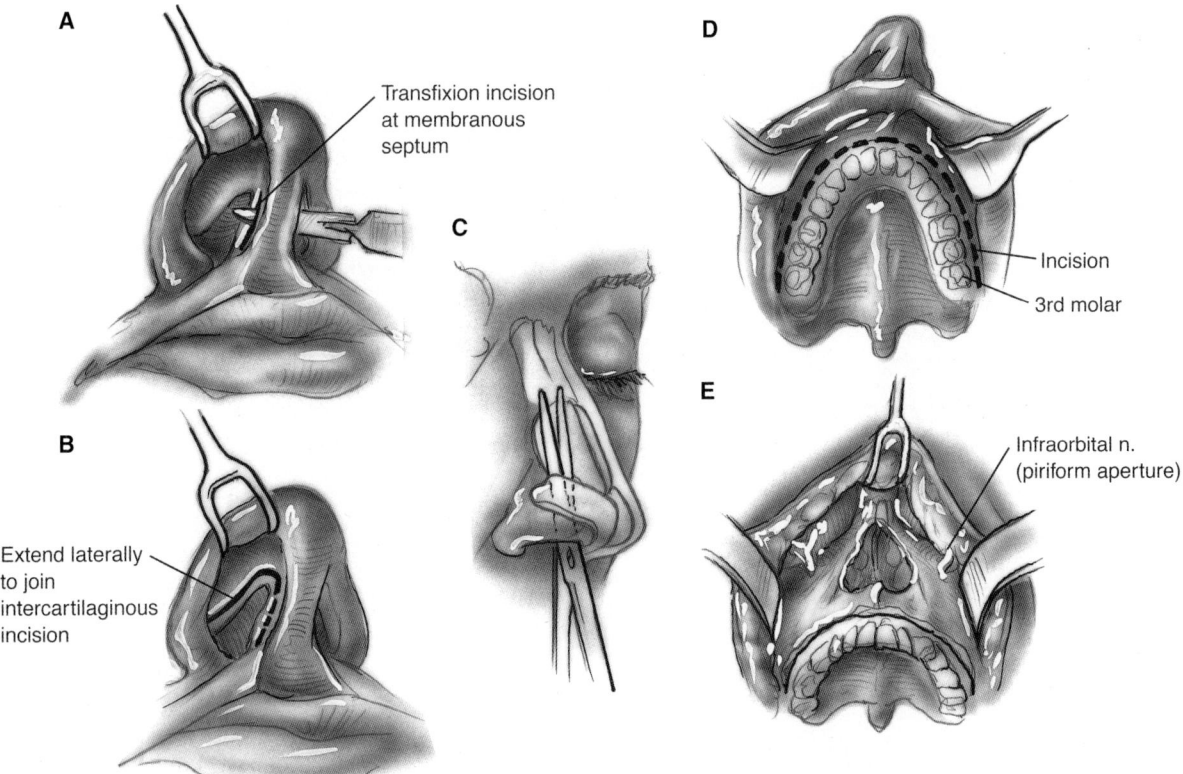

Figure 129.2 A,B: Mid-face degloving. A transfixion incision is performed at the membranous septum and is extended laterally to join a transcartilaginous incision. **C:** A gingivobuccal incision is performed, extending laterally from the midline to the maxillary tuberosities. **D:** In exposing the surgical area, tenotomy scissors are introduced through the transcartilaginous incisions to dissect the skin from the nasal skeleton. The dissection over the maxilla is carried out in a subperiosteal plane. This dissection joins the nasal degloving using sharp dissection over the piriform aperture attachments. The dissection is extended superiorly exposing the mid-face skeleton. **E:** The exposure is limited by the infraorbital neurovascular bundles. The osteotomies, removal of the specimen, reconstruction, and closure are performed as described for the lateral rhinotomy.

or the shifting of cause of failure to distant metastases spearheaded the use of systemic and even topical chemotherapy in multimodal therapy protocols. These reports, however, are very limited in nature, including small number of patients, and the studies are usually nonrandomized. Recent reports have shown a survival advantage for patients undergoing concurrent chemoradiation followed by definitive surgery. Samant et al. (22) in 2004 reported the use of high-dose intra-arterial cisplatin with concomitant radiation in patients with carcinoma of the paranasal sinuses. The overall and disease-free survival rates at 5 years were 53% (Table 129.9). Patients who represent a poor surgical risk and those who refuse surgery, should be considered for enrollment in protocols that include combinations of radiation and chemotherapy.

Treatment by Site of Origin

This section discusses the treatment of SCCA by site of origin. The management of other epithelial and mesenchymal malignancies was discussed in the pathology section.

Nasal Cavity

SCCA is the most common malignant tumor, constituting more than half of the tumors in this area. Tumors arising at the floor, lateral wall, and septum are all amenable to surgical excision. Tumors extending to the paranasal sinuses, those larger than 2 cm, and those associated with positive surgical margins have been associated with a poor prognosis for which postoperative radiation should be administered. Most series report a 5-year survival rate of above 60%.

Maxillary Antrum

The maxillary sinus is the most common site of origin for malignancies of the sinonasal tract. Early-stage SCCA may be treated by surgery or radiation. However, SCCA is usually diagnosed at advanced stages for which combination therapy seems more successful. Survival diminishes with the stage of the tumor, and complete surgical resection is required for success. The overall 5-year survival rate in large series range between 40% and 50%.

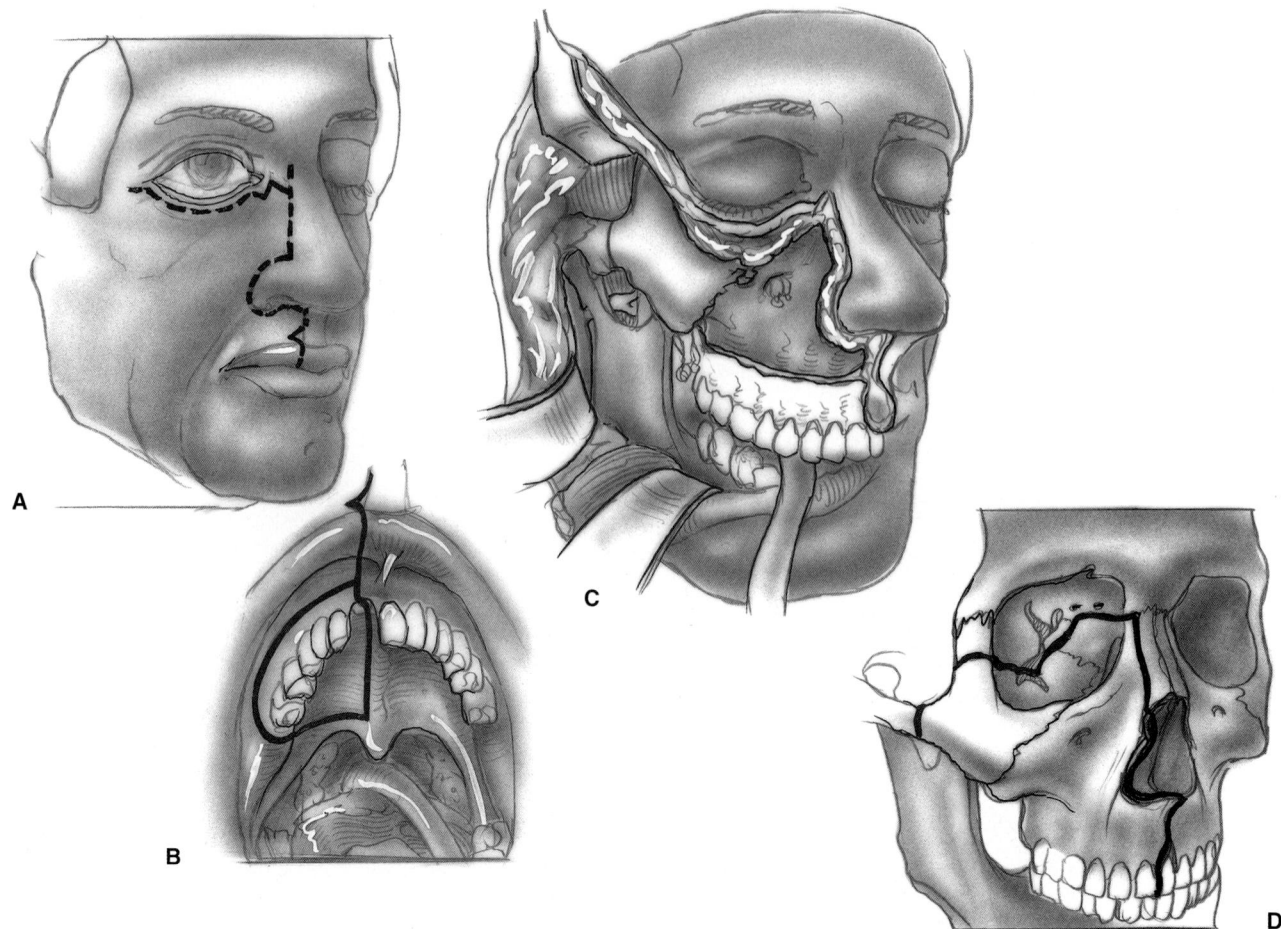

Figure 129.3 Total maxillectomy. A total maxillectomy with preservation of the orbit can be performed using incisions identical to lateral rhinotomy incisions with a lip-splitting extension. Alternatively, a lateral rhinotomy incision may be combined with an ipsilateral degloving approach. **A:** If increased exposure is necessary, the facial incisions may be modified. The superior incision begins at the lateral canthus and extends medially, passing 3 to 4 mm below the ciliary line. The eye is protected by a temporary tarsorrhaphy stitch. This incision may be substituted by a transconjunctival incision. The subciliary limb is joined to a lateral rhinotomy incision. The orbicularis oculi muscle is incised with an inferiorly directed slant, exposing the orbital septum. The gingivobuccal incision is extended laterally to the ipsilateral maxillary tuberosity. **B:** The soft palate is incised at the junction with the hard palate, and its attachments are sharply transected. The mucoperiosteum of the hard palate is incised following a paramedian line ipsilateral to the lesion. The paramedian strip of mucosa will be later imbricated over the bony edge of the hard palate to facilitate the fitting of a prosthesis. **C:** The orbital contents are dissected from the medial inferior and lateral walls, exposing the lacrimal sac, the anterior and posterior ethmoid arteries, and the infraorbital fissure. These are managed as described for a medial maxillectomy (Fig. 129.1). Osteotomies and removal of the specimen. **D:** The body and frontal process of the zygoma are divided with the saw. The maxilla is severed from the nasal bones with the saw, and the osteotomy is extended superiorly to the frontoethmoidal suture. A superior osteotomy is carried out posteriorly to a point 3 to 4 mm posterior to the posterior ethmoid artery. An osteotomy is performed connecting the lateral and medial wall osteotomies across the inferior orbital fissure. The hard palate is transected with a Gigli or sagittal saw. The maxilla is detached from the skull by tapping a chisel placed into the pterygomaxillary fissure in a posterosuperior direction. The superior attachments of the turbinates are sharply severed, as for a medial maxillectomy (Fig. 129.1). The specimen is removed by anteroinferior traction. Remnants of ethmoid sinus mucosa are removed in a piecemeal fashion. The coronoid process of the mandible is removed to avoid displacement of the prosthesis when opening the mandible. *(Continued)*

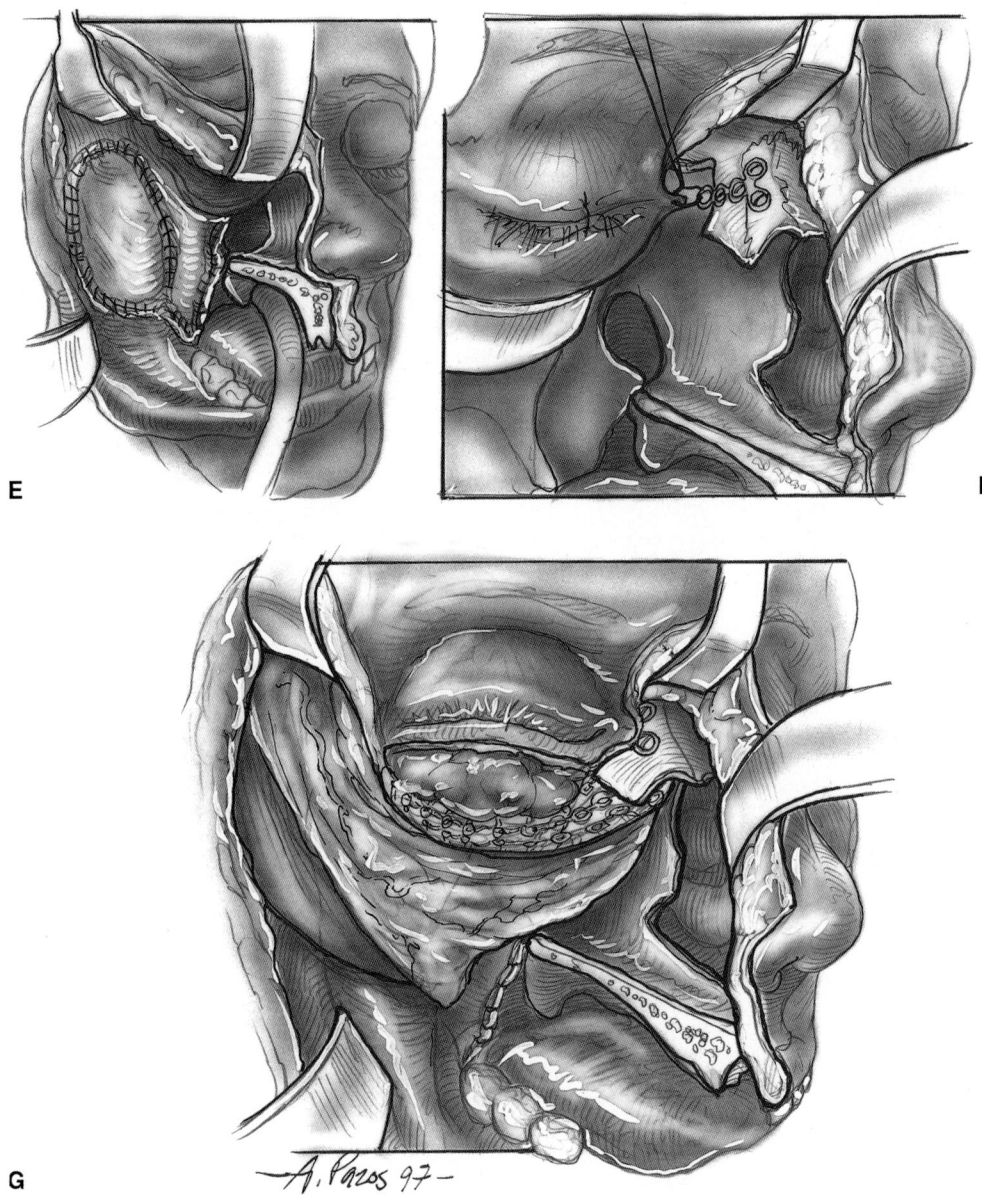

Figure 129.3 *(Continued)* **E:** The exposed facial and pterygoid muscles and periorbita are lined with a split-thickness skin graft that is 0.35 to 0.45 mm thick. The obturator or denture is wired to the remaining dentition or suspended from the zygomatic arch and piriform aperture or leg screwed to the remaining hard palate. **F:** A medial canthopexy, using a Y-shape titanium plate fixed to the nasal bones. A figure-8 nonabsorbable suture is used to medialize the medial canthal tendon. **G:** The floor and medial walls of the orbit are reconstructed with titanium mesh. This is then covered by a vertically split temporalis muscle flap. The anterior half is used for the reconstruction, and the posterior half is transposed to the anterior temporal fossa to obliterate the defect.

Ethmoid Sinus

Tumors originating in the ethmoid sinuses produce symptoms at early stages, leading to earlier diagnosis and better prognosis. SCCA continues to be the most common histologic diagnosis, but adenomatous carcinomas are more common than at other areas. Improved imaging techniques and the use of anterior craniofacial resection (see the discussion below on "Management of Advanced Tumors" of the base of skull) have improved the prognosis of previously unresectable tumors. Smaller tumor, T1 or T2, may be considered for endoscopic resection. Combined therapy with radiation is recommended for advanced stages, positive surgical margins, and recurrent tumors. The overall 5-year survival rate is 50% to 60%.

Sphenoid Sinus

Primary malignancies of the sphenoid sinus are extremely rare, making up less than 1% of malignant sinonasal tumors. En bloc surgical resection is technically difficult due to the anatomical relationships of the sphenoid

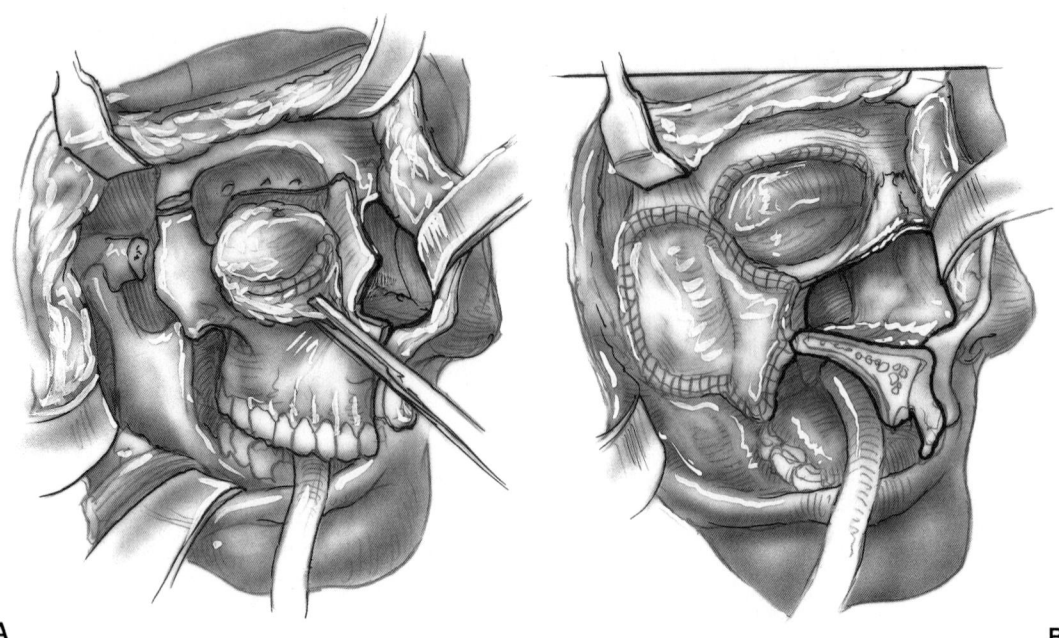

A   B

Figure 129.4 Orbital exenteration. **A**: Incisions for orbital exenteration include those described in Figure 129.3 and a supraciliary incision along the upper eyelid. These incisions allow the preservation of the lids, which can be used to line the remaining orbital cavity. If the eyelids are involved by the tumor, the incisions are modified to include their resection en bloc. The exposure proceeds as previously described (Fig. 129.3), omitting the dissection of the orbit from the inferior wall. The upper eyelid is retracted superiorly, and the periorbita is incised over the superior orbital rim. The orbit is dissected from the superior wall, identifying optic foramen and superior orbital fissure. These are infiltrated with lidocaine to block the autonomic innervation and prevent cardiac arrhythmias. The neural and vascular structures traveling through these foramina are transected after hemostasis with bipolar cautery or clamping. Inferior traction on the globe allows further visualization of the orbital floor and inferior orbital fissure. Lateral and medial wall osteotomies are connected as in Figure 129.3C. Other osteotomies are identical to Figure 129.3C. The roof of the orbit may be lined with a skin graft or left to granulate and mucosalize. Alternatively, the cavity may be filled with a temporalis muscle flap. It should be remembered that squamous epithelium tolerates trauma (e.g., prosthesis) better than mucosa. **B**: In exposing the surgical area, the facial flap is elevated subperiosteally. In the case of extension through the anterior wall of the antrum, the facial flap may be elevated in a subcutaneous plane, including the facial musculature in the specimen. The skin may also be resected en bloc, to address direct invasion by the tumor. The dissection is carried out along the lateral wall of the maxilla and the internal maxillary artery is identified at the pterygomaxillary fissure and clipped.

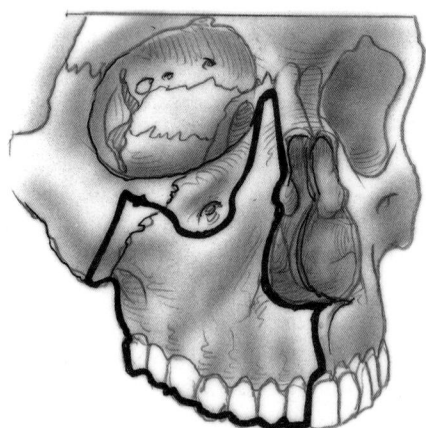

Figure 129.5 Inferior maxillectomy. Tumors confined to the floor of the antrum may be managed by partial maxillectomy. It differs from total maxillectomy on the preservation of the orbital floor and, in selected cases of the infraorbital nerve. Bilateral maxillectomy. The procedure is performed bilaterally as in Figure 129.4. The nasal septum may be sacrificed or preserved for suspension of the prosthesis or reconstructive flaps.

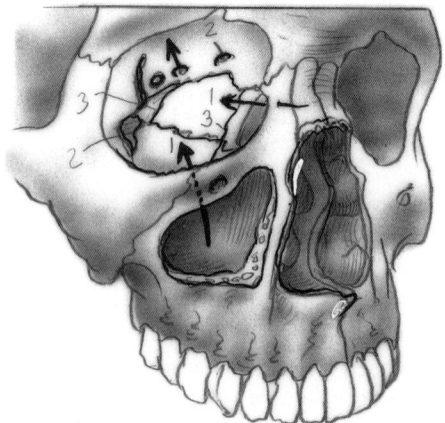

Figure 129.6 Pathways of invasion include (1) direct bony erosion (e.g., medial wall or floor), (2) perivascular or perineural invasion (e.g., infraorbital or ethmoidal neurovascular bundles), and (3) preformed pathways (e.g., infraorbital fissure, nasolacrimal duct).

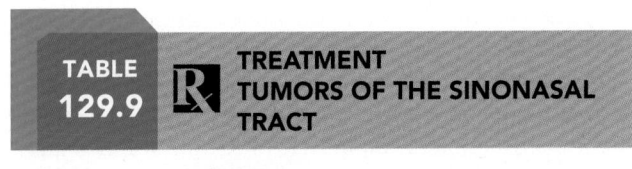

TABLE 129.9	TREATMENT TUMORS OF THE SINONASAL TRACT	

Modality	Indications
Surgery	Mainstay treatment
Radiation	Unresectable or lymphoreticular tumors, poor surgical candidates. Usually requires surgical drainage/debridement
Combination therapy	(+) margins, perineural, perivascular invasion (+) lymph nodes, recurrent tumor
Chemotherapy	Palliative role Clinical research (controlled protocols)

sinus. Gross total removal and postoperative radiation therapy is the treatment of choice for most of these tumors. Although the benefits of surgical debulking are debatable, at the very least it will provide a wide sphenoidotomy for drainage and debridement during radiation therapy. The overall prognosis at 5-year follow-up varies from 5% to 25%.

Frontal Sinus

Tumors arising in the frontal sinus, like sphenoidal tumors, are rare. The anatomical site, however, is more amenable to surgical resection. These tumors may be managed similarly to ethmoidal tumors.

MANAGEMENT OF ADVANCED TUMORS

Orbital Invasion

Sinonasal tract tumors may extend to the orbit by invasion or erosion of the bony walls, by perineural or perivascular invasion, or by following preformed pathways

(Fig. 129.6). As great as 26% of patients with sinonasal malignancies have orbital invasion at the time of presentation (23). Patients with orbital invasion rapidly develop ocular symptoms, such as proptosis, diplopia, decreased visual acuity, diminished motility, chemosis, lid edema, and epiphora. CT scanning provides evidence of bony erosion, but it is not reliable in ascertaining invasion of the soft tissues. MRI better identifies soft tissue invasion, but invasion must be confirmed during surgery.

Bone erosion does not constitute an absolute indication for orbital exenteration (24). The prognosis of patients with invasion of the periorbita is dismal; therefore, palliation is a more realistic goal (Table 129.10). Adjunctive radiation therapy, before or after surgery, does not seem to yield an improved prognosis.

Resection of the medial and inferior orbital walls produces severe enophthalmos and hypophthalmos, which is aggravated by resection of the periorbita. Rigid reconstruction of the bony orbit using titanium mesh with or without calvarial bone grafts is recommended; which is then covered with local, regional, or microvascular flaps. To better restore the orbital anatomy and to prevent lagophthalmos, due to ectropion, the lateral canthus should be reattached to the corresponding anatomical site of insertion. Ectropion may still occur due to fibrosis. The medial wall is usually resected as part of the oncologic surgery, requiring that the medial canthus be reattached to a titanium plate, as illustrated in Figure 129.5.

Cervical Metastasis

The incidence of nodal metastasis on initial presentation varies from 3% to 16%. Nodal metastases at initial presentation indicate a grim prognosis. The low incidence of nodal metastasis from sinonasal malignancies does not justify the use of elective neck dissection or radiation. Recurrence in the form of cervical metastasis ranks second after local

TABLE 129.10	META-ANALYSIS OUTCOME: INVASION OF ORBIT (NED)		
	Sparing	Exenteration	Significance
Som et al. (1971)	—	3/27 (11%)	
Perry et al. (1988)	1/2 (50%)	2/4 (50%)	
Xuexi et al. (1995)	8/23 (35%)	24/88 (27%)	
Carrau et al. (1996)	5/9 (56%)	6/12 (50%)	
Total	**14/34 (41%)**	**35/131 (27%)**	p > 0.05

This table demonstrates the lack of statistically significant difference in the survival rate of those patients in whom the orbit was preserved when compared with patients whose orbit was exenterated. The trend toward worst survival in those patients who required exenteration illustrates the aggressiveness of tumors that invade the periorbita.
Adapted from Carrau RL, Segas J, Nuss DW, et al. Squamous cell carcinoma of the sinonasal tract invading the orbit. *Laryngoscope* 109:230–235, 1999.

recurrence as a cause for treatment failure. However, an isolated recurrence to cervical nodes is rare; usually it is accompanied by recurrent disease at the primary site.

Pterygopalatine Fossa

The incidence of PtPF invasion by sinonasal tract malignancies varies from 10% to 20%. The presence of tumor in this area is considered a risk factor for local recurrence. Despite the difficulty of an en bloc resection of this area, several authors have designed approaches with sound oncologic principles, obtaining variable results. Radical surgical resection in combination with radiation therapy, however, is advised for patients with PtPF invasion.

Infratemporal Fossa and Skull Base

The skull base may be involved by tumor by direct invasion and bone erosion, by preformed pathways (e.g., cribriform plate, superior orbital fissure, foramen lacerum), or by following neural or vascular structures (e.g., V2, V3). The overall incidence of skull base invasion by sinonasal malignancies appears to be about 15%. The anterior or anterolateral craniofacial resection is a well-established procedure for sinonasal tumors invading the anterior skull (Fig. 129.7). The anterior craniofacial resection may be extended laterally to join a temporal craniotomy to include the pterygoid plates, the PtPF, the infratemporal fossa, and the floor of the middle cranial fossa en bloc. Absolute contraindications for craniofacial resection are medical or nutritional problems that would eliminate the patient as a surgical candidate, presence of distant metastases, invasion of the prevertebral fascia, invasion of the cavernous sinus by a high-grade malignancy, involvement of the carotid artery in a high-risk patient (as determined by carotid flow studies), and bilateral invasion of the optic nerves or optic chiasm. Resection of these areas is associated with an unacceptable morbidity and mortality rate, offers no significant palliation, and does not appear to improve survival. Relative contraindications include invasion of the dura and intracranial involvement of neural structures. These situations have a poor prognosis, but in selected cases craniofacial resection may offer significant palliation or local control.

Improvements in the preoperative mapping of tumors with CT scan and MRI and the use of more reliable vascularized flaps for the reconstruction of the skull base have improved the surgical mortality and morbidity. However, the overall 5-year survival rate appears unchanged at 50% to 60%.

COMPLICATIONS

Surgical

The nasolacrimal duct is sacrificed during the performance of a maxillectomy, and subsequent stenosis of the lacrimal sac opening may lead to epiphora.

A dacryocystorhinostomy at the time of definitive resection is an effective way to prevent this complication. Cannulation of the lacrimal canaliculi for 12 weeks is recommended.

Limitation of movement of the extraocular muscles may occur after trauma to the muscle or its motor innervation or upon entrapment in the craniofacial osteotomies. The latter complication should be managed by urgent surgical release. Limitations of extraocular muscle movement due to edema or neuromuscular contusion should be managed expectantly. Diplopia may be alleviated by alternating eye patching.

The optic nerve may be compressed during the mobilization of the specimen or during craniofacial resection. High-dose steroids and emergent surgical decompression are recommended.

Enophthalmos or hypophthalmos usually develop due to the loss of the inferior orbital and/or medial support. Reconstructive techniques were previously discussed.

Radiation Therapy

The incidence of radiation complications in patients with orbit preservation is close to 100% (Table 129.11). The field included in the radiation portals for sinonasal tract tumors usually includes the anterior and posterior orbital segment. When the orbit is involved by the tumor, irradiation of the entire eye is usually necessary. Complications of the anterior globe are common with full eye irradiation. A dry eye will decompensate rapidly, leading to severe keratitis, panophthalmitis, and blindness within 1 year. Enucleation is recommended for uncontrolled panophthalmitis or a painful eye.

If the anterior segment can be spared, patients will most likely experience delayed (3 to 5 years) loss of vision secondary to post-radiation retinopathy or optic neuropathy. Although the retina and optic nerve are radio resistant, their microvasculature is not. Chemotherapy, diabetes mellitus, and atherosclerosis may have an additive effect on radiation complications. The incidence of these complications is related to total dose and fractionation. The tolerance limit seems to be around 5,000 cGy with fractions of 200 cGy. Although they are rare below 3,500 cGy, their incidence is 50% to 65% with 6,000 to 7,000 cGy and above 85% with 8,000 cGy. Nevertheless, the degree of visual impairment cannot be accurately predicted and has been reported with doses considered within the safe limits. The incidence of unilateral blindness can range around 35%, while the incidence of bilateral blindness, although rarely reported, may be as high as 8% and is related to the irradiation of the contralateral posterior segment. Blindness is felt to be due to ipsilateral radiation retinopathy and contralateral optic neuropathy. However, the dose should not be compromised to diminish the complication rate if the attempted goal is cure. Conformal radiation therapy reduces the percentage of radiation received by normal tissue and may decrease the incidence of optic nerve and optic chiasm complications.

Wound Complications

Wound complications include bleeding, infection, and loss of reconstructive flaps or skin grafts (Table 129.12). Osteoradionecrosis can occur in up to 10% of patients. The most common site of osteoradionecrosis is the maxilla. Severe osteoradionecrosis can be secondary to poor dentitia or recently extracted dentitia. We recommend the routine extraction of poor dentitia with time to recover prior to postoperative radiation to avoid this complication.

Postoperative infection is rare. Cellulitis should be treated with antibiotics providing broad-spectrum coverage adjusted to the culture and sensitivity results. Venous retrograde seeding, or even direct spread in the presence of a CSF fistula can lead to meningitis or intracranial abscess. A CT scan followed by a lumbar puncture is indicated if

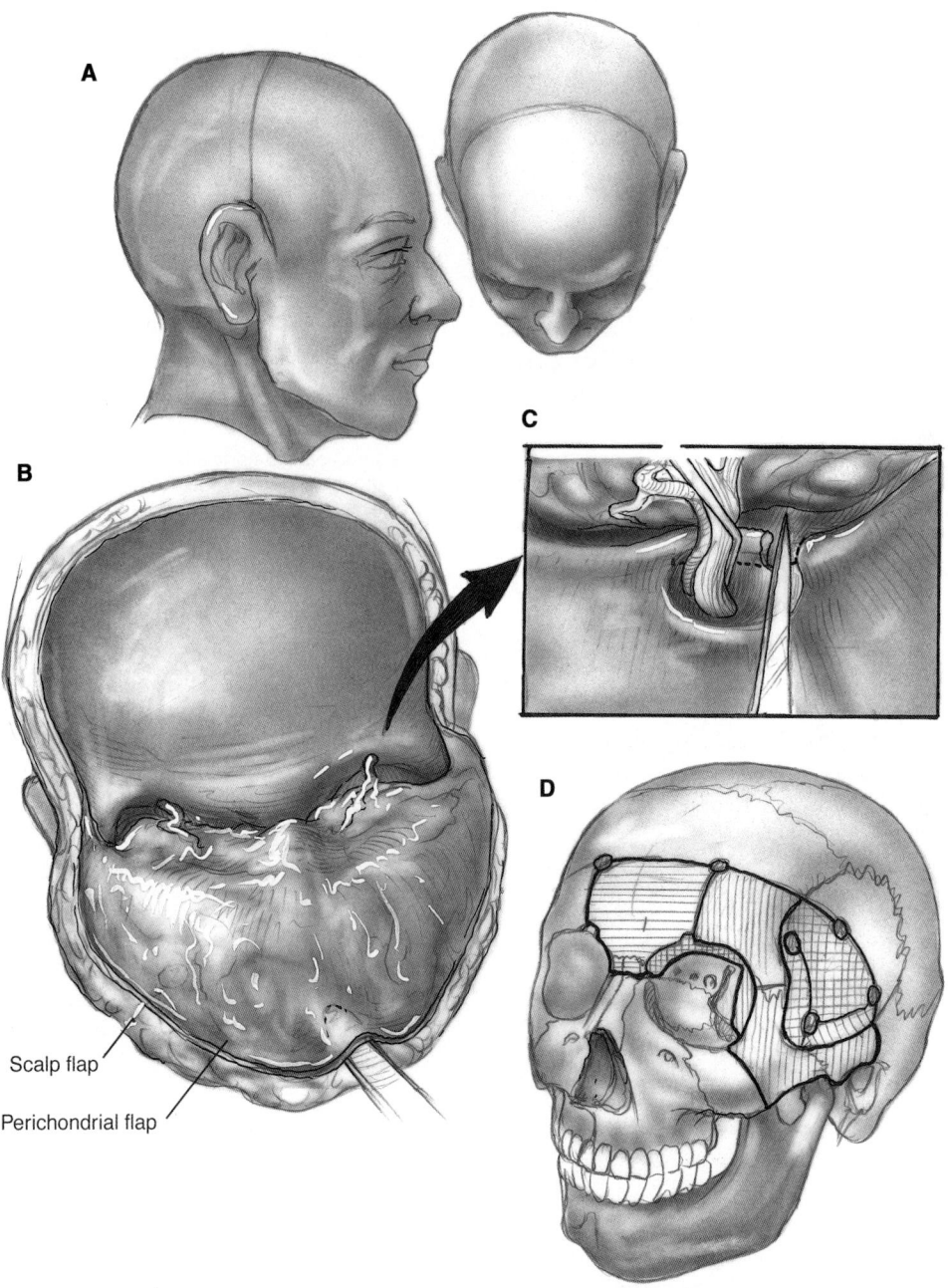

Scalp flap

Perichondrial flap

Figure 129.7 **A:** Bicoronal flap incision. **B:** The scalp flap is dissected anteriorly in a subperiosteal plane and laterally just above the superficial layer of the deep temporal fascia. Leaving the pericranial flap attached to the scalp flap prevents desiccation of the flap during the procedure. **C:** In order to expose the supraorbital rim, superior orbital cavity and nasal bones, the supraorbital neurovascular bundle is mobilized from its notch or foramen. **D:** Orbital, cranial, and zygomatic osteotomies are performed according to the required exposure. The tumor is resected en bloc with the anterior or middle fossa skull base. *(Continued)*

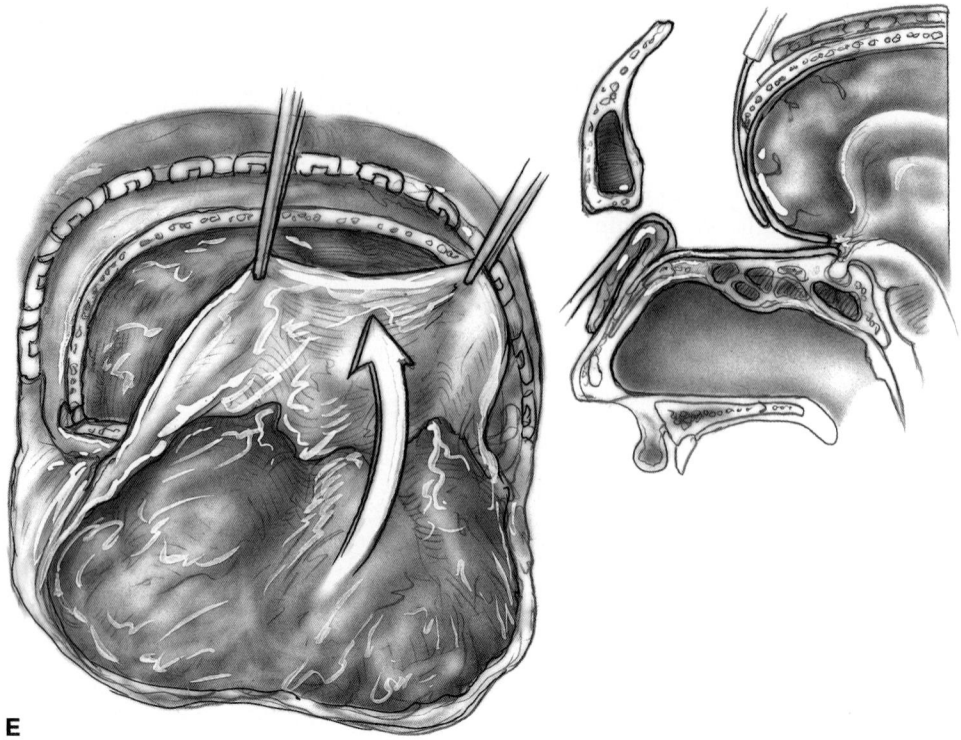

E

Figure 129.7 *(Continued)* **E:** A pericranial flap is elevated and placed under the dura of anterior lobe and over the remaining bone of the anterior fossa. The craniotomy and orbital bone grafts are replaced above the pericranial flap which separates the cranial cavity from the upper aerodigestive tract.

meningitis is suspected. Formation of crusts within the nasal cavity is a common problem and may lead to infection. Frequent irrigations with normal saline solution help with nasal hygiene.

The loss of a reconstructive flap is accompanied by necrosis and overgrowth of bacteria and is best treated by debridement and aggressive local care. A secondary reconstruction must be postponed until the defect is free of infection. However, flaps providing coverage to vital areas (e.g., carotid artery, brain) must be replaced by another vascularized flap as soon as possible. Loss of minor areas of a skin graft is usually of no consequence, since secondary epithelialization occurs rapidly. Loss of the entire skin graft, however, may lead to scarring and contraction of the cavity, healing by mucosalization, and problems in fitting a prosthesis. Treatment of local infection and debridement of necrotic tissue, followed by regrafting with internal and external splinting of the skin graft may remedy this problem.

TABLE 129.11	EFFECTS OF RADIATION ON THE EYE		
Tissue	**Effect**	**Latency**	**Dose**
Lacrimal gland	Atrophy	>6 mo	>5,000 cGy/5–6 wk
Conjunctiva	Hyperemia	1–3 wk	≥5.000 cGy/5 wk
	May lead to secondary infection		
Cornea	Edema	1–3 wk	4,000–5,000 cGy/2–3 wk
	Chronic ulceration	Several months	>6,000 cGy/5–6 wk
	Perforation	4–12 mo	>6,000 cGy/5–6 wk
Retina	Edema	Several weeks	2,000–3,500 cGy/3–4 wk
	Retinopathy	>1 y	5,000–6,000 cGy/5–6 wk
Lens	Cataract	1–20 y	≥200 cGy

Adapted from Nakissa N, Rubin P, Strohl R, et al. Ocular and orbital complications following radiation therapy of paranasal sinus malignancies and review of literature. *Cancer* 1983;51:980.

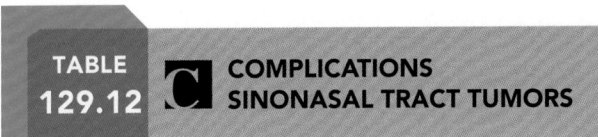

TABLE 129.12 COMPLICATIONS SINONASAL TRACT TUMORS

Problem	Treatment
Orbital	
Surgical	
Epiphora	DCR
Diplopia	Observe, release EOM if entrapped
Blindness	Perform optic nerve or orbital decompression
Enophthalmos/ hypophthalmos	Support globe with bone grafts and/or titanium mesh
Radiation	
Wound	
Bleeding	Packing, arterial ligation, or embolization
Infection	Antibiotics/debridement
Loss of reconstructive flaps or skin grafts	Debridement
Skull base	
CSF leak	Observation, bed rest Reconstructive flap for persistent leak
Meningitis	Antibiotics, correct CSF leak
Pneumocephalus	Aspiration if at tension
Osteomyelitis	Antibiotics, debridement, HBO
Other	
Serous otitis media	Ventilation tube (rule out CSF leak)

Skull Base Complications

Skull base complications include CSF leak, meningitis, intracranial abscess, tension pneumocephalus, and osteomyelitis. These complications are most commonly the result of technical errors (e.g., loss of a reconstructive flap) and are surprisingly uncommon, considering that skull base resection involves exposure of the cranial cavity to aerodigestive tract flora. Treatment includes empiric intravenous antibiotics with broad spectrum coverage, including the skin and aerodigestive flora. The antibiotics are later adjusted to the culture and sensitivity results. Further contamination or exposure of the intracranial contents to the sinonasal tract should be curtailed by the use of vascularized flaps. Free bone grafts that become infected during the early postoperative period should be removed. Late osteomyelitis or osteoradionecrosis may be managed with antibiotics and debridement limited to the affected bone. Hyperbaric oxygen treatment may be beneficial in patients with osteoradionecrosis. Intracranial abscess requires open drainage and intravenous antibiotics.

Tension pneumocephalus is treated by percutaneous aspiration and diversion of the nasal airway. The latter may be accomplished with the use of an endotracheal tube, nasal trumpets, or a tracheotomy.

EMERGENCIES ASSOCIATED WITH SINONASAL TUMORS

Bleeding

Friable or vascular tumors may lead to profuse bleeding when traumatized (e.g., biopsy), or bleeding may occur spontaneously after desiccation and breakdown of the blood vessels in the tumor (Table 129.13). Mild to moderate bleeding is managed using the principles of treatment for anterior and posterior epistaxis. Cauterization or packing is recommended. In the case of a massive tumor that completely occludes the nasal passages, angiography and embolization should be considered. This technique is also useful in vascular tumors, providing prompt hemostasis and facilitating surgical removal. If circumstances preclude the use of this technique, a transantral ligation of the internal maxillary artery and transorbital ligation of the ethmoidal arteries may control the bleeding. Ligation of the external carotid artery, although not as effective as internal maxillary artery ligation, may be necessary if the transantral approach is impossible. One should remember, however, that ligation of the external carotid artery will eliminate the possibility of embolization. A combination of these techniques may be required to prevent exsanguination. Uncontrollable hemostasis from a known malignancy may require emergency maxillectomy.

Vision Impairment

Sinonasal tumors may lead to blindness due to compression or stretching of the optic nerve, its arterial supply, or its venous drainage. Emergent treatment of the tumor with radiation or surgery may be necessary to prevent blindness, although it will be a moot point if the eye is going to be ultimately sacrificed.

Infection

Tumors of the sinonasal tract may obstruct sinus drainage and lead to acute bacterial sinusitis and possible orbital and intracranial complications. Secondary sinus infections must be treated with antibiotics providing broad aerobic

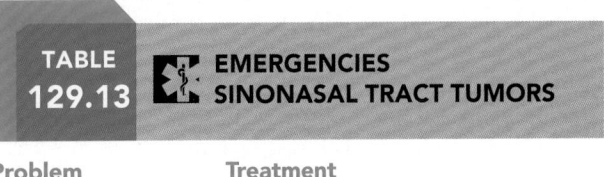

TABLE 129.13 EMERGENCIES SINONASAL TRACT TUMORS

Problem	Treatment
Bleeding	Cauterization/packing Arterial ligation/embolization Emergency extirpative surgery
Visual impairment	Decompression of orbit or optic nerve Radiation for lymphoreticular tumors
Infection	Antibiotics and drainage/debridement
CSF leak/ pneumocephalus	Definitive surgery, reconstructive flap

and anaerobic coverage. Surgical drainage by endoscopic or open technique is usually required.

CSF Leak

CSF leak may occur after destruction of the skull base and disruption of the dura mater (e.g., cribriform plate). CSF leaks are less likely to resolve spontaneously under these circumstances and therefore should be managed by prompt craniofacial resection, dural grafting, and a pericranial flap. Patients must be kept on bed rest while awaiting the operation. The use of prophylactic antibiotics is controversial. They may seem indicated in the presence of a necrotic tumor, but prolonged treatment may lead to colonization with resistant flora that will be more difficult to eradicate in case of meningitis.

HIGHLIGHTS

- The most common clinical presentation of sinonasal tumors includes symptoms that are undistinguishable from inflammatory sinus disease, namely, nasal airway obstruction, pain, and epistaxis. Abnormal V1 and/or V2 sensation strongly suggest the possibility of a tumor.
- CT or MRI is an essential component of evaluation, establishing the extent and vascularity of the tumor and its relationship to neurovascular structures.
- An understanding of the variable natural history of tumors of the sinonasal tract is crucial to patient counseling and treatment planning. A wide variety of histologies may be encountered, although SCCA is most common.
- Rehabilitation after surgical resection may be accomplished by the use of prosthodontics or reconstructive flaps.
- Radiation is a common adjuvant to surgery for patients with SCCA. The response of sinonasal tract tumors to radiation therapy varies with the stage and histology of the tumor.
- Combined intra-arterial cisplatin chemotherapy and radiation therapy before surgical resection offers a survival advantage in advanced SCCA of the paranasal sinuses.
- Bony erosion of the orbital walls does not constitute an indication for orbital exenteration.
- Patients with tumor involvement of the skull base, either in the infratemporal fossa or at the fovea ethmoidalis and cribriform plate, should be considered for craniofacial resection.
- Complications, such as CSF leak, meningitis, intracranial abscess, and tension pneumocephalus, although uncommon, are potentially devastating and need to be addressed in an emergent fashion.

REFERENCES

1. Caplan LS, Hall I, Levine RS, et al. Preventable risk factors for nasal cancer. *Ann Epidemiol* 2000;10:186–191.
2. Cantu G, Bimbi G, Miceli R, et al. Lymph node metastases in malignant tumors of the paranasal sinuses: prognostic value and treatment. *Arch Otolaryngol Head Neck Surg* 2008;134:170–177.
3. Myers EN, Fernau JL, Johnson JT, et al. Management of inverted papilloma. *Laryngoscope* 1990;100:481.
4. Weber RK, Werner JA, Hildenbrand T. Endonasal endoscopic medial maxillectomy with preservation of the inferior turbinate. *Am J Rhinol Allergy* 2010;24:132–135.
5. Philpott CM, Dharamsi A, Witheford M, et al. Endoscopic management of inverted papillomas: long-term results–the St. Paul's Sinus Centre experience. *Rhinology* 2010;48(3):358–363.
6. de Gabory L, Maunoury A, Maurice-Tison S, et al. Long-term single-center results of management of ethmoid adenocarcinoma: 95 patients over 28 years. *Ann Surg Oncol* 2010;17(4):1127–1134.
7. Rhee CS, Won TB, Lee CH, et al. Adenoid cystic carcinoma of the sinonasal tract: treatment results. *Laryngoscope* 2006;116(6):982–986.
8. Lupinetti AD, Roberts DB, Williams MD, et al. Sinonasal adenoid cystic carcinoma: the M. D. Anderson Cancer Center experience. *Cancer* 2007;110(12):2726–2731.
9. Khademi B, Bahranifard H, Nasrollahi H, et al. Primary mucosal melanoma of the sinonasal tract: report of 18 patients and analysis of 1077 patients in the literature. *Braz J Otorhinolaryngol* 2011;77(1):58–64.
10. Moreno MA, Roberts DB, Kupferman ME, et al. Mucosal melanoma of the nose and paranasal sinuses, a contemporary experience from the M. D. Anderson Cancer Center. *Cancer* 2010;116(9):2215–2223.
11. Zanation AM, Ferlito A, Rinaldo A, et al. When, how and why to treat the neck in patients with esthesioneuroblastoma: a review. *Eur Arch Otorhinolaryngol* 2010;267(11):1667–1671.
12. Kane AJ, Sughrue ME, Rutkowski MJ, et al. Posttreatment prognosis of patients with esthesioneuroblastoma. *J Neurosurg* 2010;113(2):340–351.
13. Sheikh HY, Chakravarthy RP, Slevin NJ, et al. Benign schwannoma in paranasal sinuses: a clinico-pathological study of five cases, emphasizing diagnostic difficulties. *J Laryngol Otol* 2008;122(6):598–602.
14. Hillstrom RP, Zarbo RJ, Jacobs JR. Nerve sheath tumors of the paranasal sinuses: electron microscopy and histopathologic diagnosis. *Otolaryngol Head Neck Surg* 1990;102:257.
15. Hicks J, Flaitz C. Rhabdomyosarcoma of the head and neck in children. *Oral Oncol* 2002;38:450–459.
16. Hawkins WG, Hoos A, Antonescu CR, et al. Clinicopathologic analysis of patients with adult rhabdomyosarcoma. *Cancer* 2001;91:794–803.
17. Raney RB, Meza J, Anderson JR, et al. Treatment of children and adolescents with localized parameningeal sarcoma: Experience of the intergroup rhabdomyosarcoma study group protocols IRS-II through-IV, 1978–1997. *Med Pediatr Oncol* 2002;38:22–32.
18. Harvé Alsamad A, Beautru R, Gaston A, et al. Management of sinonasal hemangiopericytomas. *Rhinology* 1999;37:153–158.
19. Kassir RR, Rassekh CH, Kinsella S, et al. Osteosarcoma of the head and neck: Meta-analysis of treatment outcomes. *Laryngoscope* 1997;107:56–61.
20. Logsdon MD, Ha CS, Kavadi VS, et al. Lymphoma of the nasal cavity and paranasal sinuses: improved outcome and altered prognostic factors with combined modality therapy. *Cancer* 1997;80:477–488.
21. Nicolai P, Battaglia P, Bignami M, et al. Endoscopic surgery for malignant tumors of the sinonasal tract and adjacent skull base: a 10-year experience. *Am J Rhinol* 2008;22(3):308–316.
22. Samant S, Robbins KT, Vang M, et al. Intra-arterial cisplatin and concomitant radiation therapy followed by surgery for advanced paranasal sinus cancer. *Arch Otolaryngol Head Neck Surg* 2004;130:948–955.
23. Gil Z, Carlson DL, Gupta A, et al. Patterns and incidence of neural invasion in patients with cancers of the paranasal sinuses. *Arch Otolaryngol Head Neck Surg* 2009;135:173–179.
24. Carrau RL, Segas J, Nuss DW, et al. Squamous cell carcinoma of the sinonasal tract invading the orbit. *Laryngoscope* 1999;109:230–235.

Orbital Tumors

130

Neda Esmaili   *Michael E. Stadler*   *Adam M. Zanation*

INTRODUCTION

In this chapter, we provide the reader with a cursory overview of orbital pathology as it may relate to the practicing Otolaryngologist. This chapter outlines the most common categories of orbital tumors and other common orbital pathologic processes. We discuss various classifications of the pathologies presented, as well as the most common associated signs/symptoms, radiographic findings, and recommended workup and treatment for these lesions. We only briefly discuss secondary lesions affecting the orbit, as these are covered in greater depth in the rhinology and skull base sections of this text. We also specifically discuss the surgical approaches that can be utilized in addressing these pathologic processes.

Classification

Orbital tumors are rare, yet constitute a wide range of lesions. They are often classified based on their origin. Primary orbital tumors originate within the bony orbit, while secondary tumors extend into the orbit from the paranasal sinuses, skin, and/or intracranial compartment. Primary tumors can further be classified based on their anatomic location, with intraconal lesions being confined within the extraocular muscle cone, and extraconal lesions occurring outside of these muscles. Lastly, metastatic orbital tumors originate from distant tissues and spread to the orbit through lymphovascular and/or hematogenous spread.

Primary orbital tumors can originate from the tissues that are present within the orbit, including vascular, lymphoid, nervous, and mesenchymal structures. Lacrimal gland tumors of epithelial and/or lymphoid origin can also present as orbital tumors. In a 40-year study of orbital tumors at the Mayo Clinic, Henderson (1) found that the five most common primary tumors of the orbit were hemangioma, non-Hodgkin lymphoma, inflammatory tumors,

meningioma, and optic nerve glioma. Similarly, in a study of 1,264 patients from the Wills Eye Institute, Shields et al. (2) showed again that there is a very wide range of pathologic types of orbital tumors and that the five most common categories of orbital lesions in their series were vasculogenic (17%), inflammatory (11%), lymphoid/leukemic (10%), lacrimal gland (9%), and optic nerve or meningeal lesions (8%).

In another large series out of MD Anderson, Shinder et al. (3) found that the five most common lesions were lymphoproliferative (25%), lacrimal (10%), inflammatory (8%), vascular (7%), and mesenchymal (7%). In a meta-analysis of five large series, Wilson and Grossniklaus (4) evaluated a total of 4,563 orbital lesions and found that the most common primary orbital tumors were meningiomas, cavernous hemangiomas, and lymphomas. While some series have shown that secondary orbital tumors can account for 33% to 45% of all orbital neoplasms (1), more recent series have found that only 11% to 26% of all orbital tumors are secondary in nature (2,3). This could be due to improved recognition and treatment of the primary processes that most often cause secondary lesions of the orbit, mainly paranasal sinus mucoceles, squamous cell carcinomas (SCCs) of the paranasal sinuses, meningiomas of the cranial base, vascular malformations, and basal cell carcinomas (BCCs) of the skin. Metastatic disease to the orbit has been found to account for anywhere between 2% and 10% of orbital tumors (1–3). (See Tables 130.1 and 130.2 for the most common orbital tumor percentages and the most common metastatic lesions.)

Interestingly, Shields et al. found that malignant lesions comprised 36% of the tumors in their series, while Shinder et al. found that 63% of their tumors were malignant (2,3). Obviously, the type of high volume referral centers where series such as these are put together largely determines the types and distribution of lesions seen, treated, and reported. Not surprisingly, the rates of malignant lesions,

TABLE 130.1 OVERALL PREVALENCE OF ORBITAL LESIONS			
Type of Lesion	**% of Orbital Tumors**	**Type of Lesion**	**% of Orbital Tumors**
Metastatic:	**5%–8%**	**Cysts:**	**6%–12%**
Breast	2%–4%	Dermoid	2%–7%
Lung	<1%	Epithelial inclusion cysts	1%
Prostate	<1%	**Mesenchymal:**	**6%–11%**
Neural:	**9%–17%**	Rhabdomyosarcoma	2%–3%
Glioma	1%–4%	Fibrous dysplasia	<1%
Meningioma	4%–10%	Solitary fibrous tumor	<1%–2%
Schwannoma	1%	Osteomas	<1%
Vascular:	**3%–10%**	Sarcomas	<1%–2.6%
Capillary hemangioma	1%–3%	**Lacrimal:**	**6%–9%**
Cavernous hemangioma	3%–6%	Lymphoid	2%–4%
Lymphangioma	1%–4%	Epithelial	4%
Inflammatory:	**7%–11%**	**Secondary:**	**11%–44%**
Pseudotumor	3%–8%	Mucoceles	3%–8%
Orbital vasculitis	1%–2%	Skin cancers	4%–11%
Thyroid-associated orbitopathy	1%–6%	Meningiomas	1%–7%
Hematopoietic:	**9%–10%**	**Pediatric:**	**n/a***
Leukemia	<1%	Rhabdomyosarcoma	
Lymphoid	2%–9%	Neuroblastoma	
Langerhans cell histiocytosis	<1%	Granulocytic sarcoma	

*Percent estimates of all orbital tumors in adults.

as a percentage of all orbital tumors, increase significantly as age increases. Most pediatric tumors are benign, with most series reporting between 10% and 30% of all pediatric orbital tumors being malignant (1,2). However, some cancer centers treat a larger proportion of pediatric malignant orbital tumors, with the MD Anderson group reporting 68% of their pediatric tumors being malignant (3).

Presentation

The volume of the orbit is roughly 30 mL, and therefore, mass occupying lesions have scant room for expansion before signs and symptoms arise. Proptosis is the cardinal clinical sign of an orbital space-occupying lesion. Direction and laterality of the proptosis are important factors that aid

TABLE 130.2 COMMON METASTATIC ORBITAL LESIONS

- Breast (adenocarcinoma): 29%–59%
- Lung (bronchogenic carcinoma): 8%–15%
- Prostate: 3%–10%
- Cutaneous melanoma: 5%–8%
- Renal cell carcinoma: 5%–7%
- Carcinoid tumors: 4%–5%
- Gastrointestinal: 2%–5%
- Sarcomas: 1%–2%
- Thyroid carcinoma: <1%

in the identification of the location, origin, and ultimate diagnosis of the lesion. Axial proptosis often occurs with lesions that exist within the intraconal space, while nonaxial proptosis tends to occur in tumors occupying an extraconal location. The timing of the proptosis also can help differentiate various processes, with acute proptosis developing over hours to days favoring inflammatory and infectious processes. Malignant tumors tend to present in a subacute time frame, while benign tumors tend to have a more indolent progression of symptoms. Age of onset can also help narrow the differential in consideration.

Diplopia and ocular motility disturbances are also common findings in patients with orbital tumors. Lesions may cause displacement of the globe with resultant diplopia. Similarly, infiltrative processes may affect the extraocular muscles and associated nerves, causing gaze restriction and diplopia. Deterioration of a patient's visual acuity, including the rate and extent, is also of importance when distinguishing between various etiologies. For example, optic nerve gliomas or meningiomas may cause significant visual acuity changes, while secondary processes affecting the nerve often cause mild symptoms related to compressive effects. Orbital pain is most often a symptom of inflammatory and/or infectious processes. However, aggressive malignant tumors and metastatic lesions can also present in this manner. Slower growing lesions more often cause a sensation of pressure rather than pain. Pupillary changes can be found when tumors invade or compress the sympathetic or parasympathetic fibers supplying the iris dilator and pupillary sphincter. Finally, while not part of the practicing otolaryngologist's clinical exam, fundus changes within the globe are common ophthalmologic exam findings and may include optic atrophy or edema, optociliary shunt vessels, retinal venous dilation, and choroidal folds (5).

Anatomy of the Orbit

Detailed knowledge of the anatomy of the orbit and peri-orbital structures is critical in developing effective surgical technique and minimizing surgical complications while operating in the tight orbital space. The following is a brief overview of orbital and eyelid anatomy.

The bony orbit (Fig. 130.1) is composed of the frontal, zygomatic, sphenoid, maxilla, lacrimal, palatine, and ethmoid bones. The adult orbit has a volume of approximately 30 mL and measures 35 mm in maximal height, 40 mm in width, and 45 mm in medial wall length. The orbital walls lie adjacent to all four paranasal sinuses: the orbital apex is located just anterolateral to the sphenoid sinus, the medial lamina papyracea borders the ethmoid sinuses, the orbital floor is adjacent to the maxillary sinus, and the roof of the orbit often forms the floor of the frontal sinus. The orbit is also intimately associated with the skull base, as the orbital roof borders the anterior cranial fossa and the orbital apex borders the middle cranial fossa. The orbit communicates with the middle cranial fossa via the superior orbital fissure and optic canal. It is contiguous with the pterygopalatine and infratemporal fossae via the inferior orbital fissure (6).

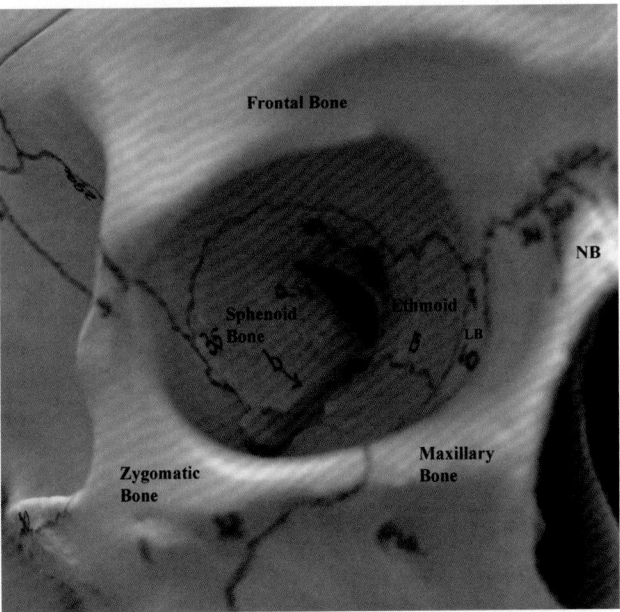

Figure 130.1 Orbital anatomy. Seven bones articulate to form the orbital vault. Six are listed; the palatine bone is not shown. LB is the lacrimal bone, and NB is the nasal bone (which is listed but does not form the orbit). The *arrow* in the apex of the orbit is pointing to the Optic Canal and "a" is the Superior Orbital Fissure and "b" is the Inferior Orbital Fissure.

The majority of the nerves of the orbit pass through the sphenoid bone. The superior orbital fissure lies between the greater and lesser wings of the sphenoid bone, with the optic canal located in the lesser wing. The annulus of Zinn, a tendinous ring at the orbital apex from which the rectus muscles arise, encircles the optic canal and separates the superior orbital fissure into two compartments at the origin of the lateral rectus muscle. The superolateral portion transmits the lacrimal, frontal and trochlear nerves, as well as the superior ophthalmic vein and occasionally the orbital branch of the middle meningeal artery. The medial portion outside of the optic canal transmits the upper and lower divisions of the oculomotor nerve (CN III), the naso-ciliary branch of CN V, and the abducens nerve (CN VI).

The intraorbital optic nerve is approximately 30 mm in length and passes through the optic canal along with the ophthalmic artery and sympathetic nerve fibers. The dura mater surrounding the nerve is continuous with the peri-osteum of the optic canal. The extraocular muscles are responsible for the movement of the eye and eyelid. All four rectus muscles (superior, medial, inferior, and lateral recti) originate posteriorly in the annulus of Zinn. The superior oblique muscle arises outside of the annulus, just supero-medial to the optic canal, and courses anteriorly to the carti-laginous trochlea prior to inserting on the globe. The levator muscle originates superior to the annulus on the lesser sphenoid wing. The inferior oblique arises in the anterior orbital floor just inferolateral to the lacrimal sac fossa and travels posterolaterally to insert onto the globe (7).

Orbital fat lies posterior to the orbital septum as intra-conal and extraconal fat. The fat pads of the eyelids are anterior extensions of the extraconal fat and lie anterior to the levator aponeurosis in the upper lid and capsulopal-pebral fascia in the lower lid. In the upper lid, there is a medial and central fat pad; the lacrimal gland lies laterally and may be mistaken for a third fat pad. In the lower lid, there is a medial, central, and lateral fat pad.

The arterial supply of the orbit arises primarily from the internal carotid artery, which gives rise to the ophthalmic artery. The ophthalmic artery lies inferolateral to the optic nerve in the optic canal, and in the majority of patients, it passes over the nerve to reach the medial orbit. As it courses anteriorly through the orbit, it gives off several branches including those to the optic nerve and retina (central reti-nal artery, posterior ciliary arteries), extraocular muscles, and lacrimal gland. Anteriorly it forms anastomoses with the external carotid arterial system to provide a rich blood supply to the eyelids and face. Venous blood is drained pri-marily by the superior ophthalmic vein, which originates in the superomedial orbit and travels posterolaterally to enter the cavernous sinus via the superior orbital fissure.

The eyelids provide a barrier for the globe against desic-cation and trauma and thus play an important role in the preservation of vision. Eyelid skin is the thinnest skin of the body and lacks subcutaneous fat. Beneath the skin lies the orbicularis oculi muscle, which is responsible for voluntary and involuntary closure of the eyelids. The orbital septum separates the eyelid anatomy from the deeper orbital contents and originates from the periosteum along the orbital rim. The orbital fat pads mentioned earlier are located posterior to the orbital septum and anterior to the upper and lower lid retractors. The main retractor of the upper lid is the levator palpebrae, which becomes the levator aponeurosis after it passes through Whitnall suspensory ligament. The capsulopebral fascia and Lockwood ligament are the analogous retractor and suspensory ligament of the lower lid. The conjunctiva is a mucous membrane that constitutes the posterior-most layer of the eyelids. The canthal tendons, which help maintain the horizontal stability of the eyelids, are fibrous bands that originate from the bony orbital walls and fuse with the upper and lower tarsal plates; the medial canthal tendon arises from the anterior and posterior lacrimal crests medially and the lateral canthal tendon originates at the lateral orbital tubercle (8).

VASCULAR TUMORS

Vascular tumors are among the most common orbital lesions in children and adults, and the majority are benign. In a recent large, 30-year series of 1,264 patients referred to an ocular oncology service for suspected orbital neoplasm, vascular tumors were the most common type of orbital lesion encountered, with an overall incidence of 17%. Of the vascular tumors, cavernous hemangioma, lymphangioma, and capillary hemangioma were the most common (2).

Capillary Hemangioma

Capillary hemangiomas are benign hamartomatous proliferations of endothelial cells. They represent 3% of all orbital lesions and are the most common orbital vascular tumors in infants (2). Lesions appear shortly after birth and rapidly enlarge for the first 6 to 12 months of life. Spontaneous involution often occurs, with 75% of lesions resolving over the following 4 years (7).

Periocular lesions occur most frequently in the superomedial quadrant of the orbit and medial upper lid, and are commonly associated with hemangiomas in other regions of the body. Periocular hemangiomas may be superficial or deep. Superficial lesions involve the skin, producing a reddish discoloration and dimpled texture known classically as the "strawberry nevus." Deeper lesions produce a bluish discoloration and may not involve the overlying skin. They are largely extraconal in location, and may even extend intracranially through the optic canal or superior orbital fissure (9).

These lesions may cause significant morbidity due to interference with visual, orbital, and facial development. Eyelid lesions may cause strabismus, anisometropia, ptosis, and subsequent amblyopia (decreased vision due to incomplete development of the visual system). Orbital lesions may lead to proptosis, globe displacement, strabismus, amblyopia, optic atrophy, and bony deformities of the orbit and face.

Diagnosis is usually made based on clinical features and orbital imaging. Since capillary hemangiomas are nonencapsulated, computed tomography (CT) shows a lobulated and diffusely infiltrating mass. Enhancement with contrast is seen on both CT and magnetic resonance imaging (MRI). MRI may demonstrate fine intralesional vascular channels separated by thin septa, as well as high blood flow from fine feeder vessels (9). Expansion of the bony walls due to mass effect can occur. Biopsy may be required in atypical cases in which malignancy is suspected. Histologically, lesions are composed of endothelial sheets that develop into capillary-caliber vascular channels.

Treatment is indicated for lesions affecting visual or orbital development. Options include topical, oral, or intralesional corticosteroid therapy. Surgical debulking can be performed for anteriorly located and well-circumscribed lesions, although complete surgical removal is generally not possible. Other treatment modalities such as interferon therapy, radiation, and pulsed-dye laser carry serious side effects and are thus reserved for life-threatening or refractory cases (7). Most recently, nonselective beta-blockers have demonstrated rapid and dramatic success in decreasing the size and symptoms of cutaneous and orbital lesions (10,11).

Cavernous Hemangioma

Cavernous hemangioma is the most common benign tumor of the orbit in adults, representing 6% of all orbital lesions (2). It occurs most frequently in middle-aged women. These lesions tend to enlarge slowly and do not involute. Patients typically present with slowly progressive, painless proptosis, although abrupt proptosis during puberty or pregnancy can occur. The lesions are often discovered incidentally on neuroimaging for symptoms such as headache. Cavernous hemangiomas tend to be isolated lesions and are often located in the lateral retrobulbar intraconal space. They may cause vision loss if located at the orbital apex, which may occur in up to 10% of cases (9).

Diagnosis can usually be made by characteristic features on orbital imaging (Fig. 130.2). CT shows a well-encapsulated, round to ovoid, hyperattenuating mass. Microcalcifications and bony remodeling may occasionally be seen (9). MRI demonstrates small intralesional vascular channels with low arterial blood flow (Fig. 130.2). Histologically, these lesions consist of large, blood-filled vascular channels lined with flattened endothelium and separated by fibrous septa containing smooth muscle. Surgical excision of the tumor and its pseudocapsule is performed if vision is threatened or proptosis results in unacceptable cosmesis. Recurrences are rare even with incomplete resection.

Lymphangioma

Lymphangiomas are benign vascular malformations that account for 4% of all orbital lesions (2). Lesions may involve the conjunctiva, eyelids, and orbit. Their origin

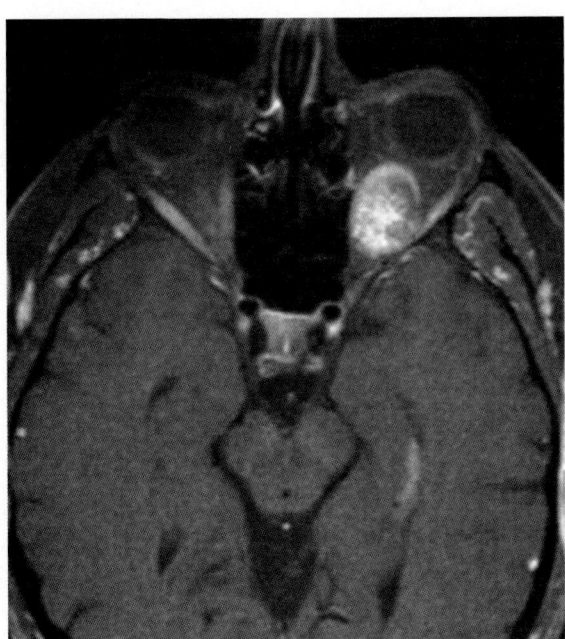

Figure 130.2 Orbital cavernous hemangioma. T1 with contrast axial MRI showing a well-circumscribed enhancing orbital lesion.

remains unclear, but they are thought to arise from embryonal elements capable of differentiating into both venous and lymphatic tissue. Histologically, these lesions are composed of endothelial-lined vascular spaces filled with lymphatic or proteinaceous fluid and a fibrotic interstitium containing follicles of lymphoid tissue.

Patients typically become symptomatic in the first decade of life. Lesions of the orbit and eyelid may present as a soft mass with bluish discoloration. Sudden proptosis may occur due to intralesional hemorrhage from fragile interstitial capillaries. This may result in significant globe displacement, strabismus, cosmetic deformity, or vision loss secondary to amblyopia, compressive optic neuropathy, or corneal exposure. These hemorrhages may occur spontaneously or after minor trauma. Hemorrhage can also occur during an upper respiratory tract infection, presumably due to the activity of lymphoid tissue in the lesions. "Chocolate cysts" refer to the subsequent collection of loculated blood breakdown products after hemorrhage (9).

MRI is the preferred imaging modality, and demonstrates characteristic findings of multiloculated cystic lesions. The presence of fluid–fluid levels due to intralesional hemorrhages is virtually pathognomonic. The lesions are isolated from the systemic circulation and thus do not enhance with IV contrast. This feature aids in distinguishing lymphangiomas from other vascular malformations such as orbital varices and arteriovenous malformations, which are distinct clinical entities requiring different management (12).

Management of lymphangiomas is challenging given their poorly circumscribed and highly infiltrative nature. As it is common for the blood-filled cysts to spontaneous

resorb, observation is recommended unless vision is threatened by optic nerve compression or exposure keratopathy. When surgical intervention is required, the cysts may be decompressed with needle aspiration or via an open surgical approach. Surgical excision may be performed on more circumscribed lesions; however, complete surgical resection is usually not possible. Recurrent hemorrhages are common, and multiple partial excisions may be required. In cases of highly infiltrative lesions with a high likelihood of a difficult and incomplete surgical excision, orbital decompression to address proptosis and globe displacement may instead be performed (7).

Multiple adjuncts to surgical resection are available and include bipolar cautery and laser ablation with carbon dioxide and Nd:YAG. These techniques may provide intraoperative hemostasis and induce shrinkage of unresectable portions of the lesion. Intralesional injections of sclerosing agents and steroids have also been utilized. Recent reports have documented benefits of intralesional fibrin glue injection, which helps delineate the walls of the lesion for more complete surgical resection and may inhibit recurrences of intralesional hemorrhages (13).

HEMATOPOIETIC TUMORS

Lymphoid Tumors

Lymphoproliferative lesions are relatively common, with an overall incidence of 20% of all orbital lesions (7). They encompass a continuum of entities of varying morphology and clinical grade, from benign reactive hyperplasia to malignant lymphoma. Non-Hodgkin lymphoma accounts for up to 90% of these lesions and is the most common orbital neoplasm in the older age group. The most common subtype is mucosa-associated lymphoid tissue (MALT) lymphoma. Other common low-grade lesions include follicular center lymphoma and small B-lymphocytic lymphoma. The most common high-grade type is diffuse large B-cell lymphoma (14).

Lymphoproliferative lesions often present as gradual painless proptosis or a slowly enlarging mass or swelling, occurring over several months. Pain and inflammation are usually minimal. Lesions may involve the orbit, lacrimal sac, eyelids, or conjunctiva. A lesion beneath the conjunctiva often gives rise to the classic salmon patch appearance on slit lamp examination. Within the orbit, the lacrimal gland, extraocular muscles, or orbital space may be involved. Whether benign or malignant, these lesions tend to mold around existing orbital structures rather than invade them. As a result, lesions may reach a large size without causing vision loss or diplopia. Imaging features on CT include indistinct margins and moderate IV contrast enhancement. Bony erosion is typically absent except in aggressive lesions. MRI shows a poorly circumscribed lesion with moderate hyperattenuation on T1- and T2-weighted images and moderate enhancement with gadolinium (15).

Once a lymphoproliferative lesion is suspected based on clinical history and imaging, an open biopsy should be performed to establish the diagnosis. Fresh tissue is analyzed with immunohistochemical, molecular genetics, and flow cytometry studies to identify monoclonal (i.e., malignant) proliferations. All patients with hypercellular lymphoproliferative lesions (including benign reactive hyperplasia) should be referred to an oncologist for evaluation of possible systemic dissemination. Evaluation may include complete blood count (CBC); bone marrow biopsy; CT scans of the chest, abdomen, and pelvis; and regular periodic follow-ups. Approximately 20% to 30% of patients with periocular lymphomas will have disseminated disease at diagnosis, and an additional 30% will develop it over 5 years. Bilateral periocular involvement confers a greater risk of systemic spread, as do certain locations; the risk is lowest with conjunctival lesions, greater with orbital lesions, and highest with eyelid lesions (7).

Low-dose radiation therapy is the treatment of choice for primary orbital lymphomas and achieves local control in most cases, with a 5-year survival rate of 90% to 100%. Surgical cure is usually not possible given the infiltrative nature of the lesions. For secondary orbital lymphomas, systemic treatment with chemotherapy is used alone or in combination with orbital radiotherapy. Recent studies have suggested an interesting link between chronic *Chlamydia psittaci* infection and orbital MALT lymphomas, based on the theory that these lesions are antigen-driven. A similar link has been previously noted in gastric MALT lymphomas and *Helicobacter pylori* infection. Treatment of orbital MALT lymphomas with doxycycline has shown to induce partial to complete response. However, other studies of orbital lymphomas have failed to detect chronic chlamydia infection, and thus suggest a possible geographic distribution of this association (15).

Leukemia

Leukemia is the most common malignancy of childhood. Leukemic infiltrates may involve the orbit, and are more common with myelogenous leukemias than lymphocytic ones. Granulocytic sarcoma (chloroma, myeloid sarcoma) is a primary tissue mass form of acute myeloid leukemia. The tumor mass is composed of granulocytic precursor cells with varying degrees of differentiation. These lesions may occur prior to the development of systemic leukemia in up to 88% of cases, with systemic involvement usually occurring within 1 year (16).

These lesions typically occur in children during the first decade of life, with a mean age of 7 years. The most common presenting clinical sign is proptosis from a rapidly enlarging mass. Eyelid swelling and ecchymosis may also occur. Lesions may involve the orbital soft tissue, lacrimal gland, and subperiosteum of the orbital bones, with a predilection for the lateral and medial walls (17).

CT scan shows a large irregular mass with possibly bony erosion. As these features may not distinguish these lesions from other pediatric orbital malignancies in cases presenting prior to systemic leukemic involvement, biopsy is often required. A greenish appearance of these lesions on biopsy has been reported in up to 70% of cases (hence the term chloroma) and is due to the exposure of myeloperoxidase to ultraviolet light (16). Touch preparations may be performed on the tissue to stain for cytoplasmic esterase (Leder stain) and myeloperoxidase. Treatment consists of local radiotherapy and systemic chemotherapy.

Langerhans Cell Histiocytosis (Histiocytosis X)

Langerhans cell histiocytosis (LCH), formerly known as Histiocytosis X, is the accumulation of proliferating monocytes and dendritic histiocytes (epidermal macrophages). The exact histogenesis is unclear, but it is thought to result from mononuclear phagocyte dysregulation. LCH encompasses a spectrum of diseases. Eosinophilic granuloma is the most common and benign entity and is characterized by unilateral, usually solitary, osseous lesions. The intermediate clinical form is called Hand-Schüller-Christian disease and classically presents as the triad of diabetes insipidus, proptosis, and multifocal lytic bone lesions. Letterer-Siwe disease is the disseminated, most aggressive form of the disease.

LCH is a rare disease, with an estimated annual incidence ranging from only 0.5 to 5.4 cases per million persons per year. The disease occurs in children and teens, with a peak incidence between 5 and 10 years of age. There is a male predilection, with male-to-female ratio of 2:1. Orbital involvement occurs in up to 20% of cases, most frequently presenting as a lytic defect of the superolateral orbit (frontal, zygomatic, or greater sphenoid bones), and causing relapsing episodes of superolateral inflammation with eyelid swelling and erythema that may initially mimic infectious orbital cellulitis. Proptosis may also occur from the enlarging bony lesion.

CT scan shows a punched-out, osteolytic bone lesion with sharp borders. Treatment of isolated orbital bone lesions consists of surgical excision, which may be curative. Intralesional steroid injection or low-dose radiotherapy may be used as adjuncts to surgery. Spontaneous remission has also been reported after biopsy. Patients with disseminated disease receive aggressive chemotherapy treatment. Prognosis depends on the degree of involvement, with unifocal disease carrying an excellent prognosis, and disseminated disease carrying a 50% mortality rate (7).

NEURAL TUMORS

Optic Nerve Gliomas

Optic nerve gliomas (juvenile pilocytic astrocytoma) are cytologically benign tumors that occur most often in childhood, with peak age of onset between 2 and 6 years. Up to 50% are associated with neurofibromatosis, and may be bilateral in this setting. Patients typically present with slowly progressive, painless, axial proptosis and profound vision loss. Eye exam findings include an afferent pupillary defect, optic atrophy, optic nerve edema, and strabismus.

Although these tumors are generally self-limited or progress slowly, some show aggressive growth. They may extend along the length of the optic nerve but typically do not invade the adjacent dura. Intracranial extension may lead to hypothalamic and pituitary dysfunction. Cystic degeneration can lead to sudden tumor enlargement and subsequent vision loss, but does not represent true tumor growth. Spontaneous improvement has also been observed but is rare (7). Characteristic orbital imaging findings are usually sufficient to establish diagnosis. Fusiform enlargement of the optic nerve is seen, with kinking or tortuosity commonly seen. Calcifications are rare. Contrast enhancement is variable on CT, and moderate to marked on MRI (18).

Treatment includes observation, resection, and radiation therapy. Close observation is indicated when the tumor remains isolated to the orbit and vision is intact. Surgical excision with free margins is indicated in cases of aggressive growth in order to prevent chiasm, contralateral optic nerve, or life-threatening intracranial extension. Radiation or chemotherapy can be used to retard growth of lesions already affecting the chiasm. Given its adverse effects on childhood development, chemotherapy is preferred over radiation.

Orbital Meningiomas

Orbital meningiomas represent up to 4% of all orbital lesions. They are the fifth most common orbital tumor (2). Meningiomas are derived from meningothelial cells of the arachnoid villi. Primary optic nerve sheath meningiomas are much less common than secondary orbital meningiomas, which arise intracranially and extend to the orbit through the optic canal, superior orbital fissure, or bone (17).

Primary optic nerve sheath meningiomas (Fig. 130.3) occur most frequently in women in the third to fourth decade of life. Slowly progressive vision loss occurs over years. Gaze-evoked transient visual obscurations, axial proptosis, and ocular motility restriction are possible. An afferent pupillary defect and visual field disturbance can be detected on exam. Ophthalmoscopic examination typically demonstrates optic nerve edema or atrophy. Optociliary shunt vessels are visible on fundus exam in up to a third of patients; these collaterals permit retinal venous outflow through the choroidal circulation and thus bypass central retinal vein obstruction secondary to tumor compression. Lesions occurring in childhood are often associated with neurofibromatosis.

Secondary meningiomas occur in a slightly older population, typically in the fifth decade of life, and also with a female preponderance. Lesions involving the greater sphenoid wing and lateral orbital wall cause proptosis, temporal fossa swelling, and lower eyelid swelling. Tumors involving the lesser sphenoid wing may lead to early vision loss and visual field defects due to optic nerve involvement (19).

Diagnosis can often be established on the basis of characteristic imaging features. Primary optic nerve meningiomas show diffuse tubular enlargement with marked contrast enhancement on both MRI and CT. Globular enlargement occurs less frequently and is the result of tumor invasion of the adjacent dura. CT demonstrates focal calcifications in 20% to 50%. Contrast-enhanced axial CT often reveals a linear central hypointense optic nerve surrounded medially and laterally by a hyperintense nerve sheath—a well-known finding termed "tram-tracking." Bony remodeling can be seen with expansive, long-standing lesions. Secondary orbital meningiomas produce bony hyperostosis. The presence of a dural tail on contrasted MRI helps distinguish meningioma from fibrous dysplasia (18). Most meningiomas are histologically benign, with aggressive forms occurring most commonly in younger patients.

Surgery is indicated for secondary meningiomas when compression of surrounding structures causes significant visual, cosmetic, or intracranial morbidity. Treatment of primary optic nerve sheath meningiomas is dictated by the degree of vision loss and the presence of intracranial extension, which occurs in up to 15% of patients. If vision loss is only moderate, patients are often observed because of the tumor's slow growth. If vision loss is progressive, vision function can be improved with radiation therapy. Surgical excision is performed when intracranial extension threatens the optic chiasm or contralateral optic nerve, or when the tumor has caused marked vision loss and significant proptosis (7).

Schwannoma (Neurilemoma)

Schwannomas are uncommon benign tumors of the peripheral nerve sheath. They arise due to proliferation of the myelin-producing Schwann cells and rarely undergo malignant transformation. They occur most commonly in adults between 20 and 60 years of age and are most often found in the superior or intraconal orbit. They can cause slowly progressive proptosis, and location at the orbital apex may cause progressive vision loss. Histopathologically, these lesions are well-encapsulated and are divided into Antoni A type (solid tissue with spindle cells arranged in whorls or palisades) or Antoni B type (loose myxoid tissue containing stellate cells). CT scan shows a dense, well-circumscribed, ovoid, or fusiform mass that enhances with contrast. Long-standing lesions may demonstrate bony remodeling, lower density areas of mucinous cystic degeneration, and calcification. Treatment consists of complete surgical excision of the tumor and capsule (17–19).

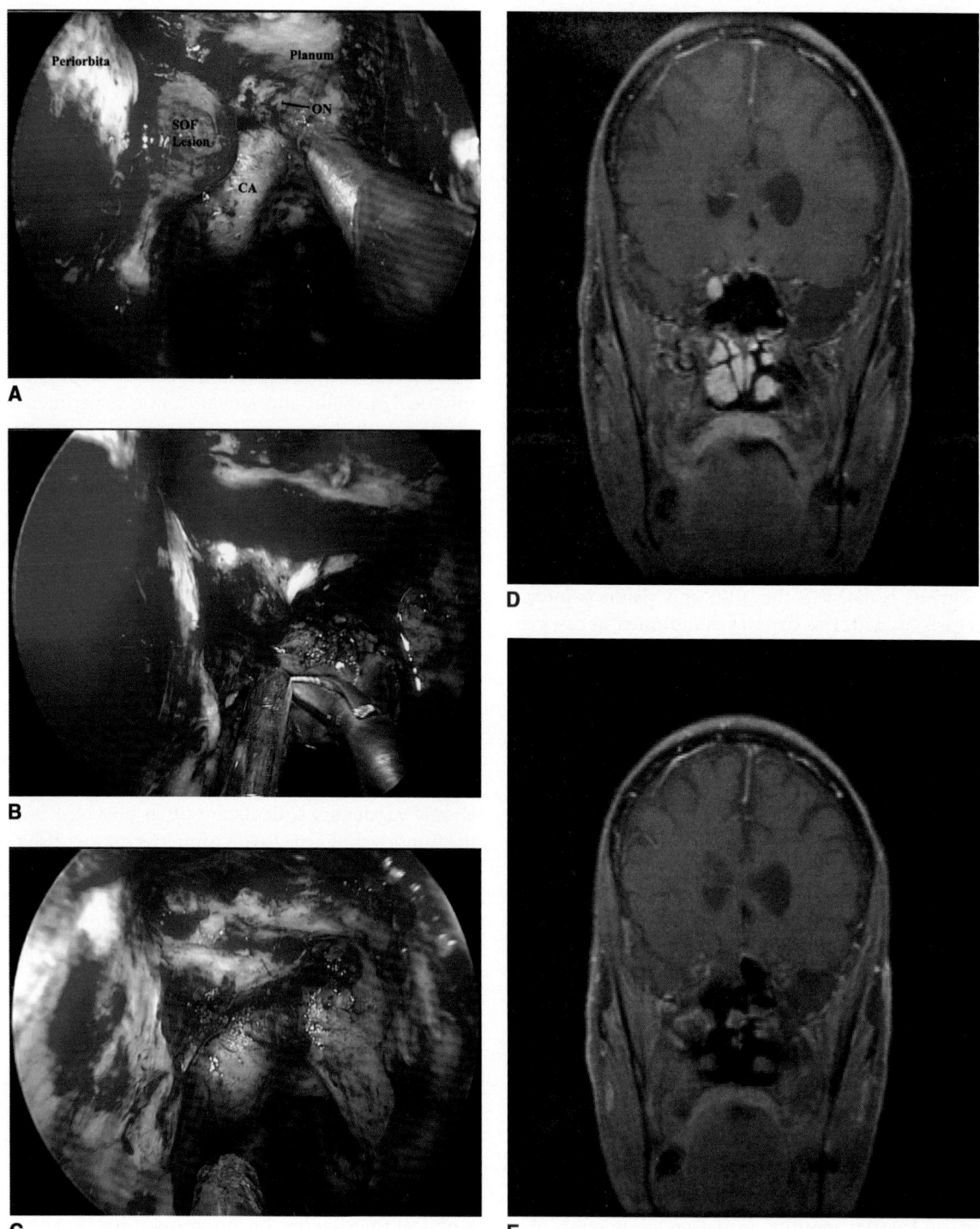

Figure 130.3 Optic canal meningioma. **A:** Tumor exposure via an endonasal endoscopic approach. **B:** Sharp dissection of the meningioma away from the optic nerve. **C:** Postresection endoscopic view with complete tumor excision. **D:** Preoperative coronal T1 MRI with contrast. **E:** Postoperative coronal T1 MRI with contrast with complete tumor removal.

INFLAMMATORY TUMORS

Idiopathic Orbital Inflammation

Idiopathic orbital inflammation (IOI), also known as orbital pseudotumor, is a nongranulomatous inflammatory disorder with a heterogeneous clinical presentation. It can occur in children and adults, and accounts for up to 11% of all orbital lesions (2). Almost any orbital structure may be involved, including one or more extraocular muscles (orbital myositis), the sclera and posterior tenons (sclerotenonitis), or the optic nerve sheath (inflammatory optic neuritis). Patients may also present with a more diffuse process involving the orbital fat, multiple orbital structures, or with extension into the sinuses or intracranial cavity.

As the anatomic site of involvement dictates the signs and symptoms, the clinical presentation of IOI is varied. Patients commonly experience deep, boring periocular pain. Ocular motility restriction, diplopia, proptosis, conjunctival inflammation, and eyelid erythema and edema may also occur. Myositis may cause pain on eye movement. Decreased vision may be seen when the optic nerve, sclera, or posterior tenons are involved. Children often present with systemic signs such as fever, emesis, abdominal pain, and lethargy. Bilateral disease is seen in up to 30% of children with IOI. In contrast, bilateral involvement in an adult signals an underlying systemic vasculitis (7).

Diagnosis is usually clinical, and often confirmed with orbital imaging. CT shows an ill-defined, heterogeneous infiltrate that enhances with contrast during the acute phase. Laboratory findings include an increase in erythrocyte sedimentation rate, peripheral blood eosinophils, and cerebrospinal fluid (CSF) pleocytosis.

First-line treatment consists of oral corticosteroids (1 mg/kg/day). A rapid and dramatic response is typically observed within a few days, and steroids are tapered slowly over several weeks to prevent rebound inflammation. Biopsy may be required in patients with atypical symptoms, imaging features, treatment failure, or recurrence off steroids. This is especially true for lacrimal gland lesions, as an aggressive malignancy may also present with inflammation. Biopsy-confirmed refractory cases may respond to low-dose radiation therapy or immunosuppressants. A sclerosing variant has been found to be less responsive to systemic steroids and radiation, and may respond to intraorbital steroid injection (20).

Orbital Vasculitis

Orbital vasculitis is an inflammatory disorder that is associated with multiple systemic vasculitides. Giant cell arteritis, polyarteritis nodosum, Wegener granulomatosis, and connective tissue disorders such as systemic lupus erythematosus, dermatomyositis, and rheumatoid arthritis may involve orbital vessels. The pathogenesis involves a type III hypersensitivity reaction to circulating immune complexes with deposition of inflammatory cells in the vessel walls and subsequent orbital ischemia. Patients may present with painful proptosis and symptoms of systemic vasculitis. In patients with no known history or symptoms of systemic disease, the presentation may be confused with IOI. For this reason, failure of corticosteroid treatment in cases of presumed IOI should prompt biopsy (7).

Thyroid-Associated Orbitopathy

Although not considered an orbital lesion, thyroid-associated orbitopathy (TAO) is a common cause of orbital inflammation and is the most common cause of unilateral and bilateral proptosis in adults. The thyroid status of patients presenting with TAO varies: 90% are hyperthyroid, 6% are euthyroid, 3% have Hashimoto thyroiditis, and 1% are hypothyroid. Smoking exacerbates the disease, with severity being dose-dependent on the number of cigarettes smoked per day. The pathogenesis of TAO involves circulating autoantibodies to thyroid-stimulating hormone receptor (TSH-R) and insulin-like growth factor receptor (IGF-1R), which cross-react with orbital fibroblasts and stimulate them to differentiate into adipocytes and produce glycosaminoglycans, with resulting increase in orbital soft tissue volume.

The most common presenting sign is eyelid retraction, often with lateral temporal flare of the palpebral fissures. Proptosis, lagophthalmos, conjunctival chemosis and hyperemia over the rectus muscle insertions, extraocular muscle restriction, and optic neuropathy may also be observed. CT scan demonstrates the classic finding of fusiform extraocular muscle enlargement, which, unlike orbital myositis, spares the tendinous muscle insertions. Treatment of the active phase of TAO is aimed at establishing a euthyroid state, which can be accomplished with radioactive iodine ablation, antithyroid medications, or total thyroidectomy. A transient worsening of TAO may be noted after radioactive iodine ablation and total thyroidectomy, likely due to the release of TSH-R antigens. Vision-threatening optic nerve compression or exposure keratopathy may be temporized with corticosteroids and/or orbital radiation therapy. Total thyroidectomy may provide further control if not already performed. Definitive treatment most often requires orbital decompression. Recent studies have shown beneficial effects of immunomodulatory agents in treating vision-threatening TAO (21).

CYSTS

Cystic lesions of the orbit are uncommon, representing only 6% of all orbital lesions (2). The majority of these lesions are dermoid cysts and epithelial inclusion cysts. Histologically, dermoid cysts and epithelial inclusion cysts are lined by epithelium and contain a central lumen filled with the secretory products of this lining. They are thought to arise from epithelial and subepithelial tissue that becomes entrapped within bony sutures during embryogenesis or becomes implanted in the orbit as the result of surgical or nonsurgical trauma.

Dermoid Cysts

Dermoid cysts are lined by keratinized stratified squamous epithelium and contain dermal appendages, such as hair shafts, sebaceous glands, and even sweat glands, in their walls. Their central lumens are filled with a mixture of keratin, oil, and occasionally hair shafts. Approximately 5% of dermoid cysts arise from conjunctival epithelium (nonkeratinized stratified squamous epithelium with goblet cells).

They are often found in the anterior superolateral orbit at the frontozygomatic suture, but can be found superomedially at the frontoethmoidal suture, or at any other bony suture. Patients often present in the first decade of life with a slowly progressive, painless, subcutaneous mass. It is typically firm to palpation, and may be freely mobile or fixed to bone. Deep orbital dermoid cysts typically present later in adulthood with proptosis and globe displacement. Dermoid cysts may also present as orbital inflammation, which is caused by an intense granulomatous reaction incited by cyst leakage. In younger patients, it is important to distinguish medial dermoid cysts from encephaloceles, mucoceles, or dacryoceles (22).

CT scan shows a round to ovoid, well-defined cystic structure with a thin wall that may contain calcifications. A dumbbell configuration may be seen with cysts that extend through the suture into the temporalis fossa, sinuses, or cranial vault. Bony remodeling or erosion may occur in long-standing cases. Fat-fluid levels may be seen on CT or MRI. Contrast may cause mild enhancement of the rim but not the lumen (18).

Treatment consists of complete surgical excision in symptomatic patients. It is important to avoid intraoperative cyst rupture. If rupture does occur, copious irrigation should be performed to avoid marked inflammatory reaction. For lesions that traverse a bony suture, complete excision may be difficult. Recurrence can occur after incomplete excision.

Epithelial Inclusion Cysts

Epithelial inclusion cysts differ from dermoid cysts in that they do not contain dermal appendages in their walls and are filled with keratin and epithelial debris. They may arise from cutaneous, conjunctival, respiratory, or apocrine gland epithelium. They may occur at any age, and are found most commonly on the eyebrow and eyelid. Orbital lesions are less common, and may represent posterior extension or a primary lesion. Unlike dermoids, epithelial inclusion cysts typically do not demonstrate fat content

or rim calcifications on CT. The clinical presentation and management of these lesions is similar to that of dermoid cysts (22).

MESENCHYMAL TUMORS

Rhabdomyosarcoma

Rhabdomyosarcoma (RMS) is the most common primary malignancy of the orbit in the pediatric population. Four types have been described, including embryonal, alveolar, pleomorphic, and botryoid types. Embryonal is the most common subtype, alveolar is the most malignant subtype, and the pleomorphic subtype carries the best prognosis. Nearly half of the primary sites of occurrence for RMS lie within the head and neck, and orbital RMS accounts for roughly one-third of these (23). Orbital RMS does not arise from the extraocular muscles, but rather from the primitive undifferentiated mesenchymal cells within the orbit, particularly within the superomedial quadrant. Metastasis does occur via hematogenous spread, mainly to the lung and bones.

The disease is nonhereditary and presents at a median age of 8, with 90% of cases being diagnosed in patients prior to the age of 13 (23). Rarely, it may occur in older adults. Males are predominantly affected with a 5:3 male-to-female ratio. Patients usually present progressive proptosis over days to weeks, with one in three children presenting with ptosis and a palpable mass. There is often marked eyelid edema and discoloration. Downward globe displacement may be observed, reflecting the predilection of this tumor for the superomedial quadrant. However, the tumor may occur in any quadrant. The alveolar subtype tends to occur more frequently in the inferior orbit.

On CT imaging, the tumor typically shows moderately well-defined to ill-defined margins and an irregular shape with moderate contrast enhancement. In roughly 40% of cases, bony destruction is also seen. It appears isointense to muscle on T1- and hyperintense to muscle on T2-weighted MRI images (23). Definitive diagnosis is usually obtained via open biopsy or CT-guided fine needle aspiration (FNA) for deeper lesions. Evaluation for systemic spread should be performed, including bone marrow biopsy, chest radiographs, CBC, liver function tests, and lumbar puncture. Once a diagnosis is confirmed by biopsy, treatment consists of primary chemoradiation therapy. With the advent and widespread use of these treatment modalities, survival rates have been found to be over 90% in most series (24,25).

Fibrous Dysplasia

Fibrous dysplasia was found to account for roughly 1% of all orbital tumors in a recent series (2). Fibrous dysplasia is a rare, nonhereditary disease of the bone that is thought to be due to hamartomatous malformations of immature bone and osteoid that replaces the normal bone with fibrous tissue. The disease may be restricted to only one site of the skeleton (monostotic) or may affect multiple skeletal areas (polyostotic). It is thought that roughly one in five cases of fibrous dysplasia involve the craniofacial bones. Most of the lesions found in the orbit are monostotic, with the orbital roof being the most common site of involvement (26). However, craniofacial involvement may accompany orbital disease in patients with McCune-Albright syndrome, which consists of a triad of polyostotic fibrous dysplasia, sexual precocity, and skin pigmentation occurring more frequently in women. Malignant transformation of this condition is quite rare but when it does occur, it is usually associated with prior irradiation (26).

While the disease has traditionally been considered a disease of childhood, it has also been found to occur well into adulthood. Lesions are usually noticed within the first two decades of life, but can remain asymptomatic and undiagnosed for extended periods of time. The clinical presentation depends upon the orbital bones involved, with most patients presenting with facial asymmetry, orbital dystopia, and proptosis. Epiphora may result from involvement of the nasolacrimal duct. Progressive narrowing of the foramina of the orbital apex can cause multiple motor and sensory cranial neuropathies, as well as vision loss from optic nerve compression in up to 50% of patients (18).

On CT imaging, the affected bone appears hyperostotic and thickened, with multiple areas of lytic spaces intermixed with "ground-glass"-like sclerotic areas (Fig. 130.4). CT imaging characteristics may resemble those of sphenoid wing meningiomas, and the lack of dural enhancement of these lesions on MRI can often be useful in further distinguishing the two. Fibrous dysplasia lesions often show an area of low-to-intermediate signal intensity and moderate to marked enhancement of contrast on MRI. Surgical treatment involves local resection or curettage and is indicated in patients with pain, marked deformity, or malignant transformation.

Solitary Fibrous Tumor

Solitary fibrous tumor (SFT) is a relatively new pathologic entity/classification. In a recent large series of 41 fibroblastic tumors with overlapping morphologic features originally diagnosed as hemangiopericytomas, fibrous histiocytomas, mixed tumors, or giant cell angiofibromas, reclassification using modern-day pathologic evaluation techniques showed that all cases were rediagnosed as SFTs (27). It is an uncommon spindle cell tumor that rarely occurs in the orbit. Previous to this recent series and likely due to previous designations, there had been only 53 cases reported worldwide since it was first described in the orbit in 1994 (28). The mean age of onset is 40 years, and patients present with proptosis and diplopia. A palpable mass with or without pain has also been observed.

SFTs are hypervascular lesions with CT scan findings of a well-circumscribed mass with moderate contrast enhancement and possible calcification and bony remodeling. On MRI, these lesions appear as an intermediate intensity mass on T1-weighted images with moderate contrast enhancement. Histologically, SFTs consist of densely arranged spindle-shaped cells in a storiform pattern with numerous

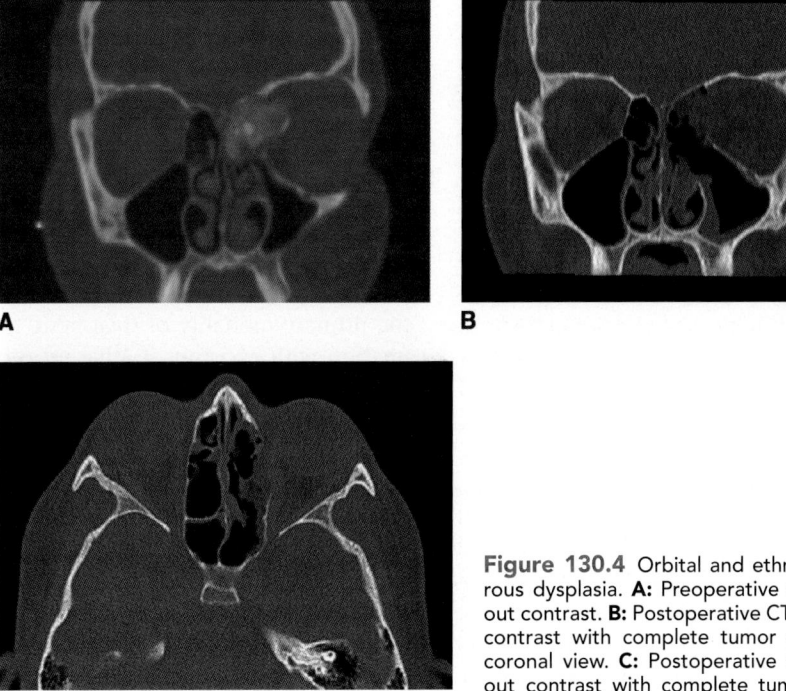

Figure 130.4 Orbital and ethmoid fibrous dysplasia. **A:** Preoperative CT without contrast. **B:** Postoperative CT without contrast with complete tumor excision, coronal view. **C:** Postoperative CT without contrast with complete tumor excision, axial view.

vascular channels (28). They share histologic similarities to fibrous histiocytoma and hemangiopericytoma lesions. However, immunohistochemical studies can differentiate between them and can be utilized to confirm the diagnosis, as SFTs stain positively for CD34. Treatment includes en bloc tumor resection, although residual tumor has been found to remain stable for some time.

Osteoma

Primary bone tumors of the orbit constitute roughly 1% of all orbital tumors and in most series, a third to a half of these lesions are benign osteomas (2,26). These lesions are often secondary orbital tumors as well, originating in the adjacent frontal, sphenoid, and/or ethmoid paranasal sinuses. The roof of the orbit is most commonly affected in primary osteomas of the orbit. These lesions are most commonly unilateral and present in adulthood. CT scan or plain films show a sessile or pedunculated smooth, rounded mass with density similar to normal cortical bone. Patients presenting with multiple lesions must be considered for Gardner syndrome, a hereditary disease associated with multiple osteomas, other soft tissue tumors, and colon polyps with nearly 100% malignant transformation. Symptoms vary depending on the location and size of the osteoma. These lesions can often be followed conservatively, while symptomatic lesions are usually resected with recurrence being rare.

Sarcomas

Malignant mesenchymal lesions such as osteosarcoma, fibrosarcoma, chondrosarcoma, and liposarcoma are exceedingly rare in the orbit, but have been reported and are known to occur in the orbit as primary malignancies. Children with a history of retinoblastoma have been shown to be at higher risk for sarcomas of the orbit even if they have not undergone treatment with radiation (7). All of these sarcomatous lesions have a very poor prognosis due to their highly malignant nature.

LACRIMAL TUMORS

Mass lesions that affect the lacrimal gland most often produce signs of proptosis and inferomedial displacement of the globe. Most lacrimal gland masses are due to idiopathic orbital inflammatory disease and are accompanied by other signs and symptoms associated with these processes. These often include lateral upper eyelid swelling, erythema, and warmth. One such diagnosis is acute dacryoadenitis, caused by either viral or bacterial infection of the lacrimal gland. Offending agents can include herpesvirus, mumps, mononucleosis, staphylococcal and/or streptococcal microorganisms. Shields et al. (2) found in their series of 1,264 patients that lacrimal gland lesions represented 9% of all space-occupying orbital lesions, with roughly 20% of these being lesions of epithelial origin. It has been said that another 20% to 30% of lacrimal gland lesions are caused by lymphoproliferative disorders with the remaining 50% to 60% of lesions being caused by inflammatory and/or infectious causes. Lymphoid lesions of the lacrimal gland include atypical and benign reactive lymphoid hyperplasia, leukemias, and malignant lymphomas.

Of the epithelial lesions, roughly 50% to 60% have been shown to be benign in nature, the vast majority of which are pleomorphic adenomas (benign mixed tumors). These usually present with slowly progressive painless proptosis with inferomedial globe displacement over a period of months to years. Upper eyelid edema may also be a presenting finding. Radiographic findings usually reveal a round well-circumscribed mass at the superolateral orbit with enlargement of the lacrimal fossa, but no bony destruction. While complete surgical excision with an intact capsule is always the goal, recent data have shown that recurrence rates remain low even when there is violation of the tumor capsule and/or when complete excision is carried out after previous incomplete excision (29).

The remaining 40% to 50% of epithelial lesions are malignant carcinomas. Of this subgroup, adenoid cystic carcinoma (ACC), carcinoma ex-pleomorphic, adenocarcinoma, and mucoepidermoid carcinoma are the most common in descending order. In ACC, the most common presenting signs are globe ptosis, dystopia, and proptosis (29). Rapidly developing pain and/or hypoesthesia are ominous signs of an aggressively behaving tumor. A basiloid histopathologic pattern has a much poorer survival when compared to nonbasaloid patterns (29). Recently, improvement in prognosis has been shown in patients with ACC that are treated with intra-arterial cytoreductive chemotherapy as an adjunct to conventional treatment of surgery and adjuvant radiation therapy, although this has not yet become standard of care (29). Other common malignant epithelial lesions include carcinoma ex-pleomorphic (aka malignant mixed cell carcinomas), adenocarcinomas, and mucoepidermoid carcinomas. All of these lesions tend to present with progressive proptosis, pain, and/or numbness in the periorbital region, and imaging findings suggest bony destruction and expansion of the lacrimal fossa. Mortality for most of these carcinomas is greater than 50%. Biopsy is indicated to establish a definitive diagnosis and if feasible, complete surgical excision of the lesion should be the primary modality of treatment, often including exenteration with excision of adjacent orbital bone and periorbital soft tissues. Adjuvant radiation therapy is nearly universally recommended as well.

SECONDARY LESIONS

With the orbit's anatomic proximity and shared borders, it is of no surprise that the majority of secondary orbital tumors arise from paranasal sinus, eyelid and periorbital skin, and intracranial primary processes. However, primary processes of the globe and conjunctiva can cause secondary orbital tumors as well. Secondary tumors accounted for roughly 44% of all tumors in Henderson Mayo Clinic series

(Henderson), while more recent large series have shown slightly lower rates of 11% to 26% (2,3). In the Mayo series, the most common secondary lesions affecting the orbit were: mucoceles, SCCs, meningiomas, BCCs, and vascular malformations (1). More recent data have shown that malignant melanomas of the skin, conjunctiva, and uvea/choroid have increased in prevalence, accounting for 45% of all secondary tumors (2). It should be noted that mucoceles were not included in this series. Regardless, primary skin lesions such as BCC, SCC, and melanoma of the eyelid and periorbital skin are an increasingly common secondary orbital lesion encountered by the modern-day physician.

Paranasal mucoceles, mainly of the frontoethmoid and sphenoid sinuses, continue to be prominent lesions secondarily involving the orbit. Similarly, the relatively rare invasive processes of the paranasal sinuses, including SCC, inverting papilloma, adenocarcinoma, ACC, mucosal melanoma, sinonasal undifferentiated carcinoma, and esthesioneuroblastoma, all have the high anatomic potential to encroach upon and invade the orbital space. Intracranial processes, most commonly meningiomas of the sphenoid ridge, also account for a substantial portion of secondary tumors of the orbit. Regardless of origin, the primary process requires treatment, often in conjunction with addressing the orbital involvement, often with a multidisciplinary team approach.

METASTATIC TUMORS

Orbital metastasis represents approximately 7% of all orbital tumors, and is therefore an important entity to consider in the differential diagnosis. Metastasis to the orbit is reported to occur in approximately 2% to 4.7% of patients with systemic cancer (30,31). Orbital metastasis may be the presenting sign of malignancy in up to 25% of patients.

The vast majority of orbital metastases are carcinomas. Breast carcinoma is the most common, accounting for 50% of metastatic orbital lesions, followed by prostate and lung carcinomas (2,30–32). Other less common metastases include gastrointestinal carcinoma, renal cell carcinoma, thyroid carcinoma, and malignant melanoma. Orbital metastasis is predominantly a condition of adulthood, with greater than 90% of cases occurring in patients aged 40 years or older. Bilateral disease is unusual, with more than 90% of cases occurring unilaterally.

The onset of symptoms is usually rapid and progressive, occurring over weeks to months. The most common presenting signs and symptoms include pain, proptosis, diplopia, decreased vision, ptosis, inflammation, and ocular motility restriction. The extraocular muscles are a common site of metastasis due to their rich blood supply. The bone marrow space of the sphenoid bone is also commonly involved given its high volume of low-flow blood, and lytic destruction of this part of the lateral orbital wall is highly suggestive of metastatic disease (7). Paradoxical enophthalmos has been well documented in metastatic scirrhous breast carcinomas due to the fibrosis and secondary contracture of orbital contents.

The most common metastatic tumor of childhood is neuroblastoma. Neuroblastoma metastasizes to the orbit in 15% of cases, presenting with the abrupt onset of unilateral or bilateral proptosis and ischemia-induced lid ecchymosis. The mean age of onset of neuroblastoma is 2 years, and metastasis often occurs late in the disease when the primary tumor can be detected in the abdomen, mediastinum, or neck (24).

Orbital imaging with CT and MRI may offer important clues to diagnosis. Metastatic lesions typically enhance on contrasted MRI. CT findings suggestive of breast carcinoma include a diffuse, infiltrative orbital mass extending along the extraocular muscles with possible bony destruction. Gastrointestinal and thyroid carcinomas may have both bony and soft tissue involvement. Prostatic carcinoma is known to metastasize to bone and produce hyperdense osteoblastic bone lesions, although osteolytic lesions may also be seen. Neuroblastoma frequently causes bony destruction of the lateral orbital wall and sphenoid marrow. Definitive diagnosis is made with tissue diagnosis by fine-needle aspiration biopsy or orbitotomy.

In general, orbital metastasis is associated with a poor prognosis (31). The goal of treatment is palliative and consists mainly of local radiation therapy. When orbital metastasis is the initial presentation of breast cancer, the orbital biopsy specimen should be analyzed for estrogen receptor expression in order to determine whether hormonal therapy would be beneficial (7,30).

SURGICAL APPROACHES

The approach that one chooses needs to be dictated by the anatomic location of the lesion, and to a lesser extent, the pathology of the lesion. An understanding of the anatomy of the orbit and the ability to correlate this with radiographic findings is also extremely important when striving to preserve form and function of the eye.

The choice of surgical approach to access orbital lesions depends on the location of the lesion, the extent of exposure required, and the goal of the surgery (biopsy, surgical debulking, or complete excision). A variety of transcutaneous and transconjunctival incisions can be used to provide transseptal, transperiosteal, or sub-Tenon's access to the extraconal and intraconal orbital space.

An anterior orbitotomy approach is used for lesions located anterior to the posterior aspect of the globe. Transcutaneous or transconjunctival incisions can be utilized to access lesions in the superior, lateral, inferior, or medial space around the eye. In the superior anterior orbit, an upper lid crease incision can be extended transseptally or subperiosteally, and provides better cosmesis than a subbrow incision. Inferiorly, a subciliary blepharoplasty incision, lower lid crease incision, or transconjunctival incision can be used. The transconjunctival approach has become the preferred approach for inferior orbitotomy, and is accomplished with an incision through the inferior palpebral conjunctiva and lower lid retractors. Access to the medial anterior orbit can be achieved through a transcutaneous frontoethmoidal (Lynch) incision, bulbar transconjunctival incision, or transcaruncular incision. Laterally, an upper lid crease incision may be combined with a lateral canthotomy incision.

Deeper extraconal lesions, intraconal lesion, and the optic nerve can be accessed via the incisions listed above with additional modifications to provide enhanced exposure. In the case of medial lesions, detachment of the medial rectus can provide access to the intraconal space. For better visualization of the posteromedial orbit, a medial orbitotomy can be combined with a lateral orbitotomy to allow lateral rotation of the globe. A full thickness vertical incision of the upper lid can also provide access to the superomedial intraconal space. In this lid-splitting technique, the incision is made at the junction of the medial and central lid and transects the tarsus and levator aponeurosis (33). The transcaruncular incision has gained popularity for access to posteromedial lesions given its improved cosmesis compared to a skin incision. The transcaruncular technique provides wide subperiosteal access to the medial wall posteriorly to the orbital apex. When combined with a transconjunctival inferior fornix incision, additional inferior and inferolateral exposure can be achieved (34). Deep inferior orbital lesions can be exposed using a Caldwell-Luc

incision to access the maxillary sinus. In this approach, an incision through the gingiva exposes the anterior wall of the maxillary sinus, an opening is created in the sinus, and the posteroinferior floor is removed (33).

A lateral orbitotomy approach provides access to the posterolateral intraconal and extraconal spaces and the optic nerve. Briefly, an upper eyelid crease or lateral canthotomy incision is used to mobilize the temporalis muscle and fascia and expose the lateral orbital wall. The bony lateral wall is removed with an oscillating saw in one piece to expose the underlying periorbita, which is excised. The lateral rectus can be retracted for intraconal access, and the bone sutured or plated back into position once excision is complete (35). Wide exposure to the posterior orbit and skull base can be achieved with extension of the bone removal to the posterior orbital wall or greater wing of the sphenoid bone. Superior extension of the bone removal provides greater access for larger lacrimal fossa lesions.

Lesions at the orbital apex, superior orbital fissure, or those that expand from the orbit into the cranial vault can be safely approached only by superior orbitotomy with frontal craniotomy. This approach requires a combined effort with neurosurgery. A frontotemporal or frontoorbitotemporal (Fig. 130.5) approach may also be used (36).

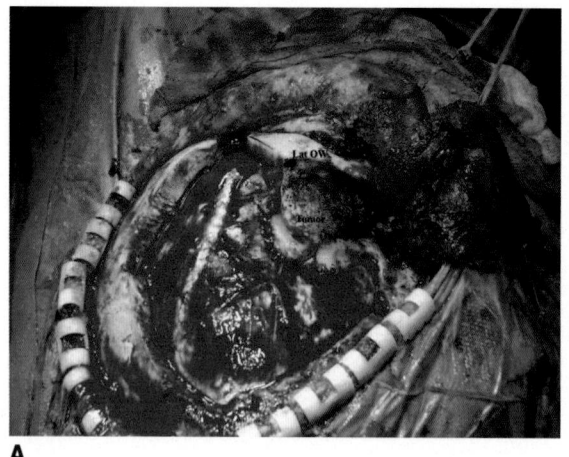

A

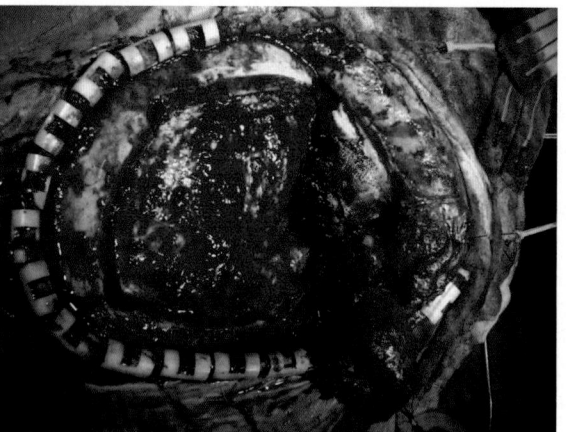

B

Figure 130.5 Frontoorbitotemporal or orbitozygomatic (OZ) craniotomy. **A:** Intraoperative view of a frontotemporal craniotomy with a view of the lateral sphenoid wing meningioma (list as Tumor). The lateral orbital wall (Lat OW) is in place. **B:** Intraoperative view of the same case with the orbitozygomatic complex removed and the Temporalis muscle retracted inferiorly. **C:** Same photograph as 5B with the Anterior Cranial Fossa, Middle Cranial Fossa and orbit color coded illustrating the extent of exposure for this approach.

C

Endoscopic skull base surgery is based upon the principle that an endonasal approach gives the operative surgeon direct access to lesions of the anterior and ventral skull base without the morbidity classically associated with approaches that traverse neurovascular boundaries. The same principle is utilized in endoscopic approaches to the orbit. The structure that needs most attention is the optic nerve, with tumors extending lateral and superior to the nerve are relatively inaccessible via the endonasal route. Conversely, lesions that are located inferomedially provide the most direct route for an endoscopic approach.

For nearly all cases, standard image guidance registration is performed, with the surgeon(s) reviewing the operative plan for that particular case. The approach first includes standard endoscopic rhinologic procedures. The uncinectomy and maxillary antrostomy are widely opened and the floor of the orbit is found. The ethmoids are traversed and the sphenoid is then opened for visualization of the carotid artery, optic nerve, planum, and sella. Dissection then proceeds anteriorly along the skull base to address the bony septations along the skull base and lamina. If orbital apex or intraconal work is required, it is best to utilize a binaural approach previously described. The ipsilateral middle turbinate, posterior septum, and the contralateral sphenoid are opened as well.

Three corridors for endoscopic endonasal intraorbital surgery for orbital tumors have previously been described (37). These include: an inferomedial approach for extraconal lesions, a transmaxillary approach for lateral extraconal lesions and a medial intraconal approach with displacement of the rectus muscles and intraconal dissection between the rectus muscles (37). The medial/inferior extraconal approach is the approach also used for endoscopic orbital and/or optic nerve decompression procedures. The medial/inferior intraconal approach utilizes a corridor between the medial and inferior rectus muscles (Fig. 130.6). This approach is best utilized after external identification, isolation, and retraction of the muscles as they insert on to the globe. This allows for a greater ease of dissection within the proposed corridor.

Transorbital neuroendoscopic surgery (TONES) is a recently described approach to lateral anterior skull base lesions, as well as to paramedian lesions that cross neurovascular structures (38). Utilization of the TONES techniques has allowed for the safe and effective repair of CSF leaks, optic nerve decompressions, repair of cranial base fractures, and removal of skull base tumors. The precaruncular (to access medial quadrant of the orbit), preseptal lower eyelid (inferior quadrant), superior eyelid crease (superior quadrant), and the lateral retrocanthal (lateral quadrant) approaches have all been described (38).

Regardless of the approach to the orbit, basic principles must be followed. First and foremost, it is critical to avoid crossing the optic nerve and ophthalmic artery. Therefore, tumors isolated to the superolateral orbit should not be approached endoscopically. Second, entry through the lamina papyracea should occur below the level of the ethmoidal foramina; therefore, limiting the risk of damage to the ethmoid arteries. Third, the extraocular muscles must be respected and handled with delicate caution. Lastly, team preoperative evaluations and planning and team surgery provides the best care for these complex lesions.

GENERAL OPERATIVE PRINCIPLES AND POSTOPERATIVE CARE

The surgeon who chooses to operate within the orbit must have a flawless knowledge of the intricate anatomy of this region. They must also utilize meticulous and deliberate technique. Respecting the delicate anatomic structures such as the vast neurovascular network within the orbit, the optic nerve and globe itself, and the extraocular muscles, is imperative. Avoiding excessive traction on these structures, while also striving for meticulous hemostasis with use of biplolar cauterization, is required. Properly utilizing dependent, and even suction, drains postoperatively is also needed. The use of the proper equipment that allows for delicate handling and dissection of tissues is needed when operating within the compact anatomy within and around the orbit. Principles such as traction/countertraction, exposure, hemostasis, and patience need to be followed at all times. Recognition of potential complications and urgent situations, both intraoperatively and postoperatively, is also important for every surgeon operating in this area. For example, realizing that extreme post-op pain, especially in association with chemosis, decreased acuity, and elevated intraocular pressures indicates a possible retroorbital hemorrhage, which can lead to permanent ischemic injury to the optic nerve. Postoperatively, head elevation and the use of ice compresses also tend to help limit the edema that is often appreciated. Also, the use of ophthalmologic-specific medications, such as bacitracin ophthalmic ointment, is also required. Similarly, if any conjunctival incisions are made, whether bulbar or palpebral, a combination steroid-antibiotic drop should be prescribed prophylactically for a week's time.

CONCLUSION

Tumors and mass lesions affecting the orbit are overall quite rare, but an awareness of the extensive array and broad scope of pathologies potentially involved is imperative for clinicians treating patients with these problems. Common presenting signs and symptoms of orbital tumors include: proptosis, diplopia, visual acuity changes, and pain/pressure. The direction of proptosis is key in helping to determine the location, and often the most likely potential pathologies, of the lesion. Imaging of the orbit plays a crucial role in the appropriate preoperative workup of patients with orbital tumors, with specific imaging characteristics often leading to a confident preliminary diagnosis prior to a true tissue diagnosis. Surgical approaches to the

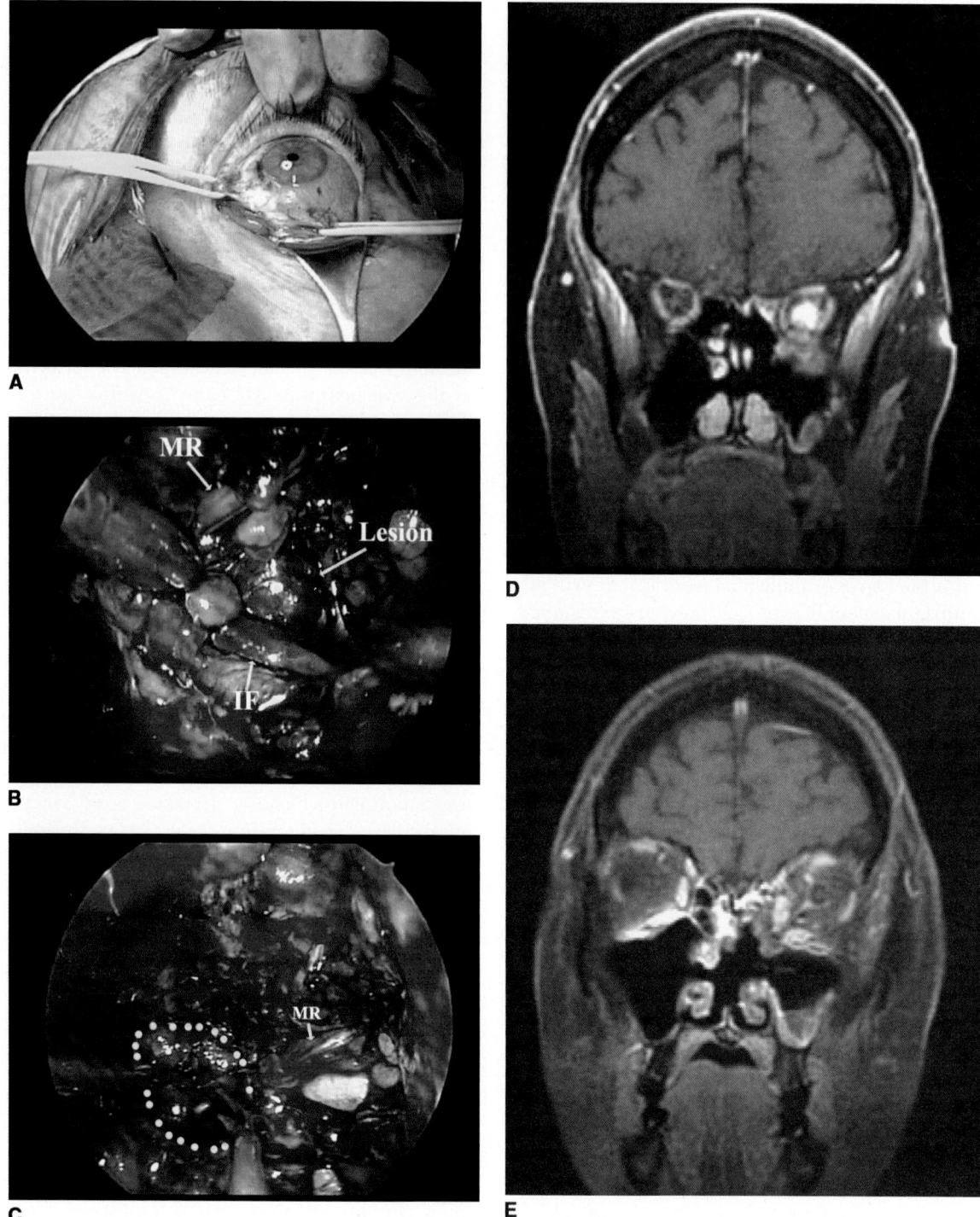

Figure 130.6 Endoscopic endonasal approach for an intraconal orbital tumor. **A:** External view of the left extraocular muscles identified and vessel looped for control. **B:** Intraconal identification and dissection of the hemangioma. MR, medial rectus, IF, inferior rectus. **C:** Lesion removed en bloc from the intraconal space. **D:** Preoperative MRI with contrast. **E:** Postoperative MRI with contrast with complete tumor excision.

orbit can be classified based on the location of the orbit that requires access. Extraorbital, transcranial, and endoscopic approaches have all been utilized in the treatment of these lesions. The choice of approach depends not only on the location of the lesion but the suspected or known pathology of the tumor, functional status of the orbit, and surgeon preference as well.

While uncommon, orbital tumors and associated diseases may present to the practicing otolaryngologist. While appropriate recognition and workup is important, if an otolaryngologist decides to treat patients with these pathologic processes, multidisciplinary teams are a tremendously important part of successful outcomes. The rarity and complexity of these cases often require Oculoplastic surgeons, Neurosurgeons, and Otolaryngologists to work together to safely and effectively treat patients. Early identification, thoughtful workup, multidisciplinary approach, meticulous technique, and appropriate postoperative care can, in some cases, prolong life and cure disease, as well as preserve or restore form and function of the orbit.

HIGHLIGHTS

- The most common benign tumors of the orbit are hemangiomas and meningiomas.
- The most common malignant tumor of the orbit is non-Hodgkin lymphoma.
- RMS is the most common primary malignancy of the orbit in the pediatric population.
- Proptosis is the initial and cardinal sign of an orbital lesion.
- Visual acuity loss is a late finding of advanced disease or a finding of a space-occupying lesion within the optic canal.
- The orbital vault is made of seven bones: frontal, zygomatic, sphenoid, maxilla, lacrimal, palatine, and ethmoid bones.
- Consideration for orbital metastases should be given for infiltrative and rapidly progressing orbital tumors. The most common primary site for metastasis in women is breast and for men is lung or prostate.
- Surgical approach needs to be dictated by the anatomic location of the lesion, the pathology of the lesion, and the primary goal for surgery (e.g., biopsy vs. resection).
- That extreme post-op pain, especially in association with chemosis, decreased acuity, and elevated intraocular pressure, indicates a possible retroorbital hemorrhage, which can lead to permanent ischemic injury to the optic nerve.
- There are several options for surgical care of orbital tumors; however, for any of these approaches team planning and surgery usually provides the best outcome.

QUESTIONS

1. A 35-year-old woman presents with a 3-month history of progressing double vision. On exam you note normal acuity but a left cranial nerve 6 palsy. What is the next step?

A. Obtain an MRI and CT	KEY
B. EMG of lateral rectus	Distracter
C. Serial clinical exam in 2 weeks	Distracter
D. Begin high dose steroids	Distracter

2. Which of these orbital bones contributes to the orbital rims?

A. Sphenoid	Distracter
B. Zygomatic	KEY
C. Palatine	Distracter
D. Lacrimal	Distracter

3. What is the main lower eyelid retractor?

A. Whitnall ligament	Distracter
B. Capsulopalpebral fascia	KEY
C. Inferior oblique muscle	Distracter
D. Orbicularis oculi	Distracter

4. A 3-year-old child presents with hypoglobus and a lesion on exam in the superior orbital rim. An FNA in clinic reveals dendritic histiocytes consistent with LCH. What is the next step in management?

A. Surgery with conservative removal	Distracter
B. Surgery with radical removal	Distracter
C. Bone survey	KEY
D. Radiation therapy	Distracter

5. Eight hours after an uneventful lateral orbitotomy for biopsy of an orbital tumor, your patient notes progressive unrelenting pain and chemosis. What must be considered as a cause for this pain?

A. Retrobulbar hematoma	KEY
B. Intraoperative traction on the inferior orbital nerve	Distracter
C. Transection of the superior orbital nerve	Distracter
D. Infection at the site of mini-plate repair	Distracter

REFERENCES

1. Henderson J. *Orbital tumors*. New York: Raven Press, 1994.
2. Shields JA, Shields CL, Scartozzi R. Survey of 1264 patients with orbital tumors and simulating lesions. *Ophthalmology* 2004;111(5): 997–1008.
3. Shinder R, Al-Zubidi N, Esmaeli B. Survey of orbital tumors at a comprehensive cancer center in the United States. *Head Neck* 2011;33(5):610–614.
4. Wilson MW, Grossniklaus HE. Orbital disease in North America. *Ophthalmol Clin N Am* 1996;9(4):539–547.
5. Darsuat TE, Lanzino G, Lopes MB, et al. An introductory overview of orbital tumors. *Neurosurg Focus* 2001;10:1–9.

6. Ellis E, Zide MF. *Surgical approaches to the facial skeleton.* Philadelphia, PA: Lippincott Williams & Wilkins, 2006.

7. Liesegang TJ, Skuta GL, Cantor LB. Orbit, eyelids, and lacrimal system. *Basic and Clinical Science Course 2007–2008.* San Francisco, CA: American Academy of Ophthalmology.

8. Dutton JJ. *Atlas of clinical and surgical orbital anatomy.* Philadelphia, PA: Saunders, 1994.

9. Smoker WRK, Gentry LR, Yee NK, et al. Vascular lesions of the orbit: more than meets the eye. *Radiographics* 2008;28:185–204.

10. Leaute-Labreze C, Dumas de la Roque E, Hubiche E, et al. Propranolol for severe hemangiomas of infancy. *N Engl J Med* 2008;358(24):2649–2651.

11. Li Y, McCahon E, Rowe NA. Successful treatment of infantile haemangiomas of the orbit with propranolol. *Clin Exp Ophthalmol* 2010;38:554–559.

12. Harris GJ. Orbital vascular malformations: a consensus statement on terminology and its clinical implications. *Am J Ophthalmol* 1999;127:453–455.

13. Boulos PR, Harrisi-Dagher M, Kavalec C, et al. Intralesional injection of Tisseel fibrin glue for resection of lymphangiomas and other thin-walled orbital cysts. *Ophthal Plast Reconstr Surg* 2005;21(3):171–176.

14. Nutting CM, Jenkins CD, Norton AJ, et al. Primary orbital lymphoma. *Hematol J* 2002;3:14–16.

15. Bernardini FP, Bazzan M. Lymphoproliferative disease of the orbit. *Curr Opin Ophthalmol* 2007;18:398–401.

16. Stockl FA, Dolmetsch AM, Saornil A, et al. Orbital granulocytic sarcoma. *Br J Ophthalmol* 1997;81:1084–1088.

17. Liesegang TJ, Skuta GL, Cantor LB. Ophthalmic pathology and intraocular tumors. *Basic and Clinical Science Course 2007–2008.* San Francisco, CA: American Academy of Ophthalmology.

18. Dutton, JJ. *Radiology of the orbit and visual pathways.* Philadelphia, PA: Saunders/Elsevier, 2010.

19. Cantore WA. Neural orbital tumors. *Curr Opin Ophthalmol* 2000;11:367–371.

20. Harris GJ. Idiopathic orbital inflammation: a pathogenetic construct and treatment strategy. *Ophthal Plast Reconstr Surg* 2006;22(2):79–86.

21. Holds JB, Buchanan AG. Thyroid eye disease. *Am Acad Ophthalmol* 2010;8(10):1–14.

22. Shields JA, Shields CL. Orbital cysts of childhood – classification, clinical features, and management. *Surv Ophthalmol* 2004;49:281–299.

23. Conneely MF, Mafee MF. Orbital rhabdomyosarcoma and simulating lesions. *Neuroimg Clin N Am* 2005;15(1):121–36.

24. Castillo BV, Kaufman L. Pediatric tumors of the eye and orbit. *Pediatr Clin N Am* 2003;50:149–172.

25. Goldberg SH, Cantore WA. Tumors of the orbit. *Curr Opin Ophthalmol* 1997;8:51–56.

26. Selva D, White VA, O'Connell JX, et al. Primary bone tumors of the orbit. *Surv Ophthalmol* 2004;49(3):328–342.

27. Furusato E, Valenzuela IA, Fanburg-Smith JC, et al. Orbital solitary fibrous tumor: encompassing terminology for hemangiopericytoma, giant cell angiofibroma, and fibrous histiocytoma of the orbit; reappraisal of 41 cases. *Hum Pathol* 2011;42:120–128.

28. Tam ES, Chen EC, Nijhawan N, et al. Solitary fibrous tumor of the orbit: a case series. *Orbit* 2008;27:426–431.

29. Bernardini FP, Devoto MH, Croxatto JO. Epithelial tumors of the lacrimal gland: an update. *Curr Opin Ophthalmol* 2008;19:409–413.

30. Ahmad SM, Esmaeli B. Metastatic tumors of the orbit and ocular adnexa. *Curr Opin Ophthalmol* 2007;18:405–413.

31. Shields JA, Shields CL, Brotman HK. Cancer metastatic to the orbit. *Ophthal Plast Reconstr Surg* 2001;17(5):346–354.

32. Char DH, Miller T, Kroll S. Orbital metastases: diagnosis and course. *Br J Ophthalmol* 1997;81:386–390.

33. Weisman RA, Kikkawa D, Moe KS, et al. Orbital tumors. *Otolaryngol Clin North Am* 2001;34(6):1157–1174, ix–x.

34. Goldberg RA, Mancini R, Demer JL. The transcaruncular approach. *Arch Facial Plast Surg* 2007;9(6):443–447.

35. Cockerham KP, Bejjani GK, Kennerdell JS, et al. Surgery for orbital tumors. Part II: transorbital approaches. *Neurosurg Focus* 2001;10(5):1–6.

36. Bejjani GK, Cockerham KP, Kennerdell JS, et al. A reappraisal of surgery for orbital tumors. Part I: extraorbital approaches. *Neurosurg Focus* 2001;10(5):1–6.

37. McKinney KA, Snyderman CH, Carrau RL, et al. Seeing the light: endoscopic endonasal intraconal orbital tumor surgery. *Otolaryngol Head Neck Surg* 2010;143(5):699–701.

38. Moe KS, Bergeron CM, Ellenbogen RG. Transorbital neuroendoscopic surgery. *Neurosurgery* 2010;67:16–28.

Cranial Base Surgery 131

Carlos D. Pinheiro-Neto *Carl H. Snyderman*
Paul A. Gardner

The cranial base is a complex anatomical region encompassing important neurovascular structures. The diversity and complexity of pathologies arising in the cranial base often require multidisciplinary evaluation and management. The collaboration between surgeons of different specialties (otolaryngology/head and neck, neurosurgery, ophthalmology, plastic and reconstructive surgery) is paramount to achieve an appropriate surgical plan. Frequently, the preoperative evaluation should include consultation with neuroradiology, radiation oncology, and medical oncology. Contributions from skilled and experienced anesthesiologists, pathologists, critical care physicians, dentists, nurses, speech pathologists, physical therapists, and other professionals are required during the intraoperative and postoperative period in order to establish good outcomes. The most effective scenario for the treatment of skull base pathologies occurs when members of these different fields are all integrated to form a skull base team.

The aim of this chapter is to provide an overview of the fundamentals of cranial base surgery. The evolution of the field in past decades is outlined. An anatomical review with clinical correlations and the evaluation and management of patients with skull base pathology are discussed. The surgical approaches for different regions of the cranial base with a discussion of complications are presented.

HISTORY

As a unique anatomical region and interface between surgical specialties, surgeries addressed to the cranial base began as sporadic procedures performed by otolaryngologists/head and neck surgeons, plastic/reconstructive surgeons, and neurosurgeons working separately. In the first decade of the 20th century, two pioneering neurosurgeons (Schloffer and Cushing) and an otorhinolaryngologist (Oskar Hirsh) were the first to reach the cranial base through the facial structures. They performed a transnasal approach to the pituitary fossa (1,2). Sixty years later, in 1967, Hardy first used the operating microscope in transsphenoidal pituitary surgery.

In 1941, Dandy (3) resected an orbital tumor using an approach through the anterior cranial fossa and ethmoid sinus. This is considered the beginning of modern craniofacial surgery (1). During the subsequent years, isolated reports were published regarding resection of cranial base lesions using intracranial and transfacial approaches. Pioneering efforts by Tessier (4) for craniofacial anomalies (e.g., orbital hypertelorism) also provided a foundation for cranial base surgery. In 1963, Ketcham et al. (5) were the first to report a series of 19 patients with sinonasal malignancies treated with anterior craniofacial resection.

In the field of lateral skull base surgery, House (6) advanced the subspecialty of neuro-otology by performing an acoustic neuroma resection via a middle fossa approach in 1961. House partnered with the neurosurgeon Doyle to form one of the first skull base teams. In the 1970s, Fisch described the resection of glomus jugulare tumors utilizing an approach through the infratemporal fossa.

The following years were characterized by the cooperation between otolaryngologists/head and neck surgeons and neurosurgeons for the development of cranial base surgery as a well-established subspecialty. A subspecialty society, the North American Skull Base Society, was established in 1989. In combination with this cooperation, advances in surgical technology especially in operative visualization, neuroimaging, powered instrumentation, anesthetic techniques, and intraoperative monitoring resulted in the incredible progress of cranial base surgery observed in the last few decades.

The introduction of endoscopes during microscopic transsphenoidal surgeries as a tool to improve visualization occurred in the late 1970s and early 1980s. In the 1990s, different groups around the world reported the use of the pure endoscopic transsphenoidal technique for pituitary surgery (7). Over the next decade, centers of excellence emerged worldwide and endoscopic endonasal techniques were further developed and applied to a wide variety of ventral skull base pathologies (8–11).

Currently, cranial base surgery encompasses a wide variety of surgical approaches and includes both external and endonasal approaches. The indications for surgery have expanded to include both benign and malignant disease and are applied to adult as well as pediatric populations.

ANATOMY

The skull base may be directly affected by a pathologic process or can be used as a pathway to approach lesions (12). Tumors and other lesions may arise intracranially or extracranially and can involve any of the intracranial fossae, nasal cavity, paranasal sinuses, orbits, pterygopalatine and infratemporal fossae, pharynx and parapharyngeal space, and craniocervical regions. Profound anatomical knowledge is the foundation for cranial base surgery and extensive dissection work in the laboratory is crucial to achieve adequate anatomical proficiency and three-dimensional mastery of the relations between the structures. The modern skull base surgeon must master both intracranial, extracranial, and endonasal surgical anatomy.

The cranial base is divided into three regions (anterior, middle, and posterior) with different anatomical relationships and distinct surgical approaches. There is an extensive connection between the intracranial and the extracranial surfaces of the cranial base through a number of foramina and canals (Table 131.1). Important neurovascular structures travel along those pathways and are a route for intracranial and extracranial spread of tumors.

Anterior Cranial Base

The intracranial surface of the anterior cranial base is formed by three different bones: frontal, ethmoid, and sphenoid (12). The frontal bones compose the majority of the anterior cranial base contributing to its lateral part. The orbital process of the frontal bone articulates posteriorly with the lesser wing of the sphenoid bone. Those two bones constitute the roof of the orbit and the optic canal, which transmits the optic nerve and the ophthalmic artery. Posterolaterally, the optic canals are bounded by the anterior clinoid processes, which are connected to the sphenoid sinus by the optic struts running under the optic nerves. The frontal sinus is located anteriorly between the external and the internal walls of the frontal bone. The internal cortical surface (posterior table of the frontal sinus) corresponds to the anterior limit of the anterior cranial base. The anterior cranial base faces the frontal lobes with the *gyri recti* medially and the orbital *gyri* laterally. In the midline, the superior sagittal sinus continues to the floor of the anterior cranial base where it connects with a small emissary vein at the foramen cecum. The fronto-orbital artery is a branch of the anterior cerebral artery that travels along the inferior and medial surface of the frontal lobe. Because of its proximity with the anterior cranial base, procedures in this region present an increased risk of injury of the

TABLE 131.1	FORAMINA OF THE BASE OF THE SKULL
Foramen	**Structures Transmitted**
Cribriform plate	Olfactory nerve (CN I)
Foramen cecum	Occasional small vein; origin of sagittal sinus
Optic canal	Optic nerve (CN II); ophthalmic artery
Superior orbital fissure	Cranial nerves III, IV, ophthalmic division of trigeminal nerve (CN V1); superior ophthalmic vein
Inferior orbital fissure	Maxillary division of trigeminal nerve (CN V2); zygomatic branch of trigeminal nerve; filaments from pterygopalatine branch of the maxillary nerve; infraorbital vessels; anastomosis between inferior ophthalmic vein and pterygoid venous plexus
Foramen rotundum	Maxillary division of trigeminal nerve (CN V2)
Foramen ovale	Mandibular division of trigeminal nerve (CN V3)
Foramen spinosum	Middle meningeal artery
Sulcus tubae auditivae	Lodges cartilaginous part of auditory (eustachian) tube
Foramen lacerum	Closed inferiorly by a fibrocartilaginous plate that contains the auditory tube; upper part traversed by the ICA
Carotid canal	Internal carotid artery
Stylomastoid foramen	Facial nerve (CN VII); stylomastoid artery
Jugular foramen	Beginning of the internal jugular vein; cranial nerves IX, X, XI
Internal acoustic meatus	Facial nerve (CN VII); vestibuloacoustic nerve (CN VIII)
Hypoglossal canal	Hypoglossal nerve (CN XII)
Foramen magnum	Spinal cord (medulla oblongata); spinal accessory nerves (CN XI); vertebral arteries; anterior and posterior spinal arteries; occipitoaxial ligament

CN, cranial nerve.

fronto-orbital branch. The olfactory bulbs are situated over the cribriform plates, and the olfactory tracts course posterolaterally over the surface of the brain as they cross over the optic nerves.

The midline of the anterior cranial base is related to the nasal cavity, ethmoid cells, and sphenoid sinus. The ethmoid bone forms the anterior two-thirds of the midline anterior cranial base. The regions of the ethmoid bone related to the intracranial surface from medial to lateral are the *crista galli*, cribriform plate, and *fovea ethmoidalis*. The crista galli separates the anterior half of the cribriform plates in the midline and is attached to the *falx cerebri*. Anterior to the crista galli, the foramen cecum transmits an emissary vein responsible for the venous drainage from the nasal cavity to the superior sagittal sinus. Besides the potential risk of intracranial dissemination of nasal infections, congenital lesions such as nasal dermoids, gliomas, and meningoceles can communicate intracranially through the foramen (13). The thin lateral lamella of the cribriform plate continues laterally as the *fovea ethmoidalis* or roof of the ethmoid sinus. The depth of the lateral lamella is an important risk factor for iatrogenic cerebrospinal fluid (CSF) leak during transethmoidal procedures. The olfactory filaments pass through the cribriform plate from the nasal cavity to the intracranial olfactory bulbs and are a route for intracranial spread of sinonasal malignancy. The posterior third of the midline anterior cranial base is formed by the *planum sphenoidale*, which corresponds to the roof of the sphenoid sinus.

At the junction of the ethmoid sinus and orbit, the anterior and posterior ethmoidal foramina along the fronto-ethmoidal suture line transmit the anterior and posterior ethmoidal arteries, respectively. The anterior ethmoid artery is located between the second and third ethmoid septations in a coronal plane that is tangential to the posterior surface of the globe. The posterior ethmoid artery is roughly at the junction of the fovea ethmoidalis and planum sphenoidale. These arteries diverge as they cross the roof of the ethmoid and often need to be identified and ligated/coagulated during procedures in the anterior cranial base.

Sphenoid Sinus

The surface anatomy of the sphenoid sinus is important for endonasal approaches to the pituitary and surrounding areas (Fig. 131.1). The degree of sphenoid pneumatization and patterns of septations vary greatly. When there are multiple septations, lateral septations always deviate toward the internal carotid artery (ICA) and care must be exercised when removing the septations. The sella is bounded by the clival recess inferiorly, cavernous sinus and ICA laterally, and optic canal superolaterally. The clival recess is bounded by the paraclival ICA and petrous apex laterally. The sixth cranial nerve courses superolaterally behind the paraclival ICA and is at risk of injury when drilling posterior to the paraclival ICA just below the sellar floor.

Middle Cranial Base

The intracranial surface of the middle cranial base is formed by the sphenoid and temporal bones. The limit between the anterior and the middle cranial bases is the sphenoid ridge joined medially by the chiasmatic sulcus. The limit between the middle and the posterior cranial bases is the petrous ridge joined medially by the *dorsum sellae* and the posterior clinoid process (12).

The intracranial surface of the middle cranial base can be divided in two regions: medial and lateral. The medial

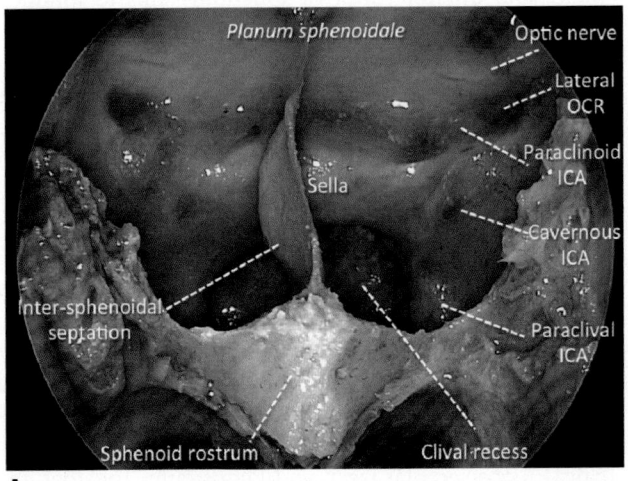

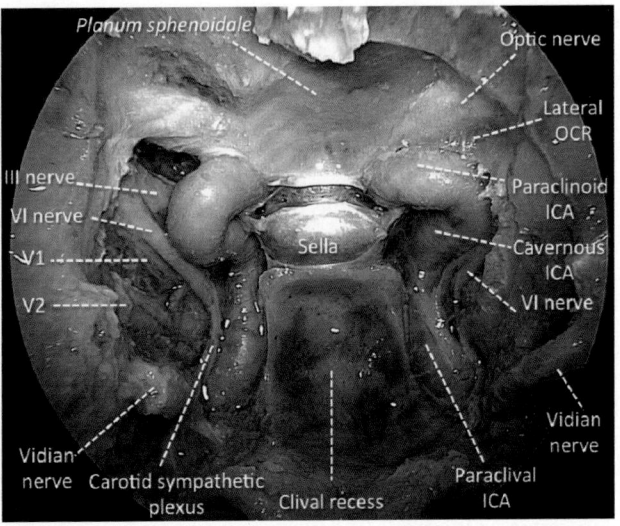

A   **B**

Figure 131.1 Endoscopic view with a 0-degree endoscope during a dissection. **A:** Surface anatomy of the sphenoid sinus after removal of the anterior wall. **B:** Surrounding structures after bony removal.

part of the middle cranial base is composed by the body of the sphenoid bone. The greater wing of the sphenoid bone and the temporal bone (squamosal and petrosal segments) form the lateral portion of the middle cranial base, containing the middle cranial fossa.

The temporal bone has a pyramidal shape, the sides of which form the middle fossa floor (superior face), the anterior limit of the posterior fossa (posterior face), muscle attachments of neck and infratemporal fossa (anteroinferior face), and the muscular–cutaneous–covered side of the head (lateral), which forms the base of the pyramid. The temporal bone consists of four embryologically distinct components: the squamous, mastoid, petrous, and tympanic part.

The greater and lesser petrosal nerves course across the upper surface of the petrous bone. The carotid canal extends upward and medially and provides passage to the ICA. Medially, Meckel's cave forms an impression on the upper surface of the petrous bone. The roof of the carotid canal opens below the trigeminal ganglion near the distal end of the carotid canal. The arcuate eminence approximates the position of the superior semicircular canal. A thin lamina of bone, the tegmen tympani, covers the middle ear and ossicles on the anterolateral side of the arcuate eminence. The internal auditory canal can be identified below the floor of the middle fossa by drilling along a line approximately 60 degrees medial to the arcuate eminence, near the middle portion of the angle between the greater petrosal nerve and arcuate eminence (12).

The area below the middle cranial fossa includes the infratemporal fossa, parapharyngeal space, infrapetrosal space, and pterygopalatine fossa. The boundaries of the infratemporal fossa are the medial pterygoid muscle and the pterygoid process medially, the mandible laterally, the posterior wall of the maxillary sinus anteriorly, the greater wing of the sphenoid superiorly, and the medial pterygoid muscle joining the mandible and the pterygoid fascia posteriorly. The fossa opens into the neck below. The infratemporal fossa contains the branches of mandibular nerve, the maxillary artery, and the pterygoid muscles and venous plexus. The mandibular nerve exits the cranial base through the foramen ovale. The pterygoid venous plexus connects through the middle fossa foramina and inferior orbital fissure with the cavernous sinus and empties into the retromandibular and facial veins (12). From a lateral infratemporal approach, a plane is formed by the lateral pterygoid plate, foramen ovale (third division of the trigeminal nerve), foramen spinosum (middle meningeal artery), and the spine of the sphenoid. On a deeper level, the eustachian tube overlays the petrous carotid canal. These are useful landmarks for locating the petrous ICA.

The pterygopalatine fossa is located between the maxillary sinus in the front, the pterygoid process behind, the palatine bone medially, and the body of the sphenoid bone above. The fossa opens laterally through the pterygomaxillary fissure into the infratemporal fossa and medially through the sphenopalatine foramen to the nasal cavity. Both the foramen rotundum for the maxillary nerve and the pterygoid canal for the vidian nerve open through the posterior wall of the fossa. The fossa contains branches of the maxillary nerve, vidian nerve, the pterygopalatine ganglion, and the pterygopalatine segment of the maxillary artery.

The parapharyngeal space is predominantly a fat-filled space, but also contains the eustachian tube, pharyngeal branches of the ascending pharyngeal and facial arteries, and branches from the glossopharyngeal nerve.

Endonasally, the medial aspect of the middle fossa (Meckel's cave) is anterior to the paraclival ICA and superior to the petrous segment of the ICA. The second division of the trigeminal nerve (foramen rotundum) and the vidian nerve (pterygoid canal) are helpful landmarks. Meckel's cave is bounded by the lateral cavernous sinus superiorly containing the third, fourth, ophthalmic branch of fifth, and sixth cranial nerves. Foramen ovale is just posterior to the pterygoid base.

Posterior Cranial Fossa and Craniocervical Junction

The posterior cranial fossa may be approached posterior, inferior, and medial to the temporal bone. The sigmoid sinus defines the posterior margin of the petrous temporal bone. The infrapetrosal space contains the jugular bulb and lower end of the inferior petrosal sinus; the branches of the ascending pharyngeal artery; the glossopharyngeal, vagus, and accessory nerves; and the opening of the carotid canal through which the carotid artery passes. Below the torcula and transverse sinuses, the occipital bone protects the posterior fossa and cerebellum down to the foramen magnum. From an endonasal view, another portion of the occipital bone, the clivus, protects the brainstem and can be divided into three segments: superior (posterior clinoid to floor of sella), middle (floor of sella to floor of sphenoid sinus), and inferior (floor of sphenoid sinus to foramen magnum). Intracranially, the superior clivus is associated with the third cranial nerve, the middle clivus is associated with the sixth cranial nerve, and the inferior clivus is associated with the lower cranial nerves. Inferolaterally, the hypoglossal foramen is bounded superiorly by the jugular tubercle and the occipital condyle inferiorly. Finally, the occipital condyle is a "ball and socket" joint that articulates with the atlas of the cervical spine.

Scalp

It is important to understand the layers of the scalp in order to preserve function and plan reconstruction with pedicled scalp flaps. The scalp has five layers designated by the acronym SCALP: Skin, subcutaneous tissues, Aponeurosis (galea), Loose areolar layer, and Periosteum. Together, the loose areolar layer and periosteum comprise the pericranial flap whereas the galeopericranial flap includes the galeal layer. The pericranial flap is supplied by the supratrochlear and supraorbital vessels, which exit from foramina or notch along the superior orbital rim. Laterally, the galea is continuous with the superficial temporal fascia. A temporoparietal flap, derived from this fascia, receives its blood supply from the superficial temporal artery. The temporalis muscle, another important reconstructive flap, is covered by the deep temporal fascia. The deep temporal arteries, terminal branches of the internal maxillary artery, supply the muscle on its deep surface.

Vascular

In many respects, surgical approaches to the skull base are determined by the vascular anatomy. The ICA has five segments: parapharyngeal, petrous, paraclival, cavernous, and supraclinoid. The ophthalmic artery branches off of the ICA just after it exits the cavernous sinus and dural rings and runs inferolateral to the optic nerve inside the optic canal. The vertebral arteries usually enter the posterior fossa through the dura between the lateral lamina of C1 (after exiting the transverse foramen) and lateral foramen magnum. The circle of Willis comprises the ICAs, anterior cerebral arteries, anterior communicating artery, posterior cerebral arteries, and posterior communicating artery. A patent circle of Willis is predictive of collateral cerebral blood flow (CBF), but anatomical variations are common.

CLINICAL DIFFERENTIAL DIAGNOSIS

Cranial base surgery is characterized by a great diversity of pathology and includes benign and malignant neoplasms, traumatic injuries, congenital lesions, inflammatory and infectious disease, and vascular pathology (Table 131.2). The differential diagnosis varies according to age group, with a preponderance of congenital lesions and benign pituitary pathology in the pediatric population. The differential diagnosis will also depend on the anatomic subsite

and can often be predicted bases on presentation, location, and radiologic appearance.

Tumors arising in the cranial base can cause an enormous variety of symptoms. Profound knowledge of skull base anatomy and cranial nerve physiology is imperative for a correct clinical topographic diagnosis. An adequate clinical examination can indicate the location and estimate extension of the tumor. However, skull base tumors can present with nonspecific symptoms such as headache, weight loss, vomiting, weakness, and loss of appetite. Anterior cranial base tumors can present with pituitary dysfunction, hyposmia/anosmia, proptosis, epiphora, nasal obstruction, epistaxis, facial deformities, personality change, diplopia, visual loss, facial numbness, or sinusitis. Middle cranial base lesions can cause trigeminal neuralgia or numbness, facial palsy, ptosis, diplopia, trismus, or eustachian tube dysfunction. When the tumor involves the temporal bone, hearing loss, tinnitus, and dizziness can occur. Symptoms associated with tumors from the posterior cranial base include tinnitus, hearing loss, balance problems, swallowing difficulties, hoarseness, speech problems, dysarthria, and shoulder weakness.

Physical examination should include a complete assessment of cranial nerve function. Nasal endoscopy should be performed on all patients with nasal/sinus or orbital symptoms but may provide valuable information for lesions in any region of the skull base. In patients with decreased olfactory function, olfaction can be objectively measured with a scratch-and-sniff test (Sensonics UPSIT test). Visual symptoms should be evaluated further by an ophthalmologist and may include visual field testing in addition to a routine funduscopic examination. Symptoms of hearing loss or vestibular dysfunction can be evaluated further with audiometric testing and vestibular tests if necessary. Lower cranial nerve dysfunction may require assessment of swallowing function and aspiration

TABLE 131.2	TOPOGRAPHIC DIFFERENTIAL DIAGNOSIS OF CRANIAL BASE PATHOLOGY	
Anterior Cranial Base/Nasal Cavity/ Maxillary Sinus/Orbit	**Middle Cranial Base/Sphenoid/Sella/ Infratemporal Fossa**	**Posterior Cranial Base**
Meningoencephalocele	Meningoencephalocele	Meningioma
Nasal dermoid	Meningioma	Chordoma
Glioma	Pituitary adenoma	Vestibular schwannoma
Mucocele	Craniopharyngioma	Epidermoid cyst
Juvenile angiofibroma	Cholesterol granuloma	Glomus jugulare
Inverted papilloma	Trigeminal schwannoma	Osteomyelitis
Meningioma	Meckel's cave adenoid cystic carcinoma	
Fibrous dysplasia	Nasopharyngeal carcinoma	
Fibro-osseous tumors		
Squamous cell carcinoma		
Esthesioneuroblastoma		
Adenocarcinoma		

TABLE 131.3	BALLOON OCCLUSION TEST OF INTERNAL CAROTID ARTERY			
Cerebral Blood Flow Test	Risk of Early Stroke	Risk of Delayed Stroke	Management Options	
Clinical neurologic deficit	High	—	ECA–ICA, high flow bypass; preservation of ICA; nonoperative therapy; subtotal resection	
Reduction of CBF (15–35 mL/110 g/min)	Low	Moderate	STA–MCA or high flow bypass; preservation of ICA; nonoperative therapy; subtotal resection	
No reduction of CBF (>35 mL/100 g/min)	Low	Low	No reconstruction (malignant tumors); consider STA–MCA or high flow bypass to prevent long term flow related aneurysms (benign tumors)	

CBF, cerebral blood flow; ECA–ICA, external carotid artery–internal carotid artery; STA–MCA, superficial temporal artery–middle cerebral artery.

risk with a functional endoscopic exam of swallowing exam or radiographic study (barium esophagram). If CSF rhinorrhea is suspected, provocative maneuvers can be performed (Valsalva maneuver). Testing of collected fluid for beta-2-transferrin or beta–trace protein will confirm the presence of CSF.

IMAGING IN CRANIAL BASE SURGERY

Computed tomography (CT) and magnetic resonance imaging (MRI) provide complementary information for the diagnosis, preoperative planning, intraoperative period, and postoperative surveillance in cranial base surgery. CT scan provides significant information regarding the bony structures. Usually the presence of bony erosion, defects, remodeling, or calcification is well recognized with the CT scan. CT angiography is particularly important for the evaluation of the vasculature within and surrounding the tumor. MRI shows better soft tissue detail and is superior for delineating intracranial or intraorbital invasion. Fluid collections (meningocele, obstructed sinus) appear bright on T2-weighted sequences, although chronic sinus obstruction with high-protein content may be dark on both T1 and T2. Fat appears bright on T1 and dark on T2 images, which explains the MRI appearance of lesions with high-lipid content such as cholesterol granulomas. Chondromatous neoplasms (clival chordomas, chondrosarcomas) characteristically enhance on T1-weighted MRI with contrast and exhibit a high signal with multiple septations on T2-weighted sequences. Special sequences such as diffusion-weighted imaging are helpful in confirming an epidermoid tumor or abscess.

The vascularity of tumors is demonstrated by tumor enhancement on contrasted CT or MRI and flow voids on MRI. For example, juvenile nasopharyngeal angiofibroma classically enlarges the pterygopalatine fossa and presents with intense contrast enhancement in both MRI and CT scan. Angiography is used to confirm the diagnosis for highly vascular tumors (angiofibroma, paraganglioma) and for preoperative embolization of feeding vessels.

Preoperative imaging (CT angio and MRI) also provides information regarding intracranial circulation and collateral CBF (patency of circle of Willis). If sacrifice of the ICA or another major vessel is anticipated or planned, preoperative balloon test occlusion with neuromonitoring is performed. Xenon-perfusion CT scan provides an objective measure of CBF. Patients can be grouped into three prognostic groups based on the results of testing and this has implications for clinical management (Table 131.3).

Positron emission tomography shows cellular activity in the body, primarily through detection of labeled glucose taken up by the tissues under examination. Although this technique eventually may be useful for identification of primary tumors, it is most appropriate for detection of metastasis and local recurrence of high-grade malignancies. This can be valuable for preoperative staging to define goals of surgical treatment.

OPERATIVE MANAGEMENT

The choice of the optimal surgical approach is contingent upon multiple factors including the diagnosis, surgical access, reconstructive options, patient comorbidities, experience of the surgical team, potential complications, and available resources. The optimal approach is one that provides good access and visualization and minimizes potential morbidity. An approach should be chosen that minimizes manipulation of neural and vascular structures, especially retraction of the brain.

Cranial base surgery is team surgery and requires close coordination of the team members. Both CT and MRI are used for intraoperative navigation, which provides accurate anatomical localization during the surgery. Scans are performed using a skull base protocol (thin, overlapping slices) that are appropriate for intraoperative navigation. Navigation is used to identify important neural and vascular structures (and avoid injury), determine tumor margins, and assess the extent of the resection. Intraoperative imaging is sometimes performed (intraoperative CT or MRI) to assess the extent of tumor resection, detect complications (hemorrhage), or to update the navigation scan if there is shift of the residual tumor.

Neurophysiologic monitoring of cortical function (somatosensory-evoked potentials) provides a global assessment of cerebral perfusion and can be adversely affected by hypotension or a subdural collection. Brainstem evoked response is used to monitor hearing during temporal bone surgery and brainstem function during surgeries of the posterior fossa. Electromyography is used to monitor motor function of cranial nerves.

APPROACHES TO THE ANTERIOR CRANIAL BASE

Surgical approaches to the cranial base can be classified based on the anatomical region (Table 131.4). External approaches can be classified by cranial fossa whereas endonasal approaches are classified into surgical modules in the sagittal and coronal planes. With open approaches, craniofacial osteotomies provide access to the cranial base and help minimize brain retraction. The classical skull base operation pioneered by Ketcham and others is the craniofacial resection and deserves special consideration as the gold standard for sinonasal malignancy.

Anterior Cranial Base: Craniofacial Resection

For many years, the craniofacial approach has been the standard surgical option for the treatment of anterior cranial base pathology and generally consists of a transcranial approach in combination with a transfacial approach. A bicoronal incision is made over the vertex of the scalp from ear to ear. The incision may be extended inferiorly in a preauricular skin crease to increase the exposure. The posterior scalp flap can be elevated in a subgaleal plane to expose extra pericranium if needed for reconstruction. Otherwise, the scalp is elevated from the underlying cranium with separation of the periosteum from the deep temporal fascia of the temporalis muscle at its margin. Laterally, the superficial layer of the deep temporal fascia is incised several centimeters above the zygomatic arch and the interfascial fat pad is elevated with the scalp to avoid injury to the temporal branches of the facial nerve.

At the level of the superior orbital rims, the supratrochlear and supraorbital neurovascular bundles are carefully dissected free from their respective foramina to preserve the blood supply of a pericranial flap; small osteotomies may be necessary if the foramina is complete. Periosteum is elevated from the orbital roofs, glabella, and nasal bones, and the scalp is retracted inferiorly.

A bifrontal craniotomy is performed encompassing the anterior and posterior tables of the frontal sinus. The inferior osteotomy is placed just above the prominence of the brow. In order to minimize brain retraction, a subfrontal approach with removal of the supraorbital bar is performed. After the frontal dura is elevated from the orbital roofs, a reciprocating saw is used to transect the orbital rims at the lateral margin of the craniotomy. The orbital contents are protected while the orbital roof is transected with a drill and the bone is drilled anterior to the crista galli. A final transverse bone cut at the level of the nasion transects the nasofrontal ducts and frees the bone segment.

The dura is separated from the crista galli and incised anterior to the cribriform plate and laterally along the medial margin of the orbit. The olfactory bulbs and tracts are dissected free from the frontal lobes, and the olfactory tracts and dura are incised posteriorly over the planum. The bone margins are then drilled to communicate with the sinuses, staying anterior to the optic canals.

Frequently the craniofacial resection combines transfacial approaches with the bifrontal craniotomy. The aim of the transfacial approaches is to provide adequate field for the dissection and resection of the lesion from the nasal cavity, paranasal sinuses, and orbit. Options include a lateral rhinotomy, midfacial degloving approach, or endoscopic endonasal approach. The lateral rhinotomy is characterized by a skin incision starting at the midpoint between the nasal dorsum and the medial canthus. The

TABLE 131.4	CRANIAL BASE APPROACHES	
Anterior Cranial Base	**Middle Cranial Base**	**Posterior Cranial Base**
Craniofacial resection	*Lateral infratemporal skull base approach*	Retrosigmoid craniotomy
Endoscopic endonasal resection of anterior cranial base	Endoscopic endonasal suprapetrous approach	Endonasal transclival and transodontoid approach
		Endonasal infrapetrous approach

incision respects facial subunits and extends along the lateral surface of the nose to the nasal ala and then curves around the nostril to the nasal sill (14,15). The incision communicates with the nasal cavity along the pyriform aperture. Additional exposure can be obtained by extending the incision with a subciliary or transconjunctival incision superiorly (Weber-Ferguson incision) or by incising the upper lip along the lateral philtrum. After exposure of the facial skeleton through these incisions, osteotomies are performed according to the location and size of the tumor.

The midfacial degloving approach avoids a facial incision and provides better bilateral exposure. A mucosal incision is made in the gingivolabial sulcus and periosteum is elevated from the anterior maxilla. The incision communicates with the nasal cavity along the pyriform aperture and the nasal soft tissues are elevated from the anterior edge of the nasal septum following a full transfixion incision. Bilateral transmaxillary antrostomies and medial maxillectomies provide additional exposure. The midfacial degloving approach may be supplemented with endoscopy to provide better visualization.

After the appropriate transfacial or endoscopic approach, the tumor is removed en bloc, if possible, by dissecting around the periphery of the neoplasm with opening of the sinuses and transection of the nasal septum. The cranial base specimen is then mobilized through the bone cuts in the cranial base and delivered transcranially.

Reconstruction of the resultant defect is necessary to provide separation of the cranial and nasal cavities and prevent CSF leak, meningitis, and pneumocephalus. The dural defect is repaired primarily. Suitable materials include synthetic dural substitutes, fascia lata, temporalis fascia, pericranial graft, or cadaveric pericardium. An inferiorly based pericranial flap is reflected posteriorly to cover the entire defect in the anterior cranial base. Rigid reconstruction using a bone graft or alloplastic material is not necessary. It is important to place the flap inferior to the replaced supraorbital bar, leaving a small gap to prevent compression of the vascular pedicle.

Endoscopic Endonasal Resection of Anterior Cranial Base

Endoscopic endonasal techniques can be used for resection of sinonasal malignancies. The intranasal portion of the tumor is first debulked to provide visualization of the margins and assess the extent of the tumor. Uninvolved sinuses are opened to allow visualization of the medial orbits, nasofrontal recesses, and sphenoid sinus. Bony landmarks (optic canals, carotid canals) are identified, and the margins of resection are defined. In most cases, this includes the posterior wall of the frontal sinus, the medial walls of the orbit, the roof of the sphenoid sinus, and the nasal septum. The nasal septum is transected inferior to the area of tumor involvement from the frontal sinus to the rostrum of the sphenoid bone. Margins from the nasal

septum mucosa are sent for frozen section analysis. If the septal mucosa is not involved by the tumor, a septal flap can be harvested for later reconstruction.

A septal flap is pedicled on the posterior septal branches of the sphenopalatine artery. The inferior incision is initiated at the superior margin of the posterior choana and extends along the posterior margin of the vomer to the nasal floor. The inferior incision continues anteriorly along the junction between the septum and nasal floor to the nasal vestibule. If additional width is needed, the nasal floor mucosa (including the inferior meatus) can be incorporated into the flap. The superior incision starts at the sphenoid ostium and connects to the superior transection margin of the septum. Anteriorly, a vertical cut is made at the mucocutaneous junction to join the superior and inferior incisions. The nasoseptal flap is elevated from the septum in a subperichondrial and subperiosteal plane to the anterior face of the sphenoid sinus, and the vascular pedicle is preserved (16,17).

After harvesting of the septal flap, bilateral frontal sinusotomies are performed with removal of the floor bilaterally (Draf III procedure). The bone of the medial orbit is removed on the side of greatest tumor involvement. The tumor is devascularized by sacrifice of the anterior and posterior ethmoid arteries bilaterally. The arteries are identified at the junction of the orbit and skull base and cauterized with bipolar electrocautery or ligated with hemoclips.

The bone of the anterior cranial base is then removed to fully expose the dura and the area of dural invasion. Thinning of the bone with a drill is followed by fracturing and elevation of the thinned bone. Bone removal extends from the *crista galli* to the *planum sphenoidale* and to the medial orbits bilaterally. The dura is then cauterized and incised lateral to the tumor. Cortical blood vessels are identified and carefully freed from the dura. The falx is cauterized and transected anteriorly to allow mobilization of the dural specimen. The olfactory bulbs are dissected from the surface of the brain and remain attached to the dural specimen. If there is a focal area of brain invasion, the surrounding cortical tissue is removed by suction dissection to achieve clear margins. The olfactory nerves are then transected posteriorly and the final posterior dural incision is made to free the specimen. Additional dural margins may be excised for frozen section analysis (18).

After complete resection of the anterior cranial base, an inlay fascial graft is placed and the septal flap is positioned to cover the defect. If a septal flap is not available because of tumor involvement or insufficient dimension, an extracranial pericranial flap is used. A bicoronal scalp incision is made and the scalp is elevated to the level of the nasal bones. The bone at the level of the nasion is removed with a drill to create a window large enough to transmit the pericranial flap (~1 × 2 cm). The flap is then transposed through the defect inferior to the frontal sinusotomy and positioned over the dural defect, maintaining a drainage pathway for the frontal sinuses on one side (Fig. 131.2).

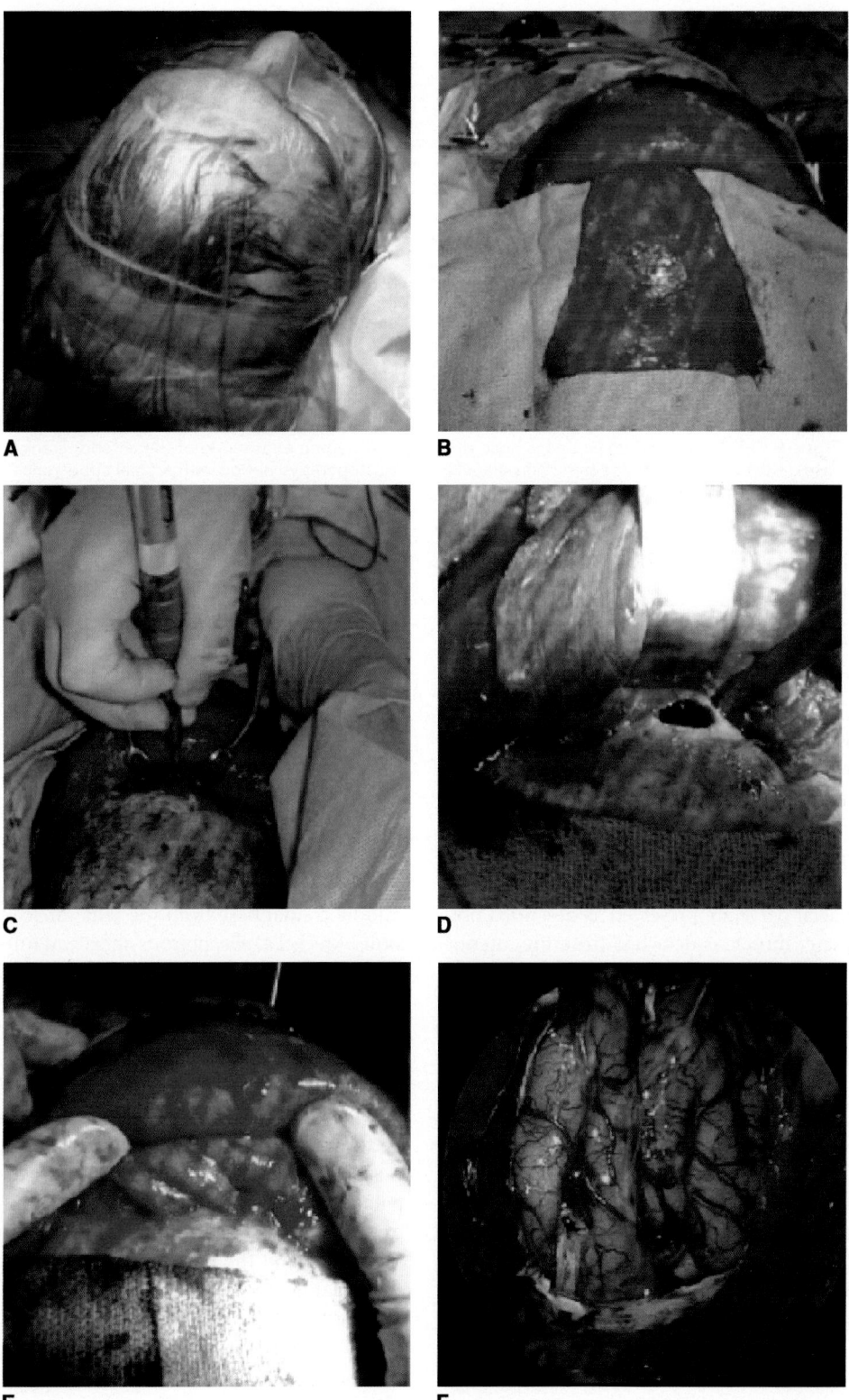

Figure 131.2 Bicoronal incision and pericranial flap transposition to the nasal cavity for reconstruction after endoscopic endonasal anterior cranial base resection. **A:** Preoperative preparation. **B:** Pericranial flap. **C:** Drilling the nasion. **D:** Nasion after osteotomy is completed. The pericranial flap is pedicled on the left supraorbital and supratrochlear arteries. **E:** Transposition of the pericranial flap to the nasal cavity. **F:** Endoscopic view with a 0-degree endoscope of the anterior cranial base defect. *(Continued)*

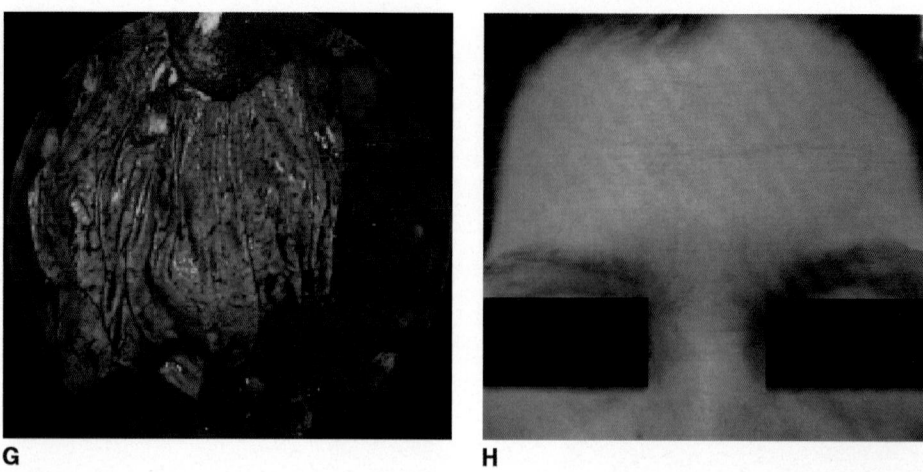

Figure 131.2 *(Continued)* **G:** Endoscopic view with a 0-degree endoscope of the anterior cranial base defect covered with the pericranial flap. **H:** Late postoperative period with normal appearance and intact sensory and motor function.

APPROACHES TO THE MIDDLE CRANIAL BASE

Open Approach: Lateral Infratemporal Skull Base Approach

The middle cranial fossa is typically accessed using a lateral transcranial approach. A bicoronal scalp incision is extended laterally in a preauricular skin crease to the inferior margin of the tragus. If transcervical exposure is required, it may be continued into the neck (parotidectomy incision). The scalp is elevated superficial to the deep temporal fascia to the level of the zygomatic arch, and the temporal branches of the facial nerve are preserved as described previously. The masseter muscle is detached from the inferior margin of the zygomatic arch and periosteum is dissected circumferentially. If a limited exposure of the infratemporal skull base is needed, the zygomatic arch is transected with a reciprocating saw anteriorly at its junction with the lateral orbit and posteriorly at the root of the zygoma.

If additional exposure is needed, an anterolateral skull base approach with orbitozygomatic osteotomies is utilized. The temporalis muscle is elevated and retracted inferiorly, and a frontotemporal craniotomy is performed. This provides access to the orbital roof. With retraction of orbital contents, an osteotomy of the superior orbital rim and roof is followed by an osteotomy from the inferior orbital fissure across the lateral orbital wall and zygoma. The capsule of the temporomandibular joint is dissected free, and osteotomies of the glenoid fossa detach the posterior end of the bone segment (Fig. 131.3).

A subtemporal craniectomy is performed and bone is removed to foramen ovale and foramen spinosum. Exposure of the petrous carotid artery requires division of the mandibular nerve and middle meningeal artery and then transgression of the eustachian tube. This approach provides access to the sphenoid sinus between the second and third divisions of the trigeminal nerve.

At the completion of the surgery, the temporalis muscle can be rotated into the defect to separate the sinuses from the cranial cavity and to protect the ICA. The orbitozygomatic bone segment is replaced and secured with titanium microplates. The temporal depression that results from transposition of the temporalis muscle can be filled with a fat graft or alloplastic material.

Endoscopic Endonasal Approach: Middle Cranial Base

The endoscopic endonasal approach permits access to the middle cranial base from the sella turcica to the cavernous sinus, Meckel's cave, petrous apex, and infratemporal fossa. The course of the petrous ICA divides the coronal plane into suprapetrous (middle fossa) and infrapetrous (posterior fossa) approaches. Key anatomical landmarks for the petrous ICA include the pterygoid canal (vidian nerve) and foramen rotundum (V2). A transpterygoid approach provides access to these structures and the middle fossa. Performing a middle meatal antrostomy and removing the posterior wall of the maxillary sinus expose the pterygopalatine space, and the contents are displaced laterally to expose the base of the pterygoids. The descending palatine artery and the greater palatine nerve run vertically in the palatine bone posterior to the antrostomy and are preserved. The vidian nerve and V2 are identified inferolaterally and superolaterally to the lateral recess of the sphenoid, and the sphenoidotomy is extended laterally. The vidian nerve can be sacrificed to provide additional exposure of the petrous ICA. The bone medial to the paraclival segment of the ICA is drilled to expose the medial petrous apex. Exposure of Meckel's cave requires removal of bone between the vidian nerve and V2 and lateral to the paraclival ICA. Foramen ovale can be accessed by following V3 from Meckel's cave or by following the lateral pterygoid plate posteriorly (19) (Fig. 131.4).

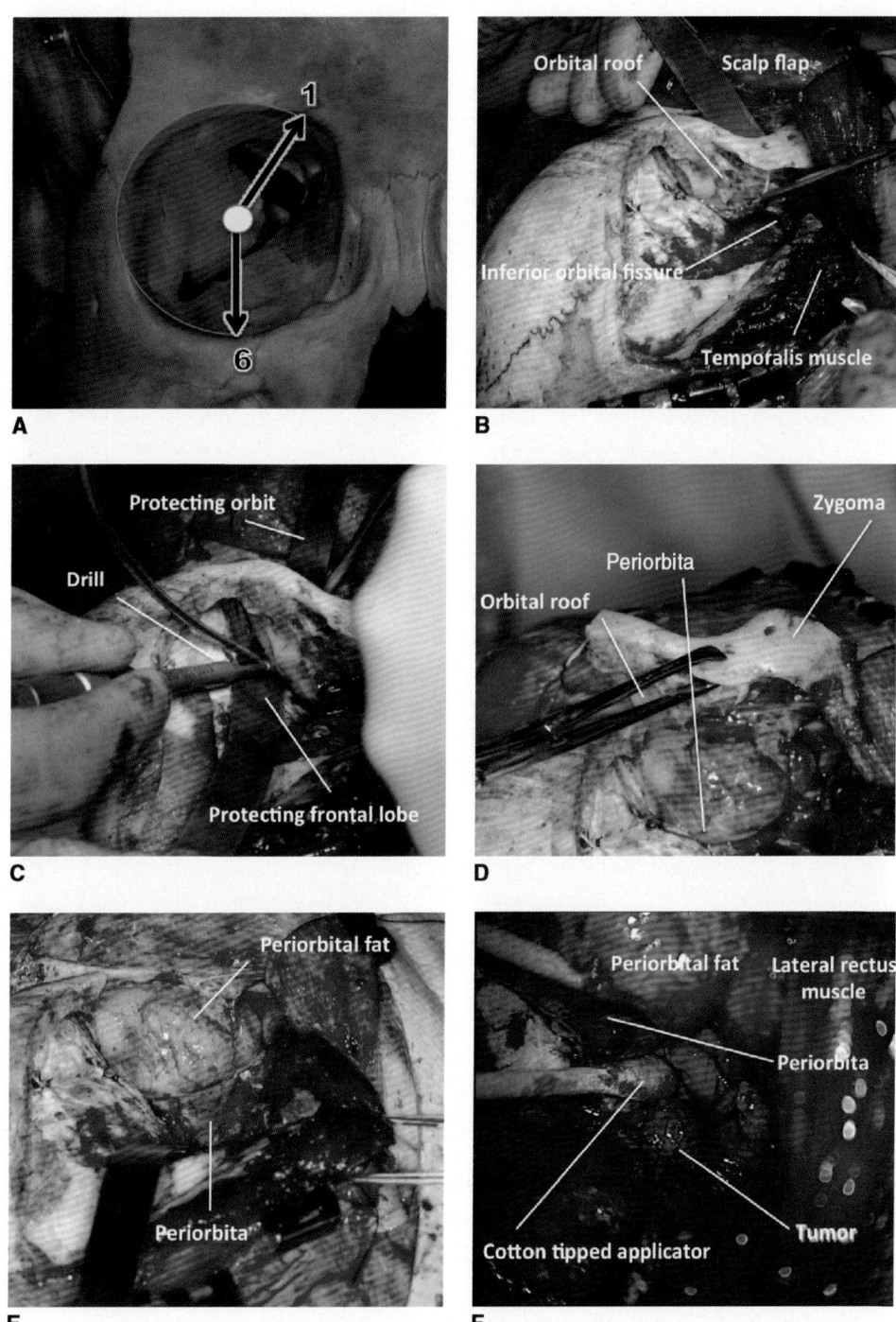

Figure 131.3 Orbitozygomatic approach for orbital apex meningioma. **A:** Right orbit in a dry skull. The highlighted area corresponds to the orbital region feasible to be reached with the orbitozygomatic approach. **B:** Exposure of the orbital lateral wall and part of the zygoma after elevation of the temporalis muscle and pterional craniotomy. **C:** Orbital burr hole. **D:** Osteotomies are performed to remove part of the zygoma and the lateral orbital rim in a single piece. **E:** Exposure of the periorbita. **F:** Microscopic view of the tumor situated between the lateral and superior rectus muscle.

More lateral access to the infratemporal skull base and masticator space is achieved with a medial maxillectomy, anteromedial maxillotomy (Denker approach), or transmaxillary approach. The lateral nasal wall is resected to the nasal floor and the lacrimal duct is sharply transected at its junction with the lacrimal sac to prevent stenosis. An endoscopic anteromedial maxillotomy requires a mucosal incision along the pyriform aperture, and periosteum is elevated from the anterior maxilla. The medial buttress is removed with a drill or bone rongeurs. Preservation of periosteum is important to minimize alar retraction postoperatively. More lateral exposure can be achieved with a

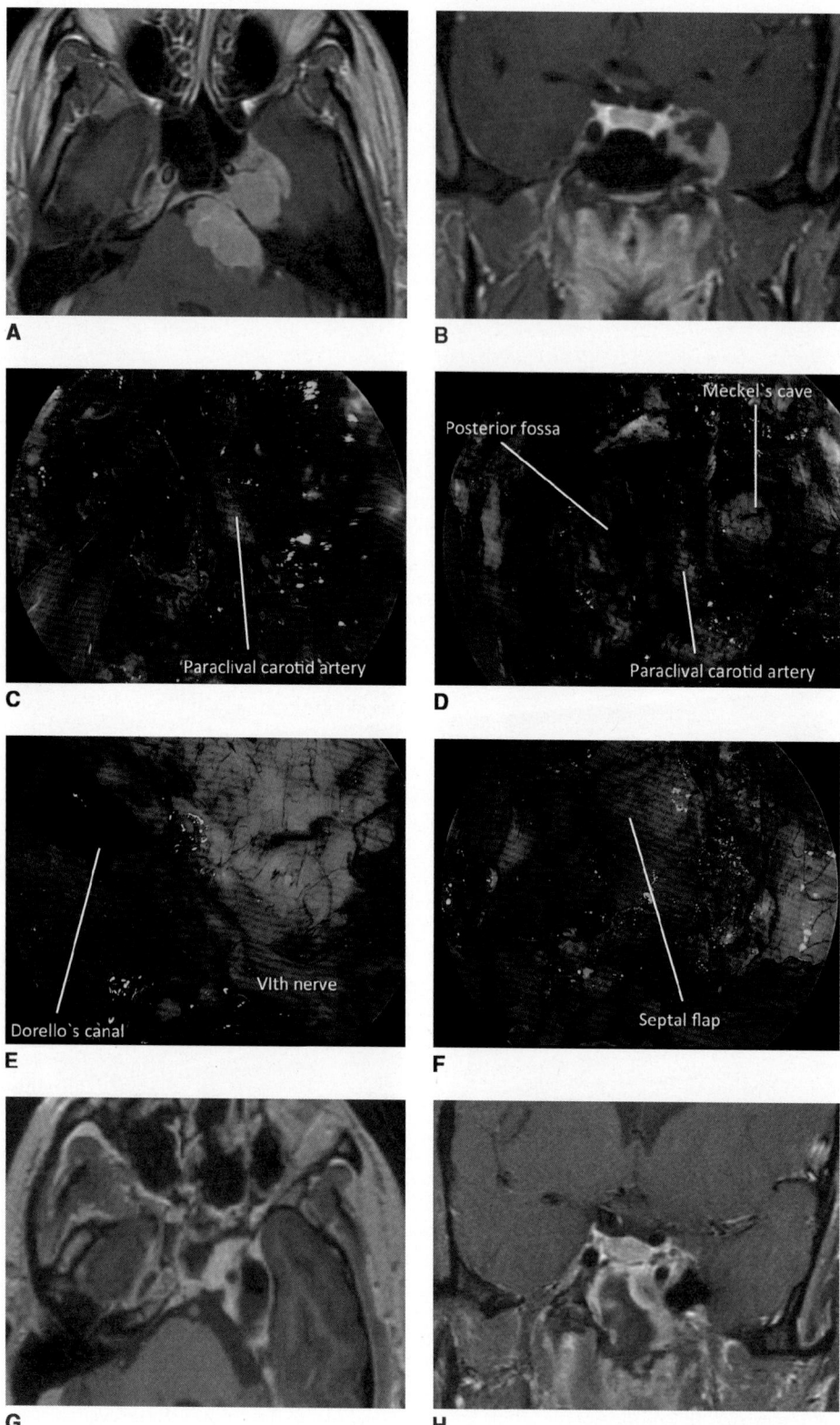

Figure 131.4 Endoscopic endonasal approach to the middle and posterior cranial fossa for resection of a left trigeminal schwannoma. **A:** Preoperative MRI T1 with contrast axial view. The tumor occupies the middle and posterior cranial fossa. **B:** Preoperative MRI T1 with contrast coronal view. Meckel's cave is filled with tumor. **C:** Endoscopic view with a 0-degree endoscope showing the resection of the tumor from the posterior cranial fossa. The paraclival carotid artery is just anterior to the anterior limit of the dissection. **D:** Endoscopic view with a 0-degree endoscope showing the posterior cranial fossa and Meckel's cave completely free of tumor. The paraclival carotid artery is seen between these two areas approached. **E:** Endoscopic close-up view of Meckel's cave with a 45-degree endoscope looking inferiorly to show the trajectory of the sixth nerve from the posterior fossa through an enlarged Dorello's canal. **F:** Right septal flap covering both cranial base defects: clival and Meckel's cave. **G:** Postoperative MRI T1 with contrast axial view and (**H**) coronal view to show the complete removal of the tumor from the middle and posterior cranial fossa.

transmaxillary approach. A sublabial mucosal incision provides exposure of the anterior maxillary wall and a maxillotomy is performed to the infraorbital nerve. The bone of the posterolateral maxilla is removed to expose the pterygoid muscles, branches of V3, and branches of the internal maxillary artery. Dissection can proceed as far as the ramus of the mandible and temporomandibular joint.

Surgical defects of the middle cranial fossa can be covered with a contralateral septal flap or with nonvascularized fascial and fat grafts. With combined endonasal and infratemporal approaches, alternative reconstructive flaps include a temporalis transposition or temporoparietal fascial flap.

APPROACHES TO THE POSTERIOR CRANIAL BASE

Open Approach: Retrosigmoid Craniotomy

A postauricular incision is made and a subperiosteal flap is elevated. The incision may be extended into the upper cervical region for control of the proximal ICA and isolation of the lower cranial nerves. The upper cervical musculature (sternocleidomastoid and trapezius muscles) is detached from the mastoid and suboccipital region, and a craniotomy is performed posterior to the mastoid and sigmoid sinus. A mastoidectomy with removal of the tip provides greater access to the jugular foramen.

If a large tumor involves the temporal bone and complete access to the extracranial ICA is needed, a Fisch type C approach provides wide exposure of the middle and posterior cranial fossae. The incision extends from the temporal area to the upper cervical region. A conchal bowl incision through the skin and cartilage allows elevation of the auricle with the skin flap; the stump of the external auditory canal remains. The facial nerve can be transposed for additional exposure or remain in situ. A transtemporal approach is then performed with dissection of the ICA to the carotid canal.

The surgical defect can be reconstructed with temporalis-muscle transposition or a posteriorly based pericranial flap (occipital artery). The craniotomy site is covered with titanium mesh or a plate and cervical musculature is reattached.

Endonasal Transclival and Transodontoid Approach

The endonasal approach provides optimal access to the clival region from the posterior clinoids to the foramen magnum. A sphenoidotomy is performed and the mucosa of the nasopharynx and underlying musculature (longus capitis muscle) is resected from the floor of the sphenoid to the ring of C1 and between the eustachian tubes. It is important to localize the parapharyngeal ICAs with image guidance to avoid injury with dissection or electrocautery. The clivus is divided into thirds. The upper third includes the posterior clinoids to the floor of the sella. Exposure of the posterior clinoids requires transposition of the pituitary gland. The

sella is opened widely and the lateral attachments of the pituitary gland are lysed with possible sacrifice of the inferior hypophyseal arteries on one or both sides. If the posterior planum is removed, the gland can be displaced into the suprasellar space with preservation of the pituitary stalk and the superior hypophyseal vessels. The middle clivus extends from the floor of the sella to the floor of the sphenoid sinus. Drilling of bone in this area is bounded by the parapharyngeal ICAs, and the sixth cranial nerve is susceptible to injury posterolateral to the vessels (20). The inferior clivus extends to the foramen magnum. The bone thins as you proceed inferiorly and intense venous bleeding from the clival plexus is often encountered. This is controlled with application of hemostatic materials (Surgifoam, Floseal). The sixth cranial nerve exits the brainstem at the level of the vertebrobasilar junction and is susceptible to injury with opening of the dura (Fig. 131.4).

If exposure of the upper cervical spine is necessary (basilar invagination, foramen magnum tumor), the anterior ring of C1 is exposed and removed. The odontoid and upper body of C2 can be drilled and ligamentous attachments are resected. Laterally, dissection is limited by the vertebral arteries.

Extradural defects of the clivus can be simply covered with fibrin glue. Septal mucosal flaps are usually inadequate in size and reach for large and deep clival defects and supplementation with fat grafts may be necessary.

Endonasal Infrapetrous Approach

The infrapetrous approach is defined by the course of the petrous and parapharyngeal ICA. A lower transclival approach is combined with a transpterygoid approach, and the location of the petrous ICA is defined using the vidian nerve as a landmark. Bone inferomedial to the pterygoid canal is carefully drilled, and the dense fibrocartilage of the foramen lacerum is exposed. The medial eustachian tube is resected and the fibrocartilage is transected inferior to foramen lacerum. This provides access to the inferior aspect of the petrous bone. Lateral dissection is limited by V3 and the parapharyngeal ICA.

At the level of the foramen magnum, removal of bone laterally exposes the hypoglossal canal and nerve. The bone superior to the hypoglossal nerve is the jugular tubercle and is bounded laterally by the jugular bulb. The occipital condyle is inferior to the hypoglossal nerve; excessive removal of this bone on both sides can destabilize the spine (21).

COMPLICATIONS

Complications associated with cranial base surgery are myriad and can be life-threatening or trivial, temporary or permanent. There is no standardized classification of skull base complications. A list of possible complications is provided in Table 131.5. For the purposes of this chapter, the more common and clinically relevant complications are discussed.

TABLE 131.5	C	COMPLICATIONS OF CRANIAL BASE SURGERY

- CSF leak
- Pneumocephalus
- Meningitis
- Epidural, subdural, or brain abscess
- ICA injury
- Stroke
- Venous thrombosis
- Thrombophlebitis
- Encephalomalacia
- Seizure
- Psychiatric disorders
- Diabetes insipidus
- Syndrome of inappropriate antidiuretic hormone secretion
- Hypopituitarism
- Cranial nerve deficit
- Flap necrosis

Pituitary: Hypopituitarism and Diabetes Insipidus

Injury to the pituitary gland and loss of function may result from aggressive resection of tumor or loss of blood supply (superior hypophyseal vessels). The effects of hypopituitarism will depend on the age of the patient but include cortisol deficiency, hypogonadism, and hypothyroidism. Endocrinologists are involved in the perioperative management of these patients and hormonal replacement therapy can be instituted. In patients who are at risk for cortisol deficiency, stress steroids are administered perioperatively.

Diabetes insipidus is a consequence of injury to the posterior gland or hypothalamus. It is characterized by a sudden increase in urine output because of impairment in the secretion of antidiuretic hormone. During the postoperative period, urine output greater than 250 mL in 2 hours is suggestive of diabetes insipidus. Manifestations include polyuria, dehydration, hypovolemia, and polydipsia. The diagnosis is confirmed if serum level of sodium exceeds 150 mEq/L, the urine is dilute with a specific gravity less than 1.005, and urine osmolality is between 50 and 150 mOsm/kg. Treatment includes fluid and electrolyte replacement. Administration of Desmopressin (DDAVP) is indicated when dehydration and electrolyte disturbances are severe or not responding to the replacement therapy. In the postoperative period, diabetes insipidus usually is a self-limited condition and pharmacologic treatment tends to be temporary.

CSF Leak/Pneumocephalus

A CSF leak occurs in up to 5% of patients undergoing endonasal cranial base surgery and is one of the most frequent major complications. Risk factors for a CSF leak include patient demographics, patient comorbidities, diagnosis, location and size of dural defect, method of reconstruction, and perioperative management. Younger and older patients appear to be at increased risk, but this may be due to other related factors. Morbidly obese patients have elevated CSF pressures. Similarly, patients presenting with a spontaneous CSF leak and those with significant mixing of blood and CSF have elevated CSF pressures postoperatively. In our experience, craniopharyngiomas have an increased risk of CSF leak that may be a consequence of a high-flow defect as well as transient hydrocephalus from the cyst contents. Large dural defects and those that communicate with CSF cisterns or ventricles pose a greater risk. Successful repair of dural defects has been achieved using a variety of nonvascularized and vascularized tissues. The use of vascularized septal flaps and pericranial flaps has decreased the incidence of postoperative CSF leaks to less than 5%. Although lumbar spinal drainage is often used to treat minor CSF leaks, the routine use of CSF diversion to prevent a postoperative CSF leak has not been convincingly demonstrated.

Usually, a postoperative CSF leak is readily apparent based on the symptoms (unilateral watery rhinorrhea, reservoir sign due to pooling of fluid in the sinuses, "double-ring" sign of blood-tinged drainage) and physical examination (endoscopic findings, Valsalva maneuver). Persistent postoperative pneumocephalus or increasing pneumocephalus imply a dural opening. In questionable cases, a postoperative CSF leak can be confirmed by testing of collected fluid for beta-2-transferrin or beta–trace protein, or with a CT cisternogram.

Aggressive management of postoperative CSF leaks is warranted to prevent the sequela of meningitis. For small leaks in the early postoperative period, a lumbar spinal drainage can allow the leak to seal. CSF diversion can increase the risk of meningitis, however, due to reversal of flow. Prophylactic antibiotic therapy for CSF leaks is not recommended due to lack of efficacy and selection of antibiotic-resistant bacteria. Following endonasal skull base surgery, aggressive management with surgical intervention within 24 hours has been an effective strategy. Lumbar drains are reserved for recurrent leaks, high-flow leaks, and patients with suspected elevated CSF pressure.

Infection/Meningitis

The incidence of meningitis following cranial base surgery is very low with reports of 0.9% to 2.5% for transcranial surgery and 1% to 2% for endonasal skull base surgery (22–24). Surprisingly, endonasal approaches through a clean–contaminated environment have not been associated with an increased risk of infection. There is no consensus for the best regimen for antibiotic prophylaxis, but a single agent with moderate CSF penetration (e.g., third- or fourth-generation cephalosporin) is sufficient. Factors that contribute to postoperative meningitis include active infection (sinusitis, wound infection), postoperative CSF leak, and use of nonvascularized tissues for reconstruction. Factors that delay healing (malnutrition, Cushing's disease, radiation therapy) may also contribute. Patients with sinusitis should be treated prior to surgery that transgresses the infected sinus. Early intervention for CSF leaks decreases the risk of delayed meningitis.

Vascular Injury

The risk of a vascular injury depends on multiple factors including the extent of the pathology, the experience of the surgeon, and the region of dissection. Vascular injury to small vessels can be as devastating as injury to the ICA. When dissecting tumors from the optic chiasm, loss of small branches of the superior hypophyseal artery can result in visual loss or hypopituitarism. Injury to small perforating vessels when dissecting tumors from the brainstem can result in stroke or hyperphagia syndrome. Tumors of the anterior cranial fossa that encase the anterior cerebral arteries pose a greater risk for dissection. Injury may result in memory and personality changes. Large tumors are internally debulked first to collapse the tumor and allow extracapsular dissection of the tumor margin without retraction. Pulling of tumor is avoided so that small vessels are not avulsed on the backside of the tumor. If tumor cannot be safely dissected from these small vessels, it is better to perform a partial resection.

Injury to the ICA is avoided with a detailed knowledge of skull base anatomy and good surgical technique. Bleeding from the ICA may result from avulsion of small branches or direct injury. Small arterioles can be sealed with bipolar electrocautery. Larger injuries should be sutured if possible or controlled with application of a crushed muscle patch. If this is not possible, intraoperative sacrifice of the ICA with packing or placement of aneurysm clips is usually necessary. Postoperative angiography should be performed in all of these patients to detect a pseudoaneurysm. Management includes insertion of a covered stent or angiographic sacrifice of the vessel. The adequacy of collateral cerebral circulation can be assessed with a combination of CT/MRI studies, angiography, and xenon-CT or single photon emission computed tomography (SPECT) balloon occlusion tests. If collateral circulation is inadequate, a bypass graft from the carotid artery to the middle cerebral artery (MCA) may be considered.

Neural Injury

Cerebral contusions are a direct consequence of brain retraction and the surgical approach should be designed to minimize retraction. The incidence of radiographic encephalomalacia is as high as 60% of patients undergoing transcranial surgery of the anterior cranial base. Risk of contusion is increased if there is preoperative cerebral edema secondary to tumor disruption of the blood–brain boundary.

Cranial nerve injury is a consequence of manipulation or ischemia. Surgical approaches should be designed to minimize manipulation of nerves and small vessels to the nerves from the cranial circulation should be preserved. The sixth cranial nerve is particularly susceptible to injury due to its long course and small diameter. It can be injured medial (brainstem) or lateral (Dorello's canal) to the paraclival segment of the ICA. Neurophysiologic monitoring of the motor component of the cranial nerves and the use of intraoperative nerve stimulation decrease the risk of permanent injury. Sacrifice of cranial nerves is often necessary due to tumor involvement. Care should be taken to avoid loss of the first division of the trigeminal nerve in association with the vidian nerve since the combination of corneal anesthesia and decreased tearing places the cornea at high risk of ulceration. Loss of the vidian nerve is generally well tolerated in young patients (loss of emotional tearing) but may contribute to a dry eye in older patients with decreased baseline tearing.

Quality of Life

Studies of postoperative quality of life (QOL) using the anterior skull base questionnaire in patients undergoing anterior craniofacial resection for sinonasal malignancy demonstrate good function across all domains (19). In patients undergoing endoscopic endonasal surgery of the skull base, excellent QOL scores are noted using the anterior skull base questionnaire (20). Limited data suggest that QOL is superior to open transcranial approaches. Nasal morbidity has been assessed in the endonasal surgical group using the SNOT-22 questionnaire, a validated instrument. As expected, increasing nasal morbidity (decreased QOL) was noted in nontransellar sagittal plane and coronal plane surgical modules compared to transellar surgery.

CONCLUSIONS

Cranial base surgery is a rapidly evolving subspecialty that requires a vast knowledge of anatomy and encompasses a wide variety of pathologies and surgical approaches. The same principles apply to pediatric and adult populations. Cranial base surgery is best practiced by teams of surgeons with expertise in open and endonasal approaches. Morbidity is acceptable and overall QOL is good following cranial base surgery. Good oncologic outcomes can be obtained for a variety of benign and malignant neoplasms.

HIGHLIGHTS

- The depth of the lateral lamella is an important risk factor for iatrogenic CSF leak during transethmoidal procedures.
- The olfactory filaments pass through the cribriform plate from the nasal cavity to the intracranial olfactory bulbs and are a route for intracranial spread of sinonasal malignancy.
- The sixth cranial nerve courses superolaterally behind the paraclival ICA and is at risk of injury when drilling posterior to the paraclival ICA just below the sellar floor.

- The arcuate eminence approximates the position of the superior semicircular canal. The internal auditory canal can be identified below the floor of the middle fossa by drilling along a line approximately 60 degrees medial to the arcuate eminence, near the middle portion of the angle between the greater petrosal nerve and arcuate eminence.

- The scalp has five layers designated by the acronym SCALP: Skin, subcutaneous tissues, Aponeurosis (galea), Loose areolar layer, and Periosteum.

- If CSF rhinorrhea is suspected, provocative maneuvers can be performed (Valsalva maneuver). Testing of collected fluid for beta-2-transferrin or beta–trace protein will confirm the presence of CSF.

- Chondromatous neoplasms (clival chordomas, chondrosarcomas) characteristically enhance on T1-weighted MRI with contrast and exhibit a high signal with multiple septations on T2-weighted sequences.

- A septal flap is pedicled on the posterior septal branches of the sphenopalatine artery and the pericranial flap is supplied by the supratrochlear and supraorbital vessels, which exit from foramina or notches along the superior orbital rim.

- During endoscopic endonasal approaches, the course of the petrous ICA divides the coronal plane into suprapetrous (middle fossa) and infrapetrous (posterior fossa) approaches. Key anatomical landmarks for the petrous ICA include the pterygoid canal (vidian nerve) and foramen rotundum (V2).

- Diabetes insipidus is a consequence of injury to the posterior gland or hypothalamus. It is characterized by a sudden increase in urine output because of impairment in the secretion of antidiuretic hormone. Treatment includes fluid, electrolyte replacement and/or administration of DDAVP.

REFERENCES

1. Donald PJ. History of skull base surgery. *Skull Base Surg* 1991;1(1):1–3.
2. Maroon JC. Skull base surgery: past, present, and future trends [Historical Article Review]. *Neurosurg Focus* 2005;19(1):E1.
3. Dandy WE. The surgical treatment of intracranial aneurysms of the internal carotid artery. *Ann Surg* 1941;114(3):336–340.
4. Tessier P. Total osteotomy of the middle third of the face for faciostenosis or for sequelae of Le Fort 3 fractures. *Plast Reconstr Surg* 1971;48(6):533–541.
5. Ketcham AS, Wilkins RH, Vanburen JM, et al. A combined intracranial facial approach to the paranasal sinuses. *Am J Surg* 1963;106:698–703.
6. House WF. Surgical exposure of the internal auditory canal and its contents through the middle, cranial fossa. *Laryngoscope* 1961;71:1363–1385.
7. Jho HD, Carrau RL. Endoscopic endonasal transsphenoidal surgery: experience with 50 patients [Clinical Trial]. *J Neurosurg* 1997;87(1):44–51.
8. Snyderman CH, Kassam AB. Endoscopic techniques for pathology of the anterior cranial fossa and ventral skull base [Comment Letter]. *J Am Coll Surg* 2006;202(3):563.
9. Snyderman CH, Kassam AB, Carrau R, et al. Endoscopic reconstruction of cranial base defects following endonasal skull base surgery. *Skull Base* 2007;17(1):73–78.
10. Stamm AC, Pignatari SS, Vellutini E. Transnasal endoscopic surgical approaches to the clivus [Review]. *Otolaryngol Clin North Am* 2006;39(3):639–56, xi.
11. Nicolai P, Castelnuovo P, Lombardi D, et al. Role of endoscopic surgery in the management of selected malignant epithelial neoplasms of the naso-ethmoidal complex. *Head Neck* 2007;29(12):1075–1082.
12. Rhoton AL Jr. The anterior and middle cranial base [Review]. *Neurosurgery* 2002;51(4 Suppl):S273–S302.
13. Pinheiro-Neto CD, Snyderman CH, Fernandez-Miranda J, et al. Endoscopic endonasal surgery for nasal dermoids. *Otolaryngol Clin North Am* 2011;44(4):981–987, ix.
14. Lueg EA, Irish JC, Katz MR, et al. A patient- and observer-rated analysis of the impact of lateral rhinotomy on facial aesthetics. *Arch Fac Plast Surg* 2001;3(4):241–244.
15. Bagatella F, Mazzoni A. Microsurgery in juvenile nasopharyngeal angiofibroma: a lateronasal approach with nasomaxillary pedicled flap. *Skull Base Surg* 1995;5(4):219–226.
16. Hadad G, Bassagasteguy L, Carrau RL, et al. A novel reconstructive technique after endoscopic expanded endonasal approaches: vascular pedicle nasoseptal flap. *Laryngoscope* 2006;116(10):1882–1886.
17. Pinheiro-Neto CD, Prevedello DM, Carrau RL, et al. Improving the design of the pedicled nasoseptal flap for skull base reconstruction: a radioanatomic study. *Laryngoscope* 2007;117(9):1560–1569.
18. Snyderman CH, Carrau RL, Kassam AB, et al. Endoscopic skull base surgery: principles of endonasal oncological surgery [Review]. *J Surg Oncol* 2008;97(8):658–664.
19. Kassam AB, Prevedello DM, Carrau RL, et al. The front door to Meckel's cave: an anteromedial corridor via expanded endoscopic endonasal approach- technical considerations and clinical series [Case Reports]. *Neurosurgery* 2009;64(3 Suppl):71–82, discussion 3.
20. Barges-Coll J, Fernandez-Miranda JC, Prevedello DM, et al. Avoiding injury to the abducens nerve during expanded endonasal endoscopic surgery: anatomic and clinical case studies [Case Reports Research Support, Non-U.S. Gov't]. *Neurosurgery* 2010;67(1):144–154, discussion 54.
21. Morera VA, Fernandez-Miranda JC, Prevedello DM, et al. "Far-medial" expanded endonasal approach to the inferior third of the clivus: the transcondylar and transjugular tubercle approaches. *Neurosurgery* 2010;66(6 Suppl Operative):211–219, discussion 9–20.
22. Korinek AM, Baugnon T, Golmard JL, et al. Risk factors for adult nosocomial meningitis after craniotomy: role of antibiotic prophylaxis. *Neurosurgery* 2006;59(1):126–133, discussion 33.
23. National Nosocomial Infections Surveillance (NNIS) System Report, data summary from January 1992 through June 2004, issued October 2004 [Research Support, U.S. Gov't, P.H.S.]. *Am J Infect Control* 2004;32(8):470–485.
24. Kono Y, Prevedello DM, Snyderman CH, et al. One thousand endoscopic skull base surgical procedures demystifying the infection potential: incidence and description of postoperative meningitis and brain abscesses. *Infect Control Hosp Epidemiol* 2011;32(1):77–83.

Odontogenic Cysts, Tumors, and Related Jaw Lesions

132

William L. Chung   **Kurt F. Summersgill**   **Mark W. Ochs**

The term *odontogenic* implies being derived from tooth-forming structures. Odontogenic cysts and tumors are a unique group of lesions due to their complex and variable history, histologic characteristics, and clinical behavior. Odontogenic cysts vary significantly in their frequency, behavior, and treatment. Odontogenic tumors are relatively uncommon lesions (1). Collectively, lesions of the jaws deserve considerable attention by surgeons because of their potential for tissue destruction and the related challenges they pose for reconstruction. This chapter reviews the more common odontogenic cysts and tumors along with several other related jaw lesions. The salient clinical, radiographic, and histologic features of each lesion will be discussed, in addition to its treatment and prognosis. Many of the odontogenic cysts and tumors share similar radiographic features, so the patient's history and eventual histopathology ultimately dictate the specific surgical therapy. Furthermore, a frozen section is not typically obtained for jaw lesions discussed in this chapter because they are not malignant lesions and a frozen section will not change the ultimate treatment plan for each lesion.

ODONTOGENIC CYSTS

In 1992, the World Health Organization (WHO) classified odontogenic cysts as either inflammatory or developmental, including odontogenic and nonodontogenic. Most cysts of the oral cavity are true cysts because they contain an epithelial lining. The lining of these cysts is derived from one of three epithelial structures: (a) reduced enamel epithelium—residual epithelium that surrounds the crown of the tooth after enamel formation is complete; (b) rests of Malassez—remnants of the Hertwig root sheath that persist in the periodontal ligament after root formation is complete; or (c) remnants of dental lamina (rests of Serres)—islands and strands of epithelium that originate from the oral epithelium and remain in tissues after inducing tooth development (2). Odontogenic cysts can become inflamed or infected, causing significant signs or symptoms.

INFLAMMATORY CYSTS

Radicular Cyst

The radicular cyst is by far the most common odontogenic cyst. It develops at the apex of an erupted tooth in response to pulpal necrosis secondary to dental caries or trauma. The cyst arises from inflammatory stimulation and proliferation of the rests of Malassez. The cyst lining forms as the epithelial elements proliferate. Cellular debris within the lumen produces an osmotic gradient, and fluid is transported across the lining. This gradient slowly increases the volume of fluid inside the lumen, ultimately expanding the cyst by hydraulic pressure from within the cyst.

Clinical and Radiographic Features

Most radicular cysts are asymptomatic and are discovered incidentally during routine radiographic evaluation (Fig. 132.1). Radicular cysts rarely exceed 1 cm in diameter except when several adjacent teeth become devitalized as a result of trauma. Radiographically, the radicular cyst is round to ovoid, well circumscribed, and contiguous with the apex of the involved tooth.

Histopathology

The cyst is lined by stratified squamous epithelium of varying thickness. The cyst wall typically supports a variable inflammatory cell infiltrate, including lymphocytes and neutrophils. The cystic lumen will frequently contain necrotic cellular debris. A small percentage of radicular cysts have crescent-shaped hyaline (Rushton) bodies within the epithelial lining. Although unique to odontogenic cysts, the biologic significance of Rushton bodies is unknown. Multinucleated foreign body giant cells, cholesterol crystal clefts, and hemosiderin may be seen throughout the connective tissue of the cyst wall.

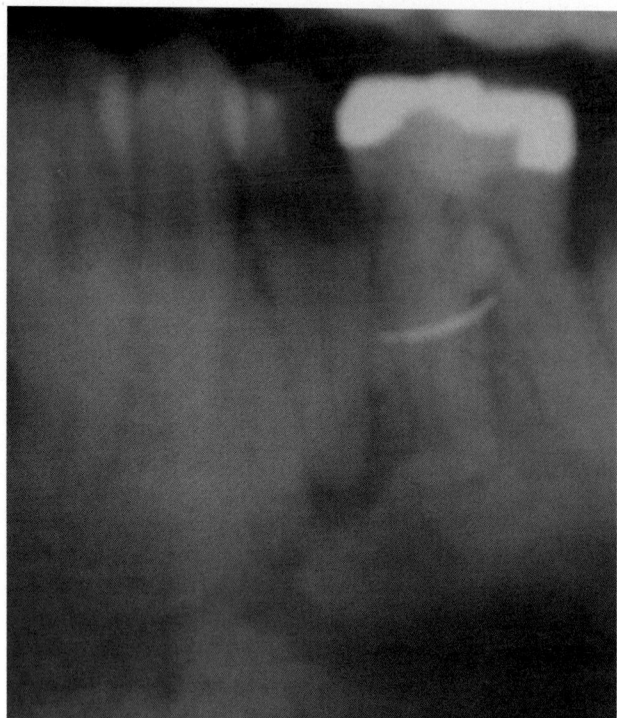

Figure 132.1 Periapical cyst. Radiograph demonstrating periapical lesion associated with grossly carious tooth # 20.

Treatment and Prognosis

These cysts are treated by extraction of the infected tooth followed by enucleation of the cyst. Extraction of the tooth without removing the cyst may allow for persistent growth of the cyst. If the cyst is incompletely removed, a *residual* cyst may develop. Complete bony healing is typically seen within 6 months if the radicular cyst has been thoroughly removed.

DEVELOPMENTAL CYSTS

Dentigerous Cyst

The dentigerous cyst is the second most common odontogenic cyst. A dentigerous cyst must be associated with the crown of an unerupted tooth (3). The cyst is attached to the cervical region of the tooth, usually a mandibular third molar. However, variants exist where the cyst is seen lateral to or completely enveloping the associated tooth. Maxillary third molars, maxillary canines, and mandibular second bicuspids are also commonly involved, as these teeth are among those frequently impacted.

Clinical and Radiographic Features

Dentigerous cysts usually occur in the second and third decades with a slight male predilection. Because they are associated with an impacted tooth, the arch will appear to be missing a tooth. The cysts usually do not produce symptoms and can achieve significant size, causing bony expansion (Fig. 132.2A and B). The dentigerous cyst is usually a well-circumscribed, unilocular, radiolucency surrounding the crown of an unerupted tooth (Fig. 132.2C). Mandibular

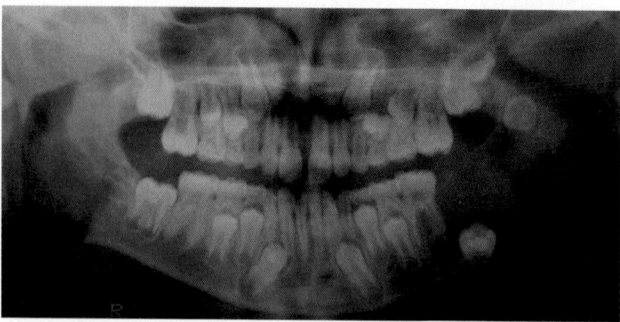

A

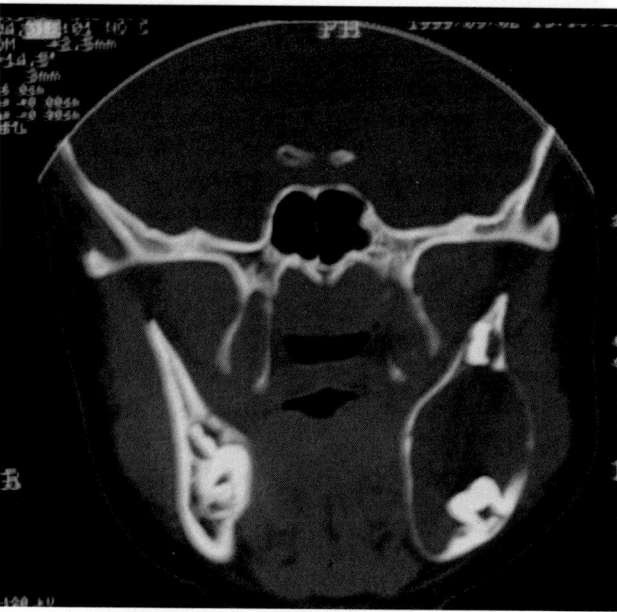

B

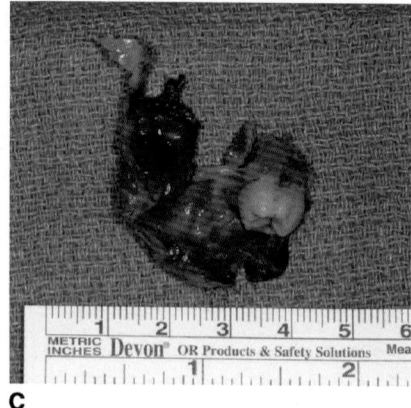

C

Figure 132.2 A,B: Dentigerous cyst. Panorex radiograph and computed tomography (CT) scan of 14-year-old who presented with facial swelling. Radiograph reveals considerable left mandibular angle and ramal involvement. Note thinning of buccal and lingual cortices and displacement of multiple permanent teeth within lesion on CT. **C:** Surgical specimen from above patient. Note adherence of cyst to permanent tooth crown.

cysts can displace the tooth into the ramus or the inferior border of the mandible, while maxillary cysts can displace the tooth into the maxillary sinus toward the orbital floor. It is important to understand that the above-stated clinical and radiographic features are not specifically diagnostic for a dentigerous cyst, although highly consistent (4). The differential diagnosis for similar-appearing radiographic lesions should include an ameloblastoma, keratocystic odontogenic tumor (KCOT), and adenomatoid odontogenic tumor (AOT).

Histopathology

The cystic lumen is lined by nonkeratinized, stratified squamous epithelium that is anywhere from 2 to 10 cell layers thick. It is common for the lining to be inflamed. The dentigerous cyst can share several microscopic features with the radicular cyst, such as Rushton bodies, cholesterol crystal clefts, and hemosiderin deposits. Chronic dentigerous cysts may exhibit areas of keratinized epithelium, which require the lesion to be differentiated from the KCOT (5). The epithelial lining of the dentigerous cyst is capable of ameloblastoma expression (3). Thus, timely diagnosis and treatment is critical.

Treatment and Prognosis

Removal of the impacted tooth along with thorough enucleation of the cyst is usually definitive therapy. When a mandibular dentigerous cyst reaches considerable size, the cyst can be marsupialized to allow for decompression and shrinkage of the cyst with compensatory bone fill prior to definitive removal of the lesion.

Calcifying Odontogenic Cyst (Gorlin Cyst)

This lesion is thought to arise from remnants of the dental lamina within the gingiva or jaws. Approximately one-fourth of all calcifying odontogenic cysts (COCs) occur extraosseously, within the gingiva anterior to the first molar in individuals older than 50 years (6).

Clinical and Radiographic Features

The COC behaves like most other odontogenic cysts, and it has little recurrence potential. The COC has a wide age range, but the peak incidence occurs in the second decade. The lesion has a predilection for females, and most are located in the anterior portion of either jaw. The extraosseous lesion may present with painless gingival expansion. These cysts are often discovered as incidental findings on routine radiographic evaluation. They initially appear lucent. As the cyst develops, calcifications may develop causing a well-circumscribed mixed radiolucent/radiopaque appearance. However, these opacities are only seen in approximately one-third to one-half of all cases.

Histopathology

These usually unilocular cysts are lined by odontogenic epithelium. The basal layer is distinct with its columnar to cuboidal cells with hyperchromatic nuclei that are polarized away from the basement membrane (Fig. 132.3). Another characteristic histologic feature of the COC is the ghost cell—an altered epithelial cell with loss of the nucleus and

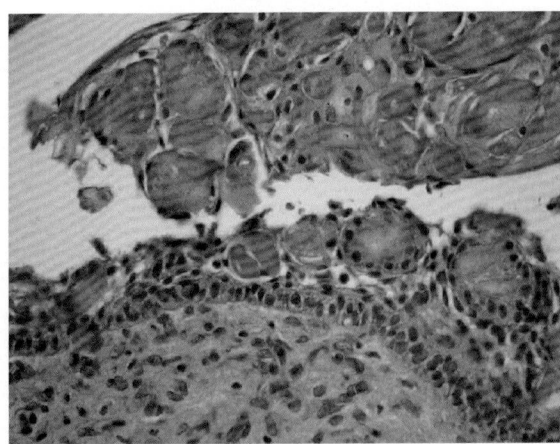

Figure 132.3 Calcifying odontogenic cyst (Gorlin cyst). Cyst lined by odontogenic epithelium. The basal cells are palisaded and columnar. Large, eosinophilic "ghost cells" are seen within and on the surface of the epithelium.

bright eosinophilic cytoplasm—that represents abnormal keratinization. With time, these ghost cells tend to become calcified, sometimes even forming calcified masses. When these cells contact the connective tissue, a foreign body reaction occurs due to the release of keratin.

Treatment and Prognosis

Surgical enucleation usually results in complete resolution. The extraosseous lesions are often associated with other odontogenic tumors and due to their low recurrence potential are managed conservatively with lesion removal only.

Glandular Odontogenic Cyst (Sialo-Odontogenic Cyst)

The glandular odontogenic cyst was first described in 1987 (7). Although only a few cases have been reported, it is worth mentioning due to its locally aggressive behavior and its propensity to recur. This lesion is generally considered odontogenic in origin with numerous mucus-secreting cells within its epithelial lining.

Clinical and Radiographic Features

This lesion occurs most commonly in middle-aged adults. The majority of glandular odontogenic cysts have been reported in the mandible especially in the anterior region. They appear as multilocular radiolucencies and may cross the midline.

Histopathology

This lesion has several unique microscopic features: (a) an epithelial lining of variable thickness and a flat epithelial–connective tissue junction; (b) small microcysts and gland-like structures within the epithelial lining; and (c) a single layer of cuboidal or columnar cells lining the gland-like structures (Fig. 132.4).

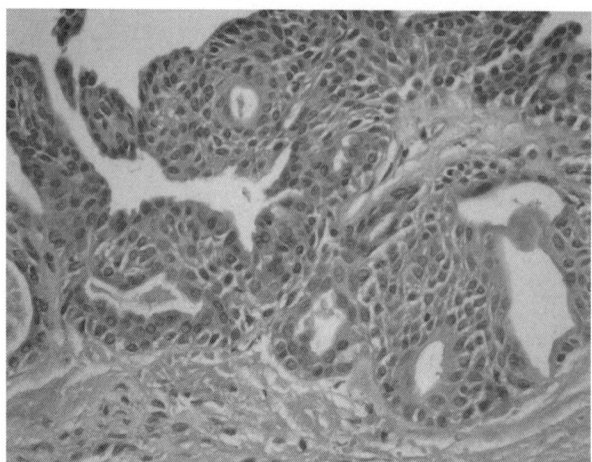

Figure 132.4 Glandular odontogenic cyst. Stratified squamous epithelium forming gland-like structures.

Treatment and Prognosis

Most glandular odontogenic cysts are amenable to enucleation and curettage. However, due to its recurrence potential, some advocate marginal resection (8). Regardless, long-term follow-up is advisable.

NONODONTOGENIC CYSTS

Nasopalatine Duct Cyst (Incisive Canal Cyst)

The nasopalatine duct cyst originates from the epithelial remnants of the two embryonic nasopalatine ducts (9). The majority of these cysts arise in the anterior maxilla near the incisive foramen.

Clinical and Radiographic Features

Men are affected twice as often as females, and this cyst occurs most frequently in the fourth to sixth decades. The nasopalatine duct cyst is either asymptomatic or presents as a soft tissue swelling in the midline of the anterior hard palate once the lesion has perforated the bone. The lesion is typically a well-circumscribed, oval-pear or heart-shaped, unilocular radiolucency in the midline of the anterior palate. If the cyst reaches large proportions, it can resorb the roots of the adjacent teeth. Some normal incisive canals are radiographically wide, which may make diagnosis of this lesion less precise. It is generally accepted that any radiographic lesion greater than 6 mm should be considered a cyst and not an enlarged incisive foramen. If no soft tissue or bony swellings are present and the patient is asymptomatic, then a diagnosis of nasopalatine duct cyst becomes unlikely.

Histopathology

The lining of this lesion can be either stratified squamous epithelium, ciliated columnar or cuboidal epithelium, or a combination of the two. This variable lining reflects whether the cyst has arrived from epithelium closer to the palate (stratified squamous) or more closely associated with the nasal cavity (ciliated columnar). The fibrous tissue contains elements of nerve and vascular tissue consistent with the surrounding incisive canal contents. Mucus glands are occasionally seen within the wall of the cyst as these glands are native to the adjacent nasal cavity.

Treatment and Prognosis

Surgical enucleation is usually curative, but may result in sacrificing the nasopalatine nerve and vessel, resulting in denervation of the mucosa of the anterior palate and maxillary incisors. Recurrence is rare.

Stafne Bone Cyst (Lingual Salivary Gland Depression, Static Bone Cyst)

The Stafne bone cyst is not a true cyst. Rather, it is a depression on the lingual aspect of the posterior body of the mandible. This condition has a pathognomonic radiographic appearance of a small ovoid, well-circumscribed radiolucency often surrounded by cortical bone, located below the inferior alveolar canal in the second or third molar region. This radiographic appearance is due to the relative thinning of the mandible. Most reported cases have occurred in males. Sialography, biopsy, and autopsy have revealed that the depression is characteristically filled with an accessory lateral lobe of the submandibular salivary gland, although occasionally connective tissue, adipose tissue, and lymphoid tissue have been seen (10). No treatment is required.

Idiopathic Bone Cavity (Traumatic Bone Cyst or Traumatic Bone Cavity)

The traumatic bone cavity is not a true cyst because it does not contain a true epithelial lining. It is usually found in the posterior mandible and presents on radiograph as a less well-defined radiolucency compared to most odontogenic cysts. These lesions are typically empty on surgical exploration or contain some straw-colored fluid. There is no lining or tissue to submit for biopsy, but exploration of the lesion will be curative, since hemorrhage within the cavity will allow for granulation tissue formation and ultimate resolution of this condition.

ODONTOGENIC TUMORS

Odontogenic tumors are collectively a rare but diverse and complicated group of lesions. They arise from epithelial or mesenchymal cells, or both, that are associated with tooth structures. Most odontogenic tumors are true neoplasms, but some behave as hamartomatous growths. Odontogenic tumors commonly present as asymptomatic swellings, which can eventually cause bone loss, tooth displacement, and jaw expansion. They rarely cause sensory nerve dysfunction. Understanding the biologic behavior of this group of lesions will assist in choosing the appropriate treatment to best attain a cure or to optimize the outcome (11,12). The tumors discussed in this chapter were selected based upon their frequency, locally aggressive behavior, and/or likelihood of recurrence.

Odontoma

Odontomas are not true neoplasms, but rather hamarto-matous growths because they form during normal tooth development and then reach a fixed size. The lesion contains elements of enamel, dentin, cementum, and pulp tissue. Depending on the degree of morphologic differentiation, an odontoma can be classified as either compound, if the lesion resembles tooth-like structures or complex, if the lesion appears as an amorphous mass.

Clinical and Radiographic Features

The odontoma is the most common odontogenic "tumor." The lesion is typically asymptomatic and is discovered in the first two decades on radiographic examination, often initiated to evaluate lack of expected eruption of a permanent tooth. Radiographically, both the compound and complex odontomas are radiopaque masses and have a well-demarcated border. The compound odontoma resembles multiple tiny tooth structures, while the complex odontoma appears as a dense irregular mass.

Histopathology

Although reduced enamel epithelium may be present, odontomas are essentially composed of enamel, dentin, cementum, and pulp tissue. Fibrous tissue is sparse.

Treatment and Prognosis

Removal of the lesion may be necessary to rule out other lesions or if the mass is impeding the eruption of a tooth. Enucleation and curettage is considered curative, and the lesion is not known to recur.

Keratocystic Odontogenic Tumor (Odontogenic Keratocyst)

The KCOT is a uni- or multicystic, intrabony lesion of odontogenic origin. It develops from remnants of the dental lamina and can occur in any location of the jaws (13,14). Its previous traditional term, odontogenic keratocyst (OKC), emphasized the benign behavior of this lesion. However, in 2005, the WHO Working Group recommended the newer term KCOT because it more accurately described its neoplastic behavior (15). These lesions mimic the radiographic appearance of any other odontogenic cyst and some odontogenic tumors. The mandibular ramus and posterior body are the most common locations for the KCOT (Fig. 132.5A and B). The KCOT in the maxilla typically favors the posterior or canine regions.

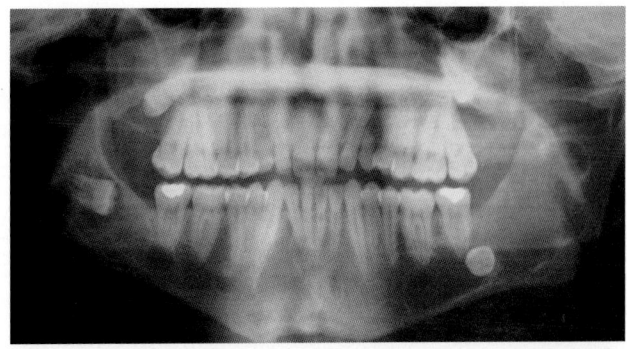

A

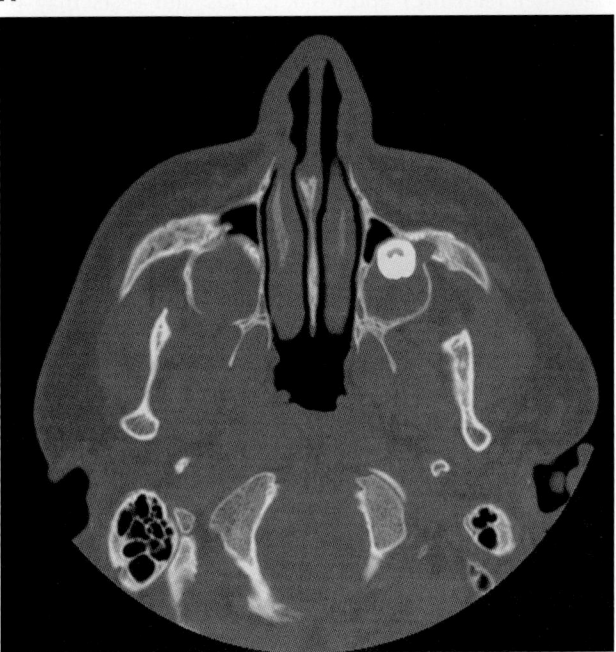

B

Figure 132.5 A: Keratocystic odontogenic tumor. Panoramic radiograph of a 18-year-old man with bilateral mandibular and maxillary KCOT. Patient also had NBCCS. **B:** Axial computed tomography (CT) scan of same patient, revealing bilateral maxillary lesions. Lesions were noted to extend to the orbital floors intraoperatively.

Clinical and Radiographic Features

The KCOT differs from other odontogenic lesions with regard to its growth potential and recurrence rate. It can display aggressive growth, causing bony expansion and destruction, and reports have shown recurrence rates from 5% to 60% (16,17). The KCOT occurs over a wide age range; however, its peak incidence is within the second and third decades. When multiple KCOTs occur in a patient, the nevoid basal cell carcinoma syndrome (NBCCS) must be considered. The mean age of patients with multiple KCOTs, with or without NBCCS, is lower than those with single, nonrecurrent KCOTs. Radiographically, the KCOT appears as a well-circumscribed radiolucency with a distinct border, and many cause bony expansion or erosion of either cortex. Involved teeth may become displaced, but root resorption rarely occurs.

Histopathology

The KCOT has the following distinct microscopic appearance: its lining is parakeratinized, stratified squamous epithelium, which is six to eight cell layers thick; the luminal surface is covered by a corrugated layer of parakeratin; the basal layer is palisaded and cuboidal, with prominent, intensely stained hyperchromatic nuclei; and a lack of rete pegs. This flat epithelial–connective tissue interface results in a separation of the epithelium on histopathologic processing. Exfoliated parakeratin often fills the cyst lumen and presents during surgery as a creamy, white material. Daughter (satellite) epithelial islands and cysts may be seen in the surrounding connective tissue and may be indicative of the NBCCS.

Treatment and Prognosis

The KCOT requires surgical enucleation and osseous curettage, and every attempt should be made to remove it in one piece (18). Modified Carnoy solution is a tissue fixative that can aid in a more complete lesion removal. Treatment of the residual bony cavity may devitalize microscopic remnants, thus decreasing the chance of recurrence (19,20). Some clinicians have advocated marginal resection to avoid recurrence (21). When large lesions are present, marsupialization may be performed to decompress the KCOT to allow for easier removal of the cyst at a later surgery (22,23). Secondary infection, need for high patient compliance, and variable results limit the use of marsupialization techniques. Most recurrences occur within 5 years, but reports of recurrence as long as 10 years later have been documented. Thus, close follow-up is mandatory. Recurrence of KCOT has been speculated based on several theories: incomplete removal of the cyst due to its thin friable membrane and adherence to adjacent tissues, residual satellite cysts following enucleation, and remnants of dental lamina not associated with the KCOT in question causing de novo cyst formation. The orthokeratinized odontogenic cyst is considered by some to be a unique cyst, and by others to be a variant of the KCOT. It is much less common than the KCOT and has a much lower recurrence rate (24). Unlike the KCOT, the orthokeratinized odontogenic cyst is lined by orthokeratinized stratified squamous epithelium. There is a prominent granular layer below a noncorrugated surface, and the basal layer is less prominent.

Nevoid Basal Cell Carcinoma Syndrome (Basal Cell Nevus Syndrome, Gorlin Syndrome)

The NBCCS is an autosomal dominant inherited condition that exhibits high penetrance and variable expressivity (25,26). It is a result of a mutation of the PTCH tumor suppressor gene located on chromosome 9q22.3-q31. Patients may manifest a combination of the following clinical and radiographic features: multiple KCOTs of the jaws, multiple basal cell carcinomas of both exposed

and non–sun-exposed areas, frontal bossing, mandibular prognathism, palmar and plantar pitting, bifid ribs, and calcification of the falx cerebri. The KCOTs associated with NBCCS should be treated in a similar manner as an isolated KCOT. However, increased vigilance with 6 month or yearly clinical follow-up and imaging (panoramic radiograph or computerized tomography) are warranted to allow early detection of new lesions. This is particularly true of children and adolescents. Once adulthood is reached, the formation of new KCOTs is less problematic, but the risk of basal cell carcinomas rises. Other than the skin lesions and those conditions that may be correctable, many of the other related abnormalities do not require any surgical intervention. Genetic counseling should be recommended to both the patient and family members due to the condition's autosomal dominant inheritance.

Ameloblastoma

With the exception of the odontoma, the ameloblastoma is the most common odontogenic tumor (27). It arises from any number of residual epithelial elements of tooth development: reduced enamel epithelium, rests of Serres, rests of Malassez, or the basal layer of the oral mucosa. The lesion can also develop from within a dental follicle or a dentigerous cyst (3). Some confusion has arisen regarding the classification schema of ameloblastomas. Most references broadly categorize ameloblastomas into one of three groups: unicystic, solid or multicystic, or peripheral ameloblastomas. A misuse of terms and/or a lack of understanding of these same terms with their overlapping meanings can lead to an inadequate treatment decision, increasing the likelihood of recurrence. One example is the term *unicystic* ameloblastoma. Unicystic ameloblastoma generally implies being amenable to enucleation and curettage. An invasive ameloblastoma may be unicystic, having just one cystic space. However, that does not suggest that this invasive lesion should be treated by enucleation and curettage merely because it was defined, properly or not, as a unicystic ameloblastoma.

Clinical and Radiographic Features

This benign, locally aggressive neoplasm is characterized by a slow growth pattern and may grow to profound proportions, causing gross facial deformities. It is usually asymptomatic and does not alter sensory nerve function. The posterior mandible appears to be a preferred site. The lesion has a very wide age range with a peak occurrence in the third and fourth decades, and it has no sex predilection. Radiographically, the lesion can appear as a unilocular or multilocular radiolucency with ill-defined borders, making it difficult to determine the exact size of the lesion. Buccal and lingual cortical expansion is common, even progressing to cortical perforation (Fig. 132.6A and B). Tooth displacement and root resorption can occur but infrequently. A variant, the desmoplastic ameloblastoma, is commonly

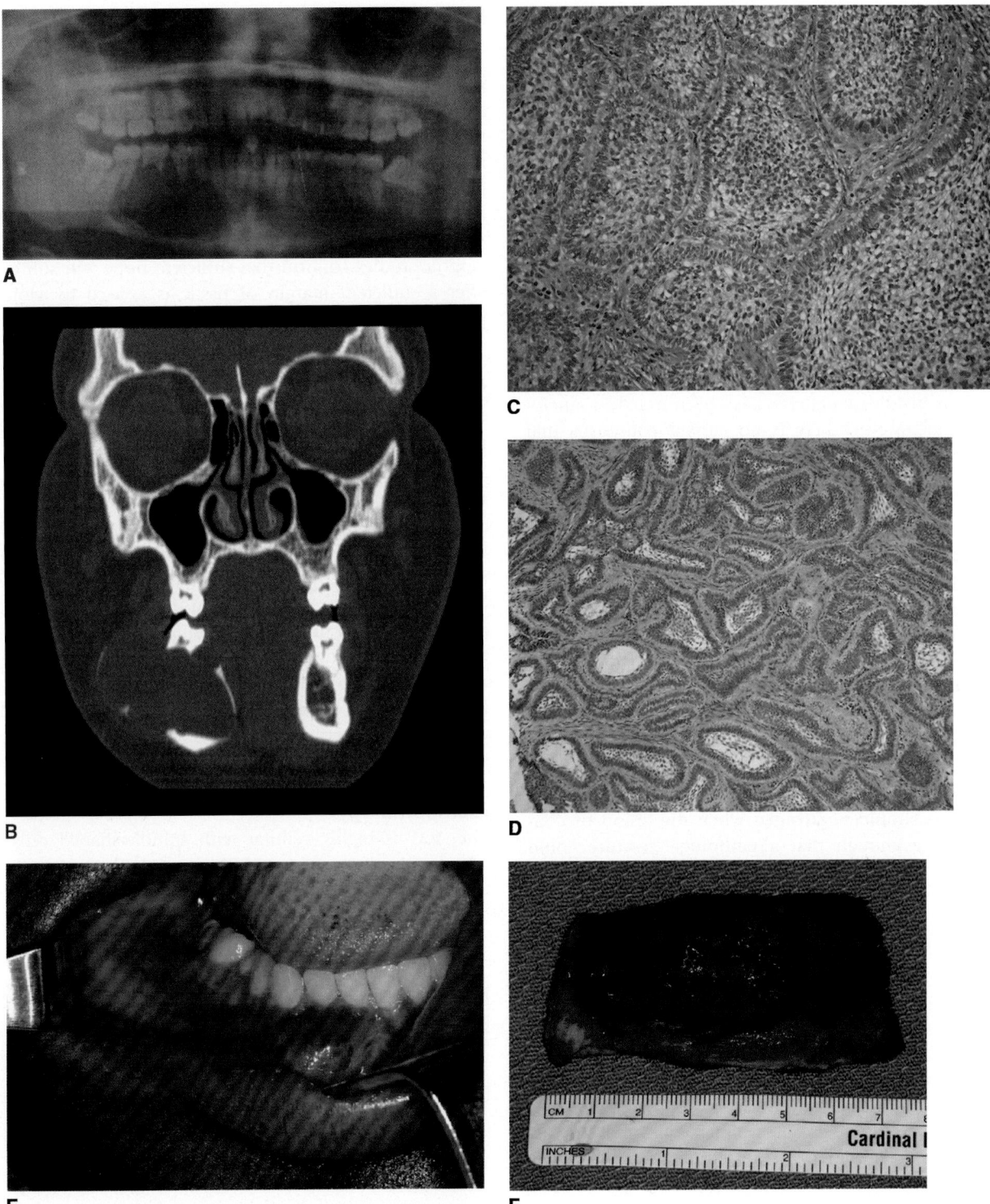

Figure 132.6 A: Ameloblastoma. Panoramic radiograph of a 17-year-old girl with unilocular ameloblastoma of right mandible. Note resorption of multiple tooth roots in right mandible. **B:** Coronal computed tomography (CT) scan of maxillofacial bones of patient from **(A)**. Note extreme buccal and lingual cortical expansion of right mandible. Focal areas of perforation were noted intraoperatively. **C:** Ameloblastoma (follicular pattern). Islands of odontogenic epithelium characterized by peripheral columnar cells exhibiting reverse polarity. The central portion of these islands resemble stellate reticulum in areas. **D:** Ameloblastoma (plexiform pattern). **E:** Preoperative photo of patient from previous images. Note significant vestibular expansion. Right mandibular teeth exhibited significant clinical mobility. **F:** A resection of the right mandible from the angle to the contralateral parasymphysis through a neck incision. Focal areas of buccal cortical perforation were noted intraoperatively. Specimen is viewed from the buccal aspect.

found in the anterior maxilla or mandible. It contains dense connective tissue, and thus has a more opaque radiographic appearance. Another variant, the peripheral ameloblastoma, is usually present on the gingival and has no radiographic features, except perhaps a "cupping" of underlying alveolar bone.

Histopathology

Ameloblastomas are histologically diverse. They may exhibit areas of focal variation, so adequate sampling must be undertaken. The ameloblastoma is unencapsulated, so it typically exhibits an infiltrative growth pattern into surrounding tissues. The basal cells in the epithelium are columnar and hyperchromatic. The nuclei are polarized away from the basement membrane ("reverse polarity"). Numerous histologic patterns have been noted in ameloblastomas; however, there is no current consensus that these different histologic patterns have different biologic behaviors (28,29). The two most frequent patterns are the follicular and plexiform (Fig. 132.6C and D).

Treatment and Prognosis

The primary treatment principle for any intrabony ameloblastoma is complete removal, regardless of the technique, due to its locally destructive potential and high risk for recurrence (30). Enucleation and curettage was once considered the recommended treatment for the unicystic ameloblastoma. However, curettage of the bone adjacent to an ameloblastoma is now discouraged because of the risk of seeding foci of ameloblastoma either deeper into the bone or into adjacent tissues. Furthermore, enucleation alone should be avoided when the lesion of concern is large enough that a pathologic fracture could occur. Recurrence rates between 15% and 35% have been reported with unicystic ameloblastomas treated by enucleation and curettage alone. A 1.0- to 1.5-cm bony margin is recommended for a unicystic ameloblastoma. When an ameloblastoma grows into or completely through the connective tissue layer surrounding the lesion, or if it recurs, then a more aggressive treatment is required. When resection is warranted, one uninvolved overlying anatomic barrier margin is advocated (Fig. 132.6E and F) (3). A bony margin of 1.5 to 2.0 cm is recommended for solid or multicystic ameloblastomas. When hard and soft tissue margins are negative, a cure rate of nearly 98% can be achieved. Recurrence rates as high as 90% have been reported when more aggressive ameloblastomas are inadvertently, or inadequately, treated with curettage. A 5-year follow-up is required, but a 10-year follow-up is prudent. When metastases have been reported, the lesions were histologically benign like the primary tumor. These lesions are referred to as *malignant ameloblastomas*, although they do not show cytologic features typically associated with malignancy. When the primary lesion is found to contain cytologic features of malignancy, it is classified as an *ameloblastic carcinoma.*

Peripheral Ameloblastoma

The peripheral variant of the ameloblastoma is a soft tissue mass involving the gingiva and mucosa that often causes separation of involved teeth (31). If radiographs confirm involvement of the underlying alveolar bone, then a block resection containing the involved mucosa, underlying periosteum, alveolar bone, and teeth, is performed. A 1.0- to 1.5-cm margin of uninvolved tissue is recommended. An en bloc resection is not necessary if supportive radiographic studies confirm that sufficient bone will still exist after a sufficient margin of tissue is excised to avoid a pathologic fracture.

Adenomatoid Odontogenic Tumor

The AOT is a benign hamartoma of odontogenic epithelium characterized by slow, progressive growth.

Clinical and Radiographic Features

The AOT typically occurs in adolescent or teen females. It has a strong predilection for the anterior maxilla and is often associated with an unerupted canine tooth (32). Most AOTs are less than 3 cm in diameter, but they can approach significant size and cause pain and displace tooth roots. Radiographically, the AOT usually is a well-circumscribed unilocular radiolucency associated with an impacted tooth. Some lesions may have radiographically evident small foci of calcifications. Root resorption is rarely seen with the AOT, and is typically mild.

Histopathology

The AOT is highly cellular with spindle-shaped cells in whorls or rosettes (Fig. 132.7). Enameloid, dentinoid, or cementum-like material can be found throughout this lesion. These calcifications suggest the lesion's development

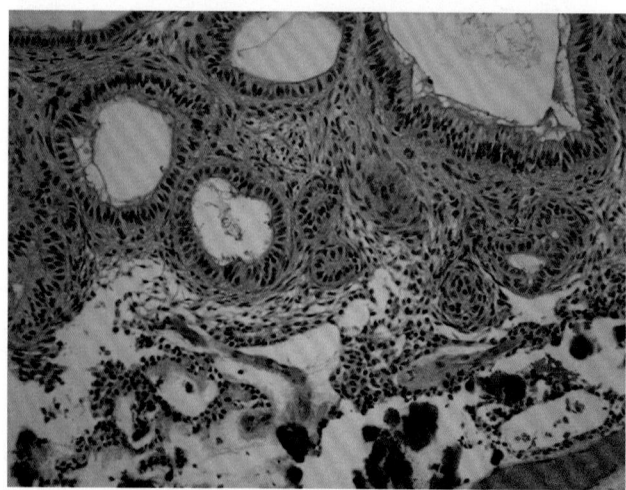

Figure 132.7 Adenomatoid odontogenic cyst. Odontogenic epithelium forming duct-like structures lined by columnar cells exhibiting reverse polarity. Calcifications, a common feature of this lesion, are seen in the lower right portion.

from Hertwig root sheath. These lesions can be mistaken for ameloblastoma by an inexperienced pathologist. If the demographic and radiographic features are not consistent with a diagnosis of ameloblastoma, a second opinion should be sought.

Treatment and Prognosis

Recurrence is not seen in this benign encapsulated lesion, so enucleation and curettage alone is curative. If the capsule is inflamed and becomes compromised during enucleation of the lesion, the surgeon should thoroughly irrigate the surgical field. Bony regeneration of the defect usually occurs in about 1 year in younger patients.

Calcifying Epithelial Odontogenic Tumor (CEOT, Pindborg Tumor)

The calcifying epithelial odontogenic tumor (CEOT) is a rare odontogenic tumor, representing less than 1% of all odontogenic tumors. It originates from the epithelial rests of the dental lamina or reduced enamel epithelium. The CEOT has distinct histologic features and a variable radiographic appearance. Like the ameloblastoma, it is considered a locally aggressive neoplasm that can be highly infiltrative and destructive and must be surgically excised (33,34).

Clinical and Radiographic Features

The CEOT has been reported in patients over a wide age range, but has a peak incidence in the fifth decade. It presents as a slow-growing, firm, painless swelling usually in the posterior mandible. The molar area is the most frequent region in either jaw. Like most other benign odontogenic tumors, the CEOT does not alter nerve function. A peripheral variant exists and typically presents as a soft tissue swelling in the anterior aspect of the mouth (35). Most of these lesions appear as diffuse radiolucent lesions, unless they are large or mature; then they will exhibit areas of faint opacities consistent with the presence of calcifications in the lesion. It is typically associated with the crown of an impacted tooth. Radiographic borders are variable, ranging from distinct lines to diffuse opacified areas fusing with adjacent bone.

Histopathology

The most common pattern of the CEOT is one of sheets or strands of polyhedral epithelial cells connected by intercellular bridges. The nuclei have prominent nucleoli, and the cells may even appear pleomorphic, but this does not imply a malignant state, and mitotic figures are not routinely found. Scattered calcifications are a distinct feature of the CEOT, and the calcifications form concentric rings referred to as *Liesegang rings*. Another histologic variant containing clear cell features has been described and associated with increased clinical aggressiveness (36). Large areas of amorphous eosinophilic material are dispersed throughout the lesion. These areas stain positive for amyloid with Congo red, crystal violet, or thioflavin T. This prominent amyloid presence is another unique characteristic feature of the CEOT (37).

Treatment and Prognosis

Much like the ameloblastoma, the CEOT is treated by resection, but no current study has stated an adequate bony margin to achieve a cure. A minimum of a 1.0-cm bony margin along with any necessary soft tissue to still achieve one layer of an uninvolved anatomic barrier is recommended unless determined otherwise by a frozen section. Recurrence has been reported, so long-term follow-up is recommended. The *peripheral* variant is treated by local excision with a 5-mm margin, which should include the underlying periosteum. The remaining wound may be closed either primarily or by local advancement flaps.

Odontogenic Myxoma

The odontogenic myxoma, although a rare tumor, is worthy of mention due to its locally aggressive behavior and high recurrence rate due to its infiltrative nature. In the jaw bones, it is derived from odontogenic ectomesenchyme that is very similar to the mesenchymal tissue of the follicular sac or dental papilla. The odontogenic myxoma only rarely occurs in non–tooth-bearing portions of the jaws or other facial bones (38).

Clinical and Radiographic Features

The odontogenic myxoma has some clinical and radiographic features in common with the ameloblastoma. It is usually asymptomatic and slow growing. It rarely displaces teeth or resorbs roots and does not alter sensory function. Although it has been reported over a wide age range, it is most commonly seen in the third decade, which is slightly younger than the peak occurrence of the ameloblastoma. The lesion has been reported in all portions of both jaws, but usually occurs in the posterior mandible. Radiographically, the lesion is radiolucent and more often multilocular, but can be unilocular (Fig. 132.8). The lesion also has been described as having a "honeycomb" appearance, with its faint, wispy trabecular bone mixed within cortical plate displacement.

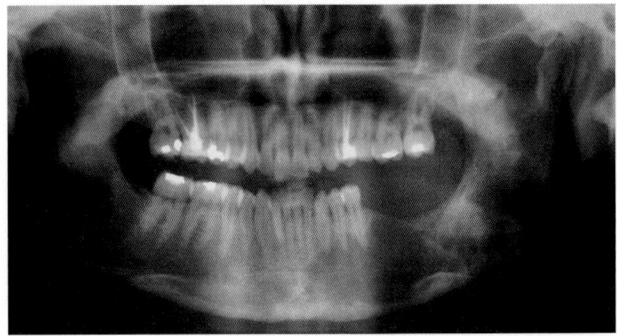

Figure 132.8 Odontogenic myxoma. Panoramic radiograph revealing diffuse, mixed radiolucent/radiopaque involvement of left hemimandible. Lesion extends from midline up to sigmoid notch.

Histopathology

The odontogenic myxoma is an infiltrative and gelatinous tumor. It contains scant, randomly arranged spindle-shaped mesenchymal cells within a myxoid ground substance, which stains predominantly basophilic with hematoxylin and eosin. When these lesions have a more significant collagenous component, they are referred to as myxofibromas or fibromyxomas. However, this classification does not alter the lesion's clinical behavior.

Treatment and Prognosis

Curative treatment requires resection with a 1.0-cm bony margin and a layer of overlying soft tissue. The lesion is unencapsulated, so infiltration into adjacent bone is common making recurrence likely if only enucleation and curettage is undertaken. Enucleation and curettage may be considered only for small, unilocular lesions (less than 1 cm in diameter), but aggressive bony curettage is recommended. The inferior alveolar nerve is not routinely sacrificed, even in large lesions that require an en bloc resection, unless the nerve has been significantly compromised by the lesion.

Ameloblastic Fibroma

The ameloblastic fibroma is a true neoplasm composed of both odontogenic epithelium and ectomesenchyme. The epithelium resembles dental lamina or ameloblastoma, and the mesenchyme resembles the developing dental papilla or myxoma.

Clinical and Radiographic Features

The ameloblastic fibroma is a tumor of young patients with rare occurrence over the age of 40. It presents as a painless swelling usually in the third molar region of the mandible. Enlargement of the affected jaw is the only frequent clinical sign. The lesion can be either a unilocular or multilocular radiolucency with a sclerotic border. It often occurs over an unerupted tooth and can displace the tooth but does not cause root resorption. The ameloblastic fibroma does not have a pathognomonic radiographic feature and can resemble a dentigerous cyst.

Histopathology

Microscopically, the tumor consists of islands of odontogenic epithelium resembling the dental lamina and cap stage of odontogenesis. This columnar epithelium is palisaded and shows striking nuclear polarity similar to that of the ameloblastoma (Fig. 132.9). The stroma is myxoid in appearance, resembling the dental papilla, a cell-rich myxoid tissue.

Treatment and Prognosis

The ameloblastic fibroma can be cured through enucleation and curettage since it is well encapsulated. Owing to its predilection for young patients, the bony defect will repair itself

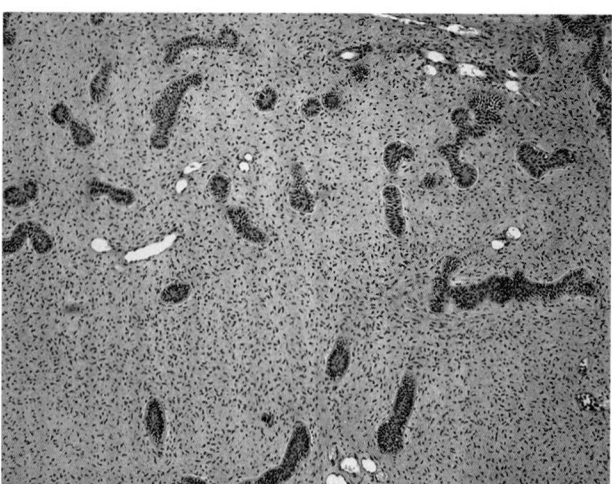

Figure 132.9 Ameloblastic fibroma. Cords of odontogenic epithelium in a background of cellular, primitive mesenchymal tissue.

within approximately 1 year. Larger lesions (greater than 5 cm) may require a resection based on the specific anatomic boundaries involved. Reported recurrences were likely due to regrowth of the tumor, which is not completely unusual for embryonal-type tumors. A diagnosis of ameloblastic fibrosarcoma should be considered if this lesion recurs.

RELATED JAW LESIONS

Various nonodontogenic lesions of the jaws are worthy of mention due to their biologic behavior as well as the diagnostic and surgical challenges they pose. Some believe that these conditions may indeed be odontogenic because many are only found in the jaws even though they do not reveal histological features consistent with odontogenic-derived structures.

Torus

A torus is a developmental overgrowth rather than a tumor or hamartoma and is thought to arise due to bone stress (39). It develops in one of two intraoral sites. When it occurs on the midline of the palate, it is termed *torus palatinus*. When tori occur on the lingual aspect of the mandible, they are typically bilateral and adjacent to the canine/bicuspid region. These are termed *torus mandibularis* or lingual tori. When a histologically similar lesion develops on the buccal aspect of either jaw, the lesion is referred to as an *exostosis*.

Clinical and Radiographic Features

The palatal torus develops after puberty. It can be found in approximately 20% of adults and has a slow growth pattern. Palatal tori can either have a smooth ovoid appearance or multiple pedunculated loculations, but both presentations should have normal pink overlying mucosa. Tori can grow to large dimensions, impairing speech or feeding or prohibiting fabrication of a maxillary prosthesis (Fig. 132.10). Also, large lesions are often prone to mucosal ulceration

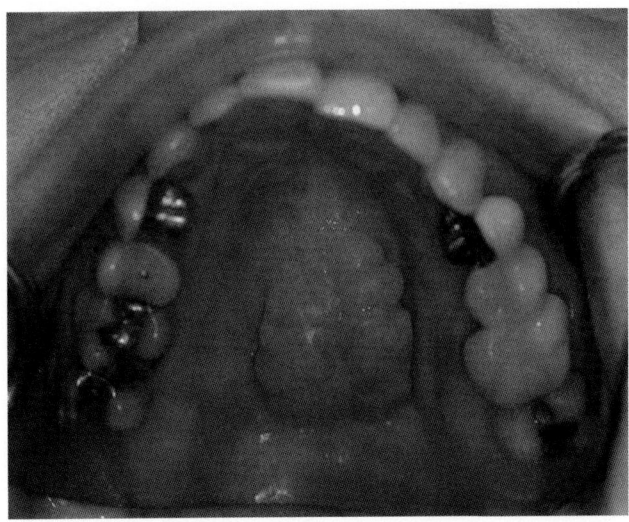

Figure 132.10 Palatal torus.

from mastication. These larger lesions may require surgical excision. Mandibular tori are commonly bilateral and also have a slow growth pattern. They too can reach sizable dimensions, adversely affecting speech or feeding or the use of a lower prosthesis.

Histopathology

Tori consist of nodular masses of dense cortical, lamellar bone with central trabecular bone containing few areas of fibrofatty marrow.

Treatment and Prognosis

Tori only require removal if they interfere with normal function or the fabrication and placement of a prosthesis such as a denture. An elliptical or double-Y-shaped mucosal incision is designed, and the lesion is taken down to the level of surrounding bone with a rotary instrument. The torus can also be scored in the shape of a cross with a surgical drill then removed with an osteotome and mallet. Care must be taken not to perforate through the nasal floor. A surgical stent can be created preoperatively so that the surgical site can be postoperatively protected from irritation from either the tongue or foods. Removal of mandibular tori requires attention to the submandibular salivary ducts when one is using an osteotome and mallet to excise these lesions. A drill can be used to make vertical cuts along the inner aspect of the torus between the lesion and the alveolus. An osteotome is then used to outfracture the torus. Then a rotary instrument is used to smooth the edges of the lingual shelf prior to closure of the flap.

Osteoma

Osteomas are hamartomas or reactive proliferations of bone and are not considered to be true tumors. They are composed of dense compact bone and arise either on the surface of bone (*periosteal osteoma*) or within bone (*endosteal*

osteoma). When multiple osteomas are present, one should consider that the patient may have *Gardner syndrome*, an autosomal dominant condition also associated with intestinal polyposis, epidermoid cysts, and desmoid tumors of the skin, impacted normal and supernumerary teeth, and odontomas (40). The formation of the osteomas will usually precede other manifestations of the syndrome. If this syndrome is suspected, the appropriate referral should be made to rule out intestinal lesions, particularly polyps, which have a high rate of malignant transformation to colorectal cancer. The frequency of malignant transformation is essentially 100% in these patients as they reach older age.

Clinical and Radiographic Features

These slow-growing, asymptomatic exophytic bony masses occur in either jaw in areas not typically affected by tori or exostoses. The mandibular angle is a common location. The lesion is usually an incidental finding on routine radiographic evaluation and appears as a well-circumscribed radiopaque mass.

Histopathology

Osteomas have similar microscopic features as tori or exostoses. The periosteum can be more active in the osteoma than the other two lesions.

Treatment and Prognosis

Asymptomatic single lesions can be followed clinically and radiographically. Those lesions requiring biopsy are surgically excised with little chance for recurrence.

Osteochondroma

Osteochondromas are benign hamartomas that develop most commonly in long bones, but also occur in the mandibular condyle or coronoid process (41). The lesion is believed to be associated with proliferation of epiphyseal cartilage into the surrounding tissues.

Clinical and Radiographic Features

The absence of this lesion in other portions of the mandible, skull, or facial bones serves to confirm its development in endochondral bone. Osteochondromas are lesions of younger patients, usually occurring in the second and third decades, and are found in twice as many males as females. The lesion is slow growing and known to cause swelling and pain along with deviation of the teeth and chin point toward the unaffected side. Radiographically, it appears as an irregular "popcorn-like" radiopaque mass on the medial side of the condyle or replacing the coronoid process (Fig. 132.11A and B).

Histopathology

Osteochondromas are bony masses that have a cartilaginous cap. Endochondral ossification is noted between the cartilage and bone (Fig. 132.11C).

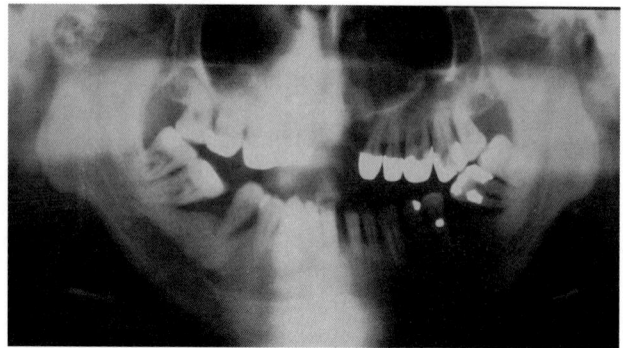

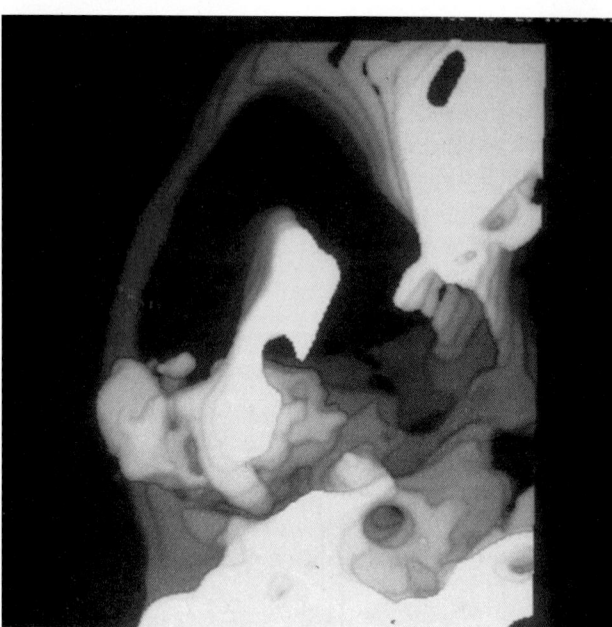

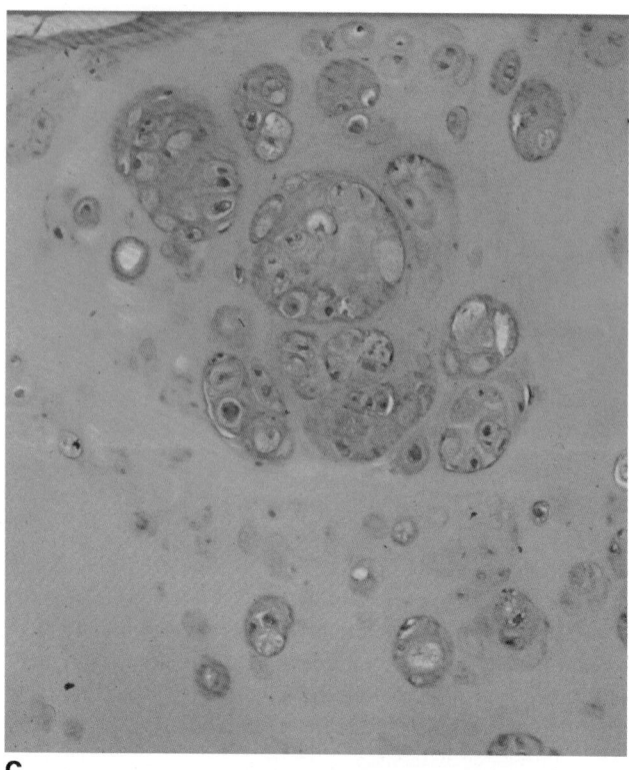

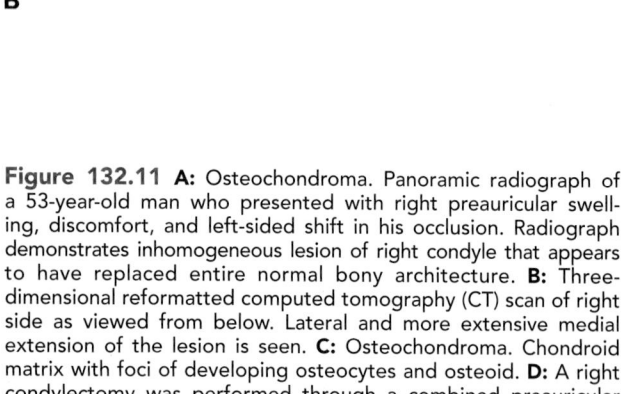

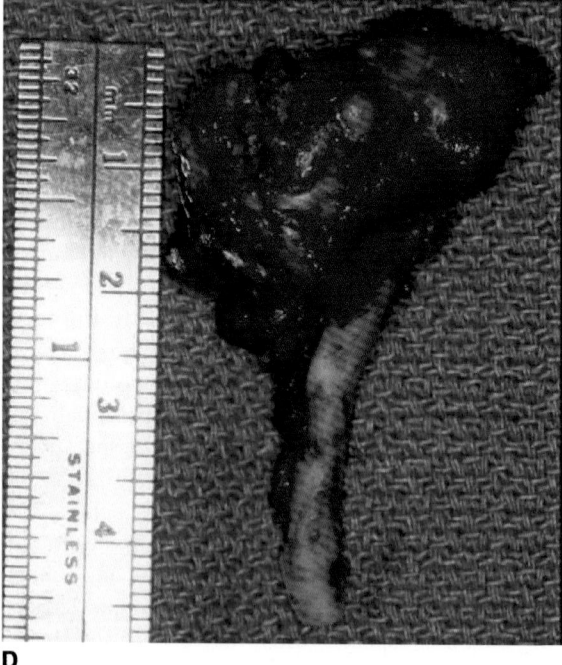

Figure 132.11 A: Osteochondroma. Panoramic radiograph of a 53-year-old man who presented with right preauricular swelling, discomfort, and left-sided shift in his occlusion. Radiograph demonstrates inhomogeneous lesion of right condyle that appears to have replaced entire normal bony architecture. **B:** Three-dimensional reformatted computed tomography (CT) scan of right side as viewed from below. Lateral and more extensive medial extension of the lesion is seen. **C:** Osteochondroma. Chondroid matrix with foci of developing osteocytes and osteoid. **D:** A right condylectomy was performed through a combined preauricular and retromandibular approach. A soft tissue capsule surrounding entire region was encountered. Specimen seen from anterior view.

Treatment and Prognosis

Lesions affecting the coronoid process are managed by a coronoidectomy with minimal removal of the attached temporalis muscle tendon. Lesions of the condyle are treated by condylectomy with a preauricular as well as a neck incision (Fig. 132.11D). Immediate reconstruction can be treatment planned with either a costochondral graft or an alloplastic condyle. Recurrence is very rare.

Ossifying Fibroma (Cementoossifying Fibroma)

Ossifying fibromas are true benign neoplasms of mesenchymal origin that have a strong predilection for the tooth-bearing portion of the jaws, although they have been reported in long bones (42). This slow-growing expansile lesion can reach enormous dimensions resulting in profound facial disfigurement.

Clinical and Radiographic Features

The typical patient with an ossifying fibroma is a woman in her second to fourth decade, although the lesion has been reported over a wide age range and in both sexes. Immature lesions initially present as a radiolucency, but become more mixed as they mature and eventually can become completely radiopaque. More aggressive lesions expand the cortices of the jaws and frequently displace adjacent structures. In the mandible, they typically appear as a mid-body growth at the inferior border, enlarging outward and downward as if "hanging off the lower lateral border" of the mandible.

Histopathology

Ossifying fibromas are well demarcated from the surrounding bone and are composed of dense cellular fibrous tissue with variable amounts of calcified trabeculae of osteoid or bone and/or spherical cementum-like structures (Fig. 132.12). The ossifying fibroma is usually well circumscribed and does not exhibit diffuse infiltration of adjacent tissues, unlike fibrous dysplasia.

Treatment and Prognosis

These lesions are amenable to enucleation and curettage if detected early, or resection for larger lesions. Because ossifying fibromas do not display aggressive infiltration of surrounding tissues, for those requiring surgical resection due to large size or problematic location, a conservative 5-mm margin is appropriate, and recurrence is rare. The juvenile (aggressive) ossifying fibroma is a rare variant of the above and is considered a more aggressive lesion, appearing at a younger age with a predilection for the maxilla.

Fibrous Dysplasia

Fibrous dysplasia is not a true neoplasm; rather, it is a genetic, tumor-like condition where normal medullary bone is replaced with fibrous connective tissue mixed with irregular bony trabeculae. Fibrous dysplasia most commonly occurs in one bone (*monostotic*), or more rarely multiple bones (*polyostotic*). Polyostotic fibrous dysplasia may be seen as a component of *McCune-Albright syndrome*, which includes café-au-lait skin macules, and multiple endocrinopathies, including hyperthyroidism and/or precocious puberty (43). Although genetically based, it is usually a sporadic condition involving a mutation in the α-subunit of a signal-transducing G protein.

Clinical and Radiographic Features

Fibrous dysplasia is a slow-growing, typically asymptomatic process that often produces a bony hard swelling (Fig. 132.13A–C). The condition can be self-limiting, beginning in the first decade and ceasing when the affected bone reaches maximum growth and maturation. It is capable of tooth displacement with resultant malocclusion. Lesions located in the paranasal sinuses can cause nasal obstruction. Fibrous dysplasia involving the midface, calvarium, or skull base can cause progressive severe facial distortion and cranial nerve dysfunction via compression. In such individuals, serial visual acuity and audiology testing correlated with 1-mm cut computerized tomography is warranted to monitor progression and guide timing of any necessary surgical intervention. Early lesions are radiolucent but become more opaque as the lesion matures. The normal medullary bone is replaced with a fine trabecular bone, giving the lesion its "ground-glass" appearance on radiographs. Fibrous dysplasia does expand the cortices but does not displace the inferior alveolar canal. The margins of the lesion are usually not well demarcated.

Histopathology

Fibrous dysplasia is seen microscopically as irregularly shaped trabeculae of woven bone in a background of a loose and cellular, fibrous connective tissue (Fig. 132.13D). Fibrous dysplasia has a distinctive microscopic picture of abnormal bone coalescing with the normal surrounding tissue, which is in contrast with the features of the ossifying fibroma.

Treatment and Prognosis

Fibrous dysplasia does not require surgery unless the lesion is disfiguring and the patient desires a more normal and esthetic appearance or rarely if there is cranial nerve dysfunction (44). Recontouring of the affected jaw or facial bone is performed rather than resection, and surgery is usually delayed until the affected bone has reached maturity (Fig. 132.13E). Reports of sarcomatous transformation have been documented, and recurrence is more likely if the lesion is treated during an active growth period.

Central Giant Cell Lesion

The central giant cell lesion (CGCL) is a locally aggressive benign lesion that occurs in both long bones and the jaws. Jaw lesions may have similar histopathologic features as

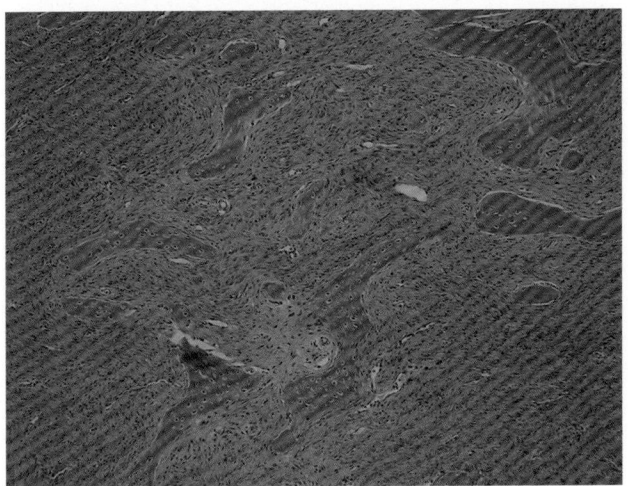

Figure 132.12 Ossifying fibroma. Irregular trabeculae of bone are seen throughout a cellular, fibrous connective tissue stroma.

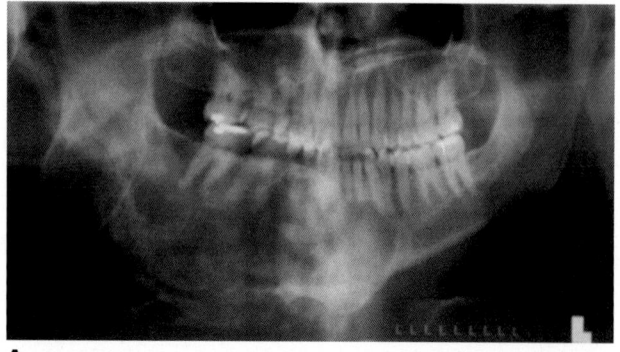

A

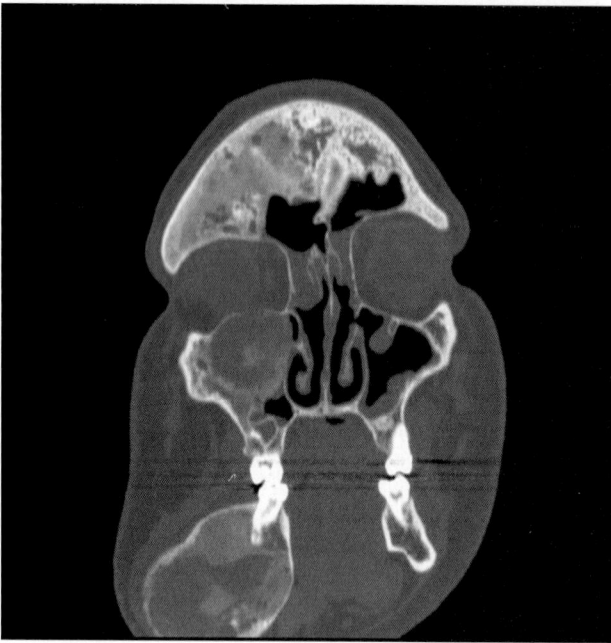

B

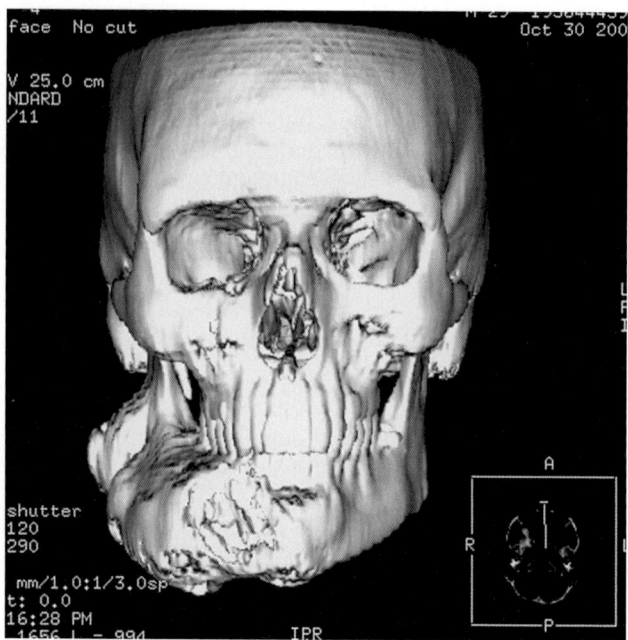

C

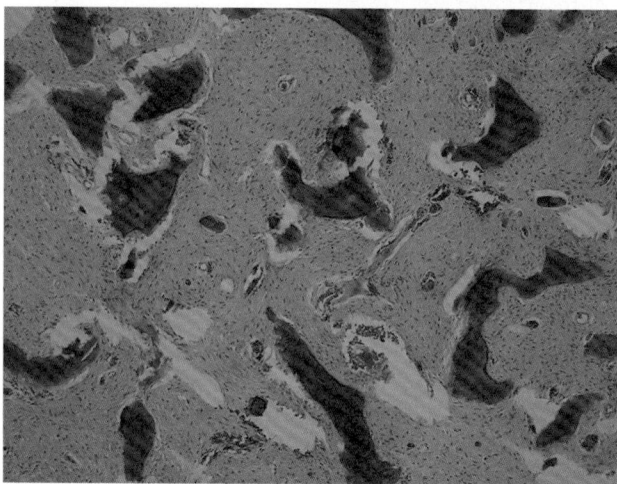

D

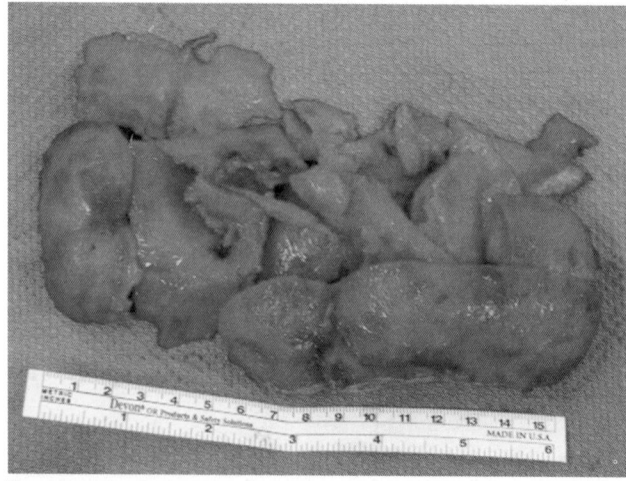

E

Figure 132.13 A: Fibrous dysplasia. Panoramic radiograph of a 28-year-old man who presented with steadily increasing right mandibular and facial enlargement, which had been monitored over several years' time. Biopsies established diagnosis of fibrous dysplasia. **B:** Coronal computed tomography (CT) scan of maxillofacial bones demonstrates frontal, maxillary, and mandibular bony involvement. **C:** Three-dimensional reformatted CT scan depicting the gross deformity of the right mandibular lesion. **D:** Fibrous dysplasia. Curvilinear portions of woven bone, without appositional osteoblasts, in a background of connective tissue stroma. **E:** Gross specimen of the fibrous dysplasia.

those that appear in long bones, but the biologic behavior differs. The CGCL is an osteolytic lesion that has been referred to as a central giant cell reparative granuloma in the past, but current understanding is that it does not represent a reparative process (45,46).

Clinical and Radiographic Features

CGCLs of the jaws most often are asymptomatic and are not recognized until they present as a painless swelling. A more aggressive form of the CGCL can cause pain or paresthesia. Clinically, the condition can appear as a bluish mass as a result of the thinning of the overlying bone and mucosa and its highly vascular nature. Most cases develop in the second to third decades, and women outnumber men 2:1. The lesion favors the anterior region of the jaws, particularly the mandible, often crossing the midline, and is occasionally seen bilaterally. The CGCL appears as either a well-circumscribed radiolucency or a multilocular radiolucency. Larger lesions can cause cortical displacement (Fig. 132.14A). The CGCL can also displace teeth, but root resorption is not typical.

Histopathology

The associated giant cells behave much like osteoclasts. Multinucleated giant cells varying in size and their number of nuclei are dispersed throughout a background of spindled mesenchymal cells. The lesion is unencapsulated, and fibrous tissue is also present to varying degrees (Fig. 132.14B). Areas of hemorrhage and hemosiderin deposits are commonly found. Immunologic studies support the biologic behavior and notion that the giant cells represent osteoclasts. Histologic features are not predictive of its biologic behavior, and the CGCL is identical to several other conditions affecting the jaws, including cherubism, the brown tumor of hyperparathyroidism, and focal areas of fibrous dysplasia. Thus, it is prudent to rule out these similar lesions if the clinical features suggest that the lesion may be something other than a CGCL.

Treatment and Prognosis

Curettage is usually curative, but recurrent or larger lesions occasionally require resection (Fig. 132.14C and D). Recurrence becomes an issue if the lesion is associated with difficult removal—attachment to multiple roots or neurovascular structures, or larger, more vascular lesions. Several nonsurgical therapies have been reported with some degree of success. Intralesional steroid injections using triamcinolone (10 mg/mL) weekly for 6 weeks is advocated by some as a first line of therapy (47). Another reported injectable therapy is calcitonin (48). The precise mechanism of action of calcitonin on the giant cell tumor is unknown, but the giant cells have been shown to have calcitonin receptors, and calcitonin somehow interferes with the progression of the tumor.

Aneurysmal Bone Cyst

The aneurysmal bone cyst (ABC) is a rare, expansile osteolytic bone lesion. It contains large blood-filled spaces that do not have an endothelial or epithelial lining, and is thus not a true cyst.

Clinical and Radiographic Features

The ABC commonly occurs in the first three decades of life. They have a predilection for the posterior portions of the jaws. They present as firm swellings that can be diffuse. Teeth may become loosened and displaced, and root resorption may occur, but the teeth remain vital. Radiographically, ABCs are expansile, often multilocular, radiolucencies. The borders are usually well demarcated, but cortical perforations with extension into the soft tissues do occur.

Histopathology

The large blood-filled spaces are separated by connective tissue septa. Hemosiderin, bone, and osteoid can be found within the septa. Osteoclast-type multinucleated giant cells, similar to those found in the CGCL, are a common feature at the periphery of the lesion. Mitoses are commonly found, but atypical forms are not.

Treatment and Prognosis

The ABC is managed by curettage, and intraoperative bleeding can become a challenge. Embolization may become necessary in select cases.

Vascular Malformations

Vascular malformations are developmental lesions that can affect soft tissue or bone. They do not present at birth like hemangiomas, which are actual neoplasms. Vascular malformations can be broadly classified as either arterial (high-flow) or venous (low-flow) malformations. Arteriovenous fistulas may also be considered high-flow lesions.

Clinical and Radiographic Features

Most vascular malformations within the jaws present as slow-growing, asymptomatic, expansile lesions (49). The associated teeth become clinically mobile and may even appear elevated. Thrills or bruits may be detectable on physical examination. When the tongue is involved, lingual veins become distended. Vascular malformations take on a variable radiographic appearance. Some may appear as well-circumscribed radiolucencies, whereas others may appear as more mixed radiolucent/radiopaque. Tooth roots may be resorbed with high-flow lesions. A CT scan or MRI should be obtained to aid in ascertaining the extent of the lesion, and angiography is performed to assist in determining the primary vascular inflow and the presence of any contralateral vascular contributions.

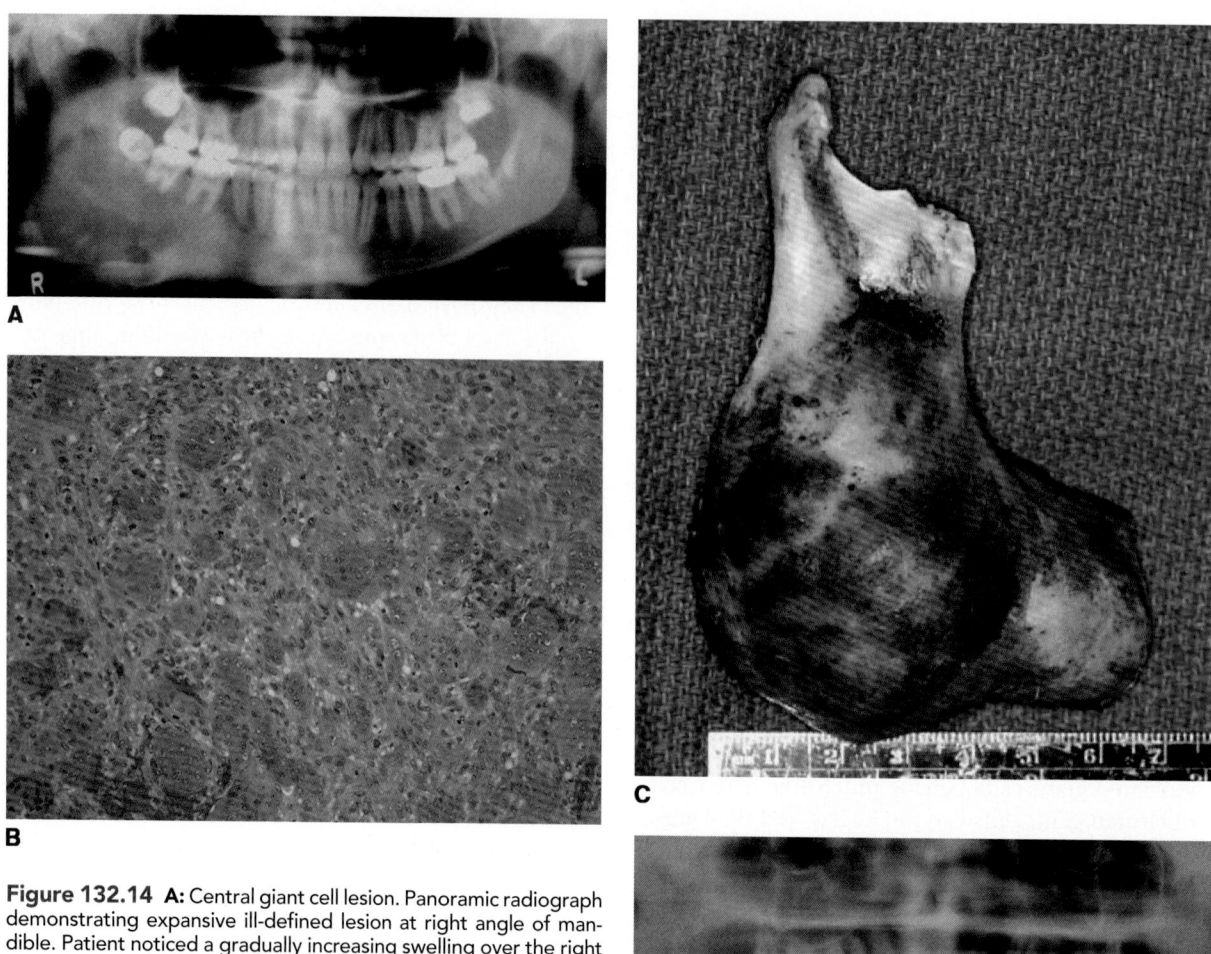

Figure 132.14 A: Central giant cell lesion. Panoramic radiograph demonstrating expansive ill-defined lesion at right angle of mandible. Patient noticed a gradually increasing swelling over the right mandible, while her occlusion was shifting to the left. **B:** CGCL. Numerous multinucleated giant cells in a background of plump, primitive mesenchymal cells. Abundant hemorrhage is seen throughout. **C:** A right hemimandibulectomy was performed via a right submandibular approach. The specimen demonstrates the well-vascularized appearance of the lesion. **D:** Post-op panoramic radiograph reveals reconstruction with an iliac crest bone graft. Endosseous implants were placed 7 months after initial graft.

Histopathology

Tortuous endothelium-lined, dilated vessels comprise the microscopic appearance of this condition. Adjacent smaller feeding vessels can also be seen in some cases.

Treatment and Prognosis

Any radiolucent lesion of the jaw, which might be clinically considered to be a vascular malformation, requires needle aspiration prior to biopsy or surgery to rule this condition out. Arterial malformations are treated with preoperative selective embolization followed by resection surgery. The purpose of embolization is to limit the blood flow to the lesion so as to minimize blood loss when the lesion is excised. A variety of materials can be used to embolize these lesions: coils, polyvinyl alcohol beads, or 100% alcohol (50). Overaggressive embolization must be avoided to prevent ischemic necrosis and sloughing of

tissues. Hypotensive anesthesia can also be used to further reduce intraoperative bleeding. Venous malformations can be treated with coils or intralesional injections of sclerosing agents. If adequate thrombosis is achieved, then the lesion can be curettaged.

CONCLUSION

Collectively, odontogenic cysts and tumors do not occur with considerable frequency. Many of these lesions are amenable to surgical enucleation and curettage. Some of the cysts and tumors possess locally aggressive behavior and are capable of great tissue distortion and/or destruction. Thus, they present challenges regarding their treatment and ultimate reconstruction. Long-term follow-up is advisable for many of these lesions, as recurrences do occur.

HIGHLIGHTS

■ The most common inflammatory cyst is the radicular cyst. Treatment is tooth extraction and enucleation.

■ All cystic lesions should be aspirated prior to performing a biopsy to rule out a vascular lesion.

■ The dentigerous cyst is associated with the crown of an unerupted tooth.

■ The WHO recommended reclassifying the OKC to KCOT to more appropriately reflect its aggressive behavior.

■ The basal cell nevus syndrome, an autosomal dominant condition, can manifest with multiple KCOTs.

■ Ameloblastoma, the most common odontogenic tumor, requires resection with one additional uninvolved margin when it grows into adjacent soft tissue.

■ Tori require removal only if they impair function or the fabrication of a prosthesis.

■ Asymptomatic osteomas need not be removed. Multiple osteomas may be indicative of Gardner syndrome.

■ Ossifying fibroma, a benign tumor, is amenable to curettage or resection with a close margin.

■ Fibrous dysplasia is not a neoplasm. Surgery is indicated in cases of disfigurement. Recontouring of the involved jaw bone may be appropriate.

■ ABC is not a true cyst. Curettage is effective.

REFERENCES

1. Daley TD, Wysocki GP, Pringle GA. Relative incidence of odontogenic tumors and oral and jaw cysts in a Canadian population. *Oral Surg* 1994;77:276–280.
2. Sapp JP, Eversole LR, Wysocki GP, eds. *Contemporary oral and maxillofacial pathology*. St. Louis, MO: Mosby-Year Book, 1997.
3. Marx RE, Stern D, eds. Odontogenic and nonodontogenic cysts. In: *Oral and maxillofacial pathology: a rationale for diagnosis and treatment*. Chicago, IL: Quintessence Publ, 2003:573–633.
4. Adelsperger J, Campbel JH, Coates DB, et al. Early soft tissue pathosis associated with impacted third molars without pericoronal radiolucency. *Oral Surg Oral Med Oral Pathol Oral Radiol Endod* 2000;89:402–406.
5. August M, Faquin WC, Traulis M, et al. Differentiation of odontogenic keratocysts from nonkeratinizing cysts by use of fine aspiration biopsy and cytokeratin-10 staining. *J Oral Maxillofac Surg* 2000;58:935–940.
6. Buchner A. The central (intraosseous) calcifying odontogenic cyst: an analysis of 215 cases. *J Oral Maxillofac Surg* 1991;49:330–339.
7. Ramer M, Montazem A, Lane SL, et al. Glandular odontogenic cyst: report of a case and review of the literature. *Oral Surg* 1987;84:54–57.
8. Kaplan H, Gal G, Amair Y, et al. Glandular odontogenic cyst: treatment and recurrence. *J Oral Maxillofac Surg* 2005;63:435–441.
9. Swanson KS, Kaugars GE, Gunsolley JC. Nasopalatine duct cyst: an analysis of 334 cases. *J Oral Maxillofac Surg* 1991;49:268–271.
10. Stafne EC. Bone cavities situated near the angle of the mandible. *J Am Dent Assoc* 1942;29:1969–1972.
11. Gold L, Williams T. Odontogenic tumors: surgical pathology and management. In: Marciani R, Carlson E, Braun T, eds. *Oral and maxillofacial surgery*, 2nd ed. Vol. 2. Philadelphia, PA: Saunders, 2009.
12. Neville B, Damm D, Allen C, Bouquot J. *Oral and maxillofacial pathology*, 2nd ed. Philadelphia, PA: Saunders, 2002.
13. Pogrel MA, Schmidt BL, eds. *The odontogenic keratocyst*. Philadelphia, PA: WB Saunders, 2003.
14. Neville BW, Damm DD, Allen CM. Odontogenic cysts and tumors. In: Gnepp D, ed. *Diagnostic surgical pathology of the head and neck*. Philadelphia, PA: Saunders, 2001.
15. Philipsen HP. Keratocystic odontogenic tumour. In: Barnes L, Everson J, Reichart P, Sidransky D, eds. *Pathology and genetics of head and neck tumors*. World Health Organization Classification of Tumours, Lyons, France: IARC Press, International Agency for Research on Cancer, 2005.
16. Shear M. Odontogenic keratocysts: clinical features. The odontogenic keratocyst. *Oral Maxillofac Clin N Am* 2003;15(3):335–345.
17. Shear M. The aggressive nature of the odontogenic keratocysts: is it a benign neoplasm? A review. Part 1. Clinical and early experimental evidence of aggressive behavior. *Oral Oncol* 2002;38:219–226.
18. Ghali GE, Connor MS. Surgical management of odontogenic keratocysts. The odontogenic keratocyst. *Oral Maxillofac Clin N Am* 2003;15(3):383–392.
19. Schmidt BL, Pogrel MA. The use of enucleation and liquid nitrogen cryotherapy in the management of odontogenic keratocysts, *J Oral Maxillofac Surg* 2001;59:720–725.
20. Schmidt BL. The use of liquid nitrogen and cryotherapy in the management of the odontogenic keratocyst. The odontogenic keratocyst. *Oral Maxillofac Clin N Am* 2003;(3):393–405.
21. Williams TP, Connor FA. Surgical management of the odontogenic keratocyst. Aggressive approach. *J Oral Maxillofac Surg* 1994;52:964–966.
22. Pogrel MA, Jordan RCK. Marsupialization as a definitive treatment for odontogenic Keratocysts, *J Oral Maxillofac Surg* 2004;62:651–2004.
23. Pogrel MA. Decompression and marsupialization as a treatment for the odontogenic Keratocyst. The odontogenic keratocyst. *Oral Maxillofac Clin N Am* 2003;(3):415–427.
24. Crowley TE, Kaugars GE, Gunsolley JC. Odontogenic keratocysts: a clinical and histologic comparison of the parakeratin and orthokeratin variants. *J Oral Maxillofac Surg* 1992;50:22–26.
25. Gorlin FJ. Nevoid basal cell carcinoma syndrome. *Medicine* 1987;66:98–113.
26. Woolgar JA, Rippin JW, Browne RM. The odontogenic keratocyst and its occurrence in the nevoid basal cell carcinoma syndrome. *Oral Surg Oral Med Oral Pathol* 1987;64:727–730.
27. Ueno S, Nakamura S, Mushimoto K, Shirasu R. A clinicopathologic study of ameloblastoma. *J Oral Maxillofac Surg* 1986;44:361–365.
28. Gardner DG. A pathologist's approach to the treatment of ameloblastoma. *J Oral Maxillofac Surg* 1984;42:161–166.
29. Gardner DG, Pecak AMJ. The treatment of ameloblastoma based on pathologic and anatomic principles. *Cancer* 1980;46:2514–2519.
30. Carlson ER, Marx RE. The ameloblastoma: primary, curative surgical management. *J Oral Maxillofac Surg* 2006;64:484.
31. Philipsen HP, Reichart PA, Nikai H, et al. Peripheral ameloblastoma: biological profile based on 160 cases from the literature. *Oral Oncol* 2001;37:17–27.
32. Poulson RC, Greer RO. Adenomatoid odontogenic tumor: clinicopathologic and ultrastructural concepts. *J Oral Maxillofac Surg* 1983;41:818–824.
33. Philipsen HP, Reichart PA. Calcifying epithelial odontogenic tumour: biologic profile based on 181 cases from the literature. *Oral Oncol* 2000;36:17–26.
34. Franklin CD, Pindborg JJ. The calcifying epithelial odontogenic tumor: a review and analysis of 113 cases. *Oral Surg* 1976;42:753–765.
35. Orsini G, Favia G, Piattelli A. Peripheral clear cell calcifying epithelial odontogenic tumor: report of a case, *J Periodontal* 2000;71:1177.
36. Cheng Y-SL, Wright JM, Walstad WR, et al. Calcifying epithelial odontogenic tumor showing microscopic features of potential malignant behavior. *Oral Surg Oral Med Oral Pathol* 2002;93:287.

37. Aviel-Ronen S, Liokumovich P, Rahima D, et al. The amyloid deposit in calcifying epithelial odontogenic tumor is immunoreactive for cytokeratins. *Arch Pathol Lab Med* 2000;124:872–876.

38. White DK, Chen SY, Mohnac AM, et al. Odontogenic myxoma: a clinical and ultrastructural study. *Oral Surg* 1975;39:901–917.

39. Carlson ER. Odontogenic cysts and tumors. In: Miloro M, ed. *Peterson's principles of oral and maxillofacial surgery*, 2nd ed. Hamilton, ON: BC Decker Inc, 2004.

40. Takeuchi T, Takenoshita Y, Kubo K, et al. Natural course of jaw lesions in Patients with familial adenomatosis coli (Gardner's syndrome). *Int J Oral Maxillofac Surg* 1993;22:226–230.

41. Vezeau PJ, Fridrich KL, Vincent SD. Osteochondroma of the mandibular condyle: literature review and report of two atypical cases. *J Oral Maxillofac Surg* 1995;53:954–963.

42. Eversole LR, Leider AS, Nelson K. Ossifying fibroma: a clinicopathologic study of sixty-four cases. *Oral Surg Oral Med Oral Pathol* 1985;60:505–511.

43. Bolger WE, Ross AT. McCune-Albright syndrome: a case report and review of the literature. *Int J Pediatr Otorhinolaryngol* 2002;65:69–74.

44. Chen YR, Noordhoff MS. Treatment of craniomaxillofacial fibrous dysplasia: how early and how extensive. *Plast Reconstr Surg* 1990;86:835–844.

45. Chuong R, Kaban LB, Kozakewich H, et al. Central giant cell lesions of the jaws: a clinicopathologic study. *J Oral Maxillofac Surg* 1986;44:708–713.

46. Ficarra G, Kaban LB, Hansen LS. Central giant cell lesions of the mandible and maxilla: a clinicopathologic and cytometric study. *Oral Surg Oral Med Oral Pathol* 1987;64:44–49.

47. Kermer C, Millesi W, Watzke IM. Local injection of corticosteroids for central giant Cell granuloma. A case report. *Int J Oral Maxillofac Surg* 1994;23:366–368.

48. deLange J, Rosenberg AJ, van den Akker HP, et al. Treatment of central giant cell Granuloma of the jaws with calcitonin. *Int J Oral Maxillofac Surg* 1999;28:372–376.

49. Kaban LB, Mulliken JB. Vascular anomalies of the maxillofacial region. *J Oral Maxillofac Surg* 1986;44:203–213.

50. Perrott D, Schmidt B, Dowd C, et al. Treatment of a high-flow arteriovenous malformation by direct puncture and coil embolization. *J Oral Maxillofac Surg* 1994;52:1083–1086.

Treatment of Thyroid Neoplasms

133

Irene Zhang   *Samantha DeMauro-Jablonski*
Robert L. Ferris

It is estimated that 45,000 new cases of thyroid cancer were diagnosed and 1,690 of them will die of this disease in 2010 (1,2). The lifetime risk of developing thyroid cancer is 0.9%, and the annual incidence has increased from 3.6 per 100,000 in 1973 to 10.2 per 100,000 in 2007 (1). This trend may be due to increasing use of neck ultrasound as well as other imaging modalities during routine physical exam. CT, MRI, or PET scans performed for other medical reasons can subsequently result in the detection of incidental benign and malignant thyroid nodules. Thyroid nodules are a common presentation of thyroid cancer. Although the prevalence of thyroid nodules is around 50% at autopsy, and up to 67% detected by ultrasonography (US), only 5% to 10% of these are malignant (3,4). The challenge exists to identify the 5% to 10% of patients with malignancy of clinical significance. Recent advances in molecular markers for thyroid cancer have improved the ability to detect subsets of cancer with aggressive behavior and to assist in the setting of indeterminate fine-needle aspiration (FNA). The diagnosis and treatment of thyroid cancer have significantly evolved over last decade, emphasizing the need for a thorough understanding of the underlying molecular pathways and risk factors, as well as the surgical anatomy, diagnostic, and treatment algorithms necessary to provide excellent care for patients with thyroid neoplasm.

SURGICAL ANATOMY AND EMBRYOLOGY

The thyroid gland originates from both primitive pharyngeal and the neural crest cells. It is the first endocrine gland to develop in the human body. The medial portion of the gland derives from the endodermal diverticulum of the first and second pharyngeal pouches at the foramen cecum. It then descends to its pretracheal position along the midline neck during 4 to 7 weeks of gestation, and the proximal portion degenerates into a fibrous stalk. If any of these portions persists, a thyroglossal duct cyst (TGDC) may result. The distal portion gives rise to the pyramidal lobe. The lateral portion of the gland derives from the fourth and fifth pharyngeal pouches, which descend to fuse with the medial portion of the gland.

Parafollicular C cells originate from the ectoderm neural crest cells as the ultimobranchial body, which secretes calcitonin. In mammals, the ultimobranchial body and medial portion of the fourth pharyngeal fuse into the lateral lobes of the thyroid. Because of this, the majority of C cells are located deep within the upper one-third of the lateral lobe, the most common location for medullary thyroid carcinoma (MTC).

Ectopic thyroid tissue can be found anywhere along the course of its developmental descent in the midline anterior neck. Lingual thyroid can be found at its origin at the foremen cecum due to failure to descend. Seventy percent of the patients with lingual thyroids have no thyroid tissue in the neck. Thyroid function should be evaluated before the surgical removal of the lingual thyroid glands. A TGDC is the most common congenital midline cervical anomaly. It may develop at any location along the thyroglossal duct tract, most commonly at the midline upper cervical location close to the hyoid bone. Rarely, this entity can occur in a lateral position. The hyoid bone divides this tract into upper and lower segments. Thus, surgical management of the TGDC (Sistrunk procedure) should remove the middle segment of hyoid bone to prevent recurrence. Preoperative imaging will aid in delineating the nature of a midline mass as well as identifying functional thyroid tissue prior to complete TGDC excision. High-resolution ultrasound, CT, and MRI are commonly used in detecting TGDC. Calcification seen in a CT scanning raises suspicion of papillary carcinoma arising from TGDC.

RISK FACTORS OF THYROID CANCER

Risk factors for thyroid cancer have been studied extensively. They include age of the patient, gender, history of previous radiation, family history, environmental exposures, and molecular genetic factors. It has been widely accepted that papillary thyroid carcinoma (PTC) is twice as common in women as in men (5). Young patients have a better prognosis than older patients. The clinical presentation differs significantly in terms of the size, extent of the cancer, the presence and the number of lymph node metastases, and response to the treatment (6). Indeed, AJCC has incorporated age as part of the staging criteria for differentiated thyroid cancer (DTC).

Although there is no clear association between dietary iodine supplementation and thyroid cancer, the pattern of thyroid cancer in iodine-sufficient areas differs significantly from iodine-deficient areas, with the shift from high proportion of follicular carcinoma to PTC (6,7).

It is well established that exposure to ionizing radiation to the head and neck region during childhood increases the risk of thyroid cancer. Radiation therapy (RT) was once a therapy for tonsil and adenoid hyperplasia, thymic enlargement, acne, hemangioma, and Hodgkin disease (mantle irradiation) to the head and neck. The risk of thyroid cancer often RT exposure is dose dependent and is greatest for children less than 15 years old. The 25-year follow-up after the Chernobyl accident demonstrated that children and adolescents exposed to radioiodine from the Chernobyl fallout have a substantial dose-related increase in thyroid cancer, with the risk greatest in those less than 18 years old at exposure (8). Fortunately, the disease-specific mortality rate in this patient population is quite low, at 1% or less (9). The increased incidence of thyroid cancer in those greater than 18 years old during the Chernobyl fallout is less definitive.

A patient with a family history of thyroid cancer has an increased risk to develop thyroid cancer, and 5% to 10% of all thyroid carcinoma cases are hereditary (10). Gardner syndrome and Peutz-Jeghers syndrome are both associated with PTC. Cowden disease is associated with follicular thyroid carcinoma (FTC). MEN IIA and MEN IIB are associated with family history of MTC (11).

MOLECULAR BASIS OF THYROID NEOPLASM

The knowledge of molecular genetics and signaling pathways in thyroid cancer has expanded in recent years. Numerous molecular alterations in thyroid cancer have been identified, and are actively studied in clinical trials as therapeutic targets for recurrent disease. Among them, four major mutations involved in development of differentiated thyroid cancer (DTC), BRAF and RAS point mutation, RET (REarranged during Transfection)/PTC, and PAX8/peroxisome proliferator-activated receptor γ (*PPARγ*)

rearrangements, seem to have most relevant clinical implications (12). Like many other malignancies, genetic alterations in the mitogen-activated protein kinase (MAPK) signaling pathway are involved in development of PTC (Fig. 133.1) (13).

PTC often carries mutually exclusive BRAF and RAS point mutations and RET/PTC rearrangements, which are activated in MAPK signaling pathway. Mutation in one of these genes presents in more than 70% of PTC (14–16).

BRAF point mutations have been reported in 40% to 45% of PTC. BRAF V600E mutation has been found in 70% to 80% of tall-cell variant of PTC and 60% of classical PTC and strongly correlated with aggressive features of this disease including extrathyroidal extension (ECE), lymph node, or distant metastases (14,17,18). BRAF V600E is not found in FTC or other benign thyroid nodules, which makes it a specific tumor marker of PTC. This association has also been reported in papillary microcarcinomas, which might have some clinical implications in the management of these tumors (19). RET/PTC rearrangements are found in 20% of adult papillary carcinomas, most commonly in patients with history of radiation (20,21). It is common in patients with history of radiation and young adults with PTC. However, it has been found in other benign thyroid lesions or hyalinizing trabecular tumors (21,22). In MTC, RET is activated by point mutation rather than chromosomal rearrangement, as found in PTC. Point mutations of the RAS genes (HRAS, KRAS, and NRAS) are found in FTC, PTC, and follicular adenoma. In thyroid carcinoma, KRAS and NRAS are the most commonly altered. RAS mutations are found in 45% of follicular carcinoma and 10% papillary carcinoma (13). In the latter, PTC with RAS mutation is almost always of the follicular variant (12). These are also found in other follicular adenomas/hyperplasia or goiters. PAX8/*PPARγ* rearrangement is present in 35% of classic follicular carcinomas. RAS mutation and PAX8/*PPARγ* rearrangement are rarely overlapping. Mutations in the RAS genes or PAX8/PPARg rearrangement occur in approximately 70% of FTC (23).

Compelling data indicate that molecular testing of thyroid FNA specimens may significantly improve the accuracy of preoperative cytologic diagnosis of thyroid nodules, especially in the subgroups including follicular lesion of indeterminate significance (FLUS), follicular neoplasm, and suspicious for malignancy. Current ATA guidelines recommend that the molecular test results may be considered for indeterminate FNA cytology to help guide the management of those patients. The feasibility and diagnostic utility of molecular testing in FNA of thyroid nodules has been reported in a recent large prospective study including 470 FNA samples. Molecular testing demonstrated 100% accuracy for malignancy in all mutation-positive FLUS cases (24). BRAF was the most common mutation and had 100% positive predictive value (PPV) for PTC, whereas RAS mutation confers 87.5% probability of malignancy (24). In light of the finding in this study, the patients with

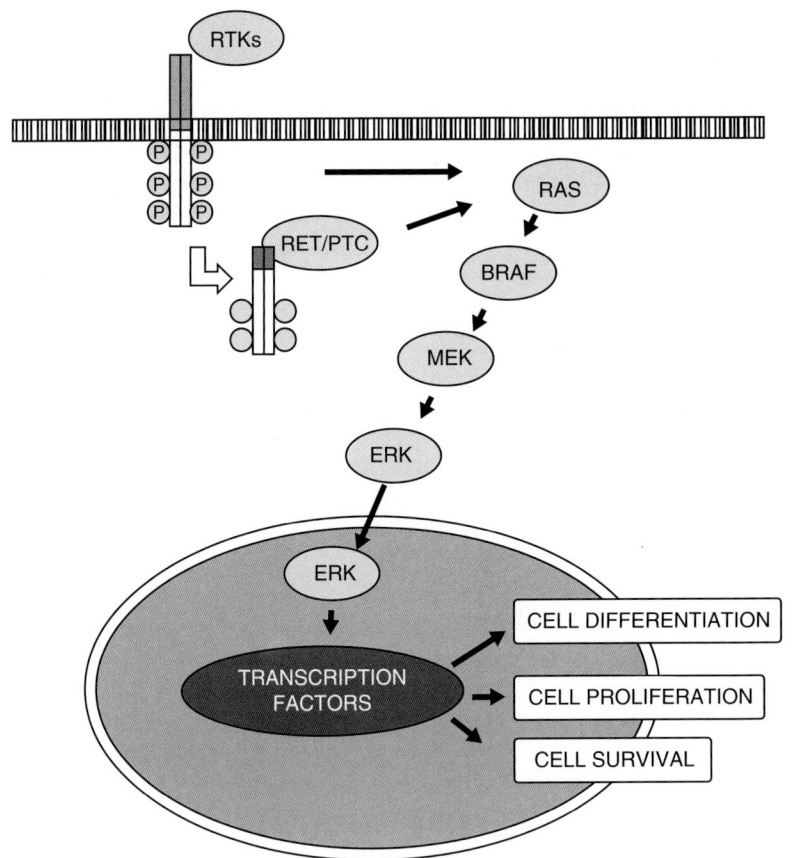

Figure 133.1 MAPK signaling pathway is activated by binding of growth factors to receptor tyrosine kinases (RTKs), such as RET. The activated receptor, via a series of adaptor proteins, leads to activation of RAS, BRAF, and subsequently MAPK/ERK pathway, which regulates cell differentiation, proliferation, and survival. Alteration of this pathway in thyroid cancer can occur at different levels as a result of BRAF and RAS point mutation or RET rearrangement. (From Nikiforov YE. Thyroid carcinoma: molecular pathways and therapeutic targets. *Mod Pathol* 2008;21:S37–S43 with permission.)

mutation-positive and cytologic indeterminate nodules are considered for total thyroidectomy, especially with BRAF mutations, to reduce the need for intraoperative pathologic consultation and to avoid a second surgery. In addition to the diagnostic value of molecular testing, the aggressive behavior of BRAF-positive PTCs provides prognostic information to refine patients' management, including consideration of central neck dissection. Although still early in clinical application, the expanding knowledge of thyroid tumor biology has started translating into clinical practice, and molecular testing in thyroid FNA will be a valuable tool for diagnosis and better prognostication of thyroid cancer.

EVALUATION OF THYROID NODULES

Most commonly thyroid neoplasms present as either palpable thyroid nodules or nonpalpable nodules incidentally found by imaging studies, so-called incidentalomas. These "incidentalomas" carry the same risk of malignancy as palpable nodules with the same size. Generally, any nodule greater than 1 cm warrants evaluation. Occasionally, subcentimeter nodules with worrisome ultrasound features, previous history of head and neck irradiation, family history of thyroid cancer, or associated neck lymphadenopathy require further evaluation. Recent studies demonstrated 27% to 42% risk of malignancy in focal or unilateral uptake in ¹⁸FDG-PET scan (25–27). The term

"PAINs" (PET-Associated Incidental Neoplasm) was introduced, and the prompt evaluation and treatment of these patients are warranted (28).

Clinical Assessment

For patients presenting with a thyroid nodule, a thorough history and physical examination should be performed. Pertinent elements increasing the possibility of malignancy in the history are previous history of irradiation to the neck, history of thyroid cancer in first-degree relatives, rapid growth, dysphasia, hoarseness, male gender, and presentation at extreme age (less than 20 or older than 70) (29).

The worrisome findings on physical examination which raise concern for malignancy are size of the nodules greater than 4 cm, lateral cervical lymphadenopathy, vocal cord immobility, and fixation of the nodule to surround structures. The accuracy of physical examination may be limited by the patient's body habitus, and further imaging may be of value for the patients with large BMI or posterior located nodules.

Laboratory Studies

Most patients with thyroid nodules are euthyroid. A serum thyroid stimulating hormone (TSH) level should be obtained as part of the evaluation. Subsequent T3, T4, and a radionuclide thyroid scan should be obtained for those with a low TSH to further evaluate the thyroid function. Thyroglobulin (Tg) level is not routinely measured as initial evaluation of thyroid nodule due to its lack of sensitivity and specificity as a screening tool. Serum calcitonin level and urine metanephrine should be obtained in patients with family history of medullary thyroid cancer or MEN IIA or IIB.

Imaging Modalities

Ultrasound

High-resolution thyroid ultrasound should be performed in all patients with thyroid nodule(s) to assess the thyroid bed, central compartment, as well as lateral neck, according to the 2009 ATA guideline. US helps to confirm the presence of a nodule corresponding to the physical examination, size of the nodule(s), presence of other nodules in the thyroid bed and/or lymphadenopathy in lateral necks, components of the nodule(s) (cystic vs. solid), and posteriorly located nodules. It also plays an important role for monitoring the interval changes of preexisting nodule(s) and posttreatment surveillance for thyroid cancer. In addition, it allows identification of certain suspicious ultrasound features suggesting malignancy. Although no single sonographic finding is pathognomonic for thyroid malignancy, certain ultrasound features of thyroid nodule are associated with higher probability of malignancy (30,31). These include hypoechogenicity, increased intranodular vascularity, irregular or infiltrated margins, presence of microcalcifications, absence of halo (for papillary carcinoma), and length greater than the width in transverse dimension. The sonographic features highly predictive of benign nodules are pure cystic, coarse calcifications, and regular margins. These features also help to select appropriate nodule(s) and/or site within the nodule (cystic vs. solid) to aspirate for fine needle aspiration biopsy (FNAB).

Radionuclide Thyroid Scan

The role of radionuclide scanning in the initial workup of a thyroid nodule is limited. It is indicated in a nodule(s) with low TSH to determine the functional status of the nodule, since the rate of malignancy in hyperfunctioning thyroid nodule is less than 1%. A hyperfunctioning nodule demonstrated on a radionuclide scan obviates the need for FNAB.

CT, MRI, and PET/CT

Unlike high-resolution, US, CT, or MRI imaging are insensitive for intrathyroid nodule(s), and routine use is rarely indicated in initial workup for thyroid nodule(s). However, both CT and MRI are excellent to evaluate the mediastinal extension or to assess, trachea, esophageal, and/or extrathyroid invasion. CT with contrast as a preoperative evaluation will delay potential postoperative radioactive iodine (RAI) therapy by roughly 3 months. Although PET/CT has been used in initial staging of oncocytic (Hurthle cell) carcinoma or poorly differentiated thyroid carcinomas, it is not indicated in initial workup for a thyroid nodule. On the other hand, PAINs deserves prompt evaluation due to its substantial risk of malignancy. Although, some suggest that PET/CT might play a role to reduce the need of diagnostic lobectomy for nodules with inconclusive cytologic results due to its high negative predictive values, further study is needed before this expensive test becomes universally accepted.

Fine-Needle Aspiration and Molecular Markers

FNA is the procedure of choice to evaluate the thyroid nodule and may be performed via palpation or via US guidance. According to 2009 ATA guideline, FNA is indicated in following situations:

1. Any nodule with high-risk history if it is greater than 5 mm, with microcalcification, or any abnormal cervical lymph nodes
2. Greater than 1-cm solid nodule
3. Greater than 1.5-cm mixed nodule with any suspicious ultrasound features
4. Greater than 2.0-cm spongiform nodules or mixed nodule without any suspicious ultrasound features

FNA is not indicated for pure cystic nodule. In case of multinodular gland, preference should be given to those hypo- or isofunctioning nodules with suspicious ultrasound features. The diagnostic accuracy is improved with US-guided FNA because of a decreased number of inadequate samples or false negative results (32). According to 2009 ATA guidelines, US-guided FNA is recommended for nonpalpable nodules, predominately cystic nodules, and posterior nodules. The cytologic results from FNA should be reported under six categories to reflect the risk of malignancy according to 2007 Bethesda system for reporting thyroid cytopathology (Table 133.1) (33). PTC can be reliably diagnosed from FNA due to its characteristic nuclear features. Benign or malignant follicular neoplasm cannot

TABLE 133.1	THE BETHESDA SYSTEM FOR REPORTING THYROID CYTOPATHOLOGY
Diagnostic Category	**Risk of Malignancy (%)**
Nondiagnostic or unsatisfactory	1–4
Benign	0–3
Atypia of undetermined significance or FLUS	5–15
Follicular neoplasm or suspicious for a follicular neoplasm	15–30
Suspicious for malignancy	60–75
Malignancy	97–99

Modified from Cibas ES, Ali SZ. The Bethesda system for reporting thyroid cytopathology. *Am J Clin Pathol* 2009;132:658–665.

be distinguished on cytology alone, because capsular or angiolymphatic invasion is required to make the diagnosis, which cannot be assessed from cytopathology.

As discussed before, recent advances in molecular testing in thyroid FNA specimens have enhanced the ability to distinguish malignant from benign nodules. The most commonly studied molecular markers in thyroid neoplasm are BRAF and RAS point mutations, as well as RET/PTC and PAX8/PPARγ rearrangements. Although the exact indications of molecular testing need to be defined, it seems that most clinical utility lies in assisting the decision making between thyroid lobectomy and total thyroidectomy when the cytology is under the category of "follicular neoplasm" or "follicular lesion of undetermined significance (FLUS)." Also, BRAF V600E-mutated cancers may be considered for central neck dissection, particularly if greater than 1 cm, to reduce the need for reoperation.

Workup

The authors have proposed the algorithm in Figure 133.2 for workup of a thyroid nodule. It is based on the 2009 American Thyroid Association guideline, 2009 Bethesda system for reporting thyroid cytopathology, and the most recent advances in thyroid FNA molecular basis of thyroid cancer.

Any symptomatic thyroid nodule should be evaluated with TSH level and diagnostic ultrasound. Thyroid uptake scan should be ordered in those with low TSH levels. The patients with hyperfunctioning nodule can be worked up by an endocrinologist, and no FNA is recommended. FNA is indicated in the patients with normal or high TSH.

A repeat FNA should be performed if FNA is reported as "unsatisfactory." Patients who have a benign FNA report can be followed. There is a 3% false negative rate. Annual US is used to monitor the nodule for growth or

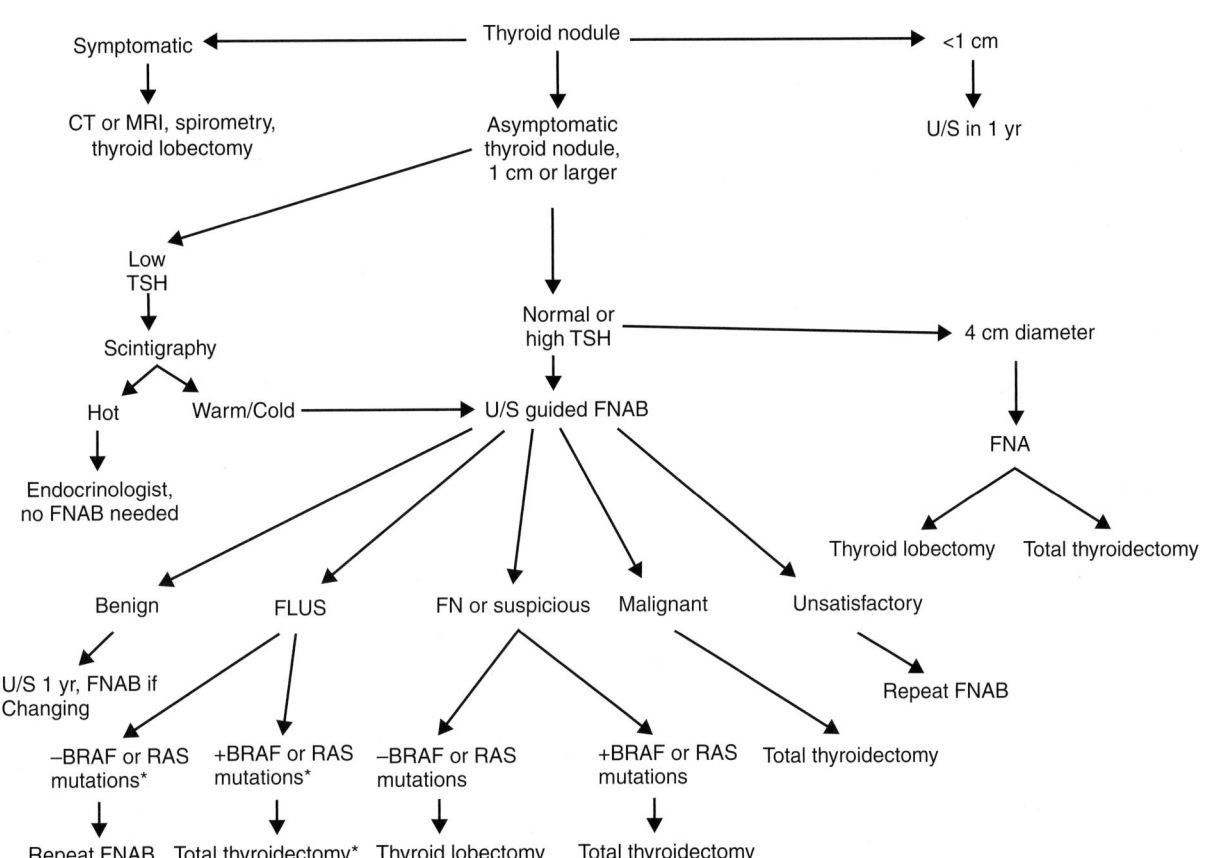

Figure 133.2 Workup of a thyroid nodule. *Asterisk* based on following data from University of Pittsburgh Medical Center:

1. Ohori NP, Nikiforova MN, Schoedel KE, et al. Contribution of molecular testing to thyroid fine-needle aspiration cytology of "follicular lesion of undetermined significance/atypia of undetermined significance". *Cancer Cytopathol* 2010;118(1):17–23.
2. Nikiforov YE, Steward DL, Robinson-Smith TM, et al. Molecular testing for mutations in improving the fine-needle aspiration diagnosis of thyroid nodules. *J Clin Endocrinol Metab* 2009;94(6):2092–2098.
3. Menta V, et al. *Head and Neck* 2012; September 13, in press.
4. Bomeli SR, LeBeau SO, Ferris RL. Evaluation of a thyroid nodule. *Otolaryngol Clin North Am* 2010;43(2):229–238.

development of suspicious sonographic features for malignancy, at which time a repeat FNA is warranted. Total thyroidectomy is recommended when the FNA report indicates malignancy. The FNA has a sensitivity of 97% to 99% (9). Recent prospective data from University of Pittsburgh Medical Center demonstrated 100% PPV and 100% specificity for BRAF-positive "follicular neoplasm" or "suspicious for malignancy" FNA (15). Another study showed 100% PPV in mutation-positive "FLUS" group, while the probability of malignancy for mutation-negative FLUS group is only 7.6% (34). The asterisk part in Figure 133.2 reflects our clinical practice based on above findings. Currently, it has not yet been fully validated or universally accepted. We believe the treatment algorithms will change in the near future as more data accumulate and molecular testing becomes more widely available.

OVERVIEW OF THYROID NEOPLASM

Thyroid Adenoma

Thyroid adenomas are true benign thyroid neoplasms, distinctly separate from surrounding thyroid tissue. They are often encapsulated and arise from normal thyroid follicular cells, in multinodular goiter or in thyroiditis. Clinically, patients usually are asymptomatic, and the nodule is often found in routine physical examination. Spontaneous bleeding into the adenoma may cause sudden increase in size and pain. Follicular adenomas are the most common. Other types include oncocytic (Hurthle cell) adenoma, hyalinizing trabecular adenoma, and nodular adenomatous goiter. Thyroid adenomas with benign FNA results warrant follow-up due to the false negative rate of 5% (35). Nodule growth during the follow-up warrants repeat FNA. The 2009 ATA guidelines recommend serial US every 6 to 18 months following initial FNA. The follow-up interval can extend up to 3 to 5 years if the nodule is stable over time. Routine TSH suppression is not recommended for benign thyroid nodules. If surgery is indicated, the minimal surgical intervention should be thyroid lobectomy.

Papillary Carcinoma

PTC is the most common type of malignant thyroid neoplasm, both in adult and children. It is twice as common in women as in men (5). The hallmark for PTC is its papillary architecture, psammoma bodies, and characteristic nuclear features. The distinct nuclear features include nuclear grooves, nuclear pseudo-inclusions, powdery chromatin, and micronucleoli. These features allow a diagnosis of PTC based on cytology of FNA. Several histologic variants of PTC have been identified, including papillary thyroid microcarcinoma, follicular variant, encapsulated variant, diffuse sclerosing variant, and oxyphilic cell variant and two aggressive types—tall cell and columnar cell variant.

Most patients present with a slow growth neck mass. Thirty-five percent PTC were found to have cervical lymph nodes involvement at the presentation. Multicentric

involvement and ECE are common. Previous exposure to ionizing radiation, especially during childhood, is well-established risk factor for papillary carcinoma. Although most of the cases are sporadic, several syndromes involving familial PTC have been described, which include Cowden syndrome and familial adenomatous polyposis coli.

Follicular Carcinoma

FTC is more aggressive compared with PTC. It is more prevalent in iodine-deficient regions. Although most radiation-induced thyroid cancers are papillary carcinoma, it also plays a role in development of FTC. There are two types of FTC: minimally invasive and widely invasive, each of which carries different prognosis. Diagnosis of FTC is based on capsular and lymphovascular invasion, which makes this entity almost impossible to diagnose based on cytology or frozen section.

The clinical presentation is similar to PTC. The incidence of nodal involvement at presentation is lower than papillary carcinoma, ranging from 15% to 20%. However, the incidence of distant metastasis at presentation is more common than PTC, ranging from 10% to 15% (36,37). The most common sites of metastasis are lung and bone.

Hurthle Cell Carcinoma

Oncocytic (formerly Hurthle cell carcinoma, HCC) is uncommon and currently considered as a variant of follicular carcinoma according to World Health Organization classification. It is twice as common in males as in females. Hurthle cells are large follicular epithelial cells with dense eosinophilic cytoplasm. Similar to follicular carcinoma, diagnosis of HCC is based on its capsular and vascular invasion. The incidence of lymph node involvement is around 6% to 9%. HCC has the highest rate of distant metastases compared to PTC and conventional type FTC. Thirty-four percent of HCC developed distant metastases, and most common sites are lung and bone (36,38).

Anaplastic Carcinoma

Anaplastic thyroid carcinoma, accounting 1% to 3% of primary thyroid malignancy, is the most aggressive thyroid neoplasm. It is more common in women than in men, affecting patients in their fifth or sixth decades. Many cases are associated with preexisting papillary or follicular carcinomas, or preexisting goiter. Thirty percent cases are found in the specimen of well-differentiated carcinoma.

Patients usually presented with rapid growing neck mass with symptoms of airway obstruction and/or dysphasia. On physical exam, the tumor is usually large, firm, and fixed to surrounding structures and may result in tracheal/esophageal invasion, unilateral or bilateral vocal cord paralysis, and carotid artery and sympathetic trunk involvement. Distal metastases are not uncommon. Anaplastic carcinoma must be differentiated from lymphoma, which presents with a similar clinical picture. Airway control is the important measure for these patients. Overall, prognosis is extensively poor. Treatment protocols include doxorubicin and external bean RT. In some situations, surgical debulking might be an option for the purpose of airway management. Surgical cure may occur when an anaplastic carcinoma is encountered prior to infiltration and metastasis.

Lymphoma

Thyroid lymphoma accounts for less than 5% of thyroid malignancy and can arise from preexisting Hashimoto thyroiditis. The majority of thyroid lymphomas are non-Hodgkin B cell lymphoma. The clinical presentation is similar to anaplastic carcinoma. Patients usually have rapid response to chemotherapy with or without radiation. The most common chemotherapy regimen is CHOP (cyclophosphamide, doxorubicin, vincristine, and prednisone). Surgery is not a primary treatment modality, and its role is limited to the diagnosis of lymphoma.

Other Forms of Thyroid Cancer

Primary squamous cell carcinoma of the thyroid has been reported. In these situations, metastases from other sites should be ruled out. Other cancers metastasizing to thyroid can occur. The primary sites include renal cell carcinoma, breast, bronchogenic carcinomas, ovarian cancer, and melanoma.

STAGING AND PROGNOSTIC CLASSIFICATIONS

Both histologic diagnosis and age were considered important factors for tumor behavior and prognosis for DTC and therefore included in the AJCC classification. Separate grouping systems are recommended for DTC (papillary and follicular), medullary, and anaplastic (or undifferentiated) thyroid carcinoma (Tables 133.2 and 133.3).

In thyroid cancer, the AJCC staging system does not include several other prognostic factors, such as histologic grade. Although many other risk stratification systems (AGES, AMES, MACIS, etc.) have been developed to address this issue, none of these prognostic classifications is able to encompass all risk factors. In addition, these classifications do not apply to patients with MTC or anaplastic carcinomas.

INITIAL SURGICAL MANAGEMENT OF DTC

Surgical Techniques

Some important steps must be taken in order to ensure a successful thyroid surgery. Preoperative laryngoscopy to

---

TABLE 133.2	TNM STAGING FOR THYROID CANCER

Primary tumor (T)

Tx	Primary tumor cannot be assessed
T0	No evidence of primary tumor
T1	Tumor 2 cm or less in greatest dimension limited to thyroid
T1a	Tumor 1 cm or less, limited to thyroid
T1b	Tumor more than 1 cm but not more than 2 cm in greatest dimension, limited to the thyroid
T2	Tumor more than 2 cm but not more than 4 cm in greatest dimension, limited to the thyroid
T3	Tumor more than 4 cm in greatest dimension limited to the thyroid, or any tumor with minimal extrathyroid extension (e.g., extension to sternothyroid muscle or perithyroid soft tissue)
T4a	Moderate advanced disease—tumor of any size extending beyond the thyroid capsule to invade subcutaneous soft tissues, larynx, trachea, esophagus, or RLN
T4b	Very advanced disease—tumor invades prevertebral fascia or encases carotid artery or mediastinal vessels
All anaplastic carcinomas are considered T4 tumors	
T4a	Intrathyroidal anaplastic carcinoma
T4b	Anaplastic carcinoma with gross extrathyroid extension

Regional lymph nodes (N)

Nx	Regional lymph nodes cannot be assessed
N0	No regional lymph node metastasis
N1	Regional lymph node metastasis
N1a	Metastasis to level VI (pretracheal, paratracheal, and prelaryngeal/Delphian lymph nodes)
N1b	Metastasis to unilateral, bilateral, or contralateral cervical (levels I, II, III, IV, or V) or retropharyngeal or superior mediastinal lymph nodes (level VII)

Distant metastases (M)

M0	No distant metastasis
M1	Distant metastasis

From American Joint Committee on Cancer: AJCC Staging Manual. 7th ed. Springer, 2009.

TABLE 133.3	STAGE GROUPINGS		

Differentiated (papillary or follicular)

Under 45 years

Stage I	Any T	Any N	M0
Stage II	Any T	Any N	M1

45 years and older

Stage I	T1	N0	M0
Stage II	T2	N0	M0
Stage III	T3	N0	M0
	T1	N1a	M0
	T2	N1a	M0
	T3	N1a	M0
Stage IVA	T4a	N0	M0
	T4a	N1a	M0
	T1	N1b	M0
	T2	N1b	M0
	T3	N1b	M0
	T4a	N1b	M0
Stage IVB	T4b	Any N	M0
Stage IVC	Any T	Any N	M1

Medullary carcinoma (all age groups)

Stage I	T1	N0	M0
Stage II	T2	N0	M0
	T3	N0	M0
Stage III	T1	N1a	M0
	T2	N1a	M0
	T3	N1a	M0
Stage IVA	T4a	N0	M0
	T4a	N1a	M0
	T1	N1b	M0
	T2	N1b	M0
	T3	N1b	M0
	T4a	N1b	M0
Stage IVB	T4b	Any N	M0
Stage IVC	Any T	Any N	M1

Anaplastic carcinoma

All anaplastic carcinomas are considered stage IV

Stage IVA	T4a	Any N	M0
Stage IVB	T4b	Any N	M0
Stage IVC	Any T	Any N	M1

From American Joint Committee on Cancer: AJCC Staging Manual. 7th ed. Springer; 2009

length and level of the incision depends on the location of the nodule and glands, habitus of the patients, and extent and approach of the surgery. Subplatysmal flaps are elevated superiorly to the level of the cricoid cartilage and inferiorly to the clavicle.

The midline cervical fascia was dissected to expose trachea, isthmus, and cricoid cartilage. The sternothyroid muscle is dissected off the thyroid gland capsule and retracted laterally to expose the entire thyroid gland. Occasionally, the strap muscle can be divided to gain access to a large superior pole nodule. This should be reapproximated toward the end of the case. An avascular plane between cricothyroid muscle and superior pole was developed, and superior vessels should be meticulously ligated and divided close to the gland to avoid the injury to superior laryngeal nerve (SLN). At this point, the thyroid gland was retracted medially and anteriorly to facilitate identification of recurrent laryngeal nerve (RLN) and parathyroid glands (Fig. 133.3).

To successfully identify and preserve the RLN, the knowledge to RLN is key to a thyroid surgeon. On the right neck, RLN loops around right subclavian artery and follows an oblique course. On the left neck, RLN traverses the ductus arteriosus and follows a more medial course, running along the tracheoesophageal groove. The RLN can be identified superiorly at the laryngeal entry point, (cricothyroid joint), at a lateral approach, at midpole level, or inferior approach where the RLN is found in the triangle bounded by trachea medially, inferior pole superiorly, and carotid sheath laterally. Preservation of the parathyroid glands is the key for thyroid surgery. The relationship between parathyroid glands and RLN is demonstrated in Figure 133.4. Superior parathyroid glands are immediately posterior and lateral to the entry point of RLN. Caution should be taken to preserve the parathyroid glands and its blood supply when we dissect RLN using superior approach. The rate of permanent RLN paralysis is 1% in experience hands. After RLN is identified, it is traced to its laryngeal entry point. The middle thyroid vein and inferior thyroid vessels are

visualize the vocal cords should be performed for every patient prior to thyroid surgery. This is especially important for revision surgery. Patients with vocal cords paralysis or symptoms of dysphagia should be thoroughly evaluated by thin-cut CT scan to assess for tracheoesophageal invasion. Patients with hyperthyroidism warrant medical management to avoid intraoperative and postoperative complications. Pheochromocytoma must be ruled out preoperatively in patients with MTC.

The patient should be placed in supine position with neck fully extended and adequate head support. A transverse incision along a skin crease below the cricoid cartilage is made and carried down to the platysma. The exact

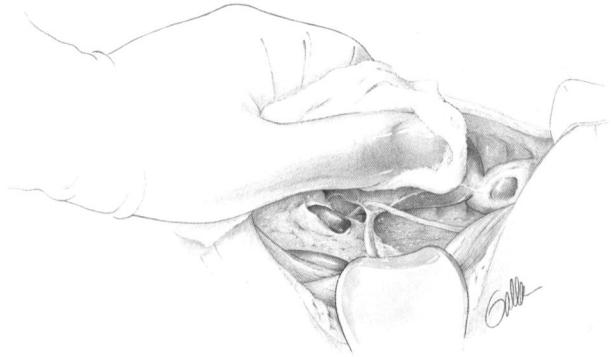

Figure 133.3 Exposure of the lateral border of the thyroid showing the relationship of the RLN to the inferior thyroid artery and parathyroid glands. (From Randolph G. *Surgery of the thyroid and parathyroid glands.* Philadelphia, PA: WB Saunders, 2003, with permission.)

The indication of routine use of RLN monitoring varies between different institutions. It may be useful if any difficulty is anticipated to identify the RLN, especially in reoperative cases, large tumor or goiters, and extensive central compartment dissection.

Novel Approaches to Thyroid Glands

With the advancement of technology, many novel approaches to thyroid surgery have developed during last decade. Among them, minimally invasive video-assisted thyroidectomy (MIVAT) has gained considerable attention and controversy (39,40). The indications for MIVAT include indeterminate nodules (less than 3.5 cm), no previous neck surgery, no evidence of metastasis, and small, low-risk PTCs (2). The oncologic efficacy of this approach continues to be debated. Other approaches including anterior chest and transaxillary approaches and transoral video-assisted thyroidectomy have been described to avoid cervical incision. These approaches are used in very limited situations for cosmetic purpose only (41,42). In recent years, transaxillary robotic thyroidectomy is evolving through extensive transaxillary approach to avoid cervical incision, which might be more important in some Asian countries for culture and cosmetic purpose (43). It is still too early to predict the level of adoption in North America. These approaches should be considered with caution to provide equal surgical outcomes in comparison to conventional open approaches.

Extent of Surgery

Surgery is the primary treatment modality for thyroid neoplasms. The goal of initial surgery is to eradicate all gross disease; to reduce local, regional, or distal recurrence; and to facilitate possible RAI therapy if required. The minimum thyroid surgery should be lobectomy. Total thyroidectomy is generally indicated in patients with thyroid cancer greater than 1 cm and some subcentimeter PTC with high-risk group and/or poor prognosis molecular alteration. Thyroid lobectomy may be sufficient for small (less than 1 cm), low-risk, and intrathyroidal papillary carcinomas. Although there is no survival benefit based on different surgical treatment for patients with less than 4 cm, intrathyroidal tumors, several studies found that the rates of recurrence are reduced by total thyroidectomy among low-risk patients (43–45).

Special Surgical Considerations

Management of the Regional Lymphatics

Regional lymph node metastases are more common in PTC and less common in FTC. Data are conflicting for the relationship between cervical lymph node metastases and overall survival. A recent SEER registry study concluded that cervical lymph node metastases conferred an independent risk of decreased survival only in patients with

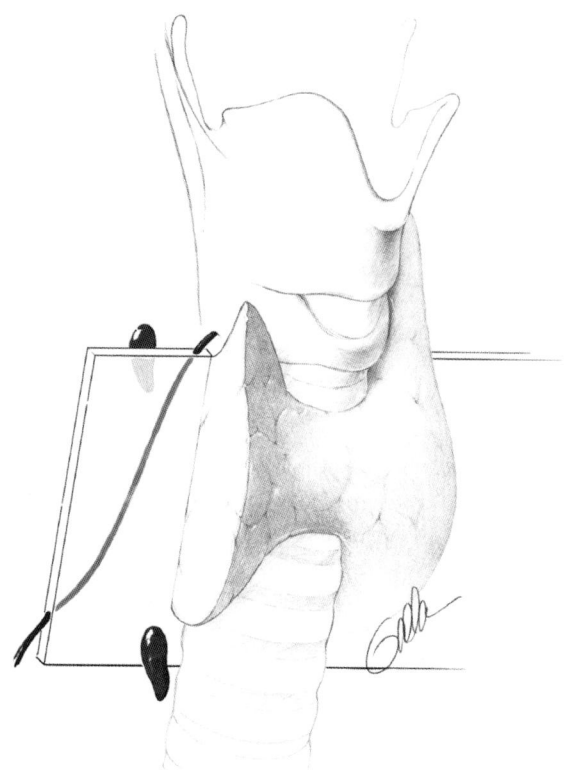

Figure 133.4 Coronal plane formed by the RLN and its relationship to parathyroid glands. (From Randolph G. *Surgery of the thyroid and parathyroid glands*. Philadelphia, PA: WB Saunders, 2003, with permission.)

dissected and ligated near the gland to preserve parathyroid blood supply. The thyroid is dissected medially from its cervical attachments after Berry ligament is carefully dissected. Dissection at this area might be difficult due to potential bleeding and close association between Berry ligament and distal course of the RLN. This is also the area where small remnant of thyroid tissue should not be left after total thyroidectomy. For a total thyroidectomy, the similar steps are repeated on the contralateral side.

Every effort must be made to preserve the function of parathyroid glands. Autotransplantation should be performed if a parathyroid gland becomes devascularized intraoperatively. A small portion of suspicious parathyroid gland is sent for frozen section to obtain histologic confirmation, especially in the situation of thyroid carcinoma. Once the confirmation is obtained, the remaining gland is minced into small pieces and autotransplanted into ipsilateral sternocleidomastoid muscle. Autotransplantation of parathyroid glands is also indicated if extensive nodule disease is seen in central neck compartment with high likelihood for reoperation.

As the specimen is removed, it should be examined carefully for the presence of any parathyroid glands before the thyroid specimen is sent to pathology. Homeostasis was then achieved meticulously, and neck should be closed with multiple layers after the strap muscles are reapproximated.

FTC and in PTC patients over 45 years of age. The 2009 ATA guidelines recommend consideration of central neck dissection for patients with clinically involved central or lateral neck lymph nodes along with total thyroidectomy or completion of thyroidectomy. Elective central neck dissection is recommended in T3 or T4 PTC patients with clinically uninvolved central neck lymph nodes and MTC patients. Therapeutic lateral neck dissection should be performed for biopsy-proven lateral cervical metastases.

Recurrent Laryngeal Nerve Invasion

Surgical sacrifice of the RLN is rare. If carcinoma of RLN by carcinoma is found intraoperatively and preoperative vocal cord paralysis is present, the RLN may be sacrificed. If the RLN is involved and preoperative nerve function is normal, it should be saved and dissected to be as free of gross disease as possible. Microscopic disease should then be treated with postoperative RAI therapy. RLN sacrifice should be considered if it is involved in MTC due to the lack of treatment response of MTC to RAI therapy.

Tracheal and/or Esophageal Invasion

For patients with tracheal and/or esophageal invasion, optimal treatment dictates surgical resection if feasible, including postoperative RAI therapy or external beam radiation. Shaving techniques can be used to remove all gross disease. In cases of intraluminal invasion, tracheal resection with anastomosis is warranted. Partial laryngectomy can be performed, and total laryngectomy is indicated in rare cases; after all, conventional treatment options fail.

Special Patient Populations

The diagnostic and therapeutic approaches to thyroid neoplasms in children are similar to adults with consideration of familial and syndromic associations. It is utmost important to balance between the potential treatment morbidity and indolent nature of the disease. MTCs in children are discussed in different sections. Thyroid nodules in pregnant women should be evaluated in the same way as nonpregnant women except that use of RAI is contraindicated. If FNA is consistent with PTC during the pregnancy, surgery is recommended and should be done before 24 weeks gestation. However, data also suggest that treatment delays for less than 1 year do not significantly affect patient outcome. A nodule with PTC diagnosed early in pregnancy should be monitored by ultrasound for growth or spread. If substantial growth is evident before 24 weeks gestation, surgery should be performed. If it is stable, or diagnosed after 24 weeks gestation, surgery may be performed after delivery.

Surgical Complications

Thyroidectomy is a safe procedure in experienced hands. Mortality rates are extremely low, and serious complications occur in less than 2%. The most common complications are injuries to RLN and parathyroid glands.

Postoperative Hematoma

Postoperative bleeding is very uncommon and usually happens during first few hours postoperatively. An expanding hematoma can lead to life-threatening airway obstruction. Airway decompression by evacuating the hematoma should be performed in urgent fashion at the bedside, and patients will then be taken back to operating room immediately for neck exploration to identify and control the bleeding.

Recurrent Laryngeal Nerve Injury

Transient RLN injury is not uncommon, but permanent paralysis should comprise approximately 1% after total thyroidectomy. All patients should undergo pre- and postoperative laryngoscopy to evaluate laryngeal function. The incidence may increase during reoperative surgery or after extensive central neck dissection. Unilateral RLN paralysis may be well compensated and asymptomatic. Symptomatic patients should be managed by vocal cord medialization including vocal cord injection or thyroplasty. Bilateral vocal cord paralysis is a devastating complication from thyroid surgery, and impending airway obstruction is the major concern in these patients. The patients may be managed using transverse cordotomy, arytenoidectomy, or tracheostomy.

Superior Laryngeal Nerve Injury

Injury to the SLN is more common than recognized, and may be temporary or permanent. Patients will have difficulty shouting. Many surgeons do not routinely visualize the SLN. However, adequate exposure and individual ligation of superior pole tributary vessels close to the glands are the keys to avoid SLN injury, in addition to nerve monitoring techniques.

Hypocalcemia

Transient hypocalcemia after total thyroidectomy is the most common complication from thyroid surgery. The rate of transient hypocalcemia has been reported to occur in up to 25% of cases, and permanent hypoparathyroidism is reported to occur in 0.4% to 13% of cases. The extent of surgery, central neck dissection, revision cases, and substernal goiter surgery all may increase the risk of hypoparathyroidism. Serum calcium level, symptoms of hypocalcemia, along with Chvostek and Trousseau signs should be closely monitored in immediate postoperative period. Symptomatic patients should be managed in timely fashion to avoid severe tetany, seizure, altered mental status, and cardiac arrhythmias. Oral and/or intravenous (IV) calcium should be given along with calcitriol. In difficult cases, an endocrinologist can be consulted to adjust the dose of IV calcium and vitamin D.

TABLE 133.4	POSTOPERATIVE RISK STRATIFICATION			
Risk stratification	Local/Distal Metastases	Tumor Invasion of locoregional tissue(s)	Aggressive Histology/ Vascular Invasion	Posttreatment Whole-Body RAI Scan (RxWBS)
Low	No	No	No	No
Intermediate	Cervical lymph node metastases	Microscopic invasion	Yes	[131]I uptake outside thyroid bed
High	Distant metastases	Macroscopic invasion	Yes/No	Tg out of proportion to uptake in RxWBS

Modified from 2009 ATA Guidelines: Cooper DS, et al. *Thyroid* 2009; 19(11):1167–1214.

POSTOPERATIVE MANAGEMENT OF DIFFERENTIATED THYROID CANCER

Postoperative Staging System and Risk Stratification

Postoperative staging is an important part of postoperative management. It allows to assess an individual patient's risk for recurrence and mortality and to tailor the decision making for RAI treatment and TSH suppression. In WDTC, the AJCC staging system is based on age and pTNM parameters to predict the risk of mortality, not recurrence. Many other schemes, including AGES, AMES, and MACIS, were developed to achieve more accurate risk stratification for recurrence. A three-level risk stratification system was suggested in the 2009 ATA guidelines to assess the risk of recurrence (Table 133.4).

In the 2009 ATA guidelines, indications for RAI treatment are based on the AJCC TNM staging. The three-level risk stratification system is also used to recommend the appropriate degree of initial TSH suppression.

RADIOACTIVE IODINE TREATMENT

The roles of RAI treatment are to facilitate postoperative staging and follow-up and to decrease the risk of recurrence and disease-specific mortality (46–48). RAI therapy is given either as remnant ablation, adjuvant therapy, or treatment of known persistent or metastatic disease. There is no therapeutic benefit observed in patients with intrathyroidal microscopic PTC, or microscopic multifocal PTC; thus, RAI ablation is not always recommended for those patients (49,50). RAI ablation is recommended for all patients with distant metastases, T4, and selective T3 disease (≥45 years old) due to decreased risks of recurrence and mortality. There remains conflicting data for 1- to 2-cm intrathyroidal T1 and T2 disease in terms of reduction of risks of recurrence. RAI ablation may be used in selective cases to facilitate staging and postoperative follow-up. There are no sufficient data to demonstrate the benefit of RAI in patients with specific aggressive histology or molecular abnormalities, and this remains the area of future research.

RAI ablation requires TSH stimulation (TSH greater than 30 mU/L) to increase iodine uptake by thyroid cancer cells. The two methods available are thyroid hormone withdrawal or rhTSH (*Thyrogen*) stimulation. Although thyroid hormone withdrawal was the gold standard, recent prospective randomized studies have demonstrated that rhTSH stimulation was equally effective as thyroid hormone withdrawal, with improved quality of life and similar short-term rates of recurrence (51,52). Thyrogen stimulation permits the patient to receive synthroid immediately postoperatively. The method used in preparation for RAI ablation is usually patient, disease status, and center specific. A low-iodine diet and avoidance of iodine exposure (e.g., IV contrast, amiodarone use) prior to RAI ablation have been suggested to prevent interference with the treatment (53).

Current guidelines recommend utilizing the minimum ^{131}I activity necessary to achieve successful remnant ablation, particularly for low-risk patients (54). Usually 30 to 100 mCi is employed. Patients with cervical or distant metastases, suspected or documented residual disease, or a more aggressive tumor histology (e.g., tall-cell variant, insular, columnar cell carcinoma), ^{131}I activity of 100 to 200 mCi was suggested (55). RAI is a relatively safe treatment modality. The side effects associated with RAI ablation include dose-dependent transient acute sialadenitis, short-term taste disturbance, GI discomfort (most commonly nausea), epiphora secondary to bilateral nasolacrimal duct obstruction, bone marrow suppression, and over time a low risk of secondary malignancies and leukemia with high dose and repeat treatments. Clinicians should ensure the benefits outweigh risks in decision making of RAI treatment.

INITIAL TSH SUPPRESSION

The initial TSH suppression therapy has been proven to decrease the risk of recurrence and improve overall survival in high-risk patients if TSH was suppressed to undetectable level (56). According to 2009 ATA guideline, targeted initial TSH suppression level is less than 0.1 mU/L for high-risk and intermediate-risk patients and 0.1 to 0.5 mU/L for low-risk patients.

EXTERNAL BEAM RADIATION THERAPY (EBRT) AND SYSTEMIC THERAPY

Role of external beam radiation therapy (EBRT) is limited, and its survival benefit is uncertain. Current recommendations suggest EBRT is indicated for gross unresectable tumor in patients over 45 years old, none operable symptomatic metastases (pain, fracture, or neurologic symptoms), or as an adjuvant therapy with surgery for selective cases of bone or brain metastases with concomitant use of glucocorticoids (57,58).

Systemic therapy in WDTC is mostly reserved for distal metastases, especially in the situations with the evidence of progression, RAI refractory diseases, or compromising organ function. Doxorubicin remains the only FDA-approved agent for metastatic thyroid carcinoma. Paclitaxel ± doxorubicin and carboplatinum with rh TSH also demonstrated partial response. With recent advances in molecular basis of WDTC, many novel targeted agents (including multi-kinase inhibitors) are in clinical trials. Among them, sorafenib in a phase II clinical trial for DTC and vandetanib in a recent phase III clinical trial for MTC showed clinical benefit (59–61).

LONG-TERM MANAGEMENT OF DTC

Methods of Follow-Up

The goals for long-term follow-up for thyroid cancer are to detect recurrent and persistent disease as well as monitor thyroxine suppression therapy. Clinical examination, serum Tg level, neck ultrasound, diagnostic whole-body RAI scans (WBS), and TSH suppression all play roles in long-term follow-up. Serum Tg level is a sensitive and specific marker to detect PTC recurrence in the absence of Tg antibodies, especially post total thyroidectomy and/or RAI ablation. Initial Tg level is measured with either thyroid hormone withdrawal or rhTSH in low-risk patients. Tg should be measured along with Tg antibodies and neck ultrasound every 6 to 12 months for intermediate- to high-risk patients and every 12 months for low-risk patients. A rising Tg level raises the suspicion for possible recurrent disease and warrants a further workup to localize the recurrence. Thyroid and lateral neck ultrasound is sensitive to detect cervical metastases (62). Tg level can be measured in the needle washout fluid in US-guided FNA sample (63). WBS performed 6 to 12 months after remnant ablation may be beneficial in high- or intermediate-risk patients. [18]FDG-PET is indicated to localize Tg positive (greater than 5 to 10 ng/mL) and RAI scan-negative tumor (64). A recent study demonstrated that PET/CT has additional benefits to detect unrecognized distant metastases and to identify non–iodine-avid metastatic lesions (65).

Long-term TSH suppression has been reported to be associated with the reduction of adverse clinical outcomes in patients with thyroid cancer (66). Current guidelines suggest maintaining TSH less than 0.1 mU/L indefinitely, for those with persistent disease, between 0.1 and 0.5 mU/L for 5 to 10 years for high-risk patients, and low-normal for low-risk disease.

Locoregional Recurrent or Persistent Disease

Studies have reported that 5% to 20% of patients treated with total thyroidectomy developed local recurrence within 10 years, 60% to 75% of which localized in the neck lymph nodes with level VI being the most common site (37,67). In patients greater than 45 years old, local regional recurrence may be associated with more morbidity than those less than 45 years old. Maintaining the balance between controlling the recurrent diseases and minimizing treatment-related morbidity is an important principle for the management of recurrent or persistent diseases. High-resolution ultrasound of the thyroid bed and bilateral necks, Tg and its antibody level, and WBS remain the important modalities to detect and follow up recurrent disease. The clinical use of serial Tg level to detect and monitor recurrent DTC is well documented. The primary role for CT and MRI in recurrent/persistent disease is to detect suspicious recurrences in unusual locations, such as supraclavicular, or superior mediastinum, and optimize the surgical planning. The use of PET scanning has been widely accepted as a modality to detect recurrence of DTC post thyroidectomy ± RAI (68). A recent study demonstrated the additional benefit of PET/CT to detect unrecognized distant metastatic disease and non–iodine-avid lesion, which led to a change in treatment plan in up to 40% of the patients (65).

REOPERATION FOR RECURRENT/ PERSISTENT DIFFERENTIATED THYROID CANCER

For recurrent or persistent DTC, a systematic approach to the thyroid bed and/or defined compartment neck dissection was reported to render a better outcome after reoperation than "berry picking" or local lymph node dissection. External beam radiation and systemic therapy are reserved for gross disease and palliation (69). To evaluate a patient for potential reoperation for recurrent or persistent disease, a thorough preoperative evaluation should encompass a detailed history, physical examination, and review of previous operative reports to obtain information of extent of the surgery and integrity of parathyroid glands, ionized calcium level, and intact PTH for lab testing. It is also crucial to evaluate vocal cord function, because clinical symptoms alone are not reliable for documenting RLN palsy (70).

Reoperative surgery in level VI places the RLN and parathyroid glands at greater risk compared with primary surgery. Early intraoperative visualization of RLN is the key to protect the integrity of RLN, and nerve monitoring can assist in the identification of RLN in reoperative settings (71).

26. Bogsrud TV, Karantanis D, Nathan MA, et al. The value of quantifying 18F-FDG uptake in thyroid nodules found incidentally on whole-body PET-CT. *Nucl Med Commun* 2007;28:373–381.

27. Kang KW, Kim SK, Kang HS, et al. Prevalence and risk of cancer of focal thyroid incidentaloma identified by 18F-fluorodeoxyglucose positron emission tomography for metastasis evaluation and cancer screening in healthy subjects. *J Clin Endocrinol Metab* 2003;88: 4100–4104.

28. Katz SC, Shaha A. PET-associated incidental neoplasms of the thyroid. *J Am Coll Surg* 2008;207:259–264.

29. Hegedus L. Clinical practice. The thyroid nodule. *N Engl J Med* 2004;351:1764–1771.

30. Frates MC, Benson CB, Doubilet PM, et al. Prevalence and distribution of carcinoma in patients with solitary and multiple thyroid nodules on sonography. *J Clin Endocrinol Metab* 2006;91: 3411–3417.

31. Moon WJ, Jung SL, Lee JH, et al. Benign and malignant thyroid nodules: US differentiation–multicenter retrospective study. *Radiology* 2008;247:762–770.

32. Danese D, Sciacchitano S, Farsetti A, et al. Diagnostic accuracy of conventional versus sonography-guided fine-needle aspiration biopsy of thyroid nodules. *Thyroid* 1998;8:15–21.

33. Cibas ES, Ali SZ. The Bethesda system for reporting thyroid cytopathology. *Am J Clin Pathol* 2009;132:658–665.

34. Ohori NP, Nikiforova MN, Schoedel KE, et al. Contribution of molecular testing to thyroid fine-needle aspiration cytology of "follicular lesion of undetermined significance/atypia of undetermined significance". *Cancer Cytopathol* 2010;118:17–23.

35. Ylagan LR, Farkas T, Dehner LP. Fine needle aspiration of the thyroid: a cytohistologic correlation and study of discrepant cases. *Thyroid* 2004;14:35–41.

36. Shaha AR, Shah JP, Loree TR. Patterns of nodal and distant metastasis based on histologic varieties in differentiated carcinoma of the thyroid. *Am J Surg* 1996;172:692–694.

37. Mazzaferri EL, Jhiang SM. Long-term impact of initial surgical and medical therapy on papillary and follicular thyroid cancer. *Am J Med* 1994;97:418–428.

38. Ruegemer JJ, Hay ID, Bergstralh EJ, et al. Distant metastases in differentiated thyroid carcinoma: a multivariate analysis of prognostic variables. *J Clin Endocrinol Metab* 1988;67:501–508.

39. Miccoli P, Berti P, Raffaelli M, et al. Comparison between minimally invasive video-assisted thyroidectomy and conventional thyroidectomy: a prospective randomized study. *Surgery* 2001;130: 1039–1043.

40. Terris DJ, Gourin CG, Chin E. Minimally invasive thyroidectomy: basic and advanced techniques. *Laryngoscope* 2006;116:350–356.

41. Inabnet WB III, Jacob BP, Gagner M. Minimally invasive endoscopic thyroidectomy by a cervical approach. *Surg Endosc* 2003;17: 1808–1811.

42. Benhidjeb T, Wilhelm T, Harlaar J, et al. Natural orifice surgery on thyroid gland: totally transoral video-assisted thyroidectomy (TOVAT): report of first experimental results of a new surgical method. *Surg Endosc* 2009;23:1119–1120.

43. Shah JP, Loree TR, Dharker D, et al. Prognostic factors in differentiated carcinoma of the thyroid gland. *Am J Surg* 1992;164: 658–661.

44. Grant CS, Hay ID, Gough IR, et al. Local recurrence in papillary thyroid carcinoma: is extent of surgical resection important? *Surgery* 1988;104:954–962.

45. Hay ID, Thompson GB, Grant CS, et al. Papillary thyroid carcinoma managed at the Mayo Clinic during six decades (1940–1999): temporal trends in initial therapy and long-term outcome in 2444 consecutively treated patients. *World J Surg* 2002;26:879–885.

46. Tsang RW, Brierley JD, Simpson WJ, et al. The effects of surgery, radioiodine, and external radiation therapy on the clinical outcome of patients with differentiated thyroid carcinoma. *Cancer* 1998;82:375–388.

47. Mazzaferri EL. Thyroid remnant 131I ablation for papillary and follicular thyroid carcinoma. *Thyroid* 1997;7:265–271.

48. Taylor T, Specker B, Robbins J, et al. Outcome after treatment of high-risk papillary and non-Hurthle-cell follicular thyroid carcinoma. *Ann Intern Med* 1998;129:622–627.

49. Hay ID, Hutchinson ME, Gonzalez-Losada T, et al. Papillary thyroid microcarcinoma: a study of 900 cases observed in a 60-year period. *Surgery* 2008;144:980–987; discussion 987–988.

50. Ross DS, Litofsky D, Ain KB, et al. Recurrence after treatment of micropapillary thyroid cancer. *Thyroid* 2009;19:1043–1048.

51. Pacini F, Ladenson PW, Schlumberger M, et al. Radioiodine ablation of thyroid remnants after preparation with recombinant human thyrotropin in differentiated thyroid carcinoma: results of an international, randomized, controlled study. *J Clin Endocrinol Metab* 2006;91:926–932.

52. Tuttle RM, Brokhin M, Omry G, et al. Recombinant human TSH-assisted radioactive iodine remnant ablation achieves short-term clinical recurrence rates similar to those of traditional thyroid hormone withdrawal. *J Nucl Med* 2008;49:764–770.

53. Pluijmen MJ, Eustatia-Rutten C, Goslings BM, et al. Effects of low-iodide diet on postsurgical radioiodine ablation therapy in patients with differentiated thyroid carcinoma. *Clin Endocrinol (Oxf)* 2003;58:428–435.

54. Cooper DS, Doherty GM, Haugen BR, et al. Management guidelines for patients with thyroid nodules and differentiated thyroid cancer. *Thyroid* 2006;16:109–142.

55. Hackshaw A, Harmer C, Mallick U, et al. 131I activity for remnant ablation in patients with differentiated thyroid cancer: a systematic review. *J Clin Endocrinol Metab* 2007;92:28–38.

56. Jonklaas J, Sarlis NJ, Litofsky D, et al. Outcomes of patients with differentiated thyroid carcinoma following initial therapy. *Thyroid* 2006;16:1229–1242.

57. McWilliams RR, Giannini C, Hay ID, et al. Management of brain metastases from thyroid carcinoma: a study of 16 pathologically confirmed cases over 25 years. *Cancer* 2003;98:356–362.

58. Brierley J, Tsang R, Panzarella T, et al. Prognostic factors and the effect of treatment with radioactive iodine and external beam radiation on patients with differentiated thyroid cancer seen at a single institution over 40 years. *Clin Endocrinol (Oxf)* 2005;63:418–427.

59. Kloos RT, Ringel MD, Knopp MV, et al. Phase II trial of sorafenib in metastatic thyroid cancer. *J Clin Oncol* 2009;27:1675–1684.

60. Cabanillas ME, Waguespack SG, Bronstein Y, et al. Treatment with tyrosine kinase inhibitors for patients with differentiated thyroid cancer: the M. D. Anderson experience. *J Clin Endocrinol Metab* 2010;95:2588–2595.

61. Wells SA Jr, Gosnell JE, Gagel RF, et al. Vandetanib for the treatment of patients with locally advanced or metastatic hereditary medullary thyroid cancer. *J Clin Oncol* 2010;28:767–772.

62. Pacini F, Molinaro E, Castagna MG, et al. Recombinant human thyrotropin-stimulated serum thyroglobulin combined with neck ultrasonography has the highest sensitivity in monitoring differentiated thyroid carcinoma. *J Clin Endocrinol Metab* 2003;88:3668–3673.

63. Snozek CL, Chambers EP, Reading CC, et al. Serum thyroglobulin, high-resolution ultrasound, and lymph node thyroglobulin in diagnosis of differentiated thyroid carcinoma nodal metastases. *J Clin Endocrinol Metab* 2007;92:4278–4281.

64. Larson SM, Robbins R. Positron emission tomography in thyroid cancer management. *Semin Roentgenol* 2002;37:169–174.

65. Razfar A, Branstetter BFT, Christopoulos A, et al. Clinical usefulness of positron emission tomography-computed tomography in recurrent thyroid carcinoma. *Arch Otolaryngol Head Neck Surg* 2010;136:120–125.

66. McGriff NJ, Csako G, Gourgiotis L, et al. Effects of thyroid hormone suppression therapy on adverse clinical outcomes in thyroid cancer. *Ann Med* 2002;34:554–564.

67. Schlumberger MJ. Diagnostic follow-up of well-differentiated thyroid carcinoma: historical perspective and current status. *J Endocrinol Invest* 1999;22:3–7.

68. Robbins RJ, Wan Q, Grewal RK, et al. Real-time prognosis for metastatic thyroid carcinoma based on 2-[18F]fluoro-2-deoxy-D-glucose-positron emission tomography scanning. *J Clin Endocrinol Metab* 2006;91:498–505.

69. Uruno T, Miyauchi A, Shimizu K, et al. Prognosis after reoperation for local recurrence of papillary thyroid carcinoma. *Surg Today* 2004;34:891–895.

70. Randolph GW, Kamani D. The importance of preoperative laryngoscopy in patients undergoing thyroidectomy: voice, vocal cord function, and the preoperative detection of invasive thyroid malignancy. *Surgery* 2006;139:357–362.

71. Dralle H, Sekulla C, Lorenz K, et al. Intraoperative monitoring of the recurrent laryngeal nerve in thyroid surgery. *World J Surg* 2008;32:1358–1366.

72. Chao TC, Jeng LB, Lin JD, et al. Reoperative thyroid surgery. *World J Surg* 1997;21:644–647.

73. Clayman GL, Shellenberger TD, Ginsberg LE, et al. Approach and safety of comprehensive central compartment dissection in patients with recurrent papillary thyroid carcinoma. *Head Neck* 2009;31:1152–1163.

74. Lin JD, Chao TC, Chou SC, et al. Papillary thyroid carcinomas with lung metastases. *Thyroid* 2004;14:1091–1096.

75. Shoup M, Stojadinovic A, Nissan A, et al. Prognostic indicators of outcomes in patients with distant metastases from differentiated thyroid carcinoma. *J Am Coll Surg* 2003;197:191–197.

76. Hundahl SA, Fleming ID, Fremgen AM, et al. A National Cancer Data Base report on 53,856 cases of thyroid carcinoma treated in the U.S., 1985–1995 [see comments]. *Cancer* 1998;83: 2638–2648.

77. Pelizzo MR, Boschin IM, Bernante P, et al. Natural history, diagnosis, treatment and outcome of medullary thyroid cancer: 37 years experience on 157 patients. *Eur J Surg Oncol* 2007;33:493–497.

78. Baloch ZW, LiVolsi VA. Prognostic factors in well-differentiated follicular-derived carcinoma and medullary thyroid carcinoma. *Thyroid* 2001;11:637–645.

79. Kloos RT, Eng C, Evans DB, et al. Medullary thyroid cancer: management guidelines of the American Thyroid Association. *Thyroid* 2009;19:565–612.

80. Carlson KM, Bracamontes J, Jackson CE, et al. Parent-of-origin effects in multiple endocrine neoplasia type 2B. *Am J Hum Genet* 1994;55:1076–1082.

81. Brandi ML, Gagel RF, Angeli A, et al. Guidelines for diagnosis and therapy of MEN type 1 and type 2. *J Clin Endocrinol Metab* 2001;86:5658–5671.

82. Mulligan LM. From genes to decisions: evolving views of genotype-based management in MEN 2. *Cancer Treat Res* 2004;122: 417–428.

Hyperparathyroidism: Evaluation and Surgery

134

Maisie L. Shindo

ABSTRACT

Primary hyperparathyroidism is characterized by autonomous hypersecretion of one or more parathyroid glands. The incidence of primary hyperparathyroidism in the United States is approximately 100,000 patients per year. Causes of hyperparathyroidism can be classified as primary hyperthyroidism, secondary hyperparathyroidism, tertiary hyperparathyroidism, familial hypocalciuric hypercalcemia (FHH), and parathyroid carcinoma. Appropriate management of these patients with hyperparathyroidism requires a thorough understanding of the pathogenesis as well as typical and atypical presentations, knowledge of laboratory tests for proper workup, and interpretation of imaging studies for localization of parathyroid adenomas. The ability to rapidly measure parathyroid hormone (PTH) level has allowed parathyroid surgeons to assess biochemical cure intraoperatively. Thus, surgical treatment of primary hyperparathyroidism has evolved primarily into minimally invasive single-gland excision. However, bilateral exploration still plays an important role in treatment of secondary and tertiary hyperparathyroidism. This chapter discusses clinical, laboratory, and radiologic evaluation of the hyperparathyroid patient as well as surgical and postoperative management.

EMBRYOLOGY AND ANATOMICAL CONSIDERATIONS

The inferior parathyroid glands are derived from the third pharyngeal pouch and descend caudally with the thyroid and thymus. The superior parathyroid glands are derived from the fourth pharyngeal pouch, attach to the posterior surface of the superior or midportion thyroid and migrate caudally with it. This pattern of migration explains the variability in the final arrest of the parathyroid glands, resulting in many possible locations of ectopic or supernumerary parathyroid glands. The limited course of the superior glands leads to less variability in location compared to the inferior gland. The inferior parathyroid glands can typically be found inferior, lateral or posterior to the inferior pole of the thyroid, anterior to a plane drawn through the recurrent laryngeal nerve. They can be quite variable in location. The superior parathyroid glands are less variable in location, the vast majority of them typically located near the cricothyroid joint, just superior to where the recurrent laryngeal nerve courses medially to enter the larynx. The blood supply to the parathyroid glands is primarily from the inferior thyroid artery, and in some there is contribution from the superior thyroid artery.

Humans typically have four parathyroid glands, two superior and two inferior. Approximately 3% to 13% of adults have supernumerary glands, and 5% have fewer than four (1). Normal parathyroid glands vary considerably in shape, size, and color. They are usually 2 to 3 mm in width, 1 to 2 mm in thickness, and 4 to 6 mm in length. Each gland weighs an average of 30 mg.

CALCIUM HOMEOSTASIS

Maintenance of extracellular calcium homeostasis involves the interaction of calcium, PTH, calcitonin, and vitamin D upon several target organs (kidney, bone, intestines, and parathyroid). Parathyroid cells respond to minute changes in the extracellular ionized calcium concentration, such that a small change in calcium concentration results in a change in the release rate of PTH in the opposite direction. This calcium-sensing property of parathyroid cells allows for the precise regulation of the extracellular ionized calcium concentration within a narrow range, normally 1.2 to 1.3 mmol/L. The calcium-sensing ability of parathyroid cells is believed to be mediated by a G-protein–coupled receptor on the parathyroid cell surface, known as calcium-sensing receptor (CaSR) (2). Hypocalcemia

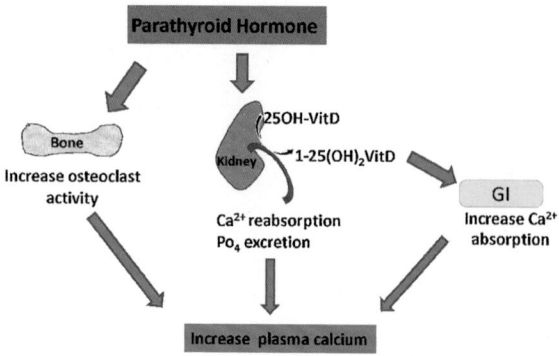

Figure 134.1 Actions of PTH.

induces PTH secretion, which raises the plasma calcium level toward normal by effecting the release of calcium from bone, increasing renal calcium reabsorption, and stimulating the production of 1,25-dihydroxyvitamin D. Vitamin D in turn increases intestinal absorption of calcium. Osteoclasts and certain cells of the renal tubule also exhibit calcium-sensing properties (Fig. 134.1).

PARATHYROID GLAND HISTOLOGY

The parenchyma of the parathyroid gland comprises primarily chief cells that are small, round, and light in color because of very weakly staining acidophilic cytoplasm. The nucleus is centrally placed. Chief cells synthesize PTH. Oxyphilic cells are less frequent, entirely lacking in small children under 6 years, and increase in number with age. Their cytoplasm is strongly acidophilic; the nucleus is small and uniformly intensely basophilic. They contain large amounts of mitochondria. These parenchymal cells are arranged in anastomosing chords surrounded by delicate connective tissue septa with abundant capillaries. A considerable number of fat cells infiltrate the gland beginning around puberty and may account for about half the weight of the parathyroid glands in adults (Fig. 134.2).

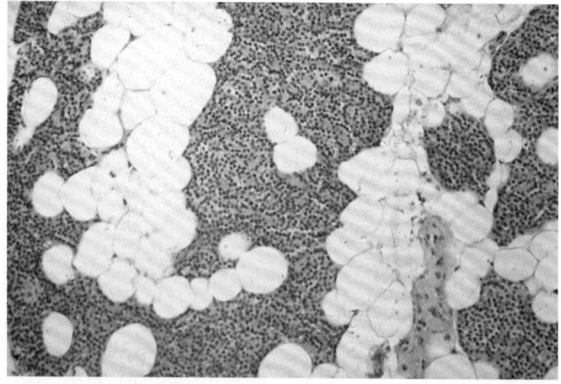

Figure 134.2 Histology of normal parathyroid gland showing chief cells and abundant fat cells.

HYPERPARATHYROIDISM

Hyperparathyroidism is classified into primary, secondary, and tertiary. Other rare causes of hyperparathyroidism include parathyroid carcinoma and FHH. It is important to understand the different causes of elevated PTH in surgical treatment considerations.

Primary Hyperparathyroidism

Primary hyperparathyroidism (1°HPT) is characterized by autonomous hypersecretion of one or more parathyroid glands. The incidence of 1°HPT in the United States is approximately 100,000 patients per year, and its prevalence is estimated to be between 0.2% and 1% (3). It predominantly affects those between the ages of 55 and 70 with a female-to-male ratio of 2:1. Recent reports from large series indicate that the etiology is a single parathyroid adenoma in 89% of cases, and hyperplasia or multiple adenomas in the remainder (4). The incidence of double adenomas ranges from 4% to 16% (5–7).

Secondary and Tertiary Hyperparathyroidism

Secondary hyperparathyroidism (2°HPT) is characterized by elevation of PTH level as a result of chronic hypocalcemia, most commonly from chronic renal failure, but it can also be caused by chronic vitamin D deficiency. In chronic renal failure, renal tubular excretion of phosphate is impaired, leading to hyperphosphatemia and binding with free calcium. In addition, renal hydroxylation of vitamin D is impaired leading to hypovitaminosis D. Vitamin D deficiency leads to decreased calcium absorption from both the gut and reabsorption of calcium in the renal tubules. The end effect is lower extracellular calcium, which in turn, stimulates the parathyroid glands to secrete PTH, resulting in hyperplasia of the parathyroid glands and elevation of PTH level. Other possible causes of elevated PTH associated with normal or low calcium are low calcium intake, inefficient calcium absorption from gastrointestinal disorders, and deficiency in intake of vitamin D; all these conditions result in low calcium and a compensatory rise in PTH level. In tertiary hyperparathyroidism, the chronically hyperplastic glands autonomously secrete PTH, which usually occurs after successful renal transplantation but can also occur after long-standing hypocalcemia of any other cause is corrected.

Parathyroid Carcinoma

Malignancy of the parathyroid gland is a very rare cause of hyperparathyroidism, representing less than 0.2% of patients with 1°HPT (7). It can rarely occur in association with hyperthyroid-jaw bone syndrome. Patients with this syndrome are carriers of the HRPT2 gene (8). This condition typically manifests with extremely high plasma calcium levels, usually greater than 13 mg/dL. Rarely a mass may be palpable (9).

Familial Hypocalciuric Hypercalcemia

FHH is an autosomal dominant genetic disorder characterized by mutations in the intracellular part of the CaSR (10,11). The result is a defect in the CaSR of the parathyroid cell resulting in a lack of PTH suppression in the setting of hypercalcemia. Genetic linkage studies have shown that chromosome 3q is the major, but not the sole, locus for FHH-causing gene (11,12). There are at least two other genetic loci, one linked to chromosome 19p and another family described in which linkage to 3q and 19q loci has been excluded but the FHH-causing gene has not yet been identified (13,14). While this condition is usually diagnosed at a younger age, it may manifest for the first time in older patients who have not sought medical attention throughout life. It typically has a benign course without the hypercalcemia-induced morbidities and is therefore generally not a surgical disease (15,16).

CLINICAL MANIFESTATIONS

The clinical presentation and complications of hyperparathyroidism depends on the degree of hypercalcemia and the rapidity in which the condition develops. The classic symptoms and manifestations of the disease are

1. Musculoskeletal: bone and joint pain, muscle pain, muscle weakness, osteopenia, osteoporosis, pseudogout, renal osteodystrophy
2. Genitourinary: nephrolithiasis, renal insufficiency, nocturia, polyuria
3. Gastrointestinal: constipation, peptic ulcers, heartburn, pancreatitis, abdominal pain, nausea
4. Neuropsychiatric: depression, anxiety, confusion, memory loss, impaired thinking or "brain fog"

A popular mnemonic for remembering these symptoms is "bones, stones, groans, and psychiatric overtones." Other manifestations that can also be seen are fatigue, calciphylaxis (soft tissue calcification), cardiocalcinosis, and band keratopathy.

EVALUATION

Evaluation of the hypercalcemic or hyperparathyroid patient starts with a good history and determination of what manifestations of the disease the patient has. Information on use of medications that can cause hypercalcemia should be elicited, specifically thiazide diuretics, lithium, dietary supplemental calcium, and vitamin D. Family history of hypercalcemia or hyperparathyroidism should be attained, as the patient may have familial hyperparathyroidism or FHH.

Laboratory Studies

The diagnosis of 1°HPT is made based on plasma calcium and PTH levels. Plasma calcium and PTH levels should be drawn on the same day. Normal range for

plasma calcium in most laboratories is 8.5 to 10.2 mg/dL (or 2.2 to 2.5 mmol/L). Since most of the body's plasma calcium is bound to albumin, a decrease in plasma albumin will lower the plasma calcium level even though the free calcium remains the same. Therefore if the albumin level is low, the plasma calcium should be corrected such that 0.8 mg/dL should be added to the total calcium for every drop in albumin of 1.0 g/dL. Alternatively, one can measure ionized calcium, which represents free calcium. Normal range for ionized calcium in most labs is 1.14 to 1.28 mmol/L. PTH is an 84 amino acid peptide chain with a C-terminal and an N-terminal. Laboratories in the past measured PTH levels by measuring the N-terminal or C-terminal. Today, the most accurate assessment of PTH level is measurement of the entire chain, known as intact PTH. Normal range for PTH in most laboratories is 15 to 72 pg/mL. The classic laboratory findings of 1°HPT are elevated plasma calcium level and high intact PTH level. Some patients may present with elevated plasma calcium levels and PTH levels only in the midrange to upper limits of normal. In the absence of 1°HPT, elevated plasma calcium should suppress the PTH level. Therefore, unsuppressed PTH in the setting of elevated plasma calcium is "inappropriate" and indicates 1°HPT. In addition to plasma calcium and intact PTH levels, it is also helpful to look at 24-hour urine calcium and serum phosphate levels. Typically in 1°HPT, the serum phosphate is low, and the 24-hour urine calcium is normal or elevated. Some patients may present with only periodic elevations of plasma calcium. In patients with mildly elevated or normal calcium, if the PTH levels are persistently elevated, the serum phosphate is low and 24-hour urine calcium is high (greater than 350 mg), the diagnosis of 1°HPT is likely. In a patient with normal or occasional mildly elevated calcium levels, intermittent mild elevation of PTH, normal phosphate and low to normal 24-hour urine calcium, the diagnosis of 1°HPT is somewhat questionable. If the diagnosis is uncertain, it would be prudent to repeat calcium and intact PTH levels and follow the laboratory values. Other than 1°HPT, the differential diagnosis of hypercalcemia includes thiazide diuretics, immobilization, and hypercalcemia of malignancy and granulomatous diseases. Contrary to 1°HTP, the PTH level is generally low in these conditions.

Elevated plasma calcium and PTH with a *low* 24-hour urine calcium is suggestive of FHH. The diagnosis of FHH should be considered if there is a family history of hypercalcemia, PTH is not markedly elevated, or the 24-hour urinary calcium is low. In that setting 24-hour urine for calcium, plasma calcium, serum creatinine and 24-hour urine creatinine levels should be obtained to calculate calcium–creatinine clearance ratio. These tests should all be performed at the same time. FHH manifests with hypercalcemia and mildly elevated or normal PTH levels (17,18). In FHH, the 24-hour urine calcium is below normal range. The calcium–creatinine clearance ratio, calculated using the following formula, is helpful in differentiating FHH from 1°HPT.

$$\frac{24\text{-hour urine calcium}}{\text{serum calcium}} \times \frac{\text{serum creatinine}}{24\text{-hour urine creatinine}}$$

A ratio that is greater than 0.01 is consistent with 1°HPT, though does not absolutely exclude FHH, and less than 0.01 is suggestive of FHH.

Some patients may also present with plasma calcium values in the mid to upper normal range but exhibit elevated ionized calcium. In recent years, a new entity known as normocalcemic hyperparathyroidism has been recognized where calcium level, including ionized calcium, is normal and PTH is elevated (19,20). It has been proposed that there is a generalized targeted tissue resistance to PTH in patients with this entity. A study by Maruani et al. (21) showed PTH-dependent functions of the kidney to be attenuated in the normocalcemic hyperparathyroid patients despite an identical primary hypersecretion of PTH. They concluded that: (a) PTH induces milder biologic bone effects than in hypercalcemic patients; (b) Calcium absorption in the renal tubular system is lower in patients with normocalcemic 1°HPT compared to that of patients with hypercalcemic form of the disease. (c) The ability of PTH to decrease tubular phosphate reabsorption and stimulate synthesis of 1,25-dihydroxyvitamin D is also blunted in the patients who remain normocalcemic, compared with those who are hypercalcemic. Normocalcemic 1°HPT can be difficult to diagnose, and 2°PTH from other conditions such as chronic vitamin D deficiency, renal insufficiency, and renal calcium leak need to be excluded first. In 2°HPT, the typical laboratory finding is elevated PTH but unlike 1°HPT, the plasma calcium level is low or normal. Those with 2°HPT from chronic renal failure also exhibit elevated blood urea nitrogen, serum creatinine, and phosphate.

Vitamin D levels should also be measured. In 1°HPT, the 25-hydroxy form will typically be low, and 1,25-hydroxy form is often elevated. Vitamin D levels are generally not used to make a diagnosis of 1°HPT but may be helpful in differentiating 2°HPT due to chronic vitamin D deficiency from "normocalcemic" 1°HPT. Since both conditions will present with normal calcium and elevated PTH, if the 25-hydroxyvitamin D level is low, one can correct the vitamin D deficiency and follow the calcium level. If the calcium level becomes elevated or the PTH level does not correct back down to normal range with vitamin D replacement, the diagnosis is likely to be 1°HPT.

Imaging Studies

While imaging studies are used primarily to localize parathyroid adenomas for surgical planning, they may also be helpful in confirming the diagnosis of 1°HPT. If the lab values are intermittently or only mildly elevated, the diagnosis of 1°HPT can be confirmed if the imaging study unequivocally detects a parathyroid adenoma. The two most commonly used imaging studies are parathyroid ultrasound and technetium-99m-sestamibi parathyroid (MIBI) scan. The sensitivity of each test varies considerably, depending on the equipment and more importantly how experienced is the individual performing or interpreting the study. In the hands of a highly experienced ultrasonographer, which can be radiologist, surgeon, or endocrinologist, the sensitivity is 80% to 85%. On ultrasound, parathyroid adenomas appear hypoechoic and hypervascular (Fig. 134.3). Generally ultrasound should be able to detect adenomas located dorsal to the esophagus. The limitation of ultrasound is detecting adenomas located retroesophageally or in the mediastinum. The principle of sestamibi parathyroid scanning is that ^{99}Tc MIBI tracer is taken up by both the thyroid and parathyroid adenoma but washes out of the thyroid faster than the parathyroid. Therefore early images at 20 minutes after injection are obtained, followed by delayed images typically at 2 hours (Fig. 134.4A). It is quite specific; however, its sensitivity

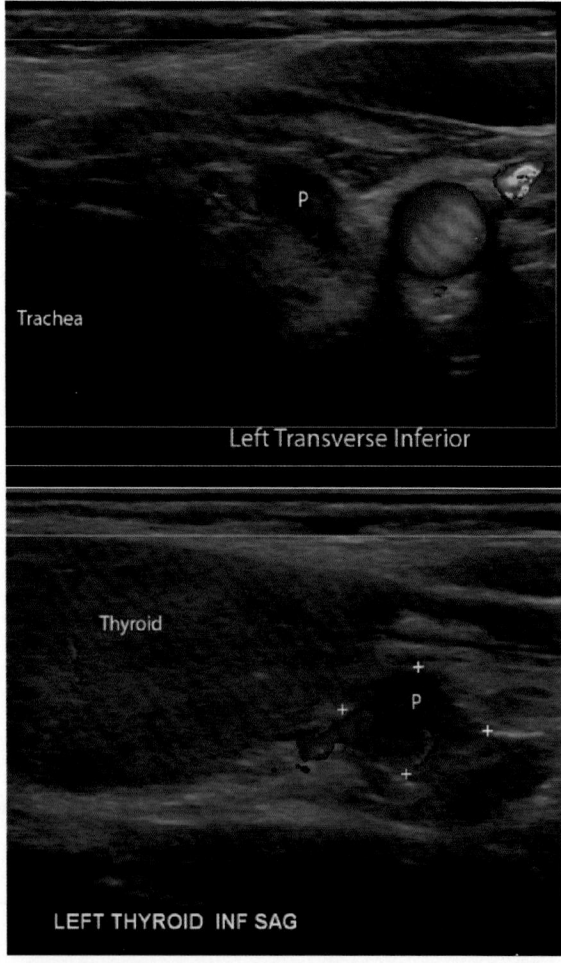

Figure 134.3 Ultrasound of left inferior parathyroid adenoma. **Top:** adenoma (P) between the trachea and carotid artery; **Bottom:** adenoma is at the inferior tip of the thyroid.

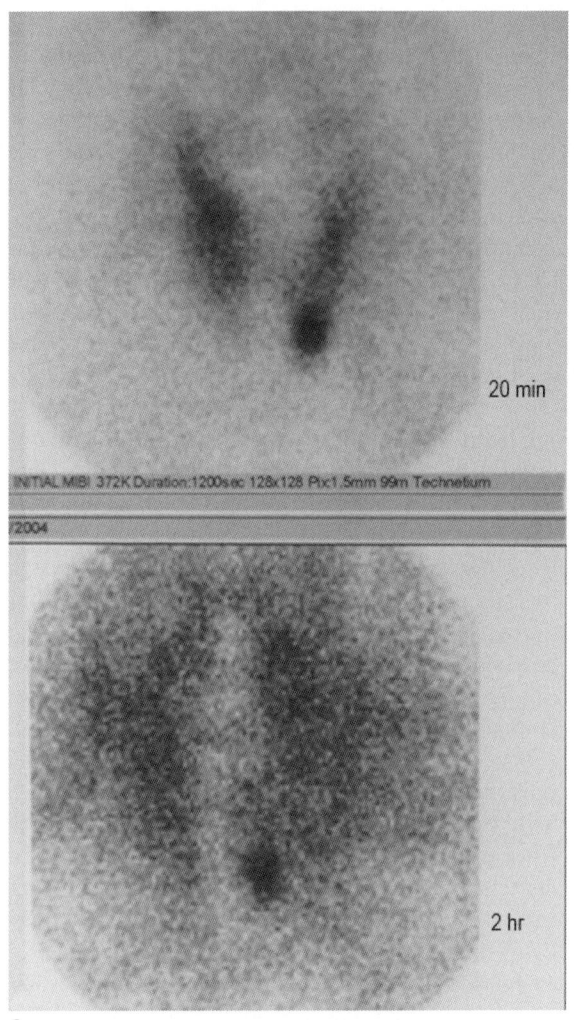

A

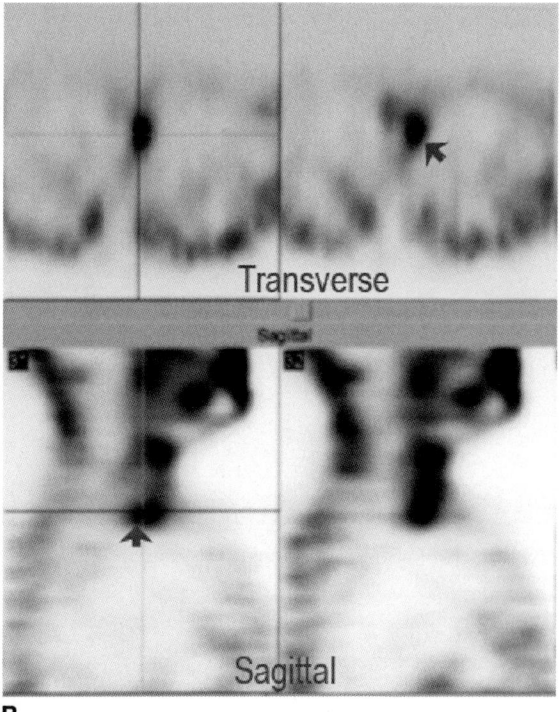

B

Figure 134.4 Sestamibi parathyroid scan. **A:** 2D planer images showing a left, inferiorly located adenoma **B:** SPECT revealing the adenoma (*arrow*) to be located posterior to the plane of the thyroid on the transverse and sagittal views.

can be low in detecting small glands. One of its limitations is that concurrent thyroid disease can result in a false-positive study. Another limitation is that the images are two-dimensional (2D) planer views and therefore do not provide information on the depth of the adenoma. This information is important for glands that are located inferior to the thyroid. On a 2D planer anterior–posterior view, without the information on the depth of the gland, a ret-roesophageal or paraesophageal gland can look virtually identical to an anteriorly located inferior gland. Oblique views or single photon emission computerized tomography (SPECT) obtained in conjunction with the 2D planer sestamibi scans can be helpful in providing informa-tion on the anterior–posterior location of the adenoma (Fig. 134.4B). Knowing this information obviates unneces-sary extensive or missed exploration. If localization with sestamibi scan and ultrasound performed in experienced hands fail, thin-cut CT with intravenous contrast may be helpful. It is especially useful in detecting ectopic glands such as paraesophageal, retroesophageal, or mediastinal glands (Fig. 134.5).

INDICATIONS FOR SURGERY

Parathyroidectomy is indicated in patients with 1°HPT who have complications of the disease, such as nephrolithiasis, hypercalcemic crisis (calcium greater than 12.5 mg/dL), or are symptomatic with musculoskeletal pain, muscle weakness, or severe neuropsychiatric dysfunction (irritabil-ity, fatigue, confusion, or insomnia). However, since the gamut of muscular and neuropsychological symptoms is broad, it is often difficult to determine if the symptoms are truly due to 1°HPT. The indications for surgery in the asymptomatic patient were first established in 1990 by a NIH sponsored consensus panel and modified in 2002 (Table 134.1) (22). In 2009, the guidelines were rereviewed at the Third International Workshop on Asymptomatic Primary Hyperparathyroidism, and the recommendations basically remained the same except for three changes: (a) hypercalciuria (24-hour urine calcium greater than 400 mg) was eliminated, (b) creatinine clearance was changed from less than 30% to less than 60 mL/min, and (c) bone density T-score at any site less than –2.5 and/or previous fracture or

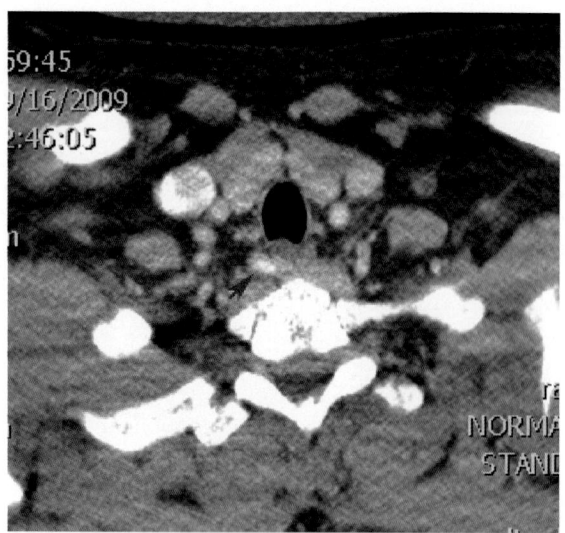

Figure 134.5 CT with contrast demonstrating a right paraesophageal adenoma (*arrow*).

bone fragility (Table 134.1) (23). Since parathyroidectomy traditionally has been performed under general anesthesia and required bilateral exploration, which has potential significant risks, many asymptomatic patients had generally been observed rather than treated surgically. However, in recent years, parathyroid surgery has evolved into minimally invasive focused exploration often under local anesthesia, with significantly lower surgical risks. Therefore, surgical consideration should be given to asymptomatic patients, even in healthy elderly patients with a reasonably long life expectancy, if they are appropriate candidates for minimally invasive parathyroidectomy (MIP).

Multiple studies in the last decade have proven the benefits of parathyroidectomy for 1°HPT. Studies on quality of life postparathyroidectomy have been performed using the

SF-36 survey, a self-ranked 36-item survey that assesses general health, as well as the Parathyroidectomy Assessment of Symptoms survey. Both have been shown to improve quickly after surgery (24–27). Furthermore, these improvements are sustained long term (24,27,28). Bone density and hyperlipidemia have also been shown to improve with parathyroidectomy (29,30).

Indications for parathyroidectomy in 2°HPT have been based mostly on presence of musculoskeletal symptoms, such as bone and joint pain, muscle weakness, or radiologic evidence of renal osteodystrophy. In recent years treatment with vitamin D and its analogs have allowed the majority of these patients to be managed by medical treatment for many years without severe symptoms of high bone turnover. Nevertheless, chronic high values of phosphate, calcium, and PTH in renal failure patients have been shown to be associated with increased mortality, mainly due to cardiovascular complications induced by ectopic calcifications (31,32). Therefore, the main indication currently for parathyroidectomy in these patients is when serum phosphate, calcium, and PTH levels cannot be maintained within target ranges with vitamin D or D-analog therapy (32,33). The introduction of cinacalcet, a new allosteric modulator of the CaSR on parathyroid cells that reduces PTH secretion, has also reduced the need for parathyroidectomy by 90% (34). Surgery is indicated when cinacalcet cannot be continued due to adverse side effects or poor compliance, or if the condition is refractory to cinacalcet therapy. Several studies have shown that parathyroidectomy in dialysis patients with advanced 2°HPT is associated with reduced incidence of major cardiovascular events and overall lower mortality (35–38).

PARATHYROIDECTOMY

Bilateral Exploration

While the majority of parathyroid surgeries today are performed using a targeted approach exploring only a single gland (see next section), surgeons still need to be thoroughly familiar with the principles of 4-gland exploration, which is essential for treatment of hyperplasia, 2°HPT, and tertiary hyperparathyroidism. Knowledge of parathyroid gland locations is the key to successful 4-gland exploration. Embryologically, the inferior parathyroid glands arise from the dorsal wing of the third pharyngeal pouch, and the ventral wing of the third brachial pouch differentiates into the thymus. The thymus then migrates caudally, pulling the parathyroids with it. Descent of the inferior parathyroid glands usually stops at the dorsal (posterior) surface of the inferior thyroid outside of its fibrous capsule. At times the inferior parathyroids may not lose its connection to the thymus and thus descend into the anterior mediastinum with the thymus. The superior parathyroid glands arise from the dorsal wing of the fourth pharyngeal pouch and descend with the thyroid. The superior parathyroids

TABLE 134.1	INDICATIONS FOR PARATHYROIDECTOMY IN ASYMPTOMATIC PATIENTS	
2002		**2009**
Ca²⁺ > 1 mg/dL above upper limit of normal		Ca²⁺ > 1 mg/dL above upper limit of normal
Creatinine clearance reduced by 30%		Creatinine clearance <60 mL/min
Reduction in bone density (hip, L Spine, Radius) T-score < −2.5		Reduction in bone density (hip, L Spine, Radius) T-score < −2.5; Previous fracture or bone fragility
Under 50 y of age		Under 50 y of age
Medical surveillance not feasible (e.g., coexistent illness) or not possible (e.g., poor follow-up)		Medical surveillance not feasible (e.g., coexistent illness) or not possible (e.g., poor follow-up)
24-h urine calcium >400 mg		

are generally located more posterior and medial than the inferior parathyroids, and their final resting point is usually on the dorsal surface of the mid or superior pole of the thyroid. However, they may also be ectopically located lateral or posterior to the esophagus. Rarely can they be located superior to the superior pole. Parathyroid glands can also be located in the carotid sheath or inside the fibrous capsule of the thyroid (intrathyroid).

When performing 4-gland exploration, it is important to search for each gland systematically moving from one quadrant to the next in the expected locations of the parathyroid glands. If the glands are not identified in the expected locations, the ectopic locations of the missing gland should then be systematically explored. For example, if a superior gland is missing, the paraesophageal and retroesophageal areas should be explored. If an inferior parathyroid is missing, exploration should be directed first at the most common ectopic location for the inferior glands—the thymus and superior mediastinum. If the missing parathyroid is not found in these locations the carotid sheath should be explored. The last location to consider is intrathyroid, in which case a hemithyroidectomy on the side of the missing gland may be necessary. An alternative to hemithyroidectomy for identifying an intrathyroid adenoma is to perform intraoperative thyroid ultrasound with a small probe. If a hypoechoic nodule adjacent to the posterior capsule is found (Fig. 134.6), needle aspiration of the lesion can be performed. The sample can be rinsed with approximately 2 mL of normal saline and a rapid PTH assay can be performed intraoperatively. The PTH level will be high if the lesion is a parathyroid adenoma.

When performing subtotal parathyroidectomy, it is important to not completely excise or devascularize each parathyroid gland as soon as it is identified. As each one is identified, it is best to biopsy part of the gland for confirmation and temporarily keep a portion *in situ*. Once all four glands are histologically confirmed, the most viable residual gland should be selected for preservation *in situ*, and then excision of the other glands can be performed. Some of the excised parathyroid glands should be cryopreserved for possible future use. Approximately 30 to 40 g of parathyroid tissue should be prepared for reimplantation. It is preferable to reimplant into the brachioradialis muscle of the patient's nondominant hand. The parathyroid tissue is incised into approximately 1 × 1 × 3 mm pieces (Fig. 134.7A) and each piece is microsurgically reimplanted into the brachioradialis muscle. Each reimplantation site should be marked with hemoclip and/or colored permanent suture for ease of identification if the need arises to someday excise hyperplastic reimplanted tissue (Fig. 134.7B).

The decision to perform subtotal versus total parathyroidectomy depends on the disease and to some extent surgeon's preference. Those with hyperplasia due to 1°HPT should undergo subtotal parathyroidectomy, with the goal for the intraoperative rapid parathyroid hormone (IOPTH) to return to the mid-normal range. Most would also

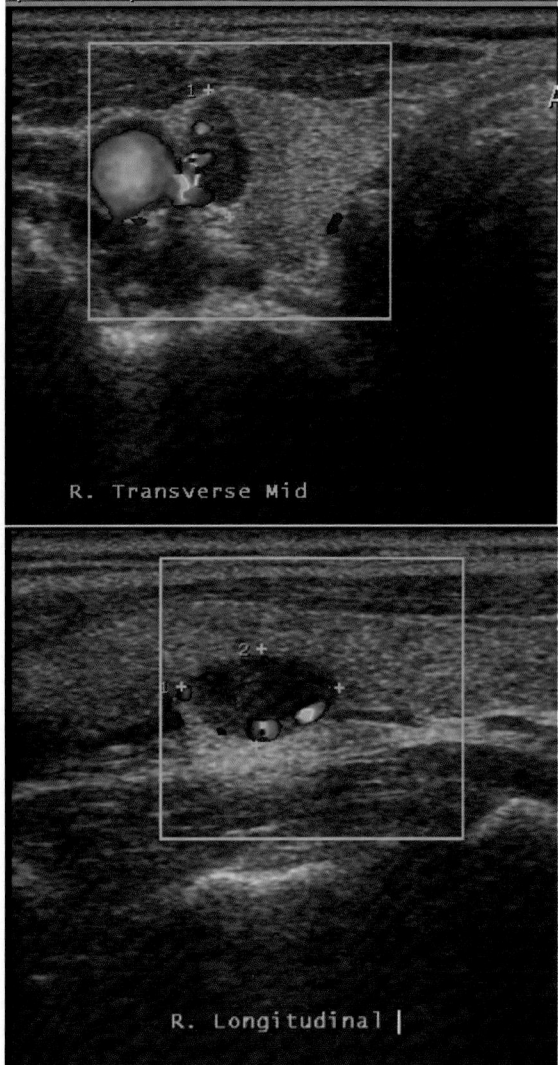

Figure 134.6 Ultrasound showing intrathyroid parathyroid.

reimplant some of the excised parathyroid tissue in the forearm, although one could argue that if the IOPTH at the end of the exploration is in midnormal range, reimplantation may not be necessary. Regardless, some of the tissue should be cryopreserved. Extent of parathyroidectomy is more controversial for 2°HPT or tertiary hyperparathyroidism. Unlike 1°HPT, chronic renal failure with hypocalcemia is a strong stimulus for parathyroid hyperplasia. Therefore, if subtotal parathyroidectomy is performed, any glandular tissue left behind can become hyperplastic again in the future in these patients. Consequently, some argue that total parathyroidectomy with reimplantation in the forearm is preferred in these patients to obviate the need for neck reexploration. Elevated preoperative calcium and post-op IOPTH levels were significant predictors for recurrent disease, while postoperative PTH less than 10 pmol/L had a positive predictive value of 97.5% for cure (39). For those who are younger patients, post kidney transplants, or candidates for kidney transplantation,

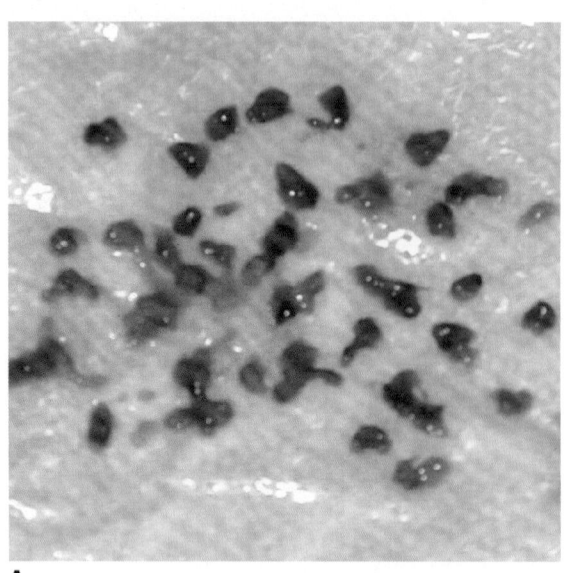
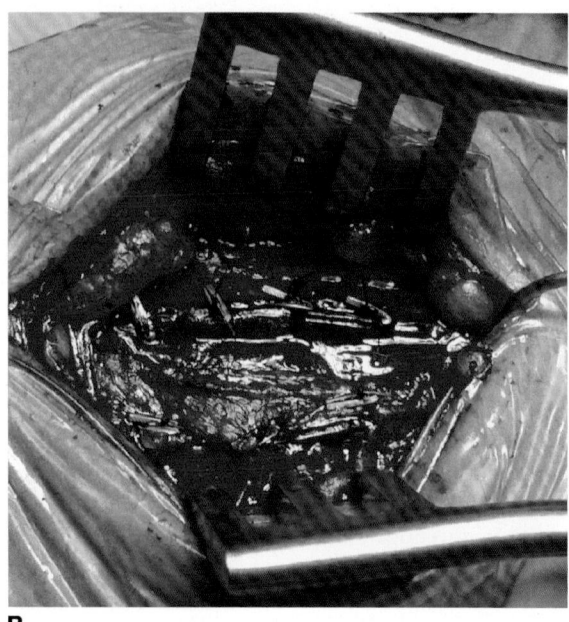

A   **B**

Figure 134.7 A: Parathyroid gland cut and prepared for reimplantation. **B:** Reimplanted sites in brachioradialis muscle marked with hemoclips.

subtotal parathyroidectomy may be appropriate, whereas total parathyroidectomy with autotransplantation may be recommended for patients expected to undergo long-term dialysis who are not candidates for transplantation (33).

Minimally Invasive Parathyroidectomy

The traditional approach for years in parathyroid surgery has been to perform bilateral exploration and examine all four parathyroid glands. With the ability to preoperatively localize an adenoma with imaging modalities unilateral exploration became acceptable, where the localized adenoma is excised and presence of another normal gland on the same side is confirmed. The limitation of this approach is that a second adenoma (double adenoma) on the contralateral side can be missed. In 1991, Irvin et al. introduced the concept of rapid measurement of intact PTH intraoperatively. The intact PTH has a very short half-life of approximately 2 to 4 minutes. Therefore, following successful removal of a single parathyroid adenoma, measurement of intact PTH level shortly after removal of an adenoma can be used to predict success of surgery. Several studies have shown that following excision of a localized adenoma, IOPTH accurately predicts presence or absence of other functioning glands (40–43). With this approach, it is no longer necessary to explore multiple glands, and the risk of missing multiglandular disease is reduced. With the ability to preoperatively localize an adenoma and use IOPTH assay, parathyroid surgery has evolved into focused exploration with single-gland excision. A 2002 study on worldwide trends in parathyroid surgery reported that 60% of surgeons perform minimally invasive single-gland

excision rather than bilateral exploration (44). Minimally invasive focused parathyroidectomy begins with a small incision in the area of a suspected adenoma. Most centers use IOPTH to confirm absence of other hyperfunctioning glands. A preexcision level is typically drawn at the time of anesthetic induction and/or right after the parathyroid adenoma is mobilized for excision. A postexcision level is then drawn 10 to 15 minutes after the adenoma is excised. A drop of more than 50% from the preexcision value is the most commonly used criteria for successful parathyroidectomy.

Pitfalls of IOPTH

Several validation studies evaluated IOPTH levels pre- and postexcision of abnormal gland(s) during conventional bilateral exploration (45–48). One pitfall of IOPTH is that the postexcision may fall below 50% of baseline yet one or more enlarged gland still remains. This is defined as a *false-positive* result. Gauger et al. (45) reported 55% false-positive rate in 20 patients during conventional bilateral exploration, all due to double adenomas. Similarly, Jaskowiak et al. (46) reported 50% false-positive and 50% true-negative rates for IOPTH when double adenomas are present. To explain this false-positive phenomenon with double adenomas, some hypothesize that the second adenoma, which is usually the smaller one, may not be hypersecretory. Therefore, if the second gland is not biochemically significant, the IOPTH value will actually drop below 50% after excision of the "active" one. Even with 4-gland hyperplasia, IOPTH may exhibit kinetics similar to that of single adenomas. For example, one study reported that in

12.5% of patients who were undergoing surgery for known hyperplasia from MEN1 syndrome, the kinetics of IOPTH was similar to that seen with a single adenoma (49).

False-positive rates have been reported to range from 2% to 13%, giving an overall specificity rate of approximately 90% (48,50,51). Thus while IOPTH significantly reduces the chances of missing multiglandular disease, operative morbidity, and length of hospital stay, it can still potentially miss multiple gland pathology, which may result in need for reoperation. Hallfeldt et al. reported that in 2 of 36 patients in whom they used the 50% criteria, but the absolute IOPTH value remained above normal range, the IOPTH levels began to elevate again postoperatively. One of these two patients were reexplored and found to have hyperplasia (48). Karakousis et al. (51) also reported that in their patients with multiglandular disease, IOPTH had a false-positive rate of 29% if the IOPTH drops by 50% but does not return to normal range, and that this would be lower if a more stringent criteria was used (51). To reduce false-positive rates, the use of a more stringent criteria has been proposed, such as postexcision level less than 50% of preexcision level and must also return within normal range (52). Therefore, if the postexcision level does not meet both of these criteria, one or more hyperfunctioning glands remain in the patient and the remaining glands should be explored systematically.

Conversely, a *false-negative* result is defined as IOPTH failing to fall below 50% when no additional enlarged glands remain. One possible mechanism for such false-negative values is that there can be a sudden rise in circulating PTH during manipulation of the adenoma; therefore, if the 5-minute postexcision value is compared to a baseline drawn before manipulation, it may not be less than 50% of baseline or sometimes can actually be higher than the baseline. For example, if the PTH level is 110 pg/dL at the time of induction and surges to 300 pg/dL after manipulation of the adenoma, a postexcision level drawn 5 minutes after removal may drop to 60 pg/dL, which is not less than 50% when compared to the 110 pg/dL preexcision level, yet it is certainly greater than a 50% drop in relation to the second level drawn. Therefore, if only the first prelevel is available for comparison, it may lead to unnecessary further exploration because technically the patient has not met the criteria for biochemical cure. Because of this some surgeons draw a second "pre" level just before excision of the adenoma and compare the postexcision level to the higher of the two preexcision levels. Another reason for false-negative results is slower kinetics for PTH clearance. To get around this problem one can delay the first postexcision draw until 10 or 15 minutes after excision of the adenoma. Another option would be to draw the IOPTH at either 10 minutes or 15 minutes after excision, at which time the values may be close to 50% of baseline. The false-negative rate ranges from 3% to 8% in the literature, giving an overall sensitivity rate of approximately 95% (50,53–55). A false-negative

result potentially can subject the patient to unnecessary additional neck exploration at the time of primary surgery.

To date, no uniform guidelines have been formulated to interpret IOPTH values. The goal is to achieve a high sensitivity and specificity. One achieves high specificity by reducing false-positive rate, and high sensitivity by lowering false-negative rate. Attempts to reduce the failure rate by adding a more stringent criterion minimizes the incidence of false-positives and increase specificity. However, this is at the expense of raising false-negative rate and thus a lower sensitivity, which results in unnecessary further explorations. Reported specificity and sensitivity rates in the literature are somewhat inconsistent, which makes it difficult to find the right balance. Lombardi proposed more than a 50% decrease from the highest preexcision level and/or an IOPTH level within the normal range 20 minutes after excision to predict surgical cure and postoperative normocalcemia. Ozimek et al. (42) also proposed more than a 50% decrease from the highest PTH level plus a decrease to the normal range within 15 minutes and reporting 97% sensitivity but reducing the specificity to 88% (42). The need for IOPTH has also been questioned in recent years (56–60). A number of authors have reported failure rates of only 1% to 3% when IOPTH was not used during MIP (57,60,61). Based on these results, a viable option when preoperative ultrasound and sestamibi studies are concordant would be *not* to measure PTH intraoperatively but to delay it until later the same day or next day in order to avoid unnecessary conversion to more extensive neck exploration. A cost analysis by Aggarwal et al. (61) showed that this approach could theoretically reduce the cost by one-third, factoring in the risk of unnecessary conversion exploration (61).

Minimally Invasive Radioguided Parathyroidectomy

Radioguided parathyroidectomy, in which technetium sestamibi is injected prior to surgery and a gamma probe is then used to compare the radioactive level before and after excision adenoma, has also been described as another way to accomplish minimally invasive targeted parathyroidectomy. Following excision of the adenoma, the radioactive counts of the adenoma as well as the background are obtained. If the *ex vivo* count on the adenoma is greater than 20% of background count, the patient is considered to have only one adenoma and surgery is deemed successful. This minimally invasive radioguided parathyroidectomy is referred to as MIRP. It should be cautioned that *ex vivo* radioactivity percentages can differentiate hyperactive parathyroid tissue from any other tissue, but they cannot differentiate adenoma from hyperplasia and thus are not helpful in ruling out multiglandular disease (62). Some surgeons also combine MIRP with the use of IOPTH to confirm biochemical cure. The cure rate with radioguided parathyroidectomy has been reported to be as high as 98% (63–65).

Outcome of Minimally Invasive Parathyroidectomy versus Bilateral Exploration

Several retrospective studies comparing the outcome of MIP with IOPTH to that of conventional bilateral exploration have shown that the success rates of the MIP were similar to or better than that of bilateral exploration (24,43,47,66–68). Furthermore complication rates tend to be lower. Burkey et al. compared the outcome of three different approaches, gamma probe ($n = 50$), IOPTH ($n = 50$), and bilateral exploration ($n = 50$). The cure rates were 98%, 100%, and 96%, respectively, and the complication rate was higher in the bilateral exploration group compared to the other two (66). Similarly, Boggs et al. (67) reported a failure rate of 1.5% when Sestamibi and IOPTH were used versus 5% when bilateral exploration was performed without IOPTH. In a study to evaluate whether or not IOPTH improves the results of parathyroidectomy, Miura et al. (43) showed that by adding IOPTH to the operation, the accuracy of Sestamibi scan improved from 83% to 92%, and the accuracy of ultrasound improved from 71% to 86%. These results were validated by Udelsman et al. (68) recently in a comparison study of a large cohort of 1,650 patients undergoing parathyroidectomy that demonstrated the superiority of MIP to bilateral exploration. The cure rate was 99.4% with a complication rate of 1.45% in the MIP group compared to conventional exploration with a cure rate of 97.1% and a complication rate of 3.10%. A prospective blinded randomized study also showed that the cure rates were similar between MIP and bilateral exploration, but MIP had lower postoperative pain, lower analgesic request rate, lower analgesic consumption, shorter scar length, better cosmetic satisfaction rate in a short time period (69).

Surgical Techniques

MIP can be performed under local anesthesia with intravenous sedation or under general anesthesia. Two approaches can be used—anterior and lateral. Most surgeons utilize the anterior approach because of familiarity from performing thyroidectomy; however, the lateral approach can also be useful.

Anterior Approach

The patient is placed in supine position and a midline curvilinear 2 to 3 cm incision is drawn at the level of the adenoma. An ultrasound can also be performed prior to marking the patient to assist in placement of the incision. The strap muscles are separated along the median raphae laterally on the side of the adenoma. When excising glands that are located inferior to the thyroid lobe or just posterior to the inferior pole the trachea or inferior thyroid pole is retracted medially and the gland should be easily identified (Fig. 134.8). For more superiorly located adenomas

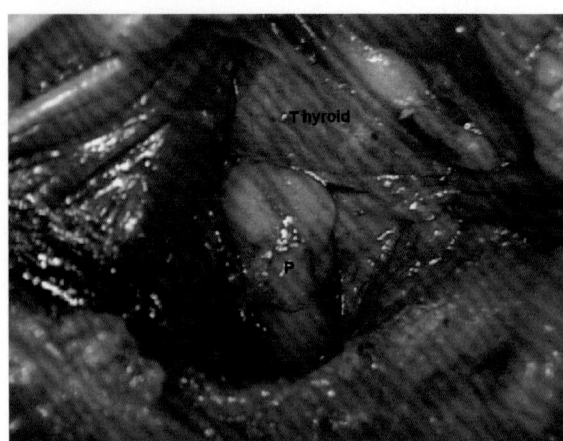

Figure 134.8 Minimally invasive parathyroidectomy using anterior approach: Right inferior parathyroid adenoma (P) identified posterior to the inferior pole of thyroid. Top of photo is cephalad.

the thyroid lobe is retracted medially and rotated to expose the posterior surface. Blunt dissect is then used to search for the adenoma. One should be cognizant of the location of the recurrent laryngeal nerve in dissecting these glands. Especially for glands located lateral or posterior to the esophagus, it is important to look for the recurrent laryngeal nerve, which often may course anterior to the adenoma. After identification of the adenoma, it is removed using blunt dissection. Small feeding vessels can be isolated and cauterized on the capsule of the parathyroid gland. Hemostasis is achieved and the incision is closed in two layers.

Lateral Approach

This approach allows better exposure to posteriorly located adenomas without having to extensively retract the thyroid lobe, thus allowing the performance of the procedure local/sedation (70). The incision is placed more laterally between the midline and the anterior border of the sternocleidomastoid muscle. The sternocleidomastoid muscle is retracted laterally to expose the strap muscles (Fig. 134.9A). The ansa hypoglossi nerve is identified coursing along the posterior edge of the strap muscles. The muscle is then retracted medially, exposing the internal jugular vein and carotid artery (Fig. 134.9B and C). The vagus nerve may also be encountered during the dissection. The vein, artery, and vagus nerve are retracted laterally, exposing the thyroid capsule (Fig. 134.9C). Again, using the ultrasound images or intraoperative ultrasound, dissection is targeted at the exact location of the adenoma (Fig. 134.9D).

Once identified, the same steps are carried out for excision and closure as described in the anterior approach. When excising adenomas located posteriorly on the prevertebral fascia, it is important to be cognizant of the recurrent laryngeal nerve (Fig. 134.10), which can course right over the adenoma or just medial to it.

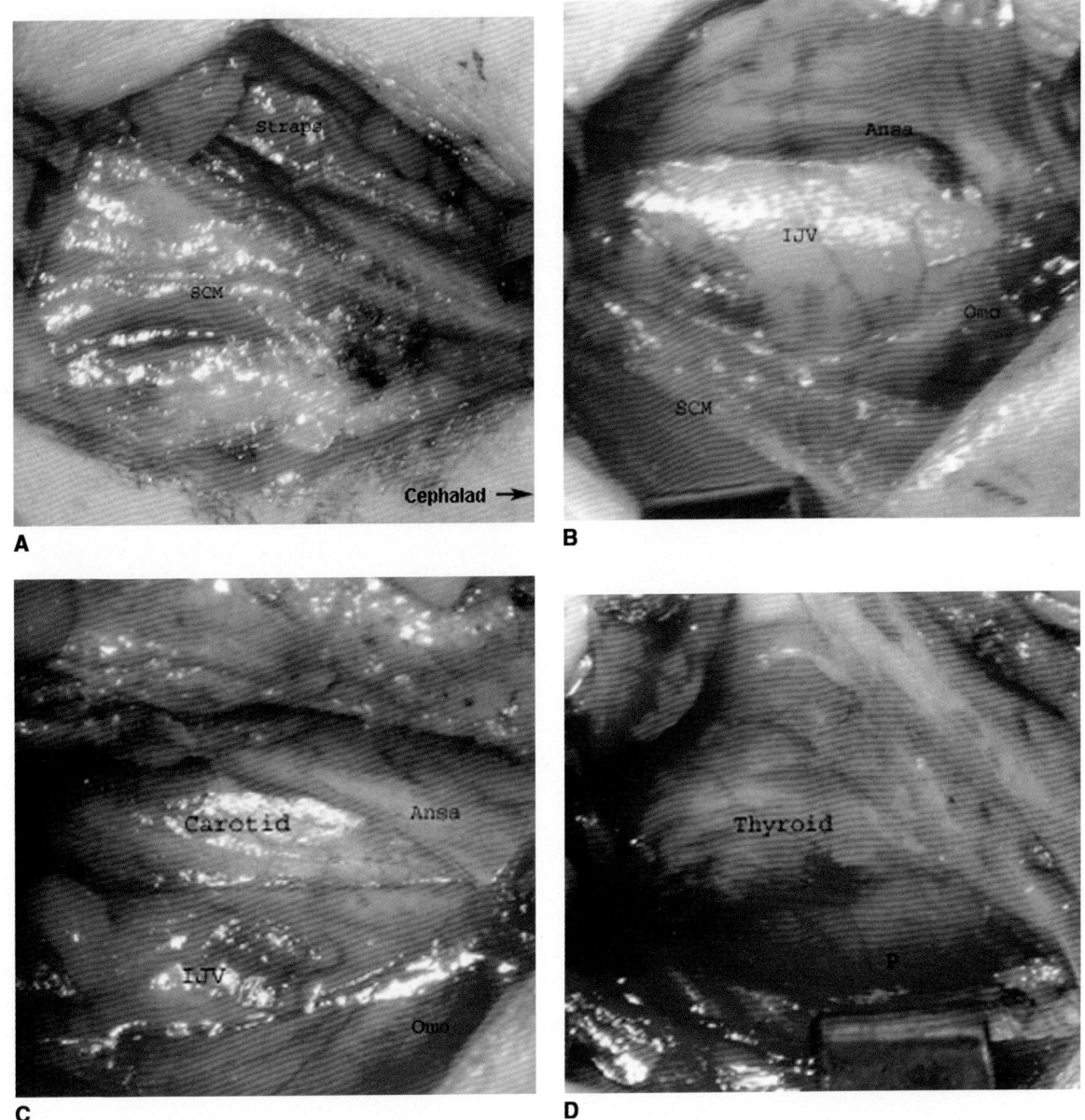

Figure 134.9 Minimally invasive parathyroidectomy using lateral approach for left superior adenoma. **A:** The sternocleidomastoid muscle (SCM) is retracted laterally and strap muscles are retracted medially; **B:** The internal jugular vein (IJV), omohyoid (OMO), and ansa hypoglossi are exposed; **C:** The carotid artery is exposed, which will be retracted laterally; **D:** After the strap muscles with the ansa are retracted medially, the thyroid is exposed with parathyroid adenoma (P) posterior to it.

MEDIASTINAL ADENOMA

Approximately 1% to 2% of parathyroid adenomas are located in the upper mediastinum. Once identified on sestamibi scan (Fig. 134.11), CT with contrast or MRI should be obtained for surgical planning. Traditionally surgical treatment required sternotomy or thoracotomy (71,72). In recent years, resection of these adenomas can be accomplished via mediastinoscopy using a suspension scope, or thorascopically through intercostals space depending on its location (73,74). Recovery and post-op complications

with these minimally invasive approaches are lower than that of traditional thoracotomy.

PARATHYROID CARCINOMA

Parathyroid carcinoma should be suspected if the patient presents with very high plasma calcium (greater than 13 mg/dL) or PTH levels, a palpable mass in the area of localized adenoma, suspicious lymphadenopathy, or high depth–width ratio of the mass on ultrasound. Intraoperatively the diagnosis of carcinoma should be

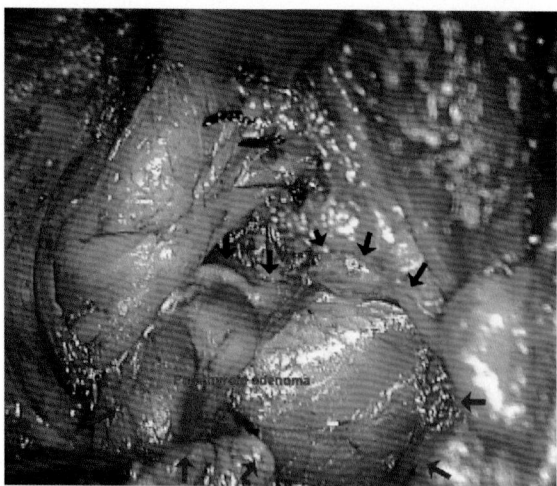

Figure 134.10 Left inferior paraesophageal adenoma (outlined by *blue arrows*) with recurrent laryngeal nerve (*black arrows*) coursing over it.

entertained if the mass is adherent to surrounding tissues, since benign parathyroid adenomas typically "shell out" easily with blunt dissection. If any of the above is present, frozen section should be performed. Making a definitive diagnosis of parathyroid carcinoma intraoperatively is extremely difficult, since the main criteria for such diagnosis are vascular invasion, perineural space invasion, capsular penetration with growth into adjacent structures, or metastases. High mitotic rate and considerable thick fibrous bands coursing throughout the gland can be seen on frozen section, but they are not diagnostic (Fig. 134.12). If the diagnosis is either confirmed or highly suspicious, complete en bloc resection, including hemithyroidectomy and paratracheal dissection, should

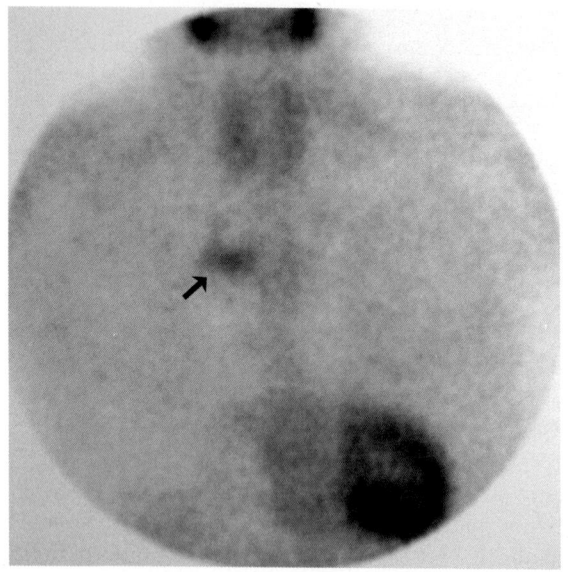

Figure 134.11 Sestamibi scan showing right superior mediastinal adenoma (*arrow*).

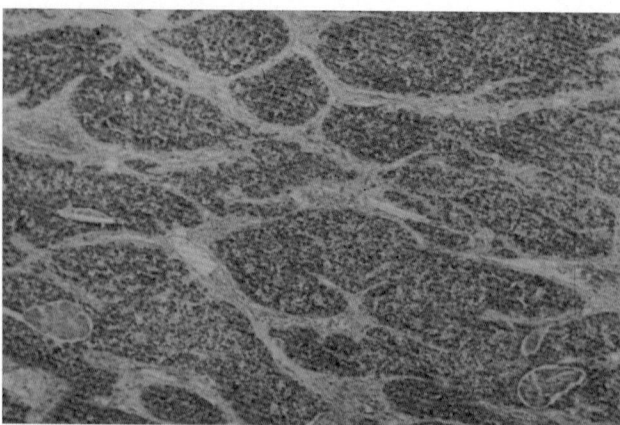

Figure 134.12 Histology of parathyroid carcinoma—Atypical chief cells with extensive fibrous bands.

be performed. Recurrence is usually in cervical nodes. The most common site of distant metastasis is lungs. Morbidity and mortality of recurrent parathyroid carcinoma usually result from unremitting hypercalcemia and its complications rather than mass effect of tumor burden. Treatment of locoregional recurrent parathyroid carcinoma is primarily surgery, since it generally responds poorly to radiation or chemotherapy. Treatment of advanced disease is primarily targeted at controlling hypercalcemia with bisphosphonate and calcimimetic agents.

POSTOPERATIVE CARE

Patients undergoing bilateral exploration may be at risk of developing hypocalcemia postoperatively and therefore have traditionally been admitted for overnight observation. Potential causes of post-op hypocalcemia after bilateral exploration and parathyroidectomy include injury and devascularization of remaining glands, calciuretic effect of intravenous fluid, decreased PTH production from the remaining suppressed parathyroids, and hungry bones syndrome. Patients who have undergone subtotal parathyroidectomy for hyperplasia are even more at risk, since the small volume of parathyroid left *in situ* may become devascularized. Virtually all who are treated with total parathyroidectomy and reimplantation for 2° HPT or tertiary hyperparathyroidism will be hypocalcemic post-op until the reimplanted tissue establishes a blood supply and regains normal function.

Those admitted for observation following 4-gland bilateral exploration should be assessed for symptoms of hypocalcemia such as paresthesias of hands, feet, or perioral region as well as muscle spasms. Early signs of hypocalcemia include: (a) Chovstek sign where tapping preauricularly elicits twitching of the ipsilateral face, and (b) Trussou sign where inflation of a blood pressure cuff elicits cramping in the extremity. Severe hypocalcemia can induce muscle cramping, tetany, seizures, and cardiac arrhythmias. Calcium levels should be checked starting the next morning, and two levels should be drawn 6 to 8 hours apart since the calcium may not drop until well beyond 24 hours after surgery. The patient can be discharged if the sequential calcium levels are stable or demonstrate an upward trend.

Another approach to facilitating safe and early discharge after bilateral exploration is routine empiric supplementation of calcium with or without calcitriol (vitamin D). Patients would then be discharged on supplementation if the plasma calcium is normal the following morning. If this approach is to be taken, the patient should be educated on symptoms of hypocalcemia and instructed to call should symptoms develop. The disadvantage of this approach with routine administration of calcium and vitamin D replacement is that measurement of postoperative calcium to ensure biochemical cure of disease may be inaccurate.

In recent years IOPTH following total thyroidectomy has been used to predict the risk of developing hypocalcemia and plan early discharge. The same concept can also be applied to management of patients following 4-gland exploration. Noordzij et al. (75) pooled results of post-thyroidectomy PTH measurements in 457 patients from 9 studies and found that the immediate post-op PTH was less than 10 pg/mL in those who became hypocalcemic. Other studies have found that the absolute value of IOPTH level at which the patient is at risk of becoming hypocalcemic ranged from 8 to 16 pg/mL (or 1.7 to 3.7 pmol/L) (76–81). Based on these studies, one can extrapolate that if the post-op PTH is greater than 16 pg/mL the patient can be safely discharged without supplements. There is no concrete algorithm for managing post-op calcium utilizing post-op IOPTH level. Figure 134.9 outlines a suggested algorithm. If post-op IOPTH is above 10 pg/mL and the morning calcium is within normal range, the patient can be discharged. If post-op IOPTH is below normal range (i.e., less than 5 pg/dL), oral calcium supplement (see below for dosage) should be initiated along with calcitriol 0.5 mcg daily. Two sequential calcium levels should be drawn 6 to 8 hours apart the next day since. The patient can be discharged if sequential calcium levels demonstrate an upward trend. If IOPTH is between 5 and 10 pg/mL, and the morning calcium level is below normal range, oral calcium supplementation should be initiated. The calcium level should be rechecked in 6 hours and monitored as described above. If the calcium is less than 7 mg/dL, or the patient experiences cramps, calcium gluconate should be administered intravenously as outlined below.

Surgeons and endocrinologists employ a variety of different postoperative regimens for treatment of hypocalcemia. While there is no consensus on this issue, there are some general principles which can guide medical management of hypocalcemic patients after parathyroidectomy.

Should symptoms develop or serum calcium values corrected for albumin drop below 8.0 mg/dL, oral calcium carbonate should be initiated at a dose of 1.5 to 4 g/d. Patients with severe hypocalcemia, that is, less than 7.0 mg/dL, or severe symptoms such as cramps and tetany require replacement with intravenous calcium gluconate. Calcium gluconate is preferred over calcium chloride for intravenous administration, as the latter is associated with increased risk of tissue necrosis. If only the chloride form is available and must be used, it should be administered via a central venous line. The initial dose for infusion is 1 g (93 mg of elemental calcium) to 2 g diluted in 250 mL of dextrose solution given over 10 to 20 minutes. If the calcium persistently remains below 7 mg/dL, a continuous intravenous infusion should be initiated. Continuous infusion is typically given as 10 g/L solution infused at a rate of 1 to 3 mg of elemental calcium/kg/h. These patients should be monitored since they can potentially develop electrocardiogram (EKG) changes. Vitamin D should be administered, as it is the mainstay of therapy in the treatment of hypoparathyroidism. A variety of vitamin D preparations are available, including ergocalciferol (vitamin D_2), cholecalciferol (vitamin D_3), and calcitriol, which is the biologically active form of vitamin D (1,25-dihydroxyvitamin D_3). Calcitriol should be used instead of the inactive forms (D_2, D_3) in hypoparathyroid patients, since there is a lack of PTH to convert the inactive form to active form. The typical dose of calcitriol is 0.25 to 0.5 mcg daily.

Special consideration should be given to management of hypocalcemia in patients with 2°HPT or tertiary hyperparathyroidism who undergo subtotal/total parathyroidectomy with reimplantation. They can develop profound hypocalcemia post-op as a result of the total parathyroidectomy and/or severe hungry bone. These patients require continuous intravenous calcium infusion with titration to maintain ionized calcium above 1.0 mmol/L. Ionized calcium levels should be monitored every 6 hours along with daily magnesium and phosphorous levels. Oral calcium and calcitriol should also be initiated simultaneously in maximum dose and then tapered when the reimplanted tissue starts to produce PTH. It is optimal to manage these patients jointly with nephrology or transplant team.

Patients undergoing minimally invasive parathyroidectomy can be discharged on the same day, since their risk of hypocalcemia is low. They may develop delayed hypocalcemia due to hungry bone syndrome, which if does occur typically will be after 2 to 3 days post-op. Therefore, patients should be instructed to call if they experience symptoms of hypocalcemia. In that setting they should be treated with oral calcium supplements and a calcium level should be checked as previously described. Some patients who have had chronically very high calcium levels in the 11 to 12 mg/dL range may experience these symptoms even though their post-op calcium is within normal range.

HIGHLIGHTS

- The most common cause of primary hyperparathyroidism is a single adenoma
- Secondary hyperparathyroidism is associated with chronic renal disease and 4-gland hypertrophy
- Serum calcium over 13 mg/dL suggests malignancy
- Symptoms of hyperparathyroidism include musculoskeletal pain, nephrolithiasis, gastrointestinal upset, and neuropsychiatric conditions ("bones, stones, groans, and psychiatric overtones")
- Hypercalcemia may be due to thiazide diuresis, immobilization, malignancy, and granulomatous diseases
- Elevate serum calcium and PTH with low 24-hour urine calcium suggests FHH
- Failure of 10 PTH to fall by over 50% into the normal range after excision of an adenoma may indicate a double adenoma
- Very low 10 PTH (below 16 pg/mL) often predicts postoperative hypocalcemia

REFERENCES

1. Ackerstrom G, Malmaeus, J, Bergstrom R. Surgical anatomy of human parathyroid glands. *Surgery* 1984;95:15–21.
2. Brown EM. Extracellular Ca2 plus sensing, regulation of parathyroid cell function, and role of Ca2 plus and other ions as extracellular (first) messengers. *Physiol Rev* 1991;7:371–411.
3. Coker LH, Rorie K, Cantley L, et al. Primary hyperparathyroidism, cognition, and health-related quality of life. *Ann Surg* 2005;242(5):642–650.
4. Ruda JM, Hollenbeak CS, Stack BC. A systematic review of the diagnosis and treatment of primary hyperparathyroidism from 1995 to 2003. *Otolaryngol Head Neck Surg* 2005;132:359–372.
5. Sipperstein A, Berber E, Barbosa GF, et al. Predicting the success of limited exploration for primary hyperparathyroidism using ultrasound, sestamibi, intraoperative parathyroid hormone. Analysis of cases 1158. *Ann Surg* 2008;248:420–428.
6. Fraker DL, Harsono H, Lewis R. Minimally invasive parathyroidectomy: benefits and requirements of localization, diagnosis and intraoperative PTH monitoring. Long-term results. *World J Surg* 2009;33:2256–2265.
7. Fraker DL. Parathyroid cancer. In: DeVita F, Rosenberg SA, Lawrence T, eds. *Cancer: principles and practice of oncology,* 2007, 8th ed. Philadelphia, PA: Lippincott, 1702–1920.
8. Shattuck TM, Valimaki S, Obara T, et al. Somatic and germ-line mutations of the HRPT2 gene in sporadic parathyroid carcinoma. *N Engl J Med* 2003;349:1722–1729.
9. Lee PK, Jarosek SL, Vimig BA, et al. Trends in the incidence and treatment of parathyroid cancer in the United States. *Cancer* 2007;109:1736–1741.
10. Cetani F, Lemmi M, Cervia D, et al. Identification and functional characterization of loss-of-function mutations of the calcium-sensing receptor in four Italian kindreds with familial hypocalciuric hypercalcemia. *Eur J Endocrinol* 2009;160(3):481–489.
11. Pollak MR, Brown EM, Estep HL, et al. Autosomal dominant hypocalcemia caused by a Ca2 plus-sensing receptor gene mutation. *Nat Genet* 1994;8:303–307.
12. Chou Y-HW, Brown EM, Levi T, et al. The gene responsible for familial hypocalciuric hypercalcemia maps to chromosome 3q in four unrelated families. *Nat Genet* 1992;1:295–299.
13. Heath H III, Jackson CE, Otterud B, et al. Genetic linkage analysis in familial benign (hypocalciuric) hypercalcemia: evidence for locus heterogeneity. *Am J Hum Genet* 1993;53:193–200.
14. Trump D, Whyte MP, Wooding C, et al. Linkage studies in a kindred from Oklahoma with familial benign (hypocalciuric) hypercalcemia (FBH) and developmental elevations in serum parathyroid hormone levels, indicate a third locus for FBH. *Hum Genet* 1995;96:183–187.
15. Marx SJ, Attie MF, Levine MA, et al. The hypocalciuric or benign variant of familial hypercalcemia: clinical and biochemical features in fifteen kindreds. *Medicine* 1981;60:397–412.
16. Law WM Jr, Heath H III. Familial benign hypercalcemia (hypocalciuric hypercalcemia). Clinical and pathogenic studies in 21 families. *Ann Intern Med* 1985;102:511–519.
17. Christensen SE, Nissen PH, Vestergaard P, et al. Plasma 25-hydroxyvitamin D, 1,25-dihydroxyvitamin D, and parathyroid hormone in familial hypocalciuric hypercalcemia and primary hyperparathyroidism. *Eur J Endocrinol* 2008;159(6):719–727.
18. Szabo E, Hellman P, Lundgren E, et al. Parathyroidectomy in familial hypercalcemia with clinical characteristics of primary hyperparathyroidism and familial hypocalciuric hypercalcemia. *Surgery* 2002;131:257–263.
19. Tordjman KM, Greenman Y, Osher E, et al. Characterization of normocalcemic primary hyperparathyroidism. *Am J Med* 2004;117:861–863.
20. Lowe H, McMahon DJ, Rubin MR, et al. Normocalcemic primary hyperparathyroidism: further characterization of a new clinical phenotype. *J Clin Endocrinol Metab* 2007;92(8):3001–3005.
21. Maruani G, Hertig A, Paillard M, et al. Normocalcemic primary hyperparathyroidism: evidence for a generalized target-tissue resistance to parathyroid hormone. *J Clin Endocrinol Metab* 2003;388:4641–4648.
22. Bilizikian JP, Potts JT Jr, Fuleihan GE-H, et al. Summary statement from a workshop on asymptomatic primary hyperparathyroidism: a perspective for the 21st century. *J Clin Endocrinol Metab* 2002;87(12):5353–5361.
23. Bilezikian JP, Khan AA, Potts JT Jr. On behalf of the Third International Workshop on the Management of Asymptomatic Primary Hyperthyroidism. Guidelines for the management of asymptomatic primary hyperparathyroidism: summary statement from the third international workshop. *J Clin Endocrinol Metab* 2009;94(2):335–339.
24. Aspinall SR, Boase S, Malycha P. Long-term symptom relief from primary hyperparathyroidism following minimally invasive parathyroidectomy. *World J Surg* 2010;34(9):2223–2227.
25. Sheldon DG, Lee FT, Neil NJ, et al. Surgical treatment of hyperparathyroidism improves health-related quality of life. *Arch Surg* 2002;137:1022–1028.
26. Greutelaers B, Kullen K, Kollias, J, et al. Pasieka illness questionnaire: its value in primary hyperparathyroidism. *ANZ J Surg* 2004;74(3):112–115.
27. Pasieka JL, Parsons LL, Demeure MJ, et al. Patient-based surgical outcome too demonstrating alleviation of symptoms following parathyroidectomy in patients with primary hyperparathyroidism. *World J Surg* 2002;26:942–924.
28. Edwards ME, Rotramel A, Beyer T, et al. Improvement in the health-related quality-of-life symptoms of hyperparathyroidism is durable on long-term follow-up. *Surgery* 2006;140:665–663.
29. Rao DS, Wallace EA, Antonelli RF, et al. Forearm bone density in primary hyperparathyroidism: long term follow-up with and without parathyroidectomy. *Clin Endocrinol* 2003;58:348–354.
30. Hagestrom E, Lundgren E, Lithell H, et al. Normalized dyslipidaemia after parathyroidectomy in mild primary hyperparathyroidism: population-based study over five years. *Clin Endocrinol* 2002;56(2):253–260.
31. Stevens LA, Djurdjev O, Cardew S, et al. Calcium, phosphate, and parathyroid hormone levels in combination and as a function of dialysis duration predict mortality: evidence for the complexity of the association between mineral metabolism and outcomes. *J Am Soc Nephrol* 2004;15:770–779.
32. Block GA, Klassen PS, Lazarus JM, et al. Mineral metabolism, mortality and morbidity in maintenance hemodialysis patients. *J Am Soc Nephrol* 2004;15:2208–2218.

33. Tominaga Y, Matsuoka S, Uno N. Surgical and medical treatment of secondary hyperparathyroidism in patients on continuous dialysis. *World J Surg* 2009;33:2335–2342.

34. Cunningham J, Danese M, Olson K, et al. Effect of the calcimimetic cinacalcet HCL on cardiovascular disease, fracture, and healthy-related quality of life in secondary hyperparathyroidism. *Kidney Int* 2005;68:1793–1800.

35. Kestenbaum B, Andress DL, Schwartz SM, et al. Survival following parathyroidectomy among United States dialysis patients. *Kidney Int* 2004;66:2010–2016.

36. Trombetti A, Stoermann C, Robert JH, et al. Survival after parathyroidectomy in patients with end-stage renal disease and severe hyperparathyroidism. *World J Surg* 2007;31:1014–1021.

37. Dussol B, Morand P, Martinat C, et al. Influence of parathyroidectomy on mortality in hemodialysis patients: a prospective observational study. *Ren Fail* 2007;29:579–586.

38. Costa-Hong V, Jorgetti V, Gowdak LHW, et al. Parathyroidectomy reduces cardiovascular events and mortality in renal hyperparathyroidism. *Surgery* 2007;142:699–703.

39. Low TH, Clark J, Gao K, et al. Outcome of parathyroidectomy for patients with renal disease and hyperparathyroidism: predictors for recurrent hyperparathyroidism. *ANZ J Surg* 2009;79:378–382.

40. Irvin GL, Prudhomme DL, Deriso GT, et al. A New approach to parathyroidectomy. *Ann Surg* 1994;219:574–581.

41. Gordon LL, Snyder WH, Wians F Jr, et al. The validity of quick intraoperative parathyroid hormone assay: an evaluation in 72 patients based on gross morphologic criteria. *Surgery* 1999;126:1030–1035.

42. Ozimek A, Gallwas J, Stocker U, et al. Validity and limits of intraoperative parathyroid hormone monitoring during minimally invasive parathyroidectomy: a 10-year experience. *Surg Endosc* 2010;24:3156–3160.

43. Miura D, Wada N, Arici C, et al. Does intraoperative quick parathyroid hormone assay improve the results of parathyroidectomy? *World J Surg* 2002;26:926–930.

44. Sackett WR, et al. Worldwide trends in the surgical treatment of primary hyperparathyroidism in the era of minimally invasive parathyroidectomy. *Arch Surg* 2002;137:1055–1059.

45. Gauger PG, Agarwal G, England BG, et al. Intraoperative parathyroid hormone monitoring fails to detect double parathyroid adenomas: a 2-institution experience. *Surgery* 2001;130:1005–1010.

46. Jaskowiak NT, Sugg SL, Helke J, et al. Pitfalls of intraoperative quick parathyroid hormone. *Arch Surg* 2002;137:659–669.

47. Carneiro DM, Irvin GL. Late parathyroid function after successful parathyroidectomy guided by intraoperative hormone assay (QPTH) compared with the standard bilateral neck exploration. *Surgery* 2000;128:925–929.

48. Hallfeldt KKJ, Trupka A, Gallwas J, et al. Minimally invasive video-assisted parathyroidectomy and intraoperative parathyroid hormone monitoring. *Surg Endosc* 2002;16:1759–1763.

49. Tonelli F, Spini S, Tommasi M, Gabbrielli G, et al. Intraoperative parathormone measurement in patients with multiple endocrine neoplasia type I syndrome and hyperparathyroidism. *World J Surg* 2000;24:556–562.

50. Caneiro DM, Solorzano CC, Nader MC, et al. Comparison of intraoperative iPTH assay (QPTH) criteria in guiding parathyroidectomy: which criterion is the most accurate? *Surgery* 2003;134:973–979.

51. Karakousis GC, Han D, Kelz RR, et al. Interpretation of intraoperative PTH changes in patients with multi-glandular primary hyperparathyroidism. *Surgery* 2007;142:845–850.

52. Lombardi CP, Rafaelli M, Traini E, et al. Intraoperative PTH monitoring during parathyroidectomy: the need for stricter criteria to detect multiglandular disease. *Langenbecks Arch Surg* 2008;393:639–645.

53. Barczynski M, Konturek A, Hubalewska-Dydejczyk A, et al. Evaluation of Halle, Miami, Rome, and Vienna intraoperative iPTH assay criteria in guiding minimally invasive parathyroidectomy. *Langenbecks Arch Surg* 2009;394:843–849.

54. Inebet WB, Dakin GF, Haber RS, et al. Targeted parathyroidectomy in the era of intraoperative parathormone monitoring. *World J Surg* 2002;26:921–925.

55. Riss P, Kaczirek K, Heinz G, et al. A "defined baseline" in PTH monitoring increases surgical success in patients with multiple gland disease. *Surgery* 2007;142:398–404.

56. Mozzon M, Mortier P-E, Jacob PM, et al. Surgical management of primary hyperparathyroidism: the case for giving up quick intraoperative PTH assay in favour of routine PTH measurement the morning after. *Ann Surg* 2004;240:949–954.

57. Gawande AA, Monchik JM, Abbruzzese TA, et al. Reassessment of parathyroid hormone monitoring during parathyroidectomy for primary hyperparathyroidism after 2 preoperative localization studies. *Arch Surg* 2006;141:381–384.

58. Ollila DW, Caudle AS, Cance WG, et al. Successful minimally invasive parathyroidectomy for primary hyperparathyroidism without using intraoperative parathyroid hormone assays. *Am J Surg* 2006;191:52–56.

59. Cassinello N, Ortega J, Lledo S. Intraoperative real-time (99m) Tc-sestamibi scintigraphy with miniature gamma camera allows minimally invasive parathyroidectomy without ioPTH determination in primary hyperparathyroidism. *Langenbecks Arch Surg* 2009;394:869–874.

60. Jacobson SR, van Heerden JA, Farley DR, et al. Focused cervical exploration for primary hyperparathyroidism without intraoperative parathyroid hormone monitoring or use of the gamma probe. *World J Surg* 2004;28:1127–1131.

61. Aggarwal G, Barakate MS, Robinson B, et al. Intraoperative quick parathyroid hormone versus same-day parathyroid hormone testing for minimally invasive parathyroidectomy: a cost effectiveness study. *Surgery* 2001;130:963–970.

62. Friedman M, Gurpinar B, Schalch P, et al. Guidelines for radioguided parathyroid surgery. *Arch Otolaryngol Head Neck Surg* 2007;133:1235–1239.

63. Adil E, Adil T, Fedok F, et al. Minimally invasive radioguided parathyroidectomy performed for primary hyperparathyroidism. *Otolaryngol Head Neck Surg* 2009;141:34–38.

64. Rubello D, Pelizzo MR, Boni G, et al. Radioguided surgery of primary hyperparathyroidism using the low-dose 99mTc-sestamibi protocol: multi-institutional experience from the Italian Study Group on Radioguided Surgery and Immunoscintigraphy (GISCRIS). *J Nucl Med* 2005;46:220–226.

65. Quillo AR, Bumpous JM, Goldstein RE, et al. Minimally invasive parathyroid surgery, the Norman 20% rule: is it valid? *Am Surg* 2011;77(4):484–487.

66. Burkey SH, Heerden JA, Farley DR, et al. Will directed parathyroidectomy utilizing the gamma probe or intraoperative parathyroid hormone assay replace bilateral cervical exploration as the preferred operation for primary hyperparathyroidism? *World J Surg* 2002;26:914–920.

67. Boggs JE, Irvin GL, Carneiro DM, et al. The evolution of parathyroidectomy failures. *Surgery* 1999;126:998–1002.

68. Udelsman R, Lin Z, Donovan P. The superiority of minimally invasive parathyroidectomy based on 1650 consecutive patients with primary hyperparathyroidism. *Ann Surg* 2011;253(3):585–591.

69. Slepavicius A, Beisa V, Janusonis V, et al. Focused versus conventional parathyroidectomy for primary hyperparathyroidism: a prospective, randomized, blinded trial. *Langenbecks Arch Surg* 2008;393(5):659–666.

70. Shindo ML, Rosenthal J. Minimal access parathyroidectomy using the focused lateral approach. *Arch Otolaryngol Head Neck Surg* 2007;133:1227–1234.

71. Conn JM, Goncalves MA, Mansour KA, et al. The mediastinal parathyroid. *Am Surg* 1991;57:62–66.

72. Russell CF, Edis AJ, Scholz DA, et al. Mediastinal parathyroid tumors: experience with 38 tumors requiring mediastinotomy for removal. *Ann Surg* 1981;193:805–809.

73. Prinz RA, Lonchyna V, Carnaille B, et al. Thoracoscopic excision of enlarged mediastinal parathyroid glands. *Surgery* 1994;116:999–1004.

74. Medrano C, Hazelrigg SR, Landreneau RJ, et al. Thoracoscopic resection of ectopic parathyroid glands. *Ann Thorac Surg* 2000;69:221–223.

75. Noordzij JP, Lee SL, Bernet VJ, et al. Early prediction of hypocalcemia after thyroidectomy using parathyroid hormone: an analysis of pooled individual patient data from nine observational studies. *J Am Coll Surg* 2007;205:748–754.

76. Kara M, Tellioglu G, Krand O, et al. Predictors of hypocalcemia occurring after a total/near total thyroidectomy. *Surg Today* 2009;39(9):752–757.

77. Jumaily JS, Noordzij JP, Dukas AG, et al. Prediction of hypocalcemia after using 1- to 6-hour postoperative parathyroid hormone and calcium levels: an analysis of pooled individual patient data from 3 observational studies. *Head Neck* 2010;32(4):427–734.

78. Lim JP, Irvine R, Bugis S, et al. Intact parathyroid hormone measurement 1 hour after thyroid surgery identifies individuals at high risk for the development of symptomatic hypocalcemia. *Am J Surg* 2009;197(5):648–653.

79. Graff AT, Miller FR, Roehm CE, et al. Predicting hypocalcemia after total thyroidectomy: parathyroid hormone level vs. serial calcium levels. *Ear Nose Throat J* 2010;89(9):462–465.

80. Fahad Al-Dhahri S, Al-Ghonaim YA, Sulieman Terkawi A. Accuracy of postthyroidectomy parathyroid hormone and corrected calcium levels as early predictors of clinical hypocalcemia. *J Otolaryngol Head Neck Surg* 2010;39(4):342–348.

81. Lombardi CP, Raffaelli M, Princi P. Early prediction of postthyroidectomy hypocalcemia by one single iPTH measurement. *Surgery* 2004;136:1236–1241.

VIII

Sleep Medicine

Ryan J. Soose   *Edward M. Weaver*

Sleep Medicine for the Otolaryngologist

135

Pell Ann Wardrop   **Kathleen L. Yaremchuk**

Otolaryngologists are frequently the portal for diagnosis and treatment of sleep disorders for patients with snoring or other airway complaints. Although sleep apnea is the most common sleep disorder encountered in an otolaryngology practice, most patients have a combination of several sleep disorders contributing to their symptomatology. Sleep affects every aspect of life from the feeling of general well-being to insulin metabolism, cardiovascular health, and cognitive functioning. Because of this gateway role, an awareness and expertise in the diagnosis and management of all sleep disorders are necessary for otolaryngologists.

OVERVIEW OF NORMAL SLEEP

The average adult needs 8.25 hours of sleep to feel rested. Normal sleep is divided into non–rapid eye movement (NREM) and rapid eye movement (REM) sleep. NREM sleep accounts for 75% to 80% of sleep time in normal sleep. NREM sleep is further divided into progressively deeper stages of sleep: stage N1, stage N2, and stage N3 (deep or delta-wave sleep) (Table 135.1). Each of these four stages of sleep has identifying patterns on electroencephalography (EEG) tracings. Sleep is entered through NREM sleep, and the normal sleep cycle is generally approximately 90 minutes in length with a period of REM sleep. Delta- or slow-wave sleep, stage N3, usually dominates the first third of the night's sleep, while REM sleep dominates the last third (Fig. 135.1). After age 55, stage N3 or slow-wave sleep decreases, and wake after sleep onset (WASO), arousals, and awakenings increase (Fig. 135.2).

OVERVIEW OF SLEEP DISORDERS—THE SLEEPY PATIENT

The International Classification of Sleep Disorders (ICSD-2) lists more than 80 specific sleep disorder diagnoses within eight major categories (Table 135.2) (1). The list demonstrates the complexity involved in making an accurate diagnosis. Review of the differential diagnosis and evaluation of the sleepy patient serve to highlight many of the common sleep disorders encountered in an otolaryngologic practice. Fatigue or excessive daytime sleepiness (EDS), defined as an Epworth Sleepiness Scale (ESS) ≥10, is one of the most common complaints among patients who present to an otolaryngologist with snoring. EDS affects approximately 12% of the general adult population. The number of affected patients climbs to 20% to 25% in the primary care physicians' practice (2). The 2008 National Sleep Foundation (NSF) survey revealed that 36% of Americans drive drowsy or have fallen asleep while driving. Sleepiness and fatigue are usually caused by voluntary sleep deprivation or by an underlying sleep disorder. Anything that disturbs or disrupts sleep can lead to sleepiness or fatigue.

Sleepiness is a presenting complaint in a wide range of sleep disorders including obstructive sleep apnea (OSA), obesity–hypoventilation syndrome (OHS), central sleep apnea (CSA), voluntary sleep restriction, poor sleep hygiene, restless legs syndrome (RLS), periodic limb movement disorder, narcolepsy, circadian rhythm disorders, and insomnia (Table 135.3). The sleepy patient can even be difficult to identify with the standard questionnaires, such as the ESS. Many patients with obstructive sleep apnea syndrome (OSAS) and other sleep disorders will complain of tiredness, fatigue, and lack of energy rather than sleepiness (3). Failure to ask about these additional symptoms may lead to a failure to diagnose a significant, treatable sleep disorder. Some sleep disorders, particularly OSAS and RLS, disrupt sleep and cause functional sleep deprivation. These patients have manifestations of sleep deprivation even if they spend adequate time in bed. Medical problems including fibromyalgia, genitourinary disorders, gastrointestinal disorders, and chronic pain may disrupt sleep. The sleep disruption may manifest in an increased arousal index in the polysomnogram (PSG). The arousal

TABLE 135.1	NORMAL SLEEP ARCHITECTURE		
Sleep Stage	Arousal Threshold	Identifying Characteristics in EEG/PSG Tracings	% of Total Sleep Time
Stage N1	Low	Theta waves on EEG Slow rolling eye movement, vertex sharp waves	1%–5%
Stage N2	High	K complexes Sleep spindles	45%–55%
Stage N3	Highest	Delta waves	20%–25%
REM or Stage R	Variable	Sawtooth waves or EEG activation, REMs and muscle atonia	20%–25%

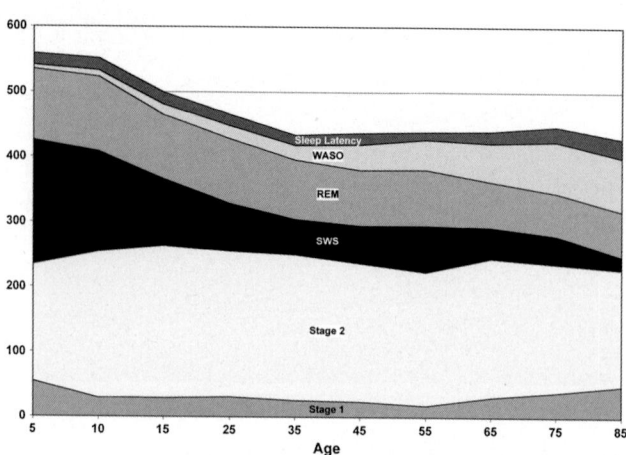

Figure 135.2 Changes in sleep with age in normal humans. (Reprinted with permission from Ohayon MM, Carskadon MA, Guilleminault C, et al. Meta-analysis of quantitative sleep parameters from childhood to old age in healthy individuals: developing normative sleep values across the human lifespan. *Sleep* 2004; 27:1255–1273.)

index represents the number of EEG arousals or partial awakenings per hour of sleep.

Sleep-Disordered Breathing

Obstructive Sleep Apnea

Sleep-disordered breathing (SDB) describes a group of disorders characterized by abnormalities of respiratory pattern (pauses in breathing) or the rate of ventilation during sleep. The spectrum of SDB includes OSA, OHS, and CSA. OSA is a common medical condition with significant adverse consequences, but OSA remains undiagnosed in many individuals. The prevalence of OSA in the United States is currently estimated to be between 5% and 10% (4). Higher prevalence rates are found among specific population subsets, such as individuals who are older, overweight, or have concomitant medical comorbidities (5). It is estimated that only 10% of the population has been adequately screened for appropriate diagnosis (6). Risk factors for the diagnosis of OSA include male gender, obesity, age over 40, history of hypertension, smoking, alcohol use, anatomic characteristics that narrow the upper airway, and a family history of sleep apnea (7).

The typical patient with OSA complains of snoring, EDS, witnessed apneas, and disrupted sleep. However, up to 75% of patients with OSA present with fatigue, tiredness, or lack of energy as their primary complaint rather than sleepiness (8). Many patients with OSA do not have a history of witnessed apneas. Younger, leaner patients and women tend to experience sleep disruptions or arousals instead of apneas during sleep (9). Patients may also present with cognitive complaints such as memory deficits or mood disorders.

Women with OSA may have different presenting symptoms than those typically described in the male population (10). Women are more likely to complain of insomnia and are more likely to have a history of depression and hypothyroid disease. They drink fewer caffeinated and alcoholic beverages than their male counterparts with OSA. Awareness of the variety of presenting complaints of patients with sleep apnea assists in timely diagnosis and treatment.

The association of cardiovascular sequelae and OSA is well documented. There is an increased risk of hypertension,

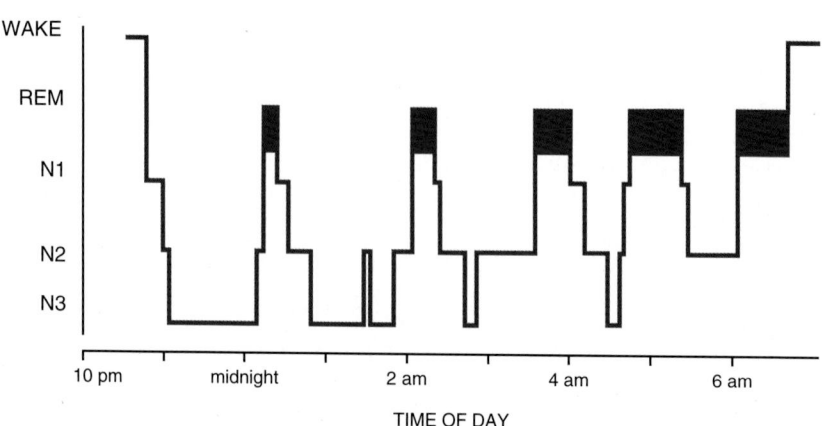

Figure 135.1 Normal young adult sleep hypnogram.

TABLE 135.2	INTERNATIONAL CLASSIFICATION OF SLEEP DISORDERS-2

I. Insomnia

Adjustment insomnia	307.41
Psychophysiologic insomnia	307.42
Paradoxical insomnia	307.42
Idiopathic insomnia	307.42
Insomnia due to mental disorder	327.02
Inadequate sleep hygiene	v69.4
Insomnia due to drug or substance	292.85
For alcohol use	291.82
Insomnia due to medical condition	327.01
Insomnia not due to substance or known physiologic condition, unspecified (*nonorganic insomnia, NOS*)	780.52
Physiologic (*organic*) insomnia, unspecified	327.00

II. Sleep-related breathing disorders

Primary CSA	327.21
Cheyne-Stokes breathing pattern	786.04
High-altitude periodic breathing	327.22
CSA due to medical condition not Cheyne-Stokes	327.27
CSA due to drug or substance	327.29
OSA, adult	327.23
Sleep-related nonobstructive alveolar hypoventilation, idiopathic	327.24
Sleep-related hypoventilation/hypoxemia Due to pulmonary parenchymal or vascular pathology	327.26
Sleep-related hypoventilation/hypoxemia Due to lower airways obstruction	327.26
Sleep-related hypoventilation/hypoxemia due to neuromuscular and chest wall disorders	327.26
Other sleep-related breathing disorders	327.20

III. Hypersomnias of central origin not due to a circadian rhythm sleep disorder, sleep-related breathing disorder, or other cause of disturbed nocturnal sleep

Narcolepsy with cataplexy	347.01
Narcolepsy without cataplexy	347.00
Narcolepsy due to medical condition without cataplexy	347.10
With cataplexy	347.11
Narcolepsy, unspecified	
Recurrent hypersomnia (*including Kleine-Levin syndrome & menstrual-related hypersomnia*)	327.13
Idiopathic hypersomnia with long sleep time	327.11
Idiopathic hypersomnia without long sleep time	327.12
Behaviorally induced insufficient sleep syndrome	307.44
Hypersomnia due to medical condition	327.14
Hypersomnia due to drug or substance (*abuse*)	292.85
For alcohol use	291.82
Hypersomnia due to drug or substance (*medications*)	292.85

Hypersomnia not due to substance or known physiologic condition	327.15
Physiologic (*organic*) hypersomnia, unspecified (*organic hypersomnia, NOS*)	327.10

IV. Circadian rhythm sleep disorders

Circadian rhythm sleep disorder, delayed sleep phase type (*delayed sleep phase disorder*)	327.31
Circadian rhythm sleep disorder, advanced sleep phase type (*advanced sleep phase disorder*)	327.32
Circadian rhythm sleep disorder, irregular sleep–wake type (*irregular sleep–wake rhythm*)	327.33
Circadian rhythm sleep disorder, free-running type (*nonentrained type*)	327.34
Circadian rhythm sleep disorder, jet lag type (*jet lag disorder*)	327.35
Circadian rhythm sleep disorder, shift work type (*shift work disorder*)	327.36
Circadian rhythm sleep disorder due to medical condition	327.37
Other circadian rhythm sleep disorder (*circadian rhythm disorder, NOS*)	327.39
Other circadian rhythm sleep disorder due to drug or substance	292.85
For alcohol use	291.82

V. Parasomnias

Confusional arousals	327.41
Sleepwalking	307.46
Sleep terrors	307.46
REM sleep behavior disorder (*Including parasomnia overlap disorder and status dissociatus*)	327.42
Recurrent isolated sleep paralysis	327.43
Nightmare disorder	307.47
Sleep-related dissociative disorders	300.15
Sleep-related groaning (*catathrenia*)	327.49
Exploding head syndrome	327.49
Sleep-related hallucinations	368.16
Sleep-related eating disorder	327.49

VI. Sleep-related movement disorders

RLS	333.99
Periodic limb movement disorder	327.51
Sleep-related leg cramps	327.52
Sleep-related bruxism	327.53

VIII. Other sleep disorders

Other physiologic (*organic*) sleep disorder	327.80
Other sleep disorder not due to substance or known physiologic condition	307.40
Environmental sleep disorder	307.48

Index of the ICSD-2 reprinted with permission.

myocardial infarction (MI), and cardiovascular accident in those with moderate to severe OSA (11). OSA syndrome significantly increases the risk of stroke or death from any cause, and the increase is independent of other risk factors, including hypertension (12). OSA is also associated with an increase in insulin resistance and metabolic syndrome (13). This association seems to be dose-related, more severe OSA, as defined by the apnea–hypopnea index (AHI), associated with more severe metabolic syndrome, and it is independent of the body mass index (BMI) (14). Physical characteristics including a BMI > 30, neck circumference greater than 17 inches in men and a BMI > 30,

TABLE 135.3	COMMON CAUSES OF EDS		
Inadequate Sleep	Poor-Quality Sleep	Central Etiology	Other
Voluntary sleep restriction	SDB	Narcolepsy	Metabolic
Insomnia	RLS/periodic limb movement disorder	Idiopathic hypersomnia	Neurologic
Circadian rhythm disorder	Pain/fibromyalgia	Posttraumatic hypersomnia	Mood disorders
Poor sleep hygiene			Infection

neck circumference greater than 14½ inches in women, retrognathia, and tonsillar hypertrophy are associated with an increased risk of OSA.

The diagnosis of OSA is made with either in-lab polysomnography or a home sleep study.

The frequency of apneas and hypopneas per hour of sleep is expressed as the "apnea–hypopnea index" or the AHI (number of apneas plus hypopneas per hour of sleep). The respiratory disturbance index (RDI) includes the total of apneas, hypopneas, and respiratory effort–related arousals (RERAs) per hour of sleep. When a portable monitor is used that does not record EEG or measure sleep, the RDI refers to the number of apneas plus hypopneas per hour of recording (15). OSA severity is defined by the AHI or the RDI as measured by a PSG or cardiorespiratory sleep study (Table 135.4).

Obesity–Hypoventilation Syndrome

OHS, historically known as the Pickwickian syndrome (16), consists of the triad of obesity, SDB, and chronic hypercapnia during wakefulness in the absence of other known causes of hypercapnia (17). Its exact prevalence is unknown, but it has been estimated that 10% to 20% of obese patients with OSA have hypercapnia (18). Of the patients with OHS, 90% have OSA, but 10% have

TABLE 135.4	CLASSIFICATION OF SLEEP APNEA SEVERITY
Classification	AHI
Mild	5–14
Moderate	15–29
Severe	≥30

AHI, apnea–hypopnea index (mean number of apneas plus hypopneas/hour of sleep).

nonobstructive hypoventilation with an AHI < 5 on polysomnography. This disorder is diagnosed in patients with an elevated body mass index (BMI > 30 kg/m²), arterial carbon dioxide level over 45 mm Hg, an increase in 10 mm Hg in the $PaCO_2$ during sleep, and hypoxemia. Over the past 20 years, the epidemic of obesity has increased exponentially in the United States. The prevalence of BMI ≥ 40 kg/m² has increased by fivefold, and the prevalence of BMI ≥ 50 has increased 10-fold. This marked increase in extreme obesity will likely result in the increase of OHS in OSA patients.

Patients with OHS have a blunted central response to hypercapnia and hypoxia and decreased lung compliance coupled with increased lung resistance, resulting in a threefold increase in the work of breathing. They have significantly increased morbidity and mortality when compared to eucapnic OSA patients; therefore, identification and prompt treatment are imperative (19).

Central Sleep Apnea/Complex Sleep Apnea

CSA is characterized by recurrent episodes of breathing cessation in sleep associated with the lack of respiratory effort. It is not a single disorder, but rather a manifestation of breathing instability that can be caused by many disorders. A form of CSA, Cheyne-Stokes breathing is a cyclical crescendo–decrescendo pattern of central apneas and hyperpneas that is seen in congestive heart failure, stroke, and renal failure. Other causes of CSA include opioid-associated central apnea, neuromuscular disorders, high-altitude periodic breathing, and brainstem lesions. Occasionally, treatment of OSA with positive airway pressure (PAP) can precipitate the emergence of central apneas or a Cheyne-Stokes pattern of breathing. This phenomenon has termed complex sleep apnea syndrome (CompSAS). Patients with CompSAS can have very disrupted breathing and fragmented sleep on continuous positive airway pressure (CPAP), with respiratory disturbances in the range typically found in patients with moderately severe sleep apnea (20).

Inadequate Sleep

The number one cause of sleepiness is self-imposed sleep restriction or inadequate time in bed. The 2008 NSF "Sleep in America" poll (21) reported that 16% of individuals obtained less than 6 hours of sleep per night on weekdays. Only 26% reported sleeping 8 hours or more per night despite the fact that this is the amount of sleep that the average individual needs to be adequately rested. This is a societal problem which, based upon the NSF annual sleep polls, appears to be increasing in prevalence.

Sleep deprivation has been shown to negatively impact cognitive functioning and performance and to increase the rate of automobile accidents and accidents in the workplace. On tests of reaction time, concentration, and memory, subjects who are experimentally sleep deprived or sleepy due to a sleep disorder perform poorly compared to subjects who are not sleep deprived or have normal sleep. To put the degree of psychomotor impairment associated with sleep deprivation in perspective, studies that compared the effects of alcohol with sleep deprivation have been conducted. In one study, sleep-deprived subjects scored similarly to those subjects with a blood alcohol level of 0.08% (22).

The cardiovascular system also is adversely affected by sleep deprivation. There are increases in inflammatory markers including C-reactive protein and an increased risk of cardiovascular events and morbidity (23). Physiologic effects of sleep deprivation include changes in circulating levels of many hormones including growth hormone, thyroid-stimulating hormone, leptin, thyroxine, cortisol, prolactin, estradiol, luteinizing hormone, adrenaline, and noradrenaline (24). Short sleep time is associated with impaired glucose tolerance and obesity (25). Alterations in immune function occur with sleep deprivation including changes in natural killer cell activity, levels of interleukin-6, antibody titers, and increased rates of some cancers (26).

Sleep deprivation or voluntary sleep restriction has significance for physicians as well as patients. There is an extensive research relative to sleep deprivation and performance relevant to resident education (27–29). This literature demonstrates decrements in cognitive function, fine motor skills, learning, judgment, and reaction time. As a result of concern about the negative effects of sleep deprivation on residents and their patients, the Accreditation Council for Graduate Medical Education began limiting work hours for residents in 1990 and implemented mandatory standards to limit work hours for resident physicians in 2003. These standards are revised intermittently, most recently in 2011, as more research on the effects of sleep deprivation on performance becomes available (30).

This issue affects attending physicians as well. Although studies have shown that older and more experienced physicians have some resistance to the effects of sleep deprivation, all physicians are susceptible to the performance and judgment decrements caused by sleep deprivation. There is a growing movement to restrict all physician work hours given the prevalence of sleep disorders in our society overall and the increase in this incidence with age (31).

Insomnia

Chronic insomnia, defined as difficulty initiating or maintaining sleep or nonrestorative sleep lasting for over a month, affects 10% to 15% of the adult population. Chronic insomnia is associated with decreased quality of life and adverse health effects, particularly an increased risk of depression. Insomnia can be the result of another sleep disorder such as sleep apnea or RLS. It can also result from poor sleep hygiene such as caffeine or alcohol intake at night, irregular sleep/wake habits, exposure to light from a computer monitor before bed, medications, other medical comorbidities, or psychiatric disorders. Patients with insomnia may complain of excessive sleepiness, feeling tired or fatigued, or an uncomfortable feeling of hyperarousal. Treatment of insomnia is important for overall patient well-being. Cognitive behavioral therapy for insomnia (CBT-I) is a specific, highly practical therapeutic approach for chronic insomnia. This is usually performed by a medical psychologist or trained therapist. CBT-I is recognized as the most effective long-term therapy of chronic insomnia (32). If the insomnia is due to a medical or psychiatric condition, treatment of the underlying cause may be beneficial. The use of hypnotics has been found to be useful only as a short-term therapeutic measure.

Circadian Rhythm Disorders

Circadian rhythm sleep disorder is a persistent or recurring pattern of sleep disruption resulting either from an altered sleep–wake schedule or a misalignment between a person's natural sleep–wake cycle and the sleep-related demands placed on him or her. These disorders, frequently overlooked by clinicians as a cause of sleep disorders, can result in excessive sleepiness, poor sleep quality, or insomnia. Frequently encountered types of circadian rhythm disorders include the following:

Shift work type—Shift work sleep disorder involves sleepiness or insomnia that occurs when the work schedule overlaps the usual wake time. There are over 6 million people in the United States working night or rotation shifts, so this is a common sleep disorder.

Delayed sleep phase type—Delayed sleep phase syndrome (DSPS) is a disorder in which the person's sleep–wake cycle is delayed by two or more hours. Patients with DSPS generally fall asleep late at night, often in the predawn hours, and wake in the late morning or in the afternoon. Furthermore, there is a striking inability to fall asleep at an earlier, more typical bedtime. This disorder, which often develops during puberty, is estimated to affect 7% to 16% of adolescents.

Jet lag type—This is caused by a mismatch of the patient's sleep–wake cycle and the time zone. The more time zones that are traveled, the greater the disruption. Eastbound travel, in which sleep–wake hours are advanced, typically causes more problems than westbound travel, in which sleep–wake hours are delayed. People who travel often and cross many time zones when they travel are most susceptible to this type.

Narcolepsy

Narcolepsy is a neurologic disorder affecting 0.05% of the US population that is characterized by EDS and abnormal manifestations of REM sleep such as cataplexy. The classic tetrad of narcolepsy, present in only 20% to 30% of patients with narcolepsy, includes EDS, cataplexy, hypnagogic hallucinations, and sleep paralysis. Patients with narcolepsy experience EDS with ESS > 14 and intermittent, uncontrollable episodes of falling asleep during the daytime. Cataplexy, a loss of muscle tone without loss of consciousness elicited by an emotional stimulus, is present in 60% of patients with narcolepsy (33). These sudden sleep attacks may occur during any type of activity at any time of the day. Symptoms generally present in the second decade of life, but the diagnosis of narcolepsy is often delayed by more than 10 years after onset of symptoms (34).

While the presence of severe EDS and cataplexy strongly supports the diagnosis of narcolepsy, diagnosis is usually made with the multiple sleep latency test (MSLT) that demonstrates two or more episodes of sleep onset REM during the five-nap study.

REM Behavior Disorder

While patients with REM behavior disorder (RBD) do have disrupted sleep and daytime sleepiness, they will usually present with the complaint of dream-enacting behavior and violent dreams. These patients can harm themselves or their bed partners during these episodes. RBD is neurologic disorder with a lack of atonia during REM sleep. The majority of patients with RBD have Parkinson disease or a related synucleinopathy; however, RBD can precede the onset of Parkinson disease by over a decade.

Restless Legs Syndrome

Patients with RLS will often complain of difficulty initiating sleep and nonrestorative sleep with daytime sleepiness. RLS is defined as an urge to move the legs, usually accompanied or caused by uncomfortable and unpleasant sensations in the legs, worse at rest, and in the evenings and relieved by movement. Eighty percent of people who have RLS also have periodic limb movements of sleep (PLMS). These are jerks of the legs or arms that occur every 20 to 30 seconds on and off throughout the night. This can cause partial awakenings or arousals that disrupt sleep. RLS is diagnosed by history. The four basic criteria for diagnosis are listed in Table 135.5 (35).

Patients with a history of nocturnal limb movements, daytime somnolence, and a lack of daytime symptoms of RLS should be studied with a full PSG to identify any leg movements leading to arousals and sleep disruption. These patients may have periodic limb movement disorder leading to daytime sleepiness, sleep maintenance insomnia, and nonrestorative sleep.

The majority of patients with sleep apnea who kick at night do not have RLS or PLMS. Their kicking is a response to their airway obstruction and is relieved by resolution of the airway obstruction. A CPAP titration study in these patients will show that the leg movements resolve with adequate CPAP pressure.

TABLE 135.5	ESSENTIAL DIAGNOSTIC CRITERIA FOR RLS

1. An urge to move the legs, usually accompanied or caused by uncomfortable and unpleasant sensations in the legs. (Sometimes the urge to move is present without the uncomfortable sensations, and sometimes the arms or other body parts are involved in addition to the legs).
2. The urge to move or unpleasant sensations begin or worsen during periods of rest or inactivity such as lying or sitting.
3. The urge to move or unpleasant sensations are partially or totally relieved by movement, such as walking or stretching, at least as long as the activity continues.
4. The urge to move or unpleasant sensations are worse in the evening or night than during the day or only occur in the evening or night. (When symptoms are very severe, the worsening at night may not be noticeable but must have been previously present).

Reprinted from Allen RP, Picchietti D, Hening WA, et al. Restless legs syndrome: diagnostic criteria, special considerations, and epidemiology: a report from the restless legs syndrome diagnosis and epidemiology workshop at the National Institutes of Health. *Sleep Med* 2003;4:101–111, with permission.

EVALUATION OF THE PATIENT WITH A SLEEP DISORDER

Although OSA is the most common sleep disorder, many of the symptoms overlap with other sleep disorders, and many patients have more than one sleep diagnosis. To make a diagnosis, it is important to spend an adequate amount of time with the patient and bed partner to ensure the right questions are being asked to ascertain the nature of a patient's particular sleep disorder (Table 135.6). It is often helpful to have a bed partner present who will be able to describe movements that occur while the patient is asleep and, may have no independent recollection of their own activities or behavior.

The evaluation of a patient with sleep apnea begins with the chief complaint that has brought the patient to the physician's office. More often than not, the patient is in the office at the direction of a bed partner who has witnessed apneas, episodes of choking, restless sleep, and/or snoring. While the condition may have been occurring for some time, it is when the patient's bed partner issues an ultimatum and ends up moving to another room to sleep that the patient seeks medical advice.

The history should include a clear description of the sleep disturbance that is bringing the patient to the office. If the problem is snoring, frequency (most nights of the week), duration (all night), and volume (can be heard outside the bedroom) should be determined. Snoring is common in the general population, with 25% of women and 45% of men reporting habitual snoring.

There is poor validity on the self-perception of snoring. A sleeping patient is often unaware of his or her snoring, with 77% unable to decide whether they snored or not.

TABLE 135.6	EVALUATION OF A PATIENT WITH A SLEEP DISORDER COVERS ISSUES OF SLEEP HYGIENE AND QUALITY

1. History
   a. Type of sleep disturbance
   b. Snoring
   c. Apneas
   d. Waking up
   e. Trouble getting to sleep and/or staying asleep
   f. Duration of symptoms
   g. Audio or video recordings
   h. Bed partner reports
2. Review of systems
   a. General
   b. Skin
   c. Head
   d. Ears
   e. Nose
   f. Throat
   g. Neck
   h. Respiratory
   i. Cardiovascular
   j. Gastrointestinal
   k. Urinary
   l. Vascular
   m. Musculoskeletal
   n. Neurologic
   o. Endocrine
   p. Psychiatric
3. Medication reconciliation
   a. Prescription
   b. Over the counter
4. ESS
5. Habits
   a. Smoking
   b. Drinking
   c. Coffee/energy drinks/caffeine
6. Sleep hygiene
   a. TV, radio, and computer in the bedroom
   b. Bed partners
      i. Bed sharing with children
      ii. Bed sharing with pets
   c. Number of times out of bed at night
   d. Time in bed to go to sleep, time of awakening, or total sleep time
   e. Naps during the day

Of the 23% who reported that they did not snore, more than half during polysomnographic objective measurements demonstrated appreciable snoring (36). The reports of snoring from bed partners are usually gathered over a longer period of time.

There is a significant positive correlation between severity of OSA and snoring intensity (37). Maimon et al. demonstrated that snoring intensity increased progressively across categories of OSA and sound levels ranged from 46 ± 3.6 dB in mild to 60 ± 6.4 dB in severe sleep apnea. Snoring intensity has also been shown to be an independent variable related to sleepiness in OSA. Snoring may explain part of sleepiness that cannot be explained by polysomnography alone (38).

Reports of apnea can also be gathered from the patient and bed partner. Often patients will have an arousal that they are aware of and can self-report the apneas. Similarly, bed partners relate stories of how they need to shake the patients to get them to breathe during prolonged periods of apnea.

Nocturnal awakening may or may not be due to an apnea, so further questioning is necessary to better delineate the problem. The second most common sleep disorder after OSA is insomnia, which can also have the symptom of EDS. Individuals with insomnia will awaken at night but will be unable to fall back asleep, which is termed sleep maintenance insomnia. The patient with OSA will awaken but return to sleep without difficulty. Either of these awakenings will, however, result in EDS but for completely different reasons.

EDS is a very common symptom of patients presenting with a sleep disorder. Although it is associated with OSA, it is also present in multiple other sleep disorders such as obesity/hypoventilation syndrome, insufficient sleep, narcolepsy, and hypersomnias.

To help differentiate between feeling tired and true sleepiness, there are multiple self-administered tools that can be used. The ESS is a subjective measurement of sleepiness completed by the patient. It has been validated in clinical populations and asks about the likelihood of falling asleep in common settings. A score greater than or equal to 10 is indicative of EDS (39) (Table 135.7).

The patient's daily schedule must be reviewed, including the time the patient gets in bed to go to sleep, an estimate of how long it takes to fall asleep, the number of awakenings during the night, and the time the patient wakes up and gets out of bed. It is important to obtain detailed sleep–wake schedules in shift workers. If the patient indicates there is great variation in the sleep–wake schedule, this may be part of the problem and causing EDS. To document, the previous day's sleep–wake activity may be sufficient to determine the usual total sleep time and assess if it is adequate in duration.

A sleep diary can be used with patients who are unable to give an accurate description of their sleep–wake habits and have symptoms of EDS (Fig. 135.3). It can be given to the patient and may be used for a week or two to determine sleep habits. It is invaluable in recognizing and documenting insufficient sleep.

It is important to determine the duration of symptoms that are causing the patient to seek treatment. If the issue is of long duration, further evaluation with clinical testing may be done sooner than if the problem is of recent onset. If the problem has been present for some time, there may be a new symptom that is causing the patient to seek help at this point in time.

If the symptoms have been present for a short amount of time, questions may be raised regarding what has changed recently in the patient's life. Sometimes a change in job or the family situation can result in changes in sleep habits that are problematic.

Because of increased access to audio and video recordings, it is not uncommon for patients and their families to bring in

TABLE 135.7	THE ESS IS A SIMPLE QUESTIONNAIRE MEASURING THE LIKELIHOOD OF FALLING ASLEEP IN DIFFERENT SITUATIONS. SCORES GREATER OR EQUAL TO 10 ARE ABNORMAL AND CORRELATE WITH EDS

The ESS—A score >10 indicates EDS

How likely are you to doze off or fall asleep in the following situations, in contrast to feeling just tired? This refers to our usual way of life in recent times. Even if you have not done some of the things recently, try to work how they would have affected you. Use the following scale to choose the most appropriate number for each situation:

0 = would never doze
1 = slight chance of dozing
2 = moderate chance of dozing
3 = high chance of dozing

Situation	Chance of dozing
1. Sitting and reading	_____
2. Watching TV	_____
3. Sitting, inactive in public place (theater or meeting)	_____
4. As a passenger in a car without a break	_____
5. Lying down to rest in the afternoon when circumstances permit	_____
6. Sitting and talking to someone	_____
7. In a car, while stopped for a few minutes in traffic	_____
8. Sitting quietly after a lunch without alcohol	_____
Total:	_____

SLEEP DIARY

Name: _____

Day/Date	At what time did you go to bed last night?	How long did it take you to fall asleep?	How many times did you wake up during the night?	For how long were you awake during the night?	At what time did you rise from bed this morning?	Did you take any sleeping pills? (name, dose & time)	How much alcohol did you drink yesterday?	How much coffee, tea cola, chocolate did you drink?	Did you nap? (number of naps, start and end times)	How did you feel this morning? Refreshed, moderate, or tired	What disturbed your sleep last night?
1											
2											
3											
4											
5											
6											
7											

FOR OFFICE USE ONLY

SOL	WAKE	WASO	TST	TIB	SE

SOL: Sleep onset latency. This is the time recorded in Column 2 and should be averaged for the week.

Wake: This is the total time the patient was awake during the sleep period and should be the sum of Columns 2 and 4 and should be averaged for the week.

WASO: Wake After Sleep Onset is the time listed in Column 4. It should be averaged for the week.

TST: Total Sleep Time. Columns (1+5)-Columns (2+4)=TST. This should be averaged for the week

TIB: Time in Bed. Columns 1-6=Time in Bed

SE: Sleep efficiency. TST/TIB= Sleep Efficiency

Figure 135.3 A sleep diary is a helpful tool for patients and physicians to evaluate sleep patterns on a daily basis. For many individuals, insufficient sleep is a primary cause for EDS and poor sleep hygiene.

recordings of snoring, or recordings of abnormal breathing patterns that may indicate suspected apneas, and videos demonstrating restless movements during sleep. These can also be helpful in determining next steps in diagnosis and treatment.

To ensure that nothing is missed during the evaluation of the patient with sleep disorders, the use of a standard intake form should be used. The form in Figure 135.4 is from Terence Davidson MD, University of California, San

SLEEP DISORDERED BREATHING

Name
MR#
DOS

Source _____ Date _____

Patient identification

Referring Physician _____

AGE	GENDER	HEIGHT	WEIGHT	BMI	Neck Circ.	BP	WHR
	☐M ☐F	cm	kg	kg/M²	inches		

Snoring: intensity (0-3) _____ frequency (0-3) _____ Apneic episodes (0-3) _____ Daytime sleepiness (0-4) _____

Co-Morbidities   **Meds:**

Yes	No			Yes	No
☐	☐	Hypertension	Heart Failure	☐	☐
☐	☐	Obesity	Diabetes	☐	☐
☐	☐	Excessiye daytime sleepiness	GERD	☐	☐
☐	☐	Coronary artery disease/MI	Asthma	☐	☐
☐	☐	Stroke	Parasomnias	☐	☐
☐	☐	Atrial fibrillation	# MVAs (in past 10 yrs.)		☐

Depression ☐ Yes ☐ No   NYHA Class _____ (I-IV)

Alcohol _____ (glasses/night)   Insomnia ☐ Yes ☐ No   Nocturia _____ x per night
Time to bed _____   Time out of bed _____   Total bed time _____ hrs

Examination *(See back for details)*   Other:
Nose (0-4) _____
Mallampati (1-4) _____   Uvula (0-4) _____
Endoscopy: Tongue base (1-4) _____   Tonsils (0-4) _____
Lingual Tonsil (1-4) _____ SNB _____ degrees   Epiglottis (0,1) _____   CT/MRI_____
Thyromental distance _____ cm   _____
                                                                  _____

Pre Sleep Test Impression: ☐Insomnia 780·52 ☐SDB 780·57 ☐OSA 327·23 ☐EDS 327·8
Plan:_____

Physician Signature/PID _____ Date _____

| Sleep Test date _____ Total sleep time _____   AHI _____   AI _____ |
| O₂ desat Index _____   LSAT _____ |
| CPAP 95th pressure _____ cm H₂0 |
| APAP Mean pressure _____ cm H₂0   Mask _____ |
| DME _____ |
| Compliance: Days/week _____ Hrs/day _____ |

Post Sleep Test
Other therapies and follow-up

D1515 (12-06)   Physician Signature/PID#   Date & Time

A

Figure 135.4 A standardized history and physical form is helpful in gathering information pertinent for patients with a sleep disorder that may be different than other otolaryngologic patients.

Snoring Sleep Examination

Snoring		Apneic Episodes	Daytime Sleepiness
Intensity	Frequency	0 = None	0 = Never
0 = None	0 = None	1 = 1 or 2/night	1 = Only after meals
1 = Mild/bedroom	1 = Occasional 1-2 d/wk	2 = 2-10/night	2 = Most days, but do not fall asleep
2 = Moderate/house	2 = Frequent 3-5 d/wk	3 = 10 or more/night	3 = Occasionally fall asleep
3 = Servere/yard	3 = Daily 6 or 7 d/wk		4 = Regularly fall asleep

Upper Respiratory Tract Sleep Examination

Nose 0-4
0 Post-op perfectly straight
1 Straight with normal cartilage/bone at floor
   <10% obstruction
2 10-50% obstruction worst side
3 50-90% obstruction worst side
4 90-100% obstruction worst side or
   obstructive nasal polyps. Allergic rhinitis-
   add one. Total not to exceed 4.

Lingual Tonsils 1-4
1 None
2 Small
3 Medium
4 Large

Mallampati 1-4
1 All of uvula and tonsils/pillars
2 Partial uvula and partial tonsils/pillars
3 Base of uvula
4 No uvula

Tonsil 0-4
0 S/P tonsillectomy
1 Inside the pillars
2 Outside the pillars,
   <25% of airway
3 25% - <75% of airway
4 75% or more of airway

Adenoids 0-4
0 Postop
1 <10% obst
2 10-50%
3 50-90%
4 >90%

Uvula 0-4
0 Absent
1 U<50 mm^2 (5 x 10mm)
2 5O>U<112.5mm^2 (7.5 x 15mm)
3 112.5>U<200mm^2 (10 x 20mm)
4 200>U

Tongue 1-4

(F.O.E.), patient sitting, mouth closed
1 Vallecula open
2 Vallecula filled with tongue base
3 Epiglottis pushed posteriorly
4 Epiglottis touching post pharyngeal wall
   secondary to tongue base pressure

Larynx 0,1 (F.Q.E.)
0 Normal
1 Any airway obstruction or deformed
   epiglottis, not covered above.

Mallampati

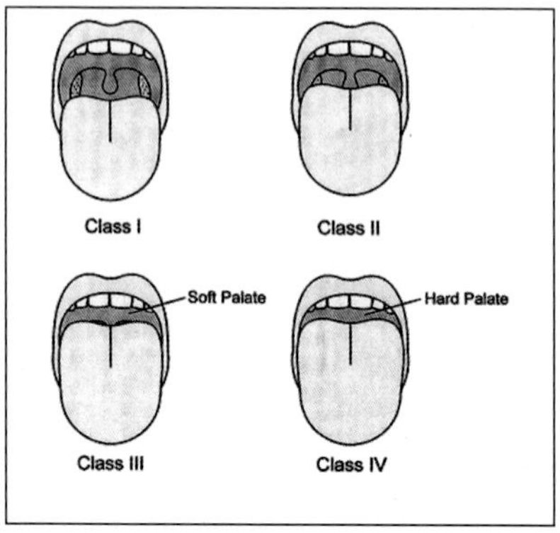

Class I   Class II
Soft Palate   Hard Palate
Class III   Class IV

Tonsil Grade

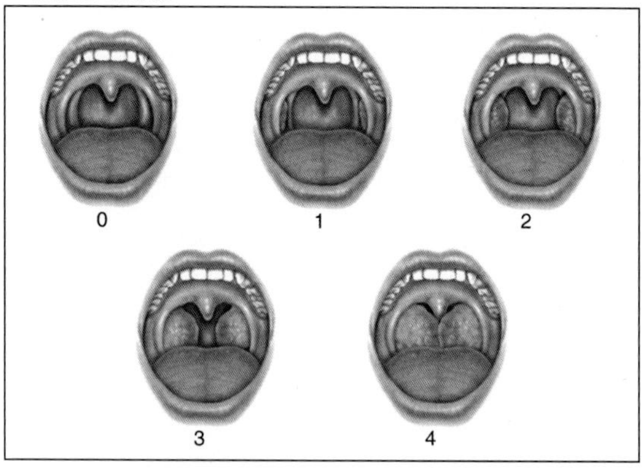

0   1   2
3   4

Waist Hip Ratio (WHR)

	acceptable		unacceptable		
	excellent	good	average	high	extreme
male	<0.85	0.85-0.9	0.9 0.95	0.95-1	>1
female	<0.75	0.75-0.8	0.8-0.85	0.85-0.9	>0.9

Depression: Yes = affirmative answer to #1 or #2
1) Over the past 2 weeks have you ever felt down, depressed, or hopeless?
2) Over the past 2 weeks, have you felt little pressure or interest in doing things?*
    (Sensitivity 96%; Specificity 57%)*

NYHA: New York Heart Association Class
Class I   - Asymptomatic
Class III - Symptomatic with little exertion

Class II - Symptomatic with moderate exertion
Class IV - Symptomatic at rest

*MP Pignone, et al: Screening for Depression in Adults: A Summary of the Evidence for the U.S. Preventive Services Task Force, Ann Intern Med 2002 136:765-776
D1515 (12-06) page 2 of 2

B

Figure 135.4 *(Continued)*

Diego Head and Neck Surgery Sleep Medicine Clinic and is comprehensive in scope (40).

Review of Systems

Many medical conditions can cause or exacerbate problems with sleep. A complete 14-point review of systems is important and should be included as part of the initial encounter with the patient (Fig. 135.5).

General—Weight loss/gain, fatigue, fever or chills, weakness, or chronic pain can lead to difficult with restorative sleep. Weight gain may exacerbate or cause OSA. Fatigue and weakness may be a symptom of a sleep disorder. There is a decreased threshold for pain when sleep is disrupted.

Nose—Nasal congestion results in increased effort for respiration. Some individuals have difficulty only at night resulting in sleep disruption. Mouth breathing causes the tongue to fall posteriorly, which results in a narrowed hypopharyngeal airway and possible obstruction. Snoring is more common in the supine position with the mouth open.

Throat—Patients with chronic mouth breathing often wake up with dryness of the throat and sometimes a swollen uvula from turbulent airflow during sleep. This can be associated with SDB and OSA.

Neck—History of a goiter, neck mass, previous tracheotomy, or radiation therapy can result in tracheal abnormalities that are manifested during sleep. Tracheomalacia is a rather uncommon site for OSA.

Checklist: Review of Symptoms

General:
☐ Weight loss or gain
☐ Fatigue
☐ Fever or chills
☐ Weakness
☐ Trouble sleeping

Skin:
☐ Rashes
☐ Lumps
☐ Itching
☐ Dryness
☐ Color changes
☐ Hair and nail changes

Head:
☐ Headache
☐ Head injury

Ears:
☐ Decreased hearing
☐ Ringing in ears (tinnitus)
☐ Earache
☐ Drainage

Nose:
☐ Stuffiness
☐ Discharge
☐ Itching
☐ Hay fever
☐ Nosebleeds
☐ Sinus pain

Throat:
☐ Teeth
☐ Gums
☐ Bleeding
☐ Dentures
☐ Sore tongue
☐ Hoarseness
☐ Thrush
☐ Non-healing sores
☐ Last dental exam

Neck:
☐ Lumps
☐ Swollen glands
☐ Pain
☐ Stiffness

Respiratory:
☐ Cough (dry or wet, productive)
☐ Sputum (color and amount)
☐ Coughing up blood (hemoptysis)
☐ Shortness of breath (dyspnea)
☐ Wheezing
☐ Painful breathing

Cardiovascular:
☐ Chest pain or discomfort
☐ Tightness
☐ Palpitations
☐ Shortness of breath with activity (dyspnea)
☐ Difficulty breathing lying down (orthopnea)
☐ Swelling (edema)
☐ Sudden awakening from sleep with shortness of breath (paroxysmal noctural dyspnea)

Gastrointestinal:
☐ Swallowing difficulties
☐ Heartburn
☐ Change in appetite
☐ Nausea
☐ Change in bowel ha
☐ Rectal bleeding
☐ Constipation
☐ Diarrhea
☐ Yellow eyes or skin (jaundice)

Urinary:
☐ Frequency
☐ Urgency
☐ Burning or pain
☐ Blood in urine (hematuria)
☐ Incontinence
☐ Change in urinary strength

Vascular:
☐ Calf pain with walking (claudication)
☐ Leg cramping

Musculoskeletal:
☐ Muscle or joint pain
☐ Stiffness
☐ Back pain
☐ Redness of joints
☐ Swelling of joints
☐ Trauma

Neurologic:
☐ Dizziness
☐ Fainting
☐ Seizures
☐ Weakness
☐ Numbness
☐ Tingling
☐ Tremor

Endocrine:
☐ Head or cold intolerance
☐ Sweating
☐ Frequent urination (polyuria)
☐ Thirst (polydypsia)
☐ Change in appetite (polyphagia)

Psychiatric:
☐ Nervousness
☐ Depression
☐ Memory loss
☐ Stress

Figure 135.5 A standardized review of systems assists in identifying comorbidities that can contribute to or exacerbate sleep disorders.

Respiratory—Coughing, choking, or wheezing can be seen in OSA as well as in individuals with gastroesophageal reflux, asthma, and chronic obstructive pulmonary disease (COPD). Recent data suggest that OSAS is an independent risk factor for asthma exacerbations (41).

Gastrointestinal—Gastroesophageal reflux has been reported to occur in 62% to 74% of patients with OSA (42). Gastroesophageal reflux, as previously mentioned, is common in OSA. The increased negative thoracic pressure results in reflux and increased complaints upon awakening.

Genitourinary—Urinary frequency is a significant issue for men, more so than women, as they grow older. Benign prostatic hypertrophy can result in men awakening multiple times a night, which prevents them from getting a good night's sleep. The sample population had a mean age of 45.8 years and was 52.6% female and 80% Caucasian. In the community sample, 31% reported greater than one void per night, and 14.2% reported greater than two voids per night. The prevalence of nocturia increased with age, with no gender differences. For over active bladder cases, 66.8% reported greater than one void per night, and 42.2% reported greater than two (43). An increase in intra-abdominal pressure, confusion associated with arousals, and increased levels of atrial natriuretic peptide have been associated with nocturia in patients with OSA. Treatment of OSA has been shown to significantly decrease nocturia.

Neurologic—About 50% of people who have had a stroke have sleep apnea (44). Sixty percent of patients with Parkinson disease have sleep problems such as sleep fragmentation, insomnia, nightmares/night terrors/nocturnal vocalizations, hallucinations, and EDS (45).

Musculoskeletal—Musculoskeletal pain syndromes such as chronic arthritis and fibromyalgia can result in poor-quality sleep and are correlated with an increase in depression, pain intensity, activity levels, and hypochondriasis (46).

Endocrine—Diabetes can result in polyuria with disruption of sleep. Any disruption of the hypothalamic–pituitary–adrenal axis will disrupt the circadian rhythm. Insomnia and OSA are associated with hypothalamic–pituitary–adrenal axis abnormalities (47). Sleep difficulty is one of the hallmarks of menopause with the primary predictor of disturbed sleep architecture being the presence of vasomotor symptoms (48).

Psychiatric—Primary psychiatric diagnoses of depression, anxiety, bipolar disease, or attention deficit disorder can contribute to sleep disturbances or daytime impairment. Many of the medications used for treatment also impact normal sleep patterns (49).

Medications—Prescription and over-the-counter medications can impact sleep and should be thoroughly covered during the visit. There are many medications which have an impact on the sleep–wake cycle. Some of the medications can induce pain (statins), cough (angiotensin converting enzyme inhibitors), restless legs symptoms (antidepressants, neuroleptics, and antihistamines), or REM sleep behavior disorder (antidepressants, monoamine oxidase type B inhibitors) and subsequently cause sleep disruptions. Tables 135.8 and 135.9 demonstrate medications that disrupt sleep and wake, respectively.

Caffeine works as a central nervous stimulant that temporarily decreases drowsiness and improves alertness. It occurs naturally in coffee, tea, and chocolate and is present in soft drinks and most energy drinks. In North America, 90% of the population consumes caffeine daily (50). Two hundred milligrams or more of caffeine, the approximate caffeine content in two cups of coffee, has been shown to improve tests of vigilance, alertness, and reaction time in US Navy SEALs after 72 hours of sleep deprivation (51). The caffeine content of some common food and beverages is listed in Table 135.10.

The nicotine in cigarettes acts as a stimulant with an average cigarette delivering 1 mg. It is distributed quickly through the bloodstream and crosses the blood–brain barrier reaching the brain within 1 to 20 seconds after inhalation. The elimination half-life of nicotine in the body is about 2 hours. Nicotine reduces total sleep time and REM sleep time in healthy control subjects. There is an increase in sleep latency and increased arousals with fragmented sleep in active smokers versus nonsmokers. About 20% of smokers experience nocturnal sleep disturbing nicotine craving that occurs with patients waking up once or more a night and are unable to fall back asleep without smoking a cigarette (52).

Alcohol has a transient sedative effect in sleepy or anxious individuals. It is the most commonly used sleeping aid by the population at large. A survey of 18- to 45-year-olds reported that 13% use alcohol to induce sleep. When taken before bedtime, it shortens sleep latency. Alcohol is metabolized rapidly at the rate of one glass of wine or beer per hour. If an individual has had several drinks before sleep, alcohol concentrations in the blood approaches zero halfway through the night. Withdrawal tends to occur at that time and causes disrupted sleep and a sympathetic arousal, which includes tachycardia and sweating (53).

Physical Examination

The age and gender of a patient are important pieces of demographic information for patients with sleep disorders. Sleep disturbances are more common in men than women until menopause when the incidence of sleep apnea in women increases.

The height and weight of a patient should be accurately measured in the office. These measurements should not be self-reported because, as a patient ages, height can decrease due to osteoporosis or because the previous height measurement was taken with the shoes on.

TABLE 135.8 **SELECTED COMMON MEDICATIONS THAT DISRUPT SLEEP**

Drug Class	Examples	Typical Indications	Patient Complaints	Mechanism	Potential Solution
Selective serotonin reuptake inhibitors	sertraline, fluoxetine, citalopram	Major depression, anxiety disorders, postmenopausal hot flashes	Restless legs symptoms, sleep-onset insomnia, nonrestorative sleep, dream enactment behavior or "sleepwalking"	Drugs may have alerting side effects.[1] Increases restless legs symptoms and periodic limb movements of sleep.[2,3] increases likelihood of REM without atonia (may lead to clinical REM behavior disorder)[4]	Reassess original indication, consider alternate agent (bupropion not associated with increased RLS symptoms)
Tricyclic antidepressants	amitriptyline, imipramine, protriptyline	Major depression, anxiety, insomnia, neuropathic pain	Restless legs symptoms, sleep-onset insomnia, nonrestorative sleep	Increases restless legs symptoms and periodic limb movements of sleep.[2] protriptyline is strongly adrenergic and has an alerting side effect profile[5,6]	Reassess original indication, consider alternate agent
ACE Inhibitors	lisinopril, enalapril	Hypertension, diabetic proteinuria, congestive heart failure	Nocturnal cough Worsening sleep apnea	Increased bradykinin production leads to airway irritation, possible increased airway edema[7]	Consider substitution with angiotensin receptor blocker or other drug class
Norepinephrine and dopamine reuptake inhibitors	venlafaxine, desvenlafaxine, bupropion	Major depression, anxiety, postmenopausal hot flashes	Sleep-onset insomnia	Increased activity of alerting neurotransmitters[8]	Reassess original indication, consider alternate agent
Beta-2 agonists	albuterol, salmeterol	Asthma, COPD	Sleep-onset insomnia Sleep maintenance insomnia	Alerting side effects of adrenergic medications[9]	Reassess original indication, educate patient regarding nocturnal use of medication, consider use of hypnotic if nocturnal usage is unavoidable
Beta-blockers	Metoprolol, propranolol	Hypertension, tachyarrhythmias, migraine prophylaxis	Nightmares	Not known, likely related to central β-adrenergic blockade, lipophilic β-blockers may be more problematic[10,12]	Consider switch to less lipophilic agent (e.g., atenolol), or alternate drug class
Corticosteroids	prednisone, methylprednisolone	Rheumatologic disorders, COPD	Sleep-onset insomnia Sleep maintenance insomnia[13] Abnormal dreams[14]	Unknown	Consider nonsteroid alternatives if medically reasonable, consider low-dose hypnotic if corticosteroid medication is medically mandatory
Nonnucleoside reverse transcriptase inhibitors (anti-retroviral)	efavirenz	HIV disease	Abnormal dreams[15]	Unknown	Consider alternate agent if severely troubling, consider low-dose hypnotic with low potential for drug–drug side effects (e.g., doxepin)[15]

(Continued)

TABLE 135.8	SELECTED COMMON MEDICATIONS THAT DISRUPT SLEEP (Continued)				
Drug Class	**Examples**	**Typical Indications**	**Patient Complaints**	**Mechanism**	**Potential Solution**
Statins	atorvastatin, simvastatin, pravastatin, rosuvastatin	Hyperlipidemia	Sleep-onset insomnia or frequent awakenings due to muscle pain	Statin-induced myopathy, possible statin-induced arthralgia[16,17]	Reassess original indication, reassess treatment goals, consider decreased dose, consider alternate agent
Opiates	methadone, oxycodone, morphine	Chronic pain, restless legs syndrome	Frequent awakenings, nocturnal breathlessness, Nonrestorative sleep	Increased risk of obstructive and central sleep apnea[18]	Consider nonopiate alternatives, consider polysomnography with positive airway pressure if sleep-disordered breathing is severe
CNS stimulants	methylphenidate, dextroamphetamine	Narcolepsy, Idiopathic CNS hypersomnia, Attention deficit hyperactivity disorder	Sleep-onset insomnia, frequent awakenings	Central stimulation of dopaminergic alerting system	Consider earlier dosing, use of immediate-release formulations for later day dosing, replacement with modafinil
Social drugs	Caffeine Tobacco/nicotine	n/a	Sleep-onset insomnia Sleep maintenance insomnia Snoring	Caffeine may have hold-over stimulatory effects lasting into the nocturnal time frame; nicotine used at night can produce CNS stimulation; heavy smokers during daytime hours can experience nocturnal withdrawal during sleep-induced abstinence, leading to physical discomfort. Smoking increases upper airway inflammation, which can worsen sleep-disordered breathing	Decrease or discontinue use
Social drugs	Alcohol	n/a	Sleep maintenance insomnia Snoring Worsening sleep apnea	Alcohol tends to worsen propensity for sleep-disordered breathing, possibly by altering upper airway tone and by increasing arousal threshold; though it shortens sleep latency, prebedtime use often results in insomnia in the second half of the night.	Decrease or discontinue use

Reprinted from McCarty DE. Beyond Ockham's razor: redefining problem-solving in clinical sleep medicine using a "five-finger" approach. *J Clin Sleep Med* 2010;6(3):292–296 (Ref. 49), with permission.

TABLE 135.9   SELECTED COMMON MEDICATIONS THAT DISRUPT WAKEFULNESS

Drug Class	Examples	Typical Indications	Patient Complaints	Mechanism	Potential Solutions
Selective serotonin reuptake inhibitors	sertraline, paroxetine	Major depression, anxiety, postmenopausal hot flashes	Daytime sleepiness	Sedating effects of medication[19]	Reassess original indication, consider taper or substitution of an agent with a more alerting side effect profile (e.g., venlafaxine or bupropion)
Tricyclic antidepressants	amitriptyline	Insomnia, major depression, anxiety, chronic neuropathic pain	Morning grogginess, nonrestorative sleep, daytime sleepiness	Sedating effects of medication Prolonged half-life for some medications leads to next-day "hangover"	Reassess original indication, consider dose decrease, consider nocturnal dosing schedule, consider alternate agent
Benzodiazepines	diazepam, clonazepam, flurazepam	Insomnia, anxiety, muscle spasms, REM behavior disorder	Morning grogginess, nonrestorative sleep, daytime sleepiness	Sedating effects of medication; prolonged half-life for some medications leads to next-day "hangover"	Reassess original diagnosis, consider alternate agent, consider addition of daytime alerting agent if agent is considered medically necessary
Anticonvulsants	gabapentin, phenytoin, levetiracetam	Seizure disorder, neuropathic pain, migraine prophylaxis	Daytime sleepiness	Sedating effects of medication	Consider dose decrease, consider alternate agent, consider addition of daytime alerting agent if agent is considered medically necessary
Neuroleptics	quetiapine, risperidone, haloperidol	Psychotic disorders, major depression, attention deficit disorder	Daytime sleepiness	Sedating effects of medication	Reassess original diagnosis, consider alternate agent, consider addition of daytime alerting agent if agent is considered medically necessary
Beta-blockers	metoprolol, propranolol, bisoprolol	Hypertension, tachyarrhythmias, migraine prophylaxis	Daytime fatigue	Central adrenergic blockade→fatigue or drowsiness[20,21]	Consider less lipophilic agent (e.g., atenolol), consider alternate drug class
Statins	atorvastatin, simvastatin, pravastatin, rosuvastatin	Hyperlipidemia	Daytime fatigue, poor exercise tolerance due to muscle pain	Statin-induced myopathy, possible statin induced arthralgia[16,17,20]	Reassess original diagnosis, reassess treatment goals, consider lower dose, consider alternate agent
Antihistamines	Diphenhydramine, hydroxyzine	Allergic reactions, anxiety, pruritic conditions, insomnia	Daytime fatigue Daytime sleepiness Poor attention and concentration[22]	Blockade of central histaminergic receptors→drowsiness, anticholinergic effects on basal forebrain decreases concentration and information processing ability	Consider lower dose, consider nonsedating alternatives, consider addition of daytime alerting agent if agent is considered medically necessary
Social drugs	Alcohol	n/a	Daytime fatigue Headaches Depression Anxiety	Alcohol can lead to daytime impairment symptoms by virtue of its effects on sleep (see Table 135.8), by direct CNS sedative effects, toxicity ("hangover") effects, or due to withdrawal symptoms.	Taper and discontinue use

Reprinted from McCarty DE. Beyond Ockham's razor: redefining problem-solving in clinical sleep medicine using a "five-finger" approach. *J Clin Sleep Med.* 2010;6(3):292–296 (Ref. 49), with permission.

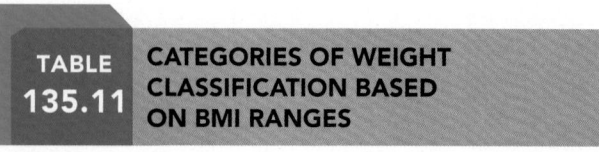

TABLE 135.10	CAFFEINE CONTENT OF SELECT COMMON FOOD, BEVERAGES, AND DRUGS	
Product	Serving Size	Caffeine per Serving (mg)
Hershey's Milk Chocolate	1 bar (1.5 oz)	10
Hershey's Special Dark (45%) cacao content	1 bar (1.5 oz)	31
Coffee, decaffeinated	7 oz	5–15
Green Tea	6 oz	30
Black Tea	6 oz	50
Coca Cola Classic	12 oz	34
Mountain Dew	12 oz	54
Red Bull Energy	8 oz	80
Starbucks Vanilla Latte	16 oz	150
Monster energy drink	16 oz	160
Dunkin Donuts Brewed Coffee	16 oz	143–206
5-h energy	2 oz	207

TABLE 135.11	CATEGORIES OF WEIGHT CLASSIFICATION BASED ON BMI RANGES	
Category	BMI (kg/m²)	
Severely underweight	<16	
Underweight	16–18.5	
Normal	18.5–25	
Overweight	25–30	
Obese Class I	30–35	
Obese Class II	35–40	
Obese Class III	>40	

Similarly, individuals frequently underestimate their weight. It may be that they are embarrassed, have not weighed themselves in some time, or do not want their spouse to be aware of it. After the height and weight have been assessed, the BMI was developed in the 1800s by Belgian Adolphe Quetelet in the development of "social physics" (54).

The BMI classification is commonly used to classify individuals as underweight, normal, overweight and obese. Obese is further grouped into class I, II, and III. The BMI should be calculated and communicated to the patient (Table 135.11). Results from the 2007 to 2008 National Health and Nutrition Examination Survey, using BMI, indicate that an estimated 34.2% of US adults aged 20 years and over are overweight, 33.8% are obese, and 5.7% are extremely obese (55) (Fig. 135.6).

BMI does not actually measure body fat. Because the BMI formula depends only upon weight and height, its assumptions about the distribution between lean mass and

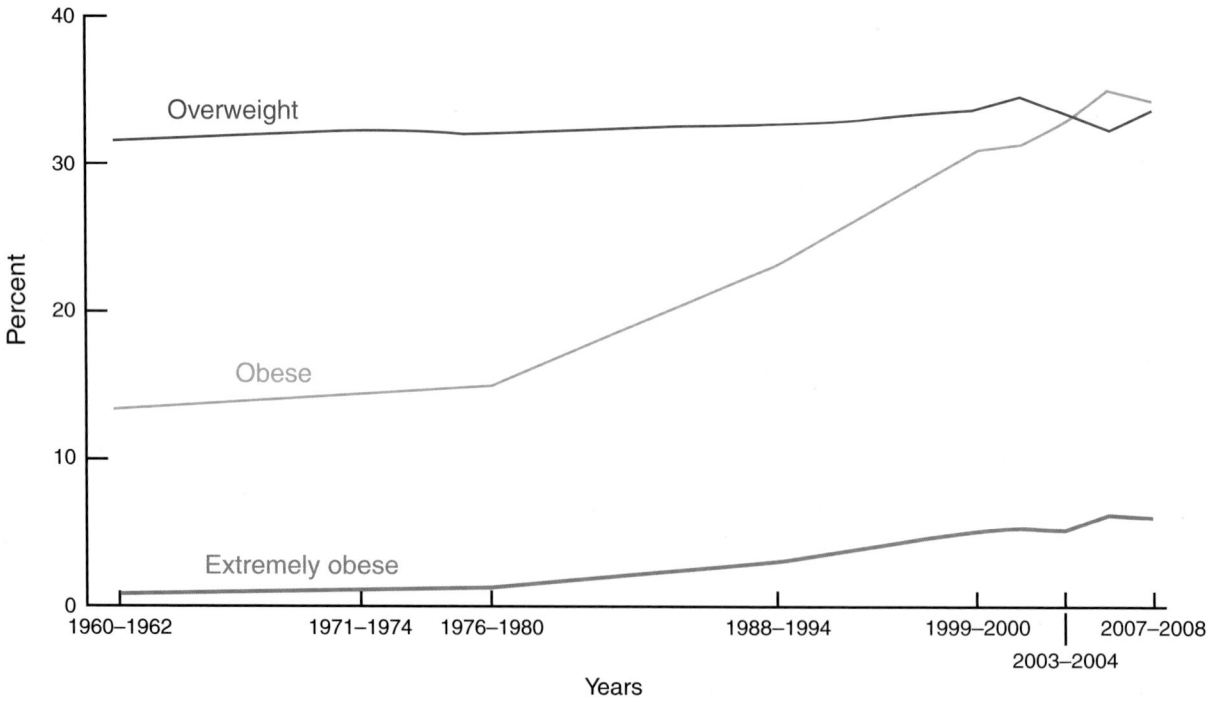

NOTE: Age-adjusted by the direct method to the year 2000 U.S. Census Bureau estimates, using the age groups 20–39, 40–59, and 60–74 years. Pregnant females were excluded. Overweight is defined as a body mass index (BMI) of 25 or greater but less than 30; obesity is a BMI greater than or equal to 30; extreme obesity is a BMI greater than or equal to 40.
SOURCE: CDC/NCHS, National Health Examination Survey cycle I (1960–1962); National Health and Nutrition Examination Survey I (1971–1974), II (1976–1980), and III (1988–1994), 1999–2000, 2001–2002, 2003–2004, 2005–2006, and 2007–2008.

Figure 135.6 Trends in overweight, obesity, and extreme obesity among adults aged 20 to 74 years: United States, 1960 to 2008. http://www.cdc.gov/NCHS/data/hestat/obesity_adult_07_08/obesity_adult_07_08.pdf

adipose tissue are not always exact. BMI sometimes overestimates adiposity on those with more lean body mass (e.g., athletes) while greatly underestimating excess adiposity on those with less lean body mass (56). There are numerous Web sites and applications that are available for handheld devices that will perform this calculation.

A complete head and neck exam should be performed with attention paid to several areas especially important to the assessment of the patient with OSA.

The nasal examination should be performed to determine if there is a septal deformity, allergic/nonallergic rhinitis, or other nasal obstruction that may lead to difficulty breathing at night. If there is nasal obstruction that results in mouth breathing at night, the mandible opens causing posterior displacement of the tongue with a narrowed glossal pharyngeal airway and increased airway resistance. Adherence to treatment of OSA with CPAP and/or oral appliances can be improved with patent nasal airways.

Mallampati rating of the oral cavity was developed by an anesthesiologist to assess the difficult airway for intubation (57). Patients are asked to open their mouths wide and to protrude their tongues forward. A modified Mallampati or Friedman palate position is performed with the mouth open and without protrusion of the tongue (58). The oropharynx is assessed, and the classification of Mallampati I to IV is made based on the degree of visualization of the posterior pharyngeal wall, uvula, soft palate, and hard palate (Fig. 135.7).

Tonsils are evaluated and categorized on a scale of 0 to 4 (Fig. 135.8). Zero is used when the tonsil has been previously surgically excised, and four would be for tonsils

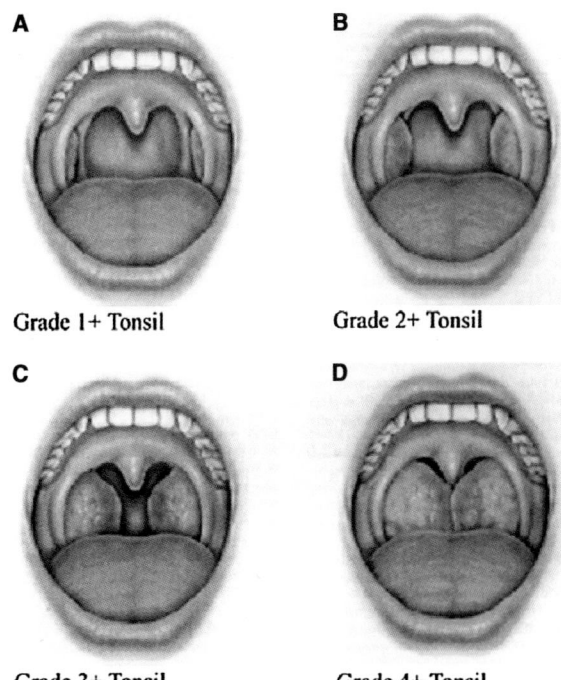

Grade 1+ Tonsil   Grade 2+ Tonsil

Grade 3+ Tonsil   Grade 4+ Tonsil

Figure 135.8 Tonsil size. **A:** Grade 1—Tonsil tissue is barely visible past anterior tonsillar pillar but not visible past posterior tonsillar pillar. **B:** Grade 2—Tonsil tissue is extending past anterior tonsillar pillar and obscuring posterior tonsillar pillar. **C:** Grade 3—Tonsil tissue is enlarged and almost obscuring pharyngeal airway. **D:** Grade 4—Tonsil tissue is meeting in the midline.

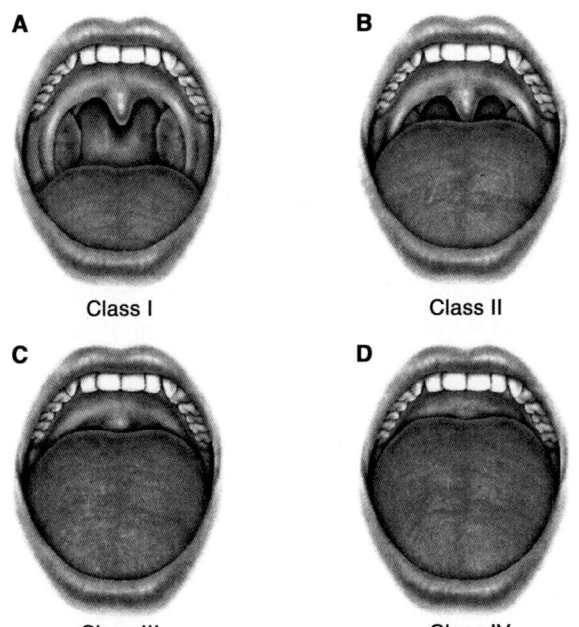

Class I   Class II

Class III   Class IV

Figure 135.7 Friedman modification of Mallampati classification. **A:** Class I: Full visibility of tonsils, uvula, soft palate, and hard palate. **B:** Class II: Visibility of hard palate, soft palate, upper portion of tonsils, and uvula. **C:** Class III: Soft palate, hard palate, and base of uvula are visible. **D:** Class IV: Only hard palate is visible.

that are "kissing" or touching in the midline. If a patient gags during the exam, the size of the tonsil may be incorrectly assessed. The tonsils will touch during the pharyngeal constriction and may be graded as touching when, in fact, this is physiologic. Removal of 3 to 4+ tonsil in some patients may result in elimination of the upper airway obstruction causing OSA.

The Friedman clinical staging system for SDB takes into consideration the modified Friedman palate position, tonsil size, and BMI. It has been used as a predictor of the success of uvulopalatopharyngoplasty (UPPP) and to determine if additional surgical procedures would be useful (59).

Dental occlusion should be assessed and recorded as Class I, II, or III (Fig. 135.9). Class I is normal occlusion with the mesial buccal cusp of the first maxillary molar positioned into the intercuspal groove of the mandibular first molar. Class II occurs when patients are retrognathic, and the mesial buccal cusp of the first maxillary molar is positioned mesial to the intercuspal groove of the mandibular first molar. Class II occlusion will have posterior displacement of the tongue and suffer from glossopharyngeal airways that have decreased anterior posterior diameter. Class III occlusion occurs with mandibular protrusion, and the mesial buccal cusp of the first maxillary molar is positioned distal to the intercuspal groove of the mandibular first molar. Maxillomandibular advancement procedures for Class II and III occlusions can be extremely successful in patients with OSA and may improve cosmesis as well (60).

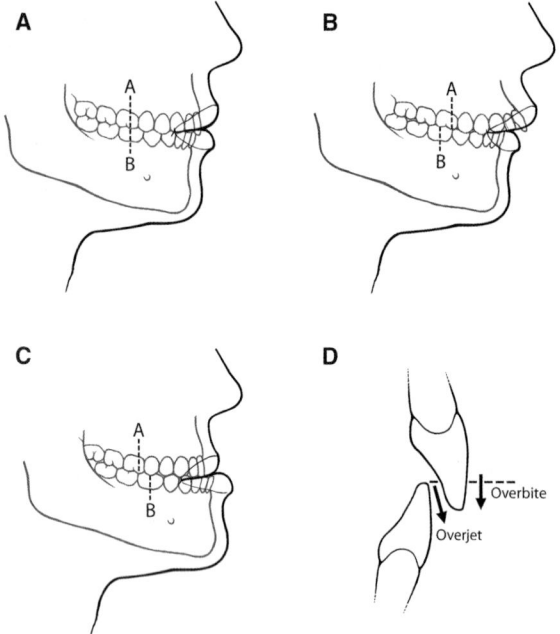

Figure 135.9 Dental occlusion is the classification between the maxillary and mandibular teeth when they come into contact during chewing or at rest. **A:** Class I molar occlusion: The mesial buccal cusp of the first maxillary molar is positioned into the intercuspal groove of the mandibular first molar and is considered normal occlusion. **B:** Class II molar occlusion is the mesial buccal cusp of the first maxillary molar positioned into the intercuspal groove of the mandibular first molar and is sometimes referred as an overbite or retrognathic. **C:** Class III molar occlusion is the mesial buccal cusp of the first maxillary molar positioned distal to the intercuspal groove of the mandibular first molar. **D:** There is normally 2 mm of overbite and overjet related to the central mandibular and central maxillary incisors.

Nasopharyngeal endoscopy with Mueller maneuver is often attempted to identify the sites of collapse in the upper airway during sleep. Introducing a flexible fiberoptic scope into the hypopharynx to obtain a view, the examiner asks the patient to inhale; patient attempts to inhale with the mouth closed and nostrils plugged, which may lead to a collapse of certain segments of the airway. This maneuver has been used to predict success of surgical treatment by guiding the surgeon to treat one or more sites of pharyngeal obstruction. However, a prospective study demonstrated that Mueller maneuvers are not predictive of surgical outcomes for UPPP (61).

Drug-induced sleep endoscopy is another diagnostic method that may help identify the specific site of obstruction during apneas more accurately than the Mueller maneuver and awake endoscopy. Described in 1991, the technique uses pharmacologic induction of sleep and the placement of a flexible fiberoptic endoscope transnasally for visualization of the upper airway (62). Sleep endoscopy is performed in an operating room or procedure room with the surgeon and with a provider administering anesthesia. During pharmacologic sleep, a fiberoptic exam includes a complete assessment of the upper airway including the palate, oropharynx, hypopharynx, and retroglossal regions (web video by Dr. Ofer Jacobowitz). There have

been attempts to correlate sleep endoscopy with surgical outcomes, but it is unclear if this technique is superior in choosing candidates for a specific surgical procedure (63).

Neck circumference has been reported to be a better predictor of OSA than BMI. The neck circumference should be measured at the level of the superior border of the cricothyroid membrane with the patient in the upright position. A male with a neck circumference of 17 inches or a female with 14½ inches or greater and a BMI greater than 30 has a 70% incidence of OSA (64).

Abdominal obesity assessed by waist measurement or waist/hip ratio is related to increased risk of all-cause mortality regardless of BMI. The waist is measured simply at the smallest circumference of the natural waist, just above the belly button, and the hip circumference is measured at its widest part of the buttocks or hip. The relative risks seem to be relatively stronger in younger than in older adults and in those with relatively low BMI compared with those with high BMI. Waist–hip ratio is a risk factor especially in severe OSA syndrome (65).

The waist–hip ratio has been found to have better predictive value for ventilation abnormalities than BMI. A ratio of more than 0.9 for men and more than 0.85 for women is abnormal. Central obesity impairs ventilation to lower lung zones, resulting in abnormally lower ventilation–perfusion ratios (66).

RADIOLOGIC EVALUATION OF THE AIRWAY IN SLEEP-DISORDERED BREATHING

Patients with OSA often have a narrower pharyngeal airway than normal individuals because of fat infiltration, increased soft tissue volume, or reduced pharyngeal muscle tone (1). Imaging techniques have been used to evaluate the sites of upper airway obstruction through static or dynamic techniques. Static techniques are x-ray cephalometry, computed tomography (CT), and magnetic resonance imaging (MRI). Dynamic techniques would be fluoroscopy, somnofluoroscopy (performed during sleep), cine CT, ultrafast CT, and MR imaging and fluoroscopic MRI. Imaging is primarily used in the planning of surgical intervention, the fitting of oral appliances, and the evaluation of treatment failures.

X-Ray Cephalometry

Lateral x-ray cephalometry is one of the standard diagnostic tools for evaluation of craniofacial skeletal abnormalities (Fig. 135.10). While it has the advantage of low cost, ready availability, and excellent demonstration of bony detail, its drawbacks include the fact that it is a static two-dimensional assessment of the airway and it is less sensitive to soft tissue interfaces.

There are multiple studies comparing differences between the upper airway and craniofacial anatomy between OSA patients and controls. The results are difficult

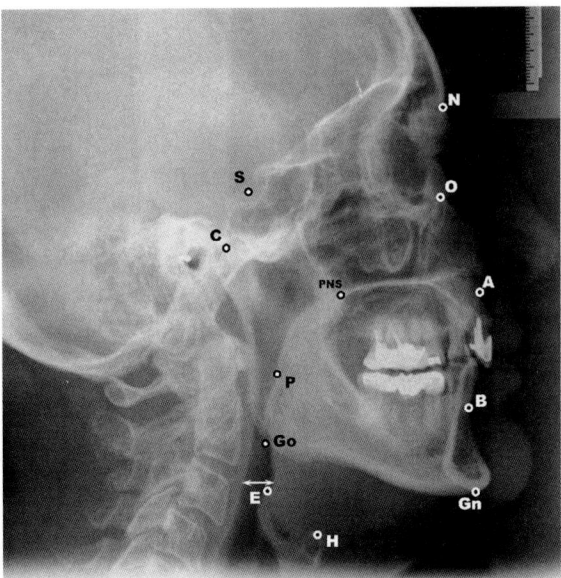

Figure 135.10 Lateral x-ray cephalogram. The cephalometric landmarks used in this study. *S* (sella), midpoint of sella; *N* (nasion), anterior point at the frontonasal suture; ANS (anterior nasal spine), most anterior point of the anterior nasal spine; *PNS* (posterior nasal spine), most posterior point of hard palate; *A* (subspinal point), deepest anterior point in concavity of the maxilla; *B* (supramental point), deepest anterior point in concavity of the mandible; *Gn* (gnathion), most inferior point of the mandibular symphysis; *H* (hyoid), most anterosuperior point of hyoid bone; *E* (epiglottis), base of epiglottis; *Go* (gonion), most posterior and inferior point of the angle of the mandible; *P* (soft palate), most inferior and posterior point of the soft palate; MP (mandibular plane), mandibular plane joining gonion with gnathion; SNA (deg), angle between nasion–sella line (NSL) and the line from A to N (measures projection, anterior or posterior of maxilla); SNB (deg), angle between NSL and the line from B and N (measures position of mandible); ANB (deg), angle between the line from A to N and the line from B to N (measures position of maxilla with mandible); PNS–ANS, linear distance between *PNS* and ANS; ANS-H, linear distance between ANS and *H*; ANS-E, linear distance between ANS and E; PNS-P, linear distance between *PNS* and P (measures length of velum of palate); MP-H, linear distance between the mandibular plane and *H*.

to compare because authors use different landmarks and calculated ratios to describe differences that were found. The reduction in mandible length and inferior displacement of the hyoid bone appears to be the most important skeletal abnormalities predisposing to OSA (67).

Fluoroscopy and Somnofluoroscopy

Fluoroscopic examination of the airway provides dynamic evaluation of the upper airway during wakefulness and sleep. Somnofluoroscopy demonstrates the dynamic events during apneas and has shown fluttering of the soft palate, which preceded airway collapse. This technique allows the examination of the sequence of events leading to airway collapse in OSA. It has also been used to determine the effect of oral appliances on airway size. Its clinical applicability is limited as this technique shows the upper airway in only two dimensions, and its use can result in high levels of radiation exposure.

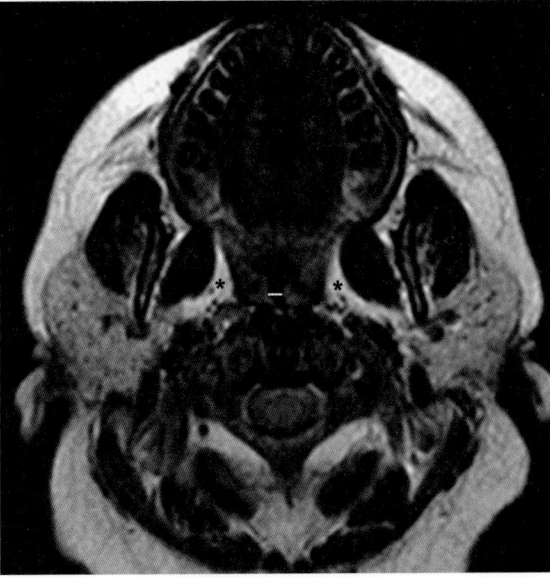

Figure 135.11 CT of patient with OSA–axial contrast-enhanced CT image at the level of the oropharynx demonstrating prominence of the lingual tonsils, which are seen to prolapse backward during sleep leading to obstruction. *Parapharyngeal fat pads.

Computed Tomography

CT scanning proves soft tissue contrast and allows precise measurements of cross-sectional areas at suspected levels of obstruction (Fig. 135.11). Newer technologies with fast scanning times allow a dynamic assessment of the upper airway during a respiratory cycle. There are scanning protocols under hypnotic sedation to replicate resting, sleep, sleep during apneas, and wakefulness (68). Concerns regarding the dose of ionized radiation remain problematic. CT images also lack soft tissue contrast particularly for adipose tissue when compared to MRI.

Magnetic Resonance Imaging

MRI offers several important advantages compared to cephalometry or CT scans. MRIs provide excellent soft tissue resolution and lack of ionizing radiation. Various studies have demonstrated the presence of parapharyngeal fat deposits in patients with OSA who are obese and anterolateral fat deposits in nonobese patients (69) (Fig. 135.12). Multiple studies have used MRI to determine structural risk factors for OSA with conflicting results. Do et al. (70) demonstrated a weak trend for larger tongues in patients with OSA; however, Schwab et al. (71), using three-dimensional MRI analysis techniques, have confirmed that the volume of the upper airway soft tissue structures, including the tongue, is enlarged in patients with sleep apnea and that this enlargement is a significant risk factor for sleep apnea. Ultrafast MRI can demonstrate dynamic three-dimensional changes in the upper airway during sleep and is used to identify site of obstruction, particularly in the pediatric population.

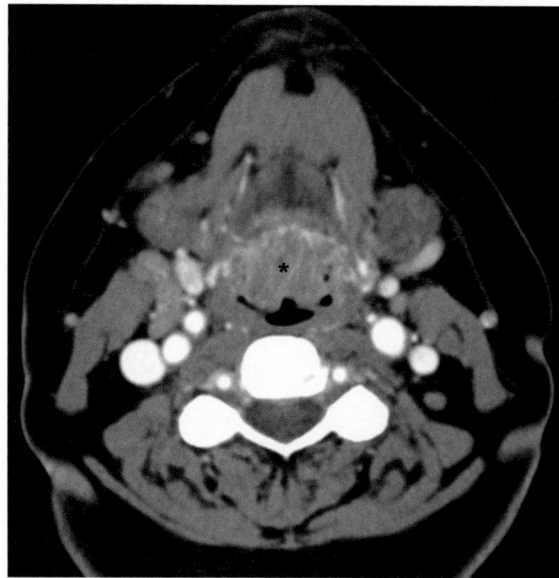

Figure 135.12 MRI demonstrating in OSA. Axial noncontrast MR image, demonstrating narrowing of the airway, which is more round than oval. In normal patients, airway is more oval with patent lateral recesses. Lateral parapharyngeal fat pads are indicated by the *asterisks* and appear larger in this apneic patient, although their role in genesis of OSA is uncertain.

DIAGNOSIS OF SLEEP DISORDERS

While the history and examination of the patient with symptoms of OSA can be highly suggestive of this diagnosis, confirmation with a sleep study is necessary. When Hoffstein and Szalai (72) studied 594 patients referred for possible OSA, they found that physician subjective impression only correctly identified 51% of the patients with OSA and 71% of the patients without OSA. The PSG is indicated in the diagnosis of SDB, positive airway titration studies, and some movement disorders of sleep (73). It consists of in-laboratory electrographic recordings of multiple physiologic parameters during drowsiness and sleep. Measurements may include EEG for sleep staging, electrooculogram (EOG) channels to measure eye movements,

TABLE 135.12	VARIABLES SCORED AND PHYSIOLOGIC PARAMETERS USED IN POLYSOMNOGRAPHY

Variable Scored	Physiologic Parameters used in Scoring
Sleep stages	EEG, EOG, EMG (atonia)
Arousals	EEG
Respiratory events	Flow (nasal pressure and thermistor), respiratory effort, oximetry
Leg movements–periodic	EMG

electromyography (EMG) measured superficially on the skin to assess for movement or atonia during REM sleep, airflow monitors including nasal pressure and thermistor, EKG leads, pulse oximetry, chest and abdominal excursion monitors to assess respiratory effort, auditory recordings of snoring, and video recording of movements in sleep (74) (Fig. 135.13). The data collected in a full night of sleep are scored in accordance with the American Academy of Sleep Medicine (AASM) guidelines (75). The variables scored in a PSG are listed in Table 135.12.

Also recorded in a PSG are data defining sleep onset, sleep efficiency, awakenings, and body position during sleep. The number of scored events is reported as an index or events per hour of sleep. The AHI is the number of apneas + hypopneas per hour of sleep. The RDI is the number of apneas + hypopneas + respiratory-related arousals per hour of sleep (Table 135.13).

Polysomnography is the traditional test for diagnosis of OSA. While many otolaryngologists interpret these studies, often physicians are called upon to treat patients based upon a sleep study interpreted by another physician. The AHI and RDI are not the only relevant and useful values contained within this report. A systematic review of the data within the PSG report will help determine the appropriate treatment for the patient. Table 135.14 contains tips for the review of polysomnographic data.

Figure 135.13 Three-hundred-second PSG recording in a 63-year-old male with snoring, hypertension, and EDS. Note snoring recorded on microphone channel apneas (*solid arrows*) and hypopneas (*dotted arrows*) on the flow channel with persistent respiratory effort and oxygen desaturations with respiratory events.

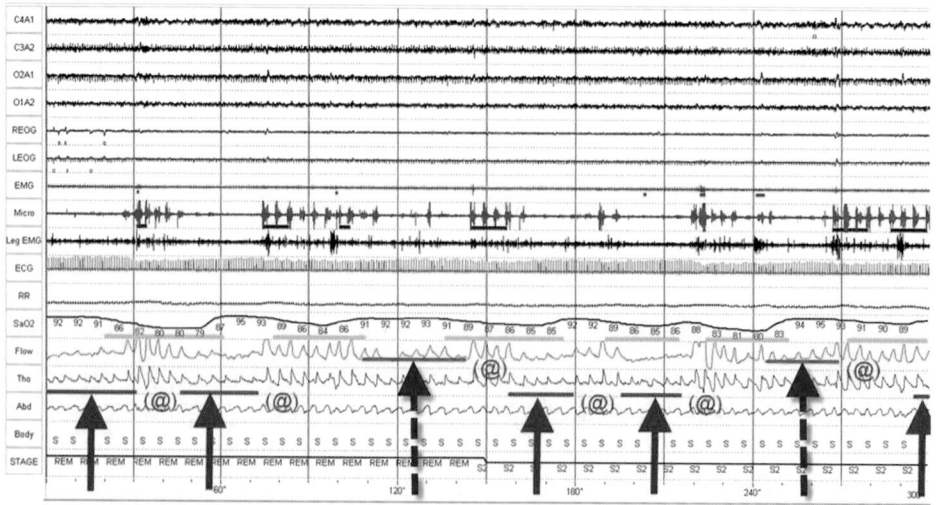

TABLE 135.13	GLOSSARY OF ADULT POLYSOMNOGRAPHY TERMS

Obstructive Apnea—Respiratory event with a drop in the respiratory signal (thermistor signal preferred) by ≥90% of baseline lasting at least 10 s associated with continued respiratory effort throughout the period of absent airflow.

Hypopnea—Respiratory event with a drop in the nasal pressure signal by ≥30% of pre-event baseline using nasal pressure or an alternative hypopnea sensor lasting at least 10 s associated with a ≥3% oxygen desaturation from pre-event baseline or an arousal.

Arousal—An abrupt change in EEG frequency >16 Hz that lasts 3 s with at least 10 s of stable sleep preceding the change. During REM sleep, a concurrent increase in submental EMG lasting at least 1 s is required.

Respiratory Effort-Related Arousal—A sequence of breaths lasting at least 10 s with a flattening of the nasal pressure waveform or increasing respiratory effort resulting in an arousal from sleep when this event does not meet criteria for an apnea or hypopnea.

AHI—Apneas + hypopneas per hour of sleep.

RDI—Apneas + hypopneas + respiratory effort-related arousals per hour of sleep.

Hypoventilation— There is an increase in the arterial PCO2 (or surrogate) to a value >55 mmHg for ≥10 min or there is a ≥10 mm Hg increase in arterial PCO2 (or surrogate) during sleep (in comparison to an awake supine value) to a value exceeding 50 mm Hg for ≥10 min.

Cheyne-Stokes Breathing— There are episodes of ≥3 consecutive central apneas and/or central hypopneas separated by a crescendo and decrescendo change in breathing amplitude with a cycle length of ≥40 s and there are ≥5 central apneas and/or central hypopneas per hour of sleep associated with the crescendo/decrescendo breathing pattern recorded over ≥2 h of monitoring.

Sleep Latency—Time in minutes from lights out until the first epoch in any sleep—usually Stage N1.

Sleep Efficiency—Total sleep time/total recording time (lights out to lights on) × 100.

REM Latency or Stage R Latency—Time in minutes from sleep onset to the first epoch of stage REM.

From Berry RB, Brooks R, Gamaldo CE, et al. *The AASM manual for the scoring of sleep and associated events: rules, terminology and technical specifications, version 2.0.* Darien, IL: American Academy of Sleep Medicine, 2012, www.aasmnet.org.

TABLE 135.14	HOW TO REVIEW A PSG REPORT

Study parameters—

Total sleep time and sleep efficiency—Review to be certain that the patient had a representative night of sleep. Normal adult sleep efficiency is 85%–90%, and sleep time in the laboratory is usually over 6 h. Very low sleep efficiency or a short sleep duration indicates a poor night of sleep that may not adequately represent the patient's usual sleep.

Sleep latency—Normal sleep latency is 10–30 min. A markedly decreased sleep latency of <10 min may signal excessive sleepiness. A sleep latency over 40 min can be secondary to a first night effect in the laboratory but may also indicate an underlying disorder such as DSPS.

REM latency—Normal REM latency is 80–110 min. A REM latency of <10 min may indicate the possibility of narcolepsy. A moderately reduced REM latency of 40–60 min can be seen in a number of conditions. It can be associated with depression, cessation of REM-suppressing drugs, alcohol withdrawal, and circadian rhythm disorders.

Sleep stages—SDB is often more prominent in REM sleep due to REM atonia. The lack of REM sleep during the study may mask or underestimate the presence or severity of SDB. Stage I (N1) sleep is a very light stage of sleep, which is normally present in 5%–10% of the night's sleep. A high percentage of N1 sleep suggests very disrupted sleep. Abnormal sleep stage distribution may also indicate medication effect, underlying sleep deprivation or other abnormalities of sleep. Since Stage N3 sleep declines with age, it is not abnormal for older adults to have little or no slow-wave sleep.

Respiratory summary—Within the respiratory summary is a detailed accounting of the number of apneas; the number and percent of each type of apnea: central, mixed, or obstructive; the number of hypopneas; and the number of RERAs. Presence of significant central apneas may indicate underlying heart failure, prior CVA, or medication effect. Also note the positional effect on the respiratory indices to determine if positional therapy may be helpful.

Arousal index—Arousals are abrupt changes of EEG frequency of 3 s or longer. These can be spontaneous, related to limb movements, or respiratory effort related. RERAs are included in the RDI, but not the AHI. A high number of spontaneous arousals may indicate an underlying medical problem such as fibromyalgia or pain. If the report does not include RERAs, the spontaneous arousals may include the respiratory arousals, and the RDI will not be reported. Studies that do not record and score arousals, including many home or portable studies, may not give a clear picture of the sleep disruption caused by SDB.

Graphic PSG data—This is a graphic representation of the data contained within the PSG report including the sleep hypnogram and graphs of the AHI, arousals, oximetry, heart rate, and body position. It is helpful in identifying associations within the study such as positional sleep apnea, REM-related events, and severely disrupted sleep.

An additional type of sleep test that determines the propensity to fall asleep during the day is an MSLT. It is recommended, with a PSG, for the diagnosis of narcolepsy or suspected idiopathic hypersomnia (76). It may also be useful in a patient with OSA who does not have resolution of EDS with adequate treatment of the OSA.

In 2007, the US Centers for Medicare and Medicaid Services (CMS) released a statement endorsing the use of certain types of portable monitoring for diagnosing OSA and initiating CPAP therapy (77). This has opened the door for the widespread use of home sleep testing or portable monitors in sleep diagnosis. This technology has the potential to provide cost savings in the diagnosis of OSA and to expedite diagnosis and treatment for patients. Portable monitoring devices generally measure airflow, oximetry, heart rate, and respiratory effort, but do not measure sleep. Some devices measure other parameters including peripheral arterial tone and pulse transit time as surrogate measures of arousals, respiratory effort, respiratory events, and sleep time. Since most portable devices do not measure sleep, the RDI reported in these devices is the number of apneas and hypopneas per hour of recording time.

A minimum of seven parameters are recorded in a PSG, and these studies require the onsite monitoring of the patient by a sleep technologist. These in-lab studies are classified as type I sleep studies. The level or type of a sleep study is determined by the number of physiologic parameters monitored (see Table 135.15).

Many patients can be successfully diagnosed with sleep apnea using portable monitoring devices. In some patients, this can be the preferred method of treatment due to issues of mobility, cognitive dysfunction away from the home environment, or safety (see Table 135.16).

There are certain medical conditions that limit the accuracy of these devices. In patients with comorbid medical conditions such as congestive heart failure, recent cerebrovascular accident (CVA), possible seizure disorder, and other sleep disorders, a PSG is recommended (78) (see Table 135.17).

TREATMENT OF SLEEP DISORDERS

Management of a patient with SDB requires a comprehensive long-term treatment plan and follow-up. Rarely does a patient have only one sleep disorder, so the entire

TABLE 135.15	CLASSIFICATION OF SLEEP STUDIES
Type 1	≥7 physiologic parameters monitored and sleep technician in attendance
Type 2	≥7 physiologic parameters monitored, unattended
Type 3	4–7 physiologic parameters monitored, unattended
Type 4	≥3 physiologic parameters monitored, unattended

TABLE 135.16	INDICATIONS FOR THE USE OF PORTABLE MONITORING IN ADULTS—AASM GUIDELINES

Patients with a high pretest probability of moderate to severe OSA

Patients for whom in-laboratory PSG is not possible by virtue of immobility, safety, or critical illness

To monitor response to non-CPAP treatments for OSA including oral appliances, upper airway surgery, and weight loss

sleep history should be considered when planning therapy. Even if the patient's SDB is successfully treated, if this patient is only sleeping 4 hours a night, the patient's chief complain of sleepiness will likely persist. Sleep hygiene issues, underlying insomnia or a circadian rhythm disorder, may require treatment to provide optimal therapy for the patient. Treatment of obesity, both with diet and lifestyle changes and with surgical intervention, has been shown to have a significant beneficial effect on OSA. A 10% loss in body weight can result in a 26% decrease in AHI (79).

OSA is a chronic disease that requires long-term follow-up. Even if symptoms are currently resolved, the patient should be made aware of the likelihood of progression of symptoms in the future and the factors that will hasten the return of these symptoms.

PAP therapy is the first line of treatment for most adult patients with SDB. Successful treatment with PAP is greatly enhanced by close support from the treating physician and staff and education for the patient about the therapy. PAP therapy is fully covered in Chapter 136. A large percentage of patients with SDB can be successfully treated with CPAP in the laboratory setting. Long-term compliance, however, is much more problematic. Adequate compliance is difficult to define and to achieve. Most studies show long-term usage by only about 50% to 65% of those patients who initially accept PAP therapy (80). Current CMS standards define successful use or adequate compliance as the use of PAP for longer than 4 hours for 70% of nights. Using this

TABLE 135.17	CONTRAINDICATIONS FOR THE USE OF PORTABLE MONITORING

Patients with significant comorbid medical conditions (moderate to severe pulmonary disease, neuromuscular disease, congestive heart failure recent cerebrovascular accident, nocturnal hypoxemia requiring oxygen therapy)

Patients suspected to have other sleep disorders (CSA, periodic limb movement disorder, insomnia, parasomnias, circadian rhythm disorders, or narcolepsy)

General screening of asymptomatic populations

definition of compliance, a patient is adequately treated when wearing CPAP less than half of their sleep time.

Patients with a fixed, surgically correctable airway obstruction, such as marked tonsillar hypertrophy or large cervical osteophytes, may be candidates for primary treatment with surgery.

For patients intolerant of CPAP therapy, sleep surgery provides a viable secondary treatment option. Factors that influence surgical success include age, health, weight, tongue size, the presence of other areas of obstruction, and severity of OSA. Resolution of OSA is not the only appropriate goal of surgical therapy in a patient with OSA. Any intervention that improves CPAP compliance can have significant benefit to the patient. A procedure that relieves nasal obstruction or allows the patient to be adequately treated at a lower, more tolerable CPAP pressure may improve the patient's CPAP compliance. Similarly, resolution of nasal obstruction may allow an OSA patient to be adequately treated with an oral appliance.

Successful diagnosis and treatment of the patient with sleep disorders are best accomplished using a thorough systematic approach. Sleep disorders affect up to 30% of the population and are associated with significant sequelae including cardiovascular and endocrine disorders, exacerbation of depression and anxiety, heightened pain perception, impaired daytime functioning, and increased motor vehicle accidents. Often a multidisciplinary approach to these complex disorders will provide optimal patient outcomes.

HIGHLIGHTS

- Sleep disorders are prevalent in the population and are associated with significant physiologic consequences.
- Inadequate sleep or sleep deprivation can impair memory, learning, judgment, fine motor skills, and reaction time.
- SDB is associated with increased risk of cardiovascular events including MI and CVA, diabetes, obesity, neurocognitive deficits, motor vehicle accidents, and an increased risk of death from all causes.
- A complete history, including a focused review of systems, and physical examination are necessary to identify patients at risk for sleep disorders.
- Diagnosis of OSA is made with either an in-lab PSG or a home sleep test.
- First-line therapy for OSA is PAP therapy. Oral appliances can also provide adequate therapy for select patients with OSA.
- Surgery for OSA is reserved for patients with a specific correctable anatomic obstruction or those who have failed PAP therapy.

REFERENCES

1. American Academy of Sleep Medicine. *The International classification of sleep disorders: diagnostic and coding manual*, 2nd ed. Westchester, IL: American Academy of Sleep Medicine, 2005.
2. Kushida CA. Symptom-based prevalence of sleep disorders in an adult primary care population. *Sleep Breath* 2000;4(1):9–14.
3. Chervin RD. Sleepiness, fatigue, tiredness, and lack of energy in obstructive sleep apnea. *Chest* 2000;118:372–379.
4. Tishler PV, Larkin EK, Schluchter MD, et al. Incidence of sleep-disordered breathing in an urban adult population: the relative importance of risk factors in the development of sleep-disordered breathing. *JAMA* 2003;289:2230–2237.
5. Al Lawati NM, Patel SR, Ayas NT. Epidemiology, risk factors, and consequences of obstructive sleep apnea and short sleep duration. *Prog Cardiovasc Dis* 2009;51(4):285–293.
6. Young T, Evans L, Finn L, et al Estimation of the clinically diagnosed proportion of sleep apnea syndrome in middle-aged men and women. *Sleep* 1997;20:705–706.
7. Punjabi NM. The epidemiology of adult obstructive sleep apnea. *Proc Am Thorac Soc* 2008;5(2):136–143.
8. Chervin RD. Sleepiness, fatigue, tiredness, and lack of energy in obstructive sleep apnea. *Chest* 2000;118:372–379.
9. Guilleminault C, Hagen CC, Huynh NT. Comparison of hypopnea definitions in lean patients with known obstructive sleep apnea hypopnea syndrome (OSAHS). *Sleep Breath* 2009;13(4):341–347.
10. Shepertycky MR, Banno K, Kryger MH. Differences between men and women in the clinical presentation of patients diagnosed with obstructive sleep apnea syndrome. *Sleep* 2005;28:309–314.
11. Marin JM, Carrizo SJ, Vincente E, et al. Long-term cardiovascular outcomes in men with obstructive sleep apnea-hypopnea with or without treatment with continuous positive airway pressure: an observational study. *Lancet* 2005;365:1046–1053.
12. Klar Yaggi H, Concato J, Kernan WN, et al. Obstructive sleep apnea as a risk factor for stroke and death. *N Engl J Med* 2005;353:2034–2041.
13. Punjabi NM, Sorkin JD, Katzel LI, et al. Sleep-disordered breathing and insulin resistance in middle-aged and overweight men. *Am J Respir Crit Care Med* 2002;165(5):677–682.
14. Peled N, Kassirer M, Shitrit D, et al. The association of OSA with insulin resistance, inflammation and metabolic syndrome. *Respir Med* 2007;101(8):1696–1701.
15. Kushida CA, Littner MR, Morgenthaler TI, et al. Practice parameters for the indications of polysomnography and related procedures. *Sleep* 2005;28(4):499–521.
16. Mokhlesi B, Kryger MH, Grunstein RR. Assessment and management of patients with obesity hypoventilation syndrome. *Proc Am Thorac Soc* 2008;5(2):218–225.
17. Littleton SW, Mokhlesi B. The pickwickian syndrome-obesity hypoventilation syndrome. *Clin Chest Med* 2009;30(3):467–478, vii–viii.
18. Mokhlesi B, Tulaimat A. Recent advances in obesity hypoventilation syndrome. *Chest* 2007;132(4):1322–1336.
19. Mokhlesi B. Obesity-hypoventilation syndrome: a state of the art review. *Respir Care* 2010;55(10):1347–1362.
20. Morgenthaler TI, Kagramanov V, Hanak V, et al. Complex sleep apnea syndrome: is it a unique clinical syndrome? *Sleep* 2006;29(9):1203–1209.
21. National Sleep Foundation. "Summary findings of the 2008 Sleep in America Poll". http://www.sleepfoundation.org/sites/default/files/2008%20POLL%20SOF.PDF
22. Arnedt JT, Wilde GJS, Munt PW, et al. How do prolonged wakefulness and alcohol compare in the decrements they produce on a simulated driving task? *Accid Anal Prev* 2001;33:337–344.
23. Nagai M, Hoshide S, Kario K. Sleep duration as a risk factor for cardiovascular disease—a review of the recent literature. *Curr Cardiol Rev* 2010;6(1):54–61.
24. Yaremchuk K, Wardrop P. Sleep Medicine. Chapter 1. San Diego: Plural Publishing, 2010:1–2.
25. Van Cauter E, Spiegel K, Tasali E, et al. Metabolic consequences of sleep and sleep loss. *Sleep Med* 2008;9(Suppl 1):S23–S28.

26. Thompson CL, Larkin EK, Patel S, et al. Short duration of sleep increases risk of colorectal adenoma. *Cancer* 2011;117:841–847.

27. Philibert I. Bibliography of articles on the effect of sleep loss on performance, ACGME, 2002. http://www.acgme.org/DutyHours/sleepdepbib.pdf. Accessed Feb 4, 2011.

28. Gerdes J, Kahol K, Smith M, et al. Jack Barney award: the effect of fatigue on cognitive and psychomotor skills of trauma residents and attending surgeons. *Am J Surg* 2008;196(6):813–820.

29. Olson EJ, Drage LA, Auger RR. Sleep deprivation, physician performance, and patient safety *Chest* 2009;136:1389–1396.

30. Accreditation Council for Graduate Medical Education. Common program requirements for duty hours. Available at: http://www.acgme-2010standards.org/pdf/Common_Program_Requirements_07012011.pdf. Accessed March 4, 2011.

31. Czeisler CA. Medical and genetic differences in the adverse impact of sleep loss on performance: ethical considerations for the medical profession. *Trans Am Clin Climatol Assoc* 2009;120:249–285.

32. National Institutes of Health. *NIH State of Science Conference Statement on Manifestations and Management of Chronic Insomnia in Adults. State-of-Science Conference Statement.* Bethesda, MD: National Institutes of Health, 2005, June 13–15.

33. Overeem S, Mignot E, Gert van Dijk J, et al. Narcolepsy: clinical features, new pathophysiologic insights, and future perspectives. *J Clin Neurophysiol* 2001;18:78–105.

34. Morrish E, King MA, Smith IE, et al. Factors associated with a delay in the diagnosis of narcolepsy *Sleep Med* 2004;5(1):37–41.

35. Allen RP, Picchietti D, Henning WA, et al. Restless legs syndrome: diagnostic criteria, special considerations, and epidemiology. A report from the restless legs syndrome diagnosis and epidemiology workshop at the National Institutes of Health. *Sleep Med* 2003;4:101–119.

36. Hoffstein V, Mateika S, Anderson D. Snoring: is it in the ear of the Beholder? *Sleep* 1994;17(6):522–526.

37. Maimon N, Hanly P. Does snoring intensity correlate with the severity of obstructive sleep apnea. *J Clin Sleep Med* 2010;6(5):475–478.

38. Nakano H, Furukawa T, Nishima S. Relationship between snoring sound intensity and sleepiness in patients with obstructive sleep apnea. *J Clin Sleep Med* 2008;4(6):551–556.

39. Johns MW. A new method for measuring daytime sleepiness: the Epworth Sleepiness Scale. *Sleep* 1991;14:540–545

40. Davidson T. Sleep medicine for surgeons. *Laryngoscope* 2008;118:915–931.

41. Alkhalil M, Schulman E, Getsy J. Obstructive sleep apnea syndrome and asthma: what are the links? *J Clin Sleep Med* 2009;5(1):71–78.

42. Senior BA, Khan M, Schwimmer C, et al. Gastroesophageal reflux and obstructive sleep apnea. *Laryngoscope* 2001;111:2144–2146.

43. Coyne KS, Zhou Z, Bhattacharrya SK, et al. The prevalence of nocturia and its effect on health-related quality of life and sleep in a community sample in the USA. *BJU Int* 2003;92(9):948–954.

44. Coyne KS, Zhou Z, Bhattacharrya SK, et al. The prevalence of nocturia and its effect on health-related quality of life and sleep in a community sample in the USA. *BJU Int* 2003;92(9):948–954.

45. Tandberg E, Larsen JP, Karlesen K. A community based study of sleep disorders in patients with Parkinson's disease. *Mov Disord* 1998;13:895–899.

46. Pilowsky I, Crettenden I, Townley M. Sleep disturbance in pain clinic patients. *Pain* 1985;23(1):27–33.

47. Buckley T, Schatzberg A. On the interactions of the hypothalamic-pituitary-adrenal axis and sleep: normal HPA axis activity and circadian rhythm, exemplary sleep disorders. *J Clin Endocrinol* 2005;90(5):3106–3114.

48. Eichling P, Sahni J. Menopause related sleep disorders. *J Clin Sleep Med* 2005;1(3):291–300.

49. McCarty D. Beyond Ockham's Razor: redefining problem solving in clinical sleep medicine using a "five-finger" approach. *J Clin Sleep Med* 2010;6(3):292–296.

50. Lovett R. Coffee: The demon drink. *New Sci* 2005;24:2518.

51. Lieberman HR, Tharion WJ, Shukitt-Hale B, et al. Effects of caffeine, sleep loss, and stress on cognitive performance and mood during U.S. Navy Seal training. *Psychopharmacology* 2002;164:250–261.

52. Jaehne A, Loessl B, Bárkai Z, et al. Effects of nicotine on sleep during consumption, withdrawal and replacement therapy. *Sleep Med Rev* 2009;13(5):363–377.

53. Madsen BW, Rossi L. Sleep and Michael-Menten elimination of ethanol. *Clin Pharmacol Ther* 1980;27:114–119.

54. Eknoyan G. Adolphe Quetelet (1796–1874)—the average man and indices of obesity. *Nephrol Dial Transplant* 2008;23(1): 47–51.

55. Ogden C, Carroll M. Prevalence of overweight, obesity, and extreme obesity among Adults: United States, trends 1976–1980 through 2007–2008. 2010; Health E-Stats. http://www.cdc.gov/NCHS/data/hestat/obesity_adult_07_08/obesity_adult_07_08.pdf

56. Romero-Corral A, Somers VK, Sierra-Johnson J, et al. Accuracy of body mass index in diagnosing obesity in the adult general population. *Int J Obes (Lond)* 2008;32(6):959–966.

57. Mallampati SR, Gatt S, Gugino LD, et al. A clinical sign to predict difficult tracheal intubation; a prospective study. *Can J Anaesth* 1985;32:429–434.

58. Friedman M, Soans R, Gurpinar B, et al. Interexaminer agreement of Friedman tongue positions for staging of obstructive sleep apnea/hypopnea syndrome. *Otolaryngol Head Neck Surg* 2008;139(3):372–377.

59. Friedman M, Ibrahim H, Bass L. Clinical staging for sleep-disordered breathing. *Otolaryngol Head Neck Surg* 2002;127:13–21.

60. Dattilo D, Drooger S. Outcome assessment of patients undergoing maxillofacial procedures for the treatment of sleep apnea: comparison of subjective and objective results. *J Oral Maxillofac Surg* 2004;62:164–168.

61. Katsantonis G, Maas C, Walsh J. The predictive efficacy of the Muller maneuver in uvulopalatopharyngoplasty. *Laryngoscope* 1989;99(7):677–680.

62. Croft CB, Pringle M. Sleep nasendoscopy: a technique of assessment in snoring and obstructive sleep apnea. *Clin Otolaryngol Allied Sci* 1991;16:504–509.

63. Kezirian E. Drug-induced sleep endoscopy. *Oper Tech Otolaryngol* 2006;17:230–232.

64. Kushida CA, Efron B, Guilleminault C. A predictive morphometric model for the obstructive sleep apnea syndrome. *Ann Intern Med* 1997;127: 581–587.

65. Seidell J. Waist circumference and waist/hip ratio in relation to all cause mortality, cancer and sleep apnea. *Eur J Clin Nutr* 2010;64(1):35–41.

66. Nieto FJ, Young TB, Lind BK. Sleep heart health study. association of sleep disordered breathing, sleep apnea and hypertension in a large community-based study. *JAMA* 2000;283: 1829–1836.

67. Miles PG, Vig PS, Weyant RJ, et al. Craniofacial structure and obstructive sleep apnea syndrome—a qualitative analysis and meta-analysis of the literature. *Am J Orthod Dentofacial Orthop* 1996;109(2):163–172.

68. Vos W, De Backer J, Devolder A, et al. Correlation between severity of sleep apnea and upper airway morphology based on advanced anatomical and functional imaging. *J Biomech* 2007;40(10):2207–2213.

69. Mortimore IL, Marshall I, Wraith PK, et al. Neck and total fat deposition in nonobese and obese patients with sleep apnea compared with that in control subjects. *Am J Respir Crit Care Med* 1998;157(1):280–283.

70. Do KL, Ferreyra H, Healy JF, et al. Does tongue size differ between patients with and without sleep-disordered breathing. *Laryngoscope* 2000;110(9):1552–1555.

71. Schwab RJ, Pasirstein M, Pierson R, et al. Identification of upper airway anatomic risk factors for obstructive sleep apnea with volumetric magnetic resonance imaging. *Am J Respir Crit Care Med* 2003;168(5):522–530.

72. Hoffstein V, Szalai JP. Predictive value of clinical features in diagnosing obstructive sleep apnea. *Sleep* 1993;16:118–122.

73. Kushida CA, Littner MR, Morgenthaler T, et al. Practice parameters for the indications for polysomnography and related procedures: an update for 2005. *Sleep* 2005;28(4):499–521.

74. Bae C, Avidan A. Evaluation and testing of the sleepy patient. In: Smith HR, Comella CL, Birgit H, eds. *Sleep medicine*. Cambridge, UK: Cambridge University Press, 2008:25–46.

75. Berry RB, Brooks R, Gamaldo CE, et al. *The AASM manual for the scoring of sleep and associated events: rules, terminology and technical specifications, version 2.0.* Darien, IL: American Academy of Sleep Medicine, 2012, www.aasmnet.org.

76. American Academy of Sleep Medicine. Standards of practice committee: practice parameters for clinical use of the multiple sleep latency tests and the maintenance of wakefulness test (sleepiness; hypersomnia; daytime wakefulness). *Sleep* 2005;28(1):113–121.

77. Agency for Healthcare Research and Quality. *Home diagnosis of obstructive sleep apnea-hypopnea syndrome (brief record)*. Rockville, MD: Agency for Healthcare Research and Quality, 2007. http://www.mrw.interscience.wiley.com/cochrane/clhta/articles/HTA-32007000609/frame.html. Accessed March 3, 2011.

78. Collop NA, Anderson WM, Boehlecke B, et al. Clinical guidelines for the use of unattended portable monitors in the diagnosis of obstructive sleep apnea in adult patients. *J Clin Sleep Med* 2007;3(7):737–747.

79. Shah N, Roux F. The relationship of obesity and obstructive sleep apnea. *Clin Chest Med* 2009;30(3):455–465.

80. Grote L, Hedner J, Grunstein R, et al. Therapy with nCPAP: incomplete elimination of sleep related breathing disorder. *Eur Respir J* 2000;16:921–927.

136 Medical Therapy for Obstructive Sleep Apnea

Ryan J. Soose   *Patrick J. Strollo*

INTRODUCTION

Obstructive sleep apnea (OSA) is a chronic condition that will require management across the lifespan. Like most chronic diseases, *prevention* of OSA remains the primary goal and most attractive treatment from a public health perspective. At this juncture, *management* of the large population of patients diagnosed with sleep-related breathing disorders (as well as those who are still undiagnosed) remains the critical focus of most sleep physicians. As with hypertension (HTN), diabetes, and other chronic conditions, the individual treatment plan is not aimed at "cure" but rather (a) symptom and quality of life improvement and (b) reduction of cardiovascular and general health risk.

Both physician and patient understanding of OSA is the cornerstone for successful management. This approach allows for customization of each individual's treatment plan depending on their symptoms, airway anatomy, disease severity, and medical comorbidities. Across the lifespan, the same patient, with the same apnea hypopnea index (AHI), may benefit from different discrete treatment options, or a combination of treatment options, depending on the clinical context at that particular stage of life.

Positive airway pressure (PAP) therapy and oral appliances comprise the foundation of OSA medical management in the majority of patients. Nevertheless, there are many other management tools that can be employed to optimize clinical results, particularly when used in combination with PAP or oral appliance therapy. An individualized approach considering all available treatment options provides the most effective long-term management strategy for many patients.

POSITIVE AIRWAY PRESSURE

Introduction

The treatment of OSA with continuous positive airway pressure (CPAP) was first described by Sullivan et al. in 1981 (1). The introduction of CPAP marked an enormous advance in the management of OSA. The first commercially available PAP systems were marketed in the mid-1980s. CPAP rapidly became the mainstay of sleep apnea therapy and is still the most widely used treatment modality today.

In the Starling resistor model of the pathophysiology of OSA (Fig. 136.1), the collapsible segment of the tube (pharynx) is bound by an upstream and downstream segment with a corresponding upstream and downstream pressure (P_{us} and P_{ds}) (2).

Airway occlusion occurs when the surrounding tissue pressure, P_{out} (comprising tongue, pharyngeal muscles, parapharyngeal fat, mucosal edema, etc.), becomes greater than the intraluminal pressure (P_{in}).

The critical closing pressure (P_{crit}) is represented by the P_{in} when airway obstruction occurs. Inspiratory airflow depends directly on the difference between P_{us} and P_{crit} and therefore, effective therapy for OSA requires widening the differential between P_{us} and P_{crit}. This goal can be accomplished in two ways: (a) increasing P_{us} or (b) reducing P_{crit}. PAP works by accomplishing the former with the application of increased pressure at the airway opening.

PAP systems for the treatment of sleep apnea consist of a generator that directs airflow downstream to the patient via tubing and an interface. Positive pressure is introduced into the upper airway providing a pneumatic splint through the entire length of the collapsible pharyngeal segment and thus maintaining airway patency and effective control of breathing. The splinting effect constitutes the primary mechanism of therapeutic action, although augmentation of lung volume may play a secondary beneficial role as well (3,4).

Modalities

Continuous Positive Airway Pressure

Continuous positive airway pressure (CPAP), or fixed-pressure CPAP, was the first modality described and still the most widely used. This modality delivers the same

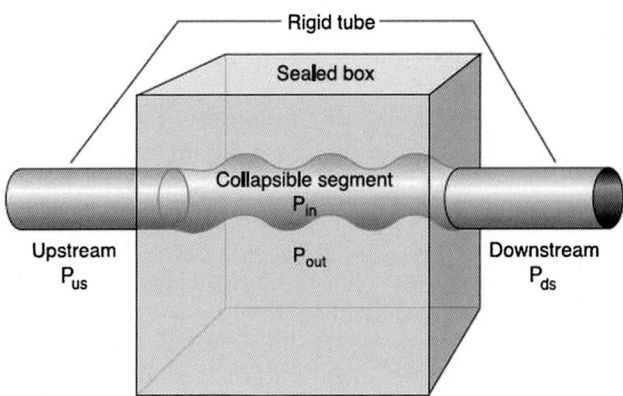

Figure 136.1 Pathophysiology of OSA: Starling resistor model of OSA depicting a collapsible tube (pharynx) with a corresponding intraluminal pressure (P_{in}) and surrounding tissue pressure (P_{out}). The upstream pressure (P_{us}) corresponds to the pressure at the nose or airway opening, and the downstream pressure corresponds (P_{ds}) to the tracheal or intrathoracic pressure. The critical closing pressure (P_{crit}) is represented by the P_{in} at which airway obstruction occurs and is directly dependent on the difference between P_{us} and P_{crit}. Successful management of OSA requires adequate increase in the P_{us} or reduction in the P_{crit}. (Reproduced from Dempsey JA, Veasey SC, Morgan BJ, et al. Pathophysiology of sleep apnea. *Physiol Rev* 2010;90:47–112, with permission.)

pressure to the patient during both inspiration and expiration and remains unchanged throughout the night.

Bilevel Positive Pressure

Bilevel positive pressure (BIPAP) provides the ability to independently adjust the inspiratory (IPAP) and expiratory (EPAP) pressure such that the pressure delivered during exhalation is lower than that delivered during inhalation (5). Several studies have confirmed the effectiveness of BIPAP in the treatment of OSA in adults (6–9).

Most BIPAP devices are used in one of two modes: spontaneous (S-mode) or spontaneous–timed (ST-mode). In S-mode, IPAP is delivered in response to a patient "trigger." In ST-mode, the patient may trigger the delivery of IPAP; in addition, the physician may set the device so that IPAP is delivered at prescribed intervals if a spontaneously triggered breath does not occur within that interval. This backup respiratory rate provided in the ST-mode is not commonly employed in the treatment of classic OSA but may be beneficial in selected patient groups with more complex sleep-disordered breathing, such as those with neuromuscular disorders, chest wall deformities, or congestive heart failure (CHF) with Cheyne-Stokes breathing.

Autotitrating Continuous Positive Airway Pressure

The pressure required to maintain airflow and control of breathing may vary throughout the night, as well as from night to night, and may be dependent on patient factors such as sleep staging, body position, and alcohol consumption. In autotitrating devices, the physician sets a prescribed pressure range, allowing the delivered pressure to vary throughout the night in order to meet the patient's changing pressure requirements in real time. Autotitrating devices employ computer algorithms to detect changes in airflow and adjust the delivered pressure accordingly. Autotitrating devices are available in both autotitrating continuous positive airway pressure (APAP) and autotitrating BIPAP (auto bilevel) forms.

One theoretical advantage of autotitrating technology is the reduction in the overall cumulative pressure exposure during the night and subsequent improvement in patient comfort and compliance. Compared to fixed CPAP, studies of APAP show similar effectiveness on both symptomatic and polysomnographic measures and a small (2 cm H_2O) average reduction in pressure. On an individual basis, some patients strongly prefer APAP over traditional fixed CPAP or BIPAP. The literature has not yet supported an improvement in adherence with autotitrating devices compared to fixed-pressure devices in CPAP naïve patients (10,11).

Methods of Titration

The traditional diagnostic and therapeutic evaluation of OSA involves two separate nights in the sleep laboratory. The first represents a full-montage attended overnight polysomnography for diagnostic purposes. If indicated, the patient then returns to the sleep lab a second night for a treatment study that again involves full-montage polysomnographic recording but in conjunction with manual PAP titration by the attendant sleep technician.

One method of improving cost-effectiveness and patient access is the consideration of a split-night study in certain clinical circumstances. A split-night study combines diagnostic polysomnography and a PAP titration in one night, rather than the traditional process of two separate nights (12,13). Proper clinical judgment in patient selection is essential, as inaccurate estimation of OSA severity and/or incomplete therapeutic titration may occur. Specific guidelines have been published by the American Academy of Sleep Medicine (AASM) for the use of split-night studies (14).

Alternatively, in-laboratory manual titration may be bypassed altogether with more recent developments in home portable monitoring and home auto-CPAP titration. Properly selected patients with a high pretest probability of OSA may undergo the initial diagnostic study at home with an unattended portable four-channel monitoring system. Additionally, the patient generally receives CPAP education and mask fitting in the clinical setting during the day. If the portable study is consistent with OSA and PAP therapy is indicated, the patient is then loaned an autotitrating device to use at home for a short period of time (e.g., 1 or 2 weeks).

The device is subsequently returned and the information downloaded with regard to effectiveness, usage, and mask leak. The patient can then receive a prescription for either fixed-pressure CPAP (usually set at the 90th percentile pressure) or an APAP as permanent therapy. At the present time, home autotitration appears to be at least as effective as traditional methods with regard to both subjective and objective outcome measures as well as adherence rates (15). Additionally, it has the potential to be associated with improved cost-savings and increased resource availability across a population.

Interfaces

A variety of types of CPAP interfaces are widely available. The most common types fall under one of three categories: nasal masks, nasal pillows, and full-face masks (Fig. 136.2). Mask selection and sizing is generally accomplished by the sleep technician addressing the patient's comfort, concerns, and facial anatomy. Proper mask fitting, patient education, and close clinical monitoring and follow-up are essential to successful long-term management.

In one randomized crossover study comparing nasal pillows and a nasal mask, investigators reported that nasal pillows were associated with less frequent adverse effects, less air leak, and less insomnia symptoms, although adherence and functional outcome measures did not differ between the groups (16).

Effectiveness

With adequate pressure application and proper usage/adherence, PAP therapy often provides effective control of sleep-disordered breathing and subsequently accomplishes the main goals of symptom/quality of life improvement and reduction of cardiovascular and general health risks.

Symptom and Quality of Life Improvement

CPAP has been shown to improve both subjective and objective measures of OSA. On polysomnography, proper CPAP titration is associated with improved sleep continuity and architecture. During the first night of treatment, some patients may manifest an unusually large percentage of rapid eye movement (REM) sleep ("REM rebound") as a result of sudden reversal of the airway obstruction and associated chronic sleep deprivation. CPAP often has a beneficial impact on other nocturnal aspects of OSA, including treatment of snoring, decreased nocturnal awakenings, and a reduction in nocturia (17–22).

In studies of patients with OSA and hypersomnia, treatment of CPAP is associated with a reduction in daytime sleepiness and improvement in neurocognitive function and quality of life measures (23,24). The effect of CPAP on objective metrics of sleep propensity during the day (e.g., multiple sleep latency test [MSLT] or maintenance of wakefulness test) is less clear, with only some studies showing an effect and a less compelling impact in patients with mild OSA (17,23,25). Nevertheless, despite some controversy with regard to the sleep laboratory results, the data on motor vehicle collisions, one of the most important public health risks associated with OSA, are much more convincing. A number of studies employing driving simulators have demonstrated improved performance

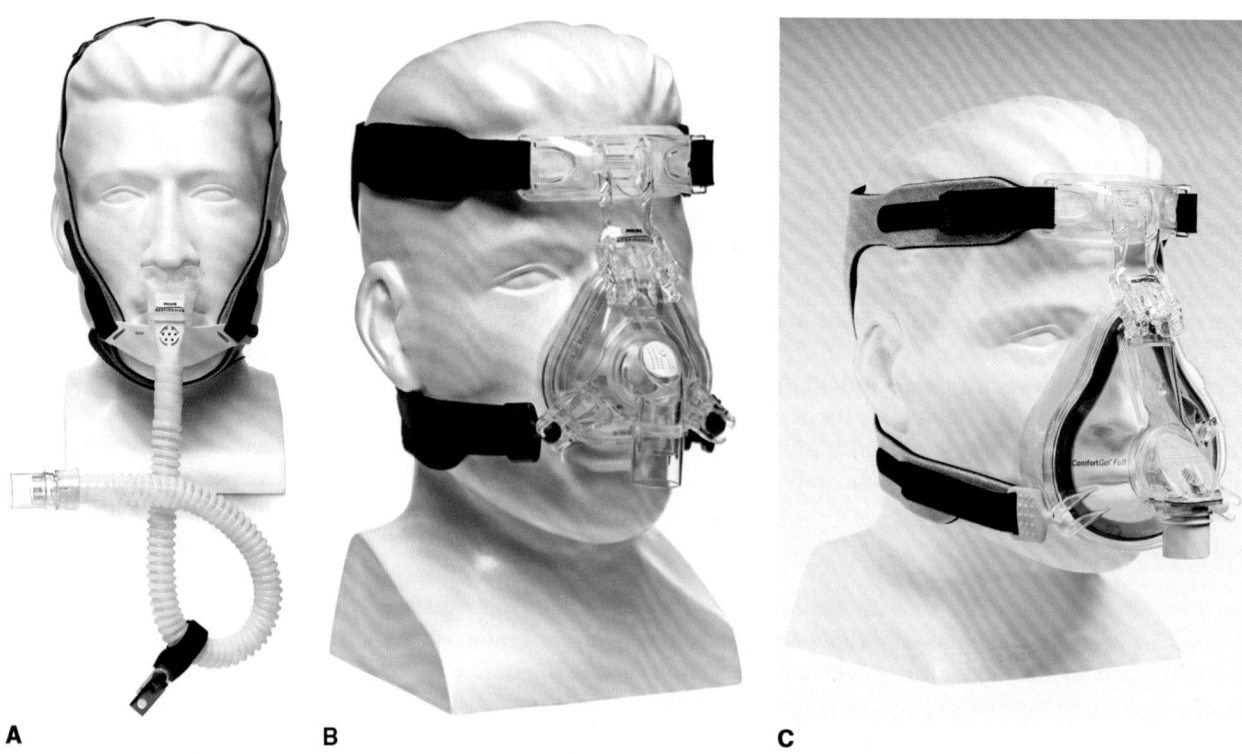

A   **B**   **C**

Figure 136.2 PAP interfaces: Examples of the three most common categories of mask interfaces for positive pressure therapy are depicted: (**A**) nasal pillows, (**B**) nasal mask, and (**C**) full-face mask.

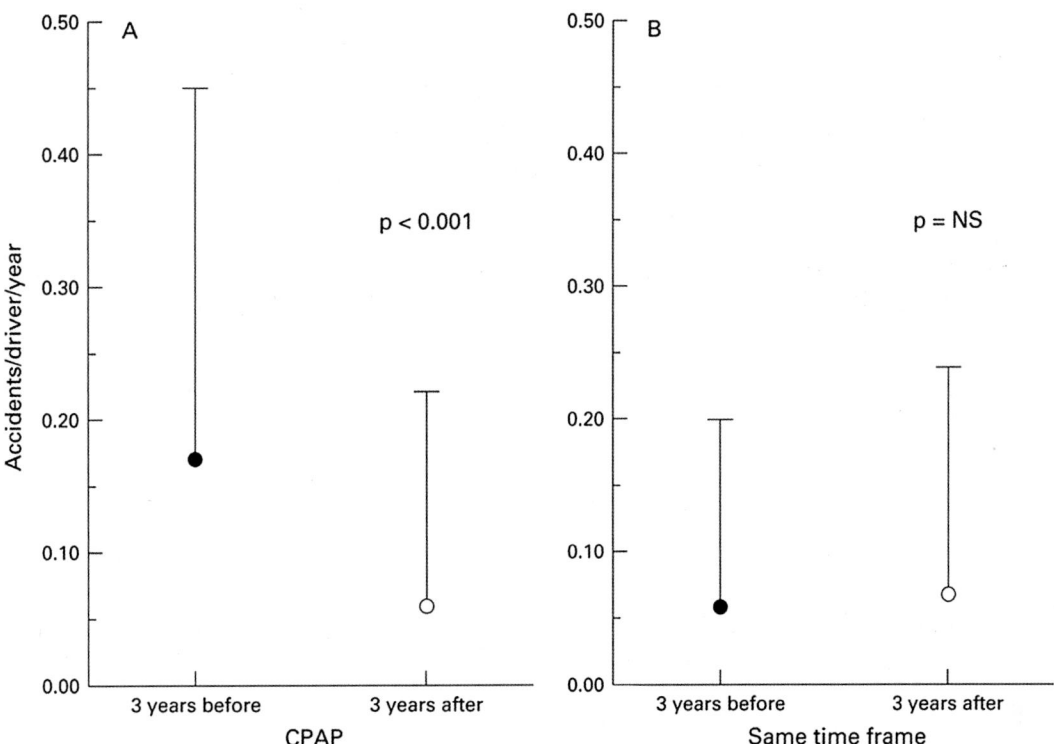

Figure 136.3 Reduction in motor vehicle collisions in patients OSA treated with CPAP: Mean motor vehicle collision rate in OSA patients during the 3-year period before CPAP treatment and the 3-year period with CPAP treatment (**A**). Mean motor vehicle collision rates in control subjects during the same time periods (**B**). (Reproduced from George CFP. Reduction in motor vehicle collisions following treatment of sleep apnea with nasal CPAP. *Thorax* 2001;56:508–512, with permission.)

following initiation of CPAP therapy (26–28). Similarly, a comparison of the number of accidents per driver per year over the 3 years before and following CPAP therapy in OSA patients demonstrated a notable reduction, reaching levels that were comparable to those in individuals without OSA (Fig. 136.3) (29).

Reduction of Cardiovascular and General Health Risks

Numerous studies have shown that OSA is associated with cardiovascular disease and that successful PAP therapy results in reduced cardiovascular mortality (30–32). In a prospective cohort from the Sleep Heart Health Study, investigators showed that sleep-disordered breathing is associated with increased overall mortality as well as mortality specifically due to coronary artery disease, particularly in those patients with severe OSA (AHI greater than 30) (Fig. 136.4) (31). A large observational study showed that men with severe OSA have an increased rate of both fatal and nonfatal cardiovascular events (32). Furthermore, treatment with PAP effectively lowered this cardiovascular risk (Fig. 136.5). Finally, Peker et al. (33) assessed incident cardiovascular events in middle-aged men with OSA over 7 years and noted that the incidence of cardiovascular events in patients who were adequately treated (by PAP, uvulopalatopharyngoplasty, or oral appliances) was about 7% in contrast to about 57% in patients who were inadequately treated.

Cardiac rhythm disturbances are common in OSA patients, and the favorable response of arrhythmias to CPAP therapy, especially in the absence of structural heart disease, reinforces the linkage between OSA and rhythm

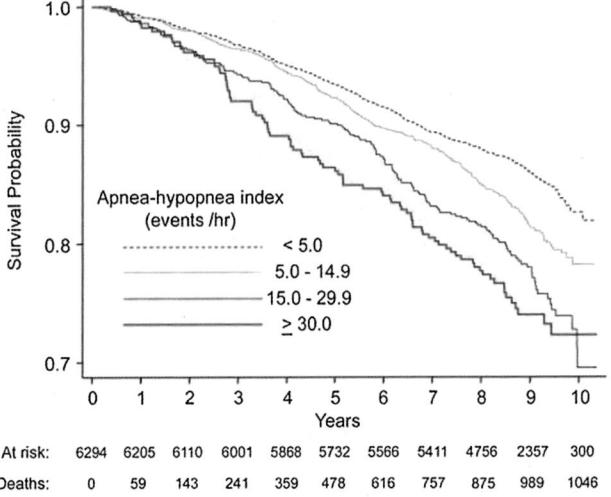

| At risk: | 6294 | 6205 | 6110 | 6001 | 5868 | 5732 | 5566 | 5411 | 4756 | 2357 | 300 |
| Deaths: | 0 | 59 | 143 | 241 | 359 | 478 | 616 | 757 | 875 | 989 | 1046 |

Figure 136.4 OSA severity and cardiovascular mortality: Prospective cohort analysis from the Sleep Heart Health Study showing that increased severity of OSA, based on AHI criteria, is associated with increased mortality from cardiovascular disease. (Reproduced from Punjabi NM, Caffo BS, Goodwin JL, et al. Sleep-disordered breathing and mortality: a prospective cohort study. *PLoS Med* 2009;6(8):e1000132, with permission.)

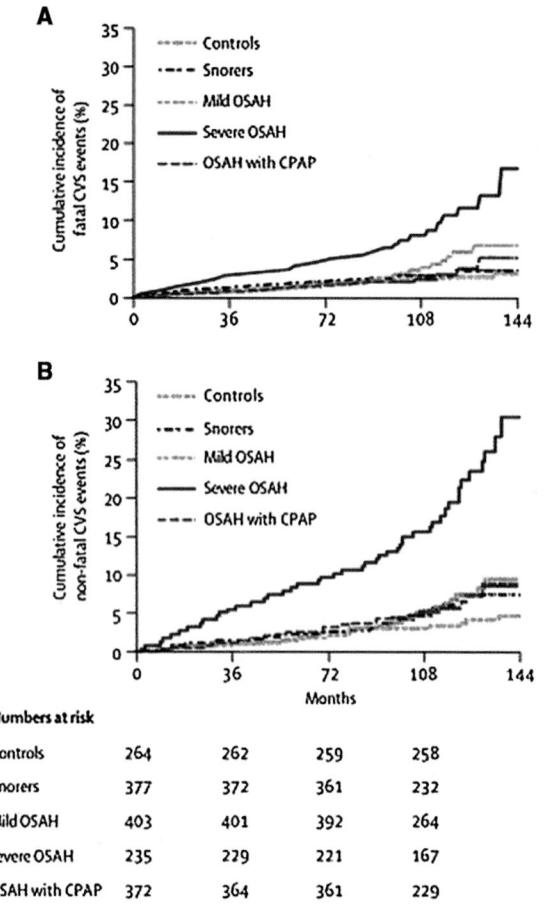

Figure 136.5 The effect of CPAP treatment on cardiovascular mortality in OSA patients: The risk of fatal (**A**) and nonfatal (**B**) cardiovascular event is increased in men with severe OSA, and that risk is significantly lowered with treatment of the OSA with positive pressure therapy. (Reproduced from Marin JM, Carrizo SJ, Vincente E, et al. Long-term cardiovascular outcomes in men with obstructive sleep apnea–hypopnea with or without treatment with continuous positive airway pressure: an observational study. *Lancet* 2005;365:1046–1053, with permission.)

disturbances (34–39). A recent randomized controlled trial reported that, after 1 month, CPAP therapy reduces the frequency of premature ventricular beats by nearly 60% in OSA patients with heart failure compared to patients who are not receiving CPAP, in whom there was no significant change (39).

Studies also support the improvement in left ventricular function after initiation of PAP therapy for patients with OSA and heart failure (40). The mechanisms by which PAP may improve cardiac function in OSA patients with heart failure include relief of sleep-related hypoxemia, elimination of cyclic increases in left ventricular afterload, reduction in sympathetic nervous system activation, and reduced inflammation.

Epidemiologic studies have provided compelling evidence that OSA is associated with increased risk for systemic HTN (41–46). Sleep apnea has been identified by the Joint National Committee on Prevention, Detection,

Evaluation and Treatment of High Blood Pressure as a risk factor for HTN (47). Although it is plausible that PAP therapy would ameliorate diurnal HTN by eliminating intermittent hypoxic exposure and sympathetic nervous system activation and improving sleep continuity, the literature provides conflicting data in this regard (48–51).

Using a randomized, placebo-controlled design to compare ambulatory blood pressure on CPAP and sham CPAP in subjectively sleepy OSA patients, Pepperell et al. (52) observed a small but significantly greater reduction in mean blood pressure during sleep in the active CPAP-treated group. Although small, the reduction in blood pressure in the active CPAP group would have a notable public health impact on cardiovascular risk. Conversely, there are a number of well-designed studies of groups of OSA patients either with or without subjective sleepiness, and with HTN, that have failed to demonstrate a significant reduction in blood pressure with PAP therapy (53–55). In summary, it is evident that further research is required to define the effect of PAP on HTN in OSA patients.

The association between sleep-disordered breathing, including OSA, and increased risk for stroke is increasingly recognized. Data from the Wisconsin Sleep Cohort indicate that, even after adjusting for age, gender, smoking, HTN, alcohol use, and body mass index (BMI), sleep-disordered breathing is associated with increased risk for prevalent stroke (56). Further, there is increasing awareness of the association between OSA, abnormal glycemic control, type 2 diabetes mellitus, and other features of the metabolic syndrome (57). Further studies are required to determine if PAP therapy of OSA reduces risk for incident stroke and improves insulin sensitivity and glycemic control.

Adherence

Despite its documented effectiveness in improving symptoms and quality of life and reduction of cardiovascular risk, acceptance of and adherence to PAP therapy remains one of the greatest challenges in treatment. In studies using at least 4 hours of average usage per night to define adherence, a wide range of 29% to 83% of patients were considered nonadherent (58). The minimal and optimal durations of usage that confer benefit are unknown and likely vary depending on the individual patient as well as the outcome measure being evaluated. It does appear that increasing duration of use is associated with increasing levels of improvement (Fig. 136.6). At least 6 hours of use per night appears to be associated with greater cardiovascular mortality risk reduction compared with fewer hours of use per night (30).

Data card monitoring, with the use of smart cards or web-based technology, has revolutionized the assessment of PAP adherence. The data card provides information over a

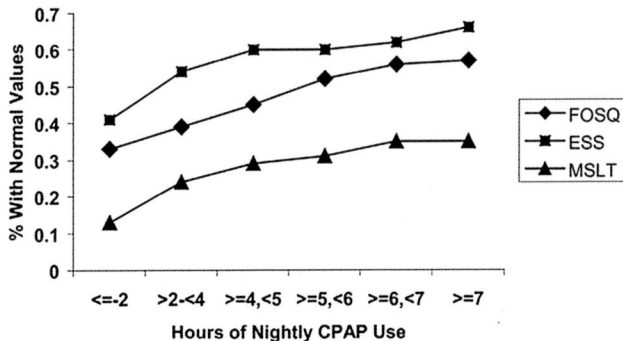

Figure 136.6 CPAP usage and dose–response of outcome measures: Cumulative proportion of participants obtaining normal threshold values on the Epworth Sleepiness Scale (ESS), MSLT, and Functional Outcomes of Sleep Questionnaire (FOSQ). (Reproduced from Weaver TE, Maislin G, Dinges DF, et al. Relationship between hours of CPAP use and achieving normal levels of sleepiness and daily functioning. *Sleep* 2007;30(6):711–719, with permission.)

selected period of time on multiple data points, including days used, hours of use per night, amount of mask leak, and a surrogate estimate of the residual AHI. Use of this technology to improve monitoring of adherence and effectiveness has the potential to dramatically improve long-term patient care. Any physician involved in the medical management of OSA should consider it part of the routine clinical practice.

Objective adherence monitoring has made it apparent that patterns of adherence, or nonadherence, are established early. CPAP use in the first week after initiating therapy often predicts long-term success or failure (59). Information regarding the degree to which a patient is adherent to PAP is essential for assessment of a suboptimal clinical response. If a patient's symptoms are inadequately resolved after the initiation of PAP treatment, possible reasons other than poor adherence include insufficient pressure delivery, mask leak, or a failure to recognize and treat a coexisting medical or sleep disorder that is also contributing to the patient's symptoms.

Since an individual's acceptance and adherence to PAP may be established shortly after initiating therapy, it stands to reason that close monitoring, education, and support during this period would be helpful. Studies have demonstrated improved adherence in conjunction with educational materials, available and knowledgeable staff, and patient support groups (60,61). Patient and family member understanding of the disease process itself, the associated functional and health implications, and the reasons and options for treatment likely contribute to more successful results.

There is increasing evidence that upper airway surgery may provide a useful adjunct to improve CPAP compliance and response to therapy. Unlike past concerns that associated traditional uvulopalatopharyngoplasty techniques result in mouth leak during CPAP use, newer, less morbid, and more effective reconstructive (rather than destructive) procedures may improve medical therapy results by lowering the critical closing pressure and reducing CPAP pressure requirements (62,63).

Side Effects and Complications

Initiation of positive pressure therapy is often associated with side effects that can impede successful management. The side effects are frequently minor and/or transient and may improve with continued use and adaptation. Others are more significant and troublesome and may negatively affect adherence and even result in discontinuation of therapy. Psychological factors, such as claustrophobia or the perceived lifestyle change associated with indefinite nightly use of a device, are common and often challenging to address (64,65). Table 136.1 provides a more comprehensive list of reported adverse events with CPAP use as well as some of the management strategies that can be employed to overcome these obstacles.

The most common adverse effects of CPAP therapy include mask leaks, rhinitis, and premature removal of the mask (66). Mask interface and proper fitting is one of the most important factors affecting adherence, and there are some data to support the potential for less side effects and improved adherence with use of a nasal pillows interface (16). Symptoms of chronic rhinitis and nasal obstruction commonly emerge or worsen with CPAP use. Empiric use of heated humidification and topical nasal steroids may be beneficial in some patients although the current literature shows variable results (67–72). A more thorough otolaryngologic approach, including endoscopic evaluation for both structural and inflammatory nasal pathology, should identify specific therapeutic targets. Surgical therapy for symptomatic structural nasal obstruction has the potential to dramatically improve PAP acceptance and adherence (73,74).

More significant morbidity and adverse health effects associated with positive pressure therapy use are *uncommon*; however, recent reports suggest some CPAP users are at risk for adverse craniofacial and ophthalmologic changes. Tsuda et al. (75) assessed craniofacial measurements in OSA patients after 2 years of CPAP therapy compared to baseline. After 2 years of CPAP, the subjects were found to have significant changes in craniofacial structure, including both maxillary and mandibular retrusion and maxillary incisor retroclination. Kiekens et al. (76) compared intraocular pressure (IOP) measurements in OSA patients before and 1 month after initiation of CPAP. The authors found a significant increase in IOP and a reduction in ocular perfusion pressure with CPAP therapy, particularly at night while CPAP was in use. As a result, they recommend routine vision screening and optic disk evaluation in patients on positive pressure.

ORAL APPLIANCES

Introduction

Oral appliances have been used for the management of snoring and OSA for last three decades, and they remain an underutilized tool in many patient populations, perhaps

TABLE 136.1	MEDICAL THERAPY FOR OBSTRUCTIVE SLEEP APNEA

Side Effects	Management Strategies
Pressure or airflow related	
Difficulty exhaling	Pressure ramp
Difficulty initiating/maintaining sleep	Mask refit
Aerophagia	Reduce expiratory pressure with bilevel therapy
Sinus or ear discomfort	
Chest wall discomfort	Reduce required pressure with adjunctive techniques (oral appliance, surgery, weight loss, positional therapy)
Device or interface related	
Nasal congestion	Mask refit
Rhinorrhea	Heated humidification
Dryness of the upper airway	Topical nasal treatments for chronic rhinitis
Epistaxis	Surgical nasal procedures to lower nasal resistance
Skin abrasion or rash of the nose/face	
Conjunctivitis from air leak	Protective skin covering
Machine noise	Longer tubing to move further from bedside
Psychological reasons	
Claustrophobia	Desensitization techniques
Cumbersomeness	Education for both patient and spouse
Travel inconvenience	Patient support group
Spousal intolerance	

due to simply a lack of familiarity of this treatment modality by the pulmonologists, neurologists, otolaryngologists, and even dentists who see patients with sleep-disordered breathing. The most commonly used appliances today fall under the general category of mandibular repositioning appliances (MRAs), also known as mandibular advancement devices (MADs). In 2006, an extensive review of the literature and practice parameters for the use of oral appliances in sleep-disordered breathing was published through the American Academy of Sleep Medicine (77,78).

Current AASM practice parameters recommend routine clinical use of oral appliances in patients with (a) primary snoring who do not respond to or are not appropriate candidates for treatment with weight loss or positional therapy or (b) mild–moderate OSA who prefer oral appliances to CPAP, are not appropriate candidates for CPAP, or do not respond to CPAP or other conservative measures. Additional data suggest that oral appliances can play a beneficial role in selected patients with severe OSA who fail or do not tolerate CPAP. A recent prospective study of patients with severe OSA and CPAP refusal showed significant improvement in objective sleep study measures as well as HTN with oral appliance as sole therapy (79). Further, in some patients with moderate–severe OSA, although data are limited, oral appliances can be combined with positive pressure or surgical therapy.

Types

Mandibular Repositioning Appliance

Also known as a MAD, it is by far the most commonly used type of oral appliance used today for sleep-disordered breathing. The MRA or MAD comes in two basic forms: a nontitratable type and a titratable type. The Thornton Adjustable Positioner (TAP) is a commonly used example of a titratable device. The TAP is composed of both a maxillary and a mandibular arch with a base and hook assembly and an internal adjustment mechanism (Fig. 136.7A).

Tongue Retaining Device

The tongue retaining device (TRD) holds the tongue forward in a suction bulb mechanism. Today, TRD's are used far less often than MRA's but may be a viable option in edentulous patients (Fig. 136.7B).

Thermoplastic Splints

Boil-and-bite appliances consist of one-piece prefabricated thermoplastic splints. They are significantly less expensive than custom-made devices and often can be ordered online and fitted directly by the patient. These cost-savings, however, must be cautiously weighed against the documented inferior efficacy, increased side effects, and lack of proper follow-up and dental monitoring compared to a custom-made MAD employed by a trained expert. A randomized, controlled, crossover trial concluded that a custom-made MAD results

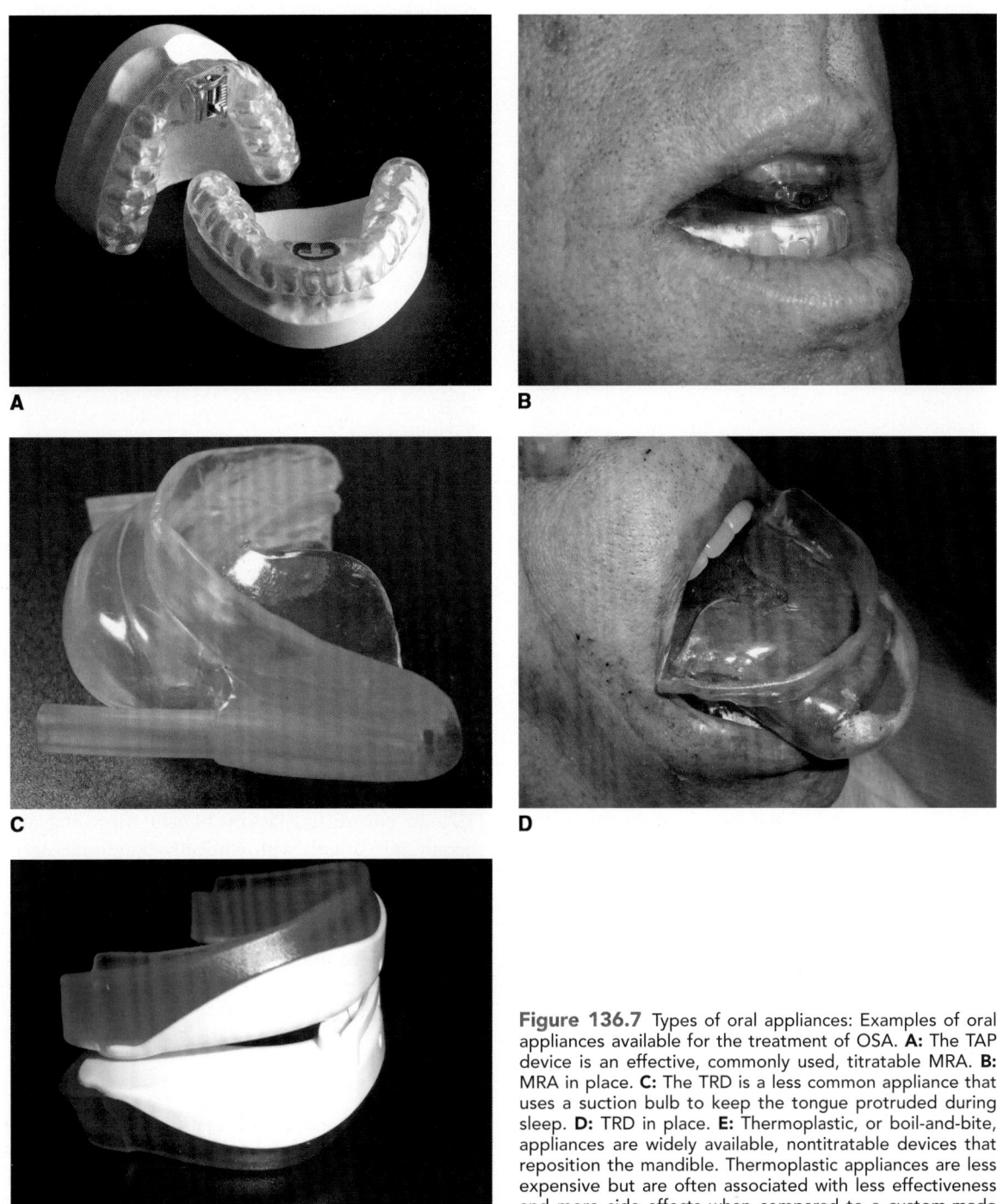

Figure 136.7 Types of oral appliances: Examples of oral appliances available for the treatment of OSA. **A:** The TAP device is an effective, commonly used, titratable MRA. **B:** MRA in place. **C:** The TRD is a less common appliance that uses a suction bulb to keep the tongue protruded during sleep. **D:** TRD in place. **E:** Thermoplastic, or boil-and-bite, appliances are widely available, nontitratable devices that reposition the mandible. Thermoplastic appliances are less expensive but are often associated with less effectiveness and more side effects when compared to a custom-made MRA. (Images courtesy of Robert Rogers, DMD, D.ABDSM, Pittsburgh Dental Sleep Medicine.)

in improved mandibular advancement, increased efficacy, and less side effects and noncompliance compared to boil-and-bite thermoplastic appliances (80) (Fig. 136.7C).

Effectiveness

In general, the mechanism of action of oral appliances, as with most successful treatments for OSA, involves enlarging the upper airway and/or reducing upper airway collapsibility (i.e., making the critical closing pressure more negative). Specifically, MRAs protrude and stabilize the mandible during sleep. MRAs have been shown to improve airway size at the level of both the palate and tongue base, including enlargement of the lateral dimension (Fig. 136.8) (81,82). Oral appliances may be used as sole therapy in some patients or in conjunction with other forms of OSA therapy including surgery, weight loss, and positive pressure.

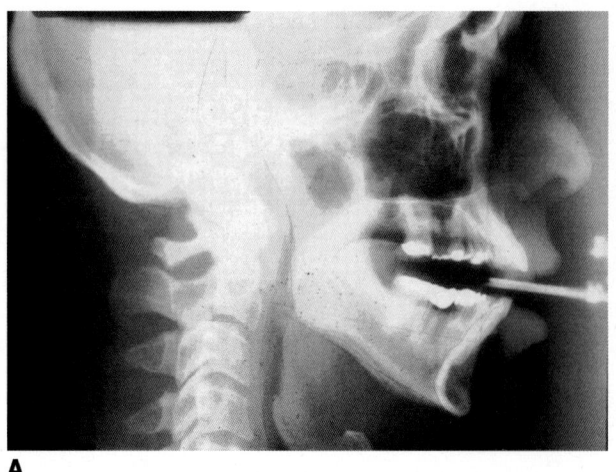
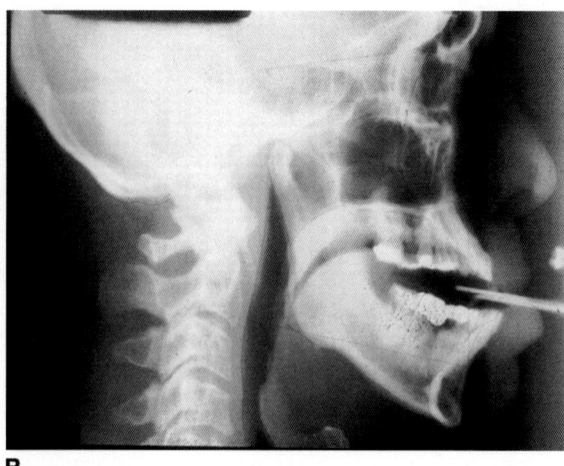

A   **B**

Figure 136.8 Effect of oral appliances on the airway: Lateral cephalometric radiograph in a patient with OSA, before (**A**) and after (**B**) application of a MAD. Note the enlargement of the pharyngeal airway with the oral appliance at both the retrolingual and retropalatal portions of the airway. (Images courtesy of Robert Rogers, DMD, D.ABDSM, Pittsburgh Dental Sleep Medicine.)

In the 2006 AASM-directed review of the literature on oral appliances, the overall effectiveness for controlling OSA based on polysomnographic criteria (defined as AHI less than 10) was 52%. This figure must be interpreted with caution, as the data reviewed as a whole represent a very heterogeneous group of patients, types of devices, titration protocols, treatment outcomes, and clinician expertise. When only the randomized, crossover, placebo-controlled studies were analyzed (five studies), the combined rate of "success" (treatment AHI less than 10) and "response" (AHI reduction of 50%) was 64% (83–88). Studies also report subjective improvement in snoring and daytime sleepiness, as well as nocturnal oxygenation, arousal index, and objective measures of sleepiness (i.e., MSLT). It must be kept in mind that these data are heterogeneous and conflicting and require further evaluation. Finally, there are three studies evaluating the effect of oral appliance therapy on HTN, and they each report a statistically significant reduction in blood pressure measurements (87,89,90).

Greater success rates may be achieved with proper patient selection and phenotyping of the individual patient anatomy and pathophysiology. At this juncture, the patient characteristics associated with more successful oral appliance therapy have not been readily established. For example, there is substantial evidence that a greater likelihood of success was achieved in patients with positional OSA (OSA primarily occurring in the supine position), although not all studies support this finding (91–93). Other studies suggest lower rates of effectiveness with increasing BMI and increasing severity of the AHI. Currently, custom-made oral appliances are reimbursed by Medicare as first-line therapy for mild OSA (AHI 5 to 14) with symptoms and moderate OSA (AHI 15 to 29) regardless of symptoms, as well as for severe OSA (AHI ≥ 30) if intolerant to PAP.

Drug-induced sleep endoscopy (DISE) represents one tool with promising potential to improve patient outcomes with oral appliance. Three recent reports used DISE to determine the likelihood of success with oral appliance therapy (94–96). The authors concluded that sleep endoscopy, with concomitant mandibular advancement to mimic treatment effect, could be a valuable prognostic indicator for successful management of both snoring and OSA. To ensure satisfactory benefit from oral appliance therapy, all patients with clinically significant sleep-disordered breathing should return for follow-up visits with a qualified sleep specialist to evaluate for symptom improvement. They should also undergo a follow-up sleep study evaluation with the oral appliance in place to assess adequate management of objective measures such as AHI and oxygen saturations (78).

Adherence

As with any device-related treatment for sleep-disordered breathing, successful management is critically dependent on usage. Assessment of adherence in the literature is complicated by heterogeneity of the types of devices and titration protocols used, patient characteristics and disease severity, and the level of clinical care and provider expertise. Further complicating matters is that the amount of usage required for improvement in subjective and objective outcome measures is unknown and likely varies between individuals. Finally, although oral appliance adherence data have relied primarily on patient self-reporting in the past, clinical trials are underway utilizing objective monitors to quantify use.

One-year subjective adherence rates range from 25% to 100%, with a median use of 77% of nights during the first year. Adherence rates tend to decrease with duration of use past 1 year (97,98). Hoffstein combined adherence reports from 21 studies evaluating over 3,000 patients and found an overall average adherence of 56% to 68% at an average of 33 months follow-up (83). In crossover studies comparing CPAP and oral appliances, adherence rates were similar between the two devices (99,100).

Side Effects and Complications

A substantial portion of nonadherent patients may discontinue oral appliance use as a result of any number of side effects or adverse events. Many of side effects are minor and do not significantly affect long-term use or morbidity. Other complications such as bite changes, malocclusion, and temporomandibular joint (TMJ) dysfunction may be permanent. This supports the notion that oral appliances should be fitted, titrated, and managed by a clinician with training and expertise in both dental care and sleep-related breathing disorders.

Commonly reported minor side effects include TMJ pain, headache or facial pain, tooth pain, excessive salivation, dry mouth, gum irritation, and morning-after occlusal changes (83). There is a wide range of reported minor side effects from 6% to 86% although many of these side effects are reported to be transient and occur with initiation of treatment (77). Most authors report frequent improvement in these side effects with regular use and occasional adjustment of the device. More severe and persistent adverse sequelae include more significant TMJ dysfunction, tooth movement, and changes in occlusion and often lead to device discontinuation. The pathophysiology of and risk factors for these more severe complications are not yet fully understood but are likely multifactorial.

OTHER FORMS OF MEDICAL THERAPY

PAP therapy, oral appliances, and surgery are considered the mainstays of directed sleep apnea therapy for OSA, but a variety of other medical options may be appropriate in properly selected patients, either as a primary management strategy or as a useful adjunct to other primary modalities. Successful management of patients with OSA requires a comprehensive sleep history, general medical evaluation, and physical examination. A number of medical conditions, medications/drugs, and lifestyle practices can place persons at increased risk for OSA or worsen existing OSA. Conversely, modification of these factors can favorably affect risk and improve treatment outcomes.

TREATMENT OF NASAL OBSTRUCTION

A number of large population-based studies have analyzed the association of nasal obstruction and subjective sleep measures, snoring, and sleep apnea. In the Wisconsin cohort of almost 5,000 patients, patients with chronic rhinitis symptoms were more likely to report habitual snoring, nonrestorative sleep, and daytime sleepiness (101). Patients with nasal congestion due to allergy were 1.8 times more likely to have moderate–severe OSA compared to allergy patients without nasal congestion. Other epidemiologic studies have confirmed that, across large populations, nasal obstruction is an independent risk factor for both snoring and OSA (102–104).

Much of the research into medical therapy for allergic rhinitis and sleep-disordered breathing has focused on the role of nasal steroids. In a group of allergic rhinitis patients with subjective nasal congestion and sleep disturbance, Craig et al. (105) demonstrated that topical nasal steroid therapy improved subjective sleep quality and daytime function. Pediatric patients with symptomatic nasal obstruction and OSA have also been shown to respond favorably to nasal steroid therapy. Brouillette et al. (106) reported a reduction in the AHI from 10.7 to 5.8 with fluticasone nasal spray in a selected group of pediatric patients. Nevertheless, long-term adherence to nasal steroids may be suboptimal and difficult to monitor, particularly in pediatric patients with parental concerns about side effects.

Nakata et al. (107) recently demonstrated that nasal surgery, in the setting of nasal obstruction and sleep apnea, improves nasal resistance, sleep architecture, and daytime sleepiness. In these patients, the observed improvement in the mean Epworth Sleepiness Scale (ESS) from 10.6 to 4.5 with nasal surgery is comparable to the improvement obtained with other forms of OSA therapy, including positive pressure. Untreated nasal obstruction may explain, at least in part, the persistent hypersomnia seen in some OSA patients with adequate CPAP adherence and objective control of the AHI. In a prospective longitudinal cohort study of patients with nasal obstruction and OSA, surgical treatment of nasal obstruction also significantly improved both disease-specific and general health (SF-36) quality of life measures (108).

Finally, treatment of nasal obstruction in OSA patients can significantly improve adherence and effectiveness of both CPAP and oral appliance therapy. Mounting evidence suggests that increased nasal resistance negatively impacts success rates and tolerance of medical therapy devices for OSA, which critically depend on regular usage to be effective. In a recent study comparing oral appliance responders and nonresponders, increased nasal resistance, particularly in the supine position, was associated with poorer treatment outcomes (109). With logistic regression analysis, Suguira et al. (73) concluded that increased nasal resistance was one of only two factors associated with nonacceptance of CPAP. Further, in patients with poor CPAP adherence and nasal obstruction, lowering nasal resistance with surgical therapy has been shown to lower average CPAP pressures and improve subsequent adherence (74).

WEIGHT LOSS

The adverse effect of obesity on the pathophysiology of OSA may be mediated through a variety of mechanisms. Histopathologic analysis of the tongue has revealed that obesity is associated with increased lingual fat deposition and increased size and weight of the tongue (110). Imaging studies have confirmed the presence of increased parapharyngeal fat in OSA patients (111). Using three-dimensional volumetric analysis MRI techniques, Welch et al. (112) showed that weight loss was associated with a significant reduction in the size of the parapharyngeal fat pads and an increase in the volume of the upper airway. In a pig animal model, enlargement of the parapharyngeal fat pad has been demonstrated to increase upper airway resistance (113). Cervical obesity may also play a pathophysiologic role via mass loading of the anterior neck and subsequent transmission of pressure changes to the airway lumen. Increased neck circumference is a well-established clinical predictor of OSA and may correlate with this hypothesis. Furthermore, velopharyngeal collapsibility appears to increase directly with increasing neck circumference in OSA patients (114). Finally, to the extent that upper airway patency is increased by greater lung volume, greater truncal obesity may contribute to OSA through a thoracic mechanism of decreasing lung volume and hypoventilation.

Numerous studies over the past three decades support the positive effect of weight loss on the treatment of OSA; however, the specific relationship between the two and the response rate may vary considerably from one patient to another. Peppard et al. (115) demonstrated that a 10% weight loss predicted a 26% reduction in the AHI (Fig. 136.9). In a randomized trial of weight loss in patients with mild OSA, those patients with more successful weight reduction achieved a more significant reduction in the AHI, compared to control subjects (116). Based on these results, the authors concluded that, in patients with mild OSA, weight loss and lifestyle intervention may be considered first-line therapy, rather than positive pressure.

The Sleep AHEAD study is a recent multicenter randomized controlled trial evaluating the effect of weight loss on sleep apnea outcomes in a population of obese type 2 diabetes mellitus patients (117). Patients were randomized either to a behavioral weight loss program (intensive lifestyle intervention) or to a control diabetes support program. The patients in the behavioral weight loss program lost significantly more weight and in turn had significant reduction in AHI.

Some patients with successful weight loss may not achieve noticeable improvement in subjective or objective measures of OSA severity, particularly because there is not a linear relationship between weight loss and AHI reduction. These nonresponders may have other predisposing risk factors for persistent OSA including genetics, craniofacial or soft tissue anatomical abnormalities, neuromuscular weakness, or other cardiopulmonary loss of ventilatory

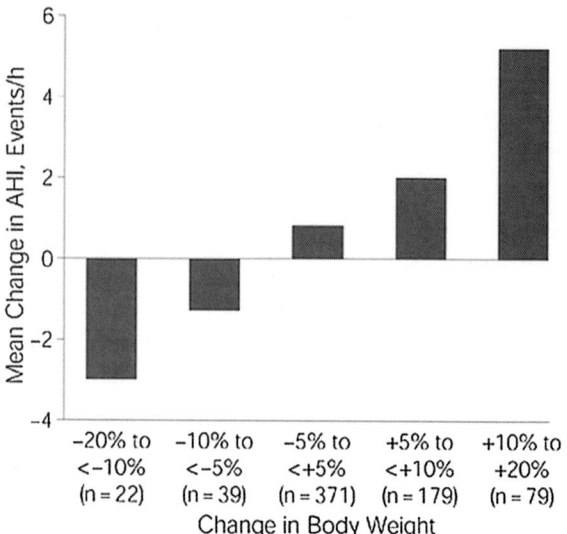

Figure 136.9 Relationship between weight change and AHI: In the Wisconsin Sleep Cohort Study, weight change across a large population was associated with change in AHI. A 10% weight gain correlated with a 32% increase in the mean AHI as well as a six-fold increased risk of developing moderate–severe OSA. A 10% weight loss was associated with a 26% decrease in the mean AHI. (Reproduced from Peppard PE, Young T, Palta M, et al. Longitudinal study of moderate weight change and sleep-disordered breathing. *JAMA* 2000;284:3015–3021, with permission.)

control. Nevertheless, a multimodality approach to weight reduction may optimize clinical results, taking into consideration dietary and lifestyle modifications, cognitive–behavioral therapy, as well as pharmacologic and surgical options (118).

For patients with severe obesity, bariatric surgery may provide more substantial and more rapid control of obesity-related medical problems, including OSA (119). One study, with longer follow-up data on bariatric surgery patients with OSA, reported a 75% reduction in the respiratory disturbance index (120).

POSITIONAL THERAPY

For some patients, the frequency of obstructive respiratory events is substantially greater in the supine position compared to the lateral or prone position. Increased probability of upper airway narrowing in the supine position is hypothesized to occur via a gravity effect that results in retrodisplacement of the tongue, soft palate, and mandible. A comprehensive sleep history should include questioning of the patient and bed partner regarding the effect of body position on snoring and subjective measures. Likewise, polysomnography interpretation should comment on the presence or absence of any significant positional dependence to the patient's AHI, oxygen saturations, and overall control of sleep-disordered breathing.

For select patients with clinically significant OSA in the supine position and essentially no significant sleep-disordered breathing in the lateral recumbent position, a number of conservative therapeutic options may obviate the need for positive pressure. The tennis ball or similar technique of placing objects in a sock that is subsequently pinned to the back of the patient's nightshirt has been recommend over the years. Newer, more user-friendly devices are now on the market to facilitate maintenance of the lateral sleeping position. One example, the Zzoma Positional Sleeper, consists of a Velcro elastic belt with a foam wedges across the lower back that prevent the patient from rolling over to the supine position. In a randomized crossover study of patients with strictly positional OSA, this device was shown to be as effective as CPAP at controlling the AHI and oxygen saturations (121). Finally, MADs may be an appropriate first-line treatment option in patients with positional OSA. Recent evidence suggests that oral appliances provide more effective control of the AHI in positional, compared to nonpositional, OSA patients (122).

Head of bed elevation, or postural therapy, is another positional method of reducing upper airway collapsibility in OSA patients. Critical closing pressure has been shown to be more negative, signifying greater upper airway stability, with 30 degrees of head of bed elevation compared to the supine position (123). Head elevation of 30 degrees may also lower the CPAP pressure requirements necessary to maintain control of breathing. Nevertheless, the ability of postural therapy alone to adequately manage OSA remains limited and highly variable from patient to patient (124).

OXYGEN THERAPY

In addition to sleep fragmentation and chronic sleep deprivation, many of the cardiopulmonary, metabolic, and neurocognitive sequelae of OSA are attributable to nocturnal intermittent hypoxemia. The current data suggest that supplemental oxygen during sleep is inadequate as a stand-alone treatment to effectively reduce apnea frequency and increase daytime alertness. There is a subgroup of patients, however, who have a relatively low AHI but experience unacceptable nocturnal oxygen desaturation. Studies suggest that desaturations of 4% were associated with fasting hyperglycemia and increased risk of cardiovascular disease (125,126). For these patients, particularly those with existing coronary artery disease or cerebrovascular disease, supplemental oxygen during sleep may be beneficial and even the primary therapeutic goal (127).

Oxygen therapy may also be combined with positive pressure therapy. Selected OSA patients with other confounding conditions such as obesity hypoventilation, CHF, or chronic obstructive pulmonary disease (COPD) may benefit from supplemental oxygen as an adjunct to other forms of directed therapy. OSA patients, who are hypoxemic during wakefulness and qualify for supplemental oxygen during the day, may meet the criteria for the addition of oxygen therapy at night, even if positive pressure therapy maintains upper airway patency. Finally, one recent small study demonstrated that high-flow (20 L/min) humidified air administered through a nasal cannula may effectively reduce the AHI (28 ± 5 to 10 ± 3) (128).

OROPHARYNGEAL EXERCISES

Recent developments in understanding the pathophysiology of OSA report that central and peripheral neuromuscular control mechanisms may have substantial impact on the disease process and evolution over time. It is well established that OSA patients have increased genioglossus muscle activity during wakefulness; however, this compensation is lost during sleep (129). More recent studies suggest that these findings are not simply a matter of compensation but rather signify neuromuscular denervation/renervation injury (130). White compared the genioglossus muscle activity in response to negative pharyngeal pressure in two patients: one with OSA and the other a normal healthy control. He found that the OSA patient did not respond with increased muscle activity as the healthy control did (131).

These findings may serve as the basis for improvement in OSA with oropharyngeal exercises. Initial anecdotal reports of reduced snoring and daytime sleepiness in students playing the didgeridoo instrument for several months lead to a randomized controlled trial. The authors concluded that regular didgeridoo playing resulted in significant improvement in subjective daytime sleepiness as well as the AHI (132). Guimaraes et al. (133) then derived a broad-based regimen of daily oropharyngeal exercises and employed them in a randomized sham-controlled trial of patients with moderate OSA. Compared to controls, patients undergoing oropharyngeal exercises had a significant improvement in AHI (22.4 to 13.7), snoring measures, daytime sleepiness, and subjective sleep quality measures. Although these findings are preliminary and the specific types and duration of exercises have not been established, oropharyngeal exercises hold promise as an effective, benign, inexpensive, and maybe more physiologically sound option for adjunctive or even sole therapy in some patients.

BEHAVIORAL MODIFICATIONS

Sleep deprivation is a well-established cause of daytime sleepiness, neurocognitive dysfunction, delayed reaction times, increased risk of motor vehicle accidents, as well as other cardiovascular, metabolic, immunologic, and general health-related negative sequelae. Additional evidence also suggests that sleep deprivation may predispose to or worsen existing OSA. The mechanism linking sleep deprivation and abnormal ventilatory control is unclear but may involve depression of the arousal threshold and blunting of chemoreceptor-mediated control of ventilation. A recent animal model suggests that sleep fragmentation attenuates the hypercapnic ventilatory response (134).

Maladaptive behaviors that may negatively impact sleep quality and quantity include untimely or excessive caffeine, alcohol or nicotine consumption, insufficient sleep duration, shift work, or a poor sleeping environment. A comprehensive sleep history, including information on evening habits, sleep times, and overall sleep hygiene, is warranted in the evaluation of all OSA patients. Likewise, counseling of patients on proper sleep hygiene and emphasis on the importance of adequate sleep duration will likely improve patient satisfaction and overall treatment outcomes.

Bed partners and family members are often the first to recognize the association between alcohol consumption and the impact on snoring and sleep disturbance. In patients with existing snoring or OSA, alcohol may increase both the frequency and duration of obstructive respiratory events. One study showed that a mean blood alcohol concentration of 0.07 g/dL in patients with mild OSA was associated with a modest increase in the AHI (135). Furthermore, compared to controls, OSA patients are more vulnerable to the detrimental effects of alcohol consumption on reaction times and simulated driving performance (136).

Smoking also has a known negative impact on sleep and potentially on sleep-disordered breathing as well. The stimulant mechanism of nicotine may explain in part why cigarette uses have more difficulty initiating and maintaining sleep (137). Smokers also have four to five times increased risk of having at least moderate sleep-disordered breathing (138). The association between OSA and smoking may be related to multiple factors including increased upper airway mucosal edema, increased laryngopharyngeal reflux, and a higher rate of cardiopulmonary disease in smokers. Although the exact effect of smoking cessation on the management of OSA is still unknown and controversial, cigarette smoking should always be discouraged for both general health as well as sleep-related reasons.

TREATMENT OF ASSOCIATED CONDITIONS

Many general medical and psychiatric conditions, as well as the medications used in their management, can directly impact sleep and also can complicate OSA management. Further, there are at least 70 other definable sleep medicine disorders that can coexist with OSA. Successful management of OSA patients and their sleep-related symptoms requires the ability to identify, and treat, these coexisting sleep and medical disorders.

Approximately one-third of patients with OSA may have another sleep disorder, such as restless legs syndrome or insomnia (139). Additional sleep pathology may be contributing to hypersomnia and other symptoms at least as much as the sleep-related breathing disorder. Therefore, persistent symptoms after apparent successful medical or surgical therapy for OSA may signify an unrecognized coexisting sleep disorder. Clinically significant insomnia is a common comorbid condition in OSA patients, and patients with both conditions may have more severe OSA as well as a higher rate of anxiety, stress, and depression (140). Furthermore, in a recent prospective crossover study of patients with both insomnia and mild OSA, Guilleminault et al. (141) found that treatment of the underlying OSA was more effective in improving insomnia than traditional cognitive–behavioral therapy for insomnia. The findings above underscore the need for a comprehensive sleep medicine history in every OSA patient.

Patients with CHF, for example, have a significantly higher risk of both obstructive and central apneas, including Cheyne-Stokes or periodic breathing. Increased venous congestion of the upper airway, high loop gain or increased central and peripheral chemoreceptor sensitivity, and decreased functional residual capacity may contribute to the increased sleep-disordered breathing seen in heart failure patients. Further, the symptoms from CHF itself, as well as commonly associated HTN, coronary artery disease, pleural effusion, pulmonary vascular congestion, and atrial fibrillation, can also negatively impact sleep and daytime function. As such, treatment of the patient with OSA and CHF often requires multimodality therapy including aggressive management of underlying heart failure, positive pressure therapy (CPAP, BIPAP, or adaptive pressure support servoventilation), cardiac pacing, supplemental oxygen, and behavioral/lifestyle modifications including diet and weight control.

COPD, asthma, interstitial lung disease, kyphoscoliosis, neuromuscular disease, and other impairments of pulmonary function are often associated with OSA and sleep disturbance. The coexistence of COPD and OSA has been termed "overlap syndrome." Hypoxemia and quality of life may be worse in patients with overlap syndrome. Careful attention to both OSA and the underlying pulmonary disease is essential to successful improvement of symptoms and quality of life as well as reduction of long-term morbidity.

HIGHLIGHTS

- PAP therapy and oral appliances provide the foundation for the medical management of OSA; however, other treatment options can play an important role as well and include weight loss, smoking cessation, behavioral modifications, positional therapy, treatment of nasal obstruction, and management of coexisting sleep disorders and/or medical conditions.
- Successful management of patients with OSA requires a comprehensive sleep history and examination, proper diagnostic evaluation, and an individualized approach that takes into account each patient's unique presentation and considers all available and applicable treatment options.

- With proper titration and acceptable adherence, positive pressure therapy has been shown to improve both subjective and objective sleep measures, improve daytime function and quality of life measures, reduce risk of motor vehicle accidents, and reduce the cardiovascular risks associated with OSA.

- Acceptance and adherence remain the greatest challenges to effective management with medical device therapy, and data card monitoring technology currently provides the best objective assessment of usage. The optimal usage that is required to achieve both sleep and health benefits is unknown and variable depending on the patient and the outcome being measured.

- A variety of side effects related to the mask/equipment, airflow/pressure, or psychological reasons may negatively impact sleep and preclude successful use of positive pressure. Proper patient education, problem identification, and early intervention can overcome many of these hurdles.

- Oral appliances can provide an effective form of medical therapy, particularly for those patients who are nonaccepting or intolerant of positive pressure. The most commonly used and most effective appliance is a custom-made titratable MAD.

- Across a population, oral appliance therapy may not provide as effective AHI reduction compared to positive pressure; however, long-term adherence may be higher resulting in comparable efficacy. Most side effects of oral appliance use are minor and transient; however, more severe and persistent adverse effects can occur and often preclude long-term use.

- Nasal obstruction is an independent risk factor for snoring, disrupted sleep, daytime sleepiness, and OSA, and it can negatively impact successful management of OSA with positive pressure and oral appliance therapy. Medical and/or surgical therapy to lower nasal resistance in patients with OSA and nasal obstruction can improve subjective and objective sleep measures as well as compliance and results with positive pressure and oral appliances.

REFERENCES

1. Sullivan CE, Issa FG, Berthon-Jones M, et al. Reversal of obstructive sleep apnoea by continuous positive airway pressure applied through the nares. *Lancet* 1981;1:862.
2. Dempsey JA, Veasey SC, Morgan BJ, et al. Pathophysiology of sleep apnea. *Physiol Rev* 2010;90:47–112.
3. Sériès F, Cormier Y, Couture J, et al. Changes in upper airway resistance with lung inflation and positive airway pressure. *J Appl Physiol* 1990;68:1075.
4. Heinzer RC, Stanchina ML, Malhotra A, et al. Lung volume and continuous positive airway pressure requirements in obstructive sleep apnea. *Am J Respir Crit Care Med* 2005;172:114.
5. Sanders MH, Kern N. Obstructive sleep apnea treated by independently adjusted inspiratory and expiratory positive airway pressures via nasal mask: physiologic and clinical implications. *Chest* 1990;98:317.
6. Laursen SB, Dreijer B, Hemmingsen C, et al. Bi-level positive airway pressure treatment of obstructive sleep apnoea syndrome. *Respiration* 1998;65:114.
7. Resta O, Guido P, Picca V, et al. Prescription of nCPAP and nBIPAP in obstructive sleep apnoea syndrome: Italian experience in 105 subjects. A prospective two centre study. *Respir Med* 1998;92:820.
8. Resta O, Guido P, Picca V, et al. The role of the expiratory phase in obstructive sleep apnoea. *Respir Med* 1999;93:190.
9. Schafer H, Hasper EE, Luderitz B. Failure of CPAP therapy in obstructive sleep apnoea syndrome: predictive factors and treatment with bilevel-positive airway pressure. *Respir Med* 1998;92:208.
10. Berry RB, Parish JM, Hartse KM. The use of auto-titrating continuous positive airway pressure for treatment of adult obstructive sleep apnea. *Sleep* 2002;25:148.
11. Ayas NT, Patel SR, Malhotra A, et al. Auto-titrating versus standard continuous positive airway pressure for the treatment of obstructive sleep apnea: results of a meta-analysis. *Sleep* 2004;27:249.
12. Strollo PJ, Sanders MH, Costantino JP, et al. Split-night studies for the diagnosis and treatment of sleep-disordered breathing. *Sleep* 1996;19(10 Suppl):S255–S259.
13. McArdle N, Grove A, Devereux G, et al. Split-night versus full-night studies for sleep apnoea/hypopnoea syndrome *Eur Respir J* 2000;15:670–675.
14. Kushida CA, Littner MR, Morgenthaler T, et al. Practice parameters for the indications for polysomnography and related procedures: an update for 2005. *Sleep* 2005;28:499.
15. West SD, Jones DR, Stradling JR. Comparison of three ways to determine and deliver pressure during nasal CPAP therapy for obstructive sleep apnoea. *Thorax* 2006;61:226.
16. Massie CA, Hart RW. Clinical outcomes related to interface type in patients with obstructive pressure sleep apnea/hypopnea syndrome who are using continuous positive airway pressure. *Chest* 2003;123:1112.
17. Barnes M, Houston D, Worsnop CJ, et al. A randomized controlled trial of continuous positive airway pressure in mild obstructive sleep apnea. *Am J Respir Crit Care Med* 2002;165:773.
18. Engleman HM, Kingshott RN, Wraith PK, et al. Randomized placebo-controlled crossover trial of continuous positive airway pressure for mild sleep apnea/hypopnoea syndrome. *Am J Respir Crit Care Med* 1999;159:461.
19. Kiely JL, Murphy M, McNicholas WT. Subjective efficacy of nasal CPAP in obstructive sleep apnoea syndrome: a prospective controlled study. *Eur Respir J* 1999;13:1086.
20. Margel D, Shochat T, Getzler O, et al. Continuous positive airway pressure reduces nocturia in patients with obstructive sleep apnea. *Urology* 2006;67:974.
21. Guilleminault C, Lin CM, Goncalves MA, et al. A prospective study of nocturia and the quality of life of elderly with obstructive sleep apnea or sleep onset insomnia. *J Psychosom Res* 2004;56:511.
22. Fitzgerald MP, Mulligan M, Parthasarathy S. Nocturic frequency is related to severity of obstructive sleep apnea, improves with continuous positive airways treatment. *Am J Obstet Gynecol* 2006;194:1399.
23. Engleman HM, Douglas NJ. Sleepiness, cognitive function, and quality of life in obstructive sleep apnoea/hypopnoea syndrome. *Thorax* 2004;59:618.
24. Marshall NS, Barnes M, Travier N, et al. Continuous positive airway pressure reduces daytime sleepiness in mild-moderate obstructive sleep apnoea: meta-analysis. *Thorax* 2006;61:430.
25. Monasterio C, Vidal S, Duran J, et al. Effectiveness of continuous positive airway pressure in mild sleep apnea-hypopnea syndrome. *Am J Respir Crit Care Med* 2001;164:939.
26. Hack M, Davies RJ, Mullins R, et al. Randomised prospective parallel trial of therapeutic versus subtherapeutic nasal continuous positive airway pressure on simulated steering performance in patients with obstructive sleep apnea. *Thorax* 2000;55:224.

27. Turkington PM, Sircar M, Saralaya D, et al. Time course of changes in driving simulator performance with and without treatment in patients with sleep apnoea hypopnoea syndrome. *Thorax* 2004;59:56.

28. Orth M, Duchna HW, Leidag M, et al. Driving simulator and neuropsychological testing in OSAS before and under CPAP therapy. *Eur Respir J* 2005;26:898.

29. George CFP. Reduction in motor vehicle collisions following treatment of sleep apnoea with nasal CPAP. *Thorax* 2001;56:508–512.

30. Campos-Rodriguez F, Pena-Grinan N, Reyes-Nunez N, et al. Mortality in obstructive sleep apnea-hypopnea patients treated with positive airway pressure. *Chest* 2005;128:624.

31. Punjabi NM, Caffo BS, Goodwin JL, et al. Sleep-disordered breathing and mortality: a prospective cohort study. *PLoS Med* 2009;6(8):e1000132.

32. Marin JM, Carrizo SJ, Vicente E, et al. Long-term cardiovascular outcomes in men with obstructive sleep apnoea hypopnoea with or without treatment with continuous positive airway pressure: an observational study. *Lancet* 2005;365:1046.

33. Peker Y, Hedner J, Norum J, et al. Increased incidence of cardiovascular disease in middle-aged men with obstructive sleep apnea: a 7-year follow-up. *Am J Respir Crit Care Med* 2002;166:159.

34. Simantirakis EN, Schizab SI, Marketoua ME, et al. Severe bradyarrhythmias in patients with sleep apnoea: the effect of continuous positive airway pressure treatment. A long-term evaluation using an insertable loop recorder. *Eur Heart J* 2004;25:1070.

35. Gami AS, Pressman G, Caples SM, et al. Association of atrial fibrillation and obstructive sleep apnea. *Circulation* 2004;110:364.

36. Alonso-Fernández A, García-Río F, Racionero MA, et al. Cardiac rhythm disturbances and ST-segment depression episodes in patients with obstructive sleep apnea-hypopnea syndrome and its mechanisms. *Chest* 2005;127:15.

37. Mehra R, Benjamin EJ, Shahar E, et al. Association of nocturnal arrhythmias with sleep-disordered breathing: the Sleep Heart Health Study. *Am J Respir Crit Care Med* 2006;173:910.

38. Gami AS, Friedman P, Chung MK, et al. Therapy Insight: interactions between atrial fibrillation and obstructive sleep apnea. *Nat Clin Pract Cardiovasc Med* 2005;2:145.

39. Ryan CM, Usui K, Floras JS, et al. Effect of continuous positive airway pressure on ventricular ectopy in heart failure patients with obstructive sleep apnea. *Thorax* 2005;60:781.

40. Mansfield DR, Gollogly NC, Kaye DM, et al. Controlled trial of continuous positive airway pressure in obstructive sleep apnea and heart failure. *Am Rev Respir Crit Care Med* 2004;169:361.

41. Davies CW, Crosby JH, Mullins RL, et al. Case-control study of 24 hour ambulatory blood pressure in patients with obstructive sleep apnoea and normal matched control subjects. *Thorax* 2000;55:736.

42. Lavie P, Herer P, Hoffstein V. Obstructive sleep apnoea syndrome as a risk factor for hypertension: population study. *BMJ* 2000;320:479.

43. Nieto FJ, Young TB, Lind BK, et al. Association of sleep-disordered breathing, sleep apnea, and hypertension in a large community-based study. Sleep Heart Health Study. *JAMA* 2000;283:1829.

44. Bixler EO, Vgontzas AN, Lin HM, et al. Association of hypertension and sleep-disordered breathing. *Arch Intern Med* 2000;160:2289.

45. Peppard PE, Young T, Palta M, et al. Prospective study of the association between sleep-disordered breathing and hypertension. *N Engl J Med* 2000;342:1378.

46. Pepperell JC, Davies RJ, Stradling JR. Systemic hypertension and obstructive sleep apnoea. *Sleep Med Rev* 2002;6:157.

47. Chobanian AV, Bakris GL, et al. H.R. for the National High Blood Pressure Program Coordinating Committee, U.S. Department of Health and Human Services, and National Heart, Lung, and Blood Institute, National Institutes of Health, et al: 7th Report of the Joint National Committee on Prevention, Detection, Evaluation and Treatment of High Blood Pressure: The JNC 7 report. *JAMA* 2003;289:2560.

48. Morrell MJ, Finn L, Kim H, et al. Sleep fragmentation, awake blood pressure, and sleep-disordered breathing in a population-based study. *Am J Respir Crit Care Med* 2000;162:2091.

49. Belozeroff V, Berry RB, Sassoon CS, et al. Effects of CPAP therapy on cardiovascular variability in obstructive sleep apnea: a closed-loop analysis. *Am J Physiol Heart Circ Physiol* 2002;282:H110.

50. Mills PJ, Kennedy BP, Loredo JS, et al. Effects of nasal continuous positive airway pressure and oxygen supplementation on norepinephrine kinetics and cardiovascular responses in obstructive sleep apnea. *J Appl Physiol* 2006;100:343.

51. Bonsignore MR, Parati G, Insalaco G, et al. Baroreflex control of heart rate during sleep in severe obstructive sleep apnoea: effects of acute CPAP. *Eur Respir J* 2006;27:128.

52. Pepperell JC, Ramdassingh-Dow S, Crosthwaite N, et al. Ambulatory blood pressure after therapeutic and subtherapeutic nasal continuous positive airway pressure for obstructive sleep apnoea: a randomised parallel trial. *Lancet* 2002;359:204.

53. Barbe F, Mayoralas LR, Duran J, et al. Treatment with continuous positive airway pressure is not effective in patients with sleep apnea but no daytime sleepiness. *Ann Intern Med* 2001;134:1015.

54. Campos-Rodriguez F, Grilo-Reina A, Perez-Ronchel J, et al. Effect of continuous positive airway pressure on ambulatory BP in patients with sleep apnea and hypertension: a placebo-controlled trial. *Chest* 2006;129:1459.

55. Robinson GV, Smith DM, Langford BA, et al. Continuous positive airway pressure does not reduce blood pressure in nonsleepy hypertensive OSA patients. *Eur Respir J* 2006;27:1229.

56. Arzt M, Young T, Finn L, et al. Association of sleep-disordered breathing and the occurrence of stroke. *Am J Respir Crit Care Med* 2005;172:1447.

57. Punjabi NM, Shahar E, Redline S, et al.; Sleep Heart Health Study Investigators. Sleep-disordered breathing, glucose intolerance, and insulin resistance. The Sleep Heart Health Study. *Am J Epidemiol* 2004;160:521.

58. Weaver TE, Maislin G, Dinges DF, et al. Relationship between hours of CPAP use and achieving normal levels of sleepiness and daily functioning. *Sleep* 2007;30(6):711–719.

59. Budhiraja R, Parthasarathy S, Drake CL, et al. Early CPAP use identifies subsequent adherence to CPAP therapy. *Sleep* 2007;30:320–324.

60. Ballard RD, Gay PG, Strollo PJ. Intervention to improve compliance in sleep apnea patients previously non-compliant with continuous positive airway pressure. *J Clin Sleep Med* 2007;3:706.

61. Hui DS, Chan JK, Choy DK, et al. Effects of augmented continuous positive airway pressure education and support on compliance and outcome in a Chinese population. *Chest* 2000;117:1410.

62. Friedman M, Soans R, Joseph N, et al. The effect of multilevel upper airway surgery on continuous positive airway pressure therapy in obstructive sleep apnea/hypopnea syndrome. *Laryngoscope* 2009;119(1):193–196.

63. Chandrashekariah R, Shaman Z, Auckley D. Impact of upper airway surgery on CPAP compliance in difficult-to-manage obstructive sleep apnea. *Arch Otolaryngol Head Neck Surg* 2008;134(9):926–930.

64. Engleman HM, Wild MR. Improving CPAP use by patients with the sleep apnoea/hypopnoea syndrome (SAHS). *Sleep Med Rev* 2003;7:81–99.

65. Olsen A, Smith S, Oei T, et al. Health belief model predicts adherence to CPAP before experience with CPAP. *Eur Resp J* 2008;31:127–131.

66. Baltzan MA, Elkholi O, Wolkove N. Evidence of interrelated side effects with reduced compliance in patients treated with nasal continuous positive airway pressure. *Sleep Med* 2009;10:198–205.

67. Ryan S, Doherty LS, Nolan GM, et al. Effects of heated humidification and topical steroids on compliance, nasal symptoms, and quality of life in patients with obstructive sleep apnea syndrome using nasal continuous positive airway pressure. *J Clin Sleep Med* 2009;5:422–427.

68. Duong M, Jayaram L, Camfferman D, et al. Use of heated humidification during nasal CPAP titration in obstructive sleep apnoea. *Eur Respir J* 2005;26:679.

69. Mador MJ, Krauza M, Pervez A, et al. Effect of heated humidification on compliance and quality of life in patients with sleep apnea using nasal continuous positive airway pressure. *Chest* 2005;128:2151.

70. Neill AM, Wai HS, Bannan SP, et al. Humidified nasal continuous positive airway pressure in obstructive sleep apnoea. *Eur Respir J* 2003;22:258.

71. Rakotonanahary D, Pelletier-Fleury N, Gagnadoux F, et al. Predictive factors for the need for additional humidification during nasal continuous positive airway pressure therapy. *Chest* 2001;119:460.

72. Brown LK. Back to Basics. If it's dry, wet it: the case for humidification of nasal continuous positive airway pressure air. *Chest* 2000;117:617.

73. Suguira T, Noda A, Nakata S, et al. Influence of nasal resistance on initial acceptance of CPAP in treatment of OSAS. *Respiration* 2007;74:56–60.

74. Nakata S, Noda A, Yagi H, et al. Nasal resistance for determinant factor of nasal surgery in CPAP failure patients with obstructive sleep apnea syndrome. *Rhinology* 2005;43:296–299.

75. Tsuda H, Almeida FR, Tsuda T, et al. Craniofacial changes after 2 years of nasal continuous positive airway pressure use in patients with obstructive sleep apnea. *Chest* 2010;138: 870–874.

76. Kiekens S, DeGroot V, Coeckelbergh T, et al. Continuous positive airway pressure therapy is associated with an increase in intraocular pressure in obstructive sleep apnea. *Invest Ophthalmol Vis Sci* 2008;49:934–940.

77. Ferguson KA, Cartwright R, Rogers R, et al. Oral appliances for snoring and sleep apnea: a review. *Sleep* 2006;29:244–262.

78. Kushida CA, Morgenthaler TI, Littner MR, et al. Practice parameters for the treatment of snoring and obstructive sleep apnea with oral appliances: an update for 2005. *Sleep* 2006;29:240–243.

79. Lam B, Sam K, Lam J, et al. The efficacy of oral appliances in the treatment of severe obstructive sleep apnea. *Sleep Breath* 2011;15(2):195–201.

80. Vanderveken OM, Devolder A, Marklund M, et al. Comparison of a custom-made and a thermoplastic oral appliance for the treatment of mild sleep apnea. *Am J Resp Crit Care Med* 2008;178: 197–202.

81. Ryan CF, Love LL, Peat D, et al. Mandibular advancement oral appliance therapy for obstructive sleep apnea: effect on awake caliber of the velopharynx. *Thorax* 199;54:972–977.

82. Chan AS, Lee RW, Srinivasan VK, et al. Nasopharyngoscopic evaluation of oral appliance therapy for obstructive sleep apnea. *Eur Resp J* 2010;35:836–842.

83. Hoffstein V. Review of oral appliances for treatment of sleep-disordered breathing. *Sleep Breath* 2007;11:1–22.

84. Mehta A, Qian J, Petocz P, et al. A randomized, controlled study of a mandibular advancement splint for obstructive sleep apnea. *Am J Resp Crit Care Med* 2001;163:1457–1461.

85. Gotsopoulos H, Chen C, Qian J, et al. Oral appliance therapy improves symptoms in obstructive sleep apnea: a randomized controlled trial. *Am J Resp Crit Care Med* 2002;166:743–748.

86. Johnston CD, Gleadhill IC, Cinnamond MJ, et al. Mandibular advancement appliances and obstructive sleep apnea: a randomized clinical trial. *Eur Resp J* 2002;24:251–262.

87. Barnes M, McEvoy RD, Banks S, et al. Efficacy of positive airway pressure and oral appliance in mild to moderate obstructive sleep apnea. *Am J Resp Crit Care Med* 2004;170:656–664.

88. Naismith SL, Winter VR, Hickie IB, et al. Effect of oral appliance therapy on neurobehavioral functioning in obstructive sleep apnea: a randomized controlled trial. *J Clin Sleep Med* 2005;1:374–380.

89. Gotsopoulos H, Kelly JJ, Cistulli PA. Oral appliance therapy reduces blood pressure in obstructive sleep apnea: a randomized controlled trial. *Sleep* 2004;27:934–941.

90. Yoshida K. Effect on blood pressure of oral appliance therapy for sleep apnea syndrome. *Int J Prosthodont* 2006;19:61–66.

91. Yoshida K. Effects of a mandibular advancement device for the treatment of sleep apnea syndrome and snoring on respiratory function and sleep quality. *Cranio* 2008;18:98–105.

92. Marklund M, Stenlund H, Franklin KA. Mandibular advancement devices in 630 men and women with obstructive sleep apnea and snoring. *Chest* 2004;125:1270–1278.

93. Marklund M, Persson M, Franklin KA. Treatment success with a mandibular advancement device is related to supine-dependent sleep apnea. *Chest* 1998;114:1630–1635.

94. Johal A, Hector MP, Battagel JM, et al. Impact of sleep nasendoscopy on the outcome of mandibular advancement splint therapy in subjects with sleep-related breathing disorders. *J Laryngol Otol* 2007;121:668–675.

95. Johal A, Battagel JM, Kotecha BT. Sleep nasendoscopy: a diagnostic tool for predicting treatment success with mandibular advancement splints in obstructive sleep apnoea. *Eur J Orthodont* 2005;27:607–614.

96. Battagel JM, Johal A, Kotecha BT. Sleep nasendoscopy as a predictor of treatment success in snorers using mandibular advancement splints. *J Laryngol Otol* 2005;119:106–112.

97. Walker-Engstrom ML, Tegelberg A, Wilhelmsson B, et al. 4-year follow-up of treatment with dental appliance or uvulopalatopharyngoplasty in patients with obstructive sleep apnea: a randomized study. *Chest* 2002;121(3):739–746.

98. Clark GT, Sohn JW, Hong CN. Treating obstructive sleep apnea and snoring: assessment of an anterior mandibular positioning device. *J Am Dent Assoc* 2000;131:765–771.

99. Ferguson KA, Ono T, Lowe AA, et al. A short term controlled trial of an adjustable oral appliance for the treatment of mild to moderate obstructive sleep apnoea. *Thorax* 1997;52:362–368.

100. Ferguson KA, Ono T, Lowe AA, et al. A randomized crossover study of an oral appliance vs nasal-continuous positive airway pressure in the treatment of mild-moderate obstructive sleep apnea. *Chest* 1996;109:1269–1275.

101. Young T, Finn L, Kim H. Nasal obstruction as a risk factor for sleep-disordered breathing. The University of Wisconsin Sleep and Respiratory Research Group. *J Allergy Clin Immunol* 1997;99:S757–S762.

102. Young T, Finn L, Palta M. Chronic nasal congestion at night is a risk factor for snoring in a population-based cohort study. *Arch Int Med* 2001;161:1514–1519.

103. Stradling JR, Crosby JH. Predictors and prevalence of obstructive sleep apnea in 1001 middle-aged men. *Thorax* 1991;46:85–90.

104. Lofaso F, Coste A, d'Ortho MP, et al. Nasal obstruction as a risk factor for sleep apnoea syndrome. *Eur Respir J* 2000;16: 639–643.

105. Craig TJ, Teets S, Lehman EB, et al. Nasal congestion secondary to allergic rhinitis as a cause of sleep disturbance and daytime fatigue and the response to topical nasal corticosteroids. *J Allergy Clin Immunol* 1998;101:633–637.

106. Brouillette RT, Manoukian JJ, Ducharme FM, et al. Efficacy of fluticasone nasal spray for pediatric obstructive sleep apnea. *J Pediatr* 2001;138:838–844.

107. Nakata S, Noda A, Yasuma F, et al. Effects of nasal surgery on sleep quality in obstructive sleep apnea syndrome with nasal obstruction. *Am J Rhinol* 2008;22:59–63.

108. Li HY, Lin Y, Chen NH, et al. Improvement in QOL after nasal surgery alone for patients with OSA and NAO. *Arch Otolaryngol Head Neck Surg* 2008;134:429–433.

109. Zeng B, Ng AT, Qian J, et al. Influence of nasal resistance on oral appliance treatment outcome in obstructive sleep apnea. *Sleep* 2008;31(4):543–547.

110. Nashi N, Kang S, Barkdull GC, et al. Lingual fat at autopsy. *Laryngoscope* 2007;117:1467–1473.

111. Schwab RJ, Gupta KB, Hoffman EA, et al. Differences in upper airway soft tissue anatomy in normal subjects and patients with sleep-disordered breathing. *Am Rev Respir Dis* 1993;147: 462–466.

112. Welch KC, Foster GD, Ritter CT, et al. A novel volumetric magnetic resonance imaging paradigm to study upper airway anatomy. *Sleep* 2002;25:532–542.

113. Winter WC, Gampper T, Gay SB, et al. Enlargement of the lateral pharyngeal fat pad space in pigs increases upper airway resistance. *J Appl Physiol* 1995;70:726–731.

114. Ryan CF, Love LL. Mechanical properties of the velopharynx in obese patients with obstructive sleep apnea. *Am J Respir Crit Care Med* 1996;154:806–812.

115. Peppard PE, Young T, Palta M, et al. Longitudinal study of moderate weight change and sleep-disordered breathing. *JAMA* 2000;284:3015–3021.

116. Tuomilehto HP, Seppa JM, Partinen MM, et al. Lifestyle intervention with weight reduction: first-line treatment in mild obstructive sleep apnea. *Am J Respir Crit Care Med* 2009;179:320–327.

117. Foster GD, Barradaile KE, Sanders MH, et al. A randomized study on the effect of weight loss on obstructive sleep apnea patients among obese patients with type 2 diabetes: the Sleep AHEAD study. *Arch Intern Med* 2009;169:1619–1626.

118. Kajaste S, Brander PE, Telakivi T, et al. A cognitive-behavioral weight reduction program in the treatment of obstructive sleep apnea syndrome with or without initial nasal CPAP: a randomized study. *Sleep Med* 2004;5:125–131.

119. Haines KL, Nelson LG, Gonzalez R, et al. Objective evidence that bariatric surgery improves obesity-related obstructive sleep apnea. *Surgery* 2007;141:354–358.

120. Guardino S, Scott JA, Ware JC, et al. The long-term results of gastric bypass on indexes of sleep apnea. *Chest* 2003;124:1615–1619.

121. Permut I, Montserrat D, Chattila W, et al. Comparison of positional therapy to CPAP in patients with positional obstructive sleep apnea. *J Clin Sleep Med* 2010;6(3):238–243.

122. Chung JW, Enciso R, Levendowski DJ, et al. Treatment outcomes of mandibular advancement devices in positional and nonpositional OSA patients. *Oral Surg Oral Med Oral Pathol Oral Radiol Endod* 2010;109(5):724–731.

123. Neill AM, Angus SM, Sajkov D, et al. Effects of sleep posture on upper airway stability in patients with obstructive sleep apnea. *Am J Respir Crit Care Med* 1997;155:199–204.

124. Skinner MA, Kingshott RN, Jones DR, et al. Elevated posture for the management of obstructive sleep apnea. *Sleep Breath* 2004;8(4):193–200.

125. Stamatakis K, Sanders M, Caffo B, et al. Fasting glycemia in sleep disordered breathing: lowering the threshold on oxyhemoglobin desaturation. *Sleep* 2008;31:1018–1024.

126. Punjabi NM, Newman AB, Young TB, et al. Sleep-disordered breathing and cardiovascular disease: an outcome-based definition of hypopneas. *Am J Respir Crit Care Med* 2008;177:1150–1155.

127. Strollo PJ. Indications for treatment of obstructive sleep apnea in adults. *Clin Chest Med* 2003;24:307–313.

128. McGinley BM, Patil SP, Kirkness JP, et al. A nasal cannula can be used to treat obstructive sleep apnea. *Am J Respir Crit Care Med* 2007;176:194–200.

129. Mezzanotte WS, et al. Waking genioglossal electromyogram in sleep apnea patients versus normal controls: a neuromuscular compensatory mechanism. *J Clin Invest* 1992;89:1571–1579.

130. Saboisky JP, et al. Neural drive to human genioglossus in obstructive sleep apnoea. *J Physiol* 2007;585:135–146.

131. White DP. Pathogenesis of obstructive and central sleep apnea. *Am J Resp Crit Care Med* 2005;172:1363–1370.

132. Puhan MA, Suarez A, Cascio CL, et al. Didgeridoo playing as alternative treatment for obstructive sleep apnoea syndrome: randomized controlled trial. *BMJ* 2005;332:266–270.

133. Guimaraes KC, Drager LF, Genta PR, et al. Effects of oropharyngeal exercises on patients with moderate obstructive sleep apnea syndrome. *Am J Resp Crit Care Med* 2009;179:962–966.

134. Liu C, Cao Y, Malhotra A, et al. Sleep fragmentation attenuates the hypercapnic (but not hypoxic) ventilatory responses via adenosine A1 receptors in awake rats. *Respir Physiol Neurobiol* 2011;175(1):29–36.

135. Scanlan MF, Roebuck T, Little PJ, et al. Effect of moderate alcohol upon obstructive sleep apnoea. *Eur Respir J* 2000;16(5):909–913.

136. Vakulin A, Baulk SD, Catcheside PG, et al. Effects of alcohol and sleep restriction on simulated driving performance in untreated patients with obstructive sleep apnea. *Ann Intern Med* 2009;151(7):447–455.

137. Phillips B, Danner F. Cigarette smoking and sleep disturbance. *Arch Intern Med* 1995;155:734–737.

138. Wetter DW, Young TB, Bidwell TR, et al. Smoking as a risk factor for sleep-disordered breathing. *Arch Intern Med* 1994;154:2219–2224.

139. Scharf AM, Tubman A, Smale P. Prevalence of concomitant sleep disorders in patients with obstructive sleep apnea. *Sleep Breath* 2005;9:50–56.

140. Smith S, Sullivan K, Hopkins W, et al. Frequency of insomnia report in patients with obstructive sleep apnoea hypopnea syndrome (OSAHS). *Sleep Med* 2004;5:449–456.

141. Guilleminault C, Davis K, Huynh NT. Prospective randomized study of patients with insomnia and mild sleep disordered breathing. *Sleep* 2008;31(11):1527–1533.

Nasal and Palatal Surgery for OSA

137

Peter D. O'Connor   Tucker Woodson

An inherent problem in obstructive sleep apnea (OSA) for any given individual is that the airway is structurally vulnerable to collapse. Multiple physiologic and anatomic factors contribute to maintain airway patency. The complex interaction between respiratory control, arousal thresholds, neuromuscular tone, and transmural pressure in the pharynx determine the patency of the airway through the respiratory cycle. Simply put, the upper airway including the pharynx and to a lesser degree the nasal cavity can be thought of as a collapsible tube. The flow of air through the upper airway is influenced by the difference in upstream, downstream, and intraluminal forces. Stabilization of airflow in an airway compromised by OSA often requires multimodality treatment.

Surgical treatments for sleep-disordered breathing (SDB) will vary depending on the structures involved and the morbidity of the intervention, severity of disease, obesity, and cost of care for many patients. The role of surgical intervention has classically been viewed as an attempt to influence the structures involved with airway collapse. An alternative and perhaps more accurate way of looking at the role of surgery is that of a reconstructive approach. The goal of airway reconstruction is to improve the patency of the tube and the flow of air. Ultimately, we want to reduce the severity of disease and sequelae. Surgical intervention is one modality that should be considered in patients presenting with SDB.

Surgical treatment often requires a combination of procedures. It is not a single unique surgery. In adults, a single anatomic structure is not usually the sole cause of obstruction, and multiple sites or levels of the airway often require treatment for optimal results. Although tracheotomy as a single procedure should be considered in certain clinical presentations of OSA, it is not practical in most cases. A vast array of surgical treatments are described and variable reported responses to them exist. This is in part due to the distinct character of each airway based on the craniofacial anatomy, neuromuscular tone, influence from other soft tissues, and physiologic elements. Understanding the pathophysiology of OSA along with the airway phenotype will aid in the selection and surgical application of procedures. Impacting only one of these factors surgically may be inadequate to achieve the desired end state. Ideally, the surgical approach is tailored to a patient rather than the application of a one method suits all approach.

The pathogenesis of SDB and luminal compromise is rarely confined to a single anatomic location. Obstruction and narrowing of both the upper pharyngeal (retropalatal) and lower pharyngeal (retroglossal) airways occurs in 70% to 80% of patients (1). Ethnic and gender variation may exist and not all sites contribute equally (2–4). Obstruction occurs in the pharynx for most events but obstruction of laryngeal tissues as a primary site is uncommon (4,5). The cause of obstruction is complex, and abnormalities of palatal and pharyngeal muscles, mucosa, lymphoid tissues, vascular structures, and other influential elements such as airway mechanoreceptors have been reported. Abnormal nasal resistance is an important but indirect cause of apnea in adults. Ultimately, the common finding is an upper airway that is structurally vulnerable to collapse. Multiple surgeries and variations of them have been described with a desired effect of improving the flow of air during sleep.

Snoring has traditionally been regarded as a social nuisance rather than a source of morbidity. It is one of the most important presenting signs in patients suspected of having OSA. When patients present with a complaint of snoring, OSA needs to be ruled out rather than assuming a diagnosis of primary snoring. Data from the Wisconsin Sleep Cohort Study showed that 31% of middle-aged females and 53% of middle-aged males had habitual snoring and an even more had nonhabitual snoring (6). Treatment of snoring to this point has emphasized the importance on bed partner quality of sleep. However, new evidence is emerging that suggests there is an association between snoring and increased mortality (7). Whether snoring is a discrete condition or there is a synergistic effect on SDB needs to be explored further.

Since surgery for sleep apnea is not a single intervention for many patients, algorithms describing planned interventions have been described. The most commonly quoted is the Stanford protocol that defines surgical procedures as being phase 1 or phase 2 procedures. Phase 1 procedures included segmental pharyngeal interventions such as uvulopalatopharyngoplasty (UPPP), genioglossal advancement, and hyoid suspension. Phase 2 procedures were maxillomandibular advancement or similar interventions (8). Others have described phased procedures using radiofrequency, lingual tonsillectomy, and glossectomy procedures as part of the phased protocol. To date, few studies have compared outcomes using different protocols. In addition to assessing how surgery may modify different structural elements of the airway, it is also important to define what the ultimate goal of surgical treatment for sleep apnea is going to be. Three general classifications for intervening may include complementing medical management (continuous positive airway pressure [CPAP] use, weight loss), salvage therapy in patients where medical management has failed, or when surgical cure is likely for select individuals. The treatment algorithm for patients may include a reassessment of prior failed therapies. It must also be recognized that OSA is a chronic disease and remittance is common. For a significant number of patients, CPAP tolerance following surgeries may be improved. Both retrospective and prospective studies suggest that nasal surgery may improve CPAP adherence and may lower CPAP pressures. Case series suggests that in some patients pharyngeal surgery may also improve CPAP use in selected patients. In the authors' anecdotal experience, a subset of patients with marked lymphoid hyperplasia or other isolated soft tissue abnormalities may benefit from surgery that has the goal of improving CPAP use. Concerns exist, however, that aggressive UPPP may worsen CPAP use in some patients by creating or worsening "mouth leak." Mouth leak occurs from over shortening of the palate, which then cannot seal against the tongue when positive pressures applied. The clinical significance of this is uncertain for most patients.

A successful outcome following surgery depends on at least three additional key elements. First, the preoperative clinical evaluation accurately defines the structures influencing the flow of air. A complementary or alternative way is describing the airway phenotype. Second, it is important to select the appropriate one or combination of procedures followed by skillful application of the procedure. The third element involves an understanding of what the potential effect of a procedure will be, the desired goal, and how the effect may change over time for a chronically, often progressive disease. An example of the latter class of patients is the nonobese pediatric patient with adenotonsillar hypertrophy and no other craniofacial or neurologic abnormalities.

In adults, positive airway pressure therapy is considered the gold standard although it does have its limitations. Certain patients are unable to tolerate positive airway pressure therapy. This is despite more sophisticated delivery methods available today. A variety of interfaces and other noninvasive pressure modalities may be beneficial for some patients. These include nasal masks including nasal pillows, masks which cover the nose and mouth, and full face masks. Varying positive pressure modalities also exist and include bilevel pressures (BiPAP), autotitrating units, devices with relaxation modes during exhalation, and newer devices with adaptive ventilation based on a continuous monitoring of flow through the device and interface.

Defining the criteria for successful outcome is also important. In the literature, this has traditionally focused on an improvement in respiratory parameters (apnea–hypopnea index [AHI], and lowest oxygen saturation [LSAT]). A threshold of treatment that defines a successful response does not exist based on current data. In addition to objective data, the subjective response should not be overlooked (9,10). Subjective improvement in sleep with reduction in nasal airway obstruction (NAO), reduction in snoring, and improved quality of life should also be elements of the treatment discussion with the patient. The remainder of the chapter focuses on nasal and palate surgery. The treatment goals and physical evaluation of a patient with sleep apnea and snoring is critical and should set the foundation for the preoperative decision making, what procedures to consider, and the postoperative management.

NASAL SURGERY

NAO is a recognized contributor to SDB. Patients with NAO report a worse quality of life, increased fatigue, and decreased quantity and quality of sleep. Some studies have shown a link between NAO and OSA (11). Population-based studies have identified chronic nocturnal nasal obstruction as being significantly more likely in individuals with SDB (12) and habitual snorers without OSA (13).

Treatments will vary depending on the pathologic findings and symptoms. Historically, the primary symptom warranting treatment was subjective nasal obstruction. The finding of such strong associations with SDB, or quality sleep, and OSA support that these are also symptoms related to nasal obstruction. Improvement in sleep quality is a major component of validated nasal treatment outcome questionnaires (nose scale). In large cohorts and randomized controlled trials, surgical therapy has been shown to significantly improve sleep architecture, subjective sleep quality, and daytime sleepiness. Studies also support that in most patients as an isolated treatment, nasal surgery does not affect the AHI. A patent nasal airway, however, has been significantly associated with patient's favorable response to treatment. A higher nasal resistance and nasal obstruction appears to decrease the use of both nasal CPAP and oral appliances, and negatively affect surgical outcomes. Use of objective data on nasal airflow is not yet common in the clinical setting. Treatments may include correction of a septal deviation, reduction in turbinate size, correcting nasal valve collapse, or removal of nasal polyps.

There are differences in the literature regarding daytime symptoms of NAO, measures of nasal resistance, and objective polysomnogram data. This is in part because nasal airflow is a complex phenomenon, and how patients perceive airflow can be quite variable at different times and from one another. The physiologic nasal cycle, controlled by the hypothalamus, alters nasal mucosa every few hours. Air entering the nasal passageway is affected by shape of turbinates, mucosal properties, and nasal cilia. The nasal mucosa, especially overlying the turbinates, has an extensive vascular bed. Expansion of the network of vessels can lead to obstruction from acute or chronic inflammation and significantly impact the level of nasal resistance.

An important distinction to consider is how nasal resistance during wakefulness compares to the resistance of the nose while lying supine during sleep. There is evidence that nasal resistance changes throughout the course of the night. Increases in nasal resistance are greater in OSA compared to non-OSA populations. Whether this is due to differences in physiology (such as vascular compliance) or anatomy of the upper airway are unknown.

Predicting how nasal obstruction will impact CPAP use is also difficult. A common complaint of patients is that they cannot tolerate their mask and may remove it during the night. Why this occurs despite a proper level of therapy is unclear. Many patients report NAO and some authors have reported an increase in nasal symptoms in certain patients after starting CPAP therapy (14).

Despite the lack of a clear understanding about the role NAO plays in SDB, it can be an important component of the overall treatment algorithm for patients. However, nasal surgery alone is not accepted as a primary treatment alone for OSA in part because a linear relationship between daytime symptoms and severity of SDB does not exist. Clinical examination for the presence of nasal obstruction remains important to rule out compromised airflow through the nasal cavity and nasopharynx.

Evaluation

Physicians currently utilize subjective surveys, visual examination with endoscopy, and computed tomography scans to help in diagnosing patients with NAO. Objective testing of the nasal airway has most commonly been done using acoustic rhinometry and rhinomanometry. Acoustic rhinometry, although still primarily used as a research tool, provides a volumetric measure of the nasal cavity (15,16). The anatomic measurement is taken during a breathhold and does not provide direct data on the flow of air through the nose. Rhinomanometry measures nasal obstruction and changes in resistance by assessing pressure and nasal airflow together during normal breathing (15).

Other methods have been utilized but to a lesser degree. These include nasal spirometry, laser Doppler velocimetry, and forced oscillation rhinomanometry to better describe nasal airflow, resistance, and potential sources of obstruction (17–23). These tests have varied acceptance and are not always practical in the clinical setting, and studies reveal differing conclusions (21,24). More recently, some investigators have begun using computational fluid dynamics to model nasal airflow (25–28).

Nasal Breathing and Impact on Sleep

NAO likely contributes to upper airway resistance through both indirect and direct mechanisms. Humans should breathe through their nose when sleeping. Nasal airflow is an important factor for maintaining neural tone and the patency of the airway. Nasal obstruction is ultimately a subjective sensation processed in the brain from numerous neurophysiologic receptors.

Use of a topical anesthetic to decrease afferent stimuli from the nasal airway has been shown to increase pharyngeal resistance resulting in an increased number of respiratory events over the course of a night (29). Decreased nasal airway flow should similarly result in a reduction of nasal afferent reflexes and subsequent decrease in muscular tone. Optimizing nasal airflow to maximize this feedback is important.

Nasal obstruction may also lead to mouth opening. Oral cavity opening leads to posterior rotation of the tongue base and displacement of the hyoid bone (30). Vertical opening with inferior displacement of the hyoid and a decrease in the hyomandibular distance results. These movements place the musculature of the tongue and pharyngeal tissues into a mechanically disadvantaged position and lead to increased upper airway collapsibility and increased hypopharyngeal obstruction. Despite mouth opening, the soft palate and tongue may remain in close apposition even if nasal breathing continues.

Additional evidence of the importance of having and maintaining nasal airflow during sleep comes via the concept of a Starling resistor. The upper airway is a collapsible tube. The larynx in humans, unlike other mammals, has a more caudal position creating a greater distance with the soft tissues of the pharynx in between. The soft tissues of the pharynx are not directly surrounded by osseous structure and are capable of collapse. The flow of air through the pharynx is influenced by upstream, downstream, and luminal forces. Tissues at multiple levels can contribute to collapse with the nasal cavity and nasopharynx providing upstream resistance. The flow of air and maximum velocity, through the collapsible segment, is inversely proportional to the upstream resistance. Areas downstream are susceptible to collapse including the retropalatal and hypopharyngeal segments. Optimization of airflow through the pharynx is impacted by reducing resistance upstream in the nasal cavity and can be extended to the nasopharynx.

TABLE 137.1	SNORING PATIENTS DIAGNOSED WITH OSA BY POLYSOMNOGRAM	
Study	**N**	**Prevalence (%)**
Viner et al. (69)	410	46
Hoffstein and Szalai (70)	594	46
Deegan and McNicholas (71)	250	54
Vaidya et al. (72)	309	73
Tami et al. (73)	94	72
Rowley et al. (74)	370	67

Weighted average = 0.597 (95% CI = 0.497–0.696).

For patients who do present with a complaint of snoring, symptoms of OSA, or disease proven by polysomnogram, it is important to explore the presence of NAO. Patients may present with a variety of findings (Table 137.1) (septal deviation, polyposis, nasal valve collapse, concha bullosa, adenoid hypertrophy, turbinate hypertrophy, choanal atresia, neoplasm, case reports of skull base, and neoplastic lesions). Chronic rhinosinusitis, allergic rhinitis, turbinate hypertrophy, polyps, and nasal septal deviation may to some degree all cause NAO (17,18,25,31). Surgical correction of an obstructing lesion is justified if there are corresponding daytime or functional symptoms or other concerns. The effect on breathing at night or the use of CPAP is less clear.

The nasal passage functions as a resistor to airflow with both dynamic and static components. The static tissues include the septum and the structural foundation of the nasal cavity and nasopharynx is the maxilla. The dynamic elements of the nasal airway include the internal and external nasal valves as well as the nasal mucosa. The internal nasal valve is the narrowest cross-sectional area of the upper airway. It can therefore have a significant impact on airflow and accounts for nearly two-thirds of the total upper airway resistance. The anatomic components which define the internal valve include the nasal septum medially, the upper lateral cartilage positioned superolateral, the anterior tip of the inferior turbinate, and the pyriform aperture inferiorly. Numerous procedures are available for improving the nasal valve function and include both grafting and suspension techniques. Recognizing the influence of the bony structures is also important because they provide the foundation for the nasal airway. To a lesser degree, the bony foundation may be modified in some patients with improvements in nasal airflow having been shown after maxillary expansion (32,33).

Investigators have attempted to produce nasal obstruction to determine its impact on respiratory parameters during sleep. Sleep disturbance has been shown in the setting of acute nasal obstruction. Following artificial simulation of NAO with catheters and balloons, an increased number of respiratory events including apneas can be seen (34,35). Some of the events include a significant increase in the number of oxygen desaturations. More recently, Friedman et al. (36) have shown that in patients with mild OSA (RDI < 15), nasal packing increased their RDI, duration of snoring, and oxygen desaturation index in the immediate postoperative period.

Nasal obstruction is also associated with poor quality sleep independent of respiratory parameters. Anecdotally, patients with symptomatic seasonal allergies or increased nasal congestion from an upper respiratory infection may present with increased complaints of snoring and CPAP intolerance during the exacerbations. Correction of chronic NAO has been shown to have a significant impact on improving quality of life and daytime somnolence measures (37,38). These findings were independent of any changes in AHI during overnight polysomnograms. This supports the notion that using a measure like AHI alone to assess the impact of nasal surgery is potentially incorrect.

Nasal Surgery

When considering nasal surgery on patients with OSA or snoring, the general categories include septoplasty, valvuloplasty, and turbinoplasty. Preoperatively, it is beneficial to contrast and compare a patient's perception of their breathing and how it correlates to physical exam findings. Knowledge about what CPAP interfaces have been tried and successful may also be beneficial. A patient with weak lower lateral cartilage and significant internal or external nasal valve collapse may do well with a nasal pillow mask if the interface stabilizes this area. Poorly fitting nasal masks can also be problematic if they cause impingement of the nasal vestibule or alar side wall. Surgical correction of increased nasal resistance can be beneficial for patients.

Most studies regarding the impact of nasal surgery on OSA have focused on septoplasty. Some authors have assessed this in combination with other procedures including turbinate reduction (37,39), UPPP (40), and sinus surgeries. Extensive study and literature addressing the nasal valves can be found elsewhere in this text. Further research into the impact of nasal valve surgery on sleep and CPAP is needed.

The ability to relieve SDB via surgery has been more difficult to demonstrate because of the complex nature of SDB and multiple structures involved. Prospective studies have shown significant changes in subjective symptoms following nasal surgery despite no significant difference on sleep parameters, AHI, or oxygen desaturation (37,41,42). One study did show a significant difference in the degree of AHI and snoring after septoplasty with or without turbinoplasty (39). Another interesting finding has been that for some patients there may be an improved tolerance of CPAP or a decrease in overall pressure required to treat their OSA following nasal surgery (37,43). This potentially could improve CPAP tolerance in patients where higher CPAP pressures are the suspected etiology for poor compliance.

The role of the nasal turbinates and the impact turbinoplasty has on OSA and snoring is another area that requires further evaluation. The ability of the nasal passage to function as a resistor depends on the ability of the turbinates to react to stimuli and change vascular tone.

In a large systematic review of the literature, Batra et al. (44) evaluated the efficacy of surgery for symptomatic adult inferior turbinate hypertrophy resulting in NAO. The majority of the studies were level 4 or 5 evidence. Of the 96 studies which met inclusion criteria for their review, 93 studies (96.9%) reported data showing a positive benefit from surgery with subjective symptom improvement in 50% or greater patients. Three studies showed no change or negative benefit. The findings reported were regardless of surgical technique utilized. In 2001, Clement and White (45) published a report on trends in research on turbinate surgery over the past four decades. They indicated a greater emphasis on technology trends rather than patient benefits in the literature. Surgical techniques utilized included turbinectomy, laser surgery, thermal techniques with predominantly radio frequency ablation and coblation, and turbinoplasty including microdebridement. Today the thermal techniques, including radiofrequency ablation and coblation, and the submucosal resection techniques with microdebridement seem to be the preferred procedures. General consensus of which is better requires more research and depends to some degree on what the surgical goal is. Some authors have shown a greater long-term benefit with powered microdebridement versus coblation or radiofrequency turbinate reduction (46–48). How these surgeries impact sleep parameters is unclear.

Objective data were reported in several studies following surgery of the inferior turbinates (44). Nasal resistance measured by rhinomanometry was improved in 83% of the studies (10 of 12) where it was performed and nasal airflow measured by acoustic rhinometry was improved in 100% (14 of 14). Unfortunately, we do not yet have a predictive mechanism to measure NAO with great specificity to determine who will tolerate and respond to CPAP or may benefit from inferior turbinate reduction.

Over a dozen techniques have been described for reduction of the inferior turbinates (49). There are some reports showing good correlation between preoperative topical decongestant and post-radiofrequency ablation of the turbinates with a visual analog score for nasal obstruction. These results have not been tested with other techniques or the impact on sleep parameters or CPAP use. Although most surgical techniques demonstrate some benefit in nasal airflow postoperatively, the most reliable technique with both sustained subjective and objective benefits is unclear. Nasal surgery can also have a large placebo effect that influences subjective scores making more research critical for this area (50).

NAO and the presence of SDB often coexist. The data supporting an improvement in subjective symptoms, decreased CPAP pressure required after nasal surgery, and improved tolerance of CPAP do not consistently correlate to the severity of disease. A beneficial outcome from surgery could be defined as improvement in both objective and subjective measures of nasal airflow. This would include improvements in sleep and a response to CPAP for patients with SDB. However, objective measurements do not always correlate with the patient's symptoms of nasal obstruction. This suggests something other than AHI and nasal airflow conductance as a link between SDB and subjective symptoms.

PALATE SURGERY

Upper airway obstruction and OSA may occur at multiple sites. The upper pharynx in the retropalatal airway is frequently a primary site of obstruction during sleep (1). Obstruction occurs due to loss of muscle tone and compensatory reflexes during sleep. The airway associated with the soft palate is particularly vulnerable since this is the smallest and most compliant portion of the pharynx. Multiple surgical procedures have been developed and advocated to treat both sleep apnea and snoring. The use of these procedures is still evolving. As a primary first-line treatment, palatal surgery is controversial. Success rates vary and causes of surgical failure are poorly understood. Failure is often attributed to obstruction at nonpalatal airway sites. Although this may contribute to failure in some patients, considerable data support that airway obstruction persists at the upper pharynx in the majority of patients (51,52). Increasingly, it is recognized that palatal surgery for sleep apnea and snoring is not a single procedure but a reconstructive approach that can be used as part of an integrated treatment plan for selected patients with OSA. The surgeon can be an important contributor to successful treatment. This requires an understanding of upper airway structure, physiology, and tools of airway reconstruction but also of upper respiratory and sleep pathophysiology and disease. In the authors' experience, understanding the airway phenotype and anatomical structures involved at the palate is important and can aid in determining which palatal procedure may be most beneficial. It is also important to recognize that many patients who fail following traditional UPPP (up to 84% in some studies) have residual retropalatal obstruction. This palatal obstruction may be in addition to hypopharyngeal collapse, further complicating decision making.

Anatomy of the Upper Pharynx

From a structural standpoint the upper pharynx and retropalatal airway is a valve. It is the smallest and most compliant segment of the pharyngeal airway in most individuals regardless of the presence or absence of OSA or snoring. This structural vulnerability combined with a loss of muscle tone to the muscles that maintain patency results in collapse and a significant risk of obstruction. The retropalatal airway is an isthmus with multiple structures determining its final configuration. There is considerable variability between individuals and anatomic structure of the upper pharyngeal airway or pharyngeal isthmus. To date there is no consensus as to how to describe this variability. Multiple anatomic elements combine to define the pharynx. Structures such as tonsil and adenoid size are well accepted as impacting the size of the pharynx. Less well recognized are how other structures such as the pharyngeal lateral walls, velum, levator palatine muscle, palatal aponeurosis, hard palate, and posterior pharyngeal wall anatomy impact the upper airway anatomy.

A number of studies have tried to use anatomic structures to predict outcomes of palatal surgery for OSA (53–56). Several approaches have been used. Methods varied based on what factors were considered to be contributing to palatal surgical failure. Traditionally, failure has been attributed to lower pharyngeal airway obstruction, and anatomy was assessed to identify obstruction at nonpalatal sites. Other studies have used pharyngeal characteristics such as tonsil size and a modified Mallampati classification (Friedman system) to predict outcomes (53,54). A third approach postulates that failure of palatal surgery is due to persistent obstruction at the palatal airway and attempts to better describe and define this portion of the airway.

Diagnosis and Evaluation

Effectiveness of UPPP varies. Its use is controversial. Because of such variability in techniques and outcomes, the effect of UPPP is still only partially understood. Failure likely occurs due to inadequate airway diagnostics, failure of technique, and failure of application. Although much of the literature in UPPP has focused on failure resulting from poor patient selection and obstruction at nonpalatal sites, more recent analysis and data suggest that much of UPPP failure is technical and failure often occurs at palatal sites following surgery. For this reason, newer more physiologic and reconstructive techniques have been advocated and developed. To date, however, these are not in widespread use.

Diagnostic prediction of UPPP has been improved by the Freidman staging system (Fig. 137.1) (53,54). This staging system has proven valuable in predicting which patients will have a greater likelihood of failure with UPPP alone. The Friedman staging system for the oral cavity and oropharyngeal portions of the upper airway defines four stages based on the following: (a) tonsil size (1 to 4+), (b) a modification of the Mallampati classification (1 to 4+), (c) presence or absence of severe obesity (> or <BMI of 40 kg/m²), and (d) major craniofacial abnormalities. The Friedman staging system identifies patients at risk for apnea who present with symptoms of snoring. It also demonstrates both positive and negative UPPP predictive values.

Friedman staging stratifies groups into favorable and unfavorable characteristics. Large tonsil size is a "favorable" (tonsil grades 3 and 4, large tonsils) surgical characteristic. Small tonsils are "unfavorable" (tonsil grades 1 and 2, small tonsils). The Mallampati classification is

	Friedman Palate Position	Tonsil Size	BMI
Stage I	1	3, 4	<40
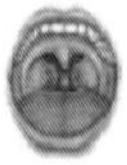	2	3, 4	<40
Stage II	1, 2	1, 2	<40
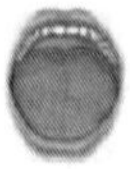	3, 4	3, 4	<40
Stage III	3	0, 1, 2	<40
	4	0, 1, 2	<40
Stage IV	1, 2, 3, 4	0, 1, 2, 3, 4	>40
All patients with significant craniofacial or other anatomic deformities.			

BMI = Body Mass Index.

Figure 137.1 Modified Friedman staging system. (Reprinted from Friedman M, Ibrahim H, Joseph NJ. Staging of obstructive sleep apnea/hypopnea syndrome: a guide to appropriate treatment. *Laryngoscope* 2004;114(3):454–459, with permission.)

"favorable" (grades 1 and 2, visualizing the free margin of the soft palate) when the tongue size is small for the mouth and "unfavorable" (grades 3 and 4, free margin of palate not visible) when the tongue is large and fills the oral cavity. Severe obesity (BMI > 40 kg/m²) is unfavorable. Using the Friedman staging system, outcomes can be better stratified (Friedman stage 1 = 70% success, stage 2 = 40% success, and stage 3 = 10% success).

Analysis of patients who failed traditional UPPP alone has been done. Localization of airway obstruction following traditional UPPP has generated interesting results. In one cohort of patients who failed following traditional UPPP, airway manometry was utilized showing 73% of the patients were found to have obstruction at the palate compared to 27% in the hypopharynx (51). The cross-sectional airway in the palatal area has also been noted to be significantly improved in responders to traditional UPPP versus patients who fail (52). The patients who failed were noted to have a persistent palatal bulge into the pharyngeal lumen. Ideally, in the preoperative setting, we could identify structures involved with airway compromise and tailor the reconstruction rather than applying a one method suits all ablative approach.

Palatal Surgery

Historically, palatopharyngoplasty was defined by UPPP as described by Fujita. Initial techniques described excision of tonsils, posterior soft palate, and uvula. Suture subsequent closure of the tonsillar pillars was then performed. Subsequently, multiple modifications have been described. Although frequently successful for the treatment of snoring, outcomes of UPPP for sleep apnea based on polysomnographic measures are variable. A 1995 review by Sher (57) identified that success rates differed by identified level of pharyngeal obstruction. In patients with obstruction isolated to the upper pharynx (Fujita type I), success rates of reducing AHI by more than 50% and to an AHI of less than 20 events/h or an apnea index (AI) of less than 10 events/h was 52.3%. In contrast, those with lower airway obstruction response using the same criteria were only 5.2%. Sher also observed that the retrospective studies reviewed had a baseline severity of disease (AHI and AI) significantly lower in the group with isolated upper pharyngeal obstruction. Using this data some authors have concluded that surgical outcomes are better for mild sleep apnea. Adequate data were not available to assess the effects of different surgical techniques or different methods of airway evaluation.

A more recent review of UPPP assessed the AHI outcomes of 15 papers, which included individual data from each subject (papers with pooled data were excluded) and demonstrated an overall reduction of AHI of 33% (58). From these studies it was not possible to assess outcomes in women, elderly, or other patient subgroups. The review also excluded what were described as "novel variations" in pharyngeal surgery such as the extended uvulopalatal flap, lateral pharyngoplasty, expansion sphincteroplasty, Z-plasty pharyngoplasty, and palatal advancement. The review also highlighted that few surgical studies have adequately evaluated non-AHI outcomes such as sleepiness, cardiovascular outcomes, or mortality.

Multiple techniques have been described for UPPP. The following procedures have been described to treat OSA by modifying the palate and retropalatal airway. The list is not comprehensive, and data supporting individual procedures vary in quality and magnitude. Few studies have attempted to objectively compare procedures on clinical outcomes, complications, or technical outcomes. Most have been reported as isolated surgical techniques or a small case series. Use of any given procedure has often been based on surgeon's preference. Techniques that have been most extensively evaluated include the extended uvulopalatal flap, lateral pharyngoplasty, expansion sphincter pharyngoplasty (ESP), Z-plasty pharyngoplasty, and palatal advancement (59–64).

A wide variety of complications have been described associated with palatopharyngoplasty for sleep apnea. The most serious risks are those associated with the surgery itself. Perioperative risk of OSA patients is increased due to commonly associated perioperative risk factors such as obesity, hypertension, difficult intubation, and hypersomnolence (65,66). Risk of mortality is uncommon with a recent Veterans Administration population review demonstrating a risk of less than 0.5% of mortality or serious cardiovascular events (67). Other side effects are common but may also be dependent on technique. Side effects include minor changes and swallowing, sensation of throat dryness, increased phlegm, increased gag, and coughing with eating.

Outcomes other than AHI are very important to consider when evaluating surgery for OSA and comparing with and against other treatments. Quality of life outcomes, measures of daytime somnolence, and mortality are a few of the parameters recently reported with a beneficial outcome following surgery (9,10,65).

Uvulopalatopharyngoplasty

UPPP is a procedure that modifies the upper pharynx and palate to reduce or eliminate obstruction during sleep and treat OSA. It is the most common of multiple palatoplasty and palatopharyngoplasty techniques used to treat OSA. Initially described by Fujita in 1981, it was the first specific procedure to treat OSA as an alternative to tracheotomy. UPPP was revolutionary not only as a less morbid surgical intervention but directed attention to the upper airway where there was not yet any consensus of upper airway pathology contributing to disease. Since its inception, UPPP similar to other procedures has evolved and technical variations have been described. In contrast to procedures that only remove or ablate tissue, UPPP involves tissue modification and primary reconstruction. Although the initial description included excision of distal soft palate, tonsils, uvula, and redundant mucosa, other reconstructive approaches are now described. These not only promise lower morbidity in many cases but preserve anatomy and are more effective in randomized clinical trials.

A small number of studies of UPPP and related procedures have been performed demonstrating it as effective in treating physiologic measures of sleep and respiration and quality of life (9). Additionally, population-based studies show that UPPP reduces risks of motor vehicle accidents and likely reduce cardiovascular risk, while large population studies support that it reduces mortality and adult OSA. Although severe complications with UPPP are infrequent (67), side effects of surgery are common. Side effects include minor difficulties and swallowing, dry throat, sensation of foreign body, and increased sensation of phlegm.

A common application of UPPP is the treatment of snoring. Various procedures including laser uvulopalatoplasty (LAUP), injection snoreplasty, placement of Pillar implants, and other stiffening procedures of the palate have been described. Outcomes of these procedures differ in short-term but not likely long-term studies. Procedures likely differ significantly in side effects. More invasive procedures may have higher short-term effectiveness but do so at the price of increasing side effects. Fortunately, the trend of recent procedures is lower side effect rates.

Adult Tonsillectomy

Tonsillectomy and adenoidectomy are common procedures in children and adults who demonstrate enlarged tonsils with OSA. In pediatric patients, the effect of this treatment can be dramatic on AHI, quality of life, and cognitive abilities. The procedure, however, should not be considered "curative." Most of the data to date is case series data in highly selected patients. Few studies have control groups. Data suggest outcomes vary by population treated, airway and facial structure, obesity, and presence of other pathologies. In adults the outcome of simple tonsillectomy is likely limited. In a subset of patients, removing isolated palatine tonsils may be definitive; however, identifying this population is difficult. Exposing an adult to the risk of two general anesthesia procedures, in order to perform isolated tonsillectomy, must be weighed against the additional morbidity of palatopharyngoplasty. Often the decision as to proceed is made intraoperatively after tonsillectomy is performed.

Evolution in Surgical Technique

Recognizing some of the technical failures of traditional UPPP to address the palatal obstruction has led to various modifications in technique. Conceptually, more aggressive

treatment of the distal soft palate may be appropriate for a few patients, but alternatively other patients need the surrounding structures modified. The transpalatal advancement and ESP are examples of two techniques which aim to address structures not directly addressed by the traditional UPPP.

The transpalatal advancement pharyngoplasty (TPA) technique (68) was developed to address the retropalatal obstruction by effecting the position of the soft palate (Fig. 137.2). It can be particularly useful to increase the retropalatal space in a patient who has a very posterior based hard, soft palate junction. Phenotypically, this airway can be described as having a *vertically* oriented soft palate.

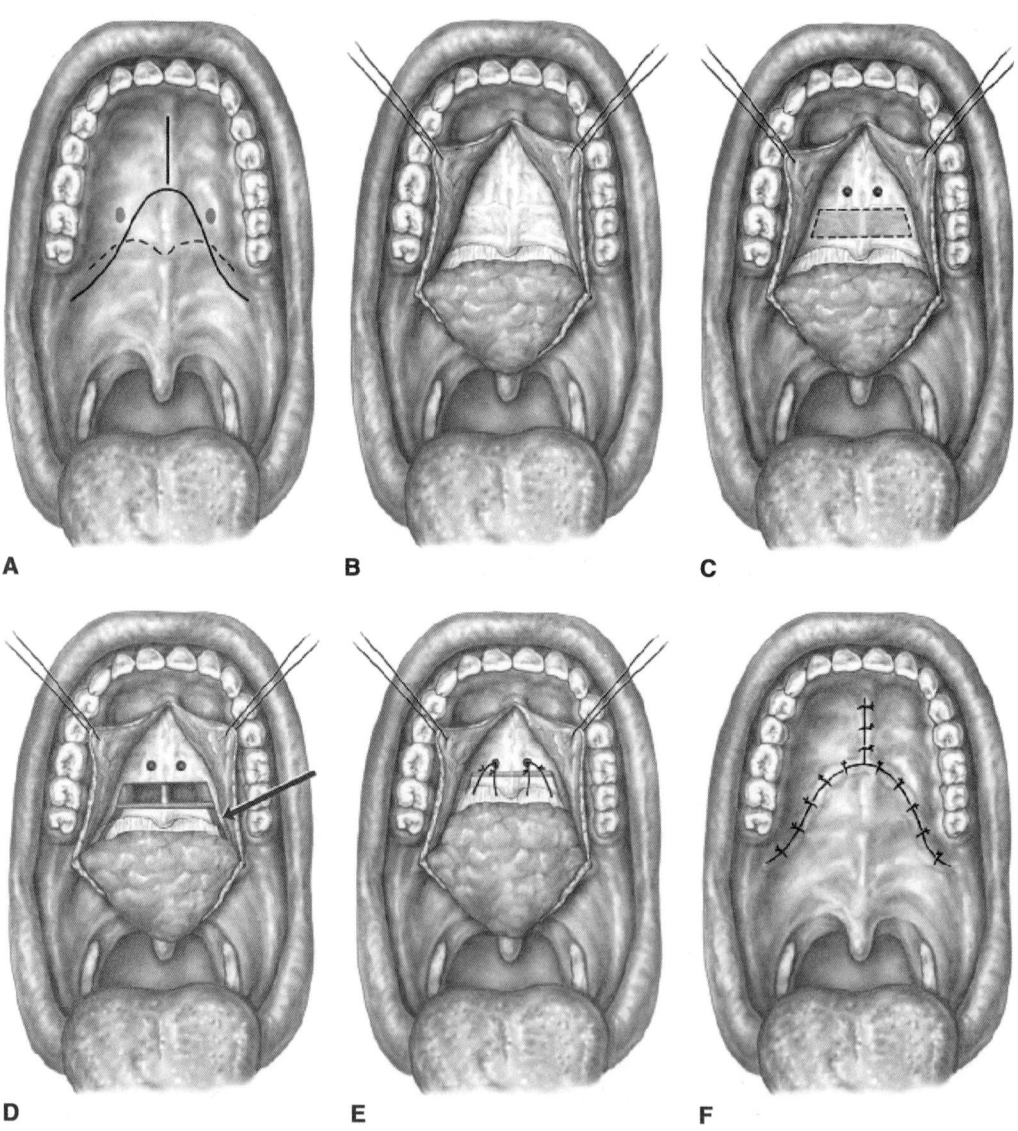

Figure 137.2 Transpalatal advancement pharyngoplasty. **A:** Palatal incision is made medial to the greater palatine foramen and extended posterior and lateral to the hamulus. **B:** Soft tissue flaps are raised exposing the hard palate. **C:** The planned osteotomy window is outlined by *dashes*. **D:** Osteotomy has been completed with 1 to 2 mm of bone preserved posteriorly. The *arrow* highlights the area for the tendolysis. **E:** Sutures are passed through the palatal drill holes and around the remaining distal hard palate and aponeurosis. **F:** The palatal incisions are closed. (Reprinted from Woodson BT. Transpalatal advancement pharyngoplasty. *Oper Tech Otolaryngol Head Neck Surg* 2007;18(1):11–16, with permission.)

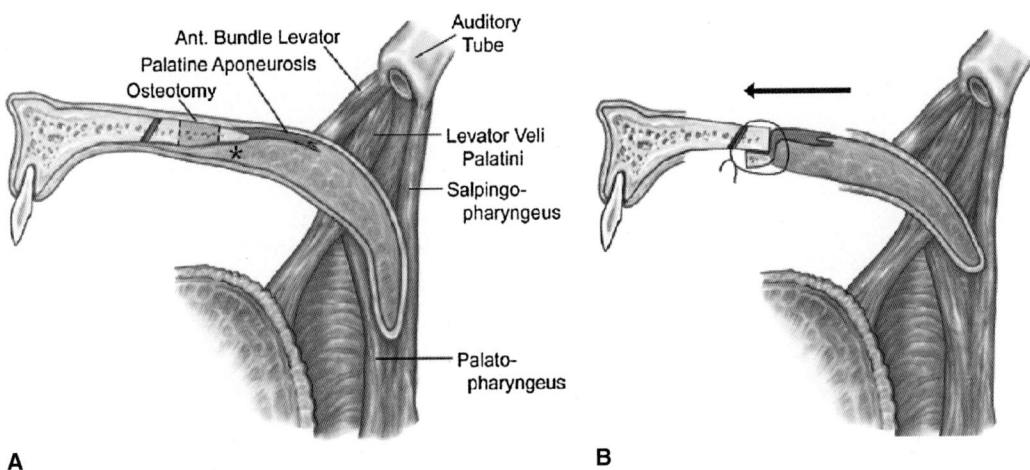

Figure 137.3 Sagittal view of a transpalatal advancement pharyngoplasty utilized to address a more *vertically* palate. **A:** The osteotomy site of the hard palate allows the soft palate to be advanced. **B:** Increased patency in the proximal nasopharynx after the soft palate is advanced creating an *obliquely* oriented palate. The uvula and distal soft palate may need to be addressed in some patients. (Reprinted from Woodson BT. Transpalatal advancement pharyngoplasty. *Oper Tech Otolaryngol Head Neck Surg* 2007;18(1):11–16, with permission.)

Specifically, the nasopharyngeal opening is narrowed in the anterior–posterior dimension at the proximal soft palate as well as distally. An *obliquely* oriented soft palate is one that has a wide proximal nasopharyngeal dimension and tapers or narrows at the distal soft palate (Fig. 137.3). During a TPA, movement of the soft palate anteriorly following osteotomy and release of the tendon aponeurosis can be beneficial to address the proximal palate where one would otherwise have to aggressively resect soft tissue with traditional UPPP methods hoping to achieve a similar result. Improvement in outcomes with TPA versus traditional UPPP has been shown in some patients (Table 137.2) (61).

The ESP (60) technique is an example of a useful technique to address the lateral wall, specifically the position of the palatopharyngeus muscles (Fig. 137.4). UPPP alone is more of a mucosal operation and does not directly affect the position of the pharyngeal muscles. Lateral pharyngeal wall collapse can play a significant role in the pathogenesis of OSA and should be recognized. The goal of ESP in airway reconstruction is to increase tension of the lateral wall and reduce lateral collapse. The technique is a modification of an earlier procedure described by Cahali (62,63) which

showed promised but resulted in significant dysphagia. The ESP technique repositions the palatopharyngeus muscles with reduced morbidity and has been shown versus UPPP to provide increased success rates (Table 137.3) (60). Additional modifications of technique to reposition the palatopharyngeus muscles and reduce lateral wall collapse are available but have not been widely utilized or studied.

Conceptually, one of the major causes of failure of palate surgery is obstruction at other nonpalatal sites. Hypopharyngeal airway narrowing has been implicated as a cause of surgical failure. Combining treatments of the hypopharyngeal airway may improve UPPP outcomes. These involve manipulation of skeletal structure as well as soft tissue. Procedures include partial glossectomy, ablational glossectomy, mandibular advancement, limited mandibular advancement, tongue and hyoid suspension procedures, lingual tonsillectomy, and limited laryngeal procedures. Only a small amount of evidence-based medicine is available on any of these procedures. Few have been compared and selection of procedure is often based on surgeon's preference. Some procedures are selected on specific anatomical abnormalities such as lingual tonsillectomy for lingual tonsil hypertrophy.

TABLE 137.2	APNEA HYPOPNEA INDEX FOR PALATAL ADVANCEMENT COMPARED WITH UPPP				
Procedure	Pre-AHI	Post-AHI	Change in AHI	P Value, Pre vs. Post	P Value Between Groups
UPPP (n = 44)	47.9 (30.0)	30.9 (24.2)	17.1 (30.1)	<0.000	
Palatal advancement (n = 30)	48.3 (24.6)	19.8 (16.8)	28.5 (25.6)	<0.000	<0.02

From Woodson BT, Robinson S, Lim HJ. Transpalatal advancement pharyngoplasty outcomes compared with uvulopalatopharyngoplasty. *Otolaryngol Head Neck Surg* 2005;133(2):211–217.

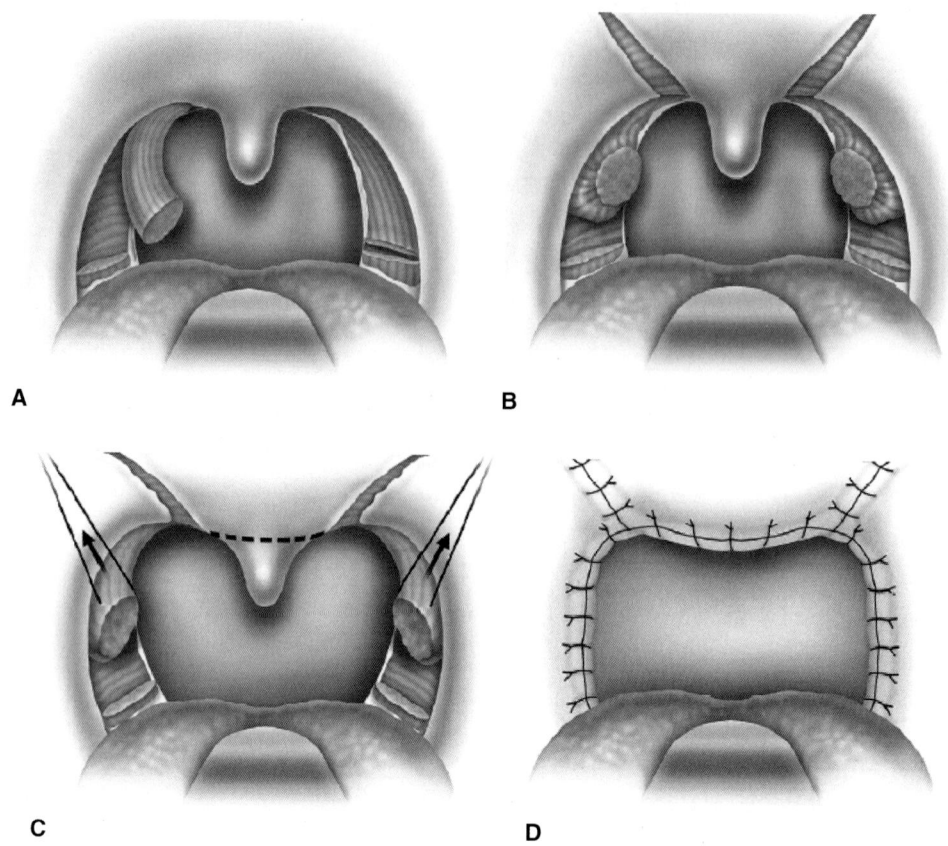

Figure 137.4 Expansion sphincter pharyngoplasty. **A:** After tonsillectomy is completed (if necessary), the palatopharyngeus muscles are isolated and transected at the inferior aspect. **B:** Mucosal incisions or submucosal tunnels are made up toward the hamulus anteriorly. **C:** A figure-eight tendon suture is placed in the cut end of the muscle to suspend it up toward the anterior soft palate and hamulus. **D:** The incisions are closed. The uvula may be preserved in some patients. (Reprinted from Pang KP, Woodson BT. Expansion sphincter pharyngoplasty in the treatment of obstructive sleep apnea. *Oper Tech Otolaryngol Head Neck Surg* 2006;17(4):223–225, with permission.)

MINIMALLY INVASIVE TECHNIQUES AND PROCEDURES FOR SNORING

Surgical therapy for snoring continues to evolve. UPPP was the first palatal procedure performed for the treatment of snoring. It continues to be an option but not frequently used because of the need for a general anesthetic and significant morbidity associated with the recovery. There has been significant interest in developing minimally invasive procedures for patients to treat SDB. In this context, we most commonly think of primary snoring as the focus of the interventions. There are a variety of reasons for this. Foremost is the fact that more invasive, multilevel, and combined therapies are required for treating OSA. Treating OSA surgically in almost all cases requires a general anesthetic in the operating room. Primary snoring on the other hand is addressed in the clinical setting were minimally invasive techniques would be ideal. Furthermore, insurance companies will often not reimburse for treatment of snoring in the operating room. Development of simple in office procedures is highly desirable. Until the 1980s, UPPP was the mainstay to treat palatal flutter snoring. In 1987, laser-assisted uvulopalatoplasty (LAUP) was performed by in Europe and later brought to the United States in 1993. The advantages over UPPP included the fact that it could be done in the office under local anesthetic with a lower incidence and severity of complications. However, significant postoperative pain was still a significant problem when treating snoring, and many patients required subsequent sessions to obtain success, if they even came

TABLE 137.3	PREOPERATIVE AND POSTOPERATIVE AHI RESULTS OF ESP AND UPPP WITH SUCCESS RATE AT AHI 50% REDUCTION AND <20	
	ESP	**UPPP**
Preoperative AHI	44.2 ± 10.2	38.1 ± 6.6
Postoperative AHI	12.0 ± 6.6	19.6 ± 7.9
P value	<0.005	<0.05
Success rate AHI reduction 50% and <20	82.60%	68.10%

From Pang KP, Woodson BT. Expansion sphincter pharyngoplasty: a new technique for the treatment of obstructive sleep apnea. *Otolaryngol Head Neck Surg* 2007;137(1):110–114.

back. Since then, less invasive and more tolerable procedures have been evolving with a goal of simple, durable, and with lasting effects. Overall, the things to consider when choosing a procedure would be presenting anatomy, short-term and long-term effectiveness based on scientific evidence, the number of sessions required for treatment, morbidity or postprocedural pain, and cost. The goal is reduce the severity and duration of snoring that is bothersome and potentially harmful without subjecting the patient to too much risk.

The most important aspect of evaluating someone with a presenting complaint of snoring would be to rule out OSA. Snoring has a prevalence of greater than 50% in the general population. Establishing the symptom as a diagnosis of primary snoring requires the AHI to be less than 5 in most cases. A review of studies evaluating snoring patients for OSA with overnight polysomnogram showed that the ability to clinically predict OSA in snoring patients is around 60% (Table 137.1) (69–74). Therefore, because of the morbidity associated with OSA and low sensitivity in predicting OSA in snoring patients on clinical exam alone, formal evaluation for OSA should be done prior to intervention for a complaint of snoring.

Snoring has traditional thought of as solely a socially bothersome problem. When evaluated against sleepiness, the importance of subjective snoring and impact on the bed partner was greater in terms of quality of life (75). This highlights the impact snoring can have socially for many patients. The impact of snoring on quality of life for the individual may be comparable to having a chronic disease (76) and may be different between certain populations (2).

More recently, snoring is being considered to have greater health impact than previously thought. There is evidence that heavy snoring is related to increased carotid artery atherosclerosis (77). An overall increase in mortality has also been identified in patients who snore despite accounting for age, sex, BMI, and AHI (7).

The sound generated during snoring is generally accepted to be from the palate in roughly 80% to 85% of patients. The remainder of patients has a pharyngeal source or a combination of areas where the snoring arises from. This is important because essentially all snoring procedures work on the principle of stabilizing or stiffening the palate. It is no coincidence therefore that palatal procedures have a reported efficacy of around 80%. Brietzke and Mair (78) explored at using acoustical analysis to predict the probability of success and showed that subjective results were positively impacted when the level of snoring could be identified.

There are a variety of factors to consider when considering procedures even if minimally invasive. They may include wound healing issues such as diabetes, the presence of a strong gag reflex, and previous snoring or OSA surgery. The use of immunosuppressant medications is also important because many of the procedures rely on the generation of scar. This could potentially be reduced with concurrent use of steroids. Lastly, occupation and hobbies of the patient should also be considered. There

are limited data on voice impact, but many vocalists and instrumentalist will be reluctant to proceed if there is any chance on negatively impacting their performance. Foodies are also another category of patients to be wary of. Taste information could theoretically be impacted by modifying receptors in the soft palate. In addition, balancing an improvement in nasal cavity airflow without deflecting too much airflow away from the olfactory tissues may be difficult when treating SDB or other NAO.

Procedures

There are a variety of procedures available in the office to treat primary snoring. Some of the same principle techniques are also being adapted for use on the nasal turbinates to improve NAO in a minimally invasive setting. In order to offer a less invasive and more tolerable following the development of UPPP and then LAUP, in 1997 Powell introduced radiofrequency tissue ablation (RFTA) of the palate for the treatment of snoring (79). Since that time additional devices and procedures have been introduced.

Radiofrequency Tissue Ablation and Coblation Techniques

RFTA, or temperature-controlled radiofrequency palatoplasty, is also done in the office under local anesthesia with the patient off any anticoagulant medications. The RF energy is delivered to the palate with a 22-gauge RF needle electrode. The generator automatically modulates the power and maintains the target temperature at 80°C to 90°C (Somnus Medical Technologies Ltd). Most patients are treated with three energy doses, one midline and two paramedian, at each treatment session. The needle is inserted in to the muscle of the soft palate with the entry point being near the junction of the hard palate. The active portion of the electrode should not extend into the base of the uvula or to the free margin of the soft palate. Most patients will require multiple treatment sessions. In a prospective, non-randomized, multicenter study of 113 patients being treated for snoring, the multiple lesion protocol was deemed most successful. However, an extended follow-up study noted that a relapse rate at 14 months was 29% (80). Terris et al. published a prospective randomized trial of LAUP versus RFTA. Twenty patients diagnosed with mild SDB were treated with LAUP achieving 86% satisfactory resolution of their snoring, and 60% of RFTA patients achieved the same results (81). Single versus multiple lesion techniques have been evaluated with multiple lesion treatments having a greater likelihood of success (82). In 2004, Stuck et al. (83) reviewed 22 studies most of which were primarily prospective, noncontrolled trials. In 345 patients, the visual analog score for snoring was significantly reduced from 8.1 ± 1.8 preoperatively to 3.5 ± 2.2 postoperatively. The primary complication noted included ulceration of mucosa (up to 43% of patients in one study). Additional findings reported were palatal fistula, uvular sloughing, and bleeding in one patient. Overall, the literature supports the possibility of a satisfactory result, but relapse has been noted long-term (84) and controlled trials are required.

Postoperative pain management is typically achieved with nonsteroidal anti-inflammatory medications such as ibuprofen and topical anesthetic lozenges. Occasionally, for any of the procedures where there is mucosal breakdown, increased analgesia may be required. If significant discomfort or palatal edema, or erythema is noted by the patient, they should be evaluated for infection and oral antibiotics considered.

Coblation, or "cold ablation," is a form of submucosal bipolar RF energy delivery. It operates at a lower energy level than RFTA (frequency range of 100 kHz and voltage of 100 to 300 V). It does require an isotonic field from saline to generate the voltage differential and subsequent reduction in tissue size by molecular disintegration. A long, thin, submucosal lesion is produced surrounding the coblation zone along the probe (*Arthrocare ENT, Sunnyvale, CA*). Palatoplasty technique can be with a single or multiple directional passes on sites in the soft palate. Comparison to other snoring procedures has been reported with comparable results and complication rates (85). Coblation techniques have also been applied to the inferior nasal turbinates with a desire for volumetric reduction and decreased NAO. Office-based use of this technique is also possible.

Injection Snoreplasty

In 2001, Drs. Brietzke and Mair (86) introduced a simple, cost-effective procedure known as snoreplasty. They found it to be highly effective in the majority of patients with easy application in the office setting. Their original procedure was developed using sodium tetradecyl sulfate (STS), but this is not always commercially available. Subsequently, other substances have been utilized including ethanol, polidocanol, and ethanolamine oleate. After the application of a topical anesthetic using spray or gel, the STS or a 50 to 50 combination of 2% lidocaine and 98% dehydrated ethanol is injected. It is typically applied as a single, midline palatal injection in the submucosal plane with a 27-gauge 1.5-inch needle. The total volume is typically 1.5 to 2.0 mL. The base of the uvula should not be injected as this may cause significant swelling. The injection should also not be in the deep muscular plane. This could theoretically lead to a greater chance of palatal fistula and increased discomfort. The submucosal plane is targeted with expected mucosal sloughing and subsequent development of scarring over the next 4 to 6 weeks. If repeat injections are needed, roughly 10% of the time, the lateral areas of the soft palate are treated approximately 6 weeks later. For patients with a strong gag reflex, they can be asked to hum, elevating their soft palate with simultaneous injection of the agent.

Postoperative management is straightforward with moderate discomfort at the most for 1 to 3 days typically. Throat lozenges, acetaminophen, or ibuprofen as needed along with regular diet as tolerated and no steroids or antibiotics are the typical instructions given. Snoring may

worsen temporarily and mucosal breakdown is expected. Follow-up is typically scheduled for 4 to 6 weeks.

An initial short-term success rate of around 80% was reported in unselected patients (86). Subsequent preoperative evaluation with acoustical analysis of snoring yielded better results with patient selection (78). Additional studies with other agents and application patterns along with comparisons to other procedures have demonstrated similar results for this simple in office procedure (87,88).

Pillar Soft Palate Implants

An additional procedure that lends itself well to the office setting with local anesthesia is the placement of Pillar implants into the soft palate. The braided polymer implants can be inserted in the office under local anesthesia. The 18 mm long by 1.5 mm round implant is designed to be placed near the junction of the hard and soft palate. The implants are deployed into the muscular layer of the soft palate using the single use delivery tool. Two additional implants are placed in parasagittal locations of the soft palate approximately 2 mm on each side. Preparation for the procedure includes the administration of a preoperative antibiotic dose and use of local anesthetic. The potential advantages with this procedure are there is potentially less pain than other palatal procedures and it could in theory have a long-term effect if extrusion does not occur. Patient selection is important. Patients with a long soft palate and uvula, narrow transverse distance between the posterior pillars, significant nasal obstruction, and snoring from the pharyngeal tissues or large tongue base would not be good candidates.

There are over a dozen articles in the literature that evaluate the response in snoring patients both with short-term and long-term follow-up. Additional studies can be found regarding the response for mild OSA and in combination with other procedures including UPPP, hypopharyngeal procedures, and CPAP use. Short-term efficacy for the reduction of snoring at 90 days was statistically significant in several studies. Long-term results defined as 12 months have also shown (89–93). An extrusion rate of 20% was noted in some of the studies; however, when this was analyzed separately, it was felt that no increase in snoring resulted if two of three implants remained in position (91,94). Despite short-term benefit which was statistically significant in several studies, a trend toward relapse has been noted long term (94,95). Studies for the treatment of mild to moderate OSA have shown limited effectiveness overall to this point (96) and of no benefit in reducing pressure needed or the improvement of compliance when combined with CPAP (97).

Anterior Palatoplasty

In 2000, the cautery-assisted palatal stiffening operation (CAPSO) was reported with a short-term efficacy of around 92% and long-term (12 months) of 77% (98). The simple office procedure for the treatment of palatal flutter snoring could be done under local anesthesia. Complications were less than 1% and included bleeding, transient velopharyngeal insufficiency (VPI), and dry mouth. Pain can be significant in some patients; however, as the demucosalized area of the soft palate heals by secondary intention.

A modification of this technique was published in 2007 for use in patients with snoring as well as mild to moderate sleep apnea (99). The procedure now known as anterior palatoplasty has been reported to have long-term benefit approximately 3 years out (100). The advantages of the procedure versus the original CAPSO are that the postoperative morbidity in one authors experience is significantly reduced. In addition, for patients with an obliquely oriented or long, redundant soft palate with extensive posterior pillar webbing and demonstrating retropalatal collapse or palatal flutter snoring, a favorable response can be achieved with low morbidity. (*For a demonstration of the procedure in the clinical setting, please refer to the online video.*)

CONCLUSION AND HIGHLIGHTS SECTION

Surgical treatments for patients with OSA continue to evolve. Select patients may benefit from a single procedure, but in the majority of adult patients, multiple sites contribute to the decreased luminal patency during sleep in patients with OSA. The nasal airway can be a critical component of airway collapse because of upstream resistance. Improved quality of sleep, compliance with other medical therapies including nasal CPAP, and improved OSA parameters have been shown in patients following nasal surgeries. A variety of palatal procedures exist for OSA and snoring. Multiple publications describe variations of the original Fujita UPPP technique and attempt to address observed anatomy among select patients. Newer techniques do provide some promising results based on improved selection of patients and airway phenotypes. Staging systems introduced by Friedman and others highlight the need for palatal surgeries to be combined with other surgeries of the airway in many cases. Snoring procedures are primarily based on reducing the social disruption from palatal flutter and vary primarily based on invasiveness, morbidity, and cost. More recent data suggest that the presence of snoring may associated with increased mortality and other health risk.

Studies evaluating a single or combination of procedures including those of the nasal and palate are difficult to compare because of wide variability in techniques. Standardization of outcomes and study parameters has been proposed to improve the understanding and role of surgery in populations of patients with OSA (101). Although the AHI and other sleep parameters are common outcome measures previously reported, newer studies have highlighted the positive impact surgery can have on quality of life (9). Additional research beyond select case series is needed to compare the effectiveness

of surgery on morbidity and mortality, outcomes from various techniques, and ability to improve outcomes based on patient selection. Outcomes beyond the traditional measures of AHI should be included. It must also be recognized that OSA is a chronic disease and remittance is common. Continued follow-up for patients is not uncommon. Improved airway phenotyping and selection systems along with identification of a genetic basis for OSA may lead to improved results in the future.

HIGHLIGHTS

- Palatal surgery for OSA continues to evolve from the original UPPP that was published by Fujita. No single procedure has proven to be successful for all patients. Limited controlled trials exist which compares the various techniques.
- The interaction between respiratory control, arousal thresholds, neuromuscular tone, and transmural pressure in the pharynx combines to effect to the patency of the airway during sleep.
- A key component of the evaluation of patients with snoring is to rule out the presence of OSA. More than half of patients who present with snoring as a complaint will have OSA.
- Surgery of the upper airway may be beneficial as a single therapy in select patients but often requires manipulation of multiple sites or levels of the airway.
- Nasal and palatal surgery may serve as an adjunctive treatment to other medical therapies including the continued use of CPAP.

REFERENCES

1. Launois SH, et al. Site of pharyngeal narrowing predicts outcome of surgery for obstructive sleep apnea. *Am Rev Respir Dis* 1993;147(1):182–189.
2. Baldwin CM, et al. Sleep disturbances, quality of life, and ethnicity: the Sleep Heart Health Study. *J Clin Sleep Med* 2010;6(2):176–183.
3. Isono S, et al. Anatomy of pharynx in patients with obstructive sleep apnea and in normal subjects. *J Appl Physiol* 1997;82(4):1319–1326.
4. Boudewyns AN, De Backer WA, Van de Heyning PH. Pattern of upper airway obstruction during sleep before and after uvulopalatopharyngoplasty in patients with obstructive sleep apnea. *Sleep Med* 2001;2(4):309–315.
5. Abdullah VJ, Wing YK, van Hasselt CA. Video sleep nasendoscopy: the Hong Kong experience. *Otolaryngol Clin North Am* 2003;36(3):461–471, vi.
6. Young T, et al. The occurrence of sleep-disordered breathing among middle-aged adults. *N Engl J Med* 1993;328(17):1230–1235.
7. Rich J, et al. An epidemiologic study of snoring and all-cause mortality. *Otolaryngol Head Neck Surg* 2011;145(2):341–346.
8. Riley RW, Powell NB, Guilleminault C. Obstructive sleep apnea syndrome: a surgical protocol for dynamic upper airway reconstruction. *J Oral Maxillofac Surg* 1993;51(7):742–747; discussion 748–749.
9. Weaver EM, et al. Studying Life Effects & Effectiveness of Palatopharyngoplasty (SLEEP) study: subjective outcomes of isolated uvulopalatopharyngoplasty. *Otolaryngol Head Neck Surg* 2011;144(4):623–631.

10. Yaremchuk K, et al. Change in Epworth Sleepiness Scale after surgical treatment of obstructive sleep apnea. *Laryngoscope* 2011;121(7):1590–1593.

11. Stull DE, et al. Relationship of nasal congestion with sleep, mood, and productivity. *Curr Med Res Opin* 2007;23(4):811–819.

12. Young T, Finn L, Kim H. Nasal obstruction as a risk factor for sleep-disordered breathing. The University of Wisconsin Sleep and Respiratory Research Group. *J Allergy Clin Immunol* 1997;99(2):S757–S762.

13. Young T, Finn L, Palta M. Chronic nasal congestion at night is a risk factor for snoring in a population-based cohort study. *Arch Intern Med* 2001;161(12):1514–1519.

14. Nilius G, et al. Upper airway complaints of patients with obstructive sleep apnea—effect of CPAP. *Pneumologie* 2007;61(1):15–19.

15. Davis SS, Eccles R. Nasal congestion: mechanisms, measurement and medications. Core information for the clinician. *Clin Otolaryngol Allied Sci* 2004;29(6):659–666.

16. Tomkinson A. Acoustic rhinometry: its place in rhinology. *Clin Otolaryngol Allied Sci* 1997;22(3):189–191.

17. Cuddihy PJ, Eccles R. The use of nasal spirometry as an objective measure of nasal septal deviation and the effectiveness of septal surgery. *Clin Otolaryngol Allied Sci* 2003;28(4):325–330.

18. Cuddihy PJ, Eccles R. The use of nasal spirometry for the assessment of unilateral nasal obstruction associated with changes in posture in healthy subjects and subjects with upper respiratory tract infection. *Clin Otolaryngol Allied Sci* 2003;28(2):108–111.

19. Realica RM, et al. A simplified pneumotachometer for the quantitative assessment of velopharyngeal incompetence. *Ann Plast Surg* 2000;44(2):163–166.

20. Doghramji K, et al. Predictors of outcome for uvulopalatopharyngoplasty. *Laryngoscope* 1995;105(3 Pt 1):311–314.

21. Parker AJ, et al. A comparison of active anterior rhinomanometry and nasometry in the objective assessment of nasal obstruction. *Rhinology* 1990;28(1):47–53.

22. Clement PA, Gordts F. Consensus report on acoustic rhinometry and rhinomanometry. *Rhinology* 2005;43(3):169–179.

23. Lenders H, Pirsig W. Diagnostic value of acoustic rhinometry: patients with allergic and vasomotor rhinitis compared with normal controls. *Rhinology* 1990;28(1):5–16.

24. Corey JP, et al. A comparison of the nasal cross-sectional areas and volumes obtained with acoustic rhinometry and magnetic resonance imaging. *Otolaryngol Head Neck Surg* 1997;117(4):349–354.

25. Bailie N, et al. An overview of numerical modelling of nasal airflow. *Rhinology* 2006;44(1):53–57.

26. Zhao K, et al. Numerical modeling of nasal obstruction and endoscopic surgical intervention: outcome to airflow and olfaction. *Am J Rhinol* 2006;20(3):308–316.

27. Yu CC, et al. Computational fluid dynamic study on obstructive sleep apnea syndrome treated with maxillomandibular advancement. *J Craniofac Surg* 2009;20(2):426–430.

28. Mosges R, et al. Computational fluid dynamics analysis of nasal flow. *B-ENT* 2010;6(3):161–165.

29. White DP, et al. The effects of nasal anesthesia on breathing during sleep. *Am Rev Respir Dis* 1985;132(5):972–975.

30. Meurice JC, et al. Effects of mouth opening on upper airway collapsibility in normal sleeping subjects. *Am J Respir Crit Care Med* 1996;153(1):255–259.

31. Rhee JS, et al. Toward personalized nasal surgery using computational fluid dynamics. *Arch Facial Plast Surg* 2011;13(5):305–310.

32. Buccheri A, Dilella G, Stella R. Rapid palatal expansion and pharyngeal space. Cephalometric evaluation. *Prog Orthod* 2004;5(2):160–171.

33. Compadretti GC, Tasca I, Bonetti GA. Nasal airway measurements in children treated by rapid maxillary expansion. *Am J Rhinol* 2006;20(4):385–393.

34. Zwillich CW, et al. Disturbed sleep and prolonged apnea during nasal obstruction in normal men. *Am Rev Respir Dis* 1981;124(2):158–160.

35. Olsen KD, Kern EB, Westbrook PR. Sleep and breathing disturbance secondary to nasal obstruction. *Otolaryngol Head Neck Surg* 1981;89(5):804–810.

36. Friedman M, et al. Impact of nasal obstruction on obstructive sleep apnea. *Otolaryngol Head Neck Surg* 2011;144(6):1000–1004.

37. Friedman M, et al. Effect of improved nasal breathing on obstructive sleep apnea. *Otolaryngol Head Neck Surg* 2000;122(1):71–74.

38. Li HY, et al. Improvement in quality of life after nasal surgery alone for patients with obstructive sleep apnea and nasal obstruction. *Arch Otolaryngol Head Neck Surg* 2008;134(4):429–433.

39. Kim ST, et al. Polysomnographic effects of nasal surgery for snoring and obstructive sleep apnea. *Acta Otolaryngol* 2004;124(3):297–300.

40. Choi JH, et al. Efficacy of single-staged modified uvulopalatopharyngoplasty with nasal surgery in adults with obstructive sleep apnea syndrome. *Otolaryngol Head Neck Surg* 2011;144(6):994–999.

41. Verse T, Maurer JT, Pirsig W. Effect of nasal surgery on sleep-related breathing disorders. *Laryngoscope* 2002;112(1):64–68.

42. Nakata S, et al. Effects of nasal surgery on sleep quality in obstructive sleep apnea syndrome with nasal obstruction. *Am J Rhinol* 2008;22(1):59–63.

43. Pirsig W, Verse T. Long-term results in the treatment of obstructive sleep apnea. *Eur Arch Otorhinolaryngol* 2000;257(10):570–577.

44. Batra PS, Seiden AM, Smith TL. Surgical management of adult inferior turbinate hypertrophy: a systematic review of the evidence. *Laryngoscope* 2009;119(9):1819–1827.

45. Clement WA, White PS. Trends in turbinate surgery literature: a 35-year review. *Clin Otolaryngol Allied Sci* 2001;26(2).124–128.

46. Cingi C, et al. Microdebrider-assisted versus radiofrequency-assisted inferior turbinoplasty: a prospective study with objective and subjective outcome measures. *Acta Otorhinolaryngol Ital* 2010;30(3):138–143.

47. Joniau S, et al. Long-term comparison between submucosal cauterization and powered reduction of the inferior turbinates. *Laryngoscope* 2006;116(9):1612–1616.

48. Lee JY, Lee JD. Comparative study on the long-term effectiveness between coblation- and microdebrider-assisted partial turbinoplasty. *Laryngoscope* 2006;116(5):729–734.

49. Hol MK, Huizing EH. Treatment of inferior turbinate pathology: a review and critical evaluation of the different techniques. *Rhinology* 2000;38(4):157–166.

50. Nease CJ, Krempl GA. Radiofrequency treatment of turbinate hypertrophy: a randomized, blinded, placebo-controlled clinical trial. *Otolaryngol Head Neck Surg* 2004;130(3):291–299.

51. Woodson BT, Wooten MR. Manometric and endoscopic localization of airway obstruction after uvulopalatopharyngoplasty. *Otolaryngol Head Neck Surg* 1994;111(1):38–43.

52. Langin T, et al. Upper airway changes in snorers and mild sleep apnea sufferers after uvulopalatopharyngoplasty (UPPP). *Chest* 1998;113(6):1595–1603.

53. Friedman M, Ibrahim H, Joseph NJ. Staging of obstructive sleep apnea/hypopnea syndrome: a guide to appropriate treatment. *Laryngoscope* 2004;114(3):454–459.

54. Friedman M, Ibrahim H, Bass L. Clinical staging for sleep-disordered breathing. *Otolaryngol Head Neck Surg* 2002;127(1):13–21.

55. Hessel NS, de Vries N. Results of uvulopalatopharyngoplasty after diagnostic workup with polysomnography and sleep endoscopy: a report of 136 snoring patients. *Eur Arch Otorhinolaryngol* 2003;260(2):91–95.

56. Woodson BT, Conley SF. Prediction of uvulopalatopharyngoplasty response using cephalometric radiographs. *Am J Otolaryngol* 1997;18(3):179–184.

57. Sher AE. Update on upper airway surgery for obstructive sleep apnea. *Curr Opin Pulm Med* 1995;1(6):504–511.

58. Caples SM, et al. Surgical modifications of the upper airway for obstructive sleep apnea in adults: a systematic review and meta-analysis. *Sleep* 2010;33(10):1396–1407.

59. Friedman M, et al. Z-palatoplasty (ZPP): a technique for patients without tonsils. *Otolaryngol Head Neck Surg* 2004;131(1):89–100.

60. Pang KP, Woodson BT. Expansion sphincter pharyngoplasty: a new technique for the treatment of obstructive sleep apnea. *Otolaryngol Head Neck Surg* 2007;137(1):110–114.

61. Woodson BT, Robinson S, Lim HJ. Transpalatal advancement pharyngoplasty outcomes compared with uvulopalatopharyngoplasty. *Otolaryngol Head Neck Surg* 2005;133(2):211–217.

62. Cahali MB. Lateral pharyngoplasty: a new treatment for obstructive sleep apnea hypopnea syndrome. *Laryngoscope* 2003;113(11):1961–1968.

63. Cahali MB, et al. Lateral pharyngoplasty versus uvulopalatopharyngoplasty: a clinical, polysomnographic and computed tomography measurement comparison. *Sleep* 2004;27(5):942–950.

64. Li HY, et al. Modified uvulopalatopharyngoplasty: the extended uvulopalatal flap. *Am J Otolaryngol* 2003;24(5):311–316.

65. Weaver EM, Maynard C, Yueh B. Survival of veterans with sleep apnea: continuous positive airway pressure versus surgery. *Otolaryngol Head Neck Surg* 2004;130(6):659–665.

66. Kezirian EJ, et al. Risk factors for serious complication after uvulopalatopharyngoplasty. *Arch Otolaryngol Head Neck Surg* 2006;132(10):1091–1098.

67. Kezirian EJ, et al. Incidence of serious complications after uvulopalatopharyngoplasty. *Laryngoscope* 2004;114(3):450–453.

68. Woodson BT, Toohill RJ. Transpalatal advancement pharyngoplasty for obstructive sleep apnea. *Laryngoscope* 1993;103(3):269–276.

69. Viner S, Szalai JP, Hoffstein V. Are history and physical examination a good screening test for sleep apnea? *Ann Intern Med* 1991;115(5):356–359.

70. Hoffstein V, Szalai JP. Predictive value of clinical features in diagnosing obstructive sleep apnea. *Sleep* 1993;16(2):118–122.

71. Deegan PC, McNicholas WT. Predictive value of clinical features for the obstructive sleep apnea syndrome. *Eur Respir J* 1996;9(1):117–124.

72. Vaidya AM, et al. Identifying obstructive sleep apnea in patients presenting for laser-assisted uvulopalatoplasty. *Laryngoscope* 1996;106(4):431–437.

73. Tami TA, Duncan HJ, Pfleger M. Identification of obstructive sleep apnea in patients who snore. *Laryngoscope* 1998;108(4 Pt 1):508–513.

74. Rowley JA, Aboussouan LS, Badr MS. The use of clinical prediction formulas in the evaluation of obstructive sleep apnea. *Sleep* 2000;23(7):929–938.

75. Woodson BT, Han JK. Relationship of snoring and sleepiness as presenting symptoms in a sleep clinic population. *Ann Otol Rhinol Laryngol* 2005;114(10):762–767.

76. Loth S, et al. Evaluation of the quality of life of male snorers using the Nottingham Health Profile. *Acta Otolaryngol* 1998;118(5):723–727.

77. Lee SA, et al. Heavy snoring as a cause of carotid artery atherosclerosis. *Sleep* 2008;31(9):1207–1213.

78. Brietzke SE, Mair EA. Acoustical analysis of snoring: can the probability of success be predicted? *Otolaryngol Head Neck Surg* 2006;135(3):417–420.

79. Powell NB, et al. Radiofrequency volumetric tissue reduction of the palate in subjects with sleep-disordered breathing. *Chest* 1998;113(5):1163–1174.

80. Li KK, et al. Radiofrequency volumetric reduction of the palate: an extended follow-up study. *Otolaryngol Head Neck Surg* 2000;122(3):410–414.

81. Terris DJ, et al. Preliminary findings from a prospective, randomized trial of two palatal operations for sleep-disordered breathing. *Otolaryngol Head Neck Surg* 2002;127(4):315–323.

82. Ferguson M, et al. Radiofrequency tissue volume reduction: multilesion vs single-lesion treatments for snoring. *Arch Otolaryngol Head Neck Surg* 2001;127(9):1113–1118.

83. Stuck BA, et al. Radiofrequency surgery of the soft palate in the treatment of snoring: a review of the literature. *Sleep* 2004;27(3):551–555.

84. Stuck BA. Radiofrequency-assisted uvulopalatoplasty for snoring: long-term follow-up. *Laryngoscope* 2009;119(8):1617–1620.

85. Back LJ, et al. Bipolar radiofrequency thermal ablation of the soft palate in habitual snorers without significant desaturations assessed by magnetic resonance imaging. *Am J Respir Crit Care Med* 2002;166(6):865–871.

86. Brietzke SE, Mair EA. Injection snoreplasty: how to treat snoring without all the pain and expense. *Otolaryngol Head Neck Surg* 2001;124(5):503–510.

87. Iseri M, Balcioglu O. Radiofrequency versus injection snoreplasty in simple snoring. *Otolaryngol Head Neck Surg* 2005;133(2):224–228.

88. Al-Jassim AH, Lesser TH. Single dose injection snoreplasty: investigation or treatment? *J Laryngol Otol* 2008;122(11):1190–1193.

89. Nordgard S, et al. Palatal implants: a new method for the treatment of snoring. *Acta Otolaryngol* 2004;124(8):970–975.

90. Ho WK, Wei WI, Chung KF. Managing disturbing snoring with palatal implants: a pilot study. *Arch Otolaryngol Head Neck Surg* 2004;130(6):753–758.

91. Maurer JT, et al. Palatal implants for primary snoring: short-term results of a new minimally invasive surgical technique. *Otolaryngol Head Neck Surg* 2005;132(1):125–131.

92. Romanow JH, Catalano PJ. Initial U.S. pilot study: palatal implants for the treatment of snoring. *Otolaryngol Head Neck Surg* 2006;134(4):551–557.

93. Gillespie MB, et al. Effectiveness of Pillar palatal implants for snoring management. *Otolaryngol Head Neck Surg* 2009;140(3):363–368.

94. Nordgard S, et al. Palatal implants for the treatment of snoring: long-term results. *Otolaryngol Head Neck Surg* 2006;134(4):558–564.

95. Catalano P, Goh YH, Romanow J. Additional palatal implants for refractory snoring. *Otolaryngol Head Neck Surg* 2007;137(1):105–109.

96. Steward DL, et al. Palate implants for obstructive sleep apnea: multi-institution, randomized, placebo-controlled study. *Otolaryngol Head Neck Surg* 2008;139(4):506–510.

97. Gillespie MB, et al. Effect of palatal implants on continuous positive airway pressure and compliance. *Otolaryngol Head Neck Surg* 2011;144(2):230–236.

98. Mair EA, Day RH. Cautery-assisted palatal stiffening operation. *Otolaryngol Head Neck Surg* 2000;122(4):547–556.

99. Pang KP, Terris DJ. Modified cautery-assisted palatal stiffening operation: new method for treating snoring and mild obstructive sleep apnea. *Otolaryngol Head Neck Surg* 2007;136(5):823–826.

100. Pang KP, et al. Anterior palatoplasty for the treatment of OSA: three-year results. *Otolaryngol Head Neck Surg* 2009;141(2):253–256.

101. Kezirian EJ, et al. Reporting results of obstructive sleep apnea syndrome surgery trials. *Otolaryngol Head Neck Surg* 2011;144(4):496–499.

138 Hypopharyngeal and Skeletal Surgery for OSA

Eric James Kezirian   Edward M. Weaver

Obstructive sleep apnea (OSA) results from a combination of numerous factors related to anatomy, airway dilator muscle activation, ventilatory control, lung volumes, and arousal threshold, with wide variation in the specific factors involved for affected individuals (1). Surgical OSA treatment is designed to alter upper airway anatomy and/or collapsibility, and a key goal of surgical evaluation is the determination of the anatomical factors that contribute substantially to obstruction in an individual patient. One approach divides the upper airway into three regions: the nasal, retropalatal, and so-called hypopharyngeal (also called retrolingual or retroglossal) (2). Another approach divides anatomy into skeletal (the box) and soft tissue (the contents) components that impact the airway. In OSA, obstruction often occurs in more than one of these regions and may be related to both bony and soft tissue components.

While all regions and components of the airway are evaluated together and integrated, this chapter presents aspects of patient evaluation relevant to hypopharyngeal procedures and skeletal surgery and then presents these procedures with their reported outcomes and risks.

OSA SURGICAL EVALUATION

A thorough history and physical examination are the foundation of any surgical examination, but there are specific components and possible additional studies that have particular relevance to hypopharyngeal and skeletal surgery. As is true for nasal and palatal surgery, the examination must evaluate the anatomical factors that can contribute substantially to upper airway obstruction. Hypopharyngeal procedures are ultimately directed at one or more of the structures that can produce hypopharyngeal obstruction: the oropharyngeal lateral walls, tongue, and epiglottis. In contrast, skeletal surgery enlarges airway dimensions along the entire length of the pharynx without a specific focus on individual structures.

The role of the history in detection of hypopharyngeal obstruction is limited, as no studies have indicated that any of the common OSA signs and symptoms are unique to hypopharyngeal obstruction. The same is true for sleep study results, as the apnea–hypopnea index (AHI) has not shown a consistent or strong association with patterns of obstruction or specific involved structures. However, these evaluations help determine the severity of OSA and its burden and, therefore, the aggressiveness of treatment.

In contrast, physical examination can identify factors that can be highly suggestive of hypopharyngeal obstruction. Table 138.1 lists some evaluation techniques that have been used for pharyngeal examination, with the goal of characterizing the pattern of airway obstruction. Because obesity and weight gain are well-established risk factors for OSA (1), measurement of the height and weight (with calculation of body mass index (BMI), a commonly used but crude measure of obesity) is an essential component of physical examination, as is questioning about changes in body weight and an association with signs or symptoms in the patient history. There are multiple mechanisms that may explain the association between increased body weight and OSA, including an increase in soft tissue mass surrounding the pharyngeal airway and decreased lung volumes that develop with increases in body weight. Magnetic resonance imaging (MRI) studies have demonstrated that weight loss results in a decrease in lateral pharyngeal wall volume (3). Increases in body weight may also result in fat deposition within the tongue base, based on a higher fat content of that tissue, relative to other portions of the tongue, shown with computed tomography (CT) (4) and a correlation between BMI and fat content of the tongue base that was notably stronger than for other parts of the tongue (5). BMI and changes in body weight are major

TABLE 138.1	AIRWAY EVALUATION TECHNIQUES

Necessary
- Awake physical examination
- Awake fiberoptic endoscopy

Adjuvant
- Plain film radiography, including lateral cephalometry
- Computed tomography
- Magnetic resonance imaging
- Airway pressure monitoring
- Acoustic techniques, including acoustic pharyngometry and flextube reflectometry
- Drug-induced sleep endoscopy

factors in treatment outcomes, and these are discussed later in this chapter.

In addition to measurement of body weight and BMI, visual examination of the oral cavity, including the tongue, tonsils, mandible, and lateral pharyngeal walls, can prove invaluable. The modified Mallampati position reflects absolute tongue size, soft palate length, and the dimensions and position of the mandible (which define the space for the tongue) (6,7). The combination of modified Mallampati position, tonsil size (according to the Brodsky classification), and BMI enables classification according to Friedman stage, which has demonstrated a stronger association with outcomes after uvulopalatopharyngoplasty (UPPP) with tonsillectomy than the AHI has (6,8). The improvement in outcomes for a combination of hypopharyngeal surgery (submucosal tongue radiofrequency) and UPPP with tonsillectomy, compared to UPPP with tonsillectomy alone, in Friedman stage II and III patients (9) suggests that these groups have at least some component of hypopharyngeal obstruction and that the Friedman stage can play an important role in considering hypopharyngeal procedures.

The position and dimensions of the mandible and dentition can contribute to OSA and affect treatment outcomes. The mandible is an important component of the bony framework housing the soft tissues surrounding the upper airway, and both retrognathia and mandibular deficiency/insufficiency compromise the airway, particularly the hypopharyngeal airway. Examination of the mandible can occur with direct inspection, indirect evaluation based on the dental occlusion, or imaging studies. Direct inspection is the simplest technique. Dental occlusion is commonly defined by the Angle classification comparing the position of the mesiobuccal cusp of the maxillary first molar to the buccal groove of the mandibular first molar. This can reflect the mandible position and size relative to the maxilla, but two limitations are that the Angle classification can be affected substantially by dental and orthodontic treatment, including dental extractions, and that relative position and size of the mandible may not be as

important as absolute measures (also true for the maxilla). Multiple imaging modalities can assist in evaluation of the mandible, and of these, lateral cephalometry has been studied most extensively in OSA. Although somewhat limited as a two-dimensional assessment of the airway, lateral cephalometry can image multiple aspects of bony and soft tissue anatomy. Individuals with OSA and normal BMI have demonstrated retrognathia (decreased sella–nasion–mandible B point angle, or SNB angle), a narrowed space between the tongue base and posterior pharyngeal wall (posterior airway space), and an increased distance between the mandible and hyoid bone (mandibular plane–hyoid distance) (10). Findings of lateral cephalometry have also demonstrated an association with outcomes after certain hypopharyngeal procedures, and these findings are discussed later in this chapter.

There is no standardized or objective assessment of the lateral pharyngeal walls during physical examination. Subjectively, certain factors may suggest a greater contribution of the lateral walls to airway obstruction: their thickness (determined indirectly by visual inspection of the pharyngeal aspect), folds or redundancy in the mucosa covering the underlying musculature (suggesting increased thickness and/or tissue laxity), and any narrowing of the transverse dimensions of the pharyngeal airway that can occur with thickened walls. MRI offers the most detailed assessment of the lateral pharyngeal walls, but currently it is used solely for research purposes. Improved methods for examination of the lateral pharyngeal walls will likely contribute substantially to understanding OSA and treatment outcomes.

Awake fiberoptic endoscopy is an invaluable tool for evaluating not only the nasal and retropalatal regions but also the hypopharyngeal region. Indirect laryngoscopy can inspect the larynx and tongue base, but its use in OSA is limited for three reasons. First, many individuals with OSA have a large tongue that impairs visualization of the hypopharynx due to physical blockage of the line of sight and/or increased likelihood of triggering a gag reflex. Second, indirect laryngoscopy requires mouth opening and tongue retraction, both of which disturb the natural anatomy of the hypopharyngeal airway. Third, it does not allow visualization of the hypopharyngeal airway under varying clinical states. Fiberoptic laryngopharyngoscopy enables a more-detailed evaluation of the hypopharyngeal airway and the individual structures surrounding it under various conditions, making it a mainstay of hypopharyngeal evaluation. The airway caliber, site of narrowing, and surrounding structures (tongue base, lateral walls, and epiglottis) can be seen under conditions such as mouth open versus closed, during snoring versus restful breathing, inspiration versus end-expiration, upright versus supine, mandible advanced forward versus neutral position, and with increased negative intrathoracic pressure (Muller maneuver). The Muller maneuver can be performed during awake endoscopy, but there are no reported studies related

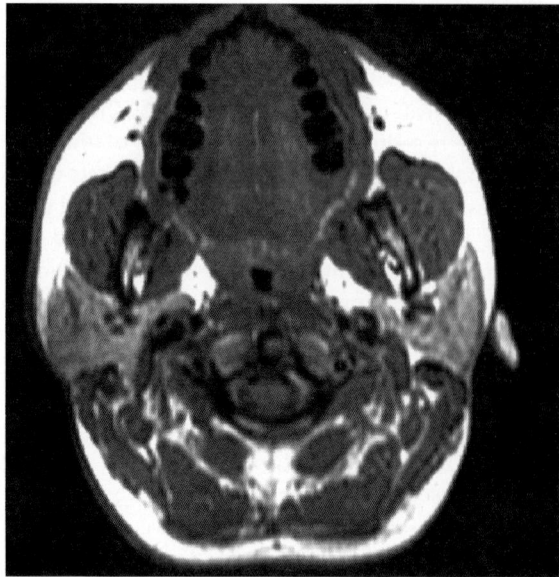

Figure 138.1 Axial T2-weighted MRI showing narrow hypopharyngeal airway posterior to the tongue base.

to hypopharyngeal procedure selection or outcomes. Subjective evaluation of airway dimensions and structures using endoscopy can provide important and useful information (11), but there are currently no commonly used, standardized, and objective measurements.

Studies based on MRI (Fig. 138.1) (12) and CT (4), in addition to a number of other modalities such as acoustic methods, airway pressure sensing, optical coherence tomography (13), and computational fluid dynamics (14), have provided a greater understanding of anatomical abnormalities among individuals with OSA and, to some extent, outcomes after palate procedures. Thus far, they have largely been limited to research purposes or surgical planning. However, these studies have important limitations for this discussion, for three reasons: most of these studies have been performed during wakefulness, they have generally characterized all hypopharyngeal region obstruction as similar without differentiation among possible subtypes, and, other than the lateral cephalogram, they have not been examined for a possible association between imaging findings and outcomes after hypopharyngeal procedures or skeletal surgery. The first two limitations are discussed here.

Airway examination during wakefulness—whether physical examination, endoscopy, or imaging—has important limitations related to the physiologic changes that occur during sleep, such as the marked decrease in genioglossus muscle tone that occurs at sleep onset (15) and the further decrease in rapid eye movement (REM) sleep (16). Of course, individuals with OSA demonstrate airway obstruction only during sleep, often with increased frequency during REM sleep. The implications for evaluation of hypopharyngeal airway obstruction (especially that related to the tongue) may be substantial. Although awake

evaluation, especially office examination, generally has relatively low cost, there are likely important differences between examinations performed during wakefulness and sleep, and further investigation will elucidate how important those differences are.

Multiple investigators have studied the airway under conditions of anesthesia, including drug-induced sleep endoscopy (DISE) (17), originally described as sleep nasendoscopy in 1991 (18). The continuum of sedation ranges from wakefulness to conscious sedation to unconscious sedation to general anesthesia, and DISE involves endoscopic examination of the pharyngeal airway during unconscious sedation. While unconscious sedation under propofol may not be a perfect simulation of natural sleep, with identical effects on upper airway collapsibility, pharyngeal dilator muscle activity during DISE appears to lie somewhere between natural non-REM and REM sleep (15,16,19,20). DISE findings have suggested that there may be multiple subtypes of hypopharyngeal region obstruction; during unconscious sedation, individuals with OSA generally have one or more of the following structures contributing to hypopharyngeal obstruction: the oropharyngeal lateral walls, tongue, and/or epiglottis (Figs. 138.2 to 138.4, respectively) (17,21). Although hypopharyngeal procedures are ultimately directed at specific structures (including these three), it remains unclear whether this diversity of patterns within the broader category of hypopharyngeal obstruction has implications for outcomes of surgical and nonsurgical treatment (i.e., whether tongue-directed procedures work better in individuals with tongue-related hypopharyngeal obstruction than in those with obstruction more related to the oropharyngeal lateral walls or epiglottis). It is possible that alleviation of one source of airway narrowing/obstruction

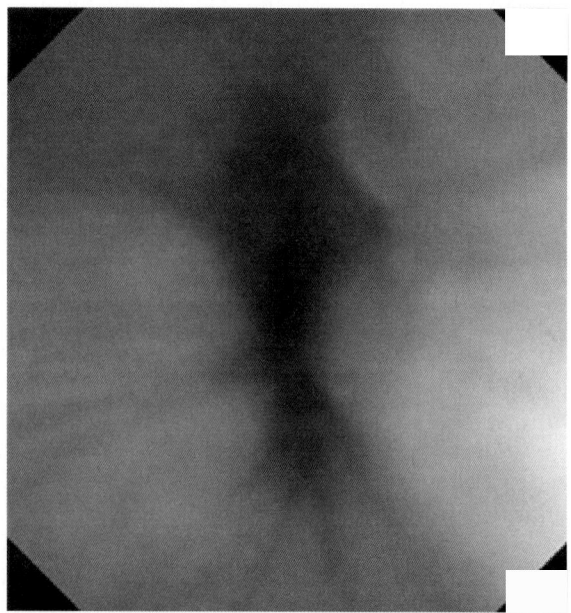

Figure 138.2 Oropharyngeal lateral wall collapse during DISE.

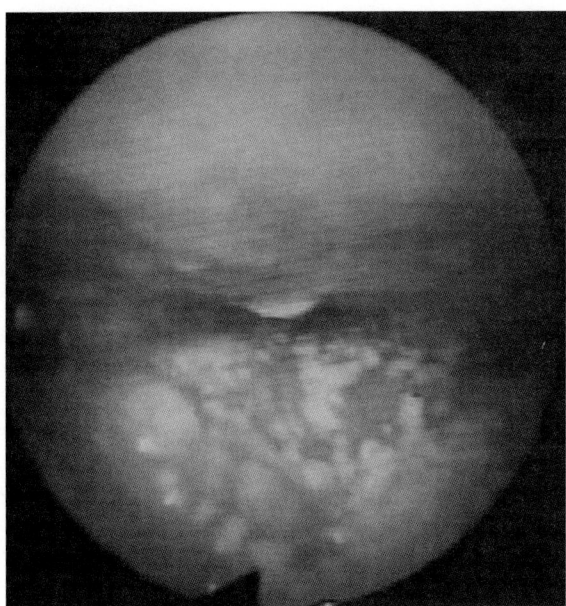

Figure 138.3 Tongue base prolapse during DISE.

may alleviate that from others, for example, by reducing resistive Bernoulli forces. Thus, the interaction of anatomy, physiology (e.g., depth of sleep, collapsibility, and ventilatory control), airflow dynamics, and conditions (e.g., body position) is complex. At a minimum, the grouping of all hypopharyngeal region obstruction together, as has occurred with most evaluation techniques, does not capture this diversity. Although DISE findings have demonstrated an association with outcomes for palate surgery (22,23), similar evaluations have not occurred for hypopharyngeal procedures.

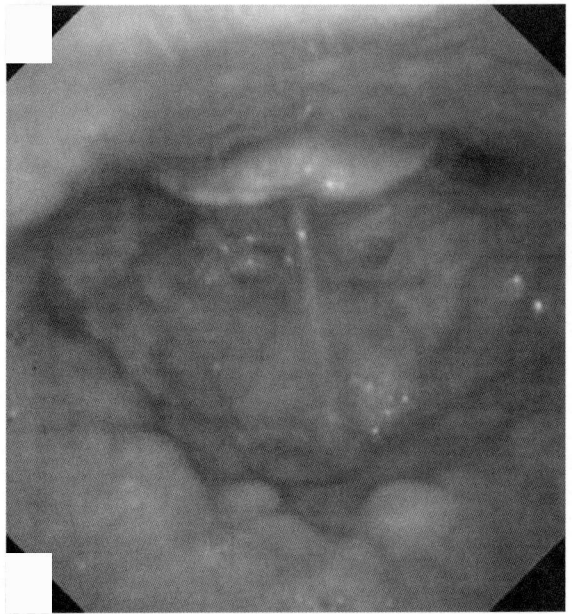

Figure 138.4 Epiglottic prolapse (anteroposterior) during DISE.

The importance of preoperative evaluation—and the association between findings of the preoperative evaluation and surgical outcomes—cannot be overemphasized. The next section discusses outcome assessment, followed by the available hypopharyngeal procedures and skeletal surgery and their reported outcomes, highlighting the factors that may be apparent during preoperative evaluation that have shown an association with outcomes, as well as their risks.

OUTCOME ASSESSMENT IN OSA SURGERY

It remains unclear how best to measure treatment outcomes for sleep apnea (24). Treatment should address primarily clinical outcomes, such as mortality, cardiovascular disease, motor vehicle crashes, daytime function, symptoms, and quality of life deficits. Surrogate measures of treatment outcome, like sleep study parameters (such as the AHI) and inflammatory markers, are important if they translate into clinically important effects. Unfortunately for patients diagnosed with sleep apnea, improvements in sleep study parameters do not necessarily translate directly into all the desired outcomes (25). Whenever possible, clinical outcomes should be measured primarily in preference to surrogate outcomes (26). Table 138.2 highlights clinically important outcomes, while Table 138.3 lists common surrogate outcome measures.

Sleep Testing Outcomes

Surgical treatment often does not physiologically cure sleep apnea (i.e., permanently normalize the AHI). This fact has left some people to suggest that surgical treatment too often fails (27–29). This view neglects the risk to patients who are otherwise inadequately treated. When considering surgical outcomes, one must view them in the context of outcomes from alternative therapies for each patient (24).

Although continuous positive airway pressure (CPAP) at the optimal pressure determined in the sleep laboratory dramatically improves physiologic measures, this is not the case for all patients (30) and often does not completely normalize the AHI (31). Moreover, the physiologic

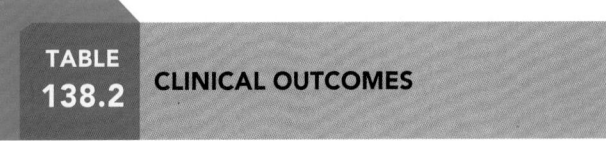

TABLE 138.2	CLINICAL OUTCOMES

- Mortality risk
- Cardiovascular disease and events
- Motor vehicle crashes
- Symptoms
- Daytime function
- Quality of life (patient and partner)

TABLE 138.3	EXAMPLES OF SURROGATE OUTCOME MEASURES

- Sleep study parameters
  - Apnea-hypopnea index
  - Oxygenation parameters
  - Arousal indexes
- Physiologic measures, such as airway collapsibility (critical airway closing pressure)
- Inflammatory markers

improvement with CPAP depends on the duration of use during sleep time. The minimum usage needed to consider CPAP physiologically successful is unknown (30). The current standard of 4 hours per night on over five nights per week (32) is probably inadequate (33). This minimum threshold amounts to 20 hours of use per week (4 hours per night × 5 nights per week), covering just 37% of the recommended 56 hours of sleep time per week (8 hours per night × 7 nights per week). Indeed, emerging data indicate a monotonically increasing dose–response relationship between the amount of average nightly CPAP use and its effect on improving clinically important outcomes like subjective sleepiness, objective sleepiness, and functional outcomes (34). Likewise, 5-year survival increases with the amount of CPAP use, with the best outcome achieved with more than 6 hours of average nightly use (35).

Because the AHI defines OSA, it is the most common primary OSA treatment end point for clinicians and in research studies. However, other sleep study parameters may be more reliable and physiologically more important (e.g., apnea index, desaturation index, percentage of sleep time with oxygen saturation below 90%). The use of AHI for outcome assessment is complicated by the variation in definitions of respiratory events (especially for hypopneas) over time and the multiplicity of definitions proposed in guidelines (36,37); the result is that notable differences exist across sleep laboratories and for different studies.

The large majority of studies for hypopharyngeal surgery and skeletal surgery are case series, and there have been attempts to compare results across procedures or, for hypopharyngeal procedures, the combination of soft palate surgery and a hypopharyngeal procedure (38–40). Because most studies of OSA surgery report AHI outcomes, these comparisons have focused largely on AHI and have examined the proportion of treated individuals who have achieved an arbitrary threshold "response" to treatment or "success," typically a reduction of at least 50% in the AHI to a level below 20 or 15 events per hour. However, this is a major oversimplification, as OSA treatment is not solely a number. Beware that the use of a single parameter in reporting trial outcomes oversimplifies the complexity of OSA disease burden and treatment outcome.

Clinical Outcomes

More important than the physiologic outcomes are the clinically important outcomes. Surgical treatment improves symptoms such as daytime sleepiness, quality of life, and daytime performance and function. One study of staged, multilevel surgical therapy compared to CPAP users showed similar symptoms and quality of life following treatment (41). Objective outcomes are possible for some clinical end points but can be cumbersome, expensive, or unavailable. Valid, reliable measures can evaluate subjective outcomes, with specific statistical and analytical approaches to evaluate potential placebo effects. Most of the research evaluating clinical outcomes in OSA surgery has focused on soft palate surgery, but there are a number of studies of hypopharyngeal surgery that have used validated measures of symptoms, daytime functioning, and sleep-related quality of life.

HYPOPHARYNGEAL PROCEDURES AND OUTCOMES

Hypopharyngeal procedures can be differentiated based on whether they are designed either to increase tissue tension to reduce collapsibility or to decrease tongue tissue volume and whether they are directed at the tongue, epiglottis, and/or, in some cases, the lateral pharyngeal walls. Overall, these procedures can be grouped into three categories, presented in Table 138.4.

Summary of reported outcomes for these procedures, generally when performed in combination with palate surgery, are presented in Table 138.5. One striking finding is that all hypopharyngeal procedures or procedure categories have a wide range of reported outcomes both for an overall case series and for individual subjects within each series. This likely reflects the importance of subject-specific characteristics that are not immediately apparent in these case series reports. This chapter discusses factors that have been associated with outcomes, but future investigations

TABLE 138.4	HYPOPHARYNGEAL PROCEDURES

- Tongue Advancement/Stabilization
  - Genioglossus advancement and mortised genioplasty
  - Hyoid suspension
  - Tongue stabilization suture
- Tongue Reduction
  - Submucosal radiofrequency reduction
  - Midline glossectomy
  - Lingualplasty
  - Hyoepiglottoplasty
  - Lingual tonsillectomy
- Epiglottis Correction
  - Hyoid suspension
  - Epiglottoplasty

| TABLE 138.5 | SUMMARY OF OUTCOMES OF HYPOPHARYNGEAL PROCEDURES[a] | | | | | |

	Response (AHI)		Range of Response Rate in Individual Series	Daytime Sleepiness	Quality of Life	Association with Outcomes
Genioglossus advancement (43–47)	57%	70/122	39%–78%			BMI
Mortised genioplasty (48)	48%	16/33				BMI, AHI
Hyoid suspension (49–55)	58%	174/300	18%–78%	Improved[a]		BMI? LSAT?
Genioglossus advancement + hyoid suspension (46,47,54,56–68)	55%	342/620	24%–78%	Improved		BMI, AHI
Tongue stabilization suture (69–79)	54%	116/216	20%–82%	Improved	Improved	BMI, technique
Submucosal tongue radiofrequency (9,70,71,80–99)	49%	408/868	20%–81%	Improved[a]	Improved[a]	Technique, FS; ±AHI
Tongue reduction procedures (other than submucosal radiofrequency) (100–112)	50%	60/121	25%–83%			BMI
Epiglottoplasty (113)	78%	21/27				

FS, Friedman stage; LSAT, lowest oxygen saturation on sleep study.
Note: Most subjects in these studies underwent previous or concurrent soft palate surgery.
[a]A single study or small minority of studies do not show improvement.
[?]Possible association with outcomes, based on some studies showing an association, with other studies showing none.

can enhance procedure selection with greater focus on examination of these factors and more standardization in the reporting of outcomes of surgical trials (42).

The tongue advancement and/or stabilization procedures include genioglossus advancement, mortised genioplasty, hyoid suspension, and the tongue stabilization suture. These can be performed in isolation or concurrently with palate or other hypopharyngeal procedures.

Genioglossus advancement (Fig. 138.5) involves creating an anterior mandibular osteotomy to capture the insertion of the genioglossus muscle at the genial tubercle, advancing the bone fragment 10 to 20 mm (often the thickness of the mandible) and thereby increasing tension on the genioglossus muscle (114). With the decrease in genioglossus muscle tone that occurs during sleep, this increased muscle tension can reduce tongue prolapse that can narrow the hypopharyngeal airway. Mortised genioplasty is a variation that includes a portion of the inferior border of the anterior mandible, advancing the bone fragment to increase tension on not only the genioglossus muscle but also the digastric and mylohyoid muscles;48 there is less advancement of the bone and muscle attachments in this procedure, as instead of advancing the osteotomized bone fragment the entire thickness of the mandible (as in genioglossus advancement), typically some bony overlap along the osteotomies is maintained to facilitate healing. Outcomes for these procedures appear to be improved in individuals with BMI below 30 kg/m² and those with lower AHI (45,46,48). Risks of genioglossus advancement and mortised genioplasty

include hematoma, incisional dehiscence and infection, dental injury, dental numbness or paresthesias, mental nerve injury, and mandible fracture (115).

The human hyoid bone is uniquely mobile, and its attachments to adjacent muscles (hyoglossus, mylohyoid, digastric, sternohyoid, thyrohyoid, and middle pharyngeal constrictor) and ligaments (hyoepiglottic and stylohyoid) led to the development of the hyoid suspension procedure. Specifically, the attachments of the hyoid bone to the inferior tongue base (hyoglossus), epiglottis (hyoepiglottic ligament), and lateral pharyngeal walls (middle pharyngeal constrictor) suggest that the hyoid suspension procedure may help stabilize the hypopharyngeal airway. The hyoid suspension procedure (Fig. 138.6) advances and stabilizes the hyoid bone to the thyroid cartilage (116) or, through some tethering material, to the inferior border of the mandible (62); it remains unclear which technique is preferable, as these have never been compared side by side. Outcomes for hyoid suspension as a sole surgical treatment for hypopharyngeal obstruction appear to be improved for subjects with BMI below 30 kg/m² (although this comes from a comparison of different studies only) and those with lower AHI (49–55). Hyoid suspension has resulted in improved control of symptoms such as daytime sleepiness, measured by the Epworth Sleepiness Scale (ESS) (49,50,52,54,55,117). Risks of hyoid suspension include seroma or hematoma, infection, dysphagia (via local edema and/or injury of the superior laryngeal or hypoglossal nerves), hyoid fracture, suspension material breakage, or pharyngocutaneous fistula (115).

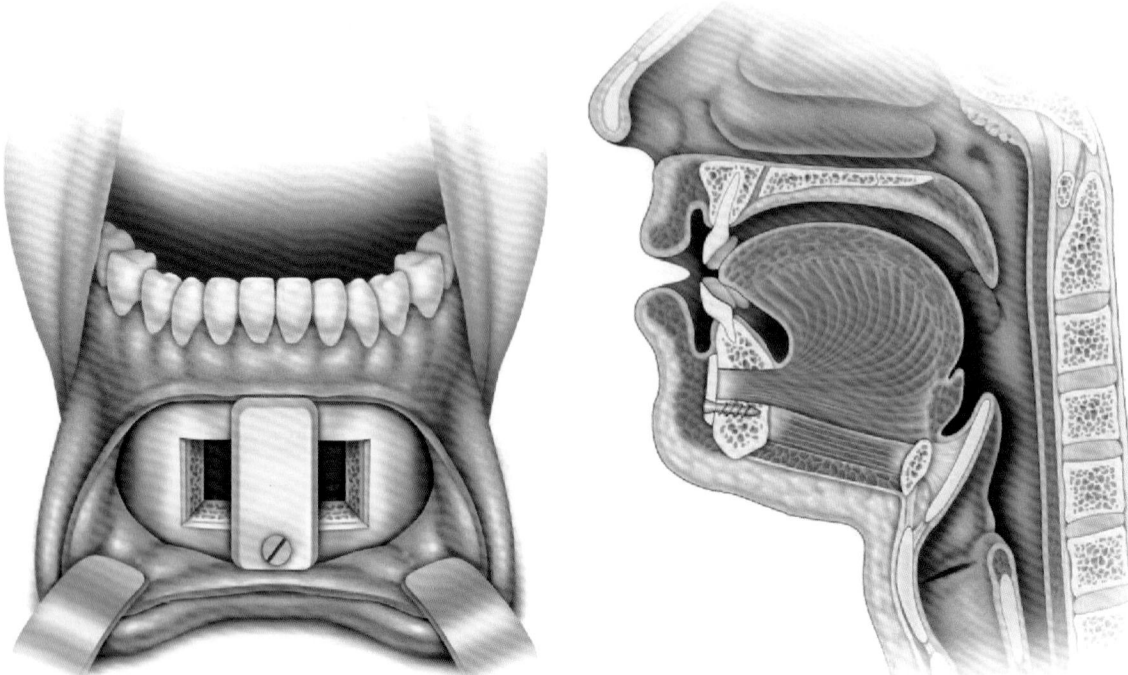

Figure 138.5 Genioglossus advancement procedure. On the **left**, an anterior view shows the mandibular osteotomy with fragment advanced, rotated, and secured inferiorly. On the **right**, a sagittal view demonstrates the advanced position of the genioglossus muscle insertion. (Reprinted with permission of www.sleep-doctor.com)

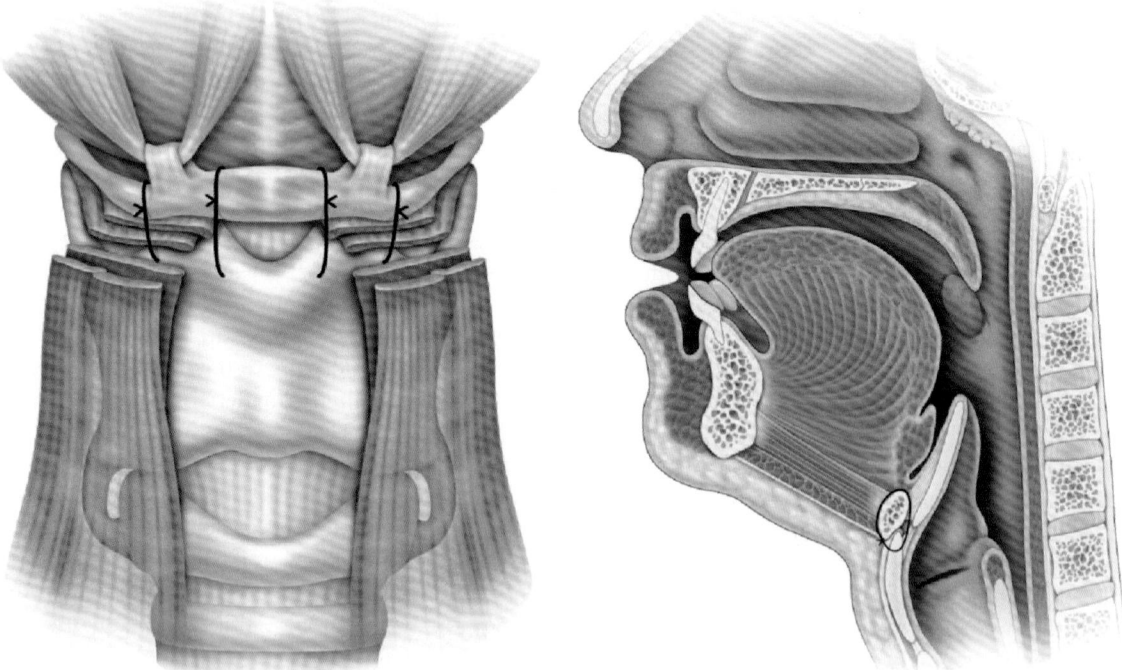

Figure 138.6 Hyoid suspension using a thyrohyoid technique. An anterior view (**left**) and sagittal view (**right**) demonstrate the use of sutures to secure the hyoid bone to the superior border of the thyroid cartilage. (Reprinted with permission of www.sleep-doctor.com)

Outcomes for the combination of genioglossus advancement and hyoid suspension as treatment of hypopharyngeal obstruction have been reported. Some studies demonstrated an association between improved outcomes in subjects with lower BMI (generally below 30 or 32 kg/m²) (47,57,59,62,66,68), lower AHI (46,47,57,59,61), and greater SNB angle on lateral cephalometry (47,60), although the associations were not seen in all studies (56,60,65,68). Concerning clinical outcomes, studies have also shown a decrease in daytime sleepiness (ESS) (56–59,61,63,65–67,97,116) and improvements in sleep-related quality of life (68).

Tongue stabilization involves securing a suture to the anterior mandible and then passing that suture though the tongue base to tether it and reduce its ability to obstruct the airway when muscle tone decreases during sleep. Outcomes appear to be improved with lower BMI (generally below 29 or 30 kg/m²) (70,76,79) and the degree of suture tightening (74). Risks include those related to placement of the fixation screw in the anterior mandible (dental injury or numbness), passage of the suture towards and through the tongue base (sialadenitis and injury to the lingual or hypoglossal nerves), or the degree of suture tightening and the related tethering of the tongue (suture breakage or migration, dysphagia, and dysarthria) (115). Tongue stabilization studies have shown a decrease in daytime sleepiness (ESS) (70,71,75,77,79,98) and improved sleep-related quality of life (98).

Tongue reduction procedures improve the retrolingual airway by decreasing tongue tissue volume. This can be accomplished either with direct tissue removal or with submucosal radiofrequency treatment that creates tissue injury and reduces tongue volume indirectly through fibrosis. Submucosal tongue radiofrequency (Fig. 138.7) involves creation of a submucosal scar with the bulk of the tongue itself that stiffens the tissue and reduces tongue volume by a mean of 17% after five treatment sessions (91); the changes in tissue characteristics that occur with fibrosis may also increase tongue tension and reduce tongue prolapse during sleep. Submucosal radiofrequency is less invasive than direct tissue resection, which translates into simpler recovery but, in general, lower effectiveness than the surgical excision techniques. Outcomes are presented in Table 138.5, and a number of studies have demonstrated that submucosal tongue radiofrequency improves daytime sleepiness (ESS) (70,71,82–85,87,89–95,98,99) and sleep-related quality of life (91,93,95,98,99).

Most published submucosal tongue radiofrequency case series studies have subjects with a mean BMI below 30 kg/m², a group that may be easier to treat due to less tongue volume at baseline (5). That being said, as opposed to other hypopharyngeal procedures for which the literature consists almost exclusively of case series or randomized pilot studies, higher-level evidence demonstrates the benefits of submucosal tongue radiofrequency. In a double-blinded, sham/placebo-controlled randomized trial of subjects with mild to moderate OSA, active submucosal tongue (combined with palate) radiofrequency produced improvements in the apnea index, daytime sleepiness, reaction time, and quality of life, with improvements similar to CPAP and even greater 2 years after treatment than at 6 months (99,118). In another study comparing isolated soft palate surgery to the combination of soft palate surgery and submucosal tongue radiofrequency, results were improved with the addition of submucosal tongue radiofrequency for both Friedman stages II and III (85). For the published case series studies, outcomes are enhanced in those with lower Friedman stage (II vs. III) (85) and BMI below 29 kg/m² (90). Risks include mucosal ulceration; hematoma; infection, including abscess; injury of the lingual or hypoglossal nerves; and sialadenitis (115). One literature review suggested that the incidence of complications of moderate or major severity was 2.7% in total, with none occurring in a series from an experienced group (119).

Multiple procedure approaches enable direct tissue excision: midline glossectomy (midline trench in the tongue base) (103), lingualplasty (extends the tongue base dissection laterally) (108), submucosal minimally invasive lingual excision (midline excision from the tongue base and posterior oral tongue) (102,120), submucosal lingualplasty (midline and lateral removal of tissue from the tongue base and posterior oral tongue) (106), and hyoepiglottoplasty (transcervical resection of tongue base tissue, with hyoid suspension to the mandible's inferior border) (101). These procedures can reduce tongue volume considerably, and the resulting scar in the tongue base also likely reduces its collapsibility. Lingual tonsillectomy (Fig. 138.8) improves the airway by removing obstructing lingual tonsil tissue without resecting tongue base musculature. In the past, these procedures were performed with lasers or electrocautery. With the newer irrigating, suctioning, bipolar instruments, bleeding and collateral tissue damage are minimized, and morbidity is decreased considerably (121). Recently, lingual tonsillectomy (alone or in combination with epiglottic procedures, such as those outlined below) has been performed as transoral robotic surgery (111). Although the reported outcomes from tongue tissue excision procedures appear to be similar to other procedures (Table 138.5), it must be noted that these case series studies generally include subjects with BMI above 30 kg/m² and with moderate to severe OSA, a group that has largely shown poorer outcomes for the alternative procedures in the table. Risks of tongue excision procedures are similar to (but more likely than) those after tongue radiofrequency (115).

Posterior displacement or retroflexion of the epiglottis impairs the airway, and there are procedures to debulk or stabilize the epiglottis. Hyoid suspension, as noted above, tethers the epiglottis indirectly through its attachment to the hyoid bone via the hyoepiglottic ligament. Epiglottoplasty resects part of the epiglottis directly and can be accomplished via a transoral approach (122) or a

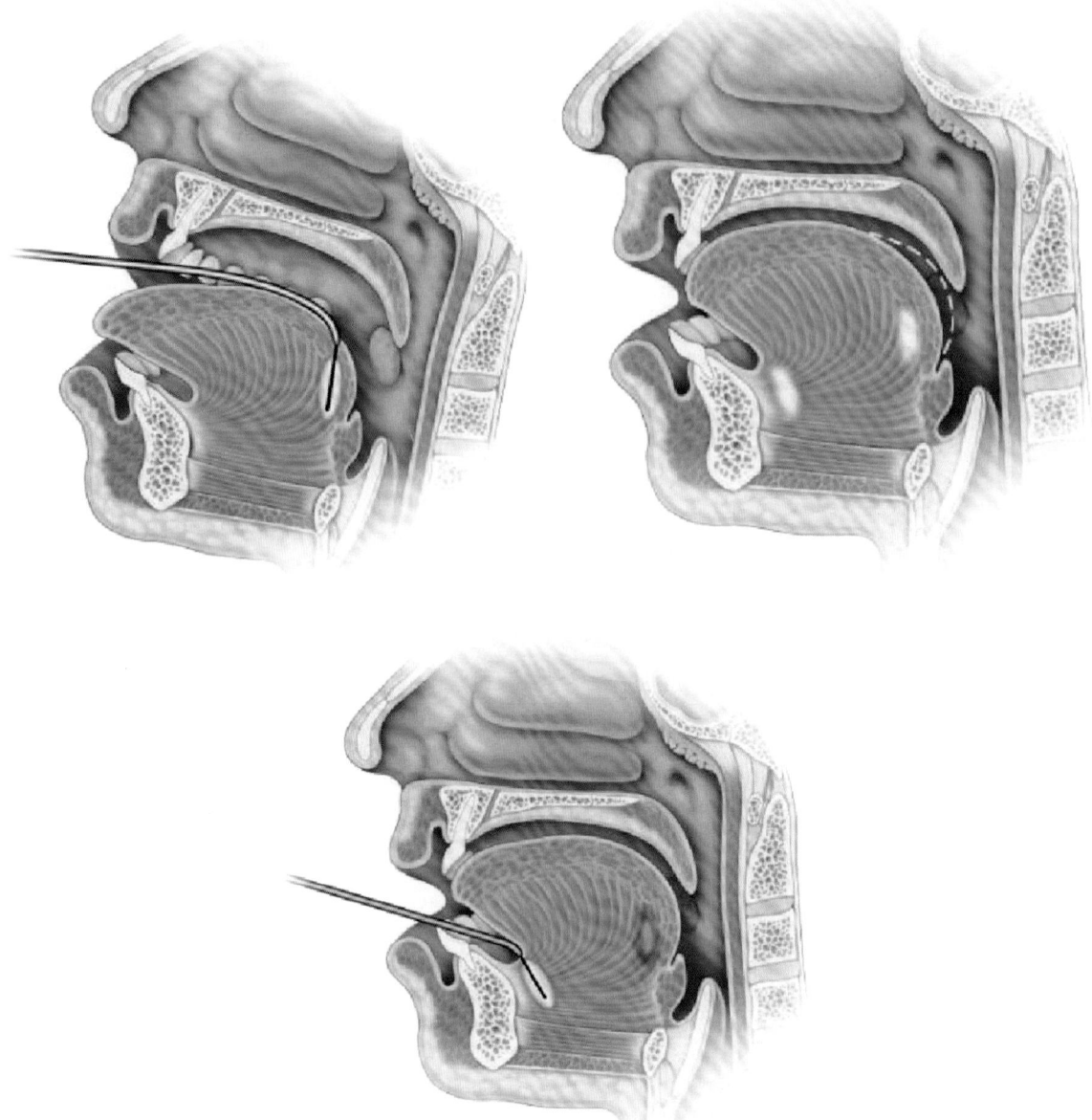

Figure 138.7 Submucosal tongue radiofrequency. Figures show the creation of tissue injury in the tongue base (**left**) and ventral tongue (**middle**), both of which heal with the development of fibrosis at these sites (**right**). (Reprinted with permission of www.sleep-doctor.com)

neck incision (typically as part of another procedure that may include tongue tissue resection, as hyoepiglottoplasty does). It is important to note that outcomes for epiglottoplasty reported in Table 138.5, while impressive, are from a single study with a highly selected group of subjects with low BMI (mean 23.4 kg/m²) and a specific finding on fiberoptic endoscopy: posterior displacement of the epiglottis away from the tongue base (113). In addition to a low risk of bleeding, the most important risk of transoral epiglottoplasty is dysphagia due to potential compromise of the epiglottis function as a protector of the airway during swallowing.

SKELETAL SURGERY AND OUTCOMES

Maxillomandibular advancement (MMA, Fig. 138.9) projects forward the entire lower facial skeleton and attached soft tissues. The dental arches are either moved in unison to maintain baseline occlusion or moved differentially to correct a malocclusion (generally requiring pre- and postoperative orthodontics). This multilevel procedure stabilizes and improves the entire pharyngeal airway and thereby treats both the retropalatal and hypopharyngeal regions of the upper airway (and all structures that can contribute to obstruction). Awake endoscopy suggests that

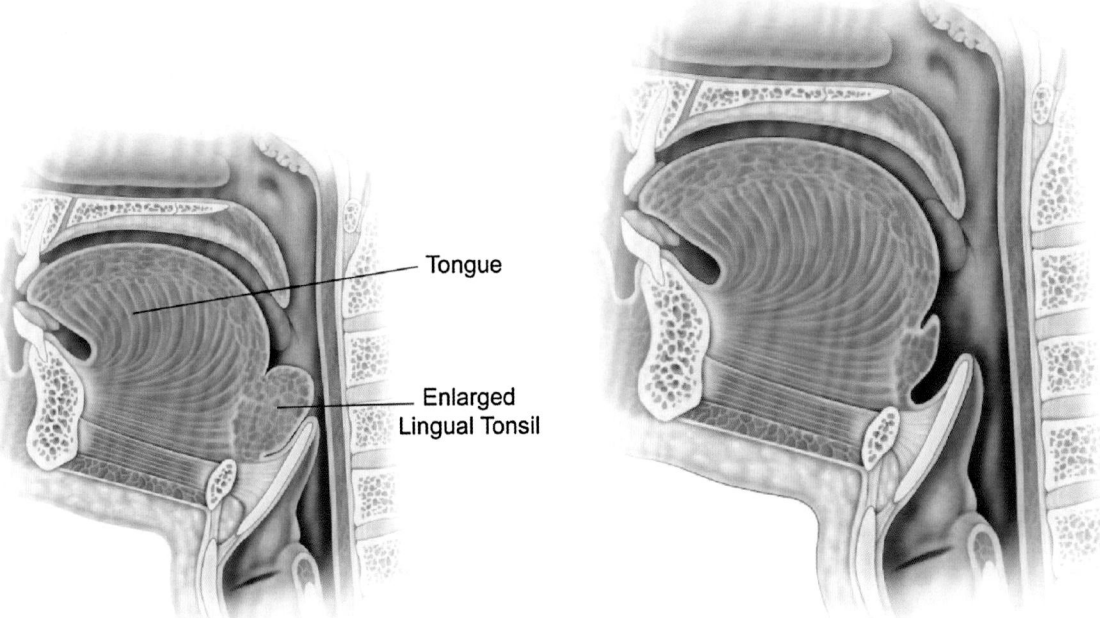

Figure 138.8 Lingual tonsillectomy. Sagittal views showing an enlarged lingual tonsil prior to excision (**left**) and following healing (**right**). (Reprinted with permission of www.sleep-doctor.com)

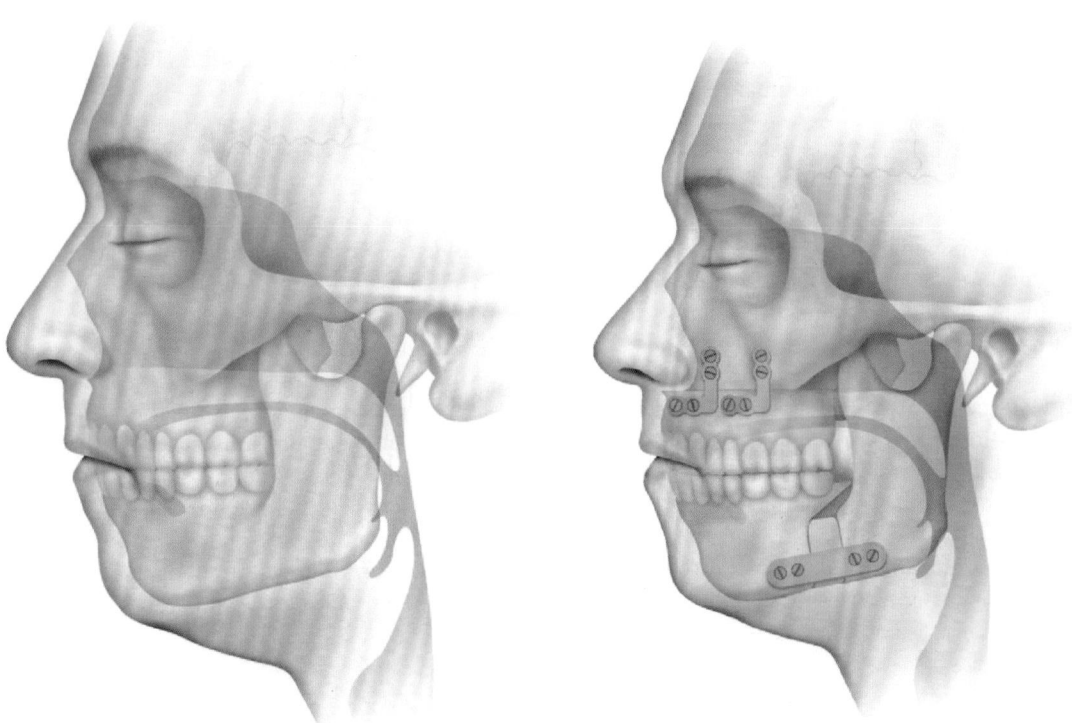

Figure 138.9 Maxillomandibular advancement. Preoperative (**left**) and postoperative (**right**) sagittal images showing the changes in the facial skeleton and pharyngeal airway. (Reprinted with permission of www.sleep-doctor.com)

this treats the lateral pharyngeal walls by placing soft tissues under tension (123).

MMA can be performed as primary surgery, although because this is a major operation, it is typically performed as a secondary procedure for patients with persistent significant OSA following other site-directed surgical treatments (124). A recent metaanalysis found that reported studies showed that MMA was associated with an 87% reduction in the AHI, whether performed as primary or secondary surgery—although MMA was performed in combination with other airway procedures in some of the included studies (125). There are no higher-level studies of MMA, but the published case series studies (44,48,56,67,124,126–136) do demonstrate a more consistent improvement in AHI (although not a cure of OSA) (137) than for hypopharyngeal procedures. As with all procedures, MMA is technique dependent, with greater degrees of advancement associated with greater improvements in airway dimensions and improved outcomes (135). Published studies suggest that the improvements in AHI do persist over a relatively long period of time, except in individuals who gain significant body weight. In a long-term follow-up of 40 patients, Riley et al. (135) showed 90% success more than 4 years from surgery. Limited data suggest that MMA also improves certain clinical outcomes, whether quality of life (138) or daytime function, with improvements similar to a group undergoing treatment with positive airway pressure therapy (127). The risks of MMA include bleeding, infection, dental injury, dental and facial numbness, malocclusion, bony malunion or nonunion, change in facial appearance, and temporomandibular disturbance.

FUTURE RESEARCH

A major challenge for the field is to conduct definitive studies to test the effectiveness of current and future surgical interventions and to develop best strategies for surgical decision making. These studies should test adjunctive surgical treatments aimed at facilitating CPAP or oral appliance therapy, and they should test comprehensive surgical approaches for definitive therapy in the absence of CPAP or oral appliance therapy, ideally measuring long-term, clinical outcomes primarily. Both observational studies and definitive trials of high quality are desirable, as they are complementary (24).

There are unique challenges to designing and conducting ethical, randomized, double-blinded, sham/placebo-controlled trials for definitive, staged, anatomically tailored, invasive surgical interventions. Examples of challenges include difficulties providing an adequate placebo, blinding the surgeon and investigators, and obtaining long-term outcomes. Recruitment, generalizability, and cost will be difficult because it is the unusual patient who is willing to be randomized to or away from invasive therapy. The feasibility of randomized trials of surgical versus nonsurgical treatment is uncertain, as studies like this have often either failed in enrollment (139) or required federal mandates preventing surgery outside the trial (140). There are competing interests of providing surgical flexibility to reflect real-world surgical decision making

(e.g., which variation of UPPP, what additional procedures to include, when and how to stage) on the one hand while standardizing the treatment protocols for methodologic purity on the other hand. Staging surgery, as is done in best practice, complicates trial design analysis by requiring repeated measures analysis and accommodating midstream crossovers. Comparing surgery to CPAP is not appropriate currently, because each treatment is offered to a different patient population in practice: CPAP is offered as first-line therapy, and surgery is offered to CPAP failures. Furthermore, testing differences between two treatments with similar effects requires particularly large sample sizes, which is especially challenging when enrollment is expected to be difficult as noted above.

These challenges are difficult, but surmountable. They will require a sophisticated group of researchers to design and conduct the studies, with major financial support and with study participation from community practitioners. Steps are underway to meet these challenges.

HIGHLIGHTS

- Individuals with OSA may experience airway obstruction in the hypopharyngeal region of the pharynx. Similarly, skeletal abnormalities may contribute substantially to OSA.
- Evaluation of the hypopharyngeal airway must include physical examination and fiberoptic laryngopharyngoscopy.
- Sleep testing outcomes are often used to measure the benefits of OSA treatment, but clinical outcomes are likely more important.
- A number of procedures are available to treat hypopharyngeal obstruction in OSA. Selection among them is based on an understanding of their mechanism of action and individual patient characteristics, among other factors.
- MMA surgery can be used as primary surgery or, more often, as a secondary procedure for those with residual OSA following previous site-directed procedures.
- High-quality observational studies or controlled clinical trials will help define the outcomes of surgical treatment for OSA. However, there are unique challenges to attempts at conducting these studies for hypopharyngeal procedures and skeletal surgery.

REFERENCES

1. White DP. Pathogenesis of obstructive and central sleep apnea. *Am J Respir Crit Care Med* 2005;172:1363–1370.
2. Fujita S, Simmons FB. Pharyngeal surgery for obstructive sleep apnea and snoring. In: Fairbanks DNF, Fujita S, Ikematsu T, et al., eds. *Snoring and obstructive sleep apnea.* New York: Raven Press, 1987:101–128.
3. Welch KC, Foster GD, Ritter CT, et al. A novel volumetric magnetic resonance imaging paradigm to study upper airway anatomy. *Sleep* 2002;25:532–542.

4. Barkdull GC, Kohl CA, Patel M, et al. Computed tomography imaging of patients with obstructive sleep apnea. *Laryngoscope* 2008;118:1486–1492.

5. Nashi N, Kang S, Barkdull GC, et al. Lingual fat at autopsy. *Laryngoscope* 2007;117:1467–1473.

6. Friedman M, Ibrahim H, Bass L. Clinical staging for sleep-disordered breathing. *Otolaryngol Head Neck Surg* 2002;127:13–21.

7. Samsoon GL, Young JR. Difficult tracheal intubation: a retrospective study. *Anaesthesia* 1987;42:487–490.

8. Friedman M, Vidyasagar R, Bliznikas D, et al. Does severity of obstructive sleep apnea/hypopnea syndrome predict uvulopalatopharyngoplasty outcome? *Laryngoscope* 2005;115:2109–2113.

9. Friedman M, Lin HC, Gurpinar B, et al. Minimally invasive single-stage multilevel treatment for obstructive sleep apnea/hypopnea syndrome. *Laryngoscope* 2007;117:1859–1863.

10. Partinen M, Guilleminault C, Quera-Salva MA, et al. Obstructive sleep apnea and cephalometric roentgenograms. The role of anatomic upper airway abnormalities in the definition of abnormal breathing during sleep. *Chest* 1988;93:1199–1205.

11. Moore KE, Phillips C. A practical method for describing patterns of tongue-base narrowing (modification of Fujita) in awake adult patients with obstructive sleep apnea. *J Oral Maxillofac Surg* 2002;60:252–260, discussion 60–61.

12. Schwab RJ, Pasirstein M, Pierson R, et al. Identification of upper airway anatomic risk factors for obstructive sleep apnea with volumetric magnetic resonance imaging. *Am J Respir Crit Care Med* 2003;168:522–530.

13. Faber CE, Grymer L. Available techniques for objective assessment of upper airway narrowing in snoring and sleep apnea. *Sleep Breath* 2003;7:77–86.

14. Mihaescu M, Mylavarapu G, Gutmark EJ, et al. Large eddy simulation of the pharyngeal airflow associated with obstructive sleep apnea syndrome at pre and post-surgical treatment. *J Biomech* 2011;44:2221–2228.

15. Fogel RB, Trinder J, White DP, et al. The effect of sleep onset on upper airway muscle activity in patients with sleep apnoea versus controls. *J Physiol* 2005;564:549–562.

16. Eckert DJ, Malhotra A, Lo YL, et al. The influence of obstructive sleep apnea and gender on genioglossus activity during rapid eye movement sleep. *Chest* 2009;135:957–964.

17. Kezirian EJ, Hohenhorst W, de Vries N. Drug-induced sleep endoscopy: the VOTE classification. *Eur Arch Otorhinolaryngol* 2011;268:1233–1266.

18. Croft CB, Pringle M. Sleep nasendoscopy: a technique of assessment in snoring and obstructive sleep apnoea. *Clin Otolaryngol Allied Sci* 1991;16:504–509.

19. Eastwood PR, Platt PR, Shepherd K, et al. Collapsibility of the upper airway at different concentrations of propofol anesthesia. *Anesthesiology* 2005;103:470–477.

20. Hillman DR, Walsh JH, Maddison KJ, et al. Evolution of changes in upper airway collapsibility during slow induction of anesthesia with propofol. *Anesthesiology* 2009;111:63–71.

21. Kezirian EJ, White DP, Malhotra A, et al. Interrater reliability of drug-induced sleep endoscopy. *Arch Otolaryngol Head Neck Surg* 2010;136:393–397.

22. Iwanaga K, Hasegawa K, Shibata N, et al. Endoscopic examination of obstructive sleep apnea syndrome patients during drug-induced sleep. *Acta Otolaryngol Suppl* 2003:36–40.

23. Hessel NS, Vries N. Increase of the apnoea-hypopnoea index after uvulopalatopharyngoplasty: analysis of failure. *Clin Otolaryngol Allied Sci* 2004;29:682–685.

24. Weaver EM. Judging sleep apnea surgery. *Sleep Med Rev* 2010;14:283–285.

25. Weaver EM, Woodson BT, Steward DL. Polysomnography indexes are discordant with quality of life, symptoms, and reaction times in sleep apnea patients. *Otolaryngol Head Neck Surg* 2005;132:255–262.

26. Fleming TR, DeMets DL. Surrogate end points in clinical trials: are we being misled? *Ann Intern Med* 1996;125:605–613.

27. Elshaug AG, Moss JR, Hiller JE, et al. Upper airway surgery should not be first line treatment for obstructive sleep apnoea in adults. *BMJ* 2008;336:44–45.

28. Elshaug AG, Moss JR, Southcott AM, et al. Redefining success in airway surgery for obstructive sleep apnea: a meta analysis and synthesis of the evidence. *Sleep* 2007;30:461–467.

29. Pepin JL, Veale D, Mayer P, et al. Critical analysis of the results of surgery in the treatment of snoring, upper airway resistance syndrome (UARS), and obstructive sleep apnea (OSA). *Sleep* 1996;19:S90–S100.

30. Grote L, Hedner J, Grunstein R, et al. Therapy with nCPAP: incomplete elimination of Sleep Related Breathing Disorder. *Eur Respir J* 2000;16:921–927.

31. Pittman SD, Pillar G, Berry RB, et al. Follow-up assessment of CPAP efficacy in patients with obstructive sleep apnea using an ambulatory device based on peripheral arterial tonometry. *Sleep Breath* 2006;10:123–131.

32. Kribbs NB, Pack AI, Kline LR, et al. Objective measurement of patterns of nasal CPAP use by patients with obstructive sleep apnea. *Am Rev Respir Dis* 1993;147:887–895.

33. Ravesloot MJ, de Vries N. Reliable calculation of the efficacy of non-surgical and surgical treatment of obstructive sleep apnea revisited. *Sleep* 2011;34:105–110.

34. Weaver TE, Maislin G, Dinges DF, et al. Relationship between hours of CPAP use and achieving normal levels of sleepiness and daily functioning. *Sleep* 2007;30:711–719.

35. Campos-Rodriguez F, Pena-Grinan N, Reyes-Nunez N, et al. Mortality in obstructive sleep apnea-hypopnea patients treated with positive airway pressure. *Chest* 2005;128:624–633.

36. Sleep-related breathing disorders in adults: recommendations for syndrome definition and measurement techniques in clinical research: the Report of an American Academy of Sleep Medicine Task Force. *Sleep* 1999;22:667–689.

37. Iber C, Ancoli-Israel S, Chesson A, et al.; for the American Academy of Sleep Medicine. *The AASM manual for the scoring of sleep and associated events: rules, terminology, and technical specifications*, 1st ed. Westchester, IL: American Academy of Sleep Medicine, 2007.

38. Kezirian EJ, Goldberg AN. Hypopharyngeal surgery in obstructive sleep apnea: an evidence-based medicine review. *Arch Otolaryngol Head Neck Surg* 2006;132:1–8.

39. Lin HC, Friedman M, Chang HW, et al. The efficacy of multilevel surgery of the upper airway in adults with obstructive sleep apnea/hypopnea syndrome. *Laryngoscope* 2008;118:902–908.

40. Sher AE, Schechtman KB, Piccirillo JF. The efficacy of surgical modifications of the upper airway in adults with obstructive sleep apnea syndrome. *Sleep* 1996;19:156–177.

41. Robinson S, Chia M, Carney AS, et al. Upper airway reconstructive surgery long-term quality-of-life outcomes compared with CPAP for adult obstructive sleep apnea. *Otolaryngol Head Neck Surg* 2009;141:257–263.

42. Kezirian EJ, Weaver EM, Criswell MA, et al. Reporting results of obstructive sleep apnea syndrome surgery trials. *Otolaryngol Head Neck Surg* 2011;144:496–499.

43. Johnson NT, Chinn J. Uvulopalatopharyngoplasty and inferior sagittal mandibular osteotomy with genioglossus advancement for treatment of obstructive sleep apnea. *Chest* 1994;105:278–283.

44. Lee NR, Givens CD Jr, Wilson J, et al. Staged surgical treatment of obstructive sleep apnea syndrome: a review of 35 patients. *J Oral Maxillofac Surg* 1999;57:382–385.

45. Liu SA, Li HY, Tsai WC, et al. Associated factors to predict outcomes of uvulopharyngopalatoplasty plus genioglossal advancement for obstructive sleep apnea. *Laryngoscope* 2005;115:2046–2050.

46. Miller FR, Watson D, Boseley M. The role of the Genial Bone Advancement Trephine system in conjunction with uvulopalatopharyngoplasty in the multilevel management of obstructive sleep apnea. *Otolaryngol Head Neck Surg* 2004;130:73–79.

47. Riley RW, Powell NB, Guilleminault C. Obstructive sleep apnea syndrome: a review of 306 consecutively treated surgical patients. *Otolaryngol Head Neck Surg* 1993;108:117–125.

48. Hendler BH, Costello BJ, Silverstein K, et al. A protocol for uvulopalatopharyngoplasty, mortised genioplasty, and maxillomandibular advancement in patients with obstructive sleep apnea: an analysis of 40 cases. *J Oral Maxillofac Surg* 2001;59:892–897, discussion 8–9.

49. Baisch A, Maurer JT, Hormann K. The effect of hyoid suspension in a multilevel surgery concept for obstructive sleep apnea. *Otolaryngol Head Neck Surg* 2006;134:856–861.

50. Benazzo M, Pagella F, Matti E, et al. Hyoidthyroidpexia as a treatment in multilevel surgery for obstructive sleep apnea. *Acta Otolaryngol* 2008;128:680–684.

51. Bowden MT, Kezirian EJ, Utley D, et al. Outcomes of hyoid suspension for the treatment of obstructive sleep apnea. *Arch Otolaryngol Head Neck Surg* 2005;131:440–445.

52. den Herder C, van Tinteren H, de Vries N. Hyoidthyroidpexia: a surgical treatment for sleep apnea syndrome. *Laryngoscope* 2005; 115:740–745.

53. Neruntarat C. Hyoid myotomy with suspension under local anesthesia for obstructive sleep apnea syndrome. *Eur Arch Otorhinolaryngol* 2003;260:286–290.

54. Vilaseca I, Morello A, Montserrat JM, et al. Usefulness of uvulo-palatopharyngoplasty with genioglossus and hyoid advancement in the treatment of obstructive sleep apnea. *Arch Otolaryngol Head Neck Surg* 2002;128:435–440.

55. Gillespie MB, Ayers CM, Nguyen SA, et al. Outcomes of hyoid myotomy and suspension using a mandibular screw suspension system. *Otolaryngol Head Neck Surg* 2011;144:225–229.

56. Bettega G, Pepin JL, Veale D, et al. Obstructive sleep apnea syndrome. Fifty-one consecutive patients treated by maxillofacial surgery. *Am J Respir Crit Care Med* 2000;162:641–649.

57. Foltan R, Hoffmannova J, Pretl M, et al. Genioglossus advancement and hyoid myotomy in treating obstructive sleep apnea syndrome–A follow-up study. *J Craniomaxillofac Surg* 2007;35:246–251.

58. Hsu PP, Brett RH. Multiple level pharyngeal surgery for obstructive sleep apnea. *Singapore Med J* 2001;42:160–164.

59. Neruntarat C. Genioglossus advancement and hyoid myotomy: short-term and long-term results. *J Laryngol Otol* 2003;117: 482–486.

60. Ramirez SG, Loube DI. Inferior sagittal osteotomy with hyoid bone suspension for obese patients with sleep apnea. *Arch Otolaryngol Head Neck Surg* 1996;122:953–957.

61. Richard W, Kox D, den Herder C, et al. One stage multilevel surgery (uvulopalatopharyngoplasty, hyoid suspension, radiofrequent ablation of the tongue base with/without genioglossus advancement), in obstructive sleep apnea syndrome. *Eur Arch Otorhinolaryngol* 2007;264:439–444.

62. Riley RW, Powell NB, Guilleminault C. Maxillary, mandibular, and hyoid advancement for treatment of obstructive sleep apnea: a review of 40 patients. *J Oral Maxillofac Surg* 1990;48:20–26.

63. Utley DS, Shin EJ, Clerk AA, et al. A cost-effective and rational surgical approach to patients with snoring, upper airway resistance syndrome, or obstructive sleep apnea syndrome. *Laryngoscope* 1997;107:726–734.

64. Verse T, Baisch A, Hormann K. Multi-level surgery for obstructive sleep apnea. Preliminary objective results. *Laryngorhinootologie* 2004; 83:516–522.

65. Yao M, Utley DS, Terris DJ. Cephalometric parameters after multilevel pharyngeal surgery for patients with obstructive sleep apnea. *Laryngoscope* 1998;108:789–795.

66. Yin SK, Yi HL, Lu WY, et al. Genioglossus advancement and hyoid suspension plus uvulopalatopharyngoplasty for severe OSAHS. *Otolaryngol Head Neck Surg* 2007;136:626–631.

67. Dattilo DJ, Drooger SA. Outcome assessment of patients undergoing maxillofacial procedures for the treatment of sleep apnea: comparison of subjective and objective results. *J Oral Maxillofac Surg* 2004;62:164–168.

68. Kezirian EJ, Malhotra A, Goldberg AN, et al. Changes in obstructive sleep apnea severity, biomarkers, and quality of life after multilevel surgery. *Laryngoscope* 2010;120:1481–1488.

69. DeRowe A, Gunther E, Fibbi A, et al. Tongue-base suspension with a soft tissue-to-bone anchor for obstructive sleep apnea: preliminary clinical results of a new minimally invasive technique. *Otolaryngol Head Neck Surg* 2000;122:100–103.

70. Fernandez-Julian E, Munoz N, Achiques MT, et al. Randomized study comparing two tongue base surgeries for moderate to severe obstructive sleep apnea syndrome. *Otolaryngol Head Neck Surg* 2009;140:917–923.

71. Fibbi A, Ameli F, Brocchetti F, et al. Tongue base suspension and radiofrequency volume reduction: a comparison between 2 techniques for the treatment of sleep-disordered breathing. *Am J Otolaryngol* 2009;30:401–406.

72. Kuhnel TS, Schurr C, Wagner B, et al. Morphological changes of the posterior airway space after tongue base suspension. *Laryngoscope* 2005;115:475–480.

73. Miller FR, Watson D, Malis D. Role of the tongue base suspension suture with The Repose System bone screw in the multilevel surgical management of obstructive sleep apnea. *Otolaryngol Head Neck Surg* 2002;126:392–398.

74. Omur M, Ozturan D, Elez F, et al. Tongue base suspension combined with UPPP in severe OSA patients. *Otolaryngol Head Neck Surg* 2005;133:218–223.

75. Sorrenti G, Piccin O, Latini G, et al. Tongue base suspension technique in obstructive sleep apnea: personal experience. *Acta Otorhinolaryngol Ital* 2003;23:274–280.

76. Terris DJ, Kunda LD, Gonella MC. Minimally invasive tongue base surgery for obstructive sleep apnoea. *J Laryngol Otol* 2002;116:716–721.

77. Thomas AJ, Chavoya M, Terris DJ. Preliminary findings from a prospective, randomized trial of two tongue-base surgeries for sleep-disordered breathing. *Otolaryngol Head Neck Surg* 2003;129:539–546.

78. Woodson BT. A tongue suspension suture for obstructive sleep apnea and snorers. *Otolaryngol Head Neck Surg* 2001;124:297–303.

79. Vicente E, Marin JM, Carrizo S, et al. Tongue-base suspension in conjunction with uvulopalatopharyngoplasty for treatment of severe obstructive sleep apnea: long-term follow-up results. *Laryngoscope* 2006;116:1223–1227.

80. Back LJ, Liukko T, Rantanen I, et al. Hypertonic saline injections to enhance the radiofrequency thermal ablation effect in the treatment of base of tongue in obstructive sleep apnea patients: a pilot study. *Acta Otolaryngol* 2009;129:302–310.

81. Blumen MB, Coquille F, Rocchicioli C, et al. Radiofrequency tongue reduction through a cervical approach: a pilot study. *Laryngoscope* 2006;116:1887–1893.

82. Ceylan K, Emir H, Kizilkaya Z, et al. First-choice treatment in mild to moderate obstructive sleep apnea: single-stage, multilevel, temperature-controlled radiofrequency tissue volume reduction or nasal continuous positive airway pressure. *Arch Otolaryngol Head Neck Surg* 2009;135:915–919.

83. Eun YG, Kim SW, Kwon KH, et al. Single-session radiofrequency tongue base reduction combined with uvulopalatopharyngoplasty for obstructive sleep apnea syndrome. *Eur Arch Otorhinolaryngol* 2008;265:1495–1500.

84. Fischer Y, Khan M, Mann WJ. Multilevel temperature-controlled radiofrequency therapy of soft palate, base of tongue, and tonsils in adults with obstructive sleep apnea. *Laryngoscope* 2003;113:1786–1791.

85. Friedman M, Ibrahim H, Lee G, et al. Combined uvulopalatopharyngoplasty and radiofrequency tongue base reduction for treatment of obstructive sleep apnea/hypopnea syndrome. *Otolaryngol Head Neck Surg* 2003;129:611–621.

86. Kao YH, Shnayder Y, Lee KC. The efficacy of anatomically based multilevel surgery for obstructive sleep apnea. *Otolaryngol Head Neck Surg* 2003;129:327–335.

87. Lin HC, Friedman M, Chang HW, et al. Z-Palatopharyngoplasty plus radiofrequency tongue base reduction for moderate/severe obstructive sleep apnea/hypopnea syndrome. *Acta Otolaryngol* 2010.

88. Nelson LM. Combined temperature-controlled radiofrequency tongue reduction and UPPP in apnea surgery. *Ear Nose Throat J* 2001;80:640–644.

89. Nelson LM, Barrera JE. High energy single session radiofrequency tongue treatment in obstructive sleep apnea surgery. *Otolaryngol Head Neck Surg* 2007;137:883–888.

90. Neruntarat C, Chantapant S. Radiofrequency surgery for the treatment of obstructive sleep apnea: short-term and long-term results. *Otolaryngol Head Neck Surg* 2009;141:722–726.

91. Powell NB, Riley RW, Guilleminault C. Radiofrequency tongue base reduction in sleep-disordered breathing: a pilot study. *Otolaryngol Head Neck Surg* 1999;120:656–664.

92. Riley RW, Powell NB, Li KK, et al. An adjunctive method of radiofrequency volumetric tissue reduction of the tongue for OSAS. *Otolaryngol Head Neck Surg* 2003;129:37–42.

93. Steward DL. Effectiveness of multilevel (tongue and palate) radiofrequency tissue ablation for patients with obstructive sleep apnea syndrome. *Laryngoscope* 2004;114:2073–2084.

94. Stuck BA, Maurer JT, Verse T, et al. Tongue base reduction with temperature-controlled radiofrequency volumetric tissue reduction for treatment of obstructive sleep apnea syndrome. *Acta Otolaryngol* 2002;122:531–536.

95. Stuck BA, Starzak K, Hein G, et al. Combined radiofrequency surgery of the tongue base and soft palate in obstructive sleep apnea. *Acta Otolaryngol* 2004;124:827–832.

96. van den Broek E, Richard W, van Tinteren H, et al. UPPP combined with radiofrequency thermotherapy of the tongue base for the treatment of obstructive sleep apnea syndrome. *Eur Arch Otorhinolaryngol* 2008;265:1361–1365.

97. Verse T, Baisch A, Maurer JT, et al. Multilevel surgery for obstructive sleep apnea: short-term results. *Otolaryngol Head Neck Surg* 2006;134:571–577.

98. Woodson BT, Nelson L, Mickelson S, et al. A multi-institutional study of radiofrequency volumetric tissue reduction for OSAS. *Otolaryngol Head Neck Surg* 2001;125:303–311.

99. Woodson BT, Steward DL, Weaver EM, et al. A randomized trial of temperature-controlled radiofrequency, continuous positive airway pressure, and placebo for obstructive sleep apnea syndrome. *Otolaryngol Head Neck Surg* 2003;128:848–861.

100. Andsberg U, Jessen M. Eight years of follow-up—uvulopalatopharyngoplasty combined with midline glossectomy as a treatment for obstructive sleep apnea syndrome. *Acta Otolaryngol Suppl* 2000;543:175–178.

101. Chabolle F, Wagner I, Blumen MB, et al. Tongue base reduction with hyoepiglottoplasty: a treatment for severe obstructive sleep apnea. *Laryngoscope* 1999;109:1273–1280.

102. Friedman M, Soans R, Gurpinar B, et al. Evaluation of submucosal minimally invasive lingual excision technique for treatment of obstructive sleep apnea/hypopnea syndrome. *Otolaryngol Head Neck Surg* 2008;139:378–384, discussion 85.

103. Fujita S, Woodson BT, Clark JL, et al. Laser midline glossectomy as a treatment for obstructive sleep apnea. *Laryngoscope* 1991;101:805–809.

104. Li HY, Wang PC, Hsu CY, et al. Same-stage palatopharyngeal and hypopharyngeal surgery for severe obstructive sleep apnea. *Acta Otolaryngol* 2004;124:820–826.

105. Mickelson SA, Rosenthal L. Midline glossectomy and epiglottidectomy for obstructive sleep apnea syndrome. *Laryngoscope* 1997;107:614–619.

106. Robinson S, Lewis R, Norton A, et al. Ultrasound-guided radiofrequency submucosal tongue-base excision for sleep apnea: a preliminary report. *Clin Otolaryngol Allied Sci* 2003;28:341–345.

107. Sorrenti G, Piccin O, Scaramuzzino G, et al. Tongue base reduction with hyoepiglottoplasty for the treatment of severe OSA. *Acta Otorhinolaryngol Ital* 2004;24:204–210.

108. Woodson BT, Fujita S. Clinical experience with lingualplasty as part of the treatment of severe obstructive sleep apnea. *Otolaryngol Head Neck Surg* 1992;107:40–48.

109. Babademez MA, Ciftci B, Acar B, et al. Low-temperature bipolar radiofrequency ablation (coblation) of the tongue base for supine-position-associated obstructive sleep apnea. *ORL J Otorhinolaryngol Relat Spec* 2010;72:51–55.

110. Elasfour A, Miyazaki S, Itasaka Y, et al. Evaluation of uvulopalatopharyngoplasty in treatment of obstructive sleep apnea syndrome. *Acta Otolaryngol Suppl* 1998;537:52–56.

111. Vicini C, Dallan I, Canzi P, et al. Transoral robotic surgery of the tongue base in obstructive sleep apnea-hypopnea syndrome: anatomic considerations and clinical experience. *Head Neck* 2011; 34:15–22.

112. Vicini C, Frassineti S, La Pietra MG, et al. Tongue Base Reduction with Thyro-Hyoido-Pexy (TBRTHP) vs. Tongue Base Reduction with Hyo-Epiglottoplasty (TBRHE) in mild-severe OSAHS adult treatment. Preliminary findings from a prospective randomised trial. *Acta Otorhinolaryngol Ital* 2010;30:144–148.

113. Golz A, Goldenberg D, Westerman ST, et al. Laser partial epiglottidectomy as a treatment for obstructive sleep apnea and laryngomalacia. *Ann Otol Rhinol Laryngol* 2000;109: 1140–1145.

114. Riley R, Guilleminault C, Powell N, et al. Mandibular osteotomy and hyoid bone advancement for obstructive sleep apnea: a case report. *Sleep* 1984;7:79–82.

115. Kezirian EJ. Complications of sleep surgery. In: Eisele DW, Smith RV, eds. *Complications in head and neck surgery.* Philadelphia, PA: Elsevier, 2009.

116. Riley RW, Powell NB, Guilleminault C. Obstructive sleep apnea and the hyoid: a revised surgical procedure. *Otolaryngol Head Neck Surg* 1994;111:717–721.

117. Neruntarat C. Genioglossus advancement and hyoid myotomy under local anesthesia. *Otolaryngol Head Neck Surg* 2003;129:85–91.

118. Steward DL, Weaver EM, Woodson BT. Multilevel temperature-controlled radiofrequency for obstructive sleep apnea: extended follow-up. *Otolaryngol Head Neck Surg* 2005;132:630–635.

119. Kezirian EJ, Powell NB, Riley RW, et al. Incidence of complications in radiofrequency treatment of the upper airway. *Laryngoscope* 2005;115:1298–1304.

120. Maturo SC, Mair EA. Submucosal minimally invasive lingual excision: an effective, novel surgery for pediatric tongue base reduction. *Ann Otol Rhinol Laryngol* 2006;115:624–630.

121. Robinson S, Ettema SL, Brusky L, et al. Lingual tonsillectomy using bipolar radiofrequency plasma excision. *Otolaryngol Head Neck Surg* 2006;134:328–330.

122. Catalfumo FJ, Golz A, Westerman ST, et al. The epiglottis and obstructive sleep apnoea syndrome. *J Laryngol Otol* 1998;112: 940–943.

123. Li KK, Guilleminault C, Riley RW, et al. Obstructive sleep apnea and maxillomandibular advancement: an assessment of airway changes using radiographic and nasopharyngoscopic examinations. *J Oral Maxillofac Surg* 2002;60:526–530, discussion 31.

124. Riley RW, Powell NB, Guilleminault C. Obstructive sleep apnea syndrome: a review of 306 consecutively treated surgical patients. *Otolaryngol Head Neck Surg* 1993;108:117–125.

125. Caples SM, Rowley JA, Prinsell JR, et al. Surgical modifications of the upper airway for obstructive sleep apnea in adults: a systematic review and meta-analysis. *Sleep* 2010;33:1396–1407.

126. Conradt R, Hochban W, Brandenburg U, et al. Long-term follow-up after surgical treatment of obstructive sleep apnea by maxillomandibular advancement. *Eur Respir J* 1997;10:123–128.

127. Conradt R, Hochban W, Heitmann J, et al. Sleep fragmentation and daytime vigilance in patients with OSA treated by surgical maxillomandibular advancement compared to CPAP therapy. *J Sleep Res* 1998;7:217–223.

128. Goh YH, Lim KA. Modified maxillomandibular advancement for the treatment of obstructive sleep apnea: a preliminary report. *Laryngoscope* 2003;113:1577–1582.

129. Gregg JM, Zedalis D, Howard CW, et al. Surgical alternatives for treatment of obstructive sleep apnoea: review and case series. *Ann R Australas Coll Dent Surg* 2000;15:181–184.

130. Hochban W, Conradt R, Brandenburg U, et al. Surgical maxillofacial treatment of obstructive sleep apnea. *Plast Reconstr Surg* 1997;99:619–626, discussion 27–28.

131. Kessler P, Ruberg F, Obbarius H, et al. Surgical management of obstructive sleep apnea. *Mund Kiefer Gesichtschir* 2007;11:81–88.

132. Li KK, Riley RW, Powell NB, et al. Maxillomandibular advancement for persistent obstructive sleep apnea after phase I surgery in patients without maxillomandibular deficiency. *Laryngoscope* 2000;110:1684–1688.

133. Prinsell JR. Maxillomandibular advancement surgery in a site-specific treatment approach for obstructive sleep apnea in 50 consecutive patients. *Chest* 1999;116:1519–1529.

134. Riley RW, Powell NB, Guilleminault C. Maxillofacial surgery and nasal CPAP. A comparison of treatment for obstructive sleep apnea syndrome. *Chest* 1990;98:1421–1425.

135. Riley RW, Powell NB, Li KK, et al. Surgery and obstructive sleep apnea: long-term clinical outcomes. *Otolaryngol Head Neck Surg* 2000;122:415–421.

136. Dekeister C, Lacassagne L, Tiberge M, et al. Mandibular advancement surgery in patients with severe obstructive sleep apnea uncontrolled by continuous positive airway pressure. A retrospective review of 25 patients between 1998 and 2004. *Rev Mal Respir* 2006;23:430–437.

137. Holty JE, Guilleminault C. Maxillomandibular advancement for the treatment of obstructive sleep apnea: a systematic review and meta-analysis. *Sleep Med Rev;*14:287–297.

138. Lye KW, Waite PD, Meara D, et al. Quality of life evaluation of maxillomandibular advancement surgery for treatment of obstructive sleep apnea. *J Oral Maxillofac Surg* 2008;66: 968–972.

139. Varner RE, Ireland CC, Summitt RL Jr, et al. Medicine or Surgery (Ms): a randomized clinical trial comparing hysterectomy and medical treatment in premenopausal women with abnormal uterine bleeding. *Control Clin Trials* 2004;25:104–118.

140. Patients at high risk of death after lung-volume-reduction surgery. *N Engl J Med* 2001;345:1075–1083.

139 Pediatric Sleep-Disordered Breathing

Stacey L. Ishman   *David F. Smith*   *Sally R. Shott*

INTRODUCTION

Sleep-disordered breathing (SDB) represents a continuum of obstructive disease that encompasses a range of specific diagnoses including snoring, upper airway resistance syndrome, obstructive hypoventilation, and obstructive sleep apnea (OSA). OSA, itself, is characterized by increasing limitation of flow through the upper airway, sometimes resulting in complete obstruction of the airway. OSA presents differently in children than it does in adolescents and adults, and identification can be hampered by the fact that children are far less likely to complain about problems with sleep than adults. In many cases, parents or guardians will be the first to express concerns about a child's sleep, and they often highlight complaints of increased fatigue or sleepiness (hypersomnia), difficulty initiating or maintaining sleep (insomnia), sleeping in strange positions and restless sleep, or other abnormal behaviors that are recognized during the sleep cycle. For this reason, a thorough history provided by the caregivers, in addition to a complete physical exam, is essential for the assessment of pediatric sleep disorders.

Epidemiology

Many epidemiologic studies have sought to accurately identify the number of children in the United States (US) with SDB and OSA, as well as to identify the risk factors associated with both; however, these figures are highly variable. In a recent study, 3.2% to 34.5% of parents reported that their children snored often to always (1), while another notes that approximately 25% of children aged 3 to 12 years old snore (2). Most population studies indicate that 1% to 4% of children in the US have OSA (1). However, OSA seems to be more prevalent in the male gender (1), and SDB is strongly associated with low socioeconomic status. This relationship may simply reflect a higher body mass index (BMI) within this subgroup (3).

Ethnicity and genetic factors are also associated with a higher risk of SDB. Black children in the US are at an increased risk of developing OSA when compared to white children (4–7). Other studies utilizing validated questionnaires, polysomnography (PSG), or cephalometric measurements have verified a higher rate of OSA in black and Asian children (8–10). Airway obstruction and OSA may be missed in children with craniofacial anomalies unless specifically addressed as parents may assume that this is "normal" for their child. One study showed more than a doubling of OSA diagnoses when using a specifically applied sleep questionnaire in a group of children with Apert, Crouzon, and Pfeiffer syndrome (11). A full list of children at higher risk for OSA is presented in Table 139.1. SDB has also been associated with specific clinical risk factors including nightly snoring, caregiver witnessed apneas, male gender, exposure to cigarette smoke, and anatomic factors including adenotonsillar hypertrophy and obesity (12,13).

Consequences of OSA

Over the last decade, studies have sought to identify the long-term complications associated with SDB and OSA. Behavioral problems that can occur as a result of untreated OSA include hyperactivity, attention-deficit disorders, aggression, and poor socialization (2). Neurocognitive disorders linked to OSA include poor school performance and variable learning disorders, such as deficits in memory, learning, and problem-solving skills (2). Much of what has been learned over the last decade suggests that children with OSA are at a much higher risk to suffer from behavioral, neurocognitive, and emotional difficulties, as well as a decrease in quality of life (QOL). In fact, both neuropsychological behavior and QOL tend to normalize after the airway obstruction has resolved (14–16). Besides the host of behavioral and neurocognitive disorders, children with OSA for prolonged periods can suffer from cardiovascular

TABLE 139.1	CONDITIONS CAUSING AN INCREASED RISK OF SDB AND OSA IN CHILDREN	
Syndromic	**Nonsyndromic**	
Apert syndrome	Achondroplasia	
Beckwith–Wiedemann syndrome	Cerebral palsy	
Crouzon syndrome	Choanal atresia	
Down syndrome	Cleft palate	
Klippel–Feil syndrome	Lymphangioma	
Pierre Robin sequence	Mucopolysaccharidosis	
Pfeiffer syndrome	Obesity	
Prader Willi syndrome	Pharyngeal flap patient	
Treacher Collins syndrome	Recurrent respiratory papillomatosis	

TABLE 139.2	FREQUENTLY WITNESSED SIGNS AND SYMPTOMS OF OSA IN CHILDREN	
Daytime Symptoms	**Nighttime Symptoms**	
Open-mouth breathing	Frequent loud snoring	
Frequent nasal obstruction	Gasping or choking	
Hyperactive behavior	Frequent nighttime sweating	
Aggressive behavior	Witnessed apneas	
Attention deficit disorder	Paradoxical breathing	
Poor school performance	Frequent position changes/restless sleep	
Daytime somnolence	Hyperextension of the neck	
	Nocturnal enuresis	

and pulmonary complications. Elevated systemic blood pressure has been found in children with OSA (17–21). More importantly, children with elevated blood pressures are more likely to suffer from hypertension and metabolic syndrome as adults (22). Although previous studies evaluating the association between primary snoring and increases in blood pressure in children have been somewhat conflicting (23–26), more recent data suggest that children with primary snoring have higher nighttime blood pressures when compared to those control patients without snoring (27). Further, a dose–response relationship exists between SDB and the severity of blood pressures in children (27). Although not fully understood, clear risks exist for those children with prolonged SDB.

DIAGNOSIS

History

The American Academy of Pediatrics (AAP) first recommended universal screening for snoring in 2002 (28). Although a PSG remains the most commonly recommended method for diagnosing SDB, a comprehensive "sleep history" is a vital clinical tool for evaluating the presence of SDB in children. This history, more often provided by caregivers, should include information about nightly hours of sleep, sleep hygiene, sleep latency, abnormal sleep behaviors, the presence and character of snoring, daytime behavior (including hypersomnia), behavioral disorders, and school performance. It is also important to understand napping behavior of children with suspected SDB.

Parents and caregivers routinely report witnessing nightly snoring, apneas, choking or gasping, increased work of breathing, hyperextension of the neck, restless sleep and night sweats, nocturnal enuresis, and parasomnias (Table 139.2). Commonly witnessed parasomnias include confusional arousals, sleep walking, and night/sleep terrors; however, the presence of these symptoms does not necessarily correlate with the presence of SDB in children. Caregivers may also report daytime symptoms including frequent mouth-breathing, chronic nasal obstruction, poor school performance, hyperactive behavior or attention deficit disorder, aggression, and less frequently, daytime somnolence (Table 139.2). Although hypersomnolence is present in some children with OSA, it is more commonly seen in adolescent and adult patients. For children with hypertrophic tonsils, caregivers may also report eating habits including avoidance of bulky foods such as meat.

While sleep questionnaires can be used in the office as a screening tool to identify children most at risk of having OSA and to acquire information about common symptoms associated with SDB and OSA (29–31), their use as a single tool to diagnose OSA has not been supported, thus they should only be used as an aid when pursuing a thorough sleep history. There are limitations to the accuracy of these data in differentiating SDB from OSA. In fact, parental reporting has been shown to be an inaccurate method of diagnosing OSA in children (30), and a recent meta-analysis of 12 articles that examined the accuracy of clinical assessment found that discrimination between primary snoring and OSA could not be precisely determined by parental reporting alone (32).

Physical Exam

Narrowing of the upper airway is the primary reason that children develop SDB and OSA. This may be the result of multiple factors including anatomic abnormalities, and thus, a complete head and neck exam is recommended. Identification of the anatomic location of the obstruction is necessary to tailor the appropriate treatment, especially in those children with multilevel obstruction.

A systematic approach to the physical examination is necessary so that no relevant findings are missed (Table 139.3). The exam should begin with evaluation of the general appearance of the patient, including height, weight, blood pressure, general craniofacial appearance, voice, and the presence or absence of mouth breathing. Voice abnormalities can be useful in identification of the location of

TABLE 139.3	SYSTEMATIC APPROACH TO THE PHYSICAL EXAMINATION IN A CHILD WITH OSA

General
    Vital signs including height, weight, blood pressure, BMI, and temperature
    General body habitus including obesity

Head and face
    Abnormal cephalic formation
    Abnormal facies

Nasal
    External deformity
    Nasal valve function
    Inferior turbinates
    Secondary areas of nasal obstruction
    Rhinorrhea
    Signs of allergic rhinitis

Oral cavity
    Dentition
    Tongue size and protrusion
    Hard and soft palate
    Uvula and posterior pharyngeal wall
    Tonsil grade
    Modified Mallampati score

Neck
    Neck size, including circumference
    Hyoid position, including submental-to-hyoid distance
    Tracheal position

Systemic
    Chest/lung exam including abnormal auscultation
    Cardiovascular examination
    Chest wall abnormalities

in children with chronic sinusitis or adenoid hypertrophy. Functional nasal valve collapse can be seen in children during deep inspiration through the nose and can contribute to obstructed flow through the nasal passages. The presence of nasal polyps is rare except in children with cystic fibrosis. Patency of the nasal cavities, information often useful in the newborn, can be determined by passing an 8 French catheter through the nose and into the oropharynx. Finally, nasal endoscopy can be used in children to evaluate multiple anomalies of the nasal cavity, such as choanal atresia or stenosis, pyriform aperture stenosis, posteriorly positioned polyps or masses, or adenoid hypertrophy.

Examination of the oral cavity and oropharynx is one of the most useful portions of the head and neck exam in a child with suspected SDB and OSA. The oropharynx, and specifically the retropalatal region, is one of the most narrow portions of the airway in normal children (34). Initial exam should assess for size and position of the mandible and dentition, including malocclusion. Tongue size and position, especially macroglossia and glossoptosis, may have a significant contribution to SDB if present. Evaluation of the palate should include inspection for overt or submucosal clefting of the hard and soft palate, a high arched or narrow palate, and palatal masses, as well as presence of a bifid uvula. The tonsils are graded based on a four-point scale as described by Brodsky et al. (35) (Fig. 139.1): 0 for surgically absent tonsils, 1 for tonsils that lie within the anterior and posterior pillars, 2 for tonsils seen just beyond the pillars, 3 for tonsils that reach beyond 50% towards the midline,

pathology. For example, a hyponasal voice can suggest enlarged adenoids, while a muffled voice can result from tonsillar hypertrophy. Care should be taken to perform a thorough cardiovascular exam including auscultation for any murmurs. Systemic findings including failure to thrive, cor pulmonale, and pectus excavatum should be considered (33). Special consideration is given to obesity and body habitus, especially in the adolescent patient. Finally, genetic and syndromal dysmorphisms should also be noted.

At the start of the exam, an overall assessment of head and neck shape and proportions should be performed. For example, midface hypoplasia is seen in Down syndrome and Crouzon syndrome, whereas mandibular hypoplasia is often seen in children with Treacher Collins or Pierre Robin sequence. Extensive cervical adipose tissue and increased neck circumference may be seen in children with obesity. Examination of the nasal cavity should include details regarding the mucosa, septum, inferior turbinates, nasal valve, and presence of polyps or masses. The nasal mucosa may be erythematous, suggesting chronic inflammation, or dusky, as is seen with allergic rhinitis. Anterior rhinoscopy can assist in identification of septal deviation and abnormalities of the inferior turbinates such as turbinate hypertrophy, contributing to nasal obstruction. Often, chronic rhinorrhea is seen

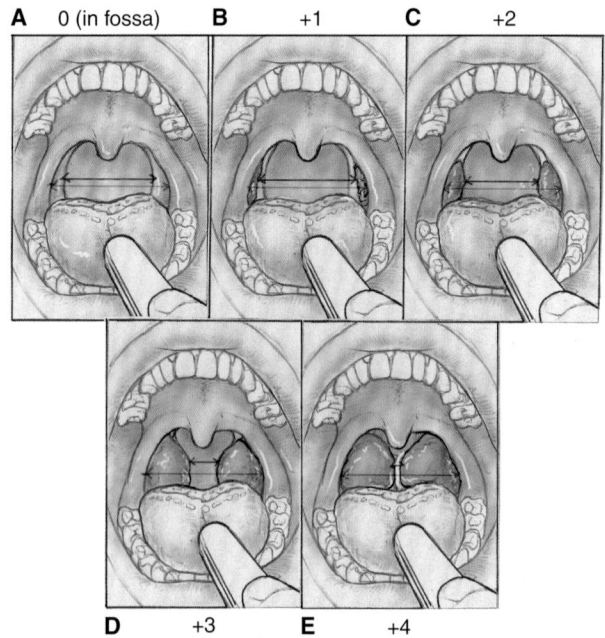

Figure 139.1 Brodsky grading of tonsil size. Tonsils are graded as: Grade 0—surgically absent (**A**), Grade 1—within the tonsillar pillars (**B**), Grade 2—just to/beyond the tonsillar pillars (**C**), Grade 3—beyond the tonsillar pillars, but not to midline (**D**), and Grade 4—touching in the midline (**E**).

and 4 for tonsils that "kiss," or approximate, in the midline. An assessment using the modified Mallampati score (36–38) can also be performed by evaluating the view of the uvula and posterior pharyngeal wall while asking the child to open his/her mouth completely while the tongue is in a resting position. Scoring is grade I when the entire uvula is visible, grade II for a partial view of the uvula, grade III when none of the uvula is visible but some of the soft palate is visible, and grade IV for a view of the hard palate only. Flexible laryngoscopy is recommended in all children under 1 year of age with OSA and when further evaluation is needed in older children. Flexible laryngoscopy allows direct visualization of the base of tongue, pharyngeal walls, vallecula, epiglottis, hypopharynx, vocal folds, and potentially, a portion of the subglottis. This procedure is useful in the evaluation of possible laryngomalacia, lingual tonsil hypertrophy, and persistent OSA despite previous tonsils and adenoids (T&A), and is also useful to document vocal cord mobility and to rule out pharyngeal/hypopharyngeal masses.

Additional Studies

Lateral neck films can be used in children that do not tolerate nasopharyngoscopy or flexible laryngoscopy. This film is most commonly used to identify adenoidal size but can also identify structural abnormalities within the nasal cavity, as well as lingual tonsil hypertrophy (39). Cine magnetic resonance imaging (MRI) has been described as a tool for assessment of the child with persistent sleep apnea despite surgical treatment with an adenotonsillectomy (40). In recent years, both pediatricians and pediatric otolaryngologists have deferred the use of airway fluoroscopy and computed tomography (CT) unless absolutely necessary, given the long-term risks of early radiation exposure. In those patients with a higher likelihood of associated cardiovascular complications from OSA, such as children with underlying congenital cardiac anomalies, electrocardiograms and echocardiograms should be considered in the workup of OSA.

Polysomnography

Polysomnography (PSG) is currently considered the traditional, and preferred, method in the evaluation and diagnosis of OSA in children (28). PSG includes the recovering of a number of different simultaneous recordings during sleep as noted in Table 139.4 (41). The results of this test provide objective measurements regarding the severity of airway obstruction in children during sleep. The apnea–hypopnea index (AHI) is obtained by averaging the number of apneas and hypopneas per hour of sleep, and this number is used to categorize the severity of OSA. Obstructive events/apneas in children are defined by continued respiratory effort with an absolute termination of airflow through the nose and mouth. A reduction in airflow of ≥30% to 50% along with either an arousal or an oxygen desaturation ≥3% from the baseline is considered a hypopnea (42).

TABLE 139.4	PARAMETERS RECORDED DURING NOCTURNAL PSG
Measurement Parameters	Electroencephalography (EEG)
	Electrooculography (EOG)
	Chin electromyography (EMG)
	End tidal CO_2
	Leg EMG
	Airflow performance
	Effort parameters
	Oxygen saturation
	Body position
Polysomnography Output	REM vs. non-REM sleep
	Apnea–hypopnea index (AHI)
	Respiratory disturbance index (RDI)
	Peak-end tidal CO_2
	Time with $CO_2 > 50$

In addition, the definition of flow limitation of apnea in children only requires an event to last for two or more consecutive breathing cycles, versus the 10-second criteria necessary for adults (42). Similar to adult evaluation, multiple series have demonstrated that the test–retest reliability, comparing multiple nights of PSG in the same child, is consistent and that PSG serves as a valid test for OSA in children (43–46).

The categories for OSA in adults are well-established; however, a standard definition of SDB disease severity does not exist for pediatric OSA, thus study interpretation may differ in their criteria used for mild, moderate, or severe OSA. One series that evaluated nonsnoring children defined a normal PSG as ≤1 obstructive apnea per hour, ≤0.9 central apneas per hour, an oxygen saturation nadir of 89% or higher, and an end tidal CO_2 greater than 45 mm Hg for 10% of the total sleep time (47). Current research definitions for OSA commonly define mild OSA when obstructive AHI is between 1 and less than 5 events per hour, moderate OSA if the AHI is 5 to less than 10, and severe OSA when the AHI is greater than 10.

While the use of PSG to diagnose OSA is widely accepted for adults, some controversy exists regarding the use of PSG in the diagnosis of pediatric OSA. It is not universally accepted that all otherwise healthy children with suspicion of OSA should undergo PSG. Issues include the fact that there are not enough sleep centers to test children in a reasonable time frame and that many sleep centers are not designed to accommodate children (i.e., with extra beds for caregivers, CO_2 monitoring, and staff specifically trained to work with children). If the PSG for a child is done in an "adult" sleep center, it is important to confirm that pediatric definitions are used in the scoring of the study. The extra cost and time to obtain a sleep study is questioned if adenotonsillectomy is planned, regardless of the PSG result.

Two recent guidelines were published in 2011 to address some of these issues. The first, by the American Academy of

Sleep Medicine (AASM), recommends that PSG is indicated when OSA is suggested by clinical assessment, and all children being considered for adenotonsillectomy for OSA should undergo PSG (48). These guidelines also recommend that PSG be used prior to decannulation in children that required tracheostomy placement, be used postoperatively in children with symptoms of persistent OSA after adenotonsillectomy as well as those with moderate to severe preoperative OSA, and those with high risk for persistent disease such as those with obesity or craniofacial abnormalities (48).

Alternatively, practice guidelines released by the American Academy of Otolaryngology—Head and Neck Surgery (AAO-HNS) recommend that all children with obesity, Down syndrome, craniofacial abnormalities, neuromuscular disorders, sickle cell disease, or mucopolysaccharidoses be referred for PSG, since these children are at the highest risk of having OSA (49). In addition, PSGs are recommended in order to determine which otherwise healthy children should be admitted after adenotonsillectomy, specifically those with severe OSA and thus high risk for respiratory distress after surgery (50). They also recommend PSGs when the need for surgery is uncertain or if the size of the tonsils found on physical exam does not correlate with the reported symptoms of SDB (49,50).

TREATMENT OF OSA

Medical Treatment

Data on the use of medicine for the treatment of OSA are relatively limited. Both nasal and oral steroids have been studied for the treatment of snoring and OSA in children. In one series looking at OSA in children, the 6-week use of nasal steroids caused a mean reduction in the respiratory disturbance index (RDI) of 25 children from 11 events per hour to 6 events per hour (51). No reduction in symptoms or the AHI by PSG was seen when children were treated with a short course of oral steroids (52). Leukotriene modifiers, such as Montelukast, may be helpful in the treatment of enlarged adenoid tissue. One study on children with mild OSA showed improvement in hypercarbia, a decrease in the AHI, and a reduction in the size of the adenoid tissue after a 16-week course of Montelukast (Fig. 139.2) (53).

Weight loss has been shown to decrease the severity of OSA, particularly in those with mild to moderate disease. In those with severe OSA, weight loss by diet and bariatric surgery can lead to a decrease in the severity, but not necessarily a full cure (54,55). Weight loss could also lower CPAP requirements, leading to better compliance of the positive pressure therapy (56).

Continuous Positive Airway Pressure

Positive airway pressure (PAP) has become a commonly accepted treatment option for children with OSA in specific circumstances. Nasal continuous positive airway pressure (CPAP) is effective in treating OSA in children, and it has been approved for use in children since 2006. It is primarily used as an adjunct therapy, especially in children that have persistent OSA after adenotonsillectomy, but it is also used in patients in whom surgery is contraindicated. CPAP is composed of a source for warm humidified air or oxygen, a generator that creates positive pressure, and a patient delivery system (for children with OSA, it is in the form of a nasal mask) (57). Ideally, CPAP titration is performed during PSG, with a minimum starting pressure of 4 cm H_2O and a maximum of 15 cm H_2O for children under the age of 12 years old (58). The goal of titration is to eliminate obstructive events with positive airflow in order to maintain airway patency (58). A large series showed that RDI was reduced and oxygen saturation increased in children aged 2 to 16 years using CPAP for OSA; however, at least 30% stopped the use of CPAP in less than 6 months (59).

As with PSG, there are certain limitations with CPAP for the treatment of OSA in children. A national survey of sleep centers found that protocols for titration varied widely between institutions, and 22% of the centers do not utilize written protocols (60). The continued use of CPAP also carries with it certain risks. Many children discontinue the use of CPAP due to the discomfort of the mask or the noise that is created by the machine. Long-term use of the mask can also lead to skin defects or potentially harmful craniofacial abnormalities, with 68% experiencing global facial flattening, 37% with maxillary retrusion, and 48% resulting in damage of the skin (61).

Pre   **Post**

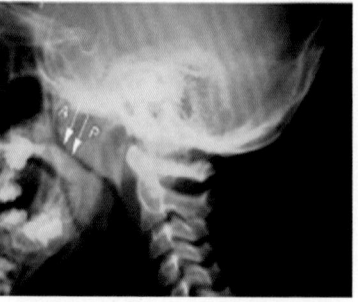 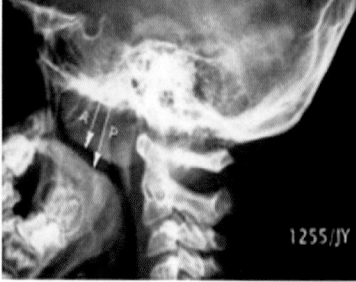

Figure 139.2 Lateral neck films showing effects of a 16-week treatment of Montelukast on adenoid size. (Reprinted from Goldbart AD, Goldman JL, et al. Leukotriene modifier therapy for mild sleep-disordered breathing in children. *Am J Respir Crit Care Med* 2005;172(3):364–370, Figure 1, with permission.)

Surgical Treatment

Adenotonsillectomy

Adenotonsillectomy is currently the first-line treatment of OSA in children. In 2009, approximately 530,000 outpatient adenotonsillectomies were performed in children in the US (62). A meta-analysis from 2006 found that resolution of OSA, defined by a postoperative RDI of less than 1 or less than 5 depending on the study, was achieved in 83% of cases (63). However, the success rate of an adenotonsillectomy is variable depending on the patient population and confounding morbidities. For example, children with morbid obesity, craniofacial abnormalities, or those with syndromes often have difficult-to-treat OSA and have incomplete resolution after adenotonsillectomy. A large study from 2009 found an overall success rate in curing OSA in 66.3% of children treated with adenotonsillectomy, but cure rates varied widely between complicated (39%) versus uncomplicated (74%) children (64). QOL measures also seem to be different after an adenotonsillectomy in obese versus normal-weight children. In a recent series, both normal-weight and obese children had overall improvements in AHI and QOL, but obese children were more likely to have persistent OSA and poor QOL scores even after adenotonsillectomy (65).

Over the years, many methods have been used and developed for the removal of the adenoids and tonsils. However, there is no universally preferred method. Common methods for performing adenotonsillectomy include "cold steel" and electrocautery, but newer techniques include coblation (Fig. 139.3), Harmonic scalpel (Ethicon, Cincinnati, OH), CO_2 laser, and microdebrider intracapsular tonsillectomy (Medtronic, Jacksonville, FL) (66). The development of these and other alternate techniques for adenotonsillectomy have been aimed at reducing postoperative pain while minimizing bleeding rates.

Although adenotonsillectomy is one of the most common surgical procedures performed in the US, the rate of complications is quite low. Potential operative and postoperative complications include hemorrhage, negative reactions to anesthesia, airway complications, electrosurgical fires, nasopharyngeal stenosis, velopharyngeal insufficiency (VPI)/incompetence, and atlantoaxial subluxation (67). Other common postoperative complications that can result in hospitalization include nausea, vomiting, and dehydration. A recent series compared postoperative complications after microdebrider, coblator, or monopolar electrocautery, and major complications, including post-tonsillectomy hemorrhage requiring an emergency department visit or surgical intervention, were studied (66). The overall major complication rates were 2.8% with coblation, 3.1% with monopolar electrocautery, and 0.7% with microdebrider (66); however, these results were confounded by multiple surgeons performing a number of different techniques (68).

Adenoidectomy

Although adenoidectomy is routinely performed with a tonsillectomy for treatment of OSA in children, some studies have looked at the use of adenoidectomy alone for OSA. Indications for adenoidectomy alone include instances where adenoids are found on either nasopharyngoscopy exam or by lateral neck x-ray to be enlarged and causing nasal obstruction, but palatine tonsils are not enlarged. Studies have shown that clinically significant regrowth of the adenoids, with recurrence of obstructive symptoms, is rare, occurring in approximately 3% of children (69,70). Regrowth is felt to be more common in younger children or in cases where "blind" adenoidectomy techniques are used with residual adenoid tissue left behind, bulging into the posterior choanae (69,71). On the other hand, another retrospective analysis of children who underwent adenoidectomy found that 38% of the children who underwent adenoidectomy alone for obstructive symptoms required subsequent surgery (72). These study results must be weighed with the risks and benefits of doing both the tonsillectomy and adenoidectomy compared to just the adenoidectomy alone.

Methods for performing adenoidectomy include curette, electrocautery, microdebrider, and coblation, but, similar to tonsillectomy, no single method is universally used. Postoperative hemorrhage requiring surgical intervention is rare and generally only seen with a tonsillectomy, and pain associated with adenoidectomy is significantly less than that seen with tonsillectomy. Less common, but concerning, risks include postoperative VPI, nasopharyngeal stenosis, and injury to the soft palate. Many suggest only removal of the superior adenoids in children at risk for postoperative VPI, including those with submucous and overt cleft palates.

PRE-, PERI-, AND POSTOPERATIVE MANAGEMENT

The preoperative evaluation of any child with OSA should include questions about a family or personal history of bleeding disorders, easy bruising, excessive bleeding during

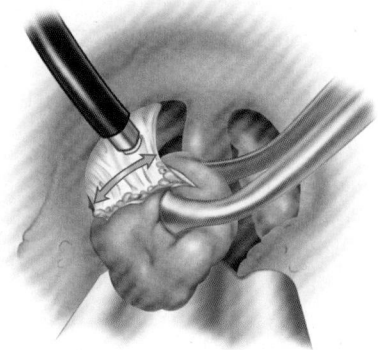

Figure 139.3 Tonsillectomy as performed with a Coblation wand (ArthroCare Corp., Sunnyvale, CA. Reprinted with permission from ArthroCare Corp.)

dental procedures, or any problems with anesthesia. If a bleeding risk is suspected, a more significant hematologic workup should be performed. In a recent study of children presenting with post-tonsillectomy bleeding, 19% of the children presented with abnormally elevated prothrombin time, partial thromboplastin time, or platelet function assays, and 4% were diagnosed with a coagulopathy (73). For those children who have other medical co-morbidities, the preoperative evaluation should be tailored to the individual. For example, for children with a higher risk of cardiovascular abnormalities/complications, including those children with long-term severe OSA, preoperative evaluation by cardiology, and/or preoperative electrocardiogram or an echocardiogram, should be considered.

Previous guidelines from the American Academy of Pediatrics note an increased risk of anesthetic complications in children with OSA (28). The AAO-HNS also advocates for detailed communication between the surgeon and anesthesiologist regarding the severity of OSA and PSG findings before surgery so that appropriate intraoperative decision making can be made (49).

Postoperatively, children with OSA should be closely monitored for hypoxemia and hypercarbia as they are at greater risk for complications compared to healthy children. Due to an increased risk of pulmonary complications, children under the age of 3 years should be monitored overnight after adenotonsillectomy (74). The 2002 AAP recommendations include postoperative admission and observation for all children in "at-risk" groups. This includes children younger than 3 years; those with severe OSA by preoperative sleep study, cardiac complications of OSA, failure to thrive, obesity, prematurity, recent respiratory infection, craniofacial anomalies; and those with neuromuscular disorders (28). The 2011 AAO-HNS recommendations include postoperative observation for children younger than 3 years of age and those with severe OSA. These recommendations also suggest that children in the "at-risk" groups "may be considered" for postoperative admission, with "at-risk" groups including those with obesity, neuromuscular or craniofacial disorders, Down syndrome, mucopolysaccharidoses, and sickle cell disease (75).

Children should have adequate pain control, either with acetaminophen, ibuprofen, or narcotics, although studies suggest that children with OSA are more sensitive to the respiratory-depressant effects of opioids, and should thus be used judiciously (76).

PERSISTENT OSA DESPITE PREVIOUS T&A

Although traditional teaching suggested that removal of the T&A successfully treated OSA and symptoms of upper airway obstruction in children who present with large T&A, studies now show that this does not occur in a significant percentage of children (63,77–79). Tauman et al. (78) showed that in a group of 110 children, only 25% had an AHI of ≤1 and

29% of the children still had an AHI greater than 5 after T&A. Obrien et al. showed in a group of 69 children, using a definition of "success" as an RDI less than 5, that only 77.5% had success after T&A. For a subgroup of obese children in this study, only 45% had success after surgery (77). Mitchell's results were somewhat better but also found a higher than expected failure rate, with 29% of the children in his study (n = 79) failing to have an AHI of ≤1 after T&A surgery. Risk factors identified in these studies include obesity, older age at the time of surgery, and severe preoperative OSA (79).

A multicenter study evaluated 560 children who underwent T&A for treatment of their sleep apnea. All children had preoperative and postoperative sleep studies. After surgery, only 27% had an AHI of less than 1, and over 21% continued to have an AHI greater than 5. Risk factors for failure included obesity, age older than 7 years, asthma in nonobese children, and more severe sleep apnea preoperatively (80).

Other populations at risk for continued OSA after T&A are those with craniofacial and mandibular anomalies. These include children with Pierre Robin sequence, cleft palate, Crouzon, Treacher Collins, achondroplasia, as well as children with cerebral palsy and genetic disorders such as Down syndrome (11,81–83). Merrell et al. showed in group of 37 children with Down syndrome who underwent T&A for treatment of sleep apnea, with an average age of 3.5 years, that only 43% had a normal AHI of ≤1 after surgery. If the persistence of hypoxemia and hypercarbia are also included in the evaluation of the postoperative sleep study, then only 29% of the children had a normal postoperative sleep study (84). Shete et al. (85) showed in a study of 11 children with Down syndrome, with an average age of 8.4 years, that only 18% had an AHI less than 2 postoperatively, significantly worse results than those seen in a group of nonsyndromic children matched for age, BMI, and degree of sleep apnea.

Evaluation of Site of Obstruction in the Oropharyngeal Airway

A PSG continues to be the most commonly used test to diagnose residual SDB after T&A. In addition to children with known higher risk factors and those with PSG-proven OSA preoperatively, PSGs should be considered for any child who continues to have persistent snoring, obstructive breathing, or oxygen desaturations following T&A (48).

If OSA is still present despite previous T&A surgery, other treatment options must be explored. Although the PSG can identify SDB and provide objective data regarding the severity of the obstruction, it does not identify at what level or levels of the airway the obstruction is occurring. Diagnosing the site(s) of obstruction in children can be more difficult compared to adults. The Mueller maneuver and the various grading systems used in adults, such as the Friedman Palate Position Grading system, the Fujita, and/or the modified Mallampati scoring methods, are not easily achieved in the pediatric population. Children are not always able to fully cooperate, and the oral cavity exam is often challenging and rarely consistent (37). The lack of sensitivity even for the oral cavity exam in evaluating tonsil size and possible OSA was recently addressed by Nolan and Brietzke. Their review assessed the association between subjective tonsil size using the 0 to 4+ scale and objective PSG data and found little, if any, association between the two, stressing the poor reliability of the physical exam in the uncooperative pediatric patient (86). In addition, even if cooperation is possible, in their critical review of the techniques of airway evaluation, Stuck and Mauer point out that the sites of obstruction detected in awake patients by the Mueller maneuver and these grading systems do not always correlate with sites of obstruction during sleep (87).

There are four anatomic sites where obstruction can potentially occur: the nose and nasopharynx, the posterior oropharynx, the lateral pharyngeal walls, and/or at the level of the hypopharynx with obstruction at the base of the tongue.

Persistent nasal airway obstruction may result from a deviated nasal septum, enlarged nasal turbinates, or polypoid changes. Studies have shown that the use of nasal steroid sprays can have a significant improvement in the severity of OSA (51). Nasal polyps are less common in children, but a proper examination should be done to rule these out. The hard palate should also be examined. Since the hard palate also represents the floor of the nose, a high arched palate may have a significant effect on nasal resistance and obstruction. Lateral wall collapse of the posterior oropharynx has also been shown to contribute to OSA (88). Edema of the posterior oropharyngeal wall, lateral banding, and/or granular pharyngitis may suggest gastroesophageal reflux, contributing to a decrease in the airway size.

Flexible endoscopy, examining the nasopharynx, posterior oropharynx, base of tongue, the lingual tonsils, and the larynx, can be performed in the office setting or in the operative room under light sedation. A study by Revell and Clark (89) showed the contribution of "late-onset" laryngomalacia to persistent OSA after T&A. Whereas the office exam does not take into account the collapsibility of the airway that occurs with muscle relaxation during sleep, the exam in the operating room may be associated with false positives because of too much muscle relaxation secondary to the anesthesia (e.g., glossoptosis is common in all undergoing general anesthesia). Drug-induced sleep endoscopy (DISE) has more routinely been used for evaluation in adult patients with OSA; however, recent studies have used sleep endoscopy in the evaluation of late-onset laryngomalacia as a means to determine the collapsibility of the airway in pediatric patients (89,90). DISE has also been used for airway evaluation during lingual tonsillectomy in pediatric patients with OSA (91). Although not prevalent in the literature, DISE is becoming a more frequently used method to characterize the specific anatomic location and pattern of obstruction in pediatric patients with SDB.

Yellon has described a staging system for epiglottic and base of tongue prolapse using flexible endoscopy. Grade 0 is normal when the entire supraglottic larynx is visible with no base of tongue prolapse. Grade 1 occurs when the epiglottis falls against the posterior pharyngeal wall but the base of tongue is not pushing up against the epiglottis. Grade 2 has both prolapse of the base of tongue and the epiglottis together, with only the tip of the epiglottis visible. Grade 3 occurs when the base of tongue prolapse is so severe that the epiglottis is no longer visible on endoscopic exam (92).

Radiographic studies can also be useful to evaluate possible sites of obstruction. A lateral neck x-ray can show regrowth of the adenoid tissues and identify enlarged lingual tonsils (93). Radiographic studies are also used for dynamic evaluations of the airway (94–96). Videofluoroscopy was initially used, but due to the high level of exposure to ionizing radiation and the poor sensitivity due to overlapping structures seen on the lateral views taken for this technique, this is rarely done today. In children with craniofacial disorders and bony abnormalities of the facial skeleton, CT scans offer better bony definition. Dynamic cine CTs can also be performed, but due to concerns of exposure to high levels of ionizing radiation, they are not commonly used (97).

Cine MRI is increasingly being utilized to provide a high-resolution examination of the dynamic airway and more accurately identify sites of upper airway obstruction in children, without the added risk of radiation exposure. It is particularly helpful in evaluation of children with multiple sites of obstruction, such as is seen in children and adults with Down syndrome and those with craniofacial anomalies. Cine images are obtained with mild sedation administered by an anesthesiologist such as dexmedetomidine, an alpha-2 agonist that works similarly to clonidine but with a higher sensitivity to the alpha-2 receptors. It mimics natural sleep with minimal respiratory depression. Other anesthetic agents that have been used include propofol, pentobarbs, and midazolam, but these drugs have a greater effect on the pharyngeal airway muscle tone (98).

In the cine MRI, 128 consecutive images are captured over 2 minutes during episodes of airway obstruction and/or oxygen desaturation. The images can then be displayed in a cine format, creating a real-time "movie" of the airway motion. Dynamic motion of the airway is evaluated in three main anatomic locations: the nasopharynx, the oropharynx, and the hypopharynx (Fig. 139.4) (99). Donnelly et al. (100) studied children with and without known OSA and found that the frequency and degree (mean change in airway diameter) of dynamic motion or collapse were statistically greater in the nasopharynx and hypopharynx in the patients with OSA. Due to the increased brightness of lymphoid tissue compared to surrounding soft tissue and muscle on T2-weighted images, the cine MRI clearly delineates adenoid regrowth or recurrence as well as lingual tonsil hypertrophy (Fig. 139.5). Adenoid enlargement

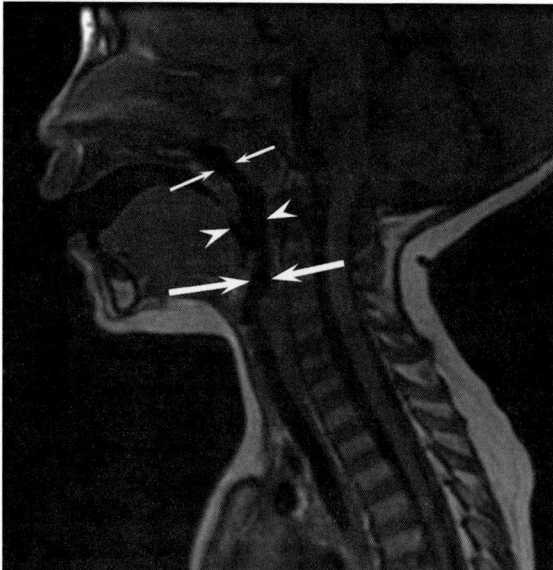

Figure 139.4 Sagittal T1-weighted MR demonstrates the anatomic regions of the supraglottic airway. The hypopharynx is behind the epiglottis (*large arrows*). The nasopharynx is between the soft palate and the adenoid tonsils (*small arrows*). The oropharynx is between the tongue base and the posterior oropharyngeal wall (*arrowheads*). (Reprinted from Shott SR, Donnelly LF. Cine magnetic resonance imaging: evaluation of persistent airway obstruction after tonsil and adenoidectomy in children with Down syndrome. *Laryngoscope* 2004;114(10):1724–1729, Figure 1, with permission.)

is reported if residual adenoid tissue is greater than 12 mm in thickness and if there is intermittent obstruction of the posterior nasopharynx seen on the sagittal cine MRIs (40). Lingual tonsil hypertrophy has been defined as tissue being thicker than 10 mm in diameter and abutting both the posterior border of the tongue and the posterior pharyngeal wall (101).

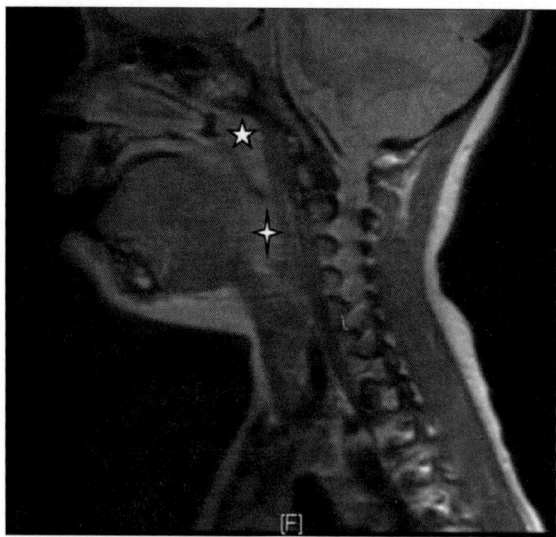

Figure 139.5 Due to increased brightness of lymphoid tissue compared to surrounding soft tissue and muscle on T2-weighted images, the cine MRI also clearly delineates adenoid regrowth (☆) or recurrence as well as lingual tonsillar hypertrophy (✛).

Unlike endoscopic examination of the airway, cine MRI allows for simultaneous assessment of multiple levels of the airway, identifying both primary and secondary sites of obstruction (40). Dynamic sagittal cine sequences can demonstrate glossoptosis, with abnormal posterior motion of the tongue during sleep (Fig. 139.6). Cine MRI axial views of the hypopharynx allow one to characterize the pattern of obstruction in either an anterior to posterior direction or more of a lateral wall movement and collapse. If there is both anterior–posterior and lateral wall collapse, a circumferential pattern of collapse is present (Fig. 139.7).

In a study evaluating 29 children with Down syndrome who had persistent OSA after T&A, cine MRIs were used to evaluate for the site(s) of residual obstruction (Table 139.5). The base of tongue, with both macroglossia and glossoptosis, was the major site of obstruction along with recurrent adenoids, each occurring in 63% to 74% of the children. Thirty percent of the children had enlarged lingual tonsils contributing to their airway obstruction (102).

TREATMENT OF PERSISTENT OSA AFTER T&A IN CHILDREN

Identification of an ideal management plan for children with residual OSA after T&A can be difficult as there is no specific treatment strategy available that is consistently effective. A multidisciplinary approach is often needed that includes sleep medicine, otolaryngology, pulmonology, and behavioral psychology to help with behavior modification and compliance issues. Many of the surgical interventions currently practiced are procedures that have been done for many years in adults, but only recently in children, thus there are few outcome studies available. Results are frequently reported via parental satisfaction reports without objective data, such as that provided by postoperative sleep studies (78).

Positive Airway Pressure Therapy

CPAP therapy continues to be a primary treatment for persistent OSA after T&A and should be offered if no obvious anatomic issue is identified. CPAP has proven to have successful therapeutic results if they are used, but unfortunately compliance is problematic in children, especially those with developmental delays or the very young. Finding appropriately sized masks can be difficult in younger children, and one study evaluating CPAP compliance in children showed that 30% stopped using within 6 months. For those who continued to use it, parents overestimated the nightly length of use by 1.8 hours (59). If CPAP is used in children, yearly retitration evaluations may be needed. One of the more serious adverse effects limiting long-term use of this treatment modality in children is the potential for craniofacial changes due to the mechanical forces applied to the maxilla from the nasal masks (61).

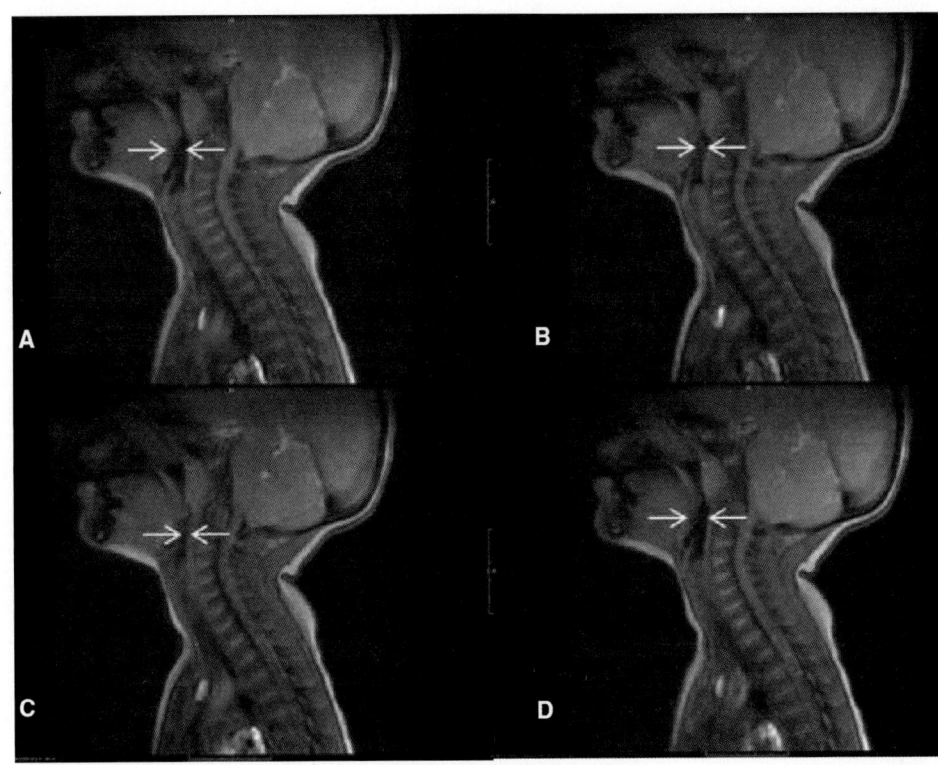

Figure 139.6 Cine MRI consecutive sagittal views showing glossoptosis. *Arrows* show area of movement of base of tongue and airway collapse (**A–D**).

Oral Appliances

Oral appliances are one of the newer advances in the treatment of pediatric OSA (103). These devices enlarge the pharyngeal airway using mechanical forces (104). The use of dental appliances to achieve nighttime mandibular advancement can be considered in older children who have all secondary dentition in place and mild OSA (105). Outcome studies on the use of oral appliances have been mainly in adults with variable success. Better results are seen in those who have mild to moderate OSA, those who are thinner, those who have a greater protrusion range, and those who have positional apnea (104). Studies have also shown a subset of patients who are better able to tolerate CPAP with the combined use of an oral appliance (106). Although useful for certain patients, these appliances, similar to the masks used for CPAP, can result in craniofacial abnormalities due to prolonged mechanical forces to the maxilla and mandible.

In children with high arched palates and mild residual OSA, rapid maxillary expansion or palate expanders are another option of treatment. In addition to the increased nasal resistance associated with a high arched palate and maxillary constriction, there can also be associated alterations in tongue posture that contribute to retroglossal airway narrowing (107). In one study evaluating 14 children undergoing rapid maxillary expansion, snoring was reduced and the AHI was decreased from a mean average of 5.8 to 1.5 events per hour (108). A recent study also showed improvement that persisted up to 24 months after treatment (109).

Weight Loss, Positional Therapy, and Medical Therapy

With the increasing number of young children and adolescents who are obese, weight loss must also be incorporated in the treatment of children with persistent OSA.

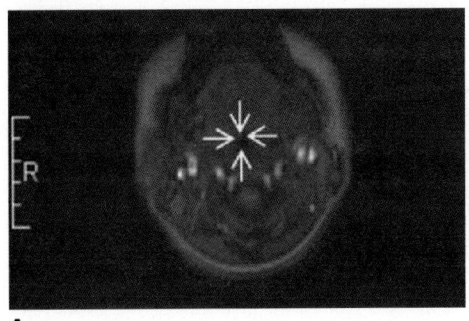

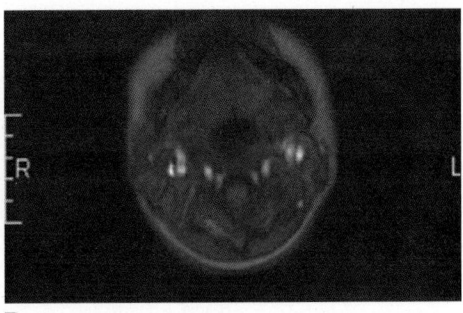

Figure 139.7 Axial view of cine MRI showing circumferential hypopharyngeal collapse of the airway with both lateral wall and anterior–posterior wall collapse (**A,B**). *Arrows* show area of collapse (**A**).

TABLE 139.5	CAUSES OF PERSISTENT OSA DESPITE PREVIOUS T&A IN CHILDREN WITH DOWN SYNDROME AS DEPICTED ON STATIC AND DYNAMIC CINE MRI

Causes of Persistent OSA in Children with Down Syndrome	
Macroglossia	74%
Glossoptosis	63%
Recurrent adenoids	63%
Enlarged lingual tonsils	30%
Hypopharyngeal collapse	22%

From Donnelly LF, Shott SR, et al. Causes of persistent obstructive sleep apnea despite previous tonsillectomy and adenoidectomy in children with down syndrome as depicted on static and dynamic cine MRI. *AJR Am J Roentgenol* 2004;183(1):175–181.

The medical treatment reviewed earlier such as nasal steroids and leukotriene inhibitors may also be considered in children with residual mild OSA (53). Positional therapy, using special shirts, pillows, or belts, is intended to keep the child sleeping on his/her side or stomach and has been shown to be effective in a subset of patients who have positional sleep apnea. Figure 139.8 shows an example of a positional belt (110).

Surgical Treatments

Patients with moderate to severe OSA will frequently obstruct at several levels. The impulse is to therefore address multiple sites at a single surgical setting, as has been advocated in the adult population (111,112). However, a study by Prager et al. (113) showed an 8.2% incidence of oropharyngeal scarring and stenosis in 48 children who underwent multilevel surgery that included lingual tonsillectomy for OSA in children. Because of this, staged surgeries are recommended. In addition, significant improvements in airway size can be accomplished with solitary surgical procedures, result in augmented airway dynamics, and reduce Bernoulli and Starling effects causing collapse at other levels (114).

The various anatomic locations of upper airway obstruction in pediatric OSA and their recommended surgical management are listed in Figure 139.9 (115). All of these surgeries have been traditionally performed in adults with varying degrees of success that rarely reach above 50% to 60% for those with moderate and severe OSA. While complete cure may not be achieved, surgery usually leads to significant improvement in the degree of OSA and may also allow for decreased CPAP pressures, facilitating improved tolerance and compliance of this treatment modality.

Nasal Surgery

Nasal obstruction that is not altered by adenoidectomy, such as seen with a deviated nasal septum or enlarged nasal turbinates, can contribute to residual OSA. Further, enlarged nasal turbinates are especially important as contributors to SDB in prepubertal children. If nasal steroid sprays or allergy treatment are not effective, surgical treatment using radiofrequency reduction of the inferior turbinates has been shown in adults to improve nasal obstruction and CPAP compliance (116). Sullivan et al. (117) evaluated children with SDB and found that children that had enlarged inferior turbinates who underwent adenotonsillectomy plus radiofrequency treatment of inferior turbinates had a significant decrease in postoperative AHI compared to children with enlarged turbinates that underwent adenotonsillectomy alone. Although nasal obstruction is not always a component of airway obstruction and SDB in children, it is an important anatomic region that requires appropriate evaluation.

Uvulopalatopharyngoplasty

Uvulopalatopharyngoplasty (UPPP) has been used in adults with variable success, ranging from 40% to 80% (118). Higher success is seen in patients with mild OSA or Stage 1 patients using the Friedman scale (119). The traditional UPPP includes submucous resection of the musculus uvulae and a portion of the distal and lateral soft palate, in addition to tonsillectomy with closure of the anterior and posterior tonsillar pillars. The concern that aggressive removal of the soft palate may lead to increased rates of postoperative VPI is elevated in children who may already

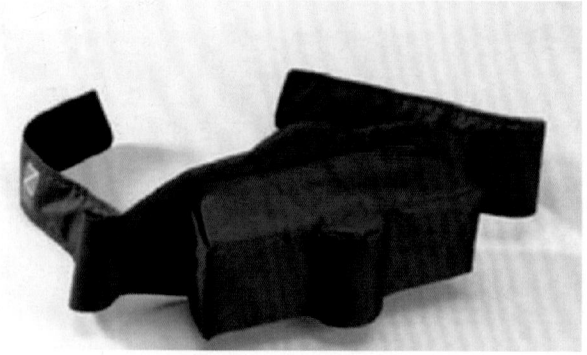
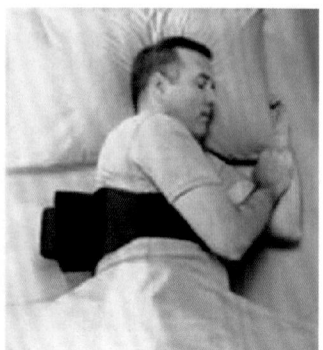

Figure 139.8 An example of a sleep belt to encourage positional treatment of OSA. (Reprinted from Permut, I, Diaz-Abad M, et al. Comparison of positional therapy to CPAP in patients with positional obstructive sleep apnea. *J Clin Sleep Med* 2010;6(3):238–243, with permission.)

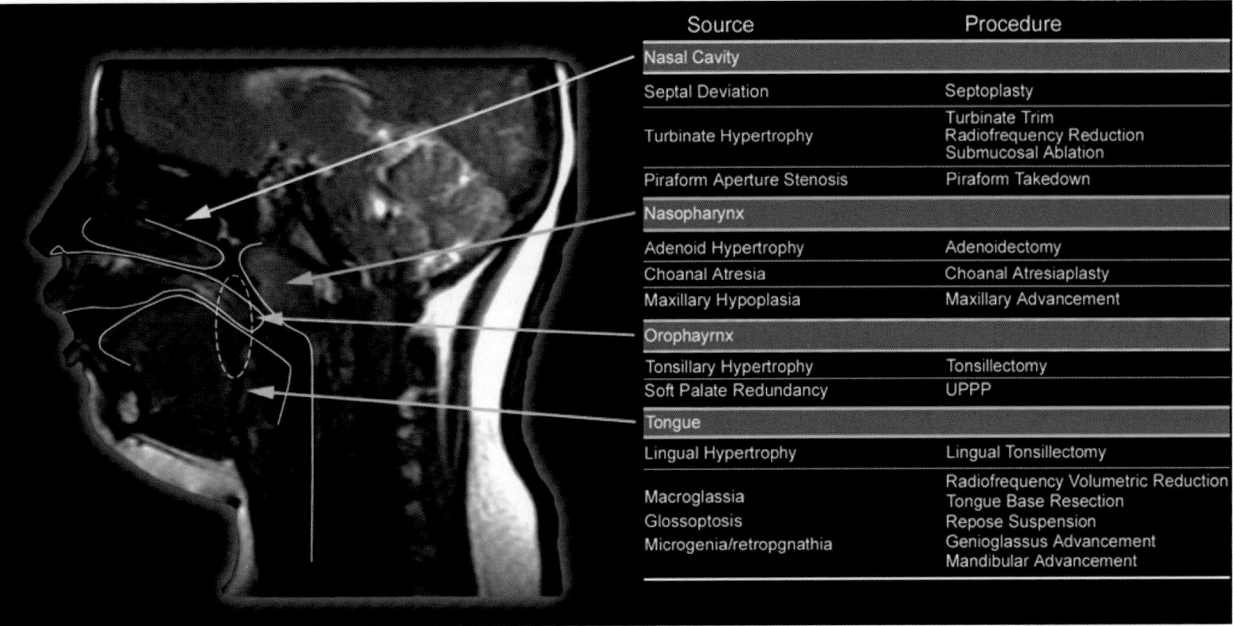

Source	Procedure
Nasal Cavity	
Septal Deviation	Septoplasty
Turbinate Hypertrophy	Turbinate Trim Radiofrequency Reduction Submucosal Ablation
Piraform Aperture Stenosis	Piraform Takedown
Nasopharynx	
Adenoid Hypertrophy	Adenoidectomy
Choanal Atresia	Choanal Atresiaplasty
Maxillary Hypoplasia	Maxillary Advancement
Orophayrnx	
Tonsillary Hypertrophy	Tonsillectomy
Soft Palate Redundancy	UPPP
Tongue	
Lingual Hypertrophy	Lingual Tonsillectomy
Macroglassia Glossoptosis Microgenia/retropgnathia	Radiofrequency Volumetric Reduction Tongue Base Resection Repose Suspension Genioglassus Advancement Mandibular Advancement

Figure 139.9 Various anatomic locations of upper airway obstruction in pediatric OSA and their recommended surgical management. (Reprinted from Shott SR, Richter GT. Chapter 8: Oral and oropharyngeal obstruction. In: Haver K, Brigger M, Hardy S, Hartnick C, eds. *Pediatric aerodigestive disorders.* San Diego, CA: Plural Publishing, 2009, Figure 8-7, page 127, with permission.)

be prone to hypernasality, such as those with submucous clefts and Down syndrome. In these cases, a more conservative excision of the soft palate, as described in the Z-pharyngoplasty procedure by Friedman, may be appropriate (120). If the exam shows more lateral wall collapse contributing to the patient's OSA, the expansion sphincter pharyngoplasty, as described by Pang and Woodson, should also be considered (88). Some have suggested the combined procedures of T&A and UPPP as first-line treatment for children in "at-risk" populations. However, no studies have shown the effectiveness of this approach with postoperative PSG data (121–125).

Lingual Tonsil Surgery

Enlarged lingual tonsils are a common site of residual obstruction in children with persistent OSA after T&A (102). Removal was initially performed with electrocautery, using an insulated blade and/or suction cautery, but this was complicated by significant postoperative pain. The use of the microdebrider allows for faster surgery but requires the use of electrocautery to control bleeding. On the other hand, the use of the coblation technique provides a good balance of speed, minimal tissue damage to surrounding areas, the ability to cauterize bleeding with the same instrument, and decreased postoperative pain. Lin and Koltai (91) reported that lingual tonsillectomy using an endoscopic coblation technique decreased the mean RDI from 14.7 to 8.1 in 26 patients, aged 3 to 20 years. This suggests that while lingual tonsils may be a significant contributor, other levels of obstruction may remain in children with residual OSA.

Base of Tongue Surgery for Macroglossia and Glossoptosis

As seen in Table 139.5, the tongue base, with associated macroglossia and glossoptosis, represents one of the most common sites of obstruction in children with Down syndrome who have persistent OSA despite previous T&A. Procedures on the base of tongue strive to either decrease the bulk of the tongue tissue or help to immobilize the tongue base in an attempt to prevent collapse of the tongue base during sleep.

The Repose system of genioglossus suspension was introduced in 1997. This is a minimally invasive technique that provides a supporting sling to the tongue base as a treatment for glossoptosis (126–129). Although originally described with a transoral approach, a submental incision and approach is much more facile in the pediatric population (Fig. 139.10). Wootten and Shott (130) reported their experience with the Repose genioglossus advancement in 31 children, with an average age of 11 years old, in 2010. Nineteen of the thirty one patients had Down syndrome. Using a "success" definition of a postoperative AHI of less than 5, no hypercarbia, and no hypoxemia less than 90%, an overall success rate of 61% was achieved. Success was higher in the children who did not have DS (66%) compared to those with DS (58%) (130).

Another method of genioglossus advancement is the midline segmental osteotomy technique (Fig. 139.11). Bone cuts through the anterior mandible create a full-thickness mandibular segment with attached genioglossus muscle. The bone is advanced anteriorly and rotated and then secured to the surrounding mandibular bone, applying anterior traction to the genioglossus muscle. Complications can

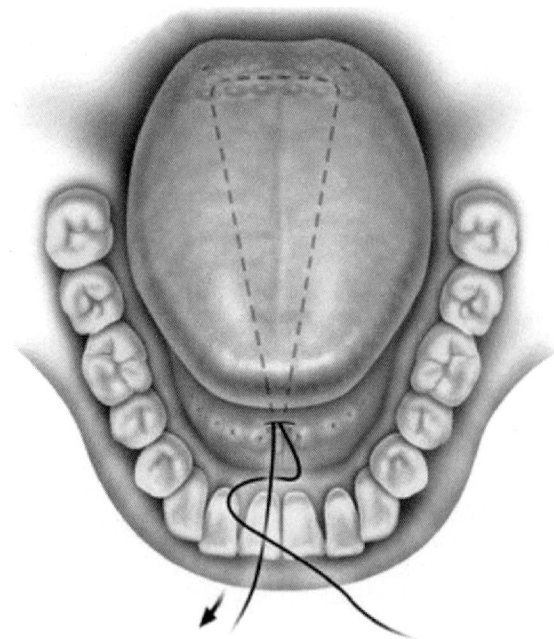

Figure 139.10 The Repose genioglossus tongue suspension applies a sling-type support to the base of the tongue to prevent hypopharyngeal collapse. (Reprinted from Pang KP, Terris D. Tongue suspension in obstructive sleep apnea. *Oper Tech Otolaryngol-HN Surg* 2006;17:252–256, Figure 6, with permission.)

include hematoma, dental and lower lip numbness, permanent injury to tooth roots and mental nerve, and infection (131). Clinical results in children have not been reported, and this surgery can only be done in older children who have already had eruption of their secondary teeth.

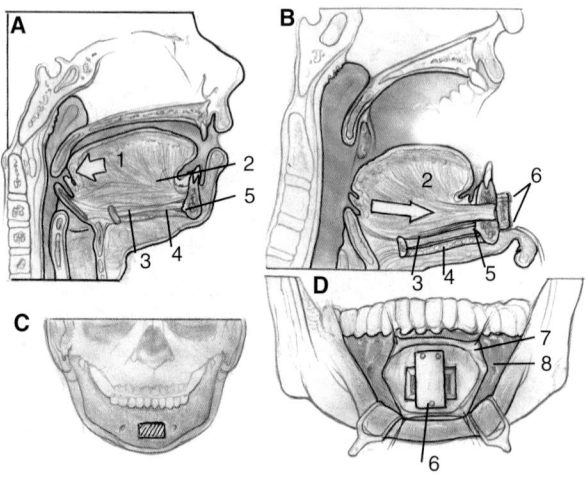

1. Enlarged tongue constricting oropharynx
2. Genioglossus m.
3. Geniohyoid m.
4. Mylohyoid m.
5. Genial tubercles
6. Screws anchor bone bloc in place
7. Periosteum
8. Mental foramen

Figure 139.11 Midline osteotomy genioglossus advancement. Bone cuts through the anterior mandible create a full-thickness mandibular segment with attached genioglossus muscle (**A**). The bone is advanced, pulling the tongue anteriorly (**B**). The window through the anterior mandible is located between the mental foramen (**C**). The bone window is anchored in place with screws (**D**).

The midline posterior glossectomy focuses on removal of tongue base muscle to decrease tissue volume that is obstructing the posterior oropharynx and hypopharynx in patients with macroglossia and glossoptosis. Techniques include midline wedge resections as well as submucosal excisions. Mickelson and Rosenthal (132) describe removal of a wedge of posterior tongue mucosa and muscle from 1 cm anterior to the posterior circumvallate papilla to the base of the epiglottis.

Because of the prolonged recovery associated with the open wound created by the wedge excision technique, submucosal excision of the tongue musculature has been described. Coblation excision is used in either open or closed techniques. For the open midline posterior glossectomy, mucosal flaps are raised after making a midline incision, and underlying muscle is then removed (Fig. 139.12). Dissection continues posteriorly into the vallecula. The mucosal incision is then closed anteriorly. Because the incision is closed, there is less pain than what is seen with the wedge resection technique.

A closed, submucosal posterior excision of the base of tongue has also been described. In the *submucosal minimally invasive lingual excision*, or "SMILE" procedure,

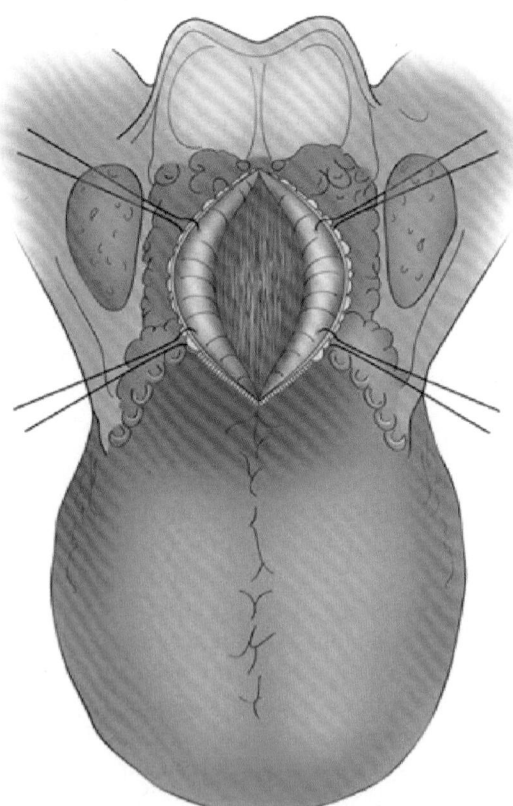

Figure 139.12 Midline posterior glossectomy: mucosal flaps are raised and posterior tongue muscle is removed with coblation wand using location of lingual arteries as margins of dissection. (Reprinted from Shott SR, Richter GT. Chapter 8: Oral and oropharyngeal obstruction. In: Haver K, Brigger M, Hardy S, Hartnick C, eds. *Pediatric aerodigestive disorders.* San Diego, CA: Plural Publishing, 2009, Figure 8-13, page 136, with permission.)

a midline incision is made on tongue dorsum, and a submucosal tunnel is made as the tongue muscle tissue is removed (133).

In both of these techniques, Doppler ultrasound is helpful to locate the lingual arteries on both sides of the midline of the tongue, providing margins for surgical safety from the more laterally sitting hypoglossal nerve. In adults, a reduction in AHI by 50% has been reported with the midline posterior glossectomy (134). Clinical studies in children are just starting to become available. Clark et al. (135) presented their initial experience with posterior midline glossectomy for treatment of macroglossia/glossoptosis at the Annual Meeting of the American Society of Pediatric Otolaryngology in 2011. In 22 patients, the success rate was 59%. Rare but reported complications include dysphagia, taste disturbances, and minor bleeding (136). Bleeding from the lingual artery, as well as the potential for hypoglossal nerve damage, should also be discussed as potential risk factors (137).

Craniofacial Surgery

In children with significant craniofacial anomalies, craniofacial surgery with mandibular and/or maxillary advancement surgery may be recommended as the primary surgical treatment.

Tracheotomy

In children with severe OSA, particularly those with associated complications of OSA such as pulmonary hypertension or cor pulmonale, tracheotomy must be considered. This may also be advisable in those with severe OSA where multilevel, staged surgeries are needed, with a recommendation to plan decannulation once surgical treatment is completed. In addition, OSA in children under 1 year old without other obvious anatomic solutions may be best treated with a tracheostomy tube.

CONCLUSION

Pediatric sleep science continues to develop and evolve while the diagnosis and management of OSA in children remain routinely debated. Because of this, clinicians must establish their own evaluation protocol with the understanding that residual OSA after T&A can be a result of obstruction at multiple sites. Endoscopic exams and radiologic evaluations, such as cine MRI, are helpful to identify the sites of obstruction. Alternatively, CPAP and BiPAP remain viable treatment options and can be successful, but compliance is difficult to achieve in the pediatric population. Despite the technique used to manage pediatric OSA, more outcomes research is needed, and currently identified surgical outcome limitations must be presented to the patients and their families. Lastly, because of the changing body size and shape that is inherent in the growing child, there is a need for continued vigilance for recurrence of the airway obstruction as the child ages.

HIGHLIGHTS

- Estimates suggest that 1% to 4% of children in the United States have OSA with snoring in 3% to 40%.
- OSA is more common in children with obesity, craniofacial anomalies, black race, and male gender.
- OSA in children commonly presents with poor school performance, snoring, daytime behavior issues, gasping and choking at night, witnessed apneas, and less frequently, daytime sleepiness.
- OSA can also result in hyperactivity, attention-deficit disorders, aggression, and poor socialization, and long-term complications include cardiovascular and pulmonary complications.
- PSG currently remains the gold standard for diagnosing OSA in children.
- The evaluation of a child with suspected OSA should include a thorough history, including a sleep history, as well as a complete head and neck exam.
- Practice Guidelines from the AAO-HNS state that PSG is recommended in children when there is a discordance in OSA severity and physical exam characteristics or is suggested by the clinical assessment, or in high-risk populations such as those with obesity, craniofacial abnormalities, sickle cell disease, and Down syndrome.
- Adenotonsillectomy is the primary treatment for OSA.
- Additional therapies to treat OSA include oral appliances, position belts, weight loss, and nasal steroids with or without leukotriene inhibitors.
- For those patients in whom surgery is contraindicated or significant OSA persists after surgery, CPAP is an appropriate alternate therapy.
- Persistent OSA occurs in a significant number of children despite a previous adenotonsillectomy.
- Children at risk for persistent OSA include those with obesity, Down syndrome, and craniofacial anomalies.
- Cine MRI is increasingly being utilized as a means to provide high-resolution examination of the dynamic airway and to identify further sites of obstruction in children with persistent OSA.
- No single specific treatment is advocated for persistent OSA in children, and often a multidisciplinary approach is appropriate.
- An array of staged surgeries, including nasal surgery, UPPP, lingual tonsil surgery, base of tongue surgery, and craniofacial surgery, can be utilized to treat persistent OSA.
- For children with severe OSA, especially in those with complications associated with OSA, a tracheotomy may be considered.

REFERENCES

1. Lumeng JC, Chervin RD. Epidemiology of pediatric obstructive sleep apnea. *Proc Am Thorac Soc* 2008;5(2):242–252.
2. Mitchell RB. Sleep-disordered breathing in children: are we underestimating the problem? *Eur Respir J* 2005;25(2):216–217.
3. Chervin RD, Clarke DF, et al. School performance, race, and other correlates of sleep-disordered breathing in children. *Sleep Med* 2003;4(1):21–27.
4. Redline S, Tishler PV, et al. Risk factors for sleep-disordered breathing in children. Associations with obesity, race, and respiratory problems. *Am J Respir Crit Care Med* 1999;159(5 Pt 1):1527–1532.
5. Rosen CL, Larkin EK. Prevalence and risk factors for sleep-disordered breathing in 8- to 11-year-old children: association with race and prematurity. *J Pediatr* 2003;142(4):383–389.
6. Johnson EO, Roth T. An epidemiologic study of sleep-disordered breathing symptoms among adolescents. *Sleep* 2006;29(9):1135–1142.
7. Montgomery-Downs HE, Gozal D. Sleep habits and risk factors for sleep-disordered breathing in infants and young toddlers in Louisville, Kentucky. *Sleep Med* 2006;7(3):211–219.
8. Ong KC, Clerk AA. Comparison of the severity of sleep-disordered breathing in Asian and Caucasian patients seen at a sleep disorders center. *Respir Med* 1998;92(6):843–848.
9. Chervin RD, Hedger K, et al. Pediatric sleep questionnaire (PSQ): validity and reliability of scales for sleep-disordered breathing, snoring, sleepiness, and behavioral problems. *Sleep Med* 2000;1(1):21–32.
10. Harding SM. Prediction formulae for sleep-disordered breathing. *Curr Opin Pulm Med* 2001;7(6):381–385.
11. Pijpers M, Poels PJ, et al. Undiagnosed obstructive sleep apnea syndrome in children with syndromal craniofacial synostosis. *J Craniofac Surg* 2004;15(4):670–674.
12. Kaditis AG, Finder J, et al. Sleep-disordered breathing in 3,680 Greek children. *Pediatr Pulmonol* 2004;37(6):499–509.
13. Vazquez JC, Montes FM, et al. Clinical predictors of sleep disordered breathing in children at moderate altitude. *Arch Med Res* 2004;35(6):525–531.
14. Beebe DW, Wells CT, et al. Neuropsychological effects of pediatric obstructive sleep apnea. *J Int Neuropsychol Soc* 2004;10(7):962–975.
15. Stewart MG, Glaze DG, et al. Quality of life and sleep study findings after adenotonsillectomy in children with obstructive sleep apnea. *Arch Otolaryngol Head Neck Surg* 2005;131(4):308–314.
16. Tran KD, Nguyen CD, et al. Child behavior and quality of life in pediatric obstructive sleep apnea. *Arch Otolaryngol Head Neck Surg* 2005;131(1):52–57.
17. Marcus CL, Greene MG, Carroll JL. Blood pressure in children with obstructive sleep apnea. *Am J Respir Crit Care Med* 1998;157:1098–1103.
18. Kohyama J, Ohinata JS, Hasegama T. Blood pressure in sleep-disordered breathing. *Arch Dis Child* 2003;88:139–142.
19. Leung LC, Ng DK, Lau MW, et al. Twenty-four-hour ambulatory BP in snoring children with obstructive sleep apnea syndrome. *Chest* 2006;130:1009–1017.
20. Enright PL, Goodwin JL, Sherrill DL, et al. Blood pressure elevations associated with sleep-related breathing disorder in a community sample of white and Hispanic children. *Arch Pediatr Adolesc Med* 2003;157:901–904.
21. Li AM, Au CT, Sung RY, et al. Ambulatory BP in children with obstructive sleep apnea: a community-based study. *Thorax* 2008;63:803–809.
22. Sun SS, Grave GD, Siervogel RM, et al. Systolic blood pressure in children predicts hypertension and metabolic syndrome later in life. *Pediatrics* 2007;119:237–246.
23. Kwok KL, Ng DK, Cheung YF. BP and arterial distensibility in children with primary snoring. *Chest* 2005;123:1561–1566.
24. Kaditis AG, Alexopoulos EI, Kostadima E, et al. Comparison of blood pressure measurements in children with and without habitual snoring. *Pediatr Pulmonol* 2005;39:408–414.
25. Verdecchia P, Porcellati C, Schillaci G, et al. Ambulatory blood pressure: an independent predictor of prognosis in essential hypertension. *Hypertension* 1994;24:793–801.
26. Amin RS, Carroll JL, Jeffries JL, et al. Twenty-four-hour ambulatory blood pressure in children with sleep-disordered breathing. *Am J Respir Crit Care Med* 2004;169:950–956.
27. Li AM, Au CT, Ho C, et al. Blood pressure is elevated in children with primary snoring. *J Pediatr* 2009;155:362–368.
28. American Academy of Pediatrics, Section of Pediatric Pulmonology. Clinical practice guideline: diagnosis and management of childhood obstructive sleep apnea syndrome. *Pediatrics* 2002;109(4):704–712.
29. Brouillette R, Hanson D, et al. A diagnostic approach to suspected obstructive sleep apnea in children. *J Pediatr* 1984;105(1):10–14.
30. Carroll JL, McColley SA, et al. Inability of clinical history to distinguish primary snoring from obstructive sleep apnea syndrome in children. *Chest* 1995;108(3):610–618.
31. Chervin RD, Weatherly RA, et al. Pediatric sleep questionnaire: prediction of sleep apnea and outcomes. *Arch Otolaryngol Head Neck Surg* 2007;133(3):216–222.
32. Brietzke SE, Katz ES, et al. Can history and physical examination reliably diagnose pediatric obstructive sleep apnea/hypopnea syndrome? A systematic review of the literature. *Otolaryngol Head Neck Surg* 2004;131(6):827–832.
33. Gozal D, O'Brien LM. Snoring and obstructive sleep apnea in children: why should we treat? *Paediatr Respir Rev* 2004;5(Suppl A):S371–S376.
34. Schwab RJ, Gupta KB, et al. Upper airway and soft tissue anatomy in normal subjects and patients with sleep-disordered breathing. Significance of the lateral pharyngeal walls. *Am J Respir Crit Care Med* 1995;152(5 Pt 1):1673–1689.
35. Brodsky L, Moore L, et al. A comparison of tonsillar size and oropharyngeal dimensions in children with obstructive adenotonsillar hypertrophy. *Int J Pediatr Otorhinolaryngol* 1987;13(2):149–156.
36. Friedman M, Tanyeri H, et al. Clinical predictors of obstructive sleep apnea. *Laryngoscope* 1999;109(12):1901–1907.
37. Friedman M, Ibrahim H, et al. Clinical staging for sleep-disordered breathing. *Otolaryngol Head Neck Surg* 2002;127(1):13–21.
38. Friedman M, Ibrahim H, et al. Combined uvulopalatopharyngoplasty and radiofrequency tongue base reduction for treatment of obstructive sleep apnea/hypopnea syndrome. *Otolaryngol Head Neck Surg* 2003;129(6):611–621.
39. Sedaghat AR, Flax-Goldenburg RB, et al. A case-control comparison of lingual tonsillar size in children with and without Down syndrome. *Laryngoscope* 2012;122(5):1165–1169.
40. Shott SR, Donnelly LF. Cine magnetic resonance imaging: evaluation of persistent airway obstruction after tonsil and adenoidectomy in children with Down syndrome. *Laryngoscope* 2004;114(10):1724–1729.
41. Kotagal S. Childhood obstructive sleep apnoea. *BMJ* 2005;330(7498):978–979.
42. Iber C, Chesson AL Jr, Quan SF. *American Academy of Sleep Medicine. Respiratory Rules. The ASSM Manual for the Scoring of Sleep and Associated Events.* Westchester, IL: American Academy of Sleep Medicine, 2007:48–49.
43. Rebuffat E, Groswasser J, et al. Polygraphic evaluation of night-to-night variability in sleep characteristics and apneas in infants. *Sleep* 1994;17(4):329–332.
44. Nieminen P, Tolonen U, et al. Snoring and obstructive sleep apnea in children: a 6-month follow-up study. *Arch Otolaryngol Head Neck Surg* 2000;126(4):481–486.
45. Katz ES, Greene MG, et al. Night-to-night variability of polysomnography in children with suspected obstructive sleep apnea. *J Pediatr* 2002;140(5):589–594.
46. Li AM, Wing YK, et al. Is a 2-night polysomnographic study necessary in childhood sleep-related disordered breathing? *Chest* 2004;126(5):1467–1472.
47. Uliel S, Tauman R, et al. Normal polysomnographic respiratory values in children and adolescents. *Chest* 2004;125(3):872–878.
48. Aurora RN, Zak RS, et al. Practice parameters for the respiratory indications for polysomnography in children. *Sleep* 2011;34(3):379–388.
49. Roland PS, Rosenfeld RM, et al. Clinical practice guideline: polysomnography for sleep-disordered breathing prior to tonsillectomy in children. *Otolaryngol Head Neck Surg* 2011;145(1 Suppl):S1–S15.

50. McColley SA, April MM, et al. Respiratory compromise after adenotonsillectomy in children with obstructive sleep apnea. *Arch Otolaryngol Head Neck Surg* 1992;118(9):940–943.

51. Brouillette RT, Manoukian JJ, et al. Efficacy of fluticasone nasal spray for pediatric obstructive sleep apnea. *J Pediatr* 2001;138(6):838–844.

52. Al-Ghamdi SA, Manoukian JJ, et al. Do systemic corticosteroids effectively treat obstructive sleep apnea secondary to adenotonsillar hypertrophy? *Laryngoscope* 1997;107(10):1382–1387.

53. Goldbart AD, Goldman JL, et al. Leukotriene modifier therapy for mild sleep-disordered breathing in children. *Am J Respir Crit Care Med* 2005;172(3):364–370.

54. Inge TH, Krebs NF, et al. Bariatric surgery for severely overweight adolescents: concerns and recommendations. *Pediatrics* 2004;114(1):217–223.

55. Mokhlesi B, Gozal D. Update in sleep medicine 2009. *Am J Respir Crit Care Med* 2010;181(6):545–549.

56. Arens R, Muzumdar H. Childhood obesity and obstructive sleep apnea syndrome. *J Appl Physiol* 2010;108(2):436–444.

57. Mahmoud RA, Roehr CC, et al. Current methods of noninvasive ventilatory support for neonates. *Paediatr Respir Rev* 2011;12(3):196–205.

58. Kushida CA, Chediak A, et al. Clinical guidelines for the manual titration of positive airway pressure in patients with obstructive sleep apnea. *J Clin Sleep Med* 2008;4(2):157–171.

59. Marcus CL, Rosen G, et al. Adherence to and effectiveness of positive airway pressure therapy in children with obstructive sleep apnea. *Pediatrics* 2006;117(3):e442–e451.

60. Stepanski EJ, Dull R, et al. CPAP titration protocols among accredited Sleep Disorder Centers. *Sleep Res* 1996;25:374.

61. Fauroux B, Lavis JF, et al. Facial side effects during noninvasive positive pressure ventilation in children. *Intensive Care Med* 2005;31(7):965–969.

62. Cullen KA, Hall MJ, et al. Ambulatory surgery in the United States, 2006. *Natl Health Stat Rep* 2009;(11):1–25.

63. Brietzke SE, Gallagher D. The effectiveness of tonsillectomy and adenoidectomy in the treatment of pediatric obstructive sleep apnea/hypopnea syndrome: a meta-analysis. *Otolaryngol Head Neck Surg* 2006;134(6):979–984.

64. Friedman M, Wilson M, et al. Updated systematic review of tonsillectomy and adenoidectomy for treatment of pediatric obstructive sleep apnea/hypopnea syndrome. *Otolaryngol Head Neck Surg* 2009;140(6):800–808.

65. Mitchell RB, Boss EF. Pediatric obstructive sleep apnea in obese and normal-weight children: impact of adenotonsillectomy on quality-of-life and behavior. *Dev Neuropsychol* 2009;34(5):650–661.

66. Gallagher TQ, Wilcox L, et al. Analyzing factors associated with major complications after adenotonsillectomy in 4776 patients: comparing three tonsillectomy techniques. *Otolaryngol Head Neck Surg* 2010;142(6):886–892.

67. Randall DA, Hoffer ME. Complications of tonsillectomy and adenoidectomy. *Otolaryngol Head Neck Surg* 1998;118(1):61–68.

68. Statham MM, Myer CM III. Complications of adenotonsillectomy. *Curr Opin Otolaryngol Head Neck Surg* 2010;18(6):539–543.

69. Buchinsky FJ, Lowry MA, et al. Do adenoids regrow after excision? *Otolaryngol Head Neck Surg* 2000;123(5):576–581.

70. Joshua B, Bahar G, et al. Adenoidectomy: long-term follow-up. *Otolaryngol Head Neck Surg* 2006;135(4):576–580.

71. Pearl AJ, Manoukian JJ. Adenoidectomy: indirect visualization of choanal adenoids. *J Otolaryngol* 1994;23(3):221–224.

72. Brietzke SE, Kenna M, et al. Pediatric adenoidectomy: what is the effect of obstructive symptoms on the likelihood of future surgery? *Int J Pediatr Otorhinolaryngol* 2006;70(8):1467–1472.

73. Sun GH, Harmych BM, et al. Characteristics of children diagnosed as having coagulopathies following posttonsillectomy bleeding. *Arch Otolaryngol Head Neck Surg* 2011;137(1):65–68.

74. Brodsky L. Adenotonsillar disease in children. In: Cotton R, ed. *Practical pediatric otolaryngology.* Philadelphia, PA: Lippincott Raven, 1999:15–39.

75. Baugh RF, Archer SM, et al. Clinical practice guideline: tonsillectomy in children. *Otolaryngol Head Neck Surg* 2011;144 (1 Suppl):S1–S30.

76. Schwengel DA, Sterni LM, et al. Perioperative management of children with obstructive sleep apnea. *Anesth Analg* 2009;109(1):60–75.

77. O'Brien LM, Sitha S, et al. Obesity increases the risk for persisting obstructive sleep apnea after treatment in children. *Int J Pediatr Otorhinolaryngol* 2006;70(9):1555–1560.

78. Tauman R, Gulliver TE, et al. Persistence of obstructive sleep apnea syndrome in children after adenotonsillectomy. *J Pediatr* 2006;149(6):803–808.

79. Mitchell RB. Adenotonsillectomy for obstructive sleep apnea in children: outcome evaluated by pre- and postoperative polysomnography. *Laryngoscope* 2007;117:1844–1854.

80. Bhattacharjee R, Kheirandish-Gozal L, et al. Adenotonsillectomy outcomes in treatment of obstructive sleep apnea in children: a multicenter retrospective study. *Am J Respir Crit Care Med* 2010;182(5):676–683.

81. Hoeve LJ, Pijpers M, et al. OSAS in craniofacial syndromes: an unsolved problem. *Int J Pediatr Otorhinolaryngol* 2003;67 (Suppl 1):S111–S113.

82. Lam DJ, Jensen CC, et al. Pediatric sleep apnea and craniofacial anomalies: a population-based case-control study. *Laryngoscope* 2010;120(10):2098–2105.

83. Robison JG, Otteson DD. Increased prevalence of obstructive sleep apnea in patients with cleft palate. *Arch Otolaryngol Head Neck Surg* 2011;137(3):269–274.

84. Merrell JA, Shott SR. OSAS in Down syndrome: T&A versus T&A plus lateral pharyngoplasty. *Int J Pediatr Otorhinolaryngol* 2007;71(8):1197–1203.

85. Shete MM, Stocks RM, et al. Effects of adeno-tonsillectomy on polysomnography patterns in Down syndrome children with obstructive sleep apnea: a comparative study with children without Down syndrome. *Int J Pediatr Otorhinolaryngol* 2010;74(3):241–244.

86. Nolan J, Brietzke SE. Systematic review of pediatric tonsil size and polysomnogram-measured obstructive sleep apnea severity. *Otolaryngol Head Neck Surg* 2011;144(6):844–850.

87. Stuck BA, Maurer JT. Airway evaluation in obstructive sleep apnea. *Sleep Med Rev* 2008;12(6):411–436.

88. Pang KP, Woodson BT. Expansion sphincter pharyngoplasty: a new technique for the treatment of obstructive sleep apnea. *Otolaryngol Head Neck Surg* 2007;137(1):110–114.

89. Revell SM, Clark WT. Late-onset laryngomalacia: a cause of pediatric obstructive sleep apnea. *Int J Pediatr Otorhinolaryngol* 2011;75(2):231–238.

90. Richter GT, Rutter MJ, deAlarcon A, et al. Late-onset laryngomalacia. *Arch Otolaryngol Head Neck Surg* 2008;134(1):75–80.

91. Lin AC, Koltai PJ. Persistent pediatric obstructive sleep apnea and lingual tonsillectomy. *Otolaryngol Head Neck Surg* 2009;141(1):81–85.

92. Yellon RF. Epiglottic and base-of-tongue prolapse in children: grading and management. *Laryngoscope* 2006;116(2):194–200.

93. Thakkar K, Yao M. Diagnostic studies in obstructive sleep apnea. *Otolaryngol Clin North Am* 2007;40(4):785–805.

94. Walsh JK, Katsantonis GP, et al. Somnofluoroscopy: cineradiographic observation of obstructive sleep apnea. *Sleep* 1985;8(3):294–297.

95. Gibson SE, Myer CM III, et al. Sleep fluoroscopy for localization of upper airway obstruction in children. *Ann Otol Rhinol Laryngol* 1996;105(9):678–683.

96. Donnelly LF, Strife JL, et al. Glossoptosis (posterior displacement of the tongue) during sleep: a frequent cause of sleep apnea in pediatric patients referred for dynamic sleep fluoroscopy. *AJR Am J Roentgenol* 2000;175(6):1557–1560.

97. Galvin JR, Rooholamini SA, et al. Obstructive sleep apnea: diagnosis with ultrafast CT. *Radiology* 1989;171(3):775–778.

98. Mahmoud M, Radhakrishman R, et al. Effect of increasing depth of dexmedetomidine anesthesia on upper airway morphology in children. *Paediatr Anaesth* 2010;20(6):506–515.

99. Donnelly LF, Casper KA, et al. Defining normal upper airway motion in asymptomatic children during sleep by means of cine MR techniques. *Radiology* 2002;223(1):176–180.

100. Donnelly LF, Surdulescu V, et al. Upper airway motion depicted at cine MR imaging performed during sleep: comparison between young patients with and those without obstructive sleep apnea. *Radiology* 2003;227(1):239–245.

101. Fricke BL, Donnelly LF, et al. Comparison of lingual tonsil size as depicted on MR imaging between children with obstructive sleep apnea despite previous tonsillectomy and adenoidectomy and normal controls. *Pediatr Radiol* 2006;36(6):518–523.

102. Donnelly LF, Shott SR, et al. Causes of persistent obstructive sleep apnea despite previous tonsillectomy and adenoidectomy in children with down syndrome as depicted on static and dynamic cine MRI. *AJR Am J Roentgenol* 2004;183(1):175–181.

103. Conley RS. Evidence for dental and dental specialty treatment of obstructive sleep apnea. Part 1: the adult OSA patient and Part 2: the paediatric and adolescent patient. *J Oral Rehabil* 2011;38(2):136–156.

104. Woodson BT. Non-pressure therapies for obstructive sleep apnea: surgery and oral appliances. *Respir Care* 2010;55(10):1314–1321; discussion 1321.

105. Holley AB, Lettieri CJ, et al. Efficacy of an adjustable oral appliance and comparison to continuous positive airway pressure for the treatment of obstructive sleep apnea syndrome. *Chest* 2011;140(6):1511–1516.

106. El-Solh AA, Moitheennazima B, et al. Combined oral appliance and positive airway pressure therapy for obstructive sleep apnea: a pilot study. *Sleep Breath* 2011;15(2):203–208.

107. Cistulli PA, Palmisano RG, et al. Treatment of obstructive sleep apnea syndrome by rapid maxillary expansion. *Sleep* 1998;21(8):831–835.

108. Villa MP, Malagola C, et al. Rapid maxillary expansion in children with obstructive sleep apnea syndrome: 12–1 month follow-up. *Sleep Med* 2007;8(2):128–134.

109. Villa MP, Rizzoli A, et al. Efficacy of rapid maxillary expansion in children with obstructive sleep apnea syndrome: 36 months of follow-up. *Sleep Breath* 2011;15(2):179–184.

110. Permut I, Diaz-Abad M, et al. Comparison of positional therapy to CPAP in patients with positional obstructive sleep apnea. *J Clin Sleep Med* 2010;6(3):238–243.

111. Jacobowitz O. Palatal and tongue base surgery for surgical treatment of obstructive sleep apnea: a prospective study. *Otolaryngol Head Neck Surg* 2006;135(2):258–264.

112. Richard W, Kox D, et al. One stage multilevel surgery (uvulopalatopharyngoplasty, hyoid suspension, radiofrequent ablation of the tongue base with/without genioglossus advancement), in obstructive sleep apnea syndrome. *Eur Arch Otorhinolaryngol* 2007;264(4):439–444.

113. Prager JD, Hopkins BS, et al. Oropharyngeal stenosis: a complication of multilevel, single-stage upper airway surgery in children. *Arch Otolaryngol Head Neck Surg* 2010;136(11):1111–1115.

114. Marcus CL, Katz ES, et al. Upper airway dynamic responses in children with the obstructive sleep apnea syndrome. *Pediatr Res* 2005;57(1):99–107.

115. Shott SR, Richter GT. Chapter 8: Oral and oropharyngeal obstruction. In: Haver K, Brigger M, Hardy S, Hartnick C, eds. *Pediatric aerodigestive disorders*. San Diego, CA: Plural Publishing, 2009.

116. Powell NB, Zonato AI, et al. Radiofrequency treatment of turbinate hypertrophy in subjects using continuous positive airway pressure: a randomized, double-blind, placebo-controlled clinical pilot trial. *Laryngoscope* 2001;111(10):1783–1790.

117. Sullivan S, Li K, Guilleminault C. Nasal obstruction in children with sleep-disordered breathing. *Ann Acad Med Singapore* 2008;37:645–648.

118. Sher AE, Schechtman KB, et al. The efficacy of surgical modifications of the upper airway in adults with obstructive sleep apnea syndrome. *Sleep* 1996;19(2):156–177.

119. Friedman M, Ibrahim H, et al. Staging of obstructive sleep apnea/hypopnea syndrome: a guide to appropriate treatment. *Laryngoscope* 2004;114(3):454–459.

120. Friedman M, Ibrahim HZ, et al. Z-palatoplasty (ZPP): a technique for patients without tonsils. *Otolaryngol Head Neck Surg* 2004;131(1):89–100.

121. Strome M. Obstructive sleep apnea in Down syndrome children: a surgical approach. *Laryngoscope* 1986;96(12):1340–1342.

122. Donaldson JD, Redmond WM. Surgical management of obstructive sleep apnea in children with Down syndrome. *J Otolaryngol* 1988;17(7):398–403.

123. Hultcrantz E, Svanholm H. Down syndrome and sleep apnea–a therapeutic challenge. *Int J Pediatr Otorhinolaryngol* 1991;21(3):263–268.

124. Kosko JR, Derkay CS. Uvulopalatopharyngoplasty: treatment of obstructive sleep apnea in neurologically impaired pediatric patients. *Int J Pediatr Otorhinolaryngol* 1995;32(3):241–246.

125. Kerschner JE, Lynch JB, et al. Uvulopalatopharyngoplasty with tonsillectomy and adenoidectomy as a treatment for obstructive sleep apnea in neurologically impaired children. *Int J Pediatr Otorhinolaryngol* 2002;62(3):229–235.

126. DeRowe A, Gunther E, et al. Tongue-base suspension with a soft tissue-to-bone anchor for obstructive sleep apnea: preliminary clinical results of a new minimally invasive technique. *Otolaryngol Head Neck Surg* 2000;122(1):100–103.

127. Miller FR, Watson D, et al. Role of the tongue base suspension suture with The Repose System bone screw in the multilevel surgical management of obstructive sleep apnea. *Otolaryngol Head Neck Surg* 2002;126(4):392–398.

128. Pang KP, Terris D. Tongue suspension in obstructive sleep apnea. *Oper Tech Otolaryngol-HN Surg* 2006;17:252.

129. Pang KP, Terris D. Modified cautery-assisted palatal stiffening operation: new method for treating snoring and mild obstructive sleep apnea. *Otolaryngol Head Neck Surg* 2007;136(5):823–826.

130. Wootten CT, Shott SR. Evolving therapies to treat retroglossal and base-of-tongue obstruction in pediatric obstructive sleep apnea. *Arch Otolaryngol Head Neck Surg* 2010;136(10):983–987.

131. Lewis MR, Ducic Y. Genioglossus muscle advancement with the genioglossus bone advancement technique for base of tongue obstruction. *J Otolaryngol* 2003;32(3):168–173.

132. Mickelson SA, Rosenthal L. Midline glossectomy and epiglottidectomy for obstructive sleep apnea syndrome. *Laryngoscope* 1997;107(5):614–619.

133. Maturo SC, Mair EA. Submucosal minimally invasive lingual excision: an effective, novel surgery for pediatric tongue base reduction. *Ann Otol Rhinol Laryngol* 2006;115(8):624–630.

134. Woodson BT, Fujita S. Clinical experience with lingualplasty as part of the treatment of severe obstructive sleep apnea. *Otolaryngol Head Neck Surg* 1992;107(1):40–48.

135. Clark S, Lam D, et al. Posterior midline glossectomy for treatment of post-adenotonsillectomy obstructive sleep apnea in children. *Abstract Presented at: American Society of Pediatric Otolaryngology Annual Meeting*, Chicago, IL, May 2011.

136. Robinson S, Lewis R, et al. Ultrasound-guided radiofrequency submucosal tongue-base excision for sleep apnea: a preliminary report. *Clin Otolaryngol Allied Sci* 2003;28(4):341–345.

137. Friedman M, Soans R, et al. Evaluation of submucosal minimally invasive lingual excision technique for treatment of obstructive sleep apnea/hypopnea syndrome. *Otolaryngol Head Neck Surg* 2008;139(3):378–384; discussion 385.

IX

Otology

Barry E. Hirsch   Robert K. Jackler

Development of the Ear

140

Michael John Wareing   **Anil K. Lalwani**   **Abbas A. Anwar**
Robert K. Jackler

The development of the structures necessary for transmission of sound information from the environment to the auditory cortex is a complex and interwoven process. An understanding of the major developmental steps and their interrelations is desirable because therein lies the key to understanding many conditions encountered by otolaryngologists. Awareness of the developmental process alerts the surgeon to anatomic associations and explains important departures from normal.

Abnormal development is important for its clinical effects, but it also has a role in unraveling the complexities of normal development. The critical period of ear development begins in the third week after fertilization, the inner ear appearing first. The inner, middle, and outer portions of the ear have different embryologic origins, and development can be arrested at any stage. The result is a range of abnormalities from mild to severe. In view of the different origins, a disorder in one part does not necessarily signify a disorder in another, but proximity in terms of time of development, originating tissue, anatomic characteristics, and function does mean that multiple malformations are possible. The disorders can be caused by an inborn genetic error, either inherited or spontaneous, or by a teratogenic influence during organogenesis. The tissues of the head and neck are derived from all three layers of the embryo—ectoderm, mesoderm, and endoderm. The neural crest cells play a special role in the head and neck, where they constitute most of the skeletal and connective tissue. These cells arise from the ectodermal layer at the junction where the neural tube begins to fold. All divisions of the ear contain some neural crest tissue. The mesodermal proportion in the head and neck is less than in the rest of the body.

The story of ear development goes back to the time life itself was in its infancy. Fish seem to be the first hearing organisms, with development of a hearing organ from an internal balance organ. Even at this early evolutionary stage, the hair-cell design now so widespread was in use.

Both amphibians and reptiles inherited the balance labyrinth of fish but went on to develop auditory labyrinths of their own, having branched from the line of fish before acquisition of a hearing organ. The need to hear in air resulted in development of a conductive apparatus to correct the impedance mismatch of sound arriving in air but having to be transmitted into the liquid of the labyrinth. Mammalian design continued from the basic reptilian design with, in particular, the addition of rows of hair cells, an independent cochlear nerve, changes in the middle-ear conduction system, and protective external auditory canals (1). Throughout this chapter, we separate development of the ear into its component parts as an aid to understanding. It is important, however, to remember that these changes occurred in a simultaneous manner. An overview of ear development is presented in Table 140.1.

AURICULAR DEVELOPMENT

In keeping with its recent evolutionary appearance, the auricle of the external ear begins its development later than do other components of the ear. From the fifth week of gestation, three hillocks arise on the first branchial (mandibular) arch (hillocks 1, 2, and 3) and three arise on the second branchial (hyoid) arch (hillocks 4, 5, and 6) on either side of the first branchial cleft (Fig. 140.1). Hillocks 1 and 6 are the first to be identifiable separately, but by the sixth week, all are distinct. The lobule also can be identified on the second arch. By the eighth week, the auricle has an identifiable structure, and the contributions of the hillocks to the adult form can be recognized: hillock 1, tragus; hillock 2, crus helicis; hillock 3, ascending helix; hillock 4, horizontal helix, upper portion of scapha, and antihelix; hillock 5, descending helix, middle portion of the scapha, and antihelix; and hillock 6, antitragus and inferior aspect of the helix (2). Although this is the majority view, there is uncertainty about the origin of the crus helicis and

TABLE 140.1	OVERVIEW OF EAR DEVELOPMENT

Fetal Age (wk)	Outer Ear	Middle Ear	Inner Ear
3			Otic placode develops. VC ganglia appear
4	EAC begins	Tubotympanic recess is apparent	Otocyst present
5	Hillocks become evident	Ossicles begin to condense in mesenchyme	Otocyst begins to divide into vestibular and cochlear areas
			Semicircular canals begin to outpouch; VC ganglion divides
6	All hillocks are distinct	Malleus and incus are identifiable as cartilaginous models	Superior SCC completed. Utricle and saccule are present; cochlear duct begins
7			Maculae present; sensory ridges in the cochlea appear
8	Auricle has identifiable structure; deep meatus is apparent as epithelial strand	Incudomalleolar and incudostapedial joints form	Ductus reuniens is identifiable; 1.5 cochlear turns; cristae present
			Vacuoles develop in vascular precartilage surrounding membranous labyrinth; cartilaginous model of otic capsule forms
9		Tympanic membrane has trilaminar structure	Nerve fibers enter sensory epithelium; oval window develops
10		Stapes loses annular form; facial nerve runs through middle ear	2.5 cochlear turns
11			Hair cells present in cochlea; synaptic connections are present
12		Tympanic ring begins to ossify	Otoconial membrane is present; cochlear duct changes to triangular shape
16		Malleus, incus, and stapes begin to ossify	Ossification of the otic capsule begins
18	Auricle has adult form		
20	Meatal plug begins to disintegrate	Tympanic cavity begins to open	Cochlear duct reaches full length; membranous labyrinth is full size
22		Antrum begins to develop	Tunnel of Corti present at all levels; basal turn of cochlea is functional
23			Otic capsule ossification is complete
24			Perilymphatic space is completed
26		Facial nerve makes second genu in adult position	
28	EAC is fully open		
30		Malleus and incus are ossified	
34		Ossicles lie within open middle ear space	
		Mastoid air cells begin to develop	

VC, vestibulocochlear; SCC, semicircular canal; EAC, external auditory canal.

ascending helix; some believe that these structures can arise from the second arch (3). By approximately 18 weeks' gestation, the auricle has achieved essentially adult form, although it continues to grow in childhood with changes continuing into late adult life.

DEVELOPMENTAL ANOMALIES

A wide spectrum of pinna deformity exists, from anotia, in which there is no development, to a small but normally formed pinna. Microtia encapsulates the wide spectrum between anotia and normality. The superior portion of the auricle usually is severely malformed or absent. The presence of a deformity of the pinna can indicate further defects of the auditory system. Although this is less common with some minor deformities, severe cases of microtia and anotia are almost always associated with atresia of the external auditory canal and defects of the middle ear (see later).

The etiology of auricular abnormalities remains unclear, but evidence has implicated both environmental and genetic factors. Environmental risk factors for microtia are numerous and include anemia, advanced maternal or paternal age, male gender, race, and multiple births. In addition, mothers with chronic type I diabetes are at significantly higher risk for having children with microtia (4). Microtia may also have genetic risk factors, as autosomal recessive and dominant forms of the deformity

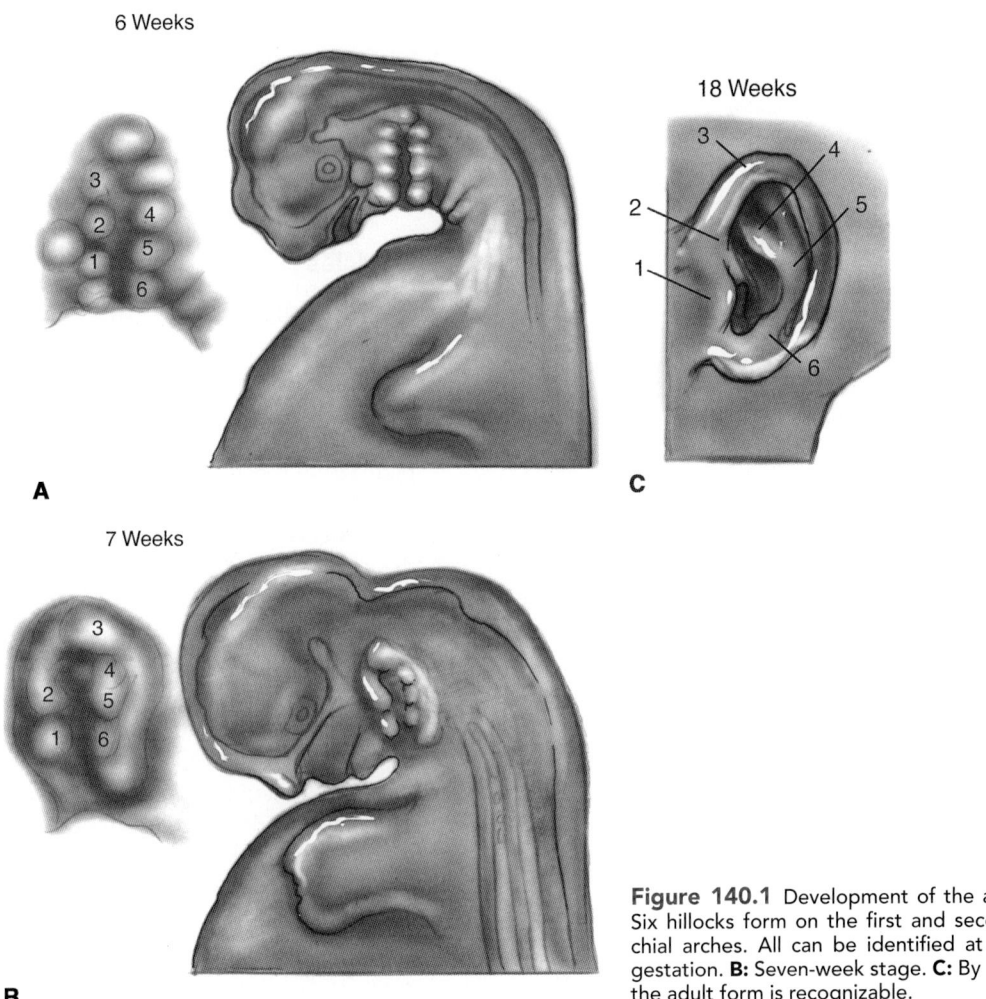

6 Weeks

7 Weeks

18 Weeks

A

B

C

Figure 140.1 Development of the auricle. **A:** Six hillocks form on the first and second branchial arches. All can be identified at 6 weeks' gestation. **B:** Seven-week stage. **C:** By 18 weeks, the adult form is recognizable.

with variable expression and incomplete penetrance have been reported. More recently, specific genes, such as the *Gsc* homeobox gene and the *BMP5* maternal peptide gene, have been implicated as possible predisposing genes for microtia (5). Auricular abnormalities also are present in all the common chromosomal abnormalities, including trisomy 13, 18, and 22 as well as chromosomal translocations and microdeletions, and thus, are useful markers of these conditions. Classification of deformities of the pinna and treatment are discussed in Chapters 190 and 191.

DEVELOPMENT OF THE EXTERNAL AND MIDDLE EAR

External Auditory Canal

The external auditory canal begins to form in the fourth week of gestation (Fig. 140.2). The first branchial cleft, between the first and second branchial arches, widens, and the ectoderm proliferates to form a pit, which comes into apposition with the endoderm of the first pharyngeal pouch. This

pit is the forerunner of the cartilaginous external auditory canal. This arrangement is temporary because mesenchymal growth separates the cleft and the pouch. The deep portion of the external auditory canal is apparent from the eighth week of gestation as a strand of epithelial cells running down to the disc-shaped precursor of the tympanic membrane (3). At approximately 28 weeks' gestation, this epithelial core has canalized from the medial to the lateral aspect to allow communication with the tympanic membrane. The epithelial core is the precursor of the bony external auditory canal.

Tympanic Membrane

The tympanic membrane has a trilaminar origin of ectoderm from the floor of the first branchial cleft laterally as the epidermal layer, endoderm of the first pharyngeal pouch medially as the mucosal layer, and neural crest mesenchyme with cephalic mesoderm interposed as the fibrous layer (6). It is almost horizontal initially but gradually tilts to lie in the adult position at approximately 3 years of age. The bone of the tympanic ring, derived from neural crest mesenchyme, begins to ossify at approximately 3 months.

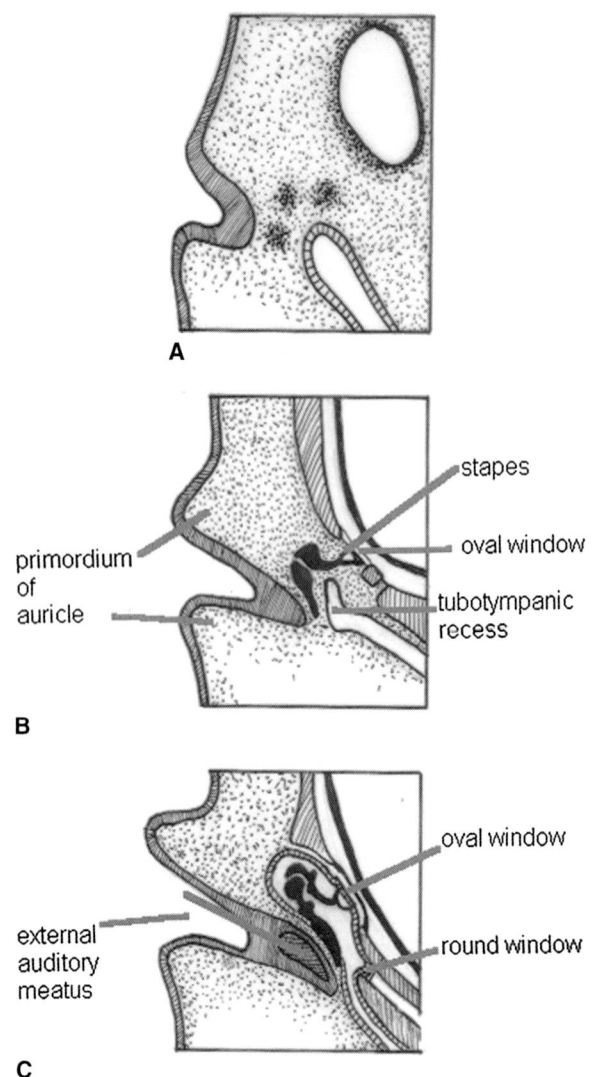

A

B

primordium
of
auricle

stapes

oval window

tubotympanic
recess

C

external
auditory
meatus

oval window

round window

Figure 140.2 Development of the middle ear and ear canal. **A:** Week 5. **B:** Week 10. **C:** Week 27.

Middle Ear Cavity

The cavity and lining of the middle ear and eustachian tube develop from the expanding terminal end of the first pharyngeal pouch with a small contribution from the second pharyngeal pouch. This is apparent in the fourth week of gestation as the tubotympanic recess, which is positioned against the ectoderm of the infolding branchial groove. In the fifth and sixth weeks, the mesenchyme between the branchial cleft and the developing inner ear has condensations destined to become the ossicles. The tympanic cavity continues to develop as the continuing expansion of the endodermal pouch surrounds the ossicles and their supporting structures. It remains a slit-like structure until the fifth month but begins to expand such that the ossicles lie within an open tympanic space by the eighth month (7). Continuation of the tympanic cavity from the epitympanum into the antrum begins at 22 weeks and is complete at birth. Formation of the mastoid air cell system begins late in fetal life, the antrum is present at birth, and continues

throughout childhood. The pattern and extent of pneumatization are highly variable. Pneumatization of the petrous pyramid, present in 30% of temporal bones, does not begin until the third year of life (8). At birth, the mastoid tip is not developed but expands through the tractional effect of the sternocleidomastoid attachment.

Ossicles

The exact origin of the ossicles has long been debated. It is certain that the main source is the neural crest mesenchyme of the first and second branchial arches—Meckel cartilage (first arch) and Reichert cartilage (second arch). The otic capsule has a role in formation of the stapes footplate (9). It is generally agreed that the head of the malleus and the body and short process of the incus are formed from Meckel cartilage and are initially continuous with the cartilaginous mandible. The mandibular branch of the trigeminal nerve is the nerve of the first arch; thus, it supplies the tensor tympani muscle, also a derivative of the first branchial arch. The long process of the incus, handle of the malleus, stapes superstructure, and tympanic surface of the stapes footplate are derived from the Reichert cartilage. The facial nerve is the nerve of the second arch; this supplies the stapedius muscle. The vestibular surface of the footplate is a derivative of the mesoderm of the otic capsule, as is the anular ligament (3) (Fig. 140.3).

The malleus and incus are first formed as cartilaginous models from the sixth week of gestation. They begin to ossify in week 16, and ossification is almost complete by week 30. The stapes appears slightly before the malleus and incus. It is initially ring shaped and penetrated by the stapedial artery, the artery of the second arch, which regresses. By 10 weeks, the stapes has already started to assume the familiar stirrup shape. By the time ossification begins from a solitary center at 16 weeks, the structure is a model of the future stapes. It is reduced in bulk throughout fetal life to develop its slender architectural form.

Maldevelopment

The spectrum of abnormal development in congenital atresia of the external auditory canal parallels the fact that the canal is present, albeit short, then is absent before achieving the adult form. In the most severe cases of atresia, a bony mass replaces the tympanic ring and forms the lateral wall of the middle ear cavity, the condyle of the mandible lying more posteriorly. In membranous atresia, which is less common, a fibrous mass replaces the external auditory canal. The mildest form of abnormality is stenosis of the external auditory canal, common in Down syndrome, which can be difficult to diagnose unless complications such as proximal cholesteatoma caused by trapped debris supervene. Congenital atresia is unilateral in 70% of cases (10).

A further consideration with atresia is the presence of coexisting abnormalities of either the pinna or the middle

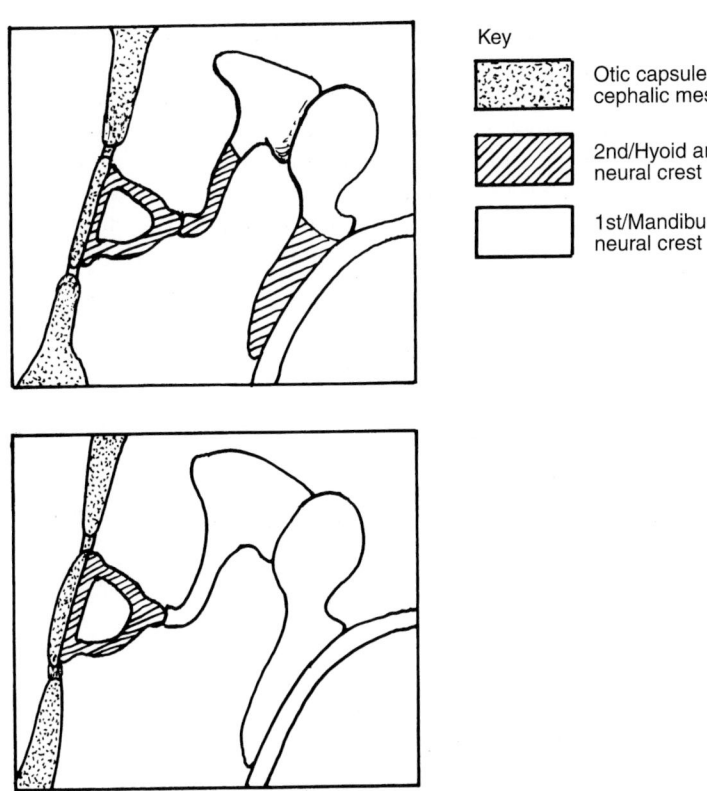

Key

Otic capsule:
cephalic mesoderm

2nd/Hyoid arch:
neural crest

1st/Mandibular arch:
neural crest

Figure 140.3 Origin of the ossicles—two interpretations.

ear. Associated auricular abnormality exists in 94% of cases of atresia, and the middle ear is frequently deranged (11), in part because all these structures are derived from the first two branchial arches and the intervening branchial cleft. Consequent are further abnormalities of branchial arch derivatives, such as the mandible. Among children with microtia or anotia, 20% to 40% have an identifiable syndromal malformation, such as hemifacial microsomia, Treacher Collins syndrome (mandibulofacial dysostosis), or Goldenhar (oculoauriculovertebral) syndrome (5,12). These syndromal malformations are discussed in Chapter 86.

Ossicular abnormalities also encompass a wide spectrum, from a rudimentary ossicular mass to minor morphologic defects. Middle ear deformities without coexisting outer ear defects are unusual, occurring among fewer than 10% of children with congenital conductive defects (13). This may, however, be an underrepresentation with cases undiagnosed or ascribed to acquired causes. The malleus is always fixed to a bony atretic plate if present, and incudomalleolar fusion or fixation is a common defect. Stapedial abnormalities are less common. In particular, the footplate can have normal mobility, even with a severe coexisting abnormality, because of its separate development from the otic capsule (14).

Persistent stapedial artery is a condition with an interesting embryologic background, although only approximately 50 cases have been reported worldwide. The stapedial artery is the remnant of the second arch artery, which courses from the aortic sac to the dorsal aorta. This artery regresses at approximately 10 weeks' gestation, and its role is assumed by the precursors of the internal and external carotid arteries. When the artery persists, a vessel

arises from the internal carotid artery in the hypotympanum, which courses through the crura of the stapes to the fallopian canal. It enters the fallopian canal and courses forward to the geniculate ganglion and to the dura. If present, a persistent stapedial artery often manifests as a pulsatile mass in the middle ear cavity, pulsatile tinnitus, and rarely, as conductive hearing loss due to stapes ankylosis. The clinical interest is in cases in which middle ear surgery has been undertaken to manage presumptive otosclerosis or for cochlear implantation, as there is an increased risk of bleeding (15). Another condition with an embryologic basis is congenital cholesteatoma. This condition is caused by failure of atrophy of epidermoid formation in the anterior mesotympanum.

Although the inner ear develops separately, there is still an approximately 10% incidence of coexisting inner and middle-outer ear abnormalities (14). Careful assessment of the auditory system is mandatory if one is alerted to problems by maldevelopment of the auricle or ear canal Classification and management of congenital atresia are discussed in Chapter 137.

DEVELOPMENT OF THE FACIAL NERVE

The facial nerve is extremely important in surgical anatomy of the ear. The complex course of the nerve is a result of development of the structures that surround it. The facioacoustic primordium appears in the third week of gestation and has split into distinct seventh and eighth cranial nerves by the fifth week. The facial nerve supplies second arch structures, in particular the muscles of facial expression. There also are secretomotor and special sensation fibers derived from the nervus intermedius, which is distinct by the seventh week. The chorda tympani has appeared in the fourth week, running to the first arch, before supplying sensation to the anterior two-thirds of the tongue. The greater superficial petrosal nerve appears in the sixth week. The nerve to the stapedius is identifiable by the seventh week (16). The first genu can be considered the result of the nerve's being pushed forward by the developing otic capsule. The fallopian canal is derived from the mesoderm of the otic capsule. More distally, the fallopian canal is formed partly by the Reichert cartilage (9). In the 10th week, the facial nerve makes its second genu in the middle ear, and its relation to the structures of the external and middle ear is far more anterior than in adults. By week 26, there is partial closure of the fallopian canal by bone, and the nerve has moved posteriorly, coming to lie in a position comparable with that in adults. In a manner similar to its being pushed forward by the otic capsule

proximally, the nerve is pulled posteriorly by the growing tympanic ring and structures of the posterior tympanum and pulled inferiorly by the developing meatus and mastoid system. The facial nerve comes to lie between the tympanic and mastoid portions of the temporal bone. Even at birth, the facial nerve, which exits through the superficially positioned stylomastoid foramen, is more superficial than it is in the final adult position, which is attained by means of growth of the mastoid tip.

Maldevelopment

In ears with congenital defects of the outer or middle ear, the implication of this pattern of development is that the facial nerve lies more anteriorly and superficially in the lateral temporal bone. Often this means that the expected position of a new external meatus is crossed by the facial nerve (Fig. 140.4). In atretic ears, the facial nerve is abnormal in as many as 50% of cases (14).

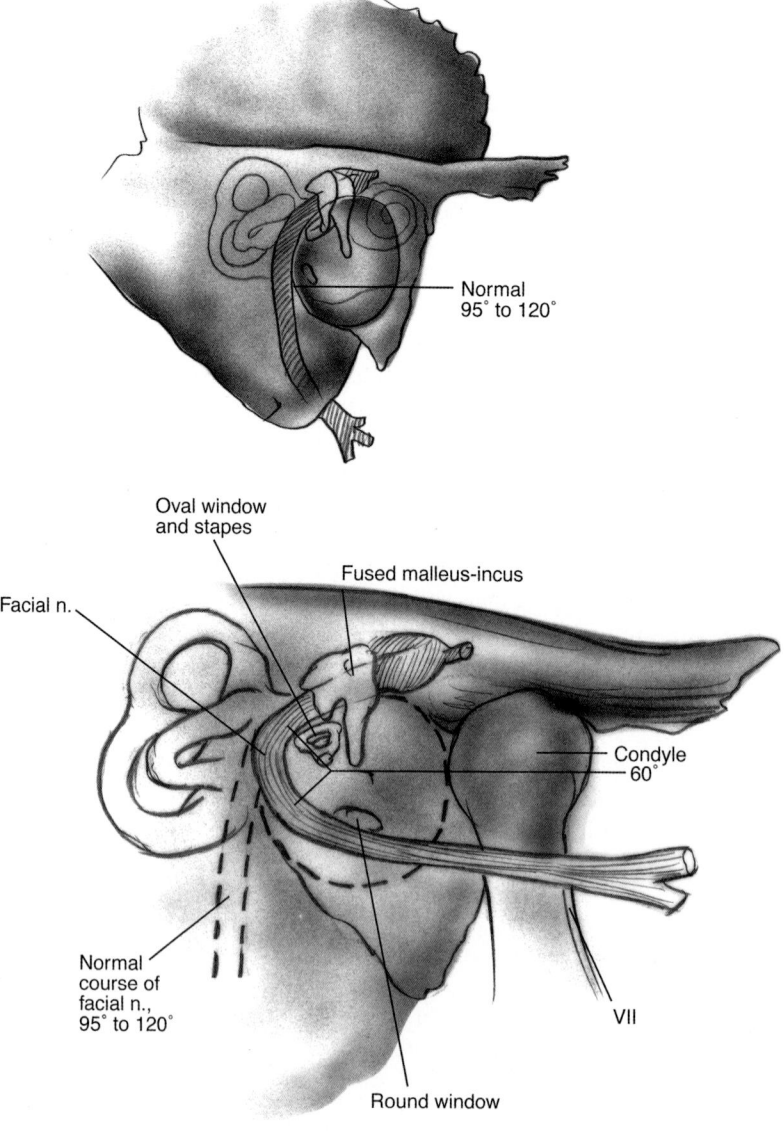

Figure 140.4 The facial nerve is anterior and superficial in atretic ears.

Some congenital disorders of the stapes are related to abnormal development of the facial nerve. Anterior displacement of the nerve at the 6-week stage can prevent the developing stapes from coming into contact with the otic capsule; the result is rudimentary formation (17). The facial nerve also can divide around the stapes. Dehiscence of the fallopian canal is common enough for it to be considered a normal variant, present in approximately 25% of temporal bones. The most common site is above the oval window, although sufficient dehiscence to allow prolapse over the oval window is much less common.

DEVELOPMENT OF THE INNER EAR

Membranous Labyrinth

The internal ear phylogenetically predates the other components of the ear and is accordingly the first part to develop. At the end of the third week of gestation, the otic placode can be differentiated on the lateral surface of the cephalic end of the embryo as a thickening of ectoderm in contact with hindbrain portion of the closing neural tube. The neural tube, also derived from ectoderm, is destined to become the central nervous system. This contact is short-lived. By the time the neural tube closes, a layer of thin ectoderm separates it from the neural epithelium. The placode invaginates itself to become a pit and a closed sac, the otocyst or otic vesicle, the precursor of the membranous labyrinth (Fig. 140.5). Positioned between the second and third branchial arches, it is predictable that the otocyst is supplied by the eighth cranial nerve. It migrates inward, changing shape and growing dramatically so that it achieves adult form by the 10th week and adult size by 20 weeks (18) (Fig. 140.6).

The otocyst lengthens more than it widens. The cranial portion becomes marked off as the developing endolymphatic duct. The caudal portion is destined to become the cochlear duct and the intermediate portion, the utriculosaccular area, is the vestibular precursor. These distinctions are discernible in the fifth week of gestation. The vestibular portion begins to take shape slightly before the cochlear portion, in keeping with its older phylogenetic status. From the utricular part of the vestibular pouch, three outpocketings appear, which are converted, through fusion of the central epithelium, into semicircular canals. The superior canal is completed first, in the sixth week. The posterior canal is next to be completed, and the lateral canal is last. The utricle and saccule start to develop in the sixth week and form the utriculosaccular duct. The cochlear duct also begins to grow from the saccule in the sixth week with recognizable narrowing of the communication; the ductus reuniens is visible by the eighth week. The cochlear duct grows rapidly, having 1.5 turns at 8 weeks and the full 2.5 turns at 10 weeks, although it does not reach full length until 20 weeks (2).

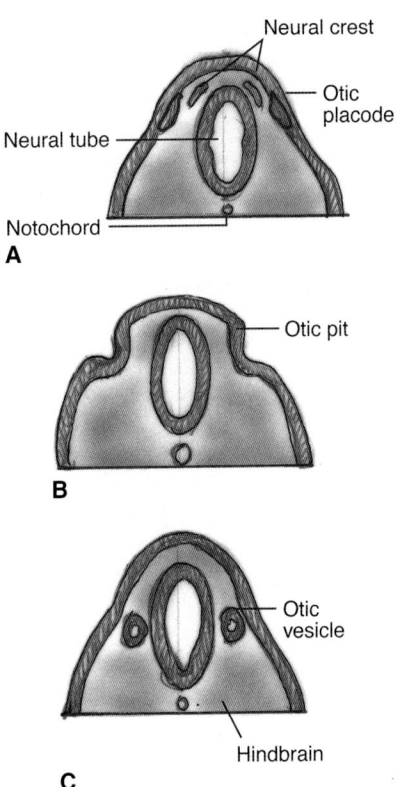

Figure 140.5 A–C: Early development of the inner ear in the third and fourth weeks of gestation—formation of the otocyst from the otic placode.

The sensory epithelia of the vestibular system, the three cristae and two maculae and the organ of Corti in the cochlea, are derived from the ectodermal epithelium of the otocyst. These six areas, which initially are close together, develop in the wall of the membranous labyrinth (3). The maculae develop in the seventh week of gestation by means of intense proliferation of the epithelium accompanied by cell differentiation. The distinctive cells and otoconial membrane are apparent by week 12. Development of the cristae parallels this event; they are distinguishable at 8 weeks and have reached adult in form at 23 weeks.

The sensory epithelium of the cochlea begins to develop in the seventh week as the duct itself grows and begins to coil. Lying on the medial wall, the layers of the epithelium organize into two ridges and spiral along the length of the cochlea. The supporting cells arise from both ridges. The larger inner ridge differentiates into the inner hair cells and tectorial membrane. The smaller outer ridge differentiates into the outer hair cells (19). *Atoh* has been identified as the earliest hair-cell-specific gene required for definitive hair cell development, as *Atoh* knockout mice show no hair-cell differentiation (20). Once differentiation begins, the hair cells become identifiable by about week 11, the inner hair cells appearing marginally before the outer hair cells at the same position along the basilar membrane (7). Hair-cell development is initially apparent in the midbasal region of the cochlea and moves

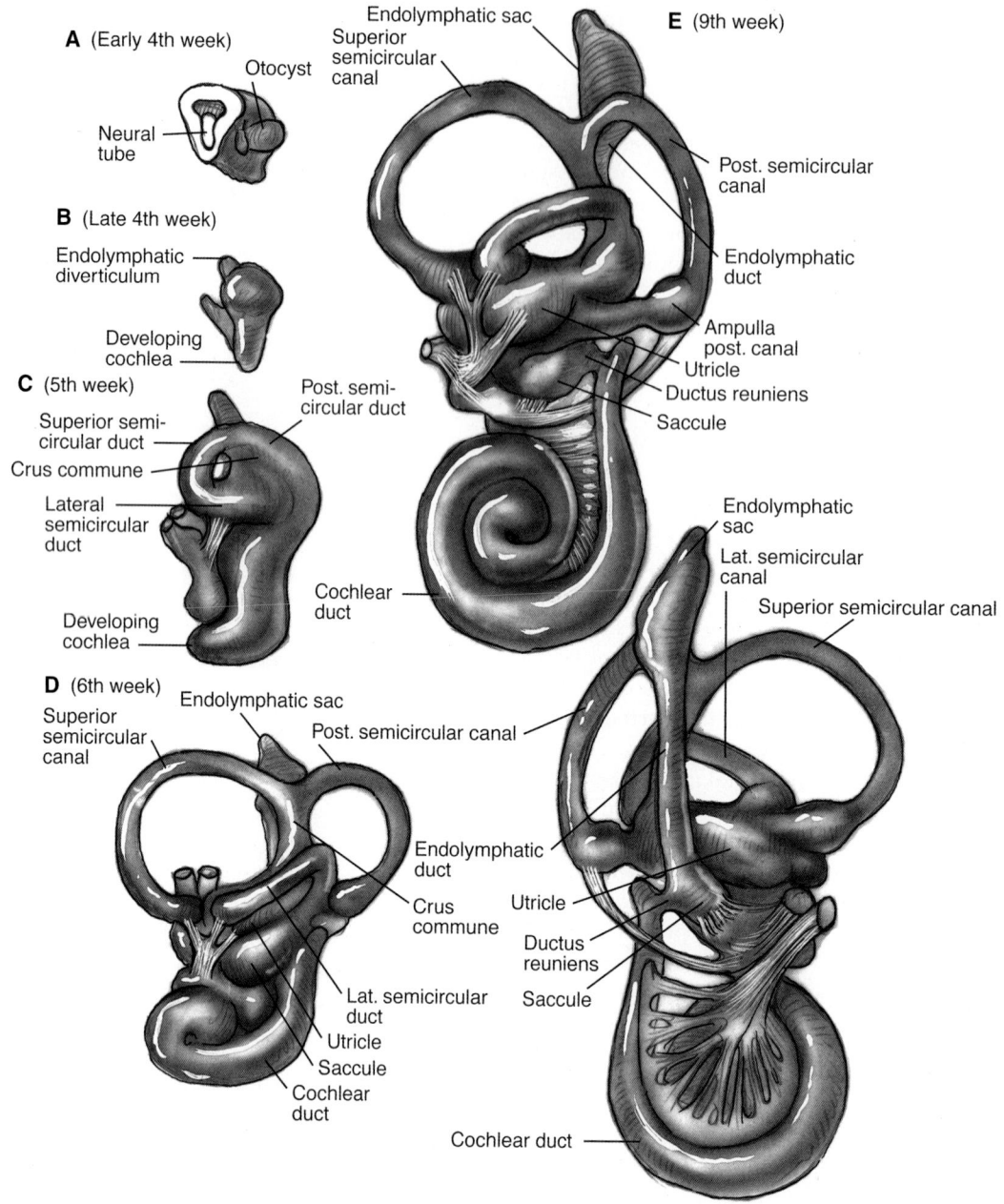

Figure 140.6 A–E: Development of the membranous labyrinth from gestational weeks 4 through 9.

toward the apex, maturation of the base preceding that of the apex by 1 to 2 weeks, although the most basal portion of the cochlear lags slightly behind the midbasal portion. The supporting cells develop in the same direction, and at the 21-week stage, the tunnel of Corti is present at all levels. At approximately this time, the organ of Corti becomes functional, at least in its basal turn (2). The shape of the cochlear duct starts changing at approximately week 12 from oval to triangular, the changes first happening in the basal turn. The surrounding mesoderm of the osseous labyrinth participates in this process. The endolymphatic duct and sac are the only parts of the inner ear that continue to grow into the third trimester. Full size is not attained until adulthood (21).

DEVELOPMENT OF INNERVATION OF THE MEMBRANOUS LABYRINTH

The facioacoustic primordium appears in the third week of gestation. It does not, however, have a uniform origin. The vestibulocochlear ganglia arise from ectoderm of the primitive otocyst, having split away from the epithelium in the third week. Although destined to innervate different portions of the inner ear, the vestibulocochlear ganglia appear to arise from a common site on the otic epithelium. The neural crest is a small additional source of supporting cells of the ganglion (6).

From the vestibulocochlear ganglia, fibers grow toward their destined target organs, the inductive process driven by the target organs and nearby tissues. While the otocyst is dividing into its vestibular and cochlear portions, the vestibulocochlear ganglion divides into a superior and an inferior division. The fibers of the superior division pass to innervate the superior and lateral ampullae of the semicircular canal and the utricle. The inferior division sends fibers to the posterior ampulla and the saccule. The remaining portion becomes the spiral ganglion of the cochlea (2). As the cochlear duct grows and coils, the ganglion follows it to give it its characteristic configuration. Recent studies have shown that, while the hair cells are the final target for the auditory fibers of the spiral ganglion, many other nonsensory tissues that are present along the pathway, such as Kolliker organ and Schwann cells, may actually provide the earliest guidance cues and survival molecules needed to direct axon growth toward the sensory epithelium. The exact signals and molecules that provide this guidance remain unclear, but there is significant evidence that *neurotrophin-3* (*NT3*) and *brain-derived neurotrophic factor* (BDNF) may play an integral role in the process, as they are required for normal innervation of the cochlea (22). Eventually, by about the ninth week, auditory nerve fibers grow to enter the sensory epithelium, and synaptic connections are identifiable as the hair cells begin to differentiate in week 11. Although differentiated hair cells are not required to successfully target auditory fibers to the sensory epithelium of the cochlea, they do appear necessary for later auditory circuit assembly, synapse formation, and ultimately, auditory neuronal survival (23). Once the hair cells differentiate, the inner hair cells are innervated before the outer hair cells, afferent innervation precedes efferent innervation, and the basal turn precedes the apex in development (19).

DEVELOPMENT OF THE OSSEOUS LABYRINTH

The most important aspect of development of the perilymph-filled osseous labyrinth is a resorptive process in the mesoderm that separates the membranous labyrinth from the developing bony otic capsule. In the eighth week of gestation, the vascular precartilage that surrounds the membranous labyrinth develops vacuoles in its structure that coalesce to leave the perilymphatic space. This process begins around the utricle and saccule and progresses outward from there. The part around the cochlear duct destined to be the scala tympani precedes the scala vestibuli, and development is farther advanced in the basal turn than in the apical turn. The perilymphatic space is completed by week 24 (9). The origin of the precartilage is cephalic mesoderm with a small contribution from neural crest cells. The cephalic mesoderm contributes to the basilar membrane, Reissner membrane, and the stria vascularis, which also has cells derived from the neural crest (24,25).

DEVELOPMENT OF THE OTIC CAPSULE

It is remarkable that the bony otic capsule achieves its adult size by week 22 of gestation. Arising from cephalic mesoderm, a precartilaginous precursor appears in the seventh week. From week 8 to week 16, the developing labyrinth is surrounded by an enlarging cartilaginous model, which ossifies in three layers over 7 weeks from a total of 14 centers (8,9). Solidification is completed in the early postnatal stage; the petrous (stony) nature of the otic capsule results from the compactness of the bone of the original ossification centers. The oval (vestibular) window is formed where the developing stapes abuts the cartilaginous model of the otic capsule in the ninth week. This section becomes the vestibular surface of the footplate. The rim of the footplate and the facing rim of the window, derivatives of the otic capsule precursor, do not turn into bone but remain cartilage; the intervening tissue becomes the annular ligament. The round (tympanic) window forms adjacent to the basal turn of the cochlea, where cartilage is not turned into bone but is converted into the fibrous tissue of the secondary tympanic membrane.

The vestibular aqueduct forms around the endolymphatic duct and sac but is late in achieving full ossification (9). The cochlear aqueduct forms in the mesoderm, which ossifies to become the otic capsule, and is first apparent as an outpouching of the subarachnoid space. Progressive ossification causes curving and lengthening of the cochlear aqueduct, which has two sections. The otic capsule section, which has a narrow cochlear opening just inside the round window membrane, becomes progressively narrower from its appearance in the fourth month to the ossification of the otic capsule at week 23. The medial petrous apex portion enlarges throughout the third trimester, and it is in this section that postnatal elongation of the cochlear aqueduct takes place. The length in a newborn infant is 3.5 mm; the average length in an adult is 10 mm (26). The internal acoustic meatus forms around the vestibulocochlear nerve and internal auditory blood vessels as well as the facial nerve. The facial nerve, however, is cranial to the eighth nerve, and its path is deflected by the growing otic capsule, although the bony fallopian canal proximal to the second genu is of otic capsule derivation. The adult position of the facial nerve in the internal acoustic meatus is in the anterosuperior quadrant.

Maldevelopment

A practical categorization divides inner ear anomalies into those affecting the osseous and membranous labyrinth and those affecting the membranous labyrinth alone (27). As many as 20% of patients with congenital sensorineural hearing loss fall into the first category, which can be identified with radiologic techniques

TABLE 140.2	CLASSIFICATION OF CONGENITAL INNER EAR MALFORMATIONS

Malformations limited to the membranous labyrinth
  Complete membranous labyrinthine dysplasia
    (Bing-Siebenmann)
  Limited membranous labyrinthine dysplasia
    Cochleosaccular dysplasia (Scheibe)
    Cochlear basal turn dysplasia
Malformations of the osseous and membranous labyrinth
  Complete labyrinthine aplasia (Michel)
  Cochlear anomalies
    Cochlear aplasia
    Cochlear hypoplasia
    Common cavity
    Incomplete partition (Mondini)
  Labyrinthine anomalies
    Semicircular canal dysplasia
    Semicircular canal aplasia
  Aqueductal anomalies
    Enlargement of the vestibular aqueduct
    Enlargement of the cochlear aqueduct
  Internal auditory canal abnormalities
    Narrow internal auditory canal
    Wide internal auditory canal

From Jackler RK. Congenital malformations of the inner ear. In: Cummings CW, Fredrickson JM, Harker LA, et al. *Otolaryngology: head and neck surgery*. St. Louis, MO: Mosby-Year Book, 1993:2576–2771, with permission.

TABLE 140.3	NOTABLE GENES IMPLICATED IN THE DEVELOPMENT OF THE INNER EAR

Structure	Genes
Cochlea	*TGF-β2, HOXA1, N-myc, Pax2, Ildr1, Tbx, Wnt, Lgr5, Six1, Eya1, Sonic hedgehog (Shh), Fgf3, Gbx2*
Vestibular labyrinth	*HOXA1, SLC4A11, GRHL2, DAN, Bmp2, Bmp4, Dlx, Hmx, Wnt, Msx1, Lmo4, Six1, Pax2, Eya1, Otx1, Fgf3, Gbx2, Lmx1a, Mafb, Foxg1, Fgfr-2*
Endolymphatic sac	*DAN, Pax2, Six1, Pds, Foxi1, Fgf3, Mafb, Otx2*
Auditory neurons	*NT3, BDNF, GDNF, Neurod1, Sox2, Npr2, Shh, TrkB, TrkC, Fgf10*
Hair cells	*GDNF, Atoh, Neurog1, Neurod1, Tbx1, Math1, Brn-3c, Tekt2, Gfi1, Lmod1, Hes/Hey, Eya1, IsK, Jag2, Lfng, Myo6, Myo7a, Tecta*

Human genes—entire gene name is in uppercase letters.
Mouse genes—first letter capitalized followed by all lowercase letters.

(28,29). In absence of histologic confirmation however, accurate categorization ultimately reflects the sensitivity of the contemporary imaging modality (30). Inner ear abnormalities can be caused by arrested or aberrant development (Table 140.2). The variable but frequent coexistence of deformities involving the component parts of the labyrinth suggests that a number of different factors can be involved: The anomaly can be genetically predetermined, an insult can occur before the fifth week, or the separate portions of the developing system can be variably susceptible to teratogenic insult; the contribution of a host of genes to the development of the inner has been determined using the modern tools of molecular genetics and mouse model of deafness (Table 140.3).

The most common histopathologic finding in congenital deafness is cochleosaccular dysplasia due to incomplete development of the caudal portion of the otocyst, the pars inferior, first described by Scheibe in 1892 (28). The organ of Corti typically is partially or completely missing, the cochlear duct and saccule are collapsed, and the stria vascularis is degenerated. The utricle and semicircular canals are normal. The normality can be explained in part by the earlier development of the vestibular system. Basal turn dysplasia is the mild end of this spectrum. Complete membranous labyrinthine dysplasia (Bing-Siebenmann) is rare and is the most severe membranous abnormality.

Most combined membranous–osseous labyrinth abnormalities appear to be caused by arrested development between the fourth and eighth weeks of gestation. The appearance of most malformed ears is in accord with the stages of labyrinthine development (Fig. 140.7). The most severe abnormality, complete aplasia (Michel malformation), is extremely rare and presumably is caused by failure

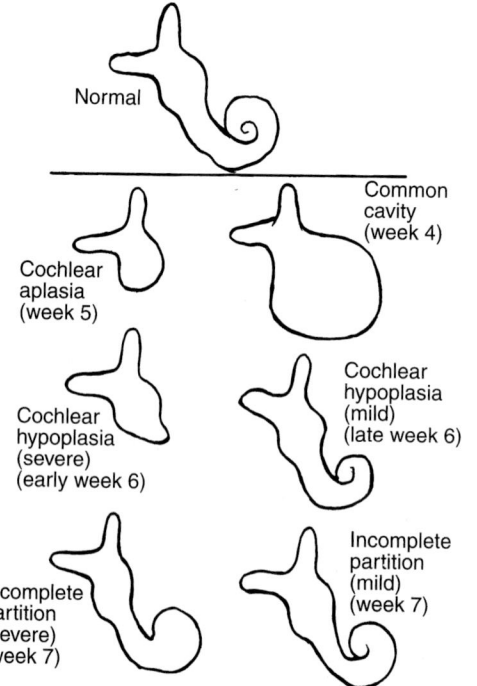

Figure 140.7 Coronal computed tomographic scan shows stages of cochlear maldevelopment.

of the otic vesicle to develop. Cochlear aplasia, hypoplasia, and incomplete partition are a spectrum occurring from arrest at gestational weeks 5, 6, and 7. The common cavity can arise from arrest at 4 weeks or can be caused by later aberrant development. Dysplasia of the semicircular canals is caused by failure of central epithelial fusion and is four times as common as aplasia of the semicircular canals. The lateral semicircular canal (LSCC) is most commonly affected because it develops later, and lateral dysplasia of the semicircular canals can occur as the sole abnormality. Approximately 40% of ears with osseous cochlear abnormalities have concomitant abnormalities of the semicircular canals (27). Bilateral involvement with osseous inner ear deformities is the rule, the same morphologic abnormality occurring in both ears (27).

An enlarged vestibular aqueduct is the most common radiologically detectable abnormality of the inner ear and may be due to acquired or genetic influences (31). The vestibular duct may be abnormally broad and short due to premature arrest of development or as a consequence of increased cerebrospinal fluid pressure. As part of the genetic Pendred syndrome, large vestibular aqueduct can be associated with disturbance of thyroid organification resulting from mutations in *SLC26A4*, a chloride–iodide transporter gene (32). In addition, recent studies have also linked mutations in *KCNJ10*, a potassium channel gene, and *FOXI1*, a transcriptional activator of *SLC26A4*, with Pendred syndrome associated with enlarged vestibular aqueduct, suggesting that it is a multigenic and complex disease (33).

Whereas the vestibular aqueduct forms around an ectodermal structure, the cochlear aqueduct is a secondary structure around a mesodermal derivative. Developmental aberrations of the otic capsule are expected to cause absence of rather than enlargement of the cochlear aqueduct. In fact, a recent study examining 400 temporal bone CT scans found no patients with enlargement of the cochlear aqueduct, suggesting that this is an exceedingly rare or even nonexistent malformation (34). Absence of the cochlear aqueduct is as yet unreported.

Of all the inner ear structures, the internal auditory canal is most variable in size, length, and configuration. Absence of bony partition between a large bulbous lateral end of the canal and the inner ear is associated with stapes gusher (DFN3). Due to a mutation in a developmental transcription factor gene POU3F4, this finding contraindicates stapedectomy for congenital stapes fixation. A narrow internal auditory canal can indicate failure of development of the eighth cranial nerve. If the internal auditory canal has a diameter less than 3 mm and there is normal facial function, it is likely that only the facial nerve is present. This condition is a contraindication to cochlear implantation (35).

The ability to identify maldevelopment of the inner ear is dependent on the sensitivity of radiologic imaging and experience of the clinician reviewing the images (36). Morphologic abnormalities of the bony labyrinth are identified in approximately 20% to 40% of patients with childhood SNHL undergoing temporal bone computerized tomography (CT) scan. While the identification of severe morphogenetic malformations such as complete labyrinthine aplasia or Michel deformity and common cavity deformity is not difficult (accounting for only 1% of abnormalities), the detection of milder radiologic abnormalities is dependent on the experience of the clinician. Nearly one-third of these less severe dysplasias are missed by simple visual inspection of the radiologic images. Introduction of standardized measurements of inner ear structures, such as the dimension of the vestibular aqueduct and the internal auditory canal, and more recently, the vertical height of the cochlea on coronal scan and of the central bony island within the LSCC on axial scan on temporal bone CT can complement visual analysis and greatly aid in the identification of inner ear malformations (Fig. 140.8) (36).

CONTROL OF EAR DEVELOPMENT

Molecular-genetic techniques with knockout and mutant animals have helped to elucidate the development of the ear. Development of both the outer and the middle ear is controlled by genes that affect first and second branchial arch identity as well as hindbrain segmentation and identity. Genetic defects range from the complete absence of structural elements to hypomorphism or duplication. The *HoxA2* gene, which is a type of developmentally critical homeobox gene, is expressed by neural crest cells that populate the first and second branchial arch and encodes a transcription factor that appears to be critical for the development of the external and middle ear. In fact, *HoxA2* knockout mice have been shown to have abnormal ear phenotypes, including transformations of middle ear bones and ectopic or duplicate malleus and incus (37). In addition, PACT, which is an RNA-binding protein expressed in the pinna, middle ear, and cochlea, may also play a crucial role in the development of the outer and middle ear, but not the inner ear, as *Pact* knockout mice express smaller external auditory canals, malformed ossicles, but normal cochlea (38). New cartilage elements can also arise from genetic defects. The phenotypes are not neatly arranged by branchial arch, reflecting functional redundancy in the system.

Invagination and inward movement of the otocyst are under control of external tissue interactions, particularly the hindbrain. Information from knockouts and mutants shows that the genes that control hindbrain segmentation, especially rhombomeres 5 and 6, and genes expressed in neural crest cells influence inner ear development. The inner ear consequently has an indirect requirement for neural genes also expressed in ear tissue. Absence of these genes can cause dramatic changes in inner ear development. For example, inactivation of the transcription factor

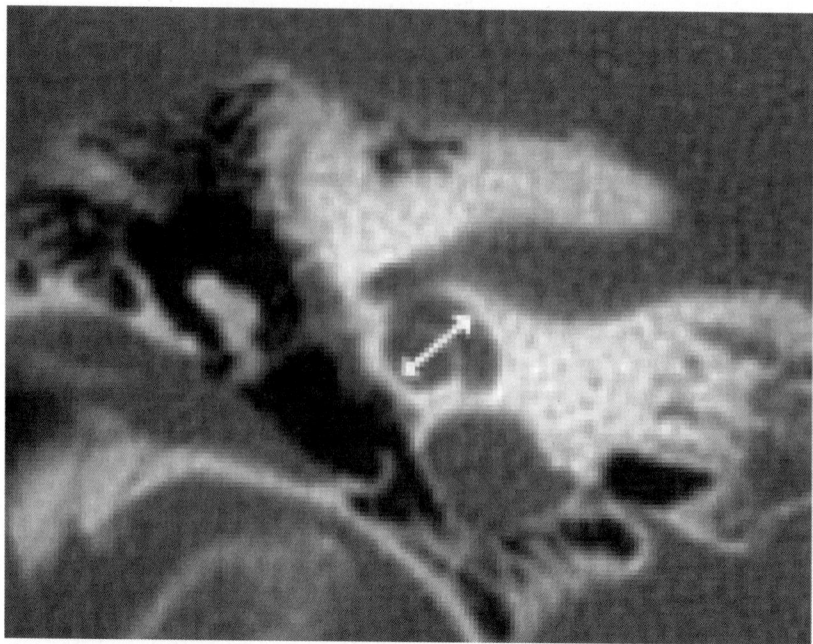

A

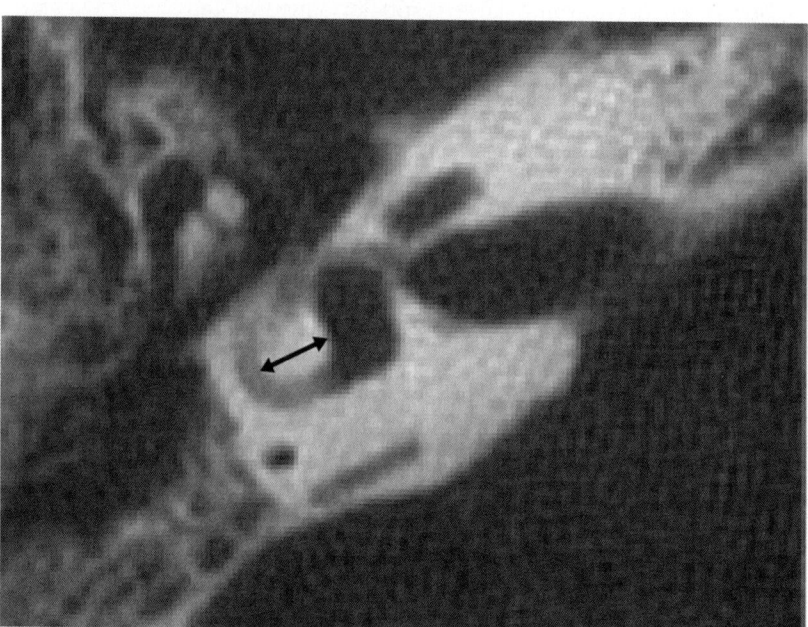

Figure 140.8 A,B: Routine measurement of the cochlear height on coronal scan and the axial measurement of the bony island of the lateral semicircular canal on CT of the temporal bone will complement visual analysis and greatly aid in the identification of inner ear malformations.

B

gene *Hoxa1* results in the complete absence or severe reduction in rhombomere 5 and produces a primitive cystic inner ear with defects of the semicircular canals and the cochlea. Furthermore, the transcription factor Pax2 also appears to be essential for inner ear development, as *Pax2* knockout mice have been shown to often lack a distinct saccule and have a fused endolymphatic duct and common crus. And although a rudimentary cochlea is always present in *Pax2* knockout mice, the organ of Corti is often absent and the formation of the spiral ganglion is frequently delayed or truncated (39). Recent studies

have even shown that the proto-oncogene *N-myc* may also play an integral role in the growth, morphogenesis, and patterning of the inner ear. For example, *N-myc* knockout mice frequently show fusion of the cochlea with the sacculus and utriculus, stunted growth of the cochlea, and absence of the LSCC (40). The LSCC seems particularly sensitive to genetic perturbations, which is in accord with it being the most commonly abnormal semicircular canal. The various structural elements of the otic vesicle are under independent genetic control for specification, morphogenesis, or both (41).

HIGHLIGHTS

- The auricle develops from six ectodermal hillocks arising from the first and second branchial arches. Most of the adult pinna is of second arch origin.

- The ectoderm of the first branchial cleft forms the external auditory canal. The cartilaginous canal forms first and the bony canal later, from medial to lateral, at 28 weeks. The outer layer of the tympanic membrane is derived from this source.

- The tympanic cavity is derived from the first pharyngeal pouch and develops from the fourth week of gestation. It remains a slit-like structure as the endodermal pouch surrounds the ossicles and their supports to the fifth month and expands so the ossicles lie in a cavity in the eighth month.

- The ossicles develop from the neural crest mesenchyme of the first and second branchial arches, except for the vestibular surface of the footplate and the annular ligament, which arise from the mesoderm of the otic capsule.

- The facial nerve only comes to lie in its adult position late in fetal life. It consequently is anterior and superficial in ears with congenital malformations of the middle or outer ear.

- The membranous labyrinth develops from the otic placode. It invaginates to become the otocyst, subdivides into vestibular and cochlear compartments, and grows and dramatically changes shape to achieve adult form at 10 weeks and adult size at 20 weeks of gestation.

- The organ of Corti becomes functional in its basal turn at approximately 20 to 24 weeks.

- The vestibulocochlear ganglia are derived from the otic placode. They innervate six areas of neuroepithelial ectoderm on the wall of the membranous labyrinth that become the three cristae, two maculae, and the spiral organ of Corti.

- The perilymphatic space forms by means of resorption of precartilage from week 8 to week 24. The cartilage model of the bony otic capsule ossifies from 14 centers between week 16 and week 23. It is adult size at 22 weeks.

- Congenital inner ear abnormalities are divided into those affecting the membranous labyrinth alone and those affecting both the bony and membranous labyrinths. The latter appear to be caused by arrested development between weeks 4 and 8 of gestation. They account for only 20% of cases of abnormality but can be diagnosed with imaging techniques.

- Molecular-genetic techniques with knockout and mutant animals have helped to elucidate the development of the ear. Specific homeobox genes and other transcription factors appear to be critical for this process. Further research may help to more clearly illustrate the roles of these genes and their specific contribution to ear development.

REFERENCES

1. Peck JE. Development of hearing, I: phylogeny. *J Am Acad Audiol* 1994;5:291–299.
2. Sulik KK. Embryology of the ear. In: Gorlin RJ, Toriello HV, Cohen MM, eds. *Hereditary hearing loss and its syndromes.* New York, NY: Oxford University Press, 1995:22–42.
3. Van De Water TR, Noden DM, Maderson PFA. Embryology of the ear: outer, middle and inner. In: Alberti PW, Ruben RJ, eds. *Otologic medicine and surgery.* New York, NY: Churchill Livingstone, 1988:3–28.
4. Alasti F, Van Camp G. Genetics of microtia and associated syndromes. *J Med Genet* 2009;46:361–369.
5. Zhang QG, Zhang J, Yu P, Shen H. Environmental and genetic factors associated with congenital microtia: a case-control study in Jiangsu, China, 2004 to 2007. *Plast Reconstr Surg* 2009;124(4):1157–1164.
6. Noden DM. Cell movements and control of patterned tissue assembly during craniofacial development. *Development* 1988;103 (Suppl):121–140.
7. Peck JE. Development of hearing, II: embryology. *J Am Acad Audiol* 1994;5:359–364.
8. Nager GT. *Pathology of the ear and temporal bone.* Baltimore, MD: Williams & Wilkins, 1993.
9. Donaldson JA, Duckert LG, Lambert PM, et al. *Anson-Donaldson surgical anatomy of the temporal bone.* New York, NY: Raven Press, 1992.
10. De La Cruz A, Linthicum FHJ, Luxford WM. Congenital atresia of the external auditory canal. *Laryngoscope* 1985;95:421–427.
11. Jafek BW, Nager GT, Strife J, et al. Congenital aural atresia: an analysis of 311 cases. *Trans Am Acad Ophthalmol Otol* 1975;80: 588–595.
12. Kaye C, Rollnick BR, Hauck WW, et al. Microtia and associated anomalies: statistical analysis. *Am J Med Genet* 1989;34: 574–578.
13. Bergstrom L. Assessment and consequence of malformation of the middle ear. In: Gorlin RJ, ed. *Morphogenesis and malformation of the ear: birth defects.* Original article series XVI(4). New York, NY: Alan R. Liss, 1980:217–241.
14. Cressman WR, Pensak MI. Surgical aspects of congenital aural atresia. *Otolaryngol Clin North Am* 1994;27:621–632.
15. Wardrop P, Kerr AIG, Moussa SA. Persistent stapedial artery preventing successful cochlear implantation. *Ann Otol Rhinol Laryngol* 1987;128(Suppl 12):443–445.
16. Sataloff RT. Embryology of the facial nerve and its clinical applications. *Laryngoscope* 1990;100:969–984.
17. Lambert PR. Congenital absence of the oval window. *Laryngoscope* 1990;100:37–40.
18. Streeter GL. The histogenesis and growth of the otic capsule and its contained periotic tissue spaces in the human embryo. *Carnegie Contrib Embryol* 1910;7:5–54.
19. Pujol R. Morphology, synaptology and electrophysiology of the developing cochlea. *Acta Otolaryngol (Stockh)* 1985;421 (Suppl):5–9.
20. Bermingham NA, Hassan BA, Price SD, et al. Math1: an essential gene for the generation of inner ear hair cells. *Science* 1999;284(5421):1837–1841.
21. Fisher NA, Curtin HD. Radiology of congenital hearing loss. *Otolaryngol Clin North Am* 1994;27:511–531.
22. Appler JM, Goodrich LV. Connecting the ear to the brain: molecular mechanisms of auditory circuit assembly. *Prog Neurobiol* 2011;93(4):488–508.

23. Fritzsch B, Matei VA, Nichols DH, et al. Atoh1 null mice show directed afferent fiber growth to undifferentiated ear sensory epithelia followed by incomplete fiber retention. *Dev Dyn* 2005; 233(2):570–583.

24. Hilding WJ, Ginzberg RD. Pigmentation of the stria vascularis. *Acta Otolaryngol (Stockh)* 1977;84:24–37.

25. Van De Water TR. Tissue interactions and cell differentiation: neuron-sensory cell interaction during otic development. *Development* 1988;103(Suppl):185–193.

26. Jackler RK, Hwang PH. Enlargement of the cochlear aqueduct: fact or fiction? *Otolaryngol Head Neck Surg* 1993;109:14–25.

27. Jackler RK, Luxford WM, House WF. Congenital malformations of the inner ear: a classification based on embryogenesis. *Laryngoscope* 1987;97(Suppl 40):2–14.

28. Jackler RK. Congenital malformations of the inner ear. In: Cummings CW, Flint PW, Harker LA, et al., eds. *Otolaryngology–head and neck surgery.* St. Louis, MO: Elsevier Mosby, 2005:4398–4421.

29. Carey JC. Inner ear. In: Stevenson RE, Hall JG, Goodman RM, eds. *Human malformations and related anomalies.* New York, NY: Oxford University Press, 1993:231–236.

30. Purcell DD, Fischbein N, Lalwani AK. Identification of previously "undetectable" abnormalities of the bony labyrinth with computed tomography measurement. *Laryngoscope* 2003;113:1908–1911.

31. Jackler RJ, De La Cruz A. The large vestibular aqueduct syndrome. *Laryngoscope* 1989;99:1238–1243.

32. Li XC, Everett LA, Lalwani AK, et al. A mutation in PDS causes non-syndromic recessive deafness. *Nat Genet* 1998;18:215–217.

33. Yang T, Gurrola Ii JG, Wu H, et al. Mutations of KCNJ10 together with mutations of SLC26A4 cause digenic nonsyndromic hearing loss associated with enlarged vestibular aqueduct syndrome. *Am J Human Genet* 2009;84(5):651–657.

34. Stimmer H. Enlargement of the cochlear aqueduct: does it exist? *Eur Arch Oto-Rhino-Laryngol* 2011:1–7.

35. Papsin BC. Cochlear implantation in children with anomalous cochleovestibular anatomy. *Laryngoscope* 2005;115(1 Pt 2, Suppl 106):1–26.

36. Purcell D, Johnson J, Fischbein N, Lalwani AK. Establishment of normative cochlear and vestibular measurements to aid in the diagnosis of inner ear malformations. *Otolaryngol Head Neck Surg* 2003;128:78–87.

37. O'Gorman S. Second branchial arch lineages of the middle ear of wild-type and Hoxa2 mutant mice. *Dev Dyn* 2005;234:124–131.

38. Rowe TM, Rizzi M, Hirose K, et al. A role of the double-stranded RNA-binding protein PACT in mouse ear development and hearing. *Proc Natl Acad Sci U S A* 2006;103:5823–5828.

39. Bouchard M, de Caprona D, Busslinger M, et al. Pax2 and Pax8 cooperate in mouse inner ear morphogenesis and innervation. *BMC Dev Biol* 2010;10:89.

40. Domínguez-Frutos E, López-Hernández I, Vendrell V, et al. N-myc controls proliferation, morphogenesis, and patterning of the inner ear. *J Neurosci* 2011;31(19):7178–7189.

41. Fekete DM. Development of the vertebrate ear: insights from knockouts and mutants. *Trends Neurosci* 1999;22:262–269.

Anatomy and Physiology of Hearing

141

Peter C. Weber　　*Samir Khariwala*

This chapter provides a brief summary of the most basic features of the anatomy and physiology of the ear. It is divided into sections on the external and middle ear, cochlea, and central nervous system (CNS). The focus is on the anatomic and physiologic bases of audition with an effort directed at functional features. Surgical anatomy, vasculature, and eustachian tube function are not discussed.

EXTERNAL EAR

The external ear consists of the pinna (auricle) and the external auditory canal (EAC) from the meatus to the tympanic membrane (Fig. 141.1). The pinna of humans is composed mostly of cartilage and has no useful muscles. The center of the pinna, the concha, leads to the external auditory meatus, which is about 2.5 cm long. The lateral third of the canal is the cartilaginous portion. It contains cerumen-producing glands and hair follicles. The remaining medial two-thirds is the bony portion, including an epithelial lining over the tympanic membrane (1).

The external ear and the head have a passive but important role in hearing because of their acoustic properties. The concha, or bowl of the auricle, has a resonance of about 5 kHz, and the irregular surface of the pinna introduces other resonances and antiresonances. These acoustic features are useful to help differentiate whether sound sources are in front of the listener or behind.

The EAC is essentially a tube that is open at one end and closed at the other; thus, the EAC behaves like a quarter-wave resonator. The resonant frequency (f_0) is determined by the length of the tube; the curvature of the tube is irrelevant. For a tube of 2.5 cm, the resonant frequency is approximately 3.5 kHz:

$$f_0 = \text{Velocity of sound @ 350 m/s}/(4 \times 2.5 \text{ cm})$$

A flat, wide-band sound measured in a sound field is changed considerably by the acoustic properties of the head and external ear. As Figure 141.2 demonstrates, a gain of about 15 dB occurs in the 3-kHz range of the human, cat, and chinchilla, and 10 dB between 2 and 5 kHz. The acoustic properties of the external ear are one of the reasons noise-induced hearing losses occur first and most prominently at the 4-kHz frequency region (boilermaker notch).

In addition to the prominence of noise-induced hearing loss in the 4-kHz region, the acoustic properties of the head and external ear have an important role in several hearing functions. In localization of sound sources, the head acts as an attenuator at frequencies at which the width of the head is greater than the wavelength of the sound. Thus at frequencies greater than 2 kHz, a *head shadow effect* occurs, in which interaural intensity differences of 5 to 15 dB are used to localize sound sources. At lower frequencies, at which the wavelength of the sound is larger than the width of the head, little attenuation is provided by the head. Interaural time differences (~0.6 ms for sound to travel across the head) are the salient cues for localization. The head-shadow effect is the reason right-handed hunters using rifles and shotguns have larger hearing losses in their left ears than in their right ears and vice versa. The muzzle of the gun, where the acoustic energy is greatest, is closer to the left ear, and the right ear is protected by the head-shadow effect.

The 10- to 15-dB gain provided by the external ear in the 3- to 5-kHz region is useful for improving the detection and recognition of low-energy, high-frequency sounds such as voiceless fricatives. The importance of the acoustic properties of the external ear and head is reflected in hearing-aid design and evaluations. Finally, the resonance of the external canal is approximately 8 kHz in infants and decreases to adult values after approximately 2.5 years of age. This developmental feature has several clinical implications, especially for sound-field testing and for hearing-aid design and evaluation of infants.

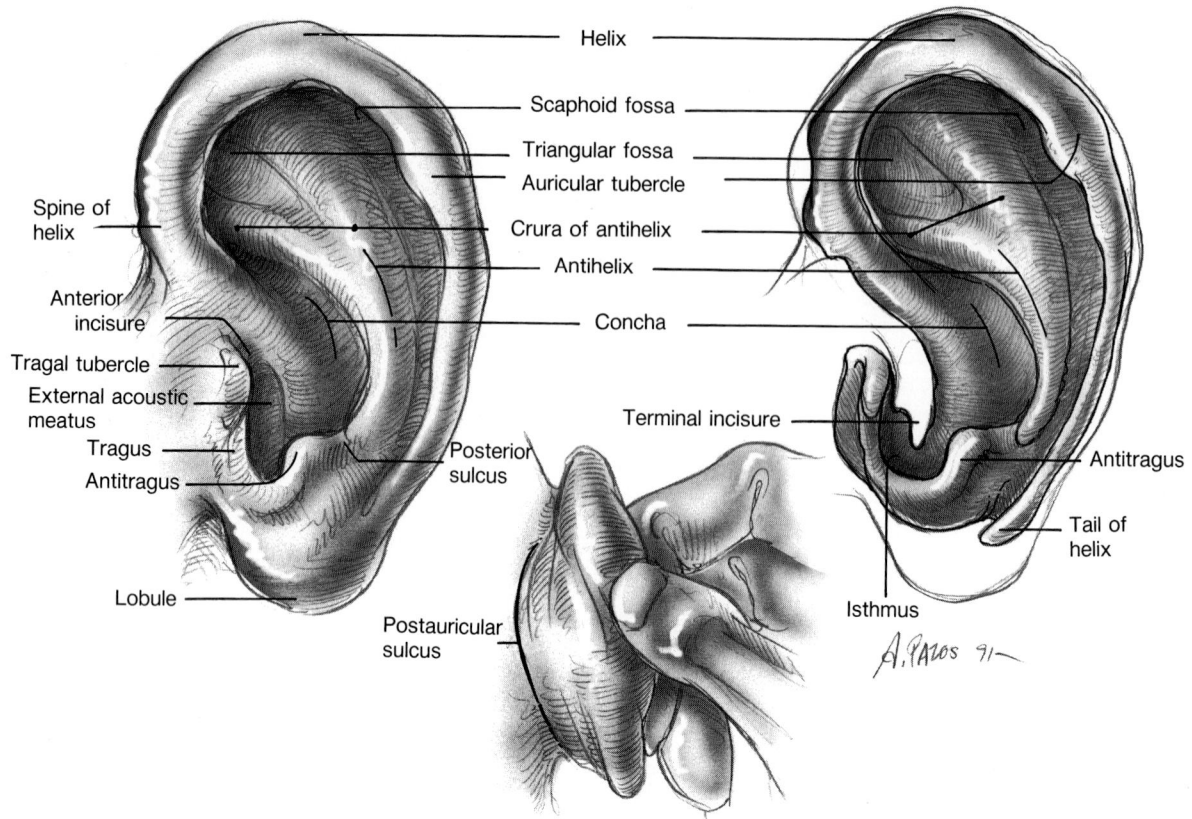

Figure 141.1 External ear.

MIDDLE EAR

The middle ear transmits acoustic energy from the air-filled EAC to the fluid-filled cochlea. It functions as an impedance-matching device inasmuch as it couples the low impedance of air to the high impedance of the fluid-filled cochlea. The impedance match is achieved in three ways. The first and most important factor is that the effective vibratory area of the tympanic membrane is approximately 17 to 20 times greater than the effective vibratory area of

the stapes footplate (Fig. 141.3). A second factor involves the lever action of the ossicular chain. The arm of the long process of the incus is shorter, by a factor of 1.3, than the length of the manubrium and neck of the malleus. A third and minor factor is the shape of the tympanic membrane. The combined result of these three factors is a pressure gain of approximately 25 to 30 dB. The variance in published

Figure 141.2 Ratio of sound pressure measured at the tympanic membrane to sound pressure measured in a sound field. Acoustic properties of the head, pinna, and external auditory meatus in three species (cat, chinchilla, and human). (From Rosowski JH. The effects of external and middle ear filters on noise-induced hearing loss. *J Acoust Soc Am* 1991;90:124, with permission.)

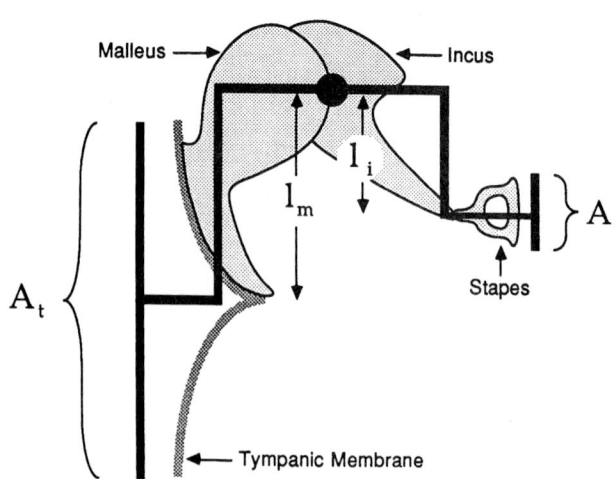

Figure 141.3 Schematic of ossicular chain and tympanic membrane shows the differences in area and vibratory pattern of the ossicles. (From Relkin EM. Introduction to the analysis of middle ear function. In: Jahn HF, Santos-Sacchi J, eds. *Physiology of the ear.* New York: Raven Press, 1988:103, with permission.)

measurements of the transformer ratio is noteworthy. With the exception of studies of acoustic impedance of the ear, most data are from studies of human cadavers, with all of their shortcomings, or of animals, usually cats. In addition to its role in the transfer of power to the inner ear, the tympanic membrane protects the middle ear space from foreign material of the ear canal and maintains the air cushion that prevents insufflation of foreign material from the nasopharynx though the eustachian tube.

The vibratory behavior of the ossicular chain is described in Figure 141.3. The transformer action of the tympanic membrane and ossicular chain provides for relatively efficient transfer of power to the inner ear, and the fidelity of sound transmission across the middle ear is outstanding. Distortion of sound signals does not occur in the middle ear, even for input signals with sound levels greater than 130 dB sound pressure level (SPL).

The middle ear, including the tympanic membrane, ossicular chain with supporting ligaments, and middle ear space, can be viewed as a passive mechanical system with both mass and compliant elements and therefore resonant properties. This linear system is coupled to the cochlea, which contributes a large resistance. The result is a middle ear system that is highly damped and linear and has a wide frequency response. The input–output function or transfer function of the middle ear is shown in Figure 141.4A. The ratio of the volume velocity of the stapes to sound pressure at the tympanic membrane increases in humans to approximately 800 to 900 Hz, which is the resonant frequency of the middle ear, and decreases at higher frequencies. Phase shift or time lag between movement of

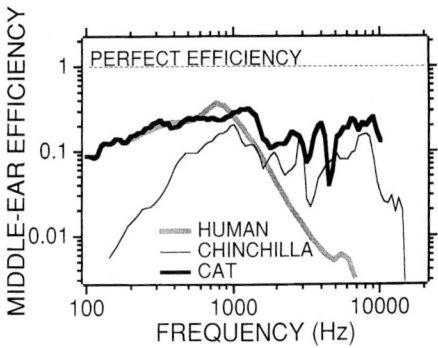

Figure 141.5 Efficiency of the transfer of power through the middle ear. For all species shown, less than half the power that enters the middle ear actually reaches the cochlea. Energy loss is caused by absorption by the tympanic membrane, ossicular ligaments, and middle ear. (From Rosowski JH. The effects of external and middle ear filters on noise-induced hearing loss. *J Acoust Soc Am* 1991;90:124, with permission.)

the tympanic membrane and the stapes generally increases with frequency (Fig. 141.4B). Although the middle ear is an impressive system in terms of frequency response, linearity, and transformer properties, considerably less than half of the power entering the middle ear actually reaches the cochlea because of the absorption of energy by the ligaments and middle ear. As shown in Figure 141.5, the human middle ear is particularly inefficient at frequencies greater than 2 kHz, especially in comparison with the ears of cats and chinchillas. It also is important to recall that a 50% loss of power is a loss of only 3 dB.

Auditory function is profoundly affected by cochlear impedance as well as the combined acoustic effects of the head, external ear, and middle ear. The combined effects of the acoustic properties of the head, external ear, and middle ear, as well the input impedance of the cochlea, have a profound effect on auditory function. For example, these factors determine the shape of the audibility curve and therefore the frequency range of human hearing (Fig. 141.6). For example, humans do not detect and recognize sounds greater than approximately 20 kHz because such high-frequency sounds are not transmitted efficiently through the middle ear to the cochlea. A second example of this sound transformation is shown in Figure 141.7, in which the spectrum of a cannon measured in a sound field is compared with the spectrum by the time it is transformed and shaped by the acoustic properties of the external ear, head, middle ear, and input impedance of the cochlea. Low-frequency energy is not transmitted to the cochlea, and the frequency region of greatest energy concentration is 3 to 4 kHz. Thus, these acoustic properties are primarily responsible for the ability of intense low-frequency sounds (measured in a sound field) to produce high-frequency hearing losses and injuries in the basal region of the cochlea.

Two striated muscles, the tensor tympani and the stapedius, are located in the middle ear. The former attaches to

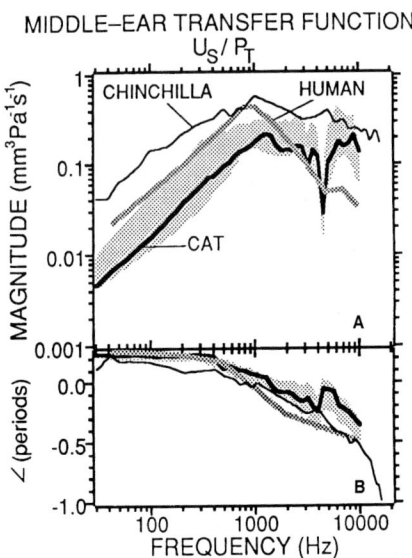

Figure 141.4 A: Transfer function of the middle ear in chinchilla, cat, and human. *Ordinate* is the ratio of the volume velocity of the stapes to sound pressure at the tympanic membrane. **B:** Phase shift of stapes footplate in relation to tympanic membrane. (From Rosowski JH. The effects of external and middle ear filters on noise-induced hearing loss. *J Acoust Soc Am* 1991;90:124, with permission.)

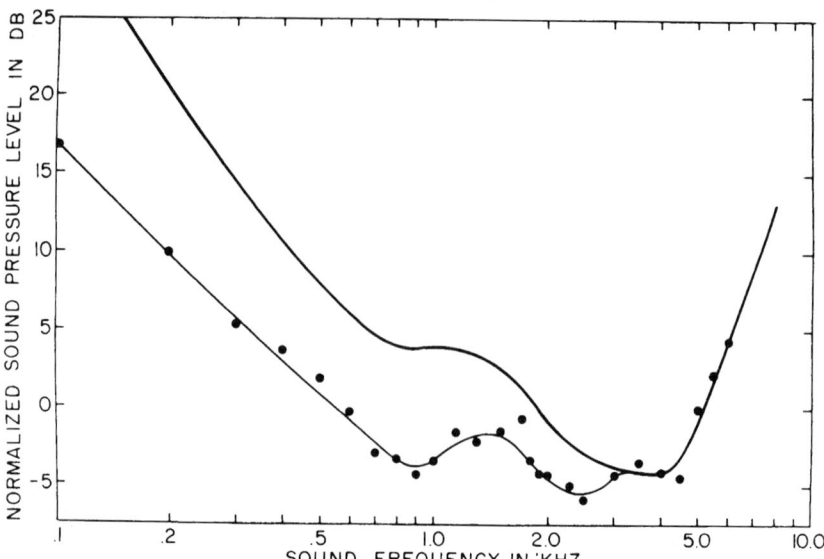

Figure 141.6 Comparison between overall outer and middle ear transfer function (*circles, lower curve*) and median threshold of audibility. (From Zwislocki JJ. The role of the external and middle ear in sound transmission. In: Turner D, ed. *The nervous system, human communication and its disorders.* Vol 3. New York: Raven Press, 1975:45, with permission.)

the malleus and is innervated by the trigeminal nerve. The stapedius muscle attaches to the stapes and is innervated by the stapedial branch of the facial nerve. Noticeably the stapedius and tensor tympani muscles are the smallest striated muscles in the body and also have a high innervation ratio, that is, nerve fibers per muscle fiber. Although no question remains that contraction of these muscles affects sound transmission through the middle ear, the details of the effect and the extent of the influence of the middle ear muscles are still not fully understood. A number of disparate functions have been attributed to the middle ear muscles.

One function of the middle ear muscles is to protect the cochlea from loud sounds (2). When sounds louder than approximately 80 dB SPL are presented monaurally

or binaurally, consensual (bilateral) reflex contraction of the stapedius muscle occurs. This contraction increases the stiffness of the ossicular chain and tympanic membrane, attenuating sounds less than approximately 2 kHz. Although the tensor tympani contracts as part of a startle response, acoustic reflex data from human subjects with neurologic involvement of cranial nerves V and VII suggest that the tensor tympani does not normally respond to intense acoustic stimulation. Laboratory and field studies of noise-induced hearing loss have shown convincingly that the stapedial reflex protects the cochlea, particularly from low-frequency (<2 kHz) sounds in excess of 90 dB. Inasmuch as the latency of the acoustic reflex is greater than 10 ms, the cochlea may be unprotected from short-duration, unanticipated impulsive sounds.

The following functions have been attributed to the middle-ear muscles. Some of these functions include providing strength and rigidity to the ossicular chain; contributing to the blood supply of the ossicular chain; reducing physiologic noise caused by chewing and vocalization; improving the signal-to-noise ratio for high-frequency signals, especially high-frequency speech sounds such as voiceless fricatives, by means of attenuating high-level, low-frequency background noise; functioning as an automatic gain control and increasing the dynamic range of the ear; and smoothing out irregularities in the middle-ear transfer function.

COCHLEA

The human cochlea is a coiled, bony tube approximately 35 mm long, divided into the scala vestibuli, scala media, and scala tympani (Fig. 141.8). The scalae vestibuli and tympani contain perilymph, an extracellular fluid-like material with a potassium concentration of 4 mEq/L and a sodium concentration of 139 mEq/L. The scala media

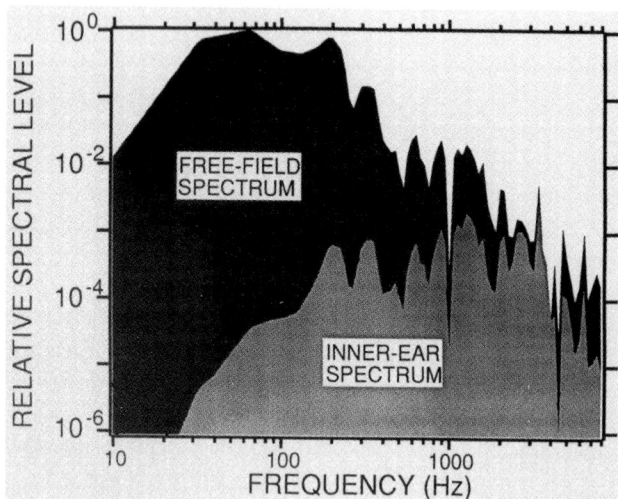

Figure 141.7 A comparison of the relative power spectra of impulses produced by a cannon and measured in a free field with the power that actually reaches the cochlea of a cat. (From Rosowski JH. The effects of external and middle ear filters on noise-induced hearing loss. *J Acoust Soc Am* 1991;90:124, with permission.)

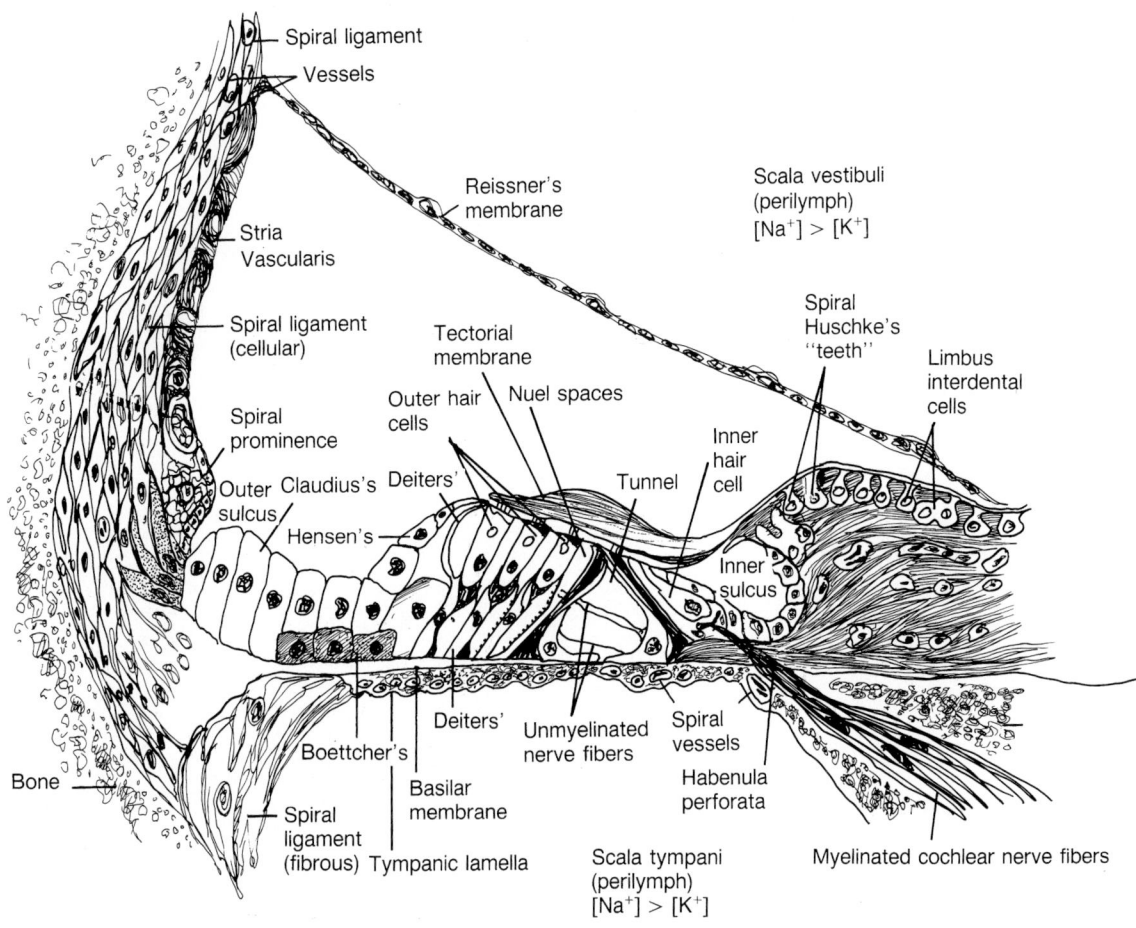

Figure 141.8 Midmodiolar view of cochlear duct. (Redrawn from Hawkins JE Jr. Hearing: anatomy and acoustics. In: Best C, Taylor NB, eds. *The physiological basis of medical practice*, 8th ed. Baltimore, MD: Williams & Wilkins, 1966:347, with permission.)

is bounded by the Reissner membrane, the basilar membrane and osseous spiral lamina, and the lateral wall. It contains endolymph, an intracellular-like fluid with a potassium concentration of 144 mEq/L and a sodium concentration of 13 mEq/L. The scala media has a positive direct current (DC) resting potential of approximately 80 mV that decreases slightly from the base to apex. This endocochlear potential is produced by the heavily vascularized stria vascularis of the lateral wall of the cochlea. The sodium-potassium-adenosine triphosphatase (Na⁺-K⁺-ATPase) pumps in a number of specialized cells of the stria vascularis contribute to this potential (3).

Acoustic energy enters the cochlea through the piston-like action of the stapes footplate on the oval window and is coupled directly to the perilymph of the scala vestibuli. The perilymph of the scala vestibuli communicates with the perilymph of the scala tympani through a small opening at the apex of the cochlea known as the *helicotrema*. The organ of Corti rests on the basilar membrane and osseous spiral lamina (Fig. 141.9). The basilar membrane is approximately 0.12 mm wide at the base and increases to approximately 0.5 mm at the apex. The major components of the organ of Corti are the outer and inner hair cells, supporting cells (Deiters, Hensen, Claudius), tectorial membrane, and the reticular lamina–cuticular plate complex (Fig. 141.10). Supporting cells provide structural and metabolic support for the organ of Corti. The phalangeal processes of the Deiters cells form tight cell junctions of the reticular lamina.

Outer and inner hair cells of the organ of Corti are important in transduction of the mechanical (acoustic) energy into electrical (neural) energy. Outer hair cells are radically different from inner hair cells. Figure 141.11 and Table 141.1 detail these differences (4). In addition to the morphologic differences between outer and inner hair cells, neural innervation is different (Fig. 141.12). The spiral ganglion, the cell body of the auditory nerve, sends axons to the cochlear nucleus of the brainstem, whereas the dendrite projects through the osseous spiral lamina. Of the 50,000 neurons that innervate the cochlea, 90% to 95% synapse directly on inner hair cells. These are called *type I neurons*. Each inner hair cell is innervated by approximately 15 to 20 type I neurons. In contrast, 5% to 10% of the 50,0000 neurons innervate the outer hair cells (*type II neurons*). Each type II neuron branches to innervate approximately 10 outer hair cells. In addition to the

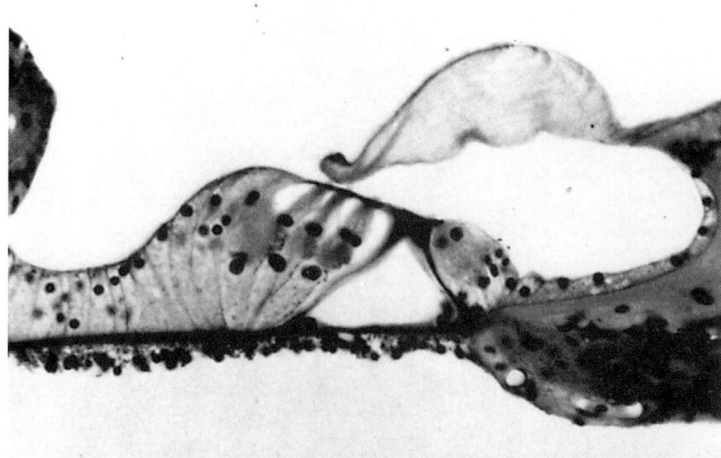

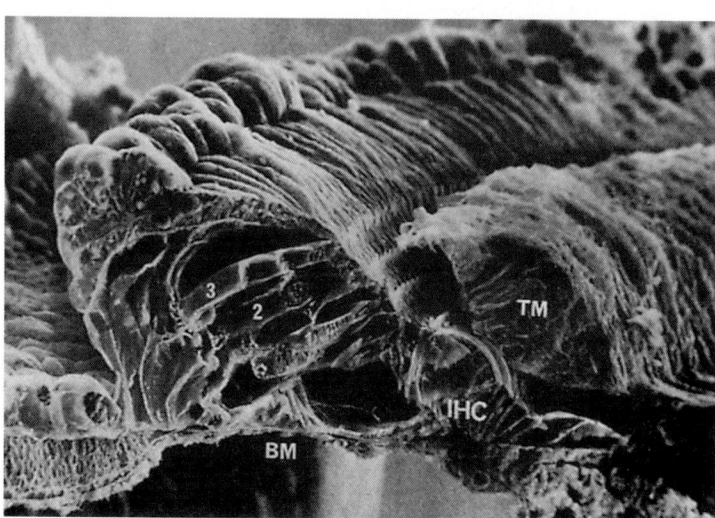

Figure 141.9 A: The organ of Corti of a cat in conventional midmodiolar section. Both sensory cells and supporting elements are evident. **B:** Photograph obtained through scanning electron microscope shows a corresponding specimen from a guinea pig. The inner hair cell (IHC) and three rows of outer hair cells (*1, 2, 3*) are visible. BM, basilar membrane; TM, tectorial membrane. (From Bredberg G, Ades W, Engstrom H. Scanning EM of the normal and pathologically altered organ of Corti: inner ear studies. *Acta Otolaryngol (Stockh)* 1972;301(suppl):48, with permission.)

afferent innervation pattern of the cochlea, approximately 1,800 efferent fibers, originating from the ipsilateral and contralateral superior olivary complex, project to the cochlea (Fig. 141.13).

Transduction is initiated by displacement of the basilar membrane in response to displacement of the stapes due to acoustic energy. The displacement pattern of the basilar membrane is a traveling wave (Fig. 141.14). The basilar membrane is stiffer at the base than in the apex. The stiffness component is distributed continuously. Therefore, the traveling wave always progresses from the base to apex. The maximal amplitude of basilar membrane displacement varies as a function of stimulus frequency. Traveling waves produced by high-frequency sounds (10 kHz) have maximal displacement near the base of the cochlea, whereas the waves to low-frequency sounds (125 Hz) have the maximum toward the apical region. Traveling waves generated by high-frequency sounds do not reach the apical regain of the cochlea, whereas waves to low-frequency sounds can travel the entire length of the basilar membrane.

In the past, the mechanical traveling wave was considered a broadly tuned response, with finer tuning introduced subsequently by transduction, the auditory nerve, and the CNS. Data obtained with sensitive recording and detection methods, however, have shown that the traveling wave has an extremely sharply tuned response (Fig. 141.15) and that many of the remarkable frequency-selective abilities of the ear can be explained by the mechanical properties of the cochlea.

The mechanism by which the sharply tuned peak is generated within the mechanical traveling wave involves an enhancement known as the *cochlear modifier*. This is an activity of the outer hair cells that enhances the motion of the basilar membrane at frequencies near the best frequency of the particular cochlear location. This enhancement contributes to the fine frequency-selective abilities of the ear and to the sensitivity of the ear and ability to detect extremely faint sounds. The notion of an active process in the cochlea, the cochlear amplifier, is supported by the phenomenon of *otoacoustic emissions*. That is, when a short-duration signal is presented to the ear, an echo emanating

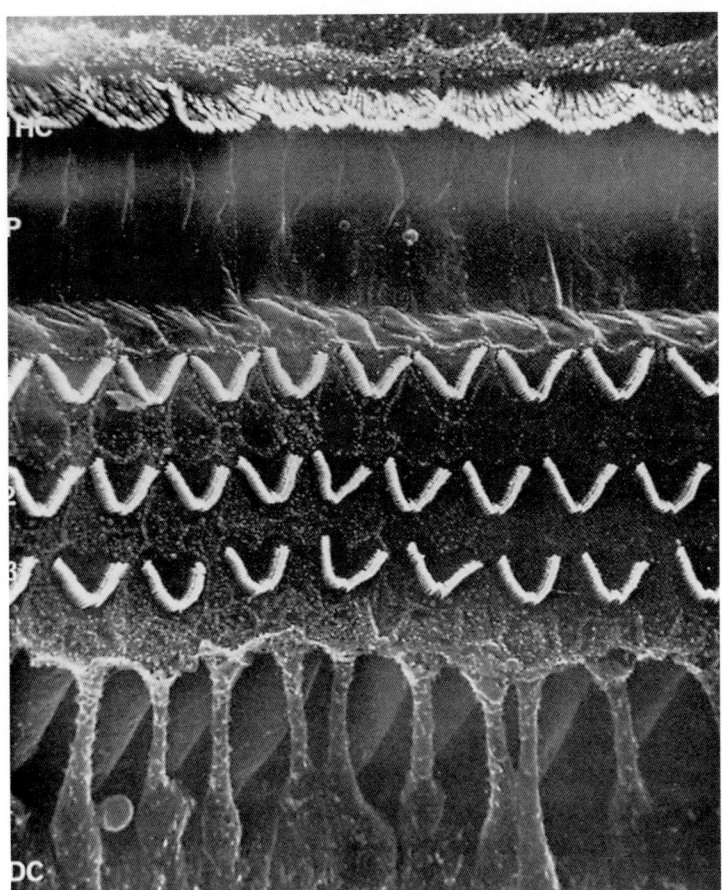

Figure 141.10 Scanning electron micrograph shows upper surface of organ of Corti with tectorial membrane removed. Modiolus is toward the *top*. Three rows of outer hair cells (*1, 2, 3*) with their characteristic V- or W-arranged stereocilia and a single row of inner hair cells (*IHC*) with slightly curved rows of stereocilia are visible. Inner and outer hair cells are separated by heads of pillar cells (*P*). Phalangeal processes of third row of Deiters cells (*DC*) are visible because Hensen cells have been removed. (From Bredberg G, Ades W, Engstrom H. Scanning EM of the normal and pathologically altered organ of Corti: inner ear studies. *Acta Otolaryngol* (*Stockh*) 1972;301(suppl):52, with permission.)

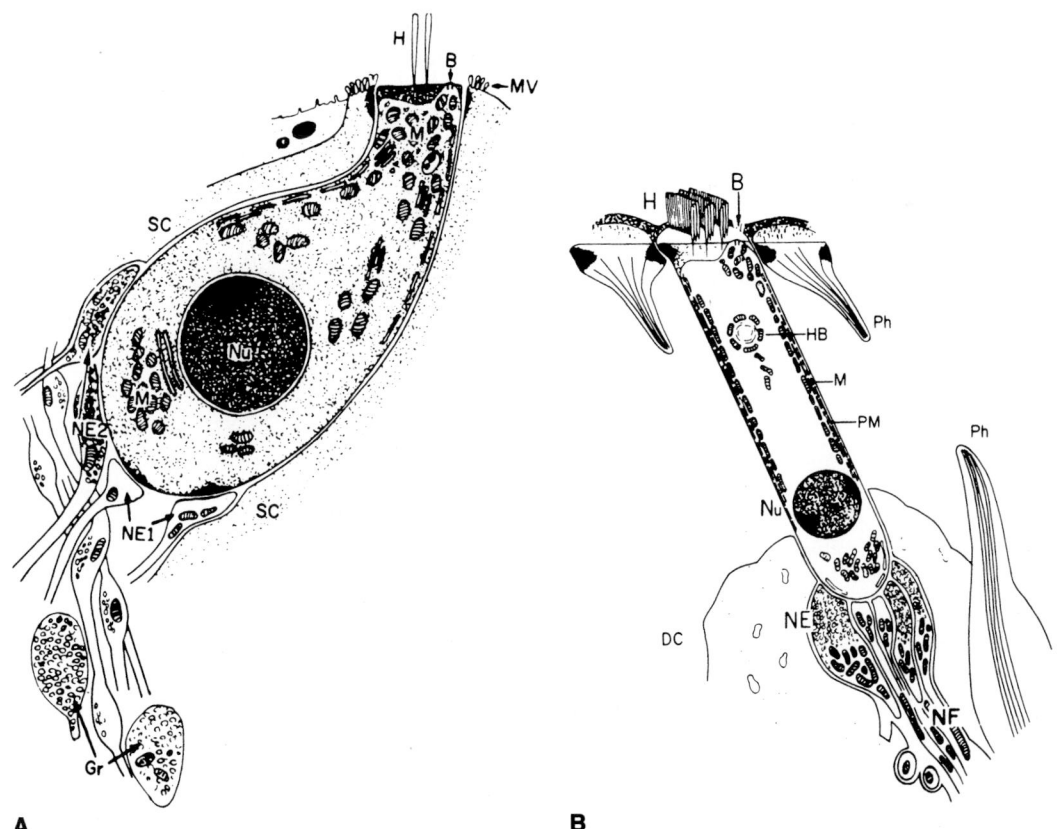

Figure 141.11 Differences in structure, ultrastructure, and innervation between inner (**A**) and outer (**B**) hair cells. B, Basal body; D, Deiters cells; H, stereocilia; M, mitochondria; MV, microvilli; NE1, afferent endings (cochlear nerve); NE2, efferent endings (olivocochlear bundle); Nu, nucleus; SC, supporting cells. (From Engstrom H, Ades HW, Hawkins JE Jr. In: Neff WD, ed. *Contribution to sensory physiology*. Vol 1. New York: Academic Press, 1965:67, with permission.)

TABLE 141.1	STRUCTURE AND INNERVATION OF INNER AND OUTER HAIR CELLS	
Characteristic	**Inner Hair Cells**	**Outer Hair Cells**
Number	3,500	12,000
Shape	Flask	Cylindrical
Stereocilia		
No. of hair cells	Few	Many
Arrangement	Three or four rows; rows slightly curved	Six or seven rows; rows arranged in V or W shape
Attachment to tectorial membrane	None or loosely connected	Longest stereocilia firmly embedded
Ultrastructure		
Position of nucleus cell body	Center	Base
Cytoplasmic organelles	Scattered	Adjacent to cell membrane
Presynaptic specializations	Large	Small or absent (synaptic bars and vesicles)
Glycogen content	Low	High
Relation to supporting cells	Completely surrounded	Supported only at surface and base
Afferent innervation		
Ganglion cells	Type I	Type II
Number of ganglion cells	27,000	2,100
Hair cell-to-ganglion cell ratio	1.8:1	5.7:1
Efferent innervation		
Source	Lateral superior olivary complex	Medial superior olivary complex
Postsynaptic target	Afferent dendrites	Base of hair cell

From Neely JG, Dennis JM, Lippe WR. Anatomy of the auditory end organ and neural pathways. In: Cummings CW, ed. *Otolaryngology–head and neck surgery*. St. Louis, MO: Mosby, 1986:2571, with permission.

from the cochlea can be recorded in the external auditory meatus. Because the energy of the echo can be greater than the energy of the short-duration signal, an active process, the cochlear amplifier, is assumed. Factors that may contribute to the cochlear amplifier include motility of outer hair cells and the mechanical properties of the stereocilia and tectorial membrane.

The stereocilia-hair cell complex is critical to transduction. Stereocilia are bundles of actin filaments that form tubes and are inserted into the cuticular plate. They also are cross-linked between themselves. Stereocilia of inner hair cells probably do not contact the tectorial membrane, but those of outer hair cells are in direct contact. Deflection of the stereocilia by the traveling wave opens and closes nonspecific ion channels at the tips of the stereocilia, resulting in a current flow (potassium) into the sensory cell. The flow of potassium ions into the sensory cell is modulated by the opening and closing of ion channels of the stereocilia. The potassium flux is caused by the endocochlear potential of +80 mV added to the negative intracellular

Figure 141.12 Schematic view from above shows the surface of the organ of Corti. The distribution of cochlear nerve fibers to inner (*IHC*) and outer (*OHC*) hair cells is evident. Basal end of cochlea is toward the *right*. Most spiral ganglion cells (*SG*) synapse with inner hair cells. Each ganglion cell innervates only one hair cell; many ganglion cells contact each hair cell. Only approximately 5% of spiral ganglion cells innervate outer hair cells. Each fiber travels basally for some distance before sending branches to several outer hair cells. (From Spoendlin H. The afferent innervation of the cochlea. In: Naunton RF, Fernandez C, eds. *Evoked electrical activity in the auditory nervous system*. New York: Academic Press, 1978:29, with permission.)

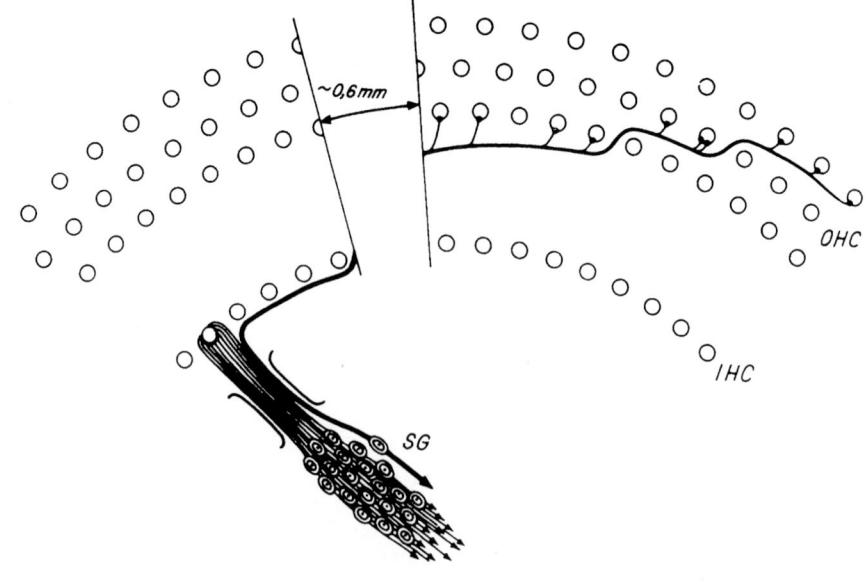

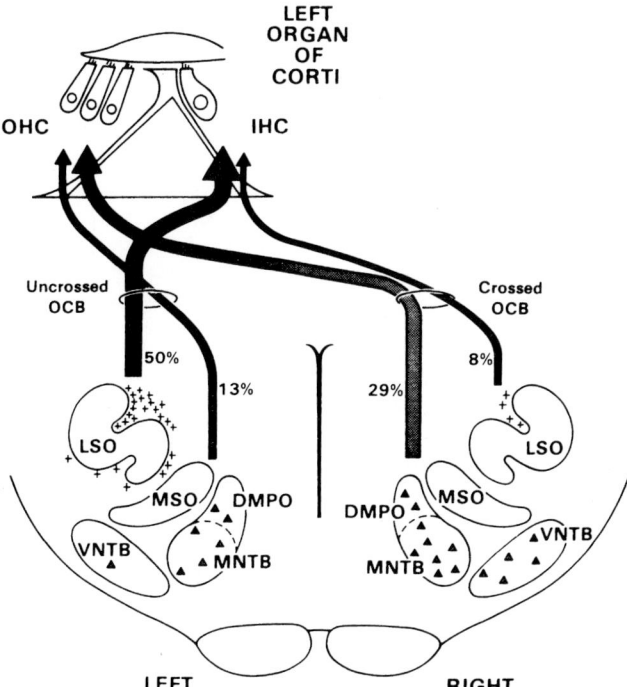

Figure 141.13 Schematic shows origin and distribution of efferent fibers of the olivocochlear bundle. *Crosses*, Small olivocochlear bundle neurons; *triangles*, large olivocochlear bundle neurons. The *number* of each kind of symbol, relative widths of *lines*, and *percentages* indicate the proportion of total olivocochlear projection to one cochlea that arises from each cell group. Efferent fibers to outer hair cells originate from large cells in the medial portion of the superior olivary complex. Approximately 70% of the projection to outer hair cells comes from the contralateral side of the brain. Projection to inner hair cells arises from small cells in the lateral region of the superior olive. Most of these fibers (85%) originate on the ipsilateral portion of the brain. Data are from studies with cats. DMPO, dorsomedial preolivary nucleus; IHC, inner hair cells; LSO, later superior olivary nucleus; MNTB, medial nucleus of the trapezoid body; MSO, medial superior olivary nucleus; OCB, olivocochlear bundle; OHC, outer hair cells; VNTB, ventral nucleus of the trapezoid body. (From Warr B. The olivocochlear bundle: its origins and terminations in the cat. In: Naunton RF, Fernandez C, eds. *Evoked electrical activity in the auditory nervous system.* New York: Academic Press, 1978:60, with permission.)

potentials of hair cells. The resulting intracellular depolarization causes an enzyme cascade involving calcium. This ultimately leads to the release of chemical transmitters, and the subsequent activation of the afferent nerve fibers.

Although the notion of the cochlea as an active rather than a passive organ is no longer debated, specific details of the cochlear amplifier and the biologic basis of its operation are under active investigation. One point of view attributes the cochlear amplifier to the ability of hair cells to contract and lengthen in response to electrical signals, a property called *somatic electromotility*. A protein named *prestin* has been identified in outer hair cells and is considered to be the motor protein of outer hair cells and the driving force of electromotility of hair cells (5). Another point of view focuses on rapidly acting potassium and calcium ion channels presumed to be the basis of the cochlear amplifier and its regulation (6). A third approach suggests that a collection of motor proteins within a hair cell can generate oscillations that depend on the elastic properties of the cell (7). The foregoing approaches are nonlinear models that involve rapidly acting calcium channels. Specification of the biologic basis of the cochlear amplifier (nonlinearity) is important inasmuch as many forms of hearing loss involve loss of the cochlear amplifier.

The neurotransmitters of the afferent and efferent systems are the subject of intense study. In regard to the afferent system, analysis of excitatory amino acid receptor expression by the techniques of reverse transcriptase–polymerase chain reaction, in situ hybridization, and immunochemical analysis indicates that glutamate is the afferent neurotransmitter. Glutamate has been detected in both spiral ganglion cells and sensory cells (8). The principal transmitter substance of cochlear efferent fibers is acetylcholine. It is possible that the organ of Corti is mechanically modified by means of motility changes of outer hair cells under the influence of the efferent system. Acetylcholine acts on receptors to produce hyperpolarization of the cell membrane

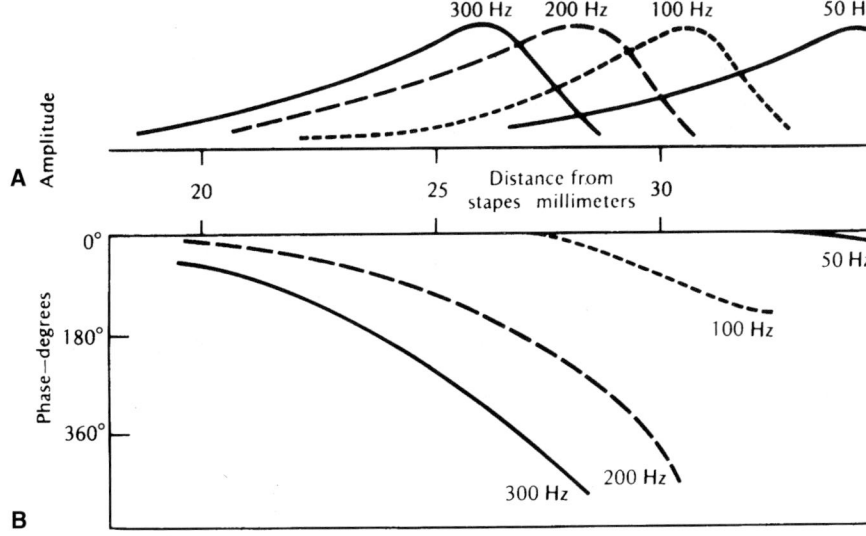

Figure 141.14 A: Amplitude of basilar membrane motion as a function of distance from the base of the cochlea to a 200-Hz tone. **Top:** instantaneous displacement of basilar membrane at successive time intervals (*solid lines*); displacement envelope (*dashed line*). **Bottom:** instantaneous velocity of basilar membrane at successive time intervals (*solid lines*); velocity envelope (*dashed line*). **B:** Relative amplitude of vibration at different points along the basilar membrane for four different frequencies. **Bottom**, phase lag at different points along the basilar membrane for four different frequencies. (From Von Bekesy G. *Experiments in hearing.* New York: John Wiley & Sons, 1960, with permission.)

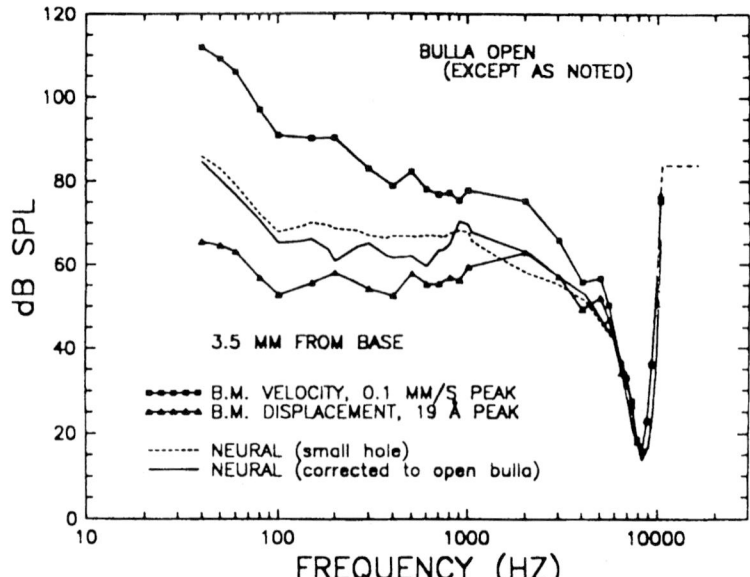

Figure 141.15 Comparison of mechanical tuning of the basilar membrane and neural tuning of an afferent fiber of the auditory nerve. (From Ruggero MA, Rich NC, Robles L, et al. Middle ear response in the chinchilla and its relationship to mechanics at the base of the cochlea. *J Acoust Soc Am* 1990;87:1612, with permission.)

and doubling of the input conductance of the cell. The acetylcholine receptor has both muscarinic and nicotinic features. In addition to acetylcholine, γ-aminobutyric acid and several neuroactive peptides are neurotransmitters for the efferent system (9–11).

GROSS COCHLEAR POTENTIALS

Four gross (extracellular) potentials can be recorded in the cochlea (12)—endolymphatic (endocochlear) potential, cochlear microphonic, summating potential, and whole-nerve action potential (Fig. 141.16). Unlike the other cochlear potentials, the endolymphatic potential is not generated in response to acoustic stimulation; rather, it is a DC potential of 80 to 100 mV recorded in the scala media. It arises from the stria vascularis of the lateral wall of the cochlea. The stria vascularis is considered to be the energy source, or "battery," of the cochlea, crucial for transduction. The nature of the energy source is the Na⁺-K⁺-ATPase pump. This pump has been localized to several types of cochlear cells, including marginal cells of the stria vascularis, outer sulcus cells, and fibrocytes near the attachment of the Reissner membrane and in the spiral ligament. Whereas Na⁺-K⁺-ATPase must play a significant role in ion transport in the cochlea, the nature of the energy source and the details of the ion exchange remain active research issues (3).

Malfunctioning of the mechanisms involved in production of endolymph and the endolymphatic potential can produce hearing loss, sometimes called *metabolic presbycusis*. When the flow of endolymph through the ductus reuniens is blocked, endolymphatic pressure increases, and hydrops occurs.

The cochlear microphonic is an alternating current (AC) voltage usually recorded within the cochlea or near

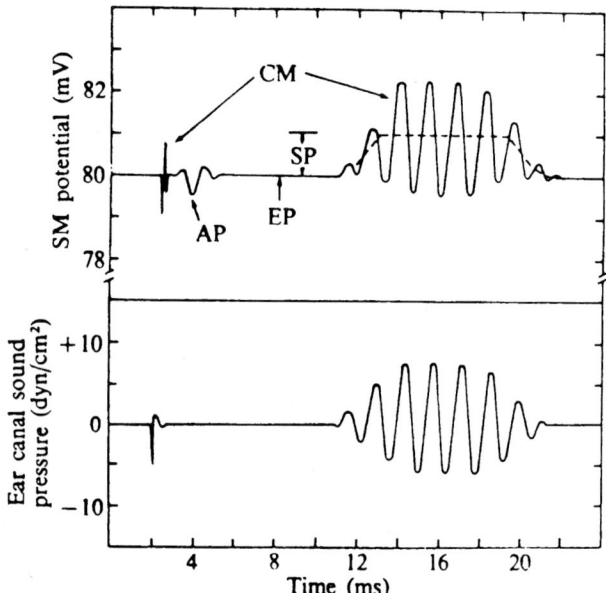

Figure 141.16 Schematic shows cochlear potentials recorded in the scala media in response to typical acoustic stimuli. All waveforms are approximately to scale. **Bottom:** Time waveforms of sound pressure in the ear canal for a click and a 750-Hz tone burst obtained with a probe-tube microphone. *Positive* and *negative* pressures refer to condensation and rarefaction, respectively, with the static value of atmospheric pressure subtracted out. An acoustic pressure of 5 dyne/cm² is equivalent to 88 dB SPL, referred to as 0.0002 dyne/cm² (20 Pa). **Top:** Resulting time waveform of the potential recorded in scala media by a single micropipette in the basal turn. The voltage is referenced to the neck of the animal. Ordinate is discontinuous to allow closer inspection of stimulus-related waveforms on the 80-mV endocochlear potential (*EP*), that is, the whole-nerve action potential (*AP*), the cochlear microphonic (*CM*), and the summating potential (*SP*). At low frequencies, the phase of the cochlear microphonic waveform leads that of the sound pressure at the eardrum. (From Schmiedt RA. Basic techniques for the measurement of cochlear potentials. In: Beagley HA, ed. *Auditory investigation: the scientific and technological basis.* Oxford: Clarendon Press, 1979:211, with permission.)

the round window. It represents the potassium ion current flow through mainly the outer hair cells; that is, the electrical resistance of outer hair cells is altered by the motion of the basilar membrane. When stereocilia are bent away from the modiolus, the resistance of the hair cells decreases. The result is an increase in current flow and a small decrease in endolymphatic potential. When stereocilia are bent toward the modiolus, resistance increases and current flow decreases with an accompanying increase in the endolymphatic potential. The corresponding voltage fluctuations, the cochlear microphonic, depend on the presence of outer hair cells. Unlike neural potentials, the waveform of the cochlear microphonic mirrors the motion of the basilar membrane. The summating potential is a DC potential recorded in the cochlea in response to sound. It follows the envelope of the stimulating sound. Recordings of this DC potential can be made in the scala tympani, media, or vestibuli and in some circumstances from a gross electrode in the human ear canal. The potential can be positive or negative, and it can reverse polarity, depending on electrode location or stimulus frequency and level. The summating potential probably has several origins, but it largely reflects the DC shifts caused by stimulus-driven intracellular potentials of outer hair cells. Inner hair cells contribute to these to a lesser extent.

The whole-nerve or compound action potential arises from the all-or-none discharge of auditory nerve fibers. The compound action potential is recorded most effectively with a gross electrode placed near the round window or auditory nerve and with high-frequency signals with rapid onsets. Such signals produce synchronous neural activity, which is summed to become the compound action potential waveform. The amplitude of the compound action potential increases with stimulus intensity over a 40- to 50-dB range, whereas latency decreases as stimulus intensity is increased. At high levels, a second peak sometimes is observed that probably reflects activity of the cochlear nucleus. The compound action potential can be clinically recorded with scalp electrodes or electrodes in the external meatus or by means of a transtympanic approach in which an electrode is placed near the round window niche. The ratio of the amplitude of the summating potential to the amplitude of the compound action potential has been used as an indicator of perilymphatic fistula, but the validity of this indicator is doubtful.

EIGHTH NERVE PHYSIOLOGY

The auditory nerve has approximately 30,000 fibers in humans and approximately 50,000 in cats. Perhaps one of the most important research findings in recent years was the observation that 90% to 95% of neurons (type I, radial fibers) innervate inner hair cells, whereas 5% to 10% (type II, outer spiral fibers) innervate to the outer hair cells (Fig. 141.12). Most, if not all, recordings from auditory nerve fibers are from the larger type I fibers in contact with

inner hair cells. These radial fibers have bipolar cell bodies in the spiral ganglion. Outer spiral fibers are monopolar and unmyelinated. Most recordings of single units of the auditory nerve are obtained by means of inserting a microelectrode into the auditory nerve where it exits the internal auditory meatus. The most basic measures of auditory nerve function are spontaneous rates, tuning curves, and intensity (rate-level) functions.

Most auditory nerve fibers in mammals discharge in the absence of acoustic stimulation. The nerve fibers have been classified into three categories on the basis of rate of spontaneous discharge—high (18 to 120 spikes per second), medium (0.5 to 18 spikes per second), and low (0 to 0.5 spikes per second). Fibers with high rates of spontaneous activity respond to auditory signals at lower levels than do fibers with medium or low rates of spontaneous activity. In other words, the most-sensitive fibers have the most-spontaneous activity. Fibers with high spontaneous rates have thick dendrites that tend to terminate on the side of inner hair cells facing outer hair cells. Fibers with low and medium spontaneous rates have thin dendrites that terminate on the side of the inner hair cell facing the modiolus. Ongoing studies indicate that fibers with high rates of spontaneous activity have different terminations in the auditory CNS (cochlear nucleus) than do fibers with low rates of spontaneous activity. In other words, spontaneous activity of nerve fibers is not random but is proving to be anatomically and functionally significant (13–16). The tuning curve of a single auditory nerve fiber is perhaps the most basic measure of auditory nerve function. A tone burst controlled in frequency and level is presented. The level is adjusted until a criterion change (one or two spikes per second) in firing rate is detected. Tone bursts covering a wide range of frequencies are used, and the lowest level of signal is recorded for a given frequency that produces a specific rate of discharge. The resulting isoresponse curve is called a *tuning curve*.

Figure 141.17 shows tuning curves for six different fibers. The sharp tip of the tuning curve identifies the best, or characteristic, frequency of the fiber. Units with low characteristic frequency innervate inner hair cells in the apical region of the cochlea, fibers with high characteristic frequency innervate inner hair cells from the basal region, and so on. Tuning curves are described according to the frequency of the tip or characteristic frequency, the high- and low-frequency side, and the tail. Fibers with a characteristic frequency less than 1 kHz are roughly V shaped. Fibers with a higher characteristic frequency have an obvious tip at the characteristic frequency and a tail that extends to the low frequencies. The high side of a tuning curve is the frequency region greater than the characteristic frequency. As characteristic frequency increases, the high side of the tuning curve becomes steeper with a slope or rejection rate that can exceed 500 dB per octave. The characteristics of tuning curves of auditory nerve fibers are strikingly similar to isoamplitude curves of a mechanical traveling wave (Fig. 141.15).

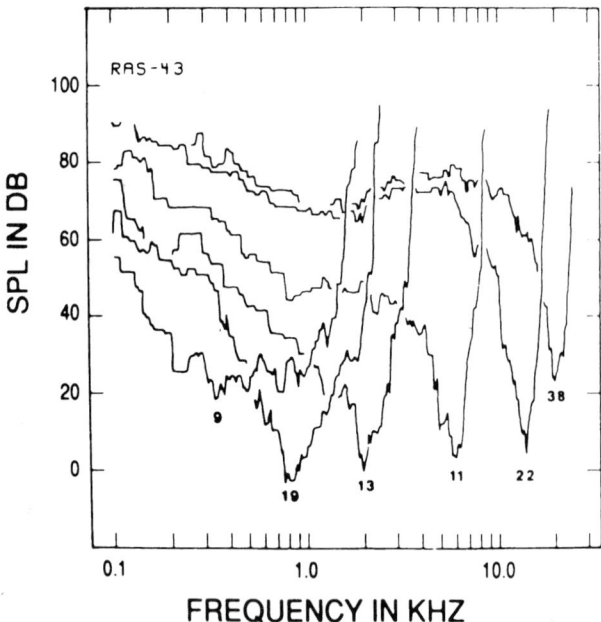

Figure 141.17 Tuning curves obtained from single fibers in the auditory nerve of a 6-month-old gerbil (CG-9) raised in quiet. Fiber numbers given in sequence during the experiment are at the *tips* of the curves. (From Schmiedt RA, Mills JH, Adams K. Tuning and suppression in auditory nerve fibers of aged gerbils raised in quiet or noise. *Hear Res* 1990;45:221, with permission.)

Injury or damage to sensory cells, including stereocilia, can alter the shape of tuning curves dramatically (Fig. 141.18). The lower right portion of the figure shows that when outer hair cells are destroyed, the tuning curve of auditory nerve fibers from normal inner hair cells is changed in several ways. The sensitive tip region is missing; that is, the threshold of the fiber is elevated by approximately 40 to 45 dB. The high-frequency side no longer has a steep slope, and the low-frequency side becomes slightly more sensitive, or hypersensitive. The characteristic frequency of the fiber appears to be much lower in frequency, and the band width of the fiber appears broader. The upper left portion of Figure 141.18 shows the consequences of partial injury to the stereocilia of outer hair cells. A threshold shift of approximately 30 dB occurs, but a short, sharply tuned tip remains, and the low-frequency tail is again hypersensitive. Irregularities in this tuning curve may explain monaural diplacusis; that is, a tone in one ear (800 Hz) has two pitches, for example, one at 800 Hz and a second at approximately 2.8 kHz.

The upper left portion of Figure 141.18 shows a tuning curve in which stereocilia of inner hair cells are damaged or in disarray, whereas most of the stereocilia of outer hair cells appear normal or nearly so. The threshold of the unit is elevated approximately 30 dB, but the tuning curve is approximately normal. The lower left portion of the figure shows responses to signals in a narrow range of frequencies only at sound levels greater than 90 dB SPL. In this case, sensory cells are present, but stereocilia of inner hair cells are

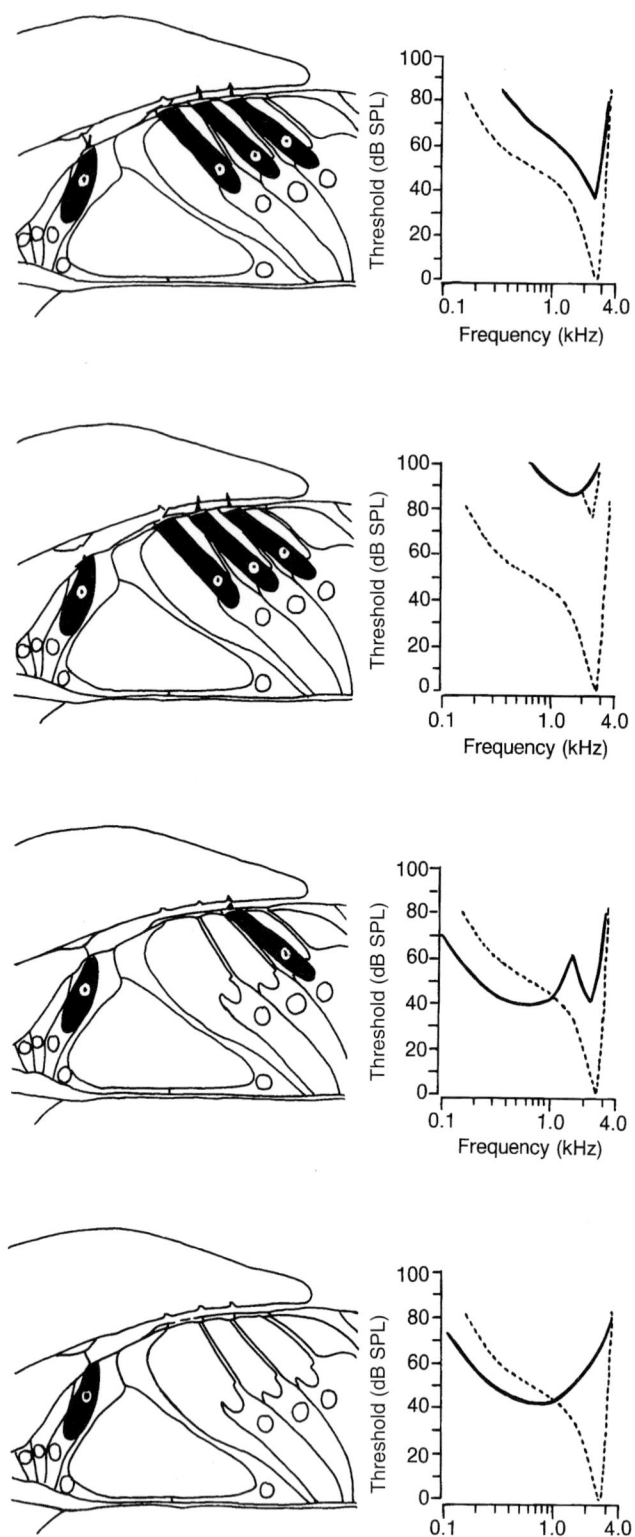

Figure 141.18 Tuning curves of single units of the auditory nerve with different degrees and types of acoustic injury to the sensory cells, including stereocilia. *Dotted line*, normal; *solid line*, after injury. (Redrawn from Liberman MC, Dodds LW. Single neuron labeling and chronic cochlear pathology III: stereocilia damage and alterations of threshold tuning curves. *Hear Res* 1984;16:55, with permission.)

destroyed, and those of outer hair cells are destroyed or in disarray. Thus normal neural activity, including sensitivity (detection of faint sounds) and frequency-resolving power, depends on intact outer hair cells and normal stereocilia.

Although thresholds of auditory nerve fibers are related to the rate of spontaneous discharge, most afferent nerve fibers (60%) have high spontaneous rates and thresholds within 20 dB greater than the thresholds for the animal. The remaining low-spontaneous fibers have thresholds that cover approximately 60 dB. The dynamic range of most auditory

nerve fibers is approximately 30 dB from threshold to saturation (Fig. 141.19), although some low-spontaneous fibers have a much wider dynamic range. Given the dynamic range of human hearing (0 dB SPL to ≥100 dB SPL), the auditory system must have neurons the thresholds of which cover a wide range and have firing rates that also cover a wide range of intensities. The ability of the human ear to respond appropriately to sounds over a 120-dB range (10,13) is remarkable. One way is with low-spontaneous fibers; another is recruitment of fibers of characteristic frequency.

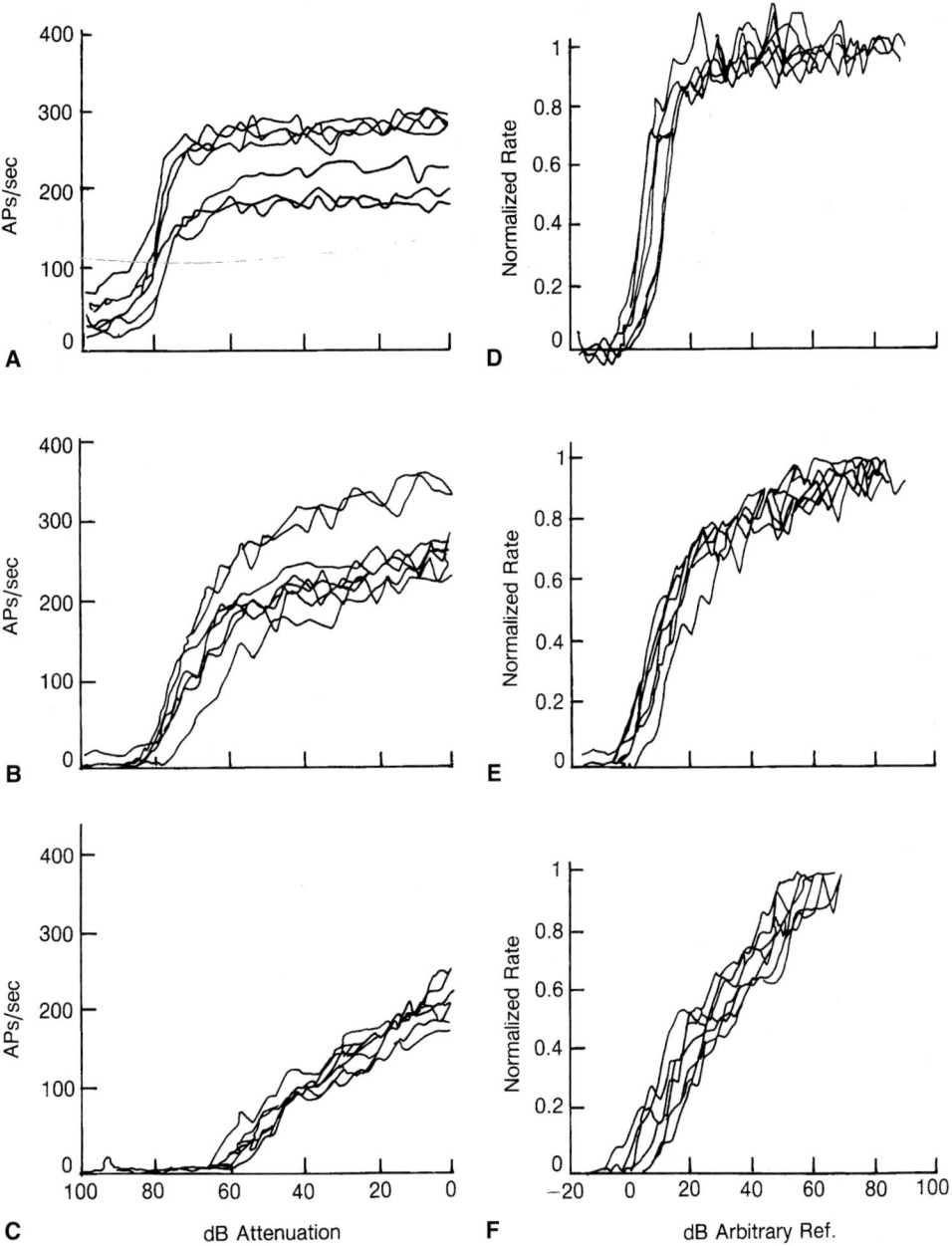

Figure 141.19 Examples of the three types of rate-intensity function. **A:** Saturating. **B:** Sloping saturation. **C:** Straight. For all units, characteristic frequency (*CF*) varies between 16 and 24 kHz, and maximum sound level varies between 104 and 115 dB SPL. **D–F:** Normalized rate–intensity functions for the fibers in **A, B,** and **C.** (Redrawn from Winter IM, Robertson D, Yabs GK. Diversity of characteristic frequency rate-intensity functions in guinea pig auditory nerve fibers. *Hear Res* 1990;45:191, with permission.)

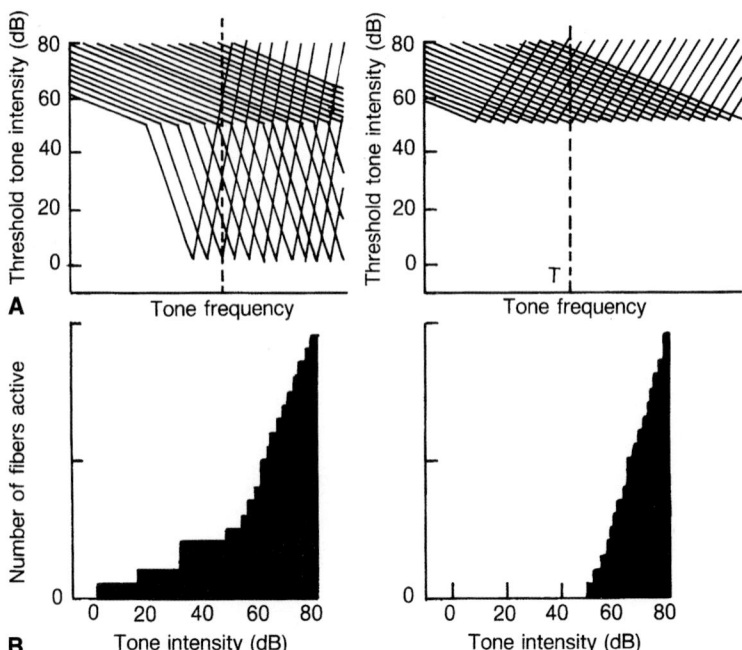

Figure 141.20 Neural explanation of one mechanism of loudness recruitment. **A:** Normal ear. **B:** Loudness in an abnormal ear grows abnormally quickly with intensity once the threshold is reached because the tips of the tuning curves are missing. (From Evans EF. The sharpening of cochlear frequency selectivity in the normal and abnormal cochlea. *Audiology* 1975;14:419, with permission.)

One of the most common features of sensorineural hearing loss is recruitment of loudness. Figure 141.20 gives an explanation. It is assumed that loudness depends on the total activity of the auditory nerve. As Figure 141.20A shows, the number of fibers activated increases slowly as intensity is increased, and only the tips of the tuning curves are activated. As the intensity increases further, the tails of the tuning curves are encountered, and the number of fibers activated increases rapidly. In the case of sensorineural hearing loss, the tips of the tuning curves are missing, and the fibers are not activated until the level of the signal is sufficient to reach the tails of the tuning curves. Abruptly, many fibers then are abruptly activated simultaneously.

NONLINEAR PROPERTIES OF THE EAR

Some of the outstanding features of the middle ear transformer are its linear properties, but the outstanding features of the cochlea and auditory nerve are the nonlinear characteristics. Perhaps the most studied nonlinearities are combination tones, described herein in relation to cochlear emissions, and two-tone rate suppression, as recorded in auditory nerve fibers.

Two-tone rate suppression is the reduction in firing rate produced by one tone when a second tone is introduced. Figure 141.21 shows a tuning curve with a suppression area outlined above the characteristic frequency of the nerve fiber and an area below the characteristic frequency of the fiber. Tones presented in the dotted or suppression areas in the figure reduce the firing rate caused by the probe tone. Both the excitor and suppressor tones are presented simultaneously, and because little or no time lag is associated with this phenomenon nor is any evidence available that

it is neurally produced, the effect is called *suppression* rather than inhibition. Two-tone suppression in single units is reflected in the compound action potential. Figure 141.21 (right) shows tuning curves of the compound action potential with suppression areas shown in the dotted areas. In this case, the amplitude of the compound action potential is altered by the suppressing signal, whereas in the single-unit case (left), the firing rate of a neuron is reduced by an arbitrary amount (20%). The single-unit and compound action potential suppression areas are similar. Inasmuch as two-tone suppression can be observed in the DC intracellular response of inner hair cells, it is probable that two-tone suppression originates in the active nature of cochlear mechanics and before the inner hair cells.

In the presence of sensorineural hearing loss caused by exposure to noise or to ototoxic drugs, two-tone rate suppression is severely affected, if at all measurable. Two-tone rate suppression appears normal or nearly so in cases of cochlear hearing loss in which the sensory cells, including stereocilia, are normal or nearly so, but in the stria vascularis is affected. The latter scenario leads to presbycusis (17).

Otoacoustic emissions (OAEs) are sounds that are detected in the ear canal when the tympanum receives vibrations transmitted through the middle ear from the cochlea. OAEs provide support for the notion that the cochlea is not just a passive receiver of acoustic energy but can also generate or amplify sounds. Several different types of OAEs are found (18). *Spontaneous* OAEs occur in the absence of acoustic stimulation and are typically highly stable pure tones of –10 to 30 dB SPL, which are found in 30% to 40% of healthy young ears (19,20). The precise frequency of a spontaneous OAE does not imply an origin at a precise place in the cochlea, but only a particular

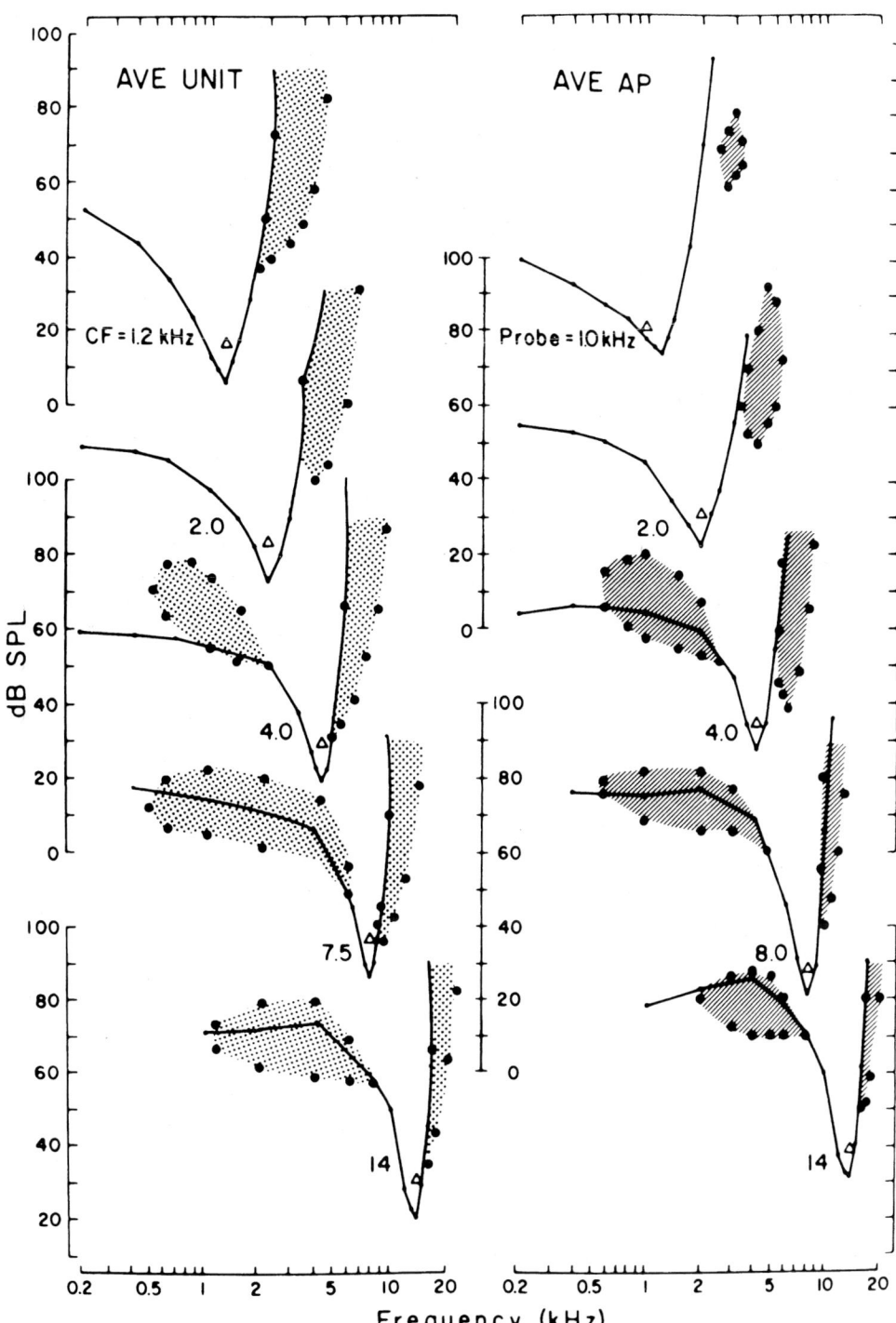

Figure 141.21 **Left:** Excitatory tuning curve (*circles*) and two-tone suppression areas (*shaded*) for a single auditory nerve fiber. Tones presented in the suppression areas decrease the firing rate to the excitatory tone. **Right:** Tuning and suppression of the compound action potential (CAP). (From Harris DM. Action potential suppression, tuning curves and thresholds: comparison with single fiber data. *Hear Res* 1979;1:133, with permission.)

coincidence of travel time and reflection from an ill-defined region of high outer cell activity. Spontaneous OAEs can be recorded over long periods with only minor but seemingly systematic variations in frequency and amplitude.

A second class of OAEs are produced after exposure to an acoustic signal. *Transient-evoked* OAEs (TEOAE) are made

via a probe placed in the ear canal. The oscillatory sound pressure waveform seen in TEOAE responses actually corresponds to the motion of the eardrum resulting from pressure fluctuations generated within the cochlea (Fig. 141.22). Although stimulatory clicks excite the entire cochlea, TEOAE responses can be used to give frequency-specific

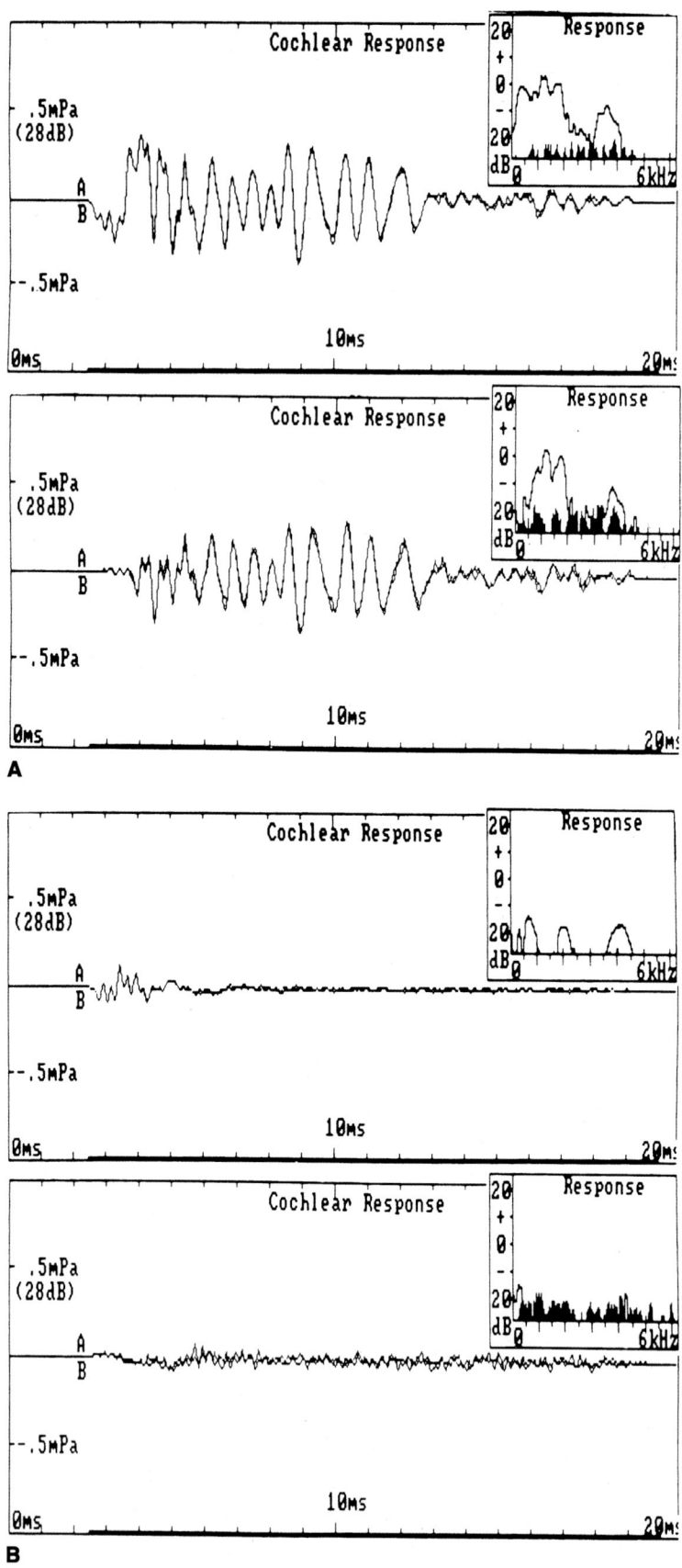

Figure 141.22 Cochlear echoes, also called *stimulated cochlear emissions*, from a normal ear (**A**) and a deaf ear (**B**). (From Kemp DT, Ryan S, Bray P. Otoacoustic emission analysis and interpretation for clinical purpose. *Adv Audio* 1990;12:77–92, with permission.)

information about the cochlea through splitting of the responses into different frequency bands. TEOAEs are highly sensitive to cochlear pathology in frequency-specific manner. Frequencies at which hearing thresholds exceed 20 to 30 dB hearing loss (HL) are typically absent in the TEOAE response (21,22). Because of their sensitivity to cochlear dysfunction, TEOAEs have found widespread application in newborn hearing screening programs (23).

Distortion-product OAEs also are used widely in clinical situations. The TEOAE and DPOAE techniques complement each other. DPOAEs offer a wider frequency range of observation with less sensitivity to minor and subclinical conditions in adults. When two primary tones, F1 and F2, are presented to the cochlea, several distortion products are produced. The most prominent of all these intermodulation distortion products is the cubic distortion tone, 2F1–F2. Measurement of DPOAEs at multiple stimulus levels can establish the OAE "growth rate." Healthy ears tend to exhibit a DPOAE growth rate of 1 dB of OAE per 1 dB of stimulus or less. Ears with some impairment show steeper growth. Single DPOAE results can be misleading, and results must be averaged across a range of frequencies. The DPOAE is easily recordable in patients with a normal middle ear system (24,25).

AUDITORY CENTRAL NERVOUS SYSTEM

The ascending and descending auditory pathways are described briefly herein in relation to auditory evoked potentials. Schematics of the afferent and efferent pathways are shown in Figures 141.13 and 141.23, respectively. These diagrams oversimplify the system but provide a rough introduction to the auditory CNS and its complexity. All eighth-nerve afferent fibers stop at the level of the cochlear nucleus. Five major cell types are found within the cochlear nucleus, each with distinct morphologic and physiologic features, such as response to stimulus onset, stimulus offset, and frequency modulation. From the cochlear nucleus, most fibers cross the brainstem to the contralateral superior olivary complex; a much smaller number of fibers run to the ipsilateral superior olivary complex.

The superior olivary complex is considered the first center in the ascending auditory system, where inputs from both ears converge. Auditory nuclei above the superior olivary complex can be excitatory or inhibitory with inputs from each ear. Stimulation of the contralateral ear typically is excitatory to cell bodies of the auditory CNS, whereas stimulation of the ipsilateral ear is inhibitory. As shown in Figure 141.13, the medial superior olivary complex is the origin of the crossed efferent fibers that terminate on outer hair cells, whereas the lateral superior olivary complex is the origin for the uncrossed efferent fibers that terminate on inner hair cells. Although many functions have been attributed to the efferent auditory system, especially protecting the cochlea from loud sounds, the functions of the system are unknown; those that have been proposed are easily debated (26,27).

The inferior colliculus is a complex nucleus with at least 18 major cell types and at least five areas of specialization. It is involved in probably all forms of auditory behavior, including differential sensitivity for frequency and intensity, loudness, and binaural hearing. The inferior colliculus is clearly more than a relay center. The medial geniculate body of the thalamus sends projections to the auditory cortex, but its specific functions are unknown.

The auditory cortex is located in the sylvian fissure of the temporal lobe; many secondary auditory areas are clustered around the primary area. In each area, the cells are tonotopically organized in a columnar manner, each column having a special attribute. The cells in one column can have different tuning at a similar characteristic frequency, whereas another column can be associated with intensity encoding, another with providing inhibitory responses to stimulation of one ear and excitatory responses of the other ear, and so on. As is common for thalamic connections with the cortex, nuclei within the medial geniculate body that send fibers to the auditory cortex also receive fibers from the same area of the cortex. Bilateral lesions of the temporal lobe have been shown to produce wide-ranging effects (cortical deafness, in which several auditory behaviors are severely affected, including speech discrimination, localization of sound, temporal processing of information, and the detection of faint, short-duration signals) (28). Another important feature of the auditory system is its tonotopic nature. From the basilar membrane to the auditory cortex, the system is organized spatially with respect to frequency. Each place on the basilar membrane responds best to a specific frequency—high-frequency sounds are localized to the base, and low-frequency sounds, to the apex. The tonotopic organization of the cochlea is preserved at the cochlear nucleus. Figure 141.24 shows that as an electrode penetrates the cochlear nucleus, fibers with different characteristic frequencies are contacted, and the characteristic frequencies form an orderly progression. Similar data exist at all nuclei of the auditory CNS, including the auditory cortex.

The most obvious clinical application of basic information on the auditory CNS involves interpretation of evoked potentials. The auditory brainstem response (ABR) is one component of auditory evoked potentials. The existence of the ABR was first reported by Sohmer and Feinmesser in 1967 (29). The ABR is recorded from electrodes attached to various positions on the head. The ABR consists of a series of seven waves occurring within about 10 milliseconds after stimulus onset. The convention in the United States is to label wave peaks with Roman numerals. It is generally accepted that the ABR is generated by the auditory nerve and subsequent fiber tracts and nuclei within the auditory brainstem pathways. It is widely believed that each wave is generated as follows: wave I and II are the eighth nerve, III is cochlear nucleus, IV is superior olive/lateral leminiscus, and V is lateral leminiscus/inferior colliculus.

The ABR is generated by a click stimulus because it yields the clearest response. The ABR is used clinically both

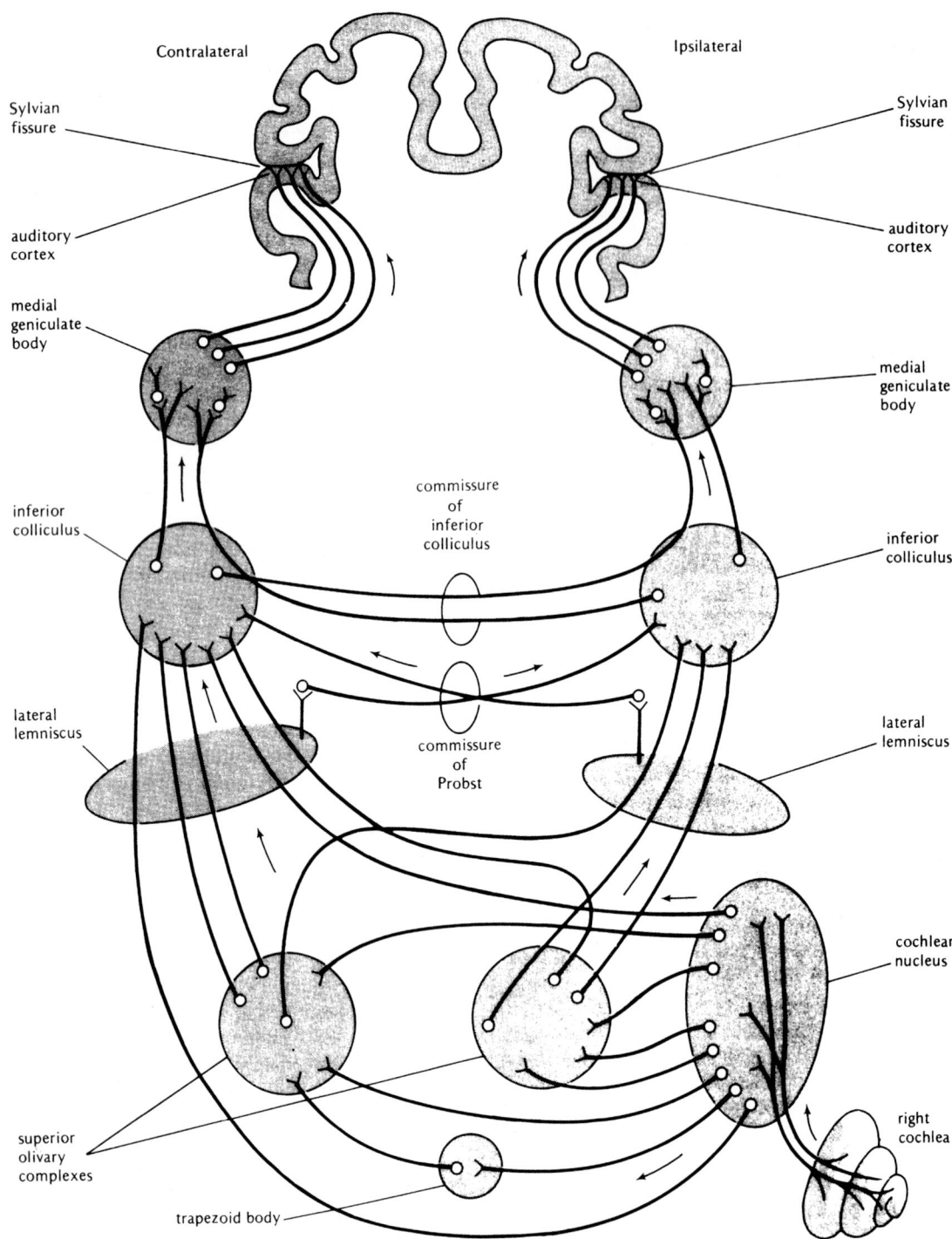

Contralateral   Ipsilateral

Sylvian fissure

auditory cortex

medial geniculate body

inferior colliculus

commissure of inferior colliculus

lateral lemniscus

commissure of Probst

superior olivary complexes

trapezoid body

Sylvian fissure

auditory cortex

medial geniculate body

inferior colliculus

lateral lemniscus

cochlear nucleus

right cochlea

Figure 141.23 Highly schematic diagram of the ascending (afferent) pathways of the central auditory system from the right cochlea to the auditory cortex. No attempt is made to show the subdivisions and connections within the various regions, cerebellar connections, or connections with the reticular formation. (From Yost WA, Neilsen *DW. Fundamentals of hearing*, 2nd ed. New York: Holt, Rinehart & Winston, 1985:121.)

in the estimation of auditory sensitivity and in otoneurologic assessment. In this way, it can be used to detect lesions along the auditory nerve and brainstem pathways. The study can be performed regardless of state of wakefulness, and the result is unaffected by most medications. As a result, children are often tested while under sedation or during sleep.

The field of clinical objective audiometry has recently gained an additional technique in the auditory evoked response battery. The *auditory steady-state response* (ASSR) promises to be a valuable study in the workup of auditory dysfunction. Unlike ABRs, which are obtained through the use of transient stimuli, ASSRs are evoked by using sustained

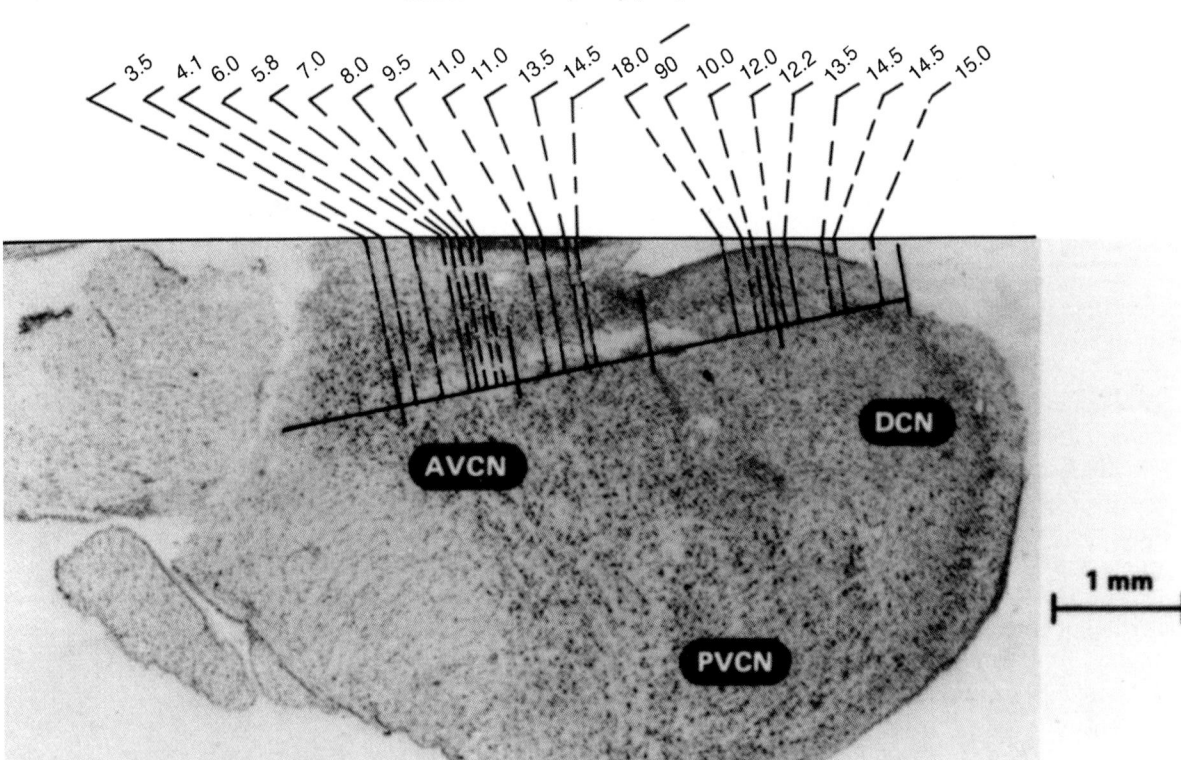

Figure 141.24 Cross section of cochlear nucleus shows the track made by electrode penetration. The characteristic frequencies of neurons recorded from various points within the anteroventral cochlear nucleus (*AVCN*) and dural cochlear nucleus (*DCN*) show that the spatial separation of frequency is maintained within those two divisions of the cochlear nucleus. PVCN, posteroventral cochlear nucleus. This tonotopic organization is maintained throughout the central auditory system. (Redrawn from Rose JE, Galambos R, Hughes JR. Microelectrode studies of the cochlear nuclei of the cat. *Bull Johns Hopkins Hosp* 1959;104:211, with permission.)

continuous tones. The tones are frequency specific because the continuous tones do not have spectral distortion problems as do brief tone bursts or click (30,31). Of note, ASSR also can be performed regardless of the state of wakefulness.

There are several advantages of ASSR over ABR. First, ASSR is a better technique for evaluating hearing aid performance because hearing aids and cochlear implants process continuous stimuli with less signal distortion than transient stimuli. Furthermore, ASSR can provide threshold information in a frequency-specific manner at intensity levels of 120 dB or greater (32,33). This allows differentiation of severe and profound hearing loss, which cannot be accomplished with ABR. This characteristic of ASSR may allow it to be used in assessing pediatric patients for cochlear implant candidacy (34). Last, ASSR has been shown to be more time efficient by determining more thresholds in a shorter time compared with ABR (35–37). Future research and clinical use are likely to solidify the status of ASSR in the audiologic armamentarium.

The neuroanatomic features of the system are complicated. Processing of neural information probably involves both parallel and serial processing. The former is anatomically described by a single fiber with ramifications to many target areas. Serial processing involves a fiber going to one target, which in turn goes to another target, and so forth. In the auditory CNS, both serial and parallel processing are involved. Because the auditory CNS is a highly redundant, complicated, and extremely powerful system, interpretation of evoked-potential data, and of other CNS neural data, is not straightforward.

HIGHLIGHTS

- The acoustic properties of the head and external ear are important, particularly because they provide cues for localizing sources of sound.
- The middle ear acts as a transformer between air and the fluid-filled cochlea and provides a sound pressure gain of 25 to 30 dB. The combined effect of the acoustic properties of the head, external ear, and middle ear, and the input impedance of the cochlea determine the frequency range of human hearing.

- The cochlea is a coiled bony tube approximately 35 mm long and divided into three compartments—the scala tympani, scala vestibuli, and scala media. The scalae tympani and vestibuli contain perilymph and are connected through the helicotrema at the apex of the cochlea. The scala media contains endolymph and has a positive DC resting potential of approximately 80 mV, which arises from Na^+-K^+-ATPase pumps in the stria vascularis.

- The auditory transducer is the organ of Corti, which contains sensory cells (three rows of outer hair cells and one row of inner hair cells). Deflection of stereocilia (hairs) of the sensory cells by a mechanical traveling wave starts transduction.

- A traveling wave, from the base toward the apex of the cochlea, arises in response to piston-like movement of the stapes. The traveling wave has a sharply tuned peak at the base for high-frequency sound that progresses toward the apex as frequency decreases.

- Deflection of stereocilia by the traveling wave opens and closes ion channels; the result is current flow (potassium ion) into the sensory cell. The potassium flux arises from the +80 mV endocochlear potential added to the negative intracellular potential of inner and outer hair cells. The resulting depolarization causes an enzyme cascade that releases chemical transmitters and activates afferent nerve fibers.

- Approximately 90% to 95% of the radial nerve fibers (type I) innervate inner hair cells. Approximately 5% to 10% (type II, outer spiral fibers) are connected to outer hair cells. Each inner hair cell is innervated by 15 to 20 type I neurons. Each type II neuron branches to innervate approximately 10 outer hair cells. Approximately 1,800 efferent fibers project to the sensory cells from the ipsilateral and contralateral superior olivary complexes.

- The most basic measure of auditory nerve function is the tuning curve of a single auditory nerve fiber. Tuning curves of single fibers of the nerve are strikingly similar to tuning curves of the mechanical traveling wave. Injury to sensory cells and stereocilia alters the features of tuning curves, including sensitivity and sharp tuning.

- The middle ear system is passive and linear in response to signals as great as 130 dB SPL, but the inner ear is an active system with its own amplifier and is nonlinear. These properties allow the inner ear to respond to a wide range of intensities and provide the basis for suppression phenomena.

- Although the efferent auditory system is well developed, the functional significance is not well understood. It may have a role in the cochlear transduction and in protecting the cochlea from overexposure to intense sound.

REFERENCES

1. Tonndorf J. The external ear. In: Jahn HF, Santos-Sacchi J, eds. *Physiology of the ear*. New York: Raven Press, 1988:4–20.
2. Moller A. The acoustic middle ear muscle reflex. In: Keidel WD, Neff WD, eds. *Handbook of sensory physiology*. New York: Springer-Verlag, 1974;5:312–329.
3. Schulte BA, Adams JC. Distribution of immunoreactive Na^+, K^+-ATPase in gerbil cochleas. *J Histochem Cytochem* 1989;37:127–135.
4. Neely JG, Dennis JM, Lippe WR. Anatomy of the auditory end organ and neural pathways. In: Cummings CW, ed. *Otolaryngology-head and neck surgery*. St. Louis, MO: Mosby, 1986.
5. Zheng J, Shen W, He DZ, et al. Prestin is the motor protein of cochlear out hair cells. *Nature* 2000;405:149–155.
6. Eguilez VM, Ospeck M Choe Y, et al. Essential nonlinearities in hearing. *Physiol Rev Lett* 2000;84:5232–5235.
7. Camalet S, Duke T, Julicher F, et al. Auditory sensitivity provided by self-tuned critical oscillations of hair cell. *Proc Natl Acad Sci USA* 2000;97:3183–3188.
8. Niedzielski AS, Safieddin S, Wenthold RJ. Molecular analysis of excitatory amino acid receptor expression in the cochlea. *Audiol Neurootol* 1997;22:79–91.
9. Sewell W. Neurotransmitters and synaptic transmission. In: Dallas P, Popper A, Fay R, eds. *The cochlea*. Berlin, Germany: Springer-Verlag, 1996:503–523.
10. Housely GD, Ryan AE. Cholinergic and purinergic neurohumoral signaling in the inner ear: a molecular physiological analysis. *Audiol Neurootol* 1997;2:92–110.
11. Roux I, Wersinger E, McIntosh JM, et al. Onset of cholinergic efferent synaptic function in sensory hair cells of the rat cochlea. *J Neurosci* 2011;31:15092–15101.
12. Schmiedt RA. Basic techniques for the measurement of cochlear potentials. In: Beagley HA, ed. *Auditory investigation: the scientific and technological basis*. Oxford, U.K.: Clarendon Press, 1979:211–232.
13. Liberman MC, Dodds LW, Pierce S. Afferent and efferent innervation of the cat cochlea: quantitative analysis with light and electron microscopy. *J Comp Neurol* 1990;301:443–451.
14. Fekete DM, Rouiller EM, Liberman MC, et al. The central projections of intercellularly labeled auditory nerve fibers in cats. *J Comp Neurol* 1984;229:432–440.
15. Leake PA, Synder RL. Topographic organization of central projections of the spiral ganglion in cats. *J Comp Neurol* 1989;281:612–629.
16. Liberman PA, Synder RL. Effects of chronic de-efferentation on auditory nerve response. *Hear Res* 1990;49:209–221.
17. Schmiedt RA, Mills JH, Adams JC. Tuning and suppression in auditory nerve fibers of aged gerbils raised in quiet or noise. *Hear Res* 1990;45:221–229.
18. Probst R. Otoacoustic emissions: new aspects of cochlear mechanics and inner ear pathophysiology. In: Pfaltz CR, ed. *Advances in otorhinolaryngology*. Basel, Switzerland: Karger, 1990.
19. Penner MJ, Zhang T. Prevalence of spontaneous otoacoustic emissions in adults revisited. *Hear Res* 1997;103:28–34.
20. Burns EM, Arehart KH, Campbell SL. Prevalence of spontaneous otoacoustic emissions in neonates. *J Acoust Soc Am* 1992;91:1571–1575.
21. Glattke TJ, Robinette MS. Transient evoked otoacoustic emissions. In: Robinette RM, Glattke T, eds. *Otoacoustic emissions: clinical applications*, 2nd ed. New York: Thieme, 2002:95–115.
22. Harris FP, Probst R. Otoacoustic emissions and audiometric outcomes. In: Robinette RM, Glattke T, eds. *Otoacoustic emissions: clinical applications*, 2nd ed. New York: Thieme, 2002:213–242.
23. Prieve BA. Otoacoustic emissions in neonatal screening. In: Robinette RM, Glattke T, eds. *Otoacoustic emissions: clinical applications*, 2nd ed. New York: Thieme, 2002:348–374.
24. Kemp DT. Otoacoustic emissions, their origin in cochlear function, and use. *Br Med Bull* 2002;63:223–241.
25. Rosner T, Kandizia F, Oswald JA. Hearing threshold estimation using concurrent measurement of DPOE and ASSR's. *J Acoust Soc Am* 2011;129:840–851.
26. Liberman MC. The olivocochlear efferent bundle and susceptibility of the inner ear to acoustic injury. *J Neurophysiol* 1991;65:123–132.

27. Graham CE, Basappa J, Tercan S, Vetter DE. The cochlear CRF signaling systems and their mechanisms of action in modulating cochlear sensitivity and protection against trauma. *Mol Neurobiol* 2011;44:383–406.

28. Jerger J, Weikers NJ, Sharbrough FW, et al. Bilateral lesions of the temporal lobe. *Acta Otolaryngol (Stockh)* 1969;258(suppl):1.

29. Sohmer H, Feinmesser M. Cochlear action potentials recorded from the external ear in man. *Ann Otol Rhinol Laryngol* 1967;76:427–436.

30. Lins OG, Picton TW. Auditory steady state responses to multiple simultaneous stimuli. *Electroencephalogr Clin Neurophysiol* 1995;95:420–432.

31. Brennen SK, Brooke RE, Stevens JC. The effect of varying stimulus phase between frequency and amplitude modulation in auditory steady state responses in neonates. *Int J Audiol* 2012;51:116–123.

32. Rans G, Dowell RC, Richards FW, et al. Steady state evoked potential and behavioral hearing thresholds in a group of children with absent click evoked auditory brainstem response. *Ear Hear* 1998;19:48–61.

33. Swanepoel D, Hugo R, Roode R. Auditory steady state responses for children with severe to profound hearing loss. *Arch Otolaryngol Head Neck Surg* 2004;130:531–535.

34. Zwolan TA. Cochlear implants. In: Katz J, ed. *Handbook of clinical audiology,* 5th ed. Baltimore, MD: Lippincott Williams & Wilkins, 2002:740–747.

35. Swanepoel D, Schmulian D, Hugo R. Establishing normal hearing with the dichotic multiple-frequency auditory steady state response compared with auditory brainstem response protocol. *Acta Otolaryngol* 2004;124:62–68.

36. Chou YF, Chen PR, Yu SH, et al. Using multistimuls suditory steady-state responses to predict hearing thresholds in high risk infants. *Eur Arch Otorhinolaryngol* 2012;269:23–29.

37. VanMaanen A, Stapells DR. Multiple ASSR thresholds in infants and young children with hearing loss. *J Am Acad Audiol* 2010;21:535–545.

142 | Assessment of Peripheral and Central Auditory Function

James W. Hall III *Patrick J. Antonelli*

New techniques and strategies for assessment of the auditory function in adults have been introduced in recent years. Pure-tone audiometry, immittance measurement (tympanometry and acoustic reflexes), and calculation of word recognition scores continue to be important for hearing assessment, and the traditional audiogram is useful in summarizing the results of basic audiologic assessment. Clinical audiology, however, now also includes other behavioral and electrophysiologic test procedures. For example, electrocochleography (ECochG) can contribute to the diagnosis of Ménière disease. Auditory brainstem response (ABR) offers a readily accessible, and relatively inexpensive, means for estimating hearing sensitivity in infants and young children and for the identification of retrocochlear auditory dysfunction. Otoacoustic emissions (OAEs), because of unique sensitivity and specificity to cochlear dysfunction, have become an integral component of the clinical audiologic test protocol. And, within recent years, the auditory steady state response (ASSR) has emerged as a valuable addition to the pediatric audiologic test battery. A variety of speech and nonspeech behavioral measures and several cortical auditory evoked responses are available for clinical assessment of central auditory nervous system dysfunction and associated auditory processing disorders (APDs).

This chapter summarizes current techniques and strategies for hearing assessment among adults. The emphasis is on use of a test battery that maximizes diagnostic accuracy and efficiency and minimizes test time and cost. A glossary of common audiologic terms and abbreviations is provided at the end of the chapter.

BASIC AUDIOLOGIC TEST BATTERY

Pure-Tone Audiometry

Pure-tone audiometry is the most common measurement of hearing sensitivity. Stimuli are pure tones (sinusoids) at octave frequencies typically from 250 Hz up to 8,000 Hz and, often, two interoctave frequencies (3,000 Hz and 6,000 Hz). Interoctave hearing loss is a characteristic of commonly encountered problems, such as noise-induced cochlear dysfunction. High-frequency audiometry for stimulus frequencies greater than 8,000 Hz (up to 20,000 Hz) is technically feasible and clinically useful to certain populations, such as patients at risk for ototoxicity. Test results in many clinics are graphed on an audiogram. Two versions of audiograms are illustrated in Figure 142.1. All audiograms include at the minimum a graph for plotting hearing threshold levels as a function of the frequency of pure-tone signals, although the exact format and symbols vary.

The unit of stimulus intensity is the decibel (dB), a logarithmic unit. The intensity of any sound is defined by the ratio of its sound pressure or sound intensity to a reference sound pressure or sound intensity. The reference sound pressure is the amount of pressure against the eardrum, caused by air molecules when a sound is present, that vibrates the eardrum and can just be detected by a normal human ear. Briefly, the relation for sound intensity is described as dB = $10 \log_{10}$ (sound intensity/reference intensity) or for sound pressure as dB = $20 \log_{10}$ (sound pressure/reference pressure). The reference sound pressure is defined as decibels sound pressure level (dBSPL) and is derived from one of two physical quantities: (a) 0.0002 dyne/cm^2 or (b) 20 micropascals root mean square (μPa) = 2×10^{-5} Pa.

Clinically, the intensity of sound is described in decibels hearing level (dB HL), a biologic reference level, rather than in sound pressure level. On an audiogram (Fig. 142.1), the decibel scale has as its reference 0 dB, which is described as audiometric 0. This is the standard for the intensity level that corresponds to the mean normal hearing threshold level, the minimal detectable intensity for each test frequency for young adults with normal hearing. Another common unit for expressing sound intensity is decibels

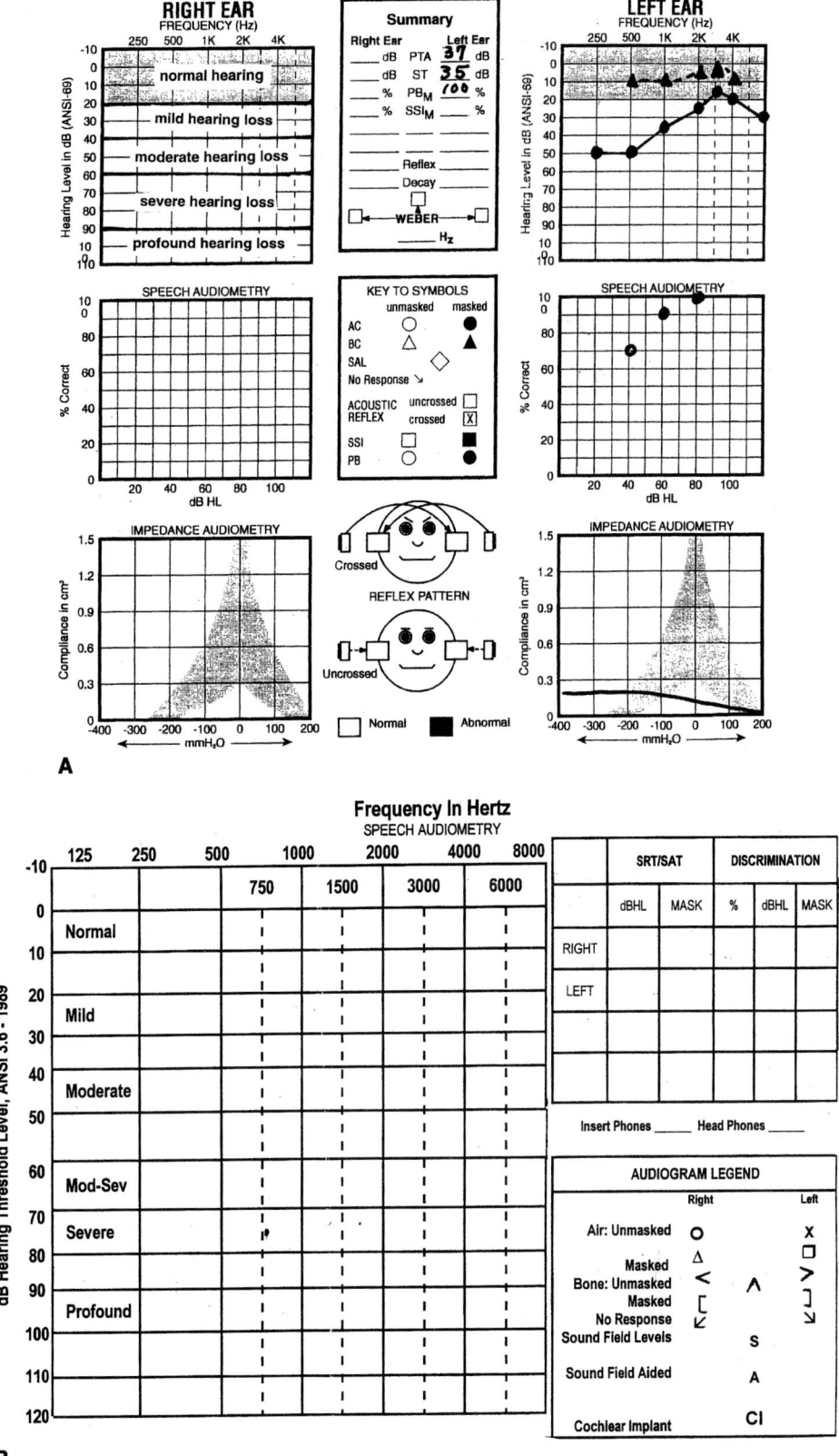

Figure 142.1 Two examples of audiographic forms. **A:** The separate ear form has sections for reporting results for pure-tone audiometry (**top**), speech audiometry (**center**), and aural immittance measurement (**bottom**). Masking is indicated by filled symbols. Categories of hearing loss of shown on the right ear graph, whereas typical findings for a conductive hearing loss are shown in the left ear graph. **B:** The traditional audiogram form utilizes symbols (see audiogram legend) for each of 13 signal presentation types. It does not permit graphic display of immittance or speech measurement findings.

sensation level (dB SL), which is intensity of the stimulus in decibels above an individual's hearing threshold. For example, a word recognition test can be administered at an intensity level of 40 dB SL (40 dB above the person's pure-tone average [PTA]).

In audiologic assessment of cooperative children and adults, hearing thresholds for tonal or speech signals are measured separately for each ear with earphones (air-conduction stimulation). Insert earphones (ER-3A) are now the transducer of choice for routine audiologic assessment. They offer distinct advantages over traditional supraaural earphones, including increased comfort, reduced likelihood of ear canal collapse, greater interaural attenuation, and greater acceptance by young children. In addition, insert earphones contribute importantly to the control of infection in a clinical setting, as the insert portion is disposable. Pure-tone audiometry can be performed with stimuli presented with a bone-conduction oscillator or vibrator placed on the mastoid bone. During pure-tone audiometry, all equipment must meet the specifications of the American National Standards Institute (ANSI). Periodic equipment calibration and validation are necessary. Testing is conducted according to clinical adaptations of psychoacoustic methods (1). Patients are instructed to listen carefully for the tones and to respond, usually by pushing a button that activates a response light on the audiometer or by raising a hand, every time they believe they hear a tone. To minimize interference by ambient background acoustic noise, pure-tone audiometry always is performed with the patient in a double-walled, sound-treated room that meets ANSI specifications.

The clinically normal region on an audiogram is 0 to 20 dB HL, although for children hearing threshold levels exceeding 15 dB should be considered abnormal. Thresholds in the 20 to 40 dB HL region constitute mild hearing loss, 40 to 60 dB HL thresholds define moderate loss, and threshold levels greater than 60 dB HL are considered severe hearing loss (2). As a reference, the intensity level of whispered speech close to the ear is less than 25 dB HL. Conversational speech is in the 40 to 50 dB HL region, and a shouted voice within 1 foot (30 cm) of the ear is at a level of about 80 dB HL. The most important frequencies for understanding speech are 500 through 4,000 Hz, although higher frequencies can contribute to discrimination between certain speech sounds. Hearing sensitivity within the speech frequency region often is summarized by means of calculation of the PTA (PTA; hearing thresholds for 500, 1,000, and 2,000 Hz divided by three and reported in decibels). A four-frequency PTA including 3,000 Hz is required by the American Academy of Otolaryngology–Head and Neck Surgery.

Audiometric results are valid only when the patient's responses are caused by stimulation of the test ear. If a sound greater than 40 dB HL is presented to one ear through air conduction with supraaural earphones and cushions (resting on the outer ear), the acoustic energy can cross over from one side of the head to the other and stimulate the ear not being tested. The main mechanism of crossover is presumed to be bone-conduction stimulation caused by vibration of the earphone cushion against the skull at high stimulus intensity levels. The amount of sound intensity needed before crossover occurs is a reflection of interaural attenuation, that is, the sound insulation between the two ears provided by the head. Interaural attenuation is usually about 50 dB for lower test frequencies and 60 dB for higher test frequencies, such as those contributing to the ABR. Interaural attenuation is considerably higher for insert earphones (2). With bone-conduction stimulation, interaural attenuation is less than 10 dB. In clinical circumstances, the examiner needs to assume conservatively that interaural attenuation for bone-conducted signals is 0 dB. In other words, even a very faint sound presented to the mastoid bone of one ear by a bone-conduction vibrator can be transmitted through the skull to either or both inner ears. Perception of this bone-conducted signal depends on the patient's sensorineural hearing sensitivity in each ear.

Masking is the audiometric technique used to eliminate participation of the ear not being tested whenever air- and bone-conduction stimulation exceeds interaural attenuation. An appropriate noise (narrow-band noise for pure-tone signals and speech noise for speech signals) is presented to the ear not being tested when the stimulus is presented to the test ear. With adequate masking, any signal crossing over to the ear not being tested is masked by the noise. The level of masking noise presented to the ear not being tested must exceed the threshold of hearing for that ear. Excess levels of masking noise must be avoided because the noise can cross back over to the ear being tested. Selection of appropriate masking can be difficult, especially when there is bilateral hearing loss (2). Indeed, patients with severe bilateral conductive hearing loss may present the "masking dilemma," that is, when enough masking to the nontest ear actually crosses over to the test ear and interferes with accurate estimation of hearing threshold. An otolaryngologist interpreting audiologic results must verify that appropriate masking was used if testing was not performed by an audiologist.

Knowledge of the type of hearing loss, determined by means of comparison of the hearing thresholds for air- and bone-conduction signals, is useful in classifying a hearing loss as sensorineural (no air–bone gap), conductive (normal bone conduction and a loss by air conduction), or mixed (loss by bone conduction with a superimposed air–bone conduction gap).

Configuration refers to hearing loss as a function of the test frequency. With a sloping configuration, hearing is better for low frequencies and then becomes poorer for higher frequencies. The most common pattern associated with sensorineural hearing loss is a deficit in thresholds for higher test frequencies. The configuration can be gently sloping from low to high frequencies, be precipitously decreasing above a high frequency cutoff, such as 2,000 Hz, or be characterized by a notching deficit within a certain frequency region, such as 4,000 Hz. A rising configuration is typified by relatively poor hearing for low-frequency stimuli and better hearing for the high frequencies. A rising configuration can be caused by varied types of middle ear abnormalities. An exception to the typical association of conductive hearing loss with rising configuration is Ménière disease (see Chapter 156). Ménière disease is one cochlear abnormality that may produce a rising configuration. A flat audiometric configuration often is recorded from patients with mixed hearing loss, that is, both sensorineural and conductive components are present. Other configurations, such as the midfrequency "cookie bite" pattern, are encountered in clinical practice. Test–retest variability in clinical pure-tone threshold estimation is typically ±5 dB.

Guidelines for Evaluation of Hearing Handicap

The results of pure-tone audiometry are adequately summarized in an audiogram and with the terms just defined, such as PTA and the degree, configuration, and type of hearing loss. It also is possible to quantify hearing loss in percentage units according to published and accepted guidelines (3). This approach sometimes is necessary in medicolegal cases or when a patient seeks compensation for hearing loss. According to the guidelines of the American Academy of Otolaryngology Committee on Hearing and Equilibrium and the American Council of Otolaryngology Committee on the Medical Aspects of Noise (3), permanent hearing impairment is defined as follows: "A change for the worse in either structure or function, outside the range of normal, is permanent impairment…. Permanent impairment is due to any anatomic or functional abnormality that produces hearing loss." This is differentiated from permanent hearing handicap, which is defined as follows: "The disadvantage imposed by an impairment sufficient to affect a person's efficiency in the activities of daily living is a permanent handicap" (3). The guidelines also detail the approach for converting hearing handicap for one or both ears into a percentage. The first step is to determine the degree of sensorineural hearing loss for four test frequencies (500, 1,000, 2,000, and 3,000 Hz) from the audiogram (Table 142.1). The next step is to follow the guidelines for computation of percentage hearing loss (3):

If the monaural percent figure is the same for both ears, that figure expresses the percent hearing handicap. If the percent monaural hearing impairments are not the same, apply the formula:

$$\left(5 \times \%\left[\text{better ear}\right]\right) + \left(1 \times \%\left[\text{poorer ear}\right]\right) / 6 = \%$$
hearing handicap

The interoctave test frequency—3,000 Hz—in the calculation of percentage of hearing handicap is very important. It is

TABLE 142.1	GUIDELINES FOR CALCULATING PERCENTAGE OF MONAURAL HEARING IMPAIRMENT[a]		
DSHL[b]	Percentage	DSHL	Percentage
100	0.0	240	52.5
105	1.9	245	54.4
110	3.8	250	56.2
115	5.6	255	58.1
120	7.5	260	60.0
125	9.4	265	61.9
130	11.2	270	63.8
135	13.1	275	65.6
140	15.0	280	67.5
145	16.9	285	69.3
150	18.8	290	71.2
155	20.6	295	73.1
160	22.5	300	75.0
165	24.4	305	76.9
170	26.2	310	78.8
175	28.1	315	80.6
180	30.0	320	82.5
185	31.9	325	84.4
190	33.8	330	86.2
195	35.6	335	88.1
200	37.5	340	90.0
205	39.4	345	93.8
210	41.2	350	93.8
215	43.1	355	95.6
220	45.0	360	97.5
225	46.9	365	99.4
230	48.9	370	100.0
235	50.6		(or greater)

[a]American Academy of Otolaryngology Committee on Hearing and Equilibrium and the American Council of Otolaryngology Committee on the Medical Aspects of Noise.
[b]From the audiogram, find the decibel sum of the hearing threshold levels (DSHL) of 500, 1,000, 2,000, and 3,000 Hz.

good clinical practice to routinely obtain hearing thresholds from each ear for the 3,000 Hz frequency. This frequency is included in the formula for hearing loss (3) because much of the spectral information vital for speech understanding is within the 2,000 to 3,000 Hz region. Percentage of binaural hearing handicap is easily calculated with a detailed tabular matrix that relates the four-frequency degree of sensorineural hearing loss for the better versus poorer ear (4).

Speech Audiometry

The purpose of speech audiometry is to determine how well a person hears and understands speech signals. Speech audiometry procedures usually are performed to measure hearing sensitivity (thresholds in decibels) for words or to estimate word recognition, such as speech discrimination, ability. Spondee reception threshold, also called speech threshold, is the softest intensity level at which a patient can correctly repeat words approximately 50% of the time. Spondee words, two syllable words with equal stress on each syllable, such as hot dog, baseball, and eardrum, are presented to the patient monaurally through earphones. The technique is comparable with the method for determining pure-tone thresholds described earlier.

Because PTA reflects hearing threshold levels in the speech frequency region and speech threshold is measured with a speech signal, one can expect close agreement between the PTA and the speech threshold. If the difference between PTA and speech threshold exceeds ±7 dB, there is reason to suspect that one or both of the measures are invalid. An unusually good speech threshold relative to PTA, such as speech threshold of 5 dB and PTA of 45 dB, immediately alerts the examiner to the possibility of nonorganic hearing loss, such as malingering. With cooperative adult patients, particularly if pure-tone hearing thresholds are within the normal region from 500 to 4,000 Hz, there is probably little or no clinical benefit in measuring speech thresholds. Test time can be saved with no loss of diagnostic information by excluding speech threshold measurement from the test battery for such patients.

Speech recognition for phonetically balanced words is a common clinical approach for estimating a person's ability to hear and understand speech (2). A list of 25 or 50 single-syllable words typically are presented to the patient through earphones at one or more fixed intensity levels. The percentage of words correctly repeated by the patient is calculated by the examiner. One ear is tested at a time. Within the list of words, specific speech sounds (phonemes) occur approximately as often as they would in everyday conversation, that is, they are phonetically balanced. These words traditionally were spoken into a microphone by the examiner while the level was monitored with a volume unit meter. The words were routed to the patient through an audiometer after selection of the test ear and desired intensity level. This is an outdated and poor clinical practice because it lacks standardization and consistency and increases the variability of test outcome. For adult patients, it almost always is possible and always is preferable to use professionally produced, commercially available speech materials presented with a tape recorder or compact disk player and an audiometer (2). Live voice probably continues to be used by many practitioners, especially in the assessment of children, because of minor efficiency gains.

Speech perception in the presence of noise is also assessed clinically. One of the most popular and well-researched procedures is the hearing in noise test, abbreviated HINT (5). Representative sentences of a standard length and phonetic complexity are presented with a low level of background noise, which is more reflective of speech understanding in real-world environments. HINT is a key measure of auditory performance used to screen hearing impaired individuals for cochlear implant candidates. The HINT is now available in over a dozen languages.

Acoustic (Aural) Immittance (Impedance) Measurement

Introduction

Aural immittance (impedance) measurement is an important part of the basic audiometric test battery. Immittance is a term derived from the terms for two related techniques for assessing middle ear function—impedance and admittance. These techniques have been used clinically since 1970 (6). The external ear canal is sealed with a soft rubber probe tip. The probe tip is connected to a device that produces a tone delivered toward the eardrum. Middle ear impedance or admittance is calculated from the intensity and other physical properties, such as phase, of the tone in the ear canal. A middle ear (tympanic membrane and ossicular system) with low impedance (higher admittance) more readily accepts the acoustic energy of the probe tone. A middle ear with abnormally high impedance (lower admittance) caused by, for example, fluid in the middle ear space tends to reject energy flow. Thus impedance (admittance) characteristics of the middle ear system can be inferred objectively with this technique and related to well-known patterns of findings for various pathologic conditions of the middle ear.

Tympanometry

Tympanometry is the dynamic recording of middle ear impedance as air pressure in the ear canal is systematically increased or decreased. The technique is a sensitive measure of the integrity of the tympanic membrane and of middle ear function (Fig. 142.2). Compliance (the reciprocal of stiffness) of the middle ear, the dominant component of immittance, is the vertical dimension of a tympanogram. Tympanometry is popular clinically because it requires little technical skill and only several seconds to perform. It is an electrophysiologic, as opposed to behavioral, method that does not depend on cooperation of the patient, and it is a highly sensitive index of middle ear function. Tympanometric patterns, in combination with audiographic patterns, allow differentiation and classification of middle ear disorders.

The most clinically widespread approach to describing tympanograms was described first by Jerger in 1970 (6). There are three general types of tympanogram—A, B, and C. A normal, or type A, tympanogram has a distinct peak in compliance within 0 to 100 mm water (dPa) in the ear canal (Fig. 142.2). To be classified as normal, the location of the compliance peak on the pressure dimension and the height of the peak must be within normal range, indicated in Figure 142.2 by the stippled area. On a type B tympanogram, there is no peak in compliance, but there is a flat pattern with little or even no apparent change in compliance as a function of pressure in the ear canal. This pattern is most often associated with the presence of fluid within the middle ear space (otitis media), although other middle ear disorders also can produce a type B tympanogram. Although a type B tympanogram can appear to be recorded from

TYMPANOMETRY

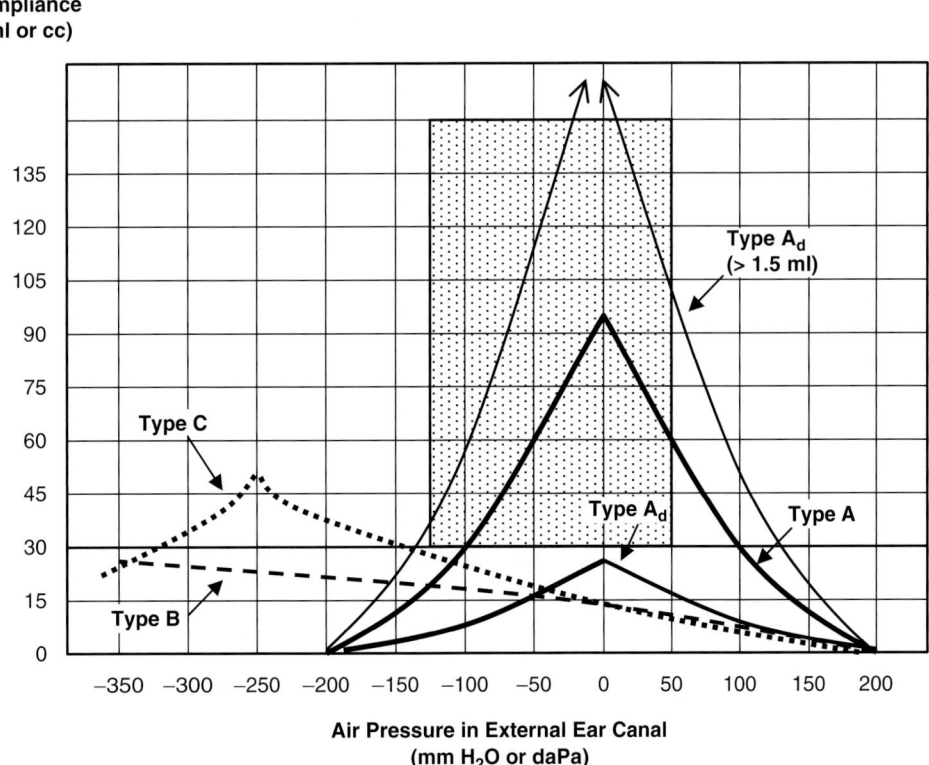

Figure 142.2 Classification system for tympanograms.

ears with perforated tympanic membranes, technically, this finding is invalid because the change in ear canal pressure needed for tympanometry is not achieved owing to the perforation. Type C tympanograms have a distinct peak in compliance as do type A recordings, but the peak is within the negative pressure region beyond approximately 100 mm water (dPa). This pattern usually occurs among patients with eustachian-tube dysfunction and inadequate ventilation of the middle ear space. It often precedes acquisition of a type B tympanogram in the development of otitis media.

A variation of a type A tympanogram is type A_s (Fig. 142. 2). The s stands for shallow. Peak compliance is less than the lower normal limit of compliance. That is, middle ear impedance is abnormally high. The type A_s pattern is common among patients with fixation of the ossicular chain, including some patients with the diagnosis of otosclerosis. In contrast, with an usually steep and high-compliance tympanogram (type A_d for deep), the peak can exceed the upper compliance limits of the equipment. A type A_d tympanogram occurs among patients with disruption of the ossicular chain, which leaves the middle ear extremely mobile and overly compliant, that is, there is little impedance. In the absence of serious hearing loss, this tympanographic pattern usually is associated with minor tympanic membrane abnormality, such as atrophy. At the beginning of a tympanometric examination, high positive or negative pressure is introduced into the ear canal. This essentially decouples the

middle ear system from the measurement. If the impedance device records an abnormally large equivalent volume of air (2 cm or more in an adult, or twice the volume recorded for the other ear) between the probe tip and presumably the eardrum at this stage in the procedure, the integrity of the eardrum is questioned. That is, the immittance device is recording not only ear canal volume but also volume of the middle ear space. This test finding is consistent with perforation of the tympanic membrane or the presence of an open (patent) middle ear ventilation tube.

Acoustic Stapedial Reflex Measurement

The stapedial muscle within the middle ear is the smallest muscle in the body. Measurement of contractions of the stapedial muscle in response to high sound intensity levels (usually 80 dB or greater) is the basis of the acoustic reflex. Acoustic reflex measurement is clinically useful for estimating hearing sensitivity and for differentiating sites of auditory disorders, including the middle ear, inner ear, eighth cranial nerve, and auditory brainstem (2,6). The afferent portion of the acoustic reflex arc is the eighth cranial nerve. Complex brainstem pathways lead from the cochlear nucleus on the stimulated side to the region of the motor nucleus of the seventh cranial (facial) nerve on both sides (ipsilateral and contralateral to the stimulus) of the brainstem. The efferent portion of the arc is the seventh cranial nerve, which innervates the stapedius muscle. The muscle contracts, causing increased stiffness (decreased compliance) of the middle ear system. The small change in compliance that follows stapedius muscle contraction within 10 ms is detected with the probe and immittance device, much as compliance changes are detected during tympanometry.

Acoustic reflex measurement is useful clinically because it quickly provides objective information on the status of the auditory system from middle ear to brainstem. Distinctive acoustic reflex patterns for ipsilateral and contralateral stimulation and measurement conditions characterize middle ear, cochlear, eighth nerve, brainstem, and even facial nerve dysfunction (lower portion of Fig. 142.1A). Comparison of acoustic reflex threshold levels—the lowest stimulus intensity level that activates the reflex—for tonal versus noise signals allows estimation of the degree of cochlear hearing loss (2). This technique is especially valuable in the care of children and difficult-to-test patients. Note, however, that even modest changes in the middle ear mechanism, often manifest by mild conductive hearing loss (e.g., otosclerosis), may lead to the loss of acoustic reflex responses. Conversely, the presence of intact reflexes in combination with a significant conductive hearing loss should be viewed as inconsistent with true pathology of the middle ear sound conduction mechanism. This could result from spurious test results or from inner ear pathology, such as canal dehiscence.

AUDITORY EVOKED RESPONSES

Auditory Brainstem Response

Auditory evoked responses are electrophysiologic recordings of responses to sounds. With proper test protocols, the responses can be recorded clinically from activation of all levels of the auditory system, from cochlea to cortex (7). Among these responses, the ABR, which neurologists often call the brainstem auditory evoked response, is used most often clinically. An ABR recording is shown schematically in Figure. 142.3. The ABR is generated with transient acoustic stimuli (clicks or tone bursts) and detected with surface electrodes (disks) placed on the forehead and near the ears (earlobe or within the external ear canal). The ABR represents minimal electrophysiologic activity (less than 1 microvolt) within electroencephalographic activity that is 100 times larger in amplitude. With a commercially available computer-based device, it is possible to present rapidly (20 to 30 per second) thousands of sound stimuli and, by means of signal averaging, to detect reliable ABR waveforms in a matter of minutes.

Extensive research has shown that the ABR wave components arise from the eighth cranial nerve and auditory regions in the caudal and rostral brainstem (Fig. 142.3). Wave I unquestionably represents the synchronously stimulated compound action potentials (APs) from the distal

(cochlear) end of the eighth cranial nerve. Wave II may arise from the eighth nerve but near the brainstem (the proximal end). Waves I and II are generated by structures ipsilateral to the stimulated ear. All later ABR waves have multiple generators within the auditory brainstem. Wave III, which usually is prominent, is generated within the caudal pons with likely contributions from the cochlear nuclei, trapezoid body, and superior olivary complex (7). The most prominent and rostral component of the ABR—wave V—is thought to arise in the region of the lateral lemniscus as it approaches the inferior colliculus, probably contralateral to the ear stimulated.

The ABR is not a test of hearing. It reflects synchronous firing of a subset of onset neurons within the auditory system. In ABR waveform analysis, the first objective is to assure that the response is reliably recorded. At the minimum, two replicated waveforms are averaged. If the response cannot be replicated, the test protocol is modified, and technical problems are considered and systematically ruled out. When the existence of a response that can be replicated is confirmed, reproducible absolute latencies for each wave component and relative (interwave) latencies between components are calculated in milliseconds. These latency data for each ear are assessed for symmetry (wave V within 0.4 ms between ears) and compared to appropriate normative data (7).

Common ABR waveform patterns are illustrated in Figure 142.4. A well-formed and clear wave I at a delayed latency value for the maximum stimulus intensity level is characteristic of conductive or mixed hearing loss. When wave I is small and poorly formed but interwave latency values are within normal limits (the wave I through V latency value less than 4.60 ms), high-frequency sensory (cochlear) hearing loss is suspected. Delayed interwave latency values are the signature of retrocochlear auditory dysfunction. Abnormal delays between the early wave components (I through III) are consistent with posterior fossa lesions that involve the eighth cranial nerve or lower brainstem, whereas prolonged latency of waves III through V suggests intraaxial auditory brainstem dysfunction.

A primary goal in any neurodiagnostic evaluation of ABR is to record a clear and reliable wave I component. Wave I is the benchmark for peripheral auditory function. Subsequent interwave latencies offer indices of retrocochlear (eighth cranial nerve and brainstem) function that are relatively unaffected by conductive or sensory hearing loss. The likelihood that wave I is recorded is enhanced through use of ear canal or tympanic membrane electrode designs and through alterations in the test protocol, such as a slower stimulus rate, rarefaction stimulus polarity, and maximum stimulus intensity level (7).

Reports on ABR dating back to the late 1970s have confirmed that waveforms evoked by high-intensity signals yield neurodiagnostic information about cochlear and retrocochlear auditory function. The data can be used in the identification of retrocochlear disorders, such as acoustic

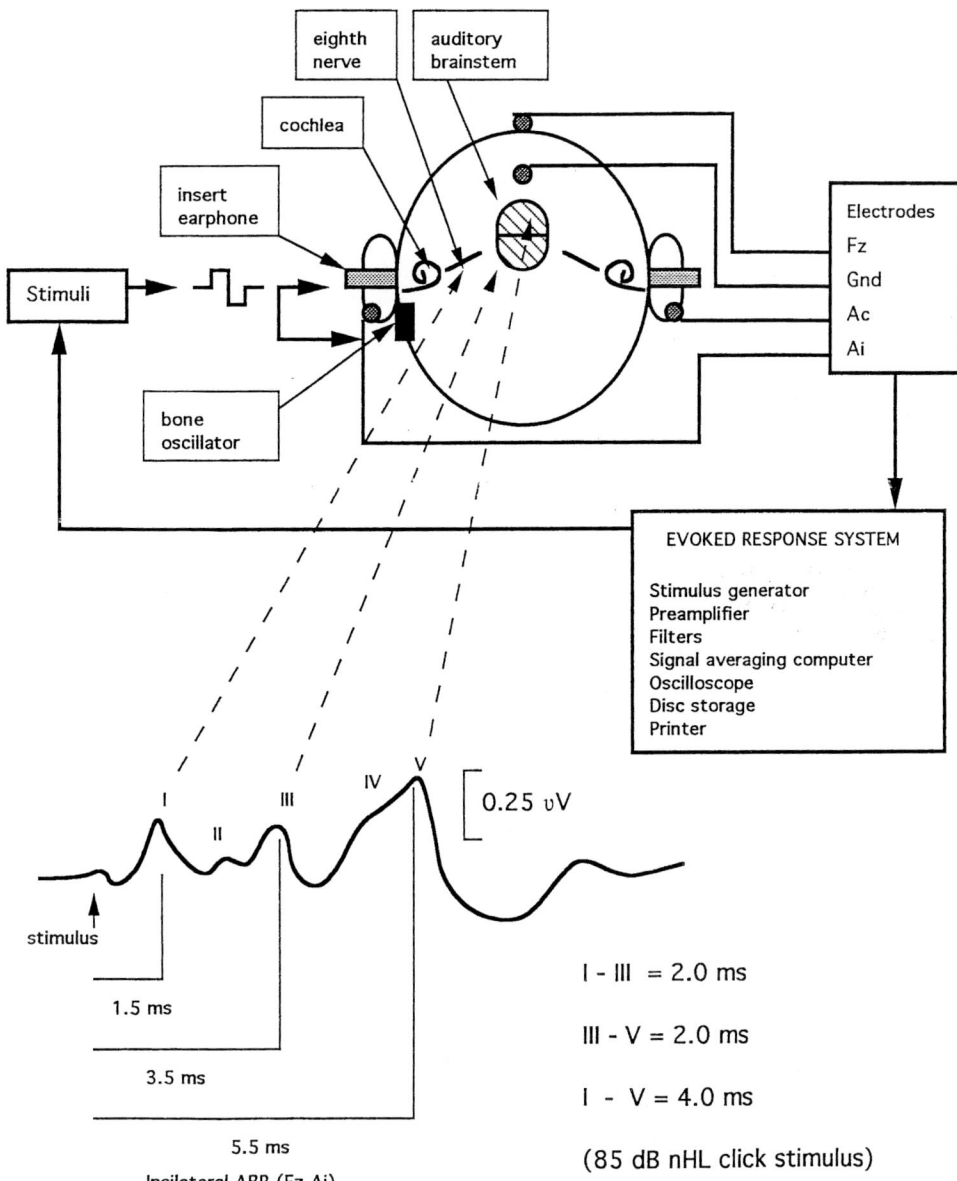

Figure 142.3 Schematic shows the instrumentation for recording the ABR and important relations between auditory anatomic features and waveform components. A simple strategy for analysis of ABR waveform in neurodiagnosis also is shown.

neuroma, with an accuracy that exceeds 95%, at least for medium to large tumors. With the development of sophisticated neuroradiologic techniques, such as magnetic resonance imaging (MRI) with enhancement, and earlier diagnosis of smaller tumors, the sensitivity of ABR has dropped (8). Inexpensive fast spin echo MRI is technically feasible and available clinically, making ABR less commonly used as a screen for retrocochlear tumors.

False-negative ABR outcomes can occur in patients at risk of retrocochlear auditory dysfunction, particularly in individuals with intracanicular vestibular schwannomas (9). The poor results are evidence of the relatively poorer sensitivity of ABR than that of MRI to mass lesions. However, false-positive outcomes of MRI also have been reported among patients with normal ABR results and no surgical evidence

of tumor (10). It must be kept in mind that ABR is a measure of function, whereas computed tomography and conventional MRI are measures of structure (see Chapter 147). Assessment of ABR continues to be a readily available, relatively inexpensive, and reasonably sensitive procedure for initial diagnostic evaluation of eighth-nerve and auditory brainstem status in the care of patients with retrocochlear signs and symptoms. ABR is particularly useful in patients for whom concerns are limited to larger tumors, the elderly, the medically infirm, and individuals who have contraindications to MRI (e.g., a pacemaker). As described in Chapter 131, assessment of ABR can also be valuable in electrophysiologic monitoring of the eighth cranial nerve and auditory brainstem function during neurotologic operations such as vestibular nerve section and posterior fossa tumor removal.

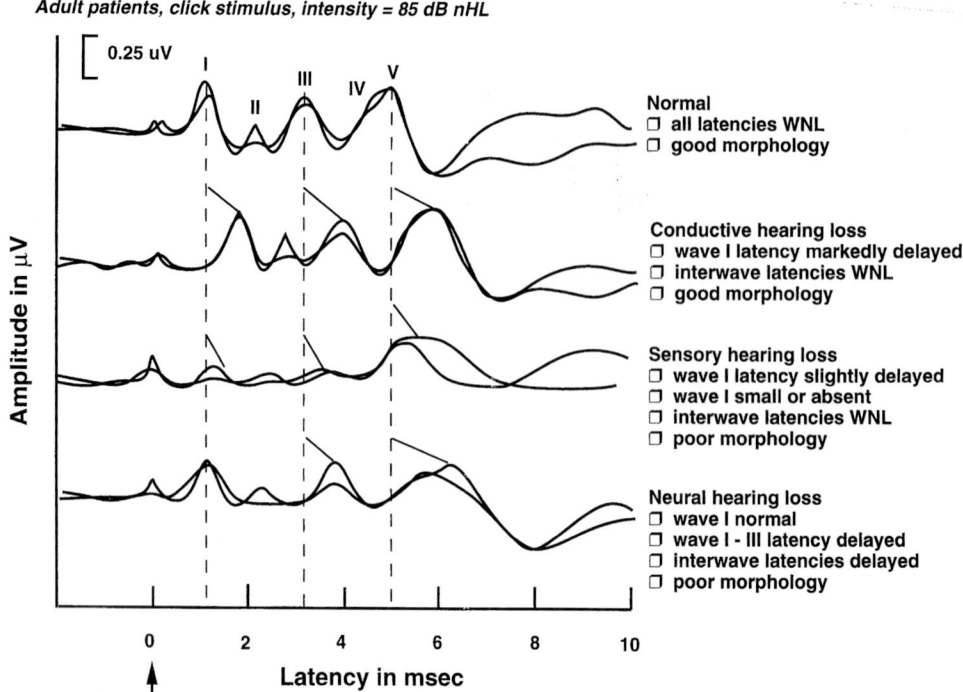

Figure 142.4 ABR patterns associated with various types of auditory dysfunction. Information about dysfunction can be inferred from the latency of specific waves and overall structure of the waveforms.

The application of ABR in the estimation of hearing sensitivity in infants and young children is now essential (7). Accurate and early hearing aid fitting is, of course, critical for infants with serious hearing loss. With the emergence of universal newborn hearing screening, children at risk for hearing loss can be routinely identified at birth. Research on the benefits of early intervention for hearing loss in infants (11) argues strongly for the diagnosis of hearing loss and the beginning of hearing aid use before a child is 6 months old. Appropriate hearing aid fitting, however, requires information on hearing sensitivity at specific frequencies within the range of hearing that is critical for understanding speech. Unfortunately, it is not possible to obtain behavioral estimates of hearing sensitivity (an audiogram) at such a young age. By performing ABR recordings with frequency-specific signals (tone bursts), hearing thresholds can be estimated electrophysiologically and infant hearing aid fitting can be accomplished within months after birth. Electrophysiologic estimation of hearing sensitivity with ABR does have one serious clinical constraint. The maximum intensity level is only about 80 dB for very brief (transient) click and tone burst signals used to elicit the ABR. Therefore, the ABR cannot be used to estimate hearing sensitivity in the severe to profound range of impairment. As with any test, false positives may occur. A small percentage of children with relatively normal hearing may have abnormal or absent ABR waveforms. ABR testing should be corroborated with other tests of auditory function, including behavioral responses.

A relatively recent clinical electrophysiologic measure, the ASSR, has proven useful for these infants (7). The ASSR is elicited with pure-tone signals (steady state signals), rather than transient signals (clicks or tone bursts). The pure tone signals are altered with rapid modulation of the amplitude and, sometimes, frequency. The pure tone signal activates the cochlea at the specific frequencies (e.g., 1,000 or 500 Hz) and provides the type of information on hearing that is available with the audiogram. In addition, energy at the modulation rate (e.g., 80 per second) is generated in the auditory system and can be detected automatically with sophisticated algorithms for signal detection. The major clinical advantage of ASSR is the ability to estimate hearing sensitivity at discrete frequencies for children with hearing loss exceeding 80 dB HL. Thus, the ABR and ASSR can be used in combination to define any degree of hearing loss in children at any age, including infants soon after birth. Analysis of ASSR findings can be particularly helpful in the earlier and more confident identification of infants who are likely candidates for cochlear implantation.

Electrocochleography

For more than 30 years, ECochG has been used to assess peripheral auditory function. The examination is performed most often for intraoperative monitoring of cochlear and eighth-nerve status and in the diagnosis of Ménière disease (7). Optimal ECochG waveforms are recorded with a small needle electrode placed through the tympanic membrane and on the promontory, although electrode placement on the tympanic membrane or, to a lesser extent, in the ear canal can be clinically useful. Stimulus and acquisition criteria for ECochG have been well defined for decades. The three major components of the ECochG are the cochlear microphonic,

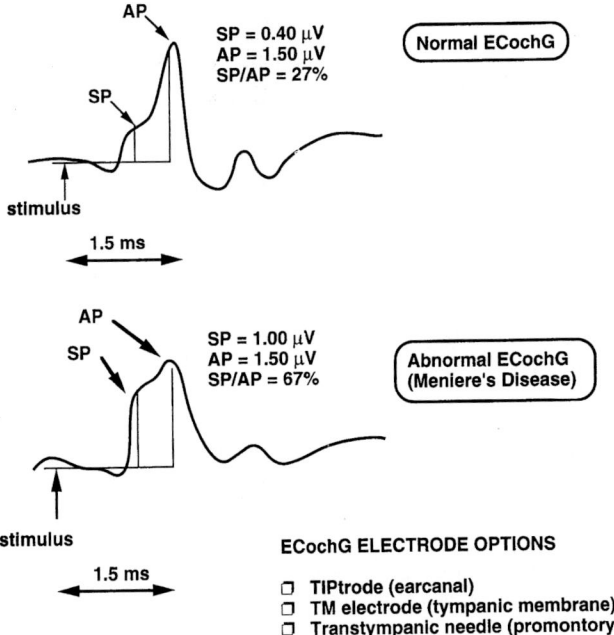

SP = 0.40 μV
AP = 1.50 μV
SP/AP = 27%

Normal ECochG

SP = 1.00 μV
AP = 1.50 μV
SP/AP = 67%

Abnormal ECochG
(Meniere's Disease)

ECochG ELECTRODE OPTIONS

- TIPtrode (earcanal)
- TM electrode (tympanic membrane)
- Transtympanic needle (promontory)

Figure 142.5 ECochG waveforms show normal relation of SP and AP and abnormally enlarged SP/AP relation for a patient with Ménière disease. Absolute and relative amplitude values for the SP and AP components and the criteria for definition of a normal response vary greatly for different electrode sites (ear canal vs. tympanic membrane vs. promontory).

summating potential (SP), and AP. The cochlear microphonic (CM) and SP reflect cochlear bioelectric activity. The AP is generated by synchronous firing of distal afferent eighth-nerve fibers and is equivalent to ABR wave I (Fig. 142.5).

The typical ECochG analysis technique in neurotology requires determination of the amplitude of the SP and the AP from a common baseline. The ratio of the SP to the AP (SP/AP) is calculated and reported as a percentage. Normal ranges and cutoffs for SP/AP ratio have been reported for each electrode type. Abnormal SP/AP ratio values are defined as more than 50% for the ear canal electrode type, more than 40% for a tympanic membrane electrode, and more than 30% for a transtympanic needle electrode (7).

Among patients with Ménière disease, the characteristic ECochG finding is abnormal enlargement of the relation between the component amplitudes of the SP and the AP. With the tympanic membrane electrode technique, the sensitivity of ECochG in the diagnosis of endolymphatic hydrops is 57%; the specificity was 94% in a series of 100 patients (12). Only 3 of 30 patients had false-positive results. Thus an abnormally enlarged SP/AP ratio is highly suggestive of endolymphatic hydrops, according to these data. In the study (10), the likelihood of an abnormal ECochG SP/AP ratio was statistically higher as hearing loss increased and when hearing loss fluctuated. Similar elevations in the SP/AP ratio have, however, been reported in perilymph fistula (13–15), autoimmune inner ear disease (16,17), and superior semicircular canal dehiscence (18).

ECochG also plays a critical role in the accurate diagnosis of auditory neuropathy spectrum disorder, or ANSD (7).

This complex assortment of auditory disorders is characterized by the absence of an ABR despite integrity of the outer hair cells (as determined by ECochG and/or OAEs). Sites of dysfunction in ANSD include the inner hair cells, the synapse between the inner hair cells and afferent auditory nerve fibers, or auditory nerve fibers (e.g., spiral ganglion). Close analysis of the pattern of ECochG findings, specifically the presence or absence of the cochlear microphonic CM, SP, and AP, permits differentiation between presynaptic dysfunction (affecting inner hair cells) and postsynaptic dysfunction (affecting auditory nerve fibers). In combination with MRI studies of the auditory nerve, ECochG provides diagnostic information important in making decisions about management of ANSD. ECochG outcome is particularly useful in determining whether cochlear implantation is an appropriate treatment option (7).

Cortical Auditory Evoked Responses

More than a dozen subtypes of auditory evoked responses can be recorded beyond the brainstem, from auditory regions of the thalamus, hippocampus, internal capsule, and cortex. Prominent among them in clinical audiology are the auditory middle latency response (AMLR), the auditory late response (ALR), and the P300 response (7). Cortical auditory evoked responses were reported as early as the 1930s. In fact, all of the above-noted responses were well described before the ABR was discovered.

Cortical auditory evoked responses are characterized by longer latencies (100 to 300 ms) than ECochG waveforms and ABR because they arise from more rostral regions of the auditory central nervous system (CNS) and depend on multisynaptic pathways. Amplitudes of the cortical responses are considerably larger (2 to 20 times) than those of the earlier responses because they reflect activity evoked from a greater number of neurons. Measurements are distinctly different for the cortical versus cochlear or brainstem responses. For example, stimulus rate must be slower and physiologic filter settings lower. As a rule, stimulus intensities are moderate, rather than high. Cortical evoked responses are best elicited with longer-duration, and therefore frequency-specific, tonal stimuli, rather than the click stimuli optimal for ECochG and ABR. The analysis time must extend beyond the expected latency of the response (more than 300 ms) for cortical responses. Recording electrode sites also are different for cortical responses. There is more emphasis on scalp sites over the hemispheres and less concern about electrode sites near the ears.

The AMLR consists of a prominent positive voltage (labeled Pa) component in the 25 to 30 ms region. When recorded with electrodes located over the temporal–parietal region, the AMLR is generated by pathways leading to the primary cortex and from this region of the temporal lobe. The ALR occurs later in time, with major peaks (N1 and P2) appearing within the time frame of 100 to 200 ms. A variety of types of signals can be used to elicit the ALR, including speech (e.g., phonemes "da"and "ga.") The AMLR and

ALR are now undergoing considerable investigation for the electrophysiologic assessment of children and adults, and for the documentation of effectiveness of intervention (e.g., auditory training, hearing aids, and cochlear implants) for communication impairment (19).

The P300 response is recorded with what is typically called the oddball paradigm. Two types of stimuli are used. One—the frequent stimulus—is presented frequently in a predictable manner. The other—the rare or deviant stimulus—is presented infrequently and pseudorandomly. The rare stimuli account for less than 20% of the total stimuli presented. The patient is instructed to ignore the frequent stimuli and to attend to the rare stimuli. The waveform for the frequent stimulus is essentially an ALR consisting of a positive peak of 5 to 10 mV within the 150 to 200 ms region. In contrast, the waveform averaged from the attended rare stimuli is characterized normally by a large positive peak in the 300 ms region, hence the term P300 response. Presumed generators of the P300 response include regions of the medial temporal lobe (hippocampus) that are important in auditory attention.

OTOACOUSTIC EMISSIONS

OAEs are low-intensity sounds produced by the cochlea either spontaneously, or more commonly, in response to an acoustic stimulus. A moderate-intensity click or an appropriate combination of two tones can evoke outer hair cell movement or motility (2,20). Outer hair cell motility affects basilar membrane biomechanics; the result is a form of intracochlear energy amplification and cochlear tuning for precise frequency resolution. Outer hair cell motility generates mechanical energy within the cochlea that is propagated outward through the middle ear system and the tympanic membrane to the ear canal. Vibration of the tympanic membrane produces an acoustic signal (the OAE), which can be measured with a sensitive microphone.

There are two broad classes of OAE—spontaneous and evoked. Spontaneous otoacoustic emissions (SOAEs) occur among only approximately 60% of persons with normal hearing. They are measured in the external ear canal when there is no external sound stimulation. A marked sex effect has been confirmed for SOAE. Women have SOAE at twice the rate of men. Evoked OAEs, elicited by moderate levels (50 to 80 dBSPL) of acoustic stimulation in the external ear canal, are generally classified according to the characteristics of the stimuli used to elicit them or the characteristics of the cochlear events that generate them. Stimulus-frequency OAEs, which are technically difficult to record, are the least studied of the evoked OAE.

Distortion-product otoacoustic emissions (DPOAEs) are produced when two pure-tone stimuli at frequencies f_1 and f_2 are presented to the ear simultaneously (Fig. 142.6). The most robust DPOAE occurs at the frequency determined by the equation $2f_1 - f_2$, whereas the actual cochlear frequency region assessed with DPOAE is between these two

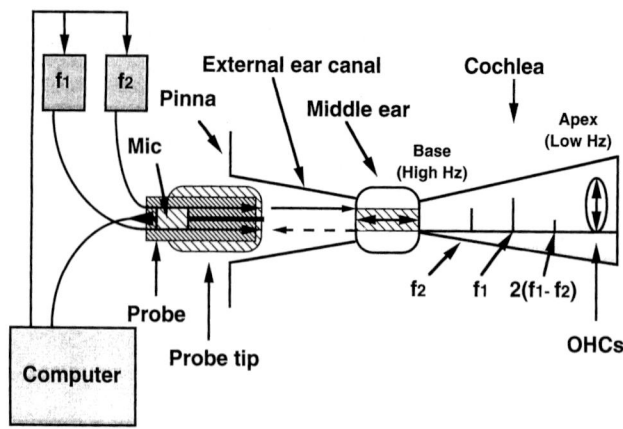

Figure 142.6 Equipment and procedure for measurement of distortion product otoacoustic emissions (DPOAEs). The two stimulus frequencies (f_1, f_2) are presented to the ear with a soft probe (*inward-pointing arrows*). The DPOAEs (at the frequency $2f_1-f_2$) produced by the outer hair cells are propagated outward through the middle ear to the external ear canal. Amplitude of DPOAE in dBSPL is plotted as a function of the frequency of the stimuli (the f_2 stimulus).

frequencies, and probably close to the f_2 stimulus for recommended test protocols (2,12). With all instruments commercially available for recording DPOAE, amplitude detected in the ear canal and described in dBSPL is plotted as a function of the frequencies of the stimuli in a DPOAEgram. Transiently evoked otoacoustic emissions (TEOAEs) are elicited with brief acoustic stimuli such as clicks or tonebursts. Although there are distinct differences in the methods for recording DPOAE and TEOAE, and the exact cochlear mechanisms responsible for generation are different, each type of evoked OAE is being incorporated into routine auditory assessment of children and adults (2,20).

When outer hair cells are structurally damaged or at least nonfunctional, OAEs cannot be evoked with acoustic stimuli. Among patients with mild cochlear dysfunction, OAEs can be recorded but amplitudes are below normal limits for some or all stimulus frequencies. Some patients with abnormal OAEs that indicate cochlear dysfunction have normal pure-tone audiograms, and OAEs provide information about auditory function at far more frequencies (up to 20 per octave) than does an audiogram. An example of these advantages is a patient with tinnitus but normal audiologic findings (20). Abnormal OAEs are expected in the frequency region represented by the tinnitus. Up to 30% of a population of outer hair cells can be damaged without substantially affecting a simple audiogram (21). In such cases, abnormal OAE findings are invariably recorded. Conversely, OAEs may be recorded in individuals with severely impaired auditory function, either as a result of mass lesion on the auditory nerve (22) or auditory neuropathy (23). OAEs are generally not detected in patients with middle ear pathology. However, OAEs can also be recorded in patients with tympanostomy tubes. Normal OAEs in such cases confirm that the tube is

TABLE 142.2	CLINICAL APPLICATIONS OF OAEs

Children

Newborn hearing screening
- Diagnostic pediatric audiology
- Monitoring ototoxicity
- Assessment of APDs
- Assessment of suspected functional (nonorganic) hearing loss

Adults

Early detection of noise-induced cochlear dysfunction
- Monitoring of cochlear status in potential ototoxicity
- Differentiation of cochlear versus retrocochlear auditory dysfunction
- Assessment in suspected functional (nonorganic) hearing loss
- Confirmation of cochlear dysfunction in patients with tinnitus

From Hall JW III. *Handbook of Otoacoustic Emissions*. San Diego, CA: Singular Publishing Group, 2000, with permission.

patent and, in addition, that outer hair cells are intact. The noninvasive nature of OAE recording, coupled with accuracy and objectivity in assessing cochlear, especially outer hair cell, function suggests diverse potential clinical applications that range from auditory screening to sensorineural diagnosis (2,20). A listing of clinical applications and their rationale is provided in Table 142.2.

ASSESSMENT OF AUDITORY PROCESSING DISORDERS

Background

Myklebust (24) in 1954 wrote, "hearing is a receptive sense ... and essential for normal language behavior." ... "the diagnostician of auditory problems in children has traditionally emphasized peripheral damage. It is desirable that he also include considerations of central damage" (24). He also explained that "central deafness (central APD) is a deficiency in transmitting auditory impulses to the higher brain centers while receptive aphasia (language disorder) is a deficiency in the interpretation of these impulses after they have been delivered" (24). During this era, Bocca et al. (25) reported that surgically confirmed central auditory system abnormalities can be detected with sufficiently sensitive audiologic procedures.

These pioneering observations and studies have since been validated by many clinical investigations. There are now a variety of behavioral and electrophysiologic techniques for the assessment of peripheral and central auditory system function, including APDs involving the peripheral or central auditory system. The term APD is used to describe a deficit in the perception or complete analysis of auditory information due to central auditory nervous system dysfunction, usually at the level of the cerebral cortex (2,26). Central auditory processing takes place before language processing or comprehension. The results

of extensive auditory neuroscience research during the past 20 years, including findings for objective assessment of CNS function like auditory evoked responses and functional MRI, have provided compelling evidence of APDs. Taken together, the substantial peer-reviewed literature on APDs confirms that "we hear with our brain."

Risk Factors for Central Auditory Nervous System Dysfunction

The Joint Committee on Infant Hearing (27) has delineated a number of indicators associated with sensorineural and conductive hearing loss among neonates and infants. Some of these indicators, such as *in utero* infection, bacterial infection, asphyxia, hyperbilirubinemia, and head trauma, as well as other neurologic insults in infancy (intraventricular hemorrhage and hydrocephalus) can be associated with central as well as peripheral auditory nervous system dysfunction. An important indicator identified by the joint committee and of interest to primary care professionals is "parent/caregiver concern regarding hearing, speech, language, and/or developmental delay" (27). Additional indications for evaluation of children for APD are teachers' concerns about hearing, recurrent middle ear disease, language impairment, attention deficit disorder with or without hyperactivity, reading delay, and learning disabilities. Central auditory nervous system dysfunction can coexist with any of these disorders. Among adults, risk factors for central auditory nervous system dysfunction include, but are not limited to, advanced age and history or clinical evidence of stroke, head injury including traumatic brain injury, brain neoplasms, Alzheimer disease, and other disorders affecting the CNS (26). It is a good clinical policy always to consider the possibility of central auditory dysfunction when a patient describes hearing problems that do not conform with audiographic findings.

APD Test Battery

The central auditory system consists of auditory regions within brainstem and midbrain, the thalamus, and the cerebral cortex, specifically the Heschl gyrus on the superior gyrus of the temporal lobe. The auditory evoked responses described earlier are useful in the assessment of the central auditory nervous system (2,7). Assessment for APD typically is conducted with a battery of behavioral tests that have proven sensitivity to central auditory dysfunction. In most cases, peripheral auditory function is normal. The overall goal is to measure reliable performance for each ear on a series of speech audiometric procedures, including a dichotic word test, such as dichotic digits, a dichotic sentence test, a speech-in-competition test (e.g., HINT or synthetic sentence identification with ipsilateral competing message, abbreviated SSI-ICM), and reliable performance with binaural stimulation on one or more nonspeech measures, such as pitch pattern sequence and duration pattern tests. Auditory evoked responses are recorded if specifically requested by the referring practitioner or if there are any concerns about the reliability or interpretation of behavioral test performance. Findings of evaluations for APD are compared with age-corrected normative data. Minimal criteria for confirmation of APD are scores less than the age-corrected normal region (more than 2.5 standard deviation below the mean) for one or both ears for at least two different procedures performed on a child with normal results of peripheral auditory tests (26).

In constructing an APD test battery, it is wise to rely on procedures not apt to be influenced by linguistic, cognitive, or attention disorders. Interpretation of APD test results is most straightforward when deficits are unilateral. The findings confirm that the patient has understood the task and that the outcome is not caused by a linguistic, cognitive, or attention disorder. A pronounced unilateral abnormality, specifically a marked left ear deficit, is one of the most common patterns of APD test battery findings. Another rather definite APD test battery pattern is reduced performance apparent only on difficult portions of a test. This finding implies an auditory as opposed to linguistic, cognitive, or strictly attentional explanation for the child's poor performance. Other important features of a clinically feasible APD test battery are (a) resistance to the influence of even slight peripheral auditory dysfunction, (b) availability of adequate age-matched normative data, and (c) use of professionally produced test materials recorded on tape or a compact disk. Earlier concerns about the usefulness of APD assessment with rudimentary procedures lacking these criteria were justifiable. Now, however, there are clinically feasible and commercially available procedures for testing children and adults (2). In addition, there is recent evidence in children with APDs of auditory nervous system development and functional improvement following the completion of computer-based and conventional auditory training programs (19,26).

INDICATIONS FOR DIAGNOSTIC AUDIOLOGIC ASSESSMENT

Children

Hearing loss, regardless of causation, affects the speech and language development of infants and young children. Communication deficits can occur within the first 6 months of life. Hearing loss among preschool and school-age children interferes with educational development. Identification of hearing loss at birth and prompt and appropriate intervention before the age of 6 months are essential if a child is to reach his or her communicative and educational potential (11). Testing a child's hearing at regular intervals during the first 5 years of life is the responsibility of pediatricians and primary care physicians (27,28). Otolaryngologists and audiologists must coordinate efforts in properly and promptly assessing and managing hearing loss among children.

Adults

The first suspicion of hearing loss among adults occurs while a medical history is being obtained. The patient cites hearing loss as the chief symptom, or close questioning reveals that the patient has difficulty in hearing, especially difficulty in understanding speech. Sometimes, this problem is apparent or is most noticeable only under specific conditions, such as when the patient is speaking on the telephone or conversing in noisy environments or conversing with certain persons, such as children or women, whose voices tend to be fainter and higher pitched than those of men. The medical history can provide other information that suggests risk of hearing loss, such as exposure to damaging levels of recreational or work-related noise or administration of ototoxic medications. Specific symptoms, such as tinnitus or vertigo, or physical findings of otologic abnormalities or of other pathologic conditions associated with auditory system involvement, also indicate the need for audiologic assessment.

STAFF TRAINING AND AUTOMATED TESTING

In some countries, such as the United States, audiometry is typically performed by clinically licensed audiologist with a graduate degree (e.g., Doctor of Audiology) from an accredited academic institution. Audiometric technicians, commonly nurses or other members of an otolaryngologist's clinic staff, have been employed to maximize availability of testing coverage and to minimize cost. Although testing by such individuals may be excellent, handling difficult situations, such as masking and interaural attenuation, may prove problematic. Similarly, self-administered, computer-automated audiometers (e.g., Otogram, Tympany, Stafford, TX) have seen tremendous growth in popularity in recent years. Early studies have shown good reliability between conventional, audiologist-administered and self-administered, computer-automated audiometry, but clinical experience with these newer modalities is limited (29,30). Results obtained with less extensively trained technicians and with automated audiometers may serve well as screening studies. Validation by more experienced and well-trained audiologists and corroboration with tuning forks should be considered before making any treatment decisions that imparts any appreciable risk to the patient. A clinician who bases treatment decisions based on audiometric assessments performed by technicians and automated audiometers implicitly takes responsibility for their diagnostic accuracy.

GLOSSARY

ABLB Alternate binaural loudness balance. A traditional diagnostic auditory procedure for detecting loudness recruitment used in differentiating cochlear from retrocochlear auditory dysfunction in unilateral hearing loss. The task is to balance the sensation of loudness for the better versus poorer hearing ear. Loudness recruitment is a cochlear auditory sign.

ABR (BAER) Auditory brainstem response (brainstem auditory evoked response). Electrical activity, evoked (stimulated) by sounds of very brief duration, that arises from the eighth cranial nerve and auditory portions of the brainstem. Usually recorded from the surface of the scalp and external ear with disk-type electrodes and processed with a fast signal averaging computer. Wave components are labeled with Roman numerals and described according to latency in milliseconds after the stimulus and amplitude in microvolts from one peak to the following trough.

AC Air conduction Audiometric signals presented through earphones to the ear canal.

Admittance An acoustic immittance measure corresponding to the ease of energy flow through the middle ear system

air–bone gap The difference in pure-tone thresholds for air-conducted versus bone-conducted signals. With calibrated audiometers, the normal ear and the sensorineurally impaired ear show no air–bone gap; conductive hearing losses are characterized by an air–bone gap.

ASSR Auditory steady state response An electrophysiologic measure similar to the ABR, but elicited with pure tone signals (vs. transient signals for ABR) that are modulated rapidly in amplitude and frequency. Electrophysiologic activity in the brain is generated by the signal modulation, and detected automatically with a sophisticated processing algorithm.

Audiologist A hearing care professional educated and trained clinically to measure the function of the auditory system and to provide nonmedical care of persons with auditory and communicative losses. Minimal educational requirements and professional credentials for audiologists are a master's degree or Doctor of Audiology (Au.D.) and state licensure.

Auditory neuropathy spectrum disorder (ANSD) A complex collection of auditory disorders that can involve various sites of dysfunction, including the inner hair cells, auditory neurotransmitters, and auditory nerve fibers. ANSD may be an early finding in patients with genetic auditory disorders, neurodegenerative diseases, and other neurological pathology.

Auditory processing disorder (APD) Dysfunction in the auditory system, including central auditory pathways and centers, that impairs effective and efficient processing of auditory information. APD may exist in persons with normal hearing sensitivity.

BC Bone conduction Audiometric signals presented to the skull, such as mastoid bone or forehead, by means of an oscillator.

BCL Békésy comfortable loudness. A Békésy audiometry procedure conducted at a comfortable loudness level as opposed to threshold level.

Békésy audiometry An audiometric procedure performed with a Békésy audiometer for differentiating cochlear and retrocochlear auditory dysfunction. Békésy audiometry is based on comparison of responses to pulsed and continuous tones varied across a wide frequency range. Four patterns of Békésy responses were classified by Jerger.

BOA Behavioral observation audiometry. A pediatric behavioral audiometry procedure in which motor responses to sounds such as eye opening and head turning are detected by a trained observer.

Configuration The shape or pattern of an audiogram. Shows how hearing loss varies as a function of the audiometric test frequency. The three main configurations are rising (low-frequency loss), sloping (high-frequency loss), and flat.

Crossover Property by which sound stimulus presented to one ear (test ear) travels around the head (by means of air conduction) or across the head (by means of bone conduction) to stimulate the other ear (nontest ear). See interaural attenuation and masking dilemma.

dB HL Decibels hearing level A decibel scale referenced to accepted standards for normal hearing (0 dB is average normal hearing for each audiometric test frequency).

dB nHL Decibels normal hearing level A decibel scale used in ABR measurement referenced to average behavioral threshold for the click stimulus of a small group of normal-hearing subjects.

dB SL Decibels sensation level Sound intensity described in reference to an individual patient's behavioral threshold for an audiometric frequency or another measure of hearing threshold, such as the speech-reception threshold.

dBSPL Decibels sound pressure level A decibel scale referenced to a physical standard for intensity, such as 0.0002 dyne/cm^2.

Dichotic Simultaneous presentation of a different sound to each ear.

DPOAEs Distortion product otoacoustic emissions Otoacoustic emissions evoked by two closely spaced pure tone frequencies that measure outer hair cell function and nonlinear activity within the cochlea

DPgram, DPOAEgram A graph of distortion product otoacoustic emission amplitude in the ear canal (dBSPL) as a function of the frequencies of the stimulus tones (Hz).

ECochG Electrocochleography Recording of evoked responses originating from the cochlea (the summating potential (SP), the cochlear microphonic (CM), and the eighth cranial nerve (the action potential, AP).

ENG Electronystagmography A test of vestibular function in which nystagmus is recorded with electrodes placed near the eyes during stimulation of the vestibular system.

ENoG Electroneurography Recording of myogenic activity of the facial muscles, usually in the nasolabial fold, in response to electrical stimulation of the facial nerve as it exits the stylomastoid foramen.

Hearing in Noise Test (HINT)   A clinical test of speech perception of sentences in noise. The sentence-to-noise difference (ratio) is manipulated during administration of the HINT.

Immittance   The word immittance is a combination of two related terms: impedance and admittance. Each term is defined in the glossary.

Impedance   An acoustic immittance measure corresponding to the resistance to energy flow through the middle ear system

Interaural attenuation   Insulation to the crossover of sound (acoustic or mechanical energy) from one ear to the other provided by the head. Varies depending on whether the signal is presented by air conduction (interaural attenuation more than 40 dB) or bone conduction (interaural attenuation less than 10 dB). Insert earphones offer maximum interaural attenuation.

Malingering   Feigning or exaggerating a hearing loss. Also called presbycusis, functional hearing loss, or nonorganic hearing loss.

Masking (masker)   A controlled background noise presented usually to the ear not being tested in an audiometric procedure to prevent a response from that ear caused by crossover when interaural attenuation is exceeded.

Masking dilemma   A problem encountered in audiometric assessment of patients with severe conductive hearing loss. The level of masking noise necessary to overcome the conductive component and adequately mask the ear not being tested exceeds interaural attenuation levels. The masking noise can cross over to the ear being tested and mask the signal, such as a pure tone or speech. In the masking dilemma, enough masking is too much masking. The masking dilemma can be reduced by the use of insert earphones. The sensory acuity level test also is helpful for measuring ear-specific bone conduction hearing thresholds for patients who present the masking dilemma.

MCL Most comfortable level   The intensity level of a sound perceived as comfortable.

MLD Masking level difference   An audiometric procedure used to compare a threshold response with masking noise presented in phase as opposed to out of phase with a pure-tone or speech signal. Release from masking is a normal phenomenon reflecting auditory brainstem integrity.

OAE Otoacoustic emissions   Sounds generated by energy produced by the outer hair cells in the cochlea and detected with a microphone placed in the external ear canal.

PB Phonetically balanced   Word lists developed in the late 1940s that contain all the phonetic elements of general American English speech that occur with the approximate frequency of occurrence in conversational speech.

PI Performance intensity   A measure of speech recognition or understanding as a function of the intensity level of the speech signal. See rollover.

PTA Pure-tone average   The arithmetic average of hearing threshold levels for 500, 1,000, and 2,000 Hz, or the speech frequency region of the audiogram. The PTA should agree within ±7 dB with the speech-reception threshold.

Rollover   A decrease in speech recognition performance, in percentage correct, at high signal intensity levels as opposed to lower levels. Rollover is an audiometric sign of retrocochlear auditory dysfunction.

SAL Sensory acuity level   An audiometric procedure developed by Jerger for assessing bone-conduction hearing among patients with serious conductive hearing loss. Air-conduction thresholds are determined without masking and with masking presented by bone conduction to the forehead. The size of the masked shift in hearing thresholds corresponds to the degree of the conductive hearing loss component.

SAT (SDT) Speech awareness threshold (speech detection threshold)   The lowest intensity level at which a person can detect the presence of a speech signal. The SAT approximates the best hearing level in the 250 to 8,000 Hz audiometric frequency region.

SISI Short increment intensity index   A clinical procedure developed by Jerger for assessing the ability to detect a 1 dB increase in intensity. A high SISI score is consistent with cochlear auditory dysfunction.

S/N Signal-to-noise ratio   The signal-to-noise ratio is the difference between the intensity level of a sound or electrical event and background acoustic or electrophysiologic energy.

SRT Speech-reception level   The lowest intensity level at which a person can accurately identify a speech signal, such as two-syllable spondee words. See PTA.

SSI Synthetic sentence identification   A measure of central auditory function that involves identification of syntactically incomplete sentences (a closed set of 10 sentences) presented simultaneously with a competing message (an ongoing story about Davy Crockett).

SSW Staggered spondaic word test   A measure of central auditory function developed by Katz in which spondee words are presented dichotically.

Tone decay test   A clinical measure of auditory adaptation in which a tone is presented continuously to an ear with a hearing loss until it becomes inaudible. There are numerous versions of tone decay tests. Excessive tone decay is a sign of retrocochlear auditory dysfunction.

TROCA Tangible reinforcement operant conditioning audiometry   A pediatric behavioral audiometry technique used to reinforce a response to auditory signals with food. TROCA is used mainly in the care of children with mental retardation or developmental delay.

UCL (LDL) Uncomfortable level (loudness discomfort level)   The intensity level of a sound perceived as too loud.

VRA Visual reinforcement audiometry   A pediatric behavioral audiometry procedure used to reinforce localization responses to acoustic signals with a visual event, such as an animal playing.

HIGHLIGHTS

- Pure-tone audiometry is the most common measure of hearing sensitivity.
- Masking is the audiometric technique used to eliminate participation of the ear not being tested whenever air- and bone-conduction stimulation exceeds interaural attenuation.
- Speech audiometry procedures usually are performed to measure hearing sensitivity (thresholds in decibels) for words or to estimate word recognition, such as speech discrimination, ability.
- Immittance is a term derived from the terms for two related techniques of assessing middle ear function (impedance and admittance), techniques that have been used clinically since 1970.
- Tympanometry is the dynamic recording of middle ear impedance as air pressure in the ear canal is systematically increased or decreased.
- Acoustic reflex measurement is useful clinically because it can quickly provide objective information about the status of the auditory system from middle ear to brainstem.
- Extensive research has shown that the ABR wave components arise from the eighth cranial nerve and auditory regions in the caudal and rostral brainstem.
- Optimal ECochG waveforms are recorded with a small needle electrode placed through the tympanic membrane onto the promontory, although placement on the tympanic membrane and to a lesser extent the ear canal also is clinically useful.
- OAEs are low-intensity sounds produced by the cochlea in response to an acoustic stimulus. OAEs are a popular technique for hearing screening of infants and older children, and for objective diagnostic confirmation of outer hair cell integrity
- Indicators of sensorineural or conductive hearing loss among neonates and infants include intrauterine infection, bacterial infection, asphyxia, hyperbilirubinemia, and head trauma, as well as neurologic insults during infancy.
- No single measure of auditory function is adequate for comprehensive hearing assessment.
- Hearing loss, regardless of causation, affects the speech and language development of infants and young children.

REFERENCES

1. Carhart R, Jerger JF. Preferred method for clinical determination of pure-tone thresholds. *J Speech Hear Disord* 1959;24:330–345.
2. Hall JW III, Mueller HG III. *Audiologists' Desk Reference.* Vol. I. San Diego, CA: Singular Publishing Group, 1997.
3. American Academy of Otolaryngology Committee on Hearing and Equilibrium and the American Council of Otolaryngology Committee on the Medical Aspects of Noise. Guide for the evaluation of hearing handicap. *JAMA* 1979;11:2055–2059.
4. Mueller HG III, Hall JW III. *Audiologists' Desk Reference.* Vol. II. San Diego, CA: Singular Publishing Group, 1998:700–714.
5. Nilsson M, Soli SD, Sullivan JA. Development of the Hearing in Noise Test for the measurement of speech reception thresholds in quiet and in noise. *J Acoust Soc Am* 1994;95:1085–1099. PubMed PMID: 8132902.
6. Jerger JF. Clinical experience with impedance audiometry. *Arch Otolaryngol* 1970;92:311–324.
7. Hall JW III. *The New Handbook of Auditory Evoked Responses.* Boston, MA: Allyn & Bacon, 2007.
8. Ruckenstein MJ, Cueva RA, Morrison DH, et al. A prospective study of ABR and MRI in the screening for vestibular schwannomas. *Am J Otol* 1996;17:317–320.
9. Schmidt RJ, Sataloff RT, Newman J, et al. The sensitivity of auditory brainstem response testing for the diagnosis of acoustic neuromas. *Arch Otolaryngol Head Neck Surg* 2001;127:19–22. PubMed PMID: 11177009.
10. Loftus B, Wazen JJ. A false-positive gadolinium-enhanced MRI: acoustic neuroma versus cochleovestibular neuritis. *Otolaryngol Head Neck Surg* 1990;103:299.
11. Yoshinaga-Itano C, Sedley AL, Coulter DK, et al. Language of early- and later-identified children with hearing loss. *Pediatrics* 1998;102:1161–1171.
12. Pou AM, Hirsch BE, Durrant JD, et al. The efficacy of tympanic electrocochleography in the diagnosis of endolymphatic hydrops. *Am J Otol* 1996;17:607–611.
13. Sass K, Densert B, Magnusson M. Transtympanic electrocochleography in the assessment of perilymphatic fistulas. *Audiol Neurootol* 1997;2:391–402.
14. Badr-el-Dine M, Gerken GM, Meyerhoff WL. Loss of perilymph affects electrocochleographic potentials in the guinea pig. *Am J Otol* 1994;15:717–722.
15. Campbell KC, Abbas PJ. Electrocochleography with postural changes in perilymphatic fistula. Animal studies. *Ann Otol Rhinol Laryngol* 1994;103:474–482.
16. Kakigi A, Sawada S, Takeda T, et al. Electrocochleographic findings in cases of autoimmune disease with sensorineural deafness. *Auris Nasus Larynx* 2003;30:349–354.
17. Bouman H, Klis SF, Meeuwsen F, et al. Experimental autoimmune inner ear disease: an electrocochleographic and histophysiologic study. *Ann Otol Rhinol Laryngol* 2000;109:457–466.
18. Arts HA, Adams ME, Telian SA, et al. Reversible electrocochleographic abnormalities in superior canal dehiscence. *Otol Neurotol* 2009;30:79–86. PubMed PMID: 19092559.
19. Hayes EA, Warrier CM, Nicol TG, et al. Neural plasticity following auditory training in children with learning problems. *Clin Neurophysiol* 2003;114:673–684.
20. Dhar S, Hall JW III. *Otoacoustic emissions: principles, procedures, and protocols.* San Diego, CA: Plural Publishing Group, 2012.
21. Bohne BA, Clark WW. Growth of hearing loss and cochlear lesion with increasing duration of noise exposure. In: Hamernik RP, Henderson D, Salvi R, eds. *New perspectives on noise-induced hearing loss.* New York: Raven Press, 1982:283–301.
22. Norman M, Thornton AR, Phillips AJ, et al. Otoacoustic emissions recorded at high rates in patients with confirmed acoustic neuromas. *Am J Otol* 1996;17:763–772.
23. Rapin I, Gravel J. "Auditory neuropathy": physiologic and pathologic evidence calls for more diagnostic specificity. *Int J Pediatr Otorhinolaryngol* 2003;67:707–728.
24. Myklebust HR. *Auditory disorders in children: a manual for differential diagnosis.* New York: Grune & Stratton, 1954.
25. Bocca E, Calearo C, Cassinari V. A new method for testing hearing in temporal lobe tumors. *Acta Otolaryngol* 1954;44:219–221.

26. American Academy of Audiology Clinical Practice Guidelines: Diagnosis, Treatment and Management of Children and Adults with Central Auditory Processing Disorder. *http://www.audiology.org/resources/documentlibrary/documents/capd%20guidelines%208-2010.pdf.* Published August 24, 2010.

27. Joint Committee on Infant Hearing. Year 2007 position statement: principles and guidelines for early hearing detection and intervention. *Pediatrics* 2007;120:898–921.

28. American Academy of Pediatrics Task Force on Newborn and Infant Hearing. Newborn infant hearing: diagnosis and intervention. *Pediatrics* 1999;103:527–529.

29. Henry JA, Flick CL, Gilbert A, et al. Reliability of computer-automated hearing thresholds in cochlear-impaired listeners using ER-4B Canal Phone earphones. *J Rehabil Res Dev* 2003;40:253–264.

30. Henry JA, Flick CL, Gilbert A, et al. Reliability of hearing thresholds: computer-automated testing with ER-4B Canal Phone earphones. *J Rehabil Res Dev* 2001;38:567–581.

Vestibular Function and Anatomy

143

J. Christopher Holt   Shawn D. Newlands

Nearly all animals have ways of monitoring their own movements and orienting themselves with respect to various sensory cues in their environment. In vertebrates, such behaviors depend heavily on a functioning vestibular system, a critical sensory system that begins in the inner ear as a collection of peripheral detectors for motion and gravity and ends among a number of higher neural centers within the central nervous system (CNS). These higher centers process and integrate incoming motion information from the periphery to inform our perception of our position in space and relative to other objects, to coordinate our movements, and to formulate appropriate reflexes (1). The vestibular system is physically linked to the peripheral auditory system through their cohabitation in the inner ear, and like the auditory system, ultimately converts mechanical forces (i.e., rotation, translation, and/ or gravitational forces rather than sound energy) into a neural code that is interpreted centrally. The ability of the vestibular system to detect movements of the head and body resides in the vestibular hair cell whose sensitivity to mechanical stimuli is coupled to a series of electrochemical processes that ultimately change the firing rate of vestibular afferent neurons. Despite the obvious necessity for the vestibular system, we often fail to appreciate its role unless it becomes deficient or defective, at which point, one becomes acutely aware of its importance. In the pages that follow, we discuss the gross anatomy of the peripheral vestibular system, the anatomy and physiology of vestibular hair cells and afferent neurons, the biophysics of sensory transduction, and the organization and functional connectivity of vestibular inputs to the CNS. This chapter serves only as an introduction to the vestibular system; for a more thorough treatment, readers are encouraged to consult dedicated texts.

GROSS ANATOMY OF THE VESTIBULAR SYSTEM

The vestibular labyrinth of vertebrates is an anatomically complex structure consisting of a series of fluid-filled tubes and sacks containing distinct sensory end organs for the detection of both angular and linear acceleration of the head and body (Fig. 143.1). In mammals, the membranous vestibular labyrinth is threaded through a bony labyrinth formed by the dense, hard bone of the otic capsule, within the petrous portion of each temporal bone. A sodium-rich, CSF-like fluid called perilymph bathes the space between the bony and membranous labyrinth, whereas the lumen of the membranous labyrinth is filled with endolymph, a potassium-rich fluid that closely resembles the normal intracellular milieu. Both the perilymphatic and endolymphatic spaces of the vestibular labyrinth are contiguous with the respective spaces of the cochlea. As such, both fluid compartments circulate between the cochlea and the vestibular labyrinth, and thus the homeostatic mechanisms for hearing discussed in Chapter 141 are crucial for vestibular function as well.

The term vestibular labyrinth generally refers to the paired right and left labyrinths together, which are essentially mirror images of each other (see Fig. 143.2A). Each side is comprised of three orthogonally arranged semicircular canals (horizontal or lateral, anterior or superior, and posterior) and two sac-like structures called the utricle and saccule. The utricle and saccule are collectively referred to as the otolith organs. Innervation for the canals, saccule, and utricle all travel in the vestibular nerve portion of cranial nerve VIII. The anterior canal, horizontal canal, utricle, and anterior one-third of the saccule receive their innervation by way of the superior division of the vestibular nerve,

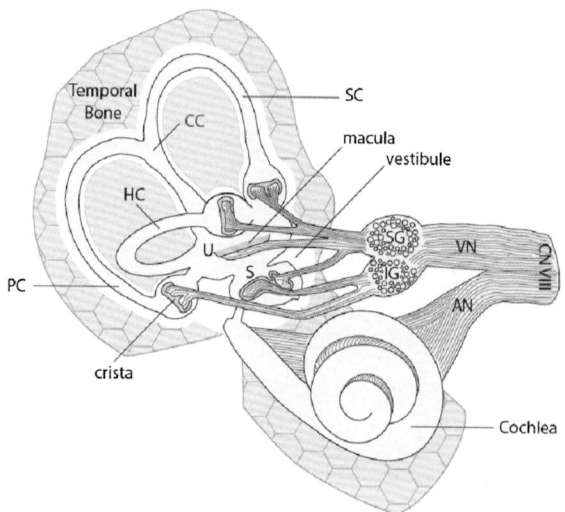

Figure 143.1 The vestibular labyrinth and its innervation. AN, auditory nerve; CC, common crus; CN VIII, cranial nerve 8; HC, horizontal canal; IG, inferior ganglion; PC, posterior vertical semicircular canal; S, saccule; SC, superior or anterior vertical semicircular canal; SG, superior ganglion; U, utricle; VN, vestibular nerve. Shaded areas at each of the nerve endings represent the sensory neuroepithelium.

whereas the inferior division innervates the posterior two-thirds of the saccule and posterior canal (Fig. 143.1). Upon reaching each end organ, the innervation terminates within the sensory portions of the membranous labyrinth. The sensory neuroepithelium of the semicircular canals and otolithic organs are called the crista and macula, respectively (Fig. 143.1).

One end of each semicircular canal is expanded to form what is called the ampulla. The ampulla is presumably enlarged to accommodate the sensory neuroepithelium and associated accessory structures. The ampulla of either the horizontal or superior semicircular canal is located at the anterior end of each canal, whereas the ampulla of the posterior semicircular canal is located more laterally. The non-ampullated ends of the posterior and superior semicircular canals join to form the common crus that subsequently enters the vestibule posteromedially. The nonampullated end of the lateral semicircular canal enters the vestibule posterolaterally.

The semicircular canals detect angular acceleration and thus are well suited for monitoring rotations of the head. A canal's greatest sensitivity to angular acceleration occurs when the head rotation is made within the plane of that canal. The anatomical organization of the three semicircular canals within the temporal bone is illustrated in Figure 143.2. Horizontal canals are pitched approximately 30 degrees above the horizontal axial plane while the head is upright. The vertical canals (i.e., anterior and posterior) are situated roughly at right angles to the horizontal canals and to each other. Thus, when one looks down at the top of the head, the plane of the anterior canal is oriented at approximately 45 degrees off the midsagittal axis and 45 degrees anterior to the interaural line. The plane of the posterior canal is also 45 degrees off the midsagittal line but aligned roughly 45 degrees behind the interaural line. Thus, the anterior canal on the left is essentially parallel to the posterior canal on the right. The right anterior canal

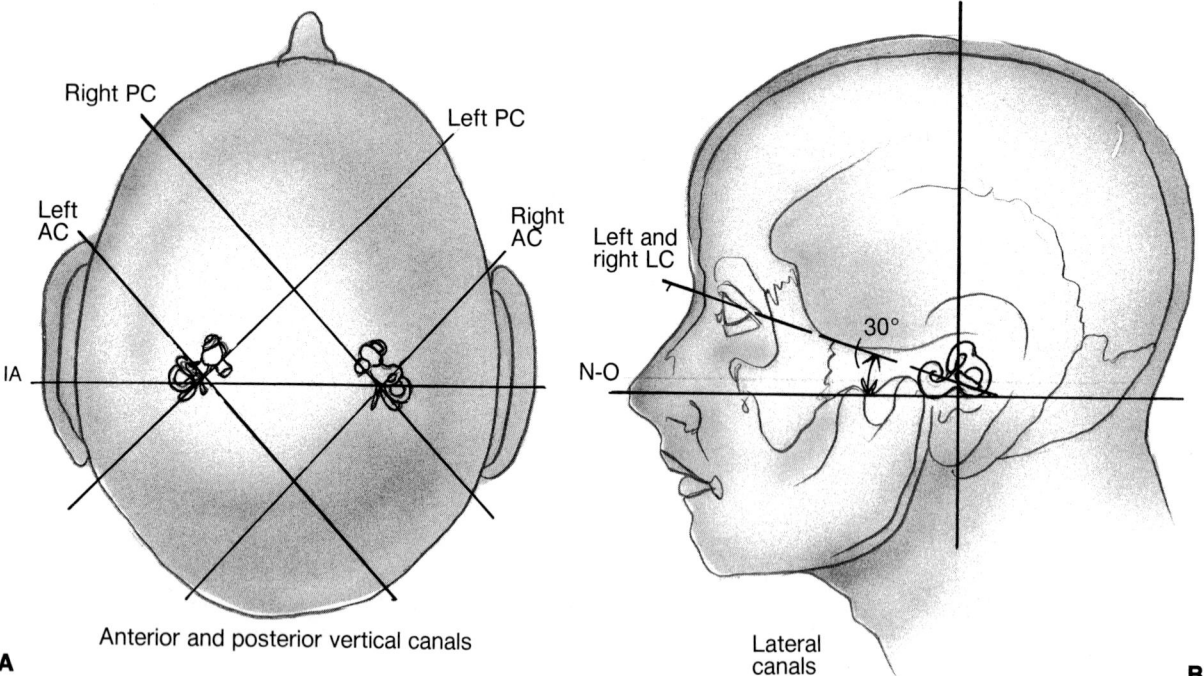

Figure 143.2 A: Orientation of the vertical canals in the human head. **B:** Plane of the lateral (horizontal) semicircular canals. AC, anterior or superior vertical semicircular canal; IA, interaural; LC, lateral or horizontal semicircular canal; N-O, nasal–occipital axis; PC, posterior vertical semicircular canal.

and the left posterior canal are similarly aligned. The plane parallel to the left anterior canal and right posterior canal passing through the center of the head is perpendicular to the horizontal canal plane and is referred to as the LARP plane. Conversely, the plane perpendicular to both the horizontal canal plane and the LARP plane, but parallel to the right anterior and left posterior plane is referred to as the RALP plane. Because of this canal pairing system (i.e., HC-HC, LA-RP, and RA-LP), movement that excites one canal will inhibit the other, which forms the basis for a push–pull system. As we discuss later, both the excitation and inhibition converge centrally to improve the sensitivity of the system.

The otolith organs, represented in most mammals and humans by the utricle and saccule, are housed in the major chamber of the vestibular labyrinth called the vestibule. In contrast to the semicircular canals, the otolith organs detect linear acceleration in the plane of each organ. Though neither organ is perfectly planar, the utricular macula is approximately aligned parallel to the earth and is roughly aligned with the ipsilateral horizontal canal (Fig. 143.3). The saccular macula is perpendicular and at right angles to the utricle. Thus, the utricle is sensitive to motion in the horizontal plane, and the saccule is sensitive to movements in the sagittal plane. Collectively, the otolith organs are anatomically organized to detect and monitor linear accelerations along three axes that are perpendicular to each other: interaural, nasal–occipital, and rostral–caudal (Figs. 143.2 and 143.3).

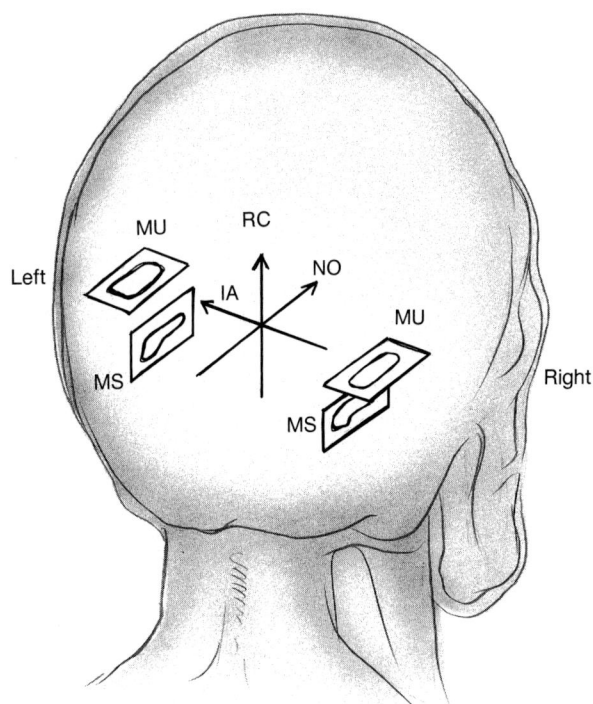

Figure 143.3 Approximate planar layout of the otolith organs. MS, Macular saccule; MU, macular utriculi; IA, interaural axis; NO, nasal–occipital axis; RC, rostral–caudal axis.

CELLULAR ANATOMY OF THE VESTIBULAR END ORGAN

In order to understand the cellular basis of how various head movements are detected and encoded by the peripheral vestibular system, further examination of the end organ is warranted. An illustration of the sensory neuro-epithelium typical of each vestibular end organ is shown in Figure 143.4A. A cross-section through either the crista or macula reveals four distinct cellular constituents: (a) hair cells, (b) supporting cells, (c) afferent nerve fibers and terminals, and (d) efferent nerve fibers and terminals. The roles that each constituent plays in vestibular physiology and function are highlighted below.

Vestibular Hair Cells

As with the auditory system, sensory transduction in the vestibular system is accomplished by a specialized neuro-epithelial cell called the hair cell, so named because of the tuft of finger-like projections located along its apical pole (Fig. 143.4A). It is this apical tuft that confers mechanical sensitivity to both auditory and vestibular hair cells. On the basis of their morphology, physiology, and afferent innervation, vestibular hair cells are classified as either type I or type II (2). The type II hair cell is a prototypical, cylindrically shaped hair cell that receives its afferent innervation as a number of bouton terminals along its basolateral edges. In contrast, the type I hair cell is flask-shaped with a rounded base and constricted apical neck, and is innervated by a cup-like, calyx afferent terminal, which almost entirely encapsulates the type I hair cell. Hair cells communicate with their respective afferent neurons by releasing the excitatory neurotransmitter glutamate from specialized presynaptic structures called synaptic ribbons. Type II hair cells are found in the vestibular end organs of all vertebrates while type I hair cells and calyx afferent neurons are restricted to amniotes (i.e., reptiles, birds, and mammals). Likely emphasizing their respective functional roles, type I and type II hair cells and their respective afferent neurons often follow zonal boundaries and thus are not evenly distributed throughout the crista or macula.

Although most of the hair cell and all of its innervation occupy the perilymphatic space, the hair bundle itself is suspended in the endolymphatic compartment. Here, it projects into a gelatinous accessory structure called the cupula in canals or the otolithic membrane in the utricle and saccule. This particular anatomical arrangement is necessary for the proper function of the hair cell and its detection of head movements. The hair bundles of vestibular hair cells are composed of a single eccentrically placed kinocilium and multiple rows of stereocilia (Fig. 143.4). There are typically 20 to 100 stereocilia per hair cell. The kinocilium is the tallest member of the hair bundle and its position at the edge of the apical surface

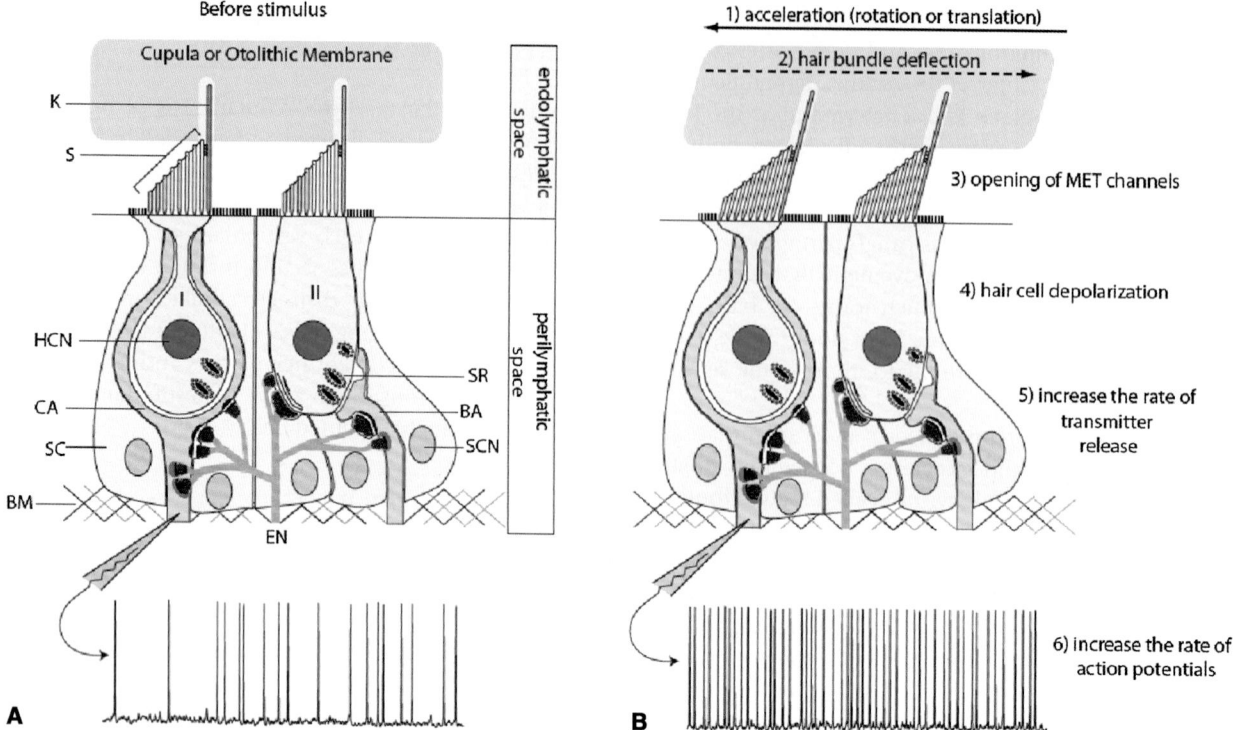

Figure 143.4 Anatomy and physiology of the sensory neuroepithelium. **A:** Cellular constituents of the sensory neuroepithelium. BA, bouton afferent; BM, basement membrane; CA, calyx afferent; EN, efferent neuron; HCN, hair cell nucleus; I, type I hair cell; II, type II hair cell; K, kinocilia; S, stereocilia; SC, supporting cell; SR, synaptic ribbon. Hair cells continuously release neurotransmitter that depolarizes afferent terminals to generate action potentials. Recording from a calyx afferent reveals the baseline discharge (**bottom**). **B:** Coupling acceleration to hair cell stimulation and afferent discharge. Rotation or translation to the left results in an inertial shift of the cupula or otoconial mass to the right. This shift deflects the hair bundle toward the kinocilium, which opens MET channels in the stereocilia to further depolarize the hair cell. Hair cells subsequently release more glutamate on to afferent terminals resulting in an increase in action potential discharge. Note the increase in the rate of action potentials (**bottom**).

indicates the orientation of the hair cell. An orderly array of adjacent stereocilia is organized in a descending staircase formation when moving away from the kinocilium. As can be seen in Figure 143.5, this particular geometrical arrangement confers a so-called morphological polarization vector (PV) or axis, which can be identified by drawing a line from the smallest stereocilia through the kinocilium. It turns out that the functional axis of the hair cell is aligned with the morphological axis. It is along this axis that a hair cell is most sensitive to displacement of the bundle. This is made possible by the expression of mechanoelectrical transduction (MET) channels along the tips of the stereocilia that open during hair bundle deflection (3). The mechanosensitivity of MET channels is provided by filamentous tip links that connect MET channels in a lower stereocilium with the membrane of its taller, adjacent neighboring sterocilium. Relative motion of the stereocilia, upon deflecting the hair bundle toward the kinocilium, exerts tension on the tip links thereby prompting the opening of MET channels. What results is an influx of potassium ions from the endolymphatic compartment into the stereocilia that subsequently depolarizes the hair cell. Conversely, deflection of stereocilia away

from the kinocilium decreases tip link tension, closes MET channels, and subsequently hyperpolarizes the hair cell. Displacement of the stereocilia perpendicular to the polarization axis, however, causes little to no response in the hair cell. In any one sensory end organ, neighboring hair cells tend to have PVs that are aligned. This is certainly true of canal hair cells whose hair bundles all face the same direction. Hair bundle orientation in otolithic maculae, however, varies considerably particularly along the striola, a line where hair bundle orientation reverses direction nearly 180 degrees (see Fig. 143.6).

Like most neurons, hair cells are able to maintain a negative resting membrane potential, which is necessary for conveying mechanical events at the bundle to vestibular afferent neurons that synapse along their basolateral edges. In the absence of a vestibular stimulus (i.e., no bundle deflection), enough MET channels are thought to remain open to sufficiently depolarize vestibular hair cells. This baseline depolarization permits the continuous release of glutamate from synaptic ribbons located along the basal pole of the hair cell. Once released, glutamate then activates postsynaptic glutamate receptors to depolarize adjacent afferent nerve terminals. Afferent

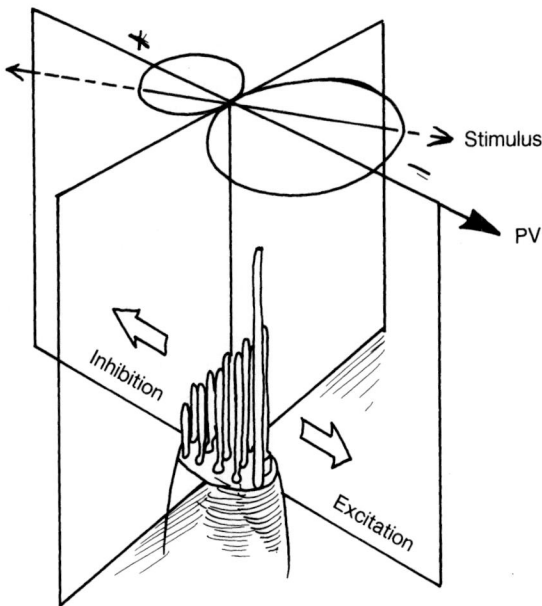

Figure 143.5 Directional sensitivity of the hair cell approximating a cosine function of stimulus direction. The output varies as the cosine of the angle between the direction of maximum sensitivity and the applied displacement varies. PV, polarization vector. (Modified from Loewenstein WR. Handbook of sensory physiology, Vol. 1. In: *Principles of receptor physiology*. New York, NY: Springer-Verlag, 1971:415, with permission.)

depolarization results in the generation of action potentials in the afferent neuron that are then transmitted to the brain (Fig. 143.4A). This type of release process is important because it allows for bidirectional modulation

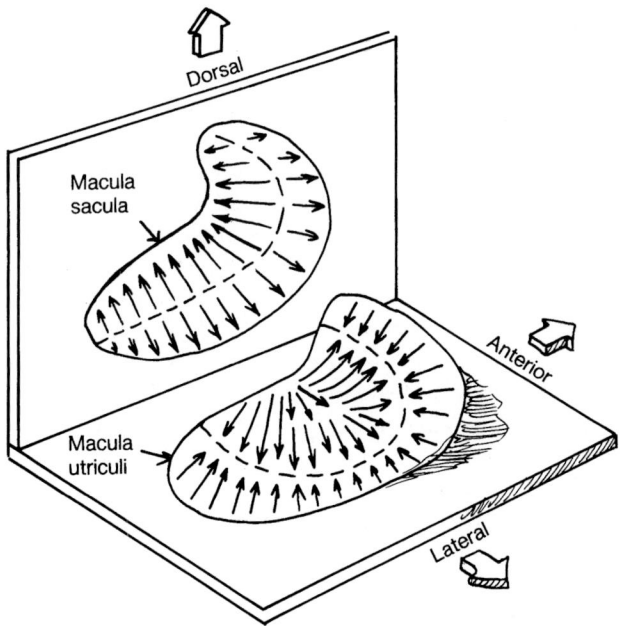

Figure 143.6 Polarization of hair cells on the otolith organs. Direction of *arrows* indicates direction of the hair bundle deflection that excites hair cells in that region of the macula. *Dashed line* represents the striola where hair bundle orientation flips by 180 degrees. (Modified from Barber HO, Stockwell CW. *Manual of electronystagmography*, 2nd ed. St. Louis, MO: Mosby, 1980:31; Fig. 2-21.)

of hair cell transmitter release as well as the downstream rate of afferent action potentials. Deflection of the hair cell bundle toward the kinocilium depolarizes the hair cell, enhances glutamate release, and increases the rate of afferent action potentials, whereas deflection of the hair cell bundle away from the kinocilium hyperpolarizes the hair cell, reduces transmitter release, and decreases the rate of action potentials. In this way, one hair cell can detect both acceleration and deceleration along the axis of their morphological PV.

Supporting Cells

In addition to hair cells, the neuroepithelium also contains other epithelial cells called supporting cells, aptly named as they provide both structural and homeostatic "support" to the sensory epithelium. The nucleus and much of the supporting cell's cytoplasm can be found between the base of hair cells and the underlying basement membrane (Fig. 143.4A). From there, they extend upward where they envelop both hair cells and afferent neurons. Along their apical margins, supporting cells combine with hair cells to form a tight barrier between the perilymphatic and endolymphatic compartments. Functions of supporting cells include glutamate uptake, potassium transport, and the synthesis and secretion of extracellular macromolecules that makeup the cupula and otolithic membrane. Another group of supporting cells called dark cells can be found at the margins of the transitional epithelium surrounding the neuroepithelium. They are critical in the production and maintenance of the ionic composition of the endolymph (4).

Vestibular Afferent Neurons

Based on of the morphology of their peripheral terminations, vestibular afferent neurons are classified as one of three distinct types: bouton, calyx, or dimorphic. As indicated earlier, calyx afferent neurons with their calyceal endings terminate exclusively on type I hair cells where they can innervate anywhere from one to five hair cells. Bouton afferent neurons end as small button-like terminals along the basolateral membrane of only type II hair cells. Dimorphic afferent neurons are a hybrid bearing both calyx endings on type I hair cells and bouton endings on type II hair cells. In mammals, dimorphic afferent neurons represent the largest proportion of afferent fibers in the vestibular nerve. Conveniently, immunohistochemical studies have also shown that antibodies against the calcium-binding protein calretinin and the intermediate filament protein peripherin can be used to identify these three afferent classes. Calretinin is only seen in calyx afferent neurons, whereas peripherin is seen only in bouton afferent neurons. Both markers, however, are not expressed in dimorphic afferent neurons.

There are other anatomical distinctions among these different afferent types. Calyx afferent neurons have characteristically thick axons, whereas bouton afferent neurons are much thinner. Dimorphic afferent neurons, however, run the gamut of thick to thin with respect to fiber diameter. Here, it is more convenient to relate the thickness of vestibular afferent neurons with their different zonal innervation patterns. The neuroepithelium of the semicircular canals (i.e., crista) can be divided concentrically into a central, intermediate, and peripheral zone with type I hair cells predominating in the central zone and type II hair cells being more common in the intermediate and peripheral zones (5,6). As such, calyx afferent endings are restricted to the central zone, whereas bouton afferent neurons terminate in the peripheral zone. Dimorphic afferent neurons innervate all three zones where their relative axonal diameter is graded from thick to thin as you move from the central to peripheral zones. A comparable organization is seen in the utricle where calyx afferent neurons terminate in the striolar region, dimorphic afferent terminals are seen throughout the macula, and bouton afferent neurons terminate peripherally. It is thought that similar regionalization occurs in the saccule as well.

One might suspect that given their different anatomical attributes, vestibular afferent neurons would likely exhibit variations in their physiology. In fact, differences in conduction velocity, discharge regularity, and sensitivity to vestibular and galvanic stimulation can also be used to identify a vestibular afferent's morphological class (i.e., calyx, dimorphic, and bouton). Calyx afferent neurons innervating the central crista zone or striolar region of otolithic organs are irregularly discharging, quite sensitive to galvanic stimulation, and yet have a low sensitivity to vestibular stimulation. Dimorphic afferent neurons vary depending on what zone they innervate. For example, dimorphic afferent neurons terminating more centrally (or within the striola) are irregularly discharging and sensitive to both galvanic and vestibular stimulation. In contrast, dimorphic and bouton afferent neurons terminating peripherally (either in the macula or crista) are regularly discharging and much less sensitive to both galvanic and natural stimulation (7). While vestibular stimuli actively engage the hair bundle's transduction apparatus, galvanic (i.e., electrical) stimulation is thought to directly interact with the afferent's spike encoder, the site of action potential generation. In this way, galvanic stimulation presumably bypasses the hair cell and provides an assessment of the afferent's response properties. Therefore, differences in hair cell input (e.g., type I vs. type II) might account for afferent neurons having similar galvanic sensitivities, but different responses to vestibular stimuli. Such is likely the case for comparisons between calyx and central dimorphic afferent neurons.

These different afferent types may be of more interest than just physiological curiosity. The high sensitivity of irregular afferent neurons makes them ideal to detect small perturbations but they are expected to display nonlinear response dynamics given that they readily silence when the head moves in the inhibitory direction. These afferent neurons may be best suited for quick, nonlinear reflexes such as vestibulospinal responses used to prevent a fall. In contrast, the linear characteristics of the thinner, more regular afferent neurons are likely more appropriate for linear vestibular reflexes, like the vestibuloocular reflex, that must work over a wide range of frequencies and peak velocities (8).

Both semicircular canal and otolith afferent neurons are cosine tuned, which means that they have one best characteristic response vector. For utricular afferent neurons, these vectors can lie anywhere in the horizontal plane and are dependent on the orientation vector of the hair cells that they innervate. The responses of afferent neurons are proportional to the cosine of the angle between the direction of stimulation and the orientation vector of the afferent neurons. Similarly, the rotational vector of maximum stimulation for semicircular canal afferent neurons is in the plane of rotation of the canal. The response of the afferent neuron decreases as a function of the cosine of the angle between the plane of rotation and the canal plane. The cosine tuning of the afferent neuron is consistent with the fact that transmitter release by hair cells is proportional to the cosine of the angle between the displacement of the hair cell bundle and the direction of stimulation (Fig. 143.5). The coding of the vestibular system is such that the direction of stimulation is determined by which afferent neurons are stimulated and the intensity of the movement is related to the intensity of the response of the stimulated afferent neuron.

Vestibular Efferent Neurons

The vestibular neuroepithelium is also innervated by vestibular efferent neurons. These predominantly cholinergic neurons originate bilaterally in the brainstem in areas adjacent to the abducens nucleus and genu of the facial nerve. They exit the brainstem and enter the vestibular periphery by way of cranial nerve VIII. Upon reaching the vestibular end organs, efferent neurons can terminate along the base of type II hair cells, on bouton afferent terminals that synapse on type II hair cells, or on the outer face and parent axon of calyx afferent neurons (Fig. 143.4A). Observations of a direct efferent innervation of type I hair cells are rare as the type I hair cell is mostly shielded by the calyx ending. Electrical stimulation of efferent neurons has been shown to hyperpolarize or depolarize hair cells as well as directly excite vestibular afferent neurons (9). The functions of the vestibular efferent system in mammals are not well understood but likely include modulating the excitability and sensitivity of both vestibular hair cells and afferent neurons to incoming vestibular stimuli.

BASIC PHYSICS OF MECHANOTRANSDUCTION

To reiterate, with respect to head motion, the utricle and saccule detect and transduce linear accelerations (i.e., translation or gravity), whereas the semicircular canals have the task of detecting and transducing angular accelerations (i.e., rotations). Now that we understand the basic principles by which vestibular hair cells operate and communicate with vestibular afferent neurons, how do we physically couple the mechanosensitivity of hair cells to the different kinds of head movements? This feat is accomplished by tethering the hair bundle to some inertial mass that is appropriately displaced during head movements. For semicircular canals, hair bundles insert into the cupula, whereas for the utricle and saccule, hair bundles are attached to the otolithic membrane. Figure 143.4A illustrates how the neuroepithelium behaves in the moments before a vestibular stimulus arrives (i.e., no acceleration). Under these circumstances, continuous release of glutamate from the hair cell helps to maintain the baseline firing of afferent action potentials. Figure 143.4B shows the sequential responses of the neuroepithelium when it is suddenly accelerated to the left. Given their inertial properties, the cupula or otolithic membrane shifts in the opposite direction to head rotation, in this case to the right. This shift deflects the hair bundles toward the kinocilium that then opens MET channels to depolarize hair cells to release more glutamate, thereby increasing the discharge rate of the afferent nerve.

To describe displacements of the cupula and otolithic membrane during head movements, it is helpful to use Newton's second law, which relates the acceleration ($\vec{a}$, a vector having both direction and amplitude) of any object of mass (m) to the force ($\vec{F}$, also a vector) needed to accelerate the said object. For the saccule and utricle, calcium carbonate crystals, or otoconia, sitting atop the otolithic membrane, provide the inertial mass. For describing linear acceleration of the otoconial mass, Newton's second law can be written as $\vec{F} = m\vec{a}$. However, the otoconial mass is also affected by gravity ($\vec{g}$, yet another vector). Thus, the total force acting on the otolithic membrane is $\vec{F} = m(\vec{a} + \vec{g})$, which shows that otoconial mass will not differentiate linear acceleration from gravity (i.e., translation vs. tilt). For describing how angular acceleration stimulates the semicircular canal, Newton's second law would be written as $\vec{T} = J \times \vec{a}$, where $\vec{a}$ is angular acceleration and $\vec{T}$ is amount of torque produced by that acceleration. J, the moment of inertia (i.e., mass equivalent), is provided by the endolymph within the membranous labyrinth. Torque is not affected by linear acceleration, which is consistent with role of the semicircular canals in detecting only head rotations.

MECHANOTRANSDUCTION IN THE SEMICIRCULAR CANALS

Recall that the semicircular canals are toroidal or doughnut-shaped (Figs. 143.1 and 143.7). As the membranous labyrinth threads its way through the temporal bone, it is anchored to the bony labyrinth in several spots. Each ampulla, in addition to containing the sensory

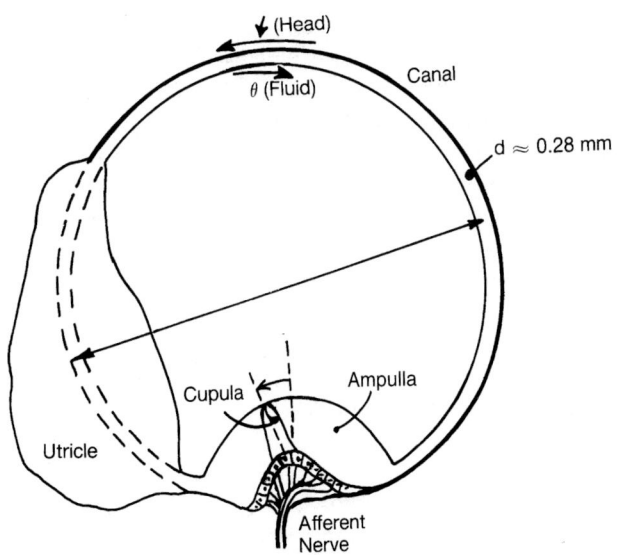

Figure 143.7 Semicircular canal. (Modified from Milsum J. *Biological control systems analysis.* New York, NY: McGraw-Hill, 1966, with permission.)

neuroepithelium, houses the cupula that practically spans the entire lumenal space beyond the apical edges of the crista to form a septum or diaphragm. Hair cells are coupled to this diaphragm by projecting their hair bundles into the cupula. As a result of this design, any rotation in the plane of the canal moves the bony and membranous labyrinth along with the head, whereby the inertia of the endolymph in the membranous canal causes deflection of the cupula in the opposite direction. As the cupula is deflected, the stereocilia bend either toward or away from the kinocilium, ultimately leading to an increase or decrease, respectively, in the firing rate of canal afferent neurons. The system is maximally sensitive to rotations made within the plane of the canal. This is because the kinocilia and resulting morphological orientation axes of hair cells are parallel to the long axis of the canal. In case of the lateral semicircular canal, hair cells are excited when endolymphatic flow deflects the cupula toward the vestibule. Hair cell excitation in the posterior and superior semicircular canals requires endolymphatic flow to deflect the cupula away from the vestibule.

Over 50 years ago, Steinhausen developed a theoretical model of the semicircular canal called the *torsion pendulum model.* By estimating the mass and viscous damping properties of the endolymph, the resetting force of the cupula, and by measuring the geometric properties of the semicircular canal, one can relate cupular deflection to rotation of the head. The model predicts that deflection of the cupula is proportional to head velocity so long as the frequency of head velocity falls between 0.1 and 10 Hz. Beyond the boundaries of this frequency range, however, the sensitivity of the semicircular canal to velocity decreases as cupular deflection under these conditions is not as great. At 0 Hz, which corresponds to constant-velocity rotation, the torsion-pendulum model predicts there will be no response. The model's prediction agrees with the perception of a person who is turned at a constant velocity around a vertical axis. Subjects can detect the initial acceleration, but in the absence of other sensory cues such as vision, they can no longer sense further rotation after 30 to 60 seconds. At this time, if subjects are suddenly brought to a full stop, they will have the distinct sensation of turning in the opposite direction. This is because of the inertia of the endolymph, which continues to rotate and now deflects the cupula in a direction opposite to that seen with the initial rotation. Reflexive eye movements measured during these steps of velocity mirror the sensation felt by the subjects and are the basis for several clinical vestibular assessments including the Bárány test and tests of the vestibuloocular reflex.

MECHANOTRANSDUCTION IN THE OTOLITH ORGANS

As with the semicircular canals, the apical bundles of hair cells in the macula of otolith organs (i.e., utricle and saccule) are also tethered overhead to a gelatinous superstructure. Instead of cupular deflections driven by the inertial mass of the endolymph during angular accelerations, the inertial mass in otolithic organs is provided by a mound of calcium carbonate crystals known as otoconia that sits atop the otolithic membrane. Located immediately underneath are the sensory hair cells whose apical bundles are in direct contact with the otolithic membrane. Such mechanical linkage allows hair cells in the otolithic organs to detect linear motion of the head and body. Here, displacement of the otolithic mass occurs due to translational motion or changes in orientation with respect to gravity, both of which involve linear acceleration.

Unlike the semicircular canals, where the PVs of each of the hair cells in the crista are directionally aligned, the PVs of hair cells in otolithic maculae are oriented in different directions, making each hair cell maximally sensitive to

acceleration in that particular direction (Fig. 143.6). A simplified otolithic organ is illustrated in Figure 143.8. Small arrows above each hair cell indicate the functional axis of that particular hair cell where the direction of maximal excitation would occur. The long arrow at the top indicates the acceleration of the otolith mass. Hair cells whose functional axes are aligned with the acceleration of the mass are excited maximally, whereas hair cells that have perpendicular PVs are not stimulated. It is from this arrangement of hair cells that the brain can estimate the magnitude and direction of linear acceleration. If all PVs were identically aligned as in the canal, it would be impossible to determine the magnitude and direction of an acceleration vector in the plane of any otolithic macula. At least two different orientations are needed to resolve the vector in two dimensions just as at least three separate orientations are needed to resolve the magnitude and direction of an acceleration vector in three dimensions.

Each otolithic organ has sensory hair cells arranged in a wide variety of orientations with respect to their PVs (Fig. 143.6). This is particularly evident within the striolar region where the orientation of hair cells on either side of the striola is roughly 180 degrees out of phase. In otolithic maculae, the striola is an approximately 100 μm zone that runs the length of the macula. The striola divides the utricular or saccular macula into medial or dorsal and lateral or ventral extrastriolar zones, respectively. PVs are oriented toward the striola in the utricular macula and away from the striola in the saccular macula. This planar geometry essentially allows detection of linear accelerations in all directions of the plane. Because of this architecture, the asymmetries inherent in the sensitivity of a single hair cell can be canceled out within one otolithic organ itself. The right and left otolithic organs, like semicircular canals, have mirror symmetry around the sagittal plane. The exact neural connections of the otolith organs have not been as extensively studied as those of the pairs of semicircular canals. Thus, the exact circuitry for resolving

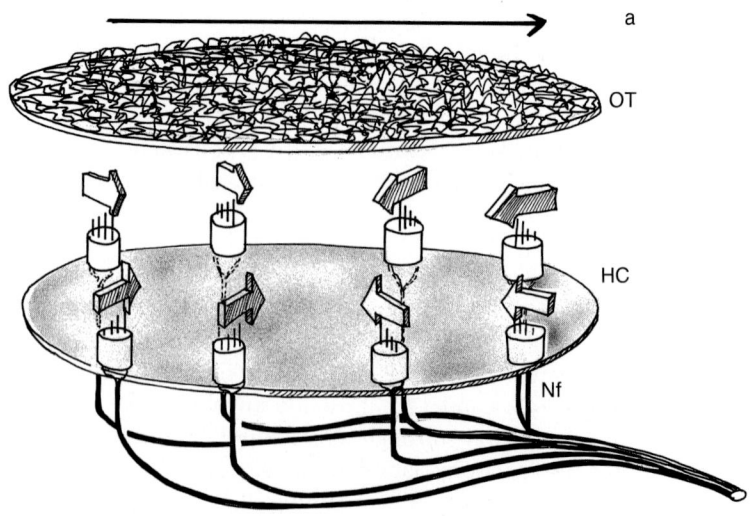

Figure 143.8 Simplified otolith organ. The otoconial mass (OT) is suspended above the sensory hair cells (HC) in an exploded view. Each hair cell is innervated by one afferent nerve fiber (Nf). These nerve fibers join together to form a branch of the vestibular nerve. Each hair cell has a *small arrow* above it that corresponds to the direction of its functional PV. This *arrow* is always pointing in the direction of the kinocilium. The *long arrow* above the otolithic mass is a linear acceleration vector. The response of hair cell depends on the cosine of the direction between its PV and linear acceleration (*a*).

linear acceleration in three-dimensional space has not been determined.

Figure 143.9 illustrates the basic principle by which two otolith organs operating in the same plane can be used to detect head tilt or translation of the head in the plane of the otolithic macula. With no acceleration in the plane of the macula, the rate of action potentials from afferent neurons innervating each otolith organ should be constant and equal. But once the head is tilted to the left, afferent discharge from the left otolithic organ will increase, while that of the right otolithic organ will decrease. This is due to the effect of gravity on the otoconial mass. Comparable responses will also be seen with translation of the head to the right where the otoconial mass will accelerate to the left. This acceleration again produces an increase of the firing rate of the left nerve and decrease in the firing rate of the right nerve. In both cases, maximum sensitivity is obtained by means of subtracting the firing rate of the right nerve from that of the left. This illustration (Fig. 143.9) shows that the asymmetry present in one hair cell innervating an otolith organ can be canceled by combining it with a signal from a hair cell that has the same polarization factor in the other side. It also shows that afferent activity from otolith organs alone cannot be used to distinguish between translation and tilt.

Einstein recognized that an ambiguity exists between linear acceleration and gravity. In aviation, this can be a real problem during the acceleration of takeoff, when pilots have trouble differentiating the acceleration of the airplane from the gravity vector. Because translational motion in one direction creates the same inertial force as gravity to tilt in the opposite direction (Fig. 143.9), this problem is known as tilt-translational ambiguity. Recent research has demonstrated that the CNS uses semicircular canal information (activated during tilt but not during translation) in combination with the otolith input to distinguish, for example, tilting the head upward versus accelerating forward as in a car, sled, or airplane (10). However, this mechanism works poorly at low frequency rotations, because the semicircular canals work poorly at low frequencies. In the circumstance where the rotational component of the motion is at low frequencies (less than 0.1 Hz), the brain uses visual or tactile information to help interpret the otolith signal. In the absence of nonotolith input, such as vision or rotation at frequencies above 0.1 Hz, the system defaults to interpreting linear acceleration as tilt (or gravity). Returning to the aviation example, fighter pilots taking off from an aircraft carrier deck at night will feel as if they are tilted backward during forward acceleration. Because of the ambiguity, the natural correction for this feeling is to steer the plane downward, which could result in disaster.

VESTIBULAR BRAINSTEM

Vestibular afferent neurons are bipolar neurons whose cell bodies reside in the inferior and superior vestibular (Scarpa) ganglion (Fig. 143.1). Following their terminations on hair cells, the peripheral (dendritic) processes of these neurons exit the sensory neuroepithelium and collect in the inferior and superior vestibular nerves. The inferior division includes neurons from the posterior canal and the posterior saccule, whereas the anterior division includes utricular, horizontal canal, and anterior canal afferent neurons as well as afferent neurons from the anterior portions of the saccular macula. Central axonal branches of primary afferent neurons ramify in the vestibular nuclei. Afferent terminals from the different end organs primarily innervate the various divisions of the vestibular nuclei, although vestibular afferent terminations are seen in the cerebellum and other brainstem nuclei as well. The precise terminations by end organ (semicircular canal or otolith) in the CNS are similar in many species (11). Not only does the brainstem region receive convergent input from different branches of the vestibular nerve, but individual neurons in the vestibular nuclei can also receive afferent input from one, two, or more end organs (canal ampullae or otolithic maculae). Thus, the vestibular nuclei have the task of integrating information from multiple ipsilateral receptors.

There are four major vestibular nuclei in the brainstem: the lateral (Deiters), superior, medial, and inferior (spinal or descending) nuclei. In addition, there are several minor vestibular nuclei that have been identified in several

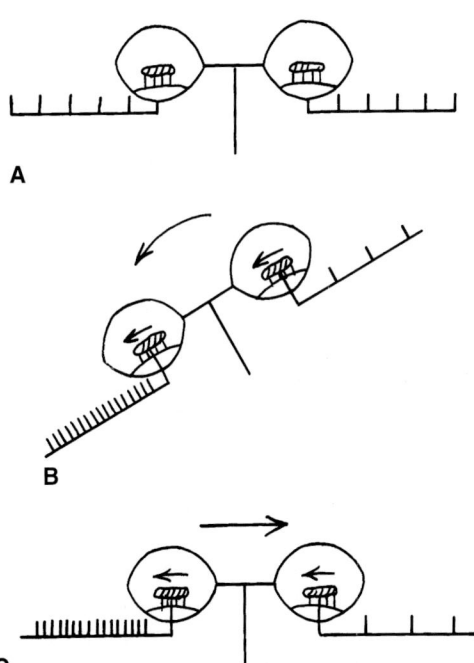

Figure 143.9 Modulation of the pulse interval by shearing of the utricular otolith membrane of the vertebrate vestibular organ. **A:** Horizontal position at rest. **B:** Tilted to the left. **C:** During linear acceleration to the right. (Modified from Barlow JS. Inertia navigation as a basis for animal navigation. *J Theor Biol* 1990;6:76, with permission.)

different species by various investigators. The vestibular nuclei not only receive vestibular information but other information pertaining to spatial orientation as well. These inputs include optokinetic signals through the accessory optic system, neck proprioceptive signals, and Purkinje cell projections from the cerebellar cortex. After leaving the vestibular nuclei, vestibular signals are passed throughout the CNS along distinct neural pathways. The primary upstream targets of the vestibular nuclei include (a) the ocular motor nuclei via the medial longitudinal fasciculus and the ascending tract of Deiters, (b) the spinal cord via the medial and lateral vestibulospinal tracts, (c) the cerebellum via the cerebellar peduncles, and (d) the contralateral vestibular nuclei by way of the vestibular commissural system. Other neural pathways connect the vestibular nuclei with the thalamus, which are involved in our perception of our orientation in space, and the autonomic system, which has implications in motion sickness and blood pressure control.

One important function of the vestibular commissural system is reciprocal inhibition. For many neurons in the central vestibular nuclei, their discharge is modulated not only by excitatory input from the ipsilateral vestibular nerve, but also by crossed inhibitory input from the contralateral side (inhibition of an inhibitory input is similar to excitation). This commissural inhibition is often modulated in phase with the paired canal from the contralateral labyrinth. Thus, a secondary neuron in the right vestibular nucleus might be driven by ipsilateral horizontal canal afferent neurons that are excitatory and increase firing for ipsilateral rotation and by inhibitory neurons that are modulated in phase with contralateral (left) rotation. This reciprocal mechanism is the basis of the so-called push–pull connection that increases the sensitivity of the system through convergence in signals between the functionally paired semicircular canals (left horizontal–right horizontal, left anterior–right posterior, left posterior–right anterior) in either ear. In this way, the paired canals complement one another and may help cancel out the asymmetries inherent in hair cell transduction mechanisms and afferent firing patterns.

The best studied vestibular reflex is the vestibuloocular reflex. Vestibuloocular reflexes are of two types: compensatory reflexes that stabilize gaze during motion and orienting reflexes that align the eye with the gravitational vector. One of the challenges for the nervous system is to translate signals from the semicircular canal planes into coordinates appropriate for effector action. Those who study the vestibular system use an external frame of reference as shown in Figure 143.3: the interaural or *pitch* axis, the nasal–occipital or *roll* axis, and the rostral–caudal or *yaw* axis. The vestibulo-oculomotor system, however, is thought to use a coordinate system based on the orientation of the three pairs of semicircular canals. Experiments have shown that stimulation of afferent branches of the vestibular nerve that come exclusively from one semicircular canal produces reflexive eye movements that tend to rotate around the axis of greatest sensitivity for that canal. The three agonist–antagonist pairs of eye muscles themselves do not produce eye movements that completely correspond to these axes of orientation of the semicircular canals. Thus, there is a distribution of signals from the semicircular canals to produce compensatory eye movement of the desired magnitude and direction. Because the orientation of the three pairs of semicircular canals roughly aligns with three pairs of extraocular eye muscles, the transformation in the CNS to coordinate eye movements is relatively simple. In contrast, control of head position and trunk position is much more complicated, and overall is not as well understood.

The nervous system can adapt its response by comparing vestibular input to other sensory input. When the head moves, the vestibuloocular reflex stabilizes the image of an object in space on the retina by producing an eye movement compensatory to the head movement. For example, the motion of the head 10 degrees to the right produces eye movement 10 degrees to the left. Provisions have been made in the nervous system for this response to adapt when necessary, owing to factors such as disease or aging. One such example is people with myopia who wear eyeglasses. If the magnification of the lens is 1.2 times, rotation of the head 10 degrees to the right produces rotation of the world as viewed by the eye 12 degrees to the left and therefore demands a corresponding reflexive eye movement 12 degrees to the left. The nervous system makes this form of adaptive change to resolve a conflict between afferent inputs, in this case vestibular and visual inputs. In this example, the nervous system can correspondingly increase the amount of eye movement produced for a given head movement so that the error between head motion input and eye motion response is reduced to nearly zero. This gain of plasticity requires participation of the flocculus of the cerebellum.

CURRENT VESTIBULAR INQUIRY

Like most fields in basic sciences, the vestibular system is actively studied in a number of excellent laboratories. Among the many actively investigated areas are the pharmacology of the vestibular periphery, interactions between active head movements and the passive vestibular reflexes, the role of vestibular signals in spatial orientation, the function of the vestibular efferent system, physiologic and cellular mechanisms of adaptation and compensation after vestibular injury, and the adaptation of the vestibular system to microgravity. In addition, efforts are ongoing to develop prosthetic devices to aid patients with vestibular deficits. This research holds the promise of improving our understanding of this vital, well-conserved, and underappreciated "sixth" sensory system.

HIGHLIGHTS

- The vestibular system is an inertial guidance system in vertebrates. It is composed of two or more sensors of linear acceleration and three or more sensors of angular acceleration in each inner ear. The right and left inner ear structures are mirror images of each other.

- Vestibular motion sensors use inertial elements connected to sensory hair cells. Both linear and angular acceleration sensors in the inner ear use a three-step process to convert accelerations of the head into useful information for the nervous system. The elements in these three steps are inertia, sensory hair cells, and nerve fibers connected to the hair cells.

- Vestibular sensory hair cells are arranged in orderly arrays. The orientation of a hair cell is defined by the orientation of its kinocilia. This orientation is known as *morphologic polarization*. A corresponding physiologic attribute is called *functional polarization*, which means the hair cell is the most sensitive to displacement along its anatomically defined PV.

- Vestibular organs are arranged by pairs in functional planes. The right and left lateral semicircular canals lie in the same plane. The other four vertical canals lie in planes nearly perpendicular to the plane of the horizontal canal pair. The anterior vertical canal on one side is in nearly the same plane as the posterior vertical canal on the other, forming a functional pairing of the semicircular canals. The otolithic organs are similarly paired.

- Head movement produces compensatory reflexive eye movement. When the head moves, the vestibuloocular reflex tends to stabilize the image of an object in space on the retina by producing eye movement compensatory to the head movement.

REFERENCES

1. Angelaki DE, Cullen KE. Vestibular system: the many facets of a multimodal sense. *Ann Rev Neurosci* 2008;31:125–150.
2. Lysakowski A, Goldberg JM. Morphophysiology of the vestibular periphery. In: Highstein SM, Popper A, Fay RR, eds. *The vestibular system.* New York: Springer-Verlag, 2004:57–152.
3. Gillespie PG, Müller U. Mechanotransduction by hair cells: models, molecules, and mechanisms. *Cell* 2009;139:33–44.
4. Zdebik AA, Wangemann P, Jentsch TJ. Potassium ion movement in the inner ear: insights from genetic disease and mouse models. *Physiology* 2009;24:307–316.
5. Merchant SN, Velazquez-Villasenor L, Tsuji K, et al. Temporal bone studies of the human peripheral vestibular system. Normative vestibular hair cell data. *Ann Otol Rhinol Laryngol Suppl* 2000;181:3–13.
6. Lysakowski A, Goldberg JM. Ultrastructural analysis of the cristae ampullares in the squirrel monkey (Saimiri sciureus). *J Comp Neurol* 2008;511:47–64.
7. Goldberg JM. Afferent diversity and the organization of central vestibular pathways. *Exp Brain Res* 2000;130:277–297.
8. Minor LB, Lasker DM, Backous DD, et al. Horizontal vestibuloocular reflex evoked by high-acceleration rotations in the squirrel monkey. I. Normal responses. *J Neurophysiol* 1999;82:1254–1270.
9. Holt JC, Lysakowski A, Goldberg JM. Efferent vestibular system. In: Ryugo DK, Fay RR, Popper AN, eds. *Springer handbook of auditory research: auditory and vestibular efferents,* Vol. 38. New York: SpringerScience+Business Media, LLC, 2011.
10. Angelaki DE, Dickman JD. Gravity or translation: central processing of vestibular signals to detect motion or tilt. *J Vestibular Res* 2003;13:245–253.
11. Newlands SD, Perachio AA. Central projections of the vestibular nerve: a review and single fiber study in the Mongolian gerbil. *Brain Res Bull* 2003;60:475–495.

144 Vestibular and Balance Laboratory Studies

Neil T. Shepard   *Kristen L. Janky*   *Jaynee A. Handelsman*

This chapter is one of the clinical companions to the preceding chapter on the vestibular function and anatomy. A clear understanding of those concepts and principles is vital to the appreciation of the information presented herein. The anatomy and physiology of the vestibular and balance systems form the basis against which interpretations of patients' presenting history, signs, symptoms and laboratory test results are developed. The nomenclature used in this chapter will follow that suggested for the International Classification of Vestibular Disorders (1). Therefore, the following are the definitions of the terms used to describe symptoms for patients reporting with vertigo, dizziness, or unsteadiness:

- Vertigo—sensation of self (internal) or environmental (external) movement when such movement is not occurring, for example, spinning, rocking, swaying, tilting, bobbing, sliding, or bouncing.
- Dizziness—sensation of disturbed or impaired spatial orientation without a sensation of self or environment movement.
- Unsteadiness—sensation of being unstable—independent of position without a directional preference.

In considering the evaluation of the patient with complaints of vertigo, unsteadiness, and dizziness or combinations of these descriptors, one must look beyond just the peripheral and central vestibular system with its oculomotor connections. The various pathways involved in postural control, only part of which have direct or indirect vestibular inputs, should be kept in mind during an evaluation. Additionally, significant variations in symptoms and test findings can be generated by migraine disorders (2) and/or anxiety disorders (3), yet these are diagnosed primarily by case history and require a specific line of questioning, not by the use of laboratory testing *per se*; however, the test helps to set up a profile.

Evaluation of the dizzy patient should be guided by the information required to make initial and subsequent management decisions. In the acute patient, the primary aim is to rule out significant cardiovascular and neurological disorders, quiet symptoms, and determine a working diagnosis. Extensive laboratory testing is generally unnecessary in the acute patient since the presenting symptoms and office examination will primarily guide initial management decisions (see chapter 165 by Joel Goebel on the clinical evaluation of the patient with vertigo in this text). In the chronic patient (defined as having symptoms that are intermittent or persistent for greater than 2 months), addressing the question of why natural central compensation has not taken place in a significant manner to reduce symptoms and establish a refined diagnosis and treatment program would be the goal. While aspects of the laboratory testing, especially caloric testing, can be of use in the acute patient, it is the exception that these would be used acutely. Therefore, for the purposes of this chapter, discussion is limited to the evaluation of the chronic patient.

For the chronic patient, a detailed neurotologic history together with a comprehensive direct vestibular office examination is as important as in the acute patient. In the chronic patient, a detailed pre-evaluation patient questionnaire combined with a focused history obtained at the start of laboratory testing can facilitate selection of appropriate laboratory tests and guide the examiner regarding what tests beyond a basic core series of evaluations are needed for any given patient. This use of a staged testing protocol effectively allows laboratory information to be collected prior to the clinician's direct office interview and examination so that all of the information can then be collectively analyzed in the context of the history and presenting symptoms (4).

Defining the role of the laboratory testing becomes an important aspect of the understanding of the benefit of the studies that are currently available.

- Determination of extent and site of lesion within the peripheral and central vestibular system
- Determination of the functional limitations in static and dynamic postural control (these may be related directly to gait abnormalities) and functional performance of the vestibuloocular reflex (VOR)
- Assessment of the status of the compensation process
- Along with symptom presentation, to aid in the prognosis and design of vestibular and balance rehabilitation

The collective use of the information is most often in the confirmation of the suspected site of lesion and diagnosis, both derived from the patient's history and direct office vestibular evaluation with audiometric evaluation. This does not imply a prioritized order to the testing versus the office visit, as with chronic dizzy patients it can be very useful to triage them to laboratory evaluations prior to the office visit.

A common misconception is that the studies will render a specific diagnosis or at a minimum drive the remainder of the investigation and help determine levels of disability. However, when the various tests listed below are reviewed and correlated with high-level activities of daily living, virtually no significant relationships exist for the chronic dizzy patient (5,6). Conversely, patient complaints cannot be used to predict the outcomes of these tests. In a limited manner, more functionally oriented evaluation tools such as computerized dynamic posturography (7) and dynamic visual acuity (DVA) testing (8) provide for correlation between test results, patient symptoms, and functional limitations (9,10). It is hypothesized that the reason for this dichotomy in test results versus functional disability and symptom complaints is the inability of the tests to adequately characterize the status of the central vestibular compensation process (9,11,12). Thus, vestibular laboratory testing is never a replacement for a detailed neurotologic history and physical examination, but needs to be interpreted in context of the history and physical examination.

LABORATORY STUDIES

The discussion to follow provides a brief description of the various laboratory studies that are available for the investigation of the patient with vertigo, dizziness, or unsteadiness. In each case, the purpose for the study, general information about administration of the test, and its general interpretations are provided. A detailed presentation of each of the studies is beyond the scope of this chapter and text. Interested readers are referred to other sources for further information (13–15). For organizational ease, the tests are divided into those in more routine use and those found only in dedicated tertiary balance centers.

Common Procedures

Electronystagmography/Videonystagmography
Electronystagmography (ENG) and videonystagmography (VNG) utilize complete computer-based systems for performing eye movement testing. During ENG testing, horizontal and vertical eye movements are recorded indirectly using electrodes via the corneoretinal potential (dipole). Electrodes are typically placed at each lateral canthus and above and below at least one eye with a common electrode on the forehead. During VNG testing, on the other hand, eye movements are recorded directly using infrared video cameras and digital video image technology. Specifically, for binocular recording, a reflected image of the eye is captured by cameras mounted above, in front of each eye or adjacent to the lateral canthi (Fig. 144.1) (16). For monocular recordings, a camera may be positioned directly in front of one eye (Fig. 144.1). Monocular recording has the disadvantage of failure to recognize and capture disconjugate eye movements. For both ENG and VNG, recording is typically limited to horizontal and vertical eye movements (three-dimensional systems are available adding the torsional movements but far from common use) and the data are recorded, digitally stored, and analyzed by the software in much the same way.

The ENG/VNG battery typically consists of a series of subtests designed to assess the function of the vestibular end organs, the central vestibuloocular pathways, and oculomotor processes, independent of vestibular input. ENG/VNG testing is useful for all patients of all ages with ongoing balance system disorders.

Oculomotor Evaluations
The availability of computerized ENG/VNG systems resulted in a transformation in the formal assessment of oculomotor function because of the ability to directly compare the timing and accuracy aspects of the eye movements with the target stimuli. The clinical utility of these tests is improved by exploiting their redundancy, such as when the results from multiple subtests point to the same site of lesion. Because oculomotor function changes with age, it is important to compare results with norms in order to minimize the number of false-positive results.

Gaze Stability Testing. The patient is typically asked to fixate on a stationary target that is positioned at eye level at a distance of 1 to 1.5 m, and the eyes are observed for the presence of nystagmus or other abnormal movements. Both horizontal and vertical eye movements are recorded. Eccentric gaze is also evaluated by moving the target from center to horizontally and vertically eccentric positions. Individuals without any peripheral or central involvement may demonstrate transient nystagmus when the eyes are at the extreme eccentric positions (referred to as end-point nystagmus, usually dies away within 5 seconds); persistent nystagmus that occurs when the targets are positioned appropriately is always considered to be abnormal.

Gaze-evoked nystagmus can originate from either the peripheral or the central vestibular system with differences in clinical presentation between the two. Nystagmus that is peripheral in origin will generally be direction fixed and

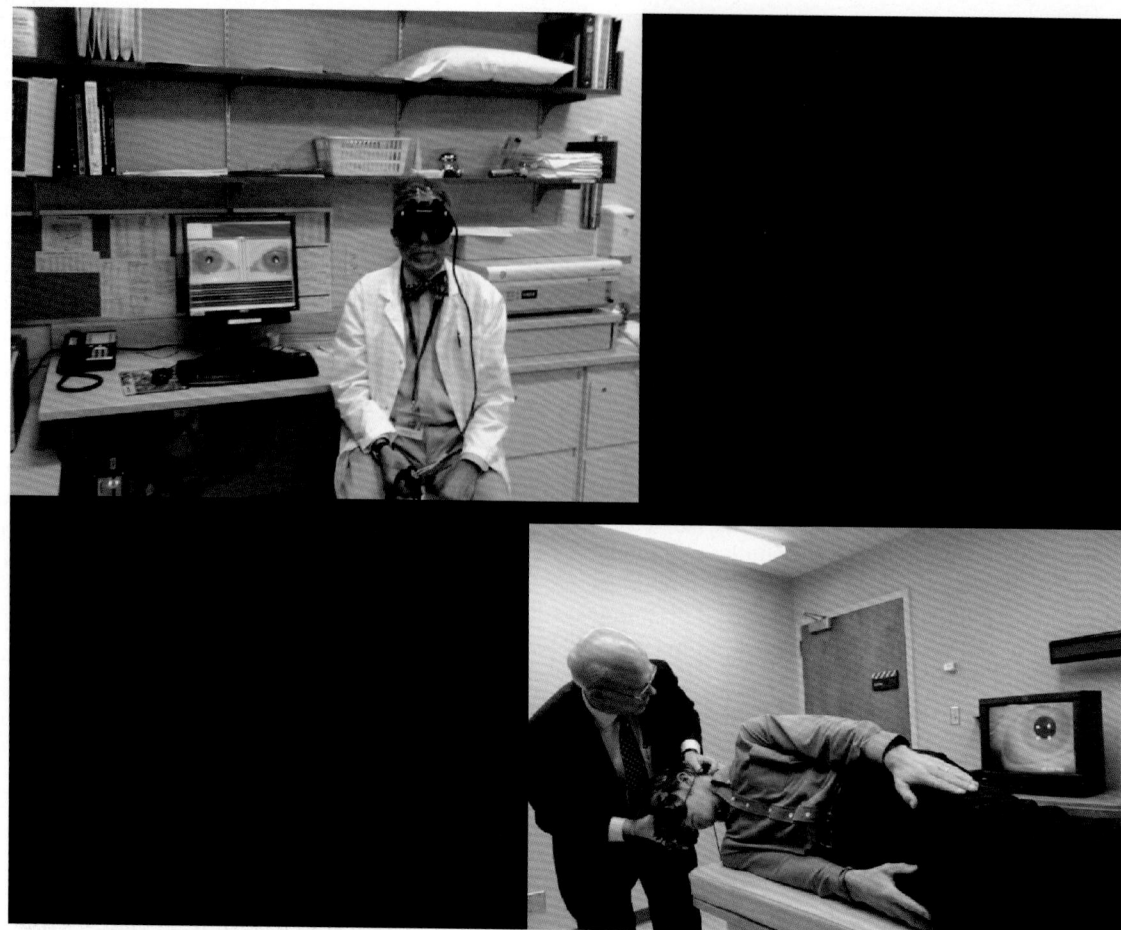

Figure 144.1 Shown are photographs that illustrate two eye movement recording techniques using VOG. The top picture shows a system with cameras mounted above reflecting see-through lenses and the display of the binocular recordings on the computer. The lower figure shows the use of monocular camera system affixed on the goggles directly in front of the right eye and the image seen on the monitor behind the subject.

enhance with fixation removed. Nystagmus is considered to be of central origin if it changes direction with change in gaze direction, if it evidences rebound, where the fast component of the nystagmus changes with the direction of the last eye movement, it enhances or does not change in intensity with fixation. In rare instances, eye movements can be consistent with both peripheral and central origin (e.g., Bruin nystagmus seen in Cerebellar-Pontine Angle mass lesions). A variety of other abnormalities may be evidenced during gaze testing such as congenital nystagmus and a variety of saccadic intrusions (special grouping of involuntary saccadic eye movements when visual fixation target is present), suggesting central vestibular system involvement (17).

Saccade Evaluation. As is the case in gaze testing, the patient is asked in saccade testing to follow a computer-controlled visual target. Random saccade testing is the paradigm that is most often included in the ENG/VNG battery. The patient's eye movements are compared by the computer to the target stimuli and the analysis typically yields measurements of saccade accuracy, latency, and velocity. Saccade accuracy generally refers to the amplitude of the eye movement relative to the target, latency refers to the delay between the onset of target movement and the initiation of eye movement, and velocity refers to the maximum sampled velocity of the saccade once it has been initiated.

The interpretation of saccade data must take into account patient variables such as age (although age-related normative data is not required), cognitive status, attention to task, visual acuity, sedation, sleep deprivation, comprehension level, and medications. Symmetrically inaccurate or slow saccades are often attributable to one or more of those variables. On the other hand, characteristic saccade abnormalities can suggest relatively specific sites of lesion and can provide for differentiating between brainstem and posterior cerebellar vermis involvement. For example, internuclear ophthalmoplegia (INO) results from a lesion in the medial longitudinal fasciculus (MLF) that causes a reduction of the neural signal to the ipsilateral medial rectus muscle (adduction) and preserved lateral-rectus-mediated movements (abduction). The resulting saccades in INO demonstrate slow velocity of adducting eye movements and overshoot for abducting eye movements. Details of the suggested lesion sites based on various combinations of abnormalities of latency, velocity, and accuracy are beyond the scope of this chapter but are available elsewhere (17).

Smooth Pursuit Tracking. Testing of smooth pursuit ability is conducted by having a patient follow a computer-controlled visual target, typically moving in a sinusoidal pattern that varies in frequency over time. Patient eye movements are evaluated qualitatively by looking for smooth eye movements. As is true with saccade testing, patient variables can negatively impact performance and interfere with interpretation. Use of age-appropriate norms is essential, as pursuit performance tends to degrade with age. The main outcome parameter is gain, which is calculated by dividing eye velocity by target velocity. Of all the oculomotor subtests, pursuit tracking has been demonstrated to be the most sensitive to central vestibular system abnormalities; however, it does not provide the same site-of-lesion localization as the remaining oculomotor subtests (17). Abnormalities with pursuit are typically taken as an indication of possible vestibulocerebellar region involvement but lesions in a variety of other areas can produce abnormalities of pursuit especially when pursuit is disrupted for both eyes moving to the right or left. Asymmetrically impaired pursuit is a more specific finding and suggests a unilateral cerebellar hemispheric or asymmetrical posterior fossa lesion (13).

Optokinetic Nystagmus. In order to truly assess the optokinetic system, use of a full-field visual stimulus and a phenomenon called "optokinetic afternystagmus" is required (13). The production of true optokinetic nystagmus involves a combination of the neurological substrate involved with smooth pursuit tracking together with areas that respond to moving visual stimuli in a full-field format but do not respond to head movement, the so-called optokinetic areas. Further, when viewing a full-field (90% or more of the visual field filled with the repeated moving targets) stimulus, the initiation of the nystagmus is dominantly a result of smooth pursuit tracking with the OKN component added as the stimulus is continued requiring seconds to fully develop. The response then continues as a combination of both smooth pursuit tracking and optokinetics. Therefore, to evaluate OKN function in isolation from smooth pursuit, one must take advantage of a perseveration of nystagmus caused by stimulation of the optokinetic system when the person is suddenly put into the dark after a minimum of 30 seconds worth of stimulation (called optokinetic after nystagmus [OKAN]). As soon as the target has been extinguished for 1 second, the smooth pursuit system no longer has any influence and the OKAN is a direct result of the activity of the optokinetic system reflected through the area of the brainstem referred to as the velocity storage system. In order to produce the OKN

stimulation through retinal input and signals transmitted via the accessory optic track, the stimulus needs to fill a minimum of 90% of the visual field and be capable of producing a circularvection effect (the illusion of circular motion when not moving).

Therefore, optokinetic nystagmus testing as a part of an ENG/VNG battery using a laser target or a traditional light bar is not a true optokinetic test but is a test dominated by smooth pursuit. Abnormal optokinetic nystagmus has a localizing value that is similar to smooth pursuit, although the sensitivity is poorer. For that reason, the cost–benefit ratio of inclusion of this test in the battery is poor.

Spontaneous Nystagmus

This test is performed with the patient sitting upright with the head straight. Eye movements are recorded while the patient is gazing straight ahead (not imagining a target) with visual fixation removed. Jerk nystagmus is the principal abnormality and is typically classified by the direction of the fast component of the nystagmus but measured by the velocity of the slow component. Clinically significant, direction-fixed nystagmus is interpreted to indicate pathology within the peripheral vestibular system if the oculomotor evaluation is normal and the nystagmus is significantly suppressed with visual fixation.

Hyperventilation Testing

The purpose of the hyperventilation test is to help diagnose, or unmask, disorders of the peripheral vestibular system and/or VIII cranial nerve (18–22). Secondly, the test can suggest possible anxiety disorder via premature symptoms without nystagmus (23). The hyperventilation test is completed by first removing fixation, either by Frenzel lenses or infrared goggles, and then having the patient take one breath per second for 30 to 90 seconds. Nystagmus induced by hyperventilation is considered significant if it persists greater than 5 seconds and if the peak slow-phase velocity is greater than 3 to 4 degrees per second, subtracting out any preexisting spontaneous nystagmus. If no nystagmus is provoked but the patient becomes symptomatic within the first 20 to 30 seconds, then anxiety issues are suspected.

Hyperventilation-induced nystagmus can beat ipsilesionally (with the fast-phase beating toward the side involved) or contralesionally (with the fast-phase beating away from the side involved). As a general rule of thumb, hyperventilation-induced nystagmus more often beats contralesionally in peripheral vestibular system lesions and ipsilesionally in VIII nerve or retrocochlear lesions: however, this relationship is not mutually exclusive.

Headshake

The headshake test also helps uncover asymmetries in peripheral and central vestibular system function and serves as an indication of dynamic central compensation. The headshake test is completed by removing fixation. The patient's head is shaken back and forth in the horizontal plane at approximately 2 to 4 Hz for 10 to 15 seconds. Post headshake nystagmus is considered clinically significant if at least three to five consecutive beats of nystagmus are present directly following the headshake and if the nystagmus peak slow-phase velocity is greater than 3 to 4 degrees per second after subtracting out any preexisting spontaneous nystagmus (20,24–26). Both vertical and horizontal headshaking can also be completed. The headshake test has relatively low sensitivity (30% to 35%) but high specificity (90% to 95%) in peripheral vestibular disorders, with the incidence of postheadshake nystagmus increasing as the severity of caloric paresis increases. Postheadshake nystagmus has also been documented in as many as 50% of normal controls (27) and in horizontal canal benign paroxysmal position vertigo (BPPV) (28). Vertical nystagmus in response to either a horizontal or vertical headshake is frequently seen in central vestibuloocular disorders (29,30).

Testing for Benign Paroxysmal Position Vertigo

Doing the Hallpike and roll tests are a common part of the VNG; however, the most common form of BPPV, posterior canal, cannot be recognized with the printouts of a typical 2-dimensional recording system since the principle movement is torsional. Therefore, in reality, these tests are clinical office tests where the examiner must watch and report the eye movements with typical recordings unnecessary. However, if a video recording is available that can be of use in reviewing the total eye movements during the performance of the Hallpike or roll tests.

Static Positional Testing

The purpose of static positional testing is to examine the effect of gravity on positional changes of the head—otolithic influence. Positional nystagmus is present if the nystagmus is provoked by taking a provocative position that produces the jerk nystagmus that represents a change from spontaneous or not present spontaneously. This is the most commonly occurring finding in ENG/VNG testing. Eye movements are recorded while the patient assumes a number of positions that involve head turning and changing the position of the head relative to gravity. Static positional testing is generally completed in the sitting, supine, body right, body left, and precaloric positions and additionally, with the head turned right and left in the sitting, supine, and head hanging positions to examine the influence of cervical region on symptoms and eye movements. Positional nystagmus is classified as either direction fixed (e.g., right beating in all positions) or direction changing (e.g., right beating in some positions and left beating in others). Direction-changing nystagmus may be further categorized as geotropic (nystagmus beating toward the earth) or apogeotropic (nystagmus beating away from the earth). Generally, positional nystagmus is nonlocalizing, needing the interpretation to be done in the context of the oculomotor findings. Pure vertical nystagmus and

nystagmus that changes direction in a fixed head position are of central origin and are the exceptions to the nonlocalizing aspect.

Caloric Irrigation Testing

Bithermal caloric testing is the only portion of the test battery that allows the examiner to evaluate individual ear function, and for that reason, it is valuable in assessing the relative responsiveness of the vestibular end organs. In caloric testing, a nonphysiologic stimulus (air or water) is utilized to induce stimulation or inhibition in the semicircular canals by creating a temperature gradient from the external auditory canal to the horizontal canal. The response is primarily the result of a pressure differential across the cupula caused by the temperature gradient coupled with placing the horizontal canal in the vertical plane, although other variables are also involved. Specifically, the head is positioned so that the horizontal canal is oriented parallel to the gravitational vector, with the nose of the patient upward and the head tilted 30 degrees upward from the horizontal plane. During a warm irrigation, the less-dense fluid attempts to rise upward. This produces a deviation of the cupula toward the utricle because of the pressure differential across the cupula, causing stimulation of the eighth nerve. The reverse action occurs for the more dense area of cooled fluid, causing inhibition. This results in the well-known mnemonic *COWS*, which refers to the direction of the fast component of the nystagmus: *Cold Opposite, Warm Same* (relative to the side of irrigation).

Typically, either water or air serves as the thermal stimulus. The stimulus temperature and duration are dependent upon stimulus type. Specifically, open-loop water irrigations are typically performed at 30°C and 44°C for cool and warm irrigations, respectively, whereas the appropriate air temperatures are 24°C and 50°C for cool and warm irrigations, respectively. Additionally, because air is a less efficient stimulus, the duration of the irrigation must be increased in order to obtain an optimal response. Recording time may also need to be increased when air calorics are used, particularly in the case of a tympanic membrane perforation. In many clinical settings, the typical stimulus duration for water irrigations is 30 to 40 seconds, while the typical stimulus duration for air is 60 to 90 seconds. Stimulus duration may be adjusted to accommodate patient needs, although in order to be able to make interear comparisons, it is essential that both ears are tested under identical conditions. Regardless of stimulus type, each ear is typically irrigated twice, alternating in such a way that the expected nystagmus direction is different for subsequent irrigations. The interstimulus interval should be sufficient to allow the response from the previous irrigation to have subsided completely.

Although the use of air is popular and has a practical advantage of being less messy, open-loop water provides a more consistent stimulus as it is impacted less by the shape or size of the external auditory meatus. With air, it is essential for the examiner to have a clear view of the tympanic membrane throughout the irrigation in order to obtain an optimal response. While that is ideal with water irrigations as well, it is not necessary because the flow rate is sufficient to reach the tympanic membrane even in the face of a narrow or bent ear canal and the temperature of water maintains itself, whereas with air, as it contacts the walls the temperature changes at a significantly greater rate. The new American National Standards Institute guidelines for performing an ENG/VNG only provide information on open-loop water caloric irrigation in part because of the technical difficulties of air (31).

The caloric test is an assessment of the horizontal semicircular canal and, subsequently, the superior branch of the VIII cranial nerve. Sensitivity and specificity of the caloric test in response to air has been reported as 82% and 82%, respectively, and in response to water as 84% and 84%, respectively (32). Since there are no other objective tests considered as sensitive as the caloric irrigation test to determine horizontal canal involvement, the use of presenting symptoms becomes the comparator of choice for these studies.

Vestibular-Evoked Myogenic Potential

The purpose of the vestibular-evoked myogenic potential (VEMP) is to provide information regarding VIII nerve and otolith organ function and to potentially separate superior from inferior vestibular nerve and likewise utricular from saccular involvement (33,34). Like the caloric test, one benefit of the VEMP is that it provides ear-specific information. There are two types of VEMP responses: the cervical VEMP (cVEMP) and the ocular VEMP (oVEMP). The cVEMP is measured at the sternocleidomastoid muscle (SCM) and is a reflection of the ipsilateral vestibulocollic reflex, measuring the pathway from the saccule, down the inferior vestibular nerve to the brainstem, and then to motorneurons in the SCM, which result in a relaxation of the contracted SCM muscle (35). The oVEMP, on the other hand, is measured at the inferior oblique muscle (directly under the eye) and is a reflection of the VOR. The pathway for the oVEMP is less well understood than that for the cVEMP; however, recent evidence suggests that this response measures the pathway from the utricle, down the superior vestibular nerve to the brainstem, and then to motor neurons of the contralateral inferior oblique muscle, which result in excitation. The innate differences between the o- and cVEMP responses are that the cVEMP arises from the saccule and is an ipsilateral, inhibiting response while the oVEMP presumably arises from the utricle and is a contralateral, excitatory response. Both the o- and cVEMP are typically obtained in response to air conduction stimuli (clicks and/or tone burst) with the best waveforms occurring in response to 500 Hz tone bursts. VEMPs are reported in terms of threshold or suprathreshold amplitude, with subsequent interaural amplitude comparisons often reported. The outcome parameter reported (threshold vs. amplitude) is generally dependent on the pathology being assessed.

VEMPs have demonstrated their effectiveness for aiding diagnosis in a variety of conditions. Most notably, VEMPs are part of a standard battery when diagnosing superior canal dehiscence syndrome (SCDS) and other third window disorders. SCDS has been characterized by significantly lower o- and cVEMP thresholds and significantly larger o- and cVEMP amplitudes (36). The o- and cVEMP can also provide complementary information in determining site-of-lesion involvement in vestibular neuritis. In the event of superior vestibular neuritis, cVEMPs have been shown to be intact with absent oVEMPs and abnormal caloric responses (33,34). Conversely, inferior vestibular neuritis has been characterized by absent cVEMP and present oVEMP with normal caloric responses (34). Because the VEMP does not induce sensations of vertigo and provides ear-specific information, VEMP testing is an excellent assessment tool for the pediatric population.

Less Commonly Available Assessment Techniques

Secondary to the more limited use of the following tests, the respective discussions are less detailed than those above.

On-Axis Total Body Rotation—Rotational Chair

The purpose of the test is to expand the investigation of the peripheral vestibular system by applying natural head movements and using three outcome parameters to characterize the peripheral vestibular system together with its central projections as to (a) the timing relationship between eye movement and steady state (sinusoidal protocol) or transient (a step test) head movement, (b) the overall responsiveness of the system to the stimulus, and (c) the responsiveness when rotating to the right versus the left. In this manner, the test expands across frequency (beyond that of stimulation by caloric irrigations) the investigation of the function of the peripheral vestibular systems. This is the only test to investigate the extent of and verification of those with bilateral peripheral system hypofunction (37,38). The test is administered by having the patient seated in a chair that is driving in a sinusoidal or fixed velocity trajectory by a motor affixed to the chair. The axis of rotation is vertical and passes through the center of the patient's head (Fig. 144.2).

Off-Axis Total Body Rotation—Unilateral Centrifugation

The class of off-axis rotational tests has been developed for assessing the otolith organs (38). Unilateral centrifugation is one protocol of the off-axis total body rotation test performed with rotary chair equipment. With unilateral centrifugation, the chair is translated laterally, which projects the vertical axis of rotation through the peripheral vestibular organ on the right or the left (Fig. 144.3). The purpose of the test is to allow for evaluation of each utricular organ individually. Investigations to date show reliable detection

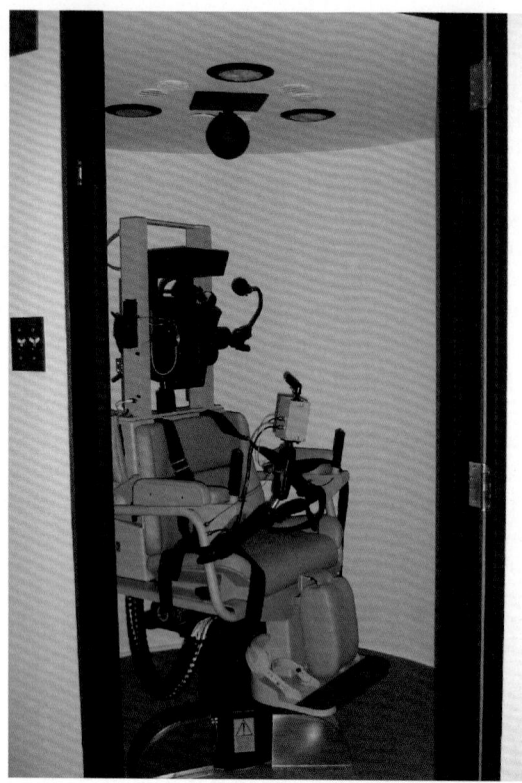

Figure 144.2 This is a photograph of a rotational chair system with the drive motor under the chair and the system enclosed in a light-tight enclosure (photo taken through the open door). The system has a means for maintaining the head secured to the chair and straps for maintaining the body still in the chair. A face camera (inferred) for visualizing the patient's face is seen on an extension coming off the right arm rest. Not shown is an inferred scene camera in the ceiling. The chair shown is able to perform lateral shifts on the drive motor to change the way the axis of rotation aligns with the head of the subject as shown in Figure 144.3.

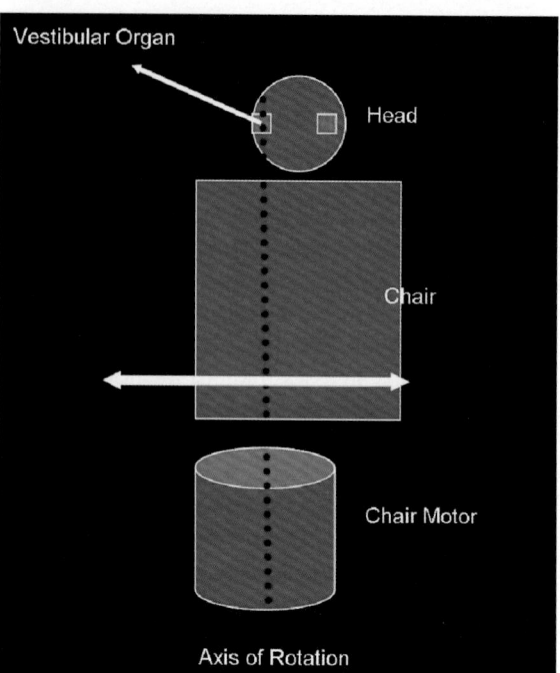

Figure 144.3 The cartoon illustrates the concept of shifting the axis of rotation to go through either the left or right (illustrated here through the right) vestibular end organ. In rotation under this condition, a specific horizontal force would be placed on the left utricular system that would cause a change in perception of vertical (tilting to the left), and when the subject is then asked to set a projected line to their perception of vertical they will set the line off to the right—a test called subjective visual vertical. During the stimulation, the eyes counter roll back to the right, and this is felt to be the basic cause for the shift in the line representing the subject's perception of vertical. The chair can then be shifted to the left and the same force placed on the right utricle and the tilt perception would be to the right and the vertical line is set to the left.

of those with surgically confirmed utricular lesions. The interested reader is referred to a recent study that provides a review of work to date contained in the introduction (39).

Head-Impulse Test

Starting as the head-thrust test for use in bedside evaluations (see chapter 165 on office evaluation by Joel Goebel), this test has expanded to be used with equipment and is referred to as the head-impulse test (HIT) (40). The test provides for a means of individually assessing the function of the VOR for the horizontal canals on the right and the left. It also provides for the assessment of the anterior and posterior canals individually. The assessment is in a different frequency range than that of the caloric test but there is a reasonable correlation between the caloric results and those of the clinical version (Head-Thrust Test) (41). Recently, with the addition of high-speed video recording devices and computer analysis, the sensitivity of the test for identification and monitoring of the function of the six individual canals has been improved (40). This improvement comes from being able to calculate the actual gain of the eye movement for a specific head movement. This technique avoids

problems with central nervous compensatory activity that cause difficulty in the simple identification of a corrective saccade when the eye is taken off the target with a head movement secondary to a deficient VOR (42).

VEMP Threshold Response Curves

The cVEMP as discussed above provides for an assessment of the status of the saccule. The function of the saccule varies over frequency. When plotting VEMP threshold across frequency, the saccule demonstrates specific tuning characteristics. The most sensitive frequency is at 500 Hz (43) (Fig. 144.4). It has been suggested (44) that in an endolymphatic condition like that of Meniere syndrome the most sensitive frequency shifts upward. Therefore, the use of the threshold response curve is being proposed as an independent study that may be able to assist in the diagnosis of Meniere syndrome or the more general condition of endolymphatic hydrops. A pilot study using this method showed sensitivity and specificity for identification of Meniere syndrome to be 48% to 50% and 79% to 88%, respectively, suggesting that while a negative test is not useful, a test showing the upward shift may add to the argument of the disorder being present (45).

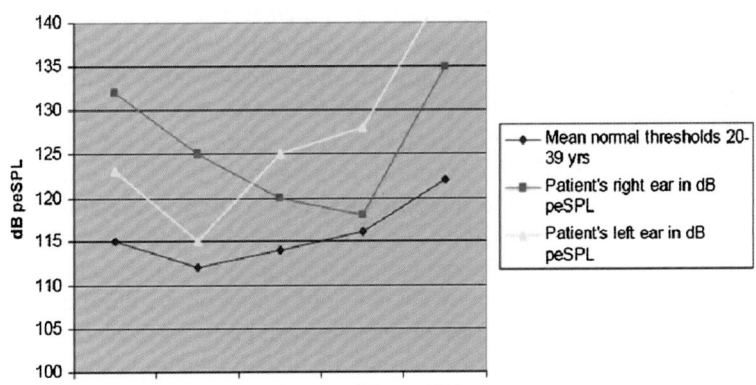

VEMP Threshold Curve

- Mean normal thresholds 20-39 yrs
- Patient's right ear in dB peSPL
- Patient's left ear in dB peSPL

Figure 144.4 The graphic shows an example of the cVEMP threshold response curves for a patient with right Meniere syndrome. The plot gives cVEMP thresholds (in dB peak SPL) as a function of tone burst stimuli at 250 to 1 kHz and then with a click stimulus. The involved right side (plotted by *squares*) shows that the most sensitive frequency has shifted from the typical at 500 Hz (shown for the normative data by the *diamonds*), whereas the uninvolved left side (plotted in *triangles*) has a configuration that parallels the normal subjects.

Dynamic Visual Acuity and Gaze Stabilization Test

All of the investigative tools discussed to this point would be classified as extent and site-of-lesion studies. DVA and gaze stabilization test (GST) however, are considered studies that provide information about the functional use of the VOR. These tests could be normal even in the presence of VOR abnormalities (i.e., caloric hypofunction) indicating the lack of functional impact of the physiologic abnormality. Both studies assess clarity of vision during head motion. For DVA, the head speed is fixed and the size of the target to be recognized is systematically changed, whereas with the GST, the target size is fixed and head speed is varied. These studies are primarily used within treatment programs of vestibular and balance rehab to help monitor progress and determine deficits on which to focus. However, in symptomatic individuals, these studies have been shown to have sensitivity (64% to 71%) and specificity (88% to 93%) performance in identifying the involved peripheral system (46). The other purpose of these studies is to provide an objective quantification of a patient's complaint of oscillopsia. Recent work has been able to demonstrate that the DVA may be used as an effective indicator of falls risk (47).

Postural Control Assessment

For a given piece of laboratory equipment (Fig. 144.5), the purpose of the study will vary from strictly functional based to strictly site-of-lesion based contingent on the protocol used and the versatility of the equipment (48). Across most commercially available equipment, a similar protocol is used for functional evaluation of maintaining of upright stance under changing sensory input conditions—Sensory Organization Test (SOT) (Fig. 144.6). The outcome measure (independent of the details of the individual manufactures analysis) is body sway in anterior–posterior/medial–lateral space. The purpose of the SOT is to determine the individual's ability to utilize visual, proprioceptive/somatosensory, and vestibular cues for maintaining quiet stance. The test is performed by manipulating the visual and foot support surface cues in a systematic manner to reduce, or for vision eliminate, the cue, forcing reliance on other than

the normal combination. The outcome of the test is related to the patient's functional ability to maintain stance as the sensory input cues are varied. This information can be used for development and monitoring of treatment programs.

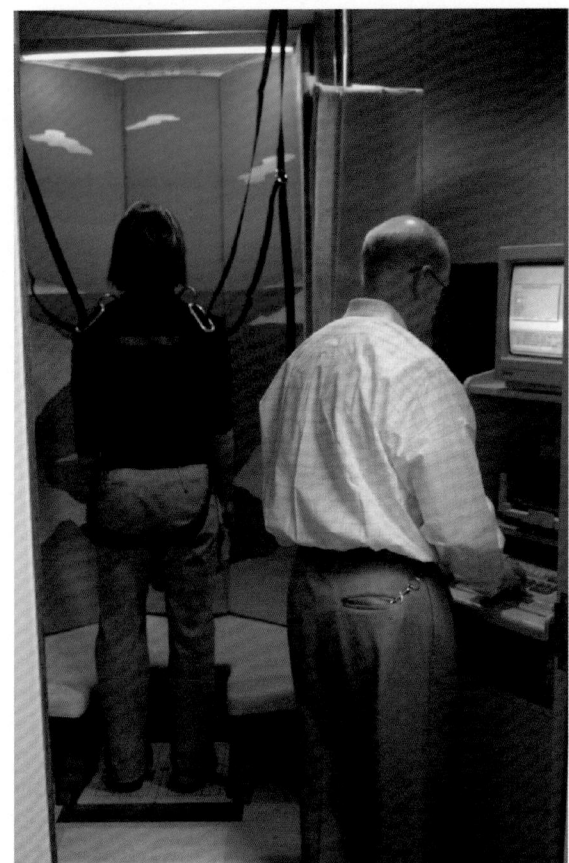

Figure 144.5 The photograph illustrates the positioning of a subject on one form of postural control platform secured from falling with the harness system. The subject is standing on a dual force plate that measures the change in the position of the force put against the right or left platform by the pressure of the foot against the floor (floor reaction force) for either the right or left foot. As the subject leans forward, the pressure under each foot shifts toward the toes. Movement of the platform on which the subject is standing and movement of the visual surround are used to perform the SOT discussed in the text, and the test conditions for the test are shown in Figure 144.6.

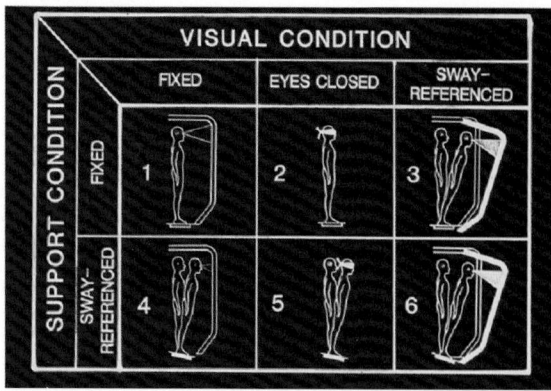

Figure 144.6 The schematic drawing shows the six conditions used in the SOT. The first three conditions provide for a stable, flat surface larger than the foot with plenty of friction to prevent slipping. Condition 1 is with eyes open, condition 2 has eyes closed, and condition 3 has eyes open but the visual surround is moving in response to the swaying of the subject on the platform so that visual information while accurate is of little or no use in knowing how the body is moving over the base of support (the feet). Conditions 4 to 6 use the same visual conditions as shown in 1 to 3 but now has the foot support surface (the force platform) moving in response to the subject's sway in the anterior/posterior plane.

The information is descriptive not diagnostic, therefore the SOT is not a site-of-lesion test (49).

Four other principle protocols are used in postural control assessment, all of which fall into the category of extent and site-of-lesion studies with the exception of #2. (a) Reaction to unexpected perturbation of the body's center of mass through tilt or linear translations, (b) protocol to determine an individual's ability to adapt to changes in surface orientation, (c) recording of distal lower limb muscles in response to sudden toes-up or down rotations around the ankle axis, and (d) quantifying an individual's sway response to changes in external auditory canal air pressure—focus on investigation of perilymphatic fistulas including canal dehiscences. Details of these tests are beyond the scope of this chapter, and the reader is referred to discussion by Shepard and Janky (50) for descriptions and list of references.

SPECIAL POPULATIONS

From the discussion above, it is clear that there are numerous tools available for the evaluation of the patient with complaints of dizziness, vertigo, and unsteadiness. There is overlap to a limited extent in the purpose such that not all studies are needed on every patient. The modest positive correlation between the various tests helps in trying to accommodate other than the otherwise normal patient with these complaints. Specifically, the child under the age 10 is better served by starting with rotational chair as an indication of possible peripheral vestibular system involvement. While most of the children above age 5 will cooperate with use of caloric irrigations, those 5 or under will not. For the child under age 2, it is unlikely the examiner would be able to obtain caloric irrigations; so again, the use of rotational chair can be very useful. If postural control is the primary focus

in a young child (5 or under), there are a variety of tools available to review the developmental status of postural control ability compared to normative ranges (51). Additionally, for the EquiTest equipment, the normative range for the SOT goes from 3 to 80 years. There are also age normative data for 3 years and above the surface EMG recordings and for cVEMPs. The main principle in testing a child is to select the tests related to the primary child or parent complaint and figure that the next test you perform (even if it is the first one) will be the last one you will obtain. Also, it is rare that video oculography (VOG) can be used on a child under 5 because of the size of the masks, and it is not likely that the child will tolerate wearing the device; therefore, any of the VNG equipment or rotational chair device used needs to be able to easily shift between electrode and video recordings.

Other groups where VOG techniques would not work would be the adults with significant ptosis, the patients who are unable to maintain eyes open in a darkened environment, or patients with significant claustrophobia. For each, the use of electrode recording is the best technique.

It would be a very rare situation that a patient with dizziness, vertigo, or balance complaints could not be tested in some manner. This may require a change in a specific protocol such as with the patient who is blind. Since they cannot see a visual stimulus, the traditional saccade and pursuit tracking tests cannot be performed. Yet, the patient can use tactile information and imagined visual targets by following the thumb for pursuit and by looking from one thumb to another to see if an approximation of pursuit and saccade performance is present. Other examples are the patients with prior mastoid surgery (especially canal wall down mastoidectomy). In that situation, caloric irrigations can be performed, but it is not necessary to have the same duration or temperatures on the left and right. The responses from right and left cannot be compared in the typical manner, so the use of the irrigation is simply to see if both sides respond. Therefore, this test on the surgical side should be performed to the patient's comfort. Irrigation time should not be longer than the duration required for symptoms to begin, if that occurs prior to the typical 30 to 40 seconds. In a normal peripheral vestibular system, symptoms in a radical mastoidectomy patient may begin in as short as just a few seconds.

A last example of a common difficulty is with the patient with significant visual acuity problems (e.g., macular degeneration or the patient with retinitis pigmentosa) who has difficulty finding a target that has suddenly changed location as in saccade testing. Instead of using a random paradigm, a fixed position with predictable timing would produce a better estimate of saccade ability.

SUMMARY AND ILLUSTRATIVE CASE EXAMPLE

The discussion above gives a brief summary of the tools available for the laboratory evaluation of the patient with vertigo, dizziness, and/or unsteadiness of central or peripheral vestibular origin. The key to the effective use of these tests is the integrated interpretation of the tests in the context of a detailed neurotologic history. In many cases, this requires a multidisciplinary approach but one in which the various specialists do not consult in isolation, but build their opinions integrated with those of the other subspecialists (audiology, neurology, psychiatry, general ENT or neurotology based on need, physical therapy). A case example is used to illustrate this concept.

A 43-year-old female presented with the primary complaint of constant internal vertigo and unsteadiness when lying, sitting, standing, and in motion. Symptoms were exacerbated with head/visual motion, visual complexity, and repeated noise exposure. The symptoms were reported to spontaneously increase in intensity without exposure to the visual or head movement stimuli. She reported hearing loss on the left with fluctuations. She was having an occasional fall without injury but not drop attacks. The patient was referred for a second opinion regarding her long-standing diagnosis of Meniere syndrome on the left.

The past medical history revealed long-standing history of migraine headaches. In 1999, she began with documented fluctuant and progressive loss of hearing on the left. Within a year, spontaneous events lasting 1 to 2 hours of external vertigo with unsteadiness, nausea, vomiting, and exacerbations in her auditory symptoms began to occur. The frequency was multiple times per month. She was diagnosed with left Meniere syndrome and started on dietary and diuretic treatment without adequate control. In 2004, an endolymphatic sac decompression procedure was performed with good control over the events of vertigo for

3 years. In 2007, the spontaneous events of external vertigo returned starting with an unusual spell where the vertigo was continuous for 4 days and then resolved. She began having recurrent events similar to those between 2000 and 2004. A distinct difference was that instead of returning to a normal baseline between the spells, she began between the spells to develop the internal vertigo and problems with unsteadiness with falls without injury provoked by visual patterns, visual motion, and visual complexity. In 2008, she underwent a left vestibular nerve section with absence of the spontaneous external vertigo and reduction in the visually provoked unsteadiness and internal vertigo but not absence. One year later, the spontaneous events of external vertigo returned. At this time, 50% of these spontaneous events were accompanied with focal headaches with migraine features and the other 50% of the events were associated with photophobia and osmophobia. Her visually provoked symptoms increased and she developed the constant nature of the internal (spinning in her head) vertigo with the always present unsteadiness. Her outside managing team was concerned that the nerve section on the left had been incomplete and offered her a left labyrinthectomy at which time the second opinion was requested.

At the time of her workup, she presented with a recent MRI of the brain without and with contrast and internal auditory canal protocol that was normal. Her audiogram is shown in Figure 144.7. Her direct office examination showed no abnormal nystagmus with or without visual fixation present. She was negative for Hallpike and roll tests. Her head thrust tests showed abnormal VOR function for all three semicircular canals on the left. Saccade

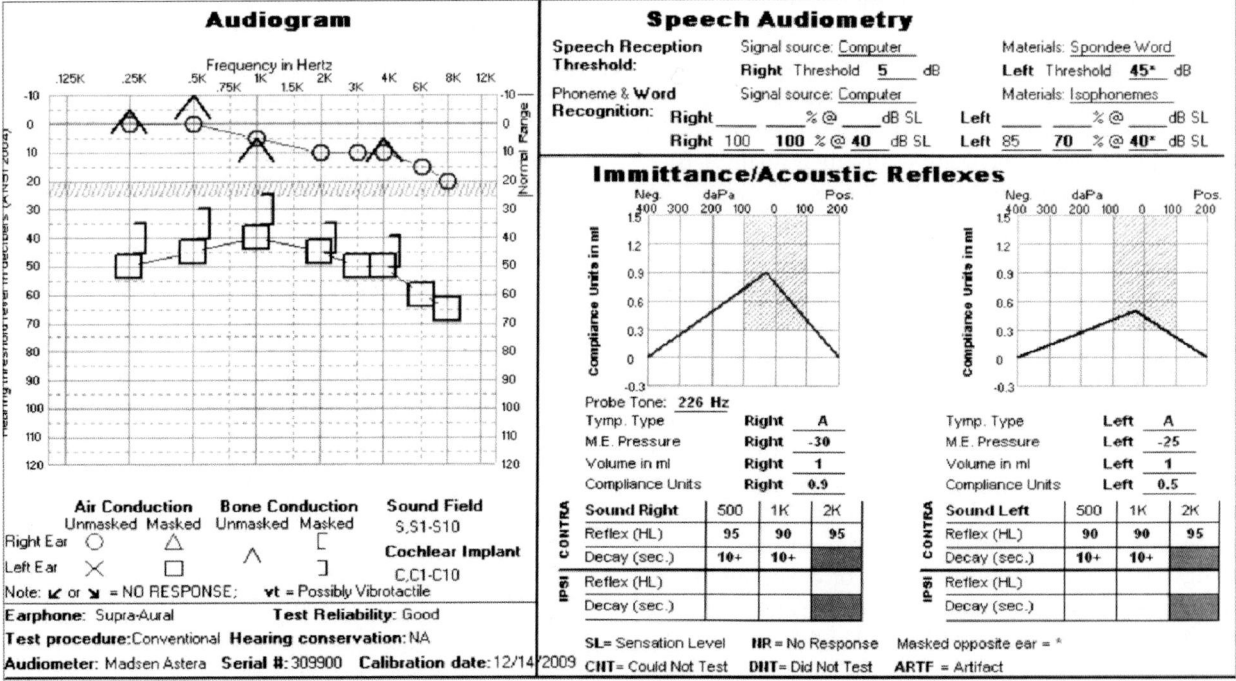

Figure 144.7 Shown is the audiogram for the case of the patient with left side Meniere syndrome, migraine-related dizziness, and chronic subjective dizziness.

function appeared normal and pursuit tracking was mildly disrupted with saccades. The VNG showed no response to warm or ice water (2°C to 3°C temperature) irrigations to the left and normal warm water irrigation to the right. Oculomotor studies were normal for saccade testing but showed that the saccadic disruption to pursuit tracking was beyond that expected or explainable for age. Rotational chair showed abnormalities consistent with peripheral unilateral involvement in a compensated state. cVEMPs were normal on the right and absent on the left. Unilateral centrifugation was normal on the right and utricular function was absent on the left. Postural control assessment showed abnormal sway with fall reactions when she was forced to rely on vestibular system cues alone and abnormal sway under all other conditions without fall reaction using a rhythmic sway—a pattern noted in patients with anxiety disorders. Finally, her Hospital Anxiety and Depression Scale test was highly positive for anxiety and depression. The summary integration of her test findings was that of a severe left peripheral vestibular hypofunction involving all semicircular canals, the saccule, and utricle on the left. The disruption in pursuit tracking was a property of her migraine headaches and not an indicator of other central system involvement given the normal MRI and neurological workup. The left hypofunction was in a partially compensated state. She was then evaluated by a neurotologist, a neurologist with subspecialty interests in dizziness and by a psychiatrist also with subspecialty interest and research activity in dizziness. The collective opinion was that while she had Meniere syndrome on the left in the past, it was now inactive and not related to her ongoing symptoms. Her 24/7 internal vertigo with unsteadiness and development of the visual sensitivities was related to anxiety disorder and the development of Chronic Subjective Dizziness Syndrome (52). Her spontaneous exacerbation in symptoms lasting hours was migraine-related dizziness. She was initiated on sequential trials of fluoxetine with a migraine prophylactic medication and then finally settled with venlafaxine and tricyclic antidepressant. Vestibular rehabilitation therapy, specifically habituation exercises for her sensitivity to head/visual motion and visual complexity with work on general balance, was used in conjunction with the medication, and no further treatment of any type was needed for her Meniere syndrome.

The case illustrates that as the presenting symptoms change over time there is need for reevaluation and likely change in diagnosis. The problem with this case was the insistence that even as the presenting symptoms and character of symptoms changed, everything was felt to be continuing as a result of Meniere syndrome. Second, the test findings were collectively supportive of a virtually compensated hypofunction other than the postural control findings that were dominantly related to her anxiety. The pursuit dysfunction with normal MRI and importantly a symptom presentation for headaches meeting international headache society criteria for migraine is what

allowed that single finding to be attributed to migraine headaches and not an unknown central disorder.

The authors note that significant portions of the above text also appear in two other recent publications by the same authors (53,54).

HIGHLIGHTS

- Vestibular and balance laboratory studies can be used for determination of the extent site of lesion and for evaluating the functional aspects of the VOR and postural control.
- The purpose of the oculomotor tests is to determine if possible central vestibular system involvement should be suspected.
- Saccade testing along with gaze-stability evaluation can be used to suggest localization of lesions within the central vestibular system.
- Positional nystagmus is the most common abnormality on an ENG/VNG but in isolation is nonlocalizing.
- Caloric irrigations by air or water evaluate only the horizontal canals and allow for comparison of left versus right side responsiveness to an exogenous stimulus.
- Rotational chair provides a means for expanding the investigation of the peripheral vestibular system.
- c- and oVEMPs and unilateral centrifugation provide tools for the evaluation of the otolith organs.
- A combination of caloric irrigations, HIT, VEMPs, and unilateral centrifugation allow for investigation of all semicircular canals and both otolith organs on left and right.
- Postural control assessment via the SOT protocol is strictly a functional evaluation.
- The key to the effective use of the laboratory studies is the integrated interpretation of the study results in the context of the presenting history.

REFERENCES

1. Bisdorff A, Von Brevern M, Lempert T, et al. Classification of vestibular symptoms: towards an international classification of vestibular disorders. *J Vestib Res* 2009;19(1-2):1–13.
2. Lempert T, Von Brevern M. Migrainous vertigo. In: Eggers DZ, Zee DS, eds. *Vertigo and imbalance: clinical neurophysiology of the vestibular system.* New York: Elsevier, 2010:440–450.
3. Staab JP. Psychological aspects of vestibular disorders. In: Eggers DZ, Zee DS, eds. *Vertigo and imbalance: clinical neurophysiology of the vestibular system.* New York: Elsevier, 2010:502–522.
4. Ruckenstein MJ, Shepard NT. Balance function testing—a rational approach. In: Shepard NT, Solomon D, eds. *Practical issues in the management of the dizzy and balance disorder patient. The Otolaryngologic Clinics of North America.* Philadelphia, PA: W.B. Saunders Co., 2000:507–518.
5. Stephens SD, Hogan S, Meredith R. The dissynchrony between complaints and signs of vestibular disorders. *Acta Oto-laryngol* 1991;111:188–192.

6. Shepard NT, Gavies S, Goldenrod N, et al. Assessment of activities of daily living in balance disorder patients—comparison to routine balance function studies and patient perceptions, *Abstract midwinter ARO meeting*, St Petersburg Beach, FL, 1997.

7. Monsell EM, Furman JM, Herdman SJ, et al. Technology assessment: computerized dynamic platform posturography. *Otolaryngol Head Neck Surg* 1997;117:394–398.

8. Herdman SJ, Tusa RJ, Blatt P, et al. Computerized dynamic visual acuity test in the assessment of vestibular deficits. *Am J Otol* 1998;19:790–796.

9. Jacobson GP, Newman CW, Hunter L, et al. Balance function test correlates of the dizziness handicap inventory. *J Am Acad Audiol* 1991;2:253–260.

10. Robertson DD, Ireland DJ. Dizziness handicap inventory correlates of computerized dynamic posturography. *Otolaryngol Head Neck Surg* 1995;24:118–124.

11. Curthoys IS, Halmagyi GM. Vestibular compensation: clinical changes in vestibular function with time after unilateral vestibular loss. In: Herdman SJ, ed. *Vestibular rehabilitation*. Philadelphia, PA: FA Davis Co., 2007:76–97.

12. Zee DS. Vestibular adaptation. In: Herdman SJ, ed. *Vestibular rehabilitation*. Philadelphia, PA: FA Davis Co., 2007:19–31.

13. Leigh R, Zee D. *The neurology of eye movements*. New York: Oxford University Press, 2006.

14. Jacobson GP, Shepard NT. *Balance function assessment and management*. San Diego, CA: Plural, 2008.

15. Eggers DZ, Zee DS. *Vertigo and imbalance: clinical neurophysiology of the vestibular system*. New York: Elsevier, 2010.

16. Jacobson GP, Shepard NT, Dundas JA, et al. Eye movement recording techniques. In: Jacobson GP, Shepard NT, eds. *Balance function assessment and management*. San Diego, CA: Plural, 2008:27–44.

17. Shepard NT, Schubert M. Interpretation and usefulness of ocular motility testing. In: Jacobson GP, Shepard NT, eds. *Balance function assessment and management*. San Diego, CA: Plural, 2008:147–170.

18. Robichaud J, DesRoches H, Bance M. Is hyperventilation-induced nystagmus more common in retrocochlear vestibular disease than in end-organ vestibular disease? *J Otolaryngol* 2002;31:140–143.

19. Park HJ, Shin JE, Lee YJ, et al. Hyperventilation-induced nystagmus in patients with vestibular neuritis in the acute and follow-up stages. *Audiol Neurootol* 2010;16:248–253.

20. Choi KD, Kim JS, Kim HJ, et al. Hyperventilation-induced nystagmus in peripheral vestibulopathy and cerebellopontine angle tumor. *Neurology* 2007;69:1050–1059.

21. Cherchi M, Hain TC. Provocative maneuvers for vestibular disorders. In: Eggers DZ, Zee DS, eds. *Vertigo and imbalance: clinical neurophysiology of the vestibular system*. New York: Elsevier, 2010:111–134.

22. Minor LB, Haslwanter T, Straumann D, et al. Hyperventilation-induced nystagmus in patients with vestibular schwannoma. *Neurology* 1999;53:2158–2168.

23. Papp LA, Klein DF, Gorman JM. Carbon dioxide hypersensitivity, hyperventilation, and panic disorder. *Am J Psychiatr* 1993;150(8):1149–1157.

24. Angeli SI, Velandia S, Snapp H. Head-shaking nystagmus predicts greater disability in unilateral peripheral vestibulopathy. *Am J Otolaryngol* 2011;32(6):522–527.

25. Harvey SA, Wood DJ, Feroah TR. Relationship of the head impulse test and head-shake nystagmus in reference to caloric testing. *Am J Otolaryngol* 1997;18:207–213.

26. Perez P, Llorente JL, Gomez JR, et al. Functional significance of peripheral head-shaking nystagmus. *Laryngoscope* 2004;114:1078–1084.

27. Hall SF, Laird ME. Is head-shaking nystagmus a sign of vestibular dysfunction? *J Otolaryngol* 1992;21:209–212.

28. Gananca FF, Gananca CF, Caovilla HH. Active head rotation in benign positional paroxysmal vertigo. *Braz J Otorhinolaryngol* 2009;75:586–592.

29. Lee JY, Lee WW, Kim JS. Perverted head-shaking and positional downbeat nystagmus in patients with multiple system atrophy. *Mov Disord* 2009;24:1290–1295.

30. Walker MF, Zee DS. Directional abnormalities of vestibular and optokinetic responses in cerebellar disease. *Ann N Y Acad Sci* 1999;871:205–220.

31. American National Standards Institute. *ANSI S3.45 – 200X American National Standards procedures for testing basic vestibular function*. New York: Acoustical Society of America, 2009.

32. Zapala DA, Olsholt KF, Lundy LB. A comparison of water and air caloric responses and their ability to distinguish between patients with normal and impaired ears. *Ear Hear* 2008;29:585–600.

33. Manzari L, Tedesco A, Burgess AM. Ocular vestibular-evoked myogenic potentials to bone-conducted vibration in superior vestibular neuritis show utricular function. *Otolaryngol Head Neck Surg* 2010;143:274–280.

34. Curthoys IS, Iwasaki S, Chihara Y, et al. The ocular vestibular-evoked myogenic potential to air-conducted sound; probable superior vestibular nerve origin. *Clin Neurophysiol* 2011;122:611–616.

35. Rosengren SM, Welgampola MS, Colebatch JG. Vestibular evoked myogenic potentials: Past, present and future. *Clin Neurophysiol* 2010;121(5):636–651.

36. Welgampola MS, Myrie OA, Minor LB, et al. Vestibular-evoked myogenic potential thresholds normalize on plugging superior canal dehiscence. *Neurology* 2008;70:464–472.

37. Brey RH, McPherson JL. Technique, interpretation and usefulness of whole body rotational testing. In: Jacobson GP, Shepard NT, eds. *Balance function assessment and management*. San Diego, CA: Plural, 2008:281–318.

38. Furman JM. Rotational testing: background, technique and interpretation. In: Eggers DZ, Zee DS, eds. *Vertigo and imbalance: clinical neurophysiology of the vestibular system*. New York: Elsevier, 2010:141–149.

39. Janky K, Shepard NT. Unilateral centrifugation: Protocol comparison. *Otol Neurotol* 2011;32(1):116–121.

40. Aw ST, Todd MJ, Halmagyi MG. Head impulse testing: angular vestibulo-ocular reflex (VOR). In: Eggers DZ, Zee DS, eds. *Vertigo and imbalance: clinical neurophysiology of the vestibular system*. New York: Elsevier, 2010:150–164.

41. Perez N, Rama-Lopez J. Head-impulse and caloric tests in patients with dizziness. *Otol Neurotol* 2003;24:913–917.

42. Schubert MC, Migliaccio AA, Della Santina CC. Modification of compensatory saccades after aVOR gain recovery. *J Vestib Res* 2006;16:285–291.

43. Janky KL, Shepard NT. Vestibular evoked myogenic potential (VEMP) testing: normative threshold response curves and effects of age. *J Am Acad Audiol* 2010;20:514–522.

44. Rauch SD, Zhou G, Kujawa SG, et al. Vestibular evoked myogenic potentials show altered tuning in patients with Meniere's disease. *Otol Neurol* 2004;25:333–338.

45. Shepard NT, McPherson JP. Sensitivity/Specificity performance of VEMP threshold response curves in Identification of Meniere's syndrome. Oral presentation, *American Balance Society Annual Meeting*, March, Scottsdale, AZ, 2011.

46. Goebel JA, Tungsiripat N, Sinks B, et al. Gaze stabilization test: A new clinical test of unilateral vestibular dysfunction. *Otol Neurotol* 2006;28:68–73.

47. Honaker JA, Shepard NT. Dynamic visual acuity: a sensitive tool for identifying falling risk. *J Vestib Res* 2011;21(5):267–276.

48. Allum JHJ, Shepard NT. An overview of the clinical use of dynamic posturography in the differential diagnosis of balance disorders. *J Vestib Res* 1999;9:223–252.

49. Shepard NT. Interpretation and usefulness of computerized dynamic posturography. In: Jacobson GP, Shepard NT, eds. *Balance function assessment and management*. San Diego, CA: Plural, 2008:359–374.

50. Shepard NT, Janky K. Background and technique of computerized dynamic posturography. In: Jacobson GP, Shepard NT, eds. *Balance function assessment and management*. San Diego, CA: Plural, 2008:339–358.

51. Rine RM. Management of the pediatric patient with vestibular hypofunction. In: Herdman SJ, ed. *Vestibular rehabilitation*. Philadelphia, PA: FA Davis Co., 2007:360–375.

52. Staab JP, Ruckenstein MJ. Expanding the differential diagnosis of chronic dizziness. *Arch Otolaryngol Head Neck Surg* 2007;133:170–176.

53. Handelsman JA, Shepard NT. Electronystagmography and videonystagmography. In: Goebel J, ed. *Practical management of the dizzy patient*, 2nd ed. Philadelphia, PA: Lippincott Williams & Wilkins, 2008.

54. Shepard NT, Janky K, Eggers SDZ. The role of vestibular laboratory testing. In: Bronstein A, ed. *Vertigo and imbalance*. Oxford: Oxford University Press, 2013.

145 Neurophysiologic Intraoperative Monitoring

Brannon D. Mangus   Betty S. Tsai   David S. Haynes

The growth of otology, neurotology, and skull base surgery has allowed the surgical extirpation of intratemporal and retrocochlear pathology while preserving the seventh and eighth cranial nerves. Along with advanced microsurgical techniques, intraoperative neurophysiologic monitoring has played an integral role in the increase in expectations of cranial nerve preservation. The primary goal of intraoperative neurophysiologic monitoring is to aid in the preservation of nerve integrity and function and, in selected applications, allow for the prediction of postoperative functional impairment. Table 145.1 describes the ideal requirements for an intraoperative neurophysiologic monitor. The purpose of this chapter is to acquaint the reader with currently available techniques of neurophysiologic monitoring, primarily as they relate to the surgical management of temporal bone and posterior fossa pathology. This chapter also explores the indications, techniques, and potential controversies of intraoperative neurophysiologic monitoring with particular focus on facial and auditory nerve monitoring.

AUDITORY SYSTEM MONITORING

The primary goal of most otologic and neurotologic procedures is the eradication of disease while minimizing morbidity. When considering vestibular schwannomas and skull base tumors, many surgeons regard the preservation of hearing a secondary, yet significant, goal even in patients with functional hearing in the contralateral ear. Advances in diagnostic capabilities, specifically the routine use of contrast-enhanced MRI, have resulted in the earlier detection of smaller tumors. This detection, coupled with advances in microsurgical techniques and intraoperative neurophysiologic monitoring, has increasingly made preservation of hearing a reasonable goal in select situations. Furthermore, the likelihood of certain disease processes, such as neurofibromatosis type II, to produce bilateral lesions highlights the benefits of attempted hearing preservation.

The characterization of the human auditory evoked potentials in 1971 by Jewett and Williston allowed for the development of the first intraoperative monitoring system of the auditory nerve, first implemented in 1978 (1,2). Since then, intraoperative eighth nerve monitoring has been used during vestibular schwannoma resection, vestibular nerve section, facial nerve exploration, and other skull base procedures in which the auditory system can be placed at risk.

Of the procedures mentioned above, vestibular schwannoma resection carries the highest risk of postoperative hearing impairment (3). Many patients with a vestibular schwannoma already present with sensorineural hearing loss, which is believed to be secondary to cochlear dysfunction induced by internal auditory artery insufficiency or by cochlear nerve dysfunction resulting from pressure, atrophy, or tumor invasion. Although surgical techniques, such as the middle fossa approach and the suboccipital (retrosigmoid) approach, have been designed to minimize the likelihood of total hearing loss associated with the translabyrinthine approach, these measures preserve some degree of hearing in only 29% to 65% of patients depending on tumor size and location (4–8). During surgery, the auditory system may be injured via direct injury to the cochlea or membranous labyrinth, through labyrinthine artery injury with resultant cochlear ischemia, via cochlear nerve stretching, compression, transection, or thermal injury from drilling, cautery, or surgical dissection, or at the brainstem. Because of the variable coverage of the central glial segment of the nerve that often extends to the internal auditory canal (IAC), the auditory nerve may be more fragile than other cranial nerves, rendering it particularly susceptible to stretch or thermal injuries (9). During vestibular schwannoma resection, the goals of intraoperative auditory monitoring are twofold: to warn the surgeon when surgical manipulation may be causing auditory system injury and to predict postoperative hearing function.

TABLE 145.1	CHARACTERISTICS OF THE IDEAL NEUROPHYSIOLOGIC MONITOR

Functions in the operating room in the presence of other electrical devices, such as air drills and anesthesia machines, with minimal dysfunction or artifact.

Functions safely so that even if dysfunction does occur, no harm to the patient can occur.

Incorporates straightforward and reproducible setup and monitoring procedures to avoid delay in preparation for the procedure and to minimize errors in data analysis, operative time, and cost.

Accurately and continuously monitors the cranial nerve (end organ, peripheral system) at risk for intraoperative injury.

Exhibits sufficient sensitivity and specificity to detect intraoperative changes in the system being monitored for surgical alterations, without unnecessary false alarms.

Rapidly alerts the surgeon in sufficient time to alter surgical technique to minimize trauma to the system at risk.

In the case of intraoperative facial nerve monitoring, allows the surgeon to receive feedback through auditory, visual (electromyographic tracing, oscilloscope), or a combination of stimuli, so that the surgeon can monitor the facial nerve without the mandatory assistance of trained personnel, if desired.

AUDITORY SYSTEM MONITORING TECHNIQUES

A number of studies, but not all, have shown that auditory monitoring may improve outcomes in neurotologic surgery. Much controversy remains concerning which monitoring technique is best (10). The evoked potentials that are generated in response to auditory stimuli provide the foundation for neurophysiologic eighth nerve monitoring. There are three primary types of intraoperative auditory monitoring: brainstem auditory evoked potentials (BAEPs), also known as auditory brainstem response (ABR); electrocochleography (ECochG); and auditory nerve compound action potential (ANCAP), also known as direct eighth nerve monitoring

(DENM) or cochlear nerve action potential (CNAP) monitoring. Each of the techniques has level-specific responses that provide useful information about auditory system integrity and function, as seen in Figure 145.1.

Although these techniques are described separately for purposes of discussion, when clinically applied to intraoperative monitoring of the auditory system, each may be used alone, or in combination with each other. They are classified as either far-field or near-field techniques based on the distance between the recording electrodes and the generators of the response (i.e., brainstem nuclei for ABR and cochlea for ECochG).

AUDITORY BRAINSTEM RESPONSE

The least invasive method of eighth nerve monitoring, ABR, is a commonly utilized far-field modality. Stimuli, often in the form of "clicks" or tone bursts, are presented to the ear through transducers or inset earphones, and responses from components of the auditory system are recorded from the scalp or external auditory canal with electroencephalogram amplifiers. When compared to near-field monitoring techniques (e.g., ECochG, CNAP), ABR has a low signal-to-noise ratio and, therefore, requires extensive, time-consuming averaging for useful interpretation.

The ABR tracing contains five peaks, moving from distal (cochlea) to proximal (brainstem) along the auditory pathway. The first two peaks (I and II) arise from activity along the distal and proximal ipsilateral cochlear nerve. The remainder of the ABR waves originate from the auditory brainstem. Wave III, which is prominent, corresponds to the cochlear nucleus; peak IV corresponds to the superior olivary nucleus; and peak V, the most prominent component of the ABR, corresponds to the lateral lemniscus and inferior colliculus, which also integrates inputs from the contralateral ear (11). Deviations from the baseline recording such as increasing latency intervals are analyzed relative to surgical manipulations. Changes in the ABR will

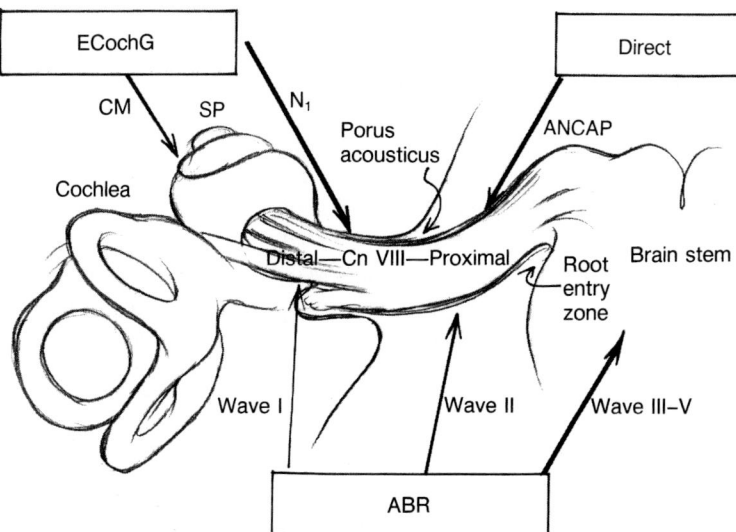

Figure 145.1 Schematic shows level-specific responses obtained with electrocochleographic, ABR, and direct ANCAP recordings.

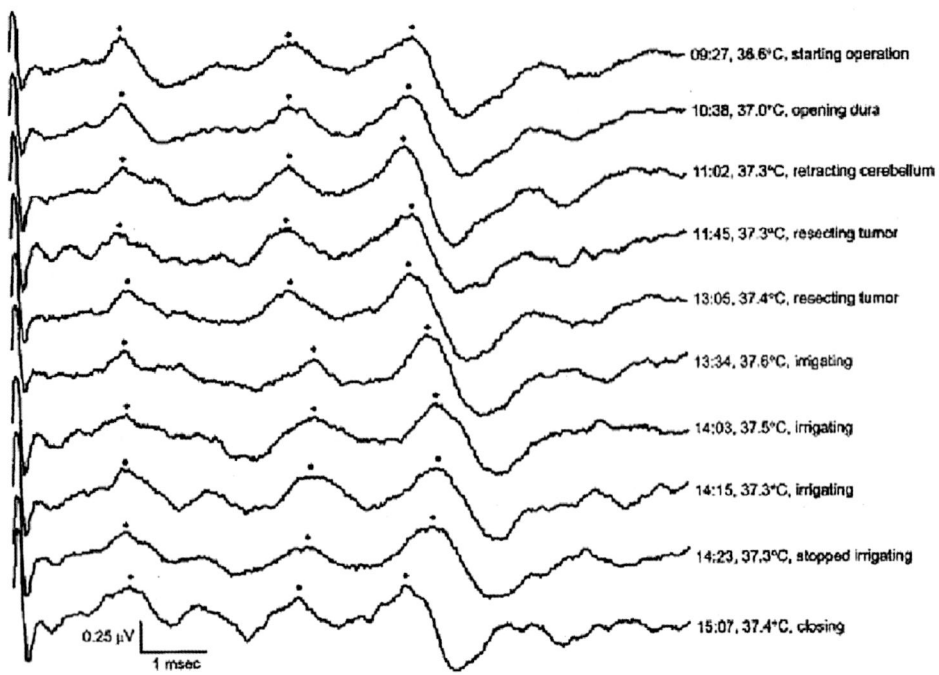

09:27, 36.6°C, starting operation

10:38, 37.0°C, opening dura

11:02, 37.3°C, retracting cerebellum

11:45, 37.3°C, resecting tumor

13:05, 37.4°C, resecting tumor

13:34, 37.6°C, irrigating

14:03, 37.5°C, irrigating

14:15, 37.3°C, irrigating

14:23, 37.3°C, stopped irrigating

15:07, 37.4°C, closing

0.25 μV

1 msec

Figure 145.2 Intraoperative ABR to right ear stimulation during surgery for a meningioma in the right cerebellopontine angle. The ABRs were stable during cerebellar retraction and tumor resection. After the tumor had been removed, copious irrigation of the surgical field with cold fluids produced a transient prolongation of the I-to-III interpeak interval, reflecting slowed neural conduction within the eighth nerve resulting from local cooling. The peak latencies of waves I, III, and V are marked by the small diamonds, and the clock times, esophageal temperatures, and surgical procedures corresponding to each of the ABR waveforms are noted at the right. (Taken from Legatt AD. Mechanisms of intraoperative brainstem auditory evoked potential changes. *J Clin Neurophysiol* 2002;19:396–408, with permission from Lippincott Williams & Wilkins.)

vary depending on the location of injury along the auditory pathway (see Fig. 145.2).

Different types of surgical manipulation can affect the intraoperative ABR in different ways. Drilling of the temporal bone can cause direct inner ear trauma or cochlear ischemia or infarction due to compromise of the internal auditory artery affecting all ABR components, including wave I. Mechanical or thermal injury to the eighth nerve will delay and potentially eliminate waves III and V, but leave wave I unaffected. Retraction of the cerebellum and brainstem stretches the eighth nerve resulting in an often reversible prolongation of the I-to-III peak interval. Similarly, vasospasm within the eighth nerve can cause potentially reversible ABR changes. Damage at or caudal to the superior olivary complex will delay or eliminate wave III, and damage to the brainstem auditory pathways at or below the level of the lateral lemniscus affect wave V in a similar fashion (9,12). Nontraumatic maneuvers such as opening the dura alters the conduction patterns of the ABR appearing as changes on the monitor; in these situations, an intraoperative baseline may need to be reestablished prior to further manipulation of the auditory system (12).

Changes to intraoperative ABR may also be caused by other physiologic mechanisms such as blood in the middle ear, certain volatile anesthetics, hypothermia, irrigation,

and acoustic masking from drilling noise. During intraoperative ABR monitoring, examination of the pattern of changes, analysis of their correlation with surgical maneuvers, and investigation for possible technical reasons can help to determine the cause of the ABR changes and provide the appropriate information to the surgical team (9).

Extensive signal averaging required in ABR monitoring result in minutes lapsing between an offensive manipulation and the appearance of changes from the baseline recording. The surgeon must then retrospectively evaluate recent operative actions and provide a corrective action, if possible. This time lag is a significant limitation to this technique. However, fast ABR, which utilizes both an analog and digital filter with enhanced software, permits interpretable ABR readings in five seconds making it more suitable for intraoperative monitoring (13). Despite recent advancements, intraoperative ABR has yet to yield improved functional outcomes (14). Being a far-field technique, intraoperative ABR has increased susceptibility to disruption by various intraoperative procedures and surgical equipment because of its poor signal-to-noise ratio and poor temporal resolution (15).

An additional disadvantage of the ABR technique is that a useful preoperative ABR is required to serve as a baseline. This is often limited in the presence of known preoperative hearing loss. However, some patients with absent preoperative

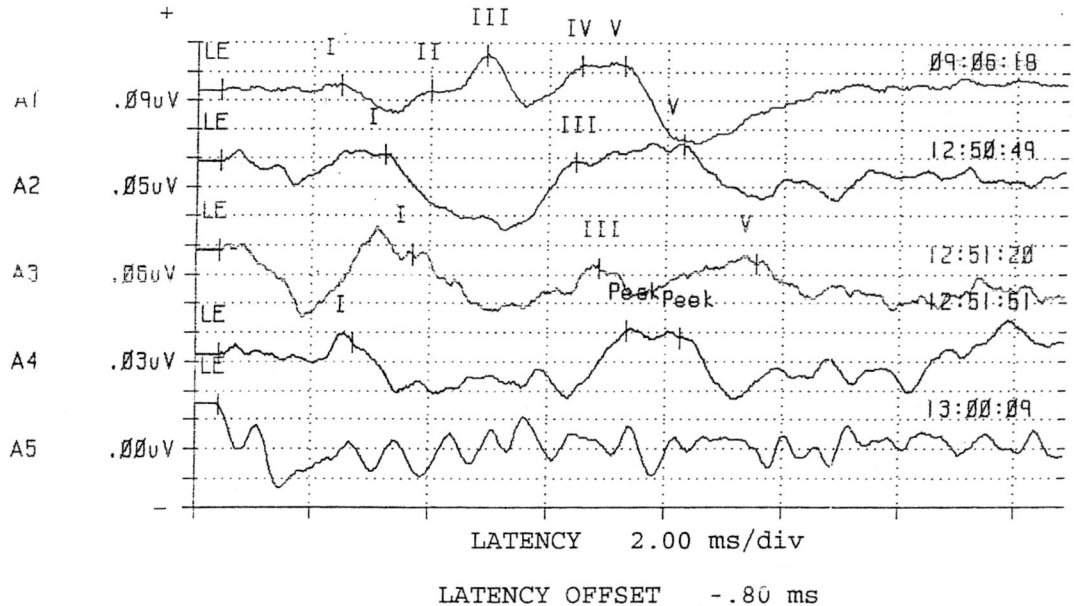

LATENCY   2.00 ms/div

LATENCY OFFSET   -.80 ms

LATENCIES (ms)

	I	II	III	IV	V	RarV	ConV	Peak	Peek	LE
A1	1.64	3.17	4.10	5.72	6.45					-.39
A2	2.39		5.64		7.46					-.39
A3	2.88		6.04		8.71					-.39
A4	1.87							6.51	7.44	-.39
A5										-.39

Figure 145.3 Intraoperative ABR tracings of a patient with preserved hearing after excision of intracanalicular acoustic neuroma. *A1*, baseline; *A2*, prolongation of I through III latency; *A3 to A5*, additional intraoperative deterioration.

ABR waveforms can be monitored with other techniques (e.g., CNAP) with a significant percentage of these patients ultimately achieving hearing preservation (16).

Despite its limitations, intraoperative ABR during vestibular schwannoma resection may be associated with improved preservation of hearing (17,18). Strauss et al. showed in a prospective, randomized fashion that the implementation of corrective actions based on ABR changes could significantly improve the rate of functional hearing preservation (19). However, Jackson et al. showed that the use of intraoperative ABR did not change their ability to preserve hearing, with an overall rate of about 60% (20).

Several studies have attempted to evaluate the prognostic value of intraoperative ABR although their significance is unclear, but certain intraoperative ABR patterns are associated with postoperative hearing outcomes (20). Persistence of wave V at the conclusion of the procedure has been associated with serviceable hearing. Similarly, complete elimination or irreversible and progressive loss of wave V indicates a high likelihood of postoperative hearing loss (12,15).

However, preservation of wave V does not guarantee maintenance of postoperative hearing, as auditory function may decline postoperatively, despite its presence in the immediate postoperative period, possibly reflecting postoperative cochlear artery spasm (21). Also, the loss of intraoperative ABR recordings does not always imply that hearing

is completely lost or unserviceable. Variable reversible loss of ABR tracings has been associated with varied hearing outcomes (15,22). Figure 145.3 shows a series of intraoperative ABR recordings on a 52-year-old male who had undergone resection of an intracanalicular vestibular schwannoma via a middle fossa approach. Tracing A1 shows a baseline intraoperative recording. During dissection of the tumor at the fundus of the IAC, there is a prolongation of wave I to III latency, seen in tracing A2. Although further tracings, A3 through A5, show progressive deterioration of the ABR recording, comparison between this patient's preoperative and postoperative audiogram showed preservation of serviceable hearing (see Figs. 145.4 and 145.5).

Intraoperative ABR monitoring has also been shown to decrease auditory morbidity during posterior fossa microvascular decompression for hemifacial spasm and trigeminal neuralgia (23–26). However, microvascular decompression for hemifacial spasm without intraoperative ABR monitoring has also been shown to provide similar postoperative auditory results (27).

ELECTROCOCHLEOGRAPHY

ECochG is a near-field technique that monitors the cochlea and the most distal portion of the auditory nerve. As such, the signal can be obtained more rapidly with fewer

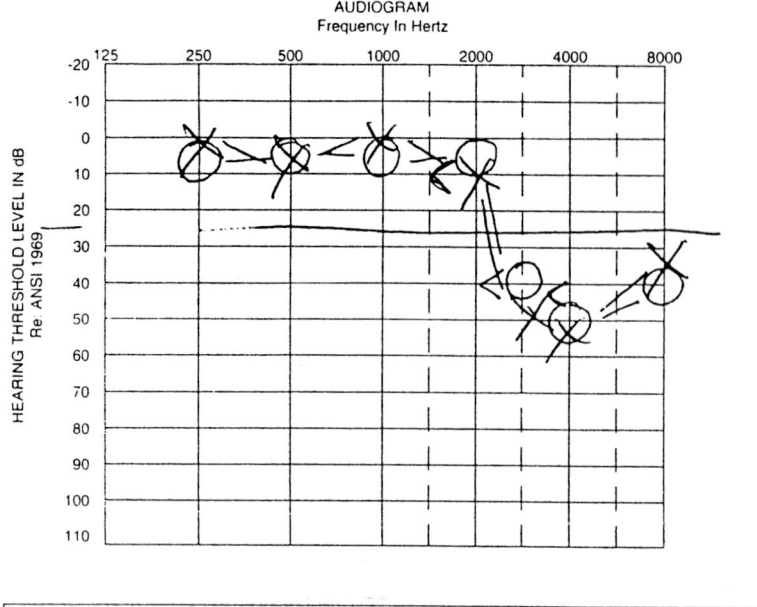

AUDIOGRAM
Frequency In Hertz

KEY	L	R
AC	X	O
AC masked	□	△
BC	>	<
BC masked	]	[
No response	↘	↙
Sound Field		S

SPEECH AUDIOMETRY						
	PTA	SRT	SDT	HL/PB	HL/PB	LIST
Right		5		65dB 96%		
Left		10		65dB 96%		
SF						

Figure 145.4 Preoperative audiometric findings for the patient in Figure 145.5.

sweeps and averaging. Auditory stimuli are delivered to the cochlea commonly in the form of a click. The two recording approaches for ECochG are transtympanic (TT) and extratympanic (ET). The TT method involves penetrating the tympanic membrane with a needle electrode so that the tip rests on the cochlear promontory. The ET method has recording sites that are peripheral to the tympanic membrane via external auditory canal electrodes. While less invasive compared to the TT counterparts, the increased distance of the ET electrodes from the recording targets minimizes the amplification advantage of this near-field technique (28). Figure 145.6 shows a typical ECochG setup, with an insulated TT recording needle electrode placed on the promontory of the middle ear. To improve stability during testing, the electrode may first be placed through the tragus. Figure 145.7 shows an ECochG tracing from a patient undergoing removal of a vestibular schwannoma. Recording electrodes placed closer to the promontory encounter less noise, resulting in more rapid signal generation (within 10 s) with less required averaging (12). ECochG monitors the cochlear microphonic (CM), as well as the summating potential (SP) and eighth nerve action potentials (APs) arising from a stimulus.

The CM and the SP represent cochlear bioelectric activity: the CM is generated by the outer hair cells in the organ

of Corti, and the SP is generated by a complex mechano-electrical transduction process within the organ of Corti. The compound action potential (AP) of the auditory nerve represents the summed response of synchronous discharges from several thousand afferent eighth nerve fibers. The first component of the AP, often referred to as N1, is analogous to wave I of the ABR (11,29). Differentiation of the SP from the AP, which are normally superimposed on each other, may be accomplished by increasing the click rate. With higher click rates, the eighth nerve AP will decrease because the stimulus frequency is shorter than the refractory period for each neuron contributing to the AP. The N1 latency is inversely related to the stimulus rate, whereas its amplitude is directly related to the stimulus rate (11).

Clinically, ECochG may be used to predict postoperative audition and is sensitive to changes in cochlear blood supply. Reduced amplitude or loss of the ECochG AP is believed to indicate direct injury to or vasopasm of the labyrinthine (internal auditory) artery (29). Change in the CM may indicate cochlear pathophysiology. Because less signal averaging is required, surgeons are alerted to damaging maneuvers or situations more quickly than with ABR (29). A comparison of monitored and nonmonitored patients undergoing vestibular schwannoma resection demonstrated a significantly improved outcome for those in the monitored group (30).

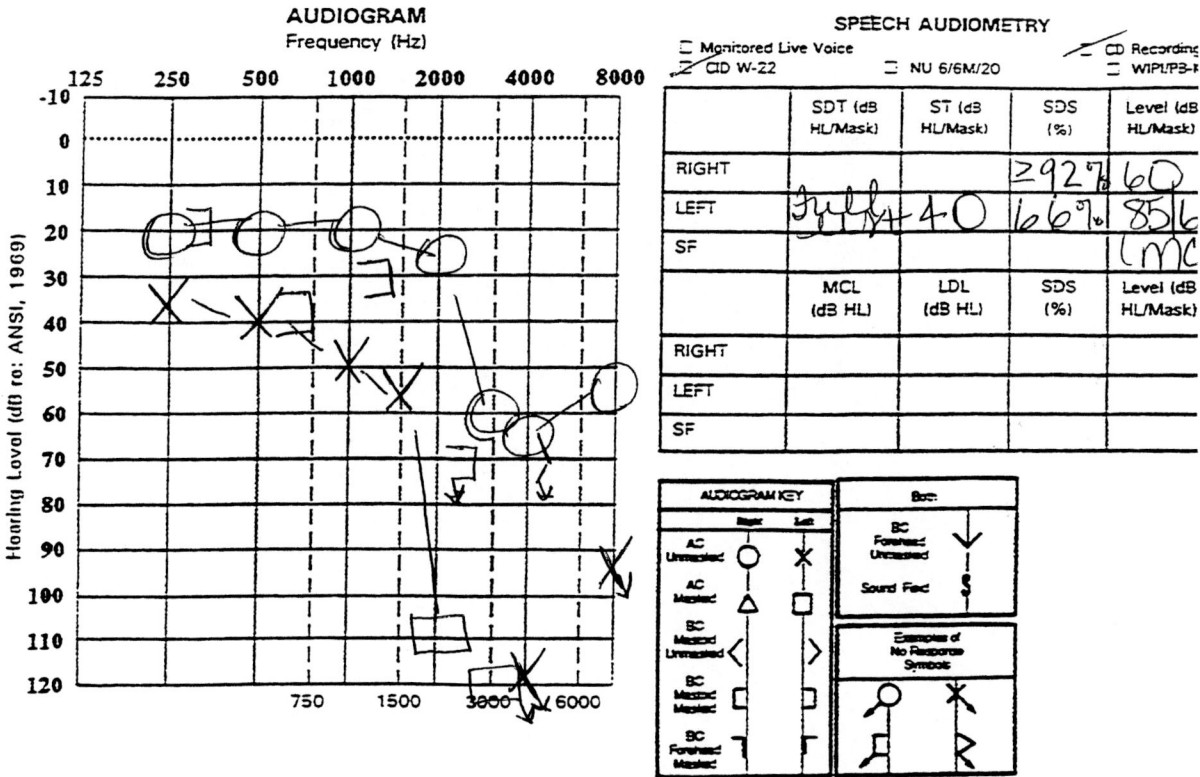

Figure 145.5 Postoperative audiometric findings for patient in Figure 145.4. SF, sound field; MCL, most comfortable loudness; LDL, loudness discomfort level; SDS, speech discrimination score; SDT, speech-detection threshold; AC, air conduction; BC, bone conduction; ST, spondee threshold.

Potential drawbacks of ECochG monitoring arise from its invasiveness, difficulty of appropriate needle placement, and potential for intraoperative dislodgement of the electrode (31). TT needle placement may increase the risk of postoperative cerebrospinal fluid otorrhea (29). More significantly, ECochG may not accurately reflect intraoperative changes that occur medially within the cerebellopontine angle (31). Persistence of ECochG signals after cochlear nerve section has been well documented. Utilizing intraoperative ECochG, Silverstein et al. demonstrated signal persistence for 25 minutes after cochlear nerve section (32), while APs have been documented 3 years after cochlear nerve resection (33). Because of limitations encountered with ECochG use and suspicion that use of ECochG alone may be less effective than other means of monitoring (12), the use of ECochG as the sole method of intraoperative monitoring has been reported with less frequency in recent years. Nevertheless, ECochG may be a useful adjunct to other monitoring techniques to provide a broader picture of the auditory pathway.

Despite its limitations, ECochG, particularly the SP, may be useful in surgery for Meniere disease, as sac decompression precipitates a decrease in previously elevated SPs in several patients (34). Although an abnormal SP/AP ratio has historically been associated with Meniere, recent studies have shown that an elevated SP/AP ratio also is a consistent finding in superior semicircular canal dehiscence

(SSCD) (35). Knowing that this SP/AP ratio normalizes after surgery suggests a potential opportunity for intraoperative monitoring with ECochG during repair of SSCD.

DIRECT EIGHTH NERVE MONITORING

Another near-field technique, direct monitoring of the CNAP or ANCAP, seeks to circumvent some of the potential problems with ABR and ECochG recording. Since its introduction by Moller and Jannetta in the 1980s, CNAP has gained increasing acceptance (36). It is the most sensitive modality to monitor the eighth cranial nerve and may be used in patients with poor or absent ABR tracings. One report described a series of nine patients with absent preoperative ABR waveforms who were successfully monitored with CNAP. Seven of the nine patients ultimately achieved hearing preservation (16).

The CNAP positive electrode is placed on the nerve proximal to the tumor or adjacent to the cochlear nucleus once exposed; hence, this type of monitoring is usually restricted to the retrosigmoid approach. However, a few authors have reported the use CNAP monitoring for middle cranial fossa approaches with some benefit (37,38). The negative electrode is placed in the contralateral mastoid tip area and the ground electrode is placed at the vertex (13). Click stimuli are administered to the ear, eliciting a characteristic waveform with an initial positive peak (N1), as in Figure 145.8. Because the compound AP is very

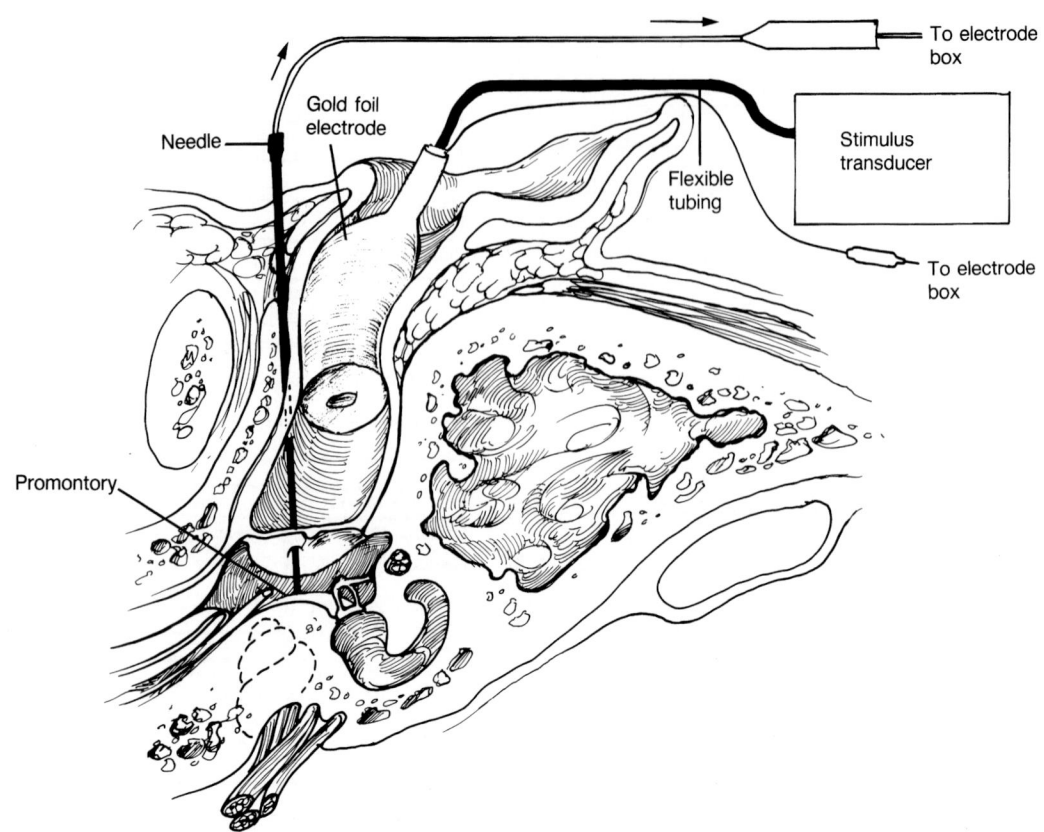

Figure 145.6 Schematic shows placement of intraoperative TT needle electrode through tragus. A gold foil electrode sound delivery system is in the distal portion of the ear canal.

large in this near-field technique, there is little to no need for signal averaging, and the feedback to the surgeon can be nearly instantaneous (12,13).

Analyzing the morphology and latency of CNAP components provides information regarding the mechanism of injury and gives the surgeon insight into which maneuvers are beneficial and which are harmful to hearing (15,39). Moderate injury to the nerve decreases CNAP amplitude, with complete loss of signal in severe contusion or transection. Stretching the nerve increases the N1 latency, and diminished N1 amplitude may be the first sign of mechanical or thermal injury to the nerve (12). Unlike

other monitoring techniques, the information provided by CNAP monitoring is presented in real time, allowing the surgeon to correct for the offending maneuver (see Fig. 145.9). Potential difficulties with securing the electrode have largely been overcome utilizing a variety of techniques (13,20). However, placement of the electrode can be challenging and sometimes not feasible when applied to tumors with cerebellopontine angle involvement where exposure may be limited (40).

CNAP monitoring is potentially a sensitive prognostic tool. Preservation of the CNAP has been associated with hearing preservation in one case series in 78% of patients

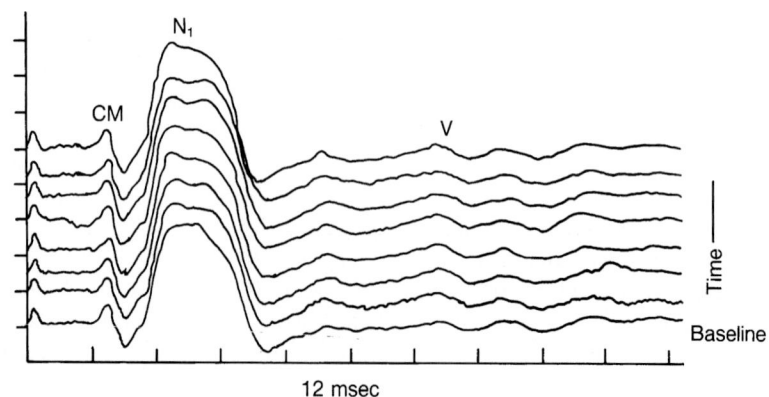

Figure 145.7 Intraoperative TT electrocochleographic recordings of a patient undergoing removal of acoustic tumor. CM, cochlear microphonic; N_1, action potential of eighth cranial nerve.

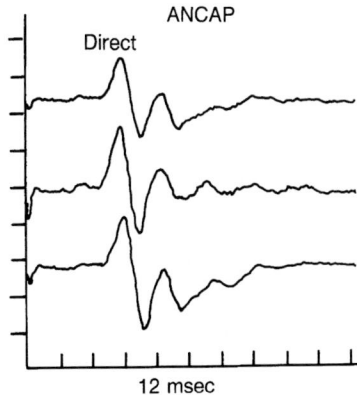

Figure 145.8 Intraoperative recording shows direct ANCAP of a patient undergoing retrolabyrinthine vestibular nerve section.

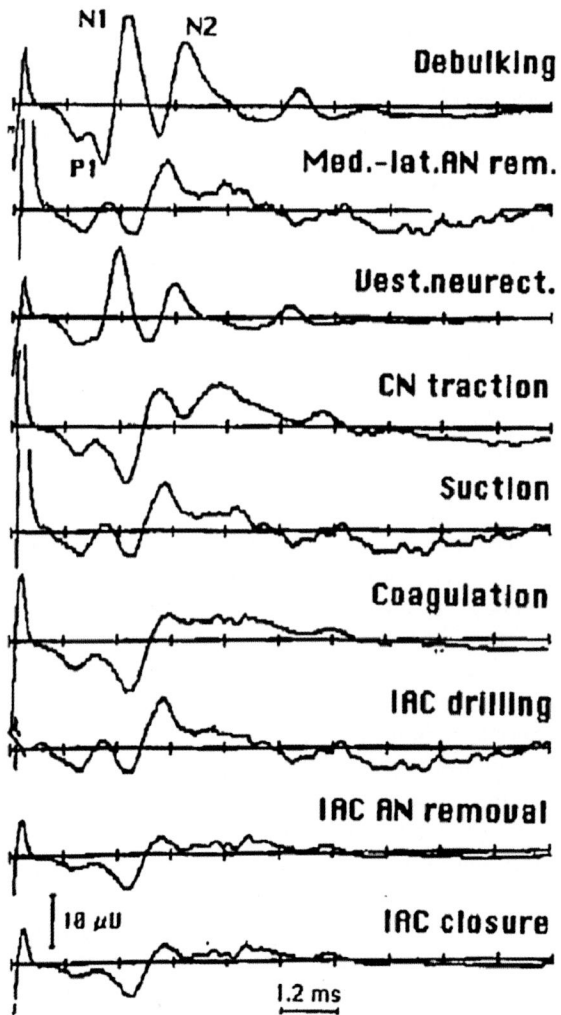

Figure 145.9 Set of CNAPs recorded during retrosigmoid-transmeatal removal of a 19-mm left vestibular schwannoma in a 33-year-old man. Preoperative hearing: PTA 26 dB; SDS 90%. The CNAP changes are shown at different surgical steps. Postoperative hearing: PTA 47 dB; SDS 70%. (Taken from Colletti V, Fiorino FG. Advances in monitoring of seventh and eighth cranial nerve function during posterior fossa surgery. *Am J Otol* 1998;19:503–512, with permission from Lippincott Williams & Wilkins.)

(20); conversely, lack of an AP response at the completion of the procedure carries a very poor prognosis for postoperative hearing preservation (12,20). However, earlier studies have shown that CNAP monitoring did not affect hearing preservation (41,42).

Despite the advantage of more instantaneous feedback with possibly improved likelihood of hearing preservation (40), some surgeons have been reluctant to embrace this technique not only because the electrode can be difficult to place but also, once placed, can become a cumbersome impediment as it lies in the surgical field.

COMPARING THE THREE MONITORING TECHNIQUES

Compared to the use of ABR and ECochG during vestibular schwannoma resection, there has been a trend toward improved hearing outcomes with CNAP monitoring. Additionally, the loss of CNAP N1 at the completion of the surgical procedure is a poor prognostic sign for hearing preservation (12). A study comparing 22 ABR-monitored patients with 44 CNAP-monitored patients reported a statistically significant improvement in hearing preservation rates, which they defined as preservation of any retained hearing in those monitored with CNAP. However, these results did not achieve statistical significance for the preservation of serviceable hearing, but the trend pointed toward CNAP monitoring (27% for ABR, 43% for CNAP) (40). It provides reliable auditory monitoring more frequently than ABR, reflects the intraoperative auditory function almost in real time, predicts postoperative hearing with excellent sensitivity and specificity, and is more useful for monitoring in the removal of small vestibular schwannomas with hearing preservation (15). Others have also concluded that CNAP monitoring offered superior monitoring and improved outcomes compared to other techniques (20,39,40). Despite the perceived superiority of CNAP monitoring, the technical difficulty of placing and operating around electrodes, as well as the limited space available in the setting of large tumors, continue to limit its acceptance (31).

The overwhelming majority of data supporting the use of intraoperative monitoring of the auditory system come from retrospective analyses (40). However, comparing the results of hearing preservation surgeries across studies or institutions is inherently difficult for a number of reasons. First, the selection criteria for patients undergoing hearing preservation surgery can differ dramatically between institutions. Tumor size, preoperative hearing ability, and the surgeon's experience in removing such tumors are other frequently encountered variables. Additionally, the intraoperative monitoring technique, the interpretation, and the surgical response are operator dependent. Lastly, the most significant limitation is how each author defines preservation of hearing. Some studies regard any detectable

TABLE 145.2	AMERICAN ACADEMY OF HEAD AND NECK SURGEONS CLASSIFICATION OF HEARING PRESERVATION SURGERY FOR VESTIBULAR SCHWANNOMA	
Class	Pure Tone Threshold	Speech Discrimination (%)
A	≤30 dB	≥70
B	>30 dB, ≤50 dB	≥50
C	>50 dB	≥50
D	Any level	<50

hearing as preservation, whereas others use more selective criteria to include only those with truly functional hearing. A recent review demonstrated that substantial variations in published rates of hearing preservation can be achieved simply by manipulating the definition of success (43). Standardized schemes for reporting results have been developed, but even these are disputed and are not uniformly applied (43,44). According to the guidelines of the American Academy of Otolaryngology–Head and Neck Surgery, hearing preservation is defined as preservation of hearing within normal and social hearing classification, that is, pure tone audiometry ≤50 dB and speech discrimination score ≥50% (10,44,45) (see Table 145.2).

Because of the increased prevalence of contrast-enhanced MRI scanning, today's surgeon encounters a greater number of small tumors and is afforded a greater opportunity to preserve hearing (46). Although comparing studies evaluating the success of hearing preservation surgery remains difficult, the use of intraoperative auditory monitoring has been associated with improved results. Many surgeons have reported monitoring to be useful, and a substantial body of literature supports the use of intraoperative auditory monitoring in the appropriate setting. Consequently, its use has become routine in hearing preservation surgery in many major centers.

COMBINED APPROACHES

Because individual cochlear nerve-monitoring modalities have limitations and weaknesses in their clinical applications, some surgeons have utilized multiple modalities. Combinations of near- and far-field techniques help create a complete picture of the auditory system, from the cochlea and the distal eighth nerve to the brainstem and higher centers. Some investigators have described the simultaneous use of ABR and ECochG to localize the origin of detected changes in the auditory system, whereas others advocate ABR and CNAP monitoring (47,48).

When monitoring patients undergoing vestibular schwannoma removal with both ABR and ECochG, Schalke et al. (29) reported an overall hearing preservation rate of 51%. The loss of ECochG signal in this study coincided with postoperative deafness (26/26 patients). However, serviceable postoperative hearing was maintained in 25% of patients with an absent postoperative ABR but preserved ECochG. Very good rates of hearing preservation have been documented when combining the use of ABR with CNAP (20,39,49). The utility of ABR in cases monitored with CNAP has been called into question, however, as multiple studies have not demonstrated any advantage with the addition of ABR monitoring compared to CNAP alone (15,20). In one study, during the microsurgical tumor removal, reliable auditory monitoring was obtained in 20 of 22 patients (91%) by CNAP and in nine of 22 (41%) by ABR. The same study showed that preserved CNAP at the completion of tumor removal predicted hearing preservation 100% sensitivity and 100% specificity; all 19 patients who had preserved CNAP at the end of the case demonstrated serviceable hearing, while one patient in whom CNAP disappeared lost hearing. It demonstrated that the loss of ABR is not specific for hearing loss; 12 of 14 patients preserved hearing despite the lack of ABR presence at the completion of the case (15).

HORIZONS

Rapid feedback and improved sensitivity of the monitoring techniques have improved the clinical applications of this technology, but all responses must be critically analyzed relative to the surgical procedure. Eighth nerve monitoring cannot serve as a replacement for preoperative planning, meticulous surgical technique, and a detailed knowledge of regional anatomy. Despite the challenges of intraoperative auditory monitoring in otologic and neurotologic procedures, expanding technologic frontiers have emerged because of information obtained from intraoperative auditory monitoring. Nimodipine has been shown to rescue traumatized cochlear neurons from degeneration in rats (50). Subsequently it was demonstrated that prophylactic vasoactive treatment consisting of nimodipine and hydroxyethyl starch (HES) provided significantly better preservation of cochlear nerve function in vestibular schwannoma surgery (6). Bischoff further showed that only patients who had reversible loss of BAEP benefitted from vasoactive treatment (51). Other monitoring techniques such as distortion product otoacoustic emissions (DPOEs) have shown some promising results (52), but further evaluation is required to assess its impact on outcomes.

Armed with an understanding of the fundamental techniques of intraoperative auditory system monitoring, the surgeon may then decide which modalities, if any, will be applicable to the planned surgical procedure. Although the future appears bright for eighth nerve monitoring, it still trails facial nerve monitoring in applications and acceptance.

INTRAOPERATIVE FACIAL NERVE MONITORING

Facial nerve injury with resultant paresis or paralysis is a devastating and one of the most feared complication of otologic surgery. It is also one of the more common reasons for malpractice litigation in otolaryngology (53). Morbidity from this injury depends on the site of the injury as well as the degree of injury to the facial nerve, ranging from a mild, partial paresis of brief duration to permanent injuries with significant sequelae. Temporary or partial paralysis may result in long-term cosmetic deformities, including synkinesis, atrophy, or bothersome facial twitching. Permanent facial paralysis may result in extensive cosmetic deformity or severe functional deficits, leading to oral incompetence and, in extreme cases, corneal injuries and blindness as well as significant psychological effects on the patient. Although facial nerve injury can occur during any otologic or neurotologic procedure, certain procedures such as vestibular schwannoma excision, revision mastoid surgery, and repair of congenital malformations carry a greater risk. While most otolaryngologists are familiar with normal facial nerve anatomy, the nerve may run an aberrant course or be obscured by tumor, fibrosis, cholesteatoma, granulation tissue, bleeding, and even spinal fluid. The incidence of facial nerve paralysis resulting from otologic and neurotologic procedures has declined over the past decades likely because of the advent of the operative microscope, high-speed surgical drill, and advanced microsurgical techniques. Prior to these advances, the incidence of facial nerve paralysis following mastoid surgery was as high as 15% (54). A more recent estimate of facial nerve paralysis found an incidence of 1.7% in 1,024 consecutive mastoidectomies (55).

The importance of facial nerve monitoring during otologic and neurotologic surgery extends beyond merely avoiding untoward outcomes. Because of its intricate involvement with the structures of the temporal bone, the facial nerve often serves as an invaluable landmark in performing certain operations. Identification of the facial nerve promotes orientation in the complex three-dimensional anatomy of the temporal bone and comprises an essential step in many otologic and neurotologic procedures.

FACIAL NERVE INJURY

There are many mechanisms by which the facial nerve can be injured during otologic and neurotologic surgery. Possible sources of trauma are listed in Table 145.3.

TABLE 145.3	TYPES OF FACIAL NERVE INJURY

Transection
Direct trauma from surgical dissection
Direct trauma from surgical drill
Stretch
Compression
Thermal damage from drilling, cautery, laser, irrigation
Vascular compromise
Direct or indirect injury from the ultrasonic aspirator
Edema of the nerve in the fallopian canal from surgical dissection

Resection of vestibular schwannomas places the facial nerve at the greatest risk, primarily because of the limited access to the intracranial facial nerve, the narrow confines of the IAC, the absence of a fibrous protective layer of epineurium, and the tendency for the tumor to splay the nerve fibers. Most facial nerve injuries during resection of vestibular schwannomas occur medial to the porus acousticus at the mid-cerebellopontine angle, where it may be injured from surgical dissection or compression by the mass (56). Additionally, bone surrounding the mastoid, tympanic, and labyrinthine segments is often thinned to maximize exposure of the IAC. In a series that looked at facial nerve injury in vestibular schwannoma resection, the facial nerve was preserved in 95% to 100% of all patients with tumors less than 1 cm, 80% to 92% of patients with tumors measuring 1 to 2 cm, and 50% to 76% of patients with tumors greater than 2 cm (6). Another study showed interruption of the facial nerve in 2% to 10% of patients who underwent resection of vestibular schwannomas (57).

Excluding vestibular schwannoma surgery, the most common site of iatrogenic injury during otologic surgery occurs in the tympanic segment followed by the mastoid segment and second genu (58). In a review of the experience at the House Ear Clinic, 57% of the iatrogenic facial nerve injuries occurred during the mastoidectomy, with or without tympanoplasty. Of note, 14% of the patients studied sustained an injury to the facial nerve during tympanoplasty, and an additional 14% were injured during the removal of bony exostoses from the ear canal (59). Intraoperative facial nerve monitoring serves as a useful adjunct to a detailed knowledge of normal and variant temporal bone anatomy, careful preoperative planning, and meticulous surgical technique to minimize the chance of inadvertent injury to the facial nerve.

HISTORY

Krause reported the first case of facial nerve monitoring during a neurotologic procedure 1898. He noted that electrical stimulation of the nerve resulted in facial movement (60). Throughout the first half of the 20th century, other surgeons used similar techniques, employing either direct observation of the facial muscles or having an assistant manually palpate the face during dissection or electrical stimulation. In 1965, Jako developed a photoelectric sensing device that detected light transmission through the cheek when placed inside the mouth, activating an audible signal (61). Some surgeons went as far as securing bells to the their patients' faces hoping that facial movement would produce an audible alert (62). Hampered by poor sensitivity and reliability, few of the early devices gained widespread acceptance.

Electromyography (EMG) was first employed as a method of facial nerve monitoring in 1979. Intraoperative stimulation of the nerve triggered responses that were detected by surface electrodes and displayed on an oscilloscope (63). To improve recognition of facial nerve stimulation, Sugita and Kobayashi devised a method to transduce facial movement into an auditory signal that could be heard by the surgeon and operating room personnel (64). In 1984, Moller and Jannetta (65) combined EMG, a constant voltage stimulator, and auditory signal in IOFNM. Combining visual and auditory signals to represent facial nerve stimulation and the use of insulated stimulator probes has not only increased the utility of facial nerve monitoring but also simplified the practical application of such technologies.

FACIAL NERVE MONITORING SYSTEMS

Several types of facial nerve monitors are currently available. Most of these systems monitor facial nerve integrity by detecting facial muscle contractions. Some systems utilize mechanical pressure sensors to detect facial muscle activity from manipulation, trauma, or directed stimulation of the nerve with a specially designed probe; others rely on video analysis of facial movements (66,67). Still others examine facial nerve APs, recorded either in an orthodromic (proximal-to-distal) or antidromic (distal-to-proximal) manner. Currently, the most common method of IOFNM measures EMG potentials, which has been shown to be more sensitive than movement sensors. By monitoring the electrical activity of the target muscles, EMG systems reflect the activity and integrity of the innervating nerve (68). Video analysis, although not as sensitive as EMG, also remains an area of active research (66,67,69). Regardless of the system used, intraoperative monitoring systems should meet certain criteria (Table 145.1) and assist in performing certain tasks (Table 145.4) (39).

ELECTROMYOGRAPHY AND EVOKED ELECTROMYOGRAPHY

EMG is performed by placing a pair of needle electrodes into a target muscle of the monitored nerve. In IOFNM, the facial musculature, typically the orbicularis oculi and orbicularis oris in the two-channel setup, is monitored; a third

TABLE 145.4	OBJECTIVES OF INTRAOPERATIVE FACIAL NERVE MONITORING

Early identification of the facial nerve in the temporal bone, IAC, cerebellopontine angle, or extratemporal portion during surgical dissection

Differentiation of the facial nerve from other structures in the surgical field, such as tumor, granulation tissue, or fibrosis

Differentiation of the facial nerve from other nerves in the cerebellopontine angle (trigeminal, cochlear, superior, and inferior vestibular nerves)

Rapid notification of the surgeon about trauma or pending trauma to the nerve

Reduction of trauma to the nerve during dissection of acoustic neuroma or cholesteatoma, as well as during procedures that require transposition or rerouting of the nerve

Early warning to the surgeon of an aberrant course of the nerve, or of unsuspected dehiscence of the nerve

Evaluation of nerve integrity at the completion of the procedure and prediction of postoperative function

Efficient identification of the site and degree of neural degeneration in patients undergoing facial nerve exploration for mass or paralysis[a]

[a]Silverstein H, Smouha EE, Jones R. Routine intraoperative facial nerve monitoring during otologic surgery. *Am J Otol* 1988;9:269–275.

channel placed in the contralateral face or the trapezius muscle may be used as a reference electrode. The potential difference between each electrode pair is subsequently amplified and displayed on an oscilloscope. Electrical activity of the muscle will appear as biphasic waveforms on the oscilloscope tracing. The motor unit potential reflects the electrical response of a single muscle fiber to a single efferent nerve fiber. When the response of an entire muscle group to an efferent motor nerve is considered, it is termed the collective action potential (CAP) or the compound muscle action potential (CMAP). Changes in neural activity may occur during operative dissection near the facial nerve and during manipulation of the nerve, altering the baseline neural activity and propagating compound action potentials that appear as deflections on the oscilloscope (56).

There are two types of electrode placement described in the literature: the bipolar technique recommends the use of electrode pairs in each muscle and the unipolar technique suggests one electrode per muscle. When these two techniques were compared during vestibular schwannoma resection, the bipolar technique was found to be significantly more sensitive to A-trains and thus recommended as the setup of choice for continuous EMG monitoring (70). Four-channel EMG, which monitors the frontalis and platysma in addition to the orbicularis oris and oculi, has been shown to improve muscular activity detection and allow a more precise determination of stimulation thresholds than the two-channel EMG (71).

Direct electrical stimulation with acoustic loudspeaker monitoring has been the technique of choice for intraoperative monitoring of the facial nerve in the last 25 years.

EMG activity can appear in a variety of forms including random muscle activity, a pulsed response coinciding with electrical stimulation, repetitive (train) activity, and nonrepetitive (burst, neurotonic discharge) activity. Train activity manifests as multiple responses from multiple motor units following a single stimulus. Such repetitive activity occurs following stretch injury or transmitted thermal injury to the nerve, actions that precipitate prolonged depolarization of the facial nerve beyond its threshold for generating an action potential. In this setting, the nerve will continue to fire until repolarization occurs or when nerve activation can no longer be sustained. In 2000, a classification system based on analysis of EMG tracings with respect to waveform characteristics, frequencies, and amplitudes was developed (68). This classification divided train activity into three subgroups. One of these particular patterns, the A-train, described as a sinusoidal pattern of high frequency and homogenous appearance, demonstrated to be the sole pattern clearly associated with postoperative paresis with high sensitivity and specificity. Additional characteristics are sudden onset and sudden termination. Its duration varies between milliseconds and several seconds. The normal amplitudes of A-trains are comparatively low, usually presenting between 100 and 200 µV (72). This study also concluded that bursts, spikes, and other train-type activities were of no significance in determining facial nerve function (68). Understanding and incorporating these waveform characteristics into monitoring technology has the potential to improve surgical outcomes by amending direct electric nerve stimulation with its real-time capabilities (68,72).

Conversely, nonrepetitive EMG activity closely follows direct mechanical or electrical stimulation, allowing otologic and neurotologic surgeons to locate and identify the facial nerve and, ideally, lead to its preservation (31). Stimulation probes deliver a stimulus of preset intensity and pulse duration to the facial nerve and are designed to function in a constantly changing surgical environment. The effects of bleeding or accumulation of other fluids such as irrigation, perilymph, endolymph, and cerebrospinal fluid may be minimized by insulating the probe flush to the tip (73). The stimulus intensity level is chosen to elicit a neuromuscular response with the least amount of delivered current. When the nerve is directly stimulated by the probe via a depolarizing current, the resulting compound action potential of the facial muscle is recorded by EMG, confirming the location of the facial nerve (see Fig. 145.10). To achieve this aim, either monopolar or bipolar stimulating probes may be used.

Bipolar probes offer the advantage of being more selective limiting the passage of current to a smaller surface area, allowing for more precise localization. Unfortunately, bipolar stimulation depends on appropriate alignment of the bipolar tip in contact with the nerve. Such precise orientation is difficult, if not impossible, to achieve in the tight confines of the posterior fossa or on a small exposed area of the intratemporal segment of the facial nerve. Despite

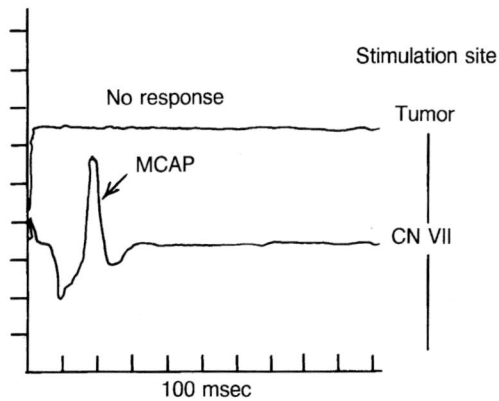

Figure 145.10 Intraoperative recordings of evoked EMG of the facial nerve in response to stimulation of the seventh cranial nerve and tumor.

the theoretical advantage, practical application of bipolar stimulators in otologic and neurotologic surgery has been limited (3,56).

Because the selectivity offered by the bipolar stimulator is not critical in surgical fields containing one, or few, nerves of interest, monopolar stimulators are more widely used in facial nerve monitoring. When stimulus intensity approximates the nerve threshold level, a monopolar electrode can achieve spatial orientation of less than 1 mm. Several methods of monopolar stimulation have been developed. A thin, malleable probe that has been insulated to the tip resembling an unsharpened pencil was fashioned to deliver a stimulus with minimal risk of collateral spread (74,75). An alternate probe with a ball electrode capping an insulated, flexible platinum–iridium tip, was developed allowing for stimulation of the nerve in obscured areas where the flush tip may not be able to gain sufficient contact with the nerve (3). A set of dissecting instruments that allow for simultaneous operating in the surgical field and stimulation of the facial nerve has also been developed (76). By applying continuous electrical current to the drill burr and insulated microsurgical instruments, the armamentarium of intraoperative facial nerve monitoring has been further advanced (77).

Stimulating probes may either have a constant current or constant voltage source. Bleeding, soft tissue, tumor, cholesteatoma, and spinal fluid may shunt current from the stimulus probe away from the nerve, creating variations in electrode impedance. To continue to depolarize the nerve, the constant current stimulator must be increased to higher levels in the face of increased resistance. Potential damage to the nerve may occur when the stimulus current remains elevated but the resistance in the operative environment is reduced by suctioning or controlling nearby bleeding. On the other hand, constant voltage systems deliver current based on the intrinsic resistance of the nerve according to the Ohm law, adjusting current accordingly and limiting the effect of shunting on these systems. Although the total current changes as the operative milieu changes, the current delivered to the nerve remains more stable in constant voltage systems (3). Despite the theoretical differences in the two systems, no specific clinical advantage of either system has been found (74).

DIRECT FACIAL NERVE MONITORING

In addition to EMG monitoring during facial nerve stimulation, techniques for direct monitoring of neural transmission exist. Unlike EMG, direct monitoring systems follow CNAPs as they progress down the nerve itself in a orthodromic, or proximal-to-distal, direction. Antidromic, or distal-to-proximal, potentials may also be monitored, allowing real-time detection of facial nerve injury or conduction blockade (78,79). Direct monitoring does, however, require the attachment of electrodes to the nerve directly, a technically challenging and potentially deleterious activity. Additionally, direct monitoring of CNAPs is limited by the smaller field potentials created by depolarization of nerve fibers, resulting in diminished sensitivity.

ANESTHESIA AND FACIAL NERVE MONITORING

In the course of general anesthesia, anesthesiologists commonly use muscle relaxants that affect the postsynaptic nicotinic receptors. These agents act as antagonists (nondepolarizing) or agonists (depolarizing) at the muscle end plate receptor. Nondepolarizing agents may be short acting or long acting. Atracurium, vecuronium, and mivacurium typically induce paralysis for up to 30 minutes, whereas effects from pancuronium and tubocurarine may last up to 1 hour. Meanwhile, succinylcholine, the most common depolarizing agent is extremely short acting, exerting its effects for 5 to 10 minutes. Paralysis from the use of these agents interferes with the recording of EMG potentials. Therefore, nondepolarizing agents are typically contraindicated in cases in which intraoperative facial nerve monitoring is planned. Succinylcholine is used for induction because of its short duration of effect with complete recovery from neuromuscular blockade within 15 minutes.

Local anesthesia can also impair the use of facial nerve monitoring. Many otologic surgeons routinely use lidocaine with epinephrine at the beginning of the procedure, both at the site of the postauricular incision and in the ear canal when indicated. The advantages of this injection are improved hemostasis and analgesia, possibly limiting the amount of narcotic analgesia required for patient comfort. To avoid potential paralysis of the facial nerve that could interfere with facial nerve monitoring, the surgeon's index finger is placed on the mastoid tip during injection to avoid deep injection of lidocaine near the stylomastoid foramen. Care is also taken to not over aggressively inject the ear canal, especially in the posteroinferior aspect. Many surgeons have encountered the unnerving transient postoperative facial paralysis that resolves within several hours that is attributed to the activity of the local anesthetic (80).

We have utilized this method of anesthesia with great success in operations in which IOFNM is used. Partial muscle paralysis is not used during monitored cases at our institution. Because a partially paralyzed muscle fatigues rapidly, multiple successive stimuli may lead to progressively smaller evoked EMG amplitudes, resulting in diminished sensitivity of the continuous EMG monitor and potential problems using the stimulus probe.

INDICATIONS FOR INTRAOPERATIVE FACIAL NERVE MONITORING

A list of surgical procedures that should be considered for intraoperative facial nerve monitoring can be found in Table 145.5. We have applied the routine use of the facial nerve monitor in all otologic and neurotologic cases, as the facial nerve is potentially at risk in all such situations. The use of IOFNM in vestibular schwannoma resection is routine at many institutions and should be employed when possible (81). A significant and substantial reduction (14.5% to 3.6%) in the frequency of facial nerve paralysis following the implementation of monitoring in cerebellpontine angle surgery has been reported (82). While the benefits of IOFNM for vestibular schwannoma surgery and posterior fossa surgery have been established, the role of monitoring in routine otologic procedures is less well defined. The use of monitoring in such cases is not universal. A recent survey of 223 American otolaryngologists showed that 66% use IOFNM at least some of the time for otologic procedures such as chronic ear surgery or stapedectomy (83). In this same survey, they found that 46% of surgeons never use facial nerve monitoring for such cases (83). Similarly, a study of surgeons in the United Kingdom similarly found that a substantial percentage of surgeons never use monitoring for mastoidectomy (38%) or stapedectomy (85%) (84). Whether IOFNM should be employed in "routine"

TABLE 145.5	POTENTIAL INDICATIONS FOR INTRAOPERATIVE FACIAL NERVE MONITORING

Acoustic neuroma and tumors of the cerebellopontine angle
Vestibular nerve section
Repair of congenital aural atresia
Skull base surgery
Microvascular decompression of the fifth, seventh, and eighth cranial nerves
Cochlear implantation
Labyrinthectomy
Endolymphatic sac surgery
Facial nerve decompression
Mastoidectomy
Tympanoplasty
Canalplasty
Stapedectomy
Parotidectomy
Excision of glomus tumors

otologic cases has been questioned. The fear that surgeons may gain a false confidence in their skills and knowledge based on their use of intraoperative facial nerve monitors reflects a broader concern from many in the otolaryngology community that overreliance on this technology could, in fact, lead to iatrogenic facial nerve injuries, particularly in situations when the monitor fails to recognize the nerve. In addition, there has been some reluctance in the otolaryngology community to declare IOFNM as the standard of care in otologic surgery. However, the use of the facial nerve monitor can never replace careful planning, experience, and a thorough knowledge of the anatomy of the temporal bone and posterior fossa. Several general principles regarding the facial nerve during otologic and neurotologic surgery should be employed:

1. Obtain and maintain thorough knowledge of the ear, temporal bone, and posterior fossa. Temporal bone lab dissection is essential in gaining this knowledge and expertise. Understand the three-dimensional anatomy of the facial nerve in the temporal bone. Appropriate courses are available throughout the United States for practicing physicians if they have no routine access to a formal temporal bone lab.
2. Treat the facial nerve as if it is dehiscent until proven otherwise, especially in the tympanic segment.
3. Expect any type of anatomic variation of the facial nerve, especially in revision cases.
4. Use meticulous technique at all times.
5. Always be well prepared—identify preoperatively cases in which the facial nerve may be at greater risk (i.e., congenital atresia).
6. Routinely examine the monitoring system to ensure that all parts are in working order, and understand the physiologic basis of your particular system.

BENEFITS AND APPLICATIONS

Numerous studies support the use of intraoperative facial nerve monitoring in performing vestibular schwannoma and skull base surgery, but the utility of this technology extends beyond the IAC and cerebellopontine angle. Facial nerve monitoring has been reported as beneficial in nearly all surgical procedures that place the facial nerve at risk. The benefits of such adaptations have been well documented.

REMOVAL OF VESTIBULAR SCHWANNOMAS AND TUMORS OF THE CEREBELLOPONTINE ANGLE

Intraoperative facial nerve monitoring allows identification of the nerve in the IAC or cerebellopontine angle before the nerve is clearly visualized through the use of stimulating probes; similar techniques allow mapping the course of the facial nerve during dissection. Based on feedback provided by the monitoring system, the surgeon may adjust the microsurgical technique to minimize injury or trauma to

the nerve. Since the advent of IOFNM, several reports have extolled the advantages of facial nerve monitoring in cerebellopontine angle surgery, each citing improved facial nerve outcome, especially in removing large tumors (82,85–87).

Additionally, IOFNM may be used to predict postoperative facial nerve function (71,88–93). After resection of the vestibular schwannoma, the facial nerve is stimulated with a facial nerve probe at the lowest stimulation threshold at the brainstem and medial to the tumor dissection. The stimulation threshold is determined by first applying 0.05 mA and increasing in 0.05-mA increments until response amplitude is obtained. The response amplitude as well as lowest stimulation threshold can then be used as a predictor of postoperative facial nerve function with lower thresholds reflecting better facial nerve function. A ratio of response amplitude recorded from stimulating the nerve both proximal and distal to the tumor dissection of 0.1 or less has been shown to correlate with a poor facial functional outcome in 75% of patients at 6 months (93). Furthermore, a small tumor size along with a stimulus threshold less than 0.05 mA has been shown to correlate with a House-Brackmann grade of III or less in 88% of patients in the initial postoperative period (88). Another study showed that a stimulus threshold of 0.05 mA or less and a response amplitude of at least 240 μV predict a House-Brackmann grade I or II facial nerve function with 98% probability (90).

The A-train has been shown to be the only intraoperative EMG pattern associated with deterioration of facial nerve function (68). Subsequent studies have investigated the correlation of intraoperative EMG parameters and their ability to predict facial nerve outcomes. Reports demonstrate a strong correlation between the length of train time and postoperative facial nerve function (94). Patients with normal preoperative facial nerve function could tolerate up to 0.5 seconds of train time. However, at 10 seconds of train time, postoperative facial nerve function could potentially deteriorate by 1 House-Brackmann grade (94).

Not only has IOFNM improved results and helped predict postoperative facial nerve function but IOFNM has given surgeons insight into which patients may benefit from intraoperative prophylactic medication. Clinical trials medicating patients who develop reversible pathognomonic intraoperative A-train EMG activity with a combination of intravenous HES, a vasoactive agent, and nimodipine have shown improvement in long-term functional facial nerve results (6,95,96).

POSTERIOR FOSSA, MIDDLE FOSSA, AND SKULL BASE PROCEDURES

Vestibular nerve section; microvascular decompression of the fifth, seventh, and eighth cranial nerves; and other lateral skull base surgical procedures constitute additional areas in which IOFNM is beneficial. Extrapolating from the benefits of identification and limited damage offered by IOFNM, Moller and Jannetta described a method of microvascular decompression of the facial nerve for hemifacial spasm that utilizes the monitoring system. The details of this procedure may be found elsewhere, but simply stated, the ongoing presence of abnormal responses to facial nerve stimulation indicates continued compromise of the nerve. Decompression, therefore, is continued until the abnormal responses abate, indicating removal of the offending vessel from the nerve (97,98). Facial nerve monitoring promotes improved identification of the offending vessel, decreasing the need for re-exploration. In addition, IOFNM has been shown to improve facial nerve function following the infratemporal fossa approach for extirpation of lesions of the lateral skull base (99,100).

CHRONIC EAR SURGERY AND REVISION MASTOID SURGERY

Previous operations and alterations in normal landmarks increase the level of difficulty in revision mastoidectomy. Cholesteatoma, otorrhea, granulation tissue, fibrosis, and other disease processes that necessitate the procedure also can obscure the facial nerve and its landmarks. The facial nerve can be dehiscent in up to 57% of patients without cholesteatoma or prior operations (101). Exposure of the nerve during prior operations or from erosion of the fallopian canal by cholesteatoma further heightens the likelihood of encountering an exposed facial nerve. Intraoperative facial nerve monitoring will alert the surgeon to the presence of dehiscent nerve segments and aid in mapping the nerve to allow focused surgical dissection (102). Some studies suggest that monitoring in this setting will often detect a dehiscence before it is visualized (103). The success of monitoring in this setting has been documented, and one group has reported 1,200 consecutive cases without facial nerve injury (102). Additionally, a recent cost-effectiveness study concluded that using facial nerve monitoring in both primary and revision surgery was the most cost-effective approach (104). Our current practice is to utilize IOFNM monitoring for all chronic ear cases, including tympanoplasty and mastoidectomy, both initial and revision.

STAPEDECTOMY

The most common site for a dehiscence in the fallopian canal occurs in the tympanic segment. The intimate relationship between the oval window and this segment of the facial nerve demands that extreme caution be exercised in performing a stapedectomy. Although a dehiscent facial nerve is not a contraindication to performing the operation, IOFNM may alert the surgeon to a dehiscent nerve during surgical dissection or laser stapedectomy. Injuries to the nerve during this procedure are rare, but have been reported (101). Any steps taken to minimize this occurrence, including IOFNM, may be beneficial to the patient. Although each individual surgeon may choose whether or not to use of IOFNM for otologic surgery, our current practice is to use facial nerve monitoring in all middle ear cases, routine or complicated, including stapedectomy.

PEDIATRIC OTOLOGY

Iatrogenic facial nerve injury is equally, if not more, devastating in the pediatric population. Although the physical consequences of such an injury are the same, the emotional damage may be magnified in children. The facial nerve occupies a similar position in children as in adults, but some subtle differences related to development exist. The development of the facial nerve is intimately related to the development of the temporal bone; therefore, the facial nerve will not typically reach its adult course until mastoid development is complete (age 2). Facial nerve development is complete by approximately age 4 (105). Any abnormality of the inner, middle, or external ear, or of the mastoid, may imply an abnormal course for the facial nerve (106). Given the potential for an aberrant nerve course, combined with the long-term consequences of an iatrogenic injury, intraoperative facial nerve monitoring may be beneficial in any pediatric otologic procedure, except in tympanostomy and tube placement.

CONGENITAL AURAL ATRESIA

Iatrogenic facial nerve injury comprises the greatest concern held by parents, patients, and surgeons during repair for congenital aural atresia. This risk, particularly in unilateral cases, dissuades many otologic surgeons from attempting these complicated operations. In these patients, the facial nerve is typically located more anterior and superior than in normal subjects. A wide range of other anomalies have also been reported (107). The incidence of iatrogenic facial paralysis in congenital aural atresia surgery ranges from 0% to 8% (108). Published reports primarily reflect the experience of the authors in their own series, most with extensive experience in this type of surgery. One surgeon describes five instances where the facial nerve is vulnerable to injury during atresia surgery (Table 145.6). From his experience, the nerve is most likely to be injured during canalplasty when drilling through the inferoposterior aspect of the dense atretic bone (108). IOFNM is routinely employed during these operations (109).

TABLE 145.6	LIKELY TIMES FOR IATROGENIC INJURY DURING REPAIR OF ATRESIA

Skin incision
Dissection in the glenoid fossa
Canalplasty with drilling of atretic bone, especially posteroinferiorly
• Transposition of the nerve to improve access to the stapes footplate and oval window
Preauricular soft tissue dissection for auricular repositioning during mastoidectomy

MONITORING OTHER CRANIAL NERVES

Although much of this chapter has focused on intraoperative monitoring of CN VII and VIII, skull base surgery can also endanger other cranial nerves, namely, CNs III, IV, V, VI, IX, X, XI, and XII. While the literature is scant, there are studies that have extended the positive experiences with IOFNM to these cranial nerves.

Cranial nerves III, IV, and VI are especially at risk during resection of tumors involving the anterior cranial fossa, the cavernous sinus, the adjacent petroclival region, and the orbit (110). Electrodes were placed into the individual extraocular muscles and spontaneous muscle activity and CMAPs were recorded, demonstrating that intraoperative EMG recordings following bipolar electrical stimulation could identify CN III in 5 out of 7 cases and CN VI in 12 out of 18 cases. However, reproducible recordings from CN IV were unable to be obtained nor were they able to predict postoperative outcomes for CN III or VI (110).

Cranial nerves IX to XII are at risk during operations on large tumors in the cerebellopontine angle, the petroclival region, the rhomboid fossa, the brainstem, the jugular foramen, and the foramen magnum. Damage to these cranial nerves can lead to dysarthria, dysphonia, dysgeusia, and dysphagia, with a potential permanent risk of aspiration (111). Similar to the study of CNs III, IV, and VI, intraoperative EMG was used to monitor these lower cranial nerves (LCN). For EMG monitoring of CN IX, a pair of electrodes was placed (at a distance of 2 to 3 mm) into the lateral aspect of the soft palate ipsilateral to the tumor. A pair of electrodes were placed into the ipsilateral vocalis muscle, trapezius, and tongue in order to monitor CNs X, XI, and XII, respectively. To allow intraoral placement of the electrodes, the patients were intubated transnasally. Intraoperative EMG monitoring proved to be a safe tool for the identification and localization of the LCNs and contributed to their anatomical and functional preservation. However, the predictive value of standard neurophysiologic parameters for functional outcome was limited (111). A study in which 123 skull base cases in which LCNs were monitored concluded that immediate feedback obtained with intraoperative monitoring helps reduce LCN morbidity and assists in gross tumor removal (112).

EMG via contact electrodes integrated into the endotracheal tube (ETT) has been used to monitor the recurrent laryngeal nerve (CN X) and has been extensively used and validated during thyroid and parathyroid surgery (113). Its ease of use makes it an attractive option for intraoperative CN X monitoring during skull base surgery. The main disadvantage of a monitoring ETT is related to the fact that the quality of recording depends on maintaining contact with the vocal cords, and if contact is lost secondary to ETT movement during surgery, the recording may not be interpretable (114). When compared to electrodes placed directly into the vocalis muscle, the monitoring ETT exhibited a lower rate of false-positive response but a lower sensitivity (115). Despite these disadvantages, intraoperative neural monitoring of CN X with a monitoring ETT has gained much support due to its familiarity by anesthesiologists and otolaryngologists during thyroid and parathyroid surgery and its ease of use.

CONCLUSIONS

Intraoperative neurophysiologic monitoring has undergone significant improvements since its nascence in the 20th century, with its applications continuing to grow. Preservation of hearing and facial nerve function is paramount in many otologic and neurotologic procedures. Although the preservation of hearing has yet to reach the same level of success achieved in preservation of the facial nerve function, the technology and our understanding of the neurophysiologic basis of hearing is advancing, and further improvement seems likely. Intraoperative monitoring of the facial and auditory nerves is now in increasing use around the world. Efficacy has been established in improving functional outcomes in cerebellopontine angle tumors and many experts favor its routine use in a wide array of both otologic and neurotologic surgeries, especially when the risk of nerve injury is considered to be high. As we expand neurophysiologic monitoring to other cranial nerves, its role in the preservation of these nerves may prove useful in quality of life outcomes and likely will play a larger role in neurotologic surgery in the future. Regardless, intraoperative neurophysiologic monitoring should serve only as an adjunct to, not a replacement for, extensive preoperative planning, a thorough knowledge of temporal bone anatomy and its common variants, and meticulous technique.

HIGHLIGHTS

- Auditory compromise during surgery can occur via direct injury to the cochlea, internal auditory artery, or the labyrinthine artery, or as a result of cochlear nerve stretching, compression, transection, or thermal injury.
- ECochG, ABR testing, and DENM, often referred to as CNAP, are all techniques used in intraoperative auditory system monitoring.
- ECochG best measures the integrity of cochlear blood supply.
- DENM, or CNAP, monitoring can be used in patients who have an absent preoperative ABR.
- ABR is a far-field technique, whereas ECochG and DENM are near-field techniques.
- Facial nerve injury may occur as a result of transection; direct trauma from drilling, using the ultrasonic aspirator, or dissection; stretch; compression; thermal injury from drilling, cautery, or the laser; vascular compromise; or edema of the nerve from regional dissection.

- The facial nerve may be monitored by mechanical pressure sensing devices, EMG, or direct monitoring of action potentials.
- The A-train as the only intraoperative EMG pattern corresponding to deterioration of facial nerve function.
- Monitoring systems may be augmented by the addition of stimulating probes and dissecting instruments that help identify and map the facial nerve.
- IOFNM should assist the surgeon in identifying the facial nerve, rapidly notify the surgeon when trauma occurs, warn the surgeon as to an aberrant nerve course, evaluate neural integrity at the conclusion of the procedure, and help predict postoperative facial nerve function.
- The use of nondepolarizing muscle relaxants during anesthesia should be avoided in cases where IOFNM is being utilized. Succinylcholine can be used for induction because of its short duration of effect with complete recovery from neuromuscular blockade within 15 minutes.
- IOFNM has proven useful in improving facial nerve outcomes during removal of acoustic neuromas and tumors of the crebellopontine angle, particularly in large tumors.
- Additional applications of IOFNM include vestibular nerve section, skull base surgery, microvascular decompression, cochlear implantation, repair of congenital aural atresia, stapedectomy, and chronic ear surgery.
- Monitoring cranial nerves other than CNs VII and VIII is effective in reducing LCN morbidity and assists in gross tumor removal.
- CN X can be monitored intraoperatively via the recurrent laryngeal nerve with a monitoring ETT.

REFERENCES

1. Jewett DL, Williston JS. Auditory-evoked far fields averaged from the scalp of humans. *Brain* 1971;94:681–696.
2. Levine RA, Montgomery WW, Ojemann RJ. Evoked potential detection of hearing loss during acoustic neuroma surgery. Abstract. *Neurology* 1978;28:339.
3. Yingling CD, Gardi JN. Intraoperative monitoring of facial and cochlear nerves during acoustic neuroma surgery. *Otolaryngol Clin North Am* 1992;25:413–448.
4. Hilton CW, Haines SJ, Agrawal A, Levine SC. Late failure rate of hearing preservation after middle fossa approach for resection of vestibular schwannoma. *Otol Neurotol* 2011;32:132–135.
5. Tringali S, Ferber-Viart C, Fuchsmann C, et al. Hearing preservation in retrosigmoid approach of small vestibular schwannomas: prognostic value of the degree of internal auditory canal filling. *Otol Neurotol* 2010;31:1469–1472.
6. Scheller C, Richter HP, Engelhardt M, et al. The influence of prophylactic vasoactive treatment on cochlear and facial nerve functions after vestibular schwannoma surgery: a prospective and open-label randomized pilot study. *Neurosurgery* 2007;61:92–97; discussion 7–8.
7. Kaylie DM, Gilbert E, Horgan MA, et al. Acoustic neuroma surgery outcomes. *Otol Neurotol* 2001;22:686–689.
8. Samii M, Gerganov V, Samii A. Improved preservation of hearing and facial nerve function in vestibular schwannoma surgery via the retrosigmoid approach in a series of 200 patients. *J Neurosurg* 2006;105:527–535.
9. Legatt AD. Mechanisms of intraoperative brainstem auditory evoked potential changes. *J Clin Neurophysiol* 2002;19:396–408.
10. Youssef AS, Downes AE. Intraoperative neurophysiological monitoring in vestibular schwannoma surgery: advances and clinical implications. *Neurosurg Focus* 2009;27:E9.
11. Hall JWI. *The new handbook of auditory evoked responses.* Boston, MA: Allyn & Bacon, 2005.
12. Battista RA, Wiet RJ, Paauwe L. Evaluation of three intraoperative auditory monitoring techniques in acoustic neuroma surgery. *Am J Otol* 2000;21:244–248.
13. Piccirillo E, Hiraumi H, Hamada M, et al. Intraoperative cochlear nerve monitoring in vestibular schwannoma surgery—does it really affect hearing outcome? *Audiol Neurootol* 2008;13:58–64.
14. Schmerber S, Lavieille JP, Dumas G, Herve T. Intraoperative auditory monitoring in vestibular schwannoma surgery: new trends. *Acta Otolaryngol* 2004;124:53–61.
15. Yamakami I, Yoshinori H, Saeki N, et al. Hearing preservation and intraoperative auditory brainstem response and cochlear nerve compound action potential monitoring in the removal of small acoustic neurinoma via the retrosigmoid approach. *J Neurol Neurosurg Psychiatry* 2009;80:218–227.
16. Roberson JB Jr, Jackson LE, McAuley JR. Acoustic neuroma surgery: absent auditory brainstem response does not contraindicate attempted hearing preservation. *Laryngoscope* 1999;109:904–910.
17. Matthies C, Samii M. Management of vestibular schwannomas (acoustic neuromas): the value of neurophysiology for evaluation and prediction of auditory function in 420 cases. *Neurosurgery* 1997;40:919–929; discussion 29–30.
18. Harper CM, Harner SG, Slavit DH, et al. Effect of BAEP monitoring on hearing preservation during acoustic neuroma resection. *Neurology* 1992;42:1551–1553.
19. Strauss C, Bischoff B, Neu M, et al. Vasoactive treatment for hearing preservation in acoustic neuroma surgery. *J Neurosurg* 2001;95:771–777.
20. Jackson LE, Roberson JB Jr. Acoustic neuroma surgery: use of cochlear nerve action potential monitoring for hearing preservation. *Am J Otol* 2000;21:249–259.
21. Schwartz DM, Gennarelli TA. Delayed sensorineural hearing loss following uncomplicated neurovascular decompression of the trigeminal root entry zone. *Am J Otol* 1990;11:95–98.
22. Neu M, Strauss C, Romstock J, et al. The prognostic value of intraoperative BAEP patterns in acoustic neurinoma surgery. *Clin Neurophysiol* 1999;110:1935–1941.
23. Lee SH, Song DG, Kim S, et al. Results of auditory brainstem response monitoring of microvascular decompression: a prospective study of 22 patients with hemifacial spasm. *Laryngoscope* 2009;119:1887–1892.
24. Polo G, Fischer C, Sindou MP, Marneffe V. Brainstem auditory evoked potential monitoring during microvascular decompression for hemifacial spasm: intraoperative brainstem auditory evoked potential changes and warning values to prevent hearing loss—prospective study in a consecutive series of 84 patients. *Neurosurgery* 2004;54:97–104; discussion -6.
25. Polo G, Fischer C. Intraoperative monitoring of brainstem auditory evoked potentials during microvascular decompression of cranial nerves in cerebellopontine angle. *Neurochirurgie* 2009;55:152–157.
26. Sindou M. Operative strategies for minimizing hearing loss associated with microvascular decompression for trigeminal neuralgia. *World Neurosurg* 2010;74:111–112.
27. Dannenbaum M, Lega BC, Suki D, et al. Microvascular decompression for hemifacial spasm: long-term results from 114 operations performed without neurophysiological monitoring. *J Neurosurg* 2008;109:410–415.
28. Ferraro JA. Electrocochleography: a review of recording approaches, clinical applications, and new findings in adults and children. *J Am Acad Audiol* 2010;21:145–152.
29. Schlake HP, Milewski C, Goldbrunner RH, et al. Combined intraoperative monitoring of hearing by means of auditory brainstem responses (ABR) and transtympanic electrocochleography

(ECochG) during surgery of intra- and extrameatal acoustic neurinomas. *Acta Neurochir (Wien)* 2001;143:985–995; discussion 95–96.

30. Nedzelski JM, Chiong CM, Cashman MZ, et al. Hearing preservation in acoustic neuroma surgery: value of monitoring cochlear nerve action potentials. *Otolaryngol Head Neck Surg* 1994;111:703–709.

31. Harper CM, Daube JR. Facial nerve electromyography and other cranial nerve monitoring. *J Clin Neurophysiol* 1998;15:206–216.

32. Silverstein H, McDaniel AB, Norrell H. Hearing preservation after acoustic neuroma surgery using intraoperative direct eighth cranial nerve monitoring. *Am J Otol* 1985;(Suppl):99–106.

33. Ohashi T, Ochi K, Kinoshita H, et al. Electrocochleogram after transection of vestibulo-cochlear nerve in a patient with a large acoustic neurinoma. *Hear Res* 2001;154:26–31.

34. Arenberg IK, Kobayashi H, Obert AD, Gibson WP. Intraoperative electrocochleography of endolymphatic hydrops surgery using clicks and tone bursts. *Acta Otolaryngol Suppl* 1993;504:58–67.

35. Arts HA, Adams ME, Telian SA, et al. Reversible electrocochleographic abnormalities in superior canal dehiscence. *Otol Neurotol* 2009;30:79–86.

36. Moller AR, Jannetta PJ. Compound action potentials recorded intracranially from the auditory nerve in man. *Exp Neurol* 1981;74:862–874.

37. Tucker A, Slattery WH III, Solcyk L, Brackmann DE. Intraoperative auditory assessments as predictors of hearing preservation after vestibular schwannoma surgery. *J Am Acad Audiol* 2001;12:471–477.

38. Meyer TA, Canty PA, Wilkinson EP, et al. Small acoustic neuromas: surgical outcomes versus observation or radiation. *Otol Neurotol* 2006;27:380–392.

39. Colletti V, Fiorino FG. Advances in monitoring of seventh and eighth cranial nerve function during posterior fossa surgery. *Am J Otol* 1998;19:503–512.

40. Danner C, Mastrodimos B, Cueva RA. A comparison of direct eighth nerve monitoring and auditory brainstem response in hearing preservation surgery for vestibular schwannoma. *Otol Neurotol* 2004;25:826–832.

41. Cohen NL, Hoffman RA. Surgical complications of multichannel cochlear implants in North America. *Adv Otorhinolaryngol* 1993;48:70–74.

42. Kveton J, Book J. A comparison of auditory nerve monitoring techniques in acoustic tumor surgery. In: Tos M, Thomsen J, eds. *Acoustic neuroma*. New York: Kugler Publications, 1992:537–542.

43. Sanna M, Khrais T, Russo A, et al. Hearing preservation surgery in vestibular schwannoma: the hidden truth. *Ann Otol Rhinol Laryngol* 2004;113:156–163.

44. Committee on Hearing and Equilibrium guidelines for the evaluation of hearing preservation in acoustic neuroma (vestibular schwannoma). American Academy of Otolaryngology-Head and Neck Surgery Foundation, INC. *Otolaryngol Head Neck Surg* 1995;113:179–180.

45. Khrais T, Sanna M. Hearing preservation surgery in vestibular schwannoma. *J Laryngol Otol* 2006;120:366–370.

46. Kanzaki J, Inoue Y, Ogawa K. The learning curve in post-operative hearing results in vestibular schwannoma surgery. *Auris Nasus Larynx* 2001;28:209–213.

47. Zappia J, Wiet RJ, O'Connor CA, Martone L. Intraoperative auditory monitoring in acoustic neuroma surgery. *Otolaryngol Head Neck Surg* 1996;115:98–106.

48. Prass RL, Kinney SE, Luders H. Transtragal, transtympanic electrode placement for intraoperative electrocochleographic monitoring. *Otolaryngol Head Neck Surg* 1987;97:343–350.

49. Yamakami I, Oka N, Yamaura A. Intraoperative monitoring of cochlear nerve compound action potential in cerebellopontine angle tumour removal. *J Clin Neurosci* 2003;10:567–570.

50. Sekiya T, Yagihashi A, Asano K, Suzuki S. Nimodipine ameliorates trauma-induced cochlear neuronal death. *Neurol Res* 2002;24:775–780.

51. Bischoff B, Romstock J, Fahlbusch R, et al. Intraoperative brainstem auditory evoked potential pattern and perioperative vasoactive treatment for hearing preservation in vestibular schwannoma surgery. *J Neurol Neurosurg Psychiatry* 2008;79:170–175.

52. Morawski K, Namyslowski G, Lisowska G, et al. Intraoperative monitoring of cochlear function using distortion product oto-acoustic emissions (DPOAEs) in patients with cerebellopontine angle tumors. *Otol Neurotol* 2004;25:818–825.

53. Savage JR, Weiner GM. Litigation in otolaryngology - trends and recommendations. *J Laryngol Otol* 2006;120:1001–1004.

54. May M, Wiet RJ. Iatrogenic injury: prevention and management. In: May M, ed. *The facial nerve*. New York: Thieme, 1986.

55. Nilssen EL, Wormald PJ. Facial nerve palsy in mastoid surgery. *J Laryngol Otol* 1997;111:113–116.

56. Selesnick SH. Optimal stimulus duration for intraoperative facial nerve monitoring. *Laryngoscope* 1999;109:1376–1385.

57. Bacciu A, Falcioni M, Pasanisi E, et al. Intracranial facial nerve grafting after removal of vestibular schwannoma. *Am J Otolaryngol* 2009;30:83–88.

58. Mancini F, Taibah AK, Falcioni M. Complications and their management in tympanomastoid surgery. *Otolaryngol Clin North Am* 1999;32:567–583.

59. Green JD, Jr, Shelton C, Brackmann DE. Iatrogenic facial nerve injury during otologic surgery. *Laryngoscope* 1994;104:922–926.

60. Krause F. *Surgery of the brain and spinal cord*. New York: Rebman, 1912.

61. Jako GJ. Facial nerve monitor. *Trans Am Acad Ophthalmol Otolaryngol* 1965;69:340–343.

62. Williams JD, Lehman R. Bells against palsy. *Am J Otol* 1988;9:81–82.

63. Delgado TE, Bucheit WA, Rosenholtz HR, Chrissian S. Intraoperative monitoring of facila muscle evoked responses obtained by intracranial stimulation of the facila nerve: a more accurate technique for facila nerve dissection. *Neurosurgery* 1979;4:418–421.

64. Sugita K, Kobayashi S. Technical and instrumental improvements in the surgical treatment of acoustic neurinomas. *J Neurosurg* 1982;57:747–752.

65. Moller AR, Jannetta PJ. Preservation of facial function during removal of acoustic neuromas. Use of monopolar constant-voltage stimulation and EMG. *J Neurosurg* 1984;61:757–760.

66. Filipo R, De Seta E, Bertoli GA. Intraoperative videomonitoring of the facial nerve. *Am J Otol* 2000;21:119–122.

67. De Seta E, Bertoli G, De Seta D, et al. New development in intraoperative video monitoring of facial nerve: a pilot study. *Otol Neurotol* 2010;31:1498–1502.

68. Romstock J, Strauss C, Fahlbusch R. Continuous electromyography monitoring of motor cranial nerves during cerebellopontine angle surgery. *J Neurosurg* 2000;93:586–593.

69. Filipo R, Pichi B, Bertoli GA, De Seta E. Video-based system for intraoperative facial nerve monitoring: comparison with electromyography. *Otol Neurotol* 2002;23:594–597.

70. Rampp S, Prell J, Rachinger JC, et al. Does electrode placement influence quality of intraoperative monitoring in vestibular schwannoma surgery? *Cen Eur Neurosurg* 2011;72:22–27.

71. Grayeli AB, Guindi S, Kalamarides M, et al. Four-channel electromyography of the facial nerve in vestibular schwannoma surgery: sensitivity and prognostic value for short-term facial function outcome. *Otol Neurotol* 2005;26:114–120.

72. Prell J, Rachinger J, Scheller C, et al. A real-time monitoring system for the facial nerve. *Neurosurgery* 2010;66:1064–1073; discussion 73.

73. Prass RL. Iatrogenic facial nerve injury: the role of facial nerve monitoring. *Otolaryngol Clin North Am* 1996;29:265–275.

74. Prass R, Luders H. Constant-current versus constant-voltage stimulation. *J Neurosurg* 1985;62:622–623.

75. Kartush JM, Niparko JK, Bledsoe SC, et al. Intraoperative facial nerve monitoring: a comparison of stimulating electrodes. *Laryngoscope* 1985;95:1536–1540.

76. Kartush JM. Electroneurography and intraoperative facial monitoring in contemporary neurotology. *Otolaryngol Head Neck Surg* 1989;101:496–503.

77. Silverstein H. Microsurgical instruments and nerve stimulator—monitor for retrolabyrinthine vestibular neurectomy. *Otolaryngol Head Neck Surg* 1986;94:409–411.

78. Richmond IL, Mahla M. Use of antidromic recording to monitor facial nerve function intraoperatively. *Neurosurgery* 1985;16:458–462.

79. Colletti V, Fiorino F, Policante Z, Bruni L. Intraoperative monitoring of facial nerve antidromic potentials during acoustic neuroma surgery. *Acta Otolaryngol* 1997;117:663–669.

80. Silverstein H, Smouha EE, Jones R. Routine intraoperative facial nerve monitoring during otologic surgery. *Am J Otol* 1988;9:269–275.

81. Acoustic neuroma. *Consens Statement* 1991;9:1–24.

82. Hammerschlag PE, Cohen NL. Intraoperative monitoring of facial nerve function in cerebellopontine angle surgery. *Otolaryngol Head Neck Surg* 1990;103:681–684.

83. Greenberg JS, Manolidis S, Stewart MG, Kahn JB. Facial nerve monitoring in chronic ear surgery: US practice patterns. *Otolaryngol Head Neck Surg* 2002;126:108–114.

84. Saravanappa N, Balfour A, Bowdler DA. Use of laser, otoendoscopy and facial nerve monitoring in otological surgery: United Kingdom survey. *J Laryngol Otol* 2003;117:751–755.

85. Nissen AJ, Sikand A, Welsh JE, et al. A multifactorial analysis of facial nerve results in surgery for cerebellopontine angle tumors. *Ear Nose Throat J* 1997;76:37–40.

86. Uziel A, Benezech J, Frerebeau P. Intraoperative facial nerve monitoring in posterior fossa acoustic neuroma surgery. *Otolaryngol Head Neck Surg* 1993;108:126–134.

87. Silverstein H, Rosenberg SI, Flanzer J, Seidman MD. Intraoperative facial nerve monitoring in acoustic neuroma surgery. *Am J Otol* 1993;14:524–532.

88. Fenton JE, Chin RY, Fagan PA, et al. Predictive factors of long-term facial nerve function after vestibular schwannoma surgery. *Otol Neurotol* 2002;23:388–392.

89. Axon PR, Ramsden RT. Assessment of real-time clinical facial function during vestibular schwannoma resection. *Laryngoscope* 2000;110:1911–1915.

90. Neff BA, Ting J, Dickinson SL, Welling DB. Facial nerve monitoring parameters as a predictor of postoperative facial nerve outcomes after vestibular schwannoma resection. *Otol Neurotol* 2005;26:728–732.

91. Isaacson B, Kileny PR, El-Kashlan H, Gadre AK. Intraoperative monitoring and facial nerve outcomes after vestibular schwannoma resection. *Otol Neurotol* 2003;24:812–817.

92. Isaacson B, Kileny PR, El-Kashlan HK. Prediction of long-term facial nerve outcomes with intraoperative nerve monitoring. *Otol Neurotol* 2005;26:270–273.

93. Goldbrunner RH, Schlake HP, Milewski C, et al. Quantitative parameters of intraoperative electromyography predict facial nerve outcomes for vestibular schwannoma surgery. *Neurosurgery* 2000;46:1140–1146; discussion 6–8.

94. Prell J, Rampp S, Romstock J, et al. Train time as a quantitative electromyographic parameter for facial nerve function in patients undergoing surgery for vestibular schwannoma. *J Neurosurg* 2007;106:826–832.

95. Scheller C, Strauss C, Fahlbusch R, Romstock J. Delayed facial nerve paresis following acoustic neuroma resection and postoperative vasoactive treatment. *Zentralbl Neurochir* 2004;65:103–107.

96. Strauss C. The facial nerve in medial acoustic neuromas. *J Neurosurg* 2002;97:1083–1090.

97. Moller AR, Jannetta PJ. Monitoring facial EMG responses during microvascular decompression operations for hemifacial spasm. *J Neurosurg* 1987;66:681–685.

98. Haines SJ, Torres F. Intraoperative monitoring of the facial nerve during decompressive surgery for hemifacial spasm. *J Neurosurg* 1991;74:254–257.

99. Leonetti JP, Brackmann DE, Prass RL. Improved preservation of facial nerve function in the infratemporal approach to the skull base. *Otolaryngol Head Neck Surg* 1989;101:74–78.

100. Chang SD, Lopez JR, Steinberg GK. Intraoperative electrical stimulation for identification of cranial nerve nuclei. *Muscle Nerve* 1999;22:1538–1543.

101. Welling DB, Glasscock ME III, Gantz BJ. Avulsion of the anomalous facial nerve at stapedectomy. *Laryngoscope* 1992;102:729–733.

102. Olds MJ, Rowan PT, Isaacson JE, Silverstein H. Facial nerve monitoring among graduates of the Ear Research Foundation. *Am J Otol* 1997;18:507–511.

103. Pensak ML, Willging JP, Keith RW. Intraoperative facial nerve monitoring in chronic ear surgery: a resident training experience. *Am J Otol* 1994;15:108–110.

104. Wilson L, Lin E, Lalwani A. Cost-effectiveness of intraoperative facial nerve monitoring in middle ear or mastoid surgery. *Laryngoscope* 2003;113:1736–1745.

105. Schaitkin BM, Shapiro A, May M. Disorders of the facial nerve. In: Lalwani AK, Grundfast KM, eds. *Pediatric otology and neurotology*. Philadelphia, PA: Lippincott-Raven, 1998:457–475.

106. Jahrsdoerfer RA. The facial nerve in congenital middle ear malformations. *Laryngoscope* 1981;91:1217–1225.

107. Schuknecht HF. Congenital aural atresia. *Laryngoscope* 1989;99:908–917.

108. Jahrsdoerfer RA, Lambert PR. Facial nerve injury in congenital aural atresia surgery. *Am J Otol* 1998;19:283–287.

109. McKinnon BJ, Jahrsdoerfer RA. Congenital auricular atresia: update on options for intervention and timing of repair. *Otolaryngol Clin North Am* 2002;35:877–890.

110. Schlake HP, Goldbrunner R, Siebert M, et al. Intra-Operative electromyographic monitoring of extra-ocular motor nerves (Nn. III, VI) in skull base surgery. *Acta Neurochir (Wien)* 2001;143:251–261.

111. Schlake HP, Goldbrunner RH, Milewski C, et al. Intra-operative electromyographic monitoring of the lower cranial motor nerves (LCN IX-XII) in skull base surgery. *Clin Neurol Neurosurg* 2001;103:72–82.

112. Topsakal C, Al-Mefty O, Bulsara KR, Williford VS. Intraoperative monitoring of lower cranial nerves in skull base surgery: technical report and review of 123 monitored cases. *Neurosurg Rev* 2008;31:45–53.

113. Randolph GW, Dralle H, Abdullah H, et al. Electrophysiologic recurrent laryngeal nerve monitoring during thyroid and parathyroid surgery: international standards guideline statement. *Laryngoscope* 2011;121(Suppl 1):S1–S16.

114. Petro ML, Schweinfurth JM, Petro AB. Transcricothyroid, intraoperative monitoring of the vagus nerve. *Arch Otolaryngol Head Neck Surg* 2006;132:624–628.

115. Jackson LE, Roberson JB, Jr. Vagal nerve monitoring in surgery of the skull base: a comparison of efficacy of three techniques. *Am J Otol* 1999;20:649–656.

Diseases of the External Ear

146

Christopher J. Linstrom   *Frank E. Lucente*

INFECTIONS OF THE EXTERNAL EAR

Otolaryngologists see many patients with infections of the external ear. The infections may be classified by location, cause, and time course as acute, subacute, and chronic. Before discussing the individual disease processes, we review the normal anatomy and physiology of the external ear.

ANATOMY AND PHYSIOLOGY

The external ear is composed of the auricle and external auditory canal (EAC). Both contain elastic cartilage derived from mesoderm and a small amount of subcutaneous tissue, covered by skin with its adnexal appendages (1,2). There is fat but no cartilage in the lobule. The auricle is derived from six hillocks, three each from branchial arches I and II (Fig. 146.1). During normal gestation, the cartilaginous hillocks merge to form the auricle, and with selective growth of the mandible, the auricle rises from its original position near the lateral commissure of the mouth to the temporal area. The tragus and antitragus form a partial barrier to the entrance of macroscopic foreign bodies.

The EAC is derived from the first ectodermal branchial groove between the mandibular (I) and hyoid (II) arches (2,3). The epithelium lining this groove contacts the endoderm of the first pharyngeal pouch, thus forming the tympanic membrane (TM), the most medial extent of EAC. Connective tissue of mesodermal origin is found between ectoderm and endoderm and becomes the fibrous layer of the TM (2). Because of its origin, the EAC, including the lateral surface of the TM, is derived from ectoderm and is lined by squamous epithelium.

The process of canalization is complete by about week 12 of gestation, at which time the canal fills with epithelial tissue. The canal ordinarily recanalizes by about week 28 of fetal life (3).

The EAC may be thought of in two sections. The outer 40% of the canal in its anterior and inferior aspect is cartilaginous and contains a thin layer of subcutaneous tissue between the skin and cartilage. The inner 60% is osseous, is formed primarily by the tympanic ring, and contains very scant soft tissue between the skin, periosteum, and bone. The average length of the adult EAC is 2.5 cm. Because of the oblique position of the TM, the posterosuperior part of the canal is about 6 mm shorter than the anteroinferior portion (1). The junction of the cartilaginous and bony portions of the canal is a narrowed section termed the isthmus.

Laterally to medially, the canal curves slightly superiorly and posteriorly in a gentle S shape. The canal can be thought of as pointing toward the nose; thus, pull the auricle gently upward, outward, and backward to straighten the canal for examination. Three macroscopic defense mechanisms protect the EAC and lateral surface of the TM: the tragus and antitragus, the skin with its cerumen coat, and the isthmus of the canal.

The skin of the cartilaginous canal contains many hair cells and sebaceous and apocrine glands such as cerumen glands (Fig. 146.2). Together, these three adnexal structures provide a protective function and are termed the *apopilosebaceous unit*. Glandular secretions combine with sloughed squamous epithelium to form an acidic coat of cerumen, one of the primary barriers to infection of the canal. An invagination of the epidermis forms the outer wall of the hair follicle, and the hair shaft forms the inner wall. The follicular canal is the space between these two structures. The alveoli of the sebaceous and apocrine glands empty into short straight excretory ducts, which drain into follicular canals. Obstruction of any part of the ductal system predisposes to infection.

The canal is normally a self-protecting and self-cleansing structure. The cerumen coat gradually works its way past the isthmus to the lateral part of the canal and

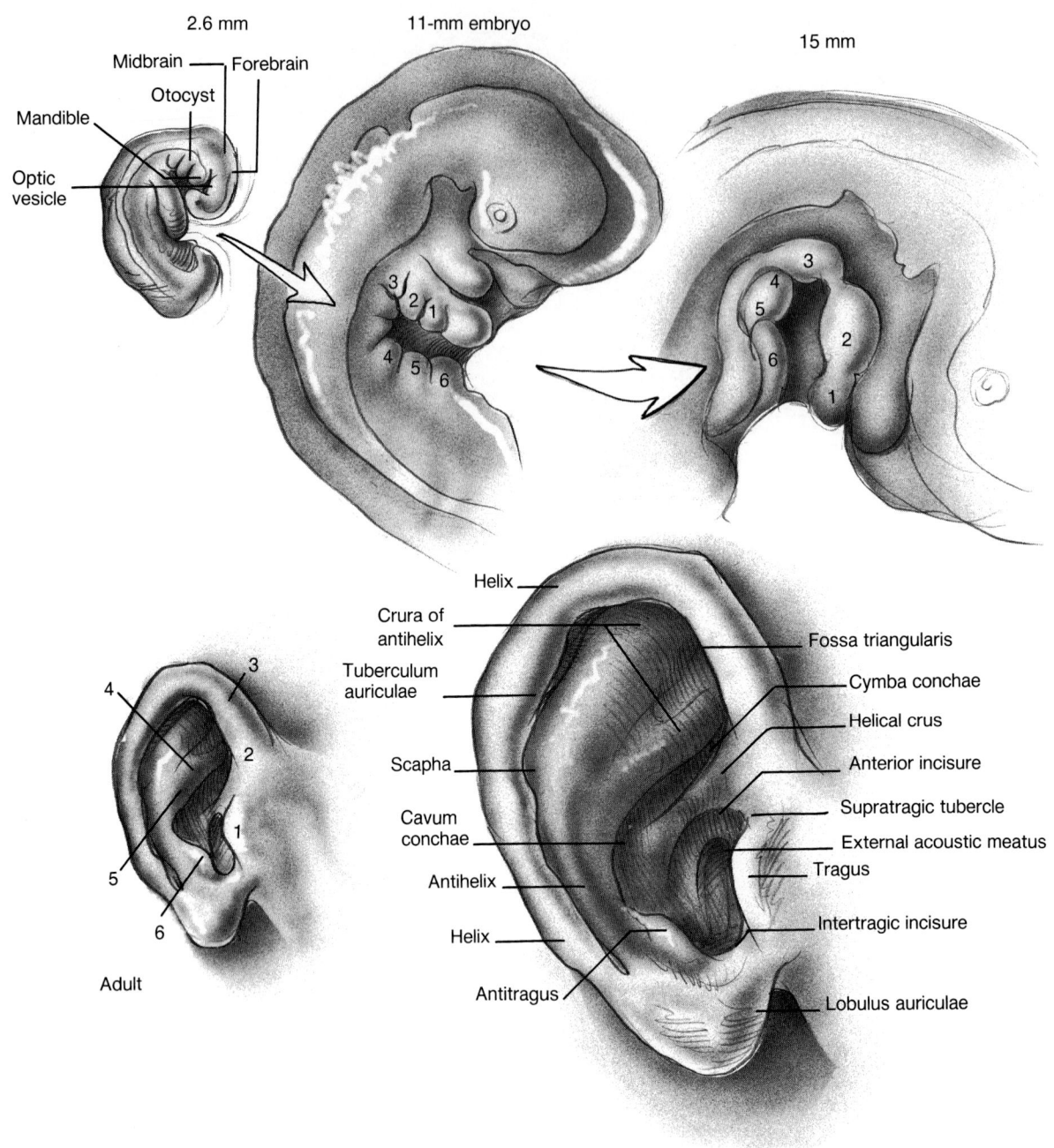

Figure 146.1 The auricle is formed from six auricular hillocks, three each from branchial arches I and II.

sloughs externally. Instrumentation and excessive cleansing of the canal disturb this primary protective barrier and may lead to infection. Individual variations in the anatomy of the canal may predispose some people to wax accumulation.

The canal interfaces on all but its lateral surface. Medially, it is bound by the TM, which when intact is a good barrier to the spread of infection. In the presence of a TM perforation, infection may spread back and forth from the middle ear cleft to the EAC. The horseshoe-shaped tympanic ring separates the canal from the middle cranial fossa. Rarely is this the direct mechanism of intracranial extension of infection. The posterior bony canal serves as the anterior boundary of the mastoid cavity. Several vessels penetrate the canal, especially along the tympanomastoid suture. These may be involved in the hematogenous extension of infection from the canal to the mastoid segment. Posterior to the cartilaginous canal lies dense connective tissue overlying the mastoid, which may become secondarily infected.

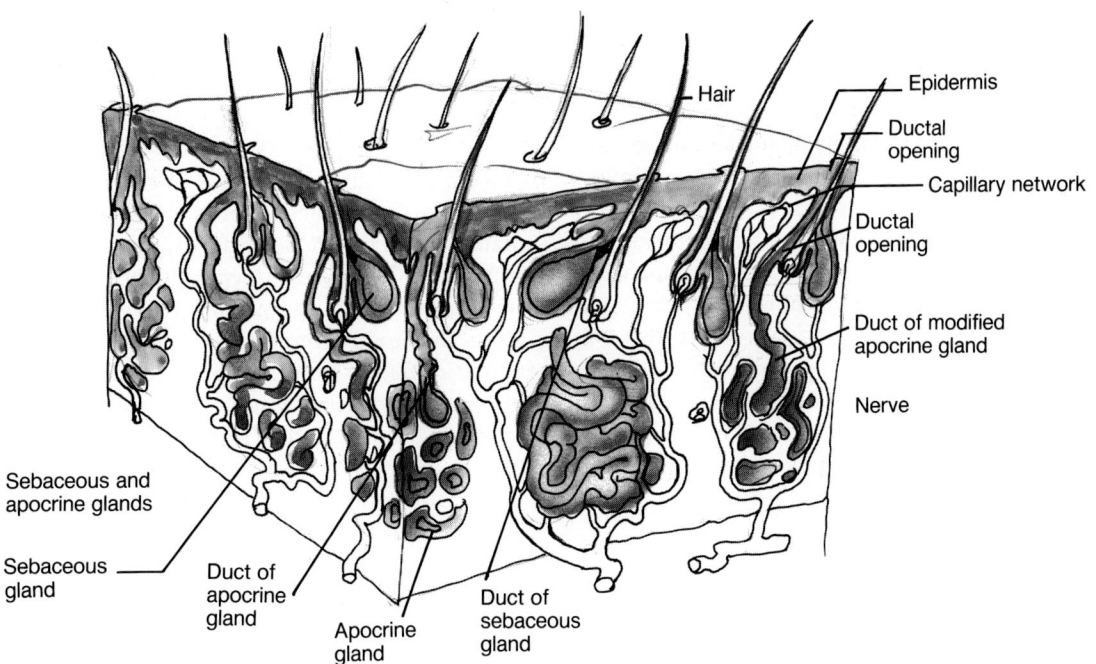

Figure 146.2 Microscopic view of the normal apopilosebaceous unit demonstrating drainage of the secretions of the sebaceous and modified apocrine glands into the follicular canal of the hair.

Superiorly, the canal is bound by the middle cranial fossa and inferiorly by the infratemporal fossa and base of the skull. Infections extending through the roof of the canal may extend into these structures. Anteriorly, the canal is bordered by the temporomandibular joint and the parotid gland.

The lymphatic drainage of the canal is an important channel for the spread of infection. Anteriorly and superiorly, the canal drains to the preauricular lymphatics in the parotid gland and the superior deep cervical nodes. The inferior portion of the canal drains into the infra-auricular nodes near the angle of the mandible. Posteriorly, the lymphatics drain into the postauricular nodes and the superior deep cervical nodes. The auricle and EAC receive their arterial supply from the superficial temporal and posterior auricular branches of the external carotid artery (1). Venous drainage from the auricle and meatus is via the superficial temporal and posterior auricular veins. The former joins the retromandibular vein, which usually divides and joins both jugular veins; the latter joins the external jugular but may also drain to the sigmoid sinus through the mastoid emissary vein (1).

Sensation to the auricle and EAC is supplied from cutaneous and cranial nerves, with contributions from the auriculotemporal branches of the trigeminal (V), facial (VII), glossopharyngeal (IX), and vagus (X) nerves and the greater auricular nerve from the cervical plexus (C2 to C3). The vestigial extrinsic muscles of the ear, anterior, superior, and posterior auricular, are supplied by the facial nerve (VII) (1).

OTITIS EXTERNA

Otitis externa is a spectrum of infection of the EAC. The appearance of the canal varies according to the time course of infection: acute, subacute, or chronic.

Acute otitis externa (AOE) is a bacterial infection of the canal caused by a break in the normal skin/cerumen protective barrier in the milieu of elevated humidity and temperature. Although commonly called "swimmer's ear," AOE may be caused by anything that results in the removal of the protective lipid film from the canal, allowing bacteria to enter the apopilosebaceous unit. It usually begins with itching in the canal and is commonly caused by instrumenting the canal with a cotton swab or fingernail. This temporarily relieves itching but allows proliferation of bacteria in locally macerated skin and sets up an itch–scratch cycle. The warm, dark, moist setting of the canal is now a perfect medium for rapid bacterial growth. Later, pain ensues as the swollen soft tissues of the canal distract the periosteal lining of the bony canal. As the disease progresses, purulent discharge begins, and the auricle and periauricular soft tissues may become involved.

In patients in whom the disease does not resolve after treatment, a subacute or chronic form may occur. This condition may be likened to eczema and is a spectrum of disease ranging from mild drying and scaling of the canal skin to complete obliteration of the canal by chronically infected hypertrophic skin.

HISTORY

The history and functional inquiry should include information regarding the length of time, the number of occurrences, the nature and severity of pain, antecedent otologic disease, previous auricular instrumentation or trauma (especially the use of cotton-tipped applicators), and any predisposing factors such as diabetes or radiotherapy or any condition causing immunosuppression. Any previous otologic or head and neck surgery is noted.

Pain, fullness, itching, and hearing loss are the four major symptoms of external otitis, although not every patient has each symptom (4). Throughout the examination, the examiner should remember the innervation of the EAC and recall that pain from other areas of the upper aerodigestive tract may be referred to the ear.

PHYSICAL EXAMINATION

On initial inspection, look at the ear itself and then at its relation to the head. Is it red, swollen, or protruding? Is there obvious discharge? Are the auricle and periauricular tissues normal in appearance or lichenified, with a heaping up of the normal epidermal architecture? Is there erythema or cellulitis spreading to the periauricular tissues, face, and neck? A gentle tug upward and backward will usually confirm the clinical suspicion. Although not an infallible rule, the patient with AOE usually will not tolerate this maneuver; patients with acute otitis media often will.

To make the correct diagnosis of infections of the external canal and to follow the clinical response to treatment, clean the canal thoroughly and examine it under good illumination. A handheld otoscope will often suffice for a quick examination, but all instrumentation of the ear is best done under the microscope with the patient lying supine in the chair in anticipation of a possible vasovagal response mediated by Arnold nerve, a branch of cranial nerve X.

Although topical and local anesthesia may be tried before cleansing, they are usually of little effect in hyperemic macerated tissue and no substitute for reassurance and patience. Using graduated specula will often ease the patient into a complete examination. The canal may be cleaned with suction, a cerumen loop, or alligator forceps. Gentleness and thoroughness in cleaning the ear are very important.

BACTERIOLOGY

The usual pathogens responsible for AOE are *Pseudomonas aeruginosa*, *Proteus mirabilis*, staphylococci, streptococci, and various gram-negative bacilli. For the mild or uncomplicated infection, culture of the canal is ordinarily not taken, because it will usually demonstrate a mixed pattern of growth. For recalcitrant infections, culture may identify a predominant organism and assist in the choice of antibiotic therapy.

STAGING

The clinical course of external otitis may be divided into the following stages: preinflammatory; acute inflammatory, which can be mild, moderate, or severe; and chronic inflammatory. Typically, the preinflammatory stage begins when the stratum corneum becomes edematous due to the removal of the protective lipid layer and acid mantle from the canal, resulting in plugging of the apopilosebaceous unit. As obstruction continues, a sense of fullness and itching begins. The disruption of the epithelial layer allows invasion of bacteria that either reside in the canal or are introduced on foreign objects inserted into the canal, such as a cotton swab or a dirty fingernail. This produces the acute inflammatory stage, which is accompanied by pain and tenderness of the auricle. In the earliest stage, the skin of the EAC shows mild erythema and minimal edema (Fig. 146.3). A small amount of clear or slightly cloudy secretion may be seen in the canal. As pain and itching increase, the patient progresses to the moderate stage, in which the canal shows more edema and a thicker more profuse exudate (Fig. 146.4). Further progression of the inflammation in the absence of treatment produces the severe inflammatory stage, characterized by increased pain and obliteration of the lumen of the canal. A profuse, purulent exudate and edema of the canal skin may obscure the TM. In addition, small white papules are often visible on the surface of the canal skin. *P. aeruginosa* or another gram-negative bacillus can almost always be cultured at this stage. In the severe stage, the physician often sees evidence of extension of infection beyond the canal to involve the adjacent soft tissues and cervical lymph nodes (Fig. 146.5).

In the chronic inflammatory stage, the patient experiences less pain but more profound itching. The skin of the external canal is thickened, and superficial flaking may be seen (Fig. 146.6). The auricle and concha often show secondary changes such as eczematization, lichenification, and superficial ulceration. This condition is likened to eczema and may range from mild drying and thickening of the canal to complete obliteration of the external canal by chronically infected, hypertrophic skin (Table 146.1).

DIFFERENTIAL DIAGNOSIS

The differential diagnosis of conditions that are similar to external otitis is large and includes necrotizing otitis externa, bullous external otitis, granular external otitis, perichondritis, chondritis, relapsing polychondritis, furunculosis, and carbunculosis, as well as many dermatoses, such as psoriasis and seborrheic dermatitis. All have features in common with acute and chronic external otitis,

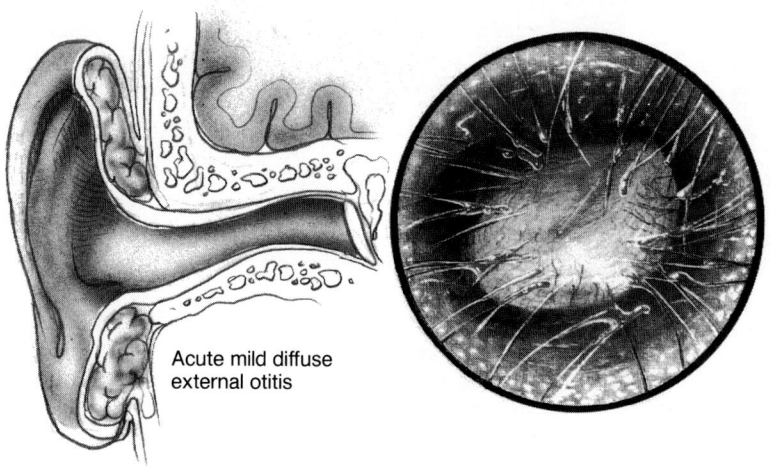

Acute mild diffuse external otitis

Figure 146.3 Otitis externa, acute inflammatory stage. Mild erythema and edema of the canal skin are seen. Clear secretions may be seen in the canal. (From Senturia BA, Marcus MD, Lucente FE. *Diseases of the external ear*, 2nd ed. New York: Grune & Stratton, 1980, with permission.)

yet have enough dissimilarities to be considered distinct clinical entities.

Carcinoma involving the EAC may present as infection and in its earliest stages is often mistaken for infection and treated inappropriately. The most common malignant neoplasm of the external ear is squamous cell carcinoma, although other primary carcinomas, such as basal cell carcinoma, malignant melanoma, ceruminous adenoma or adenocarcinoma, and adenoid cystic and metastatic carcinomas to the temporal bone with extension to the EAC such as breast, prostatic, small (oat) cell, and renal cell carcinomas, have been described. The occurrence of pain in an old previously stable mastoid cavity is the hallmark of carcinoma and must be excluded by biopsy and other investigations.

NATURAL HISTORY

The natural history of untreated AOE is one of increasing pain, swelling, and discharge from the canal. The infection may spread to the adjacent periauricular soft tissues, face,

and neck. In an immunocompromised patient, what began as an isolated superficial infection of the apopilosebaceous unit of the EAC may progress to perichondritis, chondritis, cellulitis, and erysipelas. Rich lymphatic and hematogenous drainage pathways favor the spread of infection to local and regional sites in the head and neck. Few patients progress to such an advanced stage before seeking medical attention.

The natural history of chronic otitis externa is far less dramatic than its acute counterpart. The chronic scaling and itching in the canal predispose to manipulation of the canal, excoriation, and repeated episodes of AOE. With time, the canal skin may become lichenified, and ultimately the canal may become completely obliterated.

MEDICAL TREATMENT

The four fundamental principles in the treatment of external otitis in all stages are frequent and thorough cleaning, judicious use of appropriate antibiotics, treatment of associated inflammation and pain, and recommendations

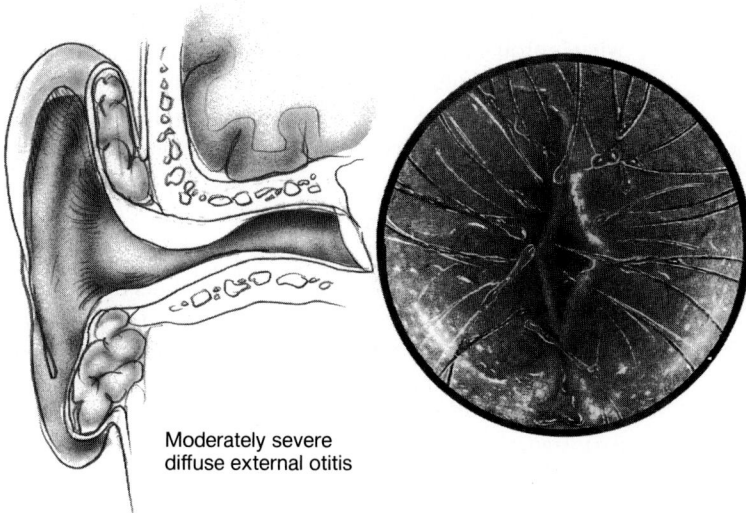

Moderately severe diffuse external otitis

Figure 146.4 Otitis externa, moderate acute inflammatory stage. The EAC is more edematous than in the acute stage, approaching obliteration of the lumen, with a more profuse exudate. (From Senturia BA, Marcus MD, Lucente FE. *Diseases of the external ear*, 2nd ed. New York: Grune & Stratton, 1980, with permission.)

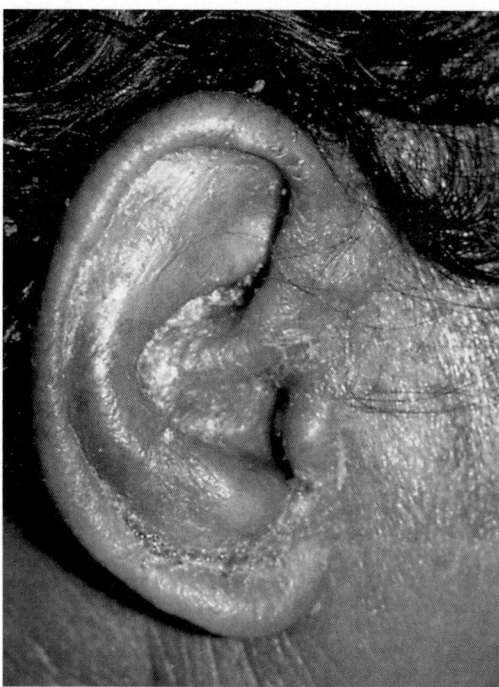

Figure 146.5 Otitis externa, severe stage. Infection extends beyond the limits of the canal to involve adjacent soft tissues and cervical lymph nodes. Erythema of the conchal skin and scaliness are secondary to profuse drainage.

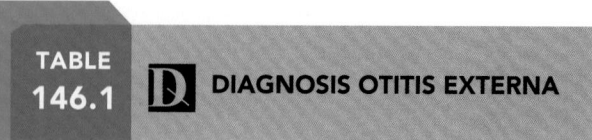

TABLE 146.1	DIAGNOSIS OTITIS EXTERNA

History
  Pain
  Fullness
  Itching
  Discharge
Physical examination
  Preinflammatory
    Mild erythema, edema
  Acute inflammatory
    Auricular tenderness
    Erythema
    Edema
    Discharge
  Chronic inflammatory
    Thickening, flaking of canal skin
    Eczematization
    Ulceration
Laboratory
  Culture
    P. aeruginosa
    P. mirabilis
    Staphylococcus sp.
    Streptococcus sp.
Radiology
  Rarely indicated

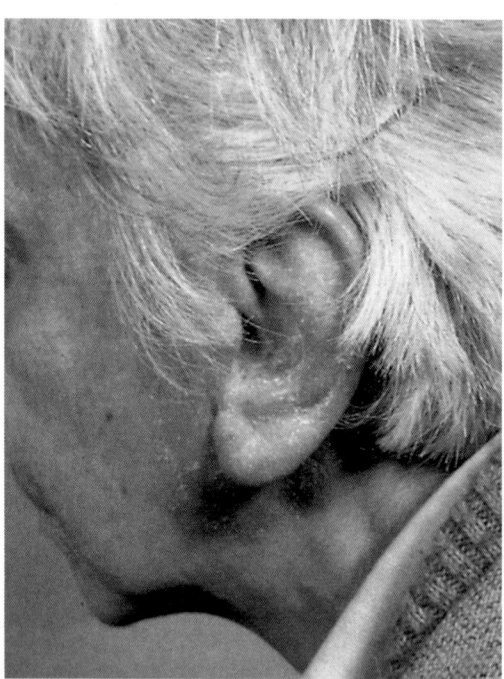

Figure 146.6 Otitis externa, chronic inflammatory stage. The skin of the external canal is thickened, and superficial flaking may be seen. The surrounding skin of the auricle may show secondary changes such as eczematization, lichenification, and superficial ulceration.

regarding the prevention of future infections. In any stage of infection, thorough cleaning is a priority. Meticulous debridement of exfoliated debris, purulence, and cerumen will do as much if not more than simply placing the patient on ear drops. In the preinflammatory stage, a complete cleaning may be all that is required. In the absence of purulence, a brief course of an acidifying drop such as aluminum sulfate–calcium sulfate (Domeboro) is efficacious in discouraging bacterial or fungal growth.

Treatment of the acute inflammatory stage varies with the extent of disease. In the mildest form, cleaning as above is indicated. An antibiotic otic drop is recommended to cover what is probably a *Pseudomonas* infection. At this stage, edema of the EAC should not be severe, and the patient should be able to instill drops into the ear by tilting the head to the side or by lying down with the involved ear upright.

MODERATE STAGE

In the moderate stage of inflammation, edema of the canal may interfere with the instillation of drops. The physician should then insert a wick into the canal and instill drops on it. Often the canal may accommodate two or even three wicks. As the wick expands, it presses the soft tissues and periosteum toward the nondistracted position; this alone may relieve pain. All instrumentation of the ear is best done under the microscope. The wick is removed by the physician at the time of reexamination. If the edema has not been significantly reduced, repacking is indicated. Antibiotic drops should be continued for at least 2 to 3 days after the cessation of pain, itching, and drainage so that complete eradication of infection may be ensured.

In the moderate stage, an oral analgesic is often prescribed because pain can be pronounced. Caution the patient to avoid manipulation of the canal. Swimmers should be taught to towel dry the concha and lateral canal, to shake water out of the canal, or to instill an acidifying drop after swimming. If the infection has not spread beyond the boundaries of the external canal, the use of oral antibiotics will be of little if any value. A final office visit is important to ensure that the infection has completely resolved and the canal is back to its normal state.

SEVERE STAGE

In the severe stage, infection usually extends beyond the limits of the canal. In addition to the cleaning, packing, and use of antibiotic drops as discussed previously, attend to any soft tissue involvement by using an oral antibiotic with broad-spectrum coverage. Successive generations of the cephalosporins widen gram-negative coverage at the expense of gram-positive coverage.

In addition to anti-*Pseudomonas* ear drops, common choices of oral antibiotics are one of the antipseudomonal fluoroquinolones such as ciprofloxacin or levofloxacin, antistaphylococcal penicillins, or cephalosporins. The fluoroquinolone antibiotics are effective against *Pseudomonas* species. In children under 12 years old, one should check with the pediatrician prior to starting oral fluoroquinolones.

Warm soaks (normal saline or a mild aluminum sulfate–calcium acetate solution) are also useful in the treatment of the crusting and edema involving the auricle and surrounding skin. Culture of the canal for aerobic bacteria and/or fungi is indicated only for the severe stage or for patients who have previously been treated without resolution. Treatment is generally continued for 10 to 14 days if there is a good response. In rare patients who do not respond to this regimen, hospitalization, vigorous daily local care, repeat culturing, and intravenous antibiotics are indicated.

CHRONIC STAGE

The chronic stage of external otitis is manifested by marked thickening of the skin of the EAC due to long-standing infection. Examination reveals flakes of dry scaly skin in the canal. Although removal of debris is recommended, this may be difficult due to the narrowing of the lumen of the canal. Repeated cleaning and instillation of antibiotics and steroids are indicated. Triamcinolone acetonide 0.25% cream or ointment (Kenalog), fluocinolone 0.01%

oil (DermOtic), or dexamethasone sodium phosphate 0.1% ophthalmic drops (Decadron, Pred Forte 1%) may be used.

In all cases of acute or chronic external otitis, instruct the patient to avoid future infections by not instrumenting the ear. Foreign objects such as Q-tips often excoriate the canal skin and push debris further into the canal rather than remove it. Patients who have repeated infections despite adhering to these measures are best advised to use an acidifying drop composed of equal measures of vinegar and water, or ethyl alcohol and water, when exposed to high humidity. One should suspect otomycosis if all other reasonable measures have failed and should treat with drying agents, especially powders. Custom-made ear molds are useful for these patients.

RECALCITRANT OTITIS EXTERNA

The physician will be able to judge very quickly which patients are responding. Prolonged antibiotic drops may suppress the normal flora of the external canal from returning and lead to a fungal superinfection. This should be suspected, especially if a grayish matted discharge is found in the ear, even if telltale hyphae are absent. A culture may have already been taken, and the result should help to direct treatment. Again, the ear must be thoroughly and meticulously cleaned, and if a fungus has been cultured such as *Candida*, this should be treated appropriately with drying agents such as powders and an antifungal drop or even systemically with an oral antifungal medication such as fluconazole. If no progress is made in the office, the rare patient may have to be admitted as an inpatient. Examine the ear under a microscope and carefully clean it frequently. Look for subtle signs of chronic middle ear disease—granulation tissue or the opening of a tiny perforation. The latter may be obscured by a swollen TM, giving a "fishmouth" appearance to the perforation. A "sewer cap" of crust on the drum may reveal a cholesteatoma underneath. Examine every part of the auricle carefully. Look for signs of underlying chondritis or perichondritis, especially diffuse crusting or exudative weeping. Culture the ear (for aerobes, anaerobes, and fungi). Examine the periauricular tissues carefully to look for signs of spreading infection. Computed tomography of the temporal bones may give additional information. Look for opacification of the mastoid and signs of bony erosion.

Place the patient on daily aural drops, preferably one covering *P. aeruginosa*, and intravenous antibiotics with gram-positive and gram-negative coverage. One may wish to try intravenous ciprofloxacin to start. In very rare cases, a cephalosporin together with an aminoglycoside is a logical combination if monotherapy does not improve the ear. Therapy should be tapered according to culture and sensitivities. Severely swollen ears may calm down with steroids.

TABLE 146.2	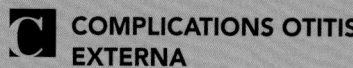	COMPLICATIONS OTITIS EXTERNA

Cellulitis
Erysipelas
Perichondritis
Chondritis
Chronic nonresolving rate

Many recalcitrant infections occur because of noncompliance or chronic instrumentation of the canal skin. The patient should be counseled to amend bad habits. The rare patient will need to be admitted for intravenous antibiotics and daily aural toilet (Tables 146.2 and 146.3).

SURGICAL MANAGEMENT OF HYPERTROPHIC CHRONIC OTITIS EXTERNA

When such local measures are insufficient to eradicate infection and reestablish the lumen of the canal, it is necessary to remove the involved canal skin and any adjacent involved cutaneous or cartilaginous tissue. This is very rarely required and may be performed through the canal but is better done through a postauricular incision, which allows visualization of the involved tissues. A generous amount of conchal cartilage is removed to effect a wide meatoplasty. The bony canal is enlarged with a drill. Take care to protect the facial nerve in its vertical segment; the use of an intraoperative facial nerve monitor facilitates this. The canal is resurfaced with a split-thickness (8:1,000 inch) skin graft that is temporarily held in place with stents or packing.

It is the experience of many otolaryngologists that even the most recalcitrant infection can be managed if the four basic principles—thorough cleaning, antibiotic treatment, pain control, and instruction of the patient—are meticulously followed. There is no substitute for thorough and repeated local care (Table 146.4).

TABLE 146.3		EMERGENCIES OTITIS EXTERNA

Unresolving pain, despite local care
  Admit to hospital
  Analgesia
  Control inflammation
Cranial neuropathy with external otitis
  Consider necrotizing external otitis

TABLE 146.4	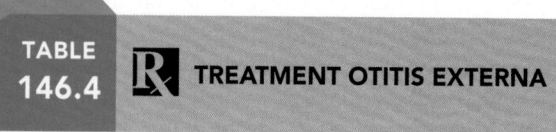	TREATMENT OTITIS EXTERNA

Medical
  Frequent thorough cleaning
  Antibiotic coverage
    Drops
    Oral
    Intravenous as needed
  Treat inflammation, pain
  Recommendations for prevention
Surgical
  Excise involved canal skin
  Perform wide meatoplasty
  Resurface canal with split-thickness skin graft

SKULL BASE OSTEOMYELITIS, FORMERLY NECROTIZING (MALIGNANT) OTITIS EXTERNA

This potentially life-threatening disease should be viewed within the larger context of osteomyelitis of the temporal bone and skull base. Thanks in large part to newer anti-*Pseudomonas* antibiotics, chief among them the fluoroquinolones, skull base osteomyelitis (SBO) is not as prevalent as it was even a decade ago. By no means is it a disease of the past, especially among diabetics, the immunocompromised, and the elderly. The otolaryngologist must still keep SBO within the differential diagnosis of a refractory external ear infection in the patient at risk.

Toulmouche (5) described a case of progressive osteomyelitis of the temporal bone in 1838 that was probably the first reported case of necrotizing external otitis (NEO). In 1959, Meltzer and Kellemen (6) described a case of progressive *Pseudomonas osteomyelitis* of the temporal bone and skull base. Chandler (7–11) is credited with the clinical description of what he termed malignant otitis externa in 1968 and thereafter. Although many early cases ended in the death of the patient, the entity does not ordinarily involve carcinoma, and thus, the more appropriate term used today is SBO, which is a proper description of the pathophysiology and clinical entity.

DIAGNOSIS

The diagnosis of SBO is made in a patient with the appropriate history, physical examination, and supporting laboratory findings. Four salient features are found (12): persistent, deep-seated severe otalgia for longer than 1 month; persistent purulent otorrhea with granulation tissue for several weeks; diabetes mellitus, another immunocompromised state, or advanced age; and cranial nerve involvement.

Other diseases to be included in the differential diagnosis include severe AOE, squamous cell carcinoma,

TABLE 146.5	**D** DIAGNOSIS NECROTIZING EXTERNAL OTITIS

History
  Persistent otalgia
  Persistent purulent otorrhea, granulations
  Diabetes mellitus, advanced age, immunocompromised state
  Cranial neuropathy(ies)
Physical examination
  Granulations in external canal
  Purulent discharge seen
  ± cranial neuropathy, especially cranial nerve VII
Culture
  Pseudomonas sp.[a]
  Pseudomonas aeruginosa[a]
Radiology
  Nuclear (gallium, technetium)
  CT with contrast
  MRI with contrast

CT, computed tomography; MRI, magnetic resonance imaging.
[a]Almost always.

glomus jugulare tumor, cholesteatoma, nasopharyngeal carcinoma, Hand-Schüller-Christian disease, eosinophilic granuloma, Wegener granulomatosis, clival chordoma, and meningeal or squamous cell carcinoma (13,14). The physician's index of suspicion should be high so that no patient is denied aggressive treatment when appropriate (Table 146.5).

CLINICAL AND RADIOGRAPHIC FINDINGS

SBO usually begins as an acute external otitis that does not resolve despite medical therapy, as described previously. The history is significant for a long-standing infection of the external canal accompanied by aural discharge and severe deep-seated pain. The disease is usually found in elderly diabetic patients in poor metabolic control, although it may be found in any chronically ill, debilitated, or immunocompromised patient (15). The HIV status of the patient should be known.

On physical examination, most patients with SBO have granulation tissue visible in the inferior aspect of the canal or even extruding from it. This may obscure the TM. It is rare to see granulation tissue in patients with routine otitis externa; however, granulations are common in an acute exacerbation of chronic otitis media with perforation of the TM. The skin of the canal is often erythematous, indurated, and sometimes macerated. Purulent secretions are common.

The causative organism is almost always *P. aeruginosa*, although other organisms such as *P. mirabilis*, *Aspergillus fumigatus*, *Proteus* sp., *Klebsiella* sp., and *Staphylococcus* sp. have been isolated (8,14).

The natural history of SBO is one of relentless progression to involve the cranial nerves, especially the facial nerve. Pain is inexorable and is deep seated. Damiani et al. (16) reported that the most commonly involved cranial nerves were VII (75%), X (70%), and XI (56%). More recent reports have estimated the facial nerve to be involved in at least one-fourth of patients, with less frequent involvement of cranial nerves IX, X, and XI (17).

Computed tomography of the temporal bone with contrast is the initial radiograph to be done, yielding excellent bony detail with less precise information about soft tissue. It may define subtle bony changes such as erosion of the anterior canal wall with involvement of the temporomandibular joint and erosion of the tympanic ring and base of the skull. It may demonstrate soft tissue thickening and mastoid clouding (18).

Magnetic resonance imaging without and with gadolinium enhancement may be advantageous in defining the medial extent of disease at the skull base. Dural enhancement and involvement of the medullary bone spaces are seen with central skull base invasion. Underlying cerebral involvement is easily visualized with gadolinium-enhanced magnetic resonance imaging. Magnetic resonance imaging yields very imprecise information about bone. The patency of the dural sinuses and great vessels of the neck may be assessed in a noninvasive fashion with magnetic resonance angiography or venography (19). Changes seen on MRI do not quickly resolve with clinical improvement. Thus, MRI is a useful diagnostic tool to assess the extent of disease but less useful to follow the clinical course of SBO (20).

Tc-99m bone scanning and Ga-67 scanning have been advocated in the evaluation of SBO (17,21). Their sensitivity for the presence of infection is far greater than their specificity for the cause. Tc-99m scanning gives excellent information about bone function but poor information about bone structure. A positive scan is thought to represent osteoblastic activity as little as 10% above normal. The scan is positive in acute and chronic osteomyelitis and in areas of active bone repair without infection, as in trauma. Its use in the evaluation of SBO is complementary to that of Ga-67 scanning. Ga-67 is thought to be incorporated into proteins and polymorphonucleocytes at sites of active infection as a Ga-67–lactoferrin complex. It will highlight an acute infective focus but not the full extent of an osteomyelitic process. As treatment progresses, the Ga-67 scan will revert to normal (negative). The Tc-99m scan will lag behind for many months. Baseline studies of both are thus recommended, and sequential imaging is used to monitor the response to therapy. Indium-111–labeled leukocyte (In-WBC) planar scintigraphy has been demonstrated to yield better results for the detection of osteomyelitis than either planar or tomographic Ga-67 and/or Tc-99m-methyline diphosphonate and may replace the former two radionuclide modalities in the evaluation of

SBO-suspected patients (17,21). It is best to consult with nuclear medicine to determine which of these various choices will be best.

MEDICAL TREATMENT

Swab and/or tissue cultures of the EAC should be obtained. If present, granulations should be biopsied and sent to rule out carcinoma or another pathologic entity. *P. aeruginosa* is almost always cultured. Because *Pseudomonas* is so frequently the predominant organism, the patient is treated with anti-*Pseudomonas* antibiotics for an extended period, often for 6 weeks or more. Two antibiotics, one an antipseudomonal antibiotic and the other an aminoglycoside, that is, each from a different class, are ordinarily chosen because of the synergy achieved with the use of two antibiotics and to avoid the emergence of a resistant strain of bacteria. Monotherapy is discouraged in the treatment of SBO. Usually two anti-*Pseudomonas* antibiotics are chosen from several alternatives, including gentamicin or tobramycin with or without ticarcillin or piperacillin. Alternative antibiotics include mezlocillin or azlocillin, ceftazidime, imipenem, aztreonam, amikacin, norfloxacin, and ciprofloxacin or any of the other appropriate anti-*Pseudomonas* fluoroquinolones (22). If an aminoglycoside is chosen, peak and trough levels and hearing must be carefully monitored. It is wise to treat in concert with an infectious disease colleague to help select those medications that will be of greatest benefit with the least toxicity.

Because of the high tissue levels seen with oral fluoroquinolones, the apparent incidence of SBO has fallen. However, the physician should not be lulled into a false sense of security. Many patients with poor microvasculature, especially diabetics, may achieve cidal concentrations of an antibiotic solely with intravenous administration. Patients refractory to intravenous administration of antibiotics may require surgical control of the infected site. Emergence of resistance to ciprofloxacin has been reported in 20% of long-term (6 weeks or more) therapy for osteomyelitis (21).

Certainly if the ear remains purulent despite adequate intravenous antibiosis and local care, repeat cultures should be taken to look for the emergence of a resistant organism.

An early clinical feature of success in treatment is the cessation of pain, and patients may be tempted to discontinue therapy once this occurs. Regardless of the choice of medication or mode of delivery, patients must understand that they will require meticulous aural toilet and antibiotic treatment for at least 6 weeks and vigorous management of the serum glucose.

Either in the hospital or in the office, the ear is debrided carefully under the microscope on a regular basis until granulations have subsided. The patient is placed on anti-*Pseudomonas* otic drops and appropriate systemic antibiotics. Diabetes is aggressively managed, usually with the aid of an internist or endocrinologist. The diet is carefully monitored with the aid of the nutritionist.

Hyperbaric oxygen has been advocated by Shupak et al. (23). Hyperbaric oxygen is thought to facilitate osteoneogenesis and to promote repair of diseased bone and thus may be of value in the most severe cases. The cost and inconvenience of hyperbaric oxygen therapy have limited its availability. Its use is recommended for advanced disease with significant skull base or intracranial involvement, recurrent disease, and infections refractory to antibiotic treatment (17,23).

Surgical Treatment

Most patients can be managed medically, and the role of surgery in SBO remains controversial. Surgical debridement of tissue and osteomyelitic bone is usually reserved for patients who do not respond to conventional therapy. Tissue may be obtained for culture in these refractive cases to look for resistant organisms or for a new organism such as an invasive fungus. Progression of pain despite aggressive medical therapy, persistence of granulations, and the development of cranial nerve involvement are all ominous signs that call for more aggressive medical therapy and possibly surgical intervention.

With the onset of clinical facial paralysis, early surgical removal of granulations and, when necessary, decompression of the descending facial nerve have given excellent return of function. The primary surgical goal is to relieve the entrapped nerve and to allow its natural return of function. Serial electroneuronography (ENOG) has been used to determine the electrical degeneration of the VII nerve in patients with clinically complete facial paralysis. An ENOG showing greater than 90% electrical degeneration of the facial nerve may support surgical decompression of the involved segment of the nerve. The entire concept of facial nerve decompression in the context of SBO remains controversial. The mainstay of therapy for SBO is medical and not surgical.

John and Cheesman (24) have advocated wide local excision of infected cartilage and soft tissues if pain persists after medical treatment or if facial palsy occurs. Reines and Schindler (25) have reported three cases in which subtotal temporal bone resection was performed to gain access to the primary focus of infection and provide adequate drainage. Surgical treatment including abscess drainage, debridement of sequestra, and more extensive resection should be individualized depending upon the patient's overall health status and response to more conservative measures (26).

The first author performed his very first mastoidectomy under *local* anesthesia in a 90-year-old lady with SBO and a large abscess of the surrounding bone and soft tissues. She had failed two previous 6-week courses of intravenous antibiotics. Her family was very involved and requested surgical intervention. She improved, was discharged, and lived another 4 years after surgery. She died of old age and not of SBO.

Mortality remains significant, especially in the immunocompromised patient. Progression of disease results in severe unremitting pain within the ear and at the base of the skull and extension of infection to the mastoid, parotid, lower cranial nerves, and transverse and sigmoid sinuses. Osteomyelitis of the skull base may lead to meningitis, brain abscess, and death. Poor prognostic factors include facial paralysis, polyneuropathy, and intracranial extension (27).

The diagnosis and management of patients with SBO remains an otolaryngologic challenge. Perhaps the greatest advance in its treatment has been the recognition of SBO as a distinct entity and a clear understanding of its pathophysiology. A team approach involving the cooperation of otolaryngology, endocrinology, and infectious disease may enhance the overall outcome (Tables 146.6 to 146.8). The devastating disease reported by Chandler (7) in his classic 1968 article has significantly changed. The advent of the fluoroquinolones and other anti-*Pseudomonas* antibiotics has significantly lowered the morbidity and mortality associated with SBO.

Conditions Related to External Otitis

Several other infectious and inflammatory diseases are included in the differential diagnosis of otitis externa.

Radiation-Induced Otitis Externa

Another form of otitis externa occasionally occurs after radiotherapy of the region of the external ear. The predominant symptoms result from the inflammation and infection that occur when radiotherapy weakens local defense mechanisms and resident bacteria flourish. When limited to the skin of the EAC, treatment measures with particular attention to water avoidance are appropriate. In the worst form of osteoradionecrosis with purulent infection,

 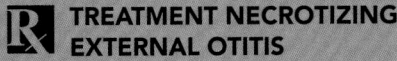

TABLE 146.6	TREATMENT NECROTIZING EXTERNAL OTITIS

Medical
  Hospital admission
  Intravenous antibiotics
  Daily cleaning, debridement
Surgical
  Excise ± granulations
    ± middle ear exploration
    ± mastoidectomy
    ± facial nerve decompression
    ± temporal bone resection if no response

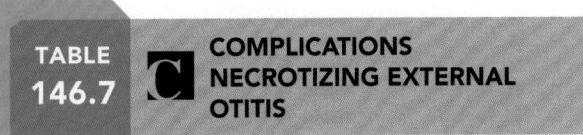

TABLE 146.7	COMPLICATIONS NECROTIZING EXTERNAL OTITIS

Cranial neuropathy (VII and lower)
Progression despite aggressive local care (to mastoid, parotid, lower cranial nerves, base of skull, dural venous sinuses, brain)
Meningitis
Brain abscess
Death

sequestra of devitalized tissue should be removed and replaced with vascularized tissue. The removal of what has become the nidus of infection is a basic surgical principle. This is fortunately a very rare thing.

Bullous External Otitis

Bullous external otitis is a very painful condition in which vesicles or bullae are noted in the bony portion of the external canal. The vesicles are commonly hemorrhagic and should not be ruptured, because secondary infection may ensue. Because *Pseudomonas* may be one of the causative organisms, appropriate otic drops are recommended. Packing and irrigation of the canal should be avoided, because they tend to prolong the course of this disease.

Granular External Otitis

Granular external otitis often resembles the earliest stage of NEO in that there may be small granular plaques or pedunculated granulations in the external canal. This condition may occur in patients who have not been fully treated for a previous episode of external otitis. It may also occur as a result of contact dermatitis, for example, exposure to hairspray. After topical or local anesthesia, removal of granulation tissue, placement of a wick in the canal, and the instillation of antibiotic drops will usually resolve the problem. Oral antibiotics should be given if the infection extends beyond the canal. If the patient is diabetic or debilitated, the diagnosis of NEO is entertained and treated appropriately.

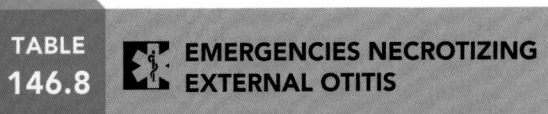

TABLE 146.8	EMERGENCIES NECROTIZING EXTERNAL OTITIS

Any complications in Table 146.7 (in living patient)
  Change antibiotic
  Increase level of daily care
  Consider surgery

Perichondritis and Chondritis

Perichondritis, inflammation of the perichondrium, and chondritis, inflammation of cartilage, may follow or complicate infections of the EAC or result from accidental or surgical trauma to the auricle. The condition is painful, and the patient often complains of severe itching deep within the canal. With time, the skin over the affected area becomes crusted with squamous debris, and the involved cartilage begins to weep. The ear is indurated and erythematous; often the canal swells shut. The surrounding soft tissues of the face and neck may become involved.

In the mildest stages, thorough debridement and treatment with topical and oral antibiotics are generally sufficient. If these measures do not succeed, the ear is debrided again, and cultures are taken. Appropriate treatment for common pathogens, especially *Pseudomonas*, is begun and tapered according to culture results. Ciprofloxacin is a logical choice for moderate stages, combined with an anti-*Pseudomonas* drops such as gentamicin or a fluoroquinolone drops.

If the infection spreads to involve regional soft tissues and lymphatics, the patient should be hospitalized and parenteral treatment with adequate coverage for *Pseudomonas* begun. In difficult cases, the ear should be cultured before starting treatment. With recalcitrant infections, the help of an infectious disease consultant is necessary. At every stage of the disease, frequent and thorough debridement of the canal is essential. The metabolic requirements of cartilage are low, and its blood supply is appropriately diminished. Once infection has become established in the perichondrium or cartilage, it is extremely difficult to treat. If subacute or chronic infection evidenced by inexorable weeping continues, surgical intervention is indicated. This is best done in the operating room under controlled conditions.

The affected area is cleansed and injected with local anesthetic containing epinephrine. Skin flaps are appropriately planned and the dissection taken down to the affected cartilage. If it has lost its normal "pearly white" appearance, it is most likely necrotic and should be excised. Often necrosis extends farther than that which can be grossly visualized. Small irrigation drains are placed beneath the flaps and sutured to the skin. The skin flaps are closed. The drainage ports are irrigated with antibiotic irrigation such as bacitracin (50,000 U of bacitracin dissolved in 250 mL of normal saline). The drains are advanced as the condition resolves. Parenteral antibiotics, otic drops, and aggressive local care continue until the infection has resolved.

Relapsing Polychondritis

Relapsing polychondritis is an intermittently progressive disease marked by inflammatory destruction of cartilage. Although thought to be an autoimmune disorder, the exact cause is unknown. Cartilage of the external ear, larynx, trachea, bronchi, and nose may be involved. Symptoms are episodic, with fever, anemia, erythema, swelling, pain, and an elevated sedimentation rate during acute episodes. As the disease progresses, symptoms of increasing respiratory obstruction become apparent. Labyrinthine disturbances are rarely present. The diagnosis is made on the basis of the history and physical examination, supported by an elevated sedimentation rate. Biopsy of involved cartilage may show necrosis, inflammation, and fibrosis. Treatment is with oral corticosteroids, rarely with intravenous steroids.

Furunculosis and Carbunculosis

Furunculosis and carbunculosis are conditions resulting from gram-positive infections, usually staphylococcal, of the hair follicles. The primary lesion is usually a small well-circumscribed pustule that may enlarge to become a furuncle or merge with several similar lesions to form a carbuncle. The infection occurs most commonly at the junction of the concha and canal skin.

For treatment to be successful, any accumulated infectious material must be removed. Spontaneous drainage can often be encouraged by the use of warm soaks, supplemented by topical and oral antibiotics and wicks if necessary. If this fails to relieve obstruction of the canal, incision and drainage (I & D) under local anesthesia are indicated.

Infectious Eczematoid Dermatitis

Infectious eczematoid dermatitis results from the drainage of contaminated or purulent material from the middle ear into the floor of the external ear and adjacent infra-auricular skin (Fig. 146.7). This drainage causes a secondary infection or an autosensitization phenomenon manifested by crusted plaques in the canal. Treatment is directed at control of the underlying middle ear infection. Supportive treatment of the external canal reaction consists of removal of accumulated debris, application of sterile saline soaks to the crusted areas, and application of an antibiotic cream or ointment.

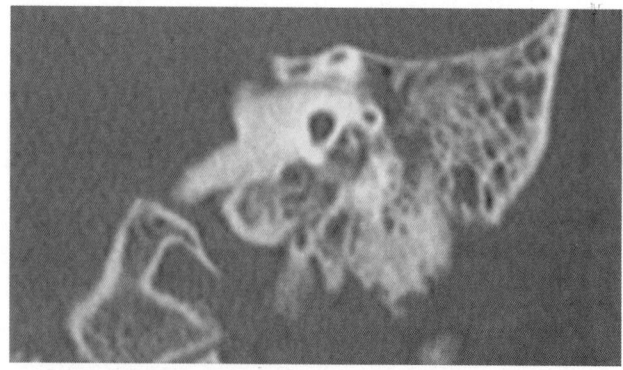

Figure 146.7 Infectious eczematoid dermatitis with inflammation and crusting of the skin of the canal and auricle secondary to drainage of purulent material through a TM perforation in a patient with chronic otitis media.

Otomycosis

Otomycosis is a fungal infection of the skin of the external canal. Although fungi may be the primary pathogens, they are usually superimposed on chronic bacterial infection of the external canal or middle ear. Secondary otomycosis tends to recur if the underlying primary infection is not controlled. All fungi have three basic growth requirements: moisture, warmth, and darkness. Altering moisture will discourage fungal growth. *Aspergillus* species are the most common, usually *A. niger*. If aural culture should grow *A. fumigatus* or *A. flavus*, one would be concerned about a more invasive infection.

Pruritus is the primary clinical complaint. The otoscopic examination commonly reveals a white, black, or dotted gray membrane. Thorough cleaning under a microscope with the patient supine to remove any fungal debris is the first and absolutely most important step in therapy. Thorough aural toilet is supplemented by the topical application of an acidifying solution such as aluminum sulfate–calcium acetate (Domeboro) or by a drying powder such as boric acid. Clotrimazole cream or solution (Lotrimin) may also be used. In the presence of a TM perforation or a patent ventilation tube, clotrimazole drops or lotion may be very painful. Thorough cleaning and drying therapies such as powders are best. Metacresyl acetate (Cresylate) may be painted on the margin of a perforation or an infected ventilation tube. This is best done under the microscope. This medication should not enter the middle ear cleft because it is quite irritating. In recalcitrant infections, a foreign body such as a ventilation tube acts as the nidus for infection and should be removed. Tympanoplasty is best performed to close a perforation that intermittently drains with a superimposed fungal infection.

Gentian violet is usually well tolerated in patients with mastoid cavities, although it is best left out of the middle ear cleft in the presence of a perforation. Because it will permanently stain skin and clothing, small amounts are used with adequate protection of the surrounding area.

Treating physicians should realize that all drops are formulated with moisture and do not persist indefinitely in an homogenized state. Eventually, the water component will separate from the precipitate of the active medical ingredient. Water is exactly what fungi need to grow. Adding drops indefinitely to an ear with otomycosis may prove counterproductive. In these cases, an acidifying powder such as boric acid or a compounded powder, as described below, will often help dry up a refractory ear.

Many patients with refractory otomycotic infections may have had previous mastoid surgery. Often the canal wall is down. Due to moderate to severe hearing loss, the patient may need to wear a hearing aid with a closed mold. This is a significant problem because the patient relies on the aid virtually all day and is reluctant to leave the instrument out. Careful instruction to the patient, meticulous debridement of the ear, and the use a drying agent such as boric acid powder, Chloromycetin–sulfanilamide–Fungizone (amphotericin B) powder or Chloromycetin–sulfanilamide–Tinactin (tolnaftate) powder will often help clean up the cavity. Ointments in cavities with closed hearing aids may promote fungal growth due to the accumulation of moisture. In refractory cases, gentian violet or metacresyl acetate (Cresylate) is used topically.

Herpes Zoster and Herpes Simplex

Herpes zoster and herpes simplex are viruses known to affect the EAC. The patient initially experiences a period of burning, pain, or localized headache, and vesicles usually appear within several days. When vesicles coalesce and rupture, crusts are formed. Herpes zoster tends to appear unilaterally in a dermatomic distribution. Involvement of the facial nerve may produce paresis or paralysis (herpes zoster oticus or Ramsay Hunt syndrome), named after Dr. James Ramsay Hunt (1872 to 1937), of late termed Hunt Syndrome. Treatment is supportive, with topical application of a drying agent, such as hydrogen peroxide for crusts. The status of the facial nerve is carefully followed; surgical decompression of the facial nerve may be a consideration if it is clinically paralyzed and electrical criteria are met by ENOG testing. Many patients excoriate the blisters, and bacitracin ointment or a suitable substitute should be applied to prevent superinfection. Acyclovir, famciclovir, and valacyclovir have been shown to ameliorate herpetic infections, especially herpes zoster oticus. The latter two have easier dosing schedules and are better absorbed orally than acyclovir. Also, famciclovir may reduce the duration of post herpetic neuralgia. However, it will cause a transitory rise in hepatic enzyme production and must be used with caution.

Dermatoses

Allergic and irritant contact dermatoses may mimic diffuse external otitis. These result when the susceptible patient comes in contact with any type of agent that can produce a cutaneous response. Irritants may be absolute, so noxious that a reaction occurs in everyone exposed (e.g., strong acids or alkalis), or relative, noxious to susceptible individuals, usually after repeated exposures (e.g., various soaps, the plastic mold of a hearing aid). Allergic contact dermatitis refers to delayed hypersensitivity reactions resulting from substances such as poison ivy, nickel compounds (earrings), and rubber compounds (headphones). The typical reaction presents as erythema, weeping, and vesiculation accompanied by itching. The patient may produce a secondary infection by scratching. Treatment consists of removal of the causative agent and the use of topical steroids and astringents. Topical or systemic antibiotics are indicated for the treatment of infection. Systemic steroids may be indicated for severe cases. In rare cases, for example, the patient with a cochlear implant and hypersensitivity to plastic, the external, ear-level receiver/stimulator may be painted with a different material or covered with a cloth casing to separate it from the skin.

External Ear Disease and HIV Infection

Among the external ear manifestations in HIV disease is Kaposi sarcoma, which presents with reddish-blue lesions typically described as hemorrhagic nodules (28). The lesions may be discrete or confluent. Although chemotherapy, radiotherapy, and interferon-α have been used for therapy, treatment of auricular and canal lesions is rarely necessary. Infections of the external ear in HIV-infected patients include both typical and atypical pathogens. Recurrent herpetic infections and *Pneumocystis carinii*–infected aural polyps have been reported in the EAC as a result of chronic otitis media (29).

Another external ear manifestation of HIV disease is seborrheic dermatitis, which tends to be more widespread and refractory to treatment than the same condition in HIV negative patients. NEO in the HIV+ patient adds another level of concern regarding its treatment. An infectious disease consultant should be involved in the overall care of the HIV+ patient. The advent of the protease inhibitor medications in the mid-1990s not only saved lives and emptied the infectious disease wards of most hospitals but also made these otologic manifestations exceedingly rare.

Traumatic Disorders of the External Ear

Blunt Injuries

Shearing forces to the auricle, commonly seen in sports such as boxing and wrestling, may disrupt the normal perichondrium of the auricular cartilaginous framework, causing seroma or hematoma formation. The lobule is composed primarily of fat covered with skin and is less susceptible to injury. Because it is malleable throughout life, auricular cartilage is more likely to be injured by shearing forces than blunt trauma. It rarely fractures.

If uninfected, a small seroma of the auricle may be observed, a larger one aspirated. If the seroma reaccumulates, it should be treated under sterile conditions with drainage and a bolster type dressing using dental rolls and through-and-through, nonabsorbable sutures placed to obliterate the potential space for reaccumulation of the seroma. If infected, there is a risk that cartilage itself may become necrotic and lost. The ear must be incised and drained with broad-spectrum antibiotic coverage; drains may need to be placed. The goal is to prevent loss of the cartilaginous frame.

The same principles apply to hematoma of the auricle, except that observation is rarely an option. Because the cartilaginous frame is at greater risk, the hematoma should be drained and a compressive dressing applied with dental rolls sutured on either side. If the hematoma reaccumulates

or is very large, drains should be placed, and the ear should be treated until the skin flaps remain flat. Preservation of the cartilaginous framework with prevention of a "cauliflower" or "boxer's" ear is the goal.

Of recent note, young male pugilists may consider a malformed auricle a "mark of prowess" (athletic, sexual, and otherwise) and will not seek medical attention for shearing injuries to the auricle. Unfortunately, once auricular cartilage has been lost and reparative scarring has begun, the auricle is doomed to reparative malformation. Intervention must be given soon after any injury if it is to be effective.

Sharp Trauma to the Auricle

Sharp trauma to the auricle may be as small as a torn ear lobe piercing to complete avulsion of the auricle, usually as a result of motor vehicular trauma. The auricle has a plentiful blood supply and as a general rule will heal if the cartilaginous and soft tissue structures remain even partly attached, less so if complete avulsion has occurred. If remnants or the entire auricle can be salvaged, these should be cleansed and an attempt made to reimplant in the acute situation.

Torn lobules may occur by gravity in which a heavy earring works its way over time through the lobule or by acute injury in which an earring is torn through the lobule. Inflammation and infection should be treated. The torn lobule may be repaired in the office; the lobule may be repierced at a later stage.

Animal and human bites of the auricle are by definition contaminated. The edges of the wound must be decontaminated with local antisepsis. Tetanus toxoid should be given. Broad-spectrum antibiotic coverage for the most likely oral flora including microaerophilic streptococci and anaerobes such as *Bacteroides* is indicated. If remnants of the auricle have been salvaged, these may be thoroughly washed, decontaminated and reattached with sutures. If only the auricular cartilage remains, it should be cleaned of soft tissue attachments, decontaminated, and buried in a subcutaneous pocket (postauricular, forearm, abdomen, etc.) for later use.

Shearing avulsions are much more difficult to treat. The auricular remnant, if found, may be mangled, torn, abraded, etc. If part or whole of it appears viable, it is worth an attempt at surgical reattachment, obeying all rules of antisepsis.

If however, it has been lost or is beyond retrieval, the edges of the EAC should be freshened, tacked away, and the canal packed with gelfoam or another material to help prevent acquired stenosis of the EAC. The patient must then be counseled regarding the main steps of auricular reconstruction (costochondral cartilage harvest, sculpture, and subcutaneous implantation; lobular transposition; auricular lateralization) as required. Another very good option in these severe cases is the insertion of osseointegrating titanium posts for the anchoring of an auricular prosthesis. A well-made auricular prosthetic for the properly selected patient is an excellent option with very acceptable cosmetic results. On the contrary, flexible hydroxyapatite (Porex), even if covered with a vascularized temporoparietal flap, has in many cases proven extremely difficult in the event of subsequent trauma or surgical manipulation of the auricle with resultant stenosis of the EAC. This type of repair must be chosen carefully with regard to the age and usual activities of the recipient.

Thermal Injuries (Thermal Burns, Frostbite)

Burns of the auricle are classified by nature of the burn (thermal, ultracooling due to frostbite) and the degree of the injury to the skin: first degree leading to erythema, second degree (blistering), and third degree (full thickness). In first- and second-degree burns, pain is present; in third-degree burns, the sensory nerve endings have been destroyed, and the affected area is anesthetic. It is of great importance to elicit a detailed history about the nature and time course of the injury.

Upon inspection, the area may be erythematous and blistered (first- and second-degree burns), blackened with eschar (third degree), or white, hard, and cold (frostbite) due to extreme vasoconstriction. It is important to suspect that the extent of the injury extends greater than that apparent on inspection. This is especially true in electrical injuries. Cooling a thermal burn should be done quickly with cold/iced compresses to waste the built-up heat within the tissue in an attempt to prevent necrosis by cell expansion and disruption. Frostbite is rewarmed more slowly with warming compresses. If frostbite extends to larger areas of the body, the patient may be placed in a warming bath or warming intravenous solutions may be used. The extremity should not be rubbed, lest shearing forces cause further damage.

Broad-spectrum antibiotic coverage against expected organisms such as *Pseudomonas* sp. and common skin flora (gram+ cocci and rods) should be given. Topical ointments and creams such as 1% silver sulfadiazine creams may be used. Surgical debridement should be delayed until the wound "declares itself" and a line of demarcation between healthy and dead tissue becomes apparent. Once this has happened, debridement of dead tissue and the application of topical antiseptic ointments may encourage healing in first- and second-degree burns. More severe burns may require split- or full-thickness grafting. There is no reason to rush into repair until the full extent of the injury is obvious. A physician or surgeon experienced in the care of burns and in reconstructive surgery is an important colleague in the care of thermal and frostbite injuries to the auricle and EAC.

Acid Burn of the EAC and Auricle

This rare occurrence causes massive denaturation of skin, surrounding soft tissue and supporting cartilage, and may result in partial or complete loss of the auricle and EAC. Acids of industrial concentration such as sulfuric acid or other fortified acids (or alkalis) are the usual agents. The injury is almost never accidental but is part of a criminal assault. As with any chemical burn, the caustic agent must be removed with copious and prolonged irrigation.

If the auricle has been severely damaged, it may ultimately undergo partial or complete autoamputation. Hypertrophic and/or keloid formation will inevitably ensue and is treated with compressive dressings and/or steroid injections (triamcinolone 10 or 40 mg/mL), as necessary. The injured auricle may be allowed to "declare itself" as with thermal and frostbite burns. It is important to inspect the EAC and the TM and to make every effort to flush any noxious agent from these areas and to attempt to salvage as much normal tissue as possible. The EAC may be packed with medicated gelfoam or another packing.

Having worked in a large inner city E.R. and burn unit, the first author's experience is that these types of injuries are almost never isolated but are often part of a much larger picture including inhalation injuries and trauma to vital internal organs and the extremities. It is important to think "beyond the ear," especially if there has been a history of smoke inhalation. These patients are properly assessed by the trauma and burn services as well as otolaryngology.

Fractures of the EAC

Foreign objects placed into the EAC may cause lacerations of the canal. These types of injuries are rare. Far more common are injuries to the EAC caused by trauma to adjacent structures. The anatomic boundaries of the EAC make it susceptible to injuries of the temporomandibular joint (e.g., a blow to the jaw) and of fractures to the temporal bone, most commonly longitudinal fractures.

Inspection of the EAC reveals a "step" deformity of the canal. A flail piece of bone may be seen, with or without an accompanying laceration. Passive movement of the jaw may cause the bone fragment to move.

The patient should be inspected for additional areas of injury, both for fractures of the jaw and for other areas of otologic injury such as traumatic perforation of the TM, damage to the ossicular chain, facial nerve injury, or injury to the vestibular labyrinth. A tuning fork test should minimally be done. If possible, at least a screening audiogram should be performed.

Radiographic studies (mandibular views, panorex, CT of the petrous temporal bones, etc.) are obtained as indicated.

Treatment is of the underlying cause: If the mandible has been fractured, this must be reduced and the patient usually placed in intermaxillary fixation (IMF), as per oral surgery protocol. Temporal bone fractures, even with CSF otorrhea, are ordinarily observed with the patient placed in bed at about 45 degrees, until CSF otorrhea subsides. The ear should not be manipulated. If there is witnessed and progressive facial nerve dysfunction, in which case the likely site of injury is at the geniculate ganglion, the nerve is followed clinically and electrically with serial ENOG and/or needle EMG studies and may need to be decompressed.

If a flail piece of bone in the EAC, usually at the scutum or tympanomastoid suture lines, becomes infected or otherwise bothersome, it may be removed. It is rarely necessary to repair soft tissue lacerations. The EAC may be packed with gelfoam moistened with otologic drops or another packing material.

Noninflammatory Lesions of the External Ear

A. *Lesions of the auricle*
  1. *Congenital lesions of the EAC*
    a. *Microtia/congenital auricular atresia*
       The reader is referred to Chapter 148, Congenital Aural Atresia, by Dr. Paul R. Lambert MD.
    b. *Preauricular skin tag(s), accessory auricular remnants*
       These consist of redundant tissue, usually comprised of skin and fat, found near or just anterior to the tragus. If the mass contains cartilage, it is a remnant of auricular tissue, left over from auricular development. It may be a duplication of one or several of the ectodermal hillocks of His. Preauricular skin tags or auricular remnants are nonfunctional, and most parents request that they be removed. However, they may carry with them cultural connotations, such as a child being "favored." Care should be taken in the excision of them. If held on with only a soft tissue stalk, the skin tag may be lassoed with a silk suture, tied at the base and allowed to necrose and fall off. If cartilage is found within the lesion, excision should be done in the operating room, with the knowledge that the facial nerve may be very superficial in young children. The patient is seen as necessary until the scar has healed. Electrocautery is rarely necessary in the excision of these lesions and should be used carefully.
    c. *Preauricular pits*
       These are depressions or sinuses lined with squamous or columnar epithelium and found in front of the anterior root of the helix. They are heritable, thought to be in an autosomal dominant fashion with variable expression; they are often bilateral. They may elaborate keratin and/or mucous and may become infected. If quiescent, they are observed. If filled with uninfected debris, they may be treated with warm compresses and the material expressed from outside the opening. If the pit or sinus becomes recurrently infected, it may require excision. It is important to remove the entire tract if it is excised.
    d. *First branchial cleft cysts, sinuses, and fistulas*
       These result from anomalous duplication of the EAC and may occur between the EAC and structures anterior or inferior to the auricle, including the neck. The classification of Work (30) is commonly accepted. Work type I anomalies contain only ectodermal derivatives and may be thought of as a "parallel" duplication of the EAC. Work type II anomalies contain both ectodermal and mesodermal derivatives and may be found extending between the EAC and the parotid, in any relationship to the extratemporal facial nerve, including bisecting the nerve. Treatment of first branchial cleft cysts, sinus, and fistulas is by excision. These anomalies may contain keratin debris that may become infected. If infected, these may require I & D, but this is not recommended if it can be avoided. The cyst, sinus, or fistula may be gently probed with a sterile, malleable lacrimal probe or another suitable instrument to map out its pathway. The opening may be gently filled with dye such as methylene blue prior to excision. A rim of tissue around the internal opening is resected with the specimen and every attempt is made to excise the tract *in toto*, leaving none of it behind. If the tract is suspected to course in any relation to the extratemporal facial nerve, the excision should be done in a more formal way. A modified Blair incision is made, and the parotid is exposed as is the facial nerve at least from the stylomastoid foramen to the *pes anserinus* and distal branching points, with the use of intraoperative facial nerve monitoring. The cyst, sinus, or fistula must be carefully dissected from the intact and stimulated facial nerve. The first attempt at excision is usually the most thorough because the anatomy of the lesion is the most preserved. With each I & D and each subsequent surgical attempt at removal, this anatomy becomes more distorted and the chance of complete resection less.
    e. *Cutaneous cysts*
       Cysts of ectodermal and sebaceous origin may be found in any relationship the auricle. If growing and painful, they should be excised by including a fusiform "stamp" of skin over the lesion as a soft tissue "handle" leading toward excision of the cyst with its tract and surrounding soft tissue. It is important to make every attempt to identify and excise every bit of the cyst lining, as there always is one. If the cyst has become acutely infected and ready to burst, the patient is treated with oral antibiotics and warm soaks. The cyst may need to be incised and drained, but this is not optimal. Once the acute infection has subsided, the cyst should be excised.

2. *Acquired lesions of the EAC*
   a. *Chondrodermatitis nodularis chronica (Winkler nodule)*
      This is a benign lesion that appears as a "punched-out crater," found most commonly in older men at the rim of the helix. It may be found in other areas of the auricle. It is thought to be caused by the breakdown of elastic fibers due to chronic sun exposure. The lesion may be painful to touch or pressure, for example, sleep in on the ear. This distinguishes it from other dermatologic lesions such as senile keratosis, keratoacanthoma, cutaneous horn, and skin cancer (squamous or basal cell), which are usually painless.

      Treatment is by full-thickness excision including supporting cartilage with reconstruction of the defect with a full-thickness skin graft or local advancement miniflaps.

   b. *Gouty tophi of the auricle*
      These are deposits of uric acid in crystalline form in the auricle, often at the helix. The patient will have hyperuricemia and should have other markings of gout: arthropathy(ies), involvement of the great toe(s), etc. Serologic markers for uric acid will confirm the suspected underlying diagnosis. If quiescent, the nodule may be observed. If painful or inflamed, it is removed under local anesthesia. Histopathologic examination will reveal fusiform, washed-out casts of monosodium urate with an accompanying inflammatory surround: polymorphoneucleocytes, histiocytes, foreign body giant cells, etc.

      The patient should be treated by the internist for gout with daily administration of allopurinol and colchicine and other antiinflammatory medications for acute exacerbations.

   c. *Keratoacanthoma*
      This is also known as a self-healing basal cell carcinoma. It is caused by actinic (sun) exposure and may arise from hair follicles. It may be rapidly growing, raised, and circular with a central crater usually containing a keratin plug. On histologic exam, this crater is seen to be filled with desquamated debris and parakeratin cells. If it is undergoing gradual resolution, it may be observed. However, because this lesion resembles other skin cancers, it will usually be biopsied to yield a definitive diagnosis.

   d. *Bacterial perichondritis*
      This is distinguished from relapsing polychondritis, which is a nonbacterial autoimmune condition treated with steroids. Bacterial perichondritis is distinguished by crusting, by weeping and exudate from the auricle, and by pus. If there are signs of bacterial infection, the ear must be treated with antibiotics.

Infection of the perichondrium of the auricle and supporting cartilage is an urgent problem and may be a sequela to otologic surgery and trauma or may follow external otitis. Predisposing factors include diabetes and any cause of relative immunosuppression. The patient presents with a swollen, painful, erythematous auricle, usually crusting and weeping. Swabs are taken for gram stain, culture, and sensitivity. The most common organism isolated is *P. aeruginosa.* Oral antibiotics with good gram-negative coverage such as fluoroquinolones should be started along with warm soaks. Treatment may begin at home, but the patient must be seen frequently, even daily, until the ear either improves or it fails to, the patient should be hospitalized, broad-spectrum intravenous antibiotics started, and drains should be placed under the skin of the auricle and irrigated with an antibiotic solution such as bacitracin. Diabetic patients must be brought under strict control, often requiring a sliding scale of insulin. Necrotic cartilage should be excised and every effort taken to save as much of the cartilaginous auricular framework as possible.

   e. *Sebaceous cysts*
      These true cystic collections occur as a result of sebaceous gland obstruction. They have a true lining and may occur anywhere in the head and neck. The scalp, nape of neck, and auricle are favored sites. If small and nonpainful, they may be observed. The acutely infected sebaceous cyst is treated with a broad-spectrum oral antibiotic and may occasionally have to be drained. If it becomes larger and painful, the sebaceous cyst is excised with care taken to remove all of the cyst lining. This is best done when the cyst is distended and noninfected. If any of the cyst lining is left behind, it will likely regrow.

   f. *Hypertrophic scars and keloids (see burns)*

   g. *Neoplasia of the auricle and EAC*
      The auricle and EAC may give rise to both benign and malignant neoplasia, based upon the cell of origin. Benign processes include actinic keratosis, papilloma, and other lesions. Cancers of the auricle and EAC include more commonly basal cell carcinoma, squamous cell carcinoma, and melanoma (melanotic and amelanotic). Rarer cancers of the auricle and EAC include Kaposi sarcoma (now seen with much less frequency in HIV disease after the advent of protease inhibitors and other reverse transcriptase inhibitors) and ceruminous adenocarcinoma (31), seen either alone or in patients with multiple cylindromas of the scalp, face, and EAC.

      Malignancies with hematogenous metastatic potential to spread to the temporal bone but not necessarily to the auricle or EAC include renal cell carcinoma, small (oat cell) adenocarcinoma of the lung, breast cancer, cancer of the prostate, and cutaneous melanoma.

In the majority of skin cancers, malignancy is an end-stage result of chronic sun (actinic) exposure. Individuals of Northern European origin with fair skin, light hair, and blue eyes or individuals who have genetic defects of skin repair are predisposed to skin cancer. The amount and longevity of sun exposure is of greatest importance. Tanning lotions with protection against the ultraviolet waves of the sun are of relative recent widespread use. Many individuals in North America over the age of 60 can recall spending long summer hours if not whole days with friends at a swimming pool or beach, scantily clad, with no thought given to protection from the damaging effects of the sun. This is where the history leading to actinic changes including skin cancer begins. A thorough history of sun exposure, work history (indoor vs. outside work), and a history of tight-fitting ear molds leading to chronic irritation of the EAC should be elicited. It is wise to enlist the help of a good dermatologist and a dermatopathologist or similarly trained individual who is proficient in Mohs chemosurgery. Many malignancies of the auricle may be treated with local, chemo-controlled excision with the defect repaired via skin grafting or local advancement flaps. Occasional malignancies may respond to topical application of 5-fluorouracil. Unless one is ready to accept all responsibility for the care and follow-up of the lesion, it is wise to refer to the appropriate authority, a dermatologist. Said physician may treat alone or may send the patient back with a biopsy-proven diagnosis and request a limited, Mohs-controlled excision. The patient is best served when the otologist works in tandem with these colleagues.

Far less frequently, advanced cancers of the auricle may occur as part of an aggressive picture of skin cancer, especially squamous cell carcinoma of high grade. Conversely, slowly growing malignancies such as basal cell cancer may persist for years before the patient seeks help. In this small number of cases, the auricle and/or skin of the EAC must be partially or completely resected, possibly with a neck dissection, possibly with a lateral temporal bone resection, and the wound closed with local, pedicled, or free vascularized flaps. The extent of the disease by clinical examination, radiographic examination, and histopathologic margins will determine the extent of the dissection. Surveillance and local control may help to avoid these more advanced cases.

The reader is referred to Chapter 147 Neoplasms of the Ear and Lateral Skull Base by Bradley P. Pickett MD.

B. *Lesions of the EAC*
  1. *Keratosis obturans*

This is an acute upon chronic condition of the external ear in which the EAC is plugged by an accumulation of dense, inspissated keratin debris leading to secondary, acute infection, swelling, pain, and hearing loss. In very advanced cases, in response to chronic irritation and infection, the normal thin architecture of the squamous epithelium lining the canal may become lichenified (heaped up) and both plugged by dense debris and secondarily stenotic. The typical patient with this problem is elderly, often in a nursing home in which care of the ear is neglected. If and when the ear becomes acutely infected, the patient will be brought to the otologist. It is important to distinguish this entity, if possible, from AOE, osteomyelitis of the skull base, and other plausible conditions. The history usually yields the answer, if it can be accurately obtained.

These ears are tough to treat, in large measure because of pain, but will usually respond well to careful, thorough cleaning. Adding yet another drop or oral antibiotic and discharging the patient back to his or her home is *not* the way to treat this problem. Cleaning should be done carefully, slowly, and thoroughly, under a microscopic vision in the office, rarely in the operating room, very rarely under general anesthesia. These ears are exquisitely painful to clean, and thus, pain must be eliminated prior to aural toilet. The patient may require a four-quadrant block of the EAC with local anesthesia. Most patients will allow the ear to be cleansed in the office. There is usually an "onion skin" appearance to the epithelial debris for it has been collecting for many months to years. Although the diagnosis is apparent with gross inspection, material should be sent for pathologic examination to assure that this is keratin debris and nothing else. The physician may not be able to completely clean the ear in one sitting and may have to bring the patient back for several sessions with the ear medicated with an appropriate acidifying solution between visits.

The important difference between this and other similar conditions such as cholesteatoma of the EAC is that, once completely cleaned and topically medicated, the ear with keratosis obturans will often slowly and gradually revert back toward a healthy appearance. The change toward health may be quite remarkable once aural toilet commences. The inciting event of dense packing of squamous debris and superinfection has been cured and the ear can now resume a more normal appearance. This does not happen with external ear cholesteatoma. Prevention of reoccurrence is via appropriate ototopic therapy and routine office-based debridement.

2. *External auditory canal cholesteatoma (EACC)*

This is a cyst of squamous debris found in the EAC. It has many features in common with primary acquired cholesteatoma: an active matrix that elaborates keratin debris. It may locally erode bone and soft tissue. Unlike keratosis obturans, it does not revert back toward a normal state once obstruction and local infection have been relieved and treated. There may be an antecedent history of trauma, prior otologic surgery, acquired stenosis, or chronic inflammation, but most patients have no identifiable cause. The tympanic ring, especially its anterior and inferior aspects is a favored site for EACC. The patient may initially present with otologic complaints due to blockage by keratin debris: hearing loss, fullness, symptoms of infection, rarely dizziness or vertigo, and most rarely involvement of the facial nerve.

An edge-enhanced CT of the temporal bones reveals features of cholesteatoma with bony erosion and scalloped edges. It is usually a localized disease process, often unilateral, bilateral in fewer patients. Depending upon the site and size of the EACC, the hearing may be normal, the hearing loss of a conductive or mixed nature, or if there has been violation of the otic capsule, anacusis. Facial nerve involvement is rare.

The mainstay of treatment is routine office-based debridement, advice to the patient about water precautions, and the judicious use of acidifying drops and/or powders as needed. If the EACC becomes obstructed, rendering the ear difficult to clean, limited localized surgery including meatoplasty may be indicated to facilitate aural toilet. Surgery to eradicate all foci of cholesteatoma has proven of little value, and hence, EACC, unlike primary and secondary cholesteatoma of the middle ear and mastoid, is managed medically and not surgically. There is really very little need for surgery in even the most advanced cases (32).

The surgeon must also have a careful mental roadmap of the problem with microscopic detail. This may be facilitated by CT imaging, but there is no substitute for careful microscopic evaluation. In very advanced cases, the jugular bulb, tympanic facial nerve, and structures of the otic capsule may be exposed. Extreme caution must be used in dealing with these most delicate structures.

Softening the squamous debris at home for several days with an organic solvent (baby oil, olive oil, docusate, etc.) prior to scheduled office debridement will greatly facilitate cleaning. If inner ear structures of the vestibular labyrinth have been exposed, the patient may experience precipitous and violent vertigo due to the caloric effect of the suction. It is best to manually debride the ear in the supine position under the microscope, using small tools such as a cerumen loop, round knife, and alligator forceps, and to use a minimal amount of suction just at the end of the cleaning. The occasional patient may bring in a hair dryer to warm the ear prior to suctioning. Because the need to clean may be as often as every 3 to 4 months, the physician and patient must work together to achieve the best system that will keep the erosive potential of EACC in check and cause the least amount of discomfort to the patient.

It is important to be aware of developmental defects in the formation of the tympanic ring, which may lead to chronic irritation, weeping, and the collection of keratin debris, mimicking cholesteatoma of the EAC and other entities. A persistent foramen tympanicum, or foramen of Huschke, is an anatomic variation of the tympanic portion of the temporal bone due to a defect in normal ossification of the tympanic ring during the first 5 years of life (33). It is not a true foramen because no neurovascular structures traverse it, but it is a defect of tympanic bone ossification due to abnormal mechanical forces during early postnatal life or due to genetic factors, thus far undefined. It is located at the anteroinferior aspect of the EAC, posteromedial to the temporomandibular joint (TMJ). From retrospective radiographic series, it has been estimated to occur in 4.6% (33) to 9.1% (34) of individuals, depending upon the method of study and inclusion criteria, with an average dimension of 4.2 mm in the axial plane and 3.6 mm in the sagittal plane. A slight female preponderance was found in one study.

The persistent foramen tympanicum or foramen of Huschke should be kept in the differential diagnosis in cases of refractory chronic otitis externa and especially cholesteatoma of the EAC. It may predispose the patient to injury of the EAC, TM, middle ear cleft, etc., during TMJ arthroscopy and may facilitate spread of infection or tumor from the EAC into the infratemporal fossa and vice versa.

CT of the temporal bone performed at thin intervals (0.6-mm section thickness, 0.3-mm section increment) with an ultra–high-resolution filter will best image this entity if it is present.

3. *Cerumen impaction*

The subject of wax impaction may seem banal, but few other conditions in our specialty can be remedied within a single office visit to the tremendous relief and satisfaction of the patient. Many patients with wax impactions will present with hearing loss, fullness, tinnitus, autophony, and rarely with imbalance or vertigo. The history and physical exam including tuning fork testing will usually confirm the diagnosis and exclude other causes. Most patients will admit to using cotton squabs and other foreign bodies in the EAC. Patients wearing tightly fitting hearing aid molds or other ear pieces may be predisposed to wax impaction. The care for and prevention of wax impaction, however nonglamorous, is fundamental to what we do, and one should develop a reliable method to care for this most common problem.

Realizing that the ear is exquisitely sensitive, especially an erstwhile normal EAC now impacted with wax, the physician must treat carefully, cautiously, *slowly*, and with reassurance. Patients can tolerate many manipulations of the ear if what will be done is explained to them and is done slowly. A few extra seconds of counsel and reassurance are well worth the effort.

A few basics:

a. Place the patient in a comfortable position. This may vary from sitting upmost to lying flat in a recumbent position. One should anticipate a vasovagal response and be prepared to treat it immediately as it may occur with any instrumentation of the EAC, just as for the treatment of epistaxis. An ounce of prevention is worth a pound of cure.

b. Use a microscope, not a handheld otoscope. It is amazing that many physicians will use advanced fiberoptic imaging techniques for the nasopharynx and larynx but will attempt to remove a cerumen impaction without a microscope. This defies logic.

c. *Explain* what one intends to do: either with curettage or suction, using the microscope. If suction is to be used, the patient must be warned that he or she may experience momentary vertigo due to the caloric effect. Anticipate nausea and/or vomiting. Reassure the patient that if the cleaning becomes painful, the physician will stop and do so if the patient so indicates.

d. Use reasonable techniques for a reasonable length of time. Procedures to the ear performed *slowly* are usually tolerated better than anything done quickly. Do not rush in cleaning: In the long run, it will save time to use caution and to proceed slowly. If the patient is tolerating the cleaning well, proceed until everything has been cleaned. It may happen quickly and the acute problem solved. Other patients may require softening with mineral oil and/or 3% hydrogen peroxide, allowing the organic solvent to work for a few minutes while the patient next door is examined. Returning to the first patient, the impaction may now have softened enough to be removed, usually with suction.

e. Avoid blind, forceful irrigation. In our age of litigation, an iatrogenic perforation of the TM due to forceful ear washing is by and large a plaintiff's verdict. Happily, this is becoming a rare event. It is simply not worth the risk of iatrogenic injury for wax. Most but not all patients can be carefully and thoroughly cleaned in one office setting. Patience, softening, and recurrent attempts to clean as described above will usually be successful.

f. Have gelfoam and alligator forceps readily available. It is not uncommon that either the physician or the hard, impacted wax may abrade the EAC as it is removed. Bleeding may ensue and this may be cumbersome if the patient is on any type of anticoagulation therapy such as aspirin or warfarin. Topical astringents such as $AgNO_3$ or 20% phenol or trichloroacetic acid may be used, but an equally effective way to control bleeding is with a few small "dots" of gelfoam strategically placed. It is very bad form to send a patient from one's office with a profusely bleeding EAC.

The patient who walks into the office with a mild impaction is quite different than the patient brought in from a nursing home a great distance away by a relative or friend with a quality of life change now causing a mixed hearing loss due to wax. The former is of course bothered by the problem, but the latter is incapacitated in terms of communication.

All reasonable attempts should be made to thoroughly clean wax impactions in *one* office visit.

After the ears have been cleaned, inspect all parts of the TM to look for other signs of disease, such as a perforation or attic retraction cholesteatoma. If the ear has been cleaned carefully under microscopic visualization, it is highly unlikely that a perforation now visualized after debridement was due to the MD's manipulations.

Patients should be counseled to avoid placing any foreign body into the ear to clean it. Doing so invites not only wax impaction but also trauma and subsequent infection to the EAC, TM, and structures of the middle ear cleft because it is done blindly. A weekly rinse of 3% hydrogen peroxide or an acidifying drop may help the ear to cleanse itself. However, a small group of patients produce either so much wax or wax with such sticky viscosity that nothing other than manual debridement at regular intervals will suffice. Ten minutes in this MD's office every 6 to 12 months is well worth it. Few other patients we treat will have such an immediate benefit from our ministrations than those with wax impaction.

4. *Foreign body*

   Foreign bodies (FB) in the EAC may be classified into "living" and "nonliving" (organic or inorganic). Several broad principles must be observed in treating a patient with a suspected or known foreign body, all based upon common sense:

   a. For young children, "if one foreign body, there may be two or three." Check the nose in addition to the ears.

   b. Living foreign bodies (usually insects) must be killed and then removed. The patient is usually quite bothered by the beating of an insect's wings or other movement. This is silenced with lidocaine or mineral oil.

   c. Batteries and acid-eluting foreign bodies must be removed as soon as possible because they may cause extensive chemical burns to the EAC. This is a rather urgent otologic situation and the patient should be treated in the office or O.R. without delay.

   d. Hygroscopic means "takes on water." Thus, it is unwise to try to irrigate out foreign objects such as beans or bugs as this may make the FB swell and compound the problem.

   e. The ear is exquisitely sensitive. If the patient is not tolerating pain, this must be controlled lest the patient suddenly move during extraction of the FB with possible injury to underlying structures such as the TM and the ossicular chain. For the uncooperative or hysterical patient, five minutes of general anesthesia is well worth the discomfort of having a swollen, impacted foreign body removed without anesthesia.

   f. In a very cooperative child, one may attempt to remove the foreign body from the EAC(s) and, if successful, have a quick look at the nose and mouth to assure that no other foreign body is present. This is usually wishful thinking and the child must be prepared and taken to the O.R.

   g. Only an experienced MD should attempt to remove any foreign body from the EAC, and it should be done with magnification. Many different instruments are ordinarily available to retrieve FBs in the office. If they are not, the patient should be taken to the operating room or referred to an MD with the requisite tools to care for the FB.

   h. A reasonable attempt to establish audition in the ear in question with at least a tuning fork test should be done prior to the removal of a densely impacted foreign body.

5. *Furuncle*

   (See "Infections of the External Ear.")

6. *Aural polyp*

   Polyps are soft tissue masses, usually circumscribed, glistening, and often obstructing the EAC. An aural polyp may be thought of as a flag: an indicator of underlying disease such as chronic otitis media or cholesteatoma with concomitant inflammation. The polyp usually arises from the middle ear mucosa (respiratory epithelium) but may arise directly from the TM as a reaction to a foreign body such as a ventilation tube.

   An aural polyp is often a physical obstruction to local medical treatment of disease in the EAC. Polyps may be treated in several ways: locally with astringents such as $AgNO_3$, trichloroacetic acid, and 20% phenol to reduce the mass of the polyp or by removal. Astringents tend to work well because of the myxedematous nature of polyps: They are inflammatory tissue and contain a lot of water. Reducing this fraction alone will shrink the mass and allow topical therapy to start working.

   Removal of an aural polyp must be done with caution. The surgeon should have a clear idea of the most likely site of origin: a perforation, a cholesteatoma, or a foreign body reaction to a tube. If there is any suspicion that the polyp could be attached to a deeper structure, such as the facial nerve, the stapes footplate, and a dehiscence of the vestibular labyrinth, or that it could in fact not by a polyp and instead a herniation of meninges and/or brain (meningoencephalocele, encephalocele), it should be left alone until definitive radiologic studies, CT and/ or MRI ± contrast, will more precisely define the anatomic site of origin.

   The polyp, once grasped with an appropriately sized instrument, should be "smeared" and never forcefully "yanked" or otherwise forcibly removed from the ear. An inflammatory polyp will easily yield to gentle manipulation. Another underlying disease process may be more resistant and should never be removed with force.

   All material removed from the body must be sent for pathologic examination and an aural polyp is no exception. Although the tissue removed may have all of the gross features of a polyp, only properly stained and examined material will definitely identify an inflammatory polyp and exclude other entities such as glial, brain, and cancer tissue. It is simply indefensible that cancer or anything other than an inflammatory polyp be missed because tissue was not sent for pathologic examination.

7. *Dermatologic conditions of the EAC*

   The EAC may be thought of as a blind pouch lined with skin. There are several differences between the skin of the EAC and skin elsewhere in the body. Specialized systems such as the apopilosebaceous unit and ceruminous glands are present in the skin of the EAC but not elsewhere. The EAC is thus susceptible to many of the dermatologic processes found elsewhere in the body. Nuanced dermatologic descriptions aside, much of what otologists treat may be generally classified as chronic otitis externa. The EAC may manifest purely local problems such as contact dermatitis and neurodermatitis (lichen simplex chronicus). The EAC may also manifest systemic conditions such as psoriasis, eczema, atopic dermatitis, seborrheic dermatitis, acne vulgaris, and sarcoidosis.

Patients typically present with itching, serous or mucous drainage, fullness, and hearing loss. The history is a key feature toward a correct diagnosis. Both ears must be given careful scrutiny under the microscope. The physician will often see a similar state in the EAC for many dermatologic conditions: very dry skin and signs of mechanical excoriation. The patient may present with an AOE. The "good" ear (if it is quiescent) will often "tell the story." The baseline problem is that the skin is too dry, leading to pruritus, scratching, and violation of the skin and its lymphatics with the resultant perfect setup for AOE: warm, moist, and dark—just what bacteria and fungi need for growth. This set of otologic problems is cyclical. The baseline is "too dry," but acute exacerbations may cause the ear to become moist and acutely infected.

As the adage goes: "If too moist, dry it; if too dry, moisten it." It is a fine tuning especially true in ladies who are taking oral birth control mediations with resultant fluctuation in hormonal homeostasis.

Drops do not stay as drops forever. Eventually, they become the residue of the drop and the liquid into which the active ingredient of the drop was dissolved. Hence, drops add fluid and often water to the ear: again, just what bacteria and fungi need to grow. Desiccating powders are often a better choice in the acutely infected, moist ear. Once the ear has reached its "baseline" (check the "good" ear), gentle moistening with steroid oils (e.g., fluocinalone 0.01% oil, prednisolone forte 1% ophthalmologic solution) or creams/ointments (triamcinolone 0.025%) once or twice a week may maintain the ear. The patient must be cautioned not to instrument the ear.

Unfortunately, chronic otitis externa is poorly understood by most general physicians and also by many otolaryngologists. The typical patient has been treated with several different drops in the hope that finding "the perfect drop" will solve the problem. This of course is illusive. Ultimately, there is no *cure* for many of these conditions, but care of acute exacerbations and the judicious use of steroids will go a long way to help care for the patient.

8. *Bacterial and fungal otitis externa* (see "Infections of the External Ear.")

9. *Osteomyelitis of the skull base* (see "Infections of the External Ear.")

10. *Osteoma and exostoses of the EAC*
    Osteoma(s) (Fig. 146.8) of the EAC are true neoplasms, often unilateral, solitary, pedunculated, and not related to cold water or air exposure. They usually occur at the tympanosquamous suture line

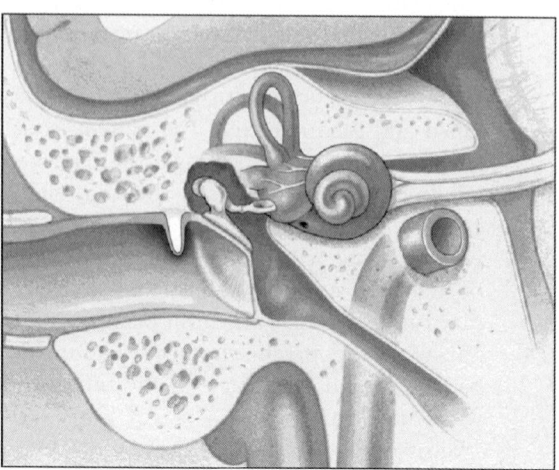

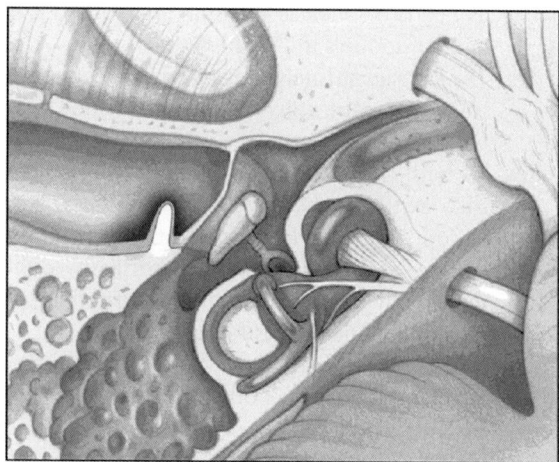

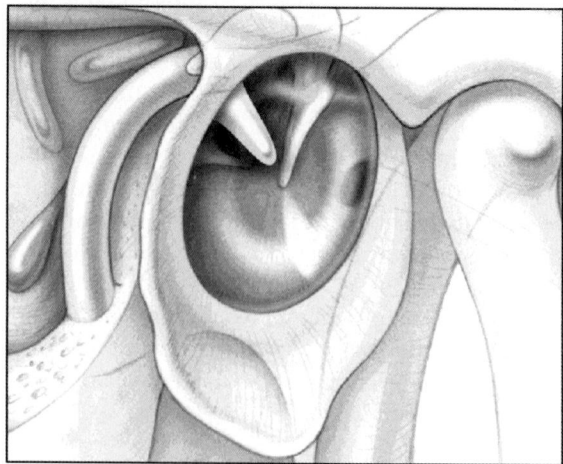

Figure 146.8 A: Coronal section of a right ear showing a single stalk of an osteoma. **B:** Axial view of left ear showing a single stalk of an osteoma. **C:** Sagittal section of a right ear showing a single stalk of an osteoma. Figure courtesy of Robert K. Jackler MD.

and are found more lateral than exostoses. A solitary, large osteoma may fill a good portion of the EAC, causing all of the problems of advanced exostoses. On CT, the osteoma may be more heterogeneous with areas of cancellous bone, less dense than an exostosis. There is usually a stalk leading to the osteoma that can be seen under microscopic exam or on CT.

Exostoses (Figs. 146.9 to 146.11) of the EAC are acquired, benign, broad-based growths of bone occurring within the EAC found most often near the tympanomastoid or tympanosquamous suture lines. They are often bilateral with one ear more advanced than the other. Exostoses are not true neoplasms. They are bony calluses or hyperostoses arising from the tympanic ring. They typically do not have a stalk. The presumed pathophysiology is refrigeration osteitis, the effect of chronic cold water or air to the bone of the EAC in activities such as swimming, surfing, skiing, or boating (35). Many but not all patients with exostoses will have a corroborating history.

If the one or several bony lesions are small and most of the TM is clearly visible, the ear is observed. There are several reasons to shave down an exostosis or to remove an osteoma:

1. Recurrent infections of the EAC. Trapped squamous debris and wax will become a nidus of recurrent EAC infections, and the obstruction should be removed.
2. Conductive hearing loss due to wax/debris impaction. With severe obstruction(s), even a small amount of wax and debris will cause conductive hearing loss.
3. The usual bony and soft tissue landmarks are becoming lost. It is not wise to wait this long because the surgeon must rely upon landmarks of the EAC to perform the surgery.
4. To allow a patient to be properly fitted with a hearing aid

Exostoses may occur along with other conditions, for example, otosclerosis. If the exostoses are too large to allow for the usual transcanal approach, the ear with the greater hearing loss should have the exostoses removed, be allowed to heal, the hearing retested, and then the stapedectomy performed.

All patients being considered for surgery must have a formal hearing test and an edge-enhanced, noncontrast CT of the temporal bones to look for landmarks around the bony lesion(s): the TM, the middle ear and ossicular chain, and the tympanic and vertical course of the facial nerve. The surgeon should have a very good idea in the preoperative preparation not only of what the ear looks like under the microscope but what radiologic landmarks will help to guide the dissection.

Surgery may be done through the EAC or through a postauricular approach. The important word is to "shave"

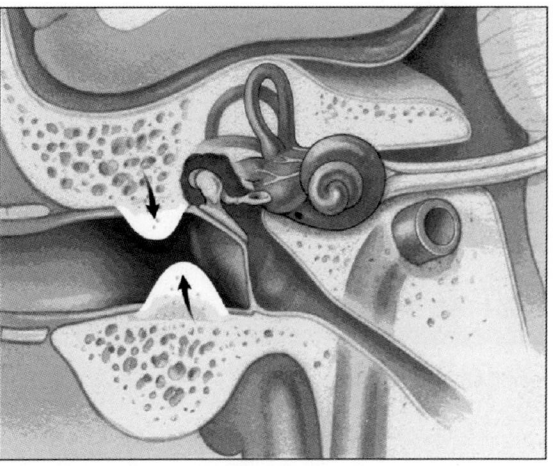

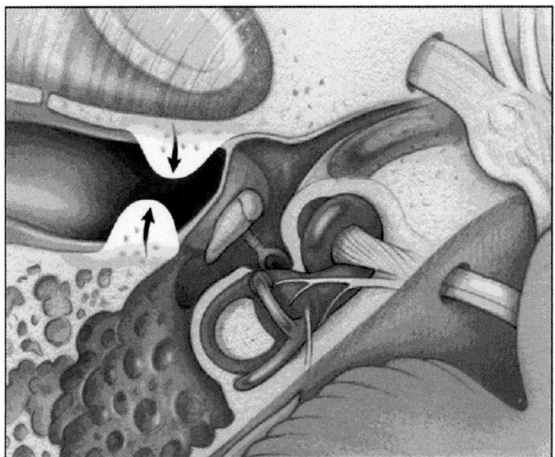

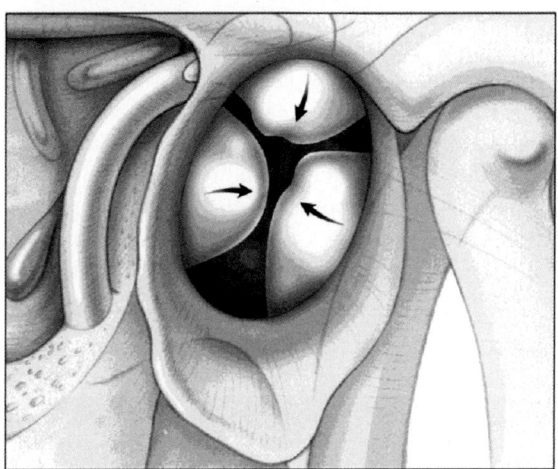

Figure 146.9 A: Coronal section of a right ear showing multiple growth centers of exostoses. **B:** Axial view of left ear showing multiple growth centers of exostoses. **C:** Sagittal section of a right ear showing multiple growth centers of exostoses. Figure courtesy of Robert K. Jackler MD.

the exostosis(es) carefully. Exostoses do not develop in a month. By the time the patient requires surgery, these lesions have been present for many years if not many decades. It is highly unlikely that they will grow back any quicker the second time than the first. Hence, there is no

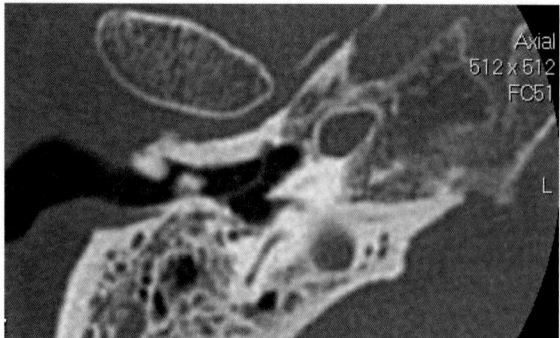

Figure 146.10 Right axial temporal bone CT showing exostoses.

need to "go for broke" and try to remove every millimeter of neo-ossification. A reasonable goal is to be able to see most of the perimeter of the TM and to know that the EAC, after it heals, will be large enough to hold an ITC (in the canal) hearing aid mold. Because of the proximity of the vertical facial nerve and of the TM, nothing more than shaving the bone need be done. Certainly the tympanic ring does not need to be "overcorrected." It is wise to perform this surgery under general anesthesia and to monitor the facial nerve with an EMG needle system. The prevention of an iatrogenic facial nerve injury is worth any and every surgical and monitoring precaution.

In extremely rare cases in which all landmarks have been lost, it is best to stay "high and anterior," that is, where the facial nerve would be unlikely to be found, to find a known landmark such as the TM and then to proceed. Approaching from behind with the vascular strip retracted with a Penrose drain or another suitable retractor may also provide landmark clues. It is usually not necessary to perform a mastoidectomy for landmarks. There are usually enough landmarks in the EAC available for the surgeon.

The surgical technique for the removal of an osteoma is somewhat more straightforward and simple than for exostoses. The lesion is ordinarily removed via a transcanal approach, but a postauricular approach may be required for extremely large osteoma. Because there is

ordinarily a stalk leading to the osteoma, it can be tapped with a 2- to 4-mm nasal osteotome and the osteoma delivered. The remaining stalk can be shaved down with a diamond burr. The remainder of the care is the same as with exostoses.

Although the patient is ordinarily consented for a split-thickness skin graft, this is almost never necessary due the redundancy of skin over the exostoses or osteoma. The skin of the EAC is incised in a horizontal fashion around the midpoint of the lesion(s) with a round knife or similar instrument and the skin is "window-shaded" fore and aft away from the bony growth, which is then shaved with an appropriately sized diamond burr or tapped out with an osteotome. Once the bony growths have been reduced and the TM easily seen, the remaining skin is placed back flat, trimmed if necessary, and the EAC is packed for about 3 to 4 weeks. (One hint to help prevent the ingrowth of soft tissue into packing material is to line the whole canal with a sleeve of moistened gelfilm or very thin silastic and then to pack the ear.) The patient must be advised that the ear will take about 6 to 8 weeks to heal properly. It is extremely rare to have to revise this type of surgery if it is done carefully and conservatively.

CONCLUSION

With a thorough knowledge of the normal embryology, anatomy, and physiology of the external ear, together with an understanding of the natural history of the various common disease processes that occur in this location, treatment of the patient with external ear disease becomes logical. However, it is not always easy. Most conditions can be managed with the recommendations outlined in this chapter. There is no substitute for patience and thoroughness.

HIGHLIGHTS

- An understanding of the various disease entities occurring in the external ear is predicated on a knowledge of the embryology, anatomy, and physiology of the canal.
- Infection and blockage of the apopilosebaceous unit are the precursors of infectious otitis externa.
- Otitis externa presents as a spectrum of disease and may be classified into preinflammatory, acute inflammatory, and chronic inflammatory stages.
- Four principles form the basis of treatment for all stages of infection of the external ear: thorough cleaning, antibiotic therapy, control of inflammation and pain, and recommendations to prevent infection. Of these, the first is the cornerstone of therapy.

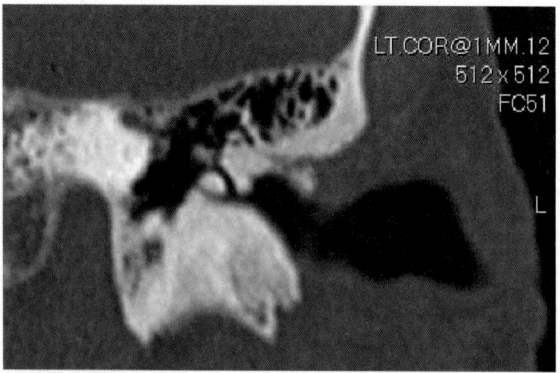

Figure 146.11 Left coronal temporal bone CT showing exostoses.

■ Recalcitrant and recurrent otitis externa must be treated aggressively with daily local care and antibiotics, often in the hospital. Patience and thoroughness are needed for successful treatment.

■ Surgery is rarely indicated for infections of the external canal but may be required to reverse the natural course of chronic disease.

■ NEO is a disease occurring in immunosuppressed patients. It must enter the differential diagnosis of any patient with nonresolving acute external otitis.

■ There are four hallmarks of NEO: persistent otalgia; persistent otorrhea and granulation tissue; diabetes mellitus, advanced age, or immunocompromised state; and cranial nerve involvement.

■ NEO must be treated aggressively with proper radiographic imaging to map the extent of disease, meticulous local care control of diabetes or immunodeficiency (when possible), and antibiotics. Surgery is rarely required. Mortality remains significant with cranial nerve involvement.

■ Many infectious and inflammatory conditions related to external otitis occur in the ear. Therapy is based on treatment of the underlying condition.

REFERENCES

1. Hollinshead WH. *Anatomy for surgeons: the head and neck,* 3rd ed. Vol. 1. Philadelphia, PA: Harper & Row, 1982:159–163.
2. Anson BJ, Donaldson JA. *Surgical anatomy of the temporal bone,* 3rd ed. Philadelphia, PA: W.B. Saunders, 1981:28.
3. Hughes GB, Pensak ML. *Textbook of clinical otology.* New York: Thieme-Stratton, 1997.
4. Lucente FE. External otitis. In: Gates GA, ed. *Current therapy in otolaryngology-head and neck surgery,* 6th ed. New York: Elsevier Science, 1997.
5. Toulmouche MA. Observations d'otorrhee cérébrale suivis des réflexions. *Gazette Med Paris* 1838;6:422–426.
6. Meltzer PE, Kellemen G. Pyocyaneus osteomyelitis of the temporal bone, mandible and zygoma. *Laryngoscope* 1959; 60:1300–1316.
7. Chandler JR. Malignant external otitis. *Laryngoscope* 1968;78:1257–1294.
8. Chandler JR. Malignant external otitis: further considerations. *Ann Otol Rhinol Laryngol* 1977;86:417–428.
9. Chandler JR. Pathogenesis and treatment of facial paralysis due to malignant otitis externa. *Ann Otol Rhinol Laryngol* 1972;81:648–656.
10. Chandler JR, Grobman L, Quencer R, et al. Osteomyelitis of the base of the skull. *Laryngoscope* 1986;96:245–251.
11. Chandler JR. Malignant external otitis and osteomyelitis of the base of the skull. *Am J Otol* 1989;10:108.
12. Kimmelman CP, Lucente FE. Use of ceftazidime for malignant external otitis. *Ann Otol Rhinol Laryngol* 1989;98:721.
13. Mattucci KF, Setzen M, Galantich P. Necrotizing otitis externa occurring concurrently with epidermoid carcinoma. *Laryngoscope* 1986;96:264–266.
14. Carfrae MJ, Kesser BW. Malignant otitis externa. *Otolaryngol Clin North Am* 2008;41:537–549, viii–ix.
15. Geerlings SE, Hoepelman AM. Immune dysfunction is patients with diabetes mellitus (DM). *FEMS Immunol Med Microbiol* 1999; 28:259–265.
16. Damiani JM, Damiani KK, Kinney FE. Malignant external otitis with multiple cranial nerve involvement. *Am J Otol* 1979;2:115.
17. Gangadar SS, Kwartler JA. Skull base osteomyelitis secondary to malignant otitis externa. *Current Opin Otol HN Surg* 2003;1:316–323.
18. Okpala NC, Siraj QH, Nilssen E, Pringle M. Radiological and radionuclide investigation of malignant otitis externa. *J Laryngol Otol* 2005;119:71–75.
19. Ismail H, Hellier WP, Batty V. Use of magnetic resonance imaging as the primary imaging modality in the diagnosis and follow-up of malignant external otitis. *J Laryngol Otol* 2004;118:576–579.
20. Grandis JR, Curton HD, Yu VL. Necrotizing (malignant) external otitis: prospective comparison of CT and MRI imaging and follow-up. *Radiology* 1995;196:499–504.
21. Weber PC, Seabold JE, Graham SM, et al. Evaluation of temporal and facial osteomyelitis by simultaneous In-WBC/Tc-99m-MDP bone SPECT scintigraphy and computed tomography scan. *Otolaryngol Head Neck Surg* 1995;113:36–41.
22. Gilbert D, Tice AD, Marsh PK, et al. Oral ciprofloxacin therapy for chronic contiguous osteomyelitis caused by aerobic gram-negative bacilli. *Am J Med* 1987;82:254.
23. Shupak A, Greenberg E, Hardoff R, et al. Hyperbaric oxygenation for necrotizing (malignant) otitis externa. *Arch Otolaryngol Head Neck Surg* 1989;115:1470.
24. John AC, Cheesman AD. Malignant otitis externa. *Hosp Update* 1979;5:589.
25. Reines JM, Schindler RA. The surgical management of recalcitrant malignant external otitis. *Laryngoscope* 1980;90:369.
26. Pedersen HB, Rosenborg J. Necrotizing external otitis: aminoglycoside and β-lactam antibiotic treatment combined with surgical treatment. *Clin Otolaryngol* 1997;22:271–274.
27. Amorosa L, Modugno GC, Pirodda A. Malignant external otitis: review and personal experience. *Acta Otolaryngol Suppl* 1996;521:3–16.
28. Gherman CR, Ward RR, Bassis ML. Pneumocystis carinii otitis media and mastoiditis as the initial manifestation of the acquired immuno-deficiency syndrome. *Am J Med* 1988;85:250.
29. Lucente FE. Acquired immunodeficiency syndrome (AIDS) In: Lucente FE, Lawson W, Novick N, eds. *The external ear.* Philadelphia, PA: W.B. Saunders, 1995:95.
30. Work WP. Newer concepts of first branchial cleft defects. *Laryngoscope* 1972;82:1581–1593.
31. Mashkevich G, Undavia S, Iacob C, et al. Malignant cylindroma of the external auditory canal. *Otol Neurotol* 2006;27:97–101.
32. Darr AE, Linstrom CJ. Conservative management of advanced external auditory canal cholesteatoma. *Otolaryngol H.N. Surg* 2010;142:278–280.
33. Lacout A, Marsot-Dupuch K, Smoker WRK, Lasjaunias P. Foramen tympanicum or Foramen of Huschke: pathologic cases and anatomic CT study. *Am J Neurorad* 2005;26:1317–1323.
34. Wang RG, Bingham B, Hawke M, et al. Persistence of the foramen of Huschke in the adult: an osteological study. *J Otolaryngol* 1991;20:251–254.
35. Van Gilse PHG. Des observations ulterieures sur la genes des exostoses du conduit externe par l'irrigations d'eau froide. *Acta Otolaryngol (Stockh)* 1938;26:343.

147 Neoplasms of the Ear and Lateral Skull Base

Bradley P. Pickett   *Brianna K. Crawley*

This chapter provides an overview of neoplasms that affect the temporal bone and the external ear. These neoplasms can be classified on the basis of their location or by their cell of origin. Classification based on location offers a relatively straightforward outline of tumor types that is useful in the differential diagnosis (Table 147.1, Fig. 147.1). Neoplasms of the pinna, the external auditory canal, the middle ear and mastoid, the temporal bone, and the cerebellopontine angle are discussed in this context. When extensive neoplasms occupy more than one anatomic location, however, or when the same pathology arises in more than one location, classification based solely on the site of origin of the neoplasm becomes confusing. In these instances, it is more appropriate to classify tumors based on the cell type that gives rise to the neoplasm. Paragangliomas and hemangiomas are examples of this type of neoplasm. Because a detailed discussion of each neoplasm is beyond the scope of this chapter, the reader is encouraged to examine the recommended readings and references. It should be borne in mind that the causes of neoplasms of the temporal bone and the external ear are in most instances unknown. Therefore, the growth patterns of neoplasms, the prognosis for individuals affected by them, and current modes of surgical and medical therapy are the principal areas of concern in this chapter.

NEOPLASMS OF CELL-SPECIFIC ORIGIN

Paraganglioma

Paragangliomas are the most common true neoplasm of the middle ear and are considered the most frequent pathologic condition involving the jugular foramen. Paragangliomas are generally slow-growing, benign neoplasms with an interval between initial symptoms and diagnosis measured in years, and an estimated doubling time of 4.2 years. The growth patterns of temporal bone

paragangliomas often follow the path of least resistance and are therefore greatly influenced by the site of tumor origin and regional anatomy. Paragangliomas that originate in the middle ear are termed glomus tympanicum tumors. Paragangliomas that originate in association in the jugular fossa are termed glomus jugulare tumors. Clinical manifestations are related to tumor extent and vascularity, as are treatment options.

Paragangliomas of the temporal bone arise from glomus bodies occupying the adventitia of the jugular bulb, along the course of the tympanic branch of the glossopharyngeal nerve (Jacobson nerve) or the auricular branch of the vagus nerve (Arnold nerve). Glomus bodies are groups of chemoreceptor cells belonging to the diffuse neuroendocrine system that are found in collections within the jugular foramen and middle ear, carotid bodies, the adrenal medulla, and along the aorta and vagus nerve. Histologically, they are identical to the carotid body and are similar to the autonomic ganglia of the adrenal medulla. Glomus bodies consist of clusters of chief cells supplied by a network of arterioles, venules, and both afferent and efferent nerve terminals. They are of neural crest derivation, migrating during embryogenesis to concentrate around autonomic ganglia. They are more accurately referred to as paraganglia, because they appear to play a role as neuromodulators or monitors of vascular activity. Chief cells have neurosecretory granules that contain norepinephrine, dopamine, and epinephrine, suggesting that the release of granule contents into the vascular system helps to regulate cardiorespiratory function, modify local blood distribution, and maintain thermoregulation. Unlike the carotid body and the adrenal medulla, however, paraganglia of the temporal bone play an uncertain role in these neuroendocrine functions. Paraganglia of the temporal bone are distinguished from other components of the diffuse neuroendocrine system, such as the adrenal medulla, by their lack of affinity for chromium salts used in certain histologic stains. They

TABLE 147.1	NEOPLASMS OF THE EAR AND LATERAL SKULL BASE

Neoplasms of cell-specific origin
Paraganglioma
    Glomus tympanicum
    Glomus jugulare
Epidermoid
    External auditory canal and middle ear (cholesteatoma)
    Internal auditory canal, petrous apex, and cerebellopontine angle
Vascular neoplasm
    Hemangioma
    Hemangiopericytoma
Hematologic malignancy
    Lymphoma
    Plasmacytoma
    Leukemia

Neoplasms of the pinna and external auditory canal
Cutaneous carcinoma
    Squamous cell carcinoma
    Basal cell carcinoma
Malignant melanoma
Glandular neoplasm
    Ceruminous adenoma
    Ceruminous adenocarcinoma
    Pleomorphic adenoma
    Adenoid cystic carcinoma
Osteoma and exostosis
Miscellaneous neoplasm
    Merkel cell carcinoma
    Squamous papilloma
    Pilomatrixoma
    Myxoma
    Auricular endochondral pseudocyst
    Chondrodermatitis nodularis chronica helicis (Winkler disease)

Neoplasms of the middle ear, mastoid, and temporal bone
Adenomatous neoplasm
    Benign middle ear adenoma
    Endolymphatic sac tumor
Langerhans cell histiocytosis
    Eosinophilic granuloma
    Hand-Schüller-Christian disease
    Letterer-Siwe disease
Sarcoma
    Rhabdomyosarcoma
    Chondrosarcoma
    Ewing sarcoma
    Osteogenic sarcoma
    Fibrosarcoma
Chordoma
Congenital neoplasm
    Dermoid
    Teratoma
    Choristoma
Cholesterol granuloma

Neoplasms of the internal auditory canal and cerebellopontine angle
Schwannoma
    Vestibular schwannoma
    Facial nerve schwannoma
    Trigeminal schwannoma
    Jugular foramen schwannoma
Meningioma
Lipoma
Metastases

are therefore categorized as nonchromaffin paraganglia. Adult temporal bones usually have only two or three paraganglia, but on occasion, there may be more, particularly during the fifth decade of life. Most paraganglia of the temporal bone are found in the anterolateral region of the jugular fossa and within the middle ear. Neoplastic transformation of paraganglia can occur in either location, indicated by local tumor invasion or metastatic spread. Metastases of head and neck paraganglioma are uncommon and are more frequently associated with non–carotid body paragangliomas of the head and neck. They occur in only 0.016% cases of paragangliomas and are most often found in the cervical lymph nodes, followed by lungs, liver, spleen, and bone (1).

Paragangliomas represent 0.6% of all head and neck tumors, with a reported incidence range of 1 in 30,000 to 100,000. They occur more frequently on the left side, and females are affected by paragangliomas more frequently than males, 4-6:1. Living at high altitude is also a risk factor. Although the peak incidence occurs during the fifth decade of life, paragangliomas may present from infancy to old age. Tumors that arise in very young patients should generate additional concern, because they tend to be more aggressive, are more commonly multifocal, and are more likely to secrete vasoactive substances (2). Approximately 5% to 10% of patients with paragangliomas eventually present with multiple tumors, but when paragangliomas occur as a familial form of an autosomal dominant disorder (about 10% of patients), multicentricity may occur in as many as 78% (3). Mutations of loci encoding succinate dehydrogenase have been implicated in the development of familial paragangliomas (4). Succinate dehydrogenase is an intracellular enzyme that plays a critical role in cellular energy production, and if the enzyme is inactive, succinate is allowed to accumulate, producing pseudohypoxic conditions that inhibit some neuroendocrine apoptotic factors. This may be the trigger that leads to proliferation of paraganglia.

On gross examination, paragangliomas are deep red, firm, rubbery masses that bleed profusely upon manipulation. The histologic appearance of paraganglioma is distinctive. Nests of argyrophilic chief cells, termed *zellballen*, are septated by a prominent fibrovascular stroma, though this characteristic appearance is occasionally not evident in temporal bone paragangliomas (Fig. 147.2). Unmyelinated nerve fibers may be identified, but they are scarce when compared with normal paraganglia. Nuclear pleomorphism and hyperchromatism are prominent in chief cells but do not appear to indicate malignant growth. Electron microscopy reveals neurosecretory granules within chief cells that store catecholamines. Variable cranial nerve invasion may occur, a feature that has significance during surgical removal of the tumor mass.

Glomus tympanicum tumors usually originate on the promontory of the cochlea. As they grow, they follow the path of least resistance. First, the tumor enlarges to fill the middle ear and to envelope the ossicles. Patients present at this stage with conductive hearing loss and

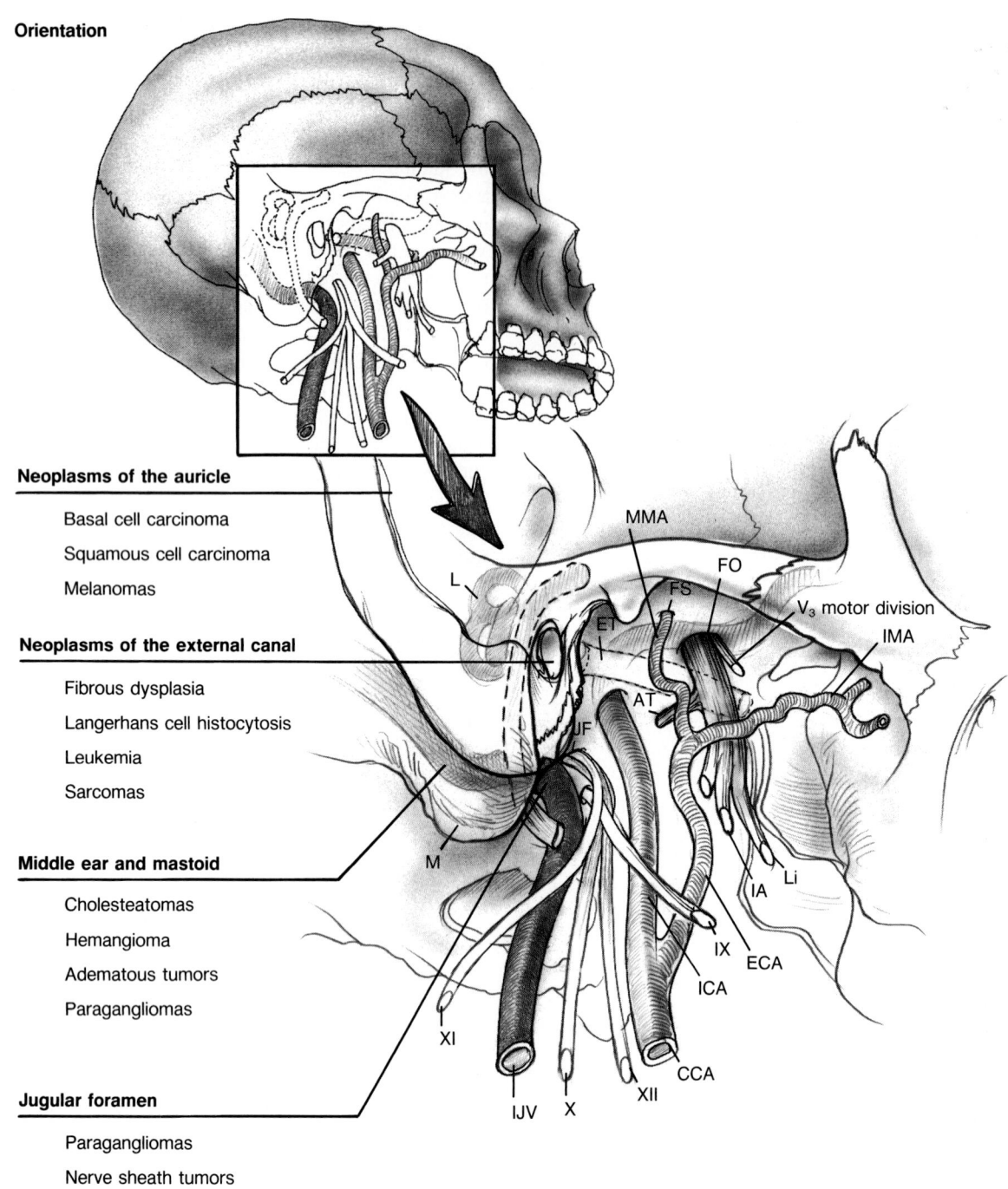

Orientation

Neoplasms of the auricle

Basal cell carcinoma

Squamous cell carcinoma

Melanomas

Neoplasms of the external canal

Fibrous dysplasia

Langerhans cell histocytosis

Leukemia

Sarcomas

Middle ear and mastoid

Cholesteatomas

Hemangioma

Adematous tumors

Paragangliomas

Jugular foramen

Paragangliomas

Nerve sheath tumors

Sarcomas

Figure 147.1 Anatomy of the lateral skull base and common locations of neoplasms found in this region. AT, auriculotemporal nerve; CCA, common carotid artery; ECA, external carotid artery; FO, foramen ovale; IA, inferior alveolar nerve; ICA, internal carotid artery; IMA, internal maxillary artery; JF, jugular foramen; JV, jugular vein; L, labyrinth; Li, lingual nerve; MMA, middle meningeal artery; IX, glossopharyngeal nerve; X, vagus nerve; XI, accessory nerve; XII, hypoglossal nerve.

pulsatile tinnitus caused by direct transmission of vascular pulsations from the highly vascularized tumor to the ossicles. Pulsatile tinnitus is the most common presenting symptom for patients with temporal bone paragangliomas. Because glomus tympanicum tumors enlarge within the middle ear cavity, patients with these tumors generally present with pulsatile tinnitus at an earlier stage than patients with glomus jugulare tumors. The tympanic membrane often remains intact as a glomus tympanicum tumor grows, but the tumor may displace the membrane laterally. If tumor extends through the tympanic membrane into the external auditory canal, patients may present with otalgia or bloody otorrhea. As glomus tympanicum tumors enlarge further, they may extend into the mastoid antrum

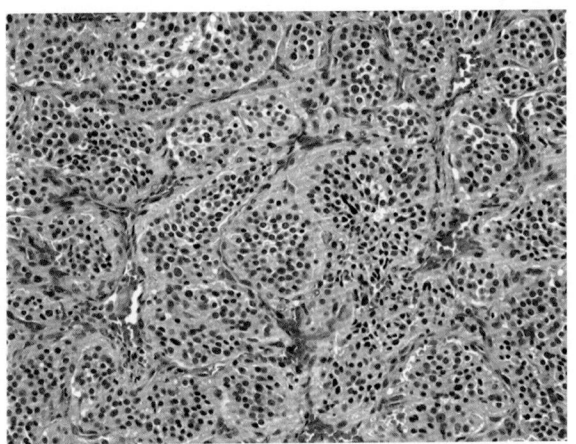

Figure 147.2 Paraganglioma: Histologic section showing tumor cells organized into nests, termed *zellballen*, separated by fibrovascular stroma.

via the aditus ad antrum, into the facial recess, or into the retrofacial air cell tract. At this stage, the tympanic and mastoid portions of the facial nerve may become involved with tumor. The tumor may grow anteriorly into the eustachian tube and inferiorly into the infralabyrinthine air cell tract. When the tumor causes bone erosion in the hypotympanum, the jugular fossa or the vertical portion of the petrous carotid artery may be exposed. It is difficult to distinguish an extensive glomus tympanicum tumor of this kind from a glomus jugulare tumor. Patients with extensive tumors may present with multiple cranial nerve neuropathies.

Glomus jugulare tumors arise in the jugular fossa and are usually large before patients become symptomatic. These are more likely to secrete catecholamines than the glomus tympanicum variety. Compression of neurovascular structures in the jugular fossa and extension medially along the skull base to the hypoglossal canal can lead to cranial nerve neuropathies manifesting as dysphagia, dysphonia, aspiration, and dysarthria. Erosion of the jugular fossa anteriorly and superiorly exposes the petrous carotid artery and allows tumor to invade the middle ear, causing conductive hearing loss and pulsatile tinnitus. Intracranial extension occurs when glomus tumors grow into the eustachian tube and extend into the peritubal air cell tract or follow the petrous carotid artery into the petrous apex, the cavernous sinus, and the middle cranial fossa, resulting in facial hypesthesia. Glomus jugulare tumors may involve the posterior cranial fossa when they extend medially along the skull base or through the infralabyrinthine air cell tract. A patient with extensive tumor that compresses the cerebellum and the brainstem in the posterior fossa may present with ataxia and imbalance.

Paragangliomas of the temporal bone can usually be diagnosed on the basis of findings on physical exam and characteristic features found on imaging studies. Otoscopic examination of a middle ear paraganglioma frequently demonstrates a reddish-blue pulsatile mass medial to the inferior tympanic membrane. Positive

pressure during pneumatic otoscopy causes blanching of the mass, a phenomenon known as the Brown sign. The pulsatile nature of the tumor can be diminished with ipsilateral carotid artery compression, a positive Aquino sign. Objective tinnitus may be apparent if auscultation over the mastoid or infra-auricular area reveals an audible bruit. When tumor extends through the tympanic membrane, otoscopic examination shows a hemorrhagic aural polyp. Tumors involving the jugular foramen can be identified when lower cranial nerve palsies develop. Jugular foramen syndrome, also termed Vernet syndrome, arises when tumor growth affects cranial nerves IX, X, and XI and causes paresis or paralysis of the muscles innervated by these nerves. Villaret syndrome is a combination of jugular foramen syndrome with Horner syndrome in patients with more extensive disease. Patients with paragangliomas that erode the carotid canal and compromise the sympathetic plexus present with Horner syndrome (miosis, ptosis, anhidrosis, and enophthalmos). If facial nerve weakness or paralysis exists, it denotes extensive involvement of the middle ear and mastoid. Tuning fork tests or complete audiometric evaluation in these patients shows conductive hearing loss and on rare occasions sensorineural hearing loss. Ataxia or rostral cranial nerve palsies are disquieting signs that indicate involvement of the posterior cranial fossa or cavernous sinus.

Although the chief cells of paragangliomas have neurosecretory granules that store catecholamines, only 1% to 3% of these tumors actively secrete norepinephrine. Catecholamines are much more likely to be secreted by glomus jugulare tumors than by glomus tympanicum tumors. Opinions vary regarding the need to screen for functionally active temporal bone paraganglioma, but all tumor patients who present with a history of flushing, frequent diarrhea, palpitations, headaches, poorly controlled hypertension, orthostasis, or excessive perspiration should have serum catecholamine levels measured and 24-hour collection of urine for analysis of vanillylmandelic acid and metanephrine.

Diagnostic imaging studies provide essential information for the evaluation of patients with temporal bone paragangliomas. These studies reveal diagnostic facts and details about tumor extent and regional anatomy that are essential in planning surgery. High-resolution computed tomography (HRCT) of the temporal bone uses a thin-section bone algorithm and is usually the first imaging study ordered to evaluate a patient suspected of having a temporal bone paraganglioma. HRCT can identify the tumor origin accurately when the bony partition between the jugular fossa and the hypotympanum is intact. In this instance, a glomus jugulare tumor that erodes the jugular fossa and involves lower cranial nerves can be distinguished from a glomus tympanicum tumor that occupies the middle ear. Without this bony partition, it may be difficult to identify the origin of a temporal bone paraganglioma. Erosion of the caroticojugular spine that separates

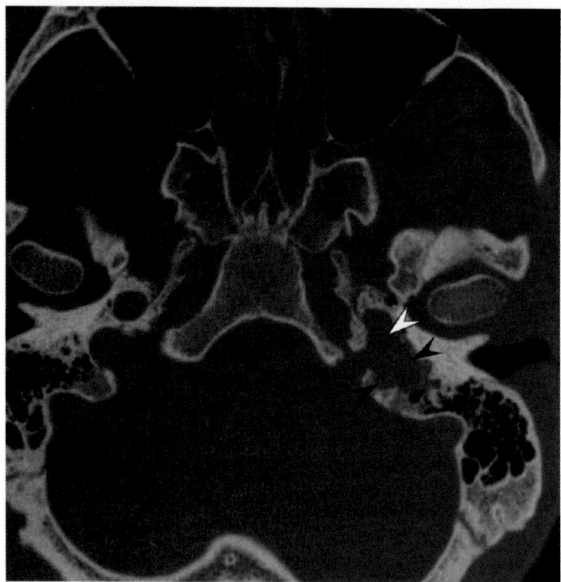

Figure 147.3 Glomus jugulare. Axial CT showing classic bony erosion of the left jugular fossa and caroticojugular spine (*black arrowheads*). The tumor abuts the posterior aspect of the vertical petrous carotid artery (*white arrowhead*).

the jugular bulb and the petrous carotid artery usually indicates a glomus jugulare tumor (Fig. 147.3). If the spine is eroded and the carotid canal is exposed, involvement of the petrous carotid artery is likely. HRCT also helps to identify other lesions that should be excluded, such as a dehiscent jugular bulb or an aberrant internal carotid artery. Obliteration of the fallopian canal indicates adherence of tumor to the facial nerve or invasion of the nerve by tumor. Multidetector CT angiography can diagnose glomus tumors with accuracy and offers information about feeding vessels, venous drainage, and jugular involvement (5). Intracranial extension can also be identified, but magnetic resonance imaging (MRI) is better than HRCT to evaluate the relationship between paraganglioma and adjacent soft tissue structures. MRI will not only identify intracranial extension, but images may help differentiate between intradural and extradural extension. MRI signal characteristics diagnostic for paragangliomas include vascular flow voids within the tumor, the so-called salt and pepper pattern. Pepper refers to the signal voids of large feeding arteries, and salt represents subacute hemorrhage within the tumor. Magnetic resonance angiography and magnetic resonance venography may demonstrate intraluminal involvement of the petrous carotid artery or occlusion of the jugular vein and sigmoid sinus. However, these studies are usually not useful for most large tumors as formal angiography will be necessary. MRI of the neck offers enough detail to screen for multicentric disease such as carotid body tumors or glomus vagale tumors, but other imaging modalities that exploit common features of neuroendocrine tissue may be useful in detecting tumors and recurrences. ^{123}I-MIBG (metaiodobenzylguanidine) scintigraphy and (18)F-DOPA

positron emission tomography can be used to detect active tumors, but somatostatin receptor scintigraphy is more reliable for paragangliomas of the head and neck (6).

The principal therapeutic modality is complete surgical excision of the tumor. Secreting tumors must be treated with adjunctive α and β blockade. If surgical therapy is deemed appropriate, small tumors isolated to the promontory can be successfully removed via the transcanal or hypotympanotomy approach. More advanced lesions of the middle ear and mastoid can be exposed with an extended facial recess approach through the mastoid. Large paragangliomas should be evaluated preoperatively with four-vessel angiography. Angiography is combined with embolization using polyvinyl alcohol or intravascular coils 1 or 2 days before surgery to decrease intraoperative blood loss, shorten duration of the procedure, and reduce postoperative morbidity. Devascularization of the entire tumor is difficult, requiring embolization of each vascular pedicle, and may prove impossible in tumors with intracranial extension (7). Sacrifice of the internal carotid artery when invaded by tumor is seldom necessary, and thus, balloon occlusion studies are rarely performed in these patients. Instead, residual mural tumor and tumor that encases the internal carotid artery after subtotal resection is observed or treated with stereotactic radiation surgery (SRS). Glomus jugulare tumors are approached via transmastoid–transcervical exposure of the jugular bulb and jugular foramen. Large tumors require limited facial nerve rerouting or formal infratemporal fossa dissection through this approach. In some cases, more extensive temporal bone dissection is necessary to eradicate tumor that has spread to the petrous apex. This may necessitate removal of part or all of the labyrinth. Intracranial extension requires a combined neurosurgical–neurotologic procedure. Postoperative cranial nerve palsies are not uncommon, and some patients require follow-up care to assist with facial reanimation, deglutition, and phonation. Alternatives to surgical therapy for primary, recurrent, or persistent disease include external beam radiation therapy, intensity-modulated radiation therapy (IMRT), and SRS. Radiation has little effect on the primary tumor cells, the chief cells, but it causes obliterative endarteritis in tumor vessels that can stop tumor growth. One recent meta-analysis suggests that SRS provides better tumor control than surgery, with diminished risk to cranial nerves, but large tumors may require surgical debulking prior to radiosurgery (8).

Epidermoid (Cholesteatoma)

Epidermoids are soft tissue masses resulting from an aberrant accumulation of keratin debris within a sac of squamous epithelium. They are customarily classified as tumors though they are not strictly cellular growths and therefore not neoplastic. Epidermoids may result from squamous epithelial entrapment during embryogenesis, mucosal metaplasia, or, most commonly, with anomalous squamous epithelial migration or deposition. The nomenclature used to describe these masses is determined based on site of origin and pathogenesis. As an example, masses that arise from congenital epithelial rests in the petrous apex, internal auditory canal, or cerebellopontine angle are generally referred to as epidermoids. Cholesteatoma is the name for epidermoids resulting from the migration of tympanic membrane epithelial cells into the middle ear or from traumatic implantation deep to the skin of the external auditory canal. Congenital cholesteatoma, in contrast, usually refers to an epithelial sac in the middle ear arising from the entrapment of congenital epithelial rests during development. Despite diversity of origin and location, all possess similar histology and growth potential.

Middle ear cholesteatomas are generally divided into two types, congenital and acquired. *Congenital* middle ear cholesteatoma occurs in the presence of an intact tympanic membrane, exclusive of any history of otorrhea, prior otologic intervention, or previous perforation. Theories advanced to explain the origin of these lesions include invagination or implantation into the middle ear, mucosal metaplasia, and epidermoid formation from retained epithelial cell rests. Though the debate persists, the latter is favored as the most likely. Histologic examination of fetal temporal bones has demonstrated epidermoid formation throughout the annular lateral wall region, not solely in the anterosuperior annular region of the tympanic cavity as previously described (9,10). *Acquired* cholesteatomas arise from the transposition of keratinizing squamous epithelium into the middle ear, epitympanum, or mastoid and are often associated with perforation or retraction of the tympanic membrane. These latter are by far the more common of the two, likely resulting from eustachian tube dysfunction or deficiencies in tympanic membrane structure, or a combination. Together, these qualities promote formation of a retraction pocket in the tympanic membrane, trapping epithelial cells within and leading to the accumulation of keratin debris in the middle ear. Acquired aural cholesteatoma may extend to the petrous bone or to the cranial cavity, but most lesions of the petrous apex and the cerebellopontine angle are thought to be of congenital origin. Cholesteatoma of the external auditory canal could conceivably result from congenital rests of tissue trapped deep to the skin of the canal, but most canal wall cholesteatomas occur after traumatic implantation of epithelium subsequent to external trauma or otologic surgery. Patients with cholesteatoma of the middle ear and external auditory canal most often present with purulent otorrhea and conductive hearing loss, while patients with congenital cholesteatoma rarely present with otorrhea as the tympanic membrane is usually intact.

Epidermoids represent approximately 1% of all intracranial tumors, and most occur in the cerebellopontine angle. Squamous metaplasia within the temporal bone or intradural space has been proposed in the histogenesis of these lesions, but it is more likely that developmental entrapment of squamous epithelium from the neural tube is the cause. As squamous epithelium located at the periphery of an epidermoid comprises its only viable proliferating tissue, it grows very slowly in comparison with solid benign neoplasms of similar dimensions. Epidermoids enlarge by expanding to fill empty spaces such as the cerebellopontine angle, the internal auditory canal, or air cells that occupy the petrous apex. These masses are infiltrative, and they grow to a relatively large size before they begin to compress or displace adjacent structures, becoming clinically detectable. Additionally, epidermoids often incite a localized inflammatory reaction that causes the lining to become densely adherent to juxtaposed brainstem or cerebellum. Local neurovascular structures become enveloped by epidermoids instead of being displaced or compressed, and neurologic function may be altered when the vascular supply of a nerve is compromised by the infiltrative process. Most patients become symptomatic in a very gradual manner, their symptoms related to the location of the mass. Patients with internal auditory canal or cerebellopontine angle epidermoids often present with imbalance and hearing loss akin to patients with vestibular schwannoma. However, epidermoids are more likely than vestibular schwannoma to cause facial weakness or hemifacial spasm. Epidermoids are also more likely to compromise the trigeminal nerve causing diminished facial sensation or facial pain. Intracranial extension of these lesions may also manifest as diplopia or headache.

All epidermoids and cholesteatomas exhibit a similar morphologic appearance. The friable lesions are either smooth and cystic with a round or oval appearance or nodular and irregular. The lining of the sac is usually white in color and spongy in consistency. Histologically, the cyst is lined with a benign keratinizing squamous epithelium consisting of three components: the sac or epithelial matrix, the perimatrix, and the contents of the cyst. Typical layers of squamous epithelium may be identified within the epithelial matrix. The contents of the cyst include fully differentiated laminated keratin. Acquired and congenital lesions can often be distinguished histologically by the thicker matrix and more vigorous proliferation of inflammatory cells within the sac and at the periphery of acquired lesions.

The diagnosis of cholesteatoma is usually made during otologic examination, while epidermoids are usually diagnosed with radiographic imaging studies. Congenital epidermoids are frequently identified as an asymptomatic mass in the anterosuperior quadrant of the middle ear. Patients with acquired disease have keratin debris, granulation polyps, or purulent material emanating from the mouth or opening of the sac. Clinical findings in patients with epidermoids include facial weakness or paralysis and sensorineural hearing loss when the lesion involves the internal auditory canal and/or the cerebellopontine angle. Facial hypesthesia and abducens nerve palsy occur when epidermoids invade the anterior petrous apex.

HRCT of the temporal bone in patients with epidermoid disease shows a well-defined homogeneous mass that occasionally contains areas of calcification or has eroded adjacent bony structures. MRI is diagnostic, revealing a well-circumscribed nonenhancing mass that has low signal intensity on T1-weighted images, high signal intensity on T2-weighted images, and hyperintensity on diffusion-weighted image sequences.

Management of cholesteatomas of the external auditory canal and middle ear is addressed in other chapters in this text. Optimal treatment of epidermoids of the skull base consists of total microsurgical resection. This often necessitates a posterior fossa or middle fossa craniotomy, but transtemporal approaches may be indicated, especially in patients with nonserviceable hearing in the ipsilateral ear. Because the capsule of the mass may be densely adherent to the brainstem or intracranial vascular structures, complete removal of skull base epidermoids is extremely difficult or even impossible. Complete excision is achieved in only half of all patients with epidermoids, and additional postoperative cranial nerve deficits are discovered in most of these patients (11). Recurrence can be expected in at least 30% of patients when subtotal removal is carried out. Malignant transformation is very rare, and only 26 cases have been reported.

Hemangioma and Hemangiopericytoma

Hemangiomas are benign vascular proliferations that arise from capillaries, arterioles, or venules. They are classified according to the type of vessel from which they originate: capillary hemangioma, cavernous hemangioma, and venous hemangioma. It is unclear whether they represent true neoplasms or hyperplastic growth of normal tissue occurring in an appropriate anatomic site. Hemangiomas are reported to occur in a variety of locations involving the external ear and lateral skull base, namely, the external auditory canal and tympanic membrane, the middle ear, the internal auditory canal, and the geniculate segment of the facial nerve. Tumors are spongy red or purple nodular masses. On microscopic examination, they show thin-walled vascular channels that contain blood and are small or intermediate in size. These channels are not surrounded by an elastic or muscular layer. Clinical presentation varies depending on tumor location. Hemangiomas of the external auditory canal and tympanic membrane have been reported when patients present with mild conductive hearing loss and aural fullness. Patients with middle ear tumors are often asymptomatic, but they can also present with conductive hearing loss, aural fullness, and pulsatile tinnitus. Otologic examination reveals a vascular intratympanic mass that can be confused with a paraganglioma, an adenomatous tumor, or an aberrant vascular anatomy. Preoperatively, hemangiomas of the internal auditory canal may be difficult to distinguish from vestibular schwannomas when patients present with unilateral sensorineural hearing loss.

However, accompanying facial nerve dysfunction is more characteristic of hemangioma, even when tumors are small. CT imaging studies help to differentiate intracanalicular lesions when hemangiomas show calcium stippling, which is characteristic of an osseous hemangioma. On MRI, they are heterogeneously hyperintense.

Geniculate hemangiomas are the most common temporal bone hemangioma and perhaps the most intriguing. They consistently arise from the superior aspect of the geniculate ganglion, probably from vascular plexuses on the surface of the facial nerve, and extend into the floor of the middle cranial fossa. Even though the tumor is generally extraneural, they sometimes infiltrate the nerve or are associated with a localized inflammatory response that causes the tumor to adhere tightly to the nerve sheath. This intimate relationship with the facial nerve accounts for the frequently associated facial nerve dysfunction, manifest by paralysis, twitching, or spasm of the facial musculature, even when tumors are very small.

Depending on their size, location, and the structures they involve, hemangiomas of the ear and temporal bone are either observed or treated with complete surgical excision. Resection of lesions from the external canal and the middle ear is usually straightforward, but it may be unnecessary in pediatric patients who are asymptomatic as these lesions often involute spontaneously. When hemangioma is associated with the facial nerve, however, proper management is controversial. If facial paralysis exists, tumor resection with nerve grafting may be appropriate. If facial nerve function is normal or only mildly compromised, early excision when the tumor can be peeled off the nerve while preserving function may be appropriate. Facial nerve monitoring is used during the surgical resection to help maintain nerve integrity. When left intact, patients generally have superior results when compared to patients who require nerve sacrifice and grafting. In patients who have undergone subtotal resection for nerve preservation, regrowth has not been detected as late as 13 years after surgery. If a cochlear fistula is noted in the setting of serviceable hearing, surgery should be delayed in order to preserve hearing for as long as possible (12). However, most case reports suggest that facial nerve integrity cannot be maintained when removing hemangiomas, and because most geniculate hemangiomas grow very slowly, observation may be the most appropriate management until severe dysfunction or facial paralysis occurs.

Hemangiopericytoma is a rare vascular tumor derived from pericytes that line the outside surface of capillary basal lamina. They can occur wherever capillaries are found. Less than 20% of hemangiopericytomas occur in the head and neck, and fewer than 10 cases have been reported where the tumor originated in the temporal bone. The middle ear, jugular fossa, and petrous bone were the apparent sites of origin of the tumors that occurred in the temporal bone. Symptoms include hearing loss, otorrhea, and cranial nerve deficits. Hemangiopericytoma can occur in patients of any age with 10% of cases occurring in children, but it is most frequent in patients aged 50 to 70, affecting males and females equally. Tumors are soft or rubbery and pale gray or white in color. The metastatic rate for primary temporal bone tumors is estimated to be 15% to 20%. On microscopic examination, hemangiopericytomas are circumscribed pseudoencapsulated cellular tumors containing thin-walled vascular spaces separated by sheets of polyhedral- and spindle-shaped cells. They do not demonstrate intratumoral calcification. Tumors with malignant behavior may display nuclear pleomorphism, lymphocytic infiltration, and lack of vascular spaces with necrosis and hemorrhage. Wide excision with or without embolization is the treatment of choice, but external beam radiation therapy, stereotactic radiosurgery, or chemotherapy may be used to treat extensive, recurrent, or inoperable tumors. Long follow-up is mandatory secondary to their propensity to recur and metastasize (13).

Lymphoma, Plasmacytoma, and Leukemia

Lymphoma is a neoplasm of the lymphoreticular system that may involve the temporal bone either as a secondary lesion after metastatic spread or as a primary lesion causing focal disease. Neoplastic infiltration of the middle ear, the facial nerve, the eighth cranial nerve, and the bone marrow of the petrous apex is not an uncommon finding during postmortem examination of temporal bones from patients with systemic lymphoma. However, most patients are asymptomatic unless lymphomatous infiltration results in middle ear effusion or hemorrhage and conductive hearing loss. Primary osseous lymphoma represents 1% to 2% of malignant lymphoma, and only 18 cases of primary temporal bone B-cell lymphoma have been reported (14). In these case reports, the most common presenting symptoms were conductive hearing loss, otalgia, aural fullness, and otorrhea. Localized swelling and pain, fevers, sensorineural hearing loss, balance disturbance, and facial and abducens palsies from perineural invasion have also been reported. Physical examination may reveal middle ear masses or effusions and facial paresis. Once diffuse lymphoma has been ruled out, most patients with primary lymphoma of the temporal bone do well after chemotherapy and/or radiation therapy. The role of surgery in these patients is to obtain tissue for diagnosis.

Extramedullary plasmacytoma of the temporal bone is a rare neoplasm that is thought to arise as a clone of malignant plasma cells in the submucosal stroma of the middle ear. These are solitary lesions that occur outside the bony medullary spaces, and they are less likely to develop into disseminated disease or into multiple myeloma when compared with solitary osseous plasmacytomas. The majority of extramedullary plasmacytomas develop in the upper aerodigestive tract with only 1% of these tumors arising in the temporal bone. Patients, more often men over 50, present with aural fullness or otalgia, hearing loss, and tinnitus,

and physical examination reveals a thickened tympanic membrane with an intratympanic mass or an aural polyp. Microscopic examination of these fleshy masses reveals sheets of monotonous round cells that are typical of plasma cells. Nuclear and cellular atypia is variable and defines tumor differentiation and grade. Tumor grade, however, is not necessarily predictive of tumor behavior. When biopsy specimens suggest the diagnosis of extramedullary plasmacytoma, patients should be evaluated for disseminated disease or multiple. This evaluation includes complete blood count with differential and smear, erythrocyte sedimentation rate, serum chemistries, creatinine, serum and urine protein analysis for monoclonal antibodies, bone marrow biopsy, and a radiographic skeletal survey. Chemotherapy is indicated for disseminated disease, but extramedullary plasmacytoma isolated to the temporal bone is usually successfully treated with external beam radiation therapy and surgery for radioresistant or very large tumors. Recurrence is rare as is dissemination to multiple myeloma, but the possibility necessitates long-term follow-up (15).

Leukemia may involve the temporal bone by infiltrating marrow spaces and the tympanomastoid cavity or by causing hemorrhage within the middle or inner ear. In leukemia patients, marrow spaces in the temporal bone are frequently infiltrated by leukemic cells, but this rarely results in clinical manifestations. Infiltration of the middle ear and mastoid air cells is less common but may result in symptomatic effusions, often misdiagnosed as otomastoiditis, as these patients are particularly susceptible to infection. Patients with acute or chronic myelogenous leukemia may develop larger consolidated infiltrates that form solid tumors known as granulocytic sarcomas or chloromas. These present with hearing loss, facial palsy, and postauricular and auditory canal swelling and are often first mistakenly treated for infection. The tumors consist of immature granulocytes and contain myeloperoxidase that gives the lesion a green hue, hence the name chloroma. Most chloromas occur in children with leukemia. Leukemic infiltrates can involve the cochlea causing sensorineural hearing loss, but inner ear injury more likely results from local hemorrhage. Diagnosis is best made with biopsy, though this is often not feasible, and MRI is the imaging modality of choice. Treatment of systemic leukemia that infiltrates the temporal bone requires appropriate high-dose chemotherapy and management by a hematologist/oncologist with consideration for radiation therapy. Prognosis is poor, especially in the setting of delayed diagnosis (16).

NEOPLASMS OF THE PINNA AND EXTERNAL AUDITORY CANAL

Cutaneous Carcinoma

Basal cell carcinoma is a cutaneous malignancy that comprises approximately one-fifth of neoplasms that involve the ear and temporal bone. This common lesion is generally discovered in adult patients and is usually diagnosed for the first time during the sixth decade of life. Most basal cell carcinomas occur on the pinna or in the periauricular area, where they are more common than squamous cell carcinoma, and only about 15% arise in the external auditory canal where squamous cell carcinoma is far more common. Actinic exposure is thought to be the primary factor responsible for initiating this neoplastic transformation because the periauricular areas and the auricular helix, which receive the most sun exposure, are especially susceptible. Males are affected approximately twice as often as females. The noduloulcerative lesion that appears on the pinna is similar to basal cell carcinomas found in other areas of the body. It is characterized by locally infiltrating nodular growth with a rolled border and a central crusting ulcer. This neoplasm appears to be well circumscribed, but there may be subcutaneous extension with indistinct clinical margins. Distant or regional metastases are extremely rare, though they are more common when lesions involve the ear. Histologic examination shows a rim of palisading basaloid cells at the tumor margin with central necrosis and ulceration. Most of the tumor is quite cellular, making it simple to make a diagnosis and to identify the tumor margin (Fig. 147.4). However, 25% of basal cell carcinomas that involve the skin of the external ear are morpheaform or sclerosing subtypes. They are distinguished from the more common noduloulcerative lesions by linear strands of basaloid cells that infiltrate the subcutaneous layers of the skin and are accompanied by a fibrous matrix. The linear strands are diffuse within the fibrous matrix, and consequently the margin of the morpheaform type of basal cell carcinoma is indistinct.

Basal cell carcinoma of the ear is a slow-growing neoplasm, and the diagnosis is readily obtained by inspection and biopsy. If untreated, these low-grade malignancies progressively enlarge and infiltrate peripherally into the periauricular tissues or medially into the external auditory canal, the middle ear, and the mastoid. Morpheaform lesions

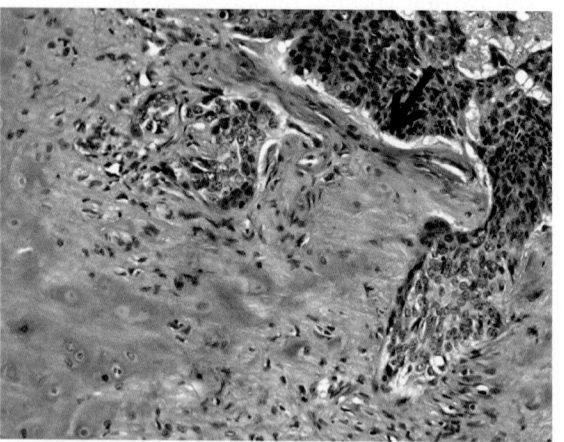

Figure 147.4 Basal cell carcinoma: Histologic section showing basophilic tumor cells invading hyaline auricular cartilage. Palisading basaloid cells are demonstrated adjacent to a clefting artifact (*arrow*).

are especially troublesome because they infiltrate along deep tissue planes. Extension into the temporal bone may remain undetected until the malignancy is far advanced. Basal cell carcinoma is best treated with complete surgical excision. However, the risk of recurrence for auricular basal cell carcinoma is high compared with other sites in the head and neck because deep invasion often occurs. Mohs micrographic surgery appears to be the most successful technique to minimize recurrence and to conserve nonneoplastic tissue. Radiation therapy is used as palliative therapy or as adjunct therapy for extensive or recurrent tumors.

Squamous cell carcinoma that involves the ear and lateral skull base is most often a cutaneous neoplasm that originates from the skin of the pinna or external auditory canal. These are aggressive tumors with prognoses affected by depth of invasion, cartilage destruction, and lymphovascular invasion. A much smaller portion of these malignancies originates from the middle ear, presumably from metaplastic middle ear mucosa. The average age at diagnosis of squamous cell carcinoma of the pinna is the late 60s, whereas primary external auditory canal lesions generally present 10 to 15 years earlier. Tumors that originate in the middle ear affect adults in an intermediate age group at an average age of 60 years. Patients with squamous cell carcinoma of the ear and temporal bone comprise 24% of patients with squamous cell carcinoma of the head and neck. Most of these tumors originate on the pinna. Like basal cell carcinoma, more than half of these occur on the helix, which receives the greatest actinic exposure. Sun exposure and cold injury certainly predispose patients to this malignancy, but other factors such as radiation exposure and chronic infection are thought to play an etiologic role. For squamous cell carcinoma that originates in the middle ear, chronic otitis media and human papillomavirus are proposed to be important elements in the pathogenesis of malignancy (17).

Squamous cell carcinoma of the pinna is a scaly, irregular, indurated maculopapular lesion. Very often, the surface of the erythematous lesion is ulcerated with either a crust or serosanguinous exudate. Patients with squamous cell carcinoma of the external auditory canal often present with hemorrhagic otorrhea that has been treated for years as otitis externa. In older patients, chronic bloody drainage and sudden onset of deep ear pain suggest an invasive malignancy. Ipsilateral facial nerve deficit is another indication of invasive malignancy. Extensive involvement of the external auditory canal or the middle ear results in conductive hearing loss, but deep invasion that extends into the internal auditory canal, the cerebellopontine angle, or the labyrinthine capsule may cause sensorineural hearing loss. Metastasis to cervical or parotid lymph nodes occurs in approximately 30% of patients with temporal bone invasion, whereas metastatic disease occurs half as often when lesions are limited to the pinna or to the membranous portion of the external auditory canal. Histologic examination shows proliferative pleomorphic spindle-shaped epidermal cells with keratin pearls and intercellular bridges that are typical features of squamous cell carcinoma. A less aggressive form of squamous cell carcinoma of the pinna, called adenoid squamous cell carcinoma, shows similar histologic features, but there is nodular proliferation of epidermoid cells that show prominent glandular patterns. These lesions are invasive but slow growing, and they rarely metastasize.

The diagnosis of squamous cell carcinoma of the pinna is easily made with a biopsy, but many middle ear and external auditory canal malignancies have advanced significantly by the time of diagnosis. Biopsy is advisable whenever middle ear or external canal infections fail to respond to appropriate medical therapy. Untreated carcinoma of the pinna will likely spread laterally to periauricular areas or medially into the external auditory canal. The prognosis worsens when external canal lesions extend medially into the tympanic bone or through the tympanic membrane and into the middle ear. Tumor in the middle ear extends anteriorly into the eustachian tube and carotid canal and posteriorly into the mastoid air cell system. From the carotid canal, squamous cell carcinoma can invade the petrous apex, the anterior skull base, and the cavernous sinus. The inner ear is generally resistant to invasion, but tumor in the mastoid may penetrate the dural plate and extend into the posterior cranial fossa.

The treatment of squamous cell carcinoma of the ear and lateral skull base, even for less advanced tumors, should be aggressive because recurrence rates are high (18). Complete surgical resection is favored whenever possible. Complete resection of lesions of the pinna is most easily achieved with Mohs micrographic surgical techniques. Carcinoma that invades the cartilaginous portion of the external auditory canal can be excised as a sleeve resection with skin grafting of the defect. Tumors that invade the bony external auditory canal require en block excision with a lateral temporal bone resection. When tumor extends through the tympanic membrane into the middle ear, expands into the mastoid air cells, or invades the otic capsule, a subtotal temporal bone resection is indicated. Parotidectomy and neck dissection may also be appropriate, and radiation therapy is recommended for patients with advanced-stage carcinoma to improve survival (19). Chemotherapy is sometimes offered as adjuvant or palliative therapy but has not yet been shown to increase survival.

Melanoma

Malignant melanoma of the external ear is a cutaneous neoplasm that originates from melanocytes in the epidermis or dermis of the pinna. Melanomas account for only 3% of malignant cutaneous neoplasms, yet approximately 75% of deaths from cutaneous malignancies are caused by melanoma. The external ear is the site of origin for approximately 10% of all primary melanomas of the head and neck and 1% of all melanomas, with the helix or antihelix being the most common location of the original lesion. Primary melanoma of the external auditory canal is extremely rare, and melanoma of the middle ear is most likely to be metastatic disease or the result of regional extension. The average age at diagnosis of melanoma of the pinna is 50 years, but this disease affects all age groups except for young children. Men are affected by melanoma at least three times more often than women, and fair-skinned individuals with blonde or red hair, blue eyes, and freckled skin are predisposed to the disease. Sun exposure, specifically repeated intense exposure causing severe solar injury, has a role in the pathogenesis of this neoplasm. Melanoma is five times more common in the southwestern United States when compared with the northeast. The incidence of melanoma in all areas of the world appears to be increasing annually. Atmospheric ozone depletion may be responsible for some of this increase, but heightened awareness of skin malignancy by patients and by medical professionals enhances the likelihood of detection. Patients may also be genetically predisposed to melanoma. First-degree relatives of patients with melanoma have twice the risk of developing this malignancy, and inherited disorders, such as familial dysplastic nevus syndrome, also increase the risk of developing melanoma.

Melanomas of the ear are divided into five subtypes based on appearance and potential for dermal invasion. *Superficial spreading melanoma* is the most common type. It starts as a regular dark pigmented macule that first grows radially throughout the epidermis and dermal–epidermal junction, becoming nodular and ulcerated with transition into its vertical growth phase. Round, pigmented epithelioid melanocytes grow in nests that invade the epidermis during the radial growth phase and the dermis during the vertical growth phase. The radial growth phase is intermediate in length and is estimated to last anywhere from 1 to 6 years. Many of these lesions will incite an inflammatory response. *Nodular melanoma* is the most aggressive of the three types. These darkly pigmented nodules invade the dermis and subcutis with minimal, if any, radial spread. On histologic examination, atypical melanocytes are both spindle shaped and epithelioid in nature, and the surrounding inflammatory response is minimal (Fig. 147.5). On immunohistochemical studies, malignant melanoma demonstrates reactivity for vimentin, S-100 protein, HMB-45, and Melan-A. *Lentigo maligna*, the third type of melanoma, is a macular lesion with variable pigmentation that tends to have a prolonged radial growth phase before dermal invasion occurs. A lentigo consists of pigmented spindle cells that are usually confined to the epidermis, and there may be a surrounding inflammatory response. *Desmoplastic melanomas* are associated with preexisting melanocytic lesions but can be amelanotic. They have a high local recurrence rate and frequent perineural involvement, but they rarely metastasize. *Mucosal melanomas* may be associated with the eustachian tube or, rarely, arise primarily from the middle ear mucosa. They are associated with a poor prognosis secondary to late stage at presentation and difficulty in obtaining adequate surgical margins.

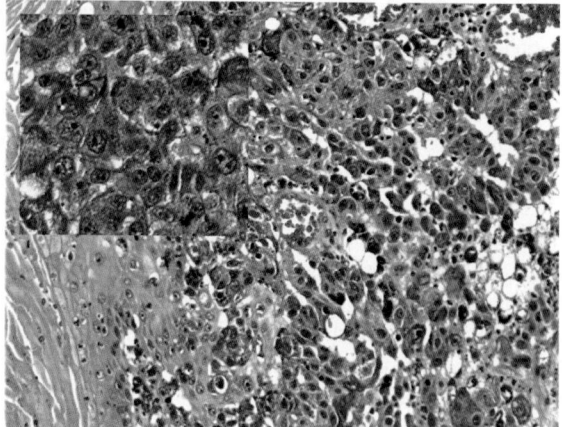

Figure 147.5 Melanoma: Histologic section showing remarkable pigmentation of malignant melanoma cells, even on standard H&E preparation. Characteristic prominent nucleoli with multiple mitotic figures are demonstrated (**inset**).

The diagnosis of melanoma is suspected when pigmented lesions change color or texture, increase rapidly in size, or ulcerate. Prompt excisional biopsy is recommended for all suspicious pigmented lesions because early melanoma is curable. Tumor thickness is critical to establish the prognosis, but nodular configuration, ulceration, and regional or distant metastases all indicate a poor prognosis. Once the dermis is invaded, the probability of regional or distant metastases increases. Unfortunately, one-third of patients have cervical node involvement at presentation. The precise location of the tumor does not appear to correlate well with metastatic patterns, but melanomas of the ear have been found to metastasize to preauricular, postauricular, anterior and posterior cervical chains, and into the parotid nodes. Elective lymph node dissection has been shown to overtreat 80% of patients without providing a survival benefit. However, waiting to perform a therapeutic lymph node dissection when metastatic disease is present may be responsible for unacceptable treatment delays. As a solution to this dilemma, sentinel node mapping using preoperative lymphoscintigraphy and intraoperative intradermal injection of marker dye and radioactive isotope has become the primary method for identification of lymph-draining nodal basins (20). Problems unique to sentinel lymph node biopsy (SLNB) in the head and neck include proximity of the sentinel node to the injection site, inaccessibility of the node (intraparotid lymph nodes), and potential for sentinel nodes that may exist in more than one region. One series demonstrated sentinel lymph nodes from primary melanomas of the auricular helix that were located in levels I to V of the neck and the parotid gland, with an average of three nodes per patient and a range of 1 to 7. Almost 90% had at least one node in level IIA (21).

The treatment of choice for malignant melanoma is complete surgical excision with at least a 1-cm margin for lesions less than 2.0 mm in depth and a 2 cm or greater margin for deeper lesions as satellite clusters can occur.

The goal of treatment is negative margins on permanent pathology. In the presence of ulceration, cartilage invasion, or recurrence, full thickness wedge resections are recommended. Sleeve resections of the external canal may be indicated for involvement, progressing to lateral temporal bone resections with more extensive disease. Reconstructions should not be performed until margins are clear. Lymphoscintigraphy with sentinel node biopsy has been recommended in appropriate surgical candidates with Breslow depth ≥0.76 mm and is becoming established as the standard of care. In the past, information about histologic features and immunohistochemical staining of lesions has been used to guide the decision regarding neck dissection for patients with clinically negative necks. However, this strategy for surgical treatment has failed to increase overall survival or influence 5-year disease-free survival (22). Completion lymphadenectomy after positive SLNB yields a superior 5-year survival rate when compared with lymphadenectomy undertaken after disease is clinically evident. In addition to its influence over the decision to proceed with lymphadenectomy, SLNB provides prognostic information, and that may determine whether adjuvant therapy is recommended (23). Though its efficacy remains controversial, interferon-alpha-2b has been shown to increase disease-free survival and may even provide overall survival benefit in subgroups of patients with high-risk melanoma. Other adjuvant therapies including immunomodulation therapy, vaccination, high-dose fractionated radiation therapy, and chemotherapy have not been shown to improve survival, but continue to be investigated (24).

Glandular Tumors

Glandular tumors of the external auditory canal are rare neoplasms that are thought to arise from the ceruminous glands of the canal. Nearly all glandular tumors of the external auditory canal arise in the lateral membranous portion of the canal where ceruminous and sebaceous glands predominate. Both ceruminous and sebaceous glands are categorized as apocrine glands, meaning that glandular cells release secretions by pinching off and liberating the secretion-rich portion of the cell. Some glandular tumors of the external ear canal, however, seem to arise from eccrine glands. These are glands that secrete by releasing secretory granules. Ceruminous glands might give rise to eccrine gland tumors if they also had some eccrine function. Electron microscopy suggests that ceruminous glands do indeed release secretory granules and may have eccrine function. They might then be better classified as apoeccrine glands and thus might be the origin of all glandular tumors of the external auditory canal.

It is possible to distinguish at least four different histologic types of glandular tumors of the external auditory canal. *Ceruminous adenoma* clearly arises from ceruminous glands. Histologically, it consists of well-differentiated proliferating ceruminous glands that form solid, cystic, and papillary patterns. The glands have a cuboidal or columnar cell layer of apocrine origin and an outer spindle-cell layer of myoepithelial origin. These tumors may be more common in males, and the average age of patients at presentation is 60 years. These nonencapsulated benign neoplasms do not invade surrounding structures. *Ceruminous adenocarcinoma*, on the other hand, is an invasive neoplasm that can metastasize to regional lymph nodes. Histologically, this tumor is nearly identical to a benign adenoma, and it may be difficult to distinguish benign and malignant forms based on microscopic anatomy. However, in some cases, microscopic examination of malignant lesions shows anaplasia, nuclear pleomorphism, mitotic figures, and perivascular or perineural invasion. The primary distinguishing features are regional metastases and invasion into surrounding tissues. Like adenomas, adenocarcinomas are more common in males, but they are diagnosed at an earlier age, averaging 48 years. *Pleomorphic adenoma* of the external auditory canal is similar to neoplasms of the salivary glands, which are eccrine glands, and consists of both epithelial and mesenchymal elements. These benign tumors affect males and females equally, and the average age at diagnosis is 51 years. *Adenoid cystic carcinoma* is the most common glandular neoplasm of the external auditory canal. The cell type that gives rise to these tumors when they occur in the external auditory canal is uncertain. Histologically, these tumors are similar to malignant salivary gland tumors. They lack a capsule and consist of small hyperchromatic cells arranged in cribriform, tubular, or solid patterns. Perineural invasion and invasion along deep tissue planes are prominent features. Regional lymph node metastases are not uncommon, and distant metastases can occur in any vascularized organ, but the lung is the most common site of distant disease. Adenoid cystic carcinoma is more common in females and is diagnosed on average at 43 years of age.

Glandular tumors usually present as asymptomatic soft tissue masses in the membranous external auditory canal. Once the canal is occluded, conductive hearing loss or secondary otitis externa may result. Malignant lesions are more likely to ulcerate or to cause otalgia. Both benign and malignant tumors grow along the path of least resistance, extending laterally out the meatus or medially through the tympanic membrane and into the middle ear. Invasive malignant tumors also extend radially through auricular cartilage and the fissures of Santorini into the parotid gland or into surrounding periauricular tissue. Medial extension with erosion of tympanic membrane or temporal bone is also indicative of malignancy. Diagnosis is made on the basis of microscopic examination of biopsy specimens. To distinguish between benign and malignant ceruminous tumors, biopsy specimens should be large enough to identify deep tissue invasion. HRCT of the temporal bone and MRI of soft tissue around the lateral skull base can be helpful in this respect also. Benign tumors are treated with wide local excision and reconstruction of the external auditory canal. Because of high recurrence rates, especially in

cases of adenoid cystic carcinoma, treatment of malignant lesions should be aggressive (25). Lateral temporal bone resection and postoperative radiation therapy are appropriate for early lesions. Larger malignant tumors require a more extensive temporal bone resection, parotidectomy, and cervical lymph node dissection in addition to postoperative radiation therapy.

Osteomata and Exostoses

Osteomata and exostoses are benign bony growths that involve the external auditory canal. Some controversy exists about whether these are separate entities or actually variations of the same pathologic process, but most sources suggest that osteoma and exostosis are clinically and histologically distinct. *Osteomata* are solitary pedunculated osseous lesions that are smooth and round and originate on the tympanosquamous and tympanomastoid suture lines inside the bony external auditory canal. Patients in almost any age group may present with these neoplasms, but most are middle-aged adults at presentation, and women appear to be affected more often than men. The etiology of osteomata is unknown. Clinically, most patients are unaware of the neoplasm until it is incidentally discovered during otologic examination. When the tumor is sufficiently large, patients may experience conductive hearing loss or recurrent bouts of otitis externa. Histologically, osteomata consist of lamellar bone around trabeculated cancellous bone that contains marrow spaces or fibrovascular tissue. The bone is lined with periosteum and keratinizing stratified squamous cell epithelium. The diagnosis is made during otologic examination when palpation reveals a pearly white or erythematous tender bony growth fixed within the bony canal. Surgical removal of symptomatic tumors requires either a transcanal or a postauricular approach for exposure. Osteomata are removed with a drill while preserving as much skin as possible. Split-thickness skin grafts are used to cover exposed tympanic bone when necessary.

Exostoses are broad-based osseous lesions that occur around the circumference of the medial aspect of the bony external auditory canal. They occur as multiple lesions and are often bilateral. Most patients are diagnosed in their teens or as young adults, and exostoses are far more common in males. The occurrence of exostoses is strongly correlated with exposure to cold water and is therefore thought to result from cold-induced periostitis. Like patients with osteomata, most are asymptomatic until the external auditory canal is occluded or nearly occluded and the diagnosis is made during otologic examination. Histologically, exostoses differ from osteomata. Exostoses consist of parallel layers of subperiosteal bone containing no or only poorly developed trabeculated fibrovascular channels. Surgical removal of exostoses is usually more challenging than removal of osteomata. Generally, a postauricular approach is required, and facial nerve monitoring is recommended because the distal mastoid portion of the facial nerve is at risk during drilling of the posteroinferior aspect of the bony canal. Skin flaps are developed to expose the bony lesions, and they are removed with a drill while preserving the skin. Split-thickness skin grafts may be necessary to prevent postoperative cicatrix formation.

Miscellaneous Neoplasms of the Pinna and External Auditory Canal

Merkel cell carcinoma is a rare but highly malignant cutaneous neuroendocrine tumor that has many characteristics in common with small cell carcinoma of the lung. Fifty percent of these tumors are found in the head and neck, and most that involve the external ear are found in the external auditory canal instead of the pinna. Lesions seem to occur on sun-exposed areas of skin or in patients who are immunosuppressed. The average patient is 65 years old and presents with a rapidly growing, firm, painless nodule that is red, pink, or blue in color. Metastases to regional lymph nodes are present in more than half of patients, and distant pulmonary, hepatic, skeletal, and neurologic metastases occur in approximately 30%. Biopsies specimens show cords, strands, and clusters of round cells in the dermis. Like small cell carcinoma of the lung, these cells have uniform basophilic oval nuclei and stain positively with labeled antibodies to vasoactive intestinal peptide and neuron-specific enolase. Merkel cell carcinoma may be distinguished from amelanotic malignant melanoma, lymphoma, or metastatic carcinoma on the basis of these immunohistochemical staining characteristics. Aggressive therapy is indicated because local recurrence rates approach 50%, metastatic potential is high, and nearly half of patients fail to survive more than 5 years (26). Wide local excision with a 2- to 3-cm margin or Mohs micrographic surgery is recommended, along with SLNB and/or therapeutic lymph node dissection, to address drainage basins in the parotid gland and in the neck. The efficacy of adjuvant therapy is uncertain, but radiation therapy is advisable in all cases. Chemotherapy, like that used for small cell carcinoma of the lung, may offer additional therapeutic benefit for patients with extensive or widely metastatic disease.

Squamous cell papilloma is a benign epithelial neoplasm that occurs in the external auditory canal and is thought to result from infection by human papillomavirus type 6 and 11 (27). Most squamous cell papillomas are fungiform lesions with narrow stalks. Microscopic examination shows well-differentiated squamous cells proliferating on the periphery of a fibrous tissue core. Papillomas are treated by complete excision or laser ablation. *Pilomatrixoma*, also termed calcifying epithelioma of Malherbe, is another benign tumor that may be found in the membranous portion of the external auditory canal or on any hair-bearing skin of the ear such as the lobule. These are solitary cystic lesions that originate from primitive hair matrix cells and are most commonly found in children. Histologically, the

wall of the tumor consists of basaloid cells interposed with connective tissue septa surrounding a central region of degenerative debris containing ghost or shadow cells, keratin, and calcified material. These lesions are easily removed and usually do not recur. *Auricular endochondral pseudocysts* are cyst-like degenerations of auricular cartilage that are thought to result from recurrent minor trauma. These are tumor-like lesions that occur in young adults and are often confused with auricular hematomas. Pathogenesis is thought to be related to minor trauma when small amounts of serous fluid collect between auricular cartilage and the perichondrium. In time, the internal surface of the perichondrium generates a layer of cartilage that encloses the serous fluid. There is no epithelial or endothelial lining and no associated inflammation. Auricular endochondral pseudocysts can be difficult to eliminate. They may require aspiration and injection of a sclerosing agent or incision and drainage with curettage and obliteration with a sclerosing agent. *Chondrodermatitis nodularis chronica helicis (Winkler disease)* is an inflammatory condition of unknown etiology. Caucasian adult males are most commonly afflicted, and the problem manifests as painful papules or nodules on the free border of the helix or on the antihelix. Within the lesions, there is a chronic inflammatory infiltration of the perichondrium, often with focal degeneration or deformity of the underlying cartilage. The lesions can be successfully treated with pressure relief strategies, wide excision with deep shave of the underlying cartilage, or intralesional injections with steroid.

NEOPLASMS OF THE MIDDLE EAR, MASTOID, AND TEMPORAL BONE

Adenomatous Tumors

Since they were first described over a century ago, classification of adenomatous tumors of the middle ear and mastoid has been the subject of controversy. The clinical course of these rare tumors is highly variable, and attempts have been made to identify tumor subtypes so that neoplastic behavior can be predicted and appropriate treatment implemented. Much of the debate about tumor classification focuses on whether the varied microscopic anatomy can be correlated with the tissue of origin (mucosal vs. neuroendocrine) and tumor growth potential. It has been suggested, based on immunohistochemical analysis, that all adenomatous tumors of the temporal bone arise from pluripotential undifferentiated neural crest cells that have migrated to the middle ear (27). This would not explain why some adenomatous lesions develop into malignant tumors, whereas others remain benign. Currently, most evidence suggests two distinct types of primary adenomatous neoplasms of the temporal bone, *benign adenoma*, which arises from the mucosa of the middle ear, and *aggressive papillary tumor*, which arises from the endolymphatic sac. Carcinoid tumors of the middle ear, which are primarily neuroendocrine derived, are either a separate clinical entity or a variant of a benign adenoma.

Benign adenomas of the middle ear are rare nonaggressive neoplasms that are most commonly found in adolescents and young adults, affecting males and females equally. As discussed above, middle ear adenomas seem to arise from the glandular elements of the middle ear mucosa, but what initiates their histogenesis is unknown. Histology of these tumors often reveals benign glandular proliferation, and it has been suggested that benign adenomas represent reactive hyperplasia and not true neoplasm. However, in most reports, there is no history of otitis media or any other source of inflammation. Adenomas are rubbery fibrous tumors that are white, gray, or reddish brown in color. Microscopic examination shows cuboidal or columnar endothelial cells arranged in single-layered glandular structures. Some tumors have trabecular or ribbon-like architecture with sheets of endothelial cells lying adjacent to one another. Nuclei are round or oval and lack mitotic figures or other features of dysplasia. Immunohistochemical staining shows positive staining for synaptophysin, chromogranin, and serotonin, suggesting a neuroectodermal origin for the tumor. Neurosecretory tumor cells predominate in carcinoid variants. Patients most often present with a middle ear mass and an intact tympanic membrane, but tumors can extend through the tympanic membrane or into the mastoid. Generally, there is no bony erosion and no other sign of malignant aggressive growth. Excisional biopsy is recommended, and recurrence is unlikely.

Endolymphatic sac tumors are rare aggressive papillary tumors of the middle ear and mastoid. Just over 100 cases have been reported since they were first described by Heffner in 1989 (28). The age of the patient at the time of diagnosis ranges from 15 to 80 years, with a mean of approximately 40 years. There appears to be no predilection for right- versus left-sided tumors, and a review of the literature suggests that they occur more frequently in females. The time between the onset of symptoms and diagnosis of the tumor is variable and ranges from 1 month to 23 years, with an average of approximately 9 years.

The association between aggressive papillary tumor of the middle ear and von Hippel-Lindau disease was first suggested by Eby et al. in 1988 (29). von Hippel-Lindau disease is an autosomal dominant disorder associated with a defect on chromosome 3p25-26 (30). The disease manifests itself as multiple hemangioblastomas of the retina and central nervous system accompanied by renal cysts, clear cell renal cell carcinoma, pheochromocytoma, and endolymphatic sac tumor. The prevalence of this disease is estimated to be 1 in 35,000 to 1 in 40,000, and the diagnosis is readily confirmed with genetic testing. Endolymphatic sac tumors associated with von Hippel-Lindau disease are clinically and histologically identical to endolymphatic sac tumors in patients without this disease. While the incidence of endolymphatic sac tumor is higher in patients with von Hippel-Lindau disease, these patients are also more likely to have bilateral tumors. Approximately 10% of patients with von Hippel-Lindau disease have endolymphatic sac tumor (31). Additionally, as many as 60% of patients with von Hippel-Lindau disease who also have hearing loss will eventually develop an endolymphatic sac tumor. Therefore, it is prudent to screen for endolymphatic sac tumor in patients with von Hippel-Lindau disease because early diagnosis allows prompt therapy.

Endolymphatic sac tumors are highly vascular friable polypoid masses. Bony invasion is characteristic of these tumors, and infiltrated bone appears to be completely replaced by fibrotic portions of the invasive tumor. On microscopic examination, endolymphatic sac tumors contain both papillary and cystic components. The cellular structure of the papillary component resembles the rugose portion of normal endolymphatic sac epithelium. The epithelial lining of an endolymphatic sac tumor consists of a single cell layer of either low cuboidal or low columnar cells. The nuclei of endolymphatic sac tumor cells are typically aligned in a uniform fashion. Nuclear pleomorphism and mitotic activity are uncommon histologic findings in these tumors. The lumen of the cystic component of the tumor contains a proteinaceous material. This material may be indistinguishable from thyroid colloid. Consequently, it is important to use thyroglobulin staining to distinguish metastatic papillary thyroid carcinoma from endolymphatic sac tumor. The underlying stroma in endolymphatic sac tumors contains an abundant capillary vascular supply that may have the appearance of a second epithelial layer. Immunohistochemical analysis of normal endolymphatic sac tissue provides additional support for the theory that adenomatous tumors of the temporal bone arise from the endolymphatic sac. Normal endolymphatic sac tissue and tissue from endolymphatic sac tumors both stain positively for S-100, a neuron-specific protein; for vimentin, an intermediate filament protein; and for neuron-specific enolase.

The clinical manifestations of endolymphatic sac tumors are best understood on the basis of tumor origin and potential routes of spread. The endolymphatic sac is located in the posteromedial plate of the petrous bone approximately midway between the sigmoid sinus and the internal auditory canal. The sac consists of both a proximal and distal segment. The proximal or rugose portion of the sac is contiguous with the endolymphatic duct and lies within the posterior portion of the petrous bone. This portion of the sac is covered in part by the bony operculum. The distal portion of the sac is located between the dura mater proper and the periosteal portion of the dura mater within the posterior cranial fossa. Both histologic and radiologic studies suggest that the proximal portion of the sac gives rise to tumors.

Endolymphatic sac tumors extend along the endolymphatic duct in the direction of the bony labyrinth. Destruction of the labyrinth results in unilateral sensorineural hearing loss, tinnitus, and vertigo. From the endolymphatic duct, an endolymphatic sac tumor may erode into the vestibule, the posterior semicircular canal, and the mastoid cavity. Once in the mastoid cavity, these tumors follow the retrofacial air cell tract to encompass the facial nerve or to involve the jugular bulb. The middle ear may become involved when tumor enveloping the facial nerve extends anteriorly. From the middle ear cavity, tumor may erode superiorly through the tegmen tympani into the middle fossa, medially to involve the otic capsule, or laterally through the tympanic membrane to involve the external auditory canal. Because of these routes of spread, involvement of the facial nerve and the middle ear space is a common clinical finding. On rare occasion, anterior extension of an endolymphatic sac tumor along the petrous ridge into the petrous apex and cavernous sinus has been reported. Anterior extension into Meckel cave and the internal auditory canal may lead to involvement of cranial nerves V, VII, and VIII. Extension into the cerebellum and into the posterior cranial fossa accounts for the high incidence of ataxia and headaches in patients with advanced lesions. Finally, inferior extension to the region of the jugular foramen accounts for the clinical findings of hoarseness, weakness of the sternocleidomastoid muscle, and palatal dysfunction.

The diagnosis of an endolymphatic sac tumor is usually made by screening audiometry in conjunction with temporal bone imaging studies. Audiograms from patients with endolymphatic sac tumors usually reveal a sensorineural hearing loss. On occasion, a conductive hearing loss may be caused by extension of the tumor into the middle ear cavity. CT shows a soft tissue mass on the posterior petrous face with erosion of adjacent regions of the temporal bone (Fig. 147.6). On bone windows, these tumors

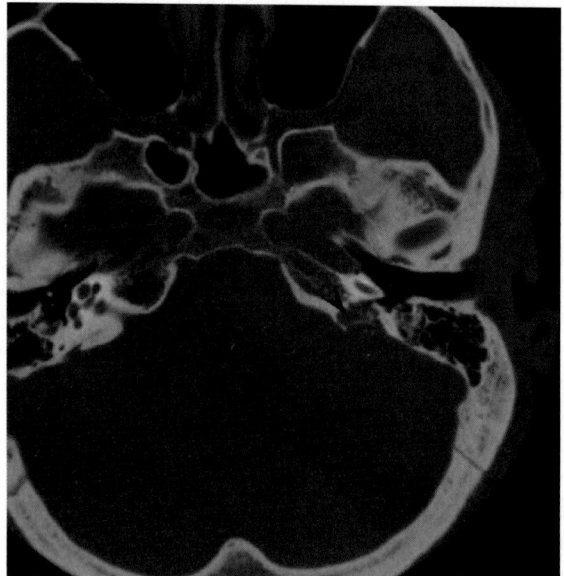

Figure 147.6 Aggressive papillary tumor of the temporal bone (endolymphatic sac tumor). Axial CT showing a left-sided tumor eroding through the posterior face of the petrous bone with invasion (*black arrowhead*) of the petrous apex adjacent to the basal turn of the cochlea. This tumor originated in the endolymphatic sac and extended inferiorly before invading the temporal bone.

commonly contain stippled, reticular, or spiculated areas of calcification. Endolymphatic sac tumors have an "expansile" appearance that helps to differentiate them from other aggressive neoplasms of the temporal bone such as metastatic tumors and high-grade chondrosarcomas that have a less regular pattern of bony destruction. Unenhanced T1-weighted images on MRI studies reveal a pattern of signal intensity that varies with tumor size. In general, endolymphatic sac tumors show increased signal intensity on T1-weighted images, but tumors greater than 3 cm in diameter display multiple intratumoral foci of increased intensity and have a "speckled" appearance. In contrast, tumors less than 3 cm in diameter often have a circumferential rim of increased signal intensity. This rim of high signal intensity is probably generated by breakdown products of subacute hemorrhage found at the periphery of tumors. This characteristic finding on unenhanced T1-weighted imaging is dissimilar to other more common tumors of the petrous apex. Endolymphatic sac tumors enhance with intravenous contrast, but the degree and type of enhancement obtained with this technique varies from tumor to tumor. On T2-weighted imaging, endolymphatic sac tumors contain scattered areas of increased signal intensity. Flow voids are found in 80% of endolymphatic sac tumors and appear to be related to tumor size.

Surgical excision of endolymphatic sac tumors is the treatment of choice, and cure may be achieved with complete resection. Most endolymphatic sac tumors, however, are quite large at the time of diagnosis and may involve the entire lateral skull base. Subtotal resection combined with regularly scheduled radiologic follow-up examinations and revision surgery for significant tumor progression is an alternate treatment option for these indolent neoplasms. However, because most patients with endolymphatic sac tumors are young adults, complete tumor resection using modern techniques in skull base surgery should be the goal. Because these tumors are quite vascular, preoperative embolization plays a role in all but the smallest tumors. Conventional radiotherapy and gamma knife radiosurgery do appear to play a role in the treatment of recurrent or unresectable disease.

Langerhans Cell Histiocytoses

Langerhans cell histiocytoses, also called Langerhans cell tumors, are a group of neoplasms characterized by idiopathic histiocytic and eosinophilic proliferation. Until recently, these tumors were discussed as three separate disease entities: Letterer-Siwe disease, Hand-Schüller-Christian disease, and eosinophilic granuloma. These disorders are now considered to represent three different manifestations of the same disease. However, the use of these names persists mainly as an aid in categorizing the location and extent of disease. In the case of eosinophilic granuloma, the mass is usually localized, whereas in Hand-Schüller-Christian disease and Letterer-Siwe disease, the disease tends to be disseminated. All forms of this disorder are characterized by proliferation of Langerhans histiocytes. These are cells that are derived from monocytes in the bone marrow, but are normally found in the epidermis. Langerhans cell histiocytes proliferation is an aggressive and sometimes malignant disease process that seems to occupy a continuum between the two extremes: histiocytic malignant lymphoma and benign reactive lymph node hyperplasia. Thus, these lesions are more accurately described as tumor-like proliferations, and the lesions may merely be the result of imbalanced immunoregulation. Eosinophils associated with histiocytosis, in cases of eosinophilic granuloma, are believed to be incidental and may be a secondary reaction that accompanies abnormal proliferation of Langerhans cells. All forms of this disease may involve the temporal bone and lateral skull base.

Eosinophilic granuloma presents as a unifocal bony lesion, usually involving the flat bones of the skull, specifically the frontal and temporal bones and the mandible. Patients are generally children and young adults with complaints of chronic or recurrent middle and external ear infection. White males are affected more frequently than other groups. The tumor is characterized by a localized collection of histiocytes, in polygonal and sheet formation, and eosinophils that cause resorption of bone, producing a radiolucent lesion. Diagnosis is confirmed by bone scan and open biopsy showing characteristic histopathology and positive immunohistochemical staining for S-100 and CD1 antigens. This disease process is considered to be the localized form of Langerhans cell histiocytosis. Treatment of eosinophilic granuloma is surgical excision, with radiation therapy for recurrent lesions.

Otologic manifestations of *Hand-Schüller-Christian disease* include chronic purulent middle and external ear disease and hearing impairment. This is also a disease of children and young adults. Typically, there are numerous bony lesions of the skull and axial skeleton. Multifocal involvement of the abdominal viscera and cutaneous lesions indicates a particularly poor prognosis. In CT images, the osteolytic lesions are described as punched-out defects or moth-eaten holes. In addition, there is triad that exists in approximately 10% of the patients, consisting of bone lesions, diabetes insipidus, and exophthalmos. Invasion of the temporal bone occurs frequently and is often bilateral. Biopsy helps establish the diagnosis, showing sheets of polygonal histiocytes admixed with eosinophils, plasma cells, and lymphocytes as the characteristic microscopic finding in these lesions. This is considered to be a chronic disseminated form of Langerhans cell histiocytosis. Treatment includes medical therapy with vinblastine and corticosteroids. Despite treatment, the mortality rate approximates 30%.

Letterer-Siwe disease affects infants and manifests as hepatosplenomegaly, lymphadenopathy, bleeding diathesis, anemia, cutaneous lesions, and multiorgan dysfunction secondary to histiocyte proliferation and infiltration.

This is the acute disseminated form of Langerhans cell histiocytosis. The temporal bone may be involved, and patients may present with ear pain and/or otorrhea. Treatment consists of chemotherapeutic agents, but the disease is almost uniformly fatal in 1 to 2 years.

Sarcoma and Chordoma

Sarcomas of the lateral skull base are exceptionally rare neoplasms; however, in children, they are the most common primary malignancy of the temporal bone. Rhabdomyosarcoma is the most common of these neoplasms, accounting for 30% of sarcomatous temporal bone tumors and 4% to 7% of all temporal bone malignancies. Ninety percent of patients with rhabdomyosarcoma are less than 10 years of age, with the average age at presentation of 4.5 years. Pluripotential mesenchymal cells in the middle ear and eustachian tube give rise to this neoplasm. Most patients present with chronic otorrhea and otalgia that fails to respond to appropriate medical therapy. Otologic examination reveals a friable aural polyp, hemorrhagic aural discharge, and/or mastoid swelling. Facial weakness or paralysis is not uncommon early in the disease process and may indicate a malignant process. Regional lymph node metastases are unusual, but distant metastases to lungs, liver, brain, and bone are present in 14% of patients at the time of presentation. Rhabdomyosarcoma is divided into several histologic types: embryonal, botryoid, alveolar, and pleomorphic. The *embryonal type* is the most common. Microscopic features of embryonal rhabdomyosarcoma are small round and spindle-shaped primitive mesenchymal cells in a loose myxoid or compact pattern. Longitudinal or cross-striations characteristic of rhabdomyosarcoma may or may not be evident in the embryonal subtype. *Alveolar rhabdomyosarcoma*, which has a poorer prognosis, consists of sheets of round, oval, or strap-like cells arranged in a trabecular pattern surrounding empty alveolar compartments. *Pleomorphic rhabdomyosarcoma* is composed of anaplastic multinucleated spindle cells that form whorls and fascicles with longitudinal striations. Most *botryoid tumors* are histologically classified as embryonal, and the term botryoid refers to their gross appearance resembling a grape cluster. Radiologic imaging of the temporal bone shows a soft tissue in the middle ear and mastoid with surrounding bony destruction. With this type of clinical presentation, the diagnosis is confirmed with biopsy specimens. Attempts at radical surgical excision rarely offer survival advantage for this highly malignant neoplasm, and therefore, current treatment includes limited surgical intervention, external beam radiation therapy, and chemotherapy. Survival has improved with the use of contemporary adjuvant therapy, and 5-year failure-free survival exceeds 60% (32).

Chondrosarcoma of the skull base is thought to arise from persistent islands of embryonal cartilage rests that occur near cranial base synchondroses. Patients in nearly all age groups can be afflicted by this relatively low-grade sarcoma, but it is most common in young adults in their fourth and fifth decades of life. Males and females are affected equally. The petroclival region near foramen lacerum and the petrous apex is perhaps the most common location of origin. Patients present with headache and symptoms suggesting cranial nerve compromise such as diplopia, hoarseness, dysphagia, facial dysesthesia, and hearing loss. Cranial nerve examination often confirms the neurologic deficits in symptomatic patients. Histologic diagnosis of sarcoma can be difficult without clinical features or radiologic findings that suggest malignancy because benign cartilage shows varying patterns of cellularity and heterogeneity that may be interpreted as anaplastic. Like rhabdomyosarcoma, there are a number of histologic subtypes of chondrosarcoma, and prognosis varies depending on histologic subtype and grade of differentiation. Imaging studies show bony destruction of the skull base lateral to the midline (Fig. 147.7) and enhancement of the tumor mass when contrast is injected. Surgical excision is the primary therapeutic modality for chondrosarcoma, but complete excision is often not possible, and recurrences are common (33). Both radiation therapy and chemotherapy are of unproven benefit.

Ewing sarcoma, osteogenic sarcoma, and fibrosarcoma are rarely reported to occur in the temporal bone. *Ewing sarcoma* of the temporal bone is an aggressive but rare malignancy that occurs in patient less than 20 years old. Patients present with signs and symptoms much like those of other temporal bone sarcomas, and imaging studies show a well-circumscribed soft tissue lesion eroding into the surrounding bone. Ewing sarcoma is a cellular tumor that is readily diagnosed during microscopic examination of biopsy specimens. Because no more than 20 cases of

Ewing sarcoma of the temporal bone have been recorded in the world literature, the prognosis is uncertain. Limited experience, however, shows that metastatic disease does not occur, and favorable outcomes can be obtained with combined temporal bone resection, radiation therapy, and chemotherapy. *Osteogenic sarcoma* of the temporal bone is highly malignant but fortunately exceedingly rare. Most patients are between the ages of 10 and 30 years, and males are affected more often than females by a ratio of 3:2. Few cases of radiation-induced osteogenic sarcoma have been reported, but in most instances, there is no clear etiology. Patients present with rapidly progressive painful swelling in the periauricular area. Temporal bone resection along with radiation therapy and chemotherapy is advocated, but this disease appears to be uniformly fatal. *Fibrosarcoma* of the temporal bone can occur in infants, and nearly one-third of infants with this neoplasm present at birth. Lymph node metastases may occur in 10% of pediatric patients, but 5-year survival rates are above 80% after surgical treatment. The prognosis for adults is not as favorable. Regional lymph node metastases occur in 50%, and radiation-induced fibrosarcoma in adults is a lethal neoplasm (34).

Skull base chordomas are low- to intermediate-grade malignancies that result from defective embryonic remnants of the notochord. During embryonic development, the cranial aspect of the notochord begins in the sphenoid bone just posterior to the sella turcica. As the notochord is followed inferiorly, it exits the bone traveling along the clivus in the soft tissue adjacent to the nasopharyngeal mucosa and reenters the basiocciput skull base before coursing inferiorly into the odontoid process and vertebral bodies. The cranial aspect of the notochord gives rise to stalks that project into the subendothelial tissue of the nasopharynx and intracranially along the ventral aspect of the brainstem. Therefore, chordoma not only occurs in the clivus but also as a primary intracranial or nasopharyngeal soft tissue tumor. Patients of all age categories may have chordomas, but they are most likely to occur in males between the ages of 35 and 45 years. On gross examination, tumors are covered with a pseudocapsule and have a characteristic lobular configuration. They are gray and semitranslucent and contain gelatinous material. Chordomas are divided into histologic subtypes, but the main microscopic features are stellate, intermediate, and vacuolated physaliphorous or soap-bubble cells in a mucoid matrix growing in nests, cords, or trabeculae. Immunohistochemical staining is positive for cytokeratin and epithelial membrane antigen, which helps to distinguish chordoma from chondrosarcoma. Metastases are unusual, and most chordomas grow slowly and insidiously, eroding the skull base and compromising regional neurovascular structures. Headache, diplopia, and visual deficits are the most common presenting complaints, and physical examination usually reveals oculomotor function abnormalities, especially abducens nerve palsy. When chordoma originates or extends into the nasopharynx, patients can present with upper airway

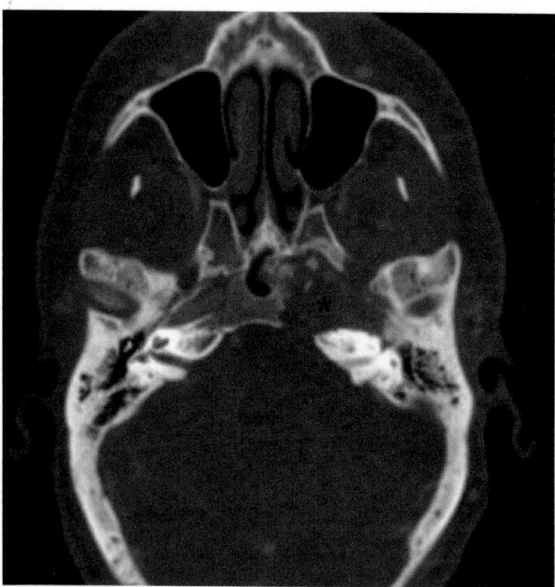

Figure 147.7 Chondrosarcoma. Axial CT showing an aggressive neoplasm eroding the left petrous apex and adjacent sphenoid bone (*asterisk*), centered at the petroclival synchondrosis.

obstruction and a nasopharyngeal mass. In many cases, the diagnosis can be obtained from imaging studies and cytologic evaluation of a transnasal fine-needle aspirate. CT images show bony erosion of the clivus or basiocciput in the midline instead of lateral erosion that is more characteristic of chondrosarcoma. The soft tissue component of the tumor is heterogeneous on MRI, usually demonstrating low signal intensity on T1-weighted images and high signal intensity on T2-weighted images. CT and MR images both show signal enhancement after injection of contrast material. The primary mode of therapy is surgical excision via transoral–transpalatal, transcondylar, or infratemporal fossa approach, but complete resection is often not feasible, and recurrence is common. Postoperative proton beam radiation therapy or stereotactic radiosurgery may improve survival and prolong disease-free intervals.

Dermoid, Teratoma, and Choristoma

Dermoids, teratomas, and choristomas are mass lesions that result from errors in fetal development. These tumors are distinguished on the basis of the embryologic germ layer from which they are derived. *Dermoids* of the temporal bone are cystic lesions derived from the ectoderm that are more correctly classified as congenital inclusions and not true neoplasms. When they occur in the middle ear, the mastoid, or the eustachian tube, they are thought to originate at a point where the first branchial cleft, the anlage of the external auditory canal, lies adjacent to the first branchial pouch, the anlage of the middle ear, and the eustachian tube. This location may be significant because it suggests that the histogenesis of dermoids is related to incomplete closure at the lines of fusion between branchial elements or to traumatic introduction of inappropriate germinal layers into the middle ear. However, dermoids may also occur in the petrous apex.

Dermoid cysts are pink or white pedunculated tumors. They have both ectodermal and mesodermal components. They are lined by keratinizing stratified squamous epithelium that contains hair follicles, sebaceous glands, smooth muscle, and adipose tissue. Most patients present as infants or children with hearing loss, otorrhea, dizziness, or upper airway obstruction, and examination reveals a middle ear mass that may extend through the eustachian tube and into the nasopharynx. The growth rate of these cysts is variable, but they eventually become symptomatic and require removal.

Teratomas of the temporal bone are extremely rare and differ significantly from dermoid cysts. They are considered to be true neoplasms that arise from pluripotential stem cells that originate near the notochord. These pluripotential cells may differentiate into types of tissue derived from any of the three embryonic germinal layers. The type of tissue into which they differentiate is generally not native to the site where they occur. Tumors are firm polypoid or cystic lesions that may contain stratified squamous

epithelium, respiratory and gastrointestinal endothelium, cartilage, skeletal muscle, glandular tissue, neural tissue, and, surprisingly, even mature teeth. Tumors are graded in relation to tissue differentiation. Malignant undifferentiated forms exist, but they have never been reported in the temporal bone. Patients present at birth or in early childhood, often with large rapidly growing tumors, and their symptoms include facial paralysis, hearing loss, and airway obstruction. Imaging studies show a heterogeneous tumor that may contain calcifications. Teratomas can be cured with complete resection, but this may require radical transtemporal or infratemporal fossa approaches to achieve adequate surgical exposure for curative resection.

Choristoma is a term that is used to describe normal tissue that occurs in a nonnative location. When choristoma occurs in the middle ear, this generally refers to salivary tissue, although sebaceous glands and neural tissue have been reported. Choristomas are probably derived from rests of salivary tissue trapped in the middle ear during development. These rests mature into small masses but have no neoplastic potential. Choristomas are pink or tan lobular masses located lateral to the long process of the incus and medial to the manubrium, and some have been associated with anomalies of the ossicles or the intratemporal portion of the facial nerve. Histologic examination reveals mature ectopic salivary gland tissue. Patients may have conductive hearing loss, but most are asymptomatic. They usually present with a middle ear mass that was incidentally discovered during routine otoscopic examination. Choristomas have little if any growth potential and only require incisional or excisional biopsy to confirm diagnosis.

Cholesterol Granuloma

Cholesterol granuloma of the petrous apex is not a true neoplasm but rather a mass lesion that results from a reactive process within the temporal bone. It can be diagnosed from imaging studies and should be included in the differential diagnosis when evaluating temporal bone masses. Cholesterol granuloma was first described more than 100 years ago as dark blue discoloration of the tympanic membrane and was called an "idiopathic hematotympanum." This condition occurred in patients with eustachian tube dysfunction and was often accompanied by chronic otitis media or cholesteatoma. It was hypothesized that cholesterol granuloma occurs as a consequence of four factors: interference with drainage of the middle ear, hemorrhage, obstruction of ventilation, and foreign body reaction to cholesterol crystals derived from hemoglobin catabolism. Evidence in support of this hypothesis has been provided by animal experiments. Cholesterol granuloma can be produced by injecting cholesterol into the middle ear or by occluding the eustachian tube (35). Cholesterol granuloma of the petrous apex, whereas not necessarily associated with otitis media or cholesteatoma, probably results from a similar pathophysiologic process. It is found in pneumatized petrous bones that occur in 30% of patients. The process starts when ventilation of petrous air cells is disrupted secondary to temporal bone trauma, eustachian tube dysfunction, or mucosal edema. Inflammation or trauma of the petrous bone may cause hemorrhage into the air cells of the petrous apex, and because there is no effective drainage pathway, detritus from the hemorrhage accumulates in the air cells. The membranes of degenerating red blood cells appear to be the primary source of cholesterol crystals, which subsequently initiate a foreign body reaction. Inflammation from the foreign body reaction increases hemorrhage and mucosal edema, promoting the inflammatory cycle and allowing the granuloma to enlarge. An alternative theory for cholesterol granuloma pathogenesis proposes these lesions result when expanding air cell tracts lined with mucosa interface with marrow spaces in the petrous apex. Coaptation between the mucosal lining and the exposed marrow results in a progressive sustained hemorrhage from the marrow spaces, and this leads to cyst formation and expansion (36). It is not surprising that histologic examination of cholesterol granuloma shows cholesterol crystals surrounded by multinucleated giant cells, round cell infiltration, and hemosiderin-laden macrophages. Cholesterol granuloma may be confined to the petrous bone and may be asymptomatic. Alternatively, it may extend into the posterior cranial fossa and cause an abducens nerve palsy, diplopia, facial pain, facial weakness or twitching, headache, dizziness, tinnitus, and hearing loss. The diagnosis of cholesterol granuloma may be made by MRI, which shows a smooth-walled, nonenhancing, expansive lesion that has high signal intensity on both T1-weighted and T2-weighted images (Fig. 147.8). The

mainstay of surgical therapy is simple drainage, allowing permanent aeration of the cavity. However, some controversy exists about whether the fibrous wall of the cyst requires removal to achieve long-term cure.

NEOPLASMS OF THE INTERNAL AUDITORY CANAL AND CEREBELLOPONTINE ANGLE

Schwannoma

Schwannomas of the temporal bone and the skull base are benign neoplasms that arise from the sheaths of cranial nerves. Available evidence suggests that these tumors arise from Schwann cells alone and not other nerve components. Therefore, terms such as acoustic neuroma are not appropriate. The etiology of schwannoma is unclear, but it has been suggested that neoplastic growth occurs preferentially at the junction between the central and peripheral components of the cranial nerves. Myelin is formed by oligodendrocytes in the intracranial portion of a cranial nerve, and as the nerve enters the skull base, there is a transition to a Schwann cell sheath. This transition occurs in a region called the Obersteiner-Redlich zone, and this zone is variable in location in different cranial nerves. It has also been proposed that schwannomas may arise in locations with the greatest concentration of Schwann cells. For vestibular schwannomas, this would be Scarpa ganglion, whereas for jugular foramen schwannomas, this would be the superior and inferior ganglia of the glossopharyngeal nerve, the jugular and nodose ganglia of the vagus nerve, or the junction of cranial and spinal components of the spinal accessory

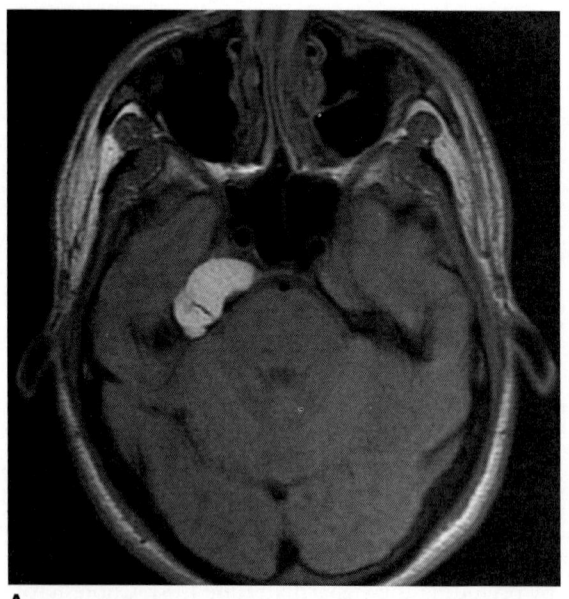
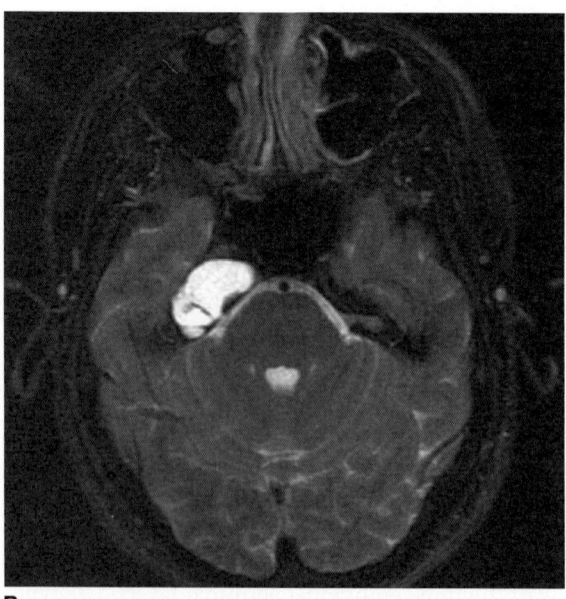

A   **B**

Figure 147.8 Cholesterol granuloma. **A:** Axial T1-weighted MRI without contrast. **B:** Axial T2-weighted MRI. These images show an expansile right petrous apex lesion with increased signal intensity on both T1- and T2-weighted images.

nerve. What causes the proliferation of Schwann cells is not known, but genetic aberrations, such as those associated with neurofibromatosis type 2 (NF2), are likely associated with this neoplastic transformation. Schwannomas in NF2 patients appear to be the result of a defect on the long arm of chromosome 22, which is responsible for the production of a tumor suppressor protein called merlin. Exactly what this protein does to inhibit Schwann cell proliferation is uncertain, but merlin interacts with many cellular proteins that regulate cell function (37). One such group of cellular proteins includes tyrosine kinase growth factor receptors, specifically a family called ErbB. NF2 is an autosomal dominant disorder, and patients may have a functioning copy of the tumor suppressor gene on their intact chromosome. However, production of merlin is terminated when a mutation occurs on the intact chromosome 22, and merlin depletion results in deregulation of ErbB receptors, which may be the event that causes NF2 patients to develop schwannomas. For the same sequence of events to occur in a patient without NF2, mutations must occur on the long arm of both chromosomes. Thus, neoplastic transformation in cases of sporadic schwannoma is a much less likely event. Other factors that may lead to neoplastic transformation of Schwann cells are under investigation. Increased genetic expression of neurotrophic factors such as brain-derived neurotrophic factor has also been observed in vestibular schwannomas when compared to peripheral nerve tissue suggesting a role in the modulation of tumor growth (38). Additionally, small RNA molecules called microRNA can regulate gene expression by inhibiting production of certain target proteins. When comparing vestibular schwannoma cells with vestibular nerve tissue, microRNA is overexpressed, which can lead to downregulation of tumor suppressor pathways (39). Genetic research looking at these pathways and others continues, but it appears likely that schwannoma growth is the result of demodulation of Schwann cell proliferation resulting in tumorigenesis.

Schwannomas of the temporal bone can be categorized as vestibular, facial, trigeminal, and jugular foramen tumors. Vestibular schwannomas are by far the most common, comprising approximately 10% of all intracranial tumors and 80% of cerebellopontine angle tumors. They occur in about 1 of 100,000 patients per year. Because they usually arise in the vicinity of the vestibular ganglion, most vestibular schwannomas begin inside the internal auditory canal. Isolated intralabyrinthine schwannomas do occur, as do cochlear schwannomas, but they are extremely rare. Vestibular schwannomas expand centrally from the internal auditory canal into the cerebellopontine angle and may compress the pontine brainstem and the cerebellum. Therefore, the most common symptoms with which patients present are unilateral hearing loss, tinnitus, and dysequilibrium. Vestibular schwannomas may also extend anteriorly within the cerebellopontine angle, compressing the trigeminal nerve and causing facial hypesthesia or paresthesia, but neuralgia is infrequent. Large tumors will eventually result in hydrocephalus with headache, visual impairment, and alterations of mental status if the tumor is left untreated.

Facial nerve schwannomas differ from vestibular schwannomas in that they can arise anywhere along the nerve from the oligodendrocyte–Schwann cell junction to the most distal aspect of the extratemporal facial nerve. Most commonly, however, they arise from the perigeniculate, tympanic, or mastoid segments of the nerve. Multiple nerve segments are usually involved by the time these lesions are diagnosed. Facial weakness or paralysis that progresses gradually over weeks or months is the most common presentation. Twenty percent of patients with facial nerve schwannoma may present with acute facial paralysis suggesting Bell palsy. Conductive hearing loss, tinnitus, or otalgia occur when neoplasms extend into the middle ear.

Trigeminal schwannomas are rare lesions that usually originate from the gasserian ganglion and may expand into posterior and/or middle cranial fossae. Patients present with facial neuralgia, paresthesia, or hypesthesia in one or more divisions of the trigeminal nerve. Retroorbital pain may be another complaint. When motor function is affected, patients describe difficulty when chewing.

Jugular foramen schwannomas arise within the jugular fossa from the sheaths of cranial nerves IX, X, and XI. Because they grow vertically along the path of least resistance, intracranial and extracranial extension of the tumor is variable. Vagus nerve origin seems most frequent, followed by glossopharyngeal origin, but it is often difficult to identify the nerve from which the tumor is derived. Patients present with dysphagia, hoarseness, or shoulder weakness. If there is significant intracranial extension, patients may note hearing loss, tinnitus, imbalance, or headache.

On gross and microscopic examination, all temporal bone schwannomas are generally the same. They are tan, yellow, or pale gray rubbery masses with varying amounts of surface vascularity. As they enlarge, schwannomas displace adjacent soft tissue structures and may become tightly adherent to these structures. They appear to have a fibrous capsule, but histologic examination shows that the capsule may be so thin that tumor cells oppose surrounding tissue directly. Tumor cells are spindle shaped and are arranged in both Antoni type A and type B patterns (Fig. 147.9). The type A pattern consists of densely packed spindle cells with aligned or palisading nuclei, termed Verocay bodies. The type B pattern, on the other hand, is characterized by spindle cells that are loosely arranged in a myxoid stroma. Cystic degeneration, necrosis, and hemorrhage are often noted, especially in larger tumors. Nuclear pleomorphism and hypercellularity might appear consistent with malignancy, but malignant degeneration of schwannomas is highly unusual.

Radiographic imaging studies may provide the diagnosis, but physical examination reveals functional deficits caused by the tumor. Otologic exam is generally normal unless a facial nerve schwannoma presents as a retrotympanic

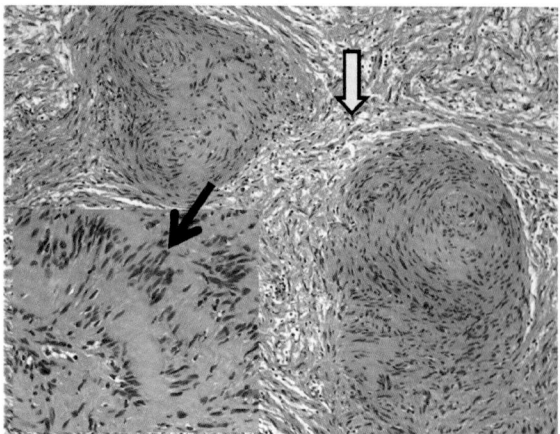

Figure 147.9 Schwannoma: Histologic section showing delicate, tightly organized wavy nuclear palisades known as Verocay bodies within the hypercellular or Antoni A regions (*solid arrow*). The characteristic pale, eosinophilic cytoplasm is more apparent in relatively hypocellular Antoni B regions (*hollow arrow*).

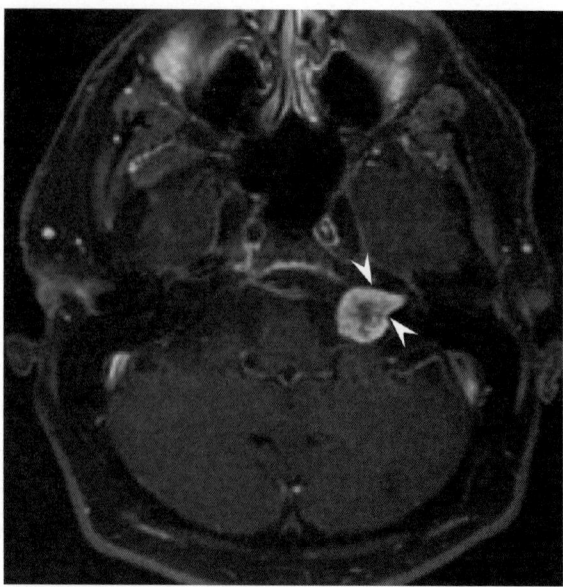

Figure 147.10 Vestibular schwannoma. Axial T1-weighed MRI with contrast enhancement showing a left-side internal auditory canal lesion that expands medially into the cerebellopontine angle. Note the expansion of the porus acusticus (*arrowheads*).

mass. In patients with cervical extension of jugular fossa schwannomas, head and neck examination may show an anterosuperior neck mass, sternocleidomastoid muscle weakness, or bulge of the lateral pharyngeal wall, suggesting a mass in the parapharyngeal space. Cranial nerve examination showing palatal weakness and vocal cord paralysis is also indicative of a jugular fossa lesion. When decreased corneal reflexes, facial hypesthesia, and masseter muscle weakness are apparent, trigeminal schwannoma or other cerebellopontine schwannomas that compress the trigeminal nerve may be the cause. Facial nerve dysfunction suggests facial nerve schwannoma rather than vestibular schwannoma, but audiometric evaluation helps to differentiate the two lesions. Sensorineural hearing loss is more common in patients with vestibular schwannoma, whereas conductive hearing loss is more common in patients with facial nerve schwannoma. The preliminary diagnosis of schwannoma is made when the deficits discovered on physical exam correlate with findings from imaging studies. MRI shows a lesion with low signal intensity on T1-weighted images that enhances during injection with intravenous contrast (Fig. 147.10). HRCT of the temporal bone shows expansion or erosion of the fallopian canal and extension into the middle ear in patients with facial nerve schwannomas. HRCT also helps to define skull base anatomy preoperatively in patients with jugular foramen schwannomas.

Details regarding the management of temporal bone schwannomas are beyond the scope of this chapter. Suffice it to say that patients generally have three therapeutic options: surgical excision, stereotactic radiation therapy, or observation. Complete surgical excision is the only curative therapy available at this time. The major disadvantage is morbidity associated with cranial nerve injury, cerebrospinal fluid leak, and central nervous system damage. Advanced technology for treating patients with schwannomas using stereotactic radiosurgery has now been available

for more than 20 years. Long-term follow-up in patients treated marginal radiation dosages of 12 to 13 Gy using highly accurate tumor targeting technology shows that complications can be minimized while tumor growth is controlled in approximately 95% (40,41). It is generally not recommended for patients with tumors greater than 3 cm in diameter or in patients who are symptomatic with significant brainstem compression. Observation as a management option is based on data suggesting that more than 60% of vestibular schwannomas, especially sporadic and intracanalicular tumors, grow very slowly, remain stable in size, or involute during an average of 4 years of follow-up (42). All three therapeutic options play a role in the management of patients with temporal bone schwannomas.

Meningioma

Meningiomas are neoplasms that arise from the arachnoid layer of the meninges. More specifically, temporal bone meningiomas arise from arachnoid cell granulations that cluster at the tips of arachnoid villi inside dural venous sinuses and at foramina, such as the internal auditory canal, the jugular fossa, the geniculate ganglion, and the bony sulci near the greater and lesser superficial petrosal nerves. Meningiomas are common neoplasms and constitute between 13% and 20% of all intracranial tumors and approximately 10% of all cerebellopontine angle tumors. The incidence of meningioma increases with age, with the highest incidence rate (40 per 100,000) in individuals older than 65 years. Children and even infants can have meningiomas, but fortunately this is rare. In children, boys are affected as often as girls, and their tumors are generally more aggressive, growing rapidly and becoming relatively large before they are diagnosed. In adults, women with meningioma outnumber men by at least 2 to 1, especially in the older age groups. The most frequent location for meningioma of the lateral skull base is on the posterior aspect of the petrous bone between the superior and inferior petrosal sinuses. Less commonly, meningioma presents as a tumor that is confined to the internal auditory canal, and in rare cases, meningioma presents as an extracranial neoplasm in the middle ear, the external auditory canal, or the infratemporal fossa.

The etiology of meningioma is the subject of controversy. The relationship between severe head injuries and subsequent development of meningioma a number of years later was first suggested by Cushing in the 1920s when he observed that meningiomas occur directly beneath a previous skull fracture. In most patients, however, there was no history of trauma, or the injury may have occurred at a site distant from the tumor. Subsequent epidemiologic studies have failed to show a causal relationship between trauma and the occurrence of meningioma. Genetic factors have some role in the pathogenesis of meningioma because inherited tumors occur in patients with NF2. In fact, aberrations involving chromosome 22 occur in almost 50% of patients with sporadic meningiomas, and abnormalities have also been identified on chromosomes 1 and 14 (43). Radiation exposure seems to be clearly linked to the occurrence of meningioma. The most convincing evidence of this is the discovery that children who were treated with low-dose radiation for tinea capitis in the 1950s were almost 10 times more likely to develop meningioma. As the radiation dose increases, the risk of developing a tumor seems to rise. Hormonal stimulation, specifically from progesterone and possibly from estrogen, is thought to have a role in the genesis and progression of meningioma. This has been suggested because meningioma is more common in women, there are estrogen and progesterone receptors in meningioma, meningiomas seem to change size during pregnancy and during the menstrual cycle, and there may be a link between meningioma and breast cancer, which also has estrogen and progesterone receptors. The details relating estrogen or progesterone release and meningioma growth are unclear, but such an association could have consequences related to prevention, detection, and treatment of this tumor.

Meningiomas are well-circumscribed, firm, rubbery, nodular masses that invade dural lining, dural sinuses, and neurovascular channels. One-fourth of these tumors are flat, so-called en plaque tumors, that invade adjacent bone and incite an osteoblastic reaction referred to as hyperostosis. Most meningiomas are benign, but approximately 5% have malignant characteristics. These tumors show anaplastic histologic features and may invade the adjacent brain. Metastatic disease is highly unusual. The clinical presentation of meningioma is variable and depends on where the tumor is located within the temporal bone or skull base.

Meningioma of the internal auditory canal is difficult to distinguish from vestibular schwannoma, which is more common. Both neoplasms present with unilateral sensorineural hearing loss and tinnitus, but auditory complaints occur more frequently in patients with vestibular schwannoma. Conversely, meningioma is more likely to cause facial twitching, weakness, or paralysis. Meningioma that originates on the posterior petrous face expands into the posterior cranial fossa, compressing the cerebellum and brainstem. These patients present with imbalance or vertigo and difficulty with fine motor movements. When these tumors become very large, they may cause hydrocephalus and elevated intracranial pressure resulting in headaches, nausea, vomiting, lethargy, and somnolence. Petrous apex lesions may extend onto the clivus, into the cavernous sinus, or through Meckel cave and into the middle cranial fossa. Extensive tumors in these locations can cause trigeminal neuralgia, facial hypesthesia, visual disturbance, and headache. Jugular fossa meningiomas may cause dysphonia, aspiration, and dysphagia, whereas physical examination shows palatal weakness, pooling of hypopharyngeal secretions, and vocal cord paresis. Geniculate ganglion and petrosal nerve tumors result in facial weakness or paralysis, and conductive hearing loss may occur when tumor extends to fill the middle ear.

The diagnosis is based on histopathologic findings and imaging characteristics that are consistent with meningioma. Histologic features that mark meningioma include polygonal- and spindle-shaped cells arranged in nests, vascular spaces, and psammoma bodies, which are spherical concretions consisting of calcium salts (Fig. 147.11). However, the microscopic appearance of meningioma is highly variable. Consequently, meningiomas are classified as endotheliomatous, fibrous, transitional, angiomatous, and sarcomatous depending on predominant cell shape, stromal content, tumor vascularity, and nuclear

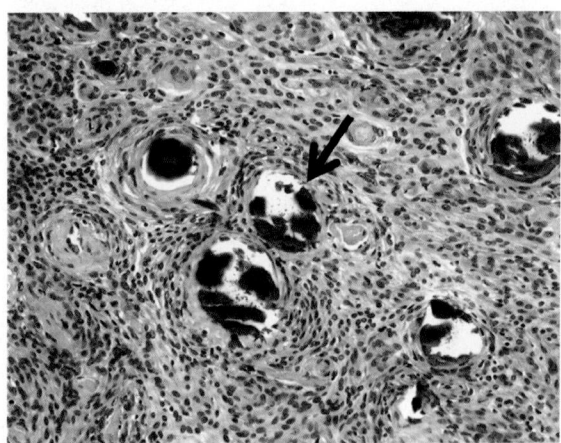

Figure 147.11 Meningioma: Histologic section demonstrating laminated calcific spheres known as psammoma bodies (*arrow*). The presence of numerous psammoma bodies indicates slow growth and a relatively favorable prognosis.

anaplasia. Further, the World Health Organization classifies meningiomas based on histologic characteristics, cellular atypia, and evidence of brain invasion. Both methods to classify meningiomas may provide prognostic information. In many cases, imaging characteristics on CT and MRI are diagnostic. Meningiomas are hyperdense or isodense compared with surrounding brain on CT images, and they exhibit homogeneous enhancement after contrast injection. Calcification within the tumor or associated hyperostosis supports the diagnosis of meningioma. Vestibular schwannomas are, on the other hand, isodense or hypodense to brain, and they exhibit inhomogeneous enhancement and lack of calcification or hyperostosis. MR images reveal the broad-based eccentric nature of meningioma and may sometimes show obvious dural or dural sinus origin (Fig. 147.12). MRI of vestibular schwannoma is more likely to show erosion of the internal auditory canal where the tumor originates and pronounced enhancement with injection of intravenous contrast. Intracanalicular lesions are difficult to distinguish on any imaging study.

Meningioma of the skull base and temporal bone can be observed with serial imaging, surgically resected, treated with radiation, or treated with a combination of subtotal resection and postoperative SRS or IMRT. Complete surgical removal is the only curative treatment available at this time. Resection is recommended for most patients with accessible tumors, especially if the patient has symptoms and there are no medical contraindications to surgery. Under ideal conditions, a Simpson grade

I resection is achieved when tumor is removed with a wide margin of meninges and adjacent. Less complete resections, Simpson grades II to VI, are associated with higher recurrence rates. Preoperative angiography helps to identify the major feeding vessels of the tumor and may be combined with embolization to reduce operative blood loss. Despite efforts at total resection, recurrence rates for meningioma are relatively high. Even with a Simpson grade I resection, meningiomas recur in almost 10% of patients. The most important features to consider when estimating the probability of surgical cure are tumor location, which may allow complete resection, and lack of malignant characteristics. For patients who are not candidates for surgery, who have residual disease after surgery, who have recurrent or unresectable disease, who have meningiomas that show malignant characteristics, or who elect for nonsurgical therapy, radiation therapy should be considered. Recent clinical studies examining the efficacy of radiosurgical treatment of skull base meningiomas are encouraging. Long-term follow-up data, excluding atypical and malignant schwannomas, show local tumor control in more than 85% of patients (44). Local control in radiosurgery patients may be better when meningiomas are treated with radiosurgery alone compared to patients treated with radiosurgery postoperatively. Current research focuses on hormonal treatment, targeted chemotherapy, gene therapy using adenovirus vectors, and other forms of medical therapy that might help to arrest tumor growth and prevent recurrences.

Lipoma

Lipomas of the internal auditory canal and the cerebellopontine angle are rare but potentially problematic tumors that may originate from the aberrant differentiation of neural crest cells into adipocytes. Bigelow et al. (45) provide the most comprehensive review of this subject in their multiinstitutional study and review of the world literature. They recorded 84 documented cases of lipoma of the internal auditory canal and cerebellopontine angle and studied the clinical findings in each case. Patients ranged in age from 7 months to 82 years with an average age of 40 years. Tumors predominated in males by a ratio of 2:1. Lipomas measured from 1 to 26 mm in diameter with a mean of 11 mm. Three patients presented with bilateral tumors. Ninety-two percent of patients were symptomatic. They most often presented with hearing loss, dizziness, tinnitus, and headache. Lipomas are fatty masses that may envelop the neurovascular structures of the internal auditory canal and cerebellopontine angle. Large lipomas may be adherent to the lateral aspect of the brainstem. Some lipomas have highly vascularized outer surfaces and are more accurately classified as angiolipomas. Biopsy specimens show benign mature adipocytes and varying amounts of fibrous tissue. Lipomas may infiltrate cranial nerves and surround component fascicles of nerve fibers.

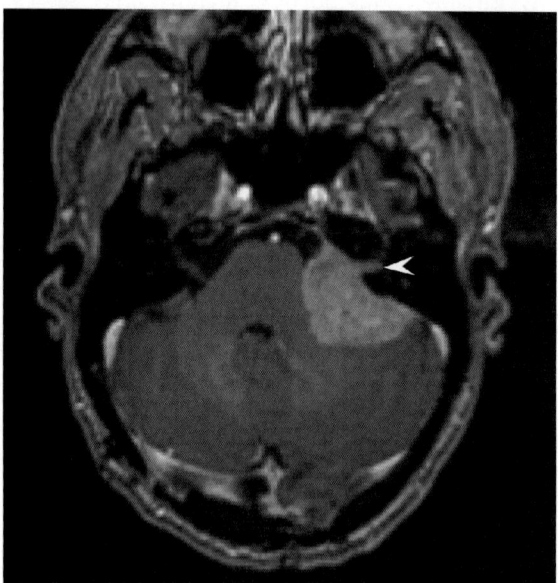

Figure 147.12 Meningioma. Axial T1-weighted image with contrast showing a left-sided tumor with its wide dural base on the posterior petrous face. There is enhancing tumor that extends laterally into the internal auditory canal (*arrowhead*), which usually indicates schwannoma, but can sometimes be seen with meningioma.

Lipomas have unique imaging characteristics. Therefore, a definitive diagnosis can be obtained from an MRI. On MRI, lipomas are similar to subcutaneous fat with high signal intensity on T1-weighted images and diminished signal intensity on T2-weighted images. T1-weighted images do not enhance with injection of intravenous contrast because the tumor signal is near saturation. MRI with fat suppression further confirms the diagnosis. Follow-up for most patients with unresected tumors has been short, and thus, the rate of growth of lipoma, thought to be very slow, is unknown. The only documented instance of the growth of a lipoma involves a patient with a 2-cm tumor that was biopsied but not removed. The tumor enlarged 15% over an 8-year period. Review of surgical outcomes shows that complete tumor resection is possible in only one-third of patients and 68% suffer postoperative neurologic deficits. Forty-three percent of postoperative patients have improvements in symptoms, but only 19% have improvement with no new neurologic deficits. From this experience, it is clear that expectant management is advisable in most cases. Surgical therapy should be reserved for patients with progressive or disabling symptoms.

METASTATIC DISEASE OF THE TEMPORAL BONE AND LATERAL SKULL BASE

Temporal bone metastases resulting from distant malignancies are an infrequent but not insignificant occurrence. In the largest series of patients with temporal bone metastases studied to date, 47 metastases to the temporal bone were documented at autopsy in a population of 212 individuals with primary nondisseminated malignant neoplasms (46). The most common sites of origin of temporal bone metastases in order of decreasing frequency are breast, lung, kidney, gastrointestinal tract, larynx, prostate gland, and thyroid gland. The incidence of bilateral involvement may exceed 50%. Metastatic involvement of the temporal bone may occur as the first evidence of distant malignant disease, first presenting as hearing loss and later as facial paralysis or dysequilibrium. There is usually a conductive hearing loss that may be accompanied by pain. More frequently, temporal bone involvement is occult and occurs late in the course of disease. Tumor cells may accumulate preferentially in area of bone with sluggish blood flow, including the marrow and aerated regions. Areas of the temporal bone that show a predilection for metastatic disease include the petrous apex, the mastoid, and the internal auditory canal. The bony labyrinth appears to resist neoplastic invasion because inner ear involvement is uncommon.

Metastatic disease should be considered as a possible cause of hearing loss in a patient with a clinical history of malignant neoplasm, especially in patients with rapidly growing temporal bone lesions associated with progressive neurological symptoms.

HIGHLIGHTS

- Paragangliomas of the temporal bone arise from nonchromaffin paraganglia, or glomus bodies, which originate from the neuroendocrine system. Glomus jugulare tumors arise within the jugular fossa, and glomus tympanicum tumors arise along the course of the tympanic branch of cranial nerve IX (Jacobson nerve) and along the course of the auricular branch of cranial nerve X (Arnold nerve).

- Temporal bone and cerebellopontine angle epidermoids are aberrant collections of keratin debris within a sac of squamous epithelium. They result from entrapment of ectodermal rests during embryogenesis and therefore are categorized as congenital lesions. Epidermoids expand to fill empty spaces and incite a localized inflammatory reaction. Thus, they are usually large and very adherent to surrounding structures by the time they are treated with surgery.

- Patients with cutaneous carcinomas of the external auditory canal may present with symptoms similar to those of patients with chronic otitis externa. Chronic bloody drainage and sudden onset of deep ear pain are indicators of a possible malignancy and indicate the need for biopsy.

- Melanoma accounts for more than 75% of deaths from cutaneous malignancies. Excisional biopsy for early diagnosis is the key first step to optimize therapeutic outcomes. Sentinel node mapping using lymphoscintigraphy is the primary method of identifying nodal drainage patterns for these neoplasms, and high-dose interferon-alpha-2b may benefit patients with high-risk disease.

- Aggressive papillary tumors of the middle ear appear to be derived from the pars rugosa portion of the endolymphatic sac. They are slow growing but aggressive tumors that erode and spread extensively throughout the temporal bone and often recur after surgical treatment. Endolymphatic sac tumors occur in more than 10% of patients with von Hippel-Lindau disease, and therefore, these patients require screening.

- Embryonal rhabdomyosarcoma accounts for 30% of sarcomatous temporal bone neoplasms and is the most common sarcoma of this region. It is derived from pluripotential mesenchymal cells that differentiate into primitive skeletal muscle cells. Most patients are less than 12 years old and present with hemorrhagic aural drainage, a friable aural polyp, mastoid swelling, and facial nerve dysfunction. Current therapy includes limited surgical intervention, external beam radiation therapy, and chemotherapy.

- Chordomas result from defective embryonic remnants of the notochord. They are semitranslucent neoplasms that contain gelatinous material and are histologically characterized by clusters of physaliphorous (soap-bubble) cells in a mucoid matrix. Most chordomas occur in the clivus, but some originate or extend laterally into the petrous apex.

- Schwannomas of the lateral skull base are neoplasms that arise from Schwann cells at the transition zone between central myelin-producing oligodendrocytes and peripheral myelin-producing Schwann cells. What initiates the growth of these neoplasms is unknown, but aberrations or mutations on the long arm of chromosome 22, such as those that occur in NF2, reduce or eliminate merlin production, and this leads to demodulation of ErbB receptors in Schwann cells.

- Microscopic examination of schwannomas is characterized by spindle-shaped cells arranged in Antoni type A and type B patterns. The type A pattern consists of densely packed cells with palisading nuclei, termed Verocay bodies. The type B pattern consists of loosely arranged spindle cells in a myxoid stroma.

- Meningiomas are neoplasms that arise from the arachnoid layer of the meninges. Imaging studies of cerebellopontine angle meningiomas show homogeneous enhancement of a broad-based eccentric neoplasm that may contain speckled calcifications and may initiate a local hyperostotic reaction. Vestibular schwannomas, conversely, often exhibit heterogeneous enhancement and are "mushroom shaped," showing internal auditory canal origin and erosion.

REFERENCES

1. Chapman DB, Lippert D, Geer CP, et al. Clinical, histopathologic, and radiographic indicators of malignancy in head and neck paragangliomas. *Otolaryngol Head Neck Surg* 2010;143(4): 531–537.
2. Heth J. The basic science of glomus jugulare tumors. *Neurosurg Focus* 2004;17(2):E2.
3. Fish JH, Klein-Weigel P, Biebl M, et al. Systematic screening and treatment evaluation of hereditary neck paragangliomas. *Head Neck* 2007;29(9):864–873.
4. Martin TPC, Irving RM, Maher ER. The genetics of paragangliomas: a review. *Clin Otolaryngol* 2007;32(1):7–11.
5. Christie A, Teasdale E. A comparative review of multidetector CT angiography and MRI in the diagnosis of jugular foramen lesions. *Clin Radiol* 2010;65(3):213–217.
6. Koopmans KP, Jager PL, Kema IP, et al. ^{111}In-octreotide is superior to ^{123}I-metaiodobenzylguanidine for scintigraphic detection of head and neck paragangliomas. *J Nucl Med* 2008;49(8): 1232–1237.
7. Suarez C, Sevilla MA, Llorente JL. Temporal paragangliomas. *Eur Arch Otorhinolaryngol* 2007;264:719–731.
8. Ivan ME, Sughrue ME, Clark AJ, et al. A meta-analysis of tumor control rates and treatment-related morbidity in patients with glomus jugulare tumors. *J Neurosurg* 2011;114(5):1299–1305.
9. Richter GT, Lee KH. Contemporary assessment and management of congenital cholesteatoma. *Curr Opin Otolaryngol Head Neck Surg* 2009;17(5):339–345.
10. Liang J, Michaels L, Wright A. Immunohistochemical characterization of the epidermoid formation in the middle ear. *Laryngoscope* 2003;113(6):1007–1014.
11. Akar Z, Tangriover N, et al. Surgical treatment of intracranial epidermoid tumors. *Neurol Med Chir (Tokyo)* 2003;43:275–281.
12. Semann MT, Slattery WH, Brackmann DE. Geniculate ganglion hemangiomas: clinical results and long-term follow-up. *Otol Neurotol* 2010;31:665–670.
13. Shaia WT, Bojrab DI, Babu S, et al. Lipomatous hemangiopericytoma of the skull base and parapharyngeal space. *Otol Neurotol* 2006;27(4):560–563.
14. Ogawa S, Tawara I, Ueno S, et al. De novo CD5-positive diffuse large B-cell lymphoma of the temporal bone presenting with an external auditory canal tumor. *Intern Med* 2006;45(11): 733–737.
15. Markou K, Karasmanis I, Goudakos JK, et al. Extramedullary plasmacytoma of temporal bone: report of 2 cases and review of literature. *Am J Otolaryngol* 2009;30(5):360–365.
16. Chang KH, Dong-Kee K, Beom-Cho J, et al. Temporal bone myeloid sarcoma. *Clin Exp Otorhinolaryngol* 2009;2(4):198–202.
17. Marioni G, Altavilla G, Busatto G, et al. Detection of human papillomavirus in temporal bone inverted papilloma by polymerase chain reaction. *Acta Otolaryngol* 2003;123:367–371.
18. Moody SA, Hirsch BE, Myers EN. Squamous cell carcinoma of the external auditory canal: an evaluation of a staging system. *Am J Otol* 2000;21:582–588.
19. Chu A, Osguthorpe JD. Nonmelanoma cutaneous malignancy with regional metastasis. *Otolaryngol Head Neck Surg* 2003;128:663–673.
20. Cochran AJ, Ohsie SJ, Binder SW. Pathobiology of the sentinel node. *Curr Opin Oncol* 2008;20:190–195.
21. Shpitzer T, Gutman H, Barnea Y, et al. Sentinel node-guided evaluation of drainage patterns for melanoma of the helix of the ear. *Melanoma Res* 2007;17(6):365–369.
22. Phan GQ, Messina JL, Sondak VK, et al. Sentinel lymph node biopsy for melanoma: indications and rationale. *Cancer Control* 2009;16(3):234–239.
23. Ravin AG, Pickett N, Johnson JL, et al. Melanoma of the ear: treatment and survival probabilities based on 199 patients. *Ann Plast Surg* 2006;57(1):70–76.
24. Verma S, Quirt I, McCready D, et al. Systematic review of systemic adjuvant therapy for patients at high risk for recurrent melanoma. *Cancer* 2006;106(7):1431–1442.
25. Dong F, Gidley PW, Ho T, et al. Adenoid cystic carcinoma of the external auditory canal. *Laryngoscope* 2008;118:1591–1596.
26. Poulsen M. Merkel-cell carcinoma of the skin. *Lancet Oncol* 2004;5:593–599.
27. Wang S, Yee H, Wen HY, et al. Papillomas of the external ear canal: report of ten cases in Chinese patients with HPV in situ hybridization. *Head Neck Pathol* 2009;3:207–211.
28. Heffner D. Low-grade adenocarcinoma of probable endolymphatic sac origin: a clinicopathologic study of 20 cases. *Cancer* 1989;64:2292–2302.
29. Eby T, Makek M, Fisch U. Adenomas of the temporal bone. *Ann Otol Rhinol Laryngol* 1988;97:605–612.
30. Choo D, Shotland L, Mastroianni M, et al. Endolymphatic sac tumors in von Hippel-Lindau disease. *J Neurosurg* 2004;100: 480–487.
31. Lonser RR, Kim HJ, Butman JA, et al. Tumors of the endolymphatic sac in von Hippel-Lindau disease. *N Engl J Med* 2004;350:2481–2486.
32. Sbeity S, Abella A, Arcand P, et al. Temporal bone rhabdomyosarcoma in children. *Int J Pediatr Otorhinolaryngol* 2007;71: 807–814.
33. Lustig LR, Sciubba J, Holliday MJ. Chondrosarcoma of the skull base and temporal bone. *J Laryngol Otol* 2007;121:725–735.
34. Daw NC, Mahmoud HH, Meyer WH, et al. Bone sarcomas of the head and neck in children: the St. Jude Children's Research Hospital experience. *Cancer* 2000;88:2172–2180.
35. Main T, Shimada T, Lim D. Experimental cholesterol granuloma. *Arch Otolaryngol* 1970;91:356–359.

36. Jackler RK, Cho M. A new theory to explain the genesis of petrous apex cholesterol granuloma. *Otol Neurotol* 2003;24:96–106.
37. Ahmad Z, Brown CM, Patel AK, et al. Merlin knockdown in human Schwann cells: clues to vestibular schwannoma tumorigenesis. *Otol Neurotol* 2010;31:460–466.
38. Kramer F, Stover T, Warnecke A, et al. BDNF mRNA expression is significantly upregulated in vestibular schwannomas and correlates with proliferative activity. *J Neurooncol* 2010;98:31–39.
39. Cioffi JA, Yue WY, Mendolia-Loffredo S, et al. MicroRNA-21 overexpression contributes to vestibular schwannoma cell proliferation and survival. *Otol Neurotol* 2010;31:1455–1462.
40. Murphy ES, Suh JH. Radiotherapy for vestibular schwannomas: a critical review. *Int J Radiat Oncol Biol Phys* 2011;79:985–997.
41. Arthurs BJ, Fairbanks RK, Demakas JJ, et al. A review of treatment modalities for vestibular schwannoma. *Neurosurg Rev* 2011;34:265–277.
42. Suryanarayanan R, Ramsden RT, Saeed SR, et al. Vestibular schwannoma: role of conservative management. *J Laryngol Otol* 2010;124:251–257.
43. Simon M, Bostrom JP, Hartmann C. Molecular genetics of meningiomas: from basic research to potential clinical applications. *Neurosurgery* 2007;60:787–789.
44. Zada G, Pagnini PG, Yu C, et al. Long-term outcomes and patterns of tumor progression after gamma knife radiosurgery for benign meningiomas. *Neurosurgery* 2010;67:322–328.
45. Bigelow D, Eisen M, Smith P, et al. Lipomas of the internal auditory canal and cerebellopontine angle. *Laryngoscope* 1998;108:1459–1469.
46. Gloria-Cruz T, Schachern P, Paparella M, et al. Metastases to temporal bones from primary nonsystemic malignant neoplasms. *Arch Otolaryngol Head Neck Surg* 2000;126:209–214.

BIBLIOGRAPHY

Jackler, RK, Driscoll, CLW. *Tumors of the ear and temporal bone.* Philadelphia, PA: Lippincott Williams & Wilkins, 2000.
Wenig, BM. *Atlas of head and neck pathology*, 2nd ed. Philadelphia, PA: Saunders Elsevier, 2007.

148 | Congenital Malformation of the Ear

Paul R. Lambert

Atresia of the ear canal with middle ear anomalies can occur in isolation or in association with microtia or craniofacial dysplasia. The reported incidence is 1 in 10,000 to 20,000 births. Genetic transmission occurs in many of the syndromes that include aural atresia (e.g., Treacher Collins syndrome), but it is rarely found in cases of isolated atresia. Aural atresia is bilateral in approximately one-third of the cases, and each side can vary in complexity (1).

The evaluation and treatment of aural atresia present a number of challenges to the otologic surgeon. First, overall hearing must be assessed and the need for immediate amplification determined. The second challenge is to formulate a long-term rehabilitation strategy. The key component of this challenge is to determine if surgical correction of the atresia is appropriate. This decision process requires the integration of results from audiometric and radiographic studies with a qualitative assessment of the patient's functional hearing status and the probability of restoring serviceable hearing. If surgery is recommended, the last challenge becomes the operative procedure itself, which is made complex by abnormal development of the temporal bone. This fact places the facial nerve and labyrinth at a greater risk than that encountered in routine temporal bone surgery and complicates the healing process, particularly for canal patency. This chapter reviews the concepts and protocols necessary to meet these challenges successfully.

EMBRYOLOGY

Placed in the context of congenital aural atresia, a general knowledge of the embryologic development of the ear is fascinating and essential for understanding the altered surgical anatomy. Development of the first pharyngeal pouch, the first and second branchial arches, the first branchial cleft, and the otic capsule must all be considered in this discussion.

External Auditory Canal

The external ear canal is derived from the first branchial groove (cleft), between the mandibular and hyoid arches. It is initially represented by a solid core of epithelial cells that extends down to the area of the tympanic ring and first pharyngeal pouch. This core of cells remains in place until the middle trimester of fetal life, a time when most structures of the inner, middle, and outer ear are well differentiated. At this point, absorption of the epithelial cells begins, progressing in a medial to lateral direction. If this canalization process is arrested prematurely, it is possible to have a more normally developed tympanic membrane and bony external ear canal associated with an atretic or very stenotic membranous canal, a situation that predisposes to canal cholesteatoma formation as the trapped squamous epithelium continues to desquamate.

The medial portion of the external ear canal is formed by the tympanic bone. This structure begins to ossify in the third embryonic month, eventually forming the tympanic ring and osseous ear canal; the latter structure continues its lateral growth during the first and second postnatal years. Malformation of the tympanic bone produces atretic bone at the level of the tympanic membrane and results in atresia of the ear canal (2). The mandibular condyle articulates with this rudimentary tympanic bone.

Mastoid and Middle Ear

The eustachian tube, middle ear, and mastoid air cells are derived from the first pharyngeal pouch. Although the middle ear cavity and mastoid air cells are smaller than normal in patients with aural atresia, no anatomic or clinical studies show impaired eustachian tube function in these ears. Pneumatization of the mastoid is a late embryologic event, starting at the seventh or eighth month and continuing into postnatal life. A well-pneumatized mastoid usually indicates good middle ear development, including size of the tympanum and formation of the ossicles. The relationship between middle ear development and degree of differentiation of the pinna is disputed (3).

The ossicles, except for the vestibular portion of the stapes footplate, are formed from the first and second branchial arches. The external ear canal and tympanic membrane are derived from the first branchial cleft. Isolated branchial arch (ossicular) or branchial cleft (external ear canal) deformities are possible, but usually these malformations occur in combination (2). Other branchial arch defects may occur, especially mandibular hypoplasia. The stapes footplate is formed in part from the otic capsule, and in most cases it is normally developed in ears with congenital atresia. It is uncommon to encounter a fixed stapes footplate in the usual major congenital ear malformation, although the superstructure is frequently deformed. This information is important, because the stapes is often partially obscured by the lateral ossicular mass or the facial nerve in atretic ears, and its normal mobility may be difficult to determine with certainty.

Absence of the stapes footplate and oval window can occur, but this is usually encountered in a patient with a patent external ear canal and normal-appearing tympanic membrane rather than in a patient with aural atresia (4). It has been suggested that this condition is caused by abnormal development of the facial nerve (5,6). By the fifth to sixth week of gestation, the horizontal and vertical segments of the facial nerve are evident (6). If anterior displacement of the facial nerve occurred at this time, the nerve could become interposed between the otic capsule and the stapes blastema, which is beginning to grow toward the otic capsule. This would interfere with further stapes development, resulting in a rudimentary ossicle attached to the incus. Continued growth of the stapes toward the otic capsule could result in the rudimentary crura becoming embedded in the displaced facial nerve (4). Because the stapes never contacts the otic capsule, an oval window does not form. With further anterior displacement of the facial nerve, it is possible for that structure to course across the promontory, inferior to the region of the oval window (4). It has been hypothesized that displacement of the facial nerve occurs because of underdevelopment of the first branchial arch (5). This results in a compensatory overshifting of the second branchial arch, and its nerve follows this shift, assuming a more anterior position.

Inner Ear

The membranous labyrinth is derived from the ectodermal otocyst. In most cases of isolated aural atresia, sensorineural and vestibular functions are normal. A comprehensive review of inner ear abnormalities in aural atresia was recently reported by Vrabec and Lin (7). Their study included aural atresia within a broad spectrum of conditions termed "craniofacial microsomia" (e.g., CHARGE, branchiootorenal

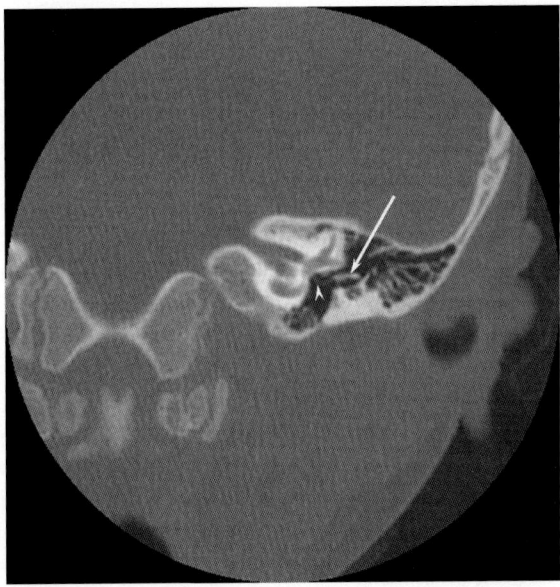

Figure 148.1 Aural atresia with inner ear dysplasia. Axial CT shows absence of the external auditory canal, incomplete partition of the upper turns of the cochlea (*arrow*), and an enlarged lateral semicircular canal (*arrowhead*).

syndrome, Treacher Collins syndrome). They noted an inner ear anomaly by computed tomography (CT) in 22% of 105 patients, with an abnormality of the horizontal semicircular canal and/or vestibule accounting for over half (Fig. 148.1). A sensorineural hearing loss, usually mild and defined as a bone-conduction threshold greater than 20 dB involving two or more frequencies, was found in 15% of patients; the sensorineural hearing loss was usually mild.

Facial Nerve

Preoperative facial nerve weakness is uncommon in isolated aural atresia, but can be seen in 10% to 15% of patients with aural atresia in association with other craniofacial anomalies (7). Facial nerve abnormalities are common in cases of aural atresia (8,9). Bony dehiscence of the fallopian canal frequently occurs, and the facial nerve may also take an anomalous course. Typically, the facial nerve makes an acute angle at the second genu, crossing the middle ear in a more anterior and lateral direction to exit into the glenoid fossa. This abnormal position of the mastoid segment of the facial nerve places it at jeopardy when drilling the posterior inferior portion of the new external ear canal. As the facial nerve exits the skull, it may lie just deep to the area of the tragus. Inadvertent injury to the nerve can occur if undermining of the auricle is necessary to better align the meatus and newly created external ear canal. A correlation between the degree of microtia and the extent of facial nerve abnormality has been observed (3,10). An association between preoperative facial nerve dysfunction and inner ear abnormality by CT has also been noted (7).

CLASSIFICATION

Patients with congenital aural atresia are classified on the basis of auricular development and external canal/middle ear development. Deformity of the auricle is straightforward and is divided into three grades (11). Grade I microtia represents a minor malformation, with the auricle being smaller than normal but with all parts discernible. In grade II microtia, the auricle is represented by a curving or vertical ridge of tissue. In grade III microtia, any resemblance to an auricle is lost, and only a small rudimentary soft tissue structure is present.

Classification of the external canal/middle ear deformity has been more problematic because of the various parameters that have been used, including clinical examination, radiographic findings, surgical observations, or histopathologic studies. Ombredanne (12) proposed dividing congenital aural atresia into two groups only, major and minor malformations. This classification scheme is attractive because of its simplicity and clinical utility. With minor modifications, the following descriptions reflect Ombredanne's criteria.

Major Malformation

In the major malformation group, the external ear canal and tympanic membrane are usually absent, although cases of severe canal stenosis are also included. A small rudimentary tympanic membrane attached to a bony septum is occasionally seen in the canal stenosis patients, but typically the stenosis prevents visualization of the medial aspect of the ear canal. The size of the middle ear space is reduced, and the malleus and incus are deformed, fused, and fixed to the atretic bone. In severe cases, the middle ear space is very hypoplastic, and ossicles are rudimentary or absent. Dehiscence or displacement of the facial nerve can be expected in most major malformations. Grade II or III microtia is common, and inner ear function is usually normal.

Minor Malformation

The significant defect in the minor malformation group involves the middle ear. A conductive hearing loss exists because of absence or deformity of one or more ossicles or fixation of the ossicular chain. Abnormalities of the stapes may be more severe in the minor malformation group than in the major group. The middle ear space and tympanic membrane are normal or only slightly smaller. The external ear canal is patent but may be mildly stenotic. Dehiscence or displacement of the facial nerve can occur, and the pinna is normally developed or only slightly deformed.

PATIENT EVALUATION

Most cases of major congenital ear malformations are evident at birth because of microtia or other craniofacial anomalies. Patients with a normal or only slightly deformed pinna and a stenotic or blindly ending external auditory canal, however, may escape diagnosis for years. Unilateral minor congenital ear malformations with a patent ear canal and normal tympanic membrane can be more difficult to diagnose and may be discovered only with routine hearing screening in school.

The evaluation of an infant or young child with congenital aural atresia must involve both the functional and cosmetic aspects of this condition. First, one must assess the overall hearing status and need for immediate amplification. Second, one must formulate a treatment plan that usually includes consultation with other specialists (e.g., plastic surgery, genetics, developmental pediatrics.)

PHYSICAL EXAMINATION

The initial focus of the physical examination is on overall craniofacial development, because abnormalities or syndromes involving the first or second branchial arch may be associated with the aural atresia. Careful palpation of the mandible may reveal a mild hemifacial microsomia not immediately obvious on inspection. Development of the palate and other intraoral structures should be assessed. The degree of microtia is observed, as is mastoid development. The caliber of the external auditory canal should be graded as normal, stenotic (i.e., mild or severe), blindly ending, or completely atretic. If possible, the tympanic membrane is examined otoscopically. Displacement of the malleus handle (usually anteriorly) or a bony shelf extending from the posterior canal wall may exist. Mobility of the tympanic membrane and malleus handle is determined. Any abnormalities of the digits, limbs, or cervical vertebra are noted.

In the case of a child, achievement of neurologic milestones, such as speech and ambulation, is assessed by history and direct observation. This information can provide insight into auditory and vestibular development. Each major division of the facial nerve is carefully examined and any weakness observed. It is rare to encounter a paresis or paralysis involving the entire hemiface, although there is occasionally involvement of the lower face or lip area. The most common anomaly of facial function is a congenital absence of the depressor anguli oris muscle.

Audiometric Evaluation

Auditory assessment in patients with unilateral atresia is usually straightforward. Behavioral audiometry can be used in most cases, although auditory brainstem response testing may be necessary in young infants or children who are difficult to test. Patients with bilateral atresia present more of a challenge because of the masking dilemma. In such cases, it is essential to determine the level of cochlear function in each ear to prevent operating on an only-hearing ear or on an ear with little or no potential for hearing improvement. It is unsafe to assume that cochlear function is normal bilaterally, even if inner ear development appears normal by CT. Objective data are needed, and bone-conduction auditory brainstem response testing can provide this (13). This testing involves placing recording electrodes near both ears to measure the responses to a bone-conduction stimulus.

Wave I of the auditory brainstem response is generated by the distal portion of the auditory nerve. There is minimal crossover of this small potential to the contralateral ear, and it is thus best measured by a recording electrode ipsilateral to the stimulated side. When recording simultaneously from both ears with surface electrodes, the presence of a wave I should represent the response from the ear being stimulated only. Although stimulation of each ear independently is not possible with a bone-conducted signal, the wave I response is ear specific, thereby allowing differential assessment of cochlear function.

If the ear canals are patent, electrocochleography can be used in a similar way to obtain ear-specific information. Instead of surface electrodes, a transtympanic, tympanic membrane, or canal electrode are possible, providing a more robust wave I response.

Computed Tomography

CT of the temporal bone is necessary in all patients being considered for surgery. It is also recommended in patients with stenosis of the external auditory canal to examine for possible cholesteatoma formation. To completely assess middle ear development, images in the axial (i.e., parallel to the line from the infraorbital rim to the external meatus) and coronal (i.e., parallel to the ramus of the mandible) planes are necessary. For example, the body of the malleus and incus, the incudostapedial joint, and the round window are best seen on axial images, but the stapes, the oval window, and the vestibule are best delineated on coronal images; both planes are necessary to follow the course of the facial nerve. Modern CT scanners can provide images in both planes without having to irradiate the patient twice. A 64-slice CT scanner (or better) is preferred to create diagnostic reformatted coronal images.

Assuming normal sensorineural function has been confirmed audiometrically, the decision to operate depends primarily on the degree of middle ear development, as reflected by the size of the tympanum and status of the ossicles. CT is also important for assessing the development of the cochlear and vestibular labyrinths because their appearance can influence middle ear surgery. For example, an enlarged vestibule and horizontal semicircular canal suggest the possibility of an abnormal communication between the perilymph and cerebrospinal fluid. In such cases, manipulation of the stapes should be avoided.

The course of the facial nerve usually can be delineated by CT. The inability to define this structure precisely, however, is not a contraindication to surgery, assuming that the other criteria for middle ear development are met.

Cholesteatoma can occur in association with congenital aural atresia. Occasionally, sufficient canalization of the external canal occurs such that a space develops in the medial end of the bony canal. Because the lateral end of the canal remains atretic or stenotic, the potential for cholesteatoma formation exists. Early in the development of this problem, symptoms such as pain or drainage from the ear canal or a fistulous track may be absent, and the diagnosis can only be made by CT.

Temporal bone CT is performed near the time of operation. Radiographic studies on infants are usually not recommended because the information is rarely applicable to immediate rehabilitative plans. In very young children, poor patient cooperation often necessitates anesthesia or results in a suboptimal study that must be repeated later. Almost all patients with cholesteatoma formation are older than 3 years, which is another reason to delay the CT evaluation until the patient is beyond that age (14).

MEDICAL MANAGEMENT

Unilateral Atresia

No immediate medical intervention is necessary in the infant discovered to have unilateral atresia, assuming there is normal hearing in the contralateral ear by ABR and OAE testing. The parents can be reassured that speech, language, and intellectual development will proceed normally. Preferential seating in school and possibly an FM system are advised, but a hearing aid is not recommended because of poor acceptance by most children. Many adults, however, find the consequences of unilateral hearing loss from atresia to be a significant aggravation at work and in social settings, and they more readily accept hearing aids. In patients with atresia of the ear canal, a bone-conduction hearing aid must be used. If the canal is only stenotic, an air-conduction aid is preferred because of cosmesis, improved sound localization (i.e., stimulation of one cochlea only), broader frequency response, less sound distortion, and comfort.

Bilateral Atresia

Early amplification within the first 3 to 4 months of life is essential in infants with bilateral atresia. Initial medical and audiologic evaluations can be completed within the first few months of life and a bone-conduction hearing aid or soft band BAHA can be fitted soon thereafter.

SURGICAL MANAGEMENT

Unilateral and Bilateral Atresia Repair

Although most otologic surgeons would consider atresia repair in bilateral cases, many are reluctant to operate on unilateral atresias. The issue is not the unilateral aspect of the hearing loss because most otologic surgeons will explore the middle ear of a child with a large unilateral conductive hearing loss due to other causes (e.g., trauma, infection). The concern is the degree and predictability of hearing improvement that can be achieved, potential lifetime care of a mastoid cavity, and the risk to the facial nerve in atresia surgery. These concerns have prompted many surgeons to recommend delaying surgery in unilateral cases until adulthood, when patients can make their own decision based on the risks and benefits.

An improvement in the hearing threshold to 25 dB or better eliminates the handicap of unilateral hearing loss. This degree of hearing improvement is not possible in all atresia patients, but it can be achieved in at least 50% of carefully selected patients. A mastoid cavity is not created if the "anterior" surgical approach is used, and risk to the facial nerve is minimized by understanding the abnormal development of this structure and by using intraoperative facial nerve monitoring. I and others contend that the benefits of binaural hearing and the possibility of achieving that goal are sufficiently great to offer corrective surgery to carefully selected children with unilateral atresia (10,15).

Patients with bilateral atresia present less of a surgical dilemma. The goal in these cases is to restore sufficient hearing so that amplification is no longer needed. In contradistinction to ear selection for other otologic disorders, the "best" (as determined by CT evaluation) ear is selected for the initial surgical procedure. Most surgeons recommend operating as the child approaches school age and, depending on the hearing result, on the second ear within the next several years. As with many conductive hearing losses (e.g., otosclerosis), the possible use of amplification with a BAHA should be discussed. The probable need for yearly or semiannual cleaning of the reconstructed ear canal should also be acknowledged.

Selection Criteria

Most patients undergoing atresia repair have a residual conductive deficit of at least 10 dB. Sensorineural function should be normal to achieve binaural hearing in unilateral cases or to obviate the need for a hearing aid in bilateral cases. Normal or near-normal sensorineural function in the contralateral ears is also important to avoid operating on the better hearing ear.

Although audiometric criteria can be defined quantitatively, the real art of patient selection is centered on the CT evaluation of the middle ear. Hypoplasia of the middle ear space, ranging from mild to severe, occurs in most cases of congenital atresia, and ossicular development can be expected to correlate directly with middle ear size. The risk of surgical complications will be minimized and the chances for a successful hearing result are increased if the middle ear and mastoid size are at least two-thirds of the normal size and if all three ossicles, although deformed, can be identified (Figs. 148.1 and 148.2). CT demonstration of the oval and round windows and a near-normal course of the facial nerve further define the ideal surgical candidate. The relationship of the facial nerve to the oval window (i.e., normally positioned or overhanging) and the position of the vertical segment are noted. Severe anterior displacement of

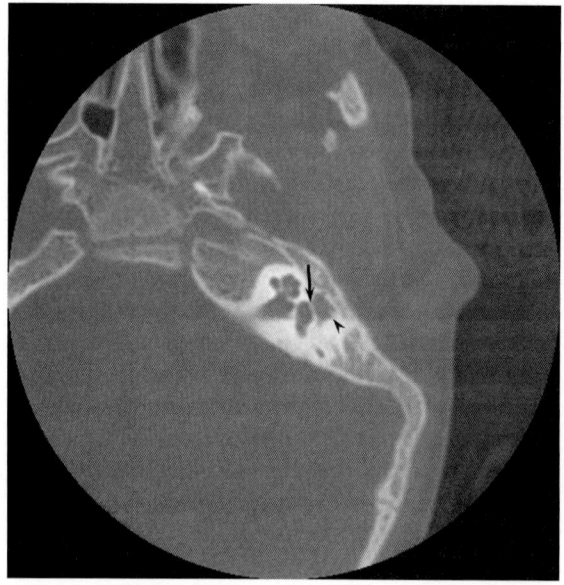
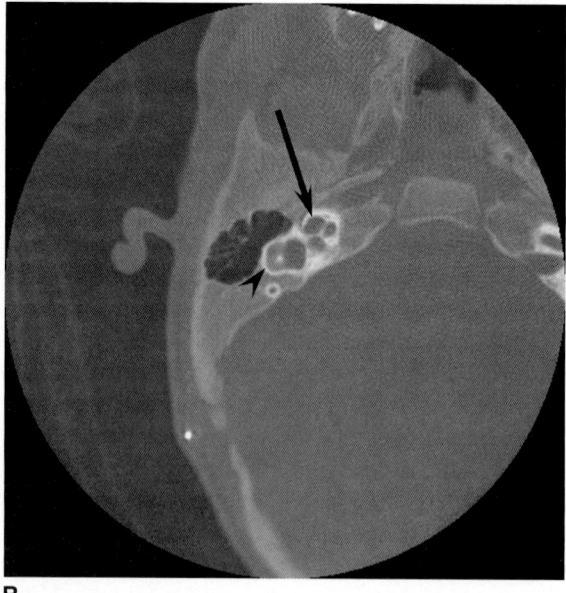

A   **B**

Figure 148.2 A: Aural atresia with mild middle ear dysplasia. Coronal CT shows an intact stapes with an intact incudostapedial joint (*arrowhead*), but the malleoincudal complex (*arrow*) is not properly formed. The tympanic segment of the facial nerve has a normal course. This patient would be a candidate for surgery. **B:** Aural atresia with severe middle ear dysplasia. Axial CT shows a diminutive middle ear cavity with no visible ossicles. The oval window is sclerosed (*arrow*), and the tympanic segment of the facial nerve is displaced laterally (*arrowhead*). This patient is not a candidate for surgery.

TABLE 148.1	JAHRSDOEFER GRADING SYSTEM FOR CONGENITAL AURAL ATRESIA

Parameter	Points[a]
Stapes present	2
Oval window patent	1
Middle ear space	1
Facial nerve	1
Malleus–incus complex	1
Mastoid pneumatization	1
Incus–stapes connection	1
Round window	1
External ear appearance	1

[a]Total points: 8, good prognosis; 7, fair prognosis; 6, marginal candidate; 5, poor prognosis.
From Jahrsdoerfer RA, Yeakley JW, Aguilar EA, et al. Grading system for the selection of patients with congenital aural atresia. *Am J Otolaryngol* 1992;13:6–12, with permission.

the vertical segment of the nerve restricts access to the middle ear space, reducing the chance for a successful hearing result and increasing the chance of facial nerve injury.

The Jahrsdoerfer grading system that quantifies the developmental status of the ear has been shown to predict postoperative hearing results (Table 148.1) (16). Specific dimensions of the mesotympanum can also be analyzed to further refine the CT analysis of atretic ears. Oliver et al. defined mesotympanic height, length, and weight measurement landmarks and showed a strong correlation with postoperative speech reception threshold (SRT) (17). Height of the mesotympanum was measured on the coronal scan from the horizontal facial nerve to the first bony prominence inferiorly (in normal ears, this would be the bony annulus). On the same coronal cut, width of the mesotympanum was measured as the distance between the oval window and the atretic bone (scutum in normal ears). Length of the mesotympanum was measured on the axial CT as the distance from the promontory to the nearest posterior lateral bone (usually the bone overlying the vertical facial nerve). If the area (height × width of the mesotympanum) was ≥ 20 mm^2, patients were six times more likely to have an SRT ≤ 25 dB. If the mesotympanum volume was ≥ 42 mm^3, patients were 24 times more likely to have an SRT ≤ 25 dB. Clearly, volume of the middle ear is a critical determinant of success in atresia surgery. This calculation will be facilitated as more sophisticated radiographic software programs designed to measure volumes of irregular shapes and contours, such as characterize the middle ear, become available.

In unilateral atresia cases, only the ideal candidates are selected; in bilateral cases, the minimal criteria are a middle ear of at least one half normal size and the presence of an ossicular mass. Overall, only about 60% of patients with aural atresia are surgical candidates.

Often the CT findings can be anticipated by the physical examination. For example, poor middle ear development

is more frequently seen in patients with craniofacial deformities than in patients with isolated aural atresia. Patients with Treacher Collins syndrome often have truly bizarre middle ear findings. In general, the better developed the auricle, the larger and better developed the middle ear.

Timing of Surgery

If elected, surgery can be performed as early as 6 to 7 years of age. By this time, accurate audiometric tests have been obtained, pneumatization of the temporal bone is well advanced, and most children are able to cooperate with postoperative care. This timing also permits microtia repair to be well under way.

In microtia patients requiring major external ear reconstruction, it is reasonable for the reconstructive surgeon to operate first. This ensures a virgin field without scars or compromised blood supply, optimizing survival of the implanted auricular framework. The overall cosmetic result should also be better without the restriction of having to reconstruct the auricle around a bony canal drilled in the temporal bone. Typically, the otologic surgery is performed midway through the multistaged microtia repair, after the auricular framework has been implanted and the lobule transposed but before the tragus is reconstructed and the auricle is elevated from the side of the head. Although the reconstructed auricle may not be centered exactly over the created bony canal, it can be repositioned with appropriate undermining so that the meatus and external canal are aligned.

Cholesteatoma

Cholesteatoma in congenital aural atresia results from squamous epithelium, which has been trapped within the medial ear canal after an arrest of the canalization process. The membranous canal may appear completely closed in these cases, but usually shows either a pinhole opening or severe stenosis. There is one reported case of a cholesteatoma appearing medial to the atretic bone in a patient with complete canal atresia (18). In this patient, an epidermoid rest in the middle ear was hypothesized as the origin of the lesion.

Cole and Jahrsdoerfer (14) reviewed a series of 50 patients (54 ears) with an average canal diameter of 4 mm or less and found that 50% of them developed a cholesteatoma. Patient age and exact canal size were important variables in predicting disease. For example, no cholesteatomas were found in patients younger than 3 years, and bone erosion and middle ear involvement from a canal cholesteatoma were not encountered in patients younger than age 12. The preponderance of cholesteatomas developed in canals 2 mm or less in diameter. Beginning in young adolescence, individuals with severe canal stenosis are at a particular risk for cholesteatoma formation (i.e., 10 of 11 ears in the series reported by Cole and Jahrsdoerfer (14)). The usual presenting symptom in these patients is drainage from the ear canal or from a fistula track postauricularly.

Patients with cholesteatoma, regardless of CT or audiometric findings, should undergo surgery to eradicate the disease process and, if possible, improve hearing. Patients with stenosis of the external canal who are at risk for cholesteatoma formation should also be considered for surgery. Given these data on the risk of canal cholesteatomas, management protocols can be set forth. Patients with stenosis extensive enough to prevent adequate cleaning of the canal and examination of the tympanic membrane should have CTs by age 4 or 5, even if there is no aural drainage. Assuming a cholesteatoma is not found, several options are available, depending on middle ear development. If the CT findings are favorable with regard to hearing improvement, canal and middle ear surgery is advised at this time. Canaloplasty alone is offered to patients with unfavorable middle ear findings. If the parents are uncomfortable with surgery, a CT should be obtained every few years to rule out cholesteatoma development. Periodic CTs are not necessary in patients with a completely atretic ear canal, given the rarity of cholesteatoma formation in that setting.

SURGICAL TECHNIQUE

There are two basic surgical approaches for repair of aural atresia: the mastoid approach and the anterior approach. In the mastoid approach, the sinodural angle is first identified and followed to the antrum (19–21). The facial recess is opened and the incudostapedial joint separated. The atretic bone is then removed. In the anterior approach, as popularized in this country by Jahrsdoerfer (3), exposure of the

mastoid air cells is limited. Drilling is confined to an area defined by the temporomandibular joint (TMJ) anteriorly, the middle cranial fossa dura superiorly, and the mastoid air cells posteriorly. An advantage of the anterior approach is that a large mastoid cavity with its attendant problems of debris accumulation and infection is avoided. There is also less surgical manipulation in the area of the mastoid segment of the facial nerve, and the more cylindrical contours of the new canal with limited mastoid exposure facilitate placement of the split-thickness skin graft. For these reasons, the anterior approach is preferred and is the technique described here. Facial nerve monitoring is used.

Incision

A postauricular incision is used to expose the mastoid bone. The soft tissues are elevated anteriorly until a depression is encountered. In most major malformations, this depression is the TMJ, although occasionally a stenotic bony ear canal may be encountered. Dissection within this area may be necessary to differentiate between the two, but the manipulation should be limited because the facial nerve frequently exits the skull into the glenoid fossa.

Drilling a Canal

In most atretic ears, a tympanic bone remnant is not identified, but occasionally it is present and clearly demarcated from the surrounding cortex (Fig. 148.3). In such instances, the atretic bone serves to direct the drilling for

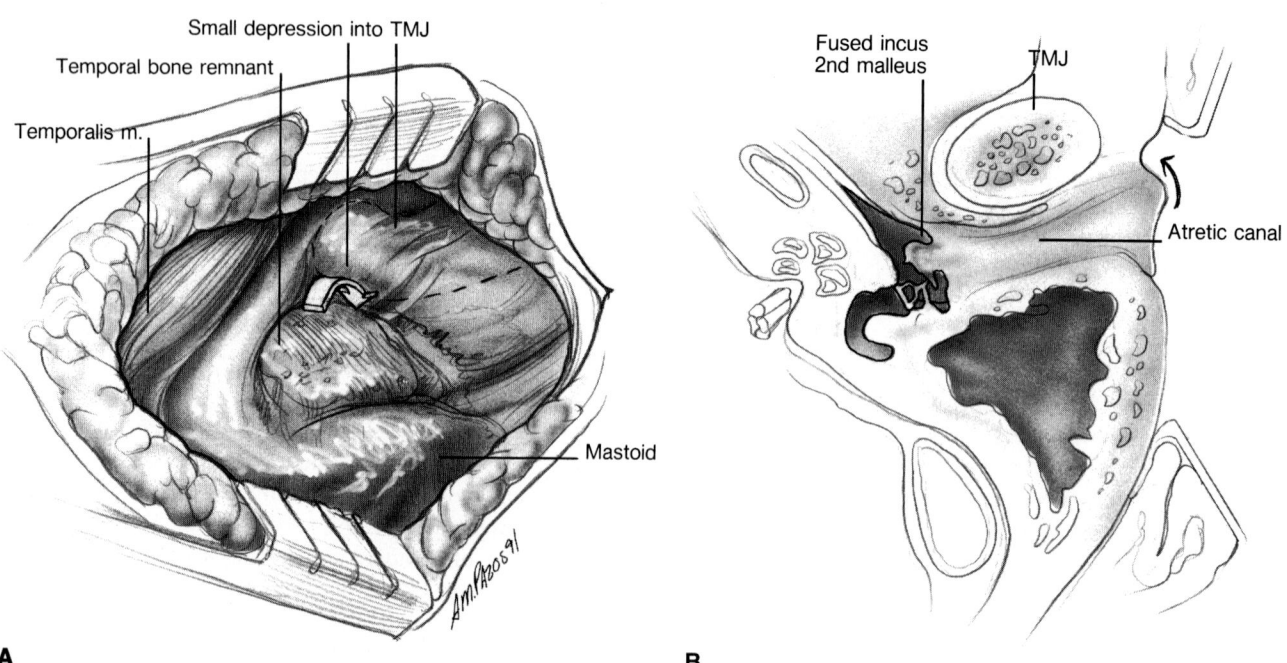

A   **B**

Figure 148.3 A: Through a postauricular incision, the soft tissues have been elevated to reveal the mastoid cortex and the atretic bone (tympanic bone remnant). Notice the depression anterior to the atretic bone, which represents the temporomandibular joint (TMJ). **B:** Axial section.

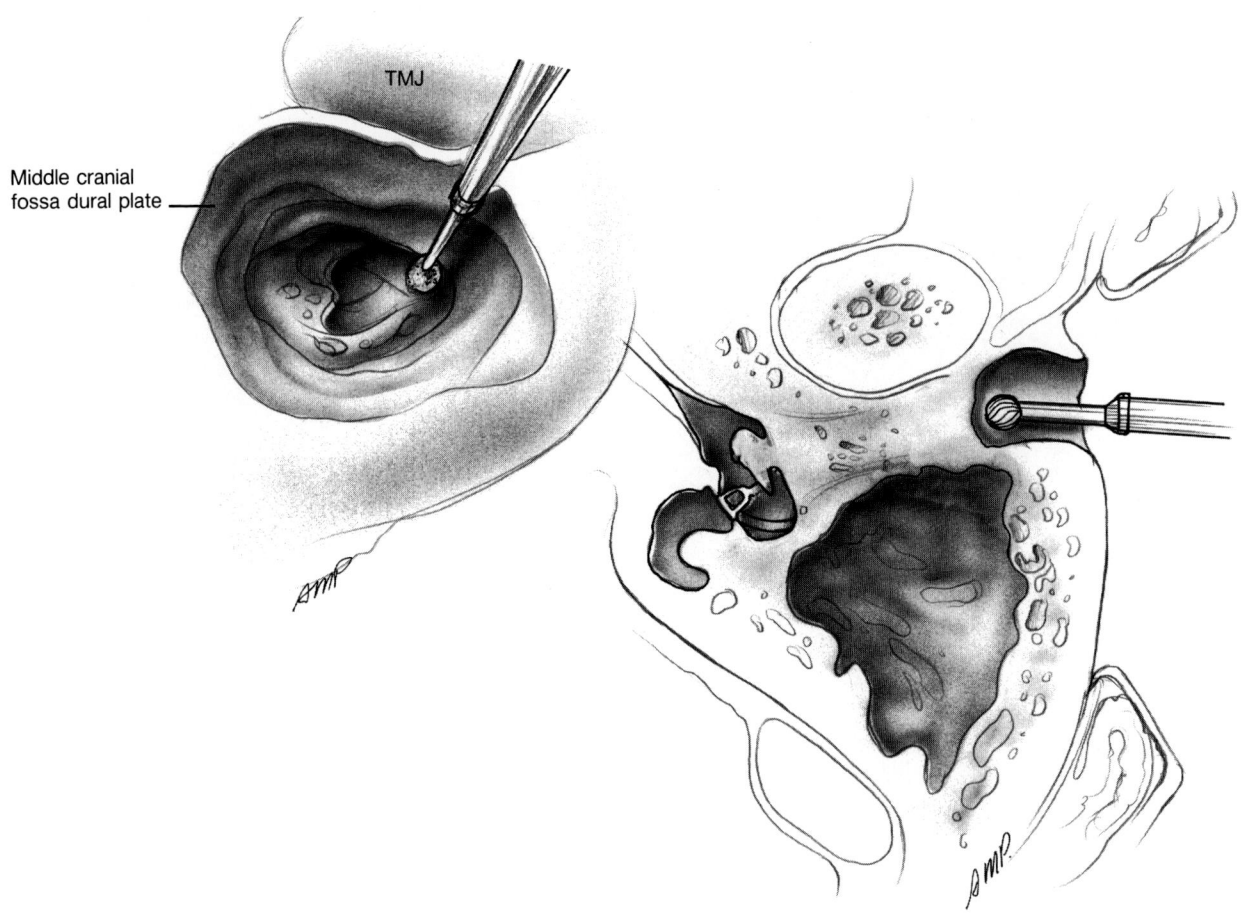

Figure 148.4 The initial stage of drilling an external auditory canal is shown. Landmarks for the canal include the middle cranial fossa dura superiorly, the temporomandibular joint (TMJ) anteriorly, and the mastoid air cells posteriorly.

the external canal. Even when not identified, there is sufficient space between the glenoid fossa anteriorly and the mastoid air cells posteriorly for a canal. Drilling is begun just slightly posterior and superior to the glenoid fossa. The tegmen is the critical landmark to define initially. Drilling toward the middle ear is accomplished by using the middle cranial fossa dura as the superior landmark and the TMJ as the anterior landmark. The bone removed is usually solid but may be cellular in areas (Fig. 148.4). The posterior wall of the glenoid fossa should be very thin to maximize anterior exposure and to limit opening into the mastoid air cells. If air cells are uncovered, they can be filled with cartilage pieces from the meatoplasty later in the procedure. As the middle cranial fossa dura plate is followed medially, the epitympanum will be entered and the fused heads of the malleus and incus identified (Fig. 148.5). Concentrating the drilling superiorly along the middle cranial fossa has the advantage of protecting the facial nerve because that structure always lies medial to the ossicular mass in the epitympanum. Because of the more acute angle the facial nerve may take at the second genu, it is vulnerable to injury as the external canal is

enlarged in the posteroinferior direction. In this area, the nerve may lie lateral to the middle ear cavity in addition to being anteriorly displaced.

Exposure of the Ossicular Chain

The malleus neck or deformed manubrium is typically fused to the atretic bone. To free the ossicular chain, this overlying bone is thinned carefully with a diamond burr and then completely removed with an incudostapedial joint knife or small hook. Periosteum underlying the atretic bone is still attached to the malleus and should be sharply excised with a microknife or microscissors, or vaporized with the laser. Care is taken to limit trauma to the inner ear by drilling or excessive manipulation of the ossicular chain. The incudostapedial joint is not routinely separated.

Except for the fossa incudis, which may be left intact, bone should be completely removed around the ossicles, leaving at least a 2- to 3-mm space between these structures and the adjacent canal wall. The atretic bone should be removed so that the ossicular mass is centered

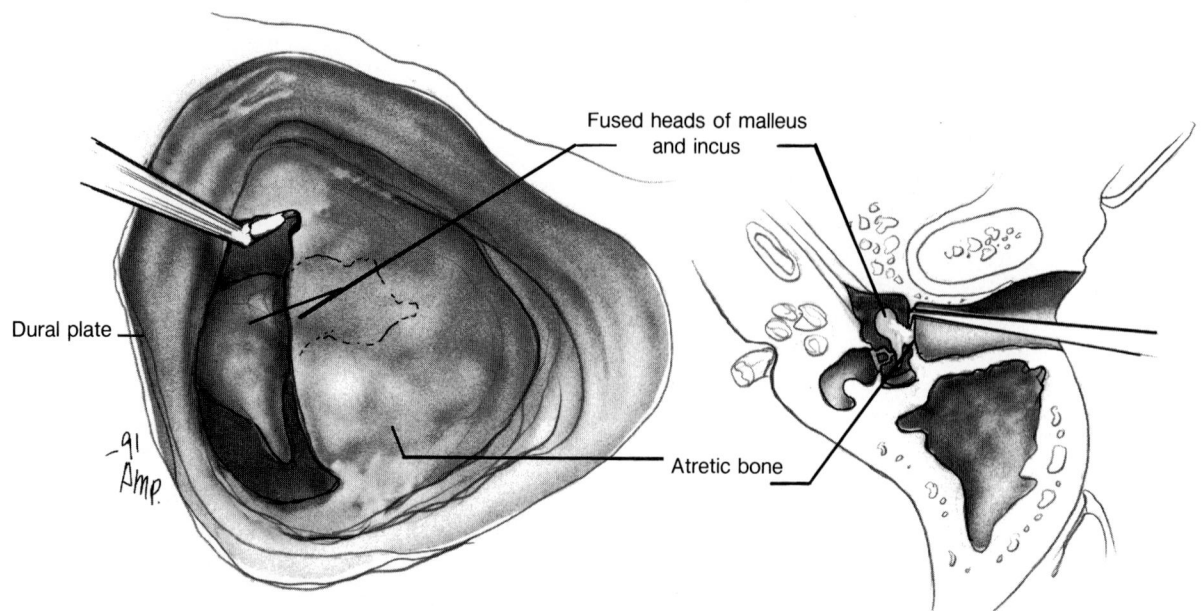

Figure 148.5 The epitympanum is entered by following the middle cranial fossa dura medially. The atretic bone over the fused malleus–incus complex is thinned with a diamond burr and removed with a right-angle hook.

in the new canal (Fig. 148.6). To ensure proper draping of the fascia and split-thickness skin graft, the canal walls should be smooth and without ledges lateral to the ossicular mass.

Middle Ear Surgery

The stapes may be partially obscured because of the contracted middle ear cavity, the malformed lateral ossicular mass, or the overlying facial nerve. Usually, enough of that ossicle can be seen to assess its mobility and the integrity of the incudostapedial joint. Although the stapes is often small, with delicate misshapen crura, a normal oval window and stapes footplate are anticipated. The lateral ossicular mass is maintained in position and not removed to obtain a better view of the stapes. In most cases, the ossicular chain, although deformed, is mobile, and hearing results may be better when the chain is left intact instead of interpositioning a prosthesis or autograft material (10,22).

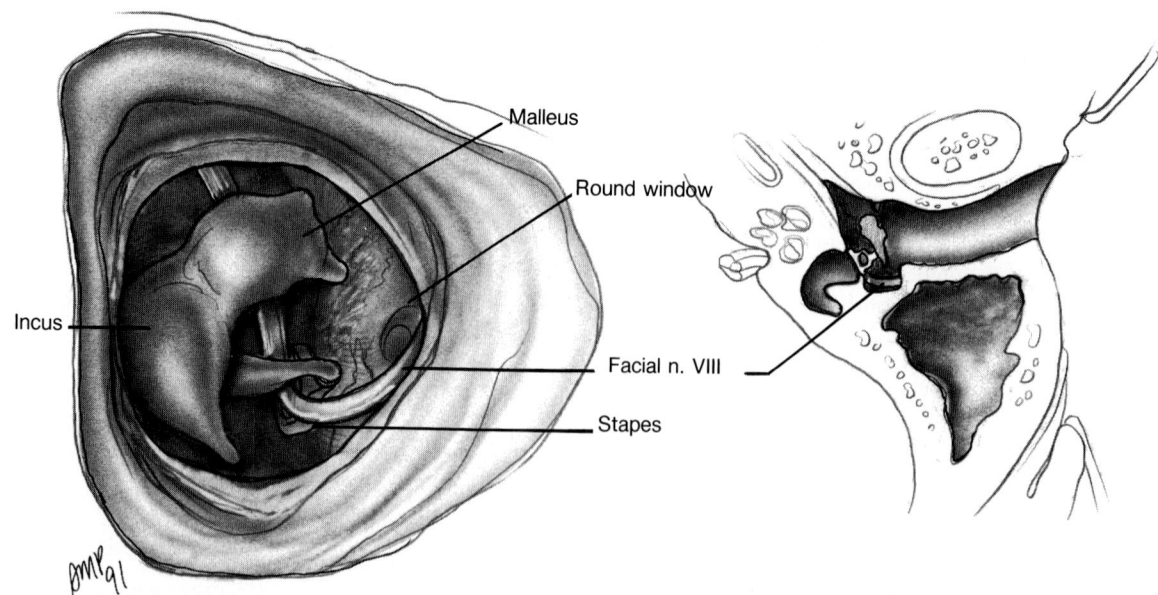

Figure 148.6 The ossicular mass is fully exposed. Notice the more acute angle of the facial nerve at its genu.

Tympanic Membrane Grafting

A thin fascia graft is placed over the mobilized ossicular chain. Because the manubrium of the malleus is either absent or very deformed, it is difficult to anchor the graft beneath the ossicular chain. Absence of a tympanic membrane remnant or annulus further predisposes to lateralization. Several techniques can be used to prevent this potential complication. First, the graft can be tucked beneath the anterior and superior bony ledges of the canal wall. If the ledges are too shallow to stabilize the graft, a sulcus several millimeters deep can be drilled in the anterior canal wall medial to the level of the ossicles. A second technique to avoid lateralization involves covering the fascia graft with the split-thickness skin graft (STSG) of the canal and then placing a silastic button that has been contoured to the circumference of the canal on top of the covered ossicles (23).

Meatoplasty

A large meatus, approximately twice normal size is created. The auricle is undermined and the deep soft tissue debulked from the approximate area of the meatus. Leaving only a small amount of subcutaneous tissue around the meatus limits the length of the membranous canal and helps prevent stenosis. When possible, an anteriorly based thin skin flap is raised over the planned meatal opening. This skin flap is subsequently noted medially into the new ear canal to cover a portion of the anterior membranous canal. The auricle is returned to its normal anatomic position to check for alignment of the meatus and the bony canal. It is secured in place by suturing its distal edge to a cuff of periosteal tissue at the bony edge of the drilled canal.

Frequently, the meatus appears to be offset anteriorly or inferiorly. In such cases, further undermining of the auricle is necessary so that it can be positioned without tension more posteriorly and superiorly. The facial nerve is vulnerable to injury if extensive soft tissue undermining is necessary because prior auricular reconstruction may have caused scarring and tethering of the extratemporal facial nerve in a more superficial position. A strip of skin can be excised from the postauricular incision to help maintain the auricle in its new location. In some cases, the framework of the auricle may need to be anchored to the periosteum to maintain proper alignment.

Skin Grafting

A skin graft 0.008 inch thick is taken from the upper thigh or upper arm and used to line the canal. To determine the proper configuration of the split-thickness skin graft, several measurements of the canal are made with a 2-0 silk suture. Typically, the resulting skin graft is shaped like a hexagon and is approximately 4 × 6 cm². To facilitate graft placement at the level of tympanic membrane and to

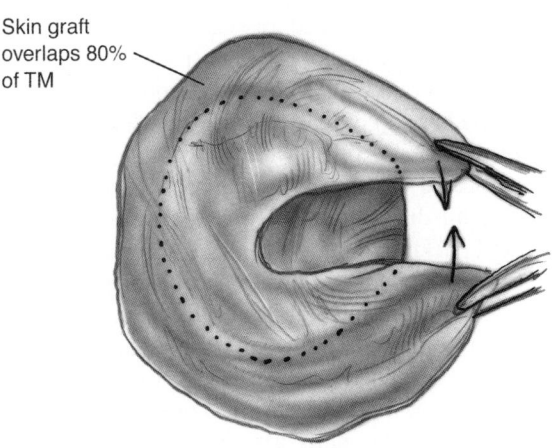

Skin graft overlaps 80% of TM

Figure 148.7 The fascia graft for the tympanic membrane has been placed and the STSG is positioned within the ear canal, overlapping the fascia.

ensure eversion of the skin edges, multiple small wedges are excised from the medial portion of the graft; the graft is also pie crusted.

With the ear retracted forward, the STSG is positioned in the bony canal so that it overlaps the fascia graft (Fig. 148.7). The seam of the graft is placed anteriorly, away from any open mastoid air cells posteriorly. Partial or substantial covering the fascia graft with the skin graft is acceptable and may facilitate epithelialization of the new tympanic membrane. A silastic disc (0.04 inches thick), approximating the diameter of the bony canal, is placed over the covered ossicles to help prevent lateralization. Stabilization of the STSG within the canal is achieved by placing Merocel wicks which are then hydrated with an antibiotic-steroid solution (Fig. 148.8). After the bony

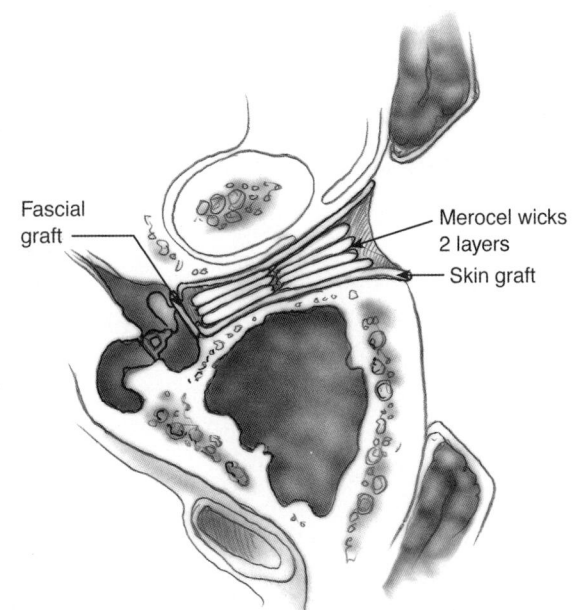

Fascial graft

Merocel wicks 2 layers

Skin graft

Figure 148.8 The fascia graft and split-thickness skin grafts are stabilized by layered packing (axial view).

canal has been fully packed, the ear is returned to its normal anatomic position, and the postauricular incision is closed with subcuticular sutures. Working through the meatus, the lateral end of the STSG is grasped and pulled through the meatal opening. It is trimmed as necessary and sutured in place. Additional packing with Merocel is used to fill the lateral soft tissue portion of the canal. The initial packing of the STSG in the bony canal prevents it from being dislodged during the final step of suturing the graft to the meatal skin. The placement of the graft in the bony canal while the ear is reflected forward provides maximal exposure, ensuring that the entire canal is covered and that the STSG has been positioned accurately relative to the fascia graft. The previously elevated skin flap from the area of the meatus is sutured to a cuff of periosteal tissue near the TMJ to cover a portion of the anterior membranous canal.

Postoperative Care

Postoperative antibiotics are not prescribed. The patient is instructed to place 10 drops of the antibiotic-steroid solution in the ear twice daily to keep the Merocel wicks moist. Approximately 10 days postoperatively, the ear canal packing and silastic disc are removed. Complete take of the STSG is anticipated at this time. If any granulation tissue is seen, antibiotic-soaked pieces of Gelfoam are placed within the canal and the patient is instructed to keep these moist for the next 7 to 10 days.

SURGICAL FINDINGS

Ossicles

In major atresia cases, the expected finding is a fused and deformed malleus–incus complex. The malleus is typically more deformed than the incus and has a short manubrium

(Fig. 148.9). The site of ossicular fixation is most commonly between the malleus neck or shortened manubrium and the atretic bone. In minor malformations, the incus and malleus are less deformed and may be completely normal. If abnormal, ossicular fixation in the epitympanum and/or a deformed manubrium or incus long process is common.

In atretic ears, the stapes is usually small and delicate with misshapen crura. Stapes fixation is uncommon. The incudostapedial joint may also appear fragile and occasionally may exist as only a fibrous connection. The facial nerve may encroach on the stapes, partially obscuring the footplate. Complete visualization of the stapes may also be impaired by the overlying ossicular mass.

Fixation of the stapes, severe deformity of the stapes, or even absence of the stapes and oval window may be encountered in minor malformation cases. These abnormalities, although rare, are more common in patients with a patent external auditory canal and normal tympanic membrane than in patients with major atresia of the ear.

Facial Nerve

Facial nerve abnormalities are common in major atresia patients. The anticipated abnormalities include complete dehiscence of the tympanic segment, inferior displacement of the tympanic segment, and anterior and lateral displacement of the mastoid segment. The last abnormality frequently obscures the round window. Although the course of the facial nerve is often aberrant, predictable abnormalities are the rule and help guide the surgeon. The degree of external ear deformity provides some indication of facial nerve development, with a higher incidence of facial nerve anomalies occurring in patients with more severe microtia (3,4).

Aberrant facial nerves are frequently encountered in ears with minor malformations, and the abnormalities

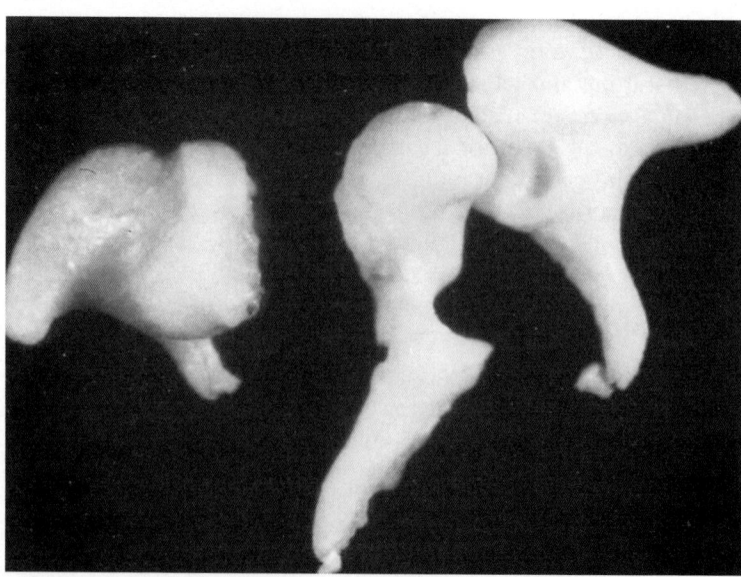

Figure 148.9 The typical appearance of a fused malleus–incus complex is shown (**left**). Notice that this complex is smaller than the normal malleus and incus (**right**) and that the malleus is more deformed than the incus.

may even be more severe than those seen in atresia cases. The most common findings include dehiscence or inferior displacement of the tympanic segment. In several cases, a facial nerve coursing across the middle portion of the promontory, well inferior to the oval window, has been observed. In all patients with a congenital conductive hearing loss, even if the pinna, external auditory canal, and tympanic membrane are normal, an abnormal facial nerve should be anticipated and appropriate facial nerve monitoring and surgical care exercised.

HEARING RESULTS

It is difficult to compare hearing results from various series because of differences in classifying congenital ears, in selection criteria, in reporting hearing results, and in the length of follow-up. In general, an initial postoperative hearing level of 30 dB or better can be achieved in approximately 50% to 75% of major congenital atresia patients; a hearing level of 20 dB or better is possible in 15% to 50% of these patients. Bellucci (2) reported a hearing level of at least 30 dB in 55% of 71 patients followed for at least 2 years. Schuknecht (24) reported similar success in 30 patients with a mean follow-up of 1.3 years. Thirty percent of Schuknecht's patients had a hearing level of 20 dB or better. Nager and Levin (19) reported that 70% of 23 patients treated over a 17-year period had a hearing level of at least 30 dB. Mattox and Fisch (25) found at least a 30-dB improvement in air-conduction thresholds in 45% of 11 patients followed a minimum of 2 years. De la Cruz and colleagues (21,26) reported 56 patients with a 6-month follow-up and observed that 53% had a conductive deficit of 20 dB or less and 73% had a deficit of 30 dB or less. In a follow-up series involving 77 ears, air-bone gap closure to less than 30 dB was achieved in 60% of cases (27). In 2003, De la Cruz and Teufert (28) reported a 30-dB or less conductive hearing loss in 58.5% of 116 ears with short-term follow-up, which decreased to 50.8% with longer-term (3.5 years) observation. Lambert (10) reported that 67% of 15 patients followed for at least 1 year had an SRT of 30 dB or better; the mean improvement in the hearing level was 30 dB. Jahrsdoerfer (3) found that 65% of 17 patients followed for 2 months to 8 years had a pure-tone average of 30 dB or less. In a more recent series of 86 patients, Jahrsdoerfer (16) reported a postoperative hearing level at 1 month of 25 dB or better in 71%.

Lambert (29) reported data comparing early (less than 1 year) and longer term (1.0 to 7.5 years, mean follow-up 2.8 years) hearing results after surgery for congenital aural atresia. This study involved 59 consecutively operated ears. In the early postoperative period, an SRT of less than 25 dB was achieved in 60% and an SRT of less than 30 dB in 70%. With longer-term follow-up, 46% of patients maintained an SRT of less than 25 dB. Digoy and Cueva reviewed less than 1 year and greater than 1 year hearing outcomes in 54 ears (30). The short-term mean SRT was 33, with 53%

of patients at 30 dB or less. For follow-ups greater than 1 year ($n = 16$), 56% of patients had an SRT of 30 dB or less (mean 32 dB).

Chang et al. reported on 100 ears (some requiring revision surgery) with a minimum follow-up of 3 years (31). The mean air-bone gap at 3 years was 30 dB, which was not statistically different from the mean value of 27 dB at 6 months postoperatively.

COMPLICATIONS

Given the fact that near-normal hearing is not universally achieved even in carefully selected atresia patients, the surgical complications must be carefully compared with the merits of atresia surgery. The two potential serious complications are sensorineural hearing loss and facial nerve paralysis. Other complications that can occur include canal stenosis, chronic infection, and recurrent conductive hearing loss.

It should be recognized that revision surgery is often required after congenital aural atresia repair (29–34). In the series by Lambert in which patients were followed for an average of 2.8 years, one-third of the patients did require revision surgery. Stenosis of the ear canal and lateralization of the tympanic membrane were the most common problems encountered. After revision surgery, approximately half of these patients did achieve an SRT of 25 dB or better with at least 1 year of follow-up.

Labyrinthine Injury

The anterior surgical approach limits exposure of mastoid air cells, thus minimizing potential injury to the horizontal semicircular canal. High-frequency sensorineural hearing loss has been noted in some patients postoperatively, although a loss in the speech frequencies is rare (10,20,24,26,35). Because the ossicular mass is connected to the atretic bone, energy from drilling will be transmitted to the inner ear in all atresia cases regardless of the approach. This may be of less consequence, however, than direct manipulation of the ossicular chain by instruments or the drill. Care in removing the final portion of atretic bone from the ossicular chain is particularly important in the anterior approach, because the incudostapedial joint is not disarticulated.

Facial Nerve Injury

The abnormal development of the temporal bone in cases of aural atresia places the facial nerve at increased vulnerability. Understanding the anomalies of the facial nerve likely to be encountered and the use of facial nerve monitoring, however, enable the surgeon to proceed with confidence. Temporary facial paralysis has occurred rarely. This complication has usually resulted from transposition of the facial nerve to gain access to the oval window (24,36).

In my series of over 200 aural atresia surgeries, facial paresis or paralysis has occurred in less than 1%. A similar incidence has been reported by Jahrsdoerfer and Lambert (37).

Potential damage to the facial nerve can be minimized by adhering to several surgical guidelines. First, as the atretic bone is removed, the drilling should be concentrated superiorly along the middle cranial fossa dural plate, entering the middle ear first in the epitympanum. The facial nerve is protected in this approach because it will always lie medial to the ossicular heads. Second, care should be exercised as the canal is enlarged in the posterior-inferior direction because of the more anterior and lateral course of the mastoid segment. Injury to the facial nerve can also occur in its extratemporal segment, as the postauricular incision is made, or as the auricle is undermined to align the soft tissue meatus and the created bony canal.

Canal Stenosis

In the reviews by Lambert (29) and Oliver et al. (32), stenosis of the membranous canal was the most common reason for revision surgery. Some degree of narrowing of the membranous canal requiring local care in the office (e.g., cauterization for granulation tissue, Kenalog injections, wick with steroid—antibiotic drops) or surgery occurs in as many as 25% of patients. If a large meatus (i.e., approximately twice normal size) has been made, this narrowing can be managed conservatively in the office. Occasionally, a significant stenosis occurs, trapping squamous epithelium and causing infection. In such cases, attempts to dilate the canal with soft or hard stents are usually ineffective, and a secondary meatoplasty with skin grafting is necessary. This potential problem can be minimized by generously debulking soft tissue from the auricle before the meatoplasty, thus decreasing the length of the membranous canal. Coverage of all exposed bone and soft tissue by the STSG is also essential to prevent granulation tissue formation and subsequent stricture. The use of the anteriorly based meatal skin flap to cover a portion of the anterior—lateral membranous canal obviates a circumferential STSG at the meatal opening and helps prevent stenosis. In addition to Kenalog injections, the application of mitomycin C has been suggested as a method to prevent or reduce excess fibrosis within the ear canal (38–40). Early results have been mixed. In a study from our laboratory, brief application of mitomycin C (0.5 mg/mL) to the middle ear of gerbils caused acute, adverse electrophysiologic changes and chronic hair cell, stria vascularis, and spiral ganglion cells damaged (41).

In some patients, the lateral canal may be narrowed by displacement of the pinna rather than by fibrous proliferation. Because the reconstructed auricle has more mass and less muscular and soft tissue support than the normal pinna, it can shift, usually anteriorly or inferiorly, after surgery. This shift causes a malalignment of the meatus and bony canal. If there is concern about proper alignment of the membranous and bony canals during the atresia surgery, a permanent suspension suture from the framework of the auricle to the mastoid periosteum or to a hole drilled in the mastoid cortex is placed.

Chronic Infection

Normal migration of keratin debris is lacking in the skin-grafted ear canal. Protective secretions from sebaceous and apocrine glands are also absent. As a consequence, the incidence of canal infections is higher than in the normal ear. A widely patent meatus and membranous canal are important for aeration and cleaning, which may be required once or twice annually. Most patients are not restricted with regard to water activities, although use of an alcohol- or acetic acid–based ear drop after swimming is often recommended.

Conductive Hearing Loss

Persistent or recurrent conductive hearing loss is the most common negative outcome in aural atresia surgery. The causes of the former are varied and include inadequate mobilization of the ossicular mass from the atretic bone, an unrecognized incudostapedial joint discontinuity, or a fixed stapes footplate. Wide exposure of the ossicular mass at surgery is necessary to ensure chain mobility and to facilitate assessment of chain integrity. Recurrence of a conductive hearing loss after an initial satisfactory improvement in air-conduction thresholds is usually secondary to refixation of the ossicular chain or to tympanic membrane lateralization. At least a 2- to 3-mm wide area of bone removal around the ossicular mass (except at the fossa incudis) is desirable, because bony regrowth can occur, especially as children enter puberty. In several male patients with initial excellent hearing results for 8 to 10 years, complete closure of the bony canal has been observed during their rapid growth spurt of adolescence. At revision surgery in these cases, the canal resembled a virgin atresia. Anchoring the fascia graft beneath a bony ledge and/or the use of a Silastic disc help minimize graft lateralization. The incidence of tympanic membrane perforation or middle ear adhesions approximates that encountered in routine tympanoplastic procedures.

Bone-Anchored Hearing Implant

A bone-anchored hearing aid is an alternative rehabilitative strategy for patients with unilateral or bilateral aural atresia, and especially for those patients who are marginal or poor surgical candidates. This approach uses an osseointegrated titanium fixture, placed in the mastoid area, to which a sound processor is attached. The osseointegration allows more efficient transfer of sound than can be achieved with a traditional bone-conduction hearing aid (42). As in patients with otosclerosis, this hearing aid option should be discussed in tandem with surgical intervention. It is also important to acknowledge that the BAHA is often associated with soft tissue infection around the titanium post. Less commonly, skin overgrowth necessitating surgical revision of the implant site and failure to osseointegrate can occur (43).

Currently, the minimum age for BAHA implantation is 5 years per FDA guidelines. A "soft band" that holds an external BAHA sound processor firmly against the skull can be worn by infants. This device provides an alternative to the traditional bone-conduction hearing aid and should be considered in children born with bilateral aural atresia.

CONCLUSIONS

The objective in congenital ear surgery is to create a functional pathway by which sound can reach the cochlear fluids. Although simple in concept, this type of surgery presents a true challenge to the otologic surgeon. A thorough knowledge of the anatomic variations that can occur with abnormal development of the temporal bone is essential, and the nuances of audiometric and radiographic interpretation must be mastered.

Hearing results that are consistently excellent cannot yet be achieved in atresia surgery, but with adherence to strict selection criteria and with further refinements in surgical technique, this goal is realistic.

HIGHLIGHTS

- During the fifth to seventh month of embryogenesis, the solid core of epithelial cells representing the external auditory canal canalizes, beginning medially and progressing laterally. If incomplete, this process can result in a stenotic membranous canal laterally, with a more normal caliber bony canal and tympanic membrane medially. This condition predisposes to cholesteatoma formation within the ear canal.
- Congenital ear malformations can be classified as major or minor. The significant defect in the minor malformation group involves the middle ear, especially the ossicular chain. In most cases of microtia and atresia of the ear canal, the cochlear and vestibular labyrinths are normally formed.
- In major atresia cases, the stapes is usually small with misshapen crura. The footplate is usually intact and mobile.
- The facial nerve is often aberrant in major congenital ear malformations. Dehiscence of the tympanic segment with or without inferior displacement is often seen. The mastoid segment of the facial nerve often makes a more acute angle at the second genu, resulting in anterior and lateral displacement; it may obscure the round window.

- Bilateral congenital atresias can present a masking dilemma during audiometric testing. Bone-conduction auditory brainstem response can provide objective data on ear-specific cochlear function in these cases and help with operative selection.
- In cases of major atresia, the middle ear space should be greater than 50% of normal size, and all three ossicles, although deformed, should be visible.
- The principal landmarks in the anterior approach for aural atresia are the middle fossa dura superiorly, the TMJ anteriorly, and the mastoid air cells posteriorly.
- With proper patient selection in cases of major atresia, it is possible to achieve a hearing level of 25 dB or better in approximately 50% to 70% of patients.
- The most frequent complications in congenital atresia surgery are canal stenosis and failure to achieve an adequate hearing level. The latter can occur because of inadequate mobilization of the ossicular mass from the atretic bone, lateralization of the tympanic membrane graft, or refixation of the ossicular chain by bony regrowth or fibrous tissue.

REFERENCES

1. Jafek BW, Nager GT, Strife J, et al. Congenital aural atresia: an analysis of 311 cases. *Trans Am Acad Ophthalmol Otolaryngol* 1975;80:588–592.
2. Bellucci RJ. Congenital aural malformations: diagnosis and treatment. *Otolaryngol Clin North Am* 1981;14:95–124.
3. Jahrsdoerfer RA. Congenital atresia of the ear. *Laryngoscope* 1978;88(Suppl 13):1–46.
4. Lambert PR. Congenital absence of the oval window. *Laryngoscope* 1990;100:37–40.
5. Gerhardt HJ, Otto HD. The intratemporal course of the facial nerve and its influence on the development of the ossicular chain. *Acta Otolaryngol* 1981;91:567–573.
6. Jahrsdoerfer RA. Embryology of the facial nerve. *Am J Otol* 1988;9:423–426.
7. Vrabec JT, Lin JW. Inner ear abnormalities in congenital aural atresia. *Otol Neurotol* 2010;31:1421–1426.
8. Crabtree JA. The facial nerve in congenital ear surgery. *Otolaryngol Clin North Am* 1974;7:505–510.
9. Jahrsdoerfer RA. The facial nerve in congenital middle ear malformations. *Laryngoscope* 1981;91:1217–1224.
10. Lambert PR. Major congenital ear malformations. *Ann Otol Rhinol Laryngol* 1988;97:641–649.
11. Marx H. Die Missblidungen des Ohres. *Handb Spez Path Anat Hist* 1926;12:620–625.
12. Ombredanne M. Chirugie des surdites congenitales par malformation ossiculaires. *Acta Otorhinolaryngol Belg* 1971;25:837–840.
13. Tucci DL, Ruth RA, Lambert PR. Use of the bone conduction ABR wave I response in determination of cochlear reserve. *Am J Otolaryngol* 1990;11:119–1124.
14. Cole RR, Jahrsdoerfer RA. The risk of cholesteatoma in congenital aural stenosis. *Laryngoscope* 1990;100:576–582.
15. Jahrsdoerfer RA. Reconstruction of the ear canal In: English GM, ed. *Otolaryngology*, Vol. 4. Philadelphia, PA: JB Lippincott, 1990:1–7.
16. Jahrsdoerfer RA, Yeakley JW, Aguilar EA, et al. Grading system for the selection of patients with congenital aural atresia. *Am J Otolaryngol* 1992;13:6–12.

17. Oliver ER, Lambert PR, Rumboldt Z, et al. Middle ear dimensions in congenital aural atresia and hearing outcomes after atresiaplasty. *Otol Neurtol* 2010;31:946–953.

18. Caughey RJ, Jahrsdoerfer RA, Kesser BW. Congenital cholesteatoma in a test of congenital aural atresia. *Otol Neurotol* 2006;27:934–936.

19. Nager GT, Levin LS. Congenital aural atresia: embryology, pathology, classification, genetics, and surgical management. In: Paparella MM, Shumrick D, eds. *Otolaryngology*. Philadelphia, PA: WB Saunders, 1980:1303–1344.

20. Glasscock ME III, Schwaber MK, Nissen AJ, et al. Management of congenital ear malformations. *Ann Otol Rhinol Laryngol* 1983;92:504–509.

21. De la Cruz A, Linthicum FH Jr, Luxford WM. Congenital atresia of the external auditory canal. *Laryngoscope* 1985;95:421–427.

22. Dobratz J, Rastogi A, Jahrsdoerfer RA, et al. Ossiculoplasty in congenital aural atresia surgery. *Laryngoscope* 2008;118:1452–1457.

23. Jahrsdoerfer RA, Cole RR, Gray LC. Advances in congenital aural atresia. In: *Advances in Otolaryngology-Head and Neck Surgery*, Vol. 5. St. Louis, MO: Mosby-Year Book, 1991:1–5.

24. Schuknecht HG. Congenital aural atresia. *Laryngoscope* 1989;99:908–917.

25. Mattox DE, Fisch U. Surgical correction of congenital atresia of the ear. *Otolaryngol Head Neck Surg* 1986;94:574–577.

26. Malony TB, De la Cruz A. Surgical approaches to congenital atresia of the external auditory canal. *Otolaryngol Head Neck Surg* 1990;103:991–1001.

27. Chandrasekhar SS, De la Cruz A. Surgery of congenital aural atresia. *Am J Otol* 1995;16:713–717.

28. De la Cruz A, Teufert KB. Congenital atresia surgery: long term results. *Otolaryngol Head Neck Surg* 2003;129:121–127.

29. Lambert PR. Congenital aural atresia: stability of surgical results. *Laryngoscope* 1998;108:1801–1805.

30. Digoyn, GP, Cueva RA. Congenital aural atresia: review of short- and long-term surgical results. *Otol Neurotol* 2007;28:54–60.

31. Chang SO, Choi BY, Hur GE. Analysis of long term hearing results after surgical repair of aural atresia. *Laryngoscope* 2006;116: 1835–1841.

32. Oliver ER, Hughley BB, Shonka DC, et al. Revision aural atresia surgery: indications and outcomes. *Otol Neurotol* 2011;32: 252–258.

33. De la Cruz A, Teufert KB. Congenital aural atresia surgery: long term results. *Otolaryngol Head Neck Surg* 2003;129:121–127.

34. Teufert, KB, De la Cruz A. Advances in congenital aural atresia surgery: effects on outcome. *Otolaryngol Head Neck Surg* 2004;131:263–270.

35. Jahrsdoerfer RA. Congenital malformation of the ear. *Ann Otol Rhinol Laryngol* 1980;89:348–352.

36. Jahrsdoerfer RA, Hall JW. Congenital malformations of the ear. *Am J Otol* 1986;7:267–269.

37. Jahsdoerfer RA, Lambert PR. Facial nerve injury and congenital aural atresia surgery. *Am J Otol* 1998;19:283–287.

38. Yoon YH, Park JY, Park YH. The preventive effect of mitomycin-C on the external auditory canal fibrosis in an experimentally induced animal model. *Am J Otolaryngol* 2010;31:9–13.

39. Battelino S, Hocevar-Boltezar I, Zargi M. Intraoperative use of mitomycin C in fibrous atresia of the external auditory canal. *Ear Nose Throat J* 2005;84:776–779.

40. Banthia V, Selesnick SH. Mitomycin-C in the postsurgical ear canal. *Otolaryngol Head Neck Surg* 2003;128:882–886.

41. Moody MW, Lang H, Spiess AC, et al. Topical application of mitomycin C to the middle ear is ototoxic in the gerbil. *Otol Neurotol* 2006;27(8):1186–1192.

42. Lustig L, Arts HA, Brackmann D, et al. Hearing rehabilitation using the BAHA bone-anchored hearing aid: results in 40 patients. *Otol Neurotol* 2001;22:328–334.

43. House JW, Cutz JW. Bone-anchored hearing aids: incidence and management of postoperative complications. *Otol Neurotol* 2007;28:213–217.

Intratemporal and Intracranial Complications of Otitis Media

149

H. Alexander Arts   *Meredith E. Adams*

Otitis media (OM) is a heterogeneous disease with a wide spectrum of presentations and natural histories. The etiology, presentation, natural history, and management of acute and chronic otitis media (AOM and COM) are discussed in detail in other chapters. In this chapter, we discuss the complications, both intratemporal and intracranial, of AOM and COM and cholesteatoma, and their management. These complications are summarized in Table 149.1.

AOM is a common infection, estimated to represent up to 5.8% of all patient visits to physicians (1,2). In the vast majority of cases, the pathologic process is self-limited, or resolves with antibiotic therapy. Indeed, although not universally agreed upon, some have recently considered observation alone for straightforward cases of AOM, with antibiotics reserved for refractory cases, or for prevention of complications in higher risk patients (3). AOM may resolve completely, resolve and recur, or evolve into one of many manifestations of COM. Complications of OM can occur directly from AOM or arise from COM. Although these complications are rare today, they occur in developed countries at approximately the same frequency as in underdeveloped countries, and are associated with high rates of serious morbidity and mortality (4). Prompt diagnosis and rapid, effective therapy are critical to minimizing these sequelae.

PATHOPHYSIOLOGY

Pathophysiology of OM

Both AOM and COM are bacterial infections involving the middle ear cleft. Risk factors can be complex and interrelated, but are primarily associated with (a) exposure to pathogens, (b) local anatomy, and (c) host response.

Exposure to pathogens can be increased or altered by exposure to day care environments, or crowded or unhygienic living situations. The specific microbiologic flora is strongly influenced by prior individual and community antibiotic treatment (5). Exposure to nasopharyngeal flora may be enhanced with patent eustachian tubes. In the case of COM, contamination by pathogens can occur via the external auditory canal via a tympanic membrane perforation or by direct contamination of debris within a cholesteatoma. The latter can be enhanced by exposure to water from swimming or bathing. Different pathogens have varying degrees of pathogenicity and disease progression. The bacteriology of OM is summarized in Table 149.2.

The primary anatomic variable affecting the development of OM is eustachian tube function. Eustachian tube function varies widely in otherwise normal individuals, but is reduced in patients with cleft palate, exposure to smoke (smokers and passive exposure), allergic rhinitis, neoplastic processes involving the cranial base, acromegaly, and many other conditions. Abnormally patent eustachian tubes result in reflux of nasopharyngeal contents into the middle ear. Mucosal disease such as nasal polyposis, ciliary dyskinesia, or cystic fibrosis results in reduced eustachian tube function. If a patient develops cholesteatoma, the local anatomy has a direct effect on how the cholesteatoma grows and what bony destruction it causes. The cholesteatoma and associated inflammation can then, in turn, directly or indirectly impact eustachian tube function.

Host response factors such as immunodeficiency, immunization status, ciliary dyskinesia, and history of bottle-feeding also play important roles in the development of OM.

Pathophysiology of Complications of OM

Similar factors influence the development of complications of OM, with the addition of many other variables. It is important to understand the anatomy in which these infections exist, their routes of spread, and the characteristic patterns of disease. Infection can spread via direct extension, via venous structures, or hematogenously. However, the primary pathogenesis seems to be a complex interaction between the specific organisms and the host (8).

TABLE 149.1	COMPLICATIONS OTITIS MEDIA

Intratemporal (extracranial)
  Mastoiditis
    Acute
    Coalescent
    Chronic
    "Masked"
    Associated with subperiosteal abscess
    Associated with deep neck abscess (Bezold abscess)
  Petrositis
  Labyrinthitis
    Serous or toxic
    Suppurative
      Otogenic
      Meningogenic
  Facial paralysis
  Labyrinthine fistula
Intracranial
  Extradural granulation tissue or abscess
  Sigmoid sinus thrombophlebitis
    Occluding
    Nonoccluding
  Brain abscess
  Otitic hydrocephalus
  Meningitis
  Subdural abscess

TABLE 149.2	BACTERIOLOGY OF OM (PATHOGENS LISTED IN ORDER OF PREVALENCE) (6,7)

Acute suppurative OM
  Streptococcus pneumoniae
  Haemophilus influenza (nontypeable)
  Moraxella catarrhalis
  Others (far less common)
    Group A Streptoccoci
    Staphylococcus aureus (infrequent)
    Gram-negative bacilli (infrequent)
Acute mastoiditis
  Streptococcus pneumonia
  Pseudomonas aeruginosa
  Group A beta-hemolytic *Streptoccoci* (e.g., *Streptococcus pyogenes*)
  Coagulase-negative *Staphylococcus* sp.
  Others (far less common)
    Staphylococcus aureus
    Proteus sp.
    Bacteroides sp.
Chronic otorrhea with or without cholesteatoma
  Mixed aerobic (also occasionally including *S. pneumonia*) and anaerobic organisms
    Foul-smelling ears (especially with cholesteatoma) may grow 5–11 organisms, always mixed aerobic and anaerobic
  Pseudomonas aeruginosa (most common aerobe)
  Staphylococcus aureus and *Staphylococcus epidermidis*
  Other aerobic organisms including *Proteus* sp., *Klebsiella* sp., *Escherichia coli*
  Various anaerobic organisms including *Bacteroides fragilis*
Intracranial abscesses (brain and subdural) of otogenic origin (mixed cultures)
  Streptococcus sp.
  Staphylococcus sp.
  Proteus sp.
  Anaerobic organisms (*Peptococcus*, *Peptostreptococcus*, *Bacteroides fragilis*)
Bacterial meningitis in children
  Streptococcus pneumonia
  Haemophilus influenzae, type B
  Neisseria meningitidis

An important host response leading to complication is the production of tissue edema and granulation tissue that subsequently becomes obstructive to drainage and aeration. This creates an environment conducive to the growth of anaerobic organisms and the destruction of bone. Important microbiologic factors seem to pivot about the synergistic pathogenicity of anaerobic organisms (9).

The epidemiology and microbiologic behavior of the organisms found in complications offer some insight into the pathogenesis and pathophysiology of these complications (Table 149.2). For example, infections with *Streptococcus pneumoniae*, nontypeable *Haemophilus influenzae*, and *Moraxella catarrhalis* are the most common causes of acute suppurative OM (3,10). Only about 4% of OM is caused by infection with *H. influenzae* type B; however, pediatric patients with OM occurring simultaneously with meningitis or other central nervous system infections were found to have an unusually high incidence of *H. influenzae* type B (10).

Uncomplicated chronic otorrhea characteristically cultures *Pseudomonas aeruginosa*, *Staphylococcus aureus*, and a variety of other Gram-negative organisms, such as *Proteus* sp., *Klebsiella* sp., and *Escherichia coli*. In contrast, mastoiditis associated with chronic suppurative otitis media (CSOM) frequently has a fetid odor and often cultures positive for *Bacteroides fragilis* (6). Multiple organisms are found in 57% of chronically draining ears with cholesteatoma, with an average of three different organisms. However, if these ears have a fetid discharge, characteristically 5 to 11 organisms are found, always including both anaerobes and aerobes. Malodorous discharge is a significant early sign of complication. Anaerobic organisms are a major cause of foul-smelling discharge.

β-Lactamase-producing organisms, such as *S. aureus*, *H. influenzae*, *B. catarrhalis*, and *Bacteroides* sp., not only survive β-lactam antibiotics but may also protect other potentially penicillin-susceptible pathogens from penicillin and other β-lactam antibiotics. Anaerobic organisms have recently been shown to play major roles in pathogenic synergism by protecting against host defenses, creating suitable environments for other organisms, and inactivating antibiotics (8,9).

Anatomic variables are tremendously important in the development of complications. Eustachian tube function plays a critical role in not only the development of the original infection and its resolution but also the development of complications. The mucosal edema resulting from OM itself impairs eustachian tube function and inhibits resolution of the infection. Highly variable factors, such as the integrity of bone over the facial nerve or dura, influence access of the infection and its products to neurovascular structures and the intracranial space. Numerous venous channels traverse the bone between the mastoid and middle ear and the dural venous sinuses, sometimes associated with arachnoid granulations. Inflammation adjacent to these veins and venules can promote thrombosis. Thrombi and infection can then propagate to the dural venous sinuses and subarachnoid space. Cholesteatoma often results in patterns of bone destruction exposing the dura or facial nerve to the infectious process. Finally, prior surgery can result in areas of entrapped squamous epithelium or deficient areas of bone that act as sources of infection and routes for the infection to spread.

GENERAL PATTERNS OF PRESENTATION

Complications of OM tend to present in predictable patterns (Table 149.3). With the exception of meningitis in children and some cases of facial paralysis, which are usually associated with AOM, most complications tend to be associated with COM. Typically, mastoiditis is the initial complication, with more severe complications developing secondarily. Petrositis (petrous apicitis), for example, almost never occurs without preceding mastoiditis. Labyrinthine fistulae virtually always develop secondary to cholesteatoma. Granulation tissue in air cells adjacent to the sigmoid sinus can result in erosion of the bone overlying the sinus, with resultant sigmoid sinus exposure and possible sigmoid sinus thrombophlebitis. If the sigmoid becomes obstructed with thrombus, intracranial hypertension, that is, otitic hydrocephalus, can result (11). Retrograde thrombophlebitis may extend intracerebrally, resulting in a brain abscess. Subdural empyema rarely occurs due to COM, but is a more typical complication of meningitis in infants.

Without a high index of suspicion, early evidence of an impending complication will be missed. Early symptoms and signs of complication are summarized in Table 149.4. Because antibiotic therapy may have a masking effect on the significant signs and symptoms of complications, a high level of clinical awareness is important for early diagnosis. Persistence of acute symptoms for 2 weeks or more or recurrence of symptoms or infection within 2 weeks is often the first sign of a potential complication. In chronically draining ears, acute exacerbation of pain or the new development of fetid drainage should be evaluated. Foul-smelling drainage that fails to respond to conservative treatment (debridement and topical antibiotics) portends an impending complication.

Once a complication has begun, signs and symptoms typically progress rapidly. Fever associated with COM

TABLE 149.3	PATTERNS OF PRESENTATION OF COMPLICATIONS OF OM

Origin of complication
  Acute infection
    Meningitis—infants and young children
    Meningitis—adults or children with occult CSF leaks
    Facial paralysis—children more commonly
    Labyrinthitis
  Subdural abscess—infants more commonly
  Subacute or chronic infection
    Mastoiditis
    Petrositis
    Facial paralysis
    Labyrinthitis
    Extradural abscess and granulations
    Sigmoid sinus thrombophlebitis
    Brain abscess
    Otitic hydrocephalus
    Meningitis
    Subdural abscess
Patterns of associated diseases and usual sequence
  Mastoiditis or petrositis
    Extradural granulation tissue and/or abscess
    Sigmoid sinus thrombophlebitis
    Brain abscess or otitic hydrocephalus
  Meningitis
    Subdural abscess—infants more commonly

TABLE 149.4	EARLY SIGNS AND SYMPTOMS OF COMPLICATIONS

Impending complication
  Persistence of acute infection for 2 weeks or more
  Recurrence of symptoms within 2 weeks after initial resolution
  Acute exacerbation of chronic infection, especially if foul-smelling
  Foul-smelling discharge during treatment
  Haemophilus influenza type B or anaerobes
Complication (associated complication)
  Fever associated with a chronic perforation (intracranial infection or extracranial cellulitis)
  Pinna displaced inferolaterally and/or edema of the posterosuperior ear canal wall skin (subperiosteal abscess)
  Retro-orbital pain (petrositis)
  Vertigo in a patient with an infected ear (labyrinthitis or labyrinthine fistula)
  Facial paralysis ipsilateral to an infected ear (facial paralysis)
  Headache and lethargy (intracranial complication of any sort)
  Meningismus (meningitis or subdural abscess)
  Focal neurologic signs or seizure (brain abscess)
  Global neurologic signs (subdural abscess or meningitis)

implies some degree of extracranial cellulitis or intracranial infection. Postauricular edema/erythema, edema of the posterior-superior external auditory canal (EAC) wall, or anterolateral displacement of the pinna indicates mastoiditis associated with subperiosteal abscess. Retro-orbital pain in an infected ear is highly suggestive of petrositis (petrous apicitis). Vertigo and nystagmus in a patient with OM may indicate serous or suppurative labyrinthitis, or possibly a labyrinthine fistula. Facial paralysis ipsilateral to an infected ear may complicate AOM, or COM with cholesteatoma. Papilledema is an obvious sign of elevated intracranial pressure, but will go undetected without a fundoscopic examination. Headache and lethargy usually accompany an intracranial infectious complication. Meningismus is associated with meningitis, and focal neurologic signs or seizures are seen in brain abscess.

SPECIFIC COMPLICATIONS

Intratemporal (Extracranial) Complications

Mastoiditis

As commonly used clinically, the term "mastoiditis" is nonspecific and often misleading. Since the mastoid air cell system is confluent with the middle ear space, any inflammatory process within the middle ear will also involve the mastoid. Although it may be pathologically correct to refer to purulent fluid within the mastoid secondary to OM as "mastoiditis," it is not clinically meaningful or helpful, and does not represent a complication of OM. An example of this clinically misleading use of the term "mastoiditis" is the radiologic diagnosis of "mastoiditis" based on the presence of opacification or increased T2 signal intensity alone. This does not imply a complication and does not require additional therapy beyond that indicated for the primary middle ear process. True mastoiditis as a complication of OM implies an invasive or persistent infection involving the mastoid bone and/or surrounding structures, distinct from AOM or OM with effusion. With this in mind, mastoiditis can be subdivided into (a) acute mastoiditis, (b) coalescent mastoiditis, (c) chronic mastoiditis, and (d) masked mastoiditis. Clinically, there is often some overlap between these diagnostic categories.

Acute Mastoiditis

Acute mastoiditis is diagnosed in the presence of postauricular pain, tenderness, erythema, swelling, and/or auricular protrusion, with or without evidence of AOM. Acute mastoiditis is most commonly seen in young children 2 to 6 days following the onset of AOM. Due to partial treatment with antibiotics, signs and symptoms may be much less obvious: antibiotic therapy obscuring the presentation but not the complication. Some authors insist on the presence of AOM for a diagnosis of acute mastoiditis; however, attic blockage may preclude otoscopic visualization (12). Most authors recommend treatment with parenteral

antibiotics, with or without simple mastoidectomy. When treated with parenteral antibiotics alone, up to one-third of patients will require mastoidectomy for failure to improve or complications (13). The most common complication is subperiosteal abscess. Other complications of acute mastoiditis include coalescent mastoiditis, facial paralysis, meningitis, and Bezold abscess. Antibiotic treatment of routine AOM has been shown to be associated with a lower incidence of acute mastoiditis (14).

Coalescent Mastoiditis

Coalescent mastoiditis implies breakdown and decalcification of the bony septa within the mastoid, progressing to bony destruction of the cortex or other aspects of the mastoid bone. Coalescent mastoiditis is what is commonly and classically referred to as "mastoiditis." This infection typically affects boys, 4 years or younger, who have previously well-aerated mastoids and little or no prior history of OM. Coalescence rarely, if ever, occurs in the setting of COM. Patients typically present with fever, otalgia, purulent otorrhea, and mastoid pain, tenderness, erythema, and/or edema. Typically, it occurs in patients who have had persistent otorrhea or otalgia for 2 weeks or more following AOM, or when these symptoms recur 10 to 14 days following AOM. Up to 25% of patients presenting with coalescent mastoiditis will have a concomitant intracranial complication. *S. pneumoniae* is the most common offending organism (15). Of those with a simultaneous intracranial complication, nearly 30% will culture positive for anaerobic organisms as well.

Diagnosis. The diagnosis is confirmed by CT imaging, demonstrating breakdown of bony septa, loss of cortical bone, and opacification of the air cell system. MR imaging should be obtained if there is any suspicion of intracranial complication.

Treatment. Treatment of coalescent mastoiditis consists of myringotomy and intravenous antibiotics, with or without simple mastoidectomy. If mastoidectomy is not performed, intravenous antibiotics should be continued for a minimum of 3 to 6 weeks. Mastoidectomy almost always results in prompt resolution of the infection and its symptoms, and is the safest and most conservative approach.

Chronic Mastoiditis

As used clinically, chronic mastoiditis is a broad term and implies chronic inflammation within the mastoid air cell system. It can occur in typical COM with tympanic membrane perforation, and results in mucosal disease and/or granulation tissue that causes otorrhea to persist in spite of antibiotic therapy. Likewise, persistent mastoid mucosal disease or granulation tissue can be a cause of tympanostomy tube otorrhea refractory to antibiotics. Mastoidectomy in either of these settings can be helpful in eradicating otorrhea. Long-term chronic mastoiditis usually results in sclerosis of the mastoid air cell system, commonly seen in CSOM. A key element in the differential diagnosis of chronic mastoiditis can be skull base osteomyelitis, otherwise known as malignant otitis externa. Malignant otitis externa is classically seen in diabetics or renal failure patients. It usually presents with a several month history of otalgia with or without otorrhea or chronic otitis externa. Focal osteomyelitis is seen adjacent to granulation tissue in the external auditory canal. CT imaging demonstrates bone destruction in the area of osteomyelitis. This topic is discussed more fully elsewhere in this text.

"Masked" Mastoiditis

This term is sometimes applied to the rare situation where granulation or mucosal disease involves some mastoid air cells when there is a normal tympanic membrane and an otherwise aerated middle ear and mastoid air cell system. Other areas of infection and inflammation respond to topical and systemic antibiotics; however, this localized area does not. Osteitis and bone erosion can occur locally at the site of the disease. Patients with masked mastoiditis have chronic mild or moderate postauricular pain and mild postauricular tenderness.

Bezold Abscess

A neck abscess secondary to mastoiditis is called a Bezold abscess. These are, typically in the upper neck, just deep to the sternocleidomastoid muscle. They occur by extension of an infection in the mastoid tip, by osteitis, bone destruction, and direct extension, or without bone erosion by venous propagation. A neck abscess can also occur by suppurated lymph nodes related to mastoid pathology, which is not a true Bezold abscess. Treatment involves surgical drainage of the neck abscess, appropriate surgical management of the temporal bone pathology, and parenteral antibiotics.

Petrositis (Petrous Apicitis)

Petrositis or petrous apicitis is, as the name implies, an infection of the apex of the petrous portion of the temporal bone and is exceptionally rare. The petrous apex is contiguous with the middle ear space, and may be aerated, sclerotic, or consist of diploic bone. Infection occurs in the petrous apex by direct extension from the middle ear and, like in the mastoid, can consist of mucosal disease, granulation tissue, purulence, or coalescence. Petrous apicitis may be associated with any of the other complications of OM. Due to its location, extension of infection from the apex may also result in cavernous sinus thrombophlebitis.

Petrous apicitis typically presents with deep, retro-orbital pain in the setting of COM. The classic triad originally described by Gradenigo consists of retro-orbital pain, otorrhea, and abducens palsy, although abducens palsy is rarely seen (16). Other manifestations can include facial paralysis, and sensory hearing loss and vertigo due to labyrinthitis.

CT imaging, with or without MR imaging, defines the nature and location of the disease (17). Treatment consists of parenteral antibiotics and surgical drainage (18). Surgical access to the petrous apex is difficult, and the route taken depends on the highly variable nature of temporal bone anatomy. Depending on the specific anatomy, access to the petrous apex may be obtained via the retrolabyrinthine, infracochlear, or subarcuate air cell tracts. In some cases, it may be necessary to perform a canal wall down mastoidectomy or possibly a middle cranial fossa approach to access this area (19).

Labyrinthine Fistula

Labyrinthine fistula consists of the erosive loss of otic capsule bone with exposure of the interior of the labyrinth (20). These fistulae occur almost exclusively secondary to cholesteatoma. The matrix of the cholesteatoma covers the exposed perilymphatic space; therefore, there is no leakage of perilymph as seen in perilymphatic fistulae. Labyrinthine fistulae from cholesteatoma most commonly involve the horizontal semicircular canal, but can involve any of the canals, the vestibule, the cochlea, or even the internal auditory canal (21). In addition to the bone of the labyrinth, cholesteatoma can erode any bone to which it comes in contact, commonly including the fallopian canal and the tegmen tympani. The mechanism of bone erosion due to cholesteatoma is the subject of considerable investigation and is discussed in other chapters of this text.

Labyrinthine fistula is frequently asymptomatic and only discovered on CT imaging or at surgery. Whenever CT demonstrates a labyrinthine fistula preoperatively, erosion of the fallopian canal or tegmen tympani should also be considered. If symptoms are present, they consist of vertigo with Valsalva or straining, motion- or position-provoked vertigo, Tullio phenomenon (vertigo secondary to auditory stimuli), vertigo with manipulation of the auricle or EAC, and varying degrees of hearing loss. Fistulae are usually clearly delineated on CT, which should always be obtained preoperatively when fistula is a consideration.

Proper management of the underlying cholesteatoma is the basis of treatment of labyrinthine fistula and is discussed elsewhere in this text (20,22,23). In brief, the matrix of the cholesteatoma can be left over the fistula when the cholesteatoma is being exteriorized. If the cholesteatoma is being removed, the matrix must be very carefully dissected from the fistula and the fistula covered with a soft tissue graft. Risks of vestibular dysfunction and hearing loss in this setting are significant. Successful management of labyrinthine fistula usually improves vestibular symptoms.

Facial Nerve Paralysis

After mastoiditis, facial nerve paralysis is the second most common complication of AOM. Less commonly, facial paralysis presents as a complication of COM—virtually always due to cholesteatoma. In either of these settings, the facial paralysis is secondary to neurapraxia. In AOM, this is due to inflammation and edema from the adjacent infection. In COM with cholesteatoma, this is usually due to compression by the cholesteatoma, with or without local inflammation. Facial paralysis can also be associated with coalescent mastoiditis, "masked" mastoiditis, or petrous apicitis.

AOM typically involves the facial nerve in its tympanic segment. Although there is no study clearly demonstrating this, it is thought that most cases of facial paralysis with AOM have dehiscent fallopian canals in the tympanic segment, which is a common finding in otherwise normal temporal bones. When facial paralysis occurs due to cholesteatoma, the site of lesion depends on the anatomy of the cholesteatoma. Most commonly, the nerve is compressed in the tympanic segment, due to bone erosion by the cholesteatoma. Other sites of injury include the geniculate ganglion region (anterior epitympanic cholesteatoma), the mastoid segment (facial recess/sinus tympani/retrofacial cholesteatoma), or the internal auditory canal (superior perilabyrinthine cholesteatoma). Cholesteatoma may not be immediately recognized as the cause of cholesteatoma in these more unusual locations.

Evaluation of facial paralysis associated with OM usually involves directed imaging. Except perhaps in very straightforward cases of facial weakness associated with AOM, dedicated temporal bone CT imaging is very useful and will likely demonstrate the pathology and site of lesion. MR imaging is helpful if lesions other than cholesteatoma are considered. Electrophysiologic facial nerve testing is sometimes useful. Electromyography (EMG), either evoked (electroneuronography) or spontaneous (standard EMG), can be helpful in predicting prognosis for recovery in some cases. This topic is fully discussed elsewhere in this text.

Management of facial paralysis associated with OM consists of aggressive treatment of the underlying OM (24). In AOM, myringotomy with cultures of the aspirate, and parenteral antibiotics are indicated. For facial paralysis due to COM with cholesteatoma, topical and systemic antibiotics followed by surgical management of the cholesteatoma are appropriate. Systemic steroid therapy is probably helpful to reduce inflammation and edema in the acute phases of facial paralysis for any type of OM. Surgical decompression of the fallopian canal, proximal and distal to the site of injury is advocated by some, and may be helpful in selected cases.

Labyrinthitis

Serous or Toxic

Serous labyrinthitis is thought to be due to alteration of the inner ear tissue fluid environment due to bacterial toxins (25). Bacterial toxins are presumed to enter the inner ear via the round or oval window, or via a labyrinthine fistula. Variable degrees of vertigo and sensory hearing loss can result. Treatment with appropriate antibiotics and steroids is probably helpful. Recovery of hearing and vestibular

function is possible in serous labyrinthitis. Endolymphatic hydrops can be seen pathologically associated with serous labyrinthitis.

Suppurative

Otogenic suppurative labyrinthitis consists of bacterial invasion of the inner ear from a suppurative process within the middle ear (25). This acute suppurative process results in rapid destruction of inner ear contents, with associated severe vertigo and sensory hearing loss. In the early phases, it is not possible to discern serous from suppurative labyrinthitis—subsequent recovery of hearing and/or vestibular function indicates that the process was serous in nature. Treatment consists of parenteral antibiotics (choose drugs with good cerebrospinal fluid penetration) and timely surgical intervention aimed at preventing additional extracranial or intracranial complications.

A particular concern with suppurative labyrinthitis is the development of meningitis. A suppurative process within the labyrinth can gain access to the subarachnoid space via the fundus of the cochlea or the cochlear aqueduct. Indeed, otogenic sources are thought to be a common etiology of bacterial meningitis in childhood. Conversely, suppurative meningitis may extend into the labyrinth and result in a secondary suppurative (meningogenic) labyrinthitis. In either direction, this phenomenon underlies the frequent association between meningitis and hearing loss. Ossification of the labyrinth (labyrinthitis ossificans) is frequently seen following suppurative labyrinthitis, particularly due to S. pneumoniae, and can complicate cochlear implantation (26). Early evaluation of hearing following meningitis and early cochlear implantation when appropriate can result in substantially better outcomes for patients with postmeningitic deafness.

Intracranial Complications

Meningitis

Bacterial meningitis presents with severe generalized headache, fever, nausea/vomiting, photophobia, and varying levels of altered mental status (ranging from irritability to unconsciousness). Patients may develop nuchal rigidity, characterized by pain and limitation of neck flexion. With progression of disease, papilledema and abnormal reflexes may develop, including Kernig sign (inability to completely extend the knee when the leg is flexed at the hip) and Brudzinski sign (passive neck forward flexion leads to active flexion of the hip and knee).

The clinician evaluating a patient with meningitis should attempt to identify the route of spread to the meninges and the organism involved. All patients with meningeal signs should undergo otoscopic examination to rule out AOM and CSOM. Most cases of otogenic meningitis in children result from hematogenous dissemination of invasive organisms during AOM (most commonly S. pneumoniae) (27). Of note, the introduction of routine vaccination against

S. pneumoniae and *H. influenzae* type B has decreased the rate of meningitis secondary to these common causative agents—recent reports suggest that brain abscess may supplant meningitis as the most common intracranial complication of OM (28). The presence of otitic meningitis, particularly if recurrent, should raise suspicion for an abnormal route of communication from the middle ear and mastoid to the CSF. The rapid onset of meningitis with AOM in a child with sensorineural hearing loss may indicate the presence of an inner ear malformation that allows communication through the oval or round windows to the vestibule, cochlea, and internal auditory canal. Accordingly, temporal bone imaging may reveal Mondini malformation, enlarged vestibular aqueduct, common cavity malformation, or congenital stapes footplate fixation. Similarly, AOM can lead to rapid onset of meningitis in patients with CSF leaks associated with tegmen dehiscences (congenital or iatrogenic), meningoencephaloceles through the middle or posterior fossae, or through a patent tympanomeningeal fissure (29). Bacterial contamination of the CSF may also occur with AOM following surgical or traumatic dural injury, stapes subluxation, or cochlear implantation (30). Patients with meningitis associated with CSOM should be suspected of having bacterial extension of infecting organisms directly through the dura. Additionally, it is possible for bacteria to enter the meninges through the labyrinth by a cholesteatoma-induced fistula.

Lumbar puncture (LP) is performed to confirm the clinical diagnosis and identify the causative organism. CT or MRI should be obtained first to identify findings suggestive of increased intracranial pressure that might predispose to herniation with LP as well as to rule out intracranial abscess, subdural empyema, or cerebritis. Meningitis typically leads to elevation of the opening pressure, and the CSF has high protein, low glucose, and an increased white blood cell content leading to a cloudy appearance. The CSF should be sent for Gram stain and culture. As cultures from the CSF and middle ear may differ, samples should also be taken at the time of myringotomy to assist in selection of antibiotic therapy. High-resolution CT of the temporal bone will delineate bony architecture and reveal inner ear malformations, tegmen defects, and destructive lesions. MRI should be obtained in all cases to identify additional intracranial complications.

Acute bacterial meningitis associated with AOM is treated with myringotomy (wide-field or with PE tube placement to maintain drainage) and intravenous antibiotics. A third-generation cephalosporin and vancomycin should be instituted empirically while awaiting culture results that will direct further therapy (31). Despite effective antibiotic treatment, about one-third of meningitis survivors suffer neurologic sequelae such as deafness, behavioral disorders, and cognitive dysfunction (32). Dexamethasone, started with or before the first dose of antibiotics, has been shown to significantly reduce the rates of death and hearing loss in patients with pneumococcal meningitis,

without interfering with antimicrobial treatment (33). While most cases do not require further surgery, inner ear malformations (Mondini) and clear sources of CSF leakage (meningoencephalocele) require repair at the conclusion of meningitis treatment to prevent further infection. Continuation of antibiotics in the perioperative period is wise in these instances.

When meningitis results from subacute or CSOM, the ear disease needs to be surgically managed. Direct disease extension into the meninges has often occurred and it is important to expose the diseased dura, remove excess dural granulation tissue, and inspect for dural defects or occult abscesses. The timing of the mastoid operation is dictated by the patient's neurologic and physiologic condition, and is generally performed once the patient is deemed stable to undergo surgery.

Extradural (Epidural) Granulation Tissue or Abscess

Granulation tissue and abscess may form between the temporal bone and adjacent dura when acute coalescent infection or chronic otitis with or without cholesteatoma erode surrounding bone. Pockets of infection then expand along the face of the posterior or middle fossae. Epidural granulation tissue and abscesses may present with headache and fever, but are often clinically silent until large (34). Contrast-enhanced CT may reveal erosion of the sigmoid plate or tegmen and, in cases of larger extradural abscesses, a rim-enhancing lentiform epidural fluid collection. Enhanced MRI is superior to CT in demonstrating small intracranial suppurative lesions. An epidural abscess appears as a crescentic fluid collection that is mildly hyperintense relative to CSF on T1-weighted images and isointense to CSF on T2-weighted images (35). Epidural abscess is often a precursor to other complications that can be identified with MRI including lateral sinus thrombophlebitis and brain abscess.

Management of extradural granulation tissue and abscess begins with intraoperative identification. Extradural abscesses may be missed unless care is taken to observe the dura of the middle and posterior fossae through thin bone. The mastoidectomy should be extended to allow for careful inspection of the dura of the tegmen tympani, tegmen mastoideum, sigmoid sinus, and posterior fossa bone medial to Trautmann triangle. Bone overlying abnormal dura should be removed until normal dura is encountered. Granulation tissue may be carefully removed with a blunt elevator, scraping parallel to the plane of the dura. A portion of granulation tissue may be left behind to avoid dural penetration and CSF contamination. If an abscess is identified, exposure via removal of the overlying bone suffices for drainage.

Brain Abscess

Otogenic brain abscesses may arise from AOM or COM. Cholesteatoma has supplanted AOM as the cause of most cases (36). The infection is typically polymicrobial with a relatively high proportion of anaerobes (37). Venous thrombophlebitis allows bacteria to spread from the mastoid to the brain parenchyma.

A brain abscess has four clinical stages (38). The first stage is invasion (initial cerebritis), during which the destructive brain infection may present with a low-grade fever, malaise, drowsiness, loss of ability to concentrate, and headache. These symptoms are subtle and frequently overlooked and may spontaneously resolve after several days. The second stage, localization (latent or quiescent abscess), when the tissue becomes necrotic and edematous, may be clinically silent and last for weeks. During the third stage, enlargement (manifest abscess), an actual abscess forms in the region of the previous cerebritis. Patients may present with high fever, headache, focal neurologic symptoms, or loss of consciousness. Abscesses of the temporal lobe may present with seizures, visual field deficits, and hemiparesis. Cerebellar abscesses may present with vertigo, nystagmus, ataxia, and dysmetria. In the fourth stage, termination (rupture of the abscess), the abscess capsule ruptures into the ventricle or into the subarachnoid space. This results in a rapidly progressive, frequently fatal, outcome.

Diagnosing a brain abscess at an early stage may be difficult and calls for a high level of clinical suspicion when confronted with signs of a possible impending complication (Table 149.4). CT and MRI with gadolinium will identify a hypointense center with a hyperintense capsule about a formed abscess. MRI offers additional precision in identifying extraparenchymal (intraventricular or subarachnoid) spread. Diffusion-weighted MR imaging may be used for abscess surveillance and to distinguish abscesses from ring-enhancing malignancies (39). Since brain abscesses can take several weeks to manifest, even if an initial MRI is negative, repeat scanning should be considered in 2 to 3 week intervals if the index of suspicion remains high.

Management of a brain abscess requires immediate broad-spectrum parenteral antimicrobial therapy and neurosurgical consultation. If surgical treatment of the brain abscess is recommended, it takes priority over management of the otologic disease. A surgical approach to treat the ear disease can be undertaken once neurologic stability has been achieved with antibiotics, aspiration, open drainage, or abscess excision.

Subdural Empyema

Subdural empyema is a purulent infection that has formed between the dura and the pia–arachnoid membranes. The subdural space may be seeded via venous channels or infection in adjacent bone or brain. It is the rarest complication of OM. Because of the mass effect and the close proximity to the cerebral cortex, symptoms progress rapidly and patients present with severe headache, marked focal neurologic deficits, seizures, and loss of consciousness. Meningeal signs are pronounced.

CT with intravenous contrast may miss early subdural abscesses but can detect larger lesions as hypodense extracerebral collections with an enhancing medial border. Contrast-enhanced MRI is more sensitive and may readily demarcate the enhancing rim and extension of infection (40). Lumbar puncture may precipitate herniation in this setting and should be avoided if the lesion is detected by imaging first.

Subdural empyema is a neurosurgical emergency. Treatment of subdural abscess requires emergent drainage and the institution of parenteral antibiotics. Treatment of the associated ear disease is accomplished after neurologic stabilization.

Sigmoid Sinus Thrombophlebitis

Sinus thrombophlebitis may develop when overlying coalescent infection, granulation tissue, or cholesteatoma incites sinus wall inflammation. The sigmoid sinus is most susceptible because of its prominent location adjacent to the mastoid air cells. Retrograde thrombosis of cerebral veins (Labbé) and sinuses (transverse, sagittal, petrosal, and cavernous) may result in dangerous degrees of intracranial hypertension, brain abscess, infarct, and death (41). The thrombus may propagate to the internal jugular vein and jugular bulb, generating septic emboli and/or a jugular foramen syndrome. While AOM remains a common inciting factor in children, COM with cholesteatoma is an increasingly frequent cause in adults and older pediatric populations. Prothrombotic factors, including elevated levels of lipoprotein apolipoprotein, antibodies to beta 2-glycoprotein and cardiolipin, and heterozygosity for factor V Leiden mutation, may predispose patients to sigmoid sinus thrombophlebitis during AOM (42).

Modern antibiotic therapy has decreased the incidence of sigmoid sinus thrombosis (43) and altered the typical clinical presentation. In regions and circumstances in which AOM and COM go untreated, sigmoid sinus thrombosis may present with the rapid onset of prominent otologic symptoms (otorrhea, otalgia, postauricular pain/erythema), severe headache, torticollis, and the classic high-spiking "picket fence" fever of sepsis with leukocytosis (44–46). When there is greater access to care, patients often have a history of AOM or COM that was treated with antibiotics in preceding weeks and may have only mild symptoms. Headache and unilateral neck pain are still common, but fevers may be low grade and leukocytosis may be absent. The symptom duration is longer (often more than 2 weeks) and neurologic symptoms are more prevalent, including diplopia from CN VI palsy and symptoms of intracranial hypertension (headache, nausea, neck stiffness, photophobia, dizziness/ataxia) (46,47). Nevertheless, the otoscopic examination is usually abnormal, revealing AOM, effusion, retraction, or signs of COM. Recent series demonstrate that bacteriology may diverge from beta-hemolytic *Streptococcus* and *S. pneumoniae* to include mixed infections with *Pseudomonas*, *Staphylococcus*, (including MRSA), *H. influenza*, *Klebsiella*, *Enterococcus*, *Proteus*, and anaerobes (46,48,49).

After a careful otologic examination, the diagnosis is confirmed with imaging studies. Head and temporal bone CT, with contrast, will reveal associated pathology in the mastoid and perisinus enhancement. The enhancement of the triangular sinus wall around nonenhancing intraluminal thrombus produces the pathognomonic "delta sign" in up to one-third of cases (49). MRI with MRV/MRA is more sensitive in detecting sigmoid sinus thrombosis and delineates the extent of the thrombus and the integrity of collateral circulation while also identifying other intracranial complications (49).

The treatment of lateral sinus thrombophlebitis entails prompt initiation of broad-spectrum antibiotics combined with surgery. A wide myringotomy is performed or a pressure equalization tube is placed. Mastoidectomy is performed to expose the inflamed sinus wall and diseased dura and to remove excess granulation tissue. Subperiosteal and epidural abscesses can be treated concomitantly. The opinions of experienced surgeons differ over the extent of additional surgery that is necessary, ranging from none to sinus resection (49). The bone over the sinus and surrounding dura may be removed and the sinus may be carefully aspirated to detect free blood flow. Venotomy may be performed for the evacuation of infected thrombus or intraluminal abscess. Some have advocated Fogarty catheter thrombectomy be used with caution to reestablish flow, after gaining control of the internal jugular (IJ) vein in the neck. The authors consider this unwise due to the potential of releasing emboli and rupturing the sinus intracranially. Ligation of the IJ may be considered in the presence of septic emboli. Recanalization has been observed in patients receiving a range of treatments, from nonsurgical medical management, mastoidectomy, and venotomy with or without thrombectomy. Currently, there is no clear evidence that a given treatment approach is superior to another in its ability to reduce recovery time and increase the likelihood of recanalization (50).

The use of anticoagulation to prevent thrombus propagation is also a matter of debate. It is unlikely to be of benefit when the thrombus is isolated to the sigmoid sinus, but it should be considered in patients with imaging evidence of thrombus progression or extension to additional sinuses, neurologic changes, embolic events, or persistent fevers despite surgical intervention (51). The risk of bleeding can be significant, particularly in the pediatric population. Thrombolytics are not recommended as they may dislodge septic emboli in infected vessel walls.

Otitic Hydrocephalus

Otitic hydrocephalus is defined as increased intracranial pressure without ventricular dilatation, meningitis, or intracranial abscess in patients with acute or chronic middle ear infection. Increased intracranial pressure may manifest with headache, nausea and vomiting, papilledema, and diplopia from ipsilateral abducens nerve (cranial nerve VI) palsy.

The etiology of otitic hydrocephalus is hypothesized to be diminished CSF resorption by arachnoid granulations secondary to thrombosis in a dominant lateral dural venous sinus (50,52). Modern imaging has demonstrated that sagittal sinus thrombosis is not a necessary precursor, but inadequate cross-communication at the torcula with occlusion of the dominant outflow tract may impair venous drainage sufficiently to raise intracranial pressure (47,52).

MRI with MRV readily identifies lateral sinus thrombosis with total occlusion. If lumbar puncture is deemed safe based on central imaging, opening pressure will be elevated, but CSF studies will reveal normal biochemistry and cytology. Patients should undergo neuro-opthalmologic examination.

Treatment of otitic hydrocephalus requires mastoidectomy appropriate for the disease, exposure of all diseased dura to normal dura, and removal of excess extradural granulation tissue. Management of sigmoid sinus thrombophlebitis is discussed above. The treatment additionally involves medically lowering intracranial hypertension and careful monitoring for reductions in visual fields and visual acuity. Initial therapy may include corticosteroids, acetazolamide, mannitol, furosemide, and/or repeat lumbar puncture. As resolution of symptoms is observed in patients even in the setting of persistent lateral sinus thrombosis, recovery from otitic hydrocephalus is purported to be secondary to development of compensatory collateral venous drainage (50,52). Thus, management often extends for months beyond the initial surgical approach to the sinus and ventriculoperitoneal shunts may be necessary to reduce intracranial hypertension on a long-term basis. Failure of these measures to reverse progressive visual deterioration necessitates fenestration of the optic nerve sheath (53).

HIGHLIGHTS

- Intratemporal (extracranial) complications of OM include
  - Mastoiditis (acute, coalescent, chronic, or "masked")
    - With or without subperiosteal abscess or Bezold abscess
  - Petrositis
  - Labyrinthitis
  - Facial paralysis
  - Labyrinthine fistula
- Intracranial complications of OM include
  - Extradural granulation tissue and/or abscess
  - Sigmoid sinus thrombophlebitis
  - Brain abscess
  - Otitic hydrocephalus
  - Meningitis
  - Subdural abscess

- Important clinical signs of impending complications include the persistence or recurrence of acute infection within 2 weeks of treatment, or the persistence of foul-smelling discharge despite treatment.
- Persistent low-intensity pain of 1 week's duration during specific antibiotic treatment for suppurative OM suggests the diagnosis of "masked mastoiditis."
- Retro-orbital pain during ear infection, a key sign of petrositis, is not always volunteered in the patient's history and must be specifically elicited.
- Extradural granulation tissue over the sigmoid sinus is predictable in mastoiditis and the key to three additional intracranial complications (sigmoid sinus thrombophlebitis, brain abscess, and otitic hydrocephalus).
- Anaerobic organisms are frequently found in masked mastoiditis or mastoiditis with subperiosteal abscess and are not found in AOM.
- The organism associated with AOM that most frequently causes meningitis is *S. pneumoniae.*
- *Streptococcus faecalis, Proteus* sp., and *B. fragilis* are the organisms most frequently found in brain abscesses.
- *Pseudomonas aeruginosa, Bacteroides* sp., and anaerobic streptococci are most commonly found in association with cholesteatoma.
- The absence of, or resolution of, a subperiosteal abscess may allow a serious intracranial complication to develop because of an unrecognized and undertreated mastoiditis.
- Proper surgical care of most intracranial and intratemporal complications requires visualization through thin bone or actual exposure of the dura of the middle cranial fossa and sigmoid sinus. Failure to do this can result in misdiagnosis and undertreatment of serous intracranial complications.
- A call to see a patient with peripheral vertigo, nystagmus, and hearing loss is a true emergency until it is established that the middle ear is normal.

REFERENCES

1. Levy C, Thollot F, Corrard F, et al. Otite moyenne aiguë en pédiatrie ambulatoire: caractéristiques épidémiologiques et cliniques après l'introduction du vaccin antpneumococcique conjugué 7 valent (PCV7). *Archives de Pédiatrie* 2011;18(6):712–718.
2. Pukander J. The demand for and cost of medical services related to acute otitis media. *Acta Otolaryngol Suppl (Stockh)* 1982;386:124–126.
3. Coker TR, Chan LS, Newberry SJ, et al. Diagnosis, microbial epidemiology, and antibiotic treatment of acute otitis media in children: a systematic review. *JAMA* 2010;304(19):2161–2169.
4. Greenberg JS, Manolidis S. High incidence of complications encountered in chronic otitis media surgery in a U.S. Metropolitan Public Hospital. *Otolaryngol Head Neck Surg* 2001;125(6):623–627.
5. Pelton SI, Leibovitz E. Recent advances in otitis media. *Pediatr Infect Dis J* 2009;28(10):S133–S137. doi:10.1097/INF.0b013e3181b6d81a.
6. Fairbanks D. *Antimicrobial therapy in otolaryngology—head and neck surgery,* 136th ed. Alexandria, VA: American Academy of Otolaryngology—Head & Neck Surgery, 2007.
7. Choi SS, Lander L. Pediatric acute mastoiditis in the post-pneumococcal conjugate vaccine era. *Laryngoscope* 2011;121(5): 1072–1080.
8. Relman D, Falkow S. A molecular perspective of microbial pathogenicity. In: Mandell G, Bennett J, Dolin R, eds. *Mandell, Douglas, and Bennett's principles and practice of infectious diseases.* Edinburgh, UK: Churchill Livingstone, 2009.
9. Cohen-Poradosu R, Kasper D. Anaerobic infections: general concepts. In: Mandell G, Bennett J, Dolin R, eds. *Mandell, Douglas, and Bennett's principles and practice of infectious diseases.* Edinburgh, UK: Churchill Livingstone, 2009.
10. Bluestone C. Clinical course, complications and sequelae of acute otitis media. *Pediatr Infect Dis J* 2000;19(5):S37–S46.
11. Agarwal A,Lowry P, Isaacson G. Natural history of sigmoid sinus thrombosis. *Ann Otol Rhinol Laryngol* 2003;112(2):191–194.
12. Quesnel S, Nguyen M, Pierrot S, et al. Acute mastoiditis in children: a retrospective study of 188 patients. *Int J Pediatr Otorhinolaryngol* 2010;74(12):1388–1392.
13. Luntz M, Brodsky A, Nusem S, et al. Acute mastoiditis—the antibiotic era: a multicenter study. *Int J Pediatr Otorhinolaryngol* 2001;57(1):1–9.
14. Van Zuijlan D, Schilder A, Van Balen F, et al. National differences in incidence of acute mastoiditis: relationship to prescribing patterns of antibiotics for acute otitis media? *Pediatr Infect Dis J* 2001;20(2):140–144.
15. Zevallos JP, Vrabec JT, Williamson RA, et al. Advanced pediatric mastoiditis with and without intracranial complications. *Laryngoscope* 2009;119(8):1610–1615.
16. American Academy of Pediatrics Subcommittee on Management of Acute Otitis Media. Diagnosis and management of acute otitis media. *Pediatrics* 2004;113:1451.
17. Hardjasudarma M. Magnetic resonance imaging features of Gradenigo's syndrome. *Am J Otolaryngol* 1995;16(4):247–250.
18. Wanna GB. Contemporary management of intracranial complications of otitis media. *Otol Neurotol* 2010;31(1):111–117.
19. Visosky AMB, Isaacson B, Oghalai JS. Circumferential petrosectomy for petrous apicitis and cranial base osteomyelitis. *Otol Neurotol* 2006;27(7):1003–1013. doi: 10.97/01.mao.0000233811.41177.48.
20. Parisier SC. Management of labyrinthine fistulas caused by cholesteatoma. *Otolaryngol Head Neck Surg* 1991;104(1):110–115.
21. Nakagawa T. Cholesteatoma extending into the internal auditory meatus. *Eur Arch Otorhinolaryngol* 1999;256(Suppl 1):S15–S17.
22. Copeland BJ. Management of labyrinthine fistulae in chronic ear surgery. *Am J Otolaryngol* 2003;24(1):51–60.
23. Ueda Y. Surgical treatment of labyrinthine fistula in patients with cholesteatoma. *J Laryngol Otol* 2009;123(Suppl 31):64–67.
24. Quaranta N, Cassano M, Quaranta A. Facial paralysis associated with cholesteatoma: a review of 13 cases. *Otol Neurotol* 2007;28(3):405–407.
25. Merchant S, Nadol J. *Schuknecht's pathology of the ear,* 3th ed. Shelton, CT: People's Medical Publishing House - USA, 2010.
26. Durisin M. Cochlear osteoneogenesis after meningitis in cochlear implant patients: a retrospective analysis. *Otol Neurotol* 2010;31(7):1072–1078.
27. Gower D, McGuirt WF. Intracranial complications of acute and chronic infectious ear disease: a problem still with us. *Laryngoscope* 1983;93(8):1028–1033.
28. Isaacson B, Mirabal C, Kutz JW Jr, et al. Pediatric otogenic intracranial abscesses. *Otolaryngol Head Neck Surg* 2010;142(3):434–437.
29. Neely JG. Classification of spontaneous cerebrospinal fluid middle ear effusion: review of forty-nine cases. *Otolaryngol Head Neck Surg* 1985;93(5):625–634.
30. Rubin LG, Papsin B. Cochlear implants in children: surgical site infections and prevention and treatment of acute otitis media and meningitis. *Pediatrics* 2010;126(2):381–391.
31. van de Beek D, de Gans J, Tunkel AR, et al. Community-acquired bacterial meningitis in adults. *N Engl J Med* 2006;354(1):44–53.
32. Rajasingham CR, Bonsu BK, Chapman JI, et al. Serious neurologic sequelae in cases of meningitis arising from infection by conjugate vaccine-related and nonvaccine-related serogroups of *Streptococcus pneumoniae. Pediatr Infect Dis J* 2008;27(9):771–775.

33. Brouwer MC, Heckenberg SG, de Gans J, et al. Nationwide implementation of adjunctive dexamethasone therapy for pneumococcal meningitis. *Neurology* 2010;75(17):1533–1539.

34. Greenberg JS, Manolidis S. High incidence of complications encountered in chronic otitis media surgery in a U.S. metropolitan public hospital. *Otolaryngol Head Neck Surg* 2001;125(6): 623–627.

35. Weingarten K, Zimmerman RD, Becker RD, et al. Subdural and epidural empyemas: MR imaging. *AJR Am J Roentgenol* 1989;152(3):615–621.

36. Sennaroglu L, Sozeri B. Otogenic brain abscess: review of 41 cases. *Otolaryngol Head Neck Surg* 2000;123(6):751–755.

37. Tandon S, Beasley N, Swift AC. Changing trends in intracranial abscesses secondary to ear and sinus disease. *J Laryngol Otol* 2009;123(3):283–288.

38. Proctor CA. Intracranial complications of otitic origin. *Laryngoscope* 1966;76(2):288–308.

39. Leuthardt EC, Wippold FJ II, Oswood MC, et al. Diffusion-weighted MR imaging in the preoperative assessment of brain abscesses. *Surg Neurol* 2002;58(6):395–402; discussion 402.

40. Komori H, Takagishi T, Otaki E, et al. The efficacy of MR imaging in subdural empyema. *Brain Dev* 1992;14(2):123–125.

41. Ozer E, Sivasli E, Bayazit YA, et al. Otogenic cerebral venous infarction: a rare complication of acute otitis media. *Int J Pediatr Otorhinolaryngol* 2003;67(9):1019–1021.

42. Oestreicher-Kedem Y, Raveh E, Kornreich L, et al. Prothrombotic factors in children with otitis media and sinus thrombosis. *Laryngoscope* 2004;114(1):90–95.

43. Teichgraeber JF, Per-Lee JH, Turner JS Jr. Lateral sinus thrombosis: a modern perspective. *Laryngoscope* 1982;92(7 Pt 1):744–751.

44. Samuel J, Fernandes CM. Lateral sinus thrombosis (a review of 45 cases). *J Laryngol Otol* 1987;101(12):1227–1229.

45. Seven H, Ozbal AE, Turgut S. Management of otogenic lateral sinus thrombosis. *Am J Otolaryngol* 2004;25(5):329–333.

46. Bales CB, Sobol S, Wetmore R, et al. Lateral sinus thrombosis as a complication of otitis media: 10-year experience at the children's hospital of Philadelphia. *Pediatrics* 2009;123(2):709–713.

47. Koitschev A, Simon C, Lowenheim H, et al. Delayed otogenic hydrocephalus after acute otitis media in pediatric patients: the changing presentation of a serious otologic complication. *Acta Otolaryngol* 2005;125(11):1230–1235.

48. Ooi EH, Hilton M, Hunter G. Management of lateral sinus thrombosis: update and literature review. *J Laryngol Otol* 2003;117(12):932–939.

49. Manolidis S, Kutz JW Jr. Diagnosis and management of lateral sinus thrombosis. *Otol Neurotol* 2005;26(5):1045–1051.

50. Neilan RE, Isaacson B, Kutz JW Jr, et al. Pediatric otogenic lateral sinus thrombosis recanalization. *Int J Pediatr Otorhinolaryngol* 2011;75(6):850–853.

51. Bradley DT, Hashisaki GT, Mason JC. Otogenic sigmoid sinus thrombosis: what is the role of anticoagulation? *Laryngoscope* 2002;112(10):1726–1729.

52. Doyle KJ, Brackmann DE, House JR III. Pathogenesis of otitic hydrocephalus: clinical evidence in support of Symonds' (1937) theory. *Otolaryngol Head Neck Surg* 1994;111(3 Pt 1):323–327.

53. Friedman DI, Jacobson DM. Idiopathic intracranial hypertension. *J Neuroophthalmol* 2004;24(2):138–145.

150 Middle Ear and Temporal Bone Trauma

Rodney C. Diaz Sally M. Kamal Hilary A. Brodie

Temporal bone trauma can result in significant morbidity and, rarely, mortality. The temporal bone houses or encapsulates many important structures, all of which are at risk of injury with trauma to the temporal bone; these include the facial nerve, vestibulocochlear nerve, cochlea and labyrinth, ossicular chain, tympanic membrane, external auditory canal, temporomandibular joint, lower cranial nerves, jugular vein, and carotid artery. Damage to each anatomic structure can lead to distinctive long- and short-term sequelae.

Adjacent intracranial structures such as the temporal lobe and meninges, abducens nerve, and brainstem may also be injured with temporal bone fracture. Fracture of the temporal bone can expose intracranial contents to the external world, resulting in cerebrospinal fluid (CSF) fistula, meningitis, and brain herniation.

In addition to inducing neurotologic manifestations by direct injury to these structures, temporal bone fractures can have associated intracranial complications such as epidural or subdural hematomas, intraparenchymal contusion or hemorrhage, cerebral edema, posttraumatic encephalopathy, and elevated intracranial pressure. Neurotologic symptoms can also result from shearing strain within the brain tissue with disruption of vessels, axons, dendrites, and synapses (1).

EPIDEMIOLOGY

Injury to the lateral skull has increased with the advent of modern technology; the leading cause of temporal bone fracture is involvement in motor vehicle accidents (2). In the past, 75% of motor vehicle accidents resulted in a head injury. The increased utilization of seat belts and the advent of frontal and side curtain airbags may, however, alter these statistics in the future. When the head trauma is of sufficient magnitude to fracture the skull, 14% to 22% of those injured sustain a temporal bone fracture (3,4). In the largest series of temporal bone fractures reported to date, 31% of the temporal bone fractures in the general population resulted from motor vehicle accidents (2). Assault was the second most common cause, followed by falls and motorcycle accidents. Pedestrian injuries, bicycle accidents, gunshot wounds, all-terrain vehicle accidents, sports injuries, and miscellaneous injuries accounted for a quarter of all cases (2) (Fig. 150.1). The most common injury etiology in temporal bone fractures specific to the pediatric population is equally divided between motor vehicle accidents and falls (between 30% and 60% each) (5–9).

Temporal bone fractures are reported to occur across all age groups with over 70% of fractures occurring in second, third, and fourth decades of life (2). These fractures occur predominantly in males, with a 3:1 to 4:1 ratio of males to females affected (2,10). The predisposition to temporal bone fractures in males is attributed not to an inherent structural weakness of the male skull versus the female skull but rather to biased involvement of males in many of the above at-risk activities. This is evidenced by the fact that head injuries in general also follow a 4:1 male-to-female ratio (10).

In a prospective study of 350 consecutive patients treated for head trauma, 10% were found to have temporal bone fractures on radiographic evaluation using helical CT, whereas only 6% manifested clinical signs of temporal bone fracture on primary evaluation (10). Large retrospective reviews at level I trauma centers have found an incidence of temporal bone fracture in 2% to 4% of consecutive head injury patients (11,12).

Eight to twenty-nine percent of patients with temporal bone fractures sustain them bilaterally (2,10,13,14).

PATHOPHYSIOLOGY

The temporal bones are pyramidal structures in the thick bone of the skull base and consequently require a great force to fracture. Early studies of static loading of the lateral

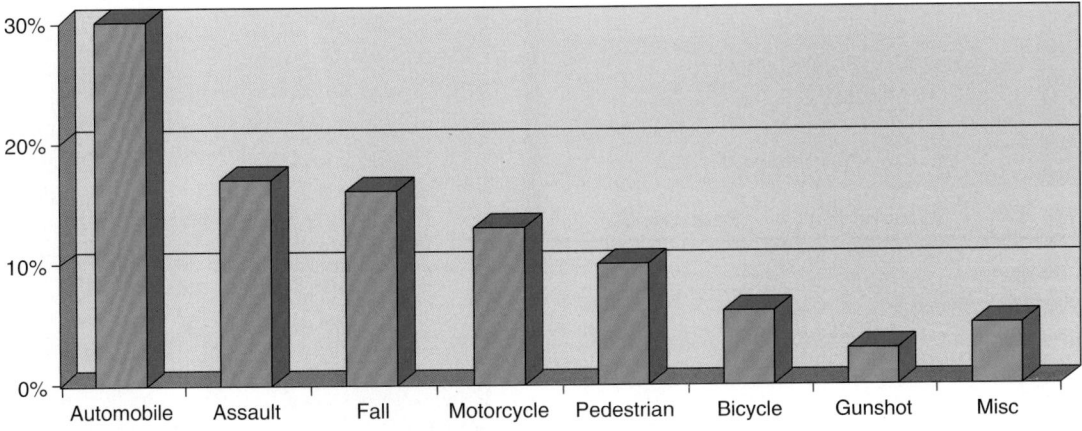

Figure 150.1 Cause of injury.

skull estimated fracture thresholds of 300 to 800 kg (15). More recent dynamic loading studies have estimated the force of lateral impact required to fracture the temporal bones of fresh cadavers at 6,000 to 8,000 N, or approximately 1,300 to 1,800 lb (16,17). Comparison of data from static versus dynamic loading experiments indicates an increase in force tolerance by a factor of two under dynamic loading (18). Such fractures typically take the path of least resistance, which is along structurally weakened points such as the various foramina perforating the skull base.

Sixty percent of temporal bone fractures are categorized as "open" fractures presenting with bloody otorrhea, brain herniation, or CSF draining from the ear canal, eustachian tube, or penetrating wound site (2). These patients are at greater risk for meningitis than those without evidence of an intracranial connection. In addition, those patients with fractures traversing the otic capsule are at even still greater risk of meningitis, sometimes delayed for years or decades, due to an inability of the otic capsule enchondral bone to remodel and heal (19–21). Pollak reported a 51-year-old man who died of meningitis who had suffered an otic capsule–disrupting fracture in childhood (20). The histopathology of his temporal bone revealed pus in the middle ear extending through an unhealed fracture line across the otic capsule. The fracture line contained a loose fibrous tissue. Membranous bone, such as that along the tegmen, has the capability to form callus and heal, whereas the enchondral bone of the otic capsule does not. Fractures through the otic capsule will generally only partially fill with fibrous tissue, although the surface may potentially seal with periosteal bone reaction (20) (Fig. 150.2).

Trauma to the temporal bone often results in one or more neurotologic complications, depending on the severity of injury and type of fracture, and can vary between adult and pediatric populations. Table 150.1 summarizes incidence of common complications of temporal bone fractures in the general and pediatric populations (2,6).

CLASSIFICATION

Temporal bone fractures have traditionally been divided into transverse and longitudinal fractures, based on the relationship of the fracture line to the axis of the petrous ridge (11,22,23). Some authors argue that the majority of fractures are actually oblique as opposed to longitudinal and/or are quite frequently mixed (24,25). This anatomical classification scheme is being replaced with a new structural scheme classifying fractures by whether they disrupt or spare the otic capsule, the bone housing the cochlea and semicircular canals (2,26,27) (Figs. 150.3–150.5).

Fractures that spare the otic capsule typically involve the squamosal portion of the temporal bone and the posterosuperior wall of the external auditory canal. The fracture passes through the mastoid air cells and middle ear and fractures the tegmen mastoideum and tegmen tympani. The fracture proceeds anterolateral to the otic capsule, typically fracturing the tegmen in the region of the facial hiatus. Otic capsule–sparing fractures typically result from a blow to the temporoparietal region.

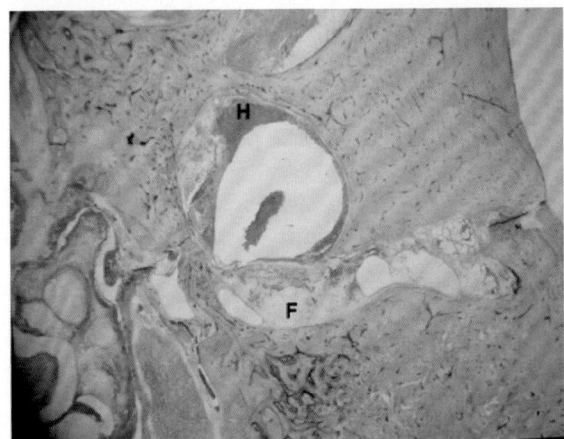

Figure 150.2 Histopathology of a patient who died of meningitis several decades following an otic capsule–disrupting temporal bone fracture. (F, fibrosis with a small amount of ossification within the fracture line in the otic capsule; H, hemorrhage and purulence.)

TABLE 150.1	INCIDENCE OF COMMON COMPLICATIONS OF TEMPORAL BONE FRACTURES IN THE GENERAL AND PEDIATRIC POPULATIONS	
Complication	General (%)	Pediatric (%)
Facial nerve injury	7	6
CSF fistula	17	28
Meningitis	2	0.7
Hearing loss	24	33
Conductive HL	21	43
Sensorineural HL	57	52
Mixed HL	22	5

Otic capsule–disrupting fractures pass through the otic capsule generally proceeding from the foramen magnum across the petrous pyramid and otic capsule. The fracture will often pass through the jugular foramen, internal auditory canal, and foramen lacerum. These fractures do not typically affect the ossicular chain or the external auditory canal (28). Otic capsule–disrupting fractures generally result from blows to the occipital region.

Longitudinal fractures are reported to constitute 70% to 90% of temporal bone fractures with the remaining 10% to 30% categorized as transverse (11,24,26,28–31). In two large series using the newer classification scheme, only 2.5% to 5.8% of fractures disrupted the otic capsule (2,25). This would suggest that many fractures that are oriented perpendicular to the petrous ridge do not actually cross the otic capsule. Many of the otic capsule–disrupting fractures are actually oriented in the longitudinal plane (25).

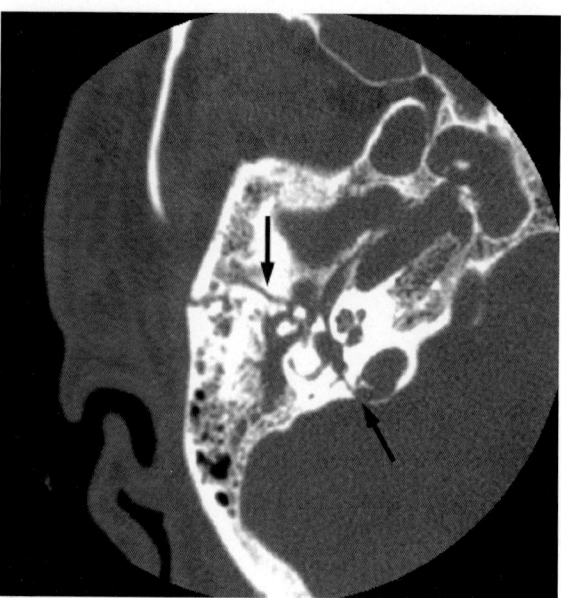

Figure 150.4 Axial bone window CT demonstrates a transverse-oriented fracture, secondary to a motor vehicle accident, disrupting the otic capsule (*arrows*).

The traditional schema of anatomical designation of fracture type was first extensively used in biomechanical studies of cadaveric skull deformation, without correlation to functional outcome (23). In contrast, the newer structural schema underscores the importance of otic capsule involvement in heralding neurotologic sequelae. Otic capsule–disrupting fractures have a much higher incidence of facial nerve paralysis than otic capsule–sparing fractures (30% to 66% vs. 6% to 13%) (2,25,32). In addition, Fisch reported a much higher incidence of nerve disruption in fractures involving the otic capsule (33). There is a two- to tenfold increase in CSF fistula in otic capsule–disrupting fractures as well as a much greater risk of intracranial injuries, compared to otic capsule–sparing fractures (2,25,27). Fractures

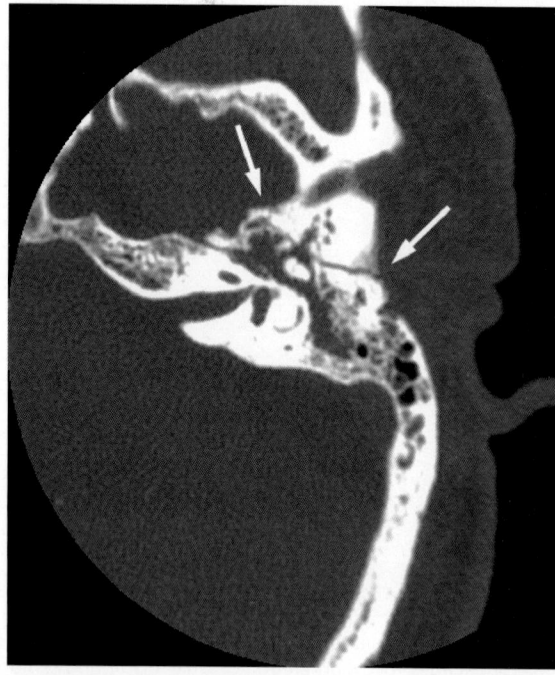

Figure 150.3 Axial bone window CT demonstrates a longitudinally oriented fracture (*arrows*) sparing the otic capsule.

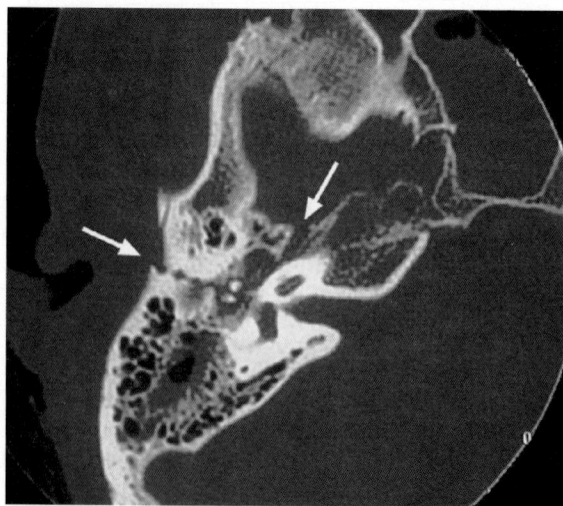

Figure 150.5 Axial bone window CT demonstrates a mixed fracture (*arrows*) that spares the otic capsule.

that disrupt the otic capsule will almost always result in a sensorineural hearing loss, although there are reported exceptions to the rule (34). Hearing loss in otic capsule–sparing fractures tends to be conductive or mixed (2,27). Historically, sensorineural hearing loss has been associated with transverse rather than longitudinal fracture type, but in a recent study, this correlation was not borne out but rather inverted: longitudinal fractures were three times as likely to be associated with sensorineural hearing loss as were transverse fractures (27). This study demonstrated a statistically significant difference in complication rates involving facial nerve injury, CSF fistula, and conductive hearing loss when 155 temporal bone fractures were categorized with the structural schema of otic capsule–sparing versus otic capsule–disrupting fracture types, while concurrently demonstrating no statistical significance when using the traditional classification schema of longitudinal versus transverse fracture types. A recent review of 30 temporal bones supported these findings and noted that otic capsule–disrupting fractures were five times more likely to have facial nerve injury, 25 times more likely to have sensorineural hearing loss, and 8 times more likely to have CSF leak (32).

The newer classification scheme emphasizes functional outcome and better prognosticates those temporal bone fractures that will exhibit neurotologic manifestations. In addition to the predictive value for various complications and comorbidities, categorization of fractures into otic capsule–sparing and otic capsule–disrupting injuries guides the indications for surgical intervention for CSF fistula and facial paralysis as well as the surgical approach to be utilized in their repair.

EVALUATION

It is uncommon for temporal bone fractures to occur in isolation of other bodily injury, and consequently the initial evaluation and management is focused on the urgent life-threatening issues of securing an airway, controlling hemorrhage, evaluating the neurologic status, and stabilizing and evaluating the cervical spine. Following or concurrent with this evaluation, the neurotologic exam is performed. It is extremely important to assess facial nerve function in the emergency room as early as possible, prior to the administration of muscle relaxants, as will be discussed below. The ear exam focuses on the condition of the auricle, ear canal, tympanic membrane, and middle ear.

Clinical Evaluation

The auricles are inspected for lacerations and hematomas. Lacerations are closed after thorough cleaning and debridement of exposed cartilage. Hematomas are drained and pressure bolsters are sutured in place to close the dead space and prevent a recollection of blood. Untreated, the auricular hematomas will result in an auricular chondropathy or "cauliflower ear."

Battle sign is seen in the presence of basilar skull fractures, including temporal bone fractures. Extravasation of blood from the mastoid emissary veins leads to ecchymosis over the mastoid bone and mastoid tip. This sign may be present in the initial clinical assessment but more often appears in a delayed fashion days after the injury.

The ear canal is inspected for fractures along the roof, CSF otorrhea, degree of hemorrhage, and the presence of brain herniation. The ear is examined as aseptically as possible. Blood and cerumen in the ear canal should never be debrided with irrigation. Following stabilization in the emergency room and transfer to the ward or intensive care unit, the ear can be more carefully examined with the aid of an operating microscope. Typical findings include fractures along the scutum and roof of the external auditory canal and/or tympanic membrane perforations. Hemotympanum or bloody otorrhea are almost invariably present and are two of the most common signs of temporal bone fracture (Figs. 150.6–150.8).

The integrity of the tympanic membrane is assessed, as is the presence of hemotympanum. Hemotympanum and any associated serous effusion generally resolve spontaneously, with resolution of concomitant conductive hearing loss, within 4 to 6 weeks and simply require observation. Traumatic tympanic membrane perforations generally heal spontaneously as well, and consequently no acute intervention is necessary.

Hearing is initially assessed clinically at the bedside with a progressively louder whispered voice. Tuning fork examination is useful in delineating conductive from sensorineural hearing loss. Pure tone and speech audiometry are not typically necessary in the acute setting and are obtained after the patient is stabilized. However, in the presence of complications of facial paralysis or CSF fistula in which surgical intervention may be necessary,

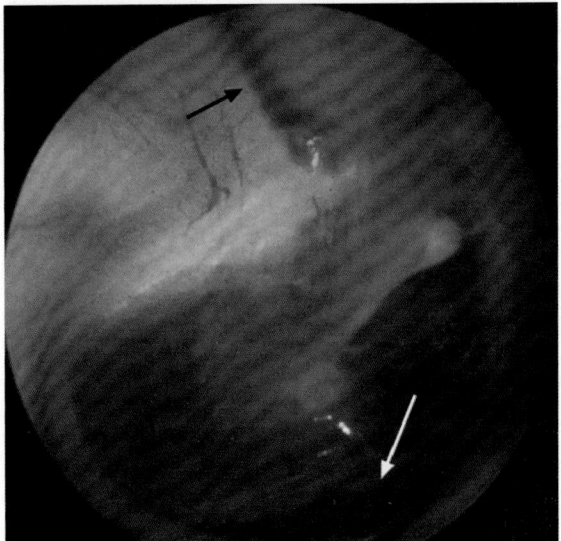

Figure 150.6 Otoscopic image demonstrating a nondisplaced fracture along the scutum (*black arrow*). Blood is layering out inferiorly (*white arrow*).

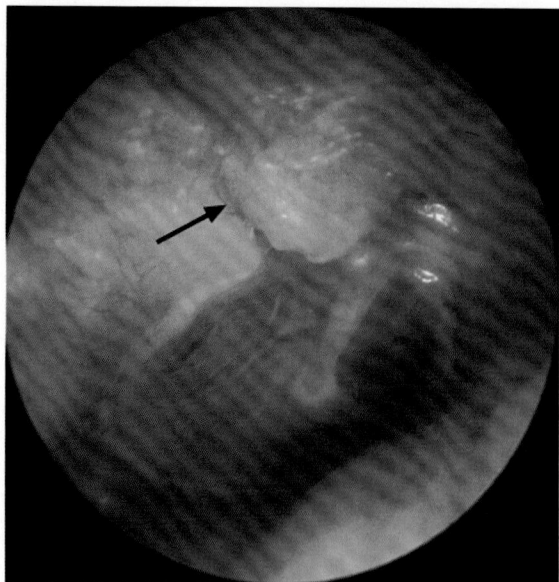

Figure 150.7 Otoscopic image demonstrating a displaced fracture along the scutum (*black arrow*).

preoperative audiometry is necessary as results will dictate the options available for management within the treatment algorithm, as is discussed below.

The neurotologic exam should note the presence or absence of nystagmus as well as the type of nystagmus. Peripheral vertigo generally manifests with horizontal or rotatory nystagmus and is suppressible with visual fixation. Central vertigo may present with vertical or direction-changing nystagmus that fails to suppress and may even enhance with fixation. The most common type of vertigo following head trauma is benign paroxysmal positional vertigo (BPPV) (35). BPPV classically manifests with

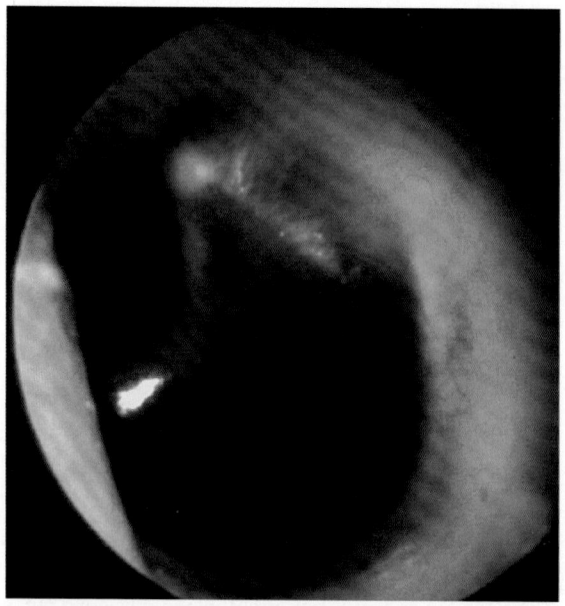

Figure 150.8 Otoscopic image demonstrating a hemotympanum.

latent-onset, transient rotatory nystagmus and concomitant vertigo with the Dix-Hallpike maneuver (35,36). The nystagmus occurs with the affected ear down. There is a 2- to 10-second latency followed by 10 to 30 seconds of rotatory nystagmus in the geotropic direction—that is, with the upper half of the globe rotating in fast phase direction towards the ground. Upon returning to an upright sitting position, a second bout of vertigo with nystagmus in the counterrotatory direction is often seen. The nystagmus is fixed in direction and is fatigable with repeated maneuvers. In contrast, central positional vertigo induces direction-changing nystagmus, which has no latency and is non-fatigable. Interestingly, the incidence of vertigo does not closely correlate with the severity of the trauma (37).

Electronystagmography (ENG) is helpful in categorizing and localizing the vestibular injury; however, as with audiometry, it is typically not obtained in the acute setting. The vast majority of posttraumatic vertigo resolves spontaneously. If the symptoms persist following discharge from the hospital, an ENG can be obtained to help clarify diagnosis on an outpatient basis.

Pneumatic otoscopy, which consists of applying positive and negative pressure in the ear canal with a pneumatic otoscope, should not be performed in the acute setting. Application of positive and negative pressure in the potential setting of CSF fistula, and/or communication with the labyrinth if the fracture is otic capsule disrupting, increases the risk of iatrogenic injury from introduction of infection or air into the intracranial space or inner ear. This risk outweighs any potential diagnostic benefit in the acute setting. If the patient continues to experience vertigo or is experiencing fluctuating or progressive hearing loss longer than 1 week after the injury, a perilymph fistula is suspected and pneumatic otoscopy can then be performed to check for nystagmus and vertigo. The continued presence of spontaneous nystagmus following traumatic injury to the temporal bone is also suggestive of a perilymph fistula. Alternobaric testing with pneumatic otoscopy should not be performed if there is evidence of a persistent CSF fistula or infection in the middle ear.

Radiographic Evaluation

Patients with severe head trauma of the magnitude required for a temporal bone fracture will generally already have had a computed tomography (CT) scan of the head to assess for intracranial hemorrhage and other intracranial injuries. Temporal bone fractures can typically be discovered on standard head CT alone and can be traditionally classified as longitudinal, transverse, or mixed, or categorized with the more clinically significant otic capsule–sparing versus otic capsule–disrupting classification, as discussed above. Intravenous contrast-enhanced CT is not necessary for the diagnosis of temporal bone fractures.

Additional imaging of the temporal bone with axial and coronal high-resolution CT scanning (HRCT) is indicated in the presence of facial paralysis, signs of CSF otorrhea or

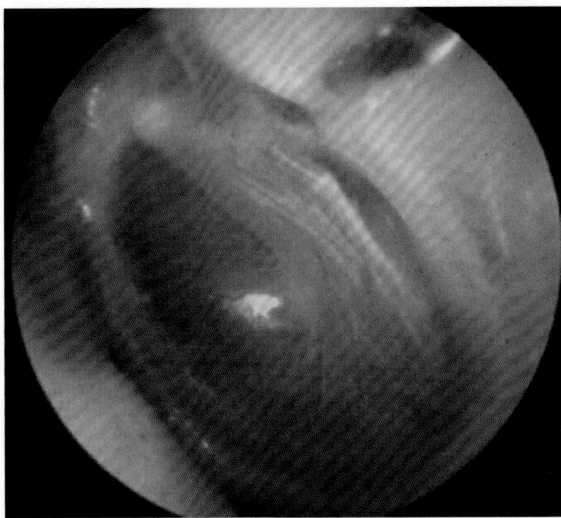

Figure 150.9 Otoscopic photograph demonstrating a distracted fracture along the roof of the external auditory canal and scutum allowing for potential in growth of canal skin.

rhinorrhea, disruption of the superior wall of the external auditory canal or scutum with potential trapping of epithelium (Fig. 150.9), or suspected vascular injury. HRCT of the temporal bones is also indicated if surgical intervention is required in the management of a neurotologic complication.

HRCT proves an invaluable tool for management decision making in the setting of immediate-onset, complete facial paralysis: A finding of bony impingement of the facial nerve and fallopian canal, either by bony spicules or by translocation of fracture components, is an indication for facial nerve exploration and decompression. In contrast, delayed-onset or incomplete facial paralysis alone does not require further radiologic evaluation with HRCT.

Hearing loss alone, whether conductive or sensorineural, in the absence of other complications also does not warrant additional temporal bone imaging in the acute setting. Demonstration of a transverse fracture or otic capsule–disrupting fracture in the setting of anacusis or profound sensorineural hearing loss will not alter the treatment plan. However, preoperative assessment with CT scanning in patients with a conductive hearing loss of sufficient magnitude to warrant exploration and ossicular reconstruction may provide useful information that may influence the surgical approach.

Ossicular discontinuity following temporal bone trauma can often be imaged on HRCT; types of discontinuities most easily identifiable on HRCT are incus dislocation and malleoincudal subluxation (38). In complete incus dislocation, in which both the malleoincudal and incudostapedial joints have been disrupted, the resulting position of the incus can be quite variable: residing in the epitympanum lateral to the malleus head (causing a "Y" configuration when viewed on coronal cuts), within the external auditory canal, or even not visible at all (presumably extruded from the body or "lost" within the mastoid air cells). Partial dislocation of the

incus and subluxation of the malleoincudal joint creates a diastasis of the malleus head "ice cream scoop" from the incus body "cone," with or without rotation of the incus body, on axial imaging. Incudostapedial subluxation and stapes fracture are difficult to ascertain on CT.

Posttraumatic sensorineural hearing loss is highly correlated with otic capsule–disrupting fractures, but many cases present with no radiologic findings. In these cases, an impulsive disruption of the membranous labyrinth, termed cochlear concussion, is theorized (39). Intralabyrinthine hemorrhage is an etiology that can be imaged and is seen as a region of signal hyperintensity within the vestibule and cochlea on noncontrast T1-weighted MR imaging if performed acutely (40,41).

Similarly, identification of perilymph fistula is usually not directly possible on radiographic imaging, but this diagnosis can be suggested when recognition is made of otic capsule–disrupting fracture, stapes fracture, loss of stapes bone, or pneumolabyrinth in the setting of persistent fluctuating hearing loss and vertigo (38,42).

The role of HRCT in the evaluation of potential carotid artery injuries is unclear. Resnick et al. reported a 5% incidence of carotid injury in basilar skull fractures if the fracture spares the carotid canal and an 18% incidence of carotid injury in patients with fractures through the carotid canal seen on HRCT (43). However, Kahn argues that, in an asymptomatic patient, HRCT demonstration of a fracture through the carotid canal yields no valuable additional information (44). Subsequent angiography performed in cases of asymptomatic carotid canal fractures yielded no evidence of carotid artery injury and provided no clinical utility (44). Consequently, in completely asymptomatic patients sustaining a temporal bone fracture, who are neurologically intact, HRCT and angiography are not required. On the other hand, if there are any transient or persistent neurologic deficits in patients with basilar skull fractures, HRCT of the temporal bone together with CT angiography is indicated (Fig. 150.10). MR angiography can also be considered for screening evaluation of the petrous carotid artery.

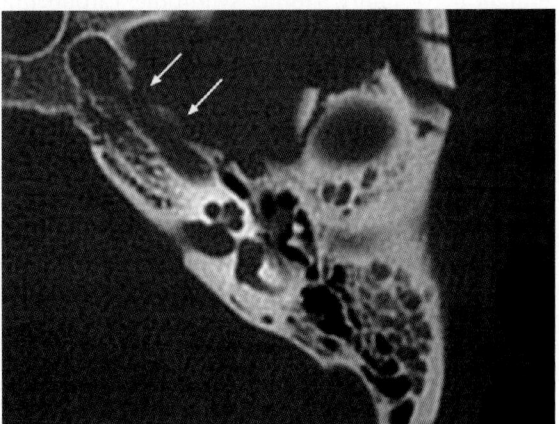

Figure 150.10 Axial bone window CT demonstrates a fracture of the carotid canal (*arrows*).

Sun et al. (45) sought to identify predictive findings of carotid artery injury on CT scan in patients who underwent angiography. Sphenoid bone fracture, petrous carotid canal fracture, and pneumocephalus were evaluated. With all three findings on CT scan, specificity of 85% and negative predictive value of 80% were obtained, while sensitivity was low. Further evaluation of correlation between CT findings and carotid artery injury is warranted.

Conventional skull radiography, including Schüller, Towne, Chamberlain, Stenvers, and basal views as well as tomograms, has been supplanted by HRCT scanning and no longer plays a role in the evaluation of patients suspected of having a temporal bone fracture.

In evaluating temporal bones for fracture on CT, care must be taken to avoid mistaking normal anatomic structures for fracture lines. Extrinsic suture lines (petro-occipital, temporo-occipital, occipitomastoid sutures), intrinsic suture lines (tympanomastoid, tympanosquamous, petrotympanic fissures), and intrinsic channels (cochlear aqueduct, vestibular aqueduct, glossopharyngeal nerve/glossopharyngeal sulcus, subarcuate artery/petromastoid canal, singular nerve/singular canal, Arnold nerve/mastoid canaliculus, Jacobson nerve/inferior tympanic canaliculus, and greater superficial petrosal nerve/facial hiatus) may all mimic fracture lines within the temporal bone (38). Knowledge of their anatomic relationships and distinction with true fracture lines is necessary to prevent incorrect interpretation of CT imaging.

MANAGEMENT

The morbidity and mortality associated with temporal bone fractures result from injuries to the structures passing through the temporal bone or abutting the temporal bone as described above. The most common complications include facial nerve injury, CSF fistula, sensorineural hearing loss, conductive hearing loss, cholesteatoma formation, and stenosis of the ear canal. In addition, rare complications may occur, including abducens nerve injury, trigeminal nerve injury, Horner syndrome, carotid injury, sigmoid sinus thrombosis, traumatic porencephalic cyst formation, and intracranial dislocation of the mandibular condyle (12,46–51).

Facial Nerve Injury

Facial paralysis is a severely disfiguring complication of temporal bone fractures. Six to seven percent of temporal bone fractures result in facial paralysis. This figure represents data based on large prospective and retrospective series of all consecutive patients treated for head injury or temporal bone fracture, thereby avoiding previous systematic bias towards overreporting of clinical complications (2,10). Of these facial nerve injuries, one-fourth are complete. The incidence of facial nerve injury in temporal bone

fractures of the pediatric population is 3% to 9%, comparable to that of the adult population (5,8,9).

The incidence of facial paralysis in the literature has previously been reported as high as 30%. However, this estimation is exaggerated due to sampling error: Simple, uncomplicated temporal bone fractures without facial nerve injury are often not referred for otolaryngologic consultation. The incidence of facial paralysis in the literature has also been overestimated by including patients in retrospective reviews who have been referred to a tertiary care center for management of complications of temporal bone fractures such as facial paresis. Since the entire pool of temporal bone fracture patients had not been included in prior statistics, the reported incidence of complications has previously been quite biased.

If head trauma patients are carefully evaluated in the emergency room upon admission, prior to the administration of muscle relaxants, 27% of facial nerve injuries will present with immediate-onset facial paralysis; 73% will have facial motion in the initial examination and subsequently deteriorate (2). The latency in onset of facial palsy ranges from 1 to 16 days. It is crucial to differentiate "delayed onset" from "delayed diagnosis." Delayed onset of facial paralysis is defined as documented facial function in the emergency room that subsequently deteriorates. A delayed diagnosis of facial paralysis occurs when the patient is given a paralytic agent and intubated prior to examination of facial function. In this situation, an assessment of facial function is delayed until extubation. These patients should be categorized as unestablished onset and treated similar to the immediate-onset patients. In one large series, 10% of patients fell into this unestablished-onset category (52).

Many aspects in the management of facial nerve injury remain controversial. One of the main issues to be resolved is the indication for surgical exploration. Since the vast majority of traumatic facial palsies resolve spontaneously, the decision of which injuries to explore is based on prognostic factors for poor outcome. The factors that are assessed in predicting recovery of facial function include timing of onset (delayed vs. immediate onset), severity of the injury (penetrating vs. nonpenetrating), and the presence of associated infection.

The delay of onset of paralysis following temporal bone fracture is the most important of the predictive factors. In one series of 37 delayed-onset facial palsies, five were lost to follow-up and the remainder recovered to a House-Brackmann grade I or II (2). McKennan and Chole (53) described their experience with 17 patients with immediate-onset facial paralysis and 19 patients with delayed-onset paralysis. Complete spontaneous recovery of facial function occurred in 94% of the patients with delayed-onset paralysis. The one remaining patient had a House-Brackmann grade II recovery. In contrast, 8 out of the 17 immediate-onset paralysis patients had facial nerve transections.

Turner reviewed a large series of traumatic facial paralysis treated conservatively (54). His paper included 36 immediate-onset and 34 delayed-onset facial palsies. Complete recovery occurred in 94% of the delayed-onset cases and 75% of immediate-onset palsies. The one patient with delayed-onset paralysis who had no recovery of function developed the facial palsy coincident with acute otitis media. Similarly, in a recent systematic review, the outcomes of 25 patients with immediate paralysis and 20 patients with delayed paralysis treated with conservative management were assessed. Eighty percent of the delayed paralysis patients had complete recovery of facial function while less than 40% of those with immediate paralysis recovered complete facial function (55). Maiman et al. (56), in contrast, found no correlation between immediate- or delayed-onset facial paralysis, treated nonsurgically, and outcome. However, 44 out of 45 of their patients (including both immediate and delayed onset) had satisfactory recovery. Review of the above literature argues strongly against surgical exploration and decompression of delayed posttraumatic and facial paralysis. The natural course of delayed facial paralysis is almost always recovery of facial function to a House-Brackmann grade I or II. There are no convincing data in the literature that demonstrate that surgical intervention in delayed-onset paralysis will increase the probability of complete recovery of function.

May describes the difficulty in differentiating immediate- from delayed-onset facial paralysis. He explored reportedly "delayed-onset" palsies and found on occasion a severed nerve (57). This observation highlights the necessity of careful examination in the emergency room prior to chemical paralysis. Even in comatose patients, painful stimuli will generally induce a symmetric grimace when both facial nerves are intact; unilateral weakness of all facial branches implies a peripheral—that is, facial nerve—lesion, whereas selective weakness of the lower branches with bilateral temporal branch sparing implies a central lesion, proximal to the facial nucleus. Admittedly, information regarding facial nerve function immediately following an injury is not always available. Sometimes the exam is omitted due to attention to other life-threatening complications or because the patient has already received muscle relaxants with intubation. Some patients are not responsive to pain and a grimace cannot be induced. The critical issue is whether or not any facial function has been identified. If facial function is present in the emergency room and subsequently deteriorates, our experience is that the patient will recover without surgical treatment. When reliable information from the emergency room is unavailable, the patient is never documented to have facial function, and the diagnosis of facial palsy is delayed by a few days, these cases must be categorized as "unknown onset" and considered with the immediate-onset group when considering management options.

The degree of facial nerve injury is also a critical factor in guiding the management algorithm. Incomplete paresis rarely fails to completely resolve spontaneously unless an additional insult to the nerve, such as infection, occurs (2). A review of 71 patients with partial facial weakness demonstrated that the overwhelming majority of patients achieved recovery to House-Brackmann grade I and no patients had House-Brackmann grade VI outcome (55). Consequently, only patients with complete paralysis of immediate or unknown onset are considered for surgical exploration.

The degree of injury can be assessed not only clinically with facial motion but also with electrodiagnostic testing using the Hilger facial nerve stimulator; evoked electromyography (EEMG), also known as electroneuronography (ENoG); and standard EMG. The role of electrodiagnostic testing is to assist the clinician in differentiating a neuropraxic injury from a neural degenerative injury and to assess the proportion of degenerated axons. Nerves sustaining a neuropraxic injury proximal to the stimulated portion of the nerve maintain electrical stimulability at all times following the injury. Partial or complete disruption of the nerve results in Wallerian degeneration and consequent decrease or loss of stimulability. However, Wallerian degeneration occurs in a delayed fashion, and the distal segment of the nerves maintains electrical stimulability for 3 to 5 days postinjury (58). Consequently, electrodiagnostic testing cannot reliably differentiate a neuropraxic injury from a laceration of the nerve for up to 3 to 5 days.

Sunderland classified nerve fiber injuries in five categories (59). The first-degree injury is an anatomically intact nerve fiber with a conduction blockade (neuropraxia). These lesions tend to recover completely. The second-degree injury transects the axons but maintains an intact endoneurium (axonotmesis). Again, these lesions also tend to resolve without subsequent deficits. The third-degree injury transects the axon and endoneurium but maintains an intact perineurium (neurotmesis). Aberrant regeneration can occur with third-degree injuries, leaving patients with some weakness and synkinesis. Fourth-degree injuries transect the entire nerve trunk but maintain an intact epineural sheath (neurotmesis). Loss of the conduit of the epineural sheath allows regenerating axons to cross into adjacent fascicles, resulting in a loss of topographic organization. A proportion of the regenerating fibers are also lost due to the healing process and scarring. These lesions result in a high incidence of residual weakness, synkinesis, and hyperkinesis. Complete transection of the entire nerve trunk and epineurium is classified as a fifth-degree injury (neurotmesis) and is associated with poor spontaneous recovery, if any, depending on the degree of diastasis of the nerve stumps. Some authors have advocated a sixth-degree injury classification in which different fascicles of the facial nerve have sustained different degrees of injury of the five traditional injury types described by Sunderland.

The Hilger facial nerve stimulator is used to perform both the minimal nerve excitability test (NET) as well as the maximal stimulation test (MST). The facial nerve is stimulated percutaneously adjacent to the stylomastoid foramen and the various distal branches. In NET, the branches of the facial nerve are stimulated on both the injured side and on the contralateral side, which serves as a control. The current used is incrementally increased just until threshold is reached, manifested by facial twitching, and this threshold level is recorded for each side individually. A threshold difference of 3.5 mA or greater between the affected and nonaffected sides of the face suggests significant neural degeneration. The test is most useful between 2 and 14 days postinjury in patients with dense facial paralysis to differentiate between neuropraxic and neurodegenerative injuries. The testing is unnecessary in incomplete paralysis in which there is almost always 100% recovery.

May et al. (60) argues that the MST provides a more reliable estimation of the degree of degeneration. In the MST, stimulation of the nonaffected, control side is performed similar to in the NET, but the intensity of the stimulus is further increased until the amount of facial contraction plateaus or is limited by patient intolerance. The affected, injured side is then stimulated with the same current amplitude, and the degree of contraction is subjectively assessed by the physician and compared with that of the unaffected side of the face. The difference in contraction is expressed as equal, mildly decreased, markedly decreased, or no response. The latter two categories are associated with poorer prognosis. Similar to NET, MST is most useful between 2 and 14 days postinjury in patients with dense facial paralysis. Again, any volitional movement of the face would indicate an intact nerve trunk and supercede any electrical testing.

Evoked electromyography (EEMG) has been popularized by Fisch and termed electroneuronography (ENoG) (61). ENoG differs from EEMG only in the use of bipolar stimulating and recording electrodes. Both techniques measure the evoked compound muscle action potential (CAP) and provide similar information to the MST but in an objective fashion. The stimulating bipolar electrodes are placed adjacent to the stylomastoid foramen, and the recording bipolar electrodes in the nasolabial crease. The peak-to-trough amplitude of the CAP is measured on both sides, and the diminution in amplitude of the CAP on the paretic side as compared to the control side is indicative of the percentage of degenerated nerve fibers. EEMG has been demonstrated to be the most accurate electrodiagnostic test for prognostic information (62). Fisch reported that patients in whom the degeneration on EEMG reaches 90% within 6 days of onset of a traumatic facial paralysis have a poorer outcome and consequently should be decompressed (63). Sillman et al. (64) demonstrated a significant association between a CAP decline of greater than 90% and poor recovery of function for idiopathic paralysis, but demonstrated no significant association between CAP decline of greater than 90% and clinical outcome in traumatic paralysis.

The value of EMG in the acute management of traumatic facial paralysis remains controversial. Standard monopolar EMG is performed by insertion of an EMG electrode into the muscle and the spontaneous electrical activity recorded. Two types of information are obtainable: voluntary activity and fibrillation potentials. If voluntary activity is present in the acute postinjury period, the patient has a very high probability of good recovery (64). However, May et al. (65) reported only 75% accuracy in predicting a poor recovery and 62% accuracy in predicting a favorable result. Fibrillation potentials result from denervation of the muscle but are delayed 2 to 3 weeks following the injury and consequently offer little additional information to guide therapy in the acute setting (66).

After defining the at-risk population for poor recovery of function, the next question to answer is: Does surgical intervention alter the outcome? Turner in 1944 reported on 69 patients with varying degrees of facial paralysis following temporal bone trauma (54). Thirty of these patients had complete facial paralysis, all of which were treated nonoperatively. This group of patients was unbiased in that none of his series underwent surgical decompression. Good recovery occurred in 63% of the patients, incomplete recovery with synkinesis in 23%, and poor recovery in 13%. Maiman et al. (56) reported on the outcome of 21 patients with posttraumatic complete facial paralysis. Full recovery occurred in 52% of the patients and incomplete recovery in 43%. One patient had a poor outcome. Brodie and Thompson (2) had eight patients with complete paralysis who met criteria for facial nerve decompression who, for a variety of reasons, did not undergo surgical exploration. Seven of the eight patients had good recovery of function and one patient had a poor outcome. The combined rate of good recovery of function with conservative, nonsurgical management, in the above three studies is 63%.

In contrast, analysis of six case series studies of patients undergoing surgical decompression for complete facial nerve paralysis revealed a combined rate of good recovery of facial function of 51%. This figure excludes severed facial nerves. The criteria to be included in the surgical groups were that the nerves were no longer stimulable with the Hilger facial nerve stimulator or demonstrated greater than 90% degeneration within 6 days or 95% degeneration within 14 days on EEMG/ENoG.

The outcomes in facial nerve function for patients who underwent conservative, nonsurgical management versus those undergoing facial nerve decompression in various series are summarized in Table 150.2 (2,52,54,56,67–70).

It is difficult to compare the recovery rates of facial nerve function in patients undergoing surgical and nonsurgical management. The patients included in the observation studies did not necessarily meet the same criteria as those included in the surgical decompression studies, thereby potentially artificially inflating the positive outcomes in patients treated nonsurgically. In an extensive review and analysis of the literature, Chang and Cass (71) concluded

TABLE 150.2	FACIAL NERVE OUTCOME FOLLOWING COMPLETE FACIAL PARALYSIS				
Treatment	n	Good (HB I or II)	Incomplete (HB III or IV)	Poor (HB V or VI)	Transected Nerve
Nonoperative					
Turner	30	19	7	4	
Maiman	21	11	9	1	
Brodie	8	7	0	1	
Rate		63%	27%	10%	
Operative					
Kamerer	62	18	15	9	20
Lambert	17	11	0	0	6
Coker	12	5	4	1	2
Brodie	6	4	0	2	0
Darrouzet	65	25	26	5	9
Yeoh	6	4	1	1	0
Rate		51%	35%	14%	(22%)

that there are no studies that prove or disprove the efficacy of facial nerve decompression.

Since Wallerian degeneration is not documented on electrodiagnostic testing for 3 to 5 days following the axonotmesis or neurotmesis, surgical intervention is delayed until several days after the nerve has degenerated. Although decompression of the facial nerve prophylactically in acoustic neuroma surgery has been proven efficacious, the decompression is performed prior to Wallerian degeneration having occurred (72). Demonstrating that decompression of a posttraumatic nonsevered nerve is efficacious remains to be proven in a randomized prospective study.

The key factor in the decision to surgically explore a facial nerve is whether the nerve is suspected of being severed, crushed, or impaled with bone fragments. The incidence of transected nerves in the largest series ranges from 6% to 45% (52,67–69,73).The high frequency of severed nerves in some of these reports is biased by patient selection, as discussed previously. Patients are referred to the tertiary centers performing nerve explorations when they fail to spontaneously recover. However, the vast majority of patients do not have a transected nerve and therefore recover spontaneously and are not referred to tertiary centers.

The probability of severing the facial nerve is actually quite low, but the outcome of a transected nerve following observation alone is poor. Therefore, an attempt should be made to identify patients with crushed, impaled, or otherwise transected nerves, as these are the patients who would most benefit from surgical intervention. Electrodiagnostic testing of nerves with complete paralysis can only differentiate injuries that have undergone Wallerian degeneration from those that have not, that is, Sunderland II–V- versus Sunderland I-degree injuries. Since one cannot differentiate a Sunderland fifth-degree injury (severed nerve) from a second-, third-, or fourth-degree injury on the basis of electrodiagnostic testing, exploration is warranted only in patients with complete, immediate-onset paralysis in whom electrical stimulability is lost; it is these patients who are at greatest risk for crushed, partially severed, or transected nerves. The site of injury to the facial nerve in temporal bone fractures is in the perigeniculate region in 80% to 93% of patients (33,67,68). Lambert and Brackmann (67) found a second lesion in 4 out of 21 patients in the mastoid segment. Accordingly, the approach utilized for the nerve exploration must expose these two regions. Fisch advocates a translabyrinthine approach for transverse fractures and a combined transmastoid/middle cranial fossa approach for longitudinal fractures (63). May described a transmastoid/supralabyrinthine approach to the region of the geniculate ganglion for facial nerve decompression (74). Goin studied this approach in cadaveric temporal bones and found that he could consistently expose the distal labyrinthine segment and geniculate ganglion (75). However, the fundus of the IAC could be exposed in only 60% of the temporal bones. Yanagihara (76) applied the transmastoid/supralabyrinthine approach in 36 patients. Only five temporal bone fractures in his series of 41 patients required a middle cranial fossa approach to expose the geniculate region.

The translabyrinthine approach is advocated for facial nerve exploration in patients with profound hearing loss. The approach provides excellent exposure for decompression, nerve rerouting with direct reanastomosis, and cable grafting. In otic capsule–sparing fractures with ossicular discontinuity, the nerve is explored via a transmastoid/supralabyrinthine approach. This approach generally requires dislocation of the incus and ossicular reconstruction at the completion of the operation. If the patient has any contralateral hearing loss or the anatomy is not conducive for supralabyrinthine exposure, a middle cranial fossa approach is utilized.

Timing of facial nerve repair has in the past been controversial. McCabe advocated repairing the nerve within the first 3 days or delaying facial nerve reanastomosis for 20 days postinjury (77). This recommendation was based on the observation that regeneration and axoplasmic flow were greatest at 3 weeks postinjury. Barrs studied the timing of facial nerve repair in micropigs and found no advantage of waiting the 3 weeks until the neuronal cell body metabolic activity was maximal (78). This animal model did not show a statistically significant difference in electrophysiologic testing between nerves grafted throughout various times within 3 months of transection.

Fisch advocates exploration when the ENoG indicates 90% degeneration occurring within 6 days (79). He argues that decompression should be performed early to minimize further degeneration. May also advocates early exploration (57). His series demonstrated a correlation between better results and shorter interval between injury and repair.

Late exploration for potentially severed nerves is still indicated, but the role of late decompression remains controversial. Quaranta et al. (80) reported on nine patients decompressed 2 to 3 months after sustaining their temporal bone fractures. Seventy-eight percent recovered to a House-Brackmann grade I or II at 1 year postdecompression. The question as to whether these patients would have recovered spontaneously to the same degree remains unanswered. Clearly, if the nerve was severed and not approximated, spontaneous recovery to a House-Brackmann grade I or II would not occur. In that scenario, a House-Brackmann grade VI would be anticipated. Sanus et al. reported on eight patients with mean time to decompression of 70 days. Six patients had nerve edema and two had bony impingement of the nerve at the time of operation. Long-term follow-up was available for six of these patients, all of whom recovered to House-Brackmann grade III (81). Again, the question remains whether these patients would have had spontaneous recovery to the same degree.

The range in latency to recovery of facial function varies from 1 day to 1 year. Fifty-nine percent of facial palsies that recover spontaneously do so within 1 month, and 88% recover by 3 months postinjury (2).

Summary of Facial Nerve Treatment Algorithm

Patients with delayed-onset facial paralysis are placed on a 2-week course of systemic corticosteroids (unless medically contraindicated) and observed. Although there are no data in the literature supporting or contradicting this recommendation, the rationale for corticosteroid use is based on antiinflammatory activity and the assumption that neural edema is the primary factor in the progression of injury in the traumatized, nontransected nerve (71) (Fig. 150.11).

Patients with complete paralysis of immediate onset are tested with the Hilger nerve stimulator between days 3 and 7 postinjury. If stimulability is present to any degree (implying a physically intact nerve), the patients are observed. If the nerve loses all stimulability within 1 week of the injury, facial nerve exploration is performed.

Facial nerve injuries occurring in an otic capsule–disrupting fracture are typically explored via a translabyrinthine approach: the translabyrinthine approach affords the most direct, complete access to the entire length of the intratemporal facial nerve, and in fractures that cause a profound sensorineural hearing loss, the approach does not engender any significant morbidity than that already sustained.

In otic capsule–sparing fractures, two surgical approaches are utilized. In patients in whom excellent intrinsic exposure of the intratemporal facial nerve can be achieved, that is, with well-aerated mastoid air cell systems or with ossicular discontinuity, a transmastoid/supralabyrinthine approach is chosen. If the patient has a poorly aerated mastoid air cell system or total facial nerve decompression cannot be achieved by the transmastoid/supralabyrinthine approach, a combined transmastoid/middle cranial fossa approach is utilized. If a severed facial nerve is encountered using the transmastoid/supralabyrinthine approach and inadequate exposure for cable grafting occurs, a middle cranial fossa approach is performed.

The transmastoid facial nerve decompression begins with a complete mastoidectomy skeletonizing the tegmen mastoideum superiorly, the sigmoid sinus posteriorly, and the posterior EAC wall anteriorly. The antrum is opened, exposing the short process of the incus and the lateral semicircular canal. The semicircular canals are then skeletonized. The facial recess is opened and the facial nerve is skeletonized from the second genu to the stylomastoid foramen. If there is any evidence of bony trauma in this region, a complete decompression is performed; however, the nerve sheath is not incised. The buttress to the incus is subsequently removed, followed by removal of the incus, and the tympanic portion of the nerve is decompressed. If there is adequate room to proceed, a supralabyrinthine decompression of the intralabyrinthine portion of the facial nerve is performed (Figs. 150.12 and 150.13). A laceration of the facial nerve in this region is cable grafted with a section of the greater auricular nerve. The cable graft is placed in the bony channel of the fallopian canal abutting the sharply incised edges of the facial nerve. To improve exposure, the tegmen can be eggshelled and retracted superiorly. If the exposure remains inadequate, a middle fossa craniotomy is performed. If the fracture involves the proximal portion of the intralabyrinthine segment of the facial nerve, a middle fossa craniotomy is performed.

To begin the middle fossa craniotomy, the squamosal portion of the temporal bone is exposed by extending the postauricular skin incision in a "lazy S" shape up towards the vertex, first extending anteriorly, then posteriorly. The temporalis fascia is reflected inferiorly and the temporalis muscle is split vertically and elevated off of the squamosal portion of the temporal bone. The soft tissue dissection and exposure should extend underneath the zygomatic arch in order to allow adequate exposure for the craniotomy. Self-retaining retractors are adjusted to hold both muscle and skin. A bone window is created

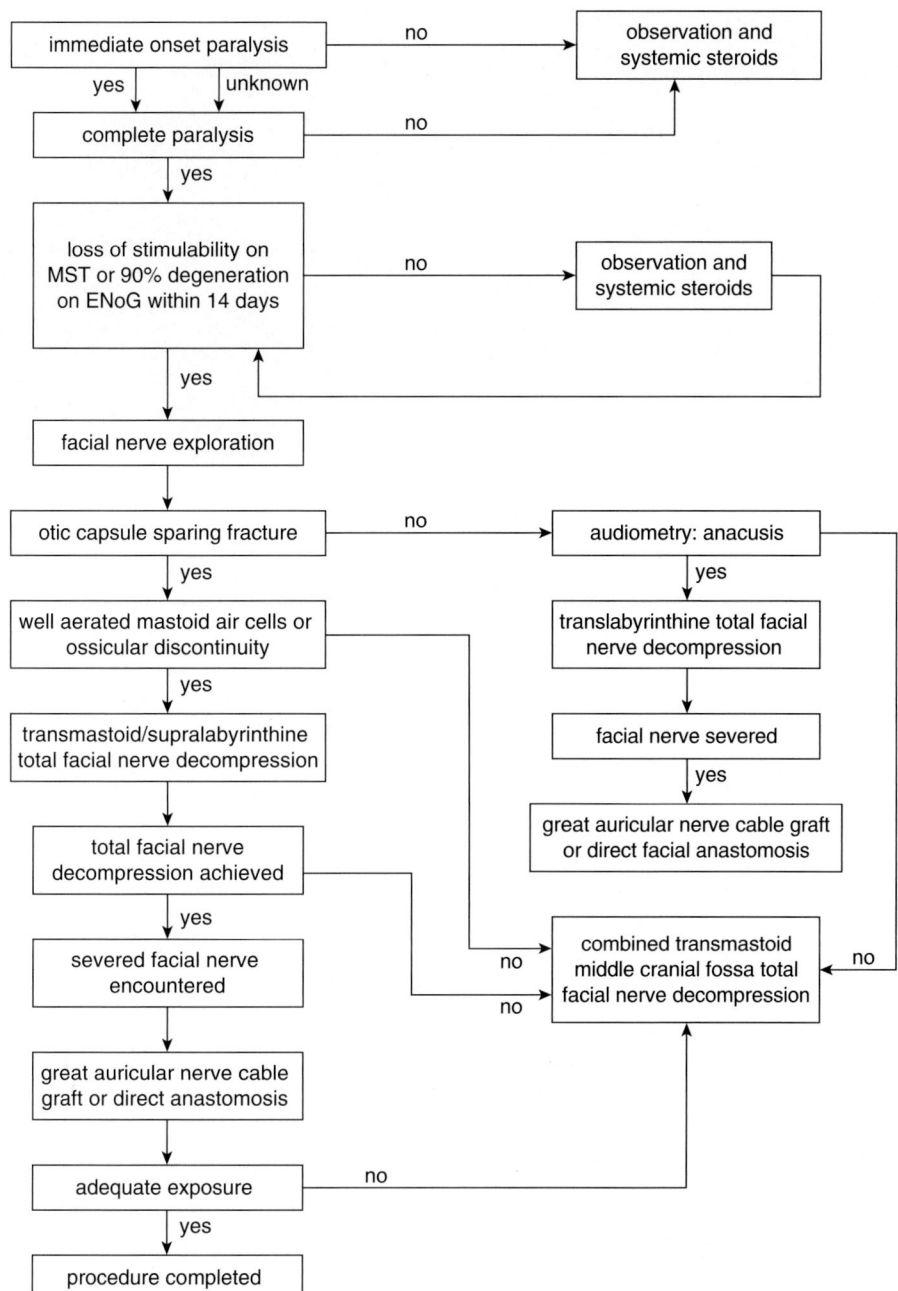

Figure 150.11 Management of traumatic facial paralysis.

with large cutting and then diamond burrs, taking care to avoid lacerating the underlying dura. This bone window is 4 by 4 cm in size and placement is set with the inferior border at the level of the zygomatic root, with two-thirds of the window anterior and one-third posterior to the vertical plane of the EAC. A rongeur is used to remove any remaining bone at the inferior edge of the craniotomy down to the level of the floor of the middle cranial fossa. This allows the optimal surgical line of site with minimal temporal lobe retraction. The House-Urban middle fossa retractor is engaged with the prongs in the edge of the craniotomy. The blade is gradually advanced, as the dura

is elevated off the floor of the middle fossa. It is common to encounter dural venous bleeding at the anterior extent of the dissection. This can usually be controlled with a hemostatic agent such as Surgicel or Oxycel. The fracture line and hematoma are generally encountered in the region of the facial hiatus, consistent with the notion of fracture lines following natural foramina within the temporal bone.

The landmarks in the middle fossa are the middle meningeal artery at the foramen spinosum, the greater superficial petrosal nerve at the facial hiatus, and the arcuate eminence. The geniculate ganglion may be exposed

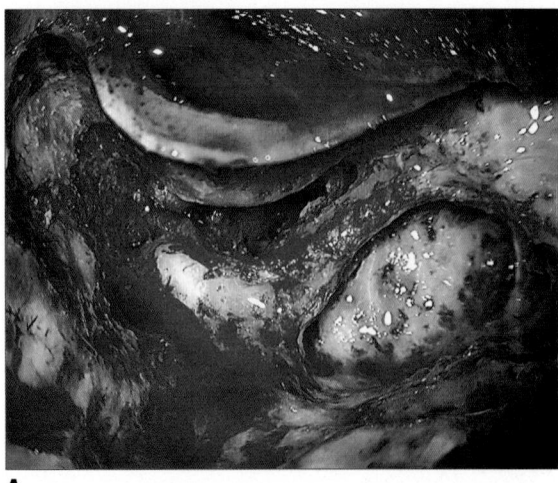

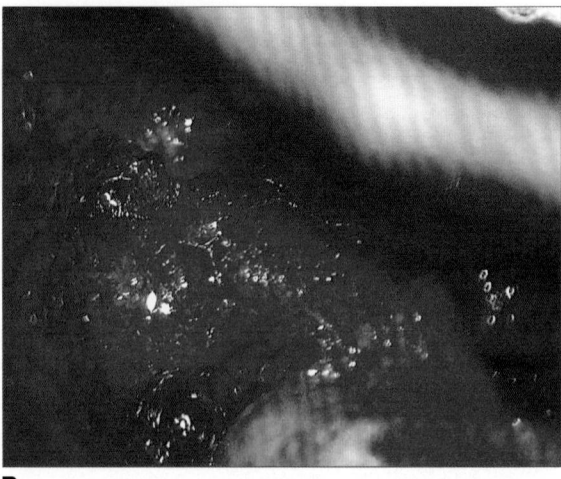

A   **B**

Figure 150.12 Transmastoid/supralabyrinthine decompression of right facial nerve in petrous temporal bone fracture. **A:** Right complete facial nerve decompression via transmastoid approach. The facial nerve is decompressed from the meatal foramen (**far left**) to the vertical segment. The incus buttress has been taken down and the incus resected. The distalmost portion of the facial nerve to the stylomastoid foramen has not yet been decompressed. Note the extremely generous retrofacial air cell tract. **B:** Close-up of supralabyrinthine component of the transmastoid decompression. The horizontal semicircular canal is at the lower border of view. The tympanic and geniculate segments are in center field of view, with the intralabyrinthine segment seen tangentially between the geniculate and horizontal semicircular canal ampulla. The fracture extended through the anterior petrous apex, with the fracture line diastasis exposing the middle fossa dura seen on the left.

without a bony covering on the floor of the middle cranial fossa, so care should be exercised during dural elevation. The landmark for the superior semicircular canal is the arcuate eminence, but the precise location of the canal does not uniformly correspond with the arcuate eminence. The canal may have very little bone coverage

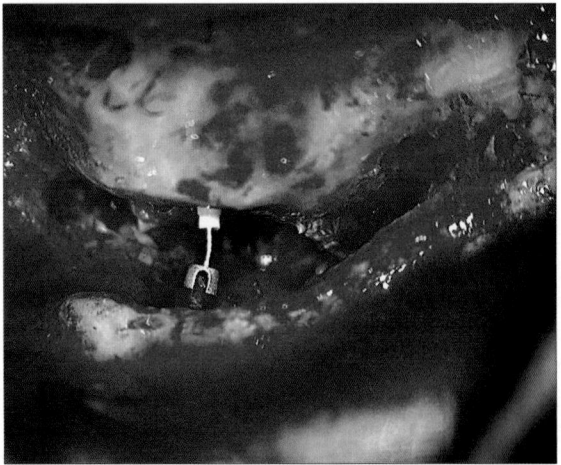

Figure 150.13 Ossicular reconstruction following supralabyrinthine decompression of the facial nerve. During transmastoid decompression, the incus may need to be resected in order to fully decompress the lateral face of the tympanic segment of the facial nerve; traumatic dislocation of the incus requires interposition ossiculoplasty, making this approach favorable. Following completion of facial nerve decompression, interposition ossiculoplasty is readily achieved through the same transmastoid approach, without the need for additional transcanal tympanoplasty, as seen here. In this case, a Bojrab Grace ALTO + HA partial ossicular prosthesis is interposed between the malleus manubrium and stapes capitulum, both easily visible from this view.

and be seen as a blue line after simple dural elevation, or there may be a large number of air cells between the canal and the surface of the tegmen. A coronal CT scan may be helpful in ascertaining this relationship: the association of the contours of the middle fossa floor to the superior semicircular canal as well as the distance between the two can be assessed.

Identification of the internal auditory canal and intralabyrinthine portion of the facial nerve can be accomplished in any of numerous ways. House and Glasscock advocated identifying the greater superficial petrosal nerve and following this to the geniculate ganglion (82,83). Fisch suggested using the relationship of the superior semicircular canal to find the internal auditory canal, which is usually offset by 60 degrees (84). Portmann et al. (85) report finding the IAC 8 to 12 mm anteromedial to the location of the superior semicircular canal in the direction parallel to the petrous ridge. The tegmen tympani may be opened with ensuing identification of the ossicles and tympanic portion of the facial nerve, which can then be followed retrograde towards the geniculate ganglion. The method of Garcia-Ibanez is a reliable, often used technique and is described (86).

The bone over the superior semicircular canal is removed using suction irrigation and diamond burrs. A light medial to lateral stroke is used until the blue line of the superior canal is identified. After the superior canal has been identified, dissection proceeds along the meatal plane, which is the line of bone bisecting the angle subtended by the greater superficial petrosal nerve and the superior semicircular canal. Drilling within the confines of this plane will reduce the risk of inadvertent injury to the cochlea. Much wider drilling may be performed medially, whereas at the lateral extent of the IAC there is very little space between the cochlea and ampulla of the superior semicircular canal. The burr should hug the line of the superior canal as bone removal progresses. The dissection will appear quite deep before the IAC is encountered. Bone should be removed 180 degrees around the IAC, from the lateral aspect of the meatus to the porus acusticus. An eggshell thickness of bone should be left over the IAC. The last step in exposure of the canal is careful removal of this bone and copious irrigation to remove bone dust.

At the most lateral extent of the IAC, the vertical crest or "Bill bar" is identified, with the facial nerve anteriorly and the superior vestibular nerve posteriorly. The dura of the IAC is incised in a longitudinal fashion, along the posterior edge, away from the facial nerve. If the facial nerve is lacerated, the proximal edge is freshened with microscissors. The nerve graft is secured proximally with a single 9-0 nylon suture and distally placed into the bony channel of the tympanic portion of the fallopian canal. A piece of temporalis fascia is placed over the graft. Bone wax is used to fill exposed air cells. A piece of temporalis muscle is placed in the bony defect, and the pedicled temporalis fascia flap is reflected over the floor of the middle cranial fossa. The temporal lobe is released, compressing the fascia over the bony defect. The bone flap is replaced within the craniotomy window, and the temporalis muscle is reapproximated, leaving a gap inferiorly where the temporalis fascia passes. Skin is closed in two layers.

Caution is advised when performing a middle fossa craniotomy for facial nerve decompression in the setting of acute trauma. In these instances, the offending temporal bone fracture may have not only caused injury to the facial nerve but also likely caused disruption of the middle fossa dura overlying the temporal bone, with potential contusion of the temporal lobe overlying these structures. Utmost care must be taken to avoid additional injury to the already disrupted middle fossa dura and contused temporal lobe during dissection, elevation, and retraction in this approach.

CSF Fistulae

CSF fistulae and the potential for meningitis are among the most serious of complications from temporal bone fractures. CSF fistulae occur in 17% of temporal bone fractures (2). CSF fistulae in otic capsule–sparing fractures typically occur through the floor of the middle cranial fossa (tegmen tympani and tegmen mastoideum) into the epitympanum, antrum, and mastoid air cell tract. The CSF will flow out the ear canal if the tympanic membrane is disrupted or into the eustachian tube, resulting in CSF rhinorrhea. In otic capsule–disrupting fractures, CSF flows from the posterior cranial fossa through the disrupted otic capsule into the middle ear.

A unique characteristic of a fracture through the otic capsule is the absence of healing. The otic capsule is adult size at birth and undergoes minimal remodeling throughout life (87). Following a fracture, fibrous tissue will partially fill the crevice, and the adjacent periosteal bone may seal off the fracture but the enchondral bone itself will not heal (19,21). This fibrous scar affords a potential tract for an infection of the middle ear cleft to spread to the intracranial space, leaving the patient at continued risk for meningitis even years after the initial injury.

The onset of CSF leakage following trauma was delayed for greater than 1 week in 28% of the 192 cases surveyed by Lewin (88). Immediate CSF leak results from separation of dural fibers in a traumatized region of dura adjacent to a fracture site. In contrast, delayed CSF leak has been theorized to occur from (a) herniation of meningocele or meningoencephalocele (often termed brain fungus or fungus cerebri) into the fracture site, followed by delayed atrophy of the brain fungus or delayed resolution of elevated intracranial pressure and retraction of brain fungus out of the fracture site or (b) resolution of hematoma previously obstructing the outflow of CSF through the fracture site.

The CSF fistula will continue to leak until fibroblastic proliferation creates a fibrous barrier, which closes the subarachnoid space or the sinus or air cell mucosa covers the bony defect (89). However, in the early stages of repair, the fibrous barrier is weak and the mucosal barrier remains fragile. If the CSF pressure gradient is greater than the healing tensile strength of these vulnerable barriers, the leak will continue. The tenuous, newly formed barrier may be easily ruptured by increased nasopharyngeal pressure or Valsalva (90). Therefore, the importance of enforcing relatively mundane precautions such as avoidance of nose blowing, avoidance of strenuous physical activity or physical therapy, keeping head of bed elevated, and scrupulous bowl care and avoidance of constipation cannot be overemphasized.

A CSF fistula is suspected when clear watery drainage is noted in the ear canal or from the nose. Otorhinorrhea will often drain down the back of the throat. The rate of flow of the discharge will usually increase with exertion or leaning forward. Consequently, when evaluating a patient for a suspected CSF fistula, the patient is asked to lean forward with the neck flexed, collecting nasal discharge into a sterile container. Patients often complain of headaches, which are dull, continuous, and bilateral. The origin of aural and nasal drainage is often obscured by concurrent bleeding or lysis of old blood clot. Once a nasal discharge is suspected of being CSF, it can be differentiated from watery rhinitis, lacrimal secretions, or serosanguinous discharge on the basis of its composition. CSF has elevated glucose, decreased protein, and decreased potassium than nasal secretions. Qualitative tests such as those utilizing glucose oxidase test strips (Clinitest) have been shown to lack specificity and result in a substantial proportion of false positives (91). Quantitative glucose, protein, and potassium determinations are more accurate in diagnosing a CSF fistula.

A noninvasive technique for identifying and localizing a CSF fistula using protein electrophoresis for beta-2 transferrin was first described by Meurman (92). The beta-2 isoform of transferrin, a protein involved in iron transport, is confined to CSF, perilymph, and aqueous humor, whereas the beta-1 isoform is found globally in serum, nasal secretions, saliva, and tears. Nasal and otic secretions with CSF contamination exhibit an additional band on immunofixation electrophoresis than noncontaminated counterparts. In addition to being noninvasive, a major advantage of this technique is the small amount of fluid specimen required for the test: recommended specimen volume is typically 0.5 mL, and beta-2 transferrin can be detected in sample specimens as small as 50 µL. False-positive results are rare and occur in patients with alcoholic cirrhosis, inborn errors of glycoprotein metabolism, or genetic transferrin variants, in which transferrin allelic variants with similar electrophoretic mobility to the beta-2 isoform are present in sera (93). In these cases, collection and electrophoresis of a concurrent serum sample—which would contain beta-1- as well as beta-2-like bands—can help avoid a falsely positive result interpretation.

Other minimally invasive techniques for detection of CSF otorrhea or rhinorrhea are currently being developed, including detection of beta–trace protein, or prostaglandin D synthase (94,95). Beta–trace protein is synthesized in the meninges and has a 20- to 40-fold increase in concentration in CSF compared to serum. Nephelometric assays of beta–trace protein are being developed and show a specificity and sensitivity of CSF detection comparable to that of current beta-2 transferrin assays (96,97). A recent study in patients with suspected CSF leak was able to quantify values of beta–trace protein in nasal secretions at which 100% positive and negative predictive values of CSF leak could be obtained (98). In addition, the nephelometric technique is comparatively inexpensive and rapid, increasing its potential for further development and use in the clinical setting.

HRCT will generally demonstrate the potential sites of a CSF fistula. When a fracture is seen but the exact site of the fistula has not been identified, CT cisternography with intrathecal contrast (Omnipaque) can be quite useful. HRCT will show a bony defect in 70% of patients with a CSF fistula (99). When a defect cannot be demonstrated by HRCT, rarely will CT cisternography or radionuclide cisternography detect a site of leakage (99). Radionuclide scans tend to lack sensitivity and specificity.

Intrathecal fluorescein is a sensitive and specific test for investigating the presence of a CSF fistula. Following a lumbar puncture, 0.5 mL of a 5% solution of fluorescein is mixed with 10 mL of the patient's CSF and reinjected. Any subsequent otorrhea or rhinorrhea can be collected on micropledgets and examined under a Wood lamp for green fluorescence. Although occasional reports of neurotoxicity (e.g., paraparesis and grand mal seizures) following intrathecal injection of fluorescein appear in the literature, these complications are very infrequent, occurred at higher doses of fluorescein than is currently recommended, and have never resulted in permanent damage (90,100,101). No persistent side effects or complications have been reported with the current recommended dosing. Fluorescein is frequently successful in localizing fistulas when all other methods have failed and can be utilized intraoperatively to aid in the actual repair of the fistula (101–103). Therefore, the continued usage of fluorescein may be justified and the risks of increased morbidity following failure to locate a CSF fistula preoperatively may outweigh the risks involved in its usage.

None of the localizing techniques described above are useful if the CSF leak is quiescent at the time of investigation.

The incidence of meningitis in patients with CSF leaks ranges from 2% to 88% (2,90,104–107). The wide range in incidence is a result of multiple factors, the most significant of which is the duration of leakage (90,105,107,108). Mincy and Leech and Patterson compared the incidence of meningitis in patients with CSF leaks continuing 7 days or less to those persisting for more than 7 days (105,107). Leech and Patterson found only a 5% incidence of meningitis in patients with CSF fistulae of less than 7 days duration, and Mincy reported a similarly low incidence of meningitis in this group of 11%. The incidence of meningitis in patients with leakage for more than 7 days in Leech and Patterson's series was 55% and in Mincy's series was 88%. Spetzler and Wilson demonstrated a 33% incidence of meningitis in persistent fistulae, and Grahne found 54% of his patients with chronic CSF leakage developed meningitis (90,108).

Many studies over the past 25 years have demonstrated no benefit of prophylactic antibiotics in temporal bone fractures in the absence of CSF fistulae (105,106,109–115). The incidence of meningitis in this group is quite low. Rathore pooled the data from many of these studies and found a 4% incidence of meningitis in patients with basilar skull fractures receiving prophylactic antibiotics and a 3% incidence in patients not receiving prophylactic antibiotics (116). Brodie and Thompson (2) demonstrated a 1% incidence of meningitis in 578 patients with temporal bone fractures and no CSF fistulae. Hoff et al. (109) conducted a prospective randomized trial assigning patients with temporal bone fractures into a prophylactic antibiotic treatment group or to a no antibiotic group. None of the patients in either group developed meningitis. All of these studies conclude that prophylactic antibiotics are not indicated, given the low incidence of meningitis in temporal bone fractures without a CSF fistula and the lack of evidence demonstrating any benefit to prophylactic antibiotics in this situation.

However, the risk of meningitis is significantly higher in patients with temporal bone fractures when CSF fistulae are present. Consequently, the role of prophylactic antibiotics must be examined in relation to this subset of trauma patients. Multiple studies over the past three decades have concluded that prophylactic antibiotics did not have a statistically significant effect on the incidence of meningitis in patients with CSF fistulae (106,108,110,111,115,117). However, the number of patients included in the various studies was inadequate for valid statistical analysis. Reevaluation of the literature over the past 25 years using a metaanalysis revealed a statistically significant reduction in meningitis using prophylactic antibiotics in patients with CSF fistula; 320 patients were included in the analysis (118). The incidence of meningitis in patients with posttraumatic CSF fistulae treated with prophylactic antibiotics was 2.1%. In patients who did not receive prophylactic antibiotics, the incidence of meningitis was significantly higher at 8.7% ($P < 0.02$). Individually, none of the studies included in the metaanalysis demonstrated a statistically significant effect of prophylactic antibiotics, which points out the pitfall of statistical analysis with inadequate numbers of patients.

In addition to the inadequate numbers of patients in these prior studies, there are significant problems inherent in this type of retrospective study. How do we define adequate prophylaxis? Do 3 days of perioperative antibiotics for repair of a concomitant open femur fracture constitute adequate prophylaxis of a CSF fistula that persists for 5 days? Do therapeutic antibiotics for a concurrent infection constitute adequate prophylaxis of a CSF fistula? One very important risk factor increasing the risk of meningitis in patients with CSF fistulae is the presence of a concurrent infection. Brodie and Thompson (2) found a 20% incidence of meningitis in patients with concurrent infection and a 3% incidence of meningitis in the absence of concurrent infection. In that study, in the absence of concurrent infection, no patients receiving prophylactic antibiotics developed meningitis within the first month postinjury.

A recent metaanalysis sought to shed light on this issue through evaluation of four randomized control trials over the past 35 years (119). It concluded that prophylactic antibiotics did not have a statistically significant effect on meningitis in the population of patients with basilar skull fractures, either with or without CSF fistulae. These results must be interpreted cautiously. Over half of the included patients were enrolled in a study where pneumocephalus was part of the inclusion criteria (120). The rate of meningitis in this study was 20%, much higher than reported rates in the literature, indicating that this patient population is unlikely representative of the population of patients with temporal bone fractures at large. Given the current lack of conclusive data, confounding variables must be controlled in a prospective multi-institutional study to adequately address the question of the efficacy of prophylactic antibiotics.

The most common infecting organisms in meningitis occurring in the presence of a CSF fistula reported in the literature are *Streptococcus pneumoniae* followed by *Streptococcus* and *Haemophilus influenzae* (106,121,122). Fifty-seven to eighty-five percent of posttraumatic fistulae, which are treated conservatively, cease leaking within 1 week (88,107). Since acute posttraumatic CSF fistulae are associated with a high probability of early spontaneous closure and a low incidence of meningitis, they can be treated conservatively for 7 to 10 days. This treatment includes total bed rest with elevation of the head of the bed; stool softeners; instructions to avoid nose blowing, sneezing, and straining; and repeat lumbar punctures or lumbar drain if the leak persists. All of these measures are directed at maintaining the CSF pressure gradient below the healing tensile strength of the healing barrier. Due to the increased risk of meningitis following persistent CSF fistulae, surgical closure of fistulae persisting greater than 7 to 10 days is recommended.

Closure of CSF Fistulae

The approach chosen to close a CSF fistula is influenced by many factors, including the status of hearing in the affected and contralateral ears, the presence of brain herniation through the tegmen, and the location of the fistula. The treatment algorithm is presented in Figure 150.12. In a patient with a fracture of the otic capsule resulting in profound sensorineural hearing loss, obliteration of the mastoid and middle ear, and canal overclosure is recommended (123,124). The ear canal, tympanic membrane, incus and malleus, and middle ear mucosa are all excised. The external auditory meatus is closed in two layers, and a complete mastoidectomy is performed. The mucosa of the eustachian tube is inverted and a muscle plug is inserted. The incus is then inserted as well, wedging the muscle into place. The eustachian tube and fracture line are covered by temporalis fascia, and the mastoid cavity and middle ear are obliterated with an abdominal fat graft.

The approach for closure of a fistula resulting from an otic capsule–sparing fracture is dictated by the location of the fracture along the floor of the middle cranial fossa, the presence of brain herniation, and the status of the ossicular chain. Fistulae, which occur laterally in the middle cranial fossa, are accessible through a complete mastoidectomy and can be repaired by sealing the mastoid cavity off from the epitympanum and middle ear by placing a temporalis fascia graft over the antrum, facial recess, and retrofacial air cell tracts. A second fascia graft is placed over the fistula and the mastoid cavity is obliterated with a fat graft.

Fistulae, which occur more medially along the tegmen tympani or are associated with brain herniation, are addressed with a combined approach. When the temporal lobe herniates through the tegmen, the damaged brain is debrided via the transmastoid approach and the remaining brain and dura are elevated back up into the middle fossa by way of the middle fossa craniotomy. Temporalis fascia is placed over the floor of the middle cranial fossa. If a bony defect is present in the tegmen, the craniotomy bone window is split or thinned with a burr and placed along the floor of the middle cranial fossa superior to the fascia to prevent subsequent prolapse. A piece of gelfilm is inserted through the mastoid cavity and antrum and placed over the top of the ossicles in the epitympanum in order to avoid adhesions and postoperative conductive hearing loss.

In the case of a fistula through the tegmen tympani in a patient with an ossicular discontinuity and the absence of brain herniation, the fistula can often be closed via a transmastoid approach alone. A tragal cartilage graft is inserted superior to the superior EAC wall extending to the tympanic portion of the facial nerve. The cartilage graft seals off the epitympanum and prevents herniation of tissue into the middle ear. The epitympanum is filled with a temporalis fascia graft.

Additional techniques have been advocated by other authors. Glasscock et al. (125) have advocated an intradural as opposed to an extradural approach for large defects, arguing that a better closure can be achieved intradurally. Kveton et al. reported on the successful closure of 13 cases of CSF leak using hydroxyapatite cement through a transmastoid approach, in addition to reporting successful closure of 106 out of 109 temporal bone defects of all types (126,127). This approach is highly successful in closing CSF leaks following translabyrinthine removal of acoustic neuromas, but care must be taken in traumatic CSF leaks where the field is much more contaminated. Placement of a foreign body in a potentially contaminated wound increases the chance of infection. One of the other potential complications of closure of tegmen CSF fistulae with hydroxyapatite cement is conductive hearing loss, which may occur if any of the cement migrates to the ossicular chain.

There is a high risk of EAC stenosis and cholesteatoma formation when the ear canal is severely traumatized, as seen with gunshot wounds to the temporal bone (128,129). In this situation, the CSF fistulae are generally closed with resection of the EAC and tympanic membrane and obliteration of the mastoid and middle ear as described above. Extreme care is taken to avoid leaving any fragments of epithelium that may subsequently lead to cholesteatoma formation. All mucosa is removed and the eustachian tube and external meatus are closed as described above (Fig. 150.14).

Hearing Loss

Temporal bone trauma can cause a conductive hearing loss, sensorineural hearing loss, or mixed loss. Otic capsule–sparing fractures extend along the roof of the EAC, often tearing the tympanic membrane in the region of the notch of Rivinus. The fracture proceeds along the tegmen tympani and in 20% of patients disrupts the ossicular chain (11). The most common injuries to the ossicular chain are subluxation of the incudostapedial joint (82%)

and dislocation of the incus (57%) followed by fracture of the stapes crura (30%) (130). The majority of stapedial fractures do not occur in isolation but are associated with incus dislocations (11). Fixation of the ossicles in the epitympanum (25%) fracture of the malleus (11%) occurs less frequently (130). One-third of the patients will have multiple concomitant middle ear pathology.

The incidence pattern of ossicular injuries can be explained by the structural features specific to each ossicle. The malleus is well supported by the tensor tympani tendon, the epitympanic ligaments, and the tympanic membrane, and the stapes, being the smallest and lightest bone in the body, is comparatively well supported by the stapedius muscle tendon and annular ligament. In contrast, the incus is relatively heavy, situated with articulating joints on both ends, and is supported by only minor posterior and superior ligaments, thereby making it the ossicle most commonly involved in posttraumatic discontinuity.

Almost universally, patients with temporal bone fractures will experience a hemotympanum with associated conductive hearing loss. Over a few days to few weeks postinjury, the middle ear will re-aerate with resolution of the hearing loss that was attributable to the middle ear fluid. Factors that increase the duration of the middle ear fluid include endotracheal intubation, associated craniofacial fractures, and the presence of a CSF leak. Eighty percent of cases of conductive hearing loss will resolve spontaneously without the need for surgical intervention (131).

Residual conductive hearing loss following resolution of the hemotympanum and healing of the tympanic membrane suggests the possibilities of ossicular fracture or discontinuity. The indications for exploratory tympanotomy and ossicular reconstruction are conductive hearing loss greater than 30 dB that persists for more than 2 months postinjury. However, if the conductive hearing loss is in an only hearing ear, surgery is contraindicated. The audiogram in a mixed hearing loss must be critically assessed to establish the true potential benefit of ossicular reconstruction. If the bone conduction thresholds are more than 30 dB worse than in the contralateral ear, reconstruction, even with an excellent closure of the conductive component of the hearing loss, will provide minimal subjective improvement. In this scenario, the patient would still require a hearing aid to attain usable hearing in the surgical ear. Consequently, unless the mixed loss is profound and the patient cannot benefit preoperatively from a hearing aid, ossicular reconstruction is not recommended.

The most conducive injury for ossicular reconstruction is a dislocation of the incudostapedial joint. In this situation an Applebaum hydroxyapatite or similar prosthesis is inserted between the long process of the incus and capitulum of the stapes, generally resulting in complete or near-complete closure of the air–bone gap. In some instances, minimal to moderate subluxation of the incus and diastasis of the incudostapedial joint can be corrected by

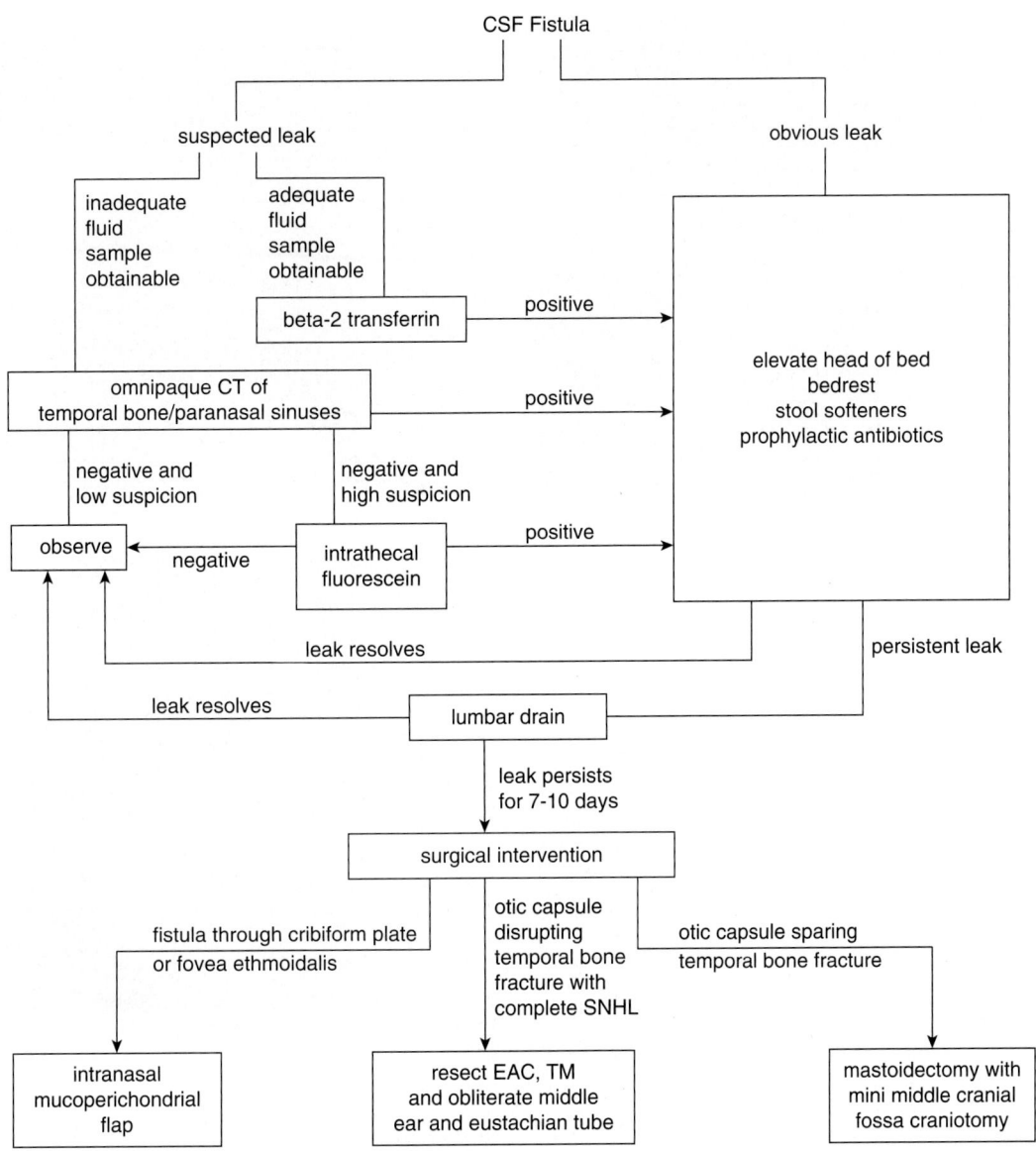

Figure 150.14   Treatment algorithm for the management of CSF fistula.

juxtaposition of the incus long process back onto the stapes capitulum and stabilization of the joint with hydroxylapatite bone cement or even just fascia. Any ossiculoplasty technique in which all three ossicles can be saved in their native orientations has the potential for complete or near-complete closure of air–bone gap (Fig. 150.15).

In contrast, cases in which the incus has been completely dislocated from the chain require interposition reconstruction, as the incus body has been completely destabilized and cannot simply be positioned back into its native orientation in a stable fashion. Dislocation of the entire incus requires bridging the gap between the stapes superstructure and the manubrium of the malleus. A sculpted incus interposition graft is preferred in this situation, although a variety of incus strut replacement and partial ossicular replacement prostheses are available and suitable for this type of reconstruction. The

incus interposition is accomplished by drilling a cup in the end of the lateral process of the incus that will fit over the capitulum of the stapes. The long process of the incus is removed and the body sculptured. The articular surface is fashioned to fit under the manubrium. If, in addition to the incus dislocation, the stapes superstructure is fractured, the long process of the incus is left intact and the body and short process sculptured. The superior surface of the body of the incus is fashioned to rest under the manubrium and the long process sits on the footplate. A variety of total ossicular replacement prostheses are available for this purpose as well.

A unique problem occurs when the stapes superstructure is fractured but the incus remains connected to the malleus. These patients are good candidates for a laser stapedotomy.

The hearing results following ossicular reconstruction for traumatic ossicular disruption are superior to those

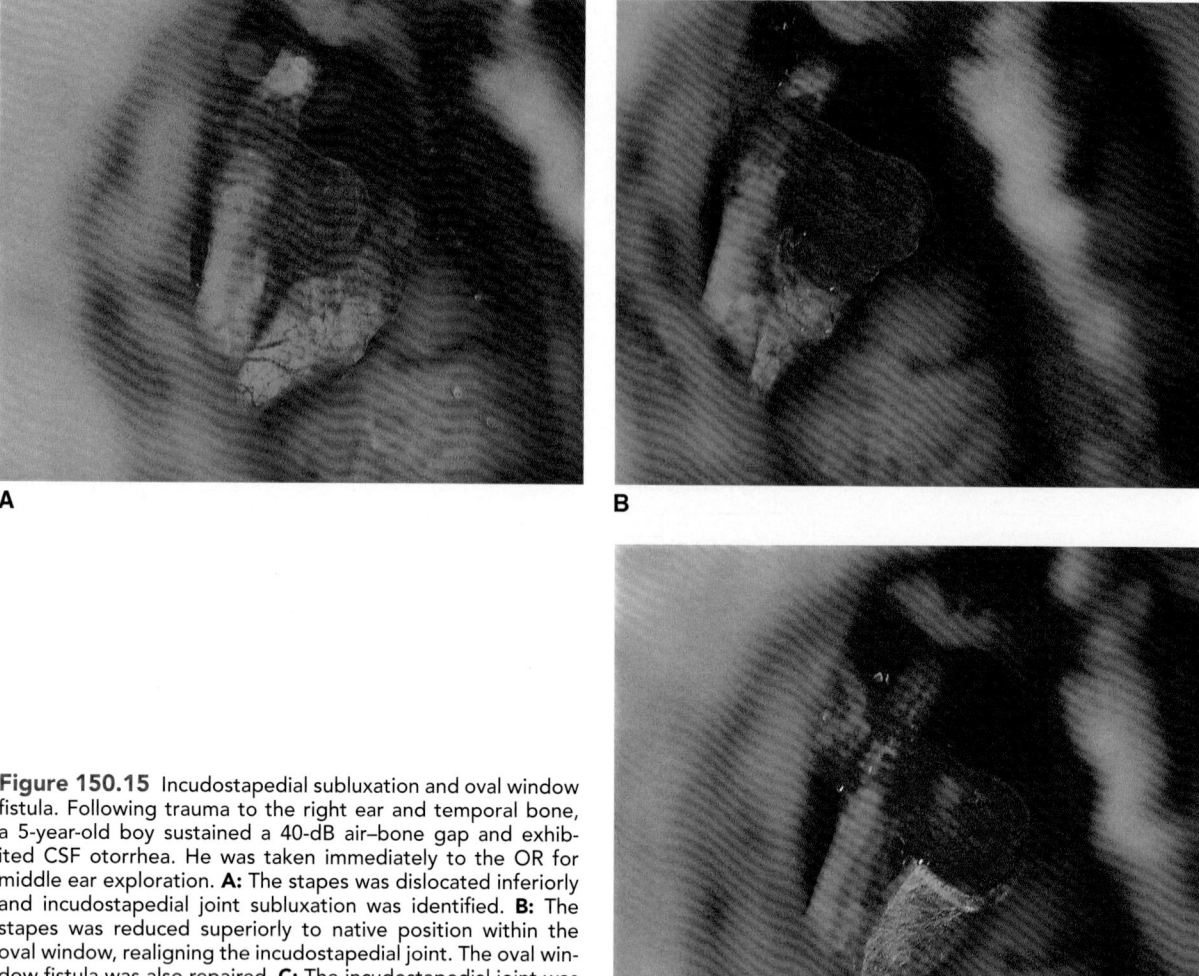

Figure 150.15 Incudostapedial subluxation and oval window fistula. Following trauma to the right ear and temporal bone, a 5-year-old boy sustained a 40-dB air–bone gap and exhibited CSF otorrhea. He was taken immediately to the OR for middle ear exploration. **A:** The stapes was dislocated inferiorly and incudostapedial joint subluxation was identified. **B:** The stapes was reduced superiorly to native position within the oval window, realigning the incudostapedial joint. The oval window fistula was also repaired. **C:** The incudostapedial joint was further stabilized with additional fascia placed circumferentially around the joint. The patient had complete closure of air–bone gap and no sensorineural hearing loss.

performed for chronic otitis media. Hough and Stuart (130) report closure of the air–bone gap to within 10 dB in 78% of patients and complete closure in 45%.

Otic capsule–disrupting fractures typically result in severe to profound sensorineural hearing loss. In addition, bilateral temporal bone fractures can also result in bilateral profound sensorineural hearing loss (132). In addition to the risk of sensorineural hearing loss from temporal bone trauma, patients who sustain closed head injuries in general, with or without temporal bone fracture, are at risk of acute sensorineural hearing loss, which can further progress with time (133). Multiple pathogenic mechanisms can contribute to posttraumatic deafness: disruption of the membranous labyrinth, avulsion or trauma to the cochlear nerve, interruption of the cochlear blood supply, hemorrhage into cochlea, and perilymphatic fistula. Another proposed mechanism is endolymphatic hydrops resulting from obstruction of the endolymphatic duct by the temporal bone fracture (134). Acoustic trauma associated with temporal bone fractures and incus dislocations frequently contributes to

a sensorineural component to a mixed hearing loss; 50% of patients with traumatic incus dislocations will have at least 10 dB of sensorineural hearing loss as well, and 18% will have more than 30 dB of loss (135). The sensorineural injury from traumatic incus dislocation appears to occur in the 2 to 4 kHz range.

High-frequency bias for cochlear acoustic injury is observed in traumatic injury to the ossicular chain, such as in cases of traumatic incus dislocation as above, as well as in iatrogenic vibrational injury to the ossicular chain as seen in cases of inadvertent drill injury to the ossicles during otologic surgery. This bias may be closely related to the phenomenon of direct acoustic injury to the cochlea seen in impulsive or severe noise-induced hearing loss, as both mechanisms involve delivery of acoustic energy through the oval window and cochlear basal turn.

Patients may suffer closed head injury (CHI) that spares the temporal bones and otic capsules of fracture yet still is of significant severity to cause sensorineural hearing loss. Such injuries to the cochlea and neurosensory hearing mechanics is sometimes referred to as cochlear concussion, when sensorineural hearing loss is clearly documented on postinjury audiogram in the absence of any fracture spanning the otic capsule or temporal bone. The traditional literature for concussive neurosensory hearing loss suggests a predilection for acoustic injury at higher frequencies, centered around 4 kHz (136,137). These older studies are limited by their small study populations, case-study-type design, and descriptive reporting of results. Additionally, results often incorporated audiometric findings years following traumatic injury, making it difficult to differentiate hearing loss resulting directly from concussive otic injury and that from age-related changes.

A recent large-scale, prospective study by Munjal et al. (138) reported the pattern of audiologic deficits measured in 290 CHI patients in comparison with 50 age- and gender-matched controls. The majority of these patients were involved in motor vehicle accidents, with the remainder suffering closed head injuries from falls or assaults. Measured hearing losses trended towards larger threshold differences and greater variability at higher frequencies; however, there was only a 5-dB average threshold difference between 250 Hz and 4 kHz for the most severe CHI patients, and there was no frequency-specific difference at all for mild and moderate CHI patients. In addition, there was a direct correlation between degree of threshold drop and severity of CHI. These findings indicate that in purely concussive cochlear injuries—such as those occurring in blunt trauma and CHI—in which there is no differential deposition of acoustic energy through the oval window, the cochlear injury is global and subsequent hearing loss flat rather than high-frequency biased and that the magnitude of such sensorineural hearing loss is directly dependent on the severity of the concussive injury.

As such, the prognosis for recovery of function in patients with anacusis or profound deafness as a result of temporal bone and cochlear trauma is extremely poor; however, patients with moderate to severe loss may have some hearing recovery (131,139). Patients who are experiencing progressive or fluctuating sensorineural hearing loss, suggestive of a possible underlying perilymphatic fistula, may benefit from middle ear exploration and repair of fistula (140).

Cholesteatoma and External Auditory Canal Stenosis

Cholesteatoma formation may occur many years after a temporal bone fracture (128,141). There are four pathogenic mechanisms responsible for posttraumatic cholesteatoma formation: (a) epithelial entrapment in the fracture line, (b) ingrowth of epithelium through the unhealed fracture line or rent in the tympanic membrane, (c) traumatic implantation of tympanic membrane skin into the middle ear, and (d) trapping of epithelium

medial to a stenosis of the EAC. The typical location for cholesteatoma resulting from epithelium trapped within the fracture line is in the epitympanum and antrum. The fracture line along the posterior superior canal wall and scutum expands and then closes trapping the canal skin. As the trapped skin grows, it expands into the epitympanum and antrum forming a cholesteatoma. The ingrowth of epithelium through a displaced fracture line may also extend into the same region. Traumatic implantation of tympanic membrane skin will result in cholesteatoma formation within the mesotympanum. Blast injuries can result in displacement of keratinizing stratified squamous epithelium into the mastoid air cells, mesotympanum, epitympanum, and even intracranium (142). The fourth mechanism of cholesteatoma formation, trapping of epithelium medial to an EAC stenosis, results in a canal cholesteatoma. Posttraumatic canal cholesteatomas are the most preventable by careful follow-up, debridement, and stenting when narrowing progresses. Early intervention with stenting at the onset of the stenosis can effectively prevent a problem that is much more difficult to address once the stenosis is mature. The ear canal can be dilated with the insertion of increasing numbers or sizes of merocel sponge packs (i.e., Pope otowick, Schindler pack, or Ambrus pack, in increasing caliber and dilational capacity) saturated with antibiotic solution, replaced every few days. Once the canal is adequately dilated, a larger merocel sponge is inserted to maintain the lumen. A large vented custom ear mold is occasionally required to maintain the lumen in the long term following severe canal injuries. The mold is used throughout the day for 3 to 6 months. When the stenosis is complete and dilation is not possible, a canalplasty and possible tympanoplasty are required. A lateral stenosis of the EAC should not be allowed to persist, even if completely benign in appearance, because of the very high probability of cholesteatoma formation.

Posttraumatic cholesteatoma involving the attic, antrum, or mastoid air cells will often grow for many years prior to detection. Until the cholesteatoma involves the ossicular chain with resultant conductive hearing loss, erodes into the labyrinth causing vertigo or sensorineural hearing loss, compresses the facial nerve resulting in facial paresis, or grows into the middle ear cleft and can be visualized on physical examination, the growth will go undetected.

Vascular Injuries

Injuries to the intratemporal carotid artery are rare but potentially life-threatening complications. Fractures that traverse the temporal bone adjacent to the carotid artery tend to involve the softer fibrocartilage of the foramen lacerum rather than the stouter, more dense bone of the carotid canal. Bloody otorrhea is a common presentation in temporal bone fractures, and the ear canal is not usually packed initially unless significant hemorrhage is present and must be controlled. In such cases, injury to the petrous portion of the carotid artery should be suspected and the patient taken immediately to either the operating room for carotid ligation or the angiography suite for balloon occlusion.

CT angiography or MR angiography is indicated in patients with focal transient or persistent neurologic deficits. In patients with significant hemorrhage from the ear or nose or with rapid neurologic deterioration, traditional interventional angiography is indicated for confirmation of carotid injury as well as immediate therapeutic intervention if necessary.

HIGHLIGHTS

- The majority of temporal bone fractures are incurred in auto accidents; multiple concurrent injuries are the rule and must be evaluated.
- The new classification system of temporal bone fracture emphasizes functional outcome: otic capsule-sparing versus otic capsule–disrupting injuries.
- The most common complications of temporal bone fractures are facial nerve injury, CSF leak, hearing loss, vertigo, cholesteatoma formation, and ear canal stenosis.
- Assessment of facial nerve function as soon as possible facilitates clinical decision making.
- Delayed-onset facial paralysis merits steroid administration and observation.
- Immediate-onset facial paralysis requires assessment of nerve stimulability. If the nerve will stimulate, observation is recommended. If the nerve will not stimulate, the nerve should be explored.
- The use of prophylactic antibiotics for temporal bone fractures is not indicated. The use of prophylactic antibiotics in the setting of CSF leak is controversial.
- Most posttraumatic CSF leaks close spontaneously. Surgical closure is required for persistent fistula.

REFERENCES

1. Makashima K, Sobel SF, Snow JB Jr. Histopathologic correlates of otoneurologic manifestations following head trauma. *Laryngoscope* 1976;86:1303–1314.
2. Brodie HA, Thompson TC. Management of complications from 820 temporal bone fractures. *Am J Otol* 1997;18:188–197.
3. Nageris B, Hansen MC, Lavelle WG, et al. Temporal bone fractures. *Am J Emerg Med* 1995;12:211–214.
4. Virapongse C, Bhimani S, Sarwar M. Radiography of the abnormal ear. In: Taveras JM, Ferrucci JT, eds. *Radiology: diagnosis-imaging-intervention*, Vol. III. Philadelphia, PA: JB Lippincott Company, 1987.
5. Lee D, Honrado C, Har-El G, et al. Pediatric temporal bone fractures. *Laryngoscope* 1998;108:816–821.
6. McGuirt WF Jr, Stool SE. Temporal bone fractures in children: a review with emphasis on long-term sequelae. *Clin Pediatr (Phila)* 1992;31:12–18.
7. Williams WT, Ghorayeb BY, Yeakley JW. Pediatric temporal bone fractures. *Laryngoscope* 1992;102:600–603.
8. Glarner H, Meuli M, Hof E, et al. Management of petrous bone fractures in children: analysis of 127 cases. *J Trauma* 1994;36:198–201.
9. Ort S, Beus K, Isaacson J. Pediatric temporal bone fractures in a rural population. *Otolaryngol Head Neck Surg* 2004;131:433–437.
10. Exadaktylos AK, Sclabas GM, Nuyens M, et al. The clinical correlation of temporal bone fractures and spiral computed tomographic scan: a prospective and consecutive study at a level I trauma center. *J Trauma* 2003;55:704–706.
11. Cannon CR, Jahrsdoerfer RA. Temporal bone fractures: review of 90 cases. *Arch Otolaryngol* 1983;109:285–288.
12. Ghorayeb BY, Rafie JJ. Fractures of the temporal bone. An evaluation of 123 cases. *J Radiol* 1989;70:703–710.
13. Tos M. Course of and sequelae to 248 petrosal fractures. *Acta Otolaryngol* 1973;75:353–354.
14. Griffin JE, Altenau MM, Schaefer SO. Bilateral longitudinal temporal bone fractures: a retrospective review of seventeen cases. *Laryngoscope* 1979;89:1432–1435.
15. Messerer O. *Uber Elasticitat und Festigkeit der Menschlichen Knochen*. Stuttgart, Germany, 1880.
16. Travis LW, Stalnaker RL, Melvin JW. Impact trauma of human temporal bone. *J Trauma* 1977;17:761–766.
17. Yoganandan N, Pintar FA, Sances AJ, et al. Biomechanics of skull fracture. *J Neurotrauma* 1995;12:659–668.
18. Yoganandan N, Pintar FA. Biomechanics of temporo-parietal skull fracture. *Clin Biomech (Bristol, Avon)* 2004;19:225–239.
19. Perlman HB. Process of healing in injuries to the capsule of labyrinth. *Arch Otolaryngol* 1939;29:287–305.
20. Pollak AM, Pauw BKH, Marion MS. Temporal bone histopathology: resident's quiz. *Am J Otol* 1991;12:56–58.
21. Sudhoff H, Linthicum FH Jr. Temporal bone fracture and latent meningitis: temporal bone histopathology study of the month. *Otol Neurotol* 2003;24:521–522.
22. Ulrich K. Verletzungen des Gehororgans bei Schadel-Basisfrakturen. *Acta Otolaryngol (Stockh)* 1926;S4:1–50.
23. Gurdjian ES, Webster JE, Lissner HR. Deformation of the skull in head injury studied by stresscoat technique. *Surg Gynecol Obstet* 1946;83:219–233.
24. Ghorayeb BY, Yeakley JW. Temporal bone fractures: longitudinal or oblique? The cases for oblique temporal bone fractures. *Laryngoscope* 1992;102:129–134.
25. Dahiya R, Keller JD, Litofsky NS, et al. Temporal bone fractures: otic capsule sparing versus otic capsule violating clinical and radiographic considerations. *J Trauma* 1999;47(6):1079–1083.
26. Kelly KE, Tami TA. Temporal bone and skull trauma. In: Jackler RK, Brackmann DE, eds. *Neurotology*. St. Louis, MO: Mosby, 1994.
27. Ishman SL, Friedland DR. Temporal bone fractures: traditional classification and clinical relevance. *Laryngoscope* 2004;114:1734–1741.
28. Wiet RJ, Valvassori GE, Kotsanis CA, et al. Temporal bone fractures. *Am J Otol* 1985;6:207–215.
29. Tos M. Course of and sequelae to 248 petrosal fractures. *Acta Otolaryngol (Stockh)* 1973;75:253–254.
30. Healy GB. Hearing loss and vertigo secondary to head injury. *N Engl J Med* 1982;306:1029–1031.
31. Fredrickson JM, Griffith AW, Lindsay JR. Transverse fractures of the temporal bone. *Arch Otolaryngol* 1963;78:770–784.
32. Little SC, Kesser BW. Radiographic classification of temporal bone fractures: clinical predictability using a new system. *Arch Otolaryngol Head Neck Surg* 2006;132:1300–1304.
33. Fisch U. Facial paralysis in fractures of the petrous bone. *Laryngoscope* 1974;84:2141–2154.
34. Vrabec JT. Otic capsule fracture with preservation of hearing and delayed-onset facial paralysis. *Int J Pediatr Otorhinolaryngol* 2001;58(2):173–177.
35. Schuknecht HF. Mechanism of inner ear injury from blows to the head. *Ann Otol Rhinol Laryngol* 1969;78:253–262.
36. Dix MR, Hallpike CS. The pathology symptomatology and diagnosis of certain common disorders of the vestibular system. *Proc R Soc Med* 1952;45:341–354.

37. Ylikoski J, Palva T, Sanna M. Dizziness after head trauma: clinical and morphologic findings. *Am J Otol* 1982;3:343–352.
38. Swartz JD. Temporal bone trauma. *Semin Ultrasound CT MR* 2001;22:219–228.
39. Morgan WE, Coker NJ, Jenkins HA. Histopathology of temporal bone fractures: implications for cochlear implantation. *Laryngoscope* 1994;104:426–432.
40. Casselman JW. Temporal bone imaging. *Neuroimaging Clin N Am* 1996;6:265–289.
41. Jang CH, Kim YH. Sudden hearing loss in intralabyrinthine haemorrhage in a child. *J Laryngol Otol* 2004;118:450–452.
42. Gross M, Ben-Yaakov A, Goldfarb A, et al. Pneumolabyrinth: an unusual finding in a temporal bone fracture. *Int J Pediatr Otorhinolaryngol* 2003;67:553–555.
43. Resnick DK, Subach BR, Marion, DW. The significance of carotid canal involvement in basilar cranial fractures. *Neurosurgery* 1997;40(6):1177–118.
44. Kahn JB, Stewart MG, Diaz-Marchan PJ. Acute temporal bone trauma: utility of high-resolution computed tomography. *Am J Otol* 2000;21(5):743–752.
45. Sun GH, Shoman NM, Samy RN, et al. Analysis of carotid artery injury in patients with basilar skull fractures. *Otol Neurotol* 2011; 32:882–886.
46. Abrunhosa J, Goncalves P, dos Santos JG, et al. Traumatic porencephalic cyst and cholesteatoma of the ear. *J Laryngol Otol* 2000; 114:864–866.
47. Ozveren MF, Uchida K, Erol FS, et al. Isolated abducens nerve paresis associated with incomplete Horner's syndrome caused by petrous apex fracture—case report and anatomical study. *Neurol Med Chir (Tokyo)* 2001;41:494–498.
48. Barron RP, Kainulainen VT, Gusenbauer AW, et al. Fracture of glenoid fossa and traumatic dislocation of mandibular condyle into middle cranial fossa. *Oral Surg Oral Med Oral Pathol Oral Radiol Endod* 2002;93:640–642.
49. Lee GY, Halcrow S. Petrous to petrous fracture associated with bilateral abducens ànd facial nerve palsies: a case report. *J Trauma* 2002; 53:583–585.
50. Spanio S, Baciliero U, Fornezza U, et al. Intracranial dislocation of the mandibular condyle: report of two cases and review of the literature. *Br J Oral Maxillofac Surg* 2002;40:253–255.
51. van der Linden WJ. Dislocation of the mandibular condyle into the middle cranial fossa: report of a case with 5 year CT follow-up. *Int J Oral Maxillofac Surg* 2003;32:215–218.
52. Darrouzet V, Duclos JY, Liguoro D, et al. Management of facial paralysis resulting from temporal bone fractures: our experience in 115 cases. *Otolaryngol Head Neck Surg* 2001;125(1):77–84.
53. McKennan KX, Chole RA. Facial paralysis in temporal bone trauma. *Am J Otol* 1992;13:167–172.
54. Turner JWA. Facial palsy in closed head injuries. *Lancet* 1944; 246:756–757.
55. Nash JJ, Friedland DR, Boorsma KJ, et al. Management and outcomes of facial paralysis from intratemporal blunt trauma: a systematic review. *Laryngoscope* 2010;120:1397–1404.
56. Maiman OJ, Cusick JF, Anderson AJ, et al. Nonoperative management of traumatic facial nerve palsy. *J Trauma* 1985;25:644–648.
57. May M. Trauma to the facial nerve. *Otolaryngol Clin North Am* 1983; 16:661–670.
58. Fisch U. Prognostic value of electrical tests in acute facial paralysis. *Am J Otol* 1984;5:494–498.
59. Sunderland S. Some anatomical and pathophysiological data relevant to facial nerve injury and repair. In: Fisch U, ed. *Facial nerve surgery*. New York: Aesculapius, 1977.
60. May M, Harvey JE, Marovitz WF, et al. The prognostic accuracy of the maximal stimulation test compared with that of the nerve excitability test in Bell's palsy. *Laryngoscope* 1971;81:931–938.
61. Fisch U. Surgery for Bell's palsy. *Arch Otolaryngol* 1981;107:1–11.
62. May M, Klein SR, Taylor FH. Idiopathic (Bell's) facial palsy: natural history defies steroid or surgical treatment. *Laryngoscope* 1985; 95:406–409.
63. Fisch U. Management of intratemporal facial nerve injuries. *J Laryngol Otol* 1980;94:129–134.
64. Sillman JS, Niparko JK, Lee SS, et al. Prognostic value of evoked and standard electromyography in acute facial paralysis. *Otolaryngol Head Neck Surg* 1992;107:377–381.
65. May M, Blumenthal F, Klein SR. Acute Bell's palsy: prognostic value of evoked electromyography, maximal stimulation, and other electrical tests. *Am J Otol* 1983;5:1–7.
66. Sittel C, Stennert E. Prognostic value of electromyography in acute peripheral facial nerve palsy. *Otol Neurotol* 2001;22: 100–104.
67. Lambert PR, Brackmann DE. Facial paralysis in longitudinal temporal bone fractures: a review of 26 cases. *Laryngoscope* 1984; 94:1022–1026.
68. Coker NJ, Kendall KA, Jenkins HA, et al. Traumatic intratemporal facial nerve injury: management rationale for preservation of function. *Otolaryngol Head Neck Surg* 1987;97:262–269.
69. Kamerer DO. Intratemporal facial nerve injuries. *Otolaryngol Head Neck Surg* 1982;90:612–615.
70. Yeoh TL, Mahmud R, Saim L. Surgical intervention in traumatic facial nerve paralysis. *Med J Malaysia* 2003;58:432–436.
71. Chang JCY, Cass S. Management of facial nerve injury due to temporal bone trauma. *Am J Otol* 1999;20:96–114.
72. Sargent EW, Kartush JM, Graham MD. Meatal facial nerve decompression in acoustic neuroma resection. *Am J Otol* 1995;16: 457–464.
73. Fisch U. Facial paralysis in fractures of the petrous bone. *Laryngoscope* 1974;84:2141–2154.
74. May M. Total facial nerve exploration: transmastoid, extralabyrinthine, and subtemporal indications and results. *Laryngoscope* 1979;89:906–917.
75. Goin OW. Proximal intratemporal facial nerve in Bell's palsy surgery: a study correlating anatomical and surgical findings. *Laryngoscope* 1982;92:263–271.
76. Yanagihara N. Transmastoid decompression of the facial nerve in temporal bone fracture. *Otolaryngol Head Neck Surg* 1982;90: 616–621.
77. McCabe BF. Facial nerve grafting. *Plast Reconstr Surg* 1970;45: 70–75.
78. Barrs DM. Facial nerve trauma: optimal timing for repair. *Laryngoscope* 1991;101:835–848.
79. Fisch U. Current surgical treatment of intratemporal facial palsy. *Clin Plast Surg* 1979;178:347–361.
80. Quaranta A, Campobasso G, Piazza F, et al. Facial nerve paralysis in temporal bone fractures: outcomes after late decompression surgery. *Acta Otolaryngol* 2001;121:652–655.
81. Sanus GZ, Tanriover N, Tanriverdi T, et al. Late decompression in patients with acute facial nerve paralysis after temporal bone fracture. *Turk Neurosurg* 2007;17:7–12.
82. House WF. Surgical exposure to the internal auditory canal and its contents through the middle cranial fossa. *Laryngoscope* 1961; 71:1363–1385.
83. Glasscock M. Middle fossa approach to the temporal bone. *Arch Otolaryngol* 1969;90:41–57.
84. Fisch U. Transtemporal surgery of the internal auditory canal. *Adv Otorhinolaryngol* 1970;17:202–239.
85. Portmann M, Cohandon F, Castel JP, Lebert G. Neurotomy of the 8th cranial pair via the temporal fossa. *Rev Laryngol Otol Rhinol (Bord)* 1969;90:700–715.
86. Garcia-Ibanez E, Garcia-Ibanez JL. Middle fossa vestibular neurectomy: a report of 373 cases. *Otolaryngol Head Neck Surg* 1980; 88:486–490.
87. Schuknecht HF, Gulya AJ. *Anatomy of the temporal bone with surgical implications*. Philadelphia, PA: Lea & Febiger, 1986.
88. Lewin W. Cerebrospinal fluid rhinorrhea in nonmissile head injuries. *Clin Neurosurg* 1964;12:237–252.
89. Hirsch D. Successful closure of cerebrospinal fluid rhinorrhea by endonasal surgery. *Arch Otolaryngol* 1952;56:1–12.
90. Grahne B. Traumatic cranionasal fistulas persistent cerebrospinal fluid rhinorrhea and their repair with frontal sinus osteoplasty. *Acta Otolaryngol* 1970;70:392–400.
91. Kogoy J, Trieff NM, Winkelmann P, et al. Glucose in nasal secretion: diagnostic significance. *Arch Otolaryngol* 1972;95:225–229.
92. Meurman OH, Irjala K, Suonpaa J, et al. A new method for the identification of cerebrospinal fluid leakage. *Acta Otolaryngol* 1979;87:366–369.
93. Sloman, AJ, Kelly RH. Transferrin allelic variants may cause false positives in the detection of cerebrospinal fluid fistulae. *Clin Chem* 1993;39:1444–1445.

94. Felgenhauer K, Schadlich HJ, Nekic M. Beta-trace protein as marker for cerebrospinal fluid fistula. *Klin Wochenschr* 1987;65:764–768.

95. Bachmann G, Nekic M, Michel O. Clinical experience with beta-trace protein as a marker for cerebrospinal fluid. *Ann Otol Rhinol Laryngol* 2000;109:1099–1102.

96. Petereit HF, Bachmann G, Nekic M, et al. A new nephelometric assay for beta-trace protein (prostaglandin D synthase) as an indicator of liquorrhea. *J Neurol Neurosurg Psychiatry* 2001;71:347–351.

97. Arrer E, Meco C, Oberascher G, et al. Beta-trace protein as a marker for cerebrospinal fluid rhinorrhea. *Clin Chem* 2002;48:939–941.

98. Sampaio MH, de Barros-Mazon S, Sakano E, et al. Predictability of quantification of beta-trace protein for diagnosis of cerebrospinal fluid leak: cutoff determination in nasal fluids with two control groups. *Am J Rhinol Allergy* 2009;23:585–590.

99. Stone JA, Castillo M, Neelon B, et al. Evaluation of CSF leaks: high-resolution CT compared with contrast-enhanced CT and radionuclide cisternography. *Am J Neuroradiol* 1999;20:706–712.

100. Briant TDR, Snell D. Diagnosis of cerebrospinal rhinorrhea and the rhinologic approach to its repair. *Laryngoscope* 1967;77:1390–1409.

101. Charles DA, Snell D. Cerebrospinal fluid rhinorrhea. *Laryngoscope* 1979;89:822–826.

102. Calcaterra TC. Extracranial surgical repair of cerebrospinal rhinorrhea. *Ann Otol* 1980;89:108–116.

103. Morley TP, Wortzman G. The importance of the lateral extensions of the sphenoidal sinus in post-traumatic cerebrospinal rhinorrhea and meningitis. *J Neurosurg* 1965;22:326–332.

104. Hughes GB, Glasscock ME III, Hays JW, et al. Cerebrospinal fluid leaks and meningitis following acoustic tumor surgery. *Otolaryngol Head Neck Surg* 1982;90:117–125.

105. Leech PI, Paterson A. Conservative and operative management of cerebrospinal fluid leakage after closed head injury. *Lancet* 1973;1:1013–1015.

106. MacGee EE, Cauthen JC, Brackett CE. Meningitis following acute traumatic cerebrospinal fluid fistula. *J Neurosurg* 1970;33:312–316.

107. Mincy JE. Post-traumatic cerebrospinal fluid fistula of the frontal fossa. *J Trauma* 1966;6:618–622.

108. Spetzler RF, Wilson CB. Management of recurrent CSF rhinorrhea of the middle and posterior fossa. *J Neurosurg* 1978;49:393–397.

109. Hoff JT, Brewin A, Sang H. Antibiotics for basilar skull fractures. *J Neurosurg* 1976;44:649.

110. Zrebeet HA, Huang PS. Prophylactic antibiotics in the treatment of fractures at the base of the skull. *Del Med J* 1986;58:741–748.

111. Frazee RC, Mucha P, Farnell MB, et al. Meningitis after basilar skull fracture. *Postgrad Med* 1988;83:267–274.

112. Einhorn A, Mizrahi EM. Basilar skull fractures in children. *Am J Dis Child* 1978;132:1121–1124.

113. Hellings TS, Evans LL, Fowler DL, et al. Infectious complications in patients with severe head injury. *J Trauma* 1988;28:1575–1577.

114. Ignelzi RJ, VanderArk GD. Analysis of the treatment of basilar skull fractures with and without antibiotics. *J Neurosurg* 1975;43:75–85.

115. Dagi TF, Meyer FB, Poletti CA. The incidence and prevention of meningitis after basilar skull fracture. *Am J Emerg Med* 1983;3:295–298.

116. Rathore MH. Do prophylactic antibiotics prevent meningitis after basilar skull fracture. *Pediatr Infect Dis J* 1991;10:87–88.

117. Klastersky J, Sadeghi M, Brihaye J. Antimicrobial prophylaxis in patients with rhinorrhea or otorrhea: a double blind study. *Surg Neurol* 1976;6:111–114.

118. Brodie HA. Prophylactic antibiotics for post-traumatic cerebrospinal fluid fistulae. A meta-analysis. *Arch Otolaryngol Head Neck Surg* 1997;123:749–752.

119. Ratilal BO, Costa J, Sampaio C. Antibiotic prophylaxis for preventing meningitis in patients with basilar skull fractures. *Cochrane Database of Systematic Reviews* 2006;Issue 1. Art. No.: CD004884, doi: 10.1002/14651858/CD004884/pub2.

120. Eftekhar B, Ghodsi M, Nejat F, et al. Prophylactic administration of ceftriaxone for the prevention of meningitis after traumatic pneumocephalus: results of a clinical trial. *J Neurosurg* 2004;101:757–761.

121. Applebaum E. Meningitis following trauma to the head and face. *JAMA* 1960;173:1818–1822.

122. Kaufman BA, Tunkel AR, Pryor JC, et al. Meningitis in the neurosurgical patient. *Infect Dis Clin North Am* 1990;4:677–701.

123. Kveton JF. Obliteration of the mastoid and middle ear for severe trauma to the temporal bone. *Laryngoscope* 1987;97:1385–1387.

124. Coker NJ, Jenkins HA, Fisch U. Obliteration of the middle ear and mastoid cleft in subtotal petrosectomy. Indications, technique and results. *Ann Otol Rhinol Laryngol* 1986;95:5–11.

125. Glasscock ME III, Dickins JRE, Jackson CG, et al. Surgical management of brain tissue herniation into the middle ear and mastoid. *Laryngoscope* 1979;89:1743–1754.

126. Kveton JF, Goravalingappa R. Elimination of temporal bone cerebrospinal fluid otorrhea using hydroxyapatite cement. *Laryngoscope* 2000;110:988–990.

127. Kveton JF, Coelho DH. Hydroxyapatite cement in temporal bone surgery: a 10 year experience. *Laryngoscope* 2004;114:33–37.

128. McKennan KX, Chole RA. Post-traumatic cholesteatoma. *Laryngoscope* 1989;99:779–782.

129. Kronenberg J, Ben-Shoshan J, Modan M, et al. Blast injury and cholesteatoma. *Am J Otol* 1988;9:127–130.

130. Hough JVD, Stuart WD. Middle ear injuries in skull trauma. *Laryngoscope* 1968;78:899–937.

131. Tos M. Prognosis of hearing loss in temporal bone fractures. *Laryngol Otol* 1971;85:1147–1159.

132. Atkin G, Watkins L, Rich P. Bilateral sensorineural hearing loss complicating basal skull fracture. *Br J Neurosurg* 2002;16:597–600.

133. Bergemalm PO. Progressive hearing loss after closed head injury: a predictable outcome? *Acta Otolaryngol* 2003;123:836–845.

134. Rizvi SS, Gibbin KP. Effect of transverse temporal bone fracture on the fluid compartment of the inner ear. *Ann Otol Rhinol Laryngol* 1979;88:741–748.

135. Dommerby H, Tos M. Sensorineural hearing loss in post-traumatic incus dislocation. *Arch Otolaryngol* 1983;109:257–261.

136. Zimmerman WD, Ganzel TM, Windmill IM, et al. Peripheral hearing loss following head trauma in children. *Laryngoscope* 1993;103:87–91.

137. Bergemalm PO, Borg E. Long-term objective and subjective audiologic consequences of closed head injury. *Arch Otolaryngol* 2001;121:724–734.

138. Munjal SK, Panda NK, Pathak A. Audiological deficits after closed head injury. *J Trauma* 2010;68:13–18.

139. Podoshin L, Fradis M. Hearing loss after head injury. *Arch Otolaryngol* 1975;101:15–18.

140. Lyos AT, Marsh MA, Jenkins HA, et al. Progressive hearing loss after transverse temporal bone fracture. *Arch Otolaryngol Head Neck Surg* 1995;121:795–799.

141. Freeman J. Temporal bone fractures and cholesteatoma. *Ann Otol Rhinol Laryngol* 1983;92:558–560.

142. Goldfarb A, Eliashar R, Gross M, et al. Middle cranial fossa cholesteatoma following blast trauma. *Ann Otol Rhino Laryngol* 2001;110:1084–1086.

Cholesteatoma

151

Ted A. Meyer *Chester L. Strunk Jr.* *Paul R. Lambert*

Cholesteatomas are expansile lesions of the temporal bone lined by stratified squamous epithelium that contain desquamated keratin. Some cholesteatomas are invaginated pouches that can develop from retraction pockets, while others are completely enclosed cysts. They most frequently involve the middle ear and mastoid, but they may develop anywhere within the pneumatized portions of the temporal bone. They may be congenital (infrequently) or acquired.

The accumulation of keratin may cause infection, otorrhea, bone destruction, hearing loss, facial nerve paralysis, a labyrinthine fistula, and intracranial complications such as epidural and subdural abscesses, parenchymal brain abscesses, meningitis, and thrombophlebitis of the dural venous sinuses.

Cholesteatoma is a misnomer originally coined by Johannes Mueller in 1838 when he described "layered pearly tumor of fat, which was distinguished from other fat tumors by the biliary fat or cholesterin that is interspersed among the sheets of polyhedral cells" (1). Cholesteatomas do not contain fat, and they do not usually contain cholesterin. Nevertheless, the term remains, despite a more appropriate term suggested by Schuknecht: keratoma.

The matrix of a cholesteatoma is composed of fully differentiated squamous epithelium resting on connective tissue. The deeper layers of the epithelium of a cholesteatoma matrix show activity in the form of downgrowths into the underlying connective tissue. Cholesteatomas have a layer of granulation tissue in contact with bone. This layer of granulation tissue elaborates various enzymes such as collagenase resulting in bone destruction.

Cholesteatomas are recidivistic by nature. The conditions or processes through which they develop are often present throughout a patient's life. Eustachian tube disease, with negative middle ear pressures, and a retracted eardrum are usually seen in patients with primary acquired cholesteatomas, and this can continue even with the complete surgical removal of a cholesteatoma. The function of the eustachian tube does not necessarily ever improve, and the patient is at risk for further cholesteatoma. If cholesteatoma is left behind surgically, either planned or unknowingly, this is considered residual disease. After being completely removed, if cholesteatoma forms again, this is considered a recurrence.

CONGENITAL CHOLESTEATOMA

Congenital cholesteatoma is defined by Derlacki and Clemis (2) as an embryonic rest of epithelial tissue in the ear without tympanic membrane perforation and without a history of ear infection. Levenson et al. (3,4) have modified the definition of a congenital cholesteatoma to include a normal pars flaccida and pars tensa, no history of prior otorrhea, and no history of prior otologic procedures. Prior episodes of otitis media without otorrhea are not criteria for excluding congenital origin. Two-thirds of the middle ear congenital cholesteatomas are seen as a white mass in the anterior–superior quadrant (Fig. 151.1). They may also be found within the tympanic membrane and in the petrous apex. The mean age at presentation for a congenital middle ear cholesteatoma is 4.5 years, with a male-to-female preponderance of 3:1 (4).

The pathogenesis of congenital cholesteatomas is incompletely understood. In a review of the development of the epibranchial organs, Teed (5) noted an ectodermal epithelial thickening that developed in proximity of the geniculate ganglion, medial to the neck of the malleus. This mass of epithelial cells soon undergoes involution to become mature middle ear lining. Teed believed that if involution failed to take place, this formation could be the source of a congenital cholesteatoma. In pursuit of this theory, Michaels (6,7) undertook a review of fetal human temporal bones and identified a squamous cell tuft present from 10 to 33 weeks of gestation in 37 of 68 specimens studied. He termed this structure the *epidermoid formation*

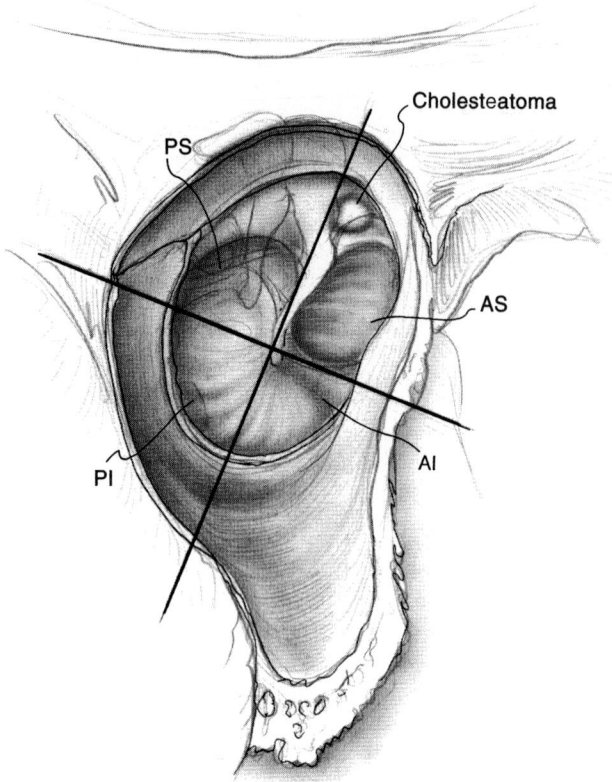

Figure 151.1 Congenital cholesteatoma of the anterior–superior quadrant. AI, anterior inferior; AS, anterior superior; PI, posterior inferior; PS, posterior superior.

and noted it to be located in the anterosuperior wall of the developing middle ear cleft. Failure of the epidermoid formation to involute could be the basis for the development of cholesteatomas in the anterior mesotympanum (8–10). Other investigators implicate ectodermal migration or even metaplasia of the middle ear mucosa in the pathogenesis of congenital cholesteatomas (11,12).

To further complicate the understanding of the development and pathogenesis of congenital cholesteatomas, they have been described as developing in or isolated to the mastoid (13,14). Staging systems and management strategies have been developed by several groups (15–17), with staged surgical procedures recommended for the more complicated or higher-stage lesions.

ACQUIRED CHOLESTEATOMA

Acquired middle ear cholesteatomas come in two varieties: primary or retraction pocket cholesteatoma and secondary cholesteatoma. Cholesteatomas that arise from retraction pockets are known as primary acquired cholesteatomas on the basis that infection has not given rise to the cholesteatoma. Several theories have been advanced to explain the formation of primary acquired or attic retraction cholesteatomas, including invagination of the pars flaccida, basal cell hyperplasia, otitis media with effusion, and perforation of the pars flaccida membrane with epithelial ingrowth

TABLE 151.1	PATHOGENESIS OF CHOLESTEATOMAS

Primary acquired cholesteatomas
  Invagination theory
  Basal cell hyperplasia theory
  Otitis media with effusion theory
  Epithelial invasion theory
Secondary acquired cholesteatomas
  Implantation theory
  Metaplasia theory
  Epithelial invasion theory

(Table 151.1). Patients with cleft palates are particularly prone to the development of primary acquired attic cholesteatomas (18–22).

The invagination theory is supported by the observations of Aschoff in 1897 and Wittmaack in 1933 (23). They proposed that an infantile sterile otitis media neonatorum or nonbacterial otitis media develops soon after birth. Before it has had time to resorb, a permanent fibrosis and thickening of the embryonic subepithelial tympanic connective tissue occurs resulting in blockage of the attic causing a localized negative pressure with retraction of the pars flaccida. The fibrosis and thickening in the attic blocks the normal process of pneumatization of the epitympanum and antrum and decreases the pneumatization of the mastoid process and petrous portions of the temporal bone throughout the patient's life. This small dimple-like retraction of the pars flaccida that cannot be reduced by inflation of the eustachian tube is the first stage in the development of an attic cholesteatoma.

A second method by which a small retraction pocket may develop is from long-standing otitis media with effusion (Fig. 151.2). Bluestone and Klein (18) demonstrated that in children with attic retractions, the eustachian tube constricts rather than dilates with swallowing. This results in impaired ventilation of the middle ear and mastoid air cell system and fluctuating or sustained high negative middle ear pressures. Negative middle ear pressure caused by eustachian tube dysfunction can result in retraction of the pars flaccida and collection of desquamated debris.

Like primary acquired cholesteatomas, several pathogenic mechanisms may contribute to the formation of secondary acquired cholesteatomas (Table 151.1). The implantation theory, the metaplasia theory, and the epithelial invasion theory have all been advanced as possible mechanisms involved in cholesteatoma formation. The implantation theory describes the formation of a cholesteatoma by the iatrogenic implantation of skin into the middle ear or eardrum as a result of surgery, a foreign body, trauma, or a blast injury. Cholesteatomas may develop secondary to a myringotomy for ventilating tube

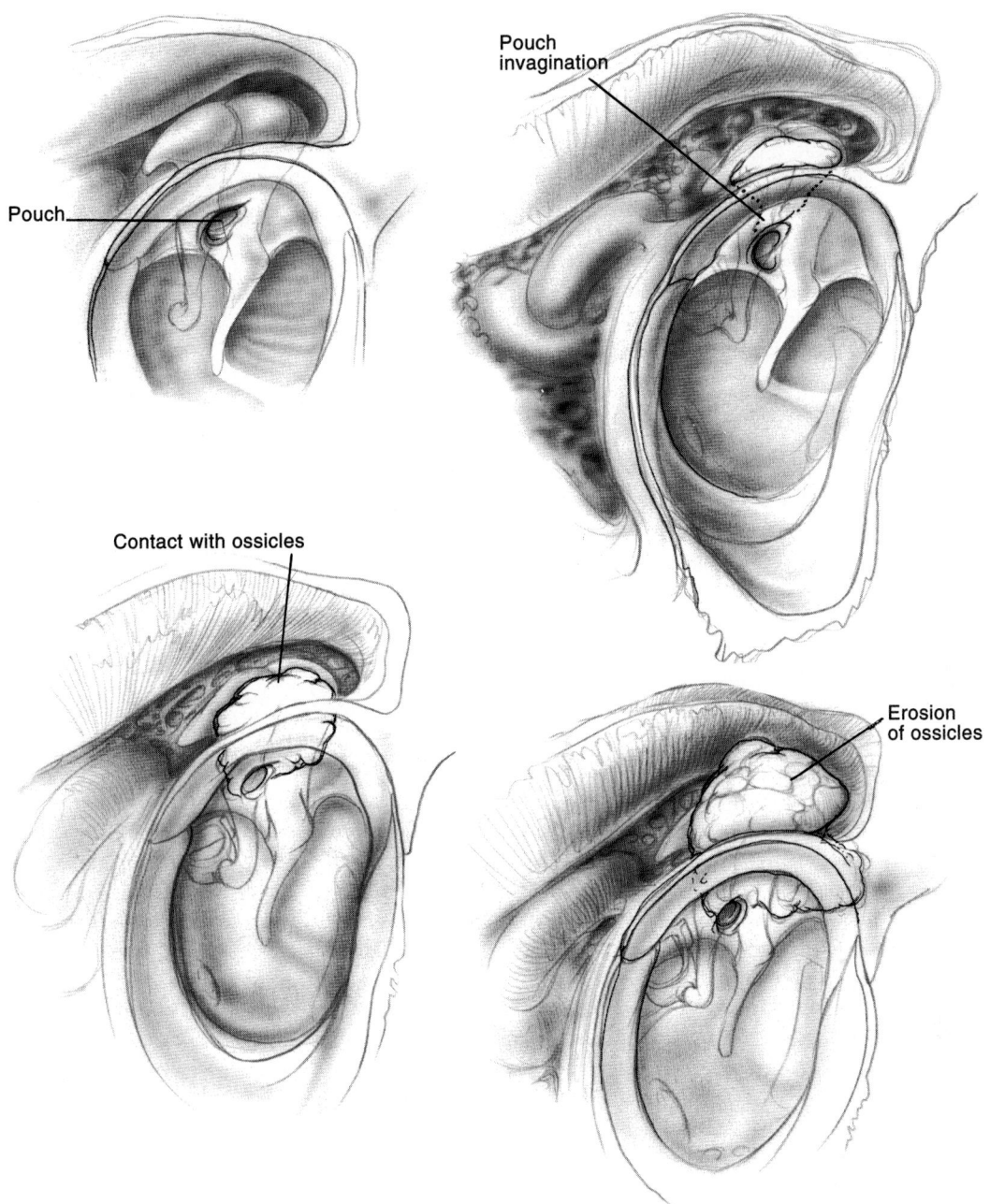

Figure 151.2 Evolution of an attic cholesteatoma.

placement or a tympanoplasty procedure. They occur as a result of epithelial migration or displacement through the myringotomy or from the displacement of a flap of the tympanic membrane into the middle ear at the time of a tympanoplasty. Secondary acquired cholesteatomas are also thought to arise from a perforation as a result of acute necrotic otitis media in childhood (24).

The metaplasia theory describes the transformation of columnar epithelium to keratinized stratified squamous epithelium secondary to chronic or recurrent otitis media. Support for this theory comes from changes that occur in the bronchi in the face of chronic irritation and infection. However, metaplasia is not thought to be a significant cause

of cholesteatoma in humans (25). The epithelial invasion theory involves the invasion of the middle ear by skin from the meatal wall of the outer drum surface through a marginal perforation or an attic perforation (26). This is supported by experimental evidence demonstrating that epithelial cells migrate along a surface until they encounter another epithelial surface, at which point they stop migrating; this is known as contact inhibition. If the middle ear mucosa were destroyed by infection, then this would allow for epithelial migration from a marginal perforation. This is the generally accepted theory for the formation of secondary acquired cholesteatomas of the posterior–superior tympanic membrane.

Cholesteatoma may also arise in the external auditory canal (27–31) often after trauma from repeated direct manipulation. Like cholesteatoma in the middle ear, epithelial migration is disrupted in external auditory canal (EAC) cholesteatoma. Patients present with otorrhea, otalgia, bony destruction, and trapped squamous debris, and some have hearing loss. Some EAC cholesteatomas have similar characteristics as keratosis obturans, but in general, surgical removal is the treatment modality of choice for EAC cholesteatoma, where patients with keratosis obturans can usually be managed by frequent office cleanings and topical therapy (32).

A unique feature that cholesteatoma and tympanic membrane epithelium have in common is migration. No other epithelium tested, including skin, vocal cord, and oral epithelium, has shown the locomotion present with tympanic membrane epithelium and cholesteatoma (33). Once a retraction pocket develops, the epithelial migratory pattern is altered and keratin accumulates. This is the second stage in the development of a cholesteatoma. The sac slowly enlarges by accumulation of keratin and other debris until the walls of the attic are reached. Once this point is reached, bone resorption occurs. Three factors appear to be involved in the process of bony resorption: (a) *mechanical*, related to pressure generated by the expansion of cholesteatoma as it accumulates increasing amounts of keratin and purulent debris (34–36); (b) *biochemical*, due to bacterial elements (endotoxins), products of the host's granulation tissue (collagenase, acid hydrolases), and substances related to the cholesteatoma itself (growth factors, cytokines) (37–49); and (c) *cellular*, predominantly induced by osteoclastic activity (50–53). It is likely that bone destruction in cholesteatoma results from a combination of these factors, but clarification is needed regarding their specific roles.

Multinucleated osteoclasts within the subepithelial matrix of a cholesteatoma release acid phosphatase, collagenase, and other proteolytic enzymes that resorb the bone products. The osteoclasts may be further activated by infection, pressure, and Langerhans cells through an immune mechanism. Cholesteatoma debris is a favorite culture medium for bacteria from the external meatus, including staphylococci, *Pseudomonas aeruginosa, Proteus, Enterobacter*, aerobic and anaerobic nonhemolytic streptococci, diphtheroid bacilli, and *Aspergillus* molds. When the cholesteatoma becomes infected from water contamination, a foul-smelling discharge ensues. An active infected cholesteatoma will resorb bone at a faster rate.

The ability of cholesteatomas to erode bone is what makes them particularly dangerous (Fig. 151.3). Their expansion is dictated by space available, their migratory tendency, and their internal desquamation. Pressure alone may cause bone resorption to take place.

SURGICAL ANATOMY

Cholesteatomas are channeled along characteristic pathways by ligaments and folds. During the third to fifth fetal months, endothelial-lined sacs develop from evaginations of

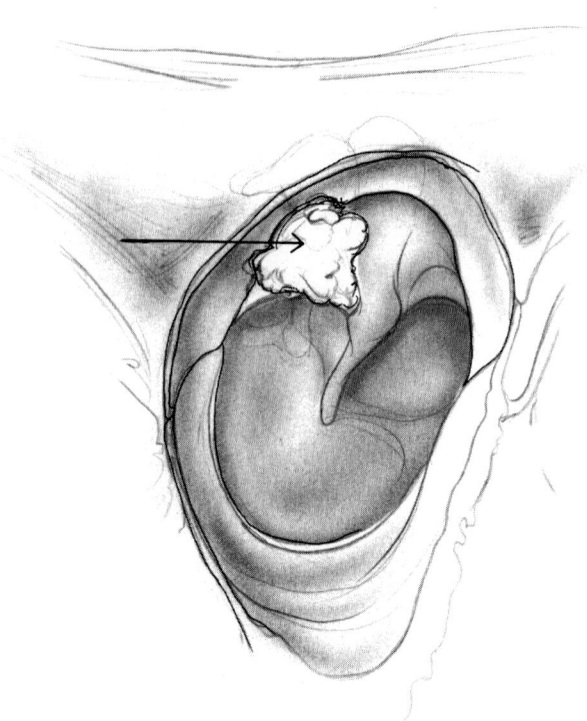

Figure 151.3 Infected cholesteatoma of the attic eroding the scutum (*arrow*).

the first brachial pouch to form the tympanic cavity mucosal folds and ossicular suspensory ligaments. These sacs contact each other, defining the various pouches, spaces, and compartments that divide the middle ear (Fig. 151.4).

The most common locations of origin of cholesteatomas in decreasing frequency are the posterior epitympanum, the posterior mesotympanum, and the anterior epitympanum (54). Epitympanum cholesteatomas originate in a shallow pocket that lies between the pars flaccida of the tympanic membrane and the neck of the malleus. This pouch, known as Prussak space, has as its floor the lateral process of the malleus and its associated mucosal folds lying in the horizontal plane. Cholesteatomas most commonly exit Prussak space by the posterior route: the cholesteatoma penetrates the superior incudal space lateral to the body of the incus. From there, it traverses the aditus ad antrum to enter the mastoid (Fig. 151.5). The cholesteatoma may reach the middle ear by descending through the floor of Prussak space into the posterior space of von Troeltsch, a pouch lying between the tympanic membrane and the posterior mallear fold, the inferior edge of which contains the chorda tympani nerve (Fig. 151.4). This pouch contains a medial, superior, and lateral wall but is open to the mesotympanum inferiorly toward the posterior mesotympanum. Cholesteatomas in this region may involve the stapes, round window, sinus tympani, and facial recess.

The second most common site of origin of cholesteatomas is the posterior mesotympanum (Fig. 151.6). The pars tensa retracts into the mesotympanum to form a cholesteatoma sac that passes medial to the malleus and the incus. Cholesteatomas in this region invade the sinus tympani

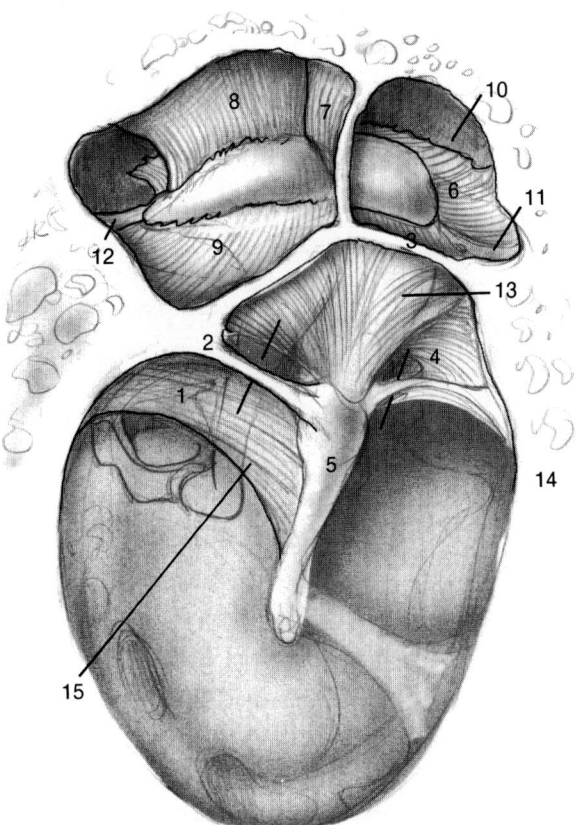

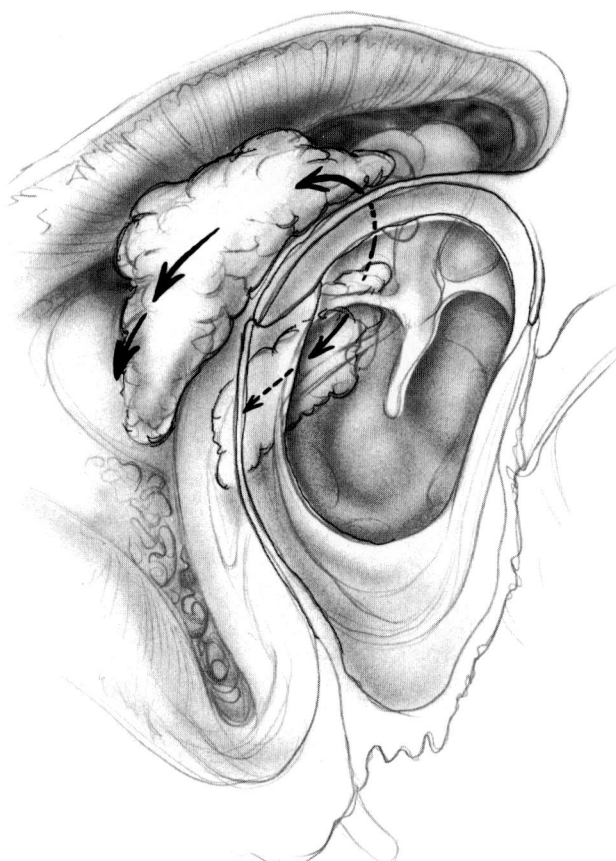

Figure 151.4 Spaces and pouches on the middle ear defined by various ligaments and folds. *1*, posterior mallear fold; *2*, posterior tympanic stria; *3*, lateral mallear fold; *4*, anterior tympanic membrane stria; *5*, malleus (short process); *6*, tensor fold; *7*, superior mallear fold; *8*, superior incudal fold; *9*, lateral incudal fold; *10*, anterior epitympanic space; *11*, anterior mallear ligament; *12*, postincudal ligament; *13*, Prussak space; *14*, anterior pouch (VT); *15*, posterior pouch of von Troeltsch.

Figure 151.5 Posterior epitympanic cholesteatoma passing through the superior incudal space and the aditus ad antrum.

PREVENTION

and facial recess. The sinus tympani lies between the facial nerve and the medial wall of the mesotympanum. The facial recess is bounded by the fossa incudis and the facial nerve posteriorly and the chorda tympani nerve anteriorly. Both areas are difficult to access surgically (Fig. 151.7) and are common sites of residual cholesteatoma.

Anterior epitympanic cholesteatomas develop as a retraction pocket anterior to the malleus head. The anterior epitympanic space or supratubal recess is limited anteriorly by the middle cranial fossa, the petrous tip, and the root of the zygoma; posteriorly by a bony ridge, termed the *cog*, extending to the cochleariform process; superiorly by the middle cranial fossa; and laterally by the tympanic bone and chorda tympani nerve. The floor of the anterior epitympanum is intimately associated with the horizontal portion of the facial nerve. Cholesteatomas in this region can therefore cause a facial paresis or paralysis (55). Anterior epitympanic cholesteatomas extend to the supratubal recess of the middle ear via the anterior pouch of von Troeltsch, a shallow pouch lying between the tympanic membrane and the anterior mallear fold (Fig. 151.8). If the area anterior to the malleus head is not explored thoroughly during tympanomastoidectomy, cholesteatomas in this region can be overlooked.

A retraction pocket secondary to eustachian tube dysfunction precedes the development of acquired cholesteatoma. It is good practice to aggressively manage such retraction pockets. A tympanostomy tube should be inserted early in an effort to resolve the negative middle ear pressure and to return the tympanic membrane to a neutral position (Fig. 151.9). However, many retraction pockets persist after tube placement. If the retraction pocket adheres to the ossicles or surrounding structures, it will not reverse. Similarly, if the tympanic membrane has been retracted for a long time and loses all its elasticity, it will not revert to a normal appearance. Tube placement is best done under general anesthesia, where the retraction pocket may be seen to distend as the patient is masked with positive-pressure ventilation. A T-tube or some other long-term ventilation tube is often necessary. If the retraction pocket does not distend with positive-pressure ventilation, then it should be examined carefully to determine the extent and depth of the pocket. Mirror examination or the use of a 90-degree telescope may be used to see hidden borders of the pocket. Most retraction pockets extend into the epitympanum or sinus tympani. If the pocket persists despite tympanostomy tube placement, then surgical exploration may be indicated.

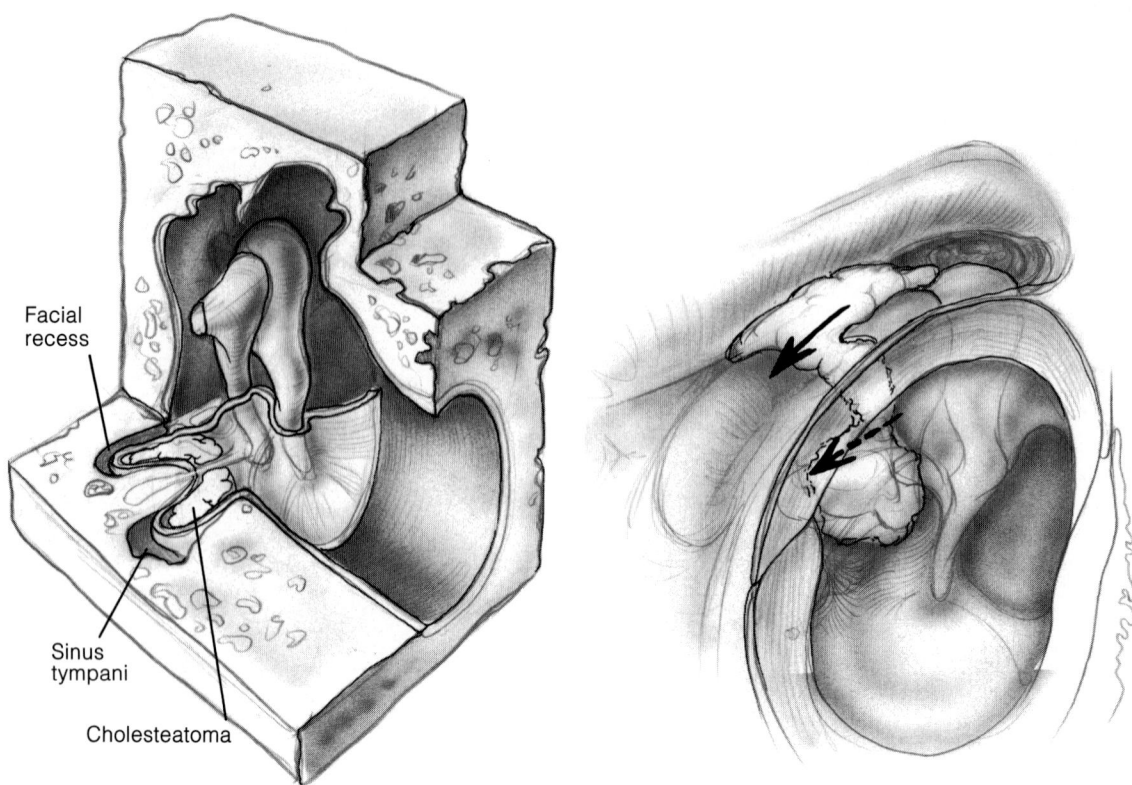

Facial recess

Sinus tympani

Cholesteatoma

Figure 151.6 Posterior mesotympanic cholesteatoma invading the sinus tympani and facial recess.

PREOPERATIVE EVALUATION

The presence of a cholesteatoma usually requires surgical management unless advanced age or poor health prohibits an operation. However, an elderly patient, with a cholesteatoma that is not infected, and is easily accessible with a microscope in the clinic, can often be managed by serial debridement. Both congenital and acquired cholesteatomas are asymptomatic during early development. Careful

questioning of a patient with a middle ear cholesteatoma often reveals many years of subtle ear symptoms, beginning with a progressive hearing loss (usually unilateral). Unilateral hearing loss may be ignored until the cholesteatoma becomes infected secondary to water contamination or an upper respiratory infection, producing a foul-smelling otorrhea. When an infected cholesteatoma is present or there is bone destruction, the purulent discharge tends to be thick, scanty, and fetid. An occasional patient will ignore the

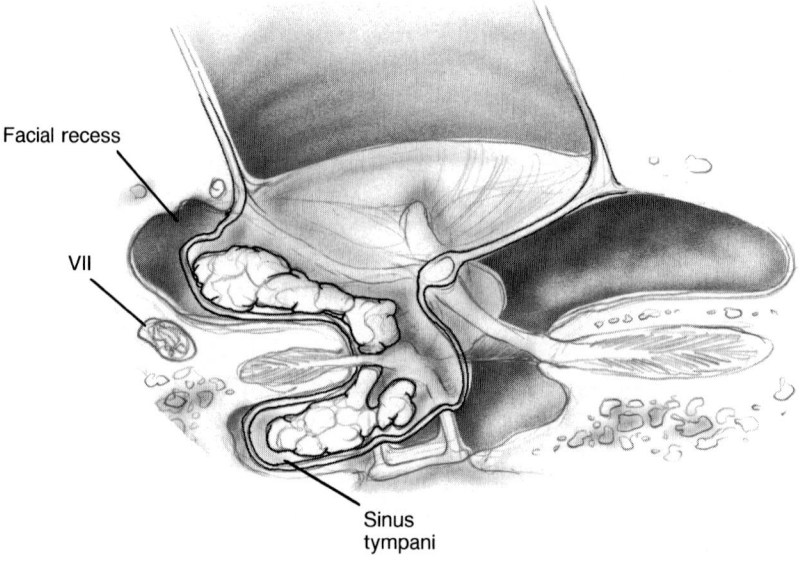

Facial recess

VII

Sinus tympani

Figure 151.7 Posterior mesotympanic cholesteatoma involving the facial recess and sinus tympani. VII, facial nerve.

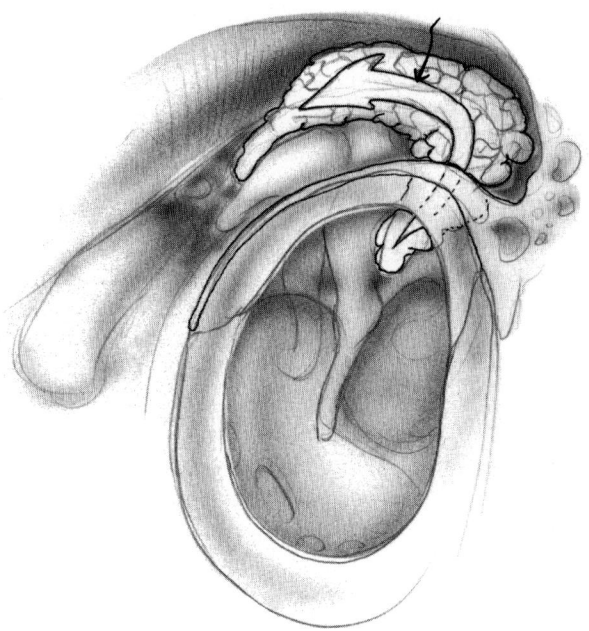

Figure 151.8 Anterior epitympanic cholesteatoma (*arrow*) with extension to the geniculate ganglion.

disease until impending complications develop, heralded by the onset of pain, bloody otorrhea, vertigo, headache, facial paresis, or the appearance of a polyp at the meatus.

The microscopic examination of the ear is the most important diagnostic maneuver in evaluating the presence of a cholesteatoma. The ear must first be meticulously cleaned with cotton-tipped applicators or suction. Acquired cholesteatomas will be noted in the attic or Shrapnell area and in the posterior–superior region, where they are usually associated with erosion of the bony canal.

Granulation tissue may arise from the diseased bone of the outer attic wall or scutum or from the posterior bony wall of the external auditory meatus, where it overhangs the facial recess. A polyp consisting of a mass of edematous granulation tissue may protrude through an attic defect. The polyp may continue to enlarge and in fact may extrude through the meatus. If the disease is very extensive, the entire attic and mastoid antrum will be filled with granulation tissue, and the underlying bone will become necrotic and friable over a wide area. General anesthesia may be required in children to perform an adequate examination. Pneumatic otoscopy should be performed in every patient with a cholesteatoma. A positive fistula response characterized by vertigo and nystagmus is very suggestive of erosion into the inner ear, especially the horizontal semicircular canal or less commonly the cochlea. Infected cholesteatomas characterized by fetid, foul-smelling otorrhea and cholesteatomas associated with polyps should be initially managed medically. Dry ears are much easier to operate on than wet, infected ears. While it is not always possible to dry a chronically infected ear with medical therapy, making an effort to calm down active purulence or drainage might make surgery easier. Polyps can be removed with great care in the clinic with microscopic visualization by using a snare, suction, or small cup forceps, or they may be cauterized. However, polyps should never be aggressively pulled out by grasping them because they may be connected to an important underlying structure such as an ossicle or the facial nerve. A vasoconstricting agent applied to a wick will control bleeding. An attic cholesteatoma may be obscured by a crust that looks like cerumen. Removing the crust reveals a whitish keratin mass typical of a cholesteatoma. Granulation tissue can be revealed under the crust as well.

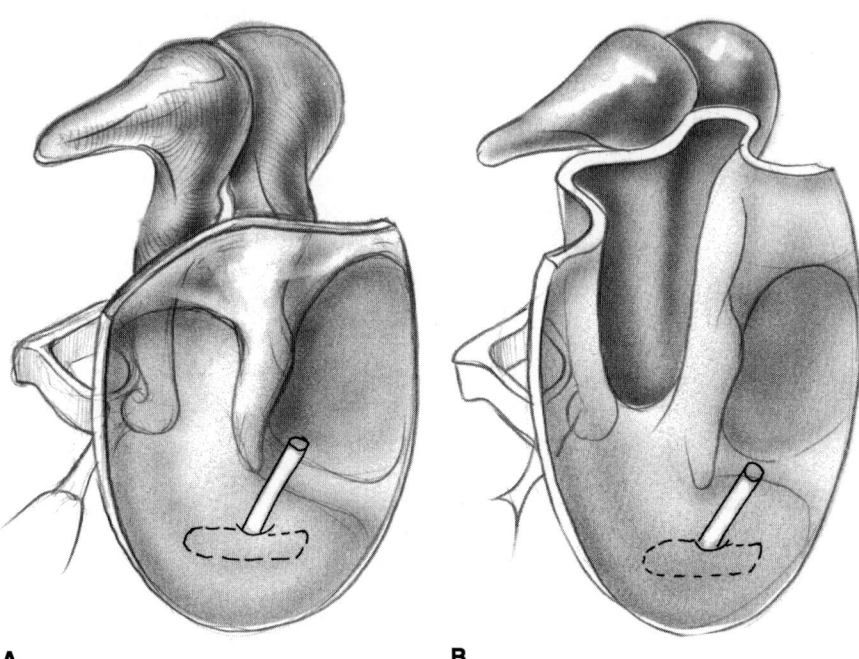

Figure 151.9 **A:** Reversal of a posterosuperior retraction pocket with a tympanostomy tube. **B:** Persistence of a retraction pocket despite tympanostomy tube placement.

A   **B**

Weber and Rinne tests using a 512-Hz tuning fork should be performed and correlated with the audiogram. Preoperative and postoperative audiometric evaluations are essential and should include air and bone thresholds, speech reception threshold, and word recognition. A conductive deficit in excess of 35 dB indicates ossicular discontinuity, usually secondary to destruction of the long process of the incus or the capitulum of the stapes. Alternatively, only a mild conductive hearing loss may be present despite incus erosion if sound is passing through the cholesteatoma directly to the stapes.

The surgical preparation of the patient with an infected cholesteatoma begins with a topical antibiotic drop. Oral quinolones such as ciprofloxacin and levofloxacin are effective with *P. aeruginosa* but are often unnecessary. For medical therapy to be effective, aural toilet is essential. Irrigating the ear with half-strength white vinegar can be effective in controlling infection.

Successful surgical management of cholesteatoma includes exteriorization and removal of all trapped keratinizing epithelium. The goals of surgery should be carefully reviewed with the patient preoperatively. The primary objectives of surgery are a safe, dry ear, with hearing improvement a secondary goal. Specific goals include the following (Table 151.2):

1. Treating complications that have already supervened (extradural abscess, brain abscess, facial nerve palsy, and labyrinthitis)
2. Removing diseased bone, mucosa, granulation polyps, and cholesteatoma to allow drainage and prevent extension of disease to vital structures
3. Stopping the discharge permanently
4. Preserving as much normal anatomy as possible (e.g., posterior canal wall)
5. Preserving or improving hearing

Patients should be carefully counseled about the possible adverse outcomes of surgery: facial paralysis, dysgeusia, vertigo, further hearing loss, tinnitus, recurrent and residual cholesteatoma, cerebrospinal fluid (CSF) leak, and meningitis. The chronic nature of the disease and the need for prolonged follow-up should be stressed. If a mastoid cavity is created, water precautions and the possible need for cavity debridement every 6 to 12 months must be mentioned. The need for second-stage procedures for residual cholesteatoma

TABLE 151.2	SURGICAL GOALS FOR CHOLESTEATOMA

Treat complications
Remove diseased tissue
Obtain a dry "safe" ear
Preserve normal anatomy
Improve hearing

or ossicular chain reconstruction should be discussed with the patient and performed when appropriate.

Thin-section (1-mm) computed tomography (CT) scans without contrast, taken in the coronal and axial projections, are often of value in the preoperative assessment of cholesteatomas. It must be emphasized that routine CT scanning is not advocated for cholesteatoma diagnosis, although several alterations of temporal bone anatomy frequently are associated with it. Among these, erosion of the scutum and expansion of the antrum within areas of air cell breakdown and soft tissue density are characteristic. Other features may include ossicular destruction, erosion of the facial canal, mastoid tegmen dehiscence, and erosion into the otic capsule, especially over the horizontal semicircular canal. CT scanning is important in complicated disease and in the evaluation of cholesteatomas and other masses behind an intact tympanic membrane or when the clinical history correlates poorly with physical findings. For example, a CT is usually obtained before surgery when the patient has facial nerve dysfunction, vertigo, or unanticipated degrees of sensorineural hearing loss. Some surgeons also obtain a CT scan when discharge persists despite medical therapy and before revision surgery to anticipate altered anatomy.

SURGICAL MANAGEMENT

Repair of the tympanic membrane is termed a tympanoplasty, and this is required in most patients with cholesteatoma. The advent of the operating microscope greatly facilitated surgery of the tympanum. Cholesteatoma limited to the middle ear can be managed with a tympanoplasty. The status of the ossicular chain must be meticulously evaluated and the extent of the cholesteatoma determined. At times, the cholesteatoma can be removed without disrupting the ossicular chain. If the lateral chain, malleus and incus, are significantly involved with cholesteatoma, the surgeon should consider separating the incus from the stapes and remove the incus. With cholesteatoma medial to the head of the malleus, the surgeon should also consider removing the head of the malleus. Cholesteatoma that is adherent to the stapes can be meticulously removed with microinstrumentation. Many surgeons at this point use a laser to remove cholesteatoma from a mobile stapes. With extensive granulation tissue, significant bleeding, or an exposed facial nerve in the tympanic segment near the stapes, the surgeon should consider leaving some cholesteatoma on the stapes and attempt to remove it at a second look procedure. In addition, cholesteatoma can be difficult to remove from the sinus tympani or from the facial nerve, and the surgeon should evaluate these areas closely at a second procedure.

Surgical treatment of the mastoid in patients with cholesteatoma has gradually evolved. Before the development of the surgical microscope and the high-speed drill, significant morbidity, including facial paralysis, profound sensorineural hearing loss, and dural tears, attended surgery of the temporal bone. Understandably, otologic surgeons of that day were reluctant to pursue complete removal of cholesteatomas, so a philosophy of exteriorization of cholesteatomas without complete removal emerged. These mastoid cavities, or bowls, led to progressive hearing loss and chronically draining ears, requiring constant supervision.

To avoid cavity problems altogether, the canal-wall-up (CWU) facial recess approach was developed. The posterior canal wall was preserved at all costs. A second stage was planned in 6 to 18 months for removal of residual disease and reconstruction of the ossicular chain. Experience with this philosophy over the past 20 years has resulted in a rethinking of this position by many prominent otologists. A high rate of recidivism approaching 36% in some series (56–62) has resulted in a more individualized approach. Instead of using the same procedure on every ear with cholesteatoma, the procedure is adapted to the extent of disease. The specific operation is determined by local ear factors, general medical factors, and the skill of the surgeon. The local ear factors include the extent of the cholesteatoma, presence of a fistula, clinical assessment of eustachian tube function, degree of mastoid pneumatization, and the degree of sensorineural hearing loss in both ears. General factors include the patient's general medical condition, occupation, and reliability (Table 151.3). The CWU procedure involves preserving the posterior canal wall with or without a posterior tympanotomy (facial recess approach). The posterior tympanotomy is performed through a triangle bounded by the fossa incudis, facial nerve, and chorda tympani nerve. The CWU procedure is indicated in patients with a well-pneumatized mastoid and middle ear space. Relative contraindications to the CWU procedure include a sclerotic mastoid, a labyrinthine fistula, an only hearing ear, and poor eustachian tube function (63–67). The choice of surgical procedure is highly dependent on the status of the opposite ear. Patients with bilateral cholesteatomas are at high risk of recurrence or recidivistic disease, and some surgeons consider a canal-wall-down (CWD) procedure more readily.

The CWD mastoidectomy involves taking down the posterior canal wall to the vertical facial nerve and marsupializing the mastoid into the external ear canal. In a CWD procedure, all accessible air cells are meticulously exenterated. CWD procedures can be divided into those in which the middle ear space is preserved (modified radical mastoidectomy) and those in which the middle ear space is eliminated and the eustachian tube plugged (radical mastoidectomy). A patient with an extensive cholesteatoma might have a large attic defect and a significant portion of the posterior canal wall destroyed from disease. Removal of disease might necessitate a further defect in the posterior ear canal. At this point, the surgeon most likely has removed the incus remnant and the head of the malleus. If reconstruction of the posterior canal is not possible or appropriate, then the surgeon should drill down the posterior ear canal wall to the level of the facial nerve. If it is appropriate to repair the tympanic membrane and create a middle ear space, this would be termed a tympanoplasty with mastoidectomy, or a modified radical mastoidectomy. If it is not appropriate to repair the tympanic membrane, then the eustachian tube can be closed off creating a radical mastoid cavity. At this point in time, a radical mastoidectomy is an uncommon procedure for the majority of otologists.

A more limited procedure is the atticotomy, which involves the removal of the lateral wall of the epitympanum (scutum) to the limits of the cholesteatoma. The atticotomy defect allows for relatively easy cleaning of a narrow epitympanic defect. However, to prevent recurrent cholesteatoma, the atticotomy defect can be blocked with cartilage; this is a variant of a canal-wall-up or canal-wall reconstruction procedure. A more extensive attic cholesteatoma that is lateral to the ossicles and accompanied by a sclerotic mastoid may be managed with a Bondy procedure. This involves the removal of the scutum and portion of the posterior canal wall with preservation of the ossicles and middle ear space. The bony defect is not reconstructed; rather, the cholesteatoma matrix is exteriorized. A patient with a cholesteatoma and poor eustachian tube function as evidenced by absence of middle ear aeration and a sclerotic mastoid should be considered for a CWD procedure (Table 151.4).

TABLE 151.3	DETERMINANTS OF OPERATIVE TECHNIQUE FOR CHOLESTEATOMA

Local factors
  Presence of a fistula
  Extent of disease
  Eustachian tube function
  Mastoid pneumatization
  Hearing status of both ears
General factors
  General medical condition
  Occupation
  Reliability
Skill and experience of the surgeon

TABLE 151.4	SURGICAL APPROACHES TO CHOLESTEATOMA

CWU
  Complete mastoidectomy
  Facial recess approach
CWD
  Modified radical mastoidectomy
  Radical mastoidectomy
Other
  Atticotomy
  Bondy procedure
  CWR
  Mastoid obliteration

Numerous variations of a canal-wall reconstruction (CWR) with or without mastoid obliteration procedures have recently been developed to improve exposure and removal of cholesteatoma as in a CWD approach while retaining the benefits of an intact canal wall (improved hearing and avoidance of the bowl cavity) (68–83). In these procedures, a complete mastoidectomy including a facial recess is performed and the posterior canal is removed. The cholesteatoma, the ossicles, and the tympanic membrane are addressed, and the posterior canal wall is replaced. Some surgeons opt to fill the mastoid cavity with bone pate or hydroxyapatite, whereas others leave it open as in a CWU procedure. These techniques have even been used to "repair" radical mastoid cavities. See Chapter 152 for a more complete description of surgical approaches to the mastoid.

With high rates of recurrence or recidivistic disease, especially with CWU or CWR procedures, monitoring the mastoid for cholesteatoma has become extremely important. If cholesteatoma is left behind in the mastoid cavity, or trapped underneath a mastoid obliteration, intracranial or vascular complications can occur even many years after the initial procedure. The advent of diffusion-weighted MRI scans have given the otologic surgeon a noninvasive mechanism to evaluate a patient's mastoid for recidivistic cholesteatoma with fairly high accuracy (84–86).

COMPLICATIONS AND EMERGENCIES

As cholesteatomas expand and become infected, they cause ossicular chain destruction, exposure of the membranous labyrinth, tegmen dehiscence, exposure of the facial nerve, erosion into the temporomandibular joint, extratemporal spread, and infection of the mastoid and intracranial spaces (Table 151.5). See Figure 151.10 for examples of complications from cholesteatoma.

Hearing Loss

Some degree of ossicular chain erosion occurs in most cases of cholesteatoma. Attic cholesteatomas involve the head of the malleus and body of the incus early. As the cholesteatoma expands inferiorly, the lenticular process of the incus and the stapes superstructure are eroded.

TABLE 151.5	COMPLICATIONS AND EMERGENCIES CHOLESTEATOMA

Conductive and sensorineural hearing loss
Labyrinthine fistula
Vertigo
Facial paralysis
Extratemporal cholesteatoma
Erosion into temporomandibular joint
Intratemporal infection
Intracranial infection
Brain herniation

Pars tensa cholesteatomas that develop from a posterior–superior retraction pocket also involve the lenticular process of the incus and the stapes superstructure. When both of these bones are involved, the hearing loss can be as great as 50 dB. However, if a natural myringostapediopexy develops, then loss may be as little as 20 dB. One should always assume that the ossicular chain is intact in a patient with a cholesteatoma. Cholesteatoma on the lateral surface of the incus can be removed using microsurgical ear instruments without disturbing the ossicular chain. Involvement of the medial surface of the incus often requires removal of the incus by first separating the incudostapedial joint, then the incudomalleolar joint. Cholesteatoma extending medial to the head of the malleus into the anterior epitympanic space (or supratubal recess) usually requires removal of the incus and the head of the malleus. Removal of cholesteatoma from the stapes should be done last by dissecting parallel with the stapedius tendon in a posterior to anterior direction to avoid dislocating the footplate and causing sensorineural hearing loss. One should avoid superior or inferior movement as well as depression of the stapes. The tympanic membrane is grafted to seal the middle ear, and Silastic sheeting is placed over the promontory to prevent adhesions. A second-stage procedure is performed in 6 to 18 months to remove residual cholesteatoma and reconstruct the ossicular chain. If cholesteatoma removal is certain and the mucosal involvement is minimal, the ossicular chain can be reconstructed at the primary procedure.

Labyrinthine Fistula

A labyrinthine fistula may be found in up to 10% of patients with long-standing cholesteatomas or in revision cases. One should suspect a fistula in patients with chronic ear disease who have sensorineural hearing loss and/or vertigo induced by noise or pressure changes in the middle ear. A positive fistula test with manipulation of the external canal may be present, although its absence does not exclude a fistula. Suppurative labyrinthitis with complete loss of hearing and vestibular function may occur secondary to a fistula from a cholesteatoma. High-resolution, thin-section CT of the temporal bone may reveal a fistula of the semicircular canals or the basal turn of the cochlea. Fistulae of the horizontal semicircular canal are most common (87). The procedure of choice in labyrinthine fistulae is a modified radical (CWD) mastoidectomy. This avoids leaving residual disease concealed in the mastoid cavity and necessitating the patient to undergo multiple procedures. Management of the matrix covering the fistula depends on several factors, including the infection status of the ear, the degree of sensorineural hearing loss in the involved ear as well as the opposite ear, the size and location of the fistula, and the surgeon's skill. In the patient with a fistula of the only hearing ear, a CWD procedure is performed and the matrix is left intact over the fistula. Attempting to remove it places the patient at significant risk for a permanent total sensorineural hearing loss. If the opposite ear has normal hearing and eustachian tube function,

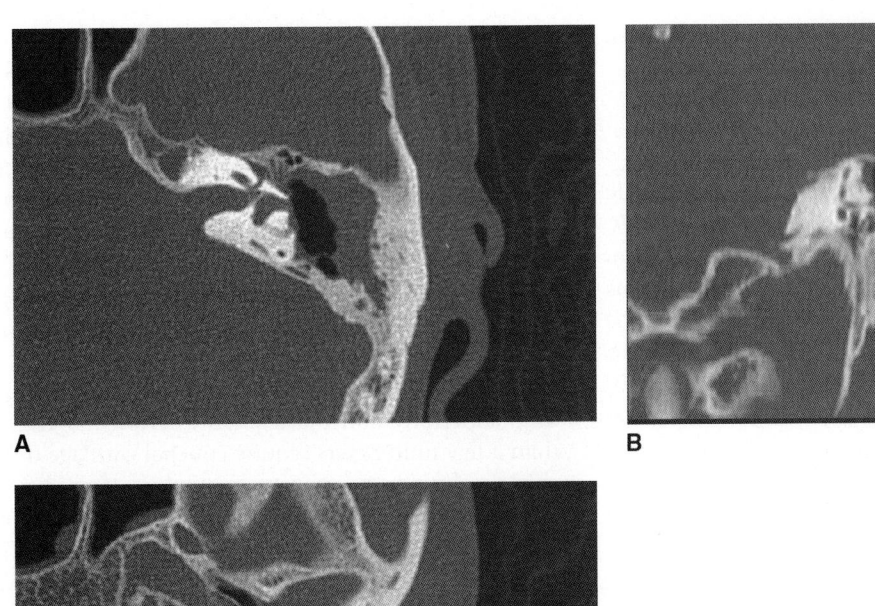

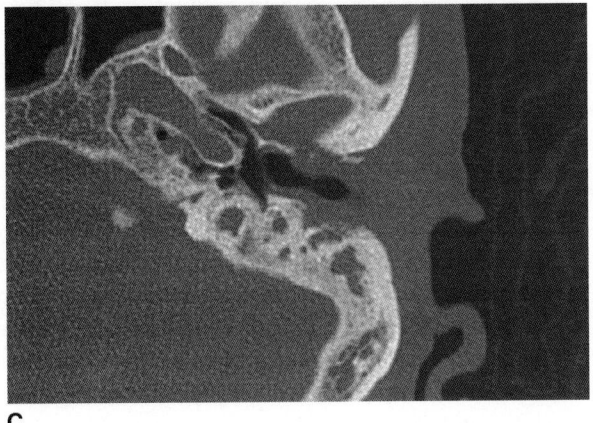

Figure 151.10 CT scan of left ear demonstrating three complications from cholesteatoma in a single patient. The patient has not had surgery. **A:** Horizontal semi-circular canal (HSCC) fistula (axial scan), **(B)** Erosion of tegmen plate (coronal scan), **(C)** Erosion into TMJ (axial scan).

then the surgeon can be more selective in management. If the fistula involves one of the semicircular canals and the mastoid is small, then a CWD mastoidectomy, leaving the matrix on the fistula, is appropriate. If there is a small semicircular canal fistula and the mastoid cavity is large, then the skillful surgeon may elect to perform an intact canal wall procedure, remove the matrix, cover the fistula with fascia, and plan a second procedure. If the hearing is normal, then the matrix covering extensive fistulae of the vestibule or cochlea should be left alone. If cochlear function is profoundly depressed, the matrix should be removed and the fistula covered with fascia. The removal of matrix over the fistula and then immediately covering it with fascia should be the last part of the procedure. Suction should not be used around the fistula site; only blunt dissection is appropriate. If the semicircular canal is inadvertently opened by a drill, then the iatrogenic fistula should be immediately covered with fascia. Parenteral antibiotics and steroids may be helpful. Postoperative vertigo is a sign of labyrinthine and cochlear trauma. A bone-conduction audiogram may be depressed immediately but may recover in 4 to 6 weeks in some cases.

Facial Paralysis

Facial paralysis in patients with cholesteatoma may develop acutely due to infection or slowly due to chronic expansion. In either case, surgery should be performed as soon as the paralysis is recognized. High-resolution, thin-section CT with both axial and coronal scanning will localize the involvement. A common site of nerve involvement is the geniculate ganglion (87). A mastoidectomy with facial recess approach will expose the horizontal and vertical portions of the facial nerve. Moody and Lambert (88) recently reviewed their cases of surgical cholesteatoma and found a high rate of dehiscence of the facial nerve. This should be expected in the case of a facial paralysis. Removing the cholesteatoma and decompressing the facial nerve are sufficient if the nerve is anatomically intact; opening the sheath of the facial nerve is unnecessary. A middle fossa approach is required for cholesteatomas involving the petrous apex. Intravenous antibiotics and high-dose steroids are helpful. The House-Brackmann facial nerve grading system should be used to assess the degree of facial paralysis, and the intraoperative use of a facial nerve stimulator/monitor is helpful. Iatrogenic injury of the facial nerve at the pyramidal turn may occur with drilling of the mastoid. The horizontal segment of the facial nerve may be injured during blunt removal of the cholesteatoma in the middle ear. Immediate repair is performed when the injury is recognized, and decompression of the facial nerve for several millimeters on either side of the injured segment is recommended. A delayed facial paralysis within a few days of surgery indicates minor trauma, with recovery expected within 6 weeks. These patients are treated like those with idiopathic facial paralysis and given high-dose steroids. Antiviral therapy may also be beneficial.

Infections

Serious infections associated with cholesteatoma include periosteal abscess, lateral sinus thrombosis, meningitis, and intracranial abscess. A high-resolution, thin-section, contrast-enhanced CT scan is performed. Infections of this nature occur in less than 1% of all cholesteatomas because of the widespread use of antibiotics and the tendency to operate earlier. The most dangerous type of infected cholesteatomas are those where drainage through the external auditory canal is obstructed by an inflamed and narrow canal. The egress may be further blocked by mucosal edema, squamous debris, or a polyp. Early intervention to remove cholesteatoma and provide adequate drainage is required.

Periosteal abscess may develop behind a cholesteatoma and inflammation that is blocking the aditus ad antrum or from an extensive cholesteatoma that erodes through the mastoid cortex. It presents as an inflamed, fluctuant postauricular mass. High-dose antibiotics are begun and adjusted according to needle aspiration culture results. Surgery is performed after 24 to 48 hours of antibiotics. It is important to be aware that the dura or lateral sinus may be exposed by disease.

Lateral sinus thrombosis may occur from an infected cholesteatoma. It presents with a characteristic high, spiking fever in a picket-fence pattern. Treatment requires high-dose antibiotics and surgery similar to management of lateral sinus thrombosis in association with acute coalescent mastoiditis. If the cholesteatoma is extensive, a CWD mastoidectomy should be performed (89).

Patients who develop headaches on the side of a cholesteatoma should have a CT scan to rule out an impending intracranial complication. Pain and headache may arise from involvement of dura by the cholesteatoma, by a developing epidural abscess, or because of loculated abscess. Cerebellar or temporal lobe abscesses may exhibit only mild symptoms such as low-grade fever, mild ataxia, or mental changes. Intracranial abscesses should be managed by the neurosurgeon after beginning intravenous antibiotics. After control of the intracranial problem, the otologist can then manage the ear disease. See Chapter 138 for more information on intracranial complications.

Brain Herniation

Brain herniation may develop following previous mastoid procedures presenting as an encephalocele or meningoencephalocele through a defect in the tegmen tympani or tegmen mastoideum. The etiology is thought secondary to aggressive drilling that exposes and traumatizes the dura during previous mastoid surgery. Subsequent brain herniation can be prevented by carefully inspecting any exposed

dura for injury. If a tegmen defect is small and the dura is intact, no further treatment is necessary. If there is a disruption in the integrity of the dura with or without a CSF leak, repair is necessary. Many of these defects can be successfully treated from the mastoid. One should circumferentially elevate the dura from the tegmen with a blunt instrument and remove 1 mm of bone from around the site of injury to expose normal-appearing dura. Bleeding is controlled with low-energy bipolar cautery rather than monopolar cautery to avoid injury and thrombosis of cerebral vessels. The surgeon should circumferentially insert temporalis fascia, cut larger than the defect, between the dura superiorly and the tegmen inferiorly. Defects larger than a few millimeters require conchal cartilage or a bone chip for support to prevent herniation. If an established encephalocele or meningoencephalocele is encountered, it should be removed. A biopsy is needed to confirm brain tissue and rule out a malignancy. One should carefully dissect the circumference of the mass to identify its site of origin. In most cases, the encephalocele in the epitympanum or mastoid is necrotic and functionless. The herniated brain tissue is removed to the level of the tegmen and dural defect and repaired as described previously. For larger defects, a mini-craniotomy is performed by making an opening in the squamosa laterally, just above the plane of the tegmen. The dura can then be elevated off the floor of the middle fossa and the defect repaired with fascia and cartilage or bone.

Extratemporal Cholesteatoma

Cholesteatoma can also escape the confines of the temporal bone after otologic surgery in rare instances (90). Concern of cholesteatoma (epidermal inclusion cyst) should arise in a patient with a lesion in or around the parotid gland with a history of prior ear surgery (Fig. 151.11).

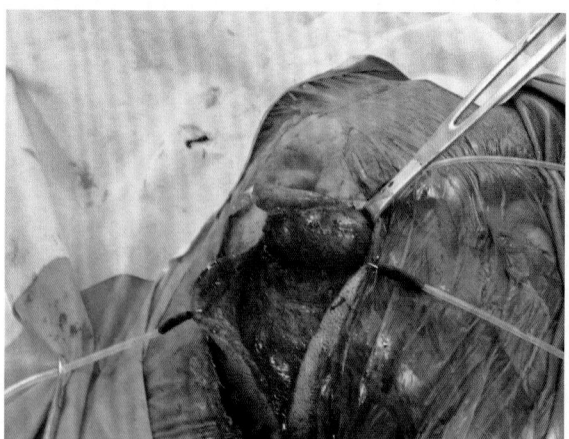

Figure 151.11 Intraoperative photograph of a patient with a cholesteatoma anterior to the left ear in the infratemporal fossa. The patient had multiple ear surgeries for cholesteatoma including a CWD tympanoplasty with mastoidectomy. Except for the mass, the patient was asymptomatic.

REFERENCES

1. Kuhn A. Das Cholesteatom des Ohres. *Zeitschr Ohrenheilk* 1891;21:231.
2. Derlacki EL, Clemis JD. Congenital cholesteatoma of the middle ear and mastoid. *Ann Otol Rhinol Laryngol* 1965;74:706–727.
3. Levenson MJ, Michaels L, Parisier SC, et al. Congenital cholesteatomas in children: an embryologic correlation. *Laryngoscope* 1988;98:949–955.
4. Levenson MJ, Michaels L, Parisier SC. Congenital cholesteatomas of the middle ear in children: origin and management. *Otolaryngol Clin North Am* 1989;22:941–954.
5. Teed FW. Cholesteatoma verum tympani (its relationship to the first epibranchial placode). *Arch Otolaryngol* 1936;24:455–474.
6. Michaels L. An epidermoid formation in the developing middle ear: possible source of cholesteatoma. *J Otolaryngol* 1986;15:169–174.
7. Michaels L. Origin of congenital cholesteatoma from a normally occurring epidermoid rest in the developing middle ear. *Int J Pediatr Otorhinolaryngol* 1988;15:51–65.
8. Karmody CS, Byahatti SV, Blevins N, et al. The origin of congenital cholesteatoma. *Am J Otol* 1998;19:292–297.
9. Lee TS, Liang JN, Michaels L, et al. The epidermoid formation and its affinity to congenital cholesteatoma. *Clin Otolaryngol Allied Sci* 1998;23:449–454.
10. Wang RG, Hawke M, Kwok P. The epidermoid formation (Michaels' structure) in the developing middle ear. *J Otolaryngol* 1987;16:327–330.
11. Aimi K. Role of the tympanic ring in the pathogenesis of congenital cholesteatoma. *Laryngoscope* 1983;93:1140–1146.
12. Fisch U. 'Congenital' cholesteatomas of the supralabyrinthine region. *Clin Otolaryngol Allied Sci* 1978;3:369–376.
13. Warren FM, Bennett ML, Wiggins RH III, et al. Congenital cholesteatoma of the mastoid temporal bone. *Laryngoscope* 2007;117:1389–1394.
14. Thakkar KH, Djalilian HR, Mafee MF. Congenital cholesteatoma isolated to the mastoid. *Otol Neurotol* 2006;27:282–283.
15. Potsic WP, Samadi DS, Marsh RR, et al. A staging system for congenital cholesteatoma. *Arch Otolaryngol Head Neck Surg* 2002;128:1009–1012.
16. Nelson M, Roger G, Koltai PJ, et al. Congenital cholesteatoma: classification, management, and outcome. *Arch Otolaryngol Head Neck Surg* 2002;128:810–814.
17. Koltai PJ, Nelson M, Castellon RJ, et al. The natural history of congenital cholesteatoma. *Arch Otolaryngol Head Neck Surg* 2002;128:804–809.
18. Bluestone CD, Klein JO. Intratemporal complications and sequelae of otitis media. In: Bluestone CD, Stool SE, eds. *Pediatric otolaryngology*. Philadelphia, PA: WB Saunders, 1990:521–526.
19. Sheahan P, Blayney AW, Sheahan JN, et al. Sequelae of otitis media with effusion among children with cleft lip and/or cleft palate. *Clin Otolaryngol Allied Sci* 2002;27:494–500.
20. Goldman JL, Martinez SA, Ganzel TM. Eustachian tube dysfunction and its sequelae in patients with cleft palate. *South Med J* 1993;86:1236–1237.
21. Dominguez S, Harker LA. Incidence of cholesteatoma with cleft palate. *Ann Otol Rhinol Laryngol* 1988;97(6 Pt 1):659–660.
22. Vartiainen E, Karja J. Bilateral chronic otitis media. *Arch Oto Rhino Laryngol* 1986;243:190–193.
23. Wittmaack K. Wie entsteht ein genuines Cholesteatom? *Arch Ohren Nasen Dehlkopfh* 1933;137:306.
24. Glasscock ME. Pathology and clinical course of inflammatory disease of the middle ear. In: Shambaugh G, Glasscock ME, eds. *Surgery of the ear*. Philadelphia, PA: WB Saunders, 1990:178.
25. Vennix PP, Kuijpers W, Tonnaer EL, et al. Cytokeratins in induced epidermoid formations and cholesteatoma lesions. *Arch Otolaryngol Head Neck Surg* 1990;116:560–565.
26. Palva T, Karma P, Makinen J. The invasion theory in cholesteatoma and mastoid surgery. In: Sade J, ed. *Cholesteatoma and mastoid surgery. Proceedings of the Second International Conference on Cholesteatoma and Mastoid Surgery.* Amsterdam, The Netherlands: Kugler Publications, 1982:249–264.
27. Yoon YH, Park CH, Kim EH, et al. Clinical characteristics of external auditory canal cholesteatoma in children. *Otolaryngol Head Neck Surg* 2008;139:661–664.
28. Dubach P, Hausler R. External auditory canal cholesteatoma: reassessment of and amendments to its categorization, pathogenesis, and treatment in 34 patients. *Otol Neurotol* 2008;29:941–948.
29. Bonding P, Ravn T. Primary cholesteatoma of the external auditory canal: is the epithelial migration defective? *Otol Neurotol* 2008;29:334–338.
30. Lee DH, Jun BC, Park CS, et al. A case of osteoma with cholesteatoma in the external auditory canal. *Auris Nasus Larynx* 2005;32:281–284.
31. Naim R, Linthicum F Jr, Shen T, et al. Classification of the external auditory canal cholesteatoma. *Laryngoscope* 2005;115:455–460.
32. Persaud RA, Hajioff D, Thevasagayam MS, et al. Keratosis obturans and external ear canal cholesteatoma: how and why we should distinguish between these conditions. *Clinic Otolaryngol Allied Sci* 2004;29:577–581.
33. Michaels L. Biology of cholesteatoma. *Otolaryngol Clin North Am* 1989;22:869–881.
34. Orisek BS, Chole RA. Pressures exerted by experimental cholesteatomas. *Arch Otolaryngol Head Neck Surg* 1987;113:386–391.
35. Wolfman DE, Chole RA. Osteoclast stimulation by positive middle-ear air pressure. *Arch Otolaryngol Head Neck Surg* 1986;112:1037–1042.
36. Chole RA, McGinn MD, Tinling SP. Pressure-induced bone resorption in the middle ear. *Ann Otol Rhinol Laryngol* 1985;94(2 Pt 1):165–170.
37. Tanaka Y, Kojima H, Miyazaki H, et al. Roles of cytokines and cell cycle regulating substances in proliferation of cholesteatoma epithelium. *Laryngoscope* 1999;109(7 Pt 1):1102–1107.

38. Yetiser S, Satar B, Aydin N. Expression of epidermal growth factor, tumor necrosis factor-alpha, and interleukin-1alpha in chronic otitis media with or without cholesteatoma. *Otol Neurotol* 2002;23:647–652.

39. Akimoto R, Pawankar R, Yagi T, et al. Acquired and congenital cholesteatoma: determination of tumor necrosis factor-alpha, intercellular adhesion molecule-1, interleukin-1-alpha and lymphocyte functional antigen-1 in the inflammatory process. *ORL J Otorhinolaryngol Relat Spec* 2000;62:257–265.

40. Albino AP, Reed JA, Bogdany JK, et al. Increased numbers of mast cells in human middle ear cholesteatomas: implications for treatment. *Am J Otol* 1998;19:266–272.

41. Albino AP, Kimmelman CP, Parisier SC. Cholesteatoma: a molecular and cellular puzzle. *Am J Otol* 1998;19:7–19.

42. Amar MS, Wishahi HF, Zakhary MM. Clinical and biochemical studies of bone destruction in cholesteatoma. *J Laryngol Otol* 1996;110:534–539.

43. Bujia J, Kim C, Ostos P, et al. Role of interleukin 6 in epithelial hyperproliferation and bone resorption in middle ear cholesteatomas. *Eur Arch Otorhinolaryngol* 1996;253(3):152–157.

44. Yan SD, Huang CC. The role of tumor necrosis factor-alpha in bone resorption of cholesteatoma. *Am J Otolaryngol* 1991;12:83–89.

45. Iino Y, Toriyama M, Ogawa H, et al. Cholesteatoma debris as an activator of human monocytes. Potentiation of the production of tumor necrosis factor. *Acta Otolaryngol* 1990;110:410–415.

46. Macias MP, Gerkin RD, Macias JD. Increased amphiregulin expression as a biomarker of cholesteatoma activity. *Laryngoscope* 2010;120:2258–2263.

47. Friedland DR, Eernisse R, Erbe C, et al. Cholesteatoma growth and proliferation: posttranscriptional regulation by microRNA-21. *Otol Neurotol* 2009;30:998–1005.

48. Olszewska E, Borzym-Kluczyk M, Olszewski S, et al. Catabolism of glycoconjugates in chronic otitis media with cholesteatoma. *J Investig Med* 2007;55:248–254.

49. Laeeq S, Faust R. Modeling the cholesteatoma microenvironment: coculture of HaCaT keratinocytes with WS1 fibroblasts induces MMP-2 activation, invasive phenotype, and proteolysis of the extracellular matrix. *Laryngoscope* 2007;117:313–318.

50. Hamzei M, Ventriglia G, Hagnia M, et al. Osteoclast stimulating and differentiating factors in human cholesteatoma. *Laryngoscope* 2003;113:436–442.

51. Jung JY, Chole RA. Bone resorption in chronic otitis media: the role of the osteoclast. *ORL J Otorhinolaryngol Relat Spec* 2002;64:95–107.

52. Chole RA. Cellular and subcellular events of bone resorption in human and experimental cholesteatoma: the role of osteoclasts. *Laryngoscope* 1984;94:76–95.

53. Jung JY, Pashia ME, Nishimoto SY, et al. A possible role for nitric oxide in osteoclastogenesis associated with cholesteatoma. *Otol Neurotol* 2004;25:661–668.

54. Jackler RK. The surgical anatomy of cholesteatoma. *Otolaryngol Clin North Am* 1989;22:883–896.

55. Chu FW, Jackler RK. Anterior epitympanic cholesteatoma with facial paralysis: a characteristic growth pattern. *Laryngoscope* 1988;98:274–279.

56. Cruz OL, Kasse CA, Leonhart FD. Efficacy of surgical treatment of chronic otitis media. *Otolaryngol Head Neck Surg* 2003;128: 263–266.

57. Silvola J, Palva T. One-stage revision surgery for pediatric cholesteatoma: long-term results and comparison with primary surgery. *Int J Pediatr Otorhinolaryngol* 2000;56:135–139.

58. Stangerup SE, Drozdziewicz D, Tos M, et al. Recurrence of attic cholesteatoma: different methods of estimating recurrence rates. *Otolaryngol Head Neck Surg* 2000;123:283–287.

59. Darrouzet V, Duclos JY, Portmann D, et al. Preference for the closed technique in the management of cholesteatoma of the middle ear in children: a retrospective study of 215 consecutive patients treated over 10 years. *Am J Otol* 2000;21:474–481.

60. Vartiainen E. Factors associated with recurrence of cholesteatoma. *J Laryngol Otol* 1995;109:590–592.

61. Rosenfeld RM, Moura RL, Bluestone CD. Predictors of residual-recurrent cholesteatoma in children. *Arch Otolaryngol Head Neck Surg* 1992;118:384–391.

62. Brown JS. A ten year statistical follow-up of 1142 consecutive cases of cholesteatoma: the closed vs. the open technique. *Laryngoscope* 1982;92:390–396.

63. Brackmann DE. Tympanoplasty with mastoidectomy: canal wall up procedures. *Am J Otol* 1993;14:380–382.

64. Dawes PJ, Leaper M. Paediatric small cavity mastoid surgery: second look tympanotomy. *Int J Pediatr Otorhinolaryngol* 2004;68:143–148.

65. McDonald TJ, Cody DTR. Surgery of the temporal bone air cell system: mastoid and petrosa. *Otolaryngol Head Neck Surg* 1986;4:3081.

66. Dodson EE, Hashisaki GT, Hobgood TC, et al. Intact canal wall mastoidectomy with tympanoplasty for cholesteatoma in children. *Laryngoscope* 1998;108:977–983.

67. Stankovic MD. Audiologic results of surgery for cholesteatoma: short- and long-term follow-up of influential factors. *Otol Neurotol* 2008;29:933–940.

68. Gantz BJ, Wilkinson EP, Hansen MR. Canal wall reconstruction typanomastoidectomy with mastoid obliteration. *Laryngoscope* 2005;115:1734–1740.

69. Babighian G. Posterior and attic wall osteoplasty: hearing results and recurrence rates in cholesteatoma. *Otol Neurotol* 2002;23(1):14–17.

70. Black B. Mastoidectomy elimination. *Laryngoscope* 1995;105(12 Pt 2 Suppl 76):1–30.

71. Dornhoffer JL. Retrograde mastoidectomy with canal wall reconstruction: a single-stage technique for cholesteatoma removal. *Ann Otol Rhinol Laryngol* 2000;109:1033–1039.

72. Grote JJ, van Blitterswijk CA. Reconstruction of the posterior auditory canal wall with a hydroxyapatite prosthesis. *Ann Otol Rhinol Laryngol Suppl* 1986;123:6–9.

73. Hartwein J, Hormann K. A technique for the reconstruction of the posterior canal wall and mastoid obliteration in radical cavity surgery. *Am J Otol* 1990;11:169–173.

74. Hosoi H, Murata K, Kimura H, et al. Long-term observation after soft posterior meatal wall reconstruction in ears with cholesteatoma. *J Laryngol Otol* 1998;112:31–35.

75. Ikeda M, Yoshida S, Ikui A, et al. Canal wall down tympanoplasty with canal reconstruction for middle-ear cholesteatoma: post-operative hearing, cholesteatoma recurrence, and status of re-aeration of reconstructed middle-ear cavity. *J Laryngol Otol* 2003;117:249–255.

76. Leatherman BD, Dornhoffer JL, Fan CY, et al. Demineralized bone matrix as an alternative for mastoid obliteration and posterior canal wall reconstruction: results in an animal model. *Otol Neurotol* 2001;22:731–736.

77. Magliulo G, Ronzoni R, Vingolo GM, et al. Reconstruction of old radical cavities. *Am J Otol* 1992;13:288–291.

78. Magliulo G, D'Amico R, Forino M. Reconstruction of the posterior auditory canal with hydroxyapatite-coated titanium. *J Otolaryngol* 2001;30:330–333.

79. Mercke U. The cholesteatomatous ear one year after surgery with obliteration technique. *Am J Otol* 1987;8:534–536.

80. Roberson JB Jr, Mason TP, Stidham KR. Mastoid obliteration: autogenous cranial bone pate reconstruction. *Otol Neurotol* 2003;24:132–140.

81. Takahashi H, Hasebe S, Sudo M, et al. Soft-wall reconstruction for cholesteatoma surgery: reappraisal. *Am J Otol* 2000;21:28–31.

82. Wiet RJ, Harvey SA, Pyle MG. Canal wall reconstruction: a newer implantation technique. *Laryngoscope* 1993;103:594–599.

83. Leatherman BD, Dornhoffer JL. The use of demineralized bone matrix for mastoid cavity obliteration. *Otol Neurotol* 2004;25:22–25.

84. De Foer B, Vercruysse JP, Spaepen M, et al. Diffusion-weighted magnetic resonance imaging of the temporal bone. *Neuroradiology* 2010;52:785–807.

85. Cimsit NC, Cimsit C, Baysal B, et al. Diffusion-weighted MR imaging in postoperative follow-up: reliability for detection of recurrent cholesteatoma. *Eur J Radiol* 2010;74:121–123.

86. Vercruysse JP, De Foer B, Pouillon M, et al. The value of diffusion-weighted MR imaging in the diagnosis of primary acquired and residual cholesteatoma: a surgical verified study of 100 patients. *Eur Radiol* 2006;16:1461–1467.

87. Farrior JB. *Surgery for cholesteatoma: complications in otolaryngology-head and neck surgery.* Toronto: BC Decker, 1986.

88. Moody MW, Lambert PR. Incidence of dehiscence of the facial nerve in 416 cases of cholesteatoma. *Otol Neurotol* 2007;28:400–404.

89. Harker LA, Koontz FP. Bacteriology of cholesteatoma: clinical significance. *Trans Sect Otolaryngol Am Acad Ophthalmol Otolaryngol* 1977;84(4 Pt 1):ORL-683–686.

90. Walshe P, Low C, Lucey D, et al. Parotid masses in patients with previous ear surgery. *Ir Med J* 2005;98:110–111.

Surgery of the Mastoid and Petrosa

152

Richard A. Chole   Hilary A. Brodie   Abraham Jacob

HISTORY

Infections of the ear were recorded as early as 380 BC in the Hippocratic canon, and surgery of the mastoid and petrosa developed as a treatment modality for suppurative ear disease. During the 16th century, Fabricius Hildanus reported a case of spontaneous drainage from a postauricular abscess, for which he advocated early incision and drainage. Riolan the Younger described a procedure akin to mastoidectomy in 1649, and John Luis Petit performed the first surgical trephination of the mastoid in 1774. Petit exposed the mastoid cortex, performed a trephination, and then enlarged the surgically created fistula. JGH Fielitz reported five similar cases in 1785; however, the procedure fell into disrepute after the sensational death of Danish physician Johanne Gust Von Berger in 1792. He died of meningitis 12 days after a mastoidectomy performed by Koelpin and Callisen. Fortunately, Schwartze repopularized the operation in 1873. Since then, technological advancements such as the operating microscope, the high-speed drill, and specialized microsurgical instruments have led to significant improvements in the treatment of mastoid disease. Regions of the skull base previously thought to be inaccessible such as the petrous apex, the complete course of the facial nerve, the endolymphatic sac, and the cerebellopontine angle were now within reach. Indications for temporal bone surgery (Table 152.1) include acute otologic infections (see Chapters 149 and 151), chronic infections with or without cholesteatoma (see Chapters 151 and 149), trauma (see Chapter 150), facial nerve disorders (see Chapter 155), vestibulopathy (see Chapter 166), and tumors of the skull base (see Chapter 147).

SURGICAL TECHNIQUE: MASTOIDECTOMY

Incisions

The two principal incisions used for access to the mastoid cortex are the postauricular incision of Wilde and the endaural incision of Lempert. The postauricular incision provides better overall exposure and allows complete access to the mastoid tip. In adults, the incision is placed 8 to 10 mm posterior to the postauricular sulcus, where it is hidden by the pinna (Fig. 152.1). This incision can be placed more posteriorly for wider exposure as might be necessary during translabyrinthine access to the cerebellopontine angle. It should not be placed directly in the postauricular crease, however, because such placement creates a deep, difficult-to-clean postauricular furrow. In children younger than 2 years, the inferior portion of this incision must be placed more posteriorly than in adults (Fig. 152.1). This is because the tympanic ring in children is underdeveloped, mastoid pneumatization is incomplete, and the stylomastoid foramen is shallow. Therefore, the facial nerve is vulnerable to injury. The surgeon should also keep in mind that congenital anomalies of the temporal bone can result in highly variable facial nerve position.

The postauricular incision is first outlined with a marking pen and infiltrated with a mixture of local anesthetic and epinephrine. The skin and subcutaneous tissues are incised sharply down to the temporalis fascia (superior to the inferior temporal line) and down to the periosteum overlying the mastoid cortex (inferior to the inferior temporal line). The ear flap is elevated anteriorly to identify the posterior edge of the external ear canal. Additional

TABLE 152.1	CLINICAL INDICATORS FOR MASTOIDECTOMY

Strategy
Indicators (one of the following)
   Persistent or recurrent otorrhea
   Persistent or recurrent ear pain
   Conductive hearing loss
   Tympanic membrane perforation and/or cholesteatoma
   Acute mastoiditis with osteitis
   Neoplasm of temporal bone
   Fracture of temporal bone with CSF leak
   Facial nerve paralysis requiring decompression of the facial nerve
Laboratory tests (as indicated)
Audiogram
Other tests (as indicated)
Type of anesthesia (as indicated)
Location of service (as indicated)

Process
Criteria for discharge
   Recovery from anesthesia
   Absence of significant vertigo
   Absence of signs of meningitis or toxic shock syndrome

Outcome
Results
Follow-up
   Healing of mastoid cavity if present
   Healing of surgical wound
   Resolution of presenting symptoms
   Evaluation of hearing

CSF, cerebrospinal fluid.
The American Academy of Otolaryngology—Head and Neck Surgery and the American Society for Head and Neck Surgery have published Clinical Indicators for surgical procedures. These Clinical Indicators are educational statements that have been drafted to assist surgeons in their practice and to promote discussion. These Indicators are not practice guidelines nor do they represent standards of practice with which individuals must conform.

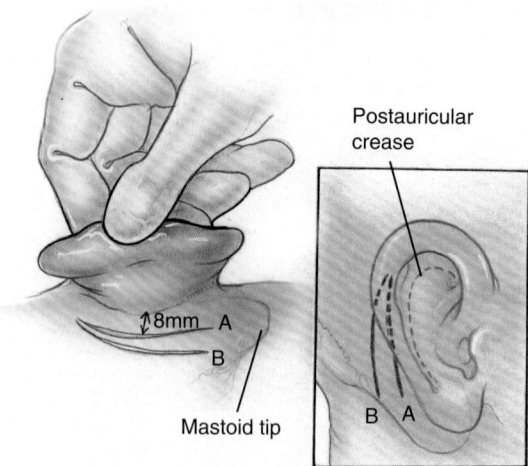

Figure 152.1 Placement of postauricular incisions in adults (*A*) and infants (*B*).

from the mastoid tip to the superior limb just described. Periosteal elevators are then used to elevate the periosteum of the mastoid cortex toward the posterior margin of the ear canal (Fig. 152.2). Superior to the ear canal, the periosteum should be elevated anteriorly along the zygomatic root. Inferior to the ear canal, the surgeon should elevate the periosteum to the anterior margin of the superior aspect of the mastoid tip. If the tip is to be removed, the surgeon must remove all the periosteum from its surface. Taking a few moments to get this anterior extension, superiorly and inferiorly, will allow the ear to be held forward easily with self-retaining retractors. The periosteum can also be elevated somewhat down the ear canal to release tension and prevent a canal laceration.

elevation superior to the ear canal exposes the root of the zygoma. Posterior to the ear canal, the postauricular muscle and pericranial soft tissues are incised and elevated in the same plane as described above. This dissection is carried to the mastoid tip. Care must be taken not to dissect anterior to the tip because this endangers the facial nerve in the stylomastoid foramen. Unless the mastoid tip is to be removed, the sternocleidomastoid muscle's insertion onto the tip should not be severed. This minimizes postoperative discomfort. Thus far, the skin and soft tissues of the pinna have been laid anteriorly, but the periosteum still remains attached to the mastoid cortex.

The mastoid cortex is now exposed to start the drilling process (Fig. 152.2). A T-shaped incision is made through the soft tissues and periosteum overlying bone. The superior limb of the "T" is placed along the inferior temporal line (inferior margin of the temporalis muscle) starting at a point just superior to the anterior–superior ear canal. This incision extends posteriorly as far as is needed for adequate exposure. An inferior limb to the "T" is fashioned

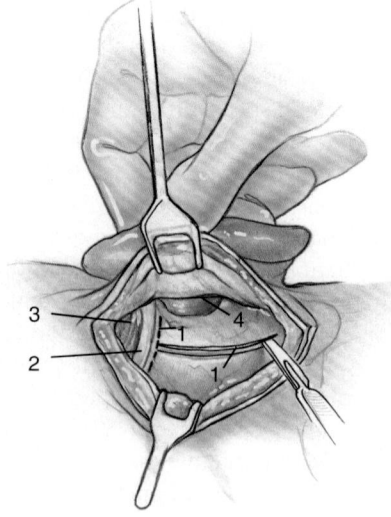

Figure 152.2 After exposure, the periosteum of the mastoid cortex is incised with a "T"-shaped or an "L"-shaped incision. The periosteum is then elevated off the mastoid cortex, exposing the posterior wall of the external auditory canal. *1*, Periosteal incisions; *2*, Temporal line; *3*, Temporalis m.; *4*, Posterior canal skin.

Self-retaining retractors should now be placed to hold the auricle forward. The suprameatal spine of Henle marks the lateral extent of the posterior–superior bony ear canal. The surgeon has raised two anteriorly based flaps: (a) the pinna and subcutaneous tissues and (b) the deeper musculoperiosteal tissues. This deeper flap can be used to partially obliterate the mastoidectomy cavity at the end of a canal-wall-down mastoidectomy. After an intact-canal-wall mastoidectomy, however, both layers should be closed to maintain a patent meatus and a properly positioned auricle.

Endaural incisions were first described by Kessel in 1885 and later popularized by Lempert (1) in 1938.

These incisions expose a limited portion of the mastoid cortex. First, a posterior canal wall incision is made from the 12-o'clock to the 6-o'clock position just medial to the bony cartilaginous junction (Lempert I incision). From the 12-o'clock position of the Lempert I incision, a medial-to-lateral incision is made into the incisura between the tragus and root of the helix (Lempert II incision). A relaxing incision is then made at the inferior margin of the Lempert I incision (in a medial-to-lateral direction) (Fig. 152.3A). This allows the posterior ear canal and conchal skin to be mobilized (Fig. 152.3A and B). Skin, soft tissues, muscle, and periosteum over the mastoid cortex are elevated using

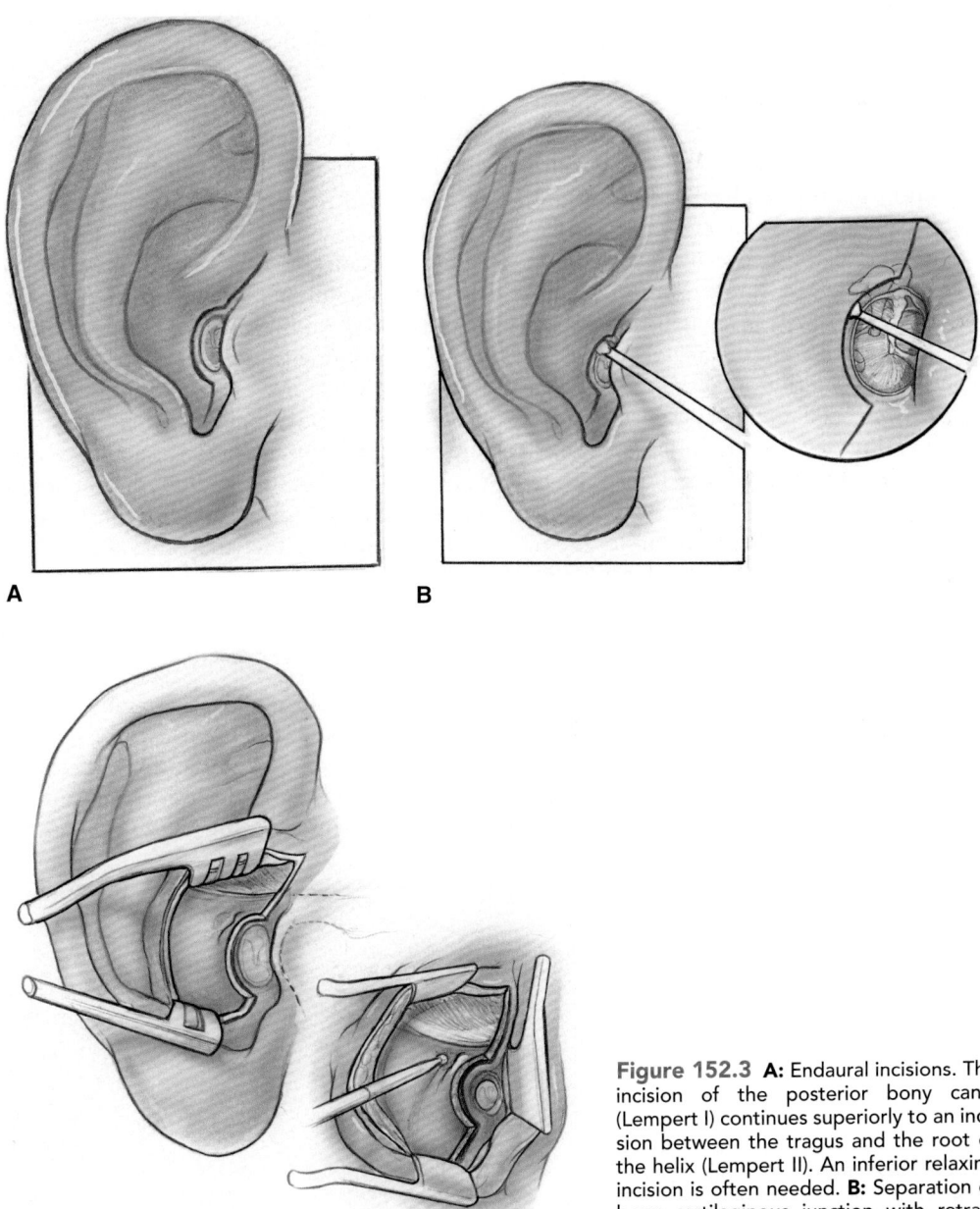

A   **B**

C

Figure 152.3 A: Endaural incisions. The incision of the posterior bony canal (Lempert I) continues superiorly to an incision between the tragus and the root of the helix (Lempert II). An inferior relaxing incision is often needed. **B:** Separation of bony cartilaginous junction with retraction. **C:** Mastoid exposure via an endaural incision.

Lempert elevators, and a self-retaining retractor is placed. Indications for this incision include simple mastoidectomy in very poorly pneumatized temporal bones, atticotomies, canaloplasties, and some tympanoplasties. The endaural incision is closed in a layered fashion approximating deep tissues and then skin.

Surface Landmarks

The inferior temporal line (linea temporalis) defines the inferior limit of the temporalis muscle and provides a topographic landmark for the approximate level of the floor of the middle cranial fossa. Inferior to the temporal line is a protuberance at the posterosuperior margin of the ear canal called the suprameatal spine of Henle. Macewen triangle (cribrose area) is a depressed pit just posterior to the spine of Henle and serves as a topographic landmark for the underlying mastoid antrum. The antrum is typically located 15 mm medial to the cribrose area. The zygomatic root is palpable anterior–superior to the ear canal. The anterior, inferior, and posterior–inferior walls of the external auditory canal are formed by the tympanic bone while the region between the tympanosquamous and tympanomastoid suture lines (i.e., the posterior–superior bony ear canal) is made of squamous bone (Fig. 152.4). The canal skin in this region is thicker and more vascular than the inferior canal skin. When creating a laterally based conchal flap, this thickened "vascular strip" is elevated and preserved. The surface anatomy of the adult and young child's temporal bone differs (Fig. 152.5). Children younger than 2 years have immature tympanic rings and poorly developed mastoids. In children or adults with canal atresia, mal-development of the tympanic bone may result in facial nerve exit directly from the mastoid cortex (2).

Types of Mastoidectomy

The ear canal is made up of a cylinder of skin contained within a bony cylinder. In the normal ear, the tympanic membrane is the medial boundary for both those cylinders.

During routine office examination, it is not possible to see the epitympanum or mastoid region when the canal wall is intact. This is because the scutum blocks the epitympanum from view, and the posterior canal wall blocks access to the mastoid cavity. Therefore, removing the superior and posterior aspects of the bony canal allows direct access to the epitympanum and mastoid. This has the advantage of more thorough postoperative examination of the ear in the office; however, it leaves patients with cavities that require lifelong maintenance.

Mastoidectomy procedures can be categorized as *canal-wall-up* and *canal-wall-down* operations. Canal-wall-up procedures include the so-called simple mastoidectomy and the complete mastoidectomy with and without a facial recess approach. Canal-wall-down operations include the radical mastoidectomy, the modified radical mastoidectomy (MRM), and the Bondy MRM. A radical mastoidectomy removes the posterior and superior bony ear canal as well as the tympanic membrane, malleus, and incus. The stapes is usually preserved. The eustachian tube is obstructed, and no middle ear space remains. The entire cavity becomes lined with squamous epithelium. The radical mastoidectomy is "modified" when the tympanic membrane is reconstructed and mucosa-lined middle ear space is created. Ossicular reconstruction can also be performed during a MRM. The Bondy MRM is performed when disease spares the middle ear and only involves the epitympanum and mastoid. The scutum and posterior bony ear canal are removed to exteriorize the antrum and epitympanum, but the middle ear is not entered. Tympanoplasty and ossicular reconstruction can be performed whether the canal wall is taken down or left intact.

Simple Mastoidectomy

A simple mastoidectomy (sometimes called a transmastoid antrotomy) has limited usefulness; it is most commonly used to drain acute mastoid infections that do not respond to antibiotics. The procedure involves removing the mastoid cortex, drilling through the lateral air cells,

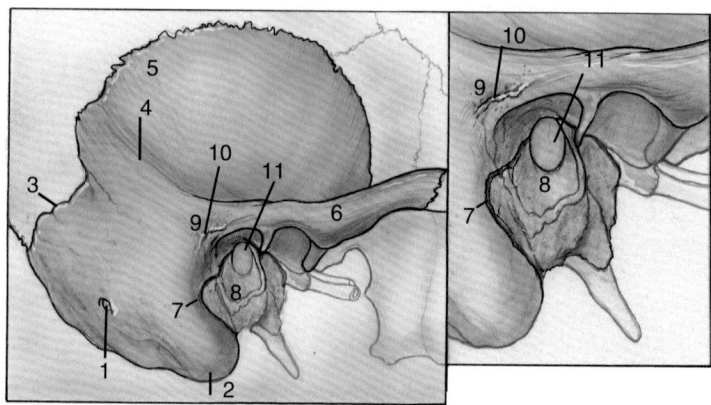

Figure 152.4 Surface anatomy of the adult temporal bone. *1,* Mastoid foramen; *2,* Mastoid tip; *3,* Petrosquamosal suture; *4,* Temporal line; *5,* Squamosa; *6,* Zygoma; *7,* Tympanomastoid suture line; *8,* Tympanic bone; *9,* Cribriform fossa; *10,* Spine of Henle; *11,* Tympanosquamous suture.

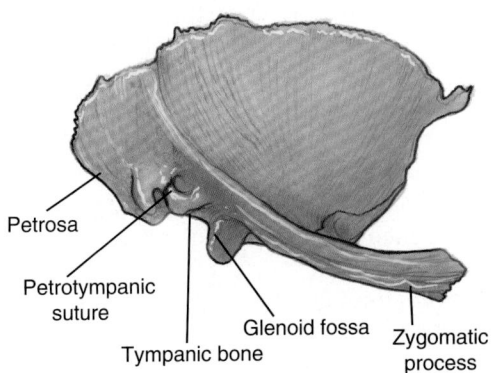

Figure 152.5 Surface anatomy of the infant temporal bone. The mastoid and the tympanic bone are disproportionately small in infants resulting in the stylomastoid foramen and facial nerve being nearer the skin surface than in adults.

and entering the antrum. The remainder of the air cell system is not exenterated. A thorough knowledge of the three-dimensional anatomy of the temporal bone is necessary for even this most direct of approaches (Fig. 152.6).

Complete Mastoidectomy

The complete mastoidectomy affords access to the antrum, attic, labyrinth, endolymphatic sac, and vertical segment of the facial nerve. All the air cells along the tegmen, sigmoid sinus, facial nerve, and semicircular canals are usually removed. The epitympanum is made accessible through the aditus ad antrum, and the incus and head of the malleus can be inspected directly. The incus and the head of the malleus may be removed for greater access to the supratubal recess in the anterior part of the attic.

Using the postauricular incision, the ear is laid forward and the mastoid cortex exposed as described above. The temporal line, spine of Henle, cribrose area, and posterior bony ear canal are used as the initial landmarks for drilling. The location of the mastoid antrum can be approximated by the intersection of a horizontal and vertical line

drawn tangential to the superior and posterior margins of the bony external auditory canal. A large cutting burr and continuous suction/irrigation are used to begin the mastoidectomy. Cortical bone is removed inferior to the middle fossa dura (tegmen mastoideum), the posterior edge of the bony ear canal is delineated, and the sigmoid sinus is identified. It is useful to widely saucerize the mastoidectomy bowl by removing any overhanging edges. This permits more light to enter the cavity and allows the surgeon to bring in his or her instruments into the operative field at an angle rather than directly along his or her line of sight. After determining the level of the tegmen, air cells lateral to the sigmoid sinus should be removed to see the blue hue of the sinus through thin bone. The sinodural angle, marking the posterior–superior limit of the mastoid cavity, is then opened. Drilling proceeds medially along the tegmen toward the epitympanum. Keeping this anterior–superior portion of the dissection as the deepest portion of the cavity avoids inadvertent injury to the facial nerve. Körner septum is a plate of bone lateral to the antrum, and it represents the posterior extension of the petrosquamous suture line within the mastoid (3) (Fig. 152.7). The superior aspect of Körner septum must be removed to enter the mastoid antrum. The floor of the antrum, which is the lateral semicircular canal, is a vital landmark that must be clearly visualized (Fig. 152.8). Otic capsule bone of the labyrinth usually appears to be a slightly lighter hue when compared with the surrounding membranous bone.

Once the antrum is entered, the bone of the posterior ear canal wall must be thinned, although excessive thinning may lead to delayed dissolution of this structure. Identifying the posterior incudal ligament (often seen as a white streak through thin bone just inferior to the fossa incudus) is a useful landmark in finding the incus. By flooding the antrum with clear irrigant, the surface of the fluid forms a lens that will bend light from the microscope and allow the surgeon to see the incus before actually coming upon it (Fig. 152.8). Touching the incus with a rotating burr must be avoided because transmission of

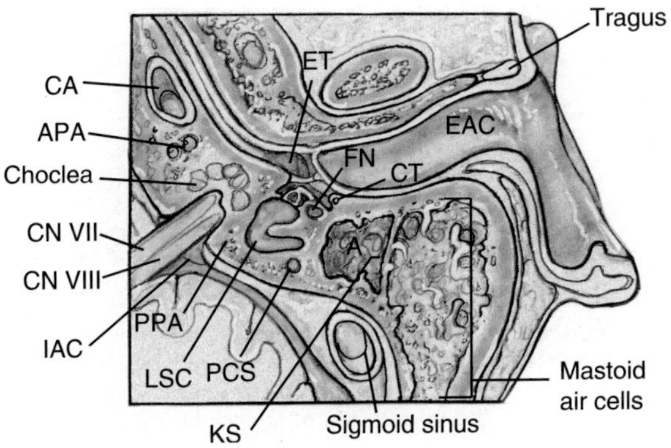

Figure 152.6 Axial section of a right adult temporal bone.

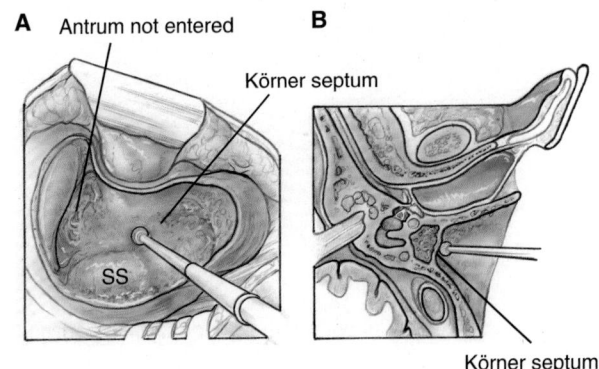

Figure 152.7 Körner septum. **A:** Axial section view of Körner septum. **B:** Lateral surgical view of Körner septum. SS, sigmoid sinus.

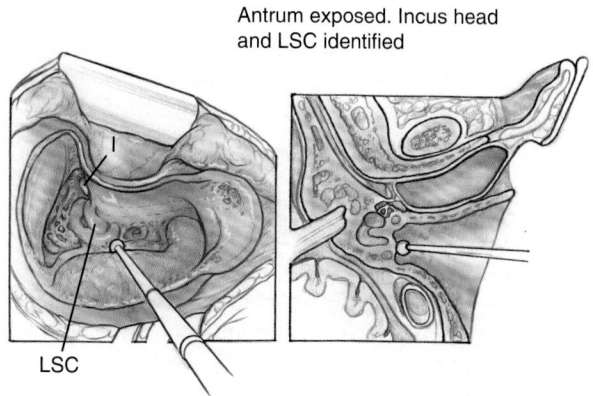

Antrum exposed. Incus head
and LSC identified

Figure 152.8 Simple mastoidectomy. **Left:** Lateral surgical view of mastoid cavity. The air cells of the mastoid have been removed back to the bone over the sigmoid sinus and the otic capsule of the bone over the lateral semicircular canal can be seen. The posterior bony canal wall and bone overlying the facial nerve (in *yellow*) are intact. **Right:** An axial section view of mastoid cavity.

high-frequency mechanical energy to the inner ear can cause sensorineural hearing loss. Once the incus body is identified, removing the bone lateral to the ossicles (between the tegmen tympani and bone of the superior ear canal) opens the epitympanum. Carrying this dissection anteriorly will expose the head of the malleus.

Having found the antrum, the horizontal semicircular canal, and the incus, attention can now be directed to identifying the facial nerve. Bony trabeculae on the bony external auditory canal are removed from a lateral to medial direction. As this dissection proceeds medially,

facial recess air cells anterior to the facial nerve will be encountered. The second genu of the facial nerve is located immediately anterior and inferior to the midpoint of the horizontal canal, just medial to the short process of the incus. Here, a 4-mm diamond burr and copious irrigation are used to make wide strokes, starting at the incus superiorly and aimed toward the stylomastoid foramen inferiorly. Adequate irrigation prevents thermal injury to the nerve. The facial nerve should be visualized through thin bone but not completely exposed. As the facial nerve is traced inferiorly, the branch-point of the chorda tympani nerve will be found (Fig. 152.9A). The chorda can then be traced anteriorly and superiorly.

All of the cells within the mastoid tip may be exenterated. The posterior belly of the digastric muscle inserts medially on the mastoid tip. Identifying the muscle through eggshelled bone is referred to as the "digastric ridge," which is actually a surgically created landmark (Fig. 152.9A). Fascia enveloping the digastric muscle is continuous with the fibrous tissue surrounding the facial nerve at the stylomastoid foramen. The stylomastoid foramen enlarges as it exits the inferior portion of the temporal bone. Following the digastric ridge anteriorly in the mastoid tip is one technique used to find the facial nerve. Infralabyrinthine (retrofacial) air cells are those cells medial to the facial nerve, superior to the jugular bulb, and inferior to the posterior semicircular canal. They should be exenterated if disease is found within them or if either the jugular bulb or endolymphatic sac needs to be exposed.

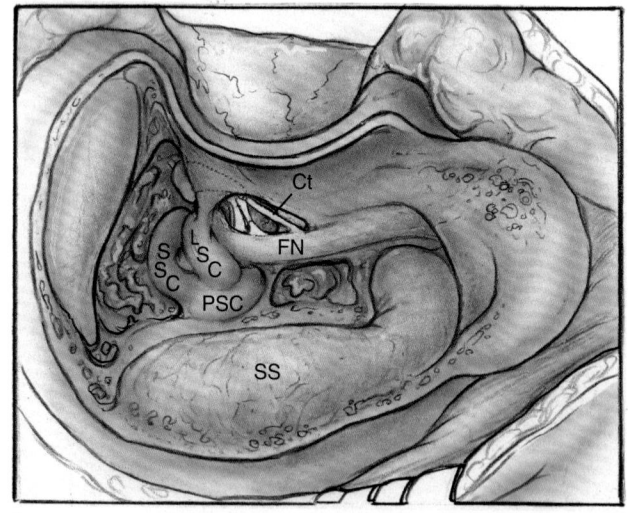

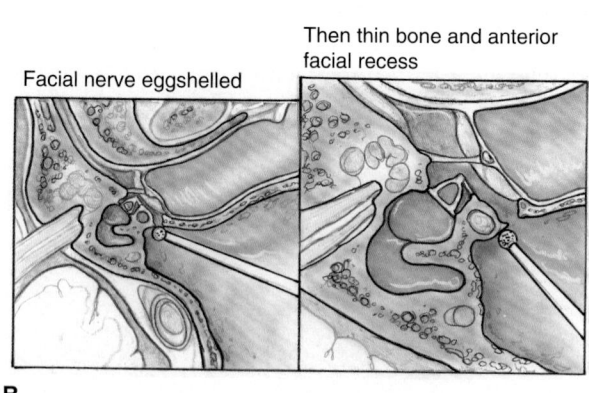

Facial nerve eggshelled

Then thin bone and anterior facial recess

A

B

Figure 152.9 Facial recess approach. **A:** Surgical view. The bone over the mastoid portion of the facial nerve and the chorda tympani is thinned. The bone between these two landmarks is removed giving access to the middle ear. **B:** An axial depiction of the facial recess approach illustrates the thinning of bone over the fallopian canal and the opening made into the middle ear between the tympanic annulus and the facial nerve. Ct, corda tympani; SSC, superior semicircular canal; LSC, lateral semicircular canal; PSC, posterior semicircular canal; SS, sigmoid sinus; FN, facial nerve.

Following a complete mastoidectomy, the surgeon should thoroughly irrigate the cavity to remove bone dust, which may otherwise cause ossicular fixation. The complete mastoidectomy cavity should consist of a well-defined tegmen tympani and tegmen mastoideum superiorly, a clearly delineated sigmoid sinus posteriorly, an open sinodural angle, well-visualized semicircular canals, an intact posterior bony ear canal wall, and the facial nerve seen through thin bone.

Complete Mastoidectomy with a Facial Recess Approach

The facial recess is an aerated extension of the posterior–superior middle ear space. Medial to the tympanic annulus and lateral to the fallopian canal, it allows access to the middle ear from the mastoid cavity without disruption of the tympanic membrane. Some surgeons use the term "posterior tympanotomy" to describe a facial recess approach. The facial recess is a triangular opening bordered posteromedially by the facial nerve, anterolaterally by the chorda tympani nerve, and superiorly by the fossa incudis (Fig. 152.9). An open facial recess provides access to the ossicles, stapedius tendon, round window, tympanic segment of the facial canal, and cochleariform process (4). Dissection of the region of the facial recess should be performed with diamond burs and copious suction irrigation to avoid mechanical or thermal damage to the nerves.

There are numerous indications for performing a posterior tympanotomy. These include transmastoid cochlear implantation, middle ear electromechanical implantation (5), presence of cholesteatoma within both the middle ear and mastoid, chronic otomastoiditis with granulation tissue or cholesterol granuloma, and tumors within the middle ear and mastoid (6).

In the anterior epitympanum, a projection of bone extending inferiorly from the tegmen tympani (the cog) can obscure disease in the supratubal recess (7). The presence of granulation tissue, cholesteatoma, or tumor in the anterior epitympanum and supratubal recess may require removal of the incus, head of the malleus, and the cog for increased exposure. If removal of the incus is necessary, the incudostapedial joint must first be disarticulated through the facial recess before removing the incus and malleus head. Opening the facial recess can also improve aeration of the mastoid by providing an alternate route for air from the eustachian tube to enter the mastoid (other than the aditus ad antrum). Inadequate aeration or loculation of the mastoid cavity may result in recurrent retraction pocket formation, mucocele formation, or chronic otomastoiditis. One way to test for adequate aeration of the mastoid cavity is to fill the middle ear with saline and watch for flow into the mastoid. When the incus has been removed, rarely is a facial recess approach required for aeration.

When thinning the posterior bony canal wall, the facial recess is encountered medially. It is first noted as a color change (darker appearing bone) anterior to the facial nerve, just inferior to its second genu. The facial nerve lies medial and inferior to the tip of the short process of the incus. The second genu of the facial nerve usually forms an angle of 95 to 125 degrees; it usually makes a gentle curve rather than an abrupt turn. The nerve may descend directly through the mastoid in a caudal direction, or it may deviate from the vertical by 5 to 35 degrees. The facial nerve travels laterally as it moves inferiorly through its vertical segment and is located lateral to the posterior–inferior tympanic annulus in 65% of cases (8).

The surgeon should be aware of potential facial nerve anomalies. Dehiscence of the facial nerve is reported to occur in 55% to 57% of temporal bones (9). The facial nerve is dehiscent approximately 50% of the time just superior to the oval window, in its tympanic segment. Other areas of possible dehiscence include the geniculate ganglion, facial recess, tympanic sinus, and the retrofacial region. Bone erosion secondary to cholesteatoma may also create dehiscence in the fallopian canal. Before encountering the nerve, the vasa nervorum can be appreciated through the eggshelled bone overlying the nerve. The most common site of injury to the facial nerve in mastoid surgery is inferior to the lateral semicircular canal just beyond the second genu (9).

At a variable point along its descent toward the stylomastoid foramen, the facial nerve gives off the chorda tympani nerve. This nerve travels in an anterior, superior, and lateral direction. Facial nerve anomalies can include a chorda that branches from the facial nerve after it exits from the stylomastoid foramen, a bifid facial nerve (10), or a nerve coursing through the middle ear space just inferior to the oval window (11). Once the chorda tympani nerve is identified, the bone between the chorda and the facial nerve may be removed with a small diamond burr and copious irrigation. This opens the facial recess (Fig. 152.9A). If additional exposure is required, an extended facial recess approach can be performed, where the chorda is sacrificed and the facial recess extended inferiorly. Care must be taken to identify the fibrous annulus of the tympanic membrane and to avoid inadvertent injury to the tympanic membrane or medial ear canal.

Intact Canal Versus Canal-Wall-Down Mastoidectomy

Both the open (canal-wall-down) and the closed (intact canal with facial recess or posterior tympanotomy) procedures have advantages and disadvantages. Judgment as to which procedure to perform depends on the nature of the disease, the reliability of the patient, and the experience of the surgeon (Table 152.2).

The intact-canal-wall approach offers several advantages over open (canal-wall-down) techniques. First, postoperatively there is no mastoid cavity to care for. Patients

| TABLE 152.2 | OPEN VERSUS CLOSED TECHNIQUES FOR MASTOIDECTOMY | |

	Advantages	Disadvantages
Intact wall	Physiologic tympanic membrane position Deep middle ear No mastoid bowl	Residual cholesteatoma may be occult Recurrent cholesteatoma may occur in attic Delayed canal breakdown Incomplete exteriorization of facial recess Second stage often required
Canal-wall-down	Residual cholesteatoma visible on follow-up Recurrent cholesteatoma is rare Total exteriorization of facial recess	Mastoid bowl maintenance can be a lifelong problem Middle ear is shallow and difficult to reconstruct Position of pinna may be altered Second stage sometimes required

with cavities often require regular office debridement, may have a difficult time fitting hearing aids, need to adhere to water precautions, and have meatoplasties that may be cosmetically unappealing. An intact-canal procedure also allows for a more physiologic ossicular reconstruction with a deeper, better-aerated middle ear. Some authors, however, have found no significant benefit in hearing results for intact-canal-wall mastoidectomy compared with canal-wall-down procedures (12,13).

There are several potential disadvantages to the intact-canal-wall approach. First, there is an increased risk of residual or recurrent disease. Widely varying results using a canal-wall-up mastoidectomy have been reported in the literature. However, most of the larger series reveal residual cholesteatoma in 20% to 35% of cases and recurrent disease in 5% to 20% (14–17). This is in contrast to results for open procedures in which there is a 2% to 17% rate of residual disease and a 0% to 10% chance for recurrence (18,19). Although uncommon, a second potential problem with the intact-canal-wall procedures is delayed breakdown of the bone of the posterior canal wall. This is due to compromised blood supply from over-thinning the bone. A third disadvantage is an inability to see the mastoid cavity in the office for surveillance. Some surgeons routinely perform "second look" operations 6 to 12 months after the initial procedure. A staged ossicular reconstruction can also be accomplished at that time. Careful patient selection is vital. Intact-canal procedures should be performed in reliable patients who plan to follow-up regularly in the office.

Radical Mastoidectomy

The radical mastoidectomy is the most aggressive of the open cavity mastoid procedures. The classic radical mastoidectomy involves a canal-wall-down mastoidectomy combined with complete removal of the tympanic membrane, annulus, malleus, incus, and all middle ear mucosa. The eustachian tube is stripped of mucosa and obliterated with packing (fascia, muscle, or bone). The goal of radical mastoidectomy is to establish a dry, open cavity devoid of

secretory epithelium. Before the advent of tympanoplasty, this radical procedure was by far the most common open procedure. However, it is rarely performed today. Most surgeons now prefer an MRM with reconstruction of a middle ear space and the sound conduction apparatus. If disease permits, a graft can be placed isolating the eustachian tube and round window from the middle ear, creating a cava minor reconstruction. However, there are still some indications for a radical mastoidectomy; these include unresectable cholesteatoma with extension into the eustachian tube, cholesteatoma with erosion into the cochlea or labyrinth, or patients who have had multiple failed MRMs.

The procedure involves performing a complete (intact bony canal) mastoidectomy with identification of all the landmarks discussed previously. The superior and posterior canal walls are then removed with a cutting burr and suction–irrigation. Prior to encountering the ossicles, the incudostapedial joint is separated and the head of the malleus as well as the incus are removed. The bone of the canal wall is lowered to the level of the mastoid portion of the fallopian canal, but the stapes is preserved. A diamond burr with copious irrigation is used to identify the facial nerve through thinned bone. All mucosa from the mastoid and middle ear is removed, and the eustachian tube is packed with fascia or bone. The mastoid tip is removed. Care should be taken to lower the facial ridge, remove overhanging edges, and lower the bone of the inferior canal wall so as to prevent creation of a dependent mastoid tip. To reduce the depth of the cavity, its perimeter is well saucerized.

Modified Radical Mastoidectomy

The radical mastoidectomy operation is termed "modified" when a middle ear space is reconstructed (Fig. 152.10). The MRM begins with a complete mastoidectomy. The decision to take the canal wall down is then based on the extent of disease (Table 152.2). Most of the bone lateral to incus can be removed quickly with a large cutting burr and the scutum made flush with the anterior canal wall. Because

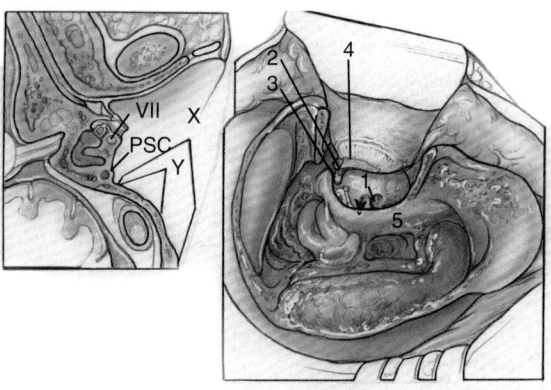

Figure 152.10 Completed canal-wall-down MRM. **Left:** Axial view demonstrating the complete removal of air cells of the mastoid and saucerization over the sigmoid sinus. X, Potential depth without saucerization; Y, Potential depth with saucerization. **Right:** Surgical view of a completed, canal-down mastoidectomy 1, Round window; 2, Tensor tympani tendon; 3, Cochleariform process; 4, Manubrium of malleus; 5, Facial ridge. *Red arrow*—sinus tympani.

the facial nerve is medial to the incus, it is protected. The bone immediately lateral to the ossicles must be removed carefully with microinstruments rather than the drill. This avoids direct contact between the rotating burr and ossicular chain. Alternately, the incudostapedial joint may be separated and the incus and head of the malleus removed. The posterior and inferior portions of the remaining bony ear canal are then removed. The bone, lateral to the facial nerve, called the "facial ridge," is drilled down to the level of the fallopian canal, leaving a thin covering of bone over the facial nerve.

A few technical points deserve mention. Once the bulk of the posterior ear canal has been removed with cutting burrs, the vertical (mastoid) segment of the facial nerve is found by lowering the facial ridge with a diamond burr. The nerve should be seen through thinned bone. Actual exposure of the facial nerve should be avoided, however, because exposure puts the nerve at risk. With radical mastoidectomies and MRMs, the mastoid cortex must be well saucerized and the mastoid tip removed. This precludes a deep cavity with overhanging edges that can be difficult to cleanse. Saucerization makes the cavity shallow by allowing surrounding soft tissues to prolapse inward. The inferior portion of the tympanic ring should be lowered so it is flush with the hypotympanum. This prevents the formation of a dependent region in the hypotympanum that may collect debris postoperatively. An anterior canal wall canaloplasty should be performed when the prominence of the anterior wall obscures the anterior tympanic sulcus. An incision is made in the anterior canal wall just lateral to the tympanic annulus, the skin is raised in a retrograde manner back to the bony cartilaginous junction, and the bone sculpted as necessary. One should use a large diamond burr with constant suction–irrigation to avoid entering the glenoid fossa.

After mastoid surgery has been completed, the middle ear space is reconstructed. Commonly a fascia or cartilage graft is laid from the anterior annulus to and over the facial ridge. The graft must be well positioned as to not adhere to the promontory. Surgeons may elect to place Silastic over the promontory to prevent adhesions between the drum and middle ear mucosa. Although the middle ear is shallow in open techniques, there is usually sufficient space to perform an ossiculoplasty.

The Bondy Modified Radical Mastoidectomy

The Bondy procedure (20), first suggested by Körner (3) in 1899, is a variation of the MRM. It can be performed through either an endaural or postauricular incision. This operation is used in cases of large attic cholesteatomas in which the middle ear has been spared of disease. An atticotomy is performed first. The entire scutum is then removed to expose the epitympanum, to marsupialize the cholesteatoma, and to debride its keratin content. The medial wall of the cholesteatoma matrix is left in place over the body of the incus and head of the malleus in the epitympanum. This seals the middle ear space. If the cholesteatoma is seen extending around the ossicles, the surgeon must be prepared to perform a traditional MRM. If involvement of the middle ear is in question preoperatively, a high-resolution computed tomography (CT) scan of the temporal bone with axial and coronal views may help determine whether a Bondy procedure is indicated. This operation is reserved for those ears with large primary acquired cholesteatomas in which hearing is preserved and the ossicular chain is free of disease. A Bondy mastoidectomy is a particularly useful technique in cases with cholesteatoma and a labyrinthine fistula, especially in an only hearing ear. After the procedure, keratin can be debrided in the office while leaving the medial matrix of the cholesteatoma intact over the fistula. The surgeon must be vigilant, however, during each office examination. If cholesteatoma appears to extend into the middle ear, this finding should be verified with CT imaging and a traditional MRM would then become necessary.

MEATOPLASTY AND MASTOID OBLITERATION

The most important factors in avoiding a chronically draining cavity are thorough removal of disease during surgery, designing a properly shaped mastoid cavity, and creating a wide external auditory meatus.

Mastoid Obliteration

Following canal-wall-down mastoidectomy, the patient is left with an open mastoid cavity. The keratinizing squamous epithelium that lines the mastoid bowl is prone to collecting debris and should be cleaned on a regular basis. Many patients must adhere to lifelong water precautions to minimize risk of infection. Some technical considerations help to limit postoperative complications in a canal-wall-down mastoidectomy. Wide saucerization of the mastoid bowl allows the surrounding soft tissues to prolapse into and partially obliterate the cavity. Lowering the bone lateral to the fallopian canal and performing a generous meatoplasty also helps. Avoiding a dependent mastoid tip prevents accumulation of debris in this difficult-to-clean area. Lowering the bony canal wall and inferior tympanic annulus flush with the hypotympanum facilitates in-office access to the dependent areas of the mastoid.

Muscle/tissue flaps. Some surgeons obliterate the mastoidectomy cavity in more formal ways. Originally described by Moser (21), the "Palva flap" has been used successfully in obliterating mastoid cavities (22,23). This flap is a laterally based postauricular musculoperiosteal flap that is rotated into cavity at the end of the procedure. Postmortem histologic examination of temporal bones from patients who underwent mastoid obliteration with the Palva flap has demonstrated viable muscle, fat, collagen, and richly vascularized tissue years after the procedure. There can be some atrophy, however, over the 5-year period after mastoidectomy. Some cavities widen as a consequence (24). Other flaps utilized for mastoid obliteration include an anteriorly based temporalis muscle flap or temporalis fascia flap based on a superficial temporal artery pedicle (the Hong Kong flap) (22). Such flaps provide bulk, cover exposed bone, recruit a blood supply, and provide a surface for epithelial migration. Palva (25) has advocated the use of bone pâté and bone chips for obliterating the mastoid defect. It is important to collect the bone pâté from cortical bone, before entering the diseased portions of the mastoid. This pâté is laid into the cavity at the end of the case and flaps rotated over it. All bone pâté must be completely covered by fascia or the Palva flap. Osteoneogenesis then results in further reduction of the size of the mastoid cavity (26) over time.

Replacement of the canal wall. Gantz et al. (27) have described carefully removing the posterior wall, exenterating disease as needed, replacing the wall, and filling the mastoid with bone chips.

Other techniques. Synthetic materials have been used for mastoid obliteration with mixed results (28,29). We recommend caution in the use of alloplastic materials for mastoid obliteration when infection is present as there have been reports of troublesome complications using hydroxyapatite preparations (30).

Meatoplasty

Enlarging the external auditory meatus is a necessary part of canal-wall-down procedures. It promotes aeration and epithelialization of the canal and cavity, facilitates effective postoperative care, and makes office debridement of the cavity much easier. An adequate meatoplasty also reduces the depth of the bowl. Several techniques to enlarge the external auditory meatus have been devised. Each involves removing some conchal cartilage and

draping the posterior meatal skin into the mastoid bowl (Fig. 152.11). An excellent meatoplasty can be performed by connecting superior and inferior Lempert endaural incisions with the postauricular incision. The superior cut is brought out laterally into the tragal incisura while the inferior cut is curved just medial to the antitragus. This creates a laterally based composite flap containing conchal cartilage and meatal skin. Varying amounts of this cartilage can be removed (through the postauricular incision), leaving behind thin conchal skin that drapes into the mastoid bowl (Fig. 152.11B) (31). Adequate resection of cartilage and appropriate positioning of the posterior canal skin are vital (Fig. 152.11C). The meatus can be maintained open by placing absorbable sutures from the remaining conchal cartilage and perichondrium to the postauricular periosteum. Three sutures are usually placed: one posterosuperiorly, one directly posterior, and the third posteroinferiorly. The sutures are not tied until all three have been properly placed. These tacking sutures prevent postoperative protrusion of the auricle and collapse of the meatus. This meatoplasty technique can be adapted to individual reconstructive needs. Permanent sutures may be used in recalcitrant cases of meatal collapse. Some have advocated suturing the medial margin of the posterior canal skin to the subcutaneous tissue posterior to the mastoidectomy defect, thereby pulling the meatus open. While this maneuver does open the meatus, it usually results in a more voluminous mastoid cavity than desired.

ENDOSCOPY

Endoscopes often see where the microscope cannot. The surgeon's view through the operating microscope depends on a clear line of sight. A 1.7- to 2.8-mm, 30-degree rigid telescope, however, can look around a corner to visualize the facial recess, sinus tympani, or epitympanum and it can be inserted through a tiny incision. It can also be used to assess the depth of retraction pockets and determine the extent of cholesteatomas. Some authors have advocated the use of endoscopes for second-look procedures following intact-canal-wall tympanomastoidectomies (32). Rosenberg et al. (33) reported that endoscopic findings correlated well with open surgical exploration in 10 out of 10 patients. The role of endoscopy will continue to expand in the otologic and neurotologic applications as surgeons become more comfortable with their use and larger studies confirm their efficacy.

ENDOLYMPHATIC SHUNT

In 1927, Guild (34) proposed that endolymph in the inner ear may flow from the cochlea to the endolymphatic sac. It was near this time that Portmann (35) first incised the endolymphatic sac in the treatment of Ménière disease. Interestingly, it was not until a decade later that Hallpike and Cairns (36) demonstrate the histopathology of endolymphatic hydrops in patients with Ménière disease.

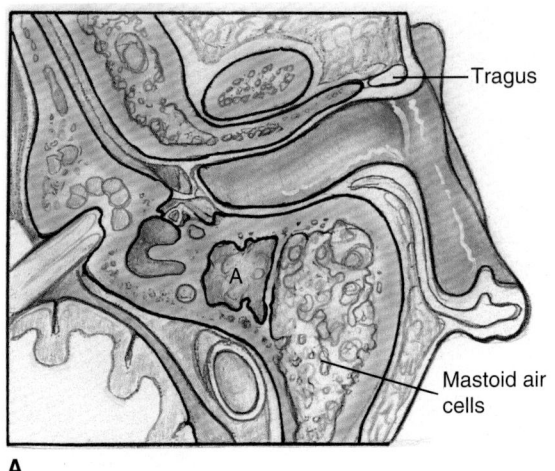

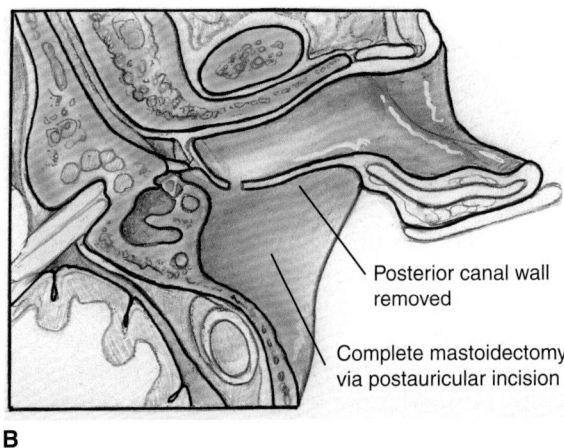

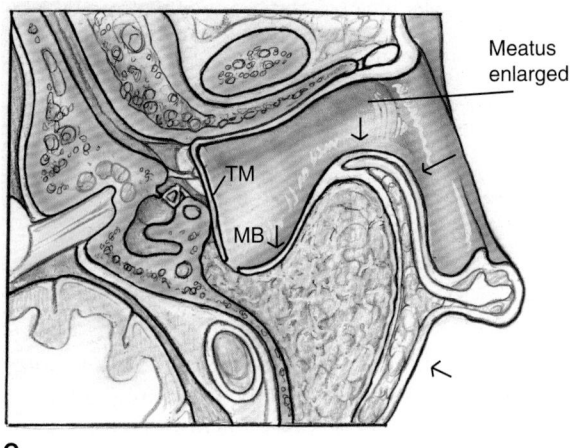

Figure 152.11 Meatoplasty following canal-wall-down mastoidectomy. **A:** Axial view of unoperated temporal bone demonstrating the physical relationships between the external auditory canal and the mastoid for comparison to (**B**) and (**C**). A, Antrum. **B:** Axial view of temporal bone after canal-wall-down mastoidectomy and removal of some of the bone of the conchal bowl. **C:** Axial view after meatoplasty and partial obliteration of mastoid bowl with muscle-periosteal flap. TM, tympanic membrane on facial ridge; MB, mastoid bowl.

Since then, multiple procedures have been designed to "shunt" or "decompress" endolymphatic sac for the treatment of intractable Ménière disease (37). Successful control of vertigo has been reported in a majority of patients regardless of the technique used, but some have questioned the efficacy of these procedures (38) (see Chapter 166).

Exposure of the endolymphatic sac requires a complete mastoidectomy. The facial nerve should be identified and traced from the second genu through its vertical segment. The otic capsule bone of the posterior semicircular canal is identified, and the posterior fossa plate between the sigmoid sinus and the posterior semicircular canal is thinned. The inferior crus of the posterior semicircular canal does not extend more than 12 mm inferior to the tip of the incus (39). The sigmoid sinus is followed inferiorly toward the jugular bulb. As the posterior fossa plate is thinned, the endolymphatic sac comes into view just posteroinferior to the posterior semicircular canal. This structure usually appears as a thickened, white area of dura. The bone overlying the sac must be removed, and its lateral wall is incised if desired (Fig. 152.12). Because the "lumen" of the endolymphatic sac is a labyrinth of small, interconnected lumina, space for the shunt is created by blunt dissection. The surgeon should place a sickle knife or similar

instrument into the sac and palpate the operculum. An anterior margin of the sigmoid sinus may obscure a direct view of the endolymphatic sac. In such cases, the sinus can be decompressed and retracted posteriorly for visualization of the sac. One should be vigilant for the presence of a high

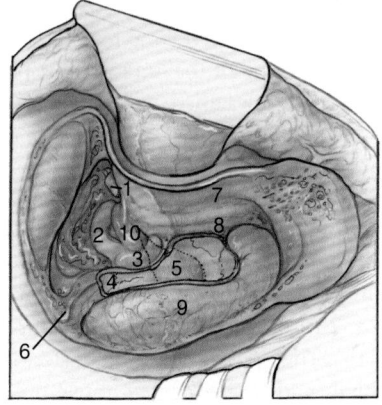

Figure 152.12 Transmastoid exposure of endolymphatic sac. The endolymphatic sac is within the posterior fossa dura generally inferior to the labyrinth and often in contact with the sigmoid sinus. 1, Incus; 2, SSC; 3, PSC; 4, Posterior fossa dura; 5, ELS; 6, SDA—sinodural angle; 7, PCW—posterior canal wall; 8, Retrofacial air cells; 9, Sigmoid sinus skeletonized; 10, LSC.

jugular bulb. This does not usually impair access to the sac, but its presence limits the amount of space available to the surgeon inferior to the posterior semicircular canal.

TRANSMASTOID BLOCKAGE OF THE SEMICIRCULAR CANALS

The posterior and superior semicircular canals can be obliterated through a mastoidectomy approach for the treatment of canalithiasis and the dehiscent superior semicircular canal syndrome. Obliteration of the posterior semicircular canal is indicated for intractable benign positional vertigo (40). With the recognition of the superior semicircular canal dehiscence (SSCD) syndrome (41), surgical approaches for its repair have been devised. Although most surgeons repair SSCD through the middle cranial fossa (42) many can be repaired by transmastoid obstruction of the superior semicircular canal (43).

Transmastoid obstruction of the semicircular canals can be achieved through a thorough mastoidectomy approach. As the bony capsule of the semicircular canals is approached, the bony trabeculae on the surface of the posterior or superior canals are removed. Once the bony labyrinth is identified, the perilymphatic space of the canal may be approached by gradually removing labyrinthine bone with a diamond burr and constant suction irrigation. The techniques to approach the posterior and superior canals vary.

In the case of canalithiasis of the posterior canal, the labyrinthine bone over the canal is thinned until a "gray line" is visible through the thinned overlying bone. This thin bone can be gently picked away to create a 1 × 3 mm opening into the perilymphatic space. Fine bone chips obtained while drilling are then placed into the canal, collapsing the contents of the canal and completely occluding it. Fibrin glue or bone wax may be used to hold the bone chips in place (40); hydroxyapatite cement may also be applied.

In the case of SSCD, the bony trabeculae between the bone of the lateral semicircular canal and the tegmen mastoideum are removed. As trabeculae are removed, the otic capsule bone of the superior semicircular canal is exposed (Fig. 152.13). The dura is often lying low, making retraction necessary. Once the bone of the anterior and posterior crus of the superior canal is identified, they can be "gray lined" as described above. There is no need to expose the middle fossa dehiscence since manipulation of the contents of the semicircular canal may damage that structure. After the bone over the anterior (ampulated) and posterior crura of the superior canal are identified by drilling with a 1 or 2 mm diamond burr, this bone may be chipped away with small picks (opening ~1 × 2 mm) and occluded with fine bone chips (see Fig. 152.13). The opening into the posterior crus of the superior canal should be performed above the junction of the posterior canal (common crus) as to avoid obstruction of the posterior semicircular canal. Fibrin glue, bone wax, or hydroxyapatite cement may be used for reinforcement (43).

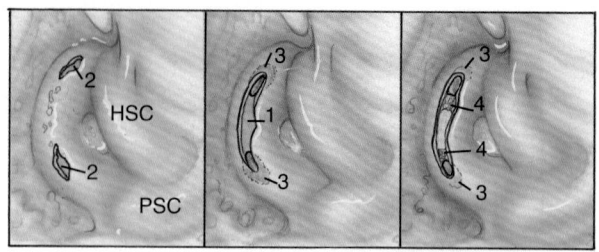

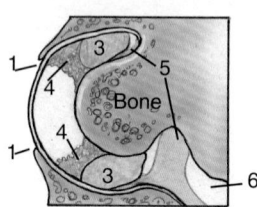

Figure 152.13 Transmastoid exposure and opening of the superior semicircular canal for obstruction of the canal. The bone over the anterior and posterior crura of the superior semicircular canal is first thinned to eggshell thickness. The canal is opened without disruption of endolymphatic membranes and both crura packed with fascia. Bone chips from drilling can be inserted over each graft to encourage osteogenesis (**lower inset**). *1*, Area of dehiscence; *2*, Eggshelled SSC; *3*, Fascia; *4*, Bone dust; *5*, Endolymph; *6*, Perilymph; HSC, horizontal semicircular canal; PSC, posterior semicircular canal.

PETROUS APICECTOMY

Infections of the mastoid and middle ear can spread to the anterior and medial segment of the temporal bone known as the petrous apex. Petrous apicitis is classically characterized by deep retro-orbital pain, abducens nerve palsy, and otorrhea (Gradenigo syndrome). Cranial nerves V, VI, and VII may become involved (44,45). Surgical access to the petrous apex becomes necessary for drainage of expanding cholesterol granulomas and mucosal cysts, exenteration of infected air cells, removal of cholesteatomas, and biopsy of various mass lesions.

The petrous apex takes the form of a truncated pyramid in the posterior skull base (Fig. 152.14A and B). It can be divided into anterior and posterior portions by a coronal plane through the internal auditory canal (Fig. 152.14C). Thirty percent of posterior petrous apices and 9% of anterior apices are pneumatized (46). The petrous tip is in close relation to Dorello canal and the trigeminal fossa anteriorly. Dorello canal, formed by the petrous apex, clivus, and petrosphenoidal (Gruber) ligament, contains the abducens nerve (Fig. 152.14B). The trigeminal fossa (Meckel cave), in the floor of the middle cranial fossa, houses the trigeminal (gasserian) ganglion (Fig. 152.14B). Given this anatomy, it is easy to see why diseases here can compromise cranial nerves V and VI.

The classic procedures designed to access the posterior petrous apex include the transmastoid infralabyrinthine approach and the translabyrinthine approach. Procedures used to access the anterior petrous apex include the

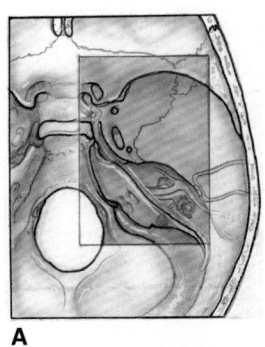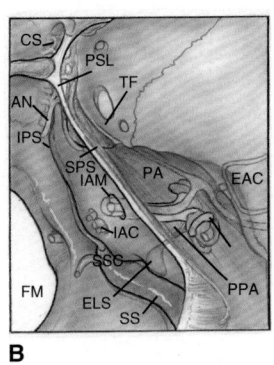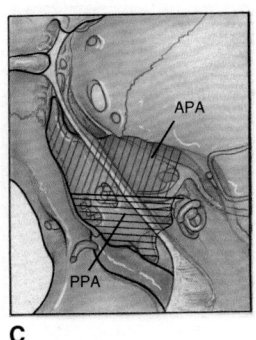

Figure 152.14 A: Superior view of base of skull indicating the position of the petrous apex in the skull base. **B:** The petrous apex with the relative location of the internal auditory canal, structures at the tip of the apex and labyrinth. **C:** Petrous apex divided into the anterior and posterior portions. IAC, internal auditory canal; IAM, internal auditory meatus; EAC, external auditory canal; SS, sigmoid sinus; SPS, superior petrosal sinus; IPS, inferior petrosal sinus; TF, trigeminal fossa; PSL, petrosphenoidal ligament; AN, abducens nerve; CS, cavernous sinus; ELS, endolymphatic sac; FM, foramen magnum; PPA, posterior petrous apex; APA, anterior petrous apex.

infracochlear approach, the transotic approach, the middle fossa approach, and an anterior approach through the glenoid fossa (Fig. 152.15). Other procedures including the transcanal anterior approach (47), endoscope-assisted approach (48), and an image-guided approach through the sphenoid sinus (49) have also been described. Sparing the otic capsule surgically is preferred in patients with serviceable hearing.

Fortunately, most lesions in the petrous apex require drainage rather than en bloc resection. An isolated middle cranial fossa approach can be used when the disease involves the anterior petrous apex but spares the middle ear and mastoid. Unfortunately, this approach does not allow for dependent drainage. In brief, a temporal craniotomy is performed, the temporal lobe of the brain is retracted superiorly, and an extradural dissection is carried out along the middle fossa floor. Key landmarks in this approach are the arcuate eminence, the geniculate ganglion, and the internal auditory canal. Bone anterior to the internal auditory canal and medial to the carotid artery is removed in order to approach the pathology.

The classic infracochlear approach provides direct surgical access to the anterior petrous apex. The ability to perform this approach depends upon aeration of the infracochlear air cell track between the cochlea and great vessels of the skull base (Fig. 152.15B–D). A postauricular incision is made and the ear retracted forward in the usual manner. A wide superiorly based tympanomeatal flap is elevated using canal incisions in the 10-o'clock and 2-o'clock positions. The flap should be relatively long so as to cover the enlarged tympanic ring created by the procedure. A canaloplasty is then performed, lowering both the inferior tympanic ring and the floor of the external auditory canal. The infracochlear air cell tract must be identified. It is initially bordered by the basal turn of the cochlea superiorly, the

ascending segment of the internal carotid artery anteriorly, and the jugular bulb posteroinferiorly (Fig. 152.15B and D). A 1- or 2-mm diamond burr and suction irrigation are used to open the air cells of this tract. Once the biopsy or drainage procedure is complete, a silastic stent can be placed into the pathway to facilitate aeration. The tympanomeatal flap is returned to its anatomic position, and the ear is closed in the usual manner. A high-riding jugular may prohibit the use of this approach.

The transmastoid, infralabyrinthine approach to the petrous apex necessitates a complete mastoidectomy and precise delineation of the facial nerve. The canal wall may be maintained in patients with adequate mastoid development and pneumatization. The infralabyrinthine air cell tract is located inferior to the posterior semicircular canal, superior to the jugular bulb, and medial to the facial nerve (Fig. 152.15B). This tract is opened in an anterior and medial direction. The route passes inferior to the internal auditory canal and through the region of the cochlear aqueduct, which, if opened, must be plugged to prevent a postoperative cerebrospinal fluid (CSF) leak. The lesion in question should be exteriorized or biopsied, and a silastic stent placed. Adequate review of preoperative high-resolution CT scans will determine whether this tract is present and of reasonable caliber for access.

Patients with large lesions and no serviceable preoperative hearing are candidates for the transotic approach. This route provides superior access for complete removal of mass lesions such as cholesteatomas. The procedure begins with a radical mastoidectomy and labyrinthectomy in which semicircular canals and cochlea are removed. Great care is taken to delineate and protect the facial nerve (superior and posterior), petrous carotid (anterior), jugular bulb (inferior), and internal auditory canal. Thinned bone should be preserved over these structures. The surgeon

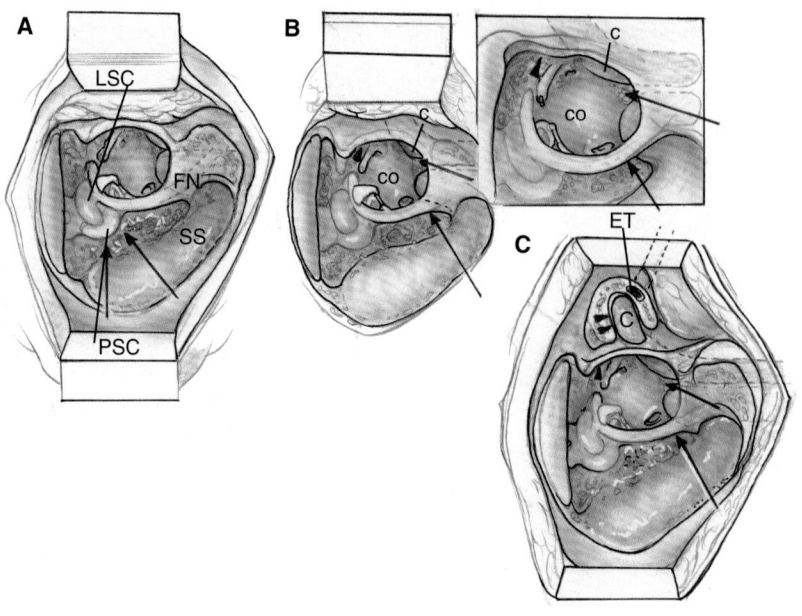

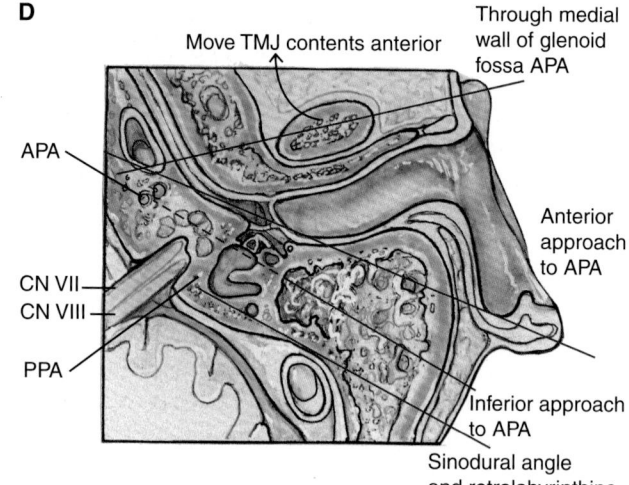

Figure 152.15 A: Access to the posterior apex air cells behind the posterior and superior semicircular canals. FN, facial nerve. **B:** Access to the petrous apex via the infralabyrinthine air cell tract accessible through the ear canal or behind the fallopian canal inferior to the labyrinth. Co, cochlea; C, carotid artery; *Arrowhead*, supracochlear access to APA; *Arrows*, infralabyrinthine access to APA. **C:** Anterior approach to the anterior petrous apex through the glenoid fossa. C, carotid artery; *Arrowhead*, supracochlear access to APA; *Arrows*, infralabyrinthine access to APA; *Double arrowhead*, direct access to APA; ET, eustachian tube. **D:** Axial view of the temporal bone demonstrating the various approaches to the petrous apex. (Adapted from Chole RA. Petrous apicitis: surgical anatomy. *Ann Otol Rhinol Laryngol* 1985;94:251, with permission.)

dissects in an anterior and medial direction. Should a patent cochlear aqueduct be encountered inferior to the basal turn of the cochlea, it must be plugged with bone chips, fascia, or bone wax at the end of the procedure. After removing the mass in question, most surgeons choose to obliterate the cavity with fat, plug the eustachian tube, and close off the external auditory canal.

Gerek et al. (47) describe a transcanal approach for drainage of limited lesions in the anterior petrous apex. Using cadaver dissections, they suggest elevation of a wide, superiorly based tympanomeatal flap followed by a generous anterior and inferior canaloplasty. The vertical segment of the petrous carotid is exposed and traced for 3 to 6 mm. The cortical bone anterior to the cochlea, between it and the internal carotid artery, is then drilled away with diamond burrs. If greater exposure of the anterior apex is required, the complete apicectomy of Ramadier and Lempert may be

performed (46,50,51). In this approach, the glenoid fossa must be exposed and the mandibular condyle can either be removed or displaced anteriorly (Fig. 152.15C and D). This provides access to the medial wall of the glenoid fossa. In the classically described procedure, the anterior external auditory canal wall is removed; however, it can be preserved in most cases. The position of the petrous carotid must be kept in mind as the medial wall of the glenoid fossa is removed using diamond burrs and suction–irrigation. All bone between the carotid artery and the dura of the middle cranial fossa is removed (Fig. 152.15C). Complete exenteration of the anterior petrous apex is impossible without performing a labyrinthectomy, but, in most cases, drainage of infected cells is sufficient to reverse the suppurative process (Fig. 152.15D). Although typically referred to as an "apicectomy," these procedures would be more accurately described by the term "petrousotomy."

ADVANCES IN TEMPORAL BONE SURGERY

Otologic surgery has had a long history of surgical innovation. Currently, many creative surgeons are suggesting further advances in surgical techniques. Robotic surgery may offer more precise control of instruments in the most delicate portions of otologic surgery (52). Technical advances in endoscopes may allow techniques of minimally invasive surgery to the discipline of temporal bone surgery (53,54). Additionally, Labadie et al. (55) have provided proof of concept studies that show that microstereotactic surgery may be applicable to the temporal bone.

COMPLICATIONS AND EMERGENCIES

Facial Nerve Injury

The facial nerve is at risk in its labyrinthine, tympanic, and mastoid segments during otologic surgery (Table 152.3). The nerve not only takes a tortuous, sometimes-anomalous course through the temporal bone, but its canal may also be dehiscent. Heat generated by a diamond burr can injure the nerve without direct mechanical trauma. Constant suction–irrigation helps dissipate thermal energy and prevents this complication. Landmarks such as the antrum, horizontal semicircular canal, short process of the incus, fossa incudis, cochleariform process, oval window, pyramidal process, chorda tympani, and digastric ridge help to locate the nerve. However, such landmarks may be absent or altered during procedures for congenital atresia or cases requiring revision surgery. Intraoperative facial nerve monitoring may be helpful in reducing the risk of iatrogenic trauma.

If the facial nerve is traumatized during surgery, the extent of injury should be assessed both by direct observation and electrical testing. The region of the suspected injury should be examined by decompressing the nerve 3 to 6 mm proximal and distal to the site of injury. It should be exposed in a 180-degree fashion. If facial muscle contraction can be elicited by stimulation with 0.5 mA or less proximal to the injured area, further treatment is unnecessary. Systemic corticosteroids may be helpful in the postoperative period to minimize swelling. If facial movement can be elicited by stimulation of the nerve distally but not proximal to the injury, the extent of nerve disruption determines the next course of action. If only a few fibers are damaged, they may simply be returned to their anatomic position. Significant disruption of the nerve, however, requires direct reanastomosis or cable grafting. When greater than 50% of the facial nerve was disrupted, Green et al. (9) obtained a House-Brackmann Grade III recovery using direct reanastomosis and Grade IV with cable grafting. Direct end-to-end repair may require facial nerve rerouting, which itself may compromise nerve function.

Unexpected facial paralysis noted postoperatively requires prompt attention. Weakness without frank paralysis has a good prognosis and can be treated with a tapering course of steroids. However, complete facial paralysis in patients where the nerve was never formally identified presents a diagnostic dilemma. Local anesthetics administered preoperatively may be responsible for immediate postoperative facial palsy. Therefore, surgical exploration should be deferred for a few hours and the patient reassessed. If complete paralysis persists, early exploration is usually indicated. High-resolution CT scanning may give additional insight into the extent and nature of the injury. The nerve must be clearly identified, and, if traumatized, the surgeon should decompress it or perform the necessary repair.

Hearing Loss

Iatrogenic hearing loss may be conductive or sensorineural. Undetected disruptions of the tympanic membrane or ossicular chain may cause a conductive hearing loss. Sensorineural hearing loss can result from a variety of causes. Acoustic trauma from a high-speed drill (56) or suction squeal may cause hearing loss. Transmission of high-frequency mechanical energy from contact between the drill and the ossicular chain also causes sensorineural hearing loss. If such contact is unavoidable, the surgeon should first disarticulate the incudostapedial joint. Inadvertent entry into the inner ear (semicircular canal, oval or round window, cochlea, etc.) and loss of perilymph/endolymph may result in hearing loss. If faced with cholesteatoma matrix overlying a semicircular canal fistula, most surgeons advise meticulous removal of the matrix and subsequent grafting with bone dust or fascia (57,58). Some recommend leaving the keratinizing epithelial cholesteatoma matrix over the fistula and perform a second operation in 6 to 12 months. At that time, the residual cholesteatoma matrix (now a small pearl) can be removed. This second procedure may be safer because the field is less inflamed and visualization improved.

TABLE 152.3	COMPLICATIONS MASTOID SURGERY

Perioperative complications
  Facial nerve injury
  Sensorineural hearing loss
  Postoperative infection
  Dysgeusia
  Brain herniation
  CSF leakage
  Bleeding
Delayed complications
  Posterior canal breakdown
  Perichondritis
  Blue-domed cyst
  Mucosalization of mastoid bowl
  Stenosis of external canal

Vestibular Injury

Injury to the labyrinth during tympanomastoid surgery can result from direct trauma or from postoperative infection. Ears affected by serous labyrinthitis often recover function over time and may benefit initially from steroid therapy. Suppurative labyrinthitis, however, usually destroys vestibular function. Complete unilateral vestibulopathy usually results in acute vertigo which resolves over the next few days to weeks as central compensation occurs. Some patients are left with mild disequilibrium that improves slowly with vestibular rehabilitation. Chronic disequilibrium may occur in the elderly and in those patients who do not undergo successful central compensation. Some patients may also experience delayed benign positional vertigo, presumably due to the mobilization of otoconia within the labyrinth and migration into the posterior semicircular canal.

Infection

Surgical procedures of the mastoid and petrosa are often necessary because of chronic recurrent and persistent infections. In chronic otitis media (59) and cholesteatoma (60) there is evidence of chronic colonization/infection with bacterial biofilms. These established colonies are highly resistant to host defenses and antibiotics. Hence, procedures are often performed in the presence of bacteria and fungi. In the presence of bacterial colonization, postoperative infection continues to pose a threat to successful outcomes in otologic surgery. Immediate concerns include dehiscence of the postauricular incision, failure of the tympanoplasty grafts, and necrosis of the external auditory canal skin flaps. In extreme cases, the cartilaginous structures of the auricle become infected. Perichondritis requires debridement of necrotic cartilage and administration of parenteral antibiotics. Other potential complications include suppurative labyrinthitis, facial nerve palsy, epidural or subdural abscess, meningitis, sigmoid sinus thrombosis, otitic hydrocephalus, and brain abscess. If an ear is grossly infected preoperatively, antibiotics may be administered based on cultures and sensitivity data. Perioperative antibiotics are generally indicated for tympanomastoid procedures done for chronic otitis although specific evidence is lacking (61). However, the use of preoperative prophylactic antibiotic therapy is not established. In a recent Cochran review by Verschuur et al. (62), they concluded that there was no role for the use of prophylactic antibiotics in clean and clean-contaminated otologic procedures.

Dysgeusia

Dysgeusia resulting from injury to the chorda tympani nerve may be quite distressing to some patients. Symptoms such as a metallic taste in the mouth usually improve with time, but patients must be warned that these taste alterations may persist. This may be of particular concern for those needing a keen sense of taste or flavor in their professions. Traumatized chorda tympani nerves tend to result in more prolonged dysgeusia than cutting the nerve.

Cerebrospinal Fluid Leakage and Encephalocele

The terms meningocele, encephalocele, and meningoencephalocele refer to herniation of meninges, brain matter, or both outside their normal confines. In the course of thinning the tegmen tympani and tegmen mastoideum during tympanomastoid surgery, areas of dura may become exposed. Approaching the dura carefully using diamond burrs rather than cutting burrs helps to prevent complications. Generally minor dural exposures are of little consequence. However, if larger areas of dura are exposed or lacerated, CSF, meninges, and brain tissue may enter into the mastoid cavity. Elderly patients are at particular risk because the dura tends to thin with advancing age. These regions may later herniate into the mastoid or epitympanum leading to delayed complications.

Myeloencephaloceles usually present with CSF otorrhea, CSF rhinorrhea, a persistent clear effusion behind an intact tympanic membrane, hearing loss due to mass effect (fluid and brain matter), or infections such as meningitis and encephalitis. A CSF leak can occur, however, without herniation of meninges or brain matter. High-resolution CT scans with axial and coronal views help define bony defects in the tegmen or posterior fossa plate, and magnetic resonance imaging (MRI), with its excellent soft tissue resolution, distinguishes brain from fluid, cholesteatoma, or cholesterol granuloma. MRI is also useful in evaluating the integrity of the dura. If fluid can be obtained, β_2-transferrin assays may help in confirming the presence of CSF.

Conservative options for managing CSF leaks in the acute phase include bed rest, stool softeners, and placement of a lumbar drain for controlled CSF removal. When such measures fail or if the patient becomes infected, surgical options are necessary. Repairing an encephalocele requires resection of devitalized tissue followed by reconstruction of the defect. If the damage is recognized during the initial procedure, the defect can be repaired at that time. Dura is elevated in a circumferential manner around the defect and a fascia graft placed intracranially between the dura and bone. Other material forms of processed collagen may be suitable as well. If the CSF leak or encephalocele is recognized postoperatively, the precise location and size of the defect dictate the surgical approach. Options include transmastoid, middle fossa, or combination techniques. Small defects may be managed through the mastoidectomy itself; use of fascia with or without bone or cartilage reinforcement may be adequate. For larger defects, a middle fossa craniotomy can be used. An extradural approach is used with temporal lobe elevation. A sheet of temporalis fascia (or other collagen material) is placed between the bone of the mastoid and the dural defect. The window of bone harvested in the craniotomy can then be thinned and inserted between the fascia and the floor of the middle cranial fossa. Use of auricular cartilage is an alternative.

Bleeding/Air Embolism

Most bleeding from the sigmoid sinus or jugular bulb can be controlled easily using gelatin foam, Surgicel pledgets covered by a small cottonoid. Hemostatic matrix preparations have also been used successfully in management of bleeds from the dural sinuses. However, a significant laceration places the patient at risk for secondary complications such as air embolism or thrombosis of the sigmoid sinus. Once the bleeding is controlled, the potential for air embolism must be entertained especially if the head is elevated. An air bubble in the venous system that becomes trapped within the right ventricle can result in cardiopulmonary arrest. The early signs of air embolism include increased end-expiratory carbon dioxide, hypotension, and abnormal cardiac sounds. The surgical field should be flooded with saline immediately and the patient should be placed in the Trendelenburg (head-down) position to minimize further ingress of air into the vascular system. Placement in the left lateral position can help to reposition the air bubble into the right atrium or vena cava. If cardiovascular compromise is still present after these maneuvers, the air must be aspirated from the vena cava using a central venous catheter.

Injury to the carotid artery during tympanomastoid surgery requires immediate hemostasis by direct compression. Once the bleeding is temporarily controlled, emergency angiography should be performed. In most cases, occlusion of the carotid artery within the temporal bone by the interventional radiologist is indicated. Occlusion of the carotid artery puts the patient at significant risk for stroke.

Delayed Complications

Other complications of mastoid surgery include delayed posterior external ear canal wall breakdown, perichondritis, cholesterol granulomas, mucosalization of the mastoid bowl, and external auditory canal stenosis.

HIGHLIGHTS

- Postauricular incisions allow excellent exposure of the mastoid cortex. The inferior portion of the incision must be placed more posteriorly in young children to avoid facial nerve injury.
- The mastoid antrum is located directly medial to Macewen triangle.
- The temporal line provides a topographic landmark for the tegmen and floor of the middle fossa.

- The surgeon must thoroughly saucerize the mastoid cavity during a canal-wall-down mastoidectomy.
- Facial nerve variations and anomalies are common within the temporal bone, especially in patients with congenital ear malformations.
- The posterior musculoperiosteal flap, known as the Palva flap (or more appropriately, the Moser flap), has been successful in obliterating mastoid cavities especially in conjunction with bone pâté.
- Saucerization, removal of the mastoid tip, obliteration techniques, and a large meatoplasty are vital to obtaining a clean, dry ear in canal-wall-down mastoidectomies.
- Disadvantages of intact-canal-wall procedures include an increased risk of occult residual and recurrent disease.
- The endolymphatic sac can be located inferiorly between the posterior semicircular canal and the sigmoid sinus.
- The anterior petrous apex can be opened through the anterior epitympanum, the hypotympanum, and the middle cranial fossa.

REFERENCES

1. Lempert J. Improvement of hearing in cases of otosclerosis: new one-stage surgical technique. *Arch Otolaryngol* 1938;77:570–580.
2. Nager GT, Proctor B. The facial canal: normal anatomy, variations and anomalies. II. Anatomical variations and anomalies involving the facial canal. *Ann Otol Rhinol Laryngol Suppl* 1982;97:45–61.
3. Körner O. *Die eitrigen erkrankungen des Schlafenbeins.* Wiesbaden: Bergmann, 1899.
4. Jackler RK. The surgical anatomy of cholesteatoma. *Otolaryngol Clin North Am* 1989;22(5):883–896.
5. Barbara M, Biagini M, Monini S. The totally implantable middle ear device 'Esteem' for rehabilitation of severe sensorineural hearing loss. *Acta Otolaryngol* 131(4):399–404.
6. Sanna M, Fois P, Pasanisi E, et al. Middle ear and mastoid glomus tumors (glomus tympanicum): an algorithm for the surgical management. *Auris Nasus Larynx* 37(6):661–668.
7. Horn KL, Brackmann DE, Luxford WM, et al. The supratubal recess in cholesteatoma surgery. *Ann Otol Rhinol Laryngol* 1986;95(1 Pt 1):12–15.
8. Litton WB, Krause CJ, Anson BA, et al. The relationship of the facial canal to the annular sulcus. *Laryngoscope* 1969;79(9):1584–1604.
9. Green JD Jr, Shelton C, Brackmann DE. Iatrogenic facial nerve injury during otologic surgery. *Laryngoscope* 1994;104(8 Pt 1):922–926.
10. Ahmed J, Chatrath P, Harcourt J. A bifid intra-tympanic facial nerve in association with a normal stapes. *J Laryngol Otol* 2006;120(5):414–415.
11. Szymanski M, Golabek W, Morshed K. Stapedectomy and variations of the facial nerve. *Ann Univ Mariae Curie Sklodowska Med* 2003;58(2):101–105.
12. Kim MB, Choi J, Lee JK, et al. Hearing outcomes according to the types of mastoidectomy: a comparison between canal wall up and canal wall down mastoidectomy. *Clin Exp Otorhinolaryngol* 2010;3(4):203–206.
13. Cook JA, Krishnan S, Fagan PA. Hearing results following modified radical versus canal-up mastoidectomy. *Ann Otol Rhinol Laryngol* 1996;105(5):379–383.
14. Roden D, Honrubia VF, Wiet R. Outcome of residual cholesteatoma and hearing in mastoid surgery. *J Otolaryngol* 1996;25(3):178–181.

15. Glasscock ME, Miller GW. Intact canal wall tympanoplasty in the management of cholesteatoma. *Laryngoscope* 1976;86(11): 1639–1657.

16. Sade J, Berco E, Brown M. Results of mastoid operations in various chronic ear diseases. *Am J Otol* 1981;3(1):11–20.

17. Charachon R, Gratacap B, Tixier C. Closed versus obliteration technique in cholesteatoma surgery. *Am J Otol* 1988;9(4):286–292.

18. Gristwood RE. Chronic otitis media with epidermoid cholesteatoma. A discussion of some points of controversy concerning surgical management. *Clin Otolaryngol Allied Sci* 1976;1(4):337–342.

19. Cody DT, McDonald TJ. Mastoidectomy for acquired cholesteatoma: follow-up to 20 years. *Laryngoscope* 1984;94(8):1027–1030.

20. Bondy G. Taoallaufmeisselung mit Erhaltung bon Trommelfull und Gehorknochelchen. *Monatsschr Ohrenheilkd* 1910;44:15.

21. Moser HP. A method of filling the excavated mastoid with a flap from the back of the auricle. *Laryngoscope* 1911;21:1158–1163.

22. Hung T, Leung N, van Hasselt CA, et al. Long-term outcome of the Hong Kong vascularized, pedicled temporalis fascia flap in reconstruction of mastoid cavity. *Laryngoscope* 2007;117(8):1403–1407.

23. Palva T. Reconstruction of ear canal and middle ear in chronic otitis. *Acta Otolaryngol* 1964;188(Suppl):228–233.

24. Palva T, Makinen J. The meatally based musculoperiosteal flap in cavity obliteration. *Arch Otolaryngol* 1979;105(7):377–380.

25. Palva T. Mastoid obliteration. *Acta Otolaryngol Suppl* 1979;360: 152–154.

26. Ojala K, Sorri M, Sipila P, et al. Correlation of postoperative ear canal volumes with obliteration material and with volume of operation cavity. *Arch Otorhinolaryngol* 1982;234(1):37–43.

27. Gantz BJ, Wilkinson EP, Hansen MR. Canal wall reconstruction tympanomastoidectomy with mastoid obliteration. *Laryngoscope* 2005;115(10):1734–1740.

28. Minoda R, Hayashida M, Masuda M, et al. Preliminary experience with beta-tricalcium phosphate for use in mastoid cavity obliteration after mastoidectomy. *Otol Neurotol* 2007;28(8):1018–1021.

29. Clark MP, Bottrill I. SerenoCem-glass ionomeric granules: a 3-year follow-up assessment of their effectiveness in mastoid obliteration. *Clin Otolaryngol* 2007;32(4):287–290.

30. Ridenour JS, Poe DS, Roberson DW. Complications with hydroxyapatite cement in mastoid cavity obliteration. *Otolaryngol Head Neck Surg* 2008;139(5):641–645.

31. Friedman CD, Wiet RJ. Meatoplasty in chronic ear disease when using an open technique. *Laryngoscope* 1987;97(1):110–111.

32. McKennan KX. Endoscopic 'second look' mastoidoscopy to rule out residual epitympanic/mastoid cholesteatoma. *Laryngoscope* 1993;103(7):810–814.

33. Rosenberg SI, Silverstein H, Hoffer M, et al. Use of endoscopes for chronic ear surgery in children. *Arch Otolaryngol Head Neck Surg* 1995;121(8):870–872.

34. Guild SR. The circulation of endolymph. *Am J Anat* 1927;39:57–81.

35. Portmann G. Vertigo: surgical treatment by opening the saccus endolymphaticus. *Arch Otolaryngol* 1927;6:309–319.

36. Hallpike CS, Cairns H. Observations on the pathology of Meniere's syndrome: (Section of Otology). *Proc R Soc Med* 1938;31(11):1317–1336.

37. Durland WF Jr, Pyle GM, Connor NP. Endolymphatic sac decompression as a treatment for Meniere's disease. *Laryngoscope* 2005;115(8):1454–1457.

38. Thomsen J, Bretlau P, Tos M, et al. Placebo effect in surgery for Meniere's disease. A double-blind, placebo-controlled study on endolymphatic sac shunt surgery. *Arch Otolaryngol* 1981;107(5): 271–277.

39. Shea DA, Chole RA, Paparella MM. The endolymphatic sac: anatomical considerations. *Laryngoscope* 1979;89(1):88–94.

40. Parnes LS, McClure JA. Posterior semicircular canal occlusion for intractable benign paroxysmal positional vertigo. *Ann Otol Rhinol Laryngol* 1990;99(5 Pt 1):330–334.

41. Minor LB, Solomon D, Zinreich JS, et al. Sound- and/or pressure-induced vertigo due to bone dehiscence of the superior semicircular canal. *Arch Otolaryngol Head Neck Surg* 1998;124(3):249–258.

42. Minor LB. Clinical manifestations of superior semicircular canal dehiscence. *Laryngoscope* 2005;115(10):1717–1727.

43. Agrawal SK, Parnes LS. Transmastoid superior semicircular canal occlusion. *Otol Neurotol* 2008;29(3):363–367.

44. Gradenigo G. Ueber die Paralyse de Nercus Abducens bei Otitis. *Arch Ohrenheilkunde Rhinolaryngol* 1907;74:149–158.

45. Chole RA, Donald PJ. Petrous apicitis. Clinical considerations. *Ann Otol Rhinol Laryngol* 1983;92(6 Pt 1):544–551.

46. Chole RA. Petrous apicitis: surgical anatomy. *Ann Otol Rhinol Laryngol* 1985;94(3):251–257.

47. Gerek M, Satar B, Yazar F, et al. Transcanal anterior approach for cystic lesions of the petrous apex. *Otol Neurotol* 2004;25(6): 973–976.

48. Mattox DE. Endoscopy-assisted surgery of the petrous apex. *Otolaryngol Head Neck Surg* 2004;130(2):229–241.

49. DiNardo LJ, Pippin GW, Sismanis A. Image-guided endoscopic transsphenoidal drainage of select petrous apex cholesterol granulomas. *Otol Neurotol* 2003;24(6):939–941.

50. Lempert J. Complete apicectomy: a preliminary report of a new technic. *New York State J Med* 1936;36:1210–1218.

51. Ramadier J. Exploration de la pointe du rocher par la coie du canal carotidien. *Ann Otol Rhinol Laryngol* 1933;4:422–444.

52. Danilchenko A, Balachandran R, Toennies JL, et al. Robotic mastoidectomy. *Otol Neurotol* 2011;32(1):11–16.

53. McKennan KX. Endoscopic transcutaneous mastoidoscopy for evaluation of residual epitympanic/mastoid cholesteatoma. *Am J Otol* 1993;14(4):369–372.

54. Marchioni D, Villari D, Alicandri-Ciufelli M, et al. Endoscopic open technique in patients with middle ear cholesteatoma. *Eur Arch Otorhinolaryngol* 2011;268(11):1557–1563.

55. Labadie RF, Balachandran R, Mitchell JE, et al. Clinical validation study of percutaneous cochlear access using patient-customized microstereotactic frames. *Otol Neurotol* 2010;31(1):94–99.

56. Karatas E, Miman MC, Ozturan O, et al. Contralateral normal ear after mastoid surgery: evaluation by otoacoustic emissions (mastoid drilling and hearing loss). *ORL J Otorhinolaryngol Relat Spec* 2007;69(1):18–24.

57. Ueda Y, Kurita T, Matsuda Y, et al. Surgical treatment of labyrinthine fistula in patients with cholesteatoma. *J Laryngol Otol Suppl* 2009;123(Suppl 31):64–67.

58. Stephenson MF, Saliba I. Prognostic indicators of hearing after complete resection of cholesteatoma causing a labyrinthine fistula. *Eur Arch Otorhinolaryngol* 2011;268(12):1705–1711.

59. Hall-Stoodley L, Hu FZ, Gieseke A, et al. Direct detection of bacterial biofilms on the middle-ear mucosa of children with chronic otitis media. *JAMA* 2006;296(2):202–211.

60. Chole RA, Faddis BT. Evidence for microbial biofilms in cholesteatomas. *Arch Otolaryngol Head Neck Surg* 2002;128(10):1129–1133.

61. Haynes DS. Perioperative antibiotics in chronic suppurative otitis media. *Ear Nose Throat J* 2002;81(8 Suppl 1):13–15.

62. Verschuur HP, de Wever WW, van Benthem PP. Antibiotic prophylaxis in clean and clean-contaminated ear surgery. *Cochrane Database Syst Rev* 2004;(3):CD003996.

Reconstruction of the Tympanic Membrane and Ossicular Chain

153

John L. Dornhoffer *Michael B. Gluth*

Seeking knowledge and expertise in the art of tympanoplasty and ossiculoplasty can be a difficult task, in part due to the overwhelming number of techniques that have been described, but also because of the plethora of dogma and surgical tradition that circulates throughout the otologic surgery community. In the following chapter, the authors seek not to champion a particular set of techniques, but to provide a broad overview of this topic with a focus on fundamental principles that apply globally. This information is delivered under the assertion that it is wise for otologists to acquire a working mastery of several techniques that may be applied in a customized manner based on pathology and conditions at hand.

DEFINITION OF TERMS

Canalplasty refers to surgical modification of the bony external auditory canal. This is often used as an adjuvant procedure in tympanoplasty to improve surgical access.

Meatoplasty refers to surgical modification of the cartilaginous external auditory canal and external auditory meatus. This is often used as an adjuvant procedure in tympanoplasty to provide improved postoperative access or to attain consistent lateral-to-medial ear canal size matching following canalplasty.

Myringoplasty refers to surgical repair of the tympanic membrane that involves work confined to the drumhead only.

Ossiculoplasty refers to surgical modification of the ossicular chain, including reconstruction and mobilization.

Tympanoplasty refers to surgical repair of the tympanic membrane in combination with work within the tympanic cleft, such as ossiculoplasty, middle ear exploration, or lysis of tympanic adhesions. Traditionally, elevation of the annulus within a tympanomeatal flap has served as a practical boundary that differentiates tympanoplasty from myringoplasty.

TYPES OF TYMPANOPLASTY AND OSSICULAR RECONSTRUCTION

Tympanoplasty techniques were classically outlined by Zollner (1) and Wullstein (2). Subsequent modifications of Wullstein's classification have been based on the underlying properties of acoustic mechanics associated with each tympanoplasty type as opposed to classification based on underlying tympanic and ossicular pathology. Understanding this classification system is helpful not only for purposes of grasping a global and historical view of tympanic membrane and ossicular chain reconstruction, but also for understanding basic principles of middle ear acoustic mechanics.

Type I Tympanoplasty

This procedure involves repair of the tympanic membrane in the setting of an intact native ossicular chain. At most, manipulation of the ossicular chain is limited to interventions aimed at improving mobility, such as lysis of tympanic adhesions or removal of tympanosclerotic foci.

Type II Tympanoplasty

This procedure involves repair of the tympanic membrane in combination with any type of ossiculoplasty procedure that preserves the integrity of the malleoincudal lever mechanism. The most common example of this is repair of a dysfunctional (eroded) incudostapedial articulation. Tympanoplasty with delayed staged ossiculoplasty consisting of an incus-grip stapedotomy could also be considered a subgroup within this category. It is perhaps worth noting that these modern depictions of type II tympanoplasty differ somewhat from the classic description that was devised to deal with the uncommon scenario of isolated malleus erosion, wherein tympanic membrane grafting is applied directly upon the intact long process of the incus.

Type III Tympanoplasty

This procedure involves repair of the tympanic membrane in combination with any type of ossiculoplasty procedure that does not preserve the integrity of the malleoincudal lever mechanism. Type III tympanoplasty includes the vast majority of techniques described for routine ossicular chain reconstruction. Accordingly, type III tympanoplasty classification has been further subdivided according to ossiculoplasty technique.

Stapes Columella Subtype

This type III tympanoplasty involves placement of a tympanic membrane graft directly onto the superstructure of the stapes *without* the use of a prosthesis or any other substantial interpositional material.

Minor Columella Subtype

This involves the use of an interpositional graft or prosthesis to establish continuity between the tympanic membrane and the superstructure of the stapes. Examples of this include the use of a synthetic partial ossicular replacement prosthesis (PORP) or sculpted ossicular (incus or malleus head) autograft. Interpositional ossiculoplasty techniques that employ a lateral contact point with the malleus manubrium also fall within this subtype.

Major Columella Subtype

This procedure is exactly the same as the minor columella subtype except that the stapes superstructure is absent; thus, with a major columella subtype the interpositional graft or prosthesis is set upon the stapes footplate. An example of this is use of a synthetic total ossicular replacement prosthesis (TORP). Tympanoplasty with delayed staged ossiculoplasty that consists of a malleus-grip stapedotomy could also be considered to fall within this subtype.

Type IV Tympanoplasty

This procedure involves repair of the tympanic membrane in such a manner that the boundary between the mucosalized middle ear space and the epithelialized lateral compartment (external auditory canal, open mastoid cavity, epitympanum) is shifted in a way that renders the stapes footplate externalized as part of the latter. As a result, the tympanic cavity is divided into a smaller-than-normal aerated space in continuity with the eustachian tube, termed the cavum minor, in which the round window is acoustically shielded, and an external component in which the mobile stapes footplate is covered by a thin epithelial layer and is directly exposed to incoming sound energy.

Type V Tympanoplasty

This procedure is the same as the type IV tympanoplasty, except that it also includes the need to address an underlying immobile stapes footplate and, therefore, is generally performed in a staged manner once active infectious disease is controlled. Historically, fenestration of the lateral semicircular canal was described as part of this procedure to counteract stapes fixation; however, total footplate removal and a soft tissue seal have generally replaced fenestration.

PHYSIOLOGY: MECHANISMS OF GAIN

The modern view of middle ear acoustic science involves two basic pathways by which sound is able to stimulate the inner ear (3,4). The first involves transmission of sound pressure through the tympanic membrane and ossicular chain via the oval window. This is known as *ossicular coupling*. This mechanism is the primary means by which the state of impedance mismatch that exists between the air in the ear canal (low impedance) and the fluid within the cochlea (high impedance) is overcome. In such a state, sound pressure is deflected during passage through the air–fluid interface, resulting in a loss of gain in the realm of 30 dB. The coupling effect of the tympanic membrane and ossicles almost overcomes this loss.

Ossicular coupling has been attributed to the collective effect of three characteristics of the tympano-ossicular mechanism traditionally known as the *acoustic transformer theory* (5). The first and most significant of these characteristics is the *hydraulic lever effect* that results from the difference between the surface area of the tympanic membrane relative to that of the oval window (usually a ratio of nearly 21:1). This effect results in compression of sound energy and increase in force at the oval window, equating to a theoretic approximate increase in gain of 26 dB. The second characteristic is the *malleoincudal lever effect* that results from the difference in length between the malleus manubrium relative to that of the long process of the incus along the axis of ossicular rotation (a ratio of 1.3:1). However, this effect only accounts for an additional 2 dB theoretical increase in gain. The final factor is the so-called *catenary lever effect* that is generated by the elastic stretching of the tympanic membrane from the annulus to the malleus manubrium—somewhat akin to the stretched strings across a tennis racquet. The specific degree of acoustic benefit derived from the catenary effect is not well understood but probably lies within a range similar to that of the malleoincudal lever.

It is important to recognize that, in reality, ossicular coupling is a much more complex phenomenon than what is suggested by these simplified traditional models as they do not account for factors such as variation in efficiency with changes in frequency or inefficiencies in sound transmission through the tympanic membrane and ossicular chain attributed to the inherent tension or laxity of the ossicular ligaments. Thus, it is perhaps not surprising that the 25 to 30 dB of gain that is predicted by the acoustic transformer theory does not equate well with experimental measurements, which suggest an actual more modest increase in the realm of just over 20 dB (6–8).

The second pathway of sound stimulation of the inner ear involves direct passage of sound pressure via the oval and round windows without involvement of the tympanic membrane or ossicular chain. This is known as *acoustic coupling* (4). Given an intact tympanic membrane and functional ossicular chain, this pathway is of only minor importance. However, in the various conditions of a diseased ear, acoustic coupling can be important. This is why, for example, a conductive hearing loss will be greater in the case of ossicular discontinuity and an intact tympanic membrane (60 dB) compared with ossicular discontinuity and an absent tympanic membrane (40 to 50 dB). With the former, the intact tympanic membrane restricts the acoustic coupling pathway by blocking direct access of sound pressure to the oval and round window membranes.

A final relevant consideration in middle ear acoustic mechanics is that of *phase*. A sound stimulus to the inner ear is detected as the net difference in sound pressures applied to the round and oval windows that results in movement of intracochlear fluids. If these sound pressures are simultaneously applied to the round and oval windows with equal amplitude and phase, they will counteract each other and no resultant intracochlear fluid displacement will occur. In the normal situation, this does not occur due to the unbalanced selective effect of ossicular coupling upon the oval window, the acoustic shielding effect of the tympanic membrane upon the round window, and the uneven anatomical positioning of the round window versus the oval widow relative to incoming sound. However, when the tympano-ossicular mechanism is absent and acoustic coupling is primarily relied upon (as in the case of a type IV or V tympanoplasty), an unshielded round window can yield significant negative acoustic consequences due to phase cancellation (4).

A simplified chart depicting the theoretic ideal acoustic effects of various tympano-ossicular scenarios is shown in Table 153.1.

PREOPERATIVE EVALUATION

When a patient is considered for tympanoplasty or ossiculoplasty, a thorough history, examination, and audiometric evaluation should be performed on both ears. Otoscopy and pneumatic insufflation under the binocular microscope, following careful removal of debris, provide a wealth of information. The results of the audiogram should always be correlated with the physical exam, including Weber and Rinne tuning fork tests, especially when a masking dilemma is present. If the audiogram and tuning fork exam do not agree, surgery should not be performed until this is reconciled.

A preoperative audiogram can be helpful in suggesting underlying pathology. Generally, a perforation will cause a conductive hearing loss between 5 and 40 dB depending on its characteristics (9). Controversy exists as to whether or not the location of a perforation impacts the degree of hearing loss, yet perforation size and underlying middle ear volume do matter (an ear with a smaller volume tends to have worse hearing than one with a larger volume, even given identical perforations).

When the tympanic membrane is intact, a conductive hearing loss greater than 35 to 40 dB strongly suggests the possibility of ossicular chain dysfunction. Furthermore, the pattern of hearing loss may be typical of particular scenarios; for example, ossicular fixation generally causes a low-tone conductive hearing loss, the degree of which is related to the extent and location of the fixation. With malleus head fixation, the low-tone air–bone gap generally closes at the higher frequencies, whereas stapes fixation tends to affect the middle and high frequencies to a relatively greater degree (10).

The status of the eustachian tube will impact surgical outcomes, yet there is no consensus on the optimal way to reliably assess its function (11). Auto-inflation using the Valsalva or Toyenbee maneuver is helpful, albeit a nonphysiologic test of tubal patency. The clinical status of the contralateral ear likewise can provide insight into tubal maturity and function in the diseased ear (12). As part of the eustachian tube evaluation, the nose should be examined so that allergy, adenoiditis, and rhinosinusitis can be treated in an effort to promote optimized tubal function (13). Furthermore, aggressive medical treatment of infection involving the ear itself should be undertaken prior to surgery, including aural toilet and ototopical agent application. When an ear will not dry with medical therapy, culture acquisition may be useful in helping to identify antimicrobial-resistant pathogens.

Once patient assessment is complete, a few general rules should be applied to surgical candidacy. First, one should avoid elective surgery on an only-hearing ear as much as is reasonably possible. Exceptions to this would be situations where surgery is primarily confined to the tympanic membrane, and drilling or significant ossicular manipulation is unlikely, or when a perforation is contributing to difficulty with hearing aid usage. Also, cases that involve disease processes that impart risk of hearing loss, such as cholesteatoma, will generally warrant intervention. Second, when bilateral disease is present, surgery should be undertaken on the worse-hearing ear in the absence of any other compelling reason to do otherwise on account of underlying disease. Finally, special consideration should be given to the timing of surgery in the pediatric patient.

Age as a prognostic factor in tympanoplasty is controversial, with contradicting reports present in the literature (14,15). The authors' approach to pediatric patients is to avoid repairing the tympanic membrane during the otitis-prone years (≤3 years). If the contralateral ear is normal, routine tympanoplasty is considered at age 4 for an ear that is dry or only occasionally drains with water

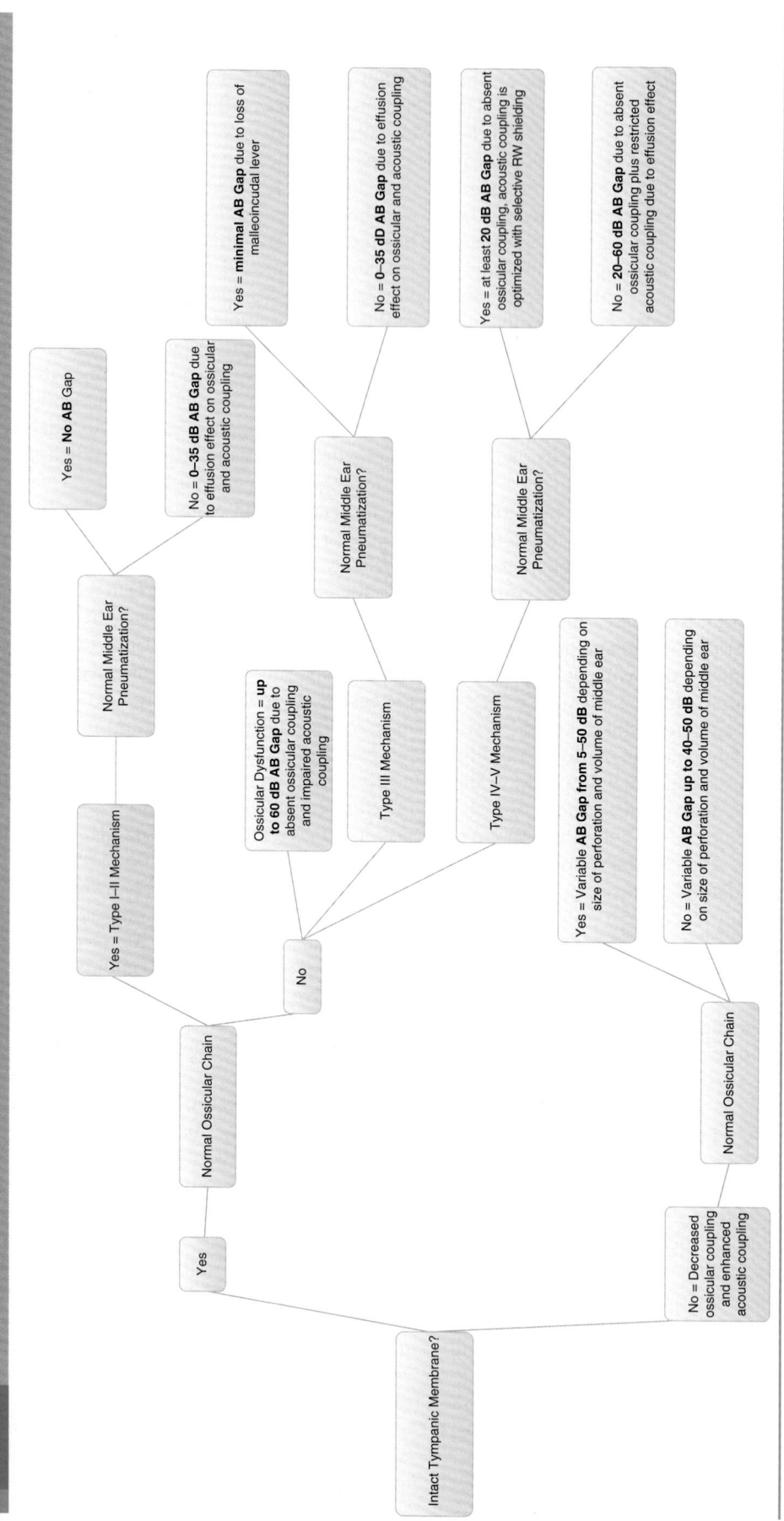

THEORETIC IDEAL ACOUSTIC EFFECTS OF VARIOUS TYMPANO-OSSICULAR SCENARIOS

Intact Tympanic Membrane?

- Yes → Normal Ossicular Chain
  - Yes = Type I–II Mechanism → Normal Middle Ear Pneumatization?
    - Yes = **No AB** Gap
    - No = **0–35 dB AB Gap** due to effusion effect on ossicular and acoustic coupling
  - No → Ossicular Dysfunction = **up to 60 dB AB Gap** due to absent ossicular coupling and impaired acoustic coupling
    - Type III Mechanism → Normal Middle Ear Pneumatization?
      - Yes = **minimal AB Gap** due to loss of malleoincudal lever
      - No = **0–35 dD AB Gap** due to effusion effect on ossicular and acoustic coupling
    - Type IV–V Mechanism → Normal Middle Ear Pneumatization?
      - Yes = at least **20 dB AB Gap** due to absent ossicular coupling, acoustic coupling is optimized with selective RW shielding
      - No = **20–60 dB AB Gap** due to absent ossicular coupling plus restricted acoustic coupling due to effusion effect

- No = Decreased ossicular coupling and enhanced acoustic coupling → Normal Ossicular Chain
  - Yes = Variable **AB Gap from 5–50 dB** depending on size of perforation and volume of middle ear
  - No = Variable **AB Gap up to 40–50 dB** depending on size of perforation and volume of middle ear

contamination (16). However, if the contralateral ear is abnormal at this time, adenoidectomy is considered and tympanoplasty is deferred until the contralateral ear reaches stable quiescence or the patient reaches age 7. If contralateral disease is still present at this time, a more aggressive technique, such as cartilage tympanoplasty, is performed on the worse-hearing ear. The second ear is repaired several months later, but only after the first ear is documented to have a stable satisfactory outcome and is not expected to require further surgery.

TYMPANOPLASTY

General Principles

Modern tympanoplasty techniques all have common ground in that they endeavor to reconstruct the deficient middle fibrous layer of a tympanic membrane perforation with graft materials that then act as a scaffold for lateral epithelial growth. Although simplified myringoplasty techniques that utilize non-grafted temporary scaffold materials, such as a thin paper patch, can be used for small perforations, they are relatively limited in application and simple to learn. Thus, patch myringoplasty techniques are not a focus of this discussion.

The common goals of tympanic membrane repair are to

- Create a barrier between the dry lateral epithelialized compartment (drumhead, external auditory canal, open mastoid cavity) and the moist medial mucosalized compartment (middle ear, eustachian tube)
- Provide reinforcement to correct tympanic membrane weaknesses in order to resist future disease processes (atelectasis, perforation)
- Create an optimized sound-conducting platform for ossicular coupling or a round window shield for acoustic coupling depending on tympanoplasty type
- Create a contour favorable for outward keratin debris migration

Applied Tympanic Membrane Mechanics

The tympanic membrane is the major element of the middle ear transformer mechanism and acts as a barrier between the sound pressure of the ear canal and middle ear. Its motion, which has been studied with laser vibrometry and stroboscopic holography, is both complex and variable depending on the frequency of stimulation (17,18). At frequencies up to 1,000 Hz, the tympanic membrane tends to vibrate in one consolidated phase, but as frequency rises further, its vibration splits into a state of phase subdivision, with overall diminished efficiency.

While it is intellectually satisfying to assert that reconstruction of the tympanic membrane must endeavor to exactly recreate these native vibratory patterns, in truth it is unknown if this is possible or even necessary. Numerous tympanic membrane graft materials have been used that are quite dissimilar to the native drumhead in rigidity and thickness, yet excellent acoustic outcomes have been attained. For example, reconstruction with large cartilage grafts has been reported to result in hearing outcomes equal to those with more pliable temporalis fascia (15,19–21), including occurrences of *complete* air–bone gap closure in the speech frequencies. Further complicating the situation is uncertainty regarding the interplay between an aphysiologic reconstructed tympanic membrane and the underlying aphysiologic reconstructed ossicular chain in collectively providing acoustic gain (22). Gaps between observed clinical outcomes and predicted tympanoplasty outcomes based on tympanic membrane acoustic models highlight the fact that there is still much to be learned.

Surgical Exposure

The importance of assuring proper visualization and exposure in order to surgically manipulate the tympanic membrane and middle ear may seem obvious, but if taken for granted, surgical results can be compromised. Line-of-sight visualization in itself does not always signify adequate exposure. The surgeon must assure that instruments are allowed to enter the microscopic field at a sufficiently open lateral angle so as not to impede binocular vision or require awkward manipulation. Although minimally invasive approaches can be desirable, these should only be utilized if they provide equally sufficient access and exposure to the surgical target. The morbidity associated with even the widest tympanoplasty access route (postauricular with canalplasty) is generally not high. Table 153.2 provides a suggested guide for choosing appropriate access for tympanic membrane repair. One noteworthy consideration is that when a perforation involves the anterior drumhead, wide exposure via a postauricular incision and, when needed, a canalplasty may be helpful.

Canal Incisions

Numerous sites for canal incisions have been described to raise a tympanomeatal flap, and generally these are chosen according to the anticipated surgical plan. Many surgeons have traditionally insisted upon preservation of the posterior–superior "vascular strip" of canal skin or avoidance of transecting the tympanic annulus. However, many of these dictums seem to be routinely ignored by accomplished otologists with little if any apparent negative consequence. In reality, quality surgical execution and careful atraumatic handling of canal skin are probably the key factors to a successful outcome regardless of how this is done (see Fig. 153.1).

Preparing the Drumhead

Prior to graft placement, the tympanic membrane should be prepared to maximize the chances of graft take and rapid epithelialization. This typically involves

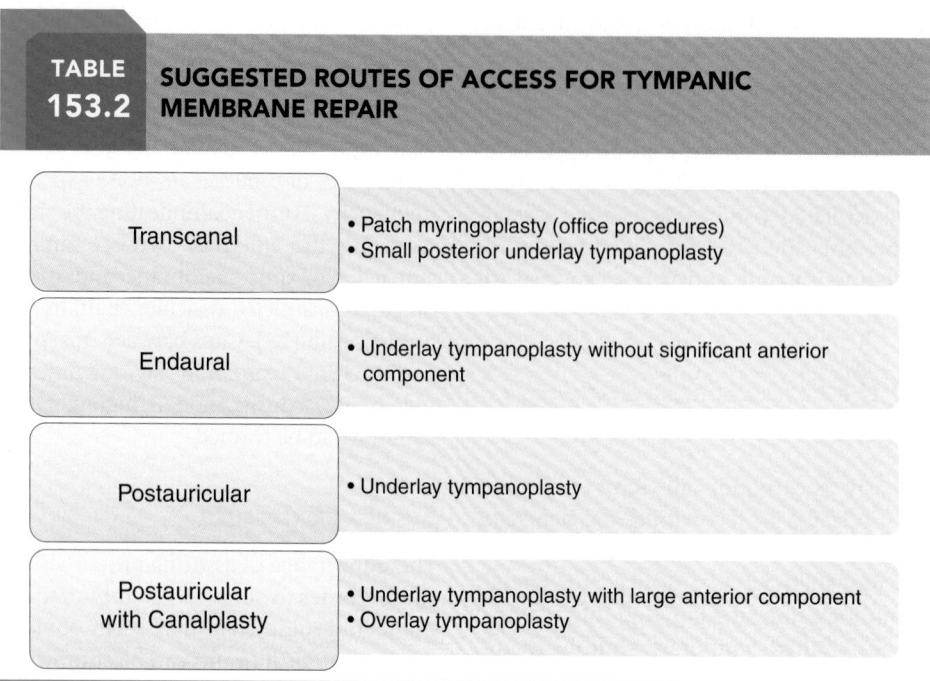

TABLE 153.2	SUGGESTED ROUTES OF ACCESS FOR TYMPANIC MEMBRANE REPAIR
Transcanal	• Patch myringoplasty (office procedures) • Small posterior underlay tympanoplasty
Endaural	• Underlay tympanoplasty without significant anterior component
Postauricular	• Underlay tympanoplasty
Postauricular with Canalplasty	• Underlay tympanoplasty with large anterior component • Overlay tympanoplasty

freshening the margins of the perforation with cold knife rim resection or laser application in order to encourage sprouting of new microvasculature. As a general rule, it is better to be aggressive in completely removing unhealthy portions of the tympanic membrane than to attempt incorporation of them into the reconstruction process. This includes myringitis (particularly important), tympanosclerotic plaque, scar, and old graft material. Pathologic adhesions between the drumhead and middle ear should also be released.

Choosing, Preparing, and Shaping the Graft

The most commonly used tympanic membrane grafting material is temporalis fascia, which is desired for its pliability. This is harvested, via either an endaural or post-auricular incision, as the glistening whitish layer of fascia immediately overlying the temporalis muscle fibers. After harvest, this is generally pressed thin and set aside for drying, which may promote ease of trimming and placement. Readily available alternatives to temporalis fascia that are also thin and pliable include pressed perichondrium, periosteum, and muscle. Cadaveric acellular dermal matrix (AlloDerm, LifeCell Corp, Branchburg, NJ) (23) has also been used with success and may be particularly useful for simple in-office tympanoplasty procedures where harvest of a tissue graft is not desired.

Auricular cartilage grafts are very useful in tympanoplasty (24,25) and may be harvested from various sites, but are typically harvested from the tragus and the cymba with the overlying perichondrium intact. These can be applied with or without perichondrium or the concurrent use of fascia; however, the authors' bias is to apply cartilage grafts

that have been stripped of perichondrium on the medial surface but have adherent perichondrium or overlying fascia on the lateral surface (26). In the authors' experience, such grafts tend to be much more resistant to involvement with postoperative middle ear adhesions than either fascia or perichondrium.

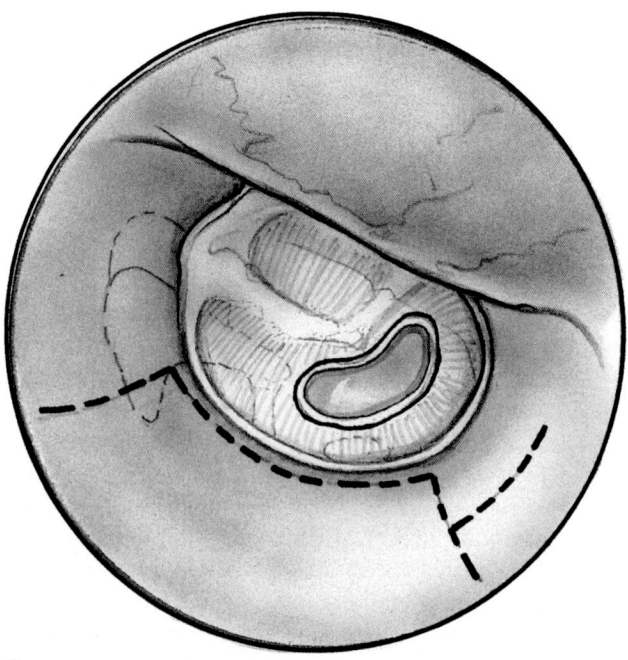

A

Figure 153.1 Canal incisions. **A:** The classic vascular strip incision involves preservation of the posterior canal skin to within a few millimeters of the annulus.

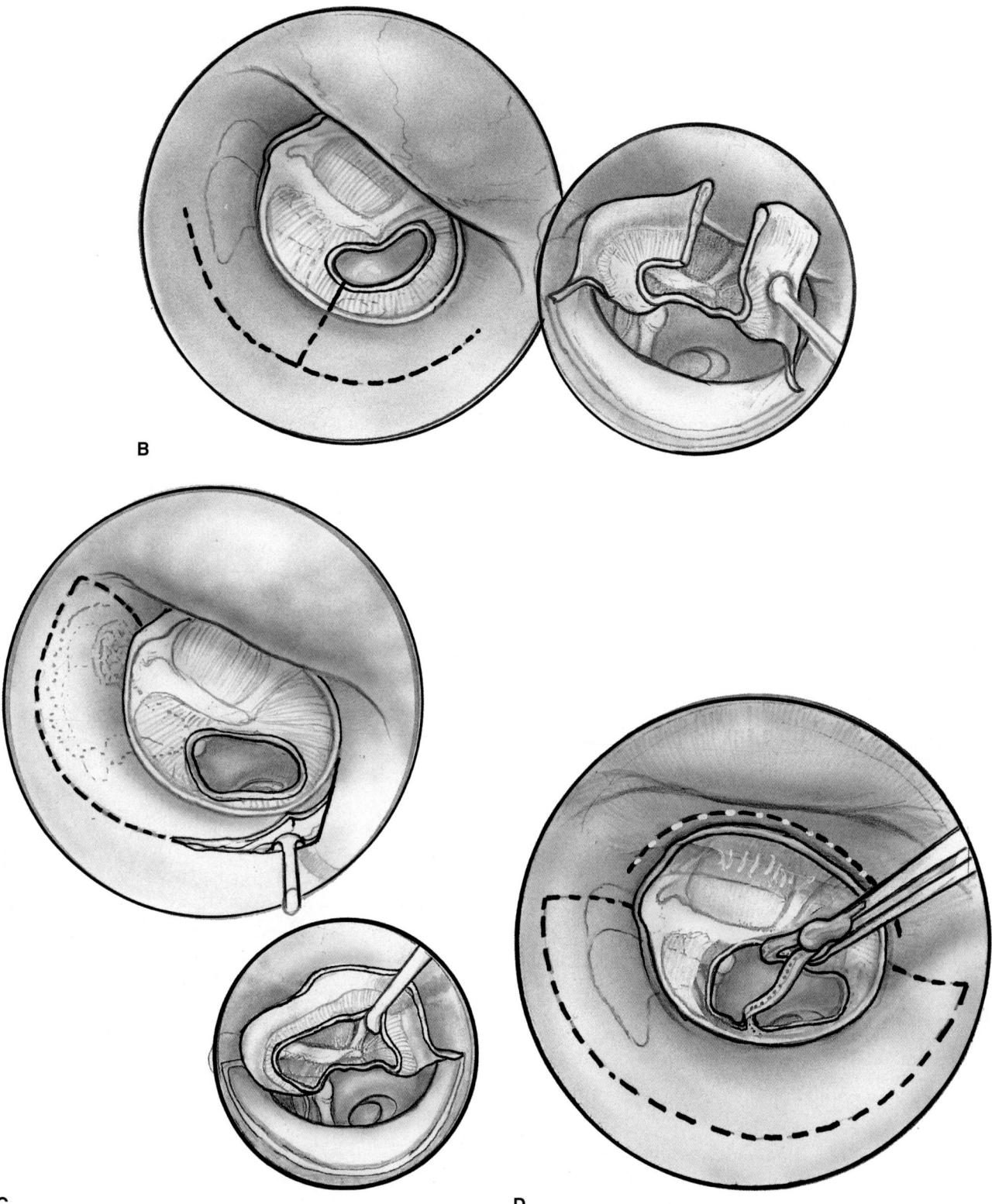

Figure 153.1 (*Continued*) **B:** A "book page" flap provides particularly good access for graft placement by dividing the annulus with an incision through the canal skin and tympanic membrane into the perforation. **C:** A "ship sail" flap is larger at the superior aspect and is particularly useful when wide curettage of scutum bone results in the need for extra tympanomeatal flap length for coverage. **D:** Modified canal incisions for underlay tympanoplasty can incorporate both a standard tympanomeatal flap as well as a separate anterior canal incision to elevate the annulus and anchor the graft. (*Continued on next page*)

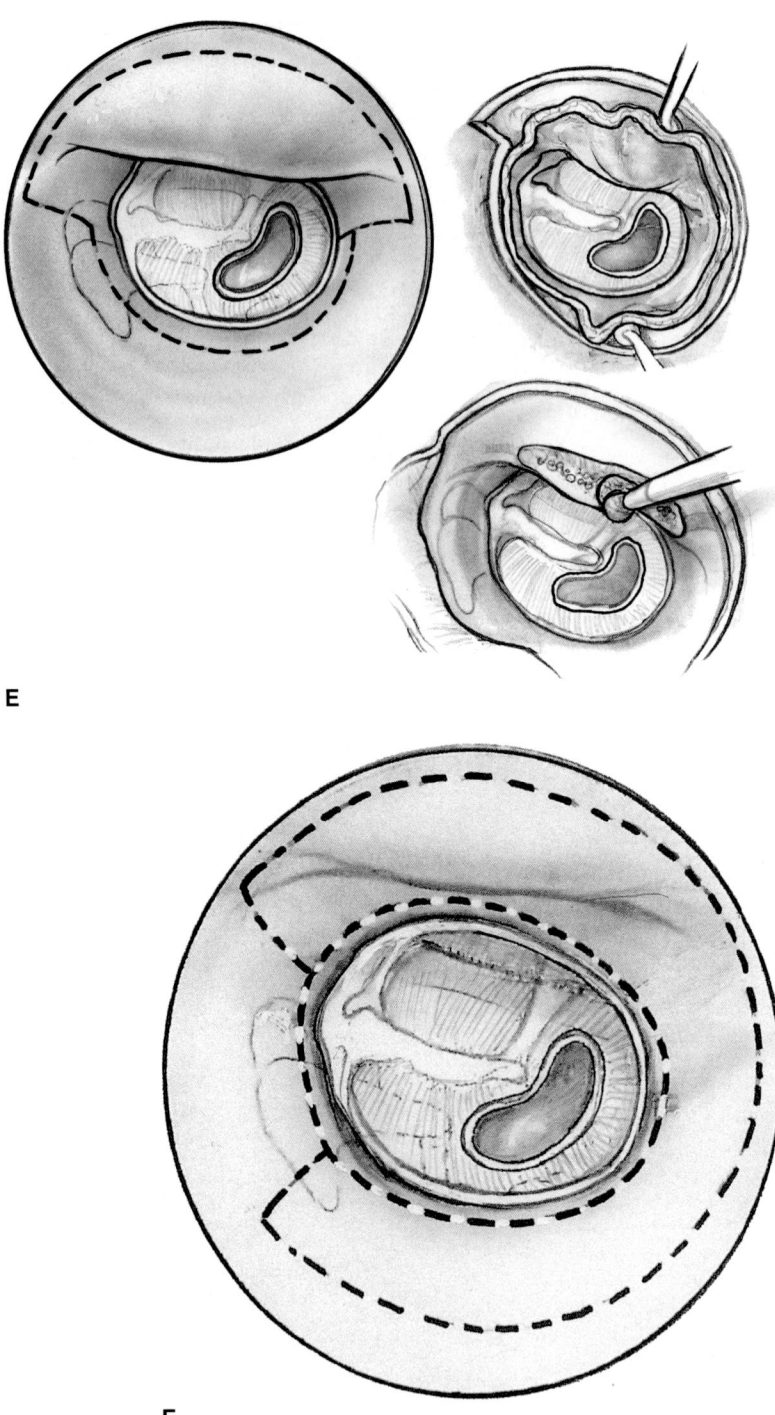

Figure 153.1 (*Continued*) **E:** Overlay tympanoplasty requires incisions that afford removal of the anterior canal wall skin to allow access for canalplasty. **F:** Overlay tympanoplasty incisions can be modified to allow wider removal of canal skin if desired.

When the use of a composite perichondrium–cartilage island graft is desired, perichondrium is usually stripped off of one side, and the remaining cartilage is cut to the desired shape as an "island" upon the preserved opposite side (see Fig. 153.2). If used for repair of a large perforation, a composite island graft is shaped into a thin circular disk 8 to 9 mm in diameter, with a notch cut to cradle the malleus manubrium and tails of perichondrium on the periphery that can be anchored on the external auditory canal wall under the annulus. For optimized acoustics,

a cartilage graft thickness of 0.7 mm or less is preferable; however, if shaved too thin, undesirable curling of the graft may occur.

The choice of graft material is made based on the complexity of the reconstruction and the activity of any underlying chronic ear disease. In higher risk situations, cartilage tympanoplasty techniques may provide more durable results (27,28). A high-risk perforation might be considered one that is larger than 50%, an anterior perforation, a perforation draining at the time of surgery, a recurrent

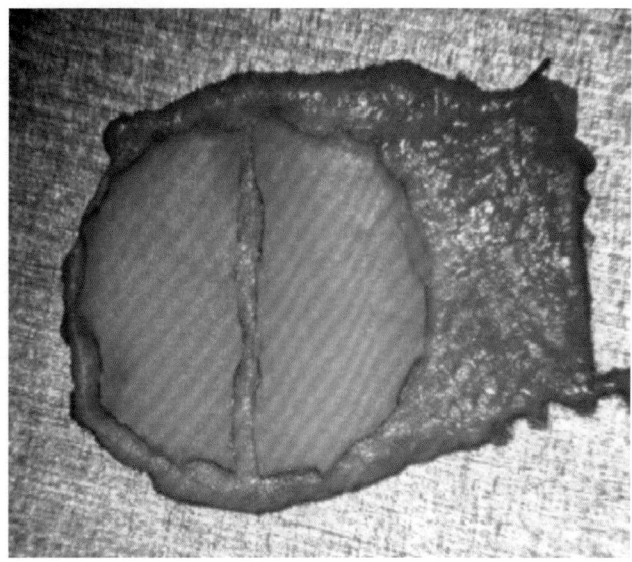

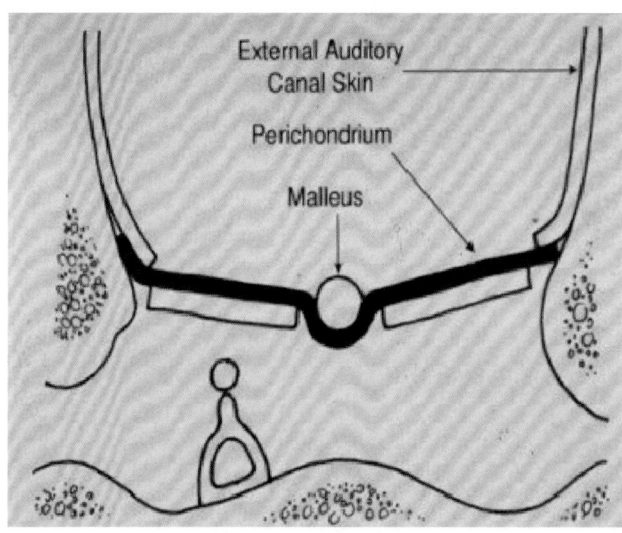

A   **B**

Figure 153.2 Composite perichondrium–cartilage island graft. **A:** A composite perichondrium–cartilage island graft is formed by stripping perichondrium off a single side of the graft. The cartilage is then cut to the desired shape and size without violating the remaining perichondrium. For total tympanic membrane reconstruction, the preferred diameter of the graft is 8 to 9 mm. A 1-mm central strip of cartilage is removed to accommodate the malleus handle and to allow posterior graft elevation for ossiculoplasty. The remaining peripheral perichondrial "apron" is set over the canal wall bone. **B:** Cross section of a perichondrium–cartilage island used as an underlay graft.

perforation (29,30), or a perforation in the setting of permanent absent eustachian tube function. Other situations where cartilage is useful are the atelectatic ear, retraction pockets, and cholesteatoma as re-atrophy and perforation are common over the long term when fascia is used solely in the reconstruction (31).

Mini split-thickness skin grafts may also be used as an adjuvant in tympanoplasty. Although it is generally not advisable to graft the entire reconstructed drumhead due to the potential for dysfunctional postoperative epithelial migration, small grafts (4 mm or less in any dimension) tend to incorporate well with adjacent native epithelium. When utilized, these grafts are best rendered very thin and positioned partially upon the intended tympanic graft target and at least partially upon adjacent healthy canal bone. Instances where mini split-thickness skin grafts may be particularly useful include correction of tympanic membrane blunting, repair of total tympanic membrane defects, removal of chronic granular myringitis, and treatment of tympanic slag injury.

Underlay Repair

Underlay tympanoplasty is the most widely used tympanic membrane repair technique and is suitable for perforations of all sizes and locations (see Fig. 153.3). The concept of underlay grafting involves placement of graft material immediately underneath the residual native drumhead in a manner that accounts for the entire defect and all perforation margins. Three forces typically support this graft.

First, medial support is obtained via absorbable middle ear packing material. Second, adhesion occurs between the graft and the undersurface of the adjacent native drumhead and between the graft and lateral packing material through the perforation. Finally, the peripheral aspect of the graft is anchored in place between the tympanic annulus/canal skin and the underlying bone of the external auditory canal. Anchoring almost always involves the posterior canal wall and tympanomeatal flap but has also been described at various anterior points (32,33).

The advantages of underlay grafting include simplicity, rapid execution, and a high rate of reported success. However, failures do occur, and these are most often related to overreliance on middle ear packing materials. If peripheral annulus anchoring is insufficient, packing may fail to prevent medial (inward) graft displacement and point separation of the graft from the perforation edge. This seems to be a particular risk when repairing an anterior or near-total perforation. In the authors' experience, large rigid cartilage grafts are less likely than fascia or perichondrium to displace medially.

Another theoretic negative consequence of underlay grafting relates to development of postoperative middle ear adhesions and tympanosclerosis. When middle ear mucosa is denuded, the large volume of middle ear packing required for underlay graft support harbors the potential to increase scar formation between the walls of the middle ear cleft and the undersurface of the drumhead. Additionally, redundant margins of underlay graft that lie in contact with the ossicular chain have the potential to adhere and negatively affect ossicular mobility.

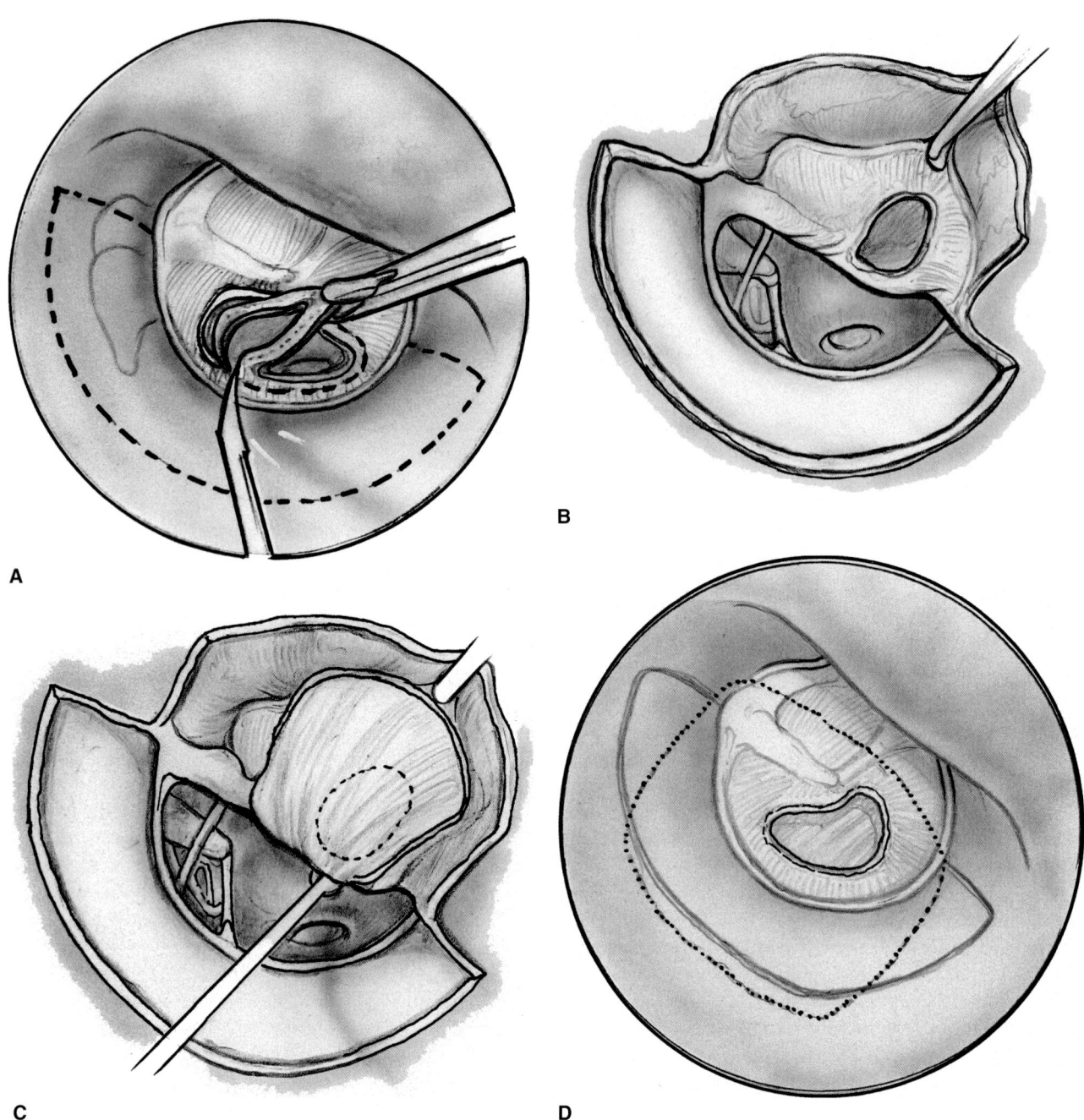

Figure 153.3 Underlay tympanoplasty. **A:** The rim of the perforation is freshened. **B:** The tympanomeatal flap is raised and middle ear work completed as needed, including palpation of the ossicular chain. **C:** The graft is set in an underlay fashion to account for all margins of the perforation. **D:** After application of middle ear packing to support the graft medially, the tympanomeatal flap is returned to the anatomical position, with perforation closure assured.

Overlay Repair

The basic concept of overlay or "lateral grafting" involves de-epithelialization of the tympanic membrane remnant while preserving what exists of the native middle fibrous layer. This preserved middle layer remnant is then used as partial medial support upon which grafting materials are set (see Fig. 153.4). Overlay techniques are robust and can be applied to all perforations, but they are especially useful in dealing with anterior and near total defects (34). They have the advantage of being relatively resistant to graft failure due to inadequate medial support and inward graft migration during the healing phase sometimes seen with underlay techniques.

Most common overlay graft techniques are combined with canalplasty to remove the bulge of the anterior canal wall. De-epithelialization of the tympanic membrane is often undertaken as part of the process of exposing the

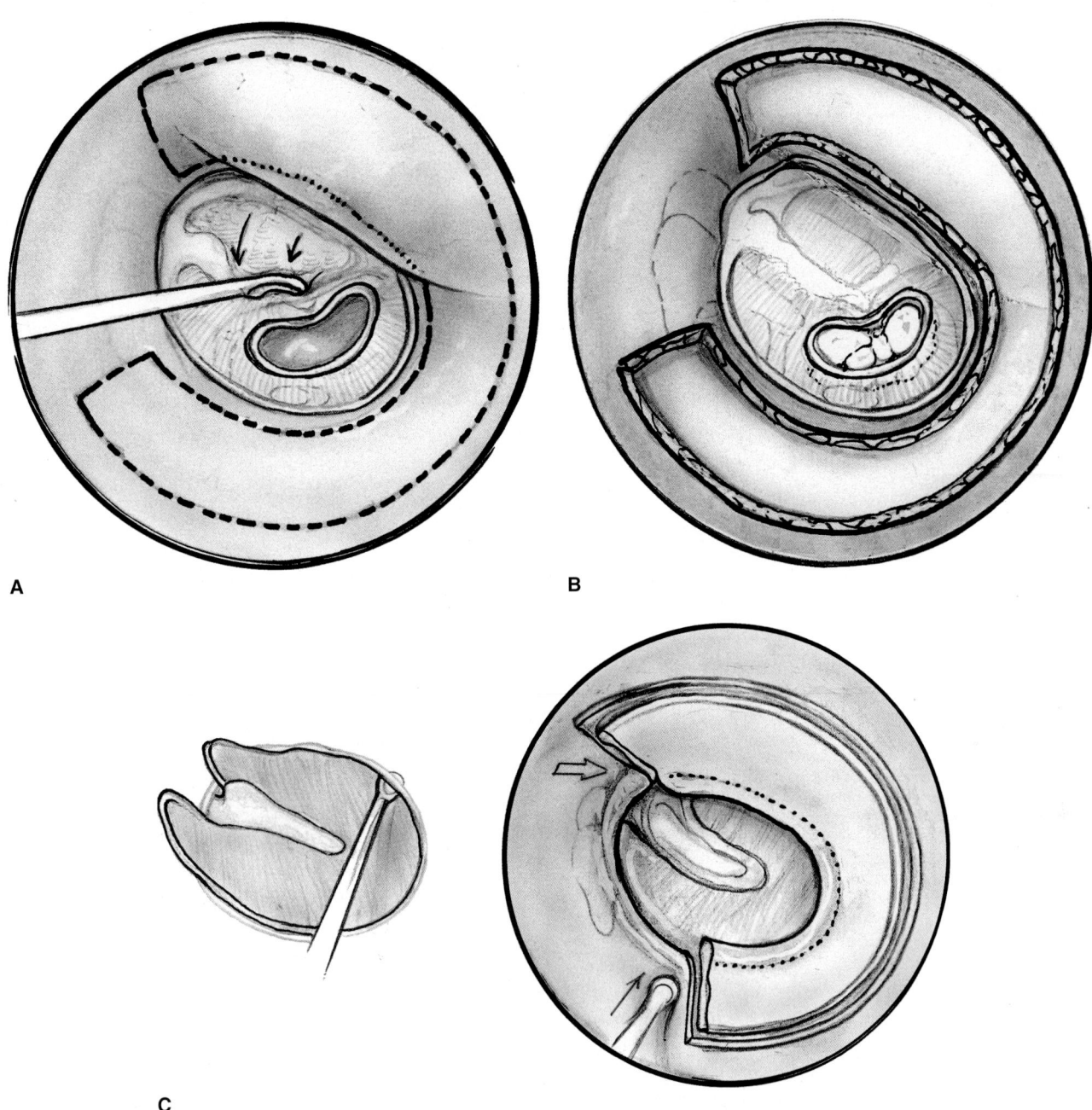

A

B

C

Figure 153.4 Overlay tympanoplasty. **A:** With exposure of the canal wall for canalplasty, all lateral epithelial components of the remnant tympanic membrane are dissected free. **B:** The graft is shaped with a notch for the malleus to account for the entire surface of the tympanic membrane. **C:** The graft is placed medial to the malleus handle to prevent lateralization and then draped over the canal wall on the periphery, lateral to the fibrous tympanic membrane remnant. *(Continued on next page)*

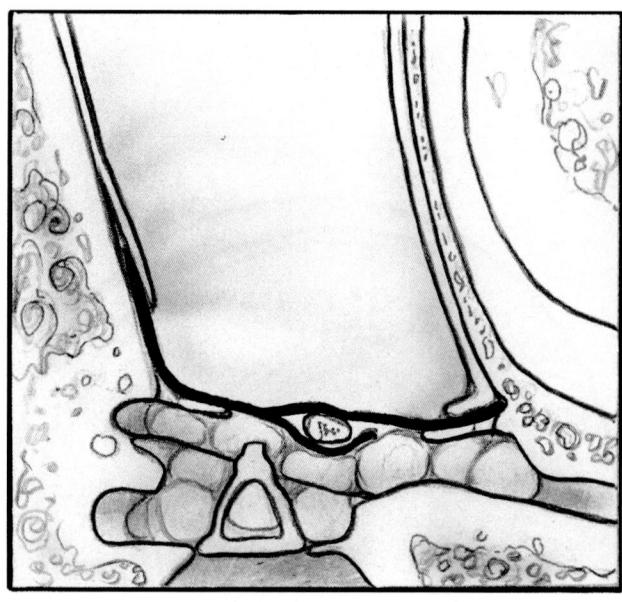

D   Ledge drilled at anterior annulus

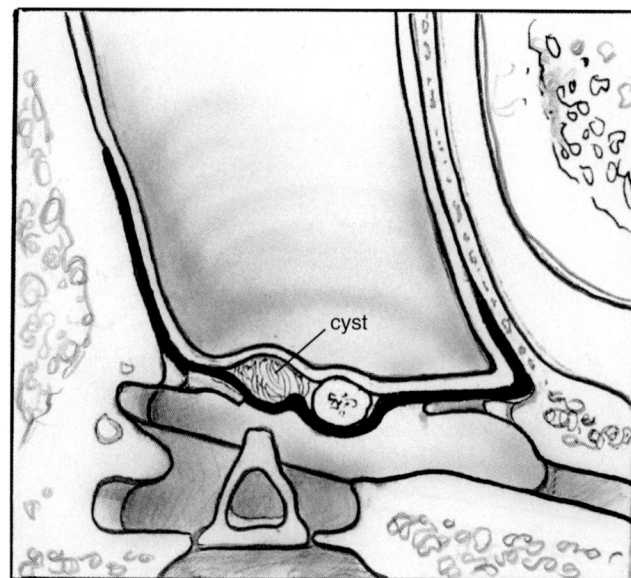

E

F

Figure 153.4 (*Continued*) **D:** Cross section of overlay graft in place. Of note, the anterior canal wall must be drilled with a groove to open the acute anterior tympanomeatal angle. This area is also tightly packed. **E:** If epithelium is left on the remnant tympanic membrane, an intratympanic keratin cyst may result. **F:** Inadequate packing or drilling of the anterior canal wall can result in blunting. Functionally, this becomes a problem when the malleus handle becomes fixed to the anterior canal wall by scar tissue.

bone of the anterior canal wall for drilling, wherein the canal skin is elevated in continuum with the epithelial remnants of the drumhead. Usually, this canal wall skin is removed and reset near the end of the surgery as a free graft. Care should be taken that all epithelial remnants have been removed prior to graft overlay in order to prevent development of intratympanic keratin inclusion cysts.

It is important to understand that canalplasty is performed with overlay grafting not only to provide adequate exposure to the anterior tympanic ring, but also to open the acute anterior tympanomeatal angle between the anterior canal wall and drumhead in an effort to prevent postoperative blunting of this area. Blunting can be functionally understood as dense scarring of the anterior tympanic membrane that results in reduction of the functional

surface area of the drumhead and "pseudo-malleus fixation" caused by adhesion between the manubrium and the anterior canal wall. This risk can be minimized not only by canalplasty, but also by strategically packing this area after graft placement.

Unique Situations

Atelectasis

Tympanic membrane atelectasis may require augmentation with an underlay graft (usually cartilage) or, rarely, drum replacement (14). As a general rule, when atelectasis is limited and has not resulted in the need for ossiculoplasty, medical management to promote eustachian tube function or tympanostomy tube placement is sufficient.

Surprisingly, even some cases of severe atelectasis will correct with the combination of nitrous oxide induction anesthesia, microsuction manipulation, tympanic intubation, and time. However, when these measures have failed and ossiculoplasty is inevitable, or when cholesteatoma risk is high due to incompletely visualized retraction pockets, tympanoplasty is generally required. One challenge unique to this scenario is that long-standing severe retractions can be quite difficult to evert and completely remove from areas such as the sinus tympani, hypotympanum, or the ossicular chain. The laser can be a useful tool for removal of disease from an intact and mobile ossicular chain in these cases. If hearing is reasonable, some surgeons prefer to watch these patients closely rather than risk generating a cholesteatoma by failing to remove all adherent tympanic membrane epithelial remnants.

Lateralized Tympanic Membrane

As a complication of tympanoplasty, it is possible for the tympanic membrane to undergo unfavorable healing and scar formation that may result in postoperative lateralization of the tympanic membrane. When this occurs, the drumhead is typically not coupled to the underlying ossicular chain, thereby resulting in a large-volume conductive hearing loss. Lateralization is particularly a concern when tympanic membrane reconstruction does not involve graft placement medial to an intact stable malleus handle or when there is a prominence of circumferential bare external auditory canal bone. Aside from anchoring the tympanic membrane graft to the malleus handle with an underlay placement, other techniques helpful in dealing with lateralization include secure underlay anchoring of the graft under the tympanic annulus. Cartilage tympanoplasty techniques have proven particularly useful in this situation as the rigid material allows precise fixation medial to the bony annulus (35). Bringing the lateralized tympanic membrane to a more normal position often involves removal of the lateralized membrane, reestablishment of a new graft using underlay techniques, and the use of small full- or split-thickness skin grafts to cover exposed external canal bone in order to promote rapid healing and minimize the scar formation that leads to lateralization.

Open Mastoid Cavity

Successful tympanic membrane repair in the setting of a canal wall–down mastoid procedure requires attention to a few unique considerations. When an open mastoid cavity is created, the epitympanum is exteriorized; thus, the anchored boundary of the tympanic membrane margin is shifted medially in the posterior and superior aspects where the bony canal wall and tympanic ring have been removed. Typically, the bony canal of the tympanic and mastoid segments of the facial nerve form convenient new marginal boundaries for the neo-tympanic membrane in these superior and posterior aspects, respectively. Ideally, this should

be achieved by complete lowering of the facial ridge of bone overlying the second genu and mastoid segment.

One oft-neglected aspect of neo-tympanic membrane creation in a canal wall–down situation is that exteriorization of the epitympanum usually involves opening the anterior supralabyrinthine communication with the supratubal recess. If this opening, located anterior to the tensor tympani tendon, is not recognized and accounted for with graft material, barrier separation between the moist middle ear mucosa and the epithelialized open mastoid cavity will not occur, and a source of moisture that acts as a *de facto* tympanic membrane perforation will lead to future open cavity instability.

A final consideration in canal wall–down neo-tympanic membrane repair relates to the resultant diminished middle ear volume, wherein much of the undersurface of the new drumhead is brought into relative proximity with the promontory and other middle ear structures. As such, postoperative negative middle ear pressure and retraction are much less well tolerated than in an intact canal wall situation as there is very little open space to buffer contact and adhesion formation. The use of cartilage grafts to resist retraction is particularly helpful in this situation. The authors favor the use of a large composite perichondrium–cartilage island graft such that residual perichondrial edges drape over the facial ridge and seal the middle ear space as part of a type III tympanoplasty with a direct stapes columella (36) or a synthetic prosthesis.

OSSICULOPLASTY

General Principles

While it is generally possible to ascertain the need for ossiculoplasty during the preoperative evaluation based on the audiogram and physical exam, one should be prepared for this contingency in every middle ear case. In addition, it should be considered routine practice to inspect the ossicular chain visually and mechanically every time the middle ear is entered. This can be performed with gentle palpation of the malleus, taking note of concomitant movement of the stapes and visualization of the round window reflex (movement of the membrane and fluid in the niche with palpation of the chain).

The goal of ossiculoplasty is to reconstruct the sound-conducting connection between the inner ear and tympanic membrane. This reconstruction should have immediate stability and long-term durability. It should also comply with as many of the gain-benefit principles of ossicular acoustic mechanics as is practical. The durability of ossiculoplasty is difficult to predict and is influenced heavily by the quality of the middle ear environment and activity of any related underlying disease process.

The timing of ossiculoplasty is controversial with respect to whether or not it should be performed primarily alongside repair of the tympanic membrane or as part of a staged process. The benefit of staged surgery is that ossicular reconstruction can be applied to a favorable environment in which the dimensions of the tympanic membrane relative to the middle ear are stable and a quiet middle ear mucosal envelope is present. When a second stage is planned after canal wall–up cholesteatoma surgery or when the middle ear environment is particularly hostile (active infection, fibrotic mucosa, revision surgery), a staged approach is logical. In such instances, temporary silastic sheeting is placed within the middle ear during primary tympanic membrane repair to prevent adhesions between the undersurface of the drumhead and the medial aspect of the middle ear. Theoretical benefits notwithstanding, the authors' preference is to perform primary ossiculoplasty alongside tympanic membrane repair in most cases. In doing so, excellent results are still typical while avoiding the cost and inconvenience of further surgery. In the rare instance of an unacceptable hearing result after primary ossiculoplasty, revision surgery can still be easily performed while utilizing the original ossicular prosthesis.

Ossiculoplasty Materials

A variety of autograft, homograft, and synthetic ossiculoplasty materials are currently used or have been tried in the past. Autologous ossicular grafting techniques have been used extensively, are the most biocompatible, and tend to maintain their configuration over time through bone substitution (37). Cortical bone grafts show good biocompatibility, but in the authors' experience, are more likely than ossicular grafts to undergo absorption over the long term, especially in a hostile middle ear environment. Autologous cartilage is biocompatible and has been used in cases when the space to be reconstructed is small; for example, this material can be used as a stapes height extender in a canal wall–down reconstruction. However, concerns about graft acquisition of chondromalacia over the long term have limited the authors' use of autologous cartilage for major reconstructions between the stapes and malleus. Homologous cadaveric bone and cartilage grafts have also been used successfully in middle ear surgery, but the cost of preparation and risk of disease transmission have made these materials progressively less popular.

Numerous synthetic materials have been used in ossicular implants (38,39). Porous high-density polyethylene was used in several early implants; however, these implants were frequently associated with processes that have negative implications, such as micro-degradation and giant cell formation. Thus, other implants have been developed using plastics, bioactive glass, stainless steel, gold, titanium, and hydroxylapatite (the last two currently being most common in the United States and Europe). Promising short-term results continue to be published for most of these materials (40–43), but the long-term histological fate is uncertain in many instances. The extrusion rates of synthetic implants are generally higher than autologous materials (44).

Applied Middle Ear Mechanics

As discussed previously, by far the most important mechanism of acoustic gain will come from reestablishment of the hydraulic lever, derived from the surface area ratio of the tympanic membrane to the oval window, by coupling the reconstructed tympanic membrane to the stapes footplate. Reestablishment of the catenary lever is also often possible by utilizing the manubrium of the malleus in the reconstruction of both the tympanic membrane and ossicular chain. Recent basic science research using infrared laser vibrometry as well as retrospective clinical studies on ossiculoplasty suggest that incorporating the malleus in the reconstruction provides increased acoustic gain (45). However, since gain derived from catenary effects is severalfold less than that derived from the hydraulic lever, these theoretic benefits should be kept in proper perspective during surgical planning. Similarly, the malleoincudal lever provides such a small theoretical increase in gain (2 to 3 dB) that it does not constitute a compelling reason to favor a type II reconstructive mechanism over one of the type III subtypes.

Specific Situations

Incus Erosion

Due to its location relative to the common pathways of development of cholesteatoma and tympanic membrane atelectasis, as well as its rather tenuous blood supply suspended between the stapes and malleus, erosion of the incus long process is the most common ossicular defect. It can be encountered in roughly one-third of cases involving a chronic posterior tympanic membrane perforation due to a variety of factors, such as pressure necrosis, inflammation, and hydrolytic enzymes produced by cholesteatoma matrix.

While an eroded incus is usually obvious during middle ear exploration, in some cases palpation is required to uncover the presence of a more subtle fibrous union between the stapes and incus. The key factor in this situation is the degree of bony contact remaining, which, if present to some reasonable degree, may compel the surgeon to leave the incus untouched. However, if contact is deficient and movement with palpation is incomplete, reconstruction is recommended.

There are basically two options for reconstruction when incus erosion is present. The first involves an attempt to reconstruct the incudostapedial joint with a type II tympanoplasty. If the defect between the incus and stapes is very small, this can be accomplished by wedging a piece of cartilage or bone between the incus and malleus. Alternatively, various cements composed of materials such as ionomer and hydroxylapatite have shown promise in small-defect joint reconstruction (46,47); however, these cements have thus far been met with somewhat limited acceptance due to concerns of toxicity (ionomer) and of excessive brittleness that may result in a tendency to dislocate or fracture (hydroxylapatite).

For larger defects, various prostheses can be utilized. The prosthesis that has been in use for the longest duration, the Applebaum prosthesis (Gyrus ENT, Bartlett, TN), is made of dense hydroxylapatite and is shaped like a block, with two divots oriented at 90 degrees from each other to engage both the stapes capitulum and the eroded lenticular process. Other metallic prostheses have been developed that tend to be similar in concept in so far as they combine an extension that heat shrinks (nitinol) or crimps (titanium) to the remnant of the long process, with a cradle that engages the stapes capitulum.

All of these type II reconstructive techniques share many of the same theoretical advantages and disadvantages. On the positive side, they reestablish the natural malleoincudal lever with minimal disruption of the normal anatomical relationships and native ossicular connections. The primary disadvantages relate to uncertain long-term durability. Little is known about the pathophysiology and natural history of incus necrosis. If erosion is related to avascular necrosis, one may speculate that the remnant of the lenticular process, if used in ossicular reconstruction, may be subject to future loss.

The second reconstructive option for incus necrosis involves removal of the incus remnant and reconstruction between the stapes and malleus (or tympanic membrane), generally as a type III minor columella mechanism. The fundamental anatomic principles governing this reconstruction are the same regardless of the graft or prostheses used. Some key relationships include the vertical height from the stapes capitulum to the plane of the neck of the malleus (2 to 2.5 mm) and the horizontal or translational distance from the capitulum to the neck of the malleus (3 to 3.5 mm) (see Fig. 153.5). Although the malleus manubrium can become rotated medially as an effect of middle ear disease processes, especially along its distal aspect, in the authors' experience, the malleus neck is spared from rotational variation and can be used in ossicular reconstruction with these distances remaining fairly consistent. This is due to the fact that the axis of malleus medial rotation lies close to the neck as the malleus is supported at the anterior malleolar spine by the fan-shaped anterior malleolar ligament and medially at the cochleariform process by the tensor tympani tendon. However, if the malleus is medially or anteriorly rotated to an extreme degree, it may be necessary to pull it laterally with a small hook, to stretch or cut the tensor tendon, or rarely, to detach it from the drumhead and translocate the manubrium while keeping ligamentous attachments intact.

If the body of the incus is not significantly eroded or at risk of harboring microscopic cholesteatoma, it can be sculpted with a drill burr and used as an incus interposition autologous graft to fit the above-noted dimensions (see Fig. 153.6). If properly executed, this technique will generate a stable, durable reconstruction that has been described extensively in the literature as having favorable hearing

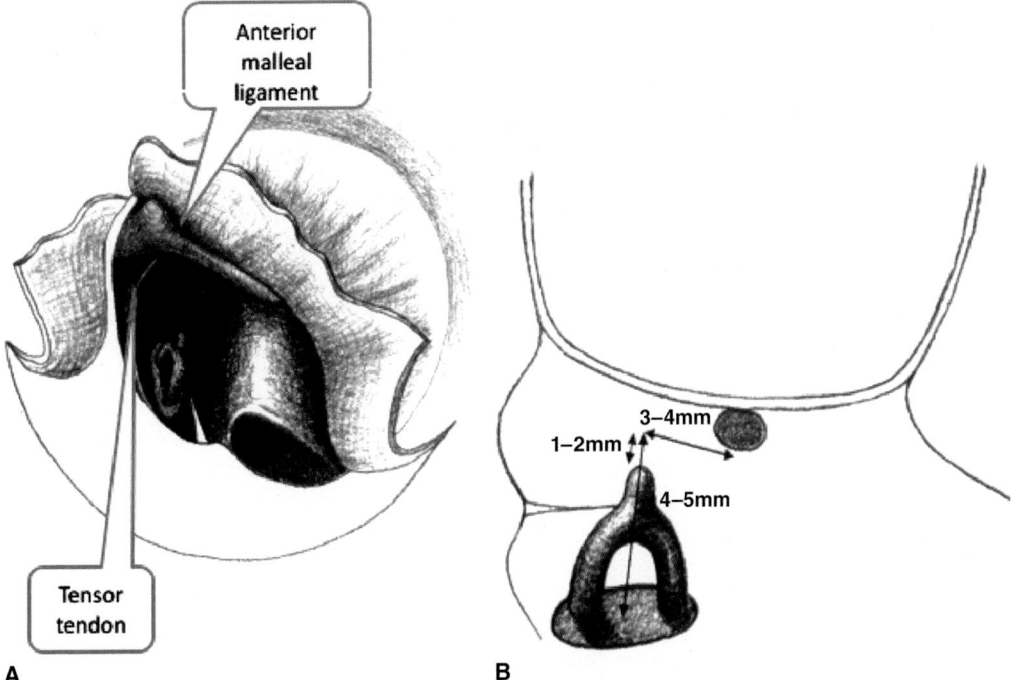

Figure 153.5 Middle ear anatomy relevant to ossiculoplasty. **A:** The tensor tympani tendon and the anterior malleal ligament anchor the malleus neck at the cochleariform process and anterior tympanic spine, respectively. These structures provide stability for tympanoplasty and ossiculoplasty procedures and should not be violated unless necessary. **B:** The stapes capitulum is typically 2 mm in height below the undersurface of the neck of the malleus, which is the proper target for the ossicular reconstruction interface. This same site is approximately 3 mm in the lateral dimension from the capitulum; thus, 3 mm of reach is generally required for a sculpted ossicular graft or synthetic prosthesis.

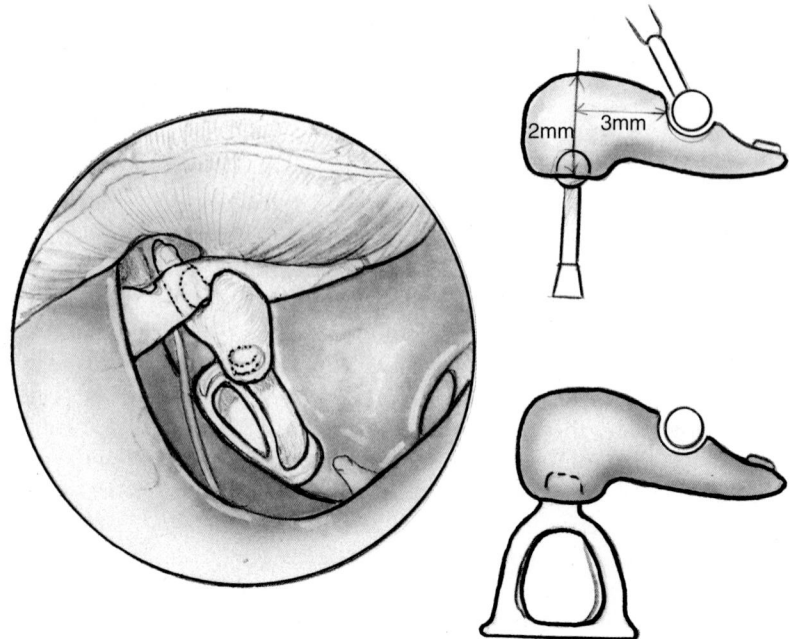

Figure 153.6 Incus interposition. Sculpted incus interposition grafts may be used to bridge the malleus handle and stapes capitulum. These should have an approximate height of 2 mm and an offset groove for the malleus interface at 3 mm.

outcomes (48). The main advantages of this technique are that it is inexpensive and there are no biocompatibility concerns. The disadvantages are that there is a low possibility of continued necrosis, the incus may not be available in all cases, and autologous ossicular grafts tend to fuse strongly to engaged native ossicles or to other adjacent structures such that revision surgery can be challenging.

If the incus is deemed unusable or if the time and work involved with autograft preparation are not embraced, most surgeons opt for the use of a synthetic PORP (49). The recommended surgical technique utilizing a PORP as a minor columella is quite similar to that described for incus interposition, keeping in mind that the vertical height should be 2 to 2.5 mm and the horizontal reach distance 3 to 3.5 mm. While many commercially prepared prostheses are produced with a wide range of lengths or are adjustable, if reconstruction is made to the malleus neck, adjustments are not often necessary. It has been the authors' experience that similar consistency in measurements to what is encountered in stapes surgery is seen in incus replacement if the proper site at the malleus neck is utilized. Thus, although it is sensible to confirm by measuring, a prosthesis with a vertical height of 2 to 2.5 mm and a horizontal reach of 3 mm can be used in almost every case as long as it is designed to engage the malleus handle and there is no stapes capitulum erosion or exaggerated inferior rotation onto the promontory.

Another important point to consider when using a PORP is that many of them have broad heads that make contact with the tympanic membrane in addition to the malleus (in contrast to the "strut-like" structure of a sculpted incus autograft that spares tympanic membrane contact). Since the tympanic membrane is a conical structure and not a flat disk, it is desirable to use a prosthesis that can be bent approximately 30 degrees at the junction of the shaft and head to

facilitate this shape (see Fig. 153.7). Doing so will encourage the superior edge of the prosthesis head under the malleus neck to become "locked" by the tensor tympani tendon.

To combat synthetic prosthesis extrusion, a cartilage graft cap is recommended at the interface between the tympanic membrane and the adjacent prosthesis head. Although it has been suggested that this barrier may be optional with a prosthesis that features a hydroxylapatite head with smooth edges, cartilage is essential with sharper titanium prosthesis heads. As opposed to host incompatibility and lateral prosthesis migration beyond the tympanic membrane, the pathophysiology of prosthesis extrusion with an appropriate-length prosthesis more often seems to involve postoperative medial retraction of the tympanic membrane around the prosthesis. Cartilage can be placed in conjunction with reconstruction of the posterior half of the tympanic membrane in order to prevent retractions or cholesteatoma formation. When the cartilage graft is reconstructed exactly in piecemeal fashion, it is known as the mosaic technique (see Fig. 153.8).

The numerous apparent benefits of incorporating the malleus into ossiculoplasty notwithstanding (45,50), some surgeons achieve favorable hearing results without engaging the malleus. Even if the malleus is not included in the reconstruction, making provisions for the conical shape of the tympanic membrane is desirable. In the end, no matter which technique is used, the goal is to create a freestanding reconstruction that fixes to the tympanic membrane and stapes head, but not to other structures, such as the tympanic ring or cochlear promontory. A limited amount of absorbable packing can be used to achieve this end, but it should be noted that its use has been implicated with postoperative middle ear fibrosis, especially when denuded mucosa is present.

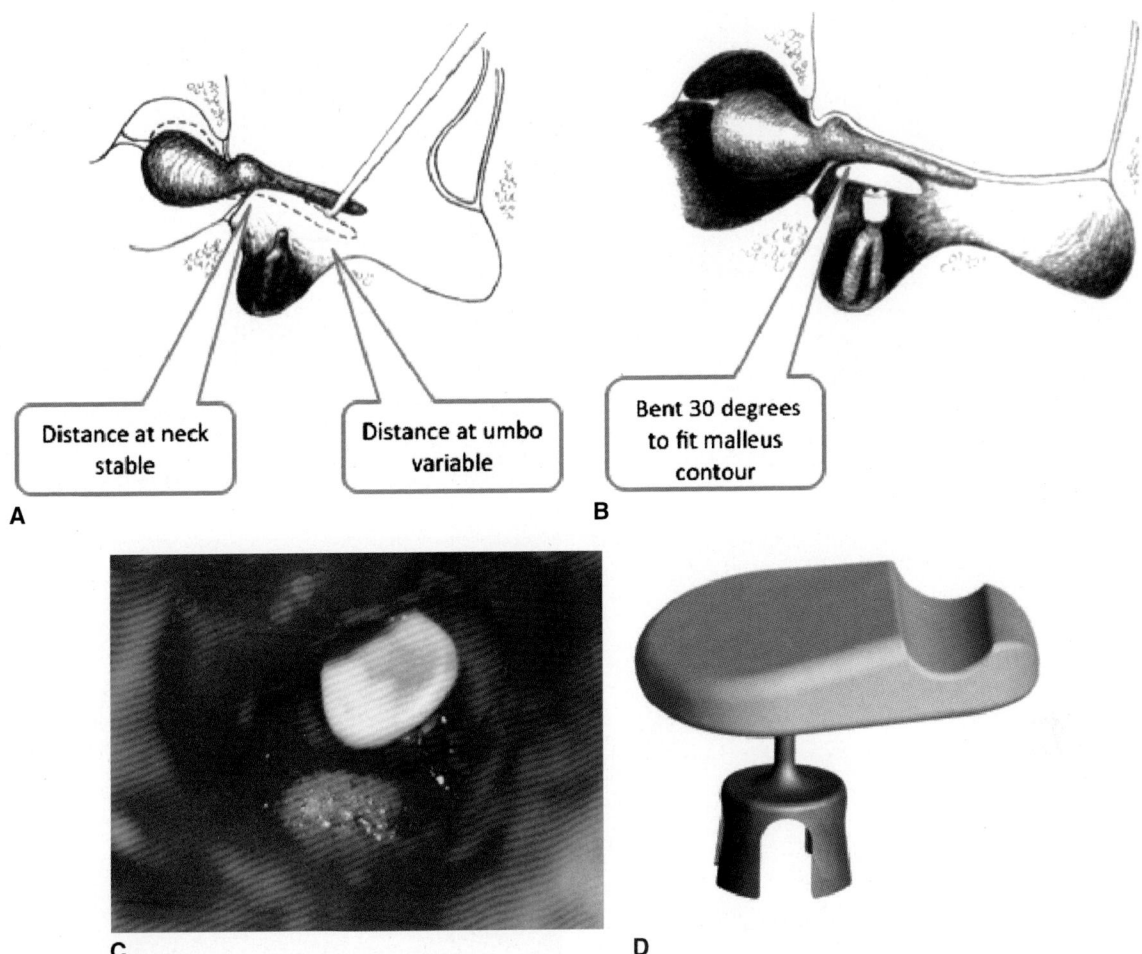

Distance at neck stable

Distance at umbo variable

A

Bent 30 degrees to fit malleus contour

B

C

D

Figure 153.7 Contour of prosthesis to malleus handle. **A:** Although retraction can result in medial displacement of the umbo, the malleus neck orientation is relatively stable due to adjacent supporting ligaments. Thus, the malleus neck, not the handle, is the most constant target for ossiculoplasty. If required, the umbo can be lateralized with a blunt hook. **B:** The prosthesis is manually contoured with a bend of 30 degrees at the interface of the shaft and head to fit properly under the malleus handle and tympanic membrane curvature. **C:** Appearance of contoured PORP in proper stable position between the stapes capitulum and malleus neck. **D:** Dornhoffer PORP with hydroxylapatite head and titanium shaft (Grace Medical, Memphis, TN). The authors assert that, if properly shaped and applied, a prosthesis 2 mm in height can be used in nearly every single case.

Incus and Stapes Absent

When both the incus and stapes superstructure are absent, common options for reconstruction include a type III major columella mechanism or a type IV tympanoplasty, the latter being suitable only in certain cases involving a canal wall–down mastoidectomy. Ossicular or cortical bone grafts are generally not ideal for use in this situation because the long process of the incus is usually eroded to less than the length required for sculpting, while cortical bone grafts tend to fix to the adjacent fallopian canal. Thus, a synthetic TORP is typically what is used as a major columella. The same basic principles of reconstruction and recognition of anatomical consistencies discussed with the use of a PORP apply to a TORP. To account for the absence of the stapes superstructure, an additional 2 to 2.5 mm is added to the vertical height recommendation. Thus, the desired TORP dimensions will be approximately 4.5 mm

in height, with 3 mm of reach in order to reconstruct to the malleus neck while maintaining the shaft oriented 90 degrees to the footplate.

One of the real challenges in this type of reconstruction relates to the lack of stability at the level of the footplate. Although the presence of the stapes superstructure offers no mechanism for acoustic gain, it does provide a convenient point for stable prosthesis fixation. The literature often shows superior hearing outcomes with a PORP versus a TORP, which is likely due to this difference in stability. The same 30-degree angled interface with the neck of the malleus and tympanic membrane is utilized for lateral stability, as described earlier. However, this alone does not ensure a stable centered footplate contact point because the forces exerted by the tympanic membrane and malleus onto the TORP head encourage the shaft to displace posteriorly. Several devices have been introduced to

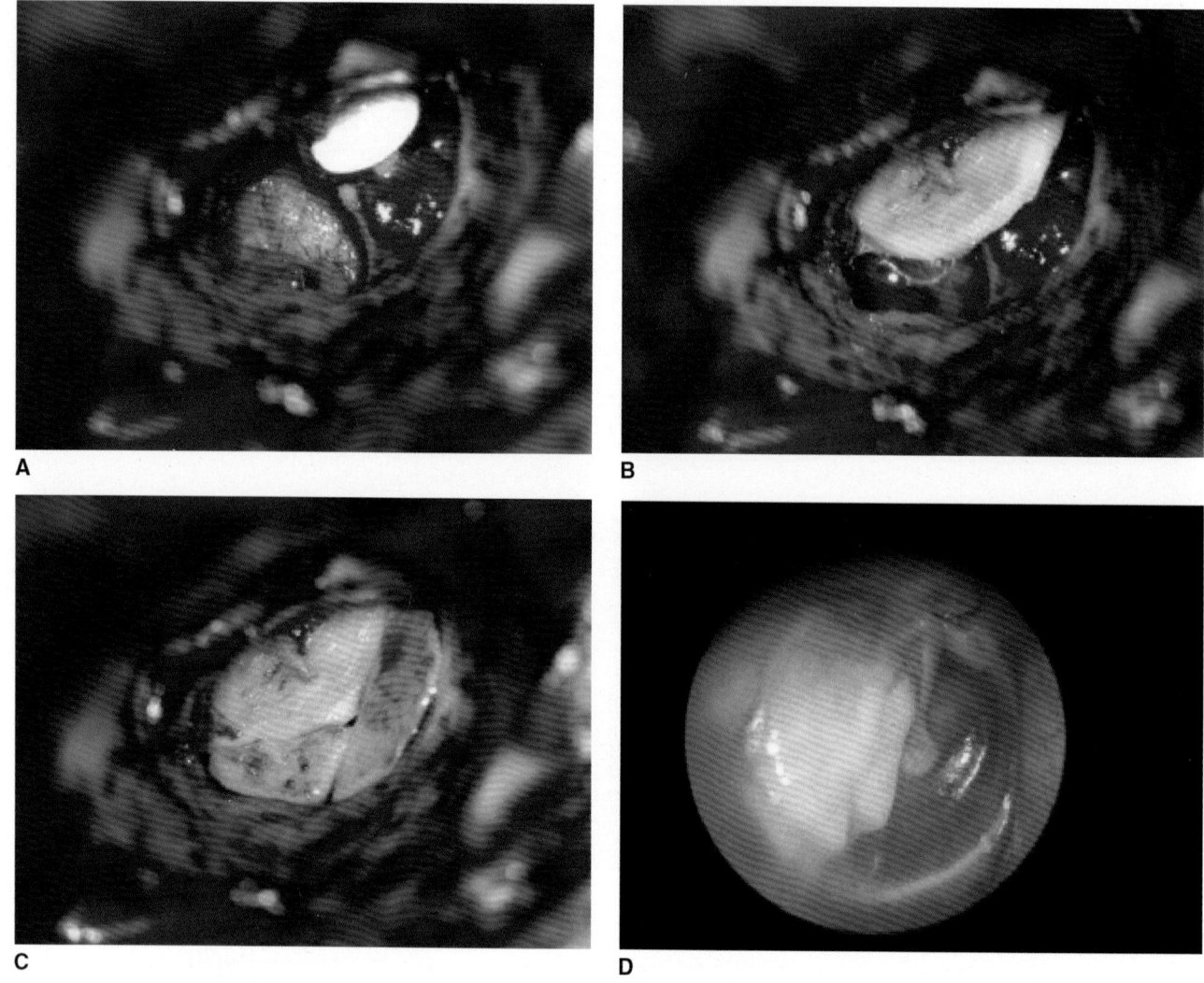

Figure 153.8 Mosaic cartilage tympanoplasty with ossiculoplasty. **A:** The PORP is set between the malleus neck and stapes capitulum. **B:** A large crescent-shaped piece of cartilage is set directly upon the prosthesis. **C:** Smaller crescent-shaped cartilage pieces are placed to form a "mosaic" of cartilage. **D:** Postoperative appearance following cartilage mosaic underlay tympanoplasty (right ear).

counteract this phenomenon, including both titanium and hydroxylapatite footplate "shoes" (see Fig. 153.9). Related techniques that utilize small oval-shaped pieces of cartilage with a central hole have also been described (51).

While it is advisable to utilize the stapes superstructure when present, inferior rotation toward the promontory due to disease or previous surgery can make a minor columella reconstruction unsuitable. In such instances, a PORP or incus interposition may produce rocking of the stapes toward the promontory instead of the desired piston motion. Therefore, a TORP placed on the footplate superior to the superstructure is a more suitable alternative that tends to rotate the stapes superiorly into a more favorable position (52).

Malleus Absent
The techniques previously described emphasize the use of the malleus for prosthesis stability and as an anatomical landmark for consistent length measurements; however, the

malleus manubrium is not always present. Some otologists believe that the malleus is such a tremendous benefit in ossiculoplasty that techniques have been developed to create a "neo-malleus" from a piece of bone or a synthetic implant that is grafted into the tympanic membrane to be used later in staged ossicular reconstruction (53). Nonetheless, several options do exist for single-stage tympano-ossicular reconstruction in the absence of a malleus manubrium (52).

The most simple of these single-stage techniques is reconstruction directly between the drumhead and stapes superstructure with a type III stapes columella mechanism (especially in a canal wall–down procedure). It is acoustically favorable to perform this type of reconstruction in combination with tympanic membrane cartilage grafting, wherein the capitulum of the stapes is in contact with a piece of cartilage that is at least 4 mm in diameter, as opposed to a stapes/drumhead interface with fascia or native drumhead only. Although it is possible to achieve

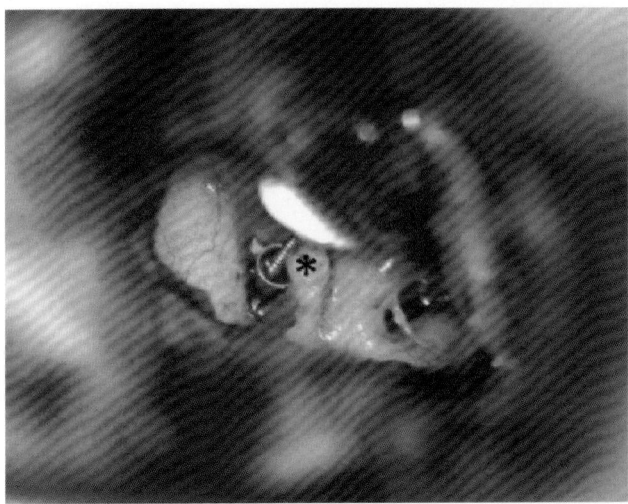

Figure 153.9 TORP with footplate shoe for rotated stapes. When unfavorable inferior rotation of the stapes superstructure is present, a TORP is often preferable to maintain an approximate perpendicular orientation between the tympanic membrane and prosthesis shaft. In this case, the TORP is stabilized at the level of the footplate by a titanium shoe. The stapes capitulum is indicated by the *asterisk*.

excellent air–bone gap closure with the stapes columella subtype of type III reconstruction (36), actual outcomes can be inconsistent or lag behind what is predicted. Various other simple modifications of type III tympanoplasty that result in a minor columella can be made when

direct contact between the drumhead and stapes is not possible but only a small gap exists. These include placement of some type of autologous interposition graft, such as a sculpted malleus head or stacked disk(s) of cartilage.

When a wider gap between the stapes and drumhead is present or when the superstructure is absent, the use of a PORP or TORP that directly contacts the drumhead (with or without the cartilage cap, depending on the prosthesis material used) is generally required. These techniques can be effective, but great care should be exercised in measuring the correct prosthesis length. It is recommended that the reconstructed drumhead be slightly tented by the prosthesis; however, a major reason for prosthesis extrusion, regardless of material, is excessive length. Because these cases involving an absent malleus harbor the potential for graft/prosthesis adherence to the undersurface of the reconstructed tympanic membrane and ossiculoplasty failure due to delayed lateralization of the capitulum or footplate as the reconstructed tympanic membrane heals and matures, many surgeons favor staged ossiculoplasty. One innovative way to accomplish this during the second stage is via the facial recess so that elevation of a tympanomeatal flap is avoided and a stable tympanic membrane measurement is afforded (54).

Finally, an alternative single-stage technique involves creation of a "pseudo-malleus" by reconstructing the tympanic membrane with a composite perichondrium–cartilage island graft that forms a creased midline ridge to act in place of the manubrium (see Fig. 153.10). This is achieved

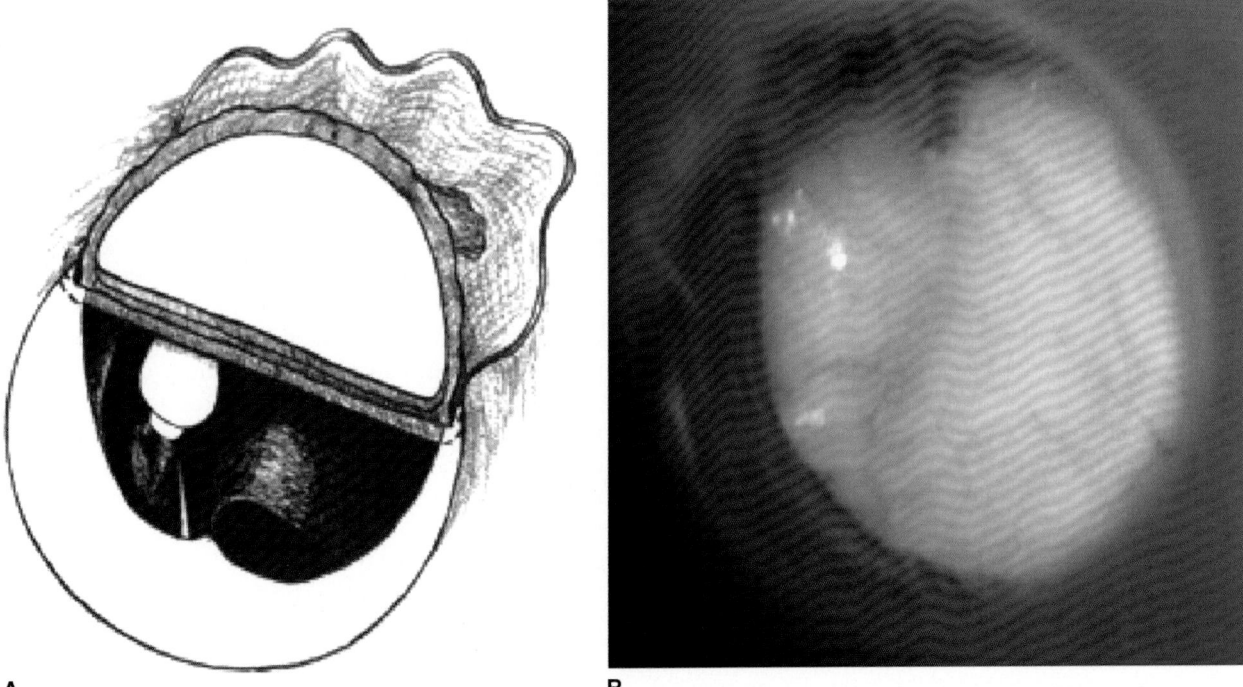

A   **B**

Figure 153.10 Tympano-ossicular reconstruction without malleus. **A:** When the malleus handle is absent, the folded ridge generated by opposing edges of a composite perichondrium–cartilage island graft can be used as a pseudo-malleus to support a prosthesis that has a notch intended for the malleus handle. **B:** Postoperative appearance of tympanic membrane after total drum reconstruction using a composite perichondrium–cartilage island graft.

by creating a circular cartilage island graft measuring 8 to 9 mm in diameter, with a 1-mm midline strip of cartilage removed from the perichondrium, bisecting the island into two half-circles. The anterior half-circle is inserted as an underlay below the tympanic ring inferiorly and anterior tympanic spine superiorly while supported medially with absorbable packing in the anterior mesotympanum. The posterior half-circle is then lifted to expose the posterior edge of the anterior island, which is placed near the position of the absent malleus handle. This pseudo-malleus ridge can then be used for ossicular reconstruction using the same lengths of prostheses described earlier.

Fixed Ossicular Chain

Tympanosclerosis involving the tympanic membrane and middle ear is common when significant otitis media has been present. When these chalky white plaques involve the tympanic membrane, little or no conductive loss is expected unless the ossicular chain is also affected. Hearing loss due to tympanosclerotic fixation can occur secondary to involvement with any component of the ossicular chain.

An isolated malleus head or incus fixation with a mobile stapes can be dealt with in two ways (10). The most common technique involves disarticulation of the incudostapedial joint followed by removal of the incus and amputation of the malleus head just above the insertion of the tensor tympani. Rarely, the malleus head is so fixed that it must be left in place; thus, a 1-mm gap is drilled between the fixed head and the mobile remnant to prevent re-fixation. Reconstruction is then accomplished with a type III minor columella as described previously.

The second technique for correcting malleus fixation involves mobilization through an atticotomy by carefully releasing the point of fixation with a diamond drill bur. While good results have been reported with this technique, great care must be taken not to contact the ossicular chain with the bur as high-frequency sensorineural hearing loss can result. Due to this and the risk of re-fixation with new bone growth, mobilization techniques are only recommended for low-complexity ossicular fixation.

Stapes fixation from tympanosclerosis represents a more complicated problem that often requires a staged approach. If fixation is secondary to a limited amount of soft tympanosclerotic plaque, it is usually possible to remove this in layers until mobilization is achieved. Unlike stapes mobilization in otosclerosis, where re-fixation is frequent, long-term mobility can be achieved with limited tympanosclerosis if otitis media is quiescent. However, if stapedial tympanosclerosis is extensive, a staged stapedotomy or the use of amplification *in lieu* of surgery is required. For stapedotomy to be considered in the setting of quiescent chronic otitis media, several criteria must be satisfied, including a healthy healed tympanic membrane, complete absence of middle ear disease and effusion for several months, and apparent eustachian tube patency (55).

During second-stage surgery standard incus-grip stapedotomy can be performed if the lateral ossicular chain is mobile although, similar to obliterative otosclerosis, this may require removal of plaque from the footplate with a laser or mechanical drill. If the lateral ossicular chain is fixed, the incus and head of the malleus can be removed so that an incus-replacement malleostapedotomy procedure can be performed. It should be noted that this is a technically challenging procedure that should be attempted only by the highly experienced otologic surgeon (56). A technically challenging alternative involves creation of a larger stapedotomy followed by placement of a tissue seal over the oval window and overlying reconstruction with a TORP (57). One must always consider that the hearing results with stapes surgery for extensive tympanosclerosis are generally not as good as for otosclerosis; thus, amplification should always be considered as an alternative to ossicular reconstruction in these instances.

RESULTS

Experienced surgeons should expect durable closure of the tympanic membrane in 85% to 95% of tympanoplasty procedures. Furthermore, although hearing results may vary, one should expect only a small air–bone gap in 90% of type I tympanoplasty cases (49). Risk factors for failure of type I tympanoplasty are not definitively understood or universally accepted; yet when viewed through the lenses of experience, common sense, and published tympanoplasty outcome data, certain themes can be recognized. First, underlying host tissue factors that negatively affect graft viability, capillary ingrowth, and nutrient supply, such as diabetes, smoking (58,59), severe malnutrition, active infection, past slag injury, or past radiation therapy, may be expected to increase the risk of failure to some degree. Furthermore, factors that increase the odds of graft displacement or migration during the healing phase, such as eustachian tube dysfunction, chronic cough, obstructive sleep apnea, or an unwillingness to adhere to recommended postoperative lifestyle guidelines, may have similar negative effects. Finally, other factors, such as the experience and skill of the surgeon, the merits and execution of the technique utilized, the size and location of the perforation, the condition of the tympanic membrane and middle ear, the presence of scar tissue or revision surgery, and the quality of the operating environment (bloodless, hypotensive), likely affect outcome.

Hearing outcomes with ossiculoplasty are more variable compared with type I tympanoplasty, and long-term results are, on average, worse than short-term results (60,61). This is likely because these procedures are more skill and technique dependent, are influenced by the inherent qualities of the prosthesis, and, on average, are associated with more advanced chronic ear disease. Traditionally, ossiculoplasty "success" has been roughly judged to be a pure tone average air–bone gap less than 30 dB for a major columella (TORP), less than 20 dB for a minor columella (PORP), and less than 10 dB for a stapedotomy (62). However, in the authors' opinion, these benchmarks are only indicative of what is minimally acceptable without the need for revision and do not necessarily portray excellence in ossiculoplasty.

Much has been discussed about the inherent qualities of a theoretically ideal ossicular replacement prosthesis (39), but assuming the material is biocompatible and is correctly placed, the qualities of the underlying middle ear environment have a far greater impact on hearing outcomes. The importance of underlying risk factor stratification has been recognized since Wullstein first reported his classification scheme. Subsequently, Bellucci (16) introduced a classification scheme based on the degree of preoperative drainage, followed by Austin (63), who introduced a classification scheme based on the ossicular defect. Kartush (64) has modified Austin's classification by adding aspects of the patient history to the surgical findings in order to develop the widely used Middle Ear Severity Index. Other modern statistics-based classification systems have since been reported by Black (65) (Surgical Prosthetic Infection Tissue Eustachian), Dornhoffer (66) (Ossiculoplasty Outcome Parameter System), and others.

As with type I tympanoplasty, there is no agreement as to which factors are most important for success in ossiculoplasty; however, review of these classification schemes does reveal certain trends (49,64–68). Specifically, revision surgery, middle ear fibrosis, mucosal disease with drainage, smoking, absence of the stapes superstructure, absence of the malleus handle, and a shallow (69) or poorly aerated middle ear cleft (7) have been cited in the majority of studies as leading to worse hearing outcomes. From a practical standpoint, understanding these factors can be helpful in predicting which patients are at risk of having a poor hearing outcome and, therefore, are perhaps more suitable for staged tympano-ossicular reconstruction.

HIGHLIGHTS

- The goal of reconstruction of the tympanic membrane and ossicular chain is to provide a stable barrier between the moist middle ear and dry lateral epithelialized compartments while optimizing the ossicular coupling properties of the tympano-ossicular mechanism.
- Cartilage grafts are especially useful in reconstructing the tympanic membrane when the risk of graft failure or reacquisition of retraction is high.
- Ossiculoplasty utilizing the malleus neck can result in prosthesis stability and may afford additional acoustic benefits.
- Underlying factors related to the middle ear environment will greatly influence ossiculoplasty outcomes, no matter which techniques are utilized.

REFERENCES

1. Zollner F. The principles of plastic surgery of the sound-conducting apparatus. *J Laryngol Otol* 1955;69(10):637–652.
2. Wullstein H. The restoration of the function of the middle ear, in chronic otitis media. *Ann Otol Rhinol Laryngol* 1956;65(4):1021–1041.
3. Merchant SN, et al. Analysis of middle ear mechanics and application to diseased and reconstructed ears. *Am J Otol* 1997;18(2):139–154.
4. Merchant SN, et al. Toynbee memorial lecture 1997. Middle ear mechanics in normal, diseased and reconstructed ears. *J Laryngol Otol* 1998;112(8):715–731.
5. Rosowski JJ. Models of external and middle ear function. In: Mcmullen TA, Hawkins HS, Popper AN, Fay RR, eds. *The Springer handbook of auditory research.* New York: Springer-Verlag, 1996:15–61.
6. Aibara R, et al. Human middle-ear sound transfer function and cochlear input impedance. *Hear Res* 2001;152(1–2):100–109.
7. Merchant SN, et al. Middle ear mechanics of Type III tympanoplasty (stapes columella): II. Clinical studies. *Otol Neurotol* 2003;24(2):186–194.
8. Puria S, Peake WT, Rosowski JJ. Sound-pressure measurements in the cochlear vestibule of human-cadaver ears. *J Acoust Soc Am* 1997;101(5 Pt 1):2754–2770.
9. Mehta RP, et al. Determinants of hearing loss in perforations of the tympanic membrane. *Otol Neurotol* 2006;27(2):136–143.
10. Vincent R, Lopez A, Sperling NM. Malleus ankylosis: a clinical, audiometric, histologic, and surgical study of 123 cases. *Am J Otol* 1999;20(6):717–725.
11. Prasad KC, et al. Assessment of eustachian tube function in tympanoplasty. *Otolaryngol Head Neck Surg* 2009;140(6):889–893.
12. Collins WO, et al. Pediatric tympanoplasty: effect of contralateral ear status on outcomes. *Arch Otolaryngol Head Neck Surg* 2003;129(6):646–651.
13. Gluth MB, et al. Management of eustachian tube dysfunction with nasal steroid spray: a prospective, randomized, placebo-controlled trial. *Arch Otolaryngol Head Neck Surg* 2011;137(5):449–455.
14. Dornhoffer JL. Surgical management of the atelectatic ear. *Am J Otol* 2000;21(3):315–321.
15. Dornhoffer JL. Hearing results with cartilage tympanoplasty. *Laryngoscope* 1997;107(8):1094–1099.
16. Bellucci RJ. Dual classification of tympanoplasty. *Laryngoscope* 1973;83(11):1754–1758.
17. Aarnisalo AA, et al. Motion of the tympanic membrane after cartilage tympanoplasty determined by stroboscopic holography. *Hear Res* 2010;263(1–2):78–84.
18. Aarnisalo AA, et al. Middle ear mechanics of cartilage tympanoplasty evaluated by laser holography and vibrometry. *Otol Neurotol* 2009;30(8):1209–1214.
19. Gerber MJ, Mason JC, Lambert PR. Hearing results after primary cartilage tympanoplasty. *Laryngoscope* 2000;110(12):1994–1999.
20. Kyrodimos E, Sismanis A, Santos D. Type III cartilage "shield" tympanoplasty: an effective procedure for hearing improvement. *Otolaryngol Head Neck Surg* 2007;136(6):982–985.
21. Ozbek C, et al. A comparison of cartilage palisades and fascia in type 1 tympanoplasty in children: anatomic and functional results. *Otol Neurotol* 2008;29(5):679–683.
22. Morris DP, Bance M, Van Wijhe RG. How do cartilage and other material overlay over a prosthesis affect its vibration transmission properties in ossiculoplasty? *Otolaryngol Head Neck Surg* 2004;131(4):423–428.
23. Downey TJ, Champeaux AL, Silva AB. AlloDerm tympanoplasty of tympanic membrane perforations. *Am J Otolaryngol* 2003;24(1):6–13.
24. Dornhoffer J. Cartilage tympanoplasty: indications, techniques, and outcomes in a 1,000-patient series. *Laryngoscope* 2003;113(11):1844–1856.
25. Tos M. Cartilage tympanoplasty methods: proposal of a classification. *Otolaryngol Head Neck Surg* 2008;139(6):747–758.
26. Dornhoffer JL. Cartilage tympanoplasty. *Otolaryngol Clin North Am* 2006;39(6):1161–1176.
27. Beutner D, et al. Cartilage plate tympanoplasty. *Otol Neurotol* 2010;31(1):105–110.

28. Cabra J, Monux A. Efficacy of cartilage palisade tympanoplasty: randomized controlled trial. *Otol Neurotol* 2010;31(4):589–595.

29. Boone RT, Gardner EK, Dornhoffer JL. Success of cartilage grafting in revision tympanoplasty without mastoidectomy. *Otol Neurotol* 2004;25(5):678–681.

30. Moore GF. Candidate's thesis: revision tympanoplasty utilizing fossa triangularis cartilage. *Laryngoscope* 2002;112(9):1543–1554.

31. Jesic SD, et al. Temporalis fascia graft perforation and retraction after tympanoplasty for chronic tubotympanic otitis and attic retraction pockets: factors associated with recurrence. *Arch Otolaryngol Head Neck Surg* 2011;137(2):139–143.

32. Jung TT, Park SK. Mediolateral graft tympanoplasty for anterior or subtotal tympanic membrane perforation. *Otolaryngol Head Neck Surg* 2005;132(4):532–536.

33. Kartush JM, et al. Over-under tympanoplasty. *Laryngoscope* 2002;112(5):802–807.

34. Angeli SI, Kulak JL, Guzman J. Lateral tympanoplasty for total or near-total perforation: prognostic factors. *Laryngoscope* 2006;116(9):1594–1599.

35. Boone R, Dornhoffer J. Surgical correction of the lateralized tympanic membrane. *Laryngoscope* 2002;112(8 Pt 1):1509–1511.

36. Chien W, Rosowski JJ, Merchant SN. Investigation of the mechanics of Type III stapes columella tympanoplasty using laser-doppler vibrometry. *Otol Neurotol* 2007;28(6):782–787.

37. Yung MW. Literature review of alloplastic materials in ossiculoplasty. *J Laryngol Otol* 2003;117(6):431–436.

38. Goldenberg RA. Ossiculoplasty with composite prostheses. PORP and TORP. *Otolaryngol Clin North Am* 1994;27(4):727–745.

39. Goode RL, Nishihara S. Experimental models of ossiculoplasty. *Otolaryngol Clin North Am* 1994;27(4):663–675.

40. Coffey CS, Lee FS, Lambert PR. Titanium versus nontitanium prostheses in ossiculoplasty. *Laryngoscope* 2008;118(9):1650–1658.

41. Hales NW, Shakir FA, Saunders JE. Titanium middle ear prostheses in staged ossiculoplasty: does mass really matter? *Am J Otolaryngol* 2007;28(3):164–167.

42. Iniguez-Cuadra R, et al. Type III tympanoplasty with titanium total ossicular replacement prosthesis: anatomic and functional results. *Otol Neurotol* 2010;31(3):409–414.

43. Neff BA, et al. Tympano-ossiculoplasty utilizing the spiggle and theis titanium total ossicular replacement prosthesis. *Laryngoscope* 2003;113(9):1525–1529.

44. House JW, Teufert KB. Extrusion rates and hearing results in ossicular reconstruction. *Otolaryngol Head Neck Surg* 2001;125(3):135–141.

45. Bance M, et al. Comparison of the mechanical performance of ossiculoplasty using a prosthetic malleus-to-stapes head with a tympanic membrane-to-stapes head assembly in a human cadaveric middle ear model. *Otol Neurotol* 2004;25(6):903–909.

46. Baglam T, et al. Incudostapedial rebridging ossiculoplasty with bone cement. *Otolaryngol Head Neck Surg* 2009;141(2):243–246.

47. Ozer E, et al. Incudostapedial rebridging ossiculoplasty with bone cement. *Otol Neurotol* 2002;23(5):643–646.

48. O'Reilly RC, et al. Ossiculoplasty using incus interposition: hearing results and analysis of the middle ear risk index. *Otol Neurotol* 2005;26(5):853–858.

49. Iurato S, Marioni G, Onofri M. Hearing results of ossiculoplasty in Austin-Kartush group A patients. *Otol Neurotol* 2001;22(2):140–144.

50. Bared A, Angeli SI. Malleus handle: determinant of success in ossiculoplasty. *Am J Otolaryngol* 2010;31(4):235–240.

51. Beutner D, Luers JC, Huttenbrink KB. Cartilage 'shoe': a new technique for stabilisation of titanium total ossicular replacement prosthesis at centre of stapes footplate. *J Laryngol Otol* 2008;122(7):682–686.

52. Vincent R, et al. Ossiculoplasty with intact stapes and absent malleus: the silastic banding technique. *Otol Neurotol* 2005;26(5):846–852.

53. Black B. Neomalleus ossiculoplasty. *Otol Neurotol* 2002;23(5):636–642.

54. Blevins NH. Transfacial recess ossicular reconstruction: technique and early results. *Otol Neurotol* 2004;25(3):236–241.

55. Gluth MB, et al. Incus replacement malleostapedotomy in quiescent chronic otitis media with a mobile stapes footplate: an alternative to TORP in select cases. *Otol Neurotol* 2011;32(2):242–245.

56. Fisch U, Acar GO, Huber AM. Malleostapedotomy in revision surgery for otosclerosis. *Otol Neurotol* 2001;22(6):776–785.

57. Vincent R, Oates J, Sperling NM. Stapedotomy for tympanosclerotic stapes fixation: is it safe and efficient? A review of 68 cases. *Otol Neurotol* 2002;23(6):866–872.

58. Becvarovski Z, Kartush JM. Smoking and tympanoplasty: implications for prognosis and the middle ear risk Index (MERI). *Laryngoscope* 2001;111(10):1806–1811.

59. Kaylie DM, et al. Effects of smoking on otologic surgery outcomes. *Laryngoscope* 2009;119(7):1384–1390.

60. Mishiro Y, et al. Long-term hearing outcomes after ossiculoplasty in comparison to short-term outcomes. *Otol Neurotol* 2008;29(3):326–329.

61. Yung M, Vowler SL. Long-term results in ossiculoplasty: an analysis of prognostic factors. *Otol Neurotol* 2006;27(6):874–881.

62. Jackson CG, et al. Ossicular chain reconstruction: the TORP and PORP in chronic ear disease. *Laryngoscope* 1983;93(8):981–988.

63. Austin DF. Reporting results in tympanoplasty. *Am J Otol* 1985;6(1):85–88.

64. Kartush JM. Ossicular chain reconstruction. Capitulum to malleus. *Otolaryngol Clin North Am* 1994;27(4):689–715.

65. Black B. Ossiculoplasty prognosis: the spite method of assessment. *Am J Otol* 1992;13(6):544–551.

66. Dornhoffer JL, Gardner E. Prognostic factors in ossiculoplasty: a statistical staging system. *Otol Neurotol* 2001;22(3):299–304.

67. De Vos C, Gersdorff M, Gerard JM. Prognostic factors in ossiculoplasty. *Otol Neurotol* 2007;28(1):61–67.

68. Pinar E, et al. Evaluation of prognostic factors and middle ear risk index in tympanoplasty. *Otolaryngol Head Neck Surg* 2008;139(3):386–390.

69. Merenda D, et al. Tympanometric volume: a predictor of success of tympanoplasty in children. *Otolaryngol Head Neck Surg* 2007;136(2):189–192.

Otosclerosis 154

Brandon Isaacson   **Joe Walter Kutz Jr.**   **Peter S. Roland**

Otosclerosis (OS) is a fibrous osteodystrophy of the human otic capsule. Its clinical manifestations are primarily conductive hearing loss (CHL), although sensorineural hearing loss (SNHL) and mixed hearing loss (MHL) can also occur. The disease process causes abnormal resorption and deposition of bone. OS is noted clinically in 1% of the Caucasian population; it is transmitted in an autosomal dominant fashion but with incomplete penetrance. Females appear to be affected twice as often as males (1).

In 1873, Schwartze described a reddish hue medial to an intact tympanic membrane (TM), which was secondary to the increased vascularity of the cochlear promontory in active OS lesions (the phase known as otospongiosis). This finding is named after him and is known as Schwartze sign. It is seen in 10% of patients with OS. In 1881, von Troltsch noted abnormalities of the middle ear mucosa in this disease and was the first to use the term OS. In 1893, Politzer described OS as a primary disease of the otic capsule, rather than a condition related to previous episodes of inflammatory ear disease, as originally thought (2).

The clinical entity of OS was further described by Bezold in 1908, when he discussed its historical, physical, and audiometric findings. In 1912, Siebenmann discussed the possibility of OS causing SNHL. Since that time, numerous etiologies of OS have been suggested, including hereditary, endocrine, biochemical, metabolic, infectious (e.g., measles), traumatic, vascular, and even autoimmune factors (3). In fact, Lopez-Gonzalez and Delgado (4) suggested that oral vaccination with type II collagen may mitigate the autoimmune reaction in those susceptible to OS through hyposensitization. It is also possible that interplay of these different factors exist and vary from individual to individual, while causing the same pathologic and clinical findings. In other words, OS may be the common, final pathway of a clinically and genetically heterogeneous group of disorders (5).

EMBRYOLOGY

The maturation of the bony labyrinth plays a role in the pathogenesis of OS. The otic capsule arises from mesenchyme surrounding the otic vesicle at 4 weeks of embryologic development. At 8 weeks, the cartilaginous framework is initiated. At 16 weeks, endochondral osseous replacement of this framework begins in 14 identifiable centers. In some people, complete bony replacement does not occur and leaves cartilage in certain locations. One of these regions, the fissula ante fenestram, is anterior to the oval window (OW) and is usually the last area of endochondral bone formation in the labyrinth. According to temporal bone studies, this region is affected in 80% to 90% of patients with OS (6). In 1985, Schuknecht and Barber (7) reported other areas of predilection for otosclerotic lesions, such as the border of the round window (RW), the apical medial wall of the cochlea, the area posterior to the cochlear aqueduct, the region adjacent to the semicircular canals, and the stapes footplate itself (which is derived from otic capsule, as opposed to the superstructure, which is a branchial arch derivative).

HISTOLOGY

There are three forms of otosclerotic lesions: otospongiosis (early phase), transitional phase, and OS (late phase). The early, active phase lesions consist of histiocytes, osteoblasts, and the most active cell group, the osteocytes. The osteocytes resorb bone around preexisting blood vessels, which causes widening of the vascular channels and dilation of the microcirculation. Otoscopic or microscopic exam can reveal the reddish hue caused by these lesions (Schwartze sign if seen on clinical examination). As osteocytes become more involved, these areas grow rich in amorphous ground substance and deficient in mature collagen, resulting in formation of new spongy bone. With hematoxylin–eosin (H&E) staining, this new spongy bone appears densely blue. This was described in 1914 by Manasse and is known as the blue mantles of Manasse. Interestingly, mantles are found in up to 20% of normal temporal bones. On electron microscopy, the foci of perivascular bony invasion coalesce as the lesions enlarge within the otic capsule (7).

The predominant finding in the late phase of OS is the formation of sclerotic, dense bone in areas of previous osseous resorption. The vascular spaces that were once dilated are narrowed due to bony deposition. Within each temporal bone containing OS, lesions can be found in early, transitional, and late phases, although the overall histologic status of the developing lesions is fairly uniform. Although OS begins in endochondral bone, as the spongiosis and sclerosis continue, the endosteal and periosteal layers also become involved (8).

BASIC SCIENCE

A number of mechanisms including autoimmune, genetic, and infectious have all been described as potential causative factors for the development of OS. Definitive evidence for an autoimmune etiology for OS is currently lacking. Conflicting evidence exists for increased levels of type II and IX collagen antibodies in patients with OS. Animal models of type II collagen autoimmunity were found to have lesions similar to OS in contrast to another nearly identical study where autoimmune mice were found to have no lesions (5).

OS has a significant genetic component with seven distinct loci reported to date. Autosomal dominant transmission with incomplete penetrance is the predominant mode of inheritance. The OS loci identified include genes that regulate growth regulation, intercellular communication; cartilage, bone, and collagen homeostasis and metabolism. Additional work is needed to identify potential candidate genes involved in the pathogenesis of OS (9).

A number of findings point toward a viral etiology for OS. Measles antigens and RNA, as well as nucleocapsid structures identical to measles virus have all been identified in otosclerotic lesions. Increased levels of measles-specific IgG have also been detected in the perilymph of OS patients undergoing stapedectomy. It is not yet certain that the measles virus is involved in the development of OS, and the pathogenesis has yet to be elucidated (9).

A more in-depth understanding of the molecular biology of bone remodeling has shed additional light on the pathogenesis of OS. The otic capsule is unique compared to the rest of the skeleton in that after the age of one, no further osseous remodeling occurs. Bone remodeling is rigorously regulated via a balance between the cytokines and receptor: osteoprotegerin (OPG), receptor activator of nuclear factor kB (RANK), and RANK ligand (RANKL). RANKL is present on the surface of osteoblasts and binds to RANK receptors on the surface of osteoclast precursor cells, which results in osteoclast differentiation, activation,

and subsequent bone remodeling. Soluble OPG competes with RANKL in binding to the RANK receptor on the surface of osteoclast precursor cells and results in decreased bone remodeling. A fine balance exists between RANKL and OPG, which regulates skeletal remodeling including the otic capsule. High levels of OPG (reduced predilection for bone turnover) have been detected in the inner ear and are secreted into perilymph by type I fibrocytes located within the spiral ligament. It has been postulated that genetic, infectious, and autoimmune mechanisms likely alter this pathway, which eventually results in OS (9).

PATHOPHYSIOLOGY

The areas of OS involvement dictate the clinical presentation. The most common type involves the stapes and accounts for those cases in which CHL is the presenting symptom. The CHL is due to fixation of the stapes footplate, usually beginning at the fissula ante fenestram (Fig. 154.1). Progressive involvement of the footplate can create a thick focus of OS that fills the OW niche (obliterative OS) (5).

If OS involves only the footplate and spares the annular ligament, minimal fixation may occur. Such a thickened footplate is called a biscuit footplate. Because of minimal fixation, biscuit footplates can become mobilized inadvertently during a stapes procedure, placing the patient at a higher risk of postoperative SNHL. The RW is involved in 30% of all clinical cases of OS; complete closure of this niche is uncommon (10).

SNHL as a result of OS is an ongoing controversial subject. Some patients with OS have a greater amount of SNHL than expected considering their age and history of noise exposure. The mechanism for the SNHL is possibly the liberation of toxic metabolites into the inner ear with resultant injury to neuroepithelium, vascular compromise, or direct extension of lesions into the cochlea, causing

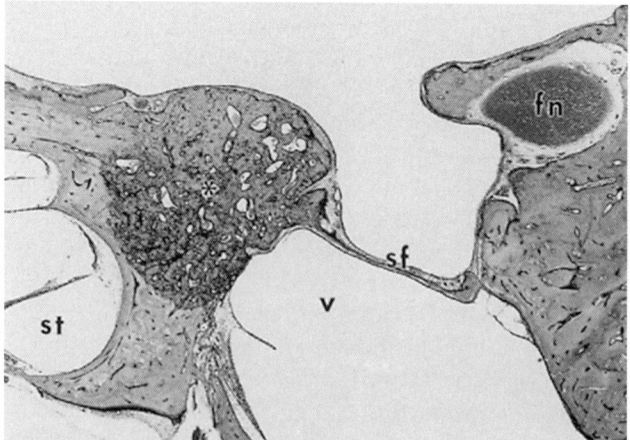

Figure 154.1 Photomicrograph of temporal bone section in a 79-year-old Caucasian male demonstrating a mature otosclerotic focus (*) involving the promontory and anterior stapes footplate (sf). st, scala tympani; v, vestibule; fn, facial nerve. (×20) (Courtesy of M.M. Paparella, director, and S. Lamey, coordinator, Otopathology Laboratory, University of Minnesota).

disruption of electrolytes and changes in basilar membrane mechanics. SNHL is usually associated with significant stapedial OS, although some otologists contend that isolated pure SNHL can be seen without associated CHL. The latter presentation is also known as cochlear OS (11).

Shambaugh (11) has suggested seven criteria to identify patients suffering from SNHL due to OS:

1. Schwartze sign in either ear
2. Family history of OS
3. Unilateral CHL consistent with OS and bilateral, symmetric SNHL
4. Audiogram with a flat or "cookie-bite" curve with excellent discrimination
5. Progressive pure cochlear loss beginning at the usual age of onset for OS
6. Computed tomography (CT) scan showing demineralization of the cochlea typical for OS
7. Stapedial reflex demonstrating the biphasic "on–off effect" seen before stapedial fixation

Vestibular symptoms occur in up to 40% of patients with OS. OS lesions have been described in the lateral semicircular canal during fenestration procedures (which have been replaced by the stapedectomy/stapedotomy). The vestibular symptoms are usually not severe, but objective evidence can be obtained with electronystagmography testing. Non-Ménière-type vertigo or disequilibrium associated with OS has been termed OS inner ear syndrome. It is important to differentiate this disorder from Ménière disease or superior semicircular canal dehiscence (SSCD). Ménière disease is an absolute contraindication for stapedectomy/stapedotomy. When the endolymphatic space is dilated (endolymphatic hydrops), the saccule may be enlarged to the point that it adheres to the undersurface of the stapes footplate. A stapes procedure can injure the saccule and result in profound SNHL. The distinction between OS inner ear syndrome and other causes of dizziness is based on differences in clinical presentation. Rarely does the inner ear syndrome of OS cause well-defined episodes of severe rotational vertigo, nausea, vomiting, and fluctuating SNHL. Dizziness in OS inner ear syndrome is milder but more persistent; low-frequency SNHL is generally not present (12).

In 2004, Mikulec et al. (13) reported on eight patients with presumed OS/unilateral CHL that did not improve after a stapes procedure. These patients were ultimately found to have SSCD. In contrast to typical SSCD patients, these patients had only CHL and no vestibular symptoms. One should keep this entity in mind, especially in a patient with CHL and pressure or sound-induced vertiginous symptoms. Intact acoustic reflexes in the setting of CHL should prompt further imaging to evaluate for an inner ear third window. SSCD, posterior and lateral semicircular canal dehiscence, enlarged vestibular aqueduct, and modiolar deficiencies (i.e., X-linked stapes gusher) can all present with a CHL or MHL with intact acoustic reflexes (13).

EPIDEMIOLOGY

OS is transmitted in an autosomal dominant fashion with incomplete penetrance (25% to 40%). The degree of penetrance is related to the distribution of lesions in the otic capsule. Some lesions are located where they cannot cause clinical symptoms. About 10% of Caucasians have histologic findings of OS. However, of those with histologic changes, only 12% have clinical symptoms; thus, overall, this represents about 1% of the Caucasian population. In the Japanese and South American populations, the incidence is 50% of that in Caucasians. The African American population has fewer cases of OS; only 1% demonstrate histologic findings of the disease. In all races, when one ear is affected, the contralateral ear shows histologic involvement 80% of the time. Generally, the lesions occur in similar anatomic locations and at similar histologic phases. The age at which symptoms become apparent is variable due to the insidious progression of hearing loss, but hearing loss often begins between the ages of 15 and 45 years. The average age at presentation is 33 years (14).

About 60% of patients with clinical OS report a family history of this condition. The remaining 40%, as suggested by Morrison and Bundey (14), make up a collection of cases that fall into one of the following categories:

1. Autosomal dominant inherited cases with failure of penetrance in other family members
2. Phenocopies (an individual expressing a trait that is environmentally as opposed to genetically induced)
3. New mutations
4. Those rare cases transmitted by alternate modes of inheritance (i.e., autosomal recessive)

OS has been reported to advance more rapidly in females than males, although no difference has been noted in age at onset. A recent study by Clayton et al. (15) examined the relationship in elderly women between osteoporosis and OS; both diseases show some similarities, including an association with the *COL1A1* gene. The study showed that a much higher percentage of women with OS also had osteoporosis as compared with a similar aged group with only presbycusis ($P < 0.007$). Juvenile OS may progress more rapidly than the adult form. Hormonal factors may play a role; some females with OS appear to have their condition worsen during pregnancy. Estrogen receptors have been noted in the OS plaques. However, more recent data minimize the association between pregnancy and worsening of OS (9).

HISTORY AND PHYSICAL EXAMINATION

Patients with OS usually present with a slowly progressive hearing loss over a period of years. Patients may describe hearing speech more easily in noisy situations. The CHL improves the signal to noise ratio by subduing background noise (paracusis of Willis). Tinnitus is present in 75% of patients. A complete head and neck examination is performed to rule out concurrent otolaryngologic abnormalities. Otomicroscopic examination with pneumatic insufflations is done of the external auditory canal (EAC) and TM to asses for the presence of a middle ear effusion or mass, cholesteatoma, or TM retraction. The physical appearance of the TM is normal in most patients with OS. A Schwartze sign (a red to pink appearance of the cochlear promontory occasionally seen in active OS through the TM) may be present.

The primary purpose of performing a tuning fork exam is to confirm the findings of the audiogram. The Rinne test should demonstrate bone conduction to be better than air conduction (Rinne negative) in patients contemplating a stapes procedure. In the initial phases of the disease, CHL may be limited to the 256-Hz tuning fork. As footplate fixation progresses, the 512- and 1,024-Hz tuning forks will "reverse" as well. The amount of air–bone gap required to reverse the tuning forks are about 10 to 15 dB for the 256-Hz tuning fork and 20 to 25 dB for the 512-Hz tuning fork. The Weber test should lateralize to the ear with the greater degree of CHL, although this test is also affected by concurrent SNHL. If the tuning fork exam does not correlate with the audiogram, repeat testing is recommended since inadequate masking may falsely lead the clinician to believe a conductive loss is present in the setting of anacusis (16).

AUDIOLOGIC TESTING

The main objective measurement in OS is the audiogram (Fig. 154.2). On the audiogram, OS is seen as a widening air–bone gap that usually begins in the low frequencies. Variable degrees of SNHL may also be present. Bone conduction may show a 20-dB loss at 2,000 Hz and a 5-dB loss at 500 and 4,000 Hz. Such an apparent depression of bone conduction at 2,000 Hz is known as Carhart notch, which is most commonly seen in OS but can be seen in other types of CHL. This notch is an artifact of the audiogram and disappears after a stapedectomy. It is secondary to stapes fixation and a resultant change in the resonance of the otic capsule (17).

Word recognition scores are usually excellent in patients with OS even in the later stages of the disease process. Impedance can show reduced TM compliance (type A or As). Stapedial reflexes are characteristically absent in the setting of CHL. Intact stapedial reflexes can occasionally be observed in the earliest stages of OS depending on the degree of fixation. With early stapes fixation, a characteristic abnormal decrease in impedance may be noted at the onset and offset of the eliciting signal. This is the on–off effect of OS. The presence of stapedial reflexes with a significant CHL warrants evaluation for an inner ear third window (i.e., SSCD). Vestibular testing should be included when dizziness is present. Although there are not characteristic findings for OS inner ear syndrome, findings or a

clinical history suggestive of SSCD or Ménière disease will alter treatment planning (17).

High-resolution CT scans can help identify or confirm patients with OS. Radiolucent areas in and around the cochlea are noted early in the course of the disease, creating the "halo sign." Diffuse sclerosis is found in mature cases (Fig. 154.3). Negative results on the CT scan are not diagnostic because some patients have disease below the capabilities of scanning protocols. The CT can rule out middle ear masses, vascular anomalies, or facial nerve abnormalities but is not an essential part of the workup. These scans can also assess the ossicular chain in addition to the osseous labyrinth (cochlea, semicircular canals) (18).

DIFFERENTIAL DIAGNOSIS

The differential diagnosis should include other causes of CHL or MHL. A history of progressive CHL or MHL in the absence of history of trauma or infection but with the presence of a normal TM limits the possibilities. However, a definitive diagnosis can only be made during exploratory tympanotomy. The most common conditions that mimic OS are those that result in ossicular discontinuity or exert a mass effect on the TM or ossicles. A history of recurrent chronic otitis media suggests an ossicular discontinuity due to incus necrosis. The TM may be normal or thickened or atrophic in cases of chronic infection. The TM in these ears is sometimes abnormally compliant, which can be manifested as a type Ad tympanogram. Fibrous union of the incudostapedial (IS) joint can produce an air–bone gap wider in the high frequencies than in the lower frequencies (16).

Fractures or displacement of the ossicular chain is not uncommon in the setting of temporal bone trauma. Hemotympanum or otorrhea is frequently encountered in the immediate period following the injury. A follow-up examination with audiometry is typically recommended in patients with temporal bone fractures to allow for resolution of hemotympanum and spontaneous healing of TM perforation. In cases of traumatic ossicular chain displacement, a fibrous union often forms with resultant resolution of CHL. Distorted TM surface landmarks occasionally provide evidence of prior temporal bone trauma that has resulted in CHL or MHL. A fracture of the stapes superstructure or incus long process may have a similar audiometric configuration as OS.

Congenital stapedial footplate fixation presents at an earlier age than does juvenile OS. De la Cruz noted in his series that congenital footplate fixation was detectable at age 3, whereas juvenile OS was not detectable until about age 10 (19). In the setting of lateral ossicular chain fixation, the malleus and/or incus become fixed in the epitympanum (usually at the superior malleolar ligament), resulting in immobility of all the ossicles; this can occur congenitally or may be acquired through tympanosclerosis. The entire ossicular chain must be examined with

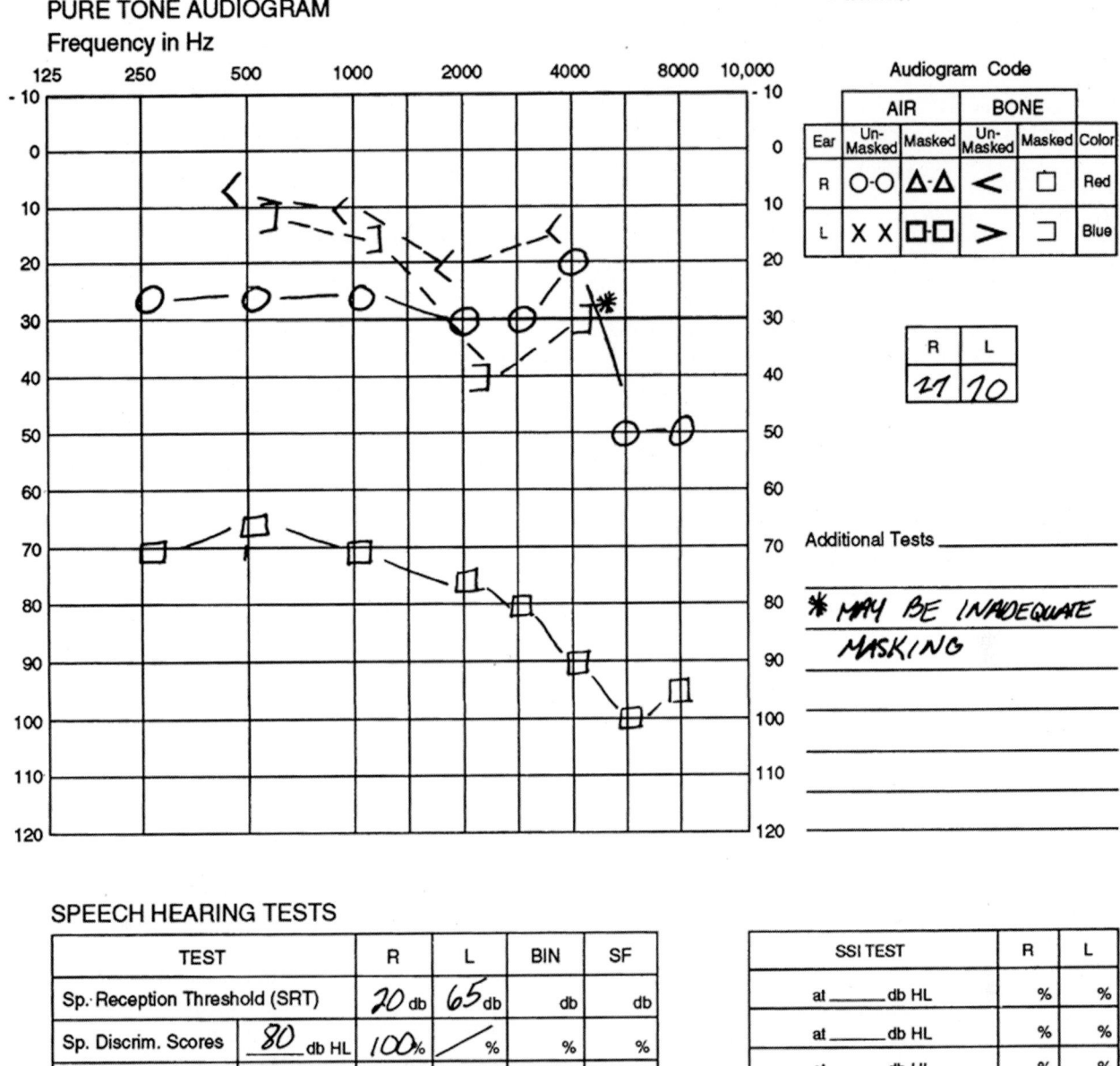

PURE TONE AUDIOGRAM
Frequency in Hz

Audiogram Code					
	AIR		**BONE**		
Ear	Un-Masked	Masked	Un-Masked	Masked	Color
R	O-O	Δ-Δ	<	☐	Red
L	X X	☐-☐	>	⊐	Blue

R	L
27	70

Additional Tests _____

* MAY BE INADEQUATE MASKING

SPEECH HEARING TESTS

TEST		R	L	BIN	SF
Sp. Reception Threshold (SRT)		20 db	65 db	db	db
Sp. Discrim. Scores	80 db HL	100%	%	%	%
(PB)	90 db HL	%	100%	%	%
	___ db HL	%	%	%	%
Most Comfortable Loudness (MCL)		db	db	db	db
Loudness Discomfort Level (LDL)		db	db	db	db

SSI TEST	R	L
at ___ db HL	%	%
at ___ db HL	%	%
at ___ db HL	%	%

Figure 154.2 An audiogram of a 27-year-old Caucasian woman with OS demonstrating a near-maximum CHL in the left ear and a Carhart notch at 2,000 Hz in both ears. Notice that discrimination remains at 100% in both ears.

every exploratory tympanotomy to avoid overlooking this lesion. Tympanosclerosis can mimic OS, but a history of recurrent otitis media or tympanostomy tubes is usually present. In addition, the TM is often thickened with associated myringosclerosis. Persistent middle ear effusion, neoplasms of the middle ear and EAC (such as glomus tumors or facial nerve tumors), and chronic suppurative otitis media with and without cholesteatoma can also cause CHL. Audiometry and physical examination should help make the diagnosis apparent (16).

Paget disease (osteitis deformans) is a disease with diffuse bony involvement that is histologically similar to OS. In contrast to OS, Paget disease begins in the periosteal layer and involves the endochondral bone last. Temporal

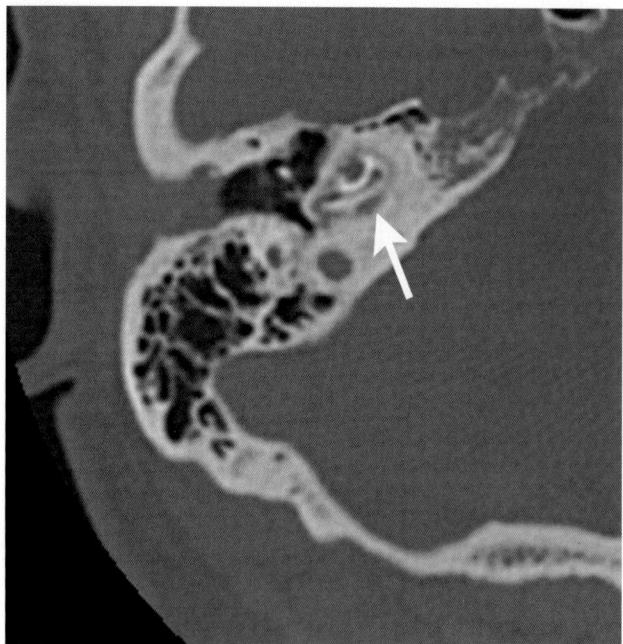

Figure 154.3 High-resolution axial temporal bone CT scan demonstrates extensive OS involving the right cochlea. A classic "halo" sign (*arrow*) surrounds the cochlea.

bone involvement can produce SNHL, but stapes involvement or fixation rarely occurs (20).

Osteogenesis imperfect (van der Hoeve-de-Kleyn syndrome) is an autosomal dominant defect of osteoblast activity resulting in multiple fractures. Stapes fixation and unique blue sclera are also found in 40% to 50% of affected patients. Stapes surgery can be performed in these patients, usually with results similar to those in patients with OS (Table 154.1) (21).

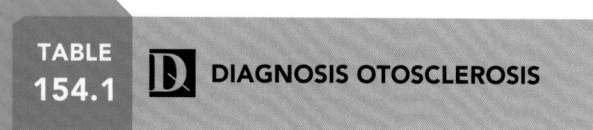

TABLE 154.1   DIAGNOSIS OTOSCLEROSIS

History
 Progressive hearing loss
 Family history of OS
 Tinnitus
 Possible vestibular symptoms (rule our Ménière or SSCD)
 Otitis media/otorrhea (absent)
 Head trauma (absent)
Physical examination
 Tympanic membrane (normal)
 Schwartze sign
 Rinne test (negative at 256 and 512 Hz)
 Weber test (lateralizes to side with greater CHL)
Ancillary studies
 Audiogram (assess for CHL, mixed HL, SNHL, Carhart notch)
 Tympanometry (type A or As; absent or on–off stapedial reflex)
 Imaging (CT scan showing radiolucent areas around bony labyrinth)

CHL, conductive hearing loss; CT, computed tomography; HL, hearing loss; SNHL, sensorineural hearing loss; SSCD, superior semicircular canal dehiscence.

MANAGEMENT

Ninety percent of patients with histologic evidence of OS are asymptomatic; active lesions usually mature without stapedial fixation or cochlear loss. In the symptomatic patient, slowly progressive CHL and SNHL usually begins between the ages of 30 and 50 years with a peak incidence in the 40s (22).The disease may advance more rapidly at times, possibly depending on environmental factors. Periods of progress may be followed by periods of quiescence. The CHL stabilizes at a maximum of 50 to 60 dB.

AMPLIFICATION

Patients with hearing loss secondary to OS should be offered the option of amplification with typical hearing aids as an alternative to observation or surgery. Unilateral or bilateral hearing aids may provide effective treatment. Some patients may not be suitable candidates for surgery, making amplification the only reasonable option. Another option is to use bone conduction hearing aid. A bone anchored hearing aid (BAHA) is another option for patients with CHL or MHL secondary to OS who cannot wear a hearing aid. Two BAHA systems are currently available in the United States (BAHA, Cochlear Corporation; PONTO, Oticon). A BAHA bypasses the ossicular chain and amplifies sound that stimulates the cochlea directly through bone conduction. McLarnon et al. (23) reported that satisfaction levels for three groups of patients receiving a BAHA was highest in patients with congenital aural atresia, followed by patients with OS, and was lowest in patients with single-sided deafness (e.g., acoustic neuroma patients).

Although amplification avoids potential risk of profound hearing loss that could occur from surgery, it is not capable of providing many of the benefits or patient satisfaction of successful stapes surgery. Hearing aids are usually not used at night. The canal occlusion effect, difficulties with feedback, and the physical sensation of the device within the EAC are disagreeable and have a negative impact on patient satisfaction. In addition, in the United States most insurance companies cover the costs of surgery but few cover the cost of hearing aids, which include batteries and a finite lifespan of 3 to 5 years.

For those with severe to profound SNHL bilaterally due to OS, cochlear implantation is an option. However, Rotteveel et al. (24) reported that partial electrode insertions, misplacement of the electrode, and inadvertent facial nerve stimulation are more likely than in patients without OS and normal cochlear anatomy.

MEDICAL MANAGEMENT

Medical therapy can be considered for all patients with OS, whether they are managed by observation, amplification, or surgery. In 1923, Escot was the first to suggest the use of

TABLE 154.2	COMPLICATIONS OTOSCLEROSIS SURGERY

Intraoperative
   Bleeding (high jugular bulb, tympanomeatal flap, persistent stapedial artery, mucoperiosteum)
   Facial nerve injury (<1%)
   Perilymph gusher
   Fracture/dislocation of incus
   Floating footplate

Postoperative
   Acute otitis media
   TM perforation
   CHL (middle ear effusion, displaced prosthesis, incus erosion)
   SNHL, vertigo, tinnitus (due to intraoperative trauma, labyrinthitis, reparative granuloma, perilymph fistula)
   Facial nerve palsy (local anesthetic, intraoperative trauma, delayed Bell palsy)

CHL, conductive hearing loss; OS, otosclerosis; SNHL, sensorineural hearing loss; TM, tympanic membrane.

calcium fluoride for the treatment of OS (25). Shambaugh (11) predicted stabilization of OS lesions with the use of sodium fluoride. Fluoride ions replace the usual hydroxyl radical, forming a more stable fluorapatite complex instead of hydroxyapatite crystal. The fluorapatite complex resists osteoclastic degradation that has been confirmed with histology. The effect of fluoride on OS remains to be elucidated, but many otologists prescribe it to stabilize active OS in an attempt to prevent progression of CHL, SNHL, and dizziness (25).

The recommended dosage of sodium fluoride is 20 to 120 mg/d. Evaluation of efficacy may be based on the disappearance of Schwartze sign (if it was present), stabilization of hearing, and improvement in the CT appearance of the otic capsule. Side effects of this therapy are usually minor. Gastrointestinal side effects (nausea) may affect patient compliance, but these effects can be minimized by lowering the dose or using enteric-coated tablets. Bone, muscle, or joint pain occasionally occurs with fluoride therapy, which usually resolves with temporary discontinuation of therapy. Rarely, fluid retention, cutaneous eruptions, and eye problems occur. Using this treatment regimen, patients may improve or show no progression of their symptoms (Table 154.2) (25).

SURGICAL MANAGEMENT

Although Rosen (8) introduced the stapes mobilization procedure in 1953, most otologists replace the stapes superstructure with a prosthesis (due to reduced risk of recurrent fixation). The stapedectomy was popularized by John Shea in the late 1950s (26). He removed the entire footplate and placed a vein graft to close off the vestibule. The stapes superstructure was reconstructed with a polyethylene prosthesis (26). This procedure has since been

modified by using a wire prosthesis with an attached piece of fat, connective tissue, or gelatin material. The use of gelatin material in replacement of the footplate is no longer advocated secondary to the increased risk of reparative granuloma formation. Partial stapedectomy and stapedotomy have also been performed (instead of a total stapedectomy). Further modifications of these procedures have been described, but the essential principles have remained the same (27).

PATIENT SELECTION AND CONTRAINDICATIONS

The clinical circumstances favoring successful stapes surgery include unacceptable CHL, reversal of the Rinne 512-Hz tuning fork exam (bone conduction greater than air conduction), and good word recognition. When maximal CHL due to OS coexists with significant SNHL, detection of the bone line and conductive component can be difficult due to the limits of the audiometer. The situation is worse with bilateral MHL. Air-conduction thresholds may be present at very low levels (90 to 100 dB) or entirely absent. A history of progressive hearing loss should raise suspicion that OS may be involved. Suspicion should be heightened if discrimination scores or the ability to function appears much better than one would expect with such a significant degree of hearing loss. The presence of As tympanograms, abnormalities of stapedial reflex, or a family history of OS should raise suspicion even further. Use of the tuning forks may also separate advanced OS from SNHL of other causes (28).

A CT scan will sometimes permit a diagnosis of advanced OS when audiometry is inconclusive. If advanced OS is suspected, exploratory tympanotomy should be considered. Stapedectomy in such a setting can produce meaningful results. Air-conduction thresholds and discrimination scores can be improved enough to allow more effective amplification (29).

Age is an important consideration when contemplating stapes surgery. A temporal bone CT scan is recommended in any patient presenting with a normal otoscopic exam and conductive or MHL present since childhood. Inner ear malformations are occasionally identified in the pediatric age group and can present with mixed or CHL. Amplification is typically recommended when an inner ear malformation is identified in patients with conductive or MHL (30). The very young patient has a higher incidence of OW reclosure after a successful initial procedure. Although revision can be performed, a secondary procedure in any patient has a reduced success rate and a greater risk for postoperative SNHL. De la Cruz noted that in addition to being manifest at an earlier age, congenital footplate fixation is less likely to have a positive family history (19). Half of the children with juvenile OS have a positive family history, but only 10% of children with congenital footplate fixation have other family members with CHL. Patients with X-linked CHL have a high incidence of poststapedectomy profound SNHL due to a perilymph (cerebrospinal fluid [CSF] leak) gusher. The incidence of congenital anomalies of the malleus and incus is substantially higher in children with congenital footplate fixation (25%) than in children with juvenile OS (3%). This difference in abnormalities of the remainder of the ossicular chain probably accounts for the poorer results. Eighty-two percent of the children with juvenile OS had closure of the air–bone gap to within 10 dB. This is in contrast to children who had congenital footplate fixation: only 44% had closure within 10 dB. Very young children with OS are also at greater risk postoperatively due to their increased incidence of otitis media and eustachian tube dysfunction (27).

Age is an important variable for surgical outcome; poorer results in the high-frequency range have been seen in older patients who have undergone stapes surgery. However, Meyer and Lambert (30) reviewed the recent literature and reported that primary and revision stapedectomy is still a reasonable option in elderly patients. Lifestyle and occupation are important factors in selecting patients for stapedectomy. Persons whose activities include repeated exposure to barometric pressure changes (e.g., scuba diver) may be at greater risk for postoperative fistula and prosthesis dislocation. Patients whose work or hobbies dictate excellent balance should be considered questionable candidates for surgery. Amplification instead of surgery is recommended in individuals whom taste is of the utmost importance (e.g., chefs, vintners), secondary to the risk of stretching or cutting the chorda tympani nerve with resultant dysgeusia (31).

Patients with otologic complaints not attributed to their OS must be carefully evaluated. For example, patients with Ménière disease and OS have a greater risk of cochlear hearing loss after stapedectomy. Patients with TM perforations and OS should have their perforations successfully repaired before attempted stapedectomy (i.e., staging of the ear). The incidence of severe to profound SNHL is much greater if stapedectomy is performed in an ear with a perforation. Patients with a history of severe eustachian tube dysfunction or a history of cholesteatoma are not good candidates for stapedectomy. Those with canal exostoses that are obstructing surgical access should have them removed before the stapedectomy. Relative contraindications for stapes surgery include the presence of an external or middle ear infection or effusion, suspected endolymphatic hydrops, active OS (positive Schwartze sign, pregnancy, and TM atelectasis). Patients with external ear infections or otitis media can undergo stapes surgery once the process has resolved. Patients presenting with OS and endolymphatic hydrops can undergo stapes surgery if they have been symptom free from their Ménière disease for at least 6 months. An absolute contraindication for stapes surgery is OS in an only hearing ear (27).

Stapes surgery should initially commence with the poorer hearing ear in patients with bilateral OS. The likelihood of achieving serviceable hearing in a unilateral MHL is an important consideration. Improved communication in such a patient may not be achieved after elimination of the CHL due to the continued SNHL. Some surgeons believe that significant high-frequency SNHL after stapedectomy in the first ear contraindicates attempting the second. A minimum of approximately 6 months should elapse before attempting surgery on the second ear due to the small but present risk of delayed postoperative hearing loss (32).

PATIENT COUNSELING

Observation, fluoride use, and a trial of hearing aid use are discussed with every patient, whether they have CHL or MHL. The patient must understand the elective nature of the procedure. The patient must be candidly informed of the risk of stapedectomy (postoperative deafness of less than 2%).

Stretching or contusion of the chorda tympani nerve is quite common and can produce alteration of taste (or rarely, dryness of the mouth). When these symptoms occur, they are usually self-limited and disappear in a few weeks or months. A severely stretched or contused chorda tympani nerve may produce more symptoms than one that is divided. Dehiscence of the fallopian canal over the OW can permit exposure or prolapse of the facial nerve. If the nerve is traumatized or injured during the stapes procedure, facial nerve palsy can result. Fortunately iatrogenic facial nerve paralysis is quite rare in the setting of stapes surgery (less than 1:1,000) (33). Facial nerve paralysis occurs less than 0.5% of the time and most commonly presents 7 to 10 days after surgery secondary to reactivation of the herpes simplex virus. Delayed facial paralysis is managed with oral prednisone, antivirals, and appropriate eye care (34).

A postoperative TM perforation may occur 2% of the time as a consequence of trauma or vascular injury to the TM flap. Acute balance disturbance is common after stapedectomy. It usually resolves in 3 to 7 days. Long-term balance disturbances or vertigo rarely occur. Sparano et al. (35) reported that 85% of patients with tinnitus improved after stapedectomy (with 52.5% reporting complete resolution, 12.5% reporting no change, and 2.5% reporting worsening of their tinnitus).

SURGICAL TECHNIQUE

A well-performed stapes procedure is gratifying for both surgeon and patient; however, stapes surgery is one of the most technically challenging procedures performed by an otologist. One concern about current resident training is the paucity of stapes surgery being performed. Prior to graduation, the average number of cases a resident performs as the operating surgeon is three. Vrabec and Coker (36) proposed that the number of surgical OS cases per surgeon could be decreasing due to the use of measles vaccination and because the number of surgeons able to perform the surgery has increased significantly over the past 30 years. The pros and cons of local versus general anesthesia must be presented to the patient. Although general anesthesia is often easier for the patient and surgeon, local anesthesia may be safer to the patient (systemically) and to hearing preservation. Local anesthesia allows the patient to provide feedback about whether any dizziness is occurring during the procedure, allowing the surgeon to terminate the procedure momentarily or permanently. The patient can also let the surgeon know about the status of hearing improvement or loss intraoperatively.

Two keys to stapes surgery are adequate exposure and hemostasis. Preoperatively, the ear canal and TM are carefully inspected for evidence of inflammation or infection that would dictate postponement of the procedure. The patient can also be consented for use of endaural or postauricular approaches if the ear canal is too small for a transcanal approach. Ear canal vibrissae may be trimmed to improved operative exposure. Trauma to the drum or the ear canal from the preparation can occur, making the procedure more difficult. The ear canal is injected with local (1% lidocaine with 1:100,000 epinephrine) for both anesthetic and vasoconstrictive effect with care being taken to avoid blebbing of the osseous canal skin. The ear is then prepped and draped in the usual sterile fashion. The largest speculum that can be placed is used; in adults, a 7-mm speculum can usually be placed. Some surgeons prefer to use a black speculum as opposed to a silver speculum; the black color absorbs light and is less likely to reflect light from the microscope back to the surgeon. It is often possible to dilate the ear canal during the procedure with progressively larger speculums. A speculum holder is used by some surgeons to reduce the technical demands of stapes surgery. A tympanomeatal flap is elevated from the 6 o'clock to 12 o'clock position superior to the level of the lateral process of the malleus. The superior exposure is important to allow inspection of the epitympanum and lateral ossicular chain if necessary. The flap is approximately 6 mm wide, as measured from the fibrous annulus. This flap must be sufficient to cover any osseous defect created by curetting the scutum (Fig. 154.4).

The TM is elevated with the fibrous annulus (Fig. 154.5). The chorda tympani nerve is identified and preserved if possible. Enough scutum (the medial most posterior–superior EAC wall) is removed to visualize the OW, pyramidal process, and the tympanic facial nerve (Fig. 154.6). The scutum may be removed either with a sharp curette or drill. Care is taken to assess whether the facial nerve has an aberrant course or if the nerve is dehiscent or herniating too much to allow the procedure to continue. Prior to assessing stapes movement, the lateral ossicular chain is assessed for normal motion; one needs to rule out other causes of preoperative CHL. The stapes superstructure and footplate are palpated. A RW reflex can also be assessed.

A stapes mobilization instead of a stapedectomy or stapedotomy can be performed in selected cases. Stapes mobilization may be performed in a select group of

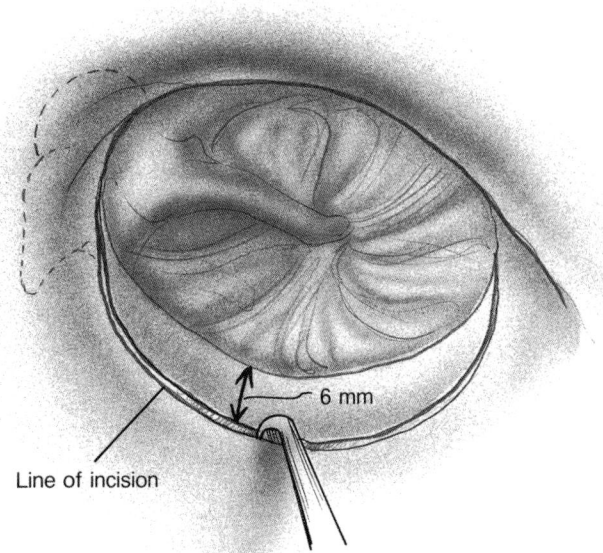

Figure 154.4 Typical design for a tympanomeatal flap.

patients, in whom a small point of fixation from OS can be seen and where improved stapes mobility can be clearly demonstrated. This technique can also be used in cases of tympanosclerosis. Poe (37) described a minimally invasive mobilization using an endoscope and the argon laser to potentially avoid the placement of a prosthesis; he called the procedure a stapedioplasty. Long-term follow-up of patients undergoing stapes mobilization frequently demonstrate refixation (38).

Anterior crurotomy with partial stapedectomy, as described by Hough in 1960, requires removal of only the anterior footplate and crus (39). This procedure is helpful in a patient with isolated anterior fixation at the fissula ante fenestram. The footplate is fractured in its midportion, and only the anterior half is removed. A

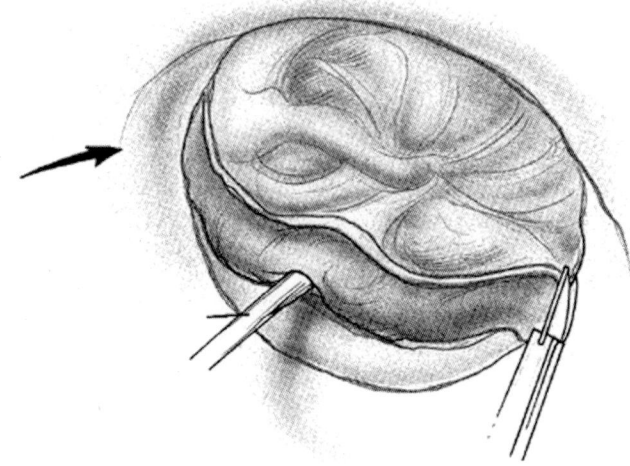

Figure 154.5 Technique for tympanomeatal flap elevation. The skin is elevated to the tympanic sulcus, and then the annulus is elevated from the sulcus.

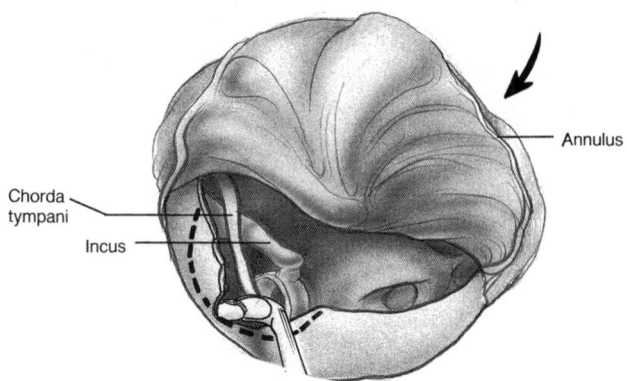

Figure 154.6 The tympanomeatal flap is now elevated. The *dotted line* indicates the area of bone removal for exposure to the OW.

connective tissue graft is then placed over the exposed area. The IS joint is not disturbed. The stapedial tendon is not divided, which makes this technique of potential benefit to patients working in a noisy environment (39). This technique has been further modified with the introduction of the laser that facilitates removal of the anterior crus and footplate (38).

Introduction of the laser has significantly reduced the technical demands of stapes surgery especially in revision cases. Perkins (40) was the first to use the laser in the treatment of OS in 1980. Since his original description, several types of lasers have been used: argon, potassium–titanyl–phosphate (KTP), erbium–YAG, and carbon dioxide. A laser provides the surgeon with a "no touch" means of transecting the stapes crura and fenestrating the stapes footplate. A CO_2 laser allows for rapid vaporization of bone and soft tissue and is the least traumatic to the membranous labyrinth medial to the stapes footplate. KTP and argon have a more favorable hemostasis profile as compared to a CO_2 laser and up until recently had

the advantage of using a handheld probe as opposed to a micromanipulator. No difference has been shown between different types of lasers in terms of safety and efficacy or between lasers and the use of a drill or microinstruments. Surgeons using the laser should become very familiar with individual laser properties and settings (power, pulse duration, pulse interval) so as to reduce the risk of thermal injuries to the facial nerve and inner ear. Irrigation, short pulse durations, and clustering laser shots all serve to reduce heat in the operative site, thus reducing the risk of thermal injuries. A retrospective study of patients undergoing argon laser or carbon dioxide laser stapedotomy (~60 patients in each group) demonstrated no difference in the incidence of postoperative complications, hearing improvement, or speech discrimination (41). The surgeon's operative experience and skill are considered the most important factors in determining the success and incidence of complications.

Surgeon preference often dictates the whether one should perform a total stapedectomy, partial stapedectomy, or stapedotomy with the current practice trending toward partial preservation of the footplate. In patients undergoing stapedectomy or stapedotomy, a measuring tool is used to assess the distance between the footplate and the distal incus long process. Placing a control hole in the stapes footplate is sometimes performed to reduce the risk of injuring the membranous labyrinth in the event that the footplate subluxes from the OW while manipulating the stapes (Fig. 154.7). Dividing the IS joint prior to transecting the stapedial tendon provides additional stability to the stapes thus reducing the chance of floating or fracturing the footplate. A laser or otologic scissors are used to divide the stapedius tendon allowing visualization of the posterior crus of the stapes. Transecting the posterior crus of the stapes with a laser reduces the chance of a floating or fractured stapes footplate. The anterior crus of the stapes, in some cases, can also be transected with a laser. The stapes superstructure is then down-fractured toward

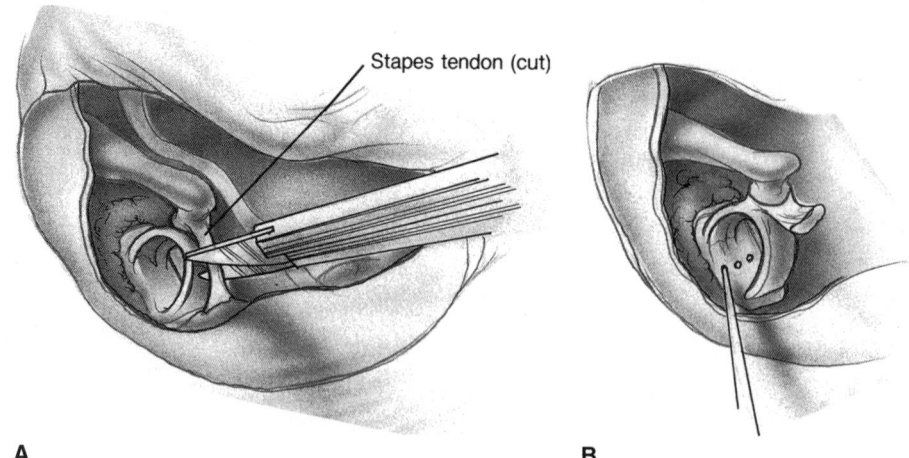

A   **B**

Figure 154.7 A: The tympanomeatal flap is now elevated, and bone has been removed. The stapedial tendon is divided by a pair of microscissors. **B:** Control holes are placed in the stapedial footplate.

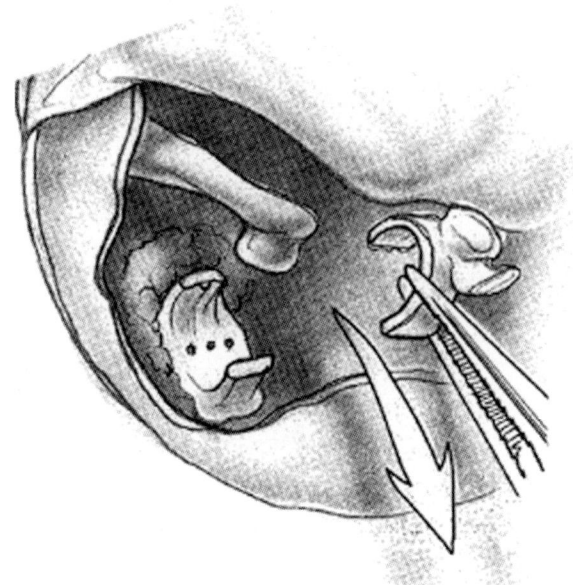

Figure 154.8 The stapedial superstructure is removed after fracturing of the anterior and posterior crus.

the promontory and is extracted (Fig. 154.8). The entire footplate is then removed in a piecemeal fashion using small right angle hooks of varying sizes for a stapedectomy (Fig. 154.9). Care is taken to avoid injuring the inner ear now that the vestibule has been exposed. Perilymph may be suctioned in an area away from the vestibule. However, one must avoid direct suctioning in the vestibule and a resultant dry vestibule, which has a risk of postoperative deafness. The OW is sealed with a graft, and the prosthesis is placed (Fig. 154.10). The most common tissue types used for grafting are the dorsal hand vein, tragal perichondrium, or fascia. Schmerber et al. (42) recently reported that use of a vein graft (as opposed to perichondrium) showed better postoperative air–bone gap closure and a lower incidence of postoperative SNHL.

Some cases of OS have formation of exuberant sclerotic bone that fills and obliterates the OW niche. Obliterative OS is encountered less commonly now than previously. When present in one ear, obliterative OS is present in the contralateral ear in 50% of cases. Obliterative OS requires thinning of the thickened footplate before creation of a fenestration and prosthesis placement. Thinning is usually accomplished with a small electrical or hand drill, which can also be used to perform the fenestration. The fenestra is usually 0.4 to 0.6 mm in diameter. A prosthesis is then placed through the fenestra into the vestibule. The vestibule is sealed by placing soft tissue around the prosthesis. However, some surgeons use just a blood seal with the stapedotomy approach. Ayache et al. (43) demonstrated a 62% success rate (with closure of the air–bone gap to 10 dB or less) in the drill-out procedure. As experience grew with the drill-out procedure for obliterative OS, some otologists began using the stapedotomy technique in all their patients with OS. The surgical technique involves creating a fenestra in the midportion of the stapes using a drill, picks, laser, or a combination thereof. The steps of a stapedotomy are identical to stapedectomy up until footplate work is initiated. A rosette pattern is created in the midportion of the footplate with a laser (Fig. 154.11). A Micropick or Skeeter drill is then used to complete the stapedotomy (Fig. 154.12). After a stapedotomy is performed, a prosthesis is then positioned over a tissue graft or the graft is positioned around the stapedotomy (Fig. 154.13). An autologous blood patch or hyaluronic acid gel can also be used to seal the OW in place of a tissue graft (43,44).

Longstanding results of the stapedotomy procedure have been comparable to a total stapedectomy. Some reports suggest a decrease in postoperative cochlear deafness and improvement in the air–bone gap closure above 2,000 Hz with stapedotomy. Stapedotomy and partial stapedectomy may show better postoperative hearing at higher frequencies (4,000 Hz) than total stapedectomy;

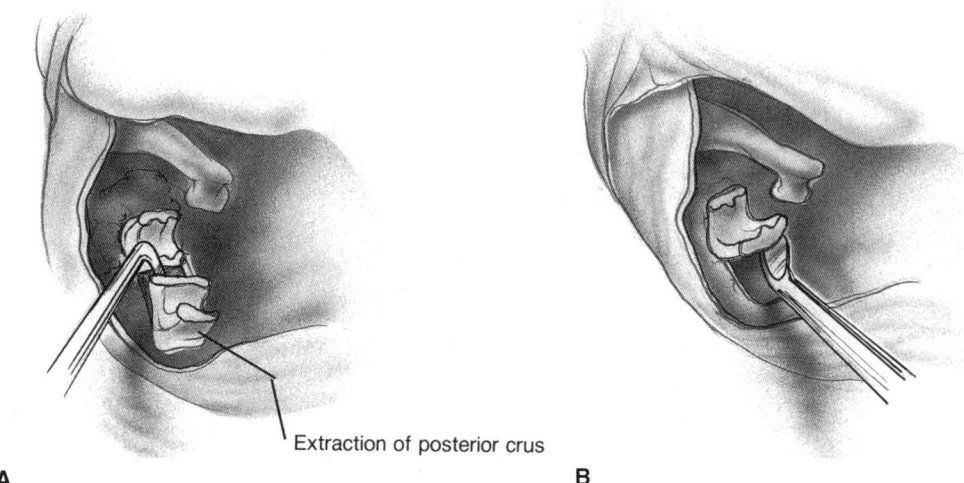

Extraction of posterior crus

A   **B**

Figure 154.9 A: The posterior half of the stapedial footplate is removed with a sharp pick. **B:** The anterior half of the stapedial footplate is removed by a joint knife or Hough hoe.

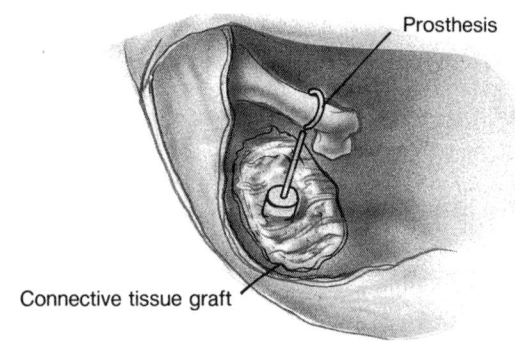

Figure 154.10 Prosthesis in place.

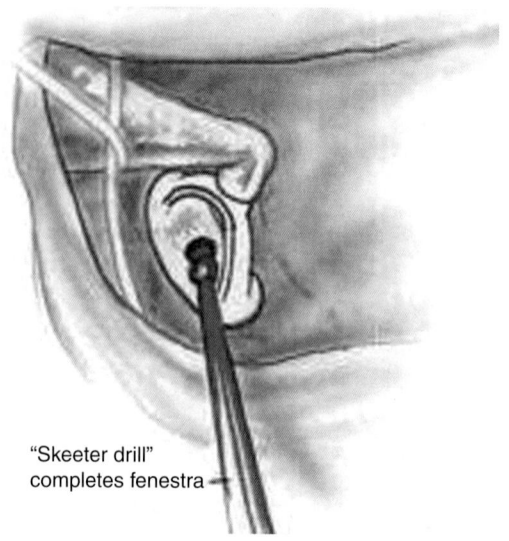

Figure 154.12 A Skeeter drill is used to complete the stapedotomy.

however, total stapedectomy may result in improved gains at lower frequencies (250 and 500 Hz) (44).

Numerous stapes prostheses have been developed since John Shea popularized the stapedectomy procedure. Early prostheses with a sharp or beveled end were found to cause a prohibitive number of postoperative fistulae. The designs that have proved most effective include a connective tissue OW graft and piston prosthesis. Tissue can be obtained from tragal perichondrium, dorsal hand vein graft, or temporalis fascia. The graft is combined with a variety of prosthetic designs, such as a wire Teflon piston or a Robinson-type bucket-handle prosthesis, which has a wire loop that is placed over the lenticular process of the incus. If the stapedotomy procedure is performed, the prosthesis is positioned, and connective tissue is placed around the prosthesis base to seal the vestibule or autologous blood is used to fill the middle ear space (Fig. 154.9). A recent addition to the variety of available stapes prostheses is a heat-activated self-crimping prosthesis, thus eliminating the crimping step necessitated by prior piston type implants. The heat-activated nitinol stapes prostheses also allow for a more uniform crimp around the incus thus reducing the risk of a loose prosthesis (45).

After completion of the desired procedure, the TM flap is returned to its normal anatomic position. The EAC may be dressed in a variety of ways (e.g., packed with gelatin sponge, antibiotic ointment), depending on the surgeon's preference. The use of perioperative antibiotics is common, despite the lack of statistical evidence of their benefits. Perioperative steroids may be used to reduce the incidence of anesthesia-induced nausea, and vomiting. In the immediate postoperative period, the patient is asked to avoid lifting and straining for about 1 month. Nose blowing should be discouraged. The patient should also cough or sneeze with the mouth open, to reduce the risk of increased middle ear pressure and displacement of the TM. The patient is kept on dry ear precautions until the TM has completely healed.

Immediate hearing improvement is noted in some patients intraoperatively when the procedure is done

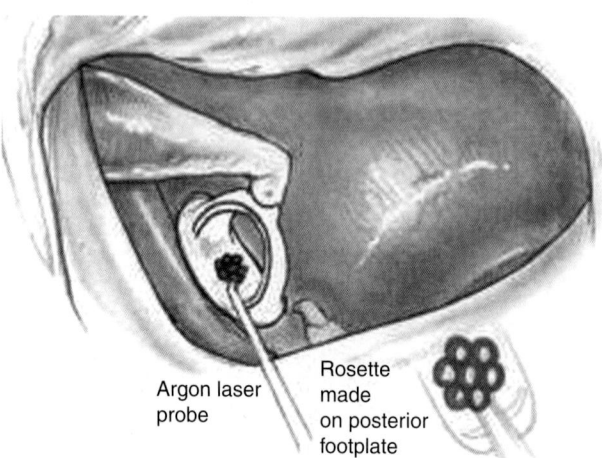

Figure 154.11 A rosette pattern is created with a laser in the midportion of the footplate. This step can be completed prior to down fracturing the stapes or after this step.

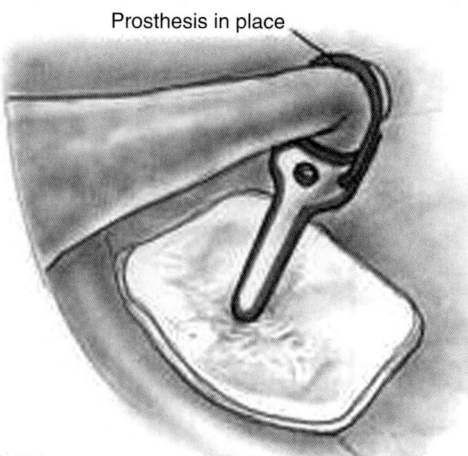

Figure 154.13 A tissue graft can be used to cover the stapedotomy prior to placement of the prosthesis to decrease the risk of a postoperative perilymph fistula. The prosthesis is then engaged between the incus lenticular process and the stapedotomy.

under local anesthesia or in the post anesthesia care unit in those undergoing a general anesthesia. Other patients report a more gradual hearing improvement with occasional associated vestibular symptoms, probably due to serous labyrinthitis. Balance disturbances usually resolve within 1 to 2 days but occasionally linger for a few weeks. A postoperative audiogram is obtained 2 to 3 months after surgery, allowing enough time for middle ear fluid and blood to resorb. Postoperative hearing results reveal closure of the air–bone gap to within 10 dB of the preoperative bone-conduction level in 90% of patients (46). About 10% of patients experience either worsening hearing or no improvement. About 2% of patients suffer persistent and profound SNHL. Recent evidence has suggested a progressive high-frequency SNHL in some poststapedectomy patients. It is unclear whether this is due to cochlear OS or long-term postsurgical effects (47).

The otolaryngologist should be aware of certain complicating factors associated with stapes surgery. Anatomic variations of the middle ear sometimes alter the surgical procedure. Occasionally, a high or dehiscent jugular bulb is encountered. If it is injured, the middle ear must be packed to tamponade the bleeding before continuing with surgery. Continued or persistent bleeding may require termination of the procedure. One must be sure that the bleeding is due to a jugular bulb and not an aberrant internal carotid artery. A persistent stapedial artery that courses in the obturator foramen of the stapes can be a complicating factor due to its bleeding potential. This artery is the embryologic remnant of the second branchial arch. To gain access to the footplate, the vessel must be divided or displaced or the procedure will need to be aborted. Blood that enters the vestibule increases the risk of postoperative SNHL (48).

Careful and complete inspection of the middle ear should be performed at each exploratory tympanotomy. Other causes of CHL, such as malleus head fixation, can be associated with OS. Malleus head fixation can be congenital or caused by immobility of the ossicular chain, allowing for ankylosis to the attic wall. Mobilization of the malleus can sometimes be accomplished through a limited atticotomy if the fixation point is at the head. Calcification of the anterior or posterior malleolar ligaments can readily be removed and is facilitated with the laser. Addressing lateral chain fixation should only proceed after the IS joint has been divided. Unfortunately, mobilization is often followed by refixation (49).

A dehiscent or inferiorly displaced fallopian canal with or without a prolapsed facial nerve can at times obscure the OW. If footplate removal and prosthesis placement can be achieved safely, surgery should continue. If the surgeon believes the nerve is in jeopardy, the procedure should be aborted.

A profuse perilymph gusher (i.e., CSF leak) is rarely encountered. A perilymph gusher is believed to be due to a patent cochlear aqueduct or more commonly a modiolar defect with communication to the fundus of the internal auditory canal. This finding is more frequently identified in patients with congenital footplate fixation. Complete stapes footplate removal in the presence of a gusher increases the risk of postoperative cochlear deafness. The fenestration (control hole) placed before footplate removal should allow for early identification of this problem. Measures to control a perilymph gusher include elevation of the head of bed, small fenestra stapedotomy, and placement of a tissue seal over the footplate defect. Wiet (10) recommended placing a prosthesis in order to hold the tissue seal in place. At times, a lumbar drain may be needed to decompress the subarachnoid space to allow for adherence of the graft to the defect in the footplate (10).

Fracture of the incus long process can occur during stapedectomy. It may follow separation of the IS joint, placement of the prosthesis, or curettage of the scutum. Usually, the prosthesis can be placed on the remaining incus, but a malleus to OW prosthesis may be needed. A notched bucket-handle prosthesis is ideally suited for short to medium incus long process defects and frequently produces excellent hearing results (50). Staging the procedure and coming back at a later time may allow the incus to heal and be utilized in the future, because a malleus to OW prosthesis is more difficult to place and typically has poorer postoperative hearing results (51).

It is difficult to remove a nonfixed (floating) stapedial footplate after the crural arches have been fractured. Attempts to manipulate the footplate may push it medially into the vestibule. This is a case in which the laser may be used to atraumatically remove or ablate the footplate. In addition, one of the purposes of the control hole made before fracturing the crura is to provide access to the footplate, if it inadvertently becomes mobilized. Small right angle hooks or needles can be placed through the hole to lift the footplate out of the vestibule. An alternative strategy for managing a floating footplate is to drill a shallow groove in the inferior part of the OW niche. A small hook can then be passed beside the footplate to remove it. If all or part of the footplate is significantly depressed into the vestibule, it is best left there. Attempts to remove it can result in significant SNHL. A connective tissue graft and prosthesis can be placed lateral to the depressed footplate. In this setting, postoperative disequilibrium can be expected but is usually self-limited (52).

The use of a local anesthetic such as lidocaine can cause intraoperative or postoperative vertigo. Lateral canal stimulation from irrigation fluids can cause vertigo, as can chemical irritation of the labyrinth from the local anesthetic. Palpation of the footplate or a long prosthesis can cause vertigo from direct mechanical stimulation of the underlying otolith organs (saccule, utricle) (53).

TM tears should be avoided. If a small tear occurs, it can be repaired with a leftover piece of the OW grafting material. Persistent postoperative perforations should be repaired within 4 to 6 weeks after surgery to prevent any

TABLE 154.3	CLINICAL INDICATORS FOR STAPEDECTOMY

Strategy

Indicators (one of the following)
   CHL without other source of conductive abnormality
   (e.g., perforated TM, serous otitis media)
Laboratory tests (required)
   Audiogram with air–bone gap, speech reception threshold,
   and discrimination scores
Other tests (as indicated)
   Impedance audiometry
Type of anesthesia (as indicated)
Location of service (as indicated)

Process

Criteria for discharge
   Recovery from anesthesia
   Absence of significant vertigo
   Ability to ambulate without assistance
   Absence of signs of infection
   Absence of significant ear drainage

Outcome

Results

Follow-up
   Improvement in hearing
   Health of TM

The American Academy of Otolaryngology-Head and Neck Surgery and the American Society for Head and Neck Surgery have published clinical indicators for surgical procedures. These clinical indicators are educational statements that have been drafted to assist surgeons in their practice and to promote discussion. These indicators are not practice guidelines nor do they represent standards of practice with which individuals must conform.
TM, tympanic membrane.

problems with transcanal contamination of the middle ear and a subsequent otitis media and SNHL (54).

The most common cause for failure of stapedectomy has been prosthesis displacement, with or without incus erosion. Other causes of failure are footplate refixation, perilymph fistula, otosclerotic regrowth, and lateralization of the OW membrane. Patients need to be informed that revision surgery is usually not as successful as primary surgery. The possibility of postoperative cochlear deafness is also more common with revision surgery. Patients who seem to achieve better results in revision procedures are those who experienced an initial improvement in hearing followed by a gradual increase of the air–bone gap over a period of months or years (Table 154.3) (55).

COMPLICATIONS/PITFALLS

Complications after stapes surgery can occur immediately or in a delayed fashion. Vertigo or disequilibrium immediately after surgery is usually due to loss of perilymph, surgical trauma, or serous labyrinthitis. This symptom generally subsides within a few days. If dizziness does not improve within the first postoperative week, the use of

corticosteroids may be of some benefit. Persistent vertigo may be due to a depressed footplate fragment, long prosthesis, OW fistula, or a reparative granuloma. Benign paroxysmal positional vertigo can also be seen during the postoperative course due to surgical injury to the utricle. This is usually self-limiting and resolves within several months (56).

Acute otitis media is a rare postoperative complication; if it does occur, it poses a serious threat to hearing in the operated ear. The newly created OW partition allows a middle ear infection to quickly involve the labyrinth (suppurative labyrinthitis) and potentially meningitis. Historically, a beveled prosthesis on a gelatin sponge appeared to increase the risk of suppurative labyrinthitis. Intensive systemic antibiotic therapy for otitis media is begun immediately; if diagnosed early, the condition may improve without significant sequelae (57).

The incidence of poststapedectomy granulation (i.e., reparative granuloma) is approximately 0.1% and usually becomes manifest within 7 to 15 days after surgery, but it can occur as late as 6 weeks postoperatively. The hallmark of poststapedectomy granulation is progressive SNHL after earlier postoperative hearing improvement. The granuloma can also be associated with vertigo, aural fullness, or tinnitus. The TM appears thickened and the posterior superior aspect is erythematous. The audiogram typically reveals an MHL or SNHL that often is most severe in the high frequencies. The discrimination score is usually significantly lower than expected from the degree of hearing loss. If this complication is suspected, early surgical intervention is warranted. A CT scan can be helpful in the diagnosis of this process and to assess the status of the prosthesis/vestibule. Findings at surgery include a significant amount of granulation tissue around the OW and possible filling the middle ear. Acute and chronic inflammation with capillaries, foreign body giant cells, chronic inflammatory cells, and fibroblastic proliferation is seen on histologic examination of the resected granuloma. Treatment involves removal of the OW seal and prosthesis with replacement using a different material. Risk factors for reparative granuloma include total stapedectomy, the use of gelatin sponge as the OW sealant, or the presence of powder on operating gloves. The overall outcome of this potentially devastating process is related to early diagnosis and treatment (58).

Perilymph fistulae may occur in the early postoperative period or may be seen many years later. The initial complaints usually include fluctuating or progressive hearing loss associated with tinnitus or vertigo. A history of sudden barometric pressure change or trauma may also be reported but is not necessarily diagnostic. Fistula testing by pneumatic otoscopy may be helpful. Audiometric testing usually reveals the expected SNHL, although fistulae rarely occur without hearing loss. The most important factor in diagnosis is a high clinical index of suspicion. If a fistula is thought to be present, conservative measures may be appropriate particularly in the immediate postoperative period, because surgical exploration is difficult. These conservative measures can include the use of acetazolamide and bed rest for 5 days. If symptoms continue, exploratory surgery with grafting of the OW is indicated. Findings at surgery may include a displaced prosthesis with or without an obvious fistula. Postoperative expectations include stabilization of the SNHL and resolution of the dizziness (55).

Persistent or progressive CHL can follow stapedectomy. Loosening or displacement of the prosthesis, resorption of the incus long process, adhesions around the prosthesis, and further OS lesions can produce postoperative CHL. Significant hearing loss may warrant surgical exploration. It must be remembered that removal of the prosthesis is associated with a higher incidence of SNHL and a reduced closure of the air–bone gap (55).

HIGHLIGHTS

- OS is a primary disease of the otic capsule that causes progressive CHL, SNHL, or MHL.
- The disease is present histologically in 8% to 10% of the Caucasian population, but only 12% of patients with histologic changes actually present with clinical symptoms.
- Histologically, the disease begins by bone resorption around vascular channels and later matures as dense, sclerotic bone.
- Patients suffering from OS typically present with a slowly progressive hearing loss over a period of years.
- The physical appearance of the TM is typically normal.
- The audiogram with acoustic immittance testing remains the key to diagnosis, revealing a CHL or MHL in most cases.
- Patients presenting with a conductive or mixed hearing loss and intact acoustic reflexes should not undergo stapes surgery as this typically represents an inner ear third window (i.e., semicircular canal dehiscence, enlarged vestibular aqueduct).
- Surgical therapy remains the mainstay of treatment for CHL from OS; however, this is an elective procedure. Patients must be given the alternative of amplification. Medical treatment can be given to all patients.
- Postoperative hearing results reveal closure of the air–bone group to within 10 dB of the preoperative bone-conduction level in 90% of patients.
- The possibility of postoperative cochlear deafness is higher with revision surgery when compared with primary stapedectomy.

REFERENCES

1. Wang PA, Merchant SN, McKenna MJ, et al. Does otosclerosis occur only in the temporal bone? *Am J Otol* 1999;20:162–165.
2. Mudry A. Adam Politzer (1835–1920) and the description of otosclerosis. *Otol Neurotol* 2006;27:276–281.
3. Hillel AD. History of stapedectomy. *Am J Otolaryngol* 1983;4: 131–140.
4. Lopez-Gonzalez MA, Delgado F. Oral vaccine in otosclerosis. *Med Hypotheses* 2000;54:216–220.
5. Chole RA, McKenna MJ. Pathophysiology of otosclerosis. *Otol Neurotol* 2001;22:249–257.
6. Guild SR. Histologic otosclerosis. *Ann Otol Rhinol Laryngol* 1944;53:246–266.
7. Schuknecht HF, Barber W. Histologic variants in otosclerosis. *Laryngoscope* 1985;95:1307–1317.
8. Rosen S. Mobilization of the stapes to restore hearing in otosclerosis. *NY J Med* 1953;53:2650–2653.
9. Stankovic KM, McKenna MJ. Current research in otosclerosis. *Curr Opin Otolaryngol Head Neck Surg* 2006;14:347–351.
10. Wiet RJ, Harvey SA, Bauer GP. Complications in stapes surgery. *Otolaryngol Clin North Am* 1993;26:471–490.
11. Shambaugh G. Clinical diagnosis of cochlear (labyrinthine) otosclerosis. *Laryngoscope* 1965;75:1558–1562.
12. Emmett JR, Shea JJ. Vestibular dysfunction associated with otosclerosis. *Trans Am Otol Soc* 1989;8:104–107.
13. Mikulec AA, McKenna MJ, Ramsey MJ, et al. Superior semicircular canal dehiscence presenting as conductive hearing loss without vertigo. *Otol Neurotol* 2004;25:121–129.
14. Morrison A, Bundey S. The inheritance of otosclerosis. *J Laryngol Otol* 1970;84:921–932.
15. Clayton AE, Mikulec AA, Mikulec KH, et al. Association between osteoporosis and otosclerosis in women. *J Laryngol Otol* 2004;118:617–621.
16. de Souza C, Glasscock ME. Physical examination and clinical evaluation of the patient with otosclerosis. In: de Souza C, Glasscock ME, eds. *Otosclerosis and stapedectomy*, 1st ed. New York: Thieme, 2004:23–29.
17. de Souza C, Glasscock ME. Audiological evaluation of the patient with otosclerosis. In: de Souza C, Glasscock ME, eds. *Otosclerosis and stapedectomy*, 1st ed. New York: Thieme, 2004:31–40.
18. Sakai O, Curtin HD, Fujita A. Otosclerosis: computed tomography and magnetic resonance findings. *Am J Otolaryngol* 2000;21: 116–118.
19. De la Cruz A, Angeli S, Slattery W. Stapedectomy in children. *Otolaryngol Head Neck Surg* 1999;120:487–492.
20. Monsell EM. The mechanism of hearing loss in Paget's disease of bone. *Laryngoscope* 2004;114:598–606.
21. Garretsen AJ, Cremers WRJ, Huygen PL. Hearing loss (in non-operated ears) in relation to age in osteogenesis imperfecta type I. *Ann Otol Rhinol Laryngol* 1997;106:575–582.
22. Niedermeyer HP, Arnold W, Schwub D, et al. Shift of the distribution of age in patients with otosclerosis. *Acta Otolaryngol* 2001;121:197–199.
23. McLarnon CM, Davison T, Johnson IJ. Bone-anchored hearing aid: comparison of benefit by patient subgroups. *Laryngoscope* 2004;114:942–944.
24. Rotteveel LJ, Proops DW, Ramsden RT, et al. Cochlear implantation in 53 patients with otosclerosis. *Otol Neurotol* 2004;25: 943–952.
25. Cruise AS, Singh A, Quiney RE. Sodium fluoride in otosclerosis treatment: review. *J Laryngol Otol* 2010;124:583–586.
26. Shea JJ. Fenestration of the oval window. *Ann Otol Rhinol Laryngol* 1958;67:932–951.
27. de Souza C, Glasscock ME. Stapedectomy. In: de Souza C, Glasscock ME, eds. *Otosclerosis and stapedectomy*. New York: Thieme, 2004:89–117.
28. Shea PF, Ge X, Shea JJ. Stapedectomy for far advanced otosclerosis. *Am J Otolaryngol* 1999;20:425–429.
29. Lagleyre S, Sorrentino T, Calmels MN, et al. Reliability of high-resolution CT scan in diagnosis of otosclerosis. *Otol Neurotol* 2009;30:1152–1159.
30. Meyer TA, Lambert P. Primary and revision stapedectomy in elderly patients. *Curr Opin Otolaryngol Head Neck Surg* 2004;12:387–392.

31. de Souza C, Glasscock ME. Hearing aids and otosclerosis. In: de Souza C, Glasscock ME, eds. *Otosclerosis and stapedectomy*, 1st ed. New York: Thieme, 2004:69–72.

32. Daniels RL, Krieger LW, Lippy WH. The other ear: findings and results in 1,800 bilateral stapedectomies. *Otol Neurotol* 2001;22:603–607.

33. Green JD Jr, Shelton C, Brackmann DE. Iatrogenic facial nerve injury during otologic surgery. *Laryngoscope* 1994;104:922–926.

34. Shea JJ, Ge X. Delayed facial palsy after stapedectomy. *Otol Neurotol* 2001;22:465–470.

35. Sparano A, Leonetti JP, Marzo S, et al. Effects of stapedectomy on tinnitus in patients with otosclerosis. *Int Tinnitus J* 2004;10(1):73–77.

36. Vrabec JT, Coker NI. Stapes surgery in the United States. *Otol Neurotol* 2004;25:465–469.

37. Poe DS. Laser-assisted endoscopic stapedectomy: a prospective study. *Laryngoscope* 2000;110(5 Pt 2 Suppl 95):1–37.

38. Silverstein H, Van Ess MJ, Alameda YA. Laser stapedotomy minus prosthesis: long-term follow-up. *Otolaryngol Head Neck Surg* 2011;144:753–757.

39. Hough N. Partial stapedectomy. *Ann Otol Rhinol Laryngol* 1960;69:571–596.

40. Perkins RC. Laser stapedotomy for otosclerosis. *Laryngoscope* 1980;90:228–240.

41. Buchman CA, Fucci MJ, Robertson JB Jr, et al. Comparison of argon and CO_2 laser stapedotomy in primary otosclerosis surgery. *Am J Otolaryngol* 2000;21:227–230.

42. Schmerber S, Cuisnier O, Charachan R, et al. Vein versus tragal perichondrium in stapedotomy. *Otol Neurotol* 2004;25:694–698.

43. Ayache D, Sleiman J, Plovin-Gaudon L, et al. Obliterative otosclerosis. *J Laryngol Otol* 1999;113:512–514.

44. House HP, Hansen MR, Al Dakhail AA, et al. Stapedectomy versus stapedotomy: comparison of results with long-term follow-up. *Laryngoscope* 2002;112:2046–2050.

45. Ying YL, Hilman TA, Chen DA. Patterns of failure in heat-activated crimping prosthesis in stapedotomy. *Otol Neurotol* 2011;32:21–28.

46. Bitterman AJ, Rovers MM, Tange RA, et al. Primary stapes surgery in patients with otosclerosis: prediction of postoperative outcome. *Arch Otolaryngol Head Neck Surg* 2011;137:780–784.

47. Vincent R, Sperling NM, Oates J, et al. Surgical findings and long-term hearing results in 3,050 stapedotomies for primary otosclerosis: a prospective study with the otology-neurotology database. *Otol Neurotol* 2006;27(8 Suppl 2):S25–S47.

48. Horn KL, Visvanathan A. Stapes surgery in the obscured oval window: management of the ptotic facial nerve and the persistent stapedial artery. *Oper Tech Otolaryngol Head Neck Surg* 1998;9:58–63.

49. Vincent R, Lopez A, Sperling NM. Malleus ankylosis: a clinical, audiometric, histologic and surgical study of 123 cases. *Am J Otolaryngol* 1999;20:717–725.

50. Lippy WH, Schuring A. Solving ossicular problems in stapedectomy. *Laryngoscope* 1983;93:1147–1150.

51. Lippy WH, Battista RA, Berenholz L, et al. Twenty-year review of revision stapedectomy. *Otol Neurotol* 2003;24:560–566.

52. de Souza C, Glasscock ME. Special conditions and complications in otosclerosis surgery. In: *Otosclerosis and stapedectomy*, 1st ed. New York: Thieme, 2004:163.

53. Lippy WH, Berenholz LP. The long prosthesis syndrome. *Otol Neurotol* 2010;31:548–549.

54. Causse JB, Causse JR, Wiet RJ, et al. Complications of stapedectomies. *Am J Otolaryngol* 1983;4:275–280.

55. Vincent R, Rovers M, Zingade N, et al. Revision stapedotomy: operative findings and hearing results. A prospective study of 652 cases from the Otology-Neurotology Database. *Otol Neurotol* 2010;31:875–882.

56. Atacan E, Sennaroglu L, Genc A, et al. Benign paroxysmal positional vertigo after stapedectomy. *Laryngoscope* 2001;111:1257–1259.

57. Ricalde RR, Portmann D. Acute infections complications in stapes surgery. *Rev Laryngol Otol Rhinol (Bord)* 2010;131:285–288.

58. Fenton JE, Turner J, Shirazi A, et al. Post-stapedectomy reparative granuloma: a misnomer. *J Laryngol Otol* 1996;110:185–188.

Acute Paralysis of the Facial Nerve

155

Jeffrey T. Vrabec   *Jerry W. Lin*

Acute facial palsy is a common diagnostic problem encountered by the otolaryngologist, but its presentation often provokes consternation on the physician's part. This reaction stems from our limited knowledge of facial nerve pathology, from the shortcomings of currently popular electrophysiologic tests in defining nerve injury, and from the controversy surrounding the management of facial palsy. This chapter presents contemporary opinions on management of acute facial palsy.

ANATOMY AND PHYSIOLOGY OF THE FACIAL NERVE

The cranial nerve VII is a complex motor/sensory nerve consisting of special visceral afferent, general visceral efferent, and special visceral efferent fibers (Fig. 155.1) (1). The special visceral afferent fibers convey the sense of taste from the sensory receptors on the anterior two-thirds of the tongue and project via the lingual and chorda tympani nerves to the geniculate ganglion and, hence, via the nervus intermedius to the tractus solitarius.

The general visceral efferent fibers constitute a parasympathetic system with three subsets of postsynaptic fibers. The preganglionic fibers arise in the superior salivatory nucleus. One subset of fibers exits the facial hiatus within the greater superficial petrosal nerve, joins the deep petrosal nerve in the vidian canal, and synapses at the sphenopalatine ganglion. Postsynaptic fibers then innervate the lacrimal and palatine glands. Another subset of preganglionic fibers within the lesser petrosal nerve synapses at the otic ganglion; the postsynaptic fibers provide secretory supply, in part, to the parotid gland. The third subset of this parasympathetic system exits the temporal bone along the chorda tympani nerve and passes along the lingual nerve to synapse at the submandibular ganglion. The postsynaptic fibers then provide the secretory supply to the submandibular and sublingual glands.

The special visceral efferent fibers arise within the facial motor nucleus and pass through the temporal bone, except for the fibers to the stapedius muscle, to exit the stylomastoid foramen and innervate the auricular, posterior belly of the digastric, stylohyoid, and platysma muscles and the superficial facial musculature.

Evidence that the sensory afferent fibers provide sensation from the external auditory canal and proprioception from the face is contradictory. These fibers are thought to account for the otalgia experienced in Bell palsy and the vesicular eruption in herpes zoster infection.

The intracranial segment of the facial nerve and the nervus intermedius exit the brainstem in a recess adjacent to the pons, cross the cerebellopontine angle ventral to the vestibuloacoustic nerve, and enter the internal auditory canal. The meatal segment of the facial nerve and the intermedius nerve occupy the anterior–superior quadrant within the canal and enter the fallopian canal at the meatal foramen superior to the crista transversa and anterior to the crista verticalis (Bill's bar). The labyrinthine segment of the nerve courses 2 to 4 mm within the narrowest part of the fallopian canal to the geniculate ganglion, where the nerve makes an acute turn of 40 to 80 degrees (external or first genu) to enter the middle ear. Coursing posteriorly and slightly inferiorly above the cochleariform process and the oval window, the tympanic segment (11 mm) curves into the second (pyramidal) turn inferior to the horizontal semicircular canal. This turn has a more obtuse angle of 110 to 120 degrees. The mastoid segment then descends 13 mm vertically to the stylomastoid foramen. There are several branches of the nerve in its intratemporal course. At the geniculate ganglion, the greater superficial petrosal nerve courses anterior and medially. The branch to the stapedius muscle arises from the proximal mastoid segment while the chorda tympani exits the distal mastoid segment. The nerve to the posterior belly of the digastric is the first branch distal to the stylomastoid foramen. The

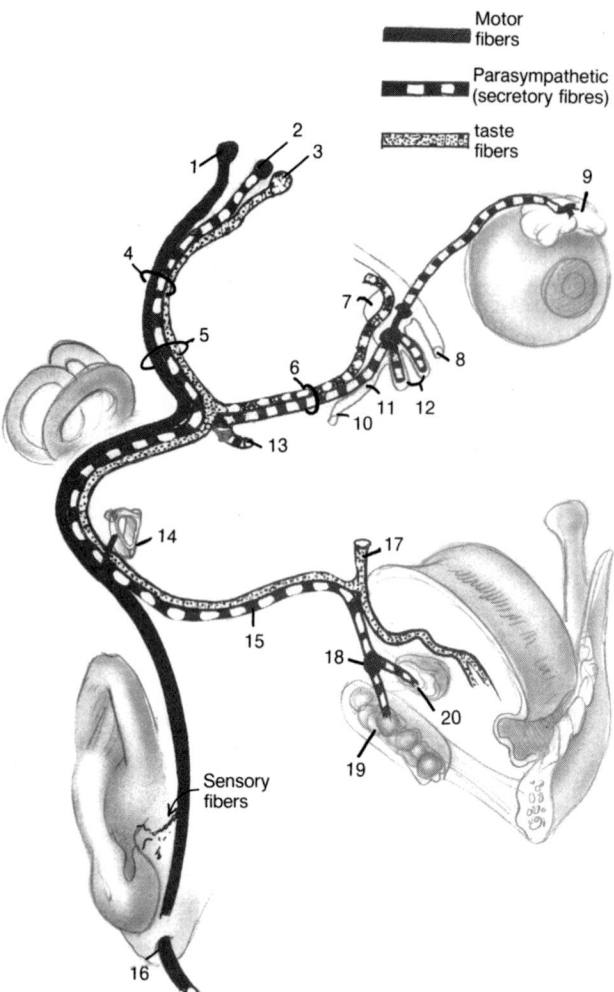

Figure 155.1 Efferent and afferent tracts of cranial nerve VII. The projection of the sensory fibers from the external auditory canal is undetermined. *1*, Nucleus of facial nerve; *2*, superior salivary nucleus; *3*, solitary tract; *4*, porus acusticus internus; *5*, meatal foramen; *6*, greater petrosal nerve; *7*, sphenopalatine ganglion; *8*, maxillary nerve; *9*, lacrimal gland; *10*, deep petrosal nerve; *11*, vidian nerve; *12*, innervation of glands of nose and palate; *13*, anastomosis with minor petrosal nerve; *14*, stapedial nerve; *15*, chorda tympani; *16*, stylomastoid foramen; *17*, lingual nerve; *18*, submandibular ganglion; *19*, submandibular gland; *20*, sublingual gland. (Modified from Miehlke A. *Surgery of the facial nerve*, 2nd ed. Baltimore, MD: Urban & Schwarzenberg, 1973:19, with permission.)

special visceral efferent fibers constituting the extracranial segment enter the posterior parotid gland and undergo secondary and tertiary branching. These fibers ultimately innervate the five regions of mimetic musculature: temporal, zygomatic, buccal, mandibular, and cervical. The peripheral branches of the nerve are the most variable in location.

Crossing nerve fibers at the level of the motor nucleus of the facial nerve in the brainstem leads to bihemispheric control of function in the upper half of the face and contralateral hemispheric control of function in the lower half of the face. Thus, forehead sparing can suggest a central versus a peripheral lesion of the facial motor pathway.

SURGICAL ANATOMY

Knowledge of the intratemporal anatomy of the facial nerve and the associated landmarks is critical to safe otologic surgery. The surgical approach to different segments of the nerve varies if middle and inner ear structures are to be preserved. When hearing is good, the meatal and labyrinthine segments of the nerve are approached via the middle cranial fossa (Fig. 155.2). This allows access to the internal auditory canal and/or geniculate ganglion. Important landmarks include the arcuate eminence, meatal plane, facial hiatus, and greater superficial petrosal nerve. The location of the internal auditory canal and meatal segment is approximated by bisection of the angle formed between the plane of the superior semicircular canal (arcuate eminence) and the greater superficial petrosal nerve. The nerve occupies the anterior quadrant of the internal auditory canal.

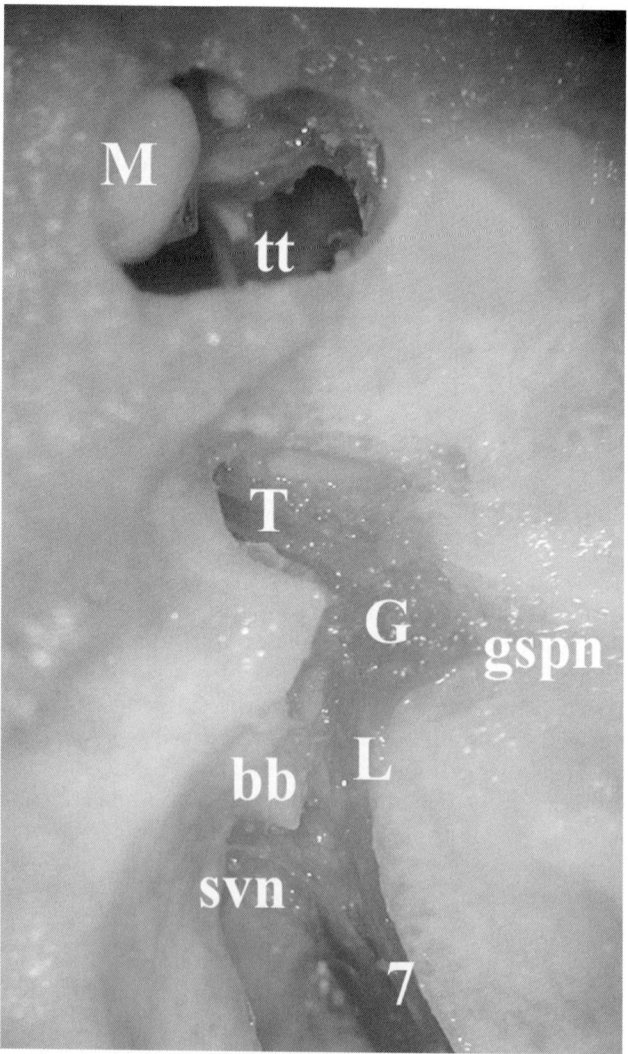

Figure 155.2 Surgical anatomy of the facial nerve in the middle cranial fossa. *7*, facial nerve in the internal auditory canal; *L*, labyrinthine segment; *G*, geniculate ganglion; *T*, tympanic segment; *M*, malleus; *tt*, tensor tympani; *bb*, Bill's bar; *svn*, superior vestibular nerve.

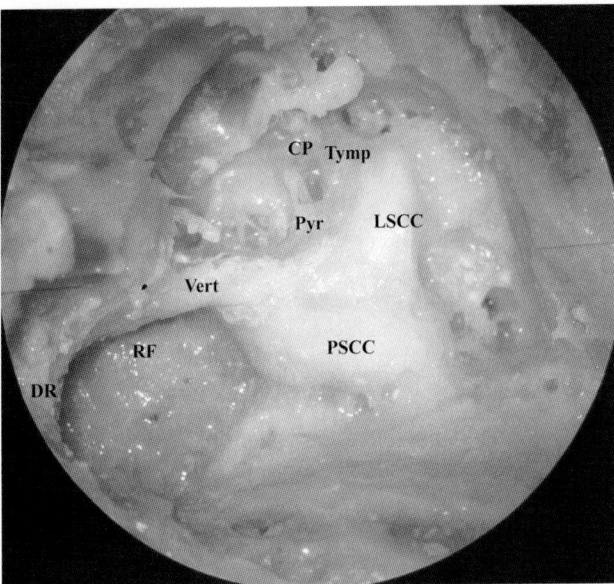

Figure 155.3 Surgical landmarks to the facial nerve in the middle ear and mastoid. *LSCC*, lateral semicircular canal; *PSCC*, posterior semicircular canal; *DR*, digastric ridge; *RF*, retrofacial air cells; *Vert*, vertical segment proximal to stylomastoid foramen; *Tymp*, tympanic segment; *CP*, cochleariform process; *Pyr*, pyramidal eminence.

Important landmarks for identification of the tympanic segment in the middle ear are the cochleariform process and the oval window. The nerve is located superior to these structures and inferior to the horizontal semicircular canal. The upper mastoid segment lies posterior and medial to the chorda tympani and medial to the facial recess air cell tract. The stapedius muscle and posterior semicirular canal are medial to the facial nerve. The lower mastoid segment is at the same level as the digastric ridge (Fig. 155.3), lateral to the retrofacial air cell tract. The mastoid segment of the nerve can be identified by removing the bone from the posterior aspect of the external auditory canal, thereby exposing the nerve on its lateral aspect. The surgeon should expect the nerve along a line drawn between the horizontal semicircular canal and digastric ridge.

When hearing preservation is not an issue, the entire intratemporal course of the nerve can be exposed via the translabyrinthine approach. The mastoid segment is defined as above. Removal of the labyrinth allows skeletonization of the tympanic segment along its superior aspect. The labyrinthine segment is located just anterior and superior to the ampulla of the superior canal. The internal auditory canal is identified medial to the vestibule. In the lateral end of the canal, the facial nerve is separated from the superior vestibular nerve by the vertical crest (Bill's bar).

Anomalies of the Facial Nerve

Anomalies of the facial nerve are rare, but their existence makes even the most experienced otologic surgeon wary. The most common "anomaly" is a dehiscence in the facial canal, which exposes the nerve to injury during temporal bone surgery. The most common location is the tympanic

segment over the oval window, followed by the geniculate ganglion and the mastoid segment adjacent to the retrofacial air cells (2). The intratemporal course of the nerve is usually constant, but variations do occur. Deviations in the labyrinthine segment are exceedingly uncommon; usually the finding in this area is a difference in the angulation of the nerve between the meatal foramen and the geniculate ganglion, which relates to the depth of the internal auditory canal below the floor of the middle fossa. In the tympanic segment, the nerve may prolapse against the arch of the stapes, bifurcate around the stapes, or course below the oval window. Below the horizontal semicircular canal, the nerve may curve more acutely, making the prominent turn more susceptible to injury during an antrotomy. In the mastoid segment, bifurcations and trifurcations are exceedingly rare, but when duplication exists, the nerves occupy separate bony canals and exit individual foramina. Anomalies of the fallopian canal are suspect in congenital atresia of the middle ear and anomalies of the otic capsule (3). Thin-section high-resolution computed tomography (CT) of the facial canal is recommended to provide as much preoperative information as possible about the course of the facial nerve.

Topographic Organization of the Facial Nerve

Topographic organization of the intracranial or intratemporal efferent and afferent fibers is not likely based on animal studies (4,5). Thus, suggestions that the site of lesion within the temporal bone can be determined according to the degree of muscle weakness in different regions of the face are inaccurate. This lack of intratemporal organization makes interfascicular repair of the nerve proximal to the stylomastoid foramen impractical and unnecessary. Synkinesis is inevitable with any reanastomosis or nerve grafting procedure.

Arterial Supply to the Facial Nerve

Both the carotid and vertebrobasilar arterial systems vascularize the intratemporal facial nerve. The labyrinthine artery, a branch of the anterior inferior cerebellar artery, provides the blood supply to the nerve within the internal auditory canal. The petrosal artery, a branch of the middle meningeal, supplies the nerve in the perigeniculate region and anastomoses with the stylomastoid artery, which feeds the mastoid and tympanic segments. The intratemporal facial nerve has a rich extrinsic anastomotic network to prevent ischemia, except in the labyrinthine segment at the junction between the carotid and vertebrobasilar systems.

EVALUATION

History

A careful history narrows the scope of the differential diagnosis and reduces the number of laboratory studies necessary to establish the cause. First, the onset of the paralysis is defined as sudden, delayed, or gradual. Sudden refers to acute deterioration of facial function over a few days, either with or without an antecedent event. Delayed refers to acute deterioration in close temporal relationship with an antecedent event, though facial function is normal immediately following the event. Gradual refers to progressive loss over a period of weeks or longer. These definitions assume normal function prior to onset. When rapid deterioration occurs in a nerve exhibiting abnormal function, the onset is considered gradual or progressive unless there has been a lengthy period of stable facial function. Recurrent refers to facial palsy that occurs after a long period of stable recovery from a previous facial palsy.

Next, the degree of paralysis is designated as complete or incomplete. This is often of great prognostic importance. Incomplete paralysis or paresis is usually associated with good prognosis for recovery, unless a neoplasm is diagnosed. Complete paralysis typically carries a guarded prognosis for return of normal facial movement, especially when accompanied by electrical evidence of complete degeneration.

Associated symptoms provide additional diagnostic clues. Numbness in the middle and lower face, otalgia, hyperacusis, diminished tearing, and an alteration in taste are common in Bell palsy and Ramsay Hunt syndrome. Intense ear pain and a vesicular eruption are the hallmarks of herpes zoster oticus. Sensorineural hearing loss and vertigo are symptoms of advanced disease involving the labyrinth, the internal auditory canal, or brainstem.

Recurrent facial palsy also may indicate a tumor, although some persistent dysfunction is likely in between episodes of worsening function. More common causes of recurrent palsy include Bell palsy and Melkersson-Rosenthal syndrome. About 7% of patients with Bell palsy develop recurrent palsy, with half of the recurrences on the ipsilateral side (6). Melkersson-Rosenthal syndrome is often familial, and the first episode of facial palsy usually occurs before 20 years (7). Associated findings include facial edema, particularly of the upper lip; fissured tongue; and migraine headaches.

Any thorough history encompasses other medical conditions that may be incriminated in the differential diagnosis of the palsy: cancer, sarcoidosis, autoimmune disorders, and previous surgeries in the posterior fossa, temporal bone, or parotid.

Physical Examination

The physical examination includes a complete head and neck evaluation with microscopic examination of the ear, a thorough assessment of the upper aerodigestive tract, and a cranial nerve assessment (III to XII) (Table 155.1). Obvious physical findings confirm many infectious, neoplastic, and traumatic diagnoses. Otorrhea, purulent middle-ear effusion, or obvious cholesteatoma indicate an infectious etiology. Slowly progressive weakness, temporal bone or parotid mass lesion, or segmental weakness (some branches paralyzed while others are spared) suggest a neoplasm.

TABLE 155.1	ASSESSMENT OF FACIAL PALSY

History
  Onset
  Duration
  Rate of progression
  Recurrent or familial
  Associated symptoms
  Major medical illness or previous surgery

Physical examination
  Complete head and neck evaluation
  Microscopic otoscopy
  Upper aerodigestive tract examination
  Cranial nerve assessment (III–XII)
  Palpation of parotid gland and neck
  Neurologic evaluation
  Cerebellar signs
  Motor
  Facial palsy
  Complete vs. incomplete (paresis)
  Segmental vs. uniform involvement
  Unilateral vs. bilateral
  Schirmer test

Laboratory studies
  Pure-tone and speech audiometry
  Electrophysiologic tests
  Nerve excitability test (NET)
  Maximal stimulation test (MST)
  Electroneurography (ENoG)
  Electromyography (EMG)
  Radiographic studies
  Computed tomography
  Magnetic resonance imaging

Other considerations
  Complete blood cell count and differential with sedimentation rate
  Serum antibody tests (Lyme titers)
  Chest x-ray radiograph
  Lumbar puncture with cerebrospinal fluid assay

Forehead sparing suggests a central motor pathway lesion. Contusion or laceration over the distribution of the extracranial nerve, Battle sign (mastoid ecchymosis), or hemotympanum are evidence of trauma. Multiple cranial nerve deficits typically indicate an advanced intracranial or skull base infection, extensive neoplasm involving the temporal bone, or a neurologic disorder, such as Guillain-Barré syndrome.

The examination focuses on the motor function of the facial nerve. Compare the range of facial movement between the affected and unaffected sides. The subject should attempt a broad range of facial expressions while the examiner watches for movement in each of the major branches of the nerve. The subject is asked to raise the eyebrows, close the eyes as tightly as possible, wrinkle the nose, smile broadly, pucker, or grimace. A common error is to attribute the movement in the upper eyelid due to the levator palpebrae superioris muscle (cranial nerve III) to

TABLE 155.2	FACIAL NERVE GRADING SCALE 2.0			

	Region			
Score	Brow	Eye	NLF	Oral
1	Normal	Normal	Normal	Normal
2	Slight weakness >75% of normal	Slight weakness >75% of normal Complete closure with mild effort	Slight weakness >75% of normal	Slight weakness >75% of normal
3	Obvious weakness >50% of normal Resting symmetry	Obvious weakness >50% of normal Complete closure with maximal effort	Obvious weakness >50% of normal Resting symmetry	Obvious weakness >50% of normal Resting symmetry
4	Asymmetry at rest <50% of normal	Asymmetry at rest <50% of normal Cannot close completely	Asymmetry at rest <50% of normal	Asymmetry at rest <50% of normal
5	Trace movement	Trace movement	Trace movement	Trace movement
6	No movement	No movement	No movement	No movement

Secondary movement (Global assessment)

Score
0 None
1 Slight synkinesis, minimal contracture
2 Obvious synkinesis, mild to moderate contracture
3 Disfiguring synkinesis, severe contracture

Reporting
Sum scores for each region and secondary movement

GRADE	Total Score
I	4
II	5–9
III	10–14
IV	15–19
V	20–23
VI	24

Legend: NLF, nasolabial fold.

facial nerve function and to misrepresent the finding as a facial paresis. Grading of the injury follows the outline in Table 155.2 (8).

The more common causes of acute facial paralysis are outlined in Table 155.3. Over half of the presentations are due to Bell palsy. Trauma is the second most common etiology, producing about 20% of cases. The palsy is not Bell's in the presence of any of the following: signs of tumor, vesicles, multiple cranial nerve involvement, temporal bone infection, trauma, palsy at birth, signs of a central nervous system lesion, and acute infectious mononucleosis. Bilateral facial nerve involvement occurs in fewer than 1% of patients who have facial palsy. Common etiologies include brainstem tumors, intracranial infection or malignancy, extensive skull base fractures, Guillain-Barré syndrome, or Lyme disease (9).

Laboratory Studies

Several studies may be indicated in the evaluation of acute facial paralysis (Table 155.1), depending on the findings in the history and physical examination. Because of numerous problems arising within the temporal bone and the proximity of the cranial nerves VII and VIII in the posterior fossa, pure tone and speech audiometry is recommended.

The once-popular topognostic testing (Schirmer test, stapedial reflex assessment, electrogustometry, and salivary flow) for determining the site of the lesion and for prognostication is obsolete. Imaging is more efficient for diagnosis and is essential in any case when the etiology is uncertain or the paralysis is recurrent or atypical. High-resolution CT of the temporal bone is the study of choice for assessment of the fallopian canal. Any potential cause of facial paralysis associated with bone destruction (mastoiditis, cholesteatoma, tumors, temporal bone trauma) is seen best on CT. MRI is most useful when infectious or neoplastic involvement of the nerve (idiopathic facial palsy, herpes zoster oticus, facial schwannoma) is suspected.

When paralysis is complete, electrophysiologic studies are done to establish the degree of degeneration and prognosis for recovery. The Schirmer test remains useful to quantitate the amount of tearing in the involved eye. Reduced tear secretion suggests the need for aggressive treatment to protect the cornea. When the diagnosis is uncertain, other laboratory studies can be considered to

TABLE 155.3	**D**	**DIFFERENTIAL DIAGNOSIS FACIAL PALSIES**

Infection
Bell palsy (herpes simplex mononeuritis)
Herpes zoster oticus (Ramsay Hunt syndrome)
Otitis media with effusion
Acute suppurative otitis media
Coalescent mastoiditis
Chronic otitis media
Malignant otitis externa (skull base osteomyelitis)
Tuberculosis
Lyme disease[a]
Acquired immunodeficiency syndrome
Infectious mononucleosis

Trauma
Temporal bone fractures[a]
Birth trauma
Facial contusions/lacerations
Penetrating wounds, face and temporal bone
Iatrogenic injury
Radiation injury

Neoplasia
Cholesteatoma
Glomus jugulare or tympanicum
Carcinoma (primary or metastatic)
Facial neuroma
Schwannoma of lower cranial nerves
Meningioma
Leukemia
Histiocytosis
Rhabdomyosarcoma

Congenital
Compression injury
Möbius syndrome
Lower lip paralysis

Idiopathic
Recurrent facial palsy
Melkersson-Rosenthal syndrome

Metabolic and systemic
Sarcoidosis[a]
Guillain-Barré syndrome[a]
Autoimmune disorders

[a]May present with bilateral palsy.

exclude blood dyscrasias, autoimmune disorders, Lyme disease, sarcoidosis, and central nervous system diseases.

PATHOPHYSIOLOGY OF NERVE INJURY

One of the greatest shortcomings in our understanding of neural degeneration and regeneration is the lack of knowledge of events occurring at the molecular level after insult. Current electrophysiologic tests cannot differentiate levels of injury; hence, prognostication is limited, which explains why a "completely degenerated" nerve can have either total recovery or none at all.

Classically, nerve injury is described in terms of neurapraxia, axonotmesis, or neurotmesis. Neurapraxia results when a lesion compresses the flow of axoplasm from the nerve cell body to the distal axons. The nerve is viable and recovers normal function when the blockade is removed. A neurapraxic nerve will demonstrate normal findings on the nerve excitability test (NET), the maximal stimulation test (MST), and electroneurography or evoked electromyography (ENoG). Electromyography (EMG), however, fails to show voluntary motor action potentials, as these cannot be conducted across the blockade.

Axonotmesis describes a state of Wallerian degeneration distal to the lesion characterized by the preservation of endoneural sheaths of the motor axons. Electrically, if the axonotmesis is complete and pure, the NET, MST, and ENoG will indicate rapid and complete degeneration. The EMG will not demonstrate voluntary motor units, and after 10 to 14 days, myogenic fibrillation potentials become evident. As long as the endoneural tubules are preserved, regeneration to the original motor end plates will proceed until recovery is total.

In neurotmesis, the lesion leads to Wallerian degeneration and the loss of endoneural tubules. Consequently, the electrophysiologic tests yield results similar to those found in axonotmesis; however, the outcome is less predictable. The regeneration process depends on the completeness of injury to all connective tissue components of the nerve, including the endoneurium, the perineurium binding the axons into fascicles, and the epineurium enclosing the fascicles into a common nerve. Endoneurium compromise disrupts axonal organization and ensures a synkinetic result if regeneration occurs. Furthermore, the growth of neurofilaments is governed by conditions at the injury site and can be hindered by ischemia and scar.

Electrophysiologic Tests

The currently popular tests used to establish prognosis for return of function are the NET, the MST, ENoG, and EMG. Serial testing can establish the end point of degeneration, but any one test given at one point in time during the paralysis provides only limited information. The tests are complementary and when used appropriately can describe the completeness of degeneration relatively accurately. The indications, interpretations, and limitations of these tests are outlined in Table 155.4.

General rules apply to the use of these tests. The NET, MST, and ENoG are most applicable in the evaluation of acute paralysis (i.e., while the nerve is in the degenerative phase). During degeneration, the NET will demonstrate increasing side-to-side threshold differences, the MST greater degrees of facial weakness, and the ENoG lower percentages of intact motor axons. The results will reach a nadir, and the nerve will enter the recovery phase. This may be evident immediately on clinical examination or may be delayed, depending on the cause and extent of nerve injury. The tests are not indicated in patients with paresis, as facial movement on examination indicates that

TABLE 155.4	ELECTROPHYSIOLOGIC TESTS		
Test	**Indication**	**Interpretation**	**Limitation**
Nerve excitability test	Complete paralysis <2 wk duration	≤3.5 mA threshold difference: prognosis good	Not useful in first 3 d after onset or during recovery
Maximal stimulation test	Same as NET	Marked weakness or no muscle contraction: advanced degeneration with guarded prognosis	Subjective
Electroneurography	Same as NET and MST	<90% degeneration: good prognosis >90%: prognosis in question	False-positive results in deblocking phase
Electromyography	Acute paralysis <1 wk duration	Active mu: intact motor axons	Cannot assess degree of degeneration of prognosis for recovery
	Chronic paralysis >3 wk duration	mu + fibrillation potentials: partial degeneration	
		Polyphasic mu: regenerating nerve	

NET, nerve excitability test; MST, maximal stimulation test; mu, motor units.

the nerve is intact, primarily neurapraxic, and the prognosis for recovery is good. The most common causes of acute facial paralysis (Bell palsy, trauma, herpes zoster oticus) produce nerve degeneration within the first 3 weeks after onset of palsy, and the NET, MST, and ENoG provide the most accurate information within this time frame. Nevertheless, when the neurapraxic axons begin recovery, asynchronous depolarization, differing conduction velocities in the motor axons, poor summation of the myogenic action potentials, and poor muscular contraction can give a false-positive report of nerve status and may even suggest that the nerve has completely degenerated.

EMG in combination with NET, MST, and ENoG greatly aids in eliminating these false-positive results, as the demonstration of voluntary active motor units confirms the integrity of intact axons in the recovery phase. This test is useful in the earliest phase of degeneration, as the presence of motor units indicates an intact nerve with incomplete injury. Within the first 3 days after onset of complete paralysis, the results of NET, MST, and ENoG yield little useful information, as Wallerian degeneration distal to the stimulation areas has not occurred; the results always indicate incomplete degeneration and good prognosis (10). Because of this limitation, the prognosis is best established by using NET, MST, or ENoG around the sixth or seventh day after onset of paralysis. The primary limitation of EMG is the inability to differentiate a totally neurapraxic nerve from a completely degenerated one in the acute phase of degeneration. Nevertheless, the EMG is complementary in the evaluation of acute paralysis and essential in the evaluation of long-standing paralysis. The presence of myogenic fibrillation potentials and the absence of voluntary motor units denote complete nerve degeneration, the coexistence of both fibrillation potentials and motor units indicates an incomplete lesion, and the appearance of polyphasic motor units signifies a regenerating nerve. The polyphasic action potentials may not be present until several weeks after the onset of paralysis.

In the NET, the current thresholds required to elicit just-visible muscle contraction on the normal side of the face are compared with those values required over corresponding sites on the side of the paralysis. The current, measured in milliamperes, is delivered percutaneously in a square-wave pulse of 0.3-ms duration at a rate of one per second over the main trunk and branches of the facial nerve. A side-to-side threshold difference is calculated for the respective sites of stimulation. A side-to-side difference of 3.0 to 3.5 mA is compatible with advanced degeneration, with an unfavorable prognosis for differences exceeding 3.5 mA (10).

The MST is a modification of the NET that uses a level of current sufficient to depolarize all motor axons underlying the stimulating probe (11). The facial muscular responses are graded subjectively according to the degree of contraction (equal, slightly decreased, markedly decreased, or absent compared with the uninvolved side). Markedly decreased or absent facial movement signifies advanced degeneration. When the response to MST remains normal for 10 days, approximately 90% of patients have complete return of facial function. If the response is decreased, most have incomplete return of function. If the response is lost, return does not begin until the fourth month (11).

Introduced by Esslen and popularized by Fisch (12), ENoG allows quantitative analysis of nerve degeneration. A supramaximal level of current applied with bipolar electrodes percutaneously over the main trunk of the facial nerve creates synchronous depolarization of the motor axons, thereby evoking a compound myogenic action potential in the facial musculature that is recorded with bipolar surface electrodes (Fig. 155.4). The peak-to-peak amplitude of this potential is directly proportional to the number of intact motor axons. Compared with the amplitude of potential evoked on the normal side, it can be used to calculate the percentage of intact axons. Greater than 90% degeneration indicates a poor prognosis for immediate or complete restoration of facial function. Traumatic injuries undergoing

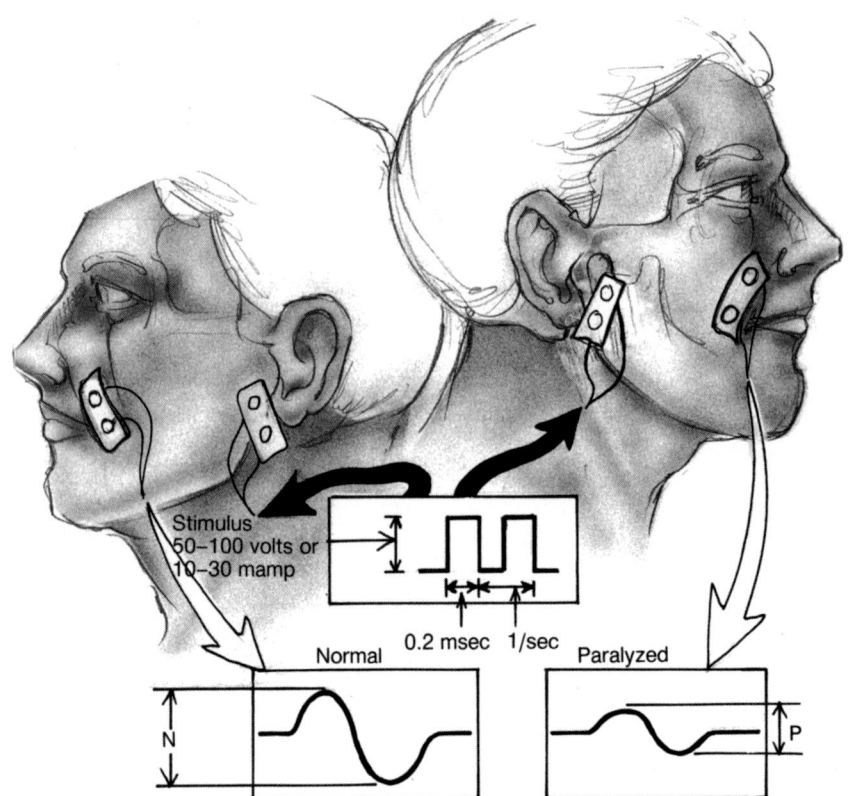

Figure 155.4 Clinical electroneurography in the assessment of acute facial paralysis. Percentage of viable motoneurons = P/N × 100. (Modified from Coker NJ, Fordice JO, Moore S. Correlation of the nerve excitability test and electroneurography in acute facial paralysis. *Am J Otol* 1992;13:127–133, with permission.)

more than 90% degeneration within 6 days of the injury represent complete lesions. In Bell palsy, patients exceeding 95% degeneration within the first 2 weeks of onset fall into the guarded prognostic category (13).

It is important for the clinician to understand potential sources of testing error. Naturally, the level of experience of the physician or technician performing the test is a significant variable. Placement of the recording electrodes can impact the test accuracy. Testing paradigms used for ENoG include standard lead placement, optimal lead placement (OLP), and the recently introduced midline electrode placement (14). The former test places recording electrodes at the same anatomic location on both sides of the face, usually at the lateral edge of the nasolabial crease and lateral and inferior to the oral commissure. The OLP technique uses repeated repositioning of recording electrodes until the maximal response is detected. A midline technique may allow recording of larger amplitude action potentials and is unlikely to be affected by masseter stimulation. The use of electrode paste and the amount of pressure applied to the stimulating and recording electrodes can influence results of any method of electrical testing. Patient factors such as age, obesity, and facial edema also influence test results.

Coker et al. (15) assessed correlation of the results of NET and ENoG testing in patients with acute facial paralysis. They found that the tests display an exponential relationship, not a linear one. The highest levels of correlation were seen when OLP technique was used in ENoG

testing. The lack of exact correlation between the two tests illustrates the inability to achieve consistent synchronous depolarization of viable axons, which the authors suggest may be explained by a deblocking phenomenon or partial demyelination. The authors concluded that the two tests are complementary in assessment of acute facial paralysis.

BELL PALSY

The term Bell palsy has been used to describe a facial paralysis of acute onset and limited duration, the etiology of which was deemed idiopathic. Contemporary studies provide convincing evidence that the herpes simplex virus (HSV) is the infecting agent in Bell palsy. The development of polymerase chain reaction techniques has allowed identification of HSV in the geniculate ganglion. Murakami et al. (16) sampled endoneurial fluid and muscle from patients undergoing decompression surgery for Bell palsy and Ramsay Hunt syndrome. Control specimens were obtained during repair of the facial nerve after trauma, excision of parotid malignancies, and facial neuromas. Samples from 10 of 13 patients who had Bell palsy were positive for HSV, whereas none of the controls showed evidence of the virus. Eight of nine patients with Ramsay Hunt syndrome had evidence of varicella zoster virus, but none had HSV.

Additional support is given by replication of the clinical syndrome in an animal model. Sugita et al. (17) produced transient facial palsy in an animal model by inoculation with HSV. In this experiment, HSV was inoculated into the auricle or lateral tongue. Paralysis developed in 56% of animals inoculated in the auricle and 20% inoculated in the tongue. The paralysis developed 6 to 9 days later and persisted for 3 to 7 days. Spontaneous resolution occurred in all cases. Histopathology revealed significant edema and inflammation about the geniculate ganglion. HSV antigens could be isolated from the nerve, geniculate ganglion, and facial motor nucleus in some of the animals that developed paralysis. Antigen could not be detected on the contralateral side in any animal.

Bell palsy is the most common diagnosis given to patients with acute facial paralysis. The incidence is between 30 and 45 cases per 1,00,000 per year (18,19). The incidence varies with age, being rare in children and increasing through the sixth decade. Women may have a slightly increased risk and incidence appears greater in arid climates and during winter months. Differences in incidence by ethnicity likely reflect differing prevalence of HSV infection within the respective populations (20).

The clinical picture is defined by rapid onset of the facial palsy, minimal associated symptoms, and spontaneous recovery. Facial nerve dysfunction developing over several weeks or months is not Bell palsy. Peitersen (19) characterized the natural history of untreated Bell palsy. Thirty percent of patients develop only a paresis, and 94% of these patients recover without sequelae. The other 70% developed a complete paralysis, with only 61% of this group achieving full recovery. Time to return of movement is associated with ultimate recovery. Some return of facial tone or movement is seen in 85% of all patients within 3 weeks. Full recovery is typically achieved by 2 months. Patients who develop complete paralysis may not have return of function for 3 to 5 months. The longer the delay until some recovery is evident, the greater the likelihood of adverse sequelae, including synkinesis, residual weakness, and muscle spasms. Other factors that are associated with poor recovery include advanced age and pain at presentation. Peitersen (19) expressed final outcome using a modification of the Jongkees grading system. Extrapolation of his findings to the more familiar (in the United States) House-Brackmann scale reveals an estimated 71% of all patients achieving grade I and 12% grade II outcome.

Histopathologic studies of patients with Bell palsy were reviewed by Liston and Kleid (21). The reported findings are not uniform, reflecting the different periods from onset of paralysis to nerve examination, methods of preparation, portion of the nerve studied, and possibly etiology of the facial paralysis. Most recent reports, however, demonstrate inflammatory infiltrates throughout the course of the facial nerve. Vascular thrombosis is generally not observed, although intraneural hemorrhage is seen occasionally.

The high rate of spontaneous recovery has made it difficult to prove efficacy of any medical or surgical intervention in patients with Bell palsy. Two recent, large, randomized trials have established the utility of oral steroids in promoting recovery (22,23). Both trials prospectively randomized patients presenting within 72 hours of onset of the facial palsy to receive oral steroids or placebo combined with antivirals or placebo. In each trial, patients receiving steroids had a significantly greater probability of full recovery. Sullivan et al. (22) studied 551 patients in Scotland. In this study, only three examiners rated all the patients using a series of four photographs for evaluation according to the House-Brackmann scale. The steroid treatment was prednisolone 500 mg (50 mg/day ×10) and the antiviral was acyclovir 2,000 mg/day for 10 days. In this study, 83% of patients displayed grade I function at 3 months when treated with prednisone versus 64% in those not receiving prednisone ($P < 0.001$). At the last assessment at 9 months, 94% of patients receiving prednisone were judged to be grade I versus 82% of those not receiving steroids.

Engström et al. (23) analyzed a group of 839 patients in Sweden and Finland. The study used both the House-Brackmann scale and the Sunnybrook scale as rating instruments. The steroid treatment was prednisolone 450 mg (60 mg/day ×5, then taper by 10 mg/day) and the antiviral was valacyclovir 3,000 mg/day for 7 days. A large number of examiners (greater than 49) were used to record the data in this study. The study found 62% of patients receiving prednisone displayed normal function (Sunnybrook score of 100) at 3 months versus 51% in the patients not receiving prednisone ($P = 0.0007$). At 12 months, the comparable figures are 72% normal in prednisone-treated patients versus 57% in those without.

The addition of antiviral medications may provide additional benefit, though conclusive evidence is lacking. It is clear that antivirals alone are not better than placebo. However, the addition of antivirals to steroid treatment may enhance recovery. Adour et al. (24) were the first to report the benefit of antivirals combined with steroid treatment in a double-blind study. Patients were randomized to receive either acyclovir 2,000 mg/day in five doses and prednisone or placebo and prednisone. All patients enrolled in this trial were within 3 days of onset of the paralysis. Only 20% of patients progressed to complete paralysis (House-Brackmann grade VI) within 2 weeks of onset, and these were evenly distributed between the two treatment groups. Acyclovir-treated patients demonstrated less evidence of degeneration as measured by MST and a lower incidence of unsatisfactory recovery (House-Brackmann grades III and IV). A meta-analysis of trials investigating efficacy of antiviral agents in Bell palsy (BP) was performed by de Almeida et al. (25). The absence of benefit of antivirals alone compared to placebo was confined. However, individuals who received antivirals combined with steroids had a relative risk of incomplete recovery of 0.75 ($P = 0.05$). Secondary analysis did not find a significant difference in outcomes according to antiviral dosage.

Selection of a medical regimen for any patient with Bell palsy must consider potential side effects of medications, concurrent illness, and the patient's wishes. Treatment must be initiated promptly for maximal efficacy. The treatment effect is greatest for those patients with complete paralysis, but waiting for a mild weakness to progress undermines the efficacy of the treatment regimen. Prednisone dosage in adults should be 450 to 500 mg administered in divided doses over 7 to 10 days. A gradual taper is optional. Antivirals can be added if treatment is initiated within the first 72 hours; beyond this time, additional efficacy is less likely. Valacyclovir is given at a dose of 1,000 mg three times daily for 7 days or famciclovir may be given at 1,500 mg daily for 7 days. Dosage adjustment in pediatric patients is indicated.

Debate continues as to how to manage best those patients who progress to severe electrical degeneration despite medical intervention. Those patients who display greater than 90% degeneration on ENoG in the first 2 weeks of the paralysis recover to House-Brackmann grade I or II function only 50% of the time (26). Although histopathologic studies demonstrate inflammatory involvement of the entire nerve, it is postulated the maximal nerve injury occurs at the meatal foramen. In this location, the nerve occupies a greater proportion of the lumen of the fallopian canal than elsewhere. Further support for this theory was given by Fisch and Esslen (12), who confirmed the presence of a conduction block proximal to the meatal foramen in 11 of 12 patients undergoing total facial nerve decompression. Surgical intervention thus is directed at unroofing the labyrinthine segment of the nerve via a middle fossa approach. Incision of the epineurium is advocated by some for additional neural decompression. Decompression of the mastoid and tympanic segments of the nerve has no effect on recovery of facial function.

Gantz et al. (26) presented the results of a prospective multi-institutional trial of middle fossa decompression. Criteria for entry into the study were development of more than 90% degeneration on ENoG (OLP technique) within 14 days of onset of the paralysis and no voluntary motor unit potentials on EMG. Patients meeting these criteria were offered middle fossa decompression. Patients self-selected treatment, choosing either surgical decompression or continued medical treatment. Good outcome (House-Brackmann grade I or II) was achieved in 91% of the surgical patients ($N = 34$) versus only 42% in the medical treatment–only group ($N = 36$). Patients who progressed to a complete paralysis but did not develop more than 90% degeneration achieved a final House-Brackmann grade I in 89% of cases. They concluded that the 90% degeneration threshold on ENoG accurately separates patients into a good or poor prognostic category. In addition, middle fossa decompression of the labyrinthine segment (including the geniculate ganglion and internal auditory canal) performed within 14 days of onset of paralysis significantly improves outcome in those patients with a poor prognosis. Decompression performed after 14 days provides no additional benefit. None of the patients in the medical treatment group received antiviral therapy; however, the potential benefit of antivirals is in preventing progression to severe degeneration. Antivirals are not expected to provide additional benefit once severe degeneration has occurred.

HERPES ZOSTER OTICUS

Varicella zoster virus establishes a latent infection in many cranial nerve ganglia at the time of the initial infection. The latent virus can be reactivated years later by an unknown mechanism. Reactivation of latent virus within the geniculate ganglion produces herpes zoster oticus or Ramsay Hunt syndrome. The patient presents with acute facial paralysis, severe ear pain, and a vesicular eruption of the external auditory canal and concha. The pain often precedes the facial paralysis by a few days. Associated symptoms of sensorineural hearing loss and vestibular dysfunction are present in more than 30% of patients.

Ramsay Hunt syndrome has an annual incidence about one-tenth that of Bell palsy. The incidence increases with age, consistent with zoster at other sites. The prognosis for spontaneous recovery of normal facial function is poorer than in Bell palsy (27). Satisfactory return of facial movement occurs in about 50% of patients; others will suffer varying grades of weakness, synkinesis, contractures, and spasm. Unlike Bell palsy, in which degeneration proceeds rapidly within the first 2 weeks after onset, degeneration of the facial nerve in herpes zoster oticus may evolve more slowly over the course of 3 weeks. When the degeneration is total, regeneration requires 3 to 6 months before facial movement becomes evident on clinical examination.

Jackson et al. (28) reported intraoperative findings in a patient with Ramsay Hunt syndrome demonstrating no return of function after 1 year. An excisional biopsy demonstrated a sharp demarcation between normal and devitalized nerve in the labyrinthine segment. Proximal and distal portions of the nerve appeared grossly normal. This observation suggests an increased susceptibility of the labyrinthine segment to inflammation-induced degeneration.

Management of herpes zoster oticus includes intervention directed at the underlying viral infection and associated complications. As stated earlier, antiviral therapy must be initiated promptly for maximal effectiveness. Antiviral medications are beneficial in treatment of herpes zoster infections, reducing pain and shortening time to resolution of skin lesions. Specific medications and dosages are the same as outlined earlier (Valacyclovir 1,000 mg tid for 7 days, or Famciclovir 500 mg tid for 7 days). Steroids are also given at the same doses as in Bell palsy. Few studies have examined the benefits of both steroids and antiviral therapy in herpes zoster oticus, but preliminary reports are encouraging (29). The role of surgical decompression remains investigational. It is difficult to identify those with a poor prognosis because electrical test data are less well established than in Bell palsy.

OTITIS MEDIA AND FACIAL PALSY

Facial palsy can present as a complication of acute suppurative otitis media, otitis media with effusion, chronic otitis media, and mastoiditis. Infection involving the fallopian canal leads to inflammation and neural edema. Immediate treatment should be directed toward eradicating the infection. When a middle-ear effusion is present, myringotomy is performed promptly to drain the middle-ear space. Cultures of the middle-ear aspirate direct antibiotic therapy against the offending organism.

The incidence of facial palsy in acute otitis media is approximately 1:20,000 cases (30). Most cases are seen in children due to the greater incidence of otitis media in the pediatric population. The prognosis of facial palsy in acute otitis media is excellent (31,32). Recovery of facial function begins rapidly in conjunction with resolution of infection. Operative management is usually limited to myringotomy and tube.

Facial paralysis in association with chronic otitis media, cholesteatoma, or skull base osteomyelitis carries a more ominous prognosis (33,34). The development of the paralysis is often more insidious, suggesting possible ischemic nerve injury. Aural toilet and antibiotics are intiated promptly. If the tympanic membrane is intact, myringotomy is performed. CT is recommended to evaluate the fallopian canal before surgery. Suspicion of intracranial complications is appropriate in this setting. Tympanomastoid surgery is usually necessary to remove infected tissue from the middle ear and mastoid. The facial nerve is inspected carefully. Granulation tissue, cholesteatoma matrix, and infected bone are removed if easily separated; however, great care is advised to avoid iatrogenic injury. Incision of the epineurium is not advised. Facial nerve function is most likely to improve in those cases where onset of paralysis is acute and treatment is prompt. Facial paralysis that has been present for several weeks or more rarely improves despite aggressive management.

TRAUMA

Facial nerve injuries occur in a variety of ways, including blunt or penetrating trauma and iatrogenic harm. Management differs according to extent of injury, though the severity of the injury is not always easy to establish. History, physical exam, imaging, and electrophysiologic testing are all important in determining the probability of spontaneous recovery.

Immediate evaluation of the motor function of the facial nerve after trauma to the head and neck provides key information. All facial nerve branches should be inspected carefully to document movement. If a paresis is present, spontaneous return of satisfactory facial function will occur without intervention. Soft tissue swelling and ecchymosis impair the assessment of facial movement; thus, repeated examinations are necessary. Immediate complete paralysis indicates a severe nerve injury and warrants surgical exploration in cases of penetrating trauma.

Electrophysiologic testing is employed when the severity of injury is uncertain. The presence of voluntary motor units on EMG establishes continuity of the nerve, and this test may be performed at any time. Evoked EMG or ENoG testing is usually deferred for several days after the injury to avoid a false positive evoked response. Severe nerve injuries lead to rapid and complete degeneration, characterized by the absence of both voluntary and evoked responses. Predicting spontaneous recovery in traumatic lesions remains imprecise; additional data correlating the rate of neural degeneration on ENoG to degree of spontaneous recovery are needed.

Pure-tone and speech audiometry is necessary for intratemporal lesions to document the type and degree of hearing loss. Imaging is usually limited to high-resolution CT scan, with the intent of defining any fractures traversing the fallopian canal. MRI or angiography is indicated if a major vascular injury is suspected, as with penetrating injuries at the skull base. Cervical spine films are requested if neck injury is suspected.

The recommended management of injuries with complete facial paralysis is outlined in Table 155.5 (35). For extracranial lacerations, the transected trunk or major branches should be repaired as soon as practical. This usually requires either direct end-to-end anastomosis or interpositional grafting, preferably at the time of soft tissue closure. Branches medial to the lateral canthus of the eye rarely need repair because of the rich cross-anastomotic connections of the nerve in the midface. Observe patients who have closed soft tissue injuries for resolution of the paralysis.

Temporal bone fractures are the most common cause of traumatic injury to the facial nerve. The fractures are categorized according to involvement of the otic capsule (36). Fewer than 5% of all temporal bone fractures involve the otic capsule. However, facial nerve injury occurs in half of all otic capsule fractures. Otic capsule sparing fractures are associated with facial paralysis in less than 10% of cases. Most injuries occur in the perigeniculate region. Less commonly, the nerve is injured in the upper mastoid segment by the fracture in the posterior osseous external auditory canal.

Once the injured segment of the nerve is identified, an operative approach is selected according to residual hearing. The middle fossa approach provides complete access to the perigeniculate region in those patients with good hearing. A transmastoid approach with a posterior tympanotomy allows examination of the tympanic and mastoid

TABLE 155.5	MANGEMENT OF TRAUMATIC INJURIES WITH COMPLETE FACIAL NERVE PARALYSIS

Mechanism of Injury	Tests	Critical Result	Management
Intratemporal Injury			
Blunt trauma (temporal bone fracture)	CT	Fracture involving fallopian canal	
	NET	>3.5 mA difference	
	ENoG	>90% degeneration	
	EMG	Absent volitional activity	Surgical exploration if all of above present
	Audiometry	Conductive loss	Transmastoid–middle fossa approach
		Sensorineural loss—severe	Translabyrinthine approach
	History	Delayed onset	Observation
Penetrating trauma	Follow algorithm above, add: Angiography	Suspicion of major vascular injury	Endovascular or open repair
Iatrogenic	History	Immediate onset	Surgical exploration
		Delayed onset (>3 d)	Observation
Extratemporal Injury			
Penetrating trauma	Physical exam		Exploration and repair
Blunt trauma	Physical exam		Observation
Iatrogenic	History	Suspected transection by report	Exploration and repair
		Nerve intact	Observation

NET, nerve excitability test; ENoG, electroneurography; EMG, electromyography.

segments of the nerve. If profound sensorineural hearing loss is present, a translabyrinthine approach allows access to all segments of the nerve.

Blunt injuries rarely result in nerve transection. The most common findings are edema and contusion (intraneural hemorrhage) (Fig. 155.5) (35). The injured segment is inspected and any bone impaling or compressing the nerve is removed. Additional decompression of the fallopian canal may be performed proximal and distal to the injury. Intraneural hematomas are evacuated after incision of the epineural sheath. Complete transection of the nerve requires rerouting of the nerve with direct end-to-end anastomosis or an interpositional graft if direct anastomosis is not feasible.

Gunshot injuries of the temporal bone produce facial nerve paralysis in more than half of all cases (37). This unique form of penetrating injury often produces severe neural damage. The nerve can be directly involved (i.e., transected) or secondarily injured by the kinetic energy imparted by the projectile or by the bony fragmentation of the temporal bone. The most common sites of injury are the mastoid and tympanic segments of the nerve. When the nerve is transected, interpositional grafting is advised. Determining extent of injury may be difficult, as the damage is often more extensive along the proximal and distal segments than anticipated. As a result, outcome of facial function is poorer than in blunt temporal bone fractures.

The incidence of facial nerve injury during middle-ear and mastoid surgery is much less than 1%. Delayed onset paresis (more than 3 days postsurgery) is more common but usually due to viral reactivation (38). The most common site of iatrogenic injury is the tympanic segment adjacent to the oval window (39). The nerve is more susceptible in this region because it is the most common site of fallopian canal dehiscence. The next most common site of injury is the mastoid segment. At times, cholesteatoma and granulation tissue obscure landmarks, increasing the risk of nerve injury. When in doubt, remove diseased tissue to confirm the location of the horizontal semicircular canal, digastric ridge, and incus to aid facial nerve dissection. Iatrogenic injury frequently results in complete transection of the nerve. Once again, end-to-end anastomosis or interpositional graft is required to restore continuity. Partial injuries, involving 50% of the diameter of the nerve or less, are best treated by decompression proximal and distal to the injury.

Nerve anastomosis is accomplished using interrupted epineural sutures of a 9-0 monofilament, such as nylon. General principles of neurorrhaphy attempt to maximize the number of regenerating axons sprouting across the anastomotic site. All neural tissue is handled atraumatically by using microinstruments designed for neural repair. Approximation of nerve endings is done best under the illumination and magnification of the operating microscope. Exact end-to-end approximation is performed without tension on the anastomosis.

Interpositional grafts are used when a direct end-to-end anastomosis creates tension or when segments of the nerve

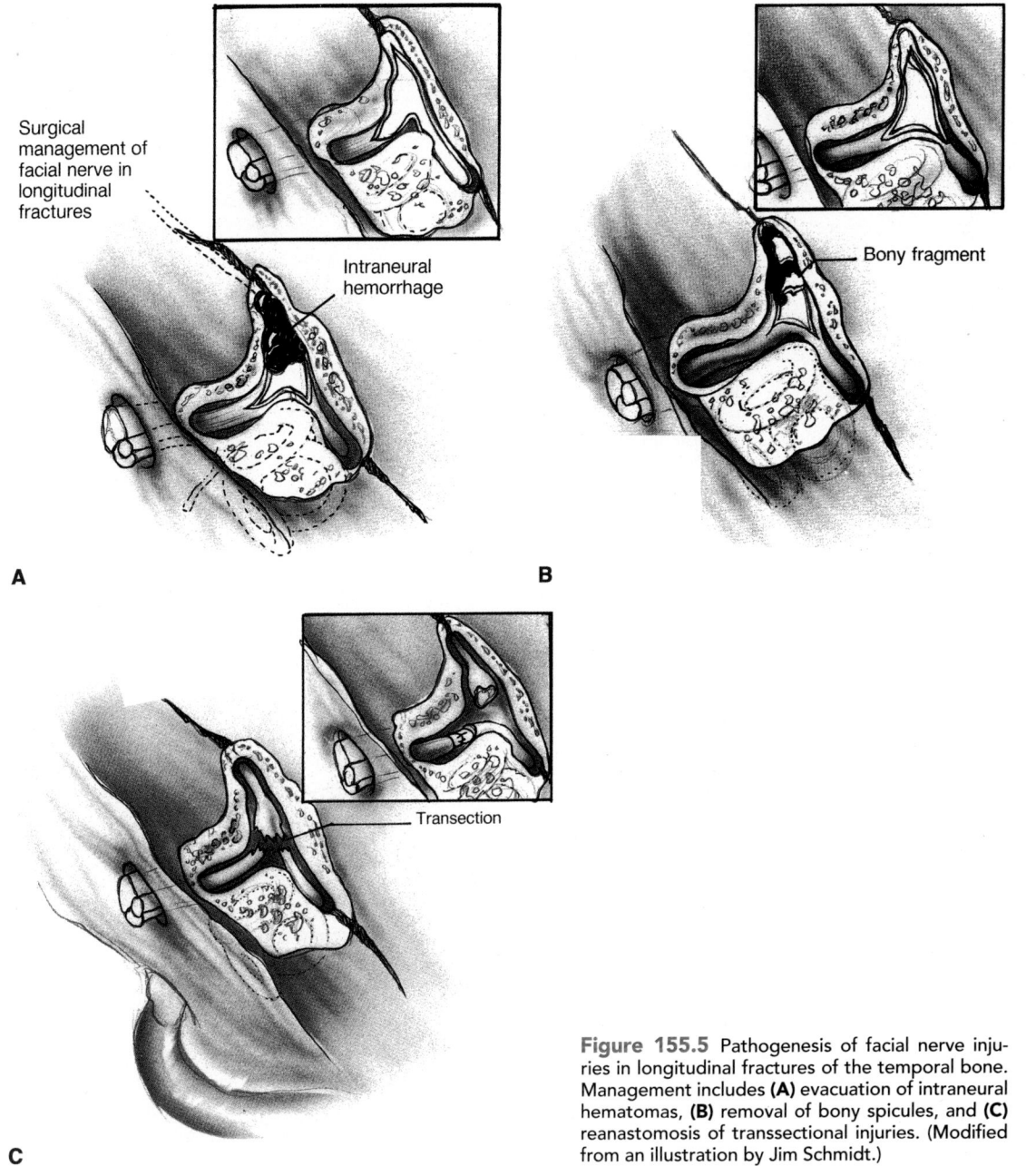

Surgical management of facial nerve in longitudinal fractures

Intraneural hemorrhage

A

Bony fragment

B

Transection

C

Figure 155.5 Pathogenesis of facial nerve injuries in longitudinal fractures of the temporal bone. Management includes **(A)** evacuation of intraneural hematomas, **(B)** removal of bony spicules, and **(C)** reanastomosis of transsectional injuries. (Modified from an illustration by Jim Schmidt.)

are missing or severely damaged. Donor nerves for use in grafting include the greater auricular, median antebrachial cutaneous, and sural nerves (Fig. 155.6). Resulting sensory deficits are modest and show some improvement with time.

TUMORS OF THE SKULL BASE AND FACIAL NERVE

Tumors rarely present with acute facial paralysis. It is estimated that only 5% of tumors involving the facial nerve present in this manner. Opinions differ on the guidelines for obtaining radiographic evaluation in patients with acute

facial paralysis, but certain circumstances do increase the probability of neoplastic discovery, including the following:

- A paresis evolving slowly over a period exceeding 3 weeks
- No return of facial function when the process has had an opportunity for regeneration
- Recurrent palsy on the same side
- Coexistence of facial twitching with an evolving paresis
- Development of chronic, unilateral eustachian tube dysfunction in a patient with no prior history of chronic middle-ear disease
- Presence of multiple cranial nerve deficits
- Presence of a neck or parotid mass
- History of cutaneous malignancy

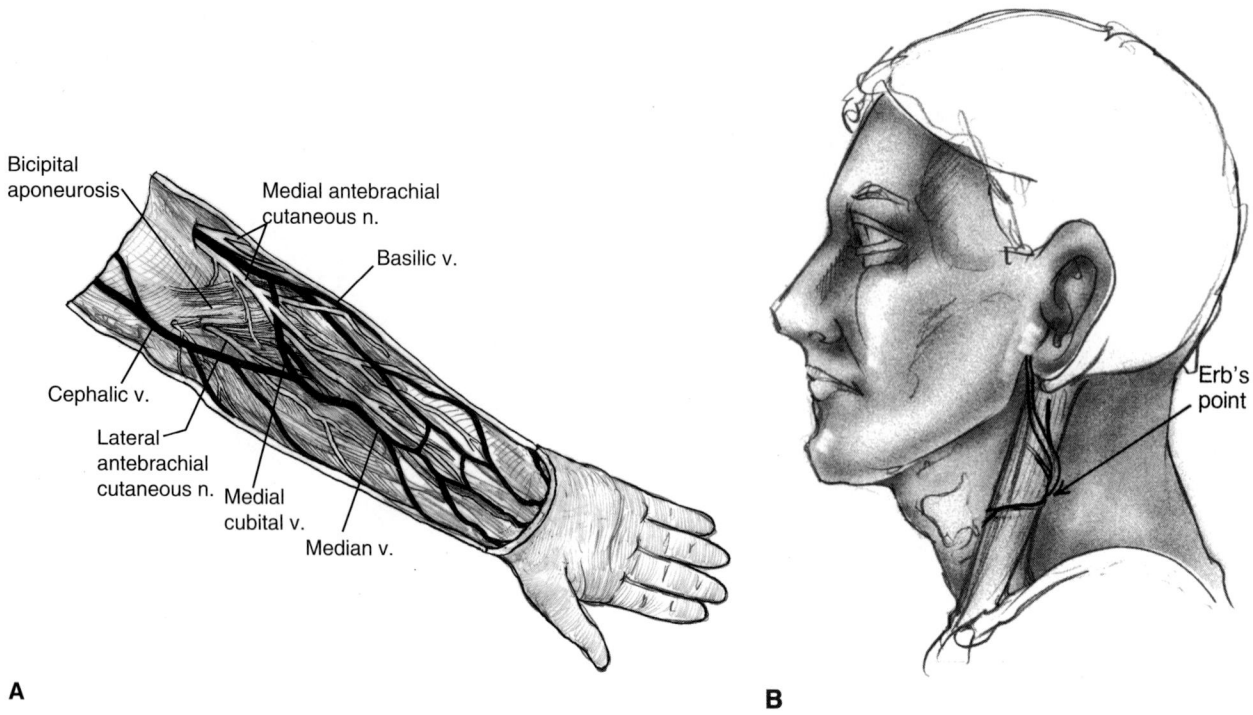

A   **B**

Figure 155.6 Popular interpositional grafts for repair of the facial nerve include the medial antebrachial cutaneous (**A**) and greater auricular (**B**) nerves.

Several benign and malignant tumors can involve the facial nerve along its intracranial, intratemporal, or extracranial course. The most common tumor of the nerve is the facial schwannoma. Initial symptoms vary, depending on the involved segment of the nerve. Tumors involving only the cerebellopontine angle or internal auditory canal portions of the nerve will present with hearing loss or tinnitus. Intratemporal tumors often present with a slowly evolving facial paralysis, middle-ear mass, or conductive hearing loss. Extratemporal tumors present as a parotid mass and rarely exhibit any facial nerve dysfunction. All segments of the nerve may be involved, although the geniculate and labyrinthine segments are most common (40). Excision usually requires the use of interpositional grafting for restoration of continuity (41). One of the most difficult decisions on discovery of the tumor is the timing of management. In the geriatric population, a small tumor with minimal facial or middle-ear involvement is best observed. In the young patient, the tumor is best resected and the nerve grafted. If the tumor is allowed to grow, more motor axons will undergo degeneration with irreversible changes in both the axons and muscle endplates, such that any neural reinnervation technique will be compromised. A grade III return of facial function is the best result anticipated from grafting, so the patient needs preparation for a less than perfect outcome.

Skull base tumors present an array of management problems regarding the facial nerve, and the otologic surgeon must be capable of any number of procedures to preserve the integrity of the nerve: transposition, rerouting, division and reanastomosis, interpositional grafting, and cranial nerve crossover. Anterior transposition of the facial nerve spares the greater superficial petrosal nerve and preserves normal tearing and is preferred for benign tumors of the infralabyrinthine compartment. Posterior transposition provides access to the petrous apex. Division and reanastomosis may aid exposure to the parapharyngeal space, but it should be avoided, as any transection of the nerve followed by neural anastomosis will result in synkinesis or mass movement. When the tumor is benign, the continuity of the nerve should be preserved by mobilization techniques. Exceptions to this rule include facial nerve schwannomas, which usually require resection of nerve with interpositional grafting; benign tumors invading the nerve (e.g., cranial nerve schwannomas, paragangliomas, cholesteatoma); and recurrent tumors adherent to the nerve, which necessitate excision of the nerve to ensure complete tumor removal.

Malignant tumors involving nerve typically require excision with a tumor-free margin. Exceptions include patients with normal or slightly impaired facial function, lymphomatous and leukemic invasion of the nerve, and low-grade malignancies of the parotid. In these cases, the tumors are removed while sparing the nerve.

FACIAL PALSY IN THE NEWBORN

Categories for facial palsy in the newborn include traumatic and congenital etiologies. Facial palsy secondary to birth trauma has an incidence of about 0.02%. Physical signs of trauma include facial contusion, ecchymosis over the mastoid or course of the extracranial nerve, or a hemotympanum. Risk factors include forceps delivery, birth weight greater than 3,500 g, and primiparity (42). Thus, the mechanism of injury is likely to be compression due to molding of the head in passage through the birth canal or to the use of forceps. Within the first 3 days of life, an infant with complete facial paralysis should undergo electrical stimulation to demonstrate muscle contraction or evoked myogenic potentials. If trauma is not so evident, the information gained from the electrical tests provides conclusive evidence of neuromuscular integrity. For later presentations, NET, MST, and ENoG should be used initially, followed by EMG if myogenic responses are absent. The EMG may demonstrate insertional muscle activity, intact motor units, fibrillation potentials, or polyphasic motor units indicative of incomplete injury. The prognosis for spontaneous regeneration is excellent and surgical exploration is not recommended unless the nerve has had an opportunity for recovery (43).

Congenital palsy most commonly presents as a unilateral weakness of the lower lip and can be associated with other anomalies. Kobayashi (44) found no relationship of this limited form of palsy to the use of teratogenic drugs, rubella, birth trauma, or hereditary factors. More rarely, congenital facial palsies can present with other physical anomalies as part of a genetic syndrome. In Mobius syndrome, paralysis can result from congenital absence of the motor portion of the facial nerve and facial musculature or agenesis of the facial motor nucleus (45). Associated findings include unilateral or bilateral and complete or incomplete facial weakness, unilateral or bilateral abducens nerve palsy, and deformities of the extremities. Congenital paralysis is best left untreated until late childhood, as muscle transfers and fascial slings are often necessary for improved cosmesis. Because of the good skin turgor, the eye does not commonly require protective measures to prevent exposure keratitis in the child.

EYE CARE

The most common complication after the onset of facial paralysis is corneal desiccation. Complete paralysis, diminished tearing, loss of corneal sensitivity due to trigeminal nerve involvement, and absent Bell phenomenon are poor prognostic signs. At the onset, the patient should be advised of the signs of corneal irritation: itching, redness, foreign-body sensation, and visual blurring. Rubbing the eye is a sure sign of corneal irritation. Measures recommended for protection include the liberal use of ophthalmic lubricants, closure of the eye with tape at night, use of moisture chambers or shielded glasses, and avoidance of wind, vents, and fans. Patient education and fastidious treatment usually prevent the development of ulcers or scarring. If symptoms persist, ophthalmologic consultation is advised. Surgical treatment of the eye is rarely necessary

in acute and temporary palsies. Patients with long-standing paralysis, corneal hypesthesia, and prior nerve repair with grafts are likely to require adjunctive management of the eye. Gold weight implants, canthoplasty, tarsorrhaphy, and upper eyelid springs are among the available surgical options.

HIGHLIGHTS

- Cranial nerve VII is composed of special visceral afferent, general visceral efferent, and special visceral efferent fibers, which provide taste, lacrimation, and mimetic functions respectively.
- The middle-ear and mastoid landmarks to the location of the facial nerve include the cochleariform process, the oval window, the horizontal semicircular canal, the chorda tympani nerve, and the digastric ridge.
- A paresis does not warrant electrophysiologic tests (NET, MST, ENoG), as the prognosis for recovery is good until the palsy is complete. Serial testing of a complete paralysis in the acute phase of degeneration provides the most accurate information on nerve injury and prognosis for recovery. EMG is the most reliable test for the evaluation of long-standing paralysis.
- Bell palsy accounts for more than half of acute facial palsy presentations. Any of the following make the diagnosis of Bell palsy less probable: a paresis evolving over a period exceeding 3 weeks, signs of neoplasia, trauma along the course of the nerve, vesicles on the head or neck, multiple cranial nerve involvement, temporal bone infection, palsy at birth, signs of central nervous system lesion, and failure to have any evidence of recovery 6 months after onset.
- Bell palsy patients demonstrate return to normal or near-normal function in 83% of cases without treatment. Experimental and clinical data implicate HSV as the likely causative agent. Medical therapy commonly includes steroids and antivirals, though the ability of these agents to alter prognosis remains controversial.
- The varicella zoster virus can produce facial paralysis. The hallmark of this infection is a vesicular eruption over the distribution of sensory afferent neurons of the cervical plexus or cranial nerves V, VII, IX, or X. The prognosis for functional recovery is poorer than in patients with Bell palsy. Antiviral therapy is recommended.
- For facial palsy presenting as a complication of infection, the immediate treatment should be directed toward eradicating the infection.

■ Temporal bone fractures are the most common cause of traumatic injury to the facial nerve. Most injuries involve the nerve in the perigeniculate region or in the tympanic segment above the oval window. The most common finding at surgical exploration is contusion.

■ The preferred order of procedures used to preserve the integrity of motor function of the facial nerve during management of skull base tumors is transposition or rerouting, division and reanastomosis, interpositional grafting, and cranial nerve crossover (XII to VII or XI to VII). Any anastomosis or grafting of the intracranial or intratemporal facial nerve will have synkinesis as a result.

REFERENCES

1. Anson BJ, Harper DG, Warpeha RL. Surgical anatomy of the facial canal and facial nerve. *Ann Otol* 1963;72:713–734.
2. Nager GT, Proctor B. Anatomical variations and anomalies involving the facial canal. *Ann Otol Rhinol Laryngol* 1982;91(Suppl):45–57.
3. Vrabec JT, Lin JW. Inner ear anomalies in congenital aural atresia. *Otol Neurotol* 2010;31:1421–1426.
4. Thomander L, Aldskogius H, Grant G. Motor fibre organization in the intratemporal portion of a cat and rat facial nerve studied with the horseradish peroxidase technique. *Acta Otolaryngol (Stockh)* 1982;93:397–405.
5. Gacek RR, Radpour S. Fiber orientation of the facial nerve: an experimental study in the cat. *Laryngoscope* 1982;92:547–556.
6. Pitts DB, Adour KK, Hilsinger RL. Recurrent Bell's palsy: analysis of 140 patients. *Laryngoscope* 1988;98:535–540.
7. Levenson MJ, Ingerman M, Grimes C, et al. Melkersson-Rosenthal syndrome. *Arch Otolaryngol* 1984;110:540–542.
8. Vrabec JT, Backous DD, Djalilian HR, et al.; Facial Nerve Disorders Committee. Facial Nerve Grading System 2.0. *Otolaryngol Head Neck Surg* 2009;140:445–450.
9. Keane JR. Bilateral seventh nerve palsy: analysis of 43 cases and review of the literature. *Neurology* 1994;44:1198–2002.
10. Lauman EPJ, Jongkees LBW. On the prognosis of peripheral facial paralysis of endotemporal origin. *Ann Otol Rhinol Laryngol* 1963;72:621–636.
11. May M, Blumenthal F, Klein SR. Acute Bell's palsy: prognostic value of evoked electromyography, maximal stimulation, and other electrical tests. *Am J Otol* 1983;5:1–7.
12. Fisch U, Esslen E. Total intratemporal exposure of the facial nerve. *Arch Otolaryngol* 1972;95:335–341.
13. Fisch U. Prognostic value of electrical tests in acute facial paralysis. *Am J Otol* 1984;5:494–498.
14. Haginomori S, Wada S, Takamaki A, et al. A novel electroneurography method in facial palsy. *Acta Otolaryngol* 2010;130:520–524.
15. Coker NJ, Fordice JO, Moore S. Correlation of the nerve excitability test and electroneurography in acute facial paralysis. *Am J Otol* 1992;13:127–133.
16. Murakami S, Mizobuchi M, Nakashiro Y, et al. Bell palsy and herpes simplex virus: identification of viral DNA in endoneurial fluid and muscle. *Ann Intern Med* 1996;124:27–30.
17. Sugita T, Murakami S, Yanagihara N, et al. Facial nerve paralysis induced by herpes simplex virus in mice: an animal model of acute and transient facial paralysis. *Ann Otol Rhinol Laryngol* 1995;104:574–581.
18. Campbell KE, Brundage JF. Effects of climate, latitude, and season on the incidence of Bell's palsy in the US Armed Forces, October 1997 to September 1999. *Am J Epidemiol* 2002;156:32–39.
19. Peitersen E. Bell's palsy: the spontaneous course of 2,500 peripheral facial nerve palsies of different etiologies. *Acta Otolaryngol Suppl* 2002;549:4–30.
20. Xu F, Sternberg MR, Kottiri BJ, et al. Trends in herpes simplex virus type 1 and type 2 seroprevalence in the United States. *JAMA* 2006;296:964–973.
21. Liston SL, Kleid MS. Histopathology of Bell's palsy. *Laryngoscope* 1989;99:23–26.
22. Sullivan FM, Swan IR, Donnan PT, et al. Early treatment with prednisolone or acyclovir in Bell's palsy. *N Engl J Med* 2007;357:1598–1607.
23. Engström M, Berg T, Stjernquist-Desatnik A, et al. Prednisolone and valacyclovir in Bell's palsy: a randomised, double-blind, placebo-controlled, multicentre trial. *Lancet Neurol* 2008;7:993–1000.
24. Adour KK, Ruboyianes JM, Von Doersten PG, et al. Bell's palsy treatment with acyclovir and prednisone compared with prednisone alone: a double-blind, randomized, controlled trial. *Ann Otol Rhinol Laryngol* 1996;105:371–378.
25. de Almeida JR, Al Khabori M, Guyatt GH, et al. Combined corticosteroid and antiviral treatment for Bell palsy: a systematic review and meta-analysis. *JAMA* 2009;302:985–993.
26. Gantz BJ, Rubinstein JT, Gidley P, et al. Surgical management of Bell's palsy. *Laryngoscope* 1999;109:1177–1188.
27. Sweeney CJ, Gilden DH. Ramsay Hunt syndrome. *J Neurol Neurosurg Psychiatry* 2001;71:149–154.
28. Jackson CG, Johnson GD, Hyams VJ, et al. Pathologic findings in the labyrinthine segment of the facial nerve in a case of facial paralysis. *Ann Otol Rhinol Laryngol* 1990;99:327–329.
29. de Ru JA, van Benthem PP. Combination therapy is preferable for patients with Ramsay Hunt syndrome. *Otol Neurotol* 2011;32:852–855.
30. Ellefsen B, Bonding P. Facial palsy in acute otitis media. *Clin Otolaryngol* 1996;21:393–395.
31. Popovtzer A, Raveh E, Bahar G, et al. Facial palsy associated with acute otitis media. *Otolaryngol Head Neck Surg* 2005;132:327–329.
32. Redaelli de Zinis LO, Gamba P, Balzanelli C. Acute otitis media and facial nerve paralysis in adults. *Otol Neurotol* 2003;24:113–117.
33. Makeham TP, Croxson GR, Coulson S. Infective causes of facial nerve paralysis. *Otol Neurotol* 2007;28:100–103.
34. Mani N, Sudhoff H, Rajagopal S, et al. Cranial nerve involvement in malignant external otitis: implications for clinical outcome. *Laryngoscope* 2007;117:907–910.
35. Coker NJ, Kendall KA, Jenkins HA, et al. Traumatic intratemporal facial nerve injury: management rationale for preservation of function. *Otolaryngol Head Neck Surg* 1987;97:262–269.
36. Brodie HA, Thompson TC. Management of complication from 820 temporal bone fractures. *Am J Otol* 1997;18:188–197.
37. Duncan NO, Coker NJ, Jenkins HA, et al. Gunshot injuries of the temporal bone. *Otolaryngol Head Neck Surg* 1986;94:47–56.
38. Vrabec JT. Delayed facial palsy following tympanomastoid surgery. *Am J Otol* 1999;20:26–30.
39. Green JD, Shelton C, Brackmann DE. Iatrogenic facial nerve injury during otologic surgery. *Laryngoscope* 1994;104:922–926.
40. Vrabec JT, Guinto FC, Nauta HJ. Recurrent facial neuromas. *Am J Otol* 1998;19:99–103.
41. Lipkin AF, Coker NJ, Jenkins HA, et al. Intracranial and intratemporal facial neuroma. *Otolaryngol Head Neck Surg* 1987;96:71–79.
42. Falco NA, Eriksson E. Facial nerve palsy in the newborn: incidence and outcome. *Plast Reconstr Surg* 1990;85:1–4.
43. Bergman I, May M, Wessle HB, et al. Management of facial palsy caused by birth trauma. *Laryngoscope* 1986;96:381–384.
44. Kobayashi T. Congenital facial palsy. In: Fisch U, ed. *Facial nerve surgery.* Birmingham: Aesculapius, 1977:578–580.
45. Nisenson A, Isaacson A, Grant S. Masklike facies with associated congenital anomalies (Möbius syndrome). *J Pediatr* 1955;46:255–261.

Otologic Manifestations of Systemic Disease: Includes Autoimmune Inner Ear Disease

156

Arnaud F. Bewley   Michael J. Ruckenstein

Numerous systemic diseases can affect the ear, causing a variety of otologic complaints including hearing loss, vestibular dysfunction, and facial nerve paresis. These diseases span a broad differential including infectious, granulomatous, autoimmune, bone, and metabolic etiologies (Table 156.1). Prior to progressing to systemic involvement, many can initially present as a process isolated to the ear. It is therefore critical that the otolaryngologist be aware of this broad differential when evaluating any otologic complaint. This chapter provides a systematic review of this differential, discussing the most pertinent examples of each etiology. The topic of autoimmune disease includes a discussion of autoimmune inner ear disease (AIED), a rare cause of sensorineural hearing loss (SNHL), given that what we know about the pathophysiology of this disease derives largely from our knowledge of how systemic autoimmune diseases affect the ear.

INFECTIOUS DISEASE

Infectious diseases are the most common type of systemic disease to manifest otologic pathology. Pathogens may infect the inner ear and auditory pathways *in utero*, resulting in congenital syndromes that often include deafness, or infection may be acquired after birth. As the fluids of the inner ear are not easily accessible for sampling, the implication of viral pathogens as the causes of otologic disease has often depended on circumstantial evidence, including an associated viral illness, like an upper respiratory infection, or demonstration of seroconversion during the time of hearing loss. In other cases, more direct evidence exists such as with CMV infection, where DNA has been amplified using PCR from perilymph obtained during cochlear implantation in children previously diagnosed with congenital infection (1).

Cytomegalovirus

Cytomegalovirus (CMV) is a large double-stranded DNA virus belonging to the herpes virus family. Its name derives from the typical appearance of infected tissues, containing massively enlarged cytomegalic inclusion cells. CMV is the most common congenital infection in the world. One percent of babies born in the United States are infected; the likely route of infection is transplacental. Of these babies, 10% will exhibit symptomatic infection, or cytomegalic inclusion disease, almost exclusively when primary maternal infection occurs during pregnancy (2). Of those babies that survive the neonatal period, the majority will have severe neurologic deficits and a severe bilateral SNHL. Possibly more significant, from an epidemiologic point of view, is hearing loss that develops in those children with apparently asymptomatic congenital CMV infection; between 7% and 15% of these infants will go on to develop SNHL. Most cases will be mild, but up to a quarter will be severe (3). Hearing loss may be unilateral or bilateral and may develop months or years after birth and be missed on routine audiometric screening. It is thought that asymptomatic CMV infection causes 20% to 30% of congenital hearing loss. In the healthy adult, CMV infection is usually asymptomatic or may cause a mononucleosis-like syndrome. In human immunodeficiency virus (HIV)-infected or transplant patients, severe multisystemic disease may ensue, but hearing loss is not common.

Rubella

Rubella is a member of the Togaviridae family. Primary maternal infection during the first trimester of pregnancy may result in congenital rubella syndrome. SNHL is the most common manifestation of this disease, seen in up to 60% of affected infants. Hearing loss may be bilateral or unilateral, may manifest as late as the second year of life, and may be the only sign of infection. Other features are ocular malformations, including cataract and retinopathy; cardiac malformations; and central nervous system (CNS) disease. Postnatal infection produces German measles, a mild viral illness (4).

TABLE 156.1	SYSTEMIC DISEASES WITH OTOLOGIC MANIFESTATIONS

Infectious diseases
  Viral infection
    Varicella-zoster
    Mumps
    Measles
    HIV
    CMV
    Rubella
  Bacterial infection
    Syphilis
    Lyme disease
Granulomatous disease
  Langerhans histiocytosis
  Sarcoidosis
  Wegener granulomatosis
Autoimmune disease
  Cogan's syndrome
  Polyarteritis nodosa
  Relapsing polychondritis
  Rheumatoid arthritis
Diseases of bone
  Paget disease
  Osteogenesis imperfecta
  Fibrous dysplasia
  Osteopetrosis
Metabolic disorders
  Mucopolysaccharidoses

Varicella-Zoster

Varicella-zoster virus (VZV) is a herpes virus that results in varicella or chickenpox with primary infection. Once the primary infection is cleared, VZV remains dormant in the dorsal root ganglia. Reactivation of the virus, often during periods of suppressed cellular immunity, results in shingles, or a dermatomal vesicular eruption. Reactivation of VZV in the geniculate ganglion results in Ramsay-Hunt syndrome, or herpes zoster oticus. Involvement of the facial nerve results in the classical presentation of deep otalgia, vesicular eruptions on the external ear and tympanic membrane, and facial palsy. Extension of the inflammatory process to involve the vestibulocochlear nerve may result in SNHL and vertigo.

Mumps and Measles

The mumps and measles viruses are members of the Paramyxoviridae family. Infection with this virus is rare in the developed world due to widespread use of vaccination, though it is still common worldwide. Mumps infection commonly presents with unilateral or bilateral parotitis and orchitis in males. The classic presentation of measles (rubeola) involves cough, coryza, conjunctivitis, white oral mucosal lesions known as Koplik spots, and a

maculopapular rash. SNHL with mumps is uncommon, affecting less than 0.05% of patients, and tends to be unilateral (5). Similarly, hearing loss is uncommon in measles infection, seen in approximately 0.1% of patients.

HIV

HIV infection is associated with a significant incidence of SNHL, though this relationship is not fully understood. The etiology is likely variable and includes a high incidence of middle-ear disease, opportunistic infections and malignancies of the CNS, viral labyrinthitis and neuritis, and ototoxicity from medications used to treat HIV infection and its complications (6).

Bacterial Infection

Most bacterial infections involving the inner ear represent extension of inflammation or infection from the middle ear or CNS. Acute otitis media can produce a sterile serous labyrinthitis secondary to the passage of bacterial toxins and inflammatory mediators into the inner ear fluids, likely through the round window or a dehiscent lateral semicircular canal in patients with chronic middle-ear disease and cholesteatoma. This typically causes a mild high-frequency hearing loss. Entrance of bacteria into the inner ear will lead to a suppurative labyrinthitis, which is heralded by severe hearing loss, vertigo, and vegetative symptoms.

Similarly, in patients with meningitis, bacteria may invade the labyrinth via the internal auditory canal or the cochlear aqueduct. SNHL is a common complication of meningitis, particularly in children. Up to a third of patients with bacterial meningitis sustain some loss of hearing. The hearing loss is typically bilateral and stable, though it may be unilateral and progressive or fluctuating. Male sex, CT scan evidence of elevated intracranial pressure, nuchal rigidity, low cerebrospinal fluid (CSF) glucose levels, and *Streptococcus pneumoniae* as the infective agent all are associated with an increased incidence of postmeningitic SNHL.

Syphilis

Syphilis was historically a common cause of otologic dysfunction though this late manifestation of the disease is uncommon today in the developed world. Syphilis is caused by infection with *Treponema pallidum*, which may be transmitted transplacentally (congenital syphilis) or through sexual contact (acquired syphilis). Though the incidence of syphilis peaked in the United States in the 1940s and has since declined, there has recently been an increase in the incidence among male homosexuals and patients with HIV (7,8). Syphilis is characterized by classic symptomatic stages interspersed with periods lacking significant symptoms. Primary syphilis is typically seen in the acquired form and is characterized by the presence of a chancre (a painless, nonpurulent, and indurated ulcer in the region of sexual contact), which usually appears 3 weeks after initial infection. Although usually solitary, multiple ulcers may be seen in HIV-infected patients (7); however, chancres may go unnoticed and may only be seen in a third of cases (9). Symptoms can last from 3 to 90 days, but often go unnoticed (10). Secondary syphilis occurs weeks after the chancre has healed and is characterized by a variety of mucosal and cutaneous lesions that appear 2 to 12 weeks after initial infection (it may overlap the primary stage in up to 75% of HIV-infected patients) as well as the presence of constitutional symptoms such as fever and malaise. Asymptomatic meningitis may occur in up to 40% of patients (10), although associated sudden progressive bilateral hearing loss and vertigo are rare (11). Other organ systems may be involved, including the liver, kidney, eyes, and joints. The latent phase follows, which is characterized by a lengthy period free of symptoms. Tertiary syphilis, which is similar to late congenital syphilis, manifests years after initial infection. It is characterized by cardiovascular, gummatous, and neurologic involvement. Approximately 15% to 40% of untreated patients will progress to the third stage (7). Neurosyphilis is composed of meningovascular and parenchymal lesions that can lead to demyelination (tabes dorsalis), motor weakness, and sensory loss.

The diagnosis of syphilis depends on clinical findings, histologic examination of lesions, and serologic testing for syphilis. The Venereal Disease Research Laboratory screening test and rapid plasma reagin are useful screening tests, but lack sufficient sensitivity for both early and late syphilis (10). Treponemal tests, such as the fluorescent treponemal antibody absorption (FTA-ABS) test or a microhemagglutination test for *T. pallidum*, have higher sensitivity and specificity, and are often required for diagnosis. In fact, routine serologic testing for otosyphilis is recommended in all cases of idiopathic progressive SNHL (12). In addition, the diagnosis of neurosyphilis may require testing of CSF (10).

The otologic manifestation of syphilis presents as both hearing and vestibular dysfunction. Sensorineural hearing is very common from both in congenital and the later stages of acquired syphilis. It can be present in up to 40% of patients with congenital syphilis and up to 80% to 90% of patients with neurosyphilis (13). In addition, many patients present with vestibular dysfunction similar to that seen with Ménière disease (14). In fact, it has been reported to be present in up to 7% on patients thought to have Ménière disease (11). Left untreated, however, otogenic syphilis has a more aggressive course than Ménière disease, commonly involving both ears and leading to profound deafness. Physical exam reveals signs consistent with SNHL and peripheral vestibular loss. Hennebert sign (vertigo and nystagmus induced with air pressure to the middle ear) and Tullio phenomenon (vertigo and nystagmus caused by loud noise) may be associated with tertiary syphilis.

The changes in the inner ear resulting from syphilis have been well described. The otic capsule may be involved during the secondary and/or tertiary stages of infection.

Involvement manifests as osteitis of the otic capsule bone. Inflammation is mediated by mononuclear cells and results in patchy bone reabsorption; these spaces are subsequently filled with fatty marrow and loose connective tissue (15). It is accompanied by an obliterative endarteritis typical of syphilitic infection. In severe cases, gumma (lymphocytic infiltrates, vascular occlusion, and central necrosis) may be noted in the otic capsule. In addition, degeneration of the labyrinthine membrane, endolymphatic hydrops, and fibrosis have been described (16). The peripheral vestibular system may also be involved during the second stage of infection, in which both the VIII cranial nerve and labyrinth are involved in fulminant meningoneurolabyrinthitis.

Penicillin-based antibiotics (or an alternate if allergic) are the treatment of choice, with duration varied by stage of disease. The use of corticosteroids in the treatment of otogenic syphilis is controversial (11,17–20). The prognosis for hearing loss in otogenic syphilis is poor, with hearing improvement seen in less than one-third of treated patients (13).

Lyme Disease

SNHL has also been reported in association with infection by another spirochete, *Borrelia burgdorferi*, the causative organism of Lyme disease. The organism is introduced into the skin by the bite of an infected tick of the genus *Ixodes*. The spirochete has particular tropism to skin, CNS, heart, joints, and the eyes. It is not fully clear which features are a result of disseminated infection and which result from the systemic inflammatory response. In the head and neck, Lyme disease is most commonly associated with facial paresis, particularly in children. There have also been reports of sudden SNHL or a Ménière-like syndrome.

GRANULOMATOUS DISEASE

Langerhans Histiocytosis

Langerhans histiocytosis (previously called histiocytosis X) describes a group of idiopathic disease caused by the abnormal proliferation of histiocytes. Histiocytes, normally benign cells found in the dermis or epidermis, accumulate in the skin, bone, lymph nodes, and visceral organs. This group is comprised of three diseases, eosinophilic granuloma, Hand-Schüller-Christian disease, and Letterer-Siwe disease, which describe progressively more aggressive and widespread manifestations of the same underlying pathology. Patients with eosinophilic granuloma develop solitary osteolytic lesions without systemic manifestations. The course of this disease is typically benign, and patients often undergo spontaneous regression of their lesions. For those who do not, local excision of the granuloma or intralesional steroids can be performed. Hand-Schüller-Christian disease typically affects patients less than 5 years old, who develop multifocal osteolytic lesions with rare extraskeletal involvement. Up to 25% of patients present with the triad of osteolytic skull lesions, exophthalmos, and diabetes insipidus. Letter-Siwe is the most aggressive of this group, presenting most commonly in children less than 3 years old, who develop disseminated disease with diffuse involvement of multiple organs. Prognosis is poor with most patients succumbing to the disease in childhood (21). Lesional biopsy for each of these diseases demonstrates characteristic tennis racket–shaped Birbeck granule on histology, the result of cytoplasmic inclusions bodies. In addition, diagnosis can be made by demonstrating the presence of the CD1 antigen with immunohistochemistry (21).

The otologic manifestations of these diseases result from the development of a granuloma within the temporal bone. As the granuloma expands, it can cause conductive hearing loss, otorrhea, facial nerve paralysis, vertigo, and SNHL depending on which anatomic structures the granuloma violates (22,23). For patients with systemic disease and a temporal bone lesion, systemic steroids are the first line of therapy, with etoposide, vincristine, and vinblastine reserved for refractory patients. For patients with disease localized to the temporal bone, surgical debulking can be performed with topical and intralesional injection of steroids. Radiation therapy has also been successful in treating temporal bone lesions refractory to resection (24).

Sarcoidosis

Sarcoidosis is a chronic multisystem disorder characterized by the presence of noncaseating granulomas. Classically, patients present with pulmonary symptoms characterized by persistent cough and hilar lymphadenopathy on chest x-ray. In addition, they can develop a granulomatous skin rash, iridocyclitis, keratoconjunctivitis, hepatosplenomegaly, myalgias, arthralgias, and neuropathies. Laboratory examination typically demonstrates hypercalcemia and an elevated angiotensin-converting enzyme level.

The otologic manifestations of sarcoidosis can result from uveoparotid fever or granulomatous disease within the middle ear or temporal bone. Uveoparotid fever, or Heerfordt syndrome, describes the constellation of parotitis, uveitis, fever, and facial nerve paralysis (25). Temporal bone or middle-ear granulomas can result in conductive or sensorineural hearing loss and vestibular dysfunction. Primary treatment of sarcoidosis is accomplished with corticosteroids. Refractory patients can benefit from methotrexate, cyclophosphamide, and number of other immunomodulatory agents (26).

Wegener Granulomatosis

Wegener granulomatosis is a systemic vasculitis of medium and small blood vessels resulting in a triad of necrotizing granulomas of the upper airway, necrotizing glomerulonephritis, and systemic necrotizing angiitis. Though Wegener granulomatosis is due to an autoimmune process, it is

included in this section on granulomatous disease given that the otologic manifestations are mostly due to granulomatous involvement of the middle ear. Necrotizing granulomas can develop within the middle ear and mastoid, compromising the ossicular chain and eustachian tube function, resulting in a conductive hearing loss. This is more common than inner ear disease, but 8% to 20% of patients with Wegener granulomatosis do develop SNHL that is likely more similar in etiology to autoimmune disease as is discussed later in this chapter (27,28).

AUTOIMMUNE DISEASE

Autoimmune inflammation of the inner ear may be part of a systemic autoimmune syndrome or may occur in isolation as an organ-specific process. The most common autoimmune diseases that affect the ear are Cogan syndrome, polyarteritis nodosa (PAN), rheumatoid arthritis, relapsing polychondritis, and Wegener granulomatosis. The clinical presentation and pathophysiology of these diseases' otologic manifestations are reviewed in this section. Several of these diseases have also been associated with cases of sudden hearing loss and histopathologic evidence of labyrinthitis (29). When autoimmune inflammation of the inner ear occurs as an organ-specific process, we refer to this as AIED, a relatively recently identified disease about which much remains unknown.

Cogan Syndrome

Cogan syndrome is a rare disease characterized by nonsyphilitic interstitial keratitis associated with vertigo, tinnitus, and hearing loss (30,31). The auditory and vestibular dysfunction resembles that seen in Ménière disease and untreated, progresses to profound deafness within weeks or months (32). The interval between ocular and otologic disease varies from a few weeks to a year; either organ may be affected first. Other forms of ocular inflammation, including uveitis, iritis, episcleritis, or conjunctivitis, may occur instead of the keratitis, in which case the disorder may be defined as atypical Cogan syndrome (33). The etiology of Cogan syndrome is unknown. While the relatively focal inflammation suggests organ-specific autoimmunity, this has not been proven. Like other vasculitides, the disease may represent a hypersensitive immune reaction to a viral infection. Vogt-Koyanagi-Harada syndrome presents with symptoms similar to those seen in Cogan syndrome. However, it also includes depigmentation of the hair and skin around the eyelashes, loss of eyelashes, and onset of aseptic meningitis. It may represent an autoimmune reaction to melanin-containing cells (34).

Polyarteritis Nodosa

Immune-mediated inner ear disease (IMIED) can also be a component of PAN (35). Postmortem temporal bone histopathologic studies on patients with PAN have demonstrated vasculitic changes within the labyrinth. PAN is a systemic vasculitis of small and medium blood vessels without glomerulonephritis. Vessel wall inflammation progresses to aneurysmal dilation, thrombosis, and tissue infraction with the manifestations of the disease being those of end-organ ischemia. There is an association with hepatitis B infection with approximately 30% of PAN patients demonstrating positive hepatitis B surface antigen.

Relapsing Polychondritis

Relapsing polychondritis describes an immune-mediated, episodic inflammation of cartilaginous structures. This inflammation can affect any of a number of cartilaginous structure including those of the ear, nose, trachea, larynx, and ribs. As with many autoimmune disorders, women are more commonly affected than men, and the age of symptom onset is typically in the fifth decade of life. Acutely, the disease manifests as local inflammation with resulting arthropathies and can be associated with weight loss, myalgia, and fever. Over time, recurrent bouts of cartilaginous inflammation result in atrophy, scarring, and anatomic distortion of cartilaginous structures. On laboratory studies, patients present with an elevated erythrocyte sedimentation rate (ESR), normochromic normocytic anemia, and positive rheumatoid factor (36).

The otologic manifestations of relapsing polychondritis affect the cartilaginous portion of the pinna. Patients present with recurrent inflammation of the pinna, characterized by erythema, tenderness, and pain that spares the lobule and the canal (37). First-line treatment is with enteral corticosteroids. Second-line therapeutic agents include dapsone, indomethacin, and salicylates.

Rheumatoid Arthritis

Rheumatoid arthritis is another immune-mediated disease that can manifest otologic pathology. It is characterized by a persistent inflammatory synovitis resulting in progressive destruction of the cartilage within joints. Like relapsing polychondritis and many other autoimmune diseases, it is more common in women and typically presents in the fifth decade of life. Acutely, this disease causes myalgias, muscular weakness, fatigue, and anorexia. Over time, patients develop joint pain, inflammation, and deformation that are typical of the disease (38). Laboratory studies mirror those of relapsing polychondritis with elevated ESR, normochromic normocytic anemia, and positive rheumatoid factor.

The otologic manifestations of rheumatoid arthritis can affect the external, middle, and inner ear. Rheumatoid nodules, painful cutaneous or subcutaneous raised lesions, can develop on the external ear. Middle-ear manifestation is typically characterized by a conductive hearing loss secondary to involvement of the ossicular suspensory ligaments and resulting abnormal middle-ear mechanics. In addition, patients have a significantly higher rate of SNHL than the general population though the pathophysiologic mechanism for this is unknown (39). First-line treatment typically involves medical therapy with aspirin or nonsteroidal anti-inflammatory drugs, though steroids and immunosuppressant are commonly used for those with refractory or more severe disease.

Autoimmune Inner Ear Disease

AIED specifically refers to the clinical presentation of idiopathic, rapidly progressive, bilateral SNHL. This condition has come to be known by a variety of names including IMIED and immune-mediated cochlea-vestibular disease. While the pathogenesis of otologic dysfunction in some systemic autoimmune diseases has been well defined, our understanding of AIED still leaves much to be discovered.

AIED was first described by McCabe in 1979 as a rapidly progressive (over a course of weeks to months) bilateral SNHL that responds to the administration of immunosuppressants (40). In his original description, McCabe describes pathology restricted to the inner ear, which is now referred to as primary AIED. Since that time, secondary AIED has come to refer to multisystemic, organ-nonspecific autoimmune diseases that also involve the inner ear.

The classification of this disease as an autoimmune or immune-mediated disorder was initially assigned given the improvement in symptoms patients achieved with immunosuppressive therapy. Autoimmune diseases result when the immune system's ability to distinguish between self and non-self is disturbed, and cytotoxic mechanisms designed to destroy foreign material and microorganisms attack the native tissue. This process is mediated by a specific antigen inherent to the targeted organ to which the immune system has become improperly sensitized. Confirming the presence of this antigen confirms the immune-mediated nature of disease and helps guide treatment. As is discussed, a large amount of research has been dedicated toward identifying such an antigen for AIED, with limited success. Despite this, AIED is still felt to most likely arise from autoimmune etiology.

Epidemiology

Primary AIED is very rare, though it is difficult to determine the exact incidence, given the lack of a definitive diagnostic test to identify affected patients. Retrospective studies estimate the incidence as less than that of sudden SNHL, which occurs with an incidence of 1 case per 5,000 to 10,000 population per year (34,41).

Pathophysiology

The pathogenesis of AIED has been the subject of extensive research guided by the goal of developing more effective therapies. Given the probable immune-mediated nature of this disorder, much of this research has focused on identifying the responsible target antigen within the inner ear that is provoking the immune response. The main contribution of this work pertains to the detection of a specific antibody that binds to a 68-kilodalton (kDa) bovine inner ear antigen on Western blot analysis. This antibody has been found in the guinea pig model, as well as in humans with AIED (42,43). The same antibody was also found to bind to the inducible form of bovine (but not human) heat shock protein 70 (HSP-70), and as a result, this protein was once considered integral to the pathogenesis of AIED. More recent data suggest that the antibody targets multiple peptides similar to those present in the highly conserved protein CTL2, which is abundantly expressed in both the guinea pig and human inner ear (44). CTL2 coprecipitates with the protein cochlin, which is one of the most expressed proteins in the inner ear. Cochlin is critical to the structure and function of the inner ear, and mutations are known to cause cochleovestibular pathology. Recent work reveals that cochlin-specific serum Ab titers are significantly elevated in those with AIED in comparison to age-matched controls (45). The same study also implicates T-cell response to this specific protein, supporting cochlin as a possible target antigen susceptible to both B-cell and T-cell influence. CTL2 and cochlin have therefore replaced HSP-70 as the most likely target of the immune target in AIED.

Clinical Presentation

The hallmark of AIED, as originally described by McCabe, is the presence of bilateral SNHL that progresses during a period of weeks to months (34). It is important to note that the hearing loss may initially be unilateral and that it may take months for the bilaterality to emerge. Fluctuations in hearing may occur, but the overall course is one of a relentless deterioration in auditory function. Approximately 50% of patients have symptoms of vestibular dysfunction, with 20% of patients experiencing episodes of vertigo consistent with those seen in Ménière disease (34).

Differential Diagnosis

Critical in the diagnosis of AIED is differentiating it from sudden idiopathic SNHL, as these two diseases can present with similar symptoms. However, AIED and idiopathic sudden SNHL are two distinct disorders. AIED is considerably more rare than sudden SNHL. AIED is by definition bilateral, while sudden hearing loss is virtually always unilateral, although, at initial presentation, AIED may not have yet affected both ears. Sudden hearing loss develops in less than 72 hours. In contrast, AIED progresses over days to months such that serial audiograms on a monthly basis will show continued decline. Sudden hearing loss is an otologic emergency with a treatment window of perhaps 2 to 4 weeks, during which a short burst and taper of corticosteroids are recommended to achieve optimal recovery.

AIED is not urgent. Patients with progression of hearing loss over a 6- to 12-month period can still achieve significant recovery with administration of a long course of high-dose corticosteroids or other immunosuppressive

drugs. Throughout the otolaryngology community, there is general awareness that some cases of SNHL are potentially reversible with corticosteroids. However, there is little awareness that these two entities are quite different in etiology, presentation, workup, and management.

The clinical presentation of AIED may closely mimic that of Ménière disease. In fact, during the first months of evaluation, the two entities may be difficult to differentiate. Both can manifest fluctuations in hearing and episodic vertigo. If corticosteroids are administered, a spontaneous recovery in hearing, as seen in Ménière disease, may be mistaken for a positive response to immunosuppressive therapy. Ultimately, the more aggressive course of AIED will allow for the differentiation of these two disorders. It has been suggested that a subgroup of patients with symptoms of Ménière disease may share a common pathophysiology with patients who have AIED. This association is based on studies that have noted that approximately one-third of patients with Ménière disease may have a positive Western blot assay for anti-HSP-70 antibodies (46,47). However, this finding was not supported by a later study, in which the commercially available assay was utilized (48).

Otosyphilis can closely mimic AIED, and must be ruled out as part of the workup. An acoustic neuroma may present with sudden or progressive unilateral SNHL. Rarely, meningitis, multiple sclerosis, or malignancy (e.g., metastatic disease, lymphoma) involving the dura may manifest as rapidly progressive bilateral hearing loss.

Diagnosis

No definitive diagnostic test exists to confirm a diagnosis of primary or secondary AIED, and identification of the disease still relies on history of clinical exam. In addition, an appropriate review of systems should include questions pertaining to recurrent or chronic ocular disease, nephritis, arthritis, pneumonitis, sinusitis, and inflammatory bowel disease in order to differentiate between primary AIED and secondary AIED.

Despite this clinical diagnosis, a number of routine serologic tests should be ordered in patients who may have suspected AIED in order to rule out other causes of otologic dysfunction. These include a complete blood count with differential white count, ESR, rheumatoid factor, antinuclear antibody test, anti–double-stranded DNA antibodies, anti-SSA/B antibodies, antiphospholipid antibodies, C3 and C4 complement levels, anti-gliadin antibodies, and Raji cell assay for circulating immune complexes. An FTA-ABS test (or a *T. pallidum* hemagglutination test) must be obtained to rule out otosyphilis. An HIV test may be considered to rule out AIDS-associated hearing loss. An MRI with paramagnetic enhancement must be obtained to rule out the retrocochlear lesions discussed earlier in this chapter.

Though not yet clinically applicable, a number of immunologic assays have been proposed to diagnose AIED. Tests of cellular immunity have been advocated by McCabe (lymphocyte migration inhibition assay) and Hughes (lymphocyte transformation test) (49). Unfortunately, these tests have never been adequately validated, and their diagnostic accuracy has not been determined. During the 1990s, attention was focused on the role of Western blotting for detection of an antibody that binds to a 68-kDa antigen derived from bovine temporal bone extract and to the inducible form of HSP-70 (50–52). As noted earlier in this chapter, these antibodies were first determined to be of significance when they were detected in both guinea pigs immunized with bovine inner ear extract and in humans manifesting AIED (52). In a prospective controlled study, with well-defined entry criteria, Moscicki and his colleagues demonstrated that 89% of patients with active, rapidly progressive hearing loss did have detectable levels of this antibody, while none of the control patients had positive Western blots (53).

There have been recent studies evaluating the use of PET scan as a tool for the diagnosis of AIED. Although initial observations suggested an association between AIED and positive PET scans, the most recent work fails to show any diagnostic benefit to PET scan (54). At this time, there is no role for PET in diagnosis of AIED.

In summary, the diagnosis of primary AIED is based on clinical evaluation, the demonstration of progressive SNHL on audiometric assessment done at monthly intervals, and most importantly, a positive response to the administration of corticosteroids. The presence of a positive Western blot may support the diagnosis of AIED but, in and of itself, can neither confirm nor rule out the diagnosis.

Treatment

Corticosteroid therapy for AIED evolved during the mid-1980s through the 1990s as a result of clinical experience. Niparko et al. (55) reported a prospective, randomized trial that showed a majority of patients with suspected AIED responded to corticosteroids, although the response was highly variable. These data seem to substantiate the current practice of most otologists. Initial therapy for adults consists of a therapeutic trial of prednisone (60 mg daily for 4 weeks). Pediatric patients receive 1 mg/kg/d of prednisone for 4 weeks. Although patients may occasionally respond early in the 4-week period, many do not begin to improve until late in the month; shorter courses of treatment usually result in relapse.

Patients' hearing is tested at the initiation of therapy and again at 4 weeks. If the threshold has improved by ≥15 dB at one frequency or 10 dB at two or more consecutive frequencies, or if the discrimination is significantly improved, patients are considered steroid responders. Nonresponders are tapered off their medication in 12 days. Responders continue full-dose therapy until monthly audiograms confirm that they have reached a plateau of recovery. Their medication is then slowly tapered over 8 weeks to a maintenance dose of 10 to 20 mg every other day. This maintenance dose is continued for a variable time. Clinical observation suggests that patients with a treatment duration of fewer than 6 months are at increased risk of relapse compared with those treated for 6 months or longer.

Patterns of response to corticosteroid therapy vary. Some patients have improvement in threshold, some in discrimination only, and some in both areas. Some patients with hearing loss fluctuation and progression before therapy show stabilization in their hearing without actual improvement. Historically, these cases have been considered nonresponders, but this issue is currently under reassessment. The majority of responders slowly taper off the steroid dose, wean from steroids, and do well. A subset of AIED patients relapse while tapering or after discontinuing steroids. In some instances, additional corticosteroid therapy is effective. In such cases, alternative immunosuppressive drugs are considered. Some patients, especially in the pediatric age group, may occasionally show steroid-dependent hearing loss. In other words, they cannot be weaned below a certain level of steroid dosage without decline in hearing. Such patients often develop unacceptable side effects of chronic steroid administration. Methotrexate has been used as part of a prednisone-sparing regimen; however, a recent randomized, prospective controlled, multicenter trial has shown methotrexate to be no better than a placebo at maintaining a remission in these patients (56).

Corticosteroid therapy has obvious limitations. Long-term administration carries a significant risk for gastritis and ulcers, fluid retention and weight gain, blood pressure lability, altered blood sugar metabolism and diabetes, avascular necrosis of the hip, mood changes or psychiatric problems, sleep disturbance, accelerated cataract formation, osteoporosis, and cushingoid habitus. Overall steroid response rate is approximately 60% in AIED patients, and patients with vestibular symptoms appear to be particularly sensitive (57). Recent research demonstrates that corticosteroid nonresponders have elevated plasma level of IL-1B and MMP-9 as compared with clinically responsive patients, suggesting that IL-1B blockade may be viable therapy for these patients (58). Although high-dose corticosteroids are associated with serious side effects, with appropriate patient selection, monitoring, and patient education, high-dose corticosteroids are safe and effective (59).

A number of alternatives to systemic corticosteroids have been proposed, including methotrexate, etanercept, and cyclophosphamide. Low-dose methotrexate appeared to be useful as an adjunct in management of steroid-dependent hearing loss (60). However, as noted earlier in this chapter, the recent large trial indicates that it may not serve an effective role as a prednisone-sparing drug. Etanercept, an inhibitor of tumor necrosis factor (TNF) alpha, has recently been used to treat AIED. Anecdotally, it appears to work well in combination with methotrexate because of its steroid-sparing effect. As seen in rheumatoid arthritis, etanercept alone does not appear nearly as effective. In both an open-label and blinded, prospective study, etanercept was shown not to be efficacious in improving hearing loss in patients with AIED (61–63).

Cyclophosphamide is a potent cytotoxic agent generally used for cancer chemotherapy and treatment of Wegener granulomatosis. Although some advocate its use as a first-line drug, the high risk of toxicity makes it a better choice as a salvage drug or treatment of last resort (64). An initial dose of 1 mg/kg/d orally for 4 to 6 weeks may be instituted. When no response is apparent, the dose is doubled to 2 mg/kg/d. Responders are treated for 6 to 12 months. Toxicity includes severe myelosuppression, opportunistic infection, hair loss, cystitis, infertility, and increased risk of malignancies. Weekly monitoring of hematologic status is mandatory. Many patients, when confronted with the risk of this medication, would rather consider cochlear implantation.

Intratympanic steroid therapy, intratympanic TNF alpha inhibitor, systemic immunoglobulin G injections, and plasmapheresis are possible treatments with sound theoretical justification (65,66). Intratympanic steroid therapy is particularly appealing because it is minimally invasive and enables direct application of the drug to the affected site with low risk of systemic effects (67). There are, however, no published series in which these treatments have been systematically applied. The best role for any of these treatment modalities remains to be determined.

Recently, researches have experimented with immunotherapy as a means of treating AIED. Studies have demonstrated that a low dose of beta-tubulin is active orally in an antigen-specific fashion and capable of inhibiting the autoimmune reactions in the inner ear by suppressing Th1 (IFN-gamma) and increasing Th2 and Th3 (IL-4, IL-5, IL-13, and TGF-beta) cytokines. Oral antigen tolerance may in the future be used to treat AIED (68).

In summary, the only drugs of proven utility in the management of AIED are the corticosteroids. All other immunosuppressants currently employed have not been systematically evaluated and carry with them serious toxicity risks. In a patient who cannot be maintained on corticosteroids because of complications, the possibility of withdrawing treatment, with the intention of inserting a cochlear implant when the hearing becomes significantly impaired, must be considered.

DISEASES OF BONE

Paget Disease

Paget disease, also known as osteitis deformans, is a chronic progressive disorder of bone metabolism of unknown etiology. It results from increased activity of osteoclasts and osteoblasts, which manifest as bony hypertrophy and remodeling. Its prevalence increases dramatically with age, with 3% of people over the age of 40 demonstrating histopathologic evidence of the disease and 11% of people over the age of 80 demonstrating histopathologic evidence of the disease (69). The disease is far more common among men than women with relative incidence of about 4:1. Patients with Paget disease typically present in their sixth decade, most commonly with complaints of an enlarging skull, progressive kyphosis,

and deformities of the pelvis, femurs, and tibia. Radiologic findings for these patients include thickening of the calvarium with ill-defined densities and poor definition of cortical margins of the inner ear and internal auditory meatus.

The otologic manifestations of Paget's typically present as a mixed conductive and SNHL, estimated to effect between 5% and 44% of patients (70). The conductive portion of this hearing loss is typically down-sloping and 20 to 30 dB in severity. The etiology of this hearing loss is not well explained and cannot be attributed to compressive etiologies as with other diseases of bone. It is believed to arise primarily from changes in bone density and geometry that interfere with normal hearing mechanisms. In addition, patients with Paget can present with tinnitus and mild vestibular complaints. Facial nerve symptoms are highly unusual.

Treatment of Paget disease relies primarily on bisphosphonate therapy, which inhibits osteoclast activity, thereby inhibiting bone reabsorption. Calcitonin has also been demonstrated to be effective in this manner. There are no surgical treatments to improve conductive hearing loss for these patients.

Osteogenesis Imperfecta

Osteogenesis imperfecta (OI), also known as Hoeve-de Kleyn syndrome, is a connective tissue disorder that manifests as a variety of types with vastly differing severity. It results from mutations in either of two genes codes for type I collagen (COL1A1 and COL1A2) (71).

Type I OI is the mildest form of the disease and is inherited in an autosomal dominant pattern. This is the classic form of the disease and is the most common type, with an incidence of 1:30,000. Clinically, patients demonstrate characteristic blue sclera and nondeforming fractures while maintaining normal stature. Type II OI is lethal with patients developing multiple fractures in utero, often resulting in stillbirth. It is inherited in an autosomal recessive pattern and has an incidence about half that of type I, 1:60,000. Type III and type IV are increasingly rare and manifest with a severity intermediate to that of type I and type II. Patients with type III OI develop multiple fractures with resulting progressive bone deformity. They also demonstrate blue sclera at a young age but this transitions to a normal white sclera later in life. This type can be inherited in an autosomal recessive or dominant pattern. Type IV OI presents with a similar clinical picture to type I but with normal, white sclera. Like type I OI, clinical manifestations can be mild, and a patient's disease can elude clinical detection.

It is estimated that 30% to 50% of patient with type I OI develop hearing loss, 50% of patients with type II OI develop hearing loss, and 10% to 30% of patient with type IV OI develop hearing loss (72). There is no demonstrated association between the severity of peripheral fractures and the presence of hearing loss. Conductive hearing loss results from fractures to the ossicles, most commonly the long process of the incus or the stapes crura. This conductive hearing loss has been addressed successfully with amplification or ossiculoplasty to replace fractured ossicles. In addition, stapedectomy can be effective but must be performed very delicately due to the fragility of the ossicles. There is some evidence to demonstrate that stapedectomy outcomes are better when performed for type I OI (73).

Fibrous Dysplasia

Fibrous dysplasia is a benign, chronic, slowly progressive disease of unknown etiology. It describes the replacement of normal cancellous bone by spicules of woven bone in a fibrous stroma. Fibrous dysplasia occurs in several forms: monostotic, polyostotic, or as part of the constellation of symptoms comprising McCune-Albright syndrome. The monostotic form is the most common. It usually presents late in childhood and then can become quiescent at puberty. The affected bone is most commonly a rib, the skull, the proximal femur, or the tibia. The polyostotic form usually presents earlier and will continue to progress throughout life (74). Skeletal lesions are multiple but usually unilateral. Radiologic findings typical of fibrous dysplasia include radiolucent areas with a well-defined smooth or scalloped edge and a ground-glass appearance.

Otologic manifestations of the disease manifest from craniofacial involvement, which occurs far more commonly in the polyostotic (50% to 100%) form than in the monostotic form (10% to 30%). Conductive hearing loss is the most common clinical manifestation, resulting from occlusion of the external auditory canal (EAC) due to painless, progressive involvement of the temporal bone. In addition, patients can develop a canal cholesteatoma or involvement of the ossicular chain (75). Facial nerve paralysis or paresis and SNHL have also been reported. Patients can benefit from medical treatment with bisphosphonates. Surgical treatment with canaloplasty, meatoplasty, or cholesteatoma resection can also benefit these patients.

Osteopetrosis

Osteopetrosis is a rare, inherited disorder of bone remodeling that results in characteristic increased bone density due to defective function of the osteoclasts. It presents in two forms, an autosomal recessive form and an autosomal dominant form. The autosomal recessive type, also called malignant osteopetrosis, is the more severe form. It is rapidly progressive, resulting in encroachment of the bone marrow and neural foramina. Patients consequently develop thrombocytopenia, hepatosplenomegaly, and cranial nerve palsies that often result in death (76). The autosomal dominant form, also known as Albers-Schönberg disease and marble bone disease, is more progressive, more indolent, and more common. It results in progressive head and mandible enlargement with clubbing of the long bones. Patients can also develop cranial neuropathies secondary to compression at neural foramina.

Otologic manifestations include SNHL from compression of the cochlear nerve and conductive hearing loss from thickening of the ossicles and the meso- and epitympanum (77). Facial nerve weakness can also develop from compression at the stylomastoid foramen. The only treatment for malignant osteopetrosis is bone marrow transplantation. Cochlear nerve decompression has also been described for SNHL resulting from the milder form of the disease.

METABOLIC DISORDERS

Mucopolysaccharidoses

Mucopolysaccharidoses are a group of diseases that result from inherited deficiencies in lysosomal enzymes needed to break down mucopolysaccharides. This results in intracellular accumulation of mucopolysaccharides and abnormally large dysfunctional cells with vacuolated cytoplasm. There have been 10 identified lysosomal enzyme deficiencies that make up this group. Examples of these include Hunter syndrome, an X-linked disease caused by an absence of L-iduronidase; Hurler syndrome, an autosomal recessive disease caused by a lack of iduronate-2-sulfate; and Morquio syndrome, caused by a lack of N-acetylgalactosamine-6-sulfate or beta-galactosidase. Diagnosis of each is made through assays that test for the presence of each of these enzymes.

The otologic manifestation of mucopolysaccharidoses typically presents as a mixed hearing loss. The conductive component is usually secondary to eustachian tube dysfunction and resulting serous otitis media. The cause of SNHL is unclear though it is thought that abnormal lipid metabolism within nerve cells may be at fault. Treatment of these patients is typically supportive with long-term tympanostomy tube placement to alleviate serous otitis media (78). Some patients respond to systemic enzyme replacement therapy. Current research is investigating the efficacy of gene therapy for these patients (79).

HIGHLIGHTS

- Infectious diseases are the most common systemic diseases to manifest otologic pathology.
- Congenital CMV infection can result in both a severe SNHL in babies presenting with symptomatic infections and a variable progressive SNHL in children with asymptomatic infections.
- Up to a third of patients with bacterial meningitis sustain some SNHL, which is typically bilateral and stable, though it may be unilateral and progressive or fluctuating.
- Otogenic syphilis can mimic Ménière disease, though it typically has a more aggressive course, involving both ears and leading to profound deafness.

- Langerhans histiocytosis can present as an isolated granuloma affecting the temporal bone (eosinophilic granuloma) or as a multifocal (Hand-Schüller-Christian disease) or disseminated (Letterer-Siwe disease) process.
- Granulomatous diseases most commonly cause conductive hearing losses, by disrupting the conductive mechanisms within the middle ear.
- AIED is a rare entity characterized by bilateral SNHL that progresses over weeks to months and is responsive to steroids.
- Diagnosis of AIED relies on clinical evaluation as well as a comprehensive assessment of immunologic markers; Western blot for an antibody to a 68-kDa protein that binds HSP-70 is not standard of care in the evaluation of AIED.
- Treatment of AIED is not urgent as there is a 6- to 12-month period in which a significant recovery of hearing loss is possible with administration of high-dose corticosteroids.
- Initial therapy for AIED is 60 mg of prednisone a day for 4 weeks. Response to steroids is variable, and treatment is tailored to initial response.
- Neither etanercept nor methotrexate has been shown to be efficacious in improving hearing loss in patients with AIED.
- Disease of bone can cause both conductive hearing loss by directly damaging the middle ear and ossicles and SNHL through compression of the cochlear nerve.
- The otologic manifestation of mucopolysaccharidoses typically presents as a mixed hearing loss, with the conductive component usually secondary to serous otitis media.

REFERENCES

1. Bauer PW, Parizi-Robinson M, Roland PS, et al. Cytomegalovirus in the perilymphatic fluid. *Laryngoscope* 2005;115(2):223–225.
2. Korver AM, Admiraal RJ, Kant SG, et al. DECIBEL-collaborative study group. *Laryngoscope* 2011;121(2):409–416.
3. Foulon I, Naessens A, Foulon W, et al. A 10-year prospective study of sensorineural hearing loss in children with congenital cytomegalovirus infection. *J Pediatr* 2008;153(1):84–88.
4. Dammeye J. Congenital rubella syndrome and delayed manifestations. *Int J Pediatr Otorhinolaryngol* 2010;74(9):1067–1070.
5. Kanra G, Kara A, Cengiz AB, et al. Mumps meningoencephalitis effect on hearing. *Pediatr Infect Dis J* 2002;21(12):1167–1169.
6. Gurney TA, Murr AH. Otolaryngologic manifestations of human immunodeficiency virus infection. *Otolaryngol Clin North Am* 2003;36(4):607–624.
7. Zetola NM, et al. Syphilis in the United States: an update for clinicians with an emphasis on HIV coinfection. [erratum appears in *Mayo Clin Proc* 2007;82(11):1434]. *Mayo Clin Proc* 2007;82(9):1091–1102.
8. Centers for Disease. Syphilis and congenital syphilis—United States, 1985–1988. *MMWR Morb Mortal Wkly Rep* 1988;37(32):486–489.
9. DiCarlo RP, Martin DH. The clinical diagnosis of genital ulcer disease in men [see comment]. *Clin Infect Dis* 1997;25(2):292–298.
10. Singh AE, Romanowski B. Syphilis: review with emphasis on clinical, epidemiologic, and some biologic features. *Clin Microbiol Rev* 1999;12(2):187–209.
11. Darmstadt GL, Harris JP. Luetic hearing loss: clinical presentation, diagnosis, and treatment. *Am J Otolaryngol* 1989;10(6):410–421.
12. Abuzeid WM, Ruckenstein MJ. Spirochetes in otology: are we testing for the right pathogens? *Otolaryngol Head Neck Surg* 2008;138(1):107–109.
13. Yimtae K, Srirompotong S, Lertsukprasert K. Otosyphilis: a review of 85 cases. *Otolaryngol Head Neck Surg* 2007;136(1):67–71.
14. Steckelberg JM, McDonald TJ. Otologic involvement in late syphilis. *Laryngoscope* 1984;94(6):753–757.
15. Allam AF. Pathology of the human spiral ligament. *J Laryngol Otol* 1970;84(8):765–779.
16. Belal A Jr, Linthicum F Jr. Pathology of congenital syphilitic labyrinthitis. *Am J Otolaryngol* 1980;1(2):109–118.
17. Linstrom CJ, Gleich LL. Otosyphilis: diagnostic and therapeutic update. *J Otolaryngol* 1993;22(6):401–408.
18. Dobbin JM, Perkins JH. Otosyphilis and hearing loss: response to penicillin and steroid therapy. *Laryngoscope* 1983;93(12):1540–1543.
19. Chan YM, Adams DA, Kerr AG. Syphilitic labyrinthitis—An update. *J Laryngol Otol* 1995;109(8):719–725.
20. Zoller M, Wilson WR, Nadol JB Jr. Treatment of syphilitic hearing loss. Combined penicillin and steroid therapy in 29 patients. *Ann Otol Rhinol Laryngol* 1979;88(2 Pt 1):160–165.
21. McClain KL. Langerhans cell histiocytosis. Version 19.2, 2011. http://www.uptodate.com
22. Cunningham MJ, Curtin HD, Jaffe R, et al. Otologic manifestations of Langerhans' cell histiocytosis. *Arch Otolaryngol Head Neck Surg* 1989;115:807.
23. Hudson WR, Kenan PD. Otologic manifestations of histiocytosis X. *Laryngoscope* 1969;79:678.
24. Irving RM, Broadbent V, Jone NS. Langerhans' cell histiocytosis in childhood: management of head and neck manifestations. *Laryngoscope* 1994;104(1 Pt 1):64–70.
25. Hybels RL, Rice DH. Neuro-otologic manifestations of sarcoidosis. *Laryngoscope* 1976;86:1873.
26. Adelola OA, Fernandex R, Ahmad R, et al. Sarcoidosis of the external ear—literature review and report of a case. *J Laryngol Otol* 2007;121:289–292.
27. Gottschlich S, Ambrosch P, Kramkowski D, et al. Head and neck manifestations of Wegener's granulomatosis. *Rhinology* 2006;44(4):227–233.
28. McDonald TJ, DeRemee RA. Wegener's granulomatosis. *Laryngoscope* 1983;93:220.
29. Stone JH, Francis HW. Immune-mediated inner ear disease. *Curr Opin Rheumatol* 2000;12(1):32–40.
30. Cogan DG. Syndrome of nonsyphilitic interstitial keratitis and vestibuloauditory symptoms. *Arch Ophthalmol* 1945;33:144.
31. Haynes BF, Kaiser-Kupfer MI, Mason P, et al. Cogan syndrome: studies in thirteen patients, long-term follow-up, and a review of the literature. *Medicine (Baltimore)* 1980;59:426.
32. Murphy G, Sullican MO, Shanahan F, et al. Cogan's syndrome: present and future directions. *Rheumatol Int* 2009;29(10):1117–1121.
33. Gluth MB, Baratz KH, Matteson EL, et al. Cogan syndrome: a retrospective review of 60 patients throughout a half century. *Mayo Clin Proc* 2006;81:483.
34. Stephens SD, Luxon L, Hinchcliffe R. Immunological disorders and auditory lesions. *Audiology* 1982;21:128.
35. Yoon TH, Paparella MM, Schachern PA. Systemic vasculitis: a temporal bone histopathologic study. *Laryngoscope* 1989;99:600.
36. Rapini RP, Warner NB. Relapsing polychondritis. *Clin Dermatol* 2006;24(6):482–485.
37. McCaffrey TV, McDonald TJ, McCaffrey LA. Head and neck manifestations of relapsing polychondritis. Review of 29 cases. *Otolaryngology* 1978;1:473–478.
38. Venables PJW, Maini RN. Clinical features of rheumatoid arthritis. Version 19.2, 2011. http://www.uptodate.com
39. Papadimitraki ED, Kyrmizakis DE, Kritkos I, et al. Ear-nose-throat manifestations of autoimmune rheumatic diseases. *Clin Exp Rheumatol* 2004;22(4):485–494.
40. McCabe BF. Autoimmune sensorineural hearing loss. *Ann Otol Rhinol Laryngol* 1979;88:585.

41. Byl F. Thirty-two cases of sudden profound hearing loss occurring in 1973: incidence and prognostic findings. *Trans Am Acad Ophthalmol Otolaryngol* 1975;80:298.

42. Harris JP. Immunology of the inner ear: response of the inner ear to antigen challenge. *Otolaryngol Head Neck Surg* 1983;91:18.

43. Harris JP. Immunology of the inner ear: evidence of local antibody production. *Ann Otol Rhinol Laryngol* 1984;93:157.

44. Nair TS, Kozma KE, Hoefling NL, et al. Identification and characterization of choline transporter-like protein 2, an inner ear glycoprotein of 68 and 72 kDa that is the target of antibody-induced hearing loss. *J Neurosci* 2004;24:1772.

45. Baek MJ, Park HM, Johnson JM, et al. Increased frequency of cochlin-specific T cells in patients with autoimmune sensorineural hearing loss. *J Immunol* 2006;177:4203.

46. Gottschlich S, Billings PB, Keithley EM, et al. Assessment of serum antibodies in patients with rapidly progressive sensorineural hearing loss and Ménière's disease. *Laryngoscope* 1995;105:1347.

47. Rauch SD, Zurakowski D, Bloch DB, et al. Anti-heat shock protein 70 antibodies in Ménière's disease. *Laryngoscope* 2000;110:1516.

48. Ruckenstein MJ, Prasthoffer A, Bigelow DC, et al. Immunologic and serologic testing in patients with Ménière's disease. *Otol Neurotol* 2002;23:517.

49. Hughes GB, Moscicki R, Barna BP, et al. Laboratory diagnosis of immune inner ear disease. *Am J Otol* 1994;15:198.

50. Billings PB, Keithley EM, et al. Evidence linking the 68 kilodalton antigen identified in progressive sensorineural hearing loss patient sera with heat shock protein 70. *Ann Otol Rhinol Laryngol* 1995;104:181.

51. Bloch DB, San Martin JE, Rauch SD, et al. Serum antibodies to heat shock protein 70 in sensorineural hearing loss. *Arch Otolaryngol Head Neck Surg* 1995;121:1167.

52. Harris JP, Sharp PA. Inner ear autoantibodies in patients with rapidly progressive sensorineural hearing loss. *Laryngoscope* 1990;100:516.

53. Moscicki RA, San Martin JE, Quintero CH, et al. Serum antibody to inner ear proteins in patients with progressive hearing loss. Correlation with disease activity and response to corticosteroid treatment. *JAMA* 1994;272:611.

54. Mazlumzadeh M, Lowe VJ, Mullan BP, et al. The utility of positron emission tomography in the evaluation of autoimmune hearing loss. *Otol Neurotol* 2003;24:201.

55. Niparko JK, Wang NY, Rauch SD, et al. Serial audiometry in a clinical trial of AIED treatment. *Otol Neurotol* 2005;26:908.

56. Harris JP, Weisman MH, Derebery JM, et al. Treatment of corticosteroid-responsive autoimmune inner ear disease with methotrexate: a randomized controlled trial. *JAMA* 2003;290:1875.

57. Dayal VS, Ellman M, Sweiss N. Autoimmune inner ear disease: clinical and laboratory findings and treatment outcome. *J Otolaryngol Head Neck Surg* 2008;37(4):591–596.

58. Pathak S, Goldofsky E, Vivas EX, et al. IL-1B is overexpressed and aberrantly regulated in corticosteroid nonresponders with autoimmune inner ear disease. *J Immunol* 2011;186(3):1870–1879.

59. Alexander TH, Weisman MH, Derebery JM, et al. Safety of high-dose corticosteroids for the treatment of autoimmune inner ear disease. *Otol Neurotol* 2009;30(4):443–448.

60. Sismanis A, Thompson T, Willis HE. Methotrexate therapy for autoimmune hearing loss: a preliminary report. *Laryngoscope* 1994;104:932.

61. Matteson EL, Choi HK, Poe DS, et al. Etanercept therapy for immune-mediated cochleovestibular disorders: a multicenter, open-label, pilot study. *Arthritis Rheum* 2005;53:337.

62. Cohen S, Shoup A, Weisman MH, et al. Etanercept treatment for autoimmune inner ear disease: results of a pilot placebo controlled study. *Otol Neurotol* 2005;26:903.

63. Wang X, Truong T, Billings PB, et al. Blockage of immune-mediated inner ear damage by etanercept. *Otol Neurotol* 2003;24:52–57.

64. Buniel MC, Geelan-Hansen K, Weber PC, et al. Immunosuppressive therapy for autoimmune inner ear disease. *Immunotherapy* 2009;1(3):425–434.

65. Garcia-Berrocal JR, Ibanez A, Rodriguez A, et al. Alternatives to systemic steroid therapy for refractory immune-mediated inner ear disease: a physiopathologic approach. *Eur Arch Otorhinolaryngol* 2006;263(11):977–982.

66. Van Wijk F, Staecker H, Keithley E, et al. Local perfusion of the tumor necrosis factor α blocker infliximab to the inner ear improves autoimmune neurosensory hearing loss. *Audiol Neurootol* 2006;11(6):357–365.

67. Yang J, Wu H, Zhang P, et al. The pharmacokinetic profiles of dexamethasone and methylprednisolone concentration in perilymph and plasma following systemic and local administration. *Acta Otolaryngol* 2008;128(5):496–504.

68. Cai Q, Du X, Zhou B, et al. Induction of tolerance by oral administration of beta-tubulin in an animal model of autoimmune inner ear disease. *ORL J Otorhinolaryngol Relat Spec* 2009;71(3):135–141.

69. Davies DG. Paget's disease of the temporal bone: a clinical and histopathological survey. *Acta Otolaryngol Suppl (Stockh)* 1968;242:1.

70. Monsell EM. The mechanism of hearing loss in Paget's disease of bone. *Laryngoscope* 2004;114:598–608.

71. Hadjipavlou AG, Gaitanis IN, Kontakis GM. Paget's disease of the bone and its management. *J Bone Joint Surg Br* 2002;84:160.

72. Paterson CR, Monk EA, MacAllion SJ. How common is hearing impairment in osteogenesis imperfect? *J Laryngol Otol* 2001;115:280.

73. Van der Rijt AJ, Cremers CW. Stapes surgery in osteogenesis imperfect: results of a new series. *Otol Neurotol* 2003;24:717–722.

74. DiCaprio MR, Enneking WF. Fibrous dysplasia: pathophysiology, evaluation, and treatment. *J Bone Joint Surg Am* 2005;87:1848–1864.

75. Lustig LR, Holliday MJ, McCarthy EF. Fibrous dysplasia involving the skill base and temporal bone. *Arch Otolaryngol Head Neck Surg* 2001;127:1239.

76. Dozier TS, Duncan IM, Klein AJ. Otologic manifestations of malignant osteopetrosis. *Otol Neurotol* 2005;26:762–766.

77. Wahab Hamed AA, Linthicum FH Jr. Temporal bone osteopetrosis. *Otol Neurotol* 2004;25:635.

78. Motamed M, Thorne S, Narula A. Treatment of OME in children with mucopolysaccharidoses. *Int J Ped Otorhinolaryngol* 2000;53:121–124.

79. Schiffmann R, Brady RO. New prospects for the treatment of lysosomal storage disease. *Drugs* 2002;62:733.

157 Noise-Induced Hearing Loss

Robert A. Dobie

Noise and aging are responsible for most cases of permanent hearing loss in the United States. Although not correctable by medical or surgical treatment, noise-induced hearing loss (NIHL) is preventable.

Otolaryngologists see patients with NIHL in many different contexts. A noise-exposed worker may be referred for preemployment examination, for evaluation of threshold shifts or other abnormalities detected by a hearing conservation program (HCP) at work, or for examination for compensation purposes at the end of his or her career. The otolaryngologist is expected to verify the existence and severity of the hearing loss, to render a differential diagnosis, to recommend treatment and rehabilitation, to counsel the worker, and to report to referring parties. Otolaryngologists also may be called on as consultants by employers designing HCPs or by attorneys involved in medicolegal and compensation disputes.

Patients with NIHL are also seen through the normal pathways of self-referral or physician referral. These patients often have occupational or nonoccupational exposures that are uncontrolled, and then the otolaryngologist's duty is to provide at least the rudiments of an HCP: periodic audiometry and counseling, including discussion of hearing protection. Unfortunately, most people with NIHL do not see otolaryngologists; thus, we should encourage primary care physicians either to refer noise-exposed patients or to provide these services themselves (1).

The goal of this chapter is to provide the otolaryngologist with most of the information needed to meet these needs.

PATHOGENESIS

Pure-Tone Threshold Shifts

Temporary Threshold Shifts

Exposure to loud noise for seconds to hours may cause a temporary sensorineural hearing loss that recovers almost completely within 24 hours. The magnitude of this temporary threshold shift (TTS) can be predicted from the acoustic parameters of the noise: its intensity, spectrum (frequency content), and temporal pattern. Obviously, more intense sounds lead to larger shifts. Pure tones cause TTSs that are greatest at and slightly above the frequencies of the exposure tones. As might be expected, the frequencies that we hear best are also the frequencies most susceptible to TTS. (See Chapter 141 for a discussion of the effects of middle-ear mechanics and ear canal resonance on thresholds for different frequencies.) Because high-frequency sounds (e.g., a 4-kHz tone) are usually more hazardous than low-frequency sounds (e.g., a 500-Hz tone) of the same intensity, risk cannot be predicted from measurements of decibel sound pressure level (dB SPL) alone. To avoid the cumbersome necessity of assessing risk separately for each of several octave bands of noise, there is an international consensus that estimates of hazard for NIHL should be based on measurements of decibels on the A scale (dBA), which gives greater weight to those frequencies most hazardous to human hearing (1 to 5 kHz) and lesser weight to higher and lower frequencies.

The effect of temporal pattern is more complex. Up to a point, longer exposures lead to increased TTS, but interrupted exposures cause less TTS than continuous exposures with the same overall duration. Presumably, recovery takes place during the rest intervals.

Permanent Threshold Shift

After repeated exposures to noises that initially cause only TTS, a worker may experience threshold changes that do not recover. This is called noise-induced permanent threshold shift (NIPTS). In a typical field study, a researcher determines the NIPTS attributable to 10 years' exposure at 100 dBA, for example, by measuring the hearing threshold levels (HTLs) of a group of workers so exposed and then subtracting the amount of hearing loss to be expected on the basis of aging. The amount of NIPTS and the frequencies involved depend primarily on the acoustic parameters of the noise, as described previously for TTS. As with TTS, intermittency has a protective effect, especially for low-frequency NIPTS (2,3).

The consensus of most experts (4,5) is that NIPTS does not progress after cessation of the offending exposure. To be precise, as people with NIPTS from a prior exposure grow older, their hearing loss does not progress more rapidly than hearing loss in people who have not been noise exposed. That consensus view has been challenged recently. Noise-exposed mice may show hearing loss that progresses more rapidly than expected after the noise stops, but this phenomenon has only been demonstrated for a single inbred strain exposed as juveniles (6). A review of serial audiograms from the Framingham Heart Study showed that middle-aged men who had 4-kHz notches (presumably due to noise exposure in most cases) experienced more threshold shift at 2 kHz in subsequent years than men whose audiograms were not notched (7). Unfortunately, there was no documentation that the men with audiometric notches had actually been noise exposed (or that those without notches had not). In addition, many if not most of these men were below retirement age at the times of their initial audiograms, and there was no documentation that their occupational and nonoccupational noise exposures (if any) had ceased. A subsequent longitudinal study from South Carolina showed no difference in age-related progression of hearing loss between retirees who had had noisy careers and those who had had quiet careers (8), in agreement with the expert consensus.

Although the acoustic reflex (contraction of the stapedius muscle in response to loud sound) evolved before firearms and industrial noise, it is probably protective against NIPTS, at least for frequencies below 2 kHz, where the acoustic reflex effectively attenuates sound. Borg et al. (9) have shown in experimental animals and in humans with Bell palsy that permanent threshold shift (PTS) and TTS increase dramatically for lower frequencies when the reflex is inactivated. The efferent innervation of the outer hair cells probably exerts a protective role as well; at least in mice and guinea pigs, strong efferent olivocochlear function is correlated with resistance to NIHL (10,11).

We have already mentioned several explanations for the familiar 4-kHz notch (which can also be at 3 or 6 kHz): the greater sensitivity of the human ear to frequencies between 1 and 5 kHz, the protective effect of the acoustic reflex below 2 kHz, and the fact that intermittency is most protective for low frequencies. Recently, another reason has been added: Outer hair cells at the base of the cochlea are especially susceptible to oxidative stress (12). However, a notch is not proof of NIHL and can be seen after head injury, after barotrauma, or even in the absence of any explanatory history (13).

In both TTS and PTS experiments in animals, the amount of threshold shift caused by a particular exposure can often be reduced by adding prior exposure at lower

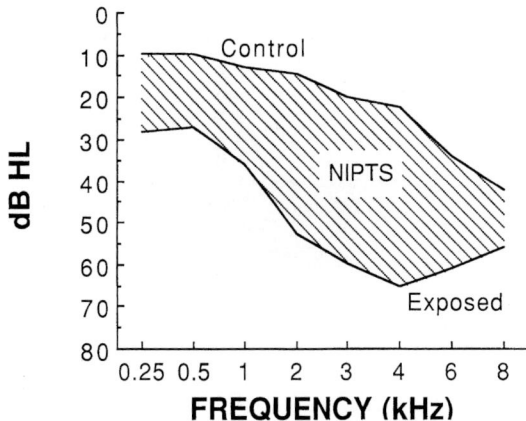

Figure 157.1 Median audiograms of retired jute weavers (exposed) and non–noise-exposed women of similar ages (control). NIPTS is estimated by subtracting HTLs expected with aging from HTLs in the exposed group.

levels; this is called "toughening" or "conditioning" the ear (14). Clearly, inner ear injury and hearing loss are not simply related to the total amount of sound energy entering the ear.

A landmark cross-sectional study of the evolution of NIHL over a working career was reported by Taylor et al. (15), in a jute-weaving factory in which noise levels (over 100 dBA) had probably been constant for generations. Figure 157.1 shows the pattern of hearing loss found in retired female weavers compared with that of age-matched female controls who had had no hazardous occupational or nonoccupational noise exposure. The shaded area indicates the estimated median NIPTS; the greatest change was at 4 kHz. Figure 157.2 shows median NIPTS curves for varying lengths of employment in the mills. As many other studies have shown, when workers are exposed to typical broad-spectrum industrial noise, the earliest changes are in the high frequencies (3 to 6 kHz). After about 10 years, loss in the high frequencies tends to plateau, but the loss continues to broaden gradually into lower frequencies.

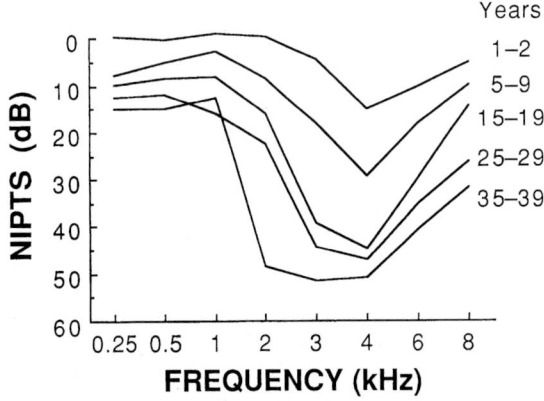

Figure 157.2 Median NIPTS as a function of audiometric frequency for different durations of exposure in jute-weaving mills (at level above 100 dBA).

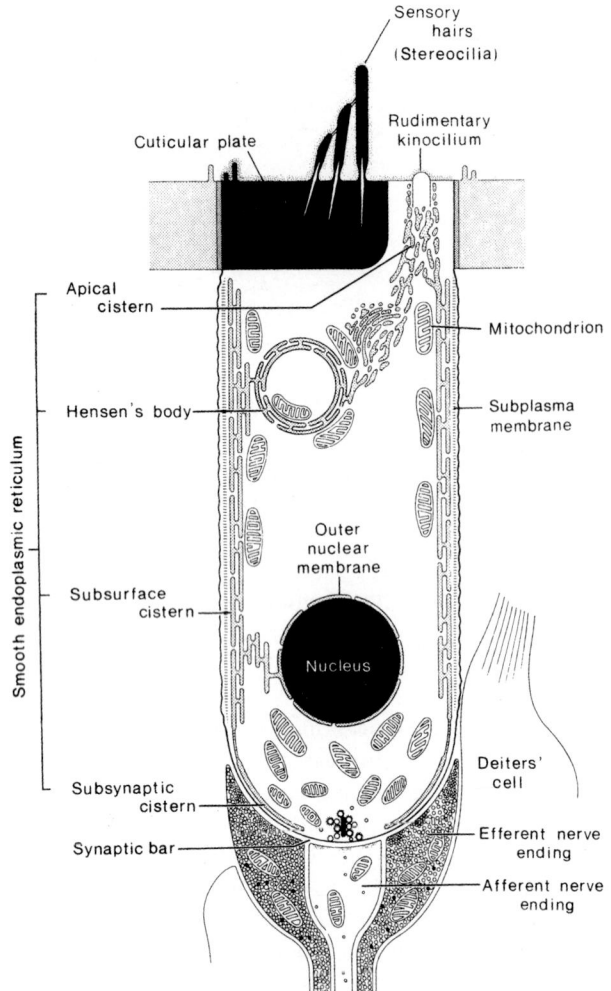

Sensory hairs (Stereocilia)

Rudimentary kinocilium

Cuticular plate

Apical cistern

Hensen's body

Mitochondrion

Subplasma membrane

Smooth endoplasmic reticulum

Outer nuclear membrane

Subsurface cistern

Nucleus

Subsynaptic cistern

Synaptic bar

Deiters' cell

Efferent nerve ending

Afferent nerve ending

Figure 157.3 Diagrammatic cross section of a normal cochlea hair cell. (Redrawn after Lim DJ. Functional structure of the organ of Corti: a review. *Hear Res* 1986;22:117, with permission.)

Pathology

Animal studies show clearly that NIHL involves the organ of Corti, especially the hair cells (Fig. 157.3). Although almost all cell types may be affected, the outer hair cells are most susceptible to damage. It has been difficult to find anatomic correlates to TTS, but it appears that the stereocilia of the outer hair cells become less stiff and therefore respond poorly to stimulation. These floppy stereocilia may recover their normal mechanical properties and function normally again. With increasing intensity and duration of exposure sufficient to cause NIPTS, more severe damage is seen with fusion of adjacent stereocilia and loss of stereocilia. The primary site of injury appears to be the rootlets that connect the stereocilia with the top of the hair cell (16). As stereocilia are lost, the hair cells themselves may die. As the severity of exposure increases, inner hair cells and supporting cells in the organ of Corti may be damaged (Fig. 157.4), and with severe hair cell loss, secondary neural degeneration is reflected in the auditory nerve and brainstem auditory nuclei. Rapid primary degeneration of VIII nerve synapses, followed by gradual loss of ganglion cells, may also occur, probably caused by glutamate excitotoxicity (17).

Acoustic Trauma

A single exposure to a very intense short-duration sound can cause a permanent hearing loss not preceded by TTS. It is generally believed that in these instances sound mechanically damages the organ of Corti, tearing membranes, rupturing cells, and allowing perilymph and endolymph to mix. This is contrasted to the gradual loss of stereocilia and hair cells seen in NIHL, preceded by TTS, and usually considered to involve both injury and metabolic repair processes. Acoustic trauma can produce losses that are more severe than those seen with NIHL, especially in the low frequencies. At extreme levels, such as with explosive or blast injury, even tympanic membrane or ossicular injury can occur, causing conductive or mixed hearing loss.

An important type of exposure that can create either NIHL or acoustic trauma is impulse noise (18). Impulses in the range of 0.2-millisecond duration have peak energy at 2 to 3 kHz, are therefore especially hazardous to human hearing, and are typical of small arms gunfire. Such impulses, when above a critical level of 140 decibels (dB) (peak), are considered potentially hazardous to human hearing (19).

Many industrial environments contain large amounts of impact noise, usually caused by collision of metal objects. These noises have high peaks and are often reverberant as well. Intense impact noises can cause acoustic trauma, but they are less likely than impulse noises to reach critical levels.

The levels at which continuous noise and tones (in contrast to impulses and impacts) cause acoustic trauma are not well defined. The earliest cordless telephones rang through the earpiece; if the person answering the phone failed to switch manually from "ring" to "talk" mode, the phone would ring directly into the ear with a 750- to 800-Hz tone at about 140 dB SPL. Dozens of cases of permanent hearing loss occurred from single-ring exposures, each probably less than 1 second in duration. At the other extreme, single 4-hour exposures below 110 dBA probably pose negligible risk of acoustic trauma (20).

Interactions

Aging

The nature of the interaction between NIPTS and age-related hearing changes has been the subject of considerable debate. Epidemiologic studies, such as those illustrated in Figure 157.2, usually assume additivity; that is, the net hearing loss is the decibel sum of the threshold shifts from aging and from noise. When this question has been addressed explicitly, the bulk of evidence favors simple additivity. For example, Macrae (21) showed that

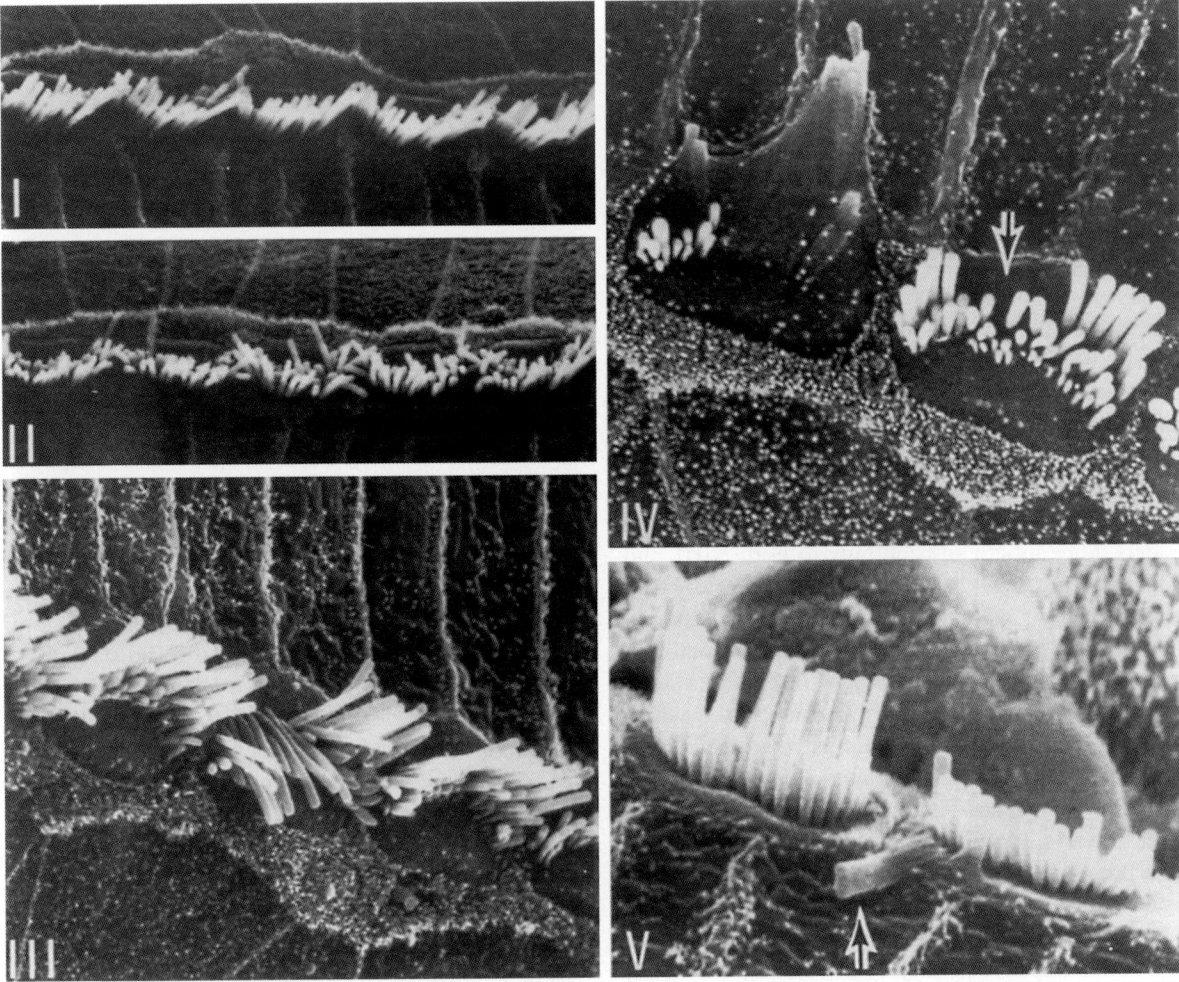

Figure 157.4 Scanning electron micrographs of cat inner hair cells that have been damaged by noise. (Redrawn after Liberman MC, Mulroy M. Acute and chronic effects of acoustic trauma: cochlear pathology and auditory nerve physiology. In: Hamernik RP, Henderson D, Salvi R, eds. *New perspectives on noise-induced hearing loss.* New York: Raven, 1982:122, with permission.)

war veterans with NIHL developed about the expected amount of additional hearing loss, based on studies of age-related hearing loss, over the ensuing years. The American National Standards Institute (ANSI) supports the theory of additivity, with a small correction factor to be used when the total hearing loss exceeds 40 dB hearing loss (22). Recent federal audiometric surveys, like those in earlier decades, show that age-related hearing loss disproportionately affects higher frequencies, especially in men; varies markedly across individuals; and accelerates in middle age (23,24).

Vibration

Czanto and Ligia (25) are among those who have shown that workers who use vibrating handheld tools, such as pneumatic hammers, grinders, and chipping tools, and who develop "vibration-induced white finger" also develop excessive NIHL. This could mean that vibration interacts with noise to damage the ear or that people who are susceptible to white finger (a peripheral vascular disorder) are also susceptible to NIHL.

Drugs and Chemicals

Humes (26) reviewed many studies and concluded that no substantial risk of hearing loss occurs from combining a noise exposure and an aminoglycoside drug when neither is present in sufficient amount to cause hearing loss on its own. Naturally, one would be reluctant to combine ototoxic drugs (primarily aminoglycosides and platinum-based antineoplastics) with hazardous noise exposures, but, with the probable exception of the newborn nursery where some borderline noise levels have been recorded, this is not a practical problem. The ototoxic drug most likely to be combined with industrial noise exposure is aspirin, but this causes a reversible hearing loss and has not been shown to potentiate or interact with NIHL.

Carbon monoxide (CO), xylene, styrene, and toluene have been reported to cause sensorineural hearing loss in rats. Workers exposed to toluene or xylene in addition to noise developed more hearing loss than those exposed to noise alone (27,28). Exposures in many of these studies were undocumented or were above Occupational Safety and Health Administration (OSHA) permissible time-weighted average (TWA) exposures, raising the question of whether exposures below OSHA limits could cause hearing loss, either alone or by interacting with occupational noise. One study (29) showed that styrene exposure below currently recommended values, plus noise, was associated with more hearing loss than noise exposure alone. Another showed that mixed solvent exposures, almost all below OSHA permissible levels, were associated with slightly elevated progression of high-frequency hearing loss (30).

Susceptibility

Persons vary widely in the degree of TTS or PTS caused by noise exposures. Efforts to predict, measure, or explain these differences in susceptibility have generally been fruitless in humans. Men often display more hearing loss in noisy occupations than do women, but this may be due to different nonoccupational exposures (especially shooting) between the genders. Mice inherit susceptibility to both NIHL and age-related hearing loss (31,32); genetic tests (33) or tests of efferent function (10) may someday permit prediction of human susceptibility to NIHL. In most experimental animals, there is a critical period in infancy, about the time of final maturation and innervation of the hair cells, in which susceptibility to NIHL is greater than at other times (34). Whether this happens in human infants is unclear.

Otoacoustic emissions (OAEs) are predictably reduced or absent in NIHL. In military studies of young men with excellent pre-noise hearing thresholds, those with baseline-reduced OAE amplitudes (of unknown etiology) were more likely to experience substantial pure-tone threshold shifts after either continuous (35) or impulsive (36) noise exposure. However, *changes* in OAE amplitude have not been shown to predict—or even to correlate with—audiometric threshold shifts.

Pathophysiology and Pathogenesis

Many investigators have wondered whether there was a vascular component to NIHL, but evidence has been conflicting. Cochlear blood flow has been shown to increase or decrease for long noise exposures, and it is unclear whether vascular disease increases susceptibility to NIHL (34).

Behavioral hearing tests in patients with NIHL can demonstrate deficits in speech recognition, in frequency and time resolution, and in other complex auditory tests. However, none of these tests has shown performance deficits specific to NIHL, and none has proved more useful than pure-tone threshold shifts for the early detection of NIHL.

EVALUATION AND DIAGNOSIS

Epidemiology

Hazardous noise exposure is common in our society; occupational noise and nonoccupational noise have each been estimated to cause 5% to 10% of the adult hearing loss burden in the United States (37). Table 157.1 shows

TABLE 157.1	NOISE EXPOSURE IN 19 US INDUSTRIES (1981)[a]	
Level (dBA)	Workers	Total (%)
<80	6,987,000	46.88
80–85	2,793,000	18.74
85–90	2,244,500	15.06
90–95	1,636,500	10.98
95–100	815,200	5.47
>100	427,700	2.87

[a]Machinery, transportation equipment, electrical machinery, fabricated metals, food, apparel, primary metals, textiles, printing and publishing, utilities, lumber and wood, rubber and plastics, stone and glass, chemicals, paper, furniture and textiles, petroleum and coal, tobacco, and leather.

the distribution of exposures in 19 industries believed by OSHA to contain most of the noisy workplaces in the United States (38): At that time, at least 5.1 million American industrial workers were exposed at levels exceeding 85 dBA, averaged over a workday (massive job losses in American manufacturing in the past two decades have almost certainly reduced those numbers). Sadly, no more recent data are available since that 1981 survey. Hazardous nonoccupational exposure is much more prevalent; the National Rifle Association estimates that 65 million Americans own guns (www.nraila.org, 2004), and many of them participate in hunting or target shooting. Significantly, firearms and occupational noise exposure often go together. The prevalence of handicapping NIHL in men has been estimated at 1.7% (39).

Damage Risk Criteria

Animal research has been essential in describing the pathogenesis of NIHL and some of its features; however, the risk of human hearing loss with various exposures can be estimated only from epidemiologic studies. The results of many such studies measuring the hearing of noise-exposed workers have been generally consistent; good summaries and professional consensus statements can be found in publications by ANSI (22) and OSHA (38).

Levels below about 80 dBA pose negligible risk to human hearing over a working lifetime. Above 85 dBA, risk grows rapidly for the high frequencies and more slowly for lower frequencies. Figure 157.5 shows the growth of NIPTS as a function of duration of employment for two frequencies (1 and 4 kHz) and two exposure levels (85 and 100 dBA) according to OSHA (38). Median threshold shifts are shown; half of all workers would show more shift, and half would show less shift than indicated. No curve is plotted for 1 kHz at 85 dBA because less than 1 dB of shift is predicted even after 40 years. Note that at 4 kHz, NIPTS grows rapidly over the first 10 years and then reaches a plateau. For 1 kHz, growth is somewhat more gradual, but more than 50% of NIPTS is accrued in the first 10 years.

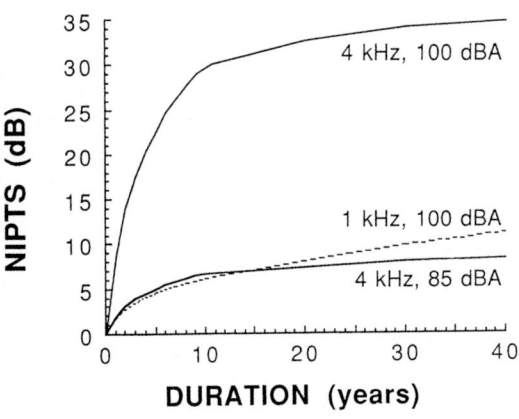

Figure 157.5 Median NIPTS as a function of exposure duration for 4 kHz (85 and 100 dBA) and 1 kHz (100 dBA).

Similar NIPTS curves are shown in Figure 157.6, using the pure-tone average (PTA) for 0.5, 1, 2, and 3 kHz (speech frequency average used in the American Medical Association [AMA] method of estimating "binaural hearing impairment" [BHI]). It is interesting to compare these curves with age-related permanent threshold shift (ARPTS) curves for men and women (Fig. 157.7), again for the 0.5, 1, 2, and 3 kHz PTA (23,24). ARPTS is an accelerating process (i.e., the rate of change of hearing loss increases with time), whereas NIPTS is a decelerating process (i.e., the rate of change decreases with time). This contrast can be helpful in determining the relative contribution of these two sources of hearing loss in individual cases.

Data like these can be used to estimate the median hearing loss for a population of workers with a given gender, age, duration, and level of exposure. The median expected hearing loss (0.5, 1, 2, and 3 kHz PTA) for 65-year-old men with 40 years of exposure at 90 dBA would be about 21 dB HL (15 dB aging plus 6 dB NIPTS), using the data from Figures 157.6 and 157.7. A greater loss than this prediction could be due to specific otologic disease, to above-average susceptibility to aging and/or noise, to undocumented noise exposure, or to a combination of factors.

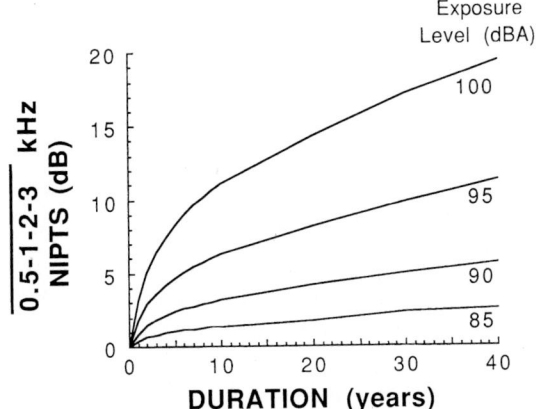

Figure 157.6 Median NIPTS for the PTA (0.5, 1, 2, and 3 kHz) as a function of exposure duration, for different exposure levels (85 to 100 dBA).

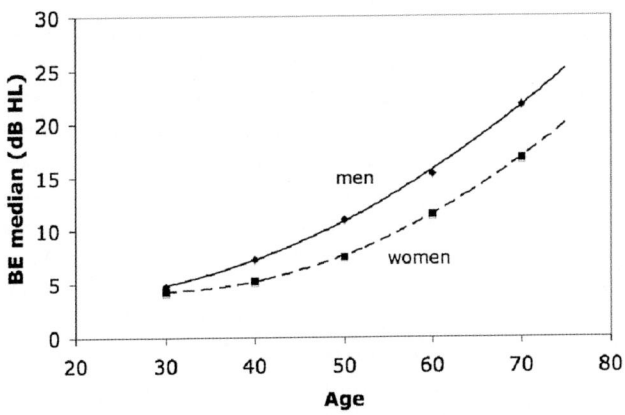

Figure 157.7 Median better-ear PTA hearing thresholds (0.5, 1, 2, and 3 kHz) for American men (*diamonds*) and women (*squares*) of different age groups (Hoffman HJ, Dobie RA, Ko Chia-Wen, et al. Hearing threshold levels at age 70 (65–74 years) in the unscreened older adult population of the United States, 1959–1962 and 1999–2006. *Ear Hear* 2012;33(3):437–440; Hoffman HJ, Dobie RA, Ko C-W, et al. Hearing threshold levels at age 70 (65–74 years) in the unscreened older adult population of the United States, 1959–1962 and 1999–2006. *Ear Hear* 2012;33(3):437–440. The smooth curves (*solid* for men, *dashed* for women) are quadratic fits to the plotted data points.

Nonoccupational Exposures

The most important nonoccupational cause of NIHL is gunfire. Impulse levels from rifles and shotguns can reach 170 dB at the shooter's ear. The left ear of a right-handed shooter is at greater risk because the right ear is somewhat protected by the head shadow. Data from the interindustry noise study showed that men in non-noisy jobs who reported hunting and shooting sustained hearing loss that was the equivalent of 20 years' occupational exposure at 89 dBA (40). Automobile airbags also produce very high impulse noise levels; they save lives but may cause acoustic trauma (41).

Exposures to leaf blowers, chain saws, and rock concerts can exceed 110 dBA. Very few people spend enough time in these exposures to cause NIPTS. The main exception is occupational exposure; thus, professional gardeners, forestry workers, and rock musicians are at considerable risk. Nonetheless, it is not unreasonable to wear hearing protection even for occasional exposures at such levels. Personal stereo systems (PSSs), including MP3 players, are capable of producing dangerous noise levels, but most users choose levels well below 90 dBA and durations below 20 hours per week. The most important risk of these devices is their use in a noisy work environment, where they can add to already-hazardous exposures.

There has been considerable media speculation about an "epidemic of hearing loss" attributable to PSSs, but scientific evidence of a link is lacking. One recent paper (42) found that teenagers in 2005 to 2006 had higher rates of hearing loss (mostly "slight," i.e., 15 to 25 dB HL) than in 1988 to 1994 and hinted that PSSs might be to blame. If PSSs had caused an increase in hearing loss, one would expect to see several additional features: an increase in audiometric notches; an increase in bilateral high-frequency, rather than unilateral and/or low-frequency losses; and perhaps most importantly, a correlation between hearing loss (especially high-frequency loss) and reported noise exposure. None of these were seen in the cited paper. Another paper comparing the same two population surveys, using different methods (43), found no overall increase in hearing loss or in noise notches in the 2005 to 2006 data, but found that while the prevalence of noise notches had decreased in boys, it had increased in girls. Once again, there was no correlation between self-reported noise exposure, including the use of PSSs, and the risk of hearing loss. While extreme use of PSSs can cause hearing loss, it appears that this does not occur frequently enough to show up in population surveys.

Diagnosis of Noise-Induced Hearing Loss

In making a diagnosis of NIHL, the otolaryngologist should consider history, physical examination, audiometric findings (ideally over a period of many years), and sometimes the results of other tests. A history of occupational or non-occupational noise exposure of hazardous intensity and duration should be sought. Noise exposure measurements from the workplace, if available, are most helpful. The history should document carefully all employment, including military service, which often includes noise exposure.

Other etiologies of sensorineural hearing loss (heredity, ototoxicity, head injury, etc.) are primarily excluded by history. Physical examination excludes external ear and middle-ear disorders and occasionally may detect cranial nerve or balance abnormalities that suggest an acoustic tumor.

The pure-tone audiogram in early cases usually shows a notch at 3, 4, or 6 kHz (not pathognomonic for NIHL); this notch is often lost over the years as loss becomes more severe and as aging changes are added to NIPTS. PTA asymmetries greater than about 15 dB suggest either another etiology or asymmetric exposures (44). Rifles and shotguns are the most common source for asymmetric NIHL. Most indoor factory environments are highly reverberant so that one ear rarely receives significantly more noise than the other. It is important to document whether hearing protectors have been used, what types were used, and when that use began.

A series of audiograms prior to employment and at intervals throughout a worker's career is most helpful. As suggested earlier, hearing loss that accelerates in middle age without any increase in noise exposure probably is due primarily to aging rather than to noise.

Laboratory and imaging tests are of no value in establishing the diagnosis of NIHL but occasionally are indicated to rule out other disorders, especially acoustic tumor, when substantial asymmetries of hearing or other findings inconsistent with NIHL are present. The American College of Occupational and Environmental Medicine (2003) has recently updated its policy statement on the diagnosis of NIHL (excerpted in Table 157.2).

TABLE 157.2	PRINCIPAL CHARACTERISTICS OF OCCUPATIONAL NOISE-INDUCED HEARING LOSS[a]

- It is always sensorineural, affecting the hair cells in the inner ear.
- Because most noise exposures are symmetric, the hearing loss is typically bilateral.
- Typically, the first sign of hearing loss due to noise exposure is a "notching" of the audiogram at 3,000, 4,000, or 6,000 Hz, with recovery at 8,000 Hz. This notching is in contrast to age-related loss, which also produces high-frequency hearing loss, but in a down-sloping pattern without recovery at 8,000 Hz.
- Noise exposure alone usually does not produce a loss >75 dB in high frequencies, and 40 dB in lower frequencies. However, individuals with superimposed age-related losses may have HTLs in excess of these values.
- The rate of hearing loss due to chronic noise exposure is greatest during the first 10–15 y of exposure and decreases as the hearing threshold increases. This is in contrast to age-related hearing loss, which accelerates over time.
- Most scientific evidence indicates that previously noise-exposed ears are not more sensitive to future noise exposure and that hearing loss due to noise does not progress (in excess of what would be expected from the addition of age-related threshold shifts) once the exposure to noise is discontinued.
- In obtaining a history of noise exposure, the clinician should keep in mind that the risk of NIHL is considered to rise significantly with chronic exposures above 85 dBA for an 8-h TWA. In general, continuous noise exposure over the years is more damaging than interrupted exposure that permits the ear to have a rest period.

[a]Occupational NIHL, as opposed to occupational acoustic trauma, is hearing loss that develops slowly over a long period (several years) as the result of exposure to continuous or intermittent loud noise. Occupational acoustic trauma is a sudden change in hearing as a result of a single exposure to a sudden burst of sound, such as an explosive blast. The diagnosis of NIHL is made clinically by a medical professional and should include a study of the noise exposure history.

Compensation

Otolaryngologists are frequently asked to evaluate workers for state workers compensation programs and for federal agencies such as the Veterans Administration and the Department of Labor. Compensation for NIHL varies widely, as do the formulas used for assessing hearing handicap (45).

Hearing handicap has been defined as a disadvantage "sufficient to affect the individual's efficiency in the activities of daily living," specifically, interference with speech communication (46). Whereas most of the acoustic power in speech is concentrated below 1,000 Hz, most of the information content is in the higher frequencies. The typical patient with a handicapping degree of NIHL or age-related hearing loss can hear speech without difficulty because of the low-frequency power in vowel sounds but has difficulty discriminating among consonants because they are relatively high-frequency, low-intensity sounds. For example, *top* and *cop* may sound alike. These problems ultimately can lead to social withdrawal and isolation, depression, and a general reduction of quality of life. Depression also may be seen with tinnitus, which commonly accompanies NIHL.

In 1979, the American Academy of Otolaryngology-Head and Neck Surgery (AAO-HNS) revised their recommended method for evaluation of hearing handicap, which was subsequently accepted by the AMA (the AMA now uses the term "binaural hearing impairment" instead of "hearing handicap"). Most states have either adopted this method explicitly or have left the determination of hearing handicap to professional judgment. The AAO-HNS/AMA 1979 method (47) is based on several assumptions and has been validated against self-report of hearing difficulties in a recent large study (48):

1. Hearing loss does not begin to be handicapping until the PTA at 0.5, 1, 2, and 3 kHz exceeds 25 dB HL.
2. Handicap (as estimated by BHI) grows at the rate of 1.5% per decibel of hearing loss beyond 25 dB.
3. Because unilateral deafness is only a mild handicap, the two ears should not be equally weighted. Specifically, a 5 to 1 weighting favoring the better ear is used.

The monaural impairment (MI) for each ear is first calculated from the four-frequency PTA:

$$MI = 1.5 \, (PTA-25) \, [\textit{Note: if PTA} < 25, MHI = 0\%]$$

BHI, ranging from 0% to 100%, is then calculated as a weighted average favoring the better ear:

$$BHI = [5(MI_b) + (MI_w)]/6$$

where MI_b and MI_w represent the MI scores of the better and worse ears.

For example, consider a person whose thresholds are as follows:

Frequency (kHz)	Right Ear (dB)	Left Ear (dB)
0.5	15	20
1	25	40
2	35	60
3	45	80

The right (better) ear PTA is $(15 + 25 + 35 + 45)/4 = 30$ dB. The better ear MI score is $(30 - 25) \, (1.5) = 7.5\%$.

The left (worse) ear PTA is $(20 + 40 + 60 + 80)/4 = 50$ dB. The worse ear MI score is $(50 - 25) \, (1.5) = 37.5\%$.

BHI is $[5(7.5) + (37.5)]/6 = 12.5\%$.

Even when no other specific otologic disease is present, elevated thresholds in noise-exposed workers can usually be thought of as containing both age-related and noise-induced components. Age correction of audiograms is not appropriate for compensation assessment purposes. It is possible, however, to make reasonable estimates of the relative contributions of noise and aging, or of separate periods of noise exposure, in individual cases (20,49).

The physician's report of a compensation examination should be complete and concise and, most importantly, should offer clear diagnostic conclusions based on clinical and scientific evidence with some explanation of the reasons for those conclusions. If a particular diagnosis is "more probable than not" (probability > 50%), it can and should be stated as a "reasonable medical certainty"; this standard, which is typical for civil and workers' compensation cases, differs substantially from the "beyond a reasonable doubt" standard used in criminal trials. The AAO-HNS (49) has published guidelines for physicians' reports in such settings.

MANAGEMENT

Hearing Conservation

Since 1970, federal law has required most employers to prevent exposures exceeding 90 dBA averaged over an 8-hour day. The detailed requirements for occupational HCPs, however, were not published until much later (50).

Many noise exposures are not steady state; the noise may fluctuate in intensity throughout the day. Other occupational exposures may be brief, as when a worker spends less than 1 hour a day in a particularly noisy part of the factory. Considerable controversy exists about how to handle such exposure variations, largely because there are only scanty epidemiologic data relating NIPTS to brief and varying exposures. If exposures containing equal sound energy were equally hazardous, one would adopt a trading rule in which the permissible exposure time would be cut in half for each 3-dB increase in exposure level (sound power, i.e., energy per unit time, doubles for each 3-dB increment). However, there is frequently a degree of intermittency in

TABLE 157.3	PERMISSIBLE NOISE EXPOSURES

Duration Per Day (h)	Sound Level (dBA)
8	90
6	92
4	95
3	97
2	100
1.5	102
1	105
0.5	110
0.25	115

occupational noise exposures, thus reducing risk. For this reason, expert consensus led OSHA to adopt a 5-dB trading rule: A 4-hour exposure at 95 dBA and a 2-hour exposure at 100 dBA are considered equally as hazardous as an 8-hour exposure at 90 dBA. Each of these exposures would be considered to be 90 dBA "time-weighted average" (exposure level that if constant for 8 hours would be expected to pose the same risk of hearing loss as the briefer exposure in question). Time-intensity trading ends at 115 dBA: Above this level, OSHA permits only exposures of less than 1 second. This relationship between sound level and duration is shown in Table 157.3.

The maximum permissible exposure (without hearing protection) under OSHA regulations is 90 dBA TWA, but HCPs must be implemented for all workers whose exposures exceed 85 dBA TWA. Impulse noise exposure is limited to a 140-dB peak level.

The essential elements of an HCP are as follows:

- Noise exposure measurements
- Engineering or administrative controls to reduce exposure
- Periodic audiometry with follow-up and referral
- Use of personal hearing protection devices (HPDs)
- Education, motivation, and counseling
- These elements should be supported by an administrative component that includes supervision, record keeping, and program evaluation.

Measurements of noise exposure may be performed with sound level meters or devices called noise dosimeters, which attach to a worker's clothing and automatically compute his or her TWA exposure. Exposures that exceed permissible limits can be reduced by noise control or by reducing the time that employees spend in the noise. In situations in which neither engineering nor administrative controls can reduce exposures below 85 dBA TWA, a program of annual audiometry must be instituted. Although workplace audiometry is less reliable than clinical testing, PTA changes of 10 dB or more usually indicate real hearing changes (51). OSHA defines a standard threshold shift (STS) as a 10-dB or greater increase in threshold for the 2-, 3-, and 4-kHz average in either ear. Unfortunately, OSHA does not mandate otologic referral, even for large or asymmetric losses, although disorders other than NIHL are often found in such cases (52). Workers who demonstrate STS or who have exposures above 90 dBA TWA must use HPDs (earplugs, earmuffs).

Although the "noise reduction ratings" on the package labels of HPDs are typically 20 to 30 dB or even higher, these numbers reflect ideal fitting in laboratory conditions. Real-world attenuation values are much lower: On the average, premolded earplugs offer about 10-dB attenuation of A-weighted levels, formable foam plugs about 15 dB, and earmuffs about 20 dB. If worn only 4 hours out of a steady 8-hour noise exposure, no HPD can provide more than 5 dB of effective attenuation. Recently, there has been great interest in electronic noise cancellation headsets, which attempt to deliver a sound wave to the ear that is exactly out of phase with the ambient noise. These devices can effectively cancel out only low-frequency noises (up to about 500 Hz), and they can thus be quite helpful in environments where the noise is predominantly low frequency, such as in private aviation. Unfortunately, the most hazardous spectral components for most occupational and recreational noises are well above 500 Hz; thus, noise cancellation has been of very little value in HCPs. In contrast, another type of electronic HPD has proved to be very useful in situations where the hazardous noise is only intermittent (such as recreational shooting): These "level-dependent" HPDs have an external microphone, an internal speaker, and circuitry that allows sounds below about 85 dB to pass into the ear while louder sounds are blocked.

The differences in protection afforded by various HPDs, when worn properly, are small compared with variations in protection that occur with improper or negligent use. Therefore, the most important factors in choosing an HPD are proper fit and acceptance by the worker. Counseling and motivation are important. Many workers fear they will miss important communications or warning signals with HPDs in place. In fact, detection of such signals is usually not impaired. Speech and other signals need to be at a high level to be heard over industrial noise anyway, and with the HPD in place, both signal and noise are equally reduced. Some workers with high-frequency hearing loss perform more poorly than normal-hearing persons in detecting and discriminating signals in noise with HPDs in place (53); this problem can often be ameliorated by using HPDs with less high-frequency attenuation, which may provide adequate protection without making high-frequency signals inaudible.

Clinical Management

Many physicians have advocated treatments, usually based on vasodilatation or hemorheologic effects, for acute acoustic trauma. Considerable recovery of hearing is part of the natural history of such events, however, and no well-controlled studies have yet demonstrated benefit for any treatment, except in animals (not human patients) given antioxidants (e.g., vitamins A, C, and E; N-acetyl L-cysteine), vasodilators (e.g., magnesium), or other drugs (e.g., furosemide) prior to or during excessive noise exposure. This continues to be an active area of research, and future studies may yet show that drugs, vitamins, and/or nutritional supplements have a role in the treatment and prevention of NIHL (54–56).

Counseling to prevent further hearing loss is crucial. Exposed workers who are not enrolled in occupational HCPs need to be scheduled for periodic monitoring audiometry and should be counseled regarding the appropriate use of HPDs. Hearing aids are helpful when hearing loss becomes handicapping, but of course they do not restore normal hearing.

Counseling hearing-impaired workers or their employers regarding fitness for continued safe and productive employment is extremely difficult. Factors to consider include not only the degree of hearing loss but also the acoustic environment at work, the communicative demands of the job, and nonauditory attributes of the worker, such as age, experience, linguistic background, and cognitive status (57).

NONAUDITORY EFFECTS

Loud noise interferes severely with speech communication at about the same levels at which hazard to hearing begins. This information can be useful in counseling and in assessing compensation claims. If a worker states that the workplace is noisy enough that he or she must speak very loudly or shout to converse at ordinary conversational distances, then, even in the absence of sound level measurements, it can be concluded that levels are probably over 80 dBA.

Other nonauditory effects of noise, including annoyance, sleep disturbance, and physiologic changes (in blood pressure, catecholamine secretion, and so on), are controversial. Certainly, annoyance and sleep disturbance may occur at levels far below any hazard for NIHL (58,59). An unwanted noise, such as a dripping faucet or a neighbor's party, even if quite faint, can be annoying and stressful. These effects are not due to the physical properties of the noise (intensity, spectrum, time) but to cognitive and psychological factors (60). It is impossible to predict these types of effects with a sound level meter. It is probably safe to say that most experts believe that no adverse long-term health effects of noise exposure have been demonstrated at exposures below those that could cause NIHL.

THE IMPORTANCE OF PREVENTION

NIHL is by far the most important preventable cause of hearing loss in adults. Noise reduction and use of HPDs, in occupational HCPs mandated since 1983, have already prevented many workers from suffering hearing impairment. Nevertheless, NIHL continues to be an important public health problem. Major coverage gaps include small employers, industries that are not currently subject to detailed OSHA regulations (construction, agriculture, oil and gas drilling), and nonoccupational noise exposure (especially shooting). Otolaryngologists can help by asking their patients about noise exposure and by providing hearing protection, counseling, and periodic audiometry for exposed patients who are not well covered at work. We should also educate our colleagues in primary care about the roles they can play in prevention of NIHL. Some have advocated more stringent hearing conservation regulations, such as lowering the permissible exposure level or the way it is calculated. But in the author's opinion, adequate enforcement of current OSHA regulations, implementation of HCPs for currently uncovered entities, and effective physician involvement would save far more hearing than any change in current OSHA regulations.

ACKNOWLEDGMENTS

Drs. Dixon Ward, William Melnick, Donald Henderson, and Jack Mills read earlier versions of the manuscript and made helpful suggestions. Michael Wilson prepared the figures; Julie Estrada and Mary Brown typed the original manuscript.

HIGHLIGHTS

- NIHL, although not medically or surgically treatable, is the major preventable cause of hearing loss in the United States.
- NIPTS grows rapidly in the high frequencies (3 to 6 kHz) and then decelerates after about 10 years.
- After about 10 years at constant exposure levels, threshold shifts at lower frequencies (especially 2 kHz) begin to predominate.
- Within the organ of Corti, the outer hair cells are most susceptible to noise-induced damage.
- Workplace exposures below 80 dBA pose negligible risk to human hearing; exposures at levels above 85 dBA may cause significant noise-induced threshold shift.
- In contrast to noise-induced loss, age-related hearing loss is an accelerating process (rate of change increases with time).
- The most important nonoccupational cause of NIHL is gunfire.
- Federal regulations forbid occupational exposures over 90 dBA TWA (8-hour equivalent) without hearing protection but require HCPs for all workers whose exposures exceed 85 dBA TWA.

- The need to shout to converse in the workplace or a worker's complaint of temporary fullness, tinnitus, or muffled hearing after work usually indicates the presence of potentially hazardous noise levels.

- Diagnosis of NIHL should not be made on the basis of audiometric contour alone, but must include a careful history of occupational and nonoccupational noise exposure.

REFERENCES

1. Yueh B, Shapiro N, MacLean CH, et al. Screening and management of adult hearing loss in primary care. *JAMA* 2003;289:1976–1985.

2. Bohne BA, Zahn SJ, Bozzay DG. Damage to the cochlea following interrupted exposure to low-frequency noise. *Ann Otol Rhinol Laryngol* 1985;94:122–128.

3. Sataloff J, Sataloff RT, Menduke H, et al. Intermittent exposure to noise: effects on hearing. *Ann Otol Rhinol Laryngol* 1983;92:623–628.

4. ACOEM Noise and Hearing Conservation Committee. ACOEM evidence-based statement: noise-induced hearing loss. *J Occup Med* 2003;45:579–581.

5. Humes LE, Joellenbeck LM, Durch JS. *Noise and military service: implications for hearing loss and tinnitus.* Washington, DC: National Academies Press, 2006.

6. Kujawa SG, Liberman MC. Acceleration of age-related hearing loss by early noise exposure: evidence of a misspent youth. *J Neuroscience* 2006;26:2115–2123.

7. Gates G, Schmid P, Kujawa S, et al. Longitudinal threshold changes in older men with audiometric notches. *Hear Res* 2000;141:220–228.

8. Lee FS, Mathews LJ, Dubno JR, et al. Longitudinal study of pure-tone thresholds in older persons. *Ear Hear* 2005;26:1–11.

9. Borg E, Nilsson R, Engström B. Effect of the acoustic reflex on inner ear damage induced by industrial noise. *Acta Otolaryngol* 1983;96:361–369.

10. Maison SF, Liberman MC. Predicting vulnerability to acoustic injury with a non-invasive assay of olivocochlear reflex strength. *J Neurosci* 2000;20:4701–4707.

11. Darrow KN, Maison SF, Liberman MC. Selective removal of lateral olivocochlear efferents increases vulnerability to acute acoustic injury. *J Neurophysiol* 2007;97:1775–1785.

12. Sha S, Taylor R, Forge A, et al. Differential vulnerability of basal and apical hair cells is based on intrinsic susceptibility to free radicals. *Hear Res* 2001;155:1–8.

13. Nondahl DM, Shi X, Cruickshanks KJ, et al. Notched audiograms and noise exposure history in older adults. *Ear Hear* 2009;30:696–703.

14. Niu X, Canlon B. Theories of sound conditioning. In Henderson D, ed. *Noise-induced hearing loss: basic mechanisms, prevention, and control.* London: NRN Publications, 2001.

15. Taylor W, Pearson J, Mair A. Study of noise and hearing in jute weaving. *J Acoust Soc Am* 1965;38:113–120.

16. Wang Y, Hirose K, Liberman M. Dynamics of noise-induced cellular injury and repair in the mouse cochlea. *J Assoc Res Otolaryngol* 2002;3:248–268.

17. Kujawa SG, Liberman MC. Adding insult to injury: cochlear nerve degeneration after "temporary" noise-induced hearing loss. *J Neuroscience* 2009;29:14077–14085.

18. Henderson D, Hamernik RP. Impulse noise: critical review. *J Acoust Soc Am* 1986;80:569–584.

19. McRobert H, Ward WD. Damage-risk criteria: the trading relation between intensity and the number of nonreverberant impulses. *J Acoust Soc Am* 1973;53:1297–1300.

20. Dobie RA. *Medical-legal evaluation of hearing loss,* 2nd ed. San Diego, CA: Singular Publishing, 2001.

21. Macrae JH. Noise-induced hearing loss and presbycusis. *Audiology* 1971;10:323–333.

22. American National Standards Institute. *Determination of occupational noise exposure and estimation of noise-induced hearing impairment.* ANSI-S3.44–1996. New York: Acoustical Society of America, 1996:27.

23. Hoffman HJ, Dobie RA, Ko C-W, et al. Americans hear as well or better today compared to 40 years ago: hearing threshold levels in the unscreened adult population of the United States, 1959–1962 and 1999–2004. *Ear Hear* 2010;31:725–734.

24. Hoffman HJ, Dobie RA, Ko C-W, et al. Hearing threshold levels at age 70 (65-74 years) in the unscreened older adult population of the United States, 1959–1962 and 1999–2006. *Ear Hear* 2012;33(3):437–440.

25. Czanto C, Ligia S. Correlation between vibration-induced white finger and hearing loss in miners. *J Occup Health* 1999;41:232–237.

26. Humes LE. Noise-induced hearing loss as influenced by other agents and by some physical characteristics of the individual. *J Acoust Soc Am* 1984;76:1318–1329.

27. Cary R, Clarke S, Delic J. Effects of combined exposure to noise and toxic substances—critical review of the literature. *Ann Occup Hyg* 1997;41:455–465.

28. Sliwinska-Kowalkska M, Zamyslowska-Szmytke E, Szymczak W, et al. Hearing loss among workers exposed to moderate concentrations of solvents. *Scand J Work Environ Health* 2001;27:335–342.

29. Morata T, Johnson A, Nylen P, et al. Audiometric findings in workers exposed to low levels of styrene and noise. *J Occup Environ Med* 2002;44:806–814.

30. Rabinowitz PM, Galusha D, Slade MD, et al. Organic solvent exposure and hearing loss in a cohort of aluminum workers. *Occup Environ Med* 2008;65:230–235.

31. Holme R, Steel K. Progressive hearing loss and increased susceptibility to noise-induced hearing loss in mice carrying a *cdh23* but not a *myo7a* mutation. *J Assoc Res Otolaryngol* 2004;5:66–79.

32. Davis R, Kozel P, Erway L. Genetic influences in individual susceptibility to noise: a review. *Noise Health* 2003;5:19–28.

33. Konings A, Van Laer L, Van Camp G. Genetic studies on noise-induced hearing loss: a review. *Ear Hear* 2009;30:151–159.

34. Saunders JC, Dear SP, Schneider ME. The anatomical consequences of acoustic injury: a review and tutorial. *J Acoust Soc Am* 1985;78:833–860.

35. Lapsley Miller JA, Marshall L, Heller LM, et al. Low-level otoacoustic emissions may predict susceptibility to noise-induced hearing loss. *J Acoust Soc Am* 2006;120:280–296.

36. Marshall L, Lapsley Miller JA, Heller LM, et al. Detecting incipient inner-ear damage from impulse noise with otoacoustic emissions. *J Acoust Soc Am* 2009;125:995–1013.

37. Dobie RA. The burdens of age-related and noise-induced hearing loss in the United States. *Ear Hear* 2008;29(4):565–565.

38. Occupational Safety and Health Administration, US Department of Labor. Occupational noise exposure: hearing conservation amendment. *Fed Regist* 1981:4078–4179.

39. Phaneuf R, Hétu R. An epidemiological perspective of the causes of hearing loss among industrial workers. *J Otolaryngol* 1990;19(1):31–40.

40. Johnson DL, Riffle C. Effects of gunfire on the hearing level of selected individuals from the Inter-Industry Noise Study. *J Acoust Soc Am* 1982;72:1311–1314.

41. Yaremchuk K, Dobie RA. Otologic injuries from airbag deployment. *Otolaryngol Head Neck Surg* 2001;125:130–134.

42. Shargorodsky J, Curhan SG, Curhan GC, et al. Change in prevalence of hearing loss in US adolescents. *JAMA* 2010;304:772–778.

43. Henderson E, Testa MA, Hartnick C. Prevalence of noise-induced hearing threshold shifts among US youths. *Pediatrics* 2011;127:e39–e46.

44. Alberti PW, Symons F, Hyde ML. Occupational hearing loss: the significance of asymmetrical hearing thresholds. *Acta Otolaryngol* 1979;87:255–263.

45. Dobie RA, Megerson SC. Workers' compensation. In: Berger EH, ed. *The noise manual,* rev. 5th ed. Fairfax, VA: American Industrial Hygiene Association, 2003.

46. American Academy of Otolaryngology—Head and Neck Surgery Foundation. *Guide for conservation of hearing in noise.* Washington, DC: American Academy of Otolaryngology—Head Neck Surgery Foundation, 1988.

47. American Medical Association (AMA). *Guides to the evaluation of permanent impairment,* 6th ed. Chicago, IL: AMA Press, 2008.

48. Dobie RA. The AMA method of estimation of hearing disability: a validation study. *Ear Hear* 2011;32(6):732–740.

49. American Academy of Otolaryngology—Head and Neck Surgery. *Evaluation of people reporting occupational hearing loss.* Alexandria, VA: American Academy of Otolaryngology—Head and Neck Surgery, 1998.

50. Occupational Safety and Health Administration, US Department of Labor. Occupational noise exposure: hearing conservation amendment; final rule (anonymous). *Fed Regist* 1983;48:9738.

51. Dobie RA. Reliability and validity of industrial audiometry: implications for hearing conservation program design (1983 Triological Society Thesis). *Laryngoscope* 1983;93:906–927.

52. Dobie RA, Archer RJ. Results of otologic referrals in an industrial hearing conservation program. *Otolaryngol Head Neck Surg* 1981;89:294–301.

53. Abel SM, Kunov H, Pichora-Fuller MK, et al. Signal detection in industrial noise: effects of noise exposure history, hearing loss, and the use of ear protection. *Scand Audiol* 1985;14:161–173.

54. Kopke R, Coleman J, Liu J, et al. Enhancing intrinsic cochlear stress defenses to reduce noise-induced hearing loss. *Laryngoscope* 2002;112:1515–1532.

55. Le Prell CL, Dolan D, Schacht J, et al. Pathways for protection from noise-induced hearing loss. *Noise Health* 2003;5:1–17.

56. Tamir S, Adelman C, Weinberger JM, et al. Uniform comparison of several drugs which provide protection from noise-induced hearing loss. *J Occup Med Toxicol* 2010;5:26–32.

57. Dobie RA, VanHemel SB, eds. National Research Council. *Hearing loss: determining eligibility for social security benefits.* Washington, DC: National Academy Press, 2004.

58. Raschke F. Arousals and aircraft noise: environmental disorders of sleep and health in terms of sleep medicine. *Noise Health* 2004;6:15–26.

59. Guski R. How to forecast community annoyance in planning noisy facilities. *Noise Health* 2004;6:59–64.

60. Ising H. Editorial. *Noise Health* 2004;6:1–2.

158 Ototoxicity

Kay W. Chang

It is important for physicians to be aware of the large number of systemic and topical agents that can cause functional impairment and cellular damage to the inner ear. Ototoxicity-induced hearing loss can result in significant disability to the affected individual, especially young children who are still in the process of speech and language development. Ototoxic effects on the vestibular system can result in significant balance disorder and impair even simple activities of daily life. Recognizing the early signs of ototoxicity may allow for discontinuation or reduction of the offending agent, thus minimizing permanent hearing and balance impairment. As our knowledge of the genetics of ototoxicity improves, it may be possible to identify patients who are at high risk of developing ototoxicity prior to exposure to the drug. Furthermore, a number of promising otoprotective agents are emerging that may also diminish or completely prevent ototoxicity.

SYSTEMIC OTOTOXICITY

Table 158.1 summarizes the major agents implicated in ototoxicity. The categories that are responsible for the majority of ototoxicity clinically observed in present-day medicine are the aminoglycosides and platinum-containing chemotherapy agents.

Aminoglycosides

Aminoglycoside antibiotics have been an important part of our antibacterial drug armamentarium since the discovery of streptomycin in 1943 by Waksman, who was awarded the Nobel Prize for this discovery. While they possess potent activity against *Pseudomonas aeruginosa* and most other aerobic gram-negative bacilli, their toxicity has resulted in restrained use in developed countries with the introduction of broad-spectrum cephalosporins, carbapenems, and fluoroquinolones. However, since many aminoglycosides are significantly cheaper than alternative drugs, aminoglycoside use remains relatively high in emerging countries in East Asia and Latin America. Aminoglycosides are also frequently utilized in patients with cystic fibrosis. In the United States, eight aminoglycosides (gentamicin, tobramycin, amikacin, streptomycin, neomycin, kanamycin, paromomycin, and spectinomycin) are approved by the FDA (1). Aminoglycosides ending in "mycin" are fermentation products or semisynthetic derivatives from *Streptomyces*, while those ending in "micin" are products of *Micromonospora* (2). Nephrotoxicity occurs in 5% to 25% of patients receiving aminoglycosides (2–7), while ototoxicity results in hearing loss in 3% to 13% (8–13), and vestibular impairment in 1% to 11% (4,9,14–17).

It is somewhat uncommon to have both vestibular and cochlear symptoms in the same patient; however, either or both may occur with any of the aminoglycosides (17). Auditory symptoms of hearing loss and tinnitus are most prevalent with neomycin, followed in order of decreasing toxicity by gentamicin, tobramycin, amikacin, and netilmicin (2,9,16,18,19). Vestibular symptoms of dizziness, imbalance, nausea, and oscillopsia are seen most with gentamicin and tobramycin, less frequent with amikacin, and least frequent with netilmicin (14,16,17). Aminoglycosides have been found to be the most common cause of bilateral vestibular dysfunction (20).

Platinum Compounds

In 1965, Barnett Rosenberg discovered that electrolysis of platinum electrodes generated a soluble platinum complex that inhibited binary fission in *Escherichia coli* (21). Cisplatin was noted to be the most active platinum complex in experimental tumor systems, and since the mid-1970s has been one of most widely used chemotherapy agents. Platinum compounds are non-cell-cycle-specific agents that inhibit deoxyribonucleic acid (DNA)

TABLE 158.1	OTOTOXIC AGENTS

Aminoglycosides
  Gentamicin
  Tobramycin
  Neomycin
  Amikacin
  Streptomycin
  Kanamycin
  Paromomycin
  Spectinomycin
  Netilmicin
  Dihydrostreptomycin
Cytotoxic agents
  Platinum compounds
    Cisplatin
    Carboplatin
    Oxaliplatin
    Others (nedaplatin, AMD-473, satraplatin)
  Vinca alkaloids
    Vincristine
    Vinblastine
    Vinorelbine
  Bleomycin
  Nitrogen mustard
Loop diuretics
  Furosemide
  Ethacrynic acid
  Bumetanide
  Others (piretanide, azosemide, triflocin, indapamide)
Macrolides
  Erythromycin
  Azithromycin
  Clarithromycin
  Ketolides (Telithromycin)
Vancomycin
  (primarily in conjunction with aminoglycosides)
Iron-chelating agents
  DFO
Anti-inflammatory agents
  Salicylates—ASA
  NSAIDs
  Quinine
Heavy metals
  Mercury
  Lead
Arsenic
Antiseptic/disinfectant agents
  Chlorhexidine
  Alcohol
Chloramphenicol
Polymyxin

replication, inducing apoptosis and/or necrosis in tumor cells. The mechanism of cisplatin ototoxicity is multifactorial with changes noted in the stria vascularis, spiral ganglion cells, and outer hair cells (OHCs) (22). In contrast, carboplatin appears to be preferentially toxic to the inner hair cells (IHCs) (23–25).

Cisplatin is associated with severe nausea and vomiting in almost all patients (26). 5-hydroxytryptamine receptor antagonists can dramatically reduce the severity of nausea and vomiting and allows cisplatin to be administered in an ambulatory care setting (27). Nephrotoxicity of cisplatin can be severe but can also be moderated with aggressive hydration with normal saline, together with infusion of hypertonic saline and mannitol-induced diuresis (28–30). Amifostine has also been shown to protect against cisplatin-induced nephrotoxicity (31) though it has not been able to protect against ototoxicity (32,33). Neurotoxicity of cisplatin includes peripheral sensory neuropathy, autonomic neuropathy (most commonly producing constipation), and ototoxicity (high-frequency hearing loss). Neuropathy can occur in 30% to 50% receiving high cumulative doses of cisplatin (34,35). Ototoxicity can occur at much lower doses, and has become the major dose-limiting toxicity of this drug, particularly in young children (36).

The reported incidence of cisplatin ototoxicity varies from 9% to 91%, due to differences in chemotherapy regimens, patient populations, the definition of ototoxicity, and variations and inconsistencies in the assessment and grading of the hearing loss (37–48). The clinical presentation of cisplatin ototoxicity includes tinnitus and a bilateral and usually symmetric high-frequency sensorineural hearing loss (SNHL) with a progression toward lower frequencies with cumulative doses. The hearing loss is permanent and usually irreversible, though occasionally recovery can be observed (49–52), as well as worsening of hearing loss following cessation of treatment (53–56). Predisposing risk factors include age extremes (particularly young children), previous or concurrent cranial irradiation, renal disease or insufficiency, IV bolus administration or high cumulative dosage of cisplatin, coadministration with aminoglycosides or loop diuretics, excessive noise exposure, poor volume status, previous history of hearing loss, and concomitant use of other ototoxic chemotherapy agents (cytarabine, bleomycin, nitrogen mustard, vincristine, and vinorelbine) (57–65).

The rate of ototoxicity when carboplatin is given alone with conventional dose regimens is generally reported in only 1% of patients. However, the incidence following high-dose or combination therapy with cisplatin rises to 33% to 82% (66–70). Nedaplatin is a second-generation platinum compound that may be less ototoxic than cisplatin, but more ototoxic than carboplatin (71–73). Oxaliplatin is a third-generation cisplatin analogue that is not associated with either nephrotoxicity or ototoxicity (74–77). However, peripheral sensory neuropathy aggravated by exposure to cold is a significant dose-limiting toxicity (78).

Vinca Alkaloids

Vinca alkaloids are antitumor drugs derived from an alkaloid obtained from the periwinkle plant *Vinca rosea* (vincristine, vinblastine) or a semisynthetic alkaloid (venorelbine)

(79). Sporadic reports suggest that vinca alkaloids are associated with risk for ototoxicity at higher doses; however, it is impossible to isolate vinca alkaloids as the responsible agent since they are typically used with other ototoxic chemotherapeutic agents (e.g., cisplatin) (57,61,80–82). A rare otolaryngologic complication of vincristine is vocal cord paralysis (83).

Loop Diuretics

Furosemide, bumetanide, and ethacrynic acid are the most commonly used loop diuretics, with ethacrynic acid reserved for those cases allergic or refractory to furosemide (84). Loop diuretics are used in the treatment of congestive heart failure, renal failure, cirrhosis, and hypertension. They are widely used in the neonatal intensive care unit in the treatment of bronchopulmonary dysplasia (85). Risk factors for ototoxicity include renal impairment, prematurity, and associated aminoglycoside use (86). The mechanism of ototoxicity appears to be a dose-related, reversible reduction in endocochlear potential (87,88).

The ototoxicity of ethacrynic acid initially was reported to be temporary (89–92); however, other reports documented permanent hearing loss in patients with impaired renal function (93–99). The incidence of ototoxicity from ethacrynic acid was estimated to be 7 patients per 1,000 treated (100). Rapid infusion (101,102) and large bolus dosings (103) of furosemide have been noted to cause a high incidence of hearing loss. While permanent hearing loss with furosemide after IV administration has been reported (104), most cases of furosemide ototoxicity have been reversible (105,106). Bumetanide is more potent but less ototoxic than furosemide (107–109); however, its higher cost appears to be a rate-limiting factor in its clinical use.

Macrolides

Erythromycin works by inhibiting protein synthesis in bacteria by reversibly binding 50S ribosomal subunits (110). Most reported ototoxicity has been reversible (111–118), though some irreversible cases have also been reported (119,120). Renal impairment (117,121–124), hepatic impairment (125), and transplant recipients (126,127) appear to have increased risk for ototoxicity. The second-generation macrolide azithromycin has been reported to cause reversible hearing loss in HIV patients (128–130) and elderly patients (131,132). There is a single case report of complete deafness (133) as well as a few of irreversible hearing loss (134,135). Clarithromycin likewise has been reported to sometimes result in ototoxicity (136–138). Telithromycin is a ketolide and represents a newer class of macrolide antibiotic with zero cases of ototoxicity reported among 2,045 patients in eight phase III trials (139).

Vancomycin

Vancomycin has been primarily associated with ototoxicity when given in conjunction with an aminoglycoside (140,141). However, in a group of patients not receiving any other ototoxic agents, 1/31 (3.2%) receiving once-daily vancomycin dosing and 5/32 (15.6%) receiving twice-daily vancomycin dosing developed hearing loss (142). Age extremes may be another risk factor. Ototoxicity after an average of 27 days of vancomycin therapy was also found in 19% of patients older than 53 years old (143). A recent study also suggested an increased risk of vancomycin ototoxicity in neonates (144).

Salicylates, Nsaids, and Quinine

Acetylsalicylic acid (ASA), commonly known as aspirin, is one of the most widely used drugs. ASA ototoxicity has been reported to occur in 11 per 1,000 patients (100,145), and results in tinnitus and a reversible mild to moderate bilaterally symmetric hearing loss (146). Recovery usually occurs 24 to 72 hours after cessation of the drug (147). Onset of tinnitus has been often used as the earliest clinical sign of salicylate toxicity (148–150). Nonsteroidal anti-inflammatory drugs (NSAIDs) share similar therapeutic actions and ototoxicity side effects with salicylates (147,151–153).

Quinine is an antimalarial drug that has been decreasing in use due to less toxic semisynthetic derivatives; however, it is still occasionally used for nocturnal leg cramps (147). Large doses of quinine produce reversible hearing loss and tinnitus, similar to salicylates (86,147,154,155). Transient vestibular effects have also been noted with quinine (156).

Iron-Chelating Agents

Deferoxamine (DFO) is an iron-chelating agent used in the treatment of acute iron intoxication and chronic iron overload secondary to multiple transfusions (157). Ototoxicity from DFO was first recognized in thalassemia major patients in the 1980s (158–162). Since then, a wide range in incidence of SNHL (12% to 56%) has been published (163–168).

Heavy Metals

Toxic levels of mercury have been reported to result in hearing loss (169–173). Lead toxicity has multisystemic toxic effects, particularly involving the peripheral and central nervous systems (174). Hearing loss has been demonstrated in both children (175,176) and lead-exposed workers (177). Experimental studies suggest that lead toxicity affects neural transmission in auditory pathways (178,179).

TOPICAL OTOTOXICITY

Ototopical Ear Drops

Animal data have demonstrated that nearly all aminoglycosides used in the middle ear as topical otic preparations are ototoxic (180). There have been long-running discussion and debate whether topically applied aminoglycosides cause similar injury in the human inner ear (181–185). The round window membrane is a potential access point between the middle ear and the inner ear, but in humans is positioned in a more protected location than in animal models and also much thicker (186–189). Furthermore, in the setting of middle ear inflammation when topical drops are likely to be applied, the round window becomes less permeable (189,190). Nonetheless, use of otic drops for extended duration in humans has been reported to result in ototoxicity (186,191,192). Furthermore, gentamicin can be topically applied to intentionally ablate vestibular function (193). A consensus AAO-HNS panel in 2004 found 54 cases of gentamicin vestibular toxicity of which 24 also had hearing loss, and 11 cases of neomycin/polymyxin auditory toxicity of which 2 had vestibular symptoms (194), and made the following recommendations (195):

1. When possible, topical antibiotic preparations free of potential ototoxicity should be used in preference to ototopical preparations that have the potential for otologic injury if the middle ear or mastoid is open.
2. If used, potentially ototoxic antibiotic preparation should be used only in infected ears. Use should be discontinued shortly after the infection has resolved.
3. If potentially ototoxic antibiotic drops are prescribed for use in the open middle ear or mastoid, the patient/parent should be warned of the risk of ototoxicity.
4. If potentially ototoxic antibiotics are prescribed, the patient should be specifically instructed to call the physician or return to his or her office if the patient develops dizziness, vertigo, hearing loss, or tinnitus.
5. If the tympanic membrane is known to be intact and the middle ear and mastoid are closed, then the use of potentially ototoxic preparations presents no risk of ototoxic injury.

The widespread availability of nonototoxic fluoroquinolone topical agents (ofloxacin, ciprofloxacin) coupled with these consensus recommendations, has resulted in a significant decrease in the clinical use of aminoglycoside otic solutions.

Other Ototoxic Topicals

Chloramphenicol has a wide antibacterial spectrum; however, its use in modern days has been limited due to significant reported ototoxicity (196,197).

Chlorhexidine has been demonstrated to have significant ototoxicity in many animal models (198–202),

though not definitively shown in humans. Likewise, ethyl alcohol has also been shown to produce ototoxicity in animals (202). Chlorhexidine and alcohol skin preparations have therefore been recommended to be avoided during ear surgery when a tympanic membrane perforation is present.

GENETICS OF OTOTOXICITY

Genetic Factors in Aminoglycoside Ototoxicity

The existence of families with multiple individuals with aminoglycoside ototoxicity has been noted since 1957 (203–207). Examination of inheritance patterns suggested a maternally transmitted mitochondrial defect as a possible etiology (203,207). The A1555G mutation in the mitochondrial 12S ribosomal ribonucleic acid (rRNA) gene was eventually implicated as the causative factor since this small rRNA had been shown to bind to aminoglycosides and to harbor resistance mutations in yeast and *Tetrahymena* (208–211). The A1555G mutation has since then been found in multiple families with aminoglycoside ototoxicity (212–219). C1494T is a different mutation in the 12S rRNA that was later identified in a large Chinese pedigree (220).

Due to their low cost and high availability, the use of aminoglycosides is widespread in China, and up to 22% of all deaf-mutes in one district could trace the cause to aminoglycoside use, 28% of them having other relatives with aminoglycoside ototoxicity (207). It is estimated that up to a third of patients with aminoglycoside ototoxicity in China have the A1555G mutation (221). In the United States, a study showed that 17% of patients with aminoglycoside ototoxicity demonstrated a mitochondrial susceptibility mutation (222).

As rapid screens for multiple mitochondrial susceptibility mutations (A1555G, C1494T, T1095C, 961delT+C(n), A827G) become more available (223), it may be possible to develop aminoglycoside treatment strategies that prevent irreversible cochlear damage, or identify patients for alternative antibiotic regimens (224). A recent screening study of 865 newborns in China identified six (0.7%) newborns with homoplasmic A1555G mutations that all passed newborn hearing screening (225). Likewise, a study of 8,974 Brazilian neonates found among 17 who failed transient-evoked otoacoustic emissions (TEOAEs), 3 individuals with A827G mutation (226).

Genetic Factors in Cisplatin Ototoxicity

An increasing number of pharmacogenomic studies investigating genetic factors in cisplatin ototoxicity have been performed. Because megalin is highly expressed in renal proximal tubular cells and marginal cells of the inner ear and also because it has been associated with the uptake of aminoglycosides, megalin was investigated for a candidate gene approach, and an association between a single nucleotide polymorphism rs2075252 of the megalin gene was found more often in those with intact hearing after cisplatin therapy (227).

Functional polymorphisms in cisplatin detoxifying enzymes such as Glutathione-S-Transferase (GST) may play also a role in protection from cisplatin ototoxicity. The genes encoding the enzymes GSTM1, GSTT1, and GSTP1 are polymorphic in humans and non-functional variants are commonly found in Caucasians. A significant association between cisplatin induced hearing loss and expression of GSTM3 was found in 39 adults (228). In a larger cohort of 173 adult testicular cancer survivors, a *GSTP1* variant was associated with protection against hearing (229). This GST genotype has also been shown to be associated with less oxaliplatin-induced neuropathy (230).

The most promising study of the role of genetics in cisplatin toxicity involved two cohorts identified through the Canadian Pharmacogenomics Network for Drug Safety. Utilizing a gene chip comprised of variants in 220 drug metabolism genes, it was found that genetic variants of TPMT (thiopurine S-methyltransferase, odds ratio = 17) and COMT (catechol O-methyltransferase, odds ratio = 5.5) were significantly associated with cisplatin-induced hearing loss. Furthermore, the number of risk alleles carried by an individual was inversely related to time to deafness (i.e., those who carried at least three out of four risk alleles had a rapid decline in their hearing, often with their first dose of cisplatin). The combination of TPMT and COMT genotypes was able to identify cisplatin-induced deafness with a positive predictive value of 92.9% and a negative predictive value of 48.6% (231).

OTOPROTECTIVE STRATEGIES

Mechanisms of Ototoxicity

There are both similarities and significant differences in the mechanisms by which cisplatin and aminoglycosides cause hearing loss and vestibular dysfunction. All ototoxic drugs induce dose-dependent death of cochlear hair cells. OHCs are more susceptible than IHCs to death caused by exposure to either cisplatin or aminoglycosides (232,233). Cochlear hair cell death becomes first evident at the base and progresses apically with continued exposure to the drug (234). Both cisplatin-induced and aminoglycoside-induced hair cell death are significantly inhibited by broad-spectrum inhibition of caspases (235–240). Cisplatin also induces degeneration of the stria vascularis, decreasing the number of marginal and intermediate cells, as well as spiral ganglion cells (241,242).

Inner ear sensory cells reside within a blood–labyrinth barrier (BLB), similar to the blood–brain barrier (BBB). Compounds essential for cellular function are transported through the endothelial cells that form the BLB. Increase in permeability between adjacent endothelial cells in the BLB rapidly induces loss of the endolymphatic potential (EP) with consequent elevation of sensory thresholds. However, ototoxins, such as aminoglycosides and cisplatin, traverse the intact BLB by trafficking mechanisms that remain poorly understood.

Antioxidants as Otoprotective Agents

Understanding the mechanisms underlying cisplatin ototoxicity has led to recognition of the role antioxidants may play in protecting the inner ear from ototoxicity. Cisplatin may permeabilize mitochondria in cochlear hair cells to release proapoptotic factors, or generate toxic levels of reactive oxygen species (ROS), each of which can initiate cell death mechanisms (243–246). ROS formation has also been implicated as a major mediator of cisplatin-induced hair cell death (247–252). Increased pools of ROS not only damage proteins and lipids but also deplete the cell's intrinsic antioxidant molecules (253,254). Cisplatin is activated by the replacement of one of its two chloride groups by a water molecule. This activated "mono aqua" cisplatin reacts preferentially with antioxidant molecules, particularly glutathione and metallothioneins. In cancer cells with very high levels of glutathione, cisplatin can be effectively bound up by the glutathione, reducing cisplatin's chemotherapeutic efficacy in these tumors (255). Cisplatin-induced ototoxicity is reduced in animal models by a variety of antioxidants, including N-acetyl-cysteine (256–258), sodium thiosulfate (259–261), D-methionine (262,263), α-lipoic acid (264,265), tocopherol (266,267), salicylate (268), ebselen (265,269), and amifostine (259,270). Antioxidant protection of cisplatin-induced ototoxicity has not been as extensively tested in humans, though amifostine does not seem to be very effective (32,33,271,272) while sodium thiosulfate has shown promising results (273–276).

Transport Mechanisms

Ototoxic drugs are able to traverse the intact BLB, yet the trafficking mechanisms by which they cross the BLB remain poorly understood. A trans-strial trafficking route from strial capillaries to marginal cells, followed by clearance into endolymph has been proposed for aminoglycosides (277). Another possible route for traversing the BLB into perilymph and subsequently into endolymph may be via transcytosis across the epithelial perilymph/endolymph barrier. For cisplatin to cross either of these trafficking routes, the positive EP (EP, +85 mV) must be overcome prior to entry of cationic cisplatin into endolymph, presumably by active trafficking.

Ototoxic aminoglycosides enter hair cells via apical endocytosis or permeation through the stereociliary mechanoelectrical transduction channels *in vitro* (278,279).

The same has not been demonstrated for cisplatin. However, a number of active copper transport mechanisms for cellular uptake of cisplatin have been proposed. Transfection of human and yeast cells with the copper transporter-like 1 (CTR1) gene to induce protein expression of CTR1 increased cellular uptake of cisplatin by 50% (280–283). Cultured cell lines with greater resistance to cisplatin toxicity have significantly lower expression of CTR1 (284,285). The copper-transporting adenosine triphosphatases 7A and 7B (ATP7A and ATP7B, respectively) have also been linked to cytoplasmic cisplatin sequestration and export out of the cell (286). Increased expression of ATP7A or ATP7B results in increased resistance to cisplatin toxicity in tumor cell lines (284,287). Following cellular uptake, ATP7B binds to cisplatin and is transported into intracellular vesicles (288).

Another transporter, OCT2, has also been associated with cisplatin excretion in the kidneys (288–290), and OCT1/2 double knockout mice are protected from cisplatin-induced ototoxicity (291). Although CTR-1 and OCT2 are present in the stria vascularis (291,292), the cellular distribution of these transporters has yet to be reported in the inner ear. CTR1, ATP7A, ATP7B, and OCT2 are all highly expressed in the choroid plexus, part of the BBB that regulates ion and substrate trafficking into and out of cerebrospinal fluids (293–295).

Several platinum-based derivatives (oxaliplatin, carboplatin) have been developed to reduce their ototoxic and nephrotoxic side effects. The reduced ototoxicity is due to the replacement of chloride ions that are integral for DNA adduct formation, thus leading to reduced platinum–DNA adduct formation in inner ear tissues. OCT2 is reported to have greater specificity for oxaliplatin (296), and a greater understanding of how transport genes such as OCT2 and CTR1 modify the uptake and trafficking of ototoxic drugs into the cochlear hair cells may result in future chemical modifications to further reduce ototoxicity (297,298).

CLINICAL MONITORING OF OTOTOXICITY

Basic audiologic assessment with pure-tone thresholds from 250 to 8,000 Hz remains an important part of ototoxicity monitoring. The basic battery should include measurement of both air and bone conduction thresholds and tympanometry if any hearing loss is identified, in order to rule out an incidental conductive involvement. Ideally, a baseline assessment prior to ototoxic drug administration is necessary to definitively demonstrate the presence of ototoxicity (299). This is especially true in the elderly population, where there exists a high incidence of preexisting high-frequency hearing loss. The pediatric oncology population may provide significant challenges, especially children developmentally younger than 3 years of age. Many of these young children can be quite sick and uncooperative to ear-specific behavioral testing (37), and the incidence of

middle ear dysfunction resulting in conductive overlays is also higher in this population.

Ototoxic drugs have been demonstrated to preferentially affect OHCs of the basal cochlear turn (8,300,301). High-frequency audiometry (HFA) of frequencies above 8,000 Hz has been shown to detect aminoglycoside-induced or cisplatin-induced ototoxic losses well before changes become evident on conventional audiometry (302–317). HFA has been shown to be efficacious in a quiet hospital room for bedside testing (318,319). High-frequency auditory brainstem response testing may also be utilized (320,321). However, HFA does require more frequent calibration and special earphones, and thus is not readily available at many institutions.

Distortion product otoacoustic emissions (DPOAEs) (322,323) or TEOAEs (324,325) are another modality for detecting ototoxicity. Otoacoustic emissions (OAEs) can be a particularly useful complement to behavioral measures in young children since they are objective and allow cross-check of behavioral responses. They may also provide some ear-specific information when insert earphones or headphones are not tolerated. Recent data suggest that DPOAEs provide evidence of whether or not there have been ototoxic changes in hearing when the highest DPOAE frequency with a robust response is used as the indicator (326,327). Widely used ototoxicity grading systems incorporating DPOAE and TEOAE do not currently exist and will need to be modified from threshold level–based systems. It is important to recognize that both DPOAE and TEOAE are exquisitely sensitive to middle ear dysfunction (328–331), and cannot be reliably used to determine ototoxicity without a normal tympanogram. Nonetheless, DPOAE and TEOAE have been found to be helpful for early detection of ototoxicity and can remain useful components of the monitoring evaluation (317,323,332–338).

The most widely used criteria to detect ototoxic change are the 1994 ASHA criteria (339), while the most widely used criteria to report adverse events in hearing are the National Cancer Institute Common Terminology Criteria for Adverse Events, Ototoxicity Grades (340) for adults, and Brock's Hearing Loss Grades in children (341). However, inconsistencies have been noted in these classification systems and it has also been demonstrated that these systems are not sensitive to obvious clinical differences in hearing loss in adult patients (276), and underreport and minimize the clinical significance of the hearing loss in children (48). Newer grading systems that more accurately characterize the clinical and functional significance of ototoxicity as specifically related to the need for intervention with assistive hearing devices have been proposed (37). As we enter a new age of otoprotective agents and strategies, coupled with greater understanding of genetic factors implicated within ototoxicity, it becomes ever more essential to develop robust audiologic assessment and classification techniques in order to design good prospective clinical studies and report outcomes in an accurate fashion (342,343).

HIGHLIGHTS

■ A large number of systemic and topical agents can cause functional impairment and cellular damage to the inner ear.

■ Symptoms of ototoxicity include hearing loss (primarily high frequency), tinnitus, and balance impairment.

■ The most commonly used drugs causing ototoxicity are the aminoglycosides and platinum-containing chemotherapy agents.

■ Topical agents are potentially ototoxic when used in the ear; therefore, nonototoxic fluoroquinolones are recommended when there is communication (e.g., open perforation, patent tube) between the ear canal and the round window membrane.

■ The A1555G mutation in mitochondrial 12S rRNA gene results in significantly increased susceptibility to aminoglycosides.

■ Genetic variants of TPMT and COMT are significantly associated with cisplatin-induced ototoxicity.

■ A number of antioxidants such as N-acetyl-cysteine and sodium thiosulfate have been shown to protect against ototoxicity. These otoprotective agents are hypothesized to lower toxic levels of ROS thus diminishing cell death mechanisms.

■ Modalities to monitor ototoxicity include standard pure-tone audiometry, HFA, and OAEs.

REFERENCES

1. American Society of Health-System Pharmacists. *Aminoglycosides in AHFS drug information 2003*. Bethesda, MD: American Society of Health-System Pharmacists Inc., 2003:61–76.
2. Gilbert DN. Aminoglycosides. In: Mandell G, Bennet JE, Dolin R, eds. *Principles and practice of infectious diseases*. 5th ed. Philadelphia, PA: Churchill Livingstone, 2000:307–336.
3. Lietman PS, Smith CR. Aminoglycoside nephrotoxicity in man. *Rev Infect Dis* 1983;5:284–293.
4. Kahlmeter G, Dahlager JI. Aminoglycoside toxicity—a review of clinical studies published between 1975 and 1982. *J Antimicrob Chemother* 1984;13(Suppl A):S9–S22.
5. Cimino MA, Rotstein C, Slaughter RL, et al. Relationship of serum antibiotic concentrations to nephrotoxicity in cancer patients receiving concurrent aminoglycoside and vancomycin therapy. *Am J Med* 1987;83:1091–1097.
6. McCormack JP, Jewesson PJ. A critical reevaluation of the "therapeutic range" of aminoglycosides. *Clin Infect Dis* 1992;14:320–329.
7. Bertino JS Jr, Booker LA, Franck PA, et al. Incidence of and significant risk factors for aminoglycoside-associated nephrotoxicity in patients dosed by using individualized pharmacokinetic monitoring. *J Infect Dis* 1993;167:173–179.
8. Fee WE. Aminoglycoside ototoxicity in the human. *Laryngoscope* 1980;90(Suppl 24):1–19.
9. Lerner AM, Cone LA, Jansen W, et al. Randomized controlled trial of the comparative efficacy, auditory toxicity and nephrotoxicity of tobramycin and nephrotoxicity of tobramycin and netilmicin. *Lancet* 1983;1:1123–1126.
10. Brummett RE, Fox KE. Aminoglycoside-induced hearing loss in humans. *Antimicrob Agents Chemother* 1989;33:797–800.
11. Munckhof WJ, Grayson ML, Turnidge JD. A meta-analysis of studies on the safety and efficacy either once daily or as divided doses. *J Antimicrob Chemother* 1996;37:645–663.
12. Hatala R, Dinh T, Cook DJ. Once-daily aminoglycoside dosing in immunocompetent adults: a meta-analysis. *Ann Intern Med* 1996;124:717–725.
13. Smyth AR, Bhatt J. Once-daily versus multiple-daily dosing with intravenous aminoglycosides for cystic fibrosis. *Cochrane Database Syst Rev* 2010;(1):CD002009.
14. Ariano RE, Zelenitsky SA, Kassum DA. Aminoglycoside-induced vestibular injury: maintaining a sense of balance. *Ann Pharmacother* 2008;42(9):1282–1289.
15. The International Antimicrobial Therapy Cooperative Group of the European Organization for Research and Treatment of Cancer. Efficacy and toxicity of single daily doses of amikacin and ceftriaxone versus multiple daily doses of amikacin and ceftazidime for injection in patients with cancer and granulocytopenia. *Ann Intern Med* 1993;119:584–593.
16. Hakashima T, Teranishi M, Hibi T, et al. Vestibular and cochlear toxicity of aminoglycosides—a review. *Acta Otolaryngol* 2000;120:904–911.
17. Black FO, Pesznecker SC. Vestibular ototoxicity: clinical considerations. *Otolaryngol Clin North Am* 1993;26:713–736.
18. Govaerts P, Van De Heyning PH, Jorens G, et al. Aminoglycoside induced ototoxicity. *Toxicol Lett* 1990;53:227–251.
19. Tange RA. Ototoxicity. *Adverse Drug React Toxicol Rev* 1998;17:75–89.
20. Zingler VC, Cnyrim C, Jahn K, et al. Causative factors and epidemiology of bilateral vestibulopathy in 255 patients. *Ann Neurol* 2007;61(6):524–532.
21. Rosenberg B, Vancamp L, Krigas T. Inhibition of cell division in Escherichia coli by electrolysis products from a platinum electrode. *Nature* 1965;205:698–699.
22. Rybak LP, Mukherjea D, Jajoo S, et al. Cisplatin ototoxicity and protection: clinical and experimental studies. *Tohoku J Exp Med* 2009;219(3):177–186.
23. Wake M, Takeno S, Ibrahim D, et al. Selective inner hair cell ototoxicity induced by carboplatin. *Laryngoscope* 1994;104(4):488–493.
24. Ding DL, Wang J, Salvi R, et al. Selective loss of inner hair cells and type-I ganglion neurons in carboplatin-treated chinchillas. Mechanisms of damage and protection. *Ann N Y Acad Sci* 1999;884:152–170.
25. Salvi RJ, Ding D, Wang J, et al. A review of the effects of selective inner hair cell lesions on distortion product otoacoustic emissions, cochlear function and auditory evoked potentials. *Noise Health* 2000;2(6):9–26.
26. Gralla RJ, Itri LM, Pisko SE, et al. Antiemetic efficacy of high-dose metoclopramide: randomized trials with placebo and prochlorperazine in patients with chemotherapy-induced nausea and vomiting. *N Engl J Med* 1981;305:905–909.
27. Marty M, Pouillart P, Scholl S, et al. Comparison of the 5-hydroxytryptamine3 (serotonin) antagonist ondansetron (GR 38032F) with high-dose metoclopramide in the control of cisplatin-induced emesis. *N Engl J Med* 1990;322:816–821.
28. Al Sarraf M, Fletcher W, Oishi N, et al. Cisplatin hydration with and without mannitol diuresis in refractory disseminated malignant melanoma: a southwest oncology group study. *Cancer Treat Rep* 1982;66:31–35.
29. Ozols RF, Corden BJ, Jacob J, et al. High-dose cisplatin in hypertonic saline. *Ann Intern Med* 1984;100:19–24.
30. Kintzel PE, Dorr RT. Anticancer drug renal toxicity and elimination: dosing guidelines for altered renal function. *Cancer Treat Rev* 1995;21:33–64.
31. Kemp G, Rose P, Lurain J, et al. Amifostine pretreatment for protection against cyclophosphamide-induced and cisplatin-induced toxicities: results of a randomized control trial in patients with advanced ovarian cancer. *J Clin Oncol* 1996;14:2101–2112.
32. Katzenstein HM, Chang KW, Krailo M, et al. Amifostine does not prevent platinum-induced hearing loss associated with the treatment of children with hepatoblastoma: a report of the intergroup hepatoblastoma study P9645 as a part of the children's oncology group. *Cancer* 2009;115(24):5828–5835.

33. Marina N, Chang KW, Malogolowkin M, et al. Amifostine does not protect against the ototoxicity of high-dose cisplatin combined with etoposide and bleomycin in pediatric germ-cell tumors: a children's oncology group study. *Cancer* 2005;104(4):841–847.

34. Cersosimo RJ. Cisplatin neurotoxicity. *Cancer Treat Rev* 1989;16: 195–211.

35. Go R, Adjei A. Review of the comparative pharmacology and clinical activity of cisplatin and carboplatin. *J Clin Oncol* 1999;17: 409–422.

36. Grewal S, Merchant T, Reymond R, et al. Auditory late effects of childhood cancer therapy: a report from the children's oncology group. *Pediatrics* 2010;125(4):e938–e950.

37. Chang KW, Chinosornvatana N. Practical grading system for evaluating cisplatin ototoxicity in children. *J Clin Oncol* 2010;28(10):1788–1795.

38. Helson L, Okonkwo E, Anton L, et al. cis-Platinum ototoxicity. *Clin Toxicol* 1978;13:469–478.

39. Aguilar-Markulis NV, Beckley S, Priore R, et al. Auditory toxicity effects of long-term cis-dichloro-diammineplatinum II therapy in genitourinary cancer patients. *J Surg Oncol* 1981;16:111–123.

40. Reddel RR, Kefford RF, Grant JM, et al. Ototoxicity in patients receiving cisplatin: importance of dose and method of drug administration. *Cancer Treat Rep* 1982;66:19–23.

41. Moroso MJ, Blair RL. A review of cis-platinum ototoxicity. *J Otolaryngol* 1983;12:365–369.

42. McHaney VA, Thibadoux G, Hayes FA, et al. Hearing loss in children receiving cisplatin chemotherapy. *J Pediatr* 1983;102(2): 314–317.

43. Brown RL, Nuss RC, Patterson R, et al. Audiometric monitoring of cis-platinum ototoxicity. *Gynecol Oncol* 1983;16:254–262.

44. Vermorken JB, Kapteijn TS, Hart AA, et al. Ototoxicity of cis-diamminedichloroplatinum (II): influence of dose, schedule and mode of administration. *Eur J Cancer Clin Oncol* 1983;19:53–58.

45. Ilveskoski I, Saarinen UM, Wiklund T, et al. Ototoxicity in children with malignant brain tumors treated with the "8 in 1" chemotherapy protocol. *Med Pediatr Oncol* 1996;27:26–31.

46. Simon T, Hero B, Dupuis W, et al. The incidence of hearing impairment after successful treatment of neuroblastoma. *Klin Padiatr* 2002;214:149–152.

47. Punnett A, Bliss B, Dupuis LL, et al. Ototoxicity following pediatric hematopoietic stem cell transplantation: a prospective cohort study. *Pediatr Blood Cancer* 2004;42(7):598–603.

48. Knight KR, Kraemer DF, Neuwelt EA. Ototoxicity in children receiving platinum chemotherapy: underestimating a commonly occurring toxicity that may influence academic and social development. *J Clin Oncol* 2005;23(34):8588–8596.

49. Truong MT, Winzelberg J, Chang KW. Recovery from cisplatin-induced ototoxicity. *Int J Pediatr Otorhinolaryngol* 2007;71(10): 1631–1638.

50. Stengs CH, Klis SF, Huizing EH, et al. Cisplatin-induced ototoxicity; electrophysiological evidence of spontaneous recovery in the albino guinea pig. *Hear Res* 1997;111(1–2):103–113.

51. Laurell G, Jungnelius U. High-dose cisplatin treatment: hearing loss and plasma concentrations. *Laryngoscope* 1990;100(7): 724–734.

52. Zuur CL, Simis YJ, Lansdaal PE, et al. Audiometric patterns in ototoxicity of intra-arterial cisplatin chemoradiation in patients with locally advanced head and neck cancer. *Audiol Neurootol* 2006;11(5):318–330.

53. Bertolini P, Lassalle M, Mercier G, et al. Platinum compound-related ototoxicity in children: long-term follow-up reveals continuous worsening of hearing loss. *J Pediatr Hematol Oncol* 2004;26(10):649–655.

54. Kolinsky DC, Hayashi SS, Karzon R, et al. Late onset hearing loss: a significant complication of cancer survivors treated with cisplatin containing chemotherapy regimens. *J Pediatr Hematol Oncol* 2010;32(2):119–123.

55. Al-Khatib T, Cohen N, Carret AS, et al. Cisplatinum ototoxicity in children: long-term follow up. *Int J Pediatr Otorhinolaryngol* 2010;74(8):913–919.

56. Jehanne M, Lumbroso-Le Rouic L, Savignoni A, et al. Analysis of ototoxicity in young children receiving carboplatin in the context of conservative management of unilateral or bilateral retinoblastoma. *Pediatr Blood Cancer* 2009;52(5):637–643.

57. Schweitzer VG. Ototoxicity of chemotherapeutic agents. *Otolaryngol Clin North Am* 1993;26:759–789.

58. Schell MJ, McHaney VA, Green AA, et al. Hearing loss in children and young adults receiving cisplatin with or without prior cranial irradiation. *J Clin Oncol* 1989;7(6):754–760.

59. Loeffler JS, Kretschmar CS, Sallan SE, et al. Pre-radiation chemotherapy for infants and poor prognosis children with medulloblastoma. *Int J Radiat Oncol Biol Phys* 1988;15:177–181.

60. Blakley BW, Gupta AK, Myers SF, et al. Risk factors for ototoxicity due to cisplatin. *Arch Otolaryngol Head Neck Surg* 1994;120: 541–546.

61. Bokemeyer C, Berger CC, Hartmann JT, et al. Analysis of risk factors for cisplatin-induced ototoxicity in patients with testicular cancer. *Br J Cancer* 1998;77:1355–1362.

62. de Jongh FE, van Veen RN, Veltman SJ, et al. Weekly high-dose cisplatin is a feasible treatment option: analysis on prognostic factors for toxicity in 400 patients. *Br J Cancer* 2003;88: 1199–1206.

63. Anthoney D, McKean M, Roberts J, et al. Bleomycin, vincristine, cisplatin/bleomycin, etoposide, cisplatin chemotherapy: an alternating, dose intense regimen producing promising results in untreated patients with intermediate or poor prognosis malignant germ-cell tumours. *Br J Cancer* 2004;90:601–606.

64. Moss PE, Hickman S, Harrison BR. Ototoxicity associated with vinblastine. *Ann Pharmacother* 1999;33:423–425.

65. Gridelli C, Gallo C, Shepherd FA, et al. Gemcitabine plus vinorelbine compared with cisplatin plus vinorelbine or cisplatin plus gemcitabine for advanced non-small-cell lung cancer: a phase III trial of the Italian GEMVIN Investigators and the National Cancer Institute of Canada Clinical Trials Group. *J Clin Oncol* 2003;21:3025–3034.

66. Alberts DS. Clinical pharmacology of carboplatin. *Semin Oncol* 1990;17:6–8.

67. Macdonald MR, Harrison RV, Wake M, et al. Oto-toxicity of carboplatin: comparing animal and clinical models at the hospital for sick children. *J Otolaryngol* 1994;23:151–159.

68. Parsons SK, Neault MW, Lehmann LE, et al. Severe ototoxicity following carboplatin-containing conditioning regimen for autologous marrow transplantation for neuroblastoma. *Bone Marrow Transplant* 1998;22:669–674.

69. Huitema AD, Spaander M, Mathjt RA, et al. Relationship between exposure and toxicity in high-dose chemotherapy with cyclophosphamide, thiotepa and carboplatin. *Ann Oncol* 2002;13:374–384.

70. Kanat O, Evrensel T, Baran I, et al. Protective effect of amifostine against toxicity of paclitaxel and carboplatin in non-small cell lung cancer: a single center randomized study. *Med Oncol* 2003;20: 237–245.

71. Horiuchi M, Miyake H, Ota K. Ototoxicity of cis-diammine glycolatoplatinum, 254-S [in Japanese]. *Gan To Kagaku Ryoho* 1992;19:1327–1332.

72. Nishida Y, Satoh Y, Nishide K, et al. Phase I study of a combination chemotherapy of nedaplatin and cisplatin [in Japanese]. *Gan To Kagaku Ryoho* 1999;26:2209–2215.

73. Vermorken JB. The integration of paclitaxel and new platinum compounds in the treatment of advanced ovarian cancer. *Int J Gynecol Cancer* 2001;11(Suppl 1):21–30.

74. Hellberg V, Wallin I, Eriksson S, et al. Cisplatin and oxaliplatin toxicity: importance of cochlear kinetics as a determinant for ototoxicity. *J Natl Cancer Inst* 2009;101(1):37–47.

75. Geoerger B, Doz F, Gentet JC, et al. Phase I study of weekly oxaliplatin in relapsed or refractory pediatric solid malignancies. *J Clin Oncol* 2008;26(27):4394–4400.

76. Spunt SL, Freeman BB III, Billups CA, et al. Phase I clinical trial of oxaliplatin in children and adolescents with refractory solid tumors. *J Clin Oncol* 2007;25(16):2274–2280.

77. Fouladi M, Blaney SM, Poussaint TY, et al. Phase II study of oxaliplatin in children with recurrent or refractory medulloblastoma, supratentorial primitive neuroectodermal tumors, and atypical teratoid rhabdoid tumors: a pediatric brain tumor consortium study. *Cancer* 2006;107(9):2291–2297.

78. Pasetto LM, D'Andrea MR, Rossi E, et al. Oxaliplatin-related neurotoxicity: how and why? *Crit Rev Oncol Hematol* 2006;59(2): 159–168.

79. *Mosby's Drug Consult*, 16th ed. St. Louis, MO: Mosby, Inc., 2006.
80. Lugassy G, Shapira A. A prospective cohort study of the effect of vincristine on audition. *Anticancer Drugs* 1996;7:525–526.
81. Tibaldi C, Pazzagli I, Berrettini S, et al. A case of ototoxicity in a patient with metastatic carcinoma of the breast treated with paclitaxel and vinorelbine. *Eur J Cancer* 1997;34:1133.
82. Moss PE, Hickman S, Harrison BR. Ototoxicity associated with vinblastine. *Ann Pharmacother* 1999;33:423–425.
83. Latiff ZA, Kamal NA, Jahendran J, et al. Vincristine-induced vocal cord palsy: case report and review of the literature. *J Pediatr Hematol Oncol* 2010;32(5):407–410.
84. Rybak LP. Ototoxicity of loop diuretics. *Otolaryngol Clin North Am* 1993;26:829–844.
85. Henley CM, Rybak LP. Developmental ototoxicity. *Otolaryngol Clin North Am* 1993;26:857–871.
86. Koegel L Jr. Ototoxicity: a contemporary review of aminoglycosides, loop diuretics, acetylsalicylic acid, quinine, erythromycin and cisplatinum. *Am J Otol* 1985;6:190–199.
87. Arnold W, Nadol JB Jr, Geidauer H. Ultrastructural histopathology in a case of human ototoxicity due to loop diuretics. *Acta Otolaryngol* 1981;91:391–414.
88. Rybak LP. Pathophysiology of furosemide ototoxicity. *Otolaryngology* 1982;11:127–133.
89. Maher JF, Schreiner GE. Studies on ethacrynic acid in patients with refractory edema. *Ann Intern Med* 1965;62:15–29.
90. Schneider WJ, Becker L. Acute transient hearing loss after ethacrynic acid therapy. *Arch Intern Med* 1966;117:715–717.
91. Matz GJ, Nauton RF. Ototoxic drugs and poor renal function. *JAMA* 1968;206:2119.
92. Hanzelik E, Peppercorn M. Deafness after ethacrynic acid. *Lancet* 1969;1(7591):416.
93. Ng PS, Conley CE, Ing TS. Deafness after ethacrynic acid. *Lancet* 1969;1(7596):673–674.
94. Matz GJ, Beal DD, Krames L. Ototoxicity of ethacrynic acid. *Arch Otolaryngol* 1969;90:152–155.
95. Pillay VK, Schwartz FD, Aimi K, et al. Transient and permanent deafness following treatment with ethacrynic acid in renal failure. *Lancet* 1969;1(7585):77–79.
96. Kohonen A, Jauhiainen T, Tarkkanen J. Experimental deafness caused by ethacrynic acid. *Acta Otolaryngol* 1970;70:187–189.
97. Meriwether WD, Mangi RJ, Serpick AA. Deafness following standard intravenous dose of ethacrynic acid. *JAMA* 1971;216:795–798.
98. McCurdy JA Jr, McCormick JG, Harrill JA. Ototoxicity of ethacrynic acid in the anuric guinea pig. *Arch Otolaryngol* 1974;100:143–147.
99. Rybak LP. Ototoxicity of ethacrynic acid (a persistent clinical problem). *J Laryngol Otol* 1988;102:518–520.
100. Boston Collaborative Drug Surveillance Program. Drug induced deafness: a cooperative study. *JAMA* 1973;224:515–516.
101. Hiedland H, Wigand ME. The effect of furosemide at high doses on auditory sensitivity in patients with uremia. *Klin Wochenschr* 1970;48:1052–1056.
102. Bosher SK. Ethacrynic ototoxicity as a general model in cochlear pathology. *Adv Otorhinolaryngol* 1977;22:81–89.
103. Venkateswaran PS. Transient deafness from high doses of furosemide. *BMJ* 1971;3:113–114.
104. Quick CA, Hoppe W. Permanent deafness associated with furosemide administration. *Ann Otol Rhinol Laryngol* 1975;84:94–101.
105. Lloyd-Mostyn RM, Lord IJ. Ototoxicity of intravenous furosemide. *Lancet* 1971;2:1156.
106. Brown CG, Ogg CS, Cameron JS, et al. High dose furosemide in acute reversible intrinsic renal failure. *Scott Med J* 1974;19(Suppl 1):35–38.
107. Bourke E. Furosemide, bumetanide and ototoxicity. *Lancet* 1976;1:917–918.
108. Brown RD. Comparative acute cochlear toxicity of intravenous bumetanide and furosemide in the pure bred beagle. *J Clin Pharmacol* 1981;21(11–12 Pt 2):620–627.
109. Halstenson CE, Matzke GR. Bumetanide a new loop diuretic (Bumex, Roche Laboratories). *Drug Intell Clin Pharm* 1983;17:786–797.
110. McGuire JM, Bunch RL, Anderson RC, et al. "Ilo-tycin," a new antibiotic. *Antibiot Chemother* 1952;2:281–284.
111. Mintz U, Amir J, Pinkhas J, et al. Transient perceptive deafness due to erythromycin lactobionate. *JAMA* 1973;225:1122–1123.
112. Eckman MR, Johnson T, Riess R. Partial deafness after erythromycin [letter]. *N Engl J Med* 1975;292:649.
113. Karmody CS, Weinstein L. Reversible sensorineural hearing loss with intravenous erythromycin lactobionate. *Ann Otol Rhinol Laryngol* 1977;86(1 Pt 1):9–11.
114. Quinnan GV Jr, McCabe WR. Ototoxicity of erythromycin. *Lancet* 1978;1:1160–1161.
115. van Marion WF, van der Meer JW, Kalff MW, et al. Ototoxicity of erythromycin. *Lancet* 1978;2:214–215.
116. Lornoy W, Steyaert J. Ototoxicity of erythromycin lactobionate. *Acta Clin Belg* 1979;34:111.
117. Thompson P, Wood RP II, Bergstrom L. Erythromycin ototoxicity. *J Otolaryngol* 1980;9:60–62.
118. Swanson DJ, Sung RJ, Fine MJ, et al. Erythromycin ototoxicity: prospective assessment with serum concentrations and audiograms in a study of patients with pneumonia. *Am J Med* 1992;92:61–68.
119. Levin G, Behrenth E. Irreversible ototoxic effect of erythromycin. *Scand Audiol* 1986;15:41–42.
120. Dylewski J. Irreversible sensorineural hearing loss due to erythromycin. *Can Med Assoc J* 1988;139:230–231.
121. Mery JP, Kanfer A. Ototoxicity of erythromycin in patients with renal insufficiency. *N Engl J Med* 1979;301:944.
122. Taylor R, Schofield IS, Ramos JM, et al. Ototoxicity of erythromycin in peritoneal dialysis patients. *Lancet* 1981;2:935–936.
123. Kroboth PD, McNeil MA, Kreeger A, et al. Hearing loss and erythromycin pharmacokinetics in a patient receiving hemodialysis. *Arch Intern Med* 1983;143:1263–1265.
124. Kanfer A, Stamatakis G, Torlotin JC, et al. Changes in erythromycin pharmacokinetics induced by renal failure. *Clin Nephrol* 1987;27:147–150.
125. Umstead GS, Neumann KH. Erythromycin ototoxicity and acute psychotic reaction in cancer patients with hepatic dysfunction. *Arch Intern Med* 1986;146:897–899.
126. Vasquez EM, Maddux MS, Sanchez J, et al. Clinically significant hearing loss in renal allograft recipients treated with intravenous erythromycin. *Arch Intern Med* 1993;153:879–882.
127. Moral A, Navasa M, Rimola A, et al. Erythromycin ototoxicity in liver transplant patients. *Transpl Int* 1994;7:62–64.
128. Wallace MR, Miller LK, Nguyen MT, et al. Ototoxicity with azithromycin. *Lancet* 1994;343:241.
129. Tseng AL, Dolovich L, Salit IE. Azithromycin-related ototoxicity in patients infected with human immunodeficiency virus. *Clin Infect Dis* 1997;24:76–77.
130. Lo SH, Kotabe S, Mitsunaga L. Azithromycin-induced hearing loss. *Am J Health Syst Pharm* 1999;56:380–383.
131. Hugues FC, Laccourreye A, Lasserre MH, et al. Cochlear toxicity of erythromycin in elderly patients. *Therapie* 1984;39:591–594.
132. Brown BA, Griffith DE, Girard W, et al. Relationship of adverse events to serum drug levels in patients receiving high-dose azithromycin for mycobacterial lung disease. *Clin Infect Dis* 1997;24:958–964.
133. Bizjak ED, Haug MT III, Schilz RJ, et al. Intravenous azithromycin-induced ototoxicity. *Pharmacotherapy* 1999;19:245–248.
134. Ress BD, Gross EM. Irreversible sensorineural hearing loss as a result of azithromycin ototoxicity: a case report. *Ann Otol Rhinol Laryngol* 2000;109:435–437.
135. Mamikoglu B, Mamikoglu O. Irreversible sensorineural hearing loss as a result of azithromycin ototoxicity: a case report. *Ann Otol Rhinol Laryngol* 2001;110:102.
136. Kolkman W, Grooneveld JH, Baur HJ, et al. Ototoxicity induced by clarithromycin [in Dutch]. *Ned Tijdschr Geneeskd* 2002;146:1743–1745.
137. Fernandez-Martin J, Leport C, Morlat P, et al. Pyrimethamine-clarithromycin combination for therapy of acute Toxoplasma encephalitis in patients with AIDS. *Antimicrob Agents Chemother* 1991;35:2049–2052.
138. Dautzenberg B, Piperno D, Diot P, et al. Clarithromycin in the treatment of mycobacterium avium lung infections in patients without AIDS. *Chest* 1995;107:1035–1040.
139. Zhanel GG, Walters M, Noreddin A, et al. The ketolides: a critical review. *Drugs* 2002;62:1771–1804.

140. Brummett RE. Ototoxicity of vancomycin and analogues. *Otolaryngol Clin North Am* 1993;26(5):821–828.

141. Gendeh BS, Gibb AG, Aziz NS, et al. Vancomycin administration in continuous ambulatory peritoneal dialysis: the risk of ototoxicity. *Otolaryngol Head Neck Surg* 1998;118(4):551–558.

142. Cohen E, Dadashev A, Drucker M, et al. Once-daily versus twice-daily intravenous administration of vancomycin for infections in hospitalized patients. *J Antimicrob Chemother* 2002;49(1):155–160.

143. Forouzesh A, Moise PA, Sakoulas G. Vancomycin ototoxicity: a reevaluation in an era of increasing doses. *Antimicrob Agents Chemother* 2009;53(2):483–486.

144. Vella-Brincat JW, Begg EJ, Robertshawe BJ, et al. Are Gentamicin and/or Vancomycin associated with ototoxicity in the neonate? A retrospective audit. *Neonatology* 2011;100(2):186–193.

145. Scott PM, Griffiths MV. A clinical review of ototoxicology. *Clin Otolaryngol* 1994;19:3–8.

146. McCabe PA, Dey DL. The effect of aspirin upon auditory sensitivity. *Ann Otol Rhinol Laryngol* 1965;74:312–325.

147. Jung TT, Rhee CK, Lee CS, et al. Ototoxicity of salicylates, non-steroidal anti-inflammatory drugs and quinine. *Otolaryngol Clin North Am* 1993;26:791–810.

148. Mongan E, Kelly P, Nies K, et al. Tinnitus as an indication of therapeutic serum salicylate levels. *JAMA* 1973;226:142–145.

149. McFadden D, Plattsmier H, Pasanen E. Aspirin can potentiate the temporary hearing loss induced by intense sounds. *Hear Res* 1983;9:295–316.

150. Day RO, Graham GG, Beiri D, et al. Concentration-response relationships for salicylate-induced ototoxicity in normal volunteers. *Br J Clin Pharmacol* 1989;28:695–702.

151. Insel PA. Analgesic-antipyretics and anti-inflammatory agents; drugs employed in treatment of rheumatoid arthritis and gout. In: Gilman AG, Goodman LS, Rall TW, et al., eds. *Goodman and Gilman's the pharmacological basis of therapeutics.* 8th ed. New York: Pergamon Press, 1990:638–681.

152. Chapman P. Naproxen and sudden hearing loss. *J Laryngol Otol* 1982;96:163–166.

153. Koopmann CF Jr, Glattke TA, Caffrey JD. Effect of ibuprofen upon hearing in the guinea pig. *Otolaryngol Head Neck Surg* 1982;90:819–823.

154. Miller JJ, ed. Antimalarial drugs. In: *CRC handbook of ototoxicity.* Boca Raton, FL: CRC Press, 1985:9–15.

155. Jastreboff PJ, Brennan JF, Sasaki CT. Quinine induced tinnitus in rats. *Arch Otolaryngol Head Neck Surg* 1991;117:1162–1166.

156. Zajtchuk JT, Mihail R, Jewell JS, et al. Electronystagmographic findings in long term low-dose quinine ingestion. *Arch Otolaryngol* 1984;110:788–791.

157. Kanno H, Yamanobe S, Rybak LP. The ototoxicity of deferoxamine mesylate. *Am J Otolaryngol* 1995;16:148–152.

158. De Virgillis S, Argiolu F, Sanna G, et al. Auditory involvement in thalassemia major. *Acta Haematol* 1979;61:209–215.

159. Marsh MN, Holbrook IB, Clark C, et al. Tinnitus in a patient with beta-thalassaemia intermedia on long-term treatment with desferrioxamine. *Postgrad Med J* 1981;57:582–584.

160. Guerin A, London G, Marchais S, et al. Acute deafness and desferrioxamine. *Lancet* 1985;2(8445):39–40.

161. Orton RB, de Veber LL, Sulh HM. Ocular and auditory toxicity of long-term, high-dose subcutaneous deferoxamine therapy. *Can J Ophthalmol* 1985;20:153–156.

162. Cases A, Campistol JM, Sabater M, et al. Desferrioxamine-induced acute neurosensorial deafness. *Nephron* 1988;48:326.

163. Olivieri NF, Buncic JR, Chew E, et al. Visual and auditory neurotoxicity in patients receiving sub-cutaneous deferoxamine infusions. *N Engl J Med* 1986;314:869–873.

164. Albera R, Pia F, Morra B, et al. Hearing loss and desferrioxamine in homozygous beta-thallasaemia. *Audiology* 1988;27:207–214.

165. Masala W, Meloni F, Gallisai D, et al. Can deferoxamine be considered an ototoxic drug? *Scand Audiol Suppl* 1988;30:237–238.

166. Triantafyllou N, Fisfis M, Sideris G, et al. Neurophysiological and neuro-otological study of homozygous beta-thalassemia under long-term desferrioxamine (DFO) treatment. *Acta Neurol Scand* 1991;83:306–308.

167. Kontzoglou G, Koussi A, Tsatra J, et al. Sensorineural hearing loss in children with thalassemia major in northern greece. *Int J Pediatr Otorhinolaryngol* 1996;35:223–230.

168. Karimi M, Asadi-Pooya AA, Khademi B, et al. Evaluation of the incidence of sensorineural hearing loss in beta-thalassemia major patients under regular chelation therapy with desferrioxamine. *Acta Haematol* 2002;108:79–83.

169. Discalzi G, Fabbro D, Meliga F, et al. Effects of occupational exposure to mercury and lead on brainstem auditory evoked potentials. *Int J Psychophysiol* 1993;14:21–25.

170. Chang YC, Yeh CY, Wang JD. Subclinical neurotoxicity of mercury vapor revealed by a multi-modality evoked potential study of chloralkali workers. *Am J Ind Med* 1995;27:271–279.

171. Counter SA, Buchanan LH, Laurell G, et al. Blood mercury and auditory neuro-sensory responses in children and adults in Nambija gold mining area of ecuador. *Neurotoxicology* 1998;19:185–196.

172. Rice DC. Age related increase in auditory impairment in monkeys exposed in utero plus postnatally to methylmercury. *Toxicol Sci* 1998;44:191–196.

173. Chuu JJ, Hsu CJ, Lin-Shiau SY. Abnormal auditory brainstem responses for mice treated with mercurial compounds: involvement of excessive nitric oxide. *Toxicology* 2001;162(1):11–22.

174. Repko JD, Corum CR. Critical review and evaluation of the neurological and behavioral sequelae of inorganic lead absorption. *CRC Crit Rev Toxicol* 1979;6:135–187.

175. Otto D, Robinson G, Bauman S, et al. Five year follow-up study of children with low to moderate lead absorption: electrophysiological evaluation. *Environ Res* 1985;38:168–186.

176. Schwartz J, Otto D. Blood lead, hearing thresholds and neurobehavioral development in children and youth. *Arch Environ Health* 1987;42:153–160.

177. Discalzi GL, Capellaro F, Bottalo L, et al. Auditory brainstem evoked potential (BAEPs) in lead-exposed workers. *Neurotoxicology* 1992;13:207–209.

178. Yamamura K, Terayama K, Yamamoto N, et al. Effects of acute lead acetate exposure on adult guinea pigs: electrophysiological study of the inner ear. *Fundam Appl Toxicol* 1989;13:509–515.

179. Lasky RE, Maeier MM, Snodgrass EB, et al. The effects of lead on otoacoustic emissions and auditory evoked potentials in monkeys. *Neurotoxicol Teratol* 1995;17:633–644.

180. Roland PS, Ryback L, Hannley M, et al. Animal ototoxicity of topical antibiotics and the relevance to clinical treatment of human subjects. *Otolaryngol Head Neck Surg* 2004; 130(3 Suppl):S57–S78.

181. Mittelman H. Ototoxicity of "ototopical" antibiotics: past, present, and future. *Trans Am Acad Ophthalmol Otolaryngol* 1972;76:1432–1443.

182. Wright CG, Meyerhoff WL. Ototopical agents: efficacy or toxicity in humans. *Ann Otol Rhinol Laryngol* 1988;97(Suppl 131): 30–32.

183. Brummett RE, Morrison RB. The incidence of aminoglycoside antibiotic-induced hearing loss. *Arch Otolaryngol Head Neck Surg* 1990;116:406–410.

184. Roland PS. Clinical ototoxicity of topical antibiotic drops. *Otolaryngol Head Neck Surg* 1994;110:598–602.

185. Pickett BP, Shinn JB, Smith MFW. Ear drop ototoxicity: reality or myth? *Am J Otol* 1997;18:782–791.

186. Nomura Y. Otological significance of the round window. *Adv Otorhinolaryngol* 1984;33:1–162.

187. Schachern PA, Paparella MM, Duvall AJ. The normal chinchilla round window membrane. *Arch Otolaryngol* 1982;108:550–554.

188. Wright CG, Halama AR, Meyerhoff WL. Ototoxicity of an ototopical preparation in a primate. *Am J Otolaryngol* 1987;8: 56–60.

189. Sahni RS, Paparella MM, Schachern PA, et al. Thickness of the human round window membrane in different forms of otitis media. *Arch Otolaryngol Head Neck Surg* 1987;113:630–634.

190. Goycoolea MV, Munchow D, Schachern P. Experimental studies on round window structure: function and permeability. *Laryngoscope* 1988;98(6 Pt 2 Suppl 44):1–20.

191. Tommerup B, Moller K. A case of profound hearing impairment following the prolonged use of framycetin ear drops. *J Laryngol Otol* 1984;98:1135–1137.

192. Podoshin L, Fradis M, Ben David J. Ototoxicity of ear drops in patients suffering from chronic otitis media. *J Laryngol Otol* 1989;103:46–50.

193. Kaplan DM, Hehar SS, Bance ML, et al. Intentional ablation of vestibular function using commercially available topical gentamicin-betamethasone eardrops in patients with meniere's disease: further evidence for topical eardrop oto-toxicity. *Laryngoscope* 2002;112:689–695.

194. Matz G, Rybak L, Roland P, et al. Ototoxicity of ototopical antibiotic drops in humans. *Otolaryngol Head Neck Surg* 2004;130 (3 Suppl):S79–S82.

195. Roland PS, Stewart MG, Hannley M, et al. Consensus panel on the role of potentially ototoxic antibiotics for topical middle ear use: introduction, methodology and recommendations. *Otolaryngol Head Neck Surg* 2004;130(3 Suppl):S51–S56.

196. Matsumuru H. A case report of anaphylaxis caused by application of 0.5% chloromycetin otic solution. *Otologica Fukuoka* 1964;10:48.

197. Supiyaphum P, Kerekhanjanarong V, Koranasophonepun J, et al. Comparison of ofloxacin otic solution with oral amoxicillin plus chloramphenicol ear drops in the treatment of chronic suppurative otitis media with acute exacerbation. *J Med Assoc Thai* 2000;83:63–68.

198. Aursnes J. Vestibular damage from chlorhexidine in guinea pigs. *Acta Otolaryngol* 1981;92:89–100.

199. Aursnes J. Cochlear damage from chlorhexidine in guinea pigs. *Acta Otolaryngol* 1981;92:259–271.

200. Igarashi Y, Suzuki J. Cochlear ototoxicity of chlorhexidine gluconate in cats. *Arch Otorhinolaryngol* 1985;242:167–176.

201. Igarashi Y, Oka Y. Vestibular ototoxicity following intratympanic applications of chlorhexidine gluconate in the cat. *Arch Otorhinolaryngol* 1988;245:210–217.

202. Perez R, Freeman S, Sohmer H, et al. Vestibular and cochlear ototoxicity of topical antiseptics assessed by evoked potentials. *Laryngoscope* 2000;110:1522–1527.

203. Higashi K. Unique inheritance of streptomycin-induced deafness. *Clin Genet* 1989;35:433–436.

204. Prazic M, Salaj B, Subotic R. Familial sensitivity to streptomycin. *J Laryngol Otol* 1964;78:1037–1043.

205. Tsuiki T, Murai S. Familial incidence of streptomycin hearing loss and hereditary weakness of the cochlea. *Audiology* 1971;10:315–322.

206. Konigsmark BW, Gorlin RJ. *Genetic and metabolic deafness.* Philadelphia, PA: WB Saunders Co., 1976:364–365.

207. Hu D-N, Qiu W-Q, Wu B-T, et al. Genetic aspects of antibiotic induced deafness: mitochondrial inheritance. *J Med Genet* 1991;28:79–83.

208. Prezant TR, Agapian JV, Bohlman MC, et al. Mitochondrial ribosomal RNA mutation associated with both antibiotic-induced and non-syndromic deafness. *Nat Genet* 1993;4: 289–294.

209. Li M, Tzagaloff A, Underbrink-Lyon K, et al. Identification of the paromomycin-resistance mutation in the 15S rRNA gene of yeast mitochondria. *J Biol Chem* 1982;257:5921–5928.

210. Spangler EA, Blackburn EH. The nucleotide sequence of the 17S ribosomal RNA gene of Tetrahymena thermophila and the identification of point mutations resulting in resistance to the antibiotics paromomycin and hygromycin. *J Biol Chem* 1985;260:6334–6340.

211. Gravel M, Melancon P, Brakier-Gingras L. Cross-linking of streptomycin to the 16S ribosomal RNA of *Escherichia coli.* *Biochemistry* 1987;26:6227–6232.

212. Hutchin T, Haworth I, Higashi K, et al. A molecular basis for human hypersensitivity to aminoglycoside antibiotics. *Nucleic Acids Res* 1993;21:4174–4179.

213. Matthijs G, Claes S, Longo-Mbenza B, et al. Non-syndromic deafness associated with a mutation and a polymorphism in the mitochondrial 12S ribosomal RNA gene in a large Zairean pedigree. *Eur J Hum Genet* 1996;4:46–51.

214. Pandya A, Xia X, Radnaabazar J, et al. Mutation in the mitochondrial 12S rRNA gene in two families from Mongolia with matrilineal aminoglycoside ototoxicity. *J Med Genet* 1997;34:169–172.

215. El-Schahawi M, deMunain L, Sarrazin AM, et al. Two large Spanish pedigrees with non-syndromic sensorineural deafness and the mtDNA mutation at nt 1555 in the 12SrRNA gene: evidence of heteroplasmy. *Neurology* 1997;48:453–456.

216. Estivill X, Govea N, Barcelo A, et al. Familial progressive sensorineural deafness is mainly due to the mtDNA A1555G mutation and is enhanced by treatment with aminoglycosides. *Am J Hum Genet* 1998;62:27–35.

217. Casano RA, Bykhovskaya Y, Johnson DF, et al. Hearing loss due to the mitochondrial A1555G mutation in Italian families. *Am J Med Genet* 1998;79:388–391.

218. Shohat M, Fischel-Ghodsian N, Legum C, et al. Aminoglycoside induced deafness in an israeli jewish family with a mitochondrial ribosomal RNA gene mutation. *Am J Otolaryngol* 1999;20:64–67.

219. del Castillo FJ, Rodriguez-Ballesteros M, Martin Y, et al. Heteroplasmy for the 1555A>G mutation in the mitochondrial 12S rRNA gene in six spanish families with non-syndromic hearing loss: implications for genetic diagnosis and counseling. *J Med Genet* 2003;40:632–636.

220. Zhao H, Li R, Wang Q, et al. Maternally inherited aminoglycoside-induced and nonsyndromic deafness is associated with the novel C1494T mutation in the mitochondrial 12S rRNA gene in a large Chinese family. *Am J Hum Genet* 2004;74(1):139–152.

221. Fischel-Ghodsian N. Genetic factors in aminoglycoside ototoxicity. In: Roland PS, Rutka JA, eds. *Ototoxicity.* Hamilton, Canada: BD Decker Inc., 2004:144–152.

222. Fischel-Ghodsian N, Prezant TR, Chaltraw W, et al. Mitochondrial gene mutations: a common predisposing factor in aminoglycoside ototoxicity. *Am J Otolaryngol* 1997;18:173–178.

223. Bardien S, Human H, Harris T, et al. A rapid method for detection of five known mutations associated with aminoglycoside-induced deafness. *BMC Med Genet* 2009;10:2.

224. Guan MX. Mitochondrial 12S rRNA mutations associated with aminoglycoside ototoxicity. *Mitochondrion* 2011;11(2):237–245.

225. Chen G, Wang X, Fu S. Prevalence of A1555G mitochondrial mutation in Chinese newborns and the correlation with neonatal hearing screening. *Int J Pediatr Otorhinolaryngol* 2011;75(4):532–534.

226. Nivoloni Kde A, da Silva-Costa SM, Pomílio MC, et al. Newborn hearing screening and genetic testing in 8974 brazilian neonates. *Int J Pediatr Otorhinolaryngol* 2010;74(8):926–929.

227. Riedemann L, Lanvers C, Deuster D, et al. Megalin genetic polymorphisms and individual sensitivity to the ototoxic effect of cisplatin. *Pharmacogenomics J* 2008;8(1):23–28.

228. Peters U, Preisler-Adams S, Hebeisen A, et al. Glutathione S-transferase genetic polymorphisms and individual sensitivity to the ototoxic effect of cisplatin. *Anticancer Drugs* 2000;11(8):639–643.

229. Oldenburg J, Kraggerud SM, Cvancarova M, et al. Cisplatin-induced long-term hearing impairment is associated with specific glutathione s-transferase genotypes in testicular cancer survivors. *J Clin Oncol* 2007;25(6):708–714.

230. Lecomte T, Landi B, Beaune P, et al. Glutathione S-transferase P1 polymorphism (Ile105Val) predicts cumulative neuropathy in patients receiving oxaliplatin-based chemotherapy. *Clin Cancer Res* 2006;12(10):3050–3056.

231. Ross CJ, Katzov-Eckert H, Dubé MP, et al. Genetic variants in TPMT and COMT are associated with hearing loss in children receiving cisplatin chemotherapy. *Nat Genet* 2009;41(12): 1345–1349.

232. Laurell G, Bagger-Sjoback D. Dose-dependent inner ear changes after i.v. administration of cisplatin. *J Otolaryngol* 1991;20(3): 158–167.

233. Ryan AF, Woolf NK, Bone RC. Ultrastructural correlates of selective outer hair cell destruction following kanamycin intoxication in the chinchilla. *Hear Res* 1980;3(4):335–351.

234. Schaefer SD, Post JD, Close LG, et al. Ototoxicity of low- and moderate-dose cisplatin. *Cancer* 1985;56(8):1934–1939.

235. Liu W, Staecker H, Stupak H, et al. Caspase inhibitors prevent cisplatin-induced apoptosis of auditory sensory cells. *Neuroreport* 1998;9(11):2609–2614.

236. Cunningham LL, Cheng AG, Rubel EW. Caspase activation in hair cells of the mouse utricle exposed to neomycin. *J Neurosci* 2002;22(19):8532–8540.

237. Matsui JI, Ogilvie JM, Warchol ME. Inhibition of caspases prevents ototoxic and ongoing hair cell death. *J Neurosci* 2002;22(4): 1218–1227.

238. Cheng AG, Cunningham LL, Rubel EW. Hair cell death in the avian basilar papilla: characterization of the in vitro model and caspase activation. *J Assoc Res Otolaryngol* 2003;4(1):91–105.

239. Shimizu A, Takumida M, Anniko M, et al. Calpain and caspase inhibitors protect vestibular sensory cells from gentamicin ototoxicity. *Acta Otolaryngol* 2003;123(4):459–465.

240. Matsui JI, Haque A, Huss D, et al. Caspase inhibitors promote vestibular hair cell survival and function after aminoglycoside treatment in vivo. *J Neurosci* 2003;23(14):6111–6122.

241. Sergi B, Ferraresi A, Troiani D, et al. Cisplatin ototoxicity in the guinea pig: vestibular and cochlear damage. *Hear Res* 2003;182(1–2):56–64.

242. Laurell G, Ekborn A, Viberg A, et al. Effects of a single high dose of cisplatin on the melanocytes of the stria vascularis in the guinea pig. *Audiol Neurootol* 2007;12(3):170–178.

243. Davis CA, Nick HS, Agarwal A. Manganese superoxide dismutase attenuates cisplatin-induced renal injury: importance of superoxide. *J Am Soc Nephrol* 2001;12(12):2683–2690.

244. Park MS, De Leon M, Devarajan P. Cisplatin induces apoptosis in LLC-PK1 cells via activation of mitochondrial pathways. *J Am Soc Nephrol* 2002;13(4):858–865.

245. Bragado P, Armesilla A, Silva A, et al. Apoptosis by cisplatin requires p53 mediated p38alpha MAPK activation through ROS generation. *Apoptosis* 2007;12(9):1733–1742.

246. Garcia-Berrocal JR, Nevado J, Ramirez-Camacho R, et al. The anticancer drug cisplatin induces an intrinsic apoptotic pathway inside the inner ear. *Br J Pharmacol* 2007;152(7):1012–1020.

247. Clerici WJ, Hensley K, DiMartino DL, et al. Direct detection of ototoxicant-induced reactive oxygen species generation in cochlear explants. *Hear Res* 1996;98(1–2):116–124.

248. Kopke RD, Liu W, Gabaizadeh R, et al. Use of organotypic cultures of Corti's organ to study the protective effects of antioxidant molecules on cisplatin-induced damage of auditory hair cells. *Am J Otol* 1997;18(5):559–571.

249. Hirose K, Westrum LE, Stone JS, et al. Dynamic studies of ototoxicity in mature avian auditory epithelium. *Ann N Y Acad Sci* 1999;884:389–409.

250. Sha SH, Schacht J. Antioxidants attenuate gentamicin-induced free radical formation in vitro and ototoxicity in vivo: D-methionine is a potential protectant. *Hear Res* 2000;142(1–2):34–40.

251. Dehne N, Lautermann J, Petrat F, et al. Cisplatin ototoxicity: involvement of iron and enhanced formation of superoxide anion radicals. *Toxicol Appl Pharmacol* 2001;174(1):27–34.

252. Banfi B, Malgrange B, Knisz J, et al. NOX3, a superoxide-generating NADPH oxidase of the inner ear. *J Biol Chem* 2004;279(44):46065–46072.

253. Rybak LP, Husain K, Morris C, et al. Effect of protective agents against cisplatin ototoxicity. *Am J Otol* 2000;21(4):513–520.

254. Rybak LP, Whitworth CA, Mukherjea D, et al. Mechanisms of cisplatin-induced ototoxicity and prevention. *Hear Res* 2007;226(1–2):157–167.

255. Kelland L. The resurgence of platinum-based cancer chemotherapy. *Nat Rev Cancer* 2007;7(8):573–584.

256. Feghali JG, Liu W, Van De Water TR. L-n-acetyl-cysteine protection against cisplatin-induced auditory neuronal and hair cell toxicity. *Laryngoscope* 2001;111(7):1147–1155.

257. Choe WT, Chinosornvatana N, Chang KW. Prevention of cisplatin ototoxicity using transtympanic N-acetylcysteine and lactate. *Otol Neurotol* 2004;25(6):910–915.

258. Dickey DT, Wu YJ, Muldoon LL, et al. Protection against cisplatin-induced toxicities by N-acetylcysteine and sodium thiosulfate as assessed at the molecular, cellular, and in vivo levels. *J Pharmacol Exp Ther* 2005;314(3):1052–1058.

259. Church MW, Kaltenbach JA, Blakley BW, et al. The comparative effects of sodium thiosulfate, diethyldithiocarbamate, fosfomycin and WR-2721 on ameliorating cisplatin-induced ototoxicity. *Hear Res* 1995;86(1–2):195–203.

260. Kaltenbach JA, Church MW, Blakley BW, et al. Comparison of five agents in protecting the cochlea against the ototoxic effects of cisplatin in the hamster. *Otolaryngol Head Neck Surg* 1997;117(5):493–500.

261. Wang J, Lloyd Faulconbridge RV, Fetoni A, et al. Local application of sodium thiosulfate prevents cisplatin-induced hearing loss in the guinea pig. *Neuropharmacology* 2003;45(3):380–393.

262. Campbell KC, Rybak LP, Meech RP, et al. D-methionine provides excellent protection from cisplatin ototoxicity in the rat. *Hear Res* 1996;102(1–2):90–98.

263. Reser D, Rho M, Dewan D, et al. L- and D-methionine provide equivalent long term protection against CDDP-induced ototoxicity in vivo, with partial in vitro and in vivo retention of antineoplastic activity. *Neurotoxicology* 1999;20(5):731–748.

264. Rybak LP, Husain K, Whitworth C, et al. Dose dependent protection by lipoic acid against cisplatin-induced ototoxicity in rats: antioxidant defense system. *Toxicol Sci* 1999;47(2):195–202.

265. Rybak LP, Whitworth C, Somani S. Application of antioxidants and other agents to prevent cisplatin ototoxicity. *Laryngoscope* 1999;109(11):1740–1744.

266. Fetoni AR, Sergi B, Ferraresi A, et al. Protective effects of alpha-tocopherol and tiopronin against cisplatin-induced ototoxicity. *Acta Otolaryngol* 2004;124(4):421–426.

267. Kalkanis JG, Whitworth C, Rybak LP. Vitamin E reduces cisplatin ototoxicity. *Laryngoscope* 2004;114(3):538–542.

268. Li G, Sha SH, Zotova E, et al. Salicylate protects hearing and kidney function from cisplatin toxicity without compromising its oncolytic action. *Lab Invest* 2002;82(5):585–596.

269. Lynch ED, Gu R, Pierce C, Kil J. Reduction of acute cisplatin ototoxicity and nephrotoxicity in rats by oral administration of allopurinol and ebselen. *Hear Res* 2005;201(1–2):81–89.

270. Hussain AE, Blakley BW, Nicolas M, et al. Assessment of the protective effects of amifostine against cisplatin-induced toxicity. *J Otolaryngol* 2003;32(5):294–297.

271. Fisher MJ, Lange BJ, Needle MN, et al. Amifostine for children with medulloblastoma treated with cisplatin-based chemotherapy. *Pediatr Blood Cancer* 2004;43(7):780–784.

272. Gallegos-Castorena S, Martínez-Avalos A, Mohar-Betancourt A, et al. Toxicity prevention with amifostine in pediatric osteosarcoma patients treated with cisplatin and doxorubicin. *Pediatr Hematol Oncol* 2007;24(6):403–408.

273. Neuwelt EA, Brummett RE, Doolittle ND, et al. First evidence of otoprotection against carboplatin-induced hearing loss with a two-compartment system in patients with central nervous system malignancy using sodium thiosulfate. *J Pharmacol Exp Ther* 1998;286(1):77–84.

274. Doolittle ND, Muldoon LL, Brummett RE, et al. Delayed sodium thiosulfate as an otoprotectant against carboplatin-induced hearing loss in patients with malignant brain tumors. *Clin Cancer Res* 2001;7(3):493–500.

275. Neuwelt EA, Gilmer-Knight K, Lacy C, et al. Toxicity profile of delayed high dose sodium thiosulfate in children treated with carboplatin in conjunction with blood-brain-barrier disruption. *Pediatr Blood Cancer* 2006;47(2):174–182.

276. Zuur CL, Simis YJ, Lansdaal PE, et al. Ototoxicity in a randomized phase III trial of intra-arterial compared with intravenous cisplatin chemoradiation in patients with locally advanced head and neck cancer. *J Clin Oncol* 2007;25(24):3759–3765.

277. Dai CF, Steyger PS. A systemic gentamicin pathway across the stria vascularis. *Hear Res* 2008;235(1–2):114–124.

278. Hashino E, Shero M. Endocytosis of aminoglycoside antibiotics in sensory hair cells. *Brain Res* 1995;704(1):135–140.

279. Marcotti W, van Netten SM, Kros CJ. The aminoglycoside antibiotic dihydrostreptomycin rapidly enters mouse outer hair cells through the mechano-electrical transducer channels. *J Physiol* 2005;567(Pt 2):505–521.

280. Ishida S, Lee J, Thiele DJ, et al. Uptake of the anticancer drug cisplatin mediated by the copper transporter Ctr1 in yeast and mammals. *Proc Natl Acad Sci U S A* 2002;99(22):14298–14302.

281. Song IS, Savaraj N, Siddik ZH, et al. Role of human copper transporter Ctr1 in the transport of platinum-based antitumor agents in cisplatin-sensitive and cisplatin-resistant cells. *Mol Cancer Ther* 2004;3(12):1543–1549.

282. Holzer AK, Samimi G, Katano K, et al. The copper influx transporter human copper transport protein 1 regulates the uptake of cisplatin in human ovarian carcinoma cells. *Mol Pharmacol* 2004;66(4):817–823.

283. Sinani D, Adle DJ, Kim H, et al. Distinct mechanisms for Ctr1-mediated copper and cisplatin transport. *J Biol Chem* 2007;282(37):26775–26785.

284. Katano K, Kondo A, Safaei R, et al. Acquisition of resistance to cisplatin is accompanied by changes in the cellular pharmacology of copper. *Cancer Res* 2002;62(22):6559–6565.

285. Zisowsky J, Koegel S, Leyers S, et al. Relevance of drug uptake and efflux for cisplatin sensitivity of tumor cells. *Biochem Pharmacol* 2007;73(2):298–307.

286. Daniel KG, Harbach RH, Guida WC, et al. Copper storage diseases: Menkes, Wilsons, and cancer. *Front Biosci* 2004;9:2652–2662.

287. Safaei R, Larson BJ, Cheng TC, et al. Abnormal lysosomal trafficking and enhanced exosomal export of cisplatin in drug-resistant human ovarian carcinoma cells. *Mol Cancer Ther* 2005;4(10):1595–1604.

288. Katano K, Safaei R, Samimi G, et al. Confocal microscopic analysis of the interaction between cisplatin and the copper transporter ATP7B in human ovarian carcinoma cells. *Clin Cancer Res* 2004;10(13):4578–4588.

289. Ciarimboli G, Ludwig T, Lang D, et al. Cisplatin nephrotoxicity is critically mediated via the human organic cation transporter 2. *Am J Pathol* 2005;167(6):1477–1484.

290. Filipski KK, Mathijssen RH, Mikkelsen TS, et al. Contribution of organic cation transporter 2 (OCT2) to cisplatin-induced nephrotoxicity. *Clin Pharmacol Ther* 2009;86(4):396–402.

291. Ciarimboli G, Deuster D, Knief A, et al. Organic cation transporter 2 mediates cisplatin-induced oto- and nephrotoxicity and is a target for protective interventions. *Am J Pathol* 2010;176(3):1169–1180.

292. More SS, Akil O, Ianculescu AG, et al. Role of the copper transporter, CTR1, in platinum-induced ototoxicity. *J Neurosci* 2010;30(28):9500–9509.

293. Jonker JW, Wagenaar E, Van Eijl S, et al. Deficiency in the organic cation transporters 1 and 2 (Oct1/Oct2 [Slc22a1/Slc22a2]) in mice abolishes renal secretion of organic cations. *Mol Cell Biol* 2003;23(21):7902–7908.

294. Kuo YM, Gybina AA, Pyatskowit JW, et al. Copper transport protein (Ctr1) levels in mice are tissue specific and dependent on copper status. *J Nutr* 2006;136(1):21–26.

295. Choi BS, Zheng W. Copper transport to the brain by the blood-brain barrier and blood-CSF barrier. *Brain Res* 2009;1248:14–21.

296. Zhang S, Lovejoy KS, Shima JE, et al. Organic cation transporters are determinants of oxaliplatin cytotoxicity. *Cancer Res* 2006;66(17):8847–8857.

297. Thomas JP, Lautermann J, Liedert B, et al. High accumulation of platinum-DNA adducts in strial marginal cells of the cochlea is an early event in cisplatin but not carboplatin ototoxicity. *Mol Pharmacol* 2006;70(1):23–29.

298. Lambert MP, Shields C, Meadows AT. A retrospective review of hearing in children with retinoblastoma treated with carboplatin-based chemotherapy. *Pediatr Blood Cancer* 2008;50(2):223–226.

299. Durrant JD, Campbell K, Fausti S, et al. American academy of audiology position statement and clinical practice guidelines: ototoxicity monitoring. http://www.audiology.org/resources/documentlibrary/Pages/OtotoxicityMonitoring.aspx. Accessed October, 2009.

300. Wright CG, Schaefer SD. Inner ear histopathology in patients treated with cisplatin. *Laryngoscope* 1982;92:1408–1413.

301. Schuknecht HF. Disorders of intoxication. In: *Pathology of the ear*. Philadelphia, PA: Lea & Febiger, 1993:255–277.

302. Jacobson EJ, Downs MP, Fletcher JL. Clinical findings in high frequency thresholds during known ototoxic drug usage. *J Aud Res* 1969;9:379–385.

303. Fausti SA, Rappaport BZ, Schechter MA, et al. Detection of aminoglycoside ototoxicity by high frequency auditory evaluation: selected case studies. *Am J Otolaryngol* 1984;5:177–182.

304. Fausti SA, Schechter MA, Rappaport BZ, et al. Early detection of cisplatin ototoxicity: selected case reports. *Cancer* 1984;53:224–231.

305. Fausti SA, Henry JA, Shaffer HI. High-frequency audiometric monitoring for early detection of aminoglycoside ototoxicity. *J Infect Dis* 1992;165:1026–1032.

306. Tange RA, Dreschler WA, van der Hulst RJ. The importance of high-tone monitoring for ototoxicity. *Arch Otorhinolaryngol* 1985;242:77–81.

307. Dreschler WA, van der Hulst RJ, Tange RA, et al. The role of high frequency audiometry in early detection of ototoxicity. *Audiology* 1985;24:387–395.

308. Dreschler WA, van der Hulst RJ, Tange RA, et al. Role of high frequency audiometry in the early detection of ototoxicity, II: clinical aspects. *Audiology* 1989;28:211–220.

309. Frank T. High-frequency hearing thresholds in young adults using a commercially available audiometer. *Ear Hear* 1990;11:450–454.

310. Frank T. High frequency (8 to 16 kHz) reference thresholds and intrasubject threshold variability relative to ototoxicity criteria using a Sennheiser HAD 200 earphone. *Ear Hear* 2001;22:161–168.

311. Feghali JG, Bernstein RS. A new approach to serial monitoring of ultra-high frequency hearing. *Laryngoscope* 1991;101:825–829.

312. Frank T, Dreisbach LE. Repeatability of high frequency thresholds. *Ear Hear* 1991;12:294–295.

313. Campbell KCM, Kelly E, Targovnik N, et al. Audiologic monitoring for potential ototoxicity in a phase I clinical trial of a new glycopeptide antibiotic. *J Am Acad Audiol* 2003;14:157–169.

314. Fausti SA, Henry JA, Helt WJ, et al. An individualized, sensitive frequency range for early detection of ototoxicity. *Ear Hear* 1999;20:497–505.

315. Fausti SA, Helt WJ, Phillips DS, et al. Early detection of ototoxicity using 1/6th-octave steps. *J Am Acad Audiol* 2003;14:444–450.

316. Sakamoto M, Kaga K, Kamio T. Extended high-frequency ototoxicity induced by the first administration of cisplatin. *Otolaryngol Head Neck Surg* 2000;122(6):828–833.

317. Knight KR, Kraemer DF, Winter C, et al. Early changes in auditory function as a result of platinum chemotherapy: use of extended high-frequency audiometry and evoked distortion product otoacoustic emissions. *J Clin Oncol* 2007;25:1190–1195.

318. Valente M, Potts LG, Valente M, et al. High frequency thresholds: sound suite versus hospital room. *J Am Acad Audiol* 1992;3:287–294.

319. Gordon JS, Phillips DS, Helt WJ, et al. The evaluation of insert earphones for high-frequency bedside oto-toxicity monitoring. *J Rehabil Res Dev* 2005;42:353–362.

320. Fausti SA, Frey RH, Henry JA, et al. Early detection of ototoxicity using high frequency, toneburst evoked auditory brainstem responses. *J Am Acad Audiol* 1992;3:397–404.

321. Fausti SA, Flick CL, Bobal AM, et al. Comparison of ABR stimuli for the early detection of ototoxicity: conventional clicks compared with high frequency clicks and single frequency tonebursts. *J Am Acad Audiol* 2003;14:239–250.

322. Arnold DJ, Lonsbury-Martin BL, Martin GK. High-frequency hearing influences distortion product otoacoustic emissions. *Arch Otolaryngol Head Neck Surg* 1999;125:215–222.

323. Ress BD, Sridhar KS, Balkany TJ, et al. Effects of cis-platinum chemotherapy on otoacoustic emissions: the development of an objective screening protocol. *Otolaryngol Head Neck Surg* 1999;121:693–701.

324. Beck A, Maurer J, Welkoborsky HJ, et al. Changes in transitory evoked otoacoustic emissions in chemotherapy and with cisplatin and 5FU. *HNO* 1992;40:123–127.

325. Allen GC, Tiu C, Koike K, et al. Transient-evoked otoacoustic emissions in children after cisplatin chemotherapy. *Otolaryngol Head Neck Surg* 1998;118:584–588.

326. Konrad-Martin D, James KE, Gordon JS, et al. Evaluation of audiometric threshold shift criteria for ototoxicity monitoring. *J Am Acad Audiol* 2010;21(5):301–314.

327. Reavis KM, McMillan G, Austin D, et al. Distortion-product otoacoustic emission test performance for ototoxicity monitoring. *Ear Hear* 2011;32(1):61–74.

328. Chang KW, Vohr BR, Norton SJ, et al. External and middle ear status related to evoked otoacoustic emission in neonates. *Arch Otolaryngol Head Neck Surg* 1993;119(3):276–282.

329. Owens JJ, McCoy MJ, Lonsbury-Martin BL, et al. Otoacoustic emissions in children with normal ears, middle ear dysfunction, and ventilating tubes. *Am J Otol* 1993;14(1):34–40.

330. Gehr DD, Janssen T, Michaelis CE, et al. Middle ear and cochlear disorders result in different DPOAE growth behaviour: implications for the differentiation of sound conductive and cochlear hearing loss. *Hear Res* 2004;193(1–2):9–19.

331. Kei J, Brazel B, Crebbin K, et al. High frequency distortion product otoacoustic emissions in children with and without middle ear dysfunction. *Int J Pediatr Otorhinolaryngol* 2007;71(1):125–133.

332. Lonsbury-Martin BL, Martin GK. Evoked otoacoustic emissions as objective screeners for ototoxicity. *Semin Hear* 2001;22(4): 377–391.

333. Stavroulaki P, Apostolopoulos N, Segas J, et al. Evoked otoacoustic emissions-an approach for monitoring cisplatin induced ototoxicity in children. *Int J Pediatr Otorhinolaryngol* 2001;59(1): 47–57.

334. Leigh-Paffenroth E, Reavis KM, Gordon JS, et al. Objective measures of ototoxicity. *ASHA special interest division 6, hearing and hearing disorders: research and diagnostics.* 2005;9:10–16.

335. Dhooge I, Dhooge C, Geukens S, et al. Distortion product otoacoustic emissions: an objective technique for the screening of hearing loss in children treated with platin derivatives. *Int J Audiol* 2006;45:337–343.

336. Coradini P, Cigana L, Selistre SG, et al. Ototoxicity from cisplatin therapy in childhood cancer. *J Pediatr Hematol Oncol* 2007;29(6):355–360.

337. Reavis K, Phillips D, Fausti S. Factors affecting sensitivity of distortion-product otoacoustic emissions to ototoxic hearing loss. *Ear Hear* 2008;29:875–893.

338. Dille MF, McMillan GP, Reavis KM, et al. Ototoxicity risk assessment combining distortion product otoacoustic emissions with a cisplatin dose model. *J Acoust Soc Am* 2010;128(3):1163–1174.

339. American Speech-Language-Hearing Association. Guidelines for the audiologic management of individuals receiving cochleotoxic drug therapy. *ASHA* 1994;36(Suppl 12):11–19.

340. National Cancer Institute. Common terminology criteria for adverse events, version 3.0 and 4.0. http://ctep.cancer.gov/protocolDevelopment/electronic_applications/ctc.htm

341. Brock PR, Bellman SC, Yeomans EC, et al. Cisplatin ototoxicity in children: a practical grading system. *Med Pediatr Oncol* 1991;19:295–300.

342. Neuwelt EA, Brock P. Critical need for international consensus on ototoxicity assessment criteria. *J Clin Oncol* 2010;28(10): 1630–1642.

343. Chang KW. Clinically accurate assessment and grading of ototoxicity. *Laryngoscope* 2011;121(12):2649–2657.

159 Cerebellopontine Angle Tumors

Matthew L. Bush   *D. Bradley Welling*

INTRODUCTION

The cerebellopontine angle (CPA) is a complex and well-guarded anatomic region of the cranial base that contains an intricate interface of the central and peripheral nervous systems. Lesions occurring within this area are diverse in etiology and may lead to significant symptoms. The otolaryngologist frequently encounters pathology of the CPA that may present a diagnostic and therapeutic dilemma. A thorough knowledge of the anatomy of the region along with a clear understanding of diagnostic and therapeutic options for tumors in this region is vital for successful management. A variety of lesions may occur in this location and the differential diagnosis is discussed.

History

Tumors occurring within the CPA were identified as early as the late 1700s (1); however, little was known about the anatomy of this region and even less was known about the physiology of the nervous system. During the 1800s, Sir Charles Bell, a surgeon and skilled anatomist, carefully documented the intricate anatomy of the brainstem and cranial nerves, and he is credited with publication of the first clinical case of a CPA tumor in 1833 (2), which was identified as a vestibular schwannoma. The first successful removal of CPA vestibular schwannoma was performed by Sir Charles Ballance in 1894; however, surgical intervention for CPA tumors carried a mortality rate near 80% (3).

Significant advances in diagnostic evaluation of brain tumors occurred during the late 1800s and early 1900s, which allowed further correlation of clinical symptoms with specific lesions (4). Subsequently, the term cerebellopontine angle tumor was introduced in 1902 (5) to describe posterior fossa tumors. With the aid of radiographic imaging and astute clinical observation, Harvey Cushing carefully described the CPA syndrome in his 1917 monograph, *Tumors of the Nervus Acusticus and the Syndrome of the Cerebellopontine Angle* (6). Furthermore, Cushing advocated surgical intervention for CPA tumors to prevent brainstem compression and death via a suboccipital craniotomy approach to facilitate subtotal tumor removal. Mortality rates for surgical intervention dropped below 30%. Walter Dandy (7) advocated complete resection of CPA tumors through a modified suboccipital approach that improved exposure through resection of the lateral third of the cerebellum.

The latter half of the 20th century led to further advances in cranial base surgery including improved imaging modalities, high-speed surgical drills, and the microscope. The translabyrinthine approach to the CPA, although previously described (8,9), was popularized by William House, who reported improved facial nerve function, tumor exposure, and reduced morbidity and mortality. In an attempt to preserve hearing, House also advocated and demonstrated the utility of the middle fossa approach in small intracanalicular tumors (10,11). Although surgical approaches to the CPA have changed little over the past several decades, technologic advances in microsurgery, stereotactic radiation, diagnostic evaluation, and perioperative care have continued to reduce morbidity and mortality.

Anatomy

The CPA is a subarachnoid space filled with cerebrospinal fluid (CSF) and contains tortuous brainstem vessels and cranial nerves (Fig. 159.1). This inverted triangular-shaped space within the lateral posterior fossa is bound superiorly by the cerebellar tentorium and inferiorly by the cerebellar tonsil. The ipsilateral cerebellar hemisphere and the brainstem form the posterior and medial borders, respectively. The posterior face of the petrous temporal bone, with its dural reflection, forms the anterior border. The CPA cistern is the space between the pons, medulla oblongata, and the cerebellum medially and the temporal bone anteriorly. It contains blood vessels, cranial nerves, and the cerebellum flocculus and choroid plexus, which are surrounded by CSF. This cistern extends into the medial aspect of the internal auditory canal (IAC) of the petrous bone, which is known as the porus acusticus. Within the superior portion of the cistern, the trigeminal nerve travels from the lateral pons to the Meckel cave. The seventh and eighth cranial nerves exit the brainstem at the lateral pontomedullary junction adjacent to the foramen of Luschka and travel prominently within the CPA and then enter the porus acusticus. Inferiorly, the ninth, tenth, and eleventh cranial

nerves extend from the medulla across the inferior lateral aspect of the CPA and enter the pars nervosa of the jugular foramen. The basilar artery lies near the midline anterior to the brainstem and gives off the anterior inferior cerebellar artery (AICA), which takes a variable course through the CPA and can loop into the porus acusticus. Adjacent to the IAC, the AICA forms a branch, the labyrinthine artery, which travels laterally in the canal to supply the cochlea and labyrinth.

Within the cistern, the seventh and eighth cranial nerves lack an epineurium and are covered by pia mater and glial tissue. The facial nerve lies inferior and then anterior to

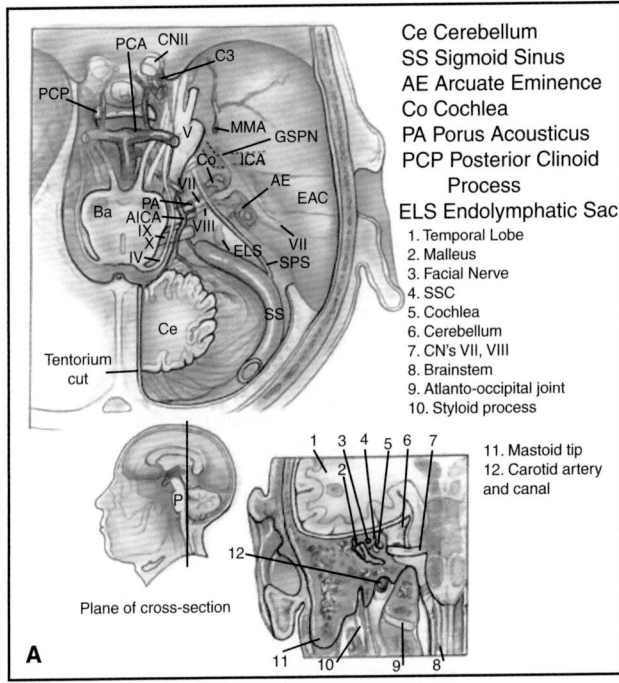

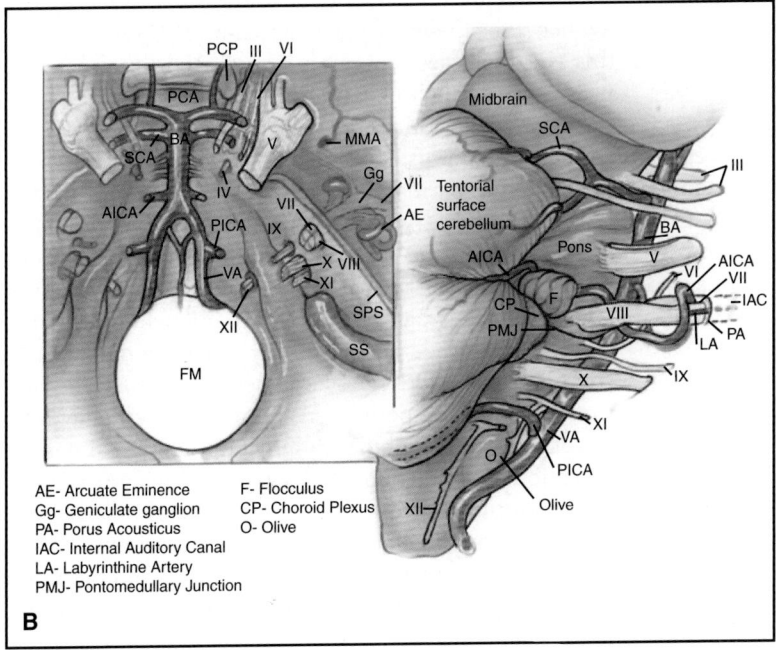

Figure 159.1 Axial and coronal **(A)** and sagittal views **(B)** through the skull at the level of the IACs and CPAs. V, trigeminal nerve; VII, facial nerve; VIII, cochleovestibular nerve; IAC, internal auditory canal. **(C)** Internal auditory canal contents.

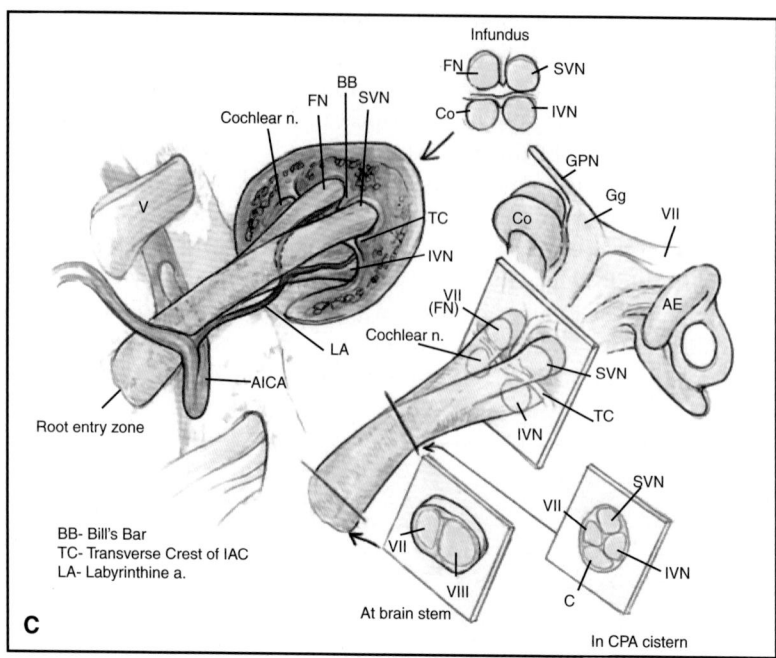

BB- Bill's Bar
TC- Transverse Crest of IAC
LA- Labyrinthine a.

Figure 159.1 *(Continued)*

the vestibulocochlear nerve complex within the cistern but rotates 90 degrees as it travels within the IAC (Fig. 159.1C). Within the canal the eighth nerve divides into its main branches, and the superior and inferior vestibular nerves fill the posterior half of the canal. The cochlear nerve resides within the anteroinferior quadrant of the canal, with the facial nerve occupying the quadrant immediately superior to the cochlear nerve and anterior to the superior vestibular nerve. The lateral aspect of the IAC, known as the fundus, possesses bony partitions of the seventh and eighth cranial nerves. The vertical crest, also known as the Bill bar, separates the facial nerve from the superior vestibular nerve, while the transverse crest separates these two superiorly located nerves from the cochlear nerve and inferior vestibular nerve.

EXTRAAXIAL LESIONS

The differential diagnosis of CPA lesions can be categorized in multiple ways based on site of origin, imaging characteristics, or histopathology. Bonneville et al. (12,13) outlined a differential diagnosis strategy for CPA tumors based on site of origin. Under this classification, lesions are categorized as extraaxial, intraaxial, or skull base in origin. Extraaxial lesions are distinct from the brain parenchyma, displace surrounding structures, and may be neural, dural, vascular, inflammatory, or infectious in nature.

Vestibular Schwannoma

Epidemiology

Vestibular schwannomas are encapsulated benign tumors that arise from the Schwann cells of the vestibular nerve. Historically, these tumors have been referred to as acoustic neuromas; however, vestibular schwannoma represents a more accurate name. Vestibular schwannomas account for approximately 6% of all intracranial tumors and 85% of all CPA tumors (14). The incidence rate is variable globally but has been increasing over the past few decades and is reported to be 1.9 tumors per 100,000 people per year (15).

Histopathology

Vestibular schwannomas may occur on either the superior or inferior nerve; however, they more commonly originate from the inferior vestibular nerve (16,17). A commonly held misconception is that tumors most often develop at the glial–Schwann cell junction known as the Obersteiner-Redlich zone. Xenellis and Linthicum (18) point out that this is a much less common site of origin than laterally near Scarpa ganglion. Tumors typically grow slowly by expanding the porus and extending into the CPA (19). Grossly, the tumors appear yellow to gray; however, larger or cystic tumors may vary in appearance due to hemorrhage or necrosis. Approximately 5% to 20% of vestibular schwannomas are cystic in nature and tend to have poorer outcomes for facial nerve preservation (20,21). Vestibular schwannomas typically slowly expand within the IAC where they invade the vestibular nerves and eventually compress the cochlear and facial nerves, as well as the labyrinthine artery. Without intervention, this eventually leads to cochlear and vestibular dysfunction. The facial nerve is exceptionally resilient to dysfunction, in spite of compression and thinning of the nerve; nevertheless, facial weakness can be present in large tumors. Extension into the CPA can lead to compression of the cerebellum and brainstem and can cause cranial neuropathy, hydrocephalus, and even death.

Histologic examination of vestibular schwannomas reveals two discrete cell arrangements. Regions of compact spindle cells with bland cytoplasm and lack of nuclear atypia along with whorls of palisading nuclei aligned in rows (Verocay bodies) are referred to as Antoni type A arrangement. Antoni type B, however, possesses a less dense and more loosely arranged cellular histology. Areas of necrosis and fibrosis may also be seen within these tumors. Due to the neural crest cell origin of Schwann cells, schwannoma cells display strong S100 immunohistochemical staining.

Molecular Biology

Vestibular schwannomas most commonly occur sporadically; however, they can also occur as part of the genetic syndrome, neurofibromatosis type 2 (NF2). This highly penetrant autosomal dominant disorder with variable expressivity presents with multiple nervous system tumors. Diagnostic criteria have been defined for NF2 (22). The presence of bilateral vestibular schwannomas establishes a diagnosis of NF2. However, NF2 patients may also develop multiple spinal and cranial nerve schwannomas, meningiomas, and ependymomas. NF2 is caused by a germ-line mutation within a tumor suppressor gene, known as *NF2*, located on chromosome 22q12. This gene, identified by both Trofatter (23) and Rouleau (24), was found to encode a cytoskeletal protein known as merlin or schwannomin that modulates cellular adhesion, proliferation, and motility (25). A variety of mutations have been identified within the NF2 gene, and disease severity appears to be at least somewhat related to the type of mutation present (26), although marked phenotypic variation can occurs within NF2 families.

The absence of merlin results in alterations in cellular signaling and promotes cellular proliferation and tumorigenesis. Merlin typically interacts with tyrosine kinase receptors, such as the ErbB receptor family (27–31), to prevent growth; therefore, these receptors have been identified as potential targets for inhibition of proliferation in merlin-deficient vestibular schwannoma cells (32–36). Merlin also prevents the pro-growth effects of the AKT/PI3 kinase signaling pathway, and AKT activation has been demonstrated in vestibular schwannomas and may be another potential target for vestibular schwannoma drug development (37,38). Vascular endothelial growth factor (VEGF) and associated receptors have been implicated in vestibular schwannoma tumorigenesis, and NF2 patients have undergone clinical trials to inhibit tumor growth with anti-VEGF medications (39–42). Although translational research has advanced our knowledge of the mechanisms of tumor growth and has provided potential treatment targets, effective medical treatments have not yet been clearly demonstrated.

Clinical Presentation

Vestibular schwannomas, when small or when they arise in the CPA rather than the confines of the IAC, may be asymptomatic. More are being diagnosed incidentally on imaging studies performed for separate indications. The majority of tumors, however, present with unilateral auditory or vestibular dysfunction. Approximately 75% of patients with vestibular schwannomas experience unilateral tinnitus as an early symptom (43). This may be severe enough to affect quality of life (44,45). Unilateral hearing loss develops in approximately 95% of vestibular schwannoma patients (46) and typically is progressive in nature (47–49). Only 5% of patients with vestibular schwannomas present with sudden sensorineural hearing loss; however, 20% to 30% of vestibular schwannoma patients may experience a sudden deterioration in their hearing during their clinical course (50,51). This asymmetric hearing loss may respond to steroid treatment; however, further evaluation is indicated to rule out retrocochlear pathology. Vestibular schwannomas gradually ablate the function of the ipsilateral vestibular system; thus patients may experience disequilibrium, although this is the presenting chief complaint in only 10% of patients (52). Tumor extension into the labyrinth may result in episodic vertigo, similar to Meniere disease. A family history of vestibular schwannomas or NF2 should be determined. A thorough neurotologic examination is warranted for any patient with suspected cranial base pathology and should include a microscopic otologic examination, evaluation of cranial nerve function, and cerebellar examination. Decreased sensation of the ear canal and conchal bowl is referred to as Hitselberger sign and is due to dysfunction of the sensory component of the facial nerve by an expanding vestibular schwannoma. Expansion of the tumor within the CPA may lead to brainstem compression and cranial nerve dysfunction and present with diplopia, facial hypesthesia, facial paralysis, dysphagia, hoarseness, hydrocephalus, and, potentially, death (45,52).

Diagnostic Evaluation

Audiologic Behavioral and Electrophysiologic Evaluation

Audiometric evaluation of hearing loss is fundamental to the evaluation of patients with vestibular schwannomas and includes, at a minimum, pure-tone audiometry and word discrimination evaluation. Patients with vestibular schwannomas typically present with unilateral sensorineural hearing loss with disproportionate asymmetric word recognition. Even when hearing loss is mild, vestibular schwannoma patients typically experience a significant degree of word recognition dysfunction. In order to report outcomes consistently, auditory function should be documented using the American Academy of Otolaryngology—Head and Neck Surgery classification (53). Acoustic reflex threshold and acoustic reflex decay have been used as a screening tool for retrocochlear pathology, but these tests are not commonly employed currently. Auditory brainstem response (ABR) may be useful for electrophysiologic assessment of auditory function. An interaural wave

V latency difference of greater than 0.2 ms, or prolonged interpeak latencies greater than 4.4 ms for I–V, 2.3 ms for I–III, or 2.1 ms for III–V raise the suspicion of a vestibular schwannoma. ABR usage is limited by the fact that a reliable waveform is absent in patients with moderately severe hearing loss. The sensitivity of ABR is greater than 90% in medium and large tumors; however, the sensitivity ranges between 60% and 80% in tumors less than 1 cm (54–56). The sensitivity of ABR has been increased to 95% with the use of a stacked ABR technique as reported by Don et al. (57).

Vestibular Assessment

Progression of vestibular schwannomas leads to eventual loss of ipsilateral vestibular function, which is most often accompanied by central compensation. Videonystagmography (VNG) may document the degree of central and peripheral vestibular dysfunction. Caloric testing is the most useful component of VNG testing in vestibular schwannoma patients, and it may identify a unilateral vestibular weakness in tumors that have affected or originate from the superior vestibular nerve. A small schwannoma of the inferior vestibular nerve may have a normal caloric response and VNG entirely. It has been suggested that VNG may add prognostic information by identifying the nerve of origin when a hearing preservation operation is considered.

Evaluation of the inferior vestibular nerve can be performed with vestibular evoked myogenic potential (VEMP) testing, which may further assist in determining the nerve of origin. A VEMP is elicited by stimulating the saccule through a high-intensity sound stimulus. Excitation through the vestibulospinal central tract leads to a biphasic reflex potential from the ipsilateral sternocleidomastoid muscle. Patients with inferior vestibular nerve tumor commonly have an absent or reduced VEMP response when the caloric testing may be normal (58,59); however, VEMP responses may be normal in the presence of an inferior vestibular nerve tumor. It is likely that the presence of a VEMP response is more closely related to the size and ensuing neural compression of a tumor within the IAC than by the nerve of origin (60).

Imaging Studies

Advancements in radiographic imaging modalities continue to improve the diagnosis of CPA tumors. Small tumors can be diagnosed with high sensitivity. Magnetic resonance imaging (MRI) is the gold standard in evaluation of patients with unilateral auditory and vestibular dysfunction. Noncontrasted T1-weighted images typically display vestibular schwannomas as hyperintense relative to CSF and iso- to hypointense to gray matter, while T2-weighted images show these tumors as hypointense to CSF and iso- to hyperintense to gray matter. These lesions typically have a component filling the IAC and may extend medially into the CPA having an "ice cream cone" or "mushroom"

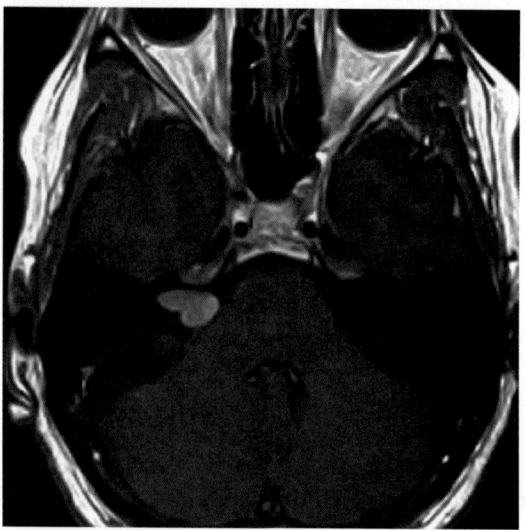

Figure 159.2 Axial T1-weighted contrast-enhanced MRI image at the level of the IAC demonstrating an enhancing right vestibular schwannoma with an "ice cream cone" or "mushroom" appearance.

appearance (Fig. 159.2). NF2 patients may develop large vestibular schwannomas that can compress the brainstem and cerebellum and lead to obstruction of the fourth ventricle (Fig. 159.3). Volumetric high-resolution T2 sequence can reveal the fluid-filled inner ear and tumor invasion into the labyrinth can be seen as a filling defect. T2 images can be useful in identifying hyperintense cystic regions within the tumor, while the solid portion of the tumor appears as a hypointense filling-defect within the CPA and/or the IAC. Additionally, the T2 images provide vital information regarding the lateral relationship of the tumor with the fundus of the IAC. CSF within the fundus of the IAC, adjacent and lateral to the tumor, is known as a "fundal cap," (Fig. 159.4) and its presence has been demonstrated to positively affect hearing preservation outcomes in middle fossa tumor resection (61).

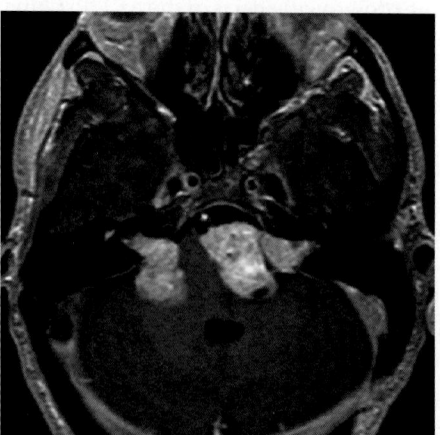

Figure 159.3 Axial T1-weighted contrast-enhanced MRI image at the level of the IAC demonstrating bilateral enhancing vestibular schwannomas with brainstem compression.

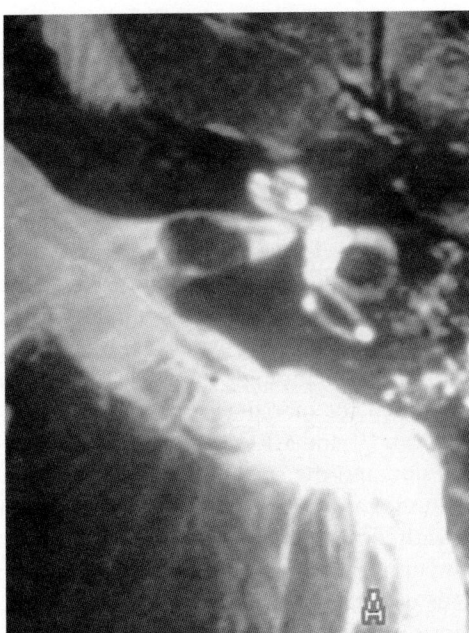

Figure 159.4 T2 fast spin-echo magnetic resonance image of a left intracanalicular vestibular schwannoma. Note the presence of CSF in the fundus lateral to the tumor.

The use of gadolinium-based contrast is standard in imaging of the CPA and the contrast-enhanced T1-weighted images of a vestibular schwannoma reveal marked tumor enhancement and can result in the detection of tumors as small as 1 to 2 mm. To reduce the expense of enhanced MRI some have advocated the use of noncontrast heavily T2-weighted fast spin echo (FSE) techniques. Comparisons of gadolinium-enhanced T1-weighted MRI with T2-weighted FSE sequences have demonstrated the reliability of T2 FSE sequences to detect mass lesions within the IAC and CPA and may be used as a screening tool for patients with sensorineural hearing loss or for those with contraindications to contrast administration (62,63).

Postimaging analysis and interpretation is vital in predicting outcomes and guiding clinical management. The standard documentation of tumor size is to record linear measurements in three dimensions; however, volumetric analysis of tumor size appears to be more sensitive in monitoring small changes of tumor growth over time (64). Prediction of hearing preservation following tumor resection has been shown to correlate with tumor volume (65).

Although MRI is the standard for diagnosis of vestibular schwannomas, patient movement causing motion artifact can limit the study resolution. Patients may not be able to tolerate the close confines of the MRI; however, mild sedatives or open MRI units may improve patient compliance. Due to the strong magnetic field, the presence of certain metallic foreign bodies or implants is a contraindication of MRI. The safety of MRI in patients with otologic or cochlear implants has been debated and concern has been raised for implant heating, malfunction, and/or displacement. Some

early stapes prostheses were made with ferromagnetic materials that would, potentially, be unsafe in an MRI. Currently, most stapes prostheses are considered safe for 1.5-Tesla magnet of MRI (66,67). NF2 patients face bilateral hearing loss and may undergo placement of cochlear or auditory brainstem implantation for rehabilitation; yet, they have a lifelong need for serial imaging. If implant magnets are removed, these patients can undergo MRI safely. Although not FDA approved, Crane et al. (68) suggest that cochlear implant patients can safely undergo MRI with the receiver magnet left in place, as long as the device is bound tightly by head wrapping prior to scanning in a low field strength magnet.

Computed tomography (CT) scanning is not ideal for CPA examination but may be used in patients who cannot undergo MRI. One-millimeter CT scanning in both the axial and coronal planes provides excellent detail of the temporal bone and IACs. Expanding vestibular schwannomas may lead to expansion of the IAC, which may be demonstrated on CT. The soft tissue resolution of CT scan, even with contrast administration, is inferior to MRI and tumors less than 1 cm can be missed on CT (69). Tumors that cause erosion of the otic capsule or large tumors that extend into the CPA and compress the brainstem are readily visible on CT. Historically, air-contrast was administered through a lumbar puncture to increase the sensitivity of CT to localize intracanalicular tumors.

Treatment Options

When considering treatment options for patients with vestibular schwannomas, the utmost priority is preservation of the patient's life, which is then followed in priority by preservation of brainstem and facial nerve function. Hearing preservation is an important objective; however, patients may be rehabilitated following the loss of hearing with contralateral routing of signals (CROS) type of hearing aids or bone-anchored devices.

Patients with vestibular schwannomas are faced with three primary treatment options: observation with serial imaging, stereotactic radiation, and microsurgical excision. Factors that affect treatment decision include patient preference, patient age/medical health, tumor size and location, auditory and vestibular function on the tumor and contralateral side, and tumor progression. The skill and experience of the treating team should also be considered. Because of the dearth of high-quality outcomes studies, patients must choose from these several options when deciding on how to manage their tumor.

Observation

Because vestibular schwannomas are most often slow-growing tumors, observation with serial imaging is recommended in 25% to 30% of our patients. At the time of diagnosis, the rate of tumor growth is unknown and somewhat unpredictable. Rates of tumor growth range widely in the literature, but meta-analyses indicate that at least 50% of vestibular schwannomas exhibit growth and growth ranges from 0.25 to 3.2 mm/y (70–72). In our patients, 66% demonstrated volumetric growth over an average follow-up of 3 years. Interestingly, NF2-associated vestibular schwannomas had an independent protective effect against deterioration of the pure tone average (73). NF2-associated vestibular schwannomas have been shown to exhibit a growth rate of 1.3 mm/y (74). Identification of predictors of tumor growth has been limited; however, patients that are younger, experience tinnitus initially, have large tumors at the time of presentation, have cystic tumors, or experience significant growth during the first year after diagnosis are more likely to have persistent tumor growth (75–77). If observation of the vestibular schwannoma is selected as the clinical path, the first follow-up MRI is recommended at 6 months and yearly thereafter if no growth is detected with volumetric measurements. Tumors may exhibit significant variability in growth and may experience precipitous increases in size with significant morbidity and even mortality (78,79); therefore, observation carries inherent risk.

Observation may allow enough time to determine the tumor growth characteristics, and if no growth is demonstrated, then no treatment may ever be necessary. If symptoms change or tumor growth is seen, then patients may undergo intervention when appropriate. If hearing is present at the time of tumor discovery, the most likely complication of observation is a decline in auditory function during the observation period. The opportunity for hearing-preservation approach may be lost. Observation is a reasonable option for patients who do not have significant brainstem compression or when the tumor affects an only-hearing ear. We are inclined to recommend observation when the patient is over 65 years of age, or if they are in poor medical health. Patients' preference certainly plays a role. In spite of the unpredictability of tumor and associated symptoms, observation may afford years of residual auditory function without the risk of radiation or surgery.

Stereotactic Radiation

Pioneered by the Swedish neurosurgeon, Lars Leksell, in the 1950s, stereotactic radiation therapy has become a vital tool in the management of a wide variety of intracranial pathology. Intracranial stereotactic radiation therapy involves the administration of radiation to a precise location so as to induce radiation damage to the target area and minimize the effect to the adjacent structures. Current modalities for radiation for vestibular schwannoma include single fraction gamma radiation therapy from an active cobalt-60 source (Gamma Knife), fractionated radiation, hypofractionated linear accelerator photon radiation therapy (XKnife, CyberKnife, Trilogy, Novalis, and SynergyS), and proton beam. The term "radiosurgery" is commonly employed to describe the precision of such radiation; however, it is a misnomer since it involves no surgery and the radiation is delivered to a closed intracranial lesion. Vestibular schwannomas are treated with a highly conformal prescribed dose of radiation under the direct supervision of a radiation treatment team, which typically consists of a surgeon (neurosurgeon or neurotologist), a radiation oncologist, and a physicist.

The goals of stereotactic radiation therapy are to provide the lowest effective dose of radiation that induces long-term tumor growth control without subjecting patients to the risk of surgical intervention and to prevent acute loss of neurologic function. The technique for stereotactic radiotherapy varies depending on the modality used. For gamma knife, patients undergo head frame placement with pretreatment MRI and/or CT imaging, which are then uploaded to the radiation dose–planning computer where the images can be examined for inaccuracies and appearance of the pathology. Both CT and MRI studies can be fused to accentuate the lesion and the surrounding structures. The margins of the tumor are outlined and then the treatment team proceeds with dose planning to contour the treatment dose to the tumor with a sharp radiation dose drop-off at the margins of the tumor (Fig. 159.5). Once all members of the team confirm the treatment plan and dose, patients are placed in the treatment suite and the head frame is immobilized on the table and advanced into the unit for treatment. The gamma knife dose used to treat vestibular schwannomas is, generally, between 12 and 13 Gray (Gy) to 50% isodose line at the periphery of the tumor to maximize tumor effect and minimize complications (80–82). The computer software calculates the time and exact positioning of the patient within the unit to achieve the treatment dose. Linear accelerators differ, in that patients do not require head frame placement or rigid fixation and they are fitted with a mask that provides immobilization. A series of real-time radiographic images are obtained during treatment to confirm correct positioning and to provide guidance during the treatment. CyberKnife treatment doses vary significantly but, typically, a total of 18 Gy is delivered over three fractions and has been reported to be safe and effective (83). Following stereotactic radiotherapy,

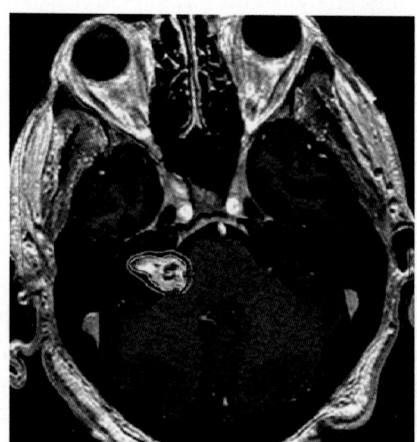

Figure 159.5 Axial T1-weighted contrast-enhanced MRI image at the level of the IAC demonstrating an enhancing right vestibular schwannoma with a conformal stereotaction radiation treatment dose plan outline.

the head frame is removed, patients are observed for a few hours and then they are discharged home. Serial MRI images are obtained over the patient's lifespan to monitor for persistent tumor growth.

Outcomes for tumor growth control and neurologic preservation vary greatly in the literature and lack uniform reporting (84). Additionally, many vestibular schwannomas do not grow over the course of time, which makes the assessment of the true efficacy of treatment difficult to determine. Nevertheless, patients who have had stereotactic radiotherapy have reported growth control rates of 90% to 100% (85–102) for gamma knife and 98% for CyberKnife (83). NF2 patients treated with gamma knife have reported actuarial tumor control rates of 71% to 85%, within declining rates with longer follow-up (103–105), while data on CyberKnife treatment of NF2 patients is limited, but has been reported to have over 90% tumor control rate in a small group of patients with short follow-up (less than 25 months) (106).

Stereotactic radiotherapy is an attractive option for many patients and has the benefit of no hospitalization and the rapid return to normal activity and work almost immediately after treatment. This treatment is indicated for those who have demonstrated tumor growth, are elderly, or have medical contraindications to microsurgery. Radiation lacks the microsurgical risks of infection and CSF leak. A wide variety of protocols have been reported that generally recommend treatment of tumors that measure less than 2.5 to 3 cm. Stereotactic radiation also is a valuable tool to treat tumor recurrence following microsurgery (107). Patients who have radiation treatment of their vestibular schwannoma rarely experience complete resolution to the mass; therefore, they are faced with a need for prolonged surveillance with repeat MRI during the course of their life.

Preservation of neurologic function is a primary goal of stereotactic radiotherapy; however, the development of adverse side effects is directly related to radiation dose. Complications of stereotactic radiotherapy are similar to microsurgical resection. Hearing loss may occur acutely following radiation, but, typically, hearing loss occurs gradually months to years later. Hearing preservation outcome reporting lacks uniformity (84); but is reported to range from 50% to 86% (108,109). This hearing loss has been linked to radiation of the cochlea and maintaining a cochlear dose less than 6.9 Gy is important in preserving residual hearing (110,111). The actuarial serviceable hearing preservation rates of NF2 patients has been reported at 73%, 59%, and 48% for 1, 2, and 5 years, respectively (105).

Facial and trigeminal cranial neuropathies due to radiation treatment are similar in incidence and are reported around 0% to 5% in sporadic vestibular schwannomas and 8% in NF2 patients; however, these rates increase with doses greater than 13 Gy (112,113). Hemifacial spasm may also occur in 2% to 4% and

may be related to a delayed insult to the facial nerve (114,115). Hydrocephalus without evidence of tumor growth may occur in up to 5% of patients and is more common in patients with larger tumors that are treated with radiotherapy and may be related to proteinaceous debris obstruction of CSF flow (116,117). Chronic vestibular dysfunction may be present in 13% to 26% of patients following stereotactic radiotherapy (114,118). Radiation has been reported to cause fibrosis of the facial nerve leading to poorer facial nerve outcomes if microsurgical resection is necessary following radiotherapy (119,120). Others, however, have reported no significant changes in facial nerve histology or functional outcomes (121). Malignant transformation and delayed oncogenesis, which is uniformly lethal, has been documented with stereotactic intracranial radiotherapy, and treatment with radiotherapy carries a 1:1,000 risk over a 5- to 30-year period (122–131).

Stereotactic radiotherapy remains a viable treatment option for patients with vestibular schwannoma. Irregularities in reporting outcomes have made it difficult to fully compare radiotherapy with microsurgical intervention. The long-term effect of radiation on tumor control and neurologic functions is not fully known and longitudinal follow-up will prove beneficial in informing patients and directing clinical management of vestibular schwannomas.

Microsurgery

Vestibular schwannomas have traditionally been treated with surgical management. Advances in microsurgical techniques and intraoperative anesthesia and monitoring have greatly reduced the morbidity and mortality in cranial base surgery. Collegial interaction and collaboration between neurosurgeons and neurotologist have greatly improved surgical management of these tumors and reduced complications. The primary surgical approaches—translabyrinthine, middle fossa, suboccipital (retrosigmoid), and combined—are described. Surgical intervention may involve complete resection, tumor debulking, or IAC decompression.

The surgical approach chosen to treat vestibular schwannomas is based on hearing function and tumor size and location. The surgery is performed under general anesthesia with neurophysiologic monitoring. In order to monitor the integrity of the facial nerve, long-acting paralytic should be avoided and facial EMG monitoring should be utilized during every procedure. Auditory function may be monitored with ABR or compound action potentials and may correlate with postoperative hearing preservation (132,133). Prophylactic doses of antibiotics along with one dose of intravenous dexamethasone are administered prior to incision. Generally, the goal for surgery is the complete resection of the tumor while preserving facial nerve and auditory function if present preoperatively. Hearing preservation can be accomplished through either the middle cranial fossa or suboccipital approaches. As a general guide, we base selection of a hearing preservation approach upon the speech discrimination being greater than 70% and the tumor being less than 1.5 cm in diameter. These criteria are not absolute and patients with poor contralateral hearing or NF2 patients may be candidates even with marginal hearing. The middle fossa approach involves a temporal craniotomy for an approach to the IAC superiorly. The approach can be chosen to remove tumors that are limited to the IAC and are less than 1.5 cm (Fig. 159.6); however, larger tumors that extend into the CPA can be accessed by ligating the superior petrosal sinus and dividing the tentorium. This approach has reported hearing preservation rates of 80% to 90% (134–136) and has the benefits of no intradural drilling and low postoperative headache rates.

The suboccipital approach, historically, has been the primary approach to the CPA and is still the approach favored by many neurosurgeons. A craniotomy is performed inferior to the transverse sinus and posterior to the sigmoid sinus and then the cerebellum retracted to gain access to the posterior fossa. Because this approach offers wide exposure of the CPA, tumors of almost any size can be resected through this approach; however, access to the lateral aspect of the IAC is limited and may be a location for recurrence of tumor. Hearing preservation is feasible with this approach as well, but compression of the brainstem may obscure the root entry zone and lateral extension into the IAC may also complicate attempts to preserve the cochlear nerve. In order to preserve hearing, this approach is, ideally, used for tumors that are confined to the medial IAC and the CPA without brainstem compression (Fig. 159.7).

At present, the translabyrinthine approach represents the most commonly used approach to vestibular schwannomas in the CPA because there is often significant

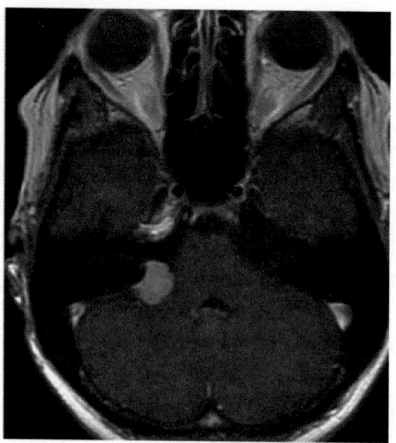

Figure 159.7 Axial T1-weighted contrast-enhanced MRI image at the level of the IAC demonstrating an enhancing lesion at the right CPA suitable for a suboccipital microsurgical resection.

hearing loss prior to tumor diagnosis, and because it gives superior exposure of the facial nerve and less retraction of the cerebellum (Fig. 159.8). This approach involves a wide mastoidectomy, labyrinthectomy, and removal of posterior fossa dura medial to the sigmoid sinus. Due to the labyrinthectomy, hearing preservation is not an option with this approach. The facial nerve is encountered early in the dissection and this approach offers visualization of, almost, the entire course of the facial nerve. The exposure of the CPA is wide and cerebellar retraction is not necessary, with the exception of exceedingly large tumors.

The combined approach typically involves a suboccipital and translabyrinthine craniotomy and is utilized to facilitate exposure and resection of CPA tumors that are greater than 4 cm (Fig. 159.9). Extension of tumor anteriorly to the petroclival region may also employ the addition of a transcochlear approach; however, the facial nerve

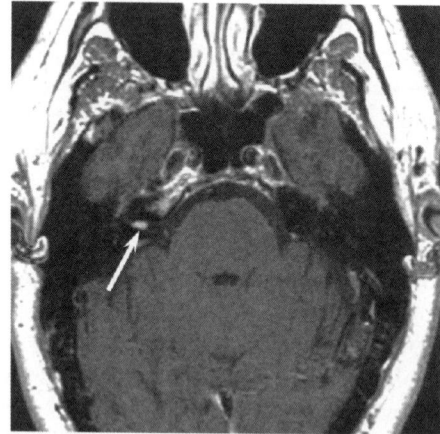

Figure 159.6 Axial T1-weighted contrast enhanced MRI image at the level of the IAC demonstrating a small enhancing intracanalicular right vestibular schwannoma (*arrow*) suitable for a middle cranial fossa microsurgical resection.

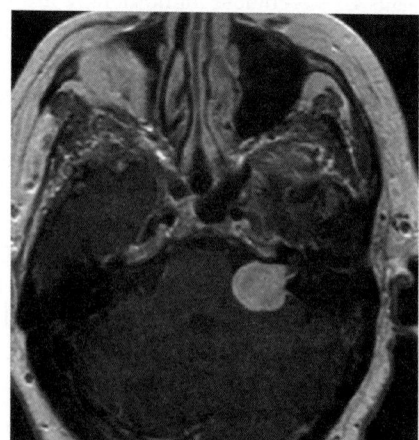

Figure 159.8 Axial T1-weighted contrast-enhanced MRI image at the level of the IAC demonstrating an enhancing left vestibular schwannoma suitable for either translabyrinthine or suboccipital microsurgical resection.

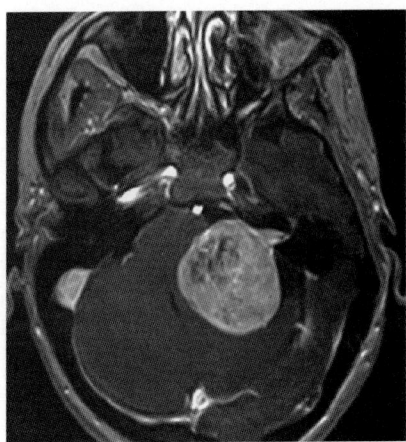

Figure 159.9 Axial T1-weighted contrast-enhanced MRI image at the level of the IAC demonstrating a large enhancing left vestibular schwannoma suitable for a combined microsurgical resection.

must be mobilized from the fallopian canal to facilitate this exposure. Hearing preservation is not feasible with combined approaches. The objective of this approach is for extensive debulking or complete resection of the tumor with decompression of the brainstem and the fourth ventricle.

Treatment planning for NF2 patients is a complex algorithm due to the complicated chronic nature of the disease. Since these patients are faced with the threat of deafness along with the loss of other special senses, preservation of hearing is vital and involves a proactive approach. Bilateral tumors also place the brainstem at greater risk of compression. Early detection and intervention may provide long-term functional hearing. Samii et al. (137) reported suboccipital resections in a series of NF2 patients and achieved total resection in 85%, preserved facial nerve anatomic integrity of 89%, and preserved useful hearing in 65% of patients. Slattery et al. (138) prefer the middle cranial fossa approach and reported 48% AAO-HNS class A hearing preservation and grade I/II facial nerve preservation in 81% of a series of pediatric patients. In NF2 patients with larger tumors, an auditory brainstem implant can be placed at the time of suboccipital or translabyrinthine tumor resection and may be utilized at a later time if the contralateral hearing declines. If the cochlear nerve can be preserved during translabyrinthine resection, cochlear implantation can be performed at the time of resection. Hearing rehabilitation is improved in patients with cochlear implants versus auditory brainstem implants, and cochlear implant patients possess higher open- and closed-set sentence understanding over time (139–141). In some NF2 cases in which hearing is declining and resection through a middle fossa approach in unlikely to preserve hearing; patients may be presented with the option of bony decompression of the IAC through a middle fossa approach. This approach does not involve any tumor

removal but alleviates the pressure of the tumor on the cochlear nerve in the IAC and allows the tumor growth to progress superiorly into the middle fossa. This may prolong functional hearing in patients that face a bleak prognosis. Early and aggressive intervention is crucial to preserved function in NF2 patients.

Middle Cranial Fossa Approach (Fig. 159.10)

As with all cranial base cases, the bed is rotated 180 degrees from the anesthesia team and facial nerve monitor electrodes are placed in the orbicularis oris and orbicularis oculi, and the integrity of the monitor is confirmed. The middle cranial fossa approach involves turning the patient's head toward the opposite the side of the lesion. The surgeon is classically seated at the head of the table with the assistant on the side of the lesion and the microscope base positioned at the opposite side of the lesion. Microscopes with a long suspension arm may be positioned behind the surgeon and brought over their head. Mannitol (0.5 to 1.0 g/kg) is given intravenously at the onset of the procedure and the CO_2 level is decreased to 25 to 28 mm Hg as the dura is approached to decrease intracranial pressure.

Following shaving, prepping, and sterile draping of the preauricular region, a skin incision is created extending 1 cm anterior to the tragus and then extending 12 cm superiorly toward the vertex of the scalp. The temporalis fascia and muscle are divided and the periosteum is widely elevated. The root of the zygoma is identified as a reference point and a craniotomy is centered on this point. A 4 cm by 4 cm craniotomy is outlined at this point and then carried out with an otologic drill or craniotome with footplate shoe. The craniotomy window extends 2 cm anterior and 2 cm posterior to the zygomatic root and the inferior rim of the craniotomy should be located immediately superior to the zygomatic root so that the floor of the middle fossa will be easily visualized. Once the bone flap is freed from the dura it is placed on the back table and will be replaced at the conclusion of the case. Exposed air cells of the mastoid or zygomatic roof are sealed with bone wax to prevent a postoperative CSF leak.

Under microscopic visualization, the temporal dura is gently elevated from the floor of the middle fossa, which is performed in a posterior to anterior direction to prevent avulsion of the greater superficial petrosal nerve. The geniculate ganglion can be dehiscent on the middle fossa floor and care should be taken not to incur trauma to this area. Anteriorly, care must be taken not to lacerate the middle meningeal artery. A meningeal venous plexus is commonly encountered anteriorly, which can cause significant bleeding, but is usually controlled with packing. The medial extent of dural elevation is the superior petrosal sinus. The arcuate eminence and greater petrosal nerve are identified. The greater petrosal nerve can be stimulated with the facial nerve stimulator probe with a 0.1 to 0.3 mA stimulus. The House-Urban middle fossa retractor is placed in position to gently retract the dura during the IAC

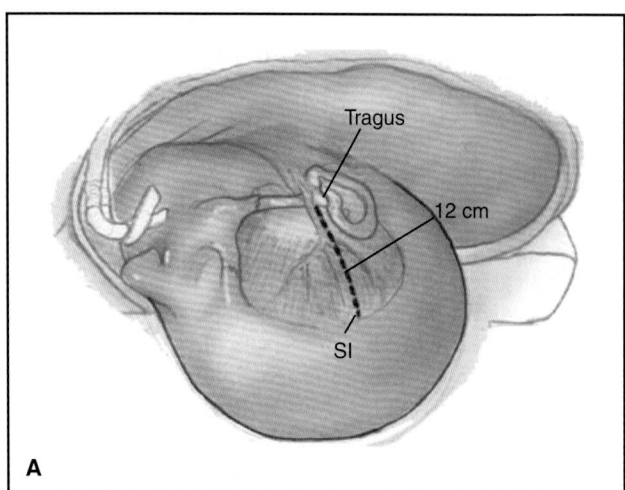

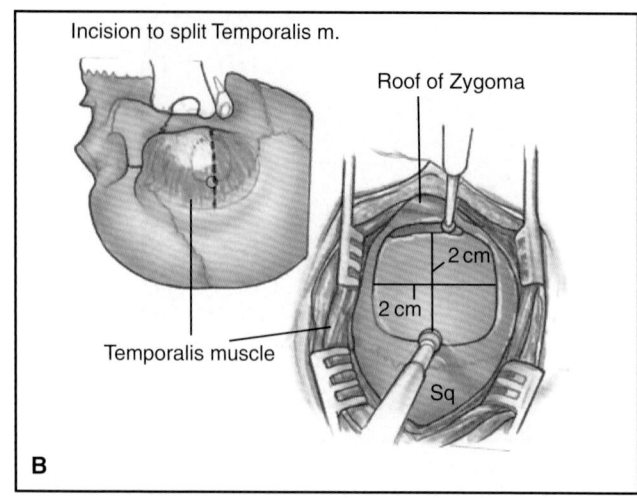

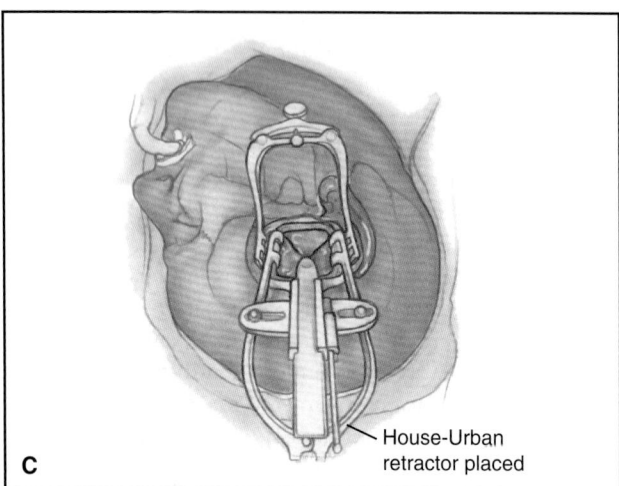

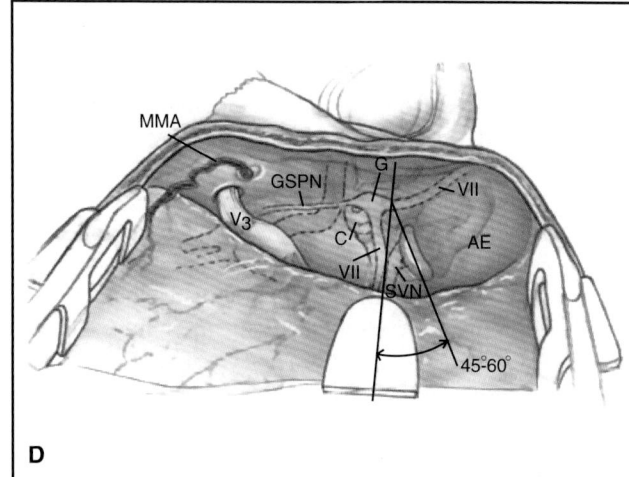

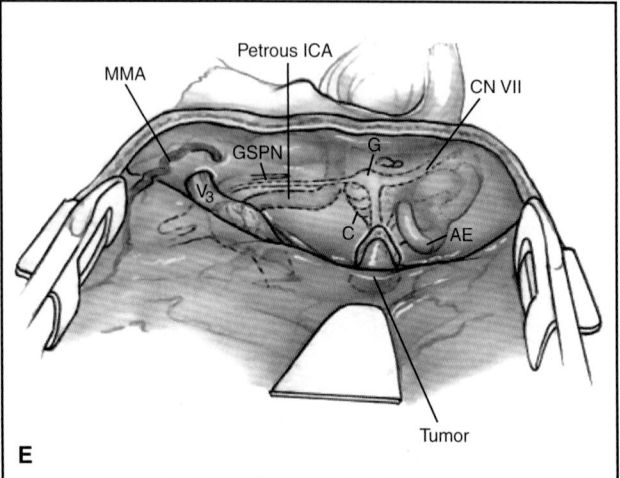

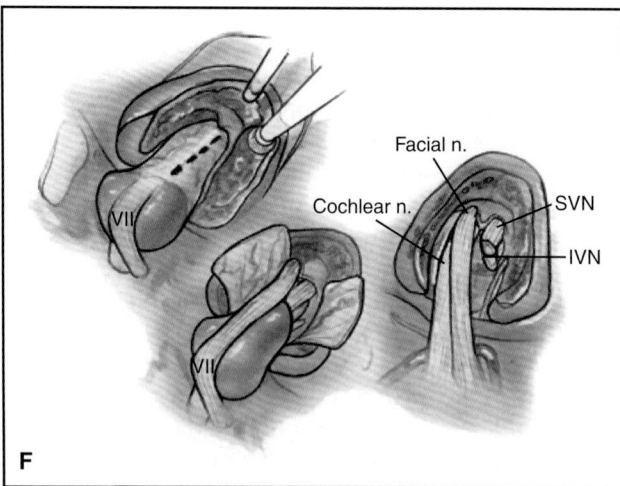

Figure 159.10 Middle fossa approach. **A** and **B:** A 12 cm incision is followed by a 4 x 4 cm crani-otomy. **C:** The retractor is positioned so that the structures of the temporal bone can be identified. With the greater superficial petrosal nerve and the arcuate eminence as guides, bone removal is be-gun and the IAC is identified. **D:** The dura then can be incised away from the facial nerve under high magnification. **E:** The internal auditory canal is identified. **F:** The dura is opened sharply avoiding the facial nerve. Fine hooks are used to separate the superior vestibular nerve from the facial nerve. The IAC is filled with fat. TL, temporal lobe; GSPN, greater superficial petrosal nerve; ICA, internal carotid artery; BB, the Bill bar; VII, facial nerve; SV, superior vestibular nerve; T, tumor; M, malleus; I, incus; SSC, superior semicircular canal; AE, arcuate eminence; G, geniculate ganglion; C, cochlea; MMA, middle meningeal artery. *(Continued on next page)*

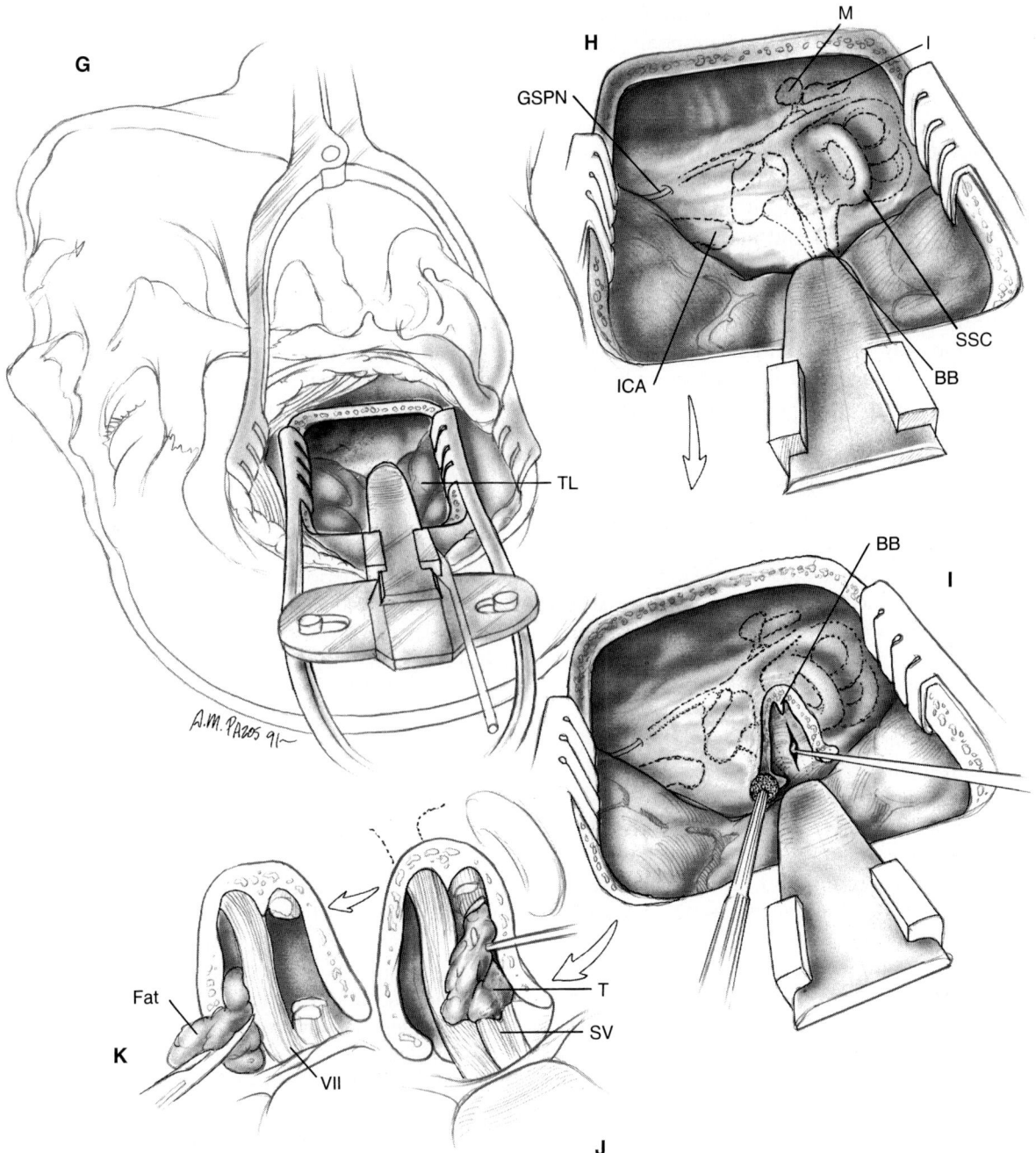

Figure 159.10 (*Continued*)

drilling and tumor resection. The location of the superior semicircular canal is confirmed by carefully thinning the bone of the arcuate eminence. The meatal plane is the approximate location of the IAC and is defined by the bisection of the angle between the superior semicircular canal and the greater superficial petrosal nerve. The bone surrounding the IAC is removed with small diamond burrs exposing approximately 180 degrees around the canal. The medial and lateral borders of dissection are the porus and vertical crest, respectively. Extreme care should be taken to avoid fenestration of the cochlea anteriorly and exposure of the labyrinthine section of the facial

nerve, which rises to form the geniculate ganglion near the middle fossa floor surface.

Once the dura is widely exposed, the posterior aspect of the dura is sharply incised and reflected anteriorly. The facial nerve is identified with the stimulator set on 0.05 mA. The facial nerve and the tumor are gently separated laterally and this plane of dissection is followed medially. The tumor is dissected from the cochlear nerve in a medial to lateral direction to prevent avulsion of the cochlear nerve from the fundus. Once this plane has been established and the tumor is free from the cochlear nerve, the superior vestibular nerve and the tumor can be avulsed from the fundus. The inferior vestibular nerve is often avulsed from the fundus as well and removed with the tumor. Once the intracanalicular tumor has been freed from the cochlear and facial nerve the medial border is identified. The medial normal vestibular nerve is sharply transected. Again, the integrity of the facial nerve is confirmed with a 0.05 mA stimulus and the IAC is occluded with a plug of temporalis muscle. Fat may also be used to occlude the IAC and may make distinguishing recurrent tumor easier on postoperative MRI. Once the retractor is removed, the dura and temporal lobe are allowed to resume their native position. The bone plate is replaced and may be fixed in position with titanium plates and screws. The wound is closed in multiple layers in watertight fashion, and a compression dressing is applied.

Suboccipital Approach (Fig. 159.11)

Positioning and setup for the suboccipital approach is similar to the other approaches, with the exception that the patient is placed in Mayfield pinions with the chin slightly tucked, the head turned laterally, and the neck slightly extended. Other options included the park bench position and the seated position. The seated position offers better visualization due to gravitational drainage of blood or fluid inferiorly; however, the risk of air embolism and lumbar disk rupture exists. Similar to the middle fossa approach, intracranial pressure is decreased with hyperventilation and intravenous mannitol.

A curvilinear incision is created approximately four fingerbreadths posterior to the postauricular crease. The incision carried down to and through the periosteum of the skull. The periosteum is widely elevated and cervical musculature attachments to the skull base are divided with electrocautery. A 4 cm by 4 cm craniotomy is then created posterior to the occipitomastoid grove, and the bone flap is placed on the back table to be replaced at the conclusion of the case. The superior and anterior borders of the craniotomy are the transverse and sigmoid sinuses, respectively. Inferiorly, bone removal can be extended to open the foramen magnum; however, care must be taken not to injure the vertebral artery as it emerges laterally from foramen transversarium.

A cruciate or "U"-shaped dural incision is performed and the dural edges are retracted with silk sutures. A nonadhesive protective collagen or gelatin sponge is placed on the lateral surface of the cerebellum to prevent desiccation. The cerebellum is gently retracted to allow egress of CSF. Placement of cottonoid strips inferiorly for 10 to 15 minutes may wick CSF effectively if elevated intracranial pressure prevents cerebellar manipulation.

Once the pressure decreases, gentle retraction of the cerebellum allows visualization of the CPA. Bands of arachnoid can be divided sharply to facilitate CPA exposure. A retractor is placed to allow full visualization of the posterior face of the tumor. The facial nerve monitor stimulating probe should be passed over the posterior face of the tumor to ensure that the facial nerve has not been displaced posteriorly. For large tumors, the posterior tumor capsule is cauterized and incised. The internal contents of the tumor are removed to facilitate circumferential extracapsular dissection. The capsule is dissected free from the cerebellum and brainstem, and the seventh and eighth nerves are identified at their root entry zone. Small tumors should be dissected away from the facial and cochlear nerves at this point.

Prior to removing the bone from the posterior IAC, cottonoid sponges or pledgets of Gelfoam are placed within the CPA to prevent bone dust dispersion. The dura overlying the posterior petrous bone is removed and small diamond burrs are utilized to the remove the posterior lip of the IAC. The posterior semicircular canal and vestibule in the otic capsule are the lateral extent of bone removal. Preoperative MRI imaging can aid in measuring the limits of lateral bony dissection. Once the dura of the IAC is exposed, it is then sharply incised. The superior and inferior vestibular nerves along with the tumor are identified and retracted inferiorly to expose the facial nerve, which is confirmed with the facial nerve stimulator. The tumor and vestibular nerves are gently avulsed from the fundus and dissected from the facial and cochlear nerves. The preferred direction of dissection is from medial to lateral to avoid avulsion of the cochlear nerve. Final tumor resection at the fundus may need to be completed in a medial to lateral fashion. The dissection around the porus continues from a lateral to medial direction until joining the dissection plane of the CPA. The medial vestibular nerves adjacent to the root entry zone are sharply divided and the tumor can be removed. A 30-degree endoscope can be used to examine the lateral IAC for any residual tumor. Special attention must be given to protect the labyrinthine artery in hearing preservation cases.

Following tumor removal, the wound is irrigated and the sponges are removed. The edges of craniotomy are inspected and air cells are sealed with bone wax. The dura is reapproximated and closed in a watertight fashion with silk suture. The bone plate is replaced and can be fixed in position with cranioplasty low-profile titanium plates and screws. The muscle and skin are closed in multiple layers in watertight fashion and a pressure dressing may be applied.

Translabyrinthine Approach (Fig. 159.12)

The translabyrinthine approach is performed with the patient in the supine position with the head turned away from the operative site. The surgical assistant is opposite the surgeon, and the microscope base is brought in at the head of the table. Once the facial nerve monitor is set up, the postauricular region is shaved, prepped, and draped in the usual fashion. Additionally, the abdominal left lower quadrant is prepared and draped for harvest of a free abdominal adipose graft for closure of the cranial base defect. The left is typically used so as to prevent confusion with an appendectomy scar.

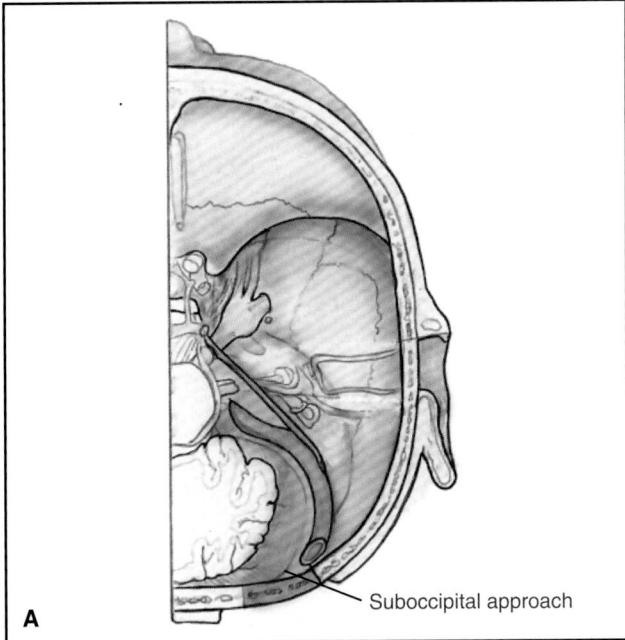

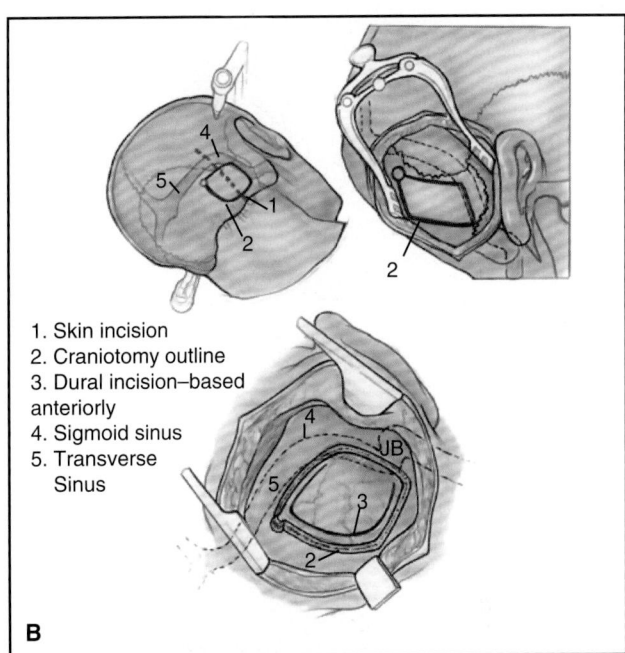

1. Skin incision
2. Craniotomy outline
3. Dural incision–based anteriorly
4. Sigmoid sinus
5. Transverse Sinus

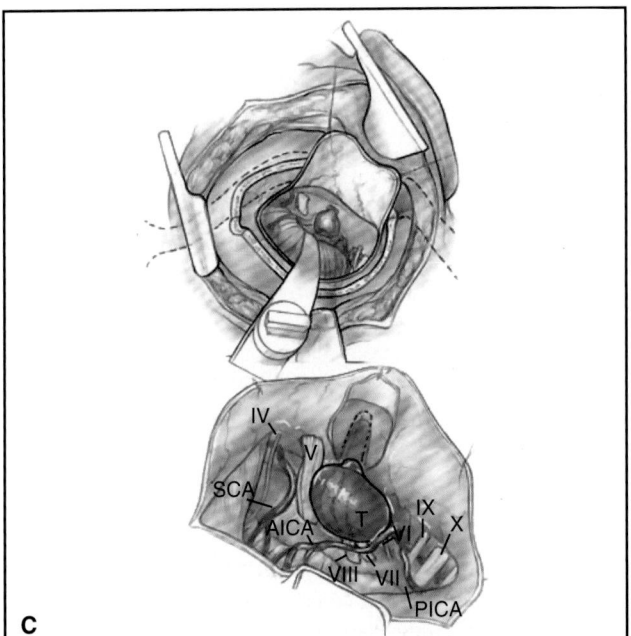

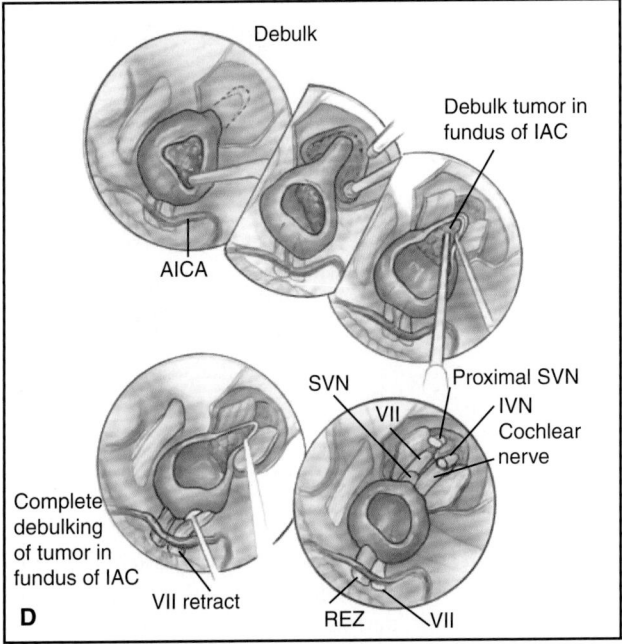

Figure 159.11 Retrosigmoid–suboccipital approach. **A:** The approach between the posterior temporal bone and cerebellum is outlined in blue. **B:** A 3 × 3-cm craniotomy is made with the cutting bur, the sigmoid sinus serving as the anterior limit and the transverse sinus as the superior limit. **C:** The cerebellum is retracted exposing the tumor and the internal auditory canal is drilled away after reflecting dura off the posterior temporal bone. **D:** The tumor is sequentially debulked and removed. SS, sigmoid sinus; TC, transverse crest; C, cochlear nerve; LA, labyrinthine artery; AICA, anterior inferior cerebellar artery; VII, facial nerve; IX, glossopharyngeal nerve; X, vagal nerve; XI, spinal accessory nerve; JB, jugular bulb; SCA, superior cerebellar artery; PICA, posterior inferior cerebellar artery; SVN, superior vestibular nerve; REZ, root entry zone. *(Continued on next page)*

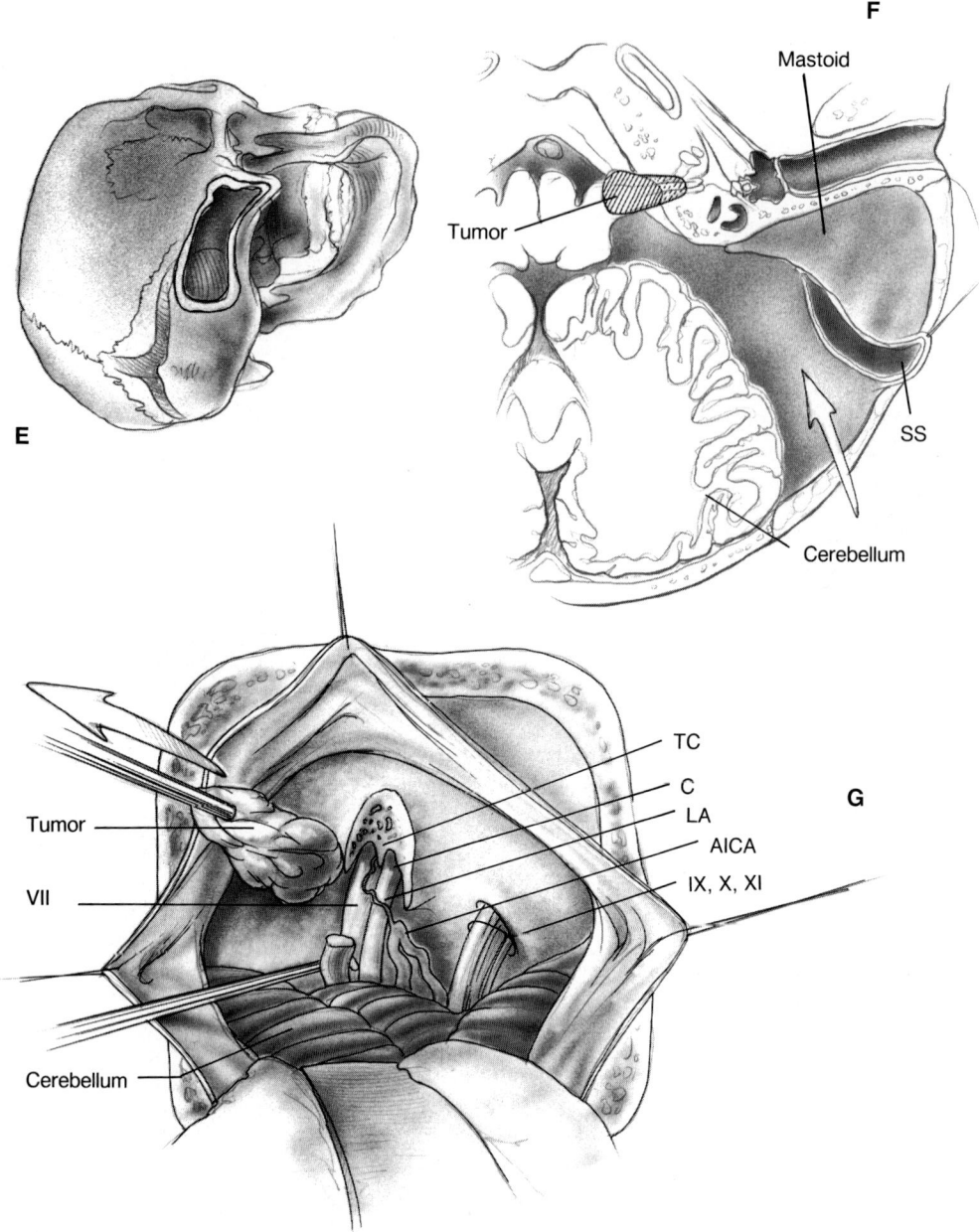

Figure 159.11 *(Continued)*

Approximately 2 to 4 cm from the postauricular crease, a C-shaped incision is performed. Dissection is performed through the dermis and the subcutaneous space is developed. Temporalis fascia and muscle are harvested and placed on the back table. A T-shaped incision is then performed through the musculoperiosteum at the linea temporalis and along the mastoid cortex. The periosteum is widely elevated to expose the mastoid. A complete mastoidectomy is carried out with wide exposure of the middle and posterior fossa dura and at least 1 cm extension posterior to the sigmoid sinus. The facial nerve is identified by removing the bone overlying the nerve at its second genu in the facial recess and the distal course of the vertical portion of the facial nerve is identified. The surgical buttress and facial recess air cells are removed and the incus is removed to facilitate visualization of the eustachian tube orifice. The dural bony plates overlying the middle and posterior fossa are removed along with the bone overlying the sigmoid sinus. Prior to opening the otic capsule, the patient's imaging studies and audiogram are checked again to confirm the correct patient and surgical site. The labyrinthectomy is performed at this point by widely opening the semicircular canals and then extending the bony dissection inferiorly through the retrofacial air cells. The jugular bulb, which is the inferior extent of the dissection, is defined and bony dissection continues through the petrous bone to

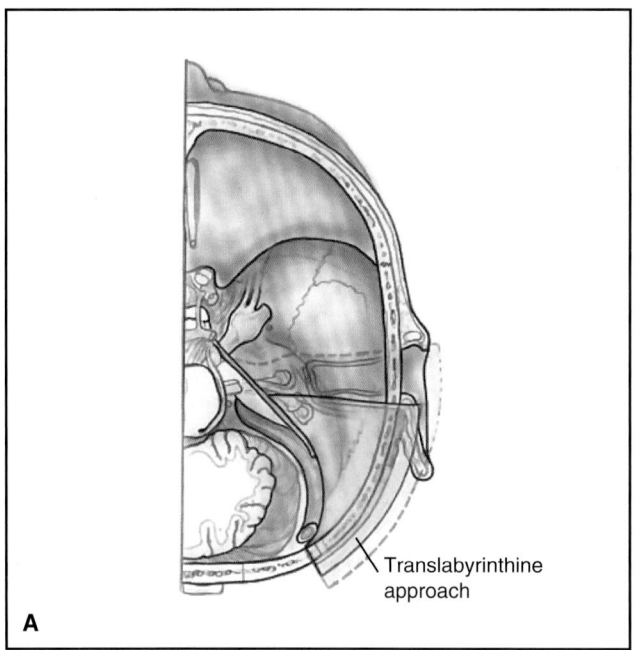

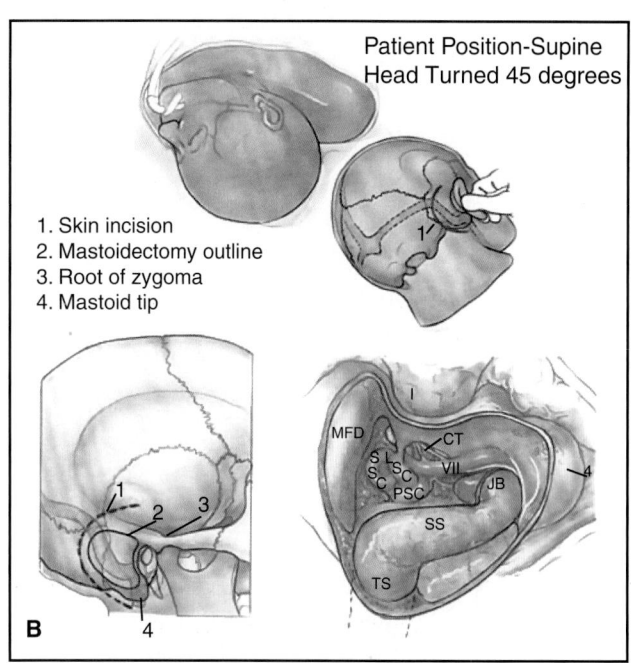

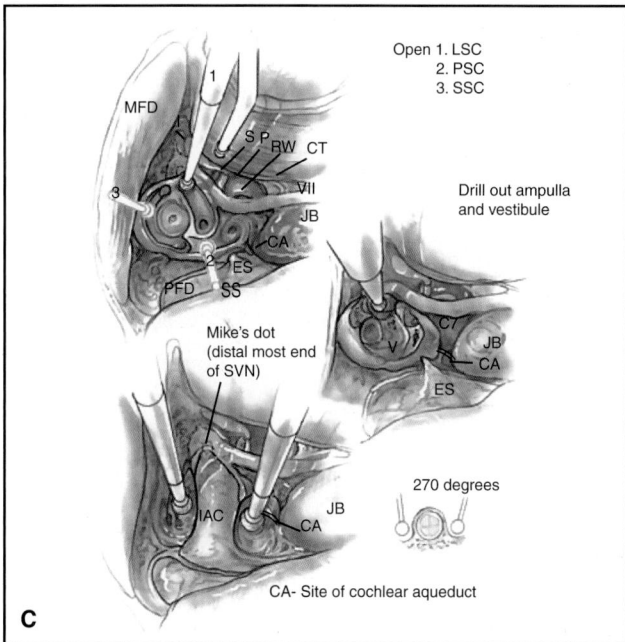

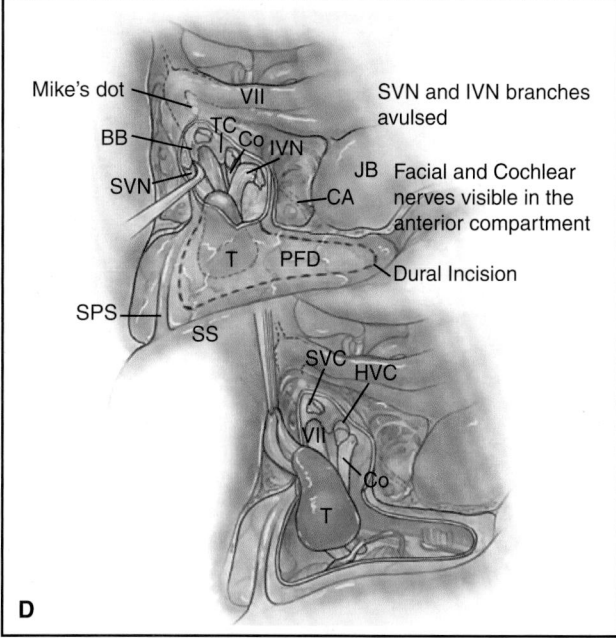

Figure 159.12 Translabyrinthine tumor removal. **A:** The tumor removal is accomplished between the posterior external auditory canal and internal auditory canal anteriorly and the sigmoid sinus posteriorly avoiding prolonged cerebellar retraction. **B:** Patient positioning and skin incision is shown with the complete mastoidectomy then carried out. **C:** Labyrinthectomy with identification of the internal auditory canal and skeletonization. **D:** Dural incision of the internal auditory canal and posterior fossa. CT, chorda tympani; MFD, middle fossa dura; SSC, superior semicircular canal; LSC, lateral semicircular canal; PSC, posterior semicircular canal; VII, facial nerve; TS, transverse sinus; SS, sigmoid sinus; JB, jugular bulb; PFD, posterior fossa dura; S, stapes; P, Promontory; RW, round window; ES, endolymphatic sac; CA, cochlear aqueduct; BB, Bill's bar; TC, transverse crest; Co, cochlear nerve; IVN, inferior vestibular nerve; T, tumor; SPS, superior petrosal sinus; SVN, superior vestibular nerve; SVC, cut superior vestibular nerve; IVC, cut inferior vestibular nerve. *(Continued on next page)*

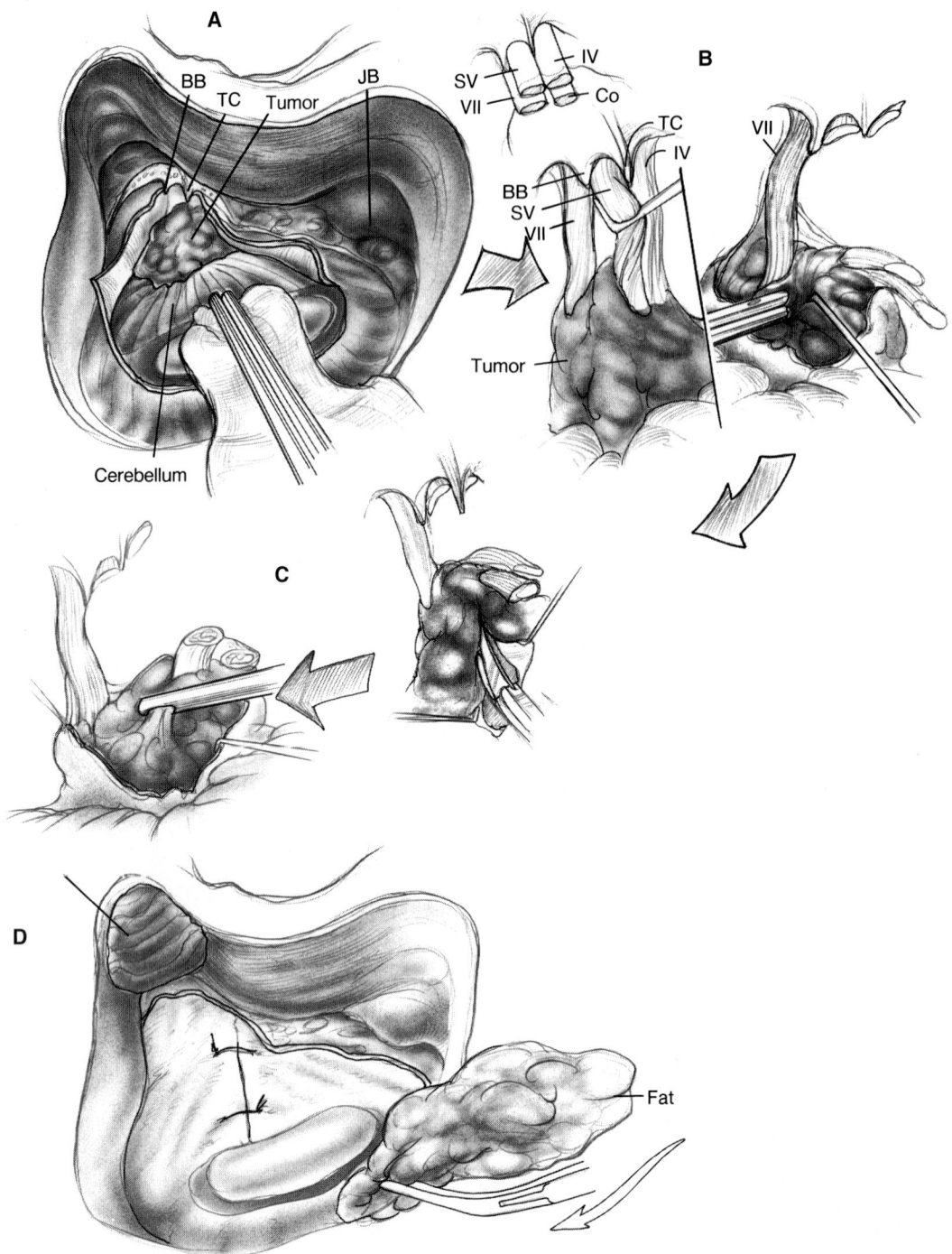

Figure 159.12 *(Continued)*

identify the IAC. The medial portion of the cochlear aqueduct is identified medial to the jugular bulb and may be opened widely to drain CSF and decompress the dura once all bone drilling is complete. Removal of bone overlying the lateral IAC will reveal the transverse crest. The macula cribrosa superioris (Mike's dot) is the landmark for the lateralmost extent of the IAC and represents the insertion of the superior vestibular nerve into the labyrinth.

When 270-degree exposure around the IAC has been obtained, the posterior fossa dura is opened widely medial to the sigmoid sinus and over the posterior face of the IAC. Collagen or gelatin foam is then placed on the cerebellum to prevent desiccation. Arachnoid bands are sharply divided, and CSF is drained from the CPA to allow cerebellar relaxation. The posterior face of the tumor is examined and stimulated to ensure that the facial nerve is not aberrantly displaced posteriorly. The capsule of the tumor is cauterized and a window is removed. The central contents of the tumor are removed to facilitate circumferential extracapsular dissection. Once the tumor has been debulked internally, dissection along the capsule is performed to gently separate the tumor from the cerebellum and brainstem while cauterizing only the vessels that are intimately attached to the capsule. Care should be taken to not dissect blindly around the tumor as such a maneuver could injure the facial nerve on the anterior surface of the tumor. Generally, the medial facial nerve can be identified at the brainstem with the assistance of the facial nerve monitor stimulator; however, following the facial nerve from the lateral end of the IAC continuously to the brainstem may be preferable as noted hereafter.

Once the tumor has been adequately debulked, the fundus of the IAC is examined. The superior and inferior vestibular nerves are avulsed and gently elevated posteriorly. The position of the facial nerve is identified with the facial nerve stimulator and adhesions between the nerve and the tumor should be sharply divided. The cochlear nerve can be preserved in its native position in the setting of NF2 where cochlear implantation may be attempted; however, the cochlear nerve is generally avulsed from the fundus and removed with the tumor as it is dissected medially. The dissection between the tumor and the facial nerve continues to the CPA. Once the tumor is free from the facial nerve, the root entry zone of the eighth cranial nerve is identified, cauterized, and sharply divided. At this point the tumor can be removed from the wound.

The closure of the translabyrinthine wound is performed meticulously to prevent postoperative CSF leak. The petrous bone adjacent to the IAC should be obliterated with bone wax. The middle ear is examined and the tensor tympani tendon is divided to allow visualization and access to the eustachian tube orifice, which is packed with muscle, bone wax, or other packing material. The middle ear is filled with pieces of temporalis muscle, and temporalis fascia is placed over the aditus ad antrum and the undersurface of the labyrinth, which is adjacent to the sinus tympani. Approximately 30 to 50 mL of abdominal fat is harvested and cut into strips. The strips are gently placed into the wound to fill the durotomy and close off the CSF egress. The remainder of the mastoid cavity is filled with the fat, and placement of a titanium mesh plate over the defect fixed with titanium screws holds the fat securely in place and prevents postoperative deformity. The periosteum and skin are closed in multiple layers in a watertight fashion and a pressure dressing is applied.

Combined Approach

The combined approach involves both translabyrinthine and suboccipital approaches as previously described and can be used to resect tumors larger than 4 cm. The procedure is complicated by prolonged operative time and involves collaboration among the surgical team. Postoperative management may include evaluation and treatment of elevated intracranial pressure and hydrocephalus. Neurosurgical consultation is beneficial. Preoperative high-dose steroid administration may help reduce edema if present. Proceeding directly to surgery with opening of the posterior fossa could lead to catastrophic brain herniation and death if the edema is not managed initially.

Surgical Results

Historically, surgery for tumors of the CPA involved high rates of mortality; however, this has dramatically dropped over the past century of cranial base surgery. The mortality rate for surgical excision of vestibular schwannoma has declined to less than 1% (142,143). Postoperative patients should be monitored initially in an ICU setting since emergencies do occur and must be dealt with promptly (Table 159.1). Recurrence of tumor is variable but is generally reported at less than 1% (144,145). Postoperative facial nerve function is dependent on the size of the tumor, the adherence to the facial nerve and the experience of the operating team (146). The translabyrinthine approach can preserve facial nerve function (House Brackmann grade I or II) in over 90% of patients with tumors less than 1.5 cm; however, this rate decreases as tumor size increases (145). The intraoperative facial nerve monitor findings can positively predict postoperative facial nerve function. A House-Brackmann grade I or II postoperative facial nerve outcome can be predicted with 98% probability when the facial nerve response is 240 mV or greater with a 0.05 mA or less stimulus (147). Hearing preservation also varies greatly and depends on the surgical approach and the size of the tumor. In small tumors, hearing can be preserved in 80% to 90% of cases with a middle cranial fossa approach. Postoperative CSF leak remains as one of the more common postoperative complications and the incidence has been reported from 1% to 10% of cases (148–150). Meningitis represents a serious concern in the postoperative period; the rate is reported between 1% and 8% of cases (151). Headache may be a primary preoperative symptom for up to 60% of vestibular schwannoma patients (152). Postoperative headaches are more common in patients who undergo a suboccipital tumor resection

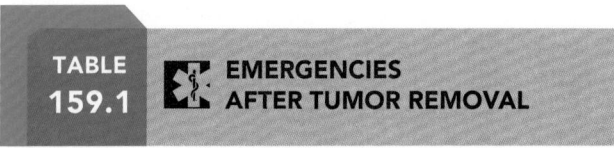

TABLE 159.1	EMERGENCIES AFTER TUMOR REMOVAL

Emergency	Management
Intracranial hemorrhage	Remove dressing and open wound, to allow rapid decompression of brainstem; move to operating room for control of hemorrhage.
Pneumocephalus	If unstable, emergency craniotomy to remove air; otherwise, discontinue lumbar drain and observe.
Meningitis	Lumbar puncture for culture and sensitivity; appropriate antibiotics intravenously; surgical closure of any CSF leak.
CSF leak	Pressure dressing; if leak persists despite lumbar drain, surgical closure.

and may be present in over 30% of patients (153). The etiology of the headache is unknown, but may be related to dural tension and persistent inflammation following closure. The majority of these patients experience resolution of their headaches over time.

NONVESTIBULAR CRANIAL NERVE SCHWANNOMAS

Schwannomas can develop on the fifth through the twelfth cranial nerves within the posterior fossa; however, they are far less common than vestibular schwannomas. Though they tend to have similar imaging characteristics to vestibular schwannomas they differ in their anatomic locations and associated symptoms. As these tumors expand within the CPA they may present similarly. Nonvestibular schwannomas account for 2% to 3% of tumors within the CPA (154) and are common in NF2 patients. Trigeminal schwannoma is the most common of nonvestibular schwannomas (12) and may involve the nerve root or the ganglion. These tumors tend to present with ipsilateral facial hypesthesia in the distribution of the trigeminal nerve. CT imaging demonstrates an enhancing expansion of the Meckel cave or the foramen lacerum. MRI imaging reveals an enhancing lesion in an anterior–posterior orientation adjacent to the Meckel cave that may be difficult to distinguish from a meningioma. Lesions extending into the Meckel cave can be treated with radiation or they can be resected through the anterolateral intradural approach (Dolenec's) and anterior petrosal approach (155).

Facial schwannomas may be difficult to distinguish from vestibular schwannomas if they are limited to the IAC. Multiple segments of the nerve may be involved, and the CPA is involved in greater than 50% of tumors (154). These slow-growing tumors present with gradual facial nerve weakness. Imaging reveals expansion of the fallopian canal within the temporal bone on CT imaging. MRI imaging may reveal an enhancing dumbbell-shaped expansion of the intratemporal facial nerve as well as enlargement and enhancement of the middle fossa geniculate ganglion region (Fig. 159.13). Patients with House-Brackmann facial nerve function I to III are managed initially with observation. Declining facial nerve function may be treated surgically with decompression of the facial nerve via a middle fossa approach or transmastoid approach depending on the location of tumor expansion. When the facial nerve becomes nonfunctional (House-Brackmann IV to VI) resection of the schwannoma may be selected followed by a greater auricular or sural nerve cable graft.

Lower cranial nerve schwannomas typically involve the inferior aspect of the posterior fossa; however, they can extend into the CPA and account for 1% of CPA lesions (154). The clinical symptoms are related to the nerve of origin but expansion of the tumor may affect all of the lower cranial nerves. MRI and CT imaging may

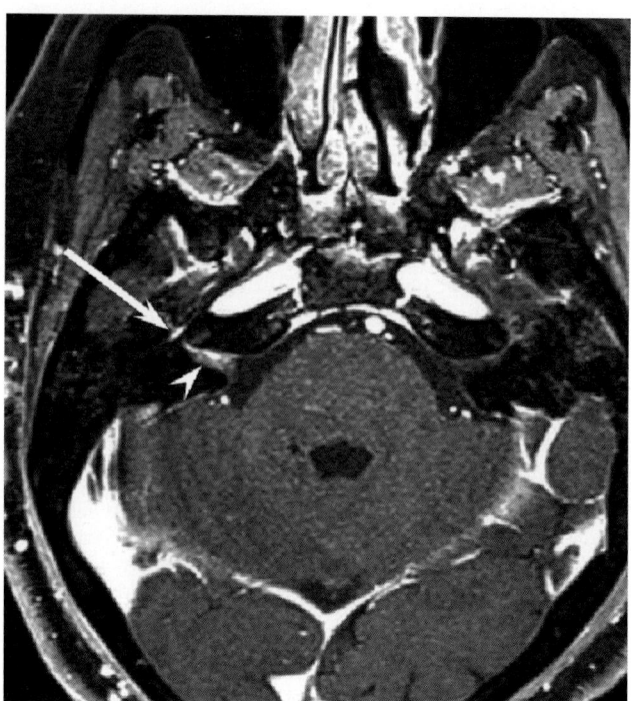

Figure 159.13 Axial T1-weighted contrast-enhanced MRI image at the level of the IAC demonstrating a right facial schwannoma. Note the enhancing mass (*arrowhead*) in the lateral IAC along with enhancement along the labyrinthine segment (*arrow*) of the facial nerve and the geniculate ganglion.

reveal an enhancing lesion of the CPA, but typically includes expansion of the jugular foramen (Fig. 159.14). Treatment of these lesions may involve surgical resection or radiation.

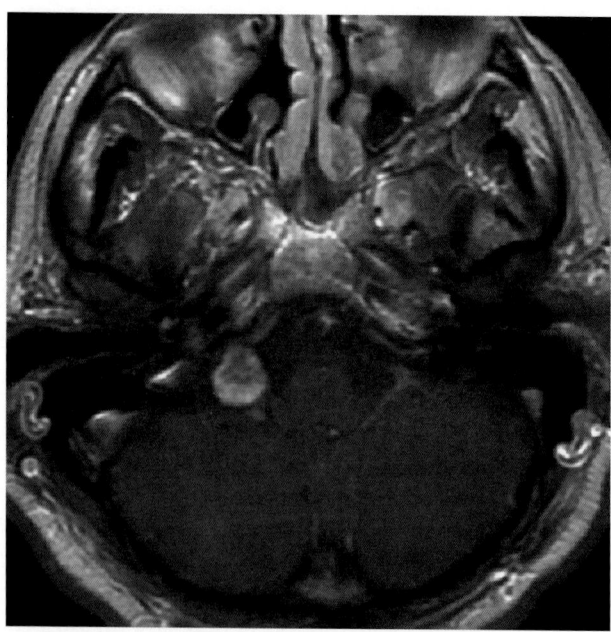

Figure 159.14 Axial T1-weighted contrast-enhanced MRI image at the level of the jugular foramen demonstrating a right glossopharyngeal nerve schwannoma. Note the enhancing mass extending from the pars nervosa of the jugular foramen into the lateral medullary cistern.

MENINGIOMA

Epidemiology

Meningiomas are the most common intracranial extraaxial tumor and account for approximately 20% of all primary intracranial tumors. The majority of these tumors occur along the convexity of the cranial vault; however, they are the second most common neoplasm of the CPA and can lead to significant morbidity when they occur along the cranial base. These tumors comprise 10% to 15% of all CPA tumors (156) and develop from the arachnoid villi cap cells adjacent to dural sinuses and may have broad dural attachments. Meningiomas are more common in middle-aged women. Sex hormone receptors and metabolism may play a role in development and progression of these tumors (154).

Histopathology

The World Health Organization has classified meningiomas as grade I (benign) (80%), while 10% to 15% are grade II or atypical, and 2% to 5% are malignant or grade III (157). Multiple histologic subtypes have been described and grade I variants include meningothelial, fibrous, transitional, psammomatous, angiomatous, microcystic, secretory, lymphoplasmacyte-rich, and metaplastic (158). Classically, grade I tumors display whorls of spindle cells with the presence of calcified psammoma bodies. Grade II tumor variants display increased cellularity, atypical nuclei, and areas of necrosis (159). Grade III tumors are anaplastic and may have papillary or rhabdoid variants and display high proliferation indices with brain invasion (158). Immunohistochemical staining is helpful in the diagnosis of meningiomas and common markers for these tumors include epithelial membrane antigen and vimentin (158). Additionally, an anti-phosphohistone H3 can help identify mitotically active areas within tumors (160).

Sporadic meningiomas are common; however, NF2 patients may develop multiple meningiomas that often lead to increased morbidity and mortality. Whether associated with NF2 or not, these benign tumor types occur along the skull base and can invade the dura, dural sinuses, skull, orbit, soft tissue, and skin. Although they may be displaced by the tumor, cranial nerves are frequently enveloped by meningiomas, thus, complicating attempts at neurologic preservation. The broad dural base and infiltrative nature of these tumors make them difficult to completely resect and recurrences are common.

Molecular Biology

Meningiomas commonly have chromosomal deletion, and may involve multiple chromosomal anomalies in grade II and III tumors (161). Mutations resulting in deletion or inactivation of the *NF2* gene are common

and occur in 30% to 70% of sporadic meningiomas (162). Additional genes are likely involved as well, such as NF1, PTCH, CREBBP, VHL, PTEN, and CDKN2A (reviewed in 163), and meningiomas have been associated with hereditary syndromes, including Cowden, Gorlin, Li-Fraumeni, Turcot, Gardener, von Hippel-Lindau, and multiple endocrine neoplasia type I (158). Meningioma development and progression has been linked to altered intracellular signaling involving p53, retinoblastoma protein interactions, and tyrosine kinase receptors such as epidermal growth factor receptor and platelet derived growth factor receptor (164–166).

Clinical Presentation

Meningiomas of the cranial base and CPA present with symptoms dependent upon their size and location. Tumors that originate along the floor of the middle cranial fossa can induce facial and/or ocular pain and diplopia from dysfunction of the trigeminal and trochlear nerves. Expansion of the tumor to compress the temporal lobe can result in seizures and sensory/motor deficits. Tumors that extend more anteriorly along the petroclival region may involve the abducens nerve, which can also result in ocular symptoms. When these lesions involve the CPA and IAC, the symptoms mirror vestibular schwannomas and may make it difficult to distinguish these tumors.

It is difficult to distinguish between vestibular schwannomas and meningiomas by audiovestibular testing. Imaging can often differentiate the two tumors. Extension of these tumors inferiorly may result in dysfunction of the lower cranial nerves with resulting dysphagia, dysphonia, shoulder weakness, and tongue hemiparalysis. Similar to vestibular schwannomas, meningioma growth within the CPA can compress the brainstem and produce hydrocephalus and, potentially, lethal brain herniation.

Diagnostic Evaluation

Audiologic and vestibular tests may reveal dysfunction of the vestibulocochlear nerve caused by meningiomas and may be indistinguishable from the dysfunction caused by vestibular schwannomas. Imaging studies are vital in the diagnosis of meningiomas. CT imaging of meningiomas may identify calcified areas and contrast enhancement of these tumors is heterogeneous. The bone adjacent to meningiomas may also be altered and have hyperostotic changes. Meningiomas appear isointense or slightly hypointense to gray matter on T1-weighted MRI sequences, with variable intensity on T2-weighted images and they display enhancement with gadolinium on T1-weighted images. The configuration of meningiomas is useful in the differential diagnosis since these tumors usually have a broad base of dural enhancement and form an obtuse angle with the underlying bone. There may also be extension of enhancement along the underlying

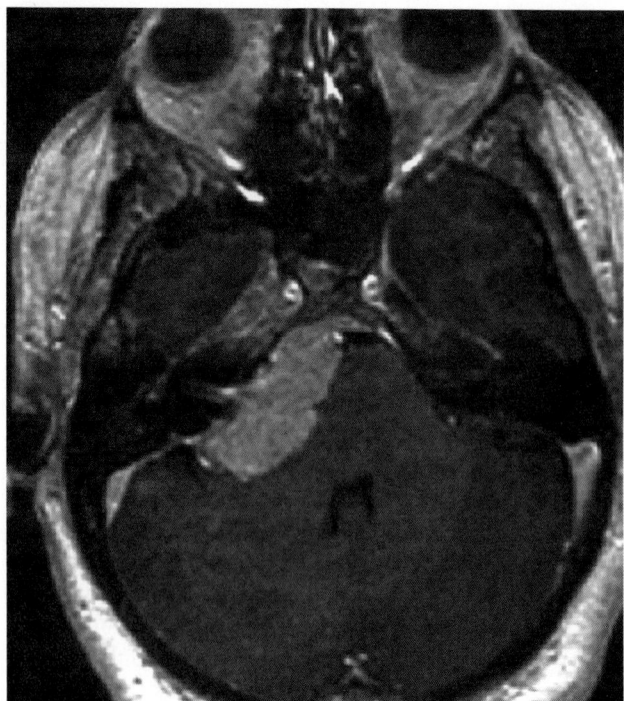

Figure 159.15 Axial T1-weighted contrast-enhanced MRI image at the level of the IAC demonstrating a right CPA meningioma with broad dural attachment and enhancement.

dural surface, which is known as a dural tail (Fig. 159.15). Meningiomas may occur adjacent to or in the IAC-like vestibular schwannomas. Tumor progression may result in erosion of bone of the cranial base and invasion of tumor into neural foramina or into the middle ear.

Treatment Options

The management of cranial base meningiomas is complex and may employ multiple modalities to preserve neurologic function and tumor control. The complex anatomy of the cranial base complicates the intervention for these tumors. The risks and benefits of each treatment option must be analyzed in terms of the surrounding structures and the natural history of the meningiomas. Although these tumors are typically benign and slow growing, they can be aggressive and resilient to eradication. The primary treatment options are the same as vestibular schwannomas and include observation, radiation therapy, and microsurgical resection.

Observation with serial imaging studies and audiometry remains a viable option for patients, especially in those of advanced age or unable to undergo surgery. The natural history of meningioma growth over an extended period of observation with serial imaging demonstrated 27% of patients with declining cranial nerve function. At 10-year follow-up, only 42% had no tumor progression. Forty percent of patients within this study eventually underwent some form of treatment (167).

Radiation therapy for meningiomas can be administered in the form of gamma photons through stereotactic radiosurgery, x-ray photons in fractionated radiotherapy, and proton beam therapy. Focused radiation techniques have gained popularity to concentrate discrete radiation doses to the tumor and minimize exposure of normal surrounding structures. Radiation can be utilized as a primary treatment or as an adjuvant modality for meningiomas and is indicated in patients in whom surgery is not desired, is not deemed safe, or is unlikely to accomplish complete resection without significant morbidity. When meningiomas impinge on sensitive neurovascular structures, debulking may relieve compression and may decrease radiation treatment complications. Additionally, radiation therapy following tumor debulking can be used to improve tumor control (168). Tumor control of 82% to 100% for cranial base meningiomas after stereotactic radiation with doses from 12 to 17 Gy has been reported. The same studies noted progressive neurologic decline from 0% to 27% (169–173).

Considering the aggressive nature of meningiomas, microsurgical resection is considered the gold standard of treatment when growth or progressive symptoms are noted. Complete resection is not always feasible but decompression of surrounding neurovascular structures may provide symptomatic relief and provide tissue for histopathologic diagnosis. The approach for microsurgical resection of meningiomas is based on the anatomic areas involved as well as the hearing status. Meningiomas isolated to the CPA with preserved hearing may be approached, as would a vestibular schwannoma. Considering the dural involvement of these tumors, it is advisable to widely excise surrounding dura to prevent recurrence. Patients with meningiomas who lack functional hearing are best managed with a translabyrinthine approach. The variable location of the facial nerve in CPA meningiomas makes the translabyrinthine approach, with its extensive facial nerve exposure, a desirable route for resection. The middle fossa approach is not commonly used to resect meningiomas; however, lesions isolated to the IAC with functional hearing can be approached in this manner. Meningiomas frequently extend anteriorly into the petroclival region that can be accessed through a transcochlear approach. This approach involves a translabyrinthine dissection followed by posterior translocation of the facial nerve from the fallopian canal. Drilling continues, in an anteromedial direction, through the cochlea using caution so as to not injure the intratemporal segment of the carotid artery. This approach provides ample exposure of the clivus and the Meckel cave; however, translocation of the facial nerve can result in its dysfunction. This region can also be approached via a transpetrosal middle fossa approach by removing intervening bone between the cochlear and internal carotid artery. The risk associated with microsurgery for meningiomas is similar to that of vestibular schwannomas and are inherent to the approach being utilized. Resection of tumors in the CPA and petroclival region can greatly reduce the risk of neurovascular compromise and facilitate adjuvant therapy; however, recurrence and iatrogenic neurologic deficit remain concerns. In a review of 150 patients with anterior CPA and petroclival meningiomas treated with microsurgery, 20% developed new neurologic deficits. Gross total resection was accomplished in 32% of patients, subtotal resection in 43% and partial resection in 25%. The mean follow up was 102 months. This review also analyzed the literature and reported total resection rates of 40% to 79% and recurrence or progression rates as 0% to 36% (174).

EPIDERMOID AND DERMOID CYSTS

Epidermoid cysts are congenital lesions that develop from sequestered ectodermal epithelial cell rests. They are synonymous with cholesteatoma; however, acquired cholesteatomas can also occur within the CPA from extension from the mastoid, middle ear, or petrous bone. This collection of squamous epithelial cells grows slowly by desquamation of cells and accumulation of keratin debris. Similar to middle ear cholesteatomas, they tend to erode surrounding bone and encase neurovascular structures. Epidermoids represent the third most common mass of the CPA, comprising approximately 5% of all masses in the region (175). Dermoid cysts develop from inclusion of cutaneous ectoderm, like epidermoids; however, these lesions differ, in that, they include fat and adnexal components. Dermoid cysts are uncommon lesions of the CPA and more commonly originate from the parasellar region (176) and contain fat, hair, calcifications, keratin debris, and products of sebaceous glands (13).

Clinically, these lesions experience extensive occult growth without causing dramatic symptoms until they are considerable in size. Symptoms are similar to other discrete tumors of the CPA; however, they may cause earlier facial neuropathy compared with lesions that only displace the nerve. CT imaging reveals remodeling of bone surrounding these lesions (Fig. 159.16A), and may identify calcifications in dermoid cysts. MRI is helpful in the diagnosis and displays epidermoid cysts as irregular nonenhancing lesions that are hypointense on T1-weighted images and hyperintense on T2-weighted images (Fig. 159.16B and C). The use of fluid-attenuated inversion recovery (FLAIR) sequences is helpful in the diagnosis, which suppresses of the signal intensity of CSF, and epidermoid cysts appear as hyperintense lesions. Additionally, diffusion-weighted imaging, which monitors the diffusion of fluid-filled structures or spaces, displays epidermoid cysts as hyperintense lesions, unlike arachnoid cysts (Fig. 159.16D). Dermoid cysts have similar characteristics and are also nonenhancing; however, they display intrinsic high T1 signal intensity due to the fatty dermal component.

The primary treatment of these lesions is microsurgical excision through one of the approaches already described. Similar to this disease process in the middle ear and mastoid, recurrences are common; thus, great care must be taken to remove all disease. The central contents of these cysts can easily be debulked with suction and blunt dissection to facilitate circumferential dissection and resection of the capsule. Cysts that envelop vital neurovascular structures can be managed with subtotal resection and monitored with imaging since these are slowing growing lesions. One recent review reported recurrence rates of 23% for epidermoid cyst total resection and 27% for subtotal resections and the majority of recurrences required surgical intervention (177).

ARACHNOID CYST

Arachnoid cysts are congenital malformation of the arachnoid that result in a pouch of sequestered normal CSF fluid. The etiology of cyst formation is unknown. These lesions comprise less than 1% of intracranial lesions and approximately 10% occur in the CPA, while most occur in the supratentorial temporal fossa (154). These lesions are typically asymptomatic but can cause compression of the seventh and eighth cranial nerve complex. MRI characteristics of arachnoids cysts are a nonenhancing lesion that is hypointense on T1-weighted images and hyperintense on T2-weighted images. These cysts displace neurovascular structures and have smooth regular borders that do no invade or envelope vital structures. Arachnoid cysts appear as a hypointense lesion on MRI FLAIR and diffusion weighted sequences. These lesions do not generally require intervention; however, they may be fenestrated via a suboccipital approach to decompress an expanding cyst (154).

LIPOMA

Lipomas of the CPA are uncommon and are due to congenital malformations resulting in hamartomatous collections of mature adipose tissue. These lesions more commonly occur in supratentorial locations and can be associated with cerebral malformations; however, lipomas of the CPA are not associated with other defects (175). These lesions tend to envelop neurovascular structures and may adhere tightly to cranial nerves. These lesions tend to grow very slowly over time but may induce similar symptoms to other CPA masses, such as facial paralysis, hearing loss, and trigeminal neuralgia. Lipomas appear as nonenhancing lesions that are hyperintense on T1-weighted images and hypointense on fat-suppressed T2-weighted images (Fig. 159.17). The diagnosis can be confirmed by performing fat suppression on unenhanced T1 sequences, which causes lipomas to appear hypointense. These lesions are typically managed with serial imaging; however, they may be treated with subtotal resection in the event of neurovascular compression.

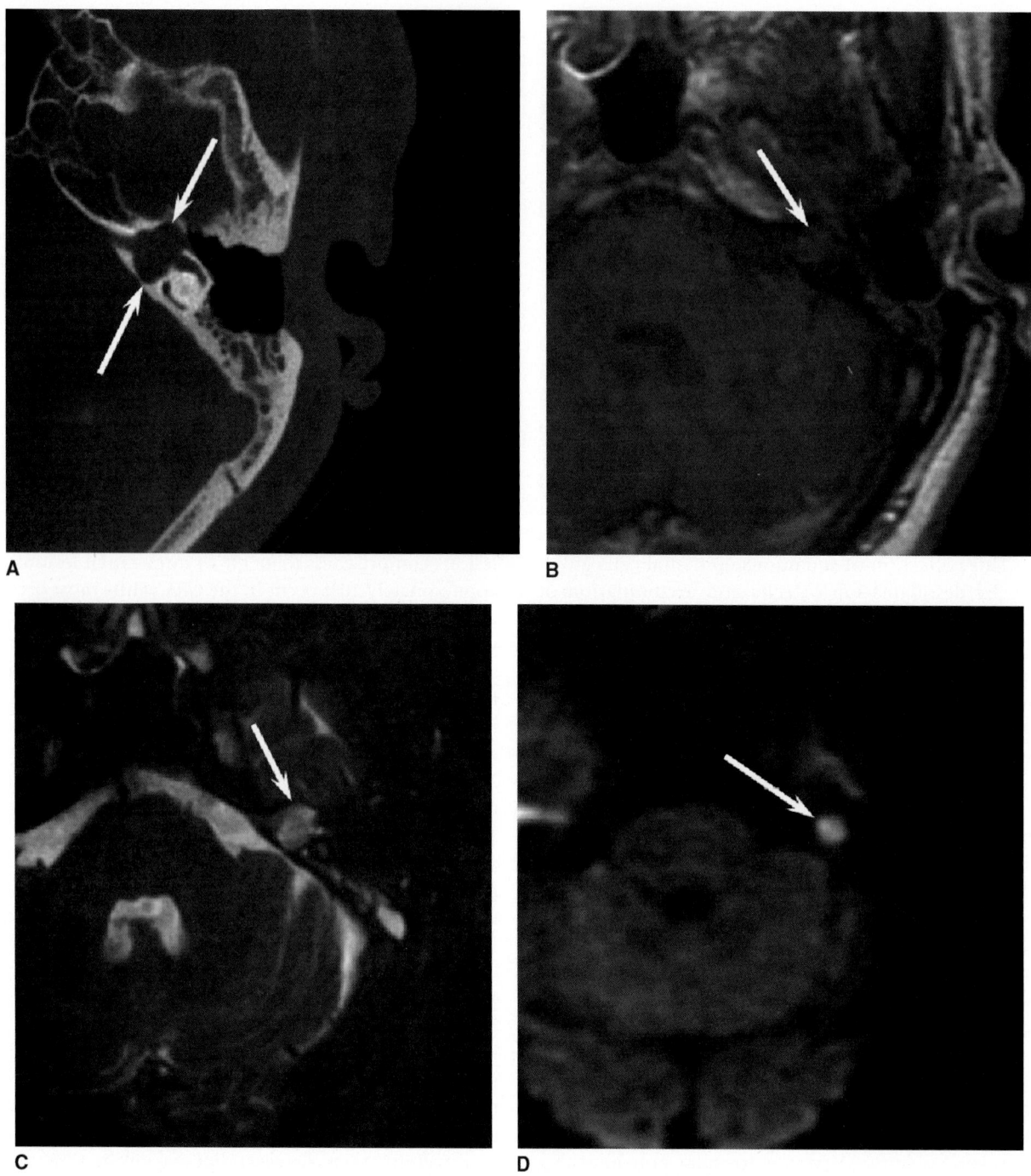

Figure 159.16 Radiographic appearance of recurrent acquired cholesteatoma. Axial CT of the temporal bone demonstrating a mastoidectomy defect with a smooth expansile mass (*arrows*) eroding the inner ear **(A)**. This mass is isointense to brain and nonenhancing on axial T1-weighted contrast-enhanced MRI image **(B)**, but hyperintense on T2-weighted images **(C)** and diffusion-weighted images **(D)**. The restricted diffusion distinguishes recurrent cholesteatoma from scar.

MISCELLANEOUS EXTRAAXIAL LESIONS

Metastases

Metastatic lesions to the CPA are uncommon and account for less than 1% of CPA lesions (178). These lesions may present as a discrete mass or as diffuse meningeal disease, also known as leptomeningeal carcinomatosis. The most common primary tumors that CPA metastases originate from are lung, breast, melanoma, and lymphoma (179). Metastases present with acute cranial neuropathies and may cause bilateral symptoms, mimicking NF2. A history of cancer should raise suspicion of metastatic disease. Diagnosis can be made with CSF cytology (180,181). Metastases typically appear as enhancing lesions on T1-weighted images and

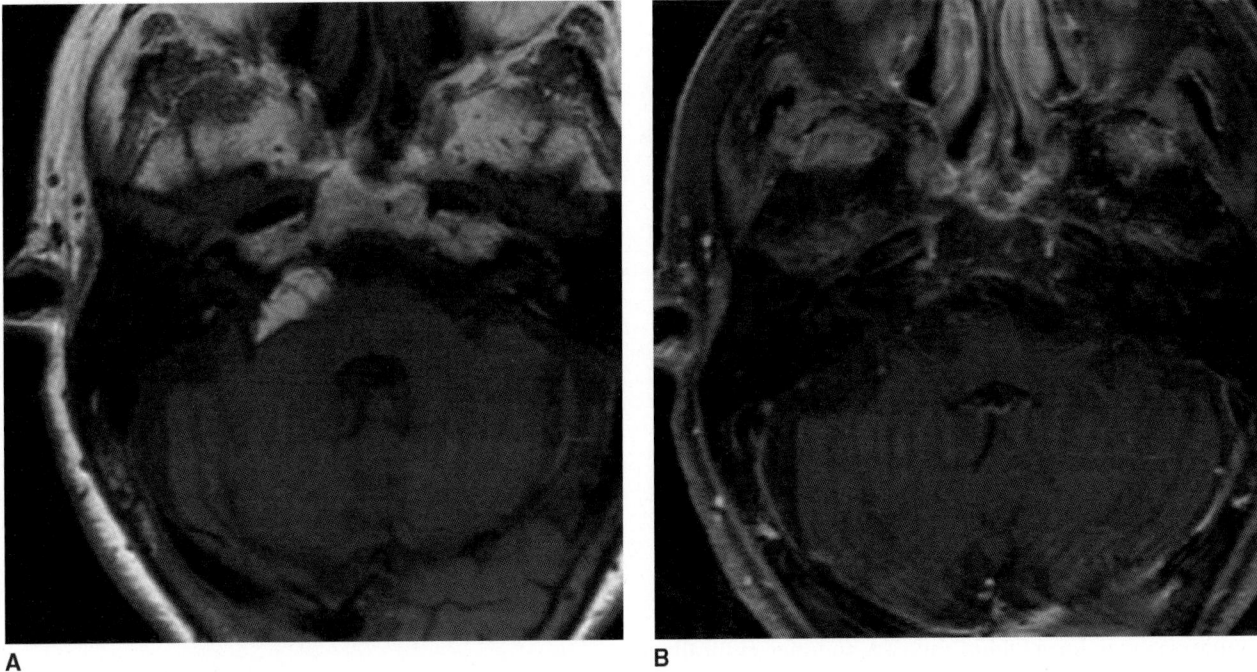

A   **B**

Figure 159.17 Axial T1-weighted unenhanced MRI image at the level of the IAC demonstrating a right CPA lipoma **(A)**. The diagnosis is confirmed with a postcontrast fat-suppressed T1 MRI image as this lesion appears dark **(B)**.

may show irregular bony destruction on CT (Fig. 159.18). Melanoma, due to the paramagnetic activity of melanin, may appear with intrinsic T1 hyperintensity, without contrast (12). A careful systematic search for the primary lesion must be undertaken when the CPA lesion is the first to be diagnosed. Treatment of these lesions is usually dictated by a multidisciplinary team of oncologists and surgeons and often involves multimodality treatment. Surgical intervention is typically reserved for palliation or for the purpose of obtaining tissue for pathologic diagnosis.

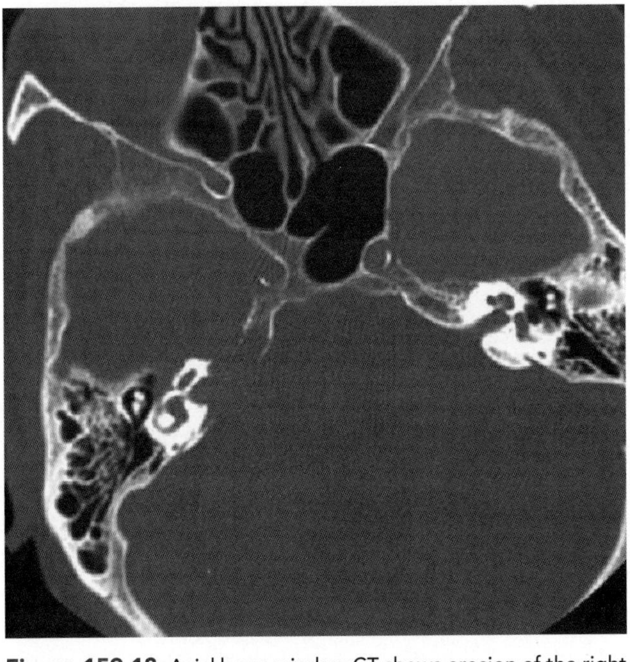

Vascular Lesions

Lesions of vascular origin account for approximately 3% of CPA and most of those are aneurysms of the vertebral arterial system, such as the AICA (182). The complex vascular system of the CPA can cause compression of the seventh to eighth cranial nerve complex when abnormal vascular loops or aneurysmal dilations develop. Aneurysms may present with subarachnoid hemorrhage and/or cranial neuropathy. These lesions may appear as discrete lesions of the CPA with flow voids and enhance with contrast administration on MRI. These lesions may be asymptomatic and are typically managed with surgical clipping through a suboccipital approach (183) or endovascular occlusion (184). Although a controversial diagnosis, ipsilateral auditory/vestibular symptoms and trigeminal neuralgia have been linked to aberrant vascular loops and can be managed with surgical decompression (185).

Hemangiomas, arteriovenous malformations (AVMs), and cavernomas can also develop with the CPA. Hemangiomas more commonly occur at the geniculate ganglion and develop from vessels that accompany the facial nerve (186). Calcifications within these lesions may be identified on CT and they appear as enhancing lesions with flow voids. An AVM is an abnormal collection of arteries and veins that, unlike other vascular malformations, have major feeding and draining vessels. These malformations may

Figure 159.18 Axial bone-window CT shows erosion of the right petrous apex from metastatic renal cell carcinoma.

result in significant hemorrhage if they rupture. These may appear similar to other vascular lesions; however, the gold standard for AVM diagnosis is cerebral angiography. These lesions may be observed if small and asymptomatic; however, they can also be managed with endovascular occlusion, surgical resection, or stereotactic radiosurgery. Cavernomas are abnormal vascular lesions that contain sinusoidal regions of blood products contained by fragile endothelial walls. Unlike AVM, these lesions do not have large feeding or draining vessels. The clinical presentation is similar to other vascular lesions and appears as enhancing heterogeneous lesions with a "popcorn" appearance with a hypointense rim on T1 and T2 sequences. Treatment is typically surgical but is dependent on the size and clinical presentation.

Sarcoidosis

This systemic disease can present with central nervous system (CNS) manifestations. Forty percent of patients with sarcoidosis have leptomeningeal enhancement (175). Granulomas may form within the CPA and may clinically mimic other lesions, although, these lesions may additionally present with signs and symptoms of meningeal inflammation. Due to the diffuse nature of this disease, diagnosis can be difficult; however, these lesions are hyperintense on CT, isointense on MRI T1 sequences, hypointense on T2 sequences, and strongly enhance with contrast administration. Neurosarcoidosis is treated with systemic immune suppression.

Tuberculosis

This disease is known to present with diverse and obscure lesions and CNS tuberculosis can include abscesses, basilar meningitis, and intraaxial tuberculomas. An extraaxial tuberculoma can closely mimic a cranial base meningioma, clinically and radiographically (187). Treatment involves systemic antimycobacterial therapy.

INTRAAXIAL LESIONS

Lesions of the brainstem may present within the CPA. As these lesions expand, normal anatomy is distorted and the fluid-filled CPA is effaced, which can complicate diagnosis. Subtle imaging findings such as an enhancing lesion without a brain–tumor interface and with peritumoral edema are indicative of an intraaxial lesion (13). These lesions are typically managed by or in conjunction with neurosurgery and oncology services.

A wide variety of neoplastic disease can develop in this region. Primary lymphoma may occur as an intraaxial and extraaxial lesion and have the same clinical and imaging characteristics. These lesions can appear hyperintense on CT, which enhance on contrast administration. They appear hypointense on T1 sequences and strongly enhance with gadolinium. These lesions are hypercellular

and result in hypointensity on T2-weighted images (13). CNS lymphoma may be the primary presentation of primary immunologic disease. Gliomas present with unilateral expansion of the brainstem with exophytic extension into the CPA; however, the imaging characteristics of glioma are not unique. Hemangioblastomas are benign lesions that are vascular in origin and develop from the cerebellum. Extension into the CPA by hemangioblastoma may mimic vestibular schwannomas (188). Most commonly these lesions are sporadic, but may occur in association with von Hippel-Lindau disease. These encapsulated lesions are strongly enhancing on MRI and may have cystic portions that appear hyperintense on T2-weighted images. Intraventricular lesions, such as ependymoma and papilloma, can extend into the CPA and MRI reveals extension of these tumors from the fourth ventricle through the foramen of Luschka. Similar to the extraaxial presentation, metastatic disease can occur within the brainstem and have similar symptoms and are managed similarly.

SKULL BASE LESIONS

Lesions that develop from or within the temporal bone may extend into the CPA. Bone erosion of the petrous bone can be extensive and CT imaging is particularly helpful in identifying extension and monitoring for recurrence or progression of disease.

Paraganglioma

Glomus tumors of the jugular foramen can extend superiorly into the CPA. These tumors develop from neuroendocrine paraganglial cells originating from neural crest cells adjacent to the ninth and tenth cranial nerves and are surrounded by a dense collection of capillaries and venules. Glomus jugulare tumors are frequently supplied by the ascending pharyngeal artery; however, that may have a variety of additional feeding vessels. Although slowly growing and benign, these lesions can aggressively erode bone and invade neurovascular structures of the cranial base. Pulsatile tinnitus is a hallmark symptom; however, disease that extends into the CPA is likely to have multiple cranial neuropathies. Less than 4% of these tumors secrete vasoactive catecholamines and produce hypertension, palpitations, diaphoresis, and arrhythmias (189). Diagnostic evaluation should involve a 24-hour urine test, if a secreting tumor is suspected, to detect vasoactive tumor products such as vanillylmandelic acid and epinephrine derivatives. CT imaging can identify irregular bony erosion of these tumors (Fig. 159.19). On MRI, these enhancing lesions typically demonstrate a "salt and pepper" pattern, which is due to flow voids within vessels of the tumor (Fig. 159.20). Angiography can also be performed to assist in diagnosis and for embolization. Treatment of glomus tumors is typically surgical; however, lesions that extend into the intracranial compartment may

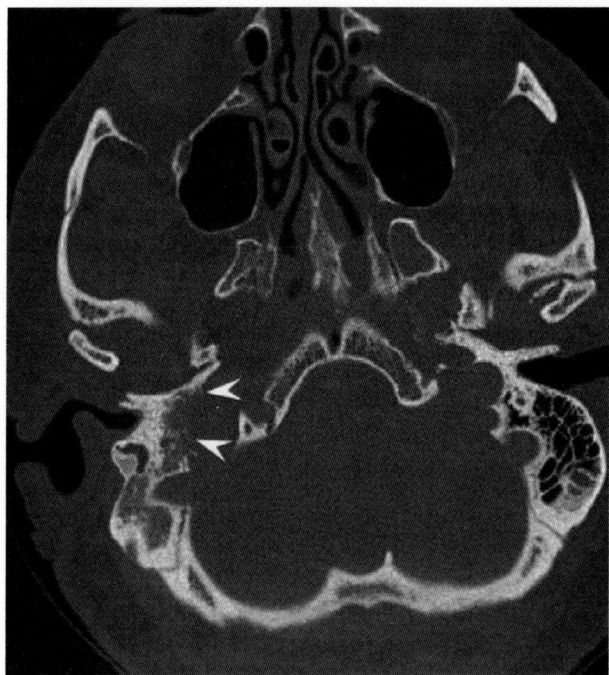

Figure 159.19 Axial temporal bone CT image at the level of the jugular foramen demonstrating permeative bony erosion (*arrowheads*) and loss of the caroticojugular spine caused by a glomus jugulare tumor.

require multiple treatment modalities. Subtotal resection with postoperative adjuvant radiotherapy useful for extensive disease. Surgical resection requires proximal and distal venous control; however, profuse bleeding may occur during resection due to the inferior petrosal sinus.

Cholesterol Granuloma

Chronic obstruction of air cells of the temporal bone may result in accumulation of secretions and hemorrhage and form cholesterol granulomas. These lesions typically occur in the petrous apex and may slowly expand into the CPA. These lesions may cause similar cranial neuropathy. CT imaging reveals smooth bony expansion of the petrous bone, which may encroach on the petrous carotid artery (Fig. 159.21). The lesions are nonenhancing and appear as hyperintense on T1 sequences and hyperintense on T2 sequences (Fig. 159.22A and B). Observation of these lesions is recommended while asymptomatic; however, drainage of these lesions and their polychromatic "crank case oil" fluid can be performed through a transsphenoidal, middle fossa or infracochlear approach.

Chondromatous Lesions

Cartilaginous components of the petroclival fissure can be the source of chondromas and chondrosarcomas of the cranial base. These lesions originate along the parasagittal petroclival suture and can extend into the CPA. CT imaging can demonstrate calcifications within the tumor as well as the degree of bone erosion. Similar to normal cartilage, chondromatous lesions have poor vascularity and are weakly enhancing. They are hypointense on T1 and hyperintense on T2 images and may have signal voids in areas of calcification (Fig. 159.23A–C). Surgical resection is the primary treatment modality as these lesions are not very radiosensitive.

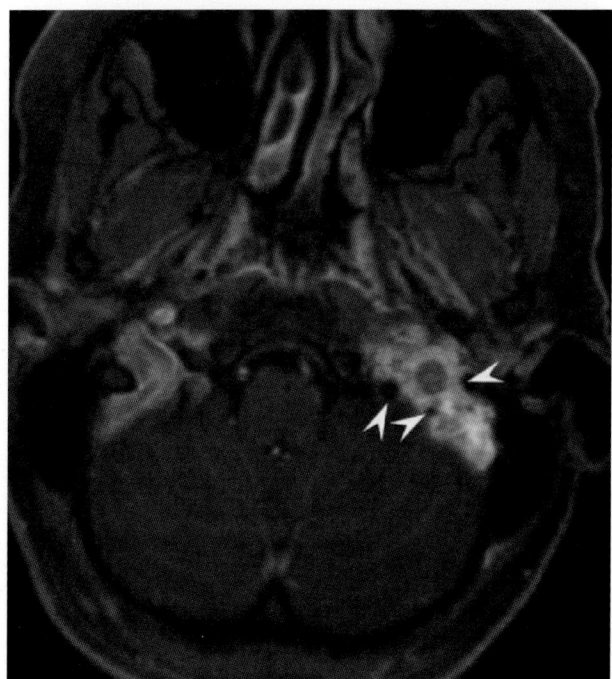

Figure 159.20 Axial T1-weighted contrast-enhanced MRI image at the level of the left jugular foramen demonstrating an enhancing glomus jugulare tumor with dark intratumoral flow voids (*arrowheads*).

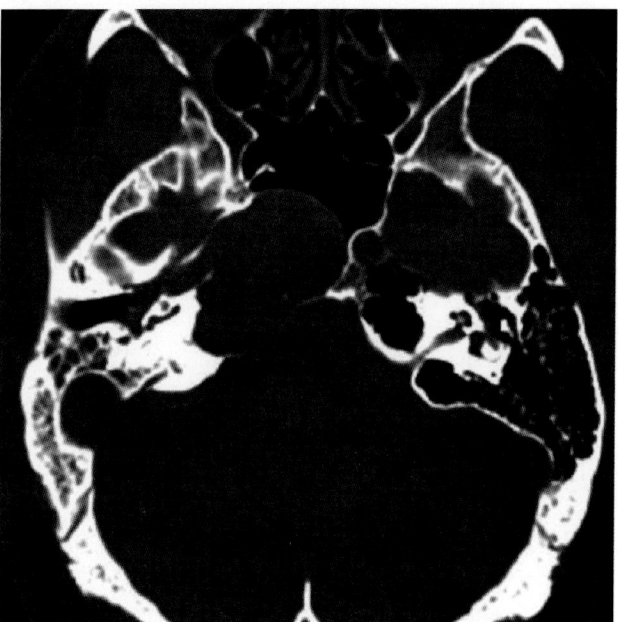

Figure 159.21 Axial temporal bone CT image at the level of the petrous apex demonstrating smooth bony expansion of the right petrous apex caused by a cholesterol granuloma. Note the loss of a distinct border between the lesion and the petrous carotid artery.

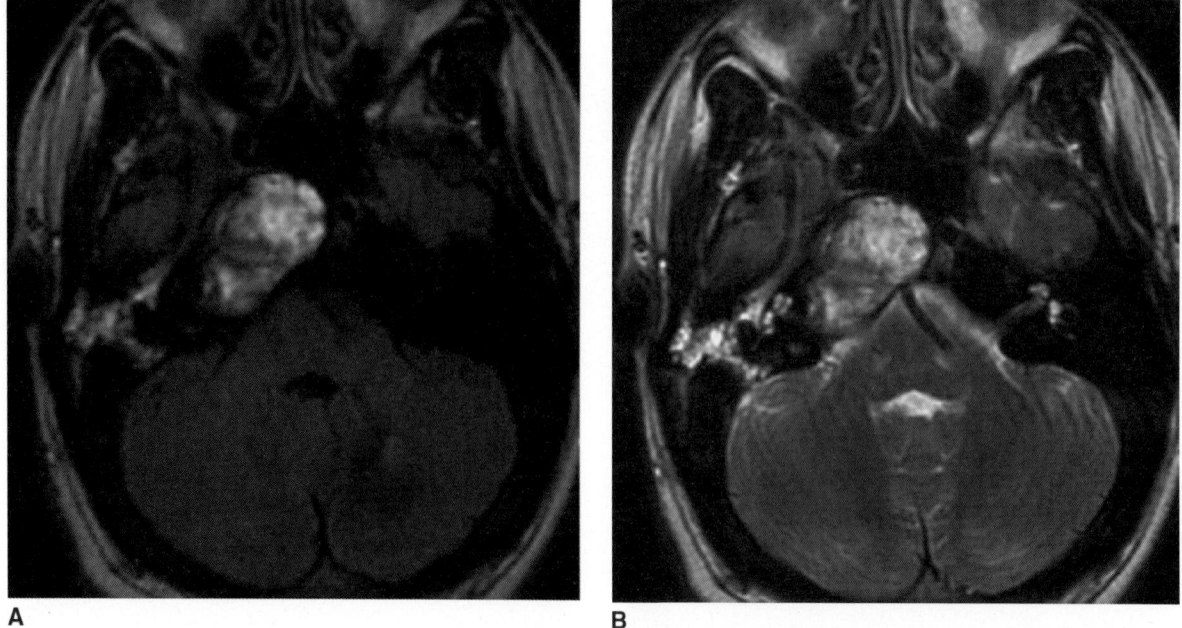

Figure 159.22 Cholesterol granuloma of the right petrous apex is hyperintense on both T1-weighted MRI images **(A)** and T2-weighted images **(B)**.

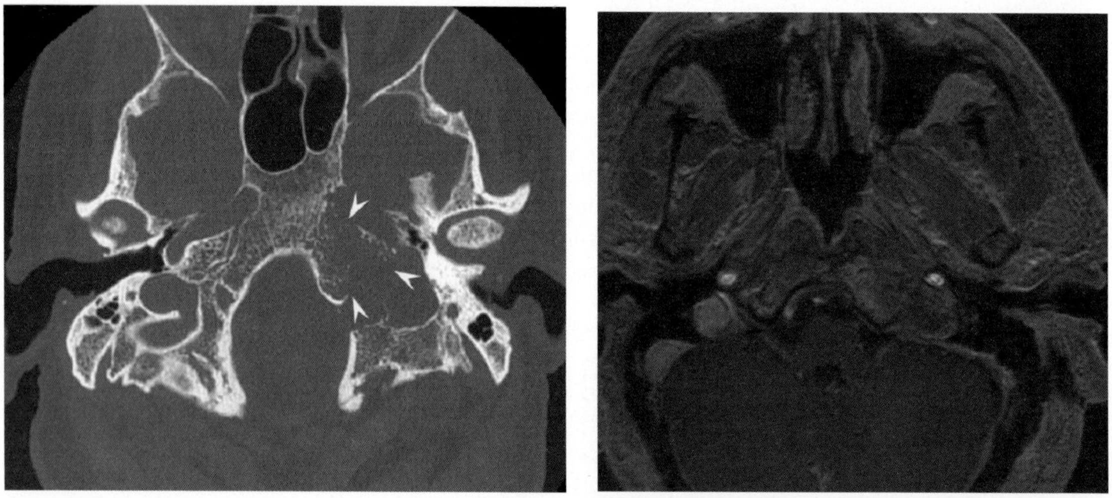

Figure 159.23 Radiographic appearance of a chondrosarcoma. Axial CT **(A)** of the temporal bone at the level of the clivus and jugular foramen demonstrates wide bony destruction (*arrowheads*) of the left cranial base. This mass is mildly enhancing and hypointense on axial T1-weighted contrast-enhanced MRI images **(B)** but hyperintense on T2-weighted images **(C)**.

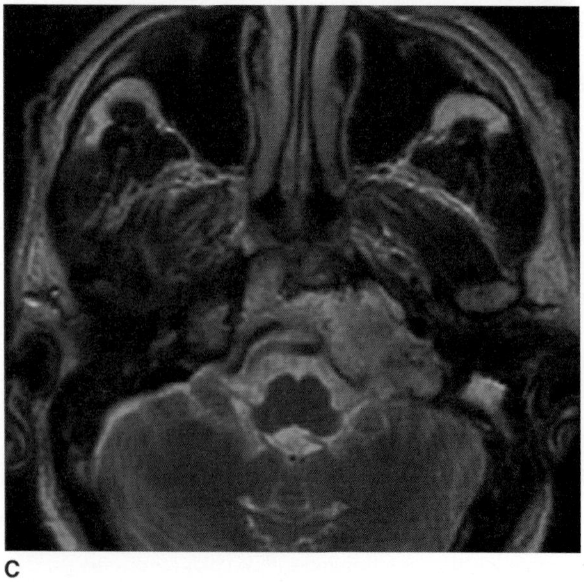

Chordoma

Chordomas are uncommon slowly growing tumors that develop from clival notochord remnants and seldom extend into the CPA; however, the chondroid chordoma variant may occur within the CPA. These lesions have a distinct histologic appearance that is characterized by the presence of physaliferous or "soap bubble" cells. These lesions appear as well-circumscribed bone-expanding midline lesions on CT and moderately enhancing lesions that appear hypointense on T1 sequences and hyperintense lesions with hypointense septations on T2 sequences (Fig. 159.24A–C). Prognosis of these lesions is poor and treatment involves surgical resection with postoperative radiotherapy.

Endolymphatic Sac Tumors

Tumors that originate from the endolymphatic sac are aggressive lesions that are papillary adenomas originating on the posterior petrous bone and may extend into the CPA. These lesions may occur sporadically but have an association with von Hippel-Lindau disease. Extensive bone erosion of the petrous bone can be identified on CT. These enhancing heterogenous masses can sequester hemorrhagic and protein-laden cysts that may be bright on T1 and T2 sequences. Treatment is surgical through a translabyrinthine approach and postoperative radiation.

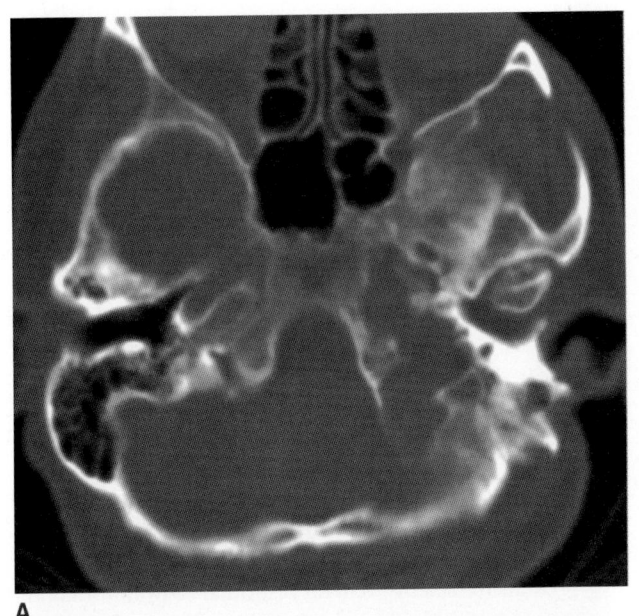

A

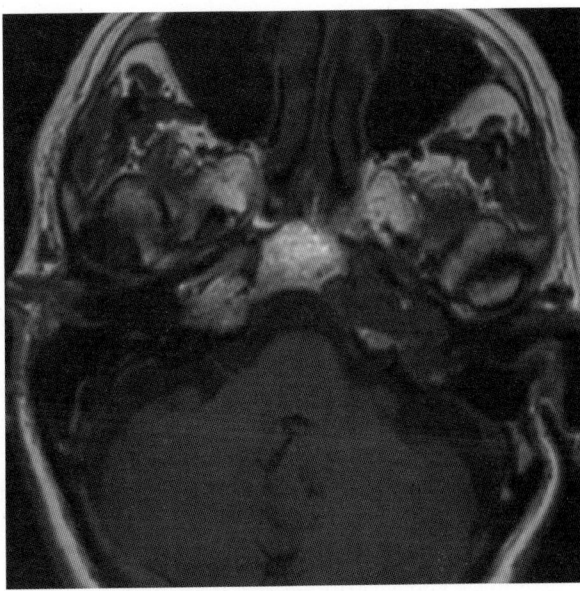

B

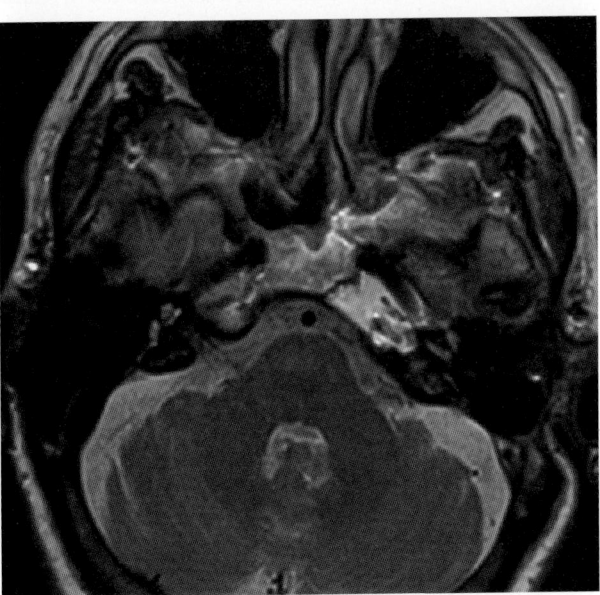

C

Figure 159.24 Radiographic appearance of a chordoma. Axial CT of the temporal bone at the level of the clivus and jugular foramen demonstrates wide bony destruction of the left cranial base **(A)**. This mass is hypointense on axial T1-weighted MRI images **(B)** but hyperintense on T2-weighted images **(C)**.

<table>
<tr><td>TABLE 159.2</td><td colspan="5">CPA LESION RADIOLOGY SUMMARY</td></tr>
</table>

Lesion	T1 (Relative to Brain)	T2 (Relative to Brain)	Contrast Enhancement	CT	Other Findings
Cranial nerve schwannoma	Isointense	Isointense, with foci of high intensity	Strong, with cystic areas	• Smooth expansion of bone (IAC, jugular foramen, fallopian canal)	Fundal cap—VS Ice cream cone—VS
Meningioma	Isointense	Isointense	Strong	• Calcifications • Hyperostosis	
Paraganglioma	Isointense	Isointense	Strong	• Permeative erosion of bone • Erosion of caroticojugular spine	Salt and pepper appearance
Endolymphatic sac tumors	Hyperintense	Hyperintense	Strong	• Extensive bony destruction	Characteristic location
Metastases	Variable	Hyperintense	Strong, but heterogeneous	• Irregular bony destruction	Melanoma—T1 hyperintensity
Chordoma	Hypointense	Hyperintense	Moderate	• Central skull base destruction	Originate at the clivus
Chondrosarcoma	Hypointense	Hyperintense	Weak	• Irregular bony destruction • Calcified central matrix	Occur along petroclival suture
Epidermoid cyst (cholesteatoma)	Hypointense	Hyperintense	None	• Erosion of bone	Bright on T2 FLAIR Bright on DWI
Dermoid cyst	Hyperintense	Hyperintense	None	• Erosion of Bone • Calcification	Bright on T2 FLAIR
Arachnoid cyst	Hypointense	Hyperintense	None	• Sculpted bone	Dark on T2 FLAIR
Lipoma	Hyperintense	Hypointense	None	• Lower density than fluid	Suppresses with fat sat
Cholesterol granuloma	Hyperintense	Hyperintense	None	• Smooth expansion of bone	

SUMMARY

A variety of lesions may develop with the CPA. Many of the lesions may grow to substantial size without causing overt symptoms. Cranial neuropathies, most commonly seventh and eighth nerves, are common with lesions of the CPA. Due to the common clinical symptoms at presentation, imaging plays a vital role in differentiating these lesions, determining the extent of disease, and planning treatment. An review of imaging characteristics of these lesions is summarized in Table 159.2. These lesions may be addressed surgically through a variety of approaches that have been developed over the last century. The role of adjuvant therapy in disease of the cranial base is evolving and a multidisciplinary team approach to the treatment of complex cranial base lesions is beneficial to patient care and outcomes.

HIGHLIGHTS

- The CPA is an inverted triangle positioned between the pons and cerebellum within the posterior fossa and may contain pathologic lesions of the 5th to 12th cranial nerves, dura, and vasculature that may be infectious, inflammatory, immunologic, or neoplastic in origin.
- Lesions of the CPA can be classified by the site of origin (extraaxial vs. intraaxial) and imaging characteristics.

- Vestibular schwannomas are the most common lesions of the CPA and may cause unilateral tinnitus, sensorineural hearing loss, disequilibrium and are best demonstrated on MRI contrasted T1 sequences.
- NF2 is caused by mutations on chromosome 22 and characterized by bilateral vestibular schwannomas and may present with multiple CNS tumors such as cranial nerve schwannomas, meningioma, and ependymoma.
- Vestibular schwannomas can be observed clinically with serial MRI scans; however, the majority of tumors exhibit growth and predictors of growth include age at presentation, presence of tinnitus initially, cystic tumors, and growth demonstrated during first year after diagnosis.
- Stereotactic radiation is a viable option for treating vestibular schwannomas and may reliably halt tumor growth; however, minimizing cochlear radiation dose is necessary to limit long-term hearing loss. Radiation treatment of NF2-associated tumors results in a higher percentage of complications.
- Microsurgical resection of vestibular schwannomas may be accomplished safely and is primarily performed through a translabyrinthine approach; however, intracanalicular tumors less than 1.5 cm can be resected through a middle fossa approach in order to preserve hearing.

- Meningiomas within the CPA possess broad dural attachments and commonly engulf or adhere to adjacent cranial nerves.
- Epidermoid and dermoid cysts are hyperintense on T2-weighted images and may be distinguished from arachnoid cysts by their bright appearance on FLAIR sequences. Additionally, dermoid cysts are hyperintense on T1-weighted images.
- Other petrous apex lesions that possess inherent T2 hyperintensity include cholesterol granuloma, chondrosarcoma, and chordoma. Cholesterol granulomas exhibit T1 hyperintensity and smooth bony expansion. Chondrosarcomas erode bone and originate from the petroclival suture while chordomas originate from the clivus and exhibit smooth bony expansion.

REFERENCES

1. Sandifort E. *Observationes anatomico-pathologicae.* Lugduni Batavorum: Apud P.v.d. Eyk et D. Vygh, 1777:116–120.
2. Bell C. *The nervous system of the human body.* Washington, DC: Green, 1833.
3. Ballance C. *Some points in the surgery of the brain and its membranes.* London, UK: Macmillan & Co., 1907.
4. House WF. A history of acoustic tumor surgery, 1900–1917: the Cushing era. In: House WF, Luetje CM, eds. *Acoustic tumors,* Vol 1. *Diagnosis.* Baltimore, MD: University Park Press, 1979.
5. Henneberg, K. Uber "Centrale" Neurofromatese und die Geschwulste des kleinhirnbruckenwinkels (Acusticus neurome). *Arch F Psychiat* 1902;36:251.
6. Cushing H. *Tumors of the nervus acusticus and the syndrome of the cerebellopontine angle.* Philadelphia, PA: WB Saunders, 1917.
7. Dandy WE. An operation for the total removal of cerebellopontine (acoustic) tumors. *Surg Gynecol Obstet* 1925;41:29.
8. Panse R. Clinical and pathological observations. IV. A glioma of the akusticus. *Arch Ohrenh* 1904;61:251.
9. Quix F. Ein Fall von operierter Acusticus-Geschwulst mit Darstellung mikrophotographischer Lichtbilder und Besprechung der Operationstechnik. *Monatsschr Ohrenh* 1915;717–718.
10. House WF. Surgical exposure of the internal auditory canal and its contents through the middle cranial fossa. *Laryngoscope* 1961;71:1363.
11. Wade PJ, House WF. Hearing preservation in patients with acoustic neuromas via the middle fossa approach. *Otolaryngol Head Neck Surg* 1984;92:184–193.
12. Bonneville F, Savatovsky J, Chiras J. Imaging of cerebellopontine angle lesions: an update. Part 1: enhancing extra-axial lesions. *Eur Radiol* 2007;17:2472–2482.
13. Bonneville F, Savatovsky J, Chiras J. Imaging of cerebellopontine angle lesions: an update. Part 2: intra-axial lesions, skull base lesions that may invade the CPA region, and non-enhancing extra-axial lesions. *Eur Radiol* 2007;17:2908–2920.
14. Hoffman S, Propp JM, McCarthy BJ. Temporal trends in incidence of primary brain tumors in the United States, 1985–1999. *Neurooncology* 2006;8(1):27–37.
15. Stangerup SE, Tos M, Thomsen J, et al. True incidence of vestibular schwannoma? *Neurosurgery* 2010;67(5):1335–1340; discussion 1340.
16. Jacob A, Robinson LL Jr, Bortman JS, et al. Nerve of origin, tumor size, hearing preservation, and facial nerve outcomes in 359 vestibular schwannoma resections at a tertiary care academic center. *Laryngoscope* 2007;117:2087–2092.
17. Khrais T, Romano G, Sanna M. Nerve origin of vestibular schwannoma: a prospective study. *J Laryngol Otol* 2008;122:128–131.
18. Xenellis JE, Linthicum FH Jr. On the myth of the glial/Schwann junction (Obersteiner-Redlich zone): origin of vestibular schwannomas. *Otol Neurotol* 2003;24:1.
19. Gruskin P, Craberry J. Pathology of acoustic tumors. In: House WF, Luetje CM, eds. *Acoustic tumors,* Vol 1. *Diagnosis.* Baltimore, MD: University Park Press, 1979.
20. Fundova P, Charabi S, Tos M, et al. Cystic vestibular schwannoma: surgical outcome. *J Laryngol Otol* 2000;114:935–939.
21. Sinha S, Sharma BS. Cystic acoustic neuromas: surgical outcome in a series of 58 patients. *J Clin Neurosci* 2008;15:511–515.
22. Baser ME, Friedman JM, Wallace AJ, et al. Evaluation of clinical diagnostic criteria for neurofibromatosis 2. *Neurology* 2002;59(11):1759–1765.
23. Trofatter JA, MacCollin MM, Rutter JL, et al. A novel moesin-, ezrin-, radixin-like gene is a candidate for the neurofibromatosis 2 tumor suppressor. *Cell* 1993;72:791–800.
24. Rouleau GA, Merel P, Lutchman M, et al. Alteration in a new gene encoding a putative membrane-organising protein causes neurofibromatosis 2. *Nature* 1993;363:515–521.
25. Welling DB, Packer MD, Chang LS. Molecular studies of vestibular schwannomas: a review. *Curr Opin Otolaryngol Head Neck Surg* 2007;15:341–346.
26. Baser ME, Kuramoto L, Woods R, et al. The location of constitutional neurofibromatosis 2 (NF2) splice site mutations is associated with the severity of NF2. *J Med Genet* 2005;24(7):540–546.
27. Stonecypher MS, Chaudhury AR, Byer SJ, et al. Neuregulin growth factors and their ErbB receptors form a potential signaling network for schwannoma tumorigenesis. *J Neuropathol Exp Neurol* 2006;65:162–175.
28. Hansen MR, Roehm PC, Chatterjee P, et al. Constitutive neuregulin-1/ErbB signaling contributes to human vestibular schwannoma proliferation. *Glia* 2006;53:593–600.
29. Hansen MR, Linthicum FH Jr. Expression of neuregulin and activation of ErbB receptors in vestibular schwannomas: possible autocrine loop stimulation. *Otol Neurotol* 2004;25:155–159.
30. Brown KD, Hansen MR. Lipid raft localization of ErbB2 in vestibular schwannoma and Schwann cells. *Otol Neurotol* 2008;29(1):79–85.
31. Doherty JK, Ongkeko W, Crawley B, et al. ErbB and Nrg: potential molecular targets for vestibular schwannoma pharmacotherapy. *Otol Neurotol* 2008;29(1):50–57.
32. Evans DG, Kalamarides M, Hunter-Schaedle K, et al. Consensus recommendations to accelerate clinical trials for neurofibromatosis type 2. *Clin Cancer Res* 2009;15:5032–5039.
33. Ammoun S, Cunliffe CH, Allen JC, et al. ErbB/HER receptor activation and preclinical efficacy of lapatinib in vestibular schwannoma. *Neuro Oncol* 2010;12(8):834–843.
34. Clark JJ, Provenzano M, Diggelmann HR, et al. The ErbB inhibitors trastuzumab and erlotinib inhibit growth of vestibular schwannoma xenografts in nude mice: a preliminary study. *Otol Neurotol* 2008;29:846–853.
35. Plotkin SR, Singh MA, O'Donnell CC, et al. Audiologic and radiographic response of NF2-related vestibular schwannoma to erlotinib therapy. *Nat Clin Pract Oncol* 2008;5(8):487–491.
36. Plotkin SR, Halpin C, McKenna MJ, et al. Erlotinib for progressive vestibular schwannoma in neurofibromatosis 2 patients. *Otol Neurotol* 2010;31(7):1135–1143.
37. Jacob A, Lee TX, Neff BA, et al. Phosphatidylinositol 3-kinase/AKT pathway activation in human vestibular schwannoma. *Otol Neurotol* 2008;29:58–68.
38. Lee TX, Packer MD, Huang J, et al. Growth inhibitory and antitumour activities of OSU-03012, a novel PDK-1 inhibitor, on vestibular schwannoma and malignant schwannoma cells. *Eur J Cancer* 2009;45(9):1709–1720.
39. Komotar RJ, et al. The role of bevacizumab in hearing preservation and tumor volume control in patients with vestibular schwannomas. *Neurosurgery* 2009;65(6):N12.
40. Mautner VF, et al. Bevacizumab induces regression of vestibular schwannomas in patients with neurofibromatosis type 2. *Neuro Oncol* 2010;12(1):14–18.
41. Plotkin SR, et al. Hearing improvement after bevacizumab in patients with neurofibromatosis type 2. *N Engl J Med* 2009;361(4):358–367.

42. Wong HK, et al. Anti-vascular endothelial growth factor therapies as a novel therapeutic approach to treating neurofibromatosis-related tumors. *Cancer Res* 2010;70(9):3483–3493.

43. Kameda K, et al. Effect of tumor removal on tinnitus in patients with vestibular schwannoma. *J Neurosurg* 2010;112(1):152–157.

44. Harner SG, Fabry DA, Beatty CW. Audiometric findings in patients with acoustic neuroma. *Am J Otol* 2000;21(3):405–411.

45. Grauvogel J, Kaminsky J, Rosahl SK. The impact of tinnitus and vertigo on patient-perceived quality of life after cerebellopontine angle surgery. *Neurosurgery* 2010;67(3):601–609; discussion 609–610.

46. Matthies C, Samii M. Management of 1000 vestibular schwannomas (acoustic neuromas): clinical presentation. *Neurosurgery* 1997;40(1):1–9.

47. Caye-Thomasen P, Dethloff T, Hansen S, et al. Hearing in patients with intracanalicular vestibular schwannomas. *Audiol Neurootol* 2007;12(1):1–12.

48. Massick DD, Welling DB, Dodson EE, et al. Tumor growth and audiometric change in vestibular schwannomas managed conservatively. *Laryngoscope* 2005;115:292–296.

49. Pennings RJE, Morris DP, Clarke L, et al. Natural history of hearing deterioration in intracanalicular vestibular schwannoma. *Neurosurgery* 2011;68(1):68–77.

50. Sauvaget E, et al. Sudden sensorineural hearing loss as a revealing symptom of vestibular schwannoma. *Acta Otolaryngol* 2005;125(6):592–595.

51. Nageris BI, Popovtzer A. Acoustic neuroma in patients with completely resolved sudden hearing loss. *Ann Otol Rhinol Laryngol* 2003;112(5):395–397.

52. Welling DB, Packer MD, Chang LS. Molecular studies of vestibular schwannomas: a review. *Curr Opin Otolaryngol Head Neck Surg* 2007;15(5):341–346.

53. American Academy of Otolaryngology–Head and Neck Surgery Foundation, INC. Committee on Hearing and Equilibrium guidelines for the evaluation of hearing preservation in acoustic neuroma (vestibular schwannoma). *Otolaryngol Head Neck Surg* 1995;113:179–180.

54. Robinette MS, Bauch CD, Olsen WO, et al. Auditory brainstem response and magnetic resonance imaging for acoustic neuromas: costs by prevalence. *Arch Otolaryngol Head Neck Surg* 2000;126:963–966.

55. Marangos N, Maier W, Merz R, et al. Brainstem response in cerebellopontine angle tumors. *Otol Neurotol* 2001;22:95–99.

56. Cueva RA. Auditory brainstem response versus magnetic resonance imaging for the evaluation of asymmetric sensorineural hearing loss. *Laryngoscope* 2004;114:1686–1692.

57. Don M, Kwong B, Tanaka C, et al. The stacked ABR: a sensitive and specific screening tool for detecting small acoustic tumors. *Audiol Neurotol* 2005;10:274–290.

58. Tsutsumi T, Tsunoda A, Noguchi Y, et al. Prediction of the nerves of origin of vestibular schwannomas with vestibular evoked myogenic potentials. *Am J Otol* 2000;21:712–715.

59. Diallo BK, Franco-Vidal V, Vasili D, et al. The neurotologic evaluation of vestibular schwannomas. Results of audiological and vestibular testing in 100 consecutive cases. *Rev Laryngol Otol Rhinol (Bord)* 2006;127:203–209.

60. Hamann C, Rudolf J, von Specht H, et al. Vestibular evoked muscle potentials dependency on neural origin and the location of an acoustic neuroma. *HNO* 2005;53:690–694.

61. Goddard JC, Schwartz MS, Friedman RA. Fundal fluid as a predictor of hearing preservation in the middle cranial fossa approach for vestibular schwannoma. *Otol Neurotol* 2010;31(7):1128–1134.

62. Daniels RL, Swallow C, Shelton C, et al. Causes of unilateral sensorineural hearing loss screened by high-resolution fast spin echo magnetic resonance imaging: review of 1,070 consecutive cases. *Am J Otol* 2000;21:173–180.

63. Annesley DJ, Laitt RD, Jenkins JP, et al. Magnetic resonance imaging in the investigation of sensorineural hearing loss: is contrast enhancement still necessary? *J Laryngol Otol* 2001;115:14–21.

64. Harris GJ, Plotkin SR, Maccollin M, et al. Three-dimensional volumetrics for tracking vestibular schwannoma growth in neurofibromatosis type II. *Neurosurgery* 2008;62(6):1314–1319.

65. Gjuric M, Mitrecic MZ, Greess H, et al. Vestibular schwannoma volume as a predictor of hearing outcome after surgery. *Otol Neurotol* 2007;28:822–827.

66. William MD, Antonelli PJ, Williams LS. Middle ear prosthesis displacement in high-strength magnetic fields. *Otol Neurotol* 2001;22:158–161.

67. Fritsch MH. MRI scanners and the stapes prosthesis. *Otol Neurotol* 2007;28(6):733–738.

68. Crane BT, Gottschalk B, Kraut M, et al. Magnetic resonance imaging at 1.5 T after cochlear implantation. *Otol Neurotol* 2010;31(8):1215–1220.

69. Welling DB, Glasscock ME III, Woods CI, et al. Acoustic neuroma: a cost-effective approach. *Otolaryngol Head Neck Surg* 1990;103(3):364–370.

70. Battaglia A, Mastrodimos B, Cueva R. Comparison of growth patterns of acoustic neuromas with and without radiosurgery. *Otol Neurotol* 2006;27(5):705–712.

71. Smouha E, Yoo M, Mohr K, et al. Conservative management of acoustic neuroma: a meta-analysis and proposed treatment algorithm. *Laryngoscope* 2005;115:450–454.

72. Raut VV, Walsh RM, Bath AP, et al. Conservative management of vestibular schwannomas: second review of a prospective longitudinal study. *Clin Otolaryngol* 2004;29:505–514.

73. Massick DD, Welling DB, Dodson EE, et al. Tumor growth and audiologic change in vestibular schwannomas managed conservatively. *Laryngoscope* 2000;110(11):1843–1849.

74. Masuda A, Fisher LM, Oppenheimer ML, et al.; Natural History Consortium. Hearing changes after diagnosis in neurofibromatosis type 2. *Otol Neurotol* 2004;25:150–154.

75. van de Langenberg R, de Bondt BJ, Nelemans PJ, et al. Predictors of volumetric growth and auditory deterioration in vestibular schwannomas followed in a wait and scan policy. *Otol Neurotol* 2011;32(2):338–344.

76. Agrawal Y, Clark JH, Limb CJ, et al. Predictors of vestibular schwannoma growth and clinical implications. *Otol Neurotol* 2010;31(5):807–812.

77. Falcioni A, Piccirillo E, Mancini F. Cystic vestibular schwannoma. *Am J Otol* 2000;21:595–596.

78. Yates CW, Weinberg M, Packer MJ, et al. Fatal case of tumor-associated hemorrhage in a large vestibular schwannoma. *Ann Otol Rhinol Laryngol* 2010;119(6):402–405.

79. Hoistad DL, Melnik G, Mamikoglu B, et al. Update on conservative management of acoustic neuroma. *Otol Neurotol* 2001;22:682–685.

80. Foote KD, Friedman WA, Buatti JM, et al. Analysis of risk factors associated with radiosurgery for vestibular schwannoma. *J Neurosurg* 2001;95(3):440–449.

81. Flickinger JC, Kindziolka D, Niramjan A, et al. Acoustic neuroma radiosurgery with marginal tumor doses of 13 to 13 Gu. *Int J Radiat Oncol Biol Phys* 2004;60(1):225–230.

82. Iwai Y, Yamanaka K, Shiotani M, et al. Radiosurgery for acoustic neuromas: results of low dose treatment. *Neurosurgery* 2003;53(2):282–288.

83. Sakamoto GT, Blevins N, Gibbs IC. Cyberknife radiotherapy for vestibular schwannoma. *Otolaryngol Clin North Am* 2009;42:665–675.

84. Bassim MK, Berliner KI, Fisher LM, et al. Radiation therapy for the treatment of vestibular schwannoma: a critical evaluation of the state of the literature. *Otol Neurotol* 2010;31(4):567–573.

85. Chung WY, Liu KD, Shiau CY, et al. Gamma Knife surgery for vestibular schwannoma: 10-year experience of 195 cases. *J Neurosurg* 2005;102(Suppl):87–96.

86. Delbrouck C, Hassid S, Massager N, et al. Preservation of hearing in vestibular schwannomas treated by radiosurgery using Leksell Gamma Knife: preliminary report of a prospective Belgian clinical study. *Acta Otorhinolaryngol Belg* 2003;57:197–204.

87. Flickinger JC, Kondziolka D, Niranjan A, et al. Results of acoustic neuroma radiosurgery: an analysis of 5 years' experience using current methods. *J Neurosurg* 2001;94:1–6.

88. Flickinger JC, Kondziolka D, Niranjan A, et al. Acoustic neuroma radiosurgery with marginal tumor doses of 12 to13 Gy. *Int J Radiat Oncol Biol Phys* 2004;60:225–230.

89. Foote KD, Friedman WA, Buatti JM, et al. Analysis of risk factors associated with radiosurgery for vestibular schwannoma. *J Neurosurg* 2001;95:440–449.

90. Harsh GR, Thornton AF, Chapman PH, et al. Proton beam stereotactic radiosurgery of vestibular schwannomas. *Int J Radiat Oncol Biol Phys* 2002;54:35–44.

91. Hasegawa T, Kida Y, Kobayashi T, et al. Long-term outcomes in patients with vestibular schwannomas treated using Gamma Knife surgery: 10-year follow up. *J Neurosurg* 2005;102:10–16.

92. Horstmann GA, Van Eck AT. Gamma Knife model C with the automatic positioning system and its impact on the treatment of vestibular schwannomas. *J Neurosurg* 2002;97:450–455.

93. Inoue HK. Low-dose radiosurgery for large vestibular schwannomas: long-term results of functional preservation. *J Neurosurg* 2005;102(Suppl):111–113.

94. Kondziolka D, Lunsford LD, Flickinger JC. Acoustic neuroma radiosurgery. Origins, contemporary use and future expectations. *Neurochirurgie* 2004;50:427–435.

95. Kondziolka D, Lunsford LD, Flickinger JC. Gamma Knife radiosurgery for vestibular schwannomas. *Neurosurg Clin North Am* 2000;11:651–658.

96. Kondziolka D, Nathoo N, Flickinger JC, et al. Long-term results after radiosurgery for benign intracranial tumors. *Neurosurgery* 2003;53:815–821.

97. Linskey ME. Stereotactic radiosurgery versus stereotactic radiotherapy for patients with vestibular schwannoma: a Leksell Gamma Knife society 2000 debate. *J Neurosurg* 2000;93(Suppl 3): 90–95.

98. Linskey ME, Johnstone PA. Radiation tolerance of normal temporal bone structures: implications for Gamma Knife stereotactic radiosurgery. *Int J Radiat Oncol Biol Phys* 2003;57:196–200.

99. Lunsford LD. Vestibular schwannomas. *Neurochirurgie* 2004;50: 151–152.

100. Lunsford LD, Niranjan A, Flickinger JC, et al. Radiosurgery of vestibular schwannomas: summary of experience in 829 cases. *J Neurosurg* 2005;102(Suppl):195–199.

101. Meijer OW, Wolbers JG, Vandertop WP, et al. Stereotactische bestraling van het vestibulair schwannoom (acusticusneurinoom). *Nederlands Tijdschrift voor Geneeskunde* 2000;144:2088–2093.

102. Petit JH, Hudes RS, Chen TT, et al: Reduced-dose radiosurgery for vestibular schwannomas. *Neurosurgery* 2001;49:1299–1306.

103. Roche PH, Robitail S, Thomassin JM, et al. Radiochirurgie Gamma Knife des schwannomes vestibulaires associes a une neurofibromatose de type 2. *Neurochirurgie* 2004;50:367–376.

104. Rowe JG, Radatz MW, Walton L, et al. Clinical experience with Gamma Knife stereotactic radiosurgery in the management of vestibular schwannomas secondary to type 2 neurofibromatosis. *J Neurol Neurosurg Psychiatry* 2003;74:1288–1293.

105. Mathieu D, Kondziolka D, Flickinger JC, et al. Stereotactic radiosurgery for vestibular schwannomas in patients with neurofibromatosis type 2: analysis of tumor control, complications, and hearing preservation rates. *Neurosurgery* 2007;60(3):460–468.

106. Ju DT, Lin JW, Lin MS, et al. Hypofractionated Cyberknife stereotactic radiosurgery for acoustic neuromas with and without association to neurofibromatosis type 2. *Acta Neurochir Suppl* 2008;101:169–173.

107. Roche PH, Robitail S, Delsanti C, et al. Radiosurgery of vestibular schwannomas after microsurgery and combined radiomicrosurgery. *Neurochirurgie* 2004;50:394–400.

108. Flickinger JC, Kondziolka D, Niranjan A, et al. Results of acoustic neuroma radiosurgery: an analysis of 5 years' experience using current methods. *J Neurosurg* 2001;94:1–6.

109. Flickinger JC, Kondziolka D, Niranjan A, et al. Acoustic neuroma radiosurgery with marginal tumor doses of 12 to 13 Gy. *Int J Radiat Oncol Biol Phys* 2004;60:225–230.

110. Paek SH, Chung HT, Jeong SS, et al. Hearing preservation after Gamma Knife stereotactic radiosurgery of vestibular schwannoma. *Cancer* 2005;104(3):580–590.

111. Massager N, Nissim O, Delbrouck C, et al. Role of intracanalicular volumetric and dosimetric parameters on hearing preservation after vestibular schwannoma radiosurgery. *Int J Radiat Oncol Biol Phys* 2006;64(5):1331–1340.

112. Yang I, Sughrue ME, Han SJ, et al. Facial nerve preservation after vestibular schwannoma Gamma Knife radiosurgery. *J Neurooncol* 2009;93(1):41–48.

113. Chopra R, Kondziolka D, Niranjan A, et al. Long-term follow-up of acoustic schwannoma radiosurgery with marginal tumor doses of 12 to 13 Gy. *Int J Radiat Oncol Bio Phys* 2007;68(3):845–851.

114. Regis J, Pellet W, Delsanti C, et al. Functional outcome after Gamma Knife surgery or microsurgery for vestibular schwannomas. *J Neurosurg* 2002;97(5):1091–1100.

115. Pollock BE. Management of vestibular schwannomas that enlarge after stereotactic radiosurgery: treatment recommendations based on a 15 year experience. *Neurosurgery* 2006;58(2):241–248.

116. Arthur BJ, Lamoreaux WT, Mackay AR, et al. Gamma knife radiosurgery for vestibular schwannomas: tumor control and functional preservation in 70 patients. *Am J Clin Oncol* 2010;34(3):265–269.

117. Yang HC, Kano H, Awan NR, et al. Gamma Knife radiosurgery for larger-volume vestibular schwannomas. *J Neurosurg* 2011;114(3):801–807.

118. Hempel JM, Hempel E, Wowra B, et al. Functional outcome after Gamma Knife treatment in vestibular schwannoma. *Eur Arch Otorhinolaryngol* 2006;263(8):714–718.

119. Friedman RA, Brackmann DE, Hitselberger WE, et al. Surgical salvage after failed irradiation for vestibular schwannoma. *Laryngoscope* 2005;115(10):1827–1832.

120. Slattery WH. Microsurgery after radiosurgery or radiotherapy for vestibular schwannomas. *Otolaryngol Clin North Am* 2009;42(4):707–715.

121. Szeifert GT, Figarella-Branger D, Roche PH, et al. Histopathological observations on vestibular schwannomas after Gamma Knife radiosurgery: the Marseille experience. *Neurochirurgie* 2004;50:327–337.

122. Bari ME, Forster DM, Kemeny AA, et al. Malignancy in a vestibular schwannoma. Report of a case with central neurofibromatosis, treated by both stereotactic radiosurgery and surgical excision, with a review of the literature. *Br J Neurosurg* 2002;16:284–289.

123. Shin M, Ueki K, Kurita H, et al. Malignant transformation of a vestibular schwannoma after Gamma Knife radiosurgery. *Lancet* 2002;360:309–310.

124. Bance M, Guha A. Radiation-induced malignant tumors after stereotactic radiosurgery. *Otol Neurotol* 2001;22:124–125.

125. Ganz JC. Gamma Knife radiosurgery and its possible relationship to malignancy: a review. *J Neurosurg* 2002;97:644–652.

126. Kaido T, Hoshida T, Uranishi R, et al. Radiosurgery induced brain tumor. Case report. *J Neurosurg* 2001;95:710–713.

127. McIver JI, Pollock BE. Radiation-induced tumor after stereotactic radiosurgery and whole brain radiotherapy: case report and literature review. *J Neurooncol* 2004;66:301–305.

128. Muracciole X, Cowen D, Régis J. Radiosurgery and brain radioinduced carcinogenesis: update. *Neurochirurgie* 2004;50:414–420.

129. Sanno N, Hayashi S, Shimura T, et al. Intracranial osteosarcoma after radiosurgery—case report. *Neurol Med Chir (Tokyo)* 2004;44:29–32.

130. Shamisa A, Bance M, Nag S, et al. Glioblastoma multiforme occurring in a patient treated with Gamma Knife surgery. Case report and review of the literature. *J Neurosurg* 2001;94:816–821.

131. Yu JS, Yong WH, Wilson D, et al. Glioblastoma induction after radiosurgery for meningioma. *Lancet* 2000;356:1576–1577.

132. Attias J, Nageris B, Ralph J, et al. Hearing preservation using combined monitoring of extra-tympanic electrocochleography and auditory brainstem responses during acoustic neuroma surgery. *Int J Audiol* 2008;47(4):178–184.

133. Phillips DJ, Kobylarz EJ, De Peralta ET, et al. Predictive factors of hearing preservation after surgical resection of small vestibular schwannomas. *Otol Neurotol* 2010;31(9):1463–1468.

134. Arts HA, Telian SA, El-Kashlan H, et al. Hearing preservation and facial nerve outcomes in vestibular schwannoma surgery: results using the middle cranial fossa approach. *Otol Neurotol* 2006;27(2):234–241.

135. Woodson EA, Dempewolf RD, Gubbels SP, et al. Long-term hearing preservation after microsurgical excision of vestibular schwannoma. *Otol Neurotol* 2010;31(7):1144–1152.

136. Sameshima T, Fukushima T, McElveen JT Jr, et al. Critical assessment of operative approaches for hearing preservation in small acoustic neuroma surgery: retrosigmoid vs middle fossa approach. *Neurosurgery* 2010;67(3):640–644.

137. Samii M, Gerganov V, Samii A. Microsurgery management of vestibular schwannomas in neurofibromatosis type 2: indications and results. *Prog Neurol Surg* 2008;21:169–175.

138. Slattery WH III, Fisher LM, Hitselberger W, et al. Hearing preservation surgery for neurofibromatosis type 2-related vestibular schwannomas in pediatric patients. *J Neurosurg* 2007;106 (4 Suppl):255–260.

139. Huy PT, Kania R, Frachet B, et al. Auditory rehabilitation with cochlear implantation in patients with neurofibromatosis type 2. *Acta Otolaryngol* 2008;18:1–5.

140. Vincenti V, Pasanisi E, Guida M, et al. Hearing rehabilitation in neurofibromatosis type 2 patients: cochlear versus auditory brainstem implantation. *Audiol Neurotol* 2008;5(1):128–136.

141. Neff BA, Wiet RM, Lasak JM, et al. Cochlear implantation in the neurofibromatosis type 2 patient: long-term follow-up. *Laryngoscope* 2007;117(6):1069–1072.

142. Charpiot A, Tringali S, Zaouche S, et al. Perioperative complications after translabyrinthine removal of large or giant vestibular schwannoma: outcomes for 123 patients. *Acta Otolaryngol* 2010;130(11):1249–1255.

143. Samii M, Gerganov VM, Samii A. Functional outcome after complete surgical removal of giant vestibular schwannomas. *J Neurosurg* 2010;112(4):860–867.

144. Bennett ML, Jackson CG, Kaufmann R, et al. Postoperative imaging of vestibular schwannomas. *Otolaryngol Head Neck Surg* 2008;138(5):667–671.

145. Brackmann DE, Cullen RD, Fisher LM. Facial nerve function after translabyrinthine vestibular schwannoma surgery. *Otolaryngol Head Neck Surg* 2007;136(5):773–777.

146. Welling DB, Slater PW, Thomas RD, et al. The learning curve in vestibular schwannoma surgery. *Am J Otol* 1999;20:644–648.

147. Neff BA, Ting J, Dickinson SL, et al. Facial nerve monitoring parameters as a predictor of postoperative facial nerve outcomes after vestibular schwannoma resection. *Otol Neurotol* 2005;26(4):728–732.

148. Goddard JC, Oliver ER, Lambert PR. Prevention of cerebrospinal fluid leak after translabyrinthine resection of vestibular schwannoma. *Otol Neurotol* 2010;31(3):473–477.

149. Merkus P, Taibah A, Sequino G, et al. Less than 1% cerebrospinal fluid leakage in 1803 translabyrinthine vestibular schwannoma surgery cases. *Otol Neurotol* 2010;31(2):276–283.

150. Selesnick SH, Liu JC, Jen A, et al. The incidence of cerebrospinal fluid leak after vestibular schwannoma surgery. *Otol Neurotol* 2004;25:387–393.

151. Harsha WJ, Backous DD. Counseling patients on surgical options for treating acoustic neuroma. *Otolaryngol Clin North Am* 2005;38(4):643–652.

152. Levo H, Blomstedt G, Hirvonen T, et al. Causes of persistent postoperative headaches after surgery for vestibular schwannoma resection. *Clin Otolaryngol* 2001;26:401–406.

153. Schaller B, Baumann A. Headache after removal of vestibular schwannoma via the retrosigmoid approach: a long-term follow-up study. *Otolaryngol Head Neck Surg* 2003;128:387–395.

154. Springborg JB, Poulsgaard L, Thomsen J. Nonvestibular schwannoma tumors in the cerebellopontine angle: a structured approach and management guidelines. *Skull Base* 2008;18:217–227.

155. Muto J, Kawase T, Yoshida K. Meckel's cave tumors: relation to the meninges and minimally invasive approaches for surgery: anatomic and clinical studies. *Neurosurgery* 2010;67(3):291–298.

156. Sarrazin JL. Infratentorial tumors. *J Radiol* 2006;87:748–763.

157. Wiemels J, Wrensch M, Claus EB. Epidemiology and etiology of meningioma. *J Neurooncol* 2010;99(3):307–314.

158. Riemenschneider MJ, Perry A, Reifenberger G. Histological classification and molecular genetics of meningiomas. *Lancet Neurol* 2006;5:1045–1054.

159. Kleihues P, Cavenee WK; International Agency for Research on Cancer. *Pathology and genetics of tumours of the nervous system.* Lyon, France: IARC Press, 2000.

160. Ribalta T, McCutcheon IE, Aldape KD, et al. The mitosis-specific antibody anti-phosphohistone-H3 (PHH3) facilitates rapid reliable grading of meningiomas according to WHO 2000 criteria. *Am J Surg Pathol* 2004;28:1532–1536.

161. Shen Y, Nunes F, Stemmer-Rachamimov A, et al. Genomic profiling distinguishes familial multiple and sporadic multiple meningiomas. *BMC Med Genomics* 2009;2:42.

162. Hansson CM, Buckley PG, Grigelioniene G, et al. Comprehensive genetic and epigenetic analysis of sporadic meningioma for macro-mutations on 22q and micro-mutations within the NF2 locus. *BMC Genomics* 2007;8:16.

163. Simon M, Bostrom JP, Hartmann C. Molecular genetics of meningiomas: from basic research to potential clinical applications. *Neurosurgery* 2007;60:787–798.

164. Bostrom J, Meyer-Puttlitz B, Wolter M, et al. Alterations of the tumor suppressor genes CDKN2A (p16(INK4a)), p14(ARF), CDKN2B (p15(INK4b)), and CDKN2C (p18(INK4c)) in atypical and anaplastic meningiomas. *Am J Pathol* 2001;159:661–669.

165. Wernicke AG, Dicker AP, Whiton M, et al. Assessment of epidermal growth factor receptor (EGFR) expression in human meningioma. *Radiat Oncol* 2010;30(5):46.

166. Yang SY, Xu GM. Expression of PDGF and its receptor as well as their relationship to proliferating activity and apoptosis of meningiomas in human meningiomas. *J Clin Neurosci* 2001;8(Suppl 1):49–53.

167. Bindal R, Goodman JM, Kawasaki A, et al. The natural history of untreated skull base meningiomas. *Surg Neurol* 2003;59(2):87–92.

168. McGregor JM, Sarkar A. Stereotactic radiosurgery and stereotactic radiotherapy in the treatment of skull base meningiomas. *Otolaryngol Clin North Am* 2009;42:677–688.

169. Zachenhofer I, Wolfsberger S, Aichholzer M, et al. Gamma-knife radiosurgery for cranial base meningiomas: experience of tumor control, clinical course, and morbidity in a follow-up of more than 8 years. *Neurosurgery* 2006;58(1):28–36.

170. Kreil W, Luggin J, Fuchs I, et al. Long term experience of Gamma Knife radiosurgery for benign skull base meningiomas. *J Neurol Neurosurg Psychiatry* 2005;76(10):1425–1430.

171. Iwai Y, Yamanaka K, Ikeda H. Gamma Knife radiosurgery for skull base meningioma: long-term results of low-dose treatment. *J Neurosurg* 2008;109(5):804–810.

172. Deinsberger R, Tidstrand J, Sabitzer H, et al. LINAC radiosurgery in skull base meningiomas. *Minim Invasive Neurosurg* 2004;47(6):333–338.

173. Hamm K, Henzel M, Gross MW, et al. Radiosurgery/stereotactic radiotherapy in the therapeutical concept for skull base meningiomas. *Zentralbl Neurochir* 2008;69(1):14–21.

174. Natarajan SK, Sekhar LN, Schessel D, et al. Petroclival meningiomas: multimodality treatment and outcomes at long-term follow-up. *Neurosurgery* 2007;60(6):965–979.

175. Lakshmi M, Glastonbury CM. Imaging of the cerebellopontine angle. *Neuroimaging Clin N Am* 2009;19(3):393–406.

176. Bonneville F, Cattin F, Marsot-Dupuch K, et al. T1 signal hyperintensity in the sellar region: spectrum of findings. *Radiographics* 2006;26:93–113.

177. Schiefer TK, Link MJ. Epidermoids of the cerebellopontine angle: a 20-year experience. *Surg Neurol* 2008;70(6):584–590.

178. Moffat DA, Saunders JE, McElveen JT Jr, et al. Unusual cerebellopontine angle tumours. *J Laryngol Otol* 1993;107:1087–1098.

179. Warren FM, Shelton C, Wiggins RH III, et al. Imaging characteristics of metastatic lesions to the cerebellopontine angle. *Otol Neurotol* 2008;29:835–838.

180. Eisen MD, Smith PG, Judy KD, et al. Cerebrospinal fluid cytology to aid the diagnosis of cerebellopontine angle tumors. *Otol Neurotol* 2006;27:553–559.

181. Eichler AF, Loeffler JS. Multidisciplinary management of brain metastases. *Oncologist* 2007;12:884–898.

182. DiMaio S, Mohr G, Dufour J. Distal mycotic aneurysms of the AICA mimicking intracanalicular acoustic neuroma. *Can J Neurol Sci* 2003;30:388–392.

183. Zotta DC, Stati G, Paulis DD, et al. Intrameatal aneurysms of the anterior inferior cerebellar artery. *J Clin Neurosci* 2011;18(4):561–563.

184. Suh SH, Kim DJ, Kim DI, et al. Management of anterior inferior cerebellar artery aneurysms: endovascular treatment and clinical outcome. *AJNR Am J Neuroradiol* 2011;32(1):159–164.

185. Shinn JB, Bush ML, Jones RO. Correlation of central auditory processing deficits and vascular loop syndrome. *Ear Nose Throat J* 2009;88(10):E34–E37.

186. Phillips CD, Bubash LA. The facial nerve: anatomy and common pathology. *Semin Ultrasound CT MR* 2002;23(3):202–217.

187. Sathyanarayana S, Baskaya MK, Fowler M, et al. Solitary tuberculoma of the cerebellopontine angle: a rare presentation. *J Clin Neurosci* 2003;10:120.

188. Bush ML, Pritchett C, Packer M, et al. Hemangioblastoma of the cerebellopontine angle. *Arch Otolaryngol Head Neck Surg* 2010;136(7):734–738.

189. Erickson D, et al. Benign paragangliomas: clinical presentation and treatment outcomes in 236 patients. *J Clin Endocrinol Metab* 2001;86(11):5210–5216.

Sudden Sensory Hearing Loss

160

Eric R. Oliver   *George T. Hashisaki*

Sudden hearing loss is a startling and unsettling experience for the patient. Fortunately, most cases of sudden hearing loss are unilateral, and the prognosis for some recovery of hearing is good. For an unlucky few, the hearing loss can be severe and bilateral. Dilemmas in diagnosis make formulating a rational treatment plan an elusive process, and unfortunately, the diagnosis is commonly delayed. Patients stricken with sudden hearing loss are often frightened and desperate for a cure. There is an emotional burden carried by the physician to provide some definitive assistance. Because sudden hearing loss is a symptom common to many diseases, sifting through the myriad possibilities is a frustrating task.

DEFINITION

Sudden sensory hearing loss is a deceptively simple term, yet the concept defies strict definition. The terms sudden hearing loss, sudden sensory hearing loss, and sudden sensorineural hearing loss (SSNHL) each imply an acute insult of the cochlea and/or retrocochlear structures. Thus, the term SSNHL is perhaps the most accurate to denote this clinical entity. Various investigators have put forth definitions based on the severity, time course, and frequency spectrum of the loss, as well as specific audiometric criteria. The most commonly used definition is a 30-decibel (dB) or greater sensorineural loss over three contiguous frequencies occurring within 3 days (1). Abrupt and rapidly progressive losses have both been encompassed under a single definition. Awakening with a hearing loss, hearing loss noted over a few days, selective low- or high-frequency loss, and distortions in speech perception have all been classified as SSNHL. Taking a broad-minded view, let us consider any noticeable and measurable loss of hearing function—pitch or speech perception—occurring over a matter of minutes to days as a sudden hearing loss. Also, SSNHL encompasses definite etiologies as well as idiopathic causes.

EPIDEMIOLOGY

Estimates of the annual incidence of sudden SSNHL range from 5 to 20 cases per 100,000 persons (2). Because many patients do not seek medical attention after spontaneous resolution, and others are misdiagnosed initially, this incidence figure is an underestimate. Likely, there is an equal distribution of female-to-male cases. Cumulative data from several studies show a slight male preponderance at 53% (1,530/2,864) (2–8); however, another large study of 1,220 patients noted a slight female preponderance, without specifying numbers (9). Gender does not seem to be a risk factor. Several studies have not delineated right versus left ears affected, other than to state an equal distribution. Curiously, from combined study data, it was found that hearing loss affected more left ears (55%) (2–5,7,10). An equal distribution between ears would be expected. Bilateral sudden hearing loss occurs in about 1% to 5% of cases (3–5,7,9–11). Sudden hearing loss occurs in all age groups, but fewer cases are reported in children or the elderly (2,5,6). Middle-aged and young adults experience similar incidence rates (2,5,6,9). The median age at presentation ranges from 40 to 54 years (3–6,8). Acute tinnitus accompanies the hearing loss in most cases, and vestibular symptoms are present in one-fourth to half of patients (3–6,8).

DIFFERENTIAL DIAGNOSIS

SSNHL can be divided into categories of defined causes and idiopathic sudden sensorineural hearing loss (ISSNHL). Defined causes of SSNHL are varied and less common (Table 160.1). Approximately 10% to 15% of cases are due to an identifiable etiology (3,5,12,13). Three main theories exist to explain ISSNHL: viral infection, vascular compromise, and intracochlear membrane rupture. There is additional evidence to support a fourth explanation:

TABLE 160.1	DIFFERENTIAL DIAGNOSIS IN SUDDEN SENSORINEURAL HEARING LOSS

Category	Etiology
Infection	Viral cochleitis, labyrinthitis, or cranial nerve VIII neuropathy
	Herpes simplex
	Mumps
	Varicella zoster (Herpes zoster oticus)
	Rubella
	Influenza
	Epstein-Barr
	Enterovirus
	Cytomegalovirus
	HIV
	Meningitis
	Syphilis
	Lyme disease
Inflammation	Autoimmune
	Cogan syndrome
	Behcet syndrome
	Systemic lupus erythematosus
	Multiple sclerosis
Trauma	Temporal bone fracture
	Acoustic trauma
	Barotrauma
	Perilymph fistula
Neoplasm	Vestibular schwannoma
	Meningioma
	Temporal bone metastasis
	Carcinomatous meningitis
Toxins	Aminoglycosides
	Aspirin
	Cisplatin
	Radiation therapy
Cardiovascular	Thromboembolism
	Macroglobulinemia
	Sickle-cell disease
	S/P coronary bypass graft surgery
	Severe acute hypotension
Otologic	Endolymphatic hydrops
	Meniere disease
Genetic	*GJB2* mutation (*DNFB1*; encoding connexin 26)
	Enlarged vestibular aqueduct in Pendred syndrome
	Branchio-otorenal syndrome
	Renal tubular acidosis
	Fabry disease

autoimmune inner ear disease. With sudden hearing loss as a symptom, a disease process could involve any of these theoretical possibilities. Each theory may explain a number of episodes of SSNHL.

VIRAL INFECTION

Considerable circumstantial evidence implicates viral infection as one cause of ISSNHL. From studies of patients with ISSNHL, this trail of evidence can be traced from reports of a high prevalence of a recent viral type of illness, through evidence of recent viral seroconversion, to temporal bone histopathology. The weakest of these links is the associated history of a recent viral illness. Noncontrolled studies report that 17% to 33% of patients recall a recent viral illness (3,9). Lest those numbers seem significant, 25% of healthy patients visiting an otolaryngology clinic had experienced a potential viral illness within a month preceding the visit (14). Wilson provided good evidence of viral seroconversion by comparing patients experiencing ISSNHL with control patients. Rates of seroconversion for the herpesvirus family were significantly higher in the sudden-hearing-loss population (15). Finally, temporal bone histopathologic studies of patients who experienced ISSNHL found damage in the cochlea consistent with viral injuries (16–19). Loss of hair cells and supporting cells, atrophy of the tectorial membrane, atrophy of the stria vascularis, and neuronal loss were seen; these patterns were similar to findings in documented cases of mumps-, measles-, and maternal rubella–related hearing loss. Viral infection can be implicated as a cause of ISSNHL, but it cannot as yet be proved.

VASCULAR COMPROMISE

The cochlea derives its blood supply from the labyrinthine artery, with no collateral vasculature. Cochlear function is exquisitely sensitive to changes in blood supply (20). Thus, vascular compromise of the cochlea caused by thrombosis, embolus, reduced blood flow, or vasospasm would seem a likely etiology for ISSNHL. The abrupt or rapid time course in sudden hearing loss correlates well with a vascular event. A reduction in oxygenation of the cochlea is the likely consequence of alterations in cochlear blood flow. Alterations in perilymph oxygen tension have been measured in response to changes in systemic blood pressure or intravascular carbon dioxide partial pressure (PCO_2) (21). Histologic evidence of cochlear damage following occlusion of the labyrinthine vessels was documented in temporal bone studies in both animals and humans (19,22). Intracochlear hemorrhage was noted as an early development; subsequently, fibrosis and ossification of the cochlea evolved. It remains unproven whether SSNHL is associated with common cardiovascular risk factors. An association between SSNHL and hypercholesterolemia was revealed in a few case-control series (23–25). SSNHL may be more common and severe in patients with diabetes (26).

INTRACOCHLEAR MEMBRANE RUPTURE

Thin membranes separate the inner ear from the middle ear, and within the cochlea, delicate membranes separate the perilymphatic and endolymphatic spaces. Rupture of either or both sets of membranes theoretically could produce a sensory hearing loss. A leak of perilymph fluid into the middle ear via the round window or oval window has been postulated to produce hearing loss by creating a state of relative endolymphatic hydrops or by producing intracochlear membrane breaks. Rupture of intracochlear membranes would allow mixing of perilymph and endolymph, effectively altering the endocochlear potential. Simmons (27) favored the theory of intracochlear membrane rupture, as did Goodhill and Harris (28); histologic evidence was documented by Gussen (29).

AUTOIMMUNE INNER EAR DISEASE

Sensorineural hearing loss induced by an autoimmune process has gained greater acceptance since the concept was introduced in 1979 by McCabe (30). Progressive sensorineural loss is seen with this condition. Whether or not SSNHL occurs with autoimmune inner ear disease is unclear, but immunologic activity in the cochlea is supported by an expanding body of evidence. The association of hearing loss in Cogan syndrome, systemic lupus erythematosus, and other autoimmune rheumatologic disorders has been well documented.

EVALUATION

Patient evaluation should proceed promptly and expeditiously. Early presentation to a physician and early institution of treatment improve the prognosis for hearing recovery (2,3,5,9). A diligent search for a treatable or defined cause of the sudden hearing loss is an immediate goal. Information about the onset, time course, associated symptoms, and recent activities may give helpful clues. Reviewing the past medical history, especially risk factors for hearing loss, is necessary. All medications, including over-the-counter products, must be delineated. A thorough head and neck examination, with special attention to the otologic and neurologic examination, is a requisite. Pneumatoscopy, in search of a fistula sign, should be included. A cardiovascular examination should also be performed to evaluate for atrial fibrillation, aortic and mitral valve pathology, and carotid bruits.

Pure tone and speech testing are mandatory components of the audiometric evaluation of SSNHL. Immittance (tympanometry and acoustic reflex) testing is recommended to assess for changes in middle ear compliance not visible on otoscopic examination. Auditory brainstem response (ABR) and otoacoustic emissions (OAEs) testing may provide additional information regarding the integrity of the auditory system. The presence of measurable OAEs indicates preservation of some outer hair cell function. The ABR reflects function of the retrocochlear neural pathways. The ABR and OAE results also may assist in diagnosing a functional hearing loss. Vestibular tests are obtained when indicated by the history and physical examination. An exhaustive set of laboratory tests would be overwhelmingly costly. One approach is to obtain those laboratory tests for which the results may influence the treatment plans (Table 160.2).

TABLE 160.2	LABORATORY TESTS AND RADIOGRAPHIC IMAGING IN SUDDEN SENSORINEURAL HEARING LOSS
Test	**Purpose**
CBC with differential	Polycythemia, leukemia, thrombocytosis
Sedimentation rate, ESR	Screen for autoimmune or inflammatory disease; follow with ANA or 68 kD Ab test
FTA-Abs or MHA-TP	Antibody test, *Treponema pallidum*, congenital or acquired
Coagulation studies	Coagulopathy (if indicated, by history)
Thyroid function tests	Hypothyroidism (if indicated, by history)
MRI	Retrocochlear lesion, multiple sclerosis, intracochlear hemorrhage
CT scan	Otic capsule abnormalities in pediatric patients

68 KD Ab, 68 kiloDalton antibody; ANA, antinuclear antibody; CBC, complete blood count; ESR, erythrocyte sedimentation rate; FTA-Abs, fluorescent treponemal antibody-absorption test; MHA-TP, microhemagglutination-*Treponema pallidum*; MRI, magnetic resonance imaging; CT, computed tomography.

At some point during the evaluation and treatment process, an imaging study of the internal auditory canal (IAC) and cerebellopontine angle (CPA) is advised. Approximately 0.8% to 4% of patients with ISSNHL have been diagnosed with IAC or CPA tumors (2,3,9,31–34). A gadolinium enhanced magnetic resonance imaging (MRI) scan is the optimal study to identify IAC and CPA lesions; alternatively, a neurodiagnostic ABR (if hearing levels permit) could be used as a screening test. In addition, MRI scanning can demonstrate evidence of demyelination, intracochlear hemorrhage, or vascular abnormalities (32–35). In younger patients, for whom there is only a small possibility of a vestibular schwannoma but a greater possibility of an anatomic abnormality, a noncontrast temporal bone computed tomography (CT) scan could be obtained. Anatomic defects such as cochlear dysplasia, Mondini malformation, or an enlarged vestibular aqueduct might account for a sudden hearing loss (36).

Because SSNHL is often accompanied with the sensation of aural fullness, the hearing loss is often attributed to the more common conditions of cerumen impaction, acute upper respiratory tract infection with associated middle ear dysfunction, or allergy by primary care providers, and no further investigation is performed. Because a delay in diagnosis and treatment can negatively impact the ultimate hearing outcome, it is essential that all health care providers are capable of differentiating SSNHL from other routine presentations of acute hearing loss. Testing with a 512 Hz tuning fork is very valuable in categorizing the hearing loss as conductive or sensorineural. Referral to an otolaryngologist and audiometric testing should proceed for any patient with a suspected SSNHL.

TREATMENT

The treatment regimens for ISSNHL are legion, and this diversity reflects both the different etiologies that may cause sudden hearing loss and the uncertainty in diagnosis. Primary treatment is guided by the specific cause, if one is identified. As discussed previously, no specific cause is identified in the vast majority of cases, and empirical treatments can be considered. These therapies can be grouped by mechanism of action: (a) anti-inflammatory agents, (b) vasodilators, (c) rheologic agents, (d) antiviral agents, (e) diuretics, (f) triiodobenzoic acid derivatives, (g) hyperbaric oxygen, and (h) surgery.

Anti-inflammatory Agents

Corticosteroids are the primary anti-inflammatory agents used to treat ISSNHL. The mechanism of action of corticosteroids in SSNHL is unknown, although reduction of cochlea and auditory nerve inflammation is the presumed pathway. The typical dosing of oral corticosteroids for SSNHL (prednisone, 1 mg/kg/d, usual maximum 60 mg/day) is tapered over a period of 10 to 14 days. Steroids may also be directly injected into the middle ear space through the tympanic membrane (intratympanic delivery) to permit perfusion into the inner ear via the round window.

Vasodilators

Theoretically, vasodilators improve the blood supply to the cochlea, reversing hypoxia. Histamine, nicotinic acid, papaverine, procaine, niacin, and carbogen have been used in attempts to improve cochlear blood flow. Carbogen (5% carbon dioxide and 95% oxygen) inhalation has been shown to increase perilymph oxygen tension (20,37).

Rheologic Agents

Altering blood viscosity to improve blood flow and oxygen delivery has been the theory behind the use of low-molecular-weight dextrans, pentoxifylline, and the anticoagulants heparin and warfarin. Dextrans cause a hypervolemic hemodilution and affect factor VIII, both effects influencing blood flow. Pentoxifylline allows greater platelet deformability, and anticoagulants interfere with the coagulation cascade.

Antiviral Agents

Acyclovir and amantadine have had limited use in treating ISSNHL, presuming a viral etiology. Famciclovir and valacyclovir are newer agents, similar in structure and activity to acyclovir. Both of these medications have a three-times-daily dosing schedule, as compared to the five-times-daily schedule for acyclovir.

Diuretics

Under the assumption that some episodes of ISSNHL are secondary to cochlear endolymphatic hydrops, diuretic therapy has been used as treatment. As in Ménière disease, the mechanism of action for diuretics in sudden hearing loss is not understood.

Triiodobenzoic Acid Derivatives

These agents are thought to affect the stria vascularis and assist in maintaining the endocochlear potential (8). Diatrizoate meglumine, an angiographic contrast agent, is the most commonly used derivative of triiodobenzoic acid.

Hyperbaric Oxygen Therapy

Therapeutic administration of 100% oxygen at environmental pressures greater than one atmosphere absolute has been proposed to improve ISSNHL by increasing the partial pressure of oxygen delivered to the inner ear. Treatments typically consists of pressurization and administration of 100% oxygen for 1 to 2 hours once or twice daily. A typical course will consist of 20 to 40 treatments (38).

Surgery

Repair of oval and round window perilymph fistulae has been used in cases of ISSNHL associated with a positive fistula test or a history of recent head trauma or barotrauma. Perilymph leaks could produce sudden hearing loss in accordance with the intracochlear membrane rupture theory. Alternatively, low perilymph pressure caused by a fistula could produce a state of relative cochlear endolymphatic hydrops.

RESULTS

Spontaneous recovery rates for SSNHL are generally good. Published rates range from 47% to 63%, combining categories of complete and good or partial recovery (1,5,39). Mattox and Simmons defined complete recovery as a pure-tone average (PTA) less than 10 dB or equaling the uninvolved ear, and good recovery as a PTA less than 40 dB or more than 50 dB improvement from the initial audiogram (5). The recovery rate for these two groups was 63%. For Wilson et al. (1), complete recovery was defined as recovery to within 10 dB of the prehearing loss speech reception threshold (SRT) or PTA. Partial recovery was defined as recovery to within 50% of the prehearing loss SRT or PTA. The unaffected ear was used to establish preexisting hearing levels for the involved ear. Fifty-two patients who had follow-up without treatment had a 58% spontaneous recovery rate. When combined with the placebo group in their study, the spontaneous recovery rate was 47%. Chen et al. (39) found similar rates of spontaneous recovery in their untreated patients, using either the criteria of Mattox and Simmons (5) or Wilson et al. (1).

A review of outcomes for the various therapeutic regimens gives conflicting results. Heterogeneity of inclusion and exclusion criteria, recovery definitions, and follow-up duration confound an accurate comparison of studies. Many studies lack control patients. Selection bias could influence measured outcomes; tertiary referral centers might accrue a different profile of patients than other practices, with some patients having a longer duration of symptoms or more severe hearing losses. Several studies using vasodilator therapy as a component of treatment failed to show significant differences from placebo (4,14); however, Fetterman et al. (3) reported their best recovery results: 63% improved to a PTA greater than 10 dB or speech discrimination greater than 15% when treatment included vasodilators. Based on controlled studies, few data support vasodilator therapy. Studies including low molecular weight dextrans or pentoxifylline did not demonstrate recovery rates better than placebo (7,10,40). Redleaf et al. (8) reported 64% of patients improving, however. They also used diatrizoate therapy, and there was no placebo arm in the study. Cochrane database systematic reviews found no significant role for vasodilator and vasoactive treatments (41), but noted an increased rate of a 25% increase in pure tone average after hyperbaric oxygen therapy (38). However, the authors urged caution when interpreting this result, due to methodologic weaknesses and low patient numbers in the included studies.

Corticosteroid therapy has shown widely varying outcomes. Published recovery rates range from 41% to 61% (1–4,10,39,40). Wilson et al. (1) demonstrated a significant improvement, finding 61% improved on oral steroids compared with a 32% improvement rate on placebo. They stratified their patient groups by audiometric patterns and determined that hearing losses between 40 and 90 dB responded better to steroid therapy; 78% in this severe loss group improved. However, the rate of improvement in the corticosteroid treated cohort was similar to the recovery rate in patients who did not receive treatment in other reports (5,40). Chen et al. (39) also found a significant benefit with oral steroids in a study of 318 patients. They found the greatest magnitude of improvement in patients with greater than 60 dB PTA hearing loss, citing a "floor effect" limiting the degree of improvement in mild hearing losses. Because of the "floor effect," a benefit of oral steroids might be present in those with mild hearing loss, but the effect could not be proven.

A recent Cochrane Review (42), systematic review (43), and meta-analysis (44) each concluded that the efficacy of oral corticosteroid therapy for SSNHL remains unproven. There are limited data comparing various doses or duration of oral corticosteroid therapy. Studies that investigated the correlation between the duration of SSNHL before treatment and hearing outcomes have reported the greatest hearing recovery when oral steroids are initiated within the first 1 to 2 weeks after hearing loss onset, and minimal to no benefit when initiated 4 or more weeks after the onset of symptoms (2,3,45).

Transtympanic steroid application has theoretical benefits of a high delivery concentration to the inner ear and low systemic concentrations. Several studies have addressed the efficacy of transtympanic steroid treatment, but because of differences in delivery technique, corticosteroid, dose, and dosing schedule, direct comparisons are difficult (46–48). Using a transtympanic injection of dexamethasone, Chandrasekhar found that 8 of 11 ears treated had some hearing improvement. The mean SRT improved by 9 dB and the mean speech discrimination or word recognition score (WRS) improved from 61.5% to 77.3% (46). Kopke et al. placed a microcatheter into the round window niche through a tympanomeatal flap and perfused the niche with methylprednisolone. For six patients treated within 4 weeks of the onset of the hearing loss, all experienced some hearing return. The mean PTA improved 50.8 dB, and the mean WRS improved from 1.3% to 62.2% (47). Gianoli and Li applied topical steroids through a ventilation tube in the tympanic membrane. Hearing improvement was seen in 44% (10 of 23 patients) (48). Applying dexamethasone through a porous wick placed inside a ventilation tube, Light and Silverstein found a 10 dB improvement in PTA for 23% and a 15% improvement in speech discrimination for 35% in a study of 48 patients. For the patients experiencing a hearing improvement, the mean PTA improved 43% and the mean WRS improved 51% (49). Haynes et al. investigated transtympanic treatment after failure of systemic oral therapy. With a definition of improvement of 20 dB PTA, the recovery rate was 27.5%. Dramatic hearing recovery in treatment failures was rarely encountered (50).

A multicenter randomized trial comparing the efficacy and safety of oral and intratympanic corticosteroids for primary therapy of unilateral ISSNHL involving 250 patients was recently completed (51). Participants were followed for 6 months. One hundred and twenty-one patients received 60 mg/day of oral prednisone for 14 days with a 5-day taper, and 129 patients received 4 doses over 14 days of 40 mg/mL of methylprednisolone injected into the middle ear. In the oral prednisone group, PTA improved by 30.7 dB compared with a 28.7-dB improvement in the intratympanic treatment group. Recovery of hearing on oral treatment at 2 months by intention-to-treat analysis was 2.0 dB greater than intratympanic treatment. The authors concluded that transtympanic therapy is not inferior to oral steroids. However, oral steroids offer a significant cost advantage over transtympanic delivery.

Given the theoretical implication of viral infection as a cause of ISSNHL, the use of antiviral therapy for ISSHL is a logical extension. A multicenter, randomized, prospective, double-blind trial comparing prednisolone against prednisolone and acyclovir did not show a significant beneficial effect of acyclovir (52). The study size was not large, having 22 patients in each arm of therapy. In patients treated with corticosteroids alone, 80% demonstrated at least a 10-dB

PTA improvement. Tucci et al. (53) did not find a significant benefit from the addition of valacyclovir to concurrent oral prednisone therapy in a larger multicenter, randomized, prospective trial. Two additional studies found no benefit from the addition of antiviral therapy (54,55). Two studies using diatrizoate were reviewed. Wilkins et al. (10) found no significant difference in recovery using diatrizoate in a multidrug regimen, compared with spontaneous recovery rates (1,5). Redleaf et al. (8), using diatrizoate and dextran, reported a beneficial effect: 64% of patients had improvement. Interestingly, using the hearing recovery criteria of Wilkins et al. (10), recalculated data from the Redleaf study indicated only a 36% recovery rate to a classification of complete or good.

Controversy regarding the results of surgical repair of perilymphatic fistulae continues. A universal standard for positive identification of a fistula has not been achieved. Without uniform standards, outcomes of surgical repair are difficult to compare.

PROGNOSIS

Prognostic factors affecting outcome have been postulated. The associated symptoms of vertigo or imbalance seem to portend a lower recovery rate (1–3,8,9). Two studies, in addition, found severe vertigo associated with more cases of high-frequency or profound hearing loss (5,6). This association could be explained anatomically by the close proximity of the basal turn of the cochlea to the vestibule (6). Patient age also may impact recovery, although there are less consistent data across studies. The youngest and the oldest patients may have lower recovery rates.

The likelihood of recovery of hearing has been reported to vary with the severity of hearing loss at presentation and the configuration of the audiogram. Patients with mild losses typically achieve complete recovery, while those with moderate losses often partially recover spontaneously, but rarely realize full recovery unless treated. Those with severe-to-profound hearing losses rarely improve spontaneously or recover fully (1,2,5). Low frequency losses and flat or downward sloping audiograms were associated with a worse prognosis in some studies (5,9,11). Patients with poorer initial WRS, lower initial thresholds at 4,000 Hz, and younger age were more likely to respond to treatments in another study (3). The prognosis for recovery of hearing seems to be worse in older patients and those with associated vestibular symptoms (2,3,5,6,9). The sooner a response is seen, the better the overall prognosis. Patients in whom there is no audiometric improvement within 2 weeks of presentation are unlikely to demonstrate much recovery (56).

CONCLUSIONS

SSNHL remains a puzzling affliction. Given the rate of spontaneous recovery, the prognosis for some hearing recovery is good. It is likely that selection bias affects most studies of ISSNHL; patients with sudden hearing loss and spontaneous recovery within a few days probably will not seek medical evaluation. The true spontaneous recovery rate is unknown.

Treatment should be based on a rational approach. Should no definite or treatable etiology be found, the treatment regimen is dictated by the most likely factors involved. Remembering that the medications used in treatment of SSNHL have potential side effects and the dictum, "Do no harm," the physician and patient must agree on the best course of action.

HIGHLIGHTS

- Sudden sensory hearing loss occurs at an annual incidence of 5 to 20 cases per 100,000 population. Some cases resolve spontaneously and medical attention is not pursued; therefore, the true incidence rate is likely higher.
- The prognosis for some recovery of the hearing loss is good. The spontaneous recovery rate may be as high as 63%.
- There are three generally accepted theories for the pathogenesis of ISSNHL. Viral infection, vascular compromise, and intracochlear membrane breaks are thought to explain most episodes that defy a clear cause. A fourth entity, autoimmune inner ear disease, also may add to the number of cases.
- The evaluation of patients with sudden hearing loss should include a thorough history and physical examination. A diligent search for treatable causes of the hearing loss is very important. Laboratory tests can be useful for this purpose.
- Because 0.8% to 4% of patients presenting with SSNHL may have a CPA mass, a retrocochlear evaluation using MRI with gadolinium or ABR is warranted.
- Many treatment regimens exist, and the rationale behind any particular therapy employed should be understood.
- Since there may be only a 2 to 4 week window for effective treatment of SSNHL, it is important to start therapy as soon as possible.
- There is no single treatment of choice for ISSNHL. Many diseases produce sudden hearing loss, and the treatment should be directed toward the most likely causes.
- Frontline health care workers who encounter patients with complaint of acute hearing loss should determine its character as either conductive or sensorineural, and carry a low threshold for audiometric testing and otolaryngology consultation.

REFERENCES

1. Wilson WR, Byl FM, Laird N. The efficacy of steroids in the treatment of idiopathic sudden hearing loss. *Arch Otolaryngol* 1980;106:772–776.
2. Byl FM. Sudden hearing loss: eight years experience and suggested prognostic table. *Laryngoscope* 1984;94:647–661.
3. Fetterman BL, Saunders JE, Luxford WM. Prognosis and treatment of sudden sensorineural hearing loss. *Am J Otol* 1996;17:529–536.
4. Grandis JR, Hirsch BE, Wagener MM. Treatment of idiopathic sudden sensorineural hearing loss. *Am J Otol* 1993;14:183–188.
5. Mattox DE, Simmons FB. Natural history of sudden sensorineural hearing loss. *Ann Otol Rhinol Laryngol* 1977;86:463–480.
6. Nakashima T, Yanagita N. Outcome of sudden deafness with and without vertigo. *Laryngoscope* 1993;103:1145–1149.
7. Probst R, Tschopp K, Ludin E. A randomized, double-blind, placebo-controlled study of dextran/pentoxifylline medication in acute acoustic trauma and sudden hearing loss. *Acta Otolaryngol (Stockh)* 1992;112:435–443.
8. Redleaf M, Bauer CA, Gantz BJ. Diatrizoate and dextran treatment of sudden sensorineural hearing loss. *Am J Otol* 1995;16:295–303.
9. Shaia FT, Sheehy JL. Sudden sensori-neural hearing impairment: a report of 1,220 cases. *Laryngoscope* 1976;86:389–398.
10. Wilkins SA, Mattox DE, Lyles A. Evaluation of a "shotgun" regimen for sudden hearing loss. *Otolaryngol Head Neck Surg* 1987;97:474–480.
11. Oh JH, Park K, Lee SJ, et al. Bilateral versus unilateral sudden sensorineural hearing loss. *Otolaryngol Head Neck Surg* 2007;136:87–91.
12. Hughes GB, Freedman MA, Haberkamp TJ, et al. Sudden sensorineural hearing loss. *Otolaryngol Clin North Am* 1996;29:393–405.
13. Jaffe BF. Sudden deafness: an otologic emergency. *Arch Otolaryngol* 1967;86:55–60.
14. Mattox DE, Lyles A. Idiopathic sudden sensorineural hearing loss. *Am J Otol* 1989;10:242–247.
15. Wilson WR. The relationship of the herpesvirus family to sudden hearing loss: a prospective clinical study and literature review. *Laryngoscope* 1986;96:870–877.
16. Khetarpal U, Nadol JB, Glynn RJ. Idiopathic sudden sensorineural hearing loss and postnatal viral labyrinthitis: a statistical comparison of temporal bone findings. *Ann Otol Rhinol Laryngol* 1990;99:969–976.
17. Vasama JP, Linthicum FH Jr. Idiopathic sudden sensorineural hearing loss: temporal bone histopathologic study. *Ann Otol Rhinol Laryngol* 2000;109:527–532.
18. Schuknecht HF, Donovan ED. The pathology of idiopathic sudden sensorineural hearing loss. *Arch Otorhinolaryngol* 1986;243:1–15.
19. Yoon TH, Paparella MM, Schachern PA. Histopathology of sudden hearing loss. *Laryngoscope* 1990;100:707–715.
20. Perlman H, Kimura R, Fernandez C. Experiments on temporary obstruction of the internal auditory artery. *Laryngoscope* 1959;69:591–612.
21. Fisch U. Management of sudden deafness. *Otolaryngol Head Neck Surg* 1983;91:3–8.
22. Belal A. Pathology of vascular sensorineural hearing impairment. *Laryngoscope* 1980;90:1831–1839.
23. Aimoni C, Bianchini C, Borin M, et al. Diabetes, cardiovascular risk factors and idiopathic sudden sensorineural hearing loss: a case-control study. *Audiol Neurootol* 2009;15:111–115.
24. Marcucci R, Alessandrello Liotta A, Cellai AP, et al. Cardiovascular and thrombophilic risk factors for idiopathic sudden sensorineural hearing loss. *J Thromb Haemost* 2005;3:929–934.
25. Capaccio P, Ottaviani F, Cuccarini V, et al. Methylenetetrahydrofolate reductase gene mutations as risk factors for sudden hearing loss. *Am J Otolaryngol* 2005;26:383–387.
26. Fukui M, Kitagawa Y, Nakamura N, et al. Idiopathic sudden hearing loss in patients with type 2 diabetes. *Diabetes Res Clin Pract* 2004;63:205–211.
27. Simmons FB. Theory of membrane breaks and sudden hearing loss. *Arch Otolaryngol* 1968;88:67–74.
28. Goodhill V, Harris I. Sudden hearing loss syndromes. In: Goodhill V, ed. *Ear diseases, dizziness, and deafness.* Hagerstown, MD: Harper & Row, 1979:664–681.
29. Gussen R. Sudden hearing loss associated with cochlear membrane rupture. *Arch Otolaryngol* 1981;107:598–600.
30. McCabe BF. Autoimmune sensorineural hearing loss. *Ann Otol Rhinol Laryngol* 1979;88:585–589.
31. Aslan A, De Donato G, Balyan FR, et al. Clinical observations on coexistence of sudden hearing loss and vestibular schwannoma. *Otolaryngol Head Neck Surg* 1997;117:580–582.
32. Schick B, Brors D, Koch O, et al. Magnetic resonance imaging in patients with sudden hearing loss, tinnitus and vertigo. *Otol Neurotol* 2001;22:808–812.
33. Fitzgerald DC, Mark AS. Sudden hearing loss: frequency of abnormal findings on contrast-enhanced MR studies. *AJNR Am J Neuroradiol* 1998;19:1433–1436.
34. Aarnisalo AA, Suoranta H, Ylikoski J. Magnetic resonance imaging findings in the auditory pathway of patients with sudden deafness. *Otol Neurotol* 2004;25:245–249.
35. Shinohara S, Yamamoto E, Saiwai S, et al. Clinical features of sudden hearing loss associated with a high signal in the labyrinth on unenhanced T1-weighted magnetic resonance imaging. *Eur Arch Otorhinolaryngol* 2000;257:480–484.
36. Jackler RK, De La Cruz A. The large vestibular aqueduct syndrome. *Laryngoscope* 1989;99:1238–1243.
37. Rahko T, Kotti V. Comparison of carbogen inhalation and intravenous heparin infusion therapies in idiopathic sudden sensorineural hearing loss. *Acta Otolaryngol Suppl* 1997;529:86–87.
38. Bennett MH, Kertesz T, Yeung P. Hyperbaric oxygen for idiopathic sudden sensorineural hearing loss and tinnitus. *Cochrane Database Syst Rev* 2007;1:CD004739.
39. Chen CY, Halpin C, Rauch SD. Oral steroid treatment of sudden sensorineural hearing loss: a ten year retrospective analysis. *Otol Neurotol* 2003;24:728–733.
40. Cinamon U, Bendet E, Kronenberg J. Steroids, carbogen or placebo for sudden hearing loss: a prospective double-blind study. *Eur Arch Otorhinolaryngol* 2001;258(9):477–480.
41. Agarwal L, Pothier DD. Vasodilators and vasoactive substances for idiopathic sudden sensorineural hearing loss. *Cochrane Database Syst Rev* 2009;4:CD003422.
42. Wei BPC, Mubiru S, O'Leary S. Steroids for idiopathic sudden sensorineural hearing loss. *Cochrane Database Syst Rev* 2006;1:CD003998.
43. Conlin AE, Parnes LS. Treatment of sudden sensorineural hearing loss: I. A systematic review. *Arch Otolaryngol Head Neck Surg* 2007;133:573–581.
44. Conlin AE, Parnes LS. Treatment of sudden sensorineural hearing loss: II. A meta-analysis. *Arch Otolaryngol Head Neck Surg* 2007;133:582–586.
45. Rauch SD. Clinical practice. Idiopathic sudden sensorineural hearing loss. *N Engl J Med* 2008;359(8):833–840.
46. Chandrasekhar SS. Intratympanic dexamethasone for sudden sensorineural hearing loss: clinical and laboratory evaluation. *Otol Neurotol* 2001;22:18–23.
47. Kopke RD, Hoffer ME, Wester D, et al. Targeted topical steroid therapy in sudden sensorineural hearing loss. *Otol Neurotol* 2001;22:475–479.
48. Gianoli GJ, Li JC. Transtympanic steroids for treatment of sudden hearing loss. *Otolaryngol Head Neck Surg* 2001;125:142–146.
49. Light JP, Silverstein H. Transtympanic perfusion: indications and limitations. *Curr Opin Otolaryngol Head Neck Surg* 2004;12:378–383.
50. Haynes DS, O'Malley M, Cohen S, et al. Intratympanic dexamethasone for sudden sensorineural hearing loss after failure of systemic therapy. *Laryngoscope* 2007;117(1):3–15.
51. Rauch SD, Halpin CF, Antonelli PJ, et al. Oral vs intratympanic corticosteroid therapy for idiopathic sudden sensorineural hearing loss. A randomized trial. *JAMA* 2011;305(20):2071–2079.
52. Stokroos RJ, Albers FWJ, Tenvergert EM. Antiviral treatment of idiopathic sudden sensorineural hearing loss: a prospective, randomized, double-blind clinical trial. *Acta Otolaryngol (Stockh)* 1998;118:488–495.

53. Tucci DL, Farmer JC Jr, Kitch RD, et al. Treatment of sudden sensorineural hearing loss with systemic steroids and valacyclovir. *Otol Neurotol* 2002;23:301–308.

54. Westerlaken BO, Stokroos RJ, Dhooge IJ, et al. Treatment of idiopathic sudden sensorineural hearing loss with antiviral therapy: a prospective, randomized, double-blind clinical trial. *Ann Otol Rhinol Laryngol* 2003;112:993–1000.

55. Uri N, Doweck I, Cohen-Kerem R, et al. Acyclovir in the treatment of idiopathic sudden sensorineural hearing loss. *Otolaryngol Head Neck Surg* 2003;128:544–549.

56. Moon IS, Kim J, Lee SY, et al. How long should the sudden hearing loss patients be followed after early steroid combination therapy? *Eur Arch Otorhinolaryngol* 2009;266:1391–1395.

Tinnitus and Hyperacusis

161

Maura K. Cosetti   *Pamela C. Roehm*

Tinnitus, or the perception of sound in the absence of an external auditory source, is a common patient complaint in otolaryngologic practices. Recent studies estimate that tinnitus may affect up to 50 million adults in the United States, with 16 million experiencing frequent or chronic tinnitus in the prior 12 months (1,2). The distinction between nonpulsatile and pulsatile tinnitus and subjective and objective tinnitus are critical in the appropriate diagnosis and management of these patients. This chapter discusses the theories of pathophysiology, epidemiology, assessment tools, and diagnostic and therapeutic considerations associated with each type of tinnitus. As hyperacusis frequently presents in conjunction with nonpulsatile subjective tinnitus, we include a discussion of this condition along with that form of tinnitus. Unfortunately, tinnitus, particularly the more common nonpulsatile subjective form, is frequently dismissed due to the mistaken belief that there is no available therapy for these patients; tinnitus patients are instructed that there is "no pill or surgery" to help them and subsequently discharged. In this chapter, we discuss the various forms of tinnitus, and rational guidelines for their diagnosis and management.

HISTORY AND PHYSICAL EXAMINATION

Classification

Although a variety of tinnitus classification systems have been proposed, there is no currently accepted system in widespread use. At present, the most clinically relevant distinction for the general otolaryngologist is the characterization of subjective versus objective and pulsatile versus nonpulsatile tinnitus. Classification of a patient's tinnitus into these different categories can aid in appropriate diagnosis and management of his or her complaint, and so the patient's history and physical examination should be structured to first determine the answers to these critical questions.

The distinction between pulsatile and nonpulsatile tinnitus is based on the patient's description of the sound that he or she perceives. Further discrimination of pulsatile sounds into arterial (pulsations following the heartbeat) or venous ("whooshing" sounds) can also be based on the patient's description. The distinction between subjective (heard only by the patient) and objective (able to be heard by patient and examiner) is also critical in diagnosis and treatment of tinnitus and is made during the physical examination (3). Objective tinnitus can occasionally be heard without other instrumentation by the clinician (as in patients with tinnitus resulting from mechanical cardiac valves). More commonly, the sound is perceived on auscultation of the periauricular region, ear canal, neck, or chest. Patient confirmation that the sound in question is identical to their tinnitus is required for definite identification. Objective tinnitus is rare and suggests an identifiable source for the acoustic stimulus underlying the tinnitus, such as a vascular bruit, vascular tumor, and palatal or tensor tympani myoclonus (4).

Pulsatile tinnitus can be either subjective or objective, while nonpulsatile tinnitus is almost exclusively subjective. Patients' descriptions of both pulsatile and nonpulsatile tinnitus can vary significantly, so clinical acumen is often required to effectively characterize the type of tinnitus. Typically, nonpulsatile tinnitus is described as "ringing," "hissing," "buzzing," or "roaring." In contrast, sounds characterized as rhythmic, concordant with the patient's pulse, modified by external movements, or altered by changes in position should be classified as "pulsatile" tinnitus.

History

A careful and accurate history of the present illness is crucial for tinnitus characterization and has important implications in both diagnosis and therapeutic management. In addition to differentiating pulsatile from nonpulsatile tinnitus, the history should clarify the location, that is, unilateral or bilateral, onset, duration, intensity, and other elements of the quality of the perceived sound. Modifying factors, such as external movements or position changes, should be identified. Patients complaining of pulsatile tinnitus should be directly asked if the pulsations of their tinnitus concords with their pulse (5). Review of systems should include questioning regarding the patient's mood and sleep patterns, particularly for patients complaining of subjective nonpulsatile tinnitus.

A complete otologic history should be obtained from every tinnitus patient, including associated symptoms of hearing loss, otalgia, otorrhea, autophony, vertigo, imbalance, disequilibrium, and other neurologic symptoms. Past medical history should include prior history of otitis media, otologic or neurosurgical procedures, head trauma, meningitis, exposure to ototoxic medications (including antibiotics, chemotherapeutic agents, and nonsteroidal anti-inflammatory medications), history of autoimmune diseases, and current or prior psychiatric disorders. A list of current medications, including vitamins, herbal supplements, and over-the-counter medications, is necessary. Finally, the clinician should inquire about pertinent family history, such as paragangliomas. Social history should include tobacco, alcohol, illicit drug usage, and intake of caffeine, all of which can cause or increase nonpulsatile tinnitus. Levels of previous noise exposure should be determined.

Physical Examination

A complete head and neck exam should be performed, including otoscopy (by binocular microscopy), pneumatic otoscopy, and tuning fork exam (both the Weber and Rinne). The tympanic membrane should be closely observed for medial and lateral excursions associated with breathing. Patients should be monitored for torsional nystagmus during pneumatic otoscopy (fistula test), preferably with Frenzel lenses in place. The patient should be questioned for vertigo induced during pneumatic insufflation of the ear canal (Hennebert symptom). Cranial nerves should be tested. Additional elements of a neurotologic examination, including cerebellar function, gait evaluation, Romberg and Fukuda testing, and positional testing, should be performed when appropriate.

For patients complaining of pulsatile tinnitus, palpation of the postauricular region, mastoid, and neck should note any thrills or vascular cords. Auscultation of periauricular region, neck, and chest should note the presence of objective tinnitus as well as the presence of any bruits, vascular hums, or murmurs. Light ipsilateral and bilateral neck compression should be performed to assess the effect of decreased jugular venous flow on presence or intensity of the pulsatile tinnitus. In young patients, carotid artery compression can also be attempted with the goal of differentiating venous from arterial causes of pulsatile tinnitus.

Careful exam of the temporomandibular joint and ipsilateral pterygoid muscles should note any tenderness, clicking, or inflammation. Palpation of the pre- and supra-auricular regions should assess for parotid abnormalities or masses. Flexible fiberoptic nasopharyngoscopy should be performed when examination of the eustachian tube (ET) orifice is warranted or when palatal myoclonus is suspected.

Diagnostic Evaluation

The initial evaluation of a patient presenting with tinnitus should include a complete audiogram, including pure-tone and spondee thresholds, word recognition scores, and tympanometry. Often it is useful to perform this test prior to evaluation in the otolaryngologist's office, as it is critical in the determination of the etiology of tinnitus and appropriate therapy. Other audiologic tests, including immittance testing, auditory brainstem responses, otoacoustic emissions, and high-frequency audiograms, may be useful in evaluation of select patients with tinnitus. Testing for vestibular function, (vestibular evoked myogenic potentials [VEMPs], videonystagmography [VNG], and rotational chair testing) may be warranted in the evaluation of patients with specific complaints and findings on physical examination, as discussed below. Similarly, imaging studies may be indicated for certain patients who present with tinnitus, but are not required for all.

SUBJECTIVE NONPULSATILE TINNITUS

Etiology

A variety of clinical entities may underlie nonpulsatile tinnitus. Most often, these conditions cause hearing loss, which is thought to be the initial step in the generation of tinnitus in these patients. Noise-induced hearing loss, presbyacusis, ototoxic medications, labyrinthitis, herpes zoster oticus, Meniere's disease, and genetic hearing losses cause inner ear hair cell damage resulting in hearing loss, which can lead to nonpulsatile tinnitus. Chronic otitis media, cholesteatoma, canal occlusion, and otosclerosis can cause a conductive hearing loss that ultimately may result in tinnitus. Lesions that affect the cochlear nerve and central nervous system (CNS) such as acoustic neuroma, meningioma, multiple sclerosis, and Charcot-Marie-Tooth disease can also induce tinnitus, typically along with a coincident hearing loss (Fig. 161.1, Table 161.1).

However, not every patient with a hearing loss will have tinnitus. Additionally, patients without a discernable hearing loss (including evaluation with a high-frequency audiogram) or other identifiable pathology may suffer from tinnitus as well. Other primary causes of tinnitus include pharmacologic or dietary stimulants, head trauma, and psychiatric disorders. Drugs or stimulants

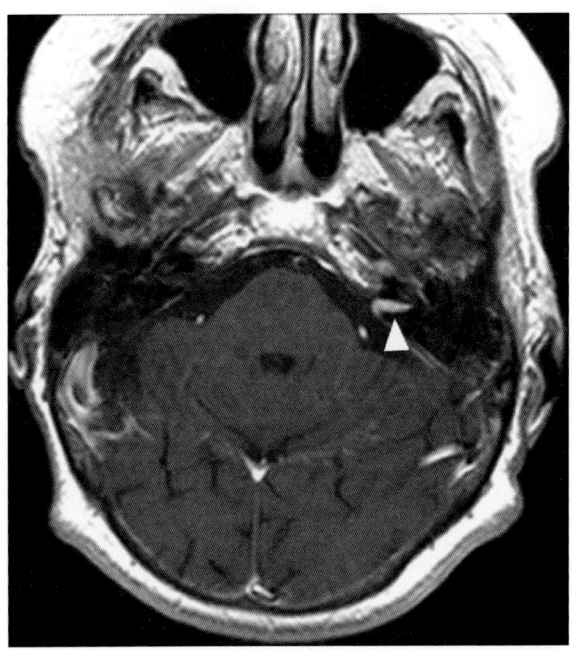

Figure 161.1 Axial contrast-enhanced MRI shows left vestibular schwannoma (*white arrowhead*) that was causing nonpulsatile tinnitus.

Initial theories of the generation of nonpulsatile tinnitus focused on the role of the cochlea, specifically the role of certain cochlear structures such as outer hair cells. These theories flowed logically from observations that subjective nonpulsatile tinnitus is frequently seen in individuals with measurable hearing loss or following known ototoxic injuries (such as ototoxic medication exposure, noise exposure, head injury). However, later findings, such as the persistence of tinnitus following truncation of the auditory nerve or ablation of the cochlea, disproved these exclusively cochleogenic etiologies for the majority of sufferers of subjective nonpulsatile tinnitus (6–8).

More recently, imaging studies on humans with tinnitus and animal studies have revealed changes in neural activity and connectivity throughout the auditory system following loss of hearing. The spontaneous firing rate of auditory neurons increases during tinnitus, a phenomenon that may generate the tinnitus sound (9,10). Another possibility is that increased synchrony of firing within auditory pathway neurons may be perceived as tinnitus (9,11). Many studies have noted a decrease in inhibitory neural input at multiple sites along the central auditory pathways, including the dorsal cochlear nucleus (12–15). This leads to a net increase in excitatory signaling in the auditory pathway and has been proposed as the neurophysiologic basis for subjective tinnitus.

Others have proposed that neuronal plasticity may lead to tinnitus. Following hearing loss, studies in animals and humans have demonstrated a change in the tonotopic map throughout the auditory system. Some have proposed that these plastic changes in the frequency representation in areas of the brain and brainstem are the origin of tinnitus, while others have suggested that these changes in the tonotopic map are merely epiphenomena of that hearing loss (16). Many other plastic changes also follow

which increase neural firing, such as aspirin, nonsteroidal anti-inflammatory medication, nicotine, ethanol, and caffeine, can cause or exacerbate nonpulsatile tinnitus (Table 161.2).

The underlying mechanism of nonpulsatile subjective tinnitus, including the generator of the noise, has not yet been described. Advances in experimental and imaging techniques have revealed significant insights into the etiology of this disorder. These insights may ultimately guide rational treatment of this form of tinnitus.

TABLE 161.1	ETIOLOGIES OF NONPULSATILE TINNITUS		
CN VIII/CNS	Charcot-Marie-Tooth Meningitis Meningioma Multiple sclerosis Vestibular schwannoma	**EAC pathology**	Acquired stenosis Cerumen Foreign body
Dietary	Caffeine Ethanol	**IHC damage**	Genetic HL HZO Labyrinthitis Meniere disease NIHL Ototoxicity Presbyacusis
Drugs	Antibiotics Antidepressants Immune modulators Nicotine	**Middle ear disease**	Cholesteatoma Chronic otitis media Otosclerosis

CN, cranial nerve; CNS, central nervous system; EAC, external auditory canal; HL, hearing loss; HZO, herpes zoster oticus; IHC, inner hair cell; NIHL, noise-induced hearing loss.

TABLE 161.2	MEDICATIONS THAT CAN CAUSE NONPULSATILE TINNITUS			
Antibiotics	Aminoglycosides Macrolides Vancomycin	**Immune modulators**	Infergen Mycophenolate Sirolimus Soriatane Tacrolimus
Antidepressants	TCAs SSRIs SNRIs	**NSAIDs**	Ibuprofen
Antimalarials	Quinine	**Salicylates**	Aspirin
Chemotherapeutics	Cisplatinin	**Misc.**	Caffeine Nicotine Prevacid
Loop diuretics	Ethacrynic acid Lasix		

Misc., miscellaneous; NSAIDs, non-steroidal anti-inflammatory drugs; SNRIs, serotonin-norepinephrine reuptake inhibitors; SSRIs, selective serotonin reuptake inhibitors; TCAs, tricyclic antidepressants.

deafferentation of areas of the auditory system, including changes in synaptic structure and firing patterns, formation of new synapses and elimination of others, and dendritic branching. All of these changes may underlie the complaint of nonpulsatile tinnitus (16).

None of these etiologies address patients with complaints of tinnitus who fall into two categories encountered in clinical practice. One is the patient who has had hearing loss for years and yet awakens suddenly with tinnitus. The other is the rare patient who has normal hearing, even in the ultra-high frequencies, no other dietary or toxic risk factors, and no psychiatric comorbidities who complains of tinnitus. For these patients, careful history-taking may uncover a traumatic or emotional event that was coincident with the onset of their tinnitus. Similarities between tinnitus and phantom limb pain have fueled the

hypothesis that both are "aversive memory networks." According to this theory, the phantom awareness (tinnitus) only becomes conscious when linked to other brain networks, and then becomes bothersome when linked by learned associations with unpleasant emotions (17).

Risk Factors

The most prevalent risk factor for subjective, nonpulsatile tinnitus is hearing loss. As discussed above, hearing loss may be the initial instigating factor underlying nonpulsatile tinnitus. Frequently this hearing loss includes significant sensorineural losses at higher frequencies; occasionally, the hearing loss can only be detected using a high-frequency audiogram (Fig. 161.2). Of note, not every patient with hearing loss will have complaints of tinnitus,

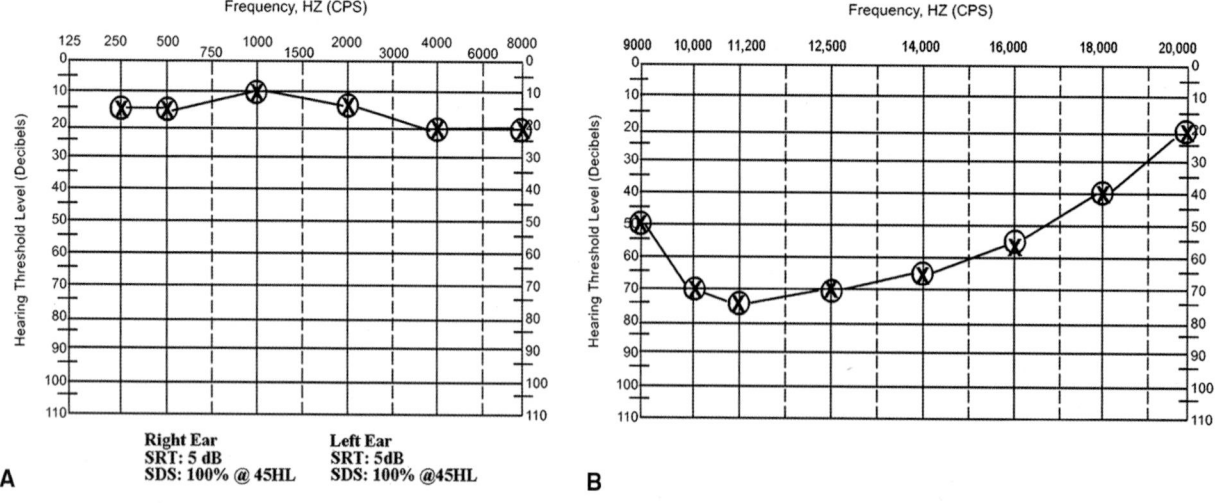

Figure 161.2 Normal **(A)** and high-frequency **(B)** audiograms of a patient with nonpulsatile tinnitus, demonstrating normal hearing from 250 to 8,000 Hz and a very-high-frequency bilateral hearing loss.

and in fact, at least 27% of patients with profound sensorineural hearing loss (SNHL) will not have tinnitus (18). Meniere's disease is associated with nonpulsatile tinnitus that typically worsens during acute vertiginous episodes. Conductive or mixed hearing loss can also be associated with tinnitus, including that caused by otosclerosis, ossicular discontinuities, or obstruction of the external auditory canal by cerumen or other factors.

Other risk factors for nonpulsatile tinnitus include intake of certain dietary, medicinal, and illicit substances. For instance, caffeine, aspirin, ibuprofen, and nicotine can cause tinnitus or exacerbate preexisting tinnitus. Even if the individual patient has used these substances previously, changes in intake patterns due to shift work, injury, or changes in metabolism due to aging can lead to worsened tinnitus.

Hyperacusis

Hyperacusis, or increased sensitivity to sound, is often seen in the context of tinnitus. Patients will complain of discomfort or pain in the presence of sounds that are typically tolerated by normal people, including car horns, sounds associated with cooking, and even loud conversations. Sometimes this sound intolerance will be limited to certain frequencies. As the patient continues to experience hyperacusis, the threshold of sound intensity required to cause discomfort may decrease. In severe cases, patients may significantly alter their behavior (wear ear muffs in public, avoid going outdoors) in order to avoid the discomfort and pain caused by exposure to these sounds. Often, hyperacusis is associated with hearing loss (19).

For patients with hearing loss, intolerance to loud sounds may result from overrepresentation of the sound frequencies bordering a hearing loss in the central auditory system (recruitment). Exposure to these sound frequencies causes intolerable overstimulation of the auditory cortex due to recruitment. A second possibility is that hyperacusis results from selective loss of efferent input to the inner ear. These efferents are critical in regulating basilar membrane excursion and firing of afferent eighth nerve fibers in response to a sound stimulus (20).

Patients may develop hyperacusis following a single exposure to a sudden loud noise (e.g., gunshot, car airbag deployment) in the absence of a detectable hearing loss. Other potential etiologies for hyperacusis in the absence of hearing loss include head trauma, migraine, depression, Bell's palsy, Ramsay Hunt Syndrome, Lyme disease, Addison's disease, and following stapes surgery (19,20). Hyperacusis is seen in over 80% of patients with Williams syndrome, a genetic disorder characterized by craniofacial and dental anomalies, mental retardation, hypertension, cardiovascular disease, and perfect pitch (21,22).

Mild hyperacusis can be managed by avoidance of sounds that stimulate an unpleasant reaction (19). Thus for hearing aid users with hyperacusis, the maximum comfort level should be utilized in programming their aids. Further treatment is required for patients with severe hyperacusis that affects their activities of daily living. For these patients, tinnitus retraining therapy (TRT) can be extremely effective in increasing their tolerance to everyday sounds (23).

Diagnostic Evaluation

Patients with nonpulsatile, subjective tinnitus should always have a standard, complete audiogram performed as the initial step in their evaluation, as discussed above. For patients with complaints of bilateral tinnitus who have a normal standard audiogram (up to and including 8,000 Hz pure tone thresholds), a high-frequency audiogram may be useful in determining the etiology of tinnitus, particularly in patients with no other risk factors.

Magnetic resonance imaging (MRI) of the brain and brainstem with gadolinium is a requisite test for patients with unilateral tinnitus (Fig. 161.3). Even in the presence of

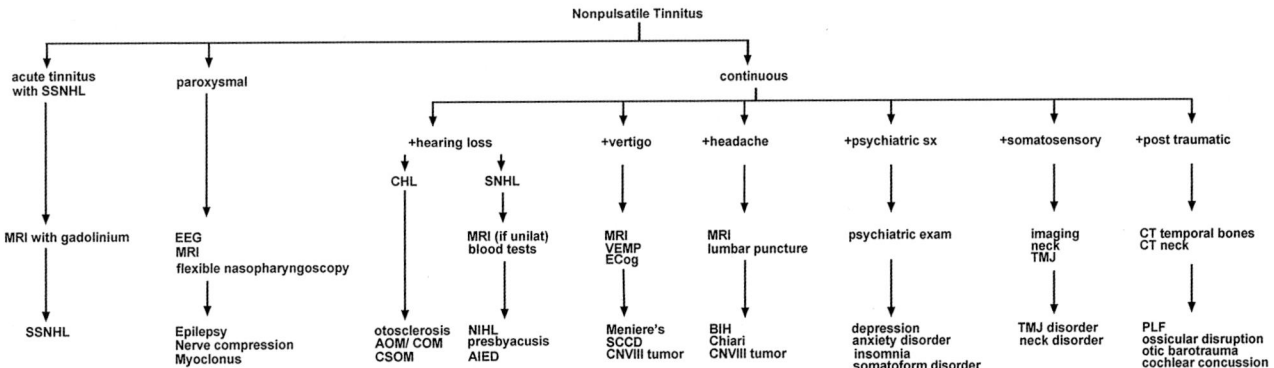

Figure 161.3 Algorithm for evaluation of nonpulsatile tinnitus. Modified from the Tinnitus Research Initiative diagnosis and treatment of tinnitus (24). AIED, autoimmune inner ear disease; AOM, acute otitis media; BIH, benign intracranial hypertension; CHL, conductive hearing loss; CN cranial nerve; COM, chronic otitis media; CSOM, chronic serous otitis media; CT, computed tomography; ECog, electrocochleography; EEG, electroencephalogram; VEMP, vestibular evoked myogenic potential; MRI, magnetic resonance image; PLF, perilymphatic fistula; SCCD, semicircular canal dehiscence; SSNHL, sudden sensorineural hearing loss; sx, symptoms; TMJ, temporomandibular joint; unilat, unilateral; NIHL, noise-induced hearing loss.

normal or symmetrical hearing, patients with unilateral tinnitus may have a vestibular schwannoma or other intracranial anomaly requiring further treatment (25) (Fig. 161.1). The complete evaluation of patients with symptoms consistent with Meniere's disease also should include an MRI.

Treatment

Occasionally, treatment of an underlying pathology causing hearing loss will alleviate nonpulsatile tinnitus. For instance, removal of cerumen or a foreign body may alleviate both the hearing loss and tinnitus associated with occlusion of the external auditory canal. Stapedectomy for a patient with otosclerosis in the absence of a significant sensorineural loss may alleviate his or her tinnitus. Decreased caffeine or aspirin intake may substantially improve or alleviate tinnitus in patients ingesting high levels of these substances.

These rapid cures are not possible for the majority of patients presenting with the primary complaint of nonpulsatile tinnitus. Management options for these patients include hearing aids, tinnitus maskers, TRT, biofeedback, electrical or magnetic stimulation, pharmacotherapy, and cochlear implantation.

Amplification

The majority of patients with subjective tinnitus have a significant hearing loss. Use of a well-fitted hearing aid can improve subjective tinnitus in 50% of patients with hearing loss and tinnitus. Hearing aids increase the ambient noise perceived by the patient, thus masking the tinnitus (26). Additionally, restoration of auditory input within the lost frequencies, particularly those matching the frequency spectrum of the tinnitus, lead to central auditory plasticity, which can decrease tinnitus. Ideally, patients with bilateral subjective tinnitus should be fitted with bilateral hearing aids that include a wide, high-frequency amplification band and open ear mold. The open mold will decrease the occlusion effect, and extend amplification at higher frequencies. Ideal hearing aid settings for a patient with hearing loss and tinnitus would include an omnidirectional microphone, a lower compression point, disabled digital noise reduction, and active digital feedback cancellation (26).

Tinnitus Masking

Nonpulsatile and pulsatile tinnitus sounds can sometimes be covered (or masked) by external sounds, thus blocking the tinnitus percept and the unpleasant sensations associated with these sounds. To use this therapy effectively, the physician or therapist needs to exclude patients for whom the tinnitus cannot be masked, the masking sound is perceived as worse than the tinnitus sound, or the tinnitus sound is tolerable as it is (27,28). For many patients, use of environmental sounds such as a noise generator or radio can effectively and inexpensively mask their tinnitus. However, in certain situations, use of such environmental

sounds may not be appropriate. Use of an ear-level tinnitus masker, a small device that makes a sound matched to the tinnitus sound the patient perceives, yields total relief for 6% of patients and partial relief for 23% to 64% of patients (27,29). The addition of masking tones to amplifications from a hearing aid can mask tinnitus sounds more effectively than a hearing aid alone (30).

For most patients, masking sounds include many of the frequencies of their hearing loss (29). Occasionally, use of masking sounds can lead to residual inhibition, or cessation of the tinnitus sound, for a period of seconds to hours (29). Residual inhibition is hypothesized to result from inhibition of synchronous activity within the auditory pathway from masking sounds that lie within the frequencies affected by hearing loss being presented above the minimal masking threshold (29). Some proponents of other therapies for tinnitus, particularly TRT, feel that tinnitus maskers may prevent habituation to the tinnitus perception and can therefore impede these patients' ultimate recovery (31). Certainly, those who benefit from tinnitus maskers require ongoing use of the masker to manage their tinnitus, especially if this is their sole treatment strategy (27,29).

Tinnitus Retraining Therapy

TRT is an effective management strategy for both subjective tinnitus and hyperacusis. TRT is based on the concept that habituation to the unpleasant stimulus can minimize the reactions that these patients experience (Fig. 161.4). Up to 80% of patients experience tinnitus without a significant unpleasant association; and tinnitus severity is not equal to the intensity of the perceived stimulus. For patients with complaints of significant tinnitus, Jastreboff hypothesized that an initial link is made between the tinnitus percept and unpleasant limbic and autonomic reactions that lead to an unconscious linkage between the tinnitus sound and the reaction (31). Since habituation to unpleasant stimuli

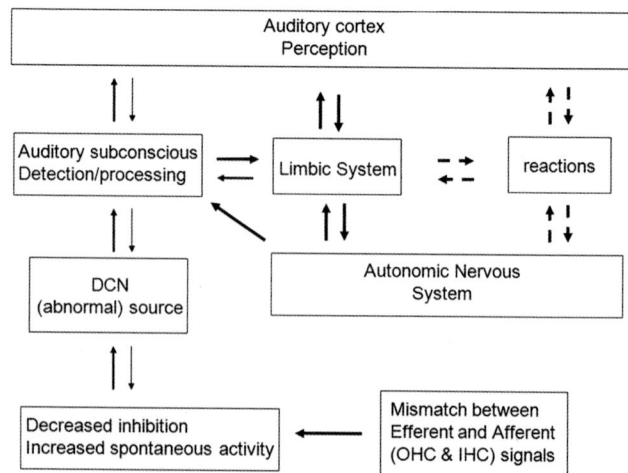

Figure 161.4 Hypothesized neural network underlying tinnitus generation according to Jastreboff (30). This pathway forms the theoretical foundation for TRT.

occurs all the time, Jastreboff surmised that habituation to tinnitus perceptions can occur as well (Fig. 161.4). Unlike other therapies for tinnitus, TRT does not seek to reduce production of the tinnitus sound but instead attempts to change the linkage between the tinnitus perception and autonomic and limbic systems using extensive counseling and sound therapy. Counseling attempts to reclassify tinnitus as a neutral stimulus and is felt to be necessary to allow habituation. Sound therapy decreases abnormal neural activity causing tinnitus and can also be an effective means to decrease hyperacusis via exposure and habituation. Studies have shown that completion of a 12-month course of TRT can decrease scores on the Tinnitus Handicap Index, a validated scale of tinnitus severity, by up to 80% (reviewed in [31]).

Neuromonics

Based on success with tinnitus maskers and counseling, investigators sought to incorporate both phenomena into treatment for tinnitus. The Neuromonics device uses sound therapy, extensive tinnitus education, and cognitive therapy to treat patients with tinnitus. Patients begin their therapy by listening to preprocessed mixed "calming music" (a combination of baroque and new age) combined with noise mixed by proprietary algorithm for 2 to 4 hours daily. The sound spectrum of this noise is shaped according to patient's audiogram to compensate for hearing loss. Over 6 to 24 months, the noise sounds are gradually decreased. The underlying rationale is that initial wide frequency stimulation will counter the auditory deprivation resulting from preexisting hearing loss, pleasant and calming sounds counter negative feedback from the limbic system, and matched tinnitus tones also incorporated into the program will lead to gradual desensitization (32). Following completion of therapy, up to 77% of patients report improvement of their tinnitus (33).

Cochlear Implantation

Up to 80% of cochlear implant recipients have moderate to severe tinnitus. All studies examining tinnitus in cochlear implant recipients show an improvement following unilateral multichannel implantation in most implantees (60% to 90%), with some recipients exhibiting improvement of contralateral tinnitus through residual inhibition (34–38). Some patients, however, experience new onset or increased severity of their tinnitus following cochlear implantation (34,35,39). Worsening of preexisting tinnitus and development of new-onset tinnitus is more common in the setting of bilateral cochlear implantation (40).

Pharmacotherapy

A wide variety of standard medications and herbal supplements have been used by patients to reduce or alleviate their tinnitus, including anesthetic agents (IV lidocaine), anticonvulsants, antidepressants, antihistamines, benzodiazepines, diuretic, GABA agonists (Baclofen), Ginko biloba

extracts, histamine, steroids, and vitamins. Of these, only a few agents have been shown to be effective agents at consistently improving patients' perceptions of their tinnitus: IV lidocaine, antidepressants, and steroids.

Lidocaine, an amine-type local anesthetic and class 1B antiarrhymic drug, blocks voltage gated sodium channels and has effects on the firing of a number of other neuronal channels. Lidocaine suppresses tinnitus in 40% to 80% of patients. Sites of action are located in both the cochlea and CNS. Intravenous lidocaine may be effective up to 4 weeks following injection, despite an elimination half-time of 90 to 120 minutes in most patients (41). Intratympanic injection of lidocaine is also effective for treatment of tinnitus, but the high incidence of vestibular side effects limit its use (42).

Antidepressants have been tested in a number of trials for the treatment of nonpulsatile tinnitus, including at least five double-blind placebo controlled studies (42,43). These studies are characterized by varying entry criteria, including the duration and severity of tinnitus, drug used, duration of its use, assessment of efficacy, and presence or absence of depression in trial participants. Often these trials were not assessed on an intention to treat basis. Drugs studied include nortriptyline, paroxetine, sertraline, and trimipramine. Overall, however, patients with anxiety, depression, and more severe tinnitus are more likely to benefit from use of these medications (42,44).

Steroids, either intratympanic or orally administered, have been described as an effective method of control of tinnitus for patients with Meniere's disease (42). However, the majority of trials of steroid therapy for Meniere's disease utilized control of vertigo as their primary outcome measure. In these trials, control of tinnitus was a secondary or tertiary outcome measure. Intratympanic steroids were shown to be ineffective for treatment of subjective tinnitus in a randomized control trial of 70 patients (45).

A number of dietary supplements and vitamins have been used to treat tinnitus, including multivitamins (A, B1, B3, B6, B9, C, E, magnesium, manganese, selenium, and zinc), antioxidants (flavonoids, Coenzyme Q, carotenoids) and herbal remedies (ginko biloba, cimicifuga racemosa, cornus officinalis, verbascum desiflorum, yoku-kan-san). Although typically considered harmless, these supplements may have significant side effects and may interact with prescription medications. Typically, there is little evidence of efficacy, and often they can be costly (42).

Microvascular Decompression

Vascular compression of the vestibulocochlear nerve (CN VIII) as a cause of nonpulsatile or pulsatile tinnitus is highly controversial. In 1975, Jannetta proposed that tinnitus, vertigo, and SNHL could be attributed to vascular compression of CN VIII from redundant loops of the anterior inferior cerebellar artery in the cerebellopontine angle (46). Recent MRI studies documenting frequent, asymptomatic contact between a vascular loop and

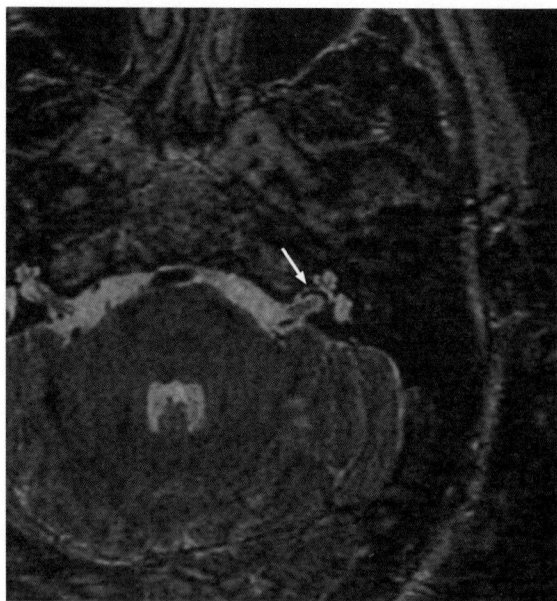

Figure 161.5 Axial MRI using CISS demonstrates a left-sided vascular loop within the IAC (*white arrow*).

TABLE 161.3	ETIOLOGIES OF PULSATILE TINNITUS		
Vascular		**Developmental**	ETD
Venous	Jugular bulb anomalies		Paget disease
	Idiopathic intra-cranial HTN		Otitis media
	Dural venous sinus aneurysm	**Infectious**	Serous otitis media
	Condylar/mastoid vein anomalies		Glomus tumors
	Transverse/ sigmoid sinus stenosis	**Neoplastic**	Hemangiomas Intracranial tumors
Arterial	Atherosclerosis	**Misc.**	SSC dehiscence
	Dural AVM		Otosclerosis
	Carotid artery anomalies		Palatal/M.E. myoclonus
	Vascular compression		
	Aneurysm		
	Hyperdynamic flow state		

AVM, arteriovenous malformations; ETD, Eustachian tube dysfunction; HTN, hypertension; ME, middle ear; SSC, semicircular canal.

CN VIII dispute the existence of this syndrome and caution against microvascular decompression surgery (47). Nevertheless, reports of efficacious microvascular decompression of the vestibulocochlear nerve suggest surgical treatment of vascular loop syndrome may be useful for some patients (48,49). Vascular loops are best identified on MRI using constructive interference in the steady state (CISS) sequences (Fig. 161.5).

Other Therapies

A variety of other therapies have been successfully used for the treatment of nonpulsatile tinnitus in studies of small groups of patients. Neurofeedback strategies can decrease perception of tinnitus sounds in patients who are able to modulate their brain activity patterns (50). Both repetitive transcranial magnetic stimulation and transcranial direct current stimulation have been demonstrated to decrease perceived tinnitus intensity in study participants in double blind placebo control studies (51,52).

PULSATILE TINNITUS

Etiology

There are numerous causes of pulsatile tinnitus. Arterial and venous etiologies are by far the most common. Vascular tumors of the temporal bone, such as tympanic and jugular paragangliomas, vascular malformations, dehiscent jugular bulb, jugular diverticula, and vascular loops of the internal auditory canal (IAC) can present with unilateral pulsatile tinnitus. Nonvascular etiologies include palatal or middle ear myoclonus, dehiscent semicircular canal (superior, lateral, or posterior), benign intracranial

hypertension, otosclerosis, middle ear effusion or ossicular abnormalities, temporomandibular joint dysfunction, and patulous ET (Table 161.3). However, for a substantial percentage of patients with pulsatile tinnitus, a definite etiology cannot be identified despite thorough evaluation. Following a brief section on diagnostic evaluation, we discuss individual etiologies of pulsatile tinnitus and their corresponding treatment options.

DIAGNOSTIC EVALUATION

Patients with complaints of tinnitus should have a behavioral audiogram including air and bone conduction with appropriate masking, speech discrimination testing, immittance testing including tympanograms and acoustic reflex testing. VEMP should be considered when a semicircular canal dehiscence (SCD) is suspected. VNG- or electronystagmography (ENG), and quantitative measurement of middle ear compliance should be employed in circumstances warranting these tests (53).

A variety of imaging techniques, including carotid Doppler ultrasonography or duplex scan, computed tomography (CT), CT angiography (CTA), MRI, MR angiography (MRA), MR venography (MRV), and the use of four-vessel angiography, have a role in the evaluation of pulsatile tinnitus. Despite combined testing with a variety of these imaging modalities, definitive diagnosis of the etiology underlying pulsatile tinnitus is possible in only 68% to 72% of patients (4,54,55).

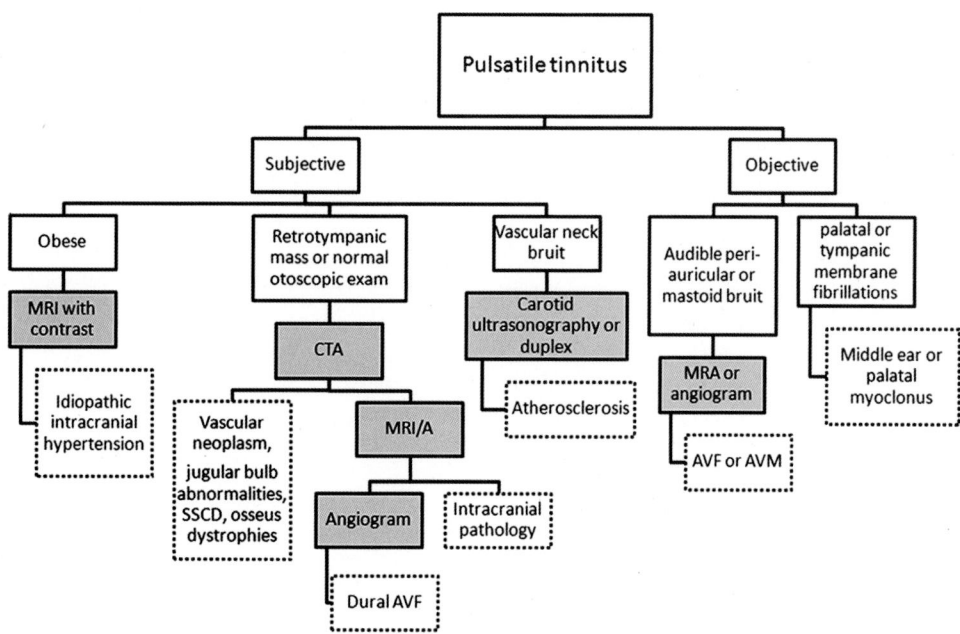

Figure 161.6 Algorithm for evaluation of pulsatile tinnitus. Modified from Mattox (4). AVF, arteriovenous fistula; AVM, arteriovenous malformation; CTA, computed tomography angiography; MRA, magnetic resonance angiography; MRI, magnetic resonance imaging.

Many algorithms have been formulated to guide use of radiologic testing. Mattox and Hudgins (4) (2008) proposed an algorithm based on patient symptoms and physical exam findings (Fig. 161.6). Patients with a visible vascular mass on otoscopic microscopy or a family history of paraganglioma should undergo CT of the temporal bone with intravenous contrast (Fig. 161.7). Patients with a normal middle ear exam and an audible vascular neck bruit should first undergo carotid Doppler ultrasonography or a CTA of the neck to assess for carotid atherosclerotic disease. Patients with suspected arterial vascular disease should still be evaluated with radiologic imaging despite a negative neck exam, because hemodynamically significant stenoses may be present without audible vascular bruits (4). Initial evaluation with CTA of the neck and temporal bones is also appropriate in patients whose tinnitus is modified by moderate neck compression suggesting a venous etiology. CTA allows evaluation of both arterial and venous vasculature as well as the fine bony structure of the temporal bone, allowing diagnosis of anatomic abnormalities such as dehiscent jugular bulb in addition to vascular etiologies. Patients presenting with symptoms of pulsatile tinnitus and autophony suggesting a diagnosis of SCD or patulous ET should be evaluated with high resolution, noncontrast CT of the temporal bone with images reformatted in coronal and Poschel's and Stenver's views (56) (Fig. 161.8). Primary use of MRA/MRV in the evaluation of patients with pulsatile tinnitus has fallen from favor as both the vascular and bony anatomy of the temporal bone is superior with CT angiography, although these tests still have a role in the evaluation of patients who are unable to receive or refuse

iodinated contrast (4,57). Because CTA is unable to identify small dural arteriovenous malformations (AVMs), negative CTA studies may be followed by four-vessel angiography (4,54,55). Use of four-vessel angiography does not guarantee diagnosis, however, and should be used judiciously due to the risks of the procedure. In a study of 54 patients with pulsatile tinnitus, 44 were definitively diagnosed on CTA. Out of the 10 patients with negative CTAs, the four-vessel angiogram identified the definitive diagnosis (carotid dissection) in only 1 patient. In obese patients presenting with pulsatile tinnitus, some authors advocate for MRI as the initial imaging study to assess for presence of benign intracranial hypertension (pseudotumor cerebri) (4).

Vascular Anomalies

Abnormalities of the intracranial venous system are the most common radiologic finding in patients with pulsatile tinnitus and a normal middle ear exam. The most commonly reported anomalies are high or dehiscent jugular bulbs and sigmoid sinus diverticula (Fig. 161.9). Cervical atherosclerotic disease is the most common arterial etiology of pulsatile tinnitus (4,5,54,55).

Anomalies of the Jugular Bulb

Jugular bulb anomalies, including dehiscent high-riding jugular bulbs and jugular bulb diverticula, are frequently associated with tinnitus of venous origin (Fig. 161.9). Anatomically, the jugular bulb represents the junction between the proximal internal jugular vein and the sigmoid sinus at the skull base. High-riding jugular bulbs

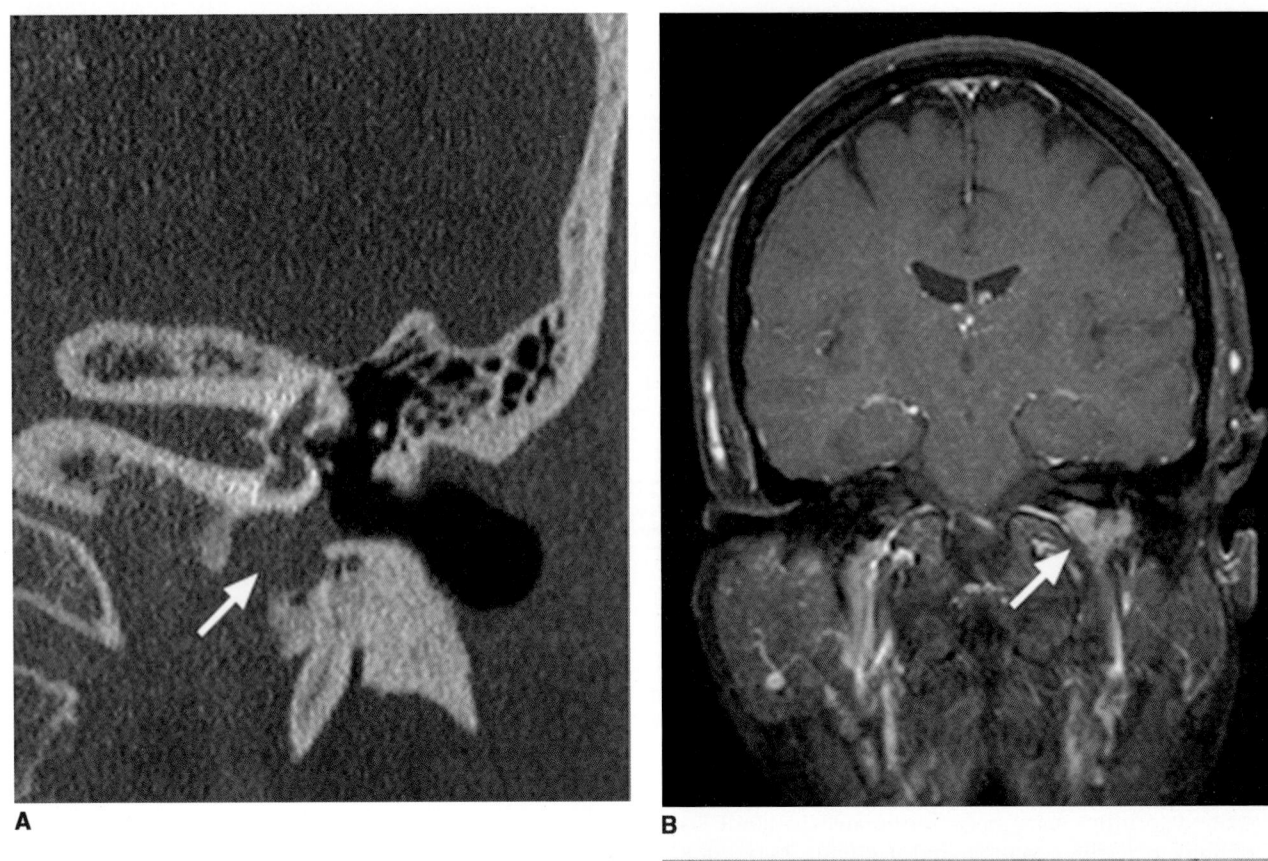

A

B

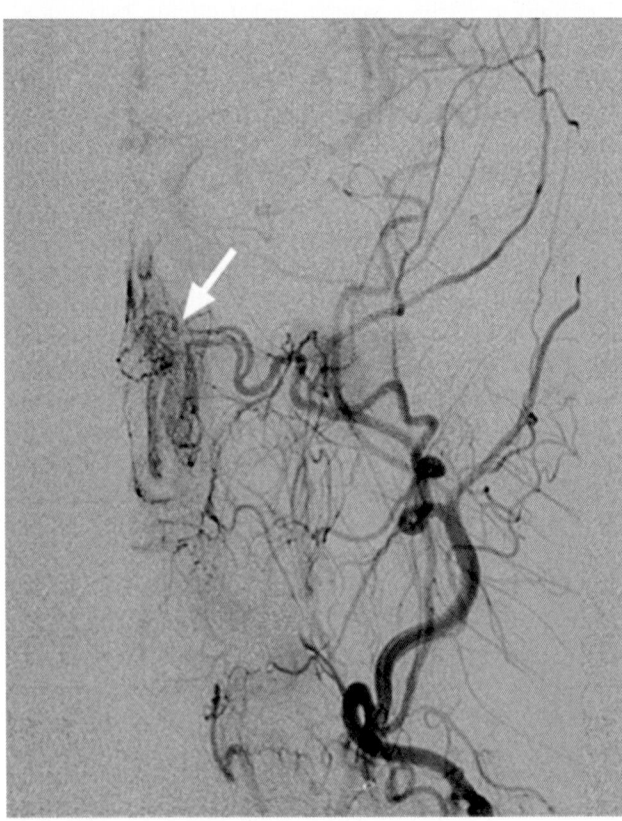

Figure 161.7 Left-sided glomus jugulare (*white arrows*) demonstrated by coronal reformatted CT **(A)**, coronal contrast-enhanced MRI **(B)**, and external carotid angiography **(C)**.

C

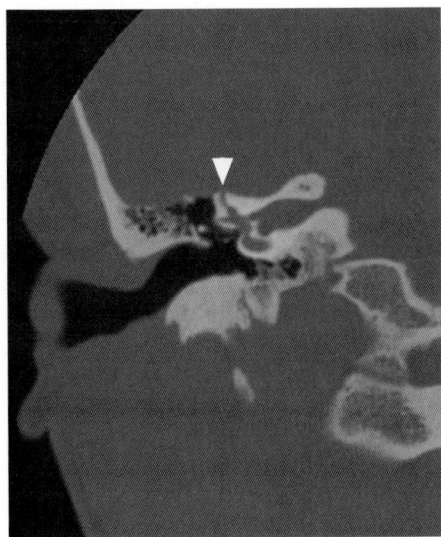

Figure 161.8 Coronal reformatted CT shows right superior SCD (*white arrowhead*).

are defined as extending above the tympanic annulus or rising to within 2 mm of the floor of the IAC (58,59). Jugular bulb diverticula represent an outpouching of the vessel wall into the middle ear, mastoid, or petrous apex. Estimates of the incidence of jugular bulb anomalies range from 4% to 20% (59,60). These anomalies may be acquired rather than congenital, as the jugular bulb does not develop until after 2 years of age. While the exact pathogenesis remains unknown, development of jugular bulb anomalies appear to be related to venous blood flow dynamics (58).

In some cases, a smooth, convex, blue mass can be visualized on otoscopy. Tinnitus of venous origin often worsens with Valsalva and decreases with compression of the ipsilateral internal jugular vein in the neck. Abnormalities of the jugular bulb are best visualized on high-resolution bone algorithm CT scans of the temporal bone (4,54,59,61) (Fig. 161.9).

Management options for symptomatic jugular bulb anomalies range from observation to surgical or endovascular intervention. Published reports describe successful improvement or elimination of pulsatile tinnitus with middle ear floor reconstruction, jugular vein ligation, and endovascular coil embolization; however, significant side effects associated with these interventions (notably benign intracranial hypertension) have limited their widespread application (60,62–64).

Sigmoid Sinus Diverticulum

Sigmoid sinus diverticula account for approximately 20% of cases of pulsatile tinnitus originating from a venous source (4,65). While the exact pathophysiology and pathogenesis remain unknown, it is hypothesized that turbulent blood within the sigmoid sinus may lead to erosion of the overlying mastoid bone with development of a venous diverticulum. As with other abnormalities of the jugular bulb, diverticula of the sigmoid sinus are best visualized on CT or CTA/Venography. Successful elimination of pulsatile symptoms has been reported with transmastoid reconstruction of the sigmoid wall and with endovascular coil embolization and stenting. In these cases, obliteration of the diverticulum was accomplished without thrombosis or occlusion of the sigmoid sinus lumen (65–67).

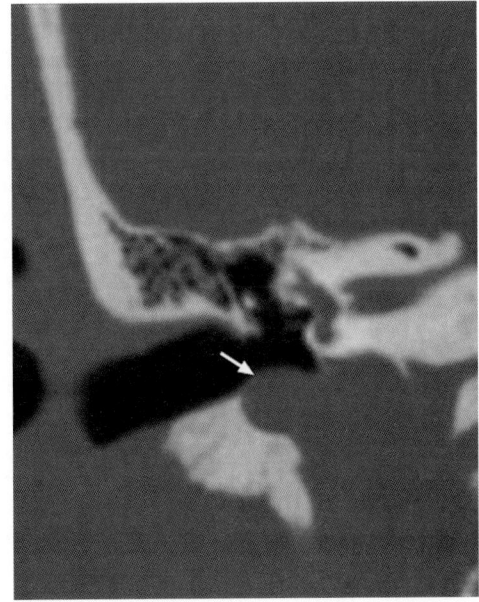
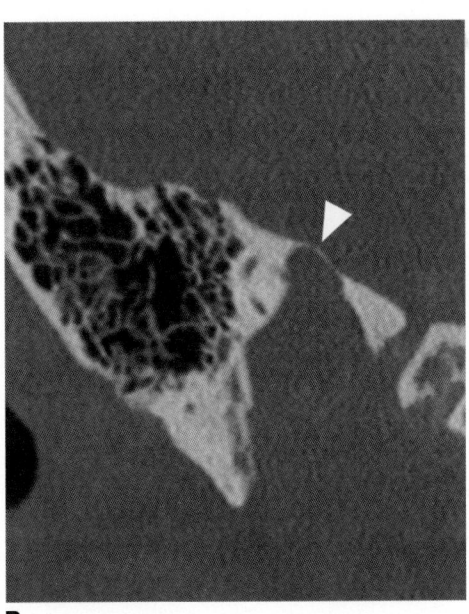

A   B

Figure 161.9 Jugular bulb anomalies associated with pulsatile tinnitus, as demonstrated on coronal CT of the temporal bones. Dehiscent jugular bulb (*white arrow*) **(A)** and a diverticulum (*white arrow head*) of the jugular bulb **(B)** from two different patients.

Dural Arteriovenous Malformation/Fistula

Dural arteriovenous fistulae (AVF) or AVMs are the most common cause of objective pulsatile tinnitus in the setting of a normal otoscopic exam (54,61,68) (Fig. 161.10). Dural AVM/F constitute 10% to 15% of all intracranial vascular malformations and typically occur along the intracranial venous sinuses, most often the transverse and sigmoid sinuses (68). AVM/F may be congenital or acquired, with symptoms precipitated by trauma, infection, puberty, or pregnancy (69). Depending on the location, size, and drainage pattern, patients may be clinically asymptomatic or present with pulsatile tinnitus, headache, neurologic compromise, or intracranial hemorrhage (68). These abnormal connections between dural arteries and venous sinuses may not be readily detectable. CT or MRI imaging and four-vessel angiography is often required for diagnosis (4,54,70). Management decisions are multifactorial and must incorporate the severity of the presenting symptoms, anatomic characteristics of the lesion, and the patient's age and comorbidities. Treatment modalities include endovascular embolization, surgical excision of the fistula and gamma knife radiosurgery (68,69,71–73).

Atherosclerotic Carotid Artery Disease

Many patients with tinnitus have at least one risk factor for atherosclerosis. Pulsatile tinnitus may be the first manifestation of atherosclerotic carotid artery disease (61,74,75). Tinnitus may result from impairment of the inner ear microcirculation due to atherosclerotic disease or from the referred sound of turbulent flow through sclerotic carotid arteries. Physical exam of a patient with tinnitus should always include bilateral auscultation of the neck; however, not all hemodynamically significant stenoses lead to audible bruits. A variety of imaging modalities can identify

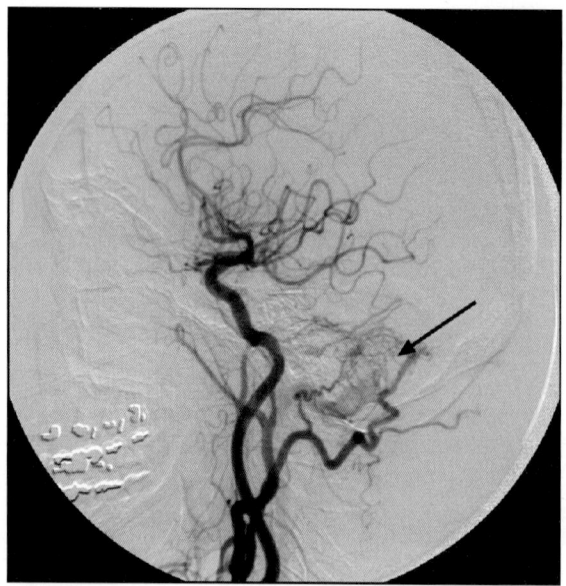

Figure 161.10 Common carotid angiogram in lateral projection demonstrates a dural arteriovenous fistula (*arrow*).

clinically significant atherosclerotic disease. Specifically, atherosclerotic plaques can be seen on ultrasonography, duplex scan, contrast-enhanced CT, CTA, MRI, and MRA; duplex scan also allows visualization of turbulent flow and increased thickness of the carotid wall (61,75,76). Symptoms of pulsatile tinnitus resulting from significant carotid stenoses typically resolve following carotid endarterectomy or intravascular stenting (77,78). Intravascular turbulence due to a torturous carotid artery may also yield a bruit. Distinction between this benign entity and significant carotid stenosis should be made with duplex scan, potentially followed by CTA or MRA as necessary.

Congenital Carotid Anomalies

Congenital anomalies of the intratemporal carotid artery, specifically an aberrant carotid artery or a persistent stapedial artery, may result in pulsatile tinnitus. In rare cases, the intrapetrous carotid artery is replaced by an enlarged inferior tympanic artery (a branch of the ascending pharyngeal). Rather than entering the skull base through the inferior tympanic canaliculus, the inferior tympanic artery anastomoses with the caroticotympanic artery in the middle ear where it is visible as a pulsating, erythematous mass. The aberrant carotid then resumes its course through the intrapetrous carotid canal. A dehiscent anatomically normal carotid artery may also present with pulsatile tinnitus and a pulsating middle ear mass (61).

Persistence of the normal fetal stapedial artery can occur in the presence of a normal or aberrant carotid artery. The stapedial artery crosses the stapes footplate through the obturator foramen, passes across the cochlear promontory and exits the middle ear adjacent to the geniculate ganglion. In the presence of a persistent stapedial artery, neither the middle meningeal artery nor the foramen spinosum develop, as stapedial arteries supply the territory of the middle meningeal artery. While the caliber of the stapedial artery is typically too small for resolution on MRI, thin cut CT allows identification of the middle ear mass, enlargement of the geniculate facial canal and absence of the foramen spinosum (61,76,79). Ligation, either via direct surgical obliteration or embolization, must be preceded by angiography to delineate any intracranial territory supplied by the persistent stapedial artery and ensure there is redundant blood supply to that region. Due to the potentially devastating consequences of intracranial ischemia and bleeding, treatment is rarely pursued (80).

Other Vascular Abnormalities and Malformations

Carotid-cavernous fistulas (CCF) can be high-flow, direct communications between the internal carotid artery and the cavernous sinus or low flow dural-based fistulae, the latter of which are minimally symptomatic. Direct CCFs classically present with chemosis, proptosis, ophthalmoplegia, and diplopia. Low-flow dural CCFs manifest with headache, isolated cranial nerve palsies and pulsatile tinnitus (81). Sudden onset of pulsatile tinnitus has also been reported with direct CCFs, most commonly as the primary presenting symptoms of spontaneous or posttraumatic CCFs (81,82).

Intracranial and extracranial aneurysms, including dilation of the intratemporal petrous carotid, vertebral artery and basilar artery in the cerebellopontine angle cistern, may present with pulsatile tinnitus. Spontaneous dissection of the internal carotid artery can also present with pulsatile tinnitus, as well as the more common symptoms of pain, cerebral ischemia, Horner's syndrome and intracranial hemorrhage (Fig. 161.11). Although fibromuscular dysplasia of the internal carotid artery most commonly presents with cerebral ischemia, it may also manifest as pulsatile tinnitus (83). These vascular abnormalities are best diagnosed with MRA or CTA. Vascular anomalies may require urgent or emergent management depending on the severity of symptoms at presentation. Acute interventions are aimed at reducing intracerebral ischemia and restoring arterial blood flood. Treatment options range from conservative management with anticoagulation and/or antiplatelet therapy to operative intervention (endovascular [intraluminal dilation or stenting] or surgical resection–anastomosis, endarterectomy or vessel reconstruction) (84–86).

Other vascular anomalies and atypical flow states can cause pulsatile tinnitus. Venous anatomic abnormalities have also been associated with pulsatile tinnitus including dural venous sinus aneurysm, dilated mastoid or condylar emissary veins, and stenosis of the dural sinuses, specifically of the transverse or sigmoid sinuses (87,88). Hyperdynamic states leading to increased cardiac output

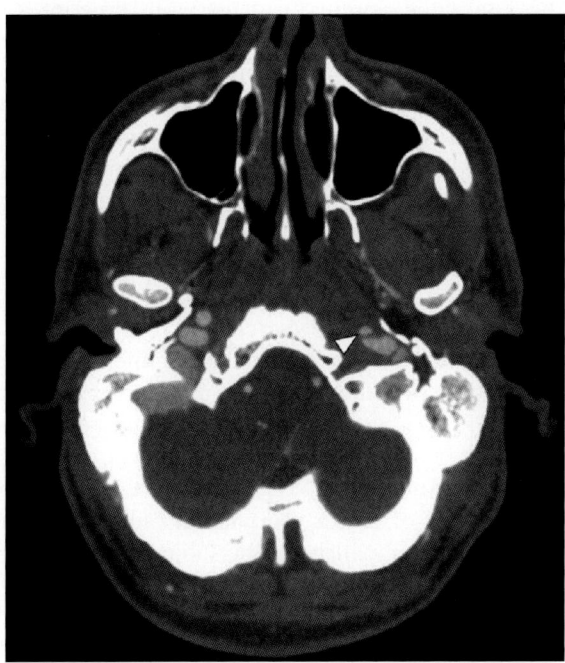

Figure 161.11 CT angiogram of the skull base shows a small, irregular left internal carotid artery (*arrowhead*) indicating internal carotid artery dissection.

can cause pulsatile tinnitus. These states include anemia, thyrotoxicosis, and pregnancy. Treatment of the underlying pathology and decrease in cardiac output will typically cure the tinnitus (5).

Vascular Neoplasms

Paragangliomas

Paragangliomas, or glomus tumors, are the most common vascular tumor of the temporal bone. Believed to arise from paraganglia on the cochlear promontory surrounding Jacobson's nerve (glomus tympanicum) or from the adventitia of the jugular bulb within the jugular foramen (glomus jugulare), these highly vascularized tumors typically present with pulsatile tinnitus (89,90). On otomicroscopy, a reddish, pulsatile mass is visualized medial to the tympanic membrane. Histologically, paragangliomas are composed of chief cells and supporting sustentacular cells surrounded by rich capillary network. Chief cells are neuroendocrine-derived chemoreceptor cells that contain neurosecretory granules capable of clinically significant catecholamine secretion, although this is rare (1% to 2% of patients) (91). Although histologically benign, rare malignant forms have been characterized by the presence of nodal or distant metastases (91). The vascular supply to paragangliomas of the temporal bone commonly originates from the external carotid system, specifically the ascending pharyngeal and occipital arteries, although it can also arise from the internal carotid (caroticotympanic branches of the intrapetrous carotid) or the vertebrobasilar system (posterior–inferior cerebellar artery).

Approximately 80% of paragangliomas are sporadic. The remainder are inherited in an autosomal dominant fashion, sometimes with maternal imprinting, are more likely to be multifocal, and present at an earlier age (91–93). A number of mutations in subunits of mitochondrial succinate dehydrogenase (SDHB, SDHC, and SDHD), which plays a critical role in the mitochondrial electron transport chain, have been identified in these families (94,95). Genetic testing is now available to identify the presence of these mutations in patients at high risk for familial inherited paraganglioma (91).

A variety of staging systems are currently employed for characterization of temporal bone paragangliomas, including those ascribed to Fisch, Glasscock-Jackson, and de la Cruz. Each attempts to characterize the tumor's locoregional extent by assessing its relationship to surrounding neurovascular, intracranial, and temporal bone structures (96–98). The size and extent of tumor can be staged based on radiologic imaging. Debate exists regarding the most appropriate initial imaging modality, although both CT and MRI are typically employed in diagnosis (Fig. 161.7). Erosion of the jugular foramen is best visualized on high-resolution CT (HRCT) of the temporal bone. Compared with CT, MRI is superior in evaluating tumor vascularity as paragangliomas enhance intensely with gadolinium.

On MRI, flow voids within the tumors are characterized by their "salt and pepper" appearance, although this feature can be missing in smaller paragangliomas (61). Additionally, MRI provides better evaluation of tumor extension and multicentricity (99). MRA can be used preoperatively to identify tumor vascular supply, while MRV can evaluate the patency of the jugular bulb, jugular vein, sigmoid and transverse sinuses. Sensitivity and specificity between MRA and standard four-vessel digital subtraction angiography are comparable at 90% and 92% respectively (99). Unlike four-vessel angiography, however, MRA does not afford the opportunity for preoperative tumor embolization.

Treatment options for temporal bone paragangliomas include observation, radiation therapy, and surgery. Currently, management decisions are based on a variety of factors, including tumor size and location, as well as patient age, comorbid conditions and preference. Surgical control rates average 80% to 95% (90,100–103). While surgical excision of glomus tympanicum tumors can be accomplished with little morbidity, removal of a glomus jugulare can risk function of CN VII, IX, X, and XI. Postoperative dysfunction of the lower cranial nerves within the jugular foramen as well as the facial nerve and sequelae resulting from ligation of the jugular vein may be significant. Both standard fractionated radiotherapy and gamma knife stereotactic radiation have been employed as primary treatment as well as adjuvant therapy following subtotal surgical resection or recurrence of glomus jugulare (101,102). Although associated with inhibition of tumor growth in greater than 90% of patients, radiation therapy is not always associated with a reduction in preoperative symptoms when used as a single modality (104–106).

Hemangiomas
Temporal bone hemangiomas, including facial nerve and cavernous hemangiomas, are rare vascular tumors of the temporal bone that can occasionally be associated with pulsatile tinnitus. Facial nerve hemangiomas are most commonly located at the geniculate ganglion, but can also be localized to the IAC. On imaging, facial hemangiomas are best diagnosed by their punctuate bone opacities and stippled appearance on bone algorithm CT scan. Cavernous hemangiomas are located predominantly in the middle ear and can resemble a glomus tympanicum on both physical exam and radiologic imaging.

Nonvascular Etiologies

Idiopathic Intracranial Hypertension
Idiopathic intracranial hypertension (IIH), also known as benign intracranial hypertension or pseudotumor cerebri, is increased intracranial pressure (ICP) in the absence of obstructive hydrocephalus or other identifiable intracranial pathology and normal sized or small symmetric ventricles, normal cerebrospinal fluid (CSF) studies and CSF pressure greater than 200 mm H_2O. Most common in young, obese women, symptoms of IIH include headache, papilledema, and visual disturbances, pulsatile tinnitus, hearing loss, and vestibular abnormalities. These symptoms may present individually or in combination. The pathophysiology of pulsatile tinnitus in IIH is currently unknown. Potentially, increased ICP compresses the intracranial venous sinuses, creating turbulence in normally laminar blood flow that may lead to unilateral or bilateral pulsatile tinnitus (107). Alternatively, stretch or edema of the vestibulocochlear nerve (CN VIII) resulting from increased ICP may account for pulsatile tinnitus (107,108). Transmission of increased pressure to the perilymph through the cochlear aqueduct leading to increased stiffness of the basilar membrane has also been implicated in the pathophysiology of tinnitus in IIH (5,107). Treatment options for IIH include lifestyle modifications, particularly weight loss, as well as medical and surgical reduction of increased ICP. Acetazolamide, corticosteroids, and diuretics have been shown to improve tinnitus resulting from IIH (109). Surgical intervention can include CSF diversion procedures or bariatric surgery for weight loss. Both are effective in reducing ICP and improving tinnitus symptoms (109,110).

Semicircular Canal Dehiscence
Initially described by Lloyd Minor in 1998 for the superior semicircular canal, SCD syndrome results from a deficiency in the bony covering overlying one of the semicircular canals (111) (Fig. 161.8). Canal dehiscence syndrome is associated with a variety of auditory and vestibular manifestations, including sound or pressure-induced vertigo (111,112). Up to 50% of patients with superior SCD complain of pulsatile tinnitus; patients with posterior canal dehiscence resulting in contact between contents of the posterior canal and the jugular bulb or sigmoid sinus may also lead to pulsatile tinnitus (113,114). The diagnosis relies on history, HRCT imaging, preservation of the ipsilateral stapedial reflex, and a lower VEMP in the affected ear (112,115,116). Management options include observation or surgical correction of the dehiscence by plugging or resurfacing the dehiscence (116).

Palatal and Middle Ear Myoclonus
Pulsatile tinnitus can arise from palatal or middle ear myoclonus and may be either subjective or objective. Although both conditions are rare, palatal spasm is more common than middle ear myoclonus and has been reported in both adults and children (117–121). Muscle spasm of the levator veli palatini or tensor veli palatini cause ET opening leading to tinnitus, which can be subjective or objective. The etiology of palatal myoclonus is unknown, but has been hypothesized to localize to the upper brainstem in the Gillian-Mollaret triangle (120). Two forms have been described: symptomatic and essential. The former is marked by intrinsic brainstem or cerebellar disease while the latter (more common) form is characterized by the absence of

visible intracranial pathology on imaging (117,120). The diagnosis is made by visualization of a rhythmic tremor of the soft palate, which often requires flexible nasopharyngoscopy (119). Children with palatal myoclonus have a benign clinical course with frequent spontaneous resolution (117). Treatment options include observation, masking techniques, muscle relaxants, ET occlusion, and local injection of botulinum neurotoxin A (Botox) (120–124). Use of oral anticonvulsant therapy for these patients has generally been abandoned due to minimal efficacy and significant side effects (119,120,129).

Middle ear myoclonus can arise from spontaneous spasm of the tensor tympani or stapedius muscles. On examination, periodic movements of the tympanic membrane often can be visualized with otomicroscopy and may be recorded with immittance testing or tympanometry. Occasionally, these spasms can produce objective tinnitus. Although typically unilateral, bilateral myoclonus of the tensor tympani and stapedius muscles have been reported (125,126). Treatment options include observation, masking techniques, lysis of the stapedial or tensor tympani tendon, and use of Botox on pledgets placed into the middle ear (126–128). Stapedius myotomy has had similar success; however, common side effects include both hyperacusis and phonophobia (126,127,129).

Patulous Eustachian Tube

Pulsatile tinnitus arising from a patulous ET originates outside the auditory pathway. Normally closed in the resting position, a patulous ET leads to symptoms of autophony, aural fullness and, in some cases, pulsatile tinnitus. Patulous ET can result from weight loss following bariatric surgery or diuresis for treatment of congestive heart failure, pregnancy, hormonal therapy, nasopharyngeal scarring/ atrophy from radiation or surgery, rheumatologic disorders, allergic disease, and craniofacial abnormalities. Approximately one-third of cases are idiopathic (113,130,131). Diagnosis can be challenging and typically depends on history. Endoscopic visualization of a longitudinal scaphoid defect in the anterolateral wall of the cartilaginous lumen can also be helpful in diagnosis (113,131). This defect may also be seen on CT and is believed to be the source of tubal incompetency in symptomatic patients. A variety of medical treatment options have been proposed, including weight gain, discontinuation of decongestants and steroid nasal sprays, mucous thickening agents, and nasal estrogen drops. Surgical interventions include myringotomy and tube insertion, endoscopic peritubal augmentation of ET valve, and surgical closure of the ET lumen (113).

Other Nonvascular Etiologies

Osseous dystrophies of the temporal bone can cause pulsatile tinnitus. Otosclerosis is an osseous dysplasia of the inner ear that leads to stapedial fixation with resulting conductive hearing loss. Cochlear otosclerosis can result in SNHL. The etiology of pulsatile tinnitus resulting from otosclerosis is unknown, but is likely related to inflammation and/or increased osseous vascularization as abnormal foci of vascular Haversian bone replace the normal endochondral layer of the otic capsule (132). Both pulsatile and nonpulsatile tinnitus may be one of the many manifestations of Paget disease of the temporal bone. Pulsatile tinnitus resulting from Paget disease is thought to arise from abnormal bony metabolism and prevalence of intraosseous arteriovenous shunts (61,133).

Abnormalities of the middle ear and tympanic membrane can be found in patients with pulsatile tinnitus, and successful management of these underlying conditions can resolve tinnitus in these patients. Serous otitis media can frequently cause pulsatile tinnitus, due to amplification of cardiac sounds by the occlusion effect induced by fluid within the middle ear space. Similarly, chronic otitis media can yield pulsatile tinnitus. Other anomalies of the middle ear, such as tympanic membrane perforation and ossicular chain abnormalities may be associated with patient complaints of pulsatile tinnitus. The clicking sounds that sometimes accompany temporomandibular joint dysfunction may also lead to rhythmic auditory precepts that can be interpreted as pulsatile tinnitus (4).

Finally, pulsatile tinnitus may be a rare manifestation of intracranial pathology, such as intraventricular cavernous hemangiomas and cerebellopontine angle pathology (including vestibular schwannomas and meningiomas) (5).

HIGHLIGHTS

- Complaints of tinnitus should be divided into subjective versus objective and nonpulsatile versus pulsatile categories to facilitate diagnosis and management.
- All patients with tinnitus should have a complete audiogram as part of their evaluation. Imaging and other studies may be indicated based on findings on history and physical examination.
- Nonpulsatile tinnitus can result from a variety of causes, including SNHL, CHL, ingestion of stimulants, head trauma, and psychiatric disease. When possible, treatment of the underlying cause can alleviate tinnitus.
- When etiology-specific management of nonpulsatile tinnitus fails or is not possible, nonspecific management of tinnitus should be attempted.
- Pulsatile tinnitus can be generated by a variety of arterial and venous causes, vascular tumors, fluid within the middle ear, otosclerosis, and tumors of the IAC. In up to one-third of these cases, no etiologic agent will be identified.
- Treatment of the underlying cause of pulsatile tinnitus, when possible, can resolve this complaint.

REFERENCES

1. Shargorodsky J, Curhan GC, Farwell WR. Prevalence and characteristics of tinnitus among US adults. *Am J Med* 2010;123:711–718.
2. Seidman MD, Standring RT, Dornhoffer JL. Tinnitus: current understanding and contemporary management. *Curr Opin Otolaryngol Head Neck Surg* 2010;18:363–368.
3. Moller AR. Pathophysiology of tinnitus. *Otolaryngol Clin North Am* 2003;36:249–266, v–vi.
4. Mattox DE, Hudgins P. Algorithm for evaluation of pulsatile tinnitus. *Acta Otolaryngol* 2008;128:427–431.
5. Sismanis A. Pulsatile tinnitus. *Otolaryngol Clin North Am* 2003;36:389–402, viii.
6. House JW, Brackmann DE. Tinnitus: surgical treatment. *Ciba Found Symp* 1981;85:204–216.
7. Silverstein H, Haberkamp T, Smouha E. The state of tinnitus after inner ear surgery. *Otolaryngol Head Neck Surg* 1986;95:438–441.
8. Harcourt J, Thomsen J, Tos M. Translabyrinthine vestibular schwannoma surgery: postoperative tinnitus and cochlear nerve integrity. *Auris Nasus Larynx* 1997;24:21–26.
9. Eggermont JJ. Pathophysiology of tinnitus. *Prog Brain Res* 2007;166:19–35.
10. Kaltenbach JA, Zhang J, Afman CE. Plasticity of spontaneous neural activity in the dorsal cochlear nucleus after intense sound exposure. *Hear Res* 2000;147:282–292.
11. Seki S, Eggermont JJ. Changes in spontaneous firing rate and neural synchony in cat primary auditory cortex after localized ton-induced hearing loss. *Hear Res* 2003;180:28–38.
12. Middleton JW, Kiritani T, Pedersen C, et al. Mice with behavioral evidence of tinnitus exhibit dorsal cochlear nucleus hyperactivity because of decreased GABAergic inhibition. *Proc Natl Acad Sci U S A* 2011;108:7601–7606.
13. Melcher JR, Levine RA, Bergevin C, et al. The auditory midbrain of people with tinnitus: abnormal sound-evoked activity revisited. *Hear Res* 2009;257:63–74.
14. Lanting CP, de Kleine E, van Dijk P. Neural activity underlying tinnitus generation: results from PET and fMRI. *Hear Res* 2009;255:1–13.
15. Kaltenbach JA. Tinnitus models and mechanisms. *Hear Res* 2010;276:52–60.
16. Moller AR. The role of neural plasticity in tinnitus. *Prog Brain Res* 2007;166:37–45.
17. De Ridder D, Elgoyhen AB, Romo R, et al. Phantom percepts: tinnitus and pain as persisting aversive memory networks. *Proc Natl Acad Sci U S A* 2011;108:8075–8080.
18. Hazell JW, McKinney CJ, Aleksy W. Mechanisms of tinnitus in profound deafness. *Ann Otol Rhinol Laryngol Suppl* 1995;166:418–420.
19. Katzenell U, Segal S. Hyperacusis: review and clinical guidelines. *Otol Neurotol* 2001;22:321–326; discussion 6–7.
20. Moller AR. Neural plasticity in tinnitus. *Prog Brain Res* 2006;157:365–372.
21. Gothelf D, Farber N, Raveh E, et al. Hyperacusis in Williams syndrome: characteristics and associated neuroaudiologic abnormalities. *Neurology* 2006;66:390–395.
22. Lenhoff HM, Wang PP, Greenberg F, et al. Williams syndrome and the brain. *Sci Am* 1997;277:68–73.
23. Jastreboff PJ, Jastreboff MM. Tinnitus retraining therapy (TRT) as a method for treatment of tinnitus and hyperacusis patients. *J Am Acad Audiol* 2000;11:162–177.
24. Beisinger E, Del Bo L, De Ridder D, et al. Algorithm for the diagnostic & therapeutic management of tinnitus. *TRI Tinnitus Clinic Network*, 2008.
25. Lustig LR, Rifkin S, Jackler RK, et al. Acoustic neuromas presenting with normal or symmetrical hearing: factors associated with diagnosis and outcome. *Am J Otol* 1998;19:212–218.
26. Del Bo L, Ambrosetti U. Hearing aids for the treatment of tinnitus. *Prog Brain Res* 2007;166:341–345.
27. Jastreboff MM. Sound therapies for tinnitus management. *Prog Brain Res* 2007;166:435–440.
28. Tyler R, Coelho C, Tao P, et al. Identifying tinnitus subgroups with cluster analysis. *Am J Audiol* 2008;17:S176–S184.
29. Roberts LE. Residual inhibition. *Prog Brain Res* 2007;166:487–495.
30. Sweetow RW, Sabes JH. Effects of acoustical stimuli delivered through hearing aids on tinnitus. *J Am Acad Audiol* 2010;21:461–473.
31. Jastreboff PJ. Tinnitus retraining therapy. *Prog Brain Res* 2007;166:415–423.
32. Hanley PJ, Davis PB. Treatment of tinnitus with a customized, dynamic acoustic neural stimulus: underlying principles and clinical efficacy. *Trends Amplif* 2008;12:210–222.
33. Wazen JJ, Daugherty J, Pinsky K, et al. Evaluation of a customized acoustical stimulus system in the treatment of chronic tinnitus. *Otol Neurotol* 2011;32:710–716.
34. Greimel KV, Meco C, Mair A, et al. How is tinnitus influenced by cochlear implantation? *HNO* 2003;51:226–231.
35. Pan T, Tyler RS, Ji H, et al. Changes in the tinnitus handicap questionnaire after cochlear implantation. *Am J Audiol* 2009;18:144–151.
36. Punte AK, Vermeire K, Hofkens A, et al. Cochlear implantation as a durable tinnitus treatment in single-sided deafness. *Cochlear Implants Int* 2011;12:26–29.
37. Amoodi HA, Mick PT, Shipp DB, et al. The effects of unilateral cochlear implantation on the tinnitus handicap inventory and the influence on quality of life. *Laryngoscope* 2011;121:1536–1540.
38. Olze H, Szczepek AJ, Haupt H, et al. The impact of cochlear implantation on tinnitus, stress and quality of life in postlingually deafened patients. *Audiol Neurootol* 2012;17:2–11.
39. Akdogan O, Ozcan I, Ozbek C, et al. Tinnitus after cochlear implantation. *Auris Nasus Larynx* 2009;36:210–212.
40. Summerfield AQ, Barton GR, Toner J, et al. Self-reported benefits from successive bilateral cochlear implantation in post-lingually deafened adults: randomised controlled trial. *Int J Audiol* 2006;45:S99–S107.
41. Trellakis S, Lautermann J, Lehnerdt G. Lidocaine: neurobiological targets and effects on the auditory system. *Prog Brain Res* 2007;166:303–322.
42. Darlington CL, Smith PF. Drug treatments for tinnitus. *Prog Brain Res* 2007;166:249–262.
43. Meeus O, De Ridder D, Van de Heyning P. Administration of the combination clonazepam-deanxit as treatment for tinnitus. *Otol Neurotol* 2011;32:701–709.
44. Robinson SK, Viirre ES, Stein MB. Antidepressant therapy in tinnitus. *Hear Res* 2007;226:221–231.
45. Topak M, Sahin-Yilmaz A, Ozdoganoglu T, et al. Intratympanic methylprednisolone injections for subjective tinnitus. *J Laryngol Otol* 2009;123:1221–1225.
46. Markowski J, Gierek T, Kluczewska E, et al. Assessment of vestibulocochlear organ function in patients meeting radiologic criteria of vascular compression syndrome of vestibulocochlear nerve–diagnosis of disabling positional vertigo. *Med Sci Monit* 2011;17:CR169–CR173.
47. Makins AE, Nikolopoulos TP, Ludman C, et al. Is there a correlation between vascular loops and unilateral auditory symptoms? *Laryngoscope* 1998;108:1739–1742.
48. Okamura T, Kurokawa Y, Ikeda N, et al. Microvascular decompression for cochlear symptoms. *J Neurosurg* 2000;93:421–426.
49. Guevara N, Deveze A, Buza V, et al. Microvascular decompression of cochlear nerve for tinnitus incapacity: pre-surgical data, surgical analyses and long-term follow-up of 15 patients. *Eur Arch Otorhinolaryngol* 2008;265:397–401.
50. Dohrmann K, Weisz N, Schlee W, et al. Neurofeedback for treating tinnitus. *Prog Brain Res* 2007;166:473–485.
51. Piccirillo JF, Garcia KS, Nicklaus J, et al. Low-frequency repetitive transcranial magnetic stimulation to the temporoparietal junction for tinnitus. *Arch Otolaryngol Head Neck Surg* 2011;137:221–228.
52. Garin P, Gilain C, Van Damme JP, et al. Short- and long-lasting tinnitus relief induced by transcranial direct current stimulation. *J Neurol* 2011;258:1940–1948.
53. McGrath AP, Michaelides EM. Use of middle ear immittance testing in the evaluation of patulous eustachian tube. *J Am Acad Audiol* 2011;22:201–207.
54. Sonmez G, Basekim CC, Ozturk E, et al. Imaging of pulsatile tinnitus: a review of 74 patients. *Clin Imaging* 2007;31:102–108.
55. Krishnan A, Mattox DE, Fountain AJ, et al. CT arteriography and venography in pulsatile tinnitus: preliminary results. *AJNR Am J Neuroradiol* 2006;27:1635–1638.
56. Mikulec AA, Poe DS, McKenna MJ. Operative management of superior semicircular canal dehiscence. *Laryngoscope* 2005;115:501–507.

57. Pirodda A, Modugno GC, Brandolini C, et al. How computed tomography may be useful in pulsatile tinnitus with normal otoscopic findings. *Arch Otolaryngol Head Neck Surg* 2005;131:728–729.

58. Friedmann DR, Eubig J, McGill M, et al. Development of the jugular bulb: a radiologic study. *Otol Neurotol* 2011;32:1389–1395.

59. Friedmann DR, Le BT, Pramanik BK, et al. Clinical spectrum of patients with erosion of the inner ear by jugular bulb abnormalities. *Laryngoscope* 2010;120:365–372.

60. El-Begermy MA, Rabie AN. A novel surgical technique for management of tinnitus due to high dehiscent jugular bulb. *Otolaryngol Head Neck Surg* 2010;142:576–581.

61. Weissman JL, Hirsch BE. Imaging of tinnitus: a review. *Radiology* 2000;216:342–349.

62. Yoon BN, Lee TH, Kong SK, et al. Management of high jugular bulb with tinnitus: transvenous stent-assisted coil embolization. *Otolaryngol Head Neck Surg* 2008;139:740–741.

63. Kondoh K, Kitahara T, Mishiro Y, et al. Management of hemorrhagic high jugular bulb with adhesive otitis media in an only hearing ear: transcatheter endovascular embolization using detachable coils. *Ann Otol Rhinol Laryngol* 2004;113:975–979.

64. Jackler RK, Brackmann DE, Sismanis A. A warning on venous ligation for pulsatile tinnitus. *Otol Neurotol* 2001;22:427–428.

65. Otto KJ, Hudgins PA, Abdelkafy W, et al. Sigmoid sinus diverticulum: a new surgical approach to the correction of pulsatile tinnitus. *Otol Neurotol* 2007;28:48–53.

66. Sanchez TG, Murao M, de Medeiros IR, et al. A new therapeutic procedure for treatment of objective venous pulsatile tinnitus. *Int Tinnitus J* 2002;8:54–57.

67. Houdart E, Chapot R, Merland JJ. Aneurysm of a dural sigmoid sinus: a novel vascular cause of pulsatile tinnitus. *Ann Neurol* 2000;48:669–671.

68. Delgado F, Munoz F, Bravo-Rodriguez F, et al. Treatment of dural arteriovenous fistulas presenting as pulsatile tinnitus. *Otol Neurotol* 2009;30:897–902.

69. Klisch J, Huppertz HJ, Spetzger U, et al. Transvenous treatment of carotid cavernous and dural arteriovenous fistulae: results for 31 patients and review of the literature. *Neurosurgery* 2003;53:836–856; discussion 56–57.

70. Prestigiacomo CJ, Niimi Y, Setton A, et al. Three-dimensional rotational spinal angiography in the evaluation and treatment of vascular malformations. *AJNR Am J Neuroradiol* 2003;24:1429–1435.

71. Carlson AP, Taylor CL, Yonas H. Treatment of dural arteriovenous fistula using ethylene vinyl alcohol (onyx) arterial embolization as the primary modality: short-term results. *J Neurosurg* 2007;107:1120–1125.

72. Pan HC, Sheehan J, Huang CF, et al. Two consecutive dural arteriovenous fistulae in a child: a case report of successful treatment with gamma knife radiosurgery. *Childs Nerv Syst* 2007;23:1185–1190.

73. Matsushige T, Nakaoka M, Ohta K, et al. Tentorial dural arteriovenous malformation manifesting as trigeminal neuralgia treated by stereotactic radiosurgery: a case report. *Surg Neurol* 2006;66:519–523; discussion 23.

74. Daneshi A, Hadizadeh H, Mahmoudian S, et al. Pulsatile tinnitus and carotid artery atherosclerosis. *Int Tinnitus J* 2004;10:161–164.

75. Fukatsu M, Yamada T, Suzuki S, et al. Tinnitus is associated with increase in the intima-media thickness of carotid arteries. *Am J Med Sci* 2011;342:2–4.

76. Marsot-Dupuch K. Pulsatile and nonpulsatile tinnitus: a systemic approach. *Semin Ultrasound CT MR* 2001;22:250–270.

77. Kirkby-Bott J, Gibbs HH. Carotid endarterectomy relieves pulsatile tinnitus associated with severe ipsilateral carotid stenosis. *Eur J Vasc Endovasc Surg* 2004;27:651–653.

78. Hartung O, Alimi YS, Juhan C. Tinnitus resulting from tandem lesions of the internal carotid artery: combined extracranial endarterectomy and intrapetrous primary stenting. *J Vasc Surg* 2004;39:679–681.

79. Thiers FA, Sakai O, Poe DS, et al. Persistent stapedial artery: CT findings. *AJNR Am J Neuroradiol* 2000;21:1551–1554.

80. Bhattacharyya N, Poe DS. Otoendoscopic view of a persistent stapedial artery. *Otolaryngol Head Neck Surg* 1999;120:923.

81. Albert GW, Dahdaleh NS, Hasan DM. Direct carotid-cavernous fistula presenting with minimal symptoms and rapid angiographic progression. *J Clin Neurosci* 2010;17:1187–1189.

82. Lerut B, De Vuyst C, Ghekiere J, et al. Post-traumatic pulsatile tinnitus: the hallmark of a direct carotico-cavernous fistula. *J Laryngol Otol* 2007;121:1103–1107.

83. Foyt D, Carfrae MJ, Rapoport R. Fibromuscular dysplasia of the internal carotid artery causing pulsatile tinnitus. *Otolaryngol Head Neck Surg* 2006;134:701–702.

84. Touze E, Oppenheim C, Trystram D, et al. Fibromuscular dysplasia of cervical and intracranial arteries. *Int J Stroke* 2010;5:296–305.

85. Lyrer P, Engelter S. Antithrombotic drugs for carotid artery dissection. *Cochrane Database Syst Rev* 2010;(10):CD000255.

86. Rao AS, Makaroun MS, Marone LK, et al. Long-term outcomes of internal carotid artery dissection. *J Vasc Surg* 2011;54:370–374.

87. Mehanna R, Shaltoni H, Morsi H, et al. Endovascular treatment of sigmoid sinus aneurysm presenting as devastating pulsatile tinnitus. A case report and review of literature. *Interv Neuroradiol* 2010;16:451–454.

88. Chauhan NS, Sharma YP, Bhagra T, et al. Persistence of multiple emissary veins of posterior fossa with unusual origin of left petrosquamosal sinus from mastoid emissary. *Surg Radiol Anat* 2011;33:827–831.

89. Jackson CG. Glomus tympanicum and glomus jugulare tumors. *Otolaryngol Clin North Am* 2001;34:941–970, vii.

90. Fayad JN, Keles B, Brackmann DE. Jugular foramen tumors: clinical characteristics and treatment outcomes. *Otol Neurotol* 2010;31:299–305.

91. Semaan MT, Megerian CA. Current assessment and management of glomus tumors. *Curr Opin Otolaryngol Head Neck Surg* 2008;16:420–426.

92. Petropoulos AE, Luetje CM, Camarata PJ, et al. Genetic analysis in the diagnosis of familial paragangliomas. *Laryngoscope* 2000;110:1225–1229.

93. Drovdlic CM, Myers EN, Peters JA, et al. Proportion of heritable paraganglioma cases and associated clinical characteristics. *Laryngoscope* 2001;111:1822–1827.

94. Baysal BE, Willett-Brozick JE, Lawrence EC, et al. Prevalence of SDHB, SDHC, and SDHD germline mutations in clinic patients with head and neck paragangliomas. *J Med Genet* 2002;39:178–183.

95. Niemann S, Muller U. Mutations in SDHC cause autosomal dominant paraganglioma, type 3. *Nat Genet* 2000;26:268–270.

96. Jackson CG, Glasscock ME III, Harris PF. Glomus tumors. Diagnosis, classification, and management of large lesions. *Arch Otolaryngol* 1982;108:401–410.

97. Fisch U. Infratemporal fossa approach for glomus tumors of the temporal bone. *Ann Otol Rhinol Laryngol* 1982;91:474–479.

98. Green JD Jr, Brackmann DE, Nguyen CD, et al. Surgical management of previously untreated glomus jugulare tumors. *Laryngoscope* 1994;104:917–921.

99. van den Berg R, Schepers A, de Bruine FT, et al. The value of MR angiography techniques in the detection of head and neck paragangliomas. *Eur J Radiol* 2004;52:240–245.

100. Forest JA III, Jackson CG, McGrew BM. Long-term control of surgically treated glomus tympanicum tumors. *Otol Neurotol* 2001;22:232–236.

101. Willen SN, Einstein DB, Maciunas RJ, et al. Treatment of glomus jugulare tumors in patients with advanced age: planned limited surgical resection followed by staged gamma knife radiosurgery: a preliminary report. *Otol Neurotol* 2005;26:1229–1234.

102. Cosetti M, Linstrom C, Alexiades G, et al. Glomus tumors in patients of advanced age: a conservative approach. *Laryngoscope* 2008;118:270–274.

103. Jackson CG, McGrew BM, Forest JA, et al. Lateral skull base surgery for glomus tumors: long-term control. *Otol Neurotol* 2001;22:377–382.

104. Hu K, Persky MS. The multidisciplinary management of paragangliomas of the head and neck, Part 2. *Oncology (Williston Park)* 2003;17:1143–1153; discussion 54, 58, 61.

105. Hu K, Persky MS. Multidisciplinary management of paragangliomas of the head and neck, Part 1. *Oncology (Williston Park)* 2003;17:983–993.

106. Foote RL, Pollock BE, Gorman DA, et al. Glomus jugulare tumor: tumor control and complications after stereotactic radiosurgery. *Head Neck* 2002;24:332–338; discussion 8–9.

107. Rudnick E, Sismanis A. Pulsatile tinnitus and spontaneous cerebrospinal fluid rhinorrhea: indicators of benign intracranial hypertension syndrome. *Otol Neurotol* 2005;26:166–168.
108. Kapoor KG. Etiology of dizziness, tinnitus, and nausea in idiopathic intracranial hypertension. *Med Hypotheses* 2008;71:310–311.
109. Jindal M, Hiam L, Raman A, et al. Idiopathic intracranial hypertension in otolaryngology. *Eur Arch Otorhinolaryngol* 2009;266:803–836.
110. Michaelides EM, Sismanis A, Sugerman HJ, et al. Pulsatile tinnitus in patients with morbid obesity: the effectiveness of weight reduction surgery. *Am J Otol* 2000;21:682–685.
111. Minor LB, Solomon D, Zinreich JS, et al. Sound- and/or pressure-induced vertigo due to bone dehiscence of the superior semicircular canal. *Arch Otolaryngol Head Neck Surg* 1998;124:249–258.
112. Minor LB. Superior canal dehiscence syndrome. *Am J Otol* 2000;21:9–19.
113. Poe DS. Diagnosis and management of the patulous eustachian tube. *Otol Neurotol* 2007;28:668–677.
114. Chi FL, Ren DD, Dai CF. Variety of audiologic manifestations in patients with superior semicircular canal dehiscence. *Otol Neurotol* 2010;31:2–10.
115. Rauch SD. Vestibular evoked myogenic potentials. *Curr Opin Otolaryngol Head Neck Surg* 2006;14:299–304.
116. Carey JP, Migliaccio AA, Minor LB. Semicircular canal function before and after surgery for superior canal dehiscence. *Otol Neurotol* 2007;28:356–364.
117. MacDonald JT. Objective tinnitus due to essential palatal tremor in a 5-year-old. *Pediatr Neurol* 2007;36:175–176.
118. Amoodi HA, Makki FM, McNeil M, et al. Transmastoid resurfacing of superior semicircular canal dehiscence. *Laryngoscope* 2011;121:1117–1123.
119. Fritsch MH, Wynne MK, Matt BH, et al. Objective tinnitus in children. *Otol Neurotol* 2001;22:644–649.
120. Krause E, Leunig A, Klopstock T, et al. Treatment of essential palatal myoclonus in a 10-year-old girl with botulinum neurotoxin. *Otol Neurotol* 2006;27:672–675.
121. Ensink RJ, Vingerhoets HM, Schmidt CW, et al. Treatment for severe palatoclonus by occlusion of the eustachian tube. *Otol Neurotol* 2003;24:714–716.
122. Penney SE, Bruce IA, Saeed SR. Botulinum toxin is effective and safe for palatal tremor: a report of five cases and a review of the literature. *J Neurol* 2006;253:857–860.
123. Abdul-Baqi KJ. Objective high-frequency tinnitus of middle-ear myoclonus. *J Laryngol Otol* 2004;118:231–233.
124. Elziere M, Roman S, Nicollas R, et al. Objective tinnitus associated with essential palatal myoclonus: report in a child. *Int Tinnitus J* 2007;13:157–158.
125. Howsam GD, Sharma A, Lambden SP, et al. Bilateral objective tinnitus secondary to congenital middle-ear myoclonus. *J Laryngol Otol* 2005;119:489–491.
126. Cohen D, Perez R. Bilateral myoclonus of the tensor tympani: a case report. *Otolaryngol Head Neck Surg* 2003;128:441.
127. Golz A, Fradis M, Martzu D, et al. Stapedius muscle myoclonus. *Ann Otol Rhinol Laryngol* 2003;112:522–524.
128. Golz A, Fradis M, Netzer A, et al. Bilateral tinnitus due to middle-ear myoclonus. *Int Tinnitus J* 2003;9:52–55.
129. Liu HB, Fan JP, Lin SZ, et al. Botox transient treatment of tinnitus due to stapedius myoclonus: case report. *Clin Neurol Neurosurg* 2011;113:57–58.
130. Doherty JK, Slattery WH III. Autologous fat grafting for the refractory patulous eustachian tube. *Otolaryngol Head Neck Surg* 2003;128:88–91.
131. Grimmer JF, Poe DS. Update on eustachian tube dysfunction and the patulous eustachian tube. *Curr Opin Otolaryngol Head Neck Surg* 2005;13:277–282.
132. Ealy M, Smith RJ. Otosclerosis. *Adv Otorhinolaryngol* 2011;70:122–129.
133. Mackenzie I, Young C, Fraser WD. Tinnitus and Paget's disease of bone. *J Laryngol Otol* 2006;120:899–902.

Aging and the Auditory and Vestibular System

162

Joe Walter Kutz Jr.   *Brandon Isaacson*   *Peter S. Roland*

The geriatric population is the fastest growing segment of the population of all industrialized nations, including the United States. As life expectancy increases and health care costs rise, the medical profession will be challenged to provide cost-effective quality care. A recent report by the Institute of Medicine (IOM) predicted the percentage of Americans older than 65 will increase by 20% and double in number from 35 million to 71 million by the year 2030 (1). Since age-related hearing loss is the fourth most common reason patients over 65 years old seek medical care and vestibular dysfunction is common in the older population, there is going to be a substantial increase in the number of outpatient visits for otologic conditions. A recent study by Lin and Bhattacharyya (2) predicted a 30% increase in annual visits to otolaryngologists for otologic diagnoses by 2020. Understanding and treating disorders of the aging auditory and vestibular systems will be more essential than ever for the otolaryngologist.

Greater than 40% of patients older than 65 years have a hearing loss that significantly impairs communication and leads to a decrease in quality of life (3). Loss of hearing negatively affects social interaction, leading to progressive isolation and withdrawal. In addition, high-frequency warning sounds such as alarms and signals may not be heard, resulting in potential harm. Although hearing loss in the geriatric population is often due to presbycusis, other causes should be sought.

Dizziness is the most common presenting complaint in patients 75 years or older and typically affects women more than men (4). Balance disturbances contribute to functional decline in the elderly. Postural stability and gait involves the complex integration of the visual, proprioceptive, somatosensory, and vestibular signals. Pathology in any of these systems can cause dizziness and, more importantly, increase the incidence of falls. It is estimated that approximately 40% of older adults living in the community have at least one fall per year. In a study by the Centers for Disease Control

(CDC), 62% of injuries presenting to the emergency department in patients older than 65 years were a direct result of a fall (5). A hip fracture is a common serious injury resulting from a fall and often leads to serious long-term consequences. Only 50% of elderly patients can return home or return to normal activity after a hip fracture (6,7).

The differential diagnosis for dizziness is extensive, sometimes making the evaluation laborious and difficult. However, 90% of the causes of dizziness can be placed in one of seven categories (Table 162.1). One recent study evaluating the cause of dizziness in 677 elderly patients identified benign paroxysmal positional vertigo (BPPV) in 42%, idiopathic vestibulopathy in 20%, migraine-associated dizziness in 13%, Meniere disease in 12%, and an acute vestibular attack in 6%, and 7% contributed to other causes (8).

AGE-RELATED CHANGES IN THE AUDITORY SYSTEM

Auditory Dysfunction

All of the usual cases of hearing loss can affect the elderly (Table 162.2). These disorders are addressed elsewhere in this textbook. With the exception of conductive loss associated with aging as described by Schuknecht, conductive hearing loss in the elderly population has the same differential diagnosis as in younger individuals.

Anatomic changes that affect hearing and balance occur because of physiologic aging. One such example involves the production of cerumen. Cerumen consists of desquamated epithelium mixed with the sebum produced from sebaceous glands and the watery secretions of modified apocrine sweat glands. Modified apocrine sweat glands atrophy with age. Without the watery component, cerumen becomes drier, harder, and less likely to be moved out the external auditory canal (EAC) by the canal's normal transport and cleansing mechanism. The tragi hairs found in adult males become coarser, larger, and more prominent with age. Their

TABLE 162.1	ETIOLOGY OF DIZZINESS

Peripheral vestibular disorders
Cardiovascular disorders
Multisensory dizziness
Brainstem cerebrovascular disease
Neurologic disorders
Psychiatric disease
Hyperventilation syndrome

presence can prevent the natural dislodgement of cerumen from the EAC, contributing to the increased incidence of cerumen impaction in the elderly male.

Presbycusis

The auditory system's durability is determined by genetic resistance and the cumulative imposed physical stress. Genetically mediated hearing loss can be difficult to distinguish from presbycusis. The ability to differentiate hearing loss caused by defective genetic material is increasing

TABLE 162.2	CAUSES OF BILATERALLY SYMMETRIC SENSORINEURAL HEARING LOSS[a]		
Ménière disease	Episodic attacks of fluctuant SNHL, vertigo, tinnitus, aural fullness or pressure; bilateral in 20%–30% of cases	History of typical attacks with symptom-free intervals; hearing loss involves low tones initially and later all frequencies, rule out neurosyphilis	Medical Diuretics and low-salt diet Surgical Decompression or shunt of endolymphatic sac; section of vestibular nerve. Penicillin and oral steroids
Luetic hearing loss (late-acquired syphilis)	Often bilateral SNHL with no characteristic audiometric pattern; speech discrimination score often worse than would be predicted on basis of pure-tone thresholds; often associated with vestibular symptoms; may mimic Ménière disease	Positive FTA-ABS test, with or without clinical history of syphilis	
Paget disease	Slowly progressive SNHL and CHL; SNHL worse in high frequencies; maximum CHL of 20–30 dB at 500 Hz	Skeletal deformities of skull and long bones of extremities, elevated serum alkaline phosphatase and urinary hydroxyproline	Calcitonin
Hypothyroidism	Slowly progressive SNHL affecting all frequencies daily	Usual clinical stigmata of hypothyroidism; decreased serum T_4	Desiccated thyroid or Synthroid mixture of T_4 and T_3
Ototoxic drugs	Hearing loss with or without vestibular dysfunction following treatment with known ototoxic drug	History	None
Hereditary progressive SNHL	Progressive SNHL beginning at earlier age than expected for presbycusis; possible positive family history	Family history	None
Noise-induced hearing loss	History of prolonged exposure to loud continuous noise or brief exposure to loud impulse noise	History; characteristic audiogram with maximum hearing loss at 4,000 Hz; may not be distinguishable from presbycusis	None; use of ear protectors may prevent further loss from noise exposure
Head trauma	Severe head injury often resulting in loss of consciousness and bilateral temporal bone fractures	History	None
Cochlear otosclerosis and far-advanced clinical otosclerosis	Far-advanced clinical otosclerosis (stapedial fixation) and cochlear otosclerosis; SNHL may appear on audiogram as severe to profound SNHL; patient will have good speech modulation (unlike in profound SNHL) and will be wearing or will have worn a bone conduction hearing aid; possibly a family history of otosclerosis	History is suggestive but surgical exploration of stapes footplate is diagnostic and therapeutic; poststapedectomy patient may be able to wear ear-level hearing aid with good results	Stapedectomy, sodium fluoride

[a]The hearing loss from any of these diseases may be improved with hearing aids unless it is of such a degree that hearing aids will be inadequate or unsatisfactory. Individuals with bilateral profound SNHL may be candidates for cochlear implant and should be evaluated by an otologist to determine their suitability for such a device.
SNHL, sensorineural hearing loss; FTA-ABS test, fluorescent treponemal antibody test, CHL, conductive hearing loss; Hz, hertz (cycles per second); dB, decibel (arbitrary unit of sound intensity).

TABLE 162.3	FACTORS CONTRIBUTING TO AGE-RELATED HEARING LOSS

Microvascular disease resulting in diminished profusion and hypoxia of labyrinthine hair cells and neurons
Effects of diet; in animals, free radical formation increases hearing loss
Noise exposure
Drug effects
Cigarette smoking

TABLE 162.4	CLINICAL MANIFESTATIONS OF PATHOLOGIC CHANGES WITHIN THE COCHLEA

Cochlear hair cell loss progresses the high-frequency hearing loss with speech discrimination preserved in the initial phases.
Neuronal loss: a nonprecipitous, generalized loss of pure-tone thresholds with speech discrimination impaired out of proportion to the threshold shift.
Atrophy of the stria: flat hearing loss with good preservation of speech discrimination.
Mechanical (cochlear conductive): gradually sloping high frequency hearing loss with speech discrimination impaired proportionate to the pure tone threshold shift.

as the types and tests of chromosomal abnormalities are identified. In any given individual, though, it is difficult to determine what component of the hearing loss is due to inherent genetic determination and what component is a consequence of stresses imposed, such as acoustic trauma, viral infections, otologic disease, vascular diseases, and ototoxic medications. Multiple variables have been evaluated that contribute to hearing loss associated with aging (Table 162.3).

A well-documented phenomenon in elderly subjects is the disproportionate deterioration of speech discrimination for any given pure-tone threshold shift (Fig. 162.1). Tests of central auditory processing include time-compressed speech (word rate per min) and overlapping or interruption of words. These tests suggest that older patients have poorer speech discrimination than younger patients because of changes in central auditory processing. Decreased cell counts in the temporal lobes, increased time required for information processing, and possibly increased transmission time in the central auditory pathways have all been identified as potential factors in central auditory processing disorders in the elderly (9). Elderly patients demonstrate mildly prolonged latencies and reduced wave I amplitudes on the auditory brainstem response (ABR) (10,11).

Schuknecht identified four categories of presbycusis based on clinical and histopathologic changes within the cochlea (Table 162.4):

1. Sensory: epithelial atrophy with loss of sensory cells and the supporting cells of the organ of Corti. Progressive hair cell reduction begins at about age 40. A precipitous decline in pure tone thresholds is seen in the high frequencies.
2. Neural: a reduction in the number of functioning cochlear neurons. Of the 35,500 cochlea neurons at birth, Schuknecht has estimated that 2,100 neurons are lost each decade. When reduction has reached 50% or more of the normal neuronal population, hearing loss develops. This spiral ganglion cell loss also results in a progressive decline in speech discrimination.
3. Strial: atrophy of the stria vascularis. A loss of 30% or more of strial tissue can result in hearing loss characterized by flat hearing loss with relative preservation of speech discrimination.
4. Conductive: alterations of the basilar membrane produce stiffening. The precise nature of these changes is partially hypothesized on the basis of conductive loss that remains otherwise unexplained.

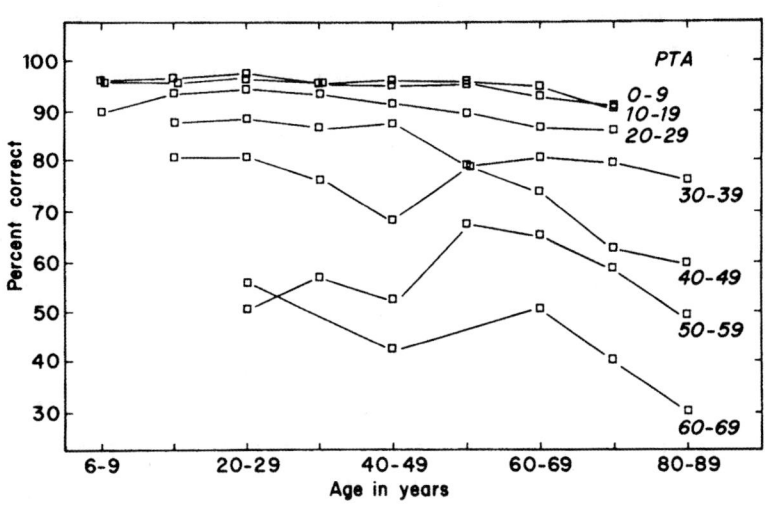

Figure 162.1 Average speech discrimination score as a function of age with the average pure-tone threshold held constant. PTA, pure-tone average. From Jerger J. Audiological findings in aging. *Adv Otorhinolaryngol* 1973;20:115–124.

Although this classification is interesting, each of the four changes may be found to various degrees in any one individual subject; consequently, the audiograms of elderly individuals rarely conform to these classic patterns.

Auditory Rehabilitation

Increased awareness of the prevalence of presbycusis is important, as those with hearing loss tend to be more socially withdrawn and isolated. Patients tend to become frustrated, as do those trying to communicate with them. The main treatment for presbycusis is amplification. Cochlear implantation is an option for some, depending on the severity of the hearing loss. Assistive listening devices (such as FM systems, speaker phones, etc.) are also beneficial. Patient should be instructed to increase the signal-to-noise ratio of their surroundings by reducing the ambient background noise in a room and having someone look directly at them.

The effective use of hearing instruments and cochlear implants is made more complicated in the elderly by commonly associated deficits. Unfortunately, only about 30% of patients who can benefit from hearing aids actually have used them. Decreased vision, cosmetic concerns (feeling "old"), manual dexterity loss, and reduced mobility can make physically removing and adjusting these devices difficult. The financial costs and willingness to wear the devices are additional deterrents for successful amplification. Cognitive deterioration and memory loss can seriously affect an individual's ability to extract maximum benefit from hearing aids or a cochlear implant. Technological advances include total or semi-implantable hearing aids, which may avoid some of the previously mentioned problems experienced with traditional amplification. Refer to Chapter 164 "Hearing aids and assistive listening devices" for a more thorough review of this topic.

AGE-RELATED CHANGES IN THE VESTIBULAR SYSTEMS

Age-related anatomic and physiologic changes to the vestibular system have been described. Age-related degeneration of neural elements in Scarpa ganglia and the vestibular end organs have been demonstrated (12,13). Degenerative changes of the otoconia and reduction in hair cells in the semicircular canals (cristae ampullares) and otolithic organs (saccule and utricle) become more marked with increasing age (14,15). This results in changes in vestibular evoked myogenic potential (VEMP) in older patients characterized by a variable and decreased VEMP amplitude (16–18). Studies evaluating the age-related changes in caloric testing and sinusoidal harmonic acceleration testing are conflicting (19–21).

The key to the evaluation of any patient with dizziness is a detailed description in the patient's own words of the sensation experienced. The subjective character of the dizziness can be classified into four broad categories (Table 162.5):

1. Vertigo (illusion of motion)
2. Presyncope (lightheadedness)
3. Disequilibrium
4. Nonspecific (often psychological disorders)

The time course of the patient's symptoms can provide additional important clues that narrow the differential diagnosis. At the simplest level, one can distinguish between episodic or continuous symptoms. It is helpful to elicit the temporal component of individual attacks as well as the entire course of the disorder:

1. Less than 1 minute: episodes of acute, rotational vertigo lasting less than 1 minute are most commonly associated with disorders of the peripheral vestibular system, such as BPPV.

TABLE 162.5	TYPES OF DIZZINESS	
Category	**Sensation**	**Diagnosis**
Vertigo	Illusion of motion, either linear or rotating (patient or environment)	Vestibular disturbance attributable to peripheral (BPPV, labyrinthitis) or central (brainstem, cerebellar disease) Cardiovascular disease
Presyncope	Impending faint	Diffuse cerebral ischemia attributable to vasovagal response, cardiac disease, or metabolic disorders
Dysequilibrium	Impaired balance and gaze	Impaired motor control due to neuromuscular disease, severe bilateral vestibular disease, stroke, multisensory deficits, or medications
Nonspecific	Light-headedness, "confusion," "wooziness," "fuzzy-headedness"	Often psychological disorders (anxiety, depression, panic), hyperventilation

2. Less than 1 hour: Vertigo lasting a few minutes to an hour or two can be secondary to Ménière disease, transient cerebral hypoperfusion, migraine headaches, or phobic/anxiety disorders.

3. Several hours to 24 hours: This type of dizziness also suggests migraine headaches or Ménière disease. Viral or vascular labyrinthitis usually presents with acute rotational vertigo of several days duration, with gradual improvement.

4. Greater than 24 hours: Migraine-associated dizziness, vestibular neuritis, chronic subjective dizziness, or other central or metabolic causes.

HISTORY AND PHYSICAL EXAMINATION

Before making a diagnosis in an elderly patient, the otologist needs to perform a thorough history and physical examination. Presbyastasis and presbycusis are diagnoses of exclusion; other pathologies must be ruled out. Associated otologic symptoms discussed with the patient include hearing loss, tinnitus, aural fullness, otorrhea, and otalgia. Patients also need to be asked about a history of significant noise exposure/trauma (e.g., loud music, gunfire, etc.), prior otologic/head and neck surgery, and a family history of hearing loss. Because of the high incidence of systemic illnesses in the elderly population, a detailed past medical and surgical history is obtained; one should inquire about the presence of neurologic or ophthalmologic diseases, which can create symptoms of dizziness. A detailed inquiry should be obtained about systemic disorders that potentially interfere with cerebral blood supply that may produce vertigo due to either focal brainstem involvement or diffuse cerebral ischemia. Cardiac abnormalities (e.g., arrhythmia, valvular regurgitation/stenosis) can cause presyncopal episodes. Systemic illnesses such as diabetes mellitus, hypothyroidism, human immunodeficiency virus infection, and sexually transmitted diseases can also result in vestibular symptoms and should be queried. The patient should be counseled to follow-up with their primary care physician for the above conditions and to meet CDC guidelines for screening tests and immunizations. Patients who present with complaints of dizziness should be asked about a prior history of falls and if they are experiencing problems with driving.

A thorough history of prescription, nonprescription, and alternative medications is assessed. A social history is critical and should include an assessment of alcohol, caffeine, salt, tobacco, and illicit drug use. Cardiovascular drugs such as diuretics, beta-blockers, and vasodilators may produce presyncope and orthostatic symptomatology. Ototoxic drugs (e.g., aminoglycosides such as gentamicin) typically cause disequilibrium and oscillopsia. Alcohol can cause postural hypotension resulting in presyncope. Psychiatric medications, muscle relaxants, and anticonvulsants also have been associated with disequilibrium (Table 162.6). Polypharmacy is a significant issue in the elderly and may be a potential cause of vestibular symptoms.

A complete neurologic examination including a peripheral vestibular assessment should be performed in patients presenting with dizziness. Refer to Chapter 165 "Clinical evaluation of the patient with vertigo" for more thorough review. Otomicroscopic exam is done to rule out middle ear disease, cholesteatoma, or temporal bone tumors. A head and neck exam is done to rule out a concomitant otolaryngologic abnormality. A directed systemic (cardiovascular) examination may also be performed. Dix-Hallpike testing with Frenzel lenses should be performed. Drachman (22) advocates the use of the Dizziness Simulation Battery in the office evaluation of dizziness (Table 162.7). The patient is asked to identify which of eight different maneuvers most closely reproduces a patient's dizziness. This test battery includes an assessment of hyperventilation, orthostatic hypotension, peripheral vestibulopathy, carotid sinus simulation, and multisensory disorders. Carotid sinus stimulation should be avoided in the clinical setting due of the risk of syncope and cardiac arrhythmias. The elderly patient with complaints of vertigo may suffer from any of the disorders found in younger individuals (e.g., BPPV, acute labyrinthitis, and Ménière disease) but more often typically has a multifactorial aspect to his or her symptoms.

TABLE 162.6	MEDICATIONS THAT CAN PRODUCE OR EXACERBATE BALANCE DISTURBANCE	
Drug Class	**Type of Dizziness**	**Mechanism**
Alcohol	Unsteady gaze, positional vertigo	Cerebellar and vestibular dysfunction
Sedatives, anxiolytics	Nonspecific lightheadedness	CNS depression
Antihypertensives	Presyncope	Orthostatic hypotension
Antiepileptics	Dysequilibrium	Cerebellar dysfunction
Aminoglycosides	Dysequilibrium, oscillopsia	Labyrinthine hair cell damage

TABLE 162.7	DIZZINESS SIMULATION BATTERY

Cardiovascular
  Orthostatic blood pressure testing
  Potentiated Valsalva maneuver (produces presyncope)
  Carotid sinus stimulation
Vestibular
  Dix-Hallpike maneuver (only produces vertigo in patients with positioning vertigo)
  Barany rotation (stimulates horizontal semicircular canals, producing vertigo in anyone who retains some vestibular function)
Multisensory
  Walk and turn
  Seated head turn
Psychiatric
  Hyperventilation (30 s)

CONDITIONS CAUSING VESTIBULAR DYSFUNCTION IN THE ELDERLY

BPPV is the most common cause of dizziness among elderly and has been reported to be the cause for vertigo in up to 39.1% of patients over 70 years old (23). A cross-sectional study found a 9% incidence of unrecognized BPPV in an elderly population (24). As in younger patients, the posterior semicircular canal is most commonly affected, although any canal can be involved. The presence of BPPV in the elderly is significant since these patients have a 78% prevalence of suffering a fall (24).

The reason for an increased incidence of BPPV in the elderly population is multifactorial. It has been demonstrated the mass and number of otoconia declines with age with the saccule affected more severely than the utricle (25). In addition, decline in calcium metabolism manifested by osteopenia and osteoporosis may have resulted in a loss of otoconia volume in the elderly (26,27). Finally, decreased vascular supply to the otolith organs is more common in the elderly population and may be associated with vertebrobasilar insufficiency or migraine headaches (28–30).

Cerebrovascular insufficiency caused by ischemia of the labyrinth or central vestibular nuclei may result in episodes of acute vertigo associated with focal neurologic deficits such as dysphagia, hemiparesis, dysarthria, headache, or blurred vision. The diagnosis is clinically based and includes the presence of focal neurologic deficits. It can arise as a consequence of reduced flow caused by arteriosclerotic disease in the vertebrobasilar system, or it can arise as a consequence of compression of the vertebral arteries from cervical osteoarthritis.

A brainstem stroke may present as paroxysmal vertigo with unremitting nausea and vomiting, but a brief neurologic examination typically will uncover other neurologic deficits. Even so, patients are occasionally released from the emergency department with an inaccurate diagnosis because the patient may only be aware of the fact that even small, brief head movements precipitate overwhelming vertigo, nausea, and vomiting. Patients may be unaware of the other neurologic deficits produced by the infarct. Fortunately cerebrovascular disease is an uncommon cause of isolated dizziness with a recent study showing an incidence of less than 1 in 500 patients having a major cerebrovascular event within a month after being discharged from the emergency department when presenting with a chief complaint of dizziness (31).

Orthostatic hypotension occurs only when the patient assumes the standing position from the supine or sitting positions. By strict criteria, orthostatic hypotension requires a 20-mm Hg decrease in systolic pressure and a10-mm Hg reduction in diastolic pressure 3 minutes after standing. The sensitivity and specificity of this test has been debated. Many patients have subjective disequilibrium, vertigo, and presyncope without ever meeting the strict definitional criteria. A cardiologist may perform tilt-table testing if the diagnosis is still suspected. Postural hypotension arises from pooling of blood in the lower extremities because of decreased tone. The chronic use of antihypertensive agents, prolonged bed rest, and autonomic dysfunction can all produce orthostatic hypotension. Vasovagal attacks (fainting) may be induced when strong emotions activate the brainstem medullary vasodepressor centers. Vagal hyperactivity causes a decreased cardiac output, leading to a decrease in cerebral blood flow. Decreased cardiac output because of arrhythmia, congestive heart failure, myocardial infarction, and valvular disease (such as aortic stenosis) may lead to the presyncopal type of lightheadedness.

Bilateral symmetric vestibular loss results in persistent unsteadiness. This type of imbalance is typically worse in the dark, when visual cues are not available to help compensate for the loss. Bilateral vestibulopathy can arise from ototoxic drug exposure but also occurs as an idiopathic degenerative disorder. Proprioceptive and somatosensory loss can produce disequilibrium that is worse in the dark. It is often secondary to peripheral neuropathy (common in patients with diabetes mellitus or renal failure).

Osteoarthritis of the cervical spine may cause disequilibrium due to spinal stenosis with spinal cord compression. Such patients often demonstrate bowel and bladder dysfunction. Degenerative disease of the cervical spine may also produce a sense of disequilibrium and imbalance because of altered proprioceptive feedback from muscle stretch receptors and position sense receptors in the muscle and joints of the cervical spine.

Lesions of the frontal lobes or basal ganglia cause disequilibrium often associated with weakness, rigidity, or tremor. Cerebellar lesions cause severe disequilibrium with or without visual cues and are often associated with visible nystagmus, a wide-based gait, and truncal ataxia.

Parkinson disease, common among the elderly, produces characteristic postural and motor abnormalities resulting in a festinating gait. These patients usually stand in a posture of flexion with the thoracic spine bent forward and the head bent down. With forward locomotion the patient takes short, shuffling steps that become successfully more rapid, and the patient may fall without assistance. This disturbance of posture and motor control often results in disequilibrium. The postural instability typically does not respond to levodopa.

Multisensory impairments are due to impaired physiologic function in several systems simultaneously and are more common in the elderly than in the young. Modest disturbances in each of these systems may synergize to produce postural instability and disequilibrium out of proportion to the individual deficits. Subjects with multisensory impairments typically present with a sense of disequilibrium during standing or walking. Multidisciplinary care involving the geriatric specialist, cardiologist, neurologist, vestibular physical therapist, and ophthalmologist may be warranted.

Hyperventilation is often a consequence of anxiety or phobic disorders. Diffuse cerebral ischemia results from constriction of the cerebral vasculature caused by decreased carbon dioxide in the blood. Anxiety and panic disorders, adjustment reactions, and depressive disorders are the most common diagnoses. Such patients often describe a chronic feeling of "wooziness." Two mechanisms have been proposed by Sloane: (a) Patients with underlying primary psychological disorders may be more susceptible to impairment by diseases affecting neurosensory systems, and (b) dizziness symptoms themselves impair function and may cause secondary psychological problems. Management consists of treating the appropriate underlying disorder when present.

DIAGNOSTIC EVALUATION

In straightforward cases (e.g., posterior canal BPPV), the diagnosis is easily determined by a careful and detailed history and physical examination. An audiogram is a relatively inexpensive but useful screening tool. In patients with vague symptoms, complicating histories, and significant comorbidities, a vestibular evaluation is recommended. This may include electronystagmography or videonystagmography, rotary chair testing, ABR, electrocochleography, VEMPs, and computerized dynamic platform posturography. Refer to Chapter 144 "Balance function tests" for a more thorough discussion of the evaluation of dizziness. Radiologic studies (CT and/or MRI scans) may be ordered as deemed necessary, especially with asymmetric otologic complaints.

MANAGEMENT

A sensation of imbalance and a fear of falling lead to a greater level of inactivity and social isolation, worsening the quality of life in a group of people who may have already lost spouses, friends, and other social support systems because of their age. When possible, treatment is directed at the underlying cause of the dizziness, as described under those conditions. Sometimes, however, the only available option is nonspecific therapy directed at symptom control. In general, medical therapy for patients with an acute loss of vestibular function is aimed at controlling the acute vestibular and autonomic symptoms. Five main classes of drugs are used: antihistamines (e.g., meclizine), phenothiazines (e.g., promethazine), anticholinergics (e.g., scopolamine), 5HT3 antagonists (e.g., ondansetron), and benzodiazepines (e.g., diazepam). All drugs should be administered sparingly and for short durations (1 to 2 weeks) because they can cause a reduction in central nervous system (CNS) compensation. Meclizine is typically administered in doses of 12.5 to 25 mg orally three times per day as needed for acute, peripheral vertigo of long duration. Benzodiazepines (usually diazepam at 2.5 to 7.5 mg daily in divided doses) suppress vestibular output of the vestibular nuclei.

Benzodiazepines are the most effective vestibular suppressants. 5HT3 antagonists may be helpful if nausea and/or vomiting are prominent symptoms. However, there is no evidence of 5HT3 receptors within the vestibular system. Phenothiazines can be administered rectally if nausea and/or vomiting does not allow oral intake of medications. All medication should be used cautiously in the elderly, to avoid CNS side effects. Many of these classes of drugs share a similar side effect profile. Antihistamines, phenothiazines, and anticholinergics all share the propensity to produce sedation, dysphoria, and disorientation. If combination therapy is used, care is taken to avoid synergy of side effects. Many geriatric patients are already taking drugs with anticholinergic or sedative side effects. The interaction of vestibular suppressants with these medications is carefully considered.

Vestibular rehabilitation has been an effective therapy for more than 50 years (32–34). In addition, it can be used in conjunction with other types of physical therapy and exercise. Many of the problems associated with aging may be due primarily to inactivity. It is thought that some of the aging process itself can be slowed by exercising and physical activity. Vestibular rehabilitation involves specific habituation exercises designed to enhance the normal adaptive mechanisms in the CNS. The benefits of vestibular rehabilitation are not affected by a patient's age (35). The goal of vestibular rehabilitation is fall prevention. One in three elderly individuals living in the community fall each year. Hospital or nursing home patients fall twice as often as those who are not in these settings. Vestibular symptoms precede falls in more than 50% of these patients. Program strategies vary depending on the patient's primary problem, but they are aimed at stabilizing gaze and posture, improving CNS adaptation, conditioning, and providing emotional and psychological support. The principal components of effective vestibular rehabilitation include gaze stabilization, balance retraining, and desensitization. Each aspect is addressed separately using different exercises.

Gaze stabilization exercises promote vestibular adaptation through exercises that stimulate the vestibuloocular reflex. Balance retraining starts with activities that progressively decrease the patient's base of support and progress to gaze exercises performed on varied surfaces (e.g., stairs, foam, balance beams). The balance system is challenged by having patients attempt to walk through crowded hallways. Strengthening exercises are prescribed to improve muscle strength and flexibility. Given the buoyancy of water, swimming pool exercises provide a safe environment in which the elderly can exercise. Repetitive head and arm movements designed to promote vertigo and unsteadiness in a safe and predictable environment enhance the CNS adaptive mechanisms. These exercises are repeated until they are well tolerated or are not providing additional meaningful improvement. Over a 6- to 8-week course, the number of repetitions is slowly increased. Vestibular rehabilitation is administered by a physical therapist with special expertise in treating vestibular disorders in the elderly. These rehabilitation strategies are effective in positional vertigo and to compensate for sudden loss of vestibular function (after recovery from an acute attack and after vegetative symptoms have disappeared). These exercises also provide improved function and mobility in patients with multisensory deficits.

ABLATIVE THERAPY

Patients who continue to suffer from incapacitating, lifestyle-limiting dizziness despite maximum medical therapy may be candidates for chemical (gentamicin) or surgical ablative therapy, such as labyrinthectomy or vestibular nerve section. Ablative therapy has very limited utility and benefit in patients without Meniere disease. Recovery from unilateral loss of vestibular function is felt to be slower and less complete in the geriatric population and postprocedure rehabilitation is recommended to optimize recovery.

SUMMARY

More than 12.5 million people over the age of 65 in the United States are thought to be significantly affected by dizziness or balance disturbances. Dizziness is the most common presenting complaint in patients over 75 years of age. The majority of the geriatric population with dizziness has multifactorial causes. It is important that one be familiar with the differential diagnosis, evaluation, and potentially multidisciplinary management of these disorders. It is inappropriate to attribute symptoms such as dizziness to the aging process alone; a complete evaluation must be performed. The otologist should be prepared to make referrals to a neurologist, audiologist, cardiologist, ophthalmologist, or psychiatrist and work in conjunction with the primary care physician to provide a full evaluation and comprehensive care.

HIGHLIGHTS

- Aging produces changes in the auditory and vestibular system that result in loss of function.
- Alterations in the physiology of the EAC lead to a dramatically increased incidence of cerumen impaction in the elderly.
- Presbycusis is multifactorial.
- Presbycusis is a diagnosis of exclusion; other causes should be sought.
- Elderly subjects with presbycusis may have degradation of speech discrimination out of proportion to pure-tone loss.
- Amplification and cochlear implantation can significantly improve the quality of life for elderly patients.
- BPPV is the most common cause of vertigo in the elderly population.
- Dizziness is the most common presenting complaint in patients over 75 years of age.
- A specific cause of dizziness and vertigo can be found in 85% of elderly patients.
- The differential diagnosis of balance disturbance in the elderly can often be rapidly narrowed by determining if they describe symptoms of true vertigo, presyncope, chronic disequilibrium, or of nonspecific complaints.

REFERENCES

1. Institute of Medicine. *Retooling for an aging America: building the health care workforce.* Washington, DC: The National Academies Press, 2008.
2. Lin HW, Bhattacharyya N. Otologic diagnoses in the elderly: current utilization and predicted workload increase. *Laryngoscope* 2011;121(7):1504–1507.
3. Ries PW. Prevalence and characteristics of persons with hearing trouble: United States, 1990–91. *Vital Health Stat 10* 1994;(188):1–75.
4. Dix MR. Rehabilitation of vertigo. In: Dix MR, Hood JD, eds. *Vertigo.* New York: Wiley, 1984:467–479.
5. Centers for Disease Control and Prevention (CDC). Public health and aging: nonfatal injuries among older adults treated in hospital emergency departments—United States, 2001. *MMWR Morb Mortal Wkly Rep* 2003;52(42):1019–1022.
6. Cooper C, Campion G, Melton LJ III. Hip fractures in the elderly: a world-wide projection. *Osteoporos Int* 1992;2(6):285–289.
7. Stevens JA, Olson S. Reducing falls and resulting hip fractures among older women. *MMWR Recomm Rep* 2000;49(RR-2):3–12.
8. Uneri A, Polat S. Vertigo, dizziness and imbalance in the elderly. *J Laryngol Otol* 2008;122(5):466–469.
9. Harris KC, Dubno JR, Keren NI, et al. Speech recognition in younger and older adults: a dependency on low-level auditory cortex. *J Neurosci* 2009;29(19):6078–6087.
10. Burkard RF, Sims D. The human auditory brainstem response to high click rates: aging effects. *Am J Audiol* 2001;10(2):53–61. [Erratum in: *Am J Audiol* 2002;11(1):12.]
11. Burkard RF, Sims D. A comparison of the effects of broadband masking noise on the auditory brainstem response in young and older adults. *Am J Audiol* 2002;11(1):13–22.

12. Park JJ, Tang Y, Lopez I, et al. Age-related change in the number of neurons in the human vestibular ganglion. *J Comp Neurol* 2001;431(4):437–443.

13. Richter E. Quantitative study of human Scarpa's ganglion and vestibular sensory epithelia. *Acta Otolaryngol* 1980;90(3–4): 199–208.

14. Merchant SN, Velázquez-Villaseñor L, Tsuji K, et al. Temporal bone studies of the human peripheral vestibular system. Normative vestibular hair cell data. *Ann Otol Rhinol Laryngol Suppl* 2000;181:3–13.

15. Rauch SD, Velazquez-Villaseñor L, Dimitri PS, et al. Decreasing hair cell counts in aging humans. *Ann N Y Acad Sci* 2001;942: 220–227.

16. Serrador JM, Lipsitz LA, Gopalakrishnan GS, et al. Loss of otolith function with age is associated with increased postural sway measures. *Neurosci Lett* 2009;465(1):10–15.

17. Janky KL, Shepard N. Vestibular evoked myogenic potential (VEMP) testing: normative threshold response curves and effects of age. *J Am Acad Audiol* 2009;20(8):514–522.

18. Su HC, Huang TW, Young YH, et al. Aging effect on vestibular evoked myogenic potential. *Otol Neurotol* 2004;25(6):977–980.

19. Maes L, Dhooge I, D'haenens W, et al. The effect of age on the sinusoidal harmonic acceleration test, pseudorandom rotation test, velocity step test, caloric test, and vestibular-evoked myogenic potential test. *Ear Hear* 2010;31(1):84–94.

20. Wall C III, Black FO, Hunt AE. Effects of age, sex and stimulus parameters upon vestibulo-ocular responses to sinusoidal rotation. *Acta Otolaryngol* 1984;98(3–4):270–278.

21. Peterka RJ, Black FO, Schoenhoff MB. Age-related changes in human vestibulo-ocular reflexes: sinusoidal rotation and caloric tests. *J Vestib Res* 1990–1991;1(1):49–59.

22. Drachman DA, Hart CW. An approach to the dizzy patient. *Neurology* 1972;22(4):323–334.

23. Katsarkas A. Dizziness in aging: a retrospective study of 1194 cases. *Otolaryngol Head Neck Surg* 1994;110(3):296–301.

24. Oghalai JS, Manolidis S, Barth JL, et al. Unrecognized benign paroxysmal positional vertigo in elderly patients. *Otolaryngol Head Neck Surg* 2000;122(5):630–634.

25. Igarashi M, Saito R, Mizukoshi K, et al. Otoconia in young and elderly persons: a temporal bone study. *Acta Otolaryngol Suppl* 1993;504:26–29.

26. Vibert D, Kompis M, Häusler R. Benign paroxysmal positional vertigo in older women may be related to osteoporosis and osteopenia. *Ann Otol Rhinol Laryngol* 2003;112(10):885–889.

27. Jeong SH, Choi SH, Kim JY, et al. Osteopenia and osteoporosis in idiopathic benign positional vertigo. *Neurology* 2009;72(12):1069–1076.

28. Ishiyama A, Jacobson KM, Baloh RW. Migraine and benign positional vertigo. *Ann Otol Rhinol Laryngol* 2000;109(4):377–380.

29. Uneri A. Migraine and benign paroxysmal positional vertigo: an outcome study of 476 patients. *Ear Nose Throat J* 2004;83(12): 814–815.

30. Baloh RW, Honrubia V, Jacobson K. Benign positional vertigo: clinical and oculographic features in 240 cases. *Neurology* 1987;37(3):371–378.

31. Kim AS, Fullerton HJ, Johnston SC. Risk of vascular events in emergency department patients discharged home with diagnosis of dizziness or vertigo. *Ann Emerg Med* 2011;57(1):34–41.

32. Jung JY, Kim JS, Chung PS, et al. Effect of vestibular rehabilitation on dizziness in the elderly. *Am J Otolaryngol* 2009;30(5):295–299.

33. Hall CD, Heusel-Gillig L, Tusa RJ, et al. Efficacy of gaze stability exercises in older adults with dizziness. *J Neurol Phys Ther* 2010;34(2):64–69.

34. McPherson D, Whitaker S, Wrobel B. DDX: disequilibrium of aging. In: Goebel JA, ed. *Practical management of the dizzy patient*, 2nd ed. Philadelphia, PA: Lippincott Williams and Wilkins, 2001:297–344.

35. Whitney SL, Wrisley DM, Marchetti GF, et al. The effect of age on vestibular rehabilitation outcomes. *Laryngoscope* 2002; 112(10):1785–1790.

163

Cochlear Implants and Other Implantable Auditory Prostheses

Oliver F. Adunka   *Craig A. Buchman*

Over the past few decades, cochlear implants and other active auditory prosthetic devices have helped revolutionize the fields of otolaryngology, audiology, and other hearing-related specialties. Generally, these prosthetic devices can be thought of as either *hair cell stimulators* when the native auditory system is driven by way of amplification of the acoustic signal or *neural stimulators* when electrical currents are applied directly to or in close proximity to the auditory neural tissues. These devices should be distinguished from prostheses that are passive conductors of acoustic energy such as ossicular reconstruction and stapes prostheses. Hair cell stimulation devices are, by design, for patients with sufficient hair cell populations and thus residual hearing. By contrast, neural stimulators are for patients with hair cell populations that are insufficient for acoustic stimulation but neural populations that are preserved. Clearly, areas of overlapping indication exist for these devices. Moreover, these concepts are beginning to be combined to achieve even greater performance for individual patients.

Hair cell stimulators activate the auditory system by increasing the transfer of acoustic energy to the inner ear through hearing aids, active middle ear implants (MEIs), and osseointegrated auditory implants. Acoustic amplification can be delivered to the tympanic membrane in the external auditory canal by conventional hearing aids. By contrast, active MEIs are placed on the ossicular chain or windows of the inner ear to deliver acoustic energy to the functional hair cells, thus bypassing the external auditory canal and tympanic membrane. Osseointegrated implants are placed distant from the otic capsule and conducting ear structures and stimulate the inner ear through osseoconductive forces delivered by setting the skull bone in motion.

Auditory neural stimulators include cochlear implants, auditory brainstem and midbrain implants. Cochlear implants are for patients with preserved auditory nerve populations and are usually placed longitudinally within the cochlear lumen, in close proximity to the distal nerve fibers. These devices rely heavily on the tonotopic arrangement of the neural fibers within the cochlea for discrete frequency-specific (i.e., place) stimulation. The auditory brainstem implant (ABI) can be used for patients in whom the auditory nerve is absent or unavailable for stimulation. This device's electrodes are applied either on the surface of or within the cochlear nucleus of the brainstem at the foramen of Luschka at the pontomedullary junction. Finally, the midbrain implant, which remains investigational, would possibly be indicated for individuals in whom the cochlear nucleus is not available for stimulation because of pathologic or surgical insults. In all three instances, speech processors are used to convert environmental acoustic signals into electrical stimulation strategies that might be appropriate for the neural tissues in question.

Clearly, cochlear implants are the most successful prosthetic solution to replace the function of a sensory organ and have helped (re)habilitate many thousands of patients with hearing loss. The success of this intervention is derived mostly from a sustained research and development effort for more than 40 years, the lack of other effective treatments for patients with severe to profound hearing loss, and the presence of a viable cochlear nerve in nearly all patients. Through auditory electrical stimulation, these devices have allowed patients with congenital and acquired deafness to obtain sound awareness and enhanced speech understanding in both quiet and noise, thereby drastically improving educational and employment opportunities, social integration, and overall quality of life. This chapter provides a detailed overview of cochlear implants and other auditory prosthetics that are currently being used in patients today.

COCHLEAR IMPLANTS

Overview

The modern cochlear implant is a device designed to convert environmental sound into electrical impulses that are delivered along a multiple electrode array situated in close proximity to the cochlear (auditory) nerve. Since the distal cochlear nerve fibers are arranged along the tonotopic, longitudinal axis of the cochlea lumen, application of discrete electrical stimulation at progressively deeper stations results in variably lower, psychophysical frequency percepts. As this paradigm does not necessarily rely upon hair cell transduction mechanisms, it is ideal for patients with significant hair cell loss. Since most patients with sensorineural hearing loss maintain some degree of functional auditory nerve fibers, these devices are particularly well adapted for most etiologies of hearing loss. Given the need for surgery and the effectiveness of hearing aids for lesser degrees of hearing impairment, the cochlear implant has been reserved for patients with significant degrees of hearing loss that are not easily rehabilitated with conventional amplification.

Outcomes for cochlear implantation can be defined in terms of sound awareness, enhancement of lipreading, improvements in speech perception, quality of life, and cost-effectiveness. Broader outcomes for adults include improvements in socialization, employment opportunities, income, and overall health and well-being (1–4). For children, extended outcomes include speech and oral language production, educational setting and achievement, the need for specialized services, and safety (5–7). Recently, expanding indications for implantation and combining the electrical stimulation of a cochlear implant with native acoustic stimulation are broadening the application of this technology.

Historical Aspects

The first electrical stimulation of the inner ear probably was performed by Count Alessandro Volta at the end of the 18th century when he placed two metal rods in his ears and connected them to the terminal of 30 or 40 electrolytic cells (~50 V). He reported the sensation of "une secousse dans la tete" or a blow on the head followed by a sound like "the boiling of a viscid liquid" (8). Djourno and Eyries are credited with the first intralabyrinthine implantation of an electrical stimulating prosthesis. This was placed through a labyrinthine fistula in a patient with chronic otitis media and cholesteatoma in Paris in 1957. Djourno was a French neurophysiologist and Eyries an established otologist. Upon stimulation, the patient described high-frequency sounds that resembled the "roulette wheel of a casino" and "crickets." Their patient was able to discern the words "pap," "mamm," and "allo" (9–11).

In 1957, a patient in Los Angeles, CA, brought William House, MD, a news article detailing the apparent success of Djourno and Eyries. By 1960 and 1961, House with his colleagues Doyle and Doyle experimented with electrical stimulation of the inner ear. House performed promontory and vestibule stimulation of patients undergoing stapedectomy surgery (12). Using a square-wave generator, he noted that patients could detect auditory percepts from electrically delivered currents better in the perilymph of the vestibule than on the promontory. Direct stimulation of the perilymph did not cause dizziness or facial stimulation above 30 Hz. In the 1960s and 1970s, numerous other groups were exploring the field of electrical stimulation of the inner ear, primarily for the purpose of hearing. Teams including F. Blair Simmons and Robert White (Stanford University); Donald Eddington (University of Utah); Robin Michelson, Michael Merzinich, and Robert Schindler (University of California at San Francisco); and Claude-Henri Chouard (France) and Graeme Clark (University of Melbourne) were most active. In contrast with House, these efforts were mostly directed at developing a multichannel electrode CI (13–18).

Blair Simmons, MD, with the assistance of Epley at Stanford (1964) implanted six electrodes in the modiolus portion of the eighth nerve near the basal cochlear fibers under local anesthesia (19). Electrical stimulation resulted in some auditory percepts. Following these initial experiments, House and Doyle implanted two adult patients with single gold electrodes for short-term stimulation of hearing. One additional patient received a 5-electrode device. All three of these devices were later removed because of compatibility issues (12). Specifically, the wires were tracked through the skin and resulted in local wound infection and irritation.

At the University of Paris as well as the Universities of Utah and California at San Francisco (UCSF), percutaneous connectors attached to intracochlear electrode arrays allowed for stimulation to be carried in a variety of ways ultimately allowing for great advances in the development of signal processing strategies (14,15,17). Ultimately, however, similar to the experiences of House and Simmons, these devices required removal because of local infection. Importantly, it was clear that the percutaneous connection was unsustainable and that an alternative method for energy and data transfer was needed.

House later teamed with engineer Jack Urban to produce the first wearable, "take home" cochlear implant, implanted in Chuck Graser in 1972 (12,20). This was possible because of the use of newer, biocompatible materials developed in the pacemaker industry. His initial device was a five-wire electrode grounded through the footplate of the stapes. He was ultimately fitted with a speech processor/stimulator that had a single electrode that delivered a 16-KHz sinusoid carrier wave. While this implant as well as the one used by Michelson (21) at UCSF failed to produce open-set speech perception, these devices proved that simple transcutaneous, inductive coupling was possible and that a percutaneous connection was not needed (21).

Dobelle et al. (22) later proposed a single radiofrequency (RF) link for both data and power transfer. In 1974, the University of Melbourne produced an electromagnetic dual link for data and power transfer that was highly efficient. This method allowed for transcutaneous, efficient transfer of power and data and is currently used in the Food and Drug Administration (FDA)-approved systems that are clinically available today in the United States (US) (23).

Creating a hermetically sealed device was a major challenge for early investigators. Graeme Clark and colleagues in Melbourne (1974) melted glass on to wires that exited a Kovar steel container that housed the circuitry (24). This was unsuccessful as fluid leakage persisted. In the pacemaker industry, epoxy resin was also unsuccessful. K. Kratochivil at Telectronics, a pacemaker company in Australia, discovered that when a blend of ceramics was sintered, it would bond to both wires and the metallic container to produce an impermeable seal. For Cochlear Corp in Australia, this technology when used in combination with a titanium package for strength produced the hermetically sealed device that is in use today. However, this construct required moving the data transmission antenna to a remote site, creating an elongated device with a susceptible antenna connection (24). After implanting their initial multichannel prototype device in 1978, great strides were made in the 1980s demonstrating the superiority of these place-coding devices over the single-channel implants of House (25–29). From this time forward, place coding using multiple electrodes situated longitudinally along the course of scala tympani to stimulate the tonotopic organization of the cochlear nerve became the preferred approach (30–32).

From Clark's work arose Cochlear Corp, the largest manufacturer of cochlear implants in the world today. In 1984, the Australian multichannel cochlear implant was introduced into the market and approved for adult usage by the FDA. In 1990, the criterion was extended to children older than 2 years of age. Over the next decade, the FDA-approved minimum criterion for age of implantation in children was lowered to 12 months.

With the help of Ingeborg and Erwin Hochmair in Vienna, Austria, Kurt Burian implanted a multichannel device in 1977. From this effort grew the company MED-EL corporation. In California, the work at UCSF by Michelson, Merzinich, and Schindler progressed to form Advanced Bionics Corporation (Sylmar, California, USA), the only US-based cochlear implant manufacturer. For both Advanced Bionics and MED-EL Corporations, a ceramic housing was chosen so the antenna and electronics were included in the same package. Unfortunately, ceramic was more brittle and susceptible to cracks in response to external trauma. The welding of ceramic to the metal header also created a relative weak point for the hermetic seal. Over time, the ceramic construct of these devices has given way to the silastic–titanium devices that are in use today by all three implant manufacturers producing FDA-approved CIs in the US.

Over the last 30 years, electrode and speech processor developments have produced more effective stimulation strategies associated with successively higher performance levels. Further miniaturization of components has resulted in small, behind-the-ear speech processors and very thin, atraumatic electrodes that preserve intracochlear structures.

In the early 2000s, bilateral cochlear implantation as well as implantation with preservation of significant acoustic residual hearing has broadened the indications for these devices. Moreover, combining acoustic stimulation with that of the electrical signal provided by the cochlear implant has begun to produce results for patients that had previously not been considered possible (33–36). Today, sound localization, hearing in noise, and even music appreciation are becoming possible.

In 2005, a totally implantable cochlear implant was developed in Sydney and implanted in Melbourne, Australia, as a part of a research project conducted by Cochlear Ltd and the University of Melbourne (37). This was the first cochlear implant system capable of functioning for sustained periods with no external components. Because this device used a subcutaneous microphone, significant attenuation of the signal and interference with bodily noise limited wide-scale application. Nonetheless, the stage has now been set for a fully implantable cochlear implant. With further advances, it seems probable that one day, normal hearing might be restored through combinations of technology without the need for visible external hardware.

In the 1960s and 1970s, considerable opposition arose within the scientific community regarding the possibility of speech understanding by patients with cochlear implants. Specifically, "auditory physiologists and histopathologists dismissed these investigations as misguided attempts by surgeons—who know little about auditory neuroscience to stimulate nerves that were already dead" (26). Moreover, the deaf community identified cochlear implants as an unacceptable intervention that "didn't work" and ultimately threatened a child's right to be deaf—a cultural right (38). Over time, combining considerable improvements in technology, indications, and results with the fact that most deaf children are born to two hearing parents who want their child to communicate in an auditory–oral way has made this opposition to cochlear implants lessen. Today, cochlear implants are widely regarded as an accepted and efficacious choice for patients who are deaf or significantly hearing-impaired.

Principles of Electric Stimulation of the Auditory System

The current cochlear implant design consists of an external device (microphone, speech processor, headpiece) and an internal, implanted device (receiver–stimulator, multichannel electrode array) that communicates across intact skin by way of RF. The internal and external device antennas are aligned for transmission by integrated magnets. The microphone detects sound and transmits the information to a signal processor. The processor includes a series of filter banks that use fast-Fourier transforms to partition the acoustic signal into the respective frequency bands and decodes the information into an electrical signal. The signal is processed according to a predefined strategy, amplified, and compressed to match the narrow, electric dynamic range of the ear and sent through the intact skin to the implanted receiver–stimulator. The electrode array that is inserted within the cochlear lumen is hardwired to the receiver–stimulator package. The longitudinal arrangement of the cochlea along a frequency spectrum (basal→apical corresponds to high pitch→low pitch regions) allows for frequency-to-place mapping. Inside the cochlea, electric impulses at the electrodes stimulate neural elements, bypassing the nonfunctioning hair cells. Thus, high-frequency information is converted to frequency pulses that are delivered to basal electrodes, while progressively lower-frequency information is relayed to more apical locations. Today, combinations of temporal and place coding account for most of the stimulation strategies in use. Temporal coding is only beginning to be implemented in newer Hilbert transformation paradigms.

Coding Strategies

The earliest speech-coding strategy used by the House-3M single-channel device employed amplitude modulation of a 16-kHz sinusoid by the bandpass-filtered audio input signal. The incoming signal needed to be compressed to cope with the limited dynamic range for electrical stimulation of the auditory nerve. Even though most of the original temporospectral information of the analog signal was preserved, the signal transfer to the auditory nerve was limited by the maximal firing frequency of the nerve in response to the electrical stimulation at a single site within the cochlea. High synchronization of nerve fibers and the neural refractory period only allowed for frequency transmission up to 1 kHz via pure temporal coding. For higher frequencies, the spectral information could not be sufficiently transferred. While these single-channel devices provided sound awareness and enhancement of lipreading, open-set speech perception was rarely achieved, thus paving the way for the frequency-place coding that is used in all of the multichannel devices on the market today (39).

The earliest multichannel place-coding devices used bandpass filters to separate frequency bands and compression to reduce the needed acoustic dynamic range in to the electrical stimulation range of the cochlear nerve (~20 dB). However, these devices remained limited by current spread and channel interaction, thereby limiting spectral resolution. Poor spectral resolution probably contributed to significant spectral mismatch between the frequency allocation to a given electrode and the perceptual consequences of stimulation. Attempts to improve this spectral

mismatch have included moving the site of electrode activation closer to the neural elements by creating modiolar conforming arrays, intraneural electrodes, light stimulation, or neurotrophic factors (40–42). Another approach has been to use multiple electrode activation at differing times (i.e., temporal coding) to avoid channel interactions, thereby improving stimulation specificity.

Today all of the modern strategies use some variation of pulsatile (on–off), interleaved stimulation of the multiple electrodes within the array in an effort to achieve specific stimulation while avoiding channel interaction, thereby improving frequency selectivity. That is, spatially separate electrodes are activated at different times to account for neural refractory times, current spread, and electrical field interaction. These strategies are commercially known as continuous interleaved sampling (CIS), advanced combination encoder (ACE), Spectral Peak (SPeak), and HiResolution (HiRes) and are individually employed by all three cochlear implant manufacturers, in their products. The primary differences among them are rate of stimulation, number of channels, the relation between the number of filters and the number of electrodes activated, as well as the details of how each channel's envelope is extracted and how much of the acoustic signals temporal information is preserved. SPeak and ACE attempt to emphasize spectral peaks in the signal by selecting a subset of filter outputs with higher energy levels. HiRes augments the envelope with temporal information by allowing higher-frequency components through the envelope detector. Although some patients can clearly perform better with one strategy than another, average speech scores across populations of patients do not clearly demonstrate superiority of a particular strategy (43).

Pathologic Basis for Success

Cochlear implantation usually results in a loss of residual acoustic hearing, presumably from intracochlear trauma induced through cochleostomy or electrode insertion, disruption of the endocochlear potential, or delayed reaction to the foreign body. A variety of evidence has demonstrated traumatic disruption of the cochlear endosteum, spiral ligament, stria vascularis, basilar membrane, osseous spiral lamina, and even modiolar fractures (44–49). Trauma and bone dust may also induce further changes in the inner ear including fibrosis and osteoneogenesis. Such intracochlear changes can potentially increase impedance values and stimulation requirements and alter psychophysical percepts. These changes might also reduce future abilities to reimplant the cochlea or the patients to consider other biologic therapies (50–55). A variety of investigations support the site of stimulation to be the spiral ganglion cell body. Moreover, most evidence demonstrates little correlation between spiral ganglion cell number and speech perception abilities using a cochlear implant. Most recently, new tissue formation in the cochlea has been associated with the degree of neurosensory element loss. These findings suggest

TABLE 163.1	CURRENT FDA APPROVED COCHLEAR IMPLANT DEVICES		
	Advanced Bionics	**Cochlear**	**MedEl**
Electrode arrays	Conforming (helix) −15.5 mm/16 contacts Lateral wall (1J) −17 mm/16 contacts	Conforming (contour advance) −15 mm/22 contacts Lateral wall (straight)[a] −16.4 mm/22 contacts	Conforming (NA) Lateral wall (Standard, Medium, Compressed)[a] −26.4, 20.9, 12.1 mm/24 contacts
Receiver stimulator	Silastic titanium (90 K)	Silastic titanium (system 5 and freedom)	Silastic titanium (concert and sonata) Ceramic (pulsar)
Processors	Ear level (harmony, auria) Body worn (platinum)	Ear level (system 5)-modular Body worn (NA)	Ear level (opus 1 & 2)-modular Body worn (NA)
Coding strategy	CIS Hi fidelity 120	ACE	Continuous interleaved sampling (CIS) Fine structure processing (FSP)
MRI compatibility	Magnet removal required	Magnet removal required	0.2 Tesla MRI
Rechargeable battery	Available	Available	Available

[a]Split array available.

that atraumatic electrodes and surgical approaches and techniques should continue to be sought in the future (48).

Current Device Technology

Currently, there are three major companies that produce cochlear implants in the US. The devices from each implant manufacturer and some of the various differences among them are outline in the Table 163.1. Comparative data between the various devices are sparse or completely lacking making efficacy claims regarding technological superiority theoretical. As these comparative data are lacking, patients are left to choose technology based on factors other than performance including reliability, aesthetics, operational characteristics, surgeon and center preference, and word-of-mouth communication amongst users.

Patient Selection

Absolute contraindications to cochlear implantation include those patients without either a cochlea (Michel aplasia) or a cochlear nerve. Relative contraindication might include those patients with active middle ear disease, severe anesthetic risk, and too much residual hearing or those who are unwilling to tolerate the surgical risks.

There are clearly patients who may require adjustment of expectations through more detailed counseling prior to considering surgery as their prognosis for attaining high-level open-set speech perception might be more limited. Patients at risk for lower level performance might include those with either anatomic disorders that can adversely affect the electrode-neural interface or central nervous system problems that result in impaired auditory processing or cognitive impairment. Examples of the former category include (a) *cochlear disorders* such as extensive cochlear obstruction from previous meningitis, otosclerosis, or

severe inner ear malformation and (b) *cochlear nerve disorders* such as cochlear nerve deficiency (CND) or tumor of the 8th cranial nerve (i.e., vestibular schwannoma). *Central nervous system disorders* that might adversely affect normal brain function and thus performance with the implant could include previous stroke, degenerative diseases such as multiple sclerosis, dementia, tumors, or infections. With these caveats in mind, it is critical to recognize that setting appropriate expectations for potentially lower levels of performance are *not contraindications* to surgery. Rather, restoration of audition through cochlear implantation can result in dramatic improvements in quality of life and daily function for these individuals but should be undertaken following appropriate counseling of expectations. In certain instances, assessment of psychological factors can be useful to better understand a patient's condition prior to considering implantation.

In the US, at least three different bodies have separate guidelines for establishing what constitutes candidacy criteria for cochlear implantation in adults and children. These include the US FDA who recognizes the results of appropriate safety and efficacy clinical trials carried out by the device manufacturers to achieve specific labeling for their product(s), insurance companies, and the Centers for Medicare and Medicaid Services. In general, adults (≥18 years) are required to have a moderate-to-profound hearing loss without medical contraindications and the desire to be a part of the hearing world. The results for aided speech perception testing vary by manufacturer and payer and are listed in Table 163.2. Prelingual children can be as young as 12 months of age, gain limited benefit from amplification, while being enrolled in an early intervention program. Older children with some degree of speech perception should also have specific speech perception testing results that are obtained while wearing appropriate amplification (Table 163.3). It is clear that candidacy criteria continue to evolve as technology improves and new

TABLE 163.2	DEVICE LABELING BASED ON SPEECH PERCEPTION TEST RESULTS IN ADULTS		
	Advanced Bionics	**Cochlear**	**MedEL**
Test materials	HINT Q	HINT Q	HINT Q
Presentation level	Not specified	70 dB SPL	Not specified
Aided condition	Appropriately fit	Binaural best-aided	Best-aided
Score	≤50%	≤50% implanted ear ≤60% best-aided	≤40% best-aided

HINT Q, Hearing in noise test administered in quiet. Presentation level 70 dB SPL.

medical discoveries uncover broadened indications. The reader should always seek up-to-date, detailed information on a case-by-case basis prior to considering candidacy.

For young children, it remains critically important to recognize the importance of early intervention in the form of appropriately fit amplification and/or cochlear implantation in the development of speech perception, speech production, and spoken language (5). While these studies clearly document the fact that earlier is better, this must be balanced against the reality that cochlear implants, in their current format, usually result in a total loss or substantial decrement in native acoustic hearing abilities in the operated ear. While electrophysiologic methods are sufficient for estimating the degree of residual hearing for the purposes of fitting amplification, there remain some patients who have no responses on auditory brainstem response (ABR) and auditory steady state response testing who can gain enough benefit from amplification for the purposes of speech and language development (56,57). With this in mind, it remains important to defer cochlear implantation until the age where developmentally appropriate behavioral audiometric results are valid (usually 7 to 9 months of age for visual reinforcement audiometry). One clear indication for very early implantation might include a history of meningitis with ongoing ossification. Irrespective of the type of intervention, early diagnostic and therapeutic auditory-based speech therapy is critical in assessing progress in spoken language development. This single factor remains of paramount importance in deciding whether to proceed with implantation in the very young, hearing-impaired child.

Temporal Bone Imaging in Cochlear Implantation

Diagnostic imaging of the temporal bone and brain is critical in patients considering cochlear implantation to (a) identify the etiology of hearing loss, (b) define surgical anatomy and the potential for complications or sequelae from surgery, and (c) identify factors that negatively impact upon prognosis for performance using the device. Even in the setting of a normal history and physical examination, it is not unusual for routine preoperative temporal bone imaging to identify conditions such as developmental labyrinthine anomalies, CND, otosclerosis, and inflammation, fibrosis, and ossification of the inner ear.

Imaging protocols for both high-resolution magnetic resonance imaging (MRI) or computed tomography (CT) of the temporal bones and brain have been described previously (58–62). From an imaging perspective, developmental labyrinthine anomalies are well-defined using either MRI or CT. However, MRI is superior to CT for identifying CND in the setting of a normal dimension internal auditory canal, inner ear luminal obstruction when ossification is lacking (i.e., fibrosis), and central nervous system disorders such as vestibular schwannoma, demyelinating disease, and stroke. Conversely, CT is better for determining

TABLE 163.3	DEVICE LABELING BASED ON SPEECH PERCEPTION TEST RESULTS IN CHILDREN		
	Advanced Bionics	**Cochlear**	**MedEL**
Pure-tone thresholds (HL)	≥90 dB HL	Bilateral profound	≥90 dB PTA (@ 1 kHz)
Hearing aid trial	3 mo if <2 y 6 mo if >2 y (NA if ossified)	3–6 mo	3–6 mo
Rehabilitation	Not mentioned	Yes	Yes
Open-set test	<20% MLNT (<4 y) <12% PBK (>4 y) <30% HINT (>4 y) (@ 70 dB SPL MLV)	≤30% MLNT	<20% MLNT or LNT

the degree of labyrinthine obstruction that is due to ossification (i.e., calcified), cochlear nerve aperture patency in the setting of a small internal auditory canal, and facial nerve location within the temporal bone (58,59,61–63). Thus, we prefer MRI to CT for patients with an uncomplicated history as this modality can identify a patent cochlea and normal cochlear nerve while avoiding radiation exposure. CT is used selectively when cochlear obstruction is present, the internal auditory canal is small, the semicircular canals are absent resulting in facial nerve anomaly, and when temporal bone pathology is present. MRI is avoided in patients with pacemakers or severe claustrophobia.

Labyrinthine anomalies have been described in detail previously (64,65). In these cases, cochlear structure can be normal, absent (Michel malformation), cystic, incompletely partitioned (IP), or hypoplastic. Semicircular canals can be either aplastic or dysplastic. The vestibular aqueduct or endolymphatic duct and sac can be enlarged (EVA) in

isolation or in association with cochlear IP. This group is referred to as the *IP-EVA spectrum*. If all cochlear partitioning is absent but there remains differentiation in to cochlear and vestibular labyrinthine compartments, this is termed as cystic cochleovestibular malformation (CCVA). Common cavity (CC) is defined as no internal differentiation of the labyrinth into either a vestibular or cochlear compartment. Examples are shown in Figure 163.1.

CND refers to a small or absent auditory nerve on high-resolution imaging and has been identified among patients with normal inner ear morphology as well as those with inner ear malformations, narrow internal auditory canals, and/or electrophysiologic characteristics of auditory neuropathy spectrum disorder (ANSD) (60,66–68). Figure 163.2 shows examples of CND in the setting of a normal and small internal auditory canal.

Cochlear obstruction can occur following previous cochlear inflammation in the setting of meningitis and

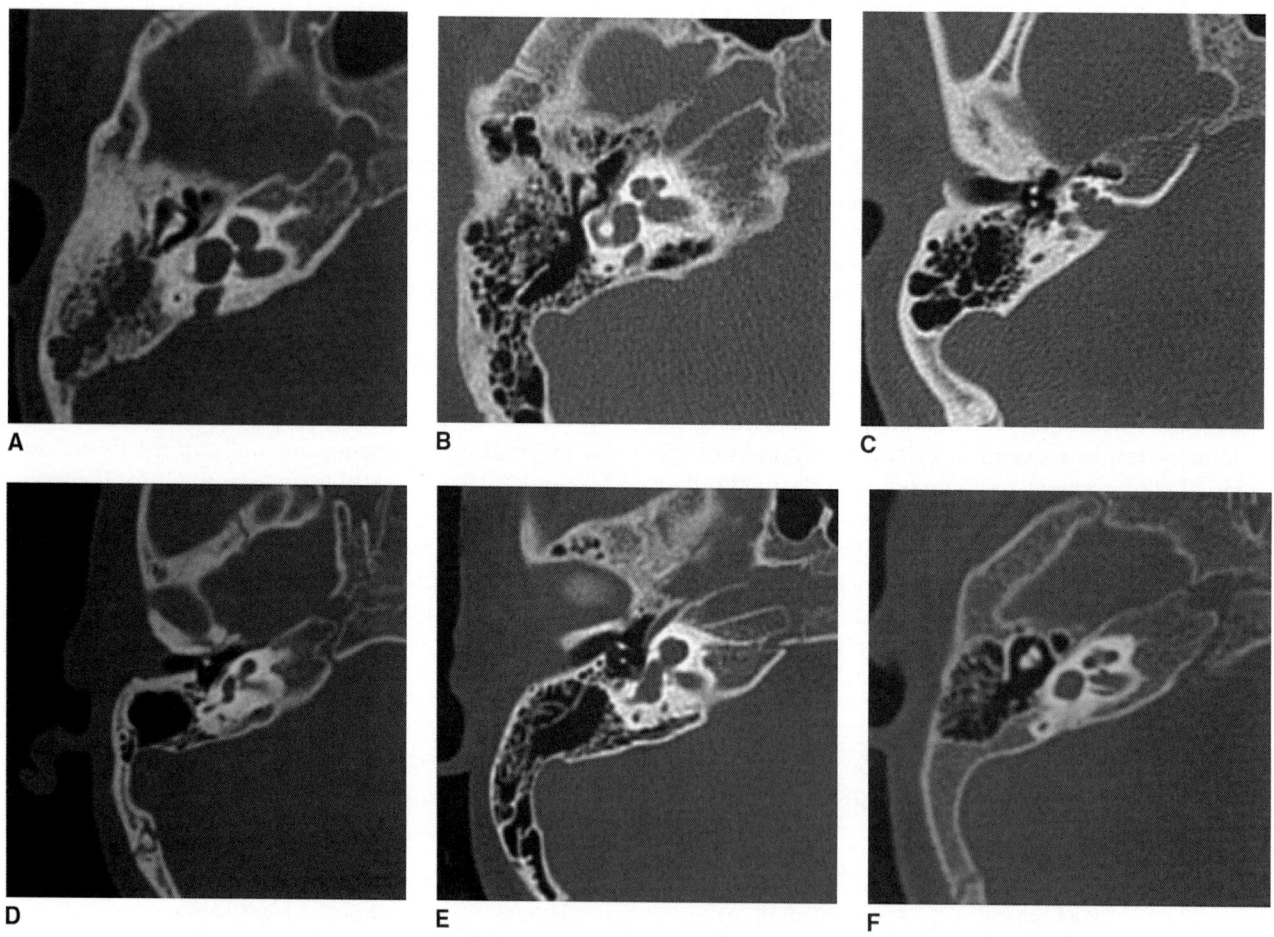

Figure 163.1 Axial CT images demonstrating various inner ear anomalies, including incomplete partition (**A–C**), cochlear hypoplasia (**D–F**), and cochleovestibular malformations (**G,H**). In incomplete partition, there are normal cochlear external dimensions, but decreased or absent partitioning. Type I (**A**) has absent internal divisions; type II (**B**) has apical fusion with a present interscalar septum (called Mondini type when the vestibular aqueduct is enlarged); type III (**C**) is X-linked stapes deafness type. Hypoplastic cochleas have smaller external dimensions: Type I (**D**) is bud-like hypoplasia; type II (**E**) is cystic hypoplasia; type III (**F**) is a cochlea with less than two turns. If all cochlear partitioning is absent but there is differentiation into cochlear and vestibular compartments, the malformation is termed a CCVA *(Conitnued)*

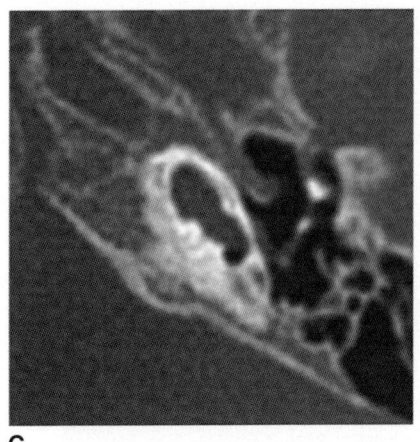

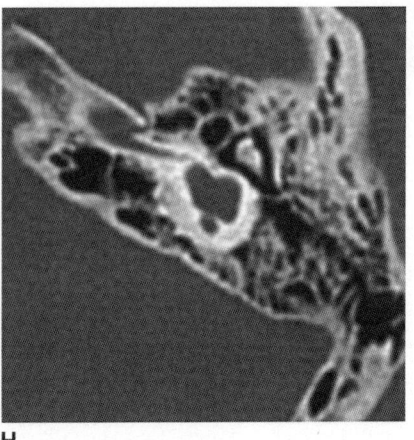

G   **H**

Figure 163.1 (*Continued*) (**G**). If there is no internal differentiation of the labyrinth into vestibular and cochlear compartments, the malformation is called a CC (**H**).

immune-mediated inner ear diseases such as Cogan syndrome or following severe cases of otitis media. Secondary ossification within the fibrotic inner ear lumen can subsequently result in solid obstruction. In such cases, neural viability can be suspect. Examples of cochlear inflammation, obstruction, and ossification are seen on both MRI and CT (Fig. 163.3).

Surgery for Cochlear Implantation

Setup

Cochlear implant surgery is performed under general anesthesia and typically takes between 1and 2 hours to complete. Patients with significant medical comorbidity should have a prior anesthetic risk assessment. Before surgery, a clear middle ear space should be confirmed through otoscopy, tympanometry, and/or temporal bone imaging to insure that the device will not be exposed to bacterial pathogens that can create future infectious complications. Facial nerve monitoring is routine for all surgeries. Perioperative antibiotics are given 30 minutes before skin incision. A first-generation cephalosporin is sufficient as ear pathogens such as *Streptococcus pneumoniae*, *Haemophilus influenzae*, and *Pseudomonas aeruginosa* should be unusual in routine cases. In instances in which common middle ear

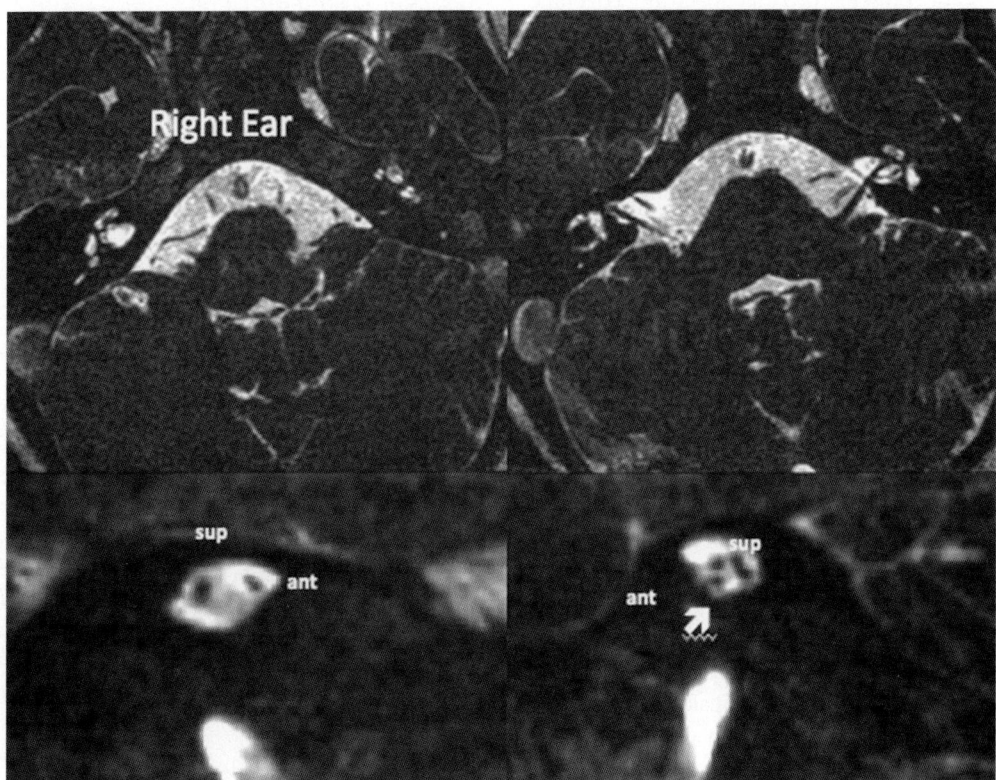

Figure 163.2 CND. High-resolution volumetric T2-weighted MRI demonstrates an absent cochlear division of cranial nerve VIII in the right ear on both the axial images and the oblique sagittal reconstructions oriented perpendicular to the internal auditory canal. The *arrow* indicates the normal contralateral cochlear nerve.

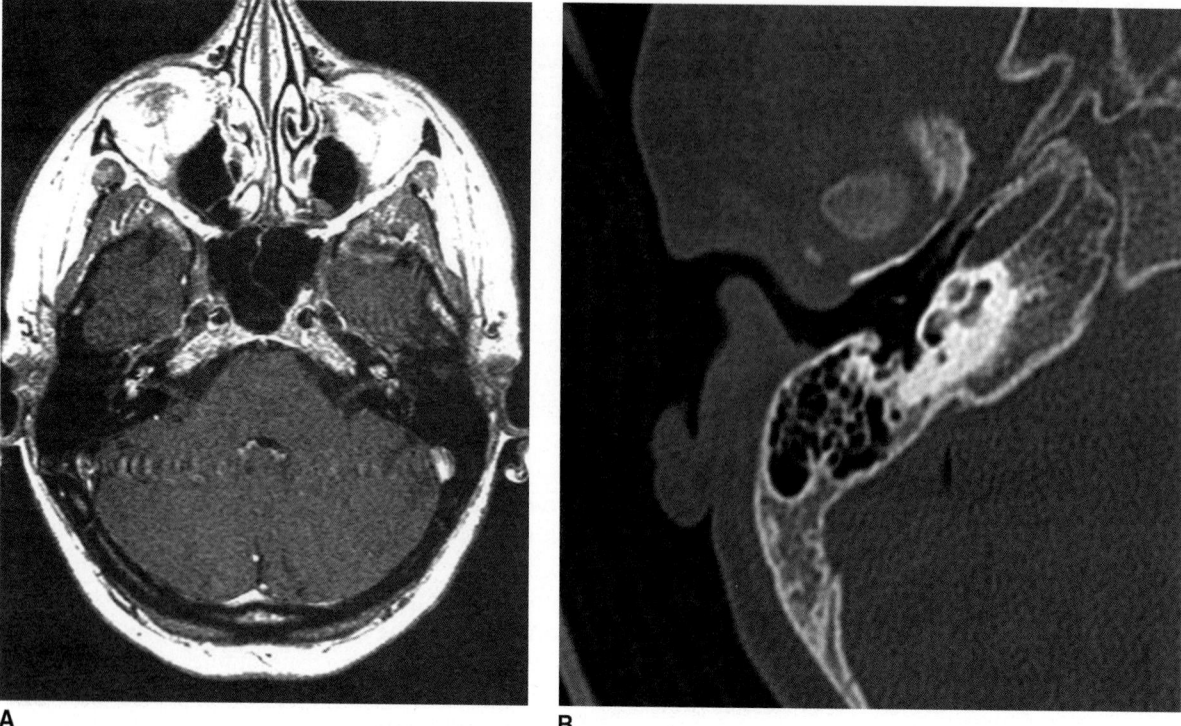

A   B

Figure 163.3 Labyrinthine obstruction. **A:** Axial-enhanced T1-weighted MRI demonstrates bilateral labyrinthine enhancement. **B:** Axial bone-window CT demonstrates postmeningitic ossification within the basal cochlear turn.

pathogens might be present, broader-spectrum coverage should be considered.

Preparation

The patient is situated in a supine position with the head turned to expose the postauricular region. Shaving of hair is mostly unnecessary. Prior to skin incision, local anesthetic with vasoconstrictor is infiltrated in the postauricular region. The skin incision is planned to achieve successful placement of the receiver–stimulator in a position that is remote from the pinna and mastoid (Fig. 163.4). Locating the receiver–stimulator too close to the pinna can result in unwanted interaction between the magnetic headpiece and the speech processor. Moreover, placement too close to the mastoid can be problematic if skin retraction in to the mastoid results in unwanted device exposure. The use of manufacturer-specific device templates prior to the incision can help locate the proper position. Focal injection of methylene blue through the skin and on to the bone allows for identification of the bony position for the internal device after skin elevation. Locating the device relative to the mastoid cavity following bony exposure can be ineffective since mastoid size varies considerably among individual of all ages. The final position of the receiver-stimulator usually is significantly superior and posterior to the pinna. The long axis of the device creates roughly a 45-degree incline from the horizontal through the zygomatic arch.

Receiver–Stimulator Placement and Fixation

Following a skin incision, a subperiosteal pocket is created in the proposed region for the internal receiver–stimulator that is bounded inferiorly by the lambdoid suture and is

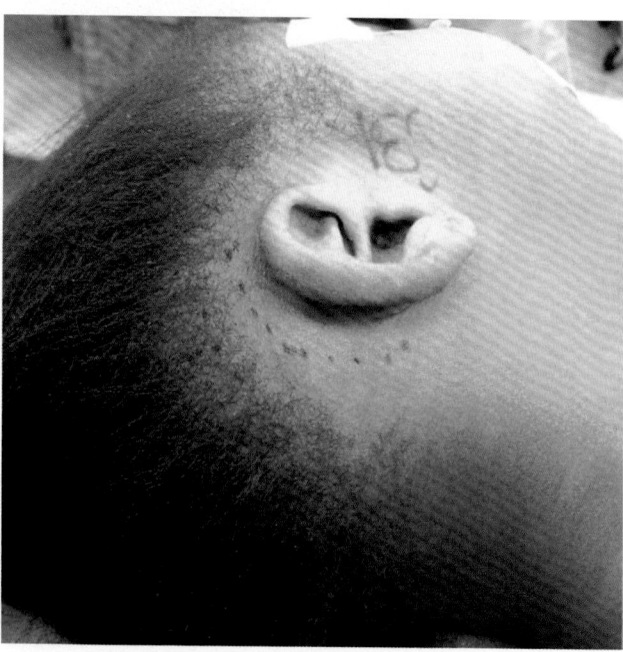

Figure 163.4 Typical skin incision used for cochlear implantation. A similar incision is used for active MEIs. Larger incisions have been used in the past but are currently not used anymore.

strictly sized for the device being implanted (69). A bony depression can be created according to the device templates and the device fixed to bone by any one of a variety of methods (70). For adults, nearly all techniques are sufficient, while for children, simple suturing of the periosteum provides rigid fixation to bone and avoids intra- or transcortical drill holes or screws that might put the underlying dura or venous sinuses at risk (71).

Approach

A standard mastoidectomy is performed. The facial recess is opened maximally using the horizontal semicircular canal, fossa incudis, chorda tympani, and facial nerve as landmarks. The facial nerve usually can be visualized through the bone without exposing it. The round window niche overhang is initially identified as a bony, rounded ridge located inferior to the oval window niche and anterior–inferior to the stapedius tendon. The niche is always located posterior to Jacobson nerve on the cochlear promontory and 1 to 2 mm inferior to the oval window. It is very important to recognize that limited opening of the facial recess can result in an inferior view towards the hypotympanum with a resulting look at the air cell system rather than the promontory and round window region. With adequate opening, the round window niche overhang is removed to expose the round window membrane, the primary landmark to scala tympani.

Cochleostomy

When describing the surgical technique for cochleostomy creation, one should keep the basic objectives in mind: open scala tympani (and not scala vestibuli), minimize collateral trauma to physiologically relevant intracochlear structures, and provide a relatively straight insertion trajectory along the longitudinal axis of the basal turn in an effort to allow for buckle-free electrode insertion. Currently, a variety of differing cochleostomy techniques exist that can be adapted to the clinical situation depending on the following: the electrode array to be used, the cochlear morphology, and the desire for hearing preservation (72).

An adaptive cochleostomy approach is used whereby electrode arrays that are long, rigid, and inserted with a stylet or rigid insertion tool are placed through a separate cochleostomy (Fig. 163.5). Such a cochleostomy is always round window related and might actually communicate with the round window membrane if higher insertion forces are not anticipated. For very long electrode arrays that are designed for complete cochlear coverage, a cochleostomy that has circumferential bony walls or a round window membrane insertion is acceptable. In these cases, cochlear length rather than cochleostomy location probably determines whether insertion resistance will be encountered. For cases in which a shorter array is to be used in a hearing-preservation capacity, openings that include the round window membrane are the rule (Fig. 163.5). The details of cochleostomy choice and creation are covered in Basura et al. (72).

Electrode Insertion

A smooth, resistance-free insertion of the proposed electrode array in to patent scala tympani is the goal of most implantations. A variety of tools exist for the various devices that are available. The reader is referred to the individual surgical manuals for details regarding usage of the various devices. In general, a standard jeweler's forceps are an excellent tool for most array insertions.

Telemetry and Imaging

Following device placement and wound closure, device interrogation is carried out using the manufacturer's software. All devices have telemetry programs that allow for measurement of electrode impedances and electrically evoked compound action potentials. Impedance measures are useful for identifying open circuits. If a substantial number of circuits are found to be open, replacement of the device should be considered to insure that an adequate number of electrodes are available for stimulation. While electrically evoked compound action potential testing is probably not useful in routine adult cases in which cochlear nerve populations are not in question (73), this technique might provide useful information in cases of possible neural compromise such as ANSD, inner ear malformations, or CND. In such cases, the result of these measures has been shown to correlate with future performance on open-set speech perception measures (67,74). Moreover, threshold determination for electrically evoked compound action potentials might identify a useful stimulation starting point for very young children.

Special Surgical Considerations

Inner Ear Malformations

Congenital inner ear malformations are common (10% to 20%) among children undergoing cochlear implantation (75). Labyrinthine anomalies have the potential to adversely affect the electrode-neural interface, reduce electrode array insertion depths, predispose to cerebrospinal fluid gusher through the cochleostomy, and be associated with facial nerve anomalies that can create access problems for scala tympani. The variety of inner ear malformations, as identified on temporal bone imaging, have been detailed above and are demonstrated in Figure 163.1 (63,65,75).

A transmastoid facial recess approach can be used in most instances of inner ear malformation except when a CC is present. In these cases, a transmastoid labyrinthotomy can be used (Fig. 163.6). Similar to cases without malformations, a round window–related cochleostomy can usually be created. A variety of electrodes are available for these special cases. In general, when a cochlear interscalar septum is lacking, modiolar conforming electrodes should probably be avoided (Fig. 163.1).

Cerebrospinal fluid gushers from the labyrinth are common is children with inner ear malformations, especially those with IP-EVA spectrum findings on imaging.

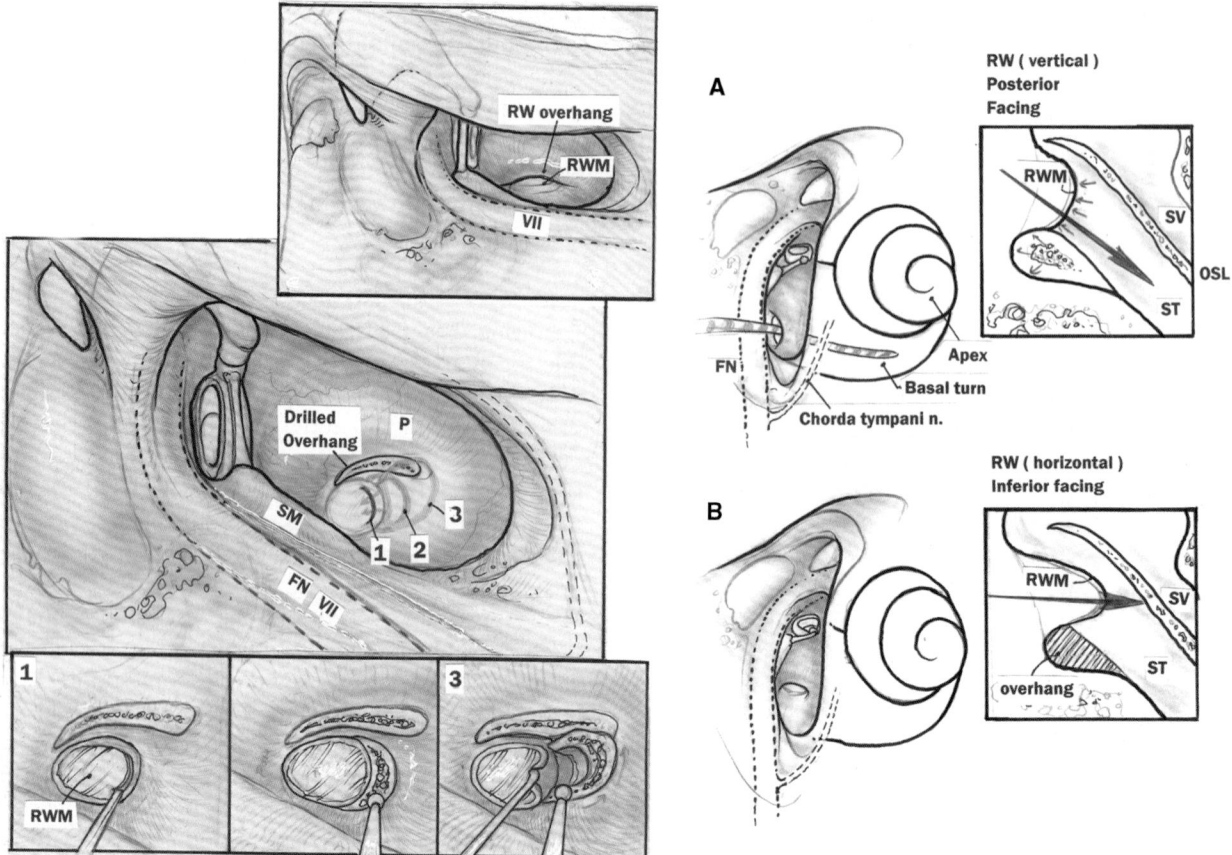

Figure 163.5 (A) Illustration demonstrating the position of the round window as seen through a typical facial recess. The bony overhang covering the actual window has to be removed to expose the actual membranous window. Also, the actual window is often covered by fibrous tissue layers making exposure more difficult. The center image shows different cochlear openings. *1:* round window incision. *2:* inferior enlargement of the round window. *3:* separate round window–related cochleostomy. The bottom images demonstrate the respective techniques. **B:** Illustration of typical insertion trajectories through the different round window alignments. Specifically, the round window membrane can assume a more vertical position (*a, top images*). In these cases, the window faces essentially posterior facilitating a direct insertion through the window. In some other temporal bones, the round window assumes a more horizontal position (*b, bottom images*), which generates a very perpendicular view onto the membrane through the facial recess. In these cases, the electrode can take a trajectory heading towards the bony modiolus.

Of interest, the cochlear morphology in most instances does not predict the gusher except when the modiolus is absent (Fig. 163.1). In such instances, creating a larger cochlear opening and tightly packing connective tissue around the electrode array is sufficient. Cerebrospinal fluid diversion is not needed if the leak is controlled intraoperatively. Electrode array insertion should be carried out only to the point of first significant resistance. Imaging that reveals a hypoplastic cochlea should be expected to have limited electrode insertion depths and for these cases, shorter arrays are helpful.

Children with absent semicircular canals or external auditory canal atresia can create significant issues for cochlear access since the facial nerve is often times displaced anteriorly. In these instances, the mastoid antrum can be indistinct, the ossicular chain malformed, the cochlea is usually hypoplastic with possible CND, and the round window niche completely obliterated by the facial

nerve. Children with CHARGE association are particularly predisposed to this situation, and special care should be exercised in considering implantation in these children. Figure 163.7 shows an intraoperative picture of such a case.

Inner Ear Obstruction
Cochlear obstruction can occur following inner ear inflammation from meningitis, immune-mediated ear disease, otitis media with labyrinthitis, or trauma. In these cases, the cochlear lumen can be narrowed or obliterated with fibrous tissue or bone. Preoperative imaging with MRI and CT will usually reveal the extent to which such obstruction exists and the approach needed for implantation. In cases of ongoing meningitis, intervention should be considered in the early stages so as to avoid total obstruction and inability to implant the ear(s) in question. Moreover, consideration should also be given to bilateral implantation at the initial surgery.

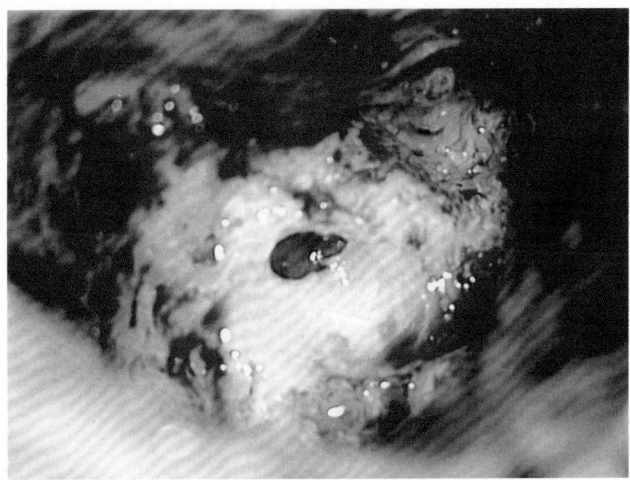

Figure 163.6 Labyrinthotomy approach for cochlear implantation in a case of a CC malformation. The lateral semicircular canal typically used as a surgical landmark cannot be used. Instead this single opening into the cavity should allow the surgeon to curl the electrode inside to generate an optimal electrode–neural interface.

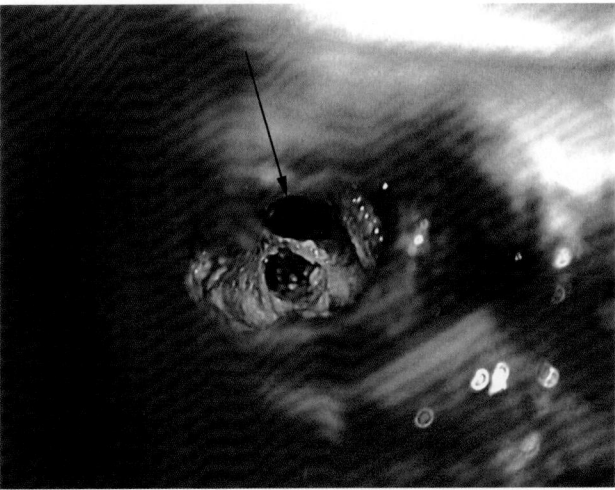

Figure 163.8 Surgical view (left ear) through the facial recess in a case of postmeningitic ossification. A cochleostomy (*arrow*) into the basal turn's scala vestibuli has been furnished superior to the initial attempt into scala tympani, which revealed ossification of the lumen.

Approach to implantation of the obstructed cochlea should be considered in a stepwise manner. Following routine round window exposure, the membrane often time appears white, indicating underlying pathology. In cases of short segment obstruction resulting from either fibrosis or bone (1 to 3 mm), a typical round window–related cochleostomy can be created by drilling through the short segment of obstruction. Array insertion can usually proceed in a normal fashion. If more than 3 mm of drilling fails to reveal a patent cochlear lumen, a scala vestibuli insertion should be considered by moving superiorly, above, and anterior to the round window region (Fig. 163.8). Usually scala vestibuli insertions can accommodate a complete electrode array. Rarely, severe first turn ossification can make both scala tympani and vestibuli inaccessible at the cochlear base. In such situations, a double array can be

used. In this situation, the trough created near the round window can be used for a short array. An apical cochleostomy is also created for an upper, retrograde insertion. This opening is made anterior to the oval window, inferior to the cochleariform process. Great care should be exercised to avoid inadvertent injury to the undersurface of the labyrinthine segment of the facial nerve. Following such insertions, communication with the individual programming the device is critical to insure that proper pitch assignment is made for the retrograde electrodes. Finally, in cases of diffuse obstruction, a circummodiolar drill out is possible (76,77).

Otitis Media

Active otitis media is a contraindication to cochlear implantation in that intracochlear or device exposure to viable bacteria can result in suppurative labyrinthitis with subsequent meningitis and ossification. Moreover, device colonization can result in subsequent wound infection, breakdown, and hardware loss.

In children, consideration of active middle ear disease is common in the winter months. The middle ear space should be assessed prior to skin incision in all cases. In cases of acute otitis media, delayed intervention is justified. If recurrent disease is probable, tympanostomy tube insertion is reasonable with delayed implantation. There are some advocates for subtotal petrousectomy with blind sac closure in the setting of otitis media to avoid future considerations for this problem. There also remains considerable dispute regarding the significance of otitis media with effusion. In cases of serous effusion, the incidence of bacterial colonization is probably very low. Conversely, in cases of mucoid effusion, delayed intervention is prudent.

Cochlear implantation in the setting of chronic suppurative otitis media with or without cholesteatoma remains

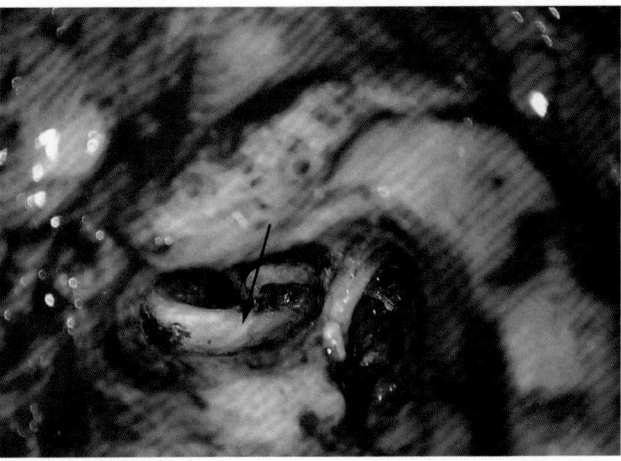

Figure 163.7 Surgical view of a left ear with a displaced facial nerve. Specifically, the nerve (*arrow*) runs over the round window niche and the cochleostomy can be seen anterior to the nerve. All semicircular canals are absent in this case.

a difficult problem. In such cases, active middle ear disease should be cleared or controlled prior to implantation. One option is to consider early blind sac closure with or without obliteration and staged implantation. This avoids the long-term issues of tympanic membrane retraction, granulation, infection, and electrode exposure within a tympanic membrane perforation.

Complications

Fortunately, complications are unusual following cochlear implantation today. Complications might be broadly categorized in to those that are *medical/surgical* in nature and those that are *device-related*. The categories are detailed in Table 163.4. Historically, medical/surgical complications were more common than device-related issues. This was primarily due to the fact that flap/wound complications were common when postauricular wounds were large, devices were rigid, and location of the receiver–stimulator was too close to the mastoid cavity. With surgical advancements, these issues have become decidedly rare. Minimal approaches to skin incisions and proper device location and immobilization have been key in reducing such complications. Careful attention to the surgical details described above can avoid or at least minimize many of the surgical complications outlined.

Common and potentially unavoidable complications include taste disturbance from chorda tympani nerve manipulation or sacrifice (~10%), transient dizziness (~10% of adults and less common in children), and subcutaneous seroma (10%) (78). The vestibular effects of cochlear implantation have long been a concern among otologic surgeons. Fortunately, complete vestibular deafferentation remains uncommon following surgery, especially when cochleostomy location is in scala tympani and attention is paid to electrode insertion vectors and force application (72,79,80). For children, the risk of vestibular loss remains quite small since most pediatric patients have limited, peripheral vestibular function preoperatively. Subcutaneous seroma, while common early after cochlear implant surgery nearly always resolves without the need for any intervention.

Device-related complications include receiver–stimulator hard failures, suspected device malfunction (i.e., soft failures), and open circuits. *Hard failure* refers to a total lack of function of the device despite properly functioning external equipment. Hard failures results from internal, receiver–stimulator problems and require revision surgery to alleviate the issue. Suspected device malfunction or *soft failure* is significantly more difficult to diagnose and refers to the situation where despite the presence of auditory percepts, the patient experiences aversive symptoms such as pain, shocking, atypical tinnitus, or a decrement in function. Following complete exchange of the external equipment and confirmation of electrode location within the cochlear lumen by imaging, an internal device problem is suspected and revision surgery considered if the symptoms are intolerable to the patient. A soft failure is also considered a clinical device failure. Open circuits can occur early or in a delayed fashion following cochlear implant surgery. A value judgment of electrode number and location is needed to insure adequate stimulation is available for performance. The details of revision cochlear implantation and reliability are often times complex. Fortunately, in most instances, revision cochlear implantation results in a functioning device that restores access to sound. In many instances, such surgery also allows for an upgrade in technology. However, it is critically important to realize that revision surgery during the formative years of a child's development can result in a significant setback in speech perception, production, and language thereby delaying educational achievement. Parents of such children should be made aware of these possible delays prior to surgery (81).

Meningitis in Cochlear Implant Recipients

The incidence of meningitis in cochlear implant recipients is greater than that of an age-matched cohort in the general population (82,83). Risk factors in this population include young age, the presence of inner ear malformations, and the use of a two-part electrode system. The risk of meningitis also appears to be higher among individuals with sensorineural hearing loss without a cochlear implant although this risk appears lower than that of implanted

TABLE 163.4	COMPLICATIONS OF COCHLEAR IMPLANTATION
Device-Related	**Medical/Surgical**
Internal Hard Failure (i.e., dead device)	Flap wound (infection, extrusion)
Internal suspected malfunction (i.e., soft failure)	CSF gusher or leak
Speech processor failure	Dural or vascular injury
Accessories malfunction (cables, headpiece, etc)	Incomplete electrode insertion
Open electrode circuits	Electrode extrusion
	Facial nerve injury

patients (84). It remains difficult to determine whether cochlear implantation *per se* confers an increase risk of meningitis in subjects without the factors cited above.

The most common organism identified in postimplantation meningitis is *S. pneumoniae*. All potential routes of spread (middle ear, inner ear, hematogenous) should be considered in such a patient. Recent animal investigations into the mechanisms of meningitis following cochlear implantation suggest that all three routes are viable sources for such an infection (85). These works also support the need to create a relatively atraumatic cochlear opening, insert the electrode array without trauma to reduce the potential for inner ear to subarachnoid space communication, and form an adequate seal at the cochleostomy with connective tissue to prevent the direct spread of infection along the array. Moreover, experimental results of pneumococcal vaccination in implanted animals support the current recommendation by the FDA and implant manufacturers for early vaccination in all cochlear implant candidates and recipients (86). Early and adequate treatment of otitis media is also important in preventing meningitis in implanted patients.

Clinical Results

Cochlear implantation is an auditory intervention that restores sound awareness for nearly all individuals that receive the device. Depending on a variety of factors and expectations, there remains a wide range of performance outcomes that are achievable through cochlear implantation. These include enhancement of lipreading and improvements in speech perception and music appreciation (87–89). Improved speech perception can result in appropriate development of spoken language and educational achievement for children and improved communication skills for adults (5,6). Many adult patients with cochlear implants can also talk on the telephone using their device (~75%). These outcomes secondarily enhance employments opportunities, socialization, and quality of life (1). Moreover, the cost-effectiveness of this intervention is astounding (1,3).

Outcomes from cochlear implantation depend heavily on the development of appropriate expectations among families and patients. A variety of patient factors, surgical factors, implant center factors, and access to appropriate rehabilitation appear to be drivers in success. Patient factors remain the single most important variable in determining outcomes. Some of the factors that should be considered include age, age of onset of hearing loss (deafness), duration of deafness, medical comorbidities, etiology of deafness, anatomic cochlear and cochlear nerve status, cognitive abilities, behavioral condition, psychological factors, parental desires and involvement, educational setting, and resources among others. Of these factors, the duration and severity of auditory deprivation prior to cochlear implantation remains the single most

important. Long-standing auditory deprivation creates a number of biologic changes within the auditory system that are not easily reversed despite restoration of auditory inputs. Timely intervention thus remains paramount for both children with congenital deafness all individuals with deafness onset later in life. For those with less than complete deafness, the degree of residual acoustic hearing also seems important at predicting outcome with a cochlear implant (90). While age at implantation appears to be associated with outcomes, this variable more than likely reflects the duration of auditory deprivation rather than being an independent factor. Thus, implantation among the elderly is not contraindicated. Other patient factors that can adversely affect outcomes include comorbidities such as cerebral palsy, psychomotor retardation, cognitive abilities, motivations, and compliance. Unfortunately, socioeconomic factors also seem to play a role in access and outcomes from this technology (91,92).

A key factor in achieving the best outcomes from cochlear implantation is the ability to create an appropriate electrode-neural interface. Both patient factors and surgical factors can alter this situation. Inner ear malformations, CND, inner ear obstruction and ossification, can reduce neural elements available for stimulation. In such instances, outcomes can be less than similar patients without these factors (67,75,93). Recently, preliminary data suggest that electrode location within the normal structure inner ear can also be important factor in performance (55,94,95). Surgeons should aspire to achieve atraumatic electrode placement in an effort to preserve neural elements and thus improve performance.

ANSD is a clinical syndrome characterized the presence of normal outer hair cell function, as revealed by the presence of otoacoustic emissions and/or cochlear microphonic on electrophysiologic testing, and aberrant or disordered neural conduction in other sites along the auditory pathway. A variety of genetic or acquired conditions can lead to the clinical phenotype. More than 50% of children with ANSD have a history of prematurity (74,96). Over the years, there has been some controversy regarding the effectiveness of hearing aids and to a lesser extent cochlear implants in children with this disorder. Recent work suggests that both hearing aids and cochlear implants can be effective in many of these children (74,97). However, there remains a subset of children with ANSD who are poor performers. These children frequently have other associated neurologic conditions such as progressive blindness, peripheral neuropathy, or evidence of CND on high-resolution imaging (74,75,98).

There are a number of potential advantages and disadvantages to bilateral cochlear implantation in both adults and children (Table 163.5). Bilateral cochlear implantation significantly improves hearing in noise and sound localization abilities in both adults and children. Moreover, bilateral implantation reduces time spent "off the air." These benefits are critical for young children who rely on

TABLE 163.5	ADVANTAGES AND DISADVANTAGES OF BILATERAL COCHLEAR IMPLANTATION

Bilateral Cochlear Implants

Advantages	Disadvantages
Always implant better ear	Two surgeries
Hearing in quiet	One or two anesthesias
Hearing in noise	Loss of acoustic hearing
Never off the air	Bathtub hearing
	CI limited frequency spectrum
	Future therapies
	Vestibular effects
	Double programming
	Economics

incidental hearing for learning. As in unilateral implantation, there also appears to be a critical period for developing binaural skills implying that second ear implantation should be considered early in young deaf patients (99). It remains to be determined whether bilateral implantation is superior to unilateral implantation in patients who can effectively use a contralateral hearing aid (i.e., bimodal hearing). Research is ongoing in this area (100–102).

Finally, cochlear implants are being placed in patients with progressively greater degrees of residual hearing using special electrode arrays and surgical techniques that allow for preservation of residual acoustic hearing. The combination of electric and acoustic stimulation in the same ear (electroacoustic stimulation or hybrid implantation) has been an active area of investigation for nearly the last decade (33,35,103). While the devices needed for this approach remain to be approved by the FDA, preliminary results seem very promising. Significant improvements in hearing are evident both in quiet and in noise when compared to similar cochlear implant recipients that have undergone conventional, non-hearing preserving implantation (104). It seems evident that the future of cochlear implantation will include hearing-preservation surgery for all patients undergoing the procedure. Challenges for this intervention will rely on making implantation with preservation of residual acoustic hearing highly reliable and precise for combining such stimulation. Areas such as automated electrode insertion and intraoperative monitoring of hearing are promising areas of investigation.

Summary

Cochlear implants are a remarkably successful prosthetic intervention for patients with sensorineural hearing loss not sufficiently managed with conventional, high gain amplification. Cochlear implants use multielectrode arrays to restore audition through auditory nerve stimulation within the tonotopic confines of the cochlea, allowing for frequency-specific stimulation. These devices can be

placed with 1 to 2 hours of surgery with relatively limited risk. Activation reliably provides sound awareness and speech understanding, thereby improving spoken language development and educational opportunities for children and communication, socialization, and (re)employment opportunities for adults. These benefits result in very favorable outcomes for cost-utility and quality of life. Future areas of investigation are focused on broadening indications, combining these devices with conventional acoustic hearing devices, totally implantable technology, and newer stimulation paradigms. Creating awareness of these devices for the general public is also seriously needed.

OSSEOINTEGRATED DEVICES

Overview

Traditional bone conduction hearing aids indirectly connect to the bony skull via the unbroken skin (105). A bone-anchored hearing system (or osteoconductive implant, generally termed the bone-anchored hearing appliance—BAHA), on the other hand, connects directly to the skull via a percutaneous attachment. Thus, the connection to the transmitting medium is provided in a much more direct fashion (106). This design allows to overcome many limitations of conventional bone conduction hearing aids. However, the abutment requires surgical placement, and while the surgery itself has evolved into a relatively straightforward procedure, minor postoperative skin complications are common (107).

Principles of Bone Conduction

Bone, like air, can conduct sound information mainly encoded via controlled oscillations. In a normal hearing person, the ear receives sound signals via air conduction mechanisms through the external and middle ears. Specifically, the tympanic membrane, the ossicles, and the stapes footplate act as an amplifier to ultimately result in peri- and endolymph oscillations of the inner ear. However, the fluid spaces of the cochlea can also receive sound information transmitted directly through vibrations of the skull. This mechanism bypasses the entire conductive apparatus of the ear (Fig. 163.9).

For patients with otherwise not correctable conductive hearing loss, a bone anchored hearing system provides a means for auditory rehabilitation. Such patients include children or adults with atretic ears, patients after failed ossiculoplasty, chronic suppurative otorrhea, or with otherwise not manageable conductive issues (106,108,109).

The other main indication for bone anchored hearing systems includes patients with unilateral deafness (110,111). Similar to the traditional indication for conductive or mixed losses, the sound signal is transferred via the skull. Due to the high tissue density of the skull, the device will always activate both cochleas. Thus, in single-sided

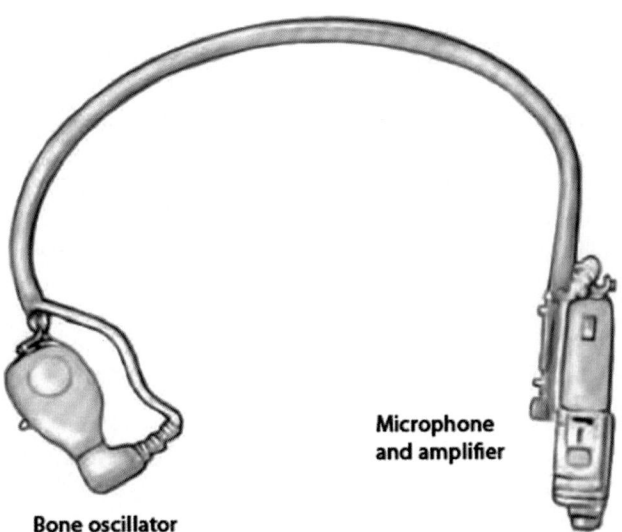

Figure 163.9 Illustration of a bone conduction hearing aid with contralateral routing of the sound signal (CROS).

deafness (SSD) candidates, the implant will help to transfer the signal through the skull to the contralateral ear. This eliminates the head shadow effect of binaural hearing. The patient will perceive spatial hearing even though only one cochlea is activated. However, the patient will not have access to the other physiologic effects of binaural hearing, as such the squelch and the binaural summation effect. They also will not be able to localize sound. Thus, the perceived hearing in these cases is pseudospatial (110).

Following this principle, binaural cochlear stimulation should be considered prior to implantation even with the traditional indication for conductive or mixed hearing losses. Specifically, unwanted contralateral stimulation might in some cases be perceived as detrimental. Adequate preoperative planning including proper estimation of the cochlear reserve and the required gain are essential.

Biologic Aspects

The main advantage of a bone-anchored hearing system is that it bypasses the conductive element of a hearing loss through direct bone conduction. Thus, it only has to provide amplification for the sensorineural component. However, in order to be able to provide adequate amplification, a minimal cochlear reserve must be met. With currently available devices, a bone conduction threshold of 65-dB HL or better should be present. Therefore, conductive or mixed hearing losses with adequate cochlear reserve and an air–bone gap or more than 30-dB HL measured at 500, 1,000, 2,000, and 4,000 Hz are among the proper indications.

With modern titanium implants, sectional imaging technologies such as CT and MRI remain feasible with the implant left *in situ*. Specifically, pure titanium produces little to no artifact on either imaging modality. Naturally, the audio processor (AP) needs to be removed prior to an MRI.

Current Device Technology

A bone anchored hearing system is typically a three-component medical device for the treatment of hearing loss. Currently available systems are manufactured by Cochlear Ltd (BAHA system, NSW, Australia) and Oticon Medical (Ponto System, Askim, Sweden). The system consists of a sound processor, an abutment, and a titanium implant (Fig. 163.10). The sound processor picks up the sound signal through a microphone. The signal is then amplified and converted into controlled oscillations. The abutment, or connector, links the sound processor and the osseointegrated titanium implant. The titanium implant is a small fixture surgically placed behind the ear, which transfers the sound information to the bony skull. As mentioned previously, the implant requires proper osseous integration to avoid failure of the system.

There are several sound processors depending on the severity and the type of hearing loss. As such, each device has different minimum bone conduction thresholds (measured at pure tone averages: 45-dB HL for the BAHA Divino, BP100 (or the Ponto/Ponto Pro); 55-dB HL for the larger Intenso (or the Ponto Pro Power); 65-dB HL for the body worn BAHA Cordelle II) to compensate for various levels of sensorineural components.

Candidacy for Bone Anchored Hearing Systems

A bone anchored hearing system is recommended for three types of hearing loss:

1. Conductive hearing loss
2. Mixed hearing loss
3. SSD

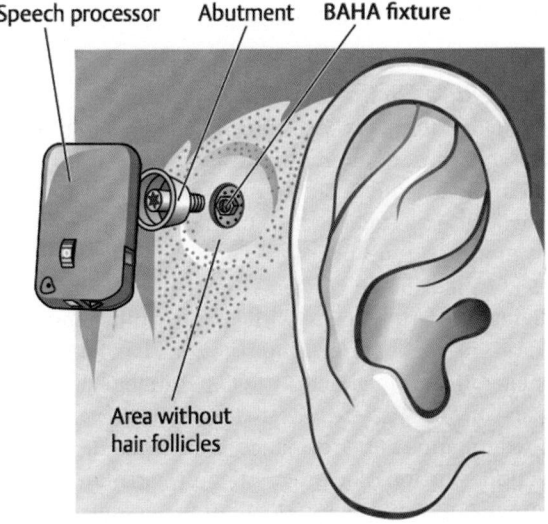

Figure 163.10 BAHA system consisting of the implant (*screw*), the abutment, and the AP.

Conductive or Mixed Hearing Losses

Various causes of conductive or mixed hearing losses have been described. They can be either congenital or acquired and the medical or surgical management mainly depends on the cause and other patient-related factors. If hearing restorative procedures are not feasible, conventional bone conduction hearing aids are the treatment of choice. These devices are available in various designs and typically include either a spring or soft headband or are included in the frame of a pair of glasses. However, traditional bone conduction hearing aids have many disadvantages. These include inconsistent coupling and resulting poor sound quality, associated reduced clarity and volume, discomfort from constant external pressure applied to the skin, poor aesthetics, and difficult placement.

A bone anchored hearing system, on the other hand, offers significantly better sound quality as the sound is transferred directly to the bone. Thus, both sound clarity and volume are preserved. It works without the application of pressure onto the skin, avoiding discomfort, headaches, and soreness typically associated with conventional bone conductors. Thus, a bone anchored hearing system offers wearing comfort, but it requires surgical placement of the implant including the percutaneous abutment.

Criteria for conductive or mixed hearing losses (for ear-level sound processors such as the BAHA Divino or Intenso) are as follows:

■ A minimum average bone conduction threshold of 45-dB HL (measured at 0.5, 1, 2 and 3 kHz) or 55-dB HL depending on the sound processor output
■ For bilateral fitting, symmetric bone conduction thresholds are recommended (i.e., there is less than a 10-dB HL difference of the PTAs [frequencies 0.5, 1, 2, and 3 kHz] or less than 15-dB HL at individual frequencies).
■ The BAHA Cordelle II body worn device is recommended for severe mixed hearing losses, but the average bone conduction thresholds of the implanted ear should be less than 65-dB HL (PTA 0.5, 1, 2, and 3 kHz).

Single-Sided Deafness

In the US alone, over 60,000 people per year suffer from SSD. The causes are multiple and include viral infections and subsequent sudden sensorineural hearing loss, Meniere disease, temporal bone fractures, and vestibular schwannomas. Multiple other causes have been described, some of them being congenital in nature. Many affected individuals learn to cope with this disability but are left without an adequate hearing solution. Previous management algorithms included a CROS (contralateral routing of signals) hearing device. These devices, however, are quite limited in terms of performance and user comfort.

A bone anchored hearing system provides an alternative treatment option for this population. As detailed above, the device transfers the acoustic information through the dense skull to the contralateral cochlea. Thus, it helps to generate an impression of binaural hearing, without actually providing the physiologic effects consistent with binaural signal processing. The head shadow effect is the sole exception, but elimination of this alone will account for the subjective benefit. Compared to CROS hearing aid, the BAHA features no occlusion effect, no need for a cable connection to transmit the signal, and overall improved sound quality through direct contact and sound transmission with the skull.

Criteria for unilateral sensorineural hearing and loss/ SSD (for ear-level sound processors such as the BAHA Divino, Intenso, Ponto, or Ponto Pro) are as follows:

■ Profound hearing loss in the implanted ear (Some candidates will have residual hearing, but these remnants should be nonfunctional in terms of speech understanding and pure tone perception.)
■ Hearing in the contralateral ear is better than or equal to 20-dB HL (measured at 0.5, 1, 2, and 3 kHz).

Pediatric Population

The sound processor of the bone anchored hearing system can be fitted to infants and children in need for amplification via bone conduction (112). The indications for a bone-anchored hearing system in children are generally the same as for adults, except that in the US, only children aged five and older are cleared by the FDA for implantation. The main reason for this is the often-insufficient thickness of the bony skull, making proper osseointegration impossible. Of note, the device's implant fixture comes in two sizes (lengths), 3 and 4 mm. Younger children may be fitted with a bone anchored hearing system using the Softband (113,114).

Surgery for Bone Anchored Hearing Systems

The implant site is generally 50 to 55 mm from the ear canal and horizontally in line with the top of the pinna (Fig. 163.11). A small amount of methylene blue dye can be used to highlight the implant site through the intact skin. Various types of skin incisions can be used. It seems, however, that a straight vertical incision has been established as the most commonly used access (115). Then, the subcutaneous tissue layers are reduced, depending on the required final thickness. Then, the periosteal layer is removed from the previously marked bony implant site, and the guide drill is used to assess the bony thickness. First, a 3-mm hole perpendicular to the skull surface is drilled followed by a 4-mm one (typically with ~ 2,000 rpm, Fig. 163.12). The 4-mm-depth drill is used after drilling with the 3-mm burr estimating there is sufficient residual cortical bone for the longer drill bit. Many children and some adults will have limited skull thickness permitting a 3-mm-long implant only. Once the adequate depth has been determined, the hole is widened using a countersink drill.

Then, the titanium implant is drilled into the previously created hole with a torque controlled drill at very low

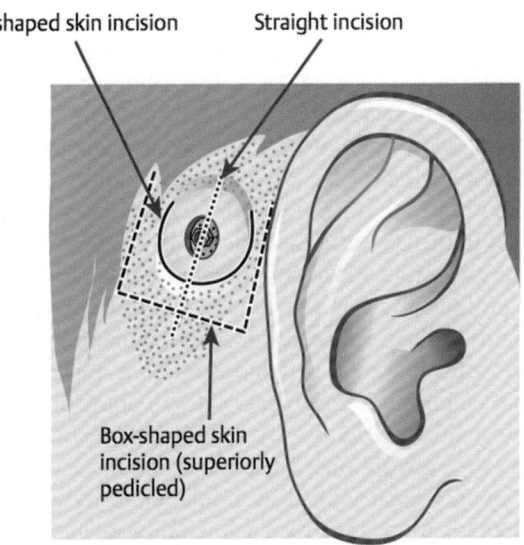

Figure 163.11 Skin incision options for placement of a BAHA. The straight incision has emerged as the preferred option used in clinical practice today.

speed. The threads of the implant will seat into the surrounding bone. For compact cortical bone, 40 to 50 Ncm of torque is typically used. Less torque is used for irradiated bone or in children. Then, the skin is closed around the abutment and the thickness of the surrounding soft tissues should be reassessed.

A healing cap is commonly placed onto the abutment, and the skin is compressed lightly using antibiotic gauze strips. The patient will follow in about 1 week to check the wound and the dressing is changed at that time. Also, the patient and his family members are carefully instructed on how to clean the abutment with its surrounding skin. The sound processor is loaded about 12 weeks postoperatively (116).

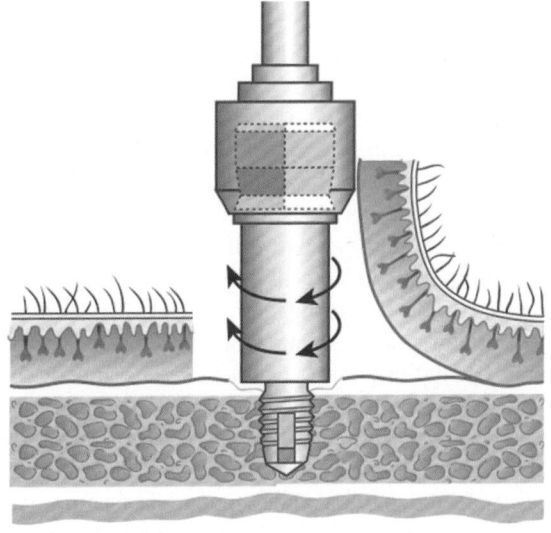

Figure 163.12 Placement of the implant into the skull. First, the thickness of the skull has to be assessed via 3- and 4-mm guide drills. Then, the site for the implant is created by enlarging the initial hole. The implant is then threaded using a torque sensitive drill.

Complications Associated with Bone Anchored Hearing Systems

The most frequently encountered complication associated with osseointegrated implants is a soft tissue reaction at the percutaneous implant site causing local infection, moisture, skin necrosis, or overgrowing over the abutment (117). Soft tissue reactions with percutaneous implants can be prevented via extensive intraoperative soft tissue reduction. Also, the skin can be tacked down to the periosteal layer to immobilize this region. Complications other than adverse skin reactions are rare. Osseointegration failure, though uncommon, is the second most common complication of this procedure.

Expected Outcomes

Overall, the bone anchored hearing system seems to offer patients with a bone conduction pure tone average of less than 45 dB a high degree of hearing rehabilitation and excellent patient satisfaction (118). This has been well documented by several clinical studies and trials. Once the initial healing phase of the skin-abutment interface has been completed, the device is reliable and the maintenance is generally low. The results for SSD have also been well documented (119). Overall, the authors encourage a trial with a bone anchored hearing system mounted in a headband so the patient can decide on whether or not proceed with implantation. As mentioned previously, a bone anchored hearing system will not provide true binaural hearing with this indication. Instead it will eliminate the head shadow effect and thus create a sensation of spatial hearing (110).

New Device Developments

The main issues associated with bone anchored hearing systems pertain to skin complications due to the percutaneous attachment. To eliminate this problem, several groups have helped to develop transcutaneous or other alternative solutions. These efforts, such as the Alpha 1 hearing system (Sophono, Boulder, CO, USA), have been approved in Europe but are currently under investigation with the FDA. Also, other efforts focus on application of the acoustic information via the jaw. Specifically, a dental appliance featuring a transducer can apply controlled oscillations to the maxilla or mandible for similar indications as conventional bone conduction devices (SoundBite, Sonitus Medical Inc., San Mateo, CA, USA).

ACTIVE MIDDLE EAR IMPLANTS

Overview

Conventional hearing aids provide amplification via the regular sound conduction apparatus of the ear. Active MEIs, on the other hand, convert acoustic information into controlled oscillations that can be transmitted either to the ossicular chain or directly to the inner ear fluid spaces (120). This method has several potential advantages over conventional hearing aids. The primary and most commonly described advantage of active MEIs is that the external auditory meatus can remain free of the actual device or an earmold. This occlusion effect is perceived as bothersome by many individuals, and some patients develop chronic otitis externa from the earmold. Acoustic distortions at the level of the tympanic membrane especially with high sound intensity levels and subsequent sound quality issues have also been described as common issues with conventional amplification. Also, many hearing aids struggle with some hearing configurations such as steeply sloping losses. In these cases, direct drive of the ossicular chain provides additional advantages over conventional technology.

New indications include conductive or mixed hearing losses (currently not FDA approved and under clinical investigation in the US). In these cases, the oscillating part of the device is placed on ossicular remnants, the round window, or other vibrating parts providing access to the fluid spaces of the inner ear (121). With these indications, active MEIs are an alternative mainly to bone anchored hearing system. In contrast to the BAHA, for example, active MEIs do not feature a percutaneous connection requiring permanent maintenance but instead use a transcutaneous link for information and energy transfer. Furthermore, active MEIs are not indicated for SSD since they do not use the bony skull for sound transmission to the contralateral ear.

Historical Aspects

Early attempts to actively stimulate the middle ear date back to the early 20th century. More concrete attempts were described in the 1970s and 1980s where piezoelectric systems were used for various hearing loss configurations. These attempts included both animal work and human implantations. Also, electromagnetic devices have been studied in both the animal model and later in humans in the 1980s. Each investigation established the feasibility of active stimulation of the conductive apparatus and the potential benefit of active stimulation to patients (122).

Most systems today feature semi-implantable technology similar to that used in modern cochlear implants. A transcutaneous link provides power and data to the internally placed demodulator and stimulating element. More recent efforts have focused on fully implantable technology with various solutions for sound sensors and implantable microphones. The first fully implantable system was the TICA (Implex AG, Germany), which featured a microphone in the subcutaneous tissue of the external auditory canal (123). It was first implanted in 1999 and feedback from the tympanic membrane required removal of parts of the ossicular chain. Due to technical difficulties, the device was eventually removed from the market.

The Vibrant Soundbridge (Symphonix, Inc., now Vibrant MED-EL, Innsbruck, Austria) was first implanted in 1996. The device has been FDA approved since 2000. Specifically, it has had FDA and CE approval for the treatment of sensorineural hearing loss and has CE approval in European countries for conductive and mixed hearing losses (121,124–126). It is currently under clinical investigation in the US for these indications.

Several issues make current fully implantable technology problematic. For one, the life of a rechargeable battery remains limited. However, new fully implantable rechargeable batteries may not demonstrate any loss of capacity for several thousand recharge cycles or about 10 years. The other main issue with fully implantable technology concerns the microphone. As detailed below, acquisition of the sound signal with fully implantable technology still underlies various inconsistencies and problems (37).

Despite the main technologic advances, active MEIs remain small in numbers when compared to conventional hearing aids or even cochlear implants. The main reasons for this seem to be financial in nature and the fact that all devices require surgical placement. Newer indications and larger patient numbers might help to improve documentation efforts and thus help provide payers and patients with better and more accurate performance and quality of life data.

Principles of Direct Ossicular or Cochlear Stimulation

Conventional hearing aids receive acoustic energy through a microphone and subsequently process and amplify the signal in a speech processor. This is then transmitted through a speaker (termed receiver in hearing aid terminology) and delivered into the external auditory canal (via a sound tube and/or an earmold) to stimulate the tympanic membrane. Active MEIs, in contrast, convert the sound signal into electrical energy and then into mechanical oscillations to amplify vibratory structures of the middle (or inner) ear.

The critical component of all MEIs is the transducer, which enables the device to deliver the sound information as a vibratory signal. This transducer can be either in direct or indirect contact with the intended structure. Two basic types of transducer technologies have been described: piezoelectric and electromagnetic (120,127). Piezoelectric devices use an amplifier featuring a piezoelectric crystal to generate oscillations. Piezoelectric materials (mostly ceramics) are dielectric materials with coupled electrical and mechanical properties. Applying a voltage across a piezoelectric rod, for example, causes it to bend or lengthen, in a precise and predictable voltage-dependent fashion. Within the implant, the sound signal acquired by a microphone is converted by the signal processor and then sent to the piezoelectric rod. As this rod vibrates in response to the converted auditory signal, it comes in direct contact with the intended structure of the sound-conducting apparatus (typically the incus or stapes). A critical feature of implants that use a piezoelectric transducer is the direct contact between the piezoelectric unit and the ossicles or the inner ear. The advantage of this type of transducer is its ability to deliver more distortion-free amplification directly to the ossicular chain and the low energy consumption.

Implantable middle ear hearing aids may also incorporate an electro-(ferro)magnetic transducer. These transducers generate a magnetic field, which then generates oscillations in a ferromagnetic medium that is nearby. Sound received from a microphone is converted by the signal processor, processed, and sent to the electromagnetic transducer. Both ferromagnetic units featuring either direct or indirect contact with the ossicular chain are available. Devices directly in contact with the target structure deliver oscillations as a result of direct attachment. Ferromagnetic transducers featuring indirect contact with the ossicular chain, on the other hand, rely on electromagnetic transmission to a ferromagnetic target unit, which is then attached to the ossicles.

The properties of the transmitting coil can influence the properties of the oscillating elements. As such, devices of 50 mg or more can influence ossicular motion and thus cause a conductive hearing loss, first affecting the high frequencies. The main downside of electromagnetic devices is the higher energy consumption when compared to piezoelectric technology.

Ossicular Attachment

Electromagnetic or piezoelectric transducers of active middle era implants are attached to various locations along the ossicular chain or the inner ear windows. The Vibrant Soundbridge attaches to the long process of the incus (Figs. 163.13 and 163.14). However, the floating mass transducer (FMT) assumes a position parallel to the stapes. Thus, the electromagnetic energy is applied in a direction mimicking the natural motion of the stapes.

The MAXUM System (Ototronix, LLC, approved by the FDA since 2009) attaches to the incudostapedial joint. It was previously approved as the SOUNDTEC Direct (Drive) Hearing System in 2001 but was ultimately withdrawn in 2004 and redesigned. The electromagnetic energy is thus applied directly to the ossicular chain in a similar fashion as with the Soundbridge. Piezoelectric systems directly attach to various portions of the ossicular chain. The Esteem system's driver provides oscillations directly to the head of the stapes (Fig. 163.15). In this system, the long process of the incus has to be removed to avoid acoustic feedback to the sensor acquiring sound information from the ossicular chain.

Various other device attachments are theoretically possible, and some have been realized in previous technology or in devices currently in clinical investigation. In this context, it seems worth mentioning that these alternate attachments include transducer placement in conjunction with

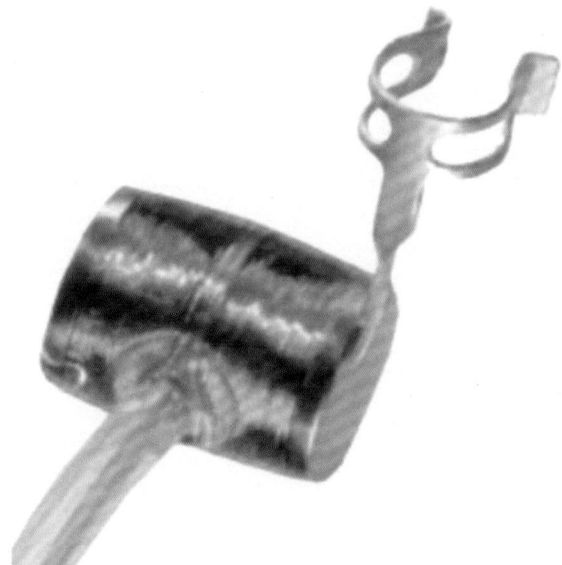

Figure 163.13 FMT of the Vibrant Soundbridge hearing system. The clip on the upper right-hand side attaches to the long process of the incus. In case of alternative placement sites such as the round window, this clip can be removed.

passive middle ear prostheses such as stapes pistons as well as partial or total ossicular replacement prostheses.

Direct Cochlear Fluid Stimulation

Stimulation paths other than via ossicular chain have been explored. The MEI transducers can be attached to the round window or oval window and directly stimulate the cochlea (Fig. 163.16). In case of a round window vibroplasty, the round window niche is drilled to accommodate the transducer, which is placed perpendicular to the round window. To improve coupling, a small piece of fascia is placed between the round window membrane and the transducer. An additional tissue such as fascia or perichondrium is

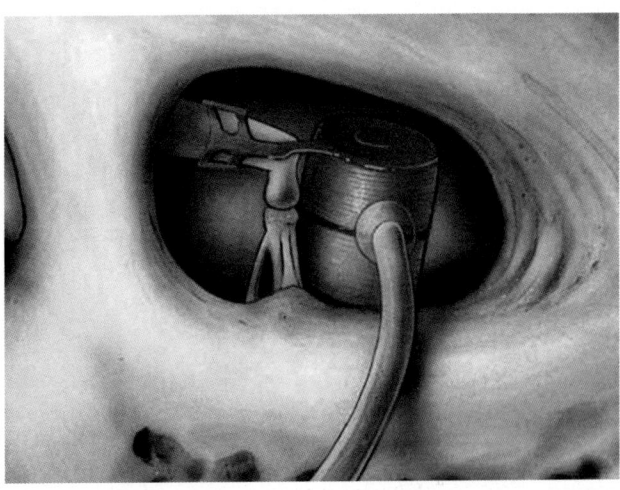

Figure 163.14 Traditional attachment of the Vibrant Soundbridge's FMT on the long process of the incus parallel to the stapes.

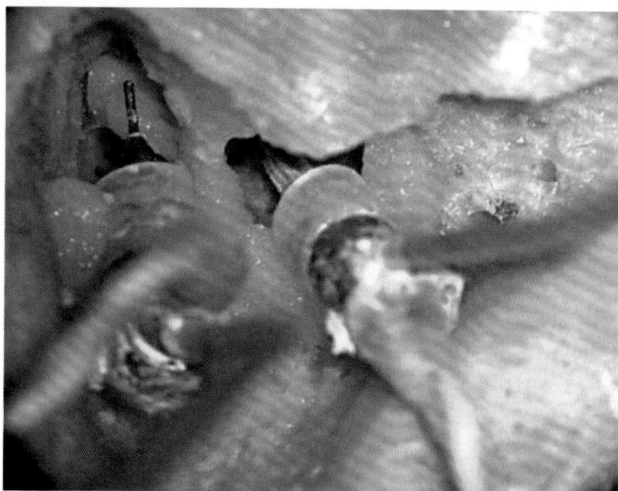

Figure 163.15 Intraoperative image (right ear) of the Envoy Esteem's transducer. The device on the left-hand side of the image depicts the transducer picking up the acoustic signal from the body of the incus. The transducer inserted through the facial recess stimulates the head of the stapes for signal delivery.

placed on the contralateral side of the transducer to secure the position.

Biologic Aspects

As with conventional hearing aids, implantable active MEIs underlie the general biologic limitations of the inner ear. Specifically, loss of inner hair cells with accompanying speech discrimination issues will limit the effectiveness of the device as much as this affects satisfaction with conventional hearing aids. As such, the devices mentioned below are mainly designed to overcome mild-to-moderate sensorineural hearing impairments with generally good discrimination abilities.

Tissue compatibility issues are theoretically possible with any implantable device. With the original attachment

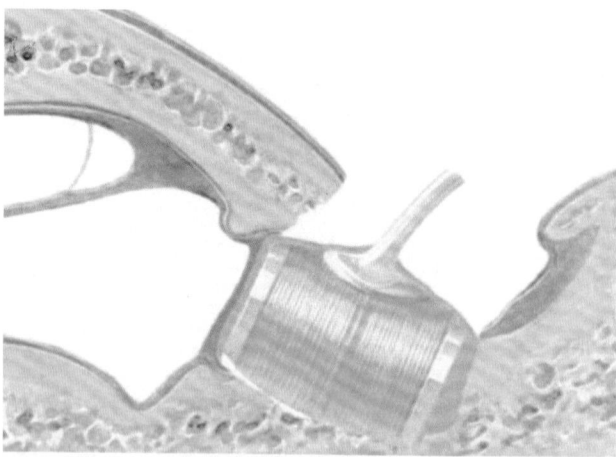

Figure 163.16 Alternate placement site of the Vibrant Soundbridge onto the round window membrane for direct cochlear stimulation.

on the long process of the incus, device fixation is typically permanent, although cases of device issues due to failure of the attachment have been described. With new indications requiring fixation on the round window niche or other parts of the labyrinth, possible device relocation issues have been described. The biology of the underlying pathology can thus not be ignored. Specifically, eustachian tube dysfunction requiring radical tympanomastoidectomy will require special surgical considerations when placing an active MEI for aural rehabilitation. In such cases, closure of the external auditory canal has been suggested to remove the potential cause for postoperative problems. This can be performed in a separate procedure before the actual device is placed.

Other potential issues can arise with retrocochlear hearing loss. At this point, the authors recommend alternative management options for this type of hearing impairment especially when the prognosis is unclear and/or if speech perception is substantially impaired.

Current Device Technology

Currently three FDA-approved active MEIs are available: the Vibrant Soundbridge (MED-EL, Innsbruck, Austria, formerly manufactured by Symphonix, Inc., initial FDA approval August 31, 2000, Fig. 163.17) (125), the fully implantable Esteem Implantable Hearing System (Envoy Medical Corp., St. Paul, MN, USA; FDA approval March 17, 2010) (128), and the MAXUM System (Ototronix, LLC, Houston, TX, USA; formerly the Direct Drive Hearing System, DDHS, SOUNDTEC, Inc., Oklahoma City, OK, USA, most recent FDA approval October 2009). All three systems are approved devices for moderate-to-severe sensorineural hearing loss. Other indications including use for conductive or mixed losses are currently under investigation in the US and/or approved in Europe. The Vibrant Soundbridge and

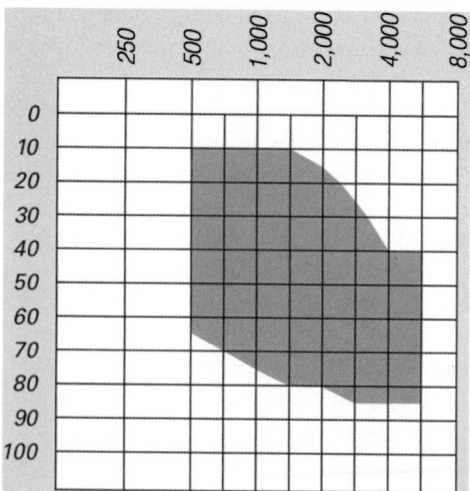

Figure 163.17 Typical audiogram template for active MEIs (in this case the Vibrant Soundbridge). Most devices are indicated with a moderate-to-severe sensorineural hearing loss with intact discrimination. Thus, the underlying biology of the sensorineural hearing loss should be carefully evaluated.

the DDHS systems are semi-implantable solutions, and the Envoy system features completely implantable technology.

Various other devices are currently under clinical investigation (Otologics Carina fully implantable system; featuring a postauricular implantable microphone and a middle ear transducer, Otologics LLC, Boulder, CO, USA).

The Vibrant Soundbridge consists of an externally worn AP and an implantable vibrating ossicular prosthesis. Similar to a cochlear implant receiver/stimulator, the latter consists of an internal coil, a magnet to secure the external components over the implant, a demodulator, a conductive link, and a so-called FMT (129,130). The FMT is the active portion of the implant and features a brace for attachment on the long process of the incus (Fig. 163.13). Several revisions of the AP have been available over the years this device has been available. The current technology uses digital sound processing as well as an external microphone and power source as part of the AP. To facilitate proper osseous integration, the device should not be activated for 8 weeks after surgery.

The MAXUM System features three components: the implant, the earmold/coil assembly (ECA), and the external amplification system or sound processor. A permanently implanted magnet is attached to the incudostapedial joint. Similar to the principle of the Vibrant Soundbridge, it provides controlled oscillations to the ossicular chain via an electromagnetic process. However, instead of a cable connection to an implantable demodulator, the implant receives its energy via the external auditory canal. Specifically, the ECA component of the device creates an alternating electromagnetic field together with the magnetic implant. The ECA therefore consists of an electromagnetic coil and an earmold/coil assembly casing. This casing is customized to the patient's external auditory canal dimensions obtained from an earmold impression. This mold can be extensively vented to minimize the external auditory canal occlusion effect. The sound processor of this system rests over the patient's external auditory canal, and it serves to convert the sound pressure into electrical signals. It consists of a microphone, a preamplifier, and a power amplifier, which has been designed to preserve battery life.

The fully implantable Esteem Implantable Hearing System features piezoelectric technology. It consists of three implantable components, external testing/programming instruments, and system accessories. Piezoelectric transducers are used to sense the acoustic sound signal from the ossicular chain and to directly drive the stapes (Fig. 163.15). The implant consists of a titanium-encased sound processor, a rechargeable battery, and two piezoelectric transducers. The sensor transducer picks up sound information from the body of the incus. It is fixated in this location with glass-ionomer cement. Similarly, the driver transducer is implanted through a facial recess approach and fixated to the head of the stapes. In order to avoid acoustic feedback via the ossicular chain, the distal tip of the long incus process has to be removed, typically via a laser. The device can be activated 6 weeks after implantation.

Candidacy for Active Middle Ear Implants

As an alternative for conventional hearing aids, active MEIs are primarily an alternative treatment option for hearing aid candidates. As such, the classical indication is mild-to-moderate sensorineural hearing loss with intact speech discrimination abilities (Fig. 163.18). Some device

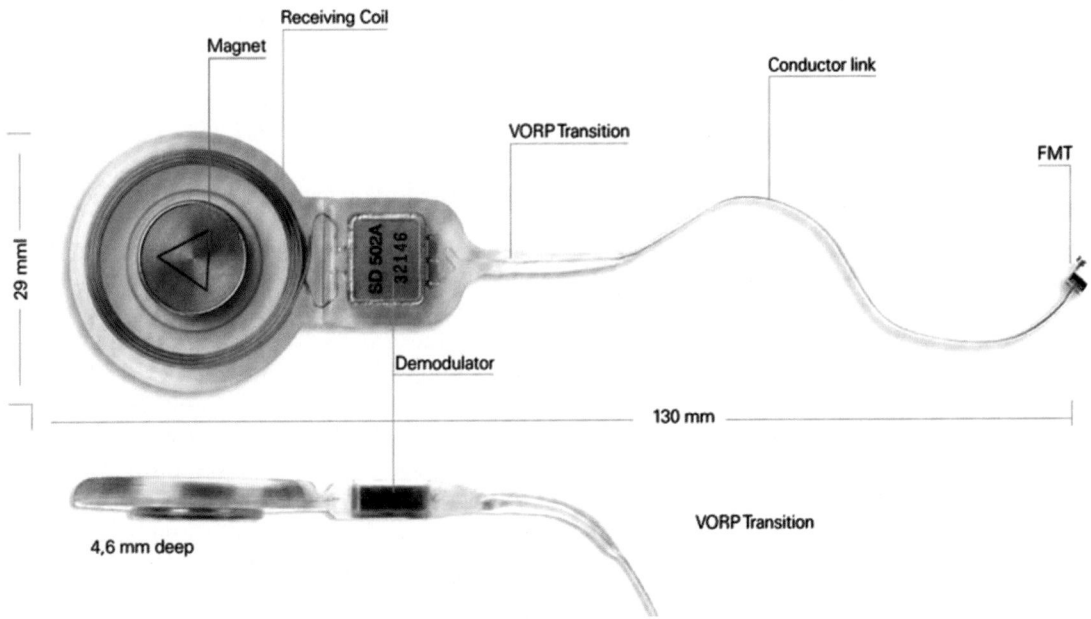

Figure 163.18 Image of the Vibrant Soundbridge implant consisting of the demodulator, the conductor link, as well as the FMT (floating mass transducer). This implant generates controlled oscillations of the ossicular chain (or the cochlear fluids) via a direct electromagnetic link.

indications include severe hearing losses. However, the clinician should keep the underlying biology of sensorineural hearing loss with potential loss of discrimination in mind. Also, indication criteria for cochlear implants continue to evolve, and many individuals with severe and some with moderate-to-severe losses are now considered cochlear implant candidates.

Many retrocochlear hearing deficits often demonstrate more severe speech discrimination problems than what would be expected from the pure tone audiogram. Thus, most manufacturers advocate a thorough trial with conventional hearing aids before proceeding with an active MEI when sensorineural hearing loss is being treated. The classic patient is an unsatisfied hearing aid candidate. Reasons for this dissatisfaction may include chronic external auditory canal issues from wearing the earmold or a bothersome occlusion effect.

Newer indications for active MEIs include conductive and mixed hearing losses. Both often require alternative attachment sites of the electromagnetic or piezoelectric transducer. For example, placement of the Vibrant Soundbridge on or near the round window has been thoroughly investigated. This site has been approved for clinical use in Europe and is currently under clinical investigation by the FDA. It allows bypassing both the external and middle ear. Thus, indication criteria include mixed or conductive losses from various causes mostly including chronic otitis media with previously failed ossiculoplasties. In case of a radical tympanomastoid cavity, it is important to provide adequate coverage of the device's components and wires. Many authors thus advocate closure of the external auditory canal either in a staged fashion or in a single operation.

Alternative attachment sites also provide other interesting applications: Atresia of the external auditory canal, for example, seems to be a perfect fit for active MEIs. Typical results after atresiaplasty are more often than not dissatisfactory for both patients as well as the clinician. Also, surgeries often have to be coordinated with reconstructive measures of the auricle. Specifically, atresiaplasty cannot precede functional reconstructive measures. A BAHA headband is often times the only option in early childhood (131). With adequate bone thickness, typically reached around age 7, an implanted BAHA might be considered. However, even in this scenario directional hearing may be compromised due to the BAHA's capacity to stimulate both inner ears simultaneously. Also, the BAHA features a percutaneous attachment requiring extensive skin care and the potential for complications.

Thus, active MEIs could provide a reasonable alternative. Previous clinical investigations have found that the procedure's scarring is minimal and will therefore not interfere with later reconstructive measures (132). As such, placement of the device may be performed at an earlier age before cosmetic reconstructive procedures are being considered. As a downside, some atretic ears feature virtually

no landmarks, no pneumatization, a very shallow middle ear space, and an aberrant position of the facial nerve. The latter can take a very anterior course in its mastoid segment making positioning of the FMT within the round window problematic. In such cases, surgery has to be carefully weighted against other options. Also, successful placement of the active portion of the device on the oval window has been described (133).

In summary, sensorineural hearing loss remains the main (and often only FDA approved) indication for active MEIs. Newer sites of attachment are very promising and have been approved in Europe. Clinical algorithms may have to be established, and more data from controlled clinical trials should enhance our understanding of direct cochlear stimulation.

Surgery for Active Middle Ear Implants

Every active MEI requires surgical placement of the transducer on the ossicular chain or an alternate site such as the round window. Except for electromagnetic devices featuring indirect transducer technology such as the MAXUM System, all other devices require implantation of other components as well. These include the demodulator and the cable connection with the transducer. Fully implantable systems also consist of a rechargeable battery, a sound processor, and a sensor device (either a subcutaneous microphone or a piezoelectric transducer as a sensor). In such cases, the surgical procedure typically includes a mastoidectomy and a (large) facial recess to access all middle ear structures necessary.

Additional hardware such as the demodulator requires a bony recess in the postauricular area. Skin incisions are adapted to the requirements of the device. With current technology, a standard postauricular incision is typically sufficient since it provides standard access to the mastoid and it allows proper placement of other device components.

Postimplantation (Re)habilitation and Fitting

After implantation, a healing period of several weeks or months is required before the device can be activated. The main underlying reason for this is proper ossicular integration of the active portion of the implant. Also, these intervals vary greatly among available devices. In any case, proper postoperative surgical follow-up should be employed. Then, device fitting is performed according to the manufacturer's specifications. Fitting software and amplification strategies are very similar to conventional hearing aids. Thus, a dispensing audiologist familiar with fitting conventional amplification will find the process intuitive.

Care must be taken not to overstimulate the cochlea. This has been reported mainly for alternative indications for conductive or mixed hearing losses. In these cases, the device gain is often too great and some patients experience a humming sound or a low-frequency noise floor. In our experience, this effect is a temporary one which did not require further surgical or audiologic action.

Proper follow-up should include annual visits with the surgeon to check for potential complications such as device extrusion, coupling issues mainly evident as performance loss of the implant, or other infectious issues. In cases in which the external auditory canal has been closed, careful follow-up should include assessment of squamous ingrowth and iatrogenic cholesteatoma formation.

Audiologic follow-up should be performed more frequently to adjust the device's fitting parameters to the patient's hearing loss. Potential progressive losses should undergo frequent testing and device adaptations. With progressive sensorineural losses, the clinician should reevaluate the patient's speech discrimination abilities to reassess suitability for the device. The authors have encountered patients who eventually required cochlear implantation due to a previously undetected progressive loss of hearing.

Expected Outcomes

Several clinical trials have now documented the beneficial effects of active MEI (125,126,134). The published data also include the benefits to the patients hearing-related quality of life (135). Overall, it appears that active MEIs provide the patients with improved sound quality and wearing comfort while offering objective hearing results equal to optimally fit conventional hearing aids. Thus, the underlying biology of the inner ear should be carefully assessed prior to implantation.

For newer indications not yet fully FDA approved, active MEIs offer an alternative treatment option. Specifically, patients with otherwise non-correctable conductive hearing loss components can be successfully rehabilitated using the Vibrant Soundbridge. The transducer (FMT in case of this device) can be placed on the round window or on ossicular remnants. Theoretically, this principle applies to other MEIs as well as long as the transducer allows proper fixation and transmission of sound energy. The Soundbridge has been approved for these types of indications in some countries outside the US. Since the device has been designed to overcome hearing loss, normal inner ear function with device placement onto the round window can sometimes be problematic. Often, the amplification has to be reduced to a minimum to avoid overstimulation. Some patients will report a humming in the initial phase after fitting. Naturally, with mixed-type hearing losses, this is less of an issue.

The results with round window vibroplasty continue to evolve. Clinical data from Europe demonstrates the hearing and quality of life benefit (121,136). For some less common indications such as for children and adults with atretic ears, the device also seems to provide a very reasonable alternative to conventional methods such as atresiaplasty or a BAHA (137,138). Compared to the latter, round window vibroplasty might offer the advantage

of true binaural hearing since the BAHA provides bilateral cochlear stimulation through the skull (110).

Complications

Since active MEIs require surgical placement, they are subject to potential complications. These are essentially what would be expected from transmastoid procedures including facial recess drilling. Specifically, most devices require a large recess. Thus, it is not surprising that chorda tympani injury has been frequently reported in clinical trials assessing active MEIs. Other surgery-related complications include skin breakdown and postoperative infection of the device and subsequent extrusion, as well as improper device placement and inadequate hearing benefit.

Device-related complications include inadvertent activation with various electromagnetic fields such as a microwave oven or the like. These events can cause various harmless but annoying auditory perceptions. Device failure, on the other hand, although rare, has been described. Failure modes are similar to cochlear implantation mainly due to failures of the hermetic seal of the demodulator. However, other components of the device could potentially be subject to failure as well.

AUDITORY CNS IMPLANTS

Overview

The ABI is a device designed to convert environmental sound into electrical impulses that are delivered along a multiple electrode array situated in close proximity to the cochlear nucleus in the brainstem. In a manner similar to the cochlear nerve, the cochlear nucleus maintains some degree of tonotopic arrangement; thus, application of discrete electrical stimulation along certain stations within the lateral recess of the fourth ventricle results in variably different, psychophysical frequency percepts. The ABI is indicated for patients in whom the cochlear nerve is absent or unavailable for stimulation bilaterally. Most commonly, patients with hearing loss secondary to neurofibromatosis type II with bilateral acoustic tumors have been the main group of patients implanted to date. Outcomes for these patients have been quite variable, but in most instances, patients gain significant sound awareness and enhanced lipreading from their devices. While open-set speech perception is unusual, occasionally individuals with ABIs can achieve such results. This section will discuss ABIs.

History

The first ABI was a single electrode device placed by William E. Hitselberger and William F. House in 1979 in Los Angeles, CA, following an acoustic neuroma removal in a patient with neurofibromatosis type II. This device provided some auditory awareness for the patient. Over the following years, with greater understanding of tonotopic awareness and multichannel stimulation with cochlear implants, a multichannel ABI was developed. The initial devices were based on the House–3M cochlear implant speech processor. Ultimately, working with Cochlear Corporation and Huntington Medical Research Institute in Pasadena, a 21-electrode array on a silicone and Dacron carrier was developed. This array when combined with the Sprint speech processor comprised the Nucleus 24 ABI. The processor is a body-worn device (Sprint processor) that performs spectral analysis (SPeak), digital processing, stimulus encoding, and transmission of commands to the implant through an RF link. The US FDA approved the Nucleus 24 ABI (Cochlear Corp, Englewood, CO) for commercial usage in 2000 (139) (Fig. 163.19). Digisonic Corp (Laboratories MXM, France) and Med-EL Corp (Austria) also manufacture ABI devices today, but these are not available for use in the US today.

Principles of Electric Stimulation of the Auditory System and Coding Strategy

As the ABI was developed from the cochlear implant, the basic tenants of stimulation are similar (see Cochlear Implants). The tonotopic arrangement of the cochlear

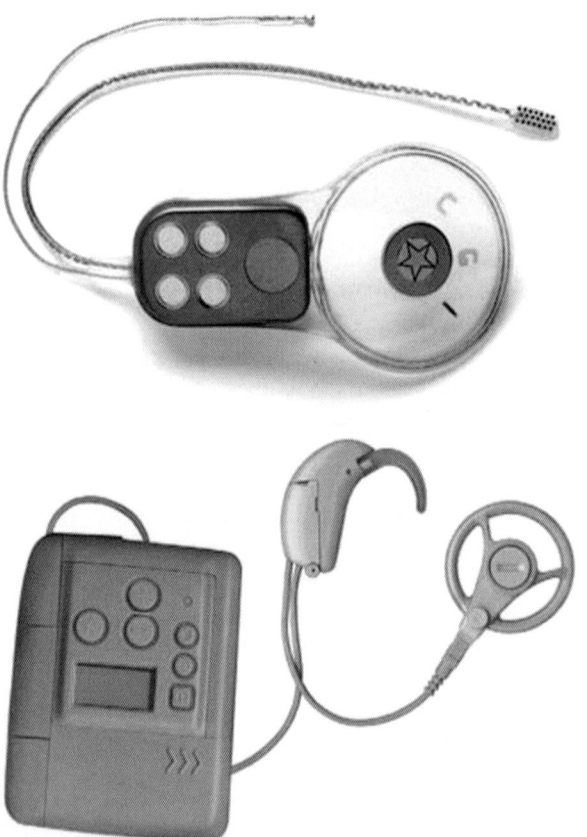

Figure 163.19 Cochlear Corporation's Auditory Brainstem Implant System. The system features a flat electrode array with 21-electrode contacts. This array is positioned on the surface of the cochlear nucleus.

nucleus, however, is somewhat more complex and less accessible in some regions. For instance, cochlear nerve fibers transmitting low-frequency sounds project mainly to the ventral portion of the cochlear nucleus, while basal cochlear nerve fibers transmitting high-frequency sounds project to the dorsal portions of each nuclear subdivision (140). This organization is best defined in the dorsal cochlear nucleus, the most superficial and exposed part, where the axis of the tonotopic gradient is oriented parallel to the brainstem surface (141). Although this issue might be a theoretical advantage for electrical stimulation, significant ascending information is processed in the deepest part of the anterior ventral cochlear nucleus, which is almost unexposed within the lateral recess area. Thus, surface stimulation might not fully be able to access the functionally important regions and might explain, in part, the relatively poor performance achieved by patients when compared to the cochlear implant. With this in mind, the penetrating auditory brainstem implant was developed in an attempt to achieve better performance. This device attained lower thresholds for stimulation, increased pitch range, and high selectivity, but these properties unfortunately did not result in improved speech recognition (142).

Indications

The primary indication for ABI is for patients with profound hearing loss and no available cochlear nerves to stimulate bilaterally. As the ABI device was originally designed for the purposes of helping patients with neurofibromatosis type II, this remains the most common indication and the only FDA-approved indication for use in the US today. There remain a number of other clinical scenarios that might be amenable to ABI, and these include congenital cochlear nerve aplasia, bilateral temporal bone fracture with cochlear nerve disruption, severe inner ear malformation, or dense ossification secondary to previous meningitis (143). In these cases, cochlear nerve integrity might be unclear, and a trial of cochlear implantation might be justified prior to undertaking an ABI operation (75).

Surgery

ABI placement is generally carried out through a posterior fossa craniotomy—either translabyrinthine or retrosigmoid. The distinct advantages of the translabyrinthine approach for ABI are (a) incision location that is more natural for receiver–stimulator placement, (b) a lack of cerebellar retraction, (c) direct line of site to the lateral recess of the 4th ventricle afforded by the presigmoid exposure, and (d) electrode path through the immobile temporal bone rather against the pulsatile cerebellar hemisphere. However, this approach can be limited in some cases by a high jugular bulb, making lower cranial nerve and recess visualization somewhat more tangential and difficult at times. Clearly, surgeons have effectively placed ABIs through both approaches with acceptable results (144,145). In cases of neurofibromatosis type II, acoustic neuroma removal precedes device placement. Cranial nerve monitoring should include facial muscle electrodes, as well as palatal and trapezius electrodes to monitor cranial nerves 9, 10, and 11. ABR monitoring electrodes include a non-inverting electrode ("active," "positive") at the vertex of the head (Cz), the inverting ("reference," "negative") electrode placed in the region of the C7, and the ground electrode at the hairline at the back of the neck (Oz). Alternatives to this electrode montage also exist.

The receiver–stimulator should be placed in a region similar to the cochlear implant, in a subperiosteal pocket. Given the extent of periosteal dissection needed for exposing the temporal bone for the approach, intraosseous tie-down holes with suture fixation can be useful for immobilizing the device. The retaining magnet is left in the device for initial placement to help retain the headpiece during intraoperative electrophysiologic testing.

The lateral recess of the fourth ventricle (i.e., foramen of Luschka) is the target for device placement. Landmarks for identifying this recess include the 8th and 9th cranial nerve root entry zones at the superior and inferior boarders of the recess, respectively. The cerebellar flocculus lies on the posterior side of the recess, and the choroid plexus can usually be identified exiting the foramen. There can be veins overlying the recess opening and careful dissection is often needed to mobilize them without disruption. As the cochlear nucleus lies on the ventral surface of the foramen superiorly, the electrode contacts should face anteriorly–superiorly. The electrode array should be advanced until the proximal most electrodes on the array are just inside the opening. Teflon can be used to pack the recess to immobilize the array. Intraoperative monitoring of the implant evoked ABR is critical for appropriate device placement (Fig. 163.20). This procedure has been detailed

previously (146). Examples of intraoperative view after electrode array placement and excellent electrophysiologic responses are shown in the figure. A postoperative CT also confirms array location (Fig. 163.21).

Complications

Surgical complications are mostly unusual from ABI surgery. In fact, most complications described in these patients result from the posterior fossa surgery indicated for removing the patient's acoustic neuroma rather than from the device placement. These might include bleeding, infection, facial nerve injury, loss of residual hearing, cerebrospinal fluid leakage, stroke, and death. Cerebrospinal fluid leakage along the electrode carrier is more common among ABI patients than typical acoustic tumor patients. These patients may also experience transient dysphonia and aspiration related to lower cranial nerve dysfunction. Inability to identify the lateral recess in large tumor or distorted anatomy cases can occur resulting in an inability to place the device. The electrode might become dislodged from the recess resulting in an absence of stimulation at activation.

During stimulation, it is common to experience nonauditory sensations that can be severe at times. In one series, 24% of individual electrodes could not be used because of nonauditory stimulation. Nonauditory sensations were usually described as tingling in the head or body. A smaller number of patients described dizziness or slight jittering of vision (147). Others symptoms can include choking, pain, vertigo, facial twitching, and potential changes in heart rate, blood pressure, and respiratory efforts. While these latter symptoms are very uncommon, special care is always taken during initial activation by having trained medical personal available for emergency resuscitation if needed (139,147–149).

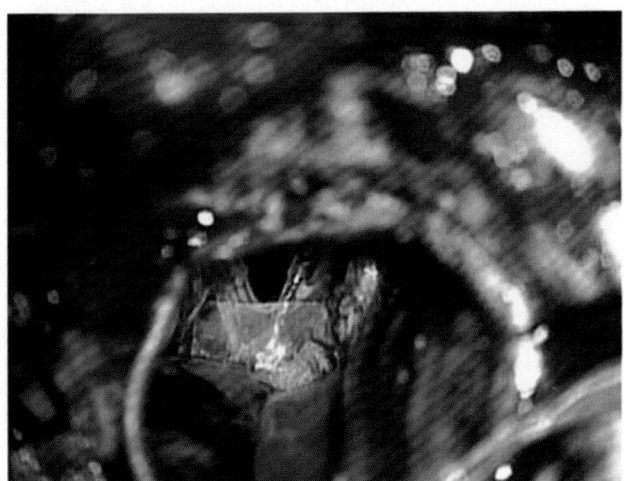 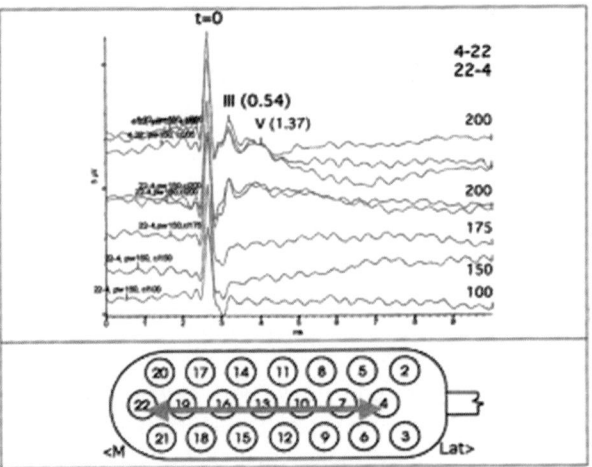

Figure 163.20 Intraoperative image (**left**) and electrically evoked auditory brainstem response (E-ABR) demonstrating proper placement of an ABR. The recording example shows evoked potentials when stimulating across the array (demonstrated below).

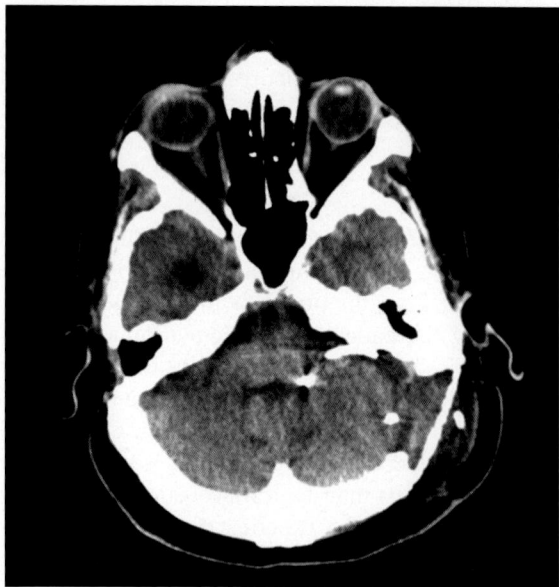

Figure 163.21 Axial head CT shows the expected postoperative appearance after placement of an ABI into the left lateral recess.

Outcomes

In general, outcomes from ABI can be described in terms of sound detection and speech perception abilities using closed- and open-set test materials with and without the addition of lipreading. In a recent review of 86 neurofibromatosis type II patients implanted with ABIs, 13 did not respond to stimulation and 1 was explanted. Of the 60 patients with available 6-month data, mean open-set speech perception scores (CUNY sentences) using the implant alone, vision alone, and both the implant and vision on CUNY sentence were less than 10%, 30%, and nearly 55% correct. However, there was a wide range of auditory abilities with some patients obtaining combined vision and sound scores of greater than 90% correct (148). Thus, in these patients, the ABI is an excellent enhancement to lipreading. For individuals that have known only spoken language throughout their entire life, this connection to the speaking world is significant, and the importance of this communication enhancement should not be underestimated.

More recently, Colletti et al. (150) in Verona, Italy, have placed ABIs in patients without neurofibromatosis type II. These non-tumor patients have had a variety of etiologies including labyrinthine ossification, cochlear nerve aplasia, temporal bone fractures, and severe inner ear malformations (150). While the results have been quite variable, some patients in this group have been able to obtain significant open-set speech perception abilities using audition alone. While these results remain to be confirmed, this report suggests that patients without neurofibromatosis type II might be better candidates for ABI. Further work is needed in this area.

ACKNOWLEDGMENTS

The authors would like to thank Dr. Benjamin Wei, MD, PhD, for his assistance preparing this manuscript. Also, we would like to acknowledge Dr. Harold C. Pillbury, MD, for his continuous support and his leadership.

REFERENCES

1. Summerfield AQ, Marshall DH, Barton GR, et al. A cost-utility scenario analysis of bilateral cochlear implantation. *Arch Otolaryngol Head Neck Surg* 2002;128:1255–1262.
2. Francis HW, Koch ME, Wyatt JR, et al. Trends in educational placement and cost-benefit considerations in children with cochlear implants. *Arch Otolaryngol Head Neck Surg* 1999;125:499–505.
3. Wyatt JR, Niparko JK, Rothman M, et al. Cost utility of the multichannel cochlear implants in 258 profoundly deaf individuals. *Laryngoscope* 1996;106:816–821.
4. Wyatt JR, Niparko JK, Rothman ML, et al. Cost-effectiveness of the multichannel cochlear implant. *Ann Otol Rhinol Laryngol Suppl* 1995;166:248–250.
5. Niparko JK, Tobey EA, Thal DJ, et al. Spoken language development in children following cochlear implantation. *JAMA* 2010;303:1498–1506.
6. Geers AE, Tobey EA, Moog JS. Editorial: long-term outcomes of cochlear implantation in early childhood. *Ear Hear* 2011;32:1S.
7. Moog JS, Geers AE. Early educational placement and later language outcomes for children with cochlear implants. *Otol Neurotol*: official publication of the *Am Otol Soc, Am Neurot Soc* [and] *Eur Acad Otol Neurot* 2010;31:1315–1319.
8. Volta A. On the electricity excited by mere contact of conducting substances of different kinds. *Phil Trans Roy Soc Phil* 1800;90:403–431.
9. Eisen MD. Djourno, Eyries, and the first implanted electrical neural stimulator to restore hearing. *Otol Neurotol*: official publication of the *Am Otol Soc, Am Neurotol Soc* [and] *Eur Acad Otol Neurotol* 2003;24:500–506.
10. Djourno A, Eyries C, Vallancien P. [Preliminary attempts of electrical excitation of the auditory nerve in man, by permanently inserted micro-apparatus]. *Bull Acad Natl Med* 1957;141:481–483.
11. Blume SS. Histories of cochlear implantation. *Soc Sci Med* 1999;49:1257–1268.
12. House W. Cochlear implants: past, present and future. *Adv Otorhinolaryngol* 1993;48:1–3.
13. Simmons FB, Dent LJ, Van Compernolle D. Comparison of different speech processing strategies on patients receiving the same implant. *Ann Otol Rhinol Laryngol* 1986;95:71–75.
14. Eddington DK. Speech discrimination in deaf subjects with cochlear implants. *J Acoust Soc Am* 1980;68:885–891.
15. Eddington DK, Dobelle WH, Brackmann DE, et al. Auditory prostheses research with multiple channel intracochlear stimulation in man. *Ann Otol Rhinol Laryngol* 1978;87:1–39.
16. Chouard CH. The surgical rehabilitation of total deafness with the multichannel cochlear implant. Indications and results. *Audiology* 1980;19:137–145.
17. Atlas LE, Herndon MK, Simmons FB, et al. Results of stimulus and speech-coding schemes applied to multichannel electrodes. *Ann N Y Acad Sci* 1983;405:377–386.
18. Clark GM, Black R, Dewhurst DJ, et al. A multiple-electrode hearing prosthesis for cochlea implantation in deaf patients. *Med Prog Technol* 1977;5:127–140.
19. Simmons FB, Epley JM, Lummis RC, et al. Auditory nerve: electrical stimulation in man. *Science* 1965;148:104–106.
20. House WF, Berliner KI, Eisenberg LS. Present status and future directions of the Ear Research Institute cochlear implant program. *Acta Otolaryngol* 1979;87:176–184.
21. Michelson RP. The results of electrical stimulation of the cochlea in human sensory deafness. *Ann Otol Rhinol Laryngol* 1971;80:914–919.
22. Dobelle WH, Mladejovsky MG. The directions for future research on sensory prostheses. *Trans Am Soc Artif Intern Organs* 1974;20B:425–429.

23. Clark GM, Black R, Forster IC, et al. Design criteria of a multiple-electrode cochlear implant hearing prosthesis [43.66.Ts, 43.66. Sr]. *J Acoust Soc Am* 1978;63:631–633.

24. Clark G. Cochlear implants in children: safety as well as speech and language. *Int J Pediatr Otorhinolaryngol* 2003;67(Suppl 1): S7–S20.

25. McCabe BF, Tyler RS, Gantz BJ, et al. Preliminary assessment of the Los Angeles, Vienna and Melbourne cochlear implants. *Acta Otolaryngol Suppl* 1984;411:247–253.

26. Tyler RS, Lowder MW, Otto SR, et al. Initial Iowa results with the multichannel cochlear implant from Melbourne. *J Speech Hear Res* 1984;27:596–604.

27. Gantz BJ, Tye-Murray N, Tyler RS. Word recognition performance with single-channel and multichannel cochlear implants. *Am J Otol* 1989;10:91–94.

28. Gantz BJ, Tyler RS, Knutson JF, et al. Evaluation of five different cochlear implant designs: audiologic assessment and predictors of performance. *Laryngoscope* 1988;98:1100–1106.

29. Gantz BJ, Tyler RS, McCabe BF, et al. Iowa cochlear implant clinical project: results with two single-channel cochlear implants and one multi-channel cochlear implant. *Laryngoscope* 1985;95:443–449.

30. von Békésy G. In: *Experiments in hearing*. New York: McGraw-Hill, 1960:745.

31. Schuknecht HF. Techniques for study of cochlear function and pathology in experimental animals; development of the anatomical frequency scale for the cat. *Arch Otolaryngol* 1953;58:377–397.

32. Greenwood DD. Critical bandwidth and consonance in relation to cochlear frequency-position coordinates. *Hear Res* 1991;54:164–208.

33. Woodson EA, Reiss LA, Turner CW, et al. The Hybrid cochlear implant: a review. *Adv Otorhinolaryngol* 2010;67:125–134.

34. Turner CW, Reiss LA, Gantz BJ. Combined acoustic and electric hearing: preserving residual acoustic hearing. *Hear Res* 2008;242:164–171.

35. von Ilberg CA, Baumann U, Kiefer J, et al. Electric-acoustic stimulation of the auditory system: a review of the first decade. *Audiol Neurootol* 2011;16(Suppl 2):1–30.

36. von Ilberg C, Kiefer J, Tillein J, et al. Electric-acoustic stimulation of the auditory system. New technology for severe hearing loss. *ORL J Otorhinolaryngol Relat Spec* 1999;61:334–340.

37. Briggs RJ, Eder HC, Seligman PM, et al. Initial clinical experience with a totally implantable cochlear implant research device. *Otology & Neurotology*: official publication of the *Am Otol Soc, Am Neurotol Soc* [and] *Eur Acad Otol Neurot* 2008;29:114–119.

38. Lane H, Bahan B. Ethics of cochlear implantation in young children. *Otolaryngol Head Neck surg*: official journal of *Am Acad Otolaryngol Head Neck Surg* 1999;121:672–675.

39. Rubinstein JT. How cochlear implants encode speech. *Curr Opin Otolaryngol Head Neck Surg* 2004;12:444–448.

40. Frijns JH, Kalkman RK, Vanpoucke FJ, et al. Simultaneous and non-simultaneous dual electrode stimulation in cochlear implants: evidence for two neural response modalities. *Acta Otolaryngol* 2009;129:433–439.

41. Huang TC, Reitzen SD, Marrinan MS, et al. Modiolar coiling, electrical thresholds, and speech perception after cochlear implantation using the nucleus contour advance electrode with the advance off stylet technique. *Otol Neurotol*: official publication of the *Am Otol Soc, Am Neurotol Soc* [and] *Eur Acad Otol Neurotol* 2006;27:159–166.

42. Richter CP, Bayon R, Izzo AD, et al. Optical stimulation of auditory neurons: effects of acute and chronic deafening. *Hear Res* 2008;242:42–51.

43. Rubinstein JT, Hong R. Signal coding in cochlear implants: exploiting stochastic effects of electrical stimulation. *Ann Otol Rhinol Laryngol Suppl* 2003;191:14–19.

44. Nadol JB Jr, Eddington DK. Histopathology of the inner ear relevant to cochlear implantation. *Adv Otorhinolaryngol* 2006;64: 31–49.

45. Nadol JB Jr, Shiao JY, Burgess BJ, et al. Histopathology of cochlear implants in humans. *Ann Otol Rhinol Laryngol* 2001;110:883–891.

46. Choi CH, Oghalai JS. Predicting the effect of post-implant cochlear fibrosis on residual hearing. *Hear Res* 2005;205:193–200.

47. Adunka O, Kiefer J. Impact of electrode insertion depth on intracochlear trauma. *Otolaryngol Head Neck Surg*: official journal of *Am Acad Otolaryngol Head Neck Surg* 2006;135:374–382.

48. Fayad JN, Linthicum FH Jr. Multichannel cochlear implants: relation of histopathology to performance. *Laryngoscope* 2006;116:1310–1320.

49. Fayad JN, Luxford W, Linthicum FH. The Clarion electrode positioner: temporal bone studies. *Am J Otol* 2000;21:226–229.

50. Fayad JN, Makarem AO, Linthicum FH Jr. Histopathologic assessment of fibrosis and new bone formation in implanted human temporal bones using 3D reconstruction. *Otolaryngol Head Neck Surg*: official journal of *Am Acad Otolaryngol Head Neck Surg* 2009;141:247–252.

51. Linthicum FH Jr, Fayad J, Otto S, et al. Inner ear morphologic changes resulting from cochlear implantation. *Am J Otol* 1991;(12 Suppl):8–10; discussion 18–21.

52. Nadol JB Jr. Patterns of neural degeneration in the human cochlea and auditory nerve: implications for cochlear implantation. *Otolaryngol Head Neck Surg*: official journal of *Am Acad Otolaryngol Head Neck Surg* 1997;117:220–228.

53. Nadol JB Jr, Eddington DK. Histologic evaluation of the tissue seal and biologic response around cochlear implant electrodes in the human. *Otol Neurotol*: official publication of the *Am Otol Soc, Am Neurot Soc* [and] *Eur Acad Otol Neurotol* 2004;25:257–262.

54. Nadol JB Jr, Eddington DK, Burgess BJ. Foreign body or hypersensitivity granuloma of the inner ear after cochlear implantation: one possible cause of a soft failure? *Otol Neurotol*: official publication of the *Am Otol Soc, Am Neurotol Soc* [and] *Eur Acad Otol Neurotol* 2008;29:1076–1084.

55. Finley CC, Holden TA, Holden LK, et al. Role of electrode placement as a contributor to variability in cochlear implant outcomes. *Otol Neurotol*: official publication of the *Am Otol Soc, Am Neurotol Soc* [and] *Eur Acad Otol Neurotol* 2008;29:920–928.

56. Holt RF, Svirsky MA. An exploratory look at pediatric cochlear implantation: is earliest always best? *Ear Hear* 2008;29:492–511.

57. Svirsky MA, Silveira A, Suarez H, et al. Auditory learning and adaptation after cochlear implantation: a preliminary study of discrimination and labeling of vowel sounds by cochlear implant users. *Acta Otolaryngol* 2001;121:262–265.

58. Adunka OF, Jewells V, Buchman CA. Value of computed tomography in the evaluation of children with cochlear nerve deficiency. *Otol Neurotol* 2007;28:597–604.

59. Adunka OF, Roush PA, Teagle HF, et al. Internal auditory canal morphology in children with cochlear nerve deficiency. *Otol Neurotol* 2006;27:793–801.

60. Glastonbury CM, Davidson HC, Harnsberger HR, et al. Imaging findings of cochlear nerve deficiency. *AJNR Am J Neuroradiol* 2002;23:635–643.

61. McClay JE, Tandy R, Grundfast K, et al. Major and minor temporal bone abnormalities in children with and without congenital sensorineural hearing loss. *Arch Otolaryngol Head Neck Surg* 2002;128:664–671.

62. Roche JP, Huang BY, Castillo M, et al. Imaging characteristics of children with auditory neuropathy spectrum disorder. *Otol Neurotol*: official publication of the *Am Otol Soc, Am Neurotol Soc* [and] *Eur Acad Otol Neurotol* 2010;31:780–788.

63. Papsin BC. Cochlear implantation in children with anomalous cochleovestibular anatomy. *Laryngoscope* 2005;115:1–26.

64. Buchman CA, Copeland BJ, Yu KK, et al. Cochlear implantation in children with congenital inner ear malformations. *Laryngoscope* 2004;114:309–316.

65. Sennaroglu L. Cochlear implantation in inner ear malformations—a review article. *Cochlear Implants Int* 2010;11:4–41.

66. Adunka OF, Roush PA, Teagle HF, et al. Internal auditory canal morphology in children with cochlear nerve deficiency. *Otol Neurotol* 2006;27:793–801.

67. Buchman CA, Roush PA, Teagle HF, et al. Auditory neuropathy characteristics in children with cochlear nerve deficiency. *Ear Hear* 2006;27:399–408.

68. Nelson EG, Hinojosa R. Aplasia of the cochlear nerve: a temporal bone study. *Otol Neurotol*: official publication of the *Am Otol Soc, Am Neurotol Soc* [and] *Eur Acad Otol Neurotol* 2001;22:790–795.

69. Balkany TJ, Whitley M, Shapira Y, et al. The temporalis pocket technique for cochlear implantation: an anatomic and clinical study. *Otol Neurotol* 2009;30:903–907.

70. Molony TB, Giles JE, Thompson TL, et al. Device fixation in cochlear implantation: is bone anchoring necessary? *Laryngoscope* 2010;120:1837–1839.

71. Adunka OF, Buchman CA. Cochlear implant fixation in children using periosteal sutures. *Otol Neurotol:* official publication of the *Am Otol Soc, Am Neurotol Soc* [and] *Eur Acad Otol Neurotol* 2007;28:768–770.

72. Basura GJ, Adunka OF, Buchman CA. Scala tympani cochleostomy for cochlear implantation. *Oper Tech Otolaryngol* 2010;21: 218–222.

73. Cosetti MK, Shapiro WH, Green JE, et al. Intraoperative neural response telemetry as a predictor of performance. *Otol Neurotol:* official publication of the *Am Otol Soc, Am Neurotol Soc* [and] *Eur Acad Otol Neurotol* 2010;31:1095–1099.

74. Teagle HF, Roush PA, Woodard JS, et al. Cochlear implantation in children with auditory neuropathy spectrum disorder. *Ear Hear* 2010;31:325–335.

75. Buchman CA, Teagle H, Roush PA, et al. Cochlear implantation in children with labyrinthine anomalies and cochlear nerve deficiency: implications for auditory brainstem implantation. *Laryngoscope* 2011;121:1979–1988.

76. Balkany T, Bird PA, Hodges AV, et al. Surgical technique for implantation of the totally ossified cochlea. *Laryngoscope* 1998;108:988–992.

77. Balkany T, Gantz B, Nadol JB Jr. Multichannel cochlear implants in partially ossified cochleas. *Ann Otol Rhinol Laryngol Suppl* 1988;135:3–7.

78. Francis HW, Buchman CA, Visaya JM, et al. Surgical factors in pediatric cochlear implantation and their early effects on electrode activation and functional outcomes. *Otol Neurotol:* official publication of the *Am Otol Soc, Am Neurotol Soc* [and] *Eur Acad Otol Neurotol* 2008;29:502–508.

79. Buchman CA, Joy J, Hodges A, et al. Vestibular effects of cochlear implantation. *Laryngoscope* 2004;114:1–22.

80. Melvin TA, Della Santina CC, Carey JP, et al. The effects of cochlear implantation on vestibular function. *Otol Neurotol:* official publication of the *Am Otol Soc, Am Neurotol Soc* [and] *Eur Acad Otol Neurotol* 2009;30:87–94.

81. Cullen RD, Fayad JN, Luxford WM, et al. Revision cochlear implant surgery in children. *Otol Neurotol:* official publication of the *Am Otol Soc, Am Neurotol Soc* [and] *Eur Acad Otol Neurotol* 2008;29:214–220.

82. Biernath KR, Reefhuis J, Whitney CG, et al. Bacterial meningitis among children with cochlear implants beyond 24 months after implantation. *Pediatrics* 2006;117:284–289.

83. Reefhuis J, Honein MA, Whitney CG, et al. Risk of bacterial meningitis in children with cochlear implants. *N Engl J Med* 2003;349:435–445.

84. Parner ET, Reefhuis J, Schendel D, et al. Hearing loss diagnosis followed by meningitis in Danish children, 1995–2004. *Otolaryngol Head and Neck Surg:* official journal of *Am Acad Otolaryngol Head Neck Surg* 2007;136:428–433.

85. Wei BP, Shepherd RK, Robins-Browne RM, et al. Pneumococcal meningitis post-cochlear implantation: potential routes of infection and pathophysiology. *Otolaryngol Head and Neck Surg:* official journal of *Am Acad Otolaryngol Head Neck Surg* 2010;143: S15–S23.

86. FDA public health notification: importance of vaccination in cochlear implant recipients. Available at: http://www.fda.gov/MedicalDevices/Safety/AlertsandNotices/PublicHealthNotifications/ucm062057.htm.

87. Bassim MK, Buss E, Clark MS, et al. MED-EL Combi40+ cochlear implantation in adults. *Laryngoscope* 2005;115:1568–1573.

88. Friedland DR, Runge-Samuelson C, Baig H, et al. Case-control analysis of cochlear implant performance in elderly patients. *Arch Otolaryngol Head Neck Surg* 2010;136:432–438.

89. Drennan WR, Rubinstein JT. Music perception in cochlear implant users and its relationship with psychophysical capabilities. *J Rehabil Res Dev* 2008;45:779–789.

90. Gomaa NA, Rubinstein JT, Lowder MW, et al. Residual speech perception and cochlear implant performance in postlingually deafened adults. *Ear Hear* 2003;24:539–544.

91. Chang DT, Ko AB, Murray GS, et al. Lack of financial barriers to pediatric cochlear implantation: impact of socioeconomic status on access and outcomes. *Arch Otolaryngol Head Neck Surg* 2010;136:648–657.

92. Stern RE, Yueh B, Lewis C, et al. Recent epidemiology of pediatric cochlear implantation in the United States: disparity among children of different ethnicity and socioeconomic status. *Laryngoscope* 2005;115:125–131.

93. Adunka OF, Jewells V, Buchman CA. Value of computed tomography in the evaluation of children with cochlear nerve deficiency. *Otol Neurotol* 2007;28:597–604.

94. Skinner MW, Holden TA, Whiting BR, et al. In vivo estimates of the position of advanced bionics electrode arrays in the human cochlea. *Ann Otol Rhinol Laryngol Suppl* 2007;197:2–24.

95. Aschendorff A, Kromeier J, Klenzner T, et al. Quality control after insertion of the nucleus contour and contour advance electrode in adults. *Ear Hear* 2007;28:75S–79S.

96. Rance G, Beer DE, Cone-Wesson B, et al. Clinical findings for a group of infants and young children with auditory neuropathy. *Ear Hear* 1999;20:238–252.

97. Rance G, Barker EJ. Speech perception in children with auditory neuropathy/dyssynchrony managed with either hearing AIDS or cochlear implants. *Otol Neurotol:* official publication of the *Am Otol Soc, Am Neurotol Soc* [and] *Eur Acad Otol Neurotol* 2008;29:179–182.

98. Miyamoto RT, Kirk KI, Renshaw J, et al. Cochlear implantation in auditory neuropathy. *Laryngoscope* 1999;109:181–185.

99. Litovsky RY, Parkinson A, Arcaroli J. Spatial hearing and speech intelligibility in bilateral cochlear implant users. *Ear Hear* 2009;30:419–431.

100. Basura GJ, Eapen R, Buchman CA. Bilateral cochlear implantation: current concepts, indications, and results. *Laryngoscope* 2009;119:2395–2401.

101. Eapen RJ, Buchman CA. Bilateral cochlear implantation: current concepts. *Curr Opin Otolaryngol Head Neck Surg* 2009;17: 351–355.

102. Eapen RJ, Buss E, Adunka MC, et al. Hearing-in-noise benefits after bilateral simultaneous cochlear implantation continue to improve 4 years after implantation. *Otol Neurotol:* official publication of the *Am Otol Soc, Am Neurotol Soc* [and] *Eur Acad Otol Neurotol* 2009;30:153–159.

103. Turner CW, Gantz BJ, Karsten S, et al. Impact of hair cell preservation in cochlear implantation: combined electric and acoustic hearing. *Otol Neurotol:* official publication of the *Am Otol Soc, Am Neurotol Soc* [and] *Eur Acad Otol Neurotol* 2010;31: 1227–1232.

104. Adunka OF, Pillsbury HC, Adunka MC, et al. Is electric acoustic stimulation better than conventional cochlear implantation for speech perception in quiet? *Otol Neurotol* 2010;31:1049–1054.

105. Christensen L, Smith-Olinde L, Kimberlain J, et al. Comparison of traditional bone-conduction hearing AIDS with the Baha system. *J Am Acad Audiol* 2010;21:267–273.

106. Tjellstrom A, Hakansson B. The bone-anchored hearing aid. Design principles, indications, and long-term clinical results. *Otolaryngol Clin North Am* 1995;28:53–72.

107. Arnold A, Caversaccio MD, Mudry A. Surgery for the bone-anchored hearing aid. *Adv Otorhinolaryngol* 2011;71:47–55.

108. Yellon RF. Atresiaplasty versus BAHA for congenital aural atresia. *Laryngoscope* 2011;121:2–3.

109. Mazita A, Fazlina WH, Abdullah A, et al. Hearing rehabilitation in congenital canal atresia. *Singapore Med J* 2009;50:1072–1076.

110. Arndt S, Aschendorff A, Laszig R, et al. Comparison of pseudobinaural hearing to real binaural hearing rehabilitation after cochlear implantation in patients with unilateral deafness and tinnitus. *Otol Neurotol:* official publication of the *Am Otol Soc, Am Neurotol Soc* [and] *Eur Acad Otol Neurotol* 2011;32:39–47.

111. Bishop CE, Eby TL. The current status of audiologic rehabilitation for profound unilateral sensorineural hearing loss. *Laryngoscope* 2010;120:552–556.

112. McDermott AL, Sheehan P. Paediatric Baha. *Adv Otorhinolaryngol* 2011;71:56–62.

113. Nicholson N, Christensen L, Dornhoffer J, et al. Verification of speech spectrum audibility for pediatric baha softband users with craniofacial anomalies. *Cleft Palate Craniofac J* 2011;48: 56–65.

114. Verhagen CV, Hol MK, Coppens-Schellekens W, et al. The Baha Softband. A new treatment for young children with bilateral congenital aural atresia. *Int J Pediatr Otorhinolaryngol* 2008;72: 1455–1459.

115. Wilkinson EP, Luxford WM, Slattery WH III, et al. Single vertical incision for Baha implant surgery: preliminary results. *Otolaryngol Head and Neck Surg:* official journal of *Am Acad Otolaryngol Head Neck Surg* 2009;140:573–578.

116. Wazen JJ, Gupta R, Ghossaini S, et al. Osseointegration timing for Baha system loading. *Laryngoscope* 2007;117:794–796.

117. Tjellstrom A, Granstrom G. How we do it: frequency of skin necrosis after BAHA surgery. *Clin Otolaryngol* 2006;31:216–220.

118. Ricci G, Della Volpe A, Faralli M, et al. Results and complications of the Baha system (bone-anchored hearing aid). *Eur Arch Otorhinolaryngol* 2010;267:1539–1545.

119. Danhauer JL, Johnson CE, Mixon M. Does the evidence support use of the Baha implant system (Baha) in patients with congenital unilateral aural atresia? *J Am Acad Audiol* 2010;21:274–286.

120. Ball GR. The vibrant soundbridge: design and development. *Adv Otorhinolaryngol* 2010;69:1–13.

121. Baumgartner WD, Boheim K, Hagen R, et al. The vibrant soundbridge for conductive and mixed hearing losses: European multicenter study results. *Adv Otorhinolaryngol* 2010;69:38–50.

122. Goode RL, Rosenbaum ML, Maniglia AJ. The history and development of the implantable hearing aid. *Otolaryngol Clin North Am* 1995;28:1–16.

123. Zenner HP. TICA totally implantable system for treatment of high-frequency sensorineural hearing loss. *Ear Nose Throat J* 2000;79:770–772, 774, 777.

124. Fisch U, Cremers CW, Lenarz T, et al. Clinical experience with the Vibrant Soundbridge implant device. *Otol Neurotol* 2001;22:962–972.

125. Luetje CM, Brackman D, Balkany TJ, et al. Phase III clinical trial results with the Vibrant Soundbridge implantable middle ear hearing device: a prospective controlled multicenter study. *Otolaryngol Head Neck Surg* 2002;126:97–107.

126. Luetje CM, Brown SA, Cullen RD. Vibrant Soundbridge implantable hearing device: critical review and single-surgeon short- and long-term results. *Ear Nose Throat J* 2010;89:E9–E14.

127. Gyo K, Yanagihara N, Araki H. Sound pickup utilizing an implantable piezoelectric ceramic bimorph element: application to the cochlear implant. *Am J Otol* 1984;5:273–276.

128. Kraus EM, Shohet JA, Catalano PJ. Envoy Esteem Totally Implantable Hearing System: phase 2 trial, 1-year hearing results. *Otolaryngol Head Neck Surg: official journal of Am Acad Otolaryngol Head Neck Surg* 2011;145:100–109.

129. Luetje CM, Brackman D, Balkany TJ, et al. Phase III clinical trial results with the Vibrant Soundbridge implantable middle ear hearing device: a prospective controlled multicenter study. *Otolaryngol Head Neck Surg: official journal of Am Acad Otolaryngol Head Neck Surg* 2002;126:97–107.

130. Snik FM, Cremers WR. The effect of the "floating mass transducer" in the middle ear on hearing sensitivity. *Am J Otol* 2000;21:42–48.

131. Hol MK, Cremers CW, Coppens-Schellekens W, et al. The BAHA Softband. A new treatment for young children with bilateral congenital aural atresia. *Int J Pediatr Otorhinolaryngol* 2005;69:973–980.

132. Frenzel H, Hanke F, Beltrame M, et al. Application of the Vibrant Soundbridge in bilateral congenital atresia in toddlers. *Acta Otolaryngol* 2010;130:966–970.

133. Huttenbrink KB, Beutner D, Zahnert T. Clinical results with an active middle ear implant in the oval window. *Adv Otorhinolaryngol* 2010;69:27–31.

134. Snik AF, Cremers CW. Vibrant semi-implantable hearing device with digital sound processing: effective gain and speech perception. *Arch Otolaryngol Head Neck Surg* 2001;127:1433–1437.

135. Sterkers O, Boucarra D, Labassi S, et al. A middle ear implant, the Symphonix Vibrant Soundbridge: retrospective study of the first 125 patients implanted in France. *Otol Neurotol* 2003;24:427–436.

136. Huber AM, Ball GR, Veraguth D, et al. A new implantable middle ear hearing device for mixed hearing loss: a feasibility study in human temporal bones. *Otol Neurotol* 2006;27:1104–1109.

137. Frenzel H, Hanke F, Beltrame M, et al. Application of the Vibrant Soundbridge to unilateral osseous atresia cases. *Laryngoscope* 2009;119:67–74.

138. Fuchsmann C, Tringali S, Disant F, et al. Hearing rehabilitation in congenital aural atresia using the bone-anchored hearing aid: audiological and satisfaction results. *Acta Otolaryngol* 2010;130:1343–1351.

139. Schwartz MS, Otto SR, Shannon RV, et al. Auditory brainstem implants. *Neurotherapeutics* 2008;5:128–136.

140. Leake PA, Snyder RL, Hradek GT. Postnatal refinement of auditory nerve projections to the cochlear nucleus in cats. *J Comp Neurol* 2002;448:6–27.

141. Kaltenbach JA, Melica RJ, Falzarano PR. Alterations in the tonotopic map of the cochlear nucleus following cochlear damage. In: Salvi J, ed. *Auditory system plasticity and regeneration.* New York: Thieme Medical Publishers, 1996:317–332.

142. Otto SR, Shannon RV, Wilkinson EP, et al. Audiologic outcomes with the penetrating electrode auditory brainstem implant. *Otol Neurotol: official publication of the Am Otol Soc, Am Neurot Soc [and] Eur Acad Otol Neurotol* 2008;29:1147–1154.

143. Colletti V, Fiorino FG, Carner M, et al. Auditory brainstem implant as a salvage treatment after unsuccessful cochlear implantation. *Otol Neurotol: official publication of the Am Otol Soc, Am Neurotol Soc [and] Eur Acad Otol Neurotol* 2004;25:485–496; discussion 496.

144. Abe H, Rhoton AL Jr. Microsurgical anatomy of the cochlear nuclei. *Neurosurgery* 2006;58:728–739; discussion 728–739.

145. Colletti V, Fiorino FG, Carner M, et al. The retrosigmoid approach for auditory brainstem implantation. *Am J Otol* 2000;21:826–836.

146. Waring MD. Intraoperative electrophysiologic monitoring to assist placement of auditory brain stem implant. *Ann Otol Rhinol Laryngol Suppl* 1995;166:33–36.

147. Otto SR, Brackmann DE, Hitselberger WE, et al. Multichannel auditory brainstem implant: update on performance in 61 patients. *J Neurosurg* 2002;96:1063–1071.

148. Schwartz MS, Otto SR, Brackmann DE, et al. Use of a multichannel auditory brainstem implant for neurofibromatosis type 2. *Stereotact Funct Neurosurg* 2003;81:110–114.

149. Colletti V. Auditory outcomes in tumor vs. nontumor patients fitted with auditory brainstem implants. *Adv Otorhinolaryngol* 2006;64:167–185.

150. Colletti V, Shannon R, Carner M, et al. Outcomes in nontumor adults fitted with the auditory brainstem implant: 10 years' experience. *Otol Neurotol: official publication of the Am Otol Soc, Am Neurotol Soc [and] Eur Acad Otol Neurotol* 2009;30:614–618.

164 Hearing Aids and Assistive Listening Devices

Catherine V. Palmer   *Barry E. Hirsch*

POPULATION

Hearing impairment is one of the most prevalent chronic disabilities in the United States. Approximately 34.25 million Americans have hearing impairments (1). The prevalence of hearing loss nearly doubled from 1965 to 1994, and the growth is predicted to continue (2). In the aging population, hearing loss is prevalent in nearly two-thirds of those over the age of 70 in the United States (3); these estimates are even higher in those with cognitive impairment such as dementia (4). Risk factors for hearing loss trend toward poor socioeconomic status, men more than women, and whites more than any other ethnicity (5). Hearing loss is associated with increased isolation (6) and functional and cognitive decline (6,7).

Hearing loss is most common in the aging population but also affects children; nearly 8% of those with permanent hearing loss are children (8). On any given day, 43% of elementary school students have a mild hearing loss (9). Congenital hearing loss affects 1 to 6 per 1,000 newborns (10). Most children with congenital hearing loss will be affected at birth and can potentially be identified by newborn hearing screening; however, some hearing losses may not be evident until later in childhood (11). Recent evidence suggests that hearing impairment in the teenage population is on the rise (12). The consequences of hearing impairment in both children and adults are detrimental to social involvement. Poor hearing leads to communication impairments and progressive social isolation that may impact overall health (13,14). Many of the health and social consequences of hearing loss can be mitigated with a comprehensive auditory (re)habilitation program of which hearing aids will be a part.

Individuals pursue hearing aids and assistive listening devices when there is no medical/surgical treatment that will resolve their hearing loss or if they are not candidates for medical/surgical intervention. For children, they may need an amplification system before they are old enough for specific surgical interventions that will later resolve conductive hearing loss. The encouraging news for individuals with permanent hearing loss is that there are treatments for all types and degrees of hearing loss at this time. The treatments will not restore normal hearing but should assist the individuals in their daily communication activities and provide a safe environment in which to function.

Pursuing amplification is a process that continues for the life of an individual. There is the initial process of selecting, fitting, and adjusting to the hearing aids and then the ongoing process of maintenance, replacement, and upgrade of the devices over time. Therefore, the patient establishes a relationship with the individual providing their amplification as part of a larger auditory (re)habilitation process. Otolaryngologists who may be managing the medical care of patients with hearing loss also will want to have a relationship with a professional they trust to take care of their patients' amplification and auditory (re) habilitation needs. The audiologist plays this role for the patient and otolaryngologist and is educated in the area of hearing assessment and hearing aid selection and fitting. The patient is provided with complete hearing health care when in the care of both the otolaryngologist and audiologist who are coordinating their services.

GOAL OF AMPLIFICATION

The reduction in hearing sensitivity produced by hearing loss results in activity limitations and participation restrictions as defined by the World Health Organization's International Classification of Functioning, Disability, and Health (15). Solutions to these challenges will come in the form of a comprehensive auditory (re)habilitation program that will include counseling, communication training, environmental modifications, speech and language development for children, and amplification.

Amplification is only one part of a complete auditory (re) habilitation program and should be viewed in the context of a larger program.

The basic goals of a hearing aid fitting are to provide audibility for the range of sounds encountered in daily life (range of intensity levels and frequencies), to allow the listener to hear in complex (noisy) situations commonly occurring in daily communication, and to do all this while being comfortable acoustically and physically. With the advent of a variety of consumer electronics designed to couple to the ear, a newer challenge is making sure these devices couple to the hearing aid that is coupled to the ear. While maintaining comfort, the properly fit amplification system makes the world of sound accessible to the user.

BASICS OF THE AMPLIFICATION SYSTEM

A basic amplification system is depicted in Figure 164.1. Every hearing aid functions in the manner described in Figure 164.1 including an acoustic input signal to the microphone, an analog/digital (A/D) converter, an amplification stage, a digital/analog (D/A) converter, and then the electric signal being converted to an acoustic signal as it leaves the receiver (loudspeaker) and enters the ear canal. The amplification stage is contained within the digital chip and may include differential amplification at various frequencies (channels). In addition, amplification may be differentially applied to certain levels of input (e.g., soft, moderate, loud) and to certain types of inputs (noise, speech, music) based on the algorithm driving the hearing aid signal processing. These details are described later in the chapter.

HEARING AID FITTING PROTOCOLS

This chapter is meant to introduce the physician to the many options and decisions that must be made when assisting patients in the selection of the appropriate amplification system for their hearing loss, communication needs, and lifestyle. In addition, the best practice components of hearing aid verification and outcome assessment are highlighted. Since the physician may be the entry point into hearing health care, the material in this chapter should better prepare them to discuss possible amplification solutions with their patients and help prepare them for the process they will encounter in order to become a successful hearing aid user. For detailed, evidence-based guidelines for the selection, fitting, verification, and outcome assessment of amplification systems for pediatric patients, the reader is referred

to the American Academy of Audiology (AAA) Pediatric Amplification Guidelines (16). For evidence-based guidelines related to the provision of hearing aids in adults, the reader is referred to the AAA Guidelines for the Audiologic Management of Adult Hearing Impairment (17).

HEARING LOSS AND CANDIDACY

The AAA Pediatric Amplification Guidelines (16) indicate, "Amplification with hearing instruments should be considered for a child who demonstrates a significant hearing loss, including sensorineural, conductive, or mixed hearing losses of any degree." (p. 2). Children are now being fit with hearing aids by the age of 6 months due to successful early identification programs and the new guidelines that suggest children should be screened for hearing loss by 1 month, diagnosed by 3 months, and fit within 1 month of diagnosis and no later than 6 months (1–3(+1)–6 goal) (18). The AAA Guideline for the Audiologic Management of Adult Hearing Impairment (17) does not specifically outline candidacy but indicates that adult amplification recommendations will be based on the hearing evaluation and the patient's reported difficulties. If an adult is having problems hearing, then he or she is a candidate for hearing assistance. A recent study (19) found that the question "On a scale from 1 to 10, 1 being the worst and 10 being the best, how would you rate your overall hearing ability?" could sort out which individuals were ready to pursue amplification (1 to 4 rating), which individuals needed more counseling (5 to 7), and which individuals were not ready to pursue amplification (8 to 10).

EVALUATION

Physical examination of the auricle, external auditory canal, tympanic membrane, and middle ear space should be conducted. It is important to recognize conditions that warrant medical or surgical intervention or findings that would preclude tolerance of a device in or over the ear. A comprehensive audiogram that includes ear-specific pure-tone air- and bone-conduction thresholds, speech reception threshold, and word recognition testing is often the starting point of the hearing aid discussion. This level of detail will not be available for an infant, and yet our goal is to fit an infant with significant hearing loss with amplification within 1 month of diagnosis. For this purpose, ear-specific thresholds (via auditory brainstem response) in one low and one high frequency will suffice to

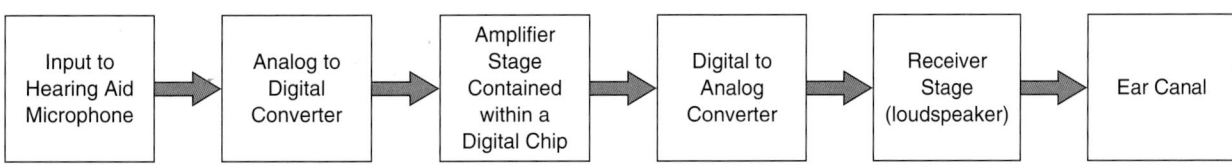

Figure 164.1 Schematic of the basic components of a hearing aid.

get the hearing aid fitting started. In the case of infants and young children, diagnostics are ongoing and the hearing aid fitting will be altered as more data related to the child's hearing loss are gathered.

With the adult patient, there are other assessments that will assist in making recommendations related to specific hearing aid configurations and technology. The quantification of frequency-specific thresholds of discomfort has been found to improve the hearing aid fitting (20). In essence, the individual's dynamic range needs to be defined in order to appropriately tune the hearing aid to produce outputs for soft, moderate, and loud sounds all within the audible but comfortable range for the individual. The lower boundary of the dynamic range is defined through threshold assessment. If thresholds of discomfort are not measured individually, then we are allowing the upper boundary of the individual's dynamic range to be defined as an average for the population. Measures of uncomfortable loudness are simple to perform and add to the precision of the hearing aid fitting. If these measures are not accomplished prior to the fitting, the clinician must be sure to verify that the individual's tolerance level has not been exceeded by use of average data through a verification procedure prior to the individual leaving the clinic.

An assessment of the individual's speech comprehension in noise also may be considered prior to recommending various amplification features. Two commonly used speech in noise tests include the Hearing in Noise Test (21) and the QuickSIN (22). A signal-to-noise ratio value is determined from these tests and can be compared to the performance of normal listeners. The QuickSIN provides ranges that relate to technology recommendations (e.g., use of directional microphones, use of assistive listening devices). In addition, the results can be very helpful in counseling the patient about realistic expectations when communicating in noise and potential environmental manipulations that may be necessary.

There is compelling evidence that if individuals want to hear in noise, they need to use two hearing aids if they have hearing loss in both ears (23). With that said, there are individuals who have binaural interference meaning that sound coming into one ear is interfering with the processing of sound from another. A dichotic test requiring hearing from both ears in order to successfully complete the test can be used to identify individuals who may be better off with one hearing aid rather than two (24). Some clinicians prefer to proceed with fitting two hearing aids allowing the individual to experience bilateral amplification and to compare that with wearing one hearing aid. This allows the hearing aid user to be part of the decision.

With these objective data in hand, the clinician will want to conduct an interview with the patient in order to assess current communication challenges, communication needs at home, in social situations, during hobbies or weekend activities, and in the workplace or school setting. In the case of a young child, the interview will be conducted with a parent or guardian. Older children should be engaged in this process. Answers to these questions may impact style, feature, and signal processing decisions as well as bring up the need for alternate solutions. For instance, if an individual is an avid bicyclist, then a style of hearing aid that can be worn comfortably with a bike helmet will be essential. In addition, the clinician may want to recommend special solutions to deal with moisture from rain and perspiration associated with this activity (see a list of special hearing aid solutions in Table 164.1). There also are systematic questionnaires available to assist in this part of the assessment including the Abbreviated Profile of Hearing Aid Benefit (25), Client Oriented Scale of Improvement (26), and the Expectations Worksheet (27). Identifying the patient's current expectations of amplification can be very helpful for creating appropriate recommendations and for motivating a conversation about realistic expectations (e.g., amplification does not return normal hearing).

PRESELECTION DECISIONS

Once the clinician is knowledgeable about the individual's hearing status, communication needs, and lifestyle, there are a variety of preselection decisions to be made. Currently, there are fewer decisions that have to be made prior to ordering the devices than in the past because many hearing aids now contain options to turn on or off various features (e.g., volume control, directionality), but some decisions continue to impact the device that will be ordered for the patient. These decisions are outlined below.

ROUTING OF THE SIGNAL

The signal from an amplification device can be delivered via air or bone conduction. In the case of a cochlear implant, the signal is electric. Cochlear implants are used by individuals with severe to profound hearing loss who do not receive benefit from traditional amplification. The needs of these patients and this technology are covered elsewhere in this text. There is evidence to encourage unilateral cochlear implant users to continue or start to use amplification on the non-implanted side (28,29). For the majority of patients with sensorineural hearing loss, an air conduction system will be recommended. Depending on the configuration of the hearing loss, various amplification arrangements may be pursued. The individual with bilateral hearing loss generally will benefit from amplification in both ears.

The individual with severe unilateral hearing loss (single-sided deafness or unaidable hearing on one side due to extremely poor clarity) may consider several recommendations that would include (a) continuing to rely on the good ear without amplification (this poses problems whenever the individual is trying to listen to someone on his/her "bad" side), (b) using a CROS (contralateral routing of signal) system where a microphone is placed on the "bad" ear and

TABLE 164.1	SPECIAL SOLUTIONS FOR HEARING AIDS							
Solution	Removing Battery	Removing Hearing Aid	Moisture	Retention and Loss	Manipulating Volume Control	Battery Ingestion	Fit Issues	Cerumen Damage
Magnet	X							
Pull string		X						
Removal notch		X						
Sweat-bands			X					
Super seals			X					
Ear gear			X	X				
Huggie aids				X				
Oto or critter clips				X				
Dri aid			X					
Dri and store			X					
Raised volume control					X			
Remote control					X			
Locking battery door						X		
Soft adhesive								X
Wax guards								X
Comply wraps							X	

Web Site addresses for products:
Ear gear www.gearforears.com
Sweat band http://www.hearingaidsweatband.com/
Superseals http://www.justbekuz.com/Super_Seals_Hearing_Aid_Covers_Moisture_Prote ction.htm
Dri aid http://hal-hen.com/cgi-bin/info.cgi?id=2579
Dry and store http://www.justbekuz.com/hearing_aid_moisture_dryers_dehumidifiers_Dry_&_Store_Moisture_Guard.htm
Huggie aids http://www.westone.com/catalog/huggie-aids
Critter clips http://hsdcstore.com/browseproducts/Critter-Clips.html
Comply http://earplugstore.stores.yahoo.net/complysnaptips.html
Ad-hear (soft adhesive) http://www.westone.com/catalog/ad-hear-plus-cerumen-guards

the signal is transferred (FM transmission) to a device that delivers the sound to the good ear, (c) a bone conduction hearing aid or device on the "bad" side that picks up sound from that side and delivers it to the "good" cochlea via bone transmission, and (d) a transcranial CROS that works in the same manner as the bone conduction aid but provides such an intense air conduction signal in the "bad" ear that the sound crosses over to the "good" cochlea via bone conduction. If the individual has some hearing loss in the "good" ear as well, a bilateral CROS (BICROS) system that not only provides a transfer of the signal from the "bad" ear but also provides amplification to the "good" ear can be used.

In the case of the bone conduction solution, this can be achieved through a bone vibrator coupled to the head on a tight band or through a bone vibrator attached to the skull with a titanium screw. There are two devices on the market currently used for this surgical solution. Both function in a similar manner. An implanted bone conduction hearing device is a type of hearing aid that transmits sound to the inner ear via bone conduction. It is appropriate to use in cases of conductive hearing loss, mixed hearing loss, or single-sided deafness. It also may be used for patients with hearing loss who cannot wear an air conduction hearing

aid due to malformations or pathologies of the outer and/or middle ear. After the patient has been identified as a candidate based on the audiologic and medical examinations, a titanium screw is surgically implanted into the mastoid region of the temporal bone. The external portion of the screw, typically referred to as the abutment, is used to anchor the bone conduction unit to the head. The titanium fixture must become osseointegrated before the bone conduction unit can be affixed. The processor converts incoming sound to vibrations that stimulate the cochlea. Another option more recently available provides an abutment free option by using an implanted magnet to affix the external sound processor to the titanium implant. This is covered in greater detail in Chapter 163.

Another device based on bone conduction transmission is attached to maxillary teeth through a dental appliance that is removable. Sound is picked up by a microphone processor, and the signal is wirelessly delivered to the oral appliance. This device also is indicated for conductive or mixed hearing loss and single-sided deafness.

The individual with conductive hearing loss who does not wish to or cannot have medical/surgical intervention may pursue amplification. An air conduction hearing aid can be used for mild-to-moderate conductive losses that are not accompanied by malformation of the outer ear or drainage. For conductive losses that are accompanied by malformations of the pinna and ear canal or that produce ongoing drainage, a bone conduction amplifier will be a better choice. In the case of pediatric patients, they may have a time period when they are waiting for their system to mature enough for surgical intervention (reconstruction) and will need to use a bone conduction hearing aid in order to keep the cochlea stimulated during this waiting period. As described above for solutions to single-sided deafness, a bone vibrator on a tight headband or an implanted bone vibrator can be used for this purpose. Currently, the FDA does not allow implantable bone vibrators for children under 5 years of age.

STYLE

For patients receiving air conduction amplification, the discussion of the style of the hearing aid will be driven by the patient's hearing loss, communication needs, lifestyle, and personal preferences. The discussion will start with defining whether the individual is interested in an extended wear option or a traditional wear option. Currently, there is one extended wear product commercially available, the Lyric hearing aid (Fig. 164.2). This hearing aid is a single-channel, analog device that is disposable. Because of this level of technology, the battery life for this hearing aid is drastically increased. The Lyric is placed deep within the ear canal by the clinician after setting the programming based on coupler measurements (a probe microphone cannot fit in the ear canal when the device is inserted). The user has a magnet that allows them some control over the volume of the device. The Lyric provides 24/7 hearing with the user being able to shower

and carry on most daily activities with the device in place. When the device stops working (this could range from a few weeks to 3 months depending on moisture, cerumen, etc.), the user has a tool that allows removal. The patient subsequently returns to the clinic or office for placement of a new device. To be a successful extended wear user, the individual needs to have reasonably cylindrical, straight ear canals. The manufacturer provides a systematic way to determine candidacy, sizing, and placement. The pricing structure of this device currently is quite different from traditional wear hearing aids and includes paying a yearly subscription fee.

Recently, several manufacturers have introduced a deep insertion traditional wear hearing aid. This provides the benefit of the sound source being right near the tympanic membrane, which provides a wider, audible high-frequency bandwidth. However, this hearing aid is removed each night and batteries are replaced when they stop functioning (as opposed to the hearing aid being disposable). A picture of the new "invisible in canal (IIC)" hearing aid is provided in Figure 164.3.

Individuals interested in traditional wear hearing aids have several styles and coupling options (connecting the hearing aid to the ear) to consider. Figure 164.4 provides pictures of the various styles of hearing aids currently available along with a list of pros and cons. Figure 164.5 provides the same type of information but focused on the pediatric patient whose outer ear will be growing over the first years of life. For pediatric patients, the behind-the-ear style is recommended because this style reduces the cost of refitting (only the earmold that couples the hearing aid to the ear needs to be replaced when the outer ear grows), provides the greatest amount of flexibility in terms of power (in case the hearing changes), offers a variety of features (ability to connect to assistive listening devices, etc.), and requires the least amount of maintenance. The final decision on style will be a balance of the clinician's recommendation and the patient's preferences.

Some of the most important changes in style recently have included the extended wear option, deep insertion

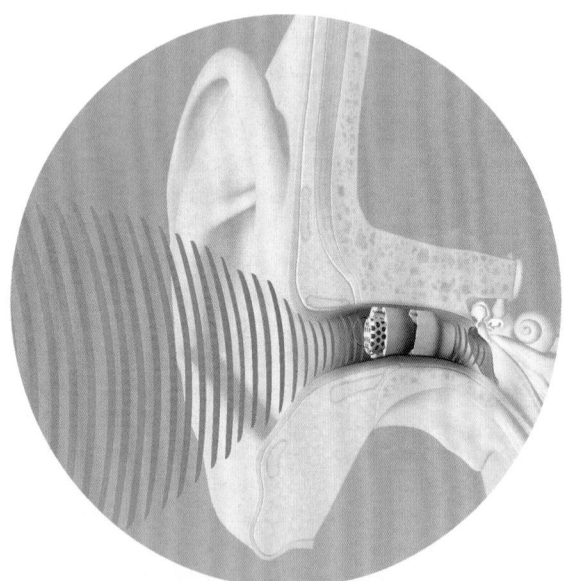

Figure 164.2 Schematic of an extended wear hearing aid. Drawing courtesy of InSound Medical Group.

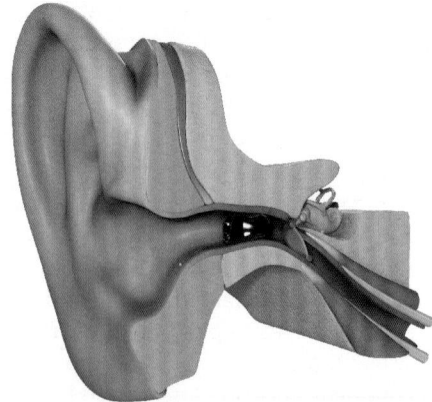

Figure 164.3 Schematic of a deep insertion completely-in-the-canal hearing aid. Drawing courtesy of Starkey Laboratories, Inc.

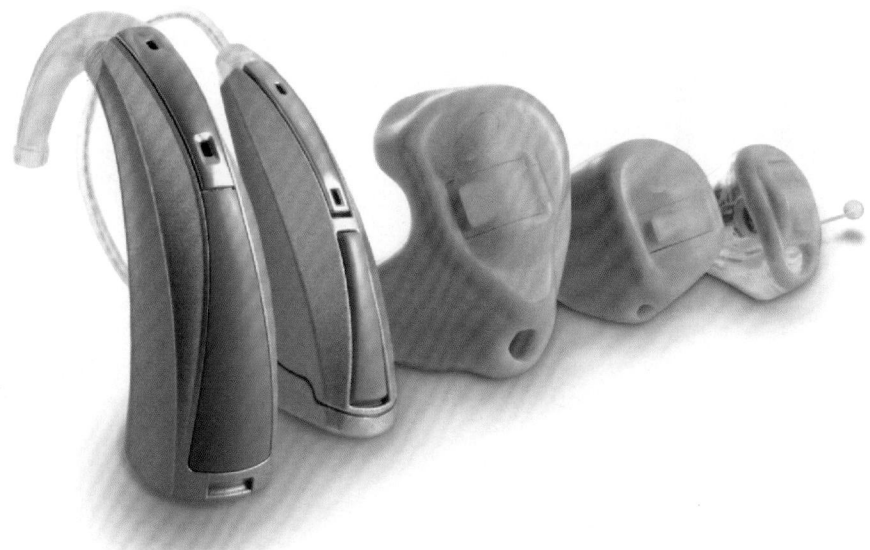

Figure 164.4 Hearing aid style chart.

	Behind-the-Ear (Standard and Mini)	In-the-Ear	In-the-Canal	Completely in-the-Canal
Fitting range	Full range	Mild-to-moderate (with some feedback control options, can fit more severe losses)	Mild-to-moderate	Mild-to-moderate
Number of features[a]	Very flexible	Depends on ear canal size	Depends on ear canal size	Few options
Advanced signal processing	Available	Available	Available	Available
Manipulation	Easy	Easy	Can be difficult	Difficult
Care	Minimal	Cerumen	Cerumen	Cerumen
Cosmetics	Depends on hair style (slim tube has made this more attractive to individuals)	Visible	Visible	Least visible
Telephone use	Good	Good	Poor	Good
Coupling to ALDs	Good	Fair	Poor	None

[a]Features refer to physical features such as volume control, program button, and multiple microphones. ALDs, assistive listening devices.

Style	High Output/ Gain	Venting Options	Cerumen Issues	Replacement Related to Growth	Coupling to the Telephone	Coupling to ALDs	Directional Microphones
Traditional BTE	+	+	+	+	+	+	+
Mini BTE	~	+	+[a]	+	+	−	~[b]
ITE	~	~	−	−	+	~	+
ITC	−	−	−	−	−	−	−
CIC	−	−	−	−	+	−	−

Key:
+ this style performs well for the feature listed
− another style may be a better choice if this feature is important
~ this style is adequate for the feature listed

[a]Receiver in the ear (RITE) in this style may increase cerumen issues
[b]If the mini BTE is coupled to the ear with an open fitting, directional benefit may be compromised

Figure 164.5 Hearing aid style chart with specific pediatric considerations.

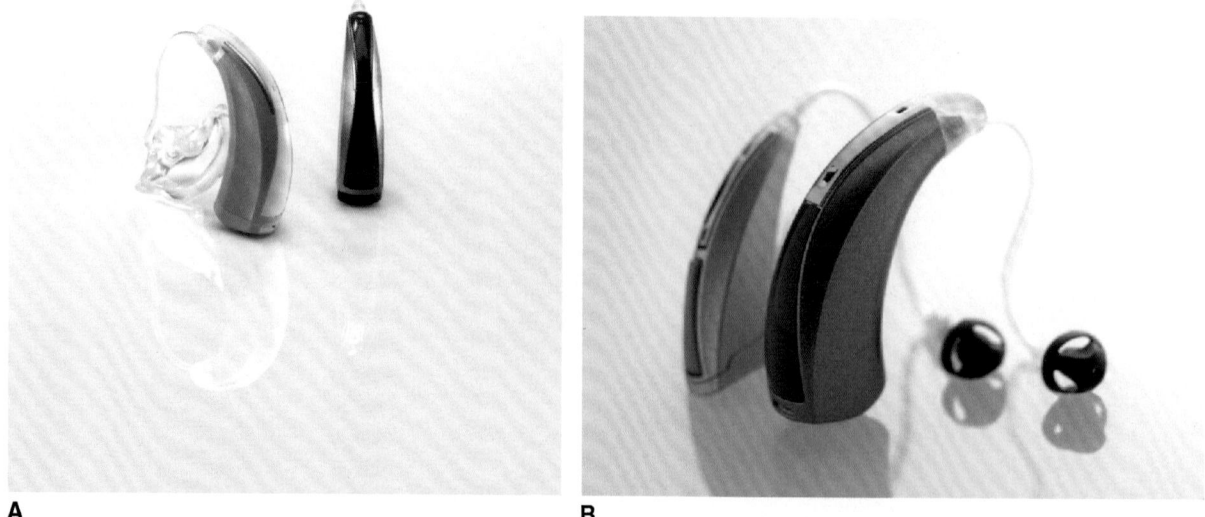

A   **B**

Figure 164.6 Behind-the-ear hearing aids coupled to a traditional earmold **(panel A)** and an open fit dome **(panel B)**. Picture courtesy of Starkey Laboratories, Inc.

completely in the canal (CIC), and ability to provide more gain in a CIC with advances in feedback management, which has allowed more users to pursue this style without operating at the limits of amplification. In addition, the behind-the-ear (BTE) hearing aid has become a popular option with adults due to miniaturization (see a mini BTE in Fig. 164.4) and the use of slim tube rather than standard tubing to couple the aid to the ear canal. In addition, with the advent of improved feedback management systems, open fit BTEs (Fig. 164.6, panel B) that leave the ear canal much more open than traditional earmolds (Fig. 164.6, panel A) have improved comfort and fit for many individuals. There has been some confusion in terminology with clinicians referring to any BTE with a slim tube as an "open fitting." The slim tube can be connected to a dome allowing for an open fit, but it also can be connected to a standard earmold producing a closed fit for individuals who have more significant hearing loss. Figure 164.7 provides the various coupling arrangements that currently are available for BTE fittings. With the goal of slimming down the BTE but maintaining a reasonable battery life (1 to 2 weeks), manufacturers have introduced the receiver in the canal (RIC) BTE. The RIC is compared to a receiver in the aid (RITA) in Figure 164.8 (RIC on the left and RITA on the right). An electrical connection from the BTE to the receiver housed inside the dome (or earmold) can be seen. By moving the receiver into the ear canal, the BTE case can be smaller while also holding a larger battery. The consequence, however, is cerumen damage to the RIC, whereas when the receiver is cased in the BTE, it is removed from potential cerumen damage. Because of this and the desire to make the CICs have a deeper insertion yet remain more dependable, cerumen guards (Fig. 164.9) are a standard on all hearing aids with receivers in the canal.

EARMOLDS

For any of the BTE styles, the hearing aid must be coupled to the ear. The clinician will make a variety of decisions related to coupling in terms of tubing size, open or closed fitting, venting within traditional earmolds, and earmold material (soft, hard, combination). These decisions will be based on the degree and configuration of hearing loss, the consistency of the individual's pinna and ear canal, and the style of hearing aid the individual would like to pursue. Venting provides an air path through the earmold to the ear canal. Venting can provide ear canal aeration and comfort with the flow of air in and out of the ear. In addition, the occlusion effect (the perception that one's own voice is loud and boomy) will be reduced with a large vent. The occlusion effect also can be reduced with a long canal portion of the earmold that reaches close to the bony portion of the ear canal. Vents are acoustic filters and will pass low frequencies both into the ear and out of the ear. Individuals with normal hearing in the low frequencies will be able to hear these frequencies naturally if a vent is provided.

For the pediatric patient, it will be most common to use a soft material that tends to reduce feedback and provides a comfortable fit. Earmolds will need to be remade every 2 months for an infant and then about every 4 months for a toddler. The young child will continue to need new earmolds every 4 to 6 months. Once the earmold is not fitting well, there is a greater chance of feedback. Feedback (whistling) is caused when amplified sound can leak out of the ear canal and reach the microphone to be re-amplified. One way to reduce this is to turn the volume down on the hearing aid. This, of course, is counter to the goal of amplification. In addition, most pediatric fittings do not activate the volume control because the clinician does not

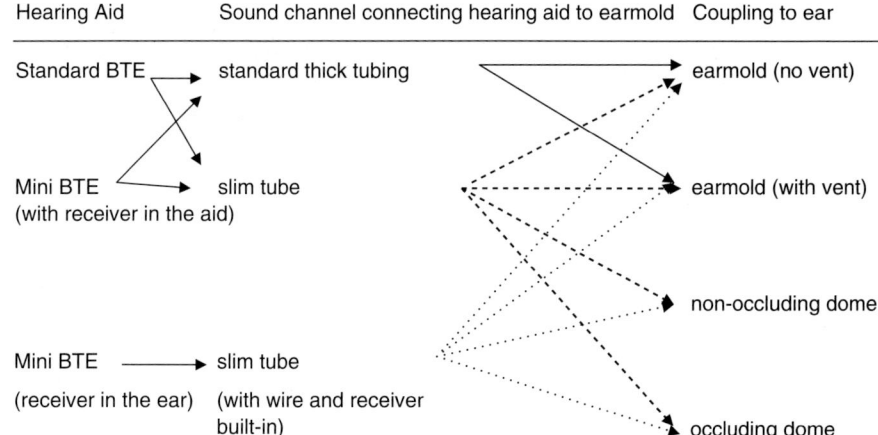

Figure 164.7 Chart of combinations of BTEs, tubing, and coupling to the ear.

want the child turning down (or off) the hearing aid. With the advent of improved feedback management strategies, some feedback will be reduced, but a poor fitting earmold cannot be compensated for by feedback management. The child should be seen proactively to replace earmolds prior to feedback problems.

TELEPHONE ACCESS

Individuals across the life span need access to telephone communication. No one should be provided with an amplification system that does not include a telephone solution. The clinician is now faced with creating solutions for landline phones, cell phones, and hands-free options. The challenge with telephones is that even with an excellent fitting earmold and the use of advanced feedback management, when a hearing aid user holds a telephone (or anything else) close to a hearing aid microphone, the hearing aid will most likely produce feedback. Landline phones emit an electromagnetic signal that can be picked up by a hearing aid telecoil circuit. When the hearing aid (BTE or ITE) is switched to the telecoil circuit, the microphone

is turned off, thereby eliminating the chance for feedback. Some hearing aids include automatic telecoils that are triggered by the magnet in the telephone when the telephone comes into proximity of the hearing aid. There is quite a bit of variability among telephones in terms of strength of electromagnetic leak and magnet. The key to successful use with a telecoil is instructing the BTE hearing aid user to hold the telephone above their ear near their hearing aid. This is strange for the individual in the beginning because they are used to holding the phone to their ear canal. The hearing aid user may need to try several phones before they find one that works well with their hearing aid. Individuals with open fit BTEs who by definition will have good low-frequency hearing may find that they can continue to use the phone successfully by holding it to their open ear canal. If this is not sufficient, they may need to simply raise the volume on the telephone slightly. Most patients including many children now use cell phones. Normally hearing individuals use cell phones by holding them to their ears or through a Bluetooth wireless connection. Depending on the style of the hearing aid, the hearing aid user also will have these options in slightly modified forms. A chart of

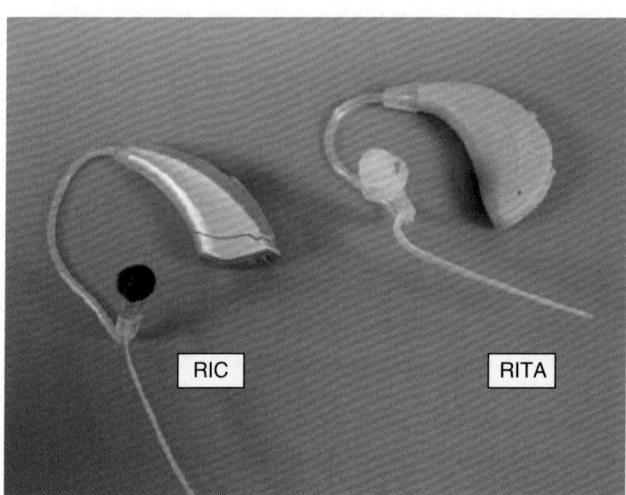

Figure 164.8 Receiver in the ear (RIC, **panel A**) and receiver in the aid (RITA, **panel B**).

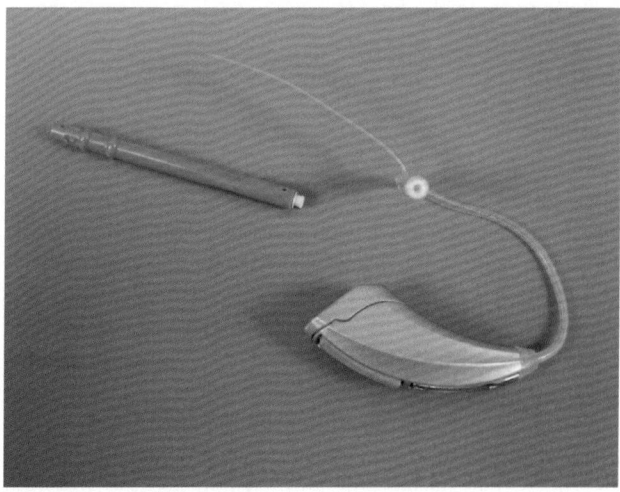

Figure 164.9 Examples of cerumen guards and their applicators.

TABLE 164.2	TELEPHONE SOLUTIONS		
Style	Landline Phone	Cell Phone[a]	Bluetooth Hands Free
Standard BTE with occluding earmold	Telecoil Speaker Phone	Hold slightly tilted from microphone to reduce feedback	Intermediary device to receive Bluetooth and transmit to hearing aid
Standard BTE with open fit	Hold normally	Hold normally	Intermediary device to receive Bluetooth and transmit to hearing aid
Mini BTE with open fit	Hold normally	Hold normally	Bluetooth receiver may fit in open ear canal
Mini BTE with occluding earmold	Hold slightly tilted from microphone to reduce feedback	Hold slightly tilted from microphone to reduce feedback	No solution
ITE	Telecoil Speaker phone	Hold slightly tilted from microphone to reduce feedback	Intermediary device to receive Bluetooth and transmit to hearing aid
ITC	Speaker phone	Speaker phone	No solution
CIC	Hold normally	Hold normally	No solution
Deep insertion	Hold normally	Hold normally	Bluetooth receiver may fit in ear canal

[a]By law, some cell phones do have an induction signal. If this is the case, then the users can use their telecoil.

possible solutions for each style of hearing aid is provided in Table 164.2.

ABILITY TO COUPLE TO OTHER SOUND SOURCES

Individuals who are pursuing hearing aids may already couple other listening devices to their ears. These might include Bluetooth phone receivers (discussed above), MP3 earphones, dictation earphones, stethoscopes, and in-ear monitors (anesthesiologists, newscasters, etc.). The variety of possible solutions are too varied to discuss in the context of this chapter, but the individual responsible for selecting the hearing aid style, earmold coupling, and technology will want to know about these devices in order to include them in the final hearing aid selection decision.

ABILITY TO COUPLE TO ASSISTIVE LISTENING DEVICES

Assistive listening devices are designed to overcome problems of noise and distance for the hearing aid user (23). The basic assistive device provides an offsite microphone (separate from the hearing aid) that is placed as close to the sound source of the signal of interest as possible. The transmitter attached to the microphone then sends this signal via a transmission technology (FM, infrared, electromagnetic) to be picked up by a receiver that will then direct the sound to the hearing aid or directly by the hearing aid with a built in receiver. Figure 164.10 provides the various iterations that are possible with current assistive listening systems. For the adult population, assistive listening devices

are often pursued if they have specific listening situations that are identified during the hearing aid selection process that cannot be solved by hearing aids or after the selection process if the individual finds they are still not communicating as well as they would like in challenging situations. The goal of the clinician is to predict the need for assistive technology, so the selected hearing aids will be compatible with receiving the transmission signal. There also are intermediary devices available that receive the signal and pass it on to the hearing aids. Not all brands or styles of hearing aids are able to couple with assistive listening devices. With the advent of Bluetooth technology, many hearing aid users would like their hearing aid to pick up a Bluetooth signal. This certainly would create a variety of universal solutions for phone, computer, and television listening. Unfortunately, at the current time Bluetooth transmission and reception creates a great deal of battery drain that cannot be supported in current hearing aids. Therefore, a Bluetooth signal must be received by an intermediary device (usually worn around the neck), and then an induction signal is passed on and received by the hearing aids.

REMOTE CONTROL

Some patients would like to have quite a bit of control over the hearing aids, and some patients want to put the hearing aids in and forget about them. This is an issue that is best defined during the preselection process. Some of the styles of hearing aids (BTE, ITE) will come with controls that are accessible on the case (i.e., program button, volume control) if the clinician orders them. Smaller hearing aids (e.g., CIC) will have very little room for controls. In these

Offsite Microphone Near Sound Source[a]	Transmission	Intermediate Receiver Worn on Body	Transmission	Hearing Aid
Microphone	FM	FM receiver	Induction loop	HA with telecoil
			DAI	HA with DAI jack or boot
Microphone	FM	→	→	HA with built in or plug in FM receiver
Microphone	Infrared	Infrared receiver	Induction loop	HA with telecoil
			DAI	HA with DAI jack or boot
Microphone	Induction area loop	→	→	HA with telecoil
Microphone	Bluetooth	Bluetooth receiver	Induction-type signal	HA

[a]Microphone near sound source or device directly plugged into sound source (e.g., television sound jack, MP3 sound jack).

Figure 164.10 Chart of assistive listening device transmissions and coupling choices.

cases, the individual may like to have a remote control. The remote control may control volume and program selection. At least one manufacturer now has an "app" for volume and program control that can be accessed through a cell phone.

BATTERIES

All hearing aids continue to need batteries in order to operate. Hearing aid battery sizes include 675, 13, 312, and 10 batteries with 10 being the smallest (generally for CICs and mini BTEs). Patients will experience a range of battery life from 3 to 5 days up to 2 weeks depending on the style of hearing aid, size of battery, and number of hours the hearing aids are used.

HEARING AID FITTING

Achieving Audibility

The challenge of fitting amplification is fitting the range of sound one encounters in day-to-day life into the reduced dynamic range of the individual with hearing loss. Figure 164.11 shows an audiogram of an individual with moderate to profound sensorineural hearing loss. The X's and O's indicate the pure-tone threshold levels at which the individual can hear sound 50% of the time. Therefore, the individual cannot hear sound below that level. In this example, we will say that the individual

will become uncomfortable when sound is presented at around 105-dB HL. So, at 1,000 Hz, an individual with normal hearing would have a dynamic range of 105 dB (0- to 105-dB HL). The individual whose hearing loss is shown in Figure 164.11 has a dynamic range of 40 dB in the right ear at 1,000 Hz (threshold of 65 and discomfort level of 105). In order to return audibility for soft, moderate, and loud sounds while maintaining comfort, the hearing aid employs expansion and compression signal processing. Compression allows gain to be differentially applied according to input level with more gain applied to soft sounds and less gain applied to loud sounds (30). For soft input levels, enough gain to achieve audibility (to produce an output greater than threshold) is applied; there will be less gain applied to a moderate sound and even less to the louder sounds. This allows for audibility across the wide range of input levels to be compressed into a much smaller range of output levels. Expansion is used to reduce circuit noise (microphone noise) and to make very low-level sounds less annoying. In essence, it is the opposite of compression and applies very little gain to extremely quiet inputs (inputs below the compression threshold) and then increases gain as the soft inputs increase. Compression and expansion signal processing are described by the threshold at which they activate (input level), the ratio of compression or expansion (e.g., a typical compression ratio for hearing aids set for a mild-to-moderate sensorineural hearing loss will be 2:1 to 3:1), and attack and release time. There is consensus regarding the need for fast attack times. The research has been less clear related to release times. The most recent study (31) indicated that there is little difference between slow and fast release times, and both may have uses for different signals. At this point, attack and release times are set by the manufacturer and are not controlled by the hearing aid fitter. Compression threshold can be manipulated in the hearing aid fitting, and compression ratio is altered whenever gain is increased differentially for soft versus loud sounds.

As can be seen in Figure 164.11, many hearing losses change across frequencies with more hearing loss in some frequency regions as opposed to other frequency regions. In order to account for these changes and the resulting need to differentially program the hearing aid gain to produce audible signals across input levels, channels are used in hearing aids. A channel is a filtered frequency area that has its own amplifier and therefore can have specific compression characteristics (threshold and ratio). In Figure 164.11, the low-frequency channel would have different compression characteristics than the mid- or high-frequency channel. In order to obtain optimum speech intelligibility, 2 to 4 channels are necessary (30). Many current hearing aids have 10 to 20 channels

available. The larger number of channels is related to their use in feedback management, which is discussed later in the chapter.

The bandwidth of a hearing aid, which is operationally defined by the lowest and highest frequency where audible output for the hearing aid user can be achieved, also contributes to audibility. Most commercially available hearing aids have output up to 4,000 to 5,000 Hz. The limits of the high-frequency bandwidth are dictated by the digital sampling used by the hearing aids. If the hearing aid is sampling at a rate of 10,000 Hz, then the bandwidth will be 5,000 Hz (half the sampling rate). Higher sampling rates would result in a wider bandwidth but also result in increased battery drain that would be unacceptable to the user. For children learning speech and language, a 5,000-Hz bandwidth is not adequate (32). A bandwidth out to 8,000 to 9,000 Hz is necessary for the correct perception of the sound /s/ for young children (33–35). Adults who can rely on context are able to fill in missing sounds and information from the amplified signal, but this requires more effort than if the signal was completely audible. The major manufacturers are all working on increasing the bandwidth of their hearing aids including the low-frequency limits that contribute to enjoyment of music.

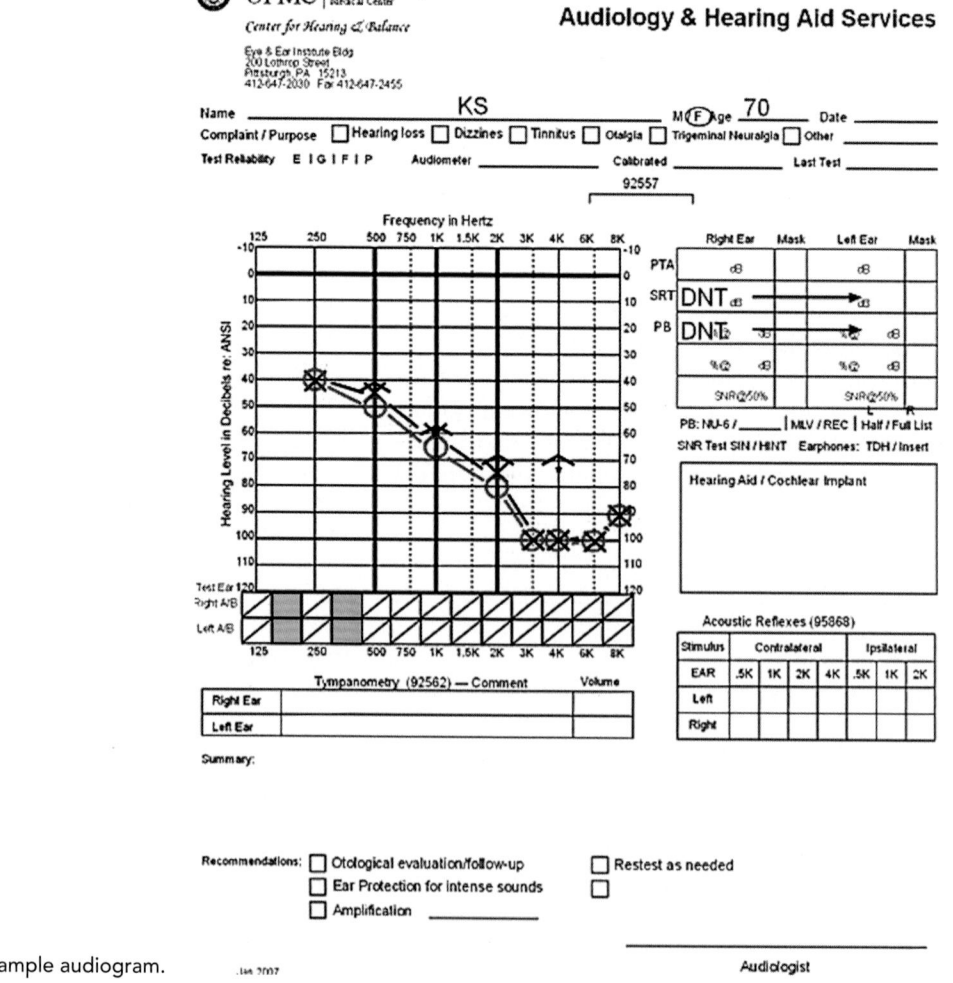

Figure 164.11 Example audiogram.

Recently, frequency lowering has been reintroduced into the hearing aid market in order to resolve audibility issues for individuals who cannot access high-frequency audibility because of the severity of their high-frequency hearing loss (severe to profound degree of loss in the high frequencies with mild-to-moderate hearing loss in the low to mid frequencies). Frequency lowering comes in three forms currently: nonlinear frequency compression, linear frequency transposition, and spectral feature identification. In nonlinear frequency compression, a cut off frequency is chosen based on the hearing loss, and the frequencies above that point are compressed into an audible range for the listener. In linear frequency transposition, the frequencies above the cut off are literally shifted down on top of other frequencies. In spectral feature identification, identifies high-frequency features in the signal and replicates those features at a lower frequency. In each case, the signal is a distortion of the original but also provides audibility to sounds that would not be audible. Success in using this signal processing has been reported with children, but the utility with adults who have not heard this type of sound previously is less clear (36–38). In either case, auditory training would be a reasonable recommendation as individuals learn to use these new sounds.

The hearing aid/cochlear implant hybrid currently under investigation also is aimed at the type of hearing loss that has no more than moderate severity in the low frequencies with profound hearing loss in the high frequencies. Once again, the new signal that combines electric and acoustic hearing will most likely require some level of auditory training to become accustomed to the signal.

Feedback management strategies also can be grouped under technologies that potentially increase audibility. The general goal of a feedback management system is to provide more usable gain prior to feedback. Manufacturers employ different strategies for feedback management, and the success of these strategies varies. Commonly, the hearing aid identifies feedback through the ongoing analysis of the incoming signal by identifying a pure-tone signal that is not commonly heard in day-to-day communication. Once this signal is identified, the gain in the specific channel that corresponds to the frequency can be temporarily reduced. Some strategies provide a matching signal that is 180 degrees out of phase in order to cancel the sound (39). Feedback management is a problem if the individual actually is trying to listen to pure tones (e.g., in some musical compositions or if the individual is a musician), and therefore many hearing aids come with a "music" program that disables the feedback and noise reduction features so music will remain intact.

HEARING IN NOISE

The majority of commercially available hearing aids are connected to a computer for programming. This includes adjusting the gain for different frequency channels as a function of input level, selecting feedback management, and frequency shifting as described above. In addition, most levels of technology come with features meant to impact the listeners experience in noise since hearing in noise is one of the most common challenges for individuals with hearing loss. The first recommendation that should be made to the hearing aid user is to wear the amplification full-time and to wear two hearing aids (23). Both of these solutions will assist the hearing aid user in hearing in noise. Individuals who try to use amplification part time often complain that sounds seem too loud and that all they hear is noise and not the signal of interest. In these cases, the brain continues to try to adjust to the new amplification without receiving a consistent, full-time signal.

The majority of hearing aids use digital signal processing. It is this processing that has allowed for more and more complex algorithms that evaluate and process the incoming signal. The clinician responsible for verifying the hearing aid fitting also will be the person setting these various parameters.

DIRECTIONAL MICROPHONES

One of the most important technology developments for tackling the problem of hearing in noise was the use of directional microphones on hearing aids (40,41). This technology continues to develop, and currently most hearing aids have a "smart" program that changes the microphone setting depending on the sound that is being sampled by the hearing aid. Because of the digital nature of the signal processing system, sound coming into the microphone can be sampled in real time. The signal processing algorithm analyzes the amplitude envelope of the incoming signal. If it determines that the amplitude envelope is steady state (little variation), it classifies the signal as primarily noise. If it identifies the amplitude envelope as varying, it identifies the signal as speech. When speech is the primary signal, the omnidirectional setting will be engaged. When noise is the primary signal, the directional microphone will be engaged. Within the directional microphone setting, various polar patterns of directionality can be implemented. Figure 164.12 provides a sample of polar plots that might be associated with a hearing aid. These polar plots will not look as organized when the hearing aid is actually in a person's ear since head and body baffle effects are present. In essence, a directional microphone is less sensitive to certain areas around the listener. In Figure 164.12, panel C, a cardioid polar plot is depicted. The individual will have less sensitivity to sound in the back and more sensitivity in the front. Successful use of directional microphones continues to demand environmental manipulation from the patient. The patient must position themselves so the signal of interest is in front and so the majority of unwanted noise is in back. Further, if the individual is trying to communicate in a highly reverberant room, the directional microphones will be of little assistance because noise will

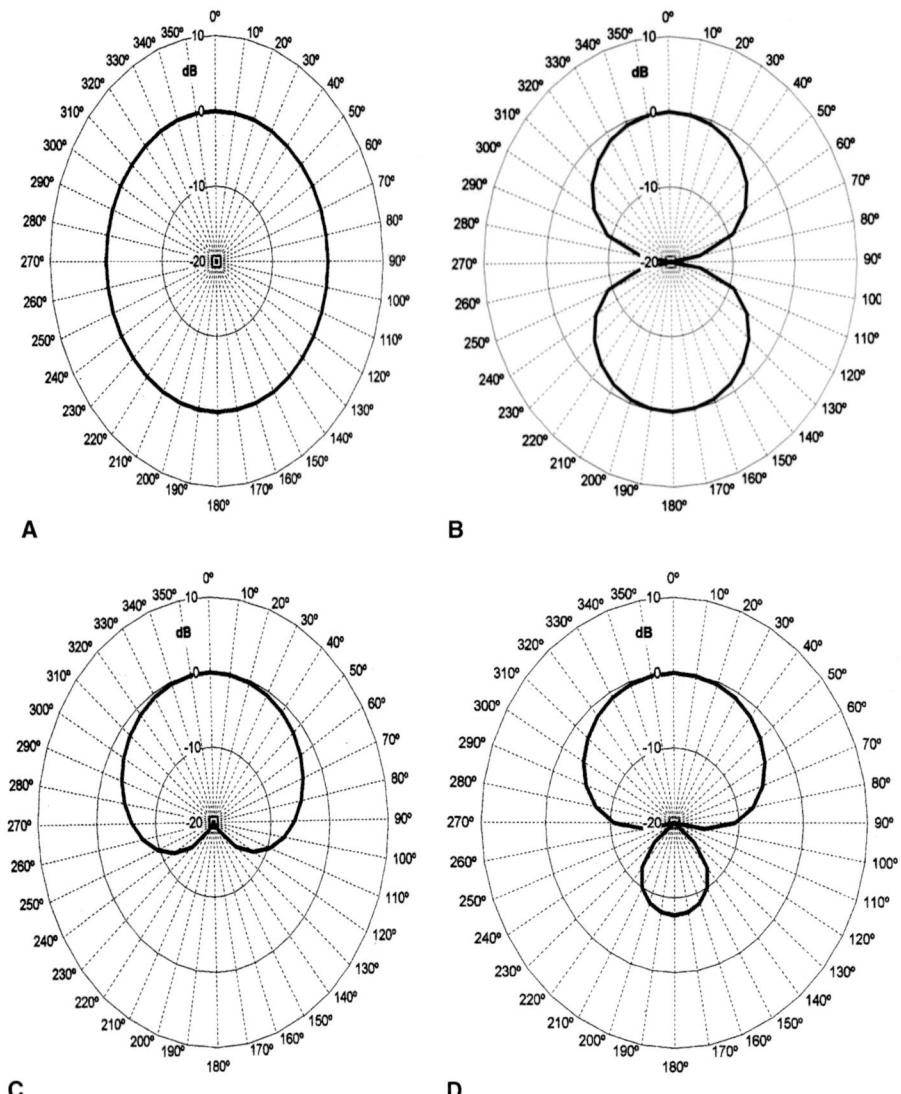

Figure 164.12 Polar patterns for **(A)** omnidirectional, **(B)** bidirectional, **(C)** cardioid, and **(D)** hyper-cardioid microphones.

be surrounding the individual as it bounces off hard surfaces. This is why investigators have found that directional microphones are considered useful in about 25% of communication situations for adults (42). The hearing aid user has to understand that the hearing aids do not know the intent of the listeners (i.e., what sound source the listener is trying to listen to) so the listeners must orient themselves to that signal.

Traditionally, directional microphones were not recommended for young children based on the philosophy that we do not want to reduce the input to the hearing aid since quite a bit of childhood learning comes through incidental listening. Two laboratories (43,44) have focused on the use of directional microphones in young children recently coming to opposite conclusions. The Australian Laboratory (44) currently recommends using directional microphones (and noise reduction signal processing) in all hearing aids regardless of age, and the US Laboratory (43) currently

does not recommend the use of directional microphones with children until they are old enough to understand and manipulate the settings (~12 years old).

DIGITAL NOISE REDUCTION

Digital noise reduction functions in the same manner as directional microphones in terms of when it is activated. If the hearing aid identifies the incoming signal as steady state, it assumes that the primary signal is noise and that the signal should be reduced. Digital noise reduction may be employed as a function of frequency channels, thereby reducing gain in some frequency regions more or less than others. The reality of the signal processing is that gain is reduced and therefore the noise and any speech are decreased in intensity. Therefore, it is not surprising that studies have not shown an increase in intelligibility when digital noise reduction is employed (45). Investigations have shown an increase in comfort and a decrease in listening effort with the use of digital noise reduction (45–48).

OTHER SETTINGS THAT CUSTOMIZE THE HEARING AID FITTING

Current technology offers a myriad of features that may be selected or deselected depending on the fitter's and patient's preference. The clinician will want to be aware of the various default settings of manufacturers, so they do not inadvertently send the new user out with signal processing or features that they did not intend to use. Many of the more advanced technology now have the option for the two hearing aids to communicate. This can be a convenience in that the hearing aid user can adjust one volume control and both hearing aids will receive the change in setting. A more sophisticated use of this same technology is to ensure that if one hearing aid switches into the directional setting, the other hearing aid will do the same. For a previous user who is not use to this, it is worth taking a few minutes to explain what is happening.

Hearing aids now are equipped with data logging that allows the clinician to see how the hearing aids have been used. Tracking data are available to determine the number of hours per day of use, whether the hearing aids are worn in situations classified as quiet or noisy by the hearing aid, and number of times the volume was manipulated or listening programs where changed. The clinician may want to describe this feature to new users, so they are not surprised when the clinician can comment on how many hours per day they have been using the devices. The newest iteration of data logging is data learning or training. When this feature is activated, the hearing aid actually changes gain and compression settings based on the user's manipulation of the volume control over time. Studies have shown that the changes the user makes will be dependent on the original settings of the hearing aid (49,50), which simply lends support to carefully setting the instruments for audibility on the day of the fitting. There is some disagreement as to whether this feature should be turned on at the time of fitting or whether new users should have an adjustment period before this "fine-tuning" feature is activated.

Hearing aids come with a variety of alerting signals to allow the user to know when a program has been changed, when the volume has been changed, and when the battery is about to die. These signals can be in the form of beeps, or they can be set so a voice indicates the change (e.g., "battery low"). It may be a surprise to the hearing aid user to hear a voice in their ear, so it is best to test these signals while the patient is in the clinic so they will know what to expect.

PRESETTING AND VERIFICATION

The output and gain of hearing aids can be measured in a coupler or in the ear of the individual. The coupler provides a standard from which various aspects of the hearing

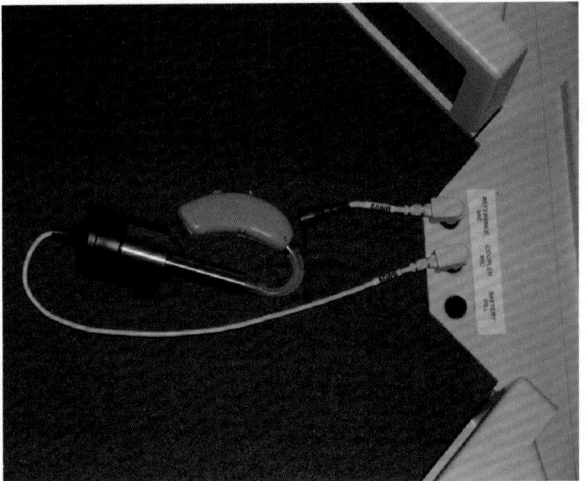

Figure 164.13 Behind-the-ear hearing aid connected to a coupler and ready to be evaluated in a test box.

aid response can be described. Figure 164.13 provides a picture of a BTE hearing aid attached to a coupler. When the test box is closed it creates a small anechoic chamber. A sound source is played from the speakers, the hearing aid microphone picks up the sound, and the output or gain of the hearing aid attached to the coupler is measured by a microphone attached to the other side of the coupler. The coupler mimics the ear canal of an average male. Figure 164.14 provides an illustration of output for a moderate input signal and maximum output measured in a coupler. A record of the hearing aid gain after the hearing aid has been programmed for the individual may be kept, so if there are any problems with the hearing aid, the response can be checked quickly and accurately. Coupler measures also can produce information about distortion in the hearing aid, circuit noise, and battery drain. For the purpose of verifying a hearing aid fitting and programming the output across frequencies and intensity levels, real ear probe microphone measures are used. In all cases of verification, the goal is to measure the output of the hearing aid that will be achieved at the individual's tympanic membrane and to compare it to evidence-based targets of the desired output.

Both the Pediatric Amplification Guidelines (16) and the Adult Amplification Guidelines (17) provide recommendations for verifying that soft, moderate, and loud signals are audible. The verification technique consists of placing a microphone in the ear canal with the hearing aid inserted. Soft, moderate, and loud speech or speech-like signals are played through a loudspeaker, and the resulting output in the ear canal is measured and displayed against the individual's frequency-specific thresholds displayed in sound pressure level (SPL). For this to be an accurate assessment of audibility, the individual's hearing thresholds have to be converted from hearing level (HL) to SPL. The real-ear-to-coupler difference (RECD) measurement is used to convert HL to SPL data (51,52).

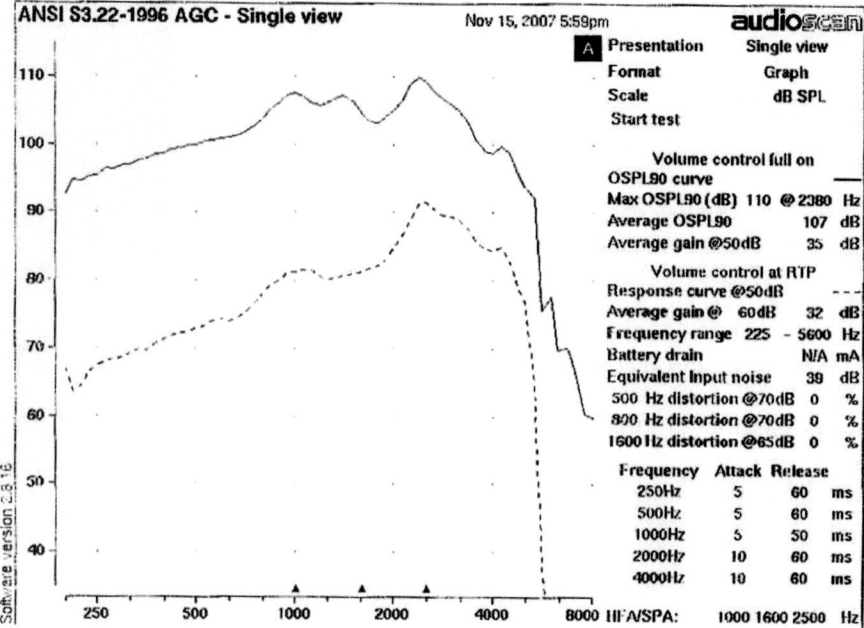

Figure 164.14 Example coupler response. The x-axis displays frequency (250 to 8,000 Hz) and the y-axis displays output (dB SPL). The *solid line* is the output for a loud signal (maximum output) and the *dashed line* is the output for a 50-dB SPL. A variety of other standard hearing aid measures are displayed on the right side of the graph.

Figure 164.15 provides the calculation used when applying RECD to HL thresholds in order to obtain SPL thresholds. Figure 164.16 provides the threshold data in SPL from the patient whose audiogram can be seen in Figure 164.11. RECD has been applied to the original HL thresholds and the resulting SPL thresholds are plotted, so the hearing aid output can be compared to the individual's dynamic range. This correction in the conversion from HL to SPL is especially critical when fitting children due to the difference in size between adult and pediatric ear canals. The average conversion data are based on average adult data. The resulting SPL thresholds are used to provide target output levels for the soft, moderate, and loud inputs across frequencies measured in the ear canal of an individual. Both the DSL (i/o) v.5 and the NAL/NL1 v.2 are evidence-based fitting formulae that will produce targets for this purpose (53–55). In the case of an infant or young child, the clinician armed with the RECD data can preset the hearing aid using coupler measurements and be able to evaluate the SPLs that will be achieved at the tympanic membrane of the individual child. The lines in Figure 164.16 show the output of a hearing aid for a child where

thresholds and RECD were used to preset the hearing aid. The hearing aid was manipulated until the output for the soft, moderate, and loud levels closely matched the DSL (i/o) v.5 targets.

During a hearing aid fitting, the hearing aid is first programmed by entering HL threshold data into the manufacturer's software. The software then makes a calculation of gain and other parameter settings (compression threshold, etc.) to provide a starting place for the fitting. Data indicate that this starting point can vary drastically between manufacturers (56–58) and will not guarantee audibility (in most cases high-frequency signals will not be audible). Therefore, measurement and tuning of the hearing aid to achieve audibility is essential, and the "first fit" from the manufacturer can only be considered a starting place.

Any features that have been selected for the hearing aid users should be verified as well. This would include directional microphones and telecoils. The directional microphone can be assessed using a front-to-back ratio, which is completed by setting the hearing aid to the directional setting and completing probe microphone measures as

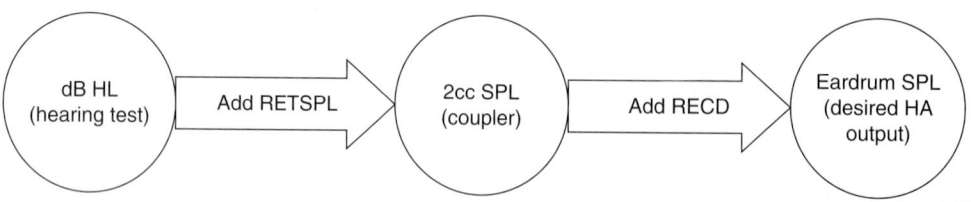

RETSPL: Reference Equivalent Threshold Sound Pressure Level
RECD: Real Ear to Coupler Difference

Figure 164.15 Converting HL to SPL thresholds using real-ear-to-coupler difference (RECD).

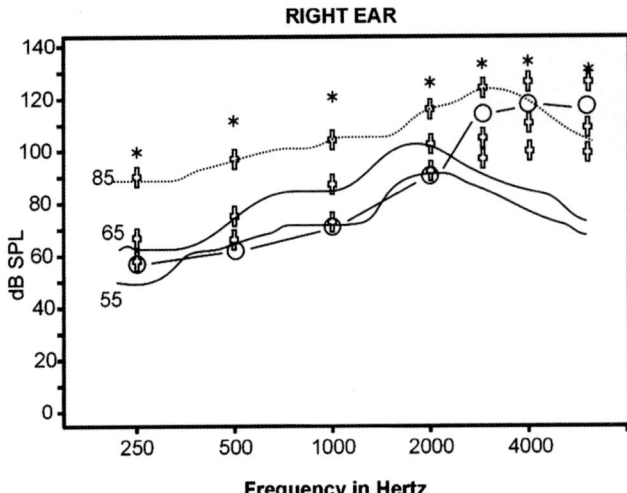

Figure 164.16 Real ear probe microphone output measures. This standard measure of hearing aid verification shows the output of the hearing aid for three input levels (55-, 65-, and 85-dB SPL). The plus signs illustrate the target output for each level across frequencies. Frequency is displayed across the x-axis, and output (dB SPL) is displayed on the y-axis. The Os represent the right hearing thresholds and the * represent the output that would be uncomfortable for this person. The range between these two symbols is the dynamic range.

TABLE 164.3	ORIENTATION CHECKLIST

Removing aids
Inserting aids
Opening the battery door
Overnight storage
Battery insertion
Battery life, storage, disposal, toxicity
On/Off function (if applicable)
Volume control (if applicable)
Telephone coupling and use
Assistive device coupling and use (if applicable)
Remote control or multimemory button (if applicable)
Cleaning and maintenance (tools)
Warranty explanation
Insurance information
Basic trouble shooting
Storage
Moisture solutions
Issues of retention
Recommended follow-up

described above. Then a second probe microphone measure is made with the speaker behind the individual. The output measurement behind the individual (with the directional microphone activated) should be less than the output measured with the speaker in front of the individual since the directional microphone should be less sensitive to sound coming from behind.

It is advisable to practice using the telephone with the new hearing aids prior to the patient leaving the clinic. The clinician may want to have the individual call a recording of the weather in order to have a signal to listen to through a landline and cell phone.

A recent study (59) found that there was a significant relationship between the testing conducted at the fitting and the patient's perceived benefit from and satisfaction with amplification. Measurement of loudness discomfort, use of real ear probe microphone measures, and some form of outcome assessment added to the individual's perceived satisfaction.

ORIENTATION

Once the hearing aid is programmed and the various settings have been selected, the new hearing aid user or parents of young children with hearing aids need to be oriented to the use and care of the amplification devices. Table 164.3 includes the various items that should be explained and practiced prior to the adult or child leaving with the hearing aids. As soon as a child is old enough to care for the hearing aids, he/she should be encouraged to do so. All of the care givers involved in a child's care need to understand the care and use of the hearing aids.

OUTCOME ASSESSMENT

Whereas verification measures that the hearing aid is producing audible signals, outcomes assessment evaluates whether the goals of the hearing aid fitting have been achieved. These goals may be related to speech and language development for a child or communicating effectively in particular situations for an adult (e.g., work, home). Several psychometrically sound instruments are available for use in outcome assessment with the adult and include the Independent Outcome Inventory for Hearing Aids (60) and the Satisfaction with Amplification in Daily Life (61). Objective tests of speech recognition are not widely recommended for outcome assessment because the testing environment in the clinic is controlled and artificial compared to the communication situations in which hearing aid users will find themselves. There are a variety of surveys currently used to assess amplification outcomes in children (62–71) that focus on various individuals in the child's communication environment including parents and teachers.

ASSISTIVE TECHNOLOGY BEYOND THE HEARING AID

Some hearing aid users may find that they require further assistance when communicating in noise or at a distance. If environmental manipulations will not solve these challenges, then the clinician may want to recommend assistive listening technology. Figure 164.11 provides examples of the types of transmission signals and coupling arrangements that can be used with assistive listening devices. Assistive listening devices consist of a microphone or direct line into a sound source. The sound is then transmitted via a wireless technology (FM, infrared, induction) that is picked up by a receiver either worn on the body of the hearing aid user or housed within the hearing aid. If the signal has been picked up by a body-worn receiver, then there is one more transfer to the hearing aid via direct audio input (hardwired) or induction. Listeners who do not use hearing aids can use earphones to receive the signal from an assistive listening device.

Adults will find these systems useful in meeting situations and restaurants where either background noise or distance is preventing them from functioning well in these challenging environments. Children will benefit from assistive listening systems in a variety of situations. For the very young child, an FM system may be used so the child can hear mom, dad, or the radio/CD while sitting in the backseat of a car. Assistive listening devices will be used in classroom situations to ensure that the child with hearing loss can hear the teacher. For children with personal hearing aids, an FM system will most often be recommended. For a child with minimal hearing loss or unilateral hearing loss, a sound field system may be recommended. Soundfield equalization systems consist of a microphone and transmitter worn by the teacher that send sounds via FM transmission to speakers placed throughout the room or to a single speaker placed on the student's desk. These systems equalize the level of sound throughout the room and create a sound environment that puts every child in the front row (with the best possible signal level and signal-to-noise ratio). Data have revealed that these systems are helpful to all of the children in the classroom. The personal system (with the speaker on the child's desk) helps only the child who is sitting at that desk, but is then portable so the child can carry the lunch box–sized device to the next classroom.

The coupling stage of these systems require that the hearing aid be compatible with the assistive listening device. Even if an assistive listening device is not ordered at the time of the hearing aid fitting, it is wise to discuss these options so the selection of the hearing aid has the potential for compatibility with assistive devices that may be pursued in the future. Currently, behind-the-ear hearing aids can have built-in FM receivers that are very attractive to users because there are no other cords and boxes to be worn.

As part of the communication assessment conducted with the adult or parents of children with hearing loss, the clinician will want to discuss the patient's ability to alert to warning signals. For the child, the clinician may want to refer to the Developmental Index of Auditory Listening (66) to get a sense of when to expect children to alert to and use various auditory signals (e.g., alarm clocks, phone use). This instrument will help guide the clinician and family in terms of what technology may allow the child to continually seek independence in using auditory signals. Important alerting signals are listed in Table 164.4. Individuals with hearing loss will need to alert to these signals when they are not wearing their hearing aids since

TABLE 164.4	SIGNALS TO WHICH INDIVIDUALS MAY NEED TO ALERT

Telephone ring
Doorbell ring or knock
Turn signal in car
Pager
Alarm clock
Smoke detector
Baby

traditional wear hearing aids are not worn during sleep. There are a variety of signals that can be used to make the person aware of an alerting signal including louder sounds, lower-frequency sounds, vibrations, lights, and fans. Choosing the best signal for the individual will be a process. Some individuals may want the alerting signals coordinated so they can wear a wristband and have a differential tactile signal depending on what signal is being triggered (i.e., baby monitor, doorbell, phone ringer, etc.).

SUMMARY

Providing complete hearing health care requires services of audiology and otolaryngology. The use of hearing aids and assistive listening devices is part of a larger auditory (re)habilitation plan that should be individually designed for the patient. The goal of amplification is to return audibility for soft, moderate, and loud sounds while maintaining comfort. There are a variety of hearing aid features and signal processing that allow the clinician to further tailor the solution to the individual. The clinician involved in the provision of amplification is challenged with monitoring developments in hearing aid technology that are introduced every 3 to 6 months. The clinician is required to be a critical consumer not only of published data (which can be three cycles behind the technology currently on the market) but also of marketing materials supplied by manufacturers. The clinician is the bridge between the evidence base and the consumer whose goal is to obtain a cost-effective solution to communication challenges. The clinician must understand the individual's hearing loss, communication needs, and listening environments in order to recommend a solution that will address the patient's needs while fitting into the individual's lifestyle. Properly fit amplification can significantly enhance the quality of life for the individual with hearing loss and the family (72–75).

ACKNOWLEDGMENTS

We would like to thank Lindsey Jorgensen and Leslie Cody for their assistance with specific content in the chapter. We would like to thank Randall Kesterson and Jenifer Fruit for their assistance with several of the figures.

REFERENCES

1. Schum D, Matthews L, Lee F. Acutal and predicted word-recognition performance of elderly hearing-impaired listeners. *J Speech Hear Res* 1991;34:636–642.
2. Wallhagen MI, Strawbridge WJ, Cohen RD, et al. Increasing prevalence of hearing impairment and associated risk factors over three decades of the Alameda County Study. *Am J Public Health* 1997;87:440–442.
3. Lin F, Thorpe R, Gordon-Salant S, et al. Hearing loss prevalence and risk factors among older adults in the United States. *J Gerontol A Biol Sci Med Sci* 2011;66A(5):582–590.
4. Yueh B, Shapiro N, MacLean C, et al. Screening and management of adult hearing loss in primary care. *JAMA* 2003;289(15): 1976–1985.
5. Cruikshanks K, Wiley T, Tweet T, et al. Prevalence of hearing loss in adults in Beaver Dam, Wisconsin. The Epidemiology of Hearing Loss Study. *Am J Epidemiol* 1998;148(9):879–886.
6. Kramer S, Kaptyen T, Kuik D, et al. The association of hearing impairment and chronic diseases with psychosocial health status in older age. *J Aging Health* 2002;14(1):122–137.
7. Uhlmann RF, Larson EB, Rees TS, et al. Relationship of hearing impairment to dementia and cognitive dysfunction in older adults. *JAMA* 1989;261(13):1916–1919.
8. Blanchfield BB. The severely to profoundly hearing-impaired population in the United States: Prevalence estimates and demographics. *J Am Acad Audiol* 2001;12:183–189.
9. Ray H. Mainstream Amplification Resource Room Study (MARRS).1992. Retrieved May 28, 2011, from Archived: Mainstream Amplification Resource Room Study (MARRS). http://www.ed.gov/pubs/EPTW/eptw12/eptw12d.html.
10. Cunningham M, Cox EO. Hearing assessment in infants and children: recommendations beyond neonatal screening. *Pediatrics* 2003;111(2):436–440.
11. Task Force on Newborn and Infant Hearing. Newborn and infant hearing loss: detection and intervention. *Pediatrics* 1999;103(2):527–530.
12. Shargorodsky J, Curhan S, Curhan G, et al. Change in prevalence of hearing loss in US adolescents. *JAMA* 2010;304(7):772–778.
13. Uchino B. Social support and health: a review of physiological processes potentially underlying links to disease outcomes. *J Behav Med* 2006;29(4):377–387.
14. Berkman L, Glass T, Brissette I, et al. From social integration to health: durkheim in the new millennium. *Soc Sci Med* 2000;51(6):843–857.
15. World Health Organization. *International classification of functioning, disability, and health (ICF)*. Geneva, Switzerland: World Health Organization, 2001.
16. American Academy of Audiology. Pediatric amplification guidelines. *Audiol Today* 2004;16(2):1–8.
17. American Academy of Audiology. *Guideline for the audiologic management of adult hearing impairment*. Reston, VA: American Academy of Audiology, 2007. Retrieved May 1, 2009 from www.audiology.org/resources/documentlibrary/documents/haguidelines.pdf.
18. American Academy of Pediatrics, Joint Committee on Infant Hearing. Year 2007 position statement: principles and guidelines for early hearing detection and intervention programs. *Pediatrics* 2007;20:898–921.
19. Palmer C, Solodar H, Hurley H, et al. Self-perception of hearing ability as a strong predictor of hearing aid purchase. *J Am Acad Audiol* 2009;20(6):341–348.
20. Mueller HG, Bentler RA. Fitting hearing aids using clinical measures of loudness discomfort levels: an evidence-based review of effectiveness. *J Am Acad Audiol* 2005;16(7):461–472.
21. Nilsson M, Soli S, Sullivan J. Development of the Hearing in Noise Test for the measurement of speech perception thresholds in quiet and in noise. *J Acoust Soc Am* 1994;95;1085–1099.
22. Etymotic Research. *The SIN Test* (compact disk). Elk Grove Village, IL; 1993.
23. Hawkins D, Yacullo W. Signal to noise ratio advantage of binaural hearing aids and directional microphones under different levels of reverberation. *Speech Hear Disord* 1984;49:278–286.
24. Kabler S, Lindbald A, Olofsson A, et al. Successful and unsuccessful users of bilateral amplification: differences and similarities in binaural performance. *Int J Audiol* 2010;49:613–627.
25. Cox R, Alexander G. The abbreviated profile of hearing aid benefit. *Ear Hear* 1995;16:176–186.
26. Dillon H, James A, Ginis J. Client oriented scale of improvement (COSI) and its relationship to several other measures of benefit and satisfaction provided by hearing aids. *J Am Acad Audiol* 1997;8:27–43.
27. Palmer C, Mormer E. Goals and expectations of the hearing aid fitting. *Trends Amplif* 1999;4(2):61–71.
28. Ching T, Incerti P, Hill M, et al. The effect of auditory experience on speech perception, localization, and functional performance of children who use a cochlear implant and a hearing aid in opposite ears. *Int J Audiol* 2005;44:677–690.
29. Ching T, Incerti P, Hill M. Binaural benefits for adults who use hearing aids and cochlear implants in opposite ears. *Ear Hear* 2004;25(1):9–21.
30. Davidson L, Skinner M. Audibility and speech perception of children using wide dynamic range compression hearing aids. *Am J Audiol* 2005;15:141–153.
31. Cox RM, Xu J. Short and long compression release times: speech understanding, real-world preferences, and association with cognitive ability. *J Am Acad Audiol* 2010;21(2):121–138.
32. Stelmachowicz P, Pittman A, Hoover B, et al. Aided perception of /s/ and /z/ by hearing-impaired children. *Ear Hear* 2002;23:316–324.
33. Stelmachowicz P, Pittman A, Hoover B, et al. Effect of stimulus bandwidth on the perception of /s/ in normal and hearing-impaired children and adults. *J Acoust Soc Am* 2001;110:2183–2190.
34. Horwitz A, Ahlstrom J, Dubno J. Factors affecting the benefits of high-frequency amplification. *J Speech Lang Hear Res* 2008;51: 798–813.

35. Ricketts T, Dittberner A, Johnson E. High-frequency amplification and sound quality in listeners with normal though moderate hearing loss. *J Speech Lang Hear Res* 2008;51:160–172.

36. Simpson A, Hersbach A, McDermott H. Frequency-compression outcomes in listeners with steeply sloping audiograms. *Int J Audiol* 2006;45(11):619–629.

37. Simpson A, Hersbach A, McDermott H. Improvements in speech perception with an experimental nonlinear frequency compression hearing device. *Intern J Audiol* 2005;44(5):281–292.

38. Robinson JD, Stainsby TH, Baer T, et al. Evaluation of a frequency transposition algorithm using wearable hearing aids. *Int J Audiol* 2009;48(6):384–393.

39. Johnson EE, Ricketts TA, Hornsby B. The effect of digital phase cancellation feedback reduction systems on amplified sound quality. *J Am Acad Audiol* 2007;18:404–416.

40. Surr R, Walden B, Cord M, et al. Influence of environmental factors on hearing aid microphone preference. *J Am Acad Audiol* 2002;13:208–322.

41. Ricketts T, Hornsby B. Directional hearing aid benefit in listeners with severe hearing loss. *Int J Audiol* 2005;45:190–197.

42. Cord M, Surr R, Walden B, et al. Performance of directional microphone hearing aids in everyday life. *J Am Acad Audiol* 2002;13:295–307.

43. Ricketts T, Galster J. Head angle and elevation in classroom environments: implications for amplification. *J Speech Lang Hear Res* 2008;51(2):516–525.

44. Ching T, O'Brien A, Dillon H, et al. Directional effects of infants and young children in real life: implications for amplification. *J Speech Hear Res* 2009;52:1241–1254.

45. Bentler R, Yu-Hsiang W, Kettel J, et al. Digital noise reduction: outcomes from laboratory and field studies. *Int J Audiol* 2008;47:447–460.

46. Palmer CV, Bentler R, Mueller HG. Amplification with digital noise reduction and the perception of annoying aversive sounds. *Trends Amplif* 2006;10(2):95–104.

47. Alcantara J, Moore B, Kuhnel V, et al. Evaluation of the noise reduction system in a commercial digital hearing aid. *Int J Audiol* 2003;42:34–42.

48. Sarampalis A, Kalluri S, Edwards B, et al. Objective measures of listening effort: effects of background noise and noise reduction. *J Speech Hear Res* 2009;52(5):1230–1240.

49. Keidser G, Dillon H, Convery E. The effect of the baseline response on self-adjustment of hearing aid gain. *J Acoust Soc* 2008;124(3):1668–1681.

50. Mueller HG, Hornsby B, Weber J. Using trainable hearing aids to examine real-world preferred gain. *J Acad Audiol* 2008;19(10):758–773.

51. Scollie S, Seewald R, Cornelisse L, et al. Validity and repeatability of level-independent HL to SPL transforms. *Ear Hear* 1998;19(5):407–413.

52. Saunders G, Morgan D. Impact on hearing aid targets of measuring thresholds in dB HL versus dB SPL. *Int J Audiol* 2003;42:319–326.

53. Byrne D, Dillon H, Ching T, et al. NAL-NL1 procedure for fitting nonlinear hearing aids: characteristics and comparisons with other procedures. *J Am Acad Audiol* 2001;12:37–51.

54. Cornelisse L, Seewald R, Jamieson D. The input/output formula: a theoretical approach to the fitting of personal amplification devices. *J Acoust Soc Am* 1995;97(3):1854–1864.

55. Scollie S, Seewald R, Cornelisse L, et al. The desired sensation level multistage input/output algorithm. *Trends Amplif* 2005;9(4):159–197.

56. Hawkins D, Cook J. Hearing aid software predictive gain values: how accurate are they? *Hear J* 2003;56(7):26–34.

57. Seewald R, Mills J, Bagatto M, et al. A comparison of manufacturer-specific prescriptive procedures for infants. *Hear J* 2008;61(11):26–34.

58. Mueller HG, Bentler RA, Wu YH. Prescribing maximum hearing aid output: differences among manufacturers found. *Hear J* 2008;61(3):30–36.

59. Kochkin S, Beck DL, Christensen LA, et al. The impact of the hearing healthcare professional on hearing aid user success. *Hear Rev* 2010;17(4):12–34.

60. Cox R, Alexander G. The international outcome inventory for hearing aids (IOI-HA): psychometric properties of the English Version. *Int J Audiol* 2002;41(1):30–35.

61. Cox R. Alexander G. Measuring satisfaction with amplification in daily life: SADL Scale. *Ear Hear* 2003;20:306–320.

62. Johnson CD, Von Almen P. Functional listening evaluation. In: Johnson CD, Benson PV, Seaton JB, eds. *Educational audiology handbook.* San Diego, CA: Singular Publishing Group, Inc, 1997:336–339.

63. Anderson KL. *Screening instrument for targeting educational risk (SIFTER).* Tampa, FL: Educational Audiology Association, 1989.

64. Anderson KL, Matkin ND. *Screening instrument for targeting educational risk in preschool children (age 3-kindergarten) (Preschool SIFTER).* Tampa, FL: Educational Audiology Association, 1996.

65. Anderson KL, Smaldino J. Listening inventory for education (LIFE), an efficacy tool. Educational Audiology Association, [online]. Available: http://www.edaud.org. 1996.

66. Palmer C, Mormer E. Goals and expectations of the hearing aid fitting. *Trends Amplif* 1999;4(2):61–71.

67. Anderson KL. Early Listening Function (ELF). Educational Audiology Association, [on-line]. Available: http://www.edaud.org. 2002.

68. Robbins AM, Renshaw JJ, Berry SW. Evaluating meaningful auditory integration in profoundly hearing impaired children. *Am J Otol* 1991;12:144–150.

69. Zimmerman S, Osberger MJ, Robbins AM. Infant-Toddler: Meaningful Auditory Integration Scale (IT-MAIS). In: Estabrooks W, ed. *Cochlear implants for kids.* Washington, DC: AG Bell Association for the Deaf, 1998.

70. Robbins AM, Svirsky MA, Osberger MJ, et al. Beyond the audiogram: the role of functional assessments. In: Bess FH, ed. *Children with hearing impairment: contemporary trends.* Nashville, TN: Bill Wilkerson Center Press, 1998:105–124.

71. Stedler-Brown A, DeConde JC. Functional auditory performance indicators: an integrated approach to auditory development [online], Colorado Department of Education, Special Education Services Unit. http://www.cde.state.co.us/cdesped/specificdisability-hearing.htm. 2001.

72. Abrams HB, Chisolm TH, McArdle R. Health related quality of life and hearing aids: a tutorial. *Trends Amplif* 2005;9(3):99–109.

73. Chisolm TH, Abrams HB, McArdle R, et al. The WHO-DAS II: psychometric properties in the measurement of functional health status in adults with acquired hearing loss. *Trends Amplif* 2005;9(3):111–126.

74. McCardle R, Chisolm T, Abrams H, et al. The WHO-DAS II: measuring outcomes of hearing aid intervention for adults. *Trends Amplif* 2005;9(3):127–143.

75. Barton GR, Bankart J, Davis AC. A comparison of the quality of life of hearing-impaired people as estimated by three different utility measures. *Int J Audiol* 2005;44(3):157–163.

Clinical Evaluation of the Patient with Vertigo

165

Courtney C. J. Voelker   *Joel A. Goebel*

INTRODUCTION

Magnitude of the Problem in Population

The diagnosis and management of the patient with dizziness and imbalance can be perplexing and challenging. Dizziness is a common symptom affecting 20% to 30% of the general population in the United States (1,2). Among patients 75 years of age and older, balance disorders are the most common reason for visiting a physician (3). In the elderly, falls caused by dizziness and poor balance are associated with morbidity and even mortality. Such falls constitute a major health care burden in our aging population (4). Early detection and intervention in these cases can result in significant improvement in the quality of life as well as in a decrease in disability and reduction in health care costs (4). It is, therefore, incumbent on those who diagnose and treat dizziness to recognize the complexity of the problem, develop a systematic and efficient process for gathering accurate historical information, perform a structured neurotologic examination, and provide a rational treatment approach that addresses all major contributing factors.

Multifactorial Nature of Dizziness

The three primary sensory inputs responsible for balance originate from the vestibular, visual, and somatosensory (proprioceptive) pathways. Maintenance of balance requires accurate integration of three processes: (a) appropriate detection of various environmental sensory inputs, (b) accurate central nervous system (CNS) integration of all sensory input and production of an appropriate neural response, and (c) performance of the correct muscle response for maintenance of postural control and gaze stability (Fig. 165.1). The vestibular labyrinth can be divided into the semicircular canals (SCCs) (horizontal, superior, and posterior) and the otolith organs (utricle and saccule). The primary function of the SCCs is to detect high-velocity, angular head movement

and to produce a compensatory eye movement via the vestibuloocular reflex (VOR) for stabilization of visual images on the retina and maintenance of acuity during head movement. In contrast, the primary function of the otolith organs is to sense linear acceleration (including gravity) and to produce compensatory postural changes in response to transient linear movements and changes via gravity through the vestibulospinal reflex (VSR) pathways. Taken together, the VOR and VSR serve to stabilize the visual world and upright stance and ambulation, respectively.

The visual tracking and fixation pathways sense movement in the visual surround and allow the individual to respond to either slowly moving (smooth pursuit, optokinetic) or novel (saccadic) objects of interest and augment the VOR for maintenance or acquisition of desired targets. With the vestibular system acting as the "gold standard" internal frame of reference, visual inputs are interpreted in combination with vestibular cues for generation of the desired eye movement for the task at hand.

The somatosensory inputs from the feet, lower limbs, and trunk serve to orient the body to contact surfaces and respond to transient perturbations by generating reflexive corrective limb movements using the ankle joint as the primary fulcrum of movement during upright stance. These cues, along with vestibular inputs, are critical for the maintenance of upright stance and gait control. The absence of accurate vestibular cues or the transmission of incorrect cues invariably leads to poor posture control and ambulation, often resulting in falls.

The second component of balance control is sensory integration, which requires the brain to interpret and weigh all sensory inputs and generate a rapid and accurate response (Fig. 165.1). In some instances, sensory cues are in conflict or ambiguous. Under these circumstances, the brain must decide which cues are appropriate for the given situation and ignore or suppress those that have an incorrect orientation. In susceptible individuals, motion sickness can result.

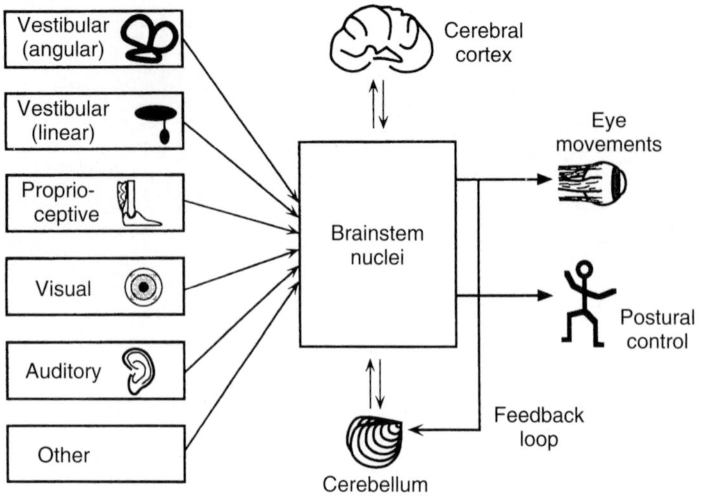

Figure 165.1 An integrated approach to the diagnosis of dizziness and imbalance. Maintaining balance requires a patient to sense the environment (via sensory afferent input), to integrate the environmental information via central processing, and to calculate the correct motor response (delivered via motor efferent output). Accurately locating the abnormality within this integrated system is crucial when a patient presents with dizziness, imbalance, or vertigo. (From Hughes GB, Pensak ML, eds. *Clinical otology*, 2nd ed. New York: Thieme Medical Publishers, 1997:44, with permission.)

The final component of posture control is generating an appropriate motor response to sensory inputs. This elaborate task requires an intact peripheral motor system and adequate musculoskeletal capability. In some cases, sensory input and central integration are intact, but inadequate motor capabilities lead to imbalance and falls. It is, therefore, important in each patient with imbalance or dizziness to decide whether or not there is a sensory deficit, a central integration problem, an inadequate musculoskeletal response, or a combination of factors leading to their symptom complex.

Importance of History

A structured and thorough discovery of all pertinent historical events is critical in the evaluation of the dizzy patient (5). In roughly 75% of cases, the history alone yields an accurate differential diagnosis, even before the physical examination or laboratory tests are performed (5). The reasons a precise history is essential are as follow: (a) Most disease processes that cause dizziness have a particular symptom pattern; (b) diseases of the inner ear and eighth cranial nerve cause distinctly different sensations than CNS, musculoskeletal, systemic, or psychogenic processes; (c) most patients are not experiencing an acute sensation of dizziness at the time of examination; and (d) the CNS has a remarkable way of compensating between episodes such that clinical examinations and laboratory findings are only seen during acute episodes or in cases of significant damage. As discussed below, development of a systematic approach to history taking allows the examiner to build a differential diagnosis even prior to performing the physical examination and further testing.

Evaluation of Sensory (Vestibular, Visual, and Somatosensory), Central Integration, and Motor Control Aspects

After obtaining a comprehensive history, the examiner then proceeds to perform a basic otolaryngologic and structured neurotologic examination. Causes of dizziness should not be overlooked at this stage and must be detected on the routine otolaryngologic head and neck examination (e.g., impacted cerumen, middle ear effusion, obstructed nasal airway, and sinus disease). Following this examination, a detailed evaluation of spontaneous and evoked eye movements, VOR and VSR functions, posture, and gait is performed. Special attention is paid to the function of each sensory input, central integration of these inputs, and the generation of an appropriate eye or trunk/limb movement for maintenance of gaze and upright stance.

Judicious Use of Laboratory Testing to Quantify Deficits

In many cases, the etiology of the patient's dizziness is clear subsequent to taking the history and performing a thorough physical examination. Further audiovestibular, radiologic, and serologic testing may be necessary to support the suspected diagnosis and to quantify the extent of the deficit prior to initiation of medical and/or surgical management. Furthermore, vestibular function tests as a whole exhibit fairly high specificity (80% to 85%), but only modest sensitivity (60% to 65%) (6). Consequently, vestibular function tests are limited in their ability to "rule out" dysfunction for most diseases affecting the labyrinth or eighth cranial nerve. It is, therefore, incumbent on the specialist who manages the dizzy patient to understand the critical role of taking a comprehensive history and performing a structured physical examination prior to ordering any further tests.

HISTORY TAKING

Methods: Questionnaire and Direct Questioning

A variety of methods exists for gathering historical information from the patient prior to the physical examination: (a) structured questionnaire mailed to the patient (see included example), (b) phone interview and verbal

Dizziness and Balance Center

Patient Name:_____ D.O.B:___/___/___ Sex: M___ F___ Date: ___/___/___

The following questions refer to your feeling of dizziness. Please answer them as "yes" or "no" and fill in all blanks.

Please describe in your own words, the sensation you feel without using the word "dizzy":

_____

_____

_____

I.	**Do you ever have any of the following sensations?**	
Yes	Spinning in circles	No
Yes	Falling to one side	No
Yes	World spinning around you	No
II.	**The following refer to a typical dizzy spells:**	
Yes	Do your dizzy spells come in attacks?	No
	How often? _____	
	How long is the attack? _____	
	Date of first spell? _____	
Yes	Are you free from dizziness between attacks?	No
Yes	Does your hearing change with an attack?	No
Yes	Are you dizzy mainly when you sit or stand up quickly?	No
Yes	Are you dizzier in certain positions?	No
	Which position? _____	
Yes	Are you nauseated during an attack?	No
Yes	Are you dizzy even when lying down?	No
Yes	Have you had a recent cold or flu preceding recent dizzy spells?	No
Yes	Have you had fullness, pressure, or ringing in your ears?	No
Yes	Have you had pain or discharge in your ear of recent onset?	No
Yes	Have you had trouble walking in the dark?	No
Yes	Are you better if you sit or lie perfectly still?	No
III.	**The following refer to other sensations you may have:**	
Yes	Do you black out or faint when dizzy?	No
	Have you had:	
Yes	Severe or recurrent headaches?	No
Yes	Light sensitivity with your headaches or dizziness?	No
Yes	Any double or blurry vision?	No
Yes	Numbness in your face or extremities?	No
Yes	Weakness or clumsiness in arms, legs?	No
Yes	Slurred or difficult speech?	No
Yes	Difficulty swallowing?	No
Yes	Tingling around your mouth?	No
Yes	Spots before your eyes?	No
Yes	Jerking of arms or legs?	No
Yes	Seizures?	No
Yes	Confusion or memory loss?	No
Yes	Recent head trauma? (If yes, please explain)	No

_____

_____

_____

IV.   <u>The following refer to your hearing. Indicate which side has been affected:</u>

Yes	Difficulty hearing in one ear?	Left	Right	Both	No
Yes	Ringing in one ear?	Left	Right	Both	No
Yes	Fullness in one ear?	Left	Right	Both	No
Yes	Change in hearing when dizzy?				No

Have you had any of the following?

Yes	Pain in ears?	Left	Right	Both	No
Yes	Discharge from ears?	Left	Right	Both	No
Yes	Hearing change?				No
Yes	Better?	Left	Right	Both	No
Yes	Worse?	Left	Right	Both	No
Yes	Exposure to loud noises?				No
Yes	Previous ear infections?				No
Yes	Previous ear surgery?				No
	What? _____				No
Yes	Family history of deafness?				No

V.   <u>The following refer to habits and lifestyle:</u>

| Yes | Is there added stress to your life recently? | No |
| Yes | Are you dizzy or unsteady constantly? | No |

Is your dizziness related to:

Yes	Moments of stress?	No
Yes	Menstrual period?	No
Yes	Overwork or exertion?	No
Yes	Do you feel lightheaded or have a swimming sensation when you are dizzy?	No
Yes	Do you find yourself breathing faster or deeper when excited or dizzy?	No
Yes	Did you recently change eyeglasses?	No
Yes	Have you ever had weakness or faintness a few hours after eating?	No
Yes	Do you drink coffee? How much? _____	No
Yes	Do you drink tea? How much? _____	No
Yes	Do you drink soft drinks? How much? _____	No
Yes	Do you drink alcohol? How much? _____	No
Yes	Do you smoke? What?_____ How much? _____	No

Past Medical History:

Please list your current medical problems and length of illness: _____

_____

_____

_____

Please list all surgery performed and approximate dates: _____

_____

_____

_____

Please list all allergies (including drugs) and reaction: _____

_____

_____

_____

Please list all medicines you currently take (including pain medicine, nonprescription medicine, nerve pills, sleeping pills, or birth control pills). _____

_____

_____

_____

Have you had any previous testing (hearing, x-rays, head scans, etc.)? _____

_____

_____

Family History:
Any family history of:

Yes	**Migraine?**	No
Yes	**High blood pressure?**	No
Yes	**Low blood pressure?**	No
Yes	**Diabetes?**	No
Yes	**Low blood sugar?**	No
Yes	**Thyroid disease?**	No
Yes	**Asthma?**	No

Please list any other diseases that run in your immediate family: _____

_____

System Review:
Check all applicable symptoms:

Constitutional:			
☐ Recent weight change	☐ Fever	☐ Fatigue	☐ N/A

Eyes:			
☐ Loss of Vision	☐ Pain	☐ Discharge/Tearing	☐ N/A
☐ Left ☐ Right ☐ Both	☐ Left ☐ Right ☐ Both	☐ Left ☐ Right ☐ Both	

Ear, Nose, Mouth, Throat:			
☐ Itchy ears	☐ Facial weakness	☐ Nasal obstruction	☐ Nasal discharge
☐ Nosebleed	☐ Sneezing	☐ "Stuffy" nose	☐ Snoring
☐ Loss of sense of smell	☐ Growth in nose	☐ Nasal bleeding	☐ Drooling
☐ Mouth growth, ulcer	☐ Chewing difficulty	☐ Lump in neck	☐ Dental problems/ Poorly fitting dentures
☐ Pain on swallowing	☐ Heartburn	☐ Sore throat	☐ Bleeding from throat
☐ Voice changes	☐ Breathing difficulty	☐ N/A	

Cardiovascular:			
☐ Chest pain	☐ Irregular heart beat	☐ Swelling of legs	☐ Leg pain with walking
☐ Leg pain with rest	☐ N/A		

Respiratory:			
☐ Wheezing	☐ Cough	☐ Shortness of breath	☐ Mucous
☐ Coughing up blood	☐ N/A		

Gastrointestinal:			☐ Difficulty swallowing (food sticks)
☐ Decrease in appetite	☐ Nausea/Vomiting	☐ Blood in stool	
☐ Diarrhea/Constipation	☐ Indigestion	☐ Food intolerance	☐ N/A

Musculoskeletal:		☐ Arthritis	
☐ Neck pain	☐ Joint pain/Stiffness	Name Joint:	☐ N/A

Skin:			
☐ Rash	☐ Jaundice	☐ Recent baldness	☐ N/A

Neurological:			
☐ Headache	☐ Blackout	☐ Seizures	☐ Paralysis
☐ Tremor	☐ N/A		

Psychiatric:		**On Medication:**	
☐ Insomnia	☐ Depression	☐ Yes ☐ No	☐ N/A

Endocrine:			
☐ Thyroid trouble	☐ Heat or cold Intolerance	☐ Excessive sweating	☐ Excessive thirst, hunger, urination
☐ N/A			

Genitourinary:			
☐ Painful urination	☐ Veneral disease	☐ Blood in urine	☐ Frequent urination at night
☐ Difficulty passing urine	☐ Incontinence	☐ N/A	

Hematologic/Lymphatic:			☐ N/A
☐ Anemia	☐ Bleeding problems	☐ Blood disorder (e.g., Sickle cell)	
	☐ Easy bruising		

Do you have anything else to tell us about your particular problem that we have not asked you on this questionnaire?

_____
_____
_____
_____

Physician Review with Patient:

_____
_____
_____
_____
_____
_____
_____
_____
_____
_____
_____

_____   _____
Physician Signature   **Date**

Rev. 01/09

gathering of information, and (c) face-to-face interview at the time of the physical examination. The advantage of a structured questionnaire is its capability to supply comprehensive data regarding the nature of the dizziness/imbalance episodes, accompanying symptoms, additional medical conditions, medications, and lifestyle. However, such questionnaires must be simplified so that it is understandable for the patient and well organized for the practitioner to efficiently interpret the data. Moreover, these questionnaires should be completed prior to the appointment rather than hurriedly filled out in the waiting room. A well constructed and thoughtfully completed questionnaire can be a valuable tool for the examiner to review prior to the patient interview. Alternatively, a medical assistant can conduct a phone interview and record the data. The disadvantages of this approach include that this method can be more time consuming and costly, and the resulting data are less comprehensive than the data from a written questionnaire. Finally, the face-to-face interview by the physician is the most important step in confirming and/or clarifying what the patient has either written in the questionnaire or told the medical assistant by phone. Using the written questionnaire as a guide allows the examiner to ask directed questions during the interview in an efficient fashion to best understand the patient's symptom complex (Table 165.1).

Components of the History

Distinction Between Vertigo, Disequilibrium, and Light-Headedness

The first important piece of information in the history is the nature or quality of the sensation experienced during their episodes. Types of dizziness can be roughly divided into three broad categories: (a) vertigo, (b) disequilibrium, and (c) light-headedness (Table 165.1). _Vertigo_ can be defined as a false sense of motion within the patient's environment and is usually described as a "spinning, whirling, tumbling, or even rhythmic rocking" feeling (7). In most instances, patients will sense that the environment is in motion around them (objective vertigo) and may describe the illusion that objects within their visual world (e.g., pictures, furniture, etc.) are actually moving in one direction or another before their eyes. In a minority of cases, the patients feel that they are in motion relative to a stationary world (subjective vertigo). In either event, the illusion of motion is distinct. Such strong sensations of environmental and/or self-motion are most often generated by a sudden asymmetry within the peripheral vestibular system (labyrinth or eighth cranial nerve) and are valuable indicators of peripheral inner ear or nerve dysfunction.

TABLE 165.1	THE HISTORY OF PRESENT ILLNESS IN A PATIENT WITH DIZZINESS

Components of the Interview	Key Historical Features
What is the character of the dizzy sensation?	Vertigo, disequilibrium, or light-headedness
What is the dizziness pattern?	Continuous or episodic
What is the time course of dizzy episodes?	Seconds, minutes, hours, days, or longer
Was there an event associated with dizziness onset?	Head/inner ear trauma, barotrauma, upper respiratory infection, ear infection, systemic illness or infection, ototoxic medication
What associated symptoms accompany the dizzy episodes?	Hearing loss, tinnitus (continuous vs. pulsatile), aural fullness, conductive hyperacusis, diplacusis, dysacusis, autophony, oscillopsia, otorrhea, otalgia, headache, facial or limb weakness, dysphagia, dysphasia, visual changes, photophobia, phonophobia, loss of consciousness, seizure
What exacerbates the dizziness?	Rapid head movement, particular head positions, increased pressure (Hennebert sign), sounds (Tullio phenomenon), hyperventilation, strong environmental stimuli (bright lights, odors, etc.), food triggers
What medications (past and present) could be involved?[a]	Antibiotics, antineoplastic, analgesics, antihypertensives, neuroleptics, antidepressants, sedatives
What is the patient's past medical history?	Migraine, endocrine (e.g., diabetes), rheumatologic, cancer, cardiovascular, systemic infections
What is the patient's past surgical history?	Focusing on otologic or brain surgery
What is the family history?	Migraine, endocrine (e.g., diabetes), rheumatologic, cancer, cardiovascular, systemic infections, genetic mutations

[a]See Table 165.2 for a more detailed discussion.

In contrast with vertigo, patients who have *disequilibrium* describe difficulty maneuvering within their physical environment often without experiencing an illusion of motion (Table 165.1). Patients with disequilibrium may use synonyms like "imbalanced, clumsy, uncoordinated, or fear of falling," and their symptoms are usually worse while standing or ambulating. A variety of CNS, peripheral neuropathic, and musculoskeletal disorders can cause disequilibrium, although slowly progressive, bilateral vestibular loss without significant asymmetry may present with this complaint.

The third category—*light-headedness*—comprises both a wide range of sensations (such as "wooziness, giddiness, feeling faint, or as if one is about to pass out") and of etiologies (including migraine, vascular, metabolic, drug-induced, endocrine, or primary psychogenic causes) (Table 165.1). Light-headedness, though, is less commonly a primary complaint of patients with damage of the peripheral vestibular pathways. Instead, light-headedness is most often comorbid with vertigo and/or disequilibrium.

Time Course

Once the nature and quality of the sensation is elucidated, the examiner then attempts to determine the duration of the symptoms (Table 165.1). The first question is whether or not the sensation is continuous or episodic and, if so, do the episodes last seconds, minutes, hours, days, or even longer. When patients complain of vertigo, this time course distinction is exceedingly valuable since the most common peripheral vestibular disease processes produce stereotypical attacks of consistent duration. For example, patients with benign paroxysmal positional vertigo (BPPV) usually complain of discrete attacks that last less than 1 minute. In contrast, patients with Ménière's disease usually describe a "spinning feeling" that can last 15 minutes to many hours. Finally, patients who develop vertigo secondary to vestibular neuritis describe attack(s) of continuous spinning lasting up to 24 hours. In patients with transient ischemic attacks involving the vertebrobasilar circulation and brainstem, attacks generally last 15 minutes, whereas brainstem infarcts and cerebellar hemorrhages exhibit acute, severe vertigo lasting hours and impact the inability to stand.

The time course of attacks in patients with disequilibrium is somewhat less stereotypical of their disease process. Frequently, patients report that symptoms persist as long as they are upright. Similarly, patients with light-headedness may have a variable symptom picture, with sensations lasting anywhere from seconds to days. Finally, patients with migraine-associated dizziness (MAD) may complain variably of all three sensations, and the duration may fluctuate from seconds to days or even longer.

Associated Events

It is crucial to elucidate associated events that occurred near the time the dizziness began, such as trauma, recent or chronic infection(s), systemic diseases (e.g., rheumatologic, autoimmune, or metabolic), or medication changes. Posttraumatic vertigo can be the result of (a) direct mechanical trauma to the head or inner ear structures (e.g., penetrating injuries damaging the inner ear, SCC dehiscence) and/or (b) barotrauma (i.e., damage caused by pressure changes). Activities associated with barotrauma may include military service with exposure to blast injuries, scuba diving, hyperbaric oxygen treatments, straining (e.g., weight lifting or childbirth), or changes in altitude (e.g., airplane flights or driving in the mountains), especially during an upper respiratory infection that causes congestion. Posttraumatic vertigo may be due to perilymphatic fistula(s) (PLF) of the oval and/or round windows (8–11), delayed endolymphatic hydrops (12), BPPV (13), migraine, or middle ear surgery (14). Furthermore, trauma may cause a dehiscence of the superior SCC if the bone covering the canal was thin prior to the injury (15–17).

Determining a history of recent infections is important. For example, vestibular neuritis is thought to be caused by viral infection, and an upper respiratory viral prodrome may occur prior to vertigo onset (18). Other infections that can cause vertigo include herpes zoster oticus (Ramsay Hunt syndrome), suppurative otitis media, human immunodeficiency virus, syphilis, Lyme disease, and tuberculosis. Additionally, recent systemic infections or cancers may have necessitated the administration of ototoxic drugs that can cause vertigo.

Finally, it is imperative to determine if the patient also has a systemic condition including a rheumatologic, autoimmune (e.g., Wegener granulomatosis, systemic lupus erythematosus), and/or metabolic (e.g., diabetes) disease that may be associated with vertigo.

Accompanying Symptoms

In many cases, accompanying symptoms assist the examiner in determining if the site of lesion is located in the labyrinth, eighth cranial nerve, brainstem, or cortical areas (Table 165.1). Hearing loss, tinnitus, aural fullness, and vertigo strongly suggest labyrinthine involvement. Fluctuations in these symptoms may suggest Ménière's disease or posttraumatic endolymphatic hydrops. On the other hand, vertigo without hearing loss may be generated by the labyrinth (e.g., BPPV), eighth cranial nerve (e.g., vestibular neuritis), brainstem (e.g., isolated vestibular nuclei infarct), and/or cerebral cortex (e.g., migraine, seizure). Patients with superior SCC dehiscence can present with conductive hyperacusis or autophony. Conductive hyperacusis includes symptoms such as hearing one's own eye movements, one's own heartbeat, and/or the impact of one's feet during walking or running in the affected ear (17,19). Associated facial weakness suggests a lesion proximal to the labyrinth, while dysphagia, dysphasia, limb weakness, and ataxia are indicators of CNS involvement. Patients with MAD frequently complain of photophobia, phonophobia, or heightened sense of smell. Finally, loss of consciousness implies a significant perfusion failure of the cerebrovascular circulation and is not associated with primary labyrinthine or eighth cranial nerve lesions.

Exacerbating Factors

Since the vestibular labyrinth is sensitive to angular motion (turning the head), transient linear motion (sudden translations), and gravity (tipping the head and body), disorders of the inner ear are frequently aggravated by head movements and changes of the head and/or body vis-a-vis gravity (Table 165.1). Patients with vestibular disorders tend to keep their head as still as possible and avoid sudden movements. Vertigo induced by very specific head positions (e.g., rolling over in bed, or tilting the head back to rinse their hair in the shower), which lasts for seconds, suggests BPPV. In cases of bilateral and uncompensated unilateral vestibular dysfunction, patients have difficulty walking in the dark or on uneven surfaces and avoid fast head movements due to bobbing or blurring of their visual field (oscillopsia). Patients with orthostasis become more symptomatic with changes in position against gravity such as arising from a bed or chair and obtain relief by lying flat.

Patients with superior SCC dehiscence may present with sound-induced vertigo (Tullio phenomenon) or pressure-induced vertigo (Hennebert sign) (17,19). Valsalva maneuvers, coughing, or sneezing can induce vertigo or oscillopsia. Furthermore, hyperventilation (e.g., exercising) may induce vertigo in peripheral (e.g., cerebellopontine angle [CPA] tumors) or central (e.g., multiple sclerosis) lesions.

In cases with MAD, exposure to visual motion, bright lights, loud sounds, or strong odors can exacerbate dizziness. Furthermore, MAD patients can, at times, identify food triggers such as caffeine, alcohol, cheese, or citrus fruits. Changes in dietary salt intake may trigger dizziness in patients with Ménière's disease.

Medications and Comorbidity

Dizziness is a common side effect of many medications, and, in some instances, the interaction of multiple medicines is the cause of a patient's symptoms (Table 165.2). Medications causing dizziness, light-headedness, and/or auditory symptoms generally are divided into three categories: those that are (a) ototoxic, (b) affect systemic blood flow, and (c) act on the CNS. Once the drug is stopped or the dose adjusted, symptoms may reverse. However, in some circumstances, the damage may be permanent. Therefore, the examiner must query the patient not only about current medications but also about previous medication usage.

Ototoxic drugs damage the peripheral vestibular system. Ototoxicity usually results in a symmetric loss of vestibular end organ function, which disables the VOR. Thus, patients loose visual stability with head movement, resulting in oscillopsia (i.e., bobbing or jiggling of the visual field). Patients with bilateral vestibular loss present with disequilibrium and have tremendous difficulty or are completely unable to maintain balance and posture in the dark. The most common ototoxic drugs are aminoglycosides and chemotherapy agents (Table 165.2). Aminoglycoside antibiotics (e.g., streptomycin, gentamicin, neomycin, tobramycin, amikacin, kanamycin) constitute a group of natural and semisynthetic compounds used to treat aerobic gram-negative bacilli and mycobacterium. Aminoglycosides inhibit bacterial protein synthesis by binding to the

TABLE 165.2	MEDICATIONS THAT MAY CAUSE DIZZINESS

Drug Class	Mechanism	Symptoms
Ototoxic		
Aminoglycosides *Gentamicin, neomycin, tobramycin, amikacin, kanamycin*	Damages vestibular type I sensory cells, outer hair cells in the organ of Corti, and cochlear and vestibular neurons Loop diuretics and vancomycin can potentiate ototoxicity	Oscillopsia from symmetric vestibular hypofunction Vertigo from asymmetric vestibular loss, sensorineural hearing loss, and tinnitus
Antineoplastic agents *Cisplatin*	Damages vestibular hair cells, outer hair cells in the organ of Corti, stria vascularis, and spiral ligament	Same symptoms as aminoglycoside damage
Analgesic agents NSAIDs *(aspirin, naproxen, indomethacin, and ibuprofen)*	Reversible outer hair cell function changes and reduced blood flow via vasoconstriction	Reversible sensorineural hearing loss, tinnitus, and rarely vertigo
Acetaminophen/hydrocodone	Permanent hair cell damage	Rapidly progressive, permanent sensorineural hearing loss, tinnitus, and rarely vertigo
Systemic Blood Flow		
Antihypertensives *Diuretics, β-blockers, vasodilators, CCB α-adrenergic blocker*	Systemic vasodilation leading to decreased peripheral vascular resistance	Light-headedness, syncope, visual changes, and fatigue
Central Nervous System		
Neuroleptics Antidepressants *Tricyclics, MAOIs, SSRIs* sedatives	Target central dopamine, serotonin, GABA, and acetylcholine neurotransmitter pathways	Light-headedness, vertigo, and ataxia

CCB, calcium channel blocker; GABA, γ-aminobutyric acid; MAOIs, monoamine oxidase inhibitor; NSAIDs, nonsteroidal anti-inflammatory drugs; SSRI, selective serotonin reuptake inhibitor.

30S ribosomal subunit and cause mRNA to be misread. While the use of systemic aminoglycosides is declining in developed nations due to their significant toxicities and the availability of better alternatives, aminoglycosides are still widely used in developing countries. This is because aminoglycosides are inexpensive and effective against diseases such as multidrug-resistant tuberculosis (20,21).

All aminoglycosides cause cochlear and vestibular damage that is usually permanent. However, individual aminoglycosides differ in their ability to produce cochlear versus vestibular toxicity. Gentamicin and streptomycin are primarily vestibulotoxic (22), whereas neomycin, amikacin, and kanamycin are more cochleotoxic. Aminoglycosides destroy vestibular type I sensory hair cells, outer hair cells in the organ of Corti (from cochlear base to apex), and cochlear and vestibular neurons (20,21). The perilymph and endolymph drug concentration is directly proportional to the plasma concentration, which in turn is directly related to renal clearance (23). Aminoglycosides persist in the inner ear tissue for 6 months or longer after administration (24). The ototoxic damage may be potentiated by concurrent administration of loop diuretics (e.g., ethacrynic acid and furosemide) or vancomycin. Patients with a mutation in the mitochondrial 12S ribosomal subunit (*MTRNR1*) are particularly susceptible to aminoglycoside ototoxicity. This mutation is associated with spontaneous as well as aminoglycoside-induced hearing loss even following a single dose. Interestingly, the

vestibular system does not have an increased susceptibility to aminoglycoside toxicity in patients with this mutation (25). In contrast, missense polymorphisms in three oxidative stress-related genes (*NOS3*, *GSTZ1*, and *GSTP1*) have increased susceptibility to gentamicin-induced vestibular dysfunction (26).

Numerous chemotherapeutic drugs are ototoxic. The alkylating agent cisplatin (*cis*-diamminedichloroplatinum II) is the most ototoxic antineoplastic drug and is used to treat various malignancies including head and neck cancers. Cisplatin targets the outer hair cells in the organ of Corti, stria vascularis, and the spiral ligament (Table 165.2) (27). Vestibular toxicity seems to occur later than auditory toxicity. Both elderly and pediatric patients are reportedly more sensitive to cisplatin ototoxicity than other age groups (28). Patient symptoms of bilateral vestibular loss will present in the same way as aminoglycoside toxicity.

There is evidence that high-dose analgesic use is ototoxic. Nonsteroidal anti-inflammatory drugs (NSAIDs) such as salicylates (aspirin) (29), naproxen (30), indomethacin, and ibuprofen are among the offending agents (31,32). High-dose salicylates (several grams per day) cause outer hair cell dysfunction and decreased blood flow to the inner ear via vasoconstriction, possibly mediated by antiprostaglandin activity. The result is reversible hearing loss and tinnitus (29,33,34). Other NSAIDs have similar ototoxic effects through reduction of blood flow (29). Acetaminophen/hydrocodone (e.g., Vicodin, Lortab, and Norco) abuse has been reported to cause permanent, rapidly progressive, sensorineural hearing loss (35–38). Although less common than auditory symptoms, vestibular symptoms (e.g., vertigo or disequilibrium) caused by high-dose analgesics can occur. When vestibular symptoms do develop, their onset can even precede tinnitus (Table 165.2) (39).

Many types of antihypertensive medications can cause dizziness (Table 165.2). Examples include diuretics, β-blockers, vasodilators, calcium channel blockers, and α-adrenergic blockers. These medications result in dizziness through persistent orthostatic hypotension or, in part, by effecting CNS neurotransmitter pathways. Symptoms can include light-headedness, syncope, visual changes, and fatigue. Often these symptoms improve or resolve completely with dose adjustments.

Drugs acting on the CNS can cause dizziness (Table 165.2). The pharmacologic targets of neuroleptics, antidepressants (e.g., tricyclics, monoamine oxidase inhibitors, and selective serotonin reuptake inhibitors), and sedatives are located in the cortex or the brainstem. Several of these drug classes affect neurotransmitters such as dopamine,

serotonin, acetylcholine, and γ-aminobutyric acid (GABA), which can lead to hypotension, light-headedness, vertigo, and ataxia. At therapeutic doses, Dilantin can often lead to ataxia, vertigo, and gaze-evoked nystagmus (GEN). The first step in diagnosis is obtaining a detailed medical history, including a thorough medication history, and determining the character of the dizziness. Medication side effects may be the sole offender or may be exacerbating an underlying vestibular pathology.

STRUCTURED NEUROTOLOGIC EXAMINATION

The most effective examination of the dizzy patient is a structured, stand-alone series of tests after the standard otolaryngologic head and neck examination has been completed. Common disorders such as serous middle ear effusion, nasal airway obstruction, and sinusitis can cause dizziness and must be excluded. Table 165.3 outlines the structure of the neurotologic examination for dizziness. In the following section, each test is described and the interpretation discussed.

TABLE 165.3	THE NEUROTOLOGIC EXAMINATION OF THE DIZZY PATIENT

Examination	Test Performance	Outcome	Interpretation of Clinical Finding
Spontaneous nystagmus	Static visual fixation	Nystagmus waveform, direction, effect of fixation	Peripheral: Horizontal–rotary jerk nystagmus, suppresses with visual fixation Central: direction changing, horizontal, vertical, torsional, or pendular nystagmus, enhances with visual fixation
Gaze-evoked nystagmus	<30° eccentric gaze	Nystagmus waveform, direction	Peripheral: Direction-fixed nystagmus, increases while gazing in the direction of the fast phase (Alexander law) Brainstem or cerebellum: Direction-changing nystagmus, fast-phase movement in the direction of gaze, or rebound nystagmus in neutral gaze CPA mass: Brun nystagmus (direction-changing nystagmus caused by a combination of central GEN and vestibular nystagmus)
Saccades	Alternate fixation on two stationary targets	Accuracy, conjugate movement, velocity, and initiation	Peripheral: normal. Abnormalities indicate a central etiology
Smooth pursuit	Track visual target	Smooth versus jerking eye movements	Normal in peripheral vestibular pathology. Abnormalities (e.g., catch-up saccades) indicate a central etiology
Fixation suppression	Rotate examination chair ± visual fixation	Effect of fixation on rotation-induced nystagmus	Normal fixation suppression in peripheral pathology. Failure of fixation suppression suggests central (flocular) dysfunction
Head impulse test (HIT)	Rotational head thrusts while maintaining visual fixation	Refixation saccade	Peripheral vestibular dysfunction: Refixation saccade generated with rotational head thrusts toward the weak side
Head heave test (HHT)	Linear head heaves while maintaining visual fixation	Refixation saccade	Otolith damage: Refixation saccade generated with linear head heaves toward the damaged side

TABLE 165.3	THE NEUROTOLOGIC EXAMINATION OF THE DIZZY PATIENT (*Continued*)

Examination	Test Performance	Outcome	Interpretation of Clinical Finding
Postheadshake nystagmus	Headshake	Nystagmus direction	Asymmetric peripheral damage: nystagmus (in plane of damaged canal with fast phase toward stronger ear). Central: cross-coupling of nystagmus
Dynamic visual acuity (DVA)	Visual acuity (static vs. head movement)	Visual acuity decline	Peripheral vestibular dysfunction: Visual acuity decline (>2 lines on Snellen chart)
Positional testing	Various static head positions	Nystagmus onset, direction, duration, effect of fixation	Peripheral: Severe vertigo, transient, and usually direction fixed. Removing visual fixation[a] enhances nystagmus. Central: Usually asymptomatic, persistent, direction changing, and may be disconjugate. Removing visual fixation[a] improves nystagmus
Positioning testing	Head movement to various head positions (e.g., *Dix-Hallpike*)	Nystagmus latency, direction, duration, fatigability, reversal	Peripheral: see Table 165.4 for details of posterior, horizontal, and superior semicircular canal BPPV. Central: Immediate (no latency), persists >1 min, no reversal nystagmus, no fatigue, direction changing, no vertigo
Limb coordination tests	Limb coordination tests[b]	Limb coordination. Arm drift with past pointing	Peripheral (vestibulospinal): All limb coordination tests, except past pointing, are normal Past pointing: excessive arm drift toward side of peripheral lesion. Central: abnormalities in any of the tests
Gait	Tandem gait, Unterberger (Fukuda) stepping test	Gait abnormalities. Rotation with stepping	Peripheral: Abnormal tandem gait with eyes closed, rotation to side of lesion with stepping test. Central: Gait abnormalities (e.g., ataxia, shuffling, etc.)
Posture	Romberg tests	Excessive sway and fall	Peripheral: Fall on tandem and foam Romberg tests (eyes closed)
Mastoid vibration	Vibration source on mastoid	Nystagmus direction	Nystagmus in the plane of the affected canal toward the stronger ear
Malleolar sign	256-Hz tuning fork on malleolus	Conductive hyperacusis	Patient hears tuning fork vibration on side of superior canal dehiscence
Pressure-evoked eye movements	Tragal compression, pneumatic otoscopy, Valsalva maneuvers	Eye movement, vertigo	Perilymph fistula, otic syphilis, or semicircular canal dehiscence
Sound-evoked eye movements	Pure tones (≈100 dB)	Eye movement, vertigo	Perilymph fistula, otic syphilis, or semicircular canal dehiscence
Hyperventilation-induced nystagmus	Hyperventilate for 90 s	Nystagmus direction	Peripheral: excitatory nystagmus toward affected ear[c]

In CNS demyelinating diseases.
[a]Frenzel lenses and infrared video goggles remove visual fixation.
[b]Finger-to-nose, finger–nose–finger, hand rapid alternating movement test, fine finger movements, heel-to-shin, past pointing test.
[c]Hyperventilation-induced nystagmus may also occur.
BPPV, benign paroxysmal positional vertigo; CPA, cerebellopontine angle.

Equipment

Figure 165.2 illustrates the minimal equipment required for the structured neurotologic examination. Three tuning forks are used (i.e., 128, 256, and 512 Hz). The 128-Hz fork is used to assess vibrotactile sensation in the lower extremities (often reduced in peripheral neuropathy). The 256 Hz is used for the malleolar test, where patients with a third-window pathology (e.g., superior SCC dehiscence) can abnormally perceive the sound in the affected ear while the fork is placed on the ankle. The 512-Hz fork is the standard auditory stimulus for Weber and Rinne testing. The Frenzel lenses allow for ocular examination without visual fixation, which can enhance peripheral vestibular nystagmus. The pneumatic otoscope (including a Siegel speculum) is used to introduce positive and negative pressures into the external auditory canal to elicit eye movement

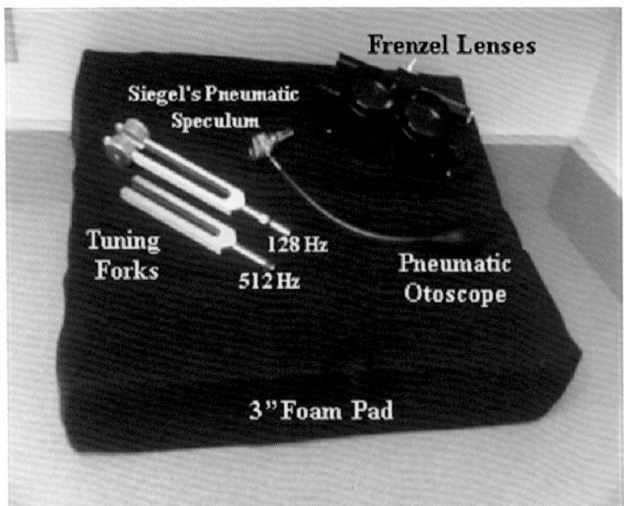
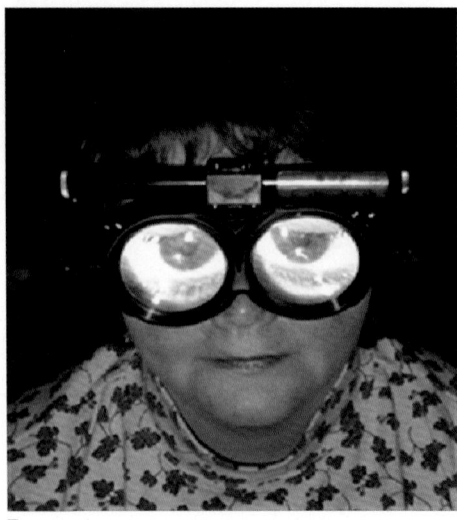

A   **B**

Figure 165.2 Tools necessary for a neurotologic examination of the dizzy patient. **A:** Tools include (1) tuning forks: 512 Hz for standard auditory stimulus (Weber and Rinne testing), 128 Hz to assess vibrotactile sensation in the lower extremities, and 256 Hz (not shown) for the malleolar test for third-window pathology, (2) a pneumatic otoscope including a Siegel pneumatic speculum to assess tympanic membrane mobility and to assess third-window pathology, (3) Frenzel lenses, and (4) a 3" foam pad for the foam Romberg test. **B:** Frenzel lenses provide magnification of the eyes and remove visual fixation. Peripheral vestibular nystagmus is enhanced and central nystagmus is suppressed when visual fixation is removed using Frenzel lenses.

associated with SCC dehiscence or PLF. Finally, the 3-inch foam pad is used to alter sensory input to the proprioceptive system during quiet stance with eyes closed to emphasize the use of vestibular cues for balance.

Spontaneous Nystagmus

At present, no clinical test can directly measure peripheral vestibular function. However, observing eye movements enables the examiner to gain important information regarding vestibular function. Under normal circumstances, when subjects are seated and gaze straight ahead, there is no rhythmic movement of the eyes. If, however, the eyes have a repetitive to-and-fro motion, then the term *nystagmus* is used to describe the abnormal, rhythmic oscillation. Characterizing nystagmus components often allows the examiner to infer the etiology of the eye movement and/or location of the lesion. The most common type of nystagmus is *jerk nystagmus* (e.g., *vestibular nystagmus*), which consists of a slow phase and a fast phase. Vestibular control of eye movements results in the slow phase, while the fast phase is caused by the rapid resetting of the eyes in the orbit. Jerk nystagmus is often named by the direction of the fast phase.

Test Performance

The patient is seated in an upright position and fixates on a stationary target in primary gaze position with best-corrected vision (with glasses or contact lenses in place if applicable). The patient should be queried about mono-vision correction because monovision can be associated with the inability to verge normally. The examiner

observes the eyes for nystagmus or rhythmic refixation eye movements. The procedure is repeated under Frenzel lenses to remove target fixation. The following nystagmus characteristics are noted: (a) Waveform. Does the nystagmus have a fast phase and slow phase (*jerk nystagmus*), or are the movements equal in both directions (*pendular nystagmus*)? Is the waveform consistent or does it change? (b) Direction. In cases of horizontal or vertical jerk nystagmus, in which direction does the fast phase beat (i.e., right, left, up, or down)? For purely torsional nystagmus, the direction of movement of the upper pole of the eye is described as either a clockwise or counterclockwise rotation from the examiner's perspective. If the nystagmus has mixed components, each feature can be described (e.g., left clockwise horizontal rotary). (c) Effect of fixation. What is the relative intensity of the nystagmus with and without visual fixation? (d) Effect of gaze. What is the effect of eccentric gaze on the quality and intensity of the spontaneous nystagmus?

Interpretation

Under normal conditions, there is no spontaneous nystagmus with visual fixation and only minimal spontaneous nystagmus if any under Frenzel lenses. Vestibular nystagmus is usually direction fixed; that is, regardless of the direction of the patient's gaze, the direction of the nystagmus does not change. Unilateral, vestibular hypofunction causes an imbalance in the tonic activity of the VOR and tends to cause eye movement in the plane of the damaged SCC. This input asymmetry usually results in a spontaneous, direction-fixed, horizontal-rotary jerk nystagmus with fast-phase movement toward the healthy ear (away from the damaged side). Removing visual fixation (e.g., placing Frenzel lenses on a patient) or gazing in the direction of the fast phase enhances the nystagmus, while gazing in the direction of the slow phase suppresses the nystagmus. This effect is called *Alexander law*. Alexander classified nystagmus as first-, second-, and third-degree nystagmus. First-degree nystagmus is the least intense and is only observed with gaze toward the fast phase. Second-degree nystagmus is more intense and is observed with the eyes in primary gaze position or when gazing toward the fast phase. Third-degree nystagmus is the most intense and is present when the eyes are in primary gaze position, gazing toward the fast phase or, gazing in the direction of the slow phase. If second- and third-degree nystagmus are present, the finding represents an acute condition or a greater disparity between the good and bad sides. Characterizing the vestibular nystagmus degree is important in determining the time course and degree of compensation for a peripheral vestibular lesion. For example, immediately after unilateral peripheral vestibular damage (e.g., vestibular ablative surgery or vestibular neuronitis), third-degree nystagmus is observed. Over the next several days, the nystagmus intensity declines passing through the stages of second- and then first-degree nystagmus. It has been postulated that the neural integrator, which is responsible for gaze-holding, is disabled when the nervous system is presented with a sudden sustained asymmetric vestibular input. The nystagmus intensity declines as the central system compensates (for a thorough description, see Ref. (40)).

In contrast, central lesions of the brainstem and cerebellum may cause direction-changing horizontal, vertical, torsional, or pendular nystagmus that may appear diminished under Frenzel lenses. Medications and alcohol may also induce a variety of nystagmus patterns. The most common form of central nystagmus is *congenital nystagmus*, which has been present since early childhood. This type of nystagmus is direction changing and waveform changing with the direction of gaze. Furthermore, there is a reduction in nystagmus with convergence, eye closure, and eccentric gaze (*null point*). Acquired forms of central nystagmus represent a failure of the central gaze-holding mechanisms in the brainstem and cerebellum or intrusions of inappropriate fast, eye movements (*saccades*) during attempted fixation. Nystagmus is reduced or absent without fixation under Frenzel lenses. *Periodic alternating nystagmus* (PAN) is a type of horizontal spontaneous nystagmus, which is also indicative of a CNS etiology. PAN is observed with the eyes in neutral gaze, and the direction of the horizontal nystagmus changes approximately every 2 minutes. Between each episode, there is often between 5 and 20 seconds where there is no nystagmus, downbeating, or upbeating nystagmus. Visual fixation has no effect on PAN and results from cerebellar pathology. It is important that the examiner observe the patient in neutral gaze for several minutes, or PAN can be missed.

Gaze-Evoked Nystagmus

GEN is a type of nystagmus that results when the eyes assume an eccentric position in the orbit. Normally, coordinated contraction of the extraocular muscles under the control of the central neural integrator is required to hold the eccentric gaze. Transient GEN is normal at extreme gaze (greater than 30 degrees from midline) and is called *end-point nystagmus*. However, any rhythmic eye movement with attempts to hold the eyes in an eccentric position within 0 to 30 degrees off midline is abnormal.

Test Performance

With the patient seated using best-corrected vision (glasses or contacts), the examiner holds his/her finger 20 to 30 degrees from the nasal root, first in the horizontal plane and then in the vertical plane, for 10 to 20 seconds in each position. The patient is asked to fixate on the examiner's fingertip. The direction and waveform of any GEN are noted. If GEN is observed with the fast phase in the direction of gaze, the examiner has the patient hold the eccentric gaze for 30 to 60 seconds, then, refixate on a fingertip held in center position. The examiner observes for a reversed fast-phase direction (*rebound nystagmus*).

Interpretation

GEN may be observed in peripheral vestibular dysfunction or in lesions of the brainstem or vestibulocerebellum. Direction-fixed GEN that increases while gazing in the direction of the fast phase (*Alexander law*) suggests unilateral peripheral vestibular dysfunction. Direction-changing GEN with fast-phase movement in the direction of gaze and/or the presence of rebound nystagmus in primary gaze indicates impairment of the brainstem or midline cerebellum (vestibulocerebellum). This observation is rarely observed in isolated peripheral vestibular injury. The vestibulocerebellum (especially the flocculonodular lobes) plays a key role in maintaining eccentric gaze. Structural lesions, degenerative conditions, CNS depressant drugs, or alcohol can give rise to GEN. However, the presence of a few transient nystagmus beats with a gaze greater than 30 degrees off midline is common and should not be confused with pathologic gaze nystagmus, which is persistent and observed at gaze angles less than 30 degrees.

Patients with a CPA mass large enough to compress the ipsilateral cerebellar flocculus may display *Brun nystagmus*. Brun nystagmus results from a combination of central (GEN) and peripheral (vestibular nystagmus). It is a gaze-dependent, direction-changing nystagmus. In primary gaze position, the patient usually does not have nystagmus. For example, if the patient has a right CPA tumor, they will have a left-beating vestibular nystagmus (small amplitude, higher frequency) with left gaze (away from the lesion). With right gaze (toward the lesion), a right-beating GEN (large amplitude, low frequency) is often observed (for a thorough description, see Ref. (40)).

Saccades

Conjugate movement of the eyes to a new visual target is generated by the command saccadic system. Saccadic eye movements involve the frontal and parietal eye fields, paramedian pontine reticular formation, medial longitudinal fasciculus, superior colliculus, and oculomotor nuclei III, IV, and VI.

Test Performance

Saccadic eye movements are examined by having the patient alternatively fixate on two stationary targets without moving their head. Using best-corrected vision and keeping the head stationary, the patient is asked to look back and forth between the examiner's nose (in neutral position) and fingertip (held 15 degrees off midline (repeat in the right and left horizontal plane as well as up and down in the vertical plane). Observe for the following eye movement characteristics: accuracy of target acquisition, conjugate movement, velocity (especially slowing), and latency of onset (initiation). Abnormalities in saccadic eye movements may be difficult to detect in the clinic examination. Videonystagmography may be necessary in order to identify subtle abnormalities.

Interpretation

Patients with peripheral vestibular pathology have normal saccadic eye movement; oculomotor abnormalities indicate ocular or CNS pathology. The midline cerebellum and fastigial nuclei control saccadic accuracy, whereas velocity, latency, and conjugate deviation are controlled by the brainstem and frontal eye fields. Abnormalities in saccadic initiation may be seen in Parkinson disease and Huntington disease. Voluntary saccades have increased latency and hypometria, whereas involuntary saccades are normal. Small-amplitude saccades are characteristic of myasthenia gravis or an abnormality in the orbit. Cortical and brainstem diseases exhibit slow saccades. Progressive supranuclear palsy (PSP) is characterized by slow vertical saccades initially as well as slow and *hypometric* (undershoot) horizontal saccades. Olivopontocerebellar atrophy (OPCA), also known as spinocerebellar ataxia (SCA), is characterized by slow saccades, especially in the horizontal direction. Inaccurate saccades (*dysmetria*) are associated with cerebellar vermis and fastigial nuclei lesions. For example, Wallenberg syndrome (i.e., lateral medullary infarction) is characterized by *hypermetria* (overshoot) toward the lesion and hypometria away from the lesion. Lesions of the frontal eye fields produce an increased latency for contralateral saccades. Pathology of the medial longitudinal fasciculus produces *internuclear ophthalmoplegia* (INO), which is frequently associated with multiple sclerosis. INO is characterized by disconjugate eye movements with slowing of the adducting eye and overshoots and/or nystagmus of the abducting eye. INO is often associated with a monocular nystagmus in the adducting eye contralateral to the lesion.

Normally, subjects can suppress saccades when visually fixating on a target. Saccadic intrusions are inappropriate movements that divert the eye from the target during attempted visual fixation. There are several types of saccadic intrusions, all of which are signs of an abnormal central process. *Square-wave jerks* are small (0.5 degrees), horizontal, involuntary saccades that take the eye off the target. After a 250-ms intersaccadic interval, a corrective saccade brings the eye back to the target. Square-wave jerks can be seen in older people. In younger individuals, square-wave jerks may be a sign of anxiety or else brainstem or cerebellar pathology. If saccades occur during visual fixation and lack an intersaccadic interval, they are termed *ocular flutter* (occur only in the horizontal direction) or *opsoclonus* (occur in all directions). Ocular flutter and opsoclonus can result from structural lesion of the pons or cerebellum, viral encephalitis, or a paraneoplastic syndrome (41).

Smooth Pursuit

Smooth pursuit is the visual tracking of moving objects caused by either target movement and/or movement of the viewer. The tracking capability of objects using foveal vision is dependent on many factors, including velocity, brightness, and predictability of the target as well as the visual acuity and age of the viewer. Smooth pursuit requires intact central optic tracts through the brainstem, visual cortices in the occipital lobes, and the flocculonodular lobes of the cerebellum. Patients must have accurate acuity (either natural or corrected) in order to perform accurate smooth pursuit. Individuals younger than 40 years of age can pursue a visual target up to 100 degrees per second with a steady decline to 60 degrees per second with advancing age. Furthermore, bright discrete targets are much easier to pursue than are dim ill-defined visual targets. The visual cortex senses relative target movement and initiates voluntary ocular tracking. The cerebellum ensures accurate pursuit by minimizing slippage of the image off the fovea. Next, the pursuit signal is compared and integrated with vestibular input in the brainstem, and a unified signal is transmitted to the oculomotor nuclei. Finally, the appropriate ocular muscle response is generated. It is clear, therefore, that abnormal ocular pursuit can arise from a variety of lesions within this complex pathway. Thus, the examiner must take many factors into consideration when testing and interpreting ocular pursuit abnormalities.

Test Performance

To assess smooth pursuit, the examiner positions his/her index finger directly in front of the patient and moves the target smoothly 20 to 30 degrees per second, first in the horizontal plane and then in the vertical plane. The testing area is restricted to the central 60 degrees of the visual field (30 degrees to the left, right, up, and down from neutral position) to avoid provoking physiologic end-gaze nystagmus. Using best-corrected vision (glasses or contacts), the patient is asked to track the examiner's finger. The examiner must assure that the patient can visualize the target clearly and is attentive to the task. The examiner performs three to five cycles in each plane, noting the degree of ocular tracking smoothness and any corrective eye movements. After testing smooth pursuit, the examiner should test vergence. The patient is asked to follow the examiner's finger as it moves toward and away from the bridge of the patient's nose. The examiner should note if the eyes move smoothly together or if there are jerking movements.

Interpretation

In the presence of adequate visual acuity as well as appropriate target speed and velocity, smooth pursuit is generally intact in patients with peripheral vestibular disease. Occasionally, patients with acute unilateral vestibular dysfunction and spontaneous nystagmus may exhibit impaired tracking when they move their eyes in the direction of the fast phase of their spontaneous nystagmus. Patients with poor visual acuity or inattention to the task demonstrate large irregular fast eye movements (*saccades*) to catch up to the target. In central lesions, a more global failure of pursuit is evident. *Catch-up saccades* refixate the eye on the visual target in order to compensate for the pursuit deficit (*saccadic pursuit*).

Most abnormalities affect smooth pursuit symmetrically. A common cause is medication, such as anticonvulsants and sedatives as well as alcohol. The examiner should be aware that smooth pursuit performance progressively deteriorates as a patient's age increases or visual acuity declines (42–45). Furthermore, smooth pursuit is impaired by neurologic conditions such as Parkinson disease, Alzheimer disease, supranuclear degeneration, and cerebellar degeneration (41). Less frequently, abnormalities in smooth pursuit may be asymmetric. Focal central lesions may include the frontal cortex (frontal eye fields) (46), posterior cortex (47), flocculus of the cerebellum, brainstem, and thalamus (41).

Vergence eye movements are disjunctive coordinated eye movements. In other words, the two eyes move in opposite directions in response to a change in gaze. As an object moves toward the nose, each eye converges. Vergence, accommodation of the lens, and pupillary constriction are necessary for maintenance of acuity during close target viewing. As the object moves away from the nose, the eyes diverge. Vergence abnormalities can occur due to lesions of the midbrain or cerebellum or in association with medication.

Fixation Suppression of Rotation-Induced Nystagmus

Fixation suppression testing yields a qualitative assessment of visual–vestibular interaction. While classically, fixation suppression has been tested after caloric stimulation, a bedside evaluation can obtain similar information. Under normal conditions, fixation suppresses both optokinetic eye movements and vestibular-induced nystagmus. Normal fixation suppression is dependent on vision and requires normal cerebellar function.

Test Performance

To test fixation suppression, the patient is seated upright in the examination chair. Using best-corrected vision, the examination chair is unlocked and rotated up to 2 Hz without fixation. The examiner observes the eyes for nystagmus. Next, the patient fixates on his/her outstretched thumb while the chair and the visual target rotate simultaneously. The examiner observes the eyes and notes whether or not there is a decrease in the visual–vestibular nystagmus compared to rotation without ocular fixation.

Interpretation

The modulation of nystagmus invoked by rotation is a CNS phenomenon that is heavily dependent on the cerebellar flocculus. When fixation suppression is normal, the eyes remain fixated on the visual target while rotating, and no nystagmus is observed. However, if the fixation suppression is abnormal, the eyes continuously slip off the visual target during rotation due to the VOR. A refixation saccade is required to realign the eyes with the target. This refixation saccade is observed as a nystagmus. Failure of fixation suppression in the presence of adequate visual acuity is related to smooth pursuit abnormalities and implies cerebellar floccular dysfunction. Patients with peripheral vestibular abnormality have normal fixation suppression.

Head Impulse Test

The head impulse test (HIT) is a bedside technique used to detect unilateral or bilateral vestibular hypofunction. To understand this test (and many of the following tests), one must understand Ewald's three laws (48). *Ewald's first law* states that the trajectory of nystagmus generated by an SCC is in the same anatomic plane of that particular SCC (48). *Ewald's second law* is based on experiments conducted on the horizontal SCC and states that ampullopetal endolymph flow (toward the ampulla) causes a greater vestibular response than ampullofugal endolymph flow (away from the ampulla) (48,49). In other words, excitatory input is a stronger vestibular stimulus than inhibitory input (50). *Ewald's third law* is based on experiments conducted on the vertical (superior and posterior) SCCs. These experiments found that ampullofugal endolymph flow produces a greater vestibular response than does ampullopetal endolymph flow (48). Therefore, ampullofugal endolymph flow is excitatory in the two vertical SCCs.

The HIT is a method of detecting asymmetries in vestibular gain from the SCCs. In patients with profound or absent SCC function, the VOR cannot produce signals to the ocular muscles for eye stabilization during high-frequency, passive angular head rotations. Consequently, the brain must generate a refixation saccade to acquire a visual target (51,52). Saccade refixation occurs in response to passive angular head movements toward the involved ear in patients with unilateral vestibular loss. Usually, symmetrical saccadic refixation occurs in patients with bilateral vestibular loss.

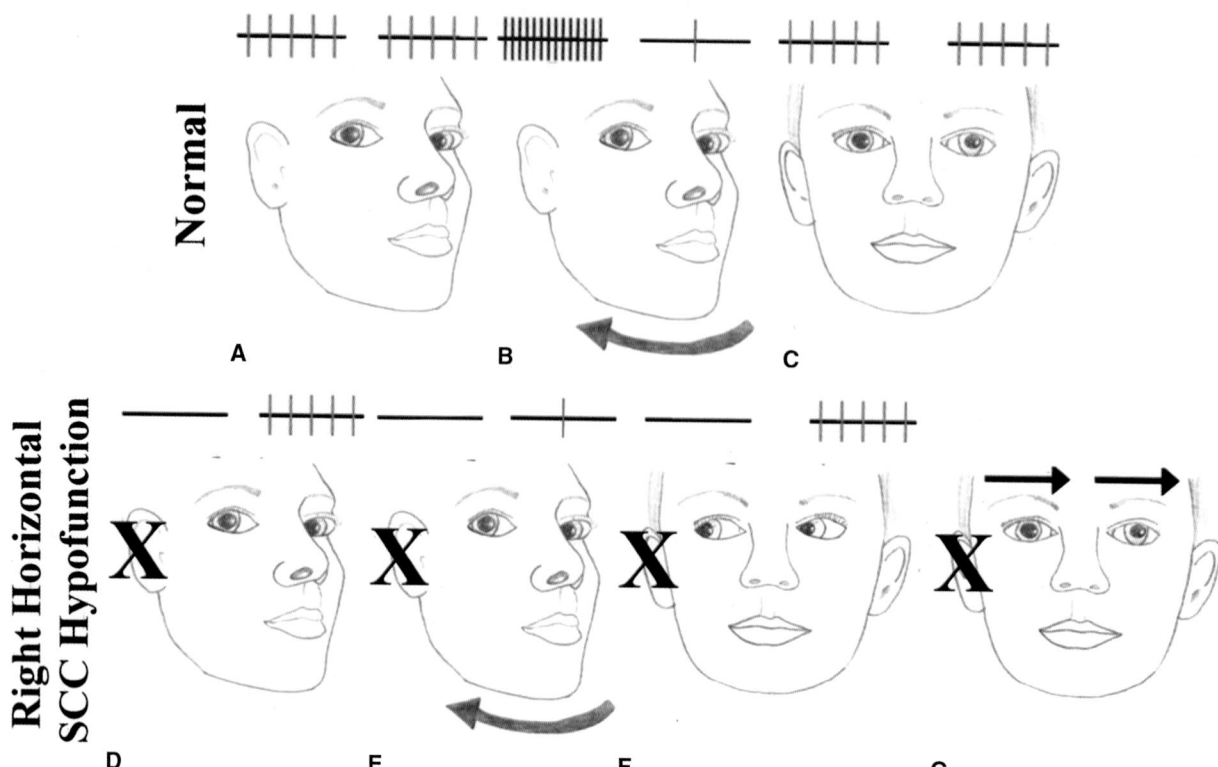

Figure 165.3 Head impulse test (HIT) in normal and unilateral vestibular dysfunction. The stages of the HIT are exemplified in a normal subject (**A–C**) and in a patient with right horizontal SCC hypofunction (**D–G**). The test begins with the patient's head at 30 degrees off midline while the patient fixates on the examiner's nose (**A, D**). **A:** In the normal subject at rest, the primary afferents of both horizontal SCCs (*green*) fire at a resting basal rate. Since the input is symmetric, the brainstem detects no motion. **B:** In the normal subject, the examiner thrusts the head rapidly (greater than 200 degrees/s or greater than 2,000 degrees/s²) to the midline (from **left** to **right**). The discharge rate of the HSCC afferents ipsilateral to the velocity vector increases (*red*, **right**). The discharge rate of the HSCC afferents contralateral to the velocity vector decreases (*blue*, **left**). With an intact VOR, the brainstem detects asymmetric input, and the eyes are driven contralateral (**left**) to the higher firing rate (*red*, **right**). **C:** Visual fixation is maintained throughout the HIT, and the HSCC afferents return to their basal firing rate. **D:** When one labyrinth is damaged (indicated with an X), the firing rate of the right afferents decreases. **E:** The head is thrust toward the damaged side (**left** to **right**). Although the firing rate in the healthy HSCC afferents (*blue*, **left**) decreases compared to the resting position, the rate is higher than that of the right damaged side. **F:** Therefore, the eyes are driven contralateral to the healthy side and ipsilateral to the damaged side (**right**). **G:** In order to reset visual fixation, a saccadic eye movement is necessary. Abbreviations: HIT, head impulse test; HSCC, horizontal semicircular canal.

However, recent studies have shown that some bilateral vestibular loss patients have covert corrective saccades (53,54). Covert saccades are small corrective saccades that occur during the actual head movement toward their affected side. These small covert saccades are difficult for the examiner to detect with their naked eye. Therefore, eye movement recordings are required to detect the abnormality (53,54). This HIT can be performed in all three canal pair orientations and has been a significant addition to the neurotologic examination in the office (51,52,55).

Test Performance
The patient is instructed to fixate on the examiner's nose while the head is impulsively and unpredictably moved 20 to 30 degrees in one direction (Fig. 165.3). The examiner observes for any indication of ocular globe slippage off the target. The velocity of the head movement must exceed

200 degrees per second, and the acceleration must exceed 2,000 degrees per square second in order to exceed smooth pursuit capacity and fully inhibit the contribution of the contralateral ear for stabilization. To avoid neck injury, it is advisable to start at slower speeds and gradually increase to the desired velocity. The HIT is best performed in the plane of paired canals (Fig. 165.4). If the horizontal SCCs canals are being tested, the head is tilted forward 30 degrees (Fig. 165.4). Hence, the movement is in the horizontal (yaw) plane, causing ampullopetal stimulation of the canal on the same side as the movement and ampullofugal inhibition of the opposite canal (Fig. 165.3). It is desirable to move the head from an eccentric position back to midline rather than from midline to the side in order to minimize patient resistance and potential neck strain. To test the vertical canals, the examiner aligns the paired canals, right anterior (superior) and left posterior (RALP) or left anterior

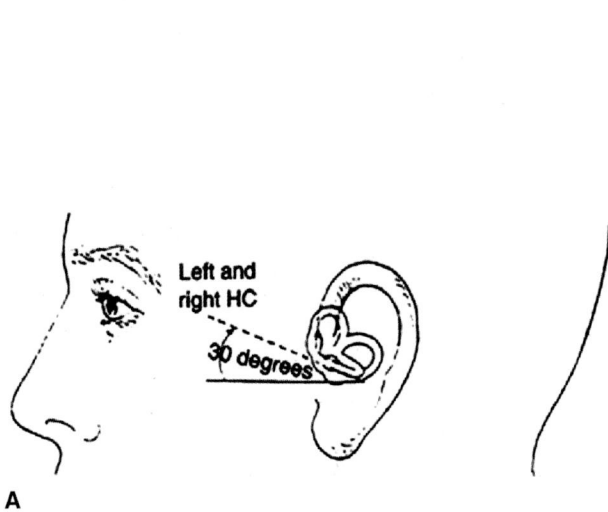

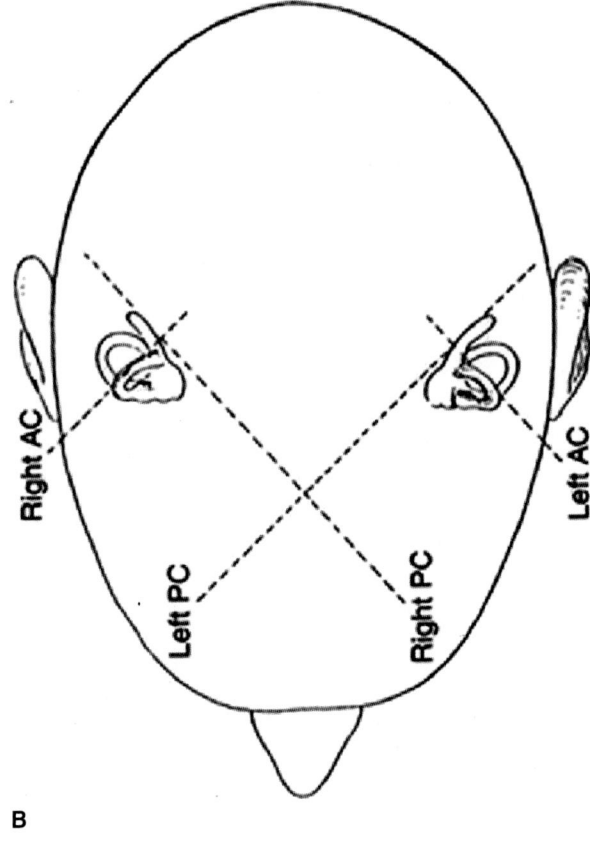

Figure 165.4 Orientation of the semicircular canals (SCCs) in the temporal bone. **A:** The horizontal SCCs are coplanar with one another and tilted 30 degrees to the horizontal plane. **B:** The vertical canals are aligned such that the anterior (superior) SCC on one side is coplanar with the posterior SCC on the other side. In other words, the right anterior (superior) and left posterior (RALP) SCCs are coplanar, and the left anterior and right posterior (LARP SCCs are coplanar. Abbreviations: AC, anterior canal; HC, horizontal canal; PC, posterior canal. (Adapted from Goebel JA (ed.). Practical anatomy and physiology. Chapter 1. In: *Practical Management of the Dizzy Patient*, 2nd ed. Philadelphia, PA: Lippincott Williams & Wilkins, 2008: 4).

and right posterior (LARP) (Fig. 165.4). HIT testing of the vertical canals involves head movements in the corresponding planes. In other words, to test the right anterior SCC, the head is turned 45 degrees to the left, and the head is thrust downward for ampullofugal stimulation. To test the left posterior SCC, the head is turned 45 degrees to the left, and the head is thrust upward causing ampullofugal stimulation (52,56). The examiner notes whether the eyes remain fixated on the target or whether the eyes travel with the head during the maneuver, and a *corrective saccade* is generated in order to refixate on the target. In general, the test is repeated 5 to 10 times to document repeatable fixation failure.

Interpretation

In healthy subjects, visual fixation is maintained during rapid head impulses, and no corrective saccades result. In cases of unilateral SCC dysfunction, head movement in the plane of the affected canal toward the lesioned side is accompanied by a repeatable eye slippage and corrective saccade in the opposite direction as the head movement. The observation of eye movement during the maneuver is a sign of decreased or absent neural input from the ipsilateral ear to the VOR. Reduced neural input results in little or no input to the VOR during rapid contralateral head movement, and the contralateral ear cannot supply enough neural activity to stabilize gaze. In such instances, the eye travels with the head during the high-velocity movement, and a refixation saccade is necessary

to refoveate the target. Bilateral refixation movements are seen frequently in cases of ototoxicity. In rare instances of a hyperactive VOR response, a corrective saccade is generated in the same direction as the head movement. In other words, the strength of the VOR response was excessive during rotation, and a corrective saccade was required to refixate the eye on the target. A positive HIT in the presence of acute vertigo and spontaneous nystagmus is suggestive of a peripheral rather than central etiology.

Head Heave Test

The otolith–ocular reflex stabilizes the retinal image by generating compensatory eye movements in response to linear head acceleration. The *head heave test (HHT)* is used to evaluate the translational VOR (57,58). The HHT is a variant of the HIT, although in this case, the HHT is used to assess utricular dysfunction (57,58).

Test Performance

For the HHT, the examiner places his/her hands over the sides of the patient's head. The patient is instructed to look at the examiner's nose, and the examiner imposes a series of quick, high-acceleration, linear, translational "heaves" along the interaural axis. The head is moved from a right lateral to midline position and then from a left lateral to midline position. Training and skill are essential to assure patient safety. The direction of refixation saccades is noted.

Interpretation

As with the HIT, in the healthy subject, the eyes remain fixed on the visual target. In a patient with unilateral utricular dysfunction, a catch-up saccade is noted during the HHT in the direction of the damaged side. This examination is difficult to perform, and there are some safety concerns as a bedside examination. However, delivering linear force via a sled in the testing laboratory offers a more practical solution and may yield information regarding otolith dysfunction (58,59).

Skew Deviation and Ocular Torsion Reaction Test

Skew deviation is a vertical misalignment of the eyes, which results from asymmetric activity along the peripheral (60–62) or central (63) pathways mediating the otolith–ocular reflex (64). Skew deviation often presents as vertical or torsional diplopia. First, the examiner must rule out that the ocular misalignment is due to extraocular muscle palsies.

Test Performance

The *alternate cover test* is used to detect skew deviation. The examiner asks the patient to fixate on a visual target and then covers one eye. The examiner then uncovers that eye and covers the contralateral eye, observing for a vertical refixation eye movement indicating a vertical misalignment.

Interpretation

In the normal condition, the eyes do not move or deviate spontaneously in the vertical plane. However, if there is skew deviation, vertical corrective saccades will occur during pursuit. Skew deviations resulting from otolith–ocular imbalance do not usually vary with eye position. Ocular tilt reaction (OTR) is an eye-head postural reaction consisting of head tilt (ear to shoulder), skew deviation, conjugated eye cyclotorsion, and alteration of vertical perception. OTR can be caused by peripheral vestibular lesions (62,65) or central lesions (63). The head usually tilts ipsilateral to the lower eye. Peripheral vestibular and vestibular nuclear lesions result in a skew deviation with the lower eye ipsilateral to the lesion (60–62,65).

Postheadshake Nystagmus Test

During head shaking, the vestibular labyrinths send neural input to the brainstem. As soon as head shaking ceases, this stored input is discharged over a short period of time (10 to 20 seconds). Unilateral damage to the peripheral vestibular organs leads to asymmetric input and discharge resulting in nystagmus. Clinical head-shaking nystagmus is useful in detecting asymmetric peripheral vestibular lesions (66–68) or asymmetric central lesions of the velocity storage mechanism.

Test Performance

To test for head-shaking nystagmus, the patient's head is tilted forward 30 degrees, and the head is either passively or actively rotated in the horizontal plane at a high frequency (2 Hz), low amplitude (20 to 30 degrees) for 20 seconds (Fig. 165.5). Then, the head is brought to an abrupt stop, and the examiner observes for the presence and direction of any postheadshake nystagmus. To avoid fixation, the

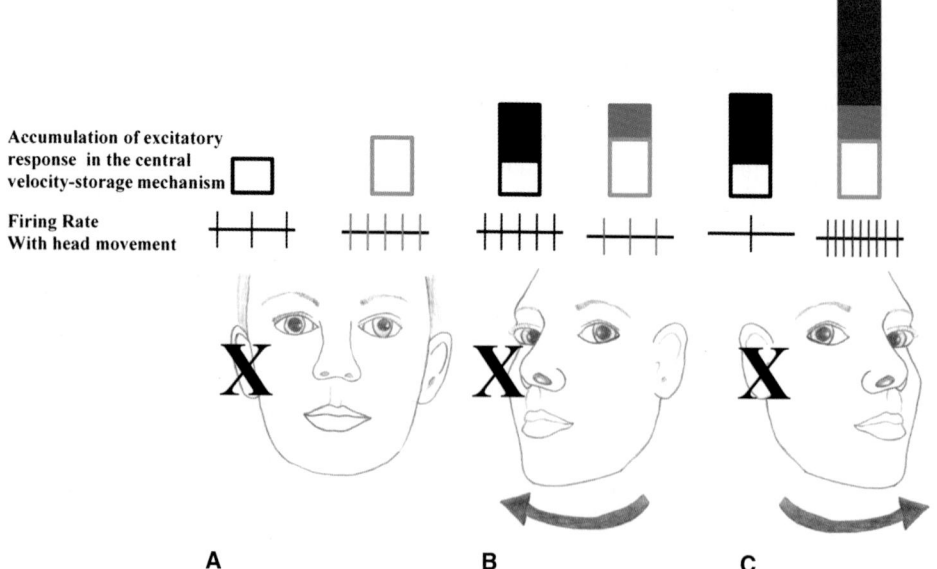

Figure 165.5 The postheadshake nystagmus test in a patient with right labyrinthine hypofunction. **A:** When the head is stationary, the asymmetry in basal firing rates between the healthy labyrinth (**left**, *green*) and the hypofunctioning labyrinth (**right**, *black*) is minimal. **B:** With head turns toward the hypofunctioning labyrinth (**right**, *black*), a weaker-than-normal excitatory response is elicited. The firing rate of the healthy labyrinth decreases (**left**, *blue*). **C:** Turning the head toward the healthy labyrinth (**left**, *red*) produces a normal excitatory response on the left. Each head rotation amplifies the asymmetry, and the activity accumulates in the central, velocity-storage mechanism. Following head shaking, stored activity is discharged from the velocity-storage center, and nystagmus results.

use of Frenzel lenses is preferred. The maneuver may be repeated in the vertical direction.

Interpretation

Postheadshake nystagmus is considered a pathologic sign of vestibular input asymmetry in the plane of rotation (66–68). If the input from the two vestibular labyrinths are symmetric (in the case of either a normal subject or an individual with symmetric, bilateral damaged), the stored vestibular activity that is discharged will cancel one another, and no nystagmus will occur. However, if the input from the vestibular labyrinths is asymmetric during head shaking (i.e., asymmetric damage to the vestibular labyrinths), then the central circuits will discharge asymmetrically, resulting in a burst of nystagmus (Fig. 165.5). Typically, a peripheral side is identified with the slow phase of nystagmus directed toward the "weaker" or abnormal ear and the fast phase directed toward the better ear. A smaller amplitude reversal of nystagmus direction is sometimes observed. Postheadshake nystagmus is not observed during an acute unilateral vestibular hypofunction because the central vestibular velocity storage system is temporarily disabled. Interpreting head-shaking nystagmus with the affected ear in Ménière's disease can be confusing as the direction depends on the excitation, paresis, or recovery phase of vestibular function following an attack. Central vestibular lesions may cause inappropriate cross-coupling of nystagmus, usually resulting in a prominent vertical nystagmus after horizontal head shaking. Signs of central etiologies can also include prolonged nystagmus and disconjugate nystagmus.

Dynamic Visual Acuity (DVA)

Maintenance of gaze stability during head movement is a complex interaction between the VOR, foveal smooth pursuit, optokinetic stimulation of the peripheral retina, and the cervico-ocular reflex. At low frequencies and peak velocities, the central oculomotor mechanisms are dominant. However, at higher frequencies and velocities, the VOR becomes the primary mechanism for maximizing visual acuity by limiting retinal slip. Standard tests of vestibular function (e.g., caloric and rotational stimulation) are useful to document deficits in low-frequency, horizontal, SCC VOR function. These tests, though, fail to assess VOR contribution to gaze stability that take place at higher frequencies and within the range of everyday head movements (1 to 4 Hz). Over the past few years, dynamic visual acuity testing (DVAT) has been developed and studied for the purpose of determining gaze stability during head movements at higher frequency (greater than 2 Hz) and peak velocity (greater than 120 degrees/s) (69–78). The DVAT compares the relative loss of visual acuity between head-still and head-moving conditions (measured in logarithmic minimal angle of resolution or logMAR). This calculation is accomplished by measuring the change in size of a visual target that a subject can accurately recognize from the resting condition (static visual acuity) to the head movement condition. The utility of the DVAT has been well documented in patients with unilateral vestibular dysfunction or bilateral vestibular loss as well as in the elderly (72,74,76,79,80).

Test Performance

With best-corrected vision, visual acuity is measured at rest using the Snellen eye chart. Visual acuity is again measured during passive horizontal head oscillations at 2 Hz. The change in visual acuity is determined. This test can also be conducted in the vertical (pitch) plane.

Interpretation

DVA is also referred to as the "dynamic illegible E test" (DIE) (71). An acuity decrease of more than two lines on the Snellen eye chart is abnormal. Excessive retinal slippage during head movement is a sign of vestibular dysfunction. In the clinical examination, the most frequent etiology is bilateral vestibular loss related to ototoxicity or aging. Poorly compensated, unilateral dysfunction can also cause loss of DVA. Nonetheless, using clinical testing, it is more challenging to identify a unilateral abnormality while simultaneously assessing DVA. During DVA assessment, it is important that the examiner shake the patient's head continually, avoiding pauses or slowing. A pause enables the patient to see the target and unconsciously attempt to compensate for their dysfunction.

Positional versus Positioning Testing

Nystagmus and vertigo can be induced by certain head postures (positional) or head movement in a specific trajectory (positioning). In other words, *positional nystagmus* is a nystagmus induced by a static head position in space. *Positioning nystagmus* is induced by the actual movement of the head from one position in space to another. The goal of positional and positioning testing is to aid in vestibular lesion localization.

Positional Testing Examination

Positional testing involves observing the eyes for nystagmus in various static head positions with and without visual fixation. Observe the eyes for at least 30 seconds in each of the following head positions: upright looking straight ahead, supine, right ear down, and left ear down. If positional nystagmus is present, it will occur approximately 30 seconds after the new head position is assumed, and the effects of positioning head movement (positioning nystagmus) have waned. The examiner should note the nystagmus direction, effect with and without visual fixation, and if it is persistent and sustained. Removing visual fixation (Frenzel lenses or infrared video goggles) worsens peripheral positional nystagmus, but central positional nystagmus improves or stays the same. Technically, true BPPV is a positioning nystagmus and occurs in the plane of the canal that is stimulated, whereas central positional nystagmus may beat in the same direction regardless of head position.

Positional Testing Interpretation

Positional nystagmus can be found in both central and peripheral pathologies. Central positional nystagmus is usually asymptomatic, persistent, and may be disconjugate. Peripheral positional nystagmus is associated with severe vertigo, transient, and usually direction fixed. A central lesion is the most likely etiology when positional nystagmus is purely vertical (up or down) or purely torsional, and visual target fixation fails to suppress nystagmus.

Positioning Testing Examination

Positioning testing is the evaluation of nystagmus in response to head movement. Positioning testing can also help distinguish central from peripheral etiologies, determine which ear is damaged, and localize the involved SCC. To perform positioning testing, the eyes are observed as the head is moved into various positions: upright, supine, right ear down, and left ear down. Preventing visual fixation (Frenzel lenses or infrared video goggles) may enhance peripheral positioning nystagmus and may diminish central positioning nystagmus. The following five nystagmus characteristics should be noted during head positioning: (a) latency, (b) direction, (c) habituation (duration), (d) fatigability (decreased nystagmus on repeated maneuvers reflects adaptation), and (e) reversal upon rising to a sitting position.

BPPV is a positioning nystagmus. The most common positioning maneuver is the Dix-Hallpike test, which is used to identify posterior canal BPPV. In other words, does BPPV indicate positional or positioning vertigo? Are the terms interchanged? (Fig. 165.6). While the patient is in a sitting position, the examination chair is unfolded, and the patient's head is turned 45 degrees toward the side to be tested. The patient's head is rapidly moved in the plane of the posterior SCC to a head-hanging, slightly extended position (120 degrees from the upright position). This position is held for 30 seconds. While keeping the head

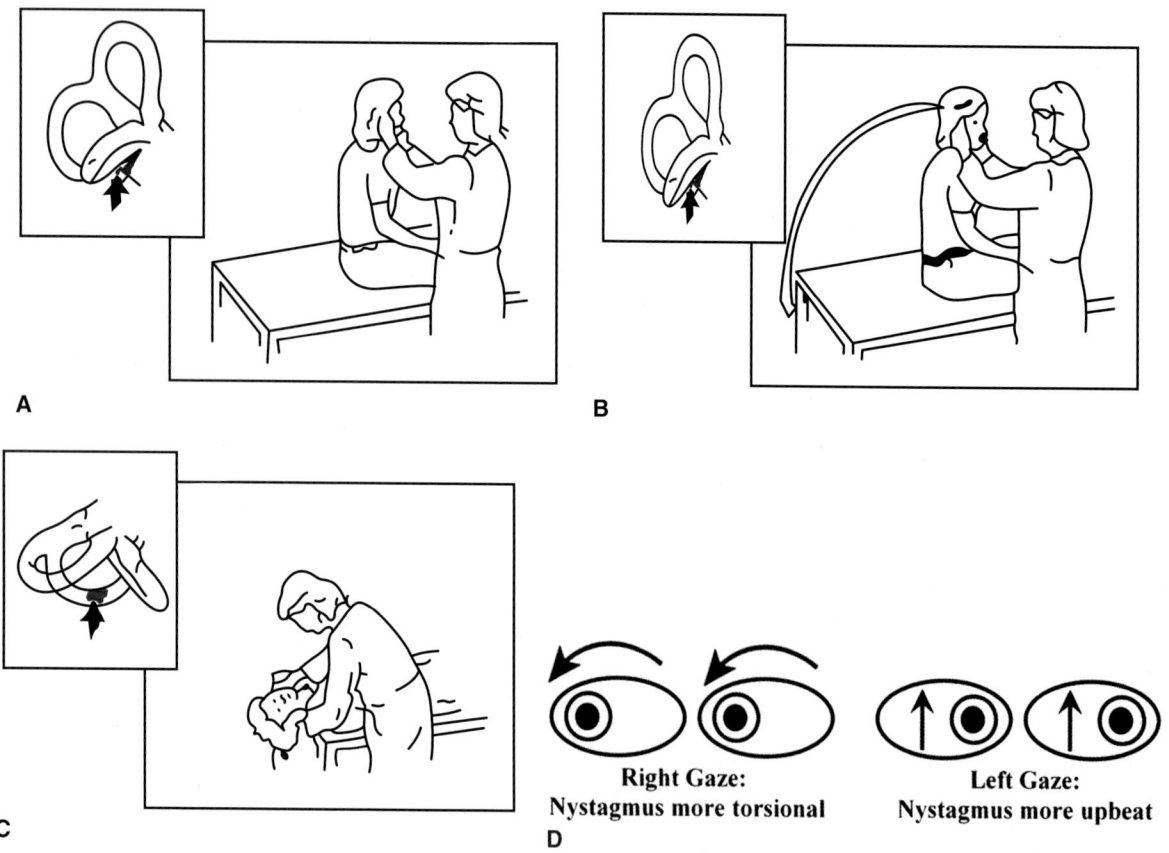

Figure 165.6 The Dix-Hallpike maneuver for diagnosing posterior SCC BPPV. The *arrow* in (**A–C**) points to the otolith debris in the right posterior SCC. **A:** While the patient is in a sitting position, the examination chair is unfolded, and the patient's head is turned 45 degrees toward the side to be tested (*right*). **B:** The patient's head is rapidly moved in the plane of the posterior SCC to a head-hanging, slightly extended position (120 degrees from the upright position). **C:** This position is held for 30 seconds, and the eyes are observed for latency, direction, duration, and fatigability of nystagmus. While keeping the head turned 45 degrees, the patient is brought back to an upright position and held for 30 seconds while the eyes are observed for reversal nystagmus. **D:** The arrows indicate the quick phase of the resulting upbeat geotropic–torsional nystagmus. With right gaze, the nystagmus is more geotropic–torsional. With left gaze, the nystagmus is more upbeat. (Adapted from Leigh RJ, Zee DS (eds.). Diagnosis and management of vestibular disorders, Chapter 11. In: *The Neurology of Eye Movements*. Oxford: Oxford University Press, 2006:572–573.)

turned 45 degrees, the patient is brought back to an upright position and held for 30 seconds while observing the eyes for nystagmus. This maneuver is then repeated on the contralateral side (Fig. 165.6). The examiner may need to perform a modified positioning maneuver in order to induce peripheral positioning nystagmus caused by horizontal SCC BPPV (81). In this maneuver, the patient is placed into the supine position, followed by turning the patient's head and body 90 degrees to the right side, back to supine, and then turn 90 degrees to the left side (82).

Positioning Testing Interpretation

BPPV is the most common cause of peripheral positioning nystagmus. BPPV is characterized by a sudden onset of episodic vertigo lasting up to 1 minute and is induced by head movement in certain positions. BPPV is caused by two mechanisms: canalithiasis (free-floating otolith debris in the endolymphatic space) or cupulolithiasis (otolith debris attached to the cupula of the SCCs) (83). The posterior SCC is affected in more than 90% of cases due to its gravity-dependent position. The horizontal SCC accounts for 6% to 8% of cases, while the superior SCC is rarely affected (less than 1%) (84,85).

For BPPV of the posterior SCC, a positive response is elicited when the head is turned toward the affected side, and the ear is positioned toward the ground. The resulting nystagmus is upbeating, geotropic torsional (upper pole of eye toward the ground). The nystagmus has a brief latency (5 to 20 seconds), less than 30 seconds duration, fatigability with repeated positioning, and in some instances, reversal nystagmus upon returning to an upright position (Table 165.4) (83). The reversal nystagmus is a downbeating, ageotropic-torsional (upper pole of eye away from the ground) nystagmus. Throughout the test, the patient is to report any vertigo sensations, which usually accompany BPPV. Vertigo without observed nystagmus may still provide a clue to the offending side and involved SCC. A positive Dix-Hallpike maneuver is diagnostic for posterior canal BPPV. Mastoid vibration may help move the otolithic debris out of the affected canal. In contrast, central positioning nystagmus is usually immediate (no latency),

persists longer than 1 minute, does not produce a reversal nystagmus, does not fatigue, is direction changing, and is not usually accompanied by vertigo.

BPPV can involve the horizontal SCC and may be spontaneous or result from a repositioning maneuver of the posterior SCC (86–88). Depending on the location of the debris within the horizontal SCC, the pattern of nystagmus is either horizontal geotropic (toward the ground) or horizontal ageotropic (away from the ground). If the debris is free-floating in the non-ampullated end of the right horizontal SCC (canalolithiasis), when the right ear is down, the debris flows toward the ampulla (ampullopetal). This results in a strong, horizontal geotropic right-beating nystagmus. When the right ear is up, the debris flows away from the right ampulla (ampullofugal), resulting in a weaker horizontal left-beating geotropic nystagmus. In contrast, if the debris is caught in the ampullated end of the right horizontal SCC (cupulolithiasis), when the right ear is down, the debris flows away from the ampulla. The result is a horizontal ageotropic left-beating nystagmus. When the right ear is up, the debris flows toward the ampulla, producing a stronger horizontal ageotropic right-beating nystagmus.

Therefore, how does the examiner decide which horizontal SCC contains the otolithic debris? In general, geotropic nystagmus is stronger when the lesioned ear is placed downward. However, when the nystagmus is ageotropic, the stronger nystagmus response occurs when the lesioned ear is placed upward. Additionally, both canalithiasis (free-floating debris) and cupulolithiasis (debris caught on the cupula) can occur in horizontal SCC BPPV. In canalithiasis, movement of the free-floating debris in the affected ear causes a more transient nystagmus, whereas with cupulolithiasis, the nystagmus duration is longer (30 to 60 seconds) (Table 165.4).

The bow and lean test (BLT) can also be used to distinguish which side contains the otolithic debris in horizontal SCC BPPV (89,90). From a seated position, the patient tips the head forward in a "bow" position and then backward into a "lean" position, and the resultant nystagmus in each position is noted. In right horizontal SCC canalolithiasis, during the bow position, the debris will fall with gravity toward the ampulla, resulting in a strong right-beating (ipsilesional) horizontal nystagmus. Conversely, when the patient tips the head backward, the debris now flows away from the ampulla, producing a weaker left-beating (contralesional) horizontal nystagmus. The opposite is true for canalolithiasis, where the nystagmus is directed toward the affected ear in the lean position and away from the affected side in the bow position.

Superior SCC BPPV is rare. Otolithic debris does not usually enter the SCC due to its anatomic position. In superior SCC BPPV, when the affected ear is away from the ground, a downbeating, ageotropic-torsional nystagmus results (Table 165.4) (91–93). However, debris in the downmost posterior SCC moving toward the cupula can produce an identical nystagmus pattern to that of the uppermost superior SCC. Therefore, special care must be taken to avoid confusing the two types.

TABLE 165.4	BPPV OF THE POSTERIOR, HORIZONTAL, AND SUPERIOR SEMICIRCULAR CANALS		
	Posterior	**Horizontal**	**Superior**
Incidence	90%	6–8%	<1%
Latency	5–20 s	0–3 s	Variable
Duration	<30 s	Variable	Variable
Direction	Upbeating, geotropic–torsional	Horizontal (geotropic or ageotropic)	Downbeating, ageotropic–torsional
Fatigability	Yes	Variable	Yes

Abbreviation: BPPV, benign paroxysmal positional vertigo.

Limb Coordination Tests

Examining limb coordination provides the examiner with important clues needed to diagnose and exclude central lesions of the cerebellum and brainstem (Table 165.5). Peripheral vestibular lesions will not cause limb coordination abnormalities. In order to examine limb coordination, the patient is observed performing a series of tasks. The right and left extremities are examined separately.

Test Performance

For the *finger-to-nose test*, the examiner asks the patient to close his/her eyes, place one arm in full horizontal arm extension, and then touch his/her own nose with the index finger of the extended hand. For the *finger–nose–finger test*, the patient should alternate touching the examiner's finger and his/her own nose. As the patient touches their nose, the examiner quickly moves their finger to a new horizontal position. This test assesses the patient's ability to accurately judge the position of a target. For the *hand rapid alternating movement test*, the examiner asks the patient to alternate hand pronation and supination by tapping the back of the hand on the thigh and then the front of the hand on the thigh in a rapid succession. To assess *fine finger movements*, the examiner asks the patient to touch their own thumb to each of their four fingers on the same hand in rapid

sequence. To test lower limb coordination, the examiner can use the *heel-to-shin test*. The patient is asked to fully extend their right leg and place their heel on the floor. The patient smoothly moves the heel of the left foot along the shin of the extended right leg. The test is repeated with the left leg extended. During each of the above tests, the examiner observes for dysmetria or dysrhythmia. For the *past pointing test*, the patient is asked to extend both arms and point to the ceiling with both index fingers. With eyes open, the patient brings the arms down into the horizontal position to touch the examiner's index fingers. This test is repeated with the patient's eyes closed. The examiner notes if he/she observes excessive drift of the arms toward the right or the left.

Interpretation

The presence of limb dysmetria or dysdiadochokinesia is a useful indicator of cerebellar disease, which may or may not accompany midline or vestibulocerebellar oculomotor dysfunction. Patients with peripheral vestibular dysfunction will not display limb coordination abnormalities. If abnormalities are noted on the limb coordination examination, the patient should undergo imaging and evaluation by a neurologist. The past pointing test assesses upper extremity tonic balance. This test is considered a bedside vestibulospinal test. While excessive drift of the extremities to the right or to the left may indicate a cerebellar (particularly a vestibulocerebellar)

TABLE 165.5	SYMPTOMS AND PHYSICAL EXAMINATION FINDINGS OF PERIPHERAL VERSUS CENTRAL NERVOUS SYSTEM DISEASE	
	Peripheral Vestibular Dysfunction	**Central Nervous System Disease**
Symptoms	Recurrent episodes of vertigo	Disequilibrium, imbalance, or vertigo
	No additional neurologic symptoms	Associated neurologic symptoms
Physical examination findings	Horizontal–rotary jerk nystagmus	Direction-changing, horizontal, vertical, torsional, or pendular nystagmus
	Nystagmus in the axis of dysfunctional SCC	Gaze-evoked nystagmus or rebound nystagmus
	Nystagmus suppressed by visual fixation	Nystagmus enhanced by visual fixation
	Nystagmus pattern follows Alexander law	
	Normal oculomotor tests[a]	Abnormal oculomotor tests[a]
	Positive head impulse test: unilateral or bilateral	Saccadic pursuit
	Positive head heave test	Dysmetric, disconjugate, slow, delayed saccades
	Positive postheadshake nystagmus tests	Postheadshake nystagmus tests: cross-coupling nystagmus[b]
	Reduced dynamic visual acuity	
	Positive positioning tests (e.g., Dix-Hallpike)[c]	Atypical positioning nystagmus
	Positive past pointing test	Limb incoordination, dysmetria, or dysdiadochokinesia
	Positive Unterberger (Fukuda) stepping test	Gait abnormalities (e.g., wide-based, shuffling, ataxic)
	Reduced stability: tandem and foam Romberg test	Failed Romberg stance
	Positive mastoid vibration test	
	Positive Valsalva maneuver tests	
	Positive tragal compression test	
	Positive pneumatic otoscopy test	
	Positive malleolar sign	
	Positive hyperventilation-induced nystagmus test	

SCC, semicircular canal.
[a]Oculomotor tests (e.g., saccades, smooth pursuit, vergence).
[b]Cross-coupling nystagmus: purely vertical nystagmus following horizontal headshakes.
[c]See Table 165.4 for more detail.

lesion, this finding is also indicative of vestibular system abnormalities. The lesion may involve either the peripheral or central vestibular system. Further evaluation is warranted.

Gait and Posture Tests

Three sensory inputs are vital for maintaining balance: (a) visual, (b) somatosensory (proprioception), and (c) vestibular. These inputs are integrated in the CNS, and the appropriate motor commands are provided to the periphery in order to maintain balance. When one of the three sensory inputs is compromised, a patient must rely on the other two inputs to maintain equilibrium. Gait and posture tests are designed to identify the location of the abnormality affecting balance.

Test Performance

The examiner first observes the patient's gait when walking into the examination room. Discrepancies with later examination observations should be noted. For the *simple gait* test, the patient is asked to walk 50 feet down a hallway, turn rapidly, and walk back without touching the walls. The examiner observes for initiation of movement, change in gait tempo/direction, stride length, arm swing, stance width, missteps, veering/deviations, shuffling, sway, ataxia, and signs of muscle weakness or skeletal abnormality (kyphoscoliosis, limb asymmetry, and limp). For the *tandem gait test*, the patient steps heel to toe in a tandem manner across the room. With the eyes open, this test assesses cerebellar function. With the eyes closed, the tandem gait better assesses vestibular function since the CNS is more reliant on the vestibular system in the absence of visual information.

The *Unterberger (Fukuda) stepping test* is used to gain insight into the vestibulospinal function (94,95). The patient is asked to march in place with eyes closed and arms extended straight out at the level of the shoulders for 1 minute. The examiner notes the degree of lateral rotation at the end of the maneuver.

The following examinations assess posture. For the *Romberg test*, the patient is asked to stand with feet together and arms at the side, first with eyes open and then with eyes closed (Fig. 165.7). The examiner observes the relative amount of sway, both with and without vision, and notes if the patient falls consistently to one side. In order to increase the sensitivity of vestibular defects, one can perform the *tandem Romberg test* or the *foam Romberg test* (Fig. 165.7). These tests are performed similarly to the original test. For the tandem Romberg test, though, the patient is asked to stand with one foot in front of the other heel to toe. For the foam Romberg test, the patient is asked to repeat the Romberg test while standing on large 3-inch dense foam.

Proprioception function relies on intact peripheral nerves and afferent pathways, which are evaluated in several ways. Firstly, the patient's reflexes are assessed in the standard manner. Secondly, the *proprioceptive movement test* is performed. The patient is asked to take off their shoes and socks. With the patient's eyes closed, the examiner moves the patient's toe up or down by grasping it on the sides to decrease pressure cues. The patient indicates in which direction the digit moved. Thirdly, the *vibration test* is performed. The examiner places a 128-Hz tuning fork on the malleolus of the ankle and compares the vibratory sensation to that at the wrist.

Interpretation

"Vestibular gait" does not define any specific manner and/or type of movement. Indeed, a broad array of characteristics can qualify a gait as abnormal. Furthermore, a number of causes can be the source(s) of the abnormal gait. If a patient suffers an acute unilateral loss of otolithic function, the patient will tend to veer toward the side of the lesion. Patients often rapidly compensate. Nevertheless, a variety of central brainstem and musculoskeletal lesions also produce lateral deviation during ambulation. Difficulties with gait initiation and turns as well as decreased arm swing can be seen in extrapyramidal disease. Gait ataxia implies cerebellar dysfunction and is distinctly different from the gait deviation associated with uncompensated peripheral vestibular disease. A shuffling gait should prompt the examiner to explore the possibility of Parkinson's disease and/or normal pressure hydrocephalus (NPH). Finally, exaggerated hip sway, rhythmic deviations, and an excessive reliance on touching the wall during ambulation may constitute signs of a functional gait disorder.

The stepping test was first described in 1938 by Unterberger (95) and later modified by Fukuda in 1959 (94). The ability to close one's eyes and step in place without turning depends on normal vestibulospinal and proprioceptive function. Most normal subjects deviate less than 30 degrees in rotation to one side during the step test, whereas some patients with uncompensated unilateral vestibular weakness deviate more than 30 degrees toward the weaker side. It is important to note that patients with chronic vestibular dysfunction that have compensated for their vestibular loss may perform normally on the Unterberger (Fukuda) stepping test (96).

The Romberg stance primarily tests somatosensation and proprioception functions and not the integrity of vestibular inputs (97). Patients compensating for bilateral vestibular loss are able to stand in the normal Romberg position with both eyes open and eyes closed because of adequate proprioception from a stable support surface. There are two ways, however, to increase this test's sensitivity to detect vestibular deficits: Instruct the patient to (a) stand in the tandem stance (tandem Romberg test) and then (b) step onto a piece of 3-inch dense foam (foam Romberg test). In the tandem stance, the support surface cues are sufficiently altered so that vestibular cues play a greater role in maintaining upright posture. Similarly, when the patient stands on a compliant support surface, such as 3-inch foam, somatosensory cues are muted, and vestibular cues become more important. Patients with vestibular dysfunction may demonstrate excessive hip sway (98,99).

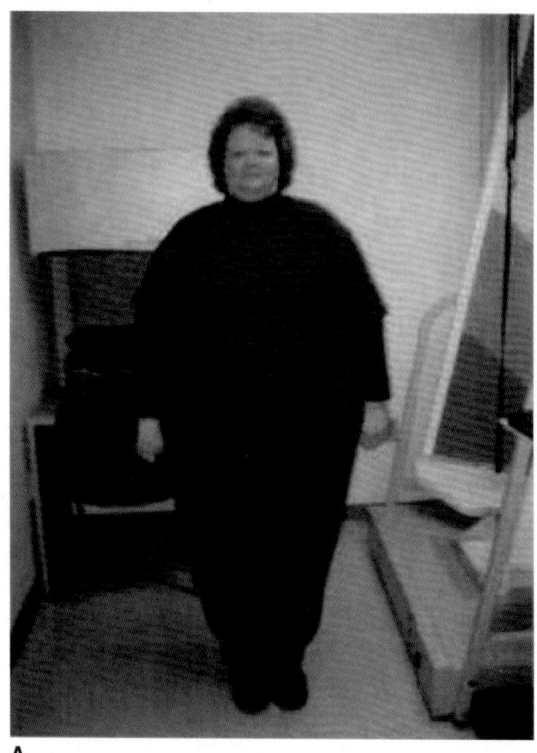

A

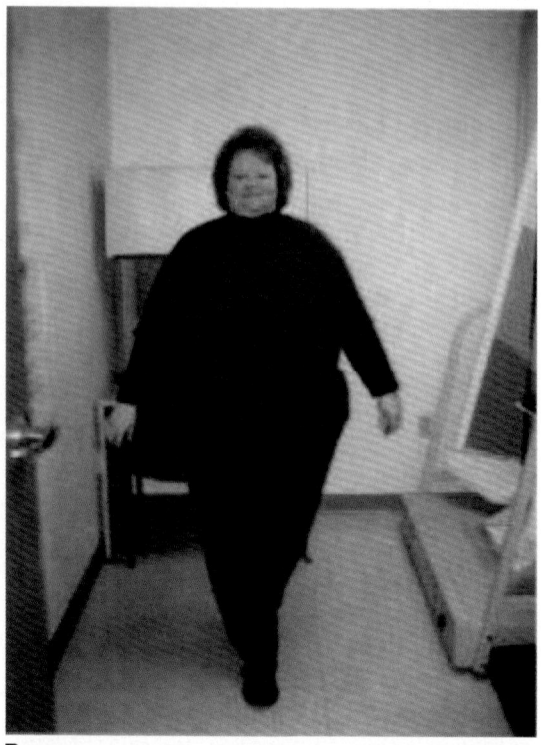

B

Figure 165.7 Romberg tests. **A:** Standard Romberg test on a firm surface. **B:** Tandem Romberg test on a firm surface. **C:** Foam Romberg test on a 3" foam pad. As proprioceptive cues are altered in (**B**) and (**C**), vestibular input to balance becomes more crucial. (Adapted from Goebel JA, White JA, Heidenreich KD. Evaluation of the vestibular system, Chapter 10. In: Snow JB, Wachym PA, Ballenger JJ. (eds.). *Ballenger's otorhino-laryngology head and neck surgery*. 17th ed. Shelton, CT: People's Medical Publishing House, 2009:131–144.).

C

Since many of the tests assessing posture and gait rely on proprioception, it is important to evaluate the peripheral nerve status. Abnormalities in reflexes, digit proprioception, and vibration sensation should provoke the examiner to investigate causes of peripheral neuropathy (e.g., diabetes) and other neurologic processes.

Additional Tests

In addition to the basic neurotologic examination, there are several other tests that can be conducted in select patients. A number of the following tests will unmask peripheral vestibular abnormalities and can provide important diagnostic clues.

Mastoid Vibration

Vibration-induced nystagmus can be used as a diagnostic tool in patients with unilateral vestibular loss or SCC dehiscence. The examiner places a vibration source on the mastoid tip and observes the patient's eyes for nystagmus under Frenzel lenses. Nystagmus produced by mastoid oscillation in patients with vestibular asymmetry was initially described by White et al. in 2007. Mastoid vibration serves as an excitatory stimulus to both labyrinths and, in some cases of asymmetry, produces a horizontal-torsional nystagmus toward the stronger ear (100–102). In patients with superior SCC dehiscence, a vertical-torsion nystagmus in the plane of the affected SCC can be induced by mastoid vibration (100–102).

Malleolar Sign

Patients with superior SCC dehiscence may have hyperacusis to bone-conducted sounds and can present with symptoms of hearing their own pulse and/or the movements of their eyes (103,104). The bone-conducted hyperacusis can be explained by the "third mobile window" effect (19,105). To assess this unique suprathreshold bone conduction, the examiner places a 256-Hz tuning fork on the patient's malleolus. A patient with superior SCC dehiscence may hear the tone in the affected ear (106).

Sound-Evoked or Pressure-Evoked Eye Movements

Consistent eye deviations or nystagmus induced by sound or pressure changes in the middle ear is abnormal. The most common involved sites are the oval window (perilymph fistula, excessive footplate movement), round window (perilymph fistula, enlarged cochlear aqueduct), lateral SCC (perilymph fistula), and superior SCC (dehiscence).

The following maneuvers can demonstrate sound-evoked and/or pressure-evoked eye movements. With Frenzel lenses in place, the examiner observes the patient's eyes for nystagmus or tonic eye deviations concurrent with symptoms of dizziness under the following test conditions: (a) steady tragal compression or insufflations through a pneumatic otoscope used to increase (or decrease) pressure in the external auditory canal, (b) Valsalva maneuvers, and (c) presentation of loud tones via a tuning fork or an audiometer.

Hennebert sign is vertigo and/or nystagmus evoked by pressure-induced movement of the tympanic membrane and may occur in patients with perilymph fistula, otic syphilis, otic capsule erosion from disease, or SCC dehiscence. Pressure changes in the middle ear can be induced by tragal compression, pneumatic otoscopy (through a Siegel speculum), or Valsalva maneuvers. A *closed-glottis Valsalva* (bearing down) results in increased intrathoracic pressure, decreased jugular venous return, and increased intracranial pressure (Fig. 165.8). The increased intracranial pressure

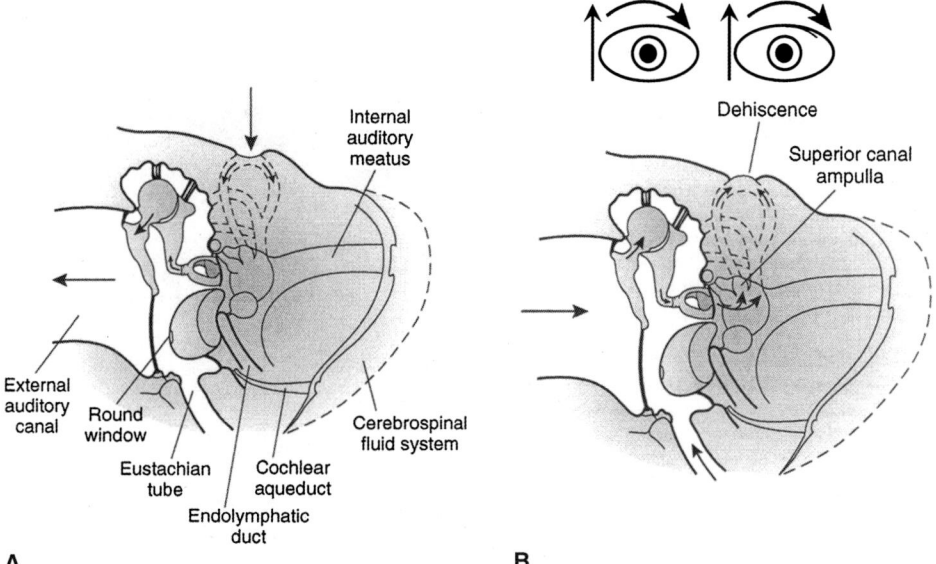

A **B**

Figure 165.8 Maneuvers for diagnosing superior SCC dehiscence. Images depict the right ear. **A:** A *closed-glottis Valsalva* (bearing down) results in increased intrathoracic pressure, decreased jugular venous return, and increased intracranial pressure. The increased intracranial pressure exerts a force directly at the site of bony dehiscence. This moves the endolymph toward the superior SCC ampulla (ampullopetal), which according to Ewald's third law is inhibitory. Upon release, the endolymph flows away from the ampulla (ampullofugal), generating stimulatory nystagmus. **B:** A pneumatic otoscope or tragal compression forces air into the external auditory canal. This surge of air increases middle ear pressure, causes inward displacement of the stapes, and moves the endolymph away from the ampulla (ampullofugal), resulting in excitation. The stimulatory nystagmus is vertical–torsional with an upward slow phase that aligns with the affected SCC, and the superior pole has torsional rotation away from the affected ear. (Adapted from Hullar TE, Zee DS, Minor LB. Evaluation of the patient with dizziness, Chapter 164. In: Cummings CW, Flint PW, Harker LA. (eds.), *Otolaryngology-head and neck surgery.* 4th ed. Philadelphia, PA: Elsevier, 2004.)

exerts a force directly at the site of bony dehiscence. This moves the endolymph toward the superior SCC ampulla (ampullopetal), which according to Ewald's third law is inhibitory. Upon release, the endolymph flows away from the ampulla (ampullofugal), generating stimulatory nystagmus. An *open-glottis Valsalva* (pressure against pinched nostrils) forces air into the middle ear through the eustachian tube (Fig. 165.8). Furthermore, a pneumatic otoscope or tragal compression forces air into the external auditory canal (Fig. 165.8). These maneuvers increase middle ear pressure and cause inward displacement of the stapes. Endolymph moves away from the ampulla (ampullofugal), resulting in excitation. The stimulatory nystagmus is vertical torsional with an upward slow phase that aligns with the affected SCC, and the superior pole has torsional rotation away from the affected ear (19,107) (Fig. 165.8). Eye movements are typically conjugate. In addition, cranial–cervical junction abnormalities (Arnold-Chiari malformation in particular) produce vertical downbeat nystagmus with any maneuver that increases intracranial pressure. *Tullio phenomenon* is the occurrence of vertigo and nystagmus with exposure to sound. The examiner introduces pure tones over a range of 250 to 4,000 Hz at intensities of 100 to 110 dB. The characteristic eye findings are similar to those resulting from increased middle ear pressure (19,106).

Hyperventilation-Induced Nystagmus

Hyperventilation may induce dizziness and light-headedness in patients with psychiatric disorders (e.g., anxiety or panic disorder), but does not result in nystagmus (108,109). Hyperventilation does induce nystagmus in demyelination of the vestibular nerve (e.g., acoustic schwannoma or microvascular nerve compression) or central demyelination conditions (e.g., multiple sclerosis) (110–112). With Frenzel lenses in place, the patient is asked to hyperventilate for 90 seconds by taking deep breaths and then inhaling and exhaling in rapid succession. The examiner inspects the patient's eyes for resulting eye movements and notes the direction and character of the nystagmus. Hyperventilation-induced nystagmus is an excitatory nystagmus with the slow phase toward the healthy ear. Hyperventilation decreases both CSF and serum PCO_2 levels (113). The alkalotic environment causes albumin to bind to calcium. The reduction in extracellular calcium levels leads to improved axonal conduction in partially demyelinated nerve fibers (114–116). Interestingly, it has been reported that after surgical resection of acoustic schwannomas, hyperventilation no longer induces nystagmus, presumably because the demyelinated nerve fibers have been removed (112).

CONCLUSION

The diagnosis and management of the patient with dizziness and imbalance can be perplexing and challenging. Therefore, it is vital that practitioners recognize the complexity of the

problem and develop a systematic and efficient approach. Taking a careful history and deciphering a true understanding of the patient's symptoms are crucial in developing a differential diagnosis. Furthermore, it is important to perform a systematic and structured neurotologic examination. Between a detailed history and a structured neurotologic examination, the physician will be best equipped to provide an accurate diagnosis and a rational treatment approach that addresses all major contributing factors.

HIGHLIGHTS

- The three primary sensory inputs responsible for balance originate from the vestibular, visual, and somatosensory (proprioceptive) pathways.
- A structured and thorough discovery of all pertinent historical events is critical in the evaluation of the dizzy patient.
- The head impulse test (HIT) is a bedside technique used to detect unilateral or bilateral vestibular hypofunction.
- Postheadshake nystagmus is considered a pathologic sign of vestibular input asymmetry in the plane of rotation.
- The dynamic visual acuity test (DVAT) has been developed and studied for the purpose of determining gaze stability during head movements at higher frequency (greater than 2 Hz) and peak velocity (greater than 120 degrees/s).
- Benign paroxysmal positional vertigo (BPPV) is characterized by a sudden onset of episodic vertigo lasting from a few seconds to several minutes that is induced by head movement in certain positions and is the most common cause of peripheral positioning nystagmus.
- It is critical to understand Ewald's laws in order to accurately interpret nystagmus resulting from peripheral vestibular pathology.

REFERENCES

1. Yardley L, Owen N, Nazareth I, et al. Prevalence and presentation of dizziness in a general practice community sample of working age people. *Br J Gen Pract* 1998;48:1131–1135.
2. Neuhauser HK, von Brevern M, Radtke A, et al. Epidemiology of vestibular vertigo: a neurotologic survey of the general population. *Neurology* 2005;65:898–904.
3. Sloane PD, Coeytaux RR, Beck RS, et al. Dizziness: state of the science. *Ann Intern Med* 2001;134:823–832.
4. Wetmore SJ, Eibling DE, Goebel JA, et al. Challenges and opportunities in managing the dizzy older adult. *Otolaryngol Head Neck Surg* 2011;144:651–656.
5. Zhao JG, Piccirillo JF, Spitznagel EL Jr, et al. Predictive capability of historical data for diagnosis of dizziness. *Otol Neurotol* 2011;32:284–290.
6. Ahmed MF, Goebel JA, Sinks BC. Caloric test versus rotational sinusoidal harmonic acceleration and step-velocity tests in

patients with and without suspected peripheral vestibulopathy. *Otol Neurotol* 2009;30:800–805.

7. Blakley BW, Goebel J. The meaning of the word "vertigo." *Otolaryngol Head Neck Surg* 2001;125:147–150.

8. Grimm RJ, Hemenway WG, Lebray PR, et al. The perilymph fistula syndrome defined in mild head trauma. *Acta Otolaryngol Suppl* 1989;464:1–40.

9. Black FO, Pesznecker S, Norton T, et al. Surgical management of perilymphatic fistulas: a Portland experience. *Am J Otol* 1992;13:254–262.

10. Black FO, Pesznecker S, Norton T, et al. Surgical management of perilymph fistulas. A new technique. *Arch Otolaryngol Head Neck Surg* 1991;117:641–648.

11. Ernst A, Basta D, Seidl RO, et al. Management of posttraumatic vertigo. *Otolaryngol Head Neck Surg* 2005;132:554–558.

12. Schuknecht HF, Suzuka Y, Zimmermann C. Delayed endolymphatic hydrops and its relationship to Meniere's disease. *Ann Otol Rhinol Laryngol* 1990;99:843–853.

13. Hoffer ME, Gottshall KR, Moore R, et al. Characterizing and treating dizziness after mild head trauma. *Otol Neurotol* 2004;25:135–138.

14. Donaldson CJ, Hoffer ME, Balough BJ, et al. Prognostic assessments of medical therapy and vestibular testing in post-traumatic migraine-associated dizziness patients. *Otolaryngol Head Neck Surg* 2010;143:820–825.

15. Carey JP, Minor LB, Nager GT. Dehiscence or thinning of bone overlying the superior semicircular canal in a temporal bone survey. *Arch Otolaryngol Head Neck Surg* 2000;126:137–147.

16. Minor LB. Superior canal dehiscence syndrome. *Am J Otol* 2000;21:9–19.

17. Minor LB. Clinical manifestations of superior semicircular canal dehiscence. *Laryngoscope* 2005;115:1717–1727.

18. Davis LE. Viruses and vestibular neuritis: review of human and animal studies. *Acta Otolaryngol Suppl* 1993;503:70–73.

19. Minor LB, Solomon D, Zinreich JS, et al. Sound- and/or pressure-induced vertigo due to bone dehiscence of the superior semicircular canal. *Arch Otolaryngol Head Neck Surg* 1998;124:249–258.

20. Chen Y, Huang WG, Zha DJ, et al. Aspirin attenuates gentamicin ototoxicity: from the laboratory to the clinic. *Hear Res* 2007;226:178–182.

21. Rybak LP, Ramkumar V. Ototoxicity. *Kidney Int* 2007;72:931–935.

22. Dobie RA, Black FO, Pezsnecker SC, et al. Hearing loss in patients with vestibulotoxic reactions to gentamicin therapy. *Arch Otolaryngol Head Neck Surg* 2006;132:253–257.

23. Henley CM III, Schacht J. Pharmacokinetics of aminoglycoside antibiotics in blood, inner-ear fluids and tissues and their relationship to ototoxicity. *Audiology* 1988;27:137–146.

24. Dulon D, Hiel H, Aurousseau C, et al. Pharmacokinetics of gentamicin in the sensory hair cells of the organ of Corti: rapid uptake and long term persistence. *C R Acad Sci III* 1993;316:682–687.

25. Fischel-Ghodsian N. Genetic factors in aminoglycoside toxicity. *Pharmacogenomics* 2005;6:27–36.

26. Roth SM, Williams SM, Jiang L, et al. Susceptibility genes for gentamicin-induced vestibular dysfunction. *J Vestib Res* 2008;18:59–68.

27. Rybak LP, Whitworth CA, Mukherjea D, et al. Mechanisms of cisplatin-induced ototoxicity and prevention. *Hear Res* 2007;226:157–167.

28. Li Y, Womer RB, Silber JH. Predicting cisplatin ototoxicity in children: the influence of age and the cumulative dose. *Eur J Cancer* 2004;40:2445–2451.

29. Jung TT, Rhee CK, Lee CS, et al. Ototoxicity of salicylate, nonsteroidal antiinflammatory drugs, and quinine. *Otolaryngol Clin North Am* 1993;26:791–810.

30. McKinnon BJ, Lassen LF. Naproxen-associated sudden sensorineural hearing loss. *Mil Med* 1998;163:792–793.

31. McFadden D, Plattsmier HS, Pasanen EG. Temporary hearing loss induced by combinations of intense sounds and nonsteroidal anti-inflammatory drugs. *Am J Otolaryngol* 1984;5:235–241.

32. Curhan SG, Eavey R, Shargorodsky J, et al. Analgesic use and the risk of hearing loss in men. *Am J Med* 2010;123:231–237.

33. Brien JA. Ototoxicity associated with salicylates. A brief review. *Drug Saf* 1993;9:143–148.

34. Stypulkowski PH. Mechanisms of salicylate ototoxicity. *Hear Res* 1990;46:113–145.

35. Yorgason JG, Kalinec GM, Luxford WM, et al. Acetaminophen ototoxicity after acetaminophen/hydrocodone abuse: evidence from two parallel in vitro mouse models. *Otolaryngol Head Neck Surg* 2010;142:814–819, 9 e1–2.

36. Friedman RA, House JW, Luxford WM, et al. Profound hearing loss associated with hydrocodone/acetaminophen abuse. *Am J Otol* 2000;21:188–191.

37. Ho T, Vrabec JT, Burton AW. Hydrocodone use and sensorineural hearing loss. *Pain Physician* 2007;10:467–472.

38. Oh AK, Ishiyama A, Baloh RW. Deafness associated with abuse of hydrocodone/acetaminophen. *Neurology* 2000;54:2345.

39. Strupp M, Jahn K, Brandt T. Another adverse effect of aspirin: bilateral vestibulopathy. *J Neurol Neurosurg Psychiatry* 2003;74:691.

40. Leigh RJ, Zee DS. *The neurology of eye movements*. New York: Oxford University Press Inc., 2006.

41. Cass SP. Performing the physical examination: ocular motor examination. In: Goebel JA, ed. *Practical management of the dizzy patient*. Philadelphia, PA: Lippincott Williams & Wilkins, 2008:75–78.

42. Knox PC, Davidson JH, Anderson D. Age-related changes in smooth pursuit initiation. *Exp Brain Res* 2005;165:1–7.

43. Paige GD. Senescence of human visual-vestibular interactions: smooth pursuit, optokinetic, and vestibular control of eye movements with aging. *Exp Brain Res* 1994;98:355–372.

44. Zackon DH, Sharpe JA. Smooth pursuit in senescence. Effects of target acceleration and velocity. *Acta Otolaryngol* 1987;104:290–297.

45. Leigh RJ, Zee DS (eds.). Smooth pursuit and visual fixation. In: *The neurology of eye movements*. Oxford: Oxford University Press, 2006:188–240.

46. Gottlieb JP, MacAvoy MG, Bruce CJ. Neural responses related to smooth-pursuit eye movements and their correspondence with electrically elicited smooth eye movements in the primate frontal eye field. *J Neurophysiol* 1994;72:1634–1653.

47. Leigh RJ. The cortical control of ocular pursuit movements. *Rev Neurol (Paris)* 1989;145:605–612.

48. Ewald JR. *Physiologische Untersuchungen über das Endorgan des Nervus octavus*. Wiesbaden, Germany: Bergmann, 1892.

49. Baloh RW, Honrubia V. *Clinical neurophysiology of the vestibular system*. Oxford: Oxford University Press, 2001.

50. Leigh RJ, Zee DS. The vestibular-optokinetic system. In: *The neurology of eye movements*. Oxford: Oxford University Press, 2006.

51. Halmagyi GM, Curthoys IS. A clinical sign of canal paresis. *Arch Neurol* 1988;45:737–739.

52. Halmagyi GM, Aw ST, Cremer PD, et al. Impulsive testing of individual semicircular canal function. *Ann N Y Acad Sci* 2001;942:192–200.

53. Weber KP, Aw ST, Todd MJ, et al. Horizontal head impulse test detects gentamicin vestibulotoxicity. *Neurology* 2009;72:1417–1424.

54. Weber KP, Aw ST, Todd MJ, et al. Head impulse test in unilateral vestibular loss: vestibulo-ocular reflex and catch-up saccades. *Neurology* 2008;70:454–463.

55. Halmagyi GM. Garnett Passe and Rodney Williams Memorial Lecture: New clinical tests of unilateral vestibular dysfunction. *J Laryngol Otol* 2004;118:589–600.

56. Cremer PD, Halmagyi GM, Aw ST, et al. Semicircular canal plane head impulses detect absent function of individual semicircular canals. *Brain* 1998;121(Pt 4):699–716.

57. Kessler P, Tomlinson D, Blakeman A, et al. The high-frequency/acceleration head heave test in detecting otolith diseases. *Otol Neurotol* 2007;28:896–904.

58. Ramat S, Zee DS, Minor LB. Translational vestibulo-ocular reflex evoked by a "head heave" stimulus. *Ann N Y Acad Sci* 2001;942:95–113.

59. Nuti D, Mandala M, Broman AT, et al. Acute vestibular neuritis: prognosis based upon bedside clinical tests (thrusts and heaves). *Ann N Y Acad Sci* 2005;1039:359–367.

60. Vibert D, Hausler R, Safran AB, et al. Diplopia from skew deviation in unilateral peripheral vestibular lesions. *Acta Otolaryngol* 1996;116:170–176.

61. Safran AB, Vibert D, Issoua D, et al. Skew deviation after vestibular neuritis. *Am J Ophthalmol* 1994;118:238–245.

62. Verhulst E, Van Lammeren M, Dralands L. Diplopia from skew deviation in Ramsey-Hunt syndrome. A case report. *Bull Soc Belge Ophtalmol* 2000;278:27–32.

63. Wong AM, Sharpe JA. Cerebellar skew deviation and the torsional vestibuloocular reflex. *Neurology* 2005;65:412–419.

64. Brandt T, Dieterich M. Pathological eye-head coordination in roll: tonic ocular tilt reaction in mesencephalic and medullary lesions. *Brain* 1987;110(Pt 3):649–666.

65. Goto F, Ban Y, Tsutumi T. Acute audiovestibular deficit with complete ocular tilt reaction and absent VEMPs. *Eur Arch Otorhinolaryngol* 2011;268:1093–1096.

66. Kamei T. Two types of head-shaking tests in vestibular examination. *Acta Otolaryngol Suppl* 1988;458:108–112.

67. Asawavichiangianda S, Fujimoto M, Mai M, et al. Significance of head-shaking nystagmus in the evaluation of the dizzy patient. *Acta Otolaryngol Suppl* 1999;540:27–33.

68. Goebel JA, Garcia P. Prevalence of post-headshake nystagmus in patients with caloric deficits and vertigo. *Otolaryngol Head Neck Surg* 1992;106:121–127.

69. Goebel JA, Tungsiripat N, Sinks B, et al. Gaze stabilization test: a new clinical test of unilateral vestibular dysfunction. *Otol Neurotol* 2007;28:68–73.

70. Burgio DL, Blakley BW, Myers SF. The high-frequency oscillopsia test. *J Vestib Res* 1992;2:221–226.

71. Longridge NS, Mallinson AI. The dynamic illegible E (DIE) test: a simple technique for assessing the ability of the vestibulo-ocular reflex to overcome vestibular pathology. *J Otolaryngol* 1987;16:97–103.

72. Tian J, Crane BT, Demer JL. Vestibular catch-up saccades in labyrinthine deficiency. *Exp Brain Res* 2000;131:448–457.

73. Demer JL, Honrubia V, Baloh RW. Dynamic visual acuity: a test for oscillopsia and vestibulo-ocular reflex function. *Am J Otol* 1994;15:340–347.

74. Tian JR, Shubayev I, Demer JL. Dynamic visual acuity during transient and sinusoidal yaw rotation in normal and unilaterally vestibulopathic humans. *Exp Brain Res* 2001;137:12–25.

75. Herdman SJ. Role of vestibular adaptation in vestibular rehabilitation. *Otolaryngol Head Neck Surg* 1998;119:49–54.

76. Herdman SJ, Tusa RJ, Blatt P, et al. Computerized dynamic visual acuity test in the assessment of vestibular deficits. *Am J Otol* 1998;19:790–796.

77. Tian JR, Shubayev I, Demer JL. Dynamic visual acuity during passive and self-generated transient head rotation in normal and unilaterally vestibulopathic humans. *Exp Brain Res* 2002;142:486–495.

78. Longridge NS, Mallinson AI. The dynamic illegible E-test. A technique for assessing the vestibulo-ocular reflex. *Acta Otolaryngol* 1987;103:273–279.

79. Herdman SJ, Schubert MC, Tusa RJ. Role of central preprogramming in dynamic visual acuity with vestibular loss. *Arch Otolaryngol Head Neck Surg* 2001;127:1205–1210.

80. Herdman SJ, Schubert MC, Das VE, et al. Recovery of dynamic visual acuity in unilateral vestibular hypofunction. *Arch Otolaryngol Head Neck Surg* 2003;129:819–824.

81. Leigh RJ, Zee DS (eds.). Diagnosis and management of vestibular disorders. In: *The neurology of eye movements*. Oxford: Oxford University Press, 2006.

82. Viirre E, Purcell I, Baloh RW. The Dix-Hallpike test and the canalith repositioning maneuver. *Laryngoscope* 2005;115: 184–187.

83. Epley JM. New dimensions of benign paroxysmal positional vertigo. *Otolaryngol Head Neck Surg* 1980;88:599–605.

84. Smullen JL, Andrist EC, Gianoli GJ. Superior semicircular canal dehiscence: a new cause of vertigo. *J La State Med Soc* 1999;151:397–400.

85. Korres S, Balatsouras DG, Kaberos A, et al. Occurrence of semicircular canal involvement in benign paroxysmal positional vertigo. *Otol Neurotol* 2002;23:926–932.

86. Hornibrook J. A newly recognised cause of vertigo: horizontal canal variant of benign positional vertigo. *N Z Med J* 2005;118:U1659.

87. Hornibrook J. Horizontal canal benign positional vertigo. *Ann Otol Rhinol Laryngol* 2004;113:721–725.

88. Herdman SJ, Tusa RJ. Complications of the canalith repositioning procedure. *Arch Otolaryngol Head Neck Surg* 1996;122: 281–286.

89. Lee JB, Han DH, Choi SJ, et al. Efficacy of the "bow and lean test" for the management of horizontal canal benign paroxysmal positional vertigo. *Laryngoscope* 2010;120:2339–2346.

90. Choung YH, Shin YR, Kahng H, et al. 'Bow and lean test' to determine the affected ear of horizontal canal benign paroxysmal positional vertigo. *Laryngoscope* 2006;116:1776–1781.

91. Yacovino DA, Hain TC, Gualtieri F. New therapeutic maneuver for anterior canal benign paroxysmal positional vertigo. *J Neurol* 2009;256:1851–1855.

92. Schratzenstaller B, Wagner-Manslau C, Strasser G, et al. Canalolithiasis of the superior semicircular canal: an anomaly in benign paroxysmal vertigo. *Acta Otolaryngol* 2005;125:1055–1062.

93. Kim YK, Shin JE, Chung JW. The effect of canalith repositioning for anterior semicircular canal canalithiasis. *ORL J Otorhinolaryngol Relat Spec* 2005;67:56–60.

94. Fukuda T. The stepping test: two phases of the labyrinthine reflex. *Acta Otolaryngol* 1959;50:95–108.

95. Unterberger S. Neue objektiv registrierbare Vestibnlaris-KSrperdrehreaktion, erhalten dm'ch Treten auf der Stelle. Der,,Tretversuch". *Archiv für Ohren Nasen und Kehlkopf Heilkunde* 1938;145:478–492.

96. Honaker JA, Boismier TE, Shepard NP, et al. Fukuda stepping test: sensitivity and specificity. *J Am Acad Audiol* 2009;20:311–314; quiz 35.

97. Romberg MH. *Lehrbuch der Nervenkrankheiten des Menschen.* Berlin: Alexander Dunckner, 1840.

98. Shupert CL, Horak FB, Black FO. Hip sway associated with vestibulopathy. *J Vestib Res* 1994;4:231–244.

99. Serrador JM, Lipsitz LA, Gopalakrishnan GS, et al. Loss of otolith function with age is associated with increased postural sway measures. *Neurosci Lett* 2009;465:10–15.

100. White JA, Hughes GB, Ruggieri PN. Vibration-induced nystagmus as an office procedure for the diagnosis of superior semicircular canal dehiscence. *Otol Neurotol* 2007;28:911–916.

101. Park H, Hong SC, Shin J. Clinical significance of vibration-induced nystagmus and headshaking nystagmus through follow-up examinations in patients with vestibular neuritis. *Otol Neurotol* 2008;29:375–379.

102. Park HJ, Shin JE, Lim YC, et al. Clinical significance of vibration-induced nystagmus. *Audiol Neurootol* 2008;13:182–186.

103. Minor LB, Cremer PD, Carey JP, et al. Symptoms and signs in superior canal dehiscence syndrome. *Ann N Y Acad Sci* 2001;942:259–273.

104. Watson SR, Halmagyi GM, Colebatch JG. Vestibular hypersensitivity to sound (Tullio phenomenon): structural and functional assessment. *Neurology* 2000;54:722–728.

105. Merchant SN, Rosowski JJ. Conductive hearing loss caused by third-window lesions of the inner ear. *Otol Neurotol* 2008;29: 282–289.

106. Minor LB, Carey JP, Cremer PD, et al. Dehiscence of bone overlying the superior canal as a cause of apparent conductive hearing loss. *Otol Neurotol* 2003;24:270–278.

107. Cremer PD, Minor LB, Carey JP, et al. Eye movements in patients with superior canal dehiscence syndrome align with the abnormal canal. *Neurology* 2000;55:1833–1841.

108. Lum JJ, Madison JR, Seto TB, et al. Management of patients with chronic kidney disease presenting with acute coronary syndrome. *Hawaii Med J* 2004;63:330–332.

109. Evans RW. Neurologic aspects of hyperventilation syndrome. *Semin Neurol* 1995;15:115–125.

110. Wilson WR, Kim JW. Study of ventilation testing with electronystagmography. *Ann Otol Rhinol Laryngol* 1981;90:56–59.

111. Bance ML, O'Driscoll M, Patel N, et al. Vestibular disease unmasked by hyperventilation. *Laryngoscope* 1998;108:610–614.

112. Minor LB, Haslwanter T, Straumann D, et al. Hyperventilation-induced nystagmus in patients with vestibular schwannoma. *Neurology* 1999;53:2158–2168.

113. Sakellari V, Bronstein AM, Corna S, et al. The effects of hyperventilation on postural control mechanisms. *Brain* 1997;120 (Pt 9):1659–1673.

114. Davies HD, Carroll WM, Mastaglia FL. Effects of hyperventilation on pattern-reversal visual evoked potentials in patients with demyelination. *J Neurol Neurosurg Psychiatry* 1986;49:1392–1396.

115. Davis FA, Becker FO, Michael JA, et al. Effect of intravenous sodium bicarbonate, disodium edetate (Na2EDTA), and hyperventilation on visual and oculomotor signs in multiple sclerosis. *J Neurol Neurosurg Psychiatry* 1970;33:723–732.

116. Bednarik J, Novotny O. Value of hyperventilation in pattern-reversal visual evoked potentials. *J Neurol Neurosurg Psychiatry* 1989;52:1107–1109.

Peripheral Vestibular Disorders

166

Yuri Agrawal   *Lloyd B. Minor*   *John P. Carey*

GENERAL PRINCIPLES

The vestibular end organ consists of five organs: three semicircular canals (anterior, posterior, and horizontal), and two otolith end organs—the saccule and the utricle. The semicircular canals detect angular head rotation, while the otolith end organs detect translational head motion and the head's orientation with respect to gravity. Hair cells in the right and left vestibular organs fire at a tonic baseline rate; if the head is turned toward the right, the hair cells of the right horizontal canal increase their firing rate while the hair cells of the left horizontal canal decrease their firing rate. The opposite changes occur with head turns to the left. Sensory input from the vestibular periphery is relayed centrally via the vestibular nerves; the superior vestibular nerve carries information from the horizontal and superior semicircular canals and the utricle while the inferior vestibular nerve transmits input from the posterior semicircular canal and saccule. The brain compares the inputs from right and left vestibular organs in order to determine that a change in head position has occurred and generates compensatory eye movements and postural changes. Collectively, the vestibular apparatus encodes information about head position and contributes to the maintenance of gaze and postural stability (via the vestibuloocular reflex (VOR) and vestibulospinal reflex respectively) (1).

In this chapter, we review peripheral vestibular disorders, which are characterized by pathology located in the peripheral vestibular end organs. The hallmark symptom of peripheral vestibular dysfunction is vertigo, which occurs if the right- and left-sided vestibular nerves fire asymmetrically *in the absence of a head movement*, creating an illusory sense of motion. We categorize peripheral vestibular disorders based on the clinical manifestations of vertigo (Table 166.1). Vertigo can be episodic, resulting from a reversible unilateral loss or gain of vestibular function, either of which can produce an asymmetry in the

firing rates of the right- and left-sided vestibular nerves. Peripheral vestibular diseases characterized by episodic disruption of vestibular function include Ménière's disease, where loss of vestibular function occurs for minutes to hours, as well as vestibular neuritis, labyrinthitis, and immune-mediated inner ear disease (IMIED), where loss of function can occur for over 24 hours. In migrainous vertigo, disruption of vestibular function may last for variable periods of time, in some events for minutes to hours, but in others for days. Peripheral vestibular disorders resulting from intermittent excitation in vestibular function include benign paroxysmal positional vertigo (BPPV) and superior canal dehiscence (SCD) syndrome. Perilymph fistulas may produce either an episodic disruption or excitation of vestibular function. A third category of peripheral vestibular disorders are those that result from chronically inadequate vestibular function. Chronic unilateral loss of vestibular function can be due to incomplete recovery after vestibular neuritis or labyrinthitis, long-term sequelae of Ménière's disease, damage from cholesteatoma or chronic otitis media, etc. Some specific other causes are discussed in other chapters, including temporal bone trauma (Chapter 150) or acoustic neuroma (Chapter 159). Chronic bilateral vestibular dysfunction typically occurs in the setting of a systemic exposure, such as to aminoglycoside antibiotics or chemotherapeutic agents, or may be genetic in origin.

BRIEF EPISODIC DISRUPTION OF UNILATERAL VESTIBULAR FUNCTION

Ménière's Disease

Ménière's syndrome is an inner ear disorder characterized by spontaneous attacks of vertigo, fluctuating low-frequency sensorineural hearing loss, aural fullness, and tinnitus. When the syndrome is idiopathic and cannot be attributed to any other cause (e.g., syphilis, IMIED, surgical trauma),

TABLE 166.1	BASIC PRESENTATIONS OF PERIPHERAL VESTIBULAR DYSFUNCTION

1. Episodic disruption of unilateral vestibular function
   Lasting minutes-hours
   - Ménière's disease
   - Perilymph fistula
   Lasting >24 h
   - Vestibular neuritis
   - Labyrinthitis
   - IMIED
   Lasting variable periods of time
   - Migrainous vertigo
2. Brief/episodic excitation of unilateral vestibular function
   - BPPV
   - SCD syndrome
   - Perilymph fistula
3. Chronically inadequate vestibular function
   Unilateral
   - Unilateral vestibular hypofunction following vestibular neuritis, trauma, etc.
   - Acoustic neuroma
   Bilateral
   - Aminoglycoside toxicity
   - Chemotherapy
   - Familial

it is referred to as Ménière's disease (2). Ménière's syndrome exhibits a relapsing–remitting pattern, with episodic attacks terminated by periods of restitution to normal auditory and vestibular function. Additionally, auditory and vestibular function may decline over time (3).

Clinical Features

The prevalence of Ménière's disease has been reported to range from 34.5 per 100,000 persons in Japan (4), 157 per 100,000 persons in the United Kingdom (5), 190 per 100,000 in the United States (6), to 513 per 100,000 in Finland (7). Disease onset typically occurs in the fourth to sixth decade of life, with a 1.3–1.9:1 female predominance (4,6). The extent to which Ménière's disease occurs bilaterally has been a subject of considerable controversy. House et al. (8) found a 24% overall prevalence of bilateral Ménière's disease, with 11% being bilateral at initial presentation, and a 14% rate of progression from unilateral to bilateral disease. The diagnosis of Ménière's disease is largely clinical at this time; there are no pathognomonic tests that confirm this diagnosis. The most widely-used guidelines to establish a diagnosis of Ménière's disease were published by the American Academy of Otolaryngology-Head and Neck Surgery (AAO-HNS), which termed "definite" Ménière's disease as two or more spontaneous episodes of vertigo, each lasting 20 minutes or longer; hearing loss documented by audiograms on at least one occasion; tinnitus or aural fullness in the affected ear; and other causes excluded (typically with gadolinium-enhanced magnetic resonance

imaging [MRI] of the cranial base) (9). The staging system established by the AAO-HNS is based on audiometric criteria, with 4-frequency pure-tone averages at 0.5, 1, 2, and 3 kHz of less than 25, 26 to 40, 41 to 70 and greater than 70 corresponding to Stages 1, 2, 3, and 4 respectively.

The presentation of Ménière's disease typically includes recurring attacks of vertigo (96.2%), with tinnitus (91.1%) and ipsilateral hearing loss (87.7%) (10). The clinical course of Ménière's disease varies considerably between patients, from long periods of remission punctuated by episodic attacks to intervals of unrelenting attacks. Longitudinal studies suggest that vertigo ceases spontaneously in 57% of cases at 2 years and 71% after 8.3 years (11). Patients classically present with a low-frequency sensorineural hearing loss that is fluctuating and progressive. With long-standing disease (greater than 10 years), the audiometric pattern flattens and the hearing loss typically stabilizes at a pure-tone average of 50 dB and a speech discrimination score of 50% (12). Profound sensorineural hearing loss occurs in 1% to 2% of patients (13); if the losses are bilateral, patients may benefit from cochlear implantation (14).

Endolymphatic Hydrops

Endolymphatic hydrops has long been held to be the pathologic basis for Ménière's disease (15–17). Endolymph, the potassium-enriched fluid in the inner ear, may be either excessively synthesized or inadequately resorbed, resulting in expansion of the endolymphatic space (17,18). Endolymphatic hydrops typically involves the pars inferior of the labyrinth (composed of the saccule and cochlea) (16,19). The pars superior (utricle and semicircular canals) may also be involved in endolymphatic hydrops, although changes tend to be less dramatic and occur less frequently.

Several mechanisms have been suggested to explain how endolymphatic hydrops may produce the spontaneous attacks of vertigo characteristic of Ménière's disease. The most prominent theory holds that hydropic distension of the endolymphatic duct causes rupture of the distended membranes, a phenomenon that has been observed throughout the labyrinth (20). Membrane rupture allows the potassium-rich endolymph to leak into the perilymphatic space and contact the basal surfaces of the hair cells as well as the eighth cranial nerve. Initial excitation and then subsequent inhibition of the hair cells manifests as a direction-changing nystagmus and may underlie episodic vertigo. Long-term declines in auditory and vestibular function may be the result of repeated exposure of the vestibular hair cells to toxic levels of potassium-enriched perilymph (21). Recent studies have challenged the primacy of endolymphatic hydrops in the pathophysiology of Ménière's disease, and have suggested that endolymphatic hydrops may be a marker of disordered cochlear homeostasis but not necessarily directly responsible for the symptoms of Ménière's disease (22).

Physiologic Tests in Ménière's Disease

The use of electrocochleography is based on endolymphatic hydrops as a presumed pathologic correlate of Ménière's disease. Electrical potentials generated by the cochlea are measured in response to repeated sound stimulation with clicks or tonebursts. The cochlear field potential responses include the cochlear microphonic potential and the summating potential (SP), both of which represent cochlear hair cell function, and the compound action potential (AP), which reflects auditory nerve activity and corresponds to wave I of the auditory brainstem reflex. The SP has been observed to be larger in response to clicks or more negative in response to tonebursts in patients with Ménière's disease. Using clicks, for example, a typical upper limit of normal for the SP/AP ratio is 0.4 (23). SP changes in Ménière's disease are thought to reflect hydropic distension of the basilar membrane into the scala tympani causing an increase in the normal asymmetry of its vibration. The sensitivity of the SP/AP ratio has been reported to be 50% to 70% (24), and efforts to augment the sensitivity have included combining the SP/AP ratio with SP amplitude, AP latency, and audiometric parameters (25). Yet while studies find that electrocochleographic findings with audiometric considerations can segregate cases of definite Ménière's disease from normals, the ability of electrocochleography to discriminate between cases of possible or probable Ménière's disease and normals is less clear (25). It is in these less-clear cases that additional information would be most helpful.

Caloric and head impulse testing are both tests of semicircular canal function. In caloric testing, bithermal irrigation is applied to the external auditory canals, which causes a convective movement of endolymph within the ipsilateral horizontal semicircular canal (26). The movement of fluid within the horizontal canal results in excitatory or inhibitory deflection of the cupula (depending upon the direction of endolymph flow). Motion of the cupula then leads to hair cell excitation or inhibition with a corresponding change in the discharge rate of vestibular-nerve afferents. Compensatory eye movements are thereby elicited (corresponding to the slow phases of nystagmus), followed by fast resetting eye movements (corresponding to the fast phase of nystagmus). The maximum velocities of the slow phases of nystagmus are compared bilaterally and used to compute unilateral weakness or caloric asymmetry. Depending on the normative data developed by individual vestibular laboratories, a caloric asymmetry of 20% or greater is usually considered indicative of unilateral peripheral vestibular hypofunction.

Head impulse (or head thrust) testing assesses the integrity of the angular vestibuloocular reflex (AVOR). Head and eye movements are recorded during high-velocity, high-acceleration rotary head impulses in the excitatory direction for each of the six semicircular canals. Normal subjects are able to maintain visual fixation on a target during rapid head movement and thus have gain values (computed as the ratio of eye velocity to head velocity) close to 1.0 (27).

A significant reduction in the caloric response of affected ears has been observed in 42% to 79% of individuals with unilateral Ménière's disease (28–34). In contrast, abnormalities of the AVOR in Ménière's disease are much less prevalent, although there appears to be a correlation between head impulse test gain asymmetry and caloric unilateral weakness percentage (29). Although caloric and head impulse testing are both measures of semicircular canal function, they may be capturing distinct phenomena. Caloric irrigation causes a slow convective flow of endolymph and provides a low frequency stimulus to the vestibular system. In contrast, high-velocity rotary head thrusts cause rapid endolymph movement and generate a high frequency input to vestibular afferents. It is possible that Ménière's disease preferentially impairs the ability of the vestibular apparatus to process low-frequency signals. It should be noted that the low-frequency caloric stimulus is a nonphysiologic input, whereas the high-frequency head thrust approximates commonly occurring stimulus frequencies to the vestibular apparatus during walking and running. Thus it is also possible that mechanisms of central adaptation can only be established for physiologic stimuli (leading to normal responses to head impulse testing) but not for inputs outside the normal range (i.e., caloric stimuli).

Vestibular-evoked myogenic potentials (VEMPs) are thought to reflect otolith function. The cervical VEMP (cVEMP) in response to air-conducted clicks or tonebursts appears to be generated by a sacculocollic reflex. In the afferent limb of this reflex pathway, acoustically-sensitive cells in the saccule respond to brief, loud, monaural sound stimuli and transmit an electrical signal centrally via the inferior vestibular nerve. The efferent limb of this reflex arc sends an inhibitory impulse to the fibers of the ipsilateral sternocleidomastoid muscle; electromyographic recordings from this muscle in response to a sound input thus reflect saccular function (35,36).

cVEMP responses to click stimuli were observed to be delayed or absent in 51% to 54% of patients with Ménière's disease (37,38) compared to the normal click-evoked response rates of 98%. Normal individuals demonstrate greatest sensitivity of their sacculocollic reflex over the 200 to 1,000 Hz frequency range (39,40); patients with Ménière's disease are noted to exhibit altered frequency tuning, such that the greatest sensitivity of the sacculocollic reflex appears to occur at higher frequencies and across a broader frequency range compared to normal subjects (41). Frequency tuning may be a function of the resonance properties of the saccule (which in part reflects the size of the saccule). Moreover, individuals with severe saccular dysfunction who experience drop attacks—otherwise known as otolithic crises of Tumarkin (42,43)—have the greatest blunting and frequency shift of their cVEMP tuning curves (44). Additionally, 27% of individuals with unilateral Ménière's disease were found to have cVEMP response abnormalities in their unaffected ear; the cVEMP tuning curves in these asymptomatic ears were noted to be intermediate in phenotype between affected and normal ears (45). cVEMP testing shows particular promise as a measure of Ménière's disease severity and in its ability to prognosticate bilateral disease.

Treatment

Given that the pathologic basis of Ménière's disease remains elusive, it follows that a curative treatment remains to be elucidated. Current therapies are directed at mitigating symptoms, particularly vertigo. First-line medical regimens include salt restriction and diuretics, aimed at alleviating endolymphatic hydrops. Betahistine, an H1-histamine receptor antagonist that increases inner ear blood flow, has been shown to reduce the frequency and severity of vertigo episodes. Betahistine is widely used in Europe in the treatment of Ménière's disease although its use is limited in the United States given insufficient evidence for its efficacy (46). Increasing evidence supports the use of corticosteroids, particularly delivered intratympanically, in the treatment of Ménière's disease. One large retrospective study found that control of vertigo symptoms was achieved in 91% of patients treated with intratympanic dexamethasone, allowing them to defer or avoid ablative therapies (47).

Medical therapy is insufficient to control vertigo symptoms in 10% of cases (48). Options for patients with refractory Ménière's disease include surgical decompression of the endolymphatic system, and surgical or chemical ablation of vestibular function. In endolymphatic sac surgery, a transmastoid approach is used to decompress the sac with or without placement of a shunt to drain endolymph. Studies demonstrate positive outcomes from endolymphatic shunt surgery in terms of hearing preservation and vertigo control (49), although a recent meta-analysis found that there is insufficient evidence showing efficacy of this procedure relative to placebo (50). Selective vestibular neurectomy via middle fossa or posterior fossa approach has been shown to relieve vertigo symptoms in over 90% of cases, although potential complications of these procedures, including hearing loss, facial nerve weakness, cerebrospinal fluid (CSF) leak, speech and language deficits (from temporal lobe retraction in the middle fossa approach), and headaches (from the posterior fossa approach) must be considered. Surgical labyrinthectomy achieves excellent vertigo control rates, although hearing in the operated ear is abolished.

Surgical procedures are increasingly being supplanted by chemical ablation of the peripheral vestibular apparatus using intratympanic gentamicin. Gentamicin is a relatively selective vestibulotoxic aminoglycoside antibiotic that is preferentially taken up by type I hair cells of the vestibular neuroepithelium (51). The use of low-dose intratympanic gentamicin has been shown to yield 70% to 90% vertigo control rates (52), and is associated with hearing loss in only 17% of cases (53). We have demonstrated that AVOR gains in Ménière's disease are typically normal before intratympanic gentamicin administration, and that they drop significantly after gentamicin, but not as much as after surgical labyrinthectomy (54). Studies in the chinchilla suggest that the lesion caused by intratympanic gentamicin primarily affects type I vestibular hair cells and may damage stereocilia on type II hair cells; however, vestibular nerve afferents continue to fire spontaneously after intratympanic gentamicin treatment (51,55). These findings suggest that a benefit of intratympanic gentamicin treatment over surgical ablation is that the gentamicin lesion is partial and does not create the kind of large static imbalance in vestibular nerve firing that accompanies surgical ablation. Therefore, adaptation to the intratympanic gentamicin lesion may be less challenging than to surgical ablation.

Migrainous Vertigo

Clinical Features

Vertigo is a common symptom of migraines, occurring in 25% of migraine patients (56). Vertigo may occur as an aura, which is a focal neurologic symptom preceding the headache. More commonly, however, attacks of vertigo occur independently and in some cases in place of the headache (57). In fact, typical migraine headaches occur with the vertigo spells in only about half of cases (58,59). Patients often report a prior history of migraine headaches that seem to have resolved. Milder head or neck pain or pressure may replace the pounding headaches and accompany the dizziness symptoms. The dizziness can be described as vertigo (spinning, rocking, swaying) or simply disequilibrium. The symptoms may be quite variable in duration, lasting minutes to days in episodic cases, or may present as constant disequilibrium lasting months. In approximately half of episodic cases the spells of vertigo or disequilibrium last more than a day (60), a feature that often helps distinguish migrainous vertigo from Ménière's disease. Photophobia, menstrual association, and nasal stuffiness at the time of attack all increase the odds that vertigo is migrainous in origin, especially if there is no history of hearing fluctuation or positional component (61). A family history of migraines may be helpful in the diagnosis, as may a history of unexplained falling spells or motion sensitivity as a child (62). Interestingly, the prevalence of migraine in patients with Ménière's disease is significantly higher than in the general population (63,64), and there may be a pathophysiologic link between the two disorders. This makes it sometimes difficult to distinguish the two in a given patient, and both may need to be treated for successful control of vertigo in some individuals.

Pathophysiology

Two pathophysiologic mechanisms have been hypothesized to cause migraine-associated vertigo: central electrical disturbances and peripheral trigeminovascular dysfunction. Functional MRI studies have demonstrated the centrifugal spread of depressed metabolic activity originating from the occipital cortex during visual aura progression (65).

This cortical spreading depression appears to represent a propagating wave of disturbed membrane ionic homeostasis; indeed, studies have linked at least one form of migraine (familial hemiplegic migraine) to several possible mutations, for example, in a calcium ion channel gene on chromosome 19 (66). Baloh (67) has suggested that the features of more common migraine syndromes resemble those of many inherited ion channelopathies. This may account for the efficacy of agents that cause an ion channel blockade, such as calcium channel blockers or beta-blockers, in the prevention and treatment of migraine. The spreading depression triggered by ion channel defects appears to affect not only cortical structures but also more caudal regions in the brainstem (68). A variety of structures may be affected by aberrant electrical activity in the tightly-packed brainstem anatomy. Involvement of the medial lemniscus, through which touch and proprioceptive fibers ascend to the thalamus, may contribute to the pain and allodynia (hypersensitivity to touch) experienced by migraineurs. Involvement of the ascending fibers of the reticular activating system, which regulate alertness, may explain the fatigue that often occurs during and after a migraine episode. Spread of the metabolic depression to the descending fibers of the brainstem that are responsible for the common integrator function of the vestibular and oculomotor systems may lead to disturbances of the VOR. The electrical disturbance may also affect the cochlear and vestibular nuclear complexes, producing the symptoms of hearing loss and vertigo. Indeed, transient sensorineural hearing loss as well as reduction in vestibular responses have been documented in patients with migraine (57,69,70).

Another possible mechanism to explain the observed labyrinthine dysfunction is activity in the trigeminovascular efferent system. Dysfunction of the trigeminal brainstem nuclei (possibly owing to spreading depression) may lead to aberrant efferent signals in the trigeminal nerve. The trigeminal nerve arborizes extensively in the head and neck, with efferents also demonstrated in the inner ear (71). Release of vasoactive compounds such as calcitonin gene-related peptide and Substance P by the trigeminal nerve may cause plasma extravasation and produce a local aseptic inflammation (72). Plasma extravasation from the spiral modiolar artery has been demonstrated after stimulation of the trigeminal ganglion, so it seems possible that a migrainous mechanism could directly affect cochlear and peripheral vestibular function (73). If so, this might explain the difficulty in separating some cases of migrainous vertigo from apparent Ménière's disease, as the peripheral effects of such trigeminovascular disturbances might mimic what we now think of as Ménière's disease.

Treatment

The treatment of migrainous vertigo can be quite successful if approached in a stepwise fashion, beginning with dietary and lifestyle modifications, and proceeding if needed to recognized migraine prophylactic agents (60).

Lifestyle changes should include regular sleep and exercise, and the identification and avoidance of migraine triggers. Stress, hormonal changes, weather and barometric pressure changes often incite migraine attacks. Common food triggers include byproducts of food aging and fermentation, such as red wine, aged cheese, yeast bread and yogurt, which contain high levels of tyramine. Foods that contain amines similar to our own neurotransmitters, such as caffeine, nitrates and other preservatives, chocolate, and various forms of glutamate including monosodium glutamate, have also been found to be migraine triggers and should be avoided. For symptoms that are constant and for which triggers cannot be identified or eliminated, the use of medications that raise the threshold above which migraines are triggered should be considered. Such prophylactic medications include calcium channel blockers, beta blockers, antidepressants such as nortriptyline or venlafaxine, and anticonvulsants including sodium valproate, gabapentin, and topiramate. Prophylactic medications should be selected based on the tolerability of their side effects in a given patient. Typically, benefits are seen after 6 to 8 weeks of therapy, and a realistic goal is to reduce symptom frequency and severity by 50% to 70%. For migraine attacks that persist despite lifestyle and dietary modifications and the use of prophylactic medications, migraine abortive medications such as the triptans can be considered. Abortive medications should not be used more than six to eight times per month, given their known rebound effects. Vestibular rehabilitation therapy has also been shown to significantly improve functional status in patients with migraine-associated vertigo (74,75).

Perilymph Fistula

Fractures of the bone of the labyrinthine capsule separating the inner ear from the middle ear and mastoid or disruption of the bone or membranes in the area of the oval or round windows can lead to a perilymph fistula with consequent sensorineural hearing loss and episodic vertigo (76,77). This diagnosis can be made with certainty following stapedectomy in which the prosthesis becomes dislodged and perilymph leaks from the open fenestra into the middle ear, and with a traumatic temporal bone fracture that allows a leakage of perilymph. In these situations, patching of the fenestration or of the area of the fracture can lead to stabilization of hearing and to eradication of vertigo. Additionally, labyrinthine fistulae, with or without leakage of perilymph, can occur in the setting of chronic otitis media, typically with cholesteatoma (78).

More ambiguous situations are encountered when a perilymph fistula is suspected in the absence of the pathologic entities described above. Potential anatomic communications between the middle and inner ears may account for the development of spontaneous perilymph fistulas (79), although these microfissures may be common in the temporal bone and not necessarily pathologic (80).

Goodhill (81) proposed that an implosive or explosive force can lead to membranous ruptures and to formation of perilymph fistula. A clear association has been reported between the Mondini deformity (partially formed cochlea lacking the normal 2½ turns) and perilymph fistula (82).

Criteria for determining when exploration for a perilymph fistula might be indicated have been difficult to establish because of the absence of an agreed upon diagnostic test that would be sensitive and specific for the identification of perilymph fistula. Studies that use electrocochleography have indicated that an abnormal ratio of SP to AP is seen in many patients with an acute leakage of perilymph (83). Fistula tests that involve positive and negative pressure in the external auditory canal and inspection for evoked eye movements (Hennebert sign) or symptoms have also been used. This testing method has been combined with platform posturography to look for increased sway in association with the pressure stimuli (84,85).

Findings at the time of middle ear exploration in patients with sudden deafness, vestibular symptoms, and/or auditory symptoms thought perhaps to be related to perilymph fistula have differed between studies and have been at times equivocal (86–88). Some patients with negative explorations have been reported to improve after surgery. The absence of an observed leakage of perilymph at the time of surgical exploration has been interpreted in different ways: that a fistula does not exist, that the fistula may be intermittent and not present at the time of surgical exploration, or that the fistula may not be detectable with conventional operative microscopy. Recommendations about how to proceed in cases in which a fistula was not identified (whether or not to patch the round and oval windows with fascia) have varied. In reports of endoscopic exploration of the middle ear when there were symptoms that could be due to spontaneous perilymph fistula, Poe and Bottrill (89) did not find evidence of a leak in any case.

The dilemmas surrounding the diagnosis and treatment of spontaneous perilymph fistula are likely to persist until a diagnostic test with high sensitivity and specificity is developed and until verification of a perilymph fistula can be definitively established at the time of surgery. Assays for beta-2 transferrin and beta-trace protein (proteins thought to be unique to perilymph and CSF) in tympanic cavity aspirates have been investigated, though the sensitivity of these analyses is low (90,91). Thus the questions posed in a comprehensive review of perilymph fistulas persist: "Can perilymph fistulas occur 'spontaneously'? What symptoms are specifically associated with such fistulas? What tests can diagnose a fistula? What is the 'gold standard' for confirming the presence of a fistula? How should a fistula be treated?" (77).

Vestibular Neuritis

Vestibular neuritis is a syndrome of sudden onset vertigo lasting for days without associated hearing loss or neurologic impairment (92). If hearing loss also occurs, this is referred to as labyrinthitis. Vestibular neuritis is thought to result from the reactivation of a latent herpes simplex virus type 1 infection in the vestibular ganglia. Histopathologic studies have demonstrated degeneration in Scarpa ganglion and the vestibular nerve after attacks of vestibular neuritis (93,94). Typically the superior division of the vestibular nerve is affected, possibly due to anatomic differences in the bony canals between the superior and inferior divisions (95,96). A reduction or loss of caloric responsiveness is the most consistent laboratory finding (97). Three-dimensional eye movement studies implicate only the horizontal and superior canals in generating the acute spontaneous nystagmus, whereas the posterior canal is still functional in many cases (98,99). The saccule continues to function in about two-thirds of patients as measured by cVEMP. About one-third of these individuals can go on to develop posterior canal BPPV, perhaps due to otolithic debris released from the damaged utricle (100).

A prospective, randomized, double-blind trial of 141 subjects with acute vestibular neuritis evaluated the relative efficacy of methylprednisolone alone, valacyclovir alone, and both methylprednisolone and valacyclovir compared to placebo in the treatment of vestibular neuritis as measured by caloric responsiveness within 3 days of the onset of symptoms and 12 months afterward (101). The study found a significant effect of methylprednisolone but not of valacyclovir on the recovery of a caloric response. The combination of methylprednisolone and valacyclovir was not superior to corticosteroid monotherapy. Steroids are thus the mainstay of treatment. Vestibular suppressants can relieve acute symptoms, but long-term use can impair compensation and should be minimized. Vestibular physical therapy should be initiated as early as possible to promote central compensation for any peripheral loss of function.

Immune-Mediated Inner Ear Disease

IMIED represents a syndrome of inner ear inflammation resulting from autoimmune mechanisms. Considerable evidence suggests that the inner ear is capable of mounting both humoral and cell-mediated immune responses (102–106). The endolymphatic sac appears to play a pivotal role in inner ear immunity; immune responses to antigenic stimulation in the cochlea were found to be significantly less robust in animals that had undergone sac obliteration (107). Temporal bone studies have demonstrated four histopathologic patterns associated with IMIED: (a) endolymphatic hydrops (or fluid-filled distension of the scala media as also seen with Ménière's disease); (b) acute labyrinthitis resulting in atrophy of hair cells and their supporting structures; (c) proliferation of fibrous tissue or bone ("neo-osteogenesis") and (d) neuronal atrophy.

IMIED may be a primary inner ear process with no evidence of associated systemic immune disease. In 15% to 30% of cases, IMIED is associated with systemic autoimmune conditions (108). It is a common feature of

Cogan syndrome, polyarteritis nodosa and relapsing polychondritis, and occurs more rarely with Wegener granulomatosis, systemic lupus erythematosus, sarcoidosis, Behçet disease and Sjögren syndrome (109). Given its association with various vasculitides, the presumed pathophysiologic mechanism for IMIED is vasculopathic changes to the labyrinthine arteries that supply the inner ear.

Clinical Features

IMIED typically presents with episodic auditory and vestibular symptoms. The onset of hearing loss in IMIED is relatively rapid, occurring over a course of weeks to months, distinguishing it from sudden sensorineural hearing loss that occurs over hours to days, and from slowly progressive hearing loss (e.g., presbycusis), which takes months to years to evolve. One ear may be affected first, followed almost invariably by decreased hearing in the contralateral ear within weeks to months. Progression to profound bilateral sensorineural hearing loss may occur in some cases. Vestibular symptoms in IMIED may also fluctuate over time, often in concert with fluctuations in hearing. Vertigo accompanies hearing loss in IMIED in over 50% of cases, while 25% to 50% of patients experience tinnitus and aural fullness associated with their hearing loss (108).

The co-occurrence of hearing loss exacerbations, vertigo, tinnitus, and aural fullness can also suggest a diagnosis of Ménière's disease. The principal method for distinguishing between these two clinical entities is by considering the time course of symptoms. In Ménière's disease, hearing loss occurs over a period of years rather than the weeks to months characteristic of IMIED. Additionally, Ménière's disease is more likely to be unilateral, with progression to the contralateral ear occurring in fewer than 50% of cases (110). It is critical to distinguish between IMIED and Ménière's disease given that IMIED is more likely to respond to the early initiation of aggressive immunosuppressive therapy. The time course of audiovestibular symptoms in IMIED can also be similar to neurosyphilis involving the inner ear (see Chapter 156 for further details); serologic testing for treponemal antibodies is critical to distinguish between these clinical entities.

A history of ocular disease in a patient with IMIED is a characteristic feature of Behçet disease, Cogan syndrome, relapsing polychondritis, and sarcoidosis. Ocular inflammation, however, may not coincide temporally with audiovestibular symptoms. Ocular inflammatory disease can take the form of conjunctivitis, keratitis (corneal inflammation), scleritis (inflammation of the white outer fibrous layer), uveitis (inflammation of the uveal layer—the iris, choroid and ciliary body), or retinal vasculitis. Ocular symptoms for any of these diseases can include redness of the eye, blurry vision, photophobia, floating spots, or eye pain. Associated clinical symptoms help to distinguish between disease entities. Behçet disease is typically accompanied by oral and genital ulcers. Cogan syndrome is defined as a triad including audiovestibular

dysfunction, interstitial keratitis (similar to that seen with syphilis) and other forms of ocular inflammation, and systemic autoimmune vasculitis. A hallmark symptom of relapsing polychondritis is inflammation of the auricular cartilages, which manifests as ear erythema, edema, and tenderness that spares the ear lobule and external auditory canal. Sarcoidosis is an idiopathic granulomatous disease associated with hilar lymphadenopathy, arthralgias, and erythema nodosum. Neurosarcoidosis refers to granulomatous involvement of the central nervous system (CNS); typical features include facial paralysis, visual changes, and hearing loss (associated with cranial neuropathies). Definitive diagnosis of neurosarcoidosis is made based on biopsy; however, given the difficulty of obtaining CNS tissue ancillary studies such as elevated serum angiotensin-converting enzyme levels or calcium levels may suggest the diagnosis. A clinical history suggestive of IMIED should prompt questioning about associated ocular symptoms.

There is no pathognomonic serologic test for IMIED; the data are perhaps most compelling for the antibody to the 68 kDa protein. In a cohort of 72 patients with idiopathic, progressive, bilateral sensorineural hearing loss, Moscicki et al. (111) found significantly higher levels of an antibody to a 68 kDa inner ear protein in patients whose hearing loss responded to corticosteroid treatment. This inner ear protein was initially thought to be heat shock protein-70, a biologically plausible hypothesis given the known role of heat shock proteins in the immune response (112,113). However, this hypothesis was not borne out in subsequent experimental analyses (114,115). More recent work has suggested that the antibody to the 68 kDa antigen is the Kresge Hearing Research Institute-3 antibody, which binds to an antigen on the supporting cells of the Organ of Corti and results in outer hair cell depletion and hearing loss (116,117). Additionally, the 68 kDa antigen itself has been identified as likely being the choline transporter-like-2 (CTL-2) protein (118). CTL-2 regulates the function of choline, which is a constituent of the neurotransmitter acetylcholine as well as of the cell membrane component phosphatidylcholine and may be required for hair cell survival. Knowing if a patient is seropositive for the antibody to the 68 kDa antigen is of potential clinical value given studies showing the increased effectiveness of steroids in these patients (119), although commercial assays for the antibody to the 68kDa protein are not widely available or well validated (120). In patients with suspected IMIED based on clinical presentation, obtaining an erythrocyte sedimentation rate or C-reactive protein may also be helpful to screen for a systemic autoimmune disease (121). Other serologic tests for IMIED have included the lymphocyte transformation test, which targets type II collagen, and the lymphocyte migration inhibition test, although the sensitivity and specificity of these tests are low and they are no longer in common clinical use. Diagnosing IMIED remains primarily based on clinical history, responsiveness to steroid therapy, and evidence of associated systemic autoimmune disease.

Treatment

IMIED is a particularly important diagnosis to make because it is one of the few causes of bilateral hearing loss or vestibulopathy that is potentially reversible. As such, IMIED is worth treating aggressively. The mainstay of treatment consists of corticosteroids; studies have shown that 60% to 70% of patients diagnosed with IMIED demonstrate clinical improvement following steroid therapy (122,123). If the patient does not respond to 2 weeks of steroids, cyclophosphamide or methotrexate may be added to the regimen. If patients show no sign of a clinical response to combined prednisone and adjunctive therapy after 3 months, therapy is discontinued to prevent treatment complications. Studies have also evaluated intratympanic application of steroids, with mixed results (124,125). The efficacy of corticosteroids in the treatment of IMIED may be derived from their glucocorticoid (anti-inflammatory) as well as mineralocorticoid effects (126). Patients who are refractory to medical therapy or who cannot be maintained on corticosteroids due to complications may benefit from hearing aids and possibly be candidates for cochlear implantation.

BRIEF EPISODIC EXCITATION OF UNILATERAL VESTIBULAR FUNCTION

Benign Paroxysmal Positional Vertigo

BPPV is the most common cause of dizziness, accounting for around 40% of vertigo complaints from patients (127). BPPV may be caused by cupulolithiasis, whereby otoconial debris are lodged in the cupula of the semicircular canals, or canalolithiasis, whereby debris are free-floating in the semicircular canal endolymphatic fluid. Typical symptoms are brief episodes of vertigo lasting less than a minute that occur after turning the head; a classic presentation is brief vertigo when rolling over in bed. The ectopic otoconia are thought to arise from the utricle, possibly following a head trauma or an ischemic injury to the inner ear. The posterior canal is usually the affected canal. Horizontal canal BPPV does occur, typically resulting from a repositioning maneuver whereby free-floating otoconia have not yet migrated back into the utricle as intended. Superior canal BPPV occurs, but even more rarely.

The diagnosis of BPPV is typically made by observing nystagmus patterns following the Dix-Hallpike positioning maneuver, whereby patients start sitting and are lowered to a supine position with the head extended and turned 45 degrees to the right or left side (Fig. 166.1) (92). The right Dix-Hallpike maneuver brings the right posterior canal into an earth-vertical plane and will cause any loose otoconia to move in an ampullofugal, or excitatory, direction. Interpreting the nystagmus of BPPV is critical to identifying the affected canal. For the posterior canal, which is normally excited by rotating the head up and rolling it toward the ipsilateral side, the appropriate nystagmus is compensatory to this perceived head movement: It has a slow phase that is downward and rolling toward the contralateral side. The fast phases of the nystagmus will beat upward and roll toward the ipsilateral side, which, being toward the ground in the Dix-Hallpike position, led to the term, "geotropic." A

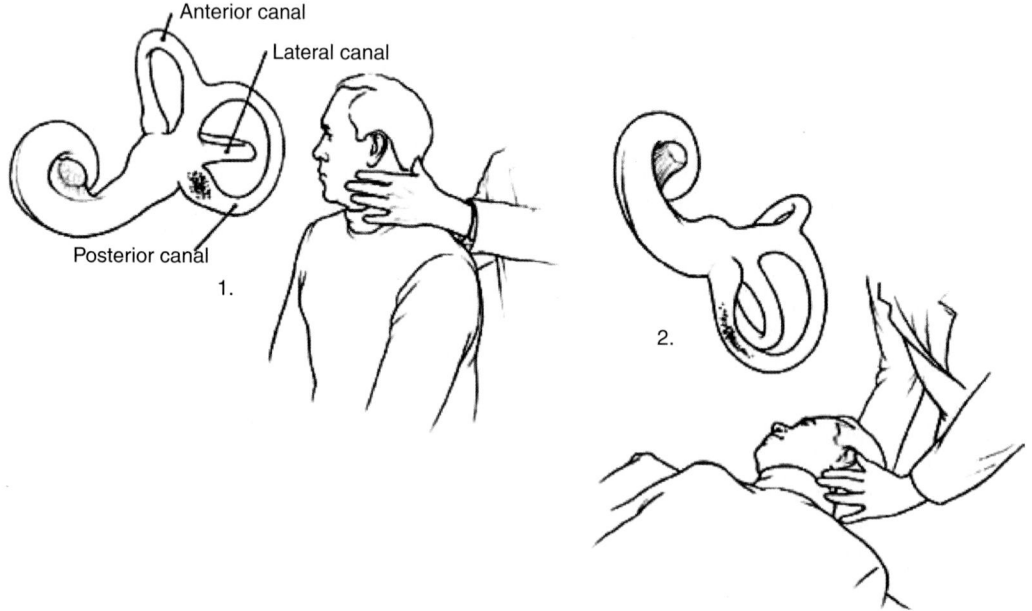

Figure 166.1 The Dix-Hallpike maneuver for identification of right posterior canal BPPV. The patient's head is turned 45 degrees to the right while sitting upright (*step 1*). Then lowering the patient to supine position with the head extended and still to the right (*step 2*) allows debris in the posterior canal to fall to a lower position in the canal. The resulting flow of endolymph away from the ampulla causes nystagmus due to deflection of the posterior canal cupula. From Hullar TE, Minor LB. The neurotologic examination. In: Jackler RK, Brackmann DE. *Neurotology*, 2nd ed. St. Louis, MO: Mosby, 2004. BPPV, benign paroxysmal positioning vertigo.

diagnosis of BPPV resulting from canalolithiasis of the posterior semicircular canal can be made with great clarity based upon the latency (2 to 10 seconds), duration (10 to 40 seconds), direction (upbeating with a torsional geotropic component beating toward the downward ear), and fatigability of the nystagmus upon repeated testing. The nystagmus with lateral canal BPPV is horizontal and may beat toward (geotropic) or away from (ageotropic) the downward ear. It often begins with a shorter latency, increases in magnitude while maintaining the test position, and is less susceptible to fatigue with repetitive testing than the nystagmus observed with posterior canal BPPV. If the nystagmus is geotropic, the particles are likely to be in the long arm of the lateral canal relatively far from the ampulla. If the nystagmus is ageotropic, the particles could be in the long arm relatively close to the ampulla, attached to the cupula, or on the opposite side of the cupula either floating within the endolymph or embedded in the cupula. This presentation is thus termed "cupulolithiasis." The difficulty in cases of cupulolithiasis arises in sorting out which horizontal canal (left or right) has the pathologic process because laying 70 degrees back toward supine with the head turned to one side will elicit ageotropic nystagmus whether the left or right horizontal canal is involved. The side that, when placed down, elicits greater symptomatic complaints and nystagmus amplitude is likely the provocative ear. These features can also lead to the nystagmus of horizontal canal BPPV being confused with a positional nystagmus arising from a central abnormality.

Canal repositioning maneuvers are designed to move otoconial particles from the semicircular canals back into the vestibule. The most commonly used maneuver to treat posterior canal canalolithiasis BPPV was described by Epley (128): Patients are first placed in the Dix-Hallpike position that provokes their vertigo; the head is then rolled 180 degrees in two steps until the affected ear is up; and finally the patient is returned to a sitting position (Fig. 166.2). Patients may experience a recurrence of their symptoms and require repetition of the Epley maneuver at home for several weeks. Other repositioning maneuvers, including the Semont liberatory maneuver and the Brandt-Daroff exercises have also been described for the treatment of BPPV that may not respond to the Epley maneuver, and specific maneuvers have also been described for the horizontal canals.

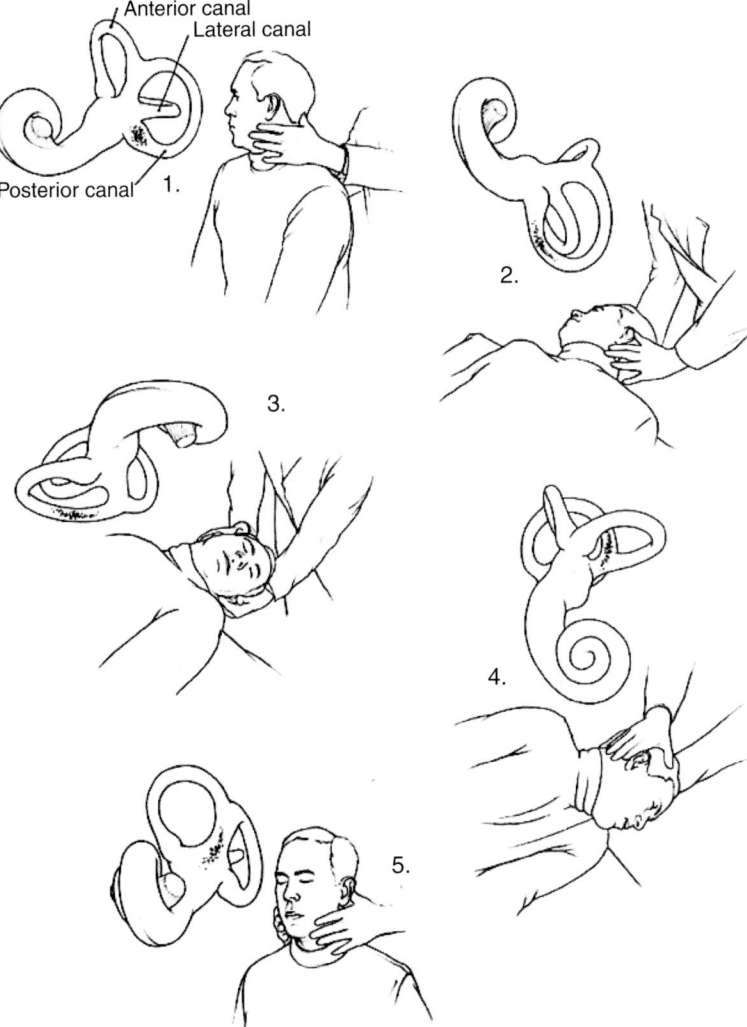

Figure 166.2 Canalith repositioning maneuver for treatment of BPPV affecting the posterior semicircular canal. In panel *1*, the patient's head is turned to the right at the beginning of the canalith repositioning maneuver. The **inset** shows the location of the otoconial debris near the ampulla of the posterior canal. The diagram of the head in each inset shows the orientation from which the labyrinth is viewed. In panel *2*, the patient is brought into the supine position with the head extended below the level of the table, that is, the Dix-Hallpike position as shown in Figure 166.1. The debris falls toward the common crus as the head is moved backward. In panel *3*, the head is rotated approximately 90 degrees to the left while keeping the neck extended with the head below the level of the table. Debris enters the common crus as the head is turned toward the contralateral side. In panel *4*, the patient's head is further rotated to the left by 90 degrees, rolling onto the left side until the patient's head faces down, and the debris begins to enter the vestibule. In panel *5*, the patient is brought back to the upright position, not turning the head until the patient is upright so that debris stays in the vestibule. Illustration by David Rini. From Hullar TE, Minor LB. Vestibular physiology and disorders of the labyrinth. In: Glasscock ME, Gulya AJ, eds. *Surgery of the ear.* 5th ed. Hamilton, ON: People's Medical Publishing House, 2003, Chapter 4. BPPV, benign paroxysmal positional vertigo.

Canalith repositioning maneuvers have been shown to control symptoms in over 90% of BPPV cases. However, a small fraction of patients continue to have refractory disabling vertigo despite multiple repositioning attempts. In these patients, surgical treatment may be considered. Section of the posterior ampullary nerve, also known as singular neurectomy, can be performed by accessing the singular nerve deep to the round window niche via a transcanal approach (129). More commonly, posterior semicircular canal occlusion is performed through a transmastoid approach, whereby the canal lumen is blocked, eliminating endolymph flow in response to the gravitational pull on canaloliths, but also dampening flow for most head movements that would normally excite the plugged canal (130).

Superior Canal Dehiscence Syndrome

In 1998, Minor et al. (131) described that dehiscence of bone overlying the superior semicircular canal can result in a clinical syndrome with symptoms and signs related to vestibular and auditory dysfunction. The vestibular abnormalities include vertigo and oscillopsia induced by loud noises or by stimuli that change middle ear or intracranial pressure. These patients may exhibit a Tullio phenomenon (eye movements induced by loud noises) or Hennebert sign (eye movements induced by pressure in the external auditory canal). They may also experience chronic disequilibrium. The auditory abnormalities include an apparent conductive hearing loss (manifested as an air–bone gap on audiometry that is not due to middle ear pathology), autophony, and pulsatile tinnitus.

The pathophysiology of SCD can be understood in terms of the effects of the dehiscence in creating a "third mobile window" into the inner ear, thereby allowing the superior canal to respond to sound and pressure stimuli (131). The finding that eye movements evoked by sound or by pressure stimuli are in the same plane as the superior canal of the affected ear was important in focusing attention on the superior canal as the cause of these abnormalities (131,132).

Clinical Features

In a study of 65 patients with SCD, the age range at the time of diagnosis was 13 to 70 (median = 41; mean = 43) years. The right ear alone was affected in 27 patients and the left ear alone in 23 patients; 10 patients had vestibular symptoms, signs, and CT findings indicative of bilateral SCD. Vestibular manifestations were present in 60 and exclusively auditory manifestations without vestibular symptoms or signs were noted in five patients (133).

The eye movements induced by sound and pressure stimuli have an important role in making the diagnosis (131,132). These stimuli often lead to nystagmus in SCD syndrome. The direction of the slow phase components of this nystagmus can be understood based upon the action of these sound and pressure stimuli on the affected superior canal. Loud sounds, positive pressure in the external auditory canal, and the Valsalva maneuver against pinched nostrils cause ampullofugal deflection of the cupula in the superior canal (Fig. 166.3). The nystagmus that is observed with these stimuli has slow phase components that are directed upward with torsional motion of the superior pole of the eye away from the affected ear. Conversely, negative pressure in the external canal, Valsalva against a closed glottis, and jugular venous compression can cause oppositely directed eye movements with slow phase components directed downward with torsional motion of the superior pole of the eye toward the affected ear.

Auditory symptoms and signs in patients with SCD have also been described (134,135). The Weber tuning fork test (512 Hz) typically lateralizes to the affected ear. Patients can experience symptoms such as hearing their pulse or hearing their eye movements, and their own voice may be perceived as distorted and too loud, a phenomenon known as autophony (136). An increased sensitivity to bone-conducted sounds, due to the low impedance for bone-conducted sound to enter the inner ear at the dehiscence, appears to be the mechanism responsible for the auditory symptoms in these patients.

Autophony can also be caused by patulous eustachian tube (137). A loss of tissue within the cartilaginous portion of the eustachian tube is thought to cause abnormal patency of the tube that results in abnormally loud perception of a person's own voice. The autophony associated with SCD tends to be unremitting from the time of onset, whereas autophony due to patulous eustachian tube may be more intermittent and especially position dependent. A further difference in the characteristics of autophony in the two conditions is that patulous eustachian tube results in autophony that is equally loud for the spoken voice and for breathing sounds, whereas autophony in SCD is typically absent for breathing sounds. Finally, on otoscopy or tympanometry patients with patulous eustachian tube who are experiencing autophony frequently will demonstrate excursions of the tympanic membrane synchronous with nasal breathing when sitting upright, especially if the contralateral nostril is closed.

Diagnostic Tests in Superior Canal Dehiscence Syndrome

Bone conduction thresholds on audiometry in patients with SCD can be less than 0 dB hearing level, that is, better than normal. An air–bone gap, therefore, can exist even when air conduction thresholds are in the normal range (134,135). These patients have heightened sensitivity for bone-conducted sounds, a phenomenon known as conductive hyperacusis. In many cases air-conduction thresholds are also elevated as well due to the loss of air-conducted sound energy at the dehiscence. The air–bone gap in patients with SCD is typically greatest at the lower frequencies (250 to 1,000 Hz).

Distinguishing an air–bone gap on audiometry due to SCD from an air–bone gap due to middle ear pathology is important in determining the appropriate

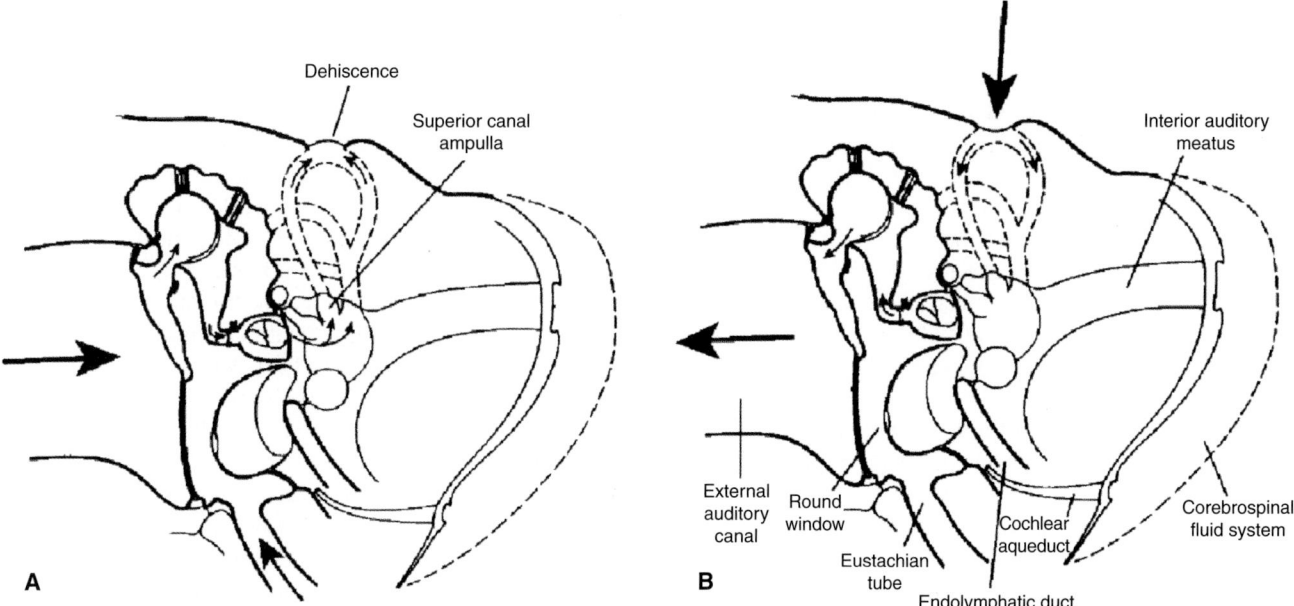

Figure 166.3 Schematic drawing of pressure changes in the middle and inner ear resulting from testing maneuvers in SCD syndrome. **A:** Sound, positive pressure in the external canal, or Valsalva maneuver against pinched nostrils move the stapes inward and result in ampullofugal endolymph flow with corresponding outward movement in the area of dehiscence. This results in excitation of vestibular-nerve afferents innervating the ampulla. **B:** Valsalva maneuver against a closed glottis, bilateral jugular venous compression, and negative pressure in the external canal result in inward movement in the area of dehiscence of the superior canal. Such pressure leads to ampullopetal deflection of the cupula and inhibition of the superior canal nerve afferents. Figure reproduced from Minor LB, Solomon D, Zinreich JS, et al. Sound-and/or pressure-induced vertigo due to bone dehiscence of the superior semicircular canal. *Arch Otolaryngol Head Neck Surg* 1998;124:249–258, with permission.

treatment options. Patients with an air–bone gap that was subsequently shown to be due to SCD but who underwent stapes surgery for presumed otosclerosis have been reported (134,135,139). Air conduction thresholds did not improve in these patients following stapes surgery. The acoustic reflex test provides a useful screening test in the identification of patients in whom the conductive hearing loss on audiometry may be due to SCD rather than to a middle ear problem such as otosclerosis. True fixation of the stapes should abolish the stapedial acoustic reflex response, whereas SCD causes conductive hearing loss but does not abolish the response. Patients with intact acoustic reflex responses and an air–bone gap on audiometry should undergo further investigation for SCD, such as a high-resolution CT scan of the temporal bones, before proceeding with surgical exploration of the middle ear.

Patients with SCDS typically have a lowered threshold for air-conducted sound to elicit the cVEMP from the ear affected by the disorder. They also have larger amplitudes for the air-conducted sound cVEMP as well as the ocular VEMP response from the affected ear (140–142). The "third mobile window" associated with the dehiscence creates a low impedance pathway that increases the sensitivity of vestibular receptors to sound and pressure stimuli. Assessment of air-conducted VEMP responses can be particularly useful in the search for the cause of an air–bone gap on audiometry. Conductive hearing loss caused by a middle ear abnormality typically results in the absence of an air-conducted VEMP response in the affected ear because the pathology decreases the amount of sound energy that is delivered to the inner ear. The presence of a VEMP response elicited at an abnormally low threshold in the setting of conductive hearing loss provides powerful evidence that middle ear mechanisms are not responsible for the air–bone gap.

High-resolution temporal bone CT scans have been used to identify dehiscence of bone overlying the superior canal. Patients with unilateral dehiscence are more likely to have thinning of the bone overlying the contralateral superior canal, suggesting an underlying developmental or congenital abnormality (143,144). Given that the onset of symptoms and signs of SCD typically occurs during adulthood, patients may develop the syndrome when an abnormally thin layer of bone is disrupted by trauma or eroded over time by pressure from the overlying temporal lobe.

Treatment

Many patients with SCD are not debilitated by the disorder and are able to avoid the stimuli that elicit the symptoms and signs. These patients may not need any specific treatment for the disorder. In other patients, symptoms such as sound- or pressure-induced vertigo, pulsatile oscillopsia, and chronic disequilibrium may be disabling. Surgical repair of SCD is typically performed through the middle cranial fossa approach (131), although a transmastoid approach has also been described (145). The dehiscent superior canal is plugged with fascia and bone, thereby obliterating the canal lumen, and the bony middle fossa plate is resurfaced with bone cement. In our experience, plugging the superior canal has been more effective in resolving SCD symptoms than canal resurfacing alone (133), and studies have demonstrated closure of the air–bone gap and normalization of VEMP responses following plugging of a dehiscent superior canal (142,146).

Chronically Inadequate Vestibular Function

Chronic loss of vestibular function typically does not present with long-standing vertigo, which is indicative of episodic disruption or excitation of vestibular activity. Acoustic neuromas, for example, cause a slow progressive decline in vestibular function, and patients infrequently present with attacks of rotary vertigo. Patients with acoustic neuromas may exhibit hyperventilation-induced nystagmus (147), whereby patients breathe heavily for 30 breaths or 30 seconds, and a nystagmus with the fast phase beating to the side of the lesion can be observed. Proposed mechanisms for this effect include transiently improving conduction in a partially demyelinated nerve leading to a relative gain in function. Acoustic neuromas are more fully discussed in Chapter 159.

Bilateral Vestibular Hypofunction

The most common cause of bilateral vestibular hypofunction is exposure to intravenous antibiotics, specifically aminoglycosides. As mentioned previously, gentamicin is an ototoxic antibiotic that damages type I vestibular hair cells (51). Following peak and trough serum gentamicin levels as well as cumulative doses may prevent ototoxicity in some but not all cases. Ideally patients on gentamicin should have daily clinical assessments of their vestibular function (using head thrust testing or dynamic visual acuity) to identify any vestibulotoxicity as soon as possible (148), as immediately halting the aminoglycoside may preserve some function (Chapter 144). Patients with poor renal function or who are receiving concomitant ototoxic medications such as loop diuretics are at increased risk of vestibular loss. The A1555G mitochondrial mutation has also been shown to confer an increased risk of gentamicin-induced ototoxicity (149). Other causes of bilateral loss of vestibular function include genetic causes, exposure to radiation or chemotherapy, autoimmune mechanisms, bilateral Ménière's disease, and neurofibromatosis-2. Oscillopsia, or gaze destabilization with head movement and a sense of motion of objects that are stationary, as well as poor postural control and gait ataxia, are typical symptoms of bilateral vestibular hypofunction. It must be emphasized that these patients tend *not* to experience episodic vertigo. Central compensation for chronic peripheral vestibular loss occurs over time in most but not all patients receiving vestibular physical therapy (150). Because of the poor performance of other ocular reflexes (visual following, cervicoocular reflex, optokinetic reflex, etc.) at high frequencies, compensation can never fully restore visual stability for high acceleration head movements as may occur with unpredictable perturbations (e.g., stepping into a pothole while walking).

Vestibular rehabilitation, or vestibular physical therapy, is currently the primary treatment modality for bilateral vestibular hypofunction (151). The goal of vestibular rehabilitation is to foster compensation for vestibular loss (152). Patients are given exercises to induce compensation via three complementary approaches: *adaptation*, whereby residual vestibular mechanisms are trained to augment their level of functioning; *substitution*, whereby patients increase their reliance on other sensory inputs such as visual or proprioceptive cues to maintain balance; and *habituation*, whereby individuals learn to decrease their sensitivity to provocative stimuli (153). The efficacy of vestibular rehabilitation in reducing symptoms of vestibular dysfunction is supported by strong and consistent evidence (Chapter 168) (154). In the future, the multi-channel vestibular prosthesis currently under development may be of significant benefit to patients with bilateral vestibular hypofunction who do not have sufficient functional abilities after vestibular rehabilitation (155).

HIGHLIGHTS

- Ménière's disease is characterized by spontaneous attacks of vertigo, fluctuating low-frequency hearing loss, aural fullness, and tinnitus. Common laboratory abnormalities include a low-frequency sensorineural hearing loss, SP/AP ratio greater than 0.4 on electrocochleography, caloric weakness, and reduced VEMP responses. First-line therapy includes salt restriction and diuretics. Next, intratympanic steroid treatment may be beneficial. Chemical or surgical vestibular ablations are options in recalcitrant cases.

- Migrainous vertigo is a syndrome of episodic vertigo that lasts for minutes to days, and may or may not be associated with classic migraine headaches. Associated symptoms frequently include photophobia, visual motion sensitivity, and nausea. The diagnosis is suggested by a history of migraine headaches or a family history of migraine. Two theories have been proposed to explain migraine-associated vertigo: central electrical disturbances and peripheral trigeminovascular dysfunction. Treatment consists of avoiding dietary and lifestyle triggers, and the use of migraine prophylactic medications.

- Perilymph fistulas are known to occur following stapes surgery, temporal bone trauma, or in the presence of a labyrinthine fistula (e.g., secondary to cholesteatoma). Patients with a Mondini deformity are at increased risk. Both a sensitive diagnostic test for perilymph fistula and clear treatment guidelines are lacking, but the fistula test (observing for eye movements during pressurization of the external auditory canal) may be helpful.

- Vestibular neuritis is a syndrome of vertigo that lasts for days, and if there is associated hearing loss this is referred to as labyrinthitis. Vestibular neuritis likely represents a reactivation of a latent herpetic infection, usually of the superior vestibular nerve, associated with caloric weakness (superior nerve test) and preservation of the cVEMP (inferior nerve test). Steroids are the mainstay of treatment, and vestibular rehabilitation should be offered routinely.

- IMIED is a syndrome of inner ear inflammation resulting from autoimmunity. Patients present with fluctuating vertigo and hearing loss, often similar to Ménière's disease, though usually bilateral and with a faster decline in audiovestibular function in IMIED. Cogan syndrome includes IMIED associated with ocular inflammation—typically interstitial keratitis—and a systemic vasculitis. The presence of antibodies to a 68 kDa protein is suggestive of IMIED. The mainstay of treatment is initial steroid therapy followed by longer-term steroid-sparing immunosuppressive agents.

- BPPV is the most common cause of vertigo. It is due to ectopic otoconia free-floating in the endolymph (canalolithiasis) or, less commonly, lodged in the cupula (cupulolithiasis). The posterior canal is most commonly affected. The diagnosis can be made by observing an upbeating, geotropic nystagmus in the Dix-Hallpike position. The majority of cases resolve with canalith repositioning maneuvers such as the Epley maneuver.

- SCD syndrome is characterized by vertigo and oscillopsia induced by loud noises or stimuli that change middle ear or intracranial pressure, owing to a "third mobile window" created by the dehiscence. Patients may also experience autophony, pulsatile tinnitus, or conductive hyperacusis. Eye movements to provocative stimuli are in the plane of the affected superior canal. Testing abnormalities include a low-frequency air–bone gap on audiometry but with intact stapedial reflexes and lowered cVEMP thresholds and elevated oVEMP amplitudes. The diagnosis is made based on high-resolution temporal bone CT. Surgical plugging of the dehiscent superior canal is the most effective treatment.

- Bilateral vestibular hypofunction most commonly results from exposure to aminoglycoside antibiotics. The risk is increased in patients with poor renal function or who are using concomitant ototoxic medications such as a loop diuretic. Patients typically experience oscillopsia and chronic disequilibrium, *not* vertigo. Vestibular rehabilitation is the mainstay of therapy.

REFERENCES

1. Schubert MC, Minor LB. Vestibulo-ocular physiology underlying vestibular hypofunction. *Phys Ther* 2004;84(4):373–385.
2. Paparella MM, Sajjadi H. Endolymphatic sac enhancement: principles of diagnosis and treatment. *Am J Otol* 1987;8(4):294–300.
3. Minor LB, Schessel DA, Carey JP. Ménière's disease. *Curr Opin Neurol* 2004;17(1):9–16.
4. Shojaku H, Watanabe Y, Fujisaka M, et al. Epidemiologic characteristics of definite Ménière's disease in Japan. A long-term survey of Toyama and Niigata prefectures. *ORL J Otorhinolaryngol Relat Spec* 2005;67(5):305–309.
5. Cawthorne T, Hewlett AB. Ménière's disease. *Proc R Soc Med* 1954;47:663–670.
6. Harris JP, Alexander TH. Current-day prevalence of Ménière's syndrome. *Audiol Neurootol* 2010;15(5):318–322.
7. Havia M, Kentala E, Pyykko I. Prevalence of Ménière's disease in general population of Southern Finland. *Otolaryngol Head Neck Surg* 2005;133(5):762–768.
8. House JW, Doherty JK, Fisher LM, et al. Ménière's disease: prevalence of contralateral ear involvement. *Otol Neurotol* 2006;27(3):355–361.
9. Monsell EM, Balkany TA, Gates GA, et al. Committee on Hearing and Equilibrium guidelines for the diagnosis and evaluation of therapy in Ménière's disease. *Otalaryngol Head Neck Surg* 1995;113:181–185.
10. Paparella MM, Mancini F. Vestibular Ménière's disease. *Otalaryngol Head Neck Surg* 1985;93(2):148–151.
11. Silverstein H, Smouha E, Jones R. Natural history vs. surgery for Ménière's disease. *Otalaryngol Head Neck Surg* 1989;100:6–16.
12. Friberg U, Stahle J, Svedberg A. The natural course of Ménière's disease. *Acta Otolaryngol Suppl (Stockh)* 1984;406:72–77.
13. Stahle J. Advanced Ménière's disease: a study of 356 severely disabled patients. *Acta Otolaryngol (Stockh)* 1976;81:113–119.
14. Lustig LR, Yeagle J, Niparko JK, et al. Cochlear implantation in patients with bilateral Ménière's syndrome. *Otol Neurotol* 2003;24(3):397–403.
15. Hallpike CS, Cairns H. Observations on the pathology of Ménière's syndrome. *J Laryngol Otol* 1938;53:625–655.
16. Schuknecht HF, Igarashi M. Pathophysiology of Ménière's disease. In: Pfaltz CR, ed. *Controversial aspects of Ménière's disease.* New York: Georg Thieme, 1986.
17. Anatoli-Candela F. The histopathology of Ménière's disease. *Acta Otolaryngol Suppl (Stockh)* 1976;340:5–42.
18. Paparella MM. The cause (multifactorial inheritance) and pathogenesis (endolymphatic malabsorption) of Ménière's disease and its symptoms (mechanical and chemical). *Acta Otolaryngol (Stockh)* 1985;99:445.
19. Schuknecht HF. Endolymphatic hydrops—can it be controlled. *Ann Otol Rhinol Laryngol* 1986;95(1):36–39.
20. Schuknecht HF. Ménière's disease: a correlation of symptomology and pathology. *Laryngoscope* 1963;73:651–665.
21. Thomsen J, Bretlau P. General conclusions. In: Pfaltz CR, ed. *Controversial aspects of Ménière's disease.* New York: Georg Thiem Verlag Stuttgart, 1986.
22. Merchant SN, Adams JC, Nadol JB Jr. Pathophysiology of Ménière's syndrome: are symptoms caused by endolymphatic hydrops? *Otol Neurotol* 2005;26(1):74–81.

23. Sass K. Sensitivity and specificiety of transtympanic electro-cochleography in Ménière's disease. *Acta Otolaryngol (Stockh)* 1998;118:150–156.

24. Adams ME, Heidenreich KD, Kileny PR. Audiovestibular testing in patients with Ménière's disease. *Otolaryngol Clin North Am* 2010;43(5):995–1009.

25. Claes GM, De Valck CF, van de Heyning P, et al. The Ménière's Disease Index: an objective correlate of Ménière's disease, based on audiometric and electrocochleographic data. *Otol Neurotol* 2011;32(5):887–892.

26. Proctor L, Dix R, Hughes D, et al. Stimulation of the vestibular receptor by means of step temperature changes during continuous aural irrigation. *Acta Otolaryngol (Stockh)* 1975;79: 425–435.

27. Aw ST, Haslwanter T, Halmagyi GM, et al. Three dimensional vector analysis of the human vestibulo–ocular reflex in response to high–acceleration head rotations I. Responses in normal subjects. *J Neurophysiol* 1996;76(6):4009–4020.

28. Stahle J, Klockhoff I. Diagnostic procedures, differential diagnosis and general conclusions. In: Pfaltz CR, ed. *Controversial aspects of Ménière's disease.* New York: George Thieme, 1986;71–86.

29. Park HJ, Migliaccio AA, Della Santina CC, et al. Search-coil head-thrust and caloric tests in Ménière's disease. *Acta Otolaryngol* 2005;125(8):852–827.

30. Black FO, Kitch R. A review of vestibular test results in Ménière's disease. *Otolaryngol Clin North Am* 1980;13(4):631–642.

31. Oosterveld WJ. Ménière's disease, signs and symptoms. *J Laryngol Otol* 1980;94(8):885–892.

32. Martin E, Perez N. Hearing loss after intratympanic gentamicin therapy for unilateral Ménière's disease. *Otol Neurotol* 2003;24(5):800–806.

33. Enander A, Stahle J. Hearing loss and caloric response in Ménière's disease. A comparative study. *Acta Otolaryngol* 1969;67(1):57–68.

34. Hone SW, Nedzelski J, Chen J. Does intratympanic gentamicin treatment for Ménière's disease cause complete vestibular ablation? [In Process Citation]. *J Otolaryngol* 2000;29(2):83–87.

35. McCue MP, Guinan JJ Jr. Acoustically responsive fibers in the vestibular nerve of the cat. *J Neurosci* 1994;14(10):6058–6070.

36. Colebatch JG, Halmagyi GM. Vestibular evoked potentials in human neck muscles before and after unilateral vestibular deafferentation. *Neurology* 1992;42:1635–1636.

37. de Waele C, Huy PT, Diard JP, et al. Saccular dysfunction in Ménière's disease. *Am J Otol* 1999;20(2):223–232.

38. Murofushi T, Shimizu K, Takegoshi H, et al. Diagnostic value of prolonged latencies in the vestibular evoked myogenic potential. *Arch Otolaryngol Head Neck Surg* 2001;127(9):1069–1072.

39. Todd NP, Cody FW, Banks JR. A saccular origin of frequency tuning in myogenic vestibular evoked potentials?: implications for human responses to loud sounds. *Hear Res* 2000;141(1-2): 180–188.

40. Welgampola MS, Colebatch JG. Characteristics of tone burst-evoked myogenic potentials in the sternocleidomastoid muscles. *Otol Neurotol* 2001;22(6):796–802.

41. Rauch SD, Zhou G, Kujawa SG, et al. Vestibular evoked myogenic potentials show altered tuning in patients with Ménière's disease. *Otol Neurotol* 2004;25(3):333–338.

42. Tumarkin A. The otolithic catastrophe: a new syndrome. *Br Med J (Clin Res)* 1936;2:175–177.

43. Baloh RW, Jacobson K, Winder T. Drop attacks with Ménière's syndrome. *Ann Neurol* 1990;28(3):384–387.

44. Timmer FC, Zhou G, Guinan JJ, et al. Vestibular evoked myogenic potential (VEMP) in patients with Ménière's disease with drop attacks. *Laryngoscope* 2006;116(5):776–779.

45. Lin MY, Timmer FC, Oriel BS, et al. Vestibular evoked myogenic potentials (VEMP) can detect asymptomatic saccular hydrops. *Laryngoscope* 2006;116(6):987–992.

46. James AL, Burton MJ. Betahistine for Ménière's disease or syndrome. *Cochrane Database Syst Rev* 2001;(1):CD001873.

47. Boleas-Aguirre MS, Lin FR, la Santina CC, et al. Longitudinal results with intratympanic dexamethasone in the treatment of Ménière's disease. *Otol Neurotol* 2008;29(1):33–38.

48. Glasscock ME III, Gulya AJ, Pensak ML, et al. Medical and surgical management of Ménière's disease. *Am J Otol* 1984;5(6): 536–542.

49. Derebery MJ, Fisher LM, Berliner K, et al. Outcomes of endolymphatic shunt surgery for Ménière's disease: comparison with intratympanic gentamicin on vertigo control and hearing loss. *Otol Neurotol* 2010;31(4):649–655.

50. Pullens B, Giard JL, Verschuur HP, et al. Surgery for Ménière's disease. *Cochrane Database Syst Rev* 2010;(1):CD005395.

51. Lyford-Pike S, Vogelheim C, Chu E, et al. Gentamicin is primarily localized in vestibular type I hair cells after intratympanic administration. *J Assoc Res Otolaryngol* 2007;8(4):497–508.

52. Chia SH, Gamst AC, Anderson JP, et al. Intratympanic gentamicin therapy for Ménière's disease: a meta-analysis. *Otol Neurotol* 2004;25(4):544–552.

53. Wu IC, Minor LB. Long-term hearing outcome in patients receiving intratympanic gentamicin for Ménière's disease. *Laryngoscope* 2003;113(5):815–820.

54. Carey JP, Minor LB, Peng GC, et al. Changes in the three-dimensional angular vestibulo-ocular reflex following intratympanic gentamicin for Ménière's disease. *J Assoc Res Otolaryngol* 2002;3(4):430–443.

55. Hirvonen TP, Minor LB, Hullar TE, et al. Effects of intratympanic gentamicin on vestibular afferents and hair cells in the chinchilla. *J Neurophysiol* 2005;93(2):643–655.

56. Kayan A, Hood J. Neuro-otological manifestations of migraine. *Brain* 1984;107:1123–1142.

57. Cutrer FM, Baloh RW. Migraine-associated dizziness. *Headache* 1992;32:300–304.

58. Aragones JM, Fortes-Rego J, Fuste J, et al. Migraine: an alternative in the diagnosis of unclassified vertigo. *Headache* 1993;33(3):125–128.

59. Parker W. Migraine and the vestibular system in adults. *Am J Otol* 1991;12(1):25–34.

60. Reploeg MD, Goebel JA. Migraine-associated dizziness: patient characteristics and management options. *Otol Neurotol* 2002;23(3):364–371.

61. Zhao JG, Piccirillo JF, Spitznagel EL Jr, et al. Predictive capability of historical data for diagnosis of dizziness. *Otol Neurotol* 2011;32(2):284–290.

62. Lanzi G, Balottin U, Fazzi E, et al. Benign paroxysmal vertigo of childhood: a long-term follow-up. *Cephalgia* 1999;14(6):458–460.

63. Rassekh CH, Harker LA. The prevalence of migraine in Ménière's disease. *Laryngoscope* 1992;102:135–138.

64. Radtke A, Lempert T, Gresty MA, et al. Migraine and Ménière's disease: is there a link? *Neurology* 2002;59(11):1700–1704.

65. Hadjikhani N, Sanchez Del RM, Wu O, et al. Mechanisms of migraine aura revealed by functional MRI in human visual cortex. *Proc Natl Acad Sci U S A* 2001;98(8):4687–4692.

66. Ophoff RA, Terwindt GM, Vergouwe MN, et al. Familial hemiplegic migraine and episodic ataxia type-2 are caused by mutations in the Ca2+ channel gene CACNL1A4. *Cell* 1996;87(3):543–552.

67. Baloh RW. Neurotology of migraine. *Headache* 1997;37:615–621.

68. Bahra A, Matharu MS, Buchel C, et al. Brainstem activation specific to migraine headache. *Lancet* 2001;357(9261):1016–1017.

69. Lipkin AF, Jenkins HA, Coker NJ. Migraine and sudden sensorineural hearing loss. *Arch Otolaryngol Head Neck Surg* 1987;113(3):325–326.

70. Viirre ES, Baloh RW. Migraine as a cause of sudden hearing loss. *Headache* 1996;36(1):24–28.

71. Vass Z, Dai CF, Steyger PS, et al. Co-localization of the vanilloid capsaicin receptor and substance P in sensory nerve fibers innervating cochlear and vertebro-basilar arteries. *Neuroscience* 2004;124(4):919–927.

72. Goadsby PJ, Lipton RB, Ferrari MD. Migraine—current understanding and treatment. *N Engl J Med* 2002;346(4):257–270.

73. Vass Z, Steyger PS, Hordichok AJ, et al. Capsaicin stimulation of the cochlea and electric stimulation of the trigeminal ganglion mediate vascular permeability in cochlear and vertebro-basilar arteries: a potential cause of inner ear dysfunction in headache. *Neuroscience* 2001;103(1):189–201.

74. Whitney SL, Wrisley DM, Brown KE, et al. Physical therapy for migraine-related vestibulopathy and vestibular dysfunction with history of migraine. *Laryngoscope* 2000;110(9):1528–1534.

75. Wrisley DM, Whitney SL, Furman JM. Vestibular rehabilitation outcomes in patients with a history of migraine. *Otol Neurotol* 2002;23(4):483–487.

76. Strohm M. Trauma of the middle ear. Clinical findings, postmortem observations and results of experimental studies. *Adv Otorhinolaryngol* 1986;35:1–254.

77. Friedland DR, Wackym PA. A critical appraisal of spontaneous perilymphatic fistulas of the inner ear. *Am J Otol* 1999;20(2): 261–276.

78. Hakuba N, Hato N, Shinomori Y, et al. Labyrinthine fistula as a late complication of middle ear surgery using the canal wall down technique. *Otol Neurotol* 2002;23(6):832–835.

79. Kohut RI, Hinojosa R, Ryu JH. The histologic characteristics of the core of the fissula ante fenestram. *Acta Otolaryngol Suppl (Stockh)* 1991;481:158–162.

80. el Shazly MA, Linthicum FH Jr. Microfissures of the temporal bone: do they have any clinical significance? *Am J Otol* 1991;12(3):169–171.

81. Goodhill V. Sudden deafness and round window rupture. *Laryngoscope* 1971;81:1462–1474.

82. Graham JM, Phelps PD, Michaels L. Congenital malformations of the ear and cochlear implantation in children: review and temporal bone report of common cavity. *J Laryngol Otol Suppl* 2000;25:1–14.

83. Arenberg IK, Ackley RS, Ferraro J, et al. ECoG results in perilymphatic fistula: clinical and experimental studies. *Otolaryngol Head Neck Surg* 1988;99(5):435–443.

84. Fitzgerald DC. Perilymphatic fistula and Ménière's disease. Clinical series and literature review. *Ann Otol Rhinol Laryngol* 2001;110(5 Pt 1):430–436.

85. Black FO, Lilly DJ, Nashner LM, et al. Quantitative diagnostic test for perilymph fistulas. *Otolaryngol Head Neck Surg* 1987;96(2):125–134.

86. Black FO, Pesznecker S, Norton T, et al. Surgical management of perilymphatic fistulas: a Portland experience. *Am J Otol* 1992;13(3):254–262.

87. Rizer FM, House JW. Perilymph fistulas: the House Ear Clinic experience. *Otalaryngol Head Neck Surg* 1991;104:239–243.

88. Shelton C, Simmons FB. Perilymph fistula: the Stanford experience. *Ann Otol Rhinol Laryngol* 1988;97:105–108.

89. Poe DS, Bottrill ID. Comparison of endoscopic and surgical explorations for perilymphatic fistulas. *Am J Otol* 1994;15(6): 735–738.

90. Buchman CA, Luxford WM, Hirsch BE, et al. Beta-2 transferrin assay in the identification of perilymph. *Am J Otol* 1999;20(2):174–178.

91. Bachmann-Harildstad G, Stenklev NC, Myrvoll E, et al. Beta-trace protein as a diagnostic marker for perilymphatic fluid fistula: a prospective controlled pilot study to test a sample collection technique. *Otol Neurotol* 2011;32(1):7–10.

92. Dix MR, Hallpike CS. The pathology, symptomatology and diagnosis of certain common disorders of the vestibular system. *Proc R Soc Med* 1952;45:341–354.

93. Ishiyama A, Ishiyama GP, Lopez I, et al. Histopathology of idiopathic chronic recurrent vertigo. *Laryngoscope* 1996;106(11): 1340–1346.

94. Schuknecht HF, Kitamura K. Second Louis H. Clerf Lecture. Vestibular neuritis. *Ann Otol Rhinol Laryngol Suppl* 1981;90 (1 Pt 2):1–19.

95. Goebel JA, O'Mara W, Gianoli G. Anatomic considerations in vestibular neuritis. *Otol Neurotol* 2001;22(4):512–518.

96. Arbusow V, Schulz P, Strupp M, et al. Distribution of herpes simplex virus type 1 in human geniculate and vestibular ganglia: implications for vestibular neuritis. *Ann Neurol* 1999;46(3): 416–419.

97. Corvera J, Davalos RL. Neurotologic evidence of central and peripheral involvement in patients with vestibular neuronitis. *Otolaryngol Head Neck Surg* 1985;93(4):524–528.

98. Ohyama Y, Yagi T, Ushio K, et al. 3D analysis of nystagmus during peripheral vertiginous attacks. *Acta Otolaryngol Suppl* 1997;528:77–79.

99. Fetter M, Dichgans J. Vestibular neuritis spares the inferior division of the vestibular nerve. *Brain* 1996;119(3):755–763.

100. Murofushi T, Halmagyi GM, Yavor RA, et al. Absent vestibular evoked myogenic potentials in vestibular neurolabyrinthitis. An indicator of inferior vestibular nerve involvement? *Arch Otolaryngol Head Neck Surg* 1996;122:845–848.

101. Strupp M, Zingler VC, Arbusow V, et al. Methylprednisolone, valacyclovir, or the combination for vestibular neuritis. *N Engl J Med* 2004;351(4):354–361.

102. Ma C, Billings P, Harris JP, et al. Characterization of an experimentally induced inner ear immune response. *Laryngoscope* 2000;110(3 Pt 1):451–456.

103. Garcia-Berrocal JR, Ramirez-Camacho R, Trinidad A, et al. Controversies and criticisms on designs for experimental autoimmune labyrinthitis. *Ann Otol Rhinol Laryngol* 2004;113(5):404–410.

104. Solares CA, Edling AE, Johnson JM, et al. Murine autoimmune hearing loss mediated by CD4+ T cells specific for inner ear peptides. *J Clin Invest* 2004;113(8):1210–1217.

105. Mogi G, Lim DJ, Watanabe N. Immunologic study on the inner ear. Immunoglobulins in perilymph. *Arch Otolaryngol* 1982;108(5):270–275.

106. Yoo TJ, Du X, Kwon SS. Molecular mechanism of autoimmune hearing loss. *Acta Otolaryngol Suppl* 2002;(548):3–9.

107. Tomiyama S, Harris JP. The role of the endolymphatic sac in inner ear immunity. *Acta Otolaryngol* 1987;103(3–4):182–188.

108. Bovo R, Aimoni C, Martini A. Immune-mediated inner ear disease. *Acta Otolaryngol* 2006;126(10):1012–1021.

109. Stone JH, Francis HW. Immune-mediated inner ear disease. *Curr Opin Rheumatol* 2000;12(1):32–40.

110. Sajjadi H, Paparella MM. Ménière's disease. *Lancet* 2008;372 (9636):406–414.

111. Moscicki RA, San Martin JE, Quintero CH, et al. Serum antibody to inner ear proteins in patients with progressive hearing loss. Correlation with disease activity and response to corticosteroid treatment. *JAMA* 1994;272(8):611–616.

112. Bloch DB, San Martin JE, Rauch SD, et al. Serum antibodies to heat shock protein 70 in sensorineural hearing loss. *Arch Otolaryngol Head Neck Surg* 1995;121(10):1167–1171.

113. Billings PB, Keithley EM, Harris JP. Evidence linking the 68 kilodalton antigen identified in progressive sensorineural hearing loss patient sera with heat shock protein 70. *Ann Otol Rhinol Laryngol* 1995;104(3):181–188.

114. Trune DR, Kempton JB, Mitchell CR, et al. Failure of elevated heat shock protein 70 antibodies to alter cochlear function in mice. *Hear Res* 1998;116(1–2):65–70.

115. Yeom K, Gray J, Nair TS, et al. Antibodies to HSP-70 in normal donors and autoimmune hearing loss patients. *Laryngoscope* 2003;113(10):1770–1776.

116. Disher MJ, Ramakrishnan A, Nair T, et al. Human autoantibodies and monoclnal antibody KHRI-3 bind to a phylogenetically conserved inner-ear-supporting cell antigen. *Ann N Y Acad Sci* 1997;830:253–265.

117. Nair TS, Raphael Y, Dolan DF, et al. Monoclonal antibody induced hearing loss. *Hear Res* 1995;83(1–2):101–113.

118. Nair TS, Kozma KE, Hoefling NL, et al. Identification and characterization of choline transporter-like protein 2, an inner ear glycoprotein of 68 and 72 kDa that is the target of antibody-induced hearing loss. *J Neurosci* 2004;24(7):1772–1779.

119. Zeitoun H, Beckman JG, Arts HA, et al. Corticosteroid response and supporting cell antibody in autoimmune hearing loss. *Arch Otolaryngol Head Neck Surg* 2005;131(8):665–672.

120. Ruckenstein MJ. Autoimmune inner ear disease. *Curr Opin Otolaryngol Head Neck Surg* 2004;12(5):426–430.

121. Hirose K, Wener MH, Duckert LG. Utility of laboratory testing in autoimmune inner ear disease. *Laryngoscope* 1999;109(11): 1749–1754.

122. Harris JP, Weisman MH, Derebery JM, et al. Treatment of corticosteroid-responsive autoimmune inner ear disease with methotrexate: a randomized controlled trial. *JAMA* 2003;290(14):1875–1883.

123. Matteson EL, Fabry DA, Facer GW, et al. Open trial of methotrexate as treatment for autoimmune hearing loss. *Arthritis Rheum* 2001;45(2):146–150.

124. Yang GS, Song HT, Keithley EM, et al. Intratympanic immunosuppressives for prevention of immune-mediated sensorineural hearing loss. *Am J Otol* 2000;21(4):499–504.

125. Garcia-Berrocal JR, Ibanez A, Rodriguez A, et al. Alternatives to systemic steroid therapy for refractory immune-mediated inner ear disease: a physiopathologic approach. *Eur Arch Otorhinolaryngol* 2006;263(11):977–982.

126. Trune DR, Kempton JB, Gross ND. Mineralocorticoid receptor mediates glucocorticoid treatment effects in the autoimmune mouse ear. *Hear Res* 2006;212(1-2):22–32.

127. Leveque M, Labrousse M, Seidermann L, et al. Surgical therapy in intractable benign paroxysmal positional vertigo. *Otolaryngol Head Neck Surg* 2007;136(5):693–698.

128. Epley JM. The canalith repositioning procedure: for treatment of benign paroxysmal positional vertigo. *Otalaryngol Head Neck Surg* 1992;107:399–404.

129. Gacek RR. Transection of the posterior ampullary nerve for the relief of benign paroxysmal positional vertigo. *Ann Otol Rhinol Laryngol* 1974;83:596–605.

130. Parnes LS, McClure JA. Posterior semicircular canal occlusion for intractable benign paroxysmal positional vertigo. *Ann Otol Rhinol Laryngol* 1990;99:330–334.

131. Minor LB, Solomon D, Zinreich JS, et al. Sound- and/or pressure-induced vertigo due to bone dehiscence of the superior semicircular canal. *Arch Otolaryngol Head Neck Surg* 1998;124:249–258.

132. Cremer PD, Minor LB, Carey JP, et al. Eye movements in patients with superior canal dehiscence syndrome align with the abnormal canal. *Neurology* 2000;55(12):1833–1841.

133. Minor LB. Clinical manifestations of superior semicircular canal dehiscence. *Laryngoscope* 2005;115(10):1717–1727.

134. Minor LB, Carey JP, Cremer PD, et al. Dehiscence of bone overlying the superior canal as a cause of apparent conductive hearing loss. *Otol Neurotol* 2003;24(2):270–278.

135. Mikulec AA, McKenna MJ, Ramsey MJ, et al. Superior semicircular canal dehiscence presenting as conductive hearing loss without vertigo. *Otol Neurotol* 2004;25(2):121–129.

136. Minor LB, Cremer PD, Carey JP, et al. Symptoms and signs in superior canal dehiscence syndrome. *Ann N Y Acad Sci* 2001;942:259–273.

137. Grimmer JF, Poe DS. Update on eustachian tube dysfunction and the patulous eustachian tube. *Curr Opin Otolaryngol Head Neck Surg* 2005;13(5):277–282.

138. Rosowski JJ, Songer JE, Nakajima HH, et al. Clinical, experimental, and theoretical investigations of the effect of superior semicircular canal dehiscence on hearing mechanisms. *Otol Neurotol* 2004;25(3):323–332.

139. Halmagyi GM, Aw ST, McGarvie LA, et al. Superior semicircular canal dehiscence simulating otosclerosis. *J Laryngol Otol* 2003;117(7):553–557.

140. Brantberg K, Bergenius J, Tribukait A. Vestibular-evoked myogenic potentials in patients with dehiscence of the superior semicircular canal. *Acta Otolaryngol* 1999;119(6):633–640.

141. Streubel SO, Cremer PD, Carey JP, et al. Vestibular-evoked myogenic potentials in the diagnosis of superior canal dehiscence syndrome. *Acta Otolaryngol Suppl* 2001;545:41–49.

142. Welgampola MS, Myrie OA, Minor LB, et al. Vestibular-evoked myogenic potential thresholds normalize on plugging superior canal dehiscence. *Neurology* 2008;70(6):464–472.

143. Hirvonen TP, Weg N, Zinreich SJ, et al. High-resolution CT findings suggest a developmental abnormality underlying superior canal dehiscence syndrome. *Acta Otolaryngol* 2003;123(4):477–481.

144. Carey JP, Minor LB, Nager GT. Dehiscence or thinning of bone overlying the superior semicircular canal in a temporal bone survey. *Arch Otolaryngol Head Neck Surg* 2000;126(2):137–147.

145. Deschenes GR, Hsu DP, Megerian CA. Outpatient repair of superior semicircular canal dehiscence via the transmastoid approach. *Laryngoscope* 2009;119(9):1765–1769.

146. Limb CJ, Carey JP, Srireddy S, et al. Auditory function in patients with surgically treated superior semicircular canal dehiscence. *Otol Neurotol* 2006;27(7):969–980.

147. Minor LB, Haslwanter T, Straumann D, et al. Hyperventilation-induced nystagmus in patients with vestibular schwannoma. *Neurology* 1999;53(9):2158–2168.

148. Halmagyi GM, Fattore CM, Curthoys IS, et al. Gentamicin vestibulotoxicity. *Otolaryngol Head Neck Surg* 1994;111:571–574.

149. Tang HY, Hutcheson E, Neill S, et al. Genetic susceptibility to aminoglycoside ototoxicity: how many are at risk? *Genet Med* 2002;4(5):336–345.

150. Gillespie MB, Minor LB. Prognosis in bilateral vestibular hypofunction. *Laryngoscope* 1999;109(1):35–41.

151. Herdman SJ, Whitney SL. Interventions for the patient with vestibular hypofunction. *Vestibular rehabilitation*, 3rd ed. Philadelphia, PA: F.A. Davis Company, 2007:309–337.

152. Schubert MC, Migliaccio AA, Clendaniel RA, et al. Mechanism of dynamic visual acuity recovery with vestibular rehabilitation. *Arch Phys Med Rehabil* 2008;89(3):500–507.

153. Herdman SJ. Role of vestibular adaptation in vestibular rehabilitation. *Otalaryngol Head Neck Surg* 1998;119:49–54.

154. Hillier SL, Hollohan V. Vestibular rehabilitation for unilateral peripheral vestibular dysfunction. *Cochrane Database Syst Rev* 2007;(4):CD005397.

155. Della Santina CC, Migliaccio AA, Hayden R, et al. Current and future management of bilateral loss of vestibular sensation—an update on the Johns Hopkins Multichannel Vestibular Prosthesis Project. *Cochlear Implants Int* 2010;11(Suppl 2):2–11.

Central Vestibular Disorders

167

Gail Ishiyama   *Akira Ishiyama*

A 48-year-old male has a 5- or 6-year history of gradually worsening gait disorder. He has had occasionally bouts of positional nystagmus that were called "benign positional vertigo." However, the modified Epley maneuver failed to resolve the positional nystagmus. He has noted increasing difficulty when walking, and recently he noted a clumsiness of his hands and arms. On examination, he has a downbeat nystagmus that is noted when looking down or to either side, and he has a saccadic pursuit. Coordination testing reveals dysdiadochokinesis and dysmetria of his extremities. He is unable to tandem walk and cannot stand in the Romberg position with eyes open or closed. A magnetic resonance imaging (MRI) demonstrates atrophy of the cerebellar vermis.

A 64-year-old woman has a history of the sudden onset of spontaneous vertigo with a persistent tilting of the body to the left as if pulled by a strong external force. She was completely unable to walk at the onset. She has a Horner's in the left pupil, large (hypermetric) saccades toward the left, and smaller (hypometric) saccades toward the right. She also had a skew deviation of the eyes with the left eye lower than the right and the upper poles rotated to the left. An MRI with diffusion-weighted imaging (DWI) was negative.

Both of these patients exhibit signs and symptoms of a central vestibular disorder. In this chapter, we discuss ways to distinguish central from peripheral vestibular disorders, the presentation of the common central vestibular disorders, the evaluation of a patient with dizziness, that is, the clinical examination, important questions to ask on history, and the audiologic and vestibular testing results in central vestibular disorders. In both patients, there are other neurologic symptoms noted in addition to the vertigo. Patient 1 has difficulty walking even when not having vertigo, and clumsiness of the extremities. Dysdiadochokinesis and dysmetria are cerebellar signs described below under cerebellar degeneration. Patient 2 has lateropulsion of the body (a sense of being pulled toward one side) and of the eye movements (bigger movements toward one side) associated with the vertigo.

From the history alone, there should be suspicion that these are not peripheral disorders. Patient 1 had been misdiagnosed with benign positional vertigo (BPV) on initial presentation, and patient 2 had been misdiagnosed with vestibular neuritis. Patient 1 had a history of cerebellar ataxia, and patient 2 had a history of a Wallenberg stroke. The negative MRI in a Wallenberg stroke may occur because the size of the stroke is too small to be detected. In central vestibular disorders, the inability to walk is oftentimes severe and cerebellar imbalance is often described as "clumsiness" or a "drunken feeling." The following chapter reviews the central and vestibular anatomy briefly, describes the specialized portions of the examination and history pertinent to evaluation of central vestibular disorders, and reviews the most common central vestibular disorders that may present to the otolaryngologist with complaints of dizziness.

THE CENTRAL AND PERIPHERAL VESTIBULAR SYSTEM

The peripheral vestibular system refers to the labyrinthine organs of the inner ear, which includes the end organs of the semicircular canals (cristae ampullares) and of the utricle and saccule (maculae) that contain the hair cells, and the innervating primary afferent neuron and nerve (Scarpa ganglia). The central vestibular system refers to the secondary vestibular neurons and their projections. The secondary neurons are the vestibular nuclei in the brainstem, divided into the superior (angular or Bechterew), the lateral (Deiters), the medial, and the descending (inferior or spinal) (1). In primates, the vestibulocerebellar and vestibuloocular connections are relatively more prominent in comparison with vestibulospinal connections. The vestibular nuclei play a large role in central compensation after a peripheral labyrinthine injury.

Vertigo that is characterized by the sense of movement of the environment can result from lesions of the labyrinth, the vestibular nerve, or the interconnecting vestibular pathways in the brainstem and cerebellum. Vertigo is an illusion of movement, often of rotation, although the movement may be described as that of linear displacement (back and forth vertigo). Lesions of the labyrinth, the vestibular nerve, the vestibular nuclei, and the visual–vestibular interaction centers in the brainstem and cerebellum can produce a spontaneous vestibular nystagmus and vertigo. The production of spontaneous nystagmus requires an imbalance of tonic activity of the vestibuloocular pathways.

A lesion of the left vestibular labyrinth or nerve will produce a right-beating nystagmus with a torsional component. In lesions of the vestibular nuclei, the direction of spontaneous nystagmus that results is not as predictable and may be toward or away from the side of the lesion. Functional brain imaging demonstrates evidence for vestibular projections to the parietotemporal cortex and the thalamus in both normative controls and subjects with peripheral and central vestibular disorders (2). Because these vestibulo-thalamo-cortical projections do not carry tonic signals, a lesion in these cortical (within the brain) pathways will not produce vertigo but can produce an alteration of the body orientation (e.g., a sense of tilt or tendency to fall).

History of the dizzy patient: differentiating between a central versus peripheral cause of vertigo (Table 167.1). It is important for the clinician to distinguish the symptoms that the patient refers to as "dizziness." This distinction can be a clinical decision of critical importance. In evaluation of the patient with dizziness, the clinician must obtain as accurate and thorough of a history as possible to aid in distinguishing probable peripheral versus central causes. Dizziness may refer to a light-headedness that feels as if nearly passing out, near faint dizziness. Typical causes include orthostatic hypotension or cardiac insufficiency, for example, aortic stenosis. Oftentimes, dizziness due to cardiac disease will worsen with exertion, and is not characterized by vertigo. When the patient describes a sense of

movement of the environment, the symptom of vertigo, it is strongly suggestive of an imbalance within the vestibular system. Vertigo can occur due to either a peripheral or a central vestibular lesion. Typically, vertigo is an episodic phenomenon, whereas a nonvestibular dizziness is more likely to be a continuous nonspecific type of dizziness. Episodes that occur only in specific places, such as walking through the store aisles, are highly unlikely to be vestibular, and are more likely related to anxiety syndromes or to a migraine-associated sensitivity to visual stimuli. Gait imbalance is often described as "dizziness," and the differential can include peripheral or central vestibular disorders, as well as neurodegenerative conditions such as Parkinson disease or spinal stenosis.

Peripheral and central spontaneous nystagmus (Table 167.2). Spontaneous nystagmus occurs when there is an imbalance of the tonic firing and signals to the oculomotor neurons. Spontaneous nystagmus is in reference to a nystagmus that occurs with the eyes in primary position, without any external stimuli. The primary position is the eyes looking forward in midposition, and the patient in the seated position. Positional nystagmus is nystagmus that is not present in the sitting position but is present in other head or body (e.g., head-hanging) position. Both spontaneous and positional nystagmus can occur secondary to either peripheral or central vestibular disorders.

The type of nystagmus can oftentimes localize the lesion. The vestibular system, both peripheral and central, is the primary source of tonic signals for most types of spontaneous nystagmus. A peripheral vestibular lesion, a lesion of the labyrinth or vestibular nerve, results in a spontaneous nystagmus with combined torsional, horizontal, and vertical components with predominantly a horizontal component. A lesion of the vestibular nucleus can cause a horizontal torsional nystagmus that appears similar to a peripheral nystagmus. However, the direction does not indicate the side of the lesion, and the nystagmus is not suppressed with fixation because of the damage to the visual–vestibular pathways (3).

Spontaneous peripheral nystagmus. Whether the lesion is of the labyrinth or the vestibular nerve, the type of nystagmus is invariable: horizontal, torsional beating toward the contralateral side, increasing in frequency and amplitude

TABLE 167.1	DISTINGUISHING CENTRAL FROM PERIPHERAL CAUSES OF DIZZINESS				
	Nausea and Vomiting	Ability to Walk	Hearing Loss	Focal Neurologic Signs and Symptoms	Associated Autonomic Symptoms (Sweating, Pallor)
Peripheral	Severe	Unsteadiness but able to walk	Common	Rare	Pronounced
Central	Moderate	Nearly incapable of walking	Rare except AICA infarct	Common	Less pronounced

TABLE 167.2	DISTINGUISHING CHARACTERISTICS OF PERIPHERAL VERSUS CENTRAL NYSTAGMUS				
	Type of Nystagmus	Effect of Fixation	Effect of Eye Position	Positional Nystagmus	Other Abnormalities on Testing
Peripheral: Labyrinth or vestibular nerve	Horizontal and torsional	Inhibited by fixation	Follows Alexander law	Latency, fatigues, torsional upbeat nystagmus, <1 min	May be associated with asymmetry of caloric response or of the VOR
Central: Brainstem or cerebellum or interconnections	Can be pure vertical, horizontal, or pure torsional	Unaffected by fixation	May be unidirectional, but if direction-changing is always central	No latency, does not fatigue, oftentimes downbeat or reversal of direction	Often associated with abnormalities of smooth pursuit, optokinetic nystagmus OKN, or saccades

on gaze to the fast component side, inhibited by fixation. A peripheral nystagmus is inhibited by fixation because the suppression requires an intact brainstem and cerebellum. The clinician should check that the nystagmus follows Alexander law: gaze in the direction of the fast component will increase the frequency and amplitude in a peripheral nystagmus, whereas gaze in the opposite direction will cause a decrease in the nystagmus (4). A peripheral nystagmus does not change direction with changes in eye position or with changes in the head or body position.

Spontaneous central nystagmus. The appearance of a central nystagmus can vary depending on the location of the lesion. Usually a central nystagmus will be prominent with or without fixation. Central spontaneous nystagmus occurs when there is an imbalance of the central vestibuloocular (VOR) or smooth pursuit pathways. In contrast to the peripheral vestibular pathways, the central horizontal and vertical pathways are separate, and thus a purely vertical or purely horizontal nystagmus is common in a central vestibular disorder. A central spontaneous nystagmus can be purely vertical, purely horizontal, or purely torsional, or some combination. Similarly to a peripheral nystagmus, gaze in the direction of the fast component may increase the amplitude and frequency of the nystagmus. However, gaze in the opposite direction will often cause a change in direction of a central vestibular nystagmus. A null region may be found several degrees off of the center beyond which the direction of the nystagmus changes. A direction-changing nystagmus is always central. An apparent direction-changing nystagmus can occur in one peripheral entity: horizontal variant of benign paroxysmal positional vertigo (5).

Positional nystagmus, central and peripheral disorders. A nystagmus that is triggered by a change in position can be either peripheral or central in etiology. BPV, a peripheral vestibular disorder due to loose otoliths, is by far the most common cause of recurrent attacks of positional vertigo. However, a positional nystagmus and vertigo can be due to a central vestibular finding. Common patterns of central

positional nystagmus include a persistent downbeat nystagmus, or a horizontal direction-changing nystagmus. The patterns of nystagmus can appear similar to an anterior canal BPV, or a horizontal canal variant BPV, respectively. The common central disorders that present with a positional nystagmus that can mimic anterior (downbeat) or horizontal (direction-changing horizontal) nystagmus include Chiari malformation, tumors of the cerebellum or around the fourth ventricle, or spinocerebellar ataxia neurodegenerative conditions. There are no central vestibular disorders that induce a nystagmus that is characteristic of the classic and most common BPV, posterior canal BPV: a burst of upbeat, torsional geotropic nystagmus with a duration usually less than 30 seconds, and always less than 1 minute.

EXAMINATION OF EYE MOVEMENTS IN CENTRAL VESTIBULAR DISORDERS

The patient should be observed in all eye positions for nystagmus (a total of eight positions): gaze 30 degrees to the left and then 30 degrees to the right, and thereafter on upgaze and downgaze to the left, to the right, and at midline, with each position held for at least 20 seconds. Traditional terms used by otolaryngologists include the following: *First degree nystagmus* is present only on gaze in the direction of the fast component. *Second degree nystagmus* is present in the primary position (midposition, looking straight ahead). *Third degree nystagmus* is present even on gaze away from the fast component. These terms are most applicable to peripheral nystagmus patterns, and may not be relevant in central vestibular nystagmus. A peripheral nystagmus should not change direction with any positional change of the body or of the eyes.

Smooth pursuit, both horizontal and vertical, should be evaluated by having the patient follow the clinician's pen or finger. The patient should be able to follow the target smoothly, without repeated "stops" that would be indicative of a "saccadic pursuit." If the eyes follow the target using a series of saccades rather than smoothly, then the central oculomotor pathway is unable to generate a smooth pursuit and is dysfunctional. A saccadic pursuit is nonspecific and can occur with normal aging, and is common in disorders such as multiple sclerosis (MS), Parkinson disease, or other neurodegenerative disorders. A severely saccadic pursuit may be seen in cerebellar conditions as in the 48-year-old patient initially described. Saccadic pursuit suggests central pathology.

Saccades. Saccadic eye movements are examined by asking the patient to fixate alternately between two fixed targets. The first target is usually in the primary position, "Look at my nose." Then, the patient is asked to look quickly to a target placed 15 degrees to the right, "Quickly look to my pen," and then placed 15 degrees to the left. Saccades that repeated "overshoot," for example, when attempting to look at a target on the right, the patient saccades further to the right, or "undershoot" is a sign of central vestibuloocular motor dysfunction (hypermetric or hypometric saccades, respectively), that usually localize to cerebellar or cerebellar peduncle lesions. Slow saccades may indicate a brainstem lesion, and delayed saccades can be seen in cerebral hemispheric lesions.

Saccadic intrusions include square wave jerks, ocular flutter, and opsoclonus. Saccadic intrusions occur when unwanted saccades disrupt steady fixation. A differential of these entities is beyond the scope of this chapter. All of these entities are associated with central vestibular pathology, and would warrant referral to a neurologic specialist. These entities are common with cerebellar lesions, progressive supranuclear palsy, Huntington disease, Friedreich ataxia, or paraneoplastic syndromes.

Ocular tilt reaction. If a normal subject tilts the head toward the right, then the eyes will reflexively counterroll and skew to allow for visual stabilization. Traditionally, a skew deviation, which clinically is described as a diplopia with two images split both slightly horizontally, and vertically, was considered to be a central finding. However, the ocular tilt reaction is a labyrinthine reflex, and can be seen by stimulation of the contralateral utricular nerve (6). The ocular tilt reaction can be seen in peripheral labyrinthine lesions (7), in which case the head tilt and lower eye are toward the ipsilateral lesion. An ocular tilt reaction can also be seen in lateral medullary infarcts (Wallenberg syndrome) (8), in which case it is also toward the ipsilateral side. In mesencephalic lesions (of the midbrain), the tilt is toward the contralateral side. Skew deviation and the ocular tilt reaction are noted following ablative procedures of the vestibular periphery (labyrinthectomy or vestibular nerve section) and in association with idiopathic sudden unilateral peripheral vestibular or cochleovestibular loss (9). This also can occur following resection of acoustic neuroma, another form of acute deafferentation. The skew deviation is often the earliest to compensate, disappearing within a few days.

Positional nystagmus. The patient should be evaluated for nystagmus in the head-hanging right and left (Dix-Hallpike maneuver). In BPV, the nystagmus fatigues, has a few seconds or more of latency, and will be a torsional upbeat nystagmus if the particles fell into the posterior semicircular canal. Positioning in a central positional nystagmus may induce a downbeat nystagmus that persists as long as the head-hanging position is held. Other central nystagmus include a direction-changing nystagmus or rebound nystagmus. Two positional maneuvers can be conducted. The Dix-Hallpike maneuver is conducted by placing the patient in right or left head-hanging position very quickly. In the side-lying test, the patient moves slowly into the side-lying position and then the clinician evaluates for a slow persistent nystagmus that would be indicative of a central vestibular disorder.

Fixation suppression means that the removal of ability to focus, as with Frenzel glasses, is associated with an increasing of the nystagmus. A peripheral nystagmus is usually inhibited by fixation. If Frenzel glasses are not available, the clinician can observe the nystagmus using an ophthalmoscope and covering the patient's other eye. If the nystagmus increases, then the nystagmus was inhibited by fixation, a characteristic of peripheral nystagmus.

Vibration-induced nystagmus. The other maneuver that can be used in the clinical setting is application of vibration to the mastoid, which can elicit a peripheral nystagmus in a compensated peripheral vestibulopathy from vestibular neuritis, Ménière disease, or anterior semicircular canal dehiscence (using vibration over the suboccipital cranium) (10,11).

Head-shaking nystagmus. The clinician should examine for head-shaking induced nystagmus. In this maneuver, the patient is asked to turn the head quickly from right to left about 20 times at 2 to 3 Hz, and the eye movements are then examined, ideally with the suppression of fixation using Frenzel lenses. Head shaking nystagmus indicates a latent asymmetry of the velocity-storage that can be due to a peripheral or a central vestibular disorder. In peripheral disorders, the nystagmus induced will be of the peripheral type: horizontal with a torsional component. In central disorders, the nystagmus induced can be vertical, downbeating or upbeating, or can be horizontal. In a study of 16 patients with lateral medullary infarction (vestibular nuclei infarction), a central vestibular disorder, head-shaking nystagmus was observed in 87.5%, and was ipsilesional in all cases. Even in patients with a contralesional nystagmus spontaneously, the head-shaking nystagmus was ipsilesional (12).

Spontaneous downbeat nystagmus. A downbeat nystagmus has a fast phase beating vertically downward and typically will increase in vertical amplitude with horizontal gaze deviation (13). A downbeat nystagmus is always a central vestibular nystagmus. Lesions of the uvula and flocculonodular lobes of the cerebellum in the monkey will induce a downbeat nystagmus (14). In humans, a downbeat nystagmus often localizes to the cervicomedullary junction, including the midline cerebellum (vermis) and associated pathologies include cerebellar ataxias, vertebrobasilar ischemia (VBI), MS, and Arnold-Chiari (AC) malformation (15). AC is a malformation associated with increased pressure on the flocculonodular region of the cerebellum (see Arnold-Chiari malformation). Decompression surgery may allow for reversal to normal (13).

Other types of central vestibular nystagmus. Other pathologic nystagmus patterns include *gaze-evoked nystagmus,* which is seen when the patient tries to move eyes away from primary (midline) position. In normal subjects, a nystagmus can be seen at the outermost peripheral positions of gaze. This normal physiologic variant is termed, "end-point nystagmus" and is normal. Typically, physiologic gaze-evoked nystagmus can be distinguished from pathologic forms in that it has lesser amplitude and frequency, is unsustained, is relatively symmetrical, and is not associated with any other ocular movement abnormalities.

However, it has been noted that a gaze-evoked nystagmus can be seen in up to 50% of the normal population (16). Furthermore, a recent study evaluating 56 subjects for gaze-evoked nystagmus reported that normal subjects have a high incidence of physiologic gaze-evoked nystagmus at even smaller angles of gaze: 93% at extreme gaze, 73% at 40 degrees, 43% at 30 degrees, and even at the lowest angle tested 21% at 10 degrees (17). In the clinical setting, the most common cause of a pathologic gaze-evoked nystagmus is drugs such as phenobarbital, phenytoin, alcohol, and benzodiazepines. Central vestibular pathologies associated with a gaze-evoked nystagmus include MS and cerebellar atrophy, and these diseases would usually be associated with other eye movement abnormalities.

Rebound nystagmus. Rebound nystagmus is a type of gaze-evoked nystagmus that disappears or reverses as the lateral gaze is held. After an attempted prolonged eccentric gaze of 20 or 30 seconds, upon returning to the primary position, a rebound nystagmus appears with the fast phase toward the center and the slow phase toward the side of attempted gaze-holding. Rebound nystagmus usually indicates cerebellar pathology, such as olivopontocerebellar atrophy (18). Tumors at the cerebellopontine angle, such as acoustic neuromas, may cause a Bruns' nystagmus. This presents with a low-frequency, large amplitude nystagmus when looking ipsilaterally, and a high-frequency, low amplitude nystagmus when looking contralaterally. In a study of 984 patients with acoustic neuroma, Bruns' nystagmus was present in 11% and was associated with larger tumor size, with 92% of patients with larger than 3.5 cm tumor having Bruns nystagmus (19).

OTHER FOCAL NEUROLOGIC EXAMINATION FINDINGS IN CENTRAL VESTIBULAR DISORDERS

1. As noted above, a careful examination of eye movements is important.
2. Examine the patient for head tilt (seen ipsilateral to a Wallenberg infarct) and the body for lateropulsion (also seen in central vestibular disorders, such as ipsilateral to a Wallenberg infarct). The lateropulsion may be so severe that the patient is unable to stand, which would usually be an indication of a central vestibular disorder. There may be concomitant lateropulsion of the eyes, with larger saccades toward the ipsilateral lesioned side in Wallenberg syndrome (20).
3. Facial weakness (CN VII): a peripheral weakness will include the upper and lower facial muscles, whereas a central weakness will spare the upper facial muscles (i.e., raising the eyebrows). Of note, both a peripheral and a central type of facial weakness can occur in association with a Wallenberg dorsolateral medullary stroke.
4. Facial sensory loss (CN V): the clinician should check the upper (V1), mid (V2), and lower chin area (V3) for light touch using a cotton wisp, and temperature sensation using a cold tuning fork (can be cooled under water). Avoid the angle of the jaw as it is innervated by upper cervical roots. Although some clinicians recommend pinprick testing, patients may find it unpleasant. Initial examination with a cotton wisp and cold tuning fork serves as a screening evaluation for additional methods of physical examination. The clinician can also check the corneal reflex which tests V1 (afferent) and VII (efferent). Ask the patient to look up and toward the opposite side and using a cotton wisp, lightly touch the cornea. This should elicit a blink response, which should be consensual. An absent corneal reflex supplements the findings of a trigeminal sensory deficit.
5. Visual fields testing the temporal and nasal upper, middle, and lower quadrants of each eye. Most infarcts in the posterior cerebral artery distribution will cause a visual field deficit.
6. Crossed sensory loss: a key indication for brainstem involvement, for example, facial sensory loss on the side ipsilateral to the infarct and extremity sensory loss on the contralateral side. A crossed sensory loss often localizes the insult to the dorsolateral medullary (Wallenberg infarct), and can be variably associated with vertigo, ipsilateral Horner's, hiccoughs, and dysarthria and dysphagia.
7. Horner syndrome consists of miosis (pupillary constriction) and ptosis, secondary to loss of sympathetic innervation. The difference in pupil size is termed anisocoria. The clinician should evaluate the patient in relative darkness since the abnormal miotic (small) pupil cannot dilate properly in a low light setting. In the Wallenberg syndrome, the Horner syndrome is ipsilateral to the infarct. Because the sympathetic pathway in the brainstem is close to the spinothalamic tract (pain and temperature) for the contralateral body, Horner syndrome due to brainstem lesions is often associated with contralateral loss of pain and temperature.
8. Head thrust test or Halmagyi maneuver (21): when positive, patients will have catch-up saccade because

they are unable to keep their eyes on the clinician's nose when the head is rapidly, passively turned to the side with the lesion. In bilateral vestibulopathy (e.g., gentamicin ototoxicity), the test will reveal catch-up saccades to both sides. In a right-sided vestibular neuritis, there may be a catch-up saccade when the head is turned passively by the clinician to the patient's right side.

9. Romberg: ask the patient to stand with the feet together with eyes open and eyes closed. A positive Romberg occurs when the patient's imbalance significantly increases with eye closure. The accentuation of imbalance with eye closure is a sign of either vestibular imbalance or proprioceptive loss. A patient with a central vestibular disorder such as a cerebellar stroke will likely be unable to stand in the Romberg position (feet together) and will be unsteady whether the eyes are open or closed. Strictly speaking, the inability to stand with the feet together (Romberg position) with the eyes open, as well as closed, is not a positive Romberg.

10. Always ask the patient to try to walk. Patients with lateropulsion will lean strongly toward one side (usually toward the lesion). Severe lateropulsion that interferes with walking or standing is usually a sign of central vestibular disorder.

11. Tandem walk: when performed with the eyes open, tandem walking is predominantly a test of cerebellar function. Vision and proprioceptive (position sense) will allow for a relatively normal tandem walk in a compensated peripheral vestibular loss (e.g., vestibular neuritis in the past). An acute vestibular lesion will usually impair the tandem walk, even with eyes open. Patients with cerebellar lesions will oftentimes have a wide-based gait and are unable to tandem walk even taking a single step.

12. Testing for coordination (cerebellar or central vestibular pathways) and other clinical manifestations of cerebellar dysfunction.
    a) Hypotonia: a diminished deep tendon reflex, oftentimes more prominent in the upper extremities or a "pendular" reflex. After tapping the patella, the patient's leg swings to and fro like a pendulum. This sign is indicative of large cerebellar hemispheric damage.
    b) Dysarthria: a slurring of the speech, abnormal articulation, and prosody (rhythm) is common in cerebellar syndromes.
    c) Eye movements as noted above. Common cerebellar eye movement findings include downbeat nystagmus, hypermetric saccades, and rebound nystagmus.
    d) Ataxia: inability to coordinate movements of the voluntary motor acts, which err in rate, range, force, and duration.
    e) Appendicular coordination: *Finger-to-nose*. Ask the patient to touch the tip of the index finger to their nose with the eyes closed. *Finger-to-finger*. Ask the patient to touch the tip of their index finger to yours. An *intention tremor* is missing the target and increasing the amplitude of tremor as the target is approached. *Dysmetria* occurs when the patient overshoots or undershoots the target.
    f) Appendicular coordination: check *rapid alternating movements*, for example, turning the hand alternating palm and back of the hand or a rhythmic slapping of the knee. An inability to conduct rapid alternating movements smoothly is called *dysdiadochokinesis*.
    g) Appendicular coordination: check *heel-to-shin*. While lying down, ask the patient to "draw" a perfectly straight line with the back of the heel, up and down the opposite shin.
    h) Tandem walk: a sensitive but nonspecific test for balance. In central vestibular disorders, the patient may be completely unable to tandem, and when severe the patient may be unable to stand. Patients with spinal stenosis or strokes causing motor weakness would also be unable to tandem walk. Similarly, patients with neurodegenerative conditions such as Parkinson disease would be unable to tandem walk. The quality of the walk can provide clues to the etiology. Spinal stenosis may be associated with a "scissoring" quality of the walk, and Parkinson may be associated with a shuffling gait and a pill-rolling tremor.

ASSOCIATED SYMPTOMS IN CENTRAL VESTIBULAR DISORDERS

In central vestibular disorders, the symptoms associated with the vertigo or onset of imbalance will be dictated by the location of the pathology. Central vestibular disorders generally localize to the brainstem or the cerebellum. Clinical examples of central vestibular disorders that can present with vertigo and imbalance include Wallenberg syndrome (an infarct of the dorsolateral medullary), MS, brainstem tumors or encephalitis, cerebellar ataxias, AC malformation, and cerebellopontine angle tumors.

Important Questions to Ask the Patient

"Do you feel as if you are about to pass out?" This would be consistent with global hypoperfusion, which can occur in orthostasis, cardiac insufficiency, or vasovagal reactions.

"If you are seated still when the dizziness occurs, do you feel as if the world or you are moving?" This would be consistent with true vertigo.

"How long is the vertigo spell, and is the onset abrupt or gradual?" Vertebrobasilar transient ischemic attacks (TIAs) often present with vertigo of abrupt onset, lasting 3 to 4 minutes in duration. The duration of the vertigo is critical in determining the differential diagnoses (see Table 167.3).

TABLE 167.3	LENGTH OF VERTIGO IN COMMON VESTIBULAR DISORDERS

Length of Vertigo Spell	Vestibular Disease Process
Seconds, always less than 1 min	Benign paroxysmal positional vertigo (22)
Minutes: 3–4	VBI (TIA) (23,24)
20 minutes to hours	Ménière disease (25)
Days	Vestibular neuritis (26)
Varies; can be seconds, minutes, or days	Migraine-associated vertigo, vestibular migraine, migranous vertigo, migraine equivalent (27)

BOX 167.1	NEUROLOGIC REVIEW OF SYSTEMS

Have you experienced any of the following symptoms? Please check yes or no and indicate if constant or in episodes.

1. Double vision, blurred vision, or blindness
2. Numbness of the face or extremities
3. Weakness in arms or legs
4. Clumsiness in arms or legs
5. Confusion or loss of consciousness
6. Difficulty with speech
7. Difficulty swallowing
8. Pain in neck or shoulder

"Are the spells provoked by positional changes of the head?" BPV is characterized by spells of vertigo induced by tilting the head back or rolling over while prone. It is important to note that vertigo of any etiology is associated with increased sensitivity to head movement.

"Have you had loss of consciousness or confusion with the spells of dizziness?" Peripheral vestibular disorders are not associated with a loss of consciousness. Some patients may have a vasovagal response to the nausea and vomiting. However, sudden spells of falls with loss of consciousness would be characteristic of vertebrobasilar insufficiency, brainstem disorders affecting the reticular activating system, or as a diagnosis of exclusion, basilar migraine.

"In between the spells of dizziness or vertigo, do you feel imbalanced when walking or clumsy with your extremities? Some but not all cerebellar disorders are characterized by spells of vertigo. However, nearly all cerebellar disorders are characterized by persistent ataxia and/or clumsiness of the extremities. Notably, a cerebellar syndrome may affect the gait (truncal ataxia) without affecting the limbs (appendicular ataxia).

"Are there accompanying otologic signs with the spells of vertigo, such as aural fullness, hearing loss, or tinnitus?" These may indicate Ménière disease, but can also be seen in basilar migraine and TIAs in the anterior inferior cerebellar artery (AICA) distribution.

"Are there accompanying focal neurologic signs with the spells of vertigo, or in isolation?" (Box 167.1). The presence of focal neurologic signs would be highly suspicious for vertebrobasilar TIAs, indicating a high risk for stroke.

"Is there a personal history of hypertension, hyperlipidemia, diabetes mellitus, cancer, coronary artery disease, peripheral vascular disease, migraines with aura or complicated migraine, strokes or TIAs in the past?" Vascular risk factors should alert the clinician to the possibility of vertebrobasilar insufficiency as the cause of spells of vertigo. Additionally, chronic nonspecific imbalance may be secondary to microvascular ischemic changes in a patient with vascular risk factors. Both require evaluation with an MRI of the brain and preventative treatment.

Imaging modalities. There are now excellent noninvasive imaging technology to evaluate the cerebrovascular arteries including the vertebrobasilar arteries, and the arch of the aorta, and takeoff of vessels. Contrast-enhanced magnetic resonance angiography (CE-MRA) can identify arterial stenosis with nearly the same sensitivity as traditional cerebral angiography (28). MRI with FLAIR (fluid-attenuated inversion recovery) imaging is especially sensitive for demyelinating lesions in MS. A sagittal MRI that includes the posterior fossa is excellent to evaluate for AC malformation. DWI is highly sensitive to ischemia or infarcts (strokes), but can be negative when the lesion is small.

VERTEBROBASILAR ISCHEMIA AND INFARCTS

Vertebrobasilar TIAs are likely to recur and to progress to stroke. It is critical to recognize the first vertebrobasilar TIA. There appears to be as high or even higher risk of stroke after VBI TIAs than after carotid TIAs. Identifying a basilar stenosis is critical as there is a very high incidence of stroke or TIA recurrence (28). Referral to a stroke center is often indicated as interventions may range from anticoagulation, stenting, angioplasty, or clot retrieval angiography.

VBI is associated with the traditional vascular risk factors. If a patient presents with vertigo or hearing loss as a TIA, then the localization is in the posterior circulation, that is, VBI. The incidence of vascular risk factors in patients with posterior circulation strokes is high. In a study of consecutive patients presenting to a large stroke center, the New England Medical Center Posterior Circulation Registry, the group of patients with extensive atherosclerotic disease involving the basilar artery had a very high incidence of stroke risk factors. Hypertension was present in 70%, and coronary artery disease was present in 60%. The incidence of stroke risk factors was also high in 300 consecutive patients presenting with posterior circulation strokes or TIAs of any cause: 58% had hypertension, 25% had diabetes mellitus, 42% tobacco abuse, 33% had coronary artery disease, 19% had hyperlipidemia. Other important modifiable lifestyle factors included alcohol abuse (13%), obesity (11%), and use of oral contraceptive pills (2%). Hyperlipidemia was more common in intracranial vertebral artery disease and basilar disease (31% and 35%, respectively) in comparison with extracranial vertebral artery disease (18%) (23).

Isolated vertigo as transient VBI. Both the central and peripheral vestibular pathways are fed by the posterior circulation: the vertebrobasilar arteries. The vertebrobasilar system represents about 20% of cerebral blood flow, and posterior circulation TIAs and strokes represent about 20% of all TIAs and strokes. In fact, isolated spells of vertigo are likely the most common presentation of vertebrobasilar TIA first described by Williams and Wilson, 1962 (Table 167.4) (29). In that study, 48% of the patients with VBI had vertigo. In the guinea pig, occlusion of the internal auditory artery causes cessation of cochlear potentials and degeneration within minutes (30). However, clinically in humans, the predominant first symptom and most common symptom reported is vertigo. In a posterior circulation TIA, the onset of vertigo is usually very abrupt and spontaneous, rather than being induced by position, and there may be a flurry of spells within a few weeks' time. The duration of the vertigo is critical. In the case of VBI, the duration of vertigo is 3 to 4 minutes in length. A comprehensive discussion of this topic is provided by the authors in another reference (31).

Some neurologists have stated that isolated vertigo is an unlikely presentation of VBI given that there are multiple neurologic structures packed closely together within the brainstem, making isolated vestibular nuclei ischemia unlikely. However, the clinical data clearly demonstrate that isolated vertigo can be a TIA in the posterior circulation. Grad and Baloh (24) reported a high incidence of isolated vertigo in patients with VBI. Sixty-two percent had

at least one episode of isolated vertigo, and in nearly one-fifth the first TIAs began with isolated vertigo. Since that report, there have been several studies demonstrating vertigo as the presentation and manifestation of VBI (32–34). It is important that clinicians and emergency room physicians are aware that transient VBI may not be evident on imaging studies, and oftentimes posterior circulation TIAs is a clinical diagnosis. In patients with VBI who had presented with vertigo, there was a high incidence of drop attacks: one out of three. There is also a very high incidence of visual symptoms of diplopia, field defects, or illusions. The visual illusions can mimic the visual aura of migraine (Table 167.5). In fact, transient ischemia within the vertebrobasilar system is a common cause of episodic nonpositional spontaneous vertigo spells in older patients.

For the clinician, there are distinguishing characteristics between the drop attacks of vertebrobasilar insufficiency and those of Ménière disease. VBI drop attacks are often described as "buckling of the knees" and a slowly crumpling downward. In a study of seven older patients with drop attacks of Ménière disease, also known as otolithic crisis, the attacks were described as forceful, and often violent, "as if being pushed by an external force." In many cases of Ménière drop attacks, there are associated injuries such as broken hip and concussions. In VBI, there may be an associated loss of consciousness. In Ménière drop attacks, there is never a loss of consciousness unless secondary to a concussion or head trauma (35).

Labyrinthine infarct. Pathologic studies following ligation of the internal auditory artery in animal studies demonstrate necrosis of the inner ear tissue with fibrous changes and osseous formation (36). Most cases of sudden hearing and vestibular loss have been associated with ischemia in the distribution of the AICA occurring with brainstem and cerebellar infarcts (37). In fact, isolated sudden

TABLE 167.4	INITIAL SYMPTOMS OF VERTEBROBASILAR INSUFFICIENCY IN 65 PATIENTS
Symptom	**No. of Patients (%)**
Vertigo	32 (48)
Visual hallucinations	7 (10)
Drop attacks or weakness	7 (10)
Visceral sensations	5 (8)
Visual field defects	4 (6)
Diplopia	3 (5)
Headaches	2 (3)
Other	5 (8)

From Williams D, Wilson TG. The diagnosis of the major and minor syndromes of basilar insufficiency. *Brain* 1962;85:741–774.

TABLE 167.5	SYMPTOMS ASSOCIATED WITH VERTIGO IN 42 PATIENTS WITH VERTEBROBASILAR INSUFFICIENCY
Symptom	**No. of Patients (%)**
Visual (diplopia, field deficits, illusions)	29 (69)
Drop attacks	14 (33)
Unsteadiness, incoordination	9 (21)
Extremity weakness	9 (21)
Confusion	7 (17)
Headache	6 (14)
Hearing loss	6 (14)
Loss of consciousness	4 (10)
Extremity numbness	4 (10)
Dysarthria	4 (10)
Tinnitus	4 (10)
Perioral numbness	2 (5)

From Grad A, Baloh RW. Vertigo of vascular origin: clinical and electronystagmographic features in 84 cases. *Arch Neurol* 1989;46:281–284.

sensorineural hearing loss or vestibular loss (presenting similar to vestibular neuritis) can be the first presentation or sole presentation of an AICA infarct (see under AICA infarct). Sudden deafness has also been associated with fat emboli (38), thromboangiitis obliterans or Buerger disease (39), and macroglobulinemia (40).

Of note, a labyrinthine infarct is too small to be seen on MRI imaging. Differentiating a labyrinthine infarct, which is presumably an infarct in the labyrinthine artery, from a viral sudden hearing loss with vertigo can be difficult. We recommend obtaining an MRI with DWI and MRA to evaluate for potentially treatable vascular pathology (see Imaging Modalities).

AICA stroke and hearing loss and vertigo. The stroke patient who is most likely to present to the otolaryngologist and the stroke patient most likely to be confused for a purely peripheral inner ear disorder is the patient with a stroke in the AICA territory. The labyrinth is fed by the internal auditory artery, an end artery with minimal collaterals from the otic capsule. The internal auditory artery is usually a branch of the AICA. The internal auditory artery perfuses the cochlea and vestibular labyrinth, and occlusion of this artery causes hearing loss and vertigo. Internal auditory artery infarction occurs mostly due to thrombotic narrowing of the AICA or the basilar artery at or near the AICA orifice (41). In fact, sudden deafness and vertigo may be the sole presentation of an AICA infarct, and could be easily mistaken for a purely inner ear disease (42).

Of importance, in a study by Lee et al. (43), patients with prodromal audiovestibular disturbances had five times higher prevalence of focal or diffuse basilar artery occlusive disease near the AICA orifice, compared with those without prodromal audiovestibular disturbance (62% vs. 13%, P < 0.001). Given the low incidence of pure auditory or pure vestibular loss, the investigators speculated that internal auditory artery ischemia seldom results in selective involvement of the anterior vestibular artery or the main cochlear artery. Conversely, there should be strong suspicion for VBI if a patient presents with acute onset of combined auditory and vestibular loss, especially in a patient with vascular risk factors (43). This contrasts with viral vestibular neuritis, which presents with only minimal or no auditory symptoms.

In a study of 12 consecutive patients with MRI confirmed AICA infarcts, one-third had vertigo and/or auditory symptoms in isolated episodes from 1 day to 2 months prior to the AICA infarct, and notably 11 out of the 12 had sensorineural hearing loss (44). Audiometric data indicate cochlear pathology primarily as the cause of deafness. A recently published (Epub) study demonstrated abnormal cervical vestibular-evoked myogenic potentials (cVEMPs) in 8 out of 16 patients with AICA infarcts (50%), an indication of saccular pathology. The abnormal cVEMP was also associated with a caloric paresis and sensorineural hearing loss, suggesting that the audiovestibular periphery is a source of vertigo and hearing loss in AICA infarcts (45).

The presence of hearing loss should be investigated in AICA infarcts as multiple publications have demonstrated this association (46,47). We recommend that any stroke or TIA associated with dizziness be formally evaluated with an audiogram as patients may be unaware of the hearing loss. We also recommend that sudden hearing loss with or without vertigo be evaluated by an MRI.

Traditionally, ischemia in the AICA territory is known to result in infarction of the dorsolateral pontomedullary region (brainstem) and the middle cerebellar peduncle. A complete AICA infarct is associated with the ipsilateral signs of a profound hearing loss, facial paralysis, cerebellar ataxia, loss of pain and temperature on the ipsilateral face, and contralateral pain/temperature loss on the body. In 82 consecutive AICA infarcts, the most common and dominant symptom was acute prolonged vertigo, lasting greater than 24 hours (98% of patients) (see Table 167.6) (43).

Posterior inferior cerebellar artery (PICA) syndrome or dorsolateral medullary syndrome: Wallenberg syndrome. An infarct in the PICA distribution causes a wedge-shaped infarct in the dorsolateral medulla, an area packed with salient neurologic nuclei. Therefore, the patient with a PICA infarct will usually have other neurologic signs. Of relevance to the otolaryngologist, in a study of 130 consecutive PICA infarcts without cerebellar involvement, only 57% presented with vertigo. However, 92% had gait ataxia, presumably from the infarct of the central vestibular nuclei and their interconnections (Table 167.7) (48). It is wise to look for a Horner's, a miotic pupil that does not dilate in darkness. The anisocoria (asymmetry of the pupils) of Horner's will be increased in darkness. In 88% of patients with Wallenberg syndrome, there was an ipsilateral Horner sign. Most of the patient exhibit severe gait ataxia. In the case report of three patients presenting with only vertigo and gait ataxia, which might be mistaken for a peripheral

TABLE 167.6	FREQUENCY OF SYMPTOMS IN 82 CONSECUTIVE PATIENTS WITH AICA INFARCTS
Symptom	**No. of Patients (%)**
Acute prolonged vertigo (>24 h)	80 (98)
Acute hearing loss	52 (63)
Limb dysmetria	55 (67)
Gait ataxia	52 (63)
Facial sensory loss	23 (28)
Facial weakness	23 (28)
Body sensory loss	5 (6)
Horner syndrome	3 (4)
Dysarthria	3 (4)
Eye motion limitation	2 (2)
Limb weakness	2 (2)

From Lee H, Kim JS, Chung EJ, et al. Infarction in the territory of anterior inferior cerebellar artery: spectrum of audiovestibular loss. *Stroke* 2009;40(12):3745–3751.

TABLE 167.7	FREQUENCY OF SYMPTOMS IN 130 CONSECUTIVE PICA INFARCTS

Symptom	No. of Patients (%)
Sensory symptoms and signs	125 (96)
Gait ataxia	120 (92)
Horner sign	114 (88)
Dysphagia	84 (65)
Dysarthria	28 (22)
Vertigo	74 (57)
Nystagmus	73 (56)
Limb ataxia	72 (55)
Nausea and vomiting	67 (52)
Headache	67 (52)
Skew deviation of eyes	53 (41)
Diplopia	41 (32)
Hiccoughs	33 (25)
Facial palsy	27 (21)

From Kim JS. Pure lateral medullary infarction: clinical-radiological correlation of 130 acute, consecutive patients. *Brain* 2003;126: 1864–1872.

vestibulopathy, the lateropulsion, a strong motor disturbance causing deviation of the trunk toward the ipsilateral side, was so strong that walking is severely impaired or impossible. The lateropulsion affects the oculomotor system, causing excessively large saccades toward the lesion, and abnormally small saccades away from the lesion (49). A PICA infarct, in contrast to vestibular neuritis, is associated with the severe motor disturbance that impairs the walking. In vestibular neuritis, the patient feels vertiginous and has some difficulty walking but will usually be able to walk. PICA infarcts, as opposed to AICA infarcts, do not present with auditory changes.

Cerebellar infarction. It has been stated that an isolated cerebellar stroke is likely sometimes mistaken for a peripheral vestibular neuritis. A recent study using MRI with DWI, a sensitive acquisition for recent ischemia, found that 75% (25 out of 33) patients with an apparent acute vestibular syndrome had a stroke, most often in the cerebellum. The study excluded patients with a recent viral illness (which occurs in about 30% of vestibular neuritis). Distinguishing characteristics of a cerebellar stroke were the inability to walk or stand, direction-changing nystagmus. Mild imbalance, characterized by the ability to stand and walk unassisted, but the inability to tandem walk, has been reported in an isolated superior cerebellar stroke (50). Cerebellar hemorrhages must be recognized promptly because of the possibility of herniation which can be fatal. A computed tomography (CT) scan can be obtained quickly, is readily available, and is highly sensitive to identify a cerebellar hemorrhage.

Vertebrobasilar ischemia and imaging. Given the similarity in presentation of some cerebellar symptoms, when seeing a patient with acute vestibular syndrome who has vascular risk factors, it is recommended to obtain an MRI

with DWI. DWI may show abnormalities (hyperintense) in the first few hours after an acute stroke syndrome that does not show up on T2-weighted imaging for several hours (51). A large burden of microvascular ischemic changes on MRI, even with a negative DWI (negative for stroke) would be indication to minimize the stroke risk factors by controlling blood pressure, providing statins and an antiplatelet agent if there is no contraindication, and modifying lifestyle factors such as diet and tobacco and ethanol abuse. The specific treatment with regards to aspirin versus aspirin-dipyridamole versus anticoagulation should be determined by a specialist such as a neurologist, given this rapidly changing field. The other consideration in the setting of a potentially acute stroke is thrombolytic treatment at a stroke center, and in some cases of vertebrobasilar stenosis, stenting may be indicated (SSYLVIA study) (52).

MIGRAINE-ASSOCIATED VERTIGO AND BASILAR MIGRAINE

Episodic vertigo spells occur in about one-fourth of patients with migraine (53). Migraine is diagnosed by the severity of the headaches and the associated symptoms (Table 167.8). Vertigo attributed to migraine is also known as vestibular migraine, migraine variant, migraine equivalent, atypical migraine, migraine-associated vertigo, benign recurrent vertigo, and previously as vestibular Ménière disease. Acephalgic migraine or atypical migraine can also occur; in this case, the patient has symptoms attributable to migraine without any headache pain. Migraine-associated vertigo is the second most common cause of recurrent vertigo after benign paroxysmal positional vertigo, and migraine-associated vertigo likely accounts for 6% to 7% of patients in clinics managing patients with dizziness (54). Benign paroxysmal vertigo of childhood is likely migrainous vertigo and is associated with the onset

TABLE 167.8	DIAGNOSTIC CRITERIA FOR MIGRAINE WITHOUT AURA (INTERNATIONAL HEADACHE SOCIETY, 2004)

At least five attacks fulfilling B-D
Headache last 4–72 h (untreated)
Headache has at least two of the following:
 – Unilateral
 – Pulsating
 – Moderate or severe (inhibits or prohibits daily activities)
 – Aggravated by walking, stairs, or similar physical activities
During headache at least one of the following:
 – Nausea and vomiting
 – Photophobia and phonophobia
Other causes of headache have been ruled out

From International Headache Society, Headache Classification Subcommittee. The international classification of headache disorders, 2nd edition. *Cephalalgia* 2004;24:1–60.

TABLE 167.9A	**PROPOSED DIAGNOSTIC CRITERIA FOR *DEFINITE* MIGRAINOUS VERTIGO**

Recurrent vestibular symptoms such as rotatory/positional vertigo, other illusory self or object motion, head motion intolerance

Current or previous history of migraine according to criteria of the International Headache Society, 2004 (59)

At least one of the following migrainous symptoms during at least two or more vertiginous attacks: migrainous headache, phonophobia, photophobia, scintillating scotoma, or other auras

Exclusion of other causes

From Lempert T, Neuhauser H. Migrainous vertigo. *Neurol Clin* 2005;23(3):715–730.

of migraine at a later age (55). The duration of vertigo in migraine-associated vertigo can vary from seconds to minutes and sometimes can last days and resemble recurrent vestibular neuritis (27). A study of 208 patients presenting to a neurotology clinic with benign recurrent vertigo demonstrated a comorbidity of migraine in 180 patients (87%) (56). Of these patients with both migraine and benign recurrent vertigo, 79% experienced the vertigo spells in isolation, unassociated with migraine symptoms. These patients would not meet the strict criteria for definite migrainous vertigo (54,57) (Tables 167.9A and 167.9B).

There is not a consensus regarding the strict definition of migrainous vertigo. Thus, a recent longitudinal follow-up of 75 patients was conducted to evaluate the reliability of diagnoses of definite or probable migrainous vertigo using the criteria of Lempert and Neuhauser (54). After a mean time of 8.75 years, definite vestibular migraine was confirmed in 85% of those previously diagnosed with definite vestibular migraine. Fifty percent of the patients with probable vestibular migraine evolved to the criteria for definite vestibular migraine, and 32% remained with diagnosis of probable vestibular migraine. Thus, there

TABLE 167.9B	**PROPOSED DIAGNOSTIC CRITERIA FOR *PROBABLE* MIGRAINOUS VERTIGO**

Recurrent vestibular symptoms such as rotatory/positional vertigo, other illusory self or object motion, head motion intolerance

Current or previous history of migraine according to criteria of the International Headache Society, 2004

Migrainous symptoms during at least two or more vertiginous attacks: headache, phonophobia, photophobia, scintillating scotoma, or other auras

Migraine precipitants of vertigo in more than 50% of attacks, such as food triggers, sleep irregularities, or hormonal changes

Response to migraine medications in more than 50% of attacks

Exclusion of other causes

From Lempert T, Neuhauser H. Migrainous vertigo. *Neurol Clin* 2005;23(3):715–730.

was very high reliability and validity of the diagnoses of probable and definite vestibular migraine. A subset evolved to have mild hearing loss, and thus met criteria for Ménière disease, but had symptoms atypical for Ménière disease (58).

Of the patients meeting the International Headache Society criteria for migraine (59), 62% of patients with migrainous vertigo met criteria for migraine with aura (56), and this percentage is significantly higher than the reported percentage of 28% of all patients with migraine that have migraine with aura (60). Migraine with aura appears to be associated with a higher frequency of infarcts than those with common migraine (migraine without aura). In the case of migraine with transient unilateral hearing loss and tinnitus as aura, the authors recommend the use of verapamil as the first-line agent, and agree that triptans would be relatively contraindicated (61). There may be a predominance of vertebrobasilar strokes associated with migrainous stroke. Bogousslavsky et al. (62) reported 9 posterior cerebral artery infarcts and 2 brainstem and cerebellar strokes among 22 migrainous strokes (41%), which is twice the ratio than general strokes of which posterior strokes reportedly represent 20% (62).

Basilar migraine. Basilar migraine is a subtype of migraine with aura characterized by recurrent headaches, oftentimes occipital in location, with focal neurologic symptoms localizing to the posterior circulation (Table 167.10) (63). The first attack in 65% of the cases was in the second or third decade. Commonly, patients with basilar migraine exhibit impaired consciousness (77%) and bilateral visual impairment (86%), as well as vertigo (63%). The impaired vision may be a blurring of the vision diffusely (69%) or flickering or wavy lines, called teichopsia (69%). The impaired consciousness ranges from coma (24%),

TABLE 167.10	**MOST COMMON SYMPTOMS IN 49 PATIENTS WITH BASILAR MIGRAINE**

Symptom	No. of Patients (%)
Headache	47 (96)
Bilateral visual impairment	42 (86)
Nausea	41 (83)
Impaired consciousness	38 (77)
Vomiting	35 (71)
Vertigo	31 (63)
Gait ataxia	31 (63)
Paresthesias (usually bilateral)	30 (61)
Dysarthria	28 (57)
Weakness (usually bilateral)	27 (55)
Tinnitus	13 (26)
Impaired hearing	10 (20)
Diplopia	8 (16)

From Bogousslavsky J, Regli F, Van Melle G. Migraine stroke. *Neurology* 1988;38:223–227.

confusion (43%), or syncope (35%). Other associated symptoms include gait ataxia, paresthesias, dysarthria, and tinnitus. The prophylactic treatment of choice in basilar migraine is calcium channel blockers. Triptans and ergots are considered relatively contraindicated in basilar migraine. Because of the similarity in presentation between basilar migraine and VBI, evaluation of the cerebrovasculature with an MRI and referral to a neurologist are warranted.

Migrainous vertigo without other symptoms does not meet criteria for basilar migraine, and has been considered to be potentially responsive to triptans. In a trial with limitation mainly from too few subjects, zolmitriptan was not associated with significantly greater relief versus placebo for migrainous vertigo. However, the study was insufficiently powered (64).

Migraine-associated vestibulopathy, hearing loss, and motion sickness. There is evidence that migraine can be associated with hearing loss, tinnitus, and auditory end organ damage (61,65). Unilateral caloric paresis has been reported to occur in 18% to 21% of migraineurs with vertigo (27,66). Migraine is also associated with Tumarkin-like falls, sudden falls with no loss of consciousness described as "being pushed by an external force," originally described in association with Ménière disease. Tumarkin-like falls were associated with vestibulopathy as demonstrated on vestibular testing in migraine patients without Ménière disease (66). Migrainous vertigo is also associated with abnormalities in vestibular evoked myogenic potentials (VEMPs) (67). These findings indicate an association of peripheral vestibular damage with migraine. A recent pilot study reported that rizatriptan pretreatment was associated with a decrease in motion sickness induced by off-vertical axis rotation in migraine patients with motion sickness (68). The effect is proposed to be mediated by serotonin receptors within the serotonergic vestibular-autonomic pathways, a central vestibular mediated pathway.

Treatment of migraine-associated vertigo. In general, the prophylaxis of migraine-associated vertigo is similar to that to prevent migraine headaches. Medications commonly used include calcium channel blockers, tricyclic amines, beta-blockers, and anticonvulsants such as topiramate or valproate. In the authors' experience, the use of acetazolamide can be effective for both the audiovestibular symptoms and the headache, especially if the disease process mimics Ménière disease (aural fullness, tinnitus, and vertigo). In the case of migraine–Ménière's, the characteristic that distinguishes it from Ménière disease is the lack of progression of hearing loss. In these cases, the tinnitus and aural fullness are oftentimes bilateral. Preventative measures should also include lifestyle changes: regular exercise (which should be introduced gradually as acutely increasing exercise may trigger a migraine), regular meals, avoidance of high-fat and high-sugar foods, moderation of caffeinated beverages or ethanol, and avoidance of tobacco. Patients should evaluate for particular food triggers including red wine, processed foods, and artificial sweeteners. Dehydration can also trigger migraine headaches or vertigo spells. Women often present with migraine symptoms near the onset of menses. It is helpful for patients to keep a headache diary and to include in the diary any potential triggers.

MULTIPLE SCLEROSIS AND NEUROTOLOGIC SYMPTOMS

MS is a demyelinating disease of the central nervous system with onset usually in the third and fourth decades of life, with a female predominance (69). Because there is evidence that early treatment with disease-modifying agents can alter and slow down the progression of this disease, it is wise for clinicians to be able to recognize MS in order to refer patients to appropriate specialists. Immune-modulating agents include β-interferon, glatiramer acetate, and second generation MS treatments may include methotrexate, azathioprine, cyclophosphamide, mitoxantrone, and recently an oral agent, fingolimod (FTY720) (70). MS is the most common cause of acquired disability in young adults in the western world with an incidence of 4 to 8 newly diagnosed patients per 100,000 per year (71). MRI is the most sensitive imaging modality to identify demyelinating disease with attention to the fluid-attenuated inversion recovery (FLAIR) sequence, ideally including a sagittal image. Neurologists use MRI to follow the progression of MS disease, and enhancement with gadolinium can be used to evaluate for active inflammatory MS disease processes.

Neurotologic signs and symptoms of MS. Hearing loss occurs in about 10% of patients with MS with no apparent relationship between the severity of MS and the severity of hearing loss (72). The clinical presentation of the hearing loss in MS varies from acute to subacute (over months) to insidious with oftentimes a partial remission of hearing loss. Vertigo is the initial symptom in about 5% of patients with MS, and is reported to occur at some time during the disease in about half of patients with MS (69). The vertigo may be secondary to demyelination of the root entry zone of the vestibular nerve, the brainstem vestibular nuclei, or the cerebellum. An acute attack of MS may be treated with intravenous Solu-Medrol to hasten the remission of symptoms and signs, and lessen the inflammatory response. Prolonged vertigo spells should be treated with antiemetics and vestibular suppressants such as benzodiazepines. Of note, there may be a higher incidence of benign paroxysmal positional vertigo in patients with MS, which can be treated with the traditional Epley maneuver.

Examination findings in MS. MS will often be associated with eye movement abnormalities, including internuclear ophthalmoplegia (INO), saccadic pursuit. An INO will manifest with an inability to adduct (move medially) the affected eye, and a dissociated nystagmus when looking to the contralateral side. The pathology is located within the medial longitudinal fasciculus (MLF), which is commonly involved in MS due to the length of the MLF. Because INO is common in MS and uncommon in other diseases, the presence of an INO should trigger an evaluation for MS (73). A history of optic neuritis is common in MS, which may be associated with a relative afferent pupillary defect. Other common findings include brisk deep tendon reflexes, ataxia or other cerebellar signs, and impaired vibratory and position sense. With regard to the neurotologic studies, VEMPs are abnormal in one-third of patients with MS (74).

Ataxia syndromes. *Friedreich ataxia* is the most common of the hereditary ataxias, with a prevalence of 2 per 100,000, which is equal to nearly all of the other dominant ataxias combined. Friedreich ataxia is a recessively inherited ataxia with presentation of progressive limb and gait ataxia, loss of position and vibration sense, onset before 25 years, and absent deep tendon reflexes in the legs. Of note, there is some variability in presentation. Friedreich ataxia is secondary to a GAA repeat in the gene frataxin, the product is a mitochondrial protein related to oxidative stress. Both auditory and vestibular loss occur commonly, but oftentimes late in the disease process (75,76). *Refsum syndrome* is an autosomal recessive ataxia syndrome characterized by retinitis pigmentosa, bilateral sensorineural hearing loss, cerebellar ataxia, and peripheral neuropathy secondary to a defect in lipid alpha oxidase.

Episodic ataxias (EA) are a rare group of disorders of the cerebellum. In general, there are episodes of ataxia with relatively normal spells in between. While these disorders are relatively rare, they may present to the otolaryngologist with complaints of "dizziness." The patient with ataxia may state that the spells are similar to the feeling of drunkenness, and they may describe a clumsiness of the extremities and slurred speech. Most of the EA are inherited and a family history should be obtained. MRI imaging of the brain and upper cervical cord can reveal a cerebellar vermis (midline) atrophy. Specific DNA tests are available for all of the trinucleotide repeat syndromes. A battery of tests can be ordered on a patient with a dominantly inherited spinocerebellar ataxia syndrome. Treatment is symptomatic. Acetazolamide is quite effective to prevent the episodic spells in patients with EA-2, and to a lesser degree, EA-1, starting with a low dose of 125 mg/d and working up to an average effective dose of between 500 and 750 mg/d (77). In EA-2, the spells of ataxia are often associated with vertigo, nausea, and vomiting. The nystagmus in between spells of vertigo/ataxia may be downbeat or gaze-evoked.

Other causes of cerebellar ataxia. Other causes include idiopathic degenerative ataxias, such as multiple system atrophy, ischemic or hemorrhagic strokes, toxins such as alcohol, heavy metals, or solvents, autoimmune conditions, and infections. Gluten ataxia occurs when gluten is ingested in a susceptible patient and is associated with antigliadin antibodies (78). The onset of gait ataxia may be insidious.

Paraneoplastic cerebellar degeneration usually presents subacutely, with the most commonly associated cancers being small-cell lung cancer, breast or ovarian cancer, and

lymphoma. The presentation of subacute cerebellar ataxia should trigger an extensive workup including imaging, and oftentimes analysis of the cerebrospinal fluid (CSF) is warranted. Paraneoplastic cerebellar ataxia is most commonly associated with small-cell lung carcinoma but many other cancers have been associated with paraneoplastic cerebellar ataxia. The underlying tumor may be unable to be detected early in the presentation of paraneoplastic disease (79). Thus, a workup for an occult malignancy is warranted in any patient with subacute cerebellar degeneration and the serum should be evaluated for antineuronal antibodies (80,81). The common antineuronal antibodies associated with paraneoplastic cerebellar ataxia include anti-Hu, anti-Yo, anti-Ri (which often has a less severe course), anti-Ma, anti-Tr, anti-CV2, anti-GAD, anti-VGKC (voltage-gated potassium channel), and anti-VGCC (voltage-gated calcium channel). These serum antibodies are identified in about one-half of patients with paraneoplastic cerebellar degeneration. An intensive search for an occult malignancy must be conducted; the first imaging modalities usually include whole-body CT and/or total body positron emission tomography (PET).

Arnold-Chiari syndrome. AC syndrome is a congenital condition characterized by a defect of the skull base that causes a herniation of the cerebellum and/or brainstem into the cervical spinal canal. The onset of symptoms usually presents in the second or third decades. AC syndromes are classified into four types. AC-I is an anomaly of congenital cerebellar tonsillar elongation with displacement through the foramen magnum. Symptomatic AC-I may present with brainstem or cerebellar signs, including downbeat nystagmus, and ataxias. Of note, herniation greater than 12 mm was invariably symptomatic. However, nearly 30% of patients with tonsillar displacements ranging from 5 to 10 mm below the foramen magnum were asymptomatic (82). Osseous abnormalities are also common including basilar invagination. The tonsillar descent is best evaluated on a sagittal T1- and T2-weighted MRI scan, which is preferred over CT. Uncomplicated AC-I may present with ataxia of gait, vertical downbeating nystagmus, which patients may describe as "oscillopsia." This is described as a visual blurring that is worse when walking on hard surfaces or when shifting the gaze. Other common features include occipital and cervical pain, ataxia of gait, and blurred vision. In symptomatic AC-I, there is nearly always pathologic nystagmus. Surgical correction by suboccipital decompression of the foramen magnum can halt the progression due to the cervical medullary compression, and can sometimes reverse the neurologic symptoms and signs. Patients with rheumatoid arthritis may be especially susceptible to cranial vertebral anomalies, and a recent series of 45 patients surgically treated for rheumatoid arthritis and cranial settling had excellent outcomes (83).

Thiamine deficiency. Wernicke's can present with eye movement paresis (ophthalmoplegia), confusion, and ataxia of gait and stance. Truncal ataxia is typically significantly worse than appendicular ataxia (testing finger to nose or heel to shin). Thus, imbalance and falls may be an early presentation of Wernicke's and may present to the otolaryngologist. Traditionally, clinicians associate thiamine deficiency with alcoholism, but thiamine deficiency is associated with bariatric surgery, chemotherapy, HIV, hyperemesis gravidarum, malabsorption syndromes, prolonged parenteral feeding, prolonged starvation, thyrotoxicosis, uremia, and cancers (84). Diabetics may be relatively susceptible to Wernicke's because insulin deficiency may cause a reduction in the rate of thiamine transport across the intestine (85). Pathologic changes are noted in the vestibular nuclei in thiamine-deficient monkeys (86). MRI may show FLAIR hyperintensities in the thalami, mammillary bodies, tectal plate, and periaqueductal area (87). However, diagnosis of Wernicke's should be a clinical diagnosis as the MRI is reported to have a sensitivity and specificity of 53% and 93%, respectively. Recovery is dependent on rapidness of institution of thiamine. Hundred milligram intravenous per day should be administered as a trial since oral absorption may be deficient, especially in gastrointestinal cancers. It is best to not wait for the thiamine levels as early treatment is important.

HIGHLIGHTS

- The history is critical in the evaluation of a patient presenting with dizziness or vertigo. Distinguishing the type of dizziness is crucial. Vertigo will present with a sensation of movement of self or the environment, and can be seen in both central and peripheral vestibular disorders.
- The characteristics of the spontaneous peripheral nystagmus in an acute vestibular syndrome are a horizontal torsional nystagmus which obeys Alexander law (increases in velocity and amplitude when looking toward the side of the fast phase) and is suppressed by visual fixation.
- Common central vestibular nystagmus patterns include downbeat nystagmus or a direction-changing nystagmus. A vertical nystagmus is always central in etiology. Central vestibular disorders are often associated with other abnormal eye movements including saccadic intrusions, abnormal saccades, and pursuit.
- VBI should be suspected in an older patient with vascular risk factors. Spontaneous vertigo with an abrupt onset and duration of 3 to 4 minutes is highly suspicious for VBI. Isolated vertigo can be a manifestation of a vertebrobasilar TIA. Because of the propensity for recurrence, prompt evaluation of the vertebrobasilar circulation is indicated using contrast-enhanced MRA and MRI. When MRI is contraindicated, a CT angiogram can be used. Treatment can include thrombolytic therapy, and in stroke centers other interventions include angio-

plasty, stenting, intra-arterial thrombolytic therapy, and the use of clot retrieval instruments.
- Sudden deafness or vertigo can be a symptom of ischemia in the AICA distribution. From one-sixth to one-third of patients who had an AICA infarct had a prodrome of vertigo or hearing symptoms in the 1 or 2 months prior.
- Migraine-associated vertigo or vestibular migraine is one of the most common central vestibular disorders presenting to the otolaryngologist. One-fourth of patients with migraine have vertigo. The duration of the vertigo can vary greatly. The Bárány Society and the International Headache Society consensus narrowed the diagnosis of definite vestibular migraine to cases having migraine features with at least 50% of the vestibular episodes (88). These criteria will likely have higher specificity, but lower sensitivity. Migraine can be associated with hearing loss, vertigo spells, Tumarkin-like falls, and BPV.
- Vertigo is the initial symptom in 5% of patients with MS and hearing loss occurs in about 10% of patients with MS. MRI with FLAIR is highly sensitive for demyelinating plaques. Other commonly associated findings include INO, optic neuritis, brisk deep tendon reflexes, and loss of vibratory sensation.
- AC-I is associated with suboccipital headache, vertigo which is oftentimes elicited by positional changes or changes of head movements, and visual complaints including blurred vision. Usually symptomatic AC-I will be associated with a pathologic nystagmus, oftentimes a downbeat nystagmus. MRI is useful to evaluate for the presence of AC malformation, and also to evaluate the volume of the posterior fossa and CSF flow dynamics. Surgical correction may halt the progression or even allow reversal of symptoms when diagnosed accurately.
- A common metabolic condition that may present with central vestibular findings is thiamine deficiency, or Wernicke encephalopathy. Ocular abnormalities, ataxia, falls, and memory impairment are common presenting symptoms. Rapid institution of thiamine can reverse the progression of the disease, which can be life threatening.
- Cerebellar syndromes often present with vertigo and ataxia. Cerebellar diseases are often associated with an abnormal nystagmus with common patterns being downbeat nystagmus or a direction-changing nystagmus. Laboratory investigations to consider include examination of the CSF, genetic panels, vitamin E, vitamin B_1, antigliadin antibodies, and evaluation for toxins. MRI is superior to CT to evaluate for cerebellar degeneration. Total body CT and/or PET may be indicated in subacute cerebellar ataxia to look for a primary tumor.

REFERENCES

1. Barmack NH. Central vestibular system: vestibular nuclei and posterior cerebellum. *Brain Res Bull* 2003;60:511.
2. Dieterich M, Brandt T. Functional brain imaging of peripheral and central vestibular disorders. *Brain* 2008;131:2538–2552.
3. Baloh RW, Spooner JW. Downbeat nystagmus: a type of central vestibular nystagmus. *Neurology* 1981;31:304.
4. Jacobson GP, McCaslin DL, Kaylie DM. Alexander's law revisited. *J Am Acad Audiol* 2008;19(8):630.
5. Baloh RW, Jacobson K, Honrubia V. Horizontal semicircular canal variant of benign positional vertigo. *Neurology* 1993;43:2542–2549.
6. Suzuki JI, Tokumasu K, Goto K. Eye movements from single utricular nerve stimulation in the cat. *Acta Otolaryngol* 1969;68:350–362.
7. Halmagyi GM, Gresty MA, Gibson WPR. Ocular tilt reaction with peripheral vestibular lesions. *Ann Neurol* 1979;6:80–83.
8. Brandt T, Dieterich M. Pathological eye head coordination in roll: tonic ocular tilt reaction in mesencephalic and medullary lesions. *Brain* 1987;110:649.
9. Vibert D, Häusler R, Safran AB, et al. Diplopia from skew deviation in unilateral peripheral lesions. *Acta Otolaryngol* 1996;116(2):170–176.
10. Park HJ, Shin JE, Lim YC, et al. Clinical significance of vibration-induced nystagmus. *Audiol Neurootol* 2008;13(3):182.
11. White JA, Hughes GB, Ruggieri PN. Vibration-induced nystagmus as an office procedure for the diagnosis of superior semicircular canal dehiscence. *Otol Neurotol* 2007;28(7):911.
12. Choi KD, Oh SY, Park SH, et al. Head-shaking nystagmus in lateral medullary infarction. *Neurology* 2007;68(17):1337–1344.
13. Spooner JW, Baloh RW. Arnold-Chiari malformation: improvement in eye movements after surgical treatment. *Brain* 1981;104:51.
14. Zee DS, Yamazaki A, Batter PH, et al. Effects of ablation of flocculus and paraflocculus on eye movements in primates. *J Neurophysiol* 1981;46:878.
15. Baloh RW, Yee RD. Spontaneous vertical nystagmus. *Rev Neurol (Paris)* 1989;145:527.
16. Leigh RJ, Zee DS. *The neurology of eye movements*, 4th ed. New York: Oxford University Press, 2006.
17. Whyte CA, Petrock AM, Rosenberg M. Occurrence of physiologic gaze-evoked nystagmus at small angles of gaze. *Invest Ophthalmol Vis Sci* 2010;51(5):2476–2478.
18. Bondar RL, Sharpe JA, Lewis AJ. Rebound nystagmus in olivocerebellar atrophy: a clinicopathological correlation. *Ann Neurol* 1984;15:474–477.
19. Lloyd SK, Baguley DM, Butler K, et al. Bruns' nystagmus in patients with vestibular schwannoma. *Otol Neurotol* 2009;30(5):625–628.
20. Baloh RW, Yee RD, Honrubia V. Eye movements in patients with Wallenberg's syndrome. *Ann N Y Acad Sci* 1981;374:600.
21. Halmagyi GM, Curthoys IS. A clinical sign of canal paresis. *Arch Neurol* 1988;45:737–739.
22. Baloh RW, Honrubia V, Jacobson K. Benign positional vertigo: clinical and oculographic features in 240 cases. *Neurology* 1987;37:371–378.
23. Caplan LR. *Posterior circulation disease: clinical findings, diagnosis and management.* Cambridge, MA: Blackwell Science, 1996, Chapter 7.
24. Grad A, Baloh RW. Vertigo of vascular origin: clinical and electronystagmographic features in 84 cases. *Arch Neurol* 1989;46:281–284.
25. American Academy of Otolaryngology-Head and Neck Surgery. Ménière's disease: criteria for diagnosis and evaluation of therapy for reporting. AAO-HNS Bulletin, July 1985.
26. Bagger-Sjöbäck D, Perols O, Bergenius J. Audiovestibular findings in patients with vestibular neuritis: a long-term follow-up study. *Acta Otolaryngol Suppl (Stockh)* 1993;503:16–17.
27. Cutrer FM, Baloh RW. Migraine-associated dizziness. *Headache* 1992;32:300–304.
28. Marquardt L, Kuker W, Chandratheva A. Incidence and prognosis of ≥50% symptomatic vertebral or basilar artery stenosis: prospective population-based study. *Brain* 2009;132:982–988.

29. Williams D, Wilson TG. The diagnosis of the major and minor syndromes of basilar insufficiency. *Brain* 1962;85:741–774.
30. Levine RA, Bu-Saba N, Brown MC. Laser-Doppler measurements and electrocochleography during ischemia of the guinea pig cochlea: implications for hearing preservation in acoustic neuroma surgery. *Ann Otol Rhinol Laryngol* 1993;102(2):127–136.
31. Ishiyama G, Ishiyama A. Vertebrobasilar infarcts and ischemia. *Otolaryngol Clin North Am* 2011;44:415–435.
32. Fife TD, Baloh RW, Duckwiler GR. Isolated dizziness in vertebrobasilar insufficiency: clinical feature, angiography and follow-up. *J Stroke Cerebrovasc Dis* 1994;4:4–12.
33. Gomez CR, Cruz-Flores S, Malkoff MD, et al. Isolated vertigo as a manifestation of vertebrobasilar ischemia. *Neurology* 1996;47(1):94–97.
34. Kim HA, Lee SR, Lee H. Acute peripheral vestibular syndrome of a vascular cause. *J Neurol Sci* 2007;254(1–2):99–101.
35. Ishiyama G, Ishiyama A, Jacobson K, et al. Drop attacks in older patients secondary to an otologic cause. *Neurology* 2001;57(6):1103–1106.
36. Kimura RS, Perlman HB. Arterial obstruction of the labyrinth. Part I: cochlear changes. *Ann Otol Rhinol Laryngol* 1958;67:5–24.
37. Lee H, Baloh RW. Sudden deafness in vertebrobasilar ischemia: clinical features, vascular topographical patterns and long-term outcome. *J Neurol Sci* 2005;228(1):99.
38. Jaffe B. Sudden deafness—a local manifestation of systemic disorders: fat emboli, hypercoagulation and infections. *Laryngoscope* 1970;80:788–801.
39. Kirikae I, Nomura Y, Shitara T, et al. Sudden deafness due to Buerger's disease. *Arch Otolaryngol* 1962;75:502–505.
40. Ruben D, Distenfeld A, Berg P, et al. Sudden sequential deafness as the presenting symptom of macroglobulinemia. *JAMA* 1969;209:1364–1365.
41. Amarenco P, Rosengart A, DeWitt LD, et al. Anterior inferior cerebellar artery territory infarcts. Mechanisms and clinical features. *Arch Neurol* 1993;50(2):154–161.
42. Lee H, Ahn BH, Baloh RW. Sudden deafness with vertigo as a sole manifestation of anterior inferior cerebellar artery infarction. *J Neurol Sci* 2004;222(1–2):105–107.
43. Lee H, Kim JS, Chung EJ, et al. Infarction in the territory of anterior inferior cerebellar artery: spectrum of audiovestibular loss. *Stroke* 2009;40(12):3745–3751.
44. Lee H, Sohn SI, Jung DK, et al. Sudden deafness and anterior inferior cerebellar artery infarction. *Stroke* 2002;33(12):2807–2812.
45. Ahn BH, Kim HA, Yi HA, et al. Abnormal cervical vestibular-evoked myogenic potential in anterior inferior cerebellar artery territory infarction: frequency, pattern and a determinant. *J Neurol Sci* 2011;307(1–2):114–119. PMID: 21571323.
46. Rajesh R, Rafeequ M, Girija AS. Anterior inferior cerebellar artery infarct with unilateral deafness. *J Assoc Physicians India* 2004;52:333–334.
47. Patzak MF, Demuth K, Kehl R, et al. Sudden hearing loss as the leading symptom of an infarction of the left anterior inferior cerebellar artery. *HNO* 2005;53(9):797–799.
48. Kim JS. Pure lateral medullary infarction: clinical-radiological correlation of 130 acute, consecutive patients. *Brain* 2003;126:1864–1872.
49. Choi KD, Kim HJ, Cho BM, et al. Saccadic adaptation in lateral medullary and cerebellar infarction. *Exp Brain Res* 2008;188(3):475.
50. Newman-Toker DE, Kattah JC, Alvernia JE, et al. Normal head impulse test differentiates acute cerebellar strokes from vestibular neuritis. *Neurology* 2008;70:2378.
51. Kitis O, Calli C, Yunten N, et al. Wallenberg's lateral medullary syndrome: diffusion-weighted imaging findings. *Acta Radiol* 2004;45(1):78.
52. SSYLVIA. Stenting of symptomatic atherosclerotic lesions in the vertebral or intracranial arteries: study results. *Stroke* 2004;35:1388.
53. Kayan A, Hood JD. Neuro-otological manifestations of migraine. *Brain* 1984;107(Pt 4):1123–1142.
54. Lempert T, Neuhauser H. Migrainous vertigo. *Neurol Clin* 2005;23(3):715–730.
55. Lanzi G, Balottin U, Fazzi E, et al. Benign paroxysmal vertigo of childhood: a long-term follow-up. *Cephalalgia* 1994;14:458–460.

56. Cha YH, Lee H, Santell LS, et al. Association of benign recurrent vertigo and migraine in 208 patients. *Cephalalgia* 2009; 29(5):550.

57. Crevits L, Bosman T. Migraine-related vertigo: towards a distinctive entity. *Clin Neurol Neurosurg* 2005;107:82–87.

58. Radtke A, Neuhauser H, von Brevern M, et al. Vestibular migraine—validity of clinical diagnostic criteria. *Cephalalgia* 2011;31(8):906–913.

59. International Headache Society, Headache Classification Subcommittee. The international classification of headache disorders, 2nd edition. *Cephalalgia* 2004;24:1–60.

60. Stewart WF, Linet MS, Delentano DD, et al. Age and sex-specific incidence rates of migraine with and without aura. *Am J Epidemiol* 1991;134:1111–1120.

61. Evans RW, Ishiyama G. Migraine with transient unilateral hearing loss and tinnitus. *Headache* 2009;49(5):756–758.

62. Bogousslavsky J, Regli F, Van Melle G. Migraine stroke. *Neurology* 1988;38:223–227.

63. Sturzenegger MH, Meienberg O. Basilar artery migraine: a follow-up of 82 cases. *Headache* 1985;25:408.

64. Neuhauser H, Radtke A, von Brevern M, et al. Zolmitriptan for treatment of migrainous vertigo: a pilot randomized placebo-controlled trial. *Neurology* 2003;60:882.

65. Viire E, Baloh RW. Migraine as a cause of sudden hearing loss. *Headache* 1996;36:24–28.

66. Ishiyama G, Ishiyama A, Baloh RW. Drop attacks and vertigo secondary to a non-Meniere's otologic cause. *Arch Neurol* 2003;60(1):71–75.

67. Baier B, Stieber N, Dieterich M. Vestibular-evoked myogenic potentials in vestibular migraine. *J Neurol* 2009;256(9):1447–1454.

68. Furman JM, Marcus DA, Balaban CD. Rizatriptan reduces vestibular-induced motion sickness in migraineurs. *J Headache Pain* 2011;12(1):81–88.

69. Courtney AM, Treadaway K, Remington G, et al. Multiple sclerosis. *Med Clin North Am* 2009;93(2):451.

70. Wipfler P, Harrer A, Pilz F, et al. Recent developments in approved and oral multiple sclerosis treatment and an update on future treatment options. *Drug Discov Today* 2011;16(1):8–21.

71. Noseworthy JH, Lucchinetti C, Rodriguez M, et al. Multiple sclerosis. *N Engl J Med* 2000;343:938–952.

72. Oh YM, Oh DH, Jeong SH, et al. Sequential bilateral hearing loss in multiple sclerosis. *Ann Otol Rhinol Laryngol* 2008;117:186.

73. Cogan DG. Internuclear ophthalmoplegia typical and atypical. *Arch Ophthalmol* 1970;84:583.

74. Patko T, Simo M, Aranyi Z. Vestibular click-evoked myogenic potentials: sensitivity and factors determining abnormality in patients with multiple sclerosis. *Mult Scler* 2007;13(2):193.

75. Fahey MC, Cremer PD, Aw ST, et al. Vestibular saccadic and fixation abnormalities in genetically confirmed Friedreich ataxia. *Brain* 2008;131:1035.

76. Lopez-Diaz-de-Leon E, Silva-Rojas A, Ysunza A, et al. Auditory neuropathy in Friedreich ataxia. A report of two cases. *Int J Pediatr Otorhinolaryngol* 2003;67(6):641.

77. Baloh RW. Periodic and progressive ataxias. In: Rose MR, Griggs R, eds. *Channelopathies of the nervous system*. London, UK: Butterworth-Heinemann, 2001.

78. Hadjivassiliou M, Sanders DS, Woodroofe N, et al. Gluten ataxia. *Cerebellum* 2008;7(3):494–498.

79. Vitaliani R, Zoccarato M, Giometto B. Diagnosis and treatment of paraneoplastic neurological syndromes. *Curr Clin Pharmacol* 2008;3(1):46.

80. Dalmau JO, Posner JB. Paraneoplastic syndromes. *Arch Neurol* 1999;56:405.

81. Linke R, Schroeder M, Helmberger T, et al. Antibody-positive paraneoplastic neurologic syndromes: value of CT and PET for tumor diagnosis. *Neurology* 2004;63:282.

82. Elster AD, Chen MYM. Chiari I malformations: clinical and radiologic reappraisal. *Radiology* 1992;183:347–353.

83. Sindou M, Gimbert E. Decompression for Chiari type I malformation (with or without syringomyelia) by extreme lateral foramen magnum opening and expansile duraplasty with arachnoid preservation: comparison with other technical modalities (Literature review). *Adv Tech Stand Neurosurg* 2009;34:85.

84. Kuo SH, Debnam JM, Fuller GN, et al. Wernicke's encephalopathy: an underrecognized and reversible cause of confusional state in cancer patients. *Oncology* 2009;76(1):10.

85. Page GLJ, Laight D, Cummings MH. Thiamine deficiency in diabetes mellitus and the impact of thiamine replacement on glucose metabolism and vascular disease. *Int J Clin Pract* 2011;65:684–690.

86. Cogan DG, Witt ED, Goldman-Rakic PS. Ocular signs in thiamine-deficient monkeys and in Wernicke's disease in humans. *Ann Ophthalmol* 1985;103:1212.

87. Zuccoli G, Pipitone N. Neuroimaging findings in acute Wernicke's encephalopathy: review of the literature. *AJR Am J Roentgenol* 2009;192(2):501–508.

88. Lempert T, Olesen J, Furman J, et al. Vestibular migraine: diagnostic criteria. *J Vestib Res* 2012;22:167–172.

Vestibular Rehabilitation

168

Susan L. Whitney   **Yael Raz**

Persons with vestibular disorders often present with complaints of dizziness, being off balance, and sometimes nausea and vomiting. They may also report falls as a result of their vestibular disorder. Dizziness is a very common complaint in an otolaryngologist's office. The diagnosis and management of persons with dizziness can be perplexing, since there are so many causes of dizziness. Medication-induced dizziness is very common as is dizziness associated with headache. Thorough history and examination, often with laboratory testing, are necessary to confirm the presence and nature of vestibular dysfunction.

Balance and dizziness disorders are generally considered to affect older adults (1), although younger people also encounter vestibular disorders (2). The prevalence of dizziness/vertigo in a 1-year period has been estimated to be approximately 29% in women and 17% in men within the German population (2). In a large US study (*n* = 5,086), it is estimated that 35% of people over the age of 40 have had vestibular dysfunction based on their ability to stand in modified Romberg on a firm and compliant surface, with active dizziness increasing the odds of falling by 12 (3). Of 546 persons presenting to the emergency room (ER) with no known cause for a fall initially, when probed, 80% had reported dizziness within the last 12 month (4), suggesting that the dizziness may be related to falls. Persons with vestibular disorders become concerned about falls, resulting in their being more sedentary and further increasing their risk of falling.

Nine percent of older adults seen for chronic medical problems in an outpatient geriatric setting for nonbalance or dizziness complaints had unrecognized benign paroxysmal positional vertigo (BPPV) (5). These older adults also had greater reports of falls and impairments of the activities of daily living (ADL) (5). Vestibular physical therapy has been used to improve balance, decrease dizziness, and improve quality of life in persons with BPPV and other central and peripheral vestibular disorders. There is mounting evidence that vestibular physical therapy is effective in the treatment of vestibular dysfunction in adults and children (6–68). Two Cochrane meta-analyses of 21 and 27 randomized trials suggested that there was moderate to strong evidence to support that vestibular rehabilitation is a safe and effective intervention for persons with peripheral vestibular disorders (38,39).

Vestibular disorders are most commonly treated by physical therapists. Other health care providers such as occupational therapists and audiologists also deliver interventional care. Knowledge related to the treatment of BPPV is commonly taught within physical therapist curricula. Standards related to the knowledge base that is critical for the identification and treatment of vestibular disorders have recently been published (69). The newly published international guidelines written by a Barany Society subgroup provide a starti ng point for therapists to determine what additional knowledge they should acquire in order to optimally treat persons with balance and vestibular dysfunction (69). The treatment of vestibular disorders in many physical therapist curricula is considered advanced knowledge beyond an entry level doctor of physical therapy degree program. Any physical therapist who is a neurologic clinical specialist should have background in specific examination and intervention techniques for persons with vestibular disorders.

Developing a relationship between physicians and physical therapists interested in treating patients with vestibular disorders is important for the patients' optimal recovery. Good communication will enhance the care that patients receive and should ultimately speed their recovery. As a physician initially seeking referral to a physical therapist, it is reasonable to ask the intended provider what his or her experience is with the treatment of persons with balance and vestibular disorders. There are advanced training options that could also further develop their skills and experience in the treatment of persons with balance and vestibular disorders if they were interested in learning more.

Medications rarely help with persons with peripheral vestibular disorders, except in the acute phase. However, chronic use of medications is often beneficial in persons with Meniere disease for long-term symptom control. As persons improve, it is optimal to taper and stop the antidizziness and antinausea medication as it may actually slow down central compensation and the recalibration process of the vestibuloocular reflex (VOR). Long-term use of antidizziness medication is not advised, especially in older adults. The drowsiness often associated with the antiemetics and vestibular suppressants might increase an older adult's risk of falling. Vestibular suppressants, which are typically used to manage symptoms in persons with acute vestibular disorders, may slow vestibular compensation (70). Venosa and Bittar (71), in a prospective trial, suggest that persons who performed exercises acutely (symptoms that began less than 5 days prior to the start of the study) were less likely to use medication at 3 weeks than those who were not provided vestibular exercises. Patients in the vestibular exercise group had a greater number of normal Fukuda step tests and normal post head shake testing. Three weeks post exercise, 13% of the vestibular exercise group and 82% of the control group were taking medication daily (71). Medication for central vestibular disorders is effective (70).

Early vestibular exercises in persons with an acute vestibular disorder resulted in better Dizziness Handicap Inventory (DHI) scores (72), less anxiety, less reliance on visual cues, and better gait (73). Quality of life scores, as measured by the Medical Outcomes Study Short Form 36, improved after vestibular rehabilitation in persons with acute vestibular disorders (8,52). Perceived dizziness also has been noted to improve after a trial of vestibular physical therapy (52). Animal studies have suggested that there may be a critical period whereby immobilization had a negative impact on recovery from a vestibular deficit (74,75). People with peripheral vestibular disorders who underwent balance exercises within 6 months of onset had much better disability scores than those who presented after 6 months (8).

Dizziness severity and quality of life measures were predicted by when the balance exercises were initiated, with earlier onset relating to less dizziness and better quality of life measures (8). A delay in the onset of Cooksey-Cawthorne (vestibular) exercises led to worse scores in all cases studied, and late onset of exercise was considered to be a negative predictor for recovery (8). Early exercise in persons with peripheral vestibular disorders resulted in fewer symptoms at 3 weeks compared to a no-exercise control group (66,73). Also, people with late intervention for BPPV were more likely to experience residual dizziness within a 3-month period (76).

In summary, early exercise appears to decrease dizziness, prevent long-term complications such as anxiety, improve quality of life, possibly decrease the patient's chance of falling, and improve balance confidence. In addition, customized exercises appear to be more effective than a generic exercise program or no exercise (28,77). Acute physical therapy intervention for the person with dizziness and balance dysfunction appears to be a safe and efficacious treatment for persons with vestibular disorders (39,66).

VESTIBULAR REHABILITATION

After the person presents to the physical therapist, an in-depth examination begins with a thorough history of the dizziness. Just as in the physician's examination, the history is critical for the physical therapist in determining the optimal interventions. Sharing pertinent health information, examination results, and laboratory findings with the treating therapist will expedite and enhance patient care. Typically, the therapist will ask the patient questions regarding the frequency, duration, timing, and intensity of the symptoms; other comorbid medical conditions; medications; requirements of work; and living status (78).

Positions or movements that increase or decrease symptoms are very important in developing the treatment plan for the person with a vestibular disorder. Often, questions are asked related to movements that increase dizziness such as bending, getting out of bed, or even walking in a grocery store. A quick neurologic exam is also performed to assess the integrity of the smooth pursuit and saccadic eye systems and cranial nerves III, IV and VI. The integrity of the VOR, VOR cancellation, and the vergence system are also clinically assessed. The therapist may perform the head thrust test (79–85), dynamic visual acuity (35–37,85–90), and vibration-induced nystagmus test (91–94). All of the above assist the therapist in treatment planning and determining if additional testing is required as some patients may be self-referred or have not seen an otolaryngologist prior to seeing the physical therapist.

Strength, range of motion, sensation, and coordination are assessed at baseline. Range of motion of the cervical spine is particularly important to determine prior to performing the Dix-Hallpike maneuver. The physical therapist performs the Dix-Hallpike and the roll test ideally with infrared goggles, to determine if the patient has BPPV. If the Dix-Hallpike or roll test are positive, the appropriate canalith repositioning maneuver (CRM) will be performed based on the patients health and medical comorbidities.

Balance testing is an integral part of the typical physical examination including Romberg, semitandem standing, and tandem standing. Semitandem standing consists of having the patient stand with one foot in front of the other but not heel to toe. It is a transitional balance test between standing feet together (Romberg position) and heel to toe (tandem standing) and is often a difficult position for older adults to maintain. The patient's gait, as described above, will be assessed, and determination will be made whether an assistive device is in order to improve gait and safety. An attempt is made to avoid providing an assistive device unless it is necessary, as many older adults will never stop using the assistive device once it has been prescribed. Persons who often do need an assistive device are those with bilateral vestibular loss because they fall frequently (95), especially on uneven surfaces or low light/no light conditions. If the person is very frail and afraid of falling, occasionally a rollator walker will be suggested. Rollators have four wheels, brakes, and a seat. The rollators allow patients to walk safely at a much faster gait speed than a standard walker. Gait speed has been shown to be an overall indicator of health (96). Walking at a more normal speed may have long-term cardiovascular and respiratory benefit. Standard canes are also used to provide support for persons with vestibular disorders and have been shown to decrease postural sway (97).

Once the examination is complete, the physical therapist will develop a plan of care. Patients are seen anywhere between one and three times per week, with frailty, depression, light sensitivity, a history of migraine, fear of falling, and anxiety being important factors in how often the patient is seen. Persons who are afraid to exercise, who are depressed, or very anxious may be unable or unwilling to perform the exercises at home without supervision/ encouragement.

Patients are provided with written home exercises to perform between visits in order to speed their recovery. Typically the number of exercises provided is kept within reason, as patients often have difficulty finding the time to perform the exercises at home, especially if they are currently working. Often the therapist will attempt to build the exercise program into the patient's daily routine, such as standing on one leg while washing the dishes. Even retired adults will complain if it takes too long for them to perform the home exercise program, so patient education and negotiation is often required in order to have the patient "buy into" performing the exercise program at home. The therapist attempts to "dose" the exercises appropriately so that the movements increase the patient's symptoms, yet do not disable them.

If the exercise prescription is too aggressive, the patient will become too dizzy or might become fearful of the falling during the exercise and will stop performing the exercises. If the program is too easy, it will not be effective at maximizing the patient's recovery. Therapist experience and dialogue with the patient will maximize the interaction resulting in an exercise program that is individualized and appropriate for the patient. Individualized exercise programs appear to be superior to generic exercise programs and better meet the needs of the patient (77).

Exercises consist of eye/head movements in every conceivable position progressing to gait, exercises that incorporate head movements during gait, and standard balance exercises. Most people are asked to begin a walking program in order to increase their endurance, strength, and tolerance to movement. Exercises can be simple or very complex. A simple example might include having a person stand on one leg progressing to standing on one leg while tossing a ball or moving the head to the right and left following a moving target with the eyes and/or head. Exercises are individualized based on the patients' comorbid medical conditions and physical/mental health.

COMMON OUTCOME MEASURES UTILIZED IN VESTIBULAR REHABILITATION

The DHI is often used to quantify subjective impairment and to report changes over time in the self-perceived handicapping effects of dizziness (72). Scores range from 0 to 100 with 0 the best score and 100 the worst score possible. Change of 18 or more has been suggested to be clinically significant (72). Scores of greater than 60 on the DHI have been related to increased reports of falling (98).

Balance confidence is also frequently reported as an outcome measure. Generally when patients feel less dizzy and have better self-reported dizziness, they are better. The Activities-specific Balance Confidence (ABC) scale is the most commonly used balance confidence measure used with persons with dizziness (99). For the ABC scale, a percentage score is reported that ranges from 0% to 100% with 100% the best score and 0% the worst score. Scores of 67% or lower on the ABC appear to represent significant fall risk (100).

Verbal and visual analog scales (101) are also frequently reported as outcome measures, which should improve as the patient begins to feel better (less dizziness, improved balance, and better quality of life). The analog scale scores can be compared across time to suggest that the patient is feeling worse, the same or better as a result of the intervention.

Measures of gait and balance often used include the dynamic gait index (DGI) (102), gait speed (96), the functional gait assessment (FGA) (103,104), the clinical test of sensory integration and balance (CTSIB) (105), the Timed Up and Go test (TUG) (106,107), the five times sit to stand test (FTSST) (108), and simple measures such as timed standing in Romberg, single-leg stance or tandem Romberg (67,78). The DGI includes eight walking tasks, two of which require head movements in the pitch and yaw planes. Scores are based on an ordinal scoring algorithm with 24 the optimal score. Scores of 19 or less have been related to increased fall risk (109,110).

Gait speed is probably the best overall gait measure, as slower gait speed has been related to increased mortality and morbidity and shortened life expectancy (96,111). According to Studenski et al. gait speed, age, and gender are the optimal combination for predicting life expectancy. Patients who walk slower are also at greater risk for falling. Often one of the goals of the physical therapist intervention is to increase gait speed.

The FGA includes many of the original DGI items but was designed to be more difficult with the inclusion of walking with eyes closed, walking backward, and walking heel to toe. Scores on the FGA vary between 0 and 30 with 30 the optimal score. Scores of ≤22 demonstrated the optimal sensitivity and specificity for fall risk (103). Scores ≤22 indicate that the person is at risk for falling.

The modified CTSIB is often performed in the physician office as well as by the physical therapist to determine fall risk and to assess vestibular function (112,113). The modified CTSIB includes standing in the Romberg position eyes open and closed plus standing on foam eyes open and closed (114). Persons who fall on foam are more likely to fall when walking on uneven surfaces. The modified CTSIB should be performed with caution because many patients fall off the foam. Careful guarding is required in order to assure that the patient and physician are safe while performing the examination. Cass et al. (114) suggested timing how long the person can maintain each of the four positions.

The TUG is a simple measure of balance that has been related to increased fall risk. The patient stands from a chair with armrests upon command and is asked to walk at their normal pace 3 m, turn, and return to sitting in the chair. Scores of 13.5 seconds or longer have been related to falling in older persons (115), and a score of 11.1 seconds has the optimal sensitivity and discriminative properties in persons with vestibular disorders (107). The TUG is extremely easy to test because one only requires 3 m of space, a chair with armrests, and a stop watch. Patients can perform the test with an assistive device (cane, walker). Generally, persons who present to the clinic with a cane or walker are more likely to have fallen, so careful guarding is advised in examining those patients who present with an assistive device.

The FTSST has been used to determine lower extremity strength and balance in persons with vestibular disorders (108). They are asked to stand as quickly as they can five times from a standard height chair (116). The test provides a good overall measure of function (116), especially in older persons with vestibular disorders.

Factors That Might Affect Recovery

Age does not seem to specially relate to recovery after vestibular insult. In a study by Jung et al. (117) persons over the age of 70 with dizziness complaints either received vestibular exercises ($n = 103$) or no treatment ($n = 46$). Significant improvements in dizziness and balance confidence were noted in the treatment group at both 3 weeks and at 3 months compared to the no intervention group. Comorbid factors often associated with aging such as diabetes, peripheral neuropathy, macular degeneration, glaucoma, impaired sensation, or restricted ability to move may affect compensation and recovery. Other factors not associated with aging that can also slow or hinder rehabilitative progress includes former eye surgery, a strabismus, a history of migraine, use of vestibular suppressants, avoidance

behavior, and certain psychiatric conditions (obsessive compulsive disorder, anxiety) (8,118–121).

Persons with migraine may have difficulty with fast head movements and become nauseous more quickly than others. A history of motion sickness early in life may be associated with subsequent migraine. Persons who are prone to motion sickness often have more difficulty performing eye/head exercises. Care must be used in order to dose the intervention to allow for adaptation but to prevent the person from becoming ill with nausea, dizziness, or vomiting during or after the exercises. People who are afraid to move are also more difficult to treat, as exercise and movement appear to be the most efficacious way to promote recovery in the person with a vestibular disorder.

Persons with anxiety can be a challenge to treat. Psychologic factors appear to influence how people respond to and perceive dizziness (122). Anxiety appears to increase dizziness and distress, especially with movement. Fear of being dizzy and anxiety can trigger autonomic reactions that are very disturbing to the patient including increased heart rate and sweating. It appears that there is a link between anxiety and dizziness (123), with anxiety increasing the patients' symptoms. At times, psychotherapy and vestibular rehabilitation are combined for optimal effectiveness. Cognitive behavioral therapy has also been shown to be effective in decreasing dizziness symptoms in persons with chronic uncompensated peripheral vestibular disorders (41).

PERIPHERAL VESTIBULAR DISORDERS

Benign Paroxysmal Positional Vertigo

In the case of BPPV, repositioning maneuvers are effective, improve quality of life, and improve gait speed in people, especially older adults (124,125). Those who had late intervention for their BPPV were more likely to experience residual dizziness within a 3-month period (76). Although BPPV often resolves within a median of 2 weeks (126), sick days, physician visits, and interruption of ADL were frequently reported (126). In some patients with BPPV, use of the CRM is the only intervention that is effective. It is unusual but we have seen people who have had BPPV for over 20 years without relief of symptoms before the appropriate diagnosis was made and treatment provided. The financial costs to make the diagnosis of BPPV can be very high. In 2000, the average cost to make the diagnosis of BPPV was $2,684 (127). Polensek and Tusa (128) reported that the number of diagnostic tests to identify BPPV had not changed even with better education about vestibular disorders, but costs had increased between 2003 and 2008. Based on two recent practice guidelines by the Academy of Head and Neck Surgery and the Academy of Neurology, repositioning maneuvers for BPPV are very effective and safe (68,129). Thus, rendering a correct diagnosis quickly with appropriate treatment obviates costly and prolonged testing.

The Epley maneuver has been clearly illustrated by Furman and Cass (130) and can be quickly performed in the office setting after a positive Dix-Hallpike maneuver had determined the involved ear. The Epley maneuver involves rotating the head 45 degrees to the involved side and extending the head 20 to 30 degrees over the edge of a bed or table. The persons head is then rotated 90 degrees to the opposite side while maintaining neck extension, then rotated toward the floor, and to complete the maneuver the person is sat up. Each position is generally maintained until the nystagmus stops. Posttreatment instruction, including head restrictions, do not appear to affect outcome as reported in a recent meta-analysis (131).

BPPV is commonly seen in older persons. Imai et al. (132) reported that the mean age of their subjects ($n = 108$) was in their sixth decade of life. Seventy-seven percent of their subjects were between 51 and 80. In persons with posterior canal BPPV, it took a mean of 39 day for resolution of their symptoms without intervention (132). Persons with horizontal canal (HC) BPPV had resolution of their symptoms within 16 days ± 19 without intervention. Imai et al. (132) also reported that more than 50% of their patients within 3 days of onset of the BPPV had a hospital ER visit associated with their symptoms, suggesting that having BPPV had a significant cost to the medical system.

There was good evidence in a recent systematic review that the Epley maneuver is effective at resolving vertigo associated with BPPV (133). In a sham versus CRM study, the CRM was more effective than the sham treatment (134). Others have suggested in a systematic review and a meta-analysis that BPPV improved with the CRM (33,135). In other randomized trials, the CRM was effective at eliminating the vertigo/dizziness associated with a change of position when compared to a control group (22,136,137).

It appears that HC BPPV may resolve spontaneously more quickly than posterior canal BPPV in a group of persons with relatively acute BPPV (1,132,138). They also noted little difference between those treated with the Lempert maneuver for HC BPPV versus those who were not treated for HC BPPV (138). HC BPPV is under 10% of the presenting cases of BPPV (68) and can occur as debris moves from the posterior canal into either the horizontal or anterior canal while performing the Epley maneuver for the posterior canal (139). Patients are highly symptomatic if the debris moves from the posterior to the HC during a repositioning with significant nystagmus and nausea reported with the canal conversion. If the debris moves from the posterior to the HC, we often finish the repositioning maneuver and attempt to have the patient return to the office the next day or within a few days, especially if they are older. They are usually too symptomatic to attempt to reposition again during the session. Generally, upon return to the clinic, the HC BPPV has resolved. Reassessment to determine if the patient has either posterior or HC BPPV is necessary in order to determine what intervention will be most efficacious.

There were significant differences in patient complaints in those treated with the modified Epley versus those who were untreated for posterior canal BPPV (138). Asawavichianginda et al. (140) reported that 84% of people with a positive Dix-Hallpike test were asymptomatic without intervention at 3 months, yet there are some patients with coexisting migraine or psychiatric disorders who continue to have psychiatric symptoms from the vestibular disorder 1 year after onset (141). Even those treated for BPPV successfully may have remaining dizziness symptoms, possibly because they have comorbid vestibular pathology (142). Those patients with remaining dizziness and balance dysfunction after the CRM who have a negative Dix-Hallpike maneuver often benefit from physical therapy intervention.

White et al. (124) reported in a systematic review that repositioning maneuvers are effective and improve quality of life, especially in older adults who experience BPPV. Immediately following repositioning therapy, many patients had resolution of disrupted perceptions of subjective visual vertigo (143) and improvement in their gait speed (125). These improvements suggest that the CRM changes a person's perception of "earth vertical" and their gait. However, persons with BPPV, especially older adults, may have disruption in their postural control system after repositioning and need a "tune up" of their balance before they are truly back to their baseline status, which may take a few days up to a few months post repositioning (10).

A recent publication suggests that after the CRM there were less reported falls 12 months post repositioning (144). Overall, the CRM performed by either the physician or the physical therapist appears to improve quality of life, decrease or eliminate dizziness, improve postural stability and gait, plus decrease the number of reported falls. Even for the physician who is very comfortable diagnosing and treating BPPV, there are certain situations in which the involvement of a vestibular physical therapist can be quite helpful. These would include persons with bilateral BPPV, morbid obesity, significant kyphosis or severe restrictions of motion in the neck, and recalcitrant BPPV with need for very frequent repositioning. While some studies suggest that CRM is equally successful in older persons (145), other studies point to a lower improvement rate in older persons and suggest that a combination of CRM and vestibular rehabilitation may improve outcome in older persons with BPPV (146).

Many patients, after repositioning, experience changes in their postural control (10). Recent evidence suggests that gait changes immediately after repositioning, yet older adults may complain of postural deficits up to 3 months post repositioning (10). A follow-up with a physical therapist is advised to ensure that the CRM was effective and that the person's balance has improved enough that the person is not at risk for falling.

Vestibular Neuritis

Exercises that promote VOR adaptation, substitution, and/ or habituation are used to facilitate recovery of the VOR in persons with vestibular dysfunction (78,147–153). It is believed that eye/head movements with a focused target creates an error signal that allows the CNS to adapt resulting in less dizziness (152). Saccadic corrections are also made to minimize the error signal (147). Habituation, whereby patients are asked to move into and out of situations that provoke their symptoms, is also utilized (153). In addition, balance, flexibility, gait exercises, patient education, plus eye/head movements as noted above are performed as part of the therapy program (15,67,78). Most patients are seen one to two times per week initially (67). Persons with central vestibular disorders appear to take longer to recover (67). Total recovery for either peripheral or central vestibular pathology is unlikely, as Bowman has reported that even well compensated persons with unilateral peripheral vestibular dysfunction continue to have some functional deficits (118).

Strupp and Brandt (83) have suggested that persons with vestibular neuritis can develop persistent postural vertigo resulting in avoidance behavior. Avoiding movement most likely slows the rehabilitative process in humans. In the baboon animal model, Lacour et al. (154) have suggested that lack of movement can inhibit vestibular compensation. In older adults, avoiding movement could create additional functional limitations beyond those associated with the original vestibular deficit. Patients who are afraid to move because it makes them dizzy may develop neck stiffness and pain, decreased physical endurance, and decreased quality of life as a result of their self-imposed sedentary lifestyle. In a randomized trial, Strupp et al. (62) reported significant differences in postural control in those enrolled in a vestibular rehabilitation program compared to a control group (66).

In a recent randomized trial in 40 persons with an acute vestibular neuritis with a positive head thrust test and third degree nystagmus on admission, Teggi et al. (73) reported that early vestibular exercises resulted in better DHI scores, less anxiety, less reliance on visual cues, and better DGI. The exercise group means DHI, anxiety, and DGI scores were all "better" than the control subjects group outcome means at 25 days post onset of the exercise program. Early rehabilitation may help to decrease secondary complication such as fear of falling, neck stiffness, and anxiety about experiencing dizziness with movement.

Meniere Disease

Persons undergoing medical management for Meniere disease who complain of being unsteady between vertiginous attacks appear to benefit from vestibular physical therapy (31). It is more difficult to treat fluctuating disorders, yet postural control can be enhanced with an exercise program. Patients undergoing surgical or chemical (intratympanic gentamicin) ablation of vestibular function for Meniere disease can also benefit from early vestibular physical therapy (13,48).

Bilateral Vestibular Hypofunction

Bilateral vestibular hypofunction is often extremely disabling (12,25,43,64). While some affected persons can derive significant benefit from vestibular physical therapy, in others improvement may be limited. Gillespie and Minor (155) studied 35 patients with bilateral vestibular hypofunction who underwent vestibular physical therapy. Improvement was noted in 18 patients (51%) and 12 (34%) showed little or no change (155). Similar findings have been reported by others (12,43). Patients are often able to be taught to stand on uneven surfaces but continue to have difficulty in low or no light conditions. Patients with bilateral vestibular loss may require the use of an assistive device such as a cane or rolling walker to stabilize their gait (12,78). Those patients with total bilateral vestibular loss will continue to have complaints of oscillopsia with head movement and fall frequently (95). New technologies such as vibrotactile stimulation (156,157) and vestibular implants (158–161). (see Innovations section below) are expected to open new avenues of treatment for this challenging disorder.

Overall, changes in dizziness, balance, gait, and quality of life have been documented post vestibular rehabilitation in persons with peripheral vestibular disorders. Table 168.1 provides a summary of vestibular rehabilitation studies with peripheral and central diagnoses reported in the literature plus subjective and objective outcomes from the vestibular rehabilitation interventions.

CENTRAL VESTIBULAR DISORDERS

In a prospective, randomized controlled trial ($n = 53$), an early customized vestibular rehabilitation exercise program in older adults (age greater than 50 years) post acoustic neuroma resection was more effective at enhancing postural control at 3 months and was maintained at 1 year compared with those who were provided general instructions. A new concept in the literature is "PREHAB," whereby Magnusson et al. (48) have suggested that they are able to get people back to work faster by initiating rehab exercises *before* vestibular ablation (179). The "PREHAB" program was first implemented in subjects undergoing gentamicin treatments for Meniere disease and then adapted for use in patients with vestibular schwannomas with residual vestibular function. The latter patients were pretreated with gentamicin and vestibular exercises prior to undergoing translabyrinthine resection of cerebellopontine-angle tumors (48,179). Separating the vestibular ablation temporally from surgical resection allowed time for vestibular compensation

TABLE 168.1	COMMON VESTIBULAR DIAGNOSIS AND OBJECTIVE/SUBJECTIVE IMPROVEMENTS THAT HAVE BEEN REPORTED IN THE LITERATURE

Patient Diagnosis	Noted Improvement with Vestibular Physical Therapy
BPPV[a]	Subjective report of vertigo (16,54,134,146,162–164), nystagmus (16,146), quality of life (162)
Unilateral vestibular disorders	Fall risk (32,109), vision (32,37,64) balance (165,166), quality of life (52)
Chronic peripheral vestibular dysfunction	VOR gain and dizziness (14,167), standing balance (28,52,168), emotional status (i.e., anxiety) (169)
Bilateral vestibular dysfunction	Postural control (7,12,43), gait speed (12,43), dizziness (7,12,43), vision (36)
Vestibular neuritis	Ocular torsion (i.e., nystagmus (62)), postural control (35,62), ambulation skills and gait (15)
Post-acoustic neuroma resection	Postural control (35,170,171), dizziness (172), motion sensitivity (35)
Meniere disease	Self-report of symptoms (31), Balance (31), Dizziness, motion sensitivity (53)
Anxiety associated with vestibular disorder	Anxiety (173), subjective report (40), postural control (163), presence of nystagmus and ability to cope with dizziness (174)
Cervical vertigo	Postural stability (42), decreased neck pain (175), intensity of dizziness (42,175), postural sway (42)
Head injury	Gait improved (29), postural stability (29,63), less dizziness (34), gaze stability (30)
Cerebellar disease and dysfunction	Self perception of symptoms (25,26), postural control (25,26), gait (25), decreased risk of falling (25,26)
Multiple sclerosis	Subjective report of dizziness and postural control (176,177)
Parkinson's disease	Subjective complaint of vertigo (178)

[a]Medline search on July 27, 2010 revealed 512 papers on the search word "BPPV." Search was limited to randomized controlled trials in the past 10 years for the same search word and 17 papers were identified. Afterward, only relevant papers were chosen. Used with permission: Airwaily M, Whitney SL. Vestibular rehabilitation of older adults with dizziness. *Otolaryngol Clin North Am* 2011;44(2):473–496.

preoperatively leading to more rapid recovery (48,179). In a different surgical study, Cohen et al. (17) found that early postoperative vestibular rehabilitation did not affect vestibular compensation following acoustic neuroma surgery.

Persons with traumatic brain injury with vestibular dysfunction appear to benefit from a vestibular rehabilitation program (173). Persons demonstrated improvements in postural control, vertigo, and anxiety symptoms plus decrease in their perceived handicap. There is recent evidence to suggest that vestibular physical therapy may be effective in persons post concussion, who complain of balance or dizziness regardless of age (6). Vestibular rehabilitation also appears to be effective in persons with migraine dizziness (120,121), stroke (180), and even in persons with cerebellar disorders (26,180).

On many occasions, otolaryngologists evaluate dizzy persons with normal central and peripheral vestibular function based on the exam and/or vestibular testing or with vestibular pathology that does not have a medical treatment, that is, disequilibrium of aging, nonspecific dizziness. It is important to recall that even in the absence of objective vestibular pathology, vestibular physical therapy and, particularly, enrollment in an exercise program, has been demonstrated to decrease symptoms and, importantly, fall risk in dizzy persons (117,181). Regardless of whether objective vestibular pathology is identified, persons with a history of muscle weakness, previous falls, gait or balance deficit, or use of assistive devices should be referred for fall risk assessment and enrolled in an exercise program (181).

INNOVATIONS IN VESTIBULAR REHABILITATION

New advances in vestibular rehabilitation include the use of vibrotactile feedback, an implantable vestibular prosthesis, and the use of virtual reality to augment recovery after a vestibular deficit. Vibrotactile feedback was designed as a prosthetic device to assist with postural control (156,157,182–186) as a result of vestibular loss, injury, or aging. The devices currently in use typically "vibrate" the person's trunk (similar to the vibration that is typically felt from a cell phone) when they have exceeded some preset limit of stability (Fig. 168.1). The prosthesis has been shown to enhance postural control during standing and some preliminary works suggests that there are improvements during gait (157,183). Persons with unilateral vestibular disorders appear to be able to process the information and demonstrated greater accuracy of stepping and reduced trunk tilt with the device on (182). More study is required to determine if this type of technology can be used during gait and out in the community. Wall et al. (157) has suggested that vibrotactile feedback may assist in falls prevention for older adults, especially for persons with bilateral vestibular dysfunction who are at greater risk for a fall.

The development and implementation of an implantable vestibular prosthesis is moving forward and will have significant implications if they are as effective as the cochlear implant. Several centers around the world are working on the technology to provide a vestibular signal to persons with vestibular dysfunction (159–161). The

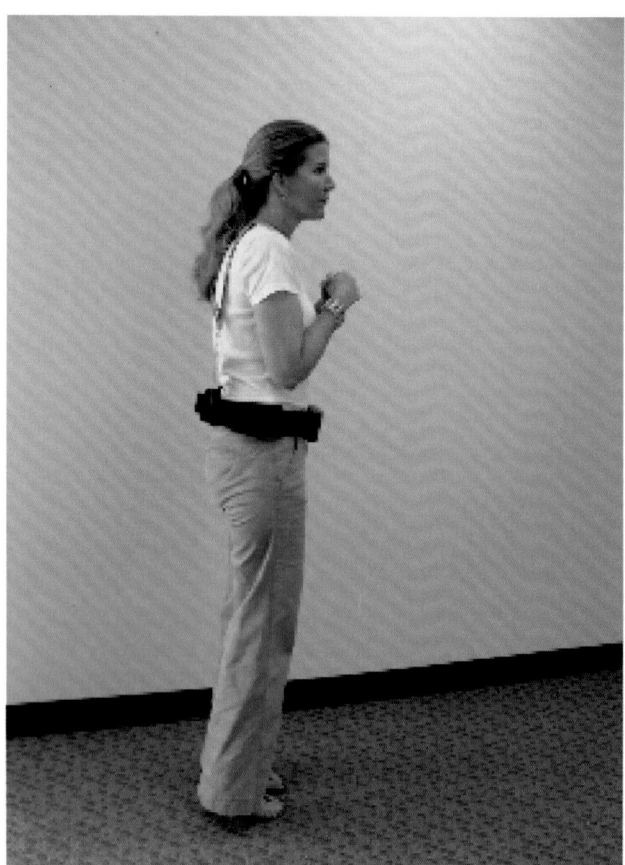

Figure 168.1 The vibrotactile device designed by Wall to provide feedback to persons lacking adequate vestibular inputs. Picture courtesy of Conrad Wall, PhD.

Hopkins Multichannel Vestibular Prosthesis (159) relies on three gyroscopes that are oriented orthogonally to capture head motion in the yaw, pitch, and roll planes. A microprocessor sends signals from the gyroscopes to electrodes implanted in the appropriate semicircular canals allowing stimulation of the ampullary nerves. Externally implanted devices have been tested in animal models with bilateral vestibular hypofunction and show promising results in terms of restoration of the VOR while preserving hearing (159,158). Challenges that remain in implementing this technology include miniaturization of the gyroscopes, enhancing the battery life and controlling current leak that leads to unwanted stimulation of adjacent ampullary nerves (159).

Recent evidence suggests that persons with vestibular disorders often complain of symptoms when there is high visual contrast and motion in the periphery (58,187). This motion-provoked dizziness phenomena has been called visual vertigo, space and motion discomfort, and also chronic subjective dizziness by various authors (188–190). Motion provoked symptoms are often seen in persons with a history of migraine and may be associated with persons who have anxiety or panic disorder (123,191–193). Staab et al. (194,195) have reported that selective serotonin

reuptake inhibitors (SSRIs) were more effective in this patient population than benzodiazepines or vestibular suppressants. It is very difficult and sometimes impossible to treat persons with space and motion discomfort without medication. They complain of having difficulty walking in certain stores, in buildings with high ceilings and walls, in large open areas, or when challenged by movement in the periphery of their vision. These environments often escalate their symptoms, and over time, because of their increased symptoms, they avoid situations that promote their dizziness. Recent evidence suggests that some patients with uncompensated vestibular disorders with chronic subjective dizziness are more difficult to treat (190). It appears that vestibular rehabilitation in combination with pharmacologic management of their motion-provoked symptoms is optimal for management (190).

There are several physical therapy treatment interventions that have been designed to attempt to address these space and motion symptoms including exposure to more compelling visual scenes (58,59), virtual reality (196–205), and even the use of a disco ball to habituate and reprogram the CNS to be able to appropriately dose the exposure without an increase in dizziness and/or anxiety. Although physical therapists are not psychotherapists, there are components of their intervention programs that are very similar to psychotherapy that are used with patients with vestibular dysfunction.

Exposure therapy is one example of a treatment intervention that is shared between the two professions. Shopping in malls and grocery stores is an example of an activity that is very difficult for many patients with space and motion symptoms—it is unclear what factors within this environment increase the patients symptoms but it often is a subjective complaint in this subset of persons with chronic uncompensated vestibular disorders (187,198). Physical therapists will often ask patients to go to the edge of a shopping mall or to push a grocery cart within a store and over time will ask them to spend more time in the provocative environment. Eventually the patient is asked to move their heads and to move into more difficult areas of the store or mall as they improve with the goal of being able to move freely about the provocative environment without symptoms.

Virtual shopping environments have been designed in order to slowly progress patients exposure to habituate the patient to the environment that provokes the symptoms (Fig. 168.2) (196,199,206). Often patients learn to avoid the situations, thereby stopping all exposure to the symptom-inducing environments. There are some patients with uncompensated vestibular disorders, that when asked, will report that they are unable to enter a grocery store or large box stores where the ceilings are very high. Virtual environments and provocative scenes may promote habituation to the symptom-provoking scenes and over time decrease their symptoms. Pavlou et al. (58) have attempted to promote symptom reduction through visually provocative scenes as part of a home exercise regimen and also with

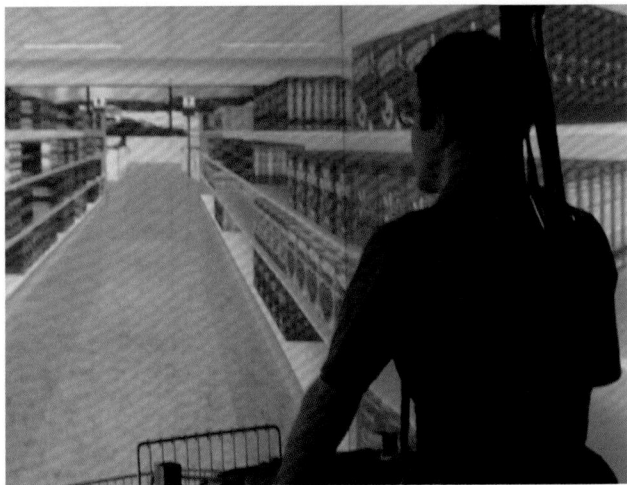

Figure 168.2 The person is ambulating in a virtual grocery store, which provides habituation of the response to the visual stimuli that increase the symptoms after a vestibular disorder.

a program where they attend sessions in the clinic and perform the exercises under the supervision of a physical therapist. The investigators have noted that even motivated persons do not comply well with a home exercise program without supervision and that patients must be slowly progressed with more provocative scenes in order for them to improve.

As with all aspects of exercises with patients with vestibular disorders, the physical therapist must carefully monitor the increase in symptoms that the exercises induce. If the patient becomes too symptomatic, the following can occur: they can become incapacitated from the symptoms and will stop exercising, they may become ill, or they become fearful of becoming ill again and limit their activity. Careful regulation of the "dose" of the exercise is required for optimal compliance and also for optimal recovery. Tool little movement may do little to nothing for the patients' recovery and too much eye/head movement may be detrimental for their well-being and recovery. If the exercise dose or exposure is too much, some patients may refuse further care or their anxiety may be increased, neither of which are good alternatives for the person with a vestibular disorder.

Working Together to Enhance Care

Patients with vestibular disorders need both good medical and physical therapy care. Working together as a team is the ideal situation for the patient, physician and physical therapist. It is not uncommon for patients to present to the physical therapist for dizziness even before seeing the physician as many physical therapists have been trained to triage for serious vestibular disorders. Developing a good working relationship can assist referrals going both ways-from the physician to the physical therapist and from the

physical therapist to the physician for testing, diagnosis, and medical management. A good relationship can assist the physician in better understanding if the medication prescribed is effective via the frequent progress reports from other team members. In addition, the physical therapist may suggest to the physician that medication might be in order for the vestibular exercises to be effective. If a patient becomes too symptomatic performing exercises, rehab will have little effect on the eye/head movement symptoms without some type of symptom control with medication.

Persons with migraine or anxiety are particularly prone to needing medication for symptom control in order to get them to move more normally after a vestibular disorder (70,194,195). Those with migraine and anxiety appear to have a tendency to move less in order to minimize their symptoms. Persons with migraine-related dizziness may also have associated depression and panic disorder, with a higher prevalence in women than men and a poorer quality of life (207–209). Through communication with the treating therapist, medication prescription and adjustment often optimizes care.

Making decisions about return to driving is also often a shared task with the treating therapist, since the physical therapist is very familiar with the patient's functional capabilities. Driving is a concern to persons with vestibular disorders, as in many societies not driving is associated with significant social isolation and severe economic consequences. Sindwani et al. (210) reported that in persons with vestibular disorders who were warned not to drive by their physician, 44% stopped driving, 52% drove more carefully and 4% drove as they usually did. Vestibular disorders do affect some person's ability to drive, especially those with uncontrolled Meniere disease. Cohen et al. (211) have reported that patients with vestibular disorders while driving report difficulty with freeways, during a rain storm (most likely from the movement of the windshield wipers), in high traffic areas, with parking, with changing lanes, and with staying in a lane while driving. If the physician is in doubt, a driver's examination may be in order. Certain physical therapists (Driving Rehabilitation specialists) can assess the appropriate automobile driving skills and safety in those with complaints of constant or intermittent dizziness. Large rehabilitation centers often have driving simulators that can assist you in determining if it is safe for the patient to be driving.

Return to work after a vestibular disorder is often one of the most difficult decisions to make as a physician. There are no clear cut criteria for return to work for the person with dizziness. The physical therapist can help with the decision about return to work. Careful consideration should be made for the following work situations: working around hazardous situations/machines, working alone, working at heights, working in deep water, working in environments that move, and when the safety of others is at risk (212). Job categories that might require special consideration include the armed forces, construction work, factory jobs that require repetitive head movement, police and fire work, long and short distance hauling of materials/driving, pilots, and working on sea or river vessels.

In summary, vestibular rehabilitation has been demonstrated to be effective in assisting in the recovery of persons with dizziness and balance disorders. A close working relationship between the physician and physical therapist facilitates expedient and effective patient care.

HIGHLIGHTS

- Vestibular rehabilitation is an effective intervention for persons with peripheral vestibular disorders.
- Early referral for persons with peripheral vestibular disorders is optimal resulting in enhanced quality of life.
- For vestibular hypofunction, anti dizziness medication may slow vestibular compensation.
- Customized exercise programs appear to be superior to a generic exercise program.
- Regardless of age, function can improve in patients with dizziness who actively participate in a program of vestibular rehabilitation.
- A tailored exercise program delivered both at home and in the clinic facilitates recovery and reduces falls.

REFERENCES

1. Uno A, Moriwaki K, Kato T, et al. [Clinical features of benign paroxysmal positional vertigo]. *Nippon Jibiinkoka Gakkai Kaiho* 2001;104:9–16.
2. Neuhauser HK, Lempert T. Vertigo: epidemiologic aspects. *Semin Neurol* 2009;29:473–481.
3. Agrawal Y, Carey JP, Della Santina CC, et al. Disorders of balance and vestibular function in US adults: data from the National Health and Nutrition Examination Survey, 2001–2004. *Arch Intern Med* 2009;169:938–944.
4. Pothula VB, Chew F, Lesser TH, et al. Falls and vestibular impairment. *Clin Otolaryngol Allied Sci* 2004;29:179–182.
5. Oghalai JS, Manolidis S, Barth JL, et al. Unrecognized benign paroxysmal positional vertigo in elderly patients. *Otolaryngol Head Neck Surg* 2000;122:630–634.
6. Alsalaheen BA, Mucha A, Morris LO, et al. Vestibular rehabilitation for dizziness and balance disorders after concussion. *J Neurol Phys Ther* 2010;34:87–93.
7. Asai M, Watanabe Y, Shimizu K. Effects of vestibular rehabilitation on postural control. *Acta Otolaryngol Suppl* 1997;528:116–120.
8. Bamiou DE, Davies RA, McKee M, et al. Symptoms, disability and handicap in unilateral peripheral vestibular disorders. Effects of early presentation and initiation of balance exercises. *Scand Audiol* 2000;29:238–244.
9. Bath AP, Walsh RM, Ranalli P, et al. Experience from a multidisciplinary "dizzy" clinic. *Am J Otol* 2000;21:92–97.
10. Blatt PJ, Georgakakis GA, Herdman SJ, et al. The effect of the canalith repositioning maneuver on resolving postural instability in patients with benign paroxysmal positional vertigo. *Am J Otol* 2000;21:356–363.
11. Brandt T, Daroff RB. Physical therapy for benign paroxysmal positional vertigo. *Arch Otolaryngol* 1980;106:484–485.
12. Brown KE, Whitney SL, Wrisley DM, et al. Physical therapy outcomes for persons with bilateral vestibular loss. *Laryngoscope* 2001;111:1812–1817.
13. Clendaniel RA, Tucci DL. Vestibular rehabilitation strategies in Meniere's disease. *Otolaryngol Clin North Am* 1997;30:1145–1158.
14. Cohen HS, Kimball KT. Increased independence and decreased vertigo after vestibular rehabilitation. *Otolaryngol Head Neck Surg* 2003;128:60–70.
15. Cohen HS, Kimball KT. Decreased ataxia and improved balance after vestibular rehabilitation. *Otolaryngol Head Neck Surg* 2004;130:418–425.
16. Cohen HS, Kimball KT. Effectiveness of treatments for benign paroxysmal positional vertigo of the posterior canal. *Otol Neurotol* 2005;26:1034–1040.
17. Cohen HS, Kimball KT, Jenkin HA. Factors affecting recovery after acoustic neuroma resection. *Acta Otolaryngol* 2002;122:841–850.
18. Cowand JL, Wrisley DM, Walker M, et al. Efficacy of vestibular rehabilitation. *Otolaryngol Head Neck Surg* 1998;118:49–54.
19. Di Girolamo S, Ottaviani F, Scarano E, et al. Postural control in horizontal benign paroxysmal positional vertigo. *Eur Arch Otorhinolaryngol* 2000;257:372–375.
20. Epley JM. The canalith repositioning procedure: for treatment of benign paroxysmal positional vertigo. *Otolaryngol Head Neck Surg* 1992;107:399–404.
21. Epley JM. Positional vertigo related to semicircular canalithiasis. *Otolaryngol Head Neck Surg* 1995;112:154–161.
22. Froehling DA, Bowen JM, Mohr DN, et al. The canalith repositioning procedure for the treatment of benign paroxysmal positional vertigo: a randomized controlled trial. *Mayo Clin Proc* 2000;75:695–700.
23. Furman JM, Whitney SL. Central causes of dizziness. *Phys Ther* 2000;80:179–187.
24. Gamiz MJ, Lopez-Escamez JA. Health-related quality of life in patients over sixty years old with benign paroxysmal positional vertigo. *Gerontology* 2004;50:82–86.
25. Gill-Body KM, Krebs DE, Parker SW, et al. Physical therapy management of peripheral vestibular dysfunction: two clinical case reports. *Phys Ther* 1994;74:129–142.
26. Gill-Body KM, Popat RA, Parker SW, et al. Rehabilitation of balance in two patients with cerebellar dysfunction. *Phys Ther* 1997;77:534–552.
27. Girardi M, Konrad HR. Vestibular rehabilitation therapy for the patient with dizziness and balance disorders. *ORL Head Neck Nurs* 1998;16:13–22.
28. Giray M, Kirazli Y, Karapolat H, et al. Short-term effects of vestibular rehabilitation in patients with chronic unilateral vestibular dysfunction: a randomized controlled study. *Arch Phys Med Rehabil* 2009;90:1325–1331.
29. Gizzi M. The efficacy of vestibular rehabilitation for patients with head trauma. *J Head Trauma Rehabil* 1995;10:60–77.
30. Gottshall KR, Hoffer ME. Tracking recovery of vestibular function in individuals with blast-induced head trauma using vestibular-visual-cognitive interaction tests. *J Neurol Phys Ther* 2010;34:94–97.
31. Gottshall KR, Hoffer ME, Moore RJ, et al. The role of vestibular rehabilitation in the treatment of Meniere's disease. *Otolaryngol Head Neck Surg* 2005;133:326–328.
32. Hall CD, Heusel-Gillig L, Tusa RJ, et al. Efficacy of gaze stability exercises in older adults with dizziness. *J Neurol Phys Ther* 2010;34:64–69.
33. Helminski JO, Zee DS, Janssen I, et al. Effectiveness of particle repositioning maneuvers in the treatment of benign paroxysmal positional vertigo: a systematic review. *Phys Ther* 2010;90:663–678.
34. Herdman SJ. Treatment of vestibular disorders in traumatically brain-injured patients. *J Head Trauma Rehabil* 1990;5:63–76.
35. Herdman SJ, Clendaniel RA, Mattox DE, et al. Vestibular adaptation exercises and recovery: acute stage after acoustic neuroma resection. *Otolaryngol Head Neck Surg* 1995;113:77–87.
36. Herdman SJ, Hall CD, Schubert MC, et al. Recovery of dynamic visual acuity in bilateral vestibular hypofunction. *Arch Otolaryngol Head Neck Surg* 2007;133:383–389.
37. Herdman SJ, Schubert MC, Das VE, et al. Recovery of dynamic visual acuity in unilateral vestibular hypofunction. *Arch Otolaryngol Head Neck Surg* 2003;129:819–824.

38. Hillier SL, Hollohan V. Vestibular rehabilitation for unilateral peripheral vestibular dysfunction. *Cochrane Database Syst Rev* 2007;(4):CD005397.

39. Hillier SL, McDonnell M. Vestibular rehabilitation for unilateral peripheral vestibular dysfunction. *Cochrane Database Syst Rev* 2011;(2):CD005397.

40. Jacob RG, Whitney SL, Detweiler-Shostak G, et al. Vestibular rehabilitation for patients with agoraphobia and vestibular dysfunction: a pilot study. *J Anxiety Disord* 2001;15:131–146.

41. Johansson M, Akerlund D, Larsen HC, et al. Randomized controlled trial of vestibular rehabilitation combined with cognitive-behavioral therapy for dizziness in older people. *Otolaryngol Head Neck Surg* 2001;125:151–156.

42. Karlberg M, Magnusson M, Malmstrom EM, et al. Postural and symptomatic improvement after physiotherapy in patients with dizziness of suspected cervical origin. *Arch Phys Med Rehabil* 1996;77:874–882.

43. Krebs DE, Gill-Body KM, Riley PO, et al. Double-blind, placebo-controlled trial of rehabilitation for bilateral vestibular hypofunction: preliminary report. *Otolaryngol Head Neck Surg* 1993;109:735–741.

44. Lopez-Escamez JA, Gamiz MJ, Fernandez-Perez A, et al. Long-term outcome and health-related quality of life in benign paroxysmal positional vertigo. *Eur Arch Otorhinolaryngol* 2005;262:507–511.

45. Lopez-Escamez JA, Gamiz MJ, Fernandez-Perez A, et al. Impact of treatment on health-related quality of life in patients with posterior canal benign paroxysmal positional vertigo. *Otol Neurotol* 2003;24:637–641.

46. Macias JD, Massingale S, Gerkin RD. Efficacy of vestibular rehabilitation therapy in reducing falls. *Otolaryngol Head Neck Surg* 2005;133:323–325.

47. Magnusson M, Kahlon B, Karlberg M, et al. Preoperative vestibular ablation with gentamicin and vestibular 'prehab' enhance postoperative recovery after surgery for pontine angle tumours—first report. *Acta Otolaryngol* 2007;127:1236–1240.

48. Magnusson M, Kahlon B, Karlberg M, et al. Vestibular "PREHAB". *Ann N Y Acad Sci* 2009;1164:257–262.

49. Mantello EB, Moriguti JC, Rodrigues-Junior AL, et al. Vestibular rehabilitation's effect over the quality of life of geriatric patients with labyrinth disease. *Braz J Otorhinolaryngol* 2008;74:172–180.

50. McGibbon CA, Krebs DE, Parker SW, et al. Tai Chi and vestibular rehabilitation improve vestibulopathic gait via different neuromuscular mechanisms: preliminary report. *BMC Neurol* 2005;5:3.

51. McGibbon CA, Krebs DE, Wolf SL, et al. Tai Chi and vestibular rehabilitation effects on gaze and whole-body stability. *J Vestib Res* 2004;14:467–478.

52. Meli A, Zimatore G, Badaracco C, et al. Vestibular rehabilitation and 6-month follow-up using objective and subjective measures. *Acta Otolaryngol* 2006;126:259–266.

53. Mruzek M, Barin K, Nichols DS, et al. Effects of vestibular rehabilitation and social reinforcement on recovery following ablative vestibular surgery. *Laryngoscope* 1995;105:686–692.

54. Munoz JE, Miklea JT, Howard M, et al. Canalith repositioning maneuver for benign paroxysmal positional vertigo: randomized controlled trial in family practice. *Can Fam Physician* 2007;53:1049–1053, 48.

55. Norre ME, Beckers A. Exercise treatment for paroxysmal positional vertigo: comparison of two types of exercises. *Arch Otorhinolaryngol* 1987;244:291–294.

56. Rine RM, Lindeblad S, Donovan P, et al. Balance and motor skills in young children with sensorineural hearing impairment: a preliminary study. *Pediatr Phys Ther* 1996;8:55–61.

57. Cooksey FS. Rehabilitation in vestibular injuries. *Proc R Soc Med* 1946;39:273–278.

58. Pavlou M. The use of optokinetic stimulation in vestibular rehabilitation. *J Neurol Phys Ther* 2010;34:105–110. 10.1097/NPT.0b013e3181dde6bf.

59. Pavlou M, Lingeswaran A, Davies RA, et al. Simulator based rehabilitation in refractory dizziness. *J Neurol* 2004;251:983–995.

60. Shepard NT, Telian SA, Smith-Wheelock M, et al. Vestibular and balance rehabilitation therapy. *Ann Otol Rhinol Laryngol* 1993;102:198–205.

61. Smith-Wheelock M, Shepard NT, Telian SA. Physical therapy program for vestibular rehabilitation. *Am J Otol* 1991;12:218–225.

62. Strupp M, Arbusow V, Maag KP, et al. Vestibular exercises improve central vestibulospinal compensation after vestibular neuritis. *Neurology* 1998;51:838–844.

63. Telian SA, Shepard NT. Update on vestibular rehabilitation therapy. *Otolaryngol Clin North Am* 1996;29:359–371.

64. Telian SA, Shepard NT, Smith-Wheelock M, et al. Bilateral vestibular paresis: diagnosis and treatment. *Otolaryngol Head Neck Surg* 1991;104:67–71.

65. Telian SA, Shepard NT, Smith-Wheelock M, et al. Habituation therapy for chronic vestibular dysfunction: preliminary results. *Otolaryngol Head Neck Surg* 1990;103:89–95.

66. Vereeck L, Wuyts FL, Truijen S, et al. The effect of early customized vestibular rehabilitation on balance after acoustic neuroma resection. *Clin Rehabil* 2008;22:698–713.

67. Whitney SL, Rossi MM. Efficacy of vestibular rehabilitation. *Otolaryngol Clin North Am* 2000;33:659–672.

68. Bhattacharyya N, Baugh RF, Orvidas L, et al. Clinical practice guideline: benign paroxysmal positional vertigo. *Otolaryngol Head Neck Surg* 2008;139:S47–S81.

69. Cohen HS, Gottshall KR, Graziano M, et al. International guidelines for education in vestibular rehabilitation therapy. *J Vestib Res* 2011;21:243–250.

70. Hain TC, Uddin M. Pharmacological treatment of vertigo. *CNS Drugs* 2003;17:85–100.

71. Venosa AR, Bittar RS. Vestibular rehabilitation exercises in acute vertigo. *Laryngoscope* 2007;117:1482–1487.

72. Jacobson GP, Newman CW. The development of the dizziness handicap inventory. *Arch Otolaryngol Head Neck Surg* 1990;116:424–427.

73. Teggi R, Caldirola D, Fabiano B, et al. Rehabilitation after acute vestibular disorders. *J Laryngol Otol* 2009;123:397–402.

74. Igarashi M, Levy JK, O-Uchi T, et al. Further study of physical exercise and locomotor balance compensation after unilateral labyrinthectomy in squirrel monkeys. *Acta Otolaryngol* 1981;92:101–105.

75. Lacour M. [Relearning and critical postoperative period in the restoration of nerve function. Example of vestibular compensation and clinical implications]. *Ann Otolaryngol Chir Cervicofac* 1984;101:177–187.

76. Seok JI, Lee HM, Yoo JH, et al. Residual dizziness after successful repositioning treatment in patients with benign paroxysmal positional vertigo. *J Clin Neurol* 2008;4:107–110.

77. Shepard NT, Telian SA. Programmatic vestibular rehabilitation. *Otolaryngol Head Neck Surg* 1995;112:173–182.

78. Herdman SJ. *Vestibular rehabilitation*, 3rd ed. Philadelphia: F.A. Davis Company, 2007:504.

79. Gilchrist DP, Curthoys IS, Cartwright AD, et al. High acceleration impulsive rotations reveal severe long-term deficits of the horizontal vestibulo-ocular reflex in the guinea pig. *Exp Brain Res* 1998;123:242–254.

80. Bartl K, Lehnen N, Kohlbecher S, et al. Head impulse testing using video-oculography. *Ann N Y Acad Sci* 2009;1164:331–333.

81. Dominguez MO, Magro JB. Bedside balance testing in elderly people. *Curr Aging Sci* 2009;2:150–157.

82. Mandala M, Nuti D, Broman AT, et al. Effectiveness of careful bedside examination in assessment, diagnosis, and prognosis of vestibular neuritis. *Arch Otolaryngol Head Neck Surg* 2008;134:164–169.

83. Strupp M, Brandt T. Vestibular neuritis. *Semin Neurol* 2009;29:509–519.

84. Weber KP, Aw ST, Todd MJ, et al. Head impulse test in unilateral vestibular loss: vestibulo-ocular reflex and catch-up saccades. *Neurology* 2008;70:454–463.

85. Halmagyi GM, Curthoys IS. A clinical sign of canal paresis. *Arch Neurol* 1988;45:737–739.

86. Badaracco C, Labini FS, Meli A, et al. Vestibular rehabilitation outcomes in chronic vertiginous patients through computerized dynamic visual acuity and Gaze stabilization test. *Otol Neurotol* 2007;28:809–813.

87. Danenbaum E, Chilingaryan G, Fung J. Effect of testing position on dynamic visual acuity. *J Otolaryngol Head Neck Surg* 2008;37:875–881.

88. Dannenbaum E, Paquet N, Chilingaryan G, et al. Clinical evaluation of dynamic visual acuity in subjects with unilateral vestibular hypofunction. *Otol Neurotol* 2009;30:368–372.

89. Demer JL, Honrubia V, Baloh RW. Dynamic visual acuity: a test for oscillopsia and vestibulo-ocular reflex function. *Am J Otol* 1994;15:340–347.

90. Goebel JA, Tungsiripat N, Sinks B, et al. Gaze stabilization test: a new clinical test of unilateral vestibular dysfunction. *Otol Neurotol* 2007;28:68–73.

91. Hamann KF, Schuster EM. Vibration-induced nystagmus—A sign of unilateral vestibular deficit. *ORL J Otorhinolaryngol Relat Spec* 1999;61:74–79.

92. Nuti D, Mandala M. Sensitivity and specificity of mastoid vibration test in detection of effects of vestibular neuritis. *Acta Otorhinolaryngol Ital* 2005;25:271–276.

93. Park H, Shin J, Shim D. Mechanisms of vibration-induced nystagmus in normal subjects and patients with vestibular neuritis. *Audiol Neurootol* 2007;12:189–197.

94. Perez N. Vibration induced nystagmus in normal subjects and in patients with dizziness. A videonystagmography study. *Rev Laryngol Otol Rhinol (Bord)* 2003;124:85–90.

95. Herdman SJ, Blatt P, Schubert MC, et al. Falls in patients with vestibular deficits. *Am J Otol* 2000;21:847–851.

96. Studenski S, Perera S, Patel K, et al. Gait speed and survival in older adults. *JAMA* 2011;305:50–58.

97. Jeka JJ. Light touch contact as a balance aid. *Phys Ther* 1997;77:476–487.

98. Whitney SL, Wrisley DM, Brown KE, et al. Is perception of handicap related to functional performance in persons with vestibular dysfunction? *Otol Neurotol* 2004;25:139–143.

99. Powell LE, Myers AM. The Activities-specific Balance Confidence (ABC) scale. *J Gerontol A Biol Sci* 1995;50A:M28–M34.

100. Lajoie Y, Gallagher SP. Predicting falls within the elderly community: comparison of postural sway, reaction time, the Berg balance scale and the Activities-specific Balance Confidence (ABC) scale for comparing fallers and non-fallers. *Arch Gerontol Geriatr* 2004;38:11–26.

101. Hall CD, Herdman SJ. Reliability of clinical measures used to assess patients with peripheral vestibular disorders. *J Neurol Phys Ther* 2006;30:74–81.

102. Shumway-Cook A, Woollacott M. *Motor control: theory and practical applications*, 1st ed. Baltimore, MD: Williams and Wilkins, 1995.

103. Wrisley DM, Kumar NA. Functional gait assessment: concurrent, discriminative, and predictive validity in community-dwelling older adults. *Phys Ther* 2010;90:761–773.

104. Wrisley DM, Marchetti GF, Kuharsky DK, et al. Reliability, internal consistency, and validity of data obtained with the functional gait assessment. *Phys Ther* 2004;84:906–918.

105. Shumway-Cook A, Horak F. Assessing the influence of sensory interaction on balance. *Phys Ther* 1986;66:1548–1550.

106. Podsiadlo D, Richardson S. The timed "Up & Go": a test of basic functional mobility for frail elderly persons. *J Am Geriatr Soc* 1991;39:142–148.

107. Whitney SL, Marchetti GF, Schade A, et al. The sensitivity and specificity of the Timed "Up & Go" and the Dynamic Gait Index for self-reported falls in persons with vestibular disorders. *J Vestib Res* 2004;14:397–409.

108. Meretta BM, Whitney SL, Marchetti GF, et al. The five times sit to stand test: responsiveness to change and concurrent validity in adults undergoing vestibular rehabilitation. *J Vestib Res* 2006;16:233–243.

109. Hall CD, Schubert MC, Herdman SJ. Prediction of fall risk reduction as measured by dynamic gait index in individuals with unilateral vestibular hypofunction. *Otol Neurotol* 2004;25:746–751.

110. Whitney SL, Hudak MT, Marchetti GF. The dynamic gait index relates to self-reported fall history in individuals with vestibular dysfunction. *J Vestib Res* 2000;10:99–105.

111. Studenski S. Bradypedia: is gait speed ready for clinical use? *J Nutr Health Aging* 2009;13:878–880.

112. Whitney SL, Wrisley DM. The influence of footwear on timed balance scores of the modified clinical test of sensory interaction and balance. *Arch Phys Med Rehabil* 2004;85:439–443.

113. Wrisley DM, Whitney SL. The effect of foot position on the modified clinical test of sensory interaction and balance. *Arch Phys Med Rehabil* 2004;85:335–338.

114. Cass SP, Borello-France D, Furman JM. Functional outcome of vestibular rehabilitation in patients with abnormal sensory-organization testing. *Am J Otol* 1996;17:581–594.

115. Shumway-Cook A, Brauer S, Woollacott M. Predicting the probability for falls in community-dwelling older adults using the Timed Up & Go test. *Phys Ther* 2000;80:896–903.

116. Lord S, Murray S, Chapman K, et al. Sit-to-stand performance depends on sensation, speed, balance, and psychological status in addition to strength in older people. *J Gerontol A Biol Sci Med Sci* 2002;57A:M539–M543.

117. Jung JY, Kim JS, Chung PS, et al. Effect of vestibular rehabilitation on dizziness in the elderly. *Am J Otolaryngol* 2009;30:295–299.

118. Bowman A. Psychological and visual-perceptual explanations of poor compensation following unilateral vestibular loss. Dissertation, University of Sydney, Sydney, 2004:506.

119. Luxon LL, Furman JM, Martini A, et al., eds. A textbook of audiological medicine: clinical aspects of hearing and balance, 1st ed. London, UK: Taylor & Francis Group, 2003:929.

120. Whitney SL, Wrisley DM, Brown KE, et al. Physical therapy for migraine-related vestibulopathy and vestibular dysfunction with history of migraine. *Laryngoscope* 2000;110:1528–1534.

121. Wrisley DM, Whitney SL, Furman JM. Vestibular rehabilitation outcomes in patients with a history of migraine. *Laryngoscope* 2002;23:483–487.

122. Kroenke K, Lucas CA, Rosenberg ML, et al. Psychiatric disorders and functional impairment in patients with persistent dizziness. *J Gen Intern Med* 1993;8:530–535.

123. Balaban CD, Jacob RG, Furman JM. Neurologic bases for comorbidity of balance disorders, anxiety disorders and migraine: neurotherapeutic implications. *Expert Rev Neurother* 2011;11:379–394.

124. White J, Savvides P, Cherian N, et al. Canalith repositioning for benign paroxysmal positional vertigo. *Otol Neurotol* 2005;26:704–710.

125. Celebisoy N, Bayam E, Gulec F, et al. Balance in posterior and horizontal canal type benign paroxysmal positional vertigo before and after canalith repositioning maneuvers. *Gait Posture* 2009;29:520–523.

126. von Brevern M, Radtke A, Lezius F, et al. Epidemiology of benign paroxysmal positional vertigo: a population based study. *J Neurol Neurosurg Psychiatry* 2007;78:710–715.

127. Li JC, Li CJ, Epley J, et al. Cost-effective management of benign positional vertigo using canalith repositioning. *Otolaryngol Head Neck Surg* 2000;122:334–339.

128. Polensek SH, Tusa R. Unnecessary diagnostic tests often obtained for benign paroxysmal positional vertigo. *Med Sci Monit* 2009;15:MT89–MT94.

129. Fife TD. Benign paroxysmal positional vertigo. *Semin Neurol* 2009;29:500–508.

130. Furman JM, Cass SP. Benign paroxysmal positional vertigo. *N Engl J Med* 1999;341:1590–1596.

131. Devaiah AK, Andreoli S. Postmaneuver restrictions in benign paroxysmal positional vertigo: an individual patient data meta-analysis. *Otolaryngol Head Neck Surg* 2010;142:155–159.

132. Imai T, Ito M, Takeda N, et al. Natural course of the remission of vertigo in patients with benign paroxysmal positional vertigo. *Neurology* 2005;64:920–921.

133. Teixeira LJ, Machado JN. Maneuvers for the treatment of benign positional paroxysmal vertigo: a systematic review. *Braz J Otorhinolaryngol* 2006;72:130–139.

134. von Brevern M, Seelig T, Radtke A, et al. Short-term efficacy of Epley's manoeuvre: a double-blind randomised trial. *J Neurol Neurosurg Psychiatry* 2006;77:980–982.

135. Woodworth BA, Gillespie MB, Lambert PR. The canalith repositioning procedure for benign positional vertigo: a meta-analysis. *Laryngoscope* 2004;114:1143–1146.

136. Lynn S, Pool A, Rose D, et al. Randomized trial of the canalith repositioning procedure. *Otolaryngol Head Neck Surg* 1995;113:712–720.

137. Yimtae K, Srirompotong S, Sae-Seaw P. A randomized trial of the canalith repositioning procedure. *Laryngoscope* 2003;113:828–832.

138. Sekine K, Imai T, Sato G, et al. Natural history of benign paroxysmal positional vertigo and efficacy of Epley and Lempert maneuvers. *Otolaryngol Head Neck Surg* 2006;135:529–533.

139. Herdman SJ, Tusa RJ. Complications of the canalith repositioning procedure. *Arch Otolaryngol Head Neck Surg* 1996;122:281–286.

140. Asawavichianginda S, Isipradit P, Snidvongs K, et al. Canalith repositioning for benign paroxysmal positional vertigo: a randomized, controlled trial. *Ear Nose Throat J* 2000;79:732–734, 36–37.

141. Best C, Eckhardt-Henn A, Tschan R, et al. Psychiatric morbidity and comorbidity in different vestibular vertigo syndromes. Results of a prospective longitudinal study over one year. *J Neurol* 2009;256:58–65.

142. Pollak L, Davies RA, Luxon LL. Effectiveness of the particle repositioning maneuver in benign paroxysmal positional vertigo with and without additional vestibular pathology. *Otol Neurotol* 2002;23:79–83.

143. Gall RM, Ireland DJ, Robertson DD. Subjective visual vertical in patients with benign paroxysmal positional vertigo. *J Otolaryngol* 1999;28:162–165.

144. Gananca FF, Gazzola JM, Gananca CF, et al. Elderly falls associated with benign paroxysmal positional vertigo. *Braz J Otorhinolaryngol* 2010;76:113–120.

145. Nunez RA, Cass SP, Furman JM. Short- and long-term outcomes of canalith repositioning for benign paroxysmal positional vertigo. *Otolaryngol Head Neck Surg* 2000;122:647–652.

146. Angeli SI, Hawley R, Gomez O. Systematic approach to benign paroxysmal positional vertigo in the elderly. *Otolaryngol Head Neck Surg* 2003;128:719–725.

147. Schubert MC, Della Santina CC, Shelhamer M. Incremental angular vestibulo-ocular reflex adaptation to active head rotation. *Exp Brain Res* 2008;191:435–446.

148. Schubert MC, Hall CD, Das V, et al. Oculomotor strategies and their effect on reducing gaze position error. *Otol Neurotol* 2010;31:228–231.

149. Schubert MC, Migliaccio AA, Clendaniel RA, et al. Mechanism of dynamic visual acuity recovery with vestibular rehabilitation. *Arch Phys Med Rehabil* 2008;89:500–507.

150. Schubert MC, Migliaccio AA, Minor LB, et al. Retention of VOR gain following short-term VOR adaptation. *Exp Brain Res* 2008;187:117–127.

151. Schubert MC, Zee DS. Saccade and vestibular ocular motor adaptation. *Restor Neurol Neurosci* 2010;28:9–18.

152. Zee DS. Adaptation to vestibular disturbances: some clinical implications. *Acta Neurol Belg* 1991;91:97–104.

153. Norré ME, De Weerdt W. Treatment of vertigo based on habituation. 2. Technique and results of habituation training. *J Laryngol Otol* 1980;94:971–977.

154. Lacour M, Roll JP, Appaix M. Modifications and development of spinal reflexes in the alert baboon (Papio papio) following an unilateral vestibular neurotomy. *Brain Res* 1976;113:255–269.

155. Gillespie MB, Minor LB. Prognosis in bilateral vestibular hypofunction. *Laryngoscope* 1999;109:35–41.

156. Wall C III, Kentala E. Control of sway using vibrotactile feedback of body tilt in patients with moderate and severe postural control deficits. *J Vestib Res* 2005;15:313–325.

157. Wall C III, Wrisley DM, Statler KD. Vibrotactile tilt feedback improves dynamic gait index: a fall risk indicator in older adults. *Gait Posture* 2009;30:16–21.

158. Dai C, Fridman GY, Della Santina CC. Effects of vestibular prosthesis electrode implantation and stimulation on hearing in rhesus monkeys. *Hear Res* 2011;277:204–210.

159. Della Santina CC, Migliaccio AA, Patel AH. A multichannel semicircular canal neural prosthesis using electrical stimulation to restore 3-d vestibular sensation. *IEEE Trans Biomed Eng* 2007;54:1016–1030.

160. Lewis RF, Haburcakova C, Gong W, et al. Vestibuloocular reflex adaptation investigated with chronic motion-modulated electrical stimulation of semicircular canal afferents. *J Neurophysiol* 2010;103:1066–1079.

161. Shkel AM, Zeng FG. An electronic prosthesis mimicking the dynamic vestibular function. *Audiol Neurootol* 2006;11:113–122.

162. Salvinelli F, Casale M, Trivelli M, et al. Benign paroxysmal positional vertigo: a comparative prospective study on the efficacy of Semont's maneuver and no treatment strategy. *Clin Ter* 2003;154:7–11.

163. Richard W, Bruintjes TD, Oostenbrink P, et al. Efficacy of the Epley maneuver for posterior canal BPPV: a long-term, controlled study of 81 patients. *Ear Nose Throat J* 2005;84:22–25.

164. Simhadri S, Panda N, Raghunathan M. Efficacy of particle repositioning maneuver in BPPV: a prospective study. *Am J Otolaryngol* 2003;24:355–360.

165. Horak FB, Jones-Rycewicz C, Black FO, et al. Effects of vestibular rehabilitation on dizziness and imbalance. *Otolaryngol Head Neck Surg* 1992;106:175–180.

166. Corna S, Nardone A, Prestinari A, et al. Comparison of Cawthorne-Cooksey exercises and sinusoidal support surface translations to improve balance in patients with unilateral vestibular deficit. *Arch Phys Med Rehabil* 2003;84:1173–1184.

167. Topuz O, Topuz B, Ardic FN, et al. Efficacy of vestibular rehabilitation on chronic unilateral vestibular dysfunction. *Clin Rehabil* 2004;18:76–83.

168. Szturm T, Ireland DJ, Lessing-Turner M. Comparison of different exercise programs in the rehabilitation of patients with chronic peripheral vestibular dysfunction. *J Vestib Res* 1994;4:461–479.

169. Meli A, Zimatore G, Badaracco C, et al. Effects of vestibular rehabilitation therapy on emotional aspects in chronic vestibular patients. *J Psychosom Res* 2007;63:185–190.

170. Cakrt O, Chovanec M, Funda T, et al. Exercise with visual feedback improves postural stability after vestibular schwannoma surgery. *Eur Arch Otorhinolaryngol* 2010;267:1355–1360.

171. Levo H, Blomstedt G, Pyykko I. Postural stability after vestibular schwannoma surgery. *Ann Otol Rhinol Laryngol* 2004;113:994–999.

172. Enticott JC, O'Leary SJ, Briggs RJ. Effects of vestibulo-ocular reflex exercises on vestibular compensation after vestibular schwannoma surgery. *Otol Neurotol* 2005;26:265–269.

173. Gurr B, Moffat N. Psychological consequences of vertigo and the effectiveness of vestibular rehabilitation for brain injury patients. *Brain Inj* 2001;15:387–400.

174. Yardley L, Beech S, Zander L, et al. A randomized controlled trial of exercise therapy for dizziness and vertigo in primary care. *Br J Gen Pract* 1998;48:1136–1140.

175. Wrisley DM, Sparto PJ, Whitney SL, et al. Cervicogenic dizziness: a review of diagnosis and treatment. *J Orthop Sports Phys Ther* 2000;30:755–766.

176. Pavan K, Marangoni BE, Schmidt KB, et al. [Vestibular rehabilitation in patients with relapsing-remitting multiple sclerosis]. *Arq Neuropsiquiatr* 2007;65:332–335.

177. Zeigelboim BS, Arruda WO, Mangabeira-Albernaz PL, et al. Vestibular findings in relapsing, remitting multiple sclerosis: a study of thirty patients. *Int Tinnitus J* 2008;14:139–145.

178. Zeigelboim BS, Klagenberg KF, Teive HA, et al. Vestibular rehabilitation: clinical benefits to patients with Parkinson's disease. *Arq Neuropsiquiatr* 2009;67:219–223.

179. Tjernstrom F, Fransson PA, Kahlon B, et al. Vestibular PREHAB and gentamicin before schwannoma surgery may improve long-term postural function. *J Neurol Neurosurg Psychiatry* 2009;80:1254–1260.

180. Brown KE, Whitney SL, Marchetti GF, et al. Physical therapy for central vestibular dysfunction. *Arch Phys Med Rehabil* 2006;87:76–81.

181. Summary of the Updated American Geriatrics Society/British Geriatrics Society clinical practice guideline for prevention of falls in older persons. *J Am Geriatr Soc* 2011;59:148–157.

182. Dozza M, Wall C III, Peterka RJ, et al. Effects of practicing tandem gait with and without vibrotactile biofeedback in subjects with unilateral vestibular loss. *J Vestib Res* 2007;17:195–204.

183. Wall C III, Oddsson LE, Horak FB, et al. Applications of vibrotactile display of body tilt for rehabilitation. *Conf Proc IEEE Eng Med Biol Soc* 2004;7:4763–4765.

184. Wall C III, Weinberg MS. Balance prostheses for postural control. *IEEE Eng Med Biol Mag* 2003;22:84–90.

185. Wall C III, Weinberg MS, Schmidt PB, et al. Balance prosthesis based on micromechanical sensors using vibrotactile feedback of tilt. *IEEE Trans Biomed Eng* 2001;48:1153–1161.

186. Wall CI. Application of vibrotactile feedback of body motion to improve rehabilitation in individuals with imbalance. *J Neurol Phys Ther* 2010;34:98–104. 10.1097/NPT.0b013e3181dde6f0.

187. Bronstein AM. Vision and vertigo: some visual aspects of vestibular disorders. *J Neurol* 2004;251:381–387.

188. Bronstein AM. Visual vertigo syndrome: clinical and posturography findings. *J Neurol Neurosurg Psychiatry* 1995;59:472–476.

189. Jacob RG, Woody SR, Clark DB, et al. Discomfort with space and motion: a possible marker of vestibular dysfunction assessed by the situational characteristics questionnaire. *J Psychopathol Behav Assess* 1993;15:299–324 check with Rolf about ALL authors.

190. Ruckenstein MJ, Staab JP. Chronic subjective dizziness. *Otolaryngol Clin North Am* 2009;42:71–77, ix.

191. Evans RW, Marcus D, Furman JM. Motion sickness and migraine. *Headache* 2007;47:607–610.

192. Furman JM, Balaban CD, Jacob RG, et al. Migraine-anxiety related dizziness (MARD): a new disorder? *J Neurol Neurosurg Psychiatry* 2005;76:1–8.

193. Marcus DA, Furman JM, Balaban CD. Motion sickness in migraine sufferers. *Expert Opin Pharmacother* 2005;6:2691–2697.

194. Staab JP, Ruckenstein MJ, Amsterdam JD. A prospective trial of sertraline for chronic subjective dizziness. *Laryngoscope* 2004;114:1637–1641.

195. Staab JP, Ruckenstein MJ, Solomon D, et al. Serotonin reuptake inhibitors for dizziness with psychiatric symptoms. *Arch Otolaryngol Head Neck Surg* 2002;128:554–560.

196. Sparto PJ, Furman JM, Whitney SL, et al. Vestibular rehabilitation using a wide field of view virtual environment. *Conf Proc IEEE Eng Med Biol Soc* 2004;7:4836–4839.

197. Sparto PJ, Whitney SL, Hodges LF, et al. Simulator sickness when performing gaze shifts within a wide field of view optic flow environment: preliminary evidence for using virtual reality in vestibular rehabilitation. *J Neuroeng Rehabil* 2004;1:14.

198. Whitney SL, Jacob RG, Sparto PJ, et al. Acrophobia and pathological height vertigo: indications for vestibular physical therapy? *Phys Ther* 2005;85:443–458.

199. Whitney SL, Sparto PJ, Hodges LF, et al. Responses to a virtual reality grocery store in persons with and without vestibular dysfunction. *Cyberpsychol Behav* 2006;9:152–156.

200. Keshner EA. Virtual reality and physical rehabilitation: a new toy or a new research and rehabilitation tool? *J Neuroeng Rehabil* 2004;1:8.

201. Kramer PD, Roberts DC, Shelhamer M, et al. A versatile stereoscopic visual display system for vestibular and oculomotor research. *J Vestib Res* 1998;8:363–379.

202. Viirre E. Vestibular telemedicine and rehabilitation. Applications for virtual reality. *Stud Health Technol Inform* 1996;29:299–305.

203. Chang CP, Hain TC. A theory for treating dizziness due to optical flow (visual vertigo). *Cyberpsychol Behav* 2008;11:495–498.

204. Keshner EA, Kenyon RV. Postural and spatial orientation driven by virtual reality. *Stud Health Technol Inform* 2009;145:209–228.

205. Virk S, McConville KM. Virtual reality applications in improving postural control and minimizing falls. *Conf Proc IEEE Eng Med Biol Soc* 2006;1:2694–2697.

206. Whitney SL, Sparto PJ, Brown KE, et al. The potential use of virtual reality in vestibular rehabilitation: preliminary findings with the BNAVE. *J Neurol Phys Ther* 2002;26:72–78.

207. Lipton RB, Stewart WF, Von Korff M. The burden of migraine. A review of cost to society. *Pharmacoeconomics* 1994;6:215–221.

208. Stewart W, Breslau N, Keck PE, Jr. Comorbidity of migraine and panic disorder. *Neurology* 1994;44:S23–S27.

209. Lipton RB, Hamelsky SW, Kolodner KB, et al. Migraine, quality of life, and depression: a population-based case-control study. *Neurology* 2000;55:629–635.

210. Sindwani R, Parnes LS, Goebel JA, et al. Approach to the vestibular patient and driving: a patient perspective. *Otolaryngol Head Neck Surg* 1999;121:13–17.

211. Cohen HS, Wells J, Kimball KT, et al. Driving disability and dizziness. *J Safety Res* 2003;34:361–369.

212. Palmer KT, Cox RA, Brown I, eds. *Fitness for work, The Medical Aspects*, New York: Oxford University Press, 2007.

Regenerative Strategies for Overcoming Deafness

169

Alan G. Cheng   **Stefan Heller**

The mammalian organ of Corti comprises a complex but organized array of mechanosensitive hair cells separated by supporting cells (see Fig. 169.1). Upon mechanical stimulation, inner hair cells transmit neural signals to innervating spiral ganglia neurons, which in turn relay neural impulses to the central nervous system in a tonopic manner. Simultaneously, outer hair cells feed back mechanical forces to augment the sensitivity and frequency selectivity of the cochlea. The integrity of all of these cell types is critical for auditory function.

Etiologies of hearing loss include genetic disorders, acoustic trauma, aging, infection, and toxins such as aminoglycoside antibiotics and the antineoplastic agent cisplatin. One common underlying pathology of hearing loss is degeneration of outer and/or inner hair cells. While hair cell–specific mutations, certain drugs (e.g., aminoglycosides and cisplatin) and noise are likely the primary cause for sensory hair cell loss, there are also scenarios in which hair cells degenerate in non–cell autonomous fashion. Such a pattern of cell loss has also been observed in lesions primarily involving the supporting cells such as gap junction gene mutations (e.g., *GJB2* encoding connexin 26) (1) or mutations that affect ion homeostasis in the stria vascularis (2). Because of the established causal relationship between hair cell loss and hearing loss, much effort has been devoted to investigate hair cell regeneration as a possible therapeutic intervention for hearing loss.

HAIR CELL REGENERATION, NONMAMMALIAN VERTEBRATES VERSUS MAMMALS

In non-mammalian vertebrates such as fish, amphibians, and birds, sensory organs have the inherent capacity to replace lost hair cells. In fish, the lateral line organs are used to detect water movement and contain hair cells that are continuously turned over and replaced (3). Likewise, in

the vestibular organs in birds, sensory hair cells degenerate and regenerate at a steady state, and the degree of regeneration increases upon damage by aminoglycoside treatment, which has been investigated in the macula of utricle (4,5), suggesting that loss of hair cells induces a repair response. A similar regenerative response exists in the avian basilar papilla (hearing organ in birds), where researchers discovered recurrence of sensory hair cells initially lost from damage caused by aminoglycoside or noise (6–8). Indeed, these newly regenerated hair cells were innervated and hearing function was restored (9). Complex cortical functions including language acquisition requires intact neural connections between the cochlear end organ to higher cortical centers. When correlates of such learning ability were examined, song birds with regenerated cochleae that had initially been lesioned with aminoglycosides learnt and sang new songs (10). These lines of evidence indicate that in non-mammalian vertebrates, hair cell regeneration is part of the inner ear's natural self-repair process.

In recent years, researchers have built on the above initial findings to delineate the mechanisms underlying hair cell regeneration. Using thymidine analogs to mark proliferating cells, the supporting cells in both the avian basilar papilla and utricles were found to generate new hair cells in two manners: via mitotic division or transdifferentiation (11). Transdifferentiation occurs when supporting cells directly acquire a hair cell phenotype without a preceding mitotic division. When the process of hair cell regeneration was examined in the avian cochlea after lesioning by aminoglycosides, both processes significantly contribute to the repopulation of lost hair cells (11,12). Inhibitors of proliferation do not affect the degree of supporting cell transdifferentiation, suggesting that the two mechanisms may operate independently of each other (12).

In the mammalian cochlea, loss of hair cells is permanent and no spontaneous regeneration of hair cells has been observed. Unlike the cochlea, limited hair cell

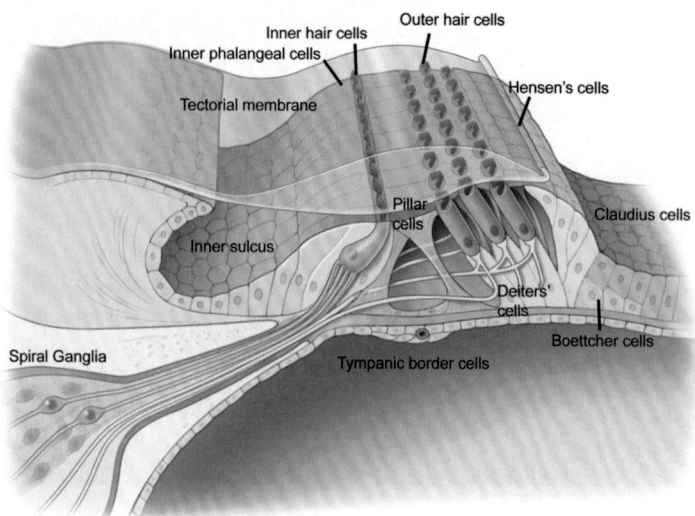

Figure 169.1 Anatomy of the mammalian organ of Corti. The hearing organ consists of three rows of outer hair cells and one row of inner hair cells. Six subtypes of supporting cells have been described (inner phalangeal, pillar, Deiters', Hensen's, Boettcher, and Claudius cells). Figure © Stanford University.

regeneration has been observed in mammalian utricles. Morphologic evidence suggests that new, immature hair cells appear after aminoglycoside damage *in vitro* (13,14), yet the lack of proliferation marker among these hair cells implies that they emerge via transdifferentiation, most likely from supporting cells. Recently, cells isolated from the mammalian utricular sensory epithelium were found to have stem cell properties, where they self-renew and were pluripotent (15), and may contribute to the regenerative capacity of utricles. Cells with stem cell properties were also found in the neonatal (see section below), but not adult cochlea (16); mechanisms underlying this fundamental difference between the mammalian auditory and balance organs are not completely understood.

In cochlea damaged as a result of aminoglycoside administration, hair cell loss is accompanied by an initial preservation of adjacent supporting cells (17). Although expression of specific markers in surviving supporting cells are mostly unaltered immediately after damage, the architecture of the sensory epithelium successively transforms from pseudostratified and complex, via an intermediate cell mound with collapsed tunnel of Corti, into to a flat, monolayered epithelium (see Fig. 169.2). A modest loss of supporting cells was noted in long deafened cochleae (17–19).

Aminoglycoside-induced hair cell loss is one of the best understood model systems for hearing loss/deafness. Studies on this model of cochlear degeneration illustrate the dynamic cellular and architectural changes following hair cell degeneration, and allow the investigation of various approaches aiming to regenerate hair cells. Yet it is important to note that this model of cochlear degeneration may differ, at least in part, from other causes of hearing loss such as those involving other cell types including mutations of the connexin or pendrin genes (1,20).

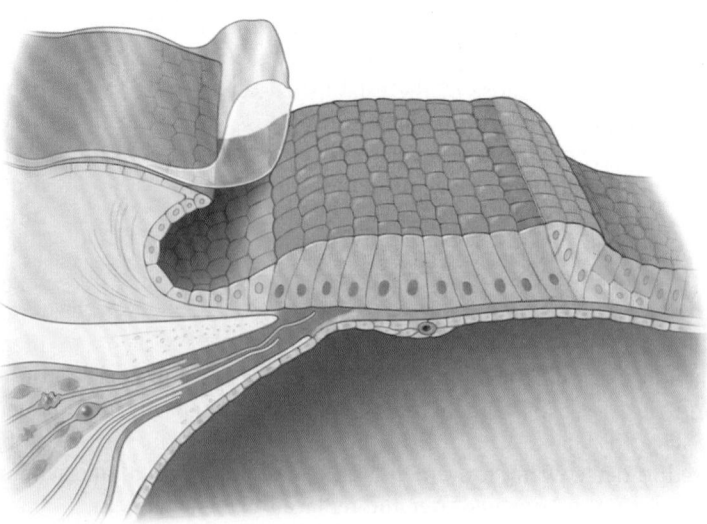

Figure 169.2 Degenerated mammalian organ of Corti. After extensive hair cell loss, the epithelial integrity is maintained by the remaining supporting cells, which morphologically transform from a complex and pseudostratified organ into a mostly simple cuboidal epithelium. Figure © Stanford University.

NOTCH PATHWAY

One key molecular pathway regulating hair cell differentiation is the Notch signaling pathway, which plays several roles during the development of many organ systems. In regenerating chicken basilar papilla, Notch ligand expression is upregulated and inhibition of Notch signaling causes excessive regeneration of hair cells (21). This finding suggests that active Notch signaling functions to suppress supporting cells from acquiring a hair cell fate. However, Notch inhibition fails to induce extra hair cell formation from quiescent supporting cells in the undamaged avian cochlea, suggesting that a separate damage-induced signal is necessary.

In the developing cochlear duct, hair cells and supporting cells share a common progenitor (22). During late embryogenesis, Notch signaling pathway regulates the mammalian cochlea through a process termed lateral inhibition (reviewed in [23]). Developing hair cells express Notch ligands (24,25), which in turn activate Notch signaling in adjacent supporting cells. Active Notch signaling in supporting cells turns on the *Hes* and *Hey* genes and represses the expression of *Atoh1*, a gene critical for hair cell differentiation (see section below). Such an interaction is important in the formation of rows of hair cells intercalated by supporting cells (26). Similar to the avian cochlea, inhibition of the Notch pathway leads to ectopic hair cell formation in the embryonic and early postnatal mouse cochlea, indicating that mammalian supporting cells have the potential to acquire a hair cell phenotype (27–30). Stringent analyses identified a subset of organ of Corti supporting cells capable of directly differentiating into hair cells in the neonatal mouse cochlea: (a) inhibition of Notch signaling leads to excessive outer hair cells at the expense of Deiters' cells, and (b) inhibition of both Notch and fibroblast growth factor (FGF) signaling causes formation of excessive inner hair cells from pillar cells (29,31). Together these experiments suggest that supporting cells can be coerced to become new hair cells, and raise the question whether they can also function to replace lost hair cells under pathologic conditions.

To gain insights into the role of Notch signaling in hair cell regeneration, researchers have studied the use of gamma secretase inhibitors, which are potent antagonists of Notch signaling by preventing cleavage and release of the intracellular domain on Notch receptors that is responsible for downstream gene regulation. In damaged chicken basilar papilla and the zebrafish lateral line system, both organs that spontaneously regenerate lost hair cells, Notch inhibition led to an increase in hair cell production (21,32). These observations suggest that events occurring during hair cell regeneration recapitulate those in development.

Whether inhibition of Notch signaling can stimulate hair cell regeneration in the mature mammalian cochlea has not been extensively examined. In one study where guinea pigs were deafened by aminoglycoside,

pharmacologic inhibition of Notch signaling has yielded limited ectopic hair cells without regeneration of outer or inner hair cells (33). Though discouraging, these results suggest that supporting cells in the mature organ of Corti have lost responsiveness to Notch inhibition. However, mechanisms underlying this loss of competence are currently unknown and warrant further investigation.

ATOH1 GENE THERAPY

The basic helix-loop-helix transcription factor Atoh1 (also known as Math1) is one of the earliest markers for hair cell differentiation (34). In mutant mice lacking *Atoh1*, hair cells fail to develop, indicating that the gene is necessary for their genesis (35,36). To investigate whether *Atoh1* is sufficient to induce hair cell formation, several groups have examined the effects of *Atoh1* overexpression in the developing and mature cochlea. When introduced in the developing otocyst *in utero*, cells transfected with *Atoh1* generated ectopic hair cells that are innervated and demonstrated mechanosensitivity, both cardinal features of functional hair cells (37). When *Atoh1*-expressing plasmids were administered to mammalian cochlear explants, independent studies have found ectopic hair cells in the greater epithelial ridge adjacent to the organ of Corti (36,38). These data suggest that defined cell populations in the embryonic and early postnatal cochlea can generate new hair cells when coerced to express *Atoh1*. Of note, new supporting cells are formed adjacent to the newly formed hair cells, likely as a result of inductive signals originating from these new hair cells (36).

Using adenovirus vehicle to force express *Atoh1*, Kawamoto et al. (39) found that limited nonsensory cells remain competent to be induced to form ectopic hair cells in the mature cochlea in guinea pigs. In a follow-up study, Izumikawa et al. (40) applied this intervention to the adult guinea pig cochleae 4 days following deafening by aminoglycoside insults, and reported hair cell regeneration and subsequent improved auditory brainstem thresholds. However, no hair cell regeneration or functional recovery was observed when the *Atoh1* gene was delivered 1 week after deafening from aminoglycoside/diuretic treatment, when the sensory epithelium was severely degenerated and on course to form a flat epithelium. While these results suggest that introducing genes important for hair cell differentiation, such as *Atoh1*, may hold promise as an intervention for deafness, the mixed outcomes of studies and the limited time window of opportunity, however, warrant further investigation to better understand this approach for future treatment.

CELL CYCLE INHIBITION

The postnatal mammalian organ of Corti is postmitotic. Studies using thymidine analog uptake have indicated that cells of the mammalian organ of Corti have gone through the last phase of mitosis between embryonic day 12.5 to 16 (41,42). Several cell cycle regulators are upregulated during this period and are thought to be important to transition the proliferative prosensory region to differentiated organ of Corti. p27^{Kip1}, a member of the cyclin-dependent kinase inhibitors, is expressed in the prosensory region (where hair cells first emerge) of the developing cochlea and becomes restricted to supporting cells in the postnatal organ of Corti (42,43). Deficiency of p27^{Kip1} leads to both increased and prolonged proliferation in the cochlea, as well as supernumerary hair cells (43,44). These mutant mice with extra hair cells have significant hearing loss and their cochleae exhibit distorted cytoarchitecture. When one of the downstream targets of cyclin-dependent kinase inhibitors, the retinoblastoma protein, is deleted (45,46), ongoing proliferation of supporting cells and hair cells were observed in the late embryonic and postnatal ages, indicating that retinoblastoma is also required for cell cycle exit in the developing cochlea. Although these overproduced hair cells are mechanosensitive, a delayed degeneration and hearing loss were observed (45–47). These results highlight two major challenges underlying hair cell regeneration: (a) preserving the intricate cellular organization and cell number in the organ of Corti is critical for its function; (b) signals inducing hair cell regeneration are probably different from those maintaining hair cell integrity. To add to this complexity, acute ablation of retinoblastoma expression fails to induce proliferation or hair cell regeneration in the adult cochlea (48), suggesting that manipulating the cell cycle pathway alone is not sufficient to awaken the mitotically quiescent cells, but the effectiveness of this approach has not been fully investigated in the damaged organ. Although supporting cells in the mature avian cochlea are likewise quiescent at rest, they are capable of reentering a proliferative state and regenerating lost hair cells as a result of noise or aminoglycoside damage. Studies on the effects of hair cell damage on the cell cycle in supporting cells are scarce, and existing evidence suggests a low level of proliferation exists as a result of hair cell loss in the mature mammalian cochlea (49). At present, our understanding of how cell cycle is regulated in the normal and damaged adult mammalian cochlea is limited and advancing it will likely be a necessary step toward inner ear regeneration.

SOMATIC STEM CELLS

In the developing cochlear duct, sensory hair cells and nonsensory supporting cells derive from common progenitor cells. During regeneration in the avian cochlea, experiments using label retention assays demonstrated that supporting cells are the source of regenerated hair cells (6–8). They behave as stem cells because they divide asymmetrically and self-renew by generating additional supporting cells, while also giving birth to daughter cells that differentiate

into *bona fide* hair cells. The mammalian cochlea, unlike its avian counterpart, does not contain supporting cells that readily proliferate upon hair cell loss nor do they spontaneously regenerate hair cells. However, recent evidence shows that the mammalian cochlea harbors cells with regenerative capacity in the early postnatal period (16,50–55).

Using a cell-based assay established to study neural stem cells, investigators have found that both the mature vestibular system and the neonatal cochlea in mice contain stem cell-like cells (15,16). They behave as stem cells in that they self-renew and also differentiate into hair cell– and supporting cell–like cells *in vitro* and upon transplantation. Recent work suggests that several cell populations in the neonatal mouse cochlea have differential potentials to proliferate and produce new hair cells (54). However, this regenerative capacity rapidly decreases during the first 3 weeks of life (16); the mechanisms underlying this loss are currently unknown. It remains to be determined whether one can rekindle these endogenous stem/progenitor cells from the developing cochlea to repair a damaged adult cochlea.

Unlike the cochlea, several mammalian organ systems continue to self-renew throughout life. These systems include the skin, hematopoietic, and intestinal organs, which contain well-characterized endogenous stem cells. While there have been several attempts at transplanting such stem cells as well as embryonic stem cells (see next section) into a damaged cochlea, results have been mixed on the success rates of cell survival, integration, and functional improvement (56–60).

EMBRYONIC STEM CELLS AND INDUCED PLURIPOTENT STEM CELLS

Embryonic stem cells originate from the inner cell mass during fetal development. They are able to self-renew and generate all cell types within the body, and are therefore an attractive resource for tissue regeneration. Induced pluripotent stem cells are similar to embryonic stem cells: they self-renew and are pluripotent. By introducing defined factors, many laboratories have reliably generated induced pluripotent stem cells from mature tissues, such as skin fibroblasts (reviewed by [61]). Several years ago, Li et al. (62) described a first protocol that guided differentiation of mouse embryonic stem cells into otic progenitor cells, which when transplanted into developing chicken otocyst, differentiated into hair cell–like cells. In a follow up study, Oshima et al. (63) refined this differentiation guidance method for both mouse embryonic stem cells and induced pluripotent stem cells so that new mechanosensitive hair cells were produced *in vitro*.

While these proofs of principle experiments have yielded encouraging results, it is unknown whether transplanting otic progenitors or more mature cochlear cell types into a deafened cochlea can regenerate hair cells and auditory function. Thus far, results on integration of transplanted otic progenitor cells derived from embryonic stem cells, like those of adult stem cells, have been mixed (see

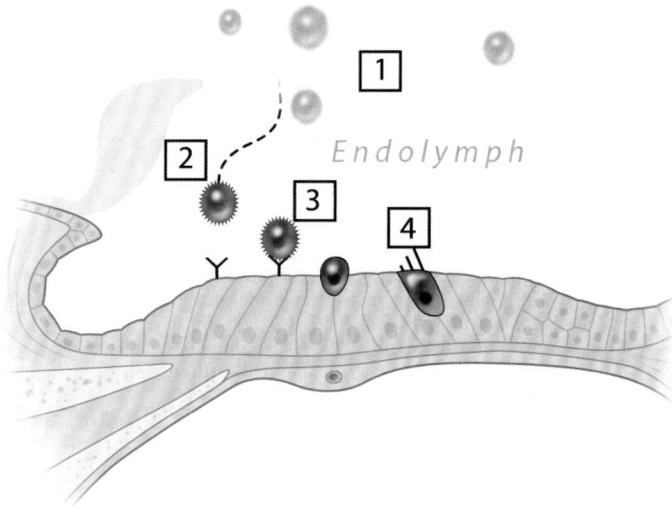

Figure 169.3 Schematic of stem cell transplantation into the inner ear. Grafting into the scala media compartment is one of several approaches to introducing cells into the inner ear. Transplanted cells will first need to survive in the endolymph fluid (*1*), then integrate into the sensory epithelium (*2–3*), and ultimately convert into functional sensory hair cells (*3*). Figure © Stanford University.

Fig. 169.3) (64–66). While some studies have reported functional recovery of deafened animals, others have observed poor survival of grafted cells and even the formation of tumors, likely teratomas. Collectively, these results highlight the challenges of cell-based therapy in treating inner ear diseases and are related to numerous factors (see Fig. 169.3): (a) the inner ear, especially the scala media housing the organ of Corti, is difficult to access for cell transplantation. Within the scala media, the electrolyte composition (high potassium) of endolymph is potentially inhospitable for grafted cells, (b) it is unclear what cell types are best suited to graft (undifferentiated stem cells, committed tissue-specific stem cells, or purified progenitor cells); (c) little is known about homing signals in the normal or damaged cochlea that may attract transplanted cells; (d) whether grafted cells will be integrated and become functional hair cells along the entire length of the cochlea is currently unclear. Without such knowledge, it is difficult to predict whether cell transplantation is a feasible route to functional recovery of the mammalian cochlea.

SUMMARY

Since the discovery of hair cell regeneration in lower vertebrates over 20 years ago, our understanding of the regenerative potentials of the mammalian cochlea has increased tremendously. In recent years, the armamentarium to investigate the mammalian cochlea has been rapidly growing and now consists of many molecular and cell-based approaches. Manipulation of the Notch and/or FGF pathways can recruit subsets of nonsensory supporting cells to generate extranumerary hair cells in the neonatal mouse cochlea, where forced expression of *Atoh1* can induce ectopic hair cell formation. Hair cells can also be produced from embryonic stem cells and induced pluripotent stem cells *in vitro*, yet many obstacles exists for cell transplantation into the inner ear. It is important to note that most studies on hair cell regeneration thus far have employed drug- or noise-induced

hair cell degeneration as model systems; however, treatment paradigms will likely differ for other causes of hearing loss, such as genetic diseases, age-related hearing loss, or auditory dyssynchrony spectrum disorder. In the coming years, new discoveries will likely continue to transform our understanding of the regenerative capacity of the mammalian cochlea. Importantly, the long-term efficacy and safety of the newly discovered interventions will need to be carefully interrogated before they are translated to new approaches to managing patients with sensorineural hearing loss.

ACKNOWLEDGMENTS

The authors would like to thank Chris Gralapp for figure illustration and Taha Jan for fruitful comments. Authors' research is supported by Akiko Yamazaki and Jerry Yang Faculty Scholar Fund, California Institute of Regenerative Medicine RN3-06529, NIDCD/NIH K08 DC011043 (to A.G.C.) and R01 DC006167 (to S.H.).

HIGHLIGHTS

- Hair cell degeneration occurs in many modes of sensorineural hearing loss.
- The mature mammalian organ of Corti lacks the ability to regenerate lost hair cells.
- The Notch signaling pathway mediates lateral inhibition and hair cell differentiation during cochlear development.
- The Atoh1 transcription factor is necessary and sufficient for hair cell differentiation.
- The neonatal mouse cochlea harbors cells with regenerative potential.
- Mouse embryonic and induced pluripotent stem cells can generate mechanosensitive hair cells *in vitro*.

REFERENCES

1. Ahmad S, et al. Restoration of connexin26 protein level in the cochlea completely rescues hearing in a mouse model of human connexin30-linked deafness. *Proc Natl Acad Sci U S A* 2007;104(4):1337–1341.
2. Heller S. Application of physiological genomics to the study of hearing disorders. *J Physiol* 2002;543(Pt 1):3–12.
3. Williams JA, Holder N. Cell turnover in neuromasts of zebrafish larvae. *Hear Res* 2000;143(1–2):171–181.
4. Matsui JI, et al. Characterization of damage and regeneration in cultured avian utricles. *J Assoc Res Otolaryngol* 2000;1(1):46–63.
5. Stone JS, et al. Progenitor cell cycling during hair cell regeneration in the vestibular and auditory epithelia of the chick. *J Neurocytol* 1999;28(10–11):863–876.
6. Corwin JT, Cotanche DA. Regeneration of sensory hair cells after acoustic trauma. *Science* 1988;240(4860):1772–1774.
7. Cruz RM, Lambert PR, Rubel EW. Light microscopic evidence of hair cell regeneration after gentamicin toxicity in chick cochlea. *Arch Otolaryngol Head Neck Surg* 1987;113(10):1058–1062.
8. Ryals BM, Rubel EW. Hair cell regeneration after acoustic trauma in adult Coturnix quail. *Science* 1988;240(4860):1774–1776.
9. Woolley SM, Wissman AM, Rubel EW. Hair cell regeneration and recovery of auditory thresholds following aminoglycoside ototoxicity in Bengalese finches. *Hear Res* 2001;153(1–2):181–195.
10. Woolley SM, Rubel EW. Vocal memory and learning in adult Bengalese Finches with regenerated hair cells. *J Neurosci* 2002;22(17):7774–7787.
11. Cafaro J, Lee GS, Stone JS. Atoh1 expression defines activated progenitors and differentiating hair cells during avian hair cell regeneration. *Dev Dyn* 2007;236(1):156–170.
12. Shang J, et al. Supporting cell division is not required for regeneration of auditory hair cells after ototoxic injury in vitro. *J Assoc Res Otolaryngol* 2010;11(2):203–222.
13. Rubel EW, Dew LA, Roberson DW. Mammalian vestibular hair cell regeneration. *Science* 1995;267(5198):701–707.
14. Warchol ME, et al. Regenerative proliferation in inner ear sensory epithelia from adult guinea pigs and humans. *Science* 1993;259(5101):1619–1622.
15. Li H, Liu H, Heller S. Pluripotent stem cells from the adult mouse inner ear. *Nat Med* 2003;9(10):1293–1299.
16. Oshima K, et al. Differential distribution of stem cells in the auditory and vestibular organs of the inner ear. *J Assoc Res Otolaryngol* 2007;8(1):18–31.
17. Oesterle EC, et al. Sox2 and JAGGED1 expression in normal and drug-damaged adult mouse inner ear. *J Assoc Res Otolaryngol* 2008;9(1):65–89.
18. Oesterle EC, Campbell S. Supporting cell characteristics in long-deafened aged mouse ears. *J Assoc Res Otolaryngol* 2009;10(4):525–544.
19. Leake PA, Hradek GT. Cochlear pathology of long term neomycin induced deafness in cats. *Hear Res* 1988;33(1):11–33.
20. Everett LA, et al. Expression pattern of the mouse ortholog of the Pendred's syndrome gene (Pds) suggests a key role for pendrin in the inner ear. *Proc Natl Acad Sci U S A* 1999;96(17):9727–9732.
21. Daudet N, et al. Notch regulation of progenitor cell behavior in quiescent and regenerating auditory epithelium of mature birds. *Dev Biol* 2009;326(1):86–100.
22. Fekete DM, Muthukumar S, Karagogeos D. Hair cells and supporting cells share a common progenitor in the avian inner ear. *J Neurosci* 1998;18(19):7811–7821.
23. Kelley MW. Cellular commitment and differentiation in the organ of Corti. *Int J Dev Biol* 2007;51(6–7):571–583.
24. Lanford PJ, et al. Expression of Math1 and HES5 in the cochleae of wildtype and Jag2 mutant mice. *J Assoc Res Otolaryngol* 2000;1(2):161–171.
25. Zine A, et al. Hes1 and Hes5 activities are required for the normal development of the hair cells in the mammalian inner ear. *J Neurosci* 2001;21(13):4712–4720.
26. Lanford PJ, et al. Notch signalling pathway mediates hair cell development in mammalian cochlea. *Nat Genet* 1999;21(3):289–292.
27. Brooker R, Hozumi K, Lewis J. Notch ligands with contrasting functions: Jagged1 and Delta1 in the mouse inner ear. *Development* 2006;133(7):1277–1286.
28. Zine A, Van De Water TR, de Ribaupierre F. Notch signaling regulates the pattern of auditory hair cell differentiation in mammals. *Development* 2000;127(15):3373–3383.
29. Yamamoto N, et al. Inhibition of Notch/RBP-J signaling induces hair cell formation in neonate mouse cochleas. *J Mol Med* 2006;84(1):37–45.
30. Takebayashi S, et al. Multiple roles of Notch signaling in cochlear development. *Dev Biol* 2007;307(1):165–178.
31. Doetzlhofer A, et al. Hey2 regulation by FGF provides a Notch-independent mechanism for maintaining pillar cell fate in the organ of Corti. *Dev Cell* 2009;16(1):58–69.
32. Ma EY, Rubel EW, Raible DW. Notch signaling regulates the extent of hair cell regeneration in the zebrafish lateral line. *J Neurosci* 2008;28(9):2261–2273.
33. Hori R, et al. Pharmacological inhibition of Notch signaling in the mature guinea pig cochlea. *Neuroreport* 2007;18(18):1911–1914.
34. Ben-Arie N, et al. Functional conservation of atonal and Math1 in the CNS and PNS. *Development* 2000;127(5):1039–1048.
35. Bermingham NA, et al. Math1: an essential gene for the generation of inner ear hair cells. *Science* 1999;284(5421):1837–1841.
36. Woods C, Montcouquiol M, Kelley MW. Math1 regulates development of the sensory epithelium in the mammalian cochlea. *Nat Neurosci* 2004;7(12):1310–1318.
37. Gubbels SP, et al. Functional auditory hair cells produced in the mammalian cochlea by in utero gene transfer. *Nature* 2008;455(7212):537–541.
38. Zheng JL, Gao WQ. Overexpression of Math1 induces robust production of extra hair cells in postnatal rat inner ears. *Nat Neurosci* 2000;3(6):580–586.
39. Kawamoto K, et al. Math1 gene transfer generates new cochlear hair cells in mature guinea pigs in vivo. *J Neurosci* 2003;23(11):4395–4400.
40. Izumikawa M, et al. Auditory hair cell replacement and hearing improvement by Atoh1 gene therapy in deaf mammals. *Nat Med* 2005;11(3):271–276.
41. Ruben RJ. Development of the inner ear of the mouse: a radioautographic study of terminal mitoses. *Acta Otolaryngol* 1967:(Suppl 220):1–44.
42. Lee YS, Liu F, Segil N. A morphogenetic wave of p27Kip1 transcription directs cell cycle exit during organ of Corti development. *Development* 2006;133(15):2817–2826.
43. Chen P, Segil N. p27(Kip1) links cell proliferation to morphogenesis in the developing organ of Corti. *Development* 1999;126(8):1581–1590.
44. Lowenheim H, et al. Gene disruption of p27(Kip1) allows cell proliferation in the postnatal and adult organ of corti. *Proc Natl Acad Sci U S A* 1999;96(7):4084–4088.
45. Sage C, et al. Essential role of retinoblastoma protein in mammalian hair cell development and hearing. *Proc Natl Acad Sci U S A* 2006;103(19):7345–7350.
46. Sage C, et al. Proliferation of functional hair cells in vivo in the absence of the retinoblastoma protein. *Science* 2005;307(5712):1114–1118.
47. Mantela J, et al. The retinoblastoma gene pathway regulates the postmitotic state of hair cells of the mouse inner ear. *Development* 2005;132(10):2377–2388.
48. Huang M, et al. Overlapping and distinct pRb pathways in the mammalian auditory and vestibular organs. *Cell Cycle* 2011;10(2):337–351.
49. Yamasoba T, Kondo K. Supporting cell proliferation after hair cell injury in mature guinea pig cochlea in vivo. *Cell Tissue Res* 2006;325(1):23–31.
50. White PM, et al. Mammalian cochlear supporting cells can divide and trans-differentiate into hair cells. *Nature* 2006;441(7096):984–987.
51. Diensthuber M, Oshima K, Heller S. Stem/progenitor cells derived from the cochlear sensory epithelium give rise to spheres with distinct morphologies and features. *J Assoc Res Otolaryngol* 2009;10(2):173–190.

52. Zhang Y, et al. Isolation, growth and differentiation of hair cell progenitors from the newborn rat cochlear greater epithelial ridge. *J Neurosci Methods* 2007;164(2):271–279.

53. Jan TA, et al. Tympanic border cells are Wnt-responsive and can act as progenitors for the postnatal mouse cochlear cells. Association of Research in Otolaryngology Midwinter Meeting, 2010;Abstract number 21.

54. Sinkkonen ST, et al. Intrinsic regenerative potential of murine cochlear supporting cells. *Sci Rep* 2011;1:26.

55. Malgrange B, et al. Proliferative generation of mammalian auditory hair cells in culture. *Mech Dev* 2002;112(1–2):79–88.

56. Hu Z, Ulfendahl M, Olivius NP. Survival of neuronal tissue following xenograft implantation into the adult rat inner ear. *Exp Neurol* 2004;185(1):7–14.

57. Ito J, Kojima K, Kawaguchi S. Survival of neural stem cells in the cochlea. *Acta Otolaryngol* 2001;121(2):140–142.

58. Tamura T, et al. Transplantation of neural stem cells into the modiolus of mouse cochleae injured by cisplatin. *Acta Otolaryngol Suppl* 2004(551):65–68.

59. Naito Y, et al. Transplantation of bone marrow stromal cells into the cochlea of chinchillas. *Neuroreport* 2004;15(1):1–4.

60. Matsuoka AJ, et al. In vivo and in vitro characterization of bone marrow-derived stem cells in the cochlea. *Laryngoscope* 2006;116(8):1363–1367.

61. Yamanaka S, Blau HM. Nuclear reprogramming to a pluripotent state by three approaches. *Nature* 2010;465(7299):704–712.

62. Li H, et al. Generation of hair cells by stepwise differentiation of embryonic stem cells. *Proc Natl Acad Sci U S A* 2003; 100(23):13495–13500.

63. Oshima K, et al. Mechanosensitive hair cell-like cells from embryonic and induced pluripotent stem cells. *Cell* 2010;141(4): 704–716.

64. Hildebrand MS, et al. Survival of partially differentiated mouse embryonic stem cells in the scala media of the guinea pig cochlea. *J Assoc Res Otolaryngol* 2005;6(4):341–354.

65. Coleman B, et al. Fate of embryonic stem cells transplanted into the deafened mammalian cochlea. *Cell Transplant* 2006; 15(5):369–380.

66. Sakamoto T, et al. Fates of mouse embryonic stem cells transplanted into the inner ears of adult mice and embryonic chickens. *Acta Otolaryngol Suppl* 2004(551):48–52.

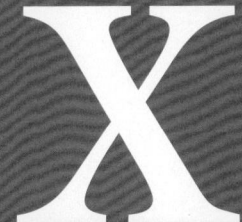

Facial Plastic and Reconstructive Surgery

Grant S. Gillman   *Jonathan M. Sykes*

Preoperative Evaluation and Facial Analysis in Facial Plastic Surgery

170

Andrew Winkler   *Justin M. Wudel*

CONCEPT OF BEAUTY AND DEFORMITY

Western civilization portrays facial beauty as flawless, young skin with ideal facial contours. Youth and beauty are pervasive in all forms of media, highlighting their significance to our culture and to humans in general (1). The value that our society places on beauty has lead to innumerable methods of enhancing one's attractiveness, including cosmetic surgery. Today, the desire to change one's appearance is considered a sufficient indication for surgery, whether or not a true "deformity" is present. The continual growth in the number of cosmetic procedures performed each year reflects the public's rapidly growing acceptance of cosmetic surgery as a means of self-improvement.

The physician and patient usually share a perception of deformity and the correction needed. Some patients, however, perceive an abnormality not readily apparent to other people. A significant difference between the perceived deformity and the surgeon's assessment of the feature raises warning flags that may warrant further evaluation. This chapter aids in defining what does and does not constitute deformity and how to elucidate whether a patient's requests are within normal limits. Psychiatric conditions that may lead to a disagreement in facial assessment between patient and surgeon are also discussed. The absolute numeric values presented in this chapter allow the surgeon to determine whether or not a feature is proportionate. However, facial features must also form a harmonious union when observed together. Harmony refers to the mind's interpretation of the facial relationships based strictly on visual observation (2). For facial beauty to exist, the proportions and architecture of the face must form a balance that is visually pleasing. When the major aesthetic masses of the face (nose, lips, ears, eyes, etc.) are individually proportionate, they are more likely to harmonize with each other to yield an aesthetically pleasing facial appearance. However, disproportionate features may also harmonize with one another, even though the feature itself falls outside of what is considered normal. Consequently, beauty is to a degree in the eye of the beholder, and aesthetic facial analysis remains a partially subjective exercise.

INITIAL CONSULTATION

Establishing a Relationship

The primary goal of the preoperative interview is to establish effective communication in order to obtain an understanding the patient's perception of the defect, the patient's motivations, and the patient's expectations from surgery (3). During the interview, the patient's thoughts and feelings about the area of concern are explored. This provides an opportunity to educate the patient about the details of potential surgery and what outcomes may be realistically achieved. The preoperative interview is also an opportunity to a review the medical history to identify conditions that may preclude surgery. Spending time with potential medical issues improves trust and rapport and may reveal issues needing further evaluation prior to undergoing elective surgery. A surgeon's mastery of the relationship-building phase of the interview results in improved patient satisfaction, reduced legal liability, and better surgical outcomes (4,5).

Preoperative Assessment

A commonsense approach to selecting candidates for surgery greatly reduces the chance of encountering an unhappy patient (6). In the preoperative interview, the surgeon seeks answers to the following questions:

- What are the patient's expectations?
- Are the expectations realistic and reasonable?
- Do I have the ability to fulfill these expectations?
- Can the patient be satisfied?

TABLE 170.1	RED FLAG SYMPTOMS. PATIENTS EXHIBITING "RED FLAGS" MAY WARRANT FURTHER INVESTIGATION

Trying to please someone else
Unrealistic expectations
Pervasively unhappy
Poor self-image
Overly flattering
Perfectionists
Rude or demanding
Know-it-all
History of doctor-shopping
History of litigation
Multiple revision surgeries

Many tools are available to aid in obtaining this information. The Sensitization, Aesthetic self-assessment, peer Group comparison and Avoidance behaviors (SAGA) tool helps to uncover patients' understanding of normal, their perception of deformity, and its impact on them (7). Sensitization refers to the point at which the patient becomes aware of and bothered by a deformity. The impetus for sensitization may be self-induced (intrinsic) or the result of extraneous remarks or teasing (extrinsic). Alternatively, the patient may not be sensitized to a deformity and may be requesting surgery to please someone else, a red flag symptom (Table 170.1).

The second concept evaluated by the SAGA tool is aesthetic self-assessment. This is the patient's private evaluation of the concerning feature in a mirror. Simply inquiring about self-assessment builds rapport and reassures the patient that this is normal behavior. The self-assessment also gives an impression of the desired improvements and whether these expectations are realistic.

Peer group comparison gives insight into patient sensitization as well as their reaction to the deformity. A patient sensitized to a feature will scrutinize others in society (7). The patient desiring to appear like that of a particular movie star reveals unrealistic expectations, and such patients are likely to blame the surgeon for perceived poor results. The patients' ability to accept the surgical result is highly correlated with the degree to which they are prepared by their surgeon. Unrealistic expectations must be discussed prior to undergoing surgery (8).

Avoidance behaviors examine the techniques and strategies used by the patient to camouflage or conceal their imperfections. This may include makeup, clothing, or a hairstyle used to cover up or draw attention away from the featured complaint. Avoidance behaviors should resolve with surgery and may provide an objective measure of success postoperatively.

The experienced surgeon develops wariness for patients who create a sense of uneasiness. Situations that raise caution flags include a history of having sued another surgeon, extreme demands of support staff, or evidence of "doctor-shopping" in search of someone who will perform the desired surgery. Such patients should be approached with extreme care and often require further evaluation (Table 170.1).

PSYCHOPATHOLOGY IN THE AESTHETIC PATIENT

It was not long ago that patients seeking aesthetic surgery were assumed to have deeply seated psychological issues. In 1960, Jacobson et al. (9), suggested that most cosmetic surgery patients required psychological evaluation because psychiatric problems were almost certainly present. As cultural norms have evolved, the level of concern about physical appearance that was once deemed psychologically abnormal is now acceptable and it is rare for a patient to require preoperative psychiatric evaluation. The rate of psychopathology in cosmetic surgery patients today approaches that of the general population. Nevertheless, only a small percentage of the population actively seeks surgery despite a continual increase in popularity. This is due to personality characteristics that differentiate those who seek cosmetic surgery from those who do not (4,10). On the extreme end of the personality spectrum are patients with diagnosable psychiatric conditions. The following section describes important pathologic conditions to consider during the initial consultation.

Depression

Traditionally, patients carrying a diagnosis of depression were rejected for facial cosmetic surgery as it was feared this would trigger deeper depression (11). In a study from 1960, patients with late-onset and prolonged depression after cosmetic procedures exhibited a causal relation between surgery and depression. This group of patients received support in the immediate postoperative period that was initially satisfying. As the sought-after attention waned, however, the patients realized that surgery had not fulfilled their desires, and they became more depressed. While a diagnosis of depression is not a contraindication to surgery, there remains a risk of depression intensifying following surgery. We now know that almost half of aesthetic surgery patients display clinically apparent postoperative depression, even with a good outcome (11,12). Despite this finding, Moss and Harris (13) demonstrated a significant improvement in patient's postoperative Beck Depression Inventory score following cosmetic surgery in comparison to their preoperative scores. It is generally accepted that patients with a preoperative diagnosis of depression can undergo cosmetic surgery without fear of long-term intensification of their symptoms, although coordination between the surgeon and psychiatrist yields the best results.

Personality Disorder

Personality disorders are psychiatric conditions in which a person's behaviors, emotions, and thoughts are markedly different from that of their culture, causing serious problems with relationships and work. Personality disorders are the most common psychopathology seen in patients seeking cosmetic surgery (14). These patients are manipulative, demanding, and difficult to please. Of all personality disorders, narcissistic and histrionic personality disorders are most commonly encountered by facial plastic surgeons (15). Although the overall prevalence of narcissistic personality disorder in the general population is 1%, up to 25% of patients who present to a plastic surgery practice display hallmarks of the diagnosis, including unexplained grandiosity accompanied by a need for admiration (14,16). Similarly, although the incidence of histrionic personality disorder in the general population is 1.8%, up to 10% of cosmetic surgery patients have this condition, marked by attention-seeking behavior, excessive emotionality, and sexual forwardness (15,16). A third personality disorder to consider is borderline personality disorder (BPD). People with BPD are uncertain about their identity, and as a result their interests and values change rapidly. These patients perceive their environment in terms of extremes, leading to rapidly shifting feelings and unstable relationships (16). The encounter with a patient who has a personality disorder can be one of frustration and aggravation. Nevertheless, an appropriate doctor-patient relationship must be established. If the surgeon is not confident that this relationship can be maintained or the patient will not cooperate, surgery should not be performed.

Body Dysmorphic Disorder

One of the most difficult challenges facing a plastic surgeon occurs when there is disagreement with a patient regarding the degree of deformity. While it is not uncommon to encounter patients who would like to have minor deformities corrected or improved, it is important to recognize patients who fall outside of the normal spectrum. The extreme example of this is body dysmorphic disorder (BDD), a condition characterized by the unhealthy obsession with one or more body parts (16). Patients with BDD have a preoccupation with some slight or perceived flaw in their physical appearance. These individuals spend an excessive amount of time thinking about their personal appearance and methods to change it. BDD is estimated to occur in approximately 1% of the general population, but the incidence is up to 16 times higher in patients desiring plastic surgery (17). When a patient demonstrates profound emotional distress and behavioral impairment out of proportion to the actual defect, the plastic surgeon is wise to refer the patient for psychiatric evaluation. The mainstay of treatment for the behavioral components of BDD is cognitive behavior therapy (18). BDD is a somatoform disorder that cannot be effectively treated with surgery and therefore these patients are not surgical candidates. BDD patients are more likely to move to litigation, and may even threaten physical violence.

FACIAL ANALYSIS

History

The desire to identify ideal facial aesthetics dates to antiquity. Greek artists sought to identify ideal facial proportions and began to formally analyze beauty. The classical Greek canons of facial balance that were developed consequently influenced anatomic scholars of the Renaissance period, and many of these form the foundation of facial analysis today.

Ricketts (19) supported the Greek concept that facial attractiveness is related to the repetition of proportions throughout the face. The ideal or "divine" proportion equates to the mathematical ratio of 1:1.618 (phi), which was believed to be the rate of mathematical progression most pleasing to the eye. The ratio refers to the point along a line at which the ratio of the smaller portion to the larger portion is the same as the ratio of the larger portion to the original line (Fig. 170.1) (20).

Farkas et al. (21) performed detailed anthropometric studies of different ethnic populations to assess the validity of the classical Greek canons for beauty and determined multiple "normal" values for various facial proportions. Measurement and memorization of normal values is cumbersome and quickly becomes impractical for everyday use by aesthetic surgeons.

Modern science defines beauty as a biologic and cross-cultural concept of attractiveness. In one study (22), infants preferred looking at aesthetically pleasing adult faces. Other studies (23) note a preference for symmetry in facial architecture (24,25). Another (26) found that test subjects preferred a composite of attractive faces to a composite of average faces, which was consistent across ethnic boundaries. Ethnic differences in aesthetic ideals exist, however, and must be considered during facial analysis to avoid inappropriate "Westernization" of ethnic features (27–31).

Defining Terms

The face is a complex balance of multiple aesthetic units that when taken together produces a unique appearance. Facial analysis uses standardized points to determine

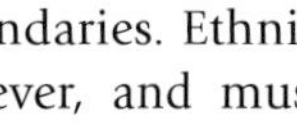

$$\frac{AB}{BC} = \frac{AC}{AB} = 1.618(\phi)$$

Figure 170.1 When the ratio of the long segment to the short segment (AB/BC) is the same as the ratio of the whole line to the long segment (AC/AB), the ratio is equivalent to the divine ratio, phi (1.618). (Adapted from Ricketts RM. Divine proportions in facial esthetics. *Clin Plast Surg* 1982;9:401–422, with permission.)

TABLE 170.2	BASIC ANATOMIC LANDMARKS AS SEEN ON FRONTAL VIEW
Trichion (Tn)	Superior margin of the forehead at the midline of the frontal hairline
Radix (R)	The region of the root of the nose
Subnasale (Sn)	Soft tissue point at the junction of the columella and upper lip in the midline
Superior and inferior vermilion border (Vs and Vi)	Mucocutaneous junction of the upper and lower lips
Stomion (St)	Midline point at the embrasure of the lips when closed
Menton (M)	Soft tissue point at the inferior-most border of the chin in the midline

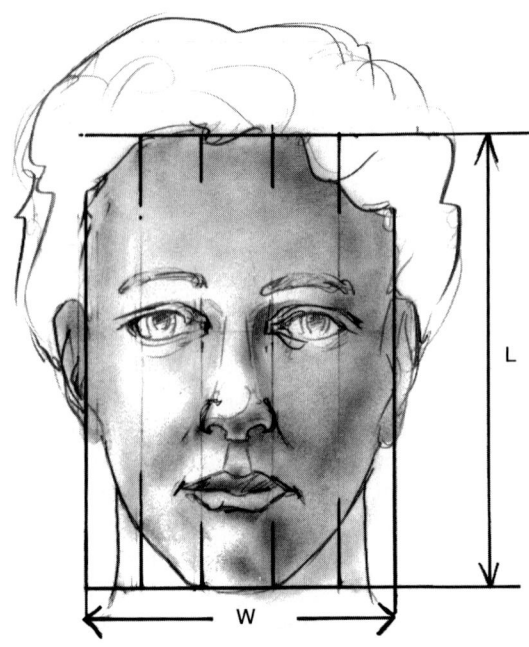

Figure 170.3 Ideal frontal symmetry and proportion is approximated by dividing the face into vertical fifths, with each fifth approximating the width of the eye. The overall width-to-length ratio should approximate 3:4.

relationships between various aesthetic masses, and to determine the proportions of each feature individually. The following tables define standard reference points used in facial analysis (Tables 170.1 and 170.2, Fig. 170.2). Using these standard points, reference angles are constructed to analyze interfacial relationships. These values serve as a general reference, but values vary from male to female and between ethnic groups. Men tend to have sharper angles and more prominent features than women. These differences help us subconsciously determine gender, as well as the degree of masculinity and femininity.

General Facial Assessment

Facial assessment begins with an evaluation of symmetry. A line drawn through the midsagittal plane on frontal view provides a side-by-side comparison of symmetry. The midline points of the forehead, nose, lips, and chin should lie on this axis. Subtle asymmetries are expected and it is helpful to point these out to the patient preoperatively.

Assessment of symmetry and proportion is further accomplished by dividing the face into vertical fifths equal to the width of one eye, or the intercanthal distance. Vertical lines at the lateral canthus should approximate the width of the neck (32). The lateral-most fifth extends from the lateral canthus to the lateral most point of the helical rim (Fig. 170.3).

Facial height is examined by dividing the face into horizontal thirds on the frontal and lateral views (Fig. 170.4). The total facial height is the distance from the trichion to the menton. However, the trichion can be an inaccurate landmark due to receding hairlines in some individuals. In these cases the trichion is approximated by marking the uppermost extent of frontalis movement. The face is

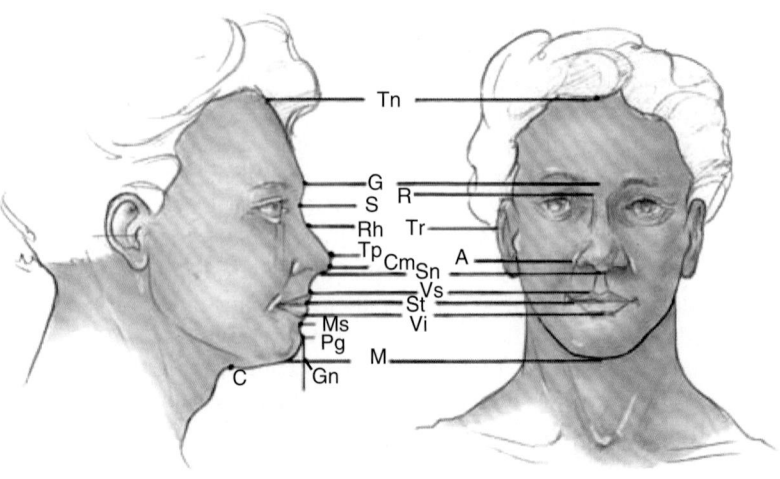

Figure 170.2 Basic anatomic landmarks for facial analysis. See Tables 170.2 and 170.3 for explanation.

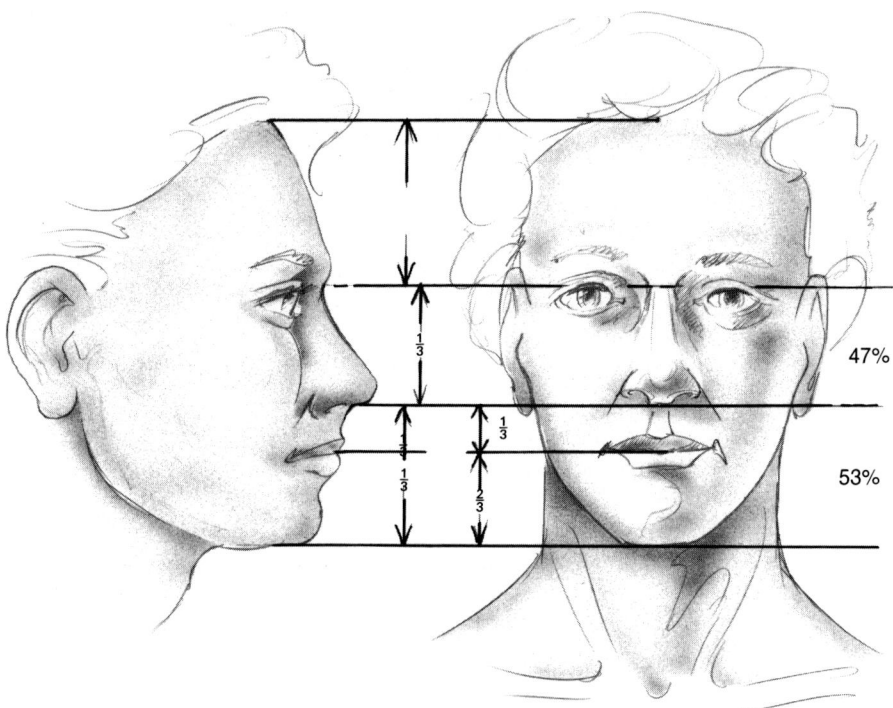

Figure 170.4 The facial thirds: trichion to glabella, glabella to subnasale, subnasale to menton. The lower face also is divided into thirds: The upper lip from subnasale to stomion is one-third, and the lower lip and chin is two-thirds. The face from nasion to subnasale is 47% and from subnasale to menton is 53% of the total height from nasion to menton. (From Powell N, Humphries B. *Proportions of the aesthetic face.* New York: Thieme-Stratton, 1984, with permission.)

then divided into horizontal thirds at the glabella and the subnasale. This creates an upper third from trichion to glabella, a middle third from the glabella to the subnasale and a lower third from subnasale to menton.

Lower facial symmetry can be further assessed by subdividing this region in thirds as well. The upper third is equal to the distance from the subnasale to the stomion, while the lower two-thirds are equal to the distance from the stomion to the menton (33).

The facial profile assessment examines the relationships of individual components to the face as a whole. Lateral view assessment begins with positioning of the patient in the Frankfort horizontal (Fig. 170.5) (Tables 170.3 and 170.4). When a line from the inferior orbital rim to the tragion is parallel to the horizon, the patient is said to be in the Frankfort horizontal. This provides a reproducible posture for comparison between patients and over time.

Gonzales-Ulloa (34) described a useful method of evaluating the aesthetic profile in relation to the Zero Meridian line. This vertical line passes through the nasion perpendicular to the Frankfort horizontal line. In the aesthetically pleasing facial profile, the outline of the midforehead, subnasale, upper and lower lips, and pogonion should rest on this line. The Zero Meridian and Frankfort horizontal line provide a framework from which to analyze the facial profile. The frontal, nasal, labial, and mandibular regions can be analyzed for protrusion or retrusion based on their relationships to these lines. In addition to providing a qualitative assessment of aesthetic units on profile view, this technique also allows the surgeon to quantify the amount of correction needed in each area.

Forehead

The forehead occupies one-third of the vertical height of the face and is a significant contributor to overall facial balance. The forehead is defined as the space between the

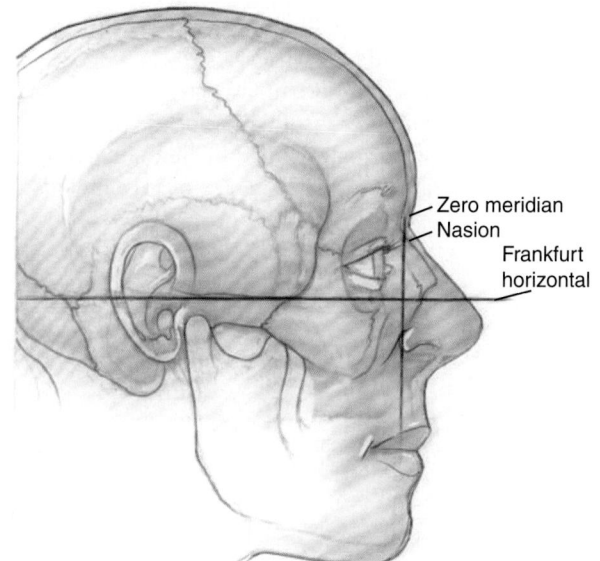

Zero meridian
Nasion
Frankfurt horizontal

Figure 170.5 The Frankfort horizontal plane connects the inferior orbital rim to the tragion and is parallel to the horizon. Gonzalez-Ulloa defined the aesthetic profile in relation to the Zero Meridian, a line perpendicular to the Frankfort horizontal plane through the nasion. In the aesthetically pleasing profile, the outline of the midforehead, subnasale, upper and lower lips, and pogonion rest on this line (From Gonzalez-Ulloa M. Quantitative principles in cosmetic surgery of the face (profi leplasty). *Plast Reconstr Surg Transplant Bull* 1962;29:186–198.).

TABLE 170.3	BASIC ANATOMIC LANDMARKS ON LATERAL VIEW
Nasion (N)	Posteriormost bony point at the root of the nose
Sellion (S)	Posteriormost soft tissue point at the root of the nose
Glabella (G)	Anteriormost point of the forehead in the midline
Rhinion (Rh)	Region at the junction of the bony and cartilaginous nasal dorsum
Tip-defining-point (Tp)	Anteriormost projection of the nasal tip, corresponding to the dome of the lower lateral cartilages
Columellar point (Cm)	Anteriormost point of the columella
Alar crease (A)	Sulcus defining the posterior border of the alar subunit of the nose
Mentolabial sulcus (Ms)	Crease between the lower lip and chin
Pogonion (Pg)	Anteriormost point of the chin in the midline
Gnathion (Gn)	Virtual point defined by the intersection of a vertical line lying tangent to the pogonion and a horizontal line that is tangent to the menton.
Cervical point (C)	Virtual point defined by the line tangent to the anterior margin of the neck and a line tangent to the menton
Tragion (Tr)	Point at the supratragal notch of the ear

trichion and the glabella, bordered by the hairline superiorly and laterally, and extending upward from the superior aspect of the eyebrows. The shape of the forehead varies between men and women, and consequently the most aesthetically pleasing contour is gender-dependent. The attractive female forehead contour has a gentle convexity on profile with its most anterior point at the supraorbital ridge lying tangent to the Zero Meridian. Men tend to have a more protruding forehead than women with a degree of supraorbital bossing. The shape of the forehead is also important in the context of the global facial appearance. A protruding forehead will draw more attention to a recessed chin or maxilla and vice versa.

One of the most important aspects of the forehead from a surgical standpoint is the nasofrontal angle (NFA). The NFA is an obtuse angle formed by lines tangent to the glabella and nasal dorsum. The vertex of this angle is the sellion, and the normal value of the NFA varies from 115 to 135 degrees (Fig. 170.6). The vertex of the NFA lies at the level of the superior limbus of the eye, though this is variable. Men tend to have a more acute NFA when compared to females, due to the increased prominence of the supraorbital rim. Thus, in men the NFA ideally measures 115 to 120 degrees whereas women ideally measure 120 to 135 degrees. Changing the position of the NFA can have dramatic effects on the harmony of surrounding structures. Additionally, the length of the nose is determined by the vertical position of the NFA; a factor that can be addressed with surgery. Moving the vertex of the NFA superiorly lengthens the nose and vice versa. The infantile nose deformity occurs when telescoping naso-orbito-ethmoid fractures result in a posterior repositioning of the NFA. This leads to a loss of nasal dorsal height that resembles the undeveloped dorsum of a child.

TABLE 170.4	PROFILE PLANES AND ANGLES USED IN FACIAL ANALYSIS
Facial Plane	Reference plane created that is tangent to the glabella and pogonion
Frankfort Horizontal	Reference line from the superior margin of the external auditory canal to the inferior border of the infraorbital rim
Zero-Meridian	Reference line perpendicular to the Frankfort Horizontal intersecting at the nasion
Nasofrontal angle (NFA)	Obtuse angle formed by lines tangent to the glabella and nasal dorsum with the vertex at the sellion
Nasofacial angle (NFcA)	Angle of inclination of the nasal dorsum from the facial plane
Nasolabial angle (NLA)	Angle of inclination between the columella and the upper lip
Lower Face-Throat Angle	Angle formed at the gnathion by the intersection of a line from the cervical point to menton with a line from the subnasale to the pogonion.
Mentocervical angle (MCA)	Angle formed by the intersection of a line from the cervical point to menton with a line from the glabella to pogonion.

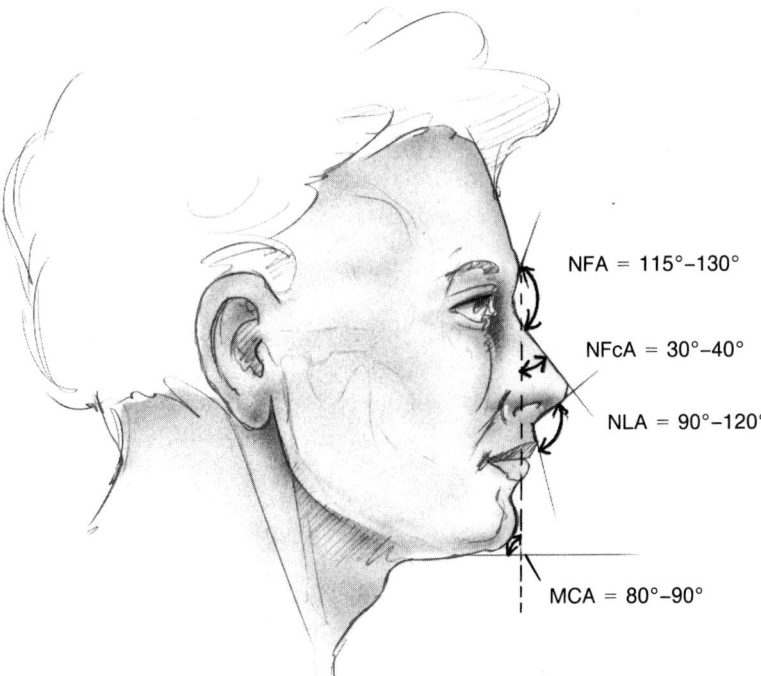

NFA = 115°–130°

NFcA = 30°–40°

NLA = 90°–120°

MCA = 80°–90°

Figure 170.6 Profile angles for facial analysis. See Table 170.4 for definitions.

Eyebrow

The eyebrows function in static protection of the eye, facial identity, and sexual dimorphism. They also convey expressions of happiness, surprise, and anger distinctly from the rest of the face (35). With aging, the brow position descends due to the affect of gravity and accumulated skin damage. Eyebrow size, position, and morphology change dramatically throughout one's life, and normative values are useful when performing an aesthetic evaluation.

The female brow is positioned at or above the supraorbital rim with an arch that peaks in the lateral third of the brow. In contrast, the male brow is positioned directly over the supraorbital rim and is relatively straight (36,37). The contemporary concept of the ideal position of the male eyebrow has remained fairly constant, but the same cannot be said for the female brow. In 1974, Westmore proposed that the aesthetic female eyebrow begins medially over the alar groove and ends laterally at a line connecting the lateral canthus and the lateral ala. The author also conjectured that the medial and lateral aspects of the eyebrow should fall in the same horizontal plane and that the apex of the eyebrow lies above the lateral limbus (36,38,39). Over the last few decades, several authors have offered modifications to Westmore's paradigm following the shifting aesthetic ideals of society. Cook et al. (40) concluded that the peak of the eyebrow belongs over the lateral canthus rather than the lateral limbus. Most recently, Roth et al. evaluated the frontal photographs of fashion models and randomly selected women. Their findings suggest that the ideal eyebrow arch position lies between the lateral limbus and lateral canthus. The authors also found that the lateral brow lies slightly superior to the medial brow in the horizontal plane (41) (Fig. 170.7).

Eyes/Eyelids

The eyes are the seat of beauty, and changes in this region, whether age-related or otherwise, often prompt patients to seek aesthetic evaluation. Appraisal of facial harmony requires close examination of the symmetry, shape, proportions, and position of the eyes. The medial limbus of the iris ideally lies on a vertical line with the oral commissures. In Caucasians, the intercanthal distance should be equal to the interalar width of the nasal base. However, this is not true for Asian or African Americans, who typically

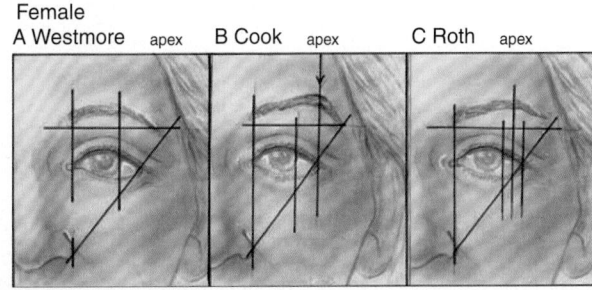

Female
A Westmore apex   **B** Cook apex   **C** Roth apex

Figure 170.7 A: The ideal brow begins at the medial canthus and ends laterally along an oblique line through the alar–facial junction and the lateral canthus. Westmore proposed that the apex of the eyebrow should reach its maximal arch along a line tangent to the lateral limbus. (Adapted from Brennan GH. Correction of the ptotic brow. *Otolaryngol Clin North Am* 1980;13:265–273, with permission.) **B:** Cook Modification: With shifting societal aesthetic ideals, the aesthetic position of the female brow has also shifted. Cook proposed that the peak of the eyebrow lies over the lateral canthus rather than the lateral limbus. **C:** Roth Modification: Most recently, Roth et al. found the ideal eyebrow arch position lies between the lateral limbus and lateral canthus and that the lateral brow lies slightly superior to the medial brow in the horizontal plane.

have a slightly wider interalar distance. The average intercanthal distance is 32 to 35 mm, whereas the average interpupillary distance is 61 to 69 mm (42). The interpupillary and intercanthal distances are approximately equal to the width of one eye (43).

The contour of the youthful upper and lower eyelids is one of smooth transitions. The upper eyelid has a definable supratarsal crease (STC) and then flows smoothly to the brow above. The lower eyelid transitions without demarcation into the malar eminence and cheek. The upper eyelid overlies the superior limbus by 2 to 3 mm, whereas the lower lid approximates or overlies the inferior limbus by 1 mm. The apex of the supratarsal plate is centered over the medial limbus, while the nadir of the lower eyelid lash line is aligned with the lateral limbus (44) The distance from lash line to lid crease on the upper lid varies from 7 to 15 mm in the non-Asian patient (32), but tends to be greater in men than in women. The lateral canthus lies 2 to 4 mm above the medial canthus (45) yielding an upward tilting intercanthal axis that is characteristic of the beautiful eye. Many anatomical variations exist based on gender, ethnicity, and body habitus. In addition, soft tissue volume is lost with aging, which disrupts the smooth transitions of the eyelid leading to dermatochalasis and periorbital wrinkles and folds (Fig. 170.8).

Ears

Ridges and concavities in the auricular cartilage framework form the distinctive shape of the external ear. The auricle reaches 80% of the adult size by age 5 (46), permitting early surgical intervention using adult normative values. When analyzing the ears, each auricle is evaluated relative to the face and individually, as deformities can be distinct between each ear.

The position of the auricle on the head contributes distinctly to overall aesthetics. The top of the ear should lie at the level of the brow and the bottom of the lobule at the nasal ala (47). The axis of the ear slants posteriorly and approximates the inclination of the nasal bridge. The helix forms the most lateral extent of the auricle on frontal view and should be just visible behind the antihelix and superior crus.

The width of the ear is approximately 55% its length. The average length and width of the male auricle is 63.5 and 35.5 mm, respectively. Corresponding measurements in the female are 59.0 and 32.5 mm (48,49). When viewed from above, the auricle protrudes 20 to 30 degrees from the skull. In assessing ear protrusion, the distance from the mastoid to the helix is recorded at the superior aspect of the helix, at the level of the external auditory canal, and at the lobule. The ideal values for these distances in the adult should be 16 to 18 mm, 14 to 16 mm, and 16 to 18 mm, respectively.

Nose

With its central location on the face, the nose is one of the most important contributors to facial aesthetics. No other feature must harmonize with other areas of the face more than the nose. Small changes to the nose can produce dramatic differences in overall facial aesthetics. For this reason, it is one of the most frequently surgically altered features and the normal proportions of the nose have been thoroughly documented. Ideal aesthetics occur when nasal proportions and angles are within normal limits and

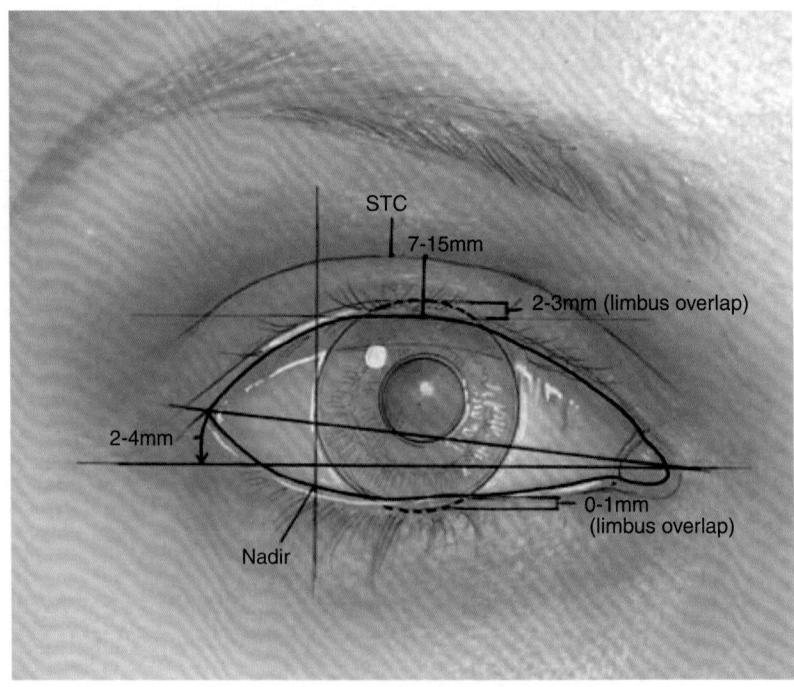

Figure 170.8 Characteristic relationships of the aesthetically pleasing eye. The upper eyelid overlaps the superior limbus of the iris by 2 to 3 mm, while the lower eyelid approximates or overlaps the inferior limbus by 1 mm. The supratarsal plate is tallest at the medial limbus. The nadir of the lower eyelid lash line is aligned with the lateral limbus. The distance from the upper eyelid lash line to the supratarsal crease (STC) varies from 7 to 15 mm. The intercanthal axis is tilted upward laterally, with the lateral limbus lying 2 to 4 mm above the medial canthus.

harmonize with other facial features. However, more than with any other facial feature, variations of the nasal proportions are accepted based on ethnicity, age, height, and gender.

Nasal Angles

Several angles are useful in defining the relationship of the nose to the face. As discussed above, the NFA is important in the aesthetics of both the nose and the forehead. It describes the superior limit of the nose and can have a dramatic effect on the overall appearance of the nose.

The nasofacial angle (NFcA) describes the relationship of the nasal dorsum to the facial plane, defined by a vertical line from the glabella to the pogonion. The NFcA is formed by the intersection of a line from the sellion to the nasal tip (drawing through any dorsal hump that may exist) with the facial plane. A NFcA of 36 degrees is aesthetically ideal and can help to determine whether to augment or reduce the nasal dorsum.

A third angle of measurement helpful in the nasal–facial aesthetics is the nasolabial angle (NLA). The NLA is formed by lines constructed from the superior vermilion border to the subnasale, and from the subnasale to the columella. This angle defines the relationship between the nose and the upper lip as well as the rotation of the nasal tip. An aesthetically pleasing NLA is 90 to 95 degrees in men and 95 to 105 degrees in women. Shorter individuals tolerate a more obtuse angle, whereas taller people require a NLA at the low end of the range for their gender (Fig. 170.6, Table 170.4).

Nasal Tip Projection

Many techniques have been proposed to define ideal nasal tip projection and controversy exists over which method is optimal. Also, one must differentiate between tip projection and rotation as they are closely related, but distinct concepts. Tip rotation is the caudal or cephalad rotational movement of the tip around the fixed point of the tragion. Nasal tip projection, on the other hand, is the anterior or posterior positioning of the nasal tip relative to the Zero Meridian (Fig. 170.9).

There are four methods commonly used to evaluate tip projection. Perhaps the simplest method was proposed by Simons in 1975 (50). He suggested that the distance from the upper lip vermilion border to the subnasale and from the subnasale to the tip defining point should be approximately equal. This method is easy to perform and takes into effect harmony with a nearby structure. However, the variable size of the upper lip length can yield inaccurate results.

Powell and Humphries described the ideal relationship between tip projection and nasal height as a 2.8:1 ratio. Height is measured from sellion to subnasale, and tip projection is measured by a line drawn perpendicular to the

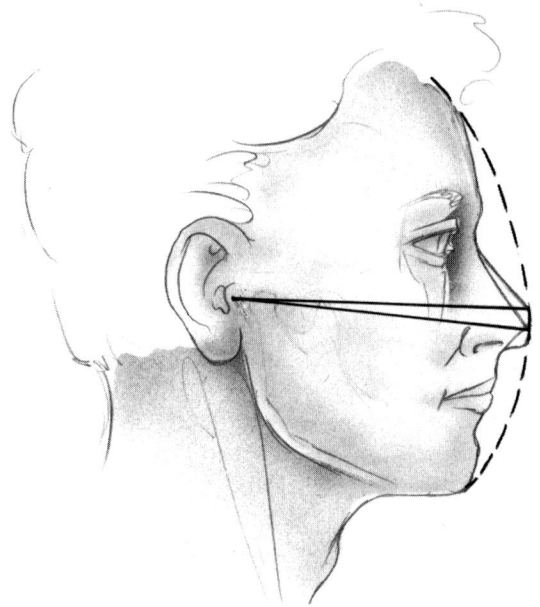

Figure 170.9 Nasal tip rotation is defined by the movement of the nasal tip on an arc around the tragion.

first line through the tip defining point (33) (Fig. 170.10). Though relatively simple, this method does not take into account the effect the length of the ala on tip projection.

Goode's method of assessing tip projection takes into account the relationship between nasal length and the alar groove. A vertical line is drawn from the sellion through the alar groove. A second perpendicular line is then drawn to the

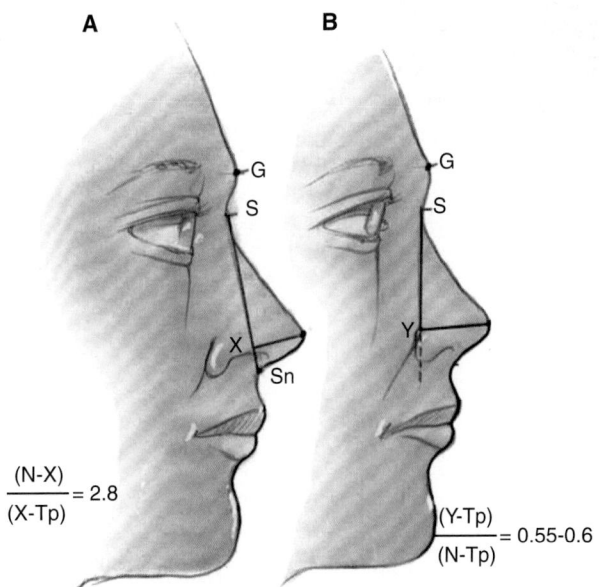

$$\frac{(N-X)}{(X-Tp)} = 2.8$$

$$\frac{(Y-Tp)}{(N-Tp)} = 0.55\text{-}0.6$$

Figure 170.10 Assessment of nasal projection. **A:** The Powell and Humphries (33) method. A line from sellion (S) to subnasale (Sn) is used to measure tip projection. The ratio of projection (X-Tp) to height (S-X) is ideally 2.8:1. **B:** The Goode (51) Method. A line from sellion (S) to the alar groove is used to measure tip projection. The ratio of projection (Y-Tp) to length (S-Tp) is ideally 0.55 to 0.6:1.

tip defining point, which effectively measures tip projection starting from the most posterior feature of the nose. Lastly, nasal length is determined using a line from the sellion to the tip (Fig. 170.10). The ideal ratio of tip projection to nasal length with the Goode method is 0.55 to 0.6:1, which produces a NFcA of 36 to 40 degrees. Crumley and Lanser (52) took this one step further by defining the relationship of tip projection, nasal length, and vertical height as a right triangle whose sides have a 3:4:5 ratio. With these parameters, the NFcA also approximates the ideal 36 degrees.

Nasal Width

The nasal width may be described as the distance between the alar grooves. The relationship of nasal base with the rest of the face is best evaluated on frontal view, where the width of nasal base should equal the width of one eye. If the distance between the medial canthi is proportionate (i.e., one eye width), then drawing a vertical line down from the medial canthus should pass through the alar groove. This technically easy evaluation can be performed during the consultation to determine if corrective surgical maneuvers are needed. A second method involves first calculating the nasal length from sellion to the tip defining point. A proportionate nasal width is estimated at 70% of the total length.

The basal view is also used to assess nasal width as well as nasal tip symmetry. On basal view, the nose should have the appearance of an equilateral triangle (53). The width of the nasal lobule should be 75% of the width of the entire nasal base. The width of the columella compared to the width of the lobule should be 2:1. The tip should comprise one-third of the total height, while the nostrils make up the remaining two-thirds on basal view (Fig. 170.11). The nostril openings are ideally ovoid and obliquely oriented toward the tip. The posterior aspect of the nostril is slightly larger and rounder, becoming more narrow anteriorly (54). Careful assessment of the individual components of the nasal base allows for a site-specific analysis of the contributors to overall nasal width and symmetry.

Lateral View Nasal Assessment

The lateral view of the nose allows one to assess the nasal profile and the ala-tip complex. On lateral view, the length of the ala and tip should be equal, though tip lobular excess is more acceptable than alar excess (53). There should be 2 to 4 mm of columellar show below the level of the nostril rim on profile view (Fig. 170.11). The elegant nasal tip profile has a "double break" produced by the tip defining point anteriorly and a subtler angulation at the junction of the tip lobule with the columella. Additionally, a supratip break exists between the nasal tip subunit and the nasal dorsum in the ideal nose. Although ethnic variations exist, a more pronounced supratip break is more acceptable in women than in men. The distance from the long axis of the nostril to the alar rim and columella should be 1 to 2 mm. Discrepancies from this ideal indicates alar or columellar retraction, or a hanging ala or columella (55).

Midface

The soft tissues of the midface provide much of the contour that gives an individual their unique facial appearance (56). While direct measurements and angles are used to define ideals in other areas, aesthetic evaluation of the midface region is more heavily reliant on symmetry and harmony with surrounding features.

The appearance of the midface is highly dependent on the underlying bone structure, fat compartments, and skin texture. The face should be widest at the zygomaticus, the most prominent portion of the zygomatic arch, and should taper down to the chin, giving the face a heart-shaped appearance. The malar eminence ideally lies within the space defined by a line from the nasal base to the tragus and a line from the oral commissure to the lateral canthus (57).

The soft tissue envelope of the midface is uniquely susceptible to solar damage, gravity, and the aging process. With

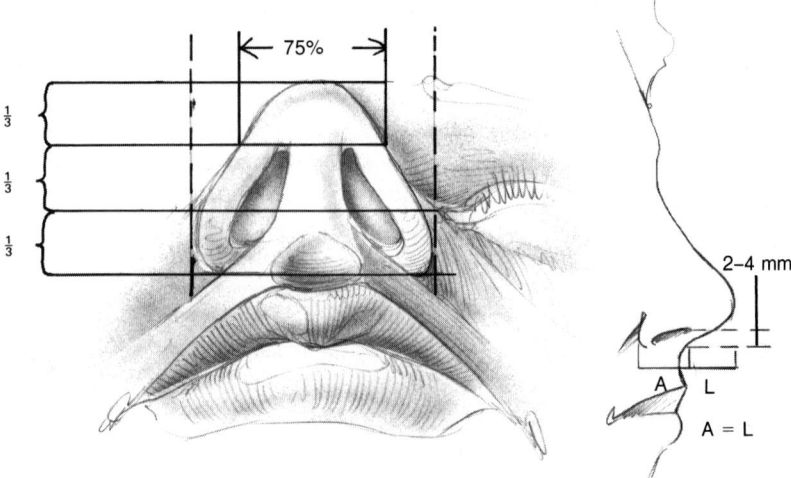

Figure 170.11 The width of the nasal lobule should be 75% of the width of the nasal base. The lobule-to-columella ratio should be 1:2. On lateral view, the ala-to-lobule ratio should be 1:1, and there should be 2 to 4 mm of columellar show.

aging, the skin and soft tissues of the midface atrophy and descend. This leads to the formation of jowls and a "squaring off" of the heart-shaped face of youth. To determine the best restorative approach for the midface, an assessment must be made of midfacial volume, skin laxity, and the prominence of the nasolabial and nasojugal folds (58,59).

Chin

The chin plays a prominent role in the balance of the facial profile. Classically, a prominent chin is associated with strength and power, whereas a retrusive chin portrays weakness. The chin extends from the mentolabial sulcus to the menton. The lower lip and chin should make up two-thirds of the total length of the lower third of the face, with the upper lip making up the other one-third. Although the chin is a distinct feature, an alteration to its architecture also changes the lower lip and neck profile.

As described above, the pogonion of the masculine chin should approximate the Zero Meridian (34). In women, the pogonion should fall just behind this line (Fig. 170.5). The relationship of the chin to the lower face is assessed with a vertical line from the lower vermilion border of the lip. In men, the pogonion is tangent to this line with the mentolabial sulcus lying 4 mm posteriorly. In women, this line should lie 2 to 3 mm anterior to the pogonion. Prognathia or retrognathia are defined by deviation of the pogonion from these positions.

Lip

The lips are an essential component of beauty and aid in the display of emotion, personality, and sexuality. In Western culture, full lips with a well-defined philtrum are associated with youth and beauty, while a thin vermilion with diminished lip highlights are signs of aging (60). The lips have an intimate relationship with the chin, nasal base, premaxilla, and teeth, which can alter their position and global facial aesthetics.

To achieve facial balance, the vertical length of the upper lip from subnasale to stomion should equal one-third of the lower facial third, whereas the lower lip and chin from stomion to menton should compose two-thirds of the lower facial third. With the lips slightly parted, there should be a maximum of 2 mm of maxillary incisoral show (61). The upper and lower lip should just appose with the teeth in occlusion and the lips relaxed. No more than two-thirds of the maxillary incisor should be exposed on full smile (62). Although gingival show was historically considered undesirable, a small amount on smile is acceptable in contemporary society (63).

The youthful projection of the lips can be determined using a line from the subnasale to the pogonion. Burstone (64) found that ideal aesthetics were obtained when the most anterior aspects of the upper and lower lips lie 3.5 and 2.2 mm anterior to this line, respectively. This provides for a subtle youthful "pout" of the lips (Fig. 170.12).

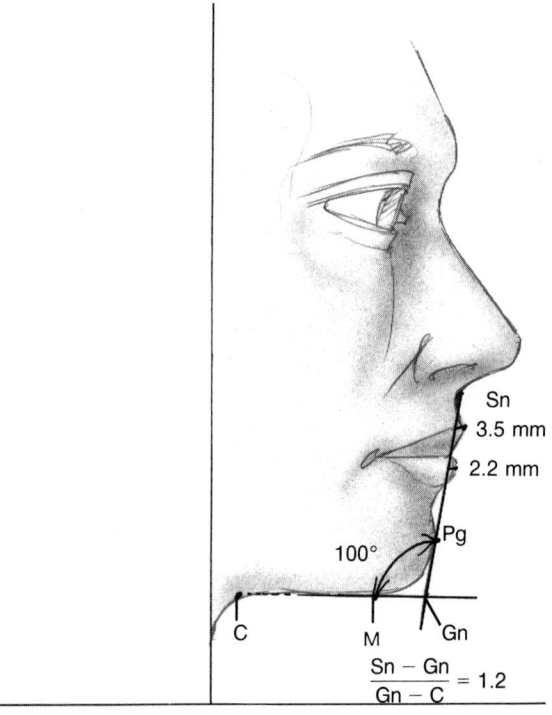

Figure 170.12 The most anterior point of the upper lip should be 3.5 mm, and that of the lower lip should be 2.2 mm, from the Sn-Pg line. Legan and Burstone (65) described the lower face–throat angle (*Sn-Gn-C*), which should be 100 degrees. The lower facial height (*Sn-Gn*) to depth (*Gn-C*) ratio should equal 1.2:1.

The height of the white upper lip, the soft tissue between the nasal base and the vermilion border, is greater in men than in women. The most prominent feature of the white lip is the philtrum (from Greek: philtron, meaning "love charm") (61). A well-defined philtrum is associated with youth and contributes to the "cupids bow" appearance of the vermillion border.

Neck

A well-contoured neckline has long been associated with elegance and beauty. The neck is intimately related to the chin, lips, and lower face and must be evaluated relative to these structures. The lower face-throat angle (65) describes the relationship of the chin to the neck. It represents the extent to which the submental tissues are tucked beneath the chin. Connecting lines from the cervical point to the menton, and from the subnasale to the pogonion forms the lower face-throat angle. The intersection of these lines is a virtual point called the gnathion. The lower face-throat angle is ideally 90 to 105 degrees. The mentocervical angle (MCA), described by Powell and Humphries, is a tool that better describes the relationship of the neck to the face. Rather than using the subnasale as a point of reference, the MCA is constructed from the glabella. This produces an angle that takes into account a broader area of the facial profile (Fig. 170.12).

The values of the MCA and lower face-throat angle are reliant on the relationship of the hyoid bone to the anterior mandible (66). The relative position of these anatomic entities to one another represents the limiting factor in attempts to surgically manipulate the neckline (67). An inferiorly and anteriorly positioned hyoid limits the amount that the submental tissues can be drawn up under the mandible. Conversely, a relatively posterior and superior position of the hyoid bone allows for a more acute MCA and lower face-throat angle, yielding a more aesthetically pleasing neckline.

Equally important in analysis of the neckline is evaluation of the neck skin and soft tissues. Blunting of the MCA is commonly caused by age-related skin laxity, proliferation of fatty deposits, and platysma muscle banding. These common culprits should be noted during consultation so that an appropriate treatment plan can be formulated (68).

METHODS OF FACIAL ANALYSIS

Cephalometrics

Orthodontists and oral maxillofacial surgeons traditionally favor the use of cephalometrics to plan treatment and evaluate their results. This method involves measurement of the maxillary, mandibular, and dental relations on lateral radiographs of the face and skull base. A cephalostat is used to hold the head in a fixed position to take the radiographs. Once obtained, soft tissue and skeletal landmarks are traced to plot points, lines, and angles, which are then used to evaluate the anterior–posterior position of the jaws and teeth in reference to the cranium and each other. Numerous systems of cephalometric analysis have been proposed and each incorporates a set of reference values for the assorted linear and angular measurements. Although the various measurements required in this method are elaborate, time-consuming, and labor intensive, it is an excellent method for evaluating craniofacial and orthognathic relationships.

Photometrics

Direct evaluation of soft tissue proportions on facial photographs, as opposed to radiographic craniofacial relations, is the method preferred by most facial plastic surgeons. In part, this is because skeletal repositioning maneuvers evaluated by cephalometric means are not absolutely correlated with a similar change in the overlying soft tissue. It is also extremely convenient to use photograph and video images to assess facial proportions and to compare the pre- and postoperative results. Similar to cephalometrics, multiple angles and ratios between the aesthetic units are calculated based on the photographic profile. An excellent summary of several cephalometric and photometric analysis systems can be found in Powell and Humphries (33) and in Chapter 171.

Three-Dimensional Photography

Facial plastic surgeons have long relied on photography for preoperative and postoperative analysis, medical-legal documentation, and communication. However, photometric techniques only allow for the measurement of two-dimensional distances, angles, and areas. Additionally, surgical outcomes are somewhat subjective because of the difficulty in quantifying three-dimensional change on a two-dimensional photograph (69).

Recently-developed three-dimensional imaging technology allows for accurate measurement of soft tissue volumetric data and surface topography (70). The technique of acquiring 3-D photographs is technically easy and can be completed in the office setting. Most camera systems utilize six cameras (3 on each side) positioned in front of the patient at oblique angles. All six cameras fire simultaneously and the images are acquired in less than 2 milliseconds. Computer software processes the images producing a mesh framework onto which the soft tissue contours and colors of the skin are applied (Fig. 170.13).

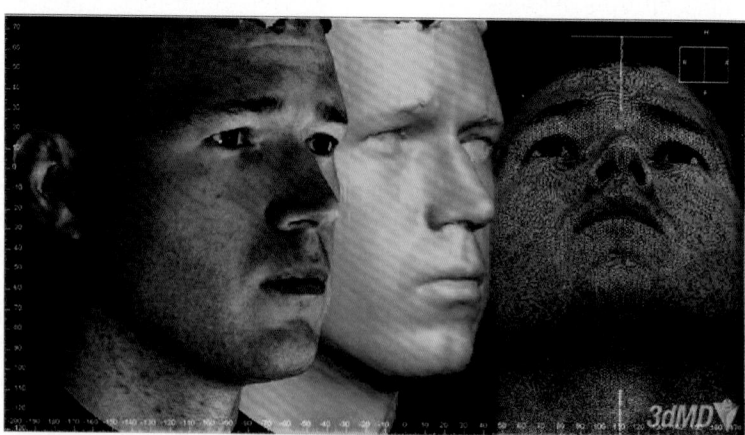

Figure 170.13 Three-dimensional photography. Three-dimensional photography allows for accurate measurement of soft tissue volume changes and surface topography. (3-D image courtesy of 3dMD (Atlanta) www.3dmd.com)

Once the image has been rendered, the physician can accurately measure angles and distances from any anatomic landmark on the face. Multiple studies have proven the accuracy of these measurements in comparison to standard techniques (71).

In addition to standard measurements, the three-dimensional aspect of the photograph allows the surgeon to evaluate changes in facial volume. The effects of aging and volume changes following surgery can therefore be quantified. By performing serial 3-D photographs and superimposing each photograph onto the original image, a topographical "color map" is created displaying changes in facial volume to cubic millimeter resolution (69). The ability to quickly and noninvasively quantify the face three dimensionally is a major advance in facial plastic surgery representing the future of aesthetic facial analysis.

CONCLUSION

Cosmetic facial surgery is more commonplace in Western society than ever before. The widespread availability of information via the Internet, social media, and other means allows today's patients to be very well informed about the procedures they seek. Now, more than ever, surgeons must be knowledgeable about what constitutes normal facial features and must be tactful in dismissing misconceptions regarding deformity and facial harmony.

During the initial consultation, establishing good rapport is necessary in order to understand the motivations for seeking plastic surgery and whether a psychiatric illness exists. Expectations from surgery are clearly identified to determine if they are realistic, reasonable, and obtainable. Once this information has been gathered, the face is analyzed from an aesthetic standpoint. Aesthetic evaluation requires an understanding of the concepts of facial harmony, proportion, and symmetry. This process begins with an overall assessment of facial symmetry, followed by a stepwise examination of the individual aesthetic masses. Each facial feature should be evaluated based on its relationship to the face globally and on feature-specific normative values. Understanding what constitutes normal helps to determine if concerns about a deformity are valid or due to psychopathology, such as BDD.

Modern facial plastic surgeons now have a variety of methods to carry out facial analysis. The traditional methods of cephalometrics and photography, though widely used are being replaced by more advanced three-dimensional photography. This technology is a major advance in facial analysis and is changing the way facial plastic surgeons analyze the face, quantify outcomes, and communicate with their patients.

HIGHLIGHTS

- Properly selecting patients for facial plastic surgery is essential to preventing unhappy patients. The surgeon must understand the patient's expectations, whether they are reasonable, and whether the desired result can be delivered.
- Although proportionate features are more likely to be aesthetically pleasing, disproportionate features can still engender a pleasing overall appearance by creating harmony with one another.
- The SAGA tool helps to uncover the patient's perception of deformity and its impact on them.
- The rate of psychopathology in cosmetic surgery patients today approaches that of the general population.
- It is generally accepted that patients with a preoperative diagnosis of depression can undergo cosmetic surgery without fear of long-term intensification of their symptoms.
- BDD is characterized by an unhealthy obsession with one or more body parts. Patients with BDD have a preoccupation with some slight or perceived flaw in their physical appearance and cannot be effectively treated with surgery.
- A system of objective measurements rather than simple subjective assessment is important in communicating the degree of deformity and surgical corrective goals with the patient.
- Facial analysis should begin with the assessment of overall facial symmetry. The face is divided into horizontal thirds and vertical fifths; asymmetries should be pointed out to the patient preoperatively.
- The profile is assessed with the patient in the Frankfort Horizontal position. The Zero Meridian line passes through the nasion perpendicular to the Frankfort horizontal line and is useful in examining profile relationships. The outline of the midforehead, subnasale, upper and lower lips should rest on this line.
- The pogonion in men should approximate the Zero Meridian and in women should fall just behind this line.
- An evaluation of the interfacial proportions of the profile involves calculating the nasofrontal, nasofacial, nasomental, and MCAs.
- The NFA is an obtuse angle formed by lines tangent to the glabella and nasal dorsum. The vertex of this angle is the sellion, and the normal value of the NFA varies from 115 to 135 degrees.
- The ideal eyebrow position is at the orbital rim in men and slightly above the rim in women. The

contemporary concept of the ideal position of the apex of the eyebrow has changed over the last several decades; it has been described in line with the medial limbus, lateral canthus, or between these two points.

■ The eyes are the seat of beauty. The medial limbus of the iris should lie on a vertical line with the oral commissures and the interpupillary and intercanthal distances are approximately equal to the width of one eye.

■ The position of the auricle contributes distinctly to overall aesthetics. The helix forms the most lateral extent of the auricle on frontal view and should be just visible behind the antihelix and superior crus.

■ Due to its central location on the face, even small changes to the nose can have dramatic effects on overall facial aesthetics. Ideal aesthetics occur when nasal proportions and angles are within normal limits and harmonize with other facial features.

■ On lateral view, the length of the ala and tip should be equal with 2 to 4 mm of columellar show below the level of the nostril rim. The elegant nasal tip profile has a "double break" produced by the tip defining point anteriorly and a subtle angulation at the junction of the tip lobule with the columella. A supratip break exists between the nasal tip subunit and the nasal dorsum.

■ On basal view, the nose ideally has the appearance of an equilateral triangle and the width of the nasal lobule is 75% of the width of the entire nasal base.

■ The soft tissue envelope of the midface is uniquely susceptible to solar damage, gravity, and the aging process. Descent of the midfacial skin and soft tissues with aging leads to the formation of jowls and a "squaring off" of the heart-shaped face of youth.

■ Though popular, cephalometric and photometric analyses lack the ability to evaluate the face in three dimensions or quantify volumetric change. Three-dimensional photo systems allow the surgeon to perform more sophisticated measurements and to quantify surgical outcomes.

REFERENCES

1. Rankin M, Borah GL. Perceived functional impact of abnormal facial appearance. *Plast Reconstr Surg* 2003;111(7):2140–2146.
2. Farkas LG, Kolar JC. Anthropometrics and art in the aesthetics of women's faces. *Clin Plast Surg* 1987;14(4):599–616.
3. Sykes JM. Managing the psychological aspects of plastic surgery patients. *Curr Opin Otolaryngol Head Neck Surg* 2009;17(4):321–325.
4. Grossbart TA, Sarwer DB. Psychosocial issues and their relevance to the cosmetic surgery patient. *Semin Cutan Med Surg* 2003;22(2):136–147.
5. Maksud DP, Anderson RC. Psychological dimensions of aesthetic surgery: essentials for nurses. *Plast Surg Nurs* 1995;15(3):137–144.
6. Honigman RJ, Phillips KA, Castle DJ. A review of psychosocial outcomes for patients seeking cosmetic surgery. *Plast Reconstr Surg* 2004;113(4):1229–1237.
7. Blackburn V, Blackburn A. Taking a history in aesthetic surgery: SAGA—the surgeon's tool for patient selection. *J Plast Reconstr Aesthet Surg* 2008;61(7):723–729.
8. Macgregor FC. Patient dissatisfaction with results of technically satisfactory surgery. *Aesthetic Plast Surg* 1981;5(1):27–32.
9. Jacobson WE, et al. Psychiatric evaluation of male patients seeking cosmetic surgery. *Plast Reconstr Surg Transplant Bull* 1960;26:356–372.
10. Sarwer DB, et al. Psychological investigations in cosmetic surgery: a look back and a look ahead. *Plast Reconstr Surg* 1998;101(4):1136–1142.
11. Goin MK, et al. A prospective psychological study of 50 female face-lift patients. *Plast Reconstr Surg* 1980;65(4):436–442.
12. Pertschuk M. Psychosocial considerations in interface surgery. *Clin Plast Surg* 1991;18(1):11–18.
13. Moss TP, Harris DL. Psychological change after aesthetic plastic surgery: a prospective controlled outcome study. *Psychol Health Med* 2009;14(5):567–572.
14. Napoleon A. The presentation of personalities in plastic surgery. *Ann Plast Surg* 1993;31(3):193–208.
15. Shridharani SM, et al. Psychology of plastic and reconstructive surgery: a systematic clinical review. *Plast Reconstr Surg* 2010;126(6):2243–2251.
16. American Psychiatric Association. *Diagnostic and Statistical Manual of Mental Disorders, Text Revision (DSM-IV-TR)*, 4th ed. Washington, DC: American Psychiatric Association, 2000.
17. Ende KH, Lewis DL, Kabaker SS. Body dysmorphic disorder. *Facial Plast Surg Clin North Am* 2008;16(2):217–223, vii.
18. Hodgkinson DJ. Identifying the body-dysmorphic patient in aesthetic surgery. *Aesthetic Plast Surg* 2005;29(6):503–509.
19. Ricketts RM. Divine proportion in facial esthetics. *Clin Plast Surg* 1982;9(4):401–422.
20. Adamson PA, Doud Galli SK. Modern concepts of beauty. *Curr Opin Otolaryngol Head Neck Surg* 2003;11(4):295–300.
21. Farkas LG, et al. Vertical and horizontal proportions of the face in young adult North American Caucasians: revision of neoclassical canons. *Plast Reconstr Surg* 1985;75(3):328–338.
22. Rubenstein AJ, Kalakanis L, Langlois JH. Infant preferences for attractive faces: a cognitive explanation. *Dev Psychol* 1999;35(3):848–855.
23. Enquist M, Arak A. Symmetry, beauty and evolution. *Nature* 1994;372(6502):169–172.
24. Penton-Voak IS, et al. Symmetry, sexual dimorphism in facial proportions and male facial attractiveness. *Proc Biol Sci* 2001;268(1476):1617–1623.
25. Pearson DC, Adamson PA. The ideal nasal profile: rhinoplasty patients vs the general public. *Arch Facial Plast Surg* 2004;6(4):257–262.
26. Perrett DI, May KA, Yoshikawa S. Facial shape and judgements of female attractiveness. *Nature* 1994;368(6468):239–242.
27. Porter JP, Lee JI. Facial analysis: maintaining ethnic balance. *Facial Plast Surg Clin North Am* 2002;10(4):343–349.
28. Erbay EF, Caniklioglu CM. Soft tissue profile in Anatolian Turkish adults: Part II. Comparison of different soft tissue analyses in the evaluation of beauty. *Am J Orthod Dentofacial Orthop* 2002;121(1):65–72.
29. Yehezkel S, Turley PK. Changes in the African American female profile as depicted in fashion magazines during the 20th century. *Am J Orthod Dentofacial Orthop* 2004;125(4):407–417.
30. Choe KS, et al. The Korean American woman's face: anthropometric measurements and quantitative analysis of facial aesthetics. *Arch Facial Plast Surg* 2004;6(4):244–252.
31. Porter JP. The average African American male face: an anthropometric analysis. *Arch Facial Plast Surg* 2004;6(2):78–81.
32. Tolleth H. Concepts for the plastic surgeon from art and sculpture. *Clin Plast Surg* 1987;14(4):585–598.
33. Powell N, Humphries B. *Proportions of the aesthetic face*. New York: Thieme-Stratton, 1984.
34. Gonzalez-Ulloa M. Quantitative principles in cosmetic surgery of the face (profileplasty). *Plast Reconstr Surg Transplant Bull* 1962;29:186–198.

35. Byrne PJ. Importance of facial expression in facial nerve rehabilitation. *Curr Opin Otolaryngol Head Neck Surg* 2004;12(4):332–335.

36. Brennan HG. Correction of the ptotic brow. *Otolaryngol Clin North Am* 1980;13(2):265–273.

37. Goldstein SM, Katowitz JA. The male eyebrow: a topographic anatomic analysis. *Ophthal Plast Reconstr Surg* 2005;21(4):285–291.

38. Westmore MG. Facial cosmetics in conjunction with surgery. Aesthetic Plastic Surgical Society Meeting, Vancouver, BC, 1974.

39. Ellenbogen R. Transcoronal eyebrow lift with concomitant upper blepharoplasty. *Plast Reconstr Surg* 1983;71(4):490–499.

40. Cook TA, et al. The versatile midforehead browlift. *Arch Otolaryngol Head Neck Surg* 1989;115(2):163–168.

41. Roth JM, Metzinger SE. Quantifying the arch position of the female eyebrow. *Arch Facial Plast Surg* 2003;5(3):235–239.

42. Barretto RL, Mathog RH. Orbital measurement in black and white populations. *Laryngoscope* 1999;109(7 Pt 1):1051–1054.

43. Mommaerts MY, Moerenhout BA. Reliability of clinical measurements used in the determination of facial indices. *J Craniomaxillofac Surg* 2008;36(5):279–284.

44. Volpe CR, Ramirez OM. The beautiful eye. *Facial Plast Surg Clin North Am* 2005;13(4):493–504.

45. Most SP, Mobley SR, Larrabee WF Jr. Anatomy of the eyelids. *Facial Plast Surg Clin North Am* 2005;13(4):487–492, v.

46. Adamson JE, Horton CE, Crawford HH. The growth pattern of the external ear. *Plast Reconstr Surg* 1965;36(4):466–470.

47. Tolleth H. Artistic anatomy, dimensions, and proportions of the external ear. *Clin Plast Surg* 1978;5(3):337–345.

48. Farkas LG. Anthropometry of normal and anomalous ears. *Clin Plast Surg* 1978;5(3):401–412.

49. Weerda H. Reconstruction of the external ear after total amputation. *Laryngorhinootologie* 2003;82(4):300–302.

50. Simons RL. Adjunctive measures in rhinoplasty. *Otolaryngol Clin North Am* 1975;8(3):717–742.

51. Goode R. A method of tip projection measurement. In: Humphries B, Powell N, eds. *Proportions of the aesthetic face*. New York: Thieme-Stratton Inc., 1984:15–39.

52. Crumley RL, Lanser M. Quantitative analysis of nasal tip projection. *Laryngoscope* 1988;98(2):202–208.

53. Bernstein L. Esthetics in rhinoplasty. *Otolaryngol Clin North Am* 1975;8(3):705–715.

54. Silver WE, Sajjadian A. Nasal base surgery. *Otolaryngol Clin North Am* 1999;32(4):653–668.

55. Gunter JP, Rohrich RJ, Friedman RM. Classification and correction of alar-columellar discrepancies in rhinoplasty. *Plast Reconstr Surg* 1996;97(3):643–648.

56. O'Connell DA, Futran ND. Reconstruction of the midface and maxilla. *Curr Opin Otolaryngol Head Neck Surg* 2010;18(4):304–310.

57. Binder WJ, Azizzadeh B. Malar and submalar augmentation. *Facial Plast Surg Clin North Am* 2008;16(1):11–32, v.

58. Rohrich RJ, Pessa JE, Ristow B. The youthful cheek and the deep medial fat compartment. *Plast Reconstr Surg* 2008;121(6):2107–2112.

59. Downs BW, Wang TD. Current concepts in midfacial rejuvenation. *Curr Opin Otolaryngol Head Neck Surg* 2008;16(4):335–338.

60. Papel ID. *Facial plastic and reconstructive surgery*, 3rd ed. New York: Everbest Printing Co., 2009:1174.

61. Wall SJ, Adamson PA. Augmentation, enhancement, and implantation procedures for the lips. *Otolaryngol Clin North Am* 2002;35(1):87–102, vi.

62. Vig KD, Ellis E III. Diagnosis and treatment planning for the surgical-orthodontic patient. *Clin Plast Surg*, 1989;16(4):645–658.

63. Sarver DM. The importance of incisor positioning in the esthetic smile: the smile arc. *Am J Orthod Dentofacial Orthop* 2001;120(2):98–111.

64. Burstone CJ. Lip posture and its significance in treatment planning. *Am J Orthod* 1967;53(4):262–284.

65. Legan HL, Burstone CJ. Soft tissue cephalometric analysis for orthognathic surgery. *J Oral Surg* 1980;38(10):744–751.

66. Wall SJ, Adamson PA. Surgical options for aesthetic enhancement of the neck. *Facial Plast Surg* 2001;17(2):109–115.

67. Sykes JM. Rejuvenation of the aging neck. *Facial Plast Surg* 2001;17(2):99–107.

68. Adamson PA, Litner JA. Surgical management of the aging neck. *Facial Plast Surg* 2005;21(1):11–20.

69. Lin SJ, et al. A new three-dimensional imaging device in facial aesthetic and reconstructive surgery. *Otolaryngol Head Neck Surg* 2008;139(2):313–315.

70. Honrado CP, Larrabee WF Jr. Update in three-dimensional imaging in facial plastic surgery. *Curr Opin Otolaryngol Head Neck Surg* 2004;12(4):327–331.

71. Ghoddousi H, et al. Comparison of three methods of facial measurement. *Int J Oral Maxillofac Surg* 2007;36(3):250–258.

171 Pictorial Documentation: Digital Imaging and Traditional Photography

Andrew K. Patel   *Amir M. Karam*   *Samuel M. Lam*

Pictorial documentation—whether film or digital based—serves multiple important purposes for the head and neck surgeon: medicolegal documentation, physician–patient communication, preoperative planning and intraoperative reference, lay and professional education, and physician self-education. In particular, the subfield of facial plastic and reconstructive surgery relies heavily on the need for standardized photographs for all of the above reasons. Photography in facial plastic surgery must be accurate, consistent, and of high quality to be useful. Photos should be free of distortion, with the greatest possible depth of field (DOF). In contrast to a studio portrait, the goal is not to make the patient appear as good as possible but rather to represent the patient as accurately as possible. Accordingly, this chapter focuses on the principles of good medical photography that relate, for the most part, to cosmetic and reconstructive facial surgery. Nevertheless, all the topics discussed can be easily applied across the broad spectrum of head and neck surgery, as indicated. The emerging and now well-established role of digital photography is also reviewed in depth and contrasted against traditional 35-mm photography to help the surgeon decide which format is better suited for his or her practice.

PRINCIPLES OF PHOTOGRAPHY

Rather than divide this section into digital and 35-mm film photography, the basic fundamental tenets that underscore good photography are universally applicable and can be discussed without reference to a chosen format. The primary spotlight will remain on good pre- and postoperative portrait photography, as this subject represents one of the most challenging and vital for the surgeon to undertake correctly. However, some practical tips on quality intraoperative photographs will also be outlined.

Informed Consent

Respect for a patient's privacy is of paramount importance for both ethical and legal grounds. Medical records should be thought of as a systemic documentation of an individual's medical history. The data contained in the physical chart or photographs is also the medical record separate from its physical embodiment. Though it may seem academic to distinguish the physical document from the information it contains, the distinction is important and relates to ownership. In the United States, patients own the information about their medical past and treatment contained in the physical form. However, the medical provider owns the physical or electronic structure that houses the information. Therefore, when discussing patient photographs, the patient actually controls the data contained in the images unless there is a legal agreement to the contrary. Use of patient photography for media or educational purposes should always be preceded with a thorough and explicit written consent. For instance, now with the rise of the Internet as a ubiquitous medium, consent forms should reflect every medium in which the surgeon intends to use the photographs, including print, television, in-office, Internet, etc. The surgeon can also state that the photograph will be used only for educational purposes and restrict the use of those photographs explicitly to scientific lectures and/or scientific articles. Further, the patient may be offered the option to camouflage his or her identity by blackening out the eyes, using only one angle of view, or cropping the image in a certain prescribed way—all of which should be stated clearly in the consent and with which the surgeon should comply. The surgeon should also guarantee in the consent that the patient's name and identity will not be further revealed unless otherwise stipulated by the patient, for example, as a testimonial.

Standardization

In order for a photograph to carry any meaningful significance, the photographs must be standardized in the following manner: same photographic media, equipment, and settings; consistent patient positioning and absence of distracting elements (makeup, jewelry, hairstyle); and identical lighting and background. Besides these considerations, the same photographer (physician or staff member) should try to take all of the photographs because slight individual interpretation of these rules can lead to dissimilar photographic results. Before taking the postoperative images, the photographer should also review the preoperative images and then alter the necessary parameters to match the preoperative photographs. For example, if the preoperative oblique view shows that the patient is turned too far laterally, the photographer should try to match the same patient positioning (albeit less than ideal) in order that the postoperative image can be meaningfully compared.

Standardized Equipment

Whether the physician ultimately decides to use film or digital media in his or her practice, the same camera should be used for all "before-and-after" photographs in order to ensure exact reproducibility in the photographic image. In addition, the same camera lens and camera settings (aperture, shutter speed, and exposure values) should be maintained, as any slight deviation can cause a quite obvious disparity in color, contrast, and shadowing. If the surgeon is using film, the exact same film stock should also be used, that is, the brand, film speed, and type (color reversal [slide, transparency] vs. negative) must be preserved.

Standardized Patient Positioning and Related Information

Proper patient positioning is the most demanding aspect of achieving reproducible photographic images. The same camera-to-subject distance must be maintained: this objective can be attained by placing the patient's stool and the camera over prescribed markings on the floor (Fig. 171.1). By using a fixed lens, that is, a lens that has no "zoom" capacity, the physician can also minimize any distortion and variability caused by altering the focal distance. The Frankfort Horizontal Plane must also be observed: the line that runs from the supratragal point through the inferior orbital rim defines the horizontal plane of the image (Fig. 171.2A–C). The Frankfort Horizontal Plane should be respected in the frontal, oblique, and lateral views. The basal view that is mandatory for rhinoplasty, malar augmentation, and midfacial trauma is defined by aligning the tip of the nose with the infrabrow line (Fig. 171.2D). On the oblique view, the patient should also be turned to a certain angle by one of two methods: (a) align the inner canthus of the eye with the oral commissure or (b) align the nasal tip with the malar eminence (Fig. 171.2).

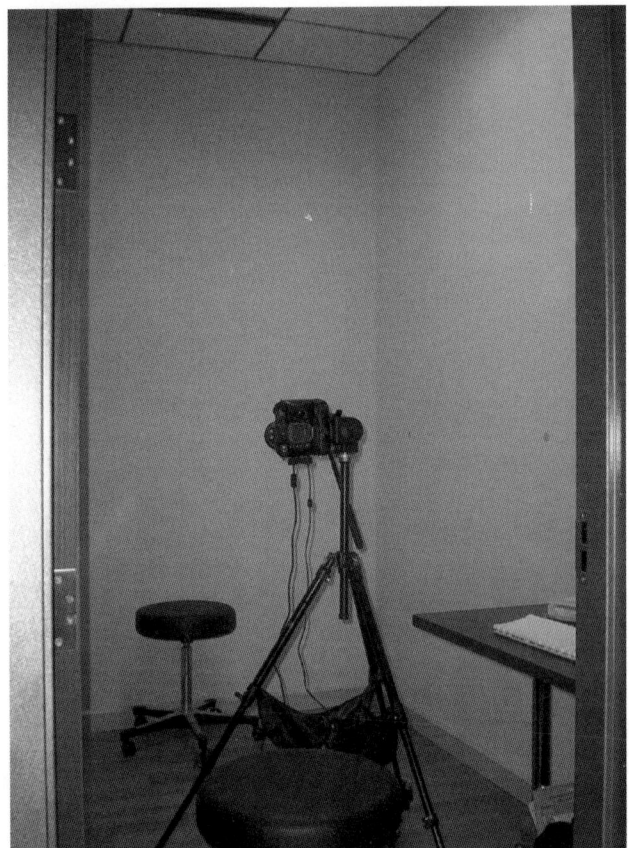

Figure 171.1 Standardized photography requires a dedicated photography room where all pre- and postoperative photographs are taken. A rotating stool with a low or no back is used to rotate the patient's entire body to the prescribed angle for each view. The digital camera is mounted on a tripod with a quick-release head that can easily adjust from a vertical to a horizontal frame position. In turn, the tripod rests on a rolling dolly to facilitate maneuverability. Markers have been placed on the wall to guide the patient how far to rotate the body in the oblique and lateral positions. In this setup, the back leg of the patient's stool contacts the wall, and the tripod's center frame is aligned with the edge of the computer table in order to maintain a standardized camera-to-subject distance. (If flash photography were used, the patient should not be so close to the wall to avoid harsh background shadows.) The back wall is painted a light blue color as a neutral background color.

Whichever method is chosen, the surgeon should attempt to rely on the same method for all images. Another reliable technique to ensure that the patient turns to the correct angle each time is to place markers on the wall that indicate where the patient should turn and face for an oblique and lateral view. When turning to the oblique and lateral positions, the patient should rotate the entire body in alignment with the face and not just turn the head to those positions, which creates neck distortion, especially in the lateral view. A rotating stool with a low back (that does not enter the frame of the image) is ideal for this goal.

One of the most common errors encountered is patient positioning with the neck tilted upward and extended, especially in the more mature patient who wants to reduce the appearance of unwanted neck-tissue redundancy. In

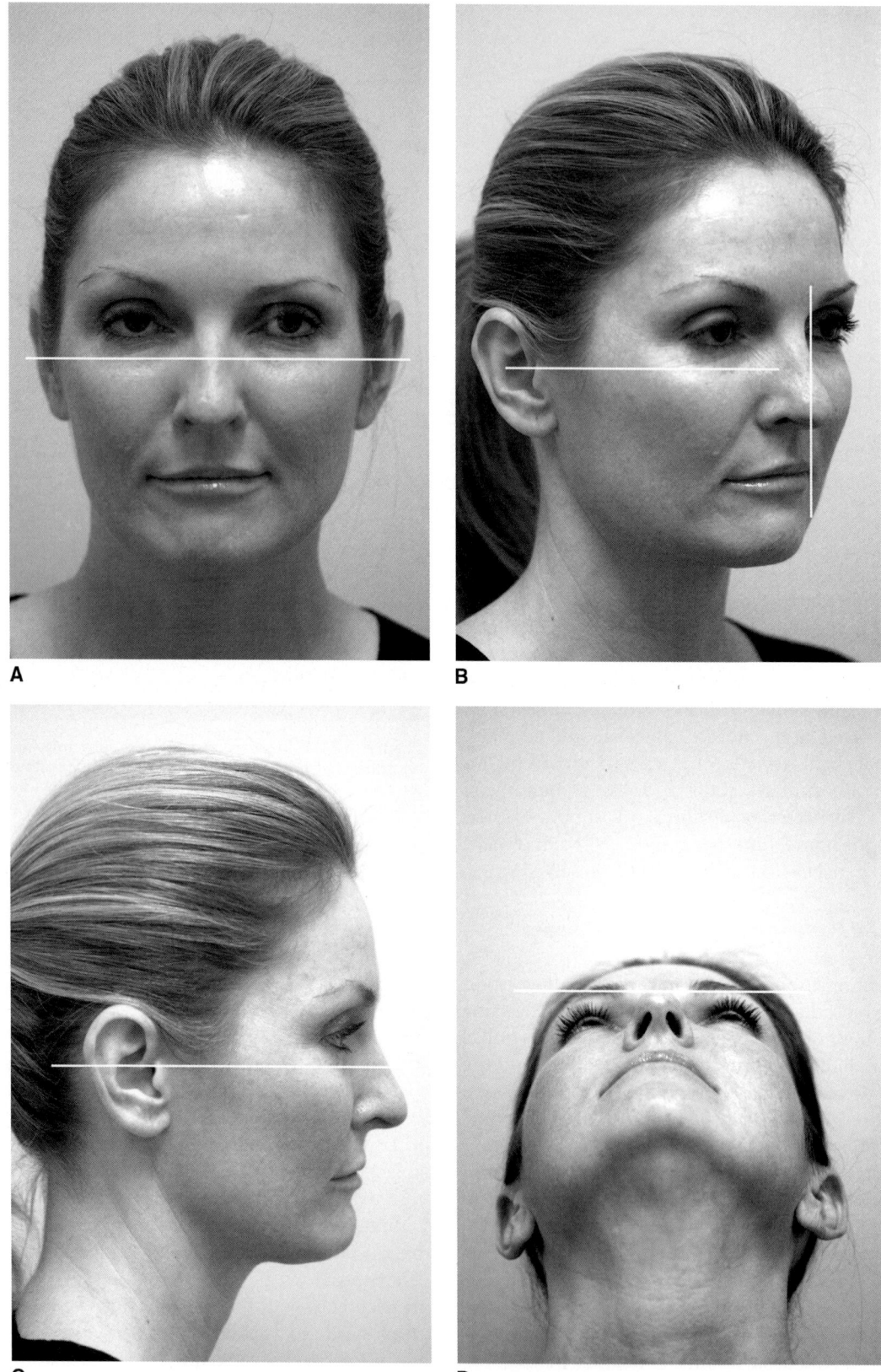

Figure 171.2 Standardized photographic views that show **(A)** frontal, **(B)** right oblique, **(C)** right lateral, and **(D)** basal of the patient. The *horizontal line* drawn in A–C indicates the Frankfort Horizontal Plane that runs through the supratragal point and the inferior orbital rim, which should be respected. The *horizontal line* in D shows the alignment of the nasal tip with the *infrabrow line*. The *vertical line* in B shows the alignment of the nasal tip with the malar eminence.

addition to distortion of the neck, over- or underrotation of the neck can cause the nose to appear erroneously rotated or derotated, respectively, and would compromise any photography for rhinoplasty (Fig. 171.3). Patients may also reflexively attempt to lift their brow if they have significant brow ptosis, making the pre- and postoperative result for browlift or upper blepharoplasty less meaningful. If the patient exhibits this behavior, the photographer should ask that the patient close his or her eyes forcefully and slowly open them until they appear fully open. This maneuver will help break the unwitting contribution of the frontalis muscle. The patient may also instinctively smile when posing for a photograph, so the photographer should gently remind the patient that no facial expression should be displayed.

Each type of planned surgical procedure mandates a different set of standardized positions with or without additional optional views (Table 171.1) (1). Besides patient positioning, distracting elements from jewelry, makeup, clothing, and hairstyling should also be minimized. All obstructive jewelry, for example, necklaces and pendulous earrings, should be removed. Turtlenecks and high-necked collars can also obstruct a straightforward view of the neck and should be pulled down or folded inward to enhance effective communication. All eyeglasses should be removed regardless of what facial surgery is being contemplated. Hairstyling ideally should be pulled back to show an unobstructed view of the eyes, nose, ears, lips, and neck and to be reduced to an unobtrusive element. Shorter hairstyles that do not interfere with any of the major facial features and the neck can be left alone or swept behind the helix of the ear as needed. All makeup should be removed, especially if any dermatologic resurfacing or scar revision is planned.

Lighting and Background

Lighting is also a critical element that should be standardized. Ambient lighting can be used alone or combined with fill lights or flash strobes. If the ambient lighting is too strong and casts a heavy shadow over the patient's facial features, then balanced fill lighting can be used to soften these harsh shadows. Hot lights positioned at

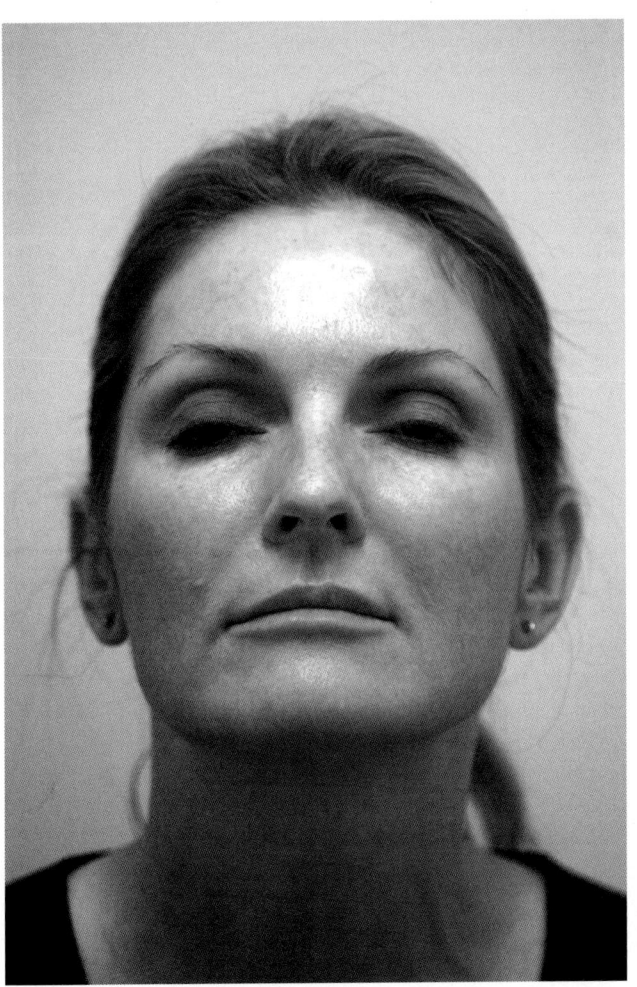
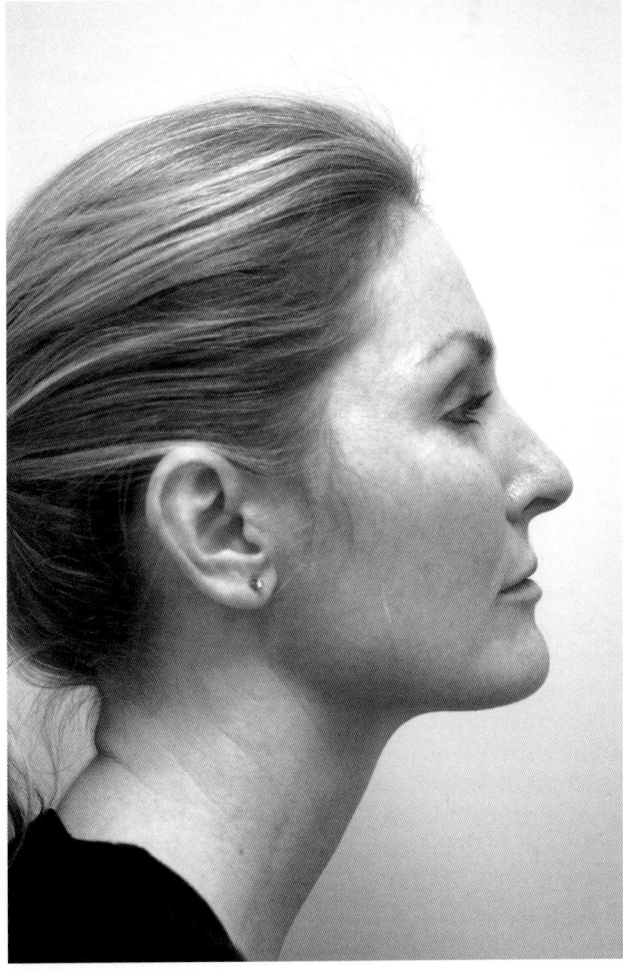

A   **B**

Figure 171.3 Poor patient positioning is shown with the neck overrotated and extended that leads to distortion of the neck as well as for the nose, as seen from the frontal view (**A**) and from the profile view (**B**).

TABLE 171.1	RECOMMENDED, STANDARDIZED PHOTOGRAPHIC VIEWS FOR SPECIFIC FACIAL PROCEDURES

Procedure	Standardized Views
Botulinum toxin (Botox)	Frontal; frontal smiling: frontal frowning: frontal brow elevation (All photographs are taken before the first session regardless of what areas will be treated in order to enhance patient dialogue should the patient complain as well as to reduce the need for further photography if the patient desires other areas treated during future sessions.)
Rhinoplasty	Frontal; basal; L/R oblique; L/R lateral; +/− dorsal (head tilted down for a crooked nose) +/− smiling laterally (If the patient has an active depressor septi muscle that alters the nasal tip position during animation.)
Blepharoplasty/browlift	Frontal; L/R oblique; L/R lateral; closeup (May also take with eyes closed and upward gaze.)
Rhytidectomy	Frontal; L/R oblique; L/R lateral
Otoplasty	Frontal; L/R oblique; L/R lateral; posterior; R/L lateral closeup (Remember to tie long hair back in a bun and/or wear a headband to lift away obstructing hair.)
Malar augmentation	Frontal; L/R oblique; L/R lateral; basal
Hair transplant	Frontal; L/R oblique; L/R lateral; posterior; posterior with head tilted back; frontal with head tilted down +/− closeup of anterior/lateral hairline (When photographing the hair, the hair should be styled in a standardized fashion and "combovers" eliminated.)
Lip augmentation	Frontal; L/R oblique; L/R lateral; closeup mouth (Remember to remove lipstick, lip liners, and other makeup that can interfere with reproducible photography.)
Scar revision	Frontal; L/R oblique; L/R lateral; closeup (Consider reducing the exposure value to highlight the scar.)

45 degrees in front on both sides of the patient can be further softened by aiming the lights away toward reflective umbrellas. A "kicker" light placed behind the patient can fill in any remaining shadows cast by the two forward placed 45-degree lamps and slaved to go off when the camera's shutter is depressed (Fig. 171.4). Placing the patient an appropriate distance away (~2 feet) from the rear wall can also minimize unwanted shadows. Generally, an on-camera flash tends to cause excessive highlights and shadows and a "washed-out" appearance to skin tones, but experimentation will determine the best balance of lighting for a particular room and camera. Rather than use fill lights or strobes, the ambient lighting and the camera's aperture/exposure can be adjusted to achieve the desired lighting objective. Furthermore, the ambient room lighting can be altered to match the color spectrum (e.g., daylight balanced) of the film used or the settings of the camera so that, for example, a green cast from fluorescent lights may be avoided. If shadows and highlights are desired in order to accentuate a scar or other contour irregularity, for example, prominent nasolabial lines for correction with a soft tissue filler, then the balanced fill lights (if used) should be turned off. In addition, the exposure value can be reduced in order to draw out the intended feature. Obviously, the same settings should be used for the postoperative views.

The background should also be uniform and light in color. Ideally, a powder blue background is preferred. Too dark a background can swallow the facial features and should be avoided. Rather than hanging a blue drape behind the patient, a smooth wall can be painted the desired blue, as a wall will remain flat and wrinkle free. Again, using the exact same room with the same lighting will aid in achieving reproducible results. Conversely, carrying a portable blue background material from room to room to photograph the patient will most likely lead to subtle, if not obvious, inconsistencies in the photography. If a wall is to be painted blue, it may be wise to record the exact shade of blue, or corresponding numeric code, so that if the physician should have to relocate the photography room in the future the same blue color can be precisely reproduced.

Intraoperative Photography

Although good pre- and postoperative photography remains the core of this section, proper techniques for superior intraoperative photography should be mentioned herein. Intraoperative photographs can be used to document medicolegally what transpired in the operating theater but primarily serve as an educational tool for other training surgeons or as part of a didactic presentation in a

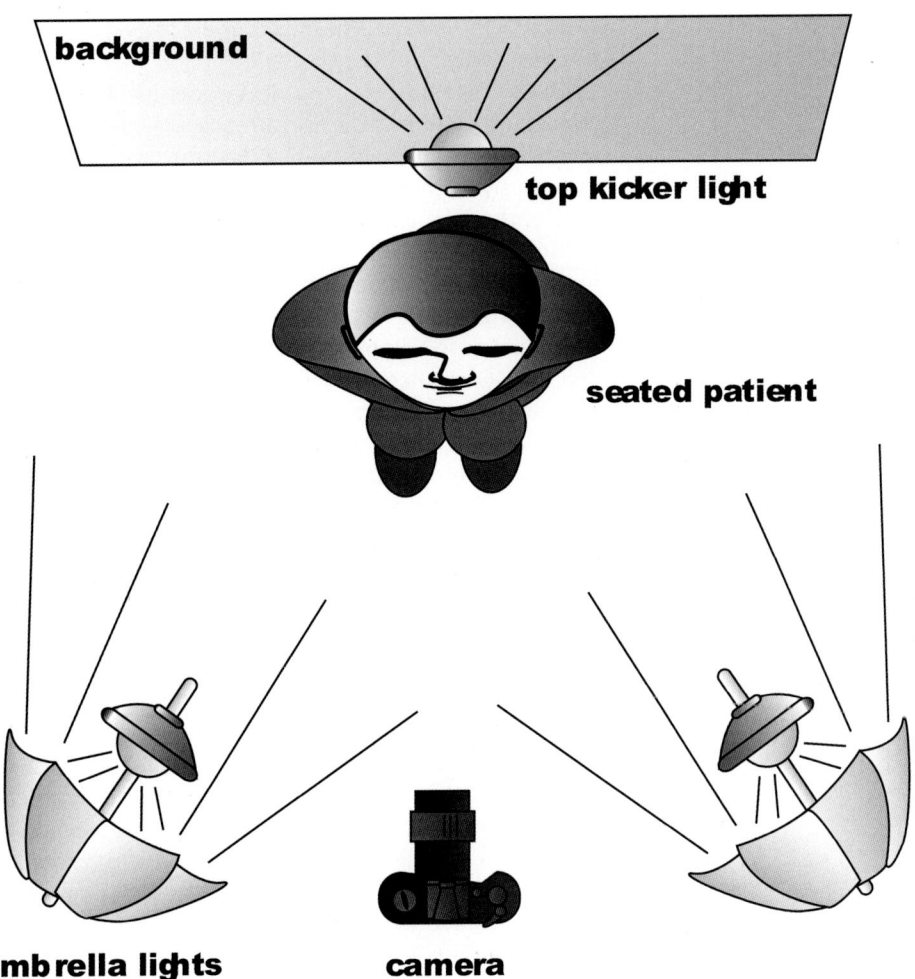

background

top kicker light

seated patient

umbrella lights   **camera**

Figure 171.4 Standardized lighting is very important for good photography. If the ambient lighting is insufficient or casts very harsh shadows, fill lights can be used to soften the shadows. Ideally, two lights placed at 45-degree angles in front of the patient can be softened with the use of reflective umbrellas, and a "kicker" light that illuminates the background positioned above and behind the patient. These lights can be triggered to strobe as a slave unit when the camera's shutter is depressed or remain constantly on to be turned off after the photographic session is over.

scientific forum. A few basic techniques that have evolved from practical experience should be mentioned to help the surgeon achieve excellent results.

First, when taking any intraoperative photograph, care should be exercised to remove all bloodstains both on the patient's tissues and on the surgeon's gloves, as these elements that may appear inconspicuous through the lens become glaringly obtrusive when the final photograph is viewed. If sequential photographs are taken to document the stepwise approach to a procedure, the same angle should be maintained to enhance the clarity of communication. If a removed specimen is to be photographed, a ruler should be placed adjacent to it in order to provide dimensional understanding of the specimen. A metallic ruler can often cast a glare and obscure the legibility of the measurements: instead, a black ruler with white measurement markings minimizes glare and is ideal, albeit possibly difficult to procure.

Although a ring flash mount may provide uniform intraoral or other facial illumination, another method may serve as a better option. The intraoperative room lights are turned off and only two dedicated overhead, directional lights are positioned at 45-degree angles to the

specific facial feature that the surgeon wants to highlight. The camera is set to spot meter off of the subject so that the surrounding background fades to a uniform black. The wrinkled blue background of a surgical gown or other drape held behind the subject always looks unprofessional and distracting. The described technique should be practiced with a particular camera's settings until the correct exposure is established (2).

TRADITIONAL PHOTOGRAPHY

Traditional, 35-mm film photography remains the "gold standard" by which the quality of digital photography is judged, though digital single lens reflex (SLR) photography offers many new advantages. Advantages of digital photography include ability to crop and adjust on a computer, instantaneous pictures, and easy storage and filing of images. The following section will discuss the various equipment needs for digital and 35-mm photography: many of the components discussed for 35-mm photography also apply to digital imaging, as camera body and lens designs for digital imaging have often been based on original 35-mm models.

Camera

Camera models can be divided into two basic types: point-and-shoot and SLR. Point-and-shoot cameras typically have the lens and body sold as one compact unit and are convenient for nonprofessional purposes like vacation photographs where portability is a priority. SLR cameras are higher-end models that usually consist only of the camera body with the lens (which can be interchanged with lenses of other focal lengths as needed) sold separately. Besides higher production quality that is characteristically associated with an SLR camera, this kind of camera also benefits from the absence of parallax error. An SLR camera avoids this distortion because the image seen through the viewfinder exactly matches what the film plate will be exposed to, as a mirror that transmits the image through the lens to the viewfinder is displaced to expose the film plate when the shutter is depressed.

With the rise of digital products, prices for 35-mm SLR cameras have plummeted. Nevertheless, many of the very advanced features that appear on an SLR camera are excessive for clinical photography, for example, high rate of frames taken per second, manual controls, etc. A basic SLR camera body that will accommodate high-quality lenses is sufficient for clinical usage.

Basic Photographic Concepts

In order to take consistently good standard photographs that will allow you to document the nuances of the human facial anatomy, an understanding to basic photography is required. One important concept is the DOF. This is the distance range in which the relevant portions of the image are in sharp focus. The focal point is the point in the image that appears sharpest. For example, if the point of interest is the nose, with the appropriate DOF, everything including the ears would be in focus on frontal view. In this case, the nose would be the focal point and therefore have the sharpest focus within the DOF. Having the correct DOF is important during facial photographic documentation. Digital SLR cameras allow manipulation of the DOF by changing three variables: the focal length of lens, the aperture size, and the distance of the subject to the photographer.

The shorter the focal length of the lens, the larger the DOF. Point-and-shoot cameras exploit this property in order to keep everything in focus. This inverse relationship between the focal length and DOF is important when using digital SLR cameras, as interchanging lenses with different focal lengths can be used to modify DOF. In some cases, distortion can occur with change in focal length; therefore, changing focal length to enhance DOF is not always ideal.

Unlike the inverse relationship between DOF and focal length, the distance between the photographer and the subject directly effects the DOF. At any given focal length, objects that are imaged at long distances will be seen with greater DOF. Space constraints in most studios often limit this possibility.

Of the three variables, the ideal way to increase the DOF is by manipulation of the aperture size (3). The DOF varies inversely with the aperture size. Aperture size is measured in f-stops, which is a value based on a calculation of the ratio of the focal length of the lens to aperture diameter in millimeters. Therefore, an f-stop of f/16 is a smaller aperture size than an f-stop of f/4. In other words, an aperture f/16 provides a greater DOF than an f-stop of f/4. With each increase in f-stop, the aperture area is roughly halved, and the DOF is therefore increased.

When changing aperture size to improve DOF, it is important to realize that exposure will be affected by changes in the aperture size (3). Increasing the DOF by increasing the f-stop will result in less light entering the camera. To maintain the correct photographic exposure when the f-stop is increased, two factors can be manipulated. The first factor is the sensitivity of the medium used to light. In 35-mm film cameras, this was measured with the American Standards Association (ASA) or International Organization for Standardization (ISO) scale. The greater the sensitivity of the medium to light, the higher the ISO (3). Digital SLR cameras have the ability to alter the ISO value. With digital SLR cameras, to maintain the correct photographic exposure when the f-stop is increased, the shutter speed needs to be reduced to prevent underexposure. Shutter speeds range from 1/60 to 1/1,000 of a second. Therefore, if increasing the f-stop is performed to increase the DOF, the shutter speed should be reduced as well.

For clinical purposes, the following basic guidelines are suggested for managing the camera settings. Four basic types of settings exist for most advanced SLR cameras: automatic, aperture priority, shutter priority, and manual. Automatic mode functions by allowing the camera's onboard computer to decide both aperture and shutter speeds. The lack of control using this setting may result in variability. Manual mode allows absolute photographic control but can be burdensome and yield poorly exposed photographs in less than professional hands. Aperture priority (A mode) allows the photographer to adjust the aperture setting while the camera's onboard computer automatically alters the shutter speed to achieve the ideal exposure given the ambient conditions; shutter priority (S mode) allows the converse, that is, control of the shutter speed, while the computer adjusts the aperture automatically. Clinically, aperture priority is the preferred mode, which ensures the appropriate exposure while achieving the best DOF. The smaller the aperture (that correlates with a higher numeric "f"-stop) yields greater DOF. It is helpful to experiment with the different aperture settings to determine the ideal DOF without excessively long shutter speeds, which can in turn lead to camera shake and a resultant blurred photographic image.

Lenses

A high-quality lens that attaches to an SLR camera is the most important element to attain distortion-free, high-quality photographs. Whether shooting with 35-mm film or digital SLR, the lens can be used interchangeably between the two systems. A reputable manufacturer, for example, Nikon or Cannon, is a reliable indicator of lens quality. Lenses are characterized based on the focal length, which is defined as the distance in millimeters from the optical center of the lens to the focal point, which is located on the film or camera sensor if the subject is in focus. The field of view (FOV) is determined by the angle of view from the lens out to the scene and can be measured either vertically or horizontally. Thirty-five-millimeter SLR cameras use larger sensors or films in order to capture a wider FOV. The FOV that is associated with a focal length is usually based on 35-mm photography. For example, in 35-mm photography, lenses with a focal length of 50 mm are called normal as they work without magnification or reduction. Lenses with a short focal length function as wide angle lenses and therefore capture more because they have a wider picture angle. Conversely, lenses with long focal length function as telephoto lenses and have a narrow picture angle.

Digital cameras on the other hand, capture images on sensors called charged coupled devices (CCDs), which are smaller than 35-mm camera frames (3). As a result, the smaller CCD sensor captures only the central portion of the information projected by the lens. This results in a cropped FOV and is the same effect as using a lens with a longer focal length (e.g., telephoto). The correction factor for the difference in size of the sensor to the traditional 35-mm window is called the focal length multiplier (FLM). This is an important concept to understand as it explains why the same lens will take different looking photos on a 35-mm SLR camera body versus a digital SLR. Specifically, at the same focal length, the digital SLR can produce a distortion of the midface (fish-eye look) as a result of the FLM. With digital SLR cameras, the FLM refers to the effective lengthening of the focal length and is equal to the diagonal of the 35-mm film (43.3 mm) divided by the diagonal of the sensor. In the example of Nikon digital SLR cameras, the FLM is 1.5, and therefore, a lens with a focal length of 60 mm would be equivalent to a 90-mm SLR lens when fitted on a digital Nikon SLR. For pictorial documentation, it is critical to use a lens that produces the least distortion and provides the largest DOF to ensure that the entire face is in focus. Macro lenses between 90 and 105 mm meet these criteria for 35-mm SLR cameras, and macro 60 mm meet these criteria for digital SLR cameras. Although a better DOF is provided by lenses with shorter focal lengths, the facial anatomy distortion becomes significant.

For 35-mm film portrait photography, a 105-mm macro lens will provide photographic images without shape distortion like a disproportionately magnified nose and reduced ears in a fish-eye look that may be present with other focal lengths. For digital photography, a 60-mm macro lens will provide the optimal photographic image for facial photography.

Data Back

An optional feature that may be worth purchasing for an SLR-type camera body is a data back, which usually replaces the hinged door on the back side of the camera used for film exchange. The data back provides the capacity of recording time and date onto the exposed film, which may serve as a useful tool for memory recall, photographic organization, and legal documentation. Digital cameras, on the other hand, do not require this feature, as the time, date, and other information are recorded with each image automatically.

Viewfinder Grid

The standard unmarked viewfinder can be replaced in many camera models with one that has vertical and horizontal markings on it. These marks help guide the photographer when following the guidelines enumerated in Figure 171.1 for good photography, for example, the Frankfort Horizontal Plane, aligning the inner canthus to the outer oral commissure on the oblique view, etc. (Electronic, on-demand grids come equipped on some high-end digital camera models that replicate this feature.)

Tripod

Speaking of camera shake, a tripod upon which a camera can be mounted promotes a stable platform for portrait photography. For intraoperative usage, setting up and using a tripod can be overly taxing and also violate sterile surgical field. If a tripod is to be used for portrait photography, several tripod features are worth acquiring. A quick-release feature on the tripod head permits the camera to be rapidly removed and taken free hand as needed. An easily adjustable tripod neck that allows rotation of the camera to achieve horizontal and vertical framing is also an important feature. Finally, wheels that can be mounted to the base of the tripod afford easy maneuverability so that the tripod can be positioned without having to lift and relocate it.

Film

Although traditional film-based photography may be divided into 35-mm, medium-, and large-format film types, 35 mm has remained the mainstay of practical clinical photography with the latter two types relegated to nonmedical, artistic endeavors. Thirty-five-millimeter film may be purchased either as negative or transparency (reversal) stock. Generally, the latter has been preferred for several reasons. Slide film produces accurate skin tones, is relatively inexpensive, is easy to project for scientific and patient communication, requires little storage space, and can have good archival preservation. Generally, if sufficient lighting is present, then a fine-grain film like 25 or 64 speed film is preferred for the high quality of the image and reproducibility of that quality when enlarged (4). If the physician prefers to remain in a film-based medium, it would be advised to consider using a digital camera or a Polaroid for immediate feedback and to ensure that the necessary image has been obtained. Also, use of a digital camera and/or Polaroid facilitates immediate patient dialogue that would otherwise be deferred due to processing time of slide film.

DIGITAL IMAGE MANAGEMENT

A few years ago, digital photography was in a nascent stage of development, and chapters described digital imaging only briefly as a tentative alternative. Today, digital photography has continued to make rapid technologic strides and has challenged 35-mm photography for its many benefits: no consumable costs of film, instant image feedback, capacity for digital morphing, no physical storage space, no processing time or expense, and easy reproducibility and backup. Nevertheless, the initial setup cost for digital photography can be quite high due to the associated hardware requirements, for example, computer, cables, software, storage, etc. Today, most offices already use computers, so few additional hardware expenditure is typically required. Moreover, the cost of technology is rapidly tumbling, and the lack of consumables will offset initial outlay very rapidly, unless every photograph is printed, for instance, on expensive inkjet paper. The primary criticism leveled against digital photography in the past concerned the purported dubious image quality as compared with the "gold standard" of 35-mm film. However, that argument is truly obsolete with the rise of 12 megapixel cameras and beyond. No accurate comparison can be made between a digital pixel and the silver-halide grain of film, but this argument really borders on arcane academic banter and lacks any practical clinical import. This section discusses input devices (digital cameras and scanners [to convert 35-mm images over to digital]), image processing and storage (compression, archiving, and morphing), and output devices (printers and projectors) (5).

Input Devices

Cameras

Like 35-mm film cameras, digital cameras may be broadly classified as point-and-shoot and SLR-type models (Fig. 171.5). Due to an SLR digital camera's expense, many consumers purchase a point-and-shoot digital model. Like 35-mm cameras, an SLR digital camera can offer higher

image quality and flexibility. Oftentimes, an SLR digital model will accommodate traditional 35-mm lenses, which can greatly save expense for the owner of these same lenses. Obviously, a high-quality, aspherical lens achieves commensurate value as in 35-mm photography. However, unlike traditional 35-mm film photography, the digital camera body contributes significantly to image quality, in terms of pixel resolution, color variation, dynamic range (i.e., the ability to capture the broad spectrum of bright whites to dark blacks), and light sensitivity. For these reasons, as mentioned for SLR cameras, it is imperative that the same digital camera and lens (not to mention the same lighting and studio) be used to attain consistent photographic results. Unlike 35-mm film in which a 105-mm macro-type lens provides a distortion-free image in portrait photography, various lenses may provide a true 1:1 image for a particular digital camera based on the size of the CCD or CMOS (complementary metal-oxide semiconductor),

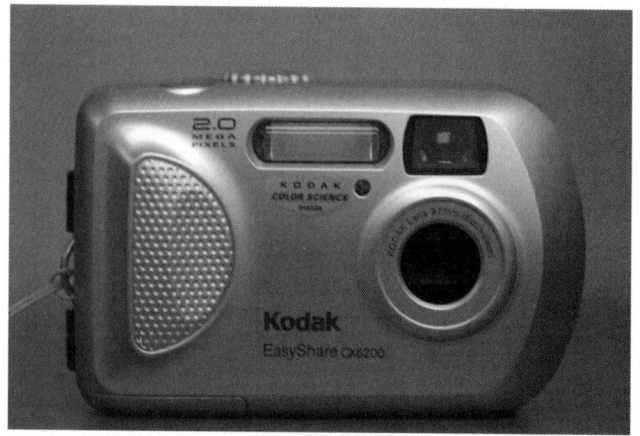

A

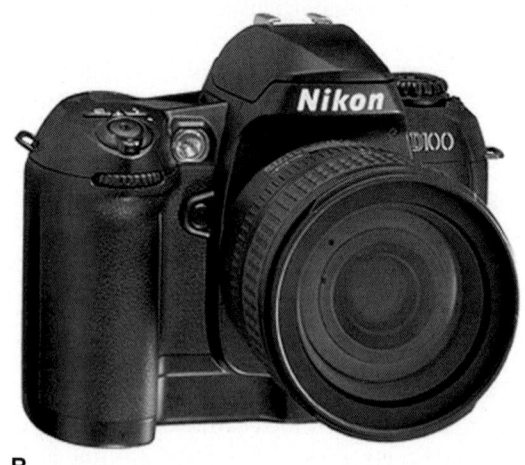

B

Figure 171.5 Like 35-mm cameras, digital cameras can be classified as point-and-shoot **(A)** and as SLR models **(B)**. Unlike 35-mm photography, the digital camera body can be as important as the quality of the lens in obtaining superlative photographic results. In general, digital SLR models have better build-out quality, but the prospective consumer should always evaluate objective reviews before any purchase.

which would be analogous to the 35-mm film plate. As reviewed above, the prospective consumer should ask the manufacturer of the SLR digital camera, which focal-length lens will provide a distortion-free 1:1 image for that specific camera model. As a general example, the 60-mm Cannon macro lens on a Cannon SLR body will achieve distortion-free photos comparable to the 105-mm macro/35-mm SLR combination. Since film is not used, ISO or ASA ratings that describe the light sensitivity of a particular film stock are not applicable for digital cameras. Nevertheless, as most consumers are familiar with what an ISO/ASA rating means, some digital cameras have adopted this terminology to describe the light sensitivity of a CCD/CMOS, with standard digital models having an ISO rating of between 50 and 200 and higher-end cameras over 400. DOF can also be different for a specific "f"-stop, as compared with a traditional 35-mm setup. Generally, a smaller numeric "f"-stop (i.e., wider aperture) will yield a greater DOF than in a 35-mm equivalent. Despite these differences, many of the principles outlined for good photography and basic equipment parallel those discussed for 35-mm photography.

Scanners

Scanners are used to convert a 35-mm library or select printed images into the digital medium. There are basically two types: flatbed and film scanners. The former consists of a specialized camera housed below a clear glass panel with a hard, opaque cover that scans an image in a linear fashion to convert it into a digital version. The flatbed scanner benefits from versatility (ability to scan multiple media, like photographs, tables, graphs, text, and—with the right adapter—even transparency or negative film) and economy (a relatively low cost). Film scanners are dedicated to scanning only slides or negatives and can do so often very quickly and at a higher resolution. Unfortunately, they also tend to cost considerably more in price. Sophisticated image correction software to repair damaged and faded slides are also featured in some high-end film scanners, like with the Nikon's series of film scanners.

Four parameters define a scanner's ultimate output quality: optical resolution, bit depth, color accuracy, and optical density (OD). Optical resolution simply refers to the number of pixels per inch (ppi) and can be achieved by a straightforward pixel per pixel output or manipulated by a process known as interpolation, which can prove to be inferior. Most scanners offer an optical resolution between 300 to 4,800 ppi and an interpolated resolution of 0 to 1,900 ppi. Generally, 300-ppi scanning is sufficient for printed materials, whereas a 72-ppi resolution is adequate for web or monitor display. Bit depth refers to the maximum number of colors that each pixel of an image can display. This numeric value is expressed as the exponential power of 2. For instance, a 1-bit image has two colors (2^1) like black and white. Although most monitors only output 24-bit images (i.e., 2^{24}, or 16.7 million

colors), scanners can exceed this value and be 30, 36, or even 42 bits. However, these higher bits are not superfluous, but the added data undergo a selection process for the best bits of color information to yield a 24-bit output product. Color accuracy refers to the scanner's ability to reproduce faithfully the original photographic image's colors. The International Color Consortium measures this accuracy with the "Delta E" value. Good Delta E values fall below 10, whereas poorer figures exceed 30. Finally, the OD usually is only a descriptor on higher-end models and denotes the brightness that a scanner can capture. OD is expressed in a logarithmic fashion so that a scanner with a 3.6 D (or OD) will have 10 times the brightness of 1 with a mere 2.8 D. If a scanner does not list an OD, the rating probably falls between 2.8 and 3.0. It is recommended to have a minimum of 3.2 D for transparencies and 3.4 D for negatives.

Image Retrieval, Storage, and Morphing

Compression

Compression refers to the mathematical algorithm used to reduce an image's overall size and therefore necessary memory allocation. Although there are many competing compression formats, the two most popular and relevant for clinical utility are TIFF (Tagged Image File Format) and JPEG (Joint Photographic Experts Group). TIFF represents a "lossless" compression, in which there is no loss in image resolution after the image is compressed. Unfortunately, due to the smaller compression ratio (typically 2:1 or 3:1), file sizes can be quite large on the order of several megabytes. JPEG images are "lossy" images that lose some quality (usually undetectable to the human eye) when compressed with reduction in file size from 10:1 to 300:1. Clearly, the more the file is compressed, the greater the loss in quality. Interestingly, every time a JPEG image is cropped or altered in any way then saved, additional loss of image quality is incurred. If the image will be manipulated numerous times, it may be wise to work from a TIFF image then convert to JPEG on the final edit.

Editing and Morphing

One of the complaints about digital imaging concerns the ability to "doctor" or alter an image unethically. This charge is a bit misguided because 35-mm film can also be digitally altered and returned to its original format. Further, some editing software like Canfield Scientific's Mirror system has built-in authentication process to detect altered images. What constitutes ethical editing? Color balancing and fine adjustment of hues and brightness, just as if you had sent film to a processing laboratory, should be considered proper. Further, cropping extraneous elements in an image so long as the image integrity has not been undermined should be deemed acceptable as well. These powerful tools underscore the strengths of the digital format. Intentional editing, or morphing, allows alteration of a digital image so that the surgeon can communicate with the patient an intended aesthetic result. Care should be taken to avoid overpromising and to remind the patient of the shortcomings in accuracy of a digitally morphed image. Morphing can be particularly effective when demonstrating to a patient the change in nasal profile and/or change in the neck and chin region for two principal reasons. First, the patient rarely if ever sees himself or herself from the side view. Second, the soft tissues are contrasted against a blue background, making image alterations relatively straightforward (as compared with moving skin over skin in a frontal view).

Archiving

The lack of physical space that a digital library takes up is also an undeniable benefit. However, the physician would be wise to select a good archiving program early so that the growing catalog of digital images can be easily organized and subsequently retrieved. There are two basic types of archiving software: browser and catalog. Browser-type software permits simple retrieval of graphic images and is usually bundled free with purchased digital cameras. On the other hand, catalog software often permits more sophisticated handling of many file types (text, graphic, video, and audio) and can attach metadata to a file. Metadata refers to the descriptive text that can be attached to a file to facilitate its retrieval, for example, "Susan Smith," "Crooked Nose," etc. It is often easier to maintain the alphanumeric name that a camera assigns to an image, for example, DSC_1789. jpg, and simply attach descriptive metadata to it. When organizing patient's images in a hierarchical folder, placement of the year, followed by the month, then the day, for example, 2005-11-6 for November 6, 2005, is preferred so that chronologic order is maintained.

Storage

Digital imaging permits infinite backup without the considerable expense associated with copying film transparencies or negatives. Backing up data should occur on a daily or weekly basis, and data should be stored both on premises and off site to ensure maximal protection. Many options exist for data storage including magnetic drives, magnetic–optical drives, optical drives, tape drives, and hard drives. Generally, tape and magnetic media are preferred for large storage backups, whereas optical media are better suited for smaller file-to-file storage.

Output Devices

Printers

Three principal types of printers exist for photographic reproduction: inkjet, dye-sublimation, and color laser. Inkjet printers comprise the majority of printer sales and can provide high-quality print resolution. They function by spraying small amounts of ink onto the paper in halftones

that are layered on top of one another. Parameters that define a high-quality printer are as follows: printer resolution expressed in dots per inch (dpi) with a good printer having upward of 1,440 dpi; the number of color inkwells (3 being a relatively low number and 6 being a favorable number); and the size of the ink droplets (3 to 4 pL are superior to 6 to 18 pL). Lightfastness refers to the printer's capacity to produce an image that retains color and avoids unfavorable color shifts over time, with some recent models being able to exceed 100 years in lightfastness. Dye-sublimation printers, or dye-subs, work by depositing vaporized ink lifted from a colored ribbon onto a specialized paper to achieve a more continuous-toned print. Unfortunately, these printers are more expensive and can only print a predetermined size, for example, 5 × 7 or 8 × 10 inch. Paper costs can also exceed that of quality inkjet paper. Color laser printers can produce high-quality images at a faster rate than inkjet printers. In addition, consumable costs can be lower, and machines are more durable. However, initial cost outlay for a laser printer can be considerably higher than a standard inkjet. Office volume and cost expenditure will dictate which printer is best suited for the job. The one major limitation that still faces the conversion of on-screen to printed digital images concerns color correction. Many digital images are created in RGB (red–green–blue) mode that is native to computer monitors. However, printers work in CMYK (cyan, magenta, yellow, and black [the "key" color]) mode. The translation from one color scheme to another can cause some color mismatch. Details for color correction lie beyond the scope of this chapter.

Projectors

Scientific, marketing, and business conferences have attested to the advent of the digital revolution: increasingly, digital projectors are preferred to traditional slide projectors for effective communication. The ability to embed animation and video footage during a digital presentation has made the digital format an unquestionably superior medium of communication. The different types of projectors that are available today include cathode ray tubes (CRTs), liquid crystal displays (LCDs), digital light projectors (DLPs), and plasma display panels. CRT projectors deliver a strictly analog signal, as compared with all of the other aforementioned types. Despite this fact, some proponents of CRTs argue that they provide as good if not superior image quality to their digital counterparts. LCD projectors may be divided into higher quality Polysilicon types and standard active-matrix styles. DLPs rely on micromirrors and have been cited to produce brighter images and have superior video capacity. However, LCDs have been thought of having better color contrast and saturation. Plasma screens work by combining pixels with CRT phosphors.

Several specific parameters should be sought when evaluating a projector's utility. Clearly, portability is important for someone seeking this option. Native resolution comes in VGA (640 × 480), SVGA (800 × 600), XGA (1,024 × 768), SXGA (1,280 × 1,024), and UXGA (1,600 × 1,200). CRTs do not have a native resolution and are deemed resolution independent, which means that they do not need to be matched to a monitor's resolution. Conversely, digital projectors should be matched to a monitor's resolution as precisely as possible. If several computers are intended for use with one projector, then the projector should be matched to the computer monitor with the highest resolution. A minimum of an SVGA projector should be acquired for straightforward graphic presentations, but an SXGA is preferable. A projector's brightness is measured in ANSI lumens with a minimum of 300 to 500 ANSI recommended for dimly lit rooms and 1,000 ANSI for a well-lit room. For an auditorium, at least 1,500 ANSI should be sought. The contrast ratio that describes the range of brightest whites to darkest blacks is also a valuable feature with a range of 100:1 (low) to 2,000:1 (high). Zoom lenses permit image size adjustment without the burden of having to move the unit. Digital keystone correction adjusts the image to reduce distortions that arise from aiming the projector at the wall from an angle. Lamp life can range from 40 to 40,000 hours, with the majority falling between 1,000 and 2,000 hours. Lamp replacement can be expensive so this factor should also be integrated into the choice of a projector.

CLOSING THOUGHTS AND THE FUTURE

Good photographic principles should be adhered to whether working in 35-mm or digital photography. Photographic documentation should always be obtained in any cosmetic or reconstructive endeavor but may also serve as a reliable tool for other types of head and neck surgical procedures on an individual case-by-case basis. The rise of digital photography has transformed the landscape of scientific and professional communication. As technology continues to evolve, digital photography will most likely entirely supplant analog 35-mm film. The next edition of this chapter will probably bear the short title "Pictorial Documentation: Digital Imaging."

REFERENCES

1. Kontis TC. Photography in facial plastic surgery. In: Papel ID, et al., eds. *Facial plastic and reconstructive surgery.* 2nd ed. New York: Thieme Medical Publishers, 2002:116–124.
2. Williams EF, Lam SM. *Comprehensive facial rejuvenation: a practical and systematic guide to surgical management of the aging face.* Philadelphia, PA: Lippincott Williams & Wilkins, 2004.
3. Swamy RS, Sykes JM, Most SP. Principles of photography in rhinoplasty for the digital photographer. *Clin Plast Surg* 2010;37(2):213–212.
4. Tardy ME. *Principles of photography in facial plastic surgery.* New York: Thieme Medical Publishers, 1992.
5. Lam SM. Digital imaging in the plastic surgical practice. *Int J Cosmet Surg Aesthetic Dermatol* 2002;4:199–212.

172 Grafts and Implants in Facial, Head, and Neck Surgery

G. Richard Holt   Christian L. Stallworth

The biotechnology of implants in otolaryngology and head and neck surgery has expanded rapidly, and facial, head, and neck implants now include autologous biomaterials, metals, polymers, synthetics, and tissue-engineered materials. Since the range of requirements for implants ranges from bone replacement and stabilization implants to soft tissue fillers, the science of surgical implantology now involves cell surface physics, molecular level biochemistry, and tissue engineering. Biomaterials, both biologic and synthetics, for osseous and soft tissue augmentation are becoming increasingly important in reconstructing defects of traumatic, congenital, extirpative, and aging etiologies.

BIOCOMPATIBILITY OF IMPLANTS

Cells do not adhere directly to the surface of implanted synthetic materials. A substance in the extracellular matrix binds the cell to the surface. This substance is essential for initial cell adhesion and proliferation. The substrate needed varies with the type of cell. Well-differentiated cells, such as chondroblasts, osteoblasts, and epithelial cells, require substrate characteristics distinct from those needed by less differentiated cells, such as fibroblasts. Focal contacts represent adhesion sites to specific extracellular matrix proteins adsorbed on the implant surface. Focal contacts typically occur in low-motility cells, such as fibroblasts and epithelial cells. The composition of the substrate (the adsorbed layer of protein on the implant surface) is crucial for tight cellular adhesion. Proteins such as fibronectin, vitronectin, cold-insoluble globulin, and possibly proteoglycans provide the necessary substrate for this adhesion.

The extracellular matrix contains collagen, elastin, and fibronectin interwoven into a hydrated network of glycosaminoglycan chains. The glycosaminoglycan chains are long, negatively charged polysaccharide chains that link proteins to form giant proteoglycan molecules. Interaction with cell membrane receptors provides linkage for cellular attachment to adsorbed extracellular matrix on the surface of a biomaterial. Tissue cells do adhere to the implant surface—not directly but by means of a complex series of protein attachments.

When implants are placed in facial soft tissue, the primary tissue reaction includes protein adsorption and cellular attachment. The predominant cell attaching to the protein layer is the fibroblast. Within the first week, the fibroblast lays down immature collagen on the implant surface, or interstices. The usual response to a soft tissue implant is production of a fibrous capsule or collagen fiber ingrowth, which secures the implant. A smooth implant such as silicone more often elicits dense capsule formation than does a porous implant. If an implant is too reactive, has surface contamination, or is biodegradable, the host tissue response usually is aggressive macrophage activity, increased vascularity, breakdown of the overlying skin, and extrusion of the implant. The presence of inflammatory cells such as neutrophils and macrophages suggests poor tissue response to the implanted material.

After placement of an implant, protein adsorption occurs. As a hole is drilled into bone to receive the implant, the bone must not be heated to more than 45°C to 50°C, or osteoblasts die. An implant in bone induces a rapid host response. The first stage is formation of a small hematoma and a cascade of chemical breakdown products. These substances act on blood vessels and attract cells from surrounding tissue. Because cortical bone is avascular, most blood products come from the marrow-containing spaces of the bone.

The second stage is tissue organization, regeneration, and repair. The duration is related to the extent of injury and implantation site geometry. Extracellular processes and cell functioning can be affected by soluble and insoluble particles from the implant and by the mechanical influence of the implant itself. The third stage of repair is remodeling, which affects the implant–host tissue interface and occurs over weeks or months. Appropriate stress levels must be imposed on the bone adjacent to the implant. Bone-binding intensity can be measured according to the shear or torque forces needed to produce failure. Bone is the main contributor to tensile strength of bonding; other tissues are less important. The basal lamina in contact with a bone implant contains type IV collagen, laminin, and proteoglycans. These constituents of the ground substance are deposited in or adjacent to the mineralized layer. Mineralization of the ground substance seems to be important for transmission of compression and for shear and tensile loads.

CHARACTERISTICS OF IMPLANTS

Implant material is characterized by composition, strength, biodegradability, and resistance to stress and fatigue (1,2). The properties of bulk material, however, can differ from those of the implant surface at the tissue–implant interface because of surface alterations by design or physicochemical reaction. The materials and clinical applications for facial, head, and neck implants are summarized in Table 172.1.

Metallic Implants

Metallic devices can be composed of a single metal or an alloy of several metals. Alloys are developed to improve qualities of the original metal by adding other metals with characteristics that improve biocompatibility or mechanical attributes. The principal metals used in facial implants are titanium, stainless steel, and tantalum. Chromium, aluminum, cobalt, copper, nickel, and tungsten are included in alloys.

Metals are crystalline materials with well-defined, orderly, three-dimensional arrangements of atoms that form a microscopic lattice characteristic of each metal. The lattice can be modified by means of heating, cooling, hardening, or altering the physical properties of the metal to achieve a particular result. Lattice defects can modify the characteristics of the metal. Large structural defects can cause failure to withstand external stresses. Metallic biomaterials are characterized by elastic modulus, tensile strength, percentage elongation, compressive strength, shear strength and modulus, and strain. Stress is the ability of a material to withstand a given load per cross-sectional area. The material must be designed to meet the functional requirements of the dental or maxillofacial implant.

TABLE 172.1   FACIAL, HEAD, AND NECK IMPLANTS

Category	Biomaterial	Clinical Application
Metals and metallic alloys	Stainless steel	Sutures, fracture wires, reconstruction bars
	Titanium and its alloys	Mandibular bone trays, osseointegrated implants, cranioplasty, orbital floor implants
	Platinum–iridium	Implantable electrodes
	Gold	Eyelid implant
Polymers	PMMA	Cranioplasty, tissue adhesive
	Cyanoacrylate	Tissue adhesive
	Silicone elastomers	Soft tissue augmentation, tissue expanders
	PTFE	Joint prosthesis covering, vocal cord injections
	ePTFA	Soft tissue augmentation, orbital floor implant
	Polyurethane	Artificial skin
	Dacron, nylon polyesters	Sutures, onlay mesh, mandibular trays
	High-density polyethylene, porous	Soft tissue augmentation, temporomandibular prosthesis
Ceramics	Bioglass	Middle ear ossicular replacement
	Hydroxylapatite	Joint prosthesis covering, bone-conduction filler, bone augmentation
	Aluminum oxide	Cranioplasty, artificial ocular prostheses
Nonceramics	HAC	Bone filler, cranioplasty, bone conduction
Biologic materials	Polyglycolic acid	Sutures, implants
	Polylactic acid	Timed-release drug delivery, implants
	Collagen	Dermal augmentation, soft tissue support
	Bone-stimulation proteins	Cartilage or bone induction
	Hyaluronic acid	Soft tissue filler
	Human acellular dermis	Soft tissue filler, augmentation

Stress versus strain curves are generated experimentally for implant materials. They provide information about the bulk material independent of shape or thickness. These can be used to predict the response of the material to mechanical forces on an implant in a particular use. The forces of shear, compression, tension, torsion, and bending must be considered in selection of a material for an implant. *In vitro* loading studies are performed to assess how a material responds to long-term wear. Most metals relax with time, and the relaxation can cause metal fatigue and implant failure. A relatively brittle metal, such as stainless steel, can function well initially but with long-term use can fail because of fatigue. All metals corrode when exposed to living tissue; the gradual result is failure of many metal implants. Stainless steel, an alloy of iron, chromium, nickel, molybdenum, and manganese, resists corrosion well. It can, however, undergo gradual plastic deformation.

Titanium and its alloys are among the most biocompatible metallic implants used today. Titanium is lightweight and corrosion resistant and has high tissue acceptance. It is rather soft and when not anchored to bone can be deformed by loading forces. Used in mandibular reconstruction and for anchoring screws in facial applications, titanium performs well. Tantalum and vanadium have been used as bone trays for mandibular reconstruction, but the mechanical properties are not as good as those of titanium. Tantalum and vanadium are not strong, can fatigue rapidly, and must be removed after the mandible heals. Some metallic implants, such as stainless steel, have a better stress response than does bone. This can cause stress shielding of the bone and impede formation of new bone. Metal implants may have to be removed after the bone is stabilized to allow growth and development.

Ceramics

Ceramics have a microscopic lattice structure. Glass ceramics, on the other hand, have an amorphous atomic structure. Most biologic implants are glass ceramics—combinations of silicon dioxide (SiO_2) and crystalline lattice materials embedded in this glass. Glass ceramics are thermally resistant and can be used when thermal shock can occur. Glass ceramics last well in the body. They are well tolerated and biocompatible. Because of a peculiar grain size and distribution, however, glass ceramics are susceptible to cracking from stress concentration. Clinically, these are considered brittle materials; they fracture rather than bend when subjected to excessive stress. This limits the use of glass ceramic implants in the head and neck to areas with minimal force loading, such as a tympanic ossicle.

Ceramics made with alumina compounds also are used in dental implants. The device is designed so the shape facilitates biomechanical stress application without fracture. Hydroxylapatite is another form of ceramic; it is characterized as bioreactive. It comes as a powder and is reconstituted as a paste for dental and bone replacement. Hydroxylapatite is resorbable and osteoconductive, and it increases bone density. It is composed of elements that exist in the ground substance of bone, that is, calcium and phosphorus. Hydroxylapatite can provide a substrate for osseointegration and osseoconduction when used as a bone replacement material for facial, head, and neck defects.

Facial augmentation with calcium hydroxylapatite (Radiesse, Merz USA, Greensboro, NC) microspheres in a gel carrier of carboxymethylcellulose can provide soft tissue enhancement for a correction period of 12 to 18 months when injected subdermally. Because the hydroxylapatite microsphere is in a gel suspension, the material can be massaged after injection into the tissues to create a smooth appearance (3). When used in porous granular form for facial skeleton augmentation, the material has been found to maintain its bony skeletal projection for at least 2 years (4).

Polymers

No synthetic implant material can exactly reproduce the biomechanical properties of bone. Ceramics and metals are stronger than human bone, and polymers are more flexible. Polymers are useful in implantation because the mechanical properties can be altered to suit the application. These properties are derived from the structural and chemical composition, which are related to length and cross-linking. Varying these two characteristics can produce a wide range of polymer properties, from soft and fragile to hard and brittle. The implant designer can choose a polymer that provides the characteristics needed for a particular situation.

The most commonly used medical polymers are polyurethanes, silicones, and polymethyl methacrylate (PMMA). These polymers are reasonably strong and biocompatible. When supplied as porous fibers (polytetrafluoroethylene [PTFE], nylon, polylactic acid, and polyglycolic acid), these materials can be woven fabric as well as suture material. Expanded PTFE (ePTFA) fabric (Gore-Tex, Gore Medical Co., Flagstaff, AZ) has excellent biocompatibility when used for soft tissue augmentation or vascular repair. Mechanical stresses on polymer implants usually are small. When used for mandibular replacement, a polymer is tested for the same mechanical tolerances as are metals, including tensile strength, modulus of elasticity, stress, and strain. Impact testing is important when a material is used for skull reconstruction. Internal defects that occur during molding and processing can cause cracks and implant failure.

Polymers are manufactured by means of thermoplastic molding (the material is formed in a heat-softened state in a mold) or by means of thermosetting (the insoluble polymers are cured by cross-linking). Suture material is formed by means of extrusion of the polymer through small holes in a die to produce a fiber thinned to the proper diameter before cooling. Used as a glue, PMMA, ethyl-2-cyanoacrylate, and butyl-2-cyanoacrylate produce histotoxic cellular reactions and an exothermic reaction. A permanent injectable polymer of cleaned microspheres of PMMA suspended in bovine collagen (ArteFill, Suneva Medical, San Diego, CA) is FDA approved for augmentation of the nasolabial folds. Serious complications such as granuloma formation have not been reported with this synthetic injectable, allegedly owing to the minimalization of the number of microspheres smaller than 20 μm (5).

Polydioxanone (PDS) is a resorbable material utilized in suture material and in thin sheets for support of osseous defects, usually an orbital wall fracture. Recently, PDS foil (PDS Flexible Plate, Mentor, San Diego, CA) has been utilized to support nasal cartilaginous structures during septoplasty and rhinoplasty, which can be particularly useful because of its low extrusion rate, structural strength during healing, and ability to support multiple free fragments of septal cartilage as a scaffold for reimplantation (6,7).

Biologic Materials

Grafts of nonhuman biologic material and xenografts are considered implants because they often are used for tissue augmentation. Bovine collagen in injectable solution or sheets (Zyderm, Allergan Medical, Irvine, CA) is enzymatically modified to diminish cutaneous sensitivity reactions and to decrease resorption time. When the macrophage system of the host identifies this collagen as foreign, immunologic defenses form antibodies to the collagen. Because collagen is similar in many ways among species, this problem can be diminished but not eliminated with biochemical alteration of unique proteins. Synthesis of components of human dermal collagen and basement membrane, such as polyglycolic acid and polylactic acid, has produced suture and implant material that is slowly resorbed by means of acid hydrolysis. These materials do not induce the intense immunologic response of animal collagen. They also are used as the carriers of sustained-release drugs in implantable drug delivery systems.

Human acellular dermis matrix, harvested from cadavers, is utilized primarily as a soft tissue augmentation material for the face. It can also serve as a "filler" or "scaffolding" for repair of a nasal septal perforation, where this material is placed between opposing flaps of nasal mucosa; if exposed, it allows for reepithelialization on its surface. Foreign antigenicity of this human allograft is achieved by leaching out the cells; however, there are "ghost channels" of preexisting vascular structures that may serve to support revascularization of the tissue. There is a tendency of this biomaterial to resorb with time in some patients.

Biodegradable (resorbable) plates and screws are not dissimilar to certain biodegradable suture materials. These firm implants are generally composed of biosynthetic polymers and copolymers of polylactide and polyglycolide and are heat malleable to fit the contour of the bony surface.

They should be especially considered in pediatric fracture patients, where metallic plates can cause stress shielding and loss of bone growth and remodeling capabilities. Such minimally invasive bioabsorbable bone plates are being increasingly utilized in facial skeleton fractures, and they have been shown to be as strong as a titanium plate when fixating fractures of the mandibular body (8). A so-called "interflex" design allows for decreasing the volume of the plate while still maintaining a low stiffness and an absorption rate that allows for gradual reduction of mechanical stability commensurate with a gradual increase in load bearing of the healing mandible.

Patient-Specific Implants

With the growing availability of three-dimensional radiographic computer modeling, surgeons can preoperatively analyze bony and soft tissue defects through virtual manipulation. This can even be done for existing defects, but also prospectively to forecast a defect that will result from an ablative procedure. With this technology comes the ability to fabricate *patient-specific implants* (PSIs). Using the patient's native contralateral anatomy or gender- and age-specific norms, implants can be constructed to replace tissue loss in multiple dimensions. Examples include preoperative fabrication of mandibular reconstruction plates to be used following composite resection of the mandible or multidimensional implants needed to replace a complex midface defect resulting from maxillectomy. In this way, manufactures are able to tailor their implant materials to precisely restore unique, patient-specific defects.

Polyetheretherketone (PEEK) (Synthes Craniomaxillofacial, West Chester, PA) is a semicrystalline polyaromatic linear polymer that is inert, nonporous, and customizable. More than 20 years of reliable use in the aerospace, automotive, and electrical industries led to its ultimate use as substitute for bone grafting and titanium cages in the treatment of cervical disc disease. PEEK has proven biocompatible, strong, and stable. It has the benefits of bone-like stiffness, can be secured with plates and screws, is lightweight, and can withstand the sterilization process. It also holds the advantage of customization (9,10). With computer modeling, a PSI can be manufactured. Digital renderings and a tangible model of the patient's skull and the fabricated implant are then provided to the surgeon for manipulation and approval preoperatively.

ASSESSMENT OF PATIENT NEEDS

As with all reconstructive procedures, it is imperative to evaluate each patient's individual needs, the goals for reconstruction, and whether or not an implant will be needed to achieve these goals. Before an implant is used, a patient's general operative candidacy must be considered. Patients with severe cardiopulmonary or other systemic diseases may be poor candidates for general anesthesia, especially if multiple stages will be required. In these cases, single-stage procedures done under monitored local anesthesia may be in the patient's best interest. The recipient's wound-healing potential and immunologic status are also assessed. Patients with diabetes, hypertension, microvascular disease, and malnutrition; those who smoke; and patients undergoing chemotherapy, radiation therapy, or taking immunosuppressive drugs are all at risk of impaired or delayed wound healing, possible infection, and eventual implant extrusion. A history of sensitivity to any component of the implant must also be sought. A thorough history and physical exam can help forecast these pitfalls and help the surgeon plan accordingly.

Once patient fitness has been established, focus turns to characteristics of the recipient site. Form and function lost at the recipient site help guide selection of an implant appropriate for the defect and compatible with the patient. Salient points include the soft, bony, or composite character of the tissue defect; the native function of the tissues lost; and their interaction with surrounding tissues. The need to bear a load, to withstand friction or other conformational stress or strain forces, or to stand up during specific activity for the patient are additional factors to consider in choosing an implant. When a young adult applies for a facial, head, or neck implant, the physician must ask about the person's usual physical activity level and sports participation. A common cause of implant loss is trauma, which causes hematoma formation, loosening of the implant, and extrusion. Patients must agree not to participate in contact sports or to delay implantation until the questionable activity is no longer a consideration.

Implants are typically used to manage bony or soft tissue defects caused by birth defects, trauma, or tumor resection. In the case of congenital defects, surrounding tissues are typical naïve and healthy, posing less risk to the implant. This is not true in many cases of traumatic or ablative defects. Traumatized tissues may have been subjected to thermal and mechanical injury that has altered surrounding tissue cellular architecture, vascularity, and pliability. Any previous infection at the site must also be considered. In the case of malignancies, patients typically have undergone some combination of surgical, radiation, and/or chemotherapies that each may adversely affect tissue viability and ultimate implant stability. Most patients with a history of irradiation of the proposed recipient sites are not good candidates for implants unless distant, nonirradiated tissues can be brought into the area. This often necessitates procedures with several stages and perioperative hyperbaric oxygen therapy for best results. Similarly, if further radiation therapy is planned after implantation, the surgeon should recognize that use of metallic implants may pose difficulties in dosimetry. In the management of deformities attributable to ablative cancer surgery, it often is prudent to delay prosthetic implantation as long as 1 year after surgery. The patient is observed for an extended period after implantation for the development of residual or recurrent disease and for rejection of the implant.

When a patient or their defects are not ideal for restoration with an implant, a prosthesis may be the ideal option. Even in these cases, though, prosthesis fixation must be considered. Fixation can be categorized as mechanical (use of a facial accessory like eyeglasses), anatomic (relying on natural facial contours for prosthesis retention), and adhesive (glues, magnets, or osseointegrated abutments). With respect to osseointegrated implants, three main factors impact retention—bone volume, local hygiene, and a history of radiation exposure to the surrounding tissue. Extraoral, skin-penetrating abutments have a long track record for successful nasal, orbital, and auricular prosthesis fixation (11).

For osseous replacement or augmentation implants, radiologic assessment of the recipient area is advisable. At minimum, computed tomography (CT) is needed. Three-dimensional CT has also become more widely available and can be linked to a computer-aided design (CAD) and fabrication system for precise manufacturing of the prosthesis. Magnetic resonance imaging is not as helpful for evaluation of osseous deformities as it is for soft tissue assessment.

Finally, the difference between functional and cosmetic implants should be noted. A functional implant is chosen to provide the best restoration and the lowest risk of complications. In cosmetic applications, emotional and psychological development is considered as well. The condition of the recipient tissues is likely to be the limiting factor in functional cases, and psychological factors count heavily in cosmetic implantation.

SURGICAL MANAGEMENT

Preoperative Counseling

It is imperative for the surgeon to discuss the risks and complications associated with alloplastic and biologic implantation with each surgical candidate. Foremost among these are infection, rejection, and extrusion of the implant. If the preoperative history and exam identify host factors that may have a deleterious effect on healing and thereby increase these risks, these must be shared with the patient (Box 172.1). In addition, patients may have personal or religious beliefs that influence their willingness to accept use of an alloplastic material, an allograft, or a xenograft. A surgeon must discuss the patient's overall surgical candidacy, the potential need for multiple reconstructive stages, and the balance of aesthetic versus functional goals, all in hopes of setting reasonable expectations regarding outcome. The authors advise against showing photographs of patients who have undergone implantation because each case is unique. Rough drawings or photographs of the patient that have undergone computerized facial analysis are helpful as long as the patient understands that there is no expressed or implied guarantee of success.

Surgical Implantation

Each region of the face, head, and neck requires an implant with unique properties. The ideal implant does not exist, but some possess many of the following qualities thought to be important:

Biocompatibility with host tissue
Noncarcinogenic nature
Simulation of the biomechanical features of the tissue it augments
Easy fabrication
Capability of being sterilized without degradation of essential properties
Capability of being resorbed or lack thereof depending on the tissue needs
Thorough investigation before use

Each region is reviewed herein, but the specific surgical techniques are found elsewhere in this book and the medical literature. Table 172.2 summarizes site-specific selection of surgical implants.

Scalp

Little has been done in the development of scalp implants. Most scalp surgery is performed for hair replacement, and grafts or flaps are used. Autologous hair follicle unit implants are commonly used both for posttraumatic defects and for genetic baldness. Over the years, the size of the follicular grafts has decreased, and microfollicular grafts, from 1 to 5 follicular units, are now used allowing for better camouflage and filling in of the defect.

Silicone tissue expanders work well in the sustained expansion of skin for reconstruction after scalp loss.

TABLE 172.2   SURGICAL IMPLANTS BY SITE

Site	Biomaterial	Clinical Application
Scalp	Silicone	Tissue expansion
Skull	Silicone, titanium tantalum, hydroxylapatite, PMMA	Cranioplasty
Ear	Silicone	Electrode covering
	Titanium	Osseointegrated implants
	Platinum–iridium	Cochlear electrodes
	Porous polyethylene	Auricular reconstruction
Orbit	Titanium	Osseointegrated implants
	Silicone hydroxylapatite, PTFE, ePTFA	Orbital volume
	Polycarbonate	Intraocular lens, artificial eye
	Methylcellular fiber silicone	Orbital floor fractures
Face	ePTFA; carbon PTFE; porous, high-density polyethylene; polyamide; hydroxylapatite	Soft tissue and osseous augmentation
	Collagen	Dermal augmentation
	Human acellular dermis	Dermal augmentation
	Calcium-based hydroxylapatite	Soft tissue filler
	Hyaluronic acid derivatives	Soft tissue filler
Mandible	Dacron polyester, nylon, titanium alloy, tantalum alloy	Reconstruction tray
	Stainless steel	Reconstruction bar
	Titanium alloy	Miniplates and screws for trauma
	Titanium	Osseointegrated implants
	Silicone	Temporomandibular meniscus
	Hydroxylapatite	Bone conduction
	Silicone, ePTFA, carbon PTFE, porous high-density polyethylene, polyamide	Mentoplasty
Neck	ePTFA	Vascular grafts and sutures
	Polyglycolic acid, polyglactin 910, polypropylene, stainless steel	Wound closure

Expansion of the generally inelastic scalp requires 6 to 8 weeks to obtain a sufficient amount of expansion, depending on the size of the defect. Large, non–hair-bearing scalp defects can be excised, and expanded hair-bearing scalp can be advanced/rotated into the deficit. Attention must be given to hair growth direction and to maintaining the appropriate anterior hairline. It should also be noted that follicular density decreases in the expanded scalp skin.

Skull

Cranioplasty with allopathic implants is one of the oldest head and neck procedures. PMMA, a common cranial implant, is formed from several monomers in the presence of a catalyst and can be molded to the defect before hardening (12). It can be drilled, sculpted, and secured to the surrounding bone. Its polymerization is exothermic, and the implant is sterile on hardening. Alloys of titanium and tantalum are available in plate or mesh-sheet form and can be cut or bent as necessary. Because they deform slowly with external trauma, malleable metal implants for skull defects are likely to protect the brain, unlike PMMA, which is brittle and can fracture with trauma.

Hydroxylapatite cement (HAC) can also be utilized for cranioplasty defects, especially in children (13). Small defects can be molded in place, utilizing fast-setting HAC. For larger defects, computer-aided design/computer-assisted manufacturing (CAD/CAM) of a larger HAC (or PMMA) can be preformed and placed into the defect with little alteration.

Ear and Temporal Bone

Reconstruction for microtia has primarily utilized rib cartilage; it is easily accessible, can be carved and sculpted, has been shown to grow with the patient, and is an autologous biomaterial. There is a slight risk of pneumothorax, hypertrophic scar, or keloid formation, and harvest may not be properly placed in females where breast development has not yet occurred. Additionally, multiple stages are generally required to achieve a good result. However, rib cartilage remains the gold standard for microtia repair.

Preformed porous polyethylene implants (Medpor, Stryker CMF, Newnan, GA) are utilized by some surgeons for a one- or two-stage ear reconstruction. This polymer implant must be covered by a temporoparietal fascial flap, and the flap, in turn, covered by a thin, full-thickness skin graft. The immediate result is good, but the risk of complications is higher than with the rib graft—loss of the fascial flap, breakdown of the skin graft, hypertrophic scar of the scalp, and potential trauma caused by the firmness of the implant. Because the implant does not grow with the patient, sizing at an early age is problematic.

Prosthetic ears are also a viable option for ear reconstruction, particularly in the case of auriculectomy from an ablative procedure. Like other regions in the head and face, the best choice for prosthetic attachment involves implantation of pure titanium fixtures into bone. In fact, the mastoid process has the most ideal bone volume for implant integration and retention (11). These fixtures osseointegrate fully with bone before loading (14). They are attached to skin-penetrating abutments and linked with a gold bridgework that contains attachment magnets for the prosthesis. Similar implants can be used to anchor a hearing aid to the temporal bone for better sound transmission than is offered by a conventional bone-conduction hearing aid, particularly in congenital canal atresia and in postsurgical chronic tympanomastoiditis where a canal-dwelling ear piece causes recurrent drainage.

In cases of conductive hearing loss, partial and total ossicular replacement prostheses may be used in middle ear reconstruction. Any number of stapes prostheses are also available for treatment of otosclerosis. For treatment of sensorineural hearing loss, cochlear implants containing an array of stimulation electrodes inserted in the cochlea may be used. They are made of platinum and iridium, two rare metals with high electrical conductance and minimal rectification at the electrode–tissue interface. They usually are coated with PTFE or silicone to diminish current loss into the tissues and to protect the electrode from corrosion.

Orbit

A diverse number of implants are frequently used for the repair of the orbital floor and lateral walls following trauma. For small fractures, thin sheets of methyl cellulose, such as Gelfilm, can be stacked and placed over the defect to serve as temporary support until scar tissue has formed and they are resorbed. Some surgeons use silicone sheets to support the orbital floor after an orbital blow-out fracture. The biocompatibility of this material is excellent, and if properly placed and sized, the implant has a low extrusion rate. Severe fractures of the orbital floor can be repaired with a size-altering titanium implant. The device is trimmed to the required size and is adjusted by means of bending to the required anatomic defect. The implant can be fixed to the orbital rim with self-tapping screws. Porous polyethylene preformed implants can also be utilized as a support for the orbital floor, either placed acutely or in a delayed reconstruction of a hypo/enophthalmic orbit. It is possible to carve some of the polyethylene implant to fit the topography of the orbital defect. Hybrid implants made from titanium mesh coated in porous polyethylene can also be used to restore larger orbital floor and wall defects.

Mesh implants made of polyglactin 910 can be used as a slowly resorbable replacement of the orbital floor. Soft tissue pads (1 to 2 mm thick) made of ePTFE fabric can be used to repair posttraumatic hypophthalmos and for temporal augmentation. The rate of infection is low, the foreign body reaction is minimal, and there is good incorporation into the tissues (15). This material is soft and pliable and easily contoured to the size and shape of the defect. Polyglactin 910 sutures (Vicryl Plus, Ethicon, Inc., Menlo Park, CA) can secure the implant to the medial and lateral orbit.

In the enophthalmic orbit following trauma, orbital volume can be restored with bone grafts or with inert substances such as PTFE, silicone beads and sheeting, Medpor (Stryker Corp, Newnan, GA), hydroxylapatite, or ePTFE fabric. Symmetric placement of the expanders, in consultation with an ophthalmologist, can diminish postoperative diplopia. Following orbital exenteration, osseointegrated implants have been used to successfully anchor orbital prostheses (Fig. 172.1). As noted previously, bone implants for patients who have undergone irradiation are less successful unless hyperbaric oxygen therapy is used. In the case of enucleation, artificial globe implants manufactured from new polymers such as polycarbonates can be designed and painted for a near-perfect match with the other eye. Intraocular lens implants also can be made of a polymer fabricated with a specific fixed focal length for patients who have undergone cataract extraction.

Gold and platinum weights are used successfully for rehabilitation of patients with facial paralysis. Use of weights can replace tarsorrhaphy in many cases. These rare metals are inert in tissue and well tolerated in the thin upper eyelid. Sutured anterior to the tarsus, a gold weight provides reversible surgical lowering of the eyelid (16). The proper weight is selected preoperatively from a "dummy" weight-sizing kit. The patient sits, and weights of varying sizes are taped to the eyelid until the desired lid position is achieved. The weight is sterilized and inserted under local anesthesia. It serves the purpose to help initiate a relaxation of the superior levator muscle of the upper eyelid and to add to the gravitational pull of the eyelid for closure.

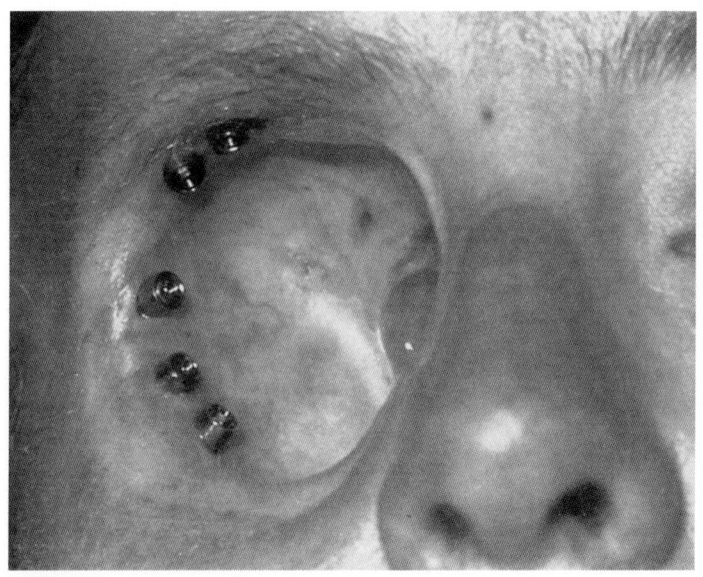

A

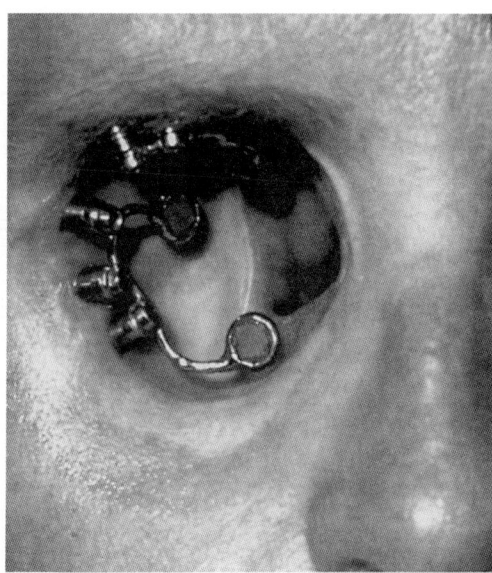

B

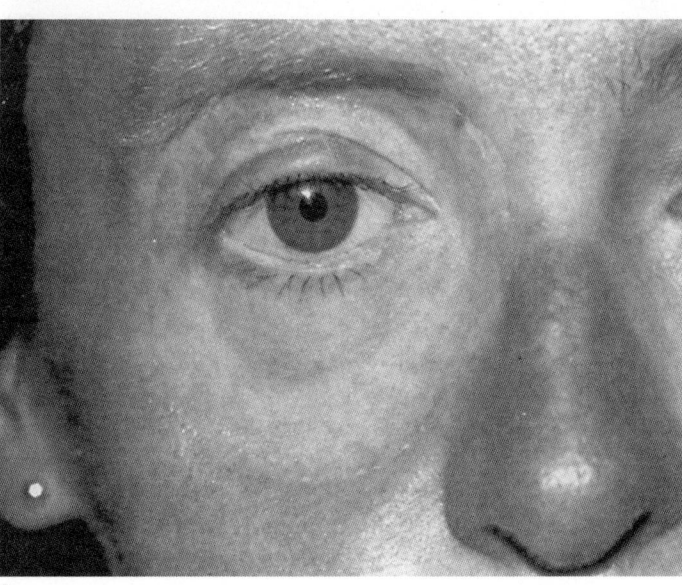

C

Figure 172.1 A: Right orbital defect in a female patient after orbital exenteration for tumor and implantation of titanium fixture. **B:** Implant bridgework in place with attached magnets. **C:** Magnetic attachment of the right orbital prosthesis secures it. (Courtesy of P.I. Branemark, MD, Branemark Implant Centers and The Institute for Experimental Biotechnology, Gothenburg, Sweden, and Stephen S. Parel, MD, The University of Texas Health Science Center, San Antonio, TX.)

Midfacial Augmentation

Augmentation of the malar region, the premaxilla, and the nasal dorsum is sometimes wanted. Although many surgeons prefer to use autogenous tissue such as cartilage or bone, alloplastic materials are being used with increasing success. Surgeons variously favor mesh (e.g., polyglactin 910, polyamide, and polyester), silicone rubber, porous polyethylene, porous PTFE or vitreous carbon fibers or aluminum oxide particles combined with PTFE, ePTFA mesh, and hydroxylapatite. Each biomaterial has advantages and disadvantages related to fiber network, pore size, inflammatory response, and ability to be secured in place. HACs come in a thick paste form and can be molded and contoured as onlay grafts.

In a fabric framework, such as ePTFE, which has a small pore size, tissue ingrowth occurs uniformly. Because of the 1- to 2-mm thickness of ePTFE, the fibroblasts can completely penetrate its depth, which is not always possible with the thicker porous implants such as porous polyethylene MedPor (Stryker Corp, Newnan, GA). All of these materials can be cut and contoured to correct the defect (Fig. 172.2). Preformed ePTFE fabric chin and malar implants are available in addition to the facial augmentation sheets. Facial augmentation can also be performed safely with ePTFE fabric.

Although it is possible to place small implants subperiosteally, large, nonyielding implants placed beneath the periosteum can cause pressure resorption of the underlying bone. The use of alloplastic materials on the dorsum and tip of the nose is controversial. Hard silicone implants are used in Asia, but they have a high rate of extrusion. ePTFA fabric (Gortex, Gore Medical, Flagstaff, AZ) has been used successfully for augmentation of the tip and the dorsum

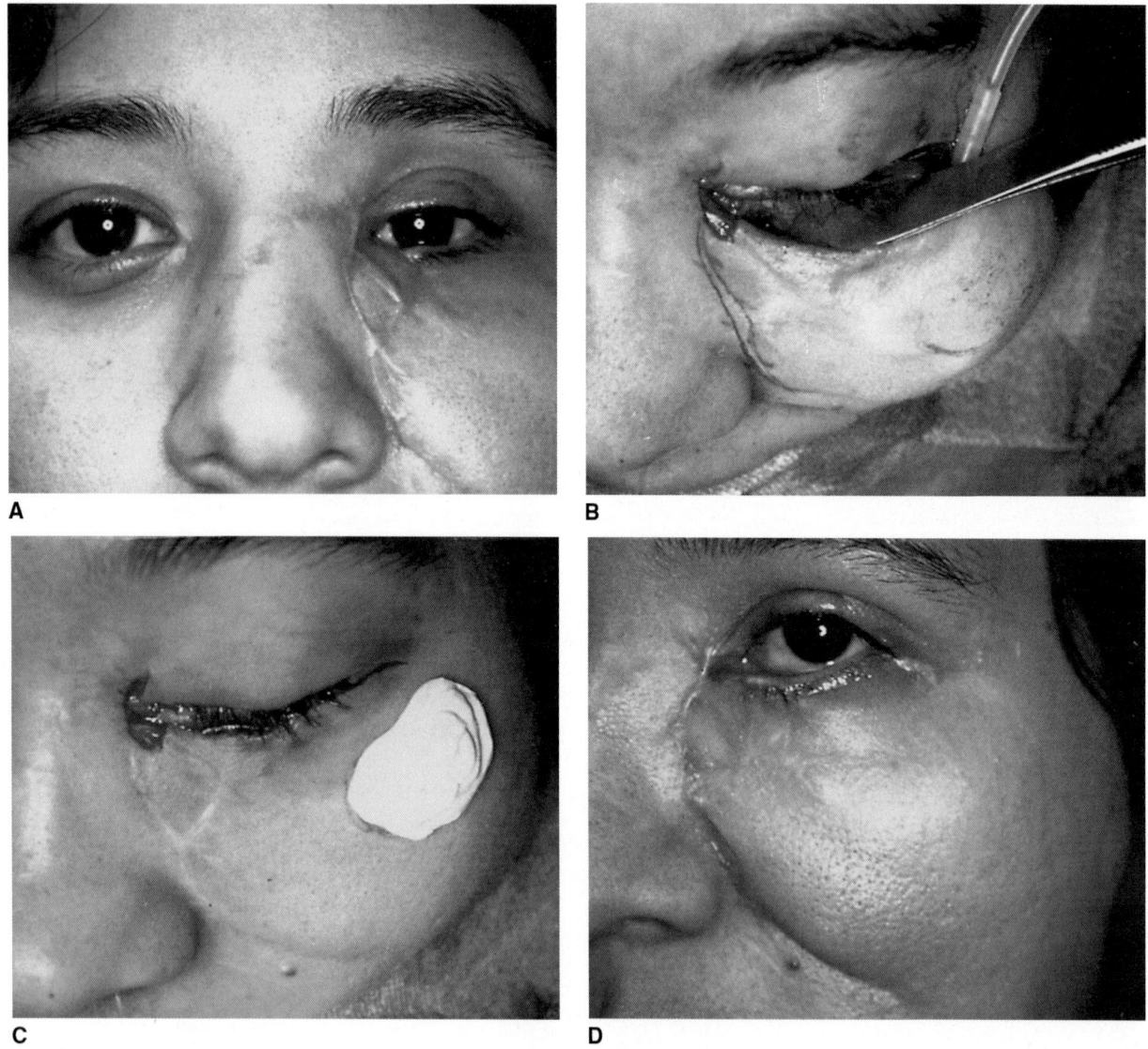

A   **B**   **C**   **D**

Figure 172.2 A: Woman with flattened left malar eminence after facial trauma. **B:** Rapid intraoperative expansion of tissue pocket to receive the implant. **C:** Layered ePTFE fabric implant is fitted to the left cheek. **D:** Augmented cheek 3 months after surgery.

of the nose. This graft seems to be easily tolerated by the thicker nasal dorsum tissues and, if secured to the periosteum, has a low rate of migration. It is soft and has a more "natural" feel than the more firm silicone. Human acellular dermis can be used as a nasal augmentation biomaterial, especially as a filler for defects when autologous cartilage is not readily available. There have been instances where it is totally resorbed, so one must be prepared for a second augmentation, should this occur. Successful immediate replacement of the alloplastic implant with autologous cartilage grafts has been reported and recommended (17).

In cases of complex bony defects of the midface, restoration of tissue volume in multiple dimensions can be challenging. For these reasons, preformed PSIs may be an ideal option for bony defects. PEEK implants fabricated with the help of three-dimensional imaging and virtual volume analysis provide a reconstructive option tailored to a patient's complex defect like that found following maxillectomy (10). If a prosthesis is the best option for a cosmetic defect, they may be anchored to underlying bone with osseointegrated implants. The growing success of endodontic implants has led some surgeons to use these for midface prosthetic fixation as well (11).

Perioral and Facial

It has become increasingly important to some patients to have perioral and facial wrinkles reduced and the lips made more plump. Facial plastic surgeons utilize a number of alloplastic and biologic materials to achieve these results. Human acellular dermis, ePTFA tubular implants, and autologous fat have been utilized for increasing the size and projection of the lips and to lessen the depth of the nasolabial folds. However, currently there is increasing use of injectable soft tissue fillers, rather than firm implants.

Fat injections, obtained from the submental region or abdomen, can also serve as a biologic filler for these areas. Some initial erythema and reaction may result from the breakdown of the fatty acids, but usually the autologous graft is well tolerated. There may be some resorption, based on technique of harvest, so overinflation is generally observed. Currently, many surgeons are beginning to investigate the use of autologous stem cell harvests from fat in order to restore soft tissue volume and enhance the longevity of results.

As collagen has presently been withdrawn from the US market (Zyplast & Cosmoplast, Allergan, Irvine, CA), newer soft tissue fillers have supplanted its use as an injectable filler for wrinkle reduction and soft tissue augmentation. Calcium hydroxylapatite–based injectable implant (Radiesse, Merz Aesthetics, San Mateo, CA) can be used in most facial wrinkles, especially perioral and glabellar lines. Immediate pain on injection and short-term erythema have been reported (18). Other fillers include various formulations of cross-linked hyaluronic acid (Juvederm, Allergan, Irvine, CA and Restylane & Perlane, Medicis Aesthetics, Scottsdale, AZ). Results vary, but in general, last for approximately 12 months. Although a cautious approach

has been advocated in the widespread use of these filling agents, their use across multiple disciplines for treatment of the aging face has become widespread. The use of injectable filler materials for facial augmentation is discussed in greater detail in Chapter 197 of this text.

Mandible

The main source of bone for mandibular reconstruction is autogenous bone. Bone pate or larger grafts can be fashioned into carrier trays made of nylon, polyester, titanium, or tantalum to hold it in position. These trays are fabricated in the shape of the mandible and trimmed to resemble the missing segment. When the tray is filled with cancellous bone, new bone forms within it. The tray can be removed after sufficient bone has formed to withstand stress and load. Stainless steel or titanium reconstruction plates can be inserted after mandibulectomy to maintain spacing. These reconstruction bars are fixed with locking screws to the proximal and distal segments to minimize motion. They may be removed when a graft is placed. In some cases, the plate itself and a regional soft tissue/muscle flap are adequate to support the bone grafts (Fig. 172.3). Many mandibular reconstructions are performed using a free flap of bone and soft tissue, often including muscle, based on the mechanical requirements of the defect, and the feasibility of vascular anastomoses.

Repair of mandible and midface fractures has been improved with miniplating and microplating systems in which a titanium alloy and self-tapping screws are used. These plates can be left in place indefinitely except when the overlying skin is thin and the plates cause discomfort. These same screws and plates can be used to secure bone grafts and other implants to the facial bones. Resorbable fixation plates are becoming a more comfortable option for some surgeons—they are typically composed of biodegradable materials, mainly polymers and copolymers of polylactide and polyglycolide. They gradually lose their strength, enabling the underlying bone to begin to remodel with stress uptake. Their application is good in the pediatric patient, in uncomplicated mandibular fracture, in non–stress-bearing fracture locations (maxilla, frontal sinus, periorbit), and also in fixating suspension sutures (endoscopic brow lift). These resorbable plates can be heat bent to the proper shape required using a thin metallic template as a guide.

The technology of osseointegrated intraoral implants has revolutionized the dental profession. Patients who could not previously wear dentures can do so with Branemark implants solidly anchored to the jaws. A single tooth, a partial denture, or a complete denture can be anchored in place with these fixtures. Fixtures can anchor augmentation bone grafts to the jaws and can be placed in a mandible reconstructed completely from autogenous cancellous bone or from a vascularized radius bone.

Mentoplasty implants are made from a variety of biomaterials—polymers (solid, gel, or mesh), carbon or

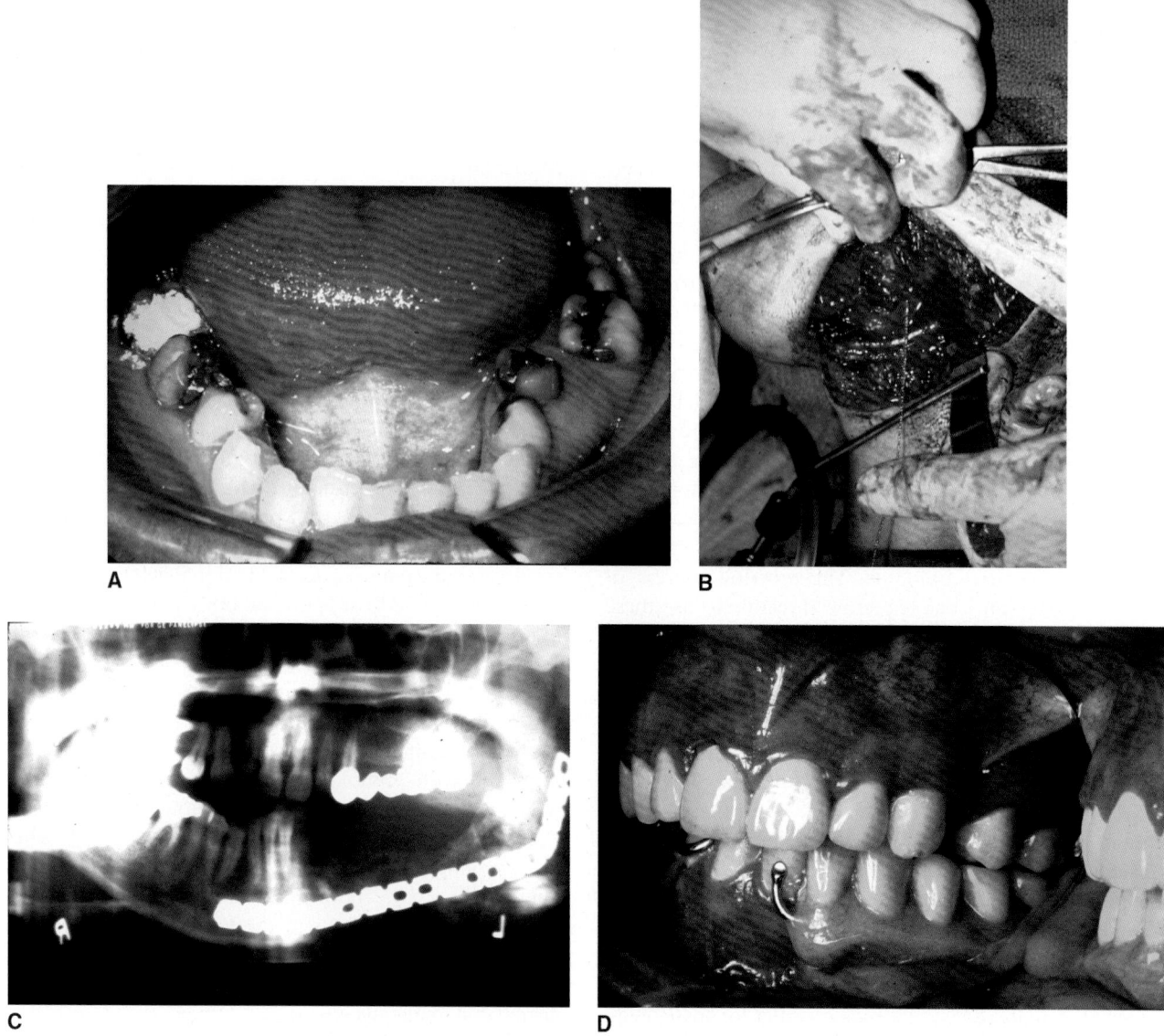

Figure 172.3 A: Preoperative view shows patient with chondrosarcoma of the left mandible. **B:** After resection of the mandible, immediate reconstruction was performed with a stainless steel reconstruction bar, autogenous iliac bone grafts, and a partial sternocleidomastoid muscle flap. **C:** Radiograph shows reconstruction bar and iliac bone grafts in place before removal. **D:** Intraoral view after removal of the reconstruction bar and healing of the mandibular grafts, with removable denture in place.

aluminum oxide combined with PTFE, high-density porous polyethylene, and ePTFE fabric. As with other sites of facial augmentation, the implants are best placed extraperiosteally and secured to the periosteum by sutures. Both extraoral and intraoral insertions can be used, and both approaches seem to work well when placed by an experienced surgeon. Most surgeons tend to anchor the implant in the midline and use subperiosteal pockets to insert and secure the lateral arms of the implant. Patient satisfaction with ePTFE chin implants has been reported as high as 97% (19).

Hydroxylapatite has been used as a bone-conduction material to provide a nonorganic framework for ingrowth of osteoactive cells to correct small defects of the mandible and maxilla. The success of this approach varies. In the future, the material may function better if combined with osseoinductive intervention. Several replacement prostheses for the temporomandibular joint have been investigated, but a single best biomaterial has not emerged. Silicone sheeting has been a reasonable substitute for the meniscus in the joint, but the articulating surfaces of most implant prostheses undergo wear and degradation.

Neck

In the field of phonosurgery, a number of laryngeal implants have been used for vocal fold medialization and augmentation. Historically, Teflon injections were used, but proved unpredictable, irreversible, and found to incite significant, long-lasting host inflammatory responses. In its place, hyaluronic acid, calcium hydroxylapatite, and autologous fat are now commonly used for injection augmentation. Medialization laryngoplasty is also performed via a thyroplasty approach. ePTFE ribbon, silicone Montgomery stents (Boston Medical Products, Westborough, MA), and surgeon-carved Silastic implants may each be used depending on surgeon preference and patient candidacy.

In vascular surgery, the use of ePTFE patches has improved the results of carotid artery surgery for stenosis, primarily because of excellent biocompatibility with the hematogenous cellular and clotting factors and because it functions as a substrate for endothelial ingrowth. Suture material for closure of neck wounds includes synthetic biosorbable sutures such as polylactic acid or polyglactin 910; ePTFE vascular sutures; stainless steel skin staples; or polypropylene sutures, which also are hemocompatible for vascular repair. Use of these materials has decreased the incidence of wound breakdown and bleeding.

Following laryngectomy, the silicone tracheoesophageal fistula prosthesis is a removable implant in the neck that has excellent surface properties in contact with aerodigestive tract secretions. A certain amount of fatigue and degradation occurs with this functional implant, and it must be replaced frequently. Use of tracheostomy tubes composed of highly surface-biocompatible silicone and PTFE with low-pressure polymer sheeting balloons have greatly reduced the complications of tracheal erosion and blockage of the tube lumen.

COMPLICATIONS AND EMERGENCIES

Bleeding, infection, traumatic injury to the implant, implant mobility, and extrusion are the primary complications of surgical implantation in the face, head, and neck. Malposition of the implant, unacceptable cosmesis or functional restoration, overcorrection or undercorrection of the defect, host inflammatory reactions, incitement of a viral flare, inappropriate selection of implant material, and overall patient dissatisfaction also affect outcome. These complications usually can be prevented through careful pairing of both patient and implant, preoperative counseling, meticulous surgical technique, and close follow-up evaluation.

Infection is a primary concern with any alloplastic implant and is a common reason for implant failure and need for removal. Most surgeons use perioperative antibiotic therapy, and all use aseptic surgical discipline. It is essential to prevent contamination of the implant before insertion. Sclafani et al. explain that risk of alloplast infection and rejection is primarily increased when bacterial contamination is present at the time of implantation and/or prior to fibrovascular tissue ingrowth. In order to prevent infection, surgeons have used a number of varied and typically unproven preimplantation techniques. These have included saline rinses, antibiotic immersions, and povidone-iodine (Betadine, Purdue Products LP, Stamford, CT) irrigations (20). Keefe and Keefe demonstrated that suction infiltration of an antibiotic solution at the time of implantation provides a statistically significant advantage to infection prophylaxis, particularly in materials with a smaller pore size. Floating or immersion techniques alone provided no inhibition to bacterial growth (21). Incorporation of antiseptic agents into the biomaterials can also minimize the risk of infection. If the implant site does become infected, high doses of broad-spectrum antibiotics are prescribed, and hot compresses are applied. Impending extrusion or failure to control an infection necessitates immediate removal of the implant.

Some liquid implants have produced histotoxic effects or hypersensitivity reactions. Ethyl-2-cyanoacrylate, a short-chain cyanoacrylate derivative, activates severe cellular toxicity, but butyl-2-cyanoacrylate, a longer-chain derivative, has minimal histotoxic effects. If it is necessary to use a tissue glue for adhesion of one hard tissue to another, butyl-2-cranoacrylate is the better choice. Silastic and methyl methacrylate have been shown to incite host foreign body reactions that increase the risk of infection and extrusion (22). Autoimmune rejection is also possible and may necessitate implant removal.

Another substance historically used widely for dermal augmentation is injectable bovine collagen. Hypersensitivity manifests as skin inflammation or gastrointestinal distress after eating beef. Each prospective patient is carefully evaluated for a history of hypersensitivity to beef products before treatment and is observed closely after collagen injections. A positive reaction to a skin test dose is an absolute contraindication to collagen injection. If a reaction occurs, it is managed medically with topical and systemic antiinflammatory agents and local skin care. The injected tissue is removed surgically if the reaction cannot be controlled conservatively. These risks are one of the underlying reasons for removal from the current market in the United States. Acellular human dermis is available in thin sheets and can be used for soft tissue augmentation. It can be used safely in most previously irradiated fields (23,24).

Other threats to implant failure include bleeding, trauma to the implant, and implant malposition. Postoperative hematoma or seroma formation must be treated as soon as possible, or at the least closely monitored. If a vascular patch or area of revascularization begins bleeding, the patient is returned immediately to the operating room for repair of the leak. Few crises are worse than vascular emergencies in surgical implants in the face, head, and neck.

Micromotion of an implant is expected and desirable, because the implant must closely simulate the characteristics of the host tissue. However, macromotion is possible unless the implant is firmly secured to the underlying tissue. Migration or malposition of an implant may

TABLE 172.3	COMPLICATIONS	
Complication	**Prevention**	**Treatment**
Infection	Perioperative antibiotics, aseptic technique	Antibiotics, hot compresses
Traumatic displacement	Patient education, implant stabilization	Surgical repositioning
Impending extrusion	Control of infection, immobilization of site	Removal of implant
Over- or undercorrection	Use of scans, photos, and measurements preoperatively	Revision according to patient's wishes
Malposition	Implant stabilization	Surgical repositioning
Bleeding	Meticulous hemostasis, compression	Surgical exploration
Patient dissatisfaction	Preoperative counseling, communication, and rapport	Reassurance and concern, revision if necessary

necessitate a second operation to realign or fixate the device. Undercorrection or overcorrection of a deformity is corrected only if the patient chooses to do so, without urging by the surgeon.

If a patient is dissatisfied with the results of a surgical implant, the surgeon reassures the patient until the swelling has subsided enough to gain an impression of the result. The patient–physician relationship is maintained with a demeanor of concern, trust, and free communication. If the patient's dissatisfaction is justified, the surgeon can discuss the possibility of surgical revision. If the patient's concern is not justified, a second opinion from a respected colleague can defuse the situation. Whatever the conditions, the physician maintains a close and empathic relationship with the patient. Table 172.3 summarizes the complications and emergencies in the use of implants as well as prevention and management.

REFERENCES

1. Holt GR. Physical characteristics and biocompatibility of implant materials. In: Glasgold AI, Silver FH, eds. *Applications of biomaterials in facial plastic surgery.* Boca Raton, FL: CRC Press, 1991:87.
2. Gosain AK, Persing JA. Biomaterials in the face: benefits and risks. *J Craniofac Surg* 1999;10:404–414.
3. Jacovella PF. Use of calcium hydroxylapatite (Radiesse®) for facial augmentation. *Clin Interv Aging* 2008;3:161–174.
4. Mendelson BC, Jacobson SR, Lavoipierre AM, et al. The fate of porous hydroxyapatite granules used in facial skeletal augmentation. *Aesthetic Plast Surg* 2010;34:455–461.
5. Lemperle G, Sadick NS, Knaplp TR, et al. ArteFill™ permanent injectable for soft tissue augmentation: II. Indications and applications. *Aesthetic Plast Surg* 2010;34:273–286.
6. James SE, Kelly MH. Cartilage recycling in rhinoplasty: polydioxanone foil as an absorbable biomechanical scaffold. *Plast Reconstr Surg* 2008;122:254–260.
7. Boenisch M, Trenite GJN. Reconstruction of the nasal septum using polydioxanone plate. *Arch Facial Plast Surg* 2010;12:4–10.
8. Gabal C, Lovald S, Baack B, et al. Minimally invasive bioabsorbable bone plates for rigid internal fixation of mandible fractures. *Arch Facial Plast Surg* 2011;13:31–35.
9. Wenz LM, Merritt K, Brown SA, et al. In vitro biocompatibility of polyetheretherketone and polysulfone composites. *J Biomed Mater Res* 1990;24:207–215.
10. Kim MM, Boahene KDO, Byrne PJ. Use of customized polyetheretherketone (PEEK) implants in the reconstruction of complex maxillofacial defects. *Arch Facial Plast Surg* 2009;11:53–57.
11. Scolozzi P, Jaques B. Treatment of midfacial defects using prostheses supported by ITI dental implants. *Plast Reconstr Surg* 2004;114:1395–1404.
12. Gibbons KJ, Hicks WL Jr, Guterman LR. A technique for rigid fixation of methyl methacrylate cranioplasty: the vault-locking method. *Surg Neurol* 1999;52:310–315.
13. Magee WP Jr, Ajkay N, Freda N, et al. Use of fast-setting hydroxyapatite cement for secondary facial contouring. *Plast Reconstr Surg* 2003;114:289–297.
14. Holt GR, Parel SM, Branemark PI. Osseointegrated titanium implants. *Facial Plast Surg* 1986;3:113.
15. Fedok FG, van Kooten DW, Levin RJ. Temporal augmentation with a layered expanded polytetrafluoroethylene implant. *Otolaryngol Head Neck Surg* 1999;120:929–933.
16. Choi HY, Hong SE, Lew JM. Long-term comparison of a newly designed gold implant with the conventional implant in facial nerve paralysis. *Plast Reconstr Surg* 1999;104:1624–1634.
17. Raghavan U, Jones NS, Romo T III. Immediate autogenous cartilage grafts in rhinoplasty after alloplastic implant rejection. *Arch Facial Plast Surg* 2004;6:192–196.
18. Tzikas TL. Evaluation of the Radiance FN soft tissue filler for facial soft tissue augmentation. *Arch Facial Plast Surg* 2004;6:234–239.
19. Godin M, Costa L, Romo T III, et al. Gore-Tex chin implants: a review of 324 cases. *Arch Facial Plast Surg* 2003;5:224–227.
20. Sclafani AP, Thomas JR, Cox AJ, et al. Clinical and histologic response of subcutaneous expanded polytetrafluoroethylene (Gore-Tex™) and porous high-density polyethylene (Medpor™) implants to acute and early infection. *Arch Otolaryngol Head Neck Surg* 1997;123:328–336.
21. Keefe MS, Keefe MA. An evaluation of the effectiveness of different techniques for intraoperative infiltration of antibiotics into alloplastic implants for use in facial reconstruction. *Arch Facial Plast Surg* 2009;11:246–251.
22. Maas CS, Merwin GE, Wilson J, et al. Comparison of biomaterials for facial bone augmentation. *Arch Otolaryngol Head Neck Surg* 1990;116:551–556.
23. Achauer BM, VanderKam VM, Celikoz B, et al. Augmentation of facial soft-tissue defects with Alloderm dermal graft. *Ann Plast Surg* 1998;41:503–507.
24. Dubin MG, Feldman M, Ibrahim HZ, et al. Allograft dermal implant (AlloDerm) in a previously irradiated field. *Laryngoscope* 2000;110:934–937.

Local Cutaneous Flaps and Grafts

173

Brian Jewett

Facial reconstruction is a challenging yet rewarding endeavor. Repair of facial defects requires an appreciation of variations in facial cutaneous tissue and the influence of these differences on use of potential reconstructive methods. Multiple factors help determine the optimal method of repair, including the size of the defect, the depth and location of the defect, and the strength of the underlying facial framework. Maintaining symmetry, contour, and function is essential for a successful facial reconstruction. Finally, of utmost importance is a thorough understanding of all appropriate reconstructive options.

SKIN ANATOMY

Skin variability in color, texture, thickness, and accessory components is demonstrated from one anatomic region to another, and an understanding of these variations is important for optimizing wound healing and soft tissue restoration. Skin consists of an epidermal component with appendages and a dermal component with neurovascular supply.

The epidermis consists of predominantly keratinocytes (80%) but also melanocytes, Langerhans cells, and Merkel cells (Table 173.1). The basal layer, spinous layer, granular layer, and cornified layer make up four distinct histologic layers, with the deepest layer, the basal layer, serving as the germinative layer. Melanocytes are dendritic, pigment-synthesizing cells of neural crest origin with clear cytoplasm, and they are confined to the basal layer. Melanin is produced by melanocytes, which is transported to adjacent basal and spinous layers for engulfment by the keratinocytes. Once engulfed, the melanin is arranged as a cover over the nuclei, serving as a protective barrier against ultraviolet irradiation. Langerhans cells are derived from bone marrow and serve to process and present antigens. These cells are found in the suprabasal epidermal layers, have dendritic processes, and contain Birbeck or Langerhans cell granules (1). Merkel cells are mechanoreceptors of neural crest origin and are primarily involved with touch sensation. Merkel cells are usually found in areas of high tactile sensitivity, where they aggregate to form tactile disks and Merkel cell–neurite complexes (2).

The dermal–epidermal junction is a critical structure that helps prevent dermal–epidermal separation, and alterations in the structure are found in diseases like epidermolysis bullosa (3). Keratin filaments within the basal keratinocyte condense and attach to an electron-dense plaque at the inferior portion of the cell membrane known as the hemidesmosome. Anchoring filaments in the lamina lucida connect hemidesmosomes to the lamina densa, which in turn is connected to the anchoring plaques in the dermis by anchoring fibrils.

Epidermal appendages include hair follicles, sebaceous glands, and eccrine and apocrine sweat glands. Pilosebaceous units contain hair follicles, sebaceous glands, arrector pili muscles, and sensory end organs. The pilosebaceous unit has motor and sensory functions, while also producing hair and sebum. On the nasal tip, the sebaceous component of the pilosebaceous unit is most prominent, while on hair-bearing surfaces, the follicular component predominates. Complete units are absent on the soils, palms, and mucous membranes. Healing of partial-thickness wounds by secondary intention is facilitated by pilosebaceous units, since reepithelialization occurs in part from the epithelial cells that line the follicular unit. Sebaceous glands connect to the hair follicle by a squamous epithelial duct, allowing the glands to secrete sebum through the duct, along the follicle, and onto the surface of the skin. Perhaps providing a protective function, sebum acts as an emollient to the hair and skin. Eccrine sweat glands contain a secretory gland in the deep reticular dermis and a coiled intraepithelial duct that opens to the skin surface. These glands are controlled by the cholinergic system, and the duct can modify the composition of sweat secretion. Apocrine sweat glands receive adrenergic

TABLE 173.1	CONTENTS OF EPIDERMIS

Keratinocytes
Melanocytes
Langerhans cells
Merkel cells

innervation and are generally found in the eyelids (Moll glands), external auditory canal (ceruminous glands), axillae, areolae, and perineum (1).

The majority of skin consists of the dermis, which contains neural and vascular networks, epidermal appendages, fibroblasts, macrophages, mast cells, and other cells (Table 173.2). The extracellular matrix consists of collagen, elastin, and amorphous substance known as the "ground substance." Skin pliability, tensile strength, and elasticity are properties attributed to the dermal component, and the dermis is divided into the papillary (superficial) and reticular (deeper) layers. Fibroblasts produce collagen, mostly type I collagen, which is responsible for the tensile strength and elasticity of skin. Type III collagen is much less common, and is found in the papillary dermis. Matrix metalloproteinases degrade collagen, allowing new collagen to replace old fibers; however, induction of collagenases by ultraviolet radiation can lead to disorganization that is clinically manifested as skin wrinkling and photoaging. Fibroblasts also produce elastin, which is degraded by elastases, allowing a continuous regenerative process. Elastin fibers are perpendicular to skin surface in the papillary dermis and parallel in the reticular dermis. Ground substance is generated by fibroblasts and consists primarily of proteoglycans, glycosaminoglycans, and filamentous glycoproteins. Ground substance is thought to help with distribution of pressure forces (1).

An abundant vascular supply is present in the skin, facilitating nutritional support and thermo regulation for the body. At the junction of the dermis and subcutaneous fat is the deep vascular plexus, whose arterioles supply the epidermal appendages and superficial vascular plexus. The superficial plexus lies in the reticular dermis and is connected to a vascular loop system in the papillary dermis, which provides nutrients to epidermal cells via diffusion.

TABLE 173.2	CONTENTS OF DERMIS

Neural and vascular networks
Epidermal appendages
Fibroblasts, macrophages, mast cells
Extracellular matrix (collagen, elastin, ground substance)

Blood vessels travel one of two ways to reach the cutaneous vascular plexus. Septocutaneous arteries travel through fascial septa, between muscular segments, parallel to the cutaneous surface. These arteries supply large areas of skin and have a pair of veins. Musculocutaneous arteries pass through muscle and are more common; however, these arteries typically supply smaller areas of cutaneous surface (Fig. 173.1) (4).

Sensory innervation includes both sensory and sympathetic nerves. Efferent nerves innervate blood vessels in the skin, and sensory nerves include dermal neural receptors known as Meissner (fine touch) and pacinian (deep pressure, vibration) corpuscles. Sensory nerves are distributed in a segmental fashion known as dermatomes.

SKIN BIOMECHANICAL PROPERTIES

The unique mechanical properties of skin influence cutaneous vascularity with tissue movement and ultimately flap survival. Skin is described as having a nonlinear stress–strain relationship, where stress represents force per unit of original cross-section and strain represents change in length divided by original length (5,6). With initial deformation, randomly oriented collagen and elastic fibers are stretched in the direction of the force, allowing extension with little force. With continued deformation, additional collagen fibers are recruited to load carrying capacity, but resistance transitions to eventual inability of further deformation with further force. At this point, no further collagen and elastic fibers can be oriented in the direction of the force and the structural integrity is protected against additional forces (7).

Skin is also characterized as being directional or anisotropic. The degree of skin tension is greatest parallel to the relaxed skin tension lines (RSTLs), a phenomenon that reflects interactions between collagen and elastic fibers at the cellular level. Lines of maximal extensibility (LME) run perpendicular to the RSTLs and represent lines of closure with the least tension (Fig. 173.2) (7–9).

Finally, skin is described as an elastic substance with lesser stress or force, but as a viscoelastic substance with higher stress loads. Higher stress loads cause skin to experience creep, which describes the increase in length with constant stress. Histologically, the increased length experienced is related to the displacement of interstitial fluid. Stress relaxation, although related to creep, defines the decrease in tension in skin overtime with constant tension (7). Larrabee showed that the effect of tension on flap survival is affected by flap length. Flaps with 3 cm base and 6 cm length showed necrosis, while flaps with the same base and 1.5 cm length all survived regardless of tension. Flaps with intermediate lengths were tension sensitive, with tension greater than 250 g tending to cause necrosis (10). Undermining is thought to reduce wound tension by releasing vertical attachments between the dermis and subcutaneous tissues, allowing less restricted movement.

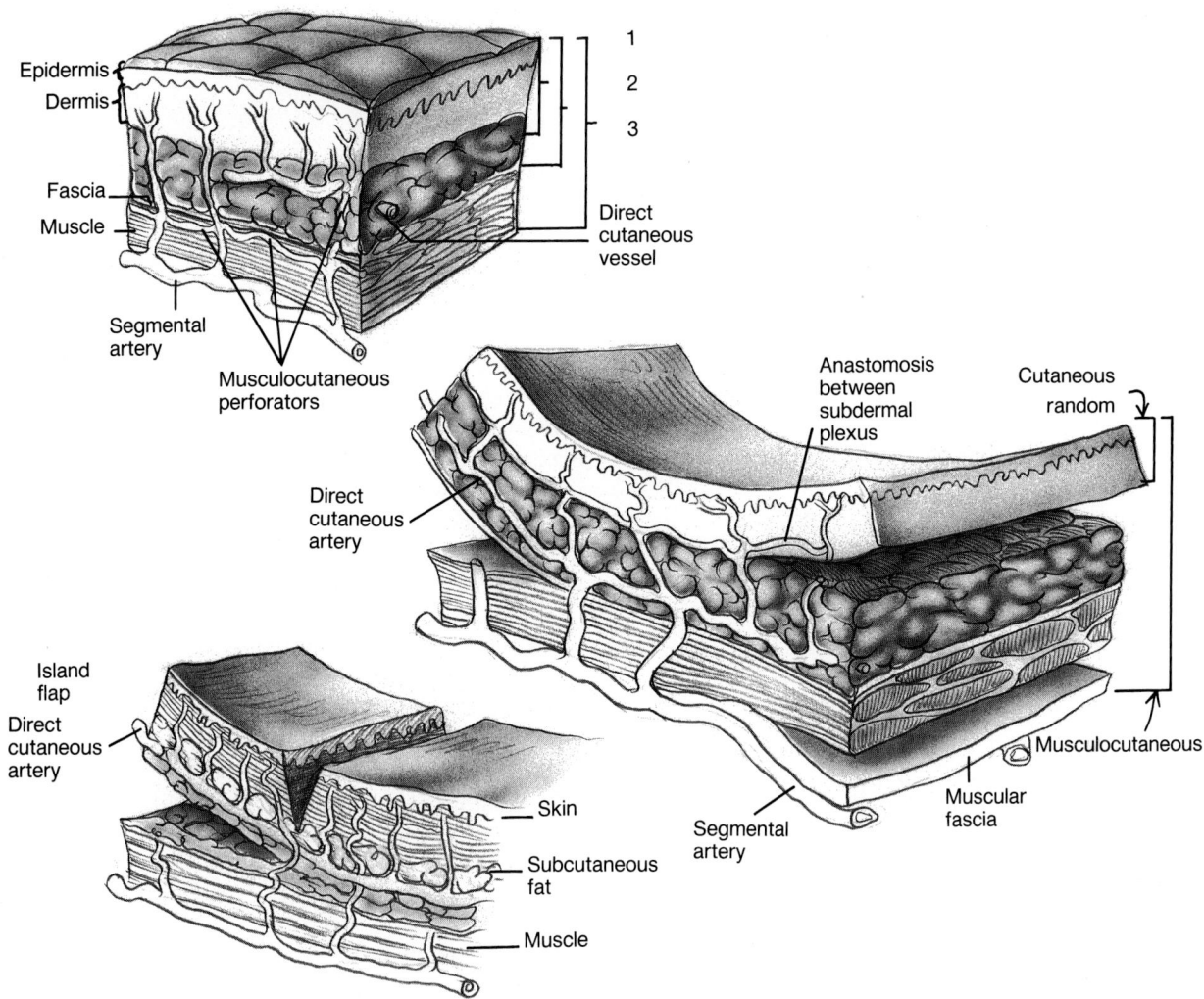

Figure 173.1 Representation of cutaneous vascular supply. Numbered parentheses delineate vascular supply for various types of flaps: *1*, random-pattern flaps; *2*, axial-pattern flaps; *3*, myocutaneous flaps.

SKIN PHYSIOLOGY

The vascular network within the skin facilitates regulation of body temperature and transfer of nutrients and other blood products, and the amount of blood flow is directly related to arteriolar pressure and flow (11). The precapillary sphincter controls the amount of nutritive blood flow to the skin (12), and this sphincter dilates with local hypoxemia (13). Preshunt sphincters, located deeper in the subcutaneous tissue, are regulated by the sympathetic nervous system, causing changes in blood flow that affects body temperature and systemic blood pressure (14). Vasodilatation can also occur with excessive body temperature, through local release of acetylcholine by sympathetic nerve fibers (4).

Revascularization is a complex process that is initiated after cutaneous injury or tissue transfer. Angiogenic stimuli lead to vasodilatation with increased vessel permeability. This is followed by dissolution of the basement membrane by proteases, allowing endothelial cells to migrate from the vascular wall toward the angiogenic stimulus. Nearby capillary sprouts anastomose with each other, forming loops. The blood vessels eventually differentiate to lay down basement membrane with type IV collagen, laminin, and proteoglycans. Some capillaries join preexisting vessels (inosculation), while others directly grow into the flap (neovascularization). Growth rate is about 0.2 mm/day, and regression of capillary loops occurs when the stimulus is discontinued after adequate vascular supply to the flap has been established (4). Revascularization adequate for detachment of a flap pedicle can be as early as 7 days (15), although waiting about 3 weeks is usually recommended.

Venous outflow is important, and venous occlusion can be more detrimental to tissue survival than adequate arterial supply. Venous outflow is generally through the subdermal plexus or with venous channels that accompany arteries within the flap. Cutaneous lymphatic drainage is also interrupted with tissue elevation, and increased

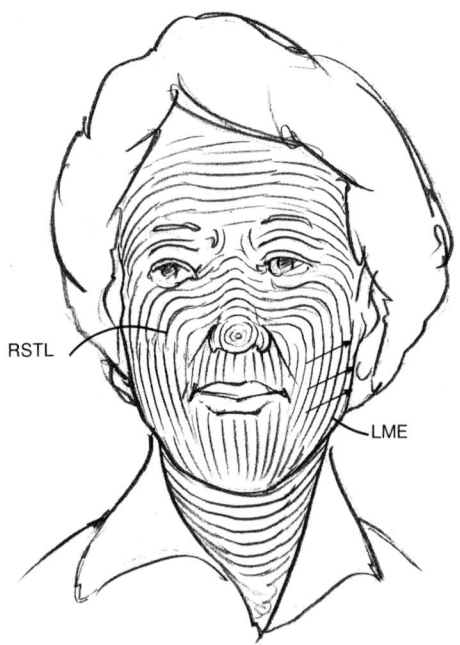

Figure 173.2 Relaxed skin tension lines (RSTLs) of the face. Notice that the lines of maximal extensibility (LME) run perpendicular to the RSTLs. Placing incisions along the RSTLs will decrease wound closure tension and optimize wound healing.

interstitial fluid pressure can affect capillary perfusion. Severing of sympathetic nerves leads to vasoconstriction (16) through the release of norepinephrine and oxygen-free radicals (17), but the depletion of neurotransmitters within 24 to 48 hours allows improvement in blood flow (18).

Delay of cutaneous flaps is thought to improve survival of the flap at the time of eventual transfer. Some theories used to explain the benefits of delay include improved blood supply after recovery from a hyperadrenergic state that is induced by sympathetic denervation (16,19) and permanent and irreversible dilation of the "choke" vessel through hyperplasia and hypertrophy (20). Both tobacco smoking and radiation have been shown to have a deleterious effect on flap survival, and delay of regional flaps is strongly considered in these patients (4).

DEFECT ANALYSIS AND PREPARATION

Analysis of a facial defect includes determining the depth of the wound, the color and texture of the missing skin, and the extent of involved aesthetic units and adjacent facial regions. In addition, the defect is inspected for any missing soft tissue, structural support, or lining. The thickness, texture, and mobility of remaining facial skin are assessed carefully; furthermore, any medical, social, and psychological issues pertaining to the patient should be considered. Finally, paramount to a successful reconstruction is appropriate assessment and treatment of any existing or potential functional compromise (i.e., nasal obstruction, eyelid malposition, oral incompetence) (Table 173.3).

TABLE 173.3	KEYPOINTS—FACIAL DEFECT ANALYSIS

Depth, size, and location of defect
Color, thickness, laxity of adjacent skin
Aesthetic units and landmarks
Nearby structures that cannot be distorted
Existing or potential functional compromise

Facial defects occasionally involve multiple areas of the face. When planning reconstructive options, it is helpful to demarcate the division between the primary and surrounding facial regions such that defects involving multiple facial regions are repaired with separate methods addressing each region. Adhering to this principle places eventual scars along boundary lines that separate each aesthetic region, which helps preserve the natural contours of the face.

Within each region, individual aesthetic units should be identified. Aesthetic units are based on variations in skin thickness and texture, as well as variations in contour created by the underlying facial framework (Fig. 173.3). Optimal repair of a facial defect may require repositioning of skin and soft tissue within an involved aesthetic unit, thereby allowing eventual scars to lie within zones of transitions between adjacent units. In addition, small defects may be enlarged to facilitate repair of an entire aesthetic unit by a single repair method.

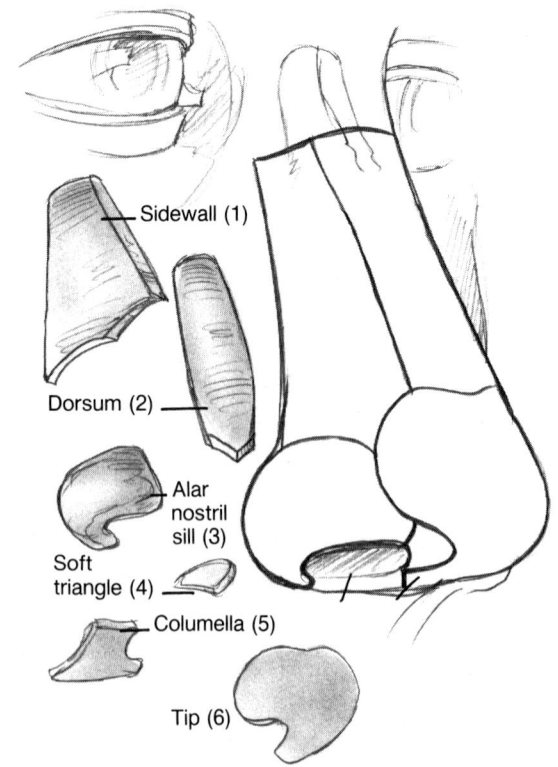

Figure 173.3 Nasal aesthetic subunits.

TABLE 173.4	LADDER OF FACIAL CUTANEOUS RECONSTRUCTIVE OPTIONS

Healing by secondary intention
Primary wound closure
Skin or composite grafts
Local cutaneous flaps
Regional cutaneous flaps
Distant tissue transfer

Establishing uniform depth, while maintaining symmetry with contralateral facial structures, is equally important. Beveled tissue at the periphery of the Mohs defect is removed if flaps are planned, in order to optimize eversion of skin edges at closure. In addition, cutaneous edges of the flap and the recipient tissue are adjusted appropriately to establish uniform thickness at the line of closure. Whenever possible, the primary defect should be deepened to establish uniformity rather than thinning the flap. One exception to removing beveled edges is when skin grafts are performed. In this circumstance, beveled edges are freshened, but maintained, to provide a gradual contour transition between recipient tissue and the skin graft. Additional techniques helpful in optimizing repair include angulation of curvilinear defects, since round defects are more likely to undergo concentric scar contraction and result in trapdoor deformity. Modifying the periphery of the defect by creating more acute angles often reduces the risk of this deformity.

Facial defects are repaired using a number of options, including healing by secondary intention, primary closure, local and regional flaps, skin grafts, composite grafts, and free tissue transfer (Table 173.4). Occasionally, cartilage grafts or subcutaneous augmentation flaps are also necessary to establish appropriate support as well as contour match with the tissue surrounding the defect. Selection of the optimal reconstructive method is influenced by the size, depth, and location of the facial defect (Table 173.5).

PATIENT PREPARATION—MEDICAL COMORBIDITIES

Systemic diseases such as diabetes, malnutrition, arteriosclerosis, hypertension, and collagen vascular disease can compromise flap vascularity and lead to necrosis and impaired wound healing. Consulting with the patient's personal physician is important to ascertain whether the patient's medical condition is optimized during the perioperative period.

Patients with a history of irradiation have subcutaneous scar tissue and decreased vascularity of the skin in the irradiated area. Cutaneous flaps from adjacent nonirradiated tissue are preferred, but even then, healing may be compromised leading to poor outcome. When interpolated flaps are transferred to an irradiated area, detachment of the flaps is best delayed until revascularization of the flap is certain. For suitable candidates, consideration is given to hyperbaric oxygen treatment to optimize tissue oxygenation levels prior to reconstruction.

Patients are questioned preoperatively concerning their use of tobacco and alcohol. Heavy alcohol consumption will dilate blood vessels, predisposing to hematoma formation. Avoidance of alcohol during the perioperative period is recommended. Ideally, tobacco and nicotine products should be avoided, at least 8 weeks before and after surgery. Even smoking cessation for 2 days before surgery and 7 days after surgery has been shown to have beneficial effects on flap survival. Smokers develop skin necrosis three times more frequently than nonsmokers, and the extent and depth of skin slough are more severe (21). Nicotine causes systemic vasoconstriction through activation of the adrenergic nervous system, which may lower tissue oxygenation pressure by greater than

TABLE 173.5	COMPARISON OF RECONSTRUCTIVE OPTIONS

Option	Advantages	Disadvantages
Healing by secondary intention	No further surgery required	Extended wound care. May result in depressed, hypopigmented scar. Contracture may distort adjacent structures.
Primary closure	Technically quick and straightforward Usually good aesthetic outcome	May require excision of additional normal skin if rounded defect Use usually limited to defects that lie along RSTLs
Cutaneous graft	Technically quick and straightforward	Donor site required Potentially poor match in cutaneous color, texture, and contour Longer wound care. Not always complete survival.
Local cutaneous flap	Easy wound care Short healing period Usually complete survival Excellent color and contour match	May be technically challenging Creates additional scars Secondary defect may cause distortion. Increased risk of bruising, swelling, trapdoor deformity Potential for greater reconstructive challenge with failure

50%. This occurs within 10 minutes of smoking a cigarette and lasts approximately 50 minutes. Smoking also produces carbon monoxide, which has a higher affinity for hemoglobin than oxygen, thereby producing high levels of carboxyhemoglobin (22–26). When possible, consideration is given to delaying surgical procedures until smoking cessation can be assured.

HEALING BY SECONDARY INTENTION

Small superficial cutaneous defects involving concave facial surfaces may granulate and epithelialize with an acceptable aesthetic result. Ideal locations for healing by secondary intention include the temple and medial canthus. It is imperative to keep wounds moist during the healing phase. Wounds are cleaned twice daily, removing fibrinous debris during each cleaning. Wounds are then covered with a topical water-based ointment containing mupirocin and nonadherent gauze for the initial 2 weeks, followed by a topical petroleum-based ointment and nonadherent gauze until complete reepithelialization occurs. For patients with larger defects or concerns for slower wound healing, wet-to-dry dressings are employed daily. These patients are instructed to place a moist, but not dripping wet, gauze to the wound in the evening, followed by removal in the morning. The morning wound care is as previously described, with topical ointment application and nonadherent gauze. Patients are counseled that wounds often take 4 to 6 weeks to heal, and massage may be indicated to address any contour irregularities. Patients may be offered resurfacing procedures if surface irregularities are persistent.

PRIMARY CLOSURE

Adjacent facial tissue provides the ideal color, thickness, and texture for repair of most facial defects. Unfortunately, scars associated with primary closure or local flaps do not always fall along borders between aesthetic units; nonetheless, the benefits gained in establishing appropriate contour and skin color may outweigh this potential disadvantage. In general, oval and linear defects along RSTLs in a patient with redundant skin are ideal defects for primary closure; in addition, an M-plasty modification can be performed to shorten the length of the anticipated scar (Fig. 173.4). Modification of underlying facial tissue or framework may facilitate wound closure (i.e., dorsal nasal framework modification), and suspension sutures may be indicated to prevent distortion of mobile structures (i.e., canthal, nasal valve, and alar suspension sutures).

Wide undermining of the skin adjacent to the defect is performed in subcutaneous plane for most facial defects; however, with nasal defects, the dissection is usually performed in a submuscular plane. Dissection in an appropriate plane minimizes bleeding and postoperative bruising,

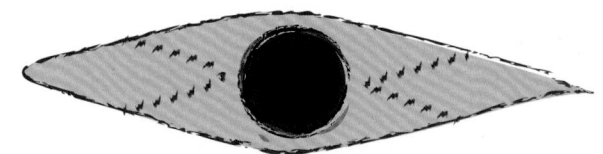

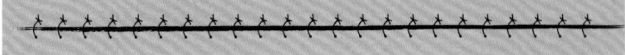

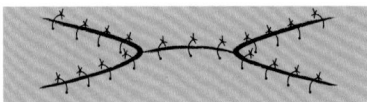

Figure 173.4 Comparison of the closure of a fusiform excision and an M-plasty excision. The straight portion of the M-plasty closure is significantly shorter than the fusiform closure.

and wide undermining helps avoid trapdoor deformity. The effect of primary closure on surrounding structures such as the nasal tip, alar margin, eyelid, canthus, oral commissure, and hairline should be evaluated. The method of repair should be reconsidered if there is significant distortion that is not expected to resolve with time and postoperative massage.

FACIAL CUTANEOUS FLAPS

When primary wound closure is not possible, local flaps from adjacent facial cutaneous tissue may be used to repair defects. Repair with local flaps may be limited by the laxity of the donor skin, and thorough analysis of blood supply, wound closure tension (Table 173.6), and strength of the underlying facial framework should be performed prior to performing a cutaneous flap. Cartilage grafting or suspension sutures may be necessary to prevent distortion of

TABLE 173.6	FACIAL CUTANEOUS FLAPS KEY DEFINITIONS
Secondary defect	Wound created when skin flap is transferred to the primary defect—goal is to place secondary defect in area of greatest tissue laxity.
Primary tissue movement	Movement of flap to defect
Secondary tissue movement	Displacement of skin surrounding defect toward center of wound usually secondary to wound closure tension and movement of tissue to close the donor site

TABLE 173.7	TYPES OF FLAP CLASSIFICATION

Location: local, regional, or distant
Vascular supply: axial or random
Flap design and method of tissue movement

TABLE 173.9	RANDOM CUTANEOUS FLAPS

Rotation flaps
Transposition flaps
Advancement flaps
Postauricular interpolation flap

mobile or weaker structures. Standing cutaneous deformities should be anticipated, and incisions should be placed along aesthetic borders or RSTLs when possible. Occasionally, flaps are combined with skin grafting for cutaneous restoration.

Flap Classification and Description

Cutaneous flaps are generally described as having skin and subcutaneous tissue with direct vascular supply and are usually transferred to an immediately adjacent or nearby location. Flaps can be classified based on (a) location, (b) vascular supply, and/or (c) flap design and method of tissue movement (Table 173.7).

Flaps may be classified based on location of flap relative to the defect. Local cutaneous flaps involve use of tissue immediately adjacent to or near the defect. Regional flap involves use of tissue from outside of the face, scalp, or neck, where arterial pedicle is sufficient to reach the facial defect (pectoralis muscle flap). Distant flaps involve harvesting of tissue from a distant location, requiring microvascular anastomosis of vessels (free flap tissue transfer).

Flaps may also be classified based on vascular supply, being described as having random or axial vascular supply (Tables 173.8 and 173.9). Random cutaneous flaps are supplied by musculocutaneous arteries near the flap base, and blood travels to the tip of the flap via the interconnecting subdermal plexus. Survival of random cutaneous flaps depends on the physical properties of the supplying vessels and the perfusion pressure (27). Flap necrosis occurs when perfusion pressure drops below the critical closing pressure of the arterioles in the subdermal plexus and there is not improved survival with a wider flap base if the arteriolar pressure remains the same (28). Axial cutaneous flaps have a greater likelihood of survival compared to random cutaneous flaps, with the survival advantage largely related to the incorporation of a septocutaneous artery within the longitudinal axis. Survival is related to the length of the

included artery, and vascular supply to the portion of skin beyond the direct arterial supply is based on the subdermal plexus, similar to a random cutaneous flap.

Flaps may be described based on the method of tissue movement and include three general types: pivotal, advancement, and hinge flaps (Table 173.10). Each of these methods will be described in more detail with the following discussion.

Pivotal Flaps

Pivotal flaps move toward the center of the wound by pivoting around a fixed point at the base of the flap pedicle, and examples include rotation, transposition, and interpolation. In general, the greater the pivot of the flap, the shorter the effective length of the flap. The effective length is reduced 5%, 15%, and 40% for flaps pivoted 45, 90, and 180 degrees, respectively (29). When designing a pivotal flap, greater degrees of pivot usually require a longer flap to account for loss of effective length, and pivoting greater than 90 degrees should be avoided. Incidentally, the greater the amount of pivot of the flap, the larger the amount of redundant tissue at the base (standing cutaneous deformity).

Rotation Flaps

Rotation flaps are pivotal flaps with curvilinear design (Fig. 173.5). In general, rotation flaps involve transfer of tissue immediately adjacent to the defect and are best used for repair of triangular defects. When rotation flaps involve pivoting of tissue only, and no advancement component, the greatest wound closure tension has been shown to be at the site perpendicular to the periphery of the flap (30).

TABLE 173.10	FLAP CLASSIFICATION BY DESIGN AND METHOD OF MOVEMENT

Pivotal flaps
  Rotation flaps
  Transposition flaps
  Interpolated flaps
Advancement flaps
  Uni-or bipedicled advancement flaps
  V-Y or Y-V advancement flaps
  Island advancement flaps
Hinge flaps

TABLE 173.8	AXIAL FLAPS WITH NAMED BLOOD SUPPLY	
Paramedian forehead flap		Supratrochlear artery
Lip crossover flap (Abbe or Estlander flap)		Orbicularis oris artery
Temporoparietal flap		Superficial temporal artery

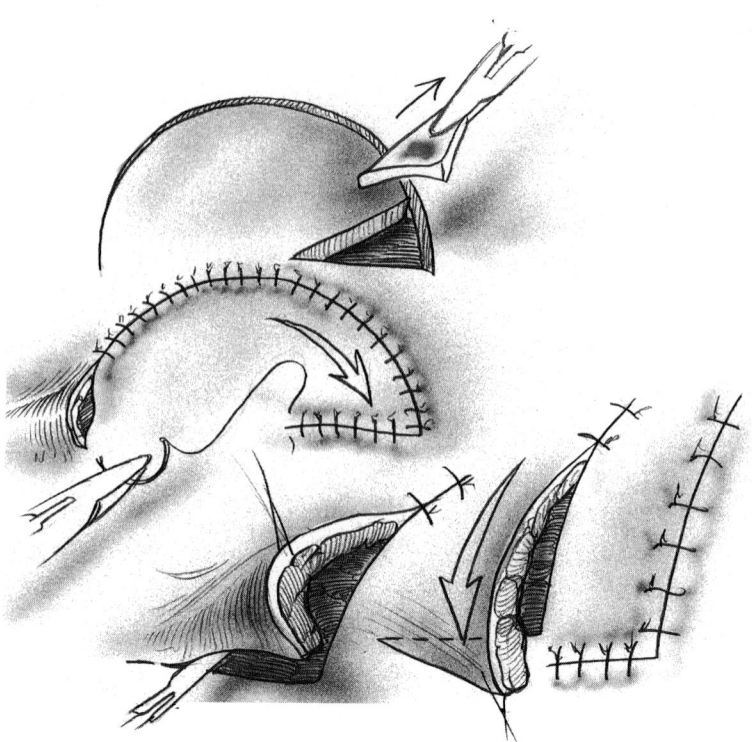

Figure 173.5 Rotation flap with semicircular design. Standing cutaneous deformity is removed at the base of the donor site.

Classically, rotation flaps are designed so that the length of the arc incision is four times the width of the defect. This configuration minimizes the need for any modifications. Rotation flaps have great flexibility in design, and position should be optimized so the flap border falls along aesthetic borders or RSTLs; in addition, flaps should be inferiorly based to facilitate lymphatic drainage. If the defect is not triangular, the defect can be modified to allow for removal of the standing cutaneous deformity at the inferior edge of the defect, thereby converting the wound to a triangular shape. Bilateral rotation flaps can be designed, with opposing flaps both transferred along curvilinear borders into the defect. When two opposing flaps are used, they result in a T-shaped scar (known as an O-to-T closure). Opposing rotation flaps can be of unequal lengths, depending on the surrounding tissue, aesthetic borders, and anatomic structures. A facial location that is particularly amenable to closure using opposing rotation flaps is the temple, with the T-shaped incision placed along the lateral canthal creases and the hairline.

When necessary, rotation flaps can be modified to reposition the standing cutaneous deformity, optimize wound closure tension, and facilitate skin redrapage. Modifications include a back cut at the base of the flap, which changes the position of the pivot point to lessen wound closure tension. In addition, this technique allows removal of the standing cutaneous deformity at the back cut, which may fall in a more optimal location such as a facial aesthetic border. Care must be taken when removing tissue at the flap base, since this may compromise the vascularity of the flap. Redundant tissue can also be removed

anywhere along the curvilinear arc, equalizing the length discrepancy between the flap's border with the adjacent defect border. Typically, the redundant tissue is removed in a triangular fashion, with excision width similar to defect width, and effort is made to place excision in an optimal position for scarring. Other modifications include changing the method of transfer from purely pivotal to include some degree of advancement as well.

Transposition Flaps

Transposition flaps transfer adjacent tissue about a pivot point but have a linear configuration (Fig. 173.6). Similar to rotation flaps, the greater the degree of pivot, the lesser the effective length of the flap and the greater the size of the standing cutaneous deformity. Wound closure tension is greatest at the closure site of the secondary defect adjacent to the base of the flap. Transposition flaps created from thick skin have limited mobility and produce larger standing cutaneous deformities and excessive wound closure tension. Design of transposition flaps with angulated borders reduces the likelihood of trapdoor deformity, which is commonly seen with curvilinear scars (31). Transposition flaps are generally pivotal but may also involve some degree of advancement. Two types of frequently used transposition flaps are rhombic flaps and bilobed flaps.

Rhombic flaps involve repair of a defect that resembles a parallelogram, having all sides equal with angles at 60 and 120 degrees opposing each other. The flap design involves extending the short diagonal of the parallelogram a distance equal to one side. Subsequently, a second incision is made parallel to one of the adjacent borders, again the same length. With this technique, with every rhombus defect, four potential flaps can be designed (Fig. 173.7). Selection of flap location relative to the defect should be considered carefully and selected based on avoidance of distortion of surrounding anatomical structures and minimizing wound closure tension by recruitment of tissue laxity. One disadvantage of the rhombic flap is the difficulty in having the majority of the scar fall within RSTLs, and for this reason, some surgeons utilize this flap less frequently in reconstruction of facial defects.

The bilobed flap is a double transposition flap with a single base (Figs. 173.8 and 173.9). The classic design involved pivoting each lobe 90 degrees, resulting in a total transposition of 180 degrees. The design was modified by Zitelli, having each lobe be 45 to 50 degrees, with total transposition under 100 degrees. This modification decreased the wound closure tension and lessened the standing cutaneous deformity (32). Similar to rhombic flaps, a disadvantage is the difficulty in having scars fall within RSTLs; however, the flap is commonly used for nasal

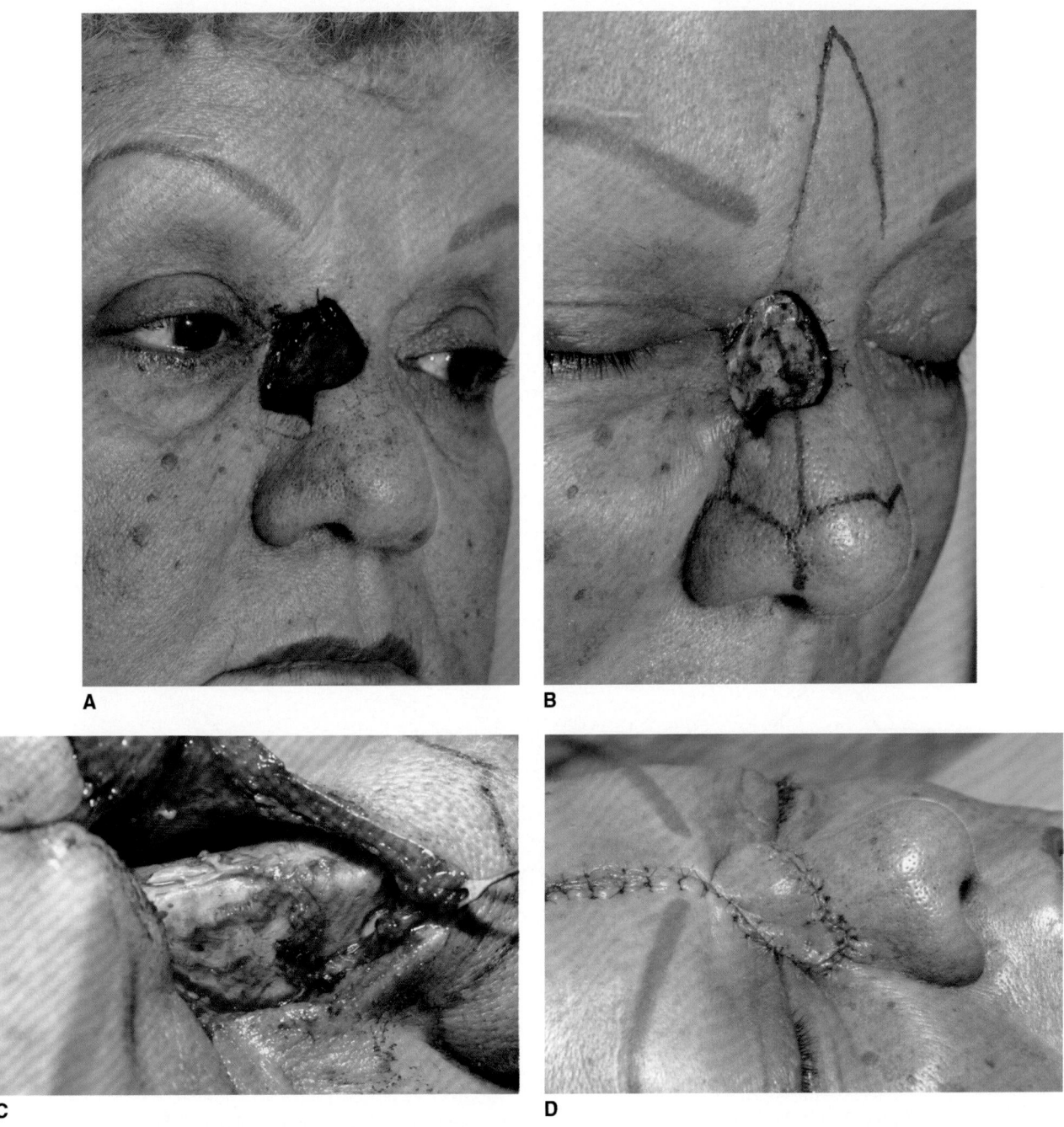

Figure 173.6 Glabellar flap. **A:** A patient with nasal defect following Mohs excision of skin cancer; **(B)** glabellar flap designed; **(C)** wide undermining of flap across nasal framework; **(D)** wound closure;

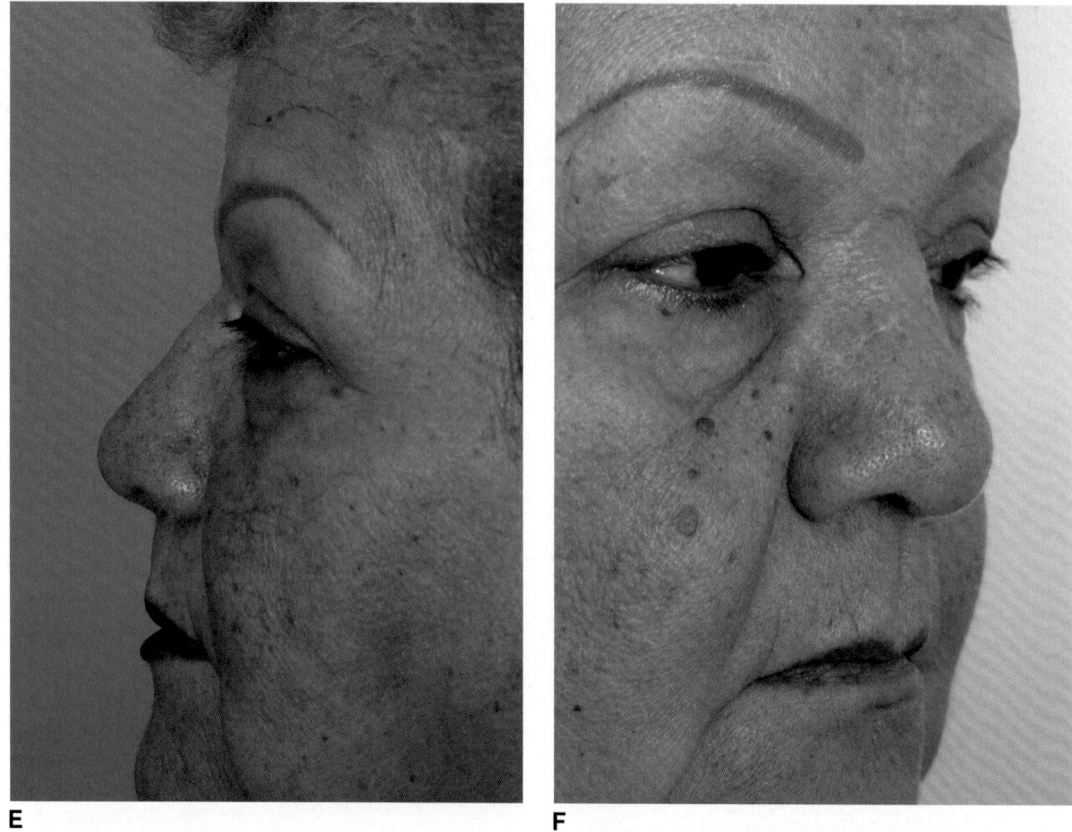

E   **F**

Figure 173.6 *(Continued)* **(E)** two-year postoperative result, lateral view; **(F)** two-year postoperative result, oblique view.

reconstruction, especially tip and supratip defects, since the double lobe design allows for recruitment of tissue from areas of greater tissue laxity such as the nasal sidewall.

The primary lobe of the bilobed flap, usually the same size as the defect, is used to restore the defect and the secondary lobe, generally 80% to 85% the size of the defect, is used to repair the donor site of the primary lobe. The donor site of the secondary lobe is closed primarily. Variations in the size of each lobe are based on differences in cutaneous thickness. If the lobe is located within an

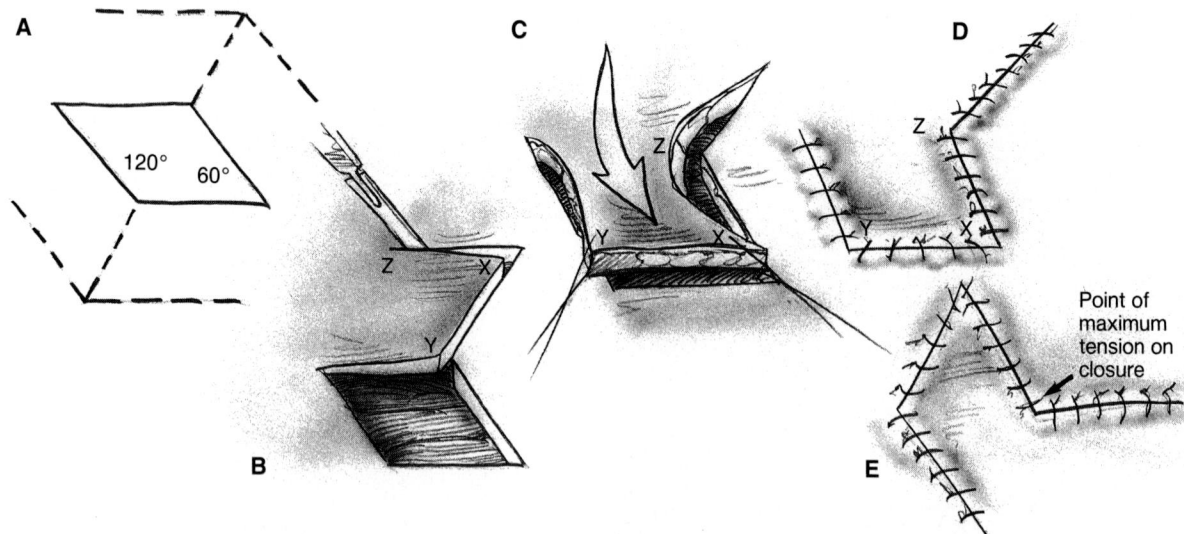

Figure 173.7 A: Classic rhomboid delineated with 60-degree and 120-degree angles with four possible limbs of tissue transfer. **B–D:** The flap is incised and transposed. **E:** Site of maximum tension demonstrated.

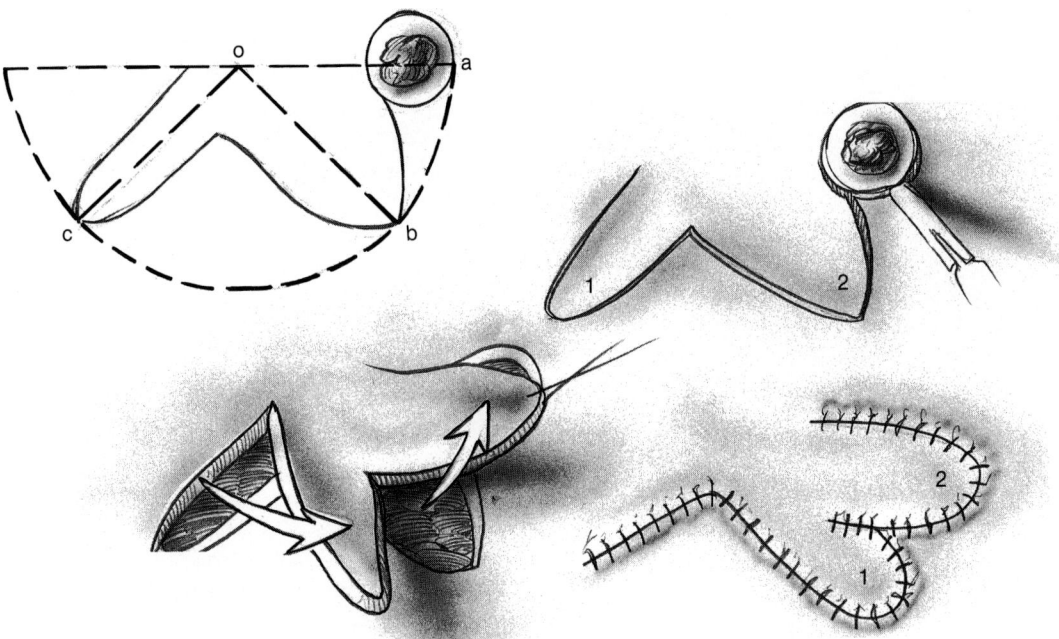

Figure 173.8 Bilobed transposition flap design. Ideal angle of flap transfer is about 90 to 100 degrees, with the angle measured between the defect and secondary lobe. Secondary lobe is placed within area of suitable tissue laxity.

area of thick, noncompliant, immobile facial tissue, it is imperative to make the lobe the same size as the defect since limited mobility and stretch is expected. Undersizing of the primary or secondary lobe will result in increased wound tension, poor scarring, and distortion of surrounding facial structures. In addition, oversizing of the flap predisposes to trapdoor deformity and uneven contours. Hence, judicious sizing is necessary and is dependent on the texture and thickness of the skin and tissue being transposed. In general, ideal patients have thin, mobile skin, while patients

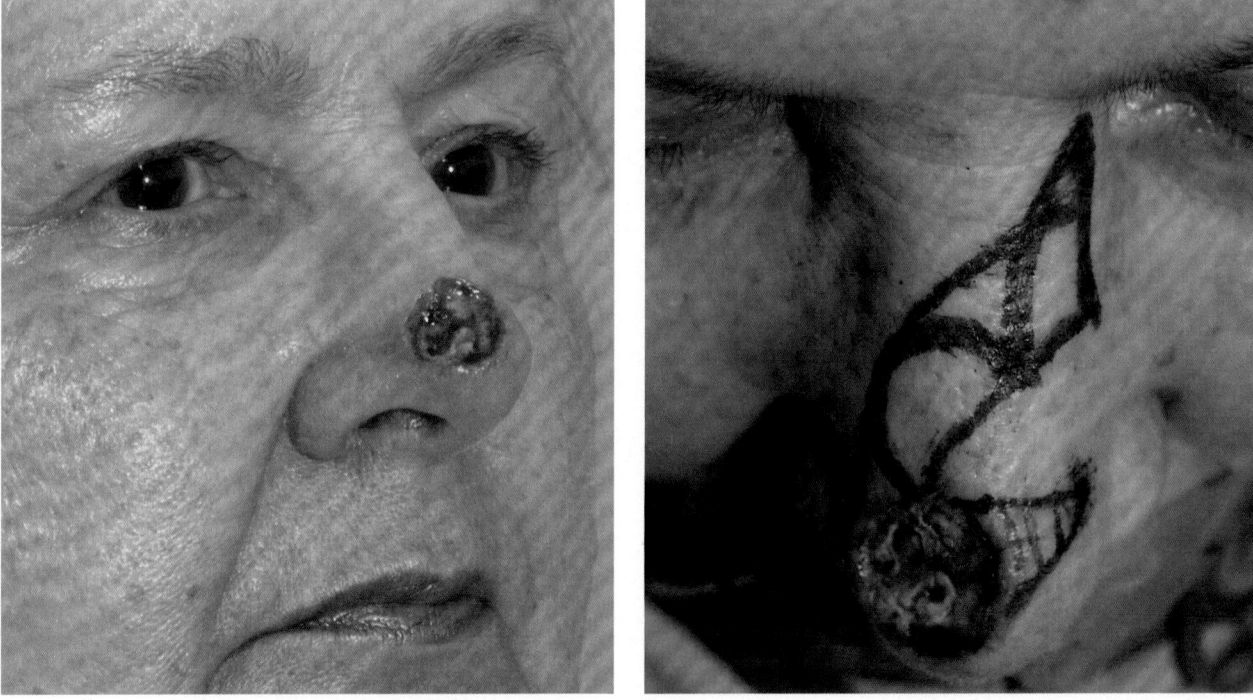

A **B**

Figure 173.9 Bilobed transposition flap. **A:** A patient with nasal defect following Mohs excision of skin cancer; **(B)** bilobed transposition delineated, with arc of rotation 100 degrees;

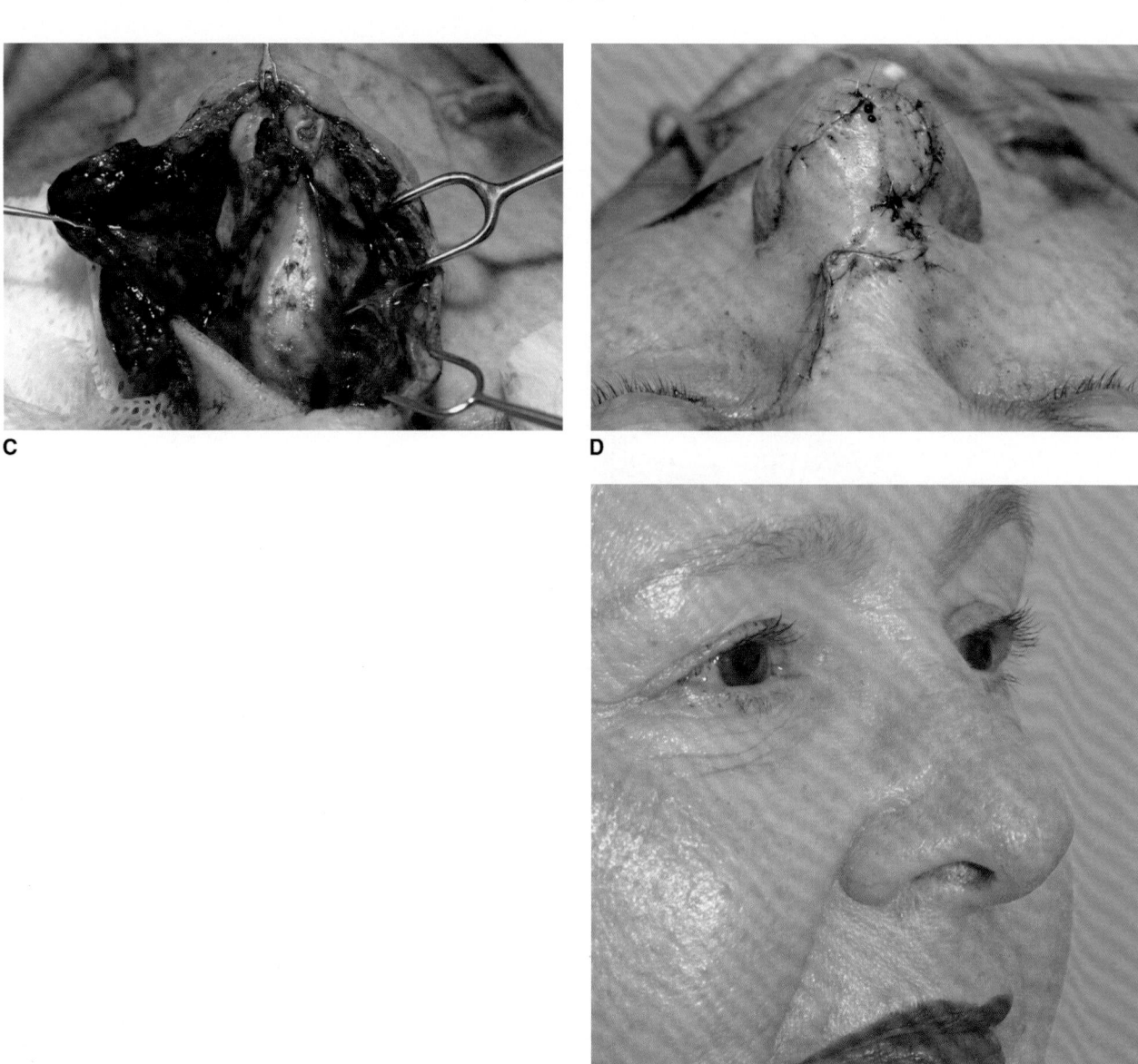

Figure 173.9 *(Continued)* **(C)** wide undermining of flap across nasal framework; **(D)** wound closure; **(E)** one-year postoperative result.

with thick, sebaceous skin have less mobility for transfer and increased risk of developing necrosis, trapdoor deformity, and depressed scars. An anticipated standing cutaneous deformity is removed, whenever possible, within an incisional line hidden along an aesthetic unit boundary.

Bilobed flaps on the nose are ideally based laterally and are best used to repair defects located on the central or lateral nasal tip that are less than 1.5 cm in diameter. When possible, the axis of the secondary lobe is placed perpendicular to the alar rim. In so doing, displacement of the alar rim by closure of the secondary lobe donor site is minimized. An ideal defect location for this technique is the zone of transition between the tip, ala, and sidewall. Use of the bilobed flap for alar reconstruction is avoided because crossing the alar groove with the pedicle causes distortion of this nasal landmark (33).

Interpolation Flaps

Interpolation flaps are similar to transposition flaps in that they have pivotal movement; however, the base of interpolated flaps is not contiguous with the defect resulting in a pedicle that spans over intervening cutaneous tissue. Interpolation flaps require secondary detachment, once recipient vascular supply to the flap has been established. Common examples of interpolation flaps include the paramedian forehead flap (Fig. 173.10) and the melolabial flap used in nasal reconstruction. Both are detailed in a separate section in this textbook and will not be further discussed in this chapter. Other examples include the lip crossover flap and the postauricular flap, both used for the repair of full-thickness defects involving the lip and ear, respectively.

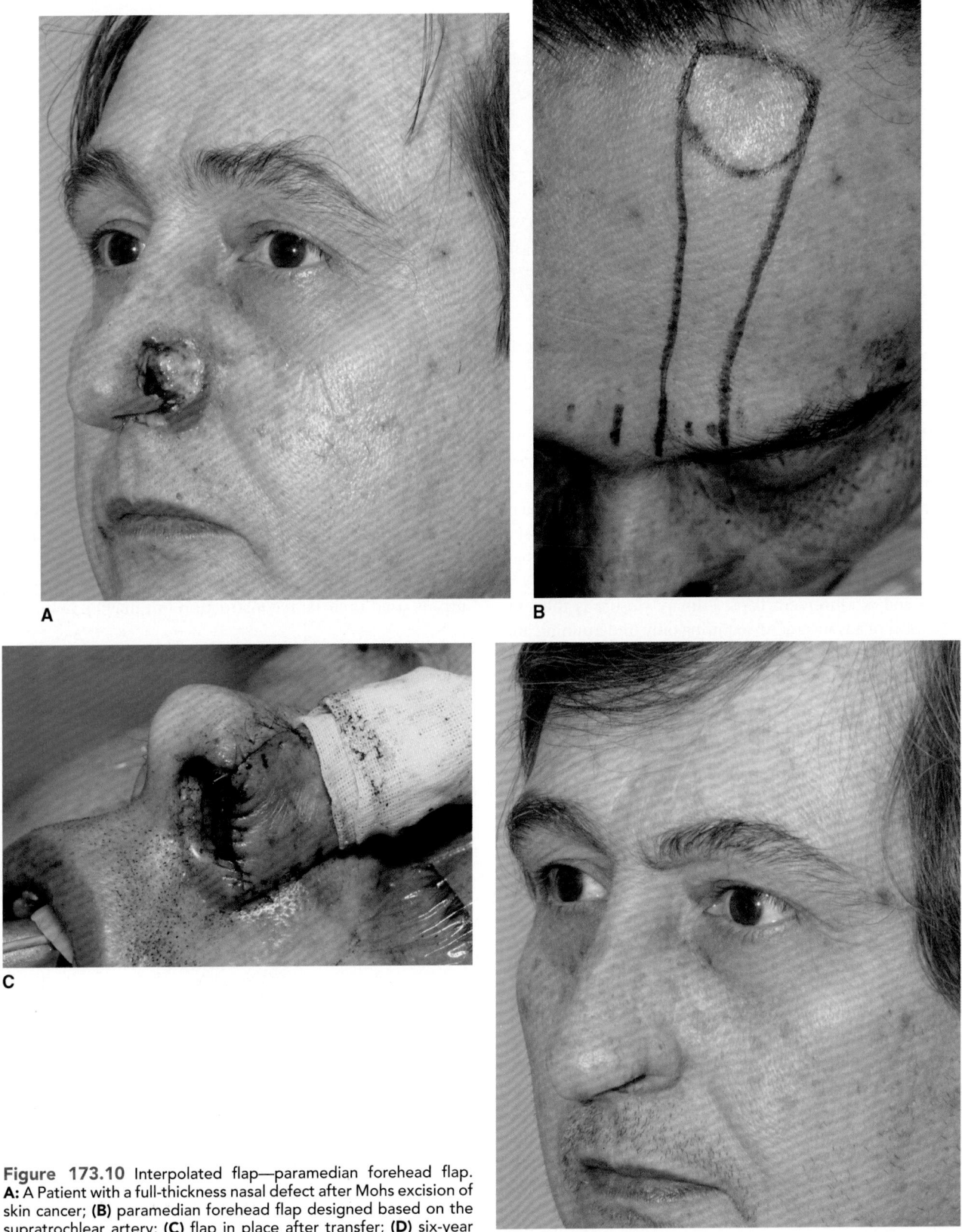

Figure 173.10 Interpolated flap—paramedian forehead flap. **A:** A Patient with a full-thickness nasal defect after Mohs excision of skin cancer; **(B)** paramedian forehead flap designed based on the supratrochlear artery; **(C)** flap in place after transfer; **(D)** six-year postoperative result.

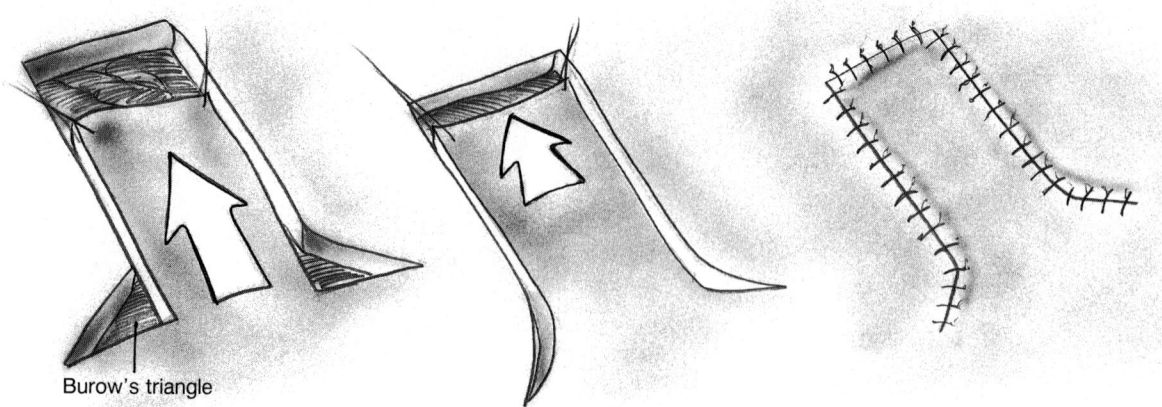

Burow's triangle

Figure 173.11 Monopedicled advancement flap. Flap is incised and transferred across the defect. Standing cutaneous deformities are excised at the base of the donor tissue.

Advancement Flaps

Advancement flaps have a linear design and are moved directly to the defect. These flaps are mobilized by undermining of tissue and inevitably have some component of "stretching" of tissue; hence, advancement flaps are most successful in areas of greatest tissue laxity and extensibility. Examples of advancement flaps include unipedicle, bipedicle, V-Y, Y-V, and island advancement flaps. Primary closure is the simplest form of advancement, requiring only undermining and advancement of tissue without releasing incisions to facilitate tissue movement. Primary closure generates standing cutaneous deformities that are ideally removed along RSTLs.

Uni- and Bipedicled Advancement Flaps

Unipedicled flaps involve parallel incisions with movement of tissue spanning over defect. Repair is completed with primary and secondary tissue movement. Given the length discrepancy between flap borders and recipient tissue, standing cutaneous deformities develop along both incisions and can be incised at any favorable point along the incision lines. Effort is made to place incisions along RSTLs, and bilateral flaps can be employed (Fig. 173.11). When two flaps are used, they are opposing and result in an H-shaped scar (Fig. 173.12). Opposing advancement flaps can be of unequal lengths, depending on the surrounding tissue laxity, aesthetic borders, and anatomic structures. Unipedicled flaps may be employed in the repair of forehead defects, where the longest portions of the H-shaped incisions are placed within the horizontal forehead creases. Bipedicled flaps involve transfer of tissue at a right angle to the defect, leaving a secondary defect that is commonly repaired with grafting. Bipedicled flaps may be used for scalp reconstruction, but more commonly, these flaps are used for vestibular lining repair of nasal alar defects.

V-Y and Y-V Advancement Flaps

V-Y advancement flaps involve "pushing" of central tissue, with closure of donor site by advancement of opposing wound borders. Wound closure tension is perpendicular to movement of central tissue, and this technique is

commonly used for release and lengthening of contracted tissue. V-Y advancement can be used to correct distorted vermillion or eyelid borders. Y-V advancement involves creation of a triangular defect, followed by "pulling" of central tissue toward the defect. Wound closure tension is parallel to the central vector of the flap and is greatest at the apex of the flap. This technique is not commonly used in facial reconstruction but may be helpful in

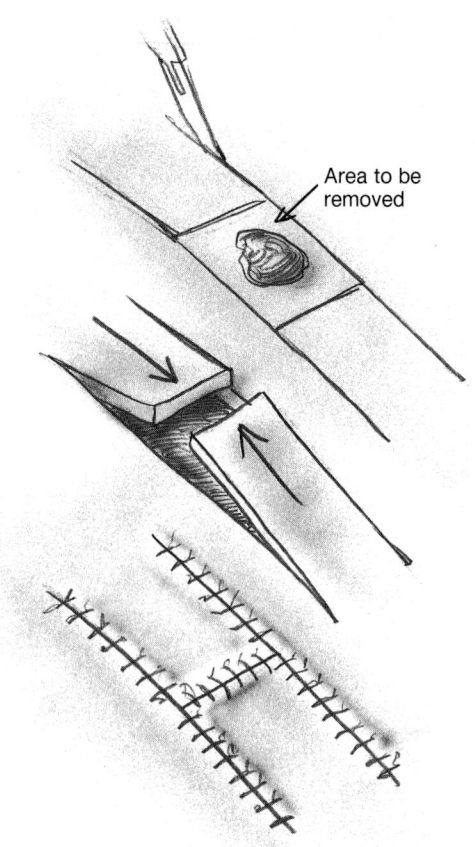

Area to be removed

Figure 173.12 Bipedicled advancement flaps. Flaps are incised and transferred across the defect. Standing cutaneous deformities are excised at the base of the donor tissue.

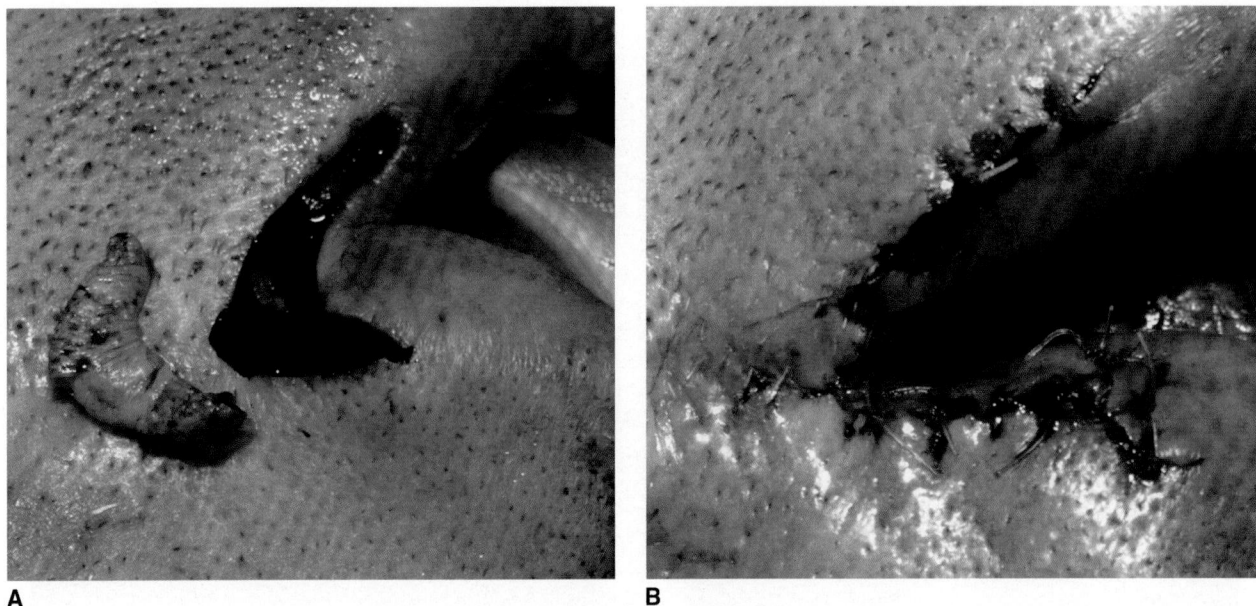

Figure 173.13 A,B: Commissuroplasty with Y to V flap.

restoring a distorted oral commissure (commissuroplasty) (Fig. 173.13).

Island Advancement Flaps

Island advancement flaps involve transfer of an "island" of cutaneous tissue, incised on all borders, with a pedicle of subcutaneous tissue containing sufficient vascular supply. Dissection is performed for the medial and lateral thirds of the flap, maintaining a central island pedicle with random arterial supply. Island advancement flaps can be rotated and/or advanced to the defect, but for facial defects, the flaps are more commonly advanced. An example of rotation would include rotation along the melolabial crease for the repair of lip or medial cheek defects (Fig. 173.14). Design of the flap is largely dependent on the shape of the defect, surrounding anatomical structures, aesthetic

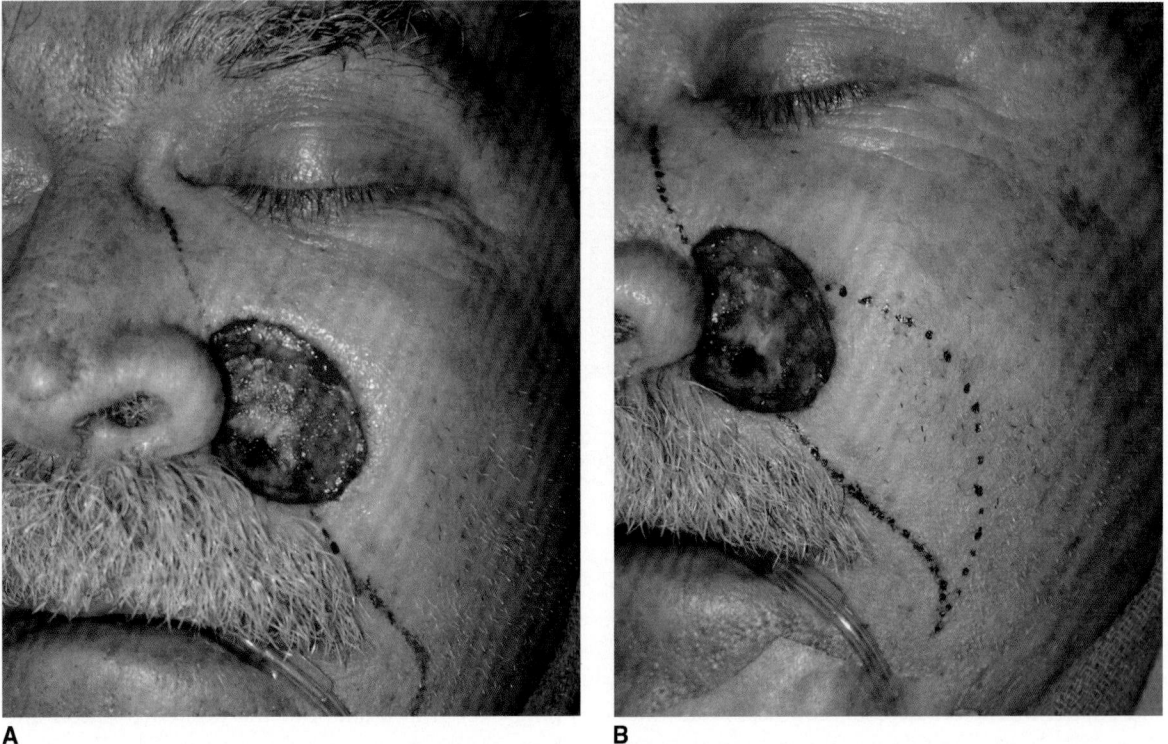

Figure 173.14 Island advancement flap. **A:** A patient with an open facial defect after Mohs resection of skin cancer; **(B)** island advancement flap designed;

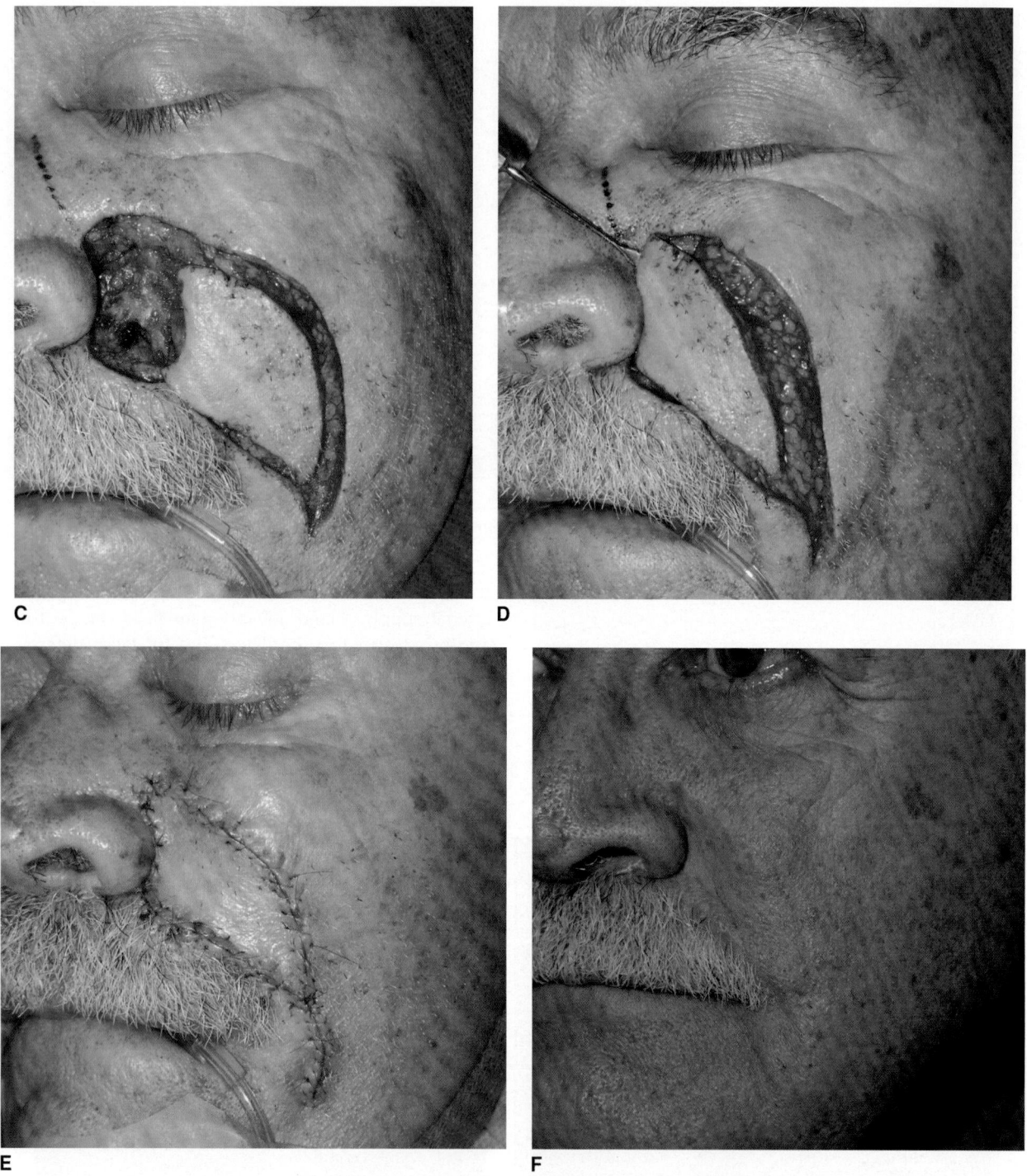

Figure 173.14 *(Continued)* **(C)** broad undermining and release of tissue; **(D)** securing the flap to medial periosteum using tacking suture; **(E)** closure; **(F)** one-year postoperative result.

borders, and RSTLs. Patients with moderate skin thickness and sufficient tissue laxity are the best candidates, and flaps may need to be oversized to avoid distortion of anatomical structures adjacent to the defect. Wide undermining of adjacent tissue decreases the likelihood of trapdoor deformity and adjacent structure deformation. Island advancement flaps may be transferred over intervening cutaneous

tissue and, thus, also be considered an interpolated flap in these circumstances.

Hinge Flaps
Cutaneous hinge flaps involve transfer of tissue by "flipping over" the tissue into the desired position and location, similar to turning the page in a book. This type of

flap may be of varied shape and is most commonly used for internal lining purposes. After transfer of the cutaneous hinge flap, the subcutaneous tissue that remains exposed is covered by a second cutaneous flap or graft. Vascularity is dependent on the tissue bordering the defect; hence, allowing the wound border to become well healed improves the vascularity of the cutaneous hinge flap. Subcutaneous hinge flaps involve transfer of only subcutaneous tissue in the same fashion and are most commonly for contour augmentation and/or coverage of cartilage grafts prior to cutaneous restoration.

Technique—Facial Cutaneous Flaps

In preparation for local flaps, the involved facial regions are injected with local anesthetic containing epinephrine in an appropriate plane to facilitate dissection and optimize hemostasis. The margins of the defect are freshened with a scalpel, removing the beveled edge from the Mohs resection. The flap is demarcated based on the size of the defect, and the flap and surrounding cutaneous tissue are elevated in an avascular plane, taking care to maintain a rich vascular supply to the flap. Wide undermining reduces trapdoor deformity and facilitates wound closure by reducing wound tension (Table 173.11).

The donor site is closed first, followed by suturing the flap in place. Polydioxanone or poliglecaprone sutures are used for subcutaneous closure, and polypropylene vertical mattress and running sutures are used for cutaneous closure. Bacitracin is applied and a compression dressing consisting of a nonadherent dressing, cotton balls, and expandable tape is placed for 24 hours. Cutaneous sutures are removed in 5 to 7 days.

Facial cutaneous flaps have the potential to distort normal facial anatomy, leading to anatomic asymmetries, retraction or distortion, and functional compromise. Careful planning and selective use of flaps minimize these potential complications; furthermore, judicious use of cartilage grafting is recommended. Cartilage grafts can be harvested from septum or the conchal bowl, and grafts are sewn in place using polyglactin mattress sutures. Cartilage grafts are commonly used along the alar rim to prevent notching. Suspension sutures may be used in the area of nasal sesamoid cartilages, spanning toward the pyriform aperture, to address any potential nasal valve collapse. Suspension

sutures may also be used at the lateral and medial canthus in the form of a canthopexy or canthoplasty, in order to address any potential eyelid malposition.

FACIAL CUTANEOUS GRAFTS

Occasionally, superficial and/or extensive facial defects are best addressed by repair with a skin or composite graft (Table 173.12). Placement of a graft obviates the need for additional scars on the face as is seen with other reconstructive methods; however, most grafts have a "patched" appearance with discrepancies in color and texture between native and grafted facial skin. Postoperative resurfacing procedures may minimize these color and texture discrepancies.

Skin graft viability depends on several factors: blood supply to the recipient site, microcirculation on the surface of the recipient site, vascularity of donor graft tissue, contact between the graft and recipient site, and certain systemic illnesses. Contact between the skin graft and recipient site is essential, and a bolster dressing prevents fluid collections and shearing forces from disrupting fibrous connections between the graft and wound bed. Systemic illnesses that may compromise graft survival include inflammatory conditions, hematologic disorders, diabetes, nutritional deficiencies, and hypoxemia (34). Use of tobacco products is also detrimental to the survival of skin grafts.

Recipient site conditions that are not favorable to graft survival include irradiated tissue, excessive fibrosis, exposed bone, cartilage, or tendon. Grafts placed over avascular defects smaller than 1 cm² may survive through nutritional support via wound edges; however, grafting over avascular wounds larger than this is unlikely to succeed (34).

Split-Thickness Grafts

Split-thickness grafts consist of epidermis and a variable portion of underlying dermis, and most surgeons harvest these grafts with a dermatome so as to contain epidermis and minimal to no dermal tissue. Because of their poor color and texture match with normal skin and their tendency to contract, split-thickness skin grafts are rarely used to replace cutaneous tissue in facial reconstruction.

TABLE 173.11	KEYPOINTS—CUTANEOUS FLAPS

Proper patient and defect selection
Orient flap tension to minimize distortion
Perpendicular incisions and wide undermining

TABLE 173.12	FACIAL CUTANEOUS GRAFTS

Split-thickness grafts
Full-thickness grafts
Staged grafts
Composite grafts

Full-Thickness Grafts

Full-thickness skin grafts consist of epidermis and full-thickness dermis. They resist contraction, have texture and pigmentation similar to normal skin, and require a well-vascularized, uncontaminated wound site for survival. Full-thickness grafts survive initially by diffusion of nutrition from fluid in the recipient site, a process known as plasma imbibition. This is followed by vascular inosculation, which usually occurs during the first 24 to 48 hours. After 48 to 72 hours, capillaries in the recipient site begin to grow into the graft to provide new circulation. By 3 to 5 days, a new blood supply has been established. Initially, full-thickness skin grafts appear blanched; however, over 3 to 7 days, a pink color develops signaling neovascularization. After 4 to 6 weeks, the pink color begins to fade, but the graft will often remain lighter than the surrounding skin, especially in darker skinned individuals.

Compared to split thickness, full-thickness grafts have the advantage of better color and texture match, less contour irregularities, no need for special equipment, and easier donor site wound care. The disadvantages may include reduced survival rate for larger grafts and longer healing time (34). The ideal facial defect to repair with a full-thickness skin graft is superficial, with loss of skin, but not underlying muscle or soft tissue. The vascularity of shallow wounds is greater than that for defects extending underlying cartilage or bone. There is a wide variation of facial skin thickness among individuals, and the overall thickness of the facial skin is an important preoperative consideration. For similar facial defects, a skin graft may provide a perfect match in terms of thickness for one person and a poor match for another.

A number of donor sites for skin grafts are available in most individuals, including the upper eyelid, forehead, melolabial fold, preauricular, postauricular, and supraclavicular areas. When selecting the donor site, the thickness and color of the recipient site skin are assessed, and the most optimal match in donor skin is determined. Skin from the postauricular area is preferred in men with skin defects of limited size because it is hairless and tends to have a similar thickness to the facial skin. Because men tend to have shorter hair than women, the postauricular skin is likely to have solar aging, which provides an improved skin color match with the facial skin. In contrast, preauricular skin is a better source for grafts in females. Preauricular skin in females is hairless and has more solar aging compared to postauricular skin, which is often covered by hair. The supraclavicular region is an excellent source for skin grafts, especially when a large graft is required. However, the supraclavicular skin is usually less sun exposed, creating a color discrepancy between the recipient skin and the skin graft. In addition, the supraclavicular skin can be much thicker than most facial skin, and judicious thinning of the graft is usually required.

There are occasions when skin grafts are used to repair defects even when it is anticipated that the graft will result in a contour depression or noticeable color discrepancy. These situations arise when caring for debilitated patients who have life-threatening illnesses. In addition, in patients who have malignancies showing aggressive growth patterns and tumor persistence or recurrence is a primary concern, skin grafts may be used as a temporary covering for a several years to facilitate tumor surveillance.

Locations particularly amenable to skin grafting include the temple, medial canthus, philtrum, and portions of the nose. The ideal nasal defects perhaps most amenable to a skin graft are separated from the free margin of the nostril by 5 mL and located in thin-skinned areas of the nose, such as the cephalic sidewalls, cephalic dorsum, and infratip lobule. Shallow wounds in these areas are typically completely filled by a full-thickness skin graft, thereby establishing confluent contour with the surrounding skin. The areas of the nose covered with thicker skin tend to heal with a contour depression and noticeable textural discrepancies between graft and adjacent facial skin. This is because the facial skin in these areas tends to have a more sebaceous nature than the graft.

If a full-thickness graft has been performed and a contour depression exists, the appearance can be improved by subsequent placement of a dermal fat graft after the skin graft has healed. Meyers et al. describe the use of dermal grafts at the time of skin graft placement to help prevent contour depression following repair of deeper defects. Their technique involves the placement of dermal tissue in linear strips within the wound bed, leaving adequate exposure of the underlying wound bed to provide nourishment to an overlying skin graft (35).

Defects located on the lateral nasal ala immediately adjacent to the nasal facial sulcus can be repaired with a number of options. If the defect extends into the cheek, the cheek component of the defect is usually repaired with a cheek advancement flap. The alar component can be repaired with a cheek or paramedian forehead flap if the defect is large. For smaller defects, especially in very young patients where preservation of regional flaps is desired, full-thickness skin grafts and composite grafts are considered for the alar portion of the defect. Full-thickness grafts are best suited for superficial defects not extending to the nostril border. In the case of deep alar defects, skin grafts do not lend any structural support, and subsequent nasal valve collapse may lead to compromise of the nasal airway. One option for patients with deep alar defects is the transfer of subcutaneous cheek tissue in the form of a hinge flap. The flap partially fills the defect and facilitates placement of an alar batten graft deep to the hinge flap. A full-thickness graft can then be placed as external covering over the hinge flap, thereby completing a single-stage reconstruction.

When defects of the nasal sidewall extend to the medial cheek, the cheek component of the defect is reconstructed with a cutaneous advancement flap. The flap is advanced and anchored in place at the nasal facial sulcus with deep sutures that pass from the medial border of the flap to the periosteum of the nasal sidewall. A full-thickness skin graft is then used to resurface the sidewall. The cheek advancement flap facilitates positioning scars along the junctional zone between the aesthetic regions of the cheek and nose.

Staged Grafts

For deeper wounds, skin grafting may be delayed until granulation tissue has filled the wound bed (2 to 3 weeks), thereby reducing the likelihood of a step-down deformity at the edges of the graft. In addition, delay provides an improved vascular recipient site for the graft (36), which is especially important in areas of exposed periosteum or perichondrium. Development of sufficient granulation tissue may be improved by initial placement of an acellular dermal graft wound matrix to facilitate healing of wound bed prior to skin grafting. The acellular dermal graft wound matrix may be placed at the time of tissue resection, and wound care is dependent on the type of acellular dermal graft employed.

Following development of sufficient granulation tissue, any epithelium is removed prior to grafting and the tissue is cross-hatched so that myofibrils are released. Granulating wounds normally contain bacteria, and bacterial counts greater than 10^5 organisms per gram of tissue often lead to graft loss (37). When delayed grafting is planned, the patient is started on a course of an antistaphylococcal antibiotic several days prior to the delayed grafting procedure.

Technique—Facial Cutaneous Grafts

All patients undergoing skin grafting receive preoperative intravenous antibiotics, followed by 1 week of oral antibiotics. The bevel of the defect after Mohs excision is freshened, taking care to maintain a bevel to the skin edge, thereby smoothing the transition between the graft and recipient skin and lessening any contour deformity (Fig. 173.15). Additional beveling of the defect may be performed if the skin graft is substantially thinner than the depth of the recipient site.

A template is made of the recipient site by outlining the periphery of the wound with a surgical marker and pressing a nonadherent dressing pad over the marking. If the defect is round, the shape is often modified by excising skin to create angulated borders, which improves the contour outcome. In addition, movement and transfer of adjacent facial skin are performed if this is found helpful in isolating the defect to a single facial aesthetic unit. Using the template,

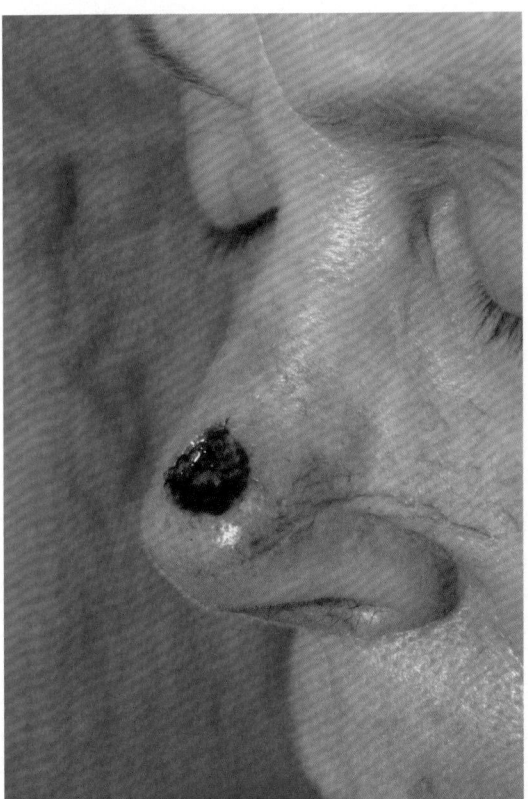

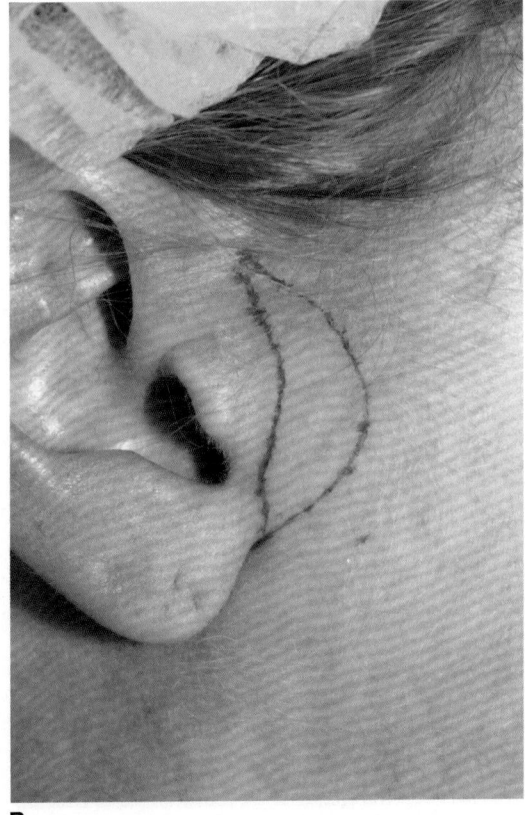

A   **B**

Figure 173.15 Cutaneous graft. A patient status post glabellar flap prior to presenting to our facility. **A:** Open nasal defect following Mohs excision of skin cancer—no nasal laxity; **(B)** preauricular donor site delineated;

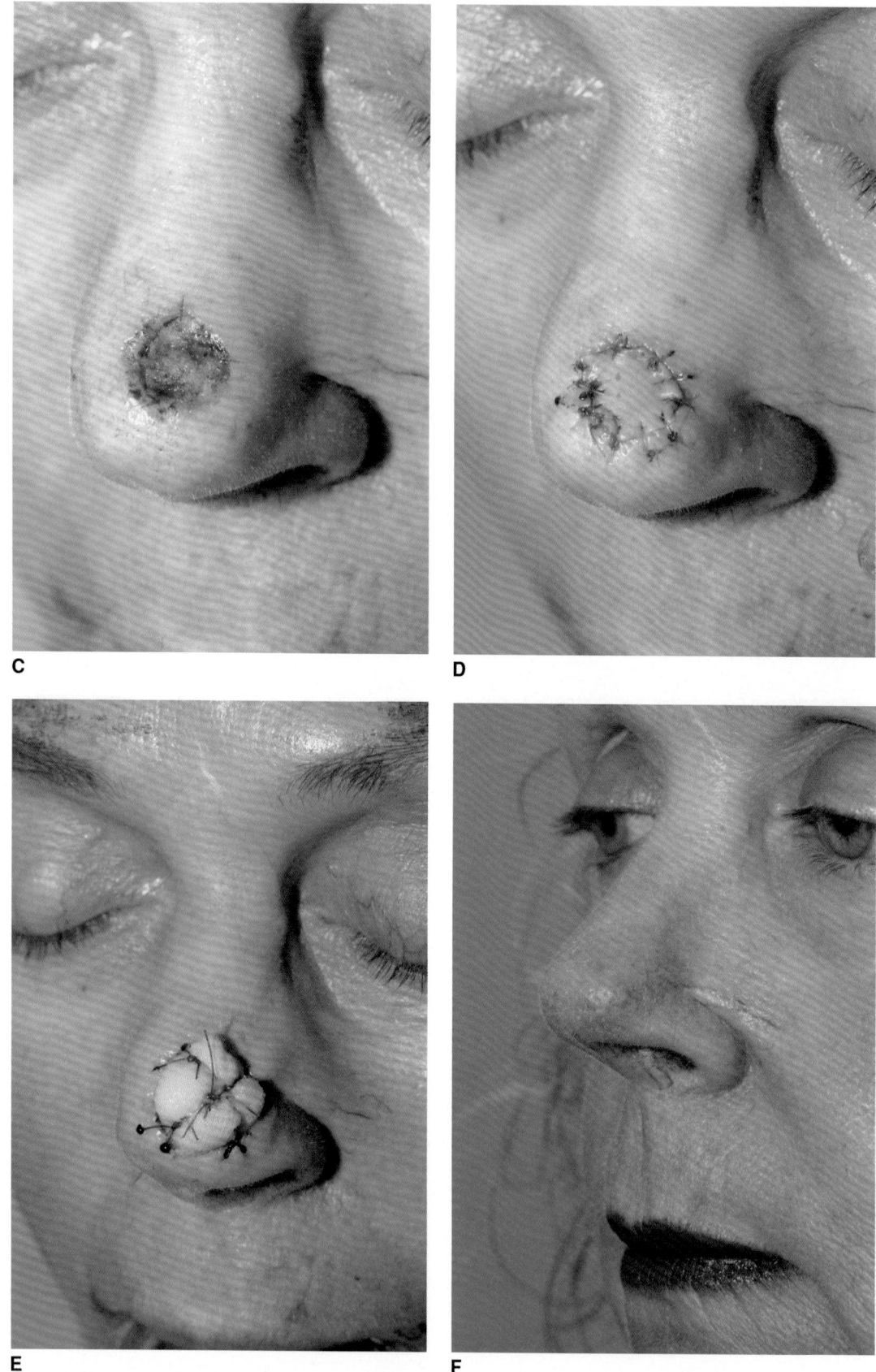

Figure 173.15 *(Continued)* **(C)** wound site preparation with angulation of borders and beveling of wound edges; **(D)** cutaneous graft inset; **(E)** bolster for skin graft placed; **(F)** one-year postoperative result.

TABLE 173.13	KEY POINTS—CUTANEOUS GRAFTS

Consider delay.
Angulate recipient site borders.
Bevel wound edges.
Optimize vascularity of wound bed.

the configuration of the graft is determined. The graft is excised and all subcutaneous tissue is removed using curved scissors. This is best accomplished by placing the graft over one's finger, epidermal side down, and trimming off excess fat until shiny dermis is visible (Table 173.13).

The graft is transferred to the recipient site and secured with absorbable sutures as well as a bolster. The bolster is removed after 5 days, and any type of shearing motion is avoided as it may disrupt vascularization of the graft. After removal of the bolster, the patient is instructed to keep the graft dry and apply topical ointment to the graft's edges only. A week or two later, when the graft has survived and is well adhered to the recipient site, the patient is allowed to bathe the area.

The graft may appear bruised during the first few days following transfer. It then transitions to a hyperemic stage, which fades over weeks to months. Occasionally, a dark graft may not survive. If the entire graft dies, it will separate from the recipient site within several weeks. More commonly, the deeper portion of the graft will survive while the more superficial portion forms an eschar, which remains fixed to the wound bed. When this occurs, reepithelialization will occur from the wound edges and from the viable deeper dermal component of the graft. Often, sufficient dermis survives to prevent the development of a depressed scar following complete healing; however, color and textural differences between facial skin and the graft are usually more apparent than when the graft survives completely.

Adjunctive procedures to optimize aesthetic appearance may be performed after grafting. Trapdoor deformities usually resolve overtime with appropriate massage. Grafts rarely require a surgical contouring procedure, but sometimes, Z-plasties may be performed at the border of the graft to enhance the transition between graft and native facial skin. Resurfacing procedures for full-thickness skin grafts are an option, and usually most of the facial skin within the aesthetic units surrounding the graft is resurfaced as well.

Facial Composite Grafts

Composite grafts contain two or more tissue layers and often are unsuccessful secondary to high metabolic demands. They obtain their nourishment through plasma imbibition during the first 24 hours after transfer, followed by vascular inosculation. Ingrowth of capillaries from the edges of the graft begins by the third day (38,39,40).

Composite grafts were first described by Konig (41), who used composite auricular grafts to repair alar defects, noting a 53% graft survival. Composite grafts have been used to repair nasal columellar defects (42,43) and deficiencies in nasal lining (44). During the first half of the 20th century, Limberg (45) advocated the cavum and cymba of the concha as the preferred donor site for repair of the nose. Symonds and Crikelair (46) also used composite auricular grafts for nasal reconstruction, reporting an 89% graft survival rate.

The auricle is an excellent source for composite grafts for facial reconstruction, especially for nasal defects, because it provides a contoured graft of skin and cartilage. Certain segments of the auricle loosely replicate the delicate topography of the columella, facet, and nostril margin where composite grafts are commonly employed. For both anatomic sites, the skin is tightly adherent to the underlying cartilage and/or fibrofatty tissue. Common auricular donor sites are helical crus, helical rim, antitragus, and fossa triangularis. The helical crus provides a good contour match for small alar rim defects and provides the option of incorporating in the graft a segment of preauricular skin.

The traditional recommendation is to limit the size of composite grafts to 1 cm or less (47). Considerably larger grafts may be successful if they are placed in a vascular recipient site and the graft is designed so that no portion is more than 1.0 cm from a wound edge (48–50). Skouge advocated a tongue and groove technique when using composite grafts. This technique involves insetting the border of the graft between two layers of tissue at the recipient site (37). This method of graft attachment has the effect of increasing surface contact between graft and recipient site by 50% (51). A hinge flap developed at the recipient site also increases the surface area for attaching a composite graft (52).

The use of perioperative corticosteroids is beneficial in enhancing survival of composite grafts in animals. Rabbits treated with preoperative and postoperative methylprednisolone demonstrated improved graft survival compared to animals receiving no steroids or postoperative doses only. Attempts to salvage compromised grafts with delayed administration of steroids were not successful (53,54). Cooling of composite grafts has also been demonstrated to improve survival. Cooling reduces biologic requirements and improves graft survival in irradiated, atrophic, or scarred recipient sites. Conley demonstrated that constant application of ice compresses for 14 days effected a fall in skin temperature from 38°F to 17°F. Grafts ranged in size from 1 × 1 cm to 2 × 2 cm. Of twelve composite grafts transferred to the nose and treated with ice compresses, ten survived completely. Five of the grafts had been placed in recipient sites with scarring or postirradiation fibrosis (55).

An ideal defect for a composite auricular graft is a small (1.0 cm or less) full-thickness defect of the nasal facet or columella. The nasal skin in these areas is extremely thin, lacking subcutaneous fat, and is tightly adherent to the underlying cartilage or fibrous connective tissue. Composite auricular grafts obtained from the helical crus provide grafts with thin skin attached to a delicate segment of cartilage, providing structural support and skin that closely resembles the adjacent nasal skin of the columella and facet.

Perhaps more commonly, composite grafts are used to repair small defects of the nasal ala, especially those extending to the alar rim. Composite grafts can be used to maintain structural integrity at the nasal valve and provide a smooth continuous border to the alar rim. Weisberg and Becker describe the use of auricular composite grafts with stabilizing struts for repair of such defects. The stabilizing struts are extensions of cartilage that are placed beneath the adjacent nasal skin in a tongue and groove fashion similar to Skouge's original description (56).

Technique—Facial Composite Grafts

Patient selection is an important consideration. The use of composite grafts is generally limited to small defects in patients who do not use tobacco and have no systemic illnesses that would compromise graft revascularization. Patients receive antibiotics and wound preparation similar to that described when performing skin grafts. In addition, prednisone is administered on the day of surgery and a steroid taper is provided postoperatively.

Improved survival rate is noted if grafting is delayed until the facial defect has partially healed by secondary intention. The facial defect is then prepared by removing any epithelium and subepithelial scar tissue, and a template is created that measures several millimeters larger than the defect in all dimensions. Harvesting a graft that is slightly larger than the defect accommodates for the inevitable contraction of the graft. Whenever possible, a flap of soft tissue hinged on a border of the defect is developed to enhance surface contact with the graft. A composite graft containing skin and cartilage is harvested from the region of the auricle that most closely matches the contour and thickness of the nose at the defect site. The graft is placed in cold saline, and the donor site is closed primarily using polydioxanone or poliglecaprone sutures to approximate the edges of the auricular cartilage and polypropylene sutures for the skin. The graft is transferred to the recipient site and secured in place with simple absorbable sutures, limiting the degree of manipulation of the graft. If the graft is small, no sutures are placed through the cartilage. Limiting the number of sutures used to fix the graft in place is thought to be beneficial in enabling earlier and more abundant vessel ingrowth.

Ice–saline compresses are applied for the first 3 to 5 days. Successful grafts transition in color during the first week: blanched at initial transfer, pink color at 6 hours, darker by 24 hours, and gradual development of a pink color in 3 to 7 days. Complications include partial or complete graft loss, contracture, pigmentary changes, and contour abnormalities. Contour abnormalities may be addressed with a debulking or scar revision procedures.

COMPLICATIONS

It is essential that surgeons become familiar with the potential complications associated with facial reconstructive surgery, anticipating these undesirable events and taking proper measures to help prevent their occurrence (Table 173.14). Establishing a consistent perioperative routine is the first step in preventing complications. Appropriate preoperative counseling of the patient will reduce the likelihood of complications, and informed consent should include an open discussion of potential problems that may occur. Immediate and regular postoperative evaluations of the patient will facilitate early recognition and treatment of complications. Some complications are reversible, and expeditious treatment may prevent a reversible complication from becoming an irreversible one. Finally, adherence to well-established surgical principles is essential for minimizing the incidence of complications when performing facial reconstructive surgery.

Bleeding

Common causes of bleeding from facial reconstruction using local flaps are drug-associated coagulopathy and inadequate hemostasis. Patients are questioned preoperatively concerning use of all prescription and over-the-counter medications that may contribute to perioperative bleeding. Discontinuation of any medications prescribed by a physician to reduce blood clotting is coordinated with the patient's medical physician or cardiovascular specialist. Bleeding may also be associated with hypertensive events, hepatic or renal failure, vomiting, straining, or alterations in the hematopoietic system.

Hemostasis is essential. Bipolar electrocoagulation is used to control bleeding from smaller vessels and larger arterial vessels are securely ligated when interrupted. Drains are rarely used with local cutaneous flaps, with the exception of extensive cervicofacial flaps or ear reconstruction.

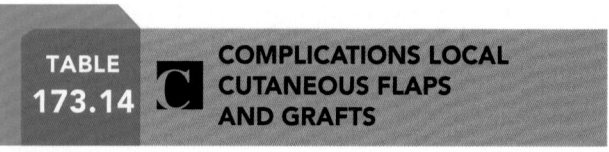

TABLE 173.14	**COMPLICATIONS LOCAL CUTANEOUS FLAPS AND GRAFTS**

Bleeding
Infection
Injury of adjacent anatomical structures
Wound dehiscence
Ischemia
Abnormal scarring
Trapdoor deformity
Distortion of facial features and boundaries

However, an appropriately sized drain is employed when a significant "potential space" is present or drainage is expected that cannot be controlled with a compression dressing. A compression dressing that conforms to the anatomical contour of the surgical site to facilitate adherence of the facial flap to the recipient site is typically left in place for 48 hours. The dressing consists of nonadherent gauze, cotton balls, and expandable mesh tape. Patients are instructed to keep their head elevated, especially at night, for the first 48 hours after surgery, and coughing and straining are to be avoided whenever possible.

Hematomas may cause compromise of local flap vascularity by inducing vasospasm, stretching the subdermal plexus, or separating the flap from the surface of the recipient site (57–59). Furthermore, iron compounds in a hematoma may promote free radical production leading to flap necrosis (60,61). Hematoma formation also predisposes to infection, which may compromise flap vascularity secondary to inflammatory edema (62,63).

If a hematoma occurs, patients usually complain of significant pain. The wound may appear mottled, pale, or bluish, and palpation of the skin in the area of the hematoma usually reveals a tight, tense flap with oozing of blood from the suture lines. Small hematomas may sometimes be aspirated through the suture line using a syringe attached to a large-bore needle. A compression dressing is then applied and the patient is reexamined in 24 hours. If the hematoma recurs, it may be necessary to return the patient to the operating room for thorough drainage and irrigation. In that setting, the wound is opened at a dependent portion, the hematoma is evacuated, bleeding vessels are controlled, and irrigation is performed. A compression dressing is reapplied with the patient being admitted or examined in clinic within 24 hours.

Infection

Fortunately, infection during facial surgery is reported to be as low at 2.8%, perhaps secondary to the rich vascularity of facial tissues (64–67). However, higher infection rates are associated with wounds that are repaired in a delayed fashion, as is often the case with facial flaps used to repair wounds created by Mohs surgery (66,68,69). Infection of a cutaneous flap is usually associated with distortion from inflammatory edema. Release of toxic substances and free radicals from inflammatory mediators leads to decreased collagen production and early degradation of suture materials with potential wound dehiscence. Necrosis of all or part of the flap may develop with the final scar being widened or thickened. Systemic dissemination of bacteria may occur if wound infections are not treated promptly (70,71).

Antiseptic solutions for skin preparation, sterile technique, proper scrubbing, and surgical attire are key elements in helping prevent infection. Avoiding crushed, charred, or excessively thinned tissue is also important. Staphylococcus aureus is the most common single pathogen causing wound infections, but streptococci,

gram-negative bacteria, and oral anaerobes may also be isolated from infected wounds (68). Antibiotics are particularly helpful when mucosal surfaces are incised, when cartilage grafting is performed, and during ear reconstruction to help prevent perichondritis. They are also employed in patients with underlying medical conditions that may predispose to infection such as diabetes and immunosuppression. In patients with open wounds greater than 3 days old, a 5-day course of oral cephalosporin is recommended prior to the surgical repair. This will decrease the bacterial colonization of the granulation tissue that may lead to graft or flap failure.

If a wound infection does develop, Gram stain and cultures of any drainage from the wound are obtained. The patient is treated with an appropriate broad-spectrum antibiotic until culture results and sensitivities are available. Any wound fluctuance is drained and the wound irrigated. The presence of excessive granulation tissue may require debridement to reduce the bacterial load. Topical antibiotic preparations may also be employed, and superficial sutures are removed to eliminate foreign bodies in the wound (72). Open wounds are allowed to heal by secondary intention. The resulting scar is addressed at a later time once the infection has been adequately treated and scarring has matured.

It is important to remember that topical allergies to antibiotic ointments and creams applied to the wound may be confused with wound infection. Topical allergic reactions manifest as erythema often with vesicle formation and exudates forming on all areas treated with the topical medication. The offending agent should be discontinued and the wound cleaned with soap and water in order to remove all residual topical medication.

Injury of Adjacent Anatomical Structures

A thorough understanding and appreciation of facial anatomy is a crucial prerequisite for performing facial reconstructive procedures, and general considerations related to protecting adjacent anatomical structures should be reviewed.

Perhaps one of the most devastating complications associated with facial surgery is injury to the facial nerve or one of its branches. Although rare, extensive dissection in the preauricular area could lead to injury to the main branch of the facial nerve. More commonly, the marginal mandibular or temporal branches of the facial nerve are injured. Familiarity with cross-sectional anatomy of the temple and mandibular regions is essential prior to surgical dissection in these areas. Sensory nerves are also susceptible to injury during facial reconstructive procedures. Extensive undermining along the superior bony orbital rim may injure the supraorbital or supratrochlear nerves leading to dysesthesias (73). Similarly, the deep branch of the supraorbital nerve runs within the galea aponeurotica and may be injured when undermining the frontalis muscle in the subgaleal plane. The great auricular nerve may be injured during subcutaneous dissection, and this nerve is identified and preserved when dissecting skin away from its attachment to the superior aspect of the sternocleidomastoid muscle.

Avoiding injury to the nasal cartilaginous framework is important for maintaining nasal symmetry and function. Inadvertent injury to these structures may lead to obvious nasal deformities including alar retraction, nasal valve collapse, and saddle nose deformity. Occasionally, preexisting structural abnormalities of the nose are corrected during reconstructive surgery of the nose, when the exposure of the nasal framework is sufficient, allowing potential improvement in aesthetic and functional outcomes. Preexisting weaknesses in the nasal structural support system may become more pronounced when cutaneous flaps are mobilized, especially when skin tension is increased across a weakened framework.

Injury to eyelid structures may lead to devastating consequences, including lagophthalmos, lacrimal duct obstruction, visual field obstruction, and vision loss. Facial surgeons should be familiar with the cross-sectional anatomy of the upper and lower eyelids, especially the connective tissue supportive apparatus. Injury to these structures is best avoided, since treatment is extremely difficult if scarring has occurred (70).

Wound Dehiscence

Wound dehiscence may develop secondary to infection, hematoma, or skin necrosis. In addition, dynamic motion or trauma to wounds may also lead to wound separation. Typically, wounds have 3% to 5% of normal skin tensile strength at 2 weeks after surgery, emphasizing the need for subcutaneous sutures. At 1 month, only 35% of the maximum wound tensile strength has been gained. However, at this point, the wound is usually able to withstand the forces of normal physical activity. Over the succeeding months, wound tensile strength increases to 80% of the strength of normal tissue. Wound separations that have been present for greater than 24 hours are best left to heal by secondary intention with scar revision reserved for the future if necessary (71,74).

Ischemia

Appropriate flap design is essential to ensure sufficient perfusion pressure of the entire flap (75). Random-pattern flaps require an intact subdermal plexus, and dissection is performed in the appropriate subcutaneous tissue plane since superficial dissection may lead to compromise of the flap's vascularity. Random-pattern flaps have a critical length beyond which the perfusion of the distal flap does not occur. Although increasing the width of a flap's pedicle potentially increases the number of vessels contained in the subdermal plexus of the flap, it does not increase the perfusion pressure to the distal portion of the flap.

Design of axial pattern flaps requires a thorough knowledge of the location and orientation of the arterial vessels supplying the skin in order to properly align the flap with the axis of the artery and to avoid inadvertent injury to the flap's blood supply. Increasing the width of the pedicle of axial flaps does not necessarily improve perfusion (76,77). Often, it is more advantageous to raise a thicker flap that contains deeper subcutaneous vessels than design the flap with a wider base.

Ischemia is defined as vascular perfusion insufficient to provide the required oxygenation of tissue (72). Cutaneous flaps are more vulnerable to tissue ischemia than wounds closed primarily given that the vascularity is isolated to the pedicle of the flap used for repair of the wound (78). This is especially true in the distal portion of the flap (28,79). Dissection of flaps causes release of catecholamines from severed sympathetic nerves, thromboxane A from platelet microthrombi, and oxygen free radicals. All of these substances cause vasoconstriction that can enhance tissue ischemia (80,81). Excessive flap thinning, electrocautery, crush injury, and wound closure tension may worsen flap ischemia. Infection is treated expeditiously since edema from inflammation may decrease tissue perfusion. When flap ischemia is evident, local wound factors and factors related to the patient are assessed and medical conditions optimized as discussed previously. In such situations, use of nicotine by the patient must be avoided.

Arterial insufficiency of a flap may be caused by kinking of the flap's pedicle, an excessively tight compression dressing or excessive wound closure tension. If these causative factors are corrected early in the postoperative period, the ischemia is usually reversible. In the case of excessive wound closure tension, sutures may be removed and/or the flap may be returned to its donor site, thereby delaying the flap that may improve blood supply to allow later transfer of the flap to the recipient site. When ischemia causes epidermolysis or skin necrosis, the tissue is allowed to demarcate since the more proximal portion of the flap is usually viable. Patients are instructed to keep the wound moist with petroleum- or water-based antibiotic ointment while the wound is allowed to heal by secondary intention. Frequent follow-up examination is essential for maintaining appropriate wound care, including wound debridement, and for providing reassurance to the patient.

Abnormal Scarring

Patients with darker skin and those with a family history of excessive scarring are prone to the development of hypertrophic scars and keloids following surgery. Intralesional triamcinolone acetonide is often helpful in reducing the volume of scar tissue within a hypertrophic or keloid scar. Injections are used to soften firm scars, lower raised keloids, and prevent their recurrence. Steroids decrease fibroblast proliferation, reduce blood vessel formation, and interfere with fibrosis by inhibiting extracellular matrix protein gene expression. Excessive steroid injection of scars may lead to skin atrophy, hypopigmentation, and telangiectasias. If the scar is responsive to the injections, surgical excision may be performed following a preoperative injection 1 week prior to surgery. Several injections are usually required postoperatively after excision for an indeterminate time interval.

Scars continue to change and improve during the remodeling phase of wound healing. Younger patients may have an exaggerated and prolonged healing reaction with increased scar erythema and hypertrophy, so scar revisions in children should be delayed as long as feasible. Immature scars tend to be erythematous, which will usually fade over time. Wounds subjected to excessive wound closure tension may result in scars that are hypopigmented and often hypertrophied. Incisions made in thick skin, especially if there is sebaceous gland hypertrophy, may heal with depressed or widened scars. Scar hyperpigmentation may be seen in patients who tan easily, particularly if the patient is exposed to excessive sun exposure during the immediate postoperative period. Hyperpigmentation improves over time and with sun avoidance. Use of topical hydroquinone gel with or without the administration of an anti-inflammatory drug may be helpful in preventing permanent discoloration of the scar (70).

Trapdoor Deformity

Trapdoor deformity may result from persistent edema and poor lymphatic drainage of flaps with curvilinear borders since the scar around the border of the flap contracts in a concentric fashion (82–84). Bilobed flaps of the nasal skin are particularly susceptible to trapdoor deformity because of the two circular lobes used for construction of the flap, especially when the nasal skin is thick and has sebaceous gland hypertrophy. Patient selection, proper flap design, and adequate tissue undermining reduce the incidence of trapdoor deformity. Presumably wide undermining reduces scar contractile vectors toward the center of the flap by enlarging the area of the underlying sheet of scar (82–84). Flaps that are superiorly based are more prone to develop trapdoor deformity than inferiorly based flaps, likely because lymphatic channels of the face drain in an inferior direction.

Trapdoor deformity usually improves with time. Steroid injections into the subcutaneous tissue plane beneath the flap may be performed using triamcinolone acetonide (10 mg/mL). If time and steroid injections are not successful, contouring of the flap with or without scar revision is necessary. This involves debulking of subcutaneous fat and scar tissue beneath the flap and redraping the skin. Excess skin is trimmed as indicated, and Z-plasties performed along the incision may be helpful in preventing recurrence.

Distortion of Facial Features and Boundaries

Scar contracture and excessive wound closure tension may lead to poor aesthetic and functional outcomes, especially in regions of the face with mobile facial structures such as the eyelids, lips, and nasal alae. This is especially problematic in the periocular and oral area where inadequate lip or eyelid closure leads to problems with eating, phonation, excessive tearing, and dry eye symptoms. Cervical facial flaps used to repair cutaneous defects near the lower

eyelids should be secured to the periosteum of the maxilla or nasal bones using a tacking suture in order to help prevent eyelid retraction secondary to excessive wound closure tension. A temporary Frost suture may also be used to limit the downward pull of the flap on the eyelid skin.

Flaps used for repair of the nose are designed sufficiently large to avoid alar retraction. For defects adjacent to the alar rim, cartilage grafting can be employed to provide a strut against the contractive forces of wound healing. The lip is also vulnerable to distortion by scars because of the mobile nature of the lips and the discreet borderline between the skin and vermilion. During healing, vertically oriented scars of the upper lip require only minimal contraction to cause notching or distortion of the vermiliocutaneous border. Such distortion is quite noticeable to the observer particularly when the vermilion is well developed. In addition to limiting wound closure tension as much as possible, precise alignment of the opposing edges of the lip wound in the vicinity of the vermiliocutaneous borders is extremely important when repairing lacerations or cutaneous defects of the lip.

Standing cutaneous deformities result from transfer of cutaneous tissue with unequal wound borders. In the majority of cases, these deformities may be safely excised at the time of wound repair. Swelling may prevent an accurate estimate of the size of the deformity and lead to a persistent standing cutaneous deformity.

It is important to respect the borders of facial aesthetic regions and units when designing cutaneous flaps in order to avoid unsightly scars. This is particularly true of the alar facial sulcus, which is an important boundary between the aesthetic regions of the nose, cheek, and upper lip. Larger defects of the ala are best reconstructed with interpolated cheek flaps that cross over the alar facial sulcus rather than using transposition or advancement cheek flaps that would obliterate this aesthetic boundary line. Cutaneous defects that extend from the nose to the medial cheek or to the upper lip are best repaired using separate flaps for each aesthetic region. This approach positions the borders of the flaps in aesthetic boundary lines that help camouflage scars and preserve the concave topography of the alar facial sulcus (70).

HIGHLIGHTS

- Skin is characterized as being directional or anisotropic, with a nonlinear stress–strain relationship.
- Delay of a cutaneous flap is thought to improve survival and is particularly helpful in patients with a history of radiation or tobacco smoking.
- Analysis of a facial defect includes determining the depth, size, and location of the wound. In addition, the color, texture, laxity, and thickness of adjacent skin should be assessed.

- Facial cutaneous flaps can be classified based on (a) location, (b) vascular supply, and/or (c) flap design and method of tissue movement.
- Examples of pivotal flaps include rotation, transposition, and interpolation flaps, and longer flaps may be required to account for loss of effective length with greater degrees of pivotal movement.
- Advancement flaps are most successful in areas of greatest tissue laxity and extensibility.
- Full-thickness cutaneous grafts have the advantage over split-thickness grafts of better color and texture match, less contour irregularities, little need for special equipment, and easier donor site wound care.
- Composite grafts contain two or more tissue layers and often are unsuccessful secondary to high metabolic demands.
- Complications of facial cutaneous flaps and grafts include bleeding, infection, injury of adjacent anatomical structures, wound dehiscence, ischemia, abnormal scarring, trapdoor deformity, and distortion of facial features and boundaries.

REFERENCES

1. Bichakjian CK, Johnson TM. Anatomy of skin. In: Baker SR, ed. *Local flaps in facial reconstruction*, 2nd ed., Philadelphia, PA: Elsevier, 2007.
2. Ogawa H. The Merkel cell as a possible mechanoreceptor cell. *Prog Neurobiol* 1996;49:317–334.
3. Uitto J, Pulkkinen L. Molecular genetics of heritable blistering disorders. *Arch Dermatol* 2001;137:1458–1461.
4. Hom DB, Goding GS. Skin flap physiology. In: Baker SR, ed. *Local flaps in facial reconstruction*, 2nd ed., Philadelphia, PA: Elsevier, 2007.
5. Daly CH, Odland GF. Age-related changes in the mechanical properties of human skin. *J Invest Dermatol* 1979;73:84–87.
6. Larrabee WF Jr, Sutton D. The biomechanics of advancement and rotation flaps. *Laryngoscope* 1981;91:726–734.
7. Larrabee WF Jr, Bloom DC. Biomechanics of skin flaps. In: Baker SR, ed. *Local flaps in facial reconstruction*, 2nd ed., Philadelphia, PA: Elsevier, 2007.
8. Pierard GE, Lapiere CM. Microanatomy of the dermis in relation to relaxed skin tension lines and Langer's lines. *Am J Dermatopathol* 1987;9:219–224.
9. Borges AF. Relaxed skin tension lines. *Dermatol Clin* 1989;7: 169–177.
10. Larrabee WF Jr, Holloway GA Jr, Sutton D. Wound tension and blood flow in skin flaps. *Ann Otol Rhinol Laryngol* 1984;93:112–115.
11. Greene N. Physiology of sympathetic denervation. *Annu Rev Med* 1962;13:87–104.
12. Guyton A. *Textbook of medical physiology*, 5th ed. Philadelphia, PA: W.B. Saunders, 1976.
13. Grange H, Goodman A, Grange N. Role of resistance and exchange vessels in local microvascular control of skeletal muscle oxygenation in the dog. *Circ Res* 1976;38:379–385.
14. Folkow B. Role of the nervous system in the control of vascular tone. *Circulation* 1960;21:760–768.
15. Tsur H, Daniller A, Strauch B. Neovascularization of skin flaps: routes and timing. *Plast Reconstr Surg* 1980;66:85–90.
16. Pang C, Forrest C, Niligan P, et al. Hemodynamics and vascular sensitivity to circulating norepinephrine in normal skin and delayed and acute random skin flaps in pig. *Plast Reconstr Surg* 1986;78:75–84.
17. Im JM, Beil RJ Jr, Wong L, et al. Effects of sympathetic denervation and oxygen free radicals on neovascularization. *Plast Reconstr Surg* 1993;92(4):736–741; discussion 742–743.
18. Jurrell G, Norberg K, Palmer B. Adrenergic nerves and the delay phenomenon. *Ann Plast Surg* 1986;17(6):493–497.
19. Pearl RM. A unifying theory of the delay phenomenon—recovery from the hyperadrenergic state. *Ann Plast Surg* 1981;7(2):102–112.
20. Dhar SC, Taylor GI. The delay phenomenon unfolds. *Plast Reconstr Surg* 1999;104:2079–2091.
21. Golminz D, Bennett RG. Cigarette smoking and flap and full thickness graft failure. *Arch Dermatol* 1991;127:1012–1015.
22. Craig S, Rees TD. The effect of smoking on experimental flaps in hamsters. *Plast Reconstr Surg* 1985;75:842–846.
23. Forrest C, Pang C, Lindsay W. Dose and time effects of nicotine treatment on the capillary blood flow and viability of random pattern flaps in the rat. *Br J Plast Surg* 1987;40:295–299.
24. Jensen JA, Goodson WH, Hopf HW, et al. Cigarette smoking decreases tissue oxygen. *Arch Surg* 1991;126:1131–1134.
25. Nolan J, Jenkins RA, Kurihara K, et al. The acute effects of cigarette exposure on experimental skin flaps. *Plast Reconstr Surg* 1985;75:544–551.
26. Kinsella JB, Rassekh CH, Wassmuth ZD, et al. Smoking increases skin flap complications. *Ann Otol Rhinol Laryngol* 1999;108: 139–142.
27. Cutting C. Critical closing and perfusion pressure in flap survival. *Ann Plast Surg* 1982;90:524.
28. Daniel RE, Kerrigan C. *The anatomy and hemodynamics of the cutaneous circulation and their influence on skin flap design*. Boston, MA: Little, Brown and Company, 1975.
29. Gorney M. Tissue dynamics and surgical geometry. In: Kernakan DA, Vistnes LM, eds. *Biological aspects of reconstructive surgery*. Boston, MA: Little, Brown and Company, 1977.
30. Larrabee WF Jr. Design of local skin flaps. *Otolaryngol Clin North Am* 1990;23:899–923.
31. Baker SR, Naficy S. *Principles of nasal reconstruction*. St. Louis, MO: Mosby, 2002, 58–70, 106.
32. Zitelli JA. Bilobe flaps. In: Baker SR, Swanson NA, eds. *Local flaps in facial reconstruction*. St Louis, MO: Mosby, 1995:165–180.
33. Jewett BS. Repair of small nasal defects. *Otolaryngol Clin North Am* 2007;40(2):337–360.
34. Glogau RG, Haas AF. Skingrafts. In: Baker SR, Swanson NA, eds. *Local Flaps in facial reconstruction*. St Louis, MO: Mosby, 1995:247–251.
35. Meyers S, Rohrer T, Grande D. Use of dermal grafts in reconstructing deep nasal defects and shaping the ala nasi. *Dermatol Surg* 2001;27(3):300–305.
36. Robinson JK, Dillig G. The advantages of delayed nasal full thickness skin grafting after Mohs micrographic surgery. *Dermatol Surg* 2002;28(9):845–851.
37. Skouge JW. *Skin grafting*. New York: Churchill Livingstone, 1991.
38. Konior RJ. Free composite grafts. *Otolaryngol Clin North Am* 1994;27(1):81–90.
39. Clairmont AA, Conley JJ. The uses and limitations of auricular composite grafts. *J Otolaryngol* 1978;7(3):249–256.
40. McLaughlin CR. Composite ear grafts and their blood supply. *Br J Plast Surg* 1954;7:274–278.
41. Konig F. Uber nasenplastik. *Beitrage Zur Klinishen Chirurgie* 1914;94: 515–529.
42. Converse JM. Reconstruction of nasolabial area by composite graft from the concha. *Plast Reconstr Surg* 1950;5:247–251.
43. Meade RJ. Composite ear grafts for construction of columella. *Plast Reconstr Surg* 1959;23:134–147.
44. Dingman RO, Walter C. Use of composite grafts in correction of the short nose. *Plast Reconstr Surg* 1969;43:117–124.
45. Limberg A. Rhinoplasty using free transplant from concha. *Sovet Khir* 1935;9:70.
46. Symonds FC, Crikelair G. Auricular composite grafts in nasal reconstruction. *Plast Reconstr Surg* 1956;37:433–437.
47. Ballantyne Dl, Converse JM. Vascularization of composite auricular grafts transplanted to the chorio-allantois of the chick embryo. *Plast Reconstr Surg* 1968;42:51.
48. Ruch M. Utilization of composite free grafts. *J Int Coll Surg* 1958;30: 274–275.
49. Becker OJ. Extended application of free composite grafts. *Trans Am Acad Ophthalmol Otolaryngol* 1960;64:649–659.

50. Avelar JM, Psillakis JM, Viterbo F. Use of large composite grafts in the reconstruction of deformities of the nose and ear. *Br J Plast Surg* 1984;37:55.

51. Davenport G, Bernard FD. Improving the take of composite grafts. *Plast Reconstr Surg* 1959;24:175–182.

52. Converse JM. *Reconstructive plastic surgery*, Vol. 2. Philadelphia, PA: WB Saunders, 1964.

53. Aden KK, Biel MA. The evaluation of pharmacologic agents on composite survival. *Arch Otolaryngol Head Neck Surg* 1992;118(2): 175–178.

54. Hartman DF, Good RL. Pharmacologic enhancement of composite graft survival. *Arch Otolaryngol Head Neck Surg* 1987;113:720–723.

55. Conley JJ, Van Fraenkel P. The principle of cooling applied to the composite graft in the nose. *Plast Reconstr Surg* 1956;17:444–451.

56. Weisberg NK, Becker DS. Repair of nasal ala defects with conchal bowl composite grafts. *Dermatol Surg* 2000;26(11):1047–105.

57. Diaz DD, Freeman SB, Wilson JF, et al. Hematoma-induced flap necrosis and free radical scavengers. *Arch Otolaryngol Head Neck Surg* 1992;118:516–518.

58. Hillelson RL, Glowacki J, Healey NA, et al. A microangiographic study of hematoma-associated flap necrosis and salvage with isoxsuprine. *Plast Reconstr Surg* 1980;66:528–533.

59. Kaufman T, Angel MF, Eichenlaub EH, et al. The salutary effects of the bed on the survival of the experimental flaps. *Ann Plast Surg* 1985;14:64–73.

60. Angel MF, Narayanan K, Swartz WM, et al. The etiologic role of free radicals in the hematoma induced flap necrosis. *Plast Reconstr Surg* 1986;77:795–803.

61. Mulliken JB, Healey NA. Pathogenesis of skin flap necrosis from an underlying hematoma. *Plast Reconstr Surg* 1979;63:540–545.

62. Krizek TJ, Davis JH. The role of the red cell in subcutaneous infection. *J Trauma* 1965;5:85–95.

63. Polk HC, Miles AA. Enhancement of bacterial infection by ferric iron. Kinetics, mechanisms and surgical significance. *Surgery* 1971;70:71–77.

64. Sylaidis P, Wood S, Murray DS. Postoperative infection following clean facial surgery. *Ann Plast Surg* 1997;39:342–346.

65. Pearl RM, Johnson D. The vascular supply to the skin: an anatomical and physiological reappraisal: Part II. *Ann Plast Surg* 1983;11:196–205.

66. Pearl RM. A vascular approach to the prevention of infection. *Ann Plast Surg* 1985;14:443–450.

67. Tran DT, Miller SH, Bucks D, et al. Potentiation of infection by epinephrine. *Plast Reconstr Surg* 1985;76:933–934.

68. Sebben JE. Prophylactic antibiotics in cutaneous surgery. *J Dermatol Surg Oncol* 1985;11:901–906.

69. Bumpous JM, Johnson JT. The infected wound and its management. *Otolaryngol Clin North Am* 1995;28:987–1001.

70. Jewett BS. Complications of local flaps. In: Baker SR, ed. *Local flaps in facial reconstruction*, 2nd ed. Philadelphia, PA: Elsevier, 2007.

71. Salische SJ. Complications of local flaps. In: Baker SR, Swanson NA, eds. *Local flaps in facial reconstruction*. New York: Mosby, 1995:545–585.

72. Vural E, Key JM. Complications, salvage, and enhancement of local flaps in facial reconstruction. *Otolaryngol Clin North Am* 2001;34(4):739–751.

73. Becker FF. *Facial reconstruction with local and regional flaps*. New York: Thieme-Stratton, 1985.

74. Edlich RF, Friedman HI, Haines PC, et al. Biology of wound repair: its influence on surgical decision. *Facial Plast Surg* 1984;1:169.

75. Kerrigan CL, Daniel FI. Monitoring acute skin flap failure. *Plast Reconstr Surg* 1983;71:519–524.

76. Milton SH. Pedicled skin flaps: the fallacy of the length:width ratio. *Br J Surg* 1970;57:502–508.

77. Daniel RK, Kerrigan CL. Skin flaps: an anatomical and hemodynamic approach. *Clin Plast Surg* 1979;6:181–200.

78. Myers B. Understanding flap necrosis. *Plast Reconstr Surg* 1986;78:813–814.

79. Suzuki S, Isshiki N, Ogawa Y, et al. The minimal requirement of circulation for survival of undelayed flaps in rats. *Plast Reconstr Surg* 1986;78:221.

80. Angel MR, Narayanan K, Swartz WM, et al. Deferoxamine increases skin flap survival: additional evidence of free radical involvement in ischemic flap surgery. *Br J Plast Surg* 1986;39:469–472.

81. Angel MF, Ramasastry SS, Swartz WM, et al. The critical relationship between free radicals and degree of ischemia: evidence for tissue intolerance of marginal perfusion. *Plast Reconstr Surg* 1988;81:233–239.

82. Hosokawa K, Susuki T, Kikui T, et al. Sheet of scar causes trapdoor deformity: a hypothesis. *Ann Plast Surg* 1990;25: 134–135.

83. Kaufman AJ, Kiene KL, Moy RL. Role of tissue undermining in the trapdoor effect of transposition flaps. *J Dermatol Surg Oncol* 1985;19:128.

84. Koopman DF. Cutaneous wound healing: an overview. *Otolaryngol Clin North Am* 1995;28:835–845.

174

Reconstructive Microsurgery of the Head and Neck

Douglas B. Chepeha

Microvascular free tissue transfer was introduced as a technique that enabled reconstruction of defects that could not otherwise be reconstructed. The viability of autogenous transplants and the long operating time were initial concerns. During the 1980s, use of regional pedicled flaps (pectoralis, trapezius, latissimus dorsi) overshadowed microvascular free tissue transfer. Regional flaps were technically much easier, required only one surgical team, and supplied nonirradiated tissue. Microvascular reconstruction continued to evolve. More donor sites were described each year, and the versatility of each site was explored and expanded. More surgeons were trained in microvascular techniques, and these surgeons became increasingly adept. As the practice of reconstructive microsurgery became more common, the success rate improved (95% to 98%), and the operative time decreased (1,2).

Controversy still exists about whether microvascular reconstruction is functionally superior to pedicled reconstruction of comparable defects. Intuition suggests that revascularized free tissue transfer is functionally superior because it allows the reconstructive surgeon to customize reconstruction of defects of the head and neck. Autogenous transplants can be designed to provide epithelium, subcutaneous tissue, muscle, nerve, and bone in proportions that closely resemble the missing tissue.

If autogenous transplantation is functionally superior, is it cost-effective? Several studies have suggested that use of pectoralis flaps is associated with longer hospital stays and higher complication rates than free tissue transfer in comparable primary reconstructions (3–5). This suggests that the costs of longer operating times associated with free autogenous transplantation may be offset by the longer hospitalizations associated with pedicled transfer.

The drive for reconstructive surgeons to provide the best functional and aesthetic reconstruction for their patients made autogenous transplantation the mainstay of head and neck reconstruction in the 1990s. In the last 10 years,

more donor sites are used, more transfers are performed, perforator-based chimeric elevations are increasing reconstructive options, indications have broadened, and operating time has been reduced (6). More research is being conducted to establish the value and exact place of these sophisticated reconstructive techniques in the various defects encountered in the head and neck.

This chapter is divided into two sections. The first section is an introduction to free tissue transfers commonly used in head and neck reconstruction (Table 174.1). Each flap is described in terms of design and use, anatomic characteristics, anatomic variations, potential morbidity, technical considerations, preoperative considerations, and postoperative management. The second section is an introduction to commonly encountered defects of the head and neck.

FASCIAL AND FASCIOCUTANEOUS AUTOGENOUS TRANSPLANTS

Radial Forearm Donor Site

Description

The radial forearm is a fasciocutaneous donor site comprised of thin skin and subcutaneous tissue based on the radial artery and its venae comitantes and the cephalic vein (Fig. 174.1). This site can be transferred as a composite transplant that contains vascularized bone, vascularized tendon, the brachioradialis muscle, and vascularized nerve. The skin of the entire forearm, from the antecubital fossa to the flexor crease of the wrist, can be transferred. The vascular pedicle can be as long as 20 cm, and the artery is 2 to 2.5 mm in diameter. The radial forearm donor site contains axial nerve supply useful for sensory reinnervation. It can be used to reconstruct small (less than 60 cm) to moderate surface area (less than 200 cm^2) defects and is a low-volume donor site. The tissue for this donor site can be folded to facilitate sophisticated reconstructions. Because

TABLE 174.1	MICROVASCULAR FREE SOFT TISSUE FLAP SELECTION IN HEAD AND NECK RECONSTRUCTION		
Flap	**Quality**	**Advantages**	**Disadvantages**
Radial forearm	Thin, pliable	Versatility, ease	Limited bulk, skin graft donor site
Lateral arm	Moderately thin	Primary closure of donor site	Small-caliber pedicle
Lateral thigh	Moderately thick	Large surface area of tissue, long pedicle	Challenging harvest
Anterolateral thigh	Thin, pliable	Long pedicle, large cutaneous component, chimeric options	Variable anatomy
Temporoparietal	Ultrathin	Can be transferred as pedicle flap	Challenging harvest, limited pedicle length, scalp skin is stiff
Rectus	Bulky	Versatility, ease of harvest, chimeric options	Risk of ventral hernia
Latissimus dorsi	Moderate bulk	Large surface area, ease of harvest	Lateral decubitus position
Gracilis	Thin muscle	Can be separated into functional units	Limited tissue available

of the increasing use of the anterolateral thigh donor site for larger defects, the radial forearm donor site is most commonly used for the reconstruction of smaller defects of the oral cavity (including central hard palate, base of the tongue, soft palate) and partial and circumferential

reconstruction of the pharynx. It also can be used to manage cutaneous defects of the eye, lip, neck, and scalp. When elevated as a fascial paddle (no cutaneous component), the radial forearm donor site can be used to manage soft tissue defects and defects of the base of the skull particularly for

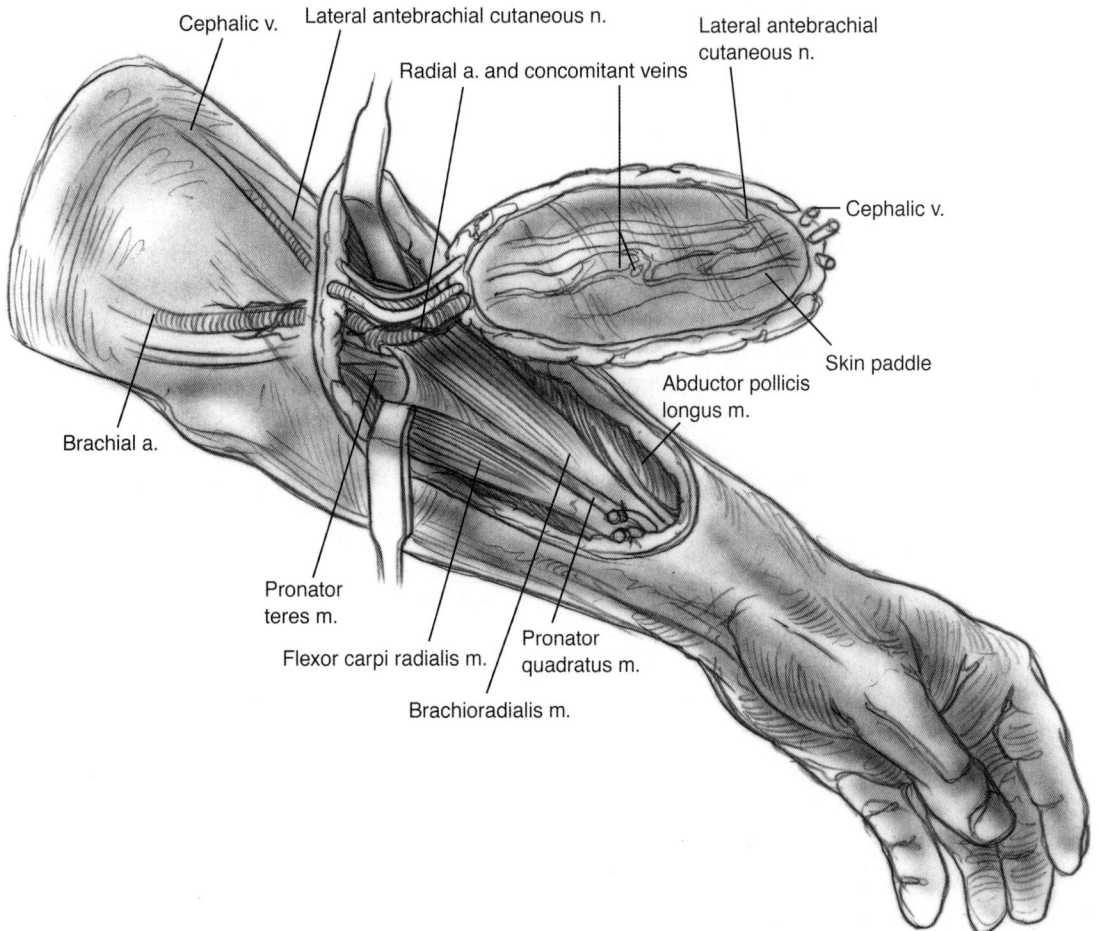

Figure 174.1 Lateral view shows left lateral forearm. The flap axis is slightly medial to the radial artery, and the flap is positioned to include the cephalic vein over the extensor compartment. Nutrient branches to the radius are immediately deep to the brachioradialis tendon. The superficial branch of the radial nerve is preserved in dissection of this flap.

a previously treated patient when local pericranial flaps are not available (7). When this donor site is elevated as an osteocutaneous flap, a segment of radius 10 to 12 cm long and as much as 40% of its circumference can be harvested with overlying fascia and skin (8). In the past, this donor site was useful for reconstruction of small-volume bone and soft tissue defects of the face, such as the periorbital tissues, particularly if the patient has undergone or is to undergo radiation therapy (9), but the thoracodorsal artery scapular tip (TDAST) has nearly replaced the use of the radial forearm donor site for patients with these mid and upper craniofacial defects. Another use of vascularized radial bone is for the prevention of plate exposure for patients who have undergone lateral mandibular resections and have low to moderate loading of the mandible (8). The disadvantage of the radial osteocutaneous transplant is the limited amount of donor bone and the risk of pathologic fracture of the radius.

Neurovascular Pedicle

The radial artery, with its two venae comitantes, courses in the lateral intermuscular septum and has several fascial branches in the forearm (10). This fascial plexus supplies most of the skin in the forearm. The length of the arterial pedicle is limited by the radial recurrent artery, which is the first major branch of the radial artery after its takeoff from the brachial artery. The site has a deep venous drainage through the paired venae comitantes and the larger superficial veins, such as the cephalic vein. Numerous connections exist between the venae comitantes and the superficial venous system; these vessels provide excellent venous drainage of this donor site. If necessary, and if proper testing of the venous drainage of this donor site is conducted after elevation, it usually is possible to drain the flap through the superficial system alone. It is nearly always possible to drain this donor site through the venae comitantes alone. The lateral antebrachial cutaneous nerve is the primary sensory nerve to the territory of forearm skin most commonly harvested. This nerve typically courses close to the cephalic vein in the upper forearm. When sensory reinnervation is needed, this nerve can be easily anastomosed to a recipient sensory nerve.

Anatomic Variations

The greatest concern during harvest of the radial forearm donor site is the integrity of the ulnar arterial supply to the hand through the palmar arches. The combination of two concurrent arterial variations, an incomplete superficial palmar arch and a lack of communication between the superficial and deep palmar arches, puts the vascular supply of the thumb and index finger in jeopardy (11). This anomaly can be detected with an Allen test. This test involves assessment of capillary refill of the thumb and index finger with the radial artery occluded. The patient is asked to clench his or her fist. The examiner uses digital pressure to occlude the radial and ulnar arteries at the wrist. The patient opens the hand to approximately 10 degrees of flexion, the examiner releases the ulnar artery, and capillary refill is assessed. If

there is uncertainty about digital blood flow during capillary refill assessment, Doppler assessment of the digital artery is performed to the thumb, and the results are definitive.

Potential Morbidity

Often the donor site cannot be closed primarily, and a skin graft is necessary, which can be unsightly. Poor take of the skin graft can be caused by inadequate immobilization of the hand or failure to preserve the paratenon over the flexor tendons. Radial osteocutaneous flaps are limited by risk of fracture of the radius and a detrimental effect on supination, wrist flexion, grip strength, and pinch strength (12). A plate can be applied to the radius bone to reduce the likelihood of radial fracture for osseocutaneous elevations (13).

Technical Considerations

The design of a radial forearm skin paddle begins with an outline of the path of the dominant subcutaneous veins and the palpable pulse of the radial artery. The skin paddle is oriented over the radial artery and cephalic vein. It is preferable not to perform the elevation over the ulnar artery. Additional subcutaneous tissue can be incorporated when needed, from the brachial fat pad, to increase the volume of the transplant. During harvest, the paratenon over the flexor tendons is preserved to facilitate skin graft healing. If necessary, the flexor tendons can be covered with turnover muscle flaps to improve the donor-site bed for skin grafting.

Preoperative Considerations

Accurate performance of an Allen test is the most important consideration in avoiding ischemia of the hand. When the Allen test results are equivocal, the opposite hand or an alternative donor site should be selected.

Postoperative Management

The forearm donor site and wrist are immobilized with a volar splint with the wrist in the position of function for 6 to 7 days. Then a removable volar plastic splint is used for an additional 3 to 5 weeks until the skin graft is healed over the donor site. After an osseocutaneous flap, the elbow and wrist are immobilized with a full arm cast with the hand in the position of function. This cast is left on for 4 weeks, then the wrist is immobilized with a forearm cast, and this is left on for an additional 2 weeks. The patient is encouraged to use the arm throughout the casting period. The underlying philosophy is to allow time for reshaping of the load lines in the radial bone. Any limb with circumferential dressing needs to be closely observed in the immediate postoperative period for signs of vascular insufficiency.

Lateral Arm Donor Site

Description

The lateral arm is a fasciocutaneous donor site that is usually thicker than the radial forearm donor site, the vascular pedicle is based on the posterior radial collateral artery and its venae comitantes, and it can be reinnervated for cutaneous sensation with the posterior cutaneous nerve of the arm (14). The donor site usually can be closed primarily when the width of harvested skin is limited to 6 to 8 cm, or one-third the circumference of the arm. Larger skin paddles can be harvested, but a skin graft will be required over the donor site. The donor site can be harvested as a fascial flap and is a good source of vascularized tissue for augmentation of subcutaneous defects caused by lateral temporal bone resection or total parotidectomy (15). The donor site can include the posterior cutaneous nerve of the forearm for use as a vascularized nerve graft, but more frequently the nerve is dissected out of the skin paddle and used as a free nerve graft because it may not be possible to properly orient the nerve and vascular pedicle when insetting. The clinical usage of the lateral arm donor site is affected by the body mass index (BMI) of the patient. In patients with a lower BMI, the lateral arm can be used for low-volume oral cavity, low-volume oropharyngeal, and low-volume cutaneous defects particularly when slightly more volume is required than the forearm donor site can provide. In patients with higher BMI, the lateral arm donor site can be used for higher-volume base of tongue, lateral oropharynx including the parapharyngeal space, anterior oral glossectomy, lateral temporal bone, and parotid and midfacial defects (16). The thickness of the skin paddle can be varied with placement because the skin over the lateral epicondyle is much thinner than the skin over the lower and mid upper arm. When estimating volume, it is important to remember that the subcutaneous tissue over the deltoid is more prone to long-term atrophy than the subcutaneous tissue over the mid lateral arm. Many of the applications of the lateral arm flap have been supplanted by the perforator-based anterolateral thigh donor site due to its larger, longer pedicle and ease of primary closure.

Neurovascular Pedicle

The vascular supply of the lateral arm skin paddle is based on the terminal branch of the profunda brachii artery and the posterior radial collateral artery and its venae comitantes. The blood supply to the skin is derived from four to five septocutaneous perforators that arise from the posterior radial collateral artery in the lateral intermuscular septum. In the region of the deltoid insertion, where the posterior radial collateral artery enters the lateral intermuscular septum, the artery has an average diameter of 1.55 mm (range, 1.25 to 1.75 mm) and a maximum pedicle length with additional dissection of 8 to 10 cm (17). Additional pedicle length and caliber can be obtained by means of extending the dissection proximally between the lateral and long heads of the triceps muscle. The muscular branches from the radial nerve to the triceps muscle must be identified and preserved when this approach is used. In practice, it is difficult to obtain more than 4 cm of pedicle length by using this proximal dissection technique without detaching a large amount of triceps and dividing the motor

branches to the triceps muscle. To accommodate the fairly short pedicle, the skin paddle can be moved to a more distal location over the lateral epicondyle. This maneuver results in a thinner skin paddle. A second superficial venous system incorporates the cephalic vein, but is rarely used in practice. Two sensory nerves are encountered during elevation of the skin paddle; each arises from the proximal portion of the radial nerve. The nomenclature of these sensory nerves is confusing. The nerve that supplies sensation to the skin paddle is the posterior cutaneous nerve of the arm (also called the lower lateral cutaneous nerve of the arm and the inferior lateral brachial cutaneous nerve). The posterior cutaneous nerve of the forearm (also called the posterior antebrachial cutaneous nerve) runs through the lateral arm flap to the forearm and can be used as a vascularized nerve graft. Harvest of the skin paddle results in a variable area of cutaneous anesthesia over the mid extensor surface of the forearm.

Anatomic Variations

Unlike the radial forearm donor site, the lateral arm elevation does not affect the circulation to the distal portion of the arm. The profunda brachii artery can be interrupted without ischemic sequelae. The incidence of duplication of the profunda brachii artery ranges from 4% to 12% in different series.

Potential Morbidity

The radial nerve, which lies in the spiral groove of the humerus, is identified and protected from injury during flap harvest. Postoperative radial nerve palsy has been attributed to constrictive dressings or tight wound closure. Use of split-thickness skin grafts is preferable to tight primary closure.

Technical Considerations

The lateral intermuscular septum is approximately 1 cm posterior to a line drawn from the insertion of the deltoid muscle and the lateral epicondyle. The central axis of the skin paddle is based on the intermuscular septum (Fig. 174.2). Closure of the donor site is important for reestablishing coverage of the radial nerve and reattachment of the insertion of the brachialis and brachioradialis muscles. The brachialis muscle is reapproximated to the triceps muscle so that 1 cm of muscle provides coverage of the radial nerve. In addition, the brachioradialis muscle needs to be sutured to the distal triceps muscle, and this is accomplished with the elbow in flexion. Recipient vessel planning is important because of the relatively short pedicle and the small caliber of the donor vessels. For patients undergoing lateral parotid and temporal reconstructions, preservation of the occipital artery as it crosses the internal jugular vein makes recipient vascular access relatively easier.

Preoperative Considerations

The thickness of the flap is assessed by means of palpation. The soft tissue of the donor site thins and becomes

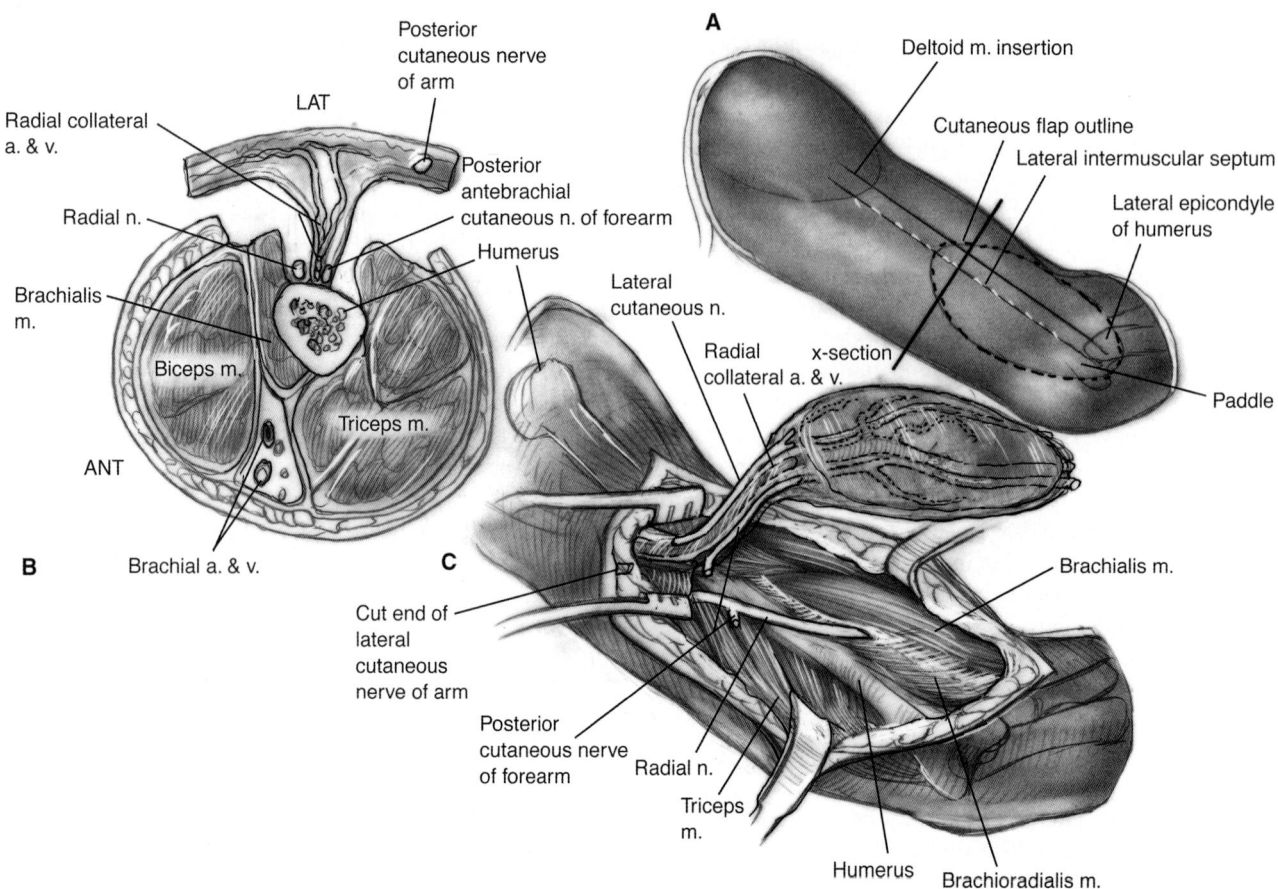

Figure 174.2 A: The flap is marked over the lateral epicondyle and 1 cm dorsal to a line drawn from the tip of the deltoid muscle to the lateral epicondyle. This position maximizes pedicle length and centers the flap over the lateral intermuscular septum. **B:** Cross section shows upper arm at the level shown in **(A)**. The lateral arm flap is elevated but still attached by the intermuscular septum to the humerus. At this level the posterior cutaneous nerve of the arm is in the subcutaneous fat, whereas the posterior cutaneous nerve of the forearm still is in the intermuscular septum. **C:** Lateral view shows lateral arm flap with the pedicle still in continuity. The radial nerve crosses the humerus and enters the cleft between the brachialis and the brachioradialis muscles.

more pliable when it is positioned more distally on the upper arm. In general, one-third of the circumference of the upper arm can be harvested. Primary closure can be assessed using a pinch test. It is best to have recipient vessels from a previously undissected neck.

Postoperative Management

A suction drain is recommended. If a skin graft is used, a volar slab is fashioned, the elbow is placed in flexion, and the donor site is managed in a manner similar to the radial forearm donor site.

Lateral Thigh

Description

The lateral thigh donor site was popularized by Hayden (18), who found it useful for pharyngeal reconstruction. For selected patients with favorable body habitus, this donor site provides a large surface area of tissue with an adequate vascular pedicle. Skin paddles as large as 25 × 14 cm

have been transferred successfully (19). This fasciocutaneous donor site ranges from thin to moderately thick depending on the patient's body habitus. Sensory reinnervation is possible with the lateral femoral cutaneous nerve. Elevation of this donor site is technically challenging and has been supplanted by the anterolateral thigh donor site, which is technically easier to harvest and has a long vascular pedicle.

Anterolateral Thigh

Description

The anterolateral thigh donor site is a septocutaneous or musculocutaneous flap based on the descending branch of the lateral circumflex femoral artery and associated venae comitantes. The elevation can be designed to include any of the structures supplied by the common pedicle of the lateral femoral circumflex vessels, which can include the tensor fascia lata, the vastus lateralis, and/or the rectus femoris. The skin paddle can be harvested as large as

20×15 cm. The skin of the anterolateral thigh is thin and pliable in most males, whereas in females, this flap can be thicker depending on the pattern of fat deposition. The anterolateral thigh donor site has become one of the workhorse donor sites for soft tissue reconstruction in the head and neck. It has many of the same characteristics as a radial forearm donor site, such as thin pliable skin and a long vascular pedicle. The anterolateral donor site is a source for larger skin paddles and more subcutaneous tissue than a radial forearm donor site and, as a result, has been nicknamed its "big brother." The nerves for sensation are the anterior femoral cutaneous and the lateral femoral cutaneous and do not run axially with the pedicle. The applications for this flap include face, neck, full-thickness buccal, hemiglossectomy, subtotal glossectomy, oropharynx, total pharyngeal, and skull base defects (20,21). The donor site is closed primarily when the skin paddle is less than 9 cm in width. The disadvantage is the variable location of the pedicle and the perforators. To overcome this disadvantage and as familiarity with this donor site has increased, more of the elevations are designed around a perforator. The dominant perforator is identified and is dissected retrograde to the lateral circumflex femoral artery. This approach has several advantages: The elevated tissue can easily be centered

on the dominant perforator, the underlying muscle is preserved, and the volume of the donor site can be controlled because the surgeon can choose to elevate muscle independent of the variation of the vascular pedicle.

Neurovascular Pedicle
The perforators from the pedicle are located on a line drawn from the anterior superior iliac spine to the lateral edge of the patella and are usually between the midpoint and the junction of the upper and middle thirds of the line. A Doppler probe is used to locate the perforators.

Anatomic Variations
There are four patterns of vascular supply to the skin paddle (22). There are two musculocutaneous types, the vertical musculocutaneous (50%) and the horizontal musculocutaneous (30%), and two septocutaneous types, the vertical septocutaneous (15%) and the horizontal septocutaneous (5%) (Fig. 174.3A and B).

Potential Morbidity
There is little morbidity reported even with harvest of large portions of the vastus lateralis. The vastus lateralis is a stabilizer of the rectus femoris (23). With more

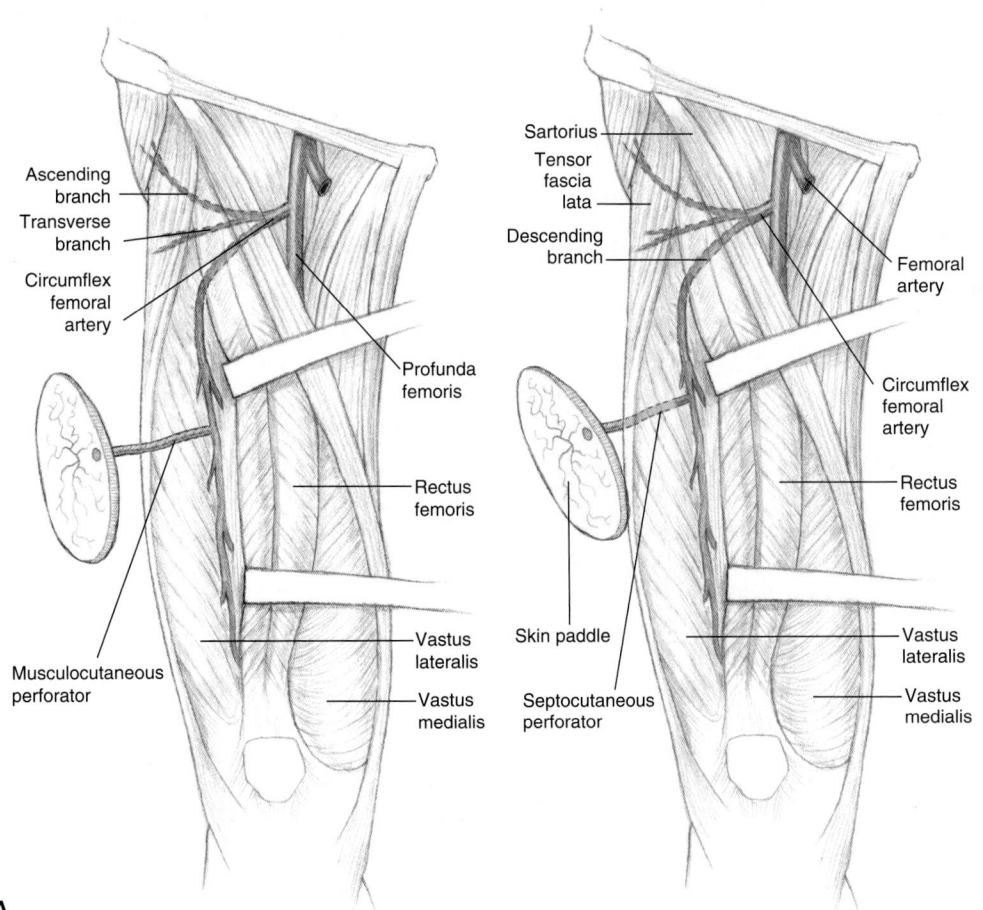

Figure 174.3 A: Type I vertical musculocutaneous perforator, which is the most common variant. **B:** Type III septocutaneous perforator.

long-term follow-up, morbidity will become better defined. Fortunately, most elevations are performed based on the perforator that spares the muscle and the nerve to the vastus lateralis, which is closely associated with vascular pedicle.

Technical Considerations

The location of the perforator is determined with a Doppler prior to elevation. Perforator-based elevation is accomplished by performing a suprafascial dissection until a perforator is located coursing through the fascia. Once located, the perforator is dissected proximally through the muscle or anterior to the muscle depending of the vascular variation that is encountered. The first incision is the medial incision over the rectus femoris. The paddle is elevated from medial to lateral until the perforator is identified. Once the perforator is identified, the dissection is carried along the perforator from lateral to medial. Multiple skin paddles and slips of muscle can be harvested based on the perforators that are present. Once the pedicle is defined, the lateral skin incision can be made to complete the elevation.

Preoperative Considerations

A history of vasculopathy with bypass grafts is a contraindication. For some reconstructions a larger muscle component may not be desirable. There is great variation of the thickness of the donor site between individuals, so skin paddle thickness needs to be assessed to be sure that it is appropriate for the recipient site.

Postoperative Management

The site can usually be closed primarily after the muscles have been approximated over a suction drain. Little rehabilitation is needed other than ambulation.

Temporoparietal

Description

In head and neck reconstruction, the fascia is most commonly transferred as a pedicled flap, but it also can be used as an autogenous transplant when the arc of rotation is inadequate. The donor site can be transferred independently or in combination with skin. The temporoparietal fascial skin can be harvested with dimensions of 17 × 14 cm with extensive scalp undermining. When skin is included, the thickness of the flap ranges from 2 to 4 mm. It is very uncommon to elevate this donor site with overlying skin except for reconstruction of the upper lip when hair is desired. As an autogenous fascial transplant, this donor site has highly specialized uses for hemilaryngeal reconstruction, or a low-volume cutaneous reconstruction when the forearm donor sites are not available. Most often it is used as a rotational flap in the midface, upper face, skull base, or lateral temporal bone to cover bone, support dural closure, or support calvarial bone grafts.

Neurovascular Pedicle

The temporoparietal scalp consists of five distinct layers (Fig. 174.4A). The temporoparietal fascia is deep to the skin and subcutaneous tissue, to which it is firmly bound. The temporoparietal fascia is superficial to the temporalis muscular fascia, which envelops the muscle. Above the superior temporal line, the temporoparietal fascia becomes the galea aponeurotica (24). The superficial temporal artery and vein, which supply this fascia and travel within the temporoparietal fascial layer, are best isolated approximately 3 cm superior to the root of the helix, where the vessels branch into frontal and parietal divisions. The flap is most commonly based on the parietal branch. The base is centered over the middle third of the superior auricular helix. The deep temporal artery arises from the proximal superficial temporal artery at the level of the zygomatic arch and supplies the temporalis muscular fascia. If the deep temporal artery is included, a two-paddled design can be raised on a single vascular pedicle (Fig. 174.4B).

Anatomic Variations

The superficial temporal artery consistently divides into two branches 3 cm above the root of the helix. Tracing the course of the posterior parietal branch with Doppler sonography helps center the fascial paddle and ensures that the planned territory of the temporoparietal fascial flap is well vascularized.

Potential Morbidity

The anterior dissection of the fascial paddle is limited by the course of the frontal branch of the facial nerve, which also is in the temporoparietal fascia. Secondary alopecia can be caused by injury to the hair follicles due to dissection that is too superficial. The venous pedicle can course with the artery or can course 2 to 3 cm posteriorly. Both the artery and vein must be included within the confines of the flap.

Technical Considerations

The superficial aspect of the fascia must be dissected first in a plane just below the hair follicles. The deep side of the donor-site elevation is a layer of loose areolar tissue that separates the temporoparietal fascia from the temporalis muscular fascia. The caudal extension of the pedicle dissection is limited by the location of the main trunk of the facial nerve.

Preoperative Considerations

Prior neck or parotid surgery, previous bicoronal incision, and external carotid embolization are relative contraindications to use of a temporoparietal fascial flap. Preoperative Doppler assessment of the patency and location of the pedicle is necessary.

Postoperative Management

The site can be primarily closed over suction drainage.

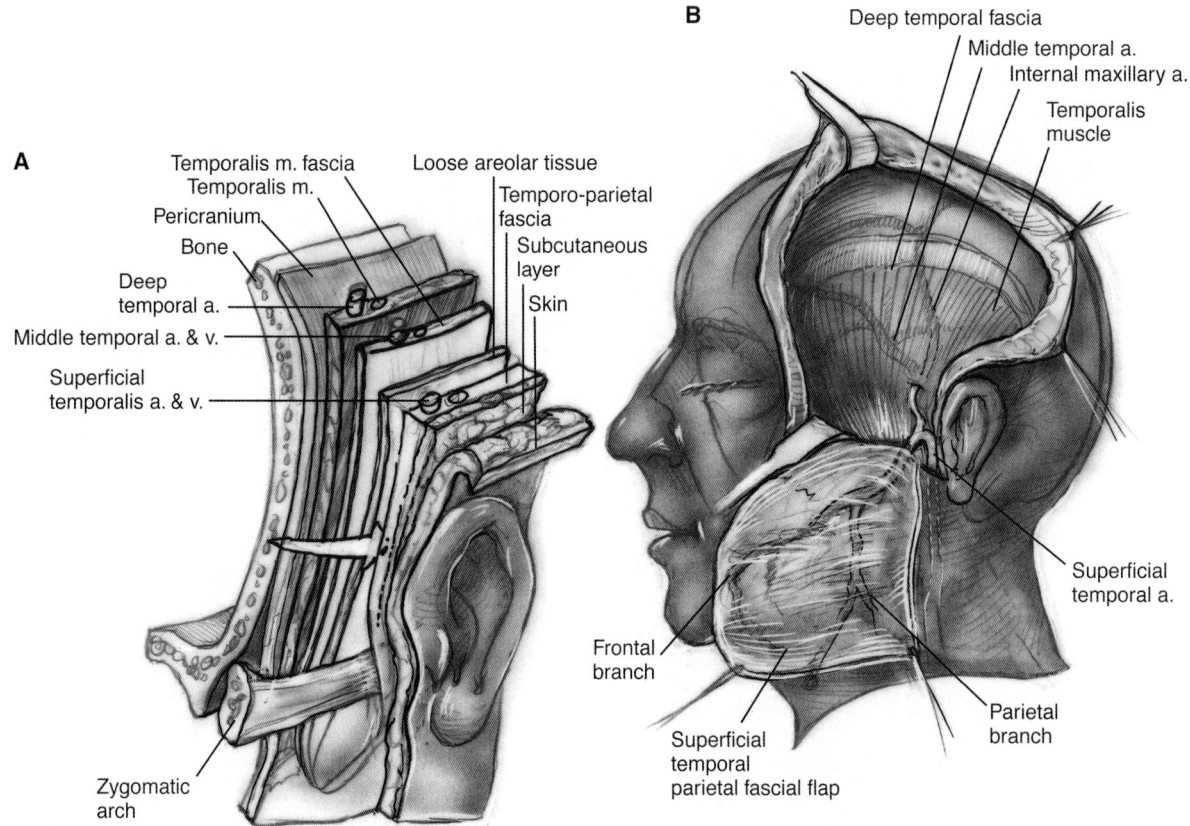

Figure 174.4 A: Cross section shows layers of the temporal scalp, superficial temporal space, and temporal skull. The superficial side of the temporoparietal facial flap is intimately associated with the subcutaneous fat of the scalp. The superficial dissection is started inferiorly just below the level of the hair follicles. As it proceeds superiorly, dissection becomes more difficult. *Arrow* denotes the deep side of the temporoparietal flap. **B:** Lateral view of the head with the temporoparietal flap folded inferiorly shows the vascular anatomic features. Dissection of the deep layer of the flap is in loose areolar tissue and is much more straightforward than is superficial dissection. Superficial dissection is completed before deep dissection.

MUSCLE AND MUSCULOCUTANEOUS AUTOGENOUS TRANSPLANTS

Rectus Abdominis

Description

The rectus abdominis donor site is relatively easy to harvest, has a long vascular pedicle, and is extremely reliable. The area of skin that can be harvested with a single rectus muscle encompasses a substantial portion of the abdomen and lower chest. Options for harvest can vary widely that include the entire muscle all the way to a cutaneous elevation that spares the muscle and is based on one to three perforators. This donor site was the most popular site for the reconstruction of most moderate- to high-volume head and neck defects. Its use is being replaced by the anterolateral thigh donor site except for the very large-volume defects or when the BMI of the patient is very low, and this is one of the remaining sites where there is ample subcutaneous fat. For many surgeons, this donor site is used to reconstruct high-volume defects such as total glossectomy defects, skull

base defects, and large cutaneous defects. At present, this donor site is one of the best alternatives for total glossectomy defects, and for patients with favorable anatomy, the rectus fascia can be sutured to the mandible to maintain the tongue mound in a position to obliterate the oral cavity. The rectus fascia can also be used to suspend the larynx to the mandible. For patients with very low BMI and very little subcutaneous fat, the rectus abdominis donor site can be used to manage moderate-volume defects such as hemiglossectomy and lateral temporal defects. For hemiglossectomy defects where the management of the reconstructed volume is critical to long-term function, a perforator-based rectus elevation may be preferable. The exclusion of the muscle facilitates better control of the volume of the reconstructed defect because muscle, which eventually undergoes atrophy, is not included. The disadvantages of this donor site are poor color match to facial skin and the development of ptosis. The versatility of the rectus abdominis donor site is based on the pattern of vascular supply from the deep inferior epigastric system of vessels, as shown in Figure 174.5.

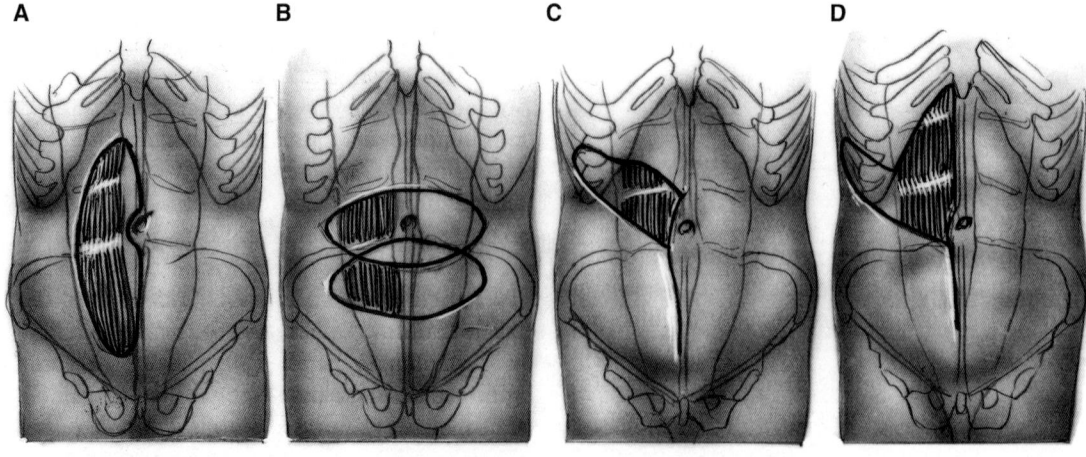

A   B   C   D

E

Above Arcuate Line

RA   Transversus aponeurosis

E.O.

IO

TA

Below Arcuate Line

Transversus aponeurosis

Transversalis fascia

S.E.

Post rectus sheath

Arcuate line

Musculocutaneous perforators

DIE A. & V.

DIE A. & V.

A.S.I.S.

Lateral vascular bundle

Rectus m. (musculotaneous flap)

Medial vascular bundle

Figure 174.5 Versatility of the rectus abdominis flap. **A:** Vertical rectus flap. **B:** Middle and lower transverse rectus abdominis flaps. **C:** Thoracoumbilical rectus flap. **D:** Combined thoracoumbilical and vertical rectus flap. **E:** The abdominal wall with the left rectus muscle reflected inferiorly to expose the arcuate line. The layers of the rectus sheath are visible above and below the arcuate line. EO, external oblique; IO, internal oblique; RA, rectus abdominis; TA, transversus abdominis.

The most commonly used configuration of the rectus donor site is the transverse rectus abdominis myocutaneous (TRAM) for breast reconstruction. This configuration can be quite useful in the head and neck particularly when large volumes of tissue are required in low-BMI patients, when the entire rectus muscle is used and can act as a separate tissue paddle, or when cosmesis is an issue (e.g., a young, low-BMI patient with a large tongue defect).

Neurovascular Pedicle

The rectus abdominis muscle has two dominant vascular pedicles, the deep superior epigastric artery and vein and the deep inferior epigastric artery and vein (25). The deep inferior epigastric artery measures an average of 3 to 4 mm in diameter, and the musculocutaneous perforators are direct branches of the deep inferior epigastric artery that passes through the overlying rectus muscle to the overlying skin. The autogenous transplant can be reinnervated with any of the lower six intercostal nerves that supply segmental motor and sensory innervation to the rectus abdominis muscle and sensory supply to the overlying skin. Unfortunately, because of the segmental innervation of this flap, it is difficult to perform effective motor or sensory reinnervation.

Anatomic Variations

Variations of the deep inferior epigastric artery and vein have been described. Sometimes the pedicle courses an unusually long distance along the lateral aspect of the muscle before taking a medial route. The perforator-based vascular anatomy is becoming more important because of the increasing use of perforator-based elevations (26).

Potential Morbidity

Removal of the rectus abdominis on one side with a portion of the overlying fascia can weaken the anterior abdominal wall and predispose the patient to ventral herniation or midline bulge. Primary closure with interrupted figure of eight with a 0.0 monofilament permanent suture on a taper needle may help decrease the likelihood of a hernia. The use of mesh to reinforce the abdominal wall is less frequent than in the past because of the high rate of infection. The time and effort needed to close the donor site and potential morbidity of the rectus donor site are other reasons that the anterolateral thigh donor site is replacing the rectus in all but the largest-volume defects.

Technical Considerations

Understanding the anatomic characteristics of the fascial envelope is perhaps more critical for rectus abdominis donor site than it is for any donor site (Fig. 174.5E). Prevention of herniation depends on restoring the integrity of the abdominal wall through effective closure of the fascial layers. An important transition occurs in the posterior sheath at the arcuate line, which is approximately at the level of the anterior superior iliac spine. Above the arcuate line, the posterior sheath is composed of contributions from the aponeuroses of the transversus abdominis and internal oblique muscles. Below the arcuate line, the aponeurotic extensions of all three muscle layers contribute to the anterior rectus sheath. The posterior sheath is composed only of transversalis fascia. The posterior rectus sheath is sufficient to prevent abdominal herniation or bulge above the arcuate line, although most surgeons reinforce this closure with closure of the anterior rectus sheath. Below the arcuate line, the anterior sheath must be reapproximated to prevent abdominal herniation. The donor site can nearly always be closed primarily. If the rectus fascia is not needed for the reconstruction, this donor site can be harvested as a perforator-based skin paddle. This technique spares the rectus muscle and the rectus sheath and avoids many of the potential morbidities of this donor site.

Preoperative Considerations

Preoperative assessment must include a careful history and physical examination of the abdomen to ensure that previous surgical procedures do not interfere with elevation of the donor site. This donor site has to be avoided in patients who have undergone inguinal herniorrhaphy or appendectomy because there can be scarring in the region of pedicle dissection. Peripheral vascular disease involving the iliac artery, particularly a history of vascular bypass, such as an aortofemoral bypass, is a contraindication to use of this donor site.

Postoperative Management

Ileus can occur in the early postoperative period. Vigorous exercise that involves the abdomen should be avoided for 3 months posttreatment although mobilization and exercise can be started before 3 months but should be done under supervision of rehab medicine or physical therapy.

Latissimus Dorsi

Description

A latissimus dorsi donor site can be used for head and neck reconstruction as either a pedicled rotation flap or an autogenous transplant. When the availability of a recipient vessel is in question, such as after radical neck dissection, this flap can be rotated onto the recipient site as a pedicled flap. When recipient vessels are available, the advantages of transferring the latissimus dorsi donor site as an autogenous transplant are as follows: there is more flexibility in positioning, the skin paddle can be inset more superiorly, and there is less risk of pedicle kinking. When the latissimus dorsi donor site is elevated as muscle alone, the muscle atrophies to a thickness of approximately 4 mm. This attribute makes it ideal for scalp reconstruction, but is poor for large-volume defects if the muscle is used to reconstitute the reconstructed volume. In the setting of massive scalp defects, which require the entire muscle, the elevation of the latissimus can be staged to recruit the distal, third angiosome. The staging procedure is performed by elevating the distal portion of the latissimus muscle and placing clips on 5 or 6 of the segmental, paravertebral, intercostal perforators from thoracic vertebrae 6 to 12 that supply the second and third angiosome. The latissimus muscle is definitively elevated 3 weeks later. For large-volume defects or large cutaneous neck defects, the latissimus dorsi muscle is transferred in a musculocutaneous paddle. For patients with total glossectomy defects, attempts have been made with little success to provide mobility of the tongue mound by reinnervating the latissimus dorsi muscle with the hypoglossal nerve.

Neurovascular Pedicle

The thoracodorsal vessels arise from the subscapular vessels or directly from the axillary artery and vein. These branches arise from the third portion of the axillary artery and vein and the vascular variations do not significantly affect pedicle length. The average diameter of the artery at its origin is 2.7 mm (range, 1.5 to 4.0 mm), the diameter of the vein is 3.4 mm (range, 1.5 to 4.5 mm), and the average length of the pedicle is 9.3 cm (range, 6.0 to 16.5 cm). One of the many appealing features of this flap is the length of the vascular pedicle. The thoracodorsal nerve provides motor innervation to the latissimus dorsi muscle. The thoracodorsal nerve usually crosses the axillary vessels approximately proximal to the subscapular artery and vein.

Anatomic Variations

The arterial supply and venous drainage of the latissimus dorsi donor site has a number of anatomic variations, but none precludes elevation or compromises pedicle length. The anatomic variations involve independent origin of the thoracodorsal vein or the thoracodorsal artery from the axillary artery or vein. When the origins are separated, the subscapular artery arises proximally in the axilla by an average of 4.2 cm (27).

Potential Morbidity

Marginal necrosis of the skin paddle can occur but the most common cause is a skin paddle that is designed too distally over the third angiosome. There is little donor-site morbidity except when a pectoralis muscle flap has been elevated on the ipsilateral side.

Technical Considerations

The patient must be carefully positioned on a beanbag in a semidecubitus position. With the patient in a 15-degree semidecubitus position, the donor site can be harvested simultaneously with the resection of the primary lesion. The anterior border of the latissimus dorsi muscle is along a line between the midpoint of the axilla and a point midway between the anterior superior iliac spine and the posterior superior iliac spine. The thoracodorsal artery and vein enter the undersurface of the muscle 8 to 10 cm below the midpoint of the axilla. The vascular branches to the serratus anterior muscle are ligated during elevation. The surgeon can harvest either a limited amount of latissimus dorsi muscle under the skin or the entire muscle, depending on reconstructive demands. A two-paddle design can be based on the medial and/or the lateral branches of the thoracodorsal vessels (Fig. 174.6). A useful elevation technique is a muscle-sparing approach that is based on the lateral branch of the thoracodorsal artery and includes only the lateral edge of the latissimus. The advantages are

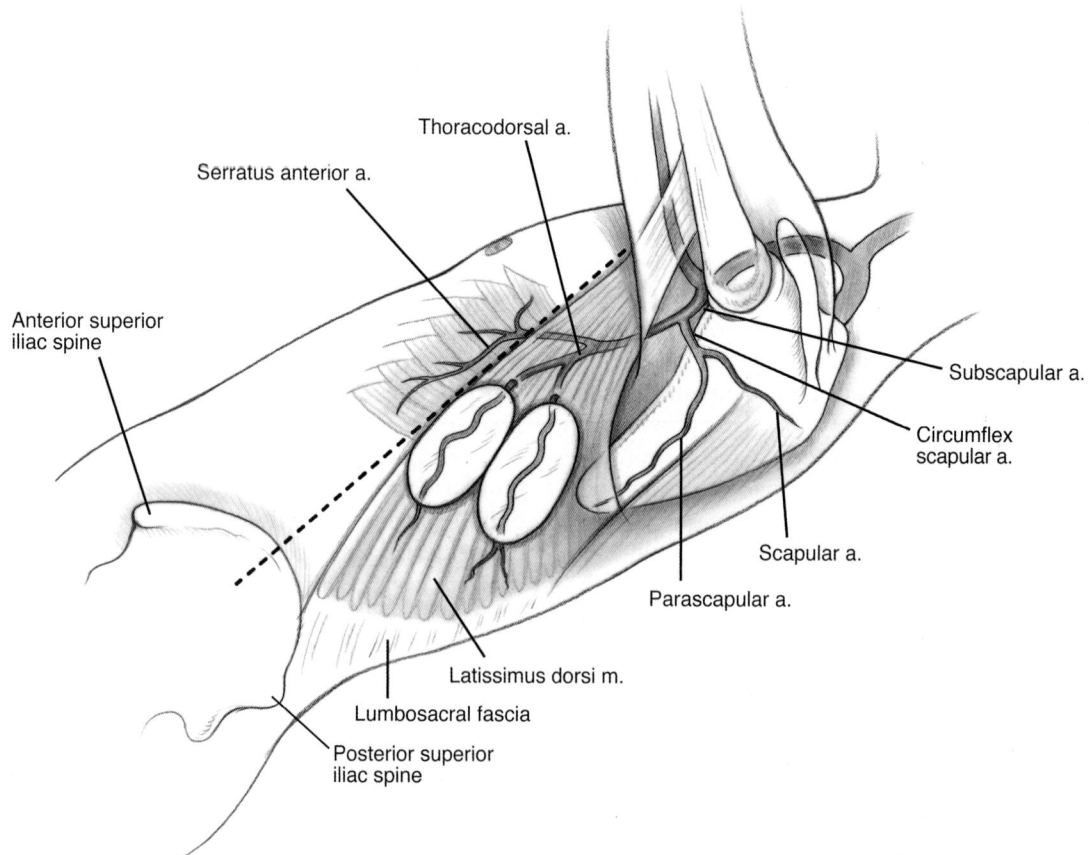

Figure 174.6 Left flank with the patient in the lateral decubitus position. The medial and lateral branches of the thoracodorsal artery are visible at the anterior edge of the muscle. The distal muscle can be used if a delay procedure that involves dividing the paraspinous perforators is performed 2 to 3 weeks before harvest. Additional pedicle length can be obtained if the circumflex scapular artery is divided.

harvest of a small volume of latissimus muscle, preservation of the innervation of the latissimus muscle from the medial branch of the thoracodorsal nerve, better control of the reconstructed volume because there is less muscle that will undergo atrophy, and less deficit in shoulder function because of preservation of innervated muscle at the donor site.

Preoperative Considerations

Previous axillary lymph node dissection is a relative contraindication to the use of the latissimus dorsi donor site. History of shoulder injury particularly of the rotator cuff is a relative contraindication.

Postoperative Management

Suction drains must be placed and left in place for several days postoperatively because of the high incidence of seroma that occurs with use of with the latissimus dorsi donor site.

Gracilis

Description

This thin myocutaneous donor site from the medial thigh was introduced by Harii et al. (28), in 1976, and was subsequently popularized as a muscle-only design for dynamic facial reanimation. The primary use of the gracilis muscle in the head and neck has been facial reanimation, in which the muscle is both revascularized and reinnervated to restore contractile activity. To restore synchronous mimetic movement when the proximal stump of the facial nerve is not available, a two-stage procedure is performed with a cross-face sural nerve graft at the initial stage. The Tinel sign is used to monitor the progression of axonal growth across the face, which usually takes 9 to 12 months after initial transfer. When the examination shows that the distal end of the sural graft has viable axons, the free muscle is transferred, revascularized, and reinnervated to the stump of the cross-face nerve graft. The advantages of this donor site for facial reanimation are its neuromuscular structure and ease of dissection.

Neurovascular Pedicle

The dominant pedicle of the gracilis donor site is the terminal branch of the adductor artery, which arises from the profunda femoris artery and runs a circuitous course between the adductor longus muscle anteriorly and the adductor brevis and magnus muscles posteriorly before entering the gracilis at the junction of the upper third and lower two-thirds. The point of entrance of the vascular pedicle into the muscle is consistently between 8 and 10 cm inferior to the pubic tubercle. The artery to the gracilis is accompanied by two venae comitantes, which either join or drain separately into the profunda femoris vein. The caliber of the artery usually is 2 mm, and the caliber of the venae comitantes measures 1.5 to 2.5 mm. The motor supply to the gracilis muscle

is the anterior branch of the obturator nerve, which enters the muscle in an oblique course approximately 2 to 3 cm cephalic to the entry point of the vascular pedicle (27).

Anatomic Variations

The main variability of the gracilis donor site is the blood supply to the overlying skin rather than the vascular or nerve supply to the muscle. Yousif et al. (29) described variations in which there are no musculocutaneous perforators from the gracilis muscle, and most of the skin supply was from septocutaneous vessels or from the inferior branch of the superior external pudendal artery. This variation is rarely important because this donor site is used as a muscle-only donor site for facial reanimation.

Technical Considerations

The branching pattern of the anterior division of the obturator nerve allows separation of the gracilis muscle into at least two functional muscular units. To minimize the bulk of muscle transferred, a single neuromuscular unit can be transferred that innervates the anterior portion of the muscle. The skin paddle, when needed, can be oriented longitudinally over the gracilis muscle. The cutaneous paddle must be centered over the dominant musculocutaneous perforator, which is 8 to 10 cm distal to the pubic tubercle (Fig. 174.7).

COMPOSITE-FREE DONOR SITES

Fibular Osteocutaneous

Description

The free fibular graft was first described by Taylor et al. in 1975 (30) for long-bone replacement after trauma or cancer. Hidalgo (31) first described the free fibular donor site for mandibular reconstruction in 1989. The fibula provides the longest possible segment of revascularized bone (25 cm) and has the thinnest associated skin paddle. This osseous donor site is the only donor site that many reconstructive surgeons use for bony reconstruction of the head and neck. The other two osseous donor sites are the iliac crest and the scapula. The iliac crest is less favored by some surgeons because of the donor-site morbidity and more difficult closure despite the excellent quality of the bone. The scapular donor site is less favored by some surgeons because the location of the scapular bone makes two-team surgery more difficult, the scapular bone is shorter, and the cross-sectional bone density is less than the fibula despite the superior selection of soft tissue options.

Due to the small volume of the fibula skin paddle, large-volume soft tissue defects may require a second revascularized flap. Although the fibula can span nearly any mandibular defect, it lacks the diameter to reconstruct many dentulous mandibles. Unless adjunctive procedures are performed such as onlay bone grafting or vertical distraction osteogenesis, it lacks the cross-sectional diameter

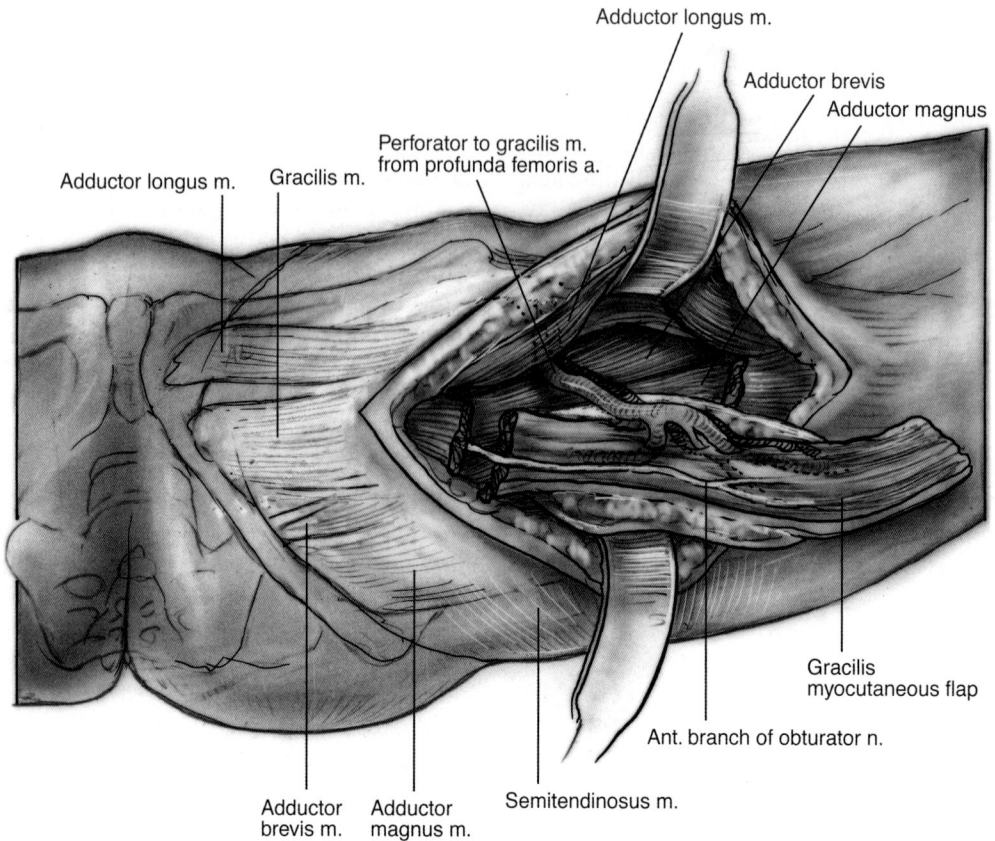

Figure 174.7 The inner thigh of the left leg with a musculocutaneous gracilis flap dissected and only attached by its pedicle. The patient is positioned with the knee flexed and the hip externally rotated. With the knee flexed, the anterior edge of the gracilis muscle is marked with a line from the adductor tubercle to the tibial tubercle. The pedicle inserts on this line approximately 8 to 10 cm from the adductor tubercle.

to reliably fix osseointegrated implants for implant bone prosthesis. The fibula is also useful for infrastructure (oral palate) maxillary reconstruction because of its long pedicle, thin associated skin paddle, and small-caliber bone stock (32). If more than 60% of the maxillary alveolus is reconstructed, vein grafting may be required. The fibula is not ideal for the reconstruction of larger maxillary defects that include the infraorbital rim because of the relative lack of soft tissue and the complex osteotomies required to reconstruct the infraorbital rim and the alveolus simultaneously. This donor site is ideal to a two-team approach and is one of the reasons for its popularity.

Neurovascular Pedicle

The peroneal artery and vein provide the primary blood supply to the fibular osteocutaneous donor site. Preoperative angiography or magnetic resonance angiography is recommended to ensure adequate arterial supply to the foot when the peroneal artery is sacrificed (33). Sensation can be variably restored when the lateral sural cutaneous nerve is used. The branches, once they supply the skin paddle, can be multiple, small, and tedious to dissect. The peroneal communicating branch can be harvested

as a vascularized nerve graft but is rarely performed in clinical practice.

Anatomic Variations

Much has been reported on the reliability of the blood supply to the skin (34). The perforators that supply the skin can course through the posterior intermuscular septum as septocutaneous perforators or can travel as musculocutaneous perforators through the flexor hallucis longus and soleus muscles. A cuff of flexor hallucis longus and soleus should be included during the elevation (Fig. 174.8A). The skin paddle is reliable if it is designed around a perforator.

Technical Considerations

When preoperative evaluation shows that either fibula is a suitable donor site, the donor site is chosen on the basis of ease of insetting. If the skin paddle is to be placed intraorally, the autogenous transplant should be harvested from the contralateral leg to the side of the inset and vascular anastomosis. If the skin paddle is to be placed extraorally, the elevation should be ipsilateral to the side of inset and vascular anastomosis. The skin paddle is centered over the posterior intermuscular septum, which is anterior to

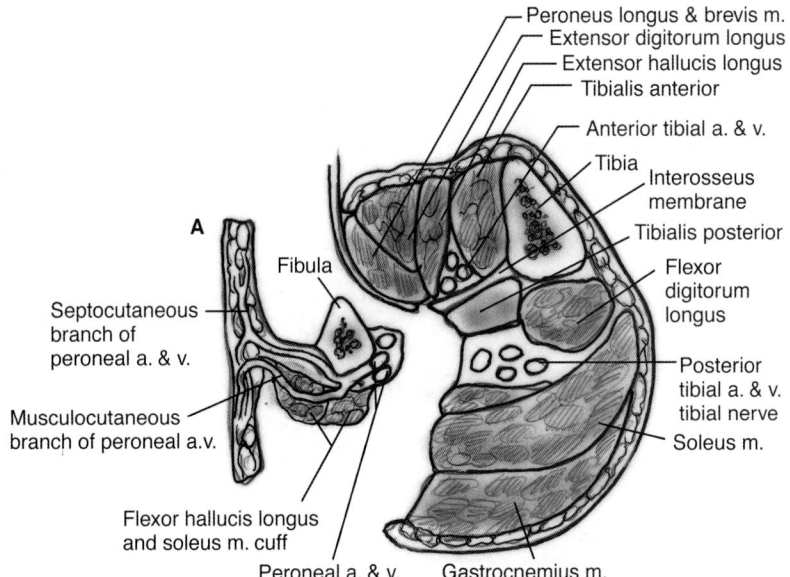

A: Peroneus longus & brevis m.
Extensor digitorum longus
Extensor hallucis longus
Tibialis anterior
Anterior tibial a. & v.
Tibia
Interosseus membrane
Tibialis posterior
Flexor digitorum longus
Posterior tibial a. & v. tibial nerve
Soleus m.
Fibula
Septocutaneous branch of peroneal a. & v.
Musculocutaneous branch of peroneal a.v.
Flexor hallucis longus and soleus m. cuff
Peroneal a. & v.
Gastrocnemius m.

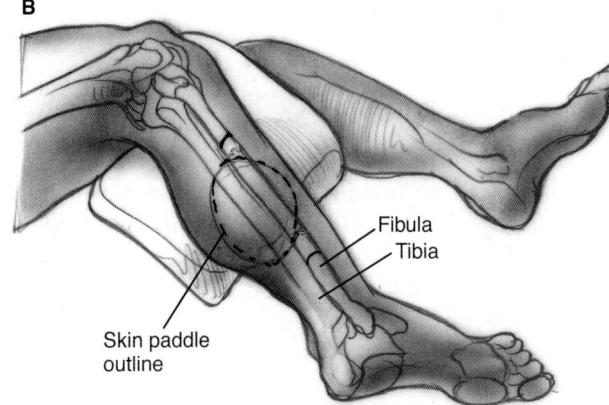

B
Fibula
Tibia
Skin paddle outline

Figure 174.8 A: Cross section of the leg shows the fibula flap is elevated, and that both musculocutaneous and septocutaneous perforators course from the peroneal artery to the skin paddle. **B:** The flap is marked on the lateral aspect of the right leg. The cutaneous paddle is marked along the posterior intermuscular septum, which is visible when the foot is flexed and inverted. Dominant cutaneous perforators can be located with a Doppler flowmeter before the flap is elevated (10 to 25 cm distal to the fibular head). The presence of septocutaneous perforators can be confirmed after the cutaneous portion of the flap over the lateral compartment is elevated. **C:** Flap detached from the vascular pedicle with the soleus muscle still attached for illustrative purposes. The anterior approach to this flap is useful for obtaining a wide cuff of flexor hallucis and soleus muscles to encompass the musculocutaneous perforators.

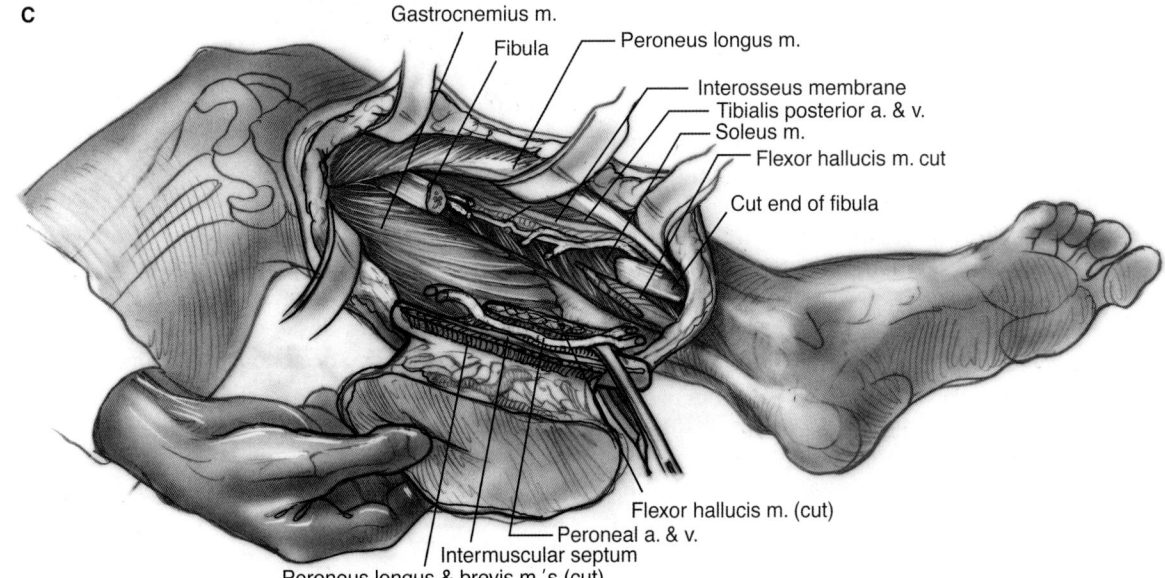

C
Gastrocnemius m.
Fibula
Peroneus longus m.
Interosseus membrane
Tibialis posterior a. & v.
Soleus m.
Flexor hallucis m. cut
Cut end of fibula
Flexor hallucis m. (cut)
Peroneal a. & v.
Intermuscular septum
Peroneus longus & brevis m.'s (cut)

the soleus muscle and posterior to the peroneus muscle (Fig. 174.8B and C). A Doppler is used to identify cutaneous perforators along the posterior septum along the distal third of the donor fibula bone. The greatest number of cutaneous perforators is present in this region. Shifting the skin paddle distally increases pedicle length. Elevation usually is performed with a thigh tourniquet inflated to 300 mm Hg. In the event that the skin paddle is inadequately perfused, a second soft tissue donor site is prepared, which is usually the radial forearm site.

Potential Morbidity

A variety of donor-site complications have been reported, including rolling out of the ankle, cold intolerance, and edema. Elevation and closure are important. The motor nerve to the lateral compartment will be exposed when the peroneal muscles are dissected from their origin on the fibula. It is not technically challenging to avoid this nerve, but knowledge of its location will facilitate identification and preservation. When reapproximating the muscles after elevation of the fibula, it is important to not injure the nerve supply to the lateral compartment and to reapproximate the flexor hallucis at an anatomic length so that it can effectively flex the toe. An 8-cm segment of fibula is preserved both proximally and distally to protect the common peroneal nerve proximally and to ensure stability of the ankle joint distally. A skin graft is often required for closure of the donor defect and is preferable to closure under excessive tension because of the risk of compartment syndrome or distal limb ischemia.

Preoperative Considerations

Assessment of the vasculature to the foot is essential before fibular transfer. MRI angiography has supplanted conventional angiography in most cases. A history of lower-extremity fracture, joint replacement, and bypass grafting directs the surgeon away from a particular extremity. Careful physical examination of the lower extremity for peripheral edema or nonhealing ulcers is advisable in selection of the donor site because diseases related to peripheral vascular compromise and peripheral neuropathy such as diabetes may direct the surgeon to alternative donor sites.

Postoperative Management

Distal pulses in the foot are monitored as closely to avoid the complication of vascular insufficiency to the foot, which can be caused by excessively tight closure or dressings. A prefabricated walking boot is fit in the operating room. It is left in position for 6 to 7 days to facilitate healing of the skin graft. After this time period, the dressing is changed daily, the patient wears the boot for another 3 to 5 weeks to allow complete healing of the skin graft and to control pain. Ambulation is initiated with partial weight bearing on the third postoperative day with the assistance of physical therapy and a walker. Full weight bearing with the assistance of a walker or a cane can take place on postoperative day 5.

Osteocutaneous and Osteomusculocutaneous Iliac Crest

Description

The iliac crest donor site can be designed as an osseous, myoosseous, or osseomyocutaneous flap. The pedicle is 5 to 6 cm long and can be lengthened if the segment of iliac crest is harvested at a more distal site. The original descriptions of the donor site (30,35) were for mandibular reconstruction. Up to 16 cm of bone can be harvested. A bone-only transplant is ideal for segmental mandibular defects with very limited soft tissue component such as those associated with odontogenic lesions. A myoosseous transplant is ideal for segmental mandibular and maxillary defects with limited associated soft tissue defects. The osseomyocutaneous transplant is excellent for defects that involve limited intraoral lining and large external skin defects. The skin paddle does not rotate easily into the oral cavity and is not particularly useful for intraoral reconstruction. If there is a large intraoral soft tissue component combined with a segmental mandibular defect, the scapula donor site or two separate donor sites may be a better alternative. The iliac crest is also the best flap for retention of osseointegrated implants as it has the largest cross-sectional area when compared to a fibular or scapular bone. Despite the excellent quality of the bone, the limitations of the soft tissue and the morbidity at the donor site limit the use of the iliac crest. Most oral cavity defects usually involve intraoral soft tissue of the tongue, cheek, or palate and would require a second flap to adequately reconstruct the soft tissue. In cases where excellent bone stock is required for osseointegrated implants and there is a complex intraoral soft tissue defect, a second soft tissue donor site will be required to adequately rehabilitate the patient.

Neurovascular Pedicle

The deep circumflex iliac artery (DCIA) arises from the lateral aspect of the external iliac artery approximately 1 to 2 cm cephalic to the inguinal ligament. The ascending branch of the DCIA supplies the internal oblique muscle in 80% of the cases. The remaining patients have multiple smaller branches supplying the internal oblique from the DCIA. This vascular pattern does not prevent use of the internal oblique muscle. The deep circumflex iliac vein usually is composed of two paired venae comitantes, which merge a variable distance lateral to the external iliac vein. The caliber of the DCIA is 2 to 3 mm. That of the deep circumflex iliac vein ranges from 3 to 5 mm. There is no easily identifiable sensory component.

Potential Morbidity

Herniation of the abdominal wall can occur in the postoperative period. Meticulous, layered closure of the abdominal wall is essential to prevent ventral hernia. The transversus abdominis muscle is approximated to the cut edge of the iliacus muscle. This layer can be reinforced by means of placing drill holes into the cut edge of the iliac bone through which sutures are placed to reinforce the deep layer of closure. The next layer of closure approximates the external oblique muscle and aponeurosis to the tensor fascia lata and gluteus medius muscles. To decrease the likelihood of direct herniation, the internal oblique muscle is retained in a position inferior to the anterior superior iliac spine. This triangle of muscle is closed back to the lateral rectus sheath, 2.0 or 0.0 Prolene is used, and a figure-of-eight suture is placed for each layer of this closure. The iliac crest donor site has robust blood supply to the bone and internal oblique muscle, but problems can occur with the blood supply to the skin. The skin is supplied by perforators from the DCIA. The perforators can be easily sheared as they pass through all three layers of the abdominal wall.

Technical Considerations

The skin paddle is centered on an axis drawn from the anterior superior iliac spine to a location on the anterior thorax where the inferior tip of the scapula is projected from the back to the anterior thorax (Fig. 174.9). Along this line, the zone of cutaneous perforators starts approximately 9 cm from the anterior superior iliac spine. The perforators are about 2.5 cm medial to the edge of the iliac crest. A generous cuff of external oblique, internal oblique, and transversus abdominis layers must be preserved as the cutaneous perforators course through these layers. This produces a bulky, relatively immobile skin paddle. The skin must not be rotated independently of the bone to avoid twisting or stretching the cutaneous perforators. This elevation also places that patient at greater risk for an incisional hernia.

Preoperative Considerations

Evidence of ventral herniation or previous inguinal herniorrhaphy can lead the surgeon to select an alternative donor site. If the patient has severe peripheral vascular disease, the surgeon needs to be sure that iliac artery bypass grafting has not been performed. For a patient who is a vasculopath and has not undergone bypass grafting, an angiography of the DCIA is performed to ensure vessel patency.

Postoperative Management

Progressive mobilization begins on the third postoperative day. On the fifth postoperative day, the patient can walk with a walker and progress to a cane and independent walking as tolerated. Rigorous abdominal exercise is avoided for 3 months after the completion of treatment including chemoradiation.

Scapular Donor Site, Subscapular and Thoracodorsal Artery

Description

The use of the scapular donor site is evolving and is different from the other commonly used osseous donor sites. The scapula bone and associated soft tissue can be harvested based on two different vascular pedicles, the circumflex scapular artery and/or the thoracodorsal artery. The unique features that make the scapular donor site useful for head and neck reconstruction include an option for a long vascular pedicle, the abundant surface area of relatively thin skin, the independent arc of rotation of the bone and the soft tissue paddles, the ability to combine the scapular flap based on the circumflex scapular artery with the latissimus dorsi based on the thoracodorsal artery, and the options

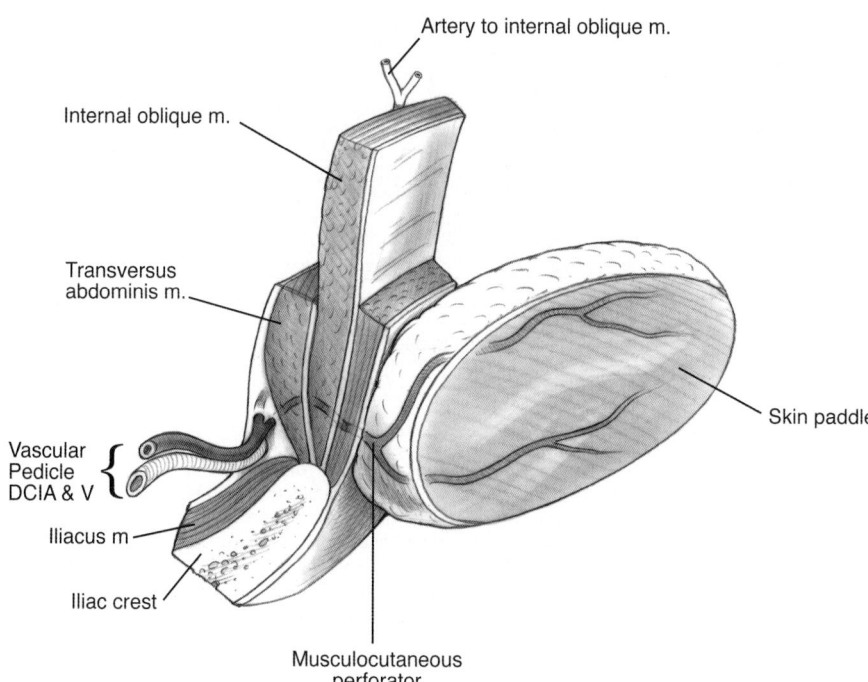

Artery to internal oblique m.

Internal oblique m.

Transversus abdominis m.

Vascular Pedicle DCIA & V

Iliacus m

Iliac crest

Musculocutaneous perforator

Skin paddle

Figure 174.9 Vascular anatomic features of the iliac crest flap. The deep circumflex iliac artery (*DCIA*) courses in the superior aspect of the iliacus muscle. After it gives off the ascending branch, the DCIA runs in the groove between the iliacus and transversus abdominis muscles before penetrating the transversus abdominis muscle and passing over the pelvic brim near the posterior superior iliac spine. The bone must be cut low enough to include the pedicle. The ascending branch can be identified on the undersurface of the internal oblique muscle and dissected proximally to help identify the DCIA. *DCIV,* deep circumflex iliac vein.

for sophisticated three-dimensional inset. The flexibility of this donor site is useful for the closure of complex multi-surfaced defects such as craniofacial and orofacial defects. Up to 10 cm of bone can be harvested from the lateral aspect of the scapula starting just inferior to the glenoid fossa based on the circumflex scapular artery. The bone stock is inadequate for the placement of osseointegrated implants for the purpose of mandibular rehabilitation without secondary onlay-free bone grafting. The fasciocutaneous skin paddle supplied by the circumflex scapular artery is an excellent source of well-vascularized, moderately thin, hairless skin. The circumflex scapular artery has two cutaneous branches that can supply two cutaneous skin paddles. The horizontally oriented scapular skin paddle is based on the transverse cutaneous branch, and the vertically oriented parascapular skin paddle is based on the descending cutaneous branch (36) (Fig. 174.10). The second vascular pedicle that supplies the tip of the scapula is the thoracodorsal, and this variation is being used with increasing frequency and is replacing the circumflex scapular-based donor site (37). The scapular tip is supplied by several branches from the thoracodorsal artery and is named the TDAST donor site (38). This variation has a long vascular pedicle, supplies the entire scapular tip, and is useful for complex multisurfaced, high-volume midface and combined orbital reconstructions. This variation can be considered a latissimus osseomyocutaneous flap and can be combined with any variation of the bone and/or soft tissue based on the circumflex scapular artery.

Neurovascular Pedicle

The parent vessels of the two scapular donor sites are the subscapular artery and vein, which arise from the third part of the axillary artery and vein. The circumflex scapular

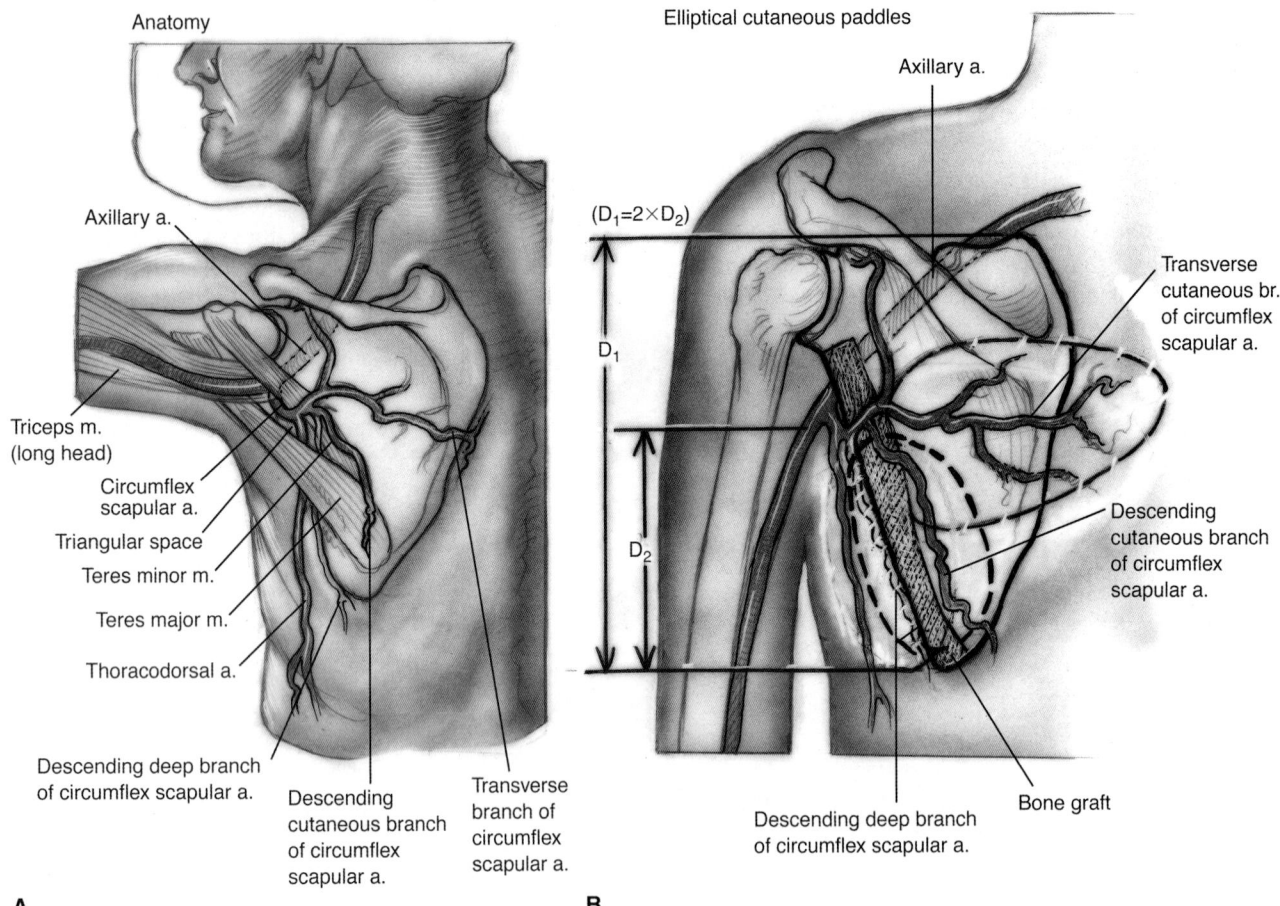

Figure 174.10 A: Vascular anatomic features of the left scapula. The subscapular artery sends the circumflex scapular branch through the triangular space to the scapular flap. The muscles that define the triangular space are palpated and marked preoperatively. The soft triangle is best approached by means of dissection over the teres major muscle at the lateral boarder of the scapula. Once the triangular space is located, the teres minor muscle can be retracted superiorly, and the pedicle can be dissected through the axillary space. **B:** The triangular space also can be located by means of marking the midpoint of the lateral aspect of the scapula. Three of the possible scapular paddles and their vascular supply are outlined. The deep branch is intimately associated with the lateral border of the scapula, which it supplies. If a bone flap is to be included, care is taken not to injure the deep branch after dissection of the cutaneous flaps.

artery and vein emerge from the triangular space defined by the teres major and teres minor muscles and the long head of the triceps muscle. The circumflex scapular artery is accompanied by paired venae comitantes, which usually join the thoracodorsal vein before entering the axillary vein. The average diameter of the circumflex scapular artery at its takeoff from the subscapular artery is 4 mm. At its origin from the axillary artery, the subscapular artery has an average diameter of 6 mm. When the circumflex scapular artery is harvested at its takeoff from the subscapular vessels, the fasciocutaneous flap has a pedicle length of 4 to 6 cm. Although a maximum pedicle length of 11 to 14 cm has been extensively quoted in the literature, in practice, the length is much closer to 8 cm. The thoracodorsal artery is described in the section on the latissimus dorsi myocutaneous donor site. The pedicle that supplies the scapular tip arises within 1 cm of the branch to the serratus muscle and can arise from the thoracodorsal artery or the artery to the serratus muscle (Fig 174.11). When skin or osseous paddles are elevated on both the circumflex scapular and the thoracodorsal pedicles, this configuration is referred to as a "mega" flap.

Anatomic Variations

There are five anatomic variations but they are of little clinical consequence from the perspective of pedicle length or viability of the transplant. The most common pattern is a single subscapular artery and a single subscapular vein branching into the circumflex scapular and the thoracodorsal pedicle supplying both the scapula and the latissimus donor sites. One of the variations is a duplicated circumflex artery. Of the remaining three variations, all are related to separate origins of the vein or artery for each of the two flaps. These variations may necessitate two recipient arteries or two recipient venous anastomoses.

Potential Morbidity

A contralateral brachial plexus neuropathy can be caused by lateral decubitus positioning during flap harvest. If the patient is positioned fully decubitus, an axillary roll is needed, as is careful attention to arm positioning. The axillary roll is to keep the thoracic cage elevated up off the bed and prevent compression of the clavicle on the brachial plexus. The scapular osteotomy must be fashioned 1 cm inferior to the glenoid fossa to avoid injury to the joint space. Harvest of the scapular osteocutaneous flap necessitates detachment of the teres major, teres minor, subscapularis, and infraspinatus, which can cause shoulder weakness and limited range of motion. These muscles must be meticulously reapproximated while the shoulder is abducted and the arm is extended.

Technical Considerations

To make two-team surgery easier, the patient can be placed in a 15-degree decubitus position with the assistance of a beanbag. Flap harvesting is technically more difficult when the patient is in a 15-degree decubitus position, but the benefit is reduction in total operative time. A separate

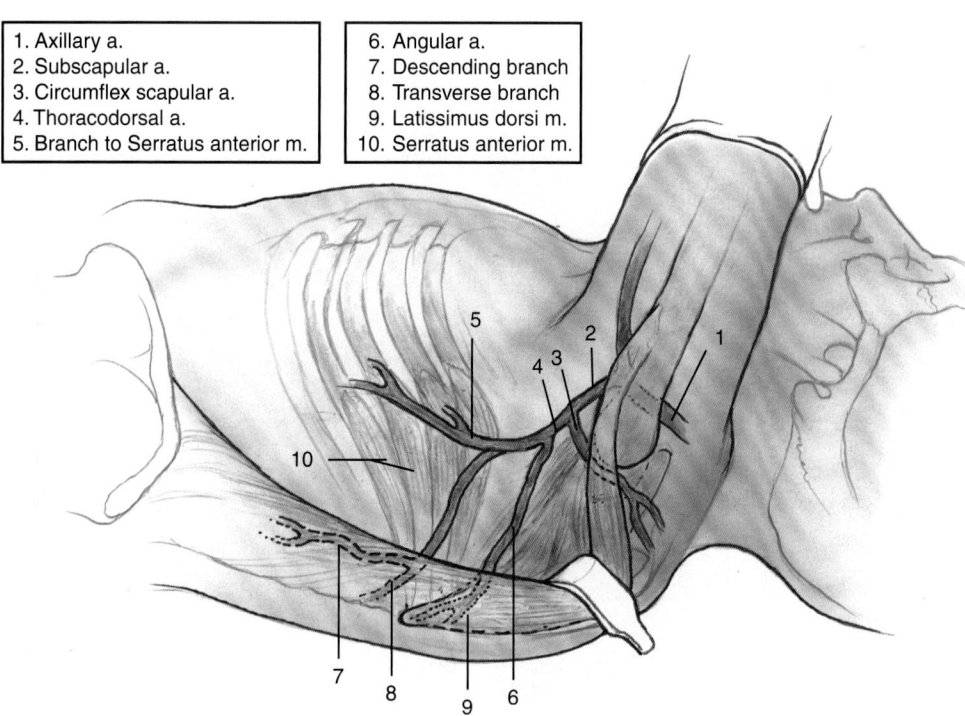

1. Axillary a.
2. Subscapular a.
3. Circumflex scapular a.
4. Thoracodorsal a.
5. Branch to Serratus anterior m.
6. Angular a.
7. Descending branch
8. Transverse branch
9. Latissimus dorsi m.
10. Serratus anterior m.

Figure 174.11 The vascular anatomy of the TDAST autogenous transplant as seen during surgical elevation with the patient in the semidecubitus position. Note that the branch to the scapular tip usually arises 1 cm distal to the serratus branch or from the serratus branch 1 cm after the serratus branch is given off from the thoracodorsal artery.

axillary incision can be helpful in dissecting the pedicle to the axillary artery and vein. If the bone of the scapula is elevated, the teres major, subscapularis, and latissimus dorsi muscles are reattached to the scapula with 2-0 PDS. Care is taken not to injure the motor nerve supply to the teres major muscle during flap elevation. Modified Kessler suture technique can be useful for optimizing reapproximation of the cut end of the teres major muscle to the scapula. If the scapular tip is harvested as part of a TDAST elevation, the insertion of the serratus should be reapproximated to stabilize the scapula. If there is enough intact latissimus muscle that is attached at the origin and the insertion, the anterior edge should be tacked to the fascia over the thoracic cage.

Preoperative Considerations

Previous axillary node dissection, shoulder reconstruction, or shoulder dislocation are contraindications to the use of fasciocutaneous and osteofasciocutaneous scapular or TDAST transplants.

Postoperative Management

If the scapular skin paddle is raised without bone, no specific limitations are necessary with active range of motion. Passive range of motion should be limited by pain. If bone is harvested, the shoulder does not have to be immobilized, but minimal mobilization and not using the axilla to move the patient in bed should continue for 5 days. Thereafter, a physical therapy program should be started that begins with active range of motion and progresses to passive range of motion.

VISCERAL DONOR SITES

Jejunum

Description

The free jejunal autogenous transplant has been successful in reconstruction of circumferential pharyngoesophageal defects. The diameter of the jejunum is a good match with the cervical esophagus and maintains a mucosal surface for food bolus transit. The graft is harvested by a transplant thoracic surgeon or a general surgeon with a simultaneous two-team approach.

Neurovascular Pedicle

Transilluminating the mesentery facilitates selection of a segment of jejunum with sufficient arborization from a single mesenteric artery and vein to supply the graft (Fig. 174.12). The second arcade of the jejunum usually is best for pharyngeal reconstruction.

Potential Morbidity

Stricture of the upper or lower anastomosis occurs in about 10% of free jejunal transfers and responds well to dilation. This rate of stricture is lower than that encountered when tubed cutaneous flaps are used. Despite the lower stricture rate and relative ease of inset, the jejunum can have long-term functional problems. The peristalsis of the jejunum produces functional obstruction during swallowing, a wet voice among patients who speak by means of tracheoesophageal puncture, and dysgeusia from the succus entericus (39). The long-term functional problems can be nearly eliminated with postoperative radiation therapy.

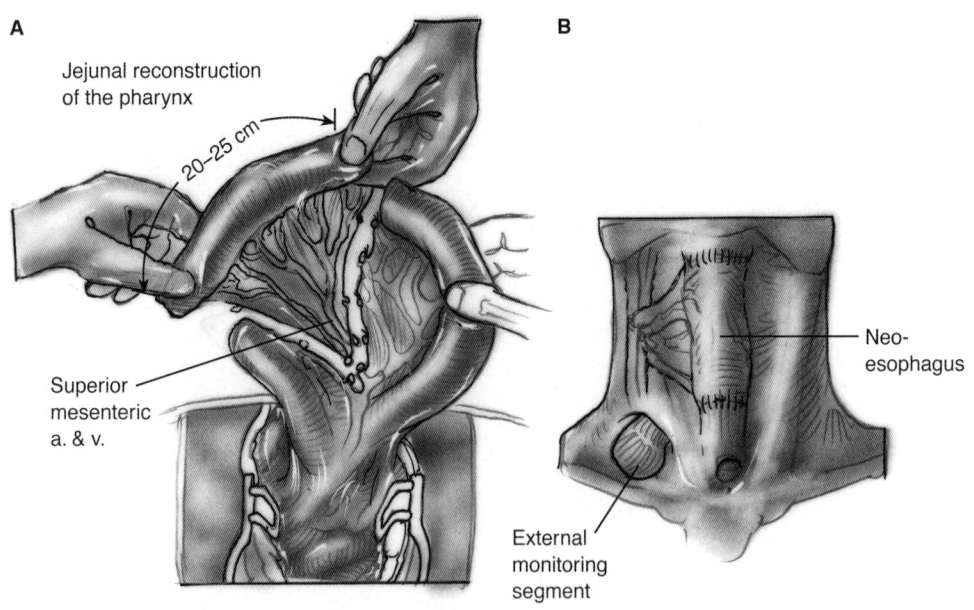

Figure 174.12 **A:** Segment of proximal jejunum of sufficient length supplied by a single arcade. **B:** The jejunum is shown as a segmental reconstruction of a total pharyngeal defect with a monitoring segment. The jejunum is inset under a minor degree of tension to reduce dysphagia.

Technical Considerations

A suture is placed at the proximal end of the graft at harvest to ensure isoperistaltic reconstruction of the pharyngoesophagus. Any redundancy of the jejunal segment is avoided to prevent dysphagia. The proximal end of the jejunum can be divided along the antimesenteric border to facilitate closure to the tongue base. The distal end of the jejunum is anastomosed in an end-to-end manner to the stump of cervical esophagus. Postoperative monitoring is facilitated by exteriorizing a monitoring segment of the jejunum. This segment is based on the same mesenteric arcade as the rest of the flap (40). This segment can be observed for peristalsis and evaluated directly with a Doppler probe.

Preoperative Considerations

Extension of disease into the proximal thoracic esophagus is an absolute indication for esophagectomy and colon interposition. The presence of ascites and chronic intestinal diseases such as Crohn disease and previous extensive abdominal surgery or intraperitoneal sepsis are all contraindications for the use of the jejunum. Patients with limited pulmonary reserve are at increased risk of morbidity after laparotomy.

Postoperative Management

The external monitoring segment of jejunum is removed at the bedside on postoperative day 7 by means of suture ligation of its mesentery.

Omentum and Gastroomentum

Description

The greater omentum is a double layer of peritoneum that hangs like a sheet from its main attachments to the greater curvature of the stomach and transverse colon (Fig. 174.13). The blood supply to this structure arises from the right and left gastroepiploic vessels, which course in the cephalic edge of the omentum where it attaches to the stomach. The omental free flap is very infrequently used in head and neck reconstruction but has been used for a variety of defects including coverage of large scalp defects,

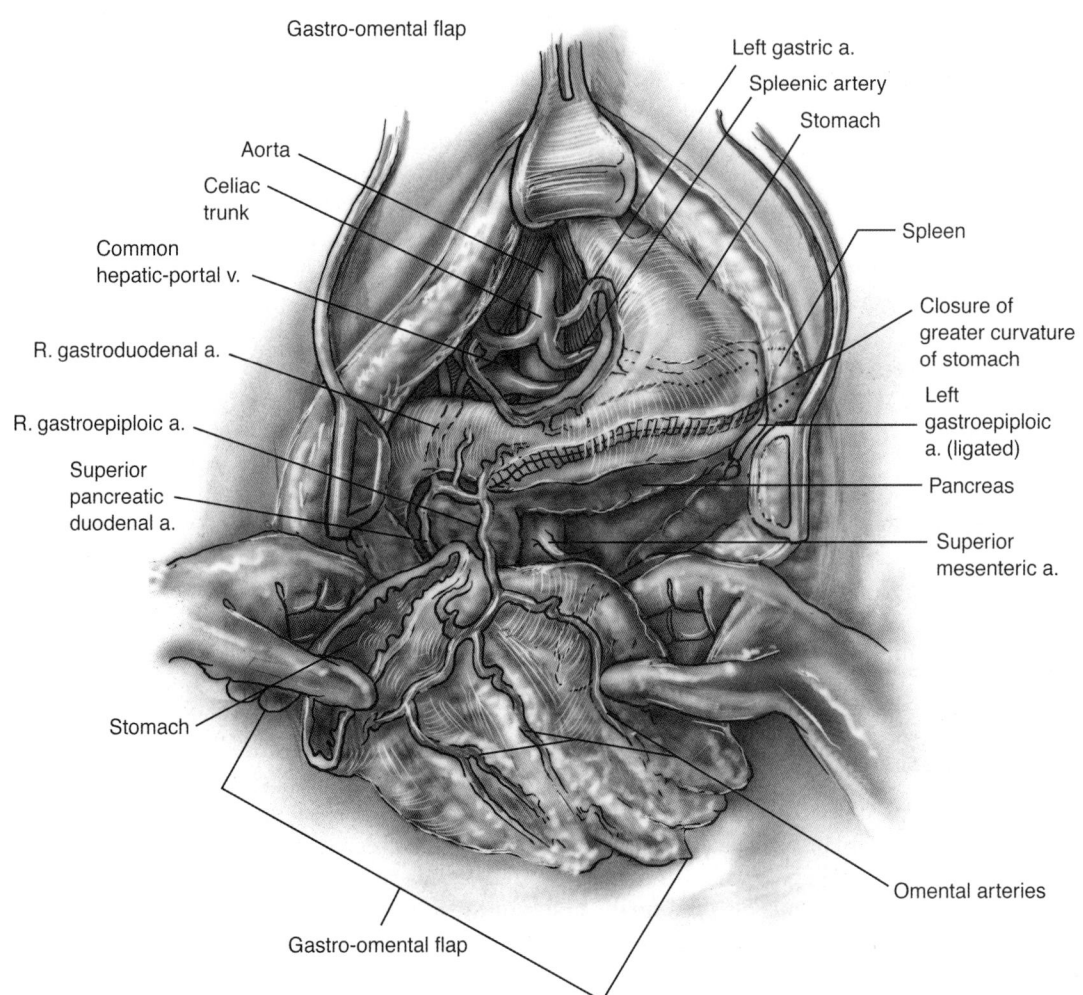

Figure 174.13 Gastroomental flap completely elevated from the greater curvature of the stomach.

repair of extensive midfacial defects with coverage of split rib or calvarial grafts, management of osteoradionecrosis and osteomyelitis in the head and neck region, and facial contouring. Although not used in North America, it has been used for severe cicatricial neck scarring after treatment of head and neck cancer with chemoradiation. Gastroomental autogenous transplants have been used for oral or pharyngeal defects; omentum is used to provide carotid coverage (41,42). The surgeon must carefully weigh the functional and aesthetic benefits of this flap against the risks of an intra-abdominal procedure. A recent application is its use as a tubed gastroomental transplant for the treatment of laryngopharyngectomy defects in patients who have failed treatment with chemoradiation. The perceived advantage is lower postoperative fistula rates, decreased neck scarring, and less postoperative structure (43).

Neurovascular Pedicle

The right gastroepiploic artery is more favorable for supplying omental flaps. The diameter of the right gastroepiploic artery ranges from 1.5 to 3.0 mm.

Potential Morbidity

A wide range of intra-abdominal complications can occur after harvest of a gastroomental free flap. The most serious is gastric leak with peritonitis and intra-abdominal abscess formation. Gastric outlet obstruction can occur if the harvest impinged *on the or is* placed too close to the pylorus.

Preoperative Considerations

A history of gastric outlet obstruction or peptic ulcer disease is a contraindication to this procedure.

MICROVASCULAR RECONSTRUCTIVE APPROACHES TO DEFECTS IN THE HEAD AND NECK

When reviewing various reconstructive approaches in the literature, it can be difficult to interpret results within a study or compare results between studies because there is no universally adopted system for coding head and neck defects. An effort has been made to classify defects on the basis of loss of epithelium, bone, nerves, and supporting musculature (44).

Pharyngoesophageal Defects

Pharyngoesophageal defects are classified according to circumferential involvement (partial, near total, and total) and whether the esophagus or a large portion of the oropharynx was included in the resection. Also important in determining the optimal reconstruction is consideration of the mechanism of postoperative voice production (tracheoesophageal puncture vs. electrolarynx) and the use of postoperative radiation therapy.

Partial pharyngoesophageal defects are divided into those that can be closed primarily with minimal risk of stricture and partial defects that require additional tissue for reconstruction to minimize the risk of stricture. In general, partial pharyngeal defects that require additional tissue for closure are those that have undergone sacrifice of at least 50% of the pharynx, such as one piriform fossa and 50% of the posterior pharyngeal wall, and primary closure cannot be performed without high risk of pharyngeal stenosis. Near-total pharyngoesophageal defects are defects in which only a thin strip of pharynx (1 cm) remains. Total pharyngeal defects are those in which there is complete absence of a segment of the pharynx and a circumferential reconstruction is required.

Partial pharyngeal defects that require additional tissue and near-total pharyngeal defects can be reconstructed with either pedicled regional flaps or free tissue transfer. The following factors are taken into account to assist in decision making: (a) There must be adequate vascular access for a free tissue transfer, (b) carotid protection is believed to be beneficial if a modified radical or radical neck dissection has been performed and a pedicled regional flap such as a pectoralis or latissimus dorsi flap can be used to provide carotid coverage, (c) for total or near-total pharyngeal defects, the soft tissue should be thinner than 2 cm.

For total pharyngoesophageal defects, four types of reconstructions are considered. A gastric transposition (this is a pedicled flap), colon interposition, autogenous jejunal transplant, and large autogenous cutaneous transplants such as radial forearm or an anterolateral thigh. It is technically possible to perform the majority of total pharyngeal reconstructions with an autogenous jejunal transplant or autogenous cutaneous transplant. If the defect extends into the mediastinum, preoperative consultation with a thoracic surgeon and planning of a colon interposition flap is appropriate. Gastric transpositions are no longer the best reconstructive option because they do not remain as well vascularized as the colon when extended up into the oropharynx and are associated with significant reflux (45).

The autogenous jejunal transplant was the first and the most commonly used donor site to reconstruct total pharyngoesophageal defects. The shortcomings are a wet voice, especially if the patient does not undergo postoperative radiation therapy, and dysphagia from autonomous peristalsis; halitosis; difficulty with reconstructing more extensive oropharyngeal defects; and the opening of the peritoneum. Cutaneous autogenous transplants (radial forearm, anterolateral thigh) have nearly replaced the jejunum as the reconstructive option of choice. The cutaneous donor sites can provide better voice, less dysphagia, and less donor-site morbidity compared to the jejunum. The trade-off with cutaneous donor sites is the higher incidence of stricture (46). Some surgeons use a salivary bypass tube at the time of surgery to reduce the likelihood of a stricture (47).

In addition to considering the size and the extent of the defect as discussed above, consideration of the quality of the tissue is important. In the situation of surgical salvage after failure of chemoradiation therapy, the fistula rate with primary hypopharyngeal closure is high. In an attempt to reduce the fistula rate, fasciocutaneous autogenous transplants are used as a pharyngeal interposition or onlay grafts. They are used to support the primary closure of hypopharyngeal defects and have been shown to decrease the fistula rate to 20% in a small case series (48). In a similar fashion, rotational muscle flaps can also be used as a source of unradiated, well-vascularized tissue to reduce the incidence of fistula. Another approach to the reduction of complications for patients undergoing salvage total laryngopharyngectomy is the autogenous gastroomental transplant. The inferior edge of the stomach is tubed for the pharyngeal reconstruction, and the omentum can be used to resurface the entire anterior neck skin as necessary.

Oral Cavity and Oropharyngeal Defects

In the oral cavity and oropharynx, microvascular reconstruction has improved function and reduced complications of the tongue and mandible (7). The sensate radial forearm autogenous transplant has become the workhorse of low-volume, soft tissue oral cavity reconstruction; the sensate lateral arm is an alternative for slightly larger-volume defects. Because of the ease of harvest and microvascular anastomosis, the anterolateral thigh has become the donor site of choice for larger-volume defects. Reconstruction of associated mandibular bony defects can compromise soft tissue reconstruction because the soft tissue associated with osseous donor sites is not as versatile as the soft tissue donor sites. When the functional results are likely to be compromised by use of the soft tissue component of an osseous transplant, two donor sites can be used. A soft tissue donor site and an osseous donor site can be combined to optimize speech, swallowing, and cosmetic results. An example is an angle-to-angle mandibular defect combined with two-thirds anterior glossectomy. A fibula autogenous transplant can be used for osseous reconstruction, and a soft tissue flap such as a perforator TRAM rectus, latissimus dorsi, anterolateral thigh, or a lateral arm can be used for the glossectomy reconstruction. For the repair of some of the largest soft tissue defects that include the entire tongue, musculocutaneous donor sites such as the rectus abdominis and latissimus dorsi are used.

The principles of oral cavity reconstruction are to obtain watertight closure; maintain mobility; provide sensation, including cable grafting of segmentally resected sensory nerves; maintain the volume of the resected tissue; maintain oral competence; and prevent medically significant aspiration. The radial forearm autogenous transplant is uniquely suited to reconstruction of the oral cavity when there is remaining functional anterior tongue. It is a thin, supple donor site of ample size to provide mobility. The antebrachial cutaneous nerve can be used to innervate the flap and provide cable grafts for the inferior alveolar or lingual nerves. Deepithelialized segments can be used to contour the reconstruction to restore the original shape of the resected tissue (49).

For total glossectomy defects a large volume of subcutaneous tissue is made into a mound to allow contact between the flap and the remaining sensate mucosa in the oral cavity. If a laryngectomy has not been performed, the hyoid bone must be resuspended to the mandible to help prevent aspiration.

Complex full-thickness defects (defects that include oral mucosa in continuity with external skin) usually are encountered in conjunction with mandibular defects. These defects can be reconstructed with a multipaddled osteocutaneous latissimus or scapula autogenous transplant or a combination of a soft tissue and a osteocutaneous fibular flap.

Midfacial Defects

Midfacial defects traditionally have been managed with a prosthesis. Revascularized free tissue transfer has been valuable in reconstructing the maxilla to maintain midfacial projection in the premaxillary, zygomatic, and infraorbital regions. It also has been useful in providing soft tissue to the cheek and orbit. The principles of midfacial reconstruction are to restore the contour and projection of the midface, to facilitate rehabilitation of an occlusal surface in the upper jaw, to provide oronasal separation, to close the orbit or provide a platform for prosthetic rehabilitation of the eye, and to maintain a functioning lacrimal system if the globe is intact. Use of a hard-palate obturator is an excellent approach to a maxillectomy defect, and that is limited to the ipsilateral secondary palate. When evaluating a patient for reconstruction of the midface, it is important to consider and coordinate the tissue transplantation with the prosthetic rehabilitation to optimize the functional and aesthetic results.

It is helpful to classify defects involving the maxilla. There are at least two classification systems that are helpful for thinking about maxillary reconstruction (50,51). These defects can be categorized first by dividing them into infrastructure (oral palate) and combined infrastructure and suprastructure defects (oral palate, maxillary buttresses, orbital rim, and orbit). Infrastructure (oral palate) defects can be approached with a wide variety of techniques. Combined infrastructure and suprastructure defects can be subdivided as follows: (a) maxillectomy with intact orbital rim, (b) maxillectomy including the infraorbital rim, (c) maxillectomy including the infraorbital rim and orbital contents, and (d) composite defects, which can include any of the other defects combined with facial skin. The principles to be addressed are midfacial projection, the infraorbital rim, orbital floor support, oral nasal separation, and a stable platform for mastication.

Maxillectomy defects with intact orbital rim that only involve two buttresses are effectively reconstructed with an obturator. The obturator provides adequate oronasal separation, a stable platform for mastication, and an anchor for additional teeth if the patient does not have an intact dental arch. Maxillectomy defects including infraorbital rim are best reconstructed with free tissue transfer, either alone or in concert with a prosthesis. An effective approach for patients without teeth or who cannot afford osseointegrated implants is vascularized bone osseocutaneous forearm autogenous transplant or a TDAST for the infraorbital rim reconstruction and orbital floor support in combination with a maxillary obturator to provide dental arch (52). For patients who can afford implants or whose remaining dentition is intact and healthy, an osseocutaneous flap such as an iliac crest, fibular, or TDAST in combination with osseointegrated implants as needed has become a more frequently used approach to avoid a maxillary obturator.

Maxillectomy defects including the infraorbital rim and orbital contents are much larger-volume defects. The principles to be addressed are the same as those for defects with an intact orbital rim with the additional issue of volume requirement for the orbital defect. A TDAST alone or an osseocutaneous radial forearm transplant in combination with a maxillary prosthesis can be used. Orbital prostheses usually are not accommodated in the primary reconstruction. A closed orbit is considered easier to manage and cosmetically superior by most but not all patients (9). Another alternative to reconstruction of these large defects is to obliterate the space with a large-volume soft tissue transplant such as an anterolateral thigh or a rectus. The approach does not restore the craniofacial skeleton or the dental arch, but it does prevent a sunken midface, provides oral nasal separation, and is much easier and reliable than the approaches with the osseous transplants (53).

The composite maxillectomy defect is relatively straightforward to reconstruct if a large soft tissue transplant is used to obliterate the resected volume. Multiple paddles are used to resurface the palate and the facial skin. If the craniofacial skeleton, the dental arch, and the soft tissue are anatomically restored for a patient with a composite maxillectomy defect, the reconstruction is much more difficult. Multiple paddles are used to resurface the palate and the facial skin. TDAST is the one of the most useful donor sites for the management of these complex defects if restoration of the craniofacial skeleton is desired (38). The osteocutaneous radial forearm is a distant second because of the small volume of bone stock and donor-site morbidity. The scapula donor site has adequate bone stock to recontour most maxillary defects, the soft tissue can be positioned independently from the bone, and there is ample subcutaneous tissue to recontour the cheek and fill the orbit as needed. This donor site is based on the subscapular and circumflex scapular artery is supplied by a pedicle that is much shorter than the latissimus dorsi artery pedicle that supplies the latissimus dorsi soft tissue and the tip of the scapula (TDAST). As a result, the TDAST is replacing the traditional subscapular/circumflex scapular donor site for the reconstruction of these defects.

Defects of the Base of the Skull

Microvascular reconstruction has been a key factor in facilitating skull base surgery. The rectus donor site has been used because of its bulk, long vascular pedicle (if the rectus muscle is included as part of the pedicle length), ability to make multiple skin islands by means of deepithelialization, and ease of patient positioning and ability to perform primary closure at the donor site. The disadvantage of use of a rectus flap is poor color match and a tendency toward ptosis. These cosmetic limitations of the myocutaneous rectus transplant decreased its use. As a result, the anterolateral thigh donor site has been used as an alternative if it can supply adequate volume to obliterate the defect. For thin patients, the rectus donor site may be the only site with adequate soft tissue. Obtaining adequate soft tissue is a common problem in breast surgery as well, and a perforator-based harvest technique borrowed from breast reconstruction that spares the rectus and reduces the problems with ptosis is useful for skull base reconstruction. It is likely that there will be increasing use of perforator-based rectus transplants for skull base reconstruction due to a long pedicle (15 to 18 cm), ample soft tissue, multiple paddles, and limited donor-site mobility. As for other craniofacial defects, the bone can be reconstructed; the functional and esthetic results are judged to be better, but these approaches are much more difficult. Calvarial defects can be reconstructed with split calvarial bone or hydroxyapatite compounds. Any area of bony projection should be reconstructed with vascularized bone if the patient has undergone or plans to undergo radiation therapy.

The principles of skull base reconstruction are to support the dural closure (separation of the cranial cavity from the upper aerodigestive tract), provide carotid coverage, obliterate dead space, support nonvascularized bone reconstruction, and restore calvarial and facial contour. The defects can be anterior or lateral defects. Anterior skull base defects that include the orbit and maxilla are best reconstructed with a large-volume flap such as a TDAST or a soft tissue flap (anterolateral thigh or rectus) if cosmesis and function are of secondary importance. Anterior defects limited to the fovea ethmoidalis or the orbitofovial defects with an intact maxilla that cannot be reconstructed with local flaps can be reconstructed with a thin, partially deepithelialized soft tissue transplant (radial forearm or anterolateral thigh). Lateral skull base defects are best reconstructed with a thick anterolateral thigh, lateral arm, or a muscle-sparing latissimus transplant. These flaps have better color match than the musculocutaneous rectus donor site and have a reduced tendency to become ptotic. The ideal donor site for color match and reduction of ptosis is the lateral arm donor site; this is also a good source of donor nerve. The challenge with the lateral arm donor site is the small short pedicle. The same principles apply to skull base reconstruction with respect to prosthetic management. It is important to have the patient see the prosthetist prior to the surgical treatment to obtain the best functional and aesthetic results.

External Soft Tissue Defects

Autogenous tissue transplantation is useful in the management of massive cutaneous defects of the scalp or skin that cannot be reconstructed with local tissue or when reconstruction with a regional pedicled rotational flap gives suboptimal cosmetic results. The optimal flap for reconstruction is based on the site of the defect. For defects of the face and neck, the anterolateral thigh, scapular and lateral arm, and muscle-sparing latissimus donor sites are used because they have an adequate amount of subcutaneous tissue to allow contouring; the contour is stable and does not become ptotic. For scalp defects, the latissimus dorsi muscle with a split-thickness skin graft is used because it is thin, is tightly adherent to the skull, and easily allows fitting of a wig. Calvarial defects are recontoured at primary reconstruction, because it is difficult to close the latissimus dorsi muscle after secondary reconstruction of the calvarium. For forehead defects, a radial forearm flap is used most often, although the color match is poor. The principles of reconstruction of large soft tissue defects are to provide coverage of critical structures (large vessels, dura, or cranial nerves), restore the skeletal contour with split calvarial bone or hydroxyapatite paste, restore soft tissue contour, allow fitting of a wig as needed, and obtain optimal color match.

- The disadvantages of free tissue transfer are complexity, need for special instrumentation and training, increased operating time, and involvement of two surgical teams.
- Radial forearm free tissue transfer has become the workhorse of head and neck reconstruction because the flap is reliable, thin, pliable, and sensate and can be contoured to the defect.
- Musculocutaneous free tissue transfers are more bulky than fasciocutaneous flaps. The flaps are used for management of larger soft tissue defects such as those caused by total glossectomy or of large skull base defects.
- Selection of the osteocutaneous flap to be used for reconstruction depends on many factors, including vascular anatomic features, vessel quality, available bone, versatility of the soft tissue, donor-site morbidity, and feasibility of simultaneous two-team surgery.
- There is no ideal osteocutaneous flap for the management of combined bone and large-volume soft tissue defects.
- Pharyngoesophageal reconstruction requires careful preoperative assessment of extent of the tumor, consideration of method of voice rehabilitation, and the planning of radiation therapy before the reconstruction and surgical team can be chosen.
- When evaluating a patient for midfacial or skull base free tissue transfer, it is important to consider the integration of prosthetics to obtain the optimal functional and aesthetic results.

HIGHLIGHTS

- Revascularized free tissue transfer is a reliable and cost-effective approach to head and neck reconstruction.
- The evolution of microvascular free tissue transfer has advanced head and neck reconstruction. The technique enables the surgeon to perform exacting and sophisticated reconstruction and primary resection in a single stage.
- Free tissue transfer is most useful for management of sophisticated oromandibular reconstruction, total pharyngeal defects, complex midfacial defects, skull base defects, and large external soft tissue defects of the head and neck.
- The advantages of free tissue transfer are reliability, vascularity, abundant supply of high-quality tissue, potential for sensory and motor reinnervation, and inset into a heavily irradiated bed if necessary.

REFERENCES

1. Brown JS, et al. Factors that influence the outcome of salvage in free tissue transfer. *Br J Oral Maxillofac Surg* 2003;41(1):16–20.
2. Nakatsuka T, et al. Analytic review of 2372 free flap transfers for head and neck reconstruction following cancer resection. *J Reconstr Microsurg* 2003;19(6):363–368; discussion 369.
3. Chepeha DB, et al. Pectoralis major myocutaneous flap vs revascularized free tissue transfer: complications, gastrostomy tube dependence, and hospitalization. *Arch Otolaryngol Head Neck Surg* 2004;130(2):181–186.
4. Funk GF, et al. Free tissue transfer versus pedicled flap cost in head and neck cancer. *Otolaryngol Head Neck Surg* 2002;127(3):205–212.
5. de Bree R, et al. Free radial forearm flap versus pectoralis major myocutaneous flap reconstruction of oral and oropharyngeal defects: a cost analysis. *Clin Otolaryngol* 2007;32(4):275–282.
6. Agarwal JP, et al. Refining the intrinsic chimera flap: a review. *Ann Plast Surg* 2009;63(4):462–467.
7. Chepeha DB, et al. Radial forearm free tissue transfer reduces complications in salvage skull base surgery. *Otolaryngol Head Neck Surg* 2004;131(6):958–963.
8. Militsakh ON, et al. Comparison of radial forearm with fibula and scapula osteocutaneous free flaps for oromandibular reconstruction. *Arch Otolaryngol Head Neck Surg* 2005;131(7):571–575.
9. Chepeha DB, et al. Restoration of the orbital aesthetic subunit in complex midface defects. *Laryngoscope* 2004;114(10):1706–1713.

10. Urken ML. Radial forearm. In: Urken ML, et al, eds. *Atlas of regional and free flaps for head and neck reconstruction.* New York: Raven Press, 1995:155.

11. Funk GF, et al. Anomalies of forearm vascular anatomy encountered during elevation of the radial forearm flap. *Head Neck* 1995;17(4):284–292.

12. Richardson D, et al. Radial forearm flap donor-site complications and morbidity: a prospective study [see comment]. *Plast Reconstr Surg* 1997;99(1):109–115.

13. Edmonds JL, et al. Torsional strength of the radius after osteofasciocutaneous free flap harvest with and without primary bone plating. *Otolaryngol Head Neck Surg* 2000;123(4):400–408.

14. Sullivan MJ, Carroll WR, Kuriloff DB. Lateral arm free flap in head and neck reconstruction. *Arch Otolaryngol Head Neck Surg* 1992;118(10):1095–1101.

15. Teknos TN, et al. Reconstruction of complex parotidectomy defects using the lateral arm free tissue transfer. *Otolaryngol Head Neck Surg* 2003;129(3):183–191.

16. Civantos FJ Jr, et al. Lateral arm microvascular flap in head and neck reconstruction. *Arch Otolaryngol Head Neck Surg* 1997;123(8):830–836.

17. Rivet D, et al. The lateral arm flap: an anatomic study. *J Reconstr Microsurg* 1987;3(2):121–132.

18. Hayden RE, Deschler DG. Lateral thigh free flap for head and neck reconstruction. *Laryngoscope* 1999;109(9):1490–1494.

19. Wei FC, et al. Have we found an ideal soft-tissue flap? An experience with 672 anterolateral thigh flaps [see comment]. *Plast Reconstr Surg* 2002;109(7):2219–2226; discussion 2227–2230.

20. Lueg EA. The anterolateral thigh flap: radial forearm's "big brother" for extensive soft tissue head and neck defects. *Arch Otolaryngol Head Neck Surg* 2004;130(7):813–818.

21. Wong CH, Wei FC. Anterolateral thigh flap. *Head Neck* 2010;32(4):529–540.

22. Shieh SJ, et al. Free anterolateral thigh flap for reconstruction of head and neck defects following cancer ablation. *Plast Reconstr Surg* 2000;105(7):2349–2357; discussion 2358–2360.

23. Hanasono MM, Skoracki RJ, Yu P. A prospective study of donor-site morbidity after anterolateral thigh fasciocutaneous and myocutaneous free flap harvest in 220 patients. *Plast Reconstr Surg* 2010;125(1):209–214.

24. Cheney ML, Varvares MA, Nadol JB Jr. The temporoparietal fascial flap in head and neck reconstruction. *Arch Otolaryngol Head Neck Surg* 1993;119(6):618–623.

25. Taylor GI, Palmer JH. The vascular territories (angiosomes) of the body: experimental study and clinical applications. *Br J Plast Surg* 1987;40(2):113–141.

26. Rozen WM, Ashton MW, Taylor GI. Reviewing the vascular supply of the anterior abdominal wall: redefining anatomy for increasingly refined surgery. *Clin Anat* 2008;21(2):89–98.

27. Strauch B, Yu H. *Atlas of Microvascular Surgery: anatomy and operative approaches.* New York: Thieme Medical Publishers, 1993:560.

28. Harii K, Ohmori K, Torii S. Free gracilis muscle transplantation, with microneurovascular anastomoses for the treatment of facial paralysis. A preliminary report. *Plast Reconstr Surg* 1976;57(2):133–143.

29. Yousif NJ, et al. The transverse gracilis musculocutaneous flap [see comment]. *Ann Plast Surg* 1992;29(6):482–490.

30. Taylor GI, Miller GD, Ham FJ. The free vascularized bone graft. A clinical extension of microvascular techniques. *Plast Reconstr Surg* 1975;55(5):533–544.

31. Hidalgo DA. Fibula free flap: a new method of mandible reconstruction. *Plast Reconstr Surg* 1989;84(1):71–79.

32. Futran ND, et al. Midface reconstruction with the fibula free flap. *Arch Otolaryngol Head Neck Surg* 2002;128(2):161–166.

33. Kelly AM, et al. Preoperative MR angiography in free fibula flap transfer for head and neck cancer: clinical application and influence on surgical decision making. *AJR Am J Roentgenol* 2007;188(1):268–274.

34. Miller ME, et al. Preoperative magnetic resonance angiography detection of septocutaneous perforators in fibula free flap transfer. *Arch Facial Plast Surg* 2011;13(1):36–40.

35. Urken ML, et al. The internal oblique-iliac crest osseomyocutaneous free flap in oromandibular reconstruction. Report of 20 cases. *Arch Otolaryngol Head Neck Surg* 1989;115(3):339–349.

36. Sullivan MJ, et al. Free scapular osteocutaneous flap for mandibular reconstruction. *Arch Otolaryngol Head Neck Surg* 1989;115(11):1334–1340.

37. Wagner AJ, Bayles SW. The angular branch: maximizing the scapular pedicle in head and neck reconstruction. *Arch Otolaryngol Head Neck Surg* 2008;134(11):1214–1217.

38. Chepeha DB et al. Thoracodorsal artery scapular tip autogenous transplant: vascularized bone with a long pedicle and flexible soft tissue. *Arch Otolaryngol Head Neck Surg* 2010;136(10):958–964.

39. Robb GL, et al. Speech and swallowing outcomes in reconstructions of the pharynx and cervical esophagus. *Head Neck* 2003;25(3):232–244.

40. Bradford CR, Esclamado RM, Carroll WR. Monitoring of revascularized jejunal autografts. *Arch Otolaryngol Head Neck Surg* 1992;118(10):1042–1044.

41. Bayles SW, Hayden RE. Gastro-omental free flap reconstruction of the head and neck. *Arch Facial Plast Surg* 2008;10(4):255–259.

42. Patel RS, Gilbert RW. Utility of the gastro-omental free flap in head and neck reconstruction. *Curr Opin Otolaryngol Head Neck Surg* 2009;17(4):258–262.

43. Patel RS, et al. Morbidity and functional outcomes following gastro-omental free flap reconstruction of circumferential pharyngeal defects. *Head Neck* 2009;31(5):655–663.

44. Urken ML, et al. Oromandibular reconstruction using microvascular composite free flaps. Report of 71 cases and a new classification scheme for bony, soft-tissue, and neurologic defects. *Arch Otolaryngol Head Neck Surg* 1991;117(7):733–744.

45. Clark JR, et al. Morbidity after flap reconstruction of hypopharyngeal defects. *Laryngoscope* 2006;116(2):173–181.

46. Yu P, et al. Comparison of clinical and functional outcomes and hospital costs following pharyngoesophageal reconstruction with the anterolateral thigh free flap versus the jejunal flap. *Plast Reconstr Surg* 2006;117(3):968–974.

47. Varvares MA, et al. Use of the radial forearm fasciocutaneous free flap and montgomery salivary bypass tube for pharyngoesophageal reconstruction. *Head Neck* 2000;22(5):463–468.

48. Teknos TN, et al. Free tissue reconstruction of the hypopharynx after organ preservation therapy: analysis of wound complications. *Laryngoscope* 2001;111(7):1192–1196.

49. Urken ML, et al. A systematic approach to functional reconstruction of the oral cavity following partial and total glossectomy. *Arch Otolaryngol Head Neck Surg* 1994;120(6):589–601.

50. Brown JS, et al. A modified classification for the maxillectomy defect. *Head Neck* 2000;22(1):17–26.

51. Okay DJ, et al. Prosthodontic guidelines for surgical reconstruction of the maxilla: a classification system of defects. *J Prosthet Dent* 2001;86(4):352–363.

52. Chepeha DB, et al. Osseocutaneous radial forearm free tissue transfer for repair of complex midfacial defects. *Arch Otolaryngol Head Neck Surg* 2005;131(6):513–517.

53. Santamaria E, Cordeiro PG. Reconstruction of maxillectomy and midfacial defects with free tissue transfer. *J Surg Oncol* 2006;94(6):522–531.

Tissue Expanders

175

Jonathan Liang   *Jonathan M. Sykes*

The reconstructive ladder is a philosophical model used in facial plastic surgery to address cutaneous and soft tissue defects. The reconstructive ladder represents a graduated approach (Fig. 175.1), with closure via secondary intention as the most basic technique and closure with a microvascular free flap as the most complex technique. Tissue expansion falls in the upper middle tier of the reconstructive ladder. It is used when there is not enough adjacent tissue to close a defect primarily or with a local flap.

Tissue expansion is a technique used by plastic and reconstructive surgeons to cause the body to grow additional skin, bone, or other tissues. Tissue expansion also occurs naturally in the human body. It can occur as a normal physiologic process—the most classic example is pregnancy, during which uterine and abdominal tissue undergo remarkable expansion and enlargement. Also, it can occur as a pathophysiologic process, such as with large tumors that lead to concurrent expansion of the overlying skin and soft tissue. Examples of tissue expansion can be seen in many cultures. Certain populations have employed forms of tissue expansion to decorate, enhance, or mutilate facial or body structures. The Mursi tribe of Ethiopia incorporates giant decorative plates in the lower lip (Fig. 175.2). The Kayan woman of Myanmar, formerly Burma wears a series of rings around the neck to enhance linear growth (Fig. 175.3). Tissue expansion is also seen in more mainstream culture with the popularity of body art and piercings. Similar to the use of large wooden spools used in the Waorani tribe of Ecuador, the youth counterculture has adopted ear gauges to widen the ear lobe as an expression of body art.

In 1905, Codvilla reported the first use of tissue expansion for medical purposes to lengthen a femur (1). In 1957, Neumann provided the first report of expanding the skin using an inflatable balloon, used in the setting to reconstruct

a helical defect (2). Tissue expansion is best known for its use in breast reconstruction. Radovan popularized tissue expansion for postmastectomy breast reconstruction (3). In the 1980s, studies investigating the histologic effects of tissue expansion elucidated the biology and physiology behind this emerging reconstructive technique (4,5). Argenta reported the first description of tissue expansion in the pediatric population in 1981 (6). Tissue expansion became a widely accepted technique in the 1980s and has continued to be a useful technique in the armamentarium of the reconstructive surgeon.

The advantages and disadvantages of tissue expansion are outlined below (Table 175.1). The ability to bring skin with near-perfect match in color and texture is a significant benefit when compared with skin grafts and pedicled or free flaps, which often transfer tissue that is not similar in texture, thickness, or color. There is also minimal or no donor site morbidity because no secondary defect occurs. Tissue expanders are also able to incorporate tissue with specialized function or adnexal characteristics. For example, tissue expansion in the setting of breast expansion is able to preserve superior sensation in the skin flaps. In the setting of tissue expansion in the scalp for treatment of alopecia, tissue expansion can incorporate hair-bearing flaps. One major disadvantage of tissue expansion is that it does involve multiple surgeries and/or office visits. There is a noticeable visible deformity during the expansion period, which can lead to physical and emotional burdens for the patient.

SKIN BIOMECHANICS AND TYPES OF EXPANSION

Human tissues exhibit dynamic effects when exposed to sustained pressure and expansion. A key understanding of the physical properties of the skin is needed to understand the changes in skin biomechanics during tissue expansion. *Tension* is a function of the elastic fiber network and varies with location and age. *Extensibility* is the response of skin

Both authors have no conflict of interest and adhere to ethical guidelines.

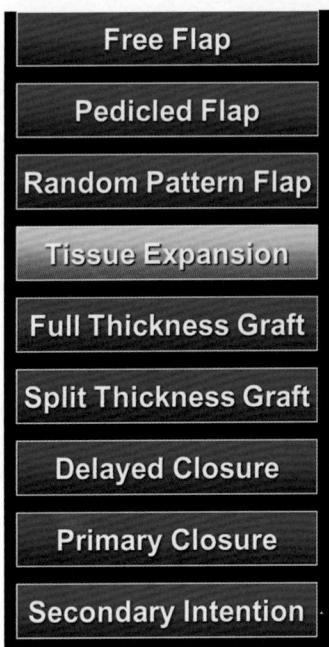

Figure 175.1 Reconstructive ladder.

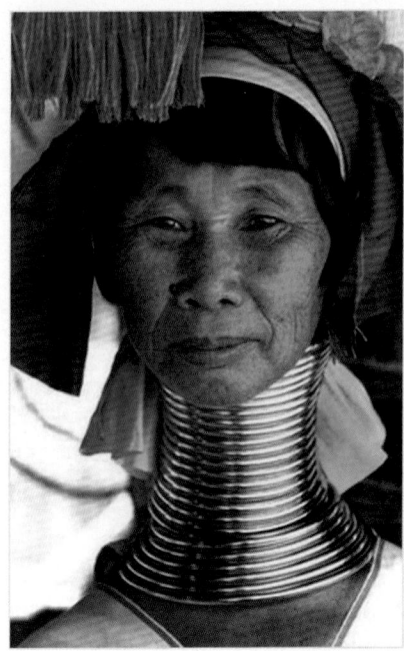

Figure 175.3 Kayan woman of Myanmar, formerly Burma with concentric rings around the neck to enhance linear growth.

to mechanical forces. *Viscoelasticity* is the function of creep and stress relaxation. *Creep* is defined as a gain in skin surface area that results when a constant load is applied. In other words, it is the tendency of a solid material to slowly move or deform permanently under the influence of stresses. *Stress relaxation* is defined as a decrease in the amount of force necessary to maintain a fixed amount of skin stretch over time (7,8).

The concept of creep is essential to understanding tissue expansion. There are different types of creep: biologic and mechanical (Table 175.2). Biologic creep involves permanent changes in the microanatomy of tissue. There is an overall increase in mitotic activity, with resultant net increase in surface area. In contrast, mechanical creep does not exhibit any change in tissue microanatomy. In mechanical creep, there is displacement of fluids and mucopolysaccharide ground substances, microfragmentation of elastic fibers, and alignment of randomly positioned collagen fibers into a more parallel position. There is no overall increase in mitotic activity and thus no net increase in surface area.

Biologic and mechanical creeps correspond to conventional long-term expansion and rapid intraoperative expansion, respectively (Table 175.3). In conventional long-term expansion, biologic creep is the underlying mechanism. It takes weeks to months to achieve and relies on physiologic and histologic changes in the tissue (9,10). Rapid

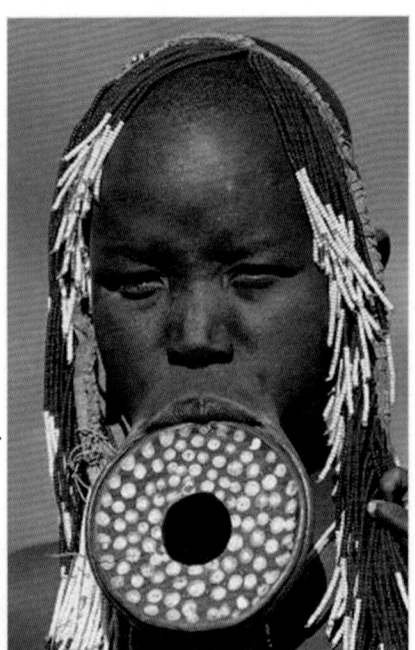

Figure 175.2 Mursi tribe woman of Ethiopia with a giant decorative plate in the lower lip.

TABLE 175.1	ADVANTAGES AND DISADVANTAGES OF TISSUE EXPANSION	
Advantages	**Disadvantages**	
Skin with near-perfect match in color and texture	Involves multiple surgeries and/or multiple office visits	
No or minimal donor site morbidity	Visible deformity	
Tissue with specialized function or adnexal characteristics	Physical and emotional burden for patient	

TABLE 175.2	TYPES OF CREEP	
Biologic Creep	**Mechanical Creep**	
Permanent changes in microanatomy	No change in microanatomy	
Increase in mitotic activity	Displaces fluid and extracellular substances; collagen fibers realign	
Net increase in surface area	No net increase in surface area	

intraoperative expansion is a more controversial method of achieving tissue expansion. The underlying mechanism that occurs during rapid intraoperative tissue expansion is mechanical creep. There is rapid cyclical stretching of the tissue, which is performed often in a single setting, and results in only mechanical changes in the tissue (10,11).

PHYSIOLOGY

Maintaining living tissues under tension causes new cells to form and the amount of tissue to increase. An understanding of the skin microanatomy will help elucidate the changes that occur with biologic creep (Fig. 175.3).

The skin is composed of epidermis, dermis, and subcutaneous tissue (hypodermis). The epidermis is the uppermost layer and contains five sublayers (in order from superficial to deep): stratum corneum, stratum lucidum, stratum granulosum, stratum spinosum, and stratum basale. The main cells found in the epidermal layer are Merkel cells, keratinocytes, melanocytes, and Langerhans cells. There are no blood vessels in the epidermis. The dermis is the middle layer and consists of a superficial papillary region and a deep reticular region. The papillary region contains loose areolar connective tissue, and the reticular region contains dense concentrations of collagen, elastic, and reticular fibers. The dermis contains many hair follicles, sweat glands, sebaceous glands, apocrine glands, lymphatics, and blood vessels. The subcutaneous tissue is

TABLE 175.3	TYPES OF EXPANSION	
Conventional Long-Term Expansion	**Rapid Intraoperative Expansion**	
Takes weeks to months to achieve	Rapid cyclical stretching performed in one setting	
Physiologic and histologic changes occur	Mechanical changes only	
Relies on *biologic creep*	Relies on *mechanical creep*	
Well accepted	Controversial	

the deepest layer of the skin and connects the dermis with the underlying bone or muscle—it supplies the underlying tissue with blood vessels and nerves. The main cell types in this layer are fibroblasts, adipocytes, and macrophages.

With conventional long-term tissue expansion, biologic creep occurs at all levels of the skin. In the epidermis, there is an increase in mitotic activity. The thickness either stays the same or is slightly increased, and the stratified structure is preserved (10,12,13). The changes are temporary, and the microscopic appearance of the skin returns to normal within a year or two after the conclusion of expansion. In the dermis, there is significant thinning of approximately 30% to 50% (10,14,15). Of note, however, the basal layer actually thickens. There is increased metabolic activity in the fibroblasts and melanocytes with enhanced collagen synthesis and melanin production, respectively. The number of hair follicles and the pattern of hair growth remain the same, but the density of hair follicles decreases. Individual follicles may be separated by a factor of two without producing noticeable hair thinning. Given normal hair density, the scalp can be expanded by two to three times its original surface area before a change in hair amount is evident. In the subcutaneous tissue, adipose tissue thins approximately 50% with loss of adipocytes (14,15). There is also some muscle thinning and atrophy (15). Vascular proliferation occurs with the growth of capillaries, venules, and arterioles (16). Nerves lengthen with conventional tissue expansion, but their function is impaired (17). A dense fibrous capsule forms around the expander and contributes to the vascularity. The capsule also contributes to contracture and shrinkage of the flap after the expander is removed (18). The expander capsule thickness does not correlate with expander volume, location, or patient age (10).

APPLICATIONS

Tissue expansion has been used in breast reconstruction, closure of abdominal wounds, decubitus ulcers, extremity defects, burn scars, and even the separation of conjoined twins. In the head and neck, common applications include use in posttraumatic or postoperative alopecia, male pattern baldness, expansion prior to major reconstruction, congenital microtia, and large or giant melanocytic nevi (19–21).

Tissue expanders have been used in the scalp, forehead, ear, nose, cheek, and neck. Table 175.4 provides general expectations for flap advancement for a given expanded flap and various areas of the head and neck (20). The measurement of expanded flap width is measured across the base of the expander. Tissue expansion works best in locations where there is solid bony support under the expander balloon device, such as the scalp and forehead. The scalp is the ideal place for tissue expansion (22,23). The tissue is thick and vascular. The solid calvarium provides an ideal base for the expander. Approximately 50% of the scalp can be reconstructed with the use of tissue expansion (24).

TABLE 175.4	EXPECTATIONS FOR FLAP ADVANCEMENT FOR AN EXPANDED FLAP IN AREAS OF THE HEAD AND NECK	
Site	Expanded Flap Width (cm)	Expected Flap Advancement (cm)
Scalp	12–16	Up to 8
Forehead	8–14	Up to 7
Midface	10–14	Up to 7
Ear	4–8	Up to 4
Neck	12–16	Up to 8

From Hoffmann JF. Tissue Expansion in the Head and Neck. *Facial Plast Surg Clin North Am* 2005;13: 315–324.

Use of tissue expanders for auricular defects is limited by the lack of adequate non–hair-bearing soft tissue in the adjacent area. Nasal reconstruction often requires an expanded midline forehead flap. The potential for contracture of an expanded flap and thickening of the tissue from the capsule may limit the application in reconstructing subunits of the nose where a thin and pliable soft tissue coverage is essential to allow the cartilaginous framework to show through. However, some surgeons do use tissue expanders in the forehead prior to elevating and transposing a forehead flap. In the cheek and neck, the skin is relatively thin and there is potential for damage to the facial nerve and underlying musculature with tissue expansion. Smaller volume expanders and longer-term expansion can be used to minimize complications. The gravitational forces in these areas can lead to the migration of expanders, and thus, the base often needs to be secured to the underlying structures.

EXPANDER DEVICES

Current tissue expanders are Silastic balloons (Fig. 175.4). Tissue expanders are defined by shape, size, and injection port.

Expanders can be rectangular-, circular-, or crescent-shaped. Custom sizes and shapes can be made for specific uses. For large scalp rotation flaps, crescent or circular expanders are ideal. For straight advancement flap, rectangular expanders are ideal. Rectangular-shaped expanders are able to achieve a gain of 38% in tissue surface area. Round or circular-shaped expanders are able to achieve a gain of 25% in tissue surface area. Crescent-shaped expanders are able to achieve a gain of 32% in tissue surface area (25).

Tissue expanders vary in size from 1 to 1,000 mL, with head and neck tissue expanders usually varying from 1 to 250 mL. The injection port can be remote, integrated, or external. For tissue expanders with an integrated injection port, a small butterfly needle (23 or 25 gauge) is commonly used for injecting the expander during the expansion phase. Most injection ports have a raised palpable ring. Some integrated expanders have a separate magnet

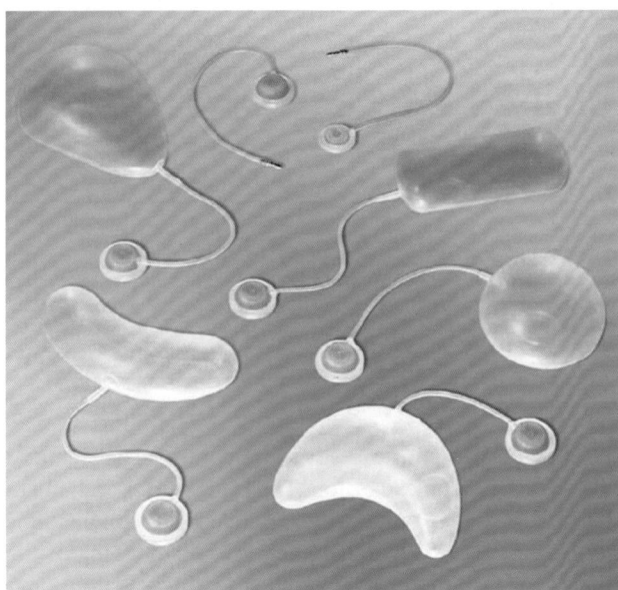

Figure 175.4 Tissue expanders. Expanders come in various shapes and sizes. These expanders have external ports, but tissue expanders with integrated ports also exist.

that helps to localize the injection port. As the volume of the implant increases, tension is distributed to the surrounding tissues, which results in their expansion over time. The advantage of internal versus external ports has been debated (26–28). The arguments for external ports are that they require less dissection, have painless port access, and allow for earlier detection of leaks.

Tissue expanders can also be classified by two-dimensional or three-dimensional expansion. Two-dimensional linear skin stretchers consist of a Dacron strip with hooks on both ends that are prestretched and placed under the previously elevated skin flaps—as the Dacron strip returns to its native size, it stretches the skin. Two-dimensional expansion creates forces by pulling the perimeter away from the central portion of skin being stretched (10). In contrast, three-dimensional expansion creates forces by pushing and compressing the skin away from a fixed perimeter (10). Three-dimensional expansion is the mainstay type of tissue expander.

SURGICAL TECHNIQUES: CONVENTIONAL LONG-TERM TISSUE EXPANSION

Strategies for use of tissue expanders vary from surgeon to surgeon. The stages of the tissue expansion process include selecting the ideal expander, inserting the expander, expanding the expander, and removing the expander with simultaneous reconstruction.

In selecting the most ideal expander for the patient, it is important to consider the size of the defect, location of the defect, and the goals of the patient. This is an important step in the preoperative assessment and preparation. General principles include using the largest possible expander, and often more than one expander may be needed for large defects. A single large expander is preferred over multiple smaller expanders because this will give the greatest gain in tissue per volume of expansion and limit the number of operative sites. The surface area of the expander base should be 2.5 to 3 times as large as the defect size (20).

The actual surgery begins with placement of the expander. The incision for the placement should be as far from the expander as possible to prevent dehiscence during expansion and exposure of the device. A small V- or U-shaped incision placed radially (perpendicularly) related to the direction of expansion is ideal (29). In the scalp, the tissue expander should be placed between the galea aponeurosis and the pericranium. In the forehead, the tissue expander should be placed deep to the frontalis muscle. In the face, the tissue expander should be placed superficial to the superficial muscular aponeurotic system. In the neck, the tissue expander should be placed superficial to the platysma muscle (30). Nevertheless, wide undermining of the pocket for the expander is important in any of these locations. The expander pocket should be dissected wider than the base of the expander in a blunt fashion to preserve the longitudinal bloody supply (4). Furthermore, the expander pocket must be large enough to allow the expander to lie completely flat without any folding, buckling, or distortion.

The expansion phase is often the most burdensome for the patient—both physically and emotionally. The interval and volume of expansion may vary by region and wound type. Typically, 2 weeks are allowed for the wounds to heal after expander placement before the expansion phase begins. Serial inflation of the expander occurs over 4 to 6 weeks. Expansion should be continued until the extended flap is approximately 20% larger than the size of the defect to account for tissue recoil during advancement. Inspection of the skin color (blanching), capillary refill, and direct palpation are routine when evaluating for further expansion. When the patient experiences any significant pain during expansion, the injection should be stopped and saline should be removed. Overinflation of the tissue expander beyond the manufacturer's recommended fill capacity is common in clinical practice (31), and one study has shown overinflation associated with lower complication rates (32).

The final step in the process involves removal of the tissue expander device and simultaneous reconstruction with the expanded flap.

Case 1

A 2-year-old girl with a hairy nevus of the anterior scalp. The lesion was present at birth and has grown proportional to the patient's growth. Examination showed a 5 × 6-cm well-circumscribed mass at the frontal hairline that is hyperpigmented (Fig. 175.5). The patient underwent conventional long-term tissue expansion. During the insertion phase, the selected tissue expander was placed in an area just

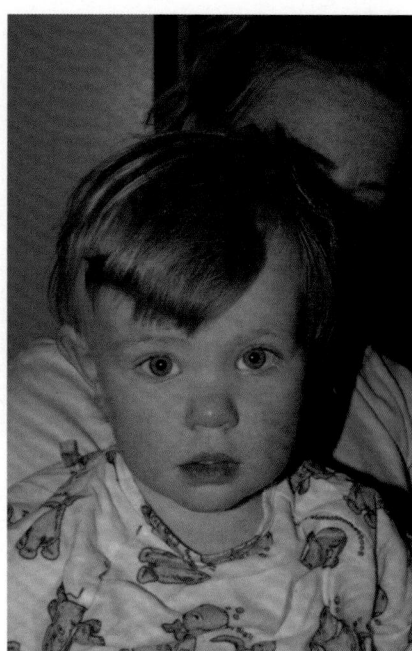

Figure 175.5 Pediatric patient with hairy nevus of anterior scalp.

posterior to the lesion between the galeal and pericranial layers of the scalp (Fig. 175.6). During the expansion phase, the patient underwent a series of five expansions over the course of 6 weeks to a final volume of 110 mL (Fig. 175.7). During the removal and reconstruction phase, the tissue expander was removed and the expanded skin was advanced to the edge of the defect site (Fig. 175.8).

Case 2

A 38-year-old woman with a neck scar from a burn injury as a child who had undergone previous revision and laser treatment with persistent scar deformity. Examination showed a horizontally oriented 10 × 3-cm hyperpigmented scar with mild wound contraction around the edges (Fig. 175.9). The patient underwent conventional long-term tissue expansion. During the insertion phase, a circular tissue expander was placed in the neck superior to the scar site in the plane above the platysma muscle. During the expansion phase, the patient underwent a series of expansions over the course of 8 weeks to a final volume of 80 mL (Fig. 175.10). During the removal and reconstruction phase, the tissue expander was removed and the expanded skin was advanced inferior over the defect site (Fig. 175.11).

SURGICAL TECHNIQUES: RAPID INTRAOPERATIVE TISSUE EXPANSION

The protocols and principles discussed above apply to conventional long term tissue expansion. The protocol for rapid intraoperative tissue expansion significantly differs. This method has been championed by Sasaki (33,34).

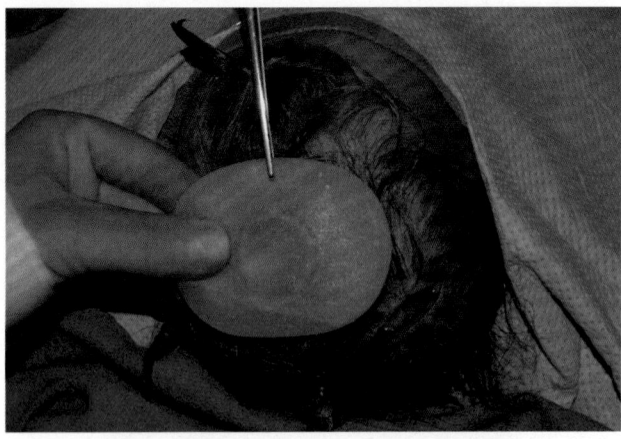 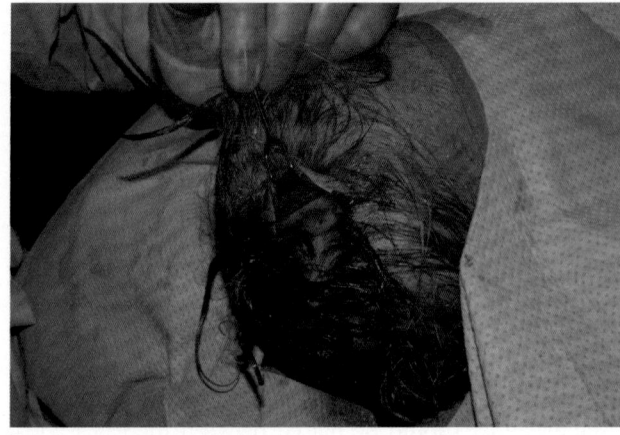

A   B

Figure 175.6 A, B: Insertion phase. An incision is made in the right posterior scalp, and a subgaleal pocket was created. A large oval-shaped tissue expander was selected to fill the planned defect site (**A**). The expander was placed in the subgaleal pocket just posterior to the lesion (**B**).

The phases are the same—selecting the ideal expander, inserting the expander, expanding the expander, and removing the expander with reconstruction. However, all this occurs in a single setting and relies on mechanical creep. There are no physiologic or metabolic changes that are seen in the setting of conventional long-term tissue expansion. A gain of 1 to 3 cm of flap length can be achieved, depending on the site of expansion. Table 175.5 provides rough estimates of the degree of lengthening one might achieve in some areas of the head and neck (34). During the expansion phase, the expander is inflated for 3 minutes and then deflated for several minutes. This process is repeated at least two more times. This is immediately followed by incision, inset, and closing of the flap. The process remains controversial. Critics of this technique have claimed that rapid intraoperative tissue expansion is simply augmented undermining and tissue rearrangement (35,36).

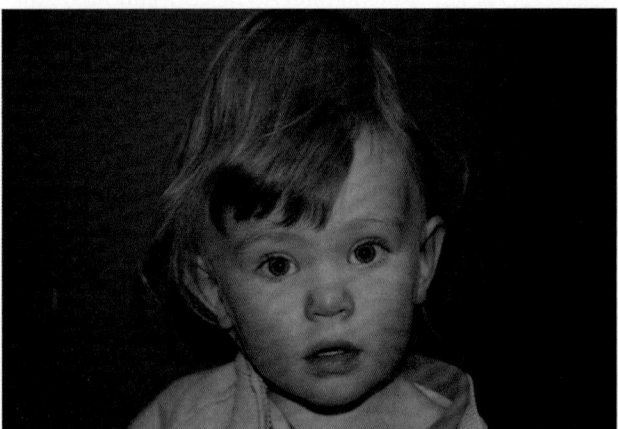

Figure 175.7 Expansion phase. The same patient during the expansion phase. The patient underwent a series of expansions for a total volume of 110 mL.

COMPLICATIONS

The reported complication rate with tissue expanders is approximately 10% (20,37,38). These complications include expander exposure or extrusion, skin necrosis or ischemia, numbness or weakness, infection, bone resorption, hematoma or seroma, and failure of the expander device. Most authors would advocate that exposed expanders can be watched, with cessation of interval expansion. However, it is often recommended that extrusion should be an indication for prompt removal. If there is evidence of skin necrosis or infection, the tissue expander should be removed, with culture and debridement of the wound. Careful antiseptic techniques should be observed to minimize infection around the devices.

CONCLUSIONS

Tissue expansion can be a useful technique in the armamentarium of a reconstructive surgeon. It can provide additional skin with similar characteristics and avoid unnecessary donor site morbidity. Tissue expanders are especially useful for reconstructing scalp and forehead defects, and its use has been described for all areas in the head and neck. The more traditional and commonplace conventional long-term tissue expansion relies on biologic creep and results in important physiologic changes at the epidermis, dermis, and subcutaneous tissue. Conventional long-term tissue expansion can be a lengthy process for both the patient and surgeon. There are many critics of rapid intraoperative expansion, but its main advantage is completing all the stages of tissue expansion in a single setting to minimize patient morbidity. There are many ongoing studies investigating new agents to help increase the rate of tissue expansion, and further research on both the mechanical and biologic properties of tissue expansion will help improve clinical outcomes of reconstruction with tissue expansion.

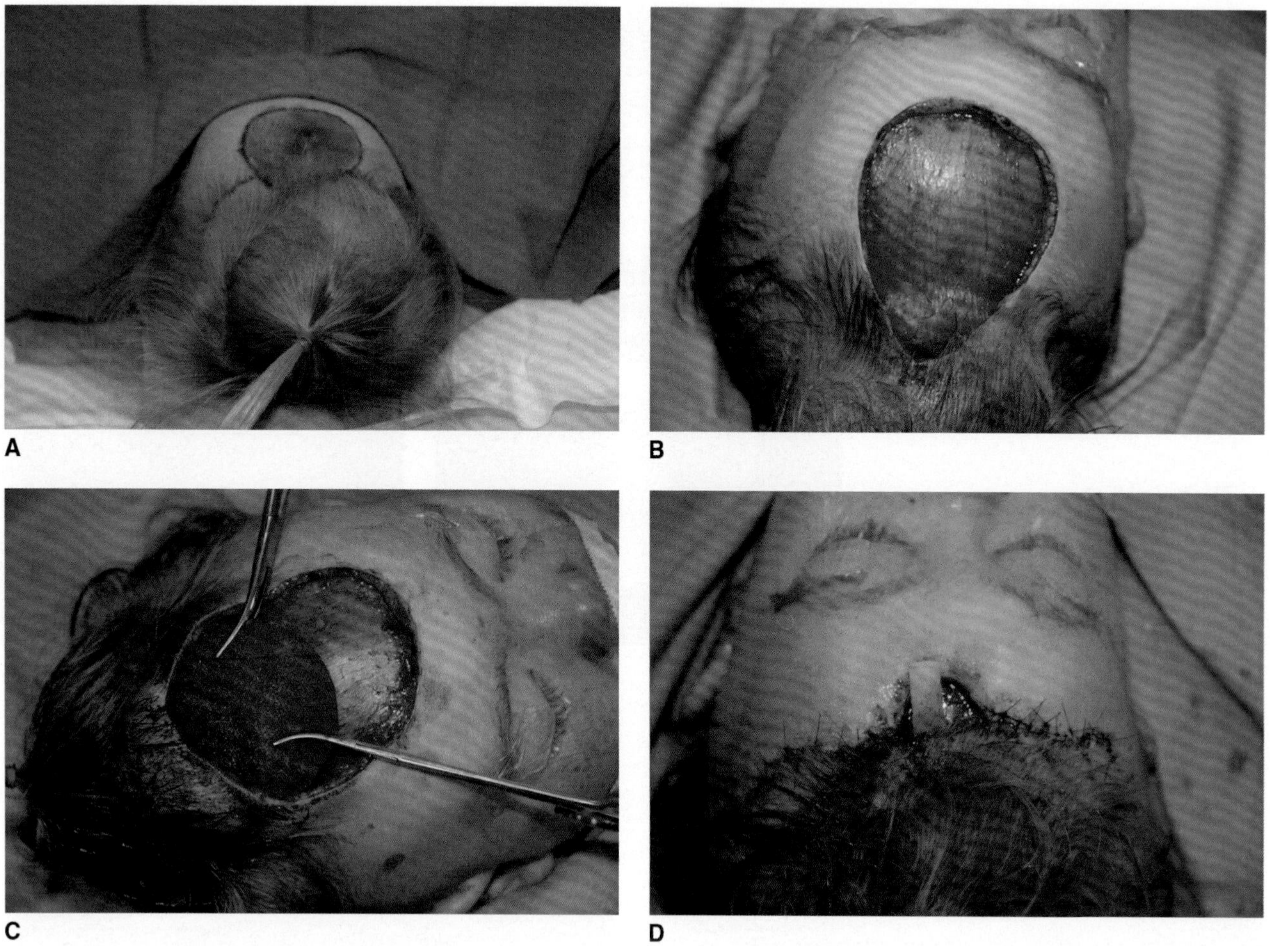

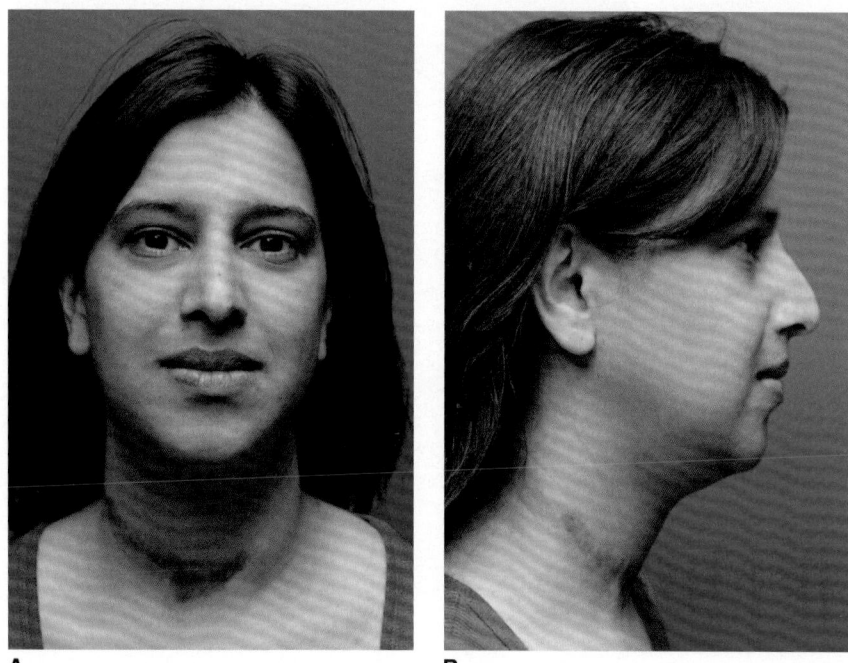

Figure 175.8 A–D: Removal and reconstructive phase. The area over the hairy nevus was shaved, and markings were made around the lesion site **(A)**. The hairy cell nevus was excised with minimal margin **(B)**. The tissue expander was dissected from the fibrous capsule, deflated, and removed **(C)**. The expanded scalp tissue was advanced to the defect size—the incision closed primarily laterally—and a small central area was left to granulate **(D)**.

Figure 175.9 A, B: Adult female patient with large neck scar on frontal view **(A)** and side view **(B)**.

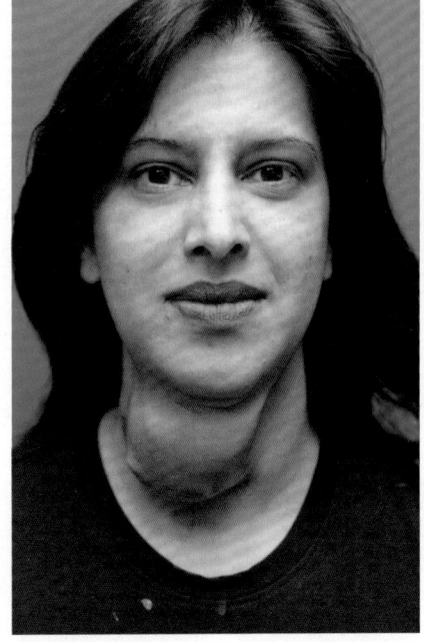
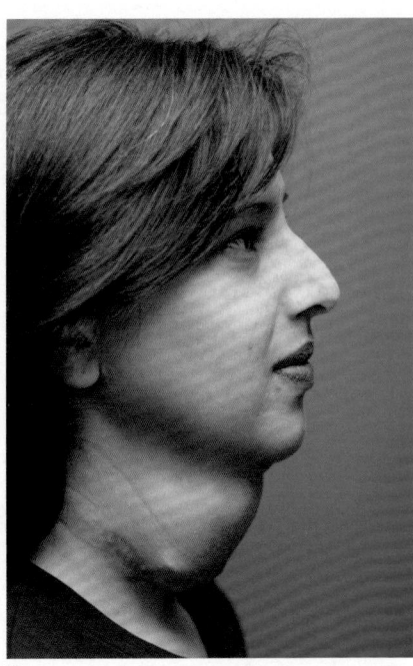

Figure 175.10 A, B: Expansion phase. The same patient during the expansion phase on frontal view **(A)** and side view **(B)**. The patient underwent a series of expansions for a total volume of 80 mL.

A

B

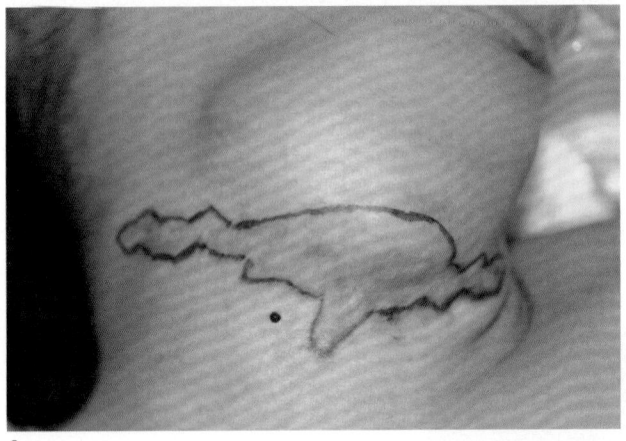
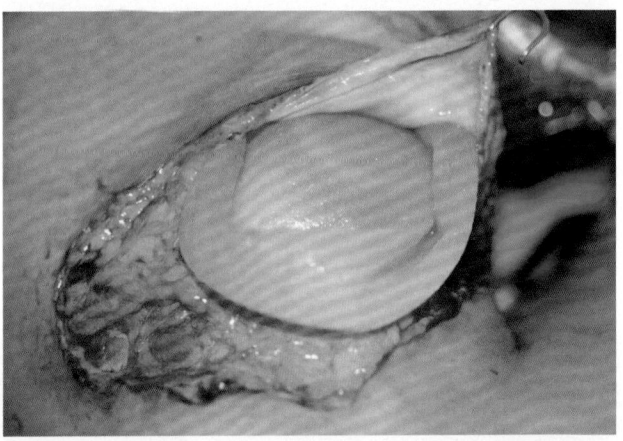

A

B

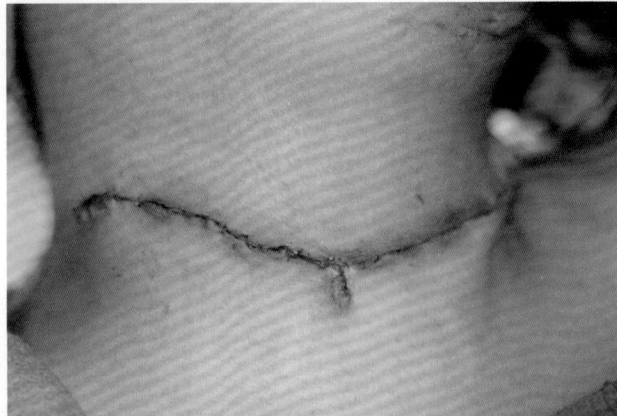

Figure 175.11 A–C: Removal and reconstructive phase. The scar was excised with irregular geometric shape pattern excision **(A)**. The tissue expander was dissected from the fibrous capsule, deflated, and removed **(B)**. The expanded neck tissue was advanced to the defect size, and the incision was closed primarily **(C)**.

C

TABLE 175.5	ESTIMATED DEGREE OF LENGTHENING IN INTRAOPERATIVE TISSUE EXPANSION

Site	Average Tissue Gain per Expander (cm)
Scalp	1.9–1.5
Forehead	1.0–2.5
Upper nose	1.0–1.5
Nasal tip	0.50–0.75
Midface	1.0–2.5
Neck	1.0–2.5

From Sasaki GH. Intraoperative sustained limited expansion as an immediate reconstructive technique. *Clin Plast Surg* 1987;14:563–573.

HIGHLIGHTS

- Tissue expansion lies in the middle rung of the reconstructive ladder. It can provide skin with similar characteristics and avoids donor site morbidity.
- Conventional long-term expansion relies on biologic creep.
- Rapid intraoperative expansion relies on mechanical creep.
- Important physiologic changes in conventional expansion include increased mitotic activity and vascular proliferation.
- Various sizes, shapes, and types of tissue expanders exist. Rectangular expanders provide the largest gain in surface area. The base of the expander should be 2.5 to 3 times the size of the defect.
- The scalp and forehead are optimal sites for reconstruction with tissue expanders.
- Stages of tissue expansion include insertion, expansion, and expander removal with simultaneous reconstruction.
- Complications occur in approximately 10% of cases, with the most common of being expander extrusion or exposure.

REFERENCES

1. Verasci A, Balkovich M. Tissue expansion: history. In: Habal M, ed. *Advances in plastic surgery*, Vol. 1. Chicago, IL: Year Book Publishers, 1984:95–102.
2. Neumann CG. The expansion of an area of skin by progressive distension of a subcutaneous balloon. *Plast Reconstr Surg* 1957;19:124–130.
3. Radovan C. Breast reconstruction after mastectomy using the temporary expander. *Plast Reconstr Surg* 1982;69:195.
4. Radovan C. Tissue expansion in soft-tissue reconstruction. *Plast Reconstr Surg* 1984;74:482.
5. Austed ED. Evolution of the concept of tissue expansion. *Facial Plast Surg* 1988;5:277–279.
6. Argenta LC, Wananabe MJ, Grabb WC. The use of tissue expansion in head and neck reconstruction. *Ann Plast Surg* 1983;11:31.
7. Gibson T, Kenedi RM. Biomechanical properties of skin. *Surg Clin North Am* 1967;47:279–294.
8. Mustoe TA, Bartell TH, Garner WL. Physical, biochemical, histologic, and biochemical effects of rapid versus conventional tissue expansion. *Plast Reconstr Surg* 1989;84(4):687–691.
9. Machida BK, Lui-Shindo M, Sasaki GH, et al. Immediate versus chronic expansion. *Ann Plast Surg* 1991;26:227–231.
10. Bascom DA, Wax MK. Tissue expansion in the head and neck: current state of the art. *Curr Opin Otolaryngol Head Neck Surg* 2002;10:273–277.
11. Suegert R, Weerda H, Hoffman S, et al. Clinical and experimental evaluation of intermittent intraoperative short-term expansion. *Plast Reconstr Surg* 1993;92:248–254.
12. Pasyk KA, Argenta LC, Hassett C. Quantitative analysis of the thickness of human skin and subcutaneous tissue following controlled expansion with a silicone implant. *Plast Reconstr Surg* 1988;81:516–523.
13. Pasyk KA, Argenta LC, Austed ED. Histopathology of human expanded tissue. *Clin Plast Surg* 1987;14:435–445.
14. Johnson TM, Lowe L, Brown MD, et al. Histology and physiology of tissue expansion. *J Dermatol Surg Oncol* 1993;19:1074–1078.
15. Sasaki GH. Reaction patterns and dysfunctional change in expanded tissue. In: *Tissue expansion in reconstructive and aesthetic surgery*. St. Louis, MO: Mosby, 1998:35–37.
16. Cherry GW, Austad E, Pasyk K, et al. Increased survival and vascularity of random pattern skin flaps elevated in controlled, expanded skin. *Plast Reconstr Surg* 1983;72:680–687.
17. Milner RH, Wilkins PR. The recovery of peripheral nerves following tissue expansion. *J Hand Surg Br* 1992;17:78–85.
18. Morris SF, Pang CY, Mohoney J, et al. Effect of capsulectomy on the hemodynamics and viability of random pattern skin flaps raised on expanded skin in the pig. *Plast Reconstr Surg* 1989;84:323–324.
19. Baker SH, Swanson NA. Clinical applications of tissue expansion in head and neck surgery. *Laryngoscope* 1990;100:313–319.
20. Hoffmann JF. Tissue expansion in the head and neck. *Facial Plast Surg Clin North Am* 2005;13:315–324.
21. Bauer BS, Few JW, Chavez CD, et al. The role of tissue expansion in the management of large congenital pigmented nevi of the forehead in the pediatric patient. *Plast Reconstr Surg* 2001;107:668–675.
22. Lee S, Rafii AA, Sykes J. Advances in scalp reconstruction. *Curr Opin Otolaryngol Head Neck Surg* 2006;14:249–253.
23. Leedy JE, Janis JE, Rohrrich RJ. Reconstruction of acquired scalp defects: an algorithmic approach. *Plast Reconstr Surg* 2005;116:54e–72e.
24. Manders ER, Schenden MJ, Furrey JA, et al. Skin expansion to eliminate large scalp defects. *Plast Reconstr Surg* 1984;74:482.
25. von Rappard JH, Molenaar J, van Doorn K, et al. Surface-area increase in tissue expansion. *Plast Reconstr Surg* 1988;82:833–839.
26. Jackson IT, Sharpe DT, Polley J, et al. Use of external reservoirs in tissue expansion. *Plast Reconstr Surg* 1987;80:266–273.
27. Lozano S, Drucker M. Use of tissue expanders with external ports. *Ann Plast Surg* 2000;44:14–17.
28. Keskin M, Kelly CP, Yavuzer R, et al. External filling ports in tissue expansion: confirming their safety and convenience. *Plast Reconstr Surg* 2006;117(5):1543–1551.
29. Wiselander JB. Tissue expansion in the head and neck. *Scand J Plast Reconstr Hand Surg* 1991;25:47–56.
30. LoGiudice J, Gosain AK. Pediatric tissue expansion: indications and complications. *J Craniofac Surg* 2003;14(6):866–872.
31. Neal HW, High RM, Billmire DA, et al. Complications of controlled tissue expansion in the pediatric burn patient. *Plast Reconstr Surg* 1988;82:840–845.
32. Hallock G. Safety of clinical overinflation of tissue expanders. *Plast Reconstr Surg* 1995;96:153–157.
33. Sasaki GH. Intraoperative sustained limited expansion as an immediate reconstructive technique. *Clin Plast Surg* 1987;14:563–573.
34. Sasaki GH. Intraoperative expansion as immediate reconstructive technique. In: *Tissue expansion in reconstructive and aesthetic surgery*. St. Louis, MO: Mosby, 1998:248.

35. Mackay DR, Saggers GC, Kotval, et al. Stretching the skin: undermining is more important than intraoperative expansion. *Plast Reconstr Surg* 1990;86:722–730.

36. Siegert R, Weerda H, Hoffman S, et al. Clinical and experimental evaluation of intermittent intraoperative short-term expansion. *Plast Reconstr Surg* 1993;92:248–254.

37. Gibstein LA, Abramson DL, Bartlett RA, et al. Tissue expansion in children: a retrospective study of complications. *Ann Plast Surg* 1997;38:358–364.

38. Manders ET, Schenden MJ, Furrey JA, et al. Soft tissue expansion: concepts and complications. *Plast Reconstr Surg* 1984;74:493–507.

Scar Camouflage

176

Shawn M. Stevens   **Krishna G. Patel**

Scar camouflage constitutes one of the primary roles of the facial plastic surgeon, and in no other location of the body does this bear such aesthetic importance. The surgeon must possess a sound understanding of prevention and tissue handling techniques, as well as a fundamental understanding of wound healing and patient-specific risk factors in scar formation. Additionally, a wide array of techniques must exist within the surgeon's armamentarium, both surgical and nonsurgical, in order to appropriately manage the high variability of scar presentations (Table 176.1).

The surgeon's goal should be to select the best technique(s) for the individual patient and scar. This constitutes a challenging decision backed by a relative paucity of high-level evidence. Well-designed, comparison-controlled trials of various interventions are lacking for reasons including the following: (a) objective markers of scar improvement (color, elevation, texture) are inconsistent between studies; (b) interpatient scar variability makes adequate controls impossible; and (c) subjective scales such as patient and physician satisfaction scores are prone to significant inter- and intragroup variability (1). Despite these difficulties, strong trends do exist within the literature regarding surgical approaches to scar camouflage. Thus, the goal of this chapter is to provide the reader with a sound, evidence-based review of the available interventions for scar camouflage.

BASIC SCIENCE

Wound Healing

The wound healing process can effectively be broken into three distinct but overlapping phases: the inflammatory phase, the proliferative phase, and the remodeling phase.

The inflammatory phase (immediate onset lasting 2 to 5 days): This initially begins with hemostasis over the first 5 to 10 minutes via vasoconstriction and activation of the clotting cascade. This includes platelet aggregation and deposition of thrombin and fibrin. Vasodilation follows and peaks at approximately 20 minutes before vascular tone returns to its baseline. Also beginning immediately, aggregating platelets and local phagocytic cells (predominantly neutrophils for the first 24 to 48 hours) release a variety of proinflammatory and chemotactic cytokines. This in turn leads to an influx of macrophages. These are the essential mediators of early wound healing and predominant cell type from 48 hours through the remainder of the inflammatory phase. The macrophages for their part phagocytize bacteria and damaged tissue and release their own milieu of cytokines, growth factors, and chemotactic agents. This subsequently promotes the arrival of fibroblasts, endothelial and epithelial cell migration, and wound contraction by myofibroblasts.

The proliferative phase (day 2 through 3 to 4 weeks): Fibroblasts enter the wound around day 2, which signifies an overlap period of the inflammatory and proliferative phases. As the inflammatory phase ends and macrophages decline in number, fibroblasts take over as the predominant cell type. Through the resulting fibroplasia, granulation tissue forms, and extracellular matrix (ECM) is deposited consisting of disorganized collagen (mostly type III), elastin, and fibronectin. Angiogenesis and wound contraction (both begin around day 4) follow and are mediated by endothelial cell migration and wound margin myofibroblasts, respectively. Wound contraction is maximal around days 12 to 15. Reepithelialization also occurs during this phase through migration of epithelial keratinocytes from the wound margins and the bases of pilosebaceous subunits preserved in the wound at the level of the dermis. The process occurs best over a moist surface of viable tissue. This underscores the importance of a moist wound environment that not only aids migration but also prevents excess scabbing that acts as a barrier to migration. Reepithelialization ceases when the opposing sheets of migrating epithelial cells meet and reestablish contact inhibition.

TABLE 176.1	UNDESIRABLE SCAR TYPES

Atrophic scars (depressed)
Hsc (protrusive)
Irregularly shaped scars
Scars with color mismatch
Scars that cross RSTL/aesthetic subunits
Contracted scars that distort surrounding tissues
Keloids

RSTL, relaxed skin tension lines.

The remodeling phase (3 weeks to 2 years): Collagen remodeling occurs with fibers becoming aligned in a more parallel fashion and type I collagen being deposited in greater proportion. Excess cells are removed via apoptosis and phagocytosis. Also during this phase, the wound's tensile strength will increase roughly according to the following progression: 15% of original strength by 3 weeks, 60% by 6 weeks, and 80% by 3 to 6 months, which is the maximum achieved (2).

Deregulation or interruptions of this wound healing process, including interventions by the surgeon, can lead to alterations in the scar that ultimately forms. Other systemic and/or external processes including malnutrition, diabetes mellitus, smoking, excessive sun exposure, and immunosuppression can severely impede this process and lead to poor wound healing and worsened outcomes.

Scar Types

Scars can be classified broadly into hypertrophic scars (Hsc)/keloids and non-Hsc (1). Hsc and keloids are quite similar in nature and represent an aberration in the wound healing process. Patients prone to these types of scars have been shown to have down-regulation of various apoptotic genes and overexpression of signaling factors such as IL-6 and TGFβ1 and β2. Resulting histologic findings include ECM overproduction and deposition of highly disorganized collagen by hypermitotic fibroblasts (2,3). Keloids, by definition, are elevated fibrous scars that extend beyond the borders of the original wound, do not regress, and usually recur after excision. They can take between 3 months and years to develop. Hsc develop quicker (within 8 weeks), are confined to the wound borders, and usually will regress over a period of 12 to 18 months (2,4). Risks for keloid formation include darkly pigmented skin (15- to 20-fold increase), familial predisposition, and high wound tension. Hsc are less likely to be related to skin pigmentation. Care must be taken by the surgeon when working with patients at risk for keloid formation as there is a very high rate of recurrence, especially when surgical excision is used alone (5).

Non-Hsc can be divided into either atrophic (depressed) scars or scars that are flat or protrude minimally above the level of the adjacent normal skin (1). While less prone to recurrence and complications than keloids and Hsc, these scars can nonetheless be disfiguring and challenging to treat. The pathophysiology of this scar type is likely related to a hypoxic wound environment, abnormal levels of cellular apoptosis, and limited angiogenesis. The ultimate result is reduced deposition of ECM and collagen and a depression of the wound bed with regard to surrounding normal skin. Similar to keloid and Hsc, excessive tension on wound edges increases risk of atrophic scar formation.

SURGICAL TECHNIQUES

Surgical Planning and Scar Relocation

Four main factors exist that cause unsatisfactory scarring. These are (a) the direction of the scar with respect to relaxed skin tension lines (RSTLs) and if there is disruption or distortion of aesthetic units; (b) the uninterrupted length of a straight scar especially if greater than 2 cm; (c) an irregular texture to the scar surface; and (d) a color mismatch between the scar and surrounding normal tissues. Many techniques exist to treat these problems. In general, the goal is to achieve relocation, excision, irregularization, and/or disruption of a scar (Table 176.2). When planning to camouflage a scar, it is of critical importance to examine the scar's relationship to the facial aesthetic units, their borders, and the general locations of RSTLs (Fig. 176.1). Facial aesthetic units include the forehead, eyelids, nose, cheeks, lips, and chin. Aesthetic borders between or at the margins of these units are excellent locations for incision placement or scar relocation and include the hairline, infraorbital rims, nasofacial grooves, melolabial folds, vermilion borders, and preauricular sulci. Careful acknowledgment of RSTLs is important, as an incision or closure that crosses these at an angle greater than 30 to 40 degrees will produce an aesthetically displeasing result. With careful planning, many scars can be excised via fusiform incision/primary closure and achieve excellent results. Thus, one of the ideal camouflage techniques is achieved by placement of incisions within existing skin folds produced by RSTLs (6–10).

Scars or defects near the center of an aesthetic unit, resting over a convexity or concavity, or of great length make simple excision less effective. If extensive undermining of surrounding tissue is necessary for tension-free closure or the anticipated closure will distort a free margin of

TABLE 176.2	CHARACTERISTICS OF AN IDEAL SCAR

Thin width
Surface flush with surrounding skin
Color matches surrounding skin
Runs parallel to RSTL or along aesthetic subunits
Irregularized if long length

RSTL, relaxed skin tension lines.

the face (lid, lip, nose) and/or cross an RSTL, alternative interventions should also be considered, such as local flap reconstruction (11).

Flaps

Flaps can be classified in a number of ways. Classification can be based on vascular supply, composition, and/or design and method of transfer (Table 176.3). Practical use often employs a combination of the above. Transposition flaps and local advancement flaps constitute the principle techniques utilized for scar camouflage. When performed correctly, these procedures can achieve excellent irregularization or disruption of a scar and provide near perfect color and texture match to surrounding healthy skin (8). The most commonly used techniques include the Z-plasty, W-plasty, and geometric broken line closure (GBLC) and will be discussed in detail below. Multiple variations of these techniques also exist and can be tailored to the individual patient and scar.

Z-plasty

One of the most common and important techniques in a surgeons' armamentarium is the Z-plasty transposition flap (Fig. 176.2). The basic Z-plasty can provide excellent cosmesis for a variety of scar revision purposes and is chiefly used to (a) lengthen a scar, (b) release a contracture, (c) disrupt a scar, or (d) realign a scar within an RSTL (Fig. 176.3). However, performing a Z-plasty also has its drawbacks. Lengthening the scar in one direction will result in shortening of the perpendicular direction, and a total of three scars must be made in the place of one.

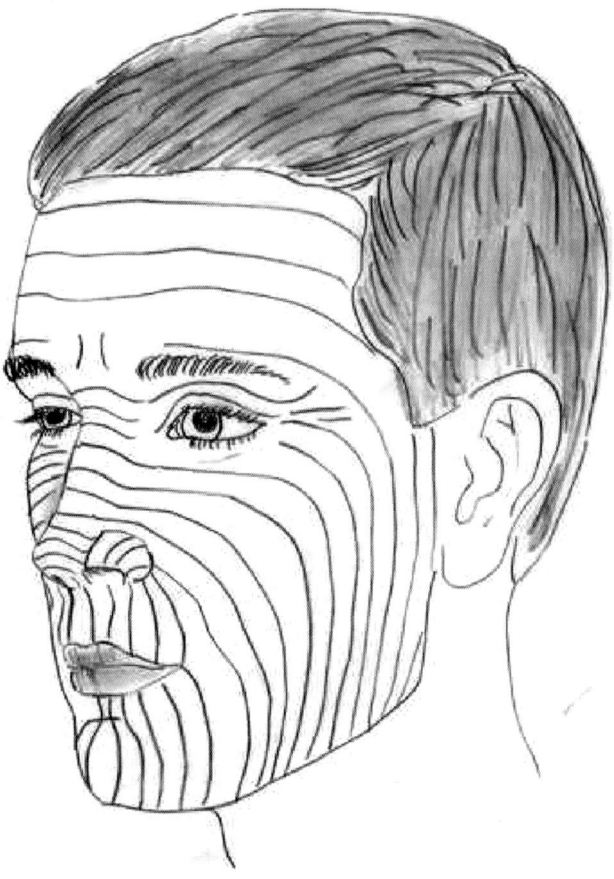

Figure 176.1 Schematic illustrating the RSTLs of the face. (Modified illustration from Larrabee WF, Sherris DA. Soft tissue biomechanics and physiology. In: Larrabee WF, Sherris DA, eds. *Principles of facial reconstruction*, Chapter 1. New York: Lippincott-Raven, 1995:3.)

TABLE 176.3	FLAP CLASSIFICATION SCHEMES		
Classification	**Subclassification**	**Subtypes**	**Examples**
Vascular supply	I. Random supply		The majority of local flaps
	II. Axial supply (by named vessel)	A. Local	a. Paramedian forehead (supratrochlear artery)
		B. Regional	b. Platysmal (branch of facial artery)
		C. Free tissue transfer	c. Pectoralis major (thoracoacromial artery)
Composition	I. Cutaneous		
	II. Fasciocutaneous		
	III. Musculocutaneous		
	IV. Osteomusculocutaneous		
Method of transfer/ design		A. Advancement flap	a. Primary fusiform closure, W-plasty, GBLC, V to Y, island, etc.
		B. Rotation flap	b. Cervicofacial, O to Z, Karapandzic, etc.
		C. Transposition flap	c. Z-plasty, bilobed, rhombic, etc.
		D. Interpolated	d. Paramedian forehead, melolabial, nasofacial, etc.
		E. Free tissue transfer	e. Latissimus, scapular, radial forearm, etc.

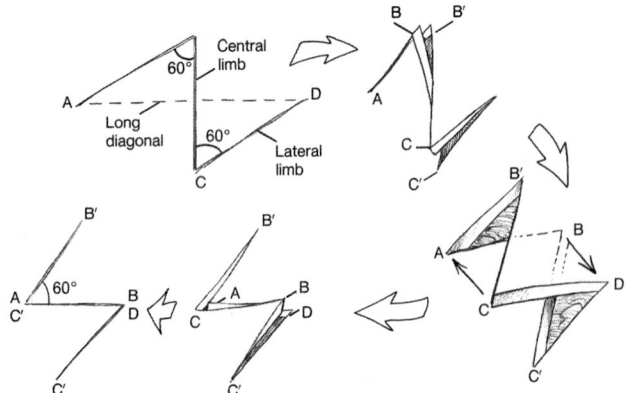

Figure 176.2 Classic design of the Z-plasty with 60 degree limbs. (From Hochman M. Scar Camouflage. In: Bailey BJ, Calhoun KH, eds. *Bailey-head and neck surgery—otolaryngology*, Chapter 166, Figure 166.3, 3rd ed., Vol. 2. New York: Lippincott Williams & Wilkins, 2001:2115.)

Technique—The traditional Z-plasty has two constant features. First, three incisions of equal length are made, one central and two limbs. The central incision, ideally, is designed to run parallel to the scar's long axis. Upon closure, the central component of the incision will achieve the greatest directional change, which makes careful planning of the central limb vital when attempting to realign the scar with an RSTL (Fig. 176.4). Most often, the defect left by a fusiform excision of the entire scar itself (or other defects such as that left by Mohs surgery) forms the central limb of the Z-plasty (11). The second feature is the two angles made by the limb incisions. In the traditional Z-plasty, these angles are equal and 60 degrees from the center. This results in the formation of two triangular skin flaps. When raised in the subcutaneous plain, the triangle tips are transposed such that the shared sides of the triangles approximate the skin side of the opposing limb incisions.

The effect achieved is a disruption of the scar itself and reorientation along the lines of the limb incisions, which do not move appreciably and should ideally be drawn within RSTLs. It is critical to note that if the initial scar was already oriented with an RSTL, the central incision will fall perpendicular to the same RSTL. Scars angling less than 40 degrees from an RSTL are often better managed with simple excision. A final important feature of the Z-plasty is that intelligent angle design allows the surgeon to anticipate the new length and degree of reorientation achieved after closure. The simple rule of thumb is that the 60-degree Z-plasty will produce a 75% increase in length and 90 degrees of rotation (Fig. 176.5). A change in angle produces predictable change of these variables (Table 176.4). If further lengthening is desired, serial Z-plasty can be performed (6,11). Of note, angles should never be less than 30 degrees as the flap tips will risk ischemia and necrosis.

A number of variations of the traditional Z-plasty exist including double-opposing Z-plasty, unequal triangle Z-plasty, four-flap Z-plasty, compound Z-plasty, and planimetric Z-plasty (6).

W-plasty

One of two common advancement flaps used for scar irregularization, the W-plasty produces a regularly irregular incision and should be used on long straight scars. Such scars reflect light homogenously and are easy for the eye to follow. Irregularization scatters that reflected light making it less visible to the observer. W-plasty is best suited for scars angling greater than 35 degrees from RSTLs or for scars that cross unforgiving areas of convexity or concavity (12). Unlike the Z-plasty, this technique does not increase the length of the scar. W-plasty is faster to perform than GBLC but forms a more predictable and conspicuous scar. As in GBLC, some normal tissue is removed, which increases overall tension on the wound.

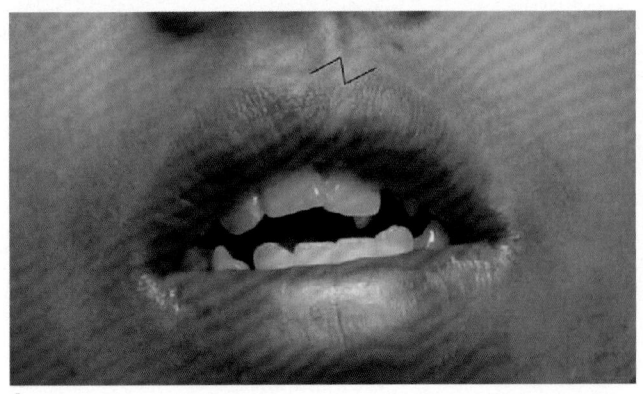
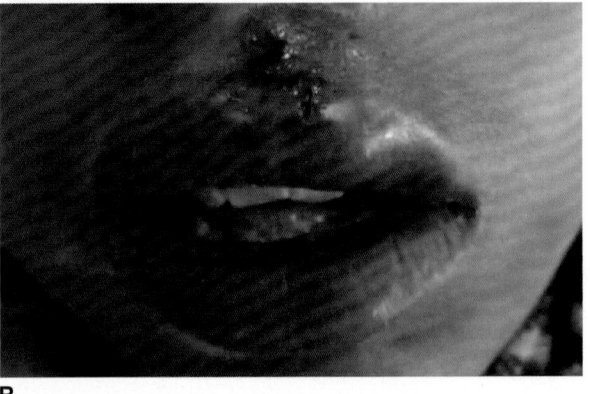

A   **B**

Figure 176.3 Patient with a history of cleft lip repair, who demonstrated a vermilion-cutaneous step-off deformity. Z-plasty technique was utilized to correct the step-off deformity and to realign the vermilion along the natural aesthetic border. **A:** Preoperative photo demonstrating the misalignment of the vermilion and skin of the upper lip disrupting the normal border of the lip vermilion subunit. Lines mark the planned limbs for the Z-plasty transposition flap. **B:** Immediate postoperative photo demonstrating the correction of the vermilion border and restoration of the natural cupids bow contour.

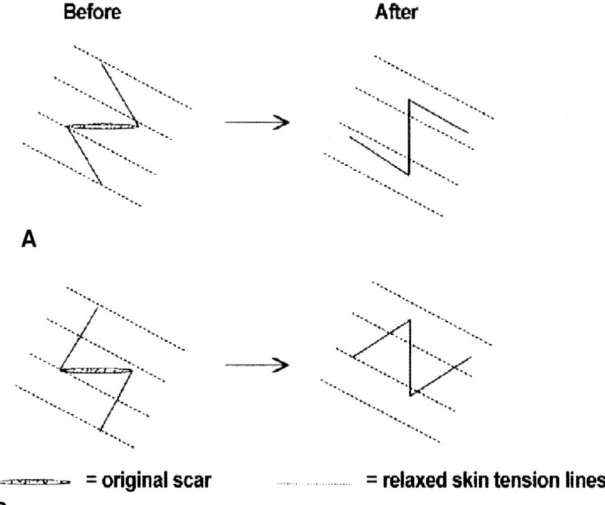

Before **After**

A

= original scar   .... = relaxed skin tension lines

B

Figure 176.4 Schematic of Z-plasty technique that illustrates the importance of limb design. **A:** Preferred limb design that allows the final incisions to mostly orient parallel with the RSTLs. **B:** Poor limb design that causes the final incisions to orient across the RSTLs. (From Shockley WW. Scar revision techniques. *Oper Tech Otolaryngol* 2011;22:84–93, Figure 7, p. 89.)

TABLE 176.4		
Z-plasty Angle	Increase Central Scar Length	Central Scar Reorientation
30°	25%	45°
45°	50%	60°
60°	75%	90°
75°	100%	–
90°	125%	–

M-plasty can also be used to avoid extending the incision further. With traction applied, the W-plasty design is excised taking both scar and normal tissue with it. Closure is performed in layers.

Geometric Broken Line Closure

More complex and time consuming than the W-plasty, GBLC produces an irregularly irregular incision that maximizes scar camouflage. This technique is ideally used on scars that are relatively long and angle 45 degrees or greater from RSTLs. While GBLC has superior camouflaging results, it also carries a high degree of technical difficulty and significantly increases operative time (Fig. 176.8).

Technique—GBLC incorporates a series of advancement flaps in the form of opposing semicircles, squares, triangles, rhomboids, and rectangles in varying order and size (Fig. 176.6). The key feature is randomness of the design, which is difficult for an observer's eye to track. As is always the case, it is important to align straight portions of the new scar with RSTLs whenever possible. Individual flap length should fall between 3 and 7 mm, as greater lengths become too visible and smaller ones become difficult to close (Fig. 176.9). Flaps should be meticulously mapped out 3 to 6 mm from the scar margins, and the triangular ends of the design should again be less than 30 degrees to avoid a standing cone deformity. The design is excised under tension taking the interposing scar and normal skin. Due to forces across the wound bed, wide undermining may be necessary to assist in tension-free closure. Closure is achieved in layers similar to the W-plasty (12).

Technique—The W-plasty is essentially a series of mirrored triangular advancement flaps (12) (Fig. 176.6). The apices of the triangles are placed 3 to 5 mm on either side of the scar, and each apex should be 5 to 6 mm apart from those adjacent. Limb length should be between 3 and 6 mm. Smaller limbs tend to not break up the scar adequately, while larger limbs form more conspicuous scars. The angle of each apex is designed individually to orient the limbs with RSTLs (Fig. 176.7). The ends of the incision are "closed" with a final set of triangles measuring 30 degrees or less. Anything larger can create a "dog ear" or "standing cone" deformity at the incisional margins. Alternatively, an

Serial Excision and Tissue Expansion

Serial Excision

This technique involves partial excision of a scar combined with undermining and advancement of the adjacent healthy skin. It requires a series of sequential procedures, but will eventually excise the scar completely. While not often used in scar camouflage, serial excision may be considered if the size and elasticity of a scar or tension

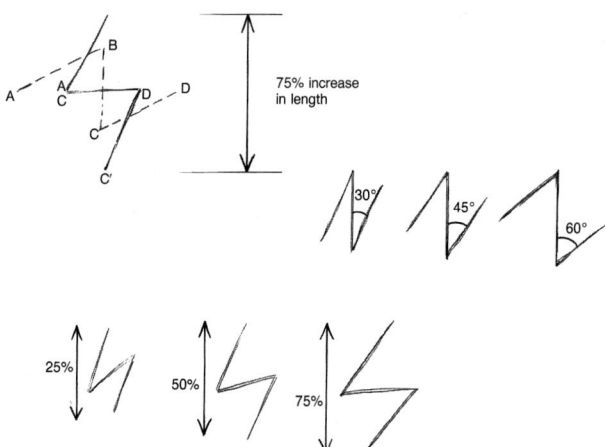

Figure 176.5 Schematic demonstrating how increasing the limb angles of a Z-plasty predictably increases the total final length of the scar. (From Hochman M. Scar Camouflage. In: Bailey BJ, Calhoun KH, eds. *Bailey-head and neck surgery—otolaryngology*, Chapter 166, Figure 166.4, 3rd ed., Vol. 2. New York: Lippincott Williams & Wilkins, 2001:2116.)

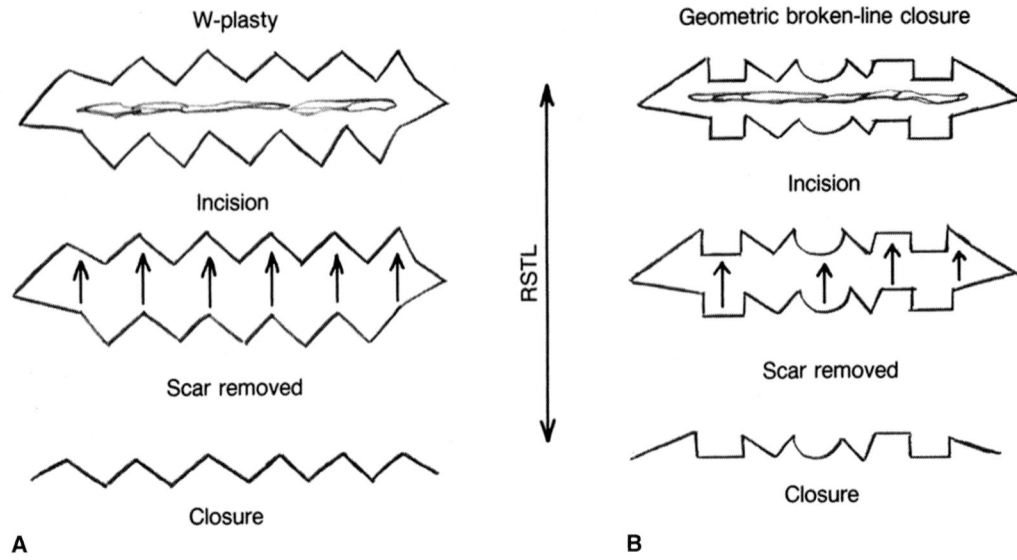

Figure 176.6 Schematic illustration of the W-plasty **(A)** and GBLC **(B)** techniques. W-plasty produces a regularly irregular incision through the advancement of serial triangular flaps. GBLC produces an irregularly irregular incision through the advancement of multiple geometric-shaped flaps. (From Hochman M. Scar Camouflage. In: Bailey BJ, Calhoun KH, eds. *Bailey-head and neck surgery—otolaryngology*, 3rd ed, Vol. 2, Chapter 166, Figure 166.6. New York: Lippincott Williams & Wilkins, 2001:2116.)

forces across the wound bed preclude a single excision and closure. The number of required excisions depends on the features of the scar. Between procedures, the available skin at the wound margin will increase via mechanisms of mechanical and biologic creep. This effectively increases the available tissue for the next stage of the excision. The primary disadvantage is the necessity for multiple operations (13).

Tissue Expansion

Tissue expansion represents another technique geared toward increasing available tissue for a planned future revision. It involves the placement of an implant under normal tissue adjacent to the scarred wound, followed by sequential office visits to expand the implant with saline injections. This in turn stretches the overlying tissue, which will again increase in area secondary to creep-related mechanisms. Even more rarely used than serial excision,

expansion mandates two procedures, multiple clinic visits, and carries risks of infection and implant extrusion. Indications are similar to those for serial excision.

Grafts

Grafts are rarely used in scar camouflage but do exist as an option for large defects not amenable to complete closure. The most common examples of grafts used in this setting are skin grafts (split-thickness, full-thickness, or dermal) or composite grafts (full-thickness skin with perichondrium with or without cartilage) (8). Important factors to consider if choosing a graft for camouflage purposes are anticipated degree of contracture at the recipient site, placement of the graft with regard to facial subunits and RSTLs, adequacy of blood supply of the recipient bed, resultant scar at the donor site, graft color, and skin thickness similarity to the surrounding normal tissue.

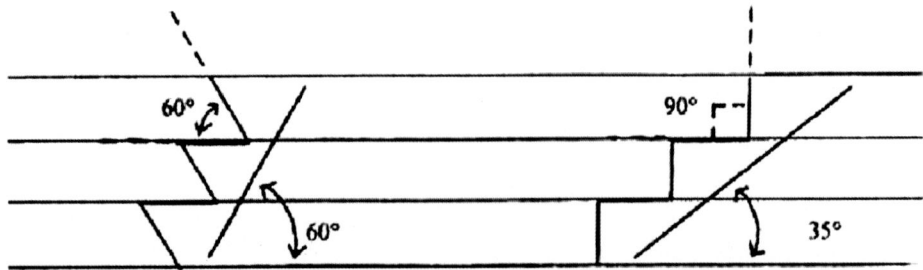

Figure 176.7 Schematic illustrating how the angle between the long axis of the scar and the RSTLs helps to predict the angles that the W-plasty limbs should be designed, in order to improve the alignment of the final incisions with the RSTLs. (From Rodgers BJ, Williams EF, Hove CR. W-plasty and geometric broken line closure. *Facial Plast Surg* 2001;17(4):239–244, Figure 2, p. 240.)

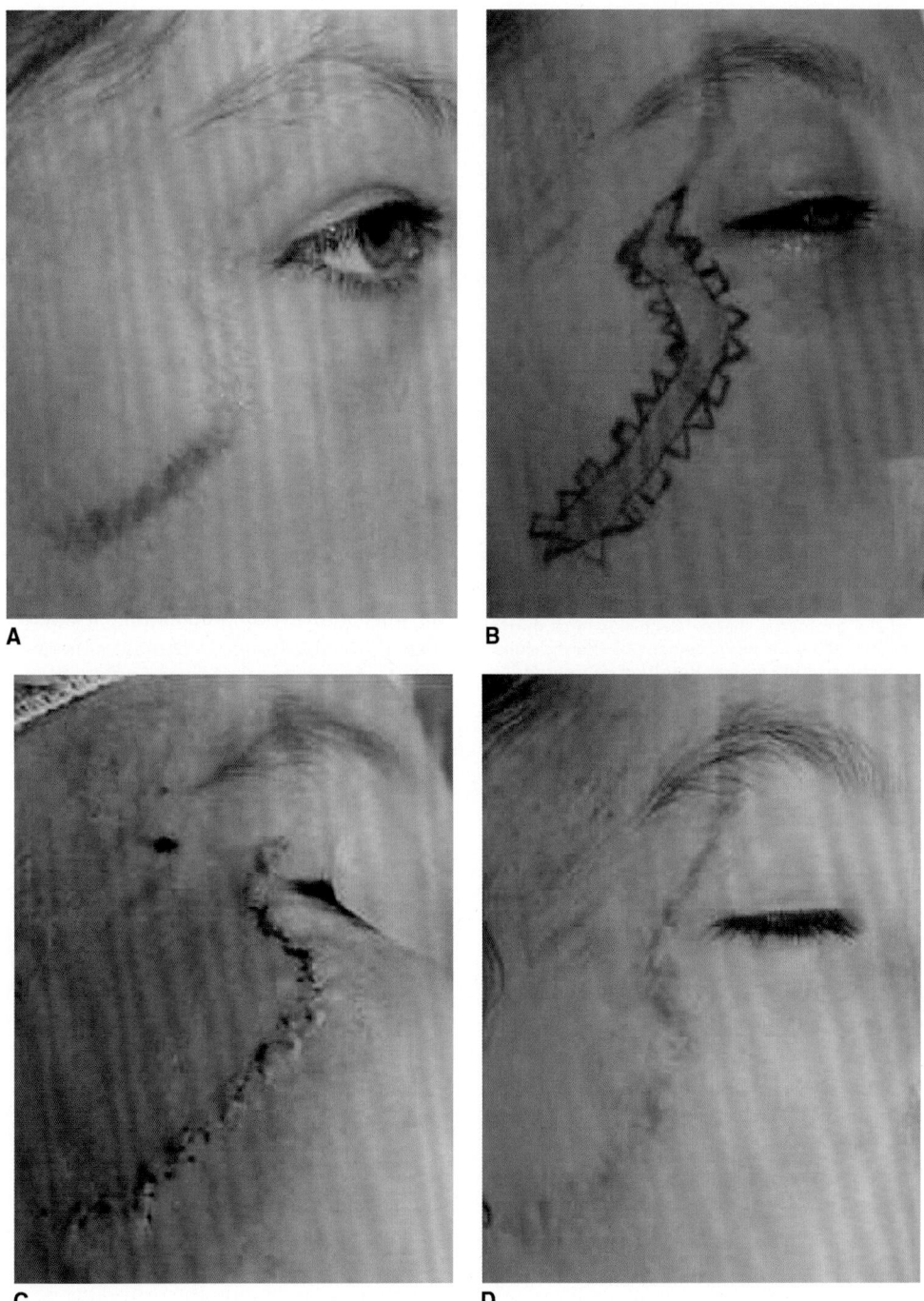

A   **B**

C   **D**

Figure 176.8 Patient with an atrophic widened scar that transgresses multiple aesthetic subunits. Serial revision was planned. Starting with repairing the lower half of the scar on the cheek. Geometric broken line closure technique was performed. **A:** Preoperative photo of the cheek portion of the scar. **B:** Intraoperative design of the GBLC. **C:** One week postoperative photo of GBLC with plans to remove sutures. **D:** Three months postoperative photo. The scar is no longer depressed and has improved width, and the irregularization makes the scar less noticeable.

Concepts in Prevention and Surgical Technique

To achieve an optimal aesthetic result after any intervention, careful surgical planning for incision placement and tissue transfer is paramount. Proper tissue handling techniques are also of critical importance and include atraumatic tissue manipulation, aseptic technique, and meticulous hemostasis (3,14,15). Careful placement of deep dermal sutures to achieve maximal wound eversion should be executed to prevent atrophic scar formation. Also of importance are the location of incisions with respect to

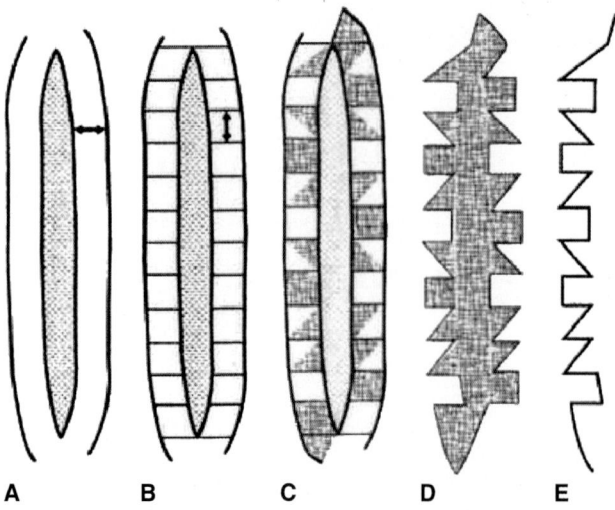

Figure 176.9 Description of the technique used to design geometric broken line advancement flaps. **A:** Lines are drawn parallel to the borders of the scar and are 5 mm beyond the borders of the scar. **B:** Horizontal lines are drawn 5 mm apart between the scar edge and the outer vertical lines. **C:** Shaded area represents the proposed excision of the geometric shapes. Each side must mirror the geometric shapes to allow for advancement of the incisions. **D:** Defect following excision of the scar. **E:** Resulting geometric line following closure. (From Shockley WW. Scar revision techniques. *Oper Tech Otolaryngol* 2011;22:84–93, Figure 11, p. 91.)

hair follicles (risk for alopecia) and proper postoperative nutrition (3). The proper timing for scar revision is variable, but most surgeons will allow a scar to mature for 6 to 12 months before considering an intervention. However, if the scar is causing significant deformity or dysfunction, earlier intervention is acceptable.

Sound postoperative wound care is also a top priority and should be tailored to the interventions performed. Proper bandaging, maintaining a moist wound environment, and early removal (if possible) of foreign surgical material all portend to superior aesthetic outcomes. Pressure dressings, intralesional injections, and topical therapies, when used correctly, can also lead to better overall cosmesis and may limit future scar formation (2,4). Investigations are showing the use of lasers immediately after primary closure may also achieve improved scar prevention (16,17). Finally, the importance of thorough patient education and avoidance of sun exposure should not be overlooked.

NONSURGICAL AND ADJUNCTIVE TECHNIQUES

While surgery is the mainstay of scar camouflage, a number of adjunctive nonsurgical interventions also exist that can augment and often improve the cosmetic outcome of a surgical intervention. These techniques can also be utilized as monotherapies in the correct settings. This section presents discussions of the various nonsurgical modalities.

Intralesional Injections

Steroids

Steroids continue to be a mainstay in scar camouflage and revision. The mechanism of action is believed to lay in suppression of inflammation and mitosis, while an increase in vasoconstriction has also been described. Corticosteroids injected intralesionally have been shown to be effective in decreasing the elevation and erythema of scars, both as a prevention tactic immediately after surgical closure and as a primary intervention. Steroids also represent a first-line agent in both the prevention and treatment of Hsc and keloids. The agent of choice is usually triamcinolone acetonide (Kenalog). Steroid injections have been shown to flatten 50% to 100% of small keloids, with a 9% to 50% rate of recurrence. These rates improve when the intralesional injection is coupled with other modalities such as silicone sheeting, cryotherapy, and/or surgical excision. Earlier injected wounds also tend to have the best outcomes in terms of scar prevention. Side effects include pain on injection, hypopigmentation, telangiectasias, atrophy, ulceration, and in rare occurrences tissue necrosis. Topical EMLA ointment or lidocaine mixed with the steroid can be used to lessen pain (4,18,19).

Agents under Investigation

A number of additional injectable agents continue to be under investigation for use in scar prevention. These include 5-fluorouracil, bleomycin, verapamil, and interferon alfa-2A among others. These agents have been shown to have limited success on scar elevation, pruritus, and erythema, especially when used to treat Hsc and keloids. All have failed to achieve the wide spread acceptance of steroids; this is likely secondary to significant side effects and theoretical risks if not administered correctly (2,4,18–26).

Resurfacing Techniques

Laser Resurfacing

The use of lasers in scar camouflage and treatment has been and remains a burgeoning area of study in recent years. Lasers can be used as monotherapy or as an adjunct to surgical intervention and other camouflaging procedures (1). Laser therapy is classified as either ablative or nonablative based on the absorption spectrum of the wavelength emitted and depth of penetration. Both classes of lasers play specific roles in scar revision and camouflage.

Ablative Resurfacing Lasers (ARL)

The most commonly used ablative lasers are the pulsed CO_2 laser and erbium: yttrium–aluminum–garnet laser (Er:YAG). The wavelengths of these lasers are primarily absorbed by intracellular water, causing an increase in thermal energy that will eventually precipitate vaporization. Pulsed CO_2 lasers are less selective in their affinity and create a high degree of contiguous thermal necrosis unless fractionated. This in turn leads to wound debulking, contraction, and stimulation of collagen remodeling. A number of studies have shown ARL to be helpful in the treatment of Hsc and keloids as a monotherapy, and improved results are often realized when used in combination with intralesional steroid injection. Er:YAG causes a lesser degree of tissue necrosis than CO_2 lasers and may better target scar margins.

Disadvantages of ablative lasers include pain, prolonged downtime, persistent erythema (described up to 3 months), hyperpigmentation, hypopigmentation, and increased risk for viral and bacterial infections. Er:YAG exhibits these effects to a lesser degree, thanks to its higher affinity for water and ability to be applied more precisely. Lesser downtimes are also described when compared to CO_2 lasers. Similarly, introduction of fractionated CO_2 laser treatments have aided in decreasing the risk profile and recovery downtime when compared to traditional CO_2 lasers.

Nonablative Resurfacing Lasers (NAR)

Common lasers in this category are the 585-nm pulsed dye laser (585nm-PDL) and neodymium: yttrium–aluminum–garnet laser (Nd:YAG) among others. These lasers work on the principle of selective photothermolysis. The emitted wavelength is absorbed primarily by oxyhemoglobin (chromophores) in the microvasculature, which leads to highly selective vaporization and subsequent tissue ischemia. Intracellular water is largely spared so the tissue necrotizing effect of ablative lasers is not observed. The end effect is a reduction in scar erythema, pruritus, and an overall leveling of the scar surface texture. Studies also show a desirable stimulatory effect on cell signaling that can increase organized collagen deposition and ECM production. Thus, nonablative lasers achieve success in the treatment of atrophic and depressed acne scars, especially when the beam is dispersed into multiple microscopic "subbeams" and the overall treatment fractionated over a series of interventions. Finally, lasers in this class can be used to treat hyperpigmented scars (1,18,27–30).

Disadvantages again include downtime, tissue erythema, pain, and infection risk, although all of these bear much less impact when compared with ablative lasers. Also of note, multiple therapies are often indicated to realize maximal outcomes with NAR. Additionally, all lasers should be used cautiously with Fitzpatrick skin types IV to VI, due to increased complication risks.

Dermabrasion

The concept behind dermabrasion is to level the skin while simultaneously promoting reepithelialization and new collagen production. This technique is typically used in the revision of acne scarring, facial rhytids, and rhinophyma, but can also be used as an adjunctive technique after surgery to smooth uneven scars (Fig. 176.10). The goal of dermabrasion is to injure the epithelium to a predetermined depth. Care is taken to extend only into the papillary dermis, with purposeful preservation of the deeper adnexal structures found in the reticular dermis. These serve as a later source of reepithelialization and migration across the abraded surface area. To determine proper depth, the surgeon must look for the appearance of punctate bleeding characteristic of the papillary dermis. Dermabrasion is performed with a high-speed diamond fraise or wire brush, and strokes must be oriented perpendicular to the direction of wheel rotation to prevent loss of control and allow for even resurfacing (Fig. 176.11). This procedure can be performed under local regional anesthesia in an office setting.

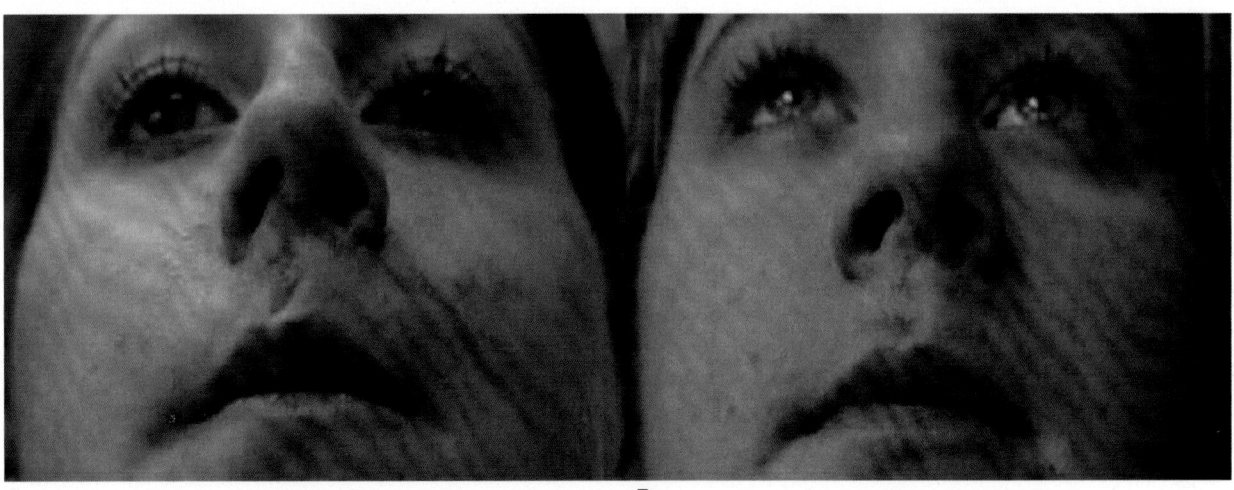

A   **B**

Figure 176.10 Photograph of dermabrasion performed on patient who sustained a severe laceration to the nose and upper lip/cheek. **A:** Preoperative photo 3 months after original injury and just prior to dermabrasion procedure. **B:** Three months after dermabrasion was performed to the upper lip/philtrum/cheek regions. The scar is less conspicuous secondary to the improved smoothness of edges and color match after dermabrasion.

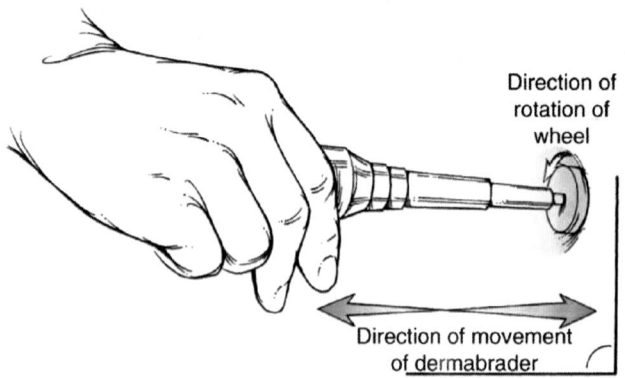

Figure 176.11 Schematic illustrating the technique of derm-abrasion. The direction of movement of the dermabrasion should be perpendicular to the rotation of the dermabrader tip. (From Thomas JR, Mobley SR. Scar revision and camouflage. In: Thomas JR, ed. *Cummings otolaryngology head and neck surgery*, 5th ed., Vol. I, Chapter 21, Figure 21–13. China: Mosby Elsevier, 2010:300.)

Cryosurgery/Cryotherapy

This modality entails the use of nitrous oxide and/or liquid nitrogen to damage both cells and microvasculature contained within the scar tissue. This in turn leads to relative vascular stasis, cell anoxia, and necrosis. The clinical affect described is usually a flattening of scar elevation and softening of the scar fibrotic matrix. The latter effect also may assist a surgeon hoping to soften dense scar tissue prior to an intralesional injection or partial excision. Used as a monotherapy, satisfactory improvement has been described in the treatment of keloid and Hsc when used over multiple sessions. In a related technique, cryoneedle probes may also be inserted intralesionally to achieve scar volume reduction (31). Side effects of cryotherapy include tissue edema, atrophy, and risk for hyperpigmentation or hypopigmentation. The latter two are of special concern in patients with darker pigmented skin types (2–4,32,33).

Direct Camouflage

Intralesional Fillers

Injectable soft tissue fillers are also well known and important in the treatment of atrophic scars (34). Types of available fillers include autologous tissue (fat), allogeneic tissue, xenographic materials, and synthetic materials. Caution must be used when injecting permanent filler products in the superficial layers of the dermis and subcutaneous tissues because this may elicit an inflammatory response leading to superficial skin changes and granuloma formation. Such secondary complications may negate the original goal of scar camouflage.

Surgical Tattooing (Dermatography)

Surgical tattooing is a sometimes overlooked modality for the camouflage of aesthetically displeasing scars and can be especially useful in hypopigmented scars and scars

involving areas of alopecia (i.e., over the eyebrow). Used in adjunct with other procedures, an improved overall outcome can usually be achieved. Risks are generally limited to pain and slight risk of infection (35).

Topical Cosmetics

Having gained widespread acceptance in the general public, use of cosmetics is logical and effective in certain camouflage scenarios. Best outcomes may be realized when used on hypo- or hyperpigmented scars to blend color tone to surrounding skin. Cosmetics can also be partially successful in leveling atrophic scars and the depressions left by severe acne.

Topical Agents

Moist Wound Dressings

Key in postoperative wound care, a moist wound environment has repeatedly been shown to improve wound healing and overall aesthetic outcomes. It is thought that maintaining a moist environment assists in keratinocyte and epithelial migration from adnexal structures and the epidermal margins of the wound. Dressings of this type can be achieved in a number of ways, but dressings impregnated with Vaseline or petroleum-based products are probably the most practical and cost-effective.

Silicone (Gels, Sheets)

A variety of silicone-based products exist on the market for scar treatment and camouflage including sheets, strips, gels, sprays, and foams. Of these, silicone impregnated elastic sheeting is probably the most extensively studied and has been shown to achieve variable levels of success. The proposed mechanism is occlusion of the wound, which increases temperature, keratinocyte hydration, and oxygen tension inside the forming scar. This in turn seems to lead to the scar softening and flattening. In concept, this is very similar to the mechanism of action of a pressure dressing. The best studied effects have been in the treatment/prevention of Hsc and keloids. One review also shows silicone to have increased efficacy when used in combination with other modalities such as intralesional steroid injections and surgical excision. Side effects are limited, but this agent should be avoided on open wounds and can be expensive. It also requires a very motivated, compliant patient, as the elastomer sheets must remain occlusive for at least 12 hours daily and for prolonged periods of up to 4 to 6 months to be effective (2,4,36,37).

Vitamin E

A popular agent in the treatment of acute and chronic dermal wounds, the effect of vitamin E is thought to be mediated by its antioxidant effects. The desired effect is to reduce wound inflammation and thus limit excessive scar tissue formation during the proliferative and remodeling phases. Research supporting efficacy of topical vitamin E, however, is relatively scant considering its popularity and has shown it to be no more effective in reduction of scar elevation, color, or appearance than other topical emollients. One important side effect is that vitamin E may reduce the tensile strength of a scar, which should be kept in consideration when planning for high-tension closures (3,4,38). Additionally, unacceptably high levels of contact dermatitis have been reported with vitamin E use.

Onion Extract (Mederma)

This is a very popular agent that has come under recent scrutiny. The active ingredient of this compound is Allium cepa, an onion extract whose derivative is a bioflavonoid called quercetin. Marketed as Mederma, this compound has demonstrated antiproliferative, antiinflammatory, and antihistaminergic effects thought to be effective in decreasing wound erythema, elevation, and pruritus. However, multiple studies have now demonstrated no statistically significant improvements regarding these parameters when compared with simple petroleum-based ointments (3,39). Similar to vitamin E topicals, contact dermatitis is a potential adverse effect.

Imiquimod 5% Cream

Part of a class of drugs called imidazoquinolines, this agent has been thought to work through immune response modulation by inducing production of a number of cytokines such as IFN alfa, IFN gamma, TNF alfa, and a number of interleukins. IFN alfa and gamma, in turn, have been shown to inhibit fibroblast collagen production in a dose-dependent fashion. Imiquimod has best been studied in the treatment and prevention of keloids and Hsc. It is applied postsurgically on alternate nights for 8 weeks and shows best results in low skin tension areas. One area of particular success is use on earlobes after surgical excision of keloids. Side effects include topical irritation and hyperpigmentation (2,4,40).

Other Interventions

Additional modalities described in less detail, or with less orientation to scar treatment and camouflage, include topical retinoids (tretinoin), tacrolimus, cyclosporin A, and mitomycin C. These agents have produced mixed results at best and portend to side effects such as photosensitivity, irritant contact dermatitis, hypertrichosis (cyclosporine), and skin atrophy.

Pressure Dressings

The utility of pressure dressings should not be overlooked. In concept similar to silicone dressings, mechanism is thought to be through occlusion of the wound. Studies have shown that pressure dressings are especially effective for preventing the recurrence of keloids and Hsc after excision.

HIGHLIGHTS

- Characteristics of an ideal scar include the following: thin width, surface is flush with surrounding skin, color matches surrounding skin, and the axis of the scar runs parallel with RSTLs or along aesthetic subunits.
- Transposition (Z-plasty) and advancement (W-plasty and GBLC) flaps are the most common types of local flap techniques employed for scar camouflage.
- Goals of Z-plasty include the following: to lengthen a scar, to release a contracture, to disrupt a scar, or to realign a scar within an RSTL.
- Although a thin scar is ideal, if long and straight, it may continue to be conspicuous and require irregularization.
- GBLC is the superior technique for irregularizing long and straight scars but is technically more challenging and time consuming when compared to Z-plasty and W-plasty techniques.
- Corticosteroids injected intralesionally have been shown to be effective in decreasing the elevation and erythema of scars, both as a prevention tactic immediately after surgical closure and as a primary intervention.
- Popular resurfacing techniques utilized for scar camouflage include dermabrasion, laser therapy, and cryotherapy.
- Resurfacing techniques extend to the depth of the papillary dermis and must preserve the deeper adnexal structures for proper wound healing and reepithelialization.
- Wounds epithelialize most quickly in a moist environment.
- Importance of thorough patient education on wound care and avoidance of sun exposure should not be underestimated.

REFERENCES

1. Lee Y. Combination treatment of surgical, post-traumatic and post-herpetic scars with ablative lasers followed by fractional laser and non-ablative laser in Asians. *Lasers Surg Med* 2009;41(2):131–140.
2. Berman B, Viera MH, Amini S, et al. Prevention and management of hypertrophic scars and keloids after burns in children. *J Craniofac Surg* 2008;19(4):989–1006.
3. Chen MA, Davidson TM. Scar management: prevention and treatment strategies. *Curr Opin Otolaryngol Head Neck Surg* 2005;13(4):242–247.
4. Juckett G, Hartman-Adams H. Management of keloids and hypertrophic scars. *Am Fam Physician* 2009;80(3):253–260.
5. Niessen FB, Spauwen PH, Schalkwijk J, et al. On the nature of hypertrophic scars and keloids: a review. *Plast Reconstr Surg* 1999;104(5):1435–1458.

6. Hove CR, Williams EF III, Rodgers BJ. Z-plasty: a concise review. *Facial Plast Surg* 2001;17(4):289–294.

7. Ulkur E, Acikel C, Evinc R, et al. Use of rhomboid flap and double Z-plasty technique in the treatment of chronic postburn contractures. *Burns* 2006;32(6):765–769.

8. Clark JM, Wang TD. Local flaps in scar revision. *Facial Plast Surg* 2001;17(4):295–308.

9. Schweinfurth JM, Fedok F. Avoiding pitfalls and unfavorable outcomes in scar revision. *Facial Plast Surg* 2001;17(4):273–278.

10. Mobley SR. Combining multiple surgical techniques for maximum scar camouflage. *Ear Nose Throat J* 2005;84(7):408–409.

11. Fader DJ, Wang TS, Johnson TM. The Z-plasty transposition flap for reconstruction of the middle cheek. *J Am Acad Dermatol* 2002;46(5):738–742.

12. Rodgers BJ, Williams EF, Hove CR. W-plasty and geometric broken line closure. *Facial Plast Surg* 2001;17(4):239–244.

13. Mostafapour SP, Murakami CS. Tissue expansion and serial excision in scar revision. *Facial Plast Surg* 2001;17(4):245–252.

14. Lee KK, Mehrany K, Swanson NA. Surgical revision. *Dermatol Clin* 2005;23(1):141–150, vii.

15. Leach J. Proper handling of soft tissue in the acute phase. *Facial Plast Surg* 2001;17(4):227–238.

16. Capon A, Iarmarcovai G, Mordon S. Laser-assisted skin healing (LASH) in hypertrophic scar revision. *J Cosmet Laser Ther* 2009;11(4):220–223.

17. Capon A, Iarmarcovai G, Gonnelli D, et al. Scar prevention using laser-assisted skin healing (LASH) in plastic surgery. *Aesthetic Plast Surg* 2010;34(4):438–446.

18. Asilian A, Darougheh A, Shariati F. New combination of triamcinolone, 5-fluorouracil, and pulsed-dye laser for treatment of keloid and hypertrophic scars. *Dermatol Surg* 2006;32(7):907–915.

19. Manuskiatti W, Fitzpatrick RE. Treatment response of keloidal and hypertrophic sternotomy scars: comparison among intralesional corticosteroid, 5-fluorouracil, and 585-nm flashlamp-pumped pulsed-dye laser treatments. *Arch Dermatol* 2002;138(9):1149–1155.

20. D'Andrea F, Brongo S, Ferraro G, et al. Prevention and treatment of keloids with intralesional verapamil. *Dermatology* 2002;204(1):60–62.

21. Skaria AM. Prevention and treatment of keloids with intralesional verapamil. *Dermatology* 2004;209(1):71.

22. Espana A, Solano T, Quintanilla E. Bleomycin in the treatment of keloids and hypertrophic scars by multiple needle punctures. *Dermatol Surg* 2001;27(1):23–27.

23. Naeini FF, Najafian J, Ahmadpour K. Bleomycin tattooing as a promising therapeutic modality in large keloids and hypertrophic scars. *Dermatol Surg* 2006;32(8):1023–1029; discussion 1029–1030.

24. Fitzpatrick RE. Treatment of inflamed hypertrophic scars using intralesional 5-FU. *Dermatol Surg* 1999;25(3):224–232.

25. Uppal RS, Khan U, Kakar S, et al. The effects of a single dose of 5-fluorouracil on keloid scars: a clinical trial of timed wound irrigation after extralesional excision. *Plast Reconstr Surg* 2001;108(5):1218–1224.

26. Berman B, Flores F. Recurrence rates of excised keloids treated with postoperative triamcinolone acetonide injections or interferon alfa-2b injections. *J Am Acad Dermatol* 1997;37(5 Pt 1):755–757.

27. Elsaie ML, Choudhary S. Lasers for scars: a review and evidence-based appraisal. *J Drugs Dermatol* 2010;9(11):1355–1362.

28. Kim S, Cho KH. Clinical trial of dual treatment with an ablative fractional laser and a nonablative laser for the treatment of acne scars in Asian patients. *Dermatol Surg* 2009;35(7):1089–1098.

29. Pham AM, Greene RM, Woolery-Lloyd H, et al. 1550-nm nonablative laser resurfacing for facial surgical scars. *Arch Facial Plast Surg* 2011;13(3):203–210.

30. Alster TS, Tanzi EL, Lazarus M. The use of fractional laser photothermolysis for the treatment of atrophic scars. *Dermatol Surg* 2007;33(3):295–299.

31. Har-Shai Y, Amar M, Sabo E. Intralesional cryotherapy for enhancing the involution of hypertrophic scars and keloids. *Plast Reconstr Surg* 2003;111(6):1841–1852.

32. Zouboulis CC, Rosenberger AD, Forster T, et al. Modification of a device and its application for intralesional cryosurgery of old recalcitrant keloids. *Arch Dermatol* 2004;140(10):1293–1294.

33. English RS, Shenefelt PD. Keloids and hypertrophic scars. *Dermatol Surg* 1999;25(8):631–638.

34. Klein AW. Skin filling. Collagen and other injectables of the skin. *Dermatol Clin* 2001;19(3):491–508, ix.

35. van der Velden EM, Defranq J, van der Dussen MF. Dermatography as an adjunctive treatment of uni- and bilateral scars in combination with pseudo-hair formation after craniosurgery. *J Craniofac Surg* 2004;15(2):270–273.

36. Berman B, Perez OA, Konda S, et al. A review of the biologic effects, clinical efficacy, and safety of silicone elastomer sheeting for hypertrophic and keloid scar treatment and management. *Dermatol Surg* 2007;33(11):1291–1302; discussion 1302–1293.

37. Mustoe TA. Evolution of silicone therapy and mechanism of action in scar management. *Aesthetic Plast Surg* 2008;32(1):82–92.

38. Baumann LS, Spencer J. The effects of topical vitamin E on the cosmetic appearance of scars. *Dermatol Surg* 1999;25(4):311–315.

39. Jackson BA, Shelton AJ. Pilot study evaluating topical onion extract as treatment for postsurgical scars. *Dermatol Surg* 1999;25(4):267–269.

40. Berman B. Imiquimod: a new immune response modifier for the treatment of external genital warts and other diseases in dermatology. *Int J Dermatol* 2002;41(Suppl 1):7–11.

Nasal Reconstruction 177

Stephen S. Park

Nasal reconstruction has evolved significantly from early, rudimentary attempts to provide covering for large nasal defects. In contemporary nasal reconstruction, surgeons combine a mastery of aesthetics and surgical techniques, to create a nose that is visually inconspicuous and functionally stable. This is expected to hold up throughout the life of the patient. Ancient methods focused on using soft tissue to fill the cavity, with little regard for structural framework, internal lining, intranasal airspace, and intrinsic contours. Nasal reconstruction in the 21st century has raised the bar to a level where the new nose may go unnoticed by the casual observer, nasal function returns to the baseline, and the patient integrates back into society without undue self-consciousness.

HISTORY OF NASAL RECONSTRUCTION

The history of nasal reconstruction dates back to antiquity when, during the fourth Egyptian dynasty (2575–2467 BC), prostheses were molded for the deceased, because "only those without physical disfigurement would enter the Kingdom of Osiris" (1). Reconstruction came into greater demand with the rise of nasal mutilation as a common form of humiliation or punishment. Around 1500 BC, when Prince Lakshmana of India deliberately amputated the nose of Lady Surpunakha, King Ravana arranged for the reconstruction of Lady Surpanakha's nose by his physicians, documenting one of the earliest accounts of nasal restoration in human history (2,3). *Sushruta Samhita*, an ancient Indian Sanskrit written during the Vedic period (600–1000 BC), describes nasal reconstruction as performed by a caste of Indian potters, using cheek tissue to cover the nasal defect (4). Early descriptions of using forehead tissue to repair a nasal defect exist in writings by the Kangiara family from 1440 AD (5). Despite the long history with this type of reconstruction, very little international exchange occurred because of the lack of maritime commerce and little communication between Europe and Asia during that period. In the 16th century, Gusparo Tagliacozzi described his success with a two-staged method of nasal reconstruction using a pedicled, cutaneous flap from the upper arm, based on the brachial vessels. This was followed by attempts with pedicled flaps from other individuals, especially slaves. Outcomes were obviously discouraging, and further progression was shortly abandoned.

In 1794, the first description of the Indian forehead flap in the English language was published in the *Madras Gazette* and later reproduced in *Gentleman's Magazine* (6). Joseph Carpue (7), an English general surgeon, is credited with the introduction of this forehead flap to the Western world when he described his experience with two successful "Indian forehead flaps" for nasal reconstruction. Subsequently, the classic forehead flap for nasal reconstruction became widespread throughout the globe and defined the standard method of repair during the early 19th century. This "classic" Indian median forehead flap was based on bilateral supratrochlear arteries with a wide pedicle that could not extend beyond the level of the brows. The wide base limited the rotation and length of the forehead flap. This limitation became more evident when it was recognized that intranasal lining left to heal by second intention resulted in significant distortion, contracture, and nasal obstruction. This restricted design could not be designed to line the intranasal defect.

Pedicled flaps moved slowly to the United States; the first American reports of forehead flaps for nasal reconstructions are from the 1940s (8,9). These early flaps were traditional "median" forehead flaps with wide pedicle bases capturing both supratrochlear vessels. Kazanjian and Converse believed that the paired arteries were needed to adequately perfuse the forehead flap. Because of the limited length of this early median forehead flap, many variations were described, largely aimed at mobilizing more tissue with greater flap length: "Gillies' up-and-down flap" (10), "New's sickle flap" (11), "Converse's scalping flap" (12), and the "Washio flap" (13). In spite of the variety of flaps attempted, none have stood the test of time primarily because of the poor quality of scalp skin in contrast to forehead skin and the significant donor site morbidity.

Millard repopularized the paramedian flap with a "seagull" design for resurfacing the nose (14–17). The primary advantage of this paramedian flap was the narrow pedicle base, which allowed for an improved arc of rotation. The inferior reach of the flap could be further extended by basing the pedicle below the level of the brow. This design created less narrowing of the brows in contrast to the original "median" forehead flap. Millard also noted that the supratrochlear artery traveled in a plane between the skin and frontalis muscle, and, consequently, the frontalis muscle could be selectively trimmed off the undersurface of the flap without jeopardizing flap vascularity. Gary Burget and Fred Menick (18) have since refined these concepts of the paramedian forehead flap design and have brought nasal reconstruction to its higher standards.

ETIOLOGY OF NASAL DEFECTS

Defects of the nose arise from a large array of causes, and, on many occasions, it is worthwhile to consider the specific etiology as it may impact the method of repair. The nose is the most common site for *de novo* cutaneous malignancies. Basal cell carcinomas predominate, and there are histologic subtypes with varying degrees of aggressiveness. The nodular subtype is most common, as characterized by a circumscribed growth pattern, and carries the most favorable prognosis. Aggressive histologic subtypes, such as the morpheaform or infiltrating, can develop small nest patterns and are more likely to involve the internal lining or to recur following surgical excision. These latter subtypes are best treated with Mohs surgery. Squamous cell carcinoma is the second most common type and also behaves aggressively, with a greater incidence of regional metastasis. Melanoma is the most serious skin tumor, warranting an aggressive surgical intervention. Recurrent skin tumors or tumors that have been previously irradiated have a less predictable vascular anatomy, which may impact flap design and closure options. Vascular and adnexal tumors of the nose are less common but often require more aggressive treatment plans. Sharp and blunt trauma to the nose, such as from motor vehicle accidents, can lead to nasal defects with associated variables for consideration. Animal or human bites are grossly contaminated, and a delay in repair is often advocated. This dogma arises from experience with extremity injuries; however, the face is characterized by such a robust vascularity that immediate repair will often be successful.

NASAL ANATOMY

A firm understanding of the normal nasal anatomy is a prerequisite for mastery of nasal reconstruction. The biomechanics of covering flaps, the importance of a firm framework, and the anatomic basis for internal lining repair are imperative concepts as one proceeds through the algorithm of reparative options.

The *external nasal skin* is variable at different areas of the nose, being thick at the nasion and tip and extremely thin along the rhinion. The thin epithelial sleeve along the alar rim and nasal facets makes these areas especially vulnerable to notching and contour irregularities following reconstruction.

There are four layers of *soft tissue* between the skin and the nasal skeleton—the superficial fatty panniculus, fibromuscular layer, deep fatty layer, and, finally, the periosteum or perichondrium. The superficial fatty panniculus is located immediately below the skin and consists of adipose tissue with interlacing vertical fibrous septi coursing from the deep dermis to the underlying fibromuscular layer. The fibromuscular layer contains the intrinsic nasal musculature and the nasal superficial musculoaponeurotic system (SMAS), which is a continuation of the facial aponeurotic system. The deep fatty layer located between the SMAS and the thin covering of the nasal skeleton contains the major superficial blood vessels and nerves. The periosteum of the nasal bones extends over the upper lateral cartilages and fuses with the periosteum of the piriform process laterally (19). Perichondrium covers the nasal cartilages, and dense fibrous interconnections can be found between the paired tip cartilages. Between the framework and the deep fatty layer is a plane of loose areolar tissue that is free of fibrous septa, making it an ideal plane for dissection and elevation of the soft tissue envelope.

The *nasal musculature* of the nose is well defined, with greatest activity along the junction of the upper lateral and alar cartilages (20). This allows for muscular dilation and stenting of the functionally critical nasal valve area. All nasal musculature is innervated by the zygomatic division of the facial nerve (21).

The nasal *blood supply* is via a predictable and consistent network of named vessels through both the internal and external carotid systems. The angular artery branches from the facial artery and is a discrete landmark along the nasofacial junction. Feeder vessels off the angular artery perforate the levator labii superioris and provide the vascular basis for the design of melolabial flaps. A medial branch off the angular artery, the lateral nasal artery, supplies the lateral surface of the caudal nose. This lateral nasal artery courses in the sulcus between the ala and nasal sidewall and is covered by the levator labii superioris alaeque nasi. It arborizes multiple times to enter the subdermal plexus covering the nostril and cheek and is the anatomic basis for many small local flaps within the lateral nasal wall, for example, bilobe flaps. The dorsal nasal artery, a branch of the ophthalmic artery, pierces the orbital septum above the medial palpebral ligament and travels inferiorly along the side of the nose to anastomose with the lateral nasal artery. The dorsal nasal artery provides a rich axial blood supply to the dorsal nasal skin and serves as the main arterial contributor to dorsal nasal flaps. The columella and tip are supplied by the paired columellar arteries, branches of the superior labial artery. The external nasal branch of the anterior ethmoidal artery, a branch of the ophthalmic artery, pierces bone on the medial wall of the orbit at the point where the lamina papyracea of the ethmoid bone articulates with the orbital portion of the frontal bone (frontoethmoid suture). The vessel enters the ethmoid sinuses to supply the mucosa and sends branches to the superior aspect of the nasal cavity. The external nasal branch of the anterior ethmoidal artery emerges between the nasal bone and the upper lateral cartilage to supply the skin covering the nasal dorsum and tip. The venous drainage of the external nose is through corresponding vessels, leading into the facial vein, the pterygoid plexus, and the valveless ophthalmic veins.

The *intranasal mucosa* has a similar number of named vessels, and they are critical when designing mucosal flaps for full-thickness nasal defects. The septal branch of the superior labial artery is a dominant feeder to the septal mucosa. In fact, a flap of the entire septal mucosa, back to the sphenoid sinus, can be based on this single vessel. The anterior and posterior ethmoidal vessels supply the superior portion of the septum. Terminal branches of the anterior ethmoidal artery cover the dorsal nasal septum, a critical region for the swinging, composite septal flaps used for internal lining and structure. Terminal branches of the sphenopalatine artery supply the posterior septum and posterior lateral nasal wall. The vasculature of the internal nose is the anatomic basis for complex nasal reconstruction.

The *sensory nerve* to the nasal skin is via the ophthalmic and maxillary divisions of the fifth cranial nerve. Branches of the supratrochlear and infratrochlear nerves supply the skin covering the radix, rhinion, and cephalic portion of the nasal sidewalls. The external nasal branch of the anterior ethmoidal nerve supplies the skin over the caudal half of the nose. The infraorbital nerve provides sensory branches to the skin of the lateral aspect of the nose.

The *structural framework* of the nose is composed of the paired nasal bones to the upper third, the nasal septum and upper lateral cartilages to the middle vault, and the paired lower lateral cartilages within the nasal tip. Dorsal support to the middle vault is primarily achieved through the rigidity of the cartilaginous septum and, to a lesser extent, the paired upper lateral cartilages. Their fusion at the midline is important clinically because of the tendency for the upper lateral cartilages to progressively contract intranasally and lead to obstruction. If a disarticulation between the septum and upper lateral cartilages occurs, the middle vault should be diligently reconstructed.

The tip is supported by the overall size and strength of the lower lateral cartilages, their ligamentous attachments to the caudal septum, the scroll with the upper lateral cartilages, and the adherence to the overlying soft tissue. Each lower lateral cartilage is subdivided into the medial, intermediate, and lateral crura. The shape, length, and angulation of the intermediate crura determine the external morphology of the tip lobule and the position of the tip-defining point. Disruption or weakening of the lateral crus predisposes to alar retraction and notching, an important consideration in nasal reconstruction when these structures may have been compromised. Laterally, small sesamoid cartilages are interconnected by a dense, fibrous connective tissue.

The *alar lobule and nasal sidewall* is a functionally pivotal area of the nose that is not often highlighted during rhinoplasty discussions but has a critical role during reconstructive surgery. This *keystone* region is located between the lateral border of the lower lateral cartilage and the bony piriform aperture. Externally, it corresponds to the supra-alar crease and is the most common location for a clinically significant, dynamic valve collapse. Beneath the skin, the area consists of a firm, fibrous-fatty aponeurosis, an occasional sesamoid cartilage, and a portion of the transverse nasalis muscle. Typically, this histologic architecture provides sufficient rigidity to prevent collapse during inspiration. If compromised, nasal function will be impaired unless it is aggressively restored with liberal grafting in a nonanatomic fashion. The *internal nasal valve* is a distinct area defined by the dorsal septum medially, upper lateral cartilage superolaterally, and the head of the inferior turbinate inferomedially. The *external nasal valve* is the cross-sectional area under the alar lobule proper. It does not entirely correlate with the lateral crus of the lower lateral cartilages. The alar rim does not have cartilage within it, and collapse or notching can readily occur. To avoid this, structural grafts to the alar rim are often needed. The junction between the ala and cheek forms an acute angle and is difficult to reconstruct; most repairs heal with gradual effacement of that alar–facial angle and may become increasingly conspicuous. If at all possible, one should try to preserve the alar–facial junction and keep incisions slightly onto the nose. The *limen vestibuli* is the junction between the internal nasal lining and the stratified squamous epithelium of the nose. It does not lie at the caudalmost border of the alar lobule but rather slightly intranasally, within the vestibule. Reconstruction of full-thickness defects of the alar rim should keep this in mind and allow the resurfacing flap to roll inward before suturing to the internal lining flap.

There is a *bony piriform platform* that surrounds the nose, and its role in tissue support is often poorly appreciated. The nasal sill, anterior nasal spine, and medial maxilla (including the frontal process of the maxilla) provide an essential platform for the nose, and resection of these structures will require a separate repair, such as with a split calvarial bone graft. Failure to rebuild this platform will often result in a soft tissue collapse and facial asymmetry.

DEFECT ANALYSIS

Analyzing a given defect and arriving at the ideal method of repair is a challenging and rewarding exercise. On occasion, the "correct" flap will be intuitive, as it appears to define itself. At other times, it can be a creative dilemma as one struggles to visualize the incisions, flap transfer, surrounding vectors of tension, and final scars. This mental challenge requires a dynamic, three-dimensional image of the nasal repair. At times, it is worthwhile to have a structured algorithm for defect analysis. Although it does not necessarily define the ideal flap, it can be very useful in avoiding errors in design. In particular, the line of questioning can guide one away from creating disfiguring mistakes such as eyelid retraction or an unnatural hairline. Once flaps are elevated and transposition is attempted, the reconstruction is committed; this is clearly not the time to discover a gross design flaw.

For every cutaneous defect, there are six questions that are reviewed prior to the first incision (Table 177.1):

1. *Immobile structures.* What surrounding landmarks must not come under any tension during flap transposition, such as the eyelid, alar margin, or upper lip? It does not necessarily mean that tissue cannot be recruited from that region but rather, adequate structure must be available in the area to fully support the adjacent flap. A common example is a cheek flap that risks lower-eyelid retraction and is vertically supported with anchors to the infraorbital rim. For the nose, there are three "immobile structures": the alar rim, nasal base symmetry, and lateral nasal wall. The immobility of the lateral nasal wall is a unique concept. Most flaps are thought of in two dimensions. The nose, as a three-dimensional structure, has an important lumen. The additional vector of tension is in this third dimension, perpendicular to the cutaneous plane. Local flaps tend to create a force perpendicular to the plane of rotation, leading to sidewall collapse and functional compromise. Recognition of this concept allows one to plan the reconstruction with prophylactic support grafts.
2. *Area of recruitment.* Given which surrounding areas are "immobile," from where can tissue be recruited without distorting those areas? Also, in what direction do the lines of maximal extensibility exist and how can the flap be designed to slide parallel with them?
3. *Facial lines.* There are numerous descriptions of facial lines that can assist with flap selection and design. Langer lines were first described by Langer (19) in 1861 as a recommendation for orienting elliptical

skin excisions. Circular defects in postmortem patients became elliptical as rigor mortis ensued, and these lines were mapped throughout the body. Clinical practice has shown that these lines do not always orient along lines for optimal healing. Relaxed skin tension lines (RSTLs) more accurately reflect the intrinsic tension within the dermis while at rest. Wounds heal under less tension when oriented along them, and they can usually assist with flap design. Lines of minimal tension (also known as skin creases) are defined by the repeated contraction of the underlying muscle as they permanently orient elastin and collagen fibers within the dermis. These lines usually run parallel with the RSTLs, but the supratip, glabella, and lateral canthal regions are in conflict. It is usually recommended to incise along lines of minimal tension rather than RSTLs.

The other "facial lines" that exist in the face are those created by the borders of *aesthetic units* and the subunits of the nose. The principle of aesthetic units is based on the fact that the human eye can only perceive things as a series of block images, thus our inability to scan a horizon without a saccadic motion. The face, or nose, is visualized as a discrete set of block images that are put together subconsciously and interpreted as a single image. These images are defined by predictable reflections of light, natural creases, and undulations in cutaneous topography. The nose has subunits defined as the nasal tip, dorsum, columella,

TABLE 177.1	DEFECT ANALYSIS

1. Immobile structures
2. Area of recruitment
3. Facial lines
4. Resultant scars
5. Nasal function
6. Depth

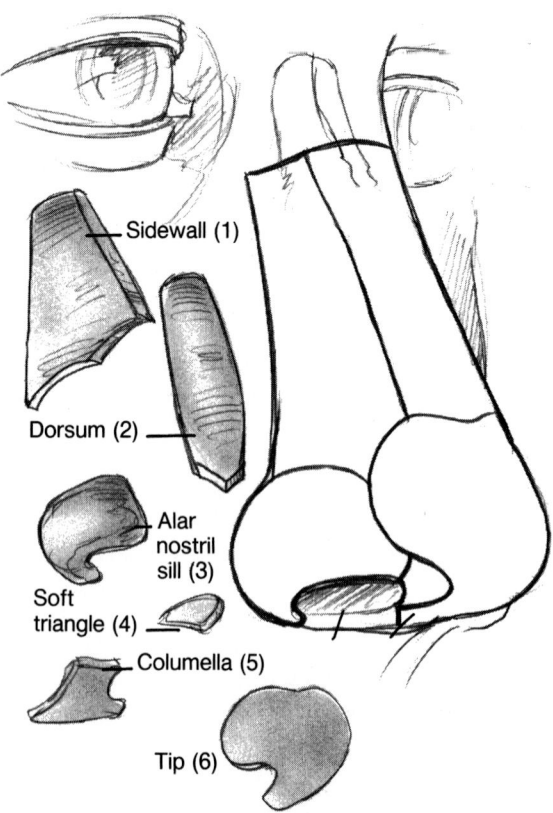

Figure 177.1 Nasal aesthetic subunits.

paired ala, sidewalls, and soft tissue facets (Fig. 177.1). Scars that are strategically placed at the border of two units will be less conspicuous than those resting within one. In order to achieve this, one usually has to modify the size/shape of the original cutaneous defect. The aesthetic subunits may require modifications with some patient groups who have other unique nasal characteristics. At times, a patient may have a significant transition from one skin type to another within the nose, such as individuals with rosacea or a rhinophyma (20).

4. *Resultant scars.* One should anticipate the final scars for each proposed flap and how they relate to preexisting facial lines. At times, this exercise is not intuitive, such as the resultant scars of a rhombic flap. This question forces the surgeon to try different orientations of flap design that might yield more favorable scars while still abiding by the previous tenets of immobile structures and area of recruitment.

5. *Function.* During the defect analysis, one of the essential considerations is the *location* in terms of function and potential lateral wall collapse. A cutaneous defect involving the critical area along the supra-alar crease will place the nasal airway at jeopardy even if the original defect does not violate native cartilage. This critical "red zone" must alert the reconstructive surgeon of the need for structural reinforcement in the form of cartilage grafting. Anatomically, it corresponds to the fibroareolar tissue immediately lateral to the lateral crus of the lower lateral cartilage and is distinct from the precise *internal* and *external nasal valves.* Similarly sized defects along the dorsum or upper third do not have the associated functional concerns.

6. *Depth.* Assessing the depth of the nasal defect is important to determine if any structural cartilage or bone is missing and to explore the internal nasal lining. Any violation of the intranasal mucosa must be recognized preoperatively, as it will alter the reconstructive plan significantly; all missing lining must be meticulously repaired prior to grafting and resurfacing. Failure to do so will risk contracture, lumen stenosis, graft exposure and resorption, and alar notching.

SMALL CUTANEOUS DEFECTS

Cutaneous defects of the nose can be found in a variety of sizes, depths, and shapes. Intuitively, the smaller ones should be more straightforward in terms of repair, but that is often not the case. Whereas large defects have a limited number of options, those less than 1.5 cm can be repaired with an array of flaps and grafts, often creating a greater intellectual challenge. Furthermore, patient expectations are generally higher with small lesions, and even small irregularities that often plague these repairs can be problematic, such as alar base asymmetry, notching, conspicuous scars, pincushioning, or valve collapse.

Pertinent Anatomy

Nasal topography during reconstruction is often discussed in terms of aesthetic subunits, but since smaller defects frequently involve only small portions of an individual site, it is more practical to discuss the defect in terms of the upper, middle, and lower thirds of the nose. The *upper third* has relatively thin skin except for the nasion region, where the subcutaneous tissue is much more prominent. The lateral borders are adjacent to the medial canthus and represent *immobile* regions that cannot be distorted, especially from contracture during second-intention healing. The area of recruitment is primarily from the glabella and, to a lesser extent, from the nasal dorsum. There is little functional concern with defects in this zone.

The *middle third* of the nose has skin that is thin medially but thicker laterally. Whereas the upper lateral cartilages support the medial portion of this zone, the lateral aspect has support only from fibroareolar tissue without native cartilage. Tissue can be recruited from multiple directions, but any vertical vector must be minimal, as ala or tip elevation can quickly occur. Functional implications are important along the lateral aspect of the middle vault, even if no native cartilage has been violated. The lateral nasal artery is found immediately cephalad to the supra-alar crease and is the basis for many local flaps of the nose.

The *lower third* of the nose consists of the nasal tip, alar lobule, columella, and soft tissue triangle. The skin is typically thicker and more sebaceous, leading to less favorable wound healing. Most defects of this region are repaired with tissue recruited from the middle vault, but great care must go into flap design and the subsequent vectors of tension. This zone is significant for its free alar margin and the fact that small degrees of wound contracture may lead to retraction and gross alar base asymmetries. The supra-alar crease and alar–facial junction are important natural landmarks that should be preserved or recreated. The alar lobule proper does not contain native cartilage, and disruption to this area predisposes to a dynamic external nasal valve collapse. Consequently, nonanatomic cartilage grafting is essential to prevent alar rim retraction and collapse.

SELECTION OF GRAFTS AND FLAPS

At times, the simplest method of repair is also the preferred one in terms of optimal aesthetic results. Second-intention healing, skin and composite grafts, and local flaps all enter the algorithm for repair of such defects, and proper selection becomes the cornerstone for a successful outcome (Table 177.2) (21). Individuals with a large nose, prominent hump, or broad nasal tip can have their nose reduced slightly, and it will not only create more tissue for recruitment but also reduce the relative size of the defect. The use of common aesthetic rhinoplasty maneuvers in the setting of nasal reconstruction can be a powerful tool. Hump reduction, cephalic trim, tip sutures, etc., all can have great

TABLE 177.2	COMMON RECONSTRUCTIVE OPTIONS FOR SMALL CUTANEOUS DEFECTS
Upper 1/3	1. Local transposition flaps 2. Full-thickness skin graft 3. Second intention
Middle 1/3	1. Primary closure (midline or paramedian) 2. Full-thickness skin graft (in combination with #1 above) 3. Bilobe transposition flap 4. Single-stage forehead flap
Lower 1/3	1. Primary closure (midline, broad tip; with/without FTSG) 2. Bilobe transposition flap 3. Composite graft (alar rim, columella) 4. Interpolated melolabial flap (ala, columella; with cartilage graft)

utility with medium size nasal defects. For many defects, this maneuver can allow the transition from a more complex repair to a simpler one with local flaps or grafts.

Upper Third

Smaller defects in this zone are readily repaired with either a full-thickness skin graft or by second-intention healing. Those larger than 1.5 cm can be resurfaced with a sliding glabellar or Rieger flap (22). Other transposition flaps recruited from the forehead and middle third of the nose are less common alternatives.

Middle Third

Small midline defects are often amenable to primary closure with wide undermining and recruitment from lateral nasal tissue; this often represents the first option for optimal repair. It will leave a vertically oriented central scar with tension evenly distributed, thus maintaining nasal symmetry. Many times, a medium-sized defect in the midline can be converted to a small defect with partial closure through bilateral advancement flaps, leaving a residual defect in the midline. The remainder can be resurfaced with a full-thickness skin graft, harvested from the standing cutaneous deformities of the primary closure. This skin is ideally suited for this because of the excellent color/texture match and lack of donor site morbidity. Small transposition flaps (rhombic, bilobe, rotation) are frequently utilized and represent another workhorse repair for this region. Skin grafts can blend in well with the thin skin of this zone, but even small contour depressions are difficult to disguise, as their shadows often remain conspicuous. If a cartilage graft is needed along the lateral wall, a

vascularized resurfacing flap is needed. Those larger than 1.5 cm often require a more elaborate flap.

Lower Third

Precise midline defects are ideally suited for primary closure, particularly when the premorbid nasal tip is somewhat bulbous and can afford to be narrowed. Like the middle vault, partial closure with skin grafting from the standing cutaneous deformity is a useful technique. A bilobe flap is often utilized for defects of the nasal tip, allowing the tension to be distributed more widely and at an adequate distance from the free alar margin. The alar lobule is often repaired with composite grafts, restoring structure and covering simultaneously. Smaller defects limited to the supra-alar crease can do well through second-intention healing, but moderately sized defects will jeopardize nasal patency. The single-stage melolabial flap can also be used; however, the supra-alar crease is often obliterated and asymmetry can result if the contralateral supra-alar crease is deep and prominent. A two-stage, interpolated melolabial flap is preferable for larger defects of the alar lobule, especially when cartilage grafts have been placed and the aesthetic unit completed. Small, full-thickness defects involving the alar margin are best repaired with a three-layered composite graft from the ear, whereas larger ones require a multilayered reconstruction involving the internal lining, structural framework, and resurfacing. The columella is characterized by a very narrow column of thin skin and lends itself well to small composite and skin grafts. For larger columellar defects, structural grafting along with a pedicled melolabial flap is most often used. The soft tissue triangle defect is ideally restored by allowing second-intention healing to occur with a natural-appearing web.

TECHNIQUES FOR GRAFTS AND FLAPS

Second-Intention Healing

Local wound care is the most important aspect when selecting this method of repair. Keeping the wound bed moist and preventing the development of a dry eschar will encourage the most prompt and favorable healing. Cytotoxic agents, especially hydrogen peroxide, should be avoided. A *guiding suture* can be employed in a similar fashion to the purse-string closures used for large defects on the scalp and face. This guiding suture partially closes a small defect and allows the remainder to heal secondarily. The greatest utility of this suture is for small defects along the alar rim. The suture can be placed horizontally, thus converting the circular defect into a vertical elliptical shape, which resists the vertical contracture that will ensue. The suture itself will often notch the alar rim inferiorly slightly, but it contracts to a normal position during healing. The suture is removed after 2 to 3 weeks. This technique will allow more defects to be managed in a conservative fashion.

Skin and Composite Grafts

Superficial defects can be immediately repaired with full-thickness skin grafts and perform well (Table 177.3). For deeper defects, or those exposing bare cartilage, it may be prudent to delay the repair for 10 days allowing a layer of granulation tissue to accumulate within the recipient bed. This enhances vascularity and fills in the depression, thereby improving surface contour. The defect shape is modified, in order to create straight lines with square corners, rather than leaving a circular defect. The entire aesthetic subunit is not necessarily completed. Wound margins are beveled toward the center of the defect in order to smooth the transition between graft and the native nasal skin. Skin grafts can be harvested from the supraclavicular fossa, periauricular skin, and melolabial area. Graft thickness is modified following harvest to best match the surrounding skin texture, especially along the nasal tip, where thicker skin is found. Small "pie crusts" can be cut into the graft to allow the egress of serous fluid, recognizing that these perforations often become discolored and remain noticeable. A bolster dressing is rarely needed on the nose as long as small tacking sutures are placed to maintain close apposition between the graft and recipient bed.

A two- or three-layered composite graft is usually taken from the ear—either the root of the helix, the conchal bowl, or the triangular fossa. Anterior auricular skin is tightly adhered to auricular cartilage and has a good success rate. The shape of the cartilage is usually concave toward the skin, and although this shape can be unfavorable for external resurfacing, it is ideal for internal lining. The auricular donor site is closed primarily with little distortion. Excising cartilage from the apices of the donor site can avoid the "cookie bite" deformity to the ear. The composite graft must be securely attached to the nose, often with through-and-through sutures or a small bolster. These grafts are ideally suited for defects along the alar rim and columella (Fig. 177.2). Many composite grafts will appear moderately dusky for a week but will usually recover during the ensuing days. Larger grafts may undergo a degree of epidermolysis, which will lead to a less favorable color and texture match. Three-layered composite grafts are kept less than 1.5 cm because the sole blood supply is from the peripheral margin. Two-layered composite grafts, on the other hand, can be designed larger because the nourishing bed is the entire surface area of the graft. When utilizing these larger, two-layered composite grafts, one can excise several small, 2-mm punch holes through the cartilage only, taking care not to puncture the overlying skin. These small perforations will allow granulation tissue to penetrate the cartilage and nourish the epithelial covering.

Primary Closure

Primary closure with wide undermining is an excellent option for many small cutaneous nasal defects, especially those located in the precise midline of the lower two-thirds of the nose and when the tip is modestly wide or bulbous to begin with. Lateral undermining over the perichondrium, and deep to the nasal SMAS layer, is essential. The elliptical design requires that the vertical apices extend further superiorly and inferiorly than the traditional 30-degree angles, in order to avoid an asymmetric narrowing of the nose. Failure to do so will narrow the nose at the site of the original defect while leaving the supratip or infratip segments disproportionately wide. Common rhinoplasty maneuvers, such as an interdomal suture and cephalic trim, are frequently utilized concomitantly in order to narrow the tip, reduce wound tension, and facilitate primary closure. These bilateral advancement flaps are very useful for medium-sized defects that are partially closed and convert the defect to a smaller one. The remainder is resurfaced with a full-thickness skin graft from the standing cutaneous deformities of the local flaps (Fig. 177.3A–H).

Defects that are off midline will leave a paramedian vertical scar and may create nasal asymmetry because of uneven recruitment and tension. In those circumstances, an "east–west" flap can be designed to control the resultant scars and move the standing cutaneous deformity to a favorable location in the midline (Fig. 177.4A–D).

Rhombic Flap

The design of the classic Limberg rhombic flap was originally described in 1946 and remains a versatile flap with predictable scars and vectors of tension (23). Because the resultant scar crosses all aesthetic units, it is difficult to orient the flaps such that scars are maximally camouflaged. In order to minimize wound tension, however, flaps are specifically designed such that the vectors of tension parallel those lines of maximal tissue recruitment. In the nose, this laxity is usually from the lateral nasal wall and medial cheek. In addition, an inferiorly based flap tends to have fewer problems with postoperative congestion and edema.

Bilobe Flap

The bilobe flap is widely used for a small nasal defect because it allows one to distribute tension further from the

TABLE 177.3	PEARLS FOR SKIN AND COMPOSITE GRAFTS

1. Consider delay for granulation tissue.
2. Square wound borders.
3. Bevel edges toward defect.
4. Minimize "pie crusts."
5. Small perforations through cartilage for larger composite grafts can help.
6. No dead space—consider a bolster or tacking sutures.

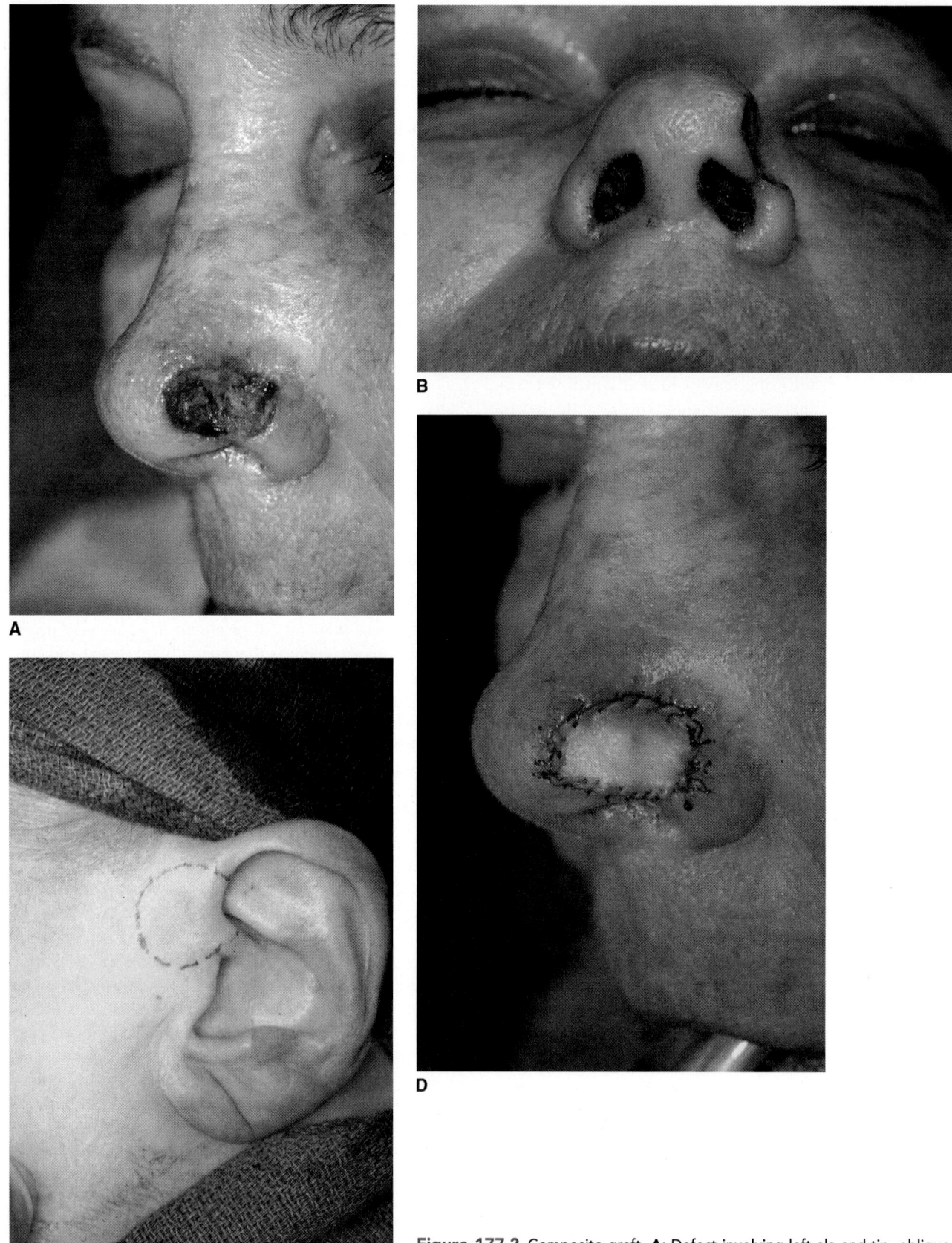

Figure 177.2 Composite graft. **A**: Defect involving left ala and tip, oblique view. **B**: Base view. **C**: Composite graft from left ear. **D**: Graft secured in defect. A tacking bolster will be secured.

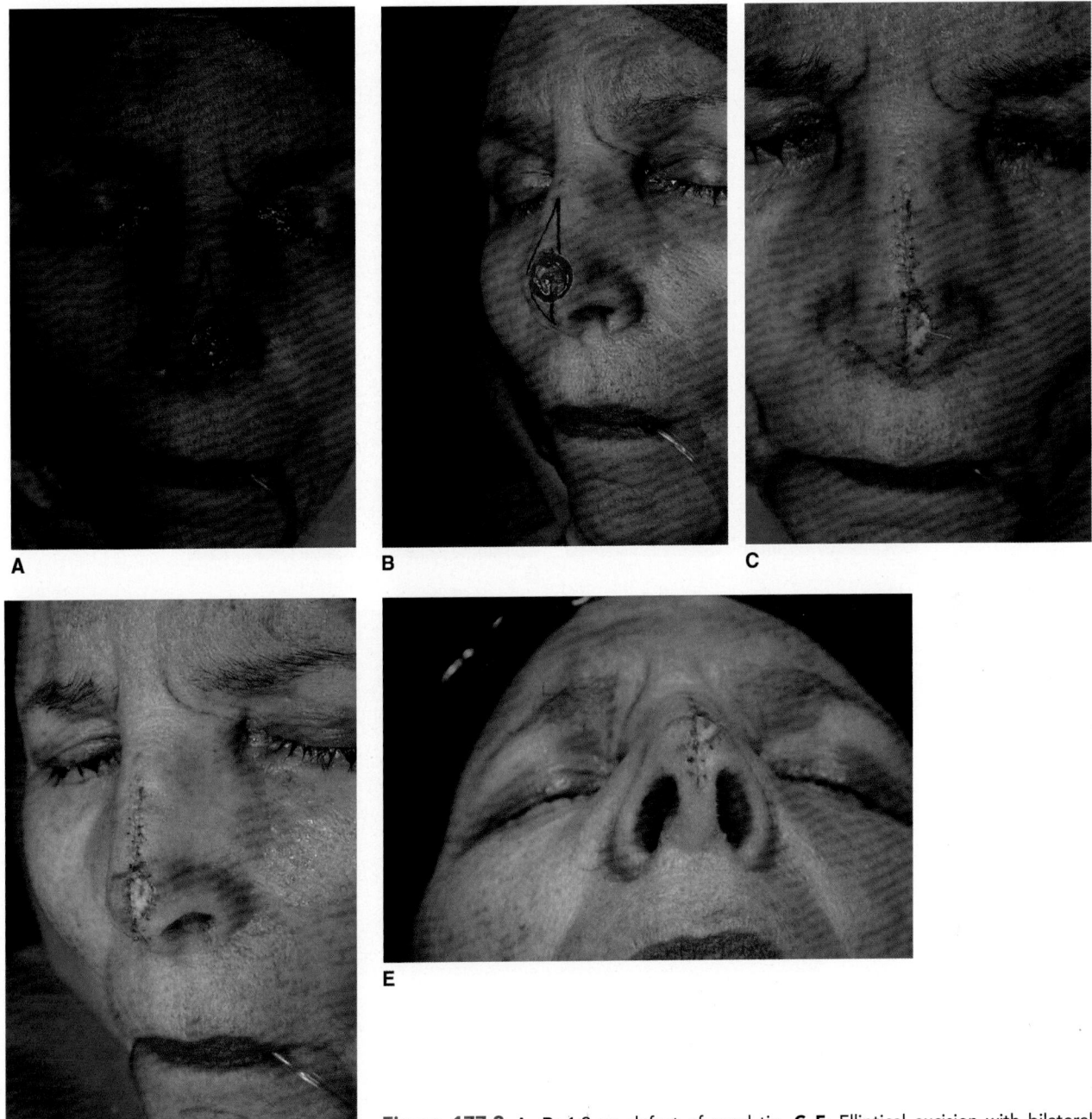

Figure 177.3 A, B: 1.2-cm defect of nasal tip. **C–E:** Elliptical excision with bilateral advancement flaps to close 80% and FTSG to cover remainder (harvested from standing cutaneous deformity of nose).

primary defect, thus controlling the degree of tension along the alar margin. Whereas early designs utilized a 180-degree arch of rotation, contemporary methods have narrowed this angle in order to minimize the standing cutaneous deformity (24). Common sequelae to these flaps include postoperative edema and "pincushioning," which can arise from several factors: (a) the curvilinear scars of the flap design will undergo natural contraction and, as they shorten, tend to bunch and lift the skin paddle of the flap; (b) a bilobe is relatively wide with respect to its pedicle, predisposing to congestion; and (c) a plane of scar tissue will form beneath

the flap and further impede lymphatic egress. In an attempt to minimize these effects, certain modifications of the bilobe can be employed. By decreasing the arc of rotation to 90 degrees, the size of the standing cutaneous deformity and the overall width of the flap are decreased. The primary flap should be aggressively debulked, removing all muscle and a majority of the subcutaneous fat. When possible, an inferiorly based flap design will be more favorable, as it permits lymphatic drainage. The entire nose is widely undermined, creating a more even plane of scar and contracture. Finally, the apex of the secondary flap can be

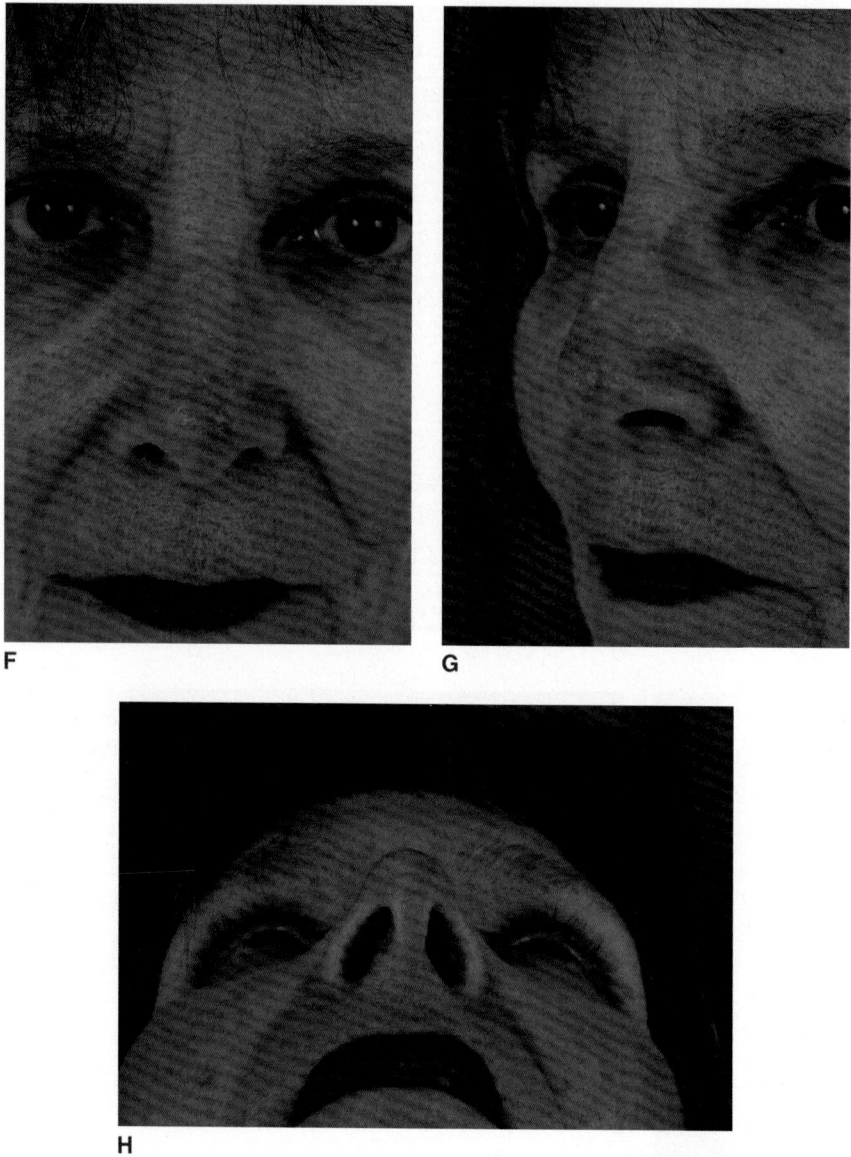

Figure 177.3 *(Continued)* **F–H**: Six-month postoperative views.

left as a triangle rather than trimming it, leaving a sharp corner that contracts less. This requires a small triangle of normal skin to be excised from the recipient normal nasal skin. Wound edges along a bilobe often become inverted and depressed. Great effort must be made to maximize skin eversion during closure with meticulous subdermal sutures. It is often possible to orient the flap such that one limb of the primary flap and the straight line from the secondary flap closure are indiscreet. One can place the Burrow triangle from the primary flap along the supra-alar crease or orient the secondary flap vertically, such that the closure of this donor site parallels the borders of aesthetic subunits (Fig. 177.5). The vector of tension from a bilobe is often counterintuitive in that there is an inferior force that can push the alar rim inferiorly. The flap border may need to be trimmed in order to pull the rim cephalad. Because of the natural convexity of the nose, the pivot point of a bilobe

also has a third-dimensional vector that is perpendicular to the plane of the flap and impinges on the airway. Most bilobes designed with the pedicle based laterally along the keystone area will compromise the valve and will require a prophylactic sidewall batten graft. Those based medially, on the other hand, tend to be more functionally forgiving and may even serve to pull the sidewall open.

Rieger Flap

The Rieger flap utilizes glabellar skin based on a unilateral medial brow/supratrochlear region. The donor site is closed primarily as the glabellar and dorsal nasal skin is advanced and rotated caudally. It is ideally suited for defects of the upper two-thirds. For lower-third defects, it is a moderately large flap that often leaves some alar base asymmetry as well as unnatural nasal creases.

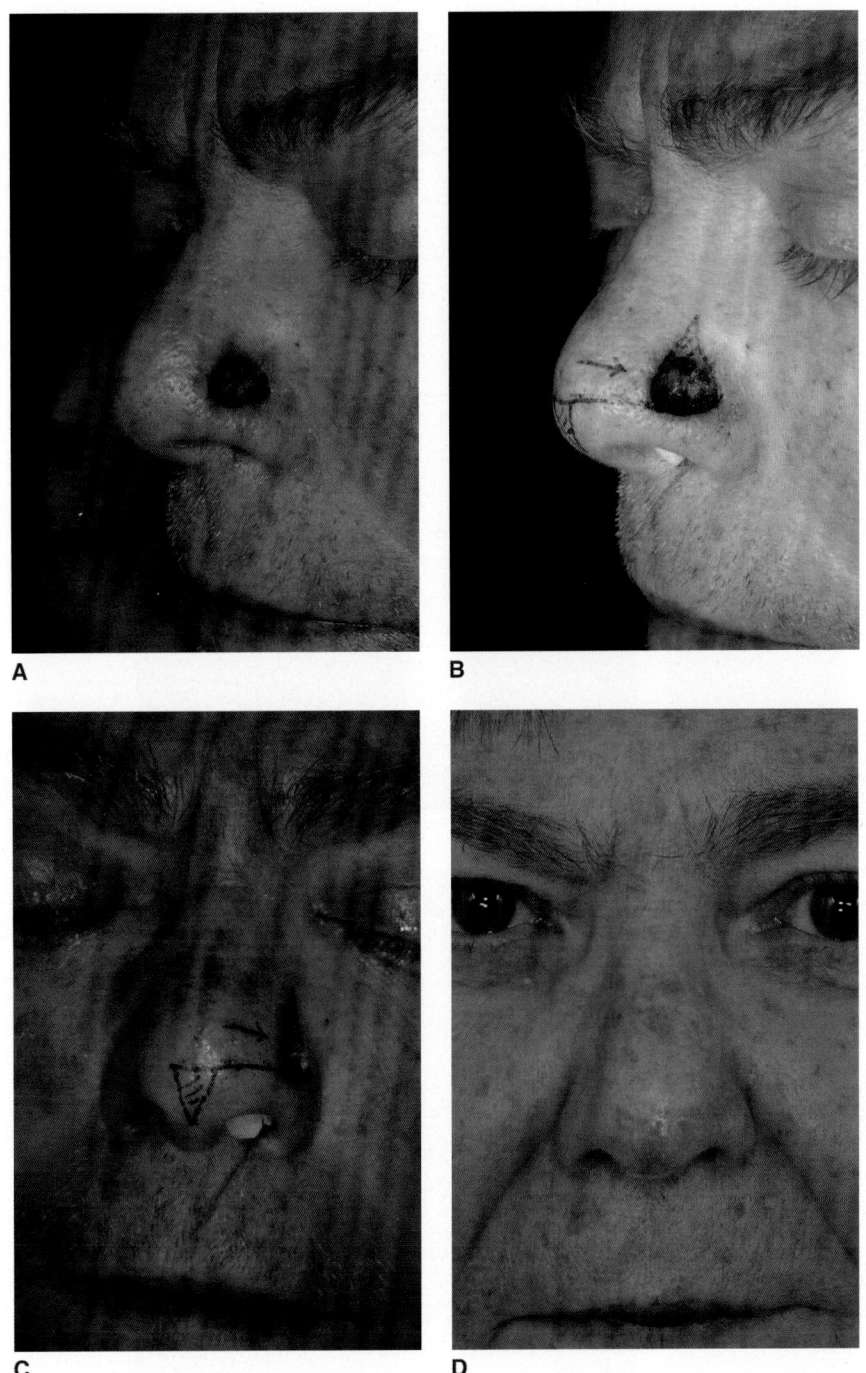

Figure 177.4 East–west flap. **A**: Left sidewall defect. **B, C**: Flap designed with standing cutaneous deformity moved to midline tip. **D**: Six-month postoperative view.

Melolabial Flap

The interpolated melolabial flap is designed with a distinct pedicle based superiorly through the perforators off the angular artery. The skin paddle is located on the medial cheek area and will have an excellent match to the normal nasal skin (Fig. 177.6). The flap is initially elevated in the subdermal plane, becoming progressively thicker as it ascends superiorly into the pedicle proper. The skin paddle must be kept thin with only a layer of subdermal fat. The pivot point for the pedicle is located along the nasal facial groove, and, although the skin incisions are narrowed superiorly to facilitate rotation, the subcutaneous portion remains thick and bulky. The vascular basis of this flap is via perforators within the subcutaneous fat and levator labii superioris, not the skin itself. After the flap is transferred, the melolabial fold is re-created with medial advancement of the cheek. Pedicle division is performed after a 3-week interval to allow for neovascularization from the recipient bed into the skin paddle. The stump of the pedicle is usually excised and donor site closed primarily, leaving a single scar along the nasofacial junction. This is done at the risk of creating subtle facial asymmetry

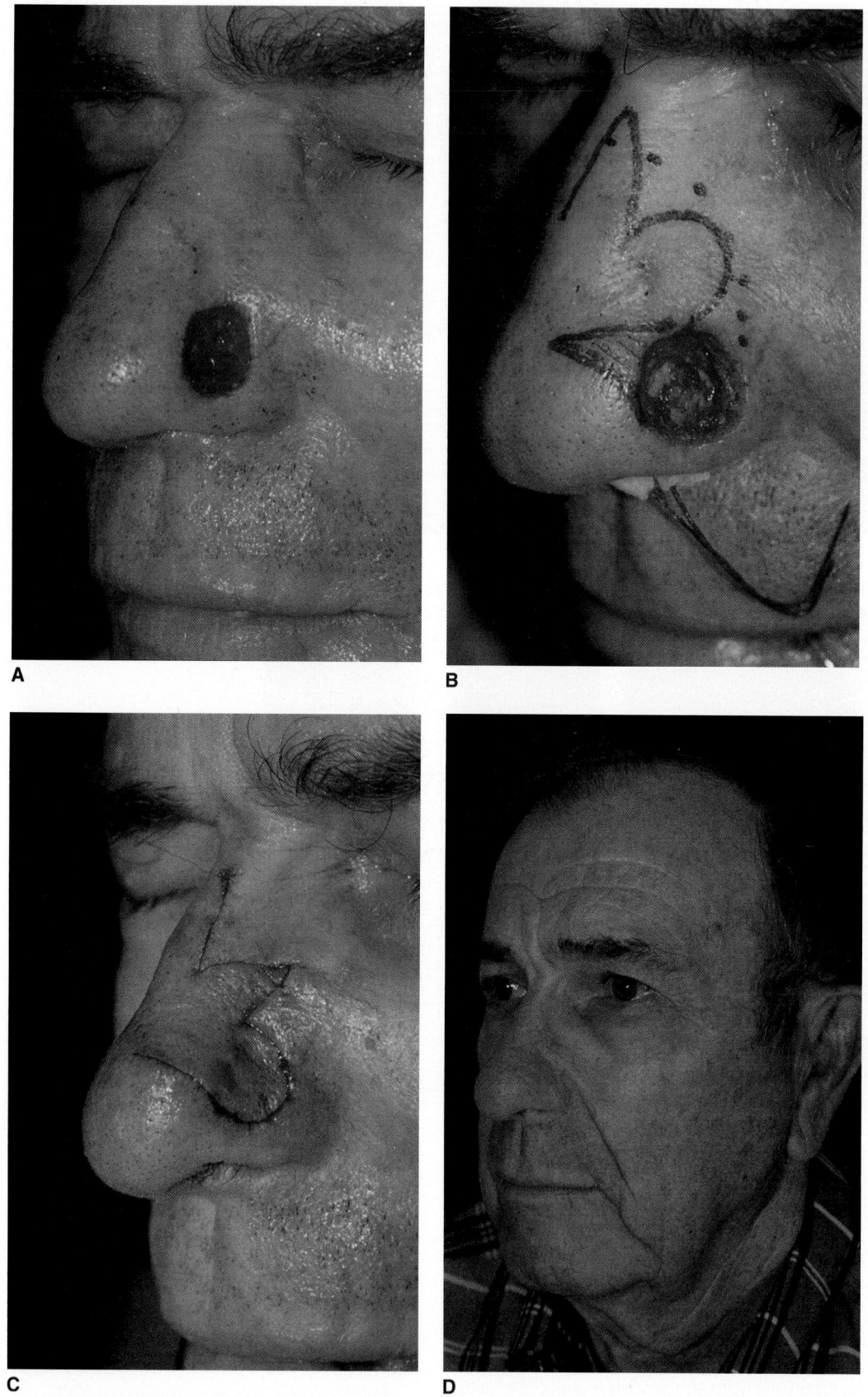

Figure 177.5 Nasal bilobe flap. **A**: 1.3-cm cutaneous defect of left ala and sidewall. **B**: Bilobe flap design. **C**: Flap transposed. Note that the secondary flap is left as a triangle rather than a curved lobe. Straight lines and sharp corners camouflage better. A cartilage batten graft was also placed (not shown). **D**: Six-month postoperative view.

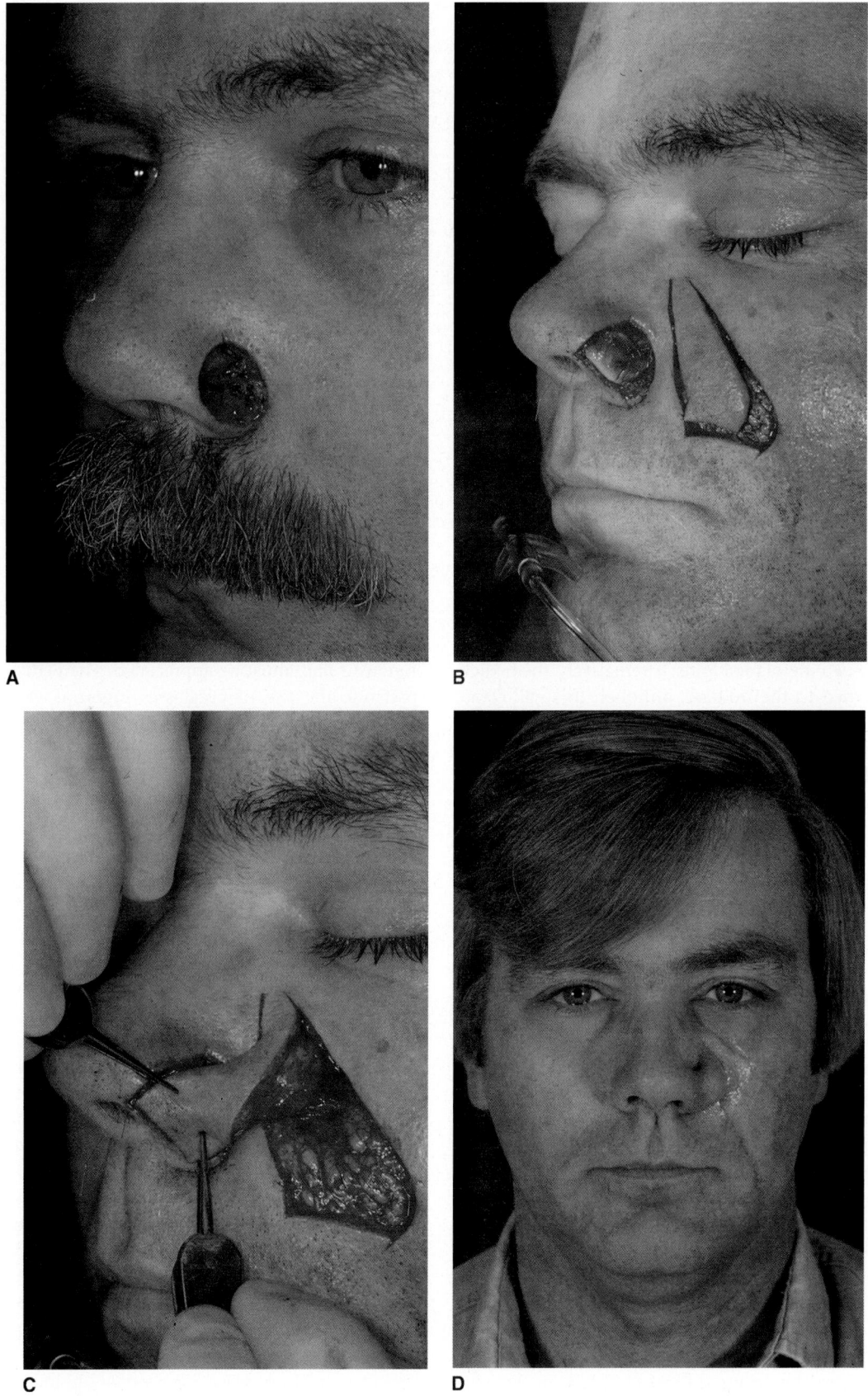

A

B

C

D

Figure 177.6 A–G: Superiorly based, interpolated melolabial flap for 1.3-cm defect of left ala. A conchal cartilage batten graft was used in the lobule to prevent collapse and retraction.

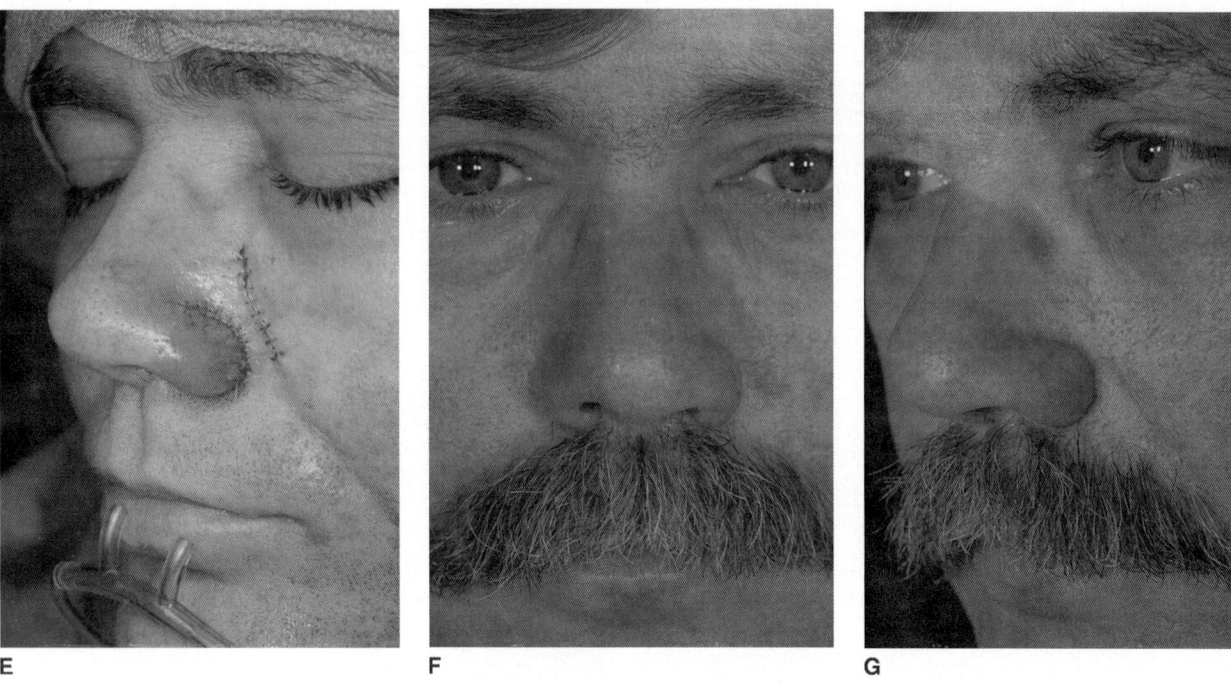

E   F   G

Figure 177.6 *(Continued)*

between the two melolabial folds. Alternatively, the pedicle can be returned to the midface, although this will create two oblique scars, one being within the cheek facial unit. The melolabial flap is ideally suited for smaller defects of the alar lobule and columella. It can be extended to the nasal sidewall and nasal tip. It brings vascularized tissue that can cover a cartilage graft. By being based on the cheek, it avoids the functional inconvenience created by a forehead flap pedicle, such as with eyeglasses.

LARGE CUTANEOUS DEFECTS

Preoperative Considerations

Most large skin defects are addressed with more elaborate, interpolated flaps, but on occasion, less invasive options can still represent the most practical means of repair. There are individual considerations that might discourage a more aggressive procedure. Advanced age, significant small-vessel disease, previous radiation therapy, and overall patient health, all might preclude a lengthy and more involved surgical intervention. A large skin graft to the nose may represent the most practical repair for select patients, and, at times, the outcomes can be surprisingly satisfactory. In addition, individual patient expectations and postoperative cooperation should be clearly defined. Although the optimal aesthetic outcome is often the surgeon's goal, patient needs may be quite different, with a much lower cosmetic concern and greater priority toward a speedy recuperation. The logistical inconveniences to the patient, especially with a staged procedure such as an interpolated

forehead flap, must be appreciated. The pedicle will often preclude the use of eyeglasses, rigorous work outdoors (which many of these patients may do), and many public positions of employment, for example, waiters, receptionists, and so on.

Simultaneously, when selecting a simpler alternative for short-term convenience purposes, it is important to communicate the aesthetic and functional sacrifices that are being made. A month of inconvenience may be small when contrasted with an outcome that is lifelong. This too must be clearly communicated. A majority of the larger nasal defects occur on a more elderly population, and one certainly needs to develop a feel for their surgical candidacy, level of support, and emotional expectations. For some individuals, a simpler covering such as a full-thickness skin graft will meet their needs as long as they do not develop significant nasal obstruction. On the other hand, there are many senescent patients who remain socially active and are entirely deserving of the optimal repair. Even patients in their eighth and ninth decade of life may have an additional life expectancy of greater than 10 years, and an aesthetic and functional repair will be borne for many meaningful years. This is especially true when weighing the total additional time and morbidity consumed by the more elaborate repair versus the simpler one; a forehead flap brings only a few additional weeks of recovery. The subtotal and total nasal reconstructions require a period of significant convalescence, irrespective of age. The chronologic age of most patients has only a minor role in the decision making for a major nasal restoration.

Forehead Flap

The most common method of nasal resurfacing for large (1.5 cm) defects is with the forehead flap. Despite its ancient origins, this flap remains the major workhorse, as it fulfills many of the criteria for the ideal facial flap. There is an excellent match in color and skin texture and sufficient donor skin to resurface the entire nose. This flap is dependable and robust, leaves an acceptable donor site morbidity, and is, in short, the gold standard for contemporary major nasal restoration (25). Several pearls can aid with the design and execution of a forehead flap (Table 177.4).

Defect Preparation

The nasal aesthetic subunits are drawn directly on the nose at the onset of surgery, irrespective of the preexisting nasal defect. Although the general topography is similar from nose to nose, each individual has intrinsic variations of their nose that must be recognized. This is especially true when there is marked dorsal asymmetry or ethnic variations. As the subunits are defined on the nose, great attention is made to preserving the sharp corners at the border of each subunit. There is a tendency to round the corners during each of the stages of repair, beginning with drawing the subunits to creating a flap that fits the modified defect. Based on the size and shape of the cutaneous defect, it is then usually modified to complete the corresponding aesthetic subunit such that the resultant scars lay along the borders of these subunits. This usually involves enlarging the existing defect. This principle is applied liberally yet not exclusively. When only a small portion of a given subunit is involved (usually 10%), it may be more practical to modify the shape by enlarging the adjacent subunit and thereby minimize excessive resection of normal tissue. This is especially true when the additional subunit will significantly lengthen or widen the skin paddle of the forehead flap. Another exception to the aesthetic subunit principle is a midline vertical scar of the upper two-thirds of the nose; although this bisects the dorsal subunit, the casual observer also sees the face and nose as two halves, and a vertical line between them can remain inconspicuous.

Asian patients, although rarely afflicted with cutaneous malignancies, have a nasal topography slightly different from most occidentals, particularly in terms of dorsal and tip projection, and the subunit principle should reflect that (26). Their nose tends to be proportionally smaller, and there may not be sufficient nasal skin to cover even defects less than 1.5 cm. Under these circumstances, one may need to complete the aesthetic subunits and resurface with a regional flap from the forehead.

The *nasal–facial junction* lies more medial on the "nose" than first impression, and it is one of the sacred borders that should not be crossed. The cheek flap should be brought up to the junction and suspended to the periosteum of the piriform aperture and even to the bone itself if necessary. Crossing the aesthetic border often creates a degree of facial asymmetry and becomes more conspicuous.

Preexisting nasal deformities can influence the surgical outcome and should be recognized with consideration for adjustment during defect preparation. Aesthetic units are defined, in large part, by the reflections of light that arise from contour changes. A twisted nose will have asymmetric and irregular subunits that do not support the aesthetic subunit principle as well, and one might consider correcting the deformity and restoring symmetry and balance to the nose. It can be an opportune time to straighten the dorsum with osteotomies, reduce a prominent hump, or refine a broad and amorphous nasal tip. Through the combination of traditional cosmetic rhinoplasty maneuvers and basic reconstructive tenets, the surgical outcome can be enhanced.

The *depth of the defect* (and the associated subunits) is always taken down to the perichondrium of the cartilaginous framework, even if the primary defect is more superficial. This allows one to shape the exposed cartilages with sutures and conservative resections. Moreover, the forehead flap is often plagued with being too thick, and increasing the depth of the nasal defect will allow a better contour match between the nose and the flap. The additional resection will also only improve the recurrence rate from the original Mohs surgery. It has been suggested that for high-risk individuals, the adjacent subunits be analyzed for occult cutaneous malignancies, as the skin has been exposed to the same degree of actinic injury (27).

Template

A precise template is made of the final cutaneous defect utilizing the aluminum package from a suture. This can be somewhat laborious but is imperative to get an accurate, *three-dimensional* map of the defect and corresponding skin paddle. One can use the contralateral side as a reference to ensure nasal symmetry. Care is taken to cut straight edges and crisp corners of this template, which is then transferred to the forehead for an accurate tracing. The vertical position of the template is determined by measuring from the medial aspect of the brow down to the nasal defect, recognizing that the length-limiting point is not always the most inferior aspect of the wound but may be the proximal, contralateral corner. The template design is precise and ensures no wasted skin from the forehead. Incisions are made along the internal margin of the markings. Murrell

TABLE 177.4	PEARLS FOR A FOREHEAD FLAP

1. Modify defect shape with consideration of subunits involved.
2. Create precise 3-D template.
3. Aggressive thinning of distal skin paddle.
4. Narrow pedicle base (<1.5cm).
5. Consider functional grafting.
6. During pedicle division, thin the upper flap and set brows at same levels.

et al. have described the application of a three-dimensional pattern using Aquaplast (WFR/Aquaplast Corporation, Wyckoff, New Jersey) to transfer a more aesthetically precise template (28). Once the template has conformed to the contour of the patient's nose, it is converted to a two-dimensional tracing on the forehead.

Anatomic Basis

The blood supply to the forehead flap is primarily through the supratrochlear artery, but not exclusively (29). This artery is a terminal branch of the ophthalmic, from the internal carotid system. It exists from the supratrochlear notch or, less frequently, foramen and courses superiorly between the corrugator muscle deep and the orbicularis oculi muscle superficially, finally piercing the orbicularis roughly 1.5 cm above the notch. The artery then anastomoses extensively with the contralateral supratrochlear and ipsilateral supraorbital vessels. The forehead vessels have a dependable axial pattern in the vertical direction, running immediately superficial to the frontalis muscles, and give this flap an axial pattern vascular basis in addition to the named pedicle artery. The pedicle is centered on the supratrochlear vessel but has more than that artery supplying it; the driving anatomic basis for this flap is the robust perfusion pressure located along the medial brow area. The terminal branch of the angular artery supplies the pedicle base and is a major contributor to the arterial supply of the forehead flap. Silicone rubber casts were created from a forehead flap after cannulation of the facial artery alone, that is, no fixative was injected in the internal carotid system. This demonstrated the extensive network of collateral vessels in the medial brow region and a significant perfusion into a forehead flap without flow from the supratrochlear artery (Fig. 177.7) (29).

Midline Versus Paramedian

The skin paddle of the forehead flap can be placed in the paramedian position, immediately centered on the supratrochlear artery (30). This has the advantage of incorporating much of the artery within the pedicle and, in theory, improves flap viability. Some individuals have a low "widow's peak," and the paramedian design can avoid it. The skin paddle can also be placed in the precise midline, creating a "midline forehead flap," with some discrete advantages (31). The pedicle is still based on a *unilateral* medial brow area, but it diverts obliquely to course in the middle of the forehead. This pedicle design will not incorporate as much of the supratrochlear artery, but the vertical axial pattern of the subdermal plexus remains. The advantage of this design is that the resultant scar will be in the exact midline of the forehead, rather than paramedian. Like the aesthetic subunits of the nose, the face is also visually divided into two halves. The midline vertical scar, despite being perpendicular to the horizontal forehead furrows, is often quite inconspicuous. There is also a natural divergence of the frontalis muscle in the superior forehead, causing the forehead furrows to be discontiguous between the left and right sides. The midline

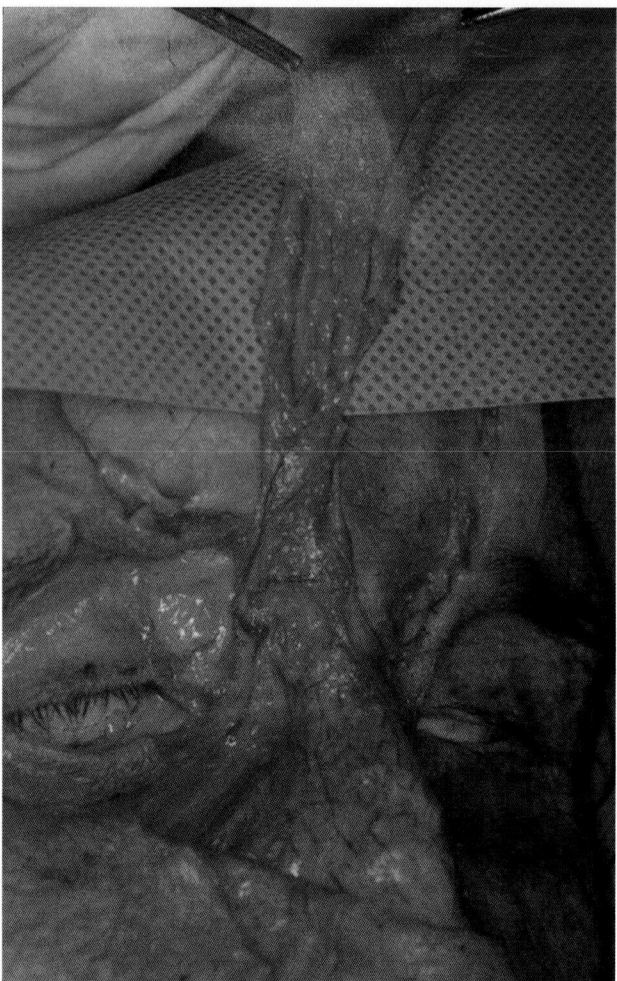

Figure 177.7 Cadaveric study with facial artery cannulated, showing perfusion of forehead flap through angular artery and collateral flow at medial brow area. No dye is from supratrochlear vessel.

vertical scar tends not to disrupt these and allows better scar camouflage. In addition, the pedicle base has a curved and oblique path rather than the straight vertical design of the paramedian flap. The former allows a slightly longer reach caudally that can be significant with a low hairline or when reaching the alar rim or columella (Fig. 177.8).

Pedicle Design

It was originally thought that the forehead flap pedicle needed to be wide enough to capture both supratrochlear vessels in order to survive. It has later been shown that this forehead flap can be raised off only a single supratrochlear artery and that the pedicle can be safely narrowed to 1.5 cm without jeopardizing viability (14–17). The pedicle for the flap can be based either ipsilateral or contralateral to the nasal defect (assuming it is not midline). Each has its unique advantages. The ipsilateral pedicle is closer to the defect and permits a shorter pedicle length, which can be very advantageous in people with a low hairline. The contralateral pedicle has a longer reach but less rotational arc, thus reducing the amount of twisting that occurs at the pedicle base and possibly

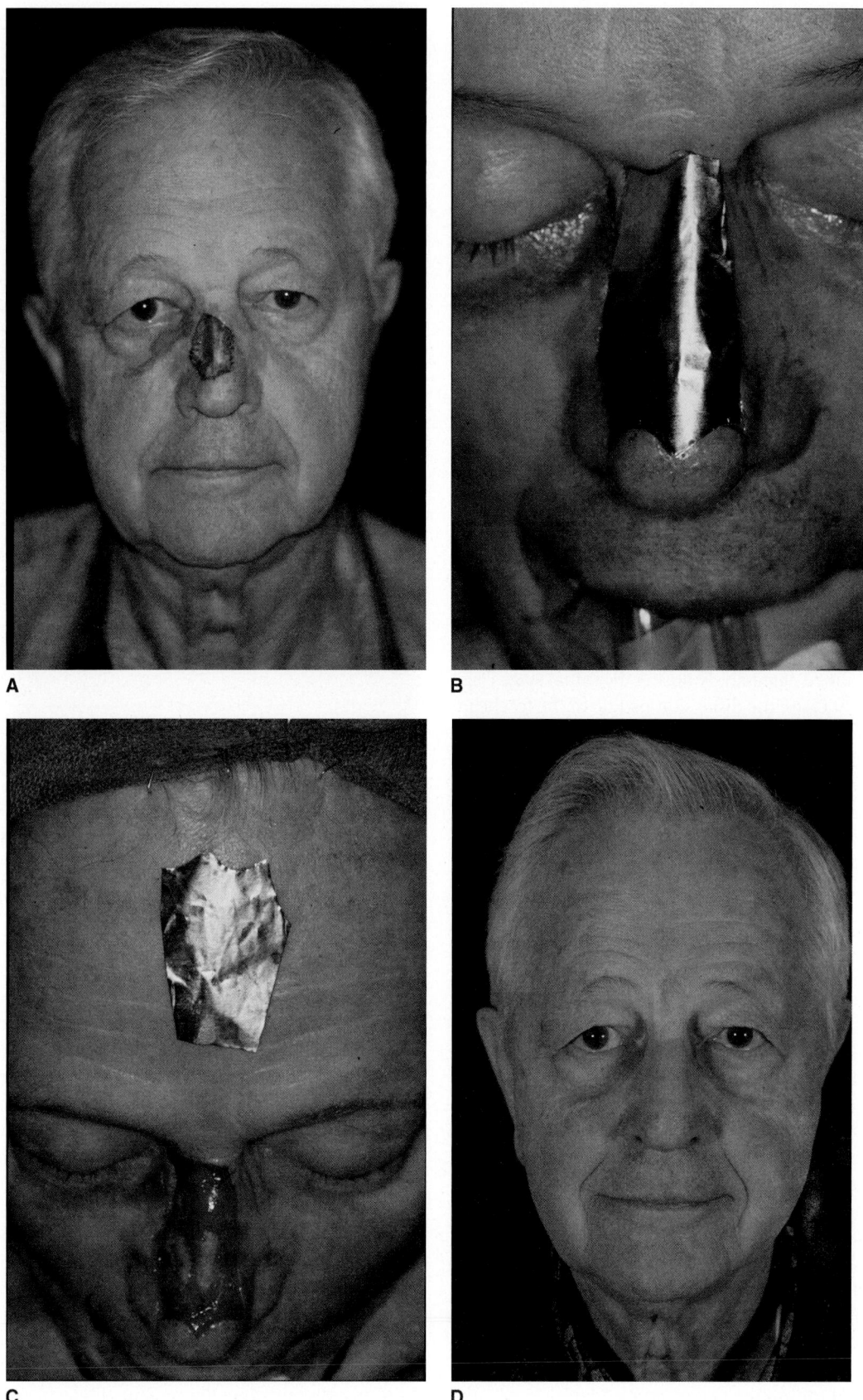

Figure 177.8 A: Nasal defect anterior view. **B**: Three-dimensional template of nasal defect (suture package). **C**: Template transferred to precise midline of forehead. **D**: Postoperative view, noting preservation of bilateral forehead furrows and brow symmetry.

improving venous return from the flap. All else being equal, the contralateral flap may be safer and more robust.

Doppler confirmation or localization of the supratrochlear artery is rarely needed, especially because the perfusion pressure and extensive collateralization is a major driving factor. The notch of the supratrochlear vessels can usually be palpated and the skin pedicle centered there. The pedicle base can also be just based on medial brow where the supraorbital rim joins the lacrimal bone. One can include a cuff of periosteum at the base of the pedicle. This serves to give the flap a small amount of additional length. It also provides some rigidity to the pedicle base.

The base of the pedicle should not exceed 1.5 cm, which provides ample vascularity yet does not strangulate the pedicle or hinder the flap rotation. Most flaps can be narrowed to closer to 1 cm at the proximal end. The pedicle can also be extended into the brow and lower glabellar area for additional length.

Skin Paddle Elevation and Thinning

One of the common problems with the forehead flap of years past was excessive bulk, often sacrificing normal nasal form for fear of compromising viability. One of the greatest modifications and advancements made with the forehead flap may be the realization that the skin paddle can, and should, be thinned aggressively during the initial stage (Fig. 177.9). In most cases, the distal skin paddle of the forehead flap is elevated in the subcutaneous plane rather than the subgaleal plane, lifting the flap off the frontalis muscle. The galea (frontalis muscle and fascia) is left down on the forehead during this initial flap elevation. This continues for approximately 25% of the skin paddle, after which the plane is dropped to the subgaleal level and continues effortlessly. The proximal part of the skin paddle will be thinned in the future, during pedicle division 3 weeks later. Once the flap is up, additional thinning is performed to match the intrinsic variations of normal nasal skin thickness. That portion corresponding to the thin rhinion skin, columella, or alar rim is further thinned directly. Axial, subdermal vessels are often encountered within the galea during this process, and the thinning can continue around them without sacrificing the vessels themselves. With healthy patients, the flap thinning will continue to the subdermal layer and fluctuate slightly to best match the variability in native skin thickness. Leaving the frontalis on the forehead donor area has the distinct advantage if the donor site cannot be closed primarily. Second-intention healing will proceed much more rapidly over the galea rather than over the periosteum.

An exception to this method of elevation is in smokers or other individuals with small-vessel disease. For these high-risk situations, the skin paddle is elevated with the bulky subgaleal layer and transferred en bloc. An *intermediate stage* is used to thin the flap (discussed later).

Donor Site

A great majority of forehead defects less than 3.5 cm can be repaired primarily through wide, subgaleal undermining

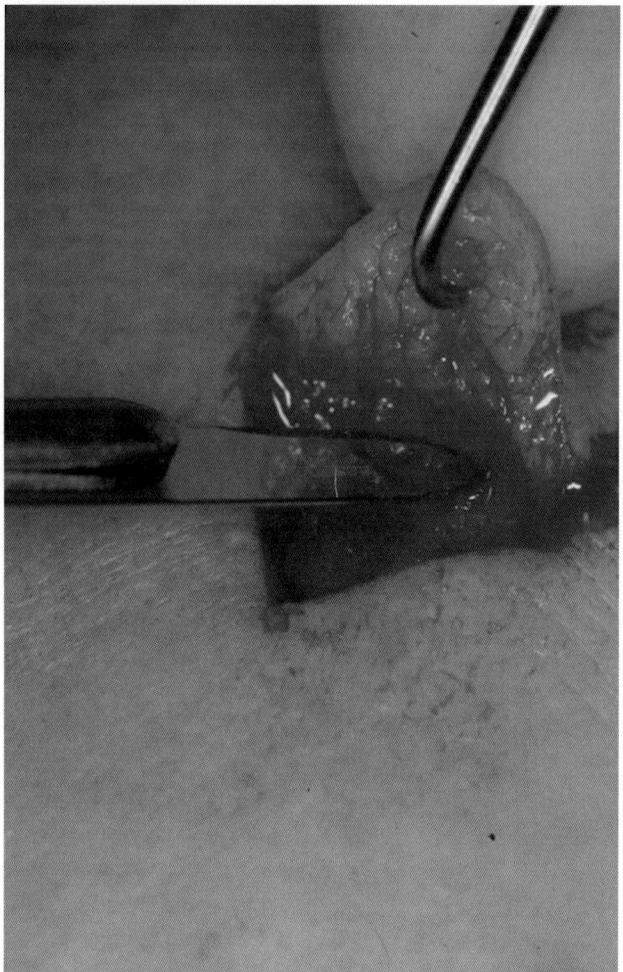

Figure 177.9 Elevation of distal forehead flap in the thin subcutaneous plane rather than subgaleal plane. Thin layer of fat is preserved under skin paddle of flap. This thinning continues only for 30% of the skin paddle and is not performed in smokers.

out to the temple areas. Deep sutures must be through the galeal layer in order to ensure sufficient strength; it is often necessary to place all the deep sutures prior to closure and tying of sutures. The standing cutaneous deformity at the superior border is directly excised in a vertical fashion with the incision extending into the frontal hair. Alternatively, the forehead can be mobilized and closed in an "O to T" fashion with a horizontal limb at the hairline. Like a trichophytic browlift, this can be closed in a running "W-plasty" to further camouflage the scar.

For wider defects, vertical galeatomies may allow additional recruitment from the sides. Any remaining defect on the forehead is allowed to heal by second intention. The resultant scar following wound contracture will generally be superior to other methods, especially when the galea has been left in place. A skin graft will allow that area to heal quickly but generally remains more noticeable. Early tissue expansion has been described as an alternative for the tight forehead or the low hairline (32). Although this does create an abundant amount of tissue and permit primary closure following wide forehead flaps, the expanded skin is less favorable in terms of flap physiology. Some flap contracture will occur, even following direct excision of the expander capsule, and will compromise the final nasal form.

Pedicle Division

The pedicle is the obligatory nutrient supply for the skin paddle until sufficient neovascularization occurs from the recipient bed into the flap itself. Vascular ingrowth is predictable and is driven, in part, by the ischemic gradient between the nasal defect and the distal flap (33). There is probably sufficient support for the flap after a 10-day period, but a 3-week interval is allowed to lapse to ensure greater fibroblast development, increased tensile strength, and adequate adherence of the flap to the nose. The pedicle is divided transversely, a few millimeters above the original nasal defect. Undermining proceeds in a superior-to-inferior direction, immediately under the dermal plane, to roughly halfway down the skin paddle. One can leave the subcutaneous portion of the pedicle intact, allowing it to provide countertraction as the skin is undermined. The bulk of the subcutaneous tissue is then removed while tapering the inferior border to smooth the transition. It is imperative to debulk this portion of the flap and allow the flap to conform to the normal nasal topography. The edges of the original nasal defect are carefully freshened and corners are squared off. Over the preceding 3 weeks, the border of the defect will have contracted and started to reepithelialize.

The superior stump of the pedicle is then trimmed accordingly and inset back into the glabellar area. There is a tendency for this portion of the pedicle to thicken and pincushion. Aggressive thinning of the corrugator muscle contained in the pedicle stump will help minimize this. It is essential to restore symmetry to the eyebrows, as the pedicle side tends to be pulled inferiorly. After the medial brow is resuspended, the new standing cutaneous deformities can be directly excised. The inferior forehead scar can be revised readily at this time. The scar in this area is often inverted and conspicuous there because a wide frontalis muscle portion is included in the pedicle. On occasion, one can dermabrade some of the scars of the nose or the forehead at this relatively early stage (Fig. 177.10).

Three Staged Forehead Flap—with Intermediate Stage

In higher-risk individuals such as smokers, the original forehead flap can be transposed as a composite of skin and frontalis muscle, without preliminary flap thinning, with a planned *intermediate stage* (34). During this step, the skin paddle is elevated from laterally on both sides, leaving the original forehead flap as a bipedicled flap, attached at the medial brow proximally and the nasal tip distally. The flap is then thinned and sculpted to the appropriate level to restore nasal form (Fig. 177.11). An additional 3 weeks are allowed to pass before the final pedicle division is performed. While this methodology leaves the pedicle intact for 6 weeks, the inconvenience is justified by improved flap

viability and better outcomes within a high-risk patient group. The flap can also be elevated more aggressively, including the distal tip. This essentially converts the forehead flap into a delayed flap.

Single-Stage Forehead Flap

The single-stage forehead flap (Table 177.5) utilizes a deepithelialized pedicle and was originally described by Converse in 1963 as a modified median forehead flap based on both supratrochlear vessels (35). It had problems with a limited arc of rotation and flap congestion and was subsequently abandoned. Utilizing what is known today about the robust vascularity of the contemporary forehead flap, one can create a single-stage, island forehead flap based on a *unilateral* medial brow area (36). This single-stage flap has a similar anatomic basis as the conventional, interpolated forehead flap but does not require a pedicle division. The advantages of accomplishing a major nasal resurfacing in a single stage can be tremendous for those patients in whom the pedicle and need for a second surgery create a hardship that is difficult to overcome. The vascularity from a subcutaneous pedicle is, however, more tenuous, and this type of forehead flap should be avoided in high-risk individuals, such as smokers and individuals with small-vessel disease.

Both a unilateral supratrochlear artery and the rich collateral supply from the angular artery provide the perfusion pressure that supports the skin paddle. It should be based on the contralateral side to avoid excessive torsion on the pedicle. This flap is converted to an island flap as the glabellar skin is carefully dissected off the pedicle. Tremendous care must be taken to avoid inadvertent changes in plane during this stage because pedicle amputation is the result. The glabellar skin is undermined widely, and the resultant tunnel is connected to the defect of the nose. Portions of the procerus muscle can be resected in order to create sufficient room to accommodate the pedicle without compression and congestion. The flap is then tunneled under the intact glabellar skin and the skin paddle delivered into the nasal defect then closed completely in a circumferential fashion. The donor site is closed primarily, often incorporating a W-plasty inferiorly that parallels the natural glabellar furrows. There is a soft tissue void where the subcutaneous pedicle was originally located, and portions of the frontalis muscles can be mobilized to fill this depression and improve glabellar contour. This flap works best for nasal defects limited to the upper two-thirds of the nose; nasal tip and alar defects require a lengthier forehead flap and may not remain viable (Fig. 177.12).

STRUCTURAL SUPPORT AND GRAFTING IN NASAL RECONSTRUCTION

In addition to the surface area of a nasal defect, it is imperative to determine its depth and location in terms of its impact on nasal function and form. Structural grafting

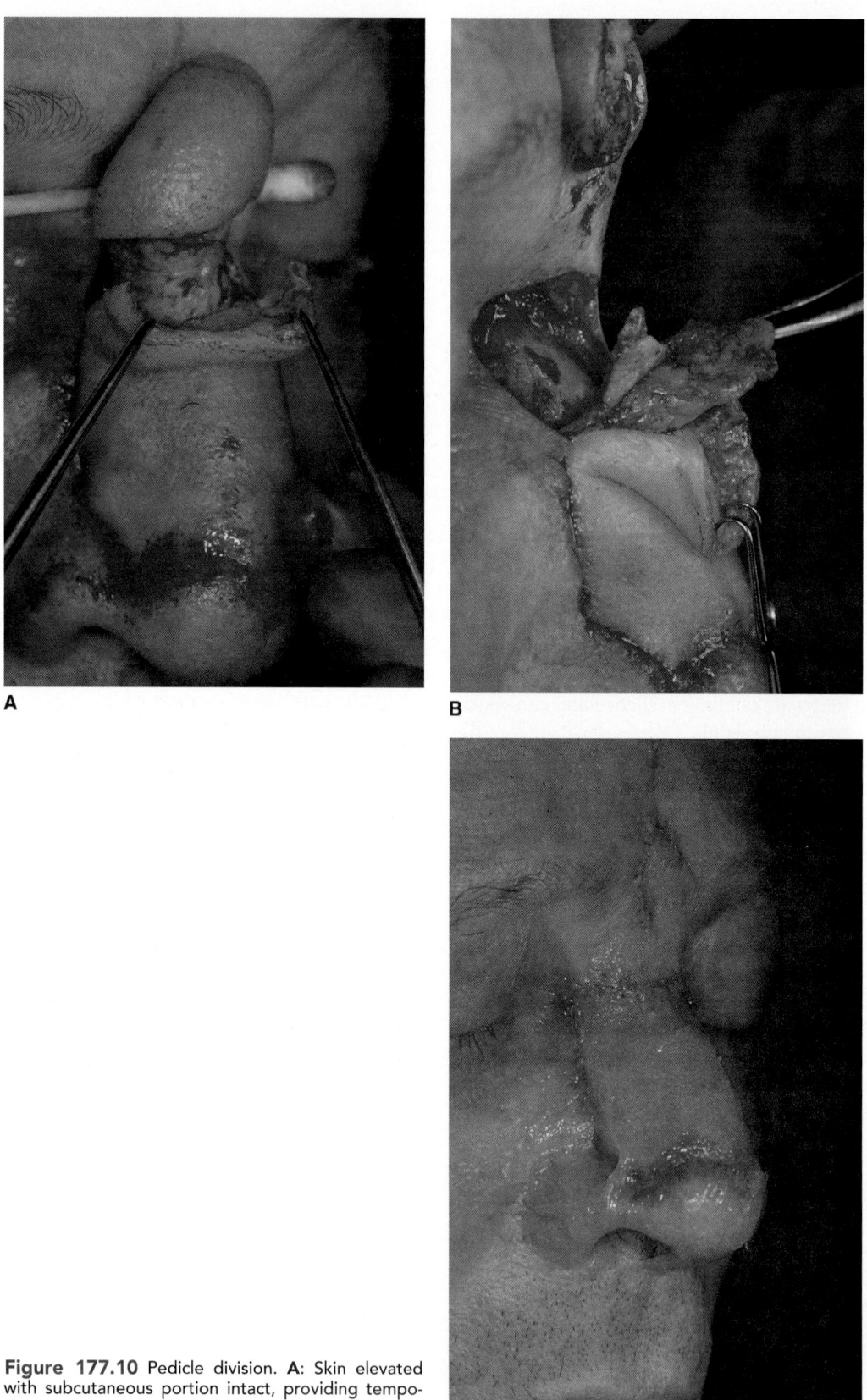

Figure 177.10 Pedicle division. **A**: Skin elevated with subcutaneous portion intact, providing temporary countertraction. **B**: Debulking subcutaneous portion. **C**: Pedicle inset with attention to brow symmetry.

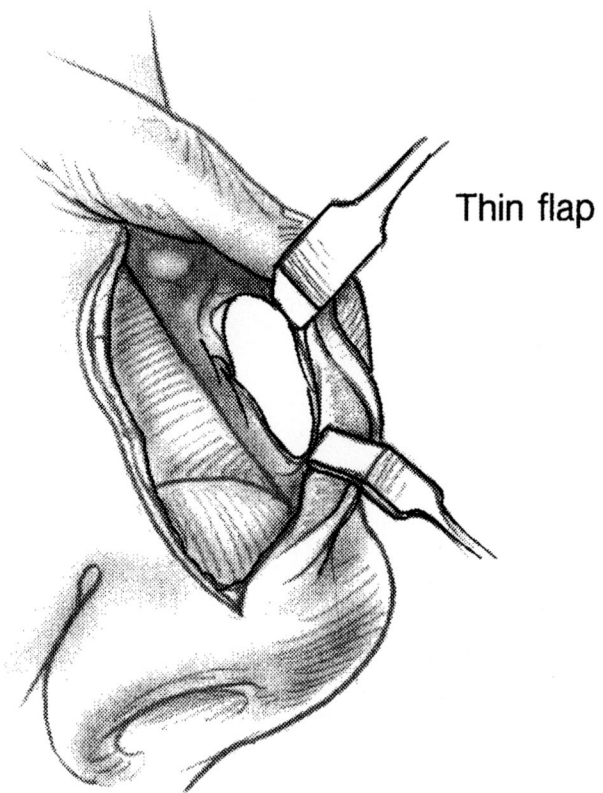

Thin flap

Figure 177.11 Intermediate stage with debulking of flap from lateral access.

is placed for three primary reasons: first, to provide rigidity to the sidewall, thus preventing collapse and nasal obstruction; second, to create or maintain form, especially along the alar rim and tip; and third, to provide dorsal support and projection. Many small and superficial defects of the lower third of the nose are repaired with composite grafts, thus providing a covering and support simultaneously. Larger and more complex defects usually require separate support grafting and an independent resurfacing flap.

Nasal Function

New onset nasal obstruction can compromise an otherwise excellent surgical outcome and be the source of significant patient dissatisfaction. Predicting those lesions that will lead to nasal obstruction is important and is influenced by

TABLE 177.5	PEARLS FOR THE SINGLE-STAGE FOREHEAD FLAP

1. Select patient carefully.
2. Create adequate room under glabellar skin.
3. Fill forehead depression with procerus and frontalis muscles.
4. Watch for flap congestion.

both the defect's depth and its location. When the depth is such that native structural support has been removed (e.g., a portion of the lateral crus), the defect will uniformly require reconstruction with some form of cartilaginous grafting. An exception is small defects of the nasal bones, albeit rare. Lesions located over the alar lobule or nasal sidewall are particularly prone to collapse and subsequent nasal obstruction at the level of the internal and external nasal valves. There is a critical area located at the junction of the two anatomic valves, corresponding to the supra-alar crease externally and the area lateral to the lateral crus internally. There may be a free-floating sesamoid cartilage in this area, which is characteristically just a firm, fibrofatty aponeurosis between the lateral crus and the bony piri-form aperture. In this area, even small defects that violate the fibroareolar tissues will tend to collapse, especially following local transposition flaps. Therefore, it is not solely the size of the defect but the depth that may be the indication for structural grafting (21). Lesions within the ala or sidewall often require a repair that involves some rigidity. Straight septal cartilage works well for support to the lateral nasal wall of the middle vault, and conchal cartilage is most often used for the alar lobule.

One can enhance nasal airflow by placement of a *flaring suture* across the upper lateral cartilages (37). The middle nasal vault is often exposed during nasal reconstruction and subject to contractile forces. Because of the concavity over the dorsum, this can lead to subtle pinching of the middle third of the nose and some degree of narrowing at the internal valve. The flaring suture placed across the dorsum serves to hold open the upper lateral cartilages during the healing process and support the airway. A long-lasting suture is placed as a horizontal mattress across each upper lateral cartilage, with the dorsal septum serving as a fulcrum. As the suture is tightened, the upper lateral cartilages will flare upward and outward, thus opening the internal nasal valve (Fig. 177.13). This can be placed during any nasal reconstruction where the upper lateral cartilages become exposed, even with smaller procedures such as a bilobe flap.

Grafting for Form

The alar rim is one of the free margins that represent an "immobile landmark" during defect analysis. Normal wound healing and contracture will tend to pull the alar rim up and create a notch deformity; preserving alar base symmetry is one of the greater challenges in nasal restoration. Any defect that encroaches on the free margin of the ala will require some form of structural support to resist the powerful wound contracture that ensues. The curve found along the inferior conchal bowl conforms well to the natural shape and curl of the alar lobule. Grafts may also be placed at the nasal tip to improve definition and form. Many of the common tip grafts used in aesthetic rhinoplasty can be employed here with equal success.

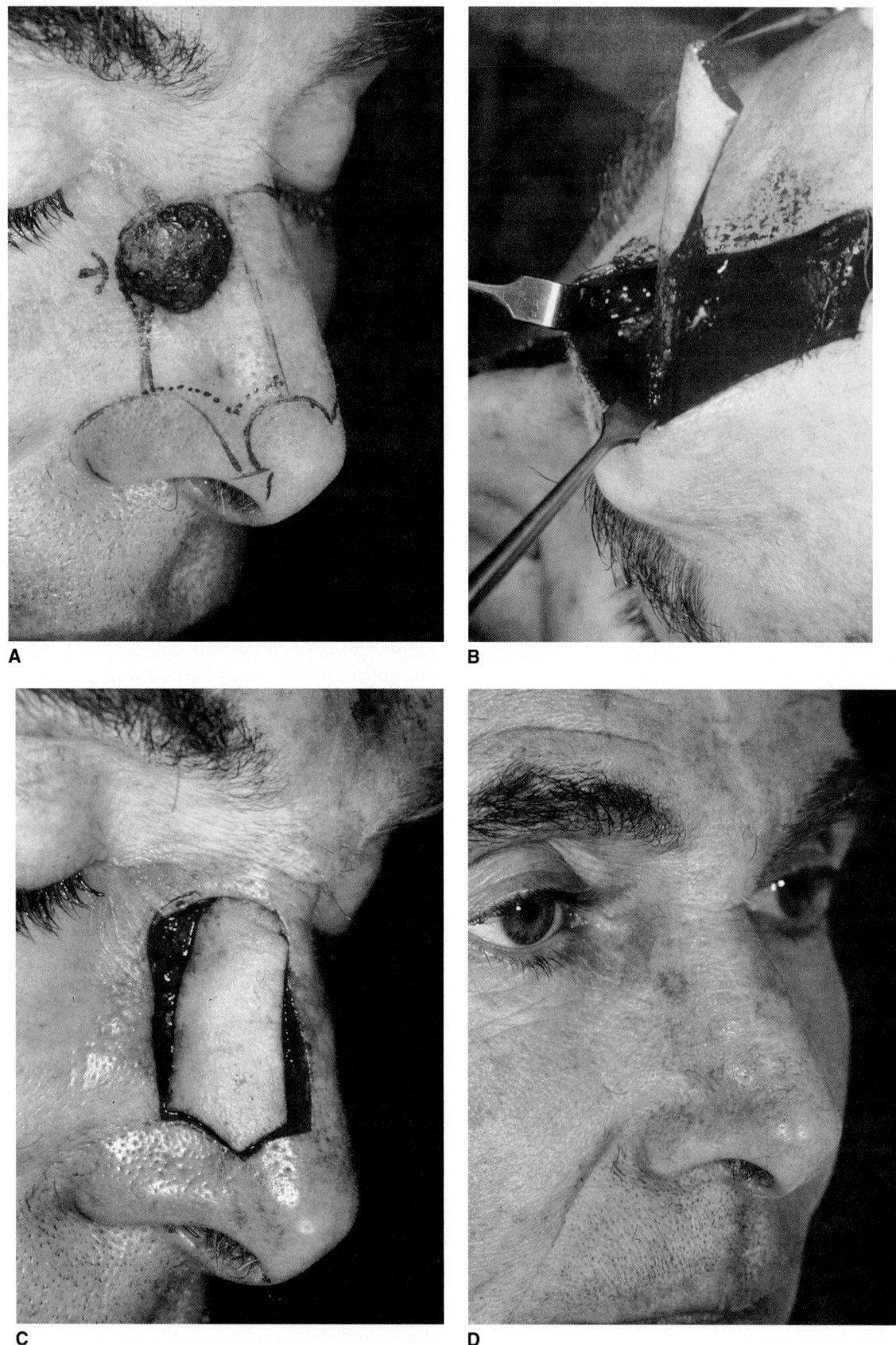

Figure 177.12 Single-stage forehead flap. **A:** Right nasal defect involving sidewall and cheek. **B:** Single-stage forehead flap elevated on subcutaneous pedicle. **C:** Flap transferred under intact glabellar skin and filling nasal defect. **D:** One-year postoperative view with some fullness at glabella.

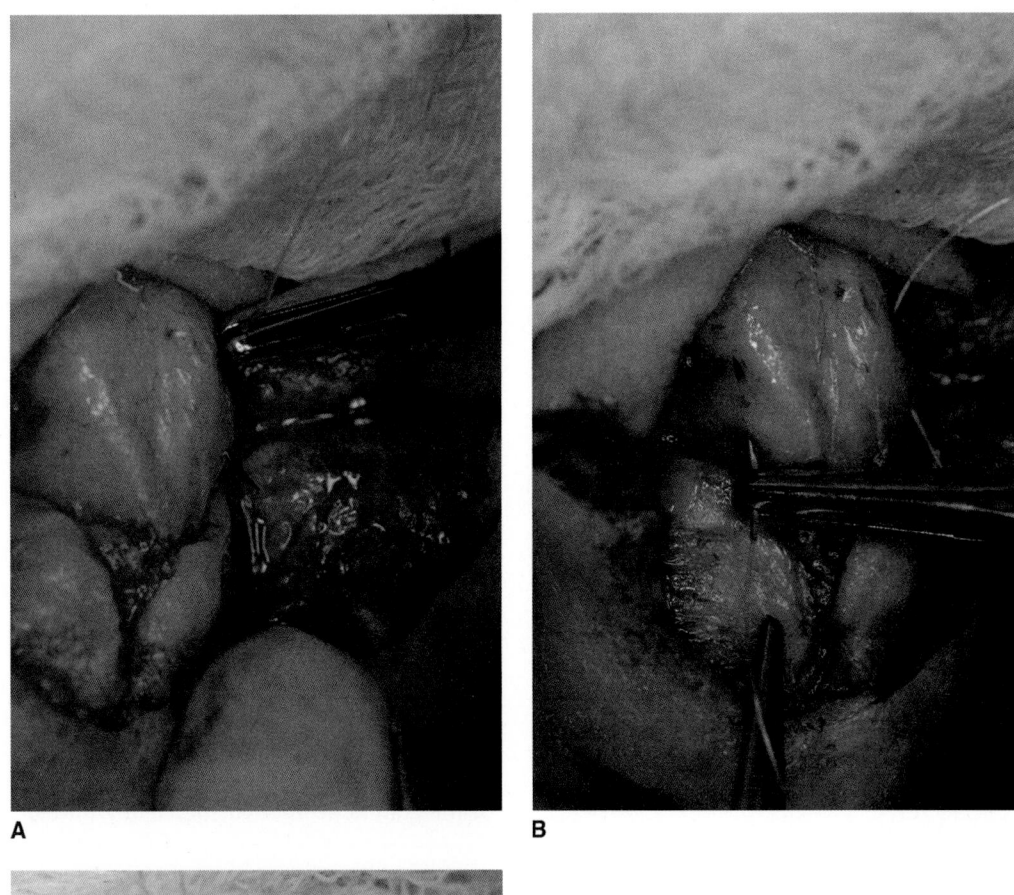

A

B

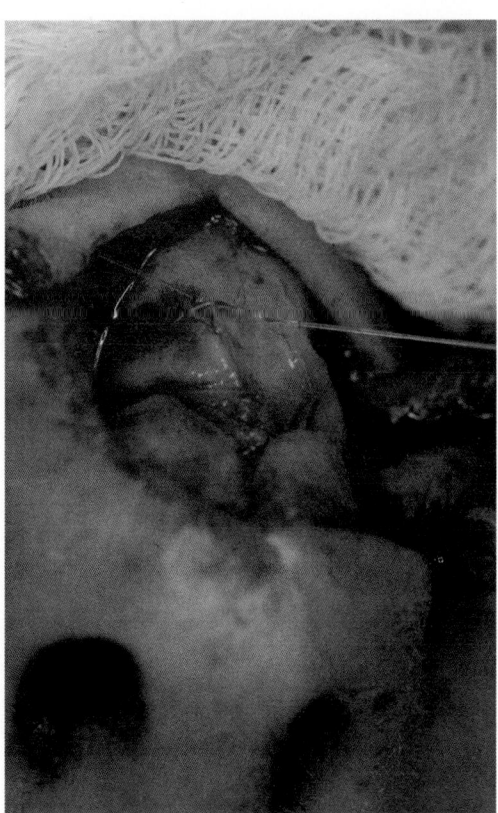

C

Figure 177.13 A: Flaring suture passed through left upper lateral cartilage. **B:** Through right upper lateral cartilage. **C:** Tied-over nasal dorsum to flare open the internal nasal valves.

Because the covering flap tends to be thicker, one can exercise tip refining measures with minimal risk of creating an unnatural "unitip." Traditional shield or cap grafts should be sutured secured to the underlying structure. Grafts to the tip can also serve to stabilize the junction of a reconstructed framework, such as the union between alar rim grafts and the midline support (e.g., columella). Bridging the junction of cartilage grafts creates substantial more stability than a primary, end-to-end union of grafts alone.

Large lesions may remove portions of the midline dorsal support, and its reconstruction can be more complex. Unlike a dorsal augmentation during the correction of a saddle nose deformity, this reconstruction must bring sufficient rigidity to support the cutaneous and *intranasal* dorsum. This can be accomplished by one of three mechanisms: septal cartilage, cantilevered split calvarial bone, or costal cartilage grafting. Some complex nasal lesions extend on to the cheek, not only cutaneously but also to involve framework. If portions of the premaxilla or lateral bony piriform aperture have been resected, they must be individually repaired in order to recreate a solid platform for the nose. Failure to do so will lead to progressive collapse of the nose. The bony aperture of the nose is an essential foundation upon which other structural grafts and flaps can be added (Fig. 177.14).

Techniques for Grafting

The *middle vault and sidewall* areas are ideally reconstructed with straight *septal cartilage*. This material is readily available and should be long enough to rest on the bony piriform aperture laterally and reach the midline dorsum. The *alar lobule* is best supported by autogenous *conchal cartilage*, but it must be carefully sculpted. It can be harvested through either the anterior or posterior approach with little risk of creating significant donor site morbidity. Like septal cartilage, the conchal cartilage graft must be sufficiently long to rest on the bony, medial buttress and extend up to the existing cartilages or close to the midline. Small discs of cartilage grafts will tend to fall intranasally and not function as the batten that is needed. For these cartilage grafts, one creates small subcutaneous pockets under the supra-alar crease or within the alar lobule, but only blunt dissection should be performed in this area in order to minimize risk of injury to the lateral nasal artery. The medial border is firmly anchored to the tip cartilages in an overlapping manner. The superior margin of the graft should be slightly more medial than the inferior margin, forcing the plane of the graft to mimic the contour of the lobule and create a supra-alar crease. In order to maintain the vertical height of the alar rim, one should ensure that the caudal border of the graft is positioned sufficiently inferior, anticipating

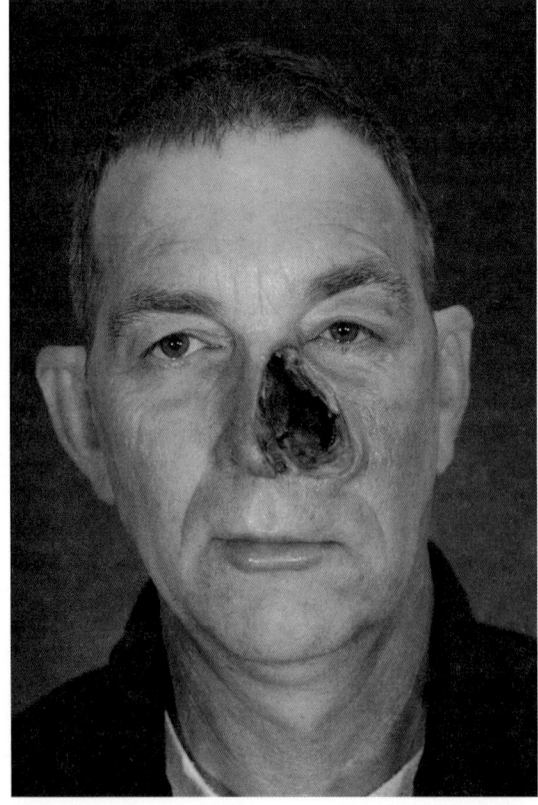
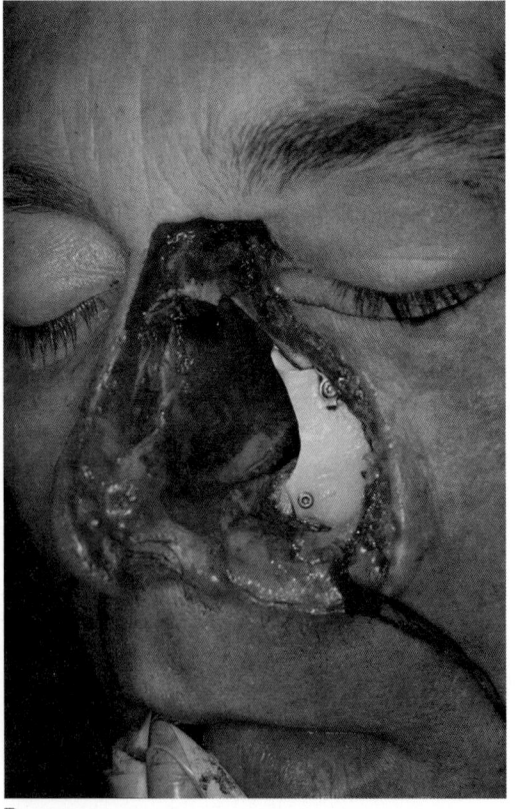

A   **B**

Figure 177.14 A: Large left heminasal and cheek defect involving maxilla. **B**: Split calvarial bone to reconstruct medial buttress, providing platform for nasal base.

the vertical contractile force of wound healing. Grafts are suture-secured to the intranasal lining with through-and-through sutures, thus pulling open the airway under the graft. The natural curvature of the cartilage holds the airway patent, even slightly over corrected. The ala will also feel unnaturally firm with respect to the contralateral side, but this is anticipated and ensures patency at the valves (Fig.177.15).

Dorsal reconstruction can be achieved through a *composite septal flap*, pivoted out of the nose with a hinge along the anterior nasal spine. A full-thickness incision is created through the nasal septum, along the dorsum superiorly, vertically posteriorly, and off the maxillary crest inferiorly. This allows the septum to hinge anteriorly and outward as a composite flap composed of cartilage and bilateral mucosal flaps, bringing structure and internal lining simultaneously. A small wedge of septal cartilage should be excised at the posterior septal angle to facilitate the outward pivot. It is imperative that the septal branch of the anterior septal artery be intact, as it is the primary blood supply to the flap. Each vessel can support the entire ipsilateral septal mucosa and underlying cartilage. Once the composite flap is rotated outward, it is secured with permanent sutures to the residual dorsum and the anterior nasal spine. Septal splints may be useful to provide additional support during the healing phase, reducing the risk of lateral displacement and nasal obstruction. By necessity, this three-layered septal composite flap will leave behind a permanent septal perforation. Although this adds to the convalescence, only rarely is it symptomatic after healing. This technique works well for reconstruction of large, complex, and full-thickness defects of the dorsum, tip, and columella (Fig. 177.16).

Costal cartilage and *split calvarial bone* are excellent structural grafts for total dorsal reconstruction. Nasal defects of this magnitude are usually associated with deficiencies of internal lining, which will always require an independent flap. Cartilage can be harvested from either the seventh, eighth, or ninth rib. Most skin incisions do not need to exceed 4 cm, and the rectus abdominis muscle can be split rather than transected, thus reducing the postoperative pain. A straight portion of the rib should be harvested and only the precise central core utilized for grafting, as eccentric portions of a rib graft will progressively warp. Graft resorption, displacement, and *in situ* warping are the more common complications that can arise. Split calvarial bone is similarly abundant and generally harvested from the straight parietal region of the skull. Its edges are carefully beveled with a drill, and it may be secured at the nasion with a lag screw technique. Both calvarial bone and costal cartilage will leave the nose feeling unnaturally rigid and immobile. It should be supported at the caudal end with an extended columellar strut graft and laterally with conchal cartilage grafts. This lateral support is essential to reduce inward collapse as well as to camouflage the lateral borders of the dorsal reconstruction graft.

INTERNAL LINING DEFICITS

The complexity of a nasal defect is dictated as much by its depth as by its overall size. Violation of the internal lining of the nose is one of the major variables that elevates the complexity and level of sophistication of the repair. It can be tempting to disregard the lining and simply address the structure and covering flap. This is misleading since the immediate result can be quite acceptable but long-term outcomes are uniformly unfavorable. Previously, a preliminary stage was performed in which grafts and internal lining were buried under the forehead as a first stage. This failed because of its lack of flexibility after the flap was transposed. The purpose of a meticulous repair of all lining defects is twofold: First, a vascularized internal covering is needed for structural grafts (e.g., conchal cartilage batten grafts), and, second, second-intention healing of intranasal areas will lead to alar notching and cicatricial stenosis, progressing to a compromise of form and function. Consequently, even small perforations of the intranasal mucosa must be addressed in some manner. Not infrequently, many options for lining repair have been eliminated by the nature of the defect, and one must proceed down an algorithm to alternative techniques. For this reason, it is imperative to be facile with a number of different grafts and flaps used for internal lining repair prior to embarking on a reconstruction of this complexity. Being able to predict the involvement of intranasal mucosa is difficult but can be useful. Certain subtypes of cutaneous malignancies are characterized by their aggressive growth patterns and propensity to extend via small isolated nests of cells beyond the gross margins, for example, morpheaform BCCA. It is prudent to recognize this propensity for intranasal involvement and plan the excision and reconstruction accordingly, including the incorporation of Mohs micrographic surgery and anticipation of a full-thickness nasal defect. In addition, one should bear in mind that the intranasal defect represents the surgical margin for the cutaneous malignancy, and close follow-up of this area is imperative. This is most accurately performed with nasal endoscopes, common to the otolaryngologist.

A very small perforation of the internal lining can often be closed primarily with a single catgut suture. It is best to close the deficit vertically rather than horizontally, in order to minimize the propensity to retract the alar rim. Larger defects will require a flap or graft and can be defined based on their tissue origin (Table 177.6). Selecting the proper internal lining flap is challenging and often based on the location of the defect; most grafts and flaps are needed for only the middle third or lower third of the nose (Table 177.7). Only rarely is an internal lining repair needed within the upper third of the nose.

Grafts

Full-thickness skin grafts require a vascularized recipient bed and, as such, will rarely be utilized for internal

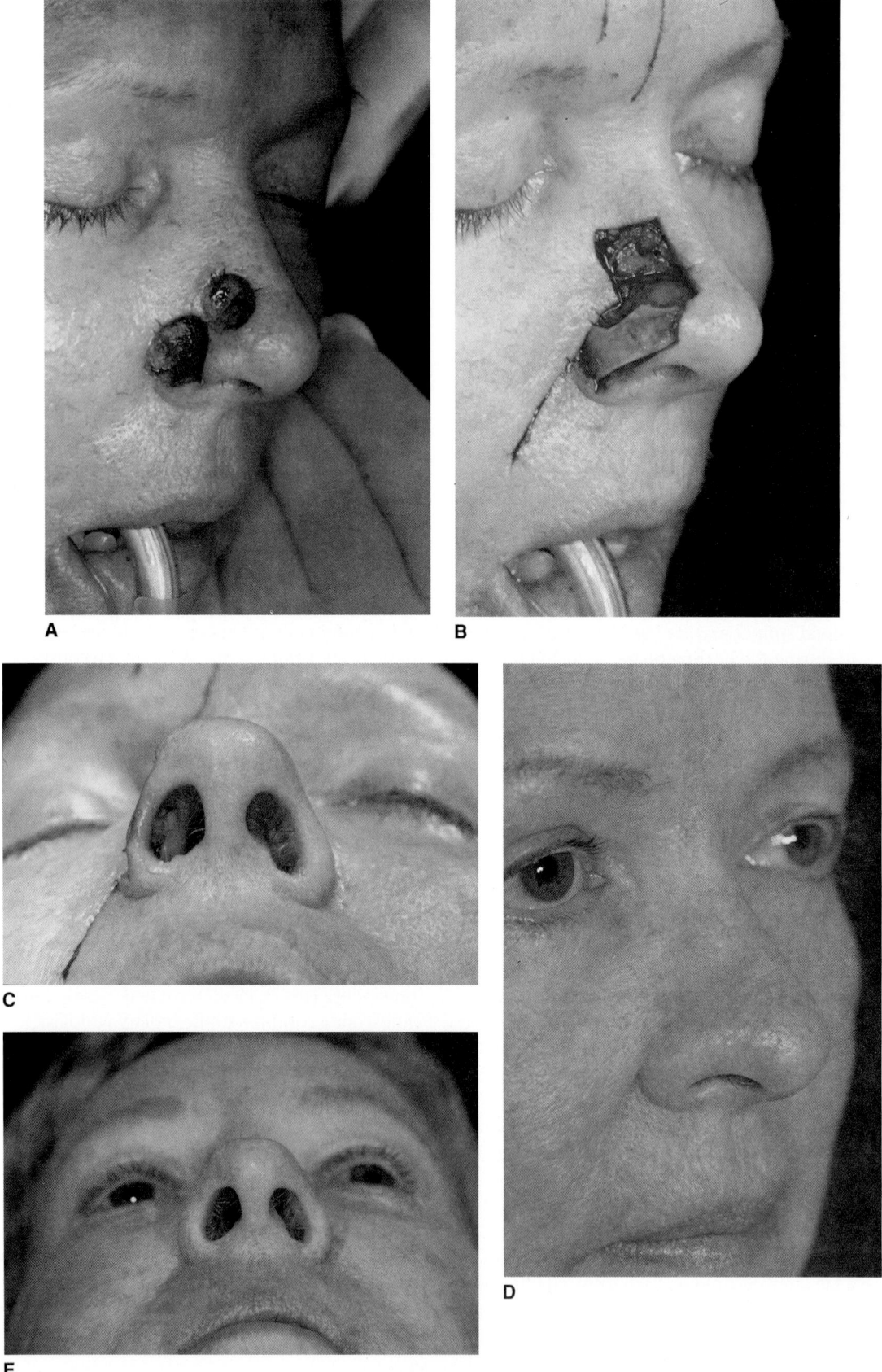

Figure 177.15 Alar batten graft. **A:** Nasal defects of right ala and sidewall. **B:** Conchal cartilage batten graft in nonanatomic position. **C:** Base view demonstrating vestibular support and patency. **D:** One year following resurfacing with a midline forehead flap. Oblique view showing alar rim contour. **E:** Base view showing vestibular patency.

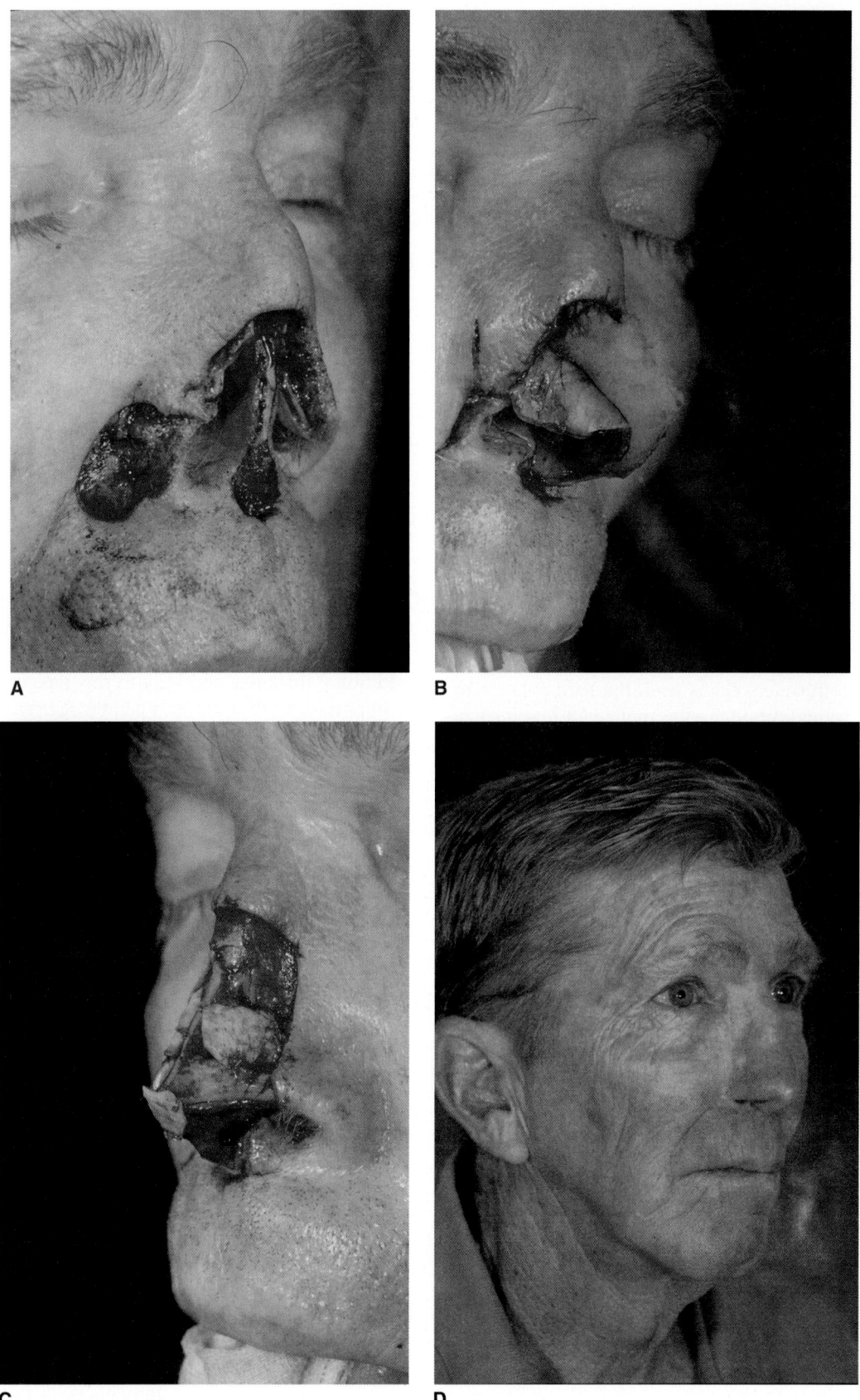

Figure 177.16 Septal mucosal flaps. **A:** Full-thickness nasal defect of distal ½ nose. **B:** Nasal septum pivoted anteriorly along posterior septal angle to provide dorsal and tip support. Bilateral septal mucosal flaps to repair internal lining deficit. **C:** Additional sidewall support from conchal cartilage grafting and shape with a tip graft. **D:** One year following resurfacing with a midline forehead flap. Dorsal support is maintained.

TABLE 177.6	OPTIONS FOR REPAIR OF INTERNAL LINING DEFECTS

1. Primary closure (vertical)
2. Grafts
   a. Skin (rare)
   b. Composite (excellent for ala)
3. Cutaneous epithelial flaps
   a. Folded, distal resurfacing flap
   b. Nasal epithelial "turn-in" flap
   c. Second cutaneous flap (melolabial, forehead)
4. Intranasal flaps
   a. Ipsilateral septal mucosa flap
   b. Contralateral swinging composite flap (excellent for middle vault)
   c. Bipedicled "bucket-handle" flap (small caudal defects only)
   d. Inferior turbinate flap
5. Labial mucosal flap (small caudal defects)
6. Pericranial flap
7. Distant microvascular flap

lining repair because of the concomitant need for structural grafts. An exception might be along the upper one-half of the nose, where collapse and contracture are much less of a concern. Many times, second-intention healing will suffice in this area. Grafts from the hard palate have more intrinsic rigidity and may be applied for intermediate size defects.

A composite graft of skin and cartilage from the ear is extremely versatile and can be liberally applied to full-thickness nasal defects. It may be the technique of choice for lining deficits of the distal one-third of the nose, especially the alar lobule, because it brings a thin epithelium to an area that is normally stratified squamous epithelium and includes a structural graft that forms well to the natural contour of the ala. Small defects of the alar rim and soft

TABLE 177.7	COMMON INTERNAL LINING TECHNIQUES FOR GIVEN NASAL REGION

Middle Vault
1. Contralateral, swinging composite septal flap
2. Epithelial "turn-in" flap
3. Inferior turbinate flap

Distal 1/3 Alar Lobule
1. Composite graft from ear
2. Bipedicled "bucket-handle" flap
3. Ipsilateral septal mucosal flap
4. Folded distal resurfacing flap (forehead flap)

Columella
1. Composite graft
2. Septal mucosal flaps
3. Folded distal resurfacing flap (melolabial flap)
4. Labial flap

tissue facet can be repaired with a composite graft harvested from the root of the helix, utilizing the skin on the inner surface of the helix, within the concha cymba. Larger defects that involve the alar lobule are best reconstructed with a composite graft from the conchal bowl. The donor site can often be closed primarily with minimal auricular deformity. Alternatively, a full-thickness skin graft can be secured to the donor site. In both cases, the skin portion of the graft is closely adhered to the cartilage with little intervening fat, thus making it an excellent option for composite grafts. The graft should be firmly secured to the undersurface of the resurfacing flap, entirely obliterating any potential dead space that might arise. A through-and-through bolster is very effective for this purpose (Fig. 177.17).

Cutaneous Epithelium

Cutaneous epithelium is an additional source for internal lining repair and has some distinct advantages. Large amounts of tissue can be mobilized to inside the nose with little morbidity. Earlier concerns regarding the nonphysiologic nature of this flap (i.e., bringing keratinizing epithelium to the intranasal space) have not borne out to be problematic. Desquamation, odor, or crusting has not been a major complaint for these patients. There is additional thickness and bulk to this type of flap, and it is important to thin the skin paddle aggressively prior to transposition. Nasal obstruction from a thick flap is difficult to correct secondarily. Perhaps the greatest concern is the mobilization of sun-exposed and potentially actinically injured skin to the intranasal portion of the nose, especially considering the high nature of recurrence or metachronous lesions. The intranasal examination postoperatively is best performed by the otolaryngologist and with a nasal endoscope.

A *second epithelial flap* can be elevated and transposed for internal lining repair. Common sites include a separate melolabial flap or second forehead flap. These are associated with extra morbidity but may represent a viable option for advanced cases (38). Distant tissue through microvascular transfer is a more dramatic means of bringing lining to within the nose. It should be viewed as a preliminary step requiring subsequent stages for thinning and sculpting (39–41).

The *distal portion of the primary resurfacing flap* can be folded on itself to wrap around a cartilage graft and provide internal lining. This utilizes cutaneous epithelium and is subject to the same guidelines in terms of risk of transferring actinically injured skin. The additional morbidity may be minimal for small lining defects since the source of skin may be the superior portion of the forehead. The skin paddle should be thinned aggressively. Moreover, this portion of the forehead flap may include the frontal hair and have to be trimmed regularly. There is concern over the vascularity of this distal part of the flap, particularly after folding it on itself, but the robust vascular perfusion appears to be

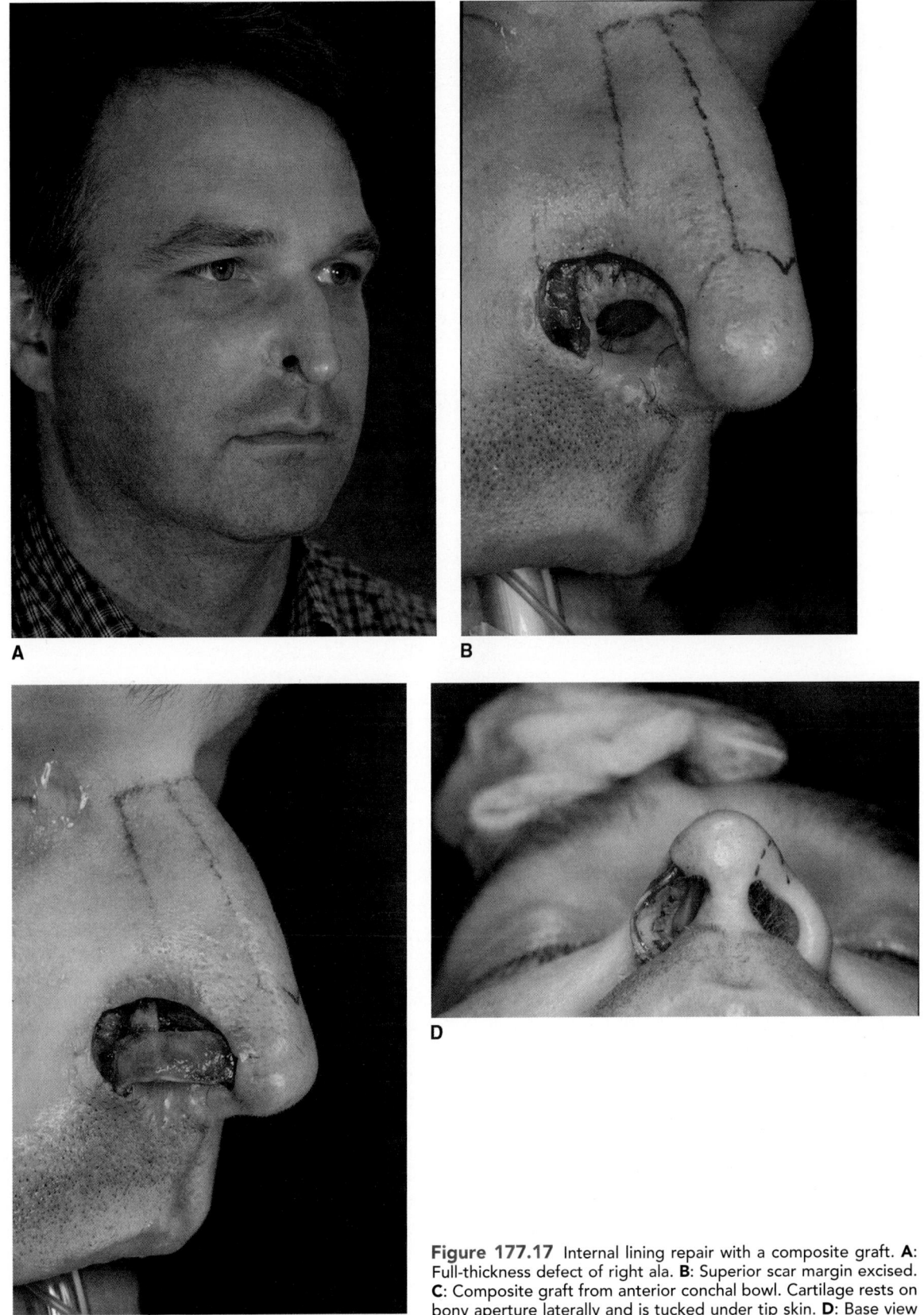

Figure 177.17 Internal lining repair with a composite graft. **A:** Full-thickness defect of right ala. **B:** Superior scar margin excised. **C:** Composite graft from anterior conchal bowl. Cartilage rests on bony aperture laterally and is tucked under tip skin. **D:** Base view demonstrating patency and support.

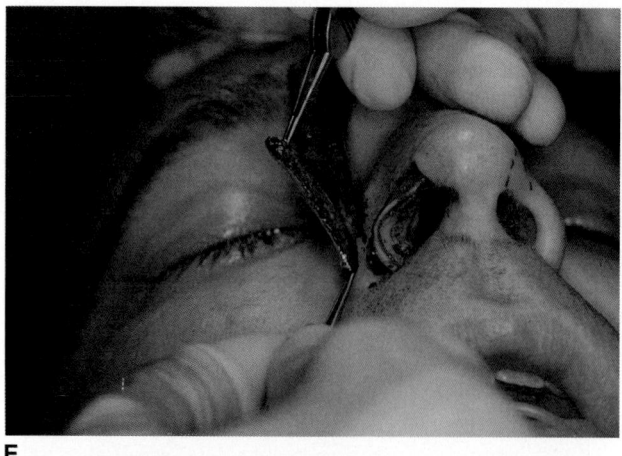

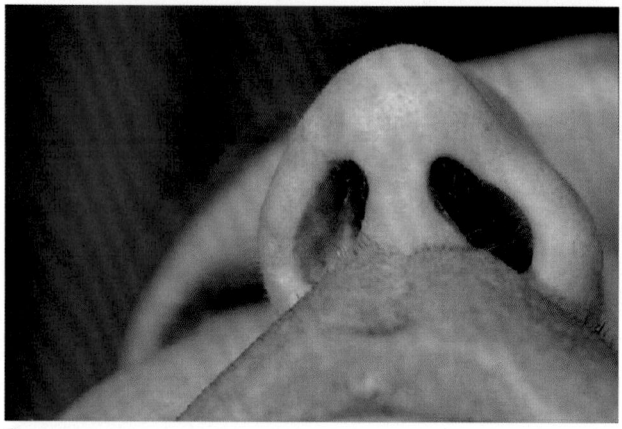

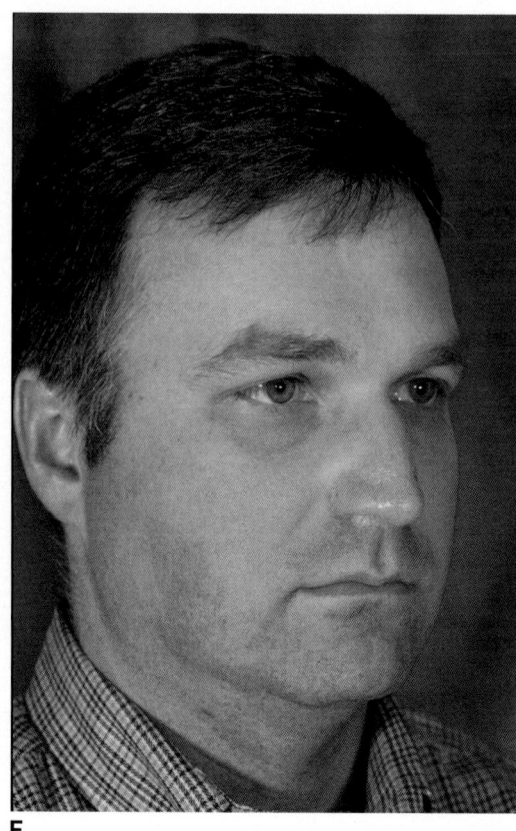

Figure 177.17 *(Continued)* **E:** Forehead flap transferred. Note aggressive thinning. **F:** One-year postoperative view showing contour at rim. **G:** Base view demonstrating vestibular patency.

adequate. Perhaps the greatest shortcoming has to do with the free margin of the ala. Although the intranasal lumen may be functionally adequate, the alar rim often takes on an unnaturally thick and straight appearance when using this method. This option is not used as often for internal lining repair.

The *epithelial "turn-in" flap* is a versatile flap for internal defects limited to the lower half of the nose, especially the middle third/lateral nasal wall (42). It utilizes the cutaneous epithelium from the upper nose and turns it in 180 degrees, so that it faces intranasally. Elevation begins superiorly in the subdermal plane and descends deeper as one proceeds inferiorly in order to create a flap with a healthy subcutaneous pedicle. The pedicle base requires careful dissection in order to avoid amputation and often leaves an area of bulk and fullness to the external nose. The ideal defect has the intranasal edge in close proximity to the skin edge, allowing for primary edge-to-edge approximation. One must closely survey the quality of the skin prior to elevation and transfer. In some cases, this flap adds no additional morbidity; at times, the "turn-in" flap represents skin that would be discarded during the completion of the nasal aesthetic subunits. It has the advantage of not disrupting the native intranasal mucosa, which can greatly

accelerate recovery. It is limited in terms of the amount of skin available and is best suited for smaller internal defects (Fig. 177.18).

Intranasal Tissue

It is ideal to replace tissue with like tissue, and intranasal mucosa has several options that provide a thin, pliable, robust, and physiologic lining for the full-thickness nasal defect. The *inferior turbinate mucosal flap* provides a modest amount of mucosa without major donor site morbidity and can be an excellent flap for defects involving the lateral aspect of the middle or lower thirds of the nose (43). It is rare for a primary cutaneous malignancy to invade so far posteriorly that it disrupts the head of the inferior turbinate. Mesenchymal tumors of the lateral nasal wall, on the other hand, can extend posteriorly to involve the turbinates or even maxillary sinus. The inferior turbinate flap is based anteriorly on its head and is best elevated by first extracting the entire turbinate, including bone, as a flap based anteriorly. The conchal bone is then dissected off and the mucosal flap mobilized to fill the lining defect as an interpolated flap. The pedicle is usually quite short and does not necessarily require revision.

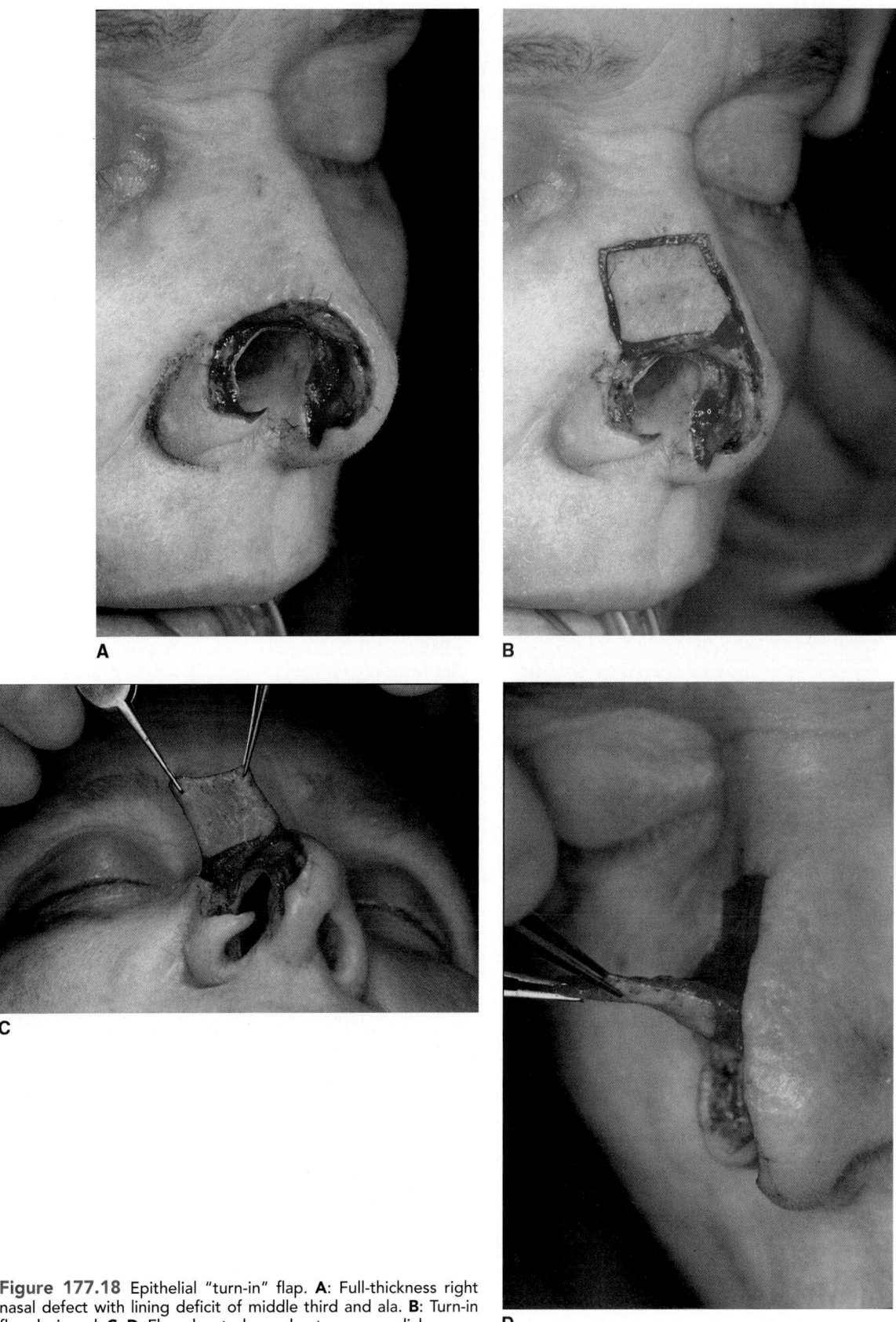

Figure 177.18 Epithelial "turn-in" flap. **A:** Full-thickness right nasal defect with lining deficit of middle third and ala. **B:** Turn-in flap designed. **C, D:** Flap elevated on subcutaneous pedicle.

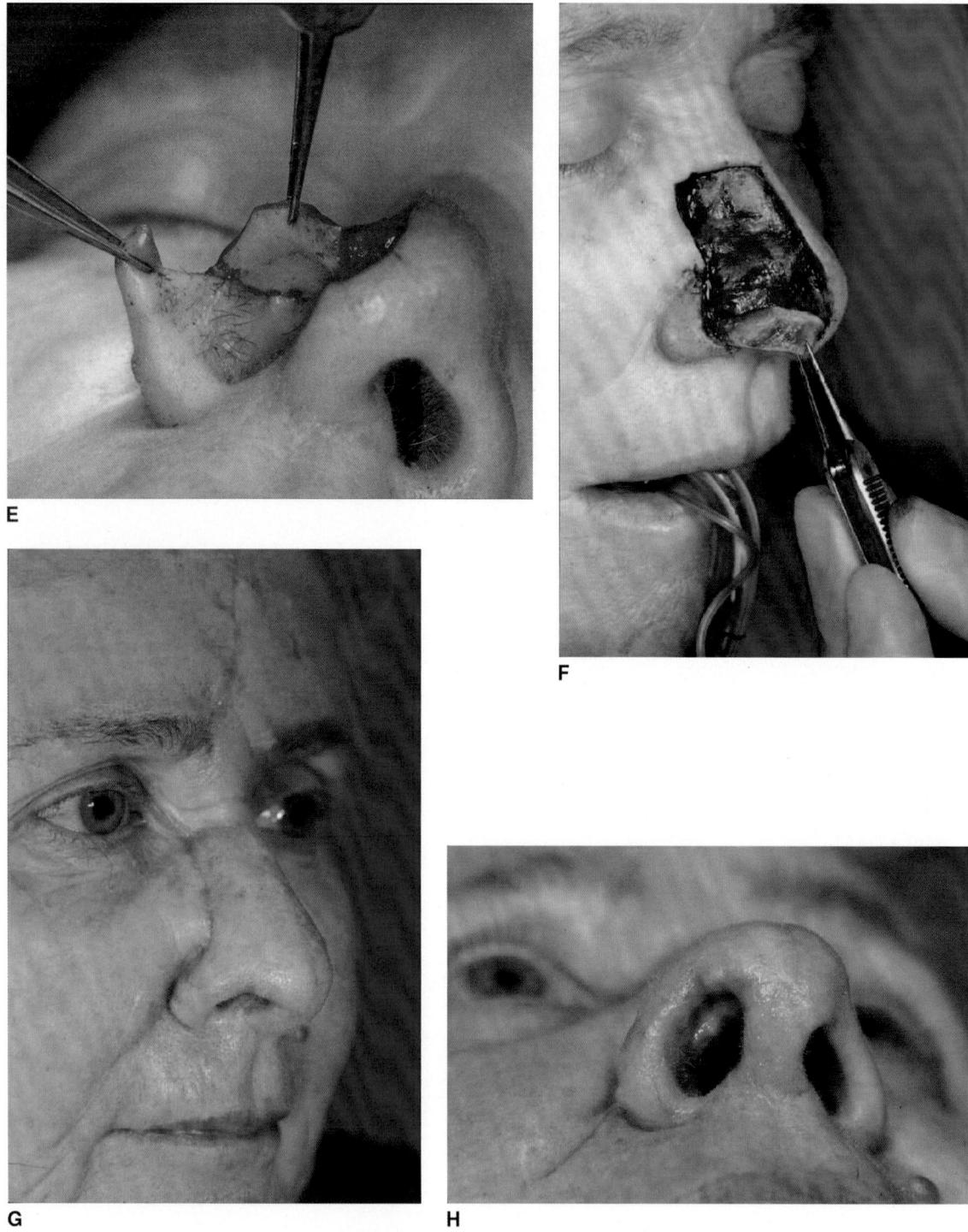

Figure 177.18 *(Continued)* **E**: Flap turned in with cutaneous epithelium facing intranasally. **F**: Two-layered composite graft to distal vestibule. **G, H**: Six months showing alar form and patency.

The *bipedicled "bucket-handle" mucosal flap* is an excellent option for relatively small lining defects along the alar lobule. It utilizes intranasal mucosa immediately above the defect and hinges it inferiorly as a flap based medially and laterally. The anterior septal artery territory does not dependably extend laterally to the sidewall, and the lateral pedicle must be maintained. Any contribution from the ethmoid system is severed by flap design. Wide undermining is critical in order to allow complete mobilization inferiorly without superior traction and recoil. A horizontal relaxing incision can be created with an angled beaver knife. The extent of undermining should be to the nasal bones, where the secondary donor site defect is allowed to heal by second intention. Placing a skin graft to this location is an alternative, but rarely necessary. Any superior retraction will inevitably lift the free alar margin and compromise the alar base symmetry.

The contralateral septal mucosa can be used via a *swinging, composite septal flap*, based on the dorsal septum and the branches of the anterior ethmoid artery. It is an excellent means of providing both intranasal lining and cartilaginous framework to the middle third of the nose. It does not have sufficient size to provide structural framework to the alar lobule. The cartilage is typically straight and can also assist with dorsal support to that area as it rests on the bony ledge of the piriform aperture. The ipsilateral septal mucosa is elevated off the septal cartilage and preserved. A full-thickness incision is then made through the septum, creating a swinging door of cartilage and contralateral septal mucosa, based on a hinge along the dorsum. The cartilage rests lateral to the bony ledge, but the mucosa is sewn directly to the internal lining margin. There is a tendency for the flap to swing back medially, and this is resisted by securing the cartilage to the boney aperture. The ipsilateral septal mucosa can be used for alar lining for larger defects or can be replaced to reconstruct the resultant septal perforation. Occasionally, this area will break down and a perforation will recur.

The ipsilateral, septal mucosa flap is a large flap for complex internal lining defects of the nose. First described by Millard (15) in 1967, it is a thin and dependable flap based on the septal branch of the superior labial artery. The entire septal mucosa is lifted off the cartilage and mobilized to line the lower two-thirds of the nose. Tremendous care should be observed to stay in the correct subperichondrial plane, especially if there coexist septal spurs or fractures. The pedicle to this mucosal flap may cross the nasal vestibule and cause nasal obstruction. This can be divided at a subsequent stage. A large septal perforation may develop but is only rarely symptomatic. The critical prerequisite for this flap is the preservation of the anterior/inferior portion of the septum and the nasal sill, as this functions as the flap base.

Pericranial Flap

The pericranial flap is a thin and versatile flap often used by neurosurgeons for anterior cranial defects. It can also be elevated for internal nasal lining and transferred as part of the forehead flap. The pericranium should be covered with a skin or mucosal graft because, although epithelialization will occur eventually, wound contracture and desiccated cartilage may present problems. The forehead flap can be elevated full thickness (i.e., with the periosteum of the forehead), then split longitudinally to excise the frontalis muscle and create a bifid flap that encapsulates the cartilage grafts of the nose. The pericranium is based on the same pedicle as the forehead flap but is more tenuous and a wider pedicle base may be needed. It can be dunked intranasally during the pedicle division at 3 weeks.

CONCLUSION

Nasal restoration in the 21st century has reached a new milestone that has brought together centuries of experiences, lessons, errors, and rewards. The bar has been set and it is nothing less than full restoration of normal function and complete aesthetic acceptance. The expectations for both minor and major nasal repair include symmetry, natural contour, excellent color and texture match, and a final product that remains inconspicuous to the casual observer. The major tenets that have been realized today include the wide application of the subunit principle, liberal and nonanatomic cartilage grafting, and addressing each of the three layers of the nose diligently and independently. The robust nature of the forehead flap has expanded its applications and lifted the outcomes of major nasal resurfacing. Anticipating resultant scars and vectors of tension are the subtle nuances of local flaps that ensure a pleasing result.

HIGHLIGHTS

- Using a reconstructive *algorithm* can assist with flap selection and avoiding pitfalls.
- Alar base symmetry must be preserved with small flaps, often requiring cartilage batten grafts and careful design.
- Consideration of the aesthetic subunit principle can improve scar camouflage.
- The forehead flap is a robust flap that remains the workhorse for resurfacing large defects.
- Full-thickness defects must address each of the three layers of the nose independently (internal lining, structure, and covering).
- Nasal function is paramount and usually addressed with nonanatomic, conchal cartilage grafts resting on the lateral nasal wall laterally.
- All internal lining defects must be meticulously repaired with flaps or grafts.

REFERENCES

1. Conroy B. The history of facial prostheses. *Clin Plast Surg* 1983;10:689–707.
2. Almast S. History and evolution of the Indian method of rhinoplasty. In: Sanvenero-Rosselli G, ed. *Transactions of the Fourth International Congress of Plastic and Reconstructive Surgery.* (Rome, 1967) Amsterdam: Excerpta Medica Foundation, 1969:49.
3. Antia NH, Daver BM. Reconstructive surgery for nasal defects. *Clin Plast Surg* 1981;8(3):535–563.
4. Sushruta S. *The Sushruta Samhita.* English translation based on original sanskrit text. Kaviraj Kunja Lal Bhishagratna, ed. Bose, Calcutta: Kaviraj Kunja Lal Bhishagratna, 1907–1916.
5. Antia NH, Daver BM. Reconstructive surgery for nasal defects. *Clin Plast Surg* 1981;8:535–563.
6. "BL." Letter to the editor. *Gentleman's Magazine.* London, October 1794:891. Reprinted in: *Plast Reconstr Surg* 1969;44:67–69.

7. Carpue J. An account of two successful operations for restoring a lost nose from the integuments of the forehead. London, UK: Longman, Hurst, Reese, Orme and Brown Publishers, 1816. Reprinted in: *Plast Reconstr Surg* 1969;44:175–185.

8. Kazanjian VH. The repair of nasal defects with the median forehead flap primary closure of the forehead wound. *Surg Gynecol Obstet* 1946;83:27–32.

9. Converse JM. New forehead flap for nasal reconstruction. *Proc R Soc Med* 1942;35:811–815.

10. Gilles HD. Experiences with the tubed pedicle flaps. *Surg Gynecol Obstet* 1935;60:291–293.

11. New GB. Sickle flaps for nasal reconstruction. *Surg Gynecol Obstet* 1945;80:497–499.

12. Converse JM. Reconstruction of the nose by the scalping flap technique. *Surg Clin North Am* 1959;39:335–364.

13. Washio H. Retroauricular temporal flap. *Plast Reconstr Surg* 1969;43:162–165.

14. Millard DR. Total reconstructive rhinoplasty and a missing link. *Plast Reconstr Surg* 1966;37:167–170.

15. Millard DR. Hemirhinoplasty. *Plast Reconstr Surg* 1967;40:440–445.

16. Millard DR. Reconstructive rhinoplasty for the lower half of the nose. *Plast Reconstr Surg* 1974;53:133–138.

17. Millard DR. Reconstructive rhinoplasty for the lower two-thirds of the nose. *Plast Reconstr Surg* 1976;57:722–728.

18. Burget GC, Menick FJ. *Aesthetic reconstruction of the nose.* St. Louis, MO: Mosby–Year Book, 1994:1–600.

19. Langer C. Zur anatomie und physiologie der haut. *Sitzungsb Acad Wissensch* 1861;45:223–229.

20. Singh DJ, Bartlett SP. Aesthetic considerations in nasal reconstruction and the role of modified nasal subunits. *Plast Reconstr Surg* 2003;111(2):639–648.

21. Woodard CR, Park SS. Reconstruction of nasal defects 1.5 cm or smaller. *Arch Facial Plast Surg* 2011;13(2):97–102.

22. Rieger RA. A local flap for repair of the nasal tip. *Plast Reconstr Surg* 1967;40:147–149.

23. Limberg AA. *Mathematical principles of local plastic procedures on the surface of the human body.* Leningrad: in-government publishing house for medical literature (Medgiz), 1946.

24. Zitelli JA. The bilobed flap for nasal reconstruction. *Arch Dermatol* 1989;125:957.

25. Oo KK, Park SS. The midline forehead flap in nasal reconstruction. *Facial Plast Surg Clin North Am* 2011;19(1):141–155.

26. Yotsuyanagi T, Yamashita K, Uroshidate S, et al. Nasal reconstruction based on aesthetic subunits in Orientals. *Plast Reconstr Surg* 2000;106(1):36–44.

27. Lang PG, Duncan IM, Hochman M. Occurrence of subclinical tumor in excised facial subunits. *Arch Facial Plast Surg* 2004;6:158–161.

28. Murrell GL, Burger GC. Aesthetically precise templates for nasal reconstruction using a new material. *Plast Reconstr Surg* 2003;112:1855–1861.

29. Park SS. Reconstruction of nasal defects larger than 1.5 cm in diameter. *Laryngoscope* 2000;110(8):1241–1250.

30. Yu D, Weng R. Anatomical study of forehead flap with its pedicle based on cutaneous branch of supratrochlear artery and its application in nasal reconstruction. *Ann Plast Surg* 2010;65(2):183–187.

31. Tardy ME, Sykes J, Kron T. The precise midline forehead flap. *Clin Plast Surg* 1985;12:481.

32. Adamson JE. Nasal reconstruction with the expanded forehead flap. *Plast Reconstr Surg* 1988;81(1):12–20.

33. Park SS, Rodeheaver G, Levine PA. Role of ischemic gradient on neovascularization of interpolated skin flaps. *Arch Otolaryngol Head Neck Surg* 1996;122(8):886–889.

34. Quetz J, Ambrosch P. Total Nasal Reconstruction: a 6-year experience with the three-stage forehead flap combined with the septal pivot flap. *Facial Plast Surg* 2011;27(3):266–275.

35. Converse JM, Wood-Smith D. Experiences with the forehead island flap with a subcutaneous pedicle. *Plast Reconstr Surg* 1963;31:521–527.

36. Park SS. Single-stage forehead flap: an alternative with advantages. *Arch Facial Plast Surg* 2002;4:32–36.

37. Park SS. The flaring suture to augment the repair of the dysfunctional nasal valve. *Plast Reconstr Surg* 1998;101(4):1120–1122.

38. Parikh S, Futran N, et al. An alternative method for reconstruction of large intranasal lining defects: the farina method revisited. *Arch Facial Plast Surg* 2010;12(5):311–314.

39. Menick FJ, Salibian A. Microvascular repair of heminasal, subtotal and total nasal defects with a folded radial forearm flap and a full-thickness forehead flap. *Plast Reconstr Surg* 2010;127(2):637–651.

40. Antunes MB, Chalian AA. Microvascular reconstruction of nasal defects. *Facial Plast Surg Clin North Am* 2011;19(1):157–162.

41. Moore EJ, Strome SA, Kasperbauer JL., et al. Vascularized radial forearm free tissue for lining in nasal reconstruction. *Laryngoscope* 2003;113(12):2078–2085.

42. Park SS, Cook TA, Wang TD. The epithelial "turn-in" flap in nasal reconstruction. *Arch Otolaryngol Head Neck Surg* 1995;121:1122–1127.

43. Murakami CS, Kriet D, et al. Nasal reconstruction using the inferior turbinate mucosal flap. *Arch Plast Surg* 1999;13:97–110.

Facial Reanimation

178

Tessa A. Hadlock

Rehabilitation of the paralyzed face remains a challenging problem for otolaryngologists, and its proper management may require input from facial plastic surgeons, head and neck reconstruction specialists, otologists, and adjunct medical personnel. Following viral nerve insult, traumatic nerve injury, or intentional sacrifice with repair or cable grafting, regenerative results vary greatly and can lead to hypofunction, hyperfunction, aberrant regeneration, or a combination of these phenomena. The functional problems related to facial paralysis are extensive. In the upper face, they include brow ptosis, leading to a visual field deficit and hygiene issues related to skin desquamation onto the cornea. In addition, loss of a blink reflex leads to corneal exposure of the affected eye, there is lacrimal gland hypo- or hyperfunction, and lower lid paralysis results in ectropion as well as poor lacrimal punctal function. In the central zone of the face, patients may suffer with unilateral nasal obstruction, upper lip ptosis, lack of oral commissure excursion with smiling, oral incompetence to both liquids and solids, and articulation problems. In the lower face, lower lip weakness also contributes to oral incompetence, and platysmal synkinesis can restrict smiling and lead to superficial torticollis symptoms. Facial paralysis also has a significant impact on nonverbal communication, and the loss of one's ability to express positive emotions on the face rivals the above-listed issues as the most dominant source of patient devastation.

Herein, we review the management of facial nerve deficits and describe the surgical management of each distinct zone of the paralyzed face, with regard to recovery potential, prognosis, and patient factors that contribute to surgical decision making. We emphasize the systematic assessment of each facial zone as a critical step to ensure comprehensive management of the paralyzed face (1).

NERVE REPAIR AND GRAFTING

Nerve Injury Classification

Nerve injuries are classified according to the level of microanatomical disruption. According to the Sunderland classification system (2), level 1 injury has no microanatomic disruption but a simple temporary dysfunction of the membrane sodium channels, resulting in transient inability of the nerve to transmit impulses. In level 2 injury, axons are disrupted, though their individual endoneurial channels are not, so that when regeneration occurs, there is little to no axonal misrouting. In level 3 injury, endoneurial sheaths are violated, though perineurium is left intact. Recovery from this type of injury occurs over months and inevitably results in some synkinesis. Level 4 injury implies total perineurial disruption, where only the outer epineurial sheath is intact, and spontaneous recovery is generally poor. Level 5 injury refers to total anatomic disruption, including the epineurium. No spontaneous recovery is expected from this injury without surgical intervention.

Management of Neural Discontinuity

In cases of complete facial nerve disruption, reestablishment of direct nerve continuity is required for restoration of muscle function. Reapproximation of freshened edges must be accomplished without placing tension across the suture line, through simple epineurial sutures. When injury occurs within the temporal bone, thorough exposure of the site of injury is recommended, and surgical repair is indicated when 50% of the diameter of the facial nerve appears to have been violated (3).

After facial nerve injury or sacrifice, if a tensionless neurorrhaphy is not possible because of a gap between the cut edges, then a nerve graft is employed to bridge the neural defect. In facial nerve reconstruction, the three most commonly employed nerve grafts are the great auricular nerve, the sural nerve, and the medial antebrachial cutaneous nerve (Fig. 178.1). For short nerve gaps in the absence of head and neck malignancy, the great auricular nerve is a convenient choice. This often does not require a separate incision from the primary facial nerve exposure incision. The resulting anesthesia to the ipsilateral auricle is well tolerated, and the nerve is of adequate diameter and caliber to provide a suitable graft. However, for nerve gaps of greater than 10 cm, the great auricular nerve does not always provide sufficient length, and the sural nerve becomes a better option. The nerve is removed from the leg via a short incision adjacent to the lateral malleolus and can be harvested

through a series of stair-step incisions, a minimally invasive stripping technique, using endoscopic equipment (Fig. 178.2). The resulting segment of anesthetic skin on the dorsum of the foot does not pose a significant clinical problem, and the nerve can yield up to 30 cm in length. For total facial nerve reconstruction from the main trunk to the peripheral branches, the medial antebrachial cutaneous nerve is most appropriate. There are at least four reliable branches, and it provides adequate length to graft the entire facial nerve, from the geniculate ganglion to the medial border of the parotid gland.

For both primary nerve repair and nerve grafting, surgery should be performed within the first 72 hours after injury or sacrifice, irrespective of the need for subsequent

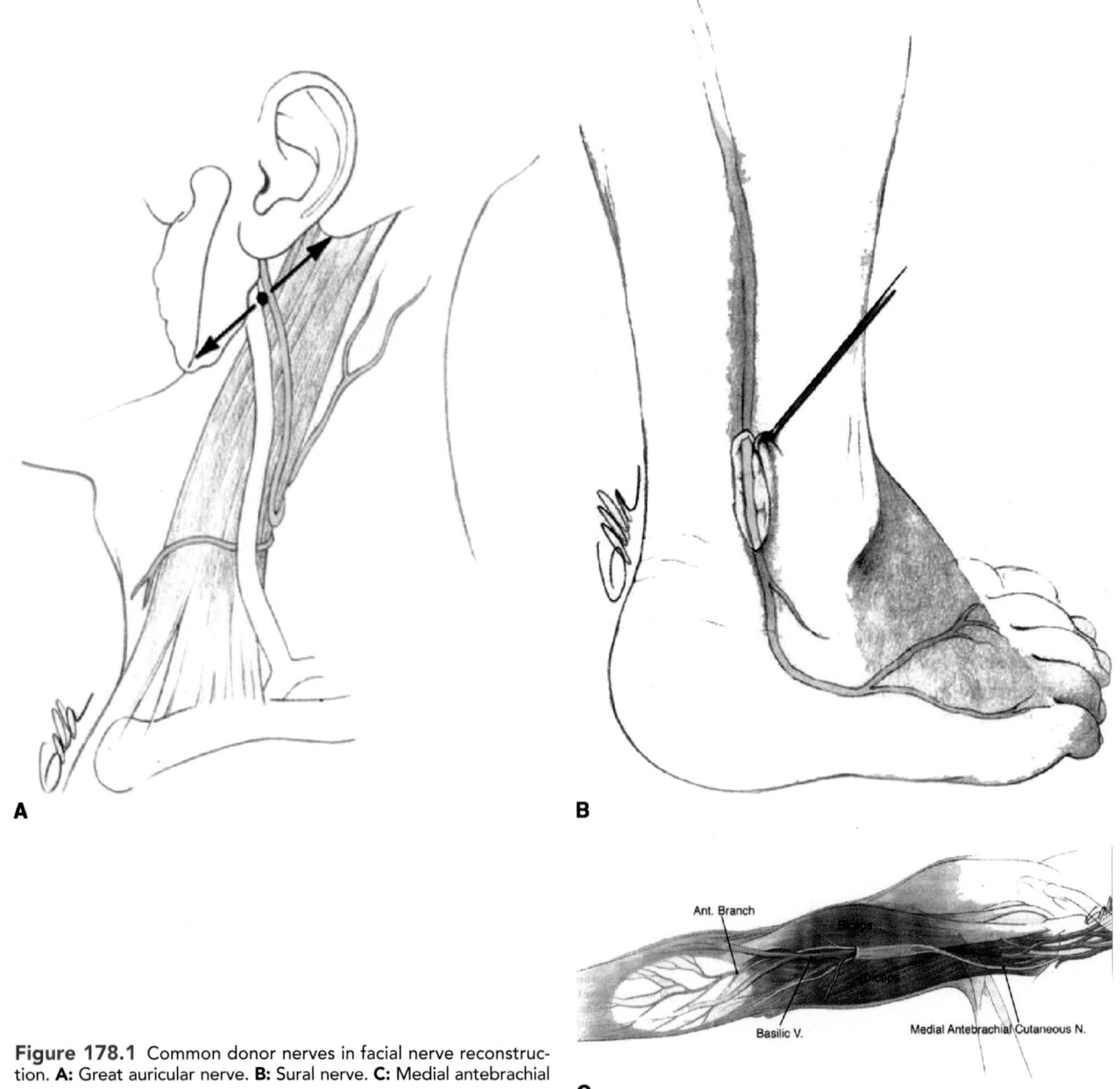

A   **B**

C

Figure 178.1 Common donor nerves in facial nerve reconstruction. **A:** Great auricular nerve. **B:** Sural nerve. **C:** Medial antebrachial cutaneous nerve.

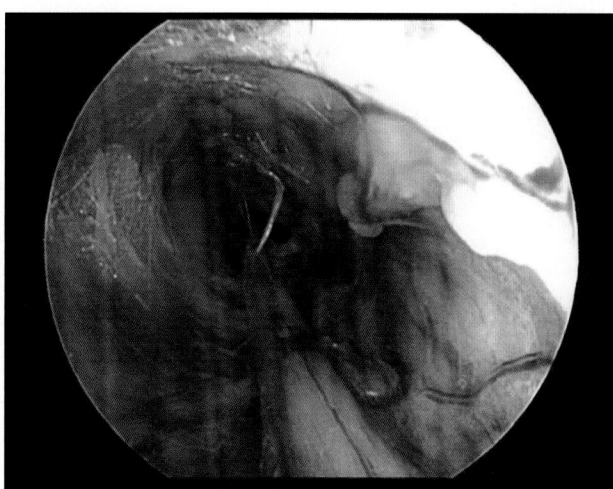

Figure 178.2 Endoscopic view of sural nerve during harvest. Note the nerve at the 6 o'clock position.

radiation therapy (4). During this time frame, the distal nerve segments retain electrical stimulability, making identification easier. Meticulous debridement and careful microsurgical technique are of paramount importance in optimizing outcome. There is debate as to the best method of nerve coaptation, as it applies to both primary and graft repair. Epineurial repair has been contrasted to fascicular repair, though no study has convincingly demonstrated improved regenerative outcome based upon fascicular facial nerve repair. Therefore, given its relative simplicity, the current standard is to perform epineurial suture repair. Though not fully established as more efficacious, it is now becoming commonplace to further reinforce the repair using fibrin glue stabilization (5).

Reinnervation Techniques

When the reestablishment of neural continuity is not possible based upon absence of an adequate proximal facial nerve stump at the brainstem, or severe comminution within the temporal bone, an alternative approach to restoring neural input to the facial musculature involves nerve substitution. This approach, also termed reinnervation, involves performing surgery to deliver neural input to the distal facial nerve and musculature via an alternative motor nerve. The hypoglossal facial transfer is most often used, though investigators have studied the utility of the spinal accessory nerve, the motor branch to the sternocleidomastoid muscle, and the masseteric branch of the trigeminal nerve as alternative inputs for the distal facial trunk. Axonal ingrowth through the distal facial nerve to the target muscles provides resting tone to the facial musculature, and voluntary movement of the tongue, shoulder, or muscle of mastication elicits facial movement. Reinnervation techniques are most commonly employed following skull base tumor resection, when the facial nerve is sacrificed at the brainstem, or when the facial nerve is

not actually sacrificed but does not appear to be reaching facial muscle targets after a 12-month waiting period, based upon clinical examination and electrophysiologic studies.

The advantages of the hypoglossal nerve as a donor for reinnervation techniques include its location, close to the extratemporal facial nerve; its dense population of motor axons; and the relative acceptability of the resultant hemitongue weakness. In the classic XII-VII transfer, the entire hypoglossal nerve is transected and reflected superiorly, and a neurorrhaphy to the facial nerve stump is performed (Fig. 178.3A). Several modifications have been described (6) (Fig. 178.3B–D), including the "split" XII-VII transfer, where approximately 30% of the width of the hypoglossal nerve is divided from the main trunk of the nerve for several centimeters, and secured to the lower division of the facial nerve (Fig. 178.3B). Another modification is the XII-VII jump graft, designed to reduce tongue morbidity by avoiding the splicing away of a significant length of the hypoglossal trunk. This involves an end-to-side neurorrhaphy between the hypoglossal nerve and a donor cable graft (usually the great auricular nerve), which in turn is sewn to the distal facial trunk (9) (Fig. 178.3C). This modification evolved from a more precise appreciation of the microanatomy of the hypoglossal nerve, which demonstrates interwoven fascicular architecture; separating a 30% segment away from the main trunk for several centimeters divides a significantly greater number of axons than if the fibers were oriented in parallel.

In circumstances where the facial nerve can be mobilized within the temporal bone and reflected inferiorly, removal of the mastoid tip has permitted direct coaptation of the facial nerve to the hypoglossal nerve, without the need for an interposition graft (see Fig. 178.3D). Elimination of the cable graft provides a theoretical regenerative advantage by reducing from two neurorrhaphies to one.

Surgical Technique

The classic XII-VII procedure is performed via a modified Blair parotidectomy incision. The main trunk of the facial nerve and the pes anserinus are identified using standard facial nerve landmarks. The hypoglossal nerve is identified deep to the posterior belly of the digastric muscle and is followed anteriorly, to just beyond the branching of the descendens hypoglossi. The hypoglossal nerve is sharply transected and reflected superiorly to meet the facial nerve. The facial nerve is transected at the stylomastoid foramen, reflected inferiorly, and secured to the hypoglossal nerve with several 10-0 nylon epineurial microsutures.

The split XII-VII transfer (Fig. 178.3B) provides many fewer axons and is therefore best utilized only for the lower segment of the face. In the jump graft procedure (Fig. 178.3C), the great auricular nerve graft is harvested and interposed between the hypoglossal nerve and the facial stump. For the facial nerve mobilization out of the

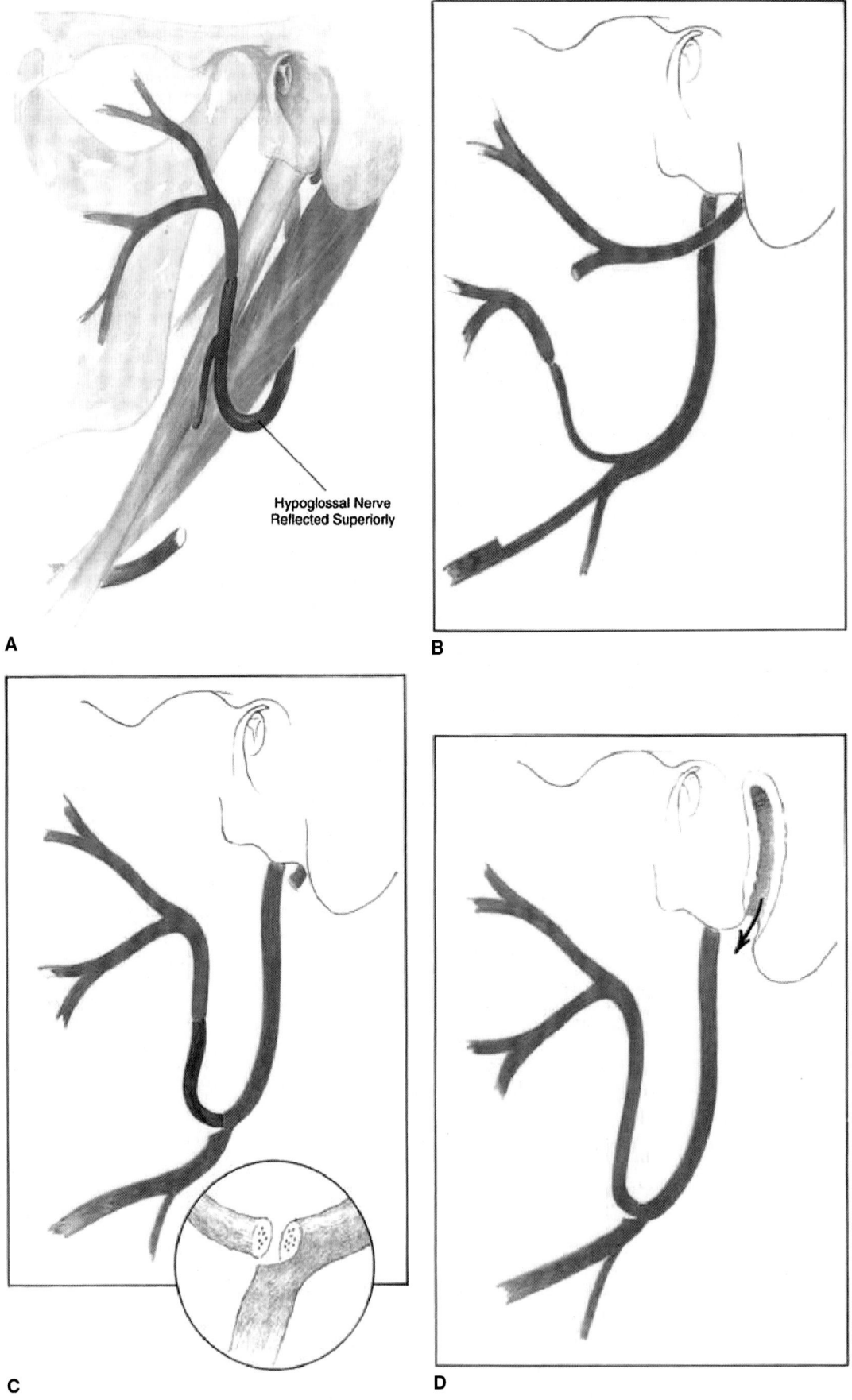

A

B

C

D

Hypoglossal Nerve
Reflected Superiorly

Figure 178.3 Hypoglossal facial nerve transfer. Hypoglossal nerve is shown in *green*, facial nerve in *orange*. **A:** Classic procedure, with entire hypoglossal nerve transected. **B:** Modification with 40% segment of nerve secured to lower division. **C:** Jump graft (*purple*) modification. Insert shows how graft is positioned to capture axons extending from the proximal aspect of the opened hypoglossal nerve. **D:** Reflection of the facial nerve out of the mastoid bone to meet the hypoglossal nerve in the neck.

temporal bone, the proximal facial nerve is mobilized from the temporal bone via mastoidectomy approach, sectioned at the second genu, and transposed into the neck by removal of the mastoid tip. The facial nerve can be further mobilized by dissecting it away from the parotid tissue beyond its bifurcation. The end-to-side neurorrhaphy is executed by removing a segment of hypoglossal epineurium, then cutting a 30% opening into the hypoglossal nerve and allowing exposure of the severed axons.

With a XII-VII transfer, good resting facial tone is achieved in over 90% of patients. When successful, the transfer allows deliberate facial movement with intentional manipulation of the tongue. Results are variable, and it is generally agreed that reinnervation must be performed within 2 years following injury, before facial muscle fibrosis and atrophy progress to a point where meaningful tone and movement are not achievable.

Two significant drawbacks of the procedure are the mass facial movement experienced by many patients and the variable tongue dysfunction, which has been categorized as "severe" in up to 25% of patients. Articulation and mastication difficulties are commonly cited. The modifications mentioned above are aimed at one or the other of these two problems. The procedure is contraindicated in patients who are likely to develop other cranial neuropathies (i.e., neurofibromatosis type II) or who have ipsilateral tenth nerve deficits, as the combined X-XII deficit can result in profound swallowing dysfunction.

VII-VII Cross-Face Grafting

Some have advocated utilizing branches of the contralateral facial nerve to drive the denervated facial musculature. It is the only donor source with the potential for mimetic function (the involuntary blink and emotive smile), and it is significantly arborized distally, so several branches may be sacrificed for use in cross-facial grafting, without adversely affecting the healthy side. Donor branches contain many fewer motor axons than the hypoglossal to power the paralyzed side, so the motor input provided by the hypoglossal nerve is distinctly superior. The use of the contralateral facial nerve strictly for reinnervation of native facial musculature has largely been replaced by cross-face nerve grafting in conjunction with free muscle transfer.

ZONAL APPROACH TO THE PARALYZED FACE

The goal of modern facial reanimation surgery is to address each specific functional and aesthetic zone of the face during the rehabilitation process (1). In order to identify specific zonal deficits, it is helpful to divide the face into upper, middle, and lower facial zones and to systematically characterize each of the issues that arise within those zones. Then, the choice as to whether to pursue a static correction of position of facial landmarks, a dynamic reconstruction that introduces movement, or alternative reanimation techniques can be made separately for each area. Below, we present approaches to each zone of the face, based upon location and functional issue.

The Upper Facial Zone

The three key regions in the paralyzed upper face are the brow, the upper eyelid, and the lower eyelid. In facial nerve dysfunction, the brow is most commonly ptotic, though it can also be in a balanced position, or be paradoxically hyperelevated. Significant brow ptosis can seriously impair peripheral vision. The upper eyelid can be superiorly malpositioned, from both paralysis of the orbicularis oculi and foreshortening of the levator palpebrae superioris (LPS) based upon the lack of periodic passive stretching of the muscle from the orbicularis oculi. The lack of passive stretch results in inappropriate cross-linking of the LPS myosin bridges, resulting in foreshortening. In chronic synkinesis (i.e., after viral facial paralysis or skull base surgery), the upper lid can also be inferiorly malpositioned and can be accompanied by acquired ptosis, likely from disinsertion of the tendon of the LPS under the chronic influence of the hyperkinetic orbicularis oculi. The flaccid lower eyelid can fall away from the globe, producing both scleral show and ectropion. Synkinesis results in superior malposition of the lower lid, with a slit-like palpebral fissure. Hyperlacrimation with eating, termed the syndrome of crocodile tears, or Bogorad syndrome, must also be assessed.

Based upon analysis of the upper facial issues, a management plan is designed. Usually, the brow and upper lid are addressed surgically, even when recovery through a graft is expected. Surgical management of the lower lid may be reserved for cases in which permanent flaccidity is clinically apparent.

Surgical Techniques

For the inferiorly positioned brow, surgical correction is ordinarily performed in the office setting. The brow can be secured into its proper position either by performing subperiosteal dissection followed by soft tissue fixation using biodegradable polymeric devices (Endotine Inc., Coapt, Palo Alto, CA) or by using suture-bearing bone pins. Additional options for brow ptosis correction include direct brow lifting and midforehead brow lifting. Alternatively, a two-stitch subcutaneous brow lift can be executed (Fig. 178.4). Using either surgical approach, excellent correction of brow position can be achieved. Recurrent brow ptosis may occur and is usually amenable to office revision.

The Upper Eyelid

There are three approaches to the flaccidly paralyzed upper eyelid: eyelid-weighting techniques, eyelid spring placement, and tarsorrhaphy. The most common and

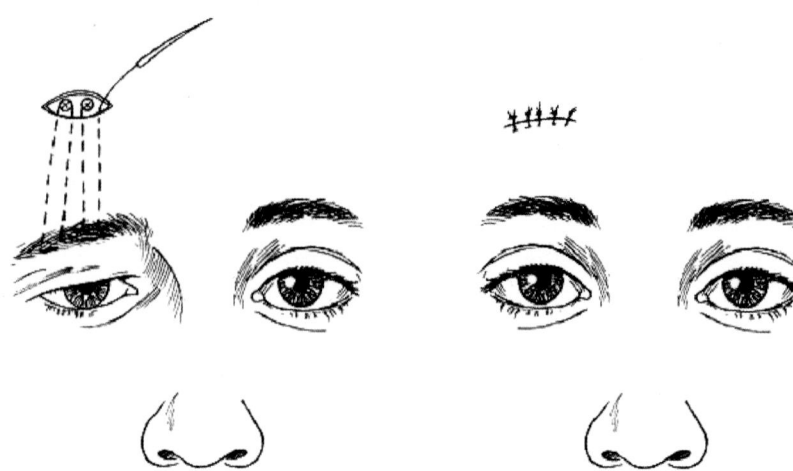

Figure 178.4 Suture-based brow lifting technique, showing placement of sutures from brow to bone pins.

predictable of these approaches is placement of a weighted implant, made of either gold or platinum. The thin profile platinum weight is preferred (7), given its higher density and the lack of reported allergic reactions, which occur up to 9% of the time using gold. The thin implants are barely visible beneath the skin, compared with thicker gold implants; the technique is straightforward and is performed under straight local anesthesia. An incision is made in the supratarsal crease, and a plane is developed deep to the orbicularis oculi, exposing the anterior surface of the tarsal plate. The implant is inserted and centered over the medial limbus. It is secured with permanent 6-0 clear nylon sutures to the tarsal plate (Fig. 178.5). If sufficient recovery to protect the cornea does occur through a nerve graft or via reinnervation, the eyelid weight is easily removed.

Eyelid springs are designed to achieve a more natural blink. However, the procedure carries a high revision rate, nearly 100%, and therefore lacks the reliability of the eyelid-weighting techniques. Tarsorrhaphy techniques (Fig. 178.6) are extremely effective at protecting the cornea but yield the least favorable aesthetic result.

For the hypertonic, inferiorly positioned upper lid seen in ocular synkinesis, lateral canthal botulinum toxin administration is effective in resolving hyperkinesis, improving quality of life, and restoring a normal palpebral fissure width (Fig. 178.7) (8). This approach involves serial treatments at 4- to 6-month intervals.

The Lower Eyelid

The weak lower eyelid may be addressed using tarsal strip procedures, in which a small segment of the lateral tarsus is removed to tighten the lower lid, though this may not have the desired long-term effect in the paralyzed eye. More long-lasting approaches include placement of a fascia lata sling from the nasal bone medially, through the lower eyelid on the lower tarsal plate, to the superolateral orbital rim (Fig. 178.8). The surgical technique involves harvesting fascia lata from the thigh and the creation of

a 0.5-cm × 10-cm strip. The fascia is secured to the nasal bone via a single bone anchor and tunneled subcutaneously with the use of a fascia needle. A small nick is made in the lateral brow, to expose a segment of the superolateral orbital rim. A through and through hole is drilled in the lateral orbital rim with a 1.5-mm otologic drill, and a suture is passed through the fascia lata and through the bone. This provides a "seat belt" for the lower lid, and tension can be very precisely set on the lower lid to achieve the proper location. This procedure provides good long-term results; however, the surgical technique possesses a steep learning curve.

Lacrimal Function

Facial nerve damage proximal to the geniculate ganglion can result in inappropriate tearing during salivation, where fibers intended for the salivary glands are misrouted to the lacrimal gland. This phenomenon is known as Bogorad syndrome (synonymous with the syndrome of crocodile tears). Hyperlacrimation with eating can be managed with botulinum toxin injection into the lacrimal gland (9). Occasionally, there is normal tear volume that masquerades as hyperlacrimation, based upon failure of the punctal system to adequately drain the fornix. Dacryocystorhinostomy, lower lid correction, and good lid hygiene can ameliorate this condition. Hypolacrimation is treated with periodic administration of artificial tears.

The Middle Facial Zone

Functional and aesthetic issues that arise in the midface include nasal base malrotation, leading to external nasal valve collapse, malposition of the nasolabial fold (NLF) (either hyperprominence or effacement), upper lip ptosis, philtral deviation, and poor excursion of the oral commissure (1). Hypertonic facial paresis, such as that seen following poorly recovered Bell palsy or Ramsay Hunt syndrome, generally leads to an overprominence of the nasolabial fold.

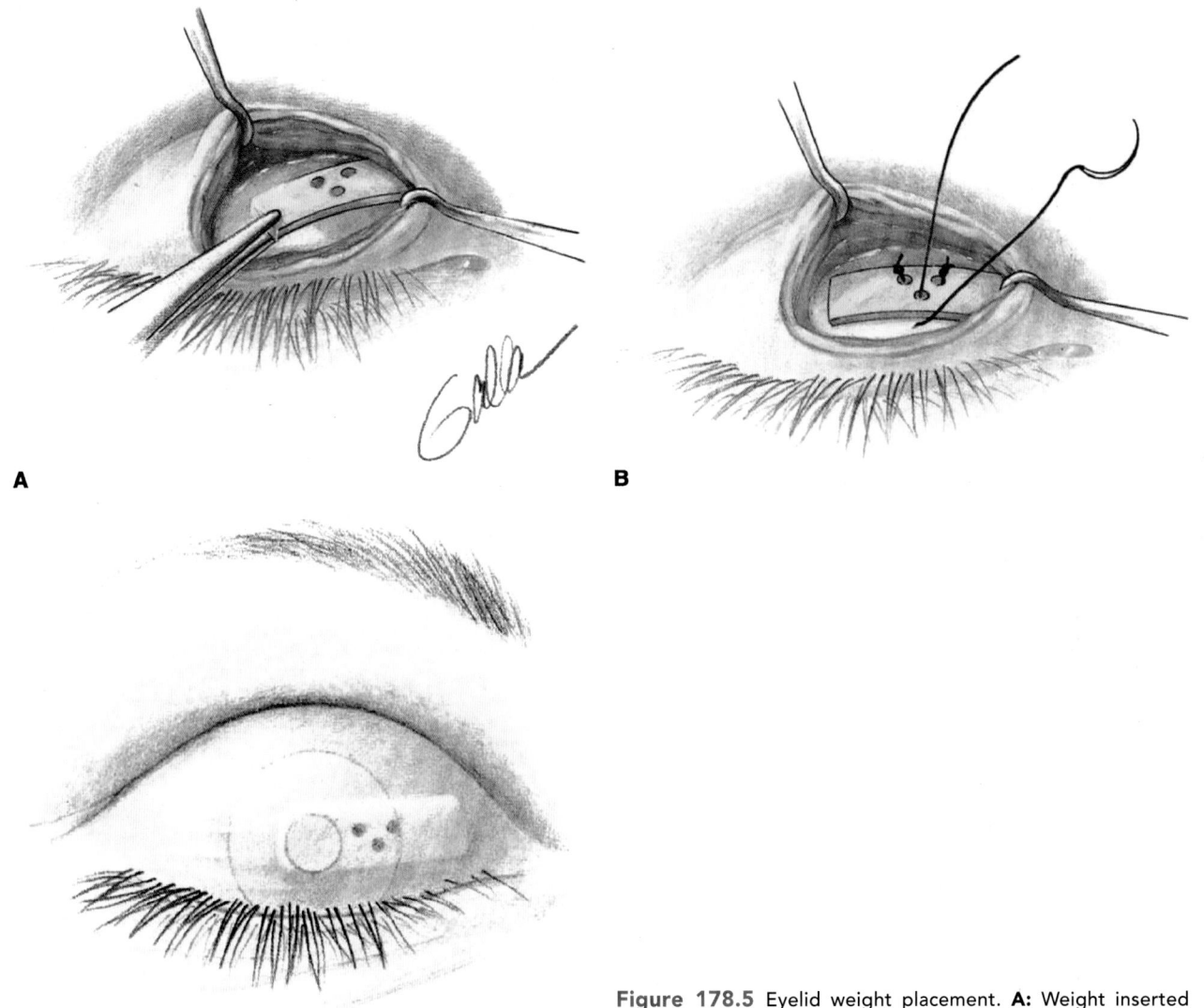

A

B

C

Figure 178.5 Eyelid weight placement. **A:** Weight inserted directly onto tarsal plate. **B:** Sutures prevent mobility of the weight. **C:** Location of weight centered over medial limbus.

Surgical Techniques

The Nose

External nasal valve collapse is addressed with a fascia lata sling technique (10). A segment of fascia lata is harvested from the lateral thigh and tunneled subcutaneously from a temporal and preauricular incision to an incision made in the alar crease. The fascia lata is secured medially to the sesamoid cartilages in the nasal ala and laterally to the true temporalis fascia (Fig. 178.9). Additional lower lateral cartilage batten grafting may help in cases of persistent valve collapse due to lower lateral cartilage in-bowing during inspiration.

The Nasolabial Fold

Nasolabial fold abnormalities are addressed according to whether there is flaccid or hypertonic facial paralysis. Suture suspension techniques analogous to those used during face lifting are placed either medial to the fold (to

define an effaced NLF) or lateral to the fold (to soften a hyperprominent NLF) (1).

Botulinum toxin chemodenervation in the midface is not helpful for nasolabial fold hyperprominence, as it frequently results in upper lip ptosis without correcting the asymmetry.

The Oral Commissure and Smile

Restoration of the smile is one of the most important goals of the facial reanimation surgeon. While every individual possesses a slightly different smile, there are three basic smile shapes (11), which are classified depending upon which muscle groups dominate during smiling (Fig. 178.10). Sixty-seven percent of individuals possess a "zygomaticus major" smile, in which the zygomaticus muscles and buccinator muscle have the strongest action during emotive smiling. In 30% of individuals, the zygomaticus and levator labii superioris muscles codominate, giving a

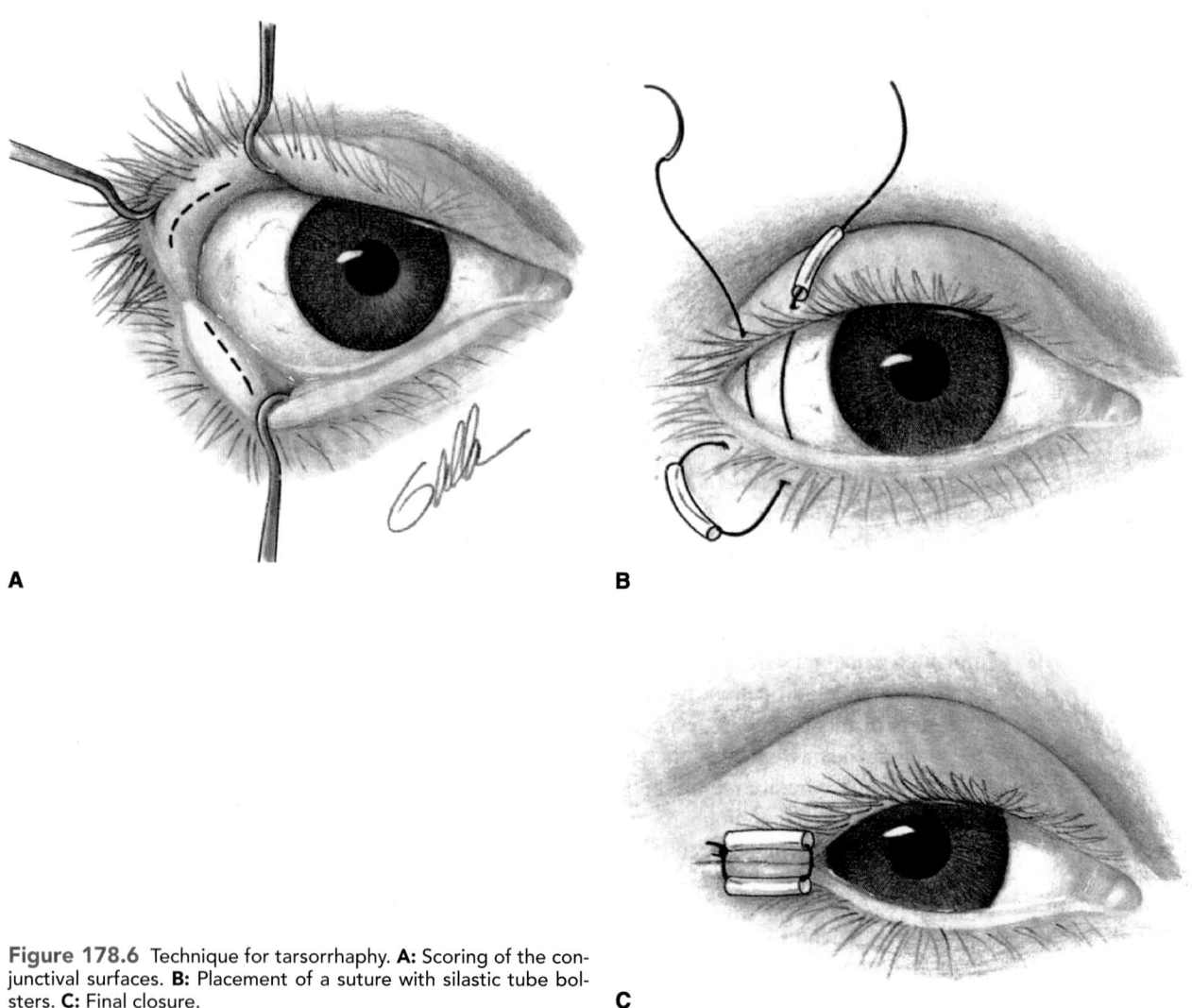

Figure 178.6 Technique for tarsorrhaphy. **A:** Scoring of the conjunctival surfaces. **B:** Placement of a suture with silastic tube bolsters. **C:** Final closure.

"canine" smile. The most infrequently encountered smile type is the "full-denture" smile, occurring in 2% of the population and characterized by equal action of both the lip elevators and depressors. It is important in patients with unilateral paralysis to observe which smile type is present, so that reconstructive efforts can most closely match the unaffected side.

Options for reanimation of the midface and oral commissure include regional or free muscle transfer for dynamic reanimation or fascia lata suspension for static reanimation. Ordinarily, static suspension is reserved for patients with a poor prognosis, in whom regional muscle transfer is not a practical option, or dynamic reanimation failures. For regional muscle, the temporalis, masseter, and digastric muscles have been utilized, but in the past decade nearly all reanimation surgeons have abandoned the use of the masseter muscle, based upon its unfavorable vector pull and the significant contour defect it leaves. The temporalis muscle is the mainstay of regional muscle transfer, based upon its surgical simplicity and its fan-shaped

architecture, permitting precise vector matching with the individual's native smile type.

Temporalis Transfer

The procedure is performed through an incision from the superior temporal line down to the attachment point of the lobule and may extend several cm below the angle of the mandible. There are two contemporary approaches to transferring the muscle. The first approach involves elevating the temporoparietal fascia off the superficial surface of the temporalis muscle, on its vascular pedicle, and rotating it posteriorly to reveal the muscle. A 1.5-cm strip of the muscle is elevated off the calvarium to the level of the zygomatic arch and reflected over the arch to reach the modiolus. The second approach, emerging in popularity in the past several years, is to expose the temporalis tendon as it attaches to the coronoid process and to remove it from the bone and secure it to the modiolus. This can be performed through a lateral incision (as above) or through a nasolabial crease incision, or intraorally.

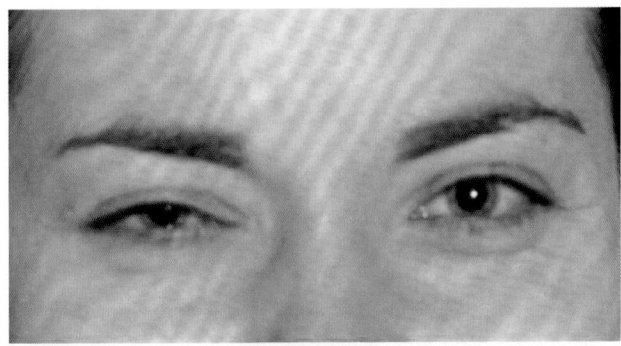

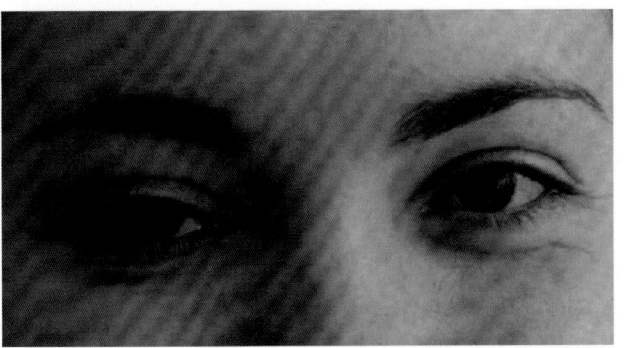

Figure 178.7 Management of periocular synkinesis with botulinum toxin. **Top:** Pretreatment view of eye while smiling. **Bottom:** Posttreatment view of same. Note more close matching of the palpebral fissure to the normal side.

Potential problems arising after temporalis muscle transfer include a visible bulge overlying the zygomatic arch (when using the first method described above), excess midfacial bulk, hollowing and/or alopecia in the temporalis fossa, and inadequate excursion of the transferred muscle. These problems can be largely avoided with meticulous surgical technique and proper candidate selection. Edentulous patients who are likely to have disuse atrophy of the muscle and those with preoperative wasting or trigeminal dysfunction are not good surgical candidates.

Free Muscle Transfer

Patients under the age of 70, in whom life expectancy is greater than 2 years, make good candidates for free muscle transfer. The most important advantage of this approach is that when it is driven by a cross-face nerve graft, it has the potential to yield an involuntary, emotive smile, and excursion is often greater than that seen using temporalis transfer. Because this approach involves microvascular anastomoses, and sometimes requires multiple operations, patients with vascular disease or other significant comorbidities are not appropriate candidates. Free muscle can alternatively be driven by the ipsilateral motor branch to the masseter muscle as a single-stage operation, which results in higher success rates and greater excursion but does not provide a completely involuntary, spontaneous emotive smile.

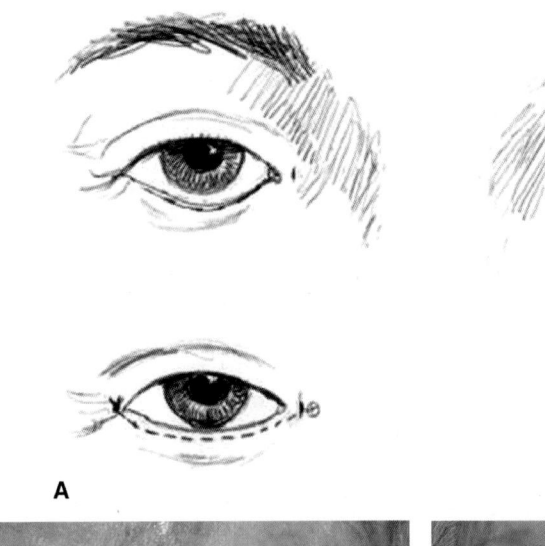

A

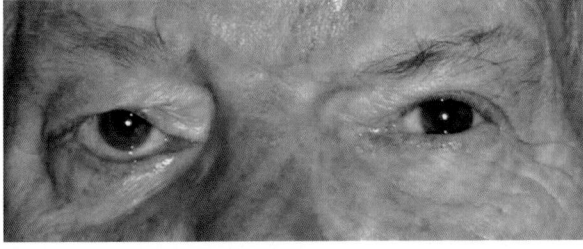

B

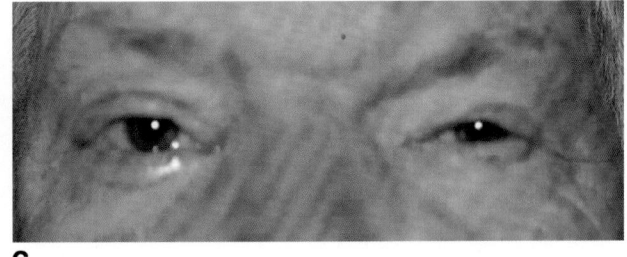

C

Figure 178.8 Fascia lata sling to lower eyelid. **A:** Schematic demonstrating technique. **B:** Preoperative view. **C:** Postoperative view.

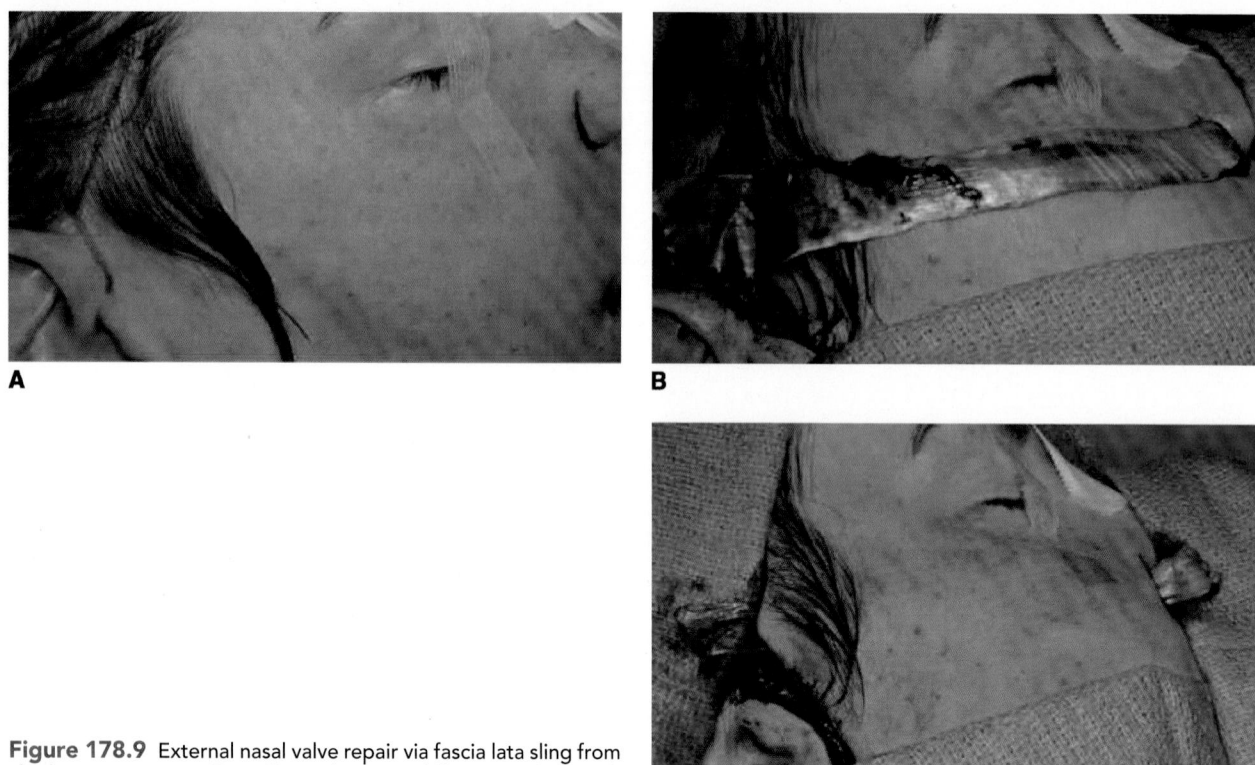

A

B

C

Figure 178.9 External nasal valve repair via fascia lata sling from alar base to zygoma. **Top:** Alar makings. **Middle:** Fascia lata graft over its tunnel. **Bottom:** Graft in place.

First-Stage Cross-Face Nerve Grafting

A preauricular incision is made on the nonparalyzed side, and a flap is raised on the parotidomasseteric fascia to the anterior border of the parotid gland. Dissection within the masseter fascia is carried out to identify several facial nerve branches. The branches yielding isolated smile movement are selected as the donor branches and transected sharply. A sural nerve graft is harvested from the leg and tunneled subcutaneously from the donor branches, across the upper lip, to the gingivobuccal sulcus on the paralyzed side, where the tip of the graft is marked with a 4-0 nylon suture. Nerve coaptation is performed between the sural nerve and the donor facial nerve branches, using 10-0 nylon sutures (Fig. 178.11). The penetration of axons into the graft is followed clinically by tapping on the graft (the Tinel sign); tingling in the zygomaticus muscle groups on the donor side indicates the presence of regenerating axons. Ordinarily, second-stage free muscle transfer ensues 6 to 9 months later.

Free Muscle Transfer

The gracilis muscle was the first muscle utilized in successful facial reanimation (12) and remains the most popular choice for this purpose, though pectoralis minor and latissimus dorsi are favored by some centers.

The gracilis muscle is harvested from the medial aspect of the thigh. An incision is made 1.5 cm posterior and parallel to a line connecting the pubic tubercle to the medial condyle of the tibia. The belly of the gracilis muscle is identified, and the vascular pedicle is located entering the deep surface of the muscle, 8 to 10 cm distal to the pubic tubercle. The obturator nerve is then identified 2 to 3 cm proximal to the vascular pedicle and similarly traced. The flap is harvested, and the length of muscle required is determined by measuring the distance from the oral commissure to the tragus and adding 2 cm. Thus, upon inset, resting length of the muscle is reestablished.

For facial inset, a preauricular incision is made and extended to just below the mandible, and the facial vessels are prepared for microvascular anastomosis. A thick skin flap is raised, extending medially to expose the orbicularis oris. In the two-stage procedure, the stump of the cross-face nerve graft is identified in the gingivobuccal sulcus for the neurorrhaphy, and in the single-stage procedure, the masseteric nerve is identified by dividing masseter fibers off the zygomatic arch to expose the nerve on the deep muscle surface. The gracilis muscle is then secured to the modiolus, stretched to its resting tension length, and secured to the temporalis fascia in the appropriate vector, taking into account the patient's healthy side smile vector. The microvascular anastomoses and the neurorrhaphy are performed, and the incisions are closed over suction drainage (Fig. 178.12).

Movement is expected starting approximately 3 months after transferring a trigeminally driven muscle and 8 to 10 months following cross-face nerve graft–driven muscle transfer (Fig. 178.13). Drawbacks include excessive

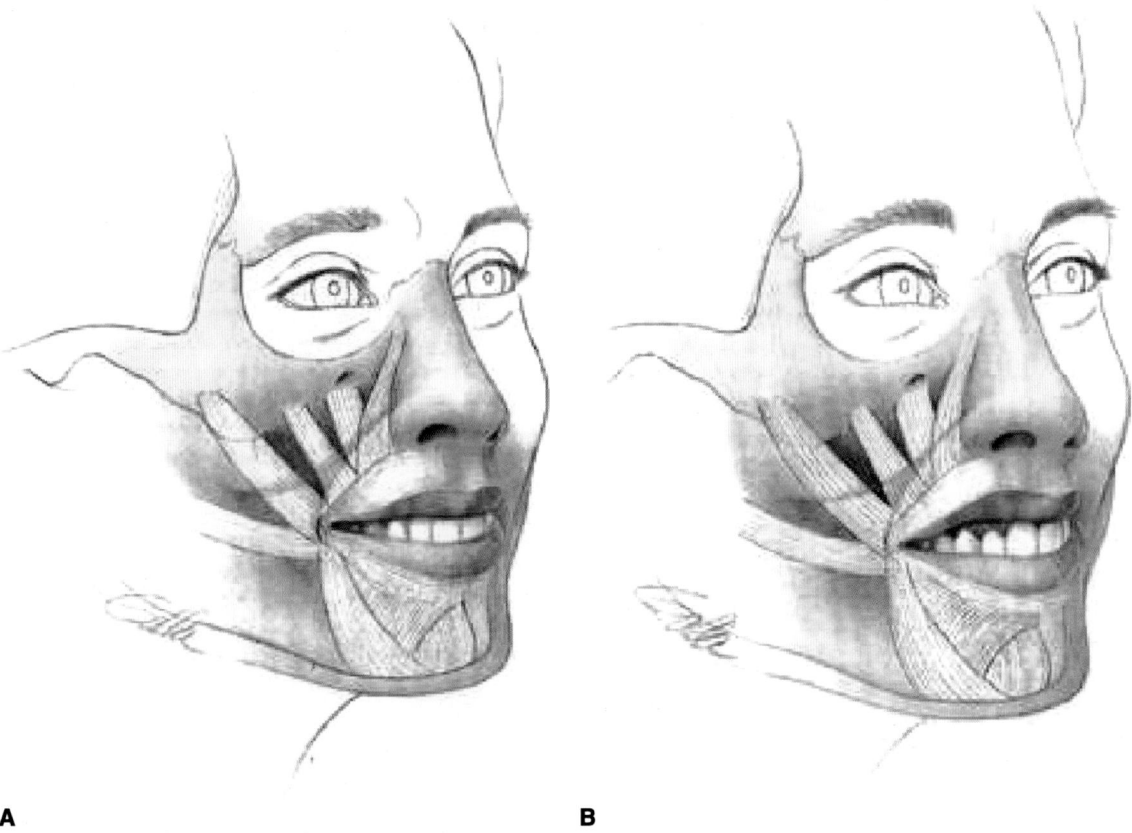

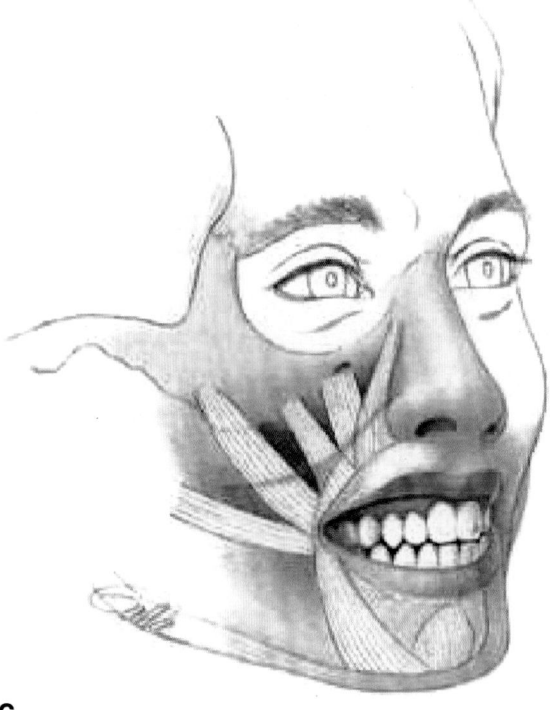

Figure 178.10 The smile types. **A:** Zygomaticus smile, dominated by zygomaticus major and minor and risorius. **B:** Canine smile, dominated by zygomaticus muscles and upper lip elevators. **C:** Full-denture smile, dominated by lip elevators and depressors.

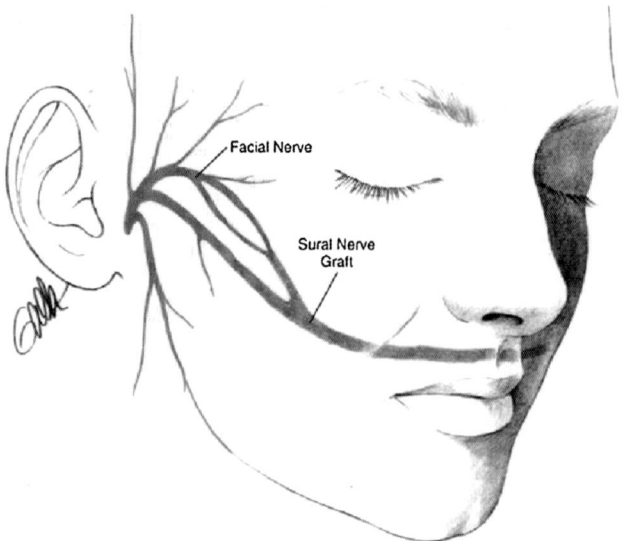

Figure 178.11 Placement of a cross-face nerve graft. Note several midface branches are sacrificed and routed into the graft.

midfacial bulk and the 8% to 30% failure rate, universally cited among those who perform this operation routinely. Failure is thought to occur secondary to poor ingrowth of the donor nerve fibers into the transferred muscle. Less commonly, microvascular failure or improper resting

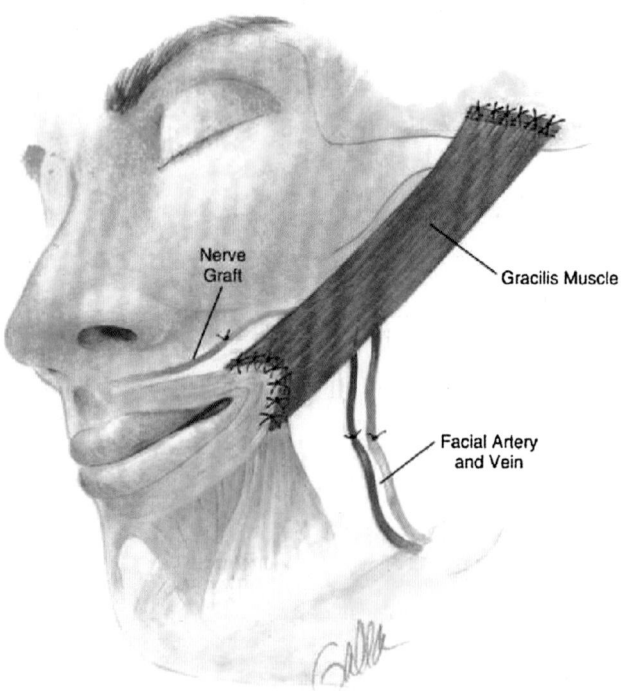

Figure 178.12 Inset of the gracilis muscle. Note the suture lines at either end of the transferred muscle.

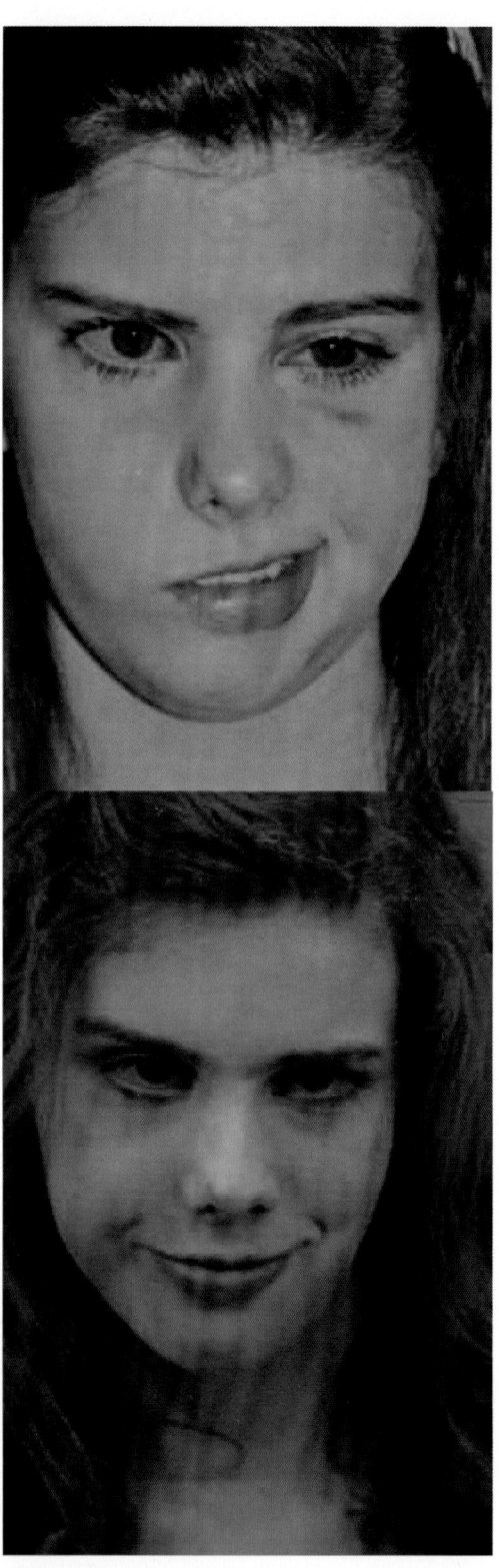

Figure 178.13 Expected result 12 months following successful free gracilis muscle transfer for flaccid facial paralysis from sacrifice during acoustic neuroma surgery. **Top:** Preoperative smile. **Bottom:** Postoperative smile.

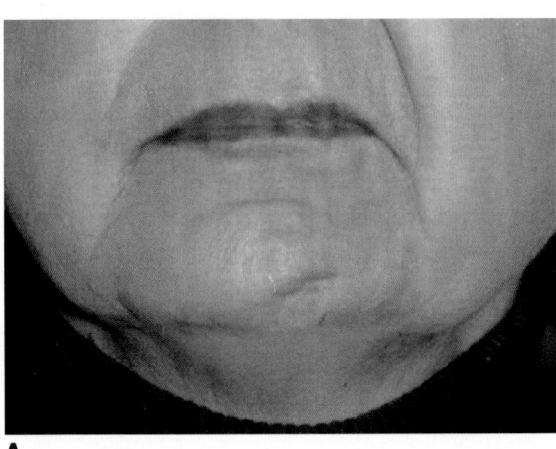
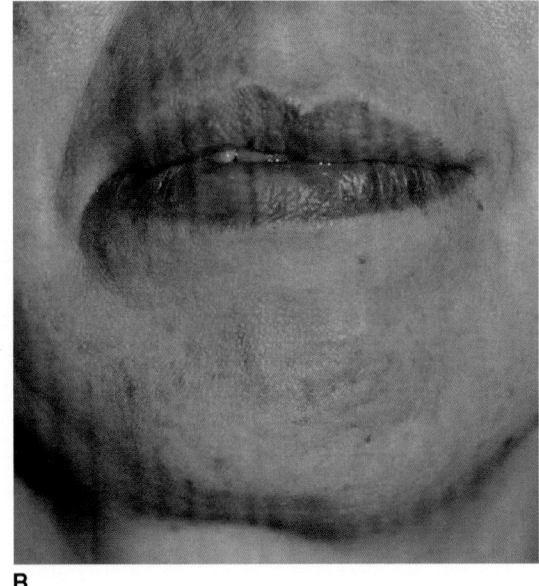

A   **B**

Figure 178.14 Hypertonic lower facial paralysis following poorly recovered Bell palsy. **A:** Classic pucker in mentalis muscle. **B:** Downturned oral commissure.

tension of the muscle may result in an unsatisfactory outcome.

The Lower Facial Zone

Within the lower face, the lower lip, the chin, and the neck require independent assessment. The lower lip tends to be superiorly displaced, based upon lack of tone from the depressor anguli oris and the depressor labii inferioris. In hypertonic facial paralysis, there may be significant hypertonicity in the mentalis muscle and the platysma, which leads to chin puckering and excessive downturning of the corner of the mouth (Fig. 178.14). Lower lip displacement can be managed by contralateral lower lip weakening

techniques, which would include either chemodenervation with botulinum toxin (Fig. 178.15) or transection of fibers of the contralateral depressor labii inferioris (13). Dynamic reanimation to the affected lower lip has been described, using digastric muscle transfer, and several surgeons have described the utility of free platysma transfer to the lower lip, though the high success rate of contralateral lower lip weakening has diminished the focus on dynamic lower lip techniques.

Mentalis dimpling is effectively managed with chemodenervation therapy, and platysmal synkinesis is eliminated either using botulinum toxin or via office-based platysmectomy (Fig. 178.16) (14).

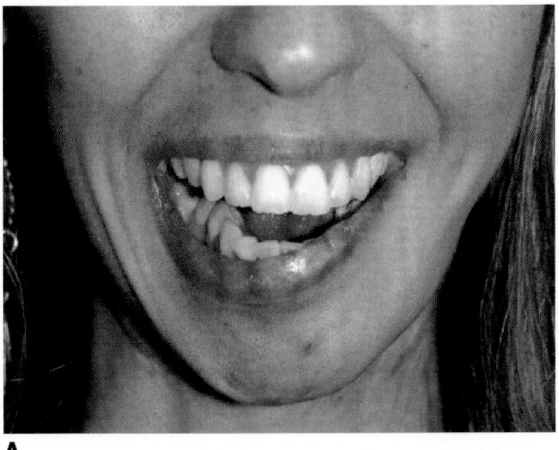
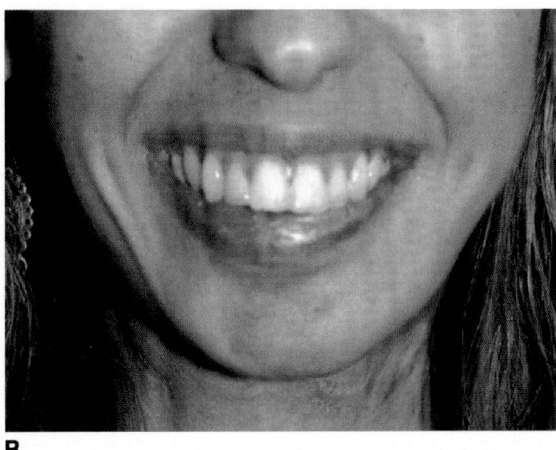

A   **B**

Figure 178.15 The effect of contralateral (**right**) lower lip chemodenervation for left lower lip weakness. **A:** Pretreatment. **B:** Posttreatment.

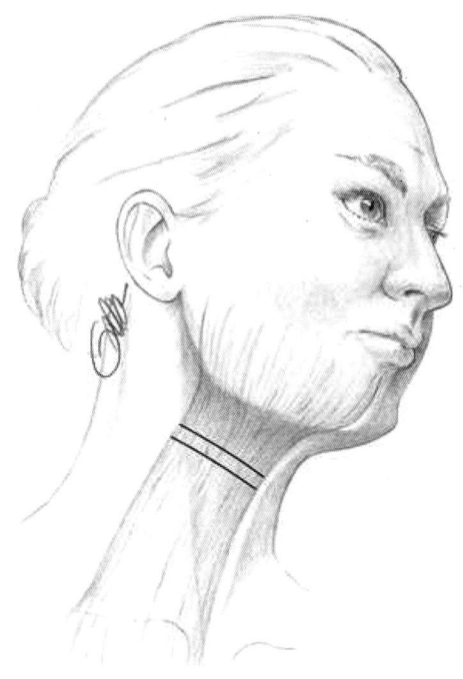

HIGHLIGHTS

- Facial paralysis has significant functional, aesthetic, and communication consequences.
- Nerve injuries are classified using the Sunderland scale according to severity, and neural discontinuity is managed with timely primary repair or nerve grafting.
- Hypoglossal–facial transfer provides global input to the facial musculature when there is no proximal facial nerve stump for grafting.
- Smile reanimation is accomplished using either free or regional muscle, and results achievable can match the excursion of normal smiling.
- Physical therapy, botulinum toxin chemodenervation, and office adjunct procedures play a critical role in thorough management of facial paralysis.

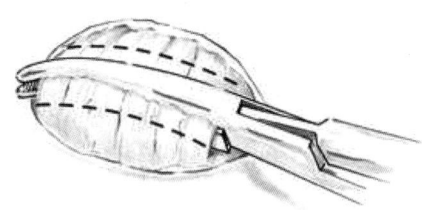

Figure 178.16 Platysmectomy. Above: Schematic outlining the 1 cm of gracilis to be removed. Below: Close-up schematic demonstrating cross-clamping of muscle prior to cautery and removal.

SUMMARY

Rehabilitation of the paralyzed face is a challenging medical, surgical, and physical therapy problem. The management strategies are determined by many critical variables, and a systematic approach to the problem is absolutely mandatory. Careful evaluation of each of the different facial zones will provide the best, most all-encompassing plan for each individual patient. In addition to surgical intervention, there is a critical role for both directed physical therapy and botulinum toxin chemodenervation (8,9,15). These adjuncts are relevant in the acutely paralyzed face (brow and lower lip), as well as the hypertonic, synkinetic face (lacrimal gland, orbicularis oculi, mentalis, and platysma). Management via a team approach, which includes neuro-otologists, facial plastic surgeons, head and neck surgical oncologists, oculoplastic surgeons, and physical therapists together, will optimize the outcome.

REFERENCES

1. Hadlock T, Greenfield L, Robinson M, et al. Multimodality approach to management of the paralyzed face. *Laryngoscope* 2006;116(8):1385–1389.
2. Sunderland S. Axon degeneration. In: *Nerve injuries and their repair.* New York: Churchill Livingstone, 1991:82–83.
3. Green JD Jr, Shelton C, Brackmann DE. Surgical management of iatrogenic facial nerve injuries. *Otolaryngol Head Neck Surg* 1994;111(5):606–610.
4. Gidley PW, Herrera SJ, Hanasono MM, et al. The impact of radiotherapy on facial nerve repair. *Laryngoscope* 2010;120(10):1985–1989.
5. Sameem M, Wood TJ, Bain JR. A systematic review on the use of fibrin glue for peripheral nerve repair. *Plast Reconstr Surg* 2011;127(6):2381–2390.
6. May M. Nerve substitution techniques. In May M, Schaitkin B, eds. *The facial nerve.* New York: Thieme Publishers, 1999:611–633.
7. Silver A, Lindsay R, Cheney M, et al. Thin profile platinum eyelid weighting: a superior option in the paralyzed eye. *Plast Reconstr Surg* 2009;123(6):1697–1703.
8. Hadlock T, Mehta R. Botulinum toxin and quality of life in patients with facial paralysis. *Arch Facial Plast Surg* 2008;10(2):84–87.
9. Boroojerdi B, Ferbert A, Schwarz M, et al. Botulinum toxin treatment of synkinesia and hyperlacrimation after facial palsy. *J Neurol Neurosurg Psychiatry* 1998;65(1):111–114.
10. Lindsay R, Smitson C, Edwards C, et al. Correction of the nasal base in the flaccidly paralyzed face: an orphaned problem in facial paralysis. *Plast Reconstr Surg* 2010;126(4):185e–186e.
11. Rubin LR, ed. *The paralyzed face.* St Louis., MO: Mosby Yearbook, 1991:11–15.
12. Harii K, Ohmori K, Torii S. Free gracilis muscle transplantation, with microneurovascular anastomoses for the treatment of facial paralysis. A preliminary report. *Plast Reconstr Surg* 1976;57(2):133–143.
13. Lindsay R, Smitson C, Cheney M, et al. A systematic algorithm for the management of lower lip asymmetry. *Am J Otolaryngol* 2011;32(1):1–7.
14. Henstrom D, Malo J, Cheney M, et al. Plastysmectomy: An effective intervention for facial synkinesis and hypertonicity. *Arch Facial Plast Surg* 2011;13(4):239–243.
15. Lindsay R, Robinson M, Hadlock T. Comprehensive facial muscle retraining improves facial function in patients with chronic facial paralysis: the MEEI five year experience. *Phys Ther* 2010;90(3):391–397.

Surgical Anatomy of the Nose: A Foundation for Rhinoplasty

179

David W. Kim   Ted Mau

GENERAL PRINCIPLES

Success in rhinoplasty depends on the surgeon's ability to create favorable functional and cosmetic changes to the nose. The operation is difficult for a number of reasons: noses are complex, three-dimensional, highly variable structures; most maneuvers attempt to alter a framework that has inherent resistance to manipulation; and the changes that are created are often subtle and subject to relentless postoperative forces of scar contracture. To overcome these challenges, the surgeon must have the ability to analyze a nose and match its variations to underlying structural correlates. Techniques may then be chosen to alter these structures into an optimal form while maintaining support and function. Finally, the maneuvers must be executed with meticulous precision. In rhinoplasty, these steps of diagnosis, selection of technique, and execution are possible only with a clear understanding of the complex anatomy.

This chapter describes sequentially the anatomy of the different regions and components of the nose. Infinite variations of these regions exist and may be the result of differences in ethnicity, gender, age, trauma, congenital deformity, or prior surgery. The unique structural characteristics of each nose underlie each individual's external appearance and may motivate that person to seek surgery. Whether or not these variations should be classified as variant anatomy is a semantic question, but because of this huge diversity, it is problematic to designate a "normal" archetypal anatomy toward which rhinoplasty surgery should aspire.

Each section in this chapter begins with general anatomic concepts, detailing the orientations and relations that are most commonly encountered. Subsequently, "variations" from normal anatomy are discussed, particularly as they pertain to rhinoplasty. A separate section focuses on the structural architecture of the nose, emphasizing how the various individual anatomic elements integrate into a stable unit. Although the chapter emphasizes anatomy predominantly, discussions on rhinoplasty philosophy, analysis, technique, and complications are included where germane.

SURFACE ANATOMY

Discussion of the surface anatomy of the nose begins within the larger contextual framework of the face. In general, the nose occupies the central horizontal third of the face, from the glabella to the subnasale, and central vertical fifth, between the medial canthi. Variations of nasal dimension and position may cause the nose to extend outside of these confines. These divergences may draw attention to the nose and may therefore be a patient's motivation to undergo rhinoplasty. Directional references and topographic landmarks are illustrated in Figures 179.1 through 179.5.

Subunits

The external topography of the nose is divided into six subunits. These consist of the nasal dorsum, sidewalls, tip, columella, ala/sill, and soft triangles (Fig. 179.6). These areas are defined by the shadows and highlights cast by incident light. Human visual processing depends on these light–dark contrasts to form a perception of the nose. The subunits do not necessarily have sharply defined boundaries and do not mirror exactly the underlying anatomic structures. Nonetheless, it is crucial for the nasal surgeon to identify them in preoperative assessment, particularly in external nasal reconstruction. During reconstruction, effort should be made to place scars within subunit borders whenever possible, as the human eye is more apt to discern a scar that traverses across a subunit than one that outlines it. This may require a surgeon to resect and replace an entire subunit (or subunits) involved, rather

Figure 179.1 Topographic key landmarks and accepted designations for **(A)** frontal and **(B)** oblique views of the nose. *1*, Glabella; *2*, nasion, nasofrontal angle; *3*, rhinion (osseocartilaginous junction); *4*, tip-defining point; *5*, infratip lobule;*6*, columella; *7*, columella–labial junction; *8*, facet; *9*, alar sidewall;*10*, alar–facial junction; *11*, medial crural footplate; *12*, supra-alar crease; *13*, alar margin; *14*, philtrum; *15*, philtral crest; *16*, supratip dorsum. (From Tardy ME. *Surgical anatomy of the nose.* New York: Raven Press, 1990, with permission.)

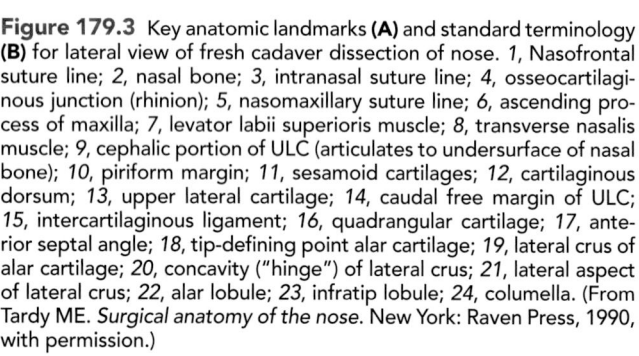

A   B

Figure 179.2 **A:** Topographic key landmarks and accepted designations for lateral view of the nose. *1*, Glabella; *2*, nasion (nasofrontal junction); *3*, rhinion (osseocartilaginous junction); *4*, tip-defining point; *5*, infratip lobule; *6*, columella; *7*, columella–labial junction; *8*, facet; *9*, alar lobule; *10*, alar–facial junction; *11*, medial crural footplate; *12*, supra-alar crease. **B:** Topographic key landmarks and accepted designations for basal view of the nose. *1*, Tip-defining point; *2*, interdomal area, alar lobule; *3*, infratip lobule; *4*, columella; *5*, medial crural footplate; *6*, columella–labial junction; *7*, philtrum; *8*, nostril aperture; *9*, facet; *10*, alar sidewall; *11*, alar–facial junction; *12*, nostril sill. (From Tardy ME. *Surgical anatomy of the nose.* New York: Raven Press, 1990, with permission.)

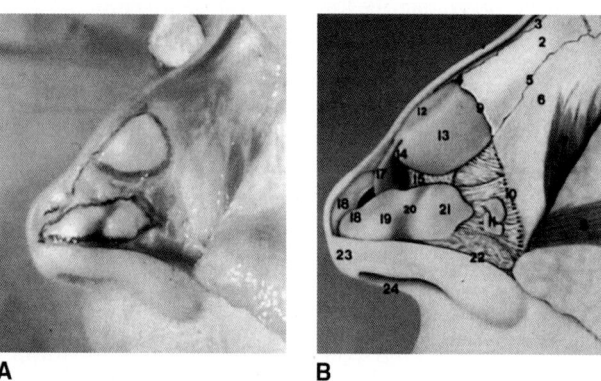

A   B

Figure 179.3 Key anatomic landmarks **(A)** and standard terminology **(B)** for lateral view of fresh cadaver dissection of nose. *1*, Nasofrontal suture line; *2*, nasal bone; *3*, intranasal suture line; *4*, osseocartilaginous junction (rhinion); *5*, nasomaxillary suture line; *6*, ascending process of maxilla; *7*, levator labii superioris muscle; *8*, transverse nasalis muscle; *9*, cephalic portion of ULC (articulates to undersurface of nasal bone); *10*, piriform margin; *11*, sesamoid cartilages; *12*, cartilaginous dorsum; *13*, upper lateral cartilage; *14*, caudal free margin of ULC; *15*, intercartilaginous ligament; *16*, quadrangular cartilage; *17*, anterior septal angle; *18*, tip-defining point alar cartilage; *19*, lateral crus of alar cartilage; *20*, concavity ("hinge") of lateral crus; *21*, lateral aspect of lateral crus; *22*, alar lobule; *23*, infratip lobule; *24*, columella. (From Tardy ME. *Surgical anatomy of the nose.* New York: Raven Press, 1990, with permission.)

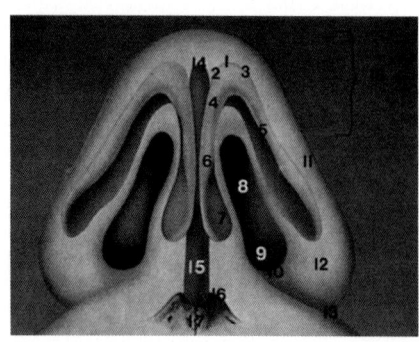 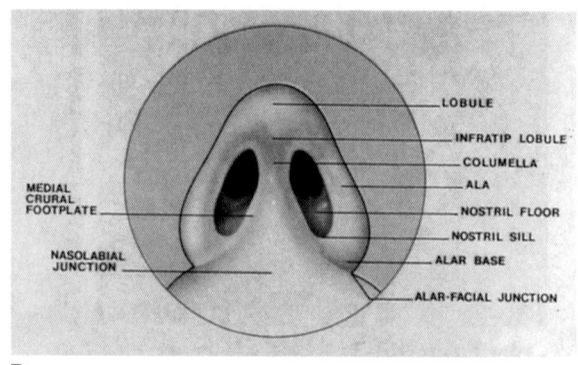

A   B

Figure 179.4 Additional anatomic landmarks **(A)** and standard nasal terminology of base of nose **(B)**. *1*, Apex of alar cartilage; *2*, medial genu; *3*, lateral genu; *4*, transitional segment; *5*, lateral crus; *6*, medial crus; *7*, medial crural footplate; *8*, nostril aperture; *9*, nostril floor; *10*, nostril sill; *11*, lateral alar sidewall; *12*, alar lobule; *13*, alar–facial junction; *14*, anterior septal angle; *15*, caudal septum; *16*, maxillary crest; *17*, nasal spine; *18*, infratip lobule. (From Tardy ME. *Surgical anatomy of the nose.* New York: Raven Press, 1990, with permission.)

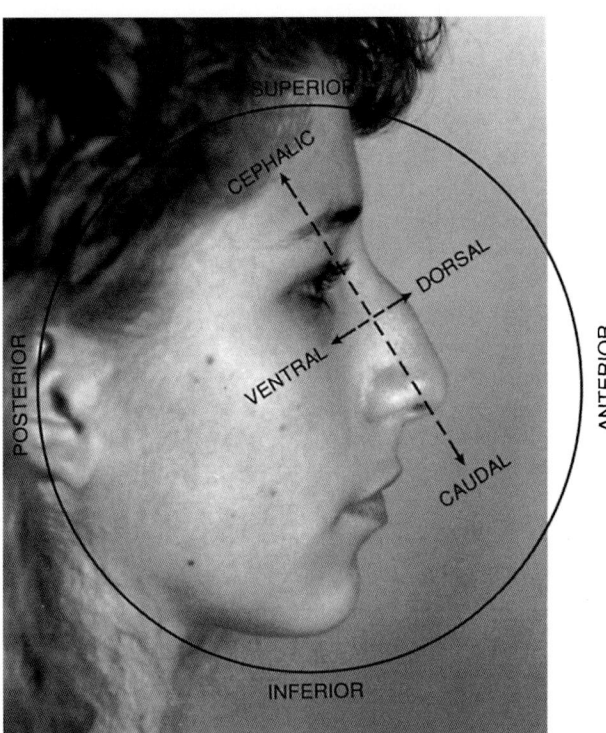

Figure 179.5 Preferred directional references applied to the nose. Note that the axes shift to lie oriented to the nasal dorsal line.

than replace only the primary defect, even if this requires removal of areas of healthy tissue. Tissue of a similar thickness, color, and consistency should be used to reconstruct these defects.

Topography

A discussion of surgical anatomy must begin with the external topography that surgery aims to alter. A detailed discussion of aesthetic facial analysis is found in Chapter 170. What follows is a limited discussion of nasal analysis and

definitions of terms with specific relevance to rhinoplasty anatomy. Correlation of nasal topography to underlying structural anatomy is introduced—details of this anatomy are discussed in greater depth in subsequent sections.

On frontal view, a gentle, unbroken curve should appear from the lateral brow to the nasal tip on each side of the nose (Fig. 179.1A). These *brow–tip aesthetic lines* should follow the normal changes of nasal width: wider cephalad at the brow/nasal root transition, narrower in the middle vault, and wider again at the tip. An irregular brow–tip aesthetic line may be correlated to bony and cartilaginous vault irregularities through palpation and close inspection with a light placed above the patient to enhance shadowing. When the upper cartilaginous vault is overly narrow, the curvature of these brow–tip lines is exaggerated.

General tip shape may be determined from the frontal and base views (e.g., bulbous, deviated, wide, amorphous, asymmetrical). The unique features of tip shape are determined by the endless variations of form, dimension, and position of the lower lateral cartilages (LLCs) and surrounding structures. Inference about the thickness of the nasal skin may be made from inspection of the contour of the tip. A tip with sharp features reflects underlying structures transmitting through thin skin. A smooth, bulbous tip is likely covered by thick skin.

The base view also provides information about the shape and size of the columella, alar base, nostrils, and infratip lobule (Figs. 179.2B and 179.4). In most noses, the frontal and base views reveal a triangular shape of the nose in which the nasal base (interface of nose and face) is wider than the tip and dorsal line. The triangularity of the tip depends on the presence of an unbroken line from a narrower nasal tip to a wider nasal base. Poor structural support along this line will manifest as alar pinching or concavity of the alar margins on frontal and base views. When the base is excessively narrow or the tip overly wide, a square or trapezoidal shape instead of triangular

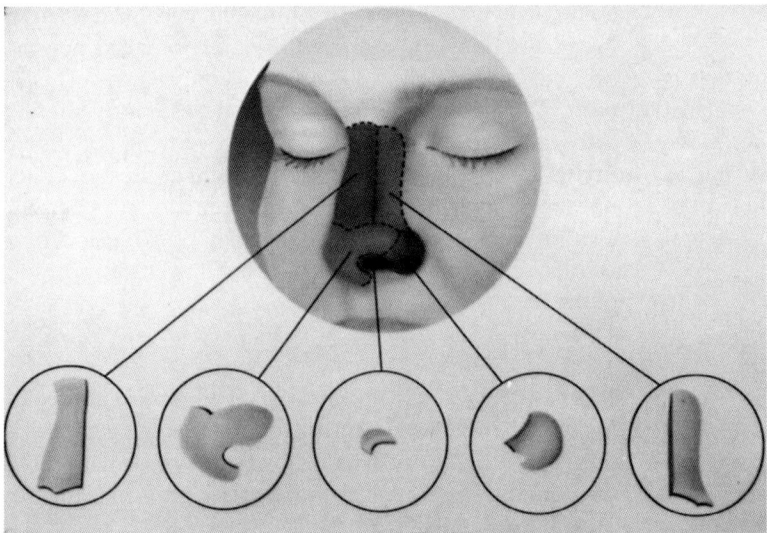

Figure 179.6 Aesthetic topographic subunits of the nasal surface. From left to right: dorsum, tip/columella, soft tissue triangle, alar lobule, and sidewall. The columella may be considered a separate distinct subunit. (From Tardy ME. *Surgical anatomy of the nose.* New York: Raven Press, 1990, with permission.)

configuration is present (1). The width of the infratip lobule reflects the underlying shape of the intermediate crura of the LLCs. Asymmetry in the columella may be caused by asymmetries of the shape or trajectory of the medial crura, deflection of the caudal edge of the cartilaginous septum, or both. The lateral flaring of the alar lobules is only indirectly determined by the shape and strength of the lateral crura of the LLCs, as the lobules themselves are composed of soft tissue only and are caudal to the lateral crura.

On lateral view, several important external landmarks may be identified (Fig. 179.2A). The nasion is the most concave point at the nasofrontal angle and corresponds anatomically to the midline of the nasofrontal suture. This angle is determined by the height of the radix, the most cephalic portion of the nasal dorsum, and the slope of the forehead. An average nasofrontal angle measures 120 degrees in the Caucasian nose. The vertical position of the nasion marks the nasal starting point and is typically between the supratarsal crease and the upper eyelid margin. The rhinion corresponds to the osseous–cartilaginous junction and often marks the location of a dorsal hump. Proceeding caudally, the presence or absence of a supratip breakpoint depends on the dorsal height of the cartilaginous septum and the projection of the domal region of the LLCs. The tip-defining point, or the pronasale, is the most anterior projection of the nose. The overall projection and rotation of the nasal tip may be assessed by using Goode's method, in which the nasal tip projection (from the alar crease to the tip-defining point) is divided by nasal length (from nasion to tip-defining point). According to Goode, the normal value should be 0.55. The nasolabial angle in men is typically between 90 and 95 degrees and in women, between 95 and 105 degrees. This angle may be affected by variations of the size and shape of the upper lip and premaxillary bone. Therefore, the nasolabial angle does not always reflect the degree of tip rotation. The lateral view of the ideal nostril is oval shaped, with 2 to 4 mm of the columella visible beneath the alar rim.

Variant Anatomy

Because the nose is a three-dimensional structure that is viewed in whole, the topographic dimensions of one area have an optical effect on the appearance of other areas. This is critical during rhinoplasty, as surgical changes to one region or parameter of the nose create the illusion of change to another. Examples as they pertain to external nasal topography follow.

Dorsal Height

The overall height of the nasal dorsum is determined predominantly by the size and development of the highly variable cartilaginous and osseous nasal septum. In general, an increased overall projection of the dorsum on the lateral view corresponds to a narrower appearance on the frontal view. Conversely, a low nasal bridge creates a wider-appearing nose from the front. This is explained by the concept that one looks down the apex of a triangle when observing a nose from the front. In a nose with a high dorsum, the sidewalls are subject to more shadowing, and the apex of the triangle appears narrower. In a nose with a low bridge, the cross-sectional triangular geometry of the nose is flattened, or if surgical hump reduction has occurred, it is truncated into a trapezoid. With less shadowing of the sidewalls, the nose appears wider on frontal view. Local differences in dorsal height create other illusions. In a normal profile, the radix, middorsum, supratip, and nasal tip are linear or nearly colinear. Because our eyes are accustomed to this norm, deviations from these relations create certain optical illusions. For instance, the presence of a mid-dorsal convexity creates an illusion of an underrotated nasal tip, irrespective of absolute tip position. A dorsal concavity, in contrast, creates a perception of increased tip rotation and a shorter nose. Before the surgeon commits to making true alterations of tip position, the effects of dorsal height and its modification must be carefully weighed.

Radix and Nasofrontal Angle

Variations in radix height have an effect on numerous aesthetic nasal parameters such as the nasal starting point, nasofrontal angle, overall dorsal profile, and apparent intercanthal distance. A low radix, as commonly seen in individuals of African or Asian descent, creates an illusion of increased intercanthal distance (see earlier explanation). If associated with tip underprojection, a low radix may create an appearance of a dorsal hump. Correction of this appearance may be accomplished with augmentation of the radix and increasing tip projection instead of reduction of the dorsum to the level of the low radix (Fig. 179.7). Maintaining a higher dorsum offers the advantages of a narrower appearance on front view and avoidance of an open-roof deformity associated with hump reduction. A high radix, in contrast, creates an appearance of decreased intercanthal distance. When excessive height at the radix blunts the nasofrontal angle, the distinction between the nose and forehead may be blurred, creating the illusion of a longer nose. This is particularly true in the presence of a posteriorly sloping forehead. Because of the abundant overlying soft tissue in this area, reduction of osseous height at the radix does not transmit well to overall profile reduction. Conversely, a more acute nasofrontal angle creates an illusion of a shorter nose, independent of the actual vertical position of the nasal starting point.

Nasolabial Angle

The nasolabial angle, formed by the upper lip and columella, is widely used as a metric for the degree of rotation of the nasal tip. This region, however, is composed of numerous anatomic components with a high degree of variation and in reality may not accurately reflect the

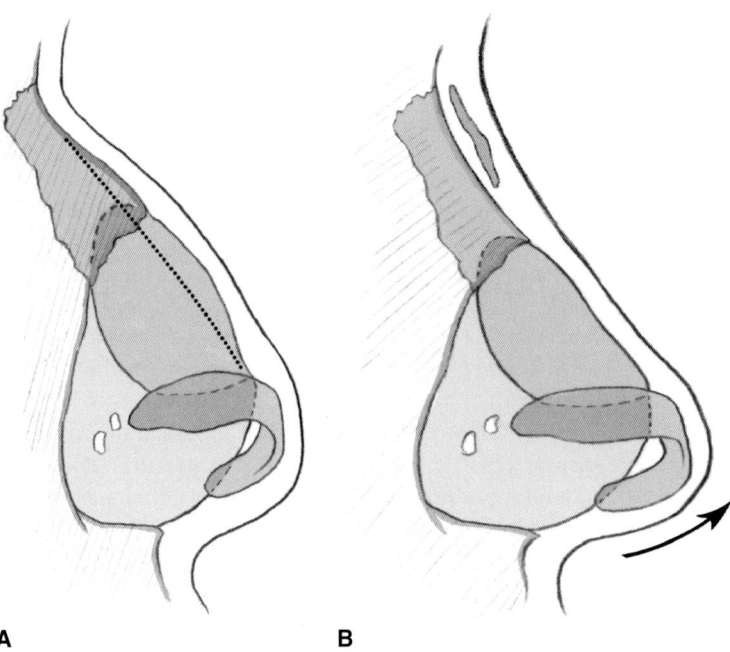

A   **B**

Figure 179.7 A: Profile view of a nose with a true dorsal hump in the region of the rhinion. Correction may involve reduction of the hump. **B**: Nose with a relative dorsal convexity due to a low radix and an underprojected nasal tip. Correction might involve elevating of the radix with a graft and increasing tip projection. Final external dorsal contour is similar in both examples.

overall degree of nasal tip rotation. Fullness in this area may be caused by an overdeveloped quadrangular cartilage in the area of the posterior septal angle, a prominent nasal spine and premaxillary bone, or tenting of the soft tissue in a projecting nose. These variations create a more obtuse angle, irrespective of the true rotational position of the nasal tip. However, even if the true rotational position of the tip is not changed, an increased nasolabial angle creates an illusion of increased tip rotation. Conversely, when these structures are less developed or retrusive, a relative deficiency on the nasolabial angle may be present, leading to a perception of counterrotation (Fig. 179.8).

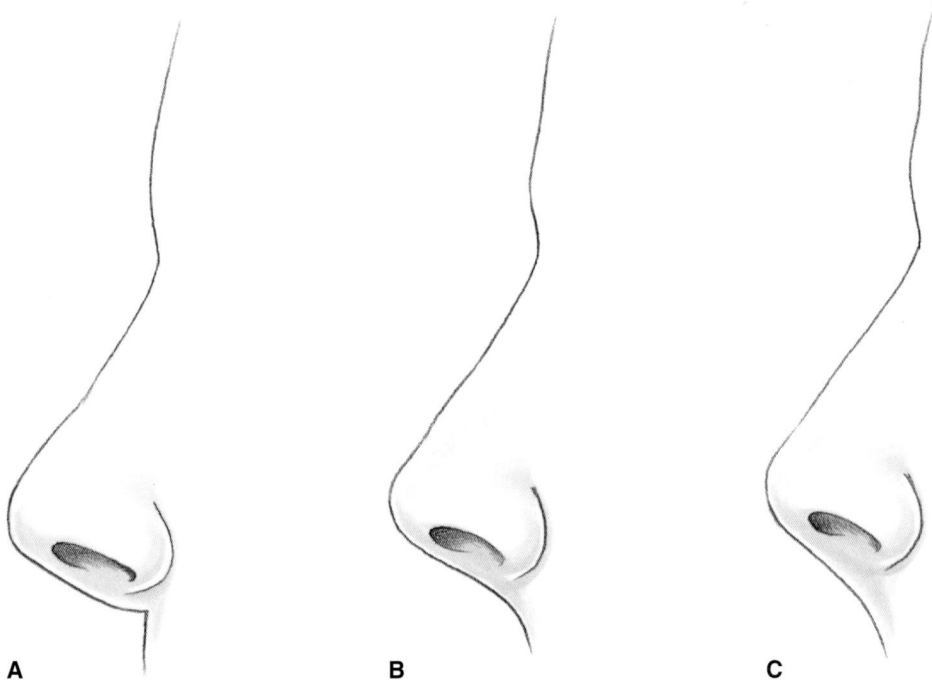

A   **B**   **C**

Figure 179.8 Lateral view of three noses with identical tip position. **A**: Relative deficiency of tissue at the nasolabial area and an acute nasolabial angle creates an illusion of underrotation of the tip. **B**: Nose with a moderate nasolabial angle. **C**: Fullness at the nasolabial area with an obtuse nasolabial angle creates an illusion of increased tip rotation.

Alar–Columellar Relation

With alar retraction or a dependent caudal edge of the cartilaginous septum, excessive columellar height is visible on the lateral view. This hanging columella may create an illusion of a ptotic nasal tip, even when tip position is normal. In contrast, a retracted caudal septum or a low alar margin may lead to a relative lack of columellar show and an associated illusion of increased tip rotation. The size, position, and interrelations of the medial crura, caudal septum, lateral crura, and alar soft tissue determine these variations.

SKIN–SOFT TISSUE ENVELOPE

The nose is constructed of a skeletal framework onto which a skin–soft tissue envelope (SSTE) is draped. Although the framework is the subject of most surgical techniques, the appearance of the nose is determined by the manner in which the SSTE drapes over the modified skeleton. An understanding of the composition of the SSTE and its variant anatomy guides the surgeon in choosing appropriate techniques for successful surgery.

Skin

The skin of the nose varies in thickness depending on its location. The skin is thickest at the nasion and thinnest at the rhinion (2). From the rhinion, the skin becomes progressively thicker as it descends along the dorsum to the tip, where a large number of sebaceous glands reside. The skin becomes thin again at the most caudal aspect of the nose along the alar margin and columella.

Understanding skin thickness variation along the dorsum aids the rhinoplasty surgeon in performing dorsal hump reduction. Because the skin is thinnest at the rhinion, a straight external profile requires a small relative convexity to remain in this region. If the dorsum is reduced so that a straight skeletal profile results, a slight concavity at the middorsum is likely to result after skin redraping (3). This may create a cartilaginous pollybeak, in which the supratip dorsum projects above the plane of the dorsum cephalad to it. To avoid this, hump reduction should be carried out incrementally, with verification of the effect of each pass on external contour through the SSTE.

Subcutaneous Tissue

The subcutaneous layer of the nose is made up of the superficial fatty layer, the fibromuscular layer, the deep fatty layer, and the periosteum or perichondrium. The superficial fatty layer is directly connected to the dermis. The fibromuscular layer comprises the nasal subcutaneous muscular aponeurotic system (SMAS) (4). The nasal SMAS is in continuity with the SMAS of the rest of the face and encases and interconnects the mimetic muscles of the nose. The deep fatty layer contains the neurovascular system of the soft tissue envelope. Dissection in the avascular plane between the deep fatty layer and the perichondrium and periosteum is met with little mechanical resistance or bleeding and results in the least postoperative scarring and contraction.

Muscles

The mimetic muscles of the nose reside within the SMAS. They are divided into four groups (5) (Table 179.1). The *elevator* muscles shorten the nose and dilate the nostrils, the *depressor* muscles lengthen the nose and dilate the nostrils, the *compressor* muscles lengthen the nose and narrow the nostrils, and the *minor dilator* muscles widen the nostrils. In addition to these individual functions, the muscles work synergistically to alter the shape of the nasal tip, alae, and dorsum. For example, simultaneous contraction of the levator labii superioris and the depressor septi nasi may depress the nasal tip, "round up" the supratip area, and lengthen the nose (6). The muscles, particularly the dilator naris (7), also serve to maintain the tone of the nostrils during inspiration, as illustrated in the patient with ipsilateral facial nerve paralysis with unilateral alar collapse (8). Dissection in the sub-SMAS layer of the soft tissue envelope allows the surgeon to avoid the nervous supply to the nasal muscles.

Although most rhinoplasty techniques do not directly address nasal muscles, division of the depressor septi nasi may correct drooping of the nasal tip and shortening of the upper lip during facial animation. The small, paired muscle that originates at the anterior nasal spine and inserts onto the medial crura footplates may be addressed through simple division (6), muscular release and plication (9), or dissection and transposition of the muscle (10). In selected patients, these techniques may reduce gingival show and nasal tip descent during smiling, elevate the nasal tip, and elongate the upper lip in the resting state.

Arterial Supply

The superficial vascular supply to the external nose derives from both the external and internal carotid systems. The

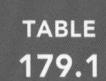

TABLE 179.1	INVESTING NASAL MUSCULATURE

Elevator muscles
   Procerus
   Levator labii superioris alaeque nasi
   Anomalous nasi
Depressor muscles
   Alar nasalis
   Depressor septi nasi
Compressor muscles
   Transverse nasalis
   Compressor narium minor
Minor dilator muscles
   Dilator naris anterior

facial artery branches into the angular artery and the superior labial artery. The lateral nasal branch of the angular artery supplies the lateral surface of the caudal nose. Branches of the superior labial artery supply the nasal sill and the base of the columella. The columellar artery, a branch of the superior labial artery, is often encountered in the transcolumellar incision used in the external rhinoplasty approach. The septal branches of the superior labial artery enter the nose on each side of the nasal spine and form the major blood supply to the anterior septum. Large septal mucosal flaps may be pedicled on the nasal spine area with these branches for reconstructive purposes.

The dorsal nasal artery, an external branch of the ophthalmic artery, anastomoses with the lateral nasal branch of the angular artery, forming an axial arterial network for the dorsal nasal skin. Arterial supply to the nasal tip derives from branches of the anterior ethmoid and angular arteries. The external nasal branch of the anterior ethmoid artery perforates the transverse nasalis muscle of the nasal sidewall and descends toward the nasal tip. The lateral nasal branch of the angular artery sends off branches from the ala anteriorly toward the nasal tip. The vascular plexus to which these arteries contribute resides predominantly in the adipose layer just deep to the SMAS. Remaining in the plane just above the perichondrium and periosteum during dissection minimizes injury to these vessels.

Sensory Nerve Supply

Sensation to the external nasal skin is supplied by branches of the ophthalmic and maxillary divisions of the trigeminal nerve. Twigs from the supratrochlear and infratrochlear branches of the ophthalmic nerve supply sensation to the skin of the radix, the rhinion, and the cephalic portion of the nasal sidewalls (11). The external nasal branch of the anterior ethmoidal nerve supplies the skin over the dorsum of the caudal nose down to and including the nasal tip. This branch emerges between the caudal edge of the nasal bone and the upper lateral cartilage (ULC) and courses in the SMAS layer. Injury to this nerve during intercartilaginous or cartilage-splitting incisions can result in tip numbness (11). Branches of the infraorbital nerve provide sensation to the side of the lower half of the nose and the lateral vestibule. The nasopalatine nerve, a branch of V2 that enters the nose through the incisive foramen, provides the major sensory supply to the posterior two-thirds of the nasal septal mucosa, maxillary gingiva, and anterior palatal mucosa. This nerve may be injured during surgery involving the maxillary crest or nasal floor and can result in temporary numbness near the incisors (12).

Inner Lining

The nasal vestibule is lined with keratinizing squamous epithelium. The surfaces of the nasal cavities, with the exception of the superior olfactory epithelium, are covered by ciliated stratified or pseudostratified respiratory epithelium (13). Because of its high vascularity, the vestibular epithelium and intranasal mucosa are excellent sources of local flaps for reconstruction of the inning lining in full-thickness nasal defects. In such procedures, a free cartilage graft is often used to rebuild structure for the nose. The rich vascular intranasal lining flap nourishes the cartilage graft from its undersurface. Common inner lining donor sites are the nasal septum or nasal vestibule. These flaps are discussed in more detail in Chapter 165. During routine rhinoplasty, care must be taken to preserve vestibular skin in the internal nasal valve area to avoid web formation and nasal valve stenosis (14).

Variant Anatomy

Thickness of the SSTE varies with ethnicity, age, and gender. Noses with thin, less sebaceous skin assume a shape that closely matches the underlying cartilaginous and osseous structure. In contrast, the underlying nasal architecture does not accurately transmit through the soft tissue envelope in thicker-skinned noses. These concepts are critical in rhinoplasty.

In the thick-skinned individual, modifications of the underlying framework, particularly reductive alterations, may not result in significant changes in external appearance because of poor redraping of the overlying SSTE. In these patients, the surgeon should consider augmenting areas of relative deficiency to create a framework that pushes and stretches the thick SSTE into a desirable shape. In such cases, overall proportion of the nose becomes more important than absolute size. Because a thick SSTE cannot conform onto the underlying structure after reduction, scar tissue may fill the resulting void. An example is the soft tissue/scar pollybeak that results after aggressive supratip hump reduction in a thick-skinned individual. Little to no external lowering of the supratip convexity occurs as the cartilaginous hump is simply replaced by scar beneath a noncompliant SSTE.

In patients with thin skin, even small irregularities of the underlying structure may become evident after surgery as the soft tissue envelope redrapes very closely to the framework below. In these cases, care must be taken to camouflage grafts, edges of bone and cartilage, and any other contour irregularities. Graft must be placed in a precise manner, and any edges that may transmit through the skin should be beveled or crushed to blend seamlessly into surrounding structures. Soft tissue or crushed cartilage onlay grafts may aid in camouflaging irregularities.

SKELETAL FRAMEWORK

The skeletal framework of the nose may be divided into thirds: the upper third consisting of the osseous vault; the middle third consisting of the upper cartilaginous vault; and the lower third consisting of the lower cartilaginous vault. The nasal septum, consisting of a bony and a cartilaginous portion, provides support in all three sections and divides the nasal cavity into two lateral halves. In this section, these structures are discussed individually, with an emphasis on anatomic forms and their variations. In a later section, the interrelations of these bodies as they pertain to nasal structural mechanics are discussed.

Septum

The nasal septum is a sagittal midline structure that divides the nose into two cavities and provides structural support to the osseous and cartilaginous vaults (15). The septum is divided into a cephalic–posterior osseous septum, composed of the perpendicular plate of the ethmoid and the vomer, and a caudal–anterior cartilaginous septum, consisting of the quadrangular cartilage.

The perpendicular plate of the ethmoid forms the dorsal aspect of the osseous septum. Its superior attachment consists of the frontal bone and its nasal spine anteriorly and the cribriform plate posteriorly. Anterosuperiorly, it articulates with the inward projection of the nasal bones in the midline. Anteroinferiorly, it borders the quadrangular cartilage, and posteroinferiorly, it borders the vomer. The thickness of the perpendicular plate of the ethmoid varies considerably, and it is rarely pneumatized. Because it is attached to the cribriform plate, aggressive lateral force high on the osseous septum may lead to fracture of the skull base and resultant cerebrospinal fluid leak or olfactory bulb injury.

The vomer, one of the bones that make up the skull, is shaped like the keel of a boat. In a midsagittal view of the skull, its superior edge forms a line connecting the sphenoid sinus to the anterior nasal spine. Superiorly, the vomer articulates with the perpendicular plate of the ethmoid. Inferiorly, it attaches to the midline nasal crest of the palatine bone posteriorly and the maxilla anteriorly. Anterior to its articulation with the vomer, the maxillary crest forms a groove into which the quadrangular cartilage sits. The posterior free edge of the vomer forms the posterior border of the choanae.

The quadrangular cartilage comprises the cartilaginous septum. This structure rests within a groove in the nasal spine and maxillary crest inferior to it. This ventral surface is typically thickened in comparison to the remainder of the structure. Dorsally, the quadrangular cartilage forms the contour of the nasal bridge externally. The ULCs articulate with the cephalic aspect of the quadrangular cartilage, forming the dorsum of the central third of the nose. The most caudal portion of the cartilage extends anterior to the nasal spine and is the least rigid portion (Fig. 179.9). Three angles may be identified at the caudal edge of the septum (Fig. 179.10). The anterior septal angle is usually the most anterior projection of the septum and forms the transition between the dorsal and caudal components of the supportive cartilaginous septal L-strut. The domal regions of the LLCs are in intimate proximity and typically project beyond the anterior septal angle, creating the external

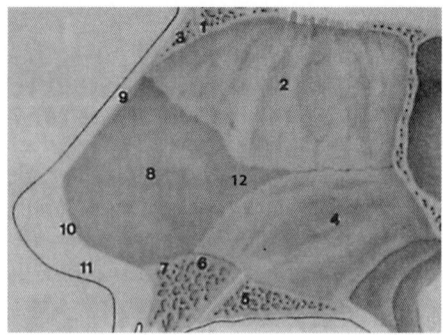

Figure 179.9 Anatomy of the typical nasal septum. *1*, Nasal process and frontal bone; *2*, perpendicular plate of ethmoid bone; *3*, nasal bone; *4*, vomer bone; *5*, palatine bone; *6*, maxillary crest; *7*, nasal spine; *8*, quadrangular cartilage; *9*, upper lateral cartilage; *10*, caudal margin quadrangular cartilage; *11*, membranous septum; *12*, posterior projection of "tongue" of quadrangular cartilage (variable length). (From Tardy ME. *Surgical anatomy of the nose.* New York: Raven Press, 1990, with permission.)

topography of the nasal tip. Because of this relation, deviations of the anterior septal angle may cause distortions of nasal tip position. The posterior septal angle is located at the quadrangular cartilage articulation with the anterior nasal spine. The intermediate septal angle lies between the anterior and posterior septal angles.

The membranous septum is the soft tissue continuation of the cartilaginous septum. Consisting of a central layer of subcutaneous areolar tissue between vestibular skin on each side, the membranous septum bridges the caudal edge of the cartilaginous septum to the medial crura and columella. Contained within it are the ligamentous attachments of the medial crura to the caudal septum. Because of a lack of cartilage, it is mobile and displaces easily with manipulation of the columella.

The septum is lined with an inner layer of perichondrium or periosteum covered by an outer layer of mucosa.

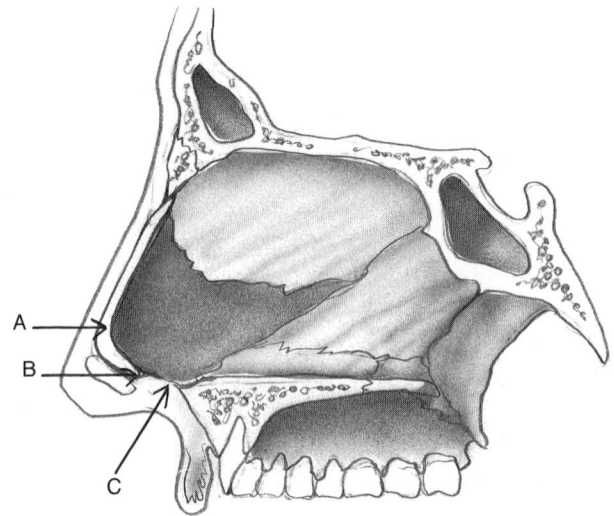

Figure 179.10 *Arrows,* The three anatomic angles composing the caudal aspect of the nasal quadrangular cartilage. *A,* Anterior septal angle; *B,* midseptal angle; *C,* posterior septal angle.

The two layers of septal lining are closely attached and together contain the vascular and nervous supply to the septum. Separation of the mucoperichondrium from the underlying cartilage, as may occur in traumatic or postsurgical septal hematoma, may lead to ischemic necrosis of the affected septum and result in a perforation or a saddle-nose deformity. When portions of septal cartilage or bone are removed during surgery, the lining flaps from each side of the septum are left to readhere and scar. Thus, during septal surgery, perforations may also result after opposing bilateral mucosal tears are created. Because the perichondrial and periosteal layers bear the majority of the biomechanical strength of the septal lining, the surgeon must remain deep to these layers during flap dissection, to maximize strength of the resulting lining flaps and reduce the risk of perforation. If the flap elevation occurs in a submucosal plane, the perichondrium or periosteum may be inadvertently resected with the septal cartilage and bone, leaving only the relatively weak mucosa and increasing the risk of perforation (16).

Variant Anatomy

Differences in the size and development of the nasal septum account for many of the functional and aesthetic variations in the nose. Because the septum is attached to the cartilages that determine nasal shape (LLCs and ULCs), its overgrowth may lead to excessive projection of these structures. In these situations, the septum pulls the cartilaginous elements of the nose under tension—the underpinnings of the so-called tension-nose deformity. Such noses are characterized by a high cartilaginous dorsum, a tip-defining point that is determined by a projecting anterior septal angle (instead of the domal angle of the LLC), and a low-hanging columella that is created by a prominent caudal septal border. In such patients, conservative trimming of the septum may be necessary to create a less conspicuous profile.

An inverse relation exists between the sizes of the cartilaginous septum and osseous septum. Patients with short nasal bones and long ULCs tend to have a greater abundance of quadrangular cartilage and less vomer and ethmoid plate. The opposite is true in noses with long nasal bones and short ULCs. This relation may help the rhinoplasty surgeon predict how much septal cartilage will be available for graft harvesting before surgery.

The septum rarely exists in a true midsagittal plane. Deviations from the midline have both functional and cosmetic implications. Particularly along the floor of the nasal airway, deviations may cause considerable airway obstruction. Most often, a combination of cartilaginous and osseous deformities contributes to the obstruction. Surgical treatment may require removing or repositioning these deviated skeletal elements. After trauma in particular, portions of the septum may be jagged and angulated. Meticulous elevation of the septal lining from these structures is required before their removal to prevent septal perforation. Uncorrected deviations of the perpendicular plate of the ethmoid and vomer may result in persistent posterior airway obstruction after septal surgery.

Deviations of the caudal and dorsal edge of the septum have cosmetic implications in addition to functional effects. From the rhinion to the anterior nasal spine, septal deviations may translate to visible external deformities. Deviation of the mid-dorsal septum, anterior septal angle, mid-caudal septum, and posterior septal angle may lead to a crooked-nose deformity at the upper cartilaginous vault, the nasal tip, the columella, or the columellar base, respectively. These irregularities may originate from a traumatic event. However, the septum will eventually develop an inherent memory to its new shape and position. Thus, the correction of a severely crooked nose may require repositioning or replacing these septal elements (17).

Osseous Vault

The osseous vault is a pyramidal structure that, together with the bony septum, provides the principal structural support for the nose. It consists of the frontal process of the maxilla and the paired nasal bones. The cephalic portion of the osseous vault articulates with the frontal bone at the nasofrontal suture line. The superior portion of the nasal bones rests on the nasal spine of the frontal bone and also derives midline support from the perpendicular plate of the ethmoid. Caudally, the free edge of the osseous vault forms the superior portion of the pyriform aperture. The caudal edge is joined by a connective tissue to the upper cartilaginous vault in the keystone area.

Each nasal bone may be thought of as an elongated quadrangle, with its lateral long edge articulating with the frontal process of the maxilla and its medial long edge articulating in the midline with its contralateral partner. The cephalic edge at the nasofrontal suture line is narrow, whereas the free caudal edge is wider. The nasal bones are thick cephalically at the nasofrontal suture line and thin progressively toward the free caudal edge. Most traumatic nasal fractures occur in the caudal, more projecting portion of the nasal bones where they are the thinnest.

The bony pyramid of the osseous vault may be mobilized with osteotomies during rhinoplasty. Medial osteotomies disconnect the two halves of the osseous vault so each may be moved independently, and lateral osteotomies free the anterior sidewall of the osseous vault from its attachment to the rest of the frontal process of the maxilla. The lateral osteotomy is made on the frontal process of the maxilla and preserves the nasomaxillary suture line. A wide range of height, length, and width of the osseous vault occurs, and this should be taken into account in the planning of osteotomies.

Variant Anatomy

The overall thickness of the nasal bones varies by age, gender, and ethnicity. As elsewhere in the body, the nasal bones are subject to age-related osteopenia and may become thinner and more fragile over time, particularly in women. Such individuals are particularly prone to nasal fractures, even with moderate-energy trauma. After such injuries, it may take these patients longer to reach stable osseous union, potentially prolonging the time window in which closed nasal reduction may be performed. Surgical osteotomies should be performed cautiously in noses with thin, fragile bone, as a higher risk exists of creating overly mobile, free-floating osseous segments. In contrast, patients with thick, rigid nasal bones may be relatively resistant to nasal fractures, may heal rapidly after fractures occur, and may require greater force to create adequate osteotomies during surgery. Often in rhinoplasty, the goal is to create a modest narrowing of the osseous vault. This may be accomplished through a controlled back-fracture of the bridge of bone that remains between the cephalic termination of the medial and lateral osteotomies. In patients with thick bone, this osseous bridge may resist back-fracture. In such cases, the area of intact bone may be weakened before back-fracture through a transcutaneous bridging osteotomy. By using a 2-mm osteotome, a series of small perforations may be made through the bone through a single entry point in the skin.

Variations in the width and medial–lateral position of the nasal bones may be hereditary or acquired. Hereditary variations are more likely to manifest as a symmetrical but unusually narrow or wide osseous vault. Gross asymmetries are more likely to be acquired traumatic injuries. In many cases, these are injuries incurred very early in life or even during the birth process. Correction of these deformities typically requires repositioning of the nasal bones through surgical osteotomies. The lateral osteotomies should lie lateral to the bony deformity so that it may be incorporated into the segment of mobilized bone. In cases in which the nasal bone has a very convex, concave, or irregular topography, the bone may need to be mobilized in more than one segment to correct the contour irregularities. In such situations, an intermediate osteotomy may be necessary between the medial and lateral osteotomies. When several osteotomies are needed, they are performed medial to lateral so that the cuts are always made on stable bone. The distance of osteotomies needed to mobilize the nasal bones is dictated by their length, which is also highly variable.

Upper Cartilaginous Vault

The upper cartilaginous vault consists of the paired, shield-like ULCs that are fused in the midline to the dorsal edge of the cartilaginous septum. The septum and the ULCs are fused early in embryonic development and form a single structural unit in this area (18). Although the cartilaginous septum provides support to the ULCs at their midline dorsal fusion, the nasal bones provide the majority

of reinforcement to the ULCs at their cephalic margin, the keystone area. Here, the ULCs overlap the caudal border of the osseous vault, extending cephalad under the bony arch for a distance of up to 11 mm. This attachment is critical in maintaining the structural integrity of the nasal framework. Vigorous downward force on the ULCs can lead to their dislocation from the nasal bones, a deformity that causes collapse of the upper cartilaginous vault. Because the nasal bones stabilize the ULCs at their cephalic aspect, the upper cartilaginous vault is less rigid and more mobile caudally.

The upper cartilaginous vault is wider cephalically where the ULCs take on a more horizontal course as they articulate with the septum. The arch of the ULCs closely follows the arch of the nasal bones in this region. Caudally, the ULCs slope more acutely away from the dorsal septum, creating a narrower dorsal line. At their caudalmost aspect, a free edge of the ULCs may diverge away laterally from the septum. This relatively narrow area of the upper cartilaginous vault corresponds intranasally to the internal nasal valve area, the region with the greatest nasal airway resistance. These regional variations are easily visualized on cross sections (Fig. 179.11).

Along with the cartilaginous septum, the ULCs determine the appearance of the middle third of the nose. The transition between these structures should be smooth and unbroken. Surgical alterations in this area, such as with hump reduction or spreader grafting, should result in a smooth, coplanar dorsal surface.

Variant Anatomy

The distance from nasion to rhinion defines the cephalic–caudal length of the osseous vault. The upper cartilaginous vault refers to the area of the nose from rhinion to the caudal edge of the ULCs. Despite their common nomenclature of upper and middle thirds of the nose, the lengths of these regions rarely occupy exactly one-third of total nasal length. The lengths of the osseous vault and upper cartilaginous vault have an inverse relation. That is, individuals with long nasal bones have a short upper cartilaginous vault and vice versa. The length of the upper cartilaginous vault typically corresponds to the length of the quadrangular septal cartilage. Thus, the presence of long nasal bones and a short upper cartilaginous vault should alert the surgeon that a relative deficiency of septal cartilage may be present.

The relative lengths of these areas have significant implications on the supportive mechanism of the internal nasal valve. Patients with long nasal bones and short ULCs tend to have more support of the internal valve area because of a greater contribution of the rigid support provided by the nasal bones. In contrast, long ULCs have less rigid osseous support and are therefore more prone to collapse, particularly at their caudal aspect in the area of the internal nasal valve (Fig. 179.12). Individuals with pre-existing narrowing in this region may already have nasal

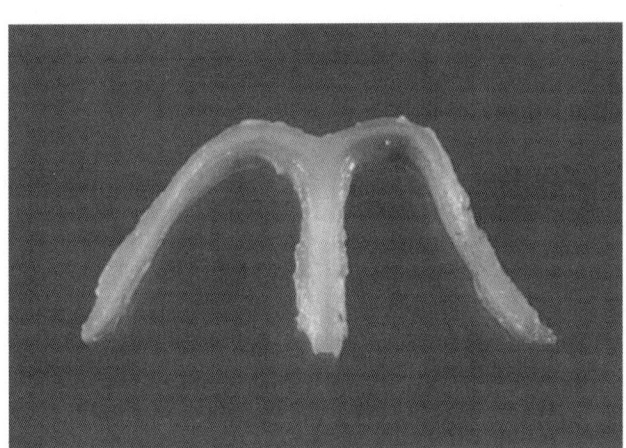

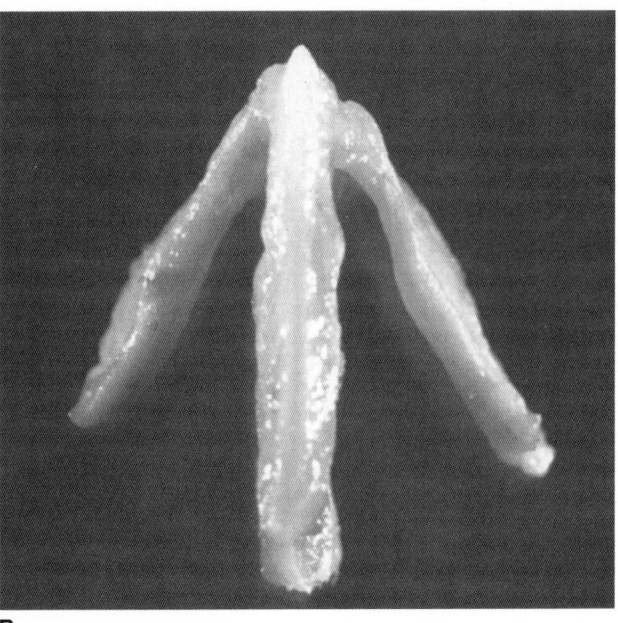

A   **B**

Figure 179.11 A: Cross section of the upper cartilaginous vault just below the rhinion. The broad arch of the ULCs closely follows the caudal margin of the nasal bones in this region. **B**: Further caudal in the area of the internal nasal valve, the structures are more flexible and a much narrower relation exists between the ULCs and nasal septum. (Photograph courtesy of Dean Toriumi.)

valve insufficiency or collapse of the ULC during inspiration. These patients are predisposed to develop postrhinoplasty nasal obstruction after dorsal hump reduction. In such cases, the articulation of the ULCs and septum is resected with the hump, leaving the ULCs unsupported along the dorsum. Ensuing inferomedial collapse of the ULCs occurs, leading to internal valve narrowing, medial pinching of the central area of the dorsal line, and the inverted-V deformity, in which cephalic ULC collapse

reveals the outline of the V-shaped caudal border of the nasal bones. To prevent such complications, the ULC should be resupported onto the septum with a technique such as spreader grafting.

Lower Cartilaginous Vault

The key elements in the lower cartilaginous vault are the paired lower lateral (or alar) cartilages. Perhaps more than

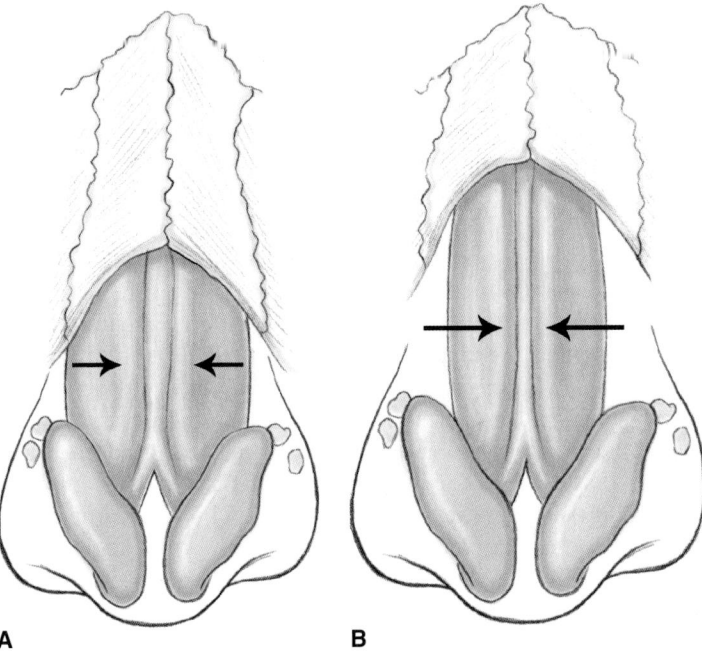

A   **B**

Figure 179.12 A: Long nasal bones create more stabilization of the caudal cartilaginous elements of the nose with less tendency for inferomedial collapse of the ULCs with inspiration or with scarring after hump reduction. **B**: Short nasal bones and a long upper cartilaginous vault may cause narrowing of the ULCs after they are separated from the nasal septum following hump reduction. Restabilization with spreader grafts may prevent this complication in such patients.

anywhere else in the nose, endless anatomic variations and divergences are found between individuals in these structures. However, the extent to which the LLCs determine the shape and configuration of the nasal tip and base is variable, depending on the thickness of the SSTE and the tensile and compressive forces imparted to these areas by the attachments to the surrounding fixed structures of the nasal septum, pyriform aperture, ULCs, and nasal bones. Nonetheless, surgical modifications of the nasal tip and base in rhinoplasty almost always involve some modification to the shape or position of the LLCs.

With the septum, the LLCs provide support to the nasal tip. Each LLC may be considered in three sections: the medial crus, the intermediate crus, and the lateral crus. The three areas are not necessarily distinct anatomic entities but transition from one to the next through a series of bends and undulations in the continuous roll of cartilage. These myriad turns and divergences create the nuances of this structure, which then form the unique external topography of each nasal tip. Two distinct angles, however, are fairly consistent in most noses and consequently are generally conceptualized as transition points that separate the three crura: the lateral genu and the medial genu (Fig. 179.4A). The subsequent discussion covers the general anatomy of each subsite of the lower lateral crura. The more commonly encountered variant anatomy is then discussed. The role of the LLCs as they pertain to mechanical stabilization of the nose is discussed subsequently.

The Medial Crus

With their connection to the caudal septum, the medial crura form the structural support of the columella. The width of the LLCs is narrowest in this region and may be as little as 4 to 5 mm. Each medial crus may be divided into an anterior columellar segment and a posterior footplate segment. On base view, each columellar segment parallels its contralateral counterpart and is connected to it and the caudal septum by fibrous tissue. The footplate segment flares posterolaterally and contributes to the normal widening of the columella at its base or pedestal. On the lateral or base view of an ideal Caucasian nose, the anterior limit of the medial crus corresponds to the columellar–lobular junction at the apex of the nostril (Fig. 179.4).

Variant Anatomy

Variation in the length and shape of the medial crus affects the appearance of the nasal base and position of the nasal tip (19). A short medial crus results in a short columella and a small anteroposterior dimension of the nostril. This tends to result in deficient nasal-tip projection and a small nostril–lobular ratio. A long medial crus that extends anteriorly beyond the apex of the nostril creates a flat, projecting nasal tip. Endless variations exist in the degree of

symmetry, curvature, flare, and smoothness of these structures. The intervening soft tissue between the columellar segments may camouflage irregularities, but a thin SSTE may lead to a bifid appearance of the columella. In general, the goals during surgery are to place the medial crura into a symmetrical, midline position. Fixation sutures to resecure the medial crura are a reliable technique to this end, but care must be taken to maintain a normal relation between the crura and surrounding structures. For instance, the medial crura should be bound together only at their cephalic borders to retain the natural flare of the caudal edges so as to maintain adequate columellar width (11). Even a small degree of malposition of the medial crura may have significant impact on nasal tip rotation, projection, columellar show, and nasolabial angle. Fixation, therefore, must be executed with enormous forethought and meticulous technique.

The width of the individual medial crura and their distance from each other determine the width of the columella. In some cases, the normal flare of the posterior medial crura (footplates) is exaggerated, leading to a wide columellar base, which may compromise airflow at the nostril aperture. Caudally positioned medial crura may result from excessive cartilaginous width, lax ligamentous attachments to the caudal septum (wide membranous septum), or caudal overgrowth of the septum, which tensions the medial crura downward. Particularly in the presence of retracted nasal ala, low medial crura will lead to excessive columellar show. Such patients may complain that their nostrils are too conspicuous. Surgical correction usually involves elevating or trimming the caudal margin of the medial crura.

The Intermediate Crus

Also called the domal segments, the intermediate crura bridge the medial and lateral crura, extending from the medial genu to the lateral genu. This structure represents the transition from the convergent and divergent portions of the paired LLCs. The region of the lateral genu is often the anteriormost projecting point of the LLC and may correspond topographically to the tip-defining point. In this region, the intermediate crus may narrow abruptly, rendering it susceptible to transection during surgery. The angle formed between the two intermediate crura as they flare away from each other laterally is termed the angle of divergence (Fig. 179.13). The ideal angle is approximately 60 degrees and provides a natural-appearing width to the infratip lobule as it transitions from the columella to the nasal tip on frontal or basal views. The intermediate crura also diverge from the medial crura in a cephalic direction by approximately 50 degrees. Externally on lateral view, this bend corresponds to the columellar–lobular angle, dividing the nasal base into the infratip lobule anteriorly and columella posteriorly—the basis of the double break.

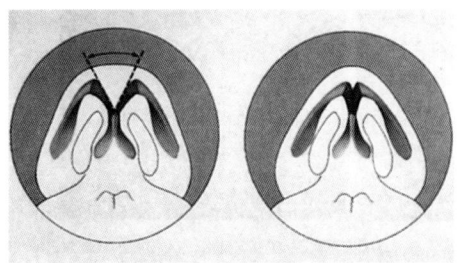

Figure 179.13 The intermediate crura bridge the lateral and medial crura of the LLCs. The angle of divergence is shown on the left. If the intermediate crura are widely bifurcated, a broad trapezoid appearance of the tip results, as shown on the left. If the intermediate crura are closely opposed, a triangular appearance results, as shown on the right.

Variant Anatomy

Variations in the length and curvature of the intermediate crura and the degree of angulation at the medial and lateral genua determine the shape of the infratip lobule on frontal and basal views. Gentle turns at the genua and a smooth convex curvature of the intermediate crus produce a convex domal segment. A broad and flat intermediate crura with angulated connections at the genua result in a "boxy" configuration. If the intermediate crura are concave, a "double-dome" segment is created (2). Variation in the angle of divergence also will affect the shape of the tip lobule. A narrow angle of divergence results in a narrow lobule and creates a more triangular appearance to the tip on base view. An angle of divergence approaching 90 degrees produces a boxy tip that appears trapezoidal on base view. These variations in the cartilage configuration may not be reflected in the shape of the tip lobule if overlying skin is thick (Fig. 179.13).

Excessive thickness or convexity of the intermediate crura in the cephalic–caudal dimension may manifest externally as bulging of the infratip lobule. On lateral view, the tip may appear rounded, transitioning to the infratip lobule with one unbroken curve, rather than as a distinct normal double break.

The Lateral Crus

The lateral crus extends from the lateral genu of the LLC posteriorly. Normally, it assumes a gentle convex shape and parallels the alar rim for its medial half, then flattens and turns posterosuperiorly for its lateral portion, ending short of the pyriform aperture. It generally becomes wider as it leaves the lateral genu and then narrows again toward its lateral termination. It is typically the broadest portion of the LLC. Although a centimeter in width is a reasonable estimate of average width, tremendous variation exists (20).

A portion of the medial cephalic borders of the lateral crura may overlap. In this region, the LLCs may be connected to each other and to the caudal border of the ULC by fibrous tissue. The connection to the ULCs is often reinforced by overlapping segments of cartilage. This scroll area is highly variable and may be thickened in comparison to other parts of the LLC (Fig. 179.14).

Variant Anatomy

The variations of lateral crus anatomy are too numerous to detail (20), but some of the more commonly seen variations are discussed herein. Variations in the width and curvature of the lateral crura greatly influence the appearance of the tip and ala. The widest portion of the lateral crus may vary from 7 to 15 mm (20). Broad convex lateral crura impart a bulbous, amorphous appearance to the tip. The concept is similar to the relation of dorsal height and the appearance of width discussed earlier. In a normal nose, the relative narrowness at the nasal tip/domes and the

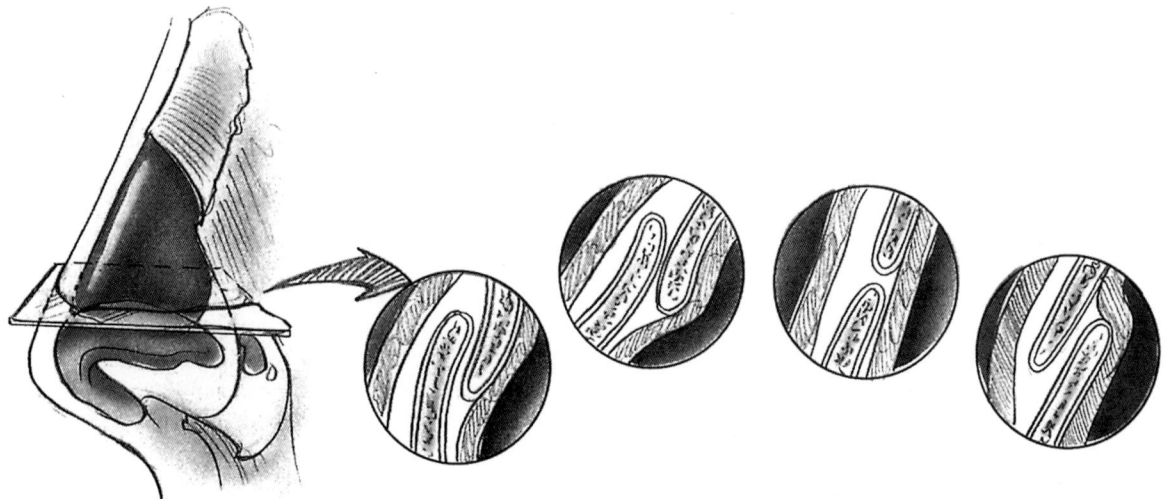

Figure 179.14 A variety of anatomic relations between the cephalic margin of the LLC and the caudal margin of the ULC is found in dissection of cadaver specimens. As individuals age, the intimate relation between the cartilages may be lost. (From Tardy ME. *Surgical anatomy of the nose.* New York: Raven Press, 1990, with permission.)

relative width at the alar base create a visual contrast that makes the tip look appropriately distinct and refined. If the transition from the tip to base is characterized by widely curving lateral crura and nasal ala, this contrast is indistinct, creating the appearance of a wide nose. Correction of such a deformity may require techniques to straighten the overly curved lateral crura, such as suture modification or structural grafting. Aggressive techniques that focus only on narrowing the domes themselves and ignore the convexity of the lateral crura may result in no improvement of the appearance of the tip while incurring structural and cosmetic complications.

Less commonly, the LLCs may be concave as they diverge away from the domes. Externally, this may manifest as a hollow, sunken appearance at the alar lobule with an exaggerated supra-alar crease. If severe, the concavity may narrow the nasal vestibule, impairing nasal airflow. Surgical correction may require structural onlay or underlay grafting, resection and graft replacement of the concave segment, or simply flipping over the concave segment through excision, inversion, and suture fixation.

The strength and thickness of the intermediate and lateral crura determine much of the inherent support of the nasal tip. Stronger cartilage is more resistant to alteration and may result in visible or palpable deformities after surgery. The surgeon must remember Tardy's admonition of the risks of bossae formation after excisional techniques to narrow the tip in patients who possess the triad of tip bifidity, thin skin, and strong LLCs. In such situations, the thick edges of cartilage gradually become apparent through the thin skin envelope as contracture distorts the disrupted tip structures. Modification through suture techniques with avoidance of LLC division is less likely to lead to bossae formation in such patients.

As discussed, the medial aspect of the cephalic border of the lateral crura may overlap for a variable distance. This degree of overlap depends on the overall cephalocaudal position of the lateral crura. In extreme cases, the trajectory of the upper border of the lateral crura is actually straight cephalad, each edge overlapping with the other in the midline over the dorsal septum. In such noses, the lateral crura may diverge from the midline only near its lateral termination. External deformities may be discernable in such patients, particularly in those with thin skin. The classic description is the parenthesis deformity, so named because the bulky outline on frontal view created by the cephalically positioned lateral crura looks as if it is framed by two parentheses on either side of the supratip—"( )." A high dorsum at the supratip on the lateral view in such patients may be misdiagnosed as overdevelopment of the quadrangular cartilage in this region when it may be caused by the overriding cephalic lateral crura. Lowering the dorsum in such patients may require trimming of the cephalic margin of the lateral crura or suture repositioning of the lateral crura instead of dorsal septal excision, the conventional approach to profile reduction. Another consequence of

cephalic lateral crura is the resultant decrease in support to the alar margin. With the lateral crus angled further cephalad, less structural reinforcement is provided to the caudal alar rim, predisposing patients to alar pinching or external nasal valve insufficiency.

Another variation of the lateral crus that may affect nasal airflow is inward (medial) recurvature of its lateral terminus. In some patients, this creates a visible or palpable mass in the lateral nasal vestibule, potentially impairing nasal airflow. In other cases, the deformity may not be apparent until after other rhinoplasty maneuvers have caused medialization of the lateral nasal wall, such as dome-narrowing or tip-projecting maneuvers. Correction may involve simple excision of this portion of the lateral crura if it is caused by overly long, redundant cartilage. Repositioning the area with a stiff underlay graft may be needed in other situations.

Asymmetries of the lateral crura may create tip irregularities and contour deformities. When these asymmetries are severe, they may create tip deviation, even in the presence of a midline caudal septum.

NASAL BASE

The main structures of the nasal base are the paired nasal alae, the nasal sills, the soft triangles, and the columella. These structures form a continuous ring around each of the nares or nostrils, the external openings of the nasal cavities. The normal Caucasian nostril should be oval, with a vertical axis less than 45 degrees from the columella and a nostril-to-infratip lobule ratio of 2:1. Ethnic differences account for significant divergences from these values.

The *nasal ala* is the most lateral wing-like portion of the nostril (21). The main body of the alar lobule is devoid of cartilaginous structure and consists of fibroareolar tissue. Because of this, the shape of the alar lobule is not typically sculpted directly in rhinoplasty. However, cartilaginous elements frame the nasal ala, and their modification alters its shape. The lateral crus of the LLC sweeps over the superomedial portion of the ala. The sesamoid cartilages are located in the soft tissue overlying the pyriform aperture above the ala. Their number is variable, with 0 to 5 cartilaginous bodies present. Interlaced with collagen and fibrous tissue, these accessory cartilages form the sesamoid complex, the connection between the mobile termination of the lateral crus to the rigid pyriform aperture rim.

The insertion of the nasal ala to the face at the junction of the lip and cheek subunits determines the width of the nasal base. Interalar width refers to the horizontal distance from one alar crease to the other. The overall width of the nostrils is also affected by the alar flare, as defined by the degree of bowing of the ala above its insertion. The insertion to the face is three-dimensional, paralleling the curved alar crease that frames the nostrils laterally. Along with the position of the columella, the vertical position of the alar insertion determines the degree of columellar show.

The *nasal sill* is the soft tissue continuation of the ala as it curves medially to join the columella at the nasal spine. It represents the floor of the nostril and is generally wider in those individuals with a large interalar width. Inadvertent injury to the thin skin in this area may lead to visible scar or contraction leading to stenosis of the nostril.

The *soft triangle* is a small base-up triangular subunit bordering the columella medially, the ala laterally, and apex of the nostril anteriorly. This area is unique in that it contains minimal subcutaneous tissue. The external nasal skin folds directly onto the internal vestibular skin, spanning across the genua of the LLC. Because of the lack of subdermal support, this delicate skin is prone to scar contracture if violated. Cicatrix in this area can also lead to reduction in the cross-sectional area of the nostril.

The *columella* is made up of the paired medial crura, which are bound together with fibrous attachments and covered with a skin envelope continuous with the membranous septum. In most individuals, the columella is fairly mobile, limited only by the attachments of the medial crura to the relatively fixed caudal border of the cartilaginous septum. The shape of the columella is determined by the paired medial crura and the most caudal edge of the cartilaginous septum. Distortions of the columella on base view often result from a deviated caudal tip of the septum, which may be easily revealed with side-to-side manipulation.

Variant Anatomy

The alar base represents one of the most highly variable regions of the nose. Width of the alar insertion is rarely within the confines of the medial canthi, as widely described, even in the leptorrhine Caucasian nose. Overall nasal alar width results from the combination of interalar width and alar flare. Patients of Asian and African descent are more likely to have greater alar base width, alar flare, a shorter columella, and more horizontally oriented nostrils. These external differences are ascribable to underlying variations of structural anatomy: weaker, flatter LLCs; thick SSTE; and deficiency of the premaxilla and nasal spine (22). Thickness of the alar wall is also inconstant and reflects the amount of subcutaneous fatty fibroareolar tissue. These variations account for a wide range of nostril orientations and resultant deviation from the "normal" nostril-to-infratip lobule ratio of 2:1. Farkas et al. (23) categorize the variants of nostril position into seven types ranging from vertical to horizontal.

It is crucial that the rhinoplasty surgeon precisely diagnose the cause of a wide alar base before surgery. Some individuals have a wide interalar distance associated with wide nasal sills as the predominant cause. Correction of such a deformity might require segmental excision and closure of a portion of the nasal sills or suture technique to narrow the sills. Other patients may have a normal alar insertion with normal interalar distance but excessive alar flare. Reduction of the ala above the insertion would then be indicated. Reduction of the sill without addressing the alar sidewalls in such patients may actually lead to an exaggeration of the flare, as the ala are forced to curve more acutely. Many patients have components of both an increased interalar width and alar flare, requiring treatment of both the sill area as well as the alar sidewalls.

In addition, the internal and external circumferences of the nostrils must be considered so that the geometry of the excision may be appropriately adjusted. Some individuals have a normal or even small inner nostril circumference but have an overall wide alar base because of thick alar walls. Such individuals benefit from a triangular or trapezoidal wedge excision such that more tissue is excised from the external rim of the nostril than is removed from the inner circumference. In extreme cases, the alar sidewall itself may be debulked and thinned through an alar rim incision.

MECHANICS AND STABILITY

Structural Elements and Relations

Considerations regarding the mechanical stability of the nose are too often overlooked in rhinoplasty. Compromise to the structures and relations that maintain the nose's architecture leads to long-term complications impairing both function and cosmesis. In this section, the regional anatomy of the nose is revisited as it pertains to the mechanical stabilization of the nose. Also discussed are several conceptual models, some of them co-opted from engineering principles, which are commonly invoked to help surgeons conceptualize the elements of nasal structural stability.

The stability of the nose derives from the strength and resiliency of its complex anatomic elements and their various interconnections. Three echelons of support may be conceptualized, each contributing various degrees of stabilization. First, the osseous framework, including the nasal bones, pyriform aperture, osseous septum, and nasal floor, provides the rigid foundation onto which the cartilaginous and soft tissue elements are built. Second, the rigid quadrangular cartilage, which is fixated to bone along its ventral and cephalic borders, directly supports the upper and lower cartilaginous vaults. And third, the intrinsic architectures of the LLCs, ULCs, and associated soft tissue, which are all supported by the osseous and septal foundations, provide much of the stability of the nasal tip and base. The extent to which these regions exert support to the nose depends on the region of the nose. Cephalad, the nasal bones and osseous septum provide nearly all of the rigid support. The middle third of the nose is supported by the nasal bones cephalically and by the quadrangular cartilage, which serves as a pillar beneath. The nasal tip and base area, farthest removed from the osseous framework, is the most flexible and dynamic region and depends most on the support of the cartilaginous buttressing of the caudal septum and the inherent strength of the LLCs.

Cantilever Concept

Sheen and Sheen (19) have described the nasal skeleton as a cantilever, in which the osseous vault is a stable extension of the skull. Like a cantilever, the upper cartilaginous vault projects as a beam, supported cephalically through the thick fibrous attachment of the keystone area, and carries the load of the dependent aspects of the nose along its length and at its distal end. The strength of this support depends on the length and thickness of the nasal bones. Longer bones impart more caudal support. The fusion of the osseous vault and the upper cartilaginous vault with the dorsal edge of the septum forms this structural I-beam that extends from the nasion toward the nasal tip. This complex forms the basis of dorsal support for the nose. Disruption of the connections between the nasal bones or of the ULCs or both to the septum greatly weakens the central support provided by the I-beam. This occurs during hump reduction in which the medial septal support element for the ULCs is resected. The ULCs then must rely only on the cephalic attachments to the nasal bones for support. Unless this medial support is reestablished, for example, with spreader grafts, the ULCs may collapse inferomedially, creating pinching, internal valve compromise and the inverted V.

Role of the Nasal Septum

The nasal septum supports the cantilever from its undersurface much as a support wall holds up a roof. Particularly at its caudal aspect, the quadrangular cartilage, functioning as a pillar, carries much of the burden of nasal tip support in most noses. Because the quadrangular cartilage is inherently rigid and sits firmly in an osseous foundation from the nasal spine along the maxillary crest and up the osseous septum to the nasal bones, it provides significant stabilization to the nose. The combination of the cantilevering dorsal element and the buttressing caudal element forms the basis of the L-shaped strut—the most structurally important aspect of the quadrangular cartilage. Compromise to the dorsal component leads to a saddle-nose deformity with ventral collapse of the upper cartilaginous vault. The classic example of this is quadrangular cartilage resorption after an untreated septal hematoma. Compromise to the caudal component may lead to nasal tip ptosis, particularly in the presence of weak medial crura. Traumatic or iatrogenic injury is most often the cause. This is shown in studies in which removal of the cartilaginous septum in cadavers has been shown to result in a significant loss in nasal tip projection (24). For these reasons, it is critical to maintain structural integrity of the L-strut during surgery. Although conventional teaching emphasizes the need to maintain an uninterrupted 1.5-cm-wide dorsal–caudal strut, malposition or deformity of the strut itself may be the cause of external deformities, particularly in the crooked nose. Correction of these problems may mandate the use of techniques that modify the septum and may require repositioning, camouflaging, or reconstruction of the L-strut itself (17).

Ligamentous Attachments

The nasal bones and the quadrangular cartilage serve as the rigid support structures of the nose. The more mobile caudal elements are reinforced onto these foundations through a network of fibrous adhesions. Although termed "ligaments," these connections do not conform to the strict definition of an attachment between an osseous origin and insertion. Rather, they bind the cartilaginous structures to each other, to the nasal septum, and to the pyriform aperture. Numerous histologic and cadaver studies have been conducted in an attempt to better characterize the nature of this tissue. Although the characteristics of these attachments are variably reported, most authors believe they impart a variable degree of structural stabilization to the nose and, in particular, the nasal tip. The ligamentous systems most commonly described are discussed later: the attachments between the ULCs and lateral crura, the intercrural ligaments, the attachments between the lateral crura and pyriform aperture, and the connection between the ULCs and nasal bones at the keystone region (discussed earlier).

The area of overlap between the caudal aspect of the ULCs and the cephalic margin of the lateral crura is commonly referred to as the *scroll region*, owing to the interlocking curved cartilaginous elements. In reality, the relation between these structures is highly variable. In the most common orientation, the upper borders of the lateral crura overlap above the ULCs. It is thought that the extent of recurvature of the ULC is determined by the tension exerted onto its cephalic margin as it is driven cephalad during fetal development (25). The angle of curvature may range from slight (less than 45 degrees) to complete (180 degrees). Other orientations exist with various relations between the cartilaginous structures (Fig. 179.14). Irrespective of the particular orientation, the cartilages are bound together within the scroll region by fibrous tissue, also described as the "intercartilaginous ligament" (26). This articulation forms a hinge mechanism around which the nasal tip is suspended and can flex (27). With advancing age, the intimate relation between the ULCs and the lateral crura may be lost as these ligamentous connections relax and the nasal tip settles caudally. In such cases, a diastasis between the upper and lower cartilaginous vaults may be present instead of a normal thickened scroll area.

The intercrural ligament, also termed "the ligamentous sling" (28), binds the medial aspect of the lateral crura, the intermediate crura, and the medial crura to each other. This ligamentous structure is thought to pull the paired LLCs into the midline. It is widely believed that fibrous attachments connect this ligament to the caudal margin of the septum in the region of the medial crura, providing additional tip support at the base of the nose. Some studies, however, dispute the existence or the importance of such connections (29–31). The contribution of the intercrural ligament in overall tip support, however, is fairly clear. After division of the intercrural ligament, nasal tip support is decreased by 25% to 35%, as measured by tensiometry (30). These studies highlight the need to restore the integrity of these attachments after they are disrupted during surgery, to prevent postoperative loss of tip support. An effective means to this end is through stabilization of the tip at the nasal base. Such techniques involve suture stabilization of the medial and intermediate crura to a stable midline foundation, such as a long nasal septum, a nasal septal caudal extension graft, or a columellar strut (1).

The connection between the lateral crura and the pyriform aperture consists of collagen fibers arranged irregularly with muscular fibers interspersed (31). This connection, which in some individuals contains embedded sesamoid cartilages, also is called the *sesamoid complex or the lateral crural complex.*

Nasal Tip Support: Tripod Concept

The nasal tip is a complex structure whose integrity is maintained by an interrelated network of supporting mechanisms made up of both the tip cartilages and the ligaments that connect them. One classic model used for understanding nasal tip support and dynamics is the tripod analogy (32). The apex of the tripod is the nasal tip, with each of the lateral crura extending cephalolaterally to form two legs of the tripod, and the conjoined medial crura together forming the third leg. Modification of the limbs of the tripod results in changes in nasal tip position. Shortening the limbs results in a loss of tip projection, whereas lengthening increases projection. Tip rotation increases as a result of either truncating the lateral limbs or extending the medial limb. The opposite maneuvers lead to decreased tip rotation. Although the tripod concept is useful to conceptualize these dynamic consequences of crural modification, the analogy falls short as a model for tip structural support. Unlike a true tripod, the LLCs do not rest on a stable surface. Rather, their "feet" are tethered by ligamentous connections to the osseous rim of the pyriform aperture and nasal spine, whereas the apex is tensioned anteriorly and cephalad by the intercrural ligament and the scroll (33). Thus, the nasal tip tripod is a dynamic unit that is suspended and supported by its rigid surrounding structures (Fig. 179.15).

Nasal Tip Support: Tardy Classification

In his classic description of nasal tip support, Tardy includes three major and six minor mechanisms (Table 179.2), each of which imparts variable degrees of support depending on individual anatomy (6). The three major mechanisms are the size, shape, thickness, and strength of the medial and lateral crura; the attachment of the medial crural footplate to the caudal border of the quadrangular cartilage; and the attachment of the caudal border of the ULCs to the cephalic border of the LLCs. The minor tip-support mechanisms are thought to augment the major ones. The classification into major and minor groups was based on clinical experience rather than on one specific structural model. Tardy advocates assessment of tip recoil through digital palpation to determine the relative importance of the various tip-support mechanisms in a given patient.

Nasal Tip Support: Other Models

Other schemas of nasal tip–support mechanisms have been reported. Based on multiple cadaver dissections, Janeke and Wright (28) proposed that the tip support is based on the fibrous connection between the ULCs and LLCs; the connection between the lateral crus to the pyriform aperture; the interdomal ligament between the paired domes of the LLCs; and the attachment of the medial crus to the caudal septum (28). Two of these are considered major tip-support mechanisms in the Tardy classification. The importance of the interdomal ligament, classified as a minor mechanism by Tardy, also is echoed by other authors who concluded that this intercrural ligament is a major tip-support mechanism and should be reconstructed during open rhinoplasty (29,34). Conversely, other authors believe that the attachment of the medial crural footplates to the septum, a major mechanism in the Tardy classification, plays only a small role in the stability of the nasal tip (33). This is supported by histologic studies of cadaveric noses showing the lack of defined attachments in this area (18,28,31). Tardy points out that minor mechanisms become major contributors (and vice versa) in certain individuals depending on their particular anatomy.

Several of the ligamentous tip-support structures have been examined in histologic detail in fresh cadaveric noses, and the results are consistent with the macroscopic findings from dissections and from clinical experience. For example, the fibrous connection between the ULCs and LLCs is shown to consist of dense collagen fibers running in the same direction and anchored firmly to each cartilage (4,7,31). This meets the histologic criteria of a true ligament.

The concept of the nasal tip as a dynamic structure is carried further in the tensegrity model of nasal tip support as proposed by Dyer (33). Applying an engineering and architectural concept to the nasal skeleton, Dyer proposed that the nasal tip may be thought of as a tensegrity structure, in which stability derives from the distribution of mechanical stress throughout all its components. Such a structure is self-stabilizing, consisting of an equilibrium of compressive and tensile elements. In the nasal tip, the LLCs and the cartilaginous septum are the compression-bearing members,

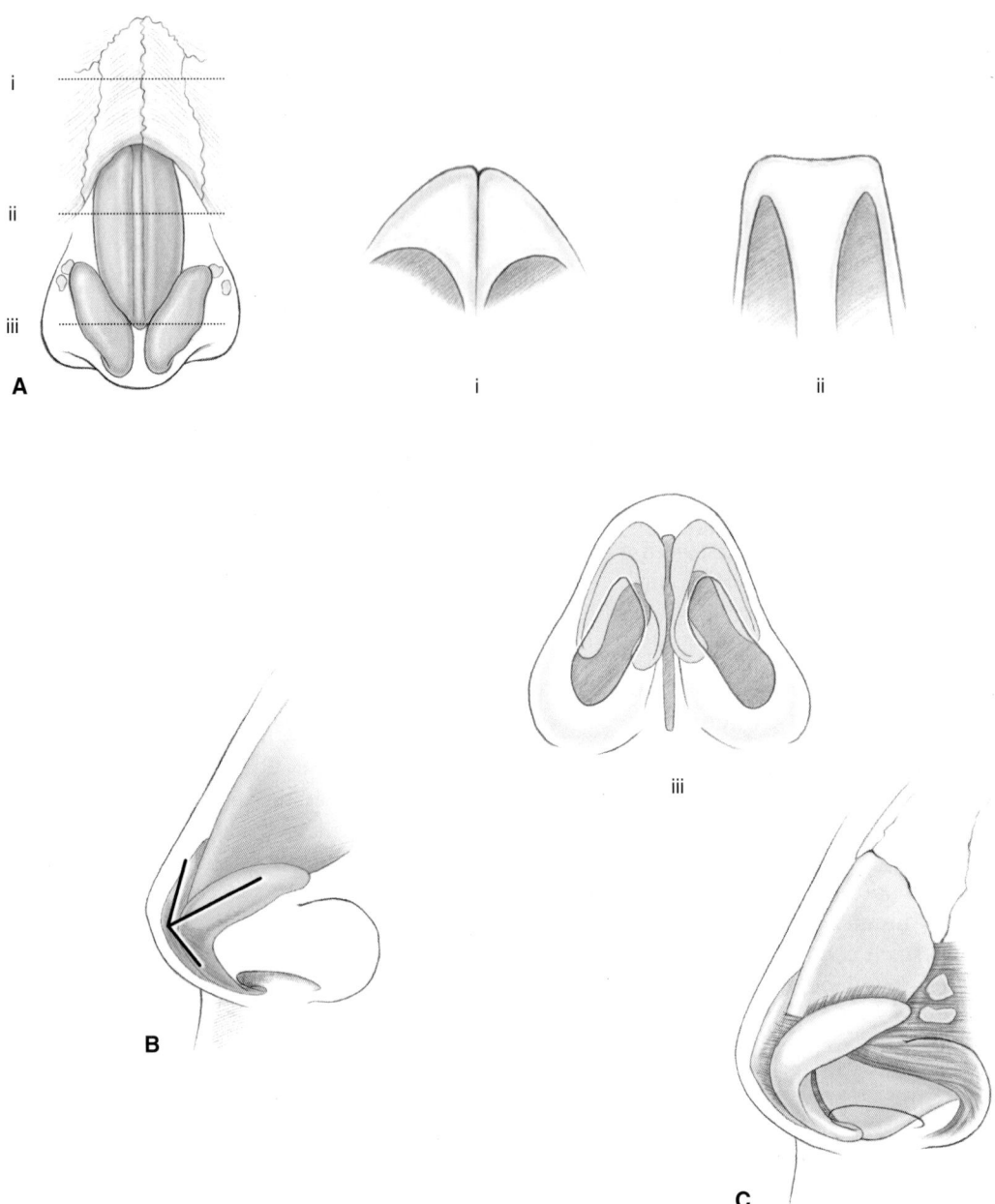

Figure 179.15 Various support mechanisms of the nose. **A:** The nasal septum functions as a supporting wall that reinforces the dorsal elements of the nose. Cross section through (*i*) osseous vault, (*ii*) upper cartilaginous vault, and (*iii*) nasal base. **B:** The two lateral crura and the conjoined medial crura create a nasal tip tripod, a model useful for understanding nasal tip dynamics. The degree to which the inherent strength of these structures contributes to nasal tip support varies significantly from individual to individual. **C:** The network of ligamentous attachments reinforce and interconnect the skeletal elements of the nose. The ULCs are connected firmly to the undersurface of the nasal bones, forming a cantilever-like support for the dorsum. The nasal tip and base are stabilized through ligamentous attachments between the lateral crura and ULC, the lateral crura and pyriform aperture, and between the two dorsal regions of each LLC.

and the fibrous, ligamentous connections are tension-bearing members. The nasal tip structure is thus viewed as an integrated structure in which disruption of one element affects the stability of the whole. Although it is difficult to test this description of nasal tip support scientifically, it is a useful concept that has already been applied to rhinoplasty techniques (33).

Areas of Structural Void

Two areas of the nose devoid of cartilaginous support are particularly susceptible to collapse in certain patients. First, the lateral nasal wall that is lateral (and often cephalad) to the termination of the lateral crura and medial to the pyriform aperture is prone to dynamic collapse with

TABLE 179.2	TIP-SUPPORT MECHANISMS

Major

Size, shape, and resilience of the medial and lateral crura

Medial crural footplate attachment to the caudal border of the quadrangular cartilage

Attachment of the upper lateral cartilages (caudal border) to the alar cartilages (cephalic border)

Minor[a]

Ligamentous sling spanning the paired domes of the alar cartilages

Cartilaginous septal dorsum

Sesamoid complex extending the support of the lateral crura to the pyriform aperture

Attachment of the alar cartilages to the overlying skin and musculature

Nasal spine

Membranous septum

[a]On occasion, because of extreme anatomic variability, a "minor" tip support may assume the importance of one of the more major supports.

inspiration. This area corresponds intranasally to the internal valve area and may require reinforcement with graft such as alar batten grafts. In the normal state, this area is supported by the dilator naris and nasalis muscles (7). A second area is the alar margin, particularly lateral to the point at which the lateral crura diverge cephalically. In patients with projecting, thin noses, the alar margins are susceptible to collapse and resultant external valve narrowing.

In summary, the stability of the nasal skeleton derives from its rigid elements, the nasal bones, pyriform aperture, and nasal septum. The dynamic caudal structures, the nasal tip and base, are stabilized largely through the lower lateral crural attachments to these anchoring structures through networks of interconnecting fibrous tissue or ligaments. The means of support may be conceptualized both as a cantilevering mechanism from the nasal bones and ULCs cephalically and a pillar-like support from the septum ventrally. Although the inherent strength and resiliency of the LLCs create a dynamic tripod and provide form and some support to the nasal tip, a significant loss of tip support is incurred if the attachments of the tripod to the surrounding rigid structures are violated. In rhinoplasty, it is therefore imperative to reconstitute tip support through methods such as suture stabilization of the medial and intermediate crura to a stable midline foundation to prevent postoperative tip instability.

Variant Anatomy

The infinite variations of form are evident in the different structural orientations encountered in different noses. As Tardy reminds us, the relative role of any of the structural component of the nose differs from person to person. For example, individuals with long, broad nasal bones are more apt to have greater stability imparted to upper cartilaginous vault and to the caudal elements of the nasal tip and base. Within the tip itself, thicker, more developed cartilage provides greater strength and has a larger role in structural support than in someone with weak, thin cartilages. These differences are important to remember when choosing rhinoplasty techniques. For instance, one traditional method to decrease projection of the tip is simply to perform a full transfixion incision and an intercartilaginous incision. Because this incision violates many of the anchoring ligamentous attachments of the tip tripod, the nasal tip may settle toward the face, thus reducing overall projection. However, in a nose in which the medial crura are long and broad, their inherent strength and resiliency may prevent the tip from moving. Methods that reposition and fixate the tip structures to stable surrounding structures are more reliable, reducing the unpredictability of results based on patient-variant anatomy (1).

FUNCTIONAL VALVULAR ANATOMY

Internal Nasal Valve

The internal nasal valve area is the narrowest portion of the nasal passage. It is framed superolaterally by the caudal border of the ULC, medially by the septum, inferiorly by the floor of the pyriform aperture, and posteriorly by the head of the inferior turbinate (35). The *internal nasal valve*, formed by the caudal border of the ULC and the septum, is a specific slit-like structure within the internal nasal valve area and is often the narrowest region of the internal valve area. The angle formed by the attachment of the ULCs to the septum is 10 to 15 degrees in the Caucasian nose and wider in the African or Asian nose. If this angle is less than 10 degrees, the patient will likely experience nasal obstruction because of the collapse of the internal valve on inspiration.

External Nasal Valve

The external nasal valve consists of the nare and the nasal vestibule. The nasal vestibule is the space just inside the external nare and is the compartment caudal to the internal valve area. The vestibule is bordered medially by the septum and columella and laterally by the alar sidewalls. The vestibule contains vibrissae, or nasal hair, on a fold of skin under the lateral crus. Functioning as a coarse filter for inspired air, the vibrissae also serve a resistive purpose to slow the inspired air current and directing it posteriorly into the nasal cavity (36).

The internal and external nasal valves are dynamic structures that function together to deliver a smooth air current to the nasal cavities for humidification. During normal, quiet inspiration, the nasal valves change little in their cross-sectional areas. On deep inspiration, the nostrils flare to increase the diameter of the external valve. With increased airflow, the intraluminal pressure in the internal valve area decreases according to the Bernoulli principle. The tendency for the valve to collapse, however, is counterbalanced by the resistance of its cartilaginous structure to deformation, as well as by isometric contraction of the alar dilator muscles to keep the lumen open. In normal nasal function, the cross-sectional area of the internal valve should be relatively unchanged during inspiration (37). Valvular collapse that occurs only during forced inspiration can be considered physiologic and does not usually require surgical correction (14).

Certain variants of normal nasal anatomy predispose people to nasal obstruction. Individuals with a narrow upper cartilaginous vault tend to have a more acute angle in the internal nasal valve and may be more susceptible to nasal obstruction, even in the resting state. Poiseuille's law states that the rate of air flow is directly proportional to the fourth power of the radius of the conduit. Therefore, even miniscule differences in airway size may have significant clinical effects. Individuals with weak ULCs or lateral nasal walls or both may have more collapse of the internal valve area during inspiration. Preexisting or traumatic septal deviation in the internal valve area also can narrow the valve and cause nasal obstruction. Collapse of the external valve on deep inspiration can result from insufficient support of the alar rim and alar lobule. Patients predisposed to such collapse have particular features that should alert the rhinoplasty surgeon: short nasal bones and a long upper cartilaginous vault (discussed earlier); narrow, projecting noses; slit-like nostrils; exaggerated supra-alar creases; visible pinching of the lateral wall with inspiration; thin cartilages and thin skin; and cephalically positioned lateral crura, which provide minimal support to the alar margins (38).

ETHNIC VARIATIONS

Three broad nasal morphology types have been used to describe ethnic variations. The *leptorrhine* ("tall and thin") nose is associated with Caucasian or Indo-European descent. The leptorrhine nose has served as the basis of aesthetic ideal in Western culture, and the specific nasal-analysis parameters associated with this ideal are discussed elsewhere in this textbook. Because it is the most extensively studied in modern nasal analysis, it also inevitably becomes the reference point for comparison when studying noses of different ethnicities. Only recently have non-Caucasian standards of nasal analysis been developed for specific ethnic groups.

The *platyrrhine* ("broad and flat") nose is associated with African descent. It is characterized by very thick skin, a low radix, a short dorsum, a bulbous and underprojected tip, and flared nostrils. An analysis of the African American female nose shows that compared with the Caucasian standard for nasal analysis, the columella-to-lobule ratio is decreased, and the alar width relative to the intercanthal distance is increased. With regard to the bulbous and underprojected tip, cadaver studies in African American males have demonstrated that the dimensions of the lateral crura are not significantly different from those of the Caucasian nose (39). However, the smallest cartilages were found among noses of the African subtype, and the largest were found in the Afro-Caucasian and Afro-Indian subtypes. This variability may underscore the effect of racial mingling on the canonic platyrrhine nose.

The *mesorrhine* ("intermediate") nose has features intermediate between the leptorrhine nose and the platyrrhine nose. The "typical" Asian or Latino nose is commonly regarded as mesorrhine, with a low radix, variable anterior dorsal projection, rounded and underprojected tip, and rounded nostrils. Note that considerable variation exists in this group. An individual from Northern China or Japan is likely to have a mesorrhine nose with strong leptorrhine characteristics, whereas another from Southeast Asia will likely share more platyrrhine features. In addition to differences in baseline characters, the types of nasal defects encountered in rhinoplasty may also depend on ethnicity. For example, Hispanic patients were more likely to have dorsal humps, saddle deformities, dependent alae, retracted columellae, and poor tip projection compared to Anglos (40).

Generalized characteristics of the canonic nasal morphology types are listed in Table 179.3 (41–43).

TABLE 179.3	GENERAL NASAL CHARACTERISTICS BY MORPHOLOGY		
	Platyrrhine	**Mesorrhine**	**Leptorrhine**
Skin type	Very thick	Moderately thick	Thin
Dorsum	Short, wide, concave	Short, wide	Long, narrow
Radix	Low	Low	High
Nasal bones	Short	Short	Long
Nasal tip	Bulbous, underprojected	Rounded, underprojected	Projected
Columella	Short	Short	Long
Nasal alar width	Wide	Intermediate	Relatively narrow
Ala	Prominent flaring	Variable	Modest flaring

Any discussion of rhinoplasty for the "non-Caucasian nose" is by its nature flawed. It is overly simplistic to classify a non-Caucasian nose as an "ethnic" nose to which "ethnic rhinoplasty" principles apply. Two noses from two different ethnic backgrounds are likely to be as different from each other as they are from a Caucasian nose. In addition, as may be expected from studies of the Caucasian nose, significant variations in facial features are found within any given ethnic group, for example, as documented in African American women (44). Intragroup differences may be as great as intergroup differences. For instance, Latinos with Caribbean ancestry are more likely to have platyrrhine noses, whereas those of Central and South American descent have more leptorrhine noses (45). It would be incorrect to apply ethnic group characteristics blindly to an individual patient based on his or her background alone. Nevertheless, an awareness of the global differences between ethnic nasal morphologies will make a rhinoplasty surgeon more sensitive to the needs of all patients in preserving desired ethnic characteristics.

CONCLUSIONS

The nose is a dynamic and inconstant structure, its anatomy varying from individual to individual. The anatomic principles and support mechanisms described in this chapter are not intended to be inflexible rules applicable to all patients. Rather, they are meant to be guidelines with which any one individual's anatomy may be assessed to understand his or her tissue characteristics, structural dynamics, and anatomic features. Selection of the appropriate surgical techniques should begin with an accurate assessment of the individual anatomy. Only then will the rhinoplasty surgeon maximize the likelihood of achieving the intended aesthetic and functional result.

HIGHLIGHTS

- Altering the topographic dimensions of one region of the nose may have a significant visual impact on the appearance of another region.
- Modifications to the underlying nasal skeleton are less accurately transmitted through a thick SSTE, particularly when they are reductive. Even small contour changes or irregularities may transmit clearly through a thin SSTE.
- An inverse relation exists between the lengths of the nasal bones and upper cartilaginous vault. Long nasal bones provide greater stabilization to the ULCs and other caudal elements of the nose than do short nasal bones.

- The tremendous variation in the size, position, shape, and contour of the LLCs accounts for much of the diversity of nasal tip form and support.
- The structural support of the nose is provided by the osseous framework, nasal septum, and the ligamentous network that attaches the cartilaginous elements to these foundations and to each other.
- Certain anatomic variations predispose patients to destabilization and valvular insufficiency after rhinoplasty: short nasal bones, narrow projecting noses, deep supra-alar creases, inspiratory pinching of the lateral wall, and cephalic LLCs.
- An understanding of individual variant nasal anatomy and the features of nasal morphology that exist for different ethnicities allow the rhinoplasty surgeon to tailor treatment for each patient's unique needs.

REFERENCES

1. Kim DW, Toriumi DM. Open rhinoplasty. In: Behrbohm H, Tardy ME, eds. *Essentials of septorhinoplasty.* New York: Thieme, 2004.
2. Lessard ML, Daniel RK. Surgical anatomy of septorhinoplasty. *Arch Otolaryngol* 1985;111:25–29.
3. Bernstein L. Surgical anatomy in rhinoplasty. *Otolaryngol Clin North Am* 1975;8:549–558.
4. Letourneau A, Daniel RK. The superficial musculoaponeurotic system of the nose. *Plast Reconstr Surg* 1988;82:48–57.
5. Griesman BL. Muscles and cartilages of the nose from the standpoint of typical rhinoplasty. *Arch Otolaryngol* 1944;39:334.
6. Tardy ME, Brown RJ. *Surgical anatomy of the nose.* New York: Raven Press, 1990.
7. Bruintjes TD, van Olphen AF, Hillen B, et al. A functional anatomic study of the relationship of the nasal cartilages and muscles to the nasal valve area. *Laryngoscope* 1998;108:1025–1032.
8. May M, West JW, Hinderer KH. Nasal obstruction from facial palsy. *Arch Otolaryngol* 1977;103:389–391.
9. De Souza Pinto EB. Relationship between tip nasal muscles and the short upper lip. *Aesthetic Plast Surg* 2003;27:381–387.
10. Rohrich RJ, Huynh B, Muzaffar AR, et al. Importance of the depressor septi nasi muscle in rhinoplasty: anatomic study and clinical application. *Plast Reconstr Surg* 2000;105:376–383.
11. Oneal RM, Beil RJ Jr, Schlesinger J. Surgical anatomy of the nose. *Clin Plast Surg* 1996;23:195–222.
12. Filippi A, Pohl Y, Tekin U. Sensory disorders after separation of the nasopalatine nerve during removal of palatal displaced canines: prospective investigation. *Br J Oral Maxillofac Surg* 1999;37:134–136.
13. Paparella MM, Shumrick DA, eds. *Otolaryngology,* 2nd ed. Philadelphia, PA: Saunders, 1980.
14. Goode RL. Surgery of the incompetent nasal valve. *Laryngoscope* 1985;95:546–555.
15. Beeson WH. The nasal septum. *Otolaryngol Clin North Am* 1987;20:743–767.
16. Kim DW, Egan KK, O'Grady K, et al. Biomechanical strength of human nasal septal lining: comparison of the constituent layers. *Laryngoscope* 2005;115:1451–1453.
17. Kim DW, Toriumi DM. Management of the post-traumatic nose: the twisted nose deformity and saddle nose deformity. *Facial Plast Surg Clin North Am* 2004;12:111–132.
18. Daniel RK, Letourneau A. Rhinoplasty: nasal anatomy. *Ann Plast Surg* 1988;20:5–13.
19. Sheen JH, Sheen AP. *Aesthetic rhinoplasty,* 2nd ed. St. Louis, MO: Quality Medical Publishing, 1998.
20. Zelnik J, Gingrass RP. Anatomy of the alar cartilage. *Plast Reconstr Surg* 1979;64:650–653.

21. Lanza DC, Kennedy DW, Koltai PJ. Applied nasal anatomy & embryology. *Ear Nose Throat J* 1991;70:416–422.

22. Brissett AE, Sherris DA. Changing the nostril shape. *Facial Plast Surg Clin North Am* 2000;8:433–445.

23. Farkas LG, Hreczko TA, Deutsch CK. Objective assessment of standard nostril types: a morphometric study. *Ann Plast Surg* 1983;11:381–389.

24. Adams WP Jr, Rohrich RJ, Hollier LH, et al. Anatomic basis and clinical implications for nasal tip support in open versus closed rhinoplasty. *Plast Reconstr Surg* 1999;103:255–261.

25. Drumheller GW. Topology of the lateral nasal cartilages: the anatomical relationship of the lateral nasal to the greater alar cartilage, lateral crus. *Anat Rec* 1973;176:321–327.

26. Dion MC, Jafek BW, Tobin CE. The anatomy of the nose: external support. *Arch Otolaryngol* 1978;104:145–150.

27. Adamson PA, Morrow TA. The nasal hinge. *Otolaryngol Head Neck Surg* 1994;111:219–231.

28. Janeke JB, Wright WK. Studies on the support of the nasal tip. *Arch Otolaryngol* 1971;93:458–464.

29. Beaty MM, Dyer WK II, Shawl MW. The quantification of surgical changes in nasal tip support. *Arch Facial Plast Surg* 2002;4:82–91.

30. Han SK, Lee DG, Kim JB, et al. An anatomic study of nasal tip supporting structures. *Ann Plast Surg* 2004;52:134–139.

31. Ordonez-Ordonez LE, Navarro-Garcia US, Angulo-Martinez ES. Nasal septum to columella attachment: a major tip support? *Otolaryngol Head Neck Surg* 2010;143:60–65.

32. Anderson JR. The dynamics of rhinoplasty. In: Bustamante GA, ed. *Proceedings of the ninth international congress in otorhinolaryngology.* Amsterdam: Excerpta Medica, 1969. Excerpta Medica, International Congress Series, No. 206:708–710.

33. Dyer WK II. Nasal tip support and its surgical modification. *Facial Plast Surg Clin North Am* 2004;12:1–13.

34. Johnson CM, Toriumi DM. *Open structure rhinoplasty.* Philadelphia, PA: WB Saunders, 1990.

35. Kasperbauer JL, Kern EB. Nasal valve physiology: implications in nasal surgery. *Otolaryngol Clin North Am* 1987;20:699–719.

36. Cottle MH. Structures and function of the nasal vestibule. *Arch Otolaryngol Head Neck Surg* 1955;62:173.

37. Cole P. The four components of the nasal valve. *Am J Rhinol* 2003;17:107–110.

38. Constantian MB. Four common anatomic variants that predispose to unfavorable rhinoplasty results: a study based on 150 consecutive secondary rhinoplasties. *Plast Reconstr Surg* 2000;105:316–331.

39. Ofodile FA, James EA. Anatomy of alar cartilages in blacks. *Plast Reconstr Surg* 1997;100:699–703.

40. Leach J. Aesthetics and the Hispanic rhinoplasty. *Laryngoscope* 2002;112:1903–1916.

41. Papel ID, Capone RB. Facial proportions and esthetic ideals. In: Behrbohm H, Tardy ME, eds. *Essentials of septorhinoplasty.* Stuttgart, AR: Thieme, 2004:65–74.

42. Rohrich RJ, Muzaffar AR. Rhinoplasty in the African-American patient. *Plast Reconstr Surg* 2003;111:1322–1339.

43. Stucker FJ, Lian T, Sanders K. African American rhinoplasty. *Facial Plast Surg Clin North Am* 2005;13:65–72.

44. Porter JP, Olson KL. Analysis of the African American female nose. *Plast Reconstr Surg* 2003;111:620–626.

45. Milgrim LM, Lawson W, Cohen AF. Anthropometric analysis of the female Latino nose: revised aesthetic concepts and their surgical implications. *Arch Otolaryngol Head Neck Surg* 1996;122:1079–1086.

Rhinoplasty: Incisions, Approaches and Analysis

180

Grant S. Gillman

A thorough and thoughtful approach to nasal analysis is the foundation upon which a successful aesthetic and functional rhinoplasty outcome is built. A consistent strategy—routinely applied—will hone one's analysis skills and minimize the likelihood of failing to address something that should have been recognized preoperatively. By studiously engaging in this practice preoperatively *and* postoperatively, one will come to better appreciate the dynamics of rhinoplasty and the anatomic and surgical correlates of one's observations and interventions.

No doubt, aesthetic ideals will vary—from patient to patient, from culture to culture, and from surgeon to surgeon (1–5). Nonetheless, the "guidelines" contained in this chapter are intended to serve as a useful, practical framework upon which to evaluate nasal aesthetics and from which to move forward to surgical planning.

ANATOMIC LANDMARKS

Familiarity with the nomenclature used for the reference points of surface anatomy facilitates improved communication between colleagues and clarity of notes and the operative record. In addition, knowing how underlying structures are reflected on the surface topography enables the surgeon to more accurately analyze, diagnose, and anticipate the pathology and thereby develop a more thoughtful surgical strategy preoperatively. Accordingly, it is appropriate to begin with terminology.

The commonly accepted terms for surface nasal anatomy, as seen from the frontal, lateral, and base views, are illustrated in Figures 180.1 to 180.3 and defined below. Nasal anatomy is also covered and reviewed in greater detail in the chapter on "Surgical Anatomy of the Nose."

Terminology

Trichion—the most anterior midline point on the hairline

Glabella—the most anterior or prominent point on the forehead (lateral view)

Nasion (aka radix)—the starting point, root, or visual takeoff of the nose, it is the deepest depression at the root of the nose in the midsagittal plane, corresponding to the nasofrontal suture. The midline junction between the frontal bone and the nasal dorsum is also known as the radix.

Rhinion—the midline junction of the nasal bones and the dorsal septum (osseocartilaginous junction)

Supratip—the point along the nasal dorsum that lies just cephalic to the nasal tip

Tip—the most anterior projecting part of the nasal profile (ideally). The tip "lobule" refers more broadly to the region bounded by the supratip superiorly, the anterior end of the alar crease laterally, and the anterior nostril margin posteroinferiorly.

Infratip lobule—the part of the nasal tip seen from the nasal base view that sits anterior to the columella and leading edge of the nares and extends to the tip-defining point

Soft tissue triangle (or soft tissue facet)—seen from the nasal base, this refers to the soft tissue skin fold that lies anterior to the apex of the nostril and just behind the caudal border of the junction of the medial and lateral crus of the lower lateral cartilage

Subnasale—midline junction of the columella and upper lip

Labrale superioris—the vermilion border of the upper lip

Stomion—the midline point at the junction of the upper and lower lips

Pogonion—the most anterior or prominent point on the chin (lateral view)

Menton—the lowest midline point on the chin

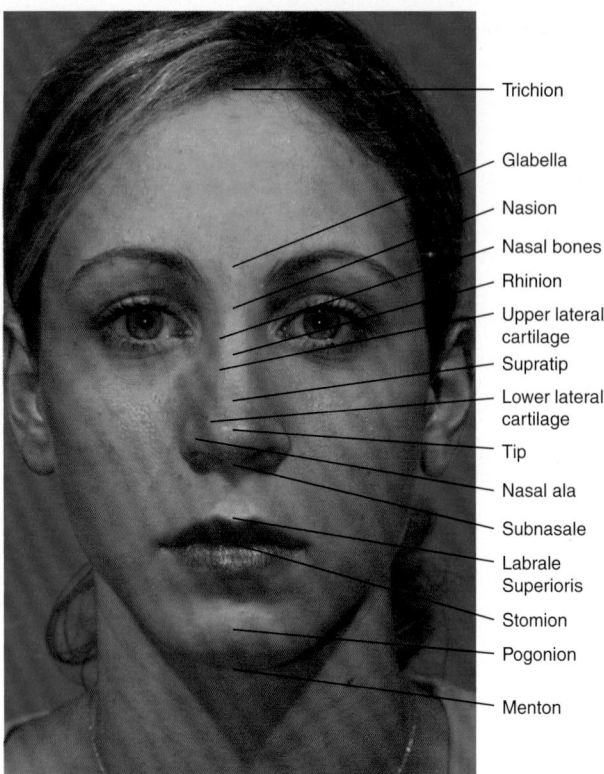

Figure 180.1 Surface anatomy nomenclature—frontal view.

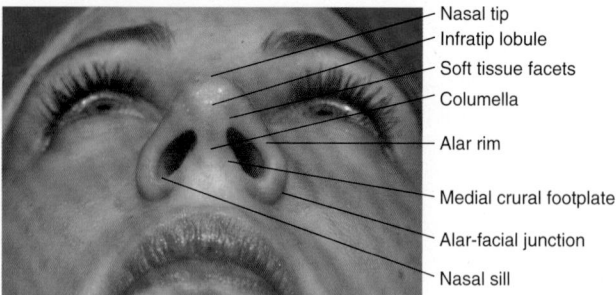

Figure 180.3 Surface anatomy nomenclature—base view.

NASAL AND FACIAL ANGLES

The most commonly referenced angles applied to nasal analysis are the nasofrontal angle, the nasofacial angle, and the nasolabial angle. Collectively these generate information on features that have some bearing on nasal–facial proportion such as tip rotation, tip projection, and nasal length, and they are very useful when evaluating the nasal profile.

The *nasofrontal angle* (Fig. 180.4) is the angle measured between a line extending from the glabella through the nasion and a second line drawn from the nasion through the nasal tip-defining point. The ideal nasofrontal angle ranges from 115 to 135 degrees. The deepest point of the nasofrontal angle is known as the nasion (or radix). Perhaps more important than the actual angle measurement itself, the position (superior vs. inferior) and depth of the nasofrontal angle and nasion have significant bearing

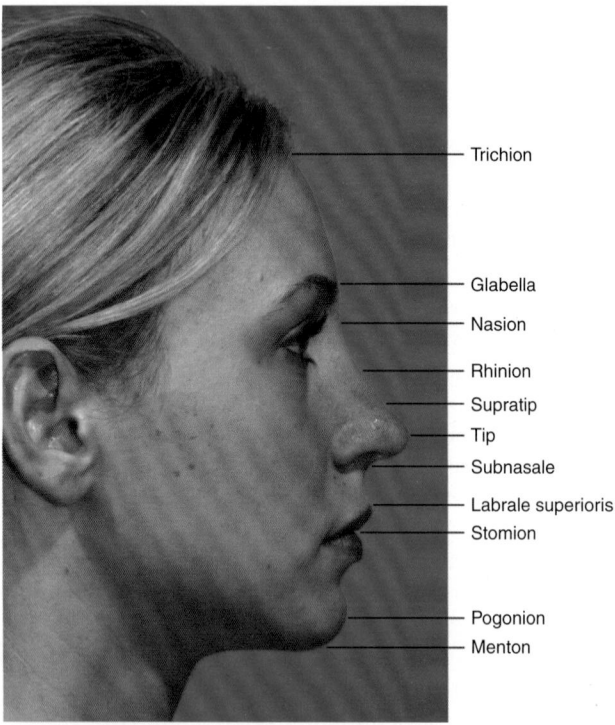

Figure 180.2 Surface anatomy nomenclature—lateral view.

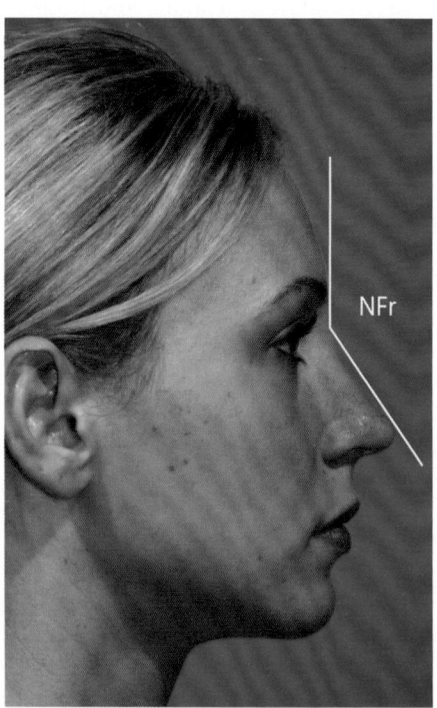

Figure 180.4 Nasofrontal angle—the normal angle measures 115 to 135 degrees.

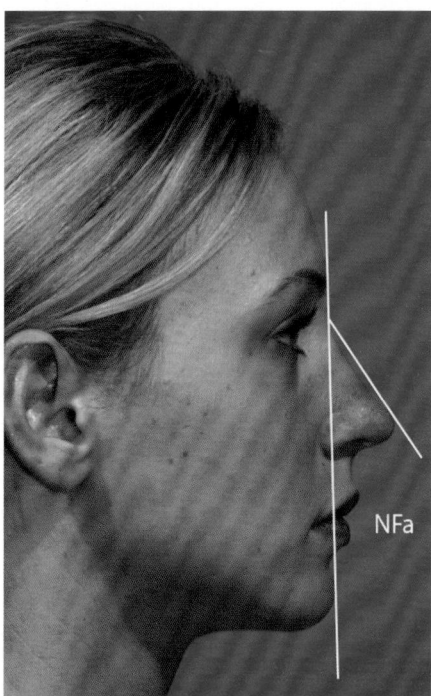

Figure 180.5 Nasofacial angle—the normal angle measures 30 to 40 degrees.

on the overall aesthetics and proportion of the nose as it relates to the rest of the face. This is discussed in greater detail in the section on nasal analysis.

The *nasofacial angle* (Fig. 180.5) is formed by a line from the glabella through the pogonion, intersecting with a line from the nasion through the nasal tip-defining point. The ideal nasofacial angle ranges from 30 to 40 degrees (ideal 36 degrees). A larger (more obtuse) angle reflects a relative increase in tip projection whereas the nasal tip would appear less projected with a more acute nasofacial angle.

The *nasolabial angle* (Fig. 180.6) is the angle formed between the upper lip (from subnasale to labrale superioris) and the plane of the columella through the subnasale. The ideal nasolabial angle ranges from 90 to 115 degrees. Males typically have a more acute nasolabial angle (90 to 105 degrees) consistent with less tip rotation, while the ideal nasolabial angle in females ranges from 100 to 115 degrees in keeping with more tip rotation.

SURGICAL INCISIONS AND APPROACHES

An important distinction is made between surgical *approaches* and *incisions*.

A surgical *approach* refers to the means of exposing the structures of interest. The approach that is chosen will then dictate the *incisions* that are used to enable that approach. The surgical approach chosen for nasal surgery will vary with the training, comfort level, experience, and preference of the operating surgeon as well as the complexity of the case. While there are a variety of surgical approaches and the preferred approach may vary from surgeon to surgeon, as a general rule, the more severe or complicated the nasal deformity in question, the more likely the surgeon is to benefit from broader exposure.

Surgical approaches can be broadly categorized into *external* or *endonasal* approaches. Endonasal approaches can be subdivided into approaches to the nasal dorsum, the nasal septum, or the nasal tip, and endonasal tip approaches can then be further divided into delivery and non-delivery approaches (Fig. 180.7).

Although no absolute indication exists for either an external or endonasal approach and multiple factors will play into the choice of the operating surgeon as noted earlier, a reasonable set of guidelines for each, which may be of benefit to the less experienced surgeon, is outlined in Table 180.1.

Incisions

Surgical incisions are made to facilitate surgical exposure, but the incisions in and of themselves, properly made, have little or no impact on the ultimate dorsal contour, tip shape, or septal position. The surgical incisions most commonly used or referred to in the literature include

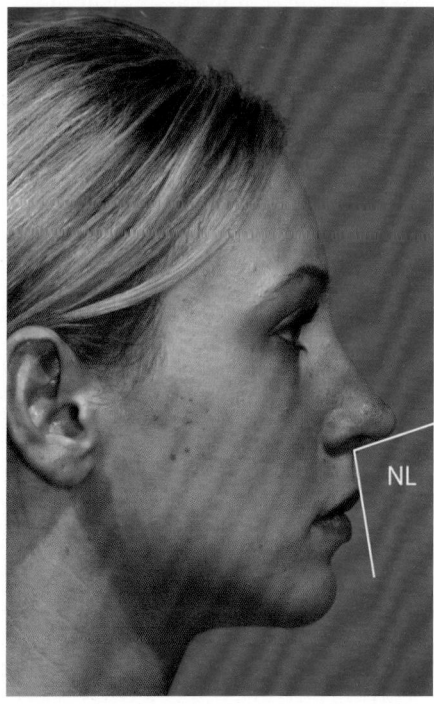

Figure 180.6 Nasolabial angle—the normal angle measures 90 to 115 degrees.

- The *marginal* (aka infracartilaginous) incision (Fig. 180.8)—an incision of variable length made along the caudal margin of the lower lateral cartilage. It may be along the caudal border of the lateral crus only in certain

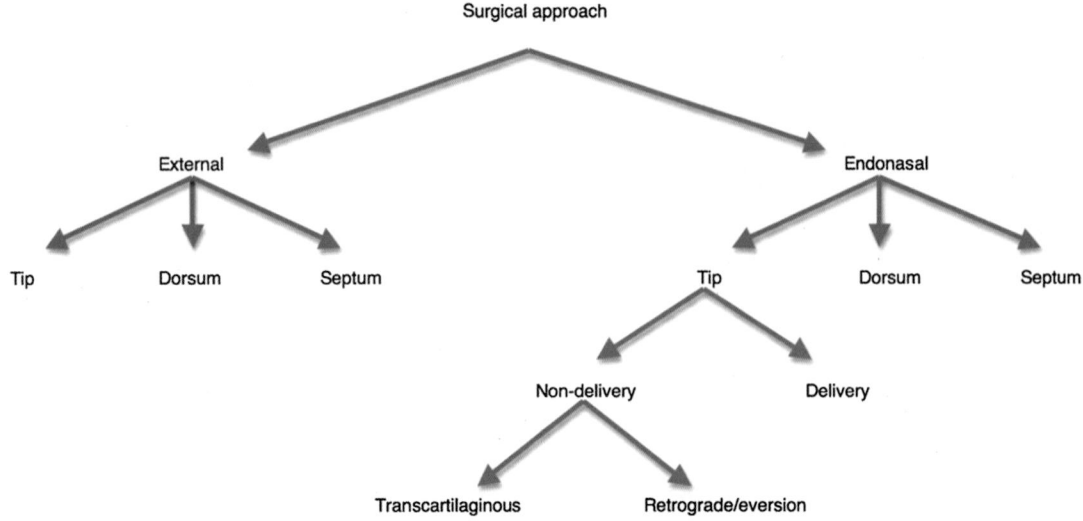

Figure 180.7 Surgical approaches to the nose.

circumstances, the medial crus only, or along the entire caudal edge of the lateral crus.

■ The *transcolumellar* incision (Fig. 180.8)—an incision made transversely across the short axis (width) of the columella, joining bilateral marginal incisions at its lateral end to facilitate the external approach to the nose. It is typically sited over the medial crura about midway back along the columella and is generally irregularized (nonlinear) in some fashion for better camouflage and less scar contracture.

■ The *intercartilaginous* incision (Fig. 180.8)—an incision made at the junction of the caudal border of the upper lateral cartilage and the cephalic border of the lower lateral cartilage (hence "inter"-cartilaginous). Alone it can provide access to the upper two-thirds of the nasal vault (bony and cartilaginous dorsum, nasal sidewall) as well as retrograde access to the lateral crura of the lower lateral cartilages. When combined with marginal incisions, it allows the surgeon to release and "deliver" the lower lateral cartilage as a bipedicled chondrocutaneous flap,

pivoting inferiorly in a bucket-handle fashion to enable tip contouring in endonasal rhinoplasty using a delivery approach.

■ The *rim* incision—an incision placed just within the nasal vestibule along the rim of the nostril margin. Owing to its proximity to the rim of the nares, any untoward healing or scar contracture with this incision carries a higher risk of visibility, retraction, notching, or irregularity along the alar margin as compared to a marginal incision, and as such, it has fallen out of favor and is less frequently used.

■ The *transcartilaginous* (or cartilage-splitting) incision (Fig. 180.8)—an incision made through the lateral crus of the lower lateral cartilage caudal to the junction of the upper and lower lateral cartilage and at least 5 to 6 mm above the caudal margin of the lateral crus of the lower lateral cartilage. Effectively this divides the lateral crus into a superior (cephalic) and inferior (caudal) segment enabling removal of the cephalic strip for volume reduction of the tip cartilage.

TABLE 180.1	GUIDELINES FOR SELECTION OF SURGICAL APPROACH

Endonasal Rhinoplasty	External Approach Rhinoplasty
• Dorsal reduction — Modest reduction, nasal bones of normal length (*not* short nasal bones with long upper lateral cartilages) — Normal width and alignment of middle third of nasal vault • Tip surgery — Primary (non-revision) surgery — To modify tip definition (boxy, wide, bifid, broad/bulbous tip) — No gross asymmetry — Modest increase/decrease in tip projection — Limited tip revision surgery • Linear deviation of nasal dorsum in need of osteotomies	• Congenital nasal deformities, for example, cleft lip rhinoplasty • Major dorsal reduction or dorsal reduction with narrow/pinched middle third of nasal vault • Major change in tip projection • Marked nasal septal deformities • Twisted nose • Need for sutured-in-place structural grafting (middle nasal vault or lower third) • Very thick skin • Large septal perforation for repair • Major secondary (revision) surgery

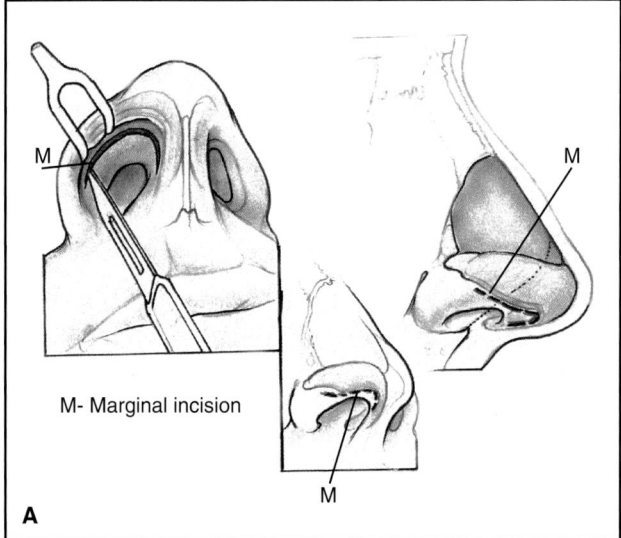

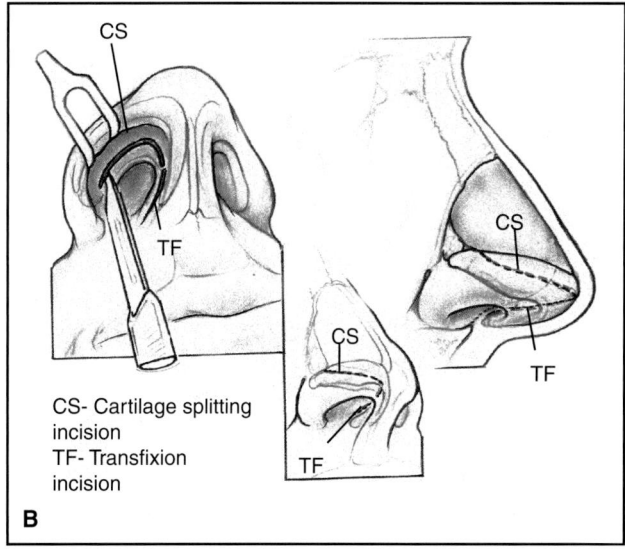

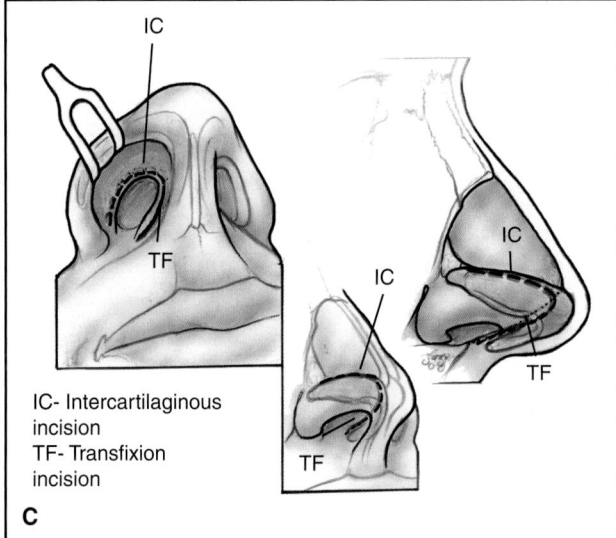

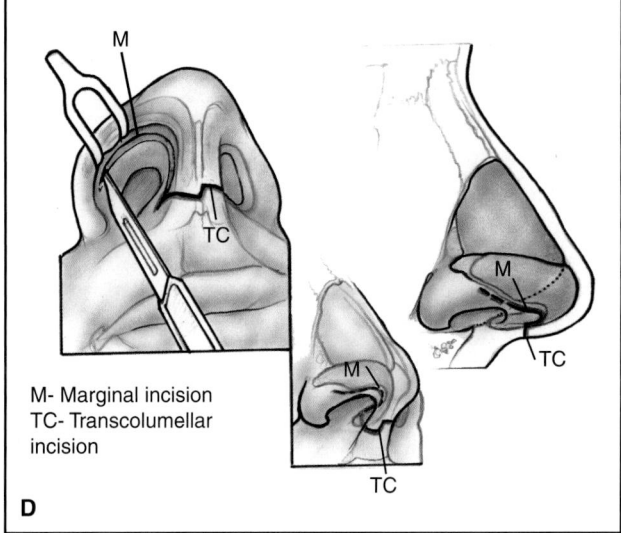

Figure 180.8 Nasal-tip incisions. **A:** Marginal incision. **B:** Cartilage splitting (trans-cartilaginous) incision and transfixion incision. **C:** Inter-cartilaginous and transfixion incision. **D:** Transcolumellar and marginal incisions.

- The *hemitransfixion* incision (Fig. 180.9)—an incision made unilaterally in the membranous septum at or just below the caudal edge of the septum. This allows access to one or both sides of the nasal septum and when combined with either an intercartilaginous or transcartilaginous incision dissection can facilitate exposure of the nasal dorsum right up to the nasion.

- The *full transfixion* incision—an incision completely across the membranous septum from one side of the nasal vestibule to the other, just below the caudal edge of the septum. This incision separates the attachment of the medial crural feet from the caudal septum. Like the hemitransfixion incision, the complete transfixion incision enables access to either side of the septum, the anterior nasal spine, and the depressor septi muscle. It may be made alone or as a continuation of either an

intercartilaginous incision (to facilitate alar delivery in combination with bilateral marginal incisions or for dissection along the nasal dorsum) or a transcartilaginous incision (to facilitate dissection along the nasal dorsum).

- The *Killian* incision (Fig. 180.9)—this incision is made through septal mucoperichondrium parallel and approximately 4 to 5 mm cephalic to the location of a hemitransfixion incision, further up in the nose proximal to the mucocutaneous junction. It is primarily a septal access incision. By virtue of its location, this incision preserves the mucosal attachment and blood supply to the most caudal aspect of the nasal septum. For septal deflections requiring modification of the caudal septum, either a hemitransfixion incision or external approach to the septum (depending on the severity of the problem) is preferred over the Killian incision.

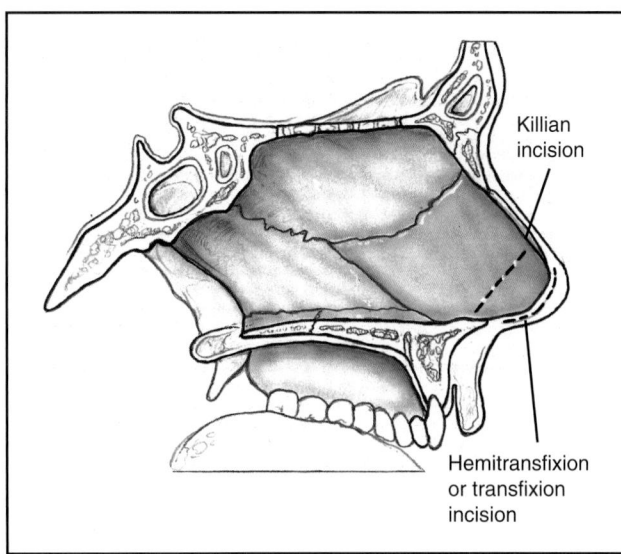

Figure 180.9 Nasal septal access incisions.

Approaches

As regards surgical approaches to the nose, the *external approach* combines bilateral marginal incisions with a transcolumellar incision as noted earlier. Dissection and elevation of the skin and soft tissue envelope can then continue in a cephalad direction right up to the nasion if need be. The primary advantage of the external approach is unparalleled exposure and the unlimited ability to modify the cartilages as need be. Optimal visualization can be particularly beneficial in circumstances where the underlying anatomy is unclear such as revision surgery or patients with gross asymmetry and provides a definite advantage when sutured-in-place cartilage grafting is desired.

Potential disadvantages of the external approach include the extent of dissection and therefore surgical trauma in situations where more limited dissection might suffice. Wider undermining with the external approach generally translates into more postoperative edema that persists longer than in the typical endonasal rhinoplasty. In circumstances where one can comfortably achieve the same or similar result through a less invasive approach, the attendant reduction in tissue trauma is desirable. Routine disruption of native cartilaginous attachments to skin may not always be necessary. Greater ligamentous disruption and skin undermining may in fact result in a greater loss of tip projection when compared to similarly applied techniques using an endonasal approach (6), thereby necessitating maneuvers to restore or reestablish tip projection. Finally, it must be said that greater exposure alone does not equate with better surgical results—failure to apply thoughtful, assiduous analysis and meticulous surgical technique will not be overcome merely by enhancing exposure.

There are a number of endonasal approaches to the nose. A *retrograde approach* utilizes an intercartilaginous incision for retrograde access to the lateral crura of the lower lateral cartilages, thereby enabling a conservative volume reduction of the cephalic portion of the lateral crus. The *transcartilaginous approach* uses a cartilage-splitting incision for removal of a predetermined amount of the cephalic portion of the lateral crus (that portion superior to where the incision is made). Like the retrograde approach, the transcartilaginous procedure has limited application, being primarily used for very moderate volume reduction of a tip which is otherwise well structured. The disadvantages of both of these two approaches are the limited ability to otherwise modify the cartilage beyond a cephalic trim, limited access to the domal area of the lower lateral cartilages, and therefore the inherent difficulty of insuring symmetry between the two sides.

The *delivery approach* is the most versatile of the endonasal approaches to the nasal tip. By using a marginal incision and an intercartilaginous incision connected to a full transfixion incision, surgical dissection will release the superior and inferior attachments of the lower lateral cartilage while maintaining attachments medially and laterally. It can thus be pivoted caudally, in a bucket-handle fashion so as to "deliver" a bipedicled chondrocutaneous flap. Broader exposure and more direct visualization of the lower lateral cartilages permits a greater range of surgical modifications to be applied than with either the retrograde or cartilage-splitting endonasal approaches. The main disadvantage with the delivery technique as compared to an external approach is the disruption or distortion of native *in situ* relationships between the lower lateral cartilages when delivered and greater technical difficulty with certain cartilage grafting techniques.

NASAL ANALYSIS

It is impossible to overstate the value of assiduous and systematic nasal analysis. Rhinoplasty surgeons may differ in terms of their own aesthetic ideal, their preferred surgical approach, instrumentation, dressings, postoperative care—in short, they may differ in almost every surgical sense. Except the value that they place on thoughtful preoperative analysis. On that they would all agree—careful and thorough preoperative analysis will promote better and more consistent outcomes, reduce revision rates, and minimize the traps that await oversight and errors of omission. Nasal surgery is not a good place for 20-20 hindsight.

Uniform and reproducible photographs are a fundamental part of the evaluation process and surgical planning, in addition to being an accurate reminder of the preoperative state. Images of consistent size, quality, lighting and positioning will facilitate an honest and accurate appraisal of postoperative changes as compared to the preoperative views. A more detailed discussion of the technical aspects of photo documentation is covered in Chapter 171 of this text.

The standard views for rhinoplasty are vertically oriented full face frontal, right and left oblique, right and left lateral views, and a base view (horizontally or vertically oriented).

Optional views include the frontal close-up (to highlight particular asymmetries or a crooked nose), a "bird's eye" or dorsal view (for a crooked nose), and a lateral smiling view (to highlight the activity of the depressor septi muscle). A lateral view with a ruler alongside the patient's face can be helpful to enable one to make life-size reproductions, which then allow for accurate preoperative measurements to be made.

All parts of the physical examination, inspection, and palpation should impart meaningful information to the examiner at each and every step. For the skilled clinician, an impressive amount of information relevant to treatment (medical or surgical) can be gleaned in only a few minutes.

Evaluation of the rhinoplasty patient begins with an overall survey of facial proportion and symmetry. Naturally there will be some variation in anthropometric norms from one race to another as alluded to earlier. The typical occidental Caucasian face can be roughly divided into equal horizontal thirds (Fig. 180.10)—from the hairline (trichion) to the glabella, from the glabella to the subnasale, and from the subnasale to the menton (chin). As there is great variability in hairline position, another way of looking at nasal and facial proportion considers the distance from the nasion to the menton (Fig. 180.11). Using this method, a nose which is in relatively good proportion to the face as measured from nasion to subnasale, is 43% of the nasion–menton distance,

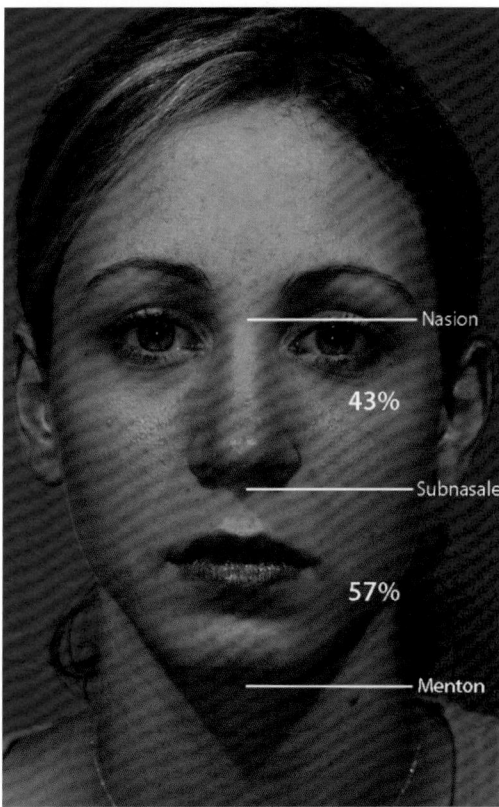

Figure 180.11 Facial proportion—lower facial two-thirds—the distance from nasion–subnasale is 43% of total nasion–menton distance, whereas the subnasale–menton distance is 57% of the total.

whereas the measurement from subnasale to menton is 57% of the total distance. The nasion-to-subnasale measurement is therefore three-fourths of the subnasale-to-menton distance. The face may also be divided into vertical fifths (Fig. 180.12), each of which equals the intercanthal distance (between medial canthi) or the width of the palpebral fissure (from medial to lateral canthus).

After an overall survey of facial proportion and symmetry is complete, inspection of the nose is carried out next from a frontal, lateral, and a base view, at rest and with normal inspiration. Any tendency of the lateral nasal wall or nasal ala to medialize or collapse on mild to moderate inspiration should be noted. Dynamic collapse of the nasal sidewall suggests instability or lack of proper structural support in that region, which should be addressed at the time of surgery.

Proper endonasal inspection of the nasal airway with a headlight and speculum further complements the information acquired from visual assessment of inspiratory stability. Ideally an endoscopic exam completes a physical examination of the nasal airway. At this point, the examiner should have a good sense of septal alignment, turbinate size, and width of the nasal valve angle (normal = 10 to 15 degrees).

Palpation of the nose follows. This gives the surgeon an indication of the thickness of the nasal skin, the presence of any palpable ridges or irregularities, the length of the

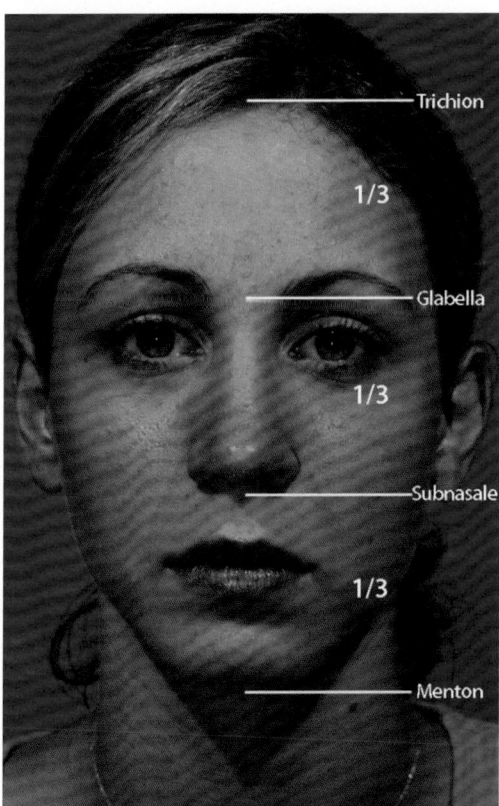

Figure 180.10 Facial proportion—the face can be roughly divided into equal horizontal thirds, from trichion (hairline) to glabella, glabella to subnasale, and subnasale to menton.

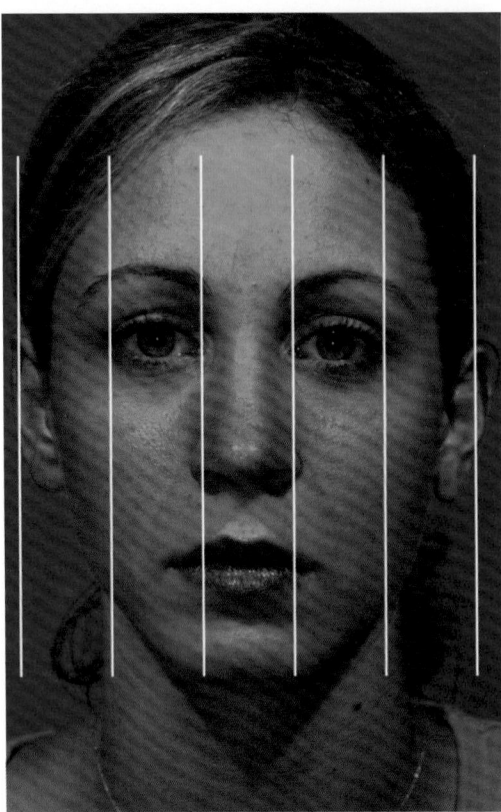

Figure 180.12 Facial proportion—the face can be divided into vertical fifths, each approximately equal to the intercanthal distance or the width of the palpebral fissure.

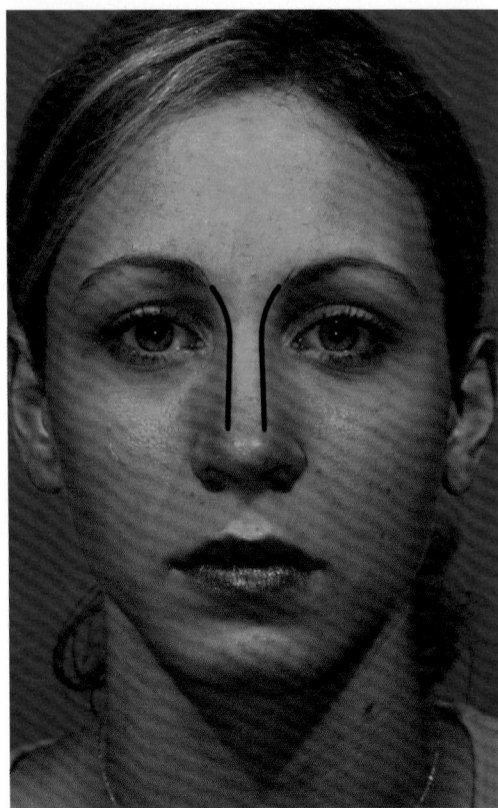

Figure 180.13 The brow–tip aesthetic lines outline the nasal dorsum.

nasal bones relative to the upper lateral cartilages along the nasal dorsum, and some sense of the intrinsic strength of the alar cartilages, tip support, and caudal septum.

Assessment is then carried out by examining the nose from a frontal view, oblique and lateral views, and base view.

On the *frontal* view the examiner should evaluate

- Overall symmetry. Asymmetries should be pointed out to the patient preoperatively.
- Alignment (straight or crooked) and where if any misalignment exists (upper one-third, middle one-third, and/or lower one-third). Problems with alignment might suggest the need for osteotomies, rasping, onlay grafts, spreader grafts, or nasal tip surgery depending on where the asymmetry is centered. This is further discussed in the chapters on tip surgery and the management of the crooked nose. Narrowing of the middle nasal vault in particular is important to recognize since medialization of the upper lateral cartilage in this region will increase airflow resistance through the internal nasal valve and may account for a functional problem that would merit spreader grafting.
- Tip definition and visible highlights or irregularities
- Width of the bony nasal pyramid (upper one-third of the nose) as well as that of the nasal base. The alar base width should fall within lines dropped from each medial canthus. The bony width should be about 75% to 80% of alar base width.

- The brow–tip aesthetic lines (Fig. 180.13)—paired, smooth, gently curving lines, which follow the curvature of the brow, continuing caudally down the lateral nasal dorsum (at the junction of the dorsum and nasal sidewall) to the tip-defining points. Deviations along this line may be seen in patients with prior trauma and crooked or twisted noses as well as in those with pinching or narrowing in the middle third of the nose where the upper lateral cartilages fuse with the dorsal septum (the internal nasal valve region).

On the *oblique* view, one should evaluate

- The brow–tip aesthetic line. The left oblique view highlights the right brow–tip line and vice versa. Often irregularities along this line are well appreciated on the oblique view.
- The height of the nasal dorsum
- Soft tissue facets

A substantial amount of information is revealed from examination of the nose in *lateral* view. Owing to the volume and complexity of what is seen from this view of the nose, it is helpful and therefore recommended to proceed in a methodical and reproducible fashion each and every time. In that respect, the author recommends first taking a broader view of the nose and how it relates to overall facial proportion and then proceeding sequentially from nasion to subnasale. In this way, one can avoid overlooking features of interest or import. Specifically, on the *lateral* view beginning at the root of the nose and moving caudally, one should evaluate

■ Radix position, radix projection, and nasofrontal angle. The ideal radix position or visual radix breakpoint should lie around the level of the supratarsal crease or between the crease and the upper eyelid margin. This will influence the height of the nose from nasion to subnasale, which should roughly equal 43% of the distance from nasion to menton. If the nasion or visual takeoff of the nose is low (a caudally positioned radix—often referred to as "low radix disproportion"), the nose will look shorter, the tip will appear to be relatively overprojected (a "bottom-heavy nose"), and the dorsal height will be somewhat exaggerated (Fig. 180.14), whereas the opposite is true when the radix is cephalically malpositioned ("high radix disproportion"). Regarding radix projection, Byrd calculates the normal radix projection to be 0.28 × ideal tip projection (see calculation under tip projection), which generally corresponds to 9 to 14 mm from the anterior corneal plane (7). An underprojected radix (deep radix) will exaggerate any apparent dorsal height and may create the illusion of a "pseudohump" when dorsal height might be appropriate (8). In addition, a deep radix, much like a low radix, will make the nose look shorter and the tip look relatively overprojected while an overprojected (shallow) radix will make the nose look longer and the tip less projected. A deep or low nasofrontal angle (deep or low radix) might warrant the need for radix grafting to bring the radix forward or higher and to improve upon relative proportions of the nose.

■ The length of the nose, from radix to the most anterior projecting point on the tip. Byrd's dimensional analysis (7) derives ideal nasal length from measurements taken from either the midface or lower face. Midfacial height (MFH) is the measured distance from the glabella to the alar base plane (a transverse line through the alar base, perpendicular to the vertical axis of the face). Using his method, ideal nasal length is two-thirds of MFH (using midfacial measurements), or equal to the distance from the stomion to the menton (using lower facial measurements). When the mandible is underdeveloped (e.g., microgenia), the midfacial guideline is preferred.

■ The height of the nasal dorsum and whether it be in need of reduction, augmentation, or neither. Height of the nasal dorsum, or lack thereof, is clearly considered relative to the radix depth and nasal-tip projection. With appropriate radix position and depth, if one were to draw a line from the nasion to the tip-defining point, the height of the dorsum would either be level with that line (male) or 1 to 2 mm below that line (female) conferring a slight supratip break so that the leading point of the nose is the tip and not the dorsum.

■ The presence or absence of a supratip break (seen when the tip projects just slightly anterior to the dorsal line in the lateral view)

■ Nasal tip projection. There are several methods to assess tip projection. Byrd calculates that ideal tip projection, measuring from the alar cheek junction to the anteriormost point on the tip, is two-thirds of ideal nasal length (as calculated above) (7). Crumley describes the nose as a right angle triangle with a 3:4:5 ratio, whereby nasal-tip projection is 60% (three-fifths) of nasal length from nasion to tip-defining point (9) (Fig. 180.15). Goode draws a vertical line from the nasion through the

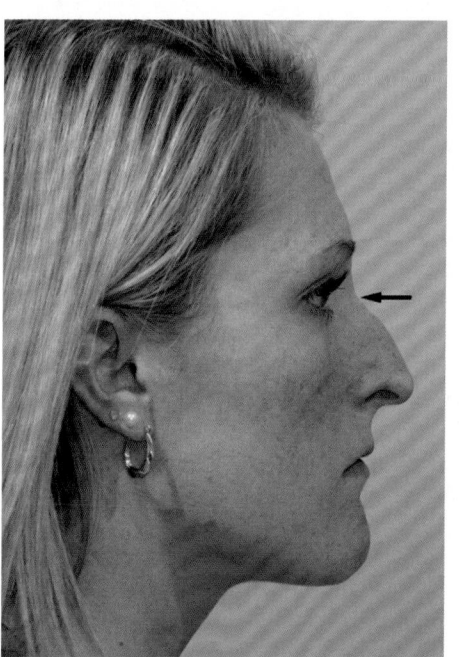
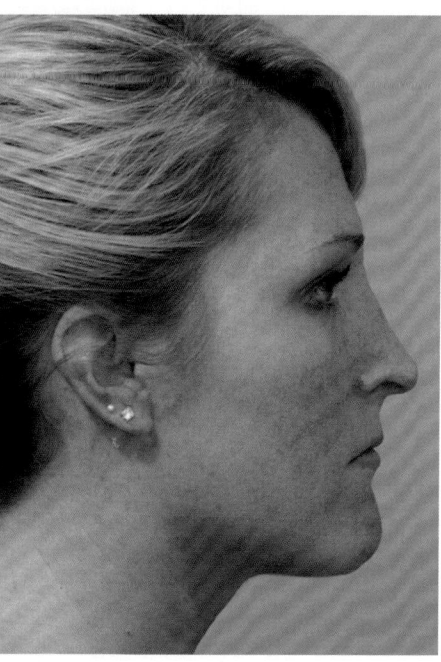

Figure 180.14 Low radix disproportion—a deep or caudally positioned radix (*arrow*) as seen preoperatively on left will make the nose appear shorter, the tip appear relatively overprojected, and the dorsal height appear exaggerated. Postoperatively on right, after radix augmentation with only conservative dorsal reduction, the radix takeoff has been moved cephalically and the nose looks better balanced and proportionate.

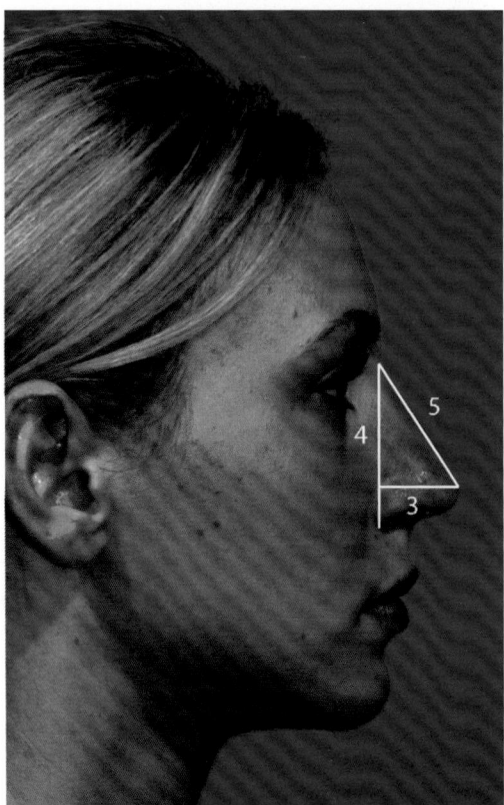

Figure 180.15 Crumley's 3:4:5 right angle triangle estimates appropriate tip projection to equal three-fifths (60%) of nasion-to-tip distance. Goode's calculations yield similar proportions.

alar cheek junction and a second line perpendicular to the first running from the alar facial junction to the nasal tip. Using his technique, this second line, which reflects tip projection, is 0.55 to 0.60 × nasion-to-tip distance (nasal length) (10). These lines essentially recreate the same 3:4:5 right angle triangle described by Crumley.

- The columellar double break—a slight change in plane along the nasal base at the transition point from the columella to the infratip lobule at the anterior nares
- The alar–columellar relationship. Normal columellar show as measured on lateral view from the highest point on the curved alar rim to the lower edge of the columella is 2 to 4 mm. Values in excess of that may be due to an overly long caudal septum, bowing of the medial crura or alar retraction. Measurements below 2 mm can be due to a retruded columella, foreshortened caudal septum or alar hooding (11).
- Tip rotation or the nasolabial angle. The ideal range is approximately 90 to 115 degrees, with men being generally more acute and women being more obtuse.
- Chin position. In men, the most anterior point of the chin (the pogonion) should lie at or just anterior to a vertical line dropped from the vermilion border of the lower lip, whereas in women the pogonion should be at or just behind that line. With obvious microgenia, a discussion of chin augmentation or advancement genioplasty is warranted to optimize overall facial balance.

On the *base* view, the examiner should evaluate

- Symmetry. Are there visible irregularities of the tip cartilages? Are the nostrils symmetric?
- Shape of the nasal base. Is it nicely triangular (isosceles) or boxy, broad, amorphous, trapezoidal, etc.?
- Bifidity (separation) of the alar domes
- Contour of the alar sidewall. Is the alar sidewall straight or slightly convex and stable, or is there any buckling/concavity of the lateral crura or alar collapse, either at rest or with inspiration (suggestive of external nasal valve compromise)?
- The position of the caudal septum
- The columella-to-lobule ratio. Ideally 2:1
- Width of the alar base

CONCLUSION

Fluency with the nomenclature, understanding the utility of the various nasal incisions and merit of different surgical approaches and having a consistent framework to apply to nasal analysis are the essential starting points for the rhinoplasty surgeon, and this chapter is intended to serve as a useful resource in that regard.

It has been said that diagnosis precedes technique. As one of the most challenging, humbling and variable procedures in facial plastic surgery, successful rhinoplasty is heavily predicated upon accurate preoperative assessment and diagnosis. It is thus incumbent upon the rhinoplasty surgeon to develop a dependable, thorough and reproducible approach to nasal analysis. In this way, more consistently successful results and greater levels of patient and surgeon satisfaction are assured.

HIGHLIGHTS

- Thoughtful, systematic and precise preoperative nasal analysis is the foundation of a well-planned and well-executed rhinoplasty.
- Fluency with proper terminology and nomenclature enables better record keeping and clearer communication between colleagues.
- Racial and anthropometric "norms" account for differences in "ideal" facial and nasal proportions and characteristics.
- Surgical approaches to the nose should be chosen based on experience, the surgical plan and complexity of the case. The goal is always maximal results with minimal surgical intervention. Once chosen, the surgical approach guides the selection of incisions.
- Each preoperative photograph conveys specific information—knowing what to look for and how to study each image is a vital skill to acquire for anyone performing rhinoplasty surgery.

REFERENCES

1. Porter JP, Olson, KL. Anthropometric facial analysis of the African American woman. *Arch Facial Plast Surg* 2001;3:191–197.
2. Sim RST, Smith JD, Chan ASY. Comparison of the aesthetic facial proportions of southern Chinese and white women. *Arch Facial Plast Surg* 2000;2:113–120.
3. Milgrim LM, Lawson W, Cohen AF. Anthropometric analysis of the female Latino nose: revised aesthetic concepts and their surgical implications. *Arch Otolaryngol Head Neck Surg* 1996;122:1079–1086.
4. Reksodiputro MH, Koento MD, Boedhihartono, et al. Facial anthropometric analysis of the Javanese female. *Arch Facial Plast Surg* 2009;11(5):347–349.
5. Adamson PA, Zavod MB. Changing perceptions of beauty: a surgeon's perspective. *Facial Plast Surg* 2006;22(3):188–193.
6. Adams WP, Rohrich RJ, Hollier LH, et al. Anatomical basis and clinical implications for nasal tip support in open vs. closed rhinoplasty. *Plast Reconstr Surg* 1999;103(1):255–261.
7. Byrd HS, Hobar PC. Rhinoplasty: a practical guide for surgical planning. *Plast Reconstr Surg* 1993;91:642–656.
8. Steiger JD, Baker SR. Nuances of profile management: the radix. *Facial Plast Surg Clin N Am* 2009;17(1):15–28.
9. Crumley RL, Lanser M. Quantitative analysis of nasal tip projection. *Laryngoscope* 1998;98:202–208.
10. Powell N, Humphreys B. *Proportions of the aesthetic face*. New York: Thieme-Stratton, 1984:23.
11. Gunter JP, Rohrich RJ, Friedman RM. Classification and correction of alar-columellar discrepancies in rhinoplasty. *Plast Reconstr Surg* 1996;97:643–648.

181 The Nasal Dorsum: Management of the Upper Two-Thirds of the Nose

Randolph B. Capone   *Ira D. Papel*

Of all the aesthetic facial units, the nose plays a predominant role in facial proportion and harmony. As a single unpaired structure occupying the midface, it serves to balance the facial thirds and fifths as well as those aesthetic units surrounding it. Seemingly small changes after rhinoplasty or traumatic injury frequently effect dramatic changes in nasal appearance. The nose is not, however, only an aesthetic structure but also a respiratory and olfactory organ. This duality of nasal form and function mandates that rhinoplasty must enhance nasal appearance and optimize the nasal airway. It is essential, therefore, that the nasal surgeon have a detailed understanding of nasal anatomy and physiology and a thorough grasp of the many interventions available in rhinoplasty. In this chapter, we discuss these issues with regard to management of the upper two-thirds of the nose, that is, the bony and cartilaginous vaults.

ANATOMY

The upper two-thirds of the nose contains the dorsum and sidewall aesthetic subunits, whereas the tip, columella, soft tissue triangles, and alae constitute the lower third of the nose (Fig. 181.1) (1). Topographically, the upper two-thirds of the nose is that portion from the *nasion* to the level of the alar groove (Fig. 181.2), where the nasion is defined as the intersection of the internasal suture with the nasofrontal suture in the midsagittal plane. The *radix* is the root of the nose and defines the most posterior point along the curve from the glabella to the nasal dorsum.

Skin and Subcutaneous Tissue

The skin overlying the upper nasal two-thirds has variable thickness. Relatively thick at the nasion (2 to 5 mm), it becomes thin and mobile over the dorsum (3.2 mm) and thinnest at the rhinion (2 to 2.2 mm) and gradually thickens

again, becoming sebaceous toward the tip (5 mm) (2). This variability is important in planning the dorsal profile because creation of a straight skeletal profile will not likely create a straight postoperative profile. When edema diminishes, the surgeon may find that the rhinion has been over-resected if no allowance for skin thickness was considered during surgery.

Beneath the skin is a thin fibrous layer designated the nasal superficial musculoaponeurotic system (SMAS) (3). Analogous to the facial SMAS, the nasal SMAS encompasses the nasal musculature and is located immediately superficial to the periosteum and perichondrium. Dissection just below the nasal SMAS provides a less traumatic and easier dissection plane during rhinoplasty, with preservation of nasal vasculature, nerves, and lymphatics that lie within the skin–soft tissue envelope (4).

Nasal Bones and Upper Lateral Cartilages

Deep to the nasal SMAS are the paired nasal bones and upper lateral cartilages. The nasal bones fuse with the frontal bone approximately 11 mm superior to the intercanthal line and are on average 2.5 cm in length (5). The length can be quite variable and represents a significant risk factor for airway compromise after rhinoplasty, for the shorter the nasal bones, the greater the proportion of cartilaginous nasal anatomy that is cantilevered and supported (6). The caudal margin of the nasal bones overlaps the cephalic margin of the upper lateral cartilages, which in turn interlock with the paired lower lateral cartilages at the *scroll* (Fig. 181.3). Each of these connections is an important structural component that contributes to nasal integrity and support.

Laterally, the caudal margin of the nasal bones and the anterior margin of the ascending processes of the maxilla form the *piriform aperture*. The lateral margin of the upper lateral cartilages fuses with dense connective tissue, and the

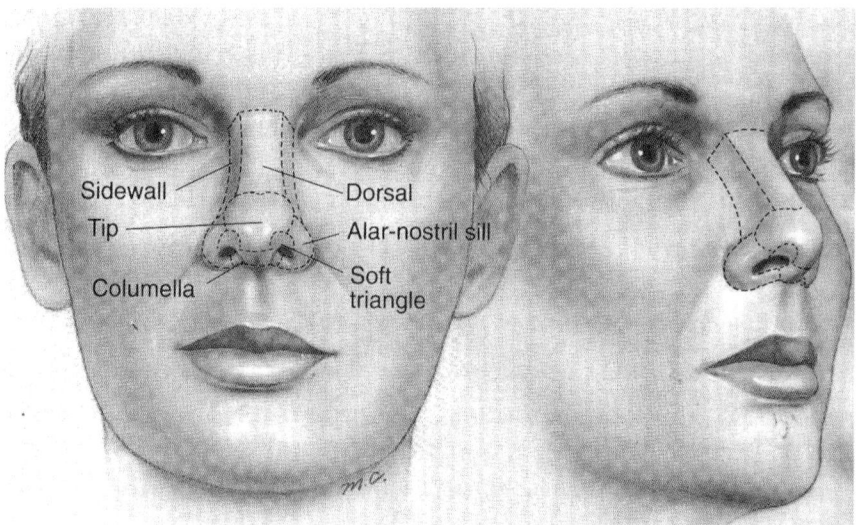

Figure 181.1 Nasal aesthetic subunits. (From Burget GC, Menick FJ. *Aesthetic reconstruction of the nose.* St. Louis, MO: Mosby, 1994:7, with permission.)

medial margin fuses with the septum superiorly but separates and is mobile inferiorly. Mucosa is tightly adherent to the internal surface of the cartilages and is continuous with the lining of the septum and lateral nasal wall.

The caudal margin of the upper lateral cartilage, the anterior head of the inferior turbinate, the proximate septum, and floor of the nose define the borders of the *internal nasal valve*. The angle between the upper lateral cartilages and the septum is the *nasal valve angle*, normally 10 to 20 degrees. The internal nasal valve typically has a cross-sectional area of 55 to 83 mm^2 and represents the site of greatest nasal resistance. It is the primary airflow-limiting segment of the nasal cavity in the human nose (7).

The Bony and Cartilaginous Vaults

The upper nasal two-thirds can be thought of as two contiguous arches, or vaults—a superior *bony vault* and an inferior *cartilaginous vault*. The nasal bones and the paired ascending processes of the maxilla comprise the bony vault, and the cartilaginous vault is composed of the upper lateral cartilages and the cartilaginous dorsal septum. The region of transition of the bony vault to the cartilaginous vault is known as the *rhinion*. The soft tissue linkage that occurs at the rhinion is comprised of upper lateral cartilage perichondrium that inserts on the undersurface of the paired nasal bones. This union allows for motion of the inferior vault relative to the superior vault.

As the name implies, nasal vaults are critical for support, distribution of forces, maintenance of dorsal height, and maintenance of nasal projection. As with any arch, the most essential support element occurs at the keystone. The nasal *keystone area* is the convergence of the caudal margin of the nasal bones, the perpendicular plate of the ethmoid bone, the cephalic margin of the upper lateral cartilages, and the cartilaginous septum. Understanding this area is critical during planning and execution of osteotomies so as to effect a change without disruption of important support mechanisms.

NASAL ANALYSIS

The face is a complex set of surfaces with tremendous variability. The goal of facial analysis is to provide a consistent framework to compare pre- and postoperative results despite this variability. Nowhere is this more important

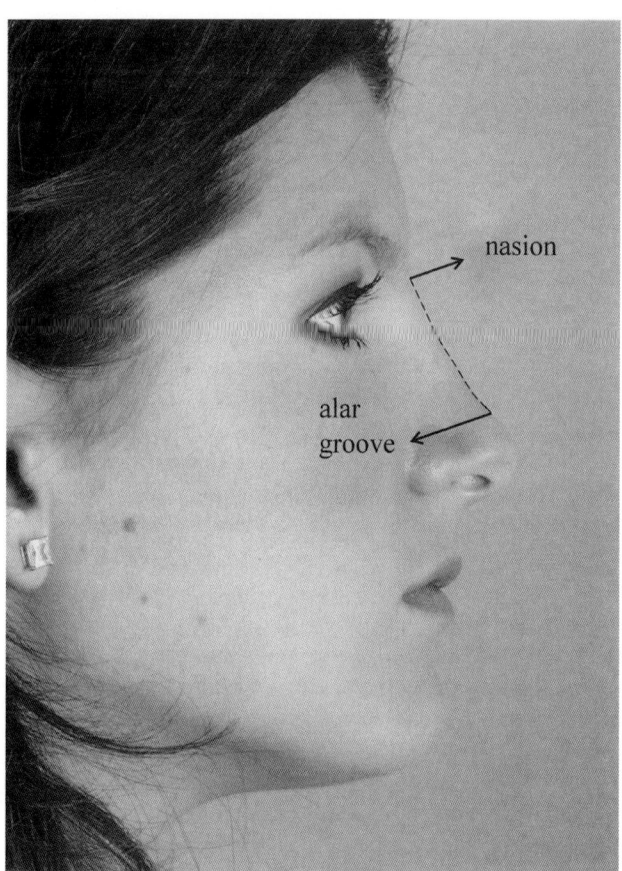

Figure 181.2 Upper nasal two-thirds: nasion to alar dorse.

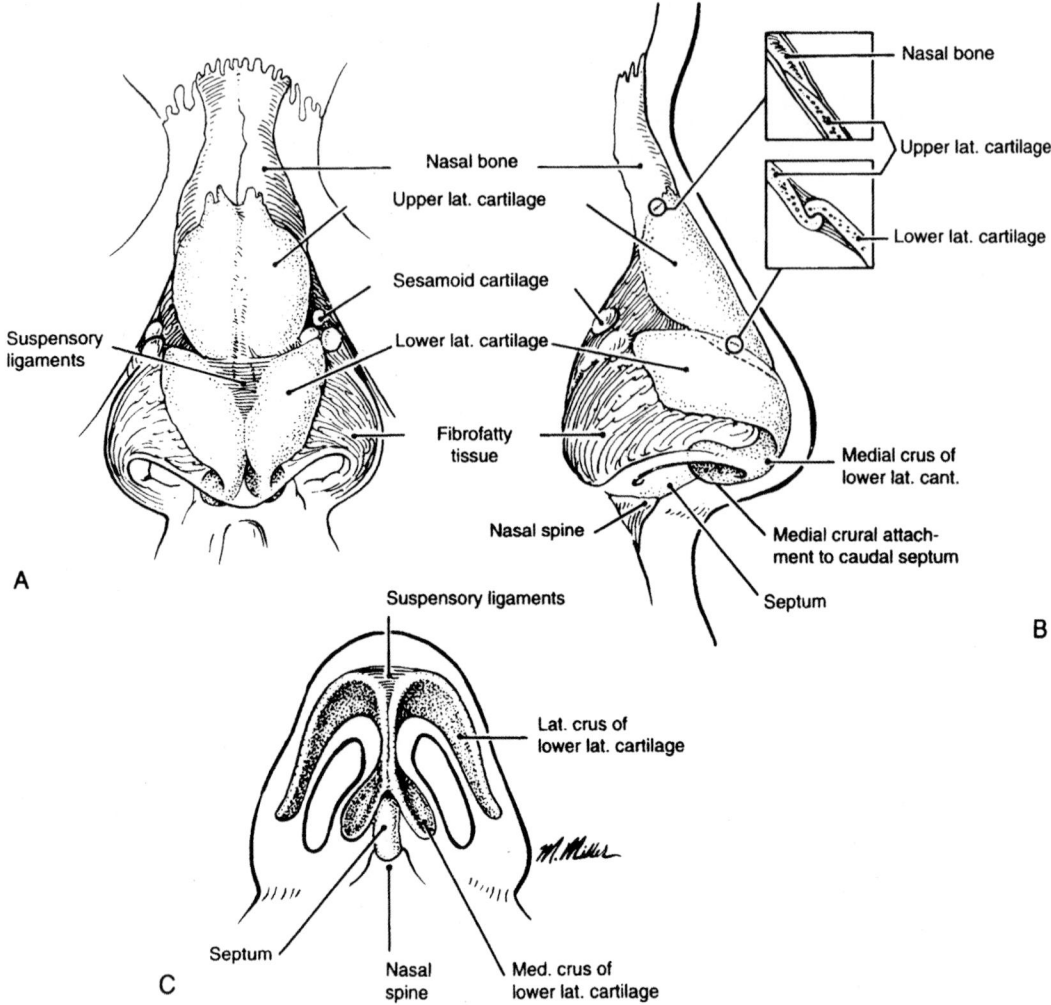

Figure 181.3 Anatomic relationships of the nasal bones, upper lateral cartilages, and lower lateral cartilages. (Modified from Papel ID. Management of the middle vault. In: Papel ID, ed. *Facial plastic and reconstructive surgery*, 2nd ed. Stuttgart, Germany: Thieme, 2002:408, with permission.)

than in rhinoplasty. Every rhinoplasty candidate should have high-quality six-view photography to facilitate analysis. In addition, an additional chin-down view is especially useful in evaluation of patients with nasal vault deformity (Fig. 181.4).

Aesthetic Angles

Analysis of the nasal aesthetic angles reveals the importance of the dorsum in evaluation of the rhinoplasty patient. Of the five facial aesthetic angles, three are determined using the geometry of the nasal dorsum: the nasofacial, the nasofrontal, and the nasomental angles. The *nasofacial angle* is the angle prescribed by the intersection of the facial plane (glabella to pogonion) and a line tangent to the nasal dorsum. Ideally, it is 36 to 40 degrees. The *nasofrontal angle* is determined by the intersection of the line connecting the nasion and glabella and the nasal dorsum tangent, ideally 115 to 130 degrees. Lastly, the *nasomental angle* is

determined by the intersection of the line connecting the tip-defining point to the pogonion and the nasal dorsum tangent. The ideal nasomental angle is 120 to 132 degrees. Each of these angles should be carefully considered during the examination and photographic evaluation of the rhinoplasty candidate.

Nasal Length

Leonardo da Vinci introduced the practice of dividing the face into equal vertical thirds and horizontal fifths for the purpose of facial analysis. Later modified by Powell and Humphreys (8), this serves as the basis for modern-day facial analysis. A method more specific to nasal analysis, however, divides the lower face into two parts using the nasion, subnasale, and menton as landmarks (9). Using this method, nasal length (nasion to subnasale) should be three-fourths the distance from the subnasale to the menton (Fig. 181.5).

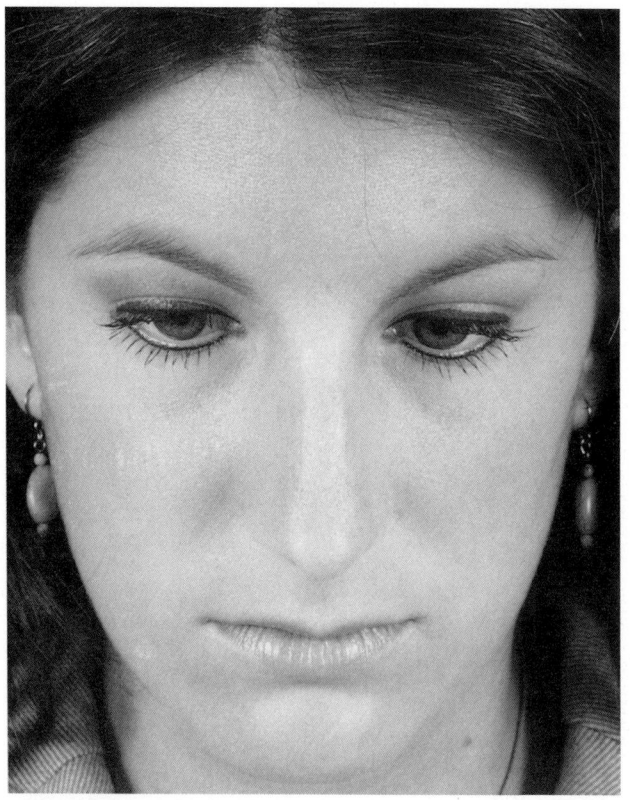

Figure 181.4 The chin-down view of nasal dorsum is useful to detect the presence of subtle radix contour irregularities or asymmetry.

Nasal Width and Radix Contours

On frontal view, nasal width should increase along its length, with a minima occurring at the intercanthal line. Maximal nasal width occurs at the alae and should equal one-fifth the width of the face. The upper nasal contour should follow a gentle curve from the medial eyebrow to the ipsilateral tip-defining point. Any irregularities in this *brow–tip aesthetic line* will quickly be noted as different from the contralateral side, thereby contributing to asymmetry and an unsightly appearance. The pair of these lines (also referred to as *radix contours*) is highlighted by the nasal light reflex and are ideally symmetric (Fig. 181.6).

Dorsal Projection

The nose projects anteriorly from the face, with its forward thrust orthogonal to the facial plane and parallel to the midsagittal plane. Quantification of nasal projection is a critical component of the rhinoplastic evaluation, yet of the many methods previously described, none specifically address *dorsal projection* (i.e., dorsal height) (10–12). Determination of proper tip projection using Crumley's method, however, utilizes the geometry of the 3:4:5 triangle; that is, projection of the nasal tip should equal three-fifths (0.6) the length from the nasion to the tip-defining point. This method can be used simultaneously to yield the ideal dorsal projection at any point along the dorsum,

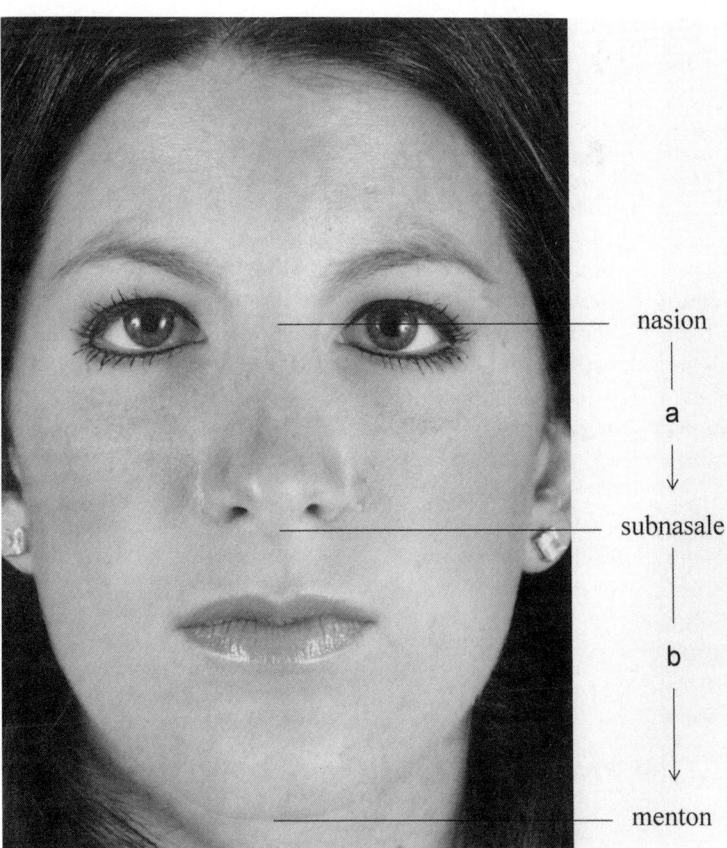

nasion

a

subnasale

b

menton

Figure 181.5 Determination of nasal length using the nasion, subnasale, and menton: ideally $a = \frac{3}{4} b$.

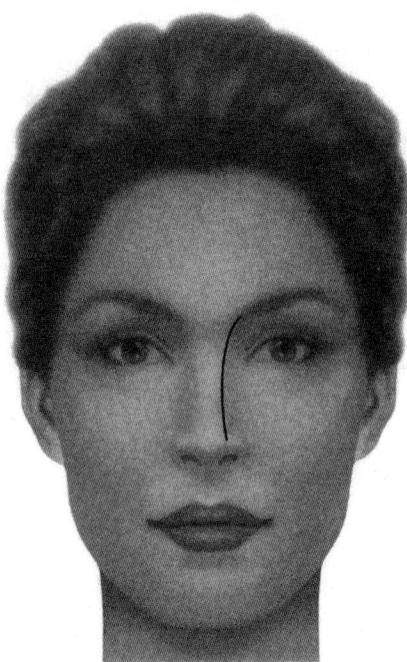

Figure 181.6 Brow–tip aesthetic line. (From Orten SS, Hilger PA. Facial analysis of the rhinoplasty patient. In: Papel ID, ed. *Facial plastic and reconstructive surgery*, 2nd ed. Stuttgart, Germany: Thieme, 2002:361, with permission.)

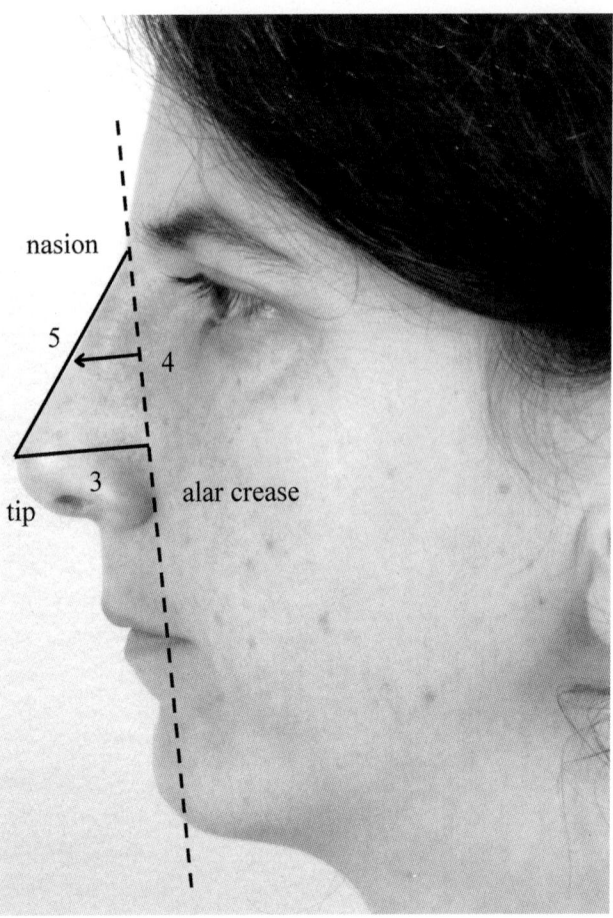

Figure 181.7 Determination of ideal dorsal projection using Crumley's tip projection analysis. At any point along the dorsum, the ratio of dorsal projection to the distance from the nasion should equal 3/5 (0.6).

because the proportions of a 3:4:5 triangle are constant (Fig. 181.7). If dorsal projection exceeds this limit (0.6), it is indicative of the presence of a dorsal hump. Because a slight dorsal concavity can be attractive, dorsal projection just less than this limit is allowable, but a significantly lower measurement could be indicative of a saddle-nose deformity.

DEFECTS OF THE NASAL VAULTS

Bony Vault Defects

Most deformities involving the bony vault arise from blunt trauma (Table 181.1). Fractured nasal bones can be comminuted and/or displaced, often resulting in an unsightly twist, depression, spur, or hump. Frequently, the skin overlying the bony dorsum is lacerated causing additional deformity by the presence of cicatrix and adherence of the dermis to the nasal bone periosteum. Severe fractures such as nasoorbital ethmoid (NOE) fractures are often quite disfiguring due to retrodisplacement of the nasal bones, deprojection and flattening of the nasal dorsum, and shortening of the nose. The resultant telescopic defect is often associated with traumatic telecanthus due to the disruption of the medial canthal tendon insertion on the nasal bones. Trauma involving the bony vault will commonly contribute to functional deficits if the keystone area, the septum, or the middle vault is also affected. Less common causes of upper vault deformity include prior rhinoplasty, neoplasia, and congenital anomalies (13,14).

Cartilaginous Vault Defects

Deformity of the middle nasal vault can be more complex than that of the bony vault because it is frequently accompanied by internal nasal deformity contributing to airway compromise. The internal nasal valve occurs near the junction of the upper lateral cartilages and the dorsal septum and is often weakened or narrowed subsequent to

TABLE 181.1	NASAL VAULT DEFECTS
Dorsal hump	Curvatures
Deep nasion	Pollybeak
Saddle nose	Bony prominences
Asymmetric nasal bones	Rocker deformity
Short/long nasal bones	Open roof deformity
Wide/narrow bony pyramid	Inverted-V deformity
Depressions	
Twists	
Partial/total rhinectomy (nasal cancer, gunshot wound)	

trauma affecting the middle vault. Furthermore, the soft tissue nature of the middle vault makes it susceptible to deformity caused by other etiologies, including unrecognized birth trauma, infections, inflammatory diseases, or autoimmune processes (15–17).

Treatment of the middle vault in rhinoplasty was for many years considered little more than removal of a hump deformity. In the 1980s, however, surgeons began to describe numerous long-term complications of this limited approach, including the inverted-V deformity, nasal valve collapse, open roof deformity, and pollybeak deformity. As a result, rhinoplasty techniques were modified to avoid these problems (18,19).

MANAGEMENT OF THE CARTILAGINOUS VAULT

Surgical correction of the middle vault involves correction of existing deformities, while ever mindful of additional deformity prevention. When certain risk factors are present, such as short nasal bones, weak upper lateral cartilages, thin skin, narrow bony pyramid, or previous trauma or surgery, preventative action may be required utilizing cartilage grafting, precise structural realignment, and fixation of nasal valve structures.

Correction of middle vault starts with septoplasty. The old saying "as the septum goes, so goes the nose" indicates the importance of straightening the central strut of the nose. With the goal of making the dorsal septum as straight as possible, the open approach is often used. Accessing the septum from above via the separation of the medial crura of the lower lateral cartilages allows better exposure than the traditional endonasal approach (20). Further separation of the upper lateral cartilages from the dorsal septum results in maximal septal exposure. The deviated portions of the quadrangular cartilage and perpendicular plate of the ethmoid bone are removed, making sure that 1 cm dorsal and caudal struts are maintained. Wide mucoperichondrial elevation, weakening incisions, wedge excisions, and sutured struts are adjuncts useful in straightening the deviated septum (21).

Spreader grafts are probably the next most common corrective modality used for middle vault rehabilitation. First described by Sheen and Sheen (22), these rectangular cartilage grafts are placed between the junctions of the upper lateral cartilages and septum to widen and stabilize the nasal valve. Spreader grafts not only lateralize the upper lateral cartilages but also strengthen the middle vault to resist the inward motion on inspiration associated with Bernoulli principle. They can be placed either through open or closed rhinoplasty techniques but are easier to stabilize with direct sutures via the open approach. Septal cartilage is the most frequently used grafting material, but auricular cartilage may be used if septum is not available. Spreader grafts can also be used for aesthetic purposes. For patients with unilateral middle vault depressions, a single spreader graft can elevate and lateralize the upper lateral cartilage to restore symmetry.

In many revision rhinoplasty cases involving middle vault pathology, separation of the septum and upper lateral cartilages has occurred due to prior hump removal. There is usually fibrous connective tissue present instead of the native cartilaginous junction. Therefore, preservation of the mucoperichondrium and creation of a pocket for graft placement through the open approach are usually preferred. If the upper lateral cartilages are fused with the septum in the internal nasal valve area, sharp dissection with an elevator will preserve the mucoperichondrium and maintain stability. In cases in which the upper lateral cartilages have been almost completely resected, conchal cartilage onlay grafts may be needed in addition to spreader grafts to augment lateral support or camouflage depressions. The grafts are carved, aligned, and fixed into position with 5-0 PDS (Polydioxanone Ethicon, Somerville, NJ) mattress sutures. Most spreader grafts are 1.5 to 2.5 cm in length and 1 to 3 mm in width. In general, the grafts should run along the dorsal septum from below the bony cartilaginous junction to the anterior septal angle. In severe cases, the grafts may be layered to provide additional bulk. Grafts of unequal width may also be used to correct asymmetries in the middle vault. Spreader grafts can also be used as internal splints to help straighten a caudal septal deflection. The technique of spreader graft placement and fixation is demonstrated in Figures 181.8 to 181.11. Placement of spreader grafts is greatly facilitated by placement of a 30-gauge needle through the cartilage complex while suturing.

A corollary to spreader grafting that deserves mention is reverse spreader grafting. This technique can be useful in patients with an overly broad middle vault, minimal nasal obstruction, and no nasal valve collapse. In these cases, patients can benefit from reduction of the horizontal width of the cartilaginous dorsum, which can be thought of as the reverse of spreader grafts (23).

Additional methods to augment the function of the nasal valve involve the placement of alar batten grafts, butterfly grafts, and various suture methods. Schlosser and Park (24) described the use of 5-0 clear nylon flaring sutures that span the upper lateral cartilages and septum horizontally. Tightening the suture theoretically increases the angle of the internal nasal valve and therefore improves nasal airflow. Their study indicated that flaring sutures used concomitantly with spreader grafts increase airflow more than the use of spreader grafts alone. Other suture techniques such as tip-lifting sutures, or valve maneuvers like internal valve M-plasty or lateral crural J-flap, can also be useful adjuncts but are outside the scope of this chapter.

Patients with saddle-nose deformity frequently have middle vault collapse without soft tissue support, commonly due to a large septal perforation. Fixation of a dorsal graft helps to enhance dorsal projection, support the soft tissues, and restore the integrity of the nasal valve. Calvarial bone secured with a lag screw or rib cartilage

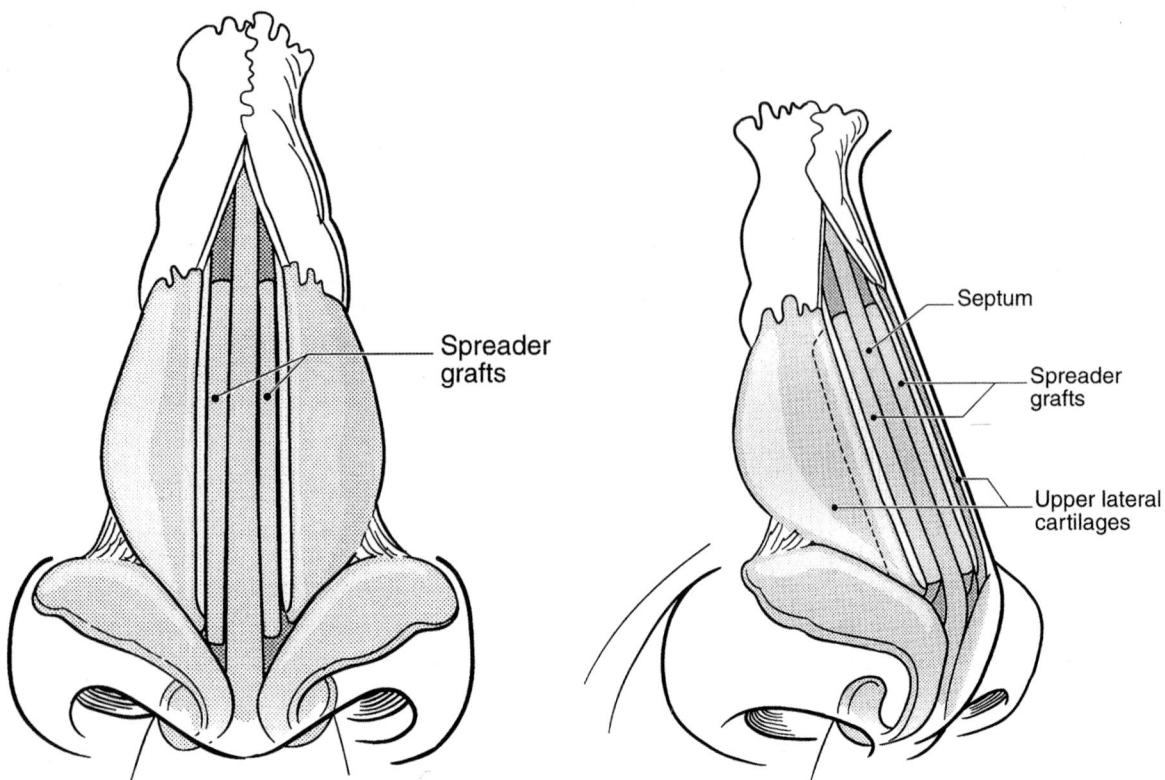

Figure 181.8 Placement of spreader grafts between septum and upper lateral cartilages. (From Papel ID. Management of the middle vault. In: Papel ID, ed. *Facial plastic and reconstructive surgery*, 2nd ed. Stuttgart, Germany: Thieme, 2002:409, with permission.)

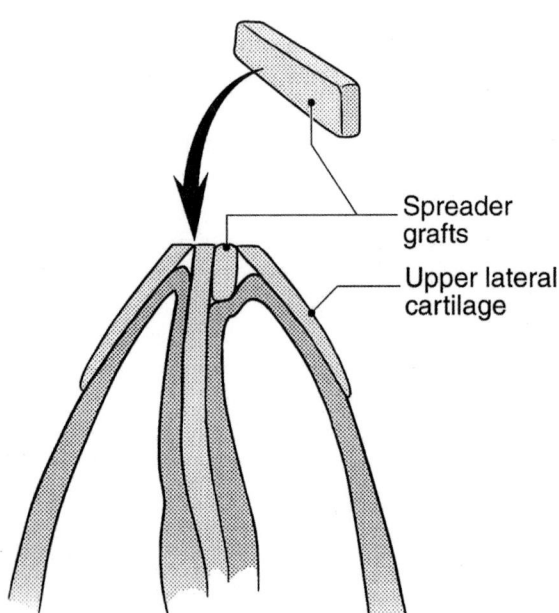

Figure 181.9 Placement of spreader graft lateralizes and elevates the upper lateral cartilage, widening the middle vault. (From Papel ID. Management of the middle vault. In: Papel ID, ed. *Facial plastic and reconstructive surgery*, 2nd ed. Stuttgart, Germany: Thieme, 2002:409, Fig. 35-5, with permission.)

secured with sutures has been very useful in these patients (25,26). In addition, dorsal calvarial grafts can serve as anchors for other reconstructive grafts (27). In some cases, the use of crushed cartilage or AlloDerm (LifeCell Corp., Branchburg, NJ) over the dorsum and graft material can help smooth an irregular profile.

The pollybeak deformity is a complex nasal deformity with multiple etiologies that deserves special mention. It is caused by *relative* underprojection of the nasal tip with regard to the projection of the dorsum. It is important to understand that a pollybeak can occur, therefore, when the tip is either *correctly projected* or *underprojected*. If tip projection is aesthetically correct but the dorsum remains overprojected, a pollybeak deformity is present. Conversely, a pollybeak results when dorsal projection is aesthetically correct but the tip is underprojected. A pollybeak deformity can occur naturally, or as the result of prior rhinoplasty, with insufficient lowering of the cartilaginous dorsum, excessive reduction of the bony dorsum, disruption of tip support without reconstitution, excessive tip deprojection, or inappropriate derotation of the tip. As such, there are different management strategies for minimizing the incidence of pollybeak, depending on the nature of the deformity. The important point is that the rhinoplasty surgeon recognizes the importance of the critical relation between tip projection and dorsal projection during rhinoplasty and maintains adequate tip projection when altering the dorsum.

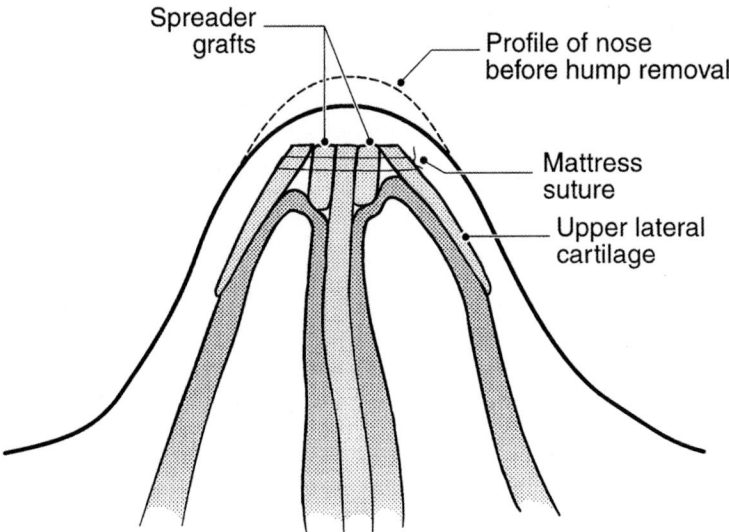

Figure 181.10 Spreader grafts in place and fixed with mattress sutures. The original dorsal height is identified. (From Papel ID. Management of the middle vault. In: Papel ID, ed. *Facial plastic and reconstructive surgery*, 2nd ed. Stuttgart, Germany: Thieme, 2002:409, with permission.)

MANAGEMENT OF THE BONY VAULT

Deformity of the upper nasal vault represents a challenge to the rhinoplasty surgeon, requiring thorough preoperative evaluation and careful surgical technique to manage. Improper or incomplete treatment of the bony vault may lead to suboptimal results, including persistence of existing defects or the creation of new ones. The presence of iatrogenic deformities listed in Table 181.1 bears witness to this. Surgical treatment of the bony vault should aim to accomplish the following: (a) establishment of appropriate dorsal projection, (b) creation of a smooth dorsal contour free of bony irregularity, (c) correction of nasal width, and (d) straightening of the crooked nose. Techniques used to accomplish these aims include hump reduction, osteotomies, and grafting.

Hump Reduction

John Orlando Roe (1848 to 1915) provided the modern age with the first account of dorsal defect correction in 1891 (Fig. 181.12) (28). Regional dorsal overprojection is managed with wide soft tissue envelope elevation and the removal of portions of the nasal bones. This can be done either through an open or closed approach. Adequate exposure must be balanced with the maintenance of soft tissue

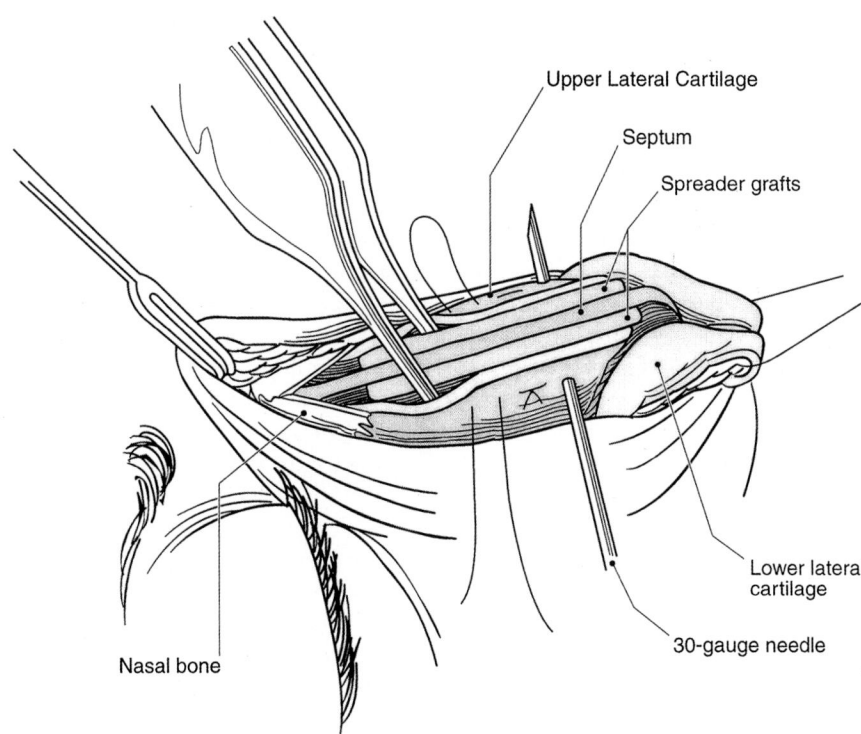

Figure 181.11 Demonstration of mattress suture fixation and use of 30-gauge needle for stabilization. (From Papel ID. Management of the middle vault. In: Papel ID, ed. *Facial plastic and reconstructive surgery*, 2nd ed. Stuttgart, Germany: Thieme, 2002:409, Fig. 35-7, with permission.)

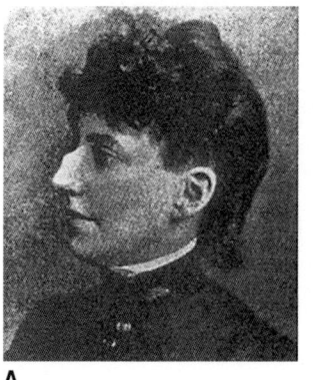 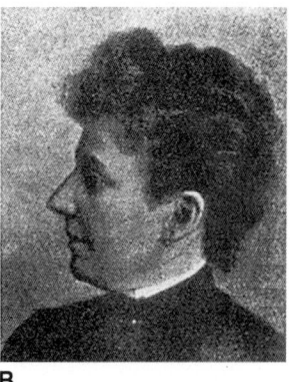

A **B**

Figure 181.12 John Orlando Roe patient: before **(A)** and after **(B)** dorsal hump removal (1891). (From Lam SM. John Orlando Roe: father of aesthetic rhinoplasty. *Arch Facial Plast Surg* 2002;4: 122–123, with permission.)

support, and it must be remembered that the upper lateral cartilages insert deep to the caudal margin of the nasal bones. Exquisite care must be taken not to disarticulate this union. The best way to avoid this is to elevate the nasal bone periosteum using a Joseph elevator starting from a point 1 to 2 mm superior to the rhinion (29). Bone removal is subsequently accomplished with a double-guarded osteotome or a carbide tungsten pull rasp, depending on the amount of bone to be removed. After sharp incision of the cartilaginous component, large humps typically require removal with the osteotome. Care should be taken to follow the planned trajectory and not make an oblique cut by straying laterally or canting the osteotome (Fig. 181.13). Refinements can then be performed by rasping just off midline in a slightly oblique manner so as not to avulse the upper lateral cartilages (30). It must always be remembered that overly aggressive bony and cartilaginous dorsal reduction can lead to a scooped nasal appearance and even *the saddle-nose deformity.*

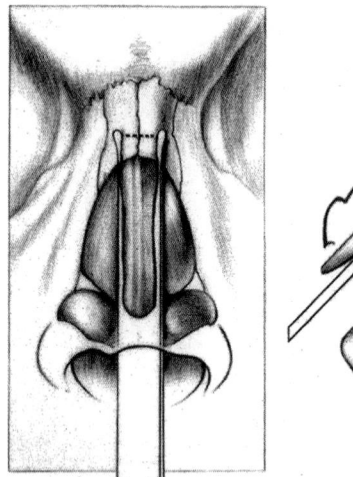 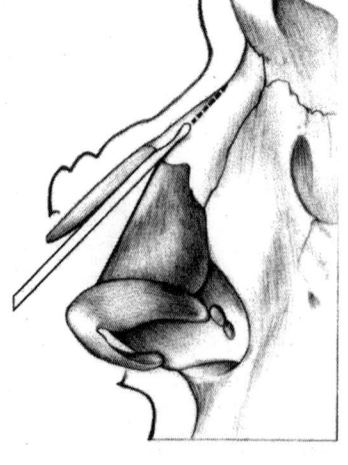

Figure 181.13 Removal of dorsal excess. (From Mostafour SP, Murakami CS, Larrabee WF Jr. Management of the bony nasal vault. In: Papel ID, ed. *Facial plastic and reconstructive surgery*, 2nd ed. Stuttgart, Germany: Thieme, 2002:403, with permission.)

Osteotomies

Osteotomies have evolved greatly since the time of Jacques Joseph (1865 to 1934), one of the rhinoplasty pioneers who touted their importance (31). Early techniques were fraught with nasal airway compromise largely due to a trajectory that caused wide disruption of periosteum and release of lower lateral cartilage lateral suspensory ligaments. Modifications have led to the emergence of modern techniques that place equal importance on preservation of the nasal airway and aesthetic improvement, in accord with the dual tenet of the rhinoplasty operation (32,33).

Osteotomies are commonly used to improve irregularities in the brow–tip aesthetic line and correct open roof deformities (diastasis of the nasal bones) associated with bony dorsum reduction. They can be performed laterally, medially, or intermediately. Lateral osteotomies should be limited to the thin bone of the pyriform aperture, lateral to the anterior margin of the ascending maxillary processes. If too far lateral, the thick bone at the nasofacial transition will be encountered, rather than the average 2.5-mm thickness typically encountered along the osteotomy path (34).

Lateral osteotomies can be linear or perforating, internal or external. The ideal trajectory is described as "high–low–high," which indicates the anteroposterior position on the nasal pyramid. A standard lateral osteotomy is a linear, internal cut that is initiated with a mucosal stab incision made just lateral to the anterior face of the inferior turbinate. The curved, guarded 4-mm osteotome is placed into the incision on the margin of the pyriform aperture, at about a 45-degree angle to the facial plane, or roughly perpendicular to the face of the aperture (Fig. 181.14). Preservation of the inferior segment of the pyriform maintains the lateral suspensory ligaments and width important for the nasal airway. Soon after the initial cut, the osteotome should be transitioned roughly parallel to the facial plane and directed toward the medial canthal area. The osteotomy should then curve anteriorly and superiorly to terminate at the level of the medial canthus, midway between the dorsal line and the medial canthus. The telltale sound of the osteotome meeting the thicker frontal bone is indicative of the proper stopping point. The osteotomy is completed with pronation and medialization of the osteotome, causing back-fracture across the superior aspect of the nasal bone. Elevation of the periosteum in this vicinity liberates the nasal bones from the soft tissue envelope, allowing the osteotomized bone to heal free of the influence of soft tissue contracture. If the back-fracture is incomplete or inadequate, it can be augmented percutaneously using a 2-mm osteotome. Alternatively, the entire back-fracture can be completed percutaneously. If the osteotomy extends superior to the medial canthus, there is greater risk of creating a *rocker deformity,* which occurs when the nasal bone inferior to the osteotomy sinks relative to the bone superior to the cut. Should this occur, steps must be taken to camouflage the step off or replace the

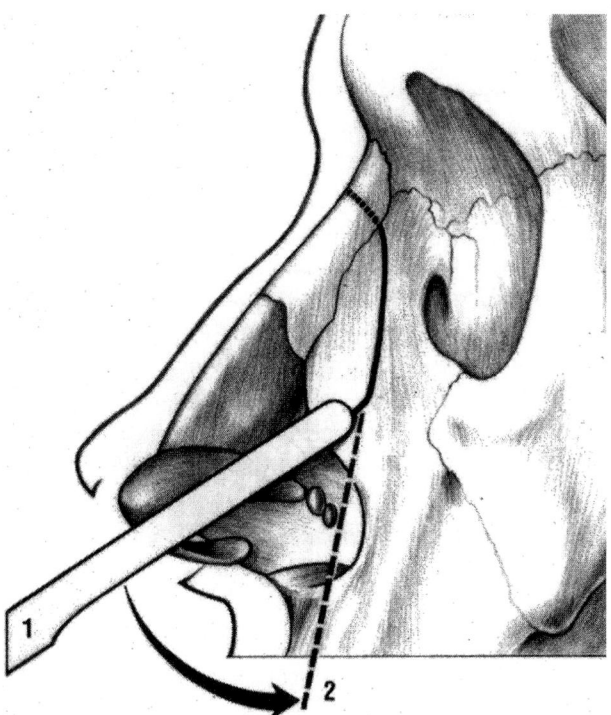

Figure 181.14 The lateral osteotomy is initiated at the anterior face of the inferior turbinate, initially perpendicular to the plane of the pyriform aperture (position *1*). The osteotomy is then transitioned (position *2*) and carried to the medial canthal area. (From Mostafour SP, Murakami CS, Larrabee WF Jr. Management of the bony nasal vault. In: Papel ID, ed. *Facial plastic and reconstructive surgery*, 2nd ed. Stuttgart, Germany: Thieme, 2002:404, with permission.)

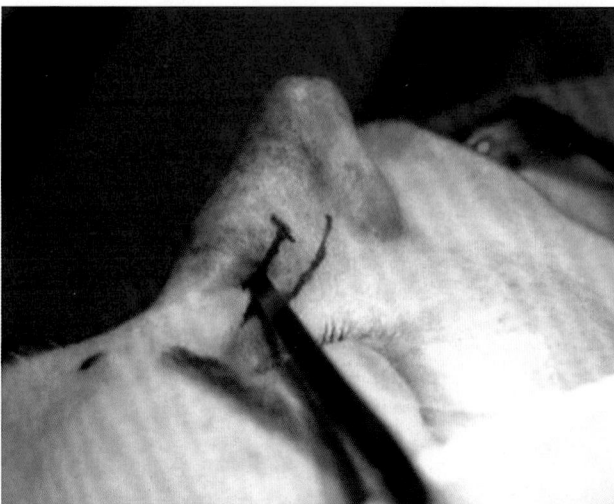

Figure 181.15 An intermediate osteotomy is marked on the skin and the inferior edge of the bone is noted. A percutaneous method is used in a perforating manner.

malpositioned bone, and wait until the bone heals before attempting further osteotomy.

Perforating lateral osteotomies can be performed either internally (transnasally) or externally (percutaneously). The perforating technique is the ideal method to complete an exact osteotomy with minimal trauma. It is preferred when maintenance of support is critical, such as in revision rhinoplasty or short nasal bones, because there is far less disruption of periosteal support and the intact periosteum stabilizes and splints the mobilized segments, enhancing precise healing (35,36). A series of perforations are made at fixed intervals along the desired fracture trajectory and then completed with minimal manual manipulation. The intranasal perforating osteotomy is useful to widen the pyriform aperture by displacing the bones laterally (37).

Medial and intermediate osteotomies should be used judiciously; however, they can be essential when the pyriform is very thick, the nose is significantly deviated, or a very large nose needs to be reduced. Both medial and intermediate osteotomies are usually performed transnasally with a 3-mm osteotome. Medial osteotomies are initiated on the medial aspect of the caudal margin of the nasal bones near the septum. This is very near the keystone area of the nasal vaults, so considerable care must be taken, for disruption of the connection between the caudal margin

of the nasal bones and the cephalic margin of the upper lateral cartilages is the cause of *the inverted-V deformity* and its accompanying nasal obstruction. The percutaneous perforation technique can be used to perform medial osteotomies to further ensure preservation of the keystone. The trajectory of the fracture is superolateral, meeting with the back-fracture of the previously performed lateral osteotomy. If further correction is needed, intermediate osteotomies can also be performed. The intermediate osteotomy is also initiated on the caudal margin of the nasal bones, intermediate to the medial and lateral osteotomies. The trajectory should parallel the lateral osteotomy and meet with the superior back-fracture. Because intermediate osteotomies are difficult to execute if the lateral bone has already been mobilized, they are best performed prior to lateral osteotomies. Figure 181.15 demonstrates a percutaneous technique for an intermediate osteotomy. Note how the bony cartilaginous margin is marked to prevent damage to the supporting system (Fig. 181.15).

It is often helpful to plan the steps needed to reshape the upper two-thirds of the nose. Drawing the lines of planned osteotomies and indicating those areas to be grafted or reduced will help guide the operation in a logical manner. This can be very helpful to keep the procedure on track, especially after edema has occurred and the original contours may not be easily visible (Fig. 181.16).

Grafts

Contemporary grafts useful in treatment of the bony vault include radix grafts, onlay grafts, and anchored bone grafts. Radix grafts serve to increase the projection of the nasofrontal trough, correcting the excessively deep nasion. If septal or auricular cartilage is readily accessible, it can be used either as a single morselized piece or multiple

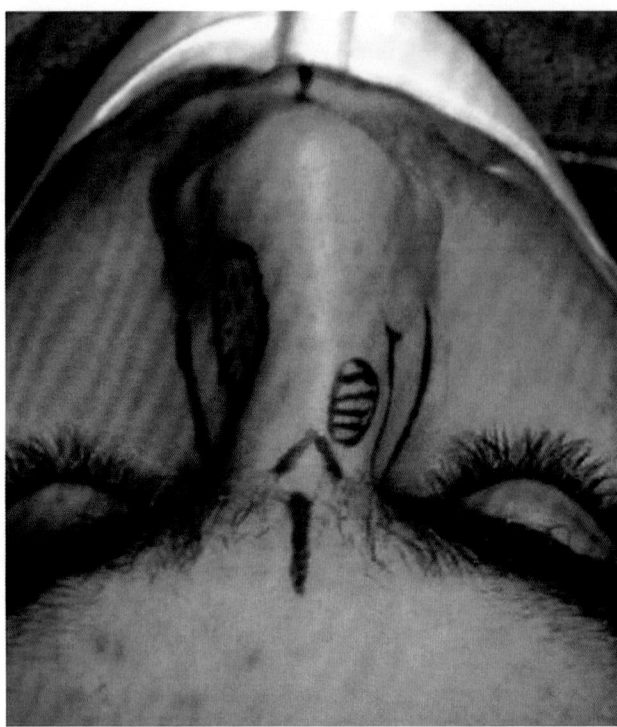

Figure 181.16 The surgical plan is marked on the skin prior to local anesthetic infiltration. Areas of grafting, reduction, and osteotomy are marked.

HIGHLIGHTS

- The internal nasal valve is located at the junction of the upper lateral cartilages and the dorsal septum.
- Spreader grafts between the upper lateral cartilages and septum may widen and stabilize the valve.
- The valve may also be augmented with batten grafts, butterfly grafts, and suture methods.
- The pollybeak deformity is relative under projection of the nasal tip relative to the dorsum.
- Upper vault deformity is managed with hump reduction, osteotomies, and grafting.
- The insertion of the upper lateral cartilages on the caudal margin of the nasal bones must not be disarticulated.

fragments sutured together as a plumping graft (38). The graft is placed either superficial or deep to the nasal bone periosteum and held in place by the overlying skin envelope. Although AlloDerm can also be used as a radix graft, it is perhaps more useful as a dorsal onlay graft to camouflage small irregularities as well as to add height. When significant bony defects are present, as after cancer resection or NOE-telescoping nasal deformity, calvarial bone grafts may be required to reconstruct the upper vault. These grafts are cantilevered off the frontal bone and anchored precisely with titanium screws.

CONCLUSION

Facial aesthetics and attractiveness rely in large part on the appearance of the nose. Deformities affecting the nasal vaults are distinct and independent from those affecting the nasal tip and contribute not only to unsightly appearance but also to improper nasal function. Building on the past experience of prior rhinoplasty surgeons, surgical techniques dealing with nasal vault deformities have evolved, ever mindful that restoration of proper anatomic vault relations significantly enhances the appearance of the nose and nasal function. The contemporary rhinoplasty surgeon must be facile with analysis and management of the bony and cartilaginous nasal vaults that comprise the upper two-thirds of the nose and be able to integrate this into management of the nasal tip for successful performance of the rhinoplasty operation.

REFERENCES

1. Burget GC, Menick FJ. *Aesthetic reconstruction of the nose*. St. Louis, MO: Mosby, 1994.
2. Behrbohm H. Preoperative management. In: Behrbohm H, Tardy ME Jr, eds. *Essentials of septorhinoplasty: philosophy, approaches, techniques*. Stuttgart, Germany: Thieme, 2004:89–106.
3. Mitz V, Peyronie M. The superficial musculo-aponeurotic system in the parotid and cheek area. *Plast Reconstr Surg* 1976;58:80.
4. Tardy ME, Brown RJ. *Surgical anatomy of the nose*. New York: Raven Press, 1995.
5. Oneal RM, Beil RJ Jr, Schlesinger J. Surgical anatomy of the nose. *Otolaryngol Clin North Am* 1999;32:145–181.
6. Guyuron B. Nasal osteotomy and airway changes. *Plast Reconstr Surg* 1998;102:856–860; discussion 861–863.
7. Papel ID. Management of the middle vault. In: Papel ID, ed. *Facial plastic and reconstructive surgery*, 2nd ed. Stuttgart, Germany: Thieme, 2002:407–413.
8. Powell N, Humphreys B. *Proportions of the aesthetic face*. New York: Thieme-Stratton, 1984.
9. Papel IP, Capone RB. Facial proportions and esthetic ideals. In: Behrbohm H, Tardy ME Jr, eds. *Essentials of septorhinoplasty: philosophy, approaches, techniques*. Stuttgart, Germany: Thieme, 2004: 65–74.
10. Simons R. Nasal tip projection, ptosis, and supratip thickening. *Ear Nose Throat J* 1982;61:44.
11. Crumley R. Quantitative analysis of nasal tip projection. *Laryngoscope* 1988;98:202–208.
12. Baum S. Introduction. *Ear Nose Throat J* 1982;61:426.
13. Dingman RO, Natvig P. The deviated nose. *Clin Plast Surg* 1977;4:145–152.
14. Vuyk HD. A review of practical guidelines for correction of the deviated, asymmetric nose. *Rhinology* 2000;38:72–78.
15. Verwoerd CDA, Verwoerd-Verhoef HL. Developmental aspects of the deviated nose. *Facial Plast Surg* 1989;6:95.
16. Fernandez-Vozmediano JM, Armario Hita JC, Gonzales Cabreriza A. Rhinoscleroma in three siblings. *Pediatr Dermatol* 2004;21:134–138.
17. Pirsig W, Pentz S, Lenders H. Repair of saddle nose deformity in Wegener's granulomatosis and ectodermal dysplasia. *Rhinology* 1993;31(2):69–72.
18. Sheen JH. Spreader graft: a method of reconstructing the roof of the middle nasal vault following rhinoplasty. *Plast Reconstr Surg* 1984;73:230–237.
19. Toriumi DM, Johnson CM. Open structure rhinoplasty: featured technical points and long-term follow-up. *Facial Plast Clin North Am* 1993;1:1–22.
20. TerKonda RP, Sykes JM. Repairing the twisted nose. *Otolaryngol Clin North Am* 1999;32:53–64.

21. Foda MTF. The role of septal surgery in management of the deviated nose. *Plast Reconstr Surg* 2005;115:406–415.
22. Sheen JH, Sheen AP. *Aesthetic rhinoplasty*. St. Louis, MO: CV Mosby, 1987.
23. Thomas JR, Prendiville S. Overly wide cartilaginous middle vault. *Facial Plast Surg Clin North Am* 2004;12:107–110.
24. Schlosser RJ, Park SS. Surgery for the dysfunctional nasal valve. *Arch Facial Plast Surg* 1999;1:105–110.
25. Frodel JL, Marentette LJ, Quatela VC, et al. Calvarial bone graft harvest: techniques, considerations, and morbidity. *Arch Otolaryngol Head Neck Surg* 1993;119:17–23.
26. Quatela VC, Jacono AA. Structural grafting in rhinoplasty. *Facial Plast Surg* 2002;18:223–232.
27. Papel ID. Augmentation rhinoplasty utilizing cranial bone grafts. *Md Med J* 1991;40:479–483.
28. Lam SM. John Orlando Roe: father of aesthetic rhinoplasty. *Arch Facial Plast Surg* 2002;4:122–123.
29. Larrabee WF Jr. Open rhinoplasty and the upper third of the nose. *Facial Plast Surg Clin North Am* 1993;1:26.
30. Mostafour SP, Murakami CS, Larrabee WF Jr. Management of the bony nasal vault. In: Papel ID, ed. *Facial plastic and reconstructive surgery*, 2nd ed. Stuttgart, Germany: Thieme, 2002:402–406.
31. Aufricht G. Joseph's rhinoplasty with some modifications. *Surg Clin North Am* 1971;51:299–316.
32. Webster RC, Davidson RC, Smith RC. Curved lateral osteotomy for airway protection in rhinoplasty. *Arch Otolaryngol* 1977;103:454–458.
33. Thomas JR, Griner NR, Remmler DJ. Steps for a safer method of osteotomies in rhinoplasty. *Laryngoscope* 1987;97:746–747.
34. Larrabee WF Jr, Murakami CS. Osteotomy techniques to correct posttraumatic deviation of the nasal pyramid: a technical note. *J Craniomaxillofac Trauma* 2000;6:43–47.
35. Tardy ME Jr. Contemporary rhinoplasty: principles and philosophy. In: Behrbohm H, Tardy ME Jr, eds. *Essentials of septorhinoplasty: philosophy, approaches, techniques*. Stuttgart, Germany: Thieme, 2004:37–63.
36. Rohrich RJ, Minoli JJ, Adams WP, et al. The lateral nasal osteotomy in rhinoplasty: an anatomic endoscopic comparison of the external versus internal approach. *Plast Reconstr Surg* 1997;99:1309–1313.
37. Byrne PJ, Walsh WE, Hilger PA. The use of inside-out lateral osteotomy to improve outcome in rhinoplasty. *Arch Facial Plast Surg* 2003;5:251–255.
38. Daniel RK, Calvert JW. Diced cartilage grafts in rhinoplasty surgery. *Plast Reconstr Surg* 2004;113:2156–2171.

182 Nasal Tip Surgery

Tatiana K. Dixon   *Dean M. Toriumi*

Creating a natural nasal tip contour is a complex task and requires a three-dimensional approach. The surgeon must have a clear understanding of what looks normal and which methods should be used to attain that natural contour. The lower third of the nose is composed of multiple subunits (tip, columella, facets, and alae), and the curvilinear surface transitions between these nasal subunits create highlights and shadows. Even the slightest concavity or asymmetry in the tip results in unnaturally positioned shadows, which detract from the person's appearance on frontal view. When contouring the nasal tip, the surgeon should focus more on creating favorable shadows and highlights and less on narrowing. Simply narrowing the nasal tip may create abnormal shadowing between the nasal tip and alae resulting in a pinched-tip look. Careful consideration of the underlying anatomic structures and proper use of suturing and repositioning techniques in combination with cartilage grafting will help create favorable, natural-appearing tip contours that will better withstand the forces of scar contracture over time (1).

ANALYSIS AND DIAGNOSIS

Analysis of the tip, which is only one component of the nasal examination, is not undertaken in isolation. For the sake of brevity, this chapter focuses only on the contribution of the tip to the form and function of the nose. The reader is encouraged to consult another source (Chapter 179) for a thorough overview of nasal analysis.

Before undertaking an intelligent analysis of the nasal tip, it is imperative to have a mastery of nasal anatomy as well as a clear understanding of the ideal contours and relationships of the nose (Figs. 182.1 to 182.6).

When evaluating the tip, the surgeon should attempt to visualize the underlying structures by inspecting the skin. The first step is to try to quantify the thickness of the skin envelope. Most surgeons classify patients into thin, medium, and thick skin categories. This can be estimated by inspection and palpation of the skin by rolling it between the thumb and index finger. When assessing skin thickness, freckles are a reliable indicator of thin skin (2). Thick skin tends to be more sebaceous and have thick nostril rims and less defined alar facets.

Understanding the implications of skin thickness should radically alter the surgical plan with an emphasis on long-term results. Thin-skinned patients require a high degree of precision and symmetry without sharp edges of bone or cartilage, lest they be visible shortly after surgery. Thin-skinned patients should also be advised that they have a greater risk of developing small, visible asymmetries than patients with thicker skin. Conversely, they will enjoy a more rapid course of healing than their thick-skinned counterparts.

Thick-skinned patients, on the other hand, have fewer surgical options than those with thin skin. It is critical that the surgeon not promise a result that is impossible to attain. For example, thick-skinned patients often request a more refined tip. Although a bulbous tip can be improved, a thick-skinned nose will not have defined soft triangles or a "chiseled" appearance postoperatively, despite the surgeon's efforts. Many thick-skinned patients also have large noses and want them made smaller. Because a thick skin envelope will not contract to any significant degree, it is a mistake to expect that cartilage resection alone will refine the contour of the tip and result in a smaller nose. Counsel these patients that, although their tip can be refined, it often necessitates the use of grafts to stretch and refine the thick tip skin and therefore requires increasing projection to achieve that definition. This increase in projection will have the added benefit of being able to keep the dorsum of the nose high, which will increase the appearance of a narrow nose. Otherwise, they risk having a loose, ptotic, poorly supported tip. Too many patients with thick skin undergo multiple revisions wherein the revising surgeon

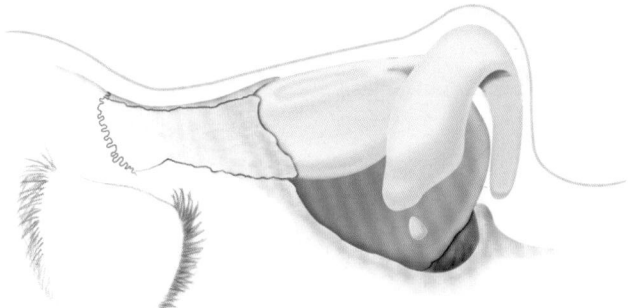

Figure 182.1 Lateral view of the structures of the nasal tip.

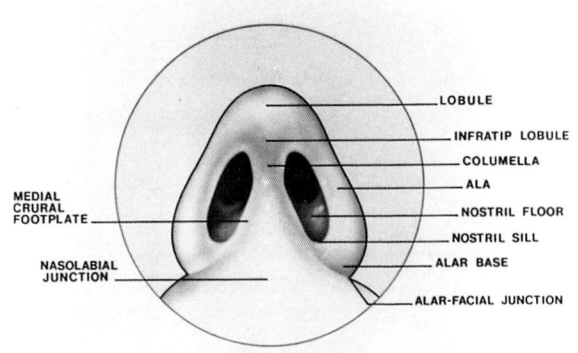

Figure 182.3 Anatomy and nomenclature of the nasal tip viewed from the basal aspect.

attempts to trim "just a little bit more," which only exacerbates the problem (Fig. 182.7).

Palpation of the tip and its ability to recoil when depressed can identify weak lower lateral cartilages or a low anterior septal angle (Fig. 182.8). The septum can also be palpated by placing the tip of the thumb and index finger in each of the nasal vestibules. This maneuver facilitates recognition of a weak or deviated caudal septum (2).

Evaluation of the tip must include assessment of the tip supporting structures. Anderson's tripod model of the nasal tip clarified the dynamics of altering tip support (3). In it, the conjoined medial crura represent one leg of the tripod and the lateral crura the other two. Tip position, therefore, is a consequence of the combined forces of the three legs of the tripod as well as the support provided by the caudal septum (Fig. 182.9). This model illustrates the variable contributions of the medial and lateral crural length when assessing projection, rotation, and the columella–labial angle.

The medial crura should be inspected by looking at the nasal base. Medial crural length has several surgical implications. Short medial crura provide little tip support and will require reinforcement to prevent postoperative loss of

projection and counterrotation. If the surgeon intends to rotate the tip by performing a cephalic trim of the lateral crura, the poor support of short medial crura will preclude any meaningful cephalic rotation. Similarly, long medial crura may provide excellent tip support, but if the nose needs to be deprojected, techniques such as a full transfixion incision will have minimal impact. These long medial crura will likely need to be modified to deproject the nose. Any deficiencies in these major tip support mechanisms need to be addressed at the time of surgery.

Important parameters to assess when analyzing the lateral view of the nasal tip are projection and rotation. Assessment of tip projection must be undertaken in the context of the entire profile. The nasofrontal angle, depth of the radix, and chin all affect the appearance of nasal projection (Fig. 182.10). When examining an abnormally projected nose, the surgeon must identify where in the nose the projection is distorted. For instance, in an overprojected nose, the medial crura may be excessively long, the domes may be too tall, or the anterior septal angle

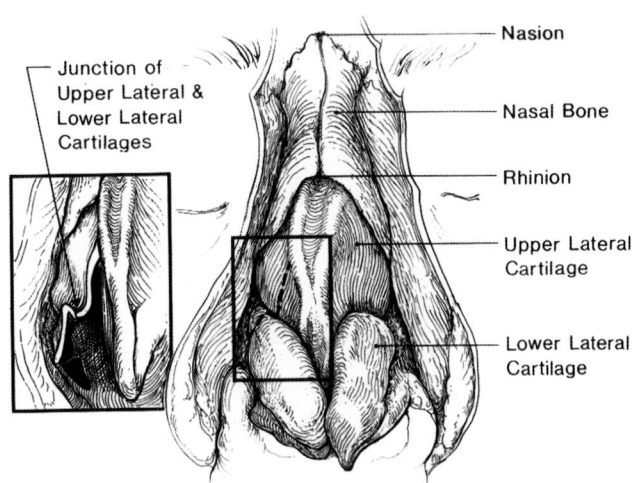

Figure 182.2 Frontal view of the underlying anatomic structures of the nasal tip.

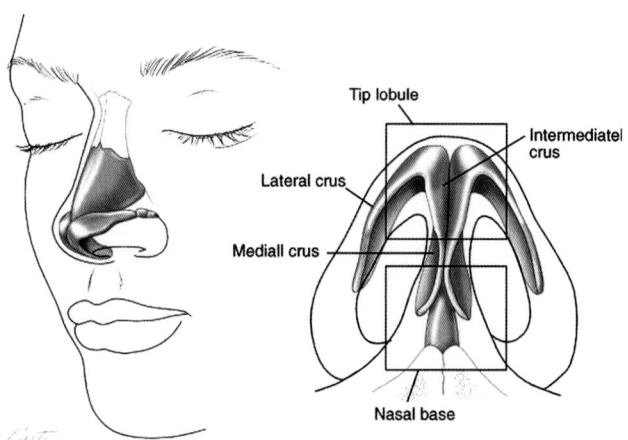

Figure 182.4 Underlying anatomic structures of the nasal base.

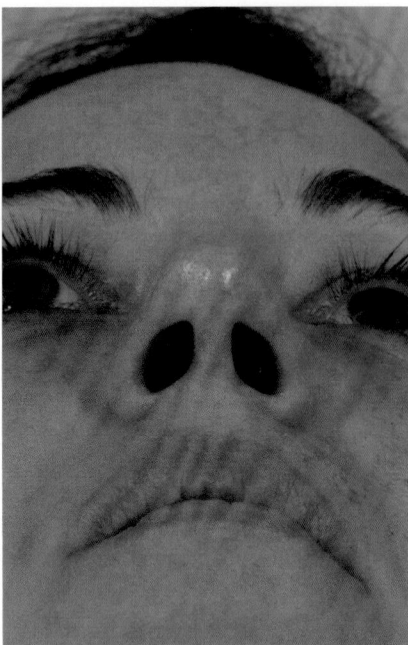

Figure 182.5 Ideal nasal tip contour. Note the triangular base view with an uninterrupted arch from alar rim to tip to alar rim.

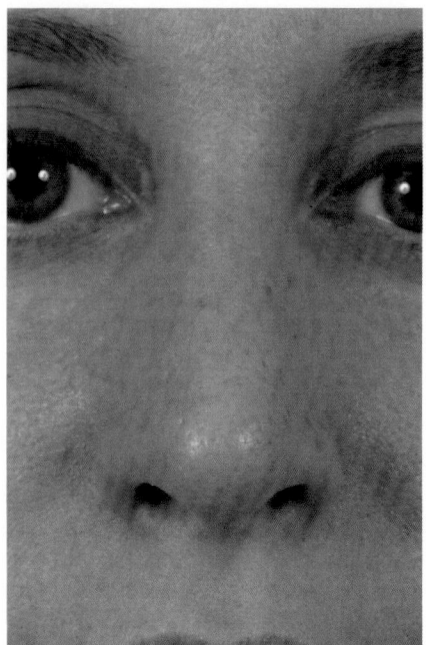

Figure 182.6 Ideal nasal tip contour with a smooth transition between the tip lobule and the well-supported nasal sidewall without bulbousness or pinching.

may be too anteriorly positioned. Similarly, short medial and lateral crura, a low anterior septal angle, flat domes, or a hypoplastic premaxilla can result in an underprojected nose. Sometimes these factors occur in combination. Therefore, although recognizing that a nose is over- or underprojected is an important first step, the appropriate

treatment options are widely divergent depending on the reason for the deformity. Unless the surgeon can identify these subtleties, good results are only a product of chance.

Ideal rotation is 90 to 100 degrees in males and 100 to 120 degrees in females. This varies according to the height of the patient as shorter patients tolerate more

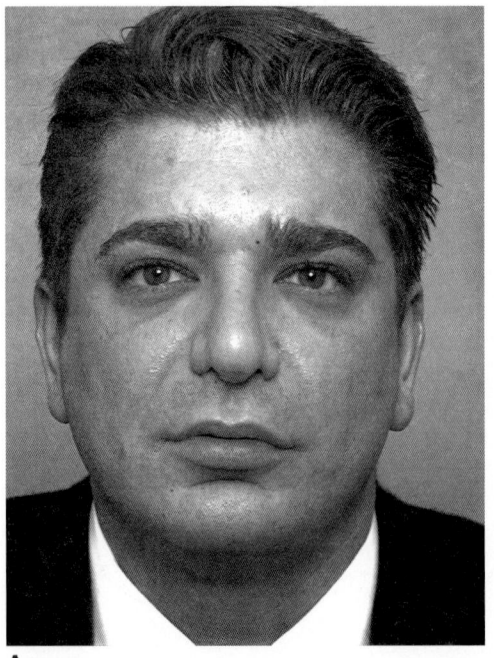

A

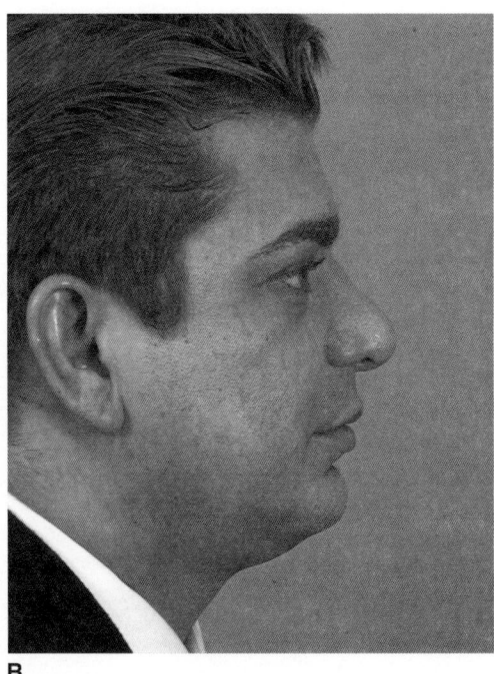

B

Figure 182.7 This patient had a bulbous tip and thick skin. After several reductive procedures, the tip is poorly supported and unrefined.

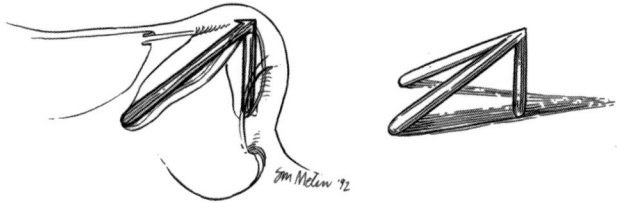

Figure 182.9 Tip position is a consequence of the combined forces of the three legs of the tripod as well as the support provided by the caudal septum.

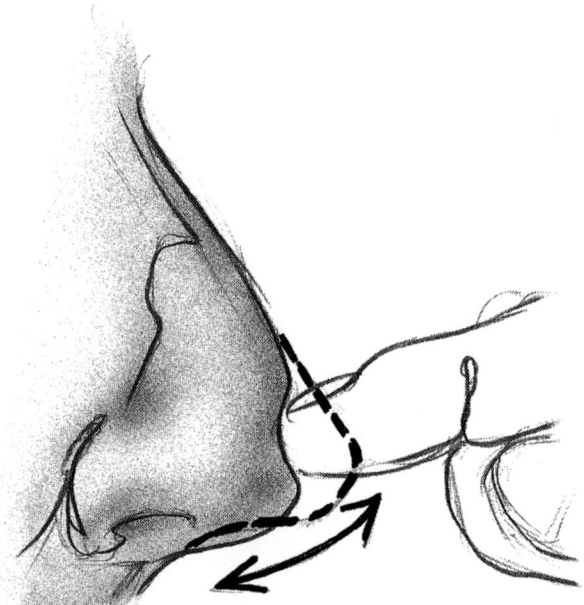

Figure 182.8 Demonstration of finger palpation of the recoil mechanism of the nasal tip. The relative resistance to deformity demonstrated by the nasal tip provides a useful indication of the integrity of nasal tip support mechanisms.

rotation and taller patients require less rotation to avoid seeing too much nostril on the frontal view. The perceived rotation is affected by the position and contour of the nasolabial angle. Another important component is the alar–columellar relationship, with approximately 2- to 4-mm columellar show being considered aesthetic. Lastly, the double break and supratip break are important components that must be maintained or created to ensure a

natural appearance of the tip. The double break is formed by the natural divergence of the intermediate crura (Fig. 182.11), and the supratip break is the transition from the tip-defining point to the dorsum.

When assessing the frontal view, subtle highlights and shadows impart a three-dimensional perspective. First, the aesthetically pleasing nasal tip has a horizontally oriented tip highlight formed by the divergence of the intermediate crura and the paired domes (Fig. 182.12). The tip highlight should gradually transition to the alae without a deep shadow (1). The average width between tip-defining points is about 8 mm, but this can vary between 6 and 14 mm based on overall facial width, base width, and cultural norms (4). Of equal importance, there is a subtle shadow in the supratip region that continues laterally into the supra-alar groove, representing the supratip break. This shadow creates the appearance of a refined tip and is caused by the transition between the most projecting point of the domes and the more posteriorly positioned septum (1).

Tip deformities and nasal obstruction can be a result of irregularities in the shape and rigidity of the lower lateral cartilages. Two important and frequently overlooked

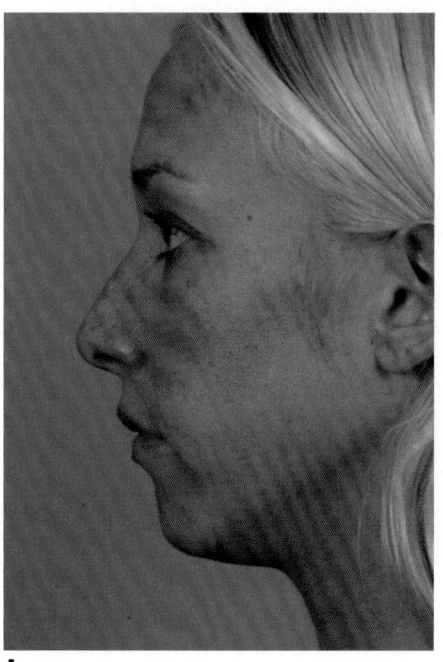

A

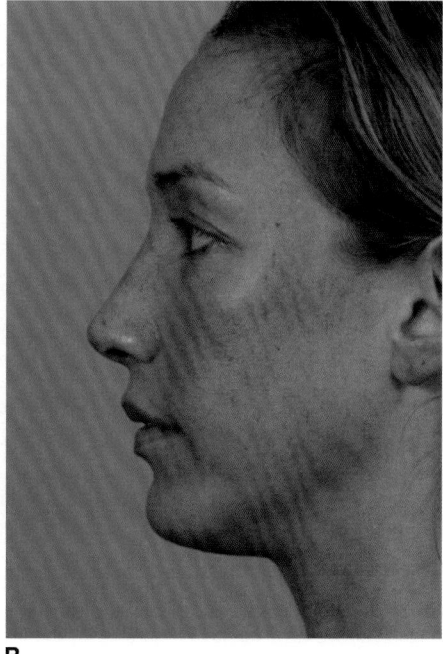

B

Figure 182.10 Demonstration of the value of chin augmentation associated with nasal tip surgery when microgenia accompanies the nasal deformity. Note how the increased postoperative chin projection helps to balance the lateral view and tip projection. The rhinoplasty involved dorsal hump reduction, nasal tip setback to decrease projection, and dome sutures with lateral crural strut grafts. **A**: Before surgery. **B**: After surgery.

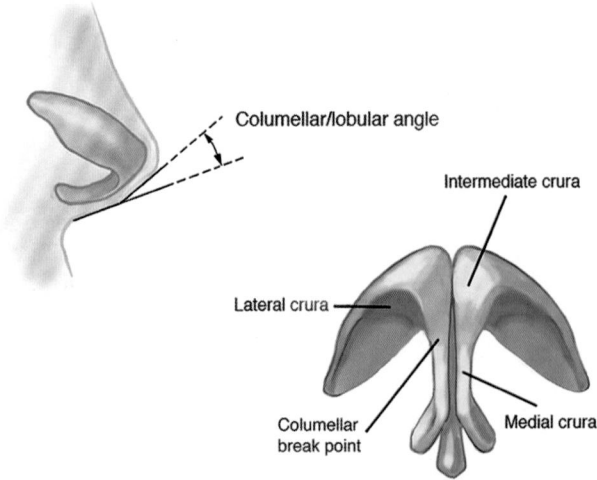

Figure 182.11 The double break is formed by the natural divergence of the intermediate crura. The columellar lobular angle is formed by the intermediate crura diverging into the lateral crura.

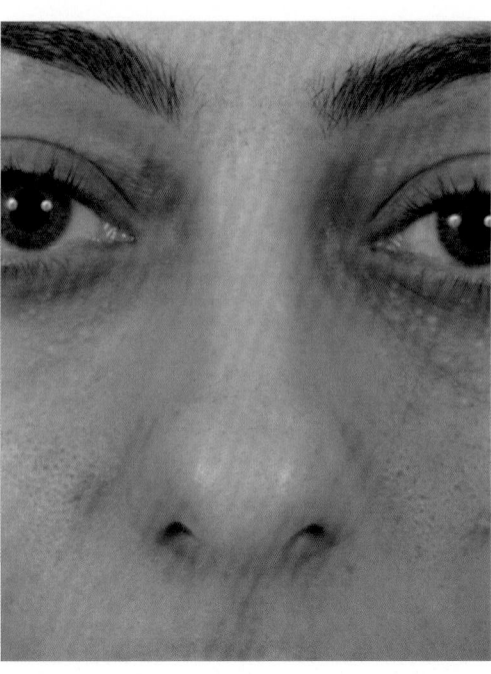

Figure 182.13 Cephalic positioning of the lateral crura often appears as a bulbous tip with a "parentheses" appearance on frontal view.

tip deformities are cephalically positioned lateral crura and internal curvature of the lateral crura. Cephalically positioned lateral crura are often the cause of a dynamic airway obstruction because of poor support of the lateral nasal wall. A hypermobile nasal sidewall is susceptible to collapse on inspiration, which narrows the internal nasal valve. Aesthetically, cephalic positioning of the lateral crura often appears as a bulbous tip with a "parentheses" appearance on frontal view (Fig. 182.13). This is because the shadow in the supratip area is lost due to

the underlying lateral crura, and due to poor lateral wall support, the horizontally oriented tip highlight does not extend onto the alae. The lateral crura may be too long and recurve into the airway creating a bulge on the internal vestibular surface of the lateral nasal wall (Fig. 182.14). This,

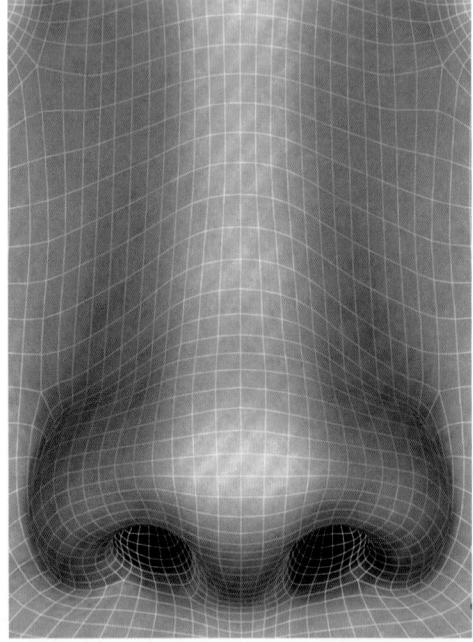

Figure 182.12 The aesthetically pleasing nasal tip has a horizontally oriented tip highlight that gradually transitions to the alae without a deep shadow. There is also a subtle shadow in the supratip region that continues laterally into the supra-alar groove, representing the supratip break.

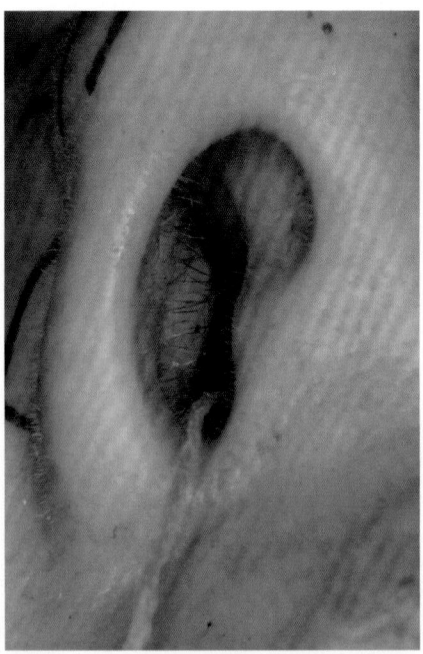

Figure 182.14 When lateral crura are too long, they can recurve into the airway, creating a bulge on the internal vestibular surface of the lateral nasal wall and cause obstruction of the nasal valve.

too, diminishes lateral wall support and can cause a static obstruction. Before formulating a plan for operating on the nasal tip, the surgeon must first accurately analyze the underlying structure that is responsible for the patient's deformity.

PREOPERATIVE PLANNING

Standardized photography is mandatory for any surgeon committed to learning from experience. It also allows the surgeon to communicate more effectively with the patient about the goals and techniques of the planned operation. Computer imaging software permits morphing or side-by-side evaluation of the preoperative and planned postoperative states. In addition, many surgeons print the manipulated images to use as a guide during surgery. Please refer to Chapter 171 for a more detailed review of the use of photography in facial plastic surgery.

In the operating room, it is helpful to mark the patient before injecting local anesthetic. The distorting effects of local anesthesia and intraoperative edema can mask many of the asymmetries and contour irregularities that should be addressed by the surgery.

SURGICAL TECHNIQUES

Stabilizing the Nasal Base

Before meaningful changes can be made to the tip lobule, the surgeon must create a stable foundation at the nasal base. The nasal base is composed of the caudal septum and its soft tissue attachments to the lower lateral cartilages. The major tip support mechanisms are (a) the strength, size, and shape of the alar cartilages; (b) the attachment of the medial crura to the septum; and (c) the attachment between the cephalic edge of the lower lateral cartilages to the upper lateral cartilages (Fig. 182.2). Patients at risk for postoperative loss of tip projection are those with weak lower lateral cartilages, a short caudal septum, and short medial crura. If the base is not stabilized, the surgeon must overcorrect projection and rotation in anticipation of postoperative loss of projection. This degree of overcorrection is based on the surgeon's best estimate of what he believes the postoperative loss in projection will be. Proper stabilization of the base enables the surgeon to place the nasal tip in the desired position and avoids postoperative loss of tip projection (1). Precise, predictable control of tip projection therefore removes much of the guesswork from rhinoplasty. The hallmark of a tip that is poorly supported is the pollybeak deformity. When the tip deprojects postoperatively, the tip–supratip relationship is reversed. The ideally concave supratip break becomes an unattractive convexity. This tempts some surgeons to overresect the septum in order to prevent this deformity. This, however, also results in an unnatural outcome where the

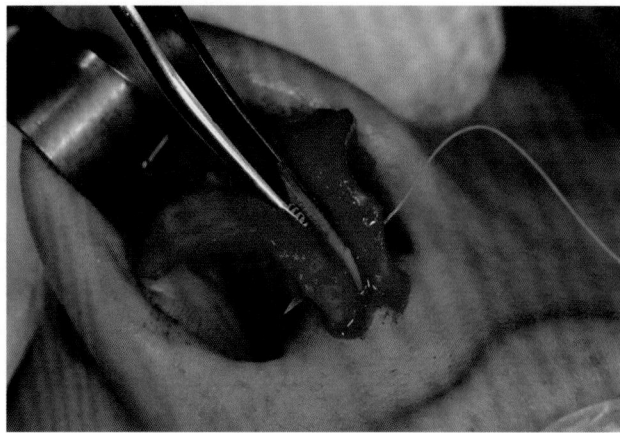

Figure 182.15 A columellar strut is placed by dissecting a pocket between the medial crura and suturing it in the midline.

nose is inadequately projected and wide or poorly defined on the frontal view.

Detailed examination of the nasal base is important to identify the necessary steps to stabilize the base and set the tip in the desired location. If the base is well supported by long medial crura, and the alar–columellar relationship is appropriate, a sutured in place columellar strut can effectively stabilize the base (4,5). This is also a good technique for reinforcing medial crura that are in good position but are buckled or warped. A columellar strut should be 5 to 12 mm in length and 3 to 6 mm wide. Ideally, a strut is less than 3 mm thick. It is placed by dissecting a pocket between the medial crura and suturing it in the midline (Fig. 182.15). The strut should not extend to the nasal spine because this can lead to clicking if it slides from side to side. A floating strut will not increase projection but will support the medial crura in their contribution to a stable nasal base.

In contrast to a floating columellar strut, an extended columellar strut is beneficial to use in patients with an underprojected tip caused by poor tip support. The extended columellar strut usually sits on the premaxilla or is suture fixated into a notch made in the nasal spine (Fig.182.16). Similarly, an extended strut can interdigitate with a premaxillary graft. This is especially helpful in patients whose poor projection is a result of inadequate tip support and a deficient premaxilla, such as those with a cleft-lip nasal deformity. The medial crura can then be advanced anteriorly and fixed in a more projected position. Often, the soft tissue over the anterior nasal spine needs to be dissected free to permit advancement of the nasal base. This also has the effect of softening the nasolabial angle. A consequence of fixing the extended columellar strut to the nasal spine is that it may prohibit upward movement of the upper lip creating a crease in the upper lip when the patient smiles. Patients with an exaggerated upward elevation of the corner of their mouth when they smile are at the highest risk for a change in their smile with an extended columellar strut.

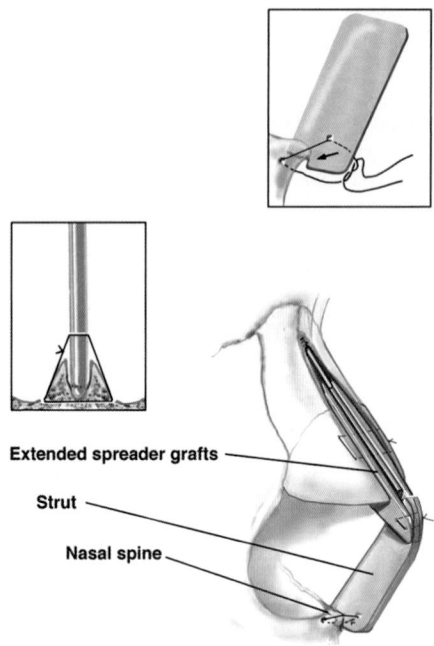

Figure 182.16 The extended columellar strut usually sits on the premaxilla or is suture fixated into a notch made in the nasal spine. The strut is placed end to end with the septum and stabilized with extended spreader grafts.

Patients who have a hanging columella and an overly long caudal septum are good candidates for fixation of the medial crura to the septum. This is done by dissecting between the medial crura to provide access to the septum. A septoplasty is easily performed through this approach by elevating bilateral mucoperichondrial flaps. The medial crura are then positioned on the caudal septum in a tongue-in-groove manner with a 4-0 chromic mattress suture (6) (Fig. 182.17). Once the tip position is satisfactory, a 5-0 polydioxanone (PDS) suture is passed through the medial surfaces of the medial crura and the septum. A 4-0 plain gut suture on a Keith needle is then used to quilt the septal mucoperichondrial flaps and redistribute any excess mucosa.

Bunching of the mucosa is a potential pitfall in patients with an overprojected tip or hanging columella. Wide undermining of the flaps around the nasal spine allows the mucosa to be moved superiorly and nearly always precludes the need to resect mucosa or vestibular skin. Fixation of the medial crura in this manner provides excellent support for the nasal tip. It also affords precise control of the tip projection, rotation, and alar–columellar relationship without having to excise mucosa or estimate the amount of postoperative tip settling. This maneuver is suited to patients with a tension-nose deformity, overprojected tip, underprojected tip, or hanging columella. If using this technique, the surgeon must avoid creating a retracted columella, obtuse columella-labial angle, or overrotated nose. These pitfalls can be avoided by restricting this technique to those patients who have an inappropriately long caudal septum that would otherwise need to be trimmed.

Alternately, if the caudal septum is short or of appropriate length but tip position must be altered or stabilized, a caudal extension graft can be used to create a septum long enough to bind to the medial crura in the midline (7). This is a graft that can be sutured end to end or overlapped with the caudal septum, depending on whether it is in the midline. End-to-end grafts are stabilized with extended spreader grafts (Figs. 182.16 and 182.18) or two sets of bilateral splinting grafts sutured with 5-0 PDS sutures. Another suture through the periosteum of the anterior nasal spine greatly improves the sturdiness of an inline graft. A slightly deviated caudal septum can be lengthened with an overlapping graft. The graft is secured to the caudal septum with horizontal mattress sutures. Regardless of the technique used, the caudal margin of the graft should be in

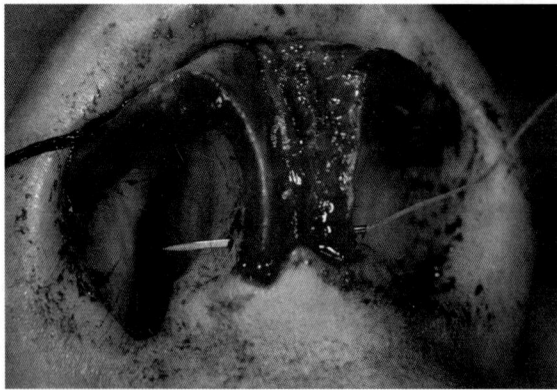

Figure 182.17 Repositioning the medial crura to set tip position and stabilize the nasal base.

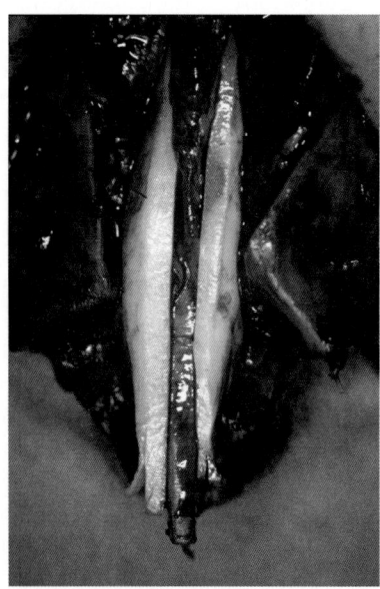

Figure 182.18 Inline caudal extension graft with splinting cartilage grafts.

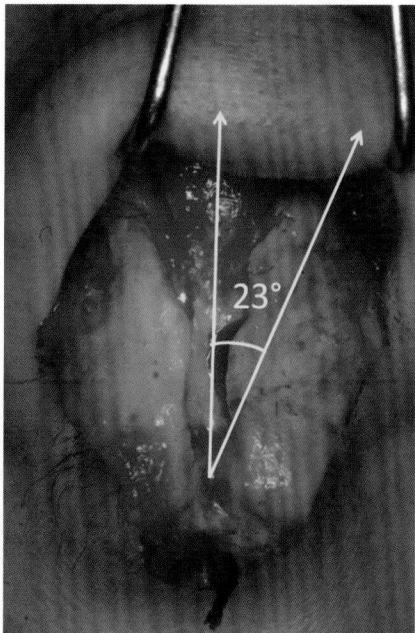
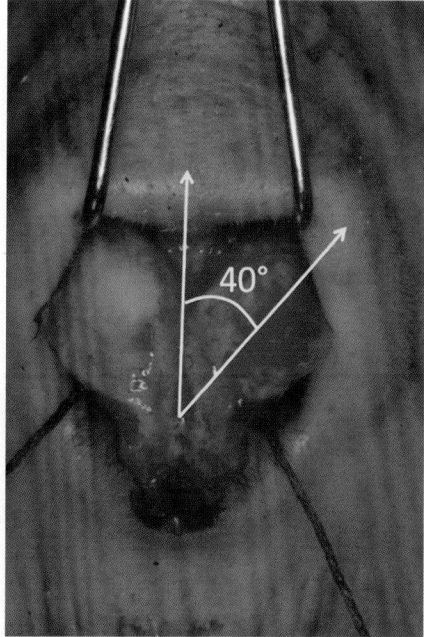

Figure 182.19 The ideal lateral crura are positioned so that they are pointing toward the lateral canthi (35 to 45 degrees off midline). Lateral crura that are oriented less than 30 degrees off of midline will tend to create a fullness in the transition point between the tip and supratip and in some patients may present with a parentheses deformity.

the midline. The lengthening of the caudal septum allows suture fixation of the medial crura to the graft to stabilize the nasal base. End-to-end grafts are preferred because they are less likely to cause deviation or airway obstruction (4). Orientation of the caudal extension graft is an important detail in its placement. If the graft is trapezoidal and has its longer edge posteriorly, it will help to open an acute nasolabial angle. A longer anterior edge will counter rotate the tip. A rectangular graft is helpful in correcting a retracted columella.

Nasal Tip Surgery

Once a solid foundation has been created at the nasal base, the tip can be modified. Following is a brief overview of some common structural techniques for improving the aesthetic contour and proportions of the nasal tip. The most important step of nasal tip surgery is the accurate assessment of the tip structures and their contribution to the tip shape. It is important to note the horizontal (dome to dome) and vertical (caudal margin to cephalic margin of the lateral crura) contributions to the tip bulbosity (1). The surgeon must also assess whether the lateral crura are oriented properly. The ideal lateral crura are positioned so that they are pointing toward the lateral canthi (35 to 45 degrees off midline) (1). Lateral crura that are oriented less than 30 degrees off of midline will tend to create a fullness in the transition point between the tip and supratip and in some patients may present with a parentheses deformity (Fig. 182.19).

If the tip cartilages are too wide in the vertical plane with normally positioned crura, there will be supratip fullness on lateral view. This can be corrected with a conservative cephalic trim of the lateral crura, leaving 8 to 10 mm of the lateral crus (4) (Fig. 182.20). The cephalic trim should be performed medially because this is the area that contributes to a bulbous tip. Trimming laterally will have little effect on the tip and will only weaken the nasal sidewall, risking supra-alar pinching with scar contracture over time (4).

Once the appropriate vertical dimensions of the nasal tip are achieved, the horizontal dimensions can be addressed. Dome-binding sutures are an excellent way to decrease horizontal width of the nasal tip in primary

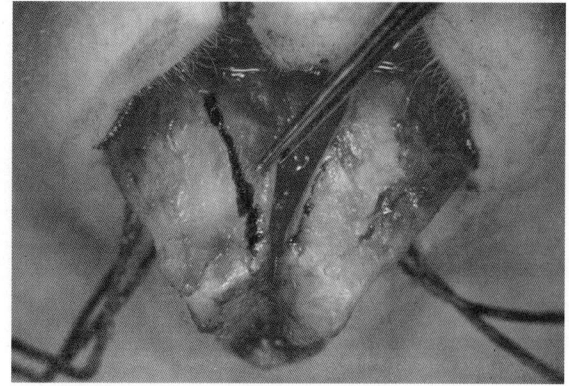

Figure 182.20 Medial-cephalic reduction of the alar cartilages, maintaining a generous residual complete strip.

rhinoplasty patients (Fig. 182.21). Using two separate dome sutures is usually preferred over a single transdomal suture, to prevent pinching of the domes together (Fig. 182.22) (1,4). The sutures are placed in a horizontal mattress fashion with the knots medially between the domes. Caution must be exercised to prevent bringing the domes too close together, as this will cause flattening of the double break on lateral view, and an excessively narrow tip with vertical orientation of the normal horizontal orientation of the nasal tip highlight (4). This will therefore give an unnatural appearance to the nasal tip. Dome sutures also have effects laterally on the lateral crura. The objective is to create flat lateral crura that will provide the desired contour between the tip lobule and the lateral alae. If the crura do not flatten properly but instead buckle or deform with placement of the suture, this can cause pinching at the junction between the tip lobule and the alar lobule. In this case, the lateral crus can be

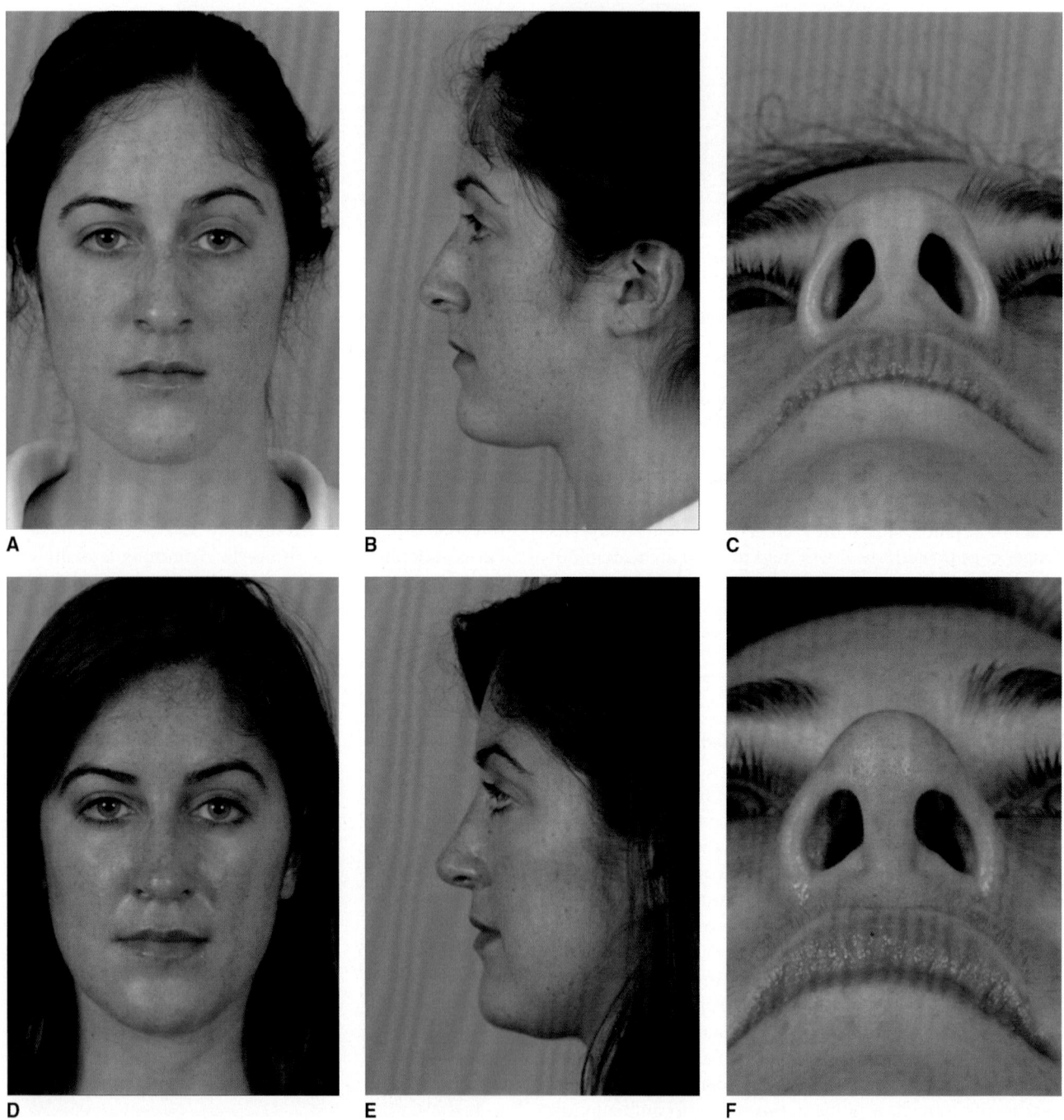

Figure 182.21 Narrowing of the tip with dome-binding sutures **(A,B,C)** before and **(D,E,F)** after procedure.

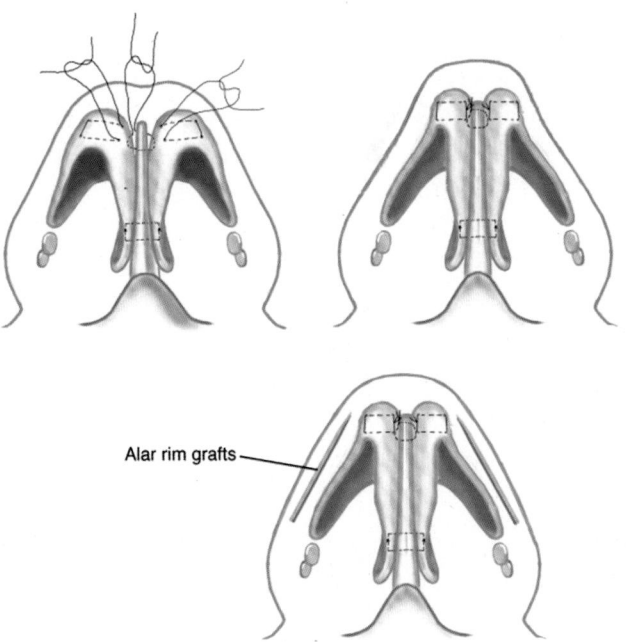

Figure 182.22 Separate dome-binding sutures are applied as shown with the knots tied between the domes. In many cases a separate interdomal suture is placed to bring the domes closer together. If necessary alar rim grafts can be placed to eliminate any pinching of the nasal tip.

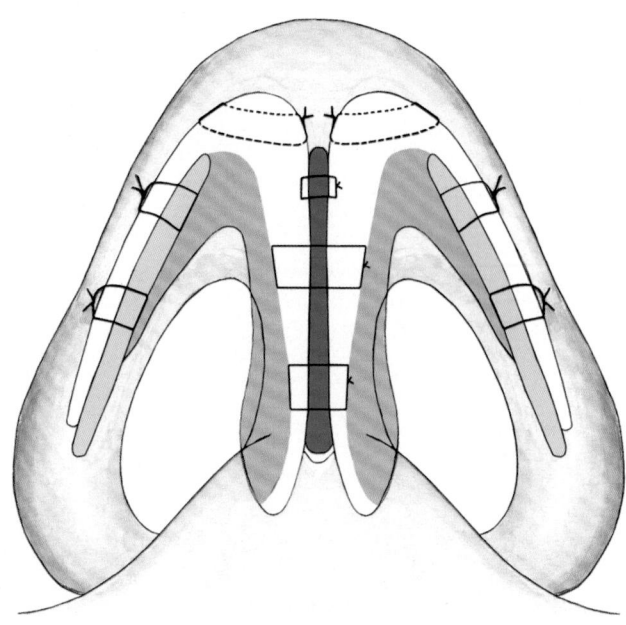

Figure 182.23 Lateral crural strut grafts (*light blue*) are placed between the undersurface of the lateral crura and the vestibular skin. The graft acts to flatten the bulbous lateral crura and also support the lateral wall of the nose. After positioning the lateral crural strut grafts bilateral dome-binding sutures are placed to set tip width.

strengthened and straightened by suturing a lateral crural strut graft onto its undersurface (Fig. 182.23) (4). This prevents nasal obstruction and creates a smooth triangular shape to the nasal base.

Lateral crural strut grafts can be used to accomplish several goals (8). They are useful in flattening lateral crura that are bulbous or intranasally blocking the internal airway (Fig. 182.24). When the lateral crura are of an appropriate length but lack the stiffness for appropriate lateral wall support, lateral crura strut grafts are a good option. Lateral crura strut grafts are usually created from stiffer cartilage from the septum or rib. Their length depends on the needs of the graft. Longer grafts are used when lateral wall collapse is a problem or when correcting alar retraction. These grafts are typically 20 to 30 mm in length, 3 to 4 mm wide, and 1 to 2 mm thick. Local anesthetic should be injected to hydrodissect the plane beneath the lateral crus. Several minutes after injection, a pocket can be dissected from the cephalic margin of the lateral crus between the cartilage and the vestibular skin. The graft is then placed in the pocket and affixed with several 5-0 PDS mattress sutures with the knots placed above the lateral crus. When reinforcing the lateral crura with lateral crural strut grafts, more of the lateral crura can be removed without compromising the support of the nose.

Often there is a lack of support lateral to the tip in the alar margin. This disruption of the favorable triangular shape of the base creates shadows that make the tip appear to be separate from the alae (Fig. 182.25).

The cause of poor support in this area can be cephalic positioning of the lateral crura or prior tip modifications. Alar rim grafts can be used to correct this pinched look (9). These are narrow cartilage grafts that are usually 5 to 8 mm in length, 2 to 3 mm in width, and 1 to 2 mm thick. They are placed in pockets along the caudal aspect of the marginal incision (Fig. 182.26). Alar rim grafts should be softer than other grafts because they are susceptible to becoming visible medially if they extend into the tip. After placing the grafts in the pockets, they are fixed with 6-0 Monocryl suture at the medial aspect. The area medial to the suture should be gently morselized with a Brown-Adson forceps to further minimize the likelihood of graft visibility. Grafts that are too stiff also tend to be visible and sometimes palpable. Alar rim grafts are also an effective way to correct external valve collapse. However, it is important to realize that alar rim grafts can cause alar flare and increase the size of the nostril. As a consequence there is an increased need for alar base reduction in patients with alar rim grafts (4).

Patients who have malpositioning of the lateral crura require a completely different approach to changing the nasal tip contour. To address the "parentheses" appearance on frontal view from bulbous cephalically positioned crura, one can perform a cephalic trim and place dome sutures with or without lateral crural strut grafts. If the lateral crura are not sufficiently flattened, then the lateral crura can be repositioned caudally. To accomplish this cephalic trim is performed followed by dissection of the

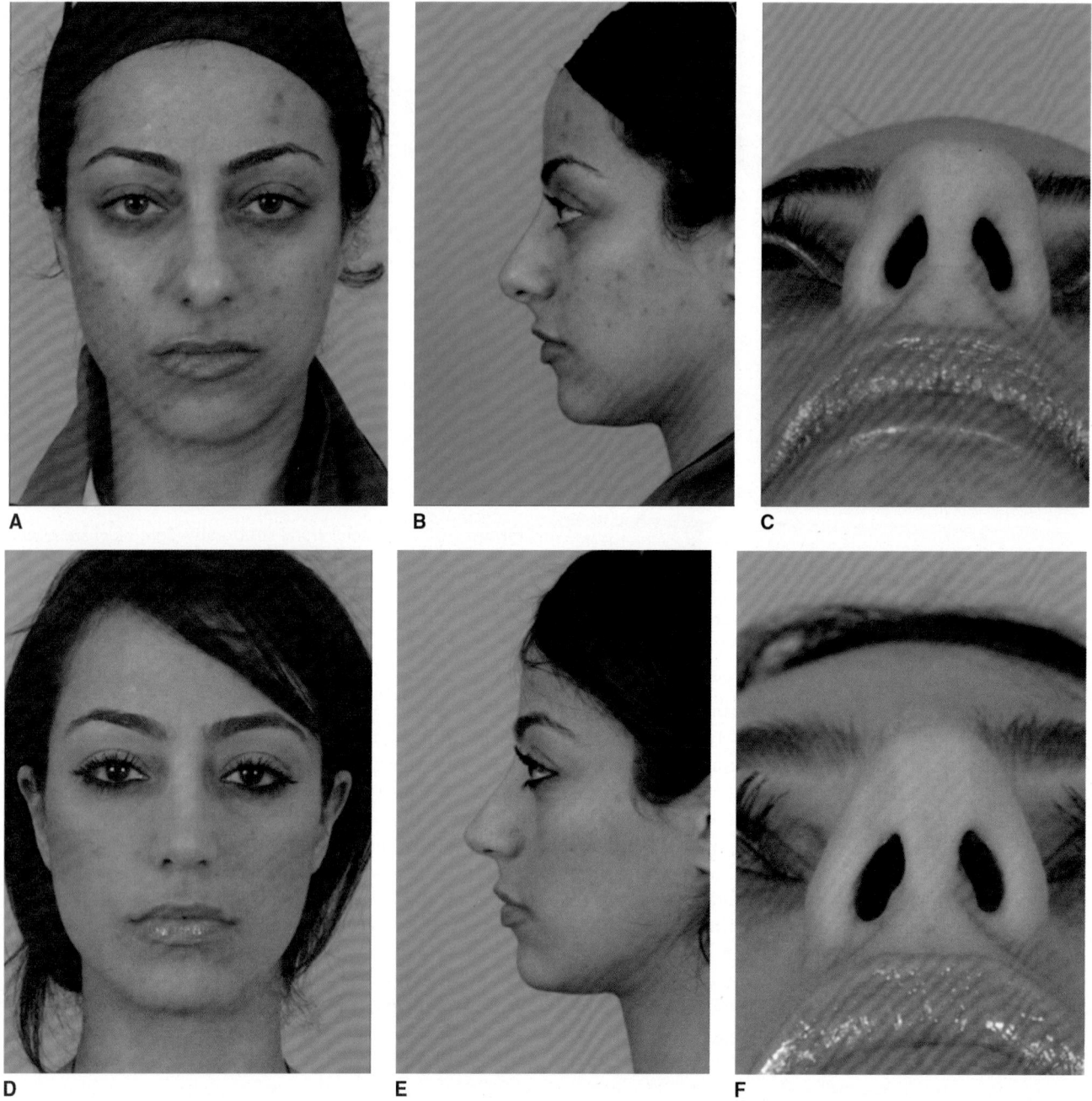

Figure 182.24 Bulbous tip **(A,B,C)** before lateral crural strut grafts and **(D,E,F)** after procedure.

lateral crura from the vestibular skin, suture lateral crural grafts to the undersurfaces of the lateral crura, and then reposition the lateral crura into caudally positioned pockets (1). This eliminates the supratip fullness and decreases fullness in the supra-alar region while increasing support along the alar margin. It also places supportive cartilage along the sidewall of the nose and prevents lateral wall collapse (1).

To provide additional tip projection and definition, tip onlay grafts can be used. These are soft cartilage grafts trimmed into a rectangular or elliptical shape to simulate the ideal tip highlight and are sutured over the domes in a horizontal orientation. It is important to gently crush the cartilage to prevent the graft from becoming visible postoperatively (4).

In some patients with weak or diminutive lower lateral cartilages that will not achieve the desired tip projection with sutures and onlay grafts, shield grafts can be used (1). Shield grafts are primarily used in secondary rhinoplasty, augmentation rhinoplasty, or in primary rhinoplasty patients who have an underprojected tip with thick skin and a deficient tip lobule (1). A shield graft is attached to the medial crura in the infratip lobule (Fig. 182.27). The posterior edge should have a shallow bevel to allow

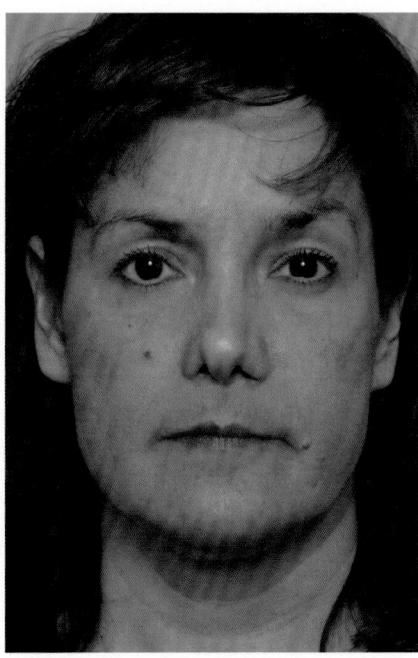

Figure 182.25 Example of alar rim and supra-alar pinching as a result of weakening the nose.

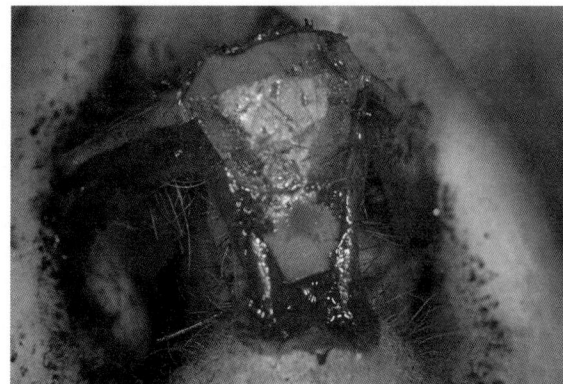

Figure 182.27 Shield graft affixed to the medial crura.

the contour of the graft to blend with the caudal edge of the medial crura. Because the purpose of the graft is to push into the tip skin to increase projection, no matter how much the anterior edge is beveled, a risk exists of the graft being visible after surgery. Because of this, the authors avoid using shield grafts in thin-skinned patients (10). Although thick-skinned patients are tolerant of shield grafts, medium-skinned patients should have some sort of camouflage of the leading edge. Perichondrium and fascia are excellent materials for softening the contours of a shield graft. Several layers can be used to prevent visibility of the graft in the long term. A buttress or cap graft is another method for camouflaging a shield graft (5,10).

This graft is a small rectangle of cartilage that is sutured to the cephalic edge of the shield graft and stabilizes it while providing a smoother transition between the shield and the domes.

Sometimes the lateral crura are so misshapen or overresected that lateral crural grafts are appropriate for reconstruction (5,10). Lateral crural grafts are also a good way to camouflage a shield graft that projects more than 3 mm above the domes, whether or not the lateral crura need structural reinforcement. These grafts create a transitional structure that bridges a shield graft to the lateral crura and simultaneously provides lateral support to the tip (Fig. 182.28). Lateral crural grafts are sutured to the anterolateral margin of a shield graft with a 6-0 Monocryl suture. A 6-0 Monocryl suture is placed laterally to secure the lateral crural graft to the existing lateral crus.

The importance of tip cartilage camouflage cannot be overemphasized. Although postoperative edema can be present for years after surgery, the surgeon should anticipate that eventually the edema will resolve and potentially reveal the underlying structure of the tip.

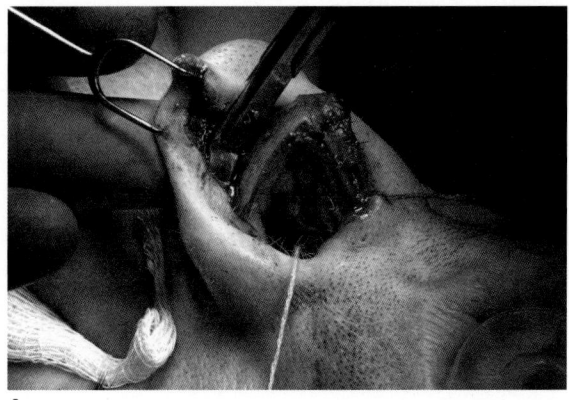

A

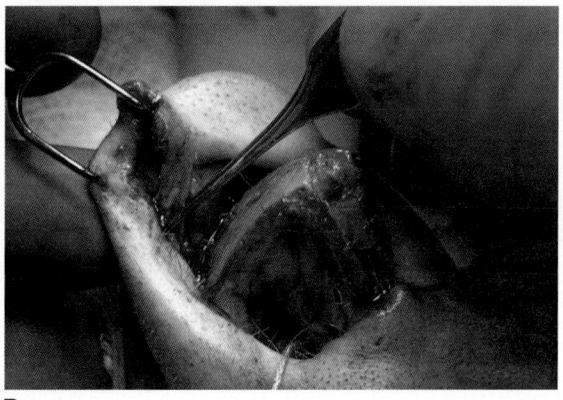

B

Figure 182.26 Proper insertion of alar rim grafts.

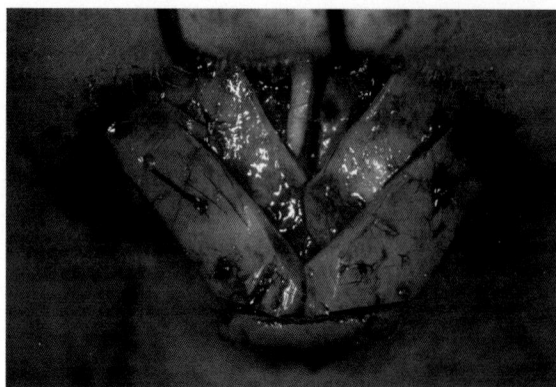

Figure 182.28 Lateral crural grafts conjoined with a shield graft.

Perichondrium from an auricular or costal cartilage graft is an excellent material for covering tip grafts (Fig. 182.29). Patients should be warned that the use of perichondrium will result in prolonged postoperative edema in the tip. In thin-skinned patients, this is favorable and should be described to patients as such. Once the postoperative edema resolves, the tip will have a soft, natural contour.

Surgery of the nasal tip is a challenging endeavor and fraught with pitfalls. Mastery of surgical technique must be paired with a clear understanding of the three-dimensional topography of the natural-appearing nasal tip. The goal should be to preserve the horizontally oriented tip highlight that transitions from tip lobule to alar lobule. This result is best accomplished by stabilizing the base of the nose, conservatively suturing the tip, and applying appropriate grafting techniques (1). These techniques will enable the surgeon to have more predictable long-term results and achieve a more natural postoperative outcome.

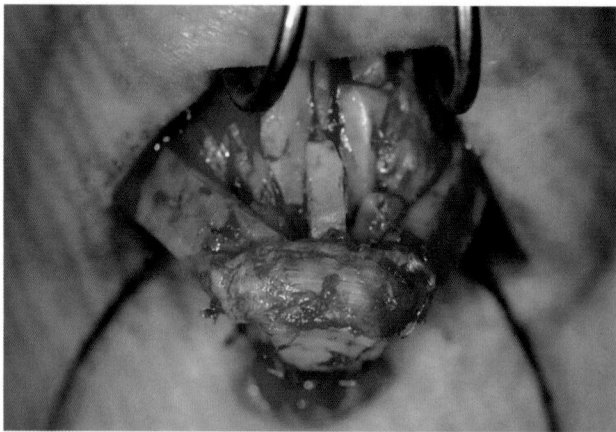

Figure 182.29 Perichondrium covering nasal tip grafts to prevent postoperative graft visibility.

HIGHLIGHTS

- The focus of nasal tip contouring should be more on creating favorable shadows and highlights and less on narrowing.
- Removal of structurally supportive tissue weakens the nose.
- Thick-skinned patients often need their tip structures projected into the skin–soft tissue envelope.
- Thin-skinned patients benefit from preservation of dome continuity and need extensive soft tissue camouflage of any cartilage grafts to prevent them from becoming visible.
- The tripod model provides the basis for understanding changes in rotation and projection.
- Before making any meaningful changes to the tip, first stabilize the nasal base.
- Vertical contributions to tip bulbosity can be addressed with a conservative cephalic trim of the lateral crura.
- Horizontal contributions to tip bulbosity can be corrected with two separate dome-binding sutures.
- Perichondrium and fascia are valuable materials for tip graft camouflage.
- Patients must understand that their noses will change over many years as the forces of scar contracture act on the supportive structures.

REFERENCES

1. Toriumi DM. New concepts in nasal tip contouring. *Arch Facial Plast Surg* 2006;8:156–185.
2. Tardy ME. Rhinoplasty: the art and the science. Philadelphia, PA: W.B. Saunders, 1996.
3. Anderson JR. The dynamics of rhinoplasty. In Proceedings of the Ninth International Congress of Otolaryngology Excerpta Medica International Congress Series, No. 206. Amsterdam, The Netherlands: Excerpta Medica, 1969:708–710.
4. Toriumi DM, Checcone MA. New concepts in nasal tip contouring. *Facial Plast Surg Clin North Am* 2009;17:55–90.
5. Johnson CM, Toriumi DM. *Open structure rhinoplasty*. Philadelphia, PA: WB Saunders, 1989;1:1–22.
6. Kridel RW, Scott BA, Foda HM. The tongue-in-groove technique in septorhinoplasty. A 10-year experience. *Arch Facial Plast Surg* 1999;1:246–256.
7. Toriumi DM. Caudal extension graft for correction of the retracted columella. *Oper Tech Otolaryngol Head Neck Surg* 1995;6:311–318.
8. Gunter JP, Friedman RM. Lateral crural strut graft: technique and clinical applications in rhinoplasty. *Plast Reconstr Surg* 1997;99:943–955.
9. Rohrich RJ, Raniere J Jr, Ha RY. The alar contour graft: correction and prevention of alar rim deformities in rhinoplasty. *Plast Reconstr Surg* 2002;109(7):2495–2505.
10. Toriumi DM, Johnson CM. Open structure rhinoplasty: featured technical points and long-term follow-up. *Facial Plast Surg Clin North Am* 1993;1:1–22.

Management of the Crooked Nose

183

Craig S. Murakami   *Richard A. Zoumalan*

The treatment of a crooked nose remains one of the most challenging problems in rhinoplasty surgery. Inadequate treatment can cause a persistent cosmetic deformity as well as problems with nasal obstruction. There are many techniques currently available for correction of the crooked nasal deformity. Regardless of the method used, revision rates remain significantly high. Patients differ in their goals for surgery, and it is essential that the surgeon understand their needs. While some patients are focused on the aesthetic outcome, others are more concerned with functional improvement. More commonly, patients have a combination of cosmetic and functional concerns.

ETIOLOGY

The crooked nose can be due to congenital, traumatic, or iatrogenic etiologies. A congenitally crooked nose is often associated with overall facial asymmetry. Sometimes the asymmetry is associated with a known syndrome. However, most patients have mild asymmetry that is nonsyndromic. The patient should be informed about these facial asymmetries preoperatively and made aware of how this may or may not affect their outcome. Treatment of the congenitally crooked nose can be difficult since the surrounding deviation of the internal and external facial framework makes it difficult to find a common midline.

Traumatic crooked noses can be the result of a low velocity force that causes a simple unilateral infracturing of the affected nasal wall or a higher velocity force that causes bilateral nasal wall deviations along with deviation of the septum. Severe nasal injuries may also be associated with deformities of the orbits or maxilla.

Iatrogenic crooked nasal deformities caused by previous surgery may be the result of poorly executed osteotomies, excessive resection of bone or cartilage, and/or poor wound healing. The nose can sometimes heal in unpredictable ways due to the effects of soft tissue contracture, cartilage memory, severe bone and cartilage asymmetries, aging, glasses, gravity, and so on.

A severely deviated nose almost always has a major septal deformity. Treating the deviated internal septum is usually necessary to facilitate correction of the deviated external nasal component (1–3). The nasal septum has a syndesmosis between the quadrangular cartilage and bones of the vomer and ethmoid that is unique in the human body. Cartilage growth occurs in the perichondrium of the anterior bony septum without eventual ossification (4). Disruption of this process *in utero* or during childhood can result in the loss of vertical growth. This disruption also has implications in pediatric nasal surgery, as violation of the posterior septum at this junction and the bony septum can have deleterious impact on the growth center of the septum.

HISTORY AND PHYSICAL

Making an accurate diagnosis is central to the management of the crooked nose, as there are many potential configurations of crooked noses. The surgeon must begin with a detailed history and physical examination, paying careful attention to all aspects of the nose. The history should include information regarding the patient's medical conditions, previous nasal surgery, nasal trauma, nasal airway, allergies, and drug and tobacco use. The mechanism of injury may be helpful to know, as it will help to separate the traumatic deviations from the congenital ones. If a patient had previous surgery, it is sometimes helpful to obtain previous operative report and radiographic studies.

To begin the examination, the surgeon should first establish the midline of the face as defined by a vertical line through the menton, the upper incisors, the philtrum, and the glabella. Figure 183.1 shows how a vertical line drawn through from the glabella, through the philtrum, and through the menton can give the doctor a sense of whether the nose is crooked. It can also help identify asymmetries

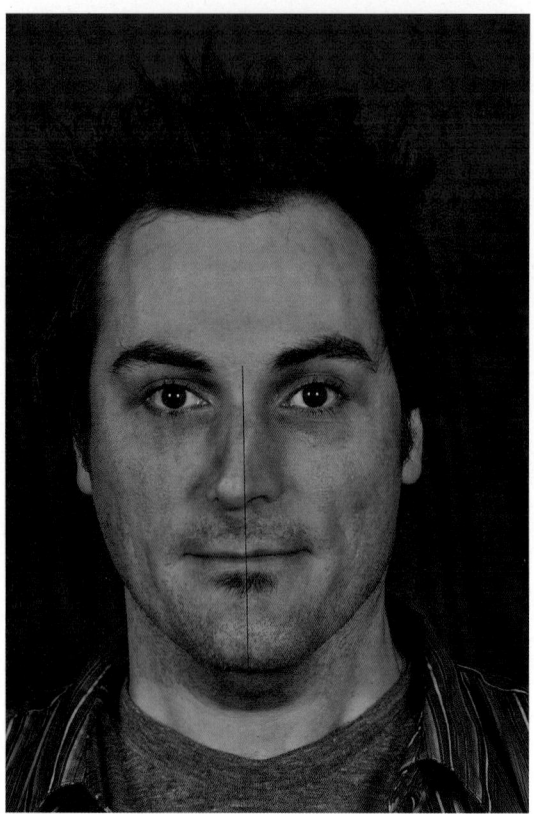

Figure 183.1 A *vertical line* is drawn from the glabella, through the philtrum, and then through the menton. This line can help identify asymmetries and deviations. One can see that the deviation of the nose lies in the middle and lower third of the nose. In this patient, the vertical lines allow the viewer to see asymmetry of the mandible and midface. His left side is stronger and has more volume than his right side.

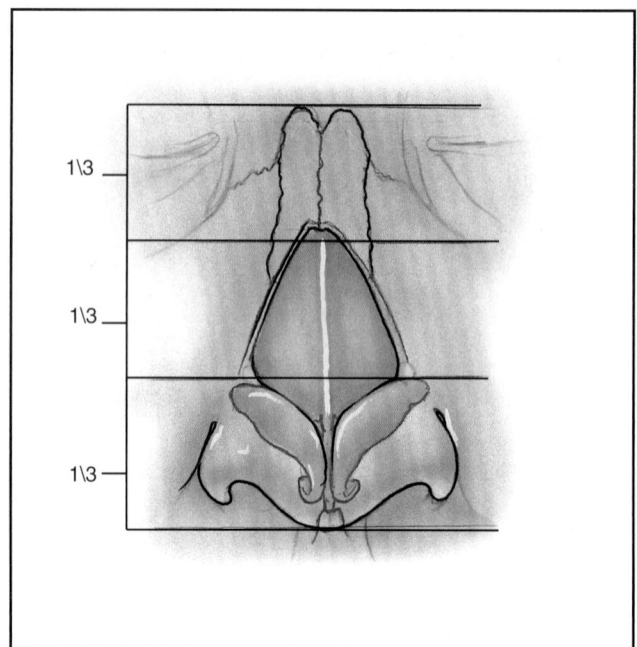

Figure 183.2 The nose can be divided into thirds. This is central to diagnosis and treatment of a crooked nose. The components of the thirds can be seen in this illustration.

A thorough endonasal exam should be completed in a systematic manner to determine the position, health, and function of the nasal septum, turbinates, the internal and external nasal valves, and nasal mucosa. The patient should be observed while taking normal and accentuated breaths through the nasal airway. The examiner will often see external evidence of nasal valve collapse, and

of the face that were previously unrecognized. The nose is then divided into thirds, that is, the upper, middle, and lower thirds (see Fig. 183.2). For the most part, we can generally say that the upper third is composed of the nasal bones, the middle third is composed of the septum and upper lateral cartilages, and the lower third is the septal angle and lower lateral cartilages. Each third is individually examined in relation to the midline or relative midline. The thirds are classified into right, left, or center of midline. Given the number of possibilities, there are theoretically 26 permutations of crooked noses. The 27th possibility is a center–center–center nose, which is a straight nose. Half of these permutations are mirror images of each other. Figure 183.3 demonstrates five of these permutations (5).

The surgeon should palpate the nose carefully to feel the thickness of the skin and the position of the bones and cartilage and determine tip strength. Convexities, concavities, and buckles in the cartilage can also be determined using palpation. Tip support is determined by manually compressing the tip. Additionally, the surgeon should feel the caudal septum and the septal angle to assess its strength and integrity, as well as the position of the septum in relation to the midline.

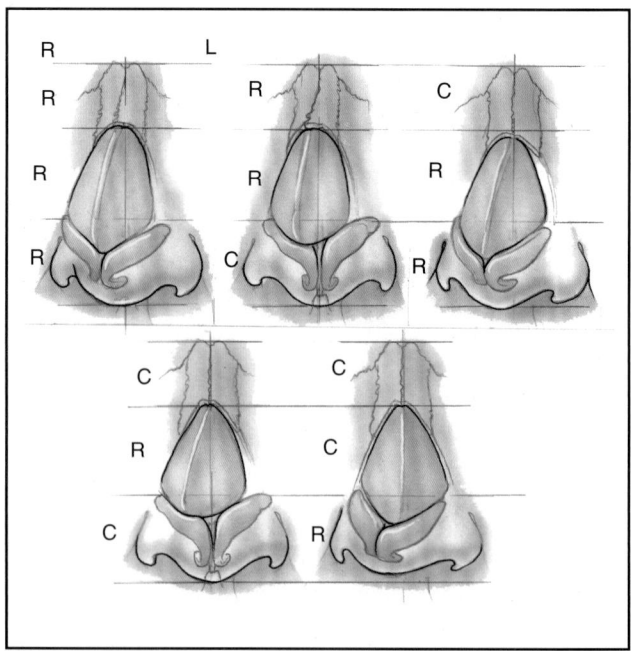

Figure 183.3 Artist-rendered images of five different permutations of crooked noses. There are 26 possible configurations.

the area of collapse should be noted. The nasal mucosa should be initially examined without decongestion. This helps assess whether there is an allergic or reactive component. Finally, the nasal mucosa must be decongested with either oxymetazoline or 0.25% Neo-Synephrine. The decongestion may reveal posterior and high dorsal septal deflections that may have been previously hidden by inflamed mucosa. If there is history of previous surgery or trauma, the septum should be palpated with a cotton tip applicator or cerumen loop to determine if the septal cartilage is missing or deficient. In a severely deviated nose, the full extent of the septum may not be able to be visualized without a fiberoptic device. The size of the turbinates must also be analyzed, as many patients can benefit from concomitant turbinoplasty. If the patient has a history that suggests chronic sinusitis, a CT scan may be of benefit.

A careful examination of the integrity of the internal and external nasal valve should be performed. When a patient inspires deeply, a weak internal valve can be seen externally by a depression just above the nasal ala or along the piriform aperture. The external valve is composed of the lateral crura, the suspensory ligaments of the lateral crura, and the fibromuscular tissue of the ala. Manually retracting the cheek laterally (the Cottle maneuver) can help assess if there is an element of valve insufficiency. This can also be done using a curette to stent open the internal and external nasal valves to independently determine where the weakness lies.

Radiographic assessment is necessary if a patient has signs and symptoms consistent with paranasal sinus disease or has polyposis. They may be also helpful in patients who previously sustained major trauma that required open reduction and internal fixation of the craniofacial skeleton. This surgical hardware will need to be identified prior to surgery, as it may need to be removed before osteotomies can be performed.

Standard rhinoplasty photographs must be taken for medical documentation and to assist with the evaluation and analysis of the patient. These views include the frontal, profile, three-quarter, and base views. The authors also like to take two additional photographs when patients have crooked noses. One is the bird's-eye view, which gives the surgeon more information on the shape of the dorsal line (see Fig. 183.4). The use of overhead flash is preferable as it most closely duplicates overhead sunlight, which accentuates deviations. The other is the three-quarter base view where the entire dorsum and nasal walls are visible in relationship to the nasal base (see Fig. 183.5). Photos must be available and easily visible in the operating room during surgery. Due to local anesthetic injections and surgical edema, asymmetries can become masked or imperceptible. Therefore, the surgeon must periodically refer to these photos during the operation. Postoperative photos are usually taken at 6-month and 1-year intervals to track healing progression.

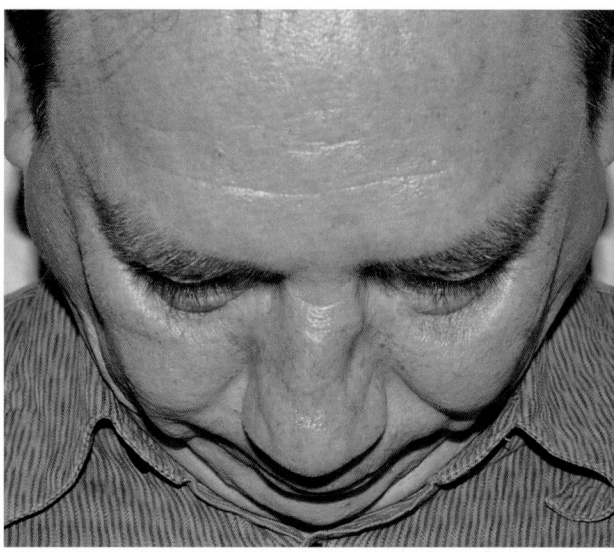

Figure 183.4 This is an example of a bird's-eye view. This allows one to see another perspective of the dorsal line.

TREATMENT STRATEGY

Surgical correction of the deviated nose can be conceptually and strategically divided into the upper third, middle third, and lower third. The upper third is composed of the nasal bones and the frontal process of the maxilla. The middle third is composed of the bony cartilaginous junction (called the keystone), the upper lateral cartilages, and the dorsal septum. The lower third is composed of the caudal septum and the lower lateral cartilages.

Septum

Septoplasty surgery in the crooked nose can be approached through a hemitransfixion incision. This incision allows easy access to both sides of the septum and facilitates easy repositioning of the caudal septum to the facial midline. To best mobilize the septum, separation of the posterior and

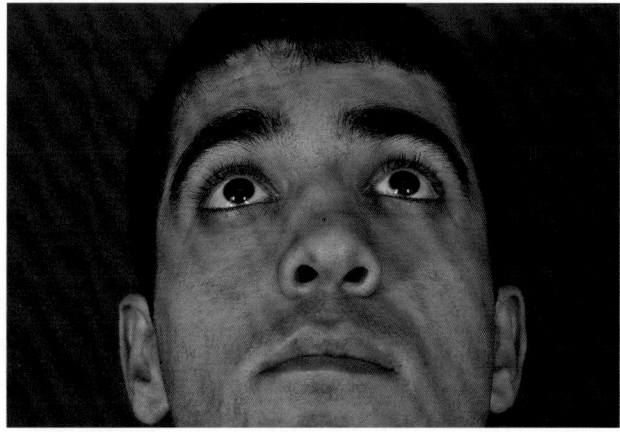

Figure 183.5 This is an example of the three-quarter base view. This view gives a view of the dorsal deviation with relation to the tip.

inferior osseocartilaginous junction plus elevation of the mucoperiosteum of the maxillary crest is often required. Releasing the attachment of the upper lateral cartilages can also help mobilize a septum that is deviated.

A dorsal and caudal "L"-shaped strut must be maintained at least 10 mm in width. The dorsal strut must maintain stable fixation at the superior bony–cartilaginous junction (the key area of the dorsum) to prevent saddling of the middle nasal vault. The caudal septum should also have support from the nasal spine and maxillary crest. Deviated cartilage is either removed or recontoured by scoring the concave side of the deviation with a scalpel. These partial thickness cuts can weaken the septum in a manner that facilitates repositioning toward the midline. Spreader grafts can also help correct deviations of the dorsal septum (see section on correction of middle third). Caudal deviations can be corrected with vertical scoring on the concave side of the septum. Retrograde soft tissue dissection behind the medial crura must be done to create a central pocket in the membranous septum. With severe deviations of the caudal septum, the mucosa is scarred toward the side of the caudal deflection. If a pocket is not made for the newly straightened caudal septum, the contracted mucosa will push the septum back toward the side of the deviation and cause a relapse of the nasal obstruction.

If the septal deviation is severe and the surgeon is unable to correct it through the endonasal or external approach without significantly compromising support to the dorsal or caudal strut, an extracorporeal septoplasty should be performed. In this procedure, the cartilaginous septum is removed, straightened, contoured, and then reimplanted (6). It is important to leave a small portion of the dorsal cartilage in the keystone area (area where the septum articulates with the nasal bones) to provide a point of suture fixation to prevent postoperative collapse of the dorsal septum. The use of a polydioxanone sheet to stabilize the cartilage grafts has been reported to facilitate the extracorporeal technique (7).

If turbinate hypertrophy is present and causing obstruction of nasal airflow, a submucous resection is performed.

Upper Third

Asymmetry of the upper third of the nose is caused by deviation of the upper bony nasal framework. The nasal bones articulate with the frontal bones superiorly and the ascending process of the maxilla laterally. They are thickest at the nasion superiorly and taper to become thinner as they approach the caudal articulations with the upper lateral cartilages. Asymmetry of the upper bony nasal dorsum is often associated with high deviations of the septum. While small deviations can be amenable to rasp reduction or small onlay grafts, osteotomies are typically needed to correct most deviations of the upper third (8). The three primary goals of osteotomies are to straighten a deviated nasal dorsum, narrow the nasal sidewalls, and close or

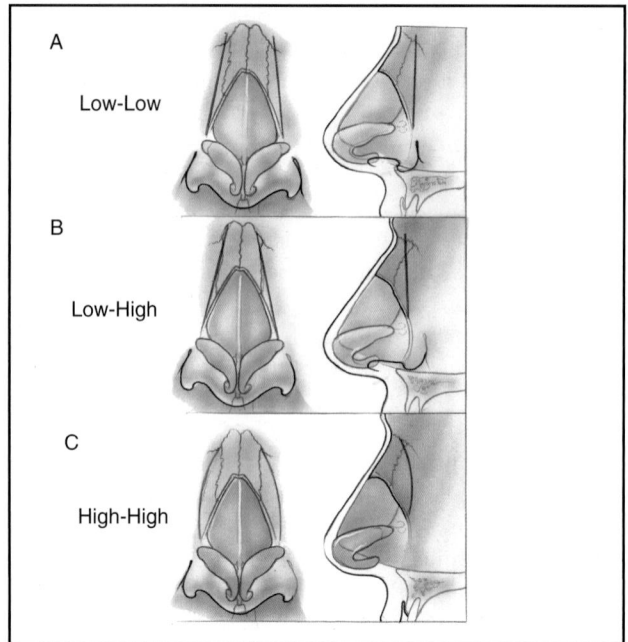

Figure 183.6 This figure shows three different types of osteotomies that can be performed. The upper image is that of a low–low osteotomies, where the osteotomy is closer to the maxilla (low) throughout its route. The middle image is that of an osteotomy that starts low and ends high (closer to the dorsum). The bottom image is that of a high–low–high route, which is the most commonly used type of osteotomy route. The midportion of the osteotomy dips closer to the maxilla (low).

open the nasal vault (9). It is important for the surgeon to know which of these goals are necessary in any given situation. There are many ways to perform osteotomies. See Figure 183.6 for three different patterns of osteotomies. If the roof is open from trauma or dorsal reduction, medial osteotomies may not be necessary (9). Lateral osteotomies are usually performed in a high–low–high fashion. However, a high deviation may require a high–low–low configuration to center the upper third. If the nasal bones are mobilized, but the upper third remains crooked, this may be due to a persistently deviated bony dorsal septum that extends into the superior septum (10). Two approaches can be taken to center the deviated superior septum. The first option is to mobilize the superior aspect of the septum with percutaneous medial osteotomies using a 2-mm chisel, taking care not to extend the fracture into the cribriform plate. The medial osteotomy can also be done as a "cross-root" osteotomy. In this technique, the osteotome is used to cut across the bony septum and the upper nasal dorsum using an endonasal approach. A curved osteotome is placed medially on the convex side of the nose at the site of a typical medial osteotomy. The curved osteotome cuts across the nasal root to the contralateral side to mobilize the central portion of the upper third. With either the percutaneous transverse or the cross-root osteotomy, the entire upper third should be easily mobilized from side to side once the lateral osteotomies have been completed.

Preserving the lateral nasal periosteum and the underlying mucosa as much as possible will avoid excessive medial or posterior displacement of the nasal walls after osteotomies are completed. This is accomplished by using small osteotomes and elevating a small tunnel of periosteum along the lateral osteotomy site prior to creation of the osteotomy.

Another option for the crooked upper nasal third is to camouflage the deviation with bony reduction on the convex side and onlay cartilage grafting on the concave side. This reduction and contralateral augmentation of the upper nasal third will help center the upper third without aggressive osteotomies. This technique works well for minor deviations when the bone is relatively thick.

Middle Third

The middle third of the nose is composed primarily of the paired upper lateral cartilages and the dorsal nasal septum. Inferiorly, the upper lateral cartilages articulate with the lower lateral cartilages via the scroll. Superiorly, both the upper lateral cartilages and the septum articulate with the nasal bones. Standard septoplasty techniques emphasize correcting deviations along the inferior aspect of the septum. Deviations along the dorsum may require separating the upper lateral cartilage from the dorsal septum, vertical scoring of the dorsal cartilage, and osteotomy techniques. However, this at times may not correct the deviation sufficiently, and other methods must be used. Two commonly used methods are the spreader graft and the onlay camouflage graft (11). The spreader graft is a cartilage graft that is placed between the upper lateral cartilage and the septum. Figure 183.7 shows bilateral spreader grafts placed to help strengthen a deviated middle third. In order to place the graft, the upper lateral cartilage must be separated from the nasal septum. The mucosa is elevated from the dorsal septum, and the spreader graft is placed between the upper lateral cartilage and septum, and it is sutured into position. Unilateral or bilateral spreader grafts can be used for this purpose. The two spreader grafts may be of unequal thickness to correct for deviations of the nasal dorsum. In Figure 183.7, bilateral spreader grafts were placed. Another option is to use the medial margin of the upper lateral cartilage as an auto-spreader graft if there is redundant cartilage after straightening the dorsum. A vertical cut is made through the redundant upper lateral cartilage 2 to 3 mm from the medial margin (preserving the mucosa) and turned inward as an auto-spreader graft (12,13). Using the redundant upper lateral cartilage saves precious septal grafting material for other parts of the nose. For noses that require dorsal augmentation and widening of the middle nasal vault, an onlay spreader graft can be used (Figs. 183.8 to 183.10). The onlay spreader is a trapezoid-shaped graft that is placed over the dorsal septum and between the upper lateral cartilages (14). The graft is 4 mm wide superiorly, 5 to 6 mm wide inferiorly, and approximately 2 cm in length and running the length of the dorsal septum.

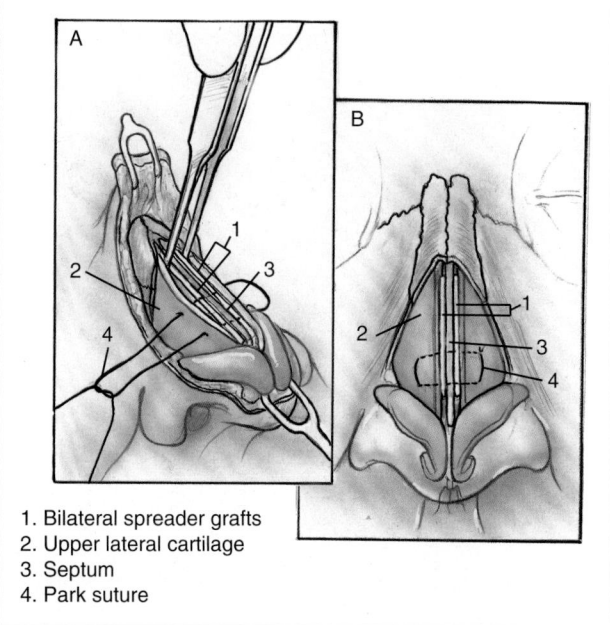

1. Bilateral spreader grafts
2. Upper lateral cartilage
3. Septum
4. Park suture

Figure 183.7 This illustration demonstrates how bilateral spreader grafts are placed. Cartilage is placed from the edge of the nasal bone and along side the septum, on each side. At least one mattress suture is placed to maintain the position of the spreader grafts in open external rhinoplasty. In endonasal rhinoplasty, suture fixation may not be necessary if properly sized pockets for the grafts are created.

It is important to avoid excising upper lateral cartilage until absolutely necessary. If the upper lateral cartilages are cut before the deviation is fixed, there may be a lack of upper lateral cartilage on the side of the deviation once the nose is shifted to the midline.

Deviations of the middle third of the nose can also be due to dislocation of the upper lateral cartilages from the caudal margin of the nasal bones. The surgeon can sometimes reapproximate the cartilages back to their anatomic position and suture-fixate them to the periosteum; otherwise, camouflage grafts can be utilized. Deviations can also be caused by depressions due to a collapse of an osteotomized or traumatically fractured lateral nasal wall. These deviations can be corrected with onlay grafts placed over the lateral nasal wall or spreader grafts. The decision to use an onlay graft versus a spreader graft is based on the patient's nasal airway, the size of the depression, and the shape of the upper lateral cartilage. If the size of the depression is small and is not affecting the internal nasal valve, a small onlay graft of crushed or precisely contoured septal cartilage suffices. If the depression is small and the nasal valves narrow, spreader grafts are preferred since they improve the airway as well as correct the depression. If the depression is large and the airway is narrow, a combination of both spreader grafts and onlay grafts over the upper lateral cartilage, dorsum, or the cephalic margin of the lower lateral cartilage may be necessary (Figs. 183.11 and 183.12).

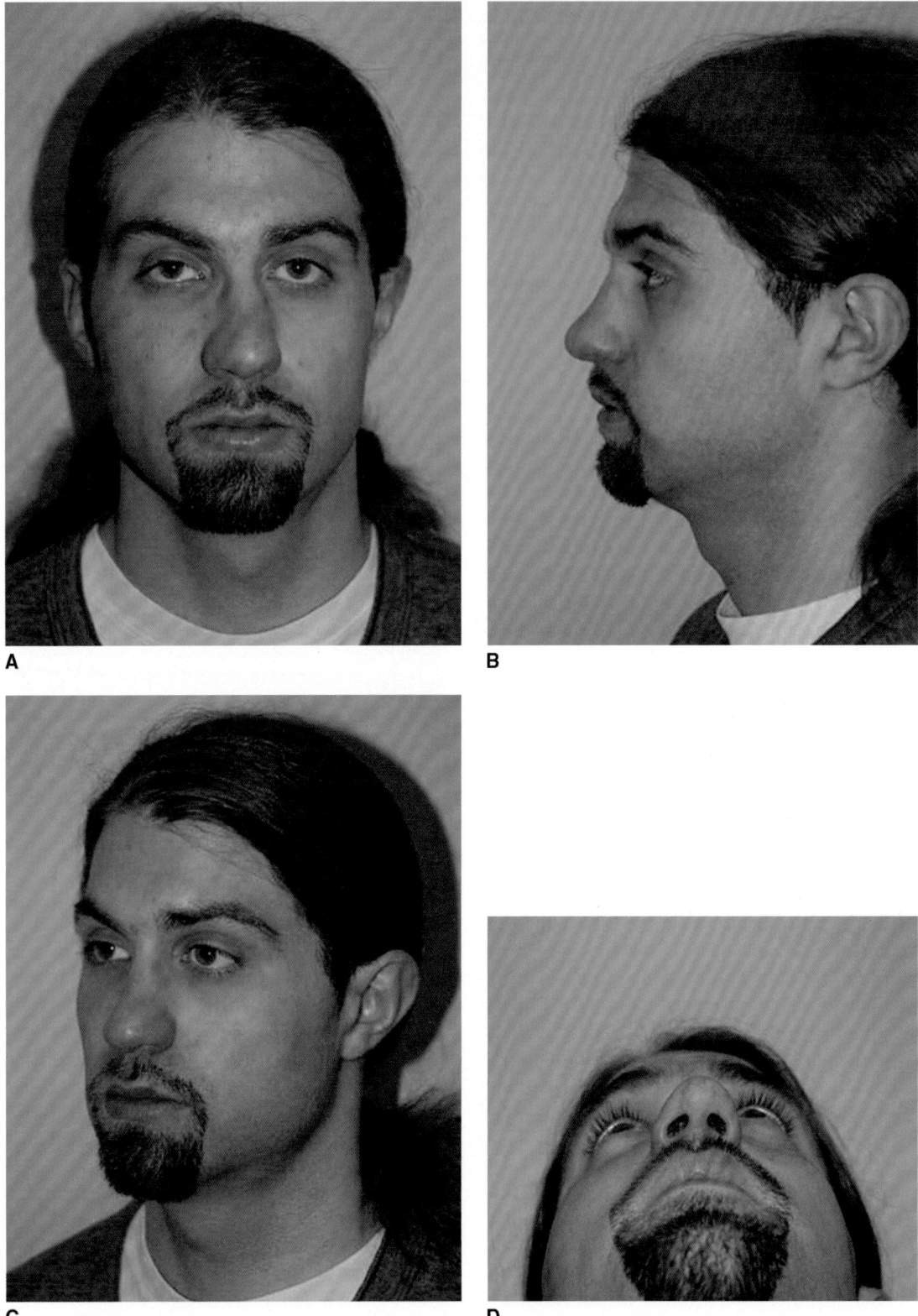

Figure 183.8 Case One. This is a 25-year-old male with a posttraumatic nasal deformity. He has a history of a prior reduction of a nasal septal fracture. He complains of persistent nasal obstruction and nasal deformity obscured by thick skin. Preoperative (**A–D,I**) and postoperative (**E–H,J**) photos can be seen here.

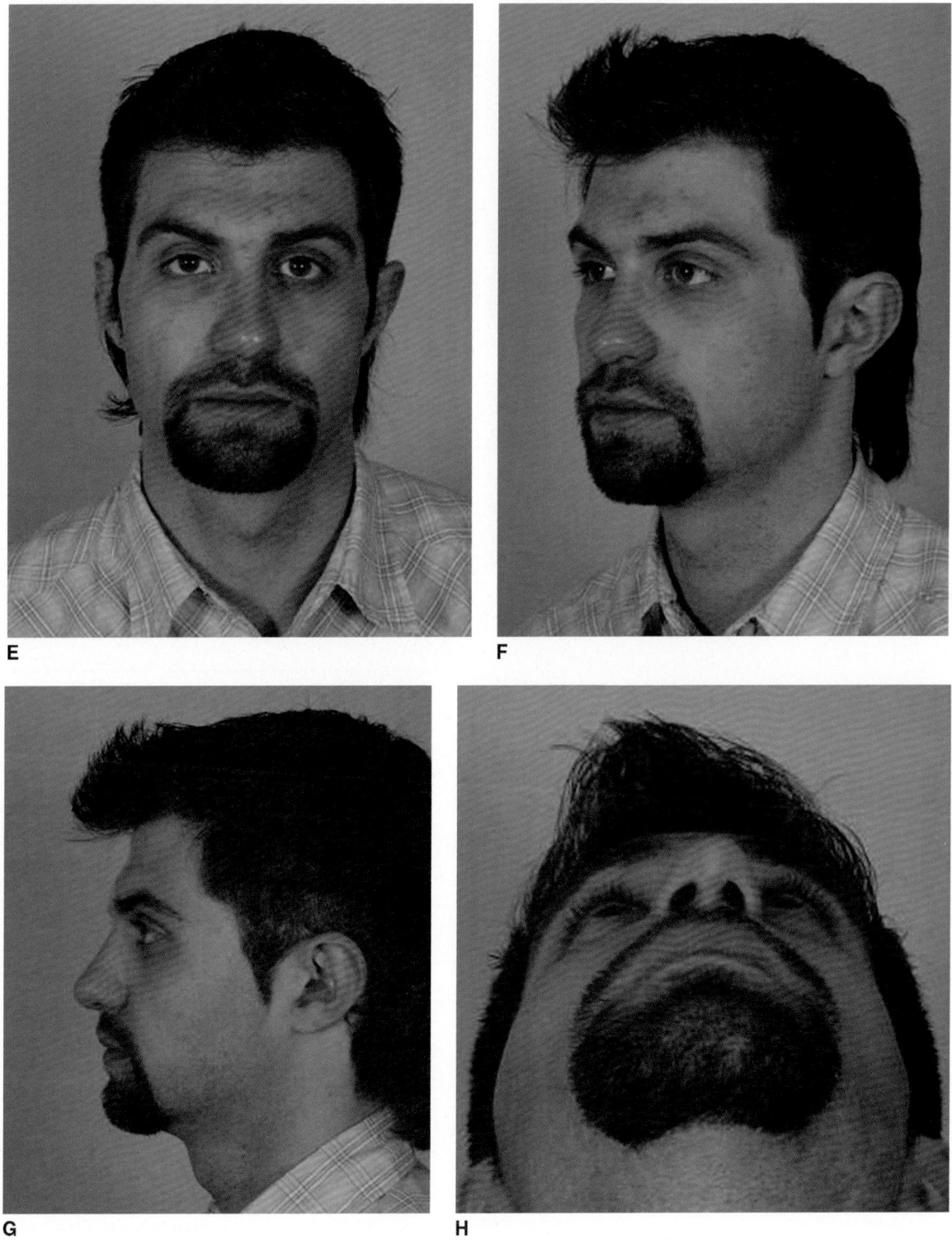

E

F

G

H

Figure 183.8 *(Continued)*

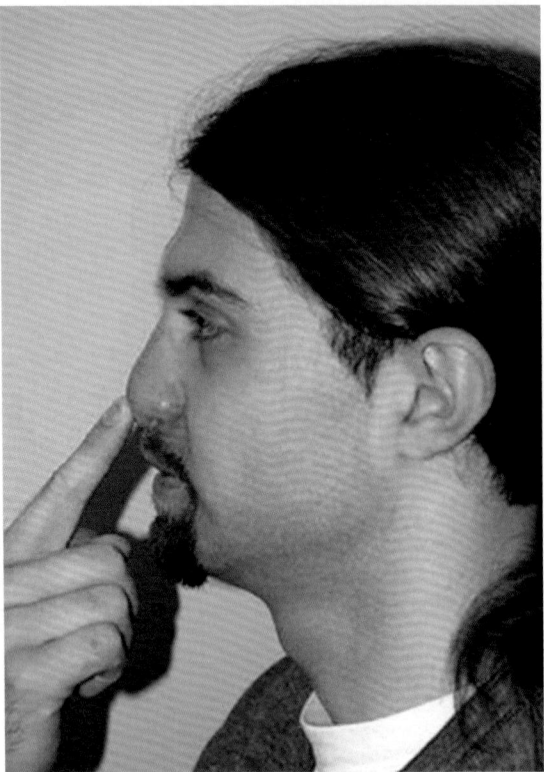

I

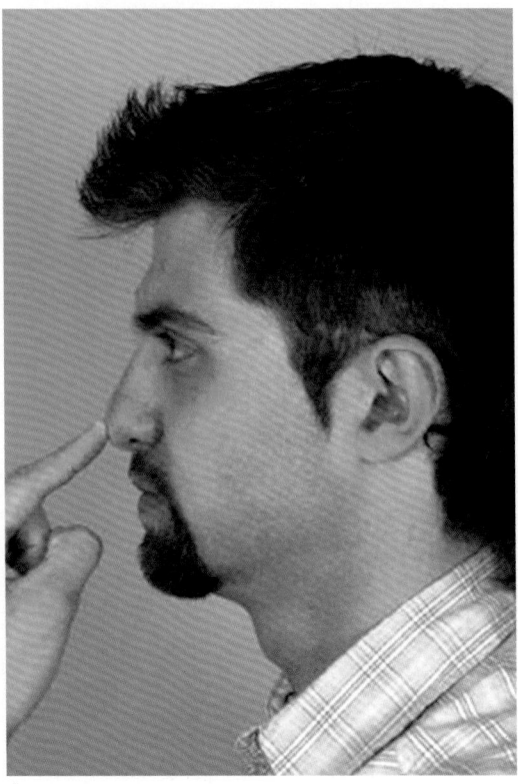

J

Figure 183.8 *(Continued)*

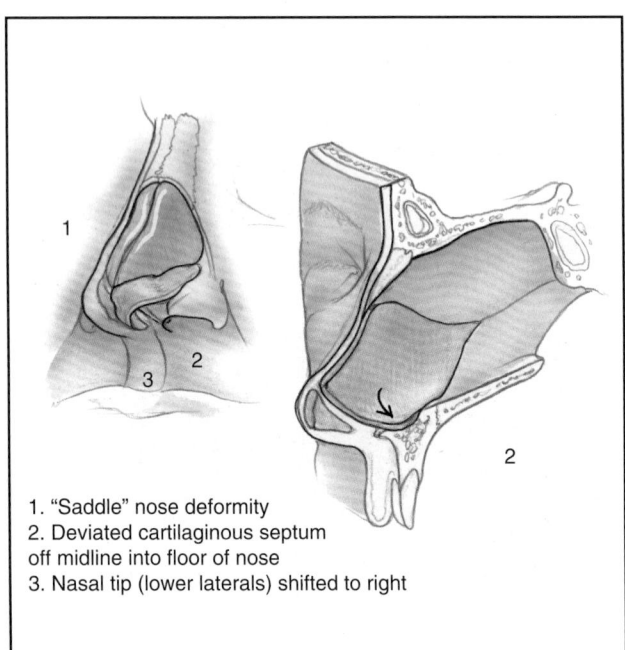

1. "Saddle" nose deformity
2. Deviated cartilaginous septum off midline into floor of nose
3. Nasal tip (lower laterals) shifted to right

Figure 183.9 The patient in Case One has a saddle deformity that is a depression of the middle third. The septum is depressed into the left nasal cavity, which causes deviation of the middle third. The lower lateral cartilages are not in contact with the septum because the tip is deviated to the right. Disarticulating the septum from the maxillary crest allows the surgeon to rotate the septum upward to increase dorsal height. This acts to reduce the saddle depression and also places the septum between the medial crura of the lower lateral cartilages. This all helps straighten the middle and lower thirds.

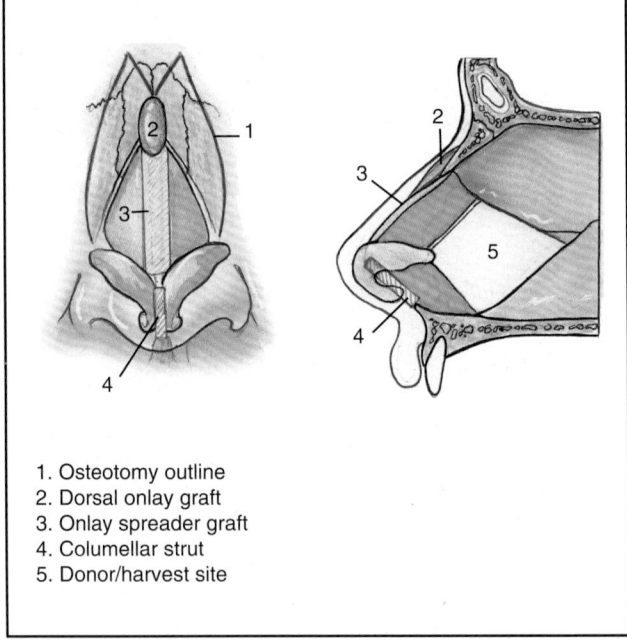

1. Osteotomy outline
2. Dorsal onlay graft
3. Onlay spreader graft
4. Columellar strut
5. Donor/harvest site

Figure 183.10 To create a nasal structure that maintains a straighter shape, the patient in Case One underwent open (external) septorhinoplasty. Autologous septal cartilage was used. The upper third was straightened with bilateral medial and bilateral lateral osteotomies. To straighten the middle third, he underwent the septal procedure described in this figure along with onlay spreader and dorsal onlay graft. The onlay spreader graft provides more dorsal augmentation to improve the saddle deformity. It also creates a higher support for the upper lateral cartilages and opens (increases) the internal nasal valve angle for better long-term breathing. The dorsal onlay graft was used for augmentation to create a uniform dorsum. To straighten the lower third, in addition to the septal procedure, a columellar strut helps keep the tip straight and supports the tip.

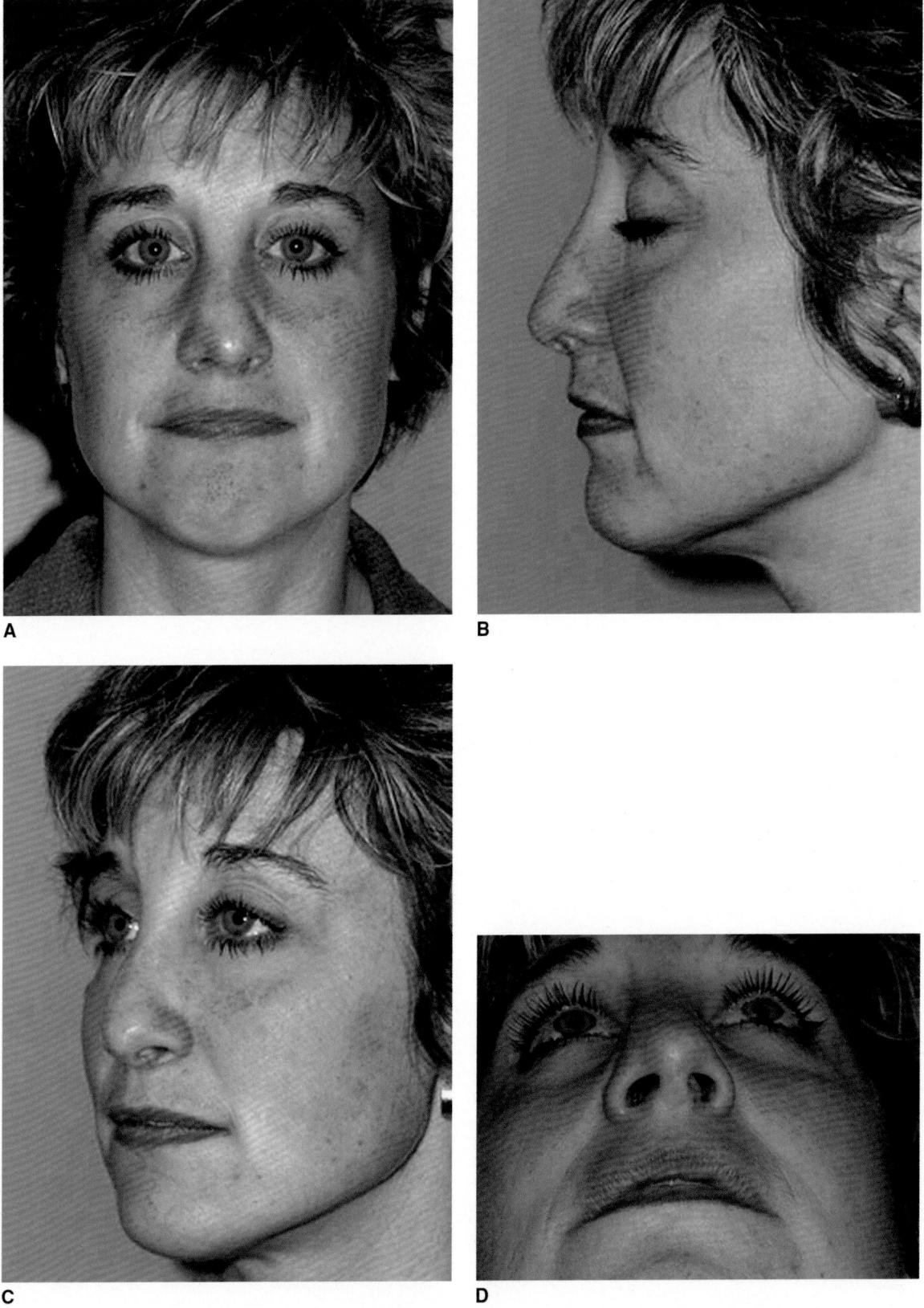

Figure 183.11 Case Two. This is a 30-year-old female patient who had childhood nasal trauma. She had a prior septorhinoplasty. She presented with a deviated nasal tip, twisted dorsum, severe caudal septal deflection to the left, concave left upper lateral cartilage, convex right upper lateral cartilage, and a buckled left lower lateral cartilage. Preoperative **(A–D)** and postoperative **(E–H)** photos can be seen here.

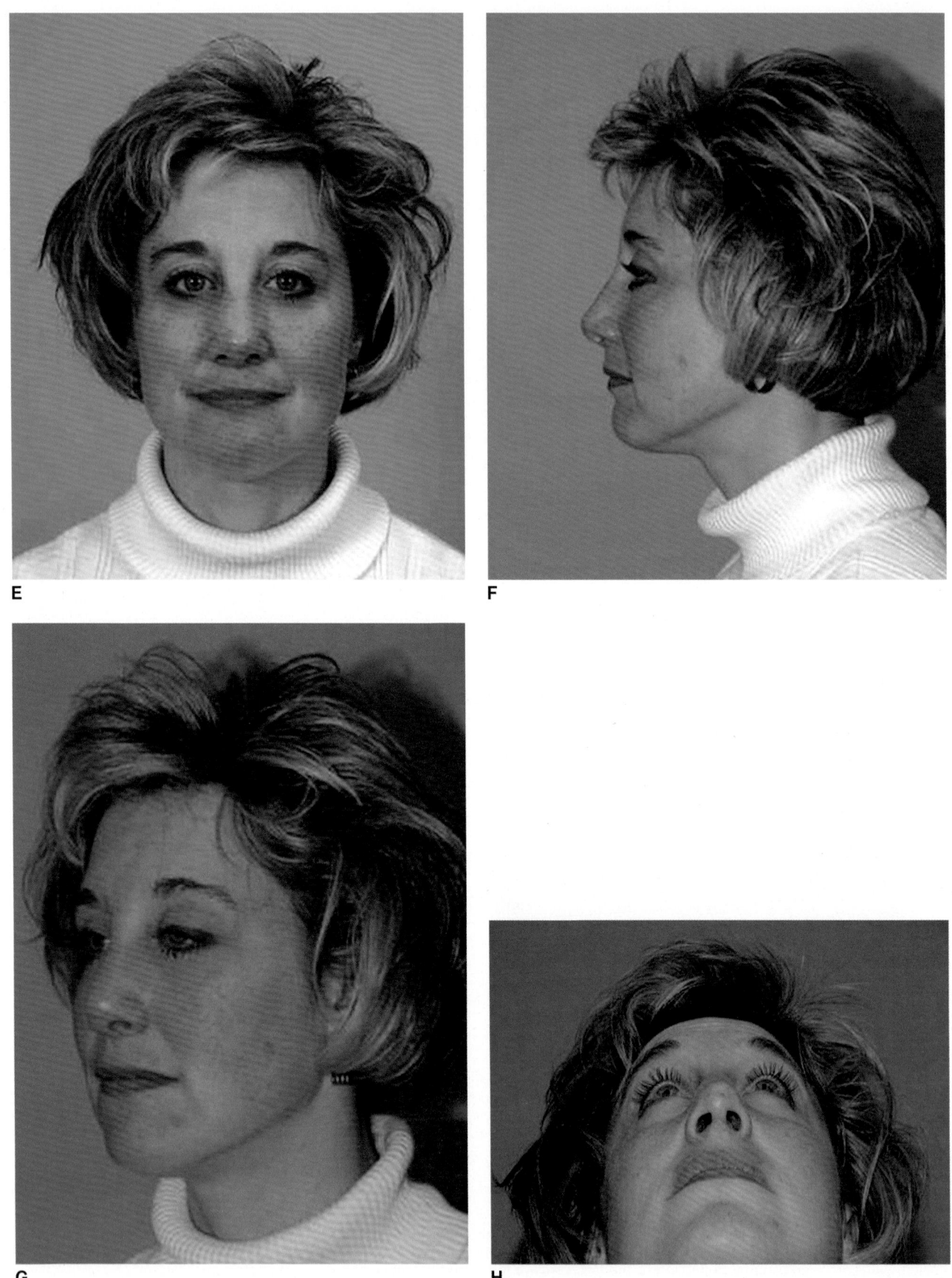

Figure 183.11 *(Continued)*

For onlay grafts, the ideal material is carved septal cartilage, followed by crushed septal or auricular cartilage, and then costal cartilage. Crushing must be kept to a minimum. The cartilage is crushed just enough to create a soft pliable layer that can be draped over the area of deficiency. It is best to place such grafts at the end of the case when the incisions are nearly closed so that the grafts do not get displaced. If necessary, the grafts can be sutured into position with either a fine monofilament absorbable or permanent suture.

Lower Third

Anatomically, the lower third of the nose consists of the paired lower lateral cartilages, the caudal nasal septum, and the nasal spine. Careful inspection and palpation can help the surgeon mentally "deglove" the nose to visualize a three-dimensional virtual image of the structures below. Palpation of the septum in relation to the maxillary spine can help determine whether the septum is dislocated from the midline. Deviations of the lower third are often due to deflections of the caudal septum or deviation of the lower lateral cartilage. However, at times, the lower lateral cartilages are asymmetrically malformed causing deviation of the nasal tip. Asymmetry of the lower lateral cartilage can be due to congenital variation, aggressive iatrogenic resection, or traumatic alterations. The two lower lateral cartilages may have significant differences in shape and size. Correction of the lower lateral cartilages to achieve symmetry can be performed with a number of methods. Many surgeons prefer the external approach for severe lower third asymmetries since the asymmetries are easier to visualize *in vitro*. Endonasal approaches can equally address the issue found in the crooked nasal deformity. Ultimately, the choice of approach depends on each surgeon's comfort and experience. The surgeon must decide whether a surgical attempt at repositioning or modifying the lower lateral cartilages back to a symmetric tripod is possible, or if it is better to use camouflage augmentation or reduction techniques to create tip symmetry.

Lower lateral cartilages that are severely distorted and asymmetric should be mobilized by releasing scar tissue and the vestibular mucosa. Some grafts such as the columellar strut and alar batten grafts (or lateral crural strut grafts) provide structural support. Once the structural integrity is returned, onlay grafts of crushed or carved cartilage can be used to improve symmetry. Suture shaping techniques, whereby a surgeon shapes the cartilages using mattress sutures, is a safe and effective way to shape the lower lateral cartilages without the risk of irrevocably damaging the cartilages if the attempt fails (15). For this reason, suture techniques have become very common. When the nasal tip is severely deviated, one often finds marked asymmetry between the two lower lateral cartilages, especially when the asymmetry is congenital or long-standing. The longer medial or lateral crura may require shortening or the shorter sides lengthening. The surgeon must balance these decisions based on the status of tip projection and rotation (Fig. 183.12). Dividing the longer crura and suturing the

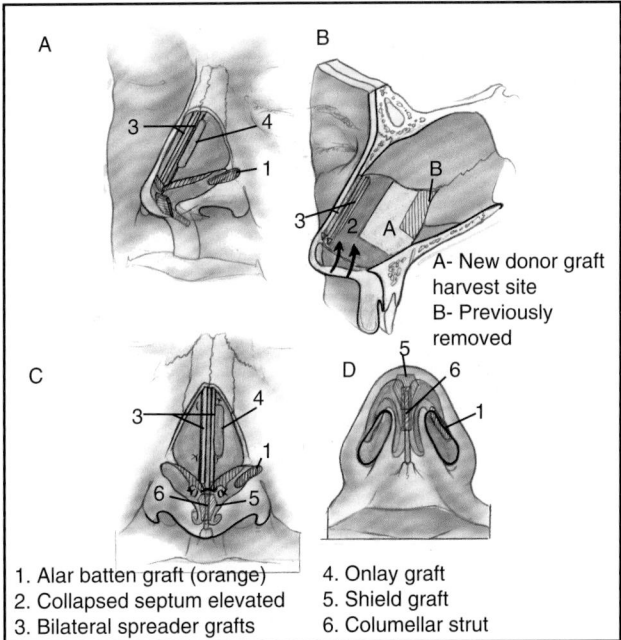

A- New donor graft harvest site
B- Previously removed

1. Alar batten graft (orange)
2. Collapsed septum elevated
3. Bilateral spreader grafts
4. Onlay graft
5. Shield graft
6. Columellar strut

Figure 183.12 The patient in Case Two underwent revision open (external) rhinoplasty. Autologous septal cartilage was used, along with ear conchal cartilage graft. The upper third was straightened using bilateral medial and bilateral low–high–low osteotomies. To straighten her middle third, bilateral spreader grafts were placed, along with a left dorsal onlay graft to account for the concavity of the upper lateral cartilage. Her collapsed septum was also elevated as in Case One (*black curved arrows*), but to a lesser degree. To straighten her lower third, a combination of suture techniques were used along with a left alar batten graft and columellar strut. Finally, a shield graft was placed for increased tip projection and definition.

overlapping segments at a length symmetrical with the contralateral lower lateral cartilage will shorten and stabilize the longer crura. The authors prefer 6-0 polypropylene suture for this purpose since they are permanent and nonreactive.

FINISHING TOUCHES

After the nose is straightened, the surgeon should view the patient from the head of the bed to ensure the nose is at midline. This view helps pick out minor asymmetries along the entire length of the nose. Final camouflage grafts may be necessary using thin pieces of crushed or lightly scored cartilage. Septal splinting may be helpful in maintaining a straight septum and preventing blood or serum collections, which can result in areas with increased thickness. An external thermoplastic splint is applied to maintain the nose at midline. It cannot be used to straighten a nose that is crooked at the end of the operation. The tape and splint stay on for 6 to 7 days. Postoperative massage may be helpful. Patients are instructed to apply gentle pressure to the lateral nasal walls using the sides of the index finger while the palms of the hand are facing outward. This is done three to four times a day while facing a mirror during the second postoperative week. Patients are then seen by the surgeon at 1, 6, and 12 months during their postoperative recovery.

HIGHLIGHTS

- Successful management of the crooked nose requires a systemic approach that begins with a clear understanding of the patient's desires and symptoms.
- Any maneuver that improves a nose aesthetically may have implications in the functionality of the airway.
- Careful thought should be given to which maneuvers can correct the deformity without destabilizing the nose.
- There are two basic approaches toward dealing with a deviation: camouflage strategy and deconstructive/reconstructive. Camouflage is best for smaller asymmetries or depressions, and deconstructive/reconstructive strategy is best for more severe deviations. Either one or a combination of the two can be used to deal with a deviation.
- Conceptually dividing the nose into anatomic thirds simplifies and organizes a planned approach for each third with a strategy to correct it individually.
- After careful consideration to what is causing the deviation of the specific third, the forces that cause the deformity must be released. In posttraumatic or post-surgical cases, releasing scar tissue and the vestibular mucosa may be necessary to improve the asymmetry.
- After release and repositioning of the structures, the structures must be resutured in a way to construct a straight and stable framework.

REFERENCES

1. Becker OJ. Problems of the septum in rhinoplastic surgery. *Arch Otolaryngol* 1951;53:622–639.
2. King E, Ashley F. The correction of the internally and externally deviated nose. *Plast Reconstr Surg* 1952;10:116–120.
3. Dingman R. Correction of nasal deformities due to defects of the septum. *Plast Reconstr Surg* 1956;18:291–304.
4. Baume L. The nasal septum: an endochondral growth center. *J Dent Res* 1961;40:625.
5. Roofe SB, Murakami CS. Treatment of the posttraumatic and postrhinoplasty crooked nose. *Facial Plast Surg Clin North Am* 2006;14(4):279–289.
6. Gubisch W. Extracorporeal septoplasty for the markedly deviated septum. *Arch Facial Plast Surg* 2005;7(4):218–226.
7. Boenisch M, Tamás H, Nolst Trenité GJ. Influence of polydioxanone foil on growing septal cartilage after surgery in an animal model: new aspects of cartilage healing and regeneration (preliminary results). *Arch Facial Plast Surg* 2003;5(4):316–319.
8. Most SP, Murakami CS. A modern approach to nasal osteotomies. *Facial Plast Surg Clin North Am* 2005;13(1):85–92.
9. Murakami CS, Larrabee WF. Comparison of osteotomy techniques in the treatment of nasal fractures. *Facial Plast Surg* 1992;8(4):209–219.
10. Foda HM. The role of septal surgery in management of the deviated nose. *Plast Reconstr Surg* 2005;115(2):406–415.
11. Sheen JH. Spreader graft: a method of reconstructing the roof of the middle nasal vault following rhinoplasty. *Plast Reconstr Surg* 1984;73(2):230–239.
12. Lerma J. The "lapel" technique. *Plast Reconstr Surg* 1998;102(6):2274–2275.
13. Oneal RM, Berkowitz RL. Upper lateral cartilage spreader flaps in rhinoplasty. *Aesthet Surg J* 1998;18(5):370–371.
14. Murakami C. Nasal valve collapse. *Ear Nose Throat J* 2004;83(3):163–164.
15. Tebbetts JB. Shaping and positioning the nasal tip without structural disruption: a new, systematic approach. *Plast Reconstr Surg* 1994;94(1):61–77.

Revision Rhinoplasty 184

Richard E. Davis

Cosmetic nasal surgery remains one of the most effective and long-lasting procedures in the cosmetic surgery arsenal. A successful rhinoplasty not only creates a more attractive nose, it diverts attention to the eyes, making for a more harmonious and thus a far more beautiful face. Yet, while cosmetic rhinoplasty ranks among the most commonly performed cosmetic operations, few if any surgeons ever fully master its numerous subtleties and peculiar nuances. Without question, the delicate and complex three-dimensional nature of nasal anatomy, the precise and unforgiving tolerances of the nasal airway, and the lofty expectations of the typical rhinoplasty consumer make cosmetic rhinoplasty an extremely challenging surgical procedure. Moreover, the profound psychological importance of the face makes rhinoplasty a tremendously high-stakes emotional endeavor in which even dramatic cosmetic improvements may sometimes fail to meet patient expectations. Nevertheless, despite the inherent technical challenges and emotional risks, the lure of a more attractive face is a powerful motivating force that is likely to ensure the popularity of cosmetic nasal surgery indefinitely.

Unfortunately, the growing popularity of cosmetic nasal surgery has also created a corresponding increase in the number of substandard rhinoplasty outcomes. While a failed rhinoplasty may occasionally result entirely from adverse tissue responses to a well-executed surgical procedure, failed surgeries are far more often the result of technical errors such as faulty cosmetic analysis, poor artistic judgment, overzealous tissue removal, and/or gross surgical ineptitude. And while *primary* (first-time) rhinoplasty is widely regarded as among the most challenging of all elective cosmetic procedures, treatment of a failed rhinoplasty, commonly known as *revision* (or *secondary*) rhinoplasty, is typically an order of magnitude more difficult. Unlike primary rhinoplasty in which the misshapen nose is devoid of surgical scarring, *every* revision rhinoplasty patient presents with previously operated tissues that have sustained varying degrees of skeletal disruption, subcutaneous fibrosis, circulatory impairment, and/or soft tissue contracture. Moreover, while the primary rhinoplasty patient is typically upbeat and excited about the prospect of a more attractive nose, the revision rhinoplasty patient is frequently burdened by apprehension, anxiety, and skepticism. Hence both the technical and psychological challenges of revision rhinoplasty are often formidable.

Without question, complex revision rhinoplasty ranks among the most technically demanding of all cosmetic surgeries and is best reserved for the revision rhinoplasty specialist. Indeed, even for the most gifted cosmetic surgeon, a near-singular devotion to nasal surgery is often necessary to develop proficiency in this extremely challenging surgical niche. And while the technical demands of revision rhinoplasty are considerable, exceptional technical skills alone are not sufficient for a successful practice. The truly effective revision surgeon must also possess a discerning, yet compassionate listening ear and a willingness to confront the myriad emotional issues that typically accompany a failed rhinoplasty. Often the patient's emotional trauma is considerable and may even lead to depression, social isolation, and impaired functioning. And since the emotional consequences of a failed rhinoplasty are often so profound, the importance of revision rhinoplasty cannot be overstated. Without question, complex revision rhinoplasty is an emotionally charged and technically demanding procedure that requires expertise, sensitivity, and exceptional technical skill.

Fortunately, contemporary techniques in revision rhinoplasty are now more effective than ever before. And while perfect restoration of the devastated nose is seldom possible, a carefully conceived and well-executed surgical treatment plan is often rewarded with considerable cosmetic and functional improvement. However, devising an effective surgical treatment plan is itself a complex and difficult undertaking. The surgeon must first correctly assess the cosmetic deformity and the corresponding tissue characteristics, and then formulate a surgical game plan that will reliably achieve the desired cosmetic goal, all while limiting risk, cost, and treatment time. Once the game plan is formulated, the surgeon must also justify the treatment rationale and disclose potential surgical risks to an often apprehensive and nervous patient. Care must be taken not to trivialize the surgical risks and generate a false sense of security; yet at the same time, equal care must be taken to avoid overemphasizing the surgical risks and needlessly alarming the already worried patient. Fortunately, for the majority of patients a single operation in competent hands results in a satisfactory, albeit slightly imperfect restoration of nasal function and beauty. For those seeking maximum improvement, staged reconstruction often yields superior overall results when tissues permit, but few patients have the inclination, time, or financial resources to undertake sequential revision surgery.

For the surgeon, successful restoration of the devastated nose is more than a technical triumph; it is an immensely rewarding endeavor in which the emotional benefits to the patient can be truly life changing. Indeed, few other elective cosmetic procedures can impact a patient so profoundly, and the heartfelt appreciation of these individuals is extremely gratifying.

POSTSURGICAL DEFORMITIES OF THE NOSE

The severity of postsurgical nasal deformities varies widely, ranging from minor to irreversible. Patients presenting with gross overresection of the skeletal framework often constitute the greatest technical challenge, especially when coupled with fibrotic nasal skin, naturally weak nasal cartilage, and/or functional airway disturbances. And technical challenges are most severe when major anatomic deficiencies are coupled with genetically unfavorable wound-healing characteristics. Although some patients may present with only mild cosmetic or functional impairment, the *complex* revision rhinoplasty patient presents with moderate to severe cosmetic deformity, often complicated by concurrent nasal airway dysfunction. Sadly, a growing number of patients are presenting with profound cosmetic deformities following multiple misguided attempts at revision surgery. In many instances, tissue limitations, such as the cumulative effects of fibrosis, contracture, and vascular impairment, prevent successful surgical restoration of the nose, even in expert hands (Fig. 184.1). Although young healthy individuals can sometimes tolerate repeated nasal surgeries and still retain effective healing responses, revision rhinoplasty becomes progressively more difficult with each successive surgery, and all noses will eventually reach a point of surgical intolerance at some time. Determining whether or not a given nose can safely tolerate further surgery is

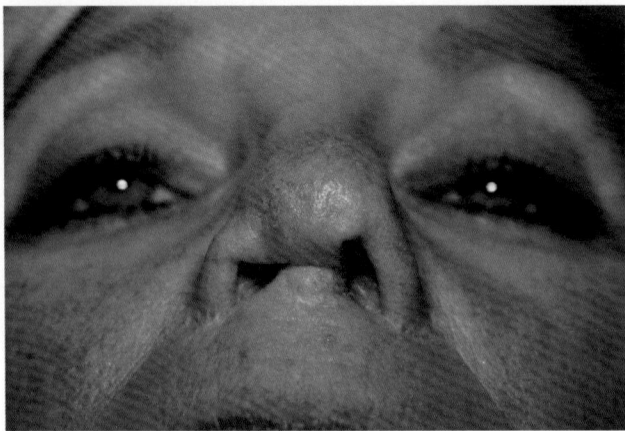

Figure 184.1 Severe nasal deformity presenting after multiple unsuccessful attempts at revision rhinoplasty.

a difficult and imprecise undertaking, and each patient must be approached cautiously in the context of potential surgical intolerance.

In deciding whether or not to pursue further surgery, a thorough physical examination of the nose is paramount. Direct physical examination is the only available means of assessing the anatomic, structural, and physiologic severity of a failed rhinoplasty, and without this critical assessment, the likelihood of a successful revision surgery is greatly diminished. Adverse physical findings such as a severely collapsed nasal framework, scarred and inelastic nasal skin, signs of borderline tissue perfusion, or dense cicatricial stenoses of the vestibular skin are the hallmarks of pending surgical intolerance, and these findings should prompt a sober reassessment of the need for further surgical treatment. In the worst-case scenario, numerous adverse physical findings combine to yield a strongly unfavorable risk-to-benefit ratio and a relative contraindication to further cosmetic surgery. On the other hand, debilitating functional impairment such as severe obstructive sleep apnea resulting from profound nasal airway obstruction may justify further intervention despite the increased surgical risk. Ironically, some seemingly intolerant noses will respond surprisingly well to a properly executed revision rhinoplasty, while some seemingly healthy noses will occasionally suffer significant wound-healing complications. Hence, the decision to reoperate is a dilemma for which there is no easy answer, and since no patient is ever fully immune from unforeseen complications, the prudent surgeon must balance the potential surgical risks against the emotional and physical burden of an untreated nasal deformity.

Although there are an infinite number of postsurgical nasal deformities that may arise following primary cosmetic rhinoplasty, cosmetic deformities can be loosely categorized as those of skeletal tissue *excess* and those of skeletal tissue *deficiency*. Postsurgical contour deformities of skeletal tissue excess are most often the result of incomplete or neglected treatment of congenital skeletal overgrowth such as a persistent dorsal hump or a persistent hanging columella. In straightforward cases of skeletal tissue excess, the prognosis is often highly favorable since revision surgery simply entails completing the primary rhinoplasty—the so-called completion rhinoplasty (see Case One).

Another common cause of skeletal tissue excess is the overzealous use of augmentation graft materials—the so-called overgrafted nose. Typically, surgical revision of the overgrafted nose is a difficult undertaking that requires reconfiguration of the nasal framework by removing, replacing, and/or modifying the existing structural elements to achieve an attractive, harmonious, and structurally sound skeletal framework. Treatment is particularly difficult when the existing nasal framework is twisted or asymmetric since extensive surgical "deconstruction"—and thus destabilization of the skeletal framework—is required. In contrast, revision of the overgrafted nose is comparatively straightforward when only superficial surface changes are required and extensive skeletal destabilization can be avoided.

Unlike postrhinoplasty deformities of skeletal tissue *excess* that are often the result of incomplete surgical treatment, postsurgical deformities of skeletal *deficiency* are commonly the result of aggressive overtreatment. In the so-called "overresected nose," excessive lowering of the nasal bridge and/or overzealous excision of the nasal tip cartilage results in a profound and often progressive collapse of the nasal framework. The cosmetic impact of surgical overresection is an unattractive and stigmatic look that is derived from an amalgamation of various characteristic nasal deformities (Fig. 184.2A–C). Surgical overresection of the alar cartilages, particularly the lateral crura, frequently leads to pinching of the nasal tip, alar retraction, bossae, and/or supra-alar pinching, while overresection of the anterior septum may lead to overrotation or excessive deprojection of the tip unit (1–3). Moreover, overresection of the anterior septum will typically weaken skeletal tip support and exacerbate the adverse effects of alar cartilage overresection (1,4). Finally, overresection of the nasal dorsum leads to a scooped dorsal profile, often accompanied by middle vault pinching, a widened and washed-out bony dorsum, and abnormal shadowing of the bony–cartilaginous junction—the so-called inverted-V deformity (3,5) (Fig. 184.3). In addition to a conspicuous and unsightly nasal appearance, the overresected nose is also emblematic of bad rhinoplasty surgery—a highly undesirable stigma that adds to the patient's emotional distress. Unfortunately the morbidity of surgical overresection is not limited to cosmetic sequelae as most overresected noses are also burdened by collapse of the internal and/or external nasal valves leading to symptomatic nasal airway obstruction (1–3). Overresection of the nasal framework is a devastating complication of cosmetic rhinoplasty that usually leads to severe nasal deformity and that likely represents the most common motivation for revision rhinoplasty.

In order to restore the overresected nose to create a sturdy, attractive, and fully functional appendage, revision rhinoplasty requires *re-expansion* of the undersized and collapsed skeletal framework—frequently against a scarred and inelastic soft tissue envelope. Unlike naturally elastic nasal skin that can stretch to accommodate full skeletal re-expansion, fibrotic and noncompliant skin may fail to permit cosmetically and functionally ideal enlargement of the nasal framework. Moreover, successful skeletal re-expansion requires a newly constructed framework of sufficient rigidity to distend the scarred and noncompliant nasal skin without invoking skeletal distortion, all while simultaneously avoiding cutaneous vascular insufficiency produced by excessive closing tension and subsequent disruption of nutrient blood flow. In patients with medical comorbidities such as cigarette smoking, diabetes, inflammatory disease, prior cocaine abuse, or any other form of preexisting vascular impairment, the risk of vascular insufficiency is greatly increased, and excessive skin tension must be carefully avoided even if the newly expanded framework must be reduced in size. Accordingly, a thorough history and physical examination is particularly important in this patient population to screen for risk factors or preexisting manifestations of impaired tissue perfusion. Although frank skin necrosis is exceedingly rare in revision rhinoplasty, vascular insufficiency may still result in wound dehiscence, incomplete revascularization of autografts, and/ or frank wound infection—any of which may potentially jeopardize the surgical outcome and produce disastrous surgical consequences. Consequently, in the overly short and underprojected nose with stubbornly noncompliant nasal skin, avoidance of vascular compromise often precludes full skeletal re-expansion and this limitation is best identified and discussed prior to surgery. Moreover, even in the absence of skeletal re-expansion, tissue perfusion is disrupted to some degree in every rhinoplasty, and proactive measures to optimize tissue perfusion are essential. Meticulous soft tissue technique, judicious use of electrocautery, appropriate use of surgical dissection planes, avoidance of overly constrictive compression dressings, careful monitoring of capillary refill, and postoperative supportive measures all serve to collectively optimize soft tissue perfusion and reduce the risk of ischemic injury. Without question, the combined skeletal and soft tissues derangements associated with the overresected nose make it one of the most technically challenging and complication-prone of all postsurgical nasal deformities.

In reality, most severe surgical deformities are a combination of overresected skeletal tissues and untreated deformities of the original nose. Coexisting nasal airway dysfunction is common, and twisting and/or asymmetry of the damaged framework is also frequently present, both of which make revision rhinoplasty considerably more complicated. And while a severely disfigured nose presents

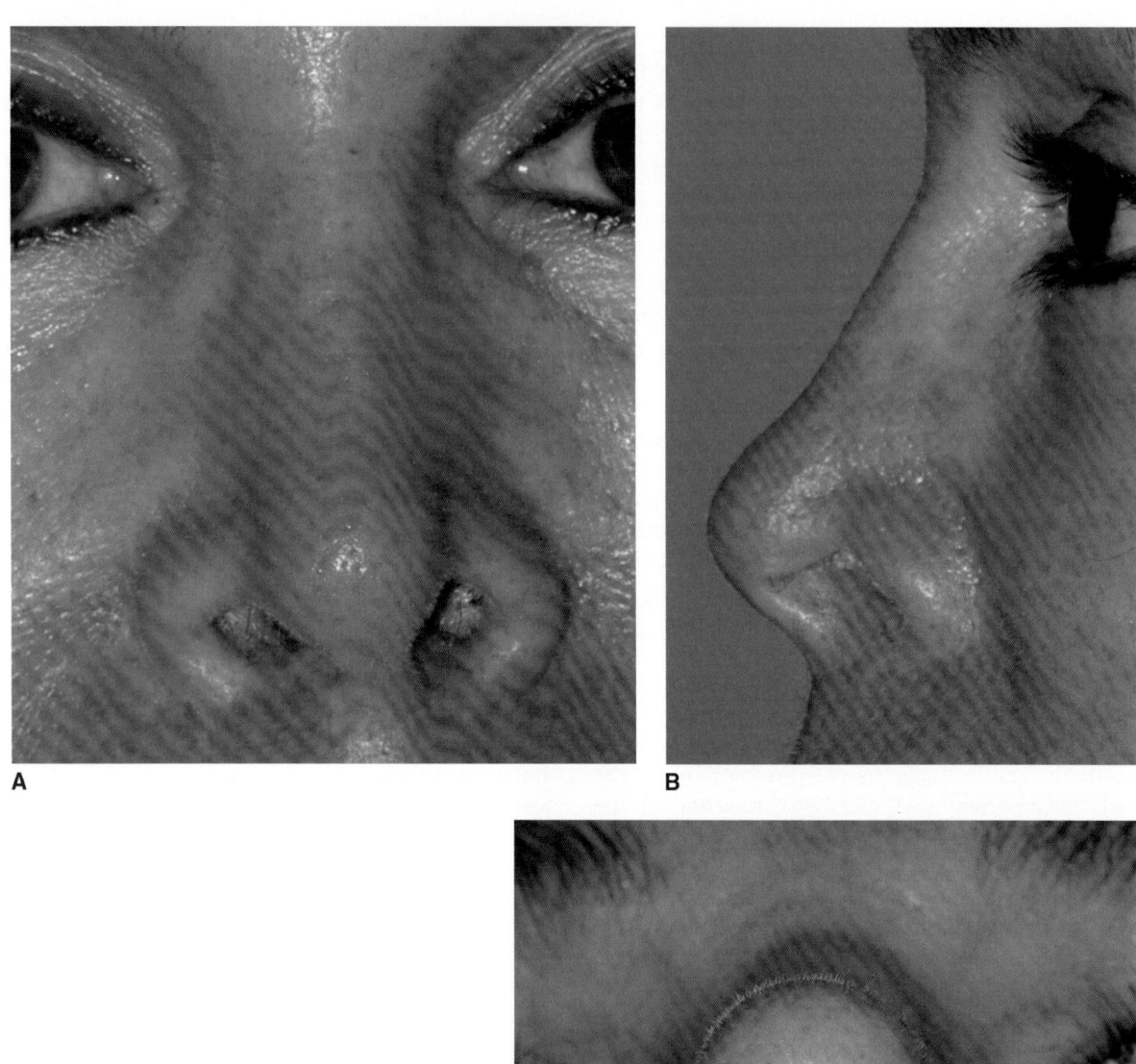

Figure 184.2 Typical cosmetic and functional stigmata of the overresected nose. **A:** Lobular pinching and alar retraction on frontal view, **(B)** severe alar retraction and poor tip projection on profile view, and **(C)** lobular pinching and nasal valve collapse on basal view.

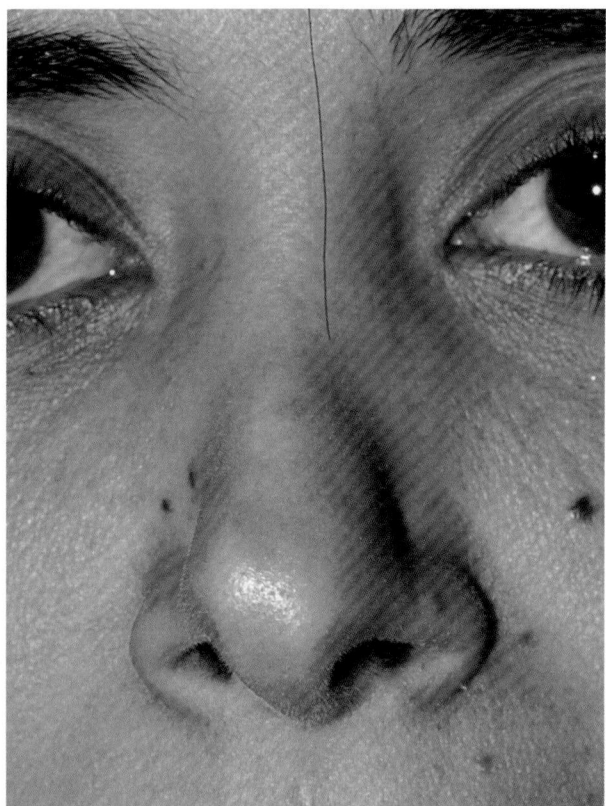

Figure 184.3 Frontal view of the "inverted-V" nasal deformity. Note disruption of the brow-tip aesthetic lines and the distinctive inverted-V shaped shadow traversing the nasal dorsum.

a formidable and sometimes insurmountable technical challenge, the presence of coexisting psychosocial issues can also greatly complicate the management of any rhinoplasty patient.

PATIENT EVALUATION AND TREATMENT PLANNING

Regardless of whether the surgical challenge is big or small, the ultimate objective of revision rhinoplasty is always the same—to create an attractive, sturdy, and fully functional nose that flatters the face and integrates naturally with the surrounding facial features. However, this task is not always easy or even medically feasible, and deciding when and how to operate is the first critical step in a successful revision rhinoplasty. Ironically, it is often the failure to properly evaluate the nose that leads to revision rhinoplasty in the first place, and the importance of the preoperative nasal history, physical examination, and cosmetic analysis cannot be overemphasized. Although the novice surgeon often focuses primarily upon the operative procedure, the accomplished surgeon will spend as much or more time on the evaluation, analysis, and treatment planning as on the operation itself. And because the end result of revision rhinoplasty depends as much upon tissue quality and healing responses as the actual

operation, *recognizing* and planning for tissue inadequacies is frequently what differentiates a favorable outcome from a disappointing one.

For the revision rhinoplasty patient, the initial nasal assessment begins with a thorough rhinoplasty history detailing the number of prior surgeries, the recovery interval between surgeries, the specific intervention for each surgery, and the subsequent tissue responses. This information serves to characterize the type and degree of prior tissue alteration and the overall wound-healing tendencies. When combined with the results of a thorough nasal examination, the rhinoplasty history will reveal the approximate anatomic and physiologic health of the nose and its likely tolerance for additional surgery. From this baseline perspective, the surgeon must then analyze the cosmetic deformity, pinpoint the desired cosmetic and functional end point, and devise an effective surgical game plan that accounts for the existing anatomic and cosmetic inadequacies. A careful assessment of the existing structural support, airway patency, nasal contour, and tissue quality will enable the surgeon to customize the surgical game plan in order to compensate for anticipated tissue deficiencies and/or adverse wound-healing responses. From the psychological standpoint, perhaps the biggest challenge in revision rhinoplasty is establishing realistic cosmetic expectations that coincide with the anticipated surgical complexity and the associated risks and limitations therein. A careful assessment of the patient's personality, underlying motives, and cosmetic objectives is also essential to reduce the likelihood of disappointment and/or confrontation stemming from unmet surgical expectations. Clearly, complex revision rhinoplasty is an intricate and complicated puzzle that can only be solved with a detailed and thorough preoperative evaluation.

PSYCHOLOGICAL ASPECTS OF REVISION RHINOPLASTY

From the moment of introduction, an evaluation of the patient's emotional health and well-being should commence. To begin the consultation, the surgeon should review the patient's social history, including the patient's education, employment, marital status, living situation, and psychiatric history. This information will help to delineate the patient's level of functioning and to define his or her emotional support network. As the consultation proceeds, the surgeon should also carefully explore the patient's justification for seeking revision rhinoplasty and the patient's concept of a satisfactory outcome. In most instances, healthy patient motives and realistic treatment expectations become increasingly evident as doctor/patient relationship develops. However, for patients with discrete emotional pathology, inappropriate motives and/or grandiose surgical expectations are often the first signs of underlying emotional illness. Unfortunately, many serious emotional disorders are not always readily apparent, and emotionally disturbed patients are often adept at concealing their symptoms. Although the majority of secondary rhinoplasty patients are not suffering from discrete emotional illness, emotional overtones are common in both emotionally unbalanced and emotionally healthy revision patients, making it difficult to properly differentiate between these fundamentally different yet outwardly similar patient groups. And because discrete emotional disorders are often more difficult to identify in the revision rhinoplasty patient, the consulting surgeon should maintain a high index of suspicion in any patient who exhibits subtle signs or symptoms suggestive of emotional pathology. Although detecting emotional illness is sometimes challenging, the importance of early identification is paramount since surgical treatment is often contraindicated in patients with discrete psychological disorders; and failure to properly screen for emotional pathology may lead to potentially catastrophic treatment complications.

As stated above, psychological evaluation of the revision rhinoplasty patient is made more challenging by the normal, yet sometimes alarming emotional overtones that typically accompany a failed rhinoplasty. While these emotional overtones manifest differently among revision rhinoplasty patients according to a variety of factors, the typical *primary* rhinoplasty patient is generally far less complicated from an emotional standpoint. For surgeons unfamiliar with the emotional by-products of a failed rhinoplasty, behavior of the typical (well-adjusted) *revision* rhinoplasty patient may occasionally seem both inappropriate and disconcerting, particularly when compared to the happy-go-lucky primary rhinoplasty patient. Consequently, understanding and appreciating the unique emotional context of the revision rhinoplasty patient is fundamental to appropriate patient selection and successful patient management.

For the typical first-time (primary) rhinoplasty patient, the prospect of an attractive and unobtrusive nose is a long-sought personal goal that is the motivating force behind surgical treatment. Characteristically, the first-time rhinoplasty patient is upbeat and excited about surgery, since it promises to beautify a nose that was often a source of insecurity, embarrassment, or social ridicule. Any fears or apprehensions generated by the anticipated discomfort or potential risks of surgery are often quickly dispelled by the prospect of an attractive new facial appearance. In fact, the typical primary rhinoplasty patient often approaches the surgery with carefree optimism, focused primarily upon the promise of a favorable cosmetic outcome.

In contrast, for the typical *revision* rhinoplasty patient, the bitter disappointment of a failed rhinoplasty gives rise to a far more pessimistic outlook dominated by apprehension, worry, and skepticism. For most revision patients, the emotional nightmare that prompted secondary rhinoplasty is not easily forgotten, and further treatment is seen through a much more ominous perspective. Frequently the prospective revision rhinoplasty patient is skeptical, indecisive, and hesitant to risk further facial deformity despite a favorable prognosis for a successful restoration. As a consequence, many patients awaiting revision surgery repeatedly second-guess their treatment decision and become increasingly more anxious as surgery approaches.

The apprehension and lack of confidence typical of the revision rhinoplasty patient is easy to understand. Rather than the attractive and natural-appearing nose that was anticipated, the revision rhinoplasty patient has been forced to contend with unexpected facial disfigurement and the array of unpleasant human emotions that naturally accompany an adverse life event. The realization that their surgeon may have been inexperienced and poorly trained, or even incompetent and deceitful, is often very difficult to accept, particularly if surgery was preceded by repeated assurances that a favorable outcome was a virtual certainty. Accordingly, confusion, bewilderment, embarrassment, resentment, anger, and mistrust often characterize the initial response to a failed cosmetic rhinoplasty. And for the emotionally frail and insecure individual who lacks strong coping skills, the psychological impact of a failed rhinoplasty is typically far more severe and disabling. Moreover, for patients with frank psychological disorders, a failed rhinoplasty may provoke considerable anger and resentment resulting in a wide range of maladaptive and aberrant behaviors. Hence the prospect of further surgery in the previously operated patient is a much different undertaking that must be approached in a far different manner.

Fortunately, most revision rhinoplasty patients are well-adjusted individuals who are reacting in a justifiable manner to an unanticipated facial deformity. And although even well-adjusted individuals must reconcile the negative human emotions that inevitably attend a failed rhinoplasty, once beyond the initial shock and disappointment of an adverse outcome, the well-balanced individual quickly rebounds and seeks appropriate restorative treatment. Eventually, anger and disappointment are channeled in a healthy and productive manner—ultimately leading to a rational plan of action and resolution of the problem.

In contrast, for those with poor coping skills, a failed rhinoplasty can become an emotionally devastating event heralded by withdrawal, self-pity, and depression. Extreme insecurity and social isolation are not uncommon in this patient population, and in severe cases may even lead to loss of employment, disruption of schooling, and/or failed interpersonal relationships. Despite their yearning for an attractive nose, the emotionally insecure patient often becomes paralyzed with apprehension and may wait years before finally deciding to undertake revision surgery. For others, the longing for a normal-looking nose is superseded by the fear of yet another failed outcome, and despite a favorable surgical prognosis, surgery is never undertaken.

Finally, a small number of revision rhinoplasty patients also suffer from underlying psychological illness. In addition to the already substantial technical challenges typical of complex revision rhinoplasty, management is further complicated by active resistance to patient counseling, a lack of rational decision making, and disregard for surgical restrictions and care requirements. In some instances, psychological disturbances may even render the patient incapable of assessing their postrhinoplasty outcome with any degree of objectivity. Regardless of whether or not these patients have legitimate cosmetic abnormalities, their inability to acknowledge previously damaged nasal tissues, subsequent treatment limitations, inherent surgical risks, and/or actual surgical improvements makes them exceedingly poor surgical candidates irrespective of their surgical prognosis. Failure to identify such individuals and to defer surgical treatment can lead to anger, confrontation, hostility, and potentially even violence against the surgeon or the surgical staff; and such problems underscore the importance of careful patient screening during the initial evaluation.

Although most revision rhinoplasty patients are well-adjusted individuals, for even the most self-assured and emotionally secure individual, the initial impact of a failed surgery is substantial and can be exacerbated by absent family support, severe disfigurement, insufficient financial resources, or limited access to appropriate medical care. Instead of enjoying the physical and emotional benefits of an attractive new nose, the failed rhinoplasty patient must contend with the prolonged public stigma of a "botched nose job," and the prospect of a second more difficult, and frequently more expensive, revision surgery. Even individuals with robust coping mechanisms and a strong emotional support network will suffer some measure of angst in this scenario, and the revision rhinoplasty surgeon must make allowances for these difficult circumstances (6). At the very least, the revision rhinoplasty surgeon should regard all prospective revision patients, including those with healthy coping skills, as emotionally traumatized, potentially labile, and justifiably distraught individuals. Without question, the addition of powerful and unpredictable emotions superimposed upon a formidable technical challenge make revision rhinoplasty patients exceptionally difficult to treat (6,7).

Perhaps one of the most difficult aspects of revision rhinoplasty is establishing a bond of trust with the apprehensive and cautious secondary rhinoplasty patient. Having previously placed their trust in a medical professional they assumed would beautify their nose, the typical revision rhinoplasty patient often finds it difficult to trust another surgeon, much less to then embark upon a more difficult and more hazardous secondary operation. Since many adverse rhinoplasty outcomes result from substandard surgical care, a cautious and skeptical approach to further surgery is clearly justified but may itself become an obstacle to the ultimate goal of nasal restoration. Furthermore, most revision rhinoplasty patients resort to the Internet for treatment advice where confusing and often erroneous recommendations are commonplace.

The Internet also provides interactions with hundreds of other unhappy rhinoplasty patients serving to underscore the prevalence of adverse outcomes and to further raise the level of patient anxiety. Sadly, the Internet often portrays rhinoplasty surgeons as uncaring and profit-driven individuals who prey upon the unsuspecting. And while the unethical and incompetent practices of some cosmetic surgeons may lend credence to these cynical viewpoints, the emotionally traumatized and gullible revision rhinoplasty patient is particularly susceptible to such distortions and may erroneously regard these views as both authoritative and trustworthy. Consequently, the prospective revision rhinoplasty patient often initially regards the treatment recommendations of the revision rhinoplasty consultant with suspicion and mistrust. Even multiple consultations with seasoned revision rhinoplasty experts may fail to provide clarity and reassurance, particularly since legitimate differences in treatment philosophy often result in contradictory treatment recommendations. Hence, while the secondary rhinoplasty patient is often eager to treat the postsurgical deformity, they are often confused and uncertain about where to turn for help.

Upon the realization that further nasal surgery is inevitable, most revision rhinoplasty patients seek to become more knowledgeable as to the methods, risks, and options for revision nasal surgery. As a result, patients occasionally demonstrate a surprising familiarity with technical rhinoplasty jargon and tout a (cursory) understanding of secondary rhinoplasty techniques. Moreover, they will often challenge the technical aspects of a proposed treatment plan based upon a naive and sometimes distorted understanding of nasal surgery. At face value, these patients may seem overly controlling and manipulative—much like the individual with narcissistic personality disorder. However, upon closer scrutiny these individuals are usually nothing more than fearful victims who are desperately trying to avoid yet another devastating surgical outcome, and the revision rhinoplasty surgeon should not necessarily be intimidated by patients seeking validation of the proposed treatment plan.

Without question, a failed rhinoplasty has numerous medical, financial, and psychosocial implications for the patient. Moreover, the task of finding a trustworthy surgeon with appropriate skills and expertise can prove a daunting and frustrating task for the gun-shy patient, particularly when conflicting opinions and misinformation abound. Since many prospective patients harbor concerns about the integrity, professionalism, and surgical competence of the revision surgeon, a compassionate listening ear and a willingness to patiently justify all treatment recommendations is the first step in earning patient trust and confidence. Failure to effectively justify the proposed treatment plan or to provide a compelling rebuttal to various misguided treatment recommendations, no matter how painstaking or time-consuming, may ultimately foster mistrust and create an emotional barrier to successful revision surgery.

And although a trusting relationship takes considerable time and effort to cultivate, it is highly improbable that a revision rhinoplasty patient will progress to surgical treatment without it.

SOMATOFORM AND PERSONALITY DISORDERS

Despite the commonly held view that cosmetic nasal surgery is merely a superficial (nontherapeutic) alteration of outward appearance, significant psychological benefits have been confirmed in well-adjusted individuals following successful primary rhinoplasty (8,9). Moreover, it is reasonable to conclude that similar therapeutic benefits are likely for the *revision* rhinoplasty patient since a successful outcome can fully eliminate the cause of emotional angst and provide analogous psychological benefits. However, roughly one-third of individuals seeking cosmetic nasal surgery also present with symptoms of mild to moderate psychiatric disease (8,9). Included among this subset of patients are those with distinct and identifiable psychological disorders such as somatoform disorders or various forms of aberrant personality disorders. In both cases, these disorders may thwart successful treatment, and the treating surgeon must be familiar with the hallmark symptoms of each disease so that appropriate precautions and/or exclusions can be implemented.

Body dysmorphic disorder (BDD) is a somatoform disorder that occurs at a far greater frequency among patients who seek cosmetic surgery (9–11). Sometimes called "imagined ugliness syndrome," BDD is a DSM-IV disorder (Diagnostic and Statistical Manual of Mental Disorder, Fourth Edition) that is defined as an irrational preoccupation with an imagined or trivial defect in appearance that results in significant emotional distress and/or impairment in daily functioning. Nearly all BDD sufferers engage in compulsive behaviors such as mirror checking or skin picking related to obsessive preoccupations with personal appearance, often spending hours each day engaged in these anxiety-producing activities (9–11). In severe forms, BDD may give rise to surgically addictive behaviors in a futile quest to eliminate imaginary flaws in body image. However, nonpsychiatric medical treatments such as cosmetic surgery seldom prove effective in eliminating symptoms of BDD (9,12). The most common form of BDD is the delusional variant in which patients lack insight or awareness regarding their obsession; whereas patients with the nondelusional variant can recognize their obsession to a variable extent (11). In the delusional form, sufferers are completely convinced that they appear ugly and grossly abnormal. Frequently BDD occurs in tandem with other psychiatric disorders including major depression, obsessive-compulsive disorder, substance abuse disorder, eating disorders, and personality disorders (9). Impaired psychosocial functioning is common in BDD and in severe cases may result in prolonged school or work absences, or

the inability to sustain interpersonal relationships (11). Clinical depression is a near-universal feature of BDD, and patients with severe BDD are at significantly increased risk for suicide (10,11). Revision rhinoplasty surgeons are also likely to encounter BDD patients with far greater frequency as the nose is one of the most common areas of concern second only to the hair and skin (10). Interestingly, BDD sufferers also frequently "doctor shop" as they relentlessly seek a surgical cure to their psychiatric illness (9,10). However, in contrast to well-balanced patients with mild but correctable complaints who will benefit from successful revision surgery, those with BDD may never achieve satisfaction regardless of the cosmetic outcome. Even exceptional cosmetic outcomes are unlikely to eliminate the patient's dissatisfaction with their nasal contour and may even trigger new obsessions with other body parts (9,10). Physical violence is also more common in distraught BDD patients and may be directed at cosmetic surgeons who fail to eliminate the perceived deformity (9–12). Because many BDD sufferers are adept at evading the screening process, the diagnosis of BDD should be entertained in any patient who dwells excessively upon a minimal or barely perceptible cosmetic defect. In a recent survey of 265 aesthetics surgeons regarding BDD, 84% failed to recognize symptoms of BDD until after surgery (12). Because surgical success rates are exceedingly poor in patients suffering from BDD, particularly delusional BDD patients in whom appropriate insight is lacking, surgery is generally contraindicated (9,11). Psychiatric evaluation and treatment is recommended for any individual in whom BDD is suspected, particularly since the delusional variant appears to respond to drug therapy with serotonin reuptake inhibitors (10,11). Psychiatric clearance is also essential for any suspected BDD patient prior to cosmetic surgical treatment (10), but surgical success rates in patients with documented BDD are notoriously poor and there is a growing consensus that BDD should be regarded as a contraindication to cosmetic treatments (9,11).

Personality disorders, defined as deeply ingrained, nonpsychotic, and maladaptive patterns of behaving and relating to others, are the most commonly encountered psychological disturbance in patients seeking cosmetic surgery (6,13). Although certain personality disorders are easily recognized, others such as borderline personality disorder may be difficult to identify since patients may initially seem normal. The borderline personality disorder is characterized by a sense of loneliness and emptiness, unpredictable mood swings, fear of abandonment, and irritability (6). Patients with borderline personality disorder may be identified as slightly "off" due to excessive flattery and premature familiarity, juxtaposed against aggressive and suspicious questioning. Despite behavior that is initially flattering, sympathetic, or seductive, stressful events such as a failed rhinoplasty (or a perceived surgical failure) may trigger acute decompensation with overt maladaptive symptoms such as postoperative depression, disordered self-image, and/or inappropriate demonstrations of anger, as individuals with borderline personality disorder look to others for cause, responsibility, and blame for their actions or circumstances (6,13).

Another commonly encountered personality disorder, the narcissistic personality disorder, is characterized by excessive arrogance and a feeling of superiority to others, regardless of actual achievements (6). Patients with narcissistic personality feel entitled to special treatment from office staff and the surgeon due to an inflated sense of self-esteem. Narcissists require continual validation of their special status and react with indifference, contempt, or even hostility to those who fail to actively reinforce their self-perceived greatness. Often they wear conspicuous flashy clothing or makeup and behave in a way that is designed to attract attention. Consequently, the narcissistic personality is typically very easy to discern in consultation. They interrupt frequently, demonstrate resistance to active listening, and show disinterest in surgical recommendations as they typically possess a preconceived notion of what procedure is best for them. While the otherwise normal but self-centered or egotistical individual may make a suitable surgical candidate when they are able to acknowledge the limitations of surgical treatment, elective cosmetic surgery is generally contraindicated in the patient with frank narcissistic personality disorder (6). Moreover, failure to meet the unrealistic cosmetic expectations of the narcissistic patient may trigger a narcissistic rage that can be disturbing, frightening, and even physically violent.

When evaluating any prospective rhinoplasty patient, it is critically important for the revision rhinoplasty surgeon to look beyond the technical aspects of surgical treatment and to closely examine the psychological health of the individual as demonstrated through the developing surgeon–patient relationship. Virtually all revision rhinoplasty patients present with some measure of recent or current emotional upheaval in response to the adverse rhinoplasty outcome, making detection of emotional pathology far more difficult. However, for the emotionally healthy individual, the normal response to a stressful adverse life event does not ultimately inhibit effective management. In contrast, for patients with various emotional disorders, the absence of insight and/or objective thinking makes attaining a satisfied patient highly improbable, and treatment is usually best avoided altogether. Failure to recognize the differentiating signs and symptoms of these emotionally troubled patients may result in significant conflict between patient and surgeon even when the surgical care is appropriate and the surgical outcome is satisfactory. In extreme cases, maladaptive behaviors may lead to confrontation, hostility, and potentially even physical violence. And with the recent popularity of Internet communication, hostility may also manifest through online slander, character assassination, and/or fictitious accounts of surgical negligence, all protected by the cloak of Internet anonymity. Clearly, a failed rhinoplasty is an emotionally charged issue, and the revision surgeon must always be mindful of the significant emotional overlay associated with treatment expectations, particularly in the presence of underlying emotional pathology.

KEY PROGNOSTIC INDICATORS IN SECONDARY RHINOPLASTY

Proper physical evaluation of the revision rhinoplasty patient includes an assessment of several key determinants that strongly impact the surgical prognosis. The importance of these determinants to successful secondary rhinoplasty merits special emphasis during the nasal examination and each of these variables is briefly highlighted below.

In addition to evaluating the psychological well-being of the patient, the initial patient evaluation should focus upon the patient's general medical health, particularly as it relates to anesthetic tolerance and surgical wound healing. Although robust general health, good exercise tolerance, and the absence of medical comorbidities are favorable indicators of physical vigor at any age, secondary nasal surgery becomes increasingly more difficult in later life. In contrast to adolescents and young adults who typically possess a dramatic and rapidly forgiving recuperative capacity, elective cosmetic nasal surgery is often far more prone to complications in middle age and beyond. While general physical vitality remains an important consideration in all patients, age alone is a major consideration in cosmetic nasal surgery, particularly in the previously operated nose. Hence, complex revision rhinoplasty should be approached with caution in the older patient since nasal healing responses often decline with age.

Another important prognostic indicator is the length of time since prior nasal surgery. Although surgically induced tissue trauma is to a large extent permanent and therefore cumulative, at least some degree of tissue injury is reversible if given adequate time for recovery. Consequently, multiple surgical procedures stacked at close intervals are highly detrimental since the nose has yet to recover from one injury before being subjected to another. In this scenario, even a young healthy patient with highly favorable recuperative powers may develop adverse wound-healing responses due to repeated uncompensated tissue trauma. Conversely, a healthy 35-year-old patient seeking revision of a failed teenage rhinoplasty has the advantage of a nearly two decade-long recovery in which all reversible injury has fully resolved. In this scenario, a well-executed revision rhinoplasty in a suitable candidate is usually followed by favorable wound-healing responses, sometimes comparable to a previously unoperated nose. Hence, noses that have been allowed a prolonged period of recovery are often far more tolerant of secondary surgery, whereas revision surgery in the face of acute swelling and inflammation may lead to increased complication rates from adverse healing responses.

Another critical factor that can dramatically impact the surgical prognosis is nasal skin quality. Without question, a smooth and healthy nasal complexion with intermediate skin thickness is best suited to cosmetic nasal surgery. In fact, a clear, smooth (nonsebaceous) complexion almost always indicates tolerant and "forgiving" nasal skin with minimal scarring tendencies and little preexisting cutaneous inflammation. On the other hand, thick oily nasal skin with large sebaceous units often responds poorly to surgical manipulation, reacting with excessive swelling, prolonged inflammation, and a tendency for heavy subcutaneous scarring. In the oversized nose, thick inelastic skin may fail to contract and properly conform to surgical reduction of the skeletal framework, whereas in the undersized nose, thick inelastic skin may limit cosmetically ideal skeletal re-expansion. Another important disadvantage of ultrathick nasal skin is the loss of surface definition created by excessive *masking* of the underlying skeletal framework. Because ultrathick nasal skin heavily obscures topographic features of the underlying nasal skeleton, the delicate surface undulations that characterize a well-defined and attractive nasal tip are lost. Moreover, a weak and underprojected nasal framework, whether acquired naturally or through surgical overresection, only serves to exacerbate the loss of desirable surface highlights. In contrast, for patients with extremely *thin* nasal skin, the atretic outer covering offers scant camouflage of underlying skeletal imperfections, and a flawless skeletal contour is required to prevent visible imperfections in the surface topography. Furthermore, both telangiectasias and dyschromias are easily provoked with repeated surgical dissection of thin nasal skin. In contrast to ultrathick or ultrathin nasal skin, intermediate skin thickness offers effective concealment of minor skeletal imperfections while still retaining a well-defined and attractive surface contour. In addition, healthy skin of intermediate thickness is usually associated with ample elasticity, prompt resolution of surgical edema with minimal subcutaneous scarring, and the capacity to rapidly conform to a surgically downsized nasal framework. When examining the previously operated nose, nasal skin quality is a crucial prognostic indicator that must be evaluated carefully. In fact, nasal skin *quality* is typically a far more reliable indicator of wound healing than is skin pigmentation, as virtually all skin tones will heal favorably when the complexion is smooth and clear. Consequently, failure to assess skin quality and to account for the intrinsic healing characteristics during surgical planning is a serious oversight in the evaluation process.

Another critical determinant of surgical success is intrinsic cartilage strength. Because the goal of any rhinoplasty is to create a permanent improvement in nasal contour via a *nondeforming* and durable skeletal framework, the biomechanical properties of the nasal cartilage are of critical importance to the long-term surgical outcome. Although cartilage strength is commonly regarded as unchanging throughout life, in reality cartilage stiffness commonly degrades over time. Age-related or disease-mediated losses in cartilage strength are inevitable in virtually every nose, and while noses blessed with naturally rigid cartilage may experience only negligible losses in structural support, in noses with naturally soft cartilage, age or disease-mediated deterioration may profoundly affect the shape and/or function of the nose over time. Moreover, even modest cartilage resection can exacerbate the age-related or disease-mediated deterioration of naturally weak nasal cartilage, producing a catastrophic effect upon long-term structural integrity. Vigorous soft tissue contraction—the so-called "shrink wrap" phenomenon—may compound the adverse impact of surgical intervention and age-related deterioration by distorting and collapsing the severely weakened nasal framework. Consequently, when evaluating the previously operated nose, baseline skeletal strength becomes a key indicator of both the existing structural support and the future susceptibility to structural failure. And since surgical restoration of the nose is only as good as the tissues used in the reconstruction, assessment of the baseline structural integrity *and* the strength of available graft materials are critical to the surgical prognosis and represent a crucial component of every new patient evaluation.

The final prognostic indicator is perhaps the most important single factor in the surgical prognosis—the body's genetically predetermined response to tissue injury. While the majority of young healthy individuals enjoy a forgiving tissue response that facilitates rapid and favorable healing, a small subset of humans appear to have tissues that respond poorly to surgical manipulation regardless of the care and precision exercised during surgical treatment. Furthermore, this sinister tendency is nearly impossible to detect with certainty in any given patient. Unlike the aforementioned prognostic indicators that can be quantified during the new patient evaluation, unfavorable wound healing responses may occasionally present without any identifying signs or symptoms. And while the majority of unsuccessful rhinoplasties are probably the result of incorrect aesthetic analysis, poor artistic judgment, technical errors, or surgical incompetence, a small subset of adverse outcomes is unquestionably the result of genetically predetermined adverse would-healing tendencies. At their worst, unfavorable healing responses may lead to prolonged inflammation, excessive fibrosis of the soft tissue envelope, excessive or inadequate soft tissue contracture, vascular insufficiency, and/or diminished immune function. The cumulative effects of these antagonistic influences may completely negate all of the surgical modifications intended to enhance nasal contour and function. Moreover, adverse wound-healing responses often become more severe with each successive nasal surgery. Although physical signs such as thick inelastic nasal skin, hypertrophic scarring, or excessive subcutaneous fibrosis often foreshadow adverse wound-healing responses, hostile healing responses can also arise in seemingly favorable surgical candidates who are devoid of discrete clinical findings.

When combined with weak skeletal anatomy in the surgically damaged nose, adverse healing responses represent an insurmountable surgical challenge in which further surgery is best avoided. Because these patients are occasionally indistinguishable from those with normal healing responses, even the accomplished surgeon will occasionally experience an adverse surgical outcome despite performing a technically appropriate and well-executed surgical procedure. Consequently the prudent surgeon should forewarn all patients about the unlikely but potentially catastrophic development of adverse healing responses, and a favorable surgical outcome should never be guaranteed even in the seemingly ideal patient. Although physical signs and symptoms are often lacking, warning signs suggestive of adverse healing responses should be sought in every new patient evaluation.

PHYSICAL ASSESSMENT OF THE NOSE

Perhaps the most commonly neglected, yet critically important component of the revision rhinoplasty assessment is physical examination of the nose. Because every secondary rhinoplasty patient presents with varying degrees of prior surgical scarring, skeletal disruption, vascular impairment, and/or structural instability; a proper revision rhinoplasty evaluation requires a thorough physical examination and *cannot* be conducted by photo review alone. Although photographic analysis of the nose is a critical component of the preoperative cosmetic assessment (5), high-resolution rhinoplasty photos fail to convey vital physical and biomechanical tissue properties like cartilage strength, tip support, sidewall rigidity, skin thickness, airway dimension, septal alignment, valve patency, or skin elasticity. In the aggregate, these tissues characteristics have a profound influence upon the method of surgical treatment and upon the probability of a successful surgical outcome. Failure to carefully examine the previously operated nose with a combination of inspection, palpation, and dynamic observation is a grave oversight that often precedes unsuccessful surgery. Hence, the present trend toward Internet consultations, while a reasonable first step in the evaluation process, should not be regarded as a suitable substitute for a proper one-on-one patient evaluation.

Surgical assessment of the nose prior to revision rhinoplasty requires a methodical physical examination designed to assess every physical characteristic that may influence the surgical outcome. The preoperative examination should be conducted in light of the patient's cosmetic and functional objectives so that a realistic treatment plan can be devised that reflects the patient's cosmetic goals and yet simultaneously recognizes and accounts for the anatomic obstacles to success. Although a proper surgical assessment cannot be performed from photographs alone, examination findings should be carefully correlated with standardized rhinoplasty photographs in order to obtain a complete and accurate cosmetic analysis. Indeed, a conventional aesthetic nasal analysis using standardized rhinoplasty photographs is an essential component of every good rhinoplasty evaluation (5). In addition to the cosmetic assessment, the preoperative nasal examination should also evaluate the structural integrity of the bony and cartilaginous skeletal framework; the thickness, elasticity, and perfusion of the inner and outer nasal lining; and the status of the entire nasal airway including the external and internal nasal valves, the nasal septum, and the nasal turbinates. In turn, this information will help to determine the associated surgical complexity, the surgical risk, and the surgical prognosis specific to each individual patient. Although this represents a time-consuming endeavor, without a comprehensive preoperative surgical evaluation the probability of a satisfactory final outcome is greatly diminished. Hence, the importance of the physical examination cannot be overemphasized.

Perhaps the most neglected aspect of the revision rhinoplasty evaluation is the functional assessment of the nose. Often the revision rhinoplasty patient is focused solely upon the cosmetic deformity and is reluctant to further complicate their management with complaints of functional impairment. However, nasal airway dysfunction is common in the revision rhinoplasty patient population and since untreated nasal airway dysfunction can lead to adverse health consequences, particular attention should be directed toward evaluating nasal airway patency. Typically, patients with nasal airway obstruction report daytime nasal congestion that becomes noticeably more severe at night. Subsequent nocturnal obstruction leads to associated symptoms of mouth breathing often accompanied by an overly dry throat, frequent awakenings from thirst or nasal obstruction, and disrupted sleep patterns with daytime fatigue. Ancillary symptoms such as rhinogenic headaches, decreased sense of smell, recurrent sinus infections, or Eustachian tube dysfunction may also be present. Symptoms of allergic rhinitis, when present, will also typically exacerbate the clinical symptoms of nasal airway dysfunction.

For a thorough cosmetic assessment, physical examination of the previously operated nose should include a careful inspection of both the external *and* internal nasal anatomy. In addition to the standard external cosmetic parameters of contour, alignment, symmetry, width, length, projection, and rotation, particular attention should also be paid to the physical and biomechanical characteristics of the outer nose, and *palpation* is an indispensible component of the physical examination. Only palpation will yield information regarding skin thickness, skin elasticity, cartilage strength, sidewall rigidity, tip support, and smoothness of the nasal dorsum. These characteristics are of considerable surgical significance as these physical properties weigh heavily upon the surgical prognosis.

Although important information is obtained through inspection and palpation of the outer nasal tissues, the external nasal attributes tell only part of the story.

Examination of the internal nasal passages is also critically important to the preoperative surgical assessment. Inspection of the nasal vestibule for the presence of cicatricial webs, valvular stenoses, prolapsed crural cartilage, recurvature of the lateral crura, or caudal septal deviations is vital to the complete preoperative assessment of the previously operated nose. In addition, observation of the nose for dynamic nasal valve collapse during normal inspiration is another important part of the physical examination. Findings of dynamic nasal valve collapse are often overlooked on speculum examination and indicate a pathologic weakness of the nasal sidewall—a more common finding in surgically overresected noses. Speculum or fiberoptic examination of the nasal cavum is also a key component of the revision rhinoplasty evaluation. Visual inspection of the nasal mucosa for excessive erythema, rhinorrhea, and edema—the triad of inflammatory findings consistent with allergic rhinitis—should not be overlooked since preoperative allergy treatment may help to reduce both intraoperative bleeding and postoperative mucosal edema. Findings of friable, dry, and heavily crusted mucosa should also be sought since these are tangible signs of decreased vascularity, such as that produced by chronic cocaine abuse, autoimmune vasculitis, or recent surgery. Similarly, visual inspection of the quadrangular cartilage for clinically significant airway obstruction and/or mucosal adhesions (synechiae) is essential since surgical treatment of these fixed anatomic deformities is required for satisfactory functional results. The presence of high (dorsal) deviations of the quadrangular septum should also be sought since a number of cosmetic and functional problems will develop if curvature of the dorsal septum is unrecognized and left untreated. Cotton-swab palpation of the quadrangular cartilage is also recommended to assess intrinsic cartilage strength and to detect potential areas of missing cartilage from previous septal surgery. Stout rigidity throughout the quadrangular septum indicates a reasonable likelihood that surplus septal cartilage is available for cartilage grafting. Septal perforations should also be sought on preoperative examination since large perforations may indicate poor vascularity and compromised structural support of the septal L-strut. While asymptomatic septal perforations do not necessarily require surgical treatment, smaller perforations are often easily eliminated during standard septal surgery and all preexisting anatomic abnormalities should be documented prior to surgical revision. Finally, visual assessment of the inferior and middle turbinates for hypertrophy and obstruction of the internal nasal airway is also necessary for proper functional assessment and treatment.

While no two revision rhinoplasty cases share identical nasal anatomy, many revision rhinoplasty patients present with a stereotypical and stigmatic nasal contour resulting from overaggressive excisional rhinoplasty. In fact, the typical revision rhinoplasty patient presents with at least some functional and cosmetic consequences of inadequate structural support stemming from overzealous skeletal resection. Characteristic stigmatic findings include low dorsal height and ill-defined sidewall shadows, pinching of the middle nasal vault and/or nasal tip with corresponding obstruction of the nasal valve, retraction of the alar rims with notching of the alar margins, and asymmetries of the nasal tip due to unequal scarification and collapse of the alar cartilage remnants. Often these deformities are interspersed with untreated deformities of the original nose such as excessive columellar protrusion, overprojection of the nasal spine, derangements in tip projection, or residual segments of dorsal overprojection such as the pollybeak deformity. Although each patient presents with a unique set of cosmetic and functional abnormalities, the vast majority of complex revision rhinoplasty patients present with varying degrees of *inadequate skeletal support* with or without simultaneous skeletal malposition.

Without question, one of the most important causes of the unsatisfactory rhinoplasty outcome is poor central tip support. In general, noses with naturally weak and/or surgically weakened central tip support are far more prone to adverse rhinoplasty outcomes and to adverse manifestations of alar cartilage overresection. In contrast, patients with vigorous central tip support suffer fewer complications of alar cartilage overresection all other factors being equal (see Case Two). While central tip support is derived in part from direct contributions of the medial crura, as well as from secondary support mechanisms from the surrounding soft tissues, the cartilaginous nasal septum is arguably the most important component of central tip support in most noses. Moreover, in the tension-nose deformity, septal support may comprise the overwhelming majority of structural tip support (14). In a fresh cadaver study examining septal contributions to nasal tip support, Adams and coworkers observed a 3.3-mm average loss in tip projection following isolated (dorsal) septal reductions of 4 mm performed through the open rhinoplasty approach (4). Moreover, even greater losses in tip projection were observed following removal of the entire quadrangular septum. The authors concluded that the septum likely plays a far more significant role in nasal tip support than previously believed, and is likely *equal* in importance to the lower lateral cartilages and their soft tissue attachments in providing nasal tip support. Consequently, assessing tip support by evaluating the intensity of tip recoil, the strength and rigidity of the anterior septum, and rigidity of the lower lateral cartilages is an essential component of the preoperative nasal exam. By the same token, restoring inadequate central support is one of the most important goals of revision rhinoplasty.

PINPOINTING THE COSMETIC OBJECTIVE WITH COMPUTER IMAGING

Without question, a thorough and methodical physical examination is requisite for a favorable surgical outcome. However, assessing the preoperative anatomy is only half of the equation. The other critical element in the preoperative assessment is the cosmetic objective—how the nose should appear as a consequence of revision surgery. The surgical prognosis will vary considerably according to the ease or difficulty of the cosmetic objective, and pinpointing the desired cosmetic outcome is an essential component of the preoperative assessment.

The ultimate goal of any rhinoplasty, whether primary or secondary, is satisfying the cosmetic desires of the patient. Aside from the formidable technical challenges of revision rhinoplasty, one of the biggest obstacles to achieving a satisfactory cosmetic outcome is obtaining a clear and unambiguous definition of the desired cosmetic objective. Since there is no universal or "ideal" nasal contour that applies equally to all faces (15), pinpointing each patient's specific cosmetic desires is a critical aspect of surgical planning. Increasingly, the typical revision rhinoplasty patient is a young adult with very strong cosmetic preferences. And while many patients have passionate opinions regarding nasal length, tip width, or dorsal contour, many patients also have difficulty effectively articulating their precise cosmetic goals. Moreover, most secondary rhinoplasty patients are seeking reassurance that their goals have been understood correctly, and few are willing to empower the surgeon merely to "do what you think is best."

The advent of computer morphing software, commonly known as preoperative *computer imaging,* is a helpful new technology that can facilitate communication between the revision surgeon and the prospective revision rhinoplasty patient (5,16). Using standardized, (high-resolution digital) rhinoplasty photographs, combined with computerized morphing software, computer imaging allows the skilled user to electronically edit (or "morph") rhinoplasty photographs in order to visually depict cosmetic surgical enhancements of the nose. Cosmetic analysis of the nose is greatly enhanced using computer imaging since individual parameters such as projection, rotation, width, or length can be altered, either independently or collectively, to determine the aesthetic impact of surgery upon the overall facial appearance. By incorporating the patient's cosmetic preferences into the editing process, lifelike simulations are created that enable the patient to "preview" various surgical changes, and ultimately to endorse the overall cosmetic objective. Because the process yields a concrete representation of the desired cosmetic outcome, a relatively unambiguous goal is established, and both the patient and surgeon are assured that the cosmetic objectives have been communicated effectively. Furthermore, the ability to electronically fade between edited images and the corresponding unedited image in real time greatly enhances the analytical power of computer imaging for surgeon and patient alike. For the patient, real-time transformation provides immediate intuitive understanding of the cosmetic deformity and greater reassurance regarding the proposed surgical correction. For the surgeon, the morphed image offers improved diagnostic insights and a mutually agreeable nasal contour from which an individualized treatment

plan can be developed and quantified. Although the benefits of computer imaging are irrefutable, computer imaging is subject to potential abuse and/or misinterpretation. Consequently, care must be taken to avoid overoptimistic simulations and to advise all patients that computer-enhanced images represent a best-case scenario, not a guaranteed outcome (5,16). Nevertheless, while exact recreation of the simulated image is virtually impossible, in skilled hands the final outcome often resembles, or even exceeds, the computer-generated simulation (17). Owing to the many benefits of this new technology, revision rhinoplasty patients now commonly request computer imaging as part of their preoperative surgical assessment.

FINALIZING THE TREATMENT PLAN

Once the cosmetic goal is determined, the final piece of the preoperative assessment is complete. The seasoned revision rhinoplasty surgeon will then carefully collate all of the available information including the patient's general health, the baseline cosmetic deformity, the biophysical tissue characteristics, the patient's cosmetic goals, the extent of functional impairment, the psychological status of the patient, and the likely healing tendencies, in order to devise an individualized surgical treatment plan and a corresponding surgical prognosis. As enumeration of the treatment plan becomes increasingly more explicit, the surgical approach (i.e., external vs. endonasal), the anesthetic options, and the choice of autologous graft materials must also be discussed and agreed upon. The surgeon must then decide if the patient's expectations are realistic and if the treatment objectives are within reach at an acceptable level of surgical risk. The patient's response to the stated surgical limitations and to the overall prognosis will help to determine if patient expectations are appropriate and sincere. Encouraging the patient to articulate and acknowledge the attendant surgical risks also helps to confirm that risk counseling was effective. Finally, the surgeon should ensure that the patient will comply with all surgical restrictions, care requirements, and follow-up appointments before assuming responsibility for surgical care.

Anesthetic Considerations

Once the decision is made to proceed with surgical treatment, preoperative preparations and restrictions are reviewed with the patient. All platelet inhibitors, including aspirin, nonsteroidal anti-inflammatory drugs, omega fish oils, high-dose vitamin E, and most herbal supplements should be discontinued at least 7 to 10 days prior to surgery to prevent drug-induced clotting disturbances. Tobacco users should be advised to discontinue all nicotine products immediately, and nasal allergies should be treated to reduce preoperative inflammation. A general medical evaluation is recommended for any patient with medical comorbidities or potential anesthetic contraindications.

While the optimal type of anesthesia remains a topic of considerable debate, the author emphatically prefers the use of general anesthesia for nasal surgery, and for revision rhinoplasty in particular. A carefully administered general anesthetic titrated to the age and body mass of the patient offers superior patient comfort, improved hemodynamic control, and optimal protection of the lower airway against the threat of aspiration. However, because secondary rhinoplasty cases are typically of a much longer duration than the average primary rhinoplasty, special precautions are required to prevent sequela of prolonged immobility during general anesthesia. All patients are placed in the semi-Fowler "beach chair" position with the feet and head elevated to facilitate peripheral venous return, and the legs are continuously massaged with sequential compression devices to minimize pooling of venous blood in the lower extremities and thereby reduce the risk of deep vein thrombosis. Pressure points on the heels and elbows are padded liberally, and the head is positioned above the heart to minimize venous back-pressure.

While the cost of general anesthesia is marginally greater, the technical advantages of general anesthesia are numerous. First, general anesthesia virtually eliminates intraoperative patient movement in response to painful stimuli. Because the depth of twilight anesthesia is limited by the need to maintain spontaneous ventilation, a partially conscious patient is often prone to unexpected movements and may even become restless, disoriented, or overtly combative. In contrast, endotracheal intubation safely permits a much deeper level of anesthesia that virtually eliminates intraoperative patient movement. Although judicious infiltration of the nose with 1% lidocaine containing epinephrine is still required for optimal hemostasis, distortion of the nose from large fluid volumes can be minimized since pain control is primarily achieved via the general anesthetic. In addition, blood pressure control is far less challenging in the absence of painful stimuli, and controlled hypotension can be used in healthy patients to improve visualization of the surgical field, to minimize extravasation of blood into the surrounding soft tissues, and to minimize operative blood loss. In contrast, patients under intravenous sedation may feel threatened as a result of anesthetic-induced disorientation and confusion. Blood pressure spikes, excessive bleeding, and defensive movements are common in this scenario and may complicate surgical management. While a skillfully administered intravenous anesthetic can often avoid these problems, susceptibility to apnea varies widely among individuals and general anesthesia eliminates this variable entirely. Finally, the presence of a cuffed endotracheal tube provides enhanced protection of the lower airway against the aspiration of blood which is an ever-present risk in upper airway surgery.

Perhaps the biggest perceived drawback to general anesthesia is the high incidence of postoperative nausea and vomiting (PONV). Moreover, PONV is more common following oral ingestion of blood, which is highly emetogenic and common following nasal surgery. In addition to being unpleasant, PONV may also lead to exacerbations in surgical site edema, ecchymosis, pain, and/or epistaxis, potentially prolonging recovery and intensifying the risk of subcutaneous fibrosis. However, a narcotic-free general anesthetic protocol can dramatically reduce the incidence of PONV (*personal observation*). After anesthetic induction with intravenous propofol (APP Pharmaceuticals LLC, Schaumburg, IL) and succinyl choline (PharMEDium Services LLC, Cleveland, MS), general anesthesia is maintained throughout the remainder of surgery on sevoflurane (Abbott Laboratories, North Chicago, IL) inhalational anesthetic. During periods of planned stimulation such as during lateral osteotomies, propofol is first administered by bolus to assist in blood pressure homeostasis and labetalol hydrochloride (Hospira Inc., Lake Forest, IL) or nicardipine hydrochloride (Sandoz Inc., Princeton, NJ) are used to supplement blood pressure and/or heart rate control. Dexamethasone sodium phosphate (APP Pharmaceuticals LLC, Schaumburg, IL) is used on induction for prophylaxis against PONV, and a single 4-mg dose of ondansetron (Baxter Healthcare Corporation, Deerfield, IL) is also used 30 minutes prior to extubation for additional PONV prophylaxis. The combined use of dexamethasone and ondansetron has been shown to be more effective at reducing severe PONV than ondansetron alone for both laparoscopic surgery and fentanyl-based patient-controlled analgesia (18,19). Moreover, by using the narcotic-free general anesthetic protocol described above, postoperative emesis is rare even when oral narcotics are used for postoperative pain control, and most patients are alert and oriented within 10 to 15 minutes of extubation. When used in combination with controlled-hypotensive anesthesia, the protocol also has a favorable impact upon postoperative swelling and ecchymosis since the intraoperative tissue extravasation of blood is greatly minimized. Patients typically perceive their surgery as lasting only a few minutes and few have recall of the operating room experience.

SURGICAL RECONSTRUCTION OF THE PREVIOUSLY OPERATED NOSE

Optimal Timing of Revision Rhinoplasty

The optimal timing of secondary rhinoplasty (and the traditional requirement to postpone surgery for 1 year) is a topic of ongoing debate. For virtually any complex secondary rhinoplasty patient, the emotional burden of a prolonged recovery is considerable, and rapid intervention would be far preferable from an emotional standpoint. However, early revision surgery in the face of *acute* postsurgical inflammation and edema is significantly more complication prone, and is generally best reserved for legitimate medical emergencies. Furthermore, even when the acute postsurgical changes have resolved, the surgically disrupted capillary and lymphatic microcirculation remains compromised, and complex revision surgery is generally best postponed until soft tissue swelling—the outward manifestation of microcirculatory impairment—has fully resolved. Although waiting a full year before correcting an unsightly postsurgical deformity can result in considerable emotional distress, a healthy microcirculation is essential to any complex secondary rhinoplasty, and the traditional recommendation to postpone revision surgery for 1 year is generally appropriate since significant microcirculatory impairment is often present in the first year after surgery. Moreover, in cases where the nose remains unacceptably large but otherwise shapely, allowing ample time for swelling and edema to resolve may obviate the need for revision surgery altogether since an acceptable cosmetic result often emerges within 12 months. And because surgical swelling is usually far more severe in patients with thick, sebaceous nasal skin, revision rhinoplasty in the ultrathick-skinned patient solely for the purpose of achieving minor size reductions is generally contraindicated for at least 18 to 24 months. Longer healing times are also necessary for patients with significant acne, allergic rhinitis, or other forms of chronic inflammation unless the inflammatory stimulus can be adequately controlled. While prolonged recovery is generally recommended for the thick-skinned or inflammation-prone patient, prolonged lymphedema may also give rise to permanent subcutaneous fibrosis, thereby tainting an otherwise satisfactory cosmetic outcome. Consequently, in patients with prolonged swelling, the judicious use of low-dose triamcinolone acetate injections is often necessary to prevent permanent iatrogenic thickening of the nasal skin (20). Although triamcinolone injections can potentially cause significant adverse side effects such as telangiectasias, dermal thinning, and even cartilage absorption, when carefully titrated, low-dose triamcinolone can greatly enhance the cosmetic outcome and obviate the need for revision surgery in the thick-skinned nose.

Although secondary surgery prior to complete healing is suboptimal, revision surgery within the first year may be preferable in a few rare circumstances. Unlike the otherwise shapely but still-swollen nose for which conservative treatment is appropriate, the overresected or twisted nose that has little hope of spontaneous improvement is sometimes best revised before progressive soft tissue contracture leads to permanent nasal collapse. In these challenging cases, nasal distortion is likely to gradually worsen in the months and years after rhinoplasty due to progressive "shrink wrap" contracture of both the inner and outer epithelial linings. Severely weakened and destabilized skeletal elements subjected to the persistent forces of soft tissue contracture often deform easily, resulting in severe buckling, pinching, retraction, and asymmetry of the cartilaginous framework. And while nonemergent reoperation during the acute phase of postoperative inflammation and edema is generally ill-advised, once the acute changes have passed and the microcirculation has recovered to a reasonable extent, early revision is reasonable—even if a full year has not elapsed—in order to prevent irreversible shrinkage of the nasal skin or mucosa. However, because early revision surgery risks unfavorable wound-healing responses and vascular insufficiency, early reoperation is best reserved for young and healthy individuals with forgiving skin and robust healing tendencies, and not for older patients or those with multiple medical comorbidities. Although the emotionally distressed patient is often seeking early revision, early intervention places additional physiologic stress upon the already damaged nasal tissues, and only the threat of permanent nasal contracture can justify the additional surgical risk. Hence, the decision to intervene early should not be taken lightly, and emotional distress alone is not justification for early surgical revision.

Another scenario in which early revision surgery is preferable is the comparatively minor anatomic deformity presenting in the patient with rapidly healing nasal skin. For the young patient with comparatively thin nasal skin and a smooth healthy complexion, surgical inflammation and swelling often resolve in far less than 12 months. In such patients, persistent skeletal deformities such as a small residual hump may be surgically corrected before the 1-year mark since further delay will not benefit surgical management. In this scenario, expeditious intervention is reasonable since the emotional impact of a flawed outcome can be remedied sooner at negligible increased risk to the patient.

In summary, the 1-year rule is an approximate guideline that is appropriate for some patients and inappropriate for others. And like most aspects of cosmetic nasal surgery, treatment decisions should be made according to the individual physical and psychological needs of the patient, and not according to broad generalizations. For the slow-healing nose, patience is often rewarded with a satisfactory cosmetic outcome in the absence of revision surgery. And while the emotionally distraught patient often pushes for early surgical intervention, sometimes accompanied by anger or hostility, appropriate treatment must not be compromised in the name of expediency. In contrast, early intervention is occasionally justified in the contracture-prone patient who exhibits signs of rapid and severe nasal contracture. However, while early intervention may come as welcome news to these challenging patients, such high-risk cases seldom lead to storybook outcomes and a thorough, candid, and well-documented informed consent is mandatory.

AUGMENTATION GRAFTING OF THE OVERRESECTED NOSE

Perhaps the most common presentation in secondary rhinoplasty is severe structural compromise resulting from overresection of the nasal framework. For most patients, the immediate postoperative deformity is characterized by a partially collapsed and noticeably less attractive nose.

However, the initial deformity often eventually gives way to progressive (delayed) contour deformity as postoperative soft tissue contracture and fibrosis further deform the surgically weakened nasal framework. And while the degree of deformity often correlates to the extent of cartilage resection, noses with soft, pliable nasal cartilage are particularly vulnerable to skeletal overexcision since naturally weak cartilage is already near the threshold for skeletal collapse. Indeed, in the susceptible patient with exceedingly soft cartilage, even modest cartilage excision can lead to severe nasal deformities. Moreover, even when the initial rhinoplasty outcome fails to exceed the threshold for skeletal collapse, age or disease-related deterioration in cartilage strength may eventually lead to failure of the surgically weakened framework and subsequent nasal deformity. Because the severity of soft tissue contracture also varies widely among individuals, those with naturally strong contractile forces—often associated with relatively thin nasal skin—are also at increased risk for delayed skeletal deformities, even when they possess comparatively strong nasal cartilage. Likewise, surgical disruption of vital secondary tip support mechanisms will also predispose to iatrogenic deformity unless secondary support mechanisms are adequately reconstituted or compensated at the time of primary rhinoplasty (4). Noses with preexisting skeletal deviations are also potentially more susceptible to overaggressive excisional techniques since aggressive surgical destabilization may exacerbate underlying imperfections of the nasal cartilage, particularly deviation of the dorsal septum. And while a large nasal tip is often equated with strong nasal cartilage, in reality, wide or bulbous alar cartilages are often exceptionally soft, making them highly susceptible to surgical overresection. Without question, durable and dependable skeletal support is fundamental to a stable and reproducible rhinoplasty outcome, and surgical techniques that imperil long-term structural support are far more susceptible to the powerful and persistent forces of wound healing.

Until recently, "excisional" rhinoplasty techniques have been the workhorse of cosmetic nasal surgery. Traditional methods for reduction of the wide nasal tip and/or rotation of the ptotic tip have relied upon aggressive resection of the lateral crura—the so-called *cephalic trim* technique. Often the cephalic trim is combined with resection of the anterior septal angle, presumably to achieve still greater tip rotation. Sadly, these techniques are more often destructive, rather than constructive, as surgical reduction in skeletal support frequently exceeds the threshold for long-term structural stability. Although excisional techniques may yield acceptable surgical outcomes in select circumstances, the practice of excising vital skeletal tissues to refine the nasal contour is a risky and unpredictable undertaking, and a disproportionate number of adverse rhinoplasty outcomes are probably the result of overaggressive cartilage excision. Indeed, aggressive destabilization of the nasal framework can severely degrade and weaken skeletal support eventually resulting in stigmatic and unsightly deformities of the nasal contour. In fact, even seemingly trivial reductions in structural support can lead to skeletal collapse in the highly predisposed patient. Yet the strong association between excisional techniques and nasal contour deformities has done little to discourage the use of excisional methods as many practitioners still perform and teach only aggressive excisional techniques. Moreover, since both the severity of soft tissue contracture and the threshold for cartilage collapse cannot be reliably determined in advance, and since arbitrary limits for cartilage excision may fail to account for age-related reductions in cartilage strength, the long-term outcome of excisional rhinoplasty is at best haphazard and unpredictable. Fortunately, an improved understanding of nasal tip dynamics and a growing recognition of the harmful effects of overzealous cartilage removal is prompting a gradual shift away from excision-based techniques and toward the adoption of safer and more reliable surgical alternatives. As a result, the unpredictable and somewhat risky practice of aggressive cartilage excision is slowly being supplanted by techniques that conserve nasal cartilage and reliably enhance tip contour with far less risk of skeletal degradation.

OPTIONS FOR SKELETAL TISSUE REPLACEMENT

In the overwhelming majority of revision rhinoplasty cases skeletal support has been severely compromised and damaged or missing skeletal tissues must be surgically reconstituted in order to restore satisfactory nasal contour and function. As a consequence, the skillful and adept use of *autologous tissue grafts* has become the mainstay of revision rhinoplasty. In addition to a familiarity with the biophysical properties and limitations of various graft materials, successful tissue grafting demands a working knowledge of the proper harvest, fabrication, and fixation of each graft material. Although accomplished rhinoplasty surgeons may use specific graft materials differently, the fundamental tenets of graft harvest and application must be followed regardless of the material selected or the specific method of application.

Despite the potential risk of infection, resorption, warping, migration, and other complications associated with autologous graft materials, autografts remain the gold standard in secondary rhinoplasty owing to their *long-term* safety and reliability. However, synthetic implant materials, while controversial, are growing in popularity as an alternative to autologous tissue grafts. In primary augmentation rhinoplasty, porous synthetic polymers, most notably expanded-polytetrafluoroethylene (Gore-Tex, W.L. Gore & Associates Inc., Flagstaff, AZ) and high-density porous polyethylene (Medpor, Porex Surgical Inc., Newnan, GA) have been used successfully for dorsal augmentation with comparatively few initial complications, particularly in comparison to traditional nonporous (silicone) implants (21–24). More recently, the use of porous polyethylene has expanded to include placement in the lower third of the nose for both functional and cosmetic purposes (25–29). Reported complication rates have generally been low, but delayed infection, extrusion, and foreign body reaction were reported in most series. Somewhat higher complication rates were observed when alloplastic materials were used in revision rhinoplasty, and increased complication rates were attributed to comorbidities such as concomitant septal perforation, prior history of cocaine abuse, cigarette smoking, and other causes of vascular compromise (22,24,30). While alloplastic materials appear to be gaining popularity in primary rhinoplasty, the use of alloplastic materials in revision rhinoplasty remains controversial due to the increased potential for delayed extrusion, infection, and/or foreign body reaction. Consequently, the use of synthetic implant materials in revision rhinoplasty remains comparatively uncommon.

As an alternative to alloplastic materials, some surgeons prefer irradiated rib homografts for complex revision rhinoplasty. While the long-standing debate regarding the longevity and efficacy of irradiated rib grafts continues, recent clinical data suggest that the performance of irradiated rib homografts may be comparable to that of autologous rib tissue (31,32). However, patient objections to cadaveric tissue grafts, the limited availability of human cadaver tissue, the increased costs, and the theoretical potential for the transmission of communicable disease make cadaver cartilage grafts a comparatively seldom-used graft material (33).

While various options such as synthetic polymers and rib homografts are now available to the contemporary revision rhinoplasty surgeon, autologous tissue grafts remain by far the most commonly used reconstructive material in revision rhinoplasty. Owing to their well-defined biomechanical characteristics, lack of toxicity, disease transmission, or foreign body reaction; and their superior long-term safety profile, autologous grafts will likely remain the material of choice for the foreseeable future, and the remainder of this chapter focuses upon autologous graft materials for use in secondary rhinoplasty.

The traditional surgical adage to "replace like with like" is particularly relevant in revision rhinoplasty. Because the nose is a naturally flexible appendage that returns to its initial shape following deformation by facial movement, the reconstructed nose should also remain flexible, yet simultaneously maintain a durable and attractive shape and provide a reliable airway conduit. Of the existing options for replacement of damaged or missing nasal cartilage, only autologous human cartilage approximates the strength, flexibility, thickness, and tolerance to movement of the original nasal tissues. Although autologous bone has previously been advocated for use in nasal reconstruction, the difficulty of harvest, combined with the associated rigidity, bulk, and susceptibility to absorption, makes bone a less commonly used option for most secondary rhinoplasty applications (3,34,35).

Owing to a wide variation in nasal morphology, particularly in the secondary rhinoplasty patient population, and the widely differing biomechanical and physical requirements within various regions of the nose, no single graft material meets all of the reconstructive requirements for every revision rhinoplasty patient. Moreover, autologous cartilage graft materials are all limited in supply, and restricted to the surplus portions of the quadrangular septum, the conchal region of the external ear, and the cartilaginous rib cage. Consequently, the choice of autologous graft materials will vary from patient to patient according to the location, size, and shape of the nasal defect, as well as the availability of cartilage from a particular donor site, the preference of the surgeon, and the willingness of the patient to authorize graft harvest. In some cases, a single graft material may enable a satisfactory surgical outcome, whereas in more complicated revision cases more than one graft type may be needed for the best reconstructive result. In the case of exceedingly large skeletal defects or the multiply-revised patient with prior depletion of both septal and conchal cartilage donor sites, rib cartilage becomes the only viable treatment option. Regardless of the graft materials chosen, the skillful application of autologous tissue grafts remains the foundation of contemporary revision rhinoplasty, and a sound working knowledge of each graft type is essential for any revision surgeon.

Septal Cartilage

Perhaps the autograft best suited to revision rhinoplasty is septal cartilage. Histologically, septal cartilage is classified as hyaline cartilage—a semisolid matrix of chondroitin sulfate embedded with chondrocytes and a network of type II collagen fibers (36,37). Scanning electron microscopy reveals a mesh-like framework of large collagen fibers yielding additional strength relative to the loosely organized and smaller collagen fibers seen in lower lateral cartilage (36). The thickness of septal cartilage also varies according to the anatomic site and ranges from 0.74 to 3.03 mm (38). Thinner portions of the nasal septum correspond closely to the 0.7-mm average thickness of the lateral crus (39,40), making septal cartilage uniquely well suited to reconstruction of the thin and lightweight lower lateral cartilages. Although the least abundant of all autologous cartilage graft materials, septal cartilage has numerous advantages over other sources of autologous tissue, including its proximity to the surgical field and its nose-like biophysical properties. Harvest of cartilage from a healthy nasal septum is generally quick and uncomplicated, but care must be taken to preserve an outer perimeter of residual cartilage to maintain structural support—the so-called septal "L-strut". Minimum width of the L-strut remains a matter of controversy and should probably be kept as wide as possible, but a 1.0-cm-wide L-strut is generally considered adequate for most noses (3). Despite preservation of a 1.0-cm L-strut, a sizeable piece of septal cartilage can still be harvested from most leptorrhine noses (Fig. 184.4A–D). Graft harvest is typically more difficult in noses with preexisting septal deformities resulting from growth disturbances,

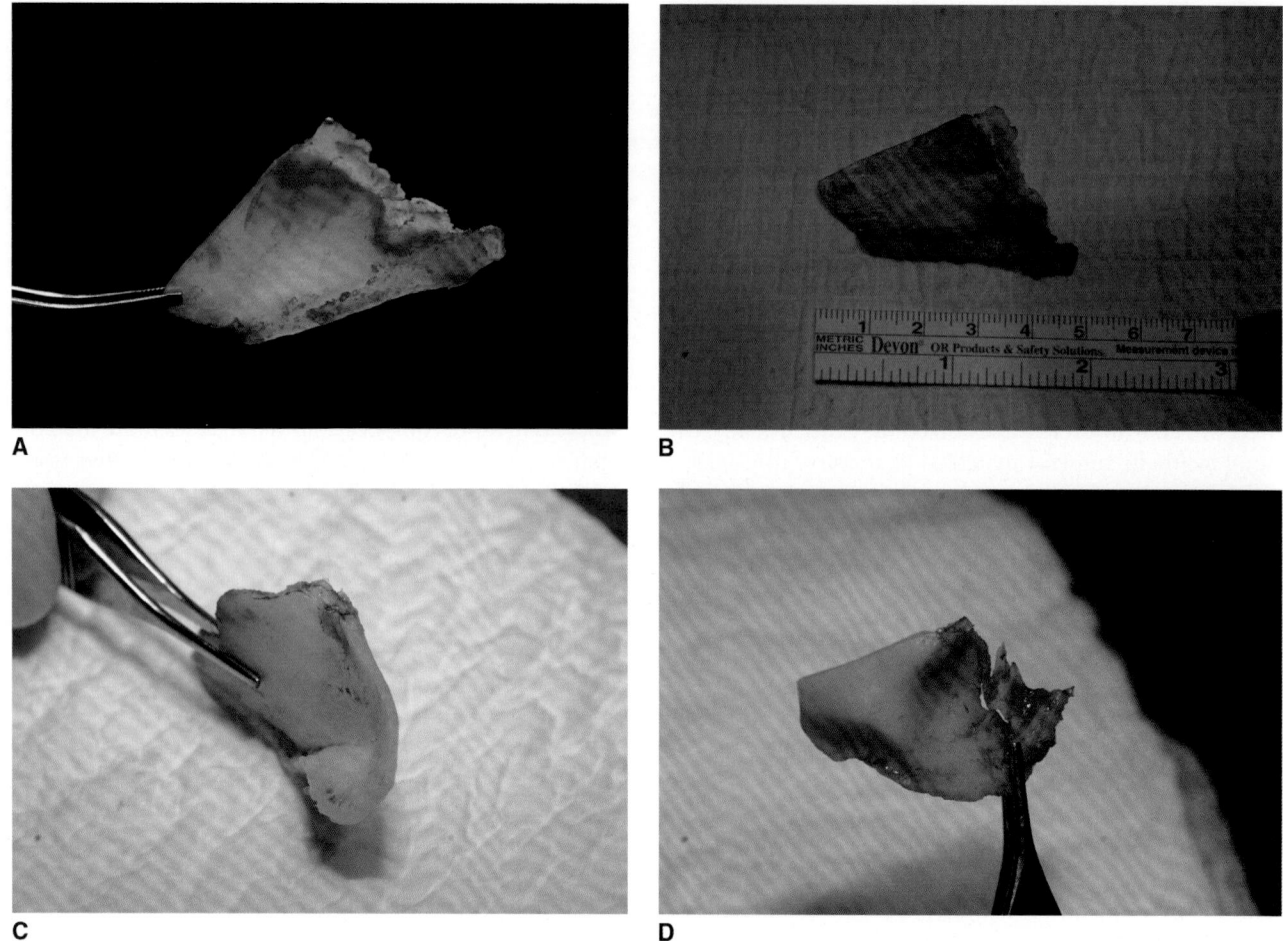

Figure 184.4 Septal cartilage graft material. **A:** Septal graft material harvested with L-strut preservation, **(B)** typical graft dimensions in the leptorrhine nose, and **(C,D)** donor graft material distorted by preexisting septal deformity.

nasal trauma, and/or prior nasal surgery, but elimination of these deformities often contributes to improved airway function. Graft yields may vary according to patient ethnicity and age (41), with larger yields in younger patients due to forward expansion of the bony ethmoid plate over time. Interestingly, graft size may not correlate with size of the external nose, making it difficult to predict the availability of septal graft material in advance (42).

Historically, septal cartilage has been regarded as a resilient graft material and is seldom associated with absorption, infection, warping, or extrusion (3,33). Owing to its combination of axial rigidity and transverse flexibility, septal cartilage is commonly used in secondary rhinoplasty for structural grafting; including struts, battens, extension grafts, spreader grafts, and various tip grafts. Similarly, because of its stability and relative ease of carving, septal cartilage can also be sculpted to create a wide variety of surface (onlay) grafts for camouflage or contour augmentation. Lightly morselized ("crushed") septal cartilage grafts can also be used for augmentation, smoothing, or camouflage with minimal risk of edge prominence or graft resorption (43).

However, like all donor tissues, septal cartilage has limitations. While convenient, harvesting septal cartilage leads to additional soft tissue trauma thereby exacerbating nasal inflammation and edema, and potentially compromising tissue perfusion. Moreover, although septal cartilage is preferred for its biomechanical properties, adequate amounts of surplus septal cartilage are not always available. In primary rhinoplasty, many flat underprojected noses lack adequate septal cartilage for significant grafting needs, and in revision cases surplus septal cartilage may be damaged or depleted from previous surgery. Efforts to generate large amounts of tissue-engineered human septal cartilage with biomechanical properties equivalent to natural septum are under way, but to date bioengineered septal cartilage is not yet clinically available (37). Interestingly, the adult human nasal septum is the preferred donor tissue for laboratory-engineered cartilage since septal chondrocytes demonstrate a greater proliferative effect in monolayer culture—a crucial preliminary step in cell culture—and they also demonstrate a better overall proliferative and chondrogenic potential relative to most other cartilage cell types (44).

Conchal Cartilage

Elastic (or hyaline-elastic) cartilage harvested from the conchal bowl of the external ear is another commonly used source of autologous cartilage. Histologically, auricular cartilage contains both type I and type II collagen and elastic fibers (37). Unlike septal cartilage that typically yields a flat uniform specimen, conchal cartilage is cupped, generally thicker, and more prone to cracking with manipulation. Moreover, conchal cartilage must be harvested from a separate and distinct surgical site, adding to surgical morbidity and time utilization. However, a single piece of conchal cartilage can be obtained from the typical ear measuring approximately 2.4 × 2.4 cm (45) (Fig. 184.5). Harvest can be performed through either an antihelical fold incision or a postauricular crease incision with minimal cutaneous scarring. When needed, harvest may also include the posterior conchal perichondrium, which can be used for tip graft camouflage or augmentation of thin nasal skin. In order to prevent postoperative auricular contour deformities following harvest of the entire conchal bowl, the antihelical fold must be fully preserved and a bolster-type dressing is required to maintain conchal contour during initial healing. Risks of conchal graft harvest include skin necrosis, scar contracture, infection, or hematoma, but these problems are exceptionally rare in experienced hands.

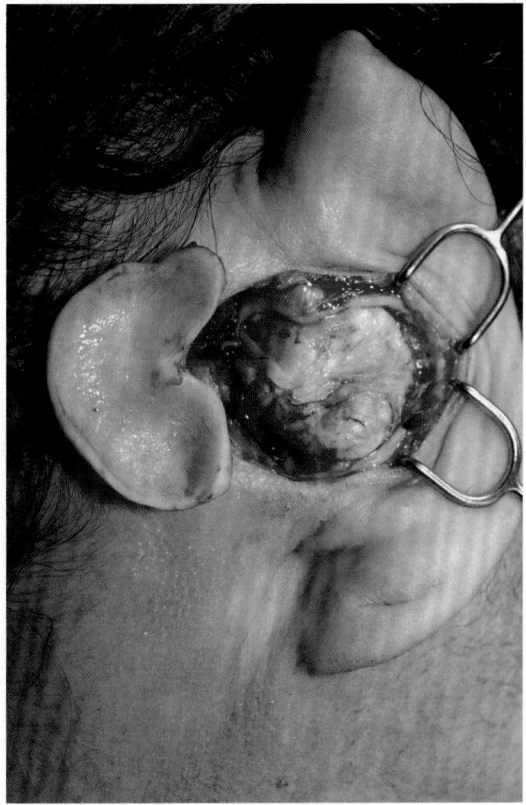

Figure 184.5 Conchal cartilage graft material harvested from the postauricular approach. Note undersurface of the conchal skin after contiguous excision of the concha cymba and cavum.

Like septal cartilage, conchal cartilage grafts are remarkably resilient and seldom succumb to infection, absorption, or extrusion making them a popular graft option in nasal surgery (3,31,45). However, conchal grafts are notoriously difficult to conceal probably as a consequence of their nonuniform shape, and warping or edge prominence are common complications with superficial placement, particularly in the absence of secure suture fixation. Moreover, beveling of graft edges on the outer surface may actually exacerbate graft edge prominence. Owing to its natural bulk and curvature, and its corresponding thickness and lack of axial rigidity, conchal cartilage is also poorly suited to the fabrication of columellar struts and septal extension grafts (SEGs). In such applications, double-layered grafts are often needed to achieve a strong and reasonably straight structural element. However, the natural graft curvature of ear cartilage is sometimes an asset in the fabrication of tip grafts, butterfly grafts, alar rim grafts, or other applications that require a gently curved surface contour (45). Placement of conchal grafts in direct contact with the dermis is ill-advised since graft prominence is common and since tenacious adherence to the skin makes removal exceedingly difficult.

In addition to standard conchal cartilage grafts, *composite* chondrocutaneous grafts are also occasionally useful in secondary rhinoplasty. Composite grafts are most commonly used to correct severe retraction of the alar rim or columella following overresection of the lateral crus or caudal septum, respectively (46,47). Small (5 × 15 mm) composite grafts can be harvested from the concha cavum while still permitting primary closure of the donor defect after undermining of the adjacent skin. Although thick, these grafts are often indispensible in correcting the aforementioned secondary nasal deformities since they replace missing vestibular skin and augment deficient skeletal support.

Costal (Rib) Cartilage

Costal cartilage is another form of hyaline cartilage containing a mix of type I and type II collagen that is mechanically stronger than either septal or conchal cartilage (37). Moreover, unlike conchal or septal cartilage, costal (rib) cartilage is also available in relative abundance. Consequently, rib cartilage is often the material of choice when large volumes of cartilage are required, or when septal or conchal donor sites have been depleted from prior surgery. However, the harvest of rib cartilage is considerably more invasive and time-consuming. Potential risks of rib graft harvest include pneumothorax, chest wall deformity, infection, hematoma/seroma, and/or intense postoperative pain. Harvest from the right chest wall is preferred to avoid inadvertent injury to the underlying left-sided cardiac tissues, and a 3.0-cm chest-wall incision typically affords adequate exposure while limiting donor site scarring. In women, an inframammary crease incision permits concealment of the scar beneath the bikini line but restricts access to the fifth, sixth, or possibly seventh ribs. Obese patients may require a longer incision for better visualization due to extra subcutaneous fat, and in older patients ossification of the rib cartilage may make harvesting and/or carving of the graft difficult (48). However, significant ossification can also occasionally occur in younger patients. The author has harvested rib on two occasions in patients less than 30 years of age who were both found to have near-complete ossification of the rib cage (*personal observation*). In one patient, this was attributed to a rare manifestation of Addison disease, while no known etiology was found for the other patient. Postoperative discomfort from rib harvest can be minimized with blunt spreading of the overlying rectus muscle, and grafts may be harvested as partial or full-thickness specimens with or without the attached perichondrium (Fig. 184.6A and B). Acute postoperative pain is greatly diminished with placement of a percutaneous bupivacaine infusion pump allowing for 4 to 5 days of postoperative donor site numbness.

While rib cartilage is available in abundance, costal cartilage has a strong propensity for warping (3,33–35,44,48–50). Soaking of the specimen in saline followed by concentric carving of the graft may help to minimize warping (51), but aggressive thinning of the graft may contribute to structural instability and eventual warping despite preventative measures. Moreover, experimental evidence suggests that saline-moistened costal grafts may continue warping for up to 4 weeks postharvest (49). Even thick dorsal onlay grafts can warp and/or migrate when the graft fails to adhere or when the graft/host interface is not sufficiently reciprocal. Some experienced rib graft surgeons feel that fixation of dorsal onlay grafts with perichondrium may help to minimize postoperative warping and migration.

In an attempt to further prevent warping of dorsal rib onlay grafts, various modifications have been advocated. Internal stabilization of costal cartilage by longitudinally skewering the graft with a Kirschner wire (K-wire) offers resistance to warping at the expense of a permanent foreign body (50). The use of a *composite* osseocartilaginous dorsal augmentation graft harvested from the sixth, seventh, or eleventh rib allows for osseointegration of the bony component to the bony substructure, promoting stabilization of the graft against migration and/or warping (34,35). Alternatively, rib cartilage may also be "diced" into 0.5- to 1.0-mm cubes and encased in a sleeve of temporalis fascia to create a malleable dorsal augmentation graft that is highly resistant to warping (52,53). The so-called diced cartilage–fascia (DC-F) graft may be used for partial or complete dorsal augmentation depending upon graft size and positioning. DC-F grafts may also be constructed from conchal or septal cartilage, but donor quantities may be insufficient for large volume defects. The harvest of temporalis fascia is generally uncomplicated and associated with minimal donor site morbidity, and the DC-F graft has proven both effective and reliable without warping or clinically significant absorption in long-term clinical application (52,53).

Soft Tissue Grafts

Although skeletal restoration is the foundation of revision rhinoplasty, thickness and uniformity of the overlying nasal skin also plays a critical role in secondary nasal surgery. Nasal skin at the extremes of thickness—extremely thick skin or exceedingly thin nasal skin—often present the greatest technical challenge in secondary rhinoplasty. For noses with extremely thick nasal skin, excessive soft tissue bulk completely obscures the skeletal contours necessary for a well-defined and attractive surface topography.

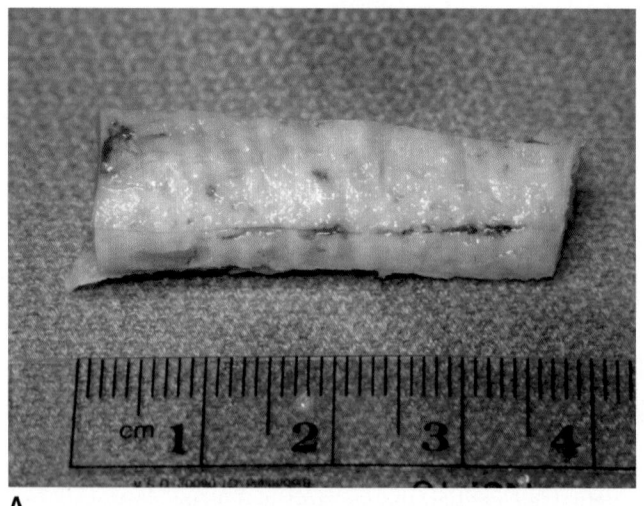

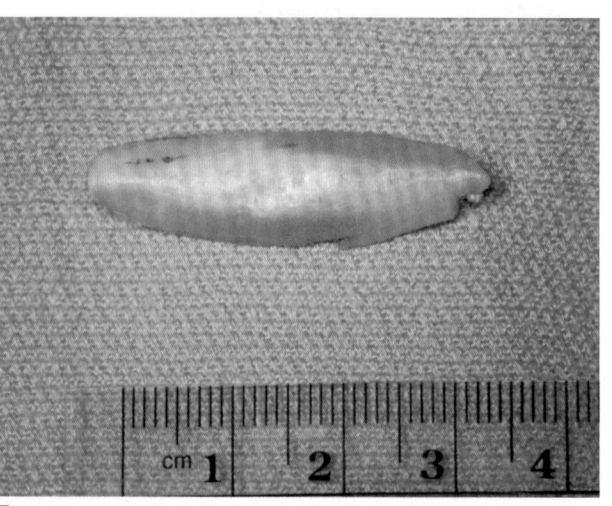

A   **B**

Figure 184.6 Rib cartilage graft material. **A:** Specimen of sixth rib following removal of perichondrium, and **(B)** solid dorsal onlay graft contoured from sixth rib specimen.

In contrast, naturally thin nasal skin provides little if any camouflage, and even minor skeletal imperfections are easily discernible beneath the ultrathin soft tissues. In the multiply operated nose with overly thin skin, surgically induced atrophy can also lead to additional thinning and still greater cosmetic deformity (Fig. 184.7A–C). Ironically,

atrophic thinning is often most severe over the rhinion and nasal tip where skeletal imperfections most commonly arise. Thin-skinned patients are also more susceptible to surgically induced erythema, which may become progressively longer lasting with each successive surgery and which may eventually fail to resolve altogether. In addition to the

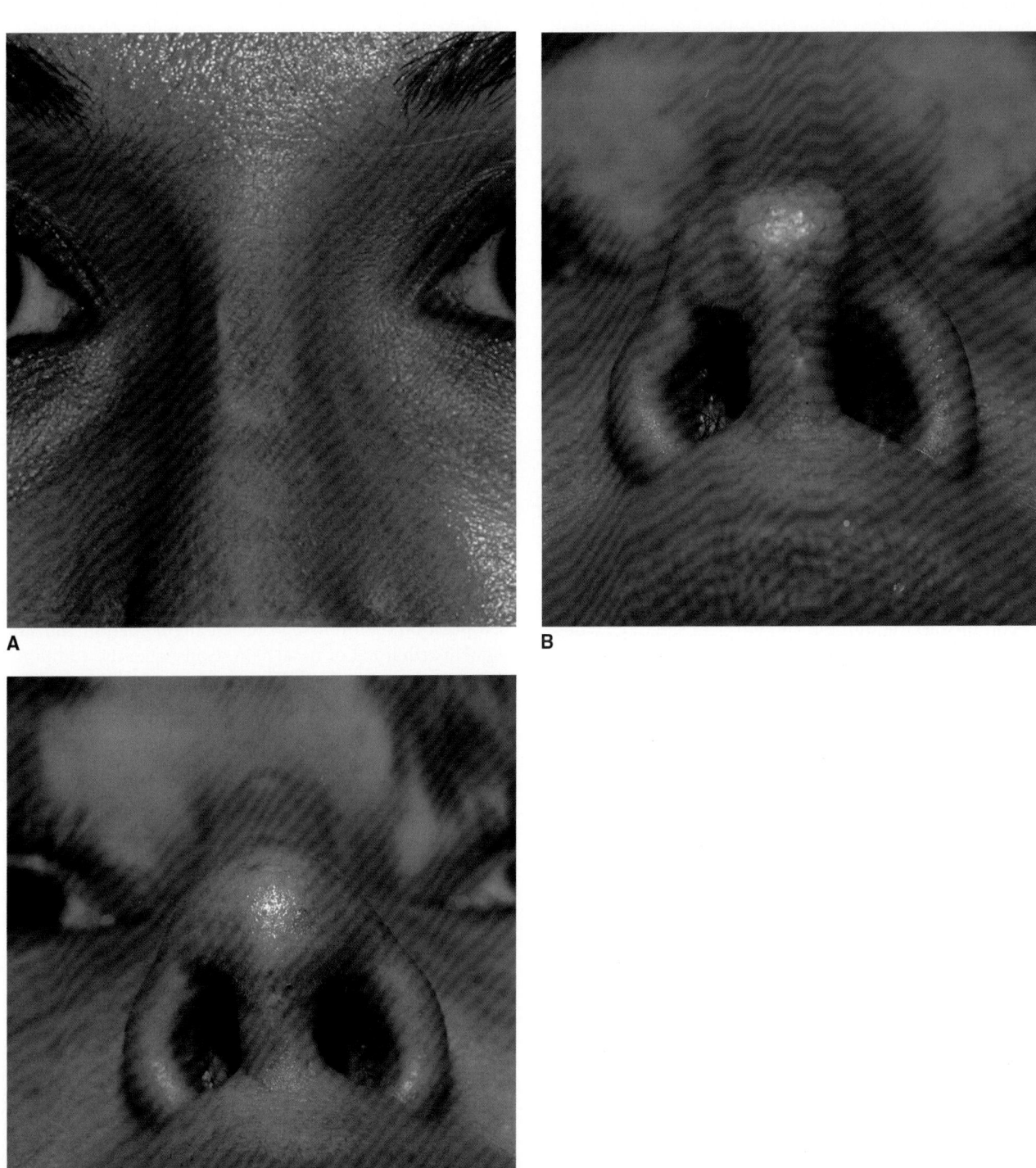

Figure 184.7 Rhinoplasty complications resulting from ultrathin nasal skin. **A:** Excessive prominence of radix graft in thin-skinned nose, **(B)** excessive tip graft prominence in the thin-skinned nose, and **(C)** nasal tip contour after camouflage with autologous (abdominal) dermal graft.

drawbacks of naturally thin nasal skin, unsightly contour irregularities can also develop in patients with intermediate nasal skin thickness as a consequence of localized surgical injury and subsequent (focal) skin atrophy. When severe, random inconsistencies in skin thickness can produce an unsightly lumpy appearance despite a smooth underlying skeletal substructure. Moreover, attempting to eliminate these surface irregularities through alteration of the underlying skeletal framework may prove exceedingly difficult and may even jeopardize skeletal integrity.

Treatment of overly thin nasal skin or focal skin inconsistencies is often best achieved using autologous soft tissue augmentation grafts. Various autologous materials have been used to augment skin thickness including dermis, perichondrium, superficial musculoaponeurosis (SMAS), and temporalis fascia. De-epithelialized dermis may be harvested from the abdomen using previous surgical scars (e.g., C-section, appendectomy) or from an elliptical Pfannenstiel-type incision below the bikini line (54) (Fig. 184.7B and C). Modest amounts of perichondrium can be obtained from the posterior conchal bowl, whereas larger amounts can be obtained from costal cartilage. A 4.0 × 5.0 cm sheet of temporalis fascia is easily obtained via a 2.0-cm temporal scalp incision placed over the mid-temporalis muscle. The nasal SMAS layer, a fibromuscular tissue layer that lies immediately deep to the subdermal fat, may be excised *en bloc* from beneath the nasal skin flap to improve tip contour, definition, and skin elasticity (55). Nasal SMAS should only be harvested from patients with exceptionally thick nasal skin and harvest is generally confined to the supratip and adjacent sidewalls where the SMAS layer is often thickest. Once removed, excised material can be reimplanted in other areas of the nose for contour enhancement (e.g., radix, rhinion, or sidewall augmentation) or for focal augmentation in areas of excessive skin thinning. Survival of autologous SMAS grafts is generally favorable in the absence of preexisting vascular insufficiency.

Since soft tissue graft survival is dependent upon an adequate recipient-site blood supply, autologous soft tissue grafts may succumb to resorption in patients with vascular insufficiency such as smokers, diabetics, or those with previously devascularized skin. While no autologous soft tissue graft is completely immune to resorption, soft tissue graft survival is generally favorable in healthy patients, especially when applied in a single layer to optimize surface contact with the recipient tissue bed. Blanketing the outer surface of the nasal framework with a single layer of autologous soft tissue can also smooth minor indentations, camouflage rough surfaces, and eliminate minor edge prominence of cartilage onlay grafts, thereby obviating the need for difficult alterations in skeletal contour. When performing either primary or revision rhinoplasty, all soft tissues removed in the course of surgical dissection should be retained in saline for possible reimplantation later in the case.

EXTERNAL RHINOPLASTY APPROACH

Surgical exposure for secondary rhinoplasty can be achieved via either the external or the endonasal rhinoplasty approach. For minor revision procedures, the endonasal (or "closed") approach is often preferable, offering minimal tissue disruption with less swelling and inflammation, and a faster return to normalcy. However, the endonasal rhinoplasty approach also restricts visibility, limits suture fixation of graft tissue, and hampers *en bloc* excision of scar tissue from beneath the nasal skin flap. Consequently, despite the requirement for a visible columellar incision, the wide-field surgical exposure afforded by the external (or "open") rhinoplasty approach is generally preferred for complex secondary rhinoplasty. The additional exposure and visibility afforded by the external rhinoplasty approach offers greater surgical exposure, increased diagnostic accuracy, and greater ease of suture graft fixation, all while preserving an intact vascularized epithelial barrier between the surgical field and the nasal cavity. Since a carefully repaired transcolumellar incision seldom creates an objectionable scar, and since various surgical techniques are precluded with the endonasal approach, external rhinoplasty is generally the procedure of choice for complex revision nasal surgery.

In the severely misshapen and previously operated nose, normal anatomic landmarks are often heavily distorted making subsequent incision placement difficult. Moreover, what may seem like appropriate incision placement at the onset of secondary surgery may later result in unfavorable scar positioning following skeletal augmentation and subsequent redraping of nasal skin. Consequently, additional care must be taken to anticipate the possible migration of incision lines and to locate the transcolumellar and marginal incisions as close to their correct (original) anatomic location as possible. Although the presence of nonanatomic cartilage grafts may make locating the lateral crural cartilage remnants difficult, marginal incisions should follow the caudal border of the lateral crus to avoid unnecessary scar visibility.

In the previously operated nose with a conspicuous transcolumellar scar, design and placement of the subsequent columellar incision can become an issue. Although the goal of surgically eliminating an unsightly columellar scar with scar excision is laudable, skin excision should be avoided unless copious skin redundancy will ensure a tensionless closure *after* skeletal re-expansion is complete. Ironically, skeletal re-expansion will often stretch the columellar skin and minimize visibility of the existing scar. Moreover, the author has found that reusing an unsightly midcolumellar scar for placement of the subsequent incision can often dramatically improve scar appearance when closed with carefully everted skin edges. Alternatively, when placing the columellar incision in previously *unoperated* columellar skin, the incision should be located over the columellar double-break—approximately halfway up the columella. In addition to providing a narrow segment and thus a shorter scar, this location is also partially concealed by the junction of two aesthetic nasal subunits. Finally, use of the traditional five-cornered "inverted-V" incision offers additional scar camouflage similar to a geometric broken line–type scar concealment, and optimizes flap alignment with an additional reference point relative to the alternative stair-step incision.

SOFT TISSUE SURGICAL TECHNIQUE

Meticulous and gentle soft tissue technique is essential in any rhinoplasty, but especially in revision rhinoplasty where nasal tissues are already partially compromised by varying degrees of scar and vascular insufficiency. Avoiding the use of crushing forceps, prolonged or aggressive tissue retraction, excessive tissue desiccation, or overzealous use of electrocautery will minimize soft tissue trauma and limit the release of harmful inflammatory mediators. While atraumatic soft tissue technique is recommended for all revision rhinoplasty patients, it is particularly important in noses with scar-prone skin or substantial vascular compromise, since aggressive tissue handling may trigger adverse wound-healing responses and ruin an otherwise successful reconstruction. Moreover, the survival of all free tissue grafts, the prevention of postoperative infection, and the viability of any surgically manipulated tissue is dependent upon an adequate and uninterrupted nutrient blood flow. While all patients suffer some degree of soft tissue swelling and inflammation, gentle soft tissue technique can mitigate surgical inflammation, minimize lymphedema, and optimize soft tissue perfusion—often determining the difference between a mediocre surgical outcome and a surprisingly good cosmetic result.

SURGICAL DECONSTRUCTION OF THE PREVIOUSLY-OPERATED NOSE

Perhaps one of the greatest technical challenges in secondary rhinoplasty is surgical *deconstruction* of the badly damaged nose. Deconstruction is the first step in dismantling and exposing the deformed, malpositioned, and/or damaged nasal components prior to surgical reconstruction. As a consequence of exposing the misshapen nasal framework, deconstruction also greatly enhances diagnostic accuracy and frequently leads to critical refinements in the surgical game plan. However, deconstruction is typically a difficult undertaking in the previously operated nose, and liberating the malpositioned and/or damaged cartilage remnants without causing further harm can prove extremely challenging in some patients (Fig. 184.8A and B). At the very least, the task of elevating the nasal skin envelope and exposing fragile cartilage remnants embedded in scar tissue, all while avoiding injury to the surrounding nasal lining, is a time-consuming endeavor that requires considerable patience and skill. Slow and tedious dissection with heavy reliance upon blunt technique is often necessary to safely deglove the weakened and distorted nasal framework.

During the course of deconstruction, skeletal remnants are often observed to have migrated from their intended position or to have transformed from their desired shape—both an unwanted consequence of scar contracture. Surgically induced contracture of the nasal lining not only leads to malpositioned and misshapen skeletal remnants, it may also result in mucosal adhesions and cartilage fixation, further adding to the difficulty of surgical deconstruction. Hence, deconstruction often involves lysis of scar adhesions to release the entrapped skeletal remnants and to permit appropriate repositioning of the displaced cartilage components.

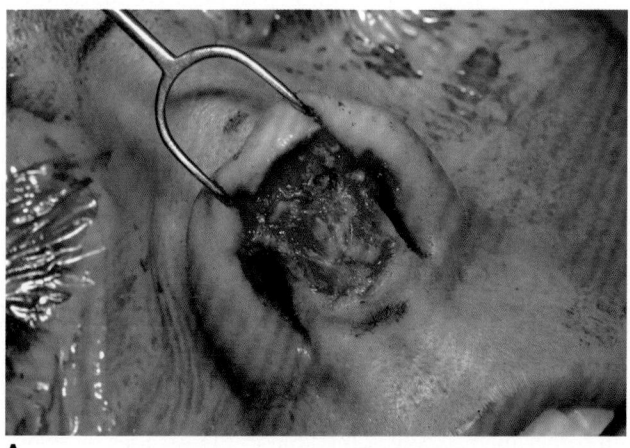

A

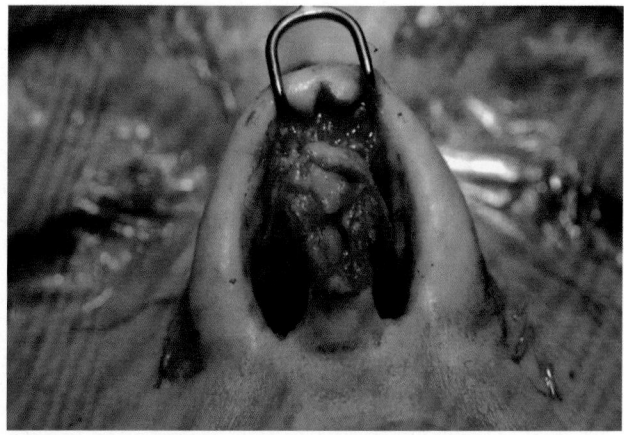

B

Figure 184.8 Examples of severe tip cartilage distortion resulting from previous cosmetic rhinoplasty. **A:** Scarred and fragmented tip cartilages prior to deconstruction, and **(B)** telescoping collapse of overresected tip cartilages prior to deconstruction.

Perhaps the most common example of contracture-mediated cartilage distortion is *retraction of the alar rim.* Alar retraction is an unsightly nasal deformity often resulting from overexcision of the lateral crus during reduction rhinoplasty. When overexcision of the cephalic crural border leaves a crural remnant that is too weak to resist deformation by scar contracture, the weakened lateral crus and the attached alar soft tissues both retract cephalically, producing a conspicuous and unsightly notching of the nostril (Fig. 184.2B). Aggressive surgical excision of the cephalic lateral crus is the basis of the *cephalic trim* maneuver, a traditional but haphazard tip refinement technique still in widespread use today. The severity of nostril retraction is largely determined by the extent of cartilage resection, since a large skeletal void is associated with both greater scar contracture and greater structural compromise. And despite the strong association of the cephalic trim maneuver with unsightly surgical tip deformities, overexcision of the cephalic margin is an almost universal intraoperative finding in most complex revision rhinoplasty cases. While successful restoration of the damaged crural cartilage is usually possible, it is frequently difficult or impossible to surgically unfurl the contractured and foreshortened epithelial lining. And in cases of irreversible scar contracture, composite (chondrocutaneous) grafts are necessary to replace the missing vestibular epithelium and to buttress the alar margin against recurrent retraction.

Despite the painstaking nature of surgical deconstruction, the time spent properly dismantling the nose is well worth the investment. Only through a methodical deconstruction are the skeletal and soft tissue components fully exposed, mobilized, and evaluated in preparation for surgical reconstruction. However, during the course of deconstruction, a number of critical decisions must be made. First, the surgeon must decide whether or not to retain the severely damaged nasal cartilages. In theory, the use of cartilage grafts to augment or replace damaged skeletal tissues can restore structural integrity and produce considerable functional and cosmetic enhancements. However, as the scope of deconstruction and replacement grafting expands, so too does the probability of unforeseen healing aberrations related to surgical inflammation and failed revascularization. Skeletal distortion resulting from graft resorption, scarring, contracture, or infection may taint the final outcome considerably, and the excessive use of graft material can also lead to a whole host of new problems. And since a shapely, rigid, and sturdy neoframework is required for predictable healing, the amount and quality of the available replacement tissue also has a profound bearing upon this decision. Because appropriate replacement tissue is sometimes in short supply, strategic intraoperative planning is also necessary to utilize limited resources wisely and to their best overall advantage. For this reason, it is generally preferable to deconstruct all problem areas of the nose first, before removing

existing skeletal elements and allocating replacement tissues. However, when the existing skeletal elements cannot be salvaged by either reshaping or repositioning, autologous cartilage grafts become the primary workhorse for strengthening, reinforcing, or sometimes completely replacing damaged skeletal components. While replacing or reinforcing critical structural elements with cartilage grafts will always have inherent risks, in the healthy individual with ample donor tissue and a robust recipient blood supply, the cosmetic and functional benefits of *structural* cartilage grafting usually *far surpass* any other surgical strategy.

In addition to damaged native nasal tissues, many complex revision rhinoplasty patients also present with previously placed tissue grafts or implants that may be contributing to unwanted functional and/or cosmetic deformities. A variety of options for treating unsightly grafts or implants are available to the revision surgeon including *in situ* modification by shaving or repositioning, camouflage, substitution, removal, or combinations therein. As part of the deconstruction process, the decision whether or not to retain these previously placed materials must take into account the overall risk-to-benefit ratio and the availability of suitable replacement materials. However, not all previously placed cartilage grafts should be discarded *per se.* Misshapen or malpositioned grafts that have no detrimental *external* cosmetic impact are often best left alone since removal may lead to unwanted external contour deformities. Moreover, contour deformities resulting from graft removal are sometimes a consequence of scarring and thickness irregularities of the nasal skin flap that are frequently very difficult to eliminate. And while the removal of unsightly skeletal components may be cosmetically justified, aggressive deconstruction of the nasal framework can also lead to significant structural instability, potentially opening the door for catastrophic consequences if the nasal soft tissues are pushed beyond their limits. In the severely ravaged nose, soft tissue linings provide both vascular and *structural* support, serving to compensate for severely weakened skeletal components. The result is sometimes a structurally borderline, yet deceptively healthy-looking appendage that belies its fragile and tenuous state. Unless the aggregate soft tissues have sufficient vascular integrity to support skeletal replacement grafts *and* to tolerate the additional stresses associated with aggressive surgical deconstruction, a far more conservative approach must be adopted intraoperatively to prevent potentially catastrophic consequences. Moreover, even in the generally healthy nose, aggressive deconstruction of the nasal framework results in progressive structural destabilization and vascular disruption, adding an element of unpredictability to the surgical outcome as the nose becomes increasingly vulnerable to the vagaries of wound healing. Hence, aggressive deconstruction is often a necessary evil, but one that is justified only when the potential benefits are likely to exceed the associated individual risks. Moreover, during surgery, the prudent surgeon will continually reassess the nasal soft tissues for telltale signs of surgical intolerance and will quickly alter the treatment plan as conditions dictate.

Another key decision confronting the revision surgeon is how large to make the neo-skeletal framework. Ideally, this decision is made early in the course of skeletal deconstruction before irreversible alterations to the existing skeletal framework are undertaken. For the overresected nose, the cosmetic ideal typically requires substantial skeletal enlargement, but the surgeon must weigh the cosmetic benefits of a larger and more attractive nasal framework against the potential hazards of an overly taut soft tissue envelope. Assessing the quality and mobility of the soft tissue envelope *prior* to surgery is paramount since noncompliant skin greatly limits skeletal re-expansion. While placing healthy elastic skin on stretch can enhance tip definition and lead to significant tip refinement, placing fibrotic inelastic skin under sufficient tension to improve surface contour may potentially impair tissue perfusion and lead to ischemic compromise (20). Consequently, patients with severely foreshortened noses coupled with severely noncompliant skin are best deferred unless skin-stretching exercises can adequately improve soft tissue elasticity. Moreover, in patients with thick inelastic skin and weak nasal cartilage, achieving a skeletal framework of sufficient strength to stretch the noncompliant skin envelope can also prove extremely challenging. In fact, the combination of thick fibrotic skin and weak central tip support is among the most challenging of all revision noses (20). In most cases, rib cartilage grafts become the only reliable means of creating a neo-framework of sufficient strength and rigidity to forcefully stretch, and subsequently thin, the dense fibrotic nasal skin. However, because long slender rib grafts under compressive load are more prone to warping, rib grafts are generally fabricated much thicker than would be cosmetically ideal. On the other hand, assuming cosmetic tolerances will permit a wider nose, the surgically distended skin produced by rib grafting often results in a more elegant and better-defined nasal contour. Nevertheless, due to the increased structural loads carried by the newly fabricated skeletal framework, coupled with the corresponding increase in tension placed upon the overlying skin, the risks of inadequate skin perfusion and/or skeletal deformation are markedly increased with this aggressive treatment strategy (20). And depending upon the extent of closing tension, the amount of postoperative swelling, and the reliability of the microcirculation, vascular insufficiency can develop even in young healthy patients. While frank skin necrosis is exceedingly rare, underperfused tissues can lead to graft resorption, wound infection, or wound dehiscence, and extreme care must be taken to minimize vascular insults when augmenting the overresected nose. Moreover, a wide and masculine nasal contour is sometimes unavoidable when using rib cartilage grafts to expand the severely foreshortened nose,

and despite the improved profile contour, significant width increases may occasionally result in patient dissatisfaction.

In the event that thick and surgically scarred nasal skin fails to accommodate optimal skeletal enlargement, judicious surgical debulking of the subcutaneous tissues can sometimes improve both skin compliance and surface definition (20,55). In histologic studies of the thick-skinned nose, Garramone et al. (56) observed that extra skin thickness is derived mostly from hypertrophy of the fibromuscular tissue layer found just beneath the subdermal fat. When scarred and thickened from prior surgery, this tissue layer can greatly inhibit skin elasticity. Because the thickened fibromuscular tissue layer—also known as the nasal SMAS (57)—can be carefully excised from the nasal tip and supratip without damaging the subdermal plexus, debulking of the nasal SMAS can greatly reduce skin thickness while simultaneously improving both skin distensibility and surface contour (55).

However, in the surgically scarred nose, SMAS excision is a potentially high-risk maneuver that may potentially reduce skin flap perfusion in a nose that may already be on the verge of vascular insufficiency. While SMAS debulking is often performed safely in revision rhinoplasty patients, previous surgical scarring may make navigation far more challenging, and the added exposure of the external rhinoplasty approach is crucial. Possible complications such as inadvertent skin perforation or ischemic skin necrosis are rare, but these risks are increased in the severely fibrotic nose with prior circulatory compromise. Hence SMAS excision should be reserved only for patients with a robust cutaneous circulation and exceedingly thick, but otherwise healthy nasal skin. In patients with nasal skin thickness of at least 5 mm, careful SMAS excision can be performed in areas where improved distensibility and surface definition are desired—usually the tip, supratip, and supra-alar sidewalls. In order to maintain a uniform flap thickness and avoid injury to the subdermal plexus, the fibromuscular SMAS layer is excised *en bloc* under direct visualization using mostly blunt dissection (55) (Fig. 184.9A–C). With careful separation of the SMAS layer, the subdermal plexus is left largely undisturbed, and the nutrient blood supply to the nasal skin is protected—a vitally important step, especially if aggressive skin stretching is also planned. However, special care must be exercised near the alar groove where the primary source of cutaneous blood supply—the lateral nasal artery—has been shown to enter the subdermal plexus (58).

In contrast to re-expansion of the undersized nose, revision of the *oversized* nose presents an entirely different set of surgical issues. While *reduction* rhinoplasty is often quite challenging in its own right, the potential for catastrophic vascular insufficiency is comparatively small since redundant nasal skin is usually generated from skeletal downsizing. As long as the redundant skin envelope shrinks promptly and adheres tightly to the smaller and more attractive skeletal framework, fibrosis of the subcutaneous

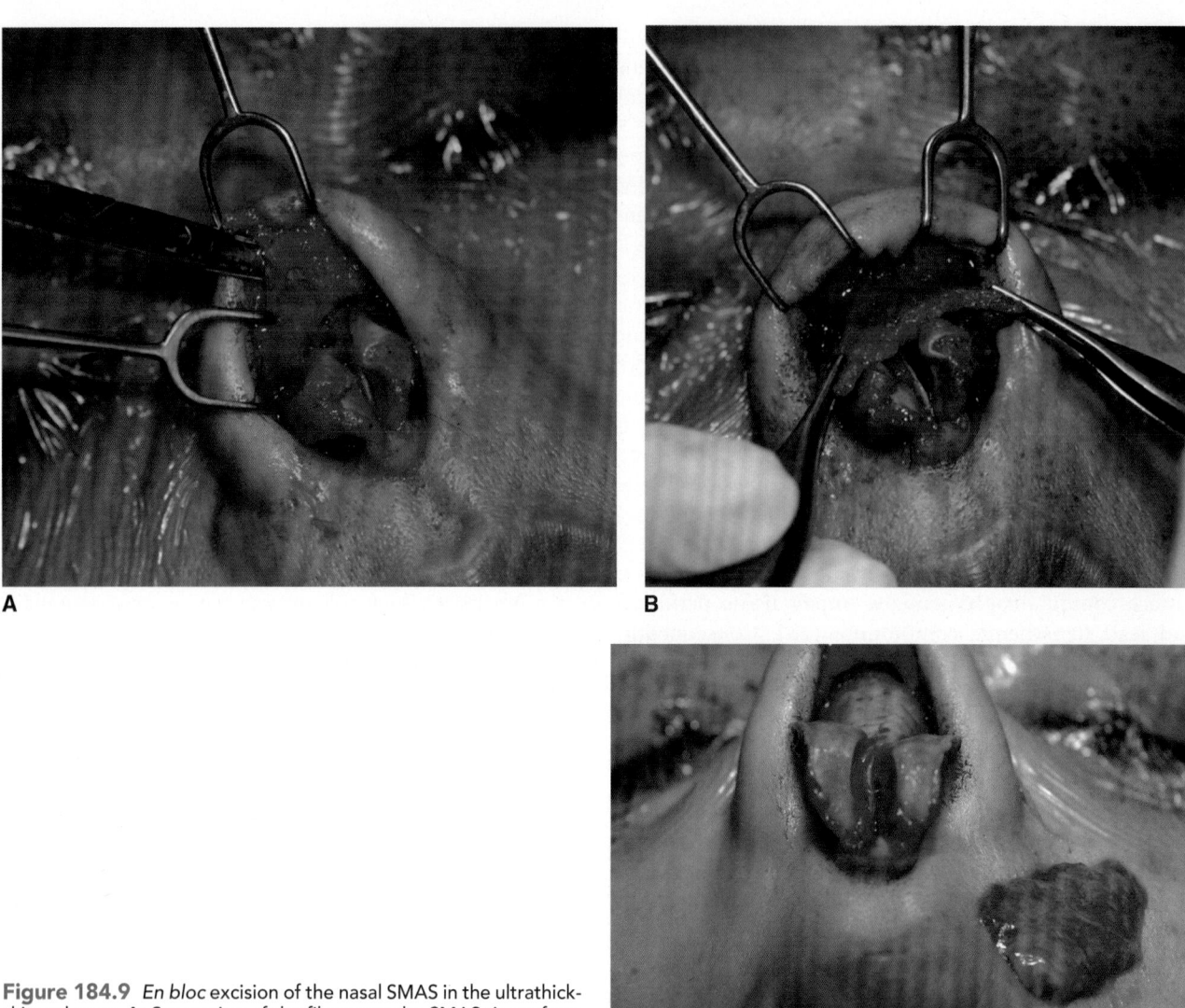

Figure 184.9 *En bloc* excision of the nasal SMAS in the ultrathick-skinned nose. **A:** Separation of the fibromuscular SMAS tissue from the subdermal fat with blunt dissection. **B:** Elevated SMAS layer prior to excision, and **(C)** excised fibromuscular tissue mass.

tissues is avoided and a well-defined and more attractive nasal contour typically ensues (see Case One). Avoiding circumstances that aggravate or prolong postoperative edema is particularly important in this patient population, since the large dead space predisposes to the formation of chronic lymphedema and subcutaneous fibrosis. In fact, the overly large nose covered with thick sebaceous nasal skin is highly susceptible to the development of dead space fibrosis, and the surgical outcome in this scenario is often a smaller, yet still unattractive nose. Consequently, it is generally preferable to avoid dramatic nasal size reductions in the oversized nose with thick, fibrotic nasal skin. Although conservative size reductions may produce a nose that is still too large for an ideal cosmetic outcome, a better-proportioned and well-defined (if still somewhat large) nose is infinitely preferable to a small, amorphous, and unattractive one.

RECONSTRUCTION OF THE SURGICALLY DEVASTATED NASAL TIP

Central Tip Support

Of all the structural elements impacting nasal tip function and aesthetics, perhaps the single most important is *central tip support*. In the naturally stable and well-supported nose, central tip support is derived from a complex and interdependent architectural system consisting of both skeletal and soft tissue components. While the paired lower lateral cartilages provide the majority of direct tip support, the anterior nasal septum also provides considerable (secondary) tip support by undergirding, suspending, and buttressing the adjacent alar cartilage complex. Ligamentous interconnections, and the enveloping inner and outer nasal linings, also serve to greatly unify and consolidate nasal tip support. However, in the overresected nose, central tip support is often severely compromised. Disrupted soft tissue support mechanisms, combined with overresection of the anterior nasal septum, typically lead to decreased tip projection and/or excessive tip rotation (4). Moreover, the loss of central septal support serves to accentuate the numerous other ill effects produced by overresection of the alar cartilages and/or nasal dorsum (1,4). Indeed, many of the unwanted stigmata of cosmetic rhinoplasty either are a direct consequence of or are markedly exacerbated by inadequate central tip support.

Not surprisingly, one of the most important objectives in restoration of the overresected nasal tip is reestablishing satisfactory central tip support. Arguably, the most effective method for achieving durable tip support is the *septal extension graft* (SEG)—a structural augmentation graft that is used to provide robust skeletal tip support (59–63). When available, septal cartilage is the preferred graft material since a thin, flat, and rigid piece of septal cartilage is ideally suited to the creation of an effective SEG. Septal cartilage is used preferentially over other graft materials since no other autologous tissue can approximate the unique

combination of vigorous axial strength, transverse flexibility, unobtrusive thickness, and dependable shape retention.

In reality, the SEG is nothing more than an enlarged columellar strut graft that is sutured to the caudal septum for added support and stability (Fig. 184.10A–F). When minor deviations of the caudal septum are present, the extension graft can be sutured to one side of the caudal septum (opposite the side of deviation) to improve alignment and to create an overlapping joint of greater stability (64). Alternatively, when the caudal septum is midline, an end-to-end joint is necessary to prevent misalignment, and figure-of-eight sutures are used for graft fixation. However, the end-to-end configuration is inherently unstable, and extended spreader grafts or splinting grafts are sometimes needed to prevent deviation of the graft from midline, particularly in the presence of high closing tension.

Although the SEG is anatomically similar to a traditional columellar strut graft, structurally the SEG is considerably more powerful, and therefore far more versatile. Unlike a conventional columellar strut graft that has no direct contact with the nasal septum, the SEG is physically joined to the caudal septum, becoming a rigid extension of the bony

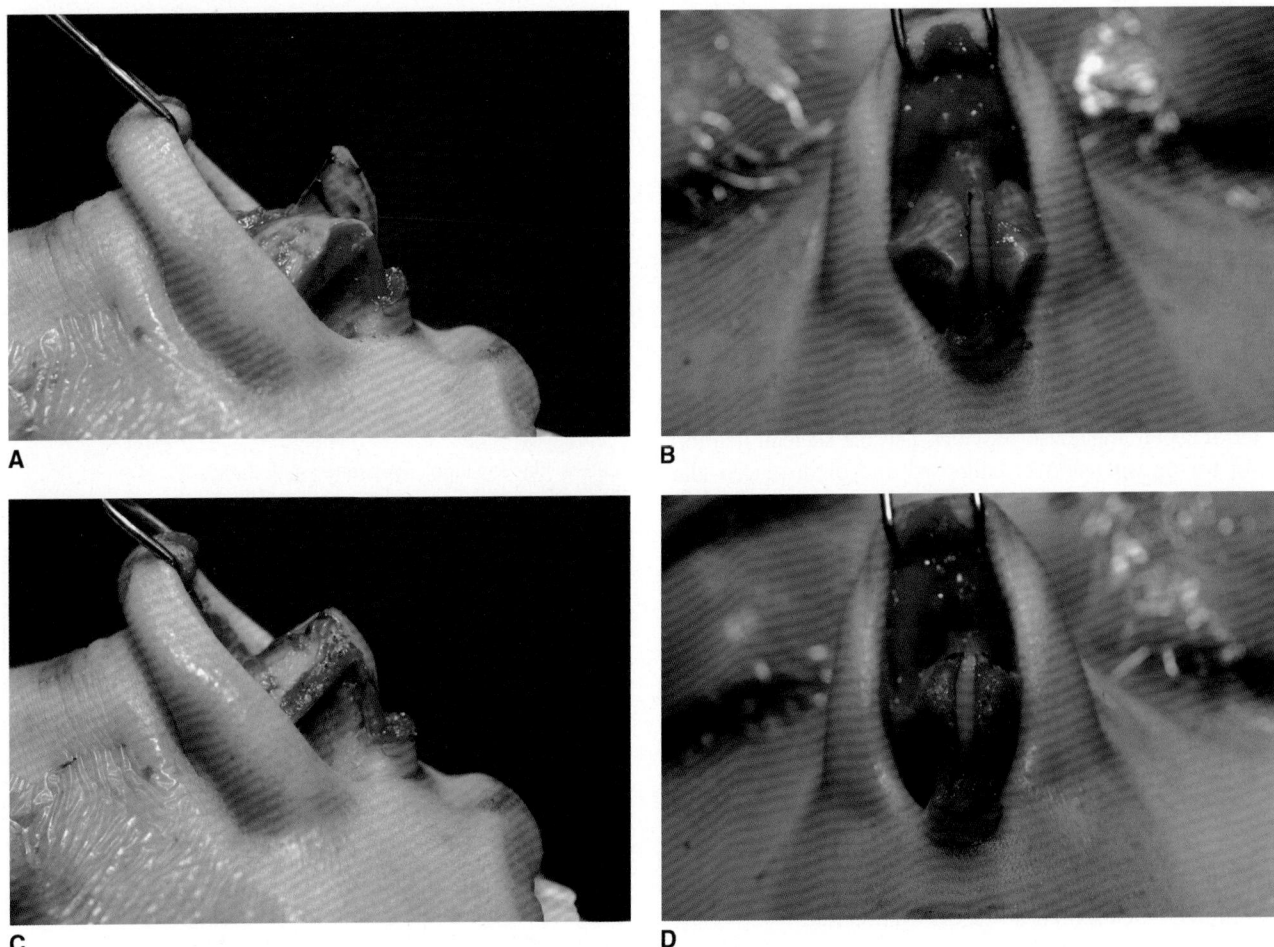

A   **B**

C   **D**

Figure 184.10 Example of SEG placement in primary rhinoplasty. **A,B:** Carved SEG placed end-to-end with the caudal septum. Note how the SEG extends beyond the weak, underprojected tip cartilages. **C,D:** Tip complex after alar cartilages are folded, advanced, and sutured to the distal SEG.

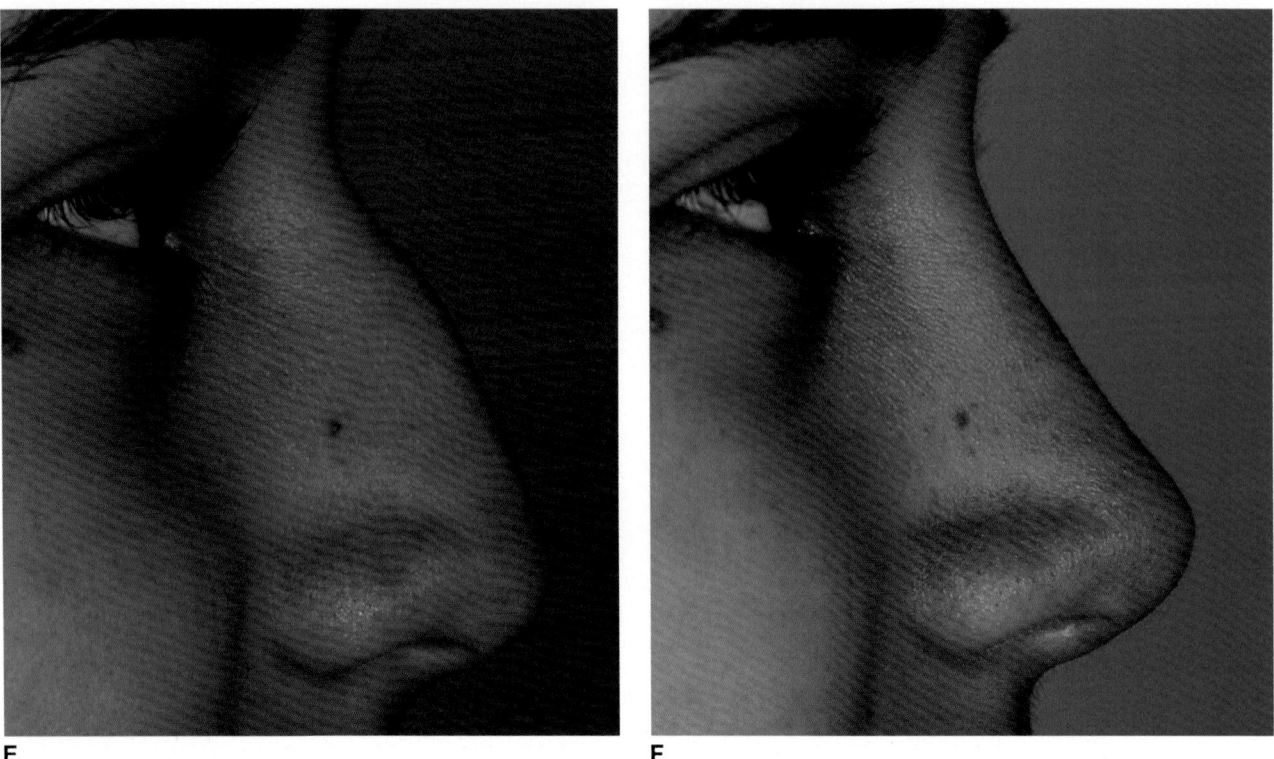

E   F

Figure 184.10 *(Continued)* **E,F:** Before and after profile views demonstrating improved tip support and contour.

facial skeleton that can forcibly stretch nasal skin to increase nasal length and/or tip projection, and thereby dramatically alter tip location (Fig. 184.11A–D). Owing to the buttressing effect of the contiguous facial skeleton, the newly lengthened nasal septum can also resist progressive "shrink wrap" contracture of the internal or external nasal lining, making the SEG a reliable means of permanently stabilizing the re-expanded nasal base. Moreover, the newly created anterior septal angle also provides a secure skeletal fixation point for resuspension of collapsed and/or displaced alar cartilages (Fig. 184.12). By engineering graft dimensions to meet the individual cosmetic needs of the patient, the SEG can theoretically pinpoint tip position anywhere along the lower nose—limited only by the amount and quality of donor graft material and the constraints of soft tissue distensibility. And by custom contouring the caudal border of the SEG, profile deformities of the columella such as an overly flat or retracted columella can also be eliminated with SEG placement (64). Finally, the SEG also compensates for weakened intercrural ligamentous support commonly disrupted with the external rhinoplasty approach. Although a SEG fashioned from septal cartilage is preferred, double-layered conchal cartilage, or concentric-carved rib cartilage can be substituted when septal cartilage is unavailable.

Unlike the underprojected and foreshortened nose in which the SEG is the preferred option for increasing central

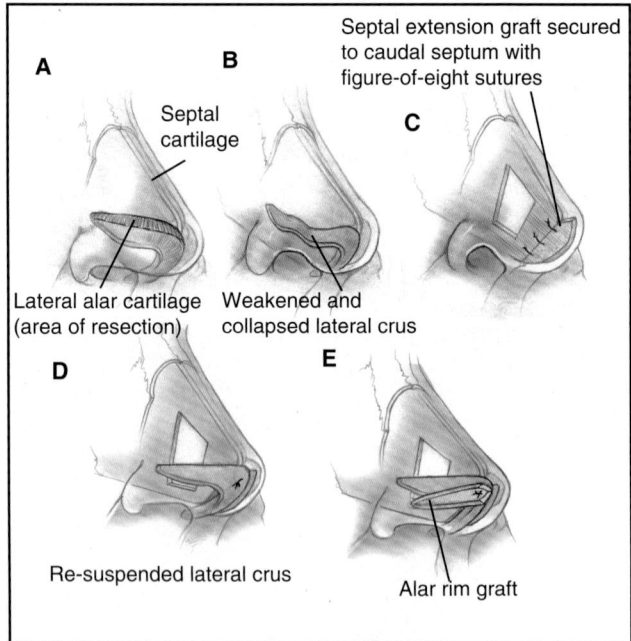

Figure 184.11 Schematic illustration showing reexpansion of the overresected nasal tip using SEG. **A:** Nasal tip complex prior to rhinoplasty. **B:** Buckled and collapsed lateral crura following overzealous cephalic trim maneuver. **C:** SEG sutured end-to-end to the caudal L-strut. **D:** Alar cartilages stretched and tightened after suspension from distal SEG. **E:** Placement of alar rim grafts to reinforce previously weakened tip complex.

tip support, in the *overly long* nose, caudal septal lengthening is contraindicated. In fact, for patients presenting with the *caudal excess nasal deformity*, characterized by an overgrown (hanging) columella, an obtuse nasolabial angle, and a short upper lip, the overgrown septum itself can

be used to provide direct central tip support (59,60,65). In this special circumstance, the medial crura are sutured directly to the caudal septum using a tongue-in-groove setback technique as described by Kridel et al. (66). In addition to improving central tip support and conserving graft

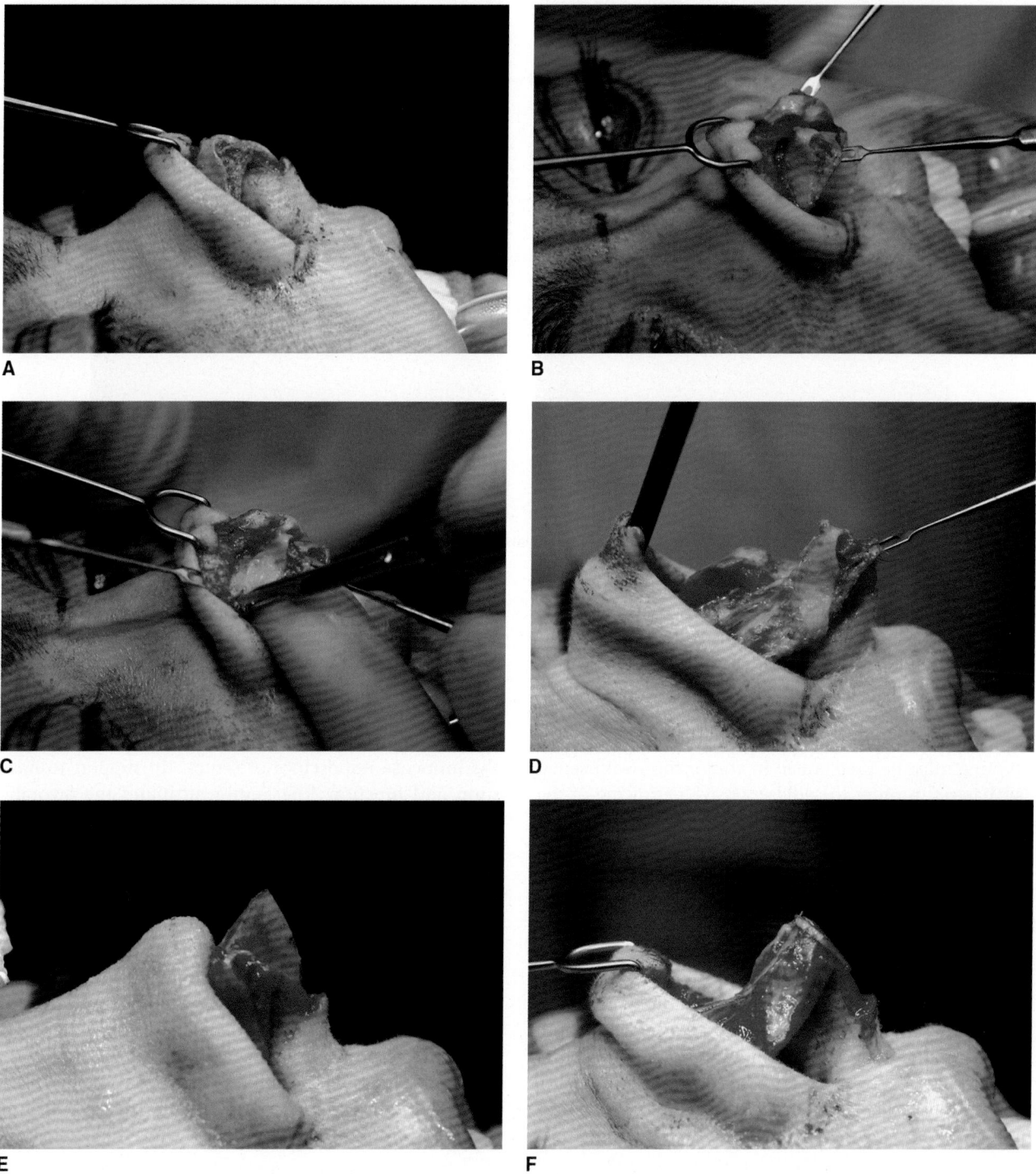

Figure 184.12 Revision of the overresected nasal tip with sidewall tensioning. **A:** Overly short nose after overzealous excisional rhinoplasty. **B:** Counterrotation of lateral crural (remnants) prevented by fibrous adhesion of cephalic margin **(C)** sharp lysis of fibrous adhesions to unfurl contractured vestibular skin and release retracted lateral crura. **D:** Improved tip cartilage mobility after lysis of fibrous adhesions. **E:** Placement of SEG to reproject, counterrotate, and tension the lateral crural remnants **(F)** counterrotated and reprojected tip cartilages after fixation to SEG.

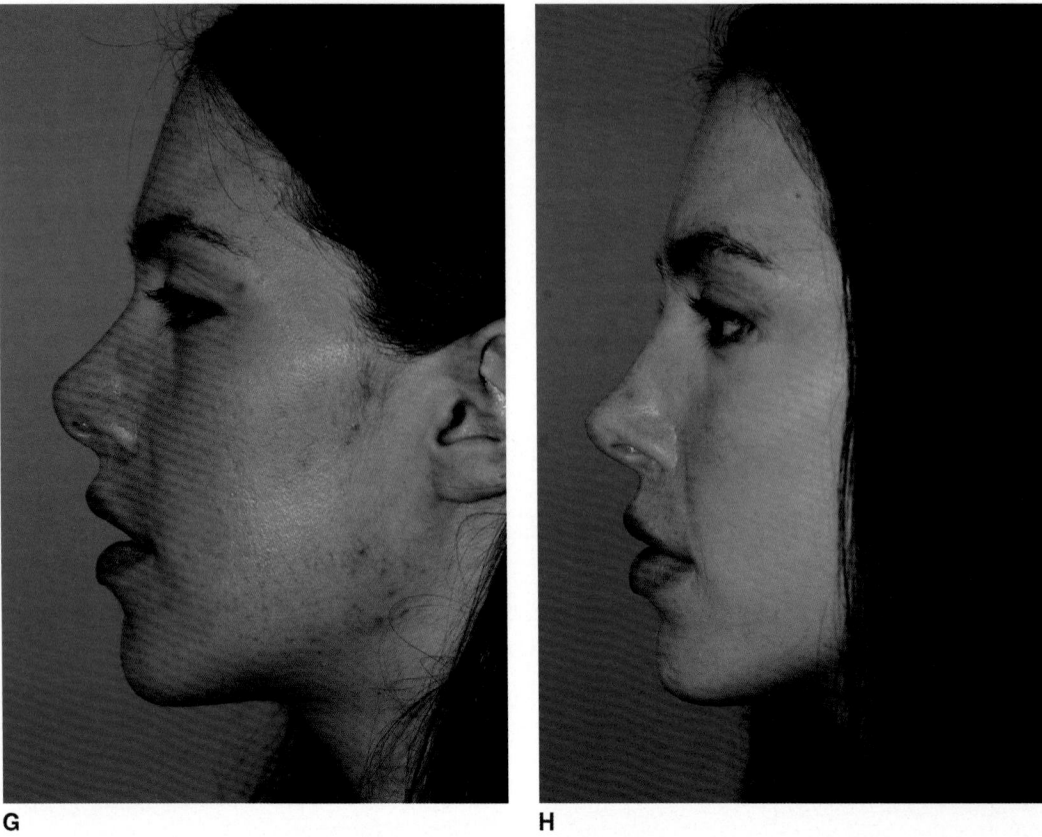

G   H

Figure 184.12 *(Continued)* **G:** Preoperative lateral view **(H)** 1-year postoperative lateral view.

material, the tongue-in-groove method can also simultaneously correct the triad of characteristic deformities comprising the caudal excess nasal deformity (65). However, in cases of extreme caudal overgrowth, the caudal septum and/or the nasal spine may require trimming to achieve the cosmetically optimal profile configuration, and septal trimming must be preplanned in conjunction with septal graft harvest in order to avoid excessive narrowing of the caudal L-strut.

The paramount importance of central tip support is perhaps best demonstrated in Case Two. In this case, a healthy middle-aged female presented 30 years after primary rhinoplasty complaining of severe nasal airway obstruction. Examination revealed a pinched and underprojected nasal tip with thick, fibrotic nasal skin (see Case Two). Surgical findings revealed subtotal resection of both lateral crura and the complete absence of both upper lateral cartilages. Only the anterior nasal septum prevented complete structural collapse of the nasal tip. While mainstream rhinoplasty techniques favor structural replacement grafts to replace the missing upper and lower lateral cartilages, this profoundly overresected nose was successfully restored using only a SEG to augment central tip support. Although nonstructural contour grafts, including a shield graft and supratip onlay graft, were also used to enhance nasal contour, the placement of a SEG permitted a forcible reprojection of the neo-tip

complex and a concomitant resuspension of both the previously unsupported vestibular skin and the inelastic outer soft tissue envelope. Consequently, despite a complete lack of skeletal sidewall support, both nasal valve patency and external nasal contour were successfully restored without structural sidewall grafts, underscoring the immense importance of central tip support to nasal form and function. The author attributes the favorable outcome to the biomechanical phenomenon of *sidewall tensioning*, an extremely useful technique made possible by rigid stability of the SEG. By first *forcibly reprojecting* the overresected nasal tip using the SEG, and then *stretching* the unfurled vestibular skin between the fixed piriform attachments laterally and the newly stabilized tip complex medially, both the inner and outer nasal linings were tightened or *tensioned*, much like a tent canvas is tightened by a large central tent pole. In addition to improved aesthetics resulting from increased nasal tip projection, improved sidewall tone and resiliency led to a demonstrable increase in (internal) nasal valve cross-sectional area and a corresponding increase in the threshold for inspiratory collapse.

Despite the theoretical benefits of sidewall tensioning, care must be taken to avoid excessive sidewall tension since excessive structural loads may exceed central tip support and lead to buckling or deviation of the septal/SEG complex. In extreme circumstances, such as a naturally weak nasal septum or severely noncompliant nasal skin, extended spreader grafts are required to increase axial rigidity and prevent distortion caused by unavoidably high compressive loads (59,61–63,67). Whenever possible, tensioning forces should also be equally distributed between the right and left side to prevent unbalanced horizontal forces from displacing the SEG.

Lateral Tip Support

While sidewall tensioning alone may not always eliminate the need for additional structural grafting, as demonstrated above, a tensioned nasal sidewall greatly improves baseline soft tissue tone and rigidity relative to a lax or collapsed nasal sidewall, even when the lateral crural cartilage has been completely excised. Moreover, when a residual strip of crural cartilage is present, tensioning of the crural remnant further enhances structural support and may potentially obviate the need for structural grafting altogether (Fig. 184.11A–E) (see Case Three). Indeed, sidewall tensioning is a near universally applicable technique for treating and/or preventing lower nasal sidewall collapse that is equally effective in both revision and primary rhinoplasty.

However, among traditional treatment options for sidewall collapse, the *lateral crural strut graft* (LCS graft) has long been the therapeutic gold standard. Originally described by Gunter and Friedman (68), the LCS graft is a long strip of autologous cartilage sutured to the undersurface of the lateral crus (or the lateral crural remnant) for permanent splinting of the collapsed crural segment. Indications for the LCS graft include treatment of alar rim retraction, alar rim collapse, concavity of the lateral crus, and lateral crural recurvature—deformities that are commonly encountered in the overresected nose. Septal cartilage is typically the preferred graft material, but conchal or rib cartilage grafts are used in cases of septal cartilage depletion, while rib cartilage is preferred by some surgeons for its extra rigidity. In modest deformities, the LCS graft is approximately the same length as, or shorter than, the lateral crus. However, when used to correct severe alar collapse, alar retraction, or cephalic malposition of the lateral crus, the LCS graft must be elongated to extend beyond the lip of the piriform aperture for added skeletal support (68).

Although the LCS graft is generally effective at eliminating external contour deformities associated with sidewall collapse (33,59,68), the sheer bulk and weight of some LCS grafts may reduce internal nasal valve patency and/or lower the threshold for inspiratory collapse (1,33). Moreover, the mass effect associated with large structural grafts, particularly LCS grafts that extend beyond the piriform aperture, may result in effacement of the superior alar crease and/or unpleasant sensations with smiling or other facial movements (*Personal observation*).

Although structural grafting is unavoidable in some patients, limiting bulk within the lower nasal sidewall is of paramount importance, particularly in the naturally narrow nose where slit-like nasal valves are already predisposed to inspiratory collapse. Since the lateral crus has an average thickness of only 0.7 mm (39,40), some structural augmentation grafts, particularly those fashioned from conchal or rib cartilage, may add considerable thickness and bulk to the lower nasal sidewall. For example, the minimum natural thickness of conchal cartilage is approximately 1.9 mm (45), which is nearly three times the thickness of the lateral crus. Depending upon the positioning, rigidity, weight, and thickness of the graft material, structural augmentation grafts may improve alar contour, but they may also reduce the cross-sectional area of the nasal valve and/or lower the threshold for dynamic nasal valve collapse. Fortunately, the requirement for bulky structural augmentation grafts can be reduced or even eliminated by tensioning the nasal sidewall, a complementary technique that raises the threshold for internal nasal valve collapse without adding the weight, bulk, or mass of structural graft material. Indeed, stretching the lateral crural remnant between two fixed points not only increases baseline rigidity, it also serves to flatten, straighten, and stiffen a buckled or retracted crural remnant, thereby minimizing or eliminating crural concavity, recurvature, or cephalic retraction—structural benefits analogous to those achieved with the LCS graft (Figs. 184.11A–E and 184.12A–G).

While sidewall tensioning is worthwhile in virtually any case of lower sidewall laxity, the need for structural augmentation grafts cannot always be eliminated with tensioning alone, and an individualized and graduated approach to sidewall reconstruction is still required. In severe cases, the goal of avoiding excessive bulk or airway encroachment and simultaneously achieving adequate sidewall tone and contour is best achieved by aggressive tensioning of the nasal sidewall followed by the judicious and step-wise application of thin, yet rigid augmentation grafts—but only when tensioning fails to provide adequate structural support. Enhancing structural support while limiting graft volume not only optimizes airway patency, it also facilitates a more delicate and refined nasal tip contour, which better suits the aesthetic preferences of the typical revision rhinoplasty patient.

One the most common problems encountered in revision of the overresected nasal tip is cephalic retraction of the alar rim following an overzealous cephalic trim procedure. The severity of iatrogenic alar retraction varies widely, ranging from mild to severe, with the worst deformities arising in patients having both a congenitally high-riding alar rim and naturally weak alar cartilage, in which aggressive cephalic resection was followed by severe scar contracture (Fig. 184.2B). In the previously operated nose with severely contracted and/or missing vestibular skin, satisfactory release and repositioning of the lateral crural remnant is rendered impossible, and auricular (chondrocutaneous) *composite grafts* are necessary to augment the deficient inner lining, and to physically buttress the alar margin against recurrent retraction (46,47). In contrast, the LCS graft remains the gold standard for correction of stubborn alar retraction in the absence of deficient nasal lining. However, a large percentage of revision rhinoplasty cases present with mild to moderate alar retraction and no significant lining deficiencies. Often these lesser deformities will respond favorably to a combination of sidewall tensioning and *alar rim grafts*, thereby obviating the need for traditional structural grafts.

The alar rim graft is a long, narrow cartilage graft that is placed (nonanatomically) in a precise pocket dissected along the alar rim (69,70) (Fig. 184.13A–E). Although diminutive in size, the alar rim graft provides increased

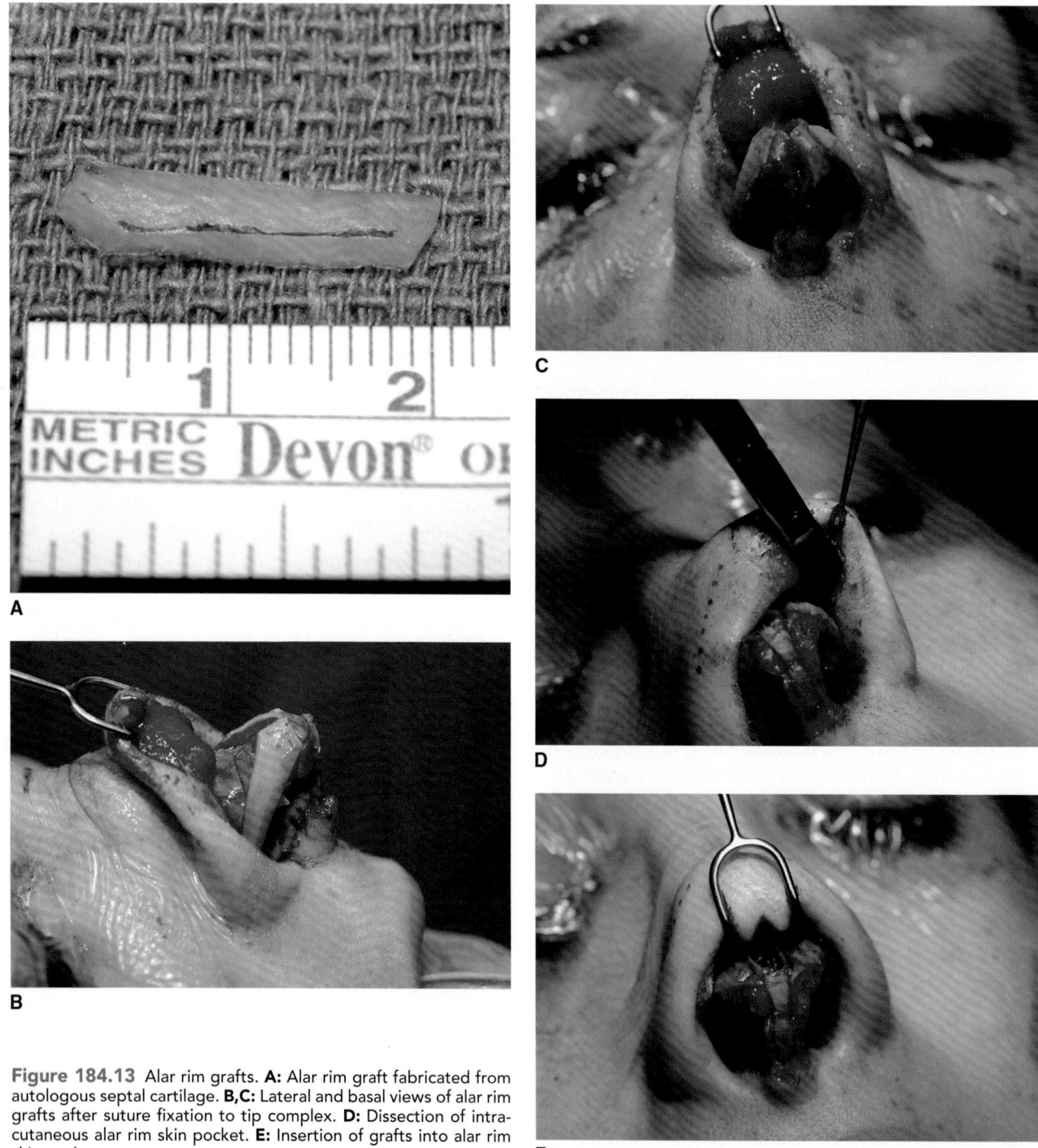

Figure 184.13 Alar rim grafts. **A:** Alar rim graft fabricated from autologous septal cartilage. **B,C:** Lateral and basal views of alar rim grafts after suture fixation to tip complex. **D:** Dissection of intracutaneous alar rim skin pocket. **E:** Insertion of grafts into alar rim skin pockets.

stability against lobular pinching and/or mild alar retraction (59,69,70). Alar rim grafts typically extend from the nasal dome medially to the mid ala laterally, and can be fashioned from septal, conchal, or costal cartilage donor material. Edges should be beveled to optimize graft camouflage and grafts wider than 3 to 4 mm are seldom necessary. Owing to the diminutive size and (nonanatomic) placement away from the internal nasal valve, airway impingement is avoided and external valve rigidity is greatly increased.

Treatment of mild alar retraction with alar rim grafts is enhanced by concomitant sidewall tensioning, which serves to tighten and straighten the lateral crural remnant and to oppose upward displacement of the alar rim. Suture fixation of the alar rim graft (medially) to the underlying tip complex is a helpful modification that stabilizes graft position to further buttress the nostril rim against cephalic displacement (Fig. 184.13B and C). In the previously operated nose, it is usually necessary to first unfurl the unsupported and contractured vestibular skin by disrupting all scar adhesions that prevent caudal repositioning of the crural remnant (Fig. 184.12A–D). If contracture release fails to permit appropriate repositioning of the crural remnant, structural augmentation grafts such as the LCS graft or the chondrocutaneous composite graft must be used to stabilize the repositioned crural remnant and to prevent recontracture.

Although alar rim grafts are often necessary in the previously operated nose, the small graft size reduces the demand for large amounts of donor cartilage. Consequently, a healthy and untouched quadrangular septum can usually provide enough graft material for fabrication of both a SEG and bilateral alar rim grafts. And by using nasal sidewall tensioning to initially stabilize and tighten the lateral crural remnants, coupled with alar rim grafts to reinforce the nostril rim against cephalic scar contracture, a large number of complex tip revisions can be effectively managed without any need for extranasal graft material. In addition to avoiding the time, expense, and potential side effects associated with the harvest and placement of extranasal structural grafts, septal donor cartilage offers the additional advantage of a structurally sound, yet characteristically delicate and slender tip contour, better suited to a narrow and refined nasal aesthetic (see Case Four).

Although sidewall tensioning is easiest when the (tensioned) crural length coincides exactly with optimal tip projection, sidewall tensioning can be accomplished in virtually any nose by first altering crural length to accommodate overprojected or underprojected alar cartilages. Alterations in crural length can be achieved through a host of conventional rhinoplasty techniques including the lateral crural steal technique for the underprojected tip (71), the lateral crural overlay or vertical lobule division technique for the overprojected tip (72,73), and the tongue-in-groove technique for both the over- and the underprojected tip (66). In conjunction with tensioning

of the crural remnants, conventional suture techniques such as dome sutures, crural spanning sutures, or crural flattening sutures can also be used to further refine alar cartilage contour, while simultaneously preserving crural volume and further reducing dependence upon large structural grafts. Unlike the cephalic trim approach, these tissue-sparing techniques are not predicated upon further narrowing of the lateral crus, and the residual structural integrity of the alar cartilage is fully preserved. Finally, a variety of nonstructural cartilage grafts are also commonly needed to optimize nasal tip contour, symmetry, and alignment in the previously operated nose. A discussion of the myriad strategies used for tip grafting used in cosmetic rhinoplasty is far beyond the scope of this chapter, but primary rhinoplasty grafting techniques are equally effective in revision nasal surgery, and contouring grafts are routinely used to finesse the final cosmetic outcome.

REVISION OF THE SURGICALLY-DEVASTATED NASAL DORSUM

In a survey of 104 consecutive patients seeking revision rhinoplasty, Yu et al. (74) found cosmetic imperfections of the nasal dorsum to be the second-most common aesthetic concern prompting revision nasal surgery, surpassed only by nasal tip asymmetry. Perhaps the most devastating dorsal deformity prompting revision rhinoplasty is overresection of the nasal dorsum, a preventable technical error that may profoundly disrupt nasal bridge aesthetics. Depending upon both the extent and location of overresection, unsightly contour deformities may involve the bony upper vault, the cartilaginous middle vault, or the entire nasal bridge. Unlike the rigid bony dorsum that tends to resist deformation from soft tissue scarring, the comparatively soft and pliable cartilages of the middle vault are particularly susceptible to pinching and collapse from progressive scar contracture. Even when dorsal hump reduction avoids profile overresection, loss of (dorsal) septal width can lead to curvature or deviation of the dorsal septum, collapse or pinching of one or both upper lateral cartilages, or combinations therein. Proactive measures to augment and stabilize middle vault architecture are generally effective in avoiding such problems, but are often neglected at the time of primary rhinoplasty. Moreover, significant functional disturbances are also a common manifestation of nasal bridge deformities. Depending upon the extent of dorsal overresection and the length of the middle vault, symptoms may range from a mild cosmetic irregularity with minimal functional disturbance to a profound nasal deformity with near-total airway obstruction (Fig. 184.14).

Although the middle vault is considerably more susceptible to postsurgical scar contracture, overaggressive reduction of the bony nasal vault may also lead to conspicuous cosmetic deformities that are especially difficult to treat.

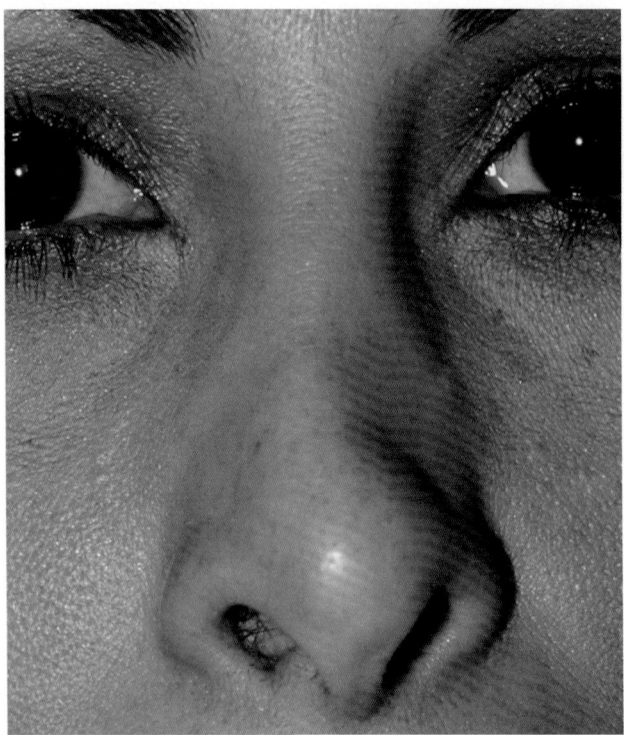

Figure 184.14 Postsurgical collapse of the nasal dorsum with severe functional impairment.

In addition to an underprojected and scooped bony profile, overaggressive reduction of the bony pyramid also leads to a widened and washed-out bony dorsum on frontal view. Variations of this characteristic appearance develop when faulty lateral osteotomies result in collapse, deviation, and/or comminution of one or both nasal bones. When combined with the wide natural variation in nasal bone morphology, a virtually limitless array of postsurgical bony vault deformities are possible, and the smooth, symmetric, and tapered configuration of a naturally elegant nasal bridge can be exceedingly difficult to recreate. Augmenting the overresected nasal dorsum such that the newly augmented segment seamlessly transitions with the underlying bony vault is indeed a formidable challenge, particularly when the underlying bony platform is also asymmetric and requires nasal bone repositioning. However, realignment of the asymmetric or deviated bony vault is a common aspect of revision rhinoplasty, and osteotomies are often essential for complete upper vault restoration. Alternatively, camouflage of bony irregularities with onlay grafts may also yield the appearance of a straight and attractive bony contour in some patients, and may be preferable to the unpredictability of widespread skeletal destabilization.

Osteotomies

Surgical modification of the bony pyramid is a challenging facet of *primary* rhinoplasty that often leads to patient dissatisfaction and revision nasal surgery. While some postsurgical bony deformities are easily corrected, severe bone deformities may prove extremely challenging, often in part due to instability from previous surgery. Even a seemingly simple task such as removing a residual bony hump or straightening a bony deviation may prove surprisingly difficult due to previous osteotomies and the potential for unpredictable bone behavior.

In general, the use of blunt-force osteotomies to modify bony architecture is more challenging in patients with a history of previous hump removal or previous nasal trauma since preexisting osteotomy or fracture lines can unexpectedly separate, collapse, or fragment with high-impact techniques. For that reason, low-impact alternatives are often less destabilizing and thus far more predictable. For resection of a residual bony hump or for smoothing of persistent dorsal surface irregularities, powered instrumentation such as a powered sagittal saw or powered reciprocating rasp (Stryker Instruments, Kalamazoo, MI) offers greater precision and less risk of excessive bone destabilization (75) (Fig. 184.15A and B). Powered instrumentation also facilitates sculpting of the bony vault that can eliminate minor bony asymmetries and potentially obviate the need for blunt-force osteotomies altogether (75). While powered instrumentation can improve accuracy and minimize bone destabilization, heat generated from powered instruments may increase bony callus formation. Callus formation is typically more common in adolescents and young adults, particularly males and athletic individuals. If left untreated, callus formation may sometimes progress to permanent osteogenesis and bony contour deformity. All patients at increased risk for callus formation should be advised about the possible need for long-term adjuvant treatment using low-dose triamcinolone injections. Although stubborn cases of callus formation may require prolonged serial injections, long-term results are usually satisfactory as long as treatment is not discontinued prematurely.

Although lateral osteotomies may behave unpredictably in the previously operated nose, revision lateral osteotomies are frequently unavoidable. Because nasal osteotomy sites or fracture lines heal slowly and initially by fibrous union, these areas of persistent bone weakness create a potential "path of least resistance" making it more difficult to control osteotome movement and to avoid opening previous osteotomy sites or fracture lines. Hence, caution should be exercised when performing revision osteotomies upon previously treated or previously fractured nasal bones. By the same token, individuals with brittle nasal bones—particularly the elderly—are also at increased risk for comminution from blunt-force osteotomies. In general, aggressive bone manipulation should be approached cautiously in the older patient since severe bone disruption may be compounded by lackluster healing responses and excessive narrowing or collapse of the bony vault. Because osteotome misdirection and excessive bone disruption are both accentuated by dull instrumentation, the use of a wet-stone–sharpened osteotome is recommended for all

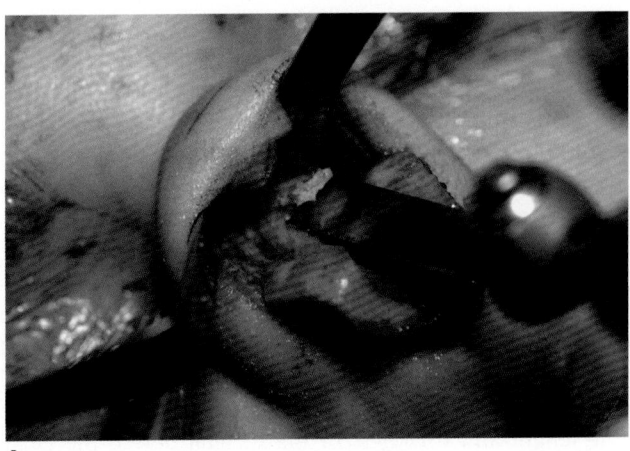
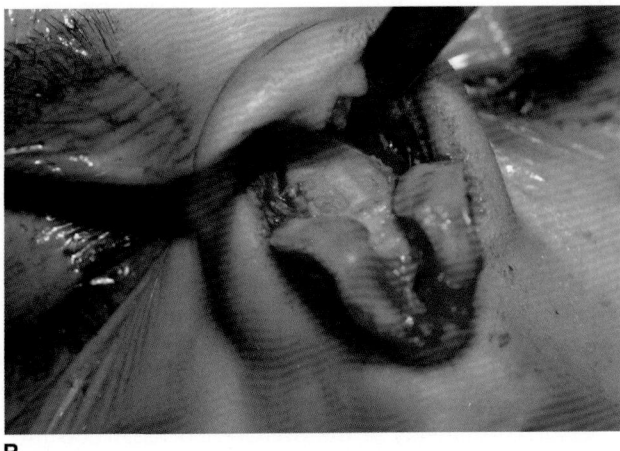

A   **B**

Figure 184.15 Removal of small bony hump using powered sagittal saw via the external rhinoplasty approach. **A:** Small bone shaving prior to complete hump removal. **B:** Smooth polished dorsum following hump removal with powered sagittal saw.

lateral osteotomies to improve osteotome control and minimize unwanted bone disruption. And while lateral osteotomies are sometimes indispensable, aggressive destabilization of the previously operated bony nasal pyramid is generally best avoided unless the potential benefits clearly outweigh the associated risks.

Perhaps the most common manifestation of the over-resected nasal dorsum is the *inverted-V deformity*. The inverted-V deformity is produced by a conspicuous width discrepancy arising between the middle and upper nasal vaults following excessive hump removal. After excessive loss of dorsal height, the comparatively stable bony vault tends to remain wide, whereas the cartilaginous middle vault tends to collapse and pinch. The resulting step-off deformity produces a characteristic upside-down V-shaped shadow along the bony–cartilaginous junction from which the deformity derives its peculiar name (Figs. 184.3 and 184.14). Treatment of an inverted-V deformity arising from dorsal overresection inevitably involves augmentation grafting to restore lost dorsal height (see Cases three and five). However, while the inverted-V deformity is a near-universal sequela of excessive hump removal, inverted-V-type shadowing of the dorsum can also occur even after a conservative hump reduction where dorsal height remains appropriate. The formation of an inverted-V deformity despite adequate dorsal height is often due to failed lateral osteotomies and a persistent bony "open roof" deformity. In this circumstance, treatment involves either narrowing the overly wide bony vault to match the slender middle vault (i.e., close the "open roof" deformity) or augmenting the middle vault with spreader grafts to restore lost septal width. However, a combination of both methods is frequently most effective in achieving a uniform and attractive nasal dorsum while also optimizing the functional outcome. Patients at greatest risk for postsurgical

deformities of the middle vault are those with short nasal bones and long slender noses, since the cartilaginous framework is disproportionately long, thin, and pliable. Prophylactic spreader grafts or equivalent measures such as upper lateral cartilage turn-in "spreader" flaps are recommended in high-risk patients at the time of primary rhinoplasty to reduce the likelihood of nasal bridge deformities and the subsequent need for revision surgery.

Dorsal Augmentation

Treatment of the overresected nasal dorsum is predicated upon restoring optimal dorsal height, as well as satisfactory contour, symmetry, and alignment. Successful dorsal restoration will produce a slender nasal bridge with smooth, parallel, and uninterrupted *brow-tip aesthetic lines* indicating a harmonious and attractive dorsal contour (59). In the absence of internal airway deformities, successful dorsal augmentation will also expand the nasal airway and produce a corresponding improvement in nasal airflow. In noses with overresection of the entire nasal dorsum, reconstruction is often achieved with simultaneous augmentation of the upper and middle vaults using a single augmentation graft spanning the entire nasal bridge. The choice between a conchal cartilage graft, a rib cartilage graft, a composite osseo-cartilaginous rib graft, or a semisolid (diced) cartilage graft varies according to the defect size, the need for structural rigidity, patient acceptance, and surgeon preference. In dorsal defects limited to 1 to 3 mm in depth, conchal cartilage can provide a satisfactory dorsal augmentation (see Case Three), but for larger dorsal defects, only rib cartilage can provide sufficient graft volume (see Case Five). When solid graft materials are chosen, proper three-dimensional graft contour is critical. In addition to a smooth and natural outer contour, the graft undersurface must be carefully sculpted to precisely complement the recipient dorsal topography.

Without a precise reciprocal interface to optimize surface contact and stability, the probability of graft displacement, mobility, and/or warping is greatly increased, particularly when using solid rib cartilage. Presoaking of the rib in saline, concentric carving of the rib cartilage, and avoidance of long thin cartilage constructs also help to prevent warping of the solid rib cartilage.

Perhaps the most reliable solid graft construct is the composite osseocartilaginous rib graft, which utilizes a large bone-on-bone interface to eliminate graft migration and warping (34,35). Osseocartilaginous grafts are harvested from the bony–cartilaginous fusion of the sixth to eleventh ribs, in order to restore the corresponding natural tissue constituents of the overresected nasal dorsum. To achieve an optimal reciprocal interface, powered instruments are used to create a flat recipient bed and to flatten the undersurface of the composite graft. Once the outer graft surface is sculpted to the desired three-dimensional contour, fixation is achieved using a percutaneous K-wire, which is removed in the office 1 week later. Owing to the large, raw bone-on-bone contact area and the secure initial immobilization provided by the K-wire, solid bone fusion

is promptly established and long-term clinical outcomes are largely free of resorption, migration, or warping (34,35). Cosmetic results are favorable as long as the graft dovetails smoothly without overhangs, step-offs, or other contour imperfections. However, as with the traditional rib graft, excessive thinning of the cartilage component may lead to an increased incidence of postoperative warping.

An alternative method of dorsal augmentation is the diced cartilage–temporalis fascia (DC-F) graft (52,53). This semisolid construct is created by encasing 0.5- to 1.0-mm cubes of finely diced autologous cartilage in a sleeve of temporalis fascia to create a malleable yet durable dorsal augmentation graft (Fig. 184.16A and B). Depending upon the length and thickness of the skeletal defect, the DC-F graft can be used to augment either a portion of the nasal bridge or the entire nasal dorsum. Although the graft has limited structural rigidity, several key advantages make this an attractive alternative to the traditional solid graft construct. Perhaps the most important advantage is the malleable nature of the graft, which automatically conforms to contour irregularities of the underlying skeletal platform. Often minor irregularities of the skeletal platform can be

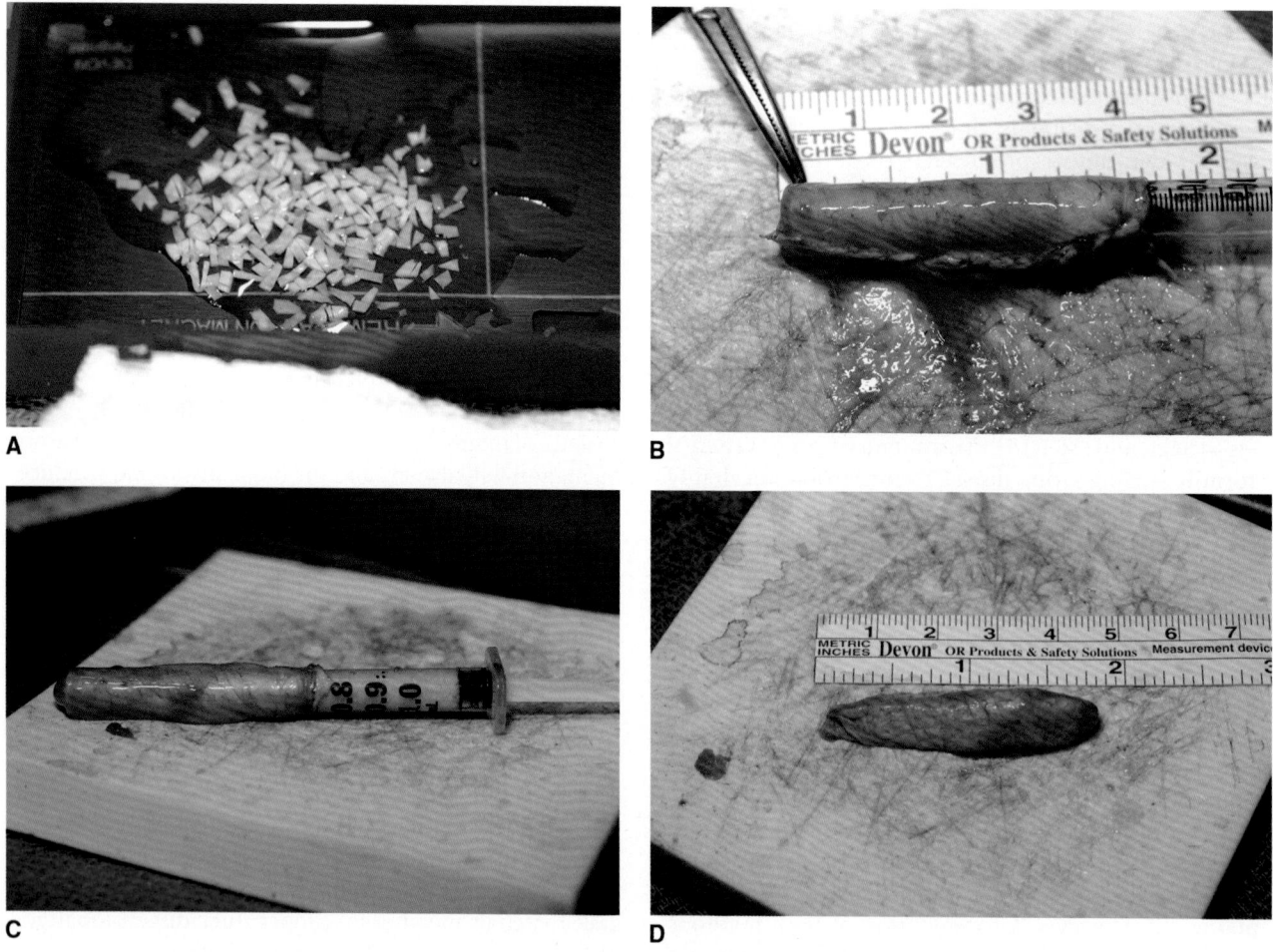

Figure 184.16 DC-F graft fabrication. **A:** Finely diced 1.0-mm cubes of autologous cartilage. **B:** Temporalis fascia sheath sewn around tuberculin syringe. **C:** Diced cartilage prior to injection into fascial sheath. **D:** DC-F graft prior to implantation.

camouflaged with the DC-F graft, creating the illusion of a straight and slender dorsum while avoiding unnecessary destabilization of the bony vault. Because the DC-F graft also provides a smooth and seamless interface with the surrounding nasal skeleton, grafts can be virtually any length or height without fear of migration, warping, or visible edge prominence. Even relatively small grafts used for radix augmentation blend seamlessly with the adjacent nasal dorsum without warping or step-off deformities. Despite rigorous sectioning of the donor cartilage, DC-F grafts have also shown excellent durability with no clinical or histologic evidence of resorption despite follow-up intervals of up to 7 years (52,53,76). In fact, owing to the clinical reliability of the DC-F graft, overcorrection is discouraged since volume loss is rare. However, long-term graft survival is contingent upon proper processing, since crushing, morselizing, or bruising of the cartilage is associated with partial necrosis and eventual loss of graft volume (77,78). Although the DC-F graft lacks structural rigidity that is typically required to lengthen a foreshortened nose, in patients with adequate skin elasticity, the DC-F graft may be combined with a SEG and extended spreader grafts to simultaneously increase dorsal height and nasal length. The growing incidence of large dorsal defects, combined with a corresponding increase in the number of graft-depleted patients, makes the DC-F graft an attractive and reliable treatment option for augmentation of the overresected nasal bridge.

Spreader Grafts

In patients with an attractive and symmetric bony vault and a satisfactory nasal profile; unsightly frontal deformities of the middle vault can still develop from isolated curvature and/or deviation of the dorsal septum. Inward collapse or pinching of one or both upper lateral cartilages can also create or aggravate middle vault deformities despite a satisfactory profile. Septal and upper lateral cartilage deformities are also a common element of more extensive dorsal deformities. Patients with long slender noses and/or short nasal bones are at greatest risk for postsurgical deformities of the middle vault following cartilage hump resection, since middle vault cartilages tend to be long, thin, and disproportionately weak.

In the absence of profile irregularities, treatment of middle vault deformities most often involves spreader graft placement. However, bilateral size-matched spreader grafts are not indicated in every patient, and a graduated and individualized approach to spreader graft placement is essential. Frequently, unilateral or partial-length spreader grafts achieve the best surgical results, and careful analysis is needed to properly individualize the treatment strategy. When using the external rhinoplasty approach, submucosal pockets are created along the dorsal septum for spreader graft insertion and suture fixation is performed at both ends of the graft for secure stabilization.

The thickness, length, and number of spreader grafts typically vary according to individual anatomic needs, but the goal is always the same: mirror-image symmetry, sagittal alignment of the dorsum, and cosmetically appropriate width of the middle vault. For C-shaped curvatures of the dorsal septum, a single spreader graft, preferably with a reciprocal C-shaped curve, can be used to straighten and strengthen the dorsal septum while adding negligible width to the middle vault. In cases of middle vault pinching (with or without septal curvature), bilateral spreader grafts are often used to restore middle vault width and to augment septal support. Typically, partial-length spreader grafts are placed bilaterally, immediately below the bony–cartilaginous junction, to eliminate step-off deformities and prevent inverted-V-type shadowing. Depending upon the width requirements, grafts fashioned from septal cartilage can be used for mild to modest width deficiencies, whereas considerably thicker grafts can be fashioned from conchal or rib donor cartilage to accommodate larger defects. For cases of sagittal deviation or canting of the dorsal septum, conventional septoplasty techniques can sometimes restore sagittal alignment after release of the upper lateral cartilage remnants. In stubborn cases, spreader grafts are sometimes needed to realign and/or camouflage misalignment of the dorsal septum (79). However, misalignment of the cartilaginous septum is sometimes due to deviation of the vertical ethmoid plate, and blunt fracture of the vertical ethmoid bone is needed in this scenario to adequately mobilize and reposition the dorsal septum. When blunt repositioning of the vertical ethmoid bone fails to provide a stable septal realignment, a spreader graft can be extended cephalically and placed beneath the nasal bone (on the side of deviation) to permanently "shim" the central ethmoid complex and maintain midline positioning. When reconstructing the pinched middle vault, suture reattachment of the collapsed upper lateral cartilages is recommended to restore middle vault width and stability, and to prevent recurrent upper lateral cartilage collapse and pinching. In patients with distal canting of the dorsal septum, the use of clocking sutures can also be helpful to realign and further stabilize the dorsal septum (79).

Although spreader grafts are unquestionably the workhorse of middle vault reconstruction, graft survival is predicated upon a robust recipient blood supply, which is sometimes lacking in the middle vault—an area that is often predisposed to vascular insufficiency following minor tissue disruption. Despite secure fixation of the graft, minimal disruption of the septal mucoperichondrium, and gentle soft tissue dissection, spreader graft resorption may develop in susceptible individuals leading to persistent middle vault deformity. Patients with saddle nose deformities arising from trauma, autoimmune vasculitis, or chronic cocaine abuse are at particular risk for resorption of middle vault cartilage grafts, as are smokers, diabetics, and patients with other forms of microvascular disease.

The adage "as goes the septum, so goes the nose" attests to the difficulty of straightening a nose without first straightening the nasal septum. While traditional (endonasal) septoplasty techniques are often successful at straightening moderate deformities of the L-strut, conventional techniques may prove inadequate for the treatment of severe telescoping or accordion-type septal deformities. In these comparatively rare and challenging cases, extracorporeal septoplasty is often needed to achieve a satisfactory long-term realignment of the L-strut (80–83). Extracorporeal septoplasty involves elevating mucoperichondrium from both sides of the quadrangular septum and surgically removing the entire cartilaginous septum, leaving only a small remnant at the keystone area for later reattachment. Following cartilage explantation, the septal partition is subdivided along fracture lines and/or spurs to obtain flat segments that can be used to rebuild the outer septal partition. Cartilage fragments are then painstakingly reassembled and sutured in a mosaic-like configuration to produce a flat, uniplanar L-strut replacement graft. Permanent autologous scaffolding, such as septal cartilage or ethmoid bone, has been traditionally used to splint the fragile construct for added structural support, but the advent of resorbable polydioxanone (PDS) plate (Mentor Worldwide, LLC, Johnson & Johnson, Inc., New Brunswick, NJ) has become a popular and effective alternative for temporary (implantable) splinting of the reconstructed septal L-strut (80–82). Once assembled, the flat PDS-reinforced L-strut is reinserted into the mucosal pocket and sutured to the nasal spine and keystone area for improved septal contour, structural support, and airway patency. Although dramatic improvements in skeletal alignment are often the result of extracorporeal septoplasty, saddle-type deformities may occasionally result if the mucoperichondrium fails to adequately reperfuse the reimplanted cartilage. Although uncommon, saddling has been observed following the use of *unperforated* PDS plate for septal splinting, presumably since it more effectively blocks revascularization of the reimplanted septal cartilage (82). No cases of saddling were observed following unilateral application of the thinner, perforated version of the PDS plate, suggesting that this modification of PDS is more conducive to prompt cartilage revascularization. In either case, the use of bilateral PDS plate is discouraged since near-complete isolation of the reimplanted cartilage greatly increases the risk of ischemic resorption.

AFTERCARE

The conclusion of surgery marks the beginning of the recovery process. And while recovery is generally beneficial for nearly all patients, the speed, extent, and quality of the healing process varies widely among individuals and is often frustratingly slow. Monitoring the healing process and treating wound-healing derangements is a crucial aspect of revision rhinoplasty that may substantially improve the final outcome. Yet despite its importance, postoperative care is frequently neglected, opening the door for healing aberrations such as subcutaneous scarring, callus formation, or scar contracture, any of which may taint the final outcome. And while some patients require nothing more than periodic assessment to confirm appropriate healing, for others, regular intervention with appropriate adjuvant therapy is required to optimize the cosmetic and/or functional result. Indeed, for a small percentage of secondary rhinoplasty patients, a well-executed surgical procedure will fail to reach its full potential without appropriate and prolonged aftercare, and potential barriers to aftercare such as travel, work, school, etc. should be reconciled prior to surgery.

For many *revision* rhinoplasty patients, postsurgical monitoring and care is a long-term commitment that may last up to several years. However, it is in the first few hours after surgery that aftercare can have its biggest and most beneficial impact. From the moment the last suture is tied, aggressive efforts to mitigate soft tissue swelling and inflammation should commence, as it is far easier to avoid adverse tissue responses than to eliminate them.

One of the most effective ways to minimize soft tissue edema is with gentle wound compression. The application of a traditional cinch dressing, followed by uniform compression of the nasal dorsum with a padded aluminum splint, serves to gently compress the outer soft tissue envelope and minimize extracellular fluid accumulation. Splinting also serves to maintain nasal alignment and to protect the unstable nasal framework in the early days following surgery. In the same manner, internal nasal packing placed within the nasal cavity serves to support and tamponade the nasal tissues from within. By tightly packing the nasal vestibule with malleable packing material, the nasal tip is firmly compressed from both inside and out, and subcutaneous dead space in the lower nose is largely eliminated. Elimination of surgical dead space is particularly important in the thick-skinned nose since accumulation of blood beneath the skin flap often leads to subcutaneous fibrosis and unwanted skin thickening. It is also critically important to secure the compression dressing well in advance of extubation, since precipitous blood pressure elevations may occur during emergence from anesthesia. Under normal circumstances, the external nasal bandage is maintained for 1 week postoperatively, but the intranasal packing can be safely discontinued the following day as the threat of subcutaneous oozing has typically resolved. While the application of a compression dressing beyond 1 week may seem logical, extended application of the external bandage is generally counterproductive since progressive irritation and inflammation of the nasal skin usually offsets any potential benefits of prolonged nasal compression. For this same reason, the bandage is occasionally removed prematurely when contact dermatitis threatens to produce severe excoriation and blistering of the nasal skin.

Although considerable debate continues regarding the need for nasal packing, the cosmetic benefits derived from immediate tamponade of the nasal tip are generally well worth the transient discomfort associated with overnight packing.

In addition to an external nasal splint, bilateral septal splints fashioned from thin silicone sheets are also occasionally beneficial in supportive aftercare. Patients with nasal bridge instability resulting from extracorporeal septoplasty, aggressive osteotomies, severe skeletal trauma, or weak nasal cartilages often benefit from silicone splints placed high in the anterior nasal cavum to support the unstable middle vault framework. Low-profile septal splints, secured with a single anterior transfixion suture, can buttress the dorsum from below and greatly benefit the weak or unstable nasal framework until fibrous consolidation increases. Septal splints also help to maintain a straight nasal septum and to minimize septal swelling. Patients at increased risk for synechiae may also benefit from septal splints, which prevent raw mucosal surfaces from making contact. When placing septal splints, care must be taken to avoid septal necrosis from overtightening of the transfixion suture.

Another essential tool for reducing ecchymosis, edema, and inflammation is the immediate and continued application of ice. Although the nasal splint initially insulates most of the nose from the direct beneficial effects of ice, cooling of the adjacent soft tissues can greatly curtail swelling, bruising, and inflammation of the surrounding face, including the nose. In addition to continuous elevation of the head to 45 degrees (or higher) and placement of a damp cloth to prevent hypothermic skin injury, application of finely crushed ice over the nasofacial grooves, inner canthi, and glabella is maintained continuously for at least 24 hours after surgery, beginning in the operating room (Fig. 184.17). Aggressive application of ice is encouraged for all patients for the first 72 hours since inflammation and swelling are most likely to increase during the first 3 days following surgery. After 72 hours, prolonged intermittent application of ice is encouraged for all patients, but continued aggressive application of ice is strongly recommended for patients with thick nasal skin and those prone to excessive bruising or scarring. Although the application of ice is most beneficial in the first few days following surgery, ice can be useful to minimize transient nasal swelling for several weeks following revision rhinoplasty, and ice is particularly beneficial to control rebound edema following splint removal. While the application of ice often becomes tiresome, the frequent and prolonged application of ice can greatly improve the final cosmetic outcome, especially in patients prone to prolonged edema and subcutaneous scarring.

In addition to the proactive measures described above, patients should be advised to avoid all activities that exacerbate swelling or delay the resolution of edema. Prolonged recumbent posture, exercise, strenuous activity,

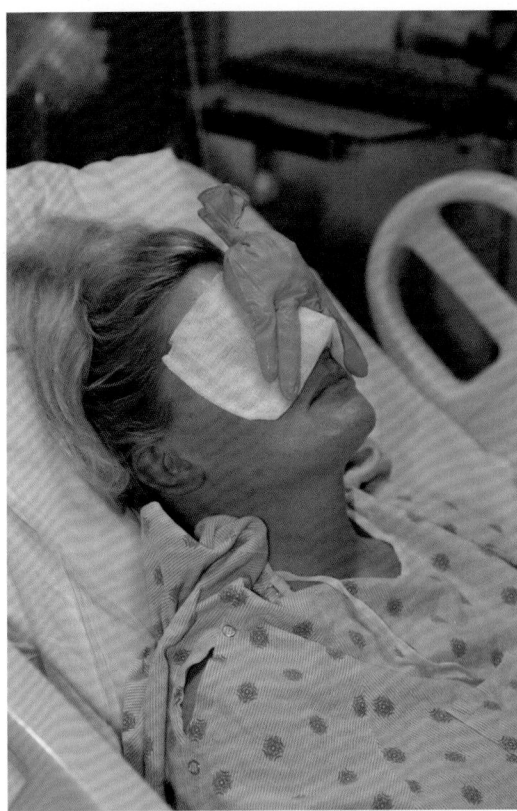

Figure 184.17 Continuous postoperative cooling using a surgical glove filled with crushed ice over a damp washcloth.

valsalva, high salt intake, and nasal sunburn should all be carefully avoided until *acute* nasal swelling subsides—usually not less than 6 weeks for patients with thin or intermediate skin thickness and longer for patients with heavy skin. While these restrictions are often unpopular with patients eager to resume their previous lifestyle, supportive measures provide an important but transient opportunity to eliminate acute edema and avoid subcutaneous scarring. Hence, missing this brief window of opportunity in exchange for a few weeks of unrestricted activity is an unwise trade-off in the long run, and patients must be continually reminded about the necessity of these vitally important restrictions.

While medically supervised aftercare is a critical aspect of revision rhinoplasty, inevitably the postoperative healing process yields a few unwelcome surprises. Typically, this takes the form of transient nasal asymmetry and/or contour misalignment resulting from a swollen and increasingly taut soft tissue envelope. Since swelling is seldom symmetric, especially when the surgical procedure may have required asymmetric tissue disruption, temporary disturbances in alignment and symmetry are common in the weeks and months following a complex revision rhinoplasty. While often disconcerting to the patient, minor asymmetries resulting from soft tissue inflammation and edema usually resolve spontaneously, and patient reassurance is appropriate. Initiation of topical nasal steroid spray

(Fluticasone) as soon as the nasal lining is fully intact, typically 2 weeks following surgery, will also help to speed the resolution of edema and inflammation and safely eliminate minor asymmetries. Compressive taping of the nasal bridge can also be used in conjunction with nasal steroids to eliminate swelling of the dorsum or supratip soft tissues. Hypoallergenic paper tape is placed firmly across the swollen area and is worn overnight, and the tape is gently removed after soaking to minimize skin irritation or skin displacement.

As with soft tissue swelling, transient contracture of the skin envelope may also result in temporary distortion of the nose. Often this problem is most noticeable in the nasal base where linear contracture of the vestibular incision lines can lead to discrepancies in nostril shape or columellar contour. In addition to topical nasal steroids, insertion of soft nostril stents to dilate and stretch the skin incisions for several hours each day can lead to considerable improvement in nasal base contour and symmetry. Asymmetries of the dorsum and widening of the bony vault are also common problems after lateral osteotomies, particularly in younger patients who are highly susceptible to lateralization of the nasal bones from periosteal contracture. Often the nasal bones are properly aligned upon bandage removal, only to be displaced weeks later by periosteal scar contracture. To prevent permanent widening or asymmetry of the bony vault, nasal compression exercises are instituted until the bony vault narrows and stabilizes. Compression exercises involve the application of firm bilateral pressure directed toward the midline using the index fingertips placed just above the lateral osteotomy site. Firm pressure is maintained for 10-second intervals and is repeated five times each day as tolerated.

Low-Dose Steroid Injection

Since minor imperfections arise in nearly all patients and since these annoying problems generally resolve with time, conservative treatment, reassurance, and close monitoring are appropriate in the early weeks after surgery. However, despite prudent measures to contain surgical inflammation, a small number of patients—often those with thick, sebaceous nasal skin—will develop a vigorous and sustained inflammatory response. In the worst case scenario, uncontrolled inflammation may result in permanent cosmetic distortion and/or airway impairment from scarring or contracture. And while postoperative steroid injections may potentially diminish the inflammatory response, early intervention and sustained treatment is paramount even at the risk of localized steroid side effects. Fortunately, most patients do not develop a fulminant inflammatory response and can be managed effectively with topical nasal steroid spray (Fluticasone or equivalent)

alone. However, even mild inflammation can lead to permanent soft tissue fibrosis if allowed to persist long enough, and additional treatment with injectable steroids is generally beneficial in any case of prolonged swelling.

In general, all patients with thick or intermediate skin thickness should be considered at risk for dead space fibrosis and permanent skin thickening, particularly following multiple prior surgeries. Although conservative treatment measures such as compression dressings, topical steroid sprays, taping, stenting, and massage are effective for the majority of primary rhinoplasty patients, the previously operated nose is far more susceptible to prolonged edema by virtue of cumulative circulatory impairment. Of all the adjunctive treatment measures available for controlling postsurgical swelling and edema, by far the most effective, yet also the most hazardous, is injection with *triamcinolone acetonide*, commonly known by its brand name Kenalog (Bristol-Myers Squibb Co., Princeton, NJ). When injected into the subcutaneous tissues, this long-acting synthetic glucocorticoid acts to reduce soft tissue edema and prevent dead space fibrosis. However, in susceptible patients this powerful anti-inflammatory agent may also result in dermal thinning, fat necrosis, cartilage graft resorption, localized infection, or telangiectasias. Unwanted side effects are more common when administered at full strength, or at frequent and prolonged intervals, but side effects can occur even at low doses in susceptible patients, particularly when administered soon after surgery. Fortunately, adverse reactions are uncommon at a starting dose of 5 to 10 mg/mL diluted in 1% lidocaine containing a 1:100,000 concentration of epinephrine, and small volumes of 0.05 to 0.1 mL are generally effective. In addition to minimizing injection site discomfort, the admixture of lidocaine with epinephrine also serves to minimize dispersal of triamcinolone from the targeted site. Because triamcinolone is typically slow-acting, assessment of the therapeutic response is delayed for a minimum of 4 weeks, at which time the initial dose can be repeated (if necessary) and/or carefully titrated to the desired effect. However, particular care should be exercised when treating callus formation in the thin-skinned rhinoplasty patient. Restricting the starting dose to 5 mg/mL and waiting 6 weeks before assessing the therapeutic response is recommended for thin-skinned patients who are at greater risk for the unwanted side effects of dermal thinning and telangiectasias. In general, triamcinolone treatment is also best avoided in the first 2 to 3 months following surgery to prevent erosion of autologous tissue grafts, unless severe fibrosis, contracture, and/or callus formation are threatening. In stubborn cases, repeated monthly injections are necessary before a sustained clinical improvement is achieved. Although low-dose triamcinolone injection is a useful adjunct in the actively healing nose, timely intervention is paramount since triamcinolone has little benefit in the fully healed nose.

Case Presentation One—"Completion Rhinoplasty"

Brief Case History

A healthy young female presents with a "bumpy," asymmetric, and oversized nose, 10 years after primary reduction rhinoplasty (see Fig. 184.19A–F). On frontal view, the bony vault is flat and asymmetric with lateral deviation of the left nasal bone. The middle vault is overly wide and both supra-alar creases are absent. The lobule is pinched, and the right ala is larger than the left. On profile, the tip is significantly overprojected and the nasolabial angle is overly obtuse. The dorsum is also overprojected, particularly in the middle vault. On oblique view, protrusions of the upper and middle vaults disrupt the dorsal line. On base view, the nose is markedly overprojected and the columellar pedestal is exceedingly wide. The caudal septum is partially obstructing the left nostril opening. The endonasal exam reveals deviation of the caudal septum into the left nasal vestibule, but the remaining septum is midline. No other endonasal pathology is observed. External revision rhinoplasty using septal and/or conchal cartilage grafts was recommended and performed.

Surgical Findings

Using the external rhinoplasty approach, the residual nasal framework was degloved. Healthy but malpositioned medial crura were encountered bilaterally, and the left alar cartilage was divided 2 mm below the dome. Both lateral crura were embedded in fibrous scar tissue and numerous blue monofilament sutures were removed from the tip and infratip. Large cephalic resections were noted bilaterally, with greater tissue excision from the right lateral crus. Crural width measured 6 mm on the right and 8 mm on the left, and both cartilages were buckled and malpositioned.

Surgical Steps (Fig. 184.18)

1. The nasal skeleton is degloved via the external approach.
2. The alar cartilage remnants are degloved and numerous blue monofilament sutures are removed from the tip and infratip.
3. The medial crura are degloved, and the distal 5 mm of cartilage (i.e., the footpods) are excised. Copious fibrous scar tissue is debulked from within the columella.
4. The membranous septum is divided, and the caudal septum and nasal spine are exposed.
5. The posterior septal angle and the nasal spine are trimmed approximately 3 mm.

6. Bilateral mucoperichondrial flaps are elevated over the caudal septum and lower ¾ of the quadrangular cartilage.
7. Septal graft material is harvested with L-strut preservation.
8. The medial crura are advanced inferiorly/posteriorly and sewn to the caudal septum ("tongue-in-groove" setback) to decrease tip projection and reduce nasolabial angle fullness.
9. The middle vault is degloved to reveal intact upper lateral cartilage/septal cartilage complex.
10. The upper lateral cartilages are sharply divided from the dorsal septum using a no. 15 blade, and after reflecting the overlying mucoperichondrium, a 4-mm pollybeak deformity is resected with straight Iris scissors.
11. A tapered (2 mm) resection of the bony hump is performed using a powered sagittal saw. Edges are rounded using a powered reciprocating rasp.
12. Bilateral (medial and lateral) osteotomies are performed to narrow the bony vault.
13. The upper lateral cartilages are sutured to the dorsal septum with running 5-0 vicryl.
14. A SEG is sewn to the right side of the caudal septum with 5-0 PDS to reproject and counterrotate the nasal tip position.

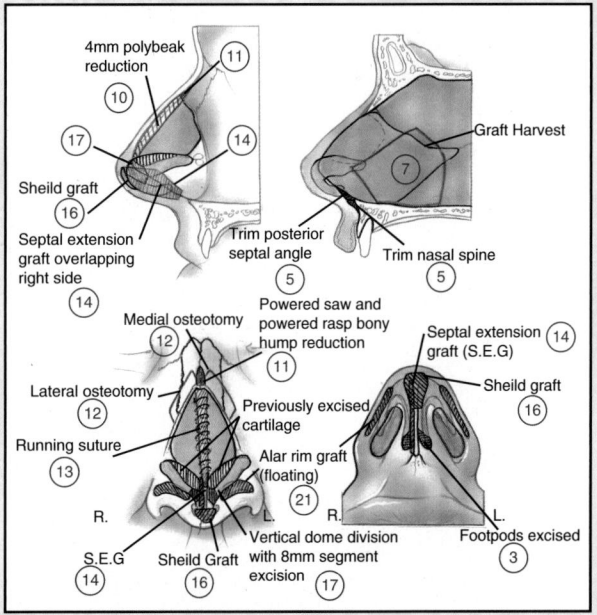

Figure 184.18 Rhinoplasty worksheet for case presentation one.

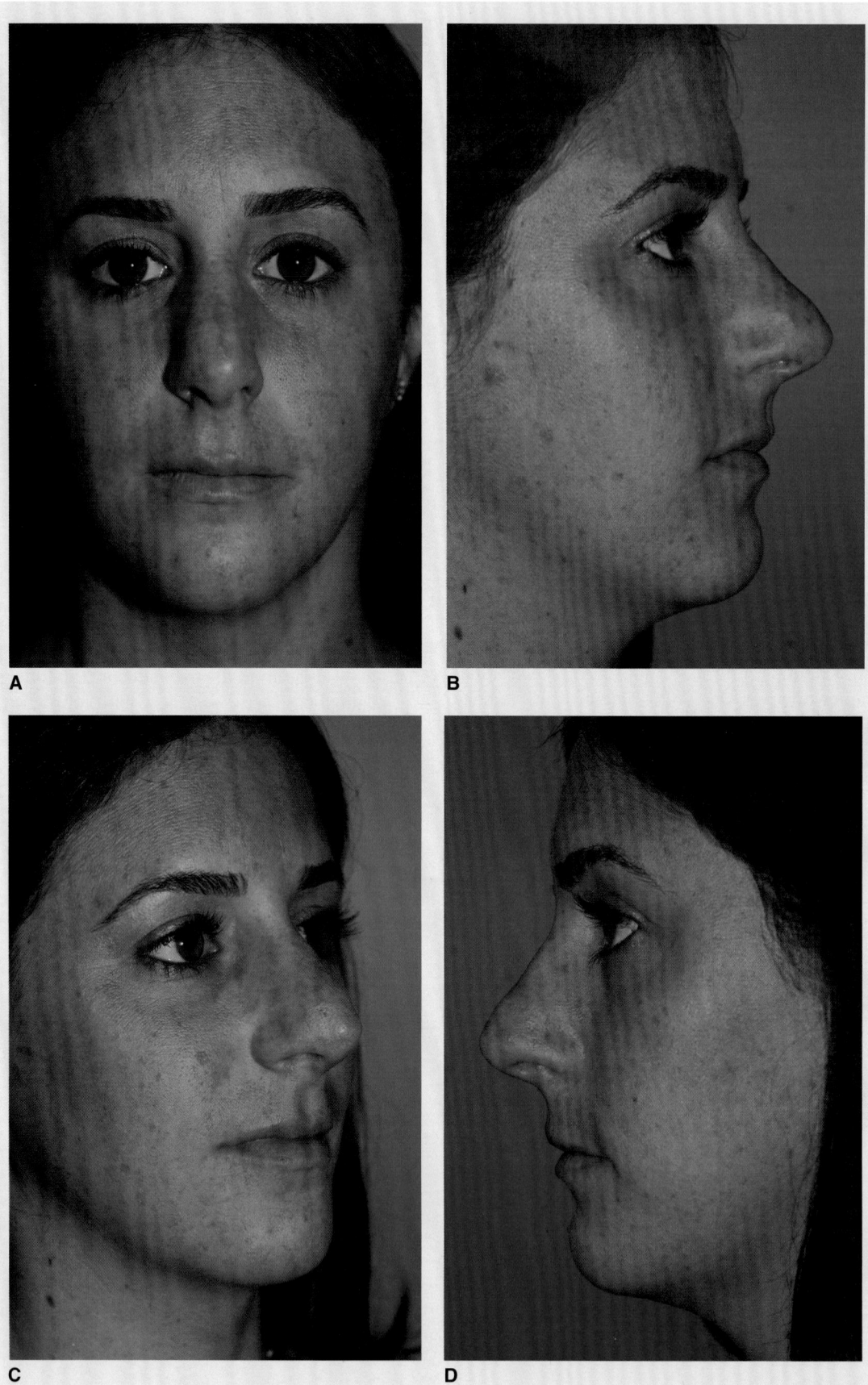

Figure 184.19 Case presentation one. **A–F:** Preoperative frontal, lateral, oblique, and basal views. **G–L:** Corresponding postoperative views.

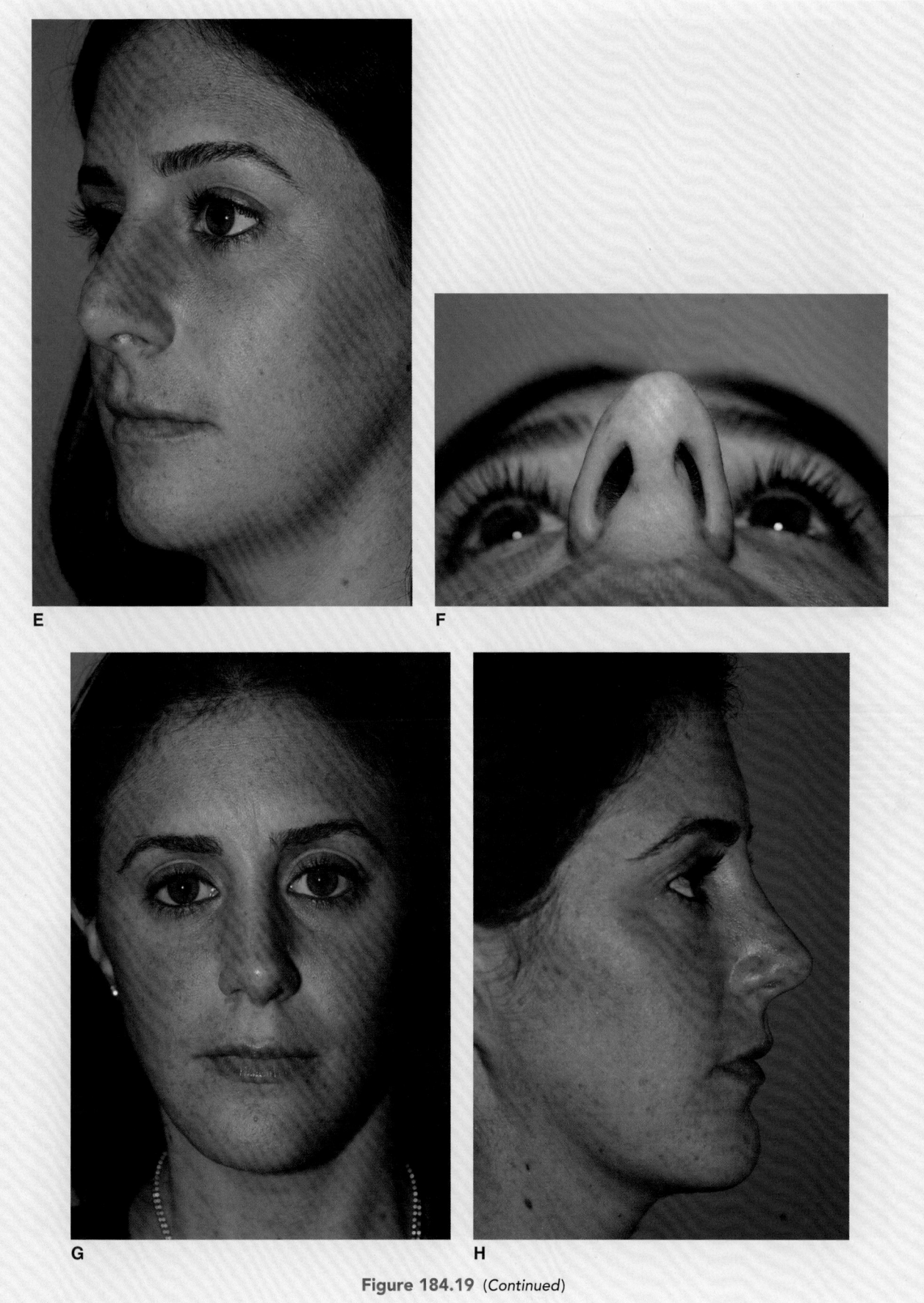

E

F

G

H

Figure 184.19 (*Continued*)

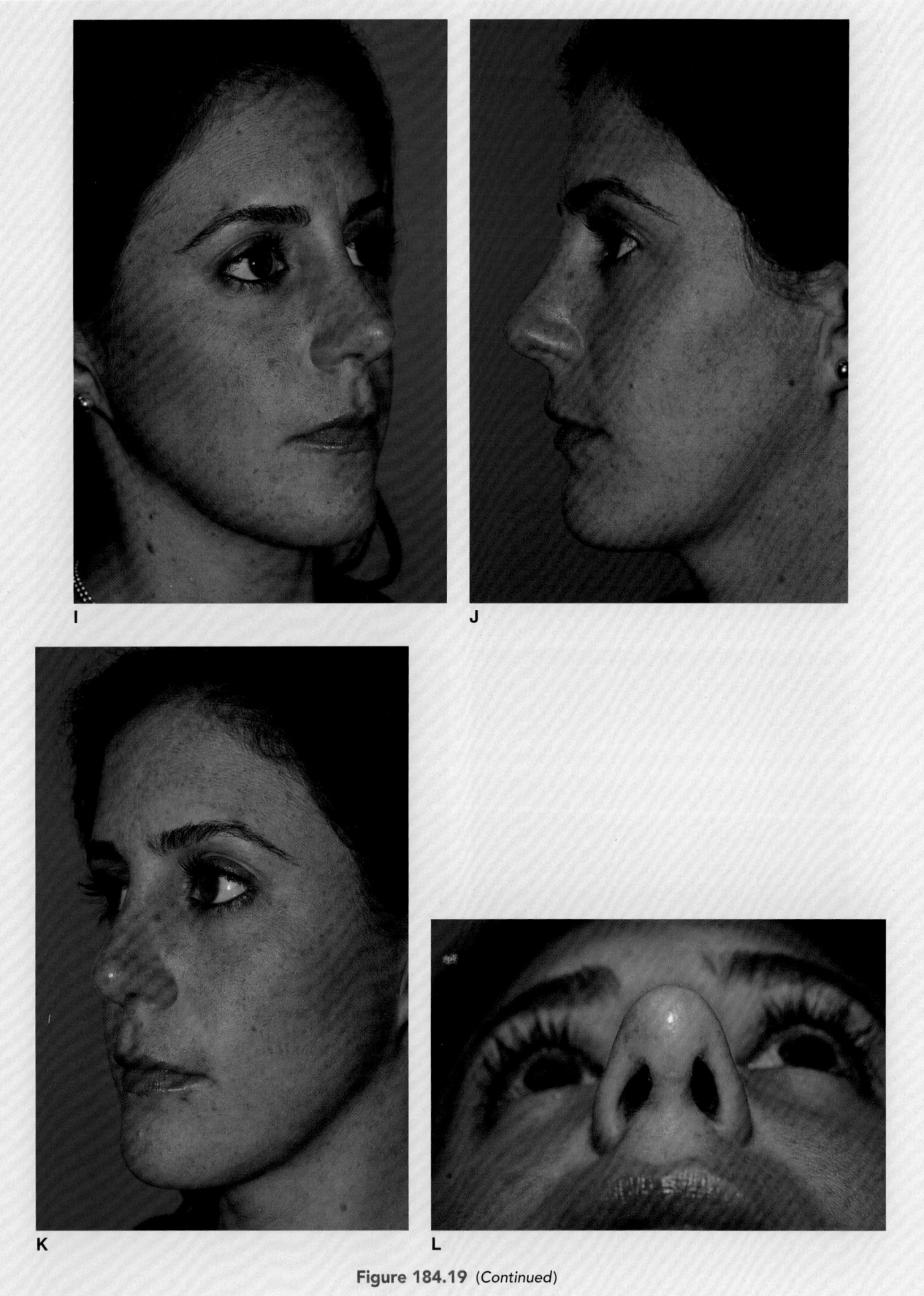

Figure 184.19 (Continued)

15. The medial crura are sutured to the caudal margin of SEG.
16. A shield graft is sutured to the infratip lobule with 5-0 PDS.
17. The domes are divided vertically, and both lateral crura are shortened by 8 mm at their cut edges. The lateral crural stumps are then folded upon themselves and sewn to the lateral shield graft with 5-0 PDS.
18. A paradomal cephalic excision is performed bilaterally to eliminate supratip fullness.
19. Lateral crural spanning sutures are placed bilaterally to flatten the lateral crural remnants.
20. A small batten graft is used to fill a concavity of the right crural cartilage.
21. Alar rim grafts are placed bilaterally (15 × 3 mm).
22. The subcutaneous pocket is irrigated with saline.
23. The skin is closed and an aluminum splint is placed.

Surgical Outcome

The postoperative nasal contour reveals a smaller, more symmetric, and more attractive nasal contour (see Fig. 184.19G–L). Despite deprojecting the nasal tip and markedly downsizing the skeletal framework, airway patency is preserved using sidewall tensioning to stretch and stiffen the overresected lateral crural cartilages.

Case Presentation Two—Restoration of Central Tip Support

Brief Case History

A healthy middle-aged female presented complaining of severe bilateral nasal airway obstruction and a pinched nasal tip. The past surgical history was remarkable for reduction rhinoplasty more than 30 years earlier. Physical examination revealed a pinched and underprojected nasal tip, and flaccid collapse of both nasal sidewalls (Fig. 184.20A–D). Palpation of the outer skin envelope revealed thick skin with moderate skin elasticity. Anterior rhinoscopy revealed a midline septum, inferior turbinate hypertrophy, swollen nasal mucosa, and bilateral nasal valve obstruction secondary to flaccid sidewall collapse. Palpation of the quadrangular septum revealed firm septal cartilage throughout. Surgical treatment with an external nasoseptal reconstruction using autologous septal cartilage and submucous resection of the inferior turbinates was recommended and performed.

Surgical Findings

Using the external rhinoplasty approach, the residual nasal framework was degloved. Healthy and intact medial crura were encountered bilaterally, but 95% of both lateral crural cartilages and 100% of both upper lateral cartilages were missing. The entire nasal septum including the dorsal septum, anterior septal angle, and quadrangular septum were fully intact.

Surgical Steps (Fig. 184.21)

1. The nasal skeleton is degloved via the external approach.
2. The membranous septum is sharply divided and bilateral mucoperichondrial flaps are elevated over the caudal septum and lower ¾ of the quadrangular cartilage.
3. Septal graft tissue is harvested with L-strut preservation.
4. An SEG (30 × 15 mm) is sutured to the caudal septum with three figure-of-8 sutures to project and counterrotate nasal tip position.
5. The medial crura are sutured to leading edge of SEG with 5-0 monocryl (percutaneous) transfixion sutures.
6. A shield graft is sutured to the infratip lobule with 5-0 PDS sutures.
7. The contractured vestibular skin is unfurled after lysis of adhesions.
8. The vestibular skin is stretched medially/anteriorly and sutured to the lateral shield graft.

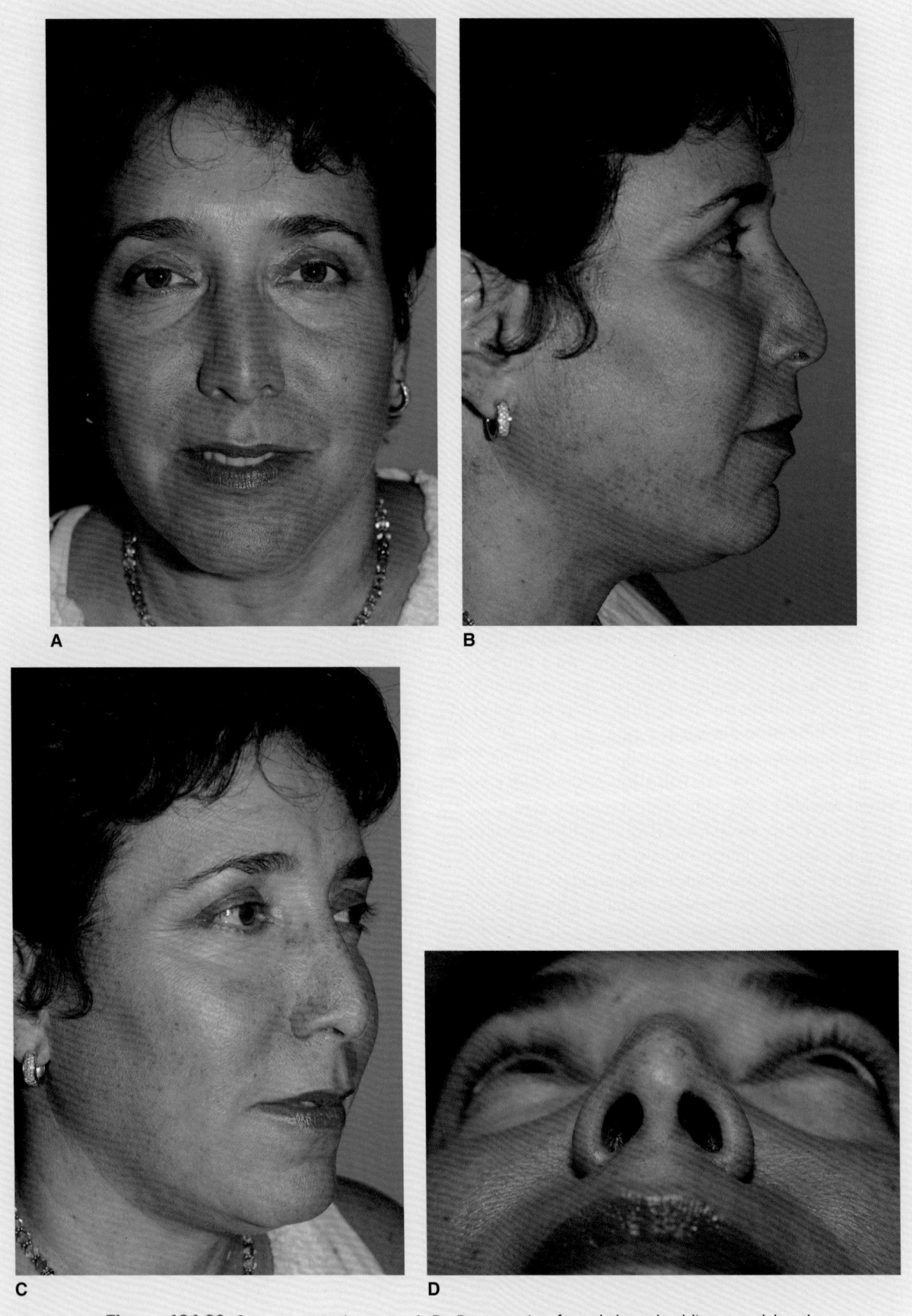

Figure 184.20 Case presentation two. **A–D:** Preoperative frontal, lateral, oblique, and basal views.

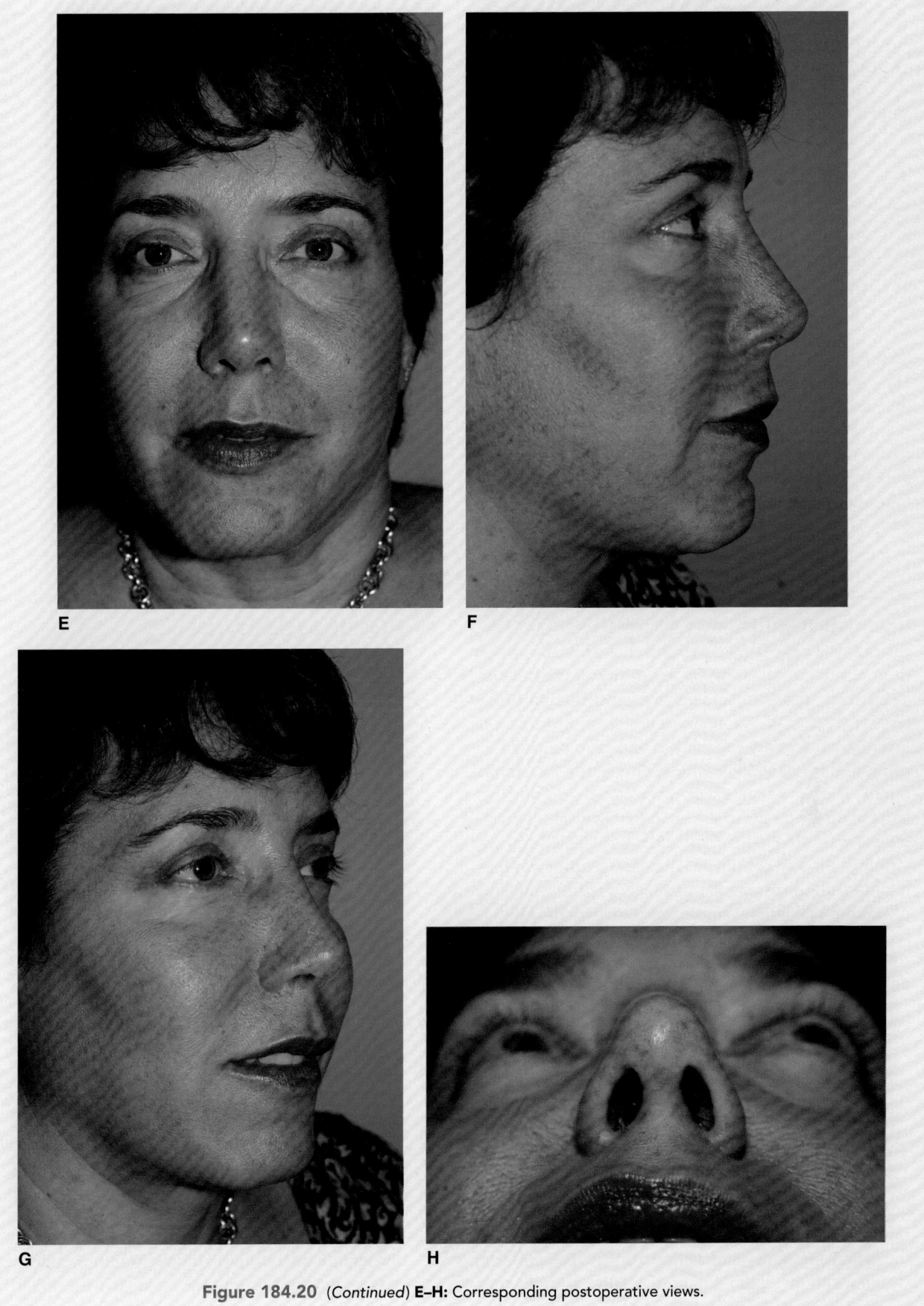

Figure 184.20 (*Continued*) **E–H:** Corresponding postoperative views.

9. A tapered middle vault onlay graft is sutured to the underlying septum to correct the small saddle indentation created by projection of the collapsed nasal tip.
10. Nasal SMAS is excised from beneath the supratip skin for improved soft tissue distensibility.
11. A cartilaginous hump (1 mm) is shaved with a no. 15 blade.
12. A small bony hump is eliminated with the power rasp obviating the need for lateral osteotomies.
13. The subcutaneous pocket is irrigated with saline.
14. The skin is closed, and an aluminum splint is placed.

Surgical Outcome

The postoperative nasal contour reveals improved tip projection and elimination of lobular pinching (Fig. 184.20E–H). In addition to a favorable cosmetic result, internal nasal valve collapse and airway dysfunction were also eliminated without structural grafting of the nasal sidewalls.

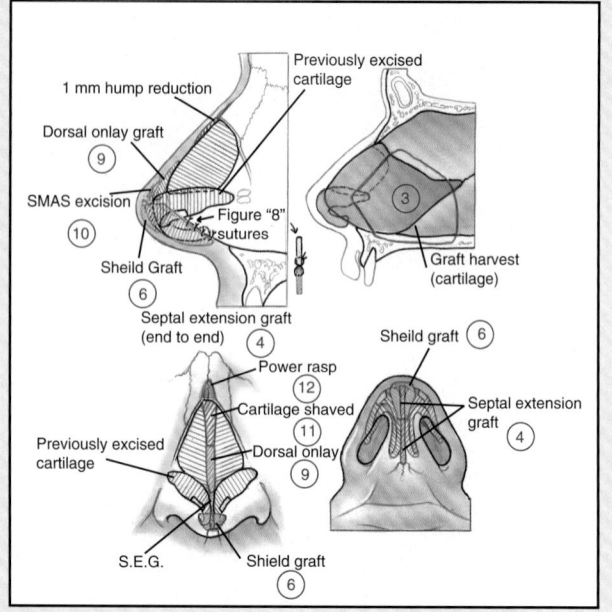

Figure 184.21 Rhinoplasty worksheet for case presentation two.

Case Presentation Three—Overresected Tip and Dorsum

Brief Case History

A healthy young female presents 1 year after primary rhinoplasty complaining of nasal airway obstruction, a "pinched" nasal tip, and an overresected nasal bridge (Fig. 184.22A–D). Examination revealed a conspicuous inverted-V deformity and marked underprojection of the rhinion, both consistent with overresection of a dorsal hump. The tip was markedly overrotated and pinched, and pinching was more severe on the right side. The columella was tilted to the right and a well-healed scar was visible at the mid columella. The nasal septum was midline and the quadrangular cartilage was fully intact to palpation. The inferior turbinates were hypertrophic.

An external nasoseptal reconstruction with septal and conchal cartilage grafts, and bilateral submucous turbinectomies was recommended and performed.

Surgical Findings

Using the external rhinoplasty approach, the residual nasal framework was surgically degloved. Overprojected, overrotated, and collapsed alar cartilages were encountered bilaterally. The right alar cartilage was previously divided vertically at the dome, and the intermediate crura were splayed by large amounts of fibrous scar tissue. The cephalic margin was also absent from both lateral crura and the crural remnants were retracted cephalically. Lysis of scar adhesions was necessary to free the crural remnants and permit caudal repositioning. Crural width measured 8 mm bilaterally, but both cartilages were buckled and malpositioned.

Surgical Steps (Fig. 184.23)

1. The nasal skeleton is degloved via the external approach.
2. The alar cartilage remnants are degloved, and fibrous scar tissue is excised from the infratip lobule.
3. Cephalic adhesions of the lateral crura are lysed to permit caudal repositioning of the crural remnants.
4. The membranous septum is divided, and the caudal septum and nasal spine are exposed.
5. Bilateral mucoperichondrial flaps are elevated over the caudal septum and lower ¾ of the quadrangular cartilage.
6. Septal graft material is harvested with L-strut preservation.
7. The middle vault is degloved to reveal overresection of the dorsal septum and upper lateral cartilages with pinching of the middle vault.
8. The nasal bones were degloved to reveal a short and overresected bony vault with bilateral open-roof deformities.
9. A fusiform-shaped conchal graft is fashioned from donor cartilage measuring 35 × 20 mm. The graft is bivalved longitudinally.
10. Submucosal pockets are developed on both sides of the dorsal septum, and the folded conchal "butterfly" graft is placed over the cartilaginous and bony septum at the rhinion and secured with 4-0 PDS mattress sutures.

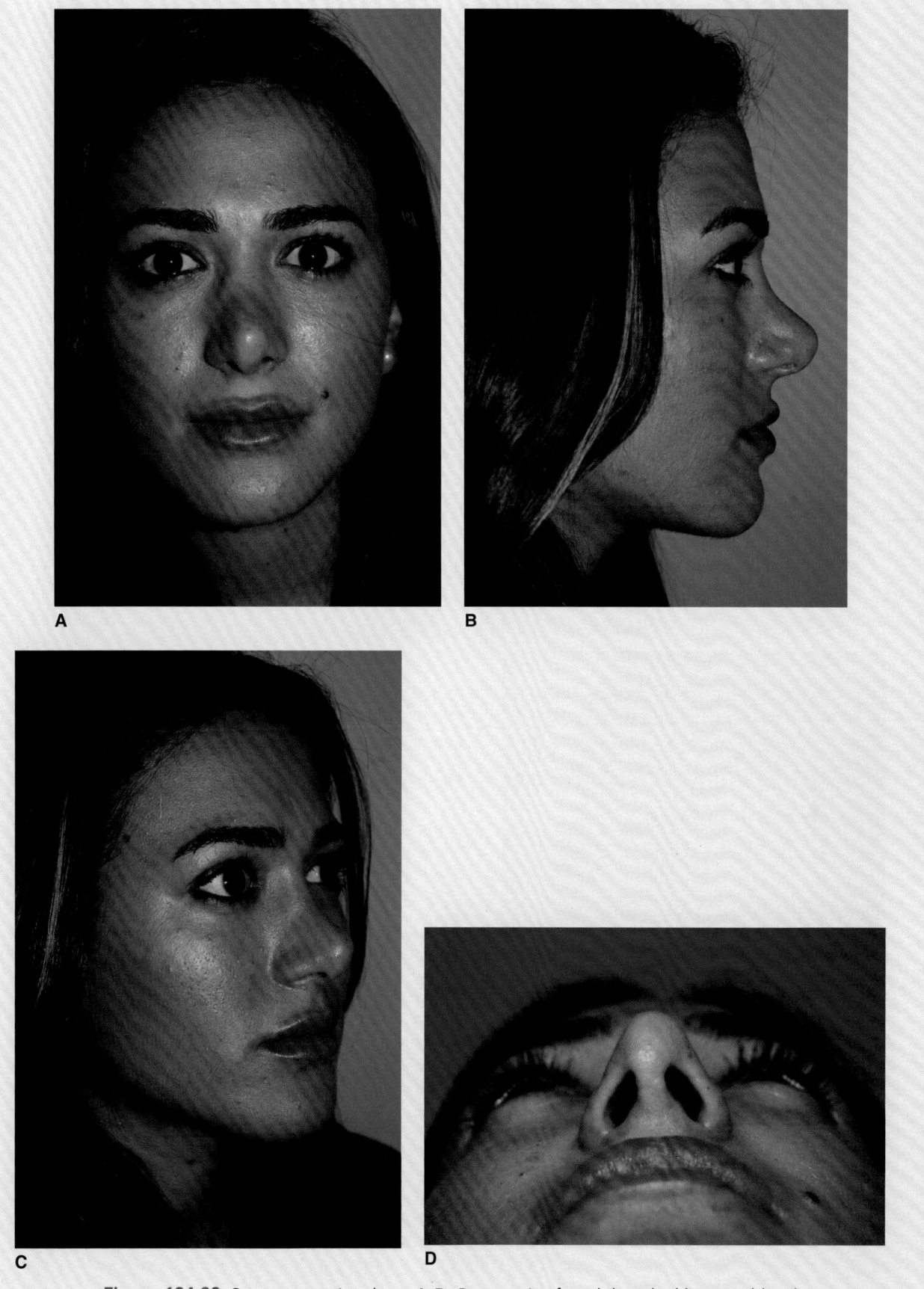

Figure 184.22 Case presentation three. **A–D:** Preoperative frontal, lateral, oblique, and basal views.

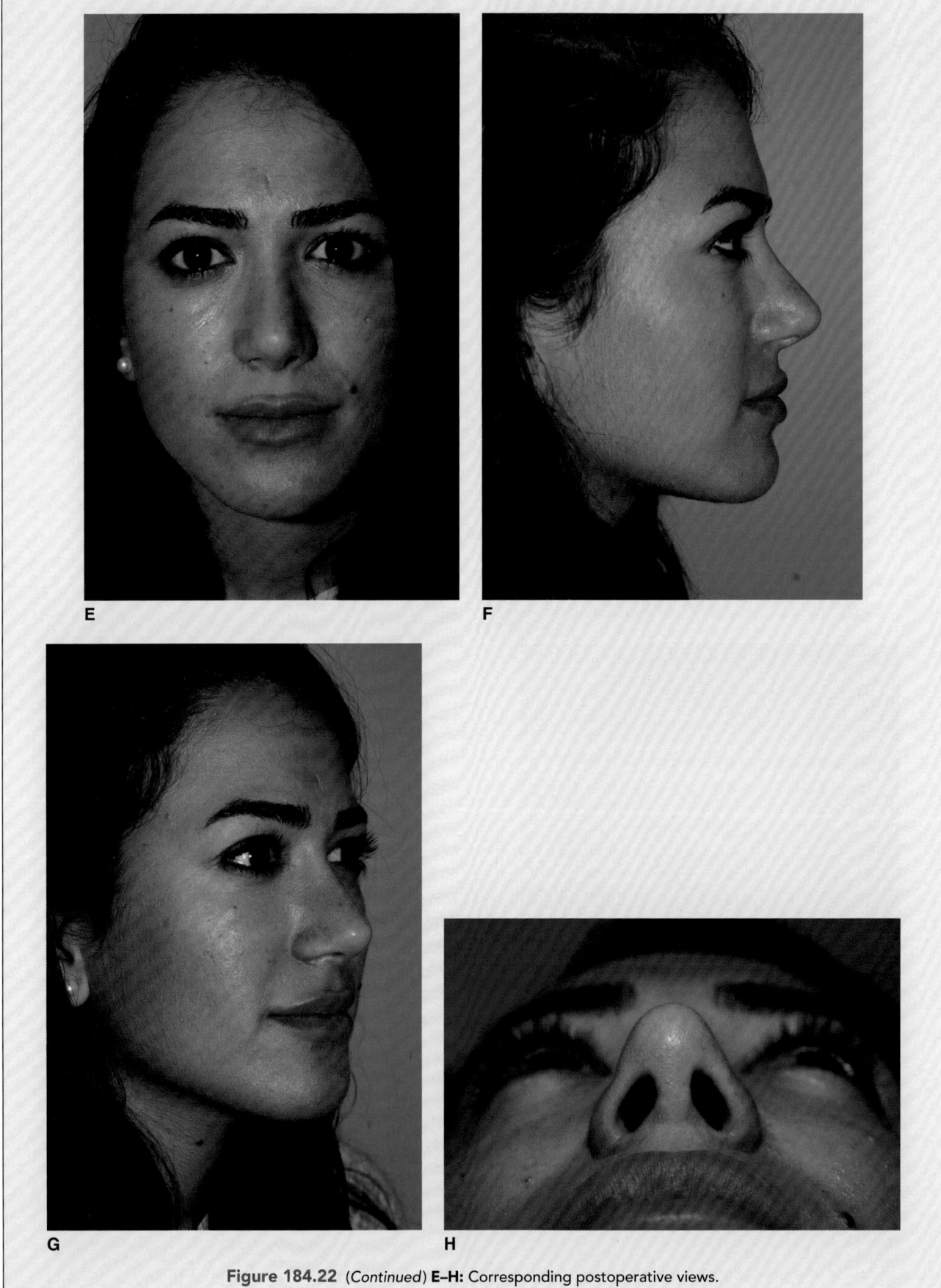

Figure 184.22 (*Continued*) **E–H:** Corresponding postoperative views.

11. Additional dorsal augmentation was achieved with a narrow septal cartilage onlay graft (with beveled edges) sutured atop the conchal butterfly graft.
12. Bilateral (medial and lateral) osteotomies are performed to narrow the bony vault.
13. The upper lateral cartilages are sutured to the outer butterfly graft with 5-0 Vicryl.
14. An SEG (septal cartilage) is sewn to the caudal septum in an end-to-end configuration using 4-0 PDS figure-of-8 sutures to lengthen the nose and counterrotate the nasal tip.
15. The medial crura are sutured to caudal margin of SEG with 5-0 Monocryl percutaneous transfixion sutures.
16. A double-layered shield graft is sutured to the infratip lobule with 5-0 PDS for additional tip counterrotation.
17. The domes are divided vertically, and both lateral crura are shortened by 5 mm at their cut edges. The lateral crural stumps are then folded upon themselves, advanced anteriorly, and sewn to the lateral shield graft with 5-0 PDS sutures to *tension* the collapsed and twisted lateral crural remnants.
18. A paradomal cephalic excision is performed bilaterally to eliminate supratip fullness produced by lateral crural advancement.
19. Alar rim grafts are placed bilaterally (15 × 3 mm).
20. The subcutaneous pocket is irrigated with saline.
21. The skin is closed, and an aluminum splint is placed.

Surgical Outcome

The postoperative contour reveals restoration of dorsal height with elimination of the inverted-V deformity and elimination of lobular pinching and tip overrotation (Fig. 184.22E–H). Nasal airway obstruction was also eliminated.

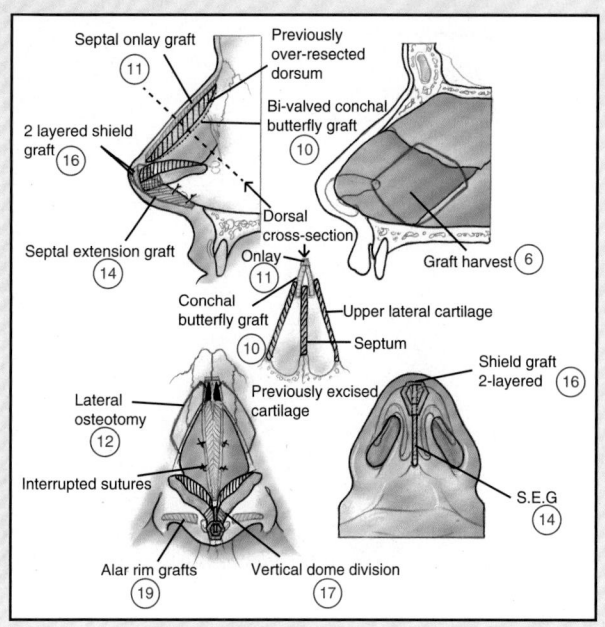

Figure 184.23 Rhinoplasty worksheet for case presentation three.

Case Presentation Four—Revision of the Narrow Nose

Brief Case History

A healthy young female presents 6 months after revision rhinoplasty complaining of nasal airway obstruction, a pinched nasal tip, and nasal asymmetry (Fig. 84.24A–D). The operative report from the primary rhinoplasty 1 year earlier described placement of bilateral lateral crural (onlay) "batten grafts" (harvested from the nasal septum) for treatment of lateral crural concavities. A second operative report from revision surgery performed 3 months later described removal of the batten grafts and placement of an interdomal suture. Frontal examination revealed a pinched lobule, flared and retracted nostrils, and a widened middle vault with effacement of the supra-alar creases. On profile examination, the columellar double-break was flattened and a persistent rhinion hump was noted. Anterior rhinoscopy revealed deviation of the caudal and quadrangular septum to the right side, constriction of both internal valves, and hypertrophy of the inferior turbinates. A membranous septum was palpable in the posterior–inferior aspect of the quadrangular cartilage. An external nasoseptal reconstruction with autologous septal cartilage and bilateral submucous inferior turbinectomies were recommended and performed.

Surgical Findings

Using the external rhinoplasty approach, the residual nasal framework was surgically degloved. The alar cartilage remnants were noted to be malpositioned, lacerated, and asymmetric (Fig. 184.25A and B). The left alar cartilage was divided vertically at the dome and again at the mid lateral crus, while the right alar cartilage remained in continuity with a vertical laceration of the right middle crus. The cephalic margin was missing from both lateral crura, and residual crural width measured approximately 8 mm, bilaterally. Despite the missing quadrangular cartilage from previous septal graft harvest, a 30 × 15 mm septal cartilage graft was removed from the upper quadrangular septum while preserving a 10- to 12-mm septal L-strut.

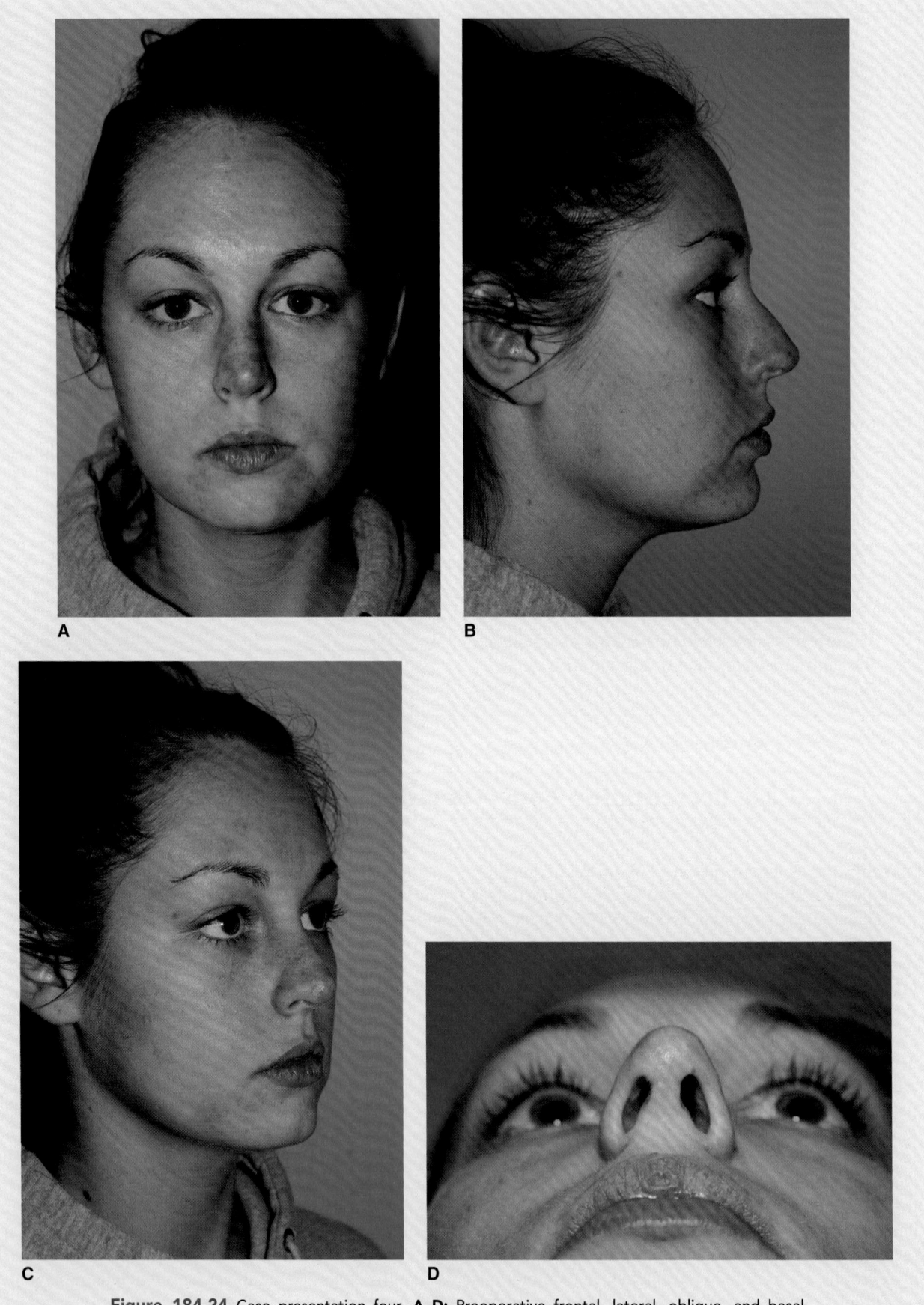

Figure 184.24 Case presentation four. **A–D:** Preoperative frontal, lateral, oblique, and basal views.

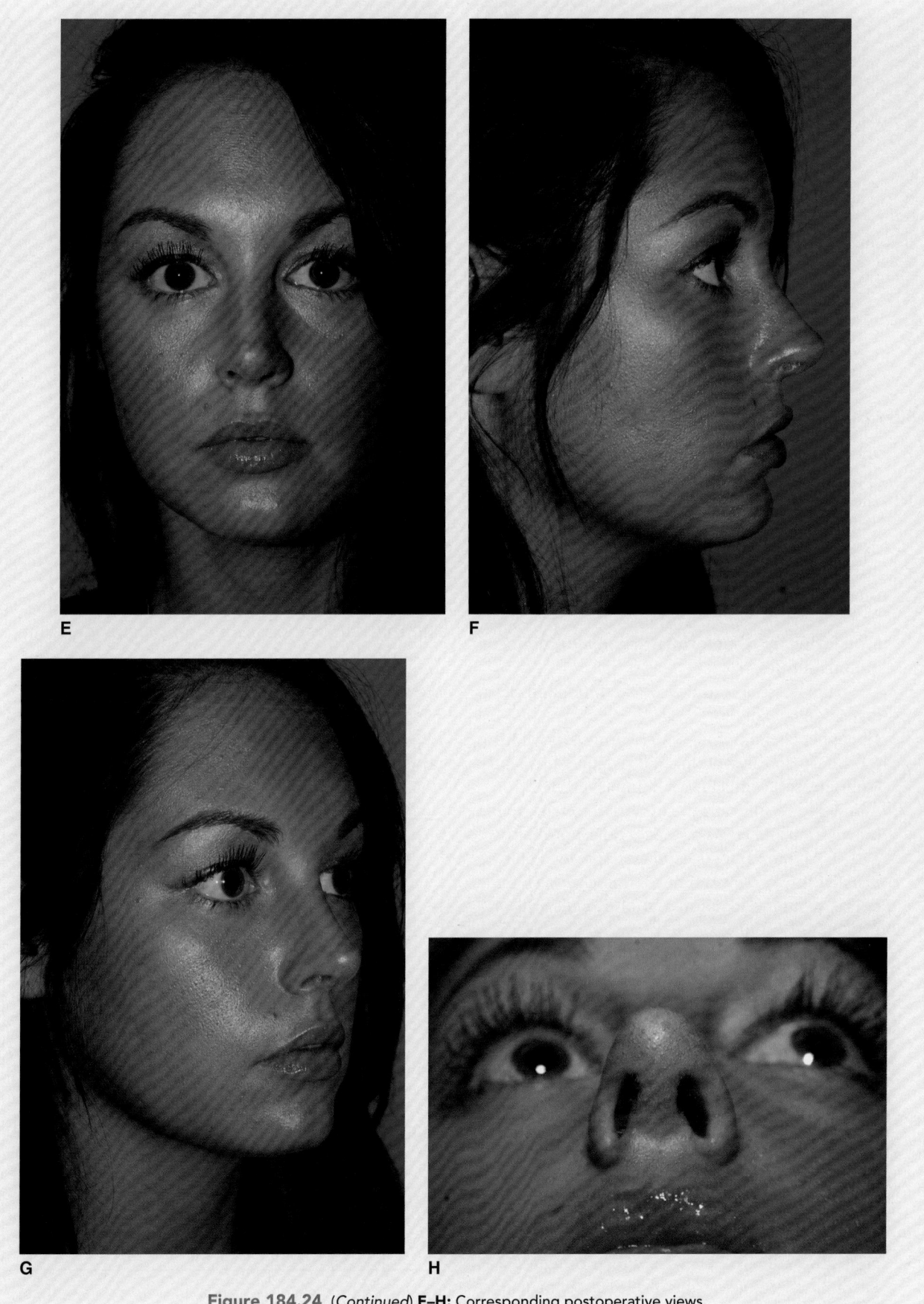

Figure 184.24 (*Continued*) **E–H:** Corresponding postoperative views.

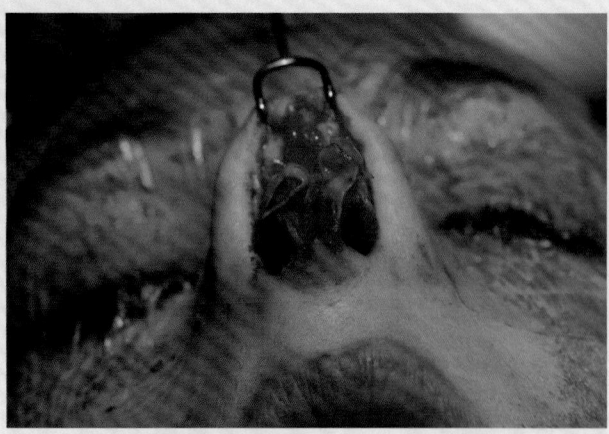

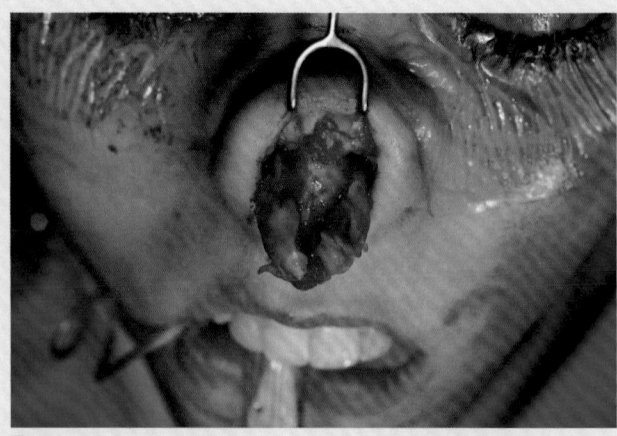

A   **B**

Figure 184.25 Intraoperative photos for case presentation four. **A,B:** Exposure of misshapen and torn alar cartilages.

Surgical Steps (Fig. 184.26)

1. The nasal skeleton is degloved via the external approach.
2. The membranous septum is sharply divided and bilateral mucoperichondrial flaps are elevated over the caudal septum and lower ¾ of the quadrangular cartilage.
3. Septal graft tissue is harvested with L-strut preservation.
4. Septal flaps are reapproximated with 5-0 monocryl quilting sutures.
5. The nasal dorsum is degloved with blunt and sharp dissection.
6. The upper lateral cartilages are sharply divided from the intact dorsal septum, and a tapered 1.5 mm (submucosal) cartilaginous hump is resected.
7. A powered reciprocating rasp is used to remove the bony hump and create a straight dorsal profile.
8. A 25 × 4 mm (septal cartilage) spreader graft is inserted into a right submucosal pocket beside the dorsal septum and sutured at both ends with 4-0 PDS mattress sutures.
9. The upper lateral cartilages are sutured to the dorsal septum with 4-0 PDS mattress sutures.
10. Medial and lateral osteotomies are performed to narrow the bony vault and close the open roof.
11. An SEG (25 × 12 mm) is sutured to the caudal septum with three figure-of-8 sutures to project and counterrotate nasal tip position.
12. The medial crura are sutured to the leading edge of SEG with 5-0 monocryl (percutaneous) transfixion sutures.
13. A shield graft is sutured to the infratip lobule with 5-0 PDS sutures.
14. The domes are divided vertically, and both lateral crura are shortened by 5 mm at their cut edges. The lateral crural stumps are then folded upon themselves and sewn to the lateral shield graft with 5-0 PDS.

15. A cap graft is fashioned from septal cartilage and sewn atop the lateral crural stumps with 5-0 PDS.
16. Fibromuscular tissue removed from the tip and infratip is placed over the lateral crura for contour enhancement.
17. A right paradomal trim is performed.
18. An alar rim graft is fashioned from septal cartilage and secured in a left intracutaneous pocket.
19. The subcutaneous pocket is irrigated with saline.
20. The skin is closed, and an aluminum splint is placed.

Surgical Outcome

The postoperative nasal contour reveals a slender, feminine, and attractive nose (Fig. 184.24E–H) with normal airway function.

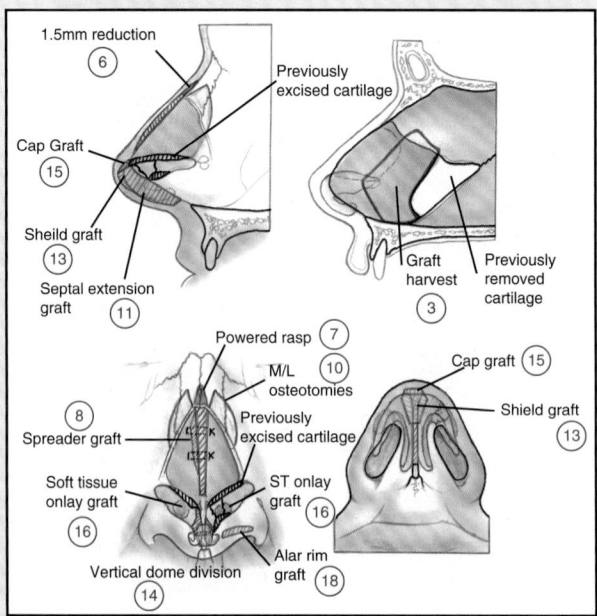

Figure 184.26 Rhinoplasty worksheet for case presentation four.

Case Presentation Five—Revision of the Severely Collapsed Nose

Brief Case History

A healthy young female presents 18 months after severe nasal trauma complaining of severe nasal obstruction and a wide, flat, and crooked nasal vault. Four weeks prior to injury, the patient underwent reduction rhinoplasty for treatment of a wide nose with severe airway obstruction. Preoperative photos reveal a naturally wide nose with adequate tip projection and a pseudo-hump from a deep radix (see Fig. 184.28A–D). Severe deviation of the caudal septum is seen on basal view. Postoperative photos reveal overresection of the rhinion, deprojection of the nasal tip, and significant additional widening of the tip and dorsum (see Fig. 184.28E–G). Upon presentation 18 months after injury, frontal examination revealed a splayed and scoliotic nose with impaction of the bony vault, pronounced rightward deviation of the dorsal septum, and a wide, amorphous nasal tip (see Fig. 184.28H–K). On profile examination, conspicuous loss of dorsal, tip, and columellar projection were evident, while the basal view revealed a severely underprojected nose with widening and impaction of the caudal septum.

Surgical Findings (see Fig. 184.29)

Using the external rhinoplasty approach, the residual nasal framework was surgically degloved. Small medial crural remnants were present in the columella, but approximately 90% of the lateral crura were missing and the remnants were noted to be embedded in scar tissue and malpositioned (see Fig. 184.29A–C). Numerous scar adhesions were lysed to unfurl the contractured vestibular skin. Upon degloving of the middle vault, the dorsal septum was found avulsed from the nasal bones, partially collapsed into the nasal cavity, and canted approximately 30 degrees to the right of midline. The caudal septum was deviated approximately 90 degrees from sagittal and was protruding into the right nasal passage. Accordion-type collapse of the left upper lateral cartilage was also observed, but the bony dorsum revealed no significant evidence of surgical or traumatic alteration.

Surgical Steps (Fig. 184.27)

1. The nasal skeleton is degloved via the external approach.
2. The alar cartilage remnants are degloved, and the contractured vestibular skin is unfurled with lysis of scar adhesions.

3. The entire cartilaginous septum, including the L-strut, is removed for donor graft material.
4. A 5-cm segment of full-thickness cartilage was harvested from the right fifth rib via an inframammary fold incision.
5. Concentric rib carving is used to create a 3.5 × 1.2 cm columellar strut graft.
6. The strut graft is notched at its base and sutured to the nasal spine with 4-0 PDS figure-of-8 suture passed through a transverse drill hole.
7. A 2.0 × 0.7 cm (dorsal) septal replacement graft was also fabricated from concentric carved rib cartilage.
8. The septal replacement graft was sutured to the upper lateral cartilages at the K-area and to the columellar strut to reconstitute the L-strut.
9. A 4 × 5 cm piece of deep temporalis fascia is harvested from the right temporal scalp.
10. Initially using a 3.0 syringe, and then a 1.0 mL syringe as templates, the temporalis fascia is sewn into a tapered cylinder measuring 4.0 cm in length. The proximal end is sewn shut.

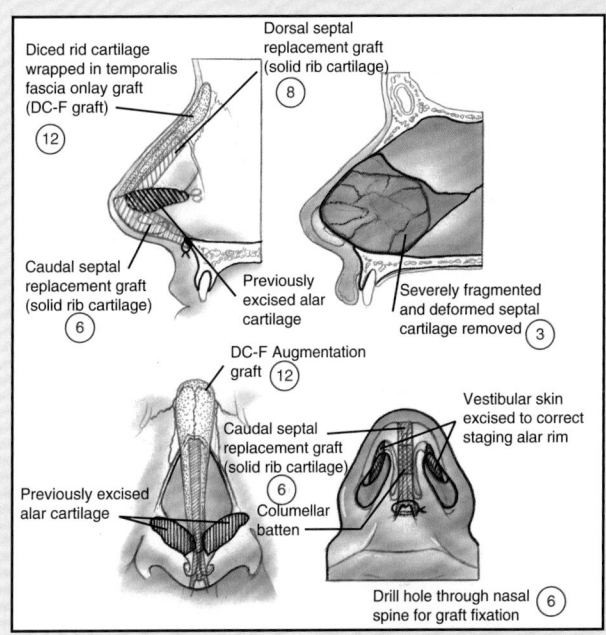

Figure 184.27 Rhinoplasty worksheet for case presentation five.

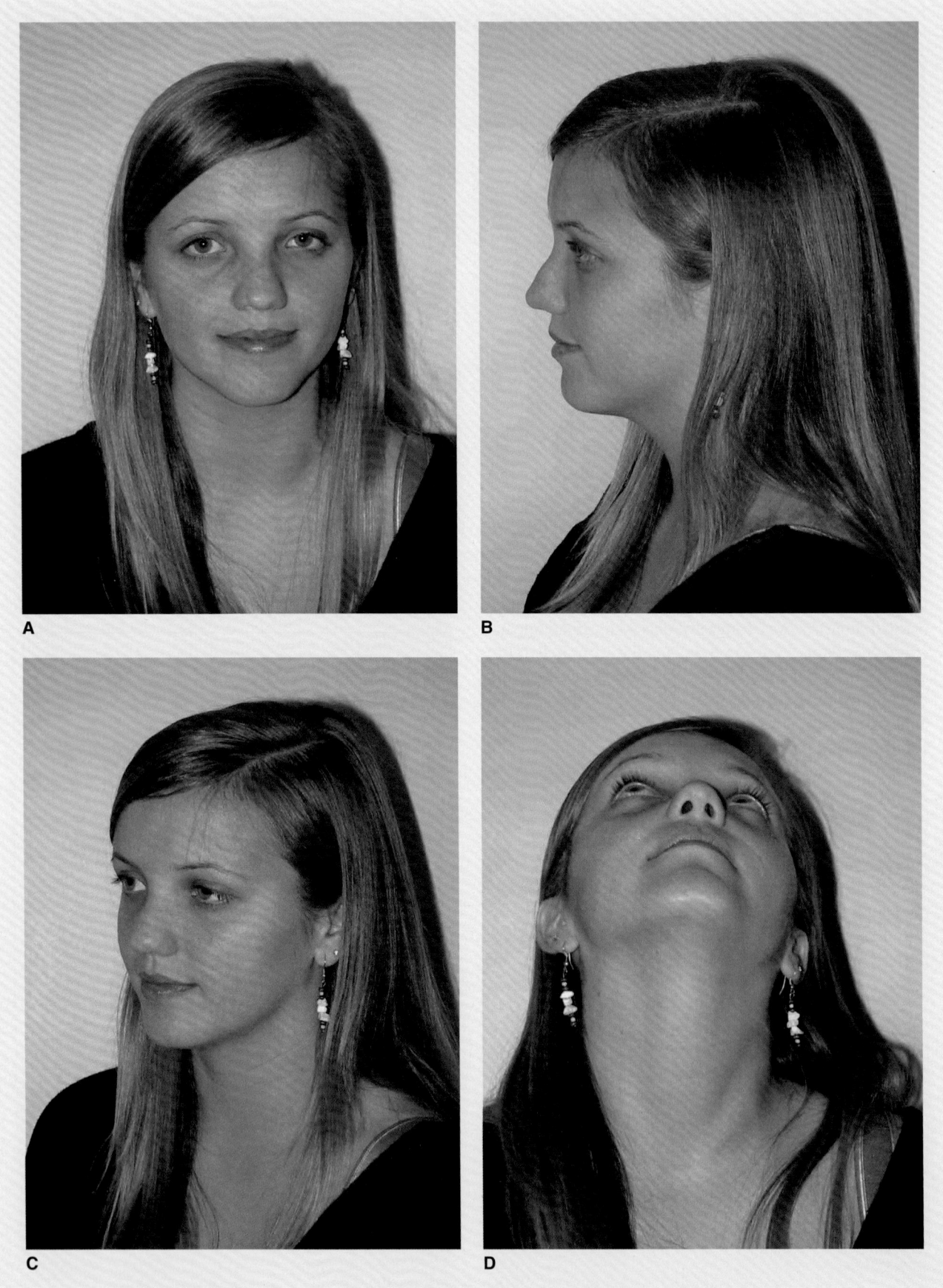

Figure 184.28 Case presentation five. **A–D:** Frontal, lateral, oblique, and basal views prior to primary rhinoplasty.

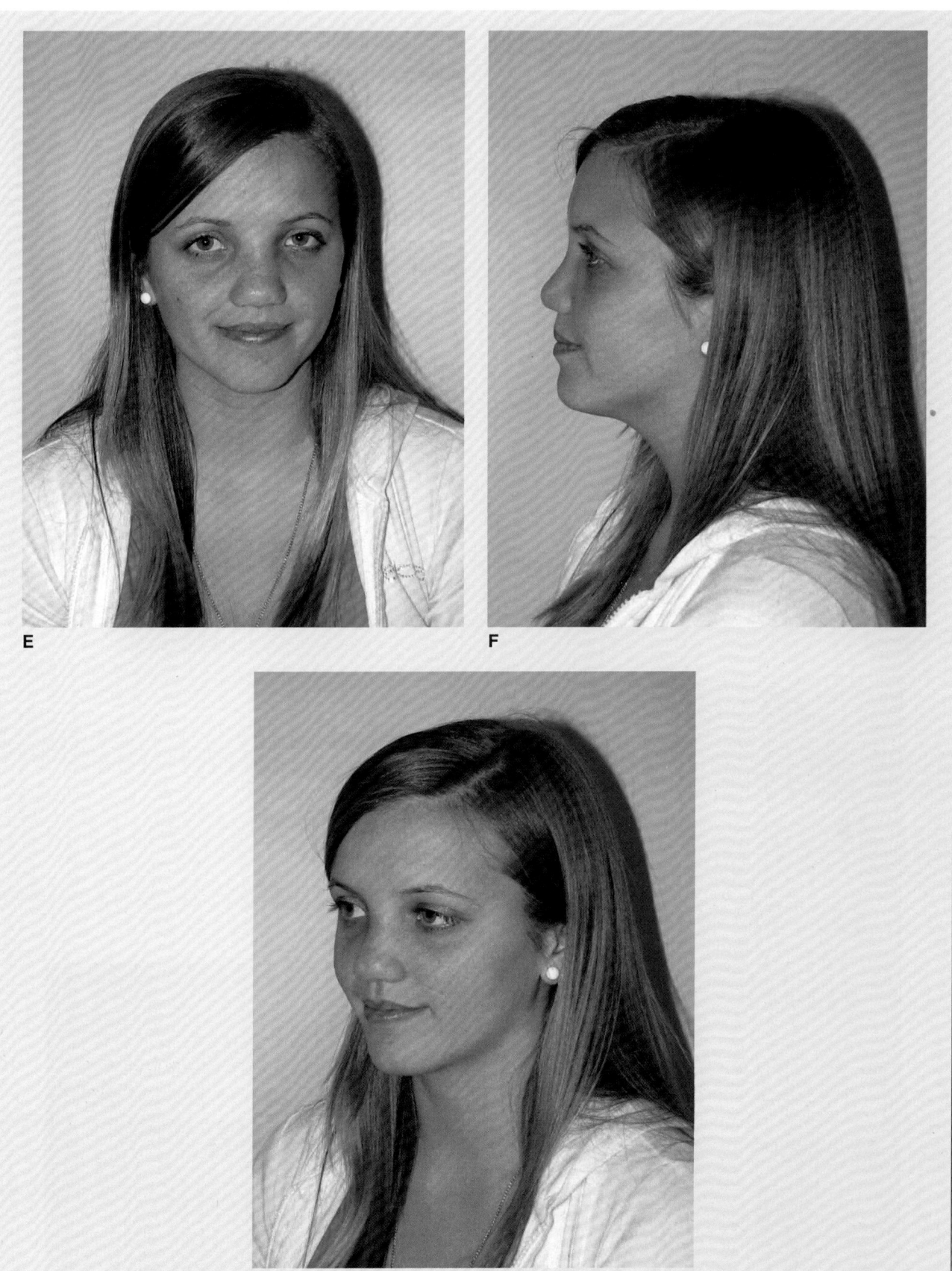

Figure 184.28 (*Continued*) **E–G:** Frontal, lateral, and oblique views 1 month after primary rhinoplasty performed elsewhere.

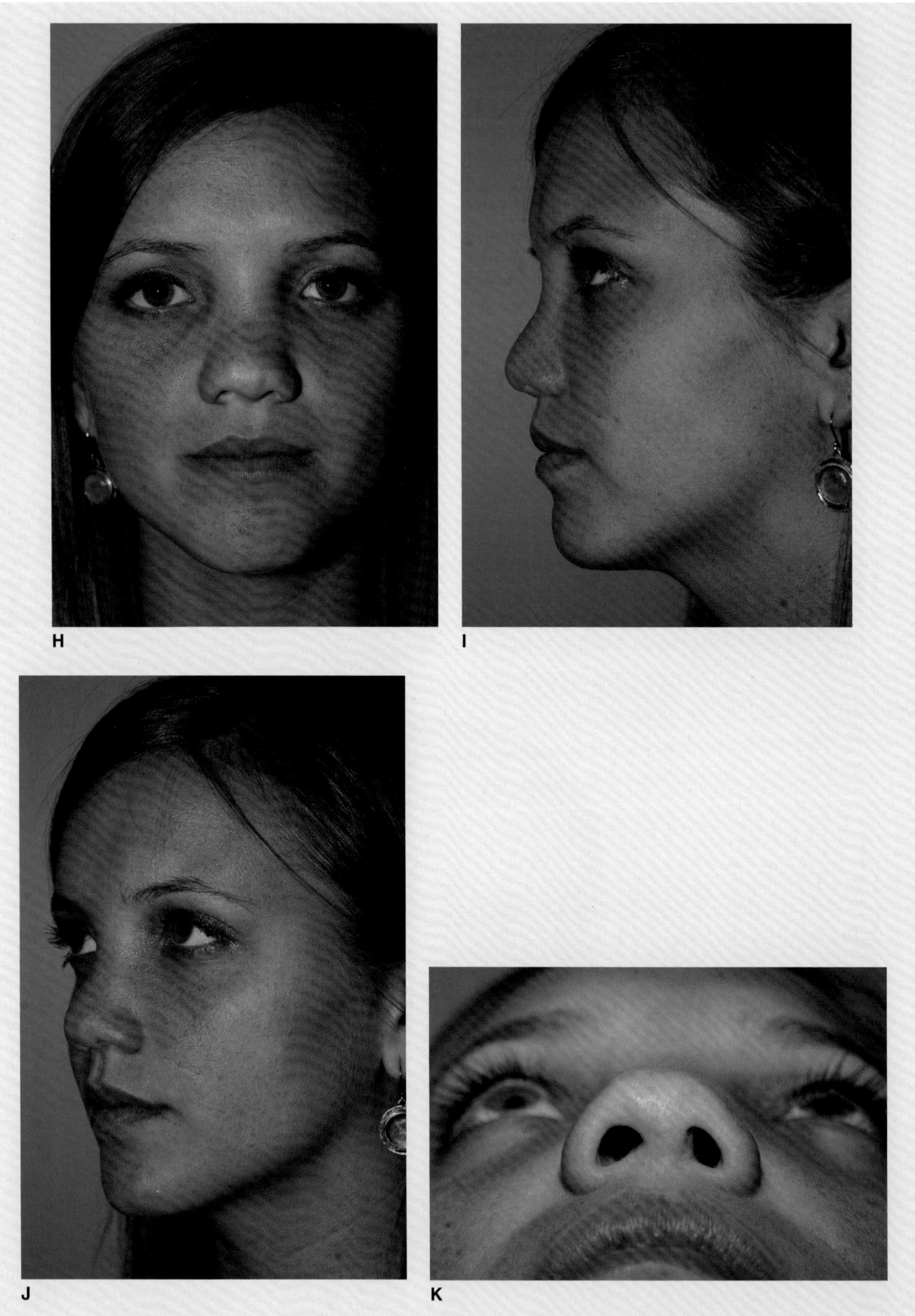

Figure 184.28 (*Continued*) **H–K:** Frontal, lateral, oblique, and basal views 18 months after blunt trauma and prior to revision rhinoplasty.

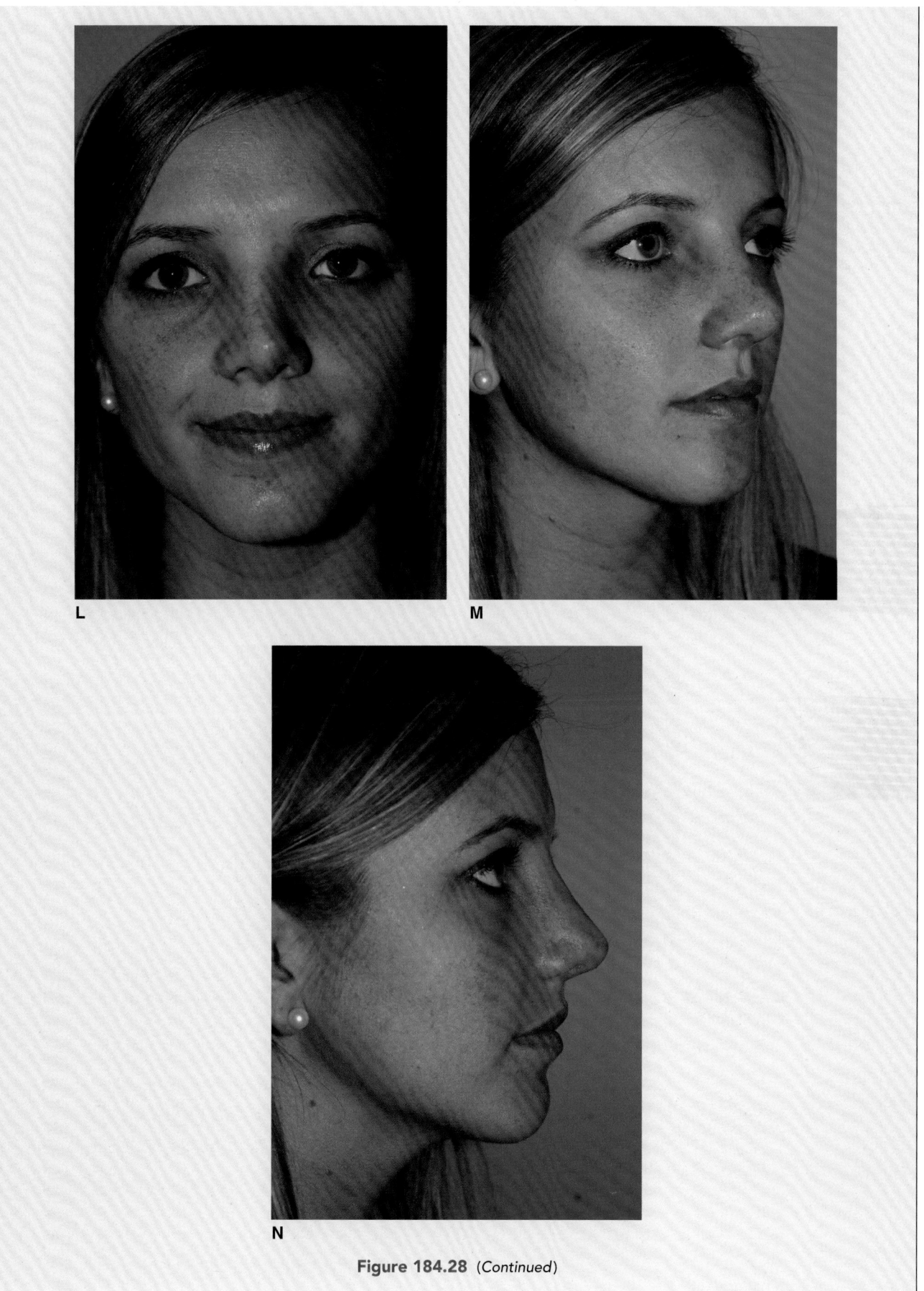

Figure 184.28 *(Continued)*

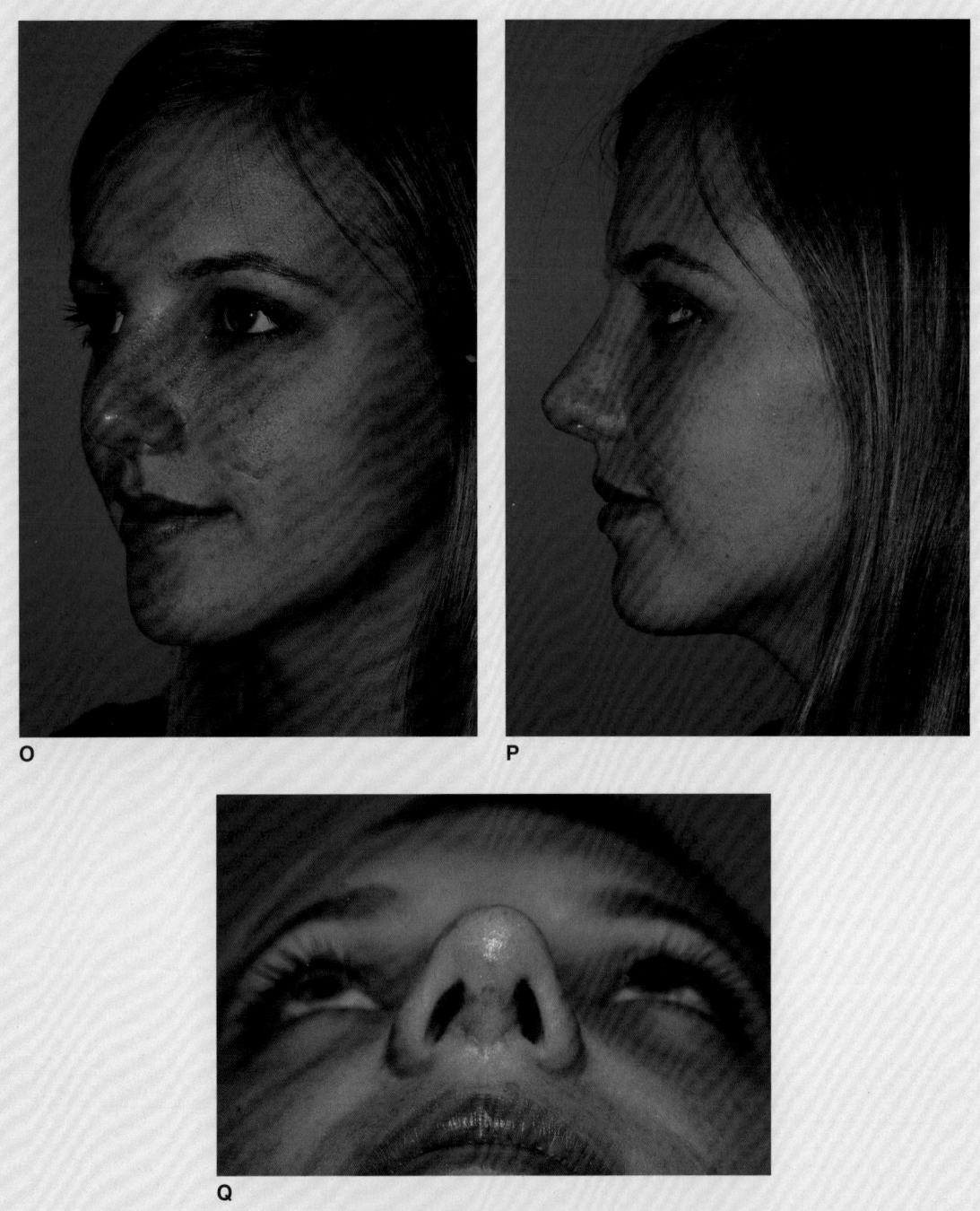

Figure 184.28 (*Continued*) **L–Q:** Corresponding postoperative views 6 weeks following rib graft reconstruction.

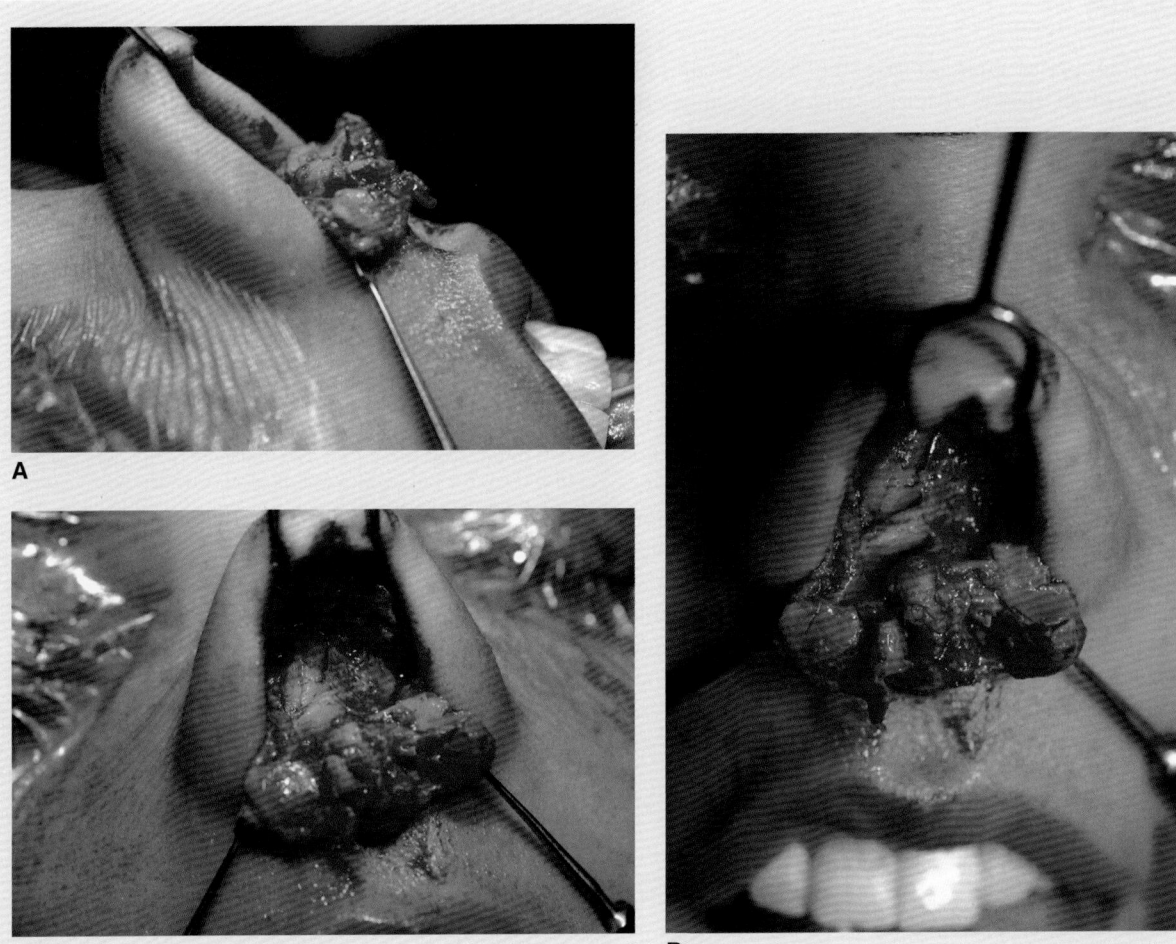

Figure 184.29 Intraoperative photos for case presentation five. **A–C:** Severe disruption and scarring of the remnant nasal cartilages.

11. The remaining rib and septal cartilage is diced into 1.0 mm³ cubes and used to fill the fascial cylinder with diced cartilage.

12. The DC-F onlay graft is inserted into a precise subcutaneous pocket overlying the nasal dorsum and lower glabella and positioned using percutaneous guiding sutures.

13. The medial crural remnants and vestibular skin are advanced anteriorly and sewn to the columella strut graft with a 5-0 PDS suture.

14. The subcutaneous pocket is irrigated with saline.

15. The nasal skin is closed under moderate tension and measured tip projection increased by 12 mm.

16. A gentle compression dressing and aluminum splint are placed.

Surgical Outcome

The postoperative contour reveals the restoration of dorsal and tip projection with a corresponding reduction in nasal width (Fig. 184.28I–M). Smooth and attractive dorsal lines are achieved with diced cartilage wrapped in temporalis fascia, while tip contour was restored using concentric-carved solid rib cartilage. Nasal airway dysfunction was also eliminated.

SUMMARY

Revision rhinoplasty ranks among the most technically demanding of all elective cosmetic surgical procedures. In addition to the technical challenges associated with profound cosmetic derangements, surgically compromised tissues and the emotional impact of an unexpected nasal deformity add to the already formidable treatment challenge. Effective treatment planning mandates a thorough assessment of the nasal tissues (both internal and external), the status of the nasal airway, and the cosmetic nasal deformity, as well as an equally careful assessment of the patient's emotional well-being and their cosmetic treatment objectives. A host of contemporary reconstructive techniques are now available for effective restoration of the complex postsurgical nasal deformity, and the efficient, skillful, and artistic application of cartilage graft material is the cornerstone of surgical restoration. Familiarity with each graft type and its unique biophysical properties is crucial to successful graft application, and an artistic sensibility to guide surgical intervention is invaluable. For most patients, the goal of an attractive, durable, and fully functional nose can be achieved when these techniques are executed successfully, and the emotional impact of a successful revision rhinoplasty can be both dramatic and immensely gratifying for patient and surgeon alike.

HIGHLIGHTS

- An in-depth review of *skeletal overresection*–perhaps the most common problem prompting complex revision rhinoplasty—including the cosmetic, functional, and anatomic sequelae of the overresected nose.
- A discussion of the unique psycho-social challenges of revision rhinoplasty, as well as several commonly encountered psychological disorders that may adversely impact patient care.
- Fundamental aspects of preoperative patient evaluation with emphasis upon tissue tolerance and the key prognostic indicators for surgical success.
- Advantages and disadvantages of various anesthetic options, surgical approaches, and potential graft materials, as well as optimal timing for favorable treatment outcomes.
- Dismantling or "deconstructing" the previously operated nose with respect to minimizing structural destabilization, vascular compromise, and soft tissue scarring.
- The strategic use of autologous graft materials for the permanent restoration of function and beauty to the upper, middle, and lower thirds of the nose.
- The importance of (postoperative) supportive care for preventing and managing adverse wound-healing responses.

REFERENCES

1. Davis RE. Nasal tip complications. *Facial Plast Surg* 2012;28(3):294–302.
2. Gubisch W, Eichhorn-Sens J. Overresection of the lower lateral cartilages: a common conceptual mistake with functional and aesthetic consequences. *Aesthetic Plast Surg* 2009;33:6–13.
3. Sajjadian A, Rubinstein R, Naghshineh N. Current status of grafts and implants in rhinoplasty: part I. autologous grafts. *Plast Reconstr Surg* 2010;125(2):40e–49e.
4. Adams WP, Rohrich RJ, Hollier LH, et al. Anatomic basis and clinical implications for nasal tip support in open versus closed rhinoplasty. *Plast Reconstr Surg* 1999;103(1):255–261.
5. Davis RE. Chapter 53: Septoplasty and rhinoplasty. In: Snow JB, Wackym PA, eds. *Ballenger's otorhinolaryngology head and neck surgery*, 17th ed. Shelton, CT: BC Decker, Inc., People's Medical Publishing House, 2009:633–659.
6. Ambro BT, Wright RJ. Psychological considerations in revision rhinoplasty. *Facial Plast Surg* 2008;24(3):288–292.
7. Davis RE, Bublik M. Psychological considerations in the revision rhinoplasty patient. *Facial Plast Surg* 2012;28(4):374–379.
8. Ercolani M, Baldaro B, Rossi N, et al. Short-term outcome of rhinoplasty for medical or cosmetic indication. *J Psychosom Res* 1999;47(3):277–281.
9. Crerand CE, Franklin ME, Sarwer DB. Body dysmorphic disorder and cosmetic surgery. *Plast Reconstr Surg* 2006;118(7):167e–180e.
10. Ende KH, Lewis DL, Kabaker SS. Body dysmorphic disorder. *Facial Plast Surg Clin North Am* 2008;16:217–223.
11. Bjornsson AS, Didie ER, Phillips KA. Body dysmorphic disorder. *Dialogues Clin Neurosci* 2010;12(2):221–232.
12. Sarwer DB. Awareness and identification of body dysmorphic disorder by aesthetic surgeons: results of a survey of American society for aesthetic plastic surgery members. *Aesthet Surg J* 2002;22(6):531–535.
13. Wright MR. Management of patient dissatisfaction with results of cosmetic procedures. *Arch Otolaryngol* 1980;106:466–471.
14. Johnson CM, Godin MS. The tension nose: open structure rhinoplasty approach. *Plast Reconstr Surg* 1995;95(1):43–51.
15. Davis RE. Rhinoplasty and concepts of facial beauty. *Facial Plast Surg* 2006;22:198–203.
16. Mehta U, Mazhar K, Frankel AS. Accuracy of preoperative computer imaging in rhinoplasty. *Arch Facial Plast Surg* 2010;12(6):394–398.
17. Adelson RT, DeFatta RJ, Bassischis BA. Objective assessment of the accuracy of computer-simulated imaging in rhinoplasty. *Am J Otolaryngol* 2008;29(3):151–155.
18. Bhattarai B, Shrestha S, Singh J. Comparison of ondansetron and combination of ondansetron and dexamethasone as a prophylaxis for postoperative nausea and vomiting in adults undergoing elective laparoscopic surgery. *J Emerg Trauma Shock* 2011;4(2):168–172.
19. Song JW, Park EY, Lee JG, et al. The effect of combining dexamethasone with ondansetron for nausea and vomiting associated with fentanyl-based intravenous patient-controlled analgesia. *Anaesthesia* 2011;66(4):263–267.
20. Davis RE. Chapter 27: The thick-skinned rhinoplasty patient. In: Azizzadeh B, Murphy M, Johnson C, et al., eds. *Master techniques in rhinoplasty*. Philadelphia, PA: Saunders Elsevier, Inc., 2011:337–345.
21. Hong JP, Yoon JY, Choi JW. Are polytetrafluoroethylene (Gore-Tex) implants an alternative material for nasal dorsal augmentation in Asians? *J Craniofac Surg* 2010;21(6):1750–1754.
22. Godin MS, Waldman SR, Johnson CM Jr. Nasal augmentation using Gore-Tex. A 10-year experience. *Arch Facial Plast Surg* 1999;1(2):118–121.
23. Peled ZM, Warren AG, Johnston P, et al. The use of alloplastic materials in rhinoplasty surgery: a meta-analysis. *Plast Reconstr Surg* 2008;121(3):85e–92e.
24. Wang TD. Gore-Tex nasal augmentation: a 26-year perspective. *Arch Facial Plast Surg* 2011;13(2):129–130.
25. Kim YH, Kim BJ, Jang TY. Use of porous high-density polyethylene (medpor) for spreader or extended septal graft in rhinoplasty:

aesthetics, functional outcomes, and long-term complications. *Ann Plast Surg* 2011;67(5):464–468.

26. Romo T III, Kwak ES, Sclafani AP. Revision rhinoplasty using porous high-density polyethylene implants to reestablish ethnic identity. *Aesthetic Plast Surg* 2006;30(6):679–684.

27. Romo T III, Sclafani AP, Sabini P. Use of porous high-density polyethylene in revision rhinoplasty and the platyrrhine nose. *Aesthetic Plast Surg* 1998;22(3):211–221.

28. Romo T III, Litner JA, Sclafani AP. Management of the severe bulbous nasal tip using porous polyethylene alloimplants. *Facial Plast Surg* 2003;19(4):341–348.

29. Mendelsohn M. Straightening the crooked middle third of the nose: using porous polyethylene extended spreader grafts. *Arch Facial Plast Surg* 2005;7(2):74–80.

30. Stelter K, Strieth S, Berghaus A. Porous polyethylene implants in revision rhinoplasty: chances and risks. *Rhinology* 2007;45(4):325–331.

31. Weber S, Cook TA, Wang TD. Irradiated homologous costal cartilage in augmentation rhinoplasty. *Operat Tech Otolaryngol Head Neck Surg* 2007;18:274–283.

32. Kridel RW, Ashoori F, Liu ES, et al. Long-term use and follow-up of irradiated homologous costal cartilage in the nose. *Arch Facial Plast Surg* 2009;11(6):378–394.

33. Weber SM, Baker SR. Alar cartilage grafts. *Clin Plast Surg* 2010;37:253–264.

34. Baek RM, Eun SC, Heo CY, et al. Rhinoplasty using rib chondro-osseous graft in Asian patients. *J Craniofac Surg* 2010;21(4):1122–1125.

35. Christophel JJ, Hilger PA. Osseocartilaginous rib graft rhinoplasty: a stable predictable technique for major dorsal reconstruction. *Arch Facial Plast Surg* 2011;13(2):78–83.

36. Holden PK, Liaw LH, Wong BJ. Human nasal cartilage ultrastructure: characteristics and comparison using scanning electron microscopy. *Laryngoscope* 2008;118(7):1153–1156.

37. Greene JJ, Watson D. Septal cartilage tissue engineering: new horizons. *Facial Plast Surg* 2010;26(5):396–404.

38. Hwang K, Huan F, Kim DJ. Mapping thickness of nasal septal cartilage. *J Craniofac Surg* 2010;21(1):243–244.

39. Patel JC, Fletcher JW, Singer D, et al. An anatomic and histologic analysis of the alar-facial crease and the lateral crus. *Ann Plast Surg* 2004;52(4):371–374.

40. Hatzis GP, Sherry SD, Hogan GM, et al. Observations of the marginal incision and lateral crura alar cartilage asymmetry in rhinoplasty: a fixed cadaver study. *Oral Surg Oral Med Oral Pathol Oral Radio Endod* 2004;97:432–437.

41. Kim J, Cho JH, Kim SW, et al. Anatomical variation of the nasal septum: correlation among septal components. *Clin Anat* 2010;23(8):945–949.

42. Kim JS, Khan NA, Song HM, et al. Intraoperative measurements of harvestable septal cartilage in rhinoplasty. *Ann Plast Surg* 2010;65(6):519–523.

43. Garg R, Shaikh M, Foulad A, et al. Chondrocyte viability in human nasal septum after morcellation. *Arch Facial Plast Surg* 2010;12(3):204–206.

44. Watson D. Tissue engineering for rhinoplasty. *Facial Plast Surg Clin North Am* 2009;17(1):157–165.

45. Mowlavi A, Pham S, Wilhelmi B, et al. Anatomical characteristics of the conchal cartilage with suggested clinical applications in rhinoplasty surgery. *Aesthet Surg J* 2010;30(4):522–526.

46. Sheen JH, Sheen AP. Chapter 6: Adjunctive techniques. In: Sheen J, Sheen A, eds. *Aesthetic rhinoplasty*, 2nd ed. St. Louis, MO: The CV Mosby Company, 1987:450–451.

47. Tardy ME, Toriumi D. Alar retraction: composite graft correction. *Facial Plast Surg* 1989;6(2):101–107.

48. Marin VP, Landecker A, Gunter JP. Harvesting rib cartilage grafts for secondary rhinoplasty. *Plast Reconstr Surg* 2008;121(4):1442–1448.

49. Adams WP, Rorich RJ, Gunter JP, et al. The rate of warping in irradiated and nonirradiated homograft rib cartilage: a controlled comparison and clinical implications. *Plast Reconstr Surg* 1999;103(1):265–270.

50. Gunter JP, Clark CP, Friedman RM. Internal stabilization of autogenous rib cartilage grafts in rhinoplasty: a barrier to cartilage warping. *Plast Reconstr Surg* 1997;100:161–169.

51. Kim DW, Shah AR, Toriumi DM. Concentric and eccentric carved costal cartilage: a comparison of warping. *Arch Facial Plast Surg* 2006;8(1):42–46.

52. Daniel RK. Diced cartilage grafts in rhinoplasty surgery: current techniques and applications. *Plast Reconstr Surg* 2008;122(6):1883–1891.

53. Daniel RK, Calvert JW. Diced cartilage grafts in rhinoplasty surgery. *Plast Reconstr Surg* 2004;113(7):2156–2171.

54. Davis RE, Guida RA, Cook TA. Autologous free dermal fat grafts: reconstruction of facial contour defects. *Arch Otolaryngol Head Neck Surg* 1995;121(1):95–100.

55. Davis RE, Wayne I. Rhinoplasty and the nasal SMAS augmentation graft: advantages and indications. *Arch Facial Plast Surg* 2004;6:124–132.

56. Garramone RR Jr, Sullivan PK, Devaney K. Bulbous nasal tip: an anatomical and histological evaluation. *Ann Plast Surg* 1995;34:288–291.

57. Letourneau A, Daniel RK. The superficial musculoaponeurotic system of the nose. *Plast Reconstr Surg* 1988;82:48–57.

58. Rohrich RJ, Gunter JP, Friedman RM. Nasal tip blood supply: an anatomic study validating the safety of the transcolumellar incision in rhinoplasty. *Plast Reconstr Surg* 1995;95:795–799.

59. Toriumi DM. New concepts in nasal tip contouring. *Arch Facial Plast Surg* 2006;8(3):156–185.

60. Byrd HS, Andochick S, Copit S, et al. Septal extension grafts: a method of controlling tip projection shape. *Plast Reconstr Surg* 1997;100:999–1010.

61. Ha RY, Byrd HS. Septal extension grafts revisited: 6-year experience in controlling nasal tip projection and shape. *Plast Reconstr Surg* 2003;112(7):1929–1935.

62. Guyuron B, Varghai A. Lengthening the nose with a tongue-and-groove technique. *Plast Reconstr Surg* 2003;111(4):1533–1539.

63. Naficy S, Baker SR. Lengthening the short nose. *Arch Otolaryngol Head Neck Surg* 1998;124(7):809–813.

64. Toriumi DM. Caudal septal extension graft for correction of the retracted columella. *Oper Tech Otolaryngol Head Neck Surg* 1995;6:311–318.

65. Davis RE. Diagnosis and surgical management of the caudal excess nasal deformity. *Arch Facial Plast Surg* 2005;7:124–134.

66. Kridel RW, Scott BA, Foda HM. The tongue-in-groove technique in septorhinoplasty. *Arch Facial Plast Surg* 1999;1:246–256.

67. Ponsky DC, Harvey DJ, Khan SW, et al. Nose elongation: a review and description of the septal extension tongue-in-groove technique. *Aesthet Surg J* 2010;30(3):335–346.

68. Gunter JP, Friedman RM. Lateral crural strut graft: techiques and clinical applications in rhinoplasty. *Plast Reconstr Surg* 1997;99(4):943–952.

69. Rorich RJ, Raniere J, Ha RY. The alar contour graft: correction and prevention of alar rim deformities in rhinoplasty. *Plast Reconstr Surg* 2002;109(7):2495–2505.

70. Boahene KDO, Hilger PA. Alar rim grafting in rhinoplasty. *Arch Facial Plast Surg* 2009;11(5):285–289.

71. Kridel RW, Konior RJ, Shumrick KA, et al. The lateral crural steal. *Arch Otolaryngol Head Neck Surg* 1989;115:1206–1212.

72. Adamson PA, Morrow TA. The nasal hinge. *Arch Otolaryngol Head Neck Surg* 1994;111:219–231.

73. Constantinides M, Liu ES, Miller PJ, et al. Vertical lobule division in rhinoplasty: maintaining and intact strip. *Arch Facial Plast Surg* 2001;3:258–263.

74. Yu K, Kim A, Pearlman SJ. Functional and aesthetic concerns of patients seeking revision rhinoplasty. *Arch Facial Plast Reconstr Surg* 2010;12(5):291–297.

75. Davis RE, Raval J. Powered instrumentation for nasal bone reduction: advantages and indications. *Arch Facial Plast Surg* 2003;5(5):384–391.

76. Calvert JW, Brenner KB, DaCosta-Iyer M, et al. Histological analysis of human diced cartilage grafts. *Plast Reconstr Surg* 2006;118:230–236.

77. Cakmak O, Bircan S, Buyuklu F, et al. Viability of crushed and diced cartilage grafts: A study in rabbits. *Arch Facial Plast Surg* 2005;7(1):21–26.

78. Buyuklu F, Hizal E, Yilmaz Z, et al. Viability of crushed human auricular and costal cartilage chondrocytes in cell culture. *J Craniomaxillofac Surg* 2011;39(3):221–225.

79. Pontius A, Leach JL. New techniques for management of the crooked nose. *Arch Facial Plast Surg* 2004;6:263–266.

80. Gubisch W. The extracorporal septum plasty: a technique to correct difficult nasal deformities. *Plast Reconstr Surg* 1995;95:672–682.

81. Heppt W, Gubisch W. Septal surgery in rhinoplasty. *Facial Plast Surg* 2011;27(2):167–178.

82. Tweedie DJ, Rowe-Jones JM. Reconstruction of the nasal septum using perforated and unperforated polydioxanone foil. *Arch Facial Plast Surg* 2010;12(2):106–113.

83. Boenisch M, Nolst Trenite GJ. Reconstruction of the nasal septum using polydioxanone plate. *Arch Facial Plast Surg* 2010;12(1):4–10.

The Aging Forehead   185

Kian Karimi   *Peter A. Adamson*

Addressing the upper third of the face is an important component of facial rejuvenation. For many patients, descent of the eyebrows leads to exacerbation of periocular aging, which is inadequately treated with blepharoplasty. Without correction of eyebrow ptosis, the aging face often conveys fatigue and even anger. Forehead rejuvenation procedures have been utilized with increasing frequency over the last several decades. The forehead lift, or the "face-lift of the upper third," is an essential tool in providing a harmonious rejuvenation in patients.

HISTORY

As examined in a recent review by Matros et al. (1), changes in eyebrow position and shape with aging have been described and refined for the past four decades. Some of the earliest descriptions of brow lifting date back to 1919 as described by Passot, Hunt, and Lexer (2). Vinas is credited for noting the difference between static and dynamic rhytids and importantly recognized that treatment would differ between the two types, including the necessity to free adhesions over the orbital rims to mobilize and elevate the brows. An important development in brow lifting occurred in 1992 with the first description of the endoscopic technique (3). Despite multiple modifications of the brow lift trending toward less invasive approaches purporting lower complication rates and higher patient acceptability, a recent review by Cilento and Johnson of over 1,000 coronal or trichophytic brow lifts demonstrated extremely high rates of patient satisfaction with an acceptably low complication rate including no permanent motor nerve dysfunction.

FOREHEAD ANATOMY

The forehead represents the upper third of the face and can be divided into vertical fifths as well, yielding five aesthetic subunits: the central forehead, lateral temporal units, and

the brows. The lower anatomic boundaries include the supraorbital rim, nasal root, and bony zygomatic arches. The supraorbital rim is usually the landmark by which brow ptosis is measured. The trichion and natural hairlines represent the upper limit. Perhaps the most important division of forehead anatomy lies on either side of the temporal line, which divides the temporal regions from the forehead and intersects with the peak of the brow in both men and women.

Branches of the external and internal carotid arteries provide the blood supply to the forehead. The external carotid artery provides the superficial temporal artery and subsequent zygomaticotemporal branch, which supply the temple region and lateral forehead. The internal carotid artery supplies the midforehead via branches of the ophthalmic artery, the supratrochlear artery medially, and the supraorbital artery laterally, typically 2.5 cm lateral to the midline (Fig. 185.1).

Sensation is provided by the supraorbital and supratrochlear nerves, which are branches of the trigeminal nerve (V). The supratrochlear nerve exits the orbit, alongside the artery, and travels through the medial corrugator supercilii, providing sensation to the medial forehead. The supraorbital nerve exits the superior orbit through a foramen along the rim in nearly 90% of patients but can also exit the orbit through a foramen up to 1.5 cm above the orbital rim (4). Laterally, sensation is provided by the lacrimal (V1), zygomaticofacial (V2), and auriculotemporal (V3) nerves. Motor innervation is provided exclusively by the notoriously fragile temporal branch of the facial nerve.

The temporal branch exits the parotid gland and courses superiorly from a point 1.5 cm below the external auditory canal, crosses the zygomatic arch approximately 2.5 cm (0.8- to 3.5-cm range) anterior to the auditory canal, and runs superomedially toward the frontalis muscle but remains 2 cm posterior to the lateral bony orbital rim. This nerve can be reliably predicted by its relation to what

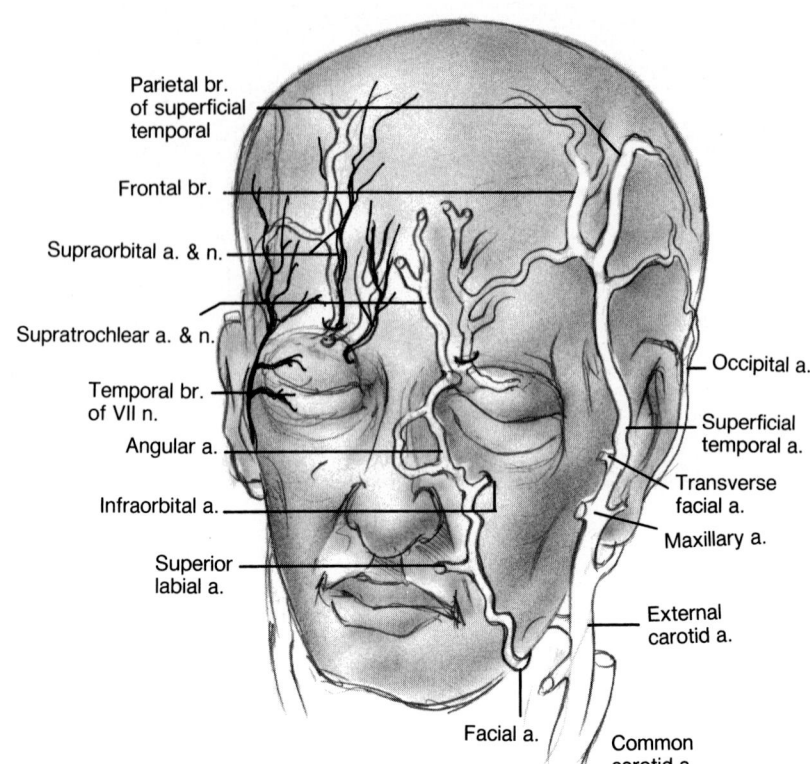

Parietal br.
of superficial
temporal

Frontal br.

Supraorbital a. & n.

Supratrochlear a. & n.

Temporal br.
of VII n.

Angular a.

Infraorbital a.

Superior
labial a.

Occipital a.

Superficial
temporal a.

Transverse
facial a.

Maxillary a.

External
carotid a.

Facial a.

Common
carotid a.

Figure 185.1 Vessels and nerves of the forehead. The major arterial and sensory innervation is through the supraorbital vessels and nerves. They arise about 2.5 cm from the midline. The temporal branch of the facial nerve is the most functionally significant.

is known as the cephalic or "sentinel vein," running just superficial to this vessel. The temporal branch remains just deep to the temporoparietal fascia and runs within the substance of this fascia, which is continuous with the superficial musculo-aponeurotic system (SMAS) inferiorly.

The forehead is an extension of the scalp and thus consists of the same layers, which, from superficial to deep, are the skin, subcutaneous tissues, galea and frontalis muscles, loose supraperiosteal areolar tissue, and pericranium (Fig. 185.2). The galea separates along the superior origin of the frontalis muscle, which divides the galea into superficial and deep layers. The posterior galea is in the same plane as the superior orbital septum. Lateral eyebrow ptosis has been described to be further exacerbated by a ptotic "galeal fat pad," which is usually fully enveloped by the deep galeal fascia but may be dehiscent in some individuals, accelerating lateral brow ptosis (4). Laterally, the galeal layer is contiguous with the superficial temporal parietal fascia, both of which fuse at the zygomatic arch. The loose subgaleal and subtemporal parietal fascial layers allow for free mobility of the galea, facilitating facial expression.

The frontalis muscle is the primary elevator of the brow and is the most significant contributor to horizontal forehead rhytids. Inferiorly, the frontalis interdigitates with the orbicularis oculi muscle, the skin of the eyebrows, and the root of the nose (Fig. 185.3). The frontalis muscle also blends with the corrugator supercilii and procerus muscles medially. The corrugator supercilius muscle, also known as the "muscle of grief," is the only muscle of facial expression

to arise from bone. After originating from the medial aspect of the supraorbital arch, it passes obliquely, deep to the frontalis and orbicularis muscles, to insert by interdigitation with these muscles throughout the medial half of the eyebrow, causing characteristic vertical and oblique rhytids. The unpaired procerus muscle is pyramid shaped and arises from the fascia over the nasal bone and upper

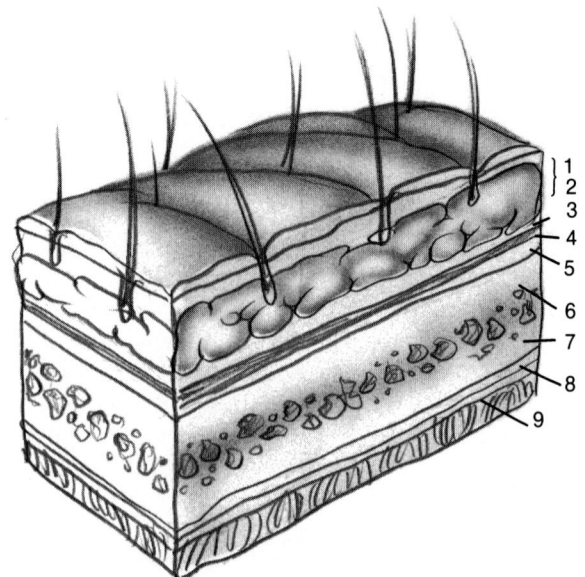

Figure 185.2 Forehead skin. "SCALP" refers to the layers of the forehead skin. *1,* Skin; *2,* subcutaneous tissue; *3,* epicranial aponeurosis (galea and frontalis m.); *4,* lax areolar tissue; *5,* pericranium; *6,* outer table; *7,* inner table; *8,* dura mater; *9,* arachnoid.

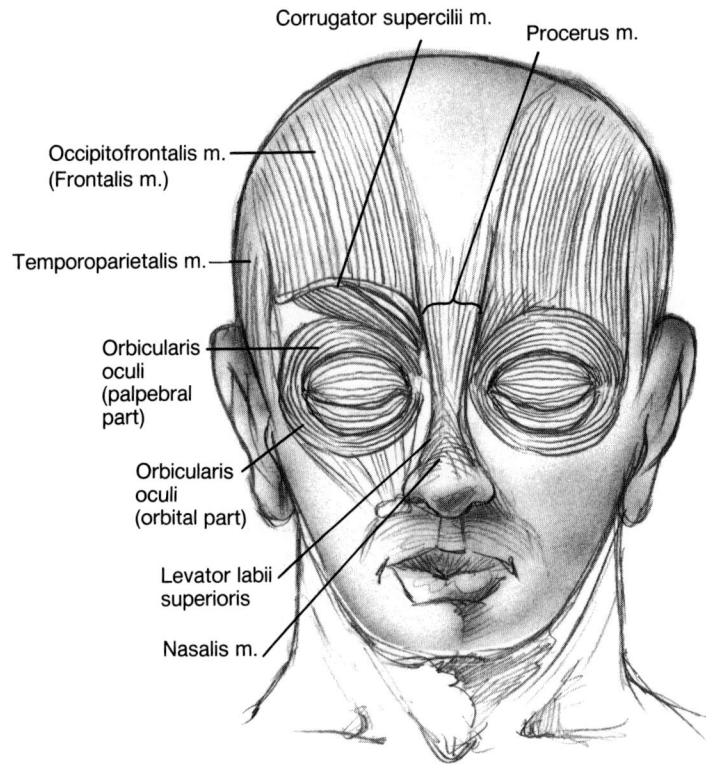

Corrugator supercilii m.   Procerus m.

Occipitofrontalis m.
(Frontalis m.)

Temporoparietalis m.

Orbicularis
oculi
(palpebral
part)

Orbicularis
oculi
(orbital part)

Levator labii
superioris

Nasalis m.

Figure 185.3 Forehead muscles. Forehead muscle activity causes the development of the rhytids associated with aging. The frontalis muscle produces horizontal forehead rhytids, the corrugator supercilius muscle vertical glabellar rhytids, and the procerus muscle horizontal glabellar rhytids.

lateral cartilages of the nose and inserts in the skin between the eyebrows, producing horizontal glabellar rhytids. The orbicularis oculi muscle also serves as a brow depressor. The depressor supercilii muscles are a minor contributor to brow depression.

In a discussion of anatomic structures that contribute to the upper face aging process, it has been recognized that superficial temporal fascia "instability" plays a role in lateral brow ptosis due to its weak adhesion between the superficial and deep temporal fascial planes, with the sole support of the superficial fascial plane being its attachment to the frontal bone along the rim of the temporal fossa in the "zone of adhesion" and a loose attachment to the superior–lateral orbital rim called the "orbital ligament," thought to represent a condensation of the superficial temporal fascia (4). It is also postulated that paucity of frontalis insertion laterally, and the stabilizing forces provided by the supraorbital and supratrochlear neurovascular bundles, explain why lateral eyebrow ptosis occurs to a far greater degree than medial or mid-brow ptosis.

PHYSIOLOGY OF AGING

In youth, the forehead, temple, and glabella are unfurrowed. The hairline is irregularly irregular, and there is no evidence of male-pattern baldness or thinning hair in women. The transition between the thicker infrabrow skin and upper eyelid skin is of particular importance. In youth, the higher brow position allows for a well-demarcated

contour of the lateral supraorbital rim above and an obvious upper eyelid fold.

With aging, the upper third of the face undertakes multiple changes (Fig. 185.4). The corrugator supercilius muscle may be the initiating factor to the aging process of the upper face by producing vertical and oblique glabellar skin lines through its transverse and oblique fibers, respectively (4). It is the interdigitation of the corrugator with the orbicularis, procerus, and depressor supercilii muscles that further causes medial eyebrow depression and glabellar rhytids. As the skin weakens over time and becomes less elastic, these rhytids become permanent. Additionally, loss of subcutaneous tissue and increased skull bone resorption is noted. Descent of the lateral third of the brow (lateral to the deep temporal fusion line) is discussed previously in this chapter. A visual field defect can result in advanced cases of lateral eyebrow ptosis, especially when compounded with upper eyelid ptosis. This "closed eye" appearance is associated with sadness, fatigue, anger, and aging.

With descent of the brows, there is a tendency of the frontalis muscle to increase activity dynamically to counteract the irritant effect of the redundant tissues on the eyelids, thereby initially creating superficial and transient rhytids that become deeper and permanent over time.

Each individual has unique facial expressions and, thus, each develops a unique pattern of upper facial rhytids and eyebrow position. The patient's skin type, photodamage, tobacco abuse, and many other factors also affect the facial parameters associated with aging.

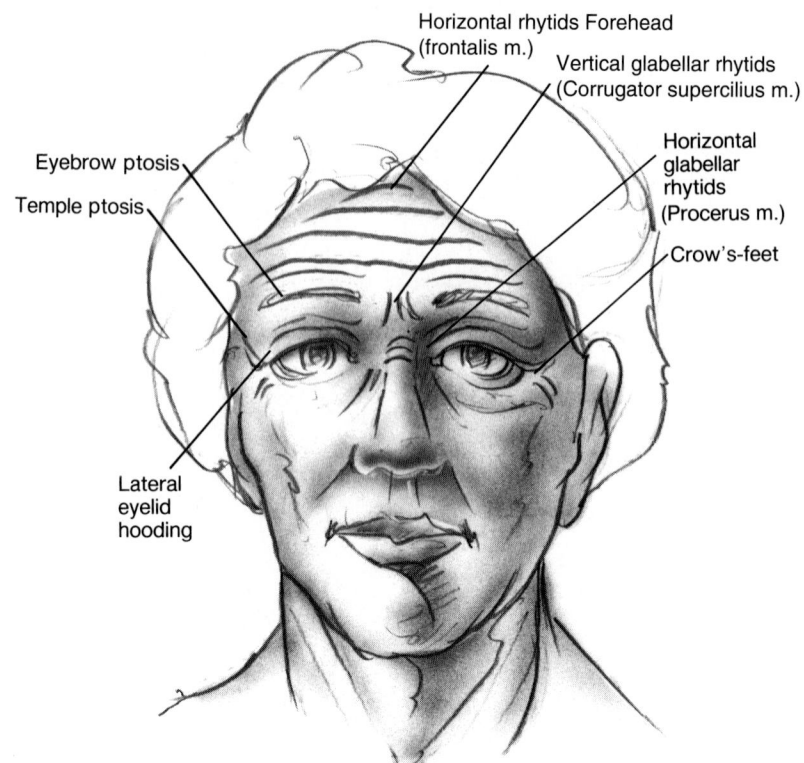

Figure 185.4 Physiology of aging. Ptosis initially occurs at the lateral brow but eventually involves the entire brow and forehead. Rhytids are caused by voluntary and involuntary muscle activity.

BROW AESTHETICS

The youthful brow, as classically described by Westmore in the 1970's, is an arch whose apex terminates above the lateral limbus of the iris, with the medial and lateral ends of the brow at the same horizontal level. With evolving concepts of beauty, the ideal brow apex has been described anywhere from the lateral limbus to the lateral canthus (5–7). A recent study found that the deep temporal fusion line is the most precise indicator of brow peak position, which makes the most sense intuitively and anatomically. The club-head–shaped medial brow should be in line with a vertical line drawn through the insertion of the ala of the nose. It arches superolaterally above the supraorbital rim to its apex somewhere between the lateral limbus and lateral canthus and tapers into a handle shape to end laterally at an oblique line drawn through the ala of the nose and the lateral canthus. The medial and lateral ends of the eyebrows should lie in the same horizontal plane. In men, the brow is ideally at the level of the supraorbital rim whereas in women the brow should peak above the supraorbital rim. The more lateral the apex of the brow, the more feminized the brow is. Eyebrow hairs are typically thicker in men and may extend in any direction. A lower, thicker brow may still be considered attractive in women, depending on its harmony with their overall facial aesthetics.

ASSESSMENT

Each patient must specify his or her particular concerns if the appropriate procedure is to be chosen for forehead rejuvenation. Oftentimes, a patient will seek correction of lateral eyelid hooding and request blepharoplasty when the ideal procedure may well be one to elevate ptotic brows. During analysis for the patient seeking facial rejuvenation, the surgeon must demonstrate the patient's own natural brow position in repose as most people with brow ptosis will unconsciously elevate their brows. A previous history of upper blepharoplasty or brow lifting procedures may produce a relative lack of upper eyelid skin for lifting procedures. Additionally, a history of laser-assisted in-situ keratomileusis surgery or dry-eye problems must be considered prior to brow lifting since a transient lagophthalmos following surgery is not uncommon. Patients with alopecia may be at an increased risk for surgical hair follicle shock. Young men with a full head of hair and who are not at risk of developing male-pattern baldness, or older men who have an established pattern of hair loss, may be candidates for coronal forehead lifts and its modifications. Hair transplantation in conjunction with a forehead lift has been described, allowing for expanded use of a pretrichial incision.

Ptosis

It is of paramount importance for the surgeon to differentiate between lateral eyelid hooding that is a result of upper eyelid skin redundancy and that due to ptosis of the eyebrow. Frontalis contraction must be eliminated by complete patient relaxation to eliminate pseudoelevation of the eyebrows. Patients with eyebrow ptosis will be disappointed with a blepharoplasty procedure without addressing the brows. Younger patients with ptotic brows and upper eyelid hooding without other signs of upper facial aging often see greater improvements with a forehead lift rather than upper eyelid blepharoplasty. Overaggressive resection of brow or eyelid skin may result in further brow ptosis and a short upper lid syndrome. The effects of the forehead lift/browlift may be demonstrated to the patient by gently elevating the forehead in the midline and laterally. The degree of surgical brow elevation required can be assessed by having the patient actively elevate the eyebrows while the surgeon holds a ruler at a predetermined landmark on the brow. This method allows for the ideal amount of brow elevation to be determined. A slightly greater excision of skin should be made to allow for a degree of stretch-back. For example, about 16 mm of skin may be excised if the real amount of aesthetic lift desired is 10 to 12 mm.

Rhytids

Static and dynamic rhytids should be assessed preoperatively. Assessment of the forehead, glabella, and temple rhytids, along with the relative degree of activity of the upper facial muscles with mimetic expression, helps to determine the extent of myoplasty required for the involved muscles. Older patients typically have more subcutaneous atrophy and thus rhytids are more pronounced due to the actions of the muscles being transmitted more directly to the skin.

Hairline Patterns

Women who have a medium or low forehead hairline are candidates for the standard coronal or endoscopic forehead lift, since both of these will elevate the height of the hairline. Women with higher hairlines most often benefit from a trichophytic lift, which not only maintains their hairline position but also reduces the vertical height of their high forehead. This eliminates the need to style their hair over their forehead to camouflage a high hairline that would result from a standard coronal lift. Older men without evidence of male-pattern balding may be candidates for a standard coronal or trichophytic lift as well.

Skin Type

Fair- and thin-skinned patients usually heal with more ideal scars than those with darker and thicker or sebaceous skin. In general, women scar better than males. Older patients often have finer scars than do younger patients because of their decreased skin elasticity.

Asymmetries

It is documented that 97% of all patients have facial asymmetries (7). Both passive and dynamic asymmetries of the eyebrows should be documented. The surgeon should not try to alter dynamic eyebrow symmetries. Additionally, the surgeon must take caution in an attempt to correct passive asymmetries as this may alter the patient's unique facial characteristics. Even when such attempts are made, the coronal forehead lift and its modification are usually unsuccessful in correcting eyebrow asymmetries because of the distance from the incision to the eyebrows. If such correction is desired, a direct eyebrow or midforehead eyebrow lift are likely to be more successful. Patients with hyperdynamic forehead muscle activity may need more aggressive myoplasties to decrease this degree of activity and minimize recurrence of forehead and glabellar rhytids. This may be achieved surgically or with neurotoxin. The clinical assessment and photographic documentation must be performed with the patient's facial muscles in repose.

Bony Contour

Women with prominent supraorbital rims and excessive forehead bossing may appear masculinized. They may benefit from bone reduction of the supraorbital rim or alloplastic augmentation in association with a coronal forehead lift (8).

PREOPERATIVE COUNSELING

It is imperative to communicate to the patient that brow lifting will have no effect on the eyes other than to improve brow position and lateral hooding. Conversely, upper blepharoplasty will not alter eyebrow position, and if overaggressive skin resection is performed, this may cause further lateral eyebrow ptosis. The lateral infrabrow skin cannot be excised during upper blepharoplasty and, thus, minimal improvement may be achieved in the patient seeking correction of lateral hooding with an upper blepharoplasty rather than with some form of eyebrow lift. Patients should be advised that rejuvenation survey will "turn the clock back" but will not stop the aging process. The patient's specific concerns in conjunction with full facial assessment must be addressed; this is the only way the correct procedures can be chosen. Patients seeking a face-lift should be advised that it will not alter the appearance of the upper face.

MANAGEMENT

During the consultation with the patient, all options—including surgical and nonsurgical options—should be discussed. Surgery may not always be indicated; other methods may be used to correct a specific defect that is of great concern to the patient or to temporize until the patient is a better candidate for surgery. Other such methods include the following:

1. Sun avoidance and protection will prevent photodamage to the skin and help prevent squinting and thus decrease vertical glabellar rhytids.
2. Judicious use of cosmetics may camouflage forehead rhytids.

3. Retin-A cream may increase the vascularity of the skin and the organization of collagen bundles and may thicken the skin, resulting in a more youthful overall appearance and improvement in fine rhytids. It does not improve deeper furrows. Chemical peels and laser resurfacing will provide a greater effect.
4. Styling the hair over the forehead will camouflage rhytids, although it usually cannot camouflage brow ptosis.
5. Injectable fillers may be used selectively for temporary effect in forehead rhytids or furrows and crow's-feet. Fillers have also been used to simulate a brow lift with some success (9).
6. Eyeglasses may camouflage both brow ptosis and glabellar rhytids.
7. Onabotulinumtoxin A (Botox®, Allergan, Inc., Irvine, CA) injections can provide several months of partial muscle paralysis with partial or complete effacement of furrows. Additionally, Botox can be injected into the lateral brows to provide several millimeters of elevation.

All patients should be counseled that the goal is improvement, not perfection. Furthermore, although rejuvenation is achieved, aging continues and cannot be stopped or reversed. Patients will appear younger than if they had not had the surgery but in time will redevelop most of the same features that were improved by the surgery. Patients must acknowledge that a specific result, a "perfect" result, or a no-risk procedure cannot be guaranteed. Each procedure will have specific effects, and patients must be aware of what will and will not be achieved with the procedures they choose. Specifically, patients should be counseled about the general and local complications associated with the procedures they are contemplating, outlining the preoperative, postoperative, and surgical protocols in detail. Literature with instructions and advice about the surgery should be given to the patient, because a well-informed patient can choose the procedure that has the highest likelihood of success for him or her. Of primary importance in forehead rejuvenation procedures are the patient's specific goals, the hairline changes involved, and the acceptability of scar placement.

SURGICAL PROCEDURE AND TECHNIQUE

Surgical rejuvenation of the upper face can be considered within three categories: the coronal forehead lift and its modifications (Fig. 185.5), the direct brow lift and its modifications (Fig. 185.6), and the endoscopic forehead lift. The indications and surgical technique for each of these follow.

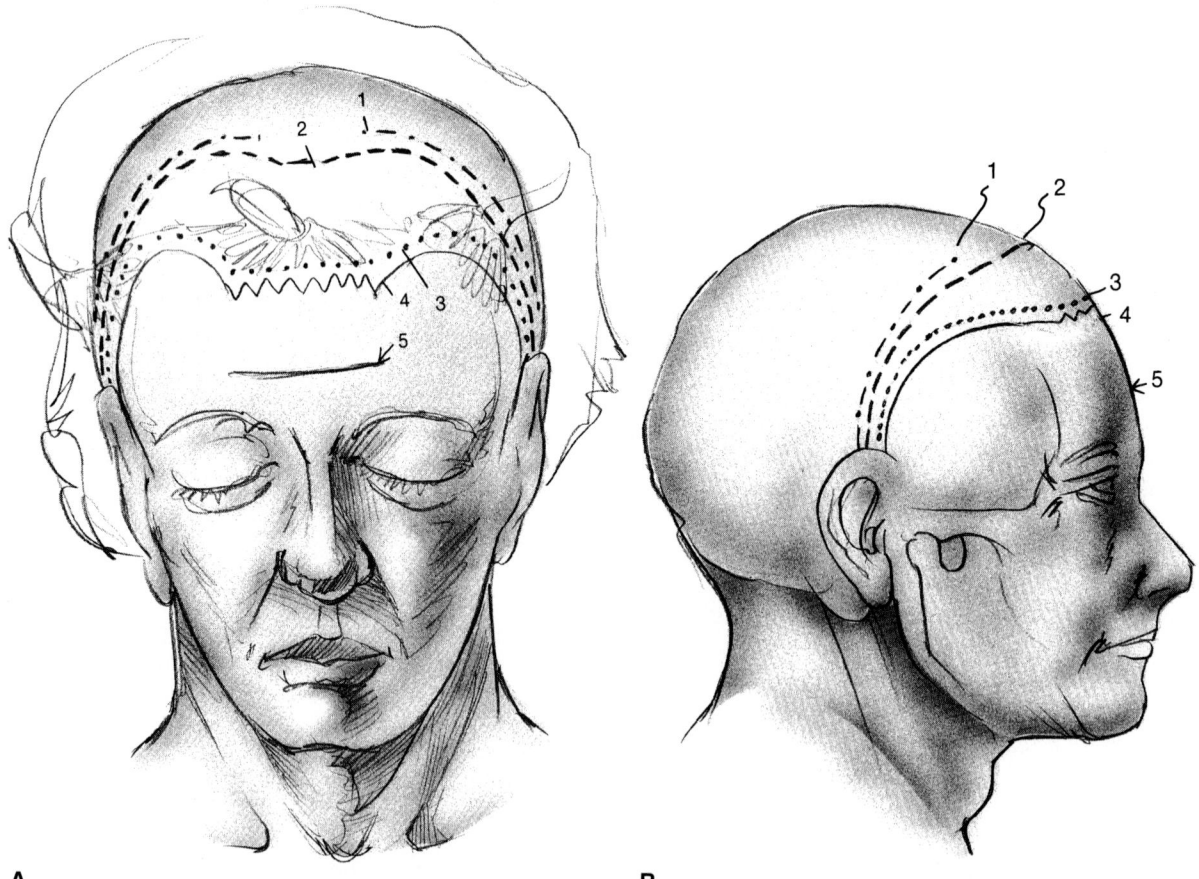

A   **B**

Figure 185.5 The coronal incision is the standard incision. Modifications may be made depending on the patient's hairline, degree of ptosis, rhytids, skin type, asymmetries, sex, and personal preference. **A:** Frontal view. **B:** Lateral view. *1*, Bilateral (temporal); *2*, coronal (forehead); *3*, trichophytic; *4*, pretrichial; *5*, midforehead.

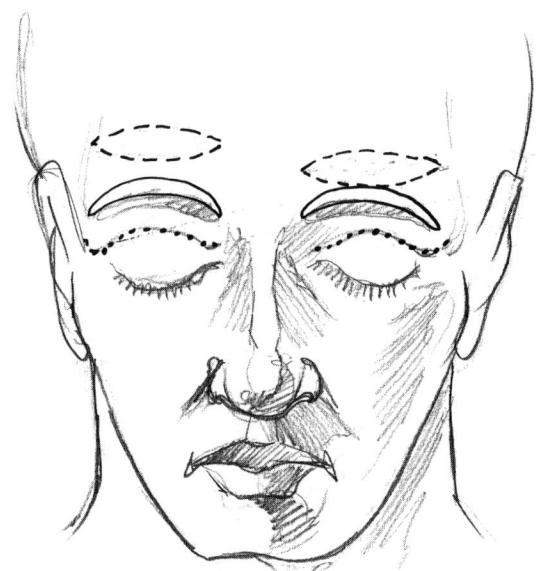

Figure 185.6 The direct brow lift (*solid lines*) is the standard incision. More recent modifications, such as the indirect brow lift (*dashes*) and browpexy (*dots*), can be useful in selected patients.

Coronal Forehead Lift

The coronal lift and its modifications are arguably the procedures of choice for rejuvenation of the upper face. Numerous recent reviews have validated its efficacy, safety, longevity, and high degree of patient satisfaction (2,10,11,12). The coronal lift is especially useful for patients who have both generalized ptosis and rhytids of the upper face and a normal or low hairline (Fig. 185.7). Relative contraindications include men with male-pattern baldness and women with high hairlines. Due to the distance between the incision and the brow, the coronal lift and its modifications are not useful to correct static or dynamic brow asymmetries. Advantages of the open lifts are the well-hidden incision within and behind the hairline and excellent exposure of the forehead musculature, allowing accurate and extensive myoplasty. Disadvantages include elevation of the frontal hairline, although this is an advantage in patients with a low frontal hairline. Other disadvantages include the temporary, and occasionally permanent, hypesthesia or paresthesia posterior to the incision line, although a recent study by Guillot et al. (13) presents good prospective and retrospective data concluding that this may not be a clinically significant disadvantage in the long term. Wide surgical undermining increases the risk for blood accumulation, and tension on the wound closure may predispose to temporary or permanent hair loss, especially if the wound is not meticulously closed in multiple layers.

Technique

The procedure is done under either local intravenous sedation or general anesthesia. General anesthesia is preferable, especially if multiple other procedures are being

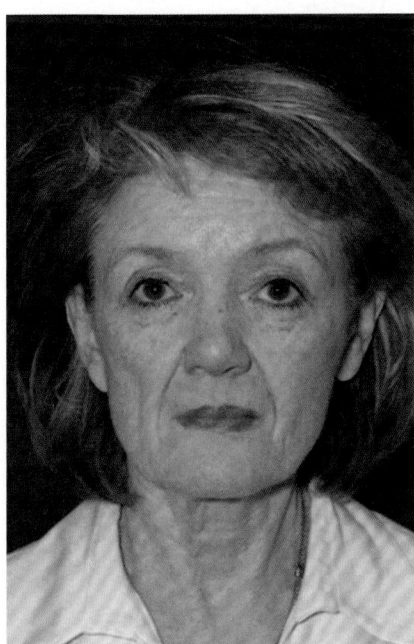
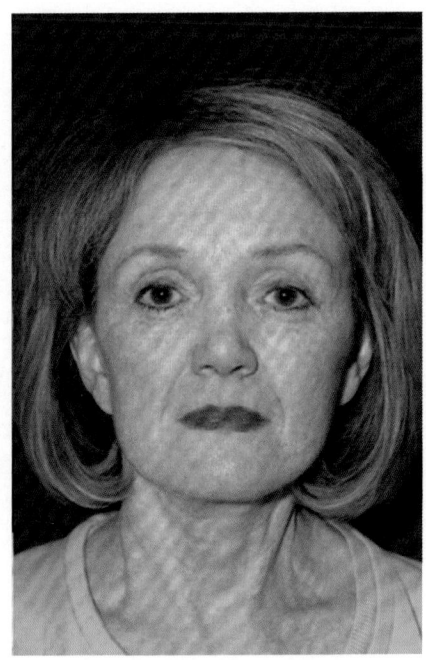
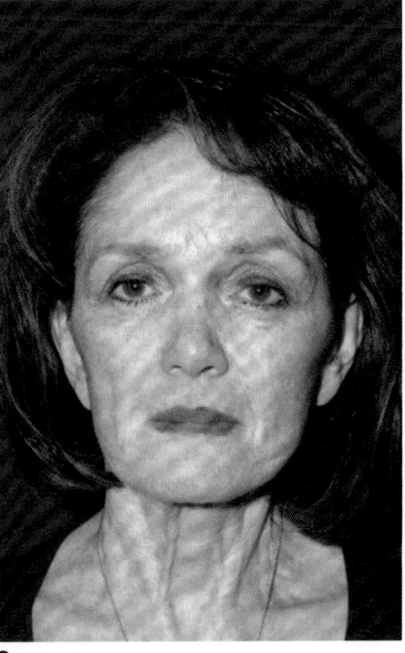

A   **B**   **C**

Figure 185.7 A: Sixty-four-year-old female with a short forehead, brow ptosis, and prominent horizontal forehead rhytids. Note the hyperdynamic elevation of the brows commonly observed in patients with brow ptosis. **B:** One year following coronal forehead lift, upper and lower blepharoplasty, and deep plane face- and neck lift. Note that the brows are now in an improved position without dynamic movement. Note the slight increase in the length of the forehead. **C:** Four years following the above-mentioned procedures—note the longevity of the open forehead lift.

performed (14,15). A curvilinear incision about 4 to 6 cm posterior to the anterior hairline is marked, and a thin strip of hair is removed along the incision line. Local infiltration of anesthesia of lidocaine 1% with epinephrine 1:100,000 and bupivacaine 0.5% with epinephrine 1:200,000 mixed in equal parts is used initially to effect a regional block at the supratrochlear and supraorbital nerves. Following this, a ring block is completed by following the supraorbital margins, the zygomas, and the scalp at the incision site. Infiltration is completed in the subgaleal plane beneath the entire area of the flap to be elevated. At least 7 minutes must be allowed for adequate vasoconstriction.

The coronal incision is beveled parallel to the shafts of the hair follicles, usually obliquely anterior at the midline and becoming more horizontal or even obliquely posterior in the temple region (Fig. 185.8). The flap is elevated with broad scalpel sweeps with a no. 10 blade in the subgaleal plane, abetting this action with firm upward traction on the flap. The pericranium is kept intact and moistened with saline gauze. Prominent vessels may be seen coursing superiorly from the supraorbital vessels about 2 to 3 cm superior to their origin. Scalpel dissection is carried inferiorly

to about 1 cm above the supraorbital rims. Dissection laterally must be carried down to the zygoma; this is most safely done with the blade handle and gentle blunt dissection just above the temporalis fascia.

Myoplasty is performed through blunt interfibrillar scissors dissection to identify and free the corrugator muscles from the supratrochlear and supraorbital nerves and vessels, which are multiple and course around the muscle. The flap is dissected over the supraorbital rims, releasing the arcus marginalis, but not so far as to expose orbital fat. In this way the brow is freed so that it may be elevated above the supraorbital rims. The muscle is cauterized with bipolar cautery at two points about 1 cm apart, and the central portion excised. Any bleeding is meticulously controlled with bipolar cautery, taking care not to injure any nerves. The procerus in the midline is identified and incised horizontally using unipolar cautery. The frontalis muscle is identified in the flap, and the unipolar cautery is used to incise the muscle and galea immediately deep to the prominent transverse forehead creases. Cauterization is maintained medial to the pupils to prevent injury to the temporal branch of the facial nerve and also to preserve some natural forehead movement through the action of

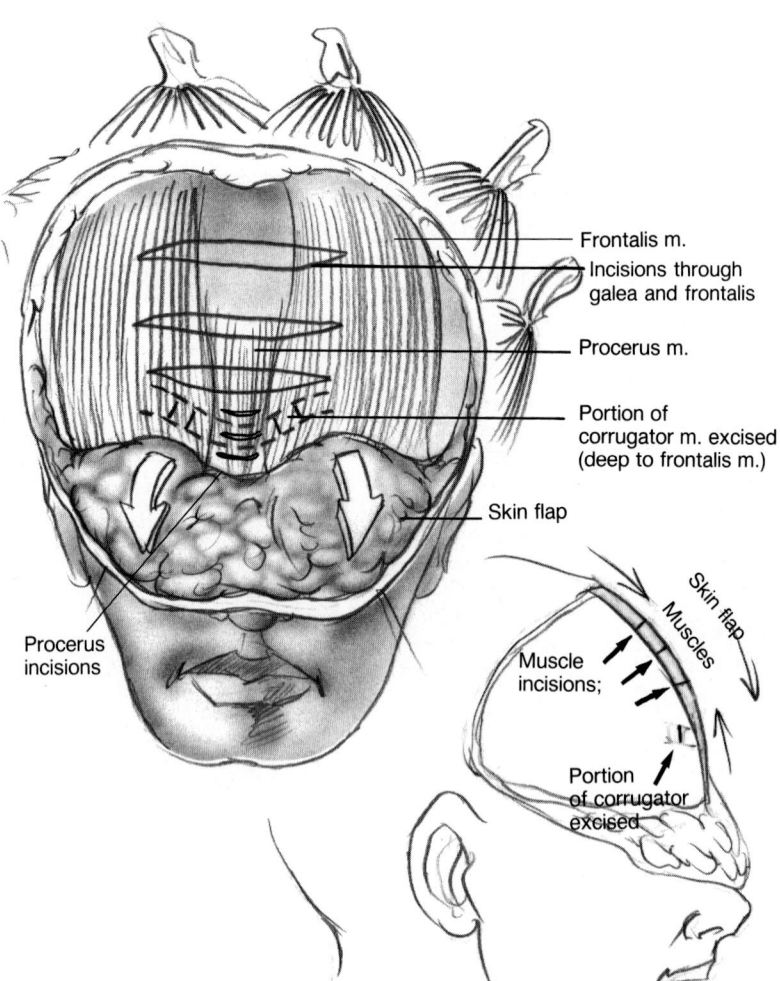

Frontalis m.

Incisions through galea and frontalis

Procerus m.

Portion of corrugator m. excised (deep to frontalis m.)

Skin flap

Procerus incisions

Muscle incisions;

Skin flap

Muscles

Portion of corrugator excised

Figure 185.8 The coronal incision is beveled parallel to the shafts of the hair follicles. The flap is elevated over the supraorbital margins and to the zygoma. A portion of the corrugator supercilius is excised, and the procerus and frontalis are incised.

the frontalis muscle laterally. Excision rather than incision of the procerus and frontalis muscles may lead to contour irregularities of the glabella and forehead.

The temporalis branch of the facial nerve is at risk in the region between the brow and the temporal hairline as it traverses this area superomedially. The nerve is deep within the parotid gland but becomes superficial in the subdermal fat as it crosses the zygomatic arch. It then courses deeply again to pierce the frontalis muscle about 2 cm from the lateral canthus (5). The frontalis muscle must not be divided in this region between the eyebrow and the temporal hairline. Absolute hemostasis is secured, paying special attention to superficial temporal artery branches in the supraauricular region. The galeal vessels are cauterized, avoiding bleeding vessels in the subcutaneous tissue so as not to damage hair follicles.

Advancement and rotation of the flap are done in a superior and posterior direction, and the appropriate portion of redundant skin parallel to the hair follicles is excised (Fig. 185.9). This amount can be determined by assessing the amount of brow elevation required and then increasing this by about 5 mm to allow for the stretch-back relaxation that inevitably occurs. Usually, about 12 to 18 mm of skin can be excised, although this will vary with each patient. Conservative excision is indicated to prevent an overelevated and frightened look. In females, more skin may be excised from the temporal region to create a more lateral, feminine lift, depending on the desired correction.

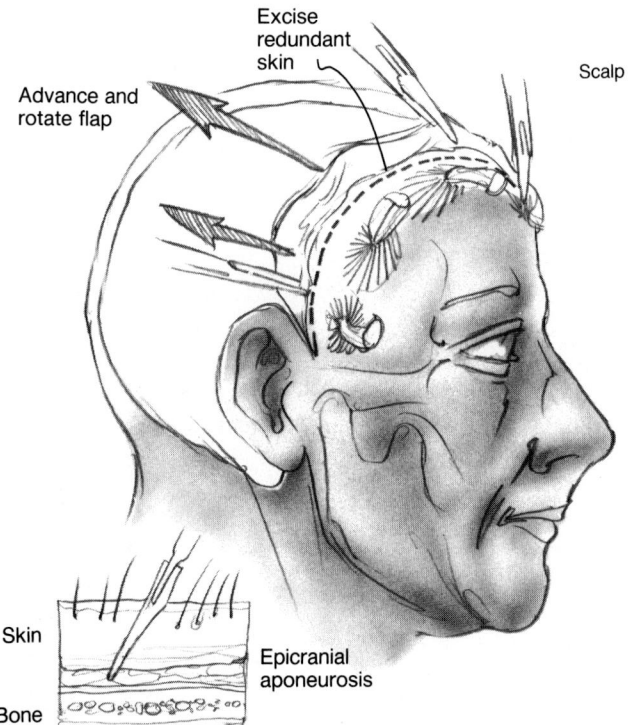

Figure 185.9 The flap is advanced and rotated in a superior and posterior direction, and the appropriate portion of redundant skin is excised parallel to the hair follicles.

The excision usually is extended laterally to 1 to 2 cm above the anterior helical root. A suction drain is placed through a separate stab incision in the temple, the galea is closed by using interrupted and inverted polyglycolic acid sutures, and the skin is closed with staples.

Ophthalmic drops and ointment are prescribed for any indications of corneal exposure. The drain is removed on the first postoperative day, and surgical staples on day 6 and day 8.

Brow Lift and Upper Blepharoplasty

A special relation exists between forehead lifting or brow lifting and upper blepharoplasty. Temporary lagophthalmos is common after brow lifting, and a concomitant upper blepharoplasty will increase the degree and duration of lagophthalmos. The brow lift should be performed first, as a more accurate assessment of the degree of eyelid skin to be excised then can be made. Conservative skin excision is advisable. If no skin must be removed, redundant upper eyelid fat can be excised through a standard excision just above the tarsal plate, taking care not to injure the insertion of the levator aponeurosis.

The eyelid margin should not be above the midpupil after surgery and usually closes within 7 to 10 days. Aggressive postoperative ocular lubrication is necessary until full closure of the palpebral fissure occurs. This is also because the blink reflex initially may be decreased, predisposing to dry eyes.

Eyelid skin can be stored as a graft for up to 3 weeks and used as a full-thickness donor graft to its original site if eyelid closure is unsatisfactory. Patients are advised that a touch-up excision of upper eyelid skin can be performed 9 to 12 months later if necessary, although in our experience this is not usually required or requested.

Patients who have had a previous upper blepharoplasty and require correction of eyebrow ptosis may be candidates for any of the brow-lifting procedures; however, the surgeon must be careful to assess the degree of redundant upper eyelid skin, the status of the tear film, and the amount of skin excised for elevation. Conservatism is advised.

Bilateral Temple Lift and Lateral Brow Lifting

The bilateral temple lift is indicated in men or women who primarily have lateral eyebrow ptosis and upper eyelid hooding. It is advantageous in that it does not elevate the central hairline, as does the full coronal forehead lift and, because of the scar position, can be used in both men and women. However, it does not allow myoplasty procedures of the forehead, and its somewhat confined exposure for elevation makes it difficult to control any bleeding vessels at the supraorbital margin, although increased adeptness with endoscopy has somewhat ameliorated this problem. Although it appears to offer good intermediate-term results, in our experience it does not appear to offer the longer-lasting results seen with the coronal forehead lift and its variations.

This procedure has essentially the same incision as the coronal forehead lift, except that the incision is carried from just above the anterior helical root up to the midpupillary line, but it does not extend completely across the midline scalp (Fig. 185.5). The incision is beveled parallel to the hair follicles, and a subgaleal dissection is carried out with blunt and sharp scissor dissection down over the supraorbital margin and to the zygoma inferiorly. The temple flap is redraped superolaterally, and the redundant skin excised; it is usually about 10 mm at its widest. The galea is closed with 3-0 polyglycolic acid antitension sutures, and the skin with surgical staples. No drain is usually placed.

The lateral browlift is indicated in patients with a lifelong appearance of downturned lateral brows. In these patients, the lateral brows are ptotic due to the lack of galeal attachment to the supraorbital rim in this region, lateral to the deep temporal fusion line (16). Other patients who may benefit from such a lift are those who suffer from lateral brow ptosis primarily as a result of excess skin.

The procedure begins with an incision 6 cm in length, 1 cm behind the hairline, designed in a curvilinear fashion in the vector of the desired elevation. Two dissection pockets are created—one lateral to the zone of fixation and one medial to it. Laterally, dissection is carried deep to the superficial temporal parietal fascia, just along the surface of the shiny deep temporal fascia. Medially, a subperiosteal pocket is developed blindly down to within 2 cm of the supraorbital rim. The two pockets are then connected from lateral to medial, using a periosteal elevator in a blind motion, sweeping superiorly. The remaining zone of adhesion, which condenses down to become the orbital ligament, is then released down to the orbital rim.

The superior and lateral attachments to the superior orbital rim must then be released either with direct visualization or with endoscopic guidance. Dissection laterally is performed similarly to the traditional endoscopic forehead techniques. Fixation can be effected with suture, bone tunnels, titanium screws, or absorbable devices. Excess scalp is excised, and tension-free closure is performed. A drain is not normally placed.

Pretrichial Lift

The primary indication for the pretrichial forehead lift is for women who have a high hairline and long vertical height to the forehead. This procedure then offers all the advantages of the coronal forehead lift but does not raise the anterior hairline to an unaesthetically high level. Furthermore, resection of the redundant forehead skin reduces the vertical height of the forehead, and this often provides improved facial balance. It is best used in women with thick hair who are prepared to wear their hair forward to camouflage the scar in the early healing stages. With scar maturation, no scar camouflage is required in the vast majority of patients (Fig. 185.10). It can be used in men who are not expected to lose more hair or who might be undergoing or willing to undergo hair transplants to camouflage the scar further, although this is rarely necessary as the incision usually heals very well and rarely needs camouflage.

Advantages of the pretrichial lift are that it allows the same wide access to the forehead musculature as the coronal lift and thus allows correction of all the components of the aging forehead. Disadvantages include the necessity for meticulous technique to obtain the finest possible scar and possibility of postoperative scar camouflage being required. A broader area of anesthesia occurs, and usually

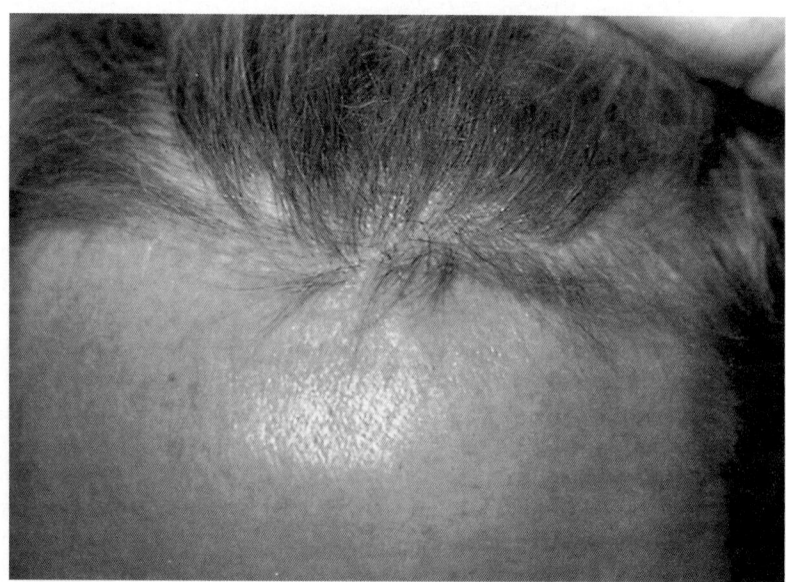

Figure 185.10 Anterior forehead hairline 3 months after W-plasty pretrichial incision in a woman.

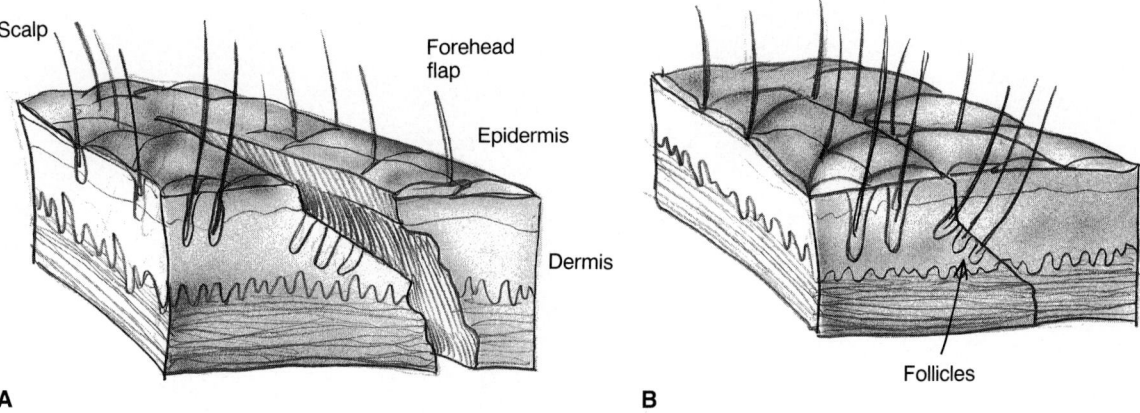

Figure 185.11 A: The trichophytic incision is an irregular beveled incision made just posterior to the anterior hairline. **B:** The follicles below the deepithelialized portion of the flap will produce hair growth through the scar.

there is a small permanent area of anesthesia just posterior to the incision. This is rarely a bother to patients, but they must be advised of this possibility preoperatively.

In this modification of the coronal forehead lift, the incision temporally remains the same but is brought anteriorly in the widow's peak region. It then follows a course just behind the anterior hairline as a W-plasty with the limbs about 5.5 mm long and at 55-degree angles that interdigitate with the anterior hairline follicles (Fig. 185.5). The forehead flap is elevated identically to the coronal lift, and myoplasty of forehead rhytids and correction of ptosis are performed. Subcutaneous variations of this lift have been described (17).

Trichophytic Forehead Lift

The trichophytic incision is currently our preferred technique when an open approach is utilized. The incision is a modification of the pretrichial incision; it is placed two or three follicles behind the anterior hairline and is therefore better camouflaged because hair follicles regrow through the scar (Fig. 185.11). It is indicated for women with high foreheads and hairlines and may be considered in men who do not have male-pattern baldness or who would agree to hair transplants should this occur (Fig. 185.12).

The incision is an irregularly irregular beveled incision made just posterior to the anterior hairline (Fig. 185.5). The superficial aspect of the incision is placed down through the epidermis only. Then it is beveled from posterior to anterior through the dermis and subcutaneous tissues to the subgaleal plane. This effectively deepithelializes about 2 mm of the leading edge of the posterior or hair-bearing flap and preserves the underlying hair follicles, although their shafts are excised. After the myoplasty procedures and redraping of the forehead flap, the redundant skin is excised from the non–hair-bearing flap in a parallel beveled fashion to allow the edge of the forehead flap to appose accurately the opposite bevel of the deepithelialized portion

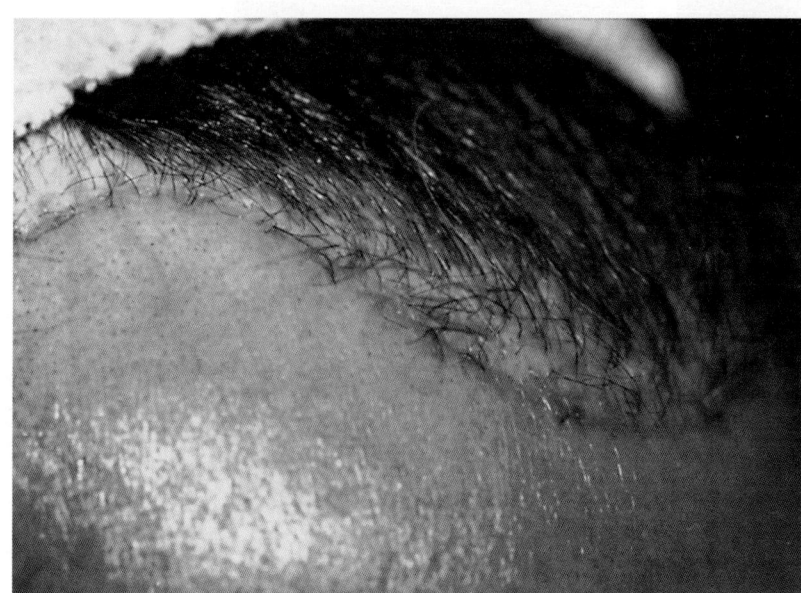

Figure 185.12 Temporal and anterior hairline of a man 3 months after a trichophytic forehead lift. Hair can be seen growing through the incision. By 6 months, this scar becomes almost imperceptible.

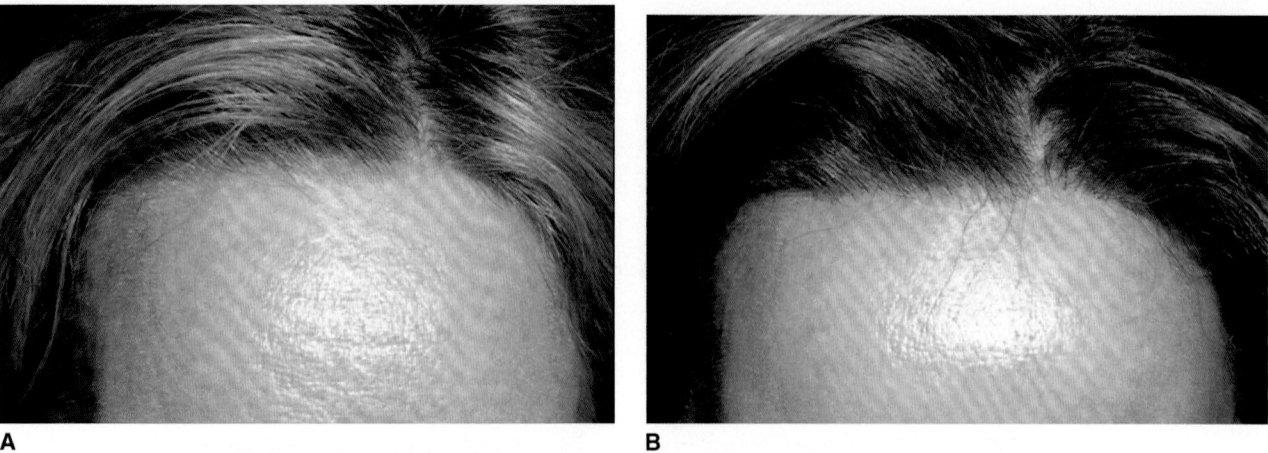

A **B**

Figure 185.13 A: Anterior hairline in a female prior to trichophytic forehead lift. **B:** Anterior hairline in same patient one year following trichophytic forehead lift. This represents an average result with near imperceptibility of the scar. Note that hair is growing through the scar. No neuromodulators were needed following surgery.

of the posterior hair-bearing flap. Galeal sutures again are used for antitension, and the wound is closed with a running 6-0 nylon suture along the forehead skin junction and with staples within the hair-bearing scalp, taking care to prevent damage to hair follicles. With further hair growth from the hair follicles below the deepithelialized portion of the posterior flap, follicles will grow through the scar itself, thus improving camouflage (Fig. 185.13).

The trichophytic incision has the advantage of providing an improved scar but again requires meticulous execution to achieve the desired result. Inaccurate incision placement or wound tension causing strangulation of the hair follicle

vasculature will compromise the result. This incision has become the preferred hairline incision. The scar heals so well that most patients can wear their hair back without scar camouflage once healing is complete. Overall, this is the commonest forehead-lifting procedure we employ today (Fig. 185.14).

Midforehead Lift

The midforehead lift, when performed in the central forehead, can be considered a modification of the coronal forehead lift because the dissection can be carried

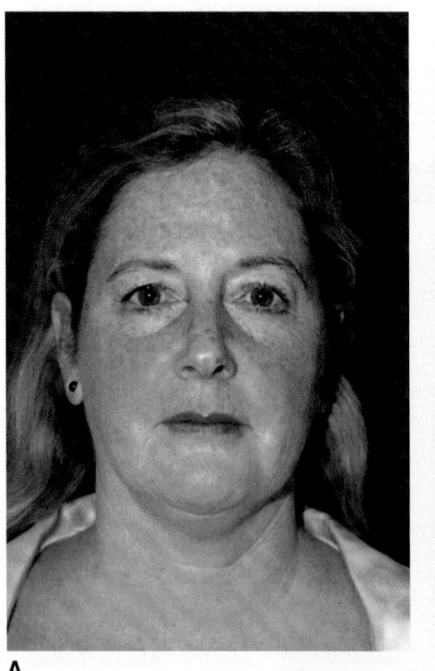
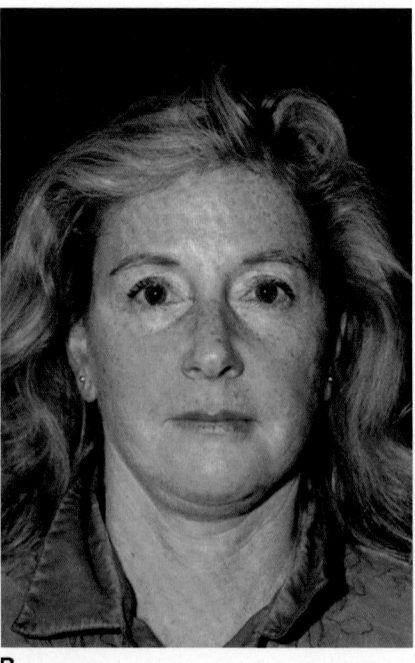

A **B**

Figure 185.14 A: Fifty-four-year-old female with a high hairline who wanted subtle elevation of brows. **B:** Three years following trichophytic forehead lift, deep plane face-lift, and neck lift.

into the subgaleal plane and myoplasty is possible. This approach is indicated in men with receding hairlines and prominent deep forehead rhytids in which the scar can be camouflaged. The incision is placed in a central midforehead crease, and subcutaneous rather than subgaleal elevation is performed down to the supraorbital margins (Fig. 185.5). This preserves the sensory supply of the forehead, which otherwise would be lost if the midforehead incision were deepened to the subgaleal plane. Access to the corrugator supercilii and procerus muscles is possible by developing a central subgaleal flap inferiorly. Myoplasty can be done if indicated, and the frontalis muscle can be divided between the supraorbital nerves. This approach does not permit the same extent of forehead muscle myoplasty as that in the coronal forehead lift. The inferior flap is redraped superiorly, and the redundant skin is excised to correct ptosis of the glabella and medial eyebrows. If the excision is extended laterally in the subcutaneous plane, some degree of elevation of the lateral eyebrows also can be achieved. In such cases, the procedure is comparable to the indirect brow lift or midforehead brow lift. Advantages of the procedure include a direct and close approach to the glabella without distortion of the hairline. It also allows myoplasty, but it does not offer improvement of the lateral brow region or upper forehead. Its major disadvantage is a potentially unsatisfactory scar and an inability to have

a satisfactory lateral brow elevation; this is minimized by making the scar irregular rather than symmetrical, as it follows the crease line. The incisions, and therefore this approach, are usually best in older patients with well-developed forehead creases and thin, nonsebaceous, lighter-colored hair.

Direct Brow Lift

The standard direct brow lift consists of selective excision of skin directly above the eyebrows, combined with suspension of the orbicularis oculi muscle to the periosteum (Fig. 185.15). Brow elevation has also been achieved through a transblepharoplasty approach through an internal brow release, excision of medial brow depressors, with or without placement a of biodegradable fixation device (18,19). This procedure is primarily indicated for men with bushy eyebrows and occasional women who are not candidates for a trichophytic or coronal forehead lift (Fig. 185.16). Because of the direct approach, it is more useful than a coronal lift to correct brow asymmetries and also can be more effective to correct marked ptosis of the lateral eyebrow. It can be used unilaterally to improve facial nerve paresis functionally with suture techniques, biodegradable devices, or with autologous fascia (20). It is relatively contraindicated in patients who have thin, light-colored eyebrows and patients who have thick sebaceous skin that may not scar well.

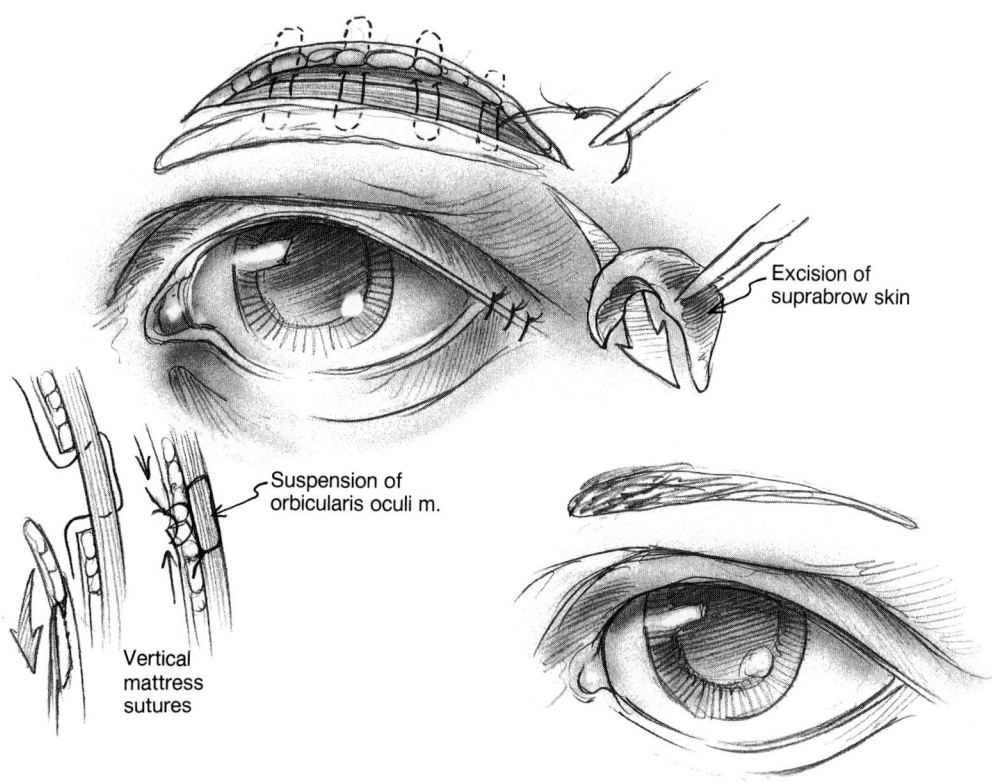

Figure 185.15 Excision of suprabrow skin and suspension of the orbicularis oculi muscle produce direct elevation of the eyebrow.

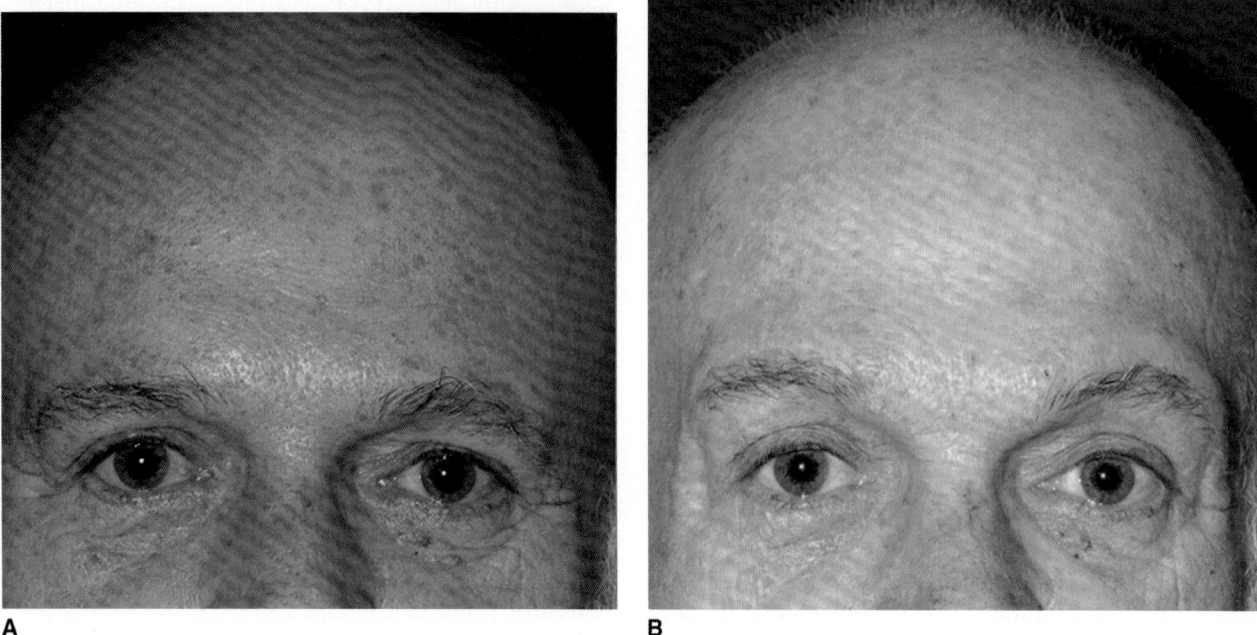

A   **B**

Figure 185.16 A: Sixty-year-old man with eyebrow ptosis, bushy eyebrows, and male-pattern baldness. **B:** One year after direct eyebrow lift and lower lid skin pinch only.

Technique

The inferior incision for the direct brow lift is placed just within the most superior growth of fine eyebrow hairs. It should not extend medial to the medial aspect of the eyebrow, as poor glabellar scarring may result. The incision should be carried lateral to the lateral eyebrow and extended horizontally laterally in a gentle arc, but not superiorly. The superior incision is carried in a gentle arch superiorly from its medial aspect to reach a high point between the lateral limbus and lateral canthus and then gently curved inferiorly to complete the excision. The superior incision defines the new position of the eyebrow, and the point of maximal height will determine the degree of masculinity (apex more medial toward the lateral limbus) or femininity (apex more lateral toward the lateral canthus) of the ultimate brow appearance. The skin is excised down to the subcutaneous plane, taking care not to injure the frontalis muscle or the supratrochlear and supraorbital nerves medially. Usually, a maximum of 10 to 12 mm of skin is excised. Minimal undermining is done inferiorly, taking care not to injure the hair follicles, with 1 to 1.5 cm of undermining in the subcutaneous plane superiorly. Four or five permanent sutures are placed through the orbicularis muscle at the level of the supraorbital margin; then this suspension suture is secured to the periosteum at the level of the superior incision. This latter suture is placed in a horizontal fashion to decrease the risk of injury to branches of the facial nerve. The apical suture

is placed first, followed by those medially and laterally. Vertical mattress 5-0 nylon sutures are used for closure and to obtain maximal skin eversion. The sutures are removed on day 4, and light laser abrasion is done, if indicated, 6 to 12 weeks postoperatively—we rarely find this necessary.

Advantages of direct brow lifting include a long-lasting lift as a result of the excellent orbicularis muscle suspension that can be achieved. It is the best technique to correct brow asymmetries or unilateral brow ptosis secondary to facial nerve paresis. More precise positioning of the eyebrow can be obtained than with the more distant coronal lifting, and less dissection is required than for coronal lifting. A significant potential disadvantage is the eyebrow scar, especially in patients who have sebaceous skin or those with thin brows or in whom meticulous technique is not applied. If the incision is not beveled parallel to the hair follicles, the superior aspect of the eyebrow may be lost in time, giving the appearance that the scar has migrated superiorly. Direct brow lifting has no effect on the forehead, glabellar, or temple ptosis and cannot be used to improve forehead or glabellar rhytids. Prominent forehead rhytids may be distorted, giving an unnatural appearance. Meticulous attention must be paid to achieving the ideal bilateral symmetry desired (Fig. 185.16).

Indirect Brow Lift

The indirect brow lift has been associated with the mid-forehead lift by some authors, and others have called it the midforehead brow lift (21). It is essentially the same procedure as the brow lift, but the skin excision is performed bilaterally at some distance above the eyebrow in the forehead. The indirect brow lift is indicated in patients with marked or asymmetrical brow ptosis and forehead furrows and those in whom a coronal forehead lift is contraindicated. The patient's skin type must be satisfactory, and the patient must be advised fully about the resultant scar. Men who have male-pattern baldness or women who have thin and light hair with a high hairline are potential candidates.

The surgical approach is similar to that for the direct brow lift, except the inferior incision is placed in a deep rhytid at a distance above the brow, and the superior incision is arched above this. This differs from the midforehead lift, in which the redundant skin is excised from below the initial crease incision rather than above. Undermining the inferior forehead flap must be maintained in the subcutaneous plane down to the supraorbital rims so as not to interfere with sensory or motor innervation. In most cases, the orbicularis muscle is suspended, as described for the direct brow lift.

Advantages of the indirect brow lift include its ability to conceal the forehead incision within a skin crease and at the same time achieve a relatively proximal suspension for the eyebrow, thus leading to a long-lasting and precise elevation. Depending on the location and extent of the skin excision, the shape of the brow also can be configured as desired. Disadvantages include its relatively selective use: it may be indicated in patients who have significant rhytids and skin that will heal well and who are not candidates for a coronal forehead lift.

Browpexy

This procedure is unique in that it is performed through an infrabrow rather than a suprabrow incision (18). It therefore can be used in association with upper blepharoplasty and may negate the need for suprabrow procedures. This procedure may be indicated in the younger woman who is primarily concerned about fullness or puffiness in the lateral portion of the upper eyelids. Other indications are women with mild to moderate eyebrow ptosis and a flatter, androgenous eyebrow appearance. Lateral prominence in the infrabrow region due to a prominent supraorbital margin or brow fat pad also may be improved with this technique. It is particularly useful in association with upper blepharoplasty. Relative contraindications include patients who have severe brow ptosis or more generalized signs of aging of the upper face.

The browplasty is performed first through an upper blepharoplasty incision. Preoperatively, the supraorbital vessels and nerves, which are identified by palpation at their exit from the supraorbital notch and the location of the lateral brow fullness, should be marked. Dissection is

extended superiorly 1 to 1.5 cm above the superior and lateral orbital rim in the submuscular plane just deep to the orbicularis oculi muscle. The redundant brow fat pad can be seen overlying the orbital margin; it is removed from the region of the central third of the superior orbital margin laterally as far as the frontozygomatic suture. The fat pad is excised in an elliptical fashion measuring about 1 to 1.5 cm in vertical dimension and tapering nasally and temporally. The underlying periosteum is left intact to prevent adhesions. If brow elevation is not required, the blepharoplasty is completed in standard fashion.

In patients requiring elevation of the central and lateral eyebrow, browpexy is performed to elevate and suspend the brow above the supraorbital margin. The eyebrow position can be fixed superiorly by using two or three permanent 4-0 Mersilene sutures. Each suture is placed transcutaneously at the level of the infrabrow hairs into the sub-brow space and then passed through the periosteum 1 cm above the supraorbital rim. It then is secured through the subeyebrow tissue at the level of the original transcutaneous suture. With tightening of the suture, the eyebrow will be elevated an appropriate amount above the supraorbital margin after the original transcutaneous suture end is drawn through the skin. The placement and tension of each suture can be used to obtain the configuration of the eyebrow and degree of elevation desired. A recent commentary by an experienced oculoplastic surgeon has recommended fixation to the deep temporal fascia laterally to prevent instability of periosteal fixation (22). The blepharoplasty procedure then is completed, removing redundant fat and upper eyelid skin.

Advantages of this technique include the single eyelid incision, which is also compatible with that made for upper blepharoplasty. It allows brow elevation with a more minimal procedure than a coronal forehead lift and allows direct access for trimming the lateral eyebrow fat pad. However, its use is restricted to patients who have only mild to moderate eyebrow ptosis, and the exposure is more difficult compared with direct eyebrow lifting. Removing the eyebrow fat pad transects the cutaneous nerves, resulting in brow anesthesia for several months over this region. Injury to the supraorbital vessels or nerves could result in heavy bleeding or forehead anesthesia. If the suspension suture is placed through the preseptal orbicularis muscle, postoperative dimpling of the thinner eyelid skin and lagophthalmos may occur secondary to eyelid tethering. Inadequate correction of brow ptosis also has been reported.

Endoscopic Forehead Lift

Endoscopic forehead-lifting techniques allow correction of brow ptosis and reduction of forehead and glabellar rhytids (23). The indications for this technique are identical to those for the conventional coronal approaches

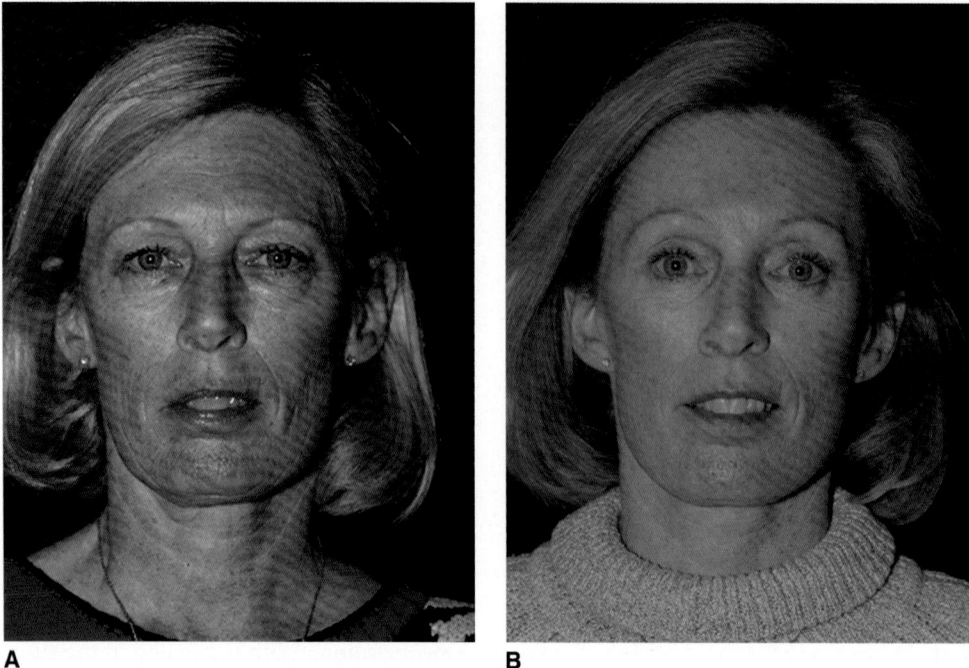

A   **B**

Figure 185.17 A: A 59-year-old woman with moderate brow ptosis, moderately marked forehead and glabellar rhytids, and moderately high forehead. **B:** The patient 3 years after endoscopic forehead lift, four-lid blepharoplasty, and deep plane face- and neck lift.

(Fig. 185.17). Direct endoscopic visualization affords the ability to identify and preserve the supraorbital and supratrochlear neurovascular bundles, although no more clearly than with the direct approach. Sensory neuropathy and scarring are decreased further because of incision size reduction, change in incision placement, and lack of skin excision in some cases. The reduction in sensory neuropathy may not be as great as was once thought, and a recent prospective and retrospective study has demonstrated that it has not made a significant difference with patient satisfaction (14). The most favorable result can be obtained in the thin-skinned patient with glabellar rhytids, minimal brow ptosis, and minimal skin redundancy. Relative contraindications include women with high hairlines, male-pattern baldness, and some Asians and Native Americans who have tight, thick skin and extensive bony attachments.

Advantages of the endoscopic approach include smaller incisions, decreased incidence of sensory neuropathy and alopecia, less bleeding, and a faster recovery period (10,11,23). Disadvantages involve the need for specialized training and experience with endoscopic techniques with a steeper learning curve than that for the other approaches and the need for confirmation of long-term lift results.

Preoperatively, the location of the supraorbital and supratrochlear neurovascular bundles is identified and marked. The amount of skin advancement to provide an adequate brow lift, usually 10 to 16 mm, is determined and marked with the patient sitting and supine. Glabellar and forehead furrows to be addressed also are marked.

This procedure may be performed with the patient under either general anesthesia or local anesthesia with intravenous sedation, depending on patient and surgeon preferences. Local infiltration with lidocaine 1% with epinephrine 1:100,000 and bupivacaine 0.5% with epinephrine 1:200,000 mixed in equal parts is used in a coronal distribution to provide vasoconstriction before the incision.

The standard endoscopic forehead lift is performed with three to six incisions, which are about 2 cm long (Fig. 185.18). A midline sagittal incision, bilateral paramedian incisions at the level of the midbrow, and bilateral coronal incisions parallel to the hair follicles are placed 1 to 1.5 cm posterior to the hairline. The location of these incisions will vary with surgeon preference. Glabellar rhytid reduction without correction of brow ptosis may be performed without the use of the temporal incisions. Y- to V-advancement flaps can be designed at the incision line if skin excision is desired. The forehead elevation is initiated by extending the vertical incisions through the pericranium. The dissection proceeds in the subperiosteal plane which, because of its decreased vascularity, permits superior visualization. Wide subperiosteal undermining of the scalp is performed in a blind fashion with a periosteal elevator, anteriorly to a level 2 cm above the supraorbital rims

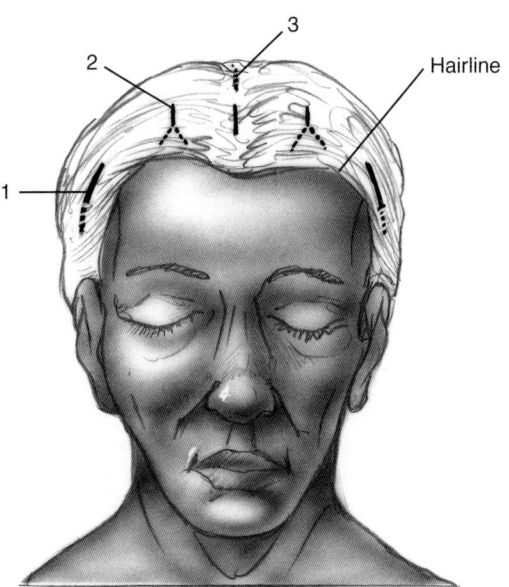

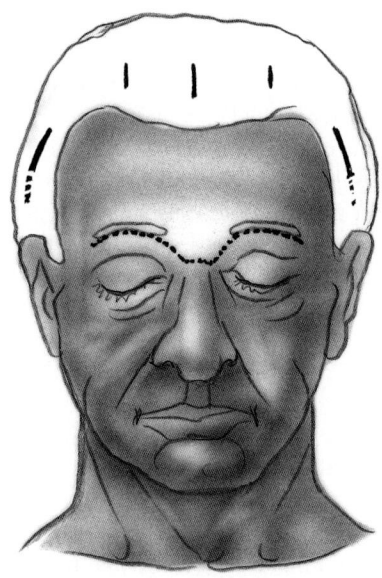

Figure 185.18 The standard endoscopic forehead lift incisions (*solid lines*) are placed 1 cm posterior to the hairline and may vary with surgeon preference. *1*, The temporal incisions may be extended to increase exposure (*dashed lines*); *2*, Y- to V-advancement flaps (*dashes*) will allow for skin excision; *3*, a central posterior vertex incision (*dashes*) provides exposure for miniplate placement.

Figure 185.19 The supraorbital dissection is performed with the 4-mm 30-degree scope in the central incision and a small endoscopic elevator in the paramedian incisions. Periosteal releasing incisions over the orbital margin and blunt elevation down to the zygomatic arch allow for flap advancement.

inferiorly and the temporal lines laterally, and posteriorly to the nuchal line. The supraorbital dissection is performed under direct endoscopic visualization. A 4-mm 30-degree scope is introduced into the central incision, and a small endoscopic elevator is used in the paramedian incisions. The supraorbital and supratrochlear nerves are identified and preserved by using blunt dissection with the endoscopic scissors. The dissection is extended inferiorly over the orbital rims and onto the nasion (Fig. 185.19).

The temporal incisions are extended through the temporoparietal fascia, preserving the superficial layer of the deep temporal fascia. The endoscope and the endoscopic periosteal elevator are used to dissect the lateral orbital rim region inferiorly to the zygomatic arch. The fused fascia planes of the galea, temporoparietal fascia, deep temporal fascia, and periosteum, which insert on the temporal line, are released with sharp dissection. The medial zygomaticotemporal vein, also known as the "sentinel vein," may be encountered 5 to 10 mm lateral to the zygomaticofrontal suture and serves as an important landmark in identifying and preserving the temporal branch of the facial nerve (4,5).

Transverse releasing incisions are made through the periosteum along the supraorbital margin to allow forehead flap advancement. The corrugator and procerus muscles are divided by using the endoscopic scissors. Frontalis muscle division, although not routinely performed, may be performed between the supraorbital neurovascular bundles. Hemostasis is obtained with cauterization.

Flap suspension and fixation are performed after advancement of the flap to predetermined levels. Several different flap-fixation techniques are described in the literature, which include the following: (a) skin staples and taping, (b) microscrew placement in the paramedian incisions of the anterior flap and fixation with skin staples posterior to the microscrew, (c) suspension sutures with cortical microscrew fixation, (d) nylon suspension sutures with fixation to a posterior vertex titanium miniplate, (e) sutures secured through cortical bone tunnels, (f) absorbable screws and cortical anchors (Endotine Coapt Systems, Palo Alto, CA), and (g) fibrin glue (24–28). A surgeon's experience or preference may determine to some degree the method of fixation used. Recent studies, though, will help confirm or deny the scientific merit of some of these techniques. More specifically, fixation methods that rely on temporary means of fixations such as fibrin glue or removable transcutaneous screws are likely to be ineffective according to studies examining the time frame for periosteal adhesion. Perhaps the best study on the subject by Sclafani et al. (29,30) demonstrated that approximately a minimum of 6 weeks is required for adhesion between the cranium and overlying periosteum. An important study by Thomas et al. (31) comparing subperiosteal versus subgaleal dissection in a rabbit model demonstrated that 8 weeks was required for the biomechanical strength of the dissected flap to match undissected controls. Thus, short-term fixation is unlikely to be adequate to maintain brow elevation. Suture fixation to a microscrew in the anterior flap incision is frequently used. Lateral forehead and brow suspension is obtained with superolateral flap advancement followed by fixation with 2.0 polydioxanone (PDS) sutures from the temporoparietal fascia to the superficial layer of the deep temporal fascia. A subperiosteal drain may be placed although this is not our practice. The scalp incisions are closed with surgical staples. A pressure dressing may be applied. The staples are removed on postoperative day 8 in the office. In general, today the commonly used fixation techniques include sutures with bone tunnels, resorbable fixation devices (i.e., Endotine device), and microscrew/suture cortical fixation.

The incidence of postoperative scarring, alopecia, and sensory neuropathy may be decreased in comparison with those after the standard coronal lift, although a recent prospective study and retrospective review has demonstrated that this does not make a clinically significant difference in objective sensory outcomes or subjective patient satisfaction (13). All other complications are similar to standard coronal-lifting techniques. The amount of forehead lifting that can be achieved and maintained has yet to be consistently confirmed. Although endoscopic forehead-lifting techniques offer distinct advantages, longer-term studies are needed to assess whether the results are comparable to those of the coronal procedures. Recent studies have demonstrated long-term efficacy of both types of lifts, with the most recent literature supporting the role of traditional open brow lifts (2,13–15,31,12).

COMPLICATIONS

Upper facial rejuvenation procedures may be performed with the patient under neuroleptic anesthesia if performed alone or under general anesthesia with more extensive facial rejuvenation procedures. The potential complications associated with any general anesthesia or surgery are present.

Diagnosis of the deformities present in the upper face poses a greater challenge for the surgeon than does that for the lower face. As such, the surgeon must specifically identify both the patient's concerns and the signs of aging that may be corrected by surgery. Such accurate diagnosis will lead to the choice of the most appropriate procedure. Patients must understand exactly what can and cannot be achieved with any given procedure, and their expectations must be realistic. Otherwise, they may be dissatisfied with a satisfactory surgical result. Specific potential complications are discussed in the following sections.

Bleeding

Significant bleeding is rare but may be encountered from the superficial temporal artery in the coronal, pretrichial, or trichophytic lifts or from the supratrochlear or supraorbital arteries in any of these procedures. In the lateral canthal region, bleeding may occur from the zygomaticotemporal artery. Absolute hemostasis with bipolar cautery is recommended. Heavy bleeding can occur from the scalp itself in the coronal forehead lift. We do not use Raney clips but believe that the vasoconstriction achieved with epinephrine in the local infiltration anesthetic is most important. Scalp vessels in the galeal plane should be cauterized, taking care to avoid hair follicles.

Sensory Nerve Injury

Temporary hypesthesia or occasionally hyperesthesia may occur because of irritation of the supratrochlear and supraorbital nerves during flap elevation over the supraorbital margin. In a recent anatomic discussion by Knize, two sites of potential injury to the supraorbital nerve are described: the deep division of the supraorbital nerve is inevitably injured with an initial incision through the galea as it runs just medial to the superior fusion line of the skull and, during subgaleal dissection, the same deep division of the supraorbital nerve may be injured more proximally where fusion between the galea and periosteum occurs at the level of the superior margin of the galeal fat pad (4).

Permanent hypesthesia or anesthesia centrally just posterior to the coronal lift incision, up to 2 cm in diameter, is not uncommon. This is usually of no concern to patients, although they should be advised of this preoperatively. The pretrichial or trichophytic lift will cause a larger area of hypesthesia posterior to the incision line, especially in the short-term period after surgery (14). The browplasty procedure results in temporary hypesthesia over the lateral eyebrow margin for several months.

Motor Nerve Injury

The temporal branch of the facial nerve is at risk primarily in the zygomatic region, probably as much from the infiltration of anesthesia as from surgical dissection. To decrease the risk of injury to this nerve laterally, the central forehead incision of the frontalis muscle should be kept between the pupils. If sharp hooks are used, they must be placed and removed judiciously, especially in the temporal region.

Lagophthalmos

It is most unlikely that lagophthalmos will occur when any of the forehead-lifting procedures is used alone. In the case of either a previous or concurrent upper blepharoplasty, however, it is important to be conservative in excising forehead skin or suspending the eyebrows to prevent inadequate upper eyelid closure, corneal exposure, and possible corneal scarring with visual loss. Inaccurate placement of the suspension sutures through the orbicularis oculi muscle in the browpexy procedure may cause temporary lagophthalmos. In most cases, the gradual resolution of the overcorrected forehead or eyebrows associated with lifting procedures results in resolution of initial mild lagophthalmos. Patient compliance in using ophthalmic drops and ointment must be obtained in these early phases.

Scar Widening

Scar widening most often occurs in the temporal region, probably as a result of the oblique nature of the hair follicles and inaccurate beveling of the initial or excisional incisions in the coronal forehead lift. Excess tension or excess electrocauterization also may contribute to loss of scalp follicles.

Alopecia

Patients may presume that they are experiencing hair loss if all hair trimmed during surgery is not combed out. True thinning resulting from follicle shock is unusual and often is preceded by a history of alopecia. If a secondary coronal lift is performed with the second incision posterior to the first, hair loss may occur between the two incisions.

Infection

Infection is rare. Its incidence is increased after hematoma development in diabetic patients and in those who have protracted surgery. Patients are covered with a single dose of a broad-spectrum antibiotic 1 hour before surgery. Irrigation of the wound with antibiotic solution can be performed. Treatment consists of incision and drainage and intravenous or oral antibiotics where indicated. If permanent sutures are used for the galeal closure, spitting of the sutures occasionally may occur.

EMERGENCIES

Hematoma

A rapidly expanding hematoma under a forehead flap could compromise vascularity of the flap or at least predispose to significant hair loss. This emergency is typically caused by branches of the superficial temporal artery at the superior helical root but also could occur from the supraorbital or supratrochlear arteries. Immediate elevation of the flap with exploration and cauterization of bleeding sites should be done and a suction drain placed. Intravenous and then oral antibiotics are given to decrease the risk of subsequent infection. A smaller, localized hematoma, as in the glabella or associated with a direct brow lift, may be managed satisfactorily by using incision and drainage, followed by a compression dressing. This is repeated daily until no further recurrence of the hematoma is seen.

Corneal Ulceration

Corneal ulceration is most likely to occur in association with a coronal or direct browlift performed at the same time as an upper blepharoplasty or if the latter was performed previously. Early recognition of exposure due to lagophthalmos is mandatory. Management includes ophthalmic drops and ointment and an eye shield or a tarsorrhaphy if necessary. Early ophthalmologic consultation is indicated.

Nerve Injury

Partial and temporary sensory nerve injuries are not rare when any manipulation is carried out in the region of the supraorbital and supratrochlear nerves, especially during subgaleal dissection at the level of the galeal fat pad (4). Expectant observation is the rule. Frontal nerve injury resulting in partial or complete paralysis of the nerve also requires only hopeful observation; however, firm patient reassurance and frequent follow-up are required in view of the cosmetic nature of these procedures. Should function not return within 3 weeks, nerve studies are performed to confirm the integrity of the nerve and to reassure the patient and surgeon. Long-term management of any residual deformity would include direct brow lifting on the affected side to improve asymmetry in repose.

DISCUSSION

The past few years have seen a tremendous increase in interest in rejuvenation of the upper face. The coronal forehead lift and direct brow lift have undergone numerous modifications to achieve more natural and superior results. This increase in surgical options mandates more accurate attention to deformity diagnosis and procedures selection. Some techniques are specific to a given indication, such as the use of the direct brow lift in a patient with unilateral forehead/eyebrow paralysis. Nonetheless, although clearly many approaches and techniques are used, the most frequently used types of forehead lift by the senior author are the trichophytic and coronal lifts. Although the 1990s and 2000s saw a heightened enthusiasm for minimally invasive and endoscopic approaches, the longevity of these approaches has not been proven in long-term studies. LaFerriere and Perkins (11,23) summarized their experience with the endoscopic brow lift as compared with open forehead lifts by concluding that no difference in the results is apparent. However, more recent analysis of long-term results suggests that the answer is not so clear. Both a national survey by Elkwood et al. (12) and a study by Baker and Chiu (10) in reviewing the results of 21 New York surgeons demonstrated complication rates that were closer to those of the open procedures than previously reported. Another recent prospective study and retrospective review by Rousso (13) demonstrates that although short-term sensory neuropathy is increased with open approaches, long-term results of objective neurosensory outcomes and subjective patient satisfaction are comparable. Johnson and Cilento (2) reported their experience with over 1,000 open browlift procedures and demonstrated excellent patient satisfaction and acceptably low rates of complications. Although a trend toward the increasing use of open approaches and a decline of endoscopic approaches have been noted in experienced facial plastic surgeons, the novice surgeon must recognize the value and utility of the endoscopic approach in the treatment of the aging forehead (32,33). However, it is an acknowledgement that each patient must be assessed as an individual, taking into account the hairline, skin type, degree of rhytids, brow position, and the individual's aesthetic goals before a surgical treatment can be recommended.

Adjuvant treatments also are an important aspect of rejuvenating the upper one-third of the face. Botox has clearly changed how this region is addressed, as it provides excellent effacement of dynamic rhytids and, thus, reduces the need to be as aggressive about performing surgical myoplasty. Filler materials based on hyaluronic acid such as Juvederm (Allergan Inc., Irvine, CA) or Restylane (Medicis Aesthetics, Scottsdale, AZ) provide a longer-lasting option to patients than did collagen, and future materials will likely continue to extend the duration of the efficacy of fillers. Finally, resurfacing techniques, whether they be chemical, laser, or light based (i.e., intense pulsed light), provide a solution to the finer rhytids of the skin. Skin surfacing serves to be synergistic with the effects of surgical treatments to the forehead. As resurfacing modalities continue to improve, so will the final results we will be able deliver to our patients.

HIGHLIGHTS

■ The eyebrow is the key landmark in forehead aesthetics. Its passive and dynamic characteristics, gender differences, and changes with aging are important factors in selecting the appropriate rejuvenation procedure.

■ The major categories of lifting procedures for upper facial rejuvenation are the coronal forehead lift, endoscopic forehead lift, and the direct eyebrow lift.

■ Modifications of each have specific indications.

■ The most commonly used techniques today are the trichophytic forehead lift, endoscopic lift, and direct brow lift.

■ Accurate diagnosis of each patient's specific complaints and findings is needed so that the correct procedure can be chosen.

■ The resultant scars should be explained in detail so that the patient can help choose the ideal procedure.

■ A complete ophthalmologic examination is required for patients who have had previous upper blepharoplasty or in whom an upper blepharoplasty is to be

performed concomitant with forehead or brow lifting. Specific attention to dry-eye problems and conservative surgery are indicated.

■ All incisions must be made to maintain hair follicle integrity and to avoid the first branch of the trigeminal nerve and the frontal branch of the facial nerve.

■ For long-lasting results, elevation of the forehead flap over the supraorbital margin and galeal suspension are required. In direct brow-lifting procedures and their modifications, the orbicularis oculi muscle must be suspended to the periosteum.

■ To maintain a smooth forehead contour, incise rather than excise the procerus and frontalis muscles.

■ When redraping, overcorrect to allow the inevitable stretch-back.

■ Forehead procedures may be indicated in patients who are not usually considered candidates, including young women who have premature ptosis of the eyebrows and men who do not have male-pattern baldness or are candidates for hair transplants.

■ Botox and fillers, especially hyaluronic acids, are excellent nonsurgical tools for rejuvenation of the aging forehead.

REFERENCES

1. Matros E, Garcia JA, Yaremchuk MJ. Changes in eyebrow position and shape with aging. *Plast Reconstr Surg* 2009;124(4): 1296–1301.
2. Cilento BW, Johnson CM Jr. The case for open forehead rejuvenation: a review of 1004 procedures. *Arch Facial Plast Surg* 2009;11(1):13–17.
3. Isse NG. Endoscopic forehead lift. Presented at: Annual Meeting of the Los Angeles County Society of Plastic Surgeons, September 12 1992, Los Angeles, CA.
4. Knize DM. Anatomic concepts for brow lift procedures. *Plast Reconstr Surg* 2009;124:2118–2126.
5. Ridgway JM, Larrabee WF. Anatomy for blepharoplasty and brow-lift. *Facial Plast Surg* 2010;26(3):177–185.
6. Pham S, Wilhelmi B, Mowlavi A. Eyebrow peak position redefined. *Aesthet Surg J* 2010;30(3):297–300.
7. Karimi K, Adamson PA. Patient analysis and selection in aging face surgery. *Facial Plast Surg* 2011;27(1):5–15.
8. Becking AG, et al. Transgender feminization of the facial skeleton. *Clin Plast Surg* 2007;34(3):557–564.
9. Carruthers JD, Carruthers A. Facial sculpting and tissue augmentation. *Dermatol Surg* 2005;31(11 Pt 2):1604–1612.
10. Chiu ES, Baker DC. Endoscopic brow lift: a retrospective review of 628 consecutive cases over 5 years. *Plast Reconstr Surg* 2003;112(2):628–633.
11. Dayan SH, Perkins SW, Vartarian AJ, et al. The forehead lift: endoscopic versus coronal approaches. *Aesthet Plast Surg* 2001;25(1):35–39.
12. Elkwood A, Matarasso A, Rankin M, et al. National plastic surgery survey: brow lifting techniques and complications. *Plast Reconstr Surg* 2001;108(7):2143–2150.
13. Guillot JM, Rousso DE, Replogle W. Forehead and scalp sensation after brow-lift: a comparison between open and endoscopic techniques. *Arch Facial Plast Surg* 2011;13(2):109–116.
14. Adamson PA, Cormier R, McGraw BL. The coronal forehead lift: modifications and results. *J Otolaryngol* 1992;21(1):25–29.

15. Adamson PA. The forehead lift: refinements in surgical technique. *J Otolaryngol* 1986;15(2):89–93.
16. Warren RJ. The modified lateral brow lift. *Aesthet Surg J* 2009;29(2):158–166.
17. Niamtu J III. The subcutaneous brow- and forehead-lift: a face-lift for the forehead and brow. *Dermatol Surg* 2008;34(10):1350–1361.
18. Georgescu D, Anderson RL, McCann JD. Brow ptosis correction: a comparison of five techniques. *Facial Plast Surg* 2010;26(3):186–192.
19. Langsdon PR, Williams GB, Rajan R, et al. Transblepharoplasty brow suspension with a biodegradable fixation device. *Aesthet Surg J* 2010;30(6):802–809.
20. Niu A, Euda K, Okazaki M, et al. New eyebrow lift technique using a semiautomatic suture device (maniceps) for patients with facial paralysis. *Ann Plast Surg* 2000;45(6):601–606.
21. Cook TA, Brownrigg PJ, Wang TD, et al. The versatile midforehead brow lift. *Arch Otolaryngol Head Neck Surg* 1989;115(2):163–168.
22. McCord C. Commentary on: browpexy through the upper lid: a new technique of lifting the brow with a standard blepharoplasty incision. *Aesthet Surg J* 2011;31(2):170.
23. Puig CM, LaFerriere KA. A retrospective comparison of open and endoscopic brow-lifts. *Arch Facial Plast Surg* 2002;4(4):221–225.
24. Bryne PJ. Efficacy and safety of endotine fixation device in endoscopic brow-lift. *Arch Facial Plast Surg* 2007;9:212–214.
25. Malata CM, Abood A. Experience with cortical tunnel fixation in endoscopic brow lift: the "bevel and slide" modification. *Int J Surg* 2009;7:510–515.
26. Morrison C, Zins J. An alternative approach to brow lift fixation: temporoparietal fascia, galeal, and periosteal imbrication. *Plast Reconstr Surg* 2007;120:1433–1434; author reply 1434–1435.
27. Pascali M, Gualdi A, Bottini DJ, et al. An original application of the Endotine Ribbon device for brow lift. *Plast Reconstr Surg* 2009;124:1652–1661.
28. Punthakee X, Keller GS, Vose JG, et al. New technologies in aesthetic blepharoplasty and brow-lift surgery. *Facial Plast Surg* 2010;26:260–265.
29. Sclafani AP, Fozo MS, Romo T III, et al. Strength and histological characteristics of periosteal fixation to bone after elevation. *Arch Facial Plast Surg* 2003;5:63–66.
30. Romo T III, Sclafani AP, Yung RT, et al. Endoscopic foreheadplasty: a histologic comparison of periosteal refixation after endoscopic versus bicoronal lift. *Plast Reconstr Surg* 2000;105:1111–1117.
31. Thomas JR, Lee AS, Patel AB. Brow-lift: subgaleal vs subperiosteal flap adherence in the rabbit model. *Arch Facial Plast Surg* 2007;9:101–105.
32. Fisher O, Zamboni WA. Endoscopic brow-lift in the male patient. *Arch Facial Plast Surg* 2010;12(1):56–59.
33. Chowdhury S, Malhotra R, Smith R, et al. Patient and surgeon experience with the endotine forehead device for brow and forehead lift. *Ophthal Plast Reconstr Surg* 2007;23(5):358–362.

186 Upper Eyelid Blepharoplasty

Jonathan M. Sykes   *Christina K. Magill*

Upper eyelid blepharoplasty is a common and often straightforward procedure; however, there are multiple considerations that need to be applied to each patient having surgery of the upper eyelid in order to ensure safety and optimal results. It is critical that the patient's underlying concerns and pathology are identified prior to surgery. A patient who desires cosmetic upper eyelid blepharoplasty must be counseled appropriately about realistic expectations, recovery time, and the details of elective surgery. The older patient who presents primarily with a complaint of decreased vision must be properly diagnosed: is there a change in visual acuity or ocular insult? Is *brow ptosis* or *blepharoptosis* contributing to the problem? Is the peripheral loss of vision primarily from excessive upper eyelid skin, also known as *dermatochalasis*? A proper assessment of the patient's desires and applied anatomy will maximize surgical outcomes and minimize complications. Success in upper eyelid blepharoplasty is guided by an understanding of surgical anatomy, patient motivational and medical history, the use of preoperative photography, appropriate surgical technique, and avoiding potential complications. This chapter outlines the preoperative considerations and surgical techniques for upper eyelid blepharoplasty.

SURGICAL ANATOMY

To perform upper eyelid blepharoplasty, a thorough understanding of the upper eyelid–brow complex, cross-sectional anatomy of the upper eyelid, and anatomic composition of the eyelid crease is necessary (Fig. 186.1) (1). The eyebrow and the upper eyelid skin constitute the *upper eyelid–brow complex*. The upper eyelid–brow complex moves the eyelid during expression and serves a functional role. The frontalis muscle acts on the brow as an elevator, and the orbicularis oculi acts on the brow as a depressor during eye closure and facial expression. When evaluating the eyebrow, it is important to evaluate brow height, inclination, and orientation (2). The brow lies along the supraorbital rim in men in a relatively straight position. In women, the hair of the brow arches above the superior orbital rim at its lateral extent. As individuals age, the frontalis muscle can become atrophic and lax, allowing the brow to descend. In some patients, placing a finger on the eyebrow and returning it to its more youthful position may correct excess upper eyelid skin or loss of peripheral vision that would not be corrected with upper eyelid blepharoplasty alone (3).

In addition to evaluation of the upper eyelid–brow complex, an understanding of the tissue layers of the upper eyelid is critical to successfully perform upper eyelid blepharoplasty. There are several tissue layers in the upper eyelid, which are (from superficial to deep) skin, *orbicularis oculi muscle, orbital septum, preaponeurotic fat*, the *levator aponeurosis, Müller muscle*, and the *tarsus* and *conjunctiva*. A sagittal section of the upper lid can help illustrate the levels and depths of the upper lid retractors, fat compartments, and the tarsal plate (Fig. 186.2) (1).

The sectional anatomy of the upper eyelid begins with the skin. The upper eyelid skin is the thinnest skin in the body and is less than 500 microns thick. The skin of the upper eyelid is the thickest superiorly and the thinnest at the ciliary margin. Excess upper eyelid skin is often what patients wish to be surgically corrected.

Beneath the thin upper eyelid skin is the orbicularis oculi muscle. This muscle has a radial, sphincter-like pattern around the eye and is considered part of the *superficial musculoaponeurotic system*, mainly innervated by the zygomatic branch of the facial nerve. The muscle acts to close the eye, narrow the palpebral opening, and squint. The lateral ocular rhytids, or smile-lines that can appear in the skin over time, are perpendicular to the underlying orbicularis oculi muscle. The orbicularis oculi muscle can be very thin and easily incised along with the skin incision. Conversely, the orbicularis oculi muscle can also

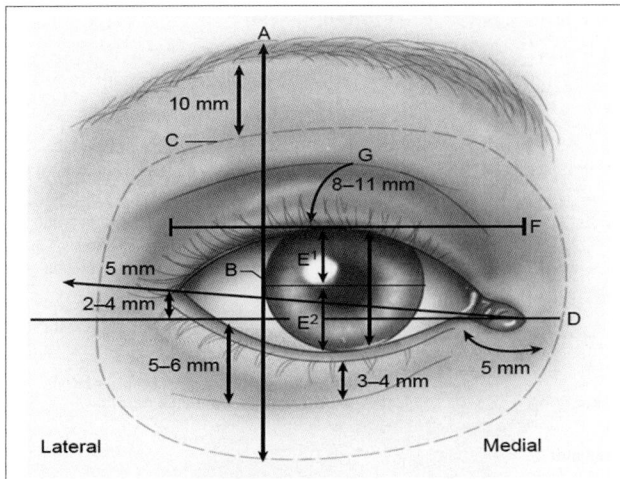

Figure 186.1 Topographic anatomy of the eyelids and eyebrow. (A) A vertical line drawn tangent to (B) the lateral limbus demarcates the highest point of the eyebrow. The inferior hair-bearing line of the eyebrow typically rests 10 mm above the superior orbital rim. (C) The orbit boundaries. (D) The lateral canthus is positioned 2 to 4 mm superior to the level of the medial canthus. (E^1) The MRD_1 is measured from the upper eyelid margin to the corneal light reflex at the level of the pupil. (E^2) The lower eyelid margin measured to the corneal light reflex is the MRD_2. The intrapalpebral distance is measured as $MRD_1 + MRD_2$ and ranges from 9 to 12 mm. (F) The palpebral width ranges from 28 to 30 mm. (G) The upper eyelid height ranges from 8 to 11 mm, depending on gender and ethnicity. (Adapted from Most SP, Mobley SR, Larrabee WF Jr. Anatomy of the eyelids. *Facial Plast Surg Clin North Am* 2005;13(4):487–492.)

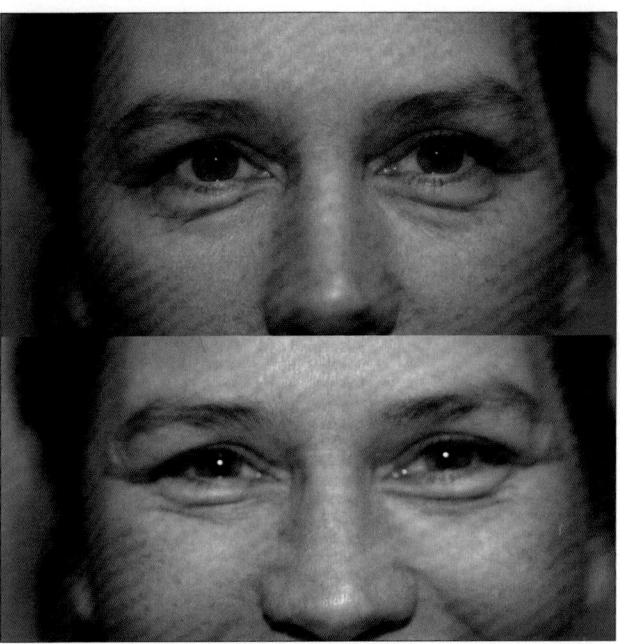

Figure 186.3 Orbicularis oculi muscle hyperfunction. Static and dynamic excess eyelid squeeze are shown.

be hypertrophic, causing lid thickening and excess eyelid squeeze (Fig. 186.3).

The tissues that lie deep to the orbicularis oculi vary from superior to inferior and include the frontal bone, orbital septum, and tarsal plate. At the level of the brow, the orbicularis oculi muscle is superficial to the frontal bone and the superior orbital rim. Inferiorly, the orbicularis oculi muscle lies superficial to the orbital septum above

and the tarsus below. Three surgical designations of the orbicularis oculi exist according to the tissue beneath the muscle: there is an *orbital*, *preseptal*, and *pretarsal* portion (Fig. 186.4) (4). The fibrous tarsal plate is approximately 8 to 9 mm in height and acts as a skeletal component that shapes and supports the arch of the lid. In addition, the tarsal plate contains *meibomian glands* at its inferior border. There are several layers of the upper eyelid that fuse and insert onto the tarsal plate, including the orbital septum and upper eyelid retractors.

The orbital septum begins superiorly at the superior orbital rim as a reflection of the frontal bone periosteum.

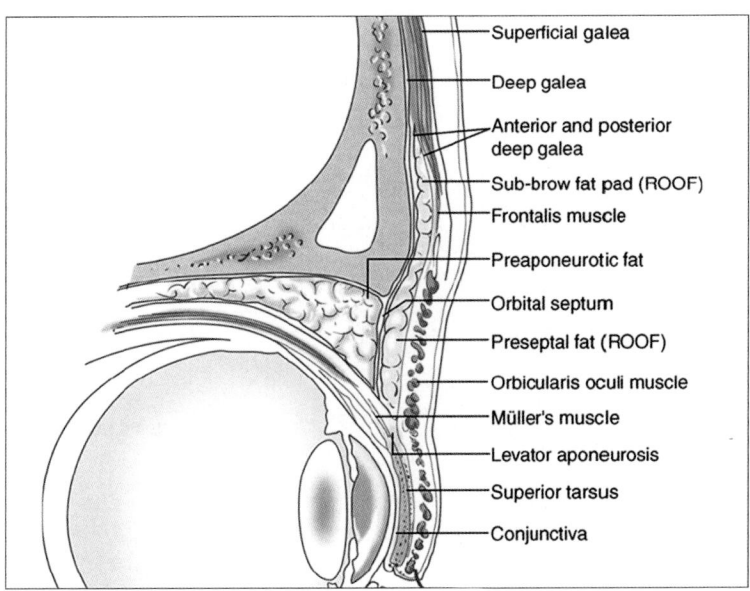

- Superficial galea
- Deep galea
- Anterior and posterior deep galea
- Sub-brow fat pad (ROOF)
- Frontalis muscle
- Preaponeurotic fat
- Orbital septum
- Preseptal fat (ROOF)
- Orbicularis oculi muscle
- Müller's muscle
- Levator aponeurosis
- Superior tarsus
- Conjunctiva

Figure 186.2 Sagittal section through orbit and upper eyelid. The superficial to deep anatomy of the upper eyelid is demonstrated. The thin upper eyelid skin overlies the orbicularis oculi muscle. Deep to the orbicularis oculi muscle is the orbital septum, which contains the preaponeurotic fat. The upper eyelid retractors are beneath the fat pad and consist of the levator aponeurosis and Müller muscle. (Adapted from Most SP, Mobley SR, Larrabee WF Jr. Anatomy of the eyelids. *Facial Plast Surg Clin North Am* 2005;13(4):487–492.)

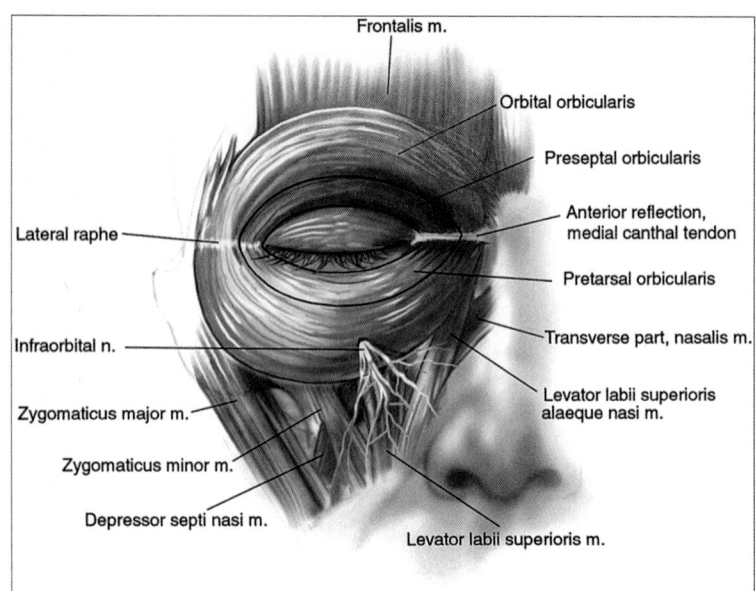

Figure 186.4 Periorbital musculature. The orbital, preseptal, and pretarsal segments of the orbicularis oculi muscle are shown. The frontalis muscle inserts at the level of the supraorbital rim and acts to elevate the eyebrow. (Adapted from Codner MA, Ford DT. Blepharoplasty. In: Thorne CH, et al, eds. *Grabb and Smith's plastic surgery.* 6th ed. Philadelphia, PA: Lippincott Williams & Wilkins, 2007.)

This reflection of the septum orbitale is called the *arcus marginalis.* The orbital septum has a white appearance (in contrast to the pink color of the orbicularis muscle) and acts as a barrier to infection. As the orbital septum becomes lax with age, underlying fat can prolapse anteriorly and inferiorly, and this can cause visible bulges beneath the thin eyelid skin.

The orbital contents contained by the orbital septum include preaponeurotic fat and the lacrimal gland. The preaponeurotic fat includes a medial fat pad and a central fat pad (Fig. 186.5) (4). The fat pads, in addition to the lacrimal gland, can all descend as the orbital septum connective tissue relaxes with aging. The prolapse of fat can create bulging beneath the thin upper eyelid skin (5). The preaponeurotic fat pads can also become prominent in *blepharochalasis,* a condition marked by intermittent eyelid edema.

Deep to the preaponeurotic fat are the muscular upper eyelid retractors. The upper eyelid retractors include the *levator palpebrae superioris muscle* (levator muscle) and *Müller muscle.* The primary upper eyelid retractor is the levator muscle, which is suspended by the superior transverse (*Whitnall ligament*). Whitnall ligament extends from the fascia of the lacrimal gland laterally to the trochlea attachment medially. The ligament conceptually suspends the levator muscle and allows it to change directions (Fig. 186.6) (4). As the levator muscle descends from its superior condensation with Whitnall ligament, it becomes a thick aponeurosis that inserts onto the anterior face of the fibrous tarsal plate. The elevation of the tarsal plate by the levator muscle is controlled by motor fibers from the oculomotor nerve (cranial nerve III).

In contrast to the levator muscle, Müller muscle is an involuntary smooth muscle lid retractor that receives

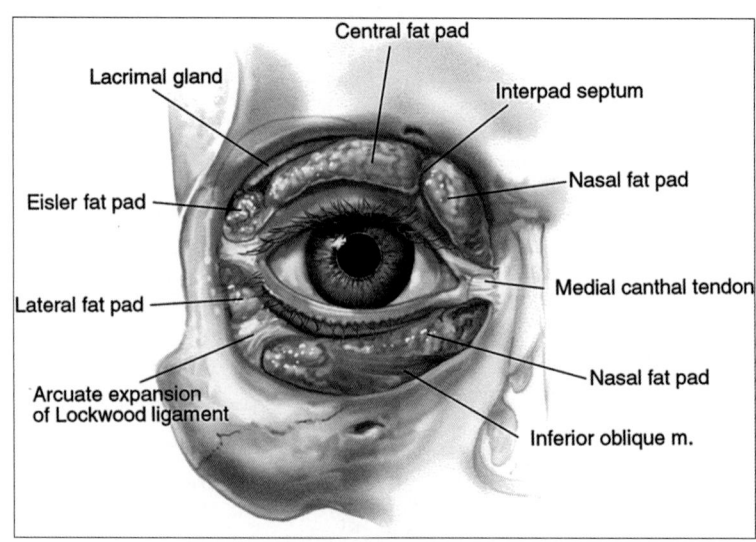

Figure 186.5 Postseptal orbital compartment. The nasal fat pad, central fat pad, and lacrimal gland are shown deep to the orbital septum. Prominent fat pads can be conservatively excised during upper eyelid blepharoplasty. (Adapted from Codner MA, Ford DT. Blepharoplasty. In: Thorne CH, et al, ed. *Grabb and Smith's plastic surgery.* 6th ed. Philadelphia, PA: Lippincott Williams & Wilkins, 2007.)

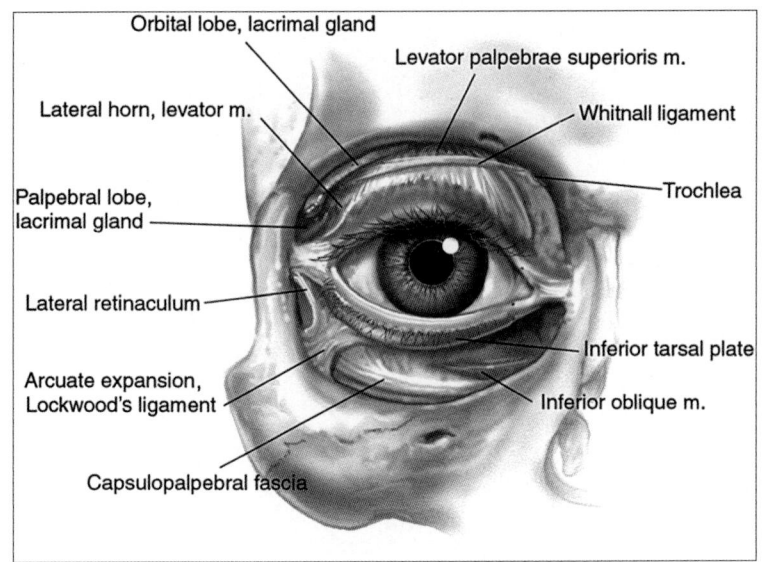

Orbital lobe, lacrimal gland

Levator palpebrae superioris m.

Lateral horn, levator m.

Whitnall ligament

Palpebral lobe, lacrimal gland

Trochlea

Lateral retinaculum

Inferior tarsal plate

Arcuate expansion, Lockwood's ligament

Inferior oblique m.

Capsulopalpebral fascia

Figure 186.6 Orbital suspensory attachments. The levator palpebrae superioris muscle is shown as it descends from Whitnall ligament to the anterior face of the tarsal plate. (Adapted from Codner MA, Ford DT. Blepharoplasty. In: Thorne CH, et al, ed. *Grabb and Smith's plastic surgery.* 6th ed. Philadelphia, PA: Lippincott Williams & Wilkins, 2007.)

sympathetic innervation. When sympathetic tone is absent, such as in *Horner syndrome*, the eyelid is noticeably ptotic by 2 mm. During dissection in the postseptal compartment of the upper eyelid, Müller muscle is found beneath the levator aponeurosis. An arcade of vessels travels on the anterior surface of Müller muscle.

The deepest layer of the upper eyelid is the conjunctiva, a clear mucous membrane that provides lubrication and protection to the sclera. The conjunctiva consists of a *tarsal* component that lines the undersurface of the eyelids, *fornix*, the apex of the orbit/eyelid junction, and a *bulbar* component that adjoins the sclera of the globe. Preserving the conjunctiva helps protect against corneal damage.

A component of the periorbital anatomy that deserves special mention is the composition of the upper eyelid crease. In Caucasian individuals, the upper eyelid crease is formed as the levator aponeurosis inserts onto the anterior surface of the tarsal plate, approximately 2 to 5 mm from its superior border, and has further insertions into the overlying skin at this level. Visually, these insertions create a fold in the upper eyelid that is usually 8 to 11 mm above the lid margin in women and 6 to 9 mm above the eyelid margin in men. In contrast to the Caucasian upper eyelid, the Asian eyelid has a crease that is much closer to the eyelid margin due to the orbital septum fusing with the levator aponeurosis above or at the level of the tarsal plate (Fig. 186.7) (6). With this difference in orbital septum insertion, in addition to lower or absent skin attachments, the fold of the upper eyelid obscures a prominent crease in the Asian eyelid.

EVALUATION

Motivational History

Patients who seek upper eyelid blepharoplasty generally have functional problems or aesthetic problems. Often,

both functional and aesthetic issues coexist. It is important to identify the goals and concerns of the patient in order to formulate the correct treatment plan.

In the patient who presents with a complaint of decreased vision, the consultation should begin with a thorough history of the problem. Patients who suffer from brow ptosis or dermatochalasis associated with aging often recount a gradual loss in their peripheral vision. Some patients will report that when they lift up their eyelids or eyebrows, they can see normally again. For other patients, visual acuity may be so poor at baseline that no manipulation of the periorbital skin improves their visual fields. For these patients, the risks of surgery may outweigh any benefits. As the visit proceeds, four patient assessment questions must be answered: (a) What is the brow position? (b) Is there any upper eyelid ptosis? (c) What is the baseline visual acuity? (d) Is the patient a candidate for elective surgery?

In addition to visual complaints, patients request upper eyelid blepharoplasty for aesthetic reasons. Communication with patients desiring a change in the appearance of their upper eyelid is of paramount importance. It is essential to understand what the patient's expectations are from the procedure and to manage these in such a way that a realistic outcome is conveyed and understood. Patients may desire a removal of excess skin or fat, or an alteration in the shape or position of the upper eyelid crease. The extra time devoted to managing the expectations of a cosmetic patient is always time well spent.

Medical History

It is important to obtain a thorough preoperative medical history. For patients undergoing blepharoplasty, it is important to evaluate for any underlying connective tissue or bleeding disorder that will affect the outcome of the surgery or lead to poor results. Patients need to be asked

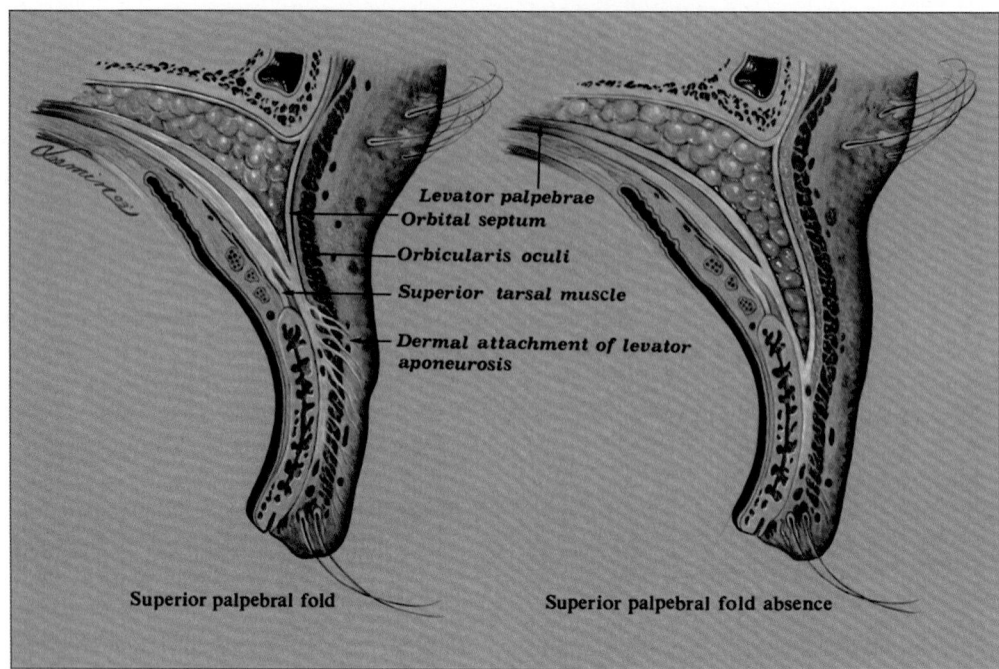

Figure 186.7 The upper eyelid crease. Anatomical variations can result in the absence of the upper eyelid crease. On the left, a sagittal section represents the Caucasian upper eyelid, with dermal attachments extending from the levator aponeurosis to the skin, resulting in an upper eyelid crease. On the right, the lower insertion of the orbital septum on the levator aponeurosis and lack of extensions into the dermis result in the absence of the upper eyelid crease. (Adapted from Chen SH, Mardini S, Chen HC, et al. Strategies for a successful corrective Asian blepharoplasty after previously failed revisions. *Plast Reconstr Surg* 2004;114(5):1270–1277.)

about a history of bleeding with prior surgeries and blood pressure control and asked to stop any elective anticoagulant medication 5 days prior to the operation. Any herbal medications known to have an anticoagulant effect must also be stopped 2 weeks prior to surgery. Patients must discontinue supplements containing vitamin E, ginkgo, fish oil, garlic, and any substance that may pose extra risk. A smoking history is also important to obtain, as cigarette smokers are at higher risk for poor wound healing.

An ocular history must also be included in the evaluation of a patient seeking blepharoplasty. This includes any previous eye surgeries, refractive eye surgery, and a history of glaucoma, cataracts, or ocular trauma. If the patient has a known "dry eye syndrome," this is also important to note, as this may place them at higher risk for postoperative corneal abrasion and serious eye exposure problems. Patients who have undergone a previous blepharoplasty will have expectant scar tissue and mandate a conservative approach to avoid excessive *lagophthalmos* or scleral show.

Physical Exam

Upper blepharoplasty is an elective procedure. Any physical exam of a patient desiring blepharoplasty should begin with a global assessment of the patient's general health and well-being, and the examiner should draw a conclusion about the patient's candidacy for elective surgery. The physician should assess the character of the facial skin

and global changes of aging. It is also important to note the solar changes of the skin and to note any suspicious skin lesions over the face that may warrant further attention. The physical exam should proceed with evaluation of visual acuity and a neurologic exam. Following this, a periocular exam should be done, including an evaluation of symmetry, brow position, eyelid skin, upper eyelid height, fat prolapse, and levator function. As one examines each of these factors, a treatment plan can be formulated.

Assessing visual fields and visual acuity are an important part of the preoperative exam. Patients will often report a change in their visual fields from drooping of the brow or upper eyelid. Documenting visual field changes is important prior to upper eyelid blepharoplasty. A superior visual field loss of 20% or 15 degrees is often required for insurance coverage. Patients can undergo visual field testing in a neutral position and then with their eyelids or brows suspended upward with tape to document potential gains from the surgery. Methods of visual field testing can include using an automated visual field technique or tangent screen technique in which a patient is seated 3 feet from a target that is advanced closer to the patient until it comes into view for the tested eye. These exams can be done in conjunction with the patient's ophthalmologist (7).

The patient's vision prior to surgery may determine their candidacy for elective upper eyelid blepharoplasty. If a patient is legally blind or has dismal visual acuity at the time of consultation, the functional improvements from performing the surgery may be nominal. Any previously undiagnosed or undocumented changes in visual acuity or baseline vision should be formally assessed by an ophthalmologist prior to any elective surgery.

Along with an assessment of vision, the patient should undergo a standard neurological exam, with attention to pupillary reaction and extraocular muscle function. Lid tone and movement should be carefully examined, with care to note any ptosis, or the presence of poor eyelid closure or scleral show from a weakness in the facial nerve. Sensation of the eye can be tested by performing a corneal reflex exam.

In addition to an assessment of vision and a neurologic evaluation, a periocular exam is done to formulate a treatment plan for the patient and identify what pathology is present. A periocular exam includes the evaluation of symmetry, brow position, quality of the eyelid skin, upper eyelid height, fat prolapse, and levator function.

Upper eyelid symmetry is important aesthetically and functionally. The surgeon can strive to measure and create symmetric upper eyelid height and to create bilateral scars that are of equal length and position. The patient and surgeon should discuss facial asymmetries before surgery and understand that baseline asymmetries may persist after the operation.

As part of the periocular exam, the brow position needs to be carefully noted. In men, the maximal point of brow height should occur in the midpupillary line, and the brow should be oriented relatively straight along the superior orbital rim. In women, the maximal brow height should occur at the level of the lateral limbus, with the brow lying slightly above the superior orbital rim and having a temporal arch. Noting the brow position helps to diagnose what changes and underlying conditions are contributing to a patient's decrease in peripheral vision or what is causing them to have excess skin laxity of the upper eyelid. If raising the brow to its natural anatomic or youthful position improves an individual's visual fields or cosmetic complaints, the patient may benefit the most from a brow lift alone or a brow lift in conjunction with upper eyelid blepharoplasty.

Following an exam of the brow, the quality of the upper eyelid skin is assessed. Excess and atrophic skin is common in the senile upper eyelid. The removal of redundant skin should not alter the position of the upper eyelid margin. Conversely, some patients may have limited upper eyelid skin, a preexisting condition causing lagophthalmos, or scleral show. Removal of skin in these patients may cause problems associated with corneal exposure.

An assessment of the upper eyelid height and crease is an important part of the periocular exam. The upper eyelid can be obscured by excess skin, can have an absent crease, or can be excessively long or blunted. The ideal upper eyelid crease height is 8 to 11 mm in women and 6 to 9 mm in men. In patients who have an absent crease, such as in the Asian eyelid, the underlying orbital septum may insert at the superior edge of the tarsus, or low along the tarsal border, and the levator aponeurosis may lack any dermal attachments (Fig. 186.7). These anatomic relationships can be altered surgically to create a crease. An excessively long or blunted crease can be a result of underlying ptosis, previous blepharoplasty, or loss of fat and periorbital volume.

The periorbital fat can bulge and prolapse beneath the thin upper eyelid skin as the orbital septum weakens with age. The removal of fat depends on the patient's anatomy and the goals of the operation. A "hollowed" look can often result from overaggressive fat excision. In contrast to the lower eyelid, which has a medial, central, and lateral fat compartment, the upper eyelid has only a medial and central compartment, with the lateral space occupied by the lacrimal gland. Any one of these compartments, and the lacrimal gland itself, may contribute to the appearance of excessive skin and volume descent in the upper eyelid. The assessment of prolapsed fat and possible asymmetries between the upper eyelid fat compartments should be noted with the patient preoperatively, and expectations and goals should be clarified.

In addition to fat prolapse, the position and mobility of the eyelid margin needs to be examined. It is important to assess any level of upper eyelid ptosis and the levator function in all patients undergoing upper blepharoplasty. Many patients who desire upper blepharoplasty or are referred for decreased central and/or peripheral vision will suffer from blepharoptosis (ptosis). The otolaryngologist needs to know how to assess both the degree and amount of ptosis and the function of the levator mechanism. In broad terms, ptosis is an abnormally low upper eyelid margin with the eye in primary gaze. Ptosis can be either congenital, in which the levator muscle usually does not function properly, or acquired, in which the levator aponeurosis has become dehiscent, or has lax insertions to the anterior tarsal plate. In acquired or involutional ptosis, the muscle will still function, but will not provide the level of lid lift to accommodate the patient's visual fields.

The physical examination for ptosis and levator function begins with a measurement of the relationship of the upper eyelid margin to the central corneal light reflex. A penlight can be used to create the reflex, and a measuring tape can be used to assess the *marginal reflex distance* (MRD_1), or the distance between the edge of the upper eyelid and the reflex. In patients without ptosis, a normal measurement for this is approximately 4 to 5 mm. The distance between the optimal eyelid level and the actual level is the amount of ptosis. The MRD_2 is the distance from the lower eyelid margin to the central corneal reflex, and it is by adding the MRD_1 and MRD_2 together that the opening of the eye or *palpebral fissure* can be measured. The average palpebral fissure will measure approximately 9 mm.

Activation of the levator muscle results in retraction of the upper eyelid, with a resultant increase in the palpebral opening. Levator function can be measured by holding the eyebrow in place to isolate the eyelid retractors and asking the patient to close the eye or look down, followed by performing an extreme upgaze (Fig. 186.8). A measuring tape can be used in the extreme upgaze position to document the distance between downgaze and upgaze. The maximal excursion of the upper lid, or levator function, is normally greater than 15 mm. Levator function between 12 and 15 mm is considered good, and less than 9 mm of function is poor. If the levator function is abnormal, a diagnosis other than acquired/involutional ptosis needs to be considered, and the differential diagnosis includes an extended list of neurological, autoimmune, neoplastic, endocrine, genetic, and connective tissue disorders. The assessment of levator function and the diagnosis of ptosis is a critical part of the

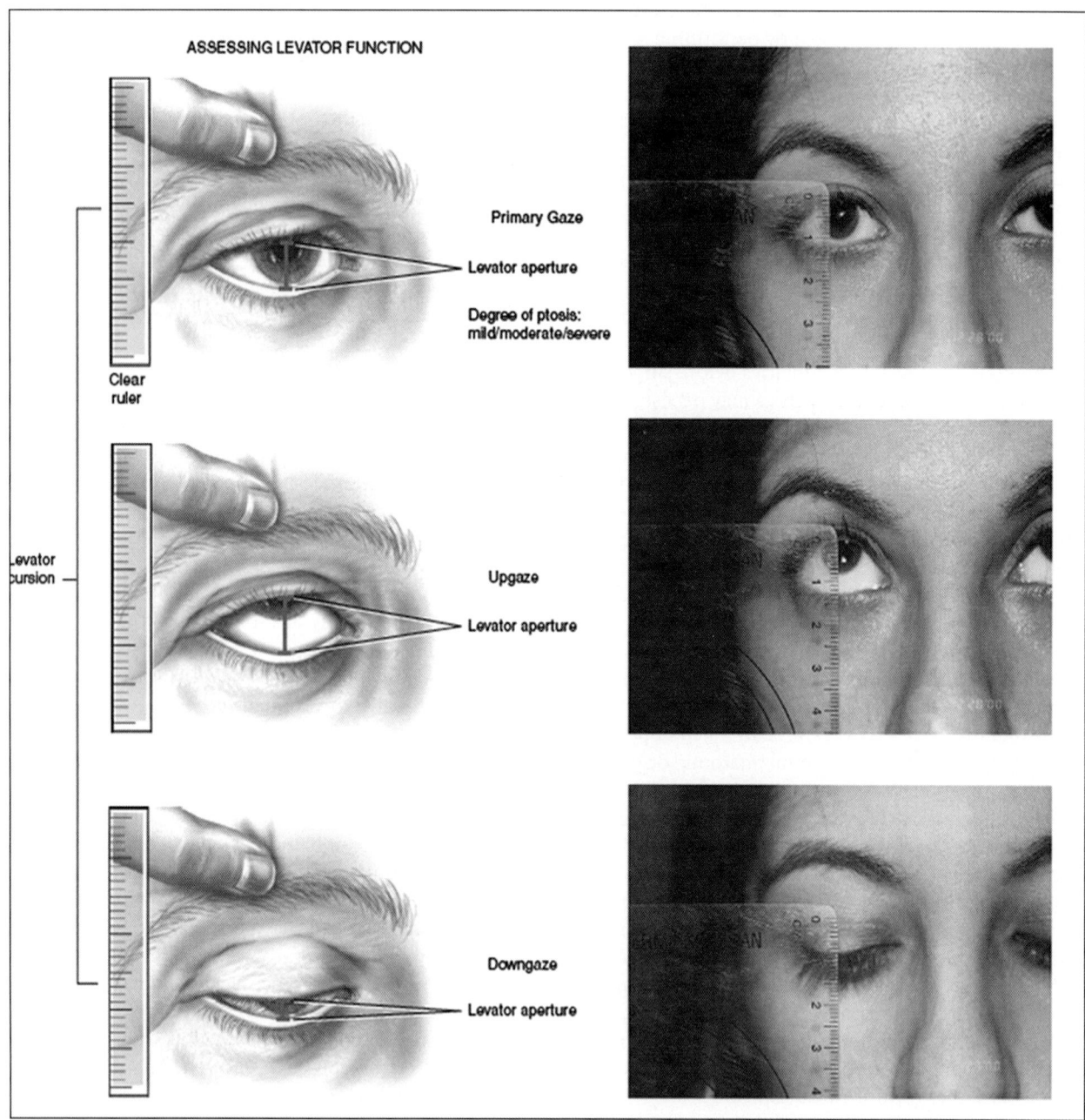

Figure 186.8 Testing levator function. In order to correctly diagnose and treat the underlying cause of ptosis, levator function is assessed. This is done by measuring the palpebral aperture in neutral position, downgaze, and upgaze. The maximal excursion of the upper lid, or levator function, is normally greater than 15 mm. (Adapted from Newman ML, Spinelli HM. Reconstruction of the eyelids, correction of ptosis, and canthoplasty. In: Thorne CH, et al. eds. *Grabb and Smith's plastic surgery.* 6th ed. Philadelphia, PA: Lippincott Williams & Wilkins, 2007. From Spinelli HM. Ptosis and upper eyelid retraction. In: Spinelli HM, ed. *Atlas of aesthetic eyelid and periocular surgery.* Philadelphia, PA: Elsevier, 2004:96.)

ocular physical exam. The surgical correction for ptosis is markedly different than simply performing an upper eyelid blepharoplasty and may involve reinsertion of the levator aponeurosis onto the anterior surface of the tarsal plate to achieve the desired result.

PHOTOGRAPHY

Preoperative photography not only aids the surgeon in devising the operative plan but may also be a prerequisite for insurance carriers. Photographs should include a frontal view of the face, in addition to standard lateral and oblique views. Close-up photos of the eyes in open and closed position help to document skin excess and fat prolapse, in addition to palpebral fissure and levator function. There are often preexisting asymmetries in the eyelids and periorbital fat that are obscured after the infiltration of local anesthetic, and preoperative photographs help to document these.

THE OPERATION

Every eyelid surgery should preoperatively define what the goals are, which may be to remove extra skin, change the skin contour, address excess muscle, remove or transpose fat, elevate the level of the upper eyelid margin, or alter the upper eyelid crease. The surgical techniques employed are organized around the goals. Upper eyelid blepharoplasty will not correct asymmetric brow or brow ptosis, lateral ocular rhytids or "crow's-feet," malar or cheek fat pad descent, or fine lines and wrinkles around the eye. These complaints can be addressed with a brow lift, the use of selective botulinum toxin (Fig. 186.9), midfacial or malar implants, deep plane facelifts, or skin resurfacing.

Surgical Technique

In patients who have the chief complaint of skin excess, the amount of extra skin removed is determined by a patient's anatomy. A 12-mm height of infrabrow skin needs to remain intact to allow adequate eyelid closure and to avoid eyelid margin malposition. The upper eyelid crease can be marked in the preoperative holding area or with the patient sitting up to achieve the greatest accuracy. The surgical markings should start with a central mark above the pupil at the level of the desired upper eyelid height. A second mark is made in the midpupillary line, directly above the initial mark which will determine the amount of skin removed. Between these two points is skin to be excised. It is critical that at least 20 mm of skin is left from the upper lid margin to the brow line or superior orbital rim in order to avoid lagophthalmos and preserve independent upper lid movement from the frontalis muscle.

After the two central marks are made, an ellipse is drawn out with medial and lateral limbs. The medial and lateral limbs should be checked for distance from the upper eyelid

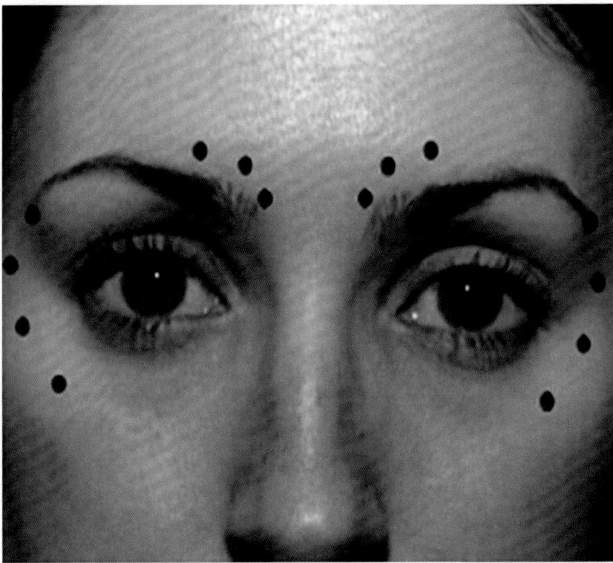

Figure 186.9 Sites of botulinum toxin injection for periocular rejuvenation. The *black dots* signify potential injection sites for botulinum toxin to treat glabellar rhytids and "crow's-feet," which are not addressed by surgery of the upper eyelid. (Adapted from Hetzler L, Sykes J. The brow and forehead in periocular rejuvenation. *Facial Plast Surg Clin North Am* 2010;18(3):375–384.)

margin, so that the distance along the inferior aspect of the incision stays relatively equidistant from the upper eyelid margin. A medial upcut or lateral triangulation can be included in the marking, according to surgeon preference, in order to aid in cosmetic closure. The lateral extent of the skin marking should remain medial to the lateral orbital rim and can be placed in a rhytid. After completing the skin markings, it is important to reexamine each mark for symmetry and to assure that adequate skin will remain after the skin excision is completed. It is at this time that moderate modifications of skin markings should be made. The patient can be asked to open and close the eyes to assess the markings for accuracy and symmetry (Fig. 186.10).

Monitored anesthesia care and local anesthetic are adequate for most patients undergoing upper eyelid blepharoplasty. The eyelid skin can be injected with 1% lidocaine, 1:100,000 epinephrine loaded into a 1-mL syringe with a 30-gauge needle. The tip of the needle is gently inserted into the upper eyelid with the goal of injecting between the skin and the muscle to avoid a hematoma. Small aliquots of local anesthetic can be delivered in the area to be excised, and pressure can be held over the injected area with gauze. The upper eyelid skin is very thin, and the injection should be very shallow. Approximately 1 to 1.5 mL of local anesthetic is injected into each upper eyelid.

Following the injection of local anesthesia, the patient is prepped and draped while the surgeon scrubs. The entire face should be included in the surgical field. A head wrap is placed, and the neck is toweled off. Because the upper eyelid skin is thin and lax, it can be difficult to make accurate incisions. For this reason, tension and countertension on the skin must be made by the surgeon and assistant to facilitate precise skin incision. The surgeon stands or sits at the patients head and makes the lower incision first with an assistant providing gentle countertraction on the upper lid. The skin incision can be made with a scalpel which provides clean wound edges. The upper limb is then incised, with an assistant providing gentle inferior countertraction on the area to be excised. If needed, the medial and lateral corners can be completed with scissors at the beginning of the dissection. After the skin is incised, the lateral corner of the incision is grasped with fine-tipped forceps. Using scissors, a plane directly beneath the skin is established. In addition to grasping forceps, the long finger of the nondominant hand can be used to provide medial pressure on the skin to be excised in order to facilitate the development of the proper plane. As the skin excision reaches its medial extent, a small upcut can be made at the corner of the ellipse to facilitate skin redraping for the closure (Fig. 186.10).

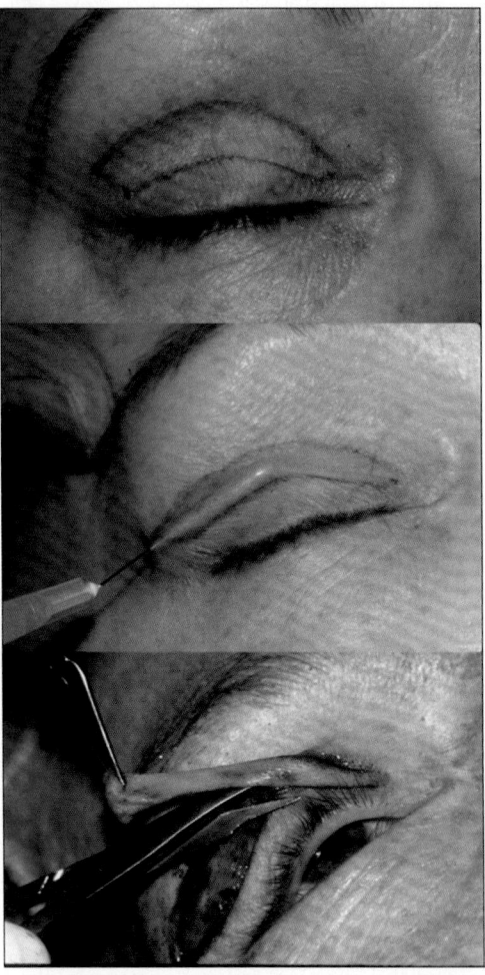

Figure 186.10 Operative technique in upper eyelid blepharoplasty. A right upper eyelid surgical marking is shown. There is a minimum of 12 mm of infrabrow skin preserved. Marking of the upper eyelid precedes the injection of local anesthestic, which is shown in the middle image. The strip of upper eyelid skin is then sharply excised **(bottom image)**, with care to preserve the underlying orbicularis oculi muscle.

In addition to the removal of skin, some patients may also need a strip of muscle excised. Many authors think that minimal or no muscle should be removed because muscle excision can cause dysfunction of the orbicularis oculi. However, in rare instance, muscle can be hypertrophic, causing excess squeeze on the upper eyelid and thickening (Fig. 186.3). In these cases, a strip of muscle can be removed.

Patients may have prolapsed upper eyelid fat pads that need to be addressed. Fat excision is accomplished after the excision of skin and begins with identifying the orbital septum. The orbital septum is beneath the orbicularis oculi muscle and contains the medial and central fat pads. A conservative approach is advised in order to avoid an aged or hollow appearance. The orbital septum can be opened over the fat pad of interest. The orbital septum is thin and pale and can be difficult to identify in some patients. If there is doubt about the location of the orbital septum, it is best to work superiorly instead of inferiorly to avoid damage to the levator aponeurosis at the level of the tarsus. Gentle pressure can be placed on the globe to exaggerate fat prolapse and identify the fat to be excised. The septum can be delicately teased off of the enderlying fat pad. The fat can be gently mobilized inferiorly and also superiorly toward the superior orbital rim. The central fat can be dissected off of the underlying levator aponeurosis. The fat pad is often covered by a delicate, thin capsule. This can be incised to reveal prominent yellow fat tissue. Patients will often require further injection with local anesthetic during this portion of the case. The base of the fat to be excised should be cauterized to avoid retraction of bleeding tissue. It is important not to remove all of the visible fat pad and to avoid excess traction on the fat as it is excised. This traction can cause trauma to deep vessels which may retract and later cause intraorbital hematoma. Traction on the orbital fat also misleads the surgeon into thinking deeper orbital fat needs resection. To remove fat from the medial compartment, the orbital septum can be opened medially with care to avoid the medial palpebral artery, which can cause brisk bleeding.

The levator aponeurosis lies beneath the orbital fat, and this can be repositioned in patients who desire a change in lid margin height or in the creation of an upper eyelid crease. For patients with involutional ptosis, whose upper eyelid margin is encroaching over the aperture of the pupil, the elevation of the upper eyelid may markedly improve vision. This is accomplished by identifying the preaponeurotic fat beneath the orbital septum and gently reflecting this superiorly. The levator aponeurosis will be visible under the fat, as a thickened, white condensation of muscle that travels inferiorly toward the tarsal plate. The patient can be asked to open the eye to confirm its location, as it will retract superiorly. At this point, if the levator aponeurosis is dehiscent from the tarsal plate, it can be reattached using medial, central, and lateral 4-0 Vicryl sutures. The suture can be thrown in a horizontal mattress fashion from the edge of the aponeurosis, to the anterior upper third of the tarsal plate. It is important not to pass any suture deep through the conjunctiva. The amount of lid elevation can be confirmed before the suture is secured by asking the patient to open the eye and examining the amount of distance achieved from the pupil and lid margin. The levator aponeurosis can also be sutured to the deep dermis at the level of a desired upper eyelid crease in Asian upper eyelid blepharoplasty (Fig. 186.11).

After all aspects of the upper eyelid blepharoplasty have been performed, the incisions are closed (Fig. 186.12). Due to the very thin nature of the upper eyelid skin, healing is usually rapid and results in a minimally visible scar. Despite the various type of surgical closures and suture materials, upper blepharoplasty incisions result in excellent scars. The overarching goal of closure is to facilitate good wound healing with a low risk of dehiscence and visible scar. The closure will create the neo-lid crease and can be done with a 7-0 nylon running suture with minimal grasp of the wound edges by the suture. Any areas of questionable strength can be reinforced with an interrupted stitch. Alternately, the wound can be closed with a running 6-0 fast gut suture with a central interrupted 6-0 suture placed for extra insurance against dehiscence. The suture line can be very delicate, and too much manipulation

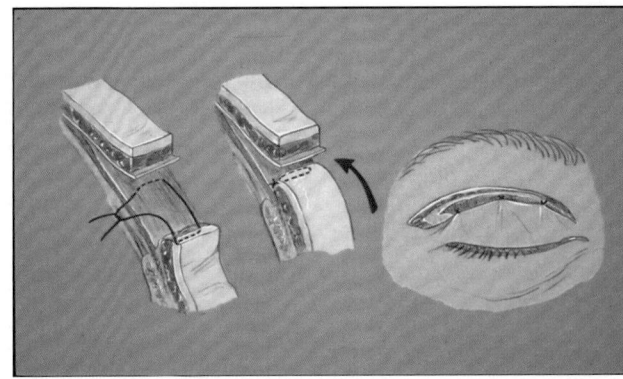

Figure 186.11 Creation of an upper eyelid crease. A sectioned upper eyelid is shown on the far left. The skin, orbicularis oculi muscle, and orbital septum have been dissected away from the levator aponeurosis. A horizontal mattress stitch has been placed superiorly in the levator aponeurosis and inferiorly in the deep dermis. In the middle image, the suture has been tightened. The image on the far right demonstrates the formation of the new upper eyelid crease after suturing.

postoperatively can lead to wound problems. Patients are advised to avoid rubbing the eyes and to abstain from vigorous physical activity in the postoperative period. Ice can help with bruising and swelling.

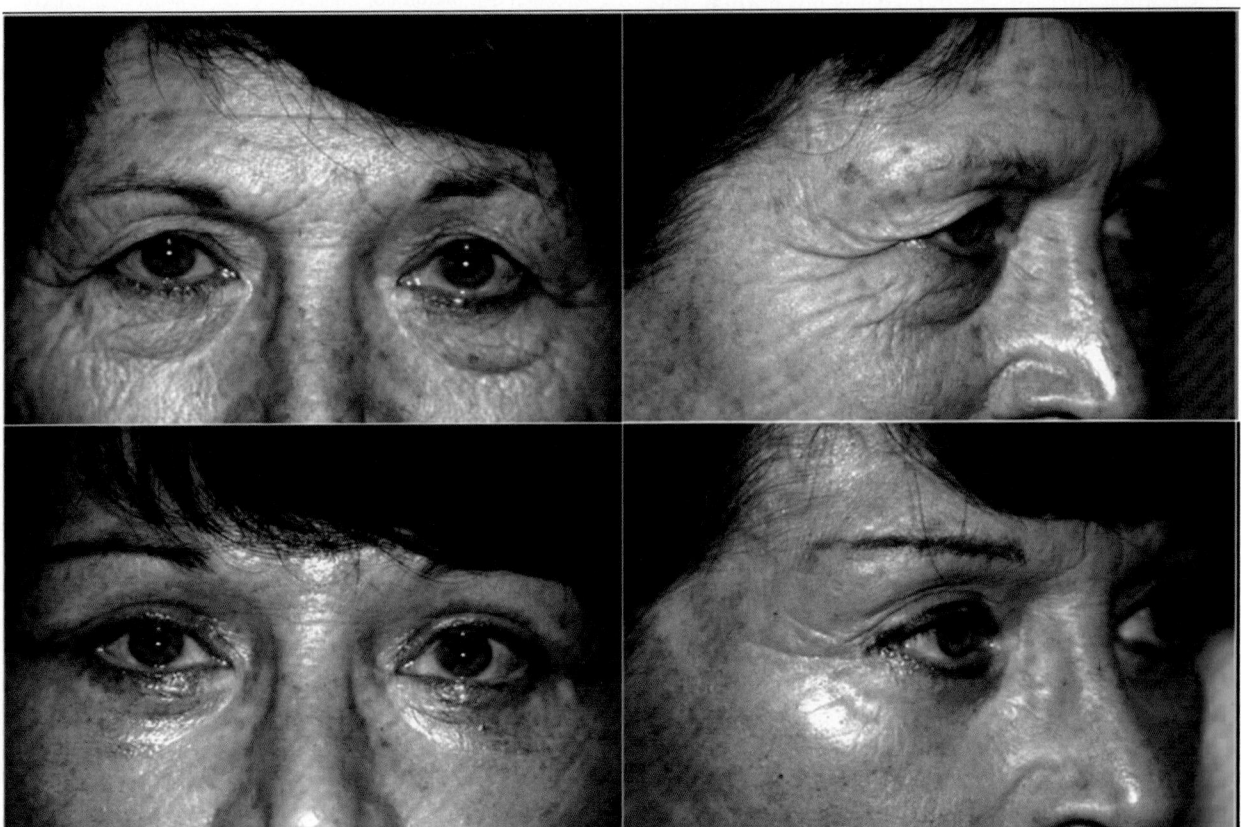

Figure 186.12 Preoperative and postoperative photographs after blepharoplasty. **(Top)** Preoperative frontal and oblique views of the eyes are shown, demonstrating dermatochalasis and global changes of aging. **(Bottom)** There is youthful restoration of the periorbital skin following bilateral upper and lower blepharoplasties.

COMPLICATIONS

Complications of upper eyelid blepharoplasty are rare and include bleeding, infection, and the need for revision surgery (8). Asymmetry between the two upper eyelids is the most common complication, and this is best avoided with careful preoperative markings. Preexisting asymmetries in lid position or brow position may contribute to postoperative asymmetry. The interruption of the orbicularis oculi can occasionally contribute to corneal exposure problems, which usually resolve as the muscle regains functionality. In the interim, corneal protection can include the use of eye lubricants and gentle massage. The presence of corneal exposure from lagophthalmos can be the result of over aggressive skin excision, which is especially problematic in revision upper blepharoplasty or in patients with known dry eye syndrome. In extreme cases, this can be treated with skin grafting, but at the expense of an ideal cosmetic result. Blindness following upper lid blepharoplasty is extremely rare and can result from postoperative hematoma formation. If recognized in a timely fashion, it may be possible to evacuate the hematoma and restore vision.

In managing and diagnosing complications, it is important that the patient have easy access to medical care and examination. The patient should be counseled about what is normal after surgery and what is not normal. It is expected that the patient will experience tenderness at the surgical site and some blurry vision from any ointment used. Abnormal postoperative events would be for the eye to swell shut, for pain to be severe, or for there to be any true vision change or loss.

CONCLUSION

Upper eyelid blepharoplasty can be a very rewarding operation for the surgeon and patient, alike. It is critical to properly diagnose any underlying brow descent or ptosis prior to upper blepharoplasty in order to offer patients the correct surgical treatment for their complaint. Taking a careful preoperative history and performing an attentive physical examination is important to ensure good outcomes. The expectations of the patient must be clearly understood and managed. Careful diagnosis and attention to detail will help avoid any untoward complications and minimize patient dissatisfaction.

REFERENCES

1. Most SP, Mobley SR, Larrabee WF Jr. Anatomy of the eyelids. *Facial Plast Surg Clin North Am* 2005;13(4):487–492.
2. Hetzler L, Sykes J. The brow and forehead in periocular rejuvenation. *Facial Plast Surg Clin North Am* 2010;18:375–384.
3. Nerad JA, Carter KD, Alford MA. Brow ptosis. In: Duker JS, Macsai MS, eds. *Rapid diagnosis in ophthalmology—oculoplastic and reconstructive surgery*. Philadelphia, PA: Mosby Elsevier; 2008.
4. Codner M, Ford DT. Blepharoplasty. In: Thorne CH, ed. *Grabb and Smith's plastic surgery*. 6th ed. Philadelphia, PA: Lippincott Williams & Wilkins; 2007:486–498.
5. Aiache AE, Ramirez OH. The suborbicularis oculi fat pads: an anatomic and clinical study. *Plast Reconstr Surg* 1995;95: 37–42.
6. Chen SH, Mardini S, Chen HC, et al. Strategies for a successful corrective Asian blepharoplasty after previously failed revisions. *Plast Reconstr Surg* 2004;114(5):1270–1277.
7. Burke AJ, Wang T. Should formal ophthalmologic evaluation be a preoperative requirement prior to blepharoplasty? *Arch Otolaryngol Head Neck Surg* 2001;127:719–722.
8. Campbell JP, Lisman RD. Complications of blepharoplasty. *Facial Plast Surg* 2000;8:303.

Lower Eyelid Blepharoplasty

187

Stephen W. Perkins   *Jess Prischmann*

Lower eyelid blepharoplasty is one of the most common and technically challenging procedures in facial plastic surgery. Unlike upper eyelid blepharoplasty, surgery on the lower eyelid has a lower threshold for error and a higher potential for complications. Most blepharoplasty surgeons will encounter unexpected postoperative outcomes. Because of this, an intimate understanding of anatomy, methodical evaluation of patients, obsessional intraoperative treatment of tissue planes, and prompt recognition of complications are required for success in this detail-driven and rewarding procedure.

LOWER EYELID ANATOMY

The upper and lower eyelids contain analogous structures. Knowledge of upper eyelid anatomy begets understanding of its lower counterpart.

The eyelids are divided into lamellae. The anterior lamella is composed of skin and the orbicularis oculi muscle. While the skin of the eyelid is the thinnest in the body, the thickness of the orbicularis is variable. The posterior lamella is composed of the tarsal plates, capsulopalpebral fascia, and palpebral conjunctiva. The capsulopalpebral fascia is part of the lower eyelid retractor and is an extension of the inferior rectus muscle. The middle lamella refers to the orbital septum (Fig. 187.1).

The lower eyelid is critical in creating a natural "almond" shape to the palpebral fissure. It is most commonly angled slightly upward, with the lateral canthus being 2 mm higher than the medial canthus. Variations exist, as the palpebral fissure can be angled downward or neutral. The lower eyelid margin should rest at the inferior limbus of the iris. Maintaining these topographical relationships is important in blepharoplasty.

The lower eyelid has three described fat pads: medial, central, and lateral. The inferior oblique muscle separates the medial and central fat pads. The central and lateral fat pads are separated by the arcuate expansion of Lockwood ligament. The medial fat pad is most commonly transposed to efface the "tear trough deformity" (as described below).

The inferior oblique muscle can be vulnerable to injury during lower lid blepharoplasty. It originates from the orbital floor lateral to the nasolacrimal canal. It takes a posterolateral course, passes inferior to the inferior rectus muscle, and inserts on the globe. Injury to the inferior oblique can result in a range of disability, from transient diplopia to permanent strabismus. This complication can largely be avoided by only transecting fat that protrudes anterior to the orbital septum (1).

The blood supply to the lower eyelid is through rich anastomoses between the internal and external carotid artery systems. The major arteries include the dorsal nasal, angular, infraorbital, transverse facial, zygomaticofacial, and medial palpebral. From a surgical perspective, the plane between the orbital septum and orbicularis is relatively avascular. However, meticulous hemostasis is required when dissection proceeds anteroinferiorly (as performed in fat transposition) or posteriorly (as performed during routine access to fat pockets).

The sensation to the lower eyelid is from branches of the infraorbital nerve, a terminal branch of the maxillary division of the trigeminal nerve. The motor innervation is through the oculomotor and facial nerves.

IMPORTANT TERMINOLOGY

Knowledge of a few basic terms is required for effective communication with regard to lower eyelid blepharoplasty.

Orbital fat pseudoherniation or palpebral bags: Bulging of orbital fat that is seen in conjunction with a weakened orbital septum and/or relaxation of Lockwood ligament. Visible pseudoherniation of orbital fat disrupts the normally smooth transition between the eyelid and cheek subunits and creates an "aged" or "tired" appearance.

Anatomy of the Lower Eyelid

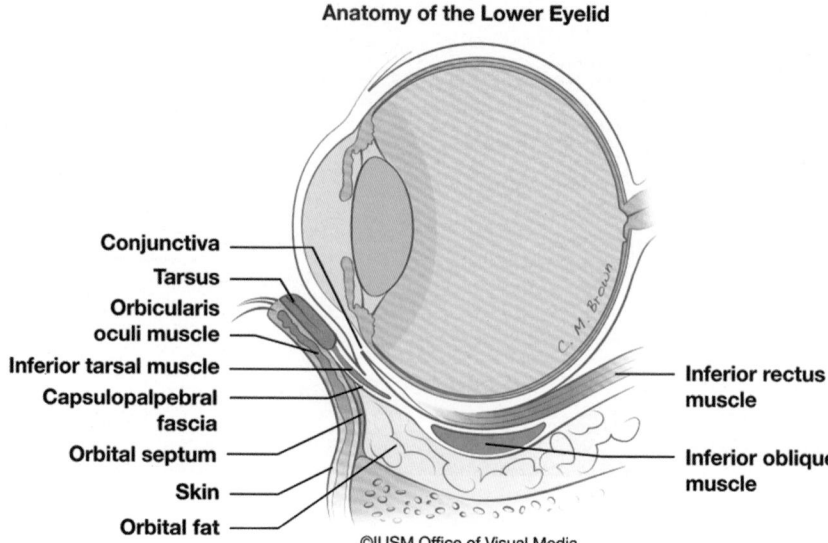

Conjunctiva
Tarsus
Orbicularis oculi muscle
Inferior tarsal muscle
Capsulopalpebral fascia
Orbital septum
Skin
Orbital fat

Inferior rectus muscle

Inferior oblique muscle

©IUSM Office of Visual Media

Figure 187.1 Anatomy of the lower eyelid.

It is considered to be the most common indication for lower eyelid blepharoplasty (Fig. 187.2).

Dermatochalasis: Excess skin of the eyelid (Fig. 187.3). Dermatochalasis should not be confused with "blepharochalasis," which is a rare inflammatory disorder of the eyelids characterized by recurrent edema.

Orbicularis hypertrophy: Increased thickness of the preseptal or preorbital portions of the orbicularis oculi muscle (Fig. 187.4). This sign is often mistaken for orbital fat pseudoherniation.

Scleral show: The measurement of white (sclera) show between the inferior limbus of the iris and the margin of the lower eyelid when the head is in the Frankfort horizontal plane (Fig. 187.5).

Negative vector: Seen when the anteriormost point of the cornea projects beyond the inferior orbital rim. Most commonly recognized on profile view (Fig. 187.6).

Lower eyelid laxity: Horizontal excess of the lower eyelid that occurs as the result of aging. Clinically determined by the snap and/or distraction tests (Fig. 187.7).

Ectropion: Outward turning of the eyelid margin away from the globe (Fig. 187.8).

Entropion: Inward turning of the eyelid margin toward the globe.

Tear trough deformity: The soft tissue surface depression seen along the medial inferior orbital rim, often accentuated by orbital fat pseudoherniation (2) (Fig. 187.9).

Double convexity deformity: The contour deformity that results from descent of the suborbicularis oculi fat pad below the arcus marginalis and weakening/bowing of the orbital septum above the arcus. Most commonly seen on three-quarters or profile view. This deformity is considered an indication for fat repositioning in lower eyelid blepharoplasty or midface lift (3) (Fig. 187.10).

Festoons: Redundant folds of lax skin and orbicularis muscle that hang in a hammock-like fashion from canthus to canthus (4) (Fig. 187.11).

Malar mounds or bags: The soft tissue convexity seen between the orbicularis retaining ligament and the zygomaticocutaneous ligament. As aging occurs, the "fixed"

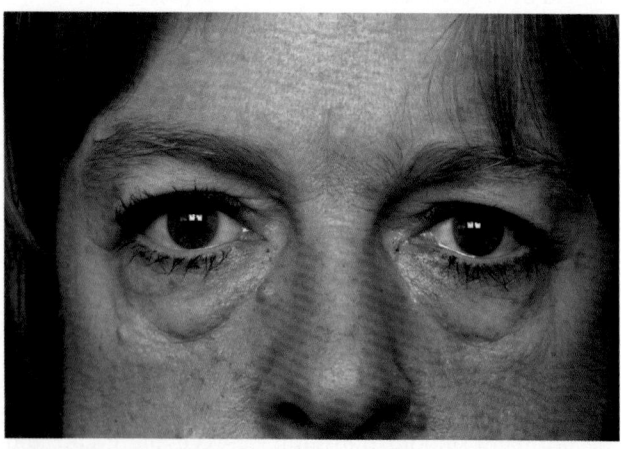

Figure 187.2 Orbital fat pseudoherniation, considered the most common indication for lower eyelid blepharoplasty.

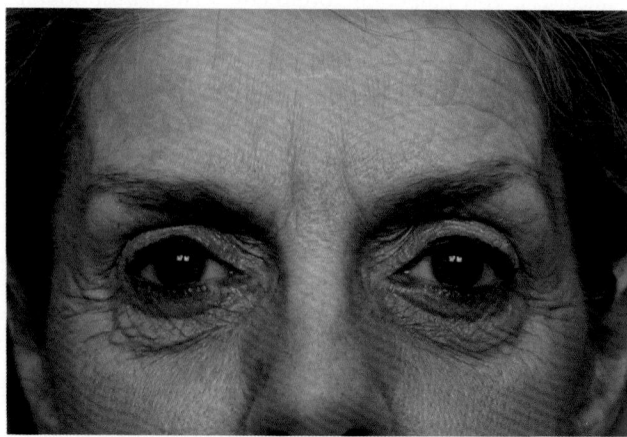

Figure 187.3 Lower eyelid dermatochalasis.

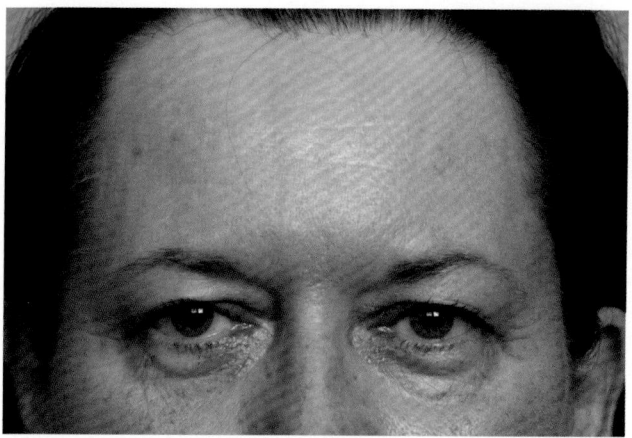

Figure 187.4 Orbicularis hypertrophy of the lower eyelid. Note the thickness of the orbicularis without pseudoherniation of orbital fat.

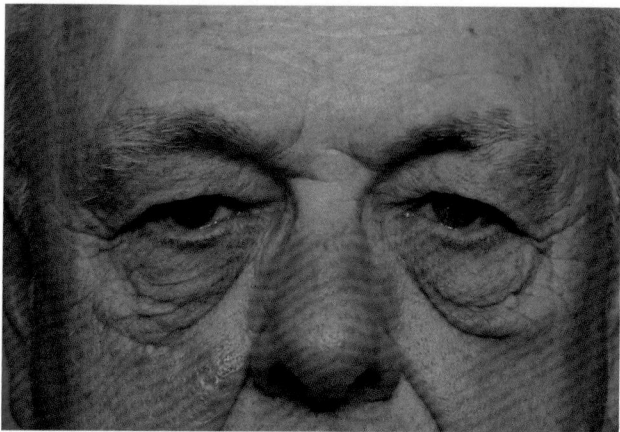

Figure 187.7 Lower eyelid laxity. Blepharoplasty in patients with this finding necessitates lid-supporting adjunctive procedures.

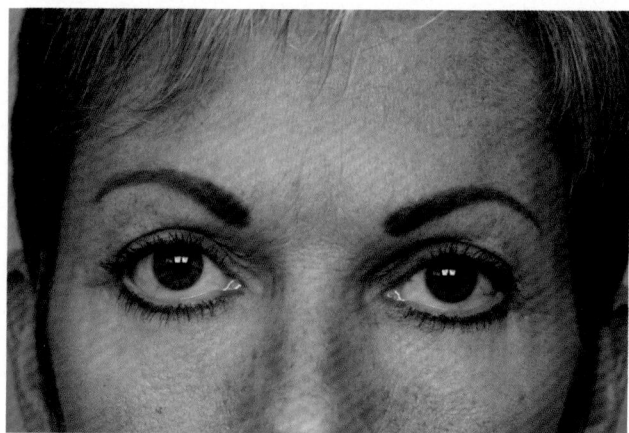

Figure 187.5 Scleral show. Note that the lid margin rests below the lower limbus of the iris.

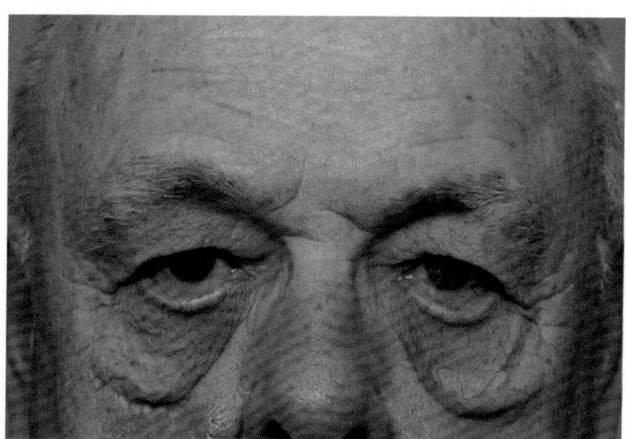

Figure 187.8 Ectropion. Note the outward turning of the lid margin away from the globe. Blepharoplasty in patients with this finding necessitates lid-supporting adjunctive procedures.

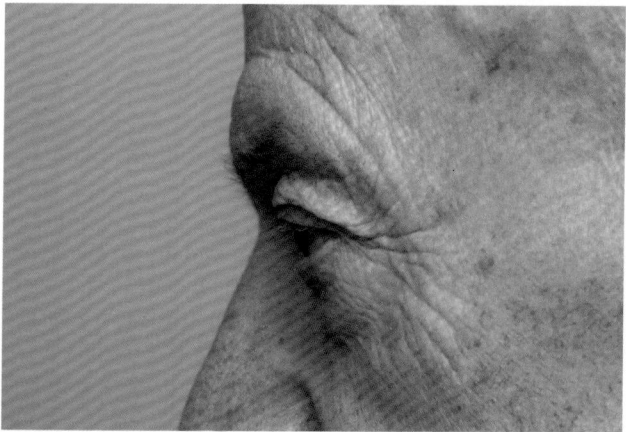

Figure 187.6 Negative vector orbit. Note that the anteriormost projecting point of the cornea projects beyond the inferior orbital rim.

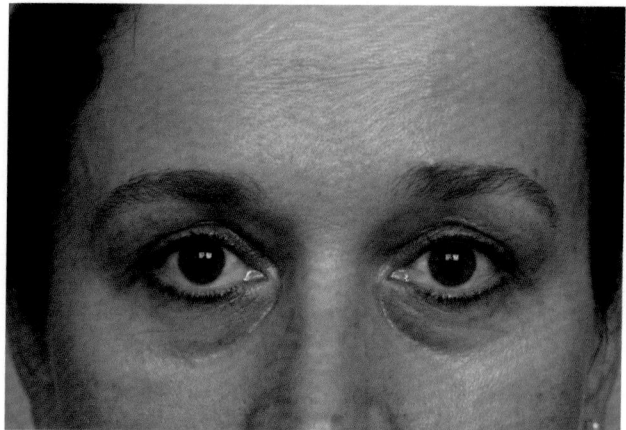

Figure 187.9 "Tear trough" deformity.

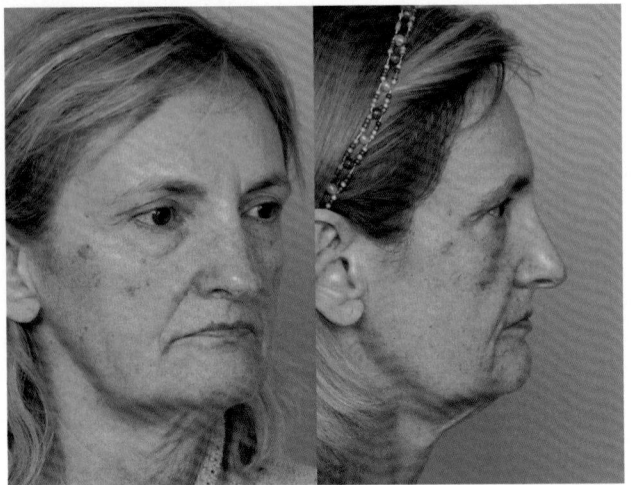

Figure 187.10 "Double convexity" deformity. Note the contour deformity that results from bowing of the orbital septum above the arcus marginalis and descent of the suborbicularis oculi fat pad below the arcus.

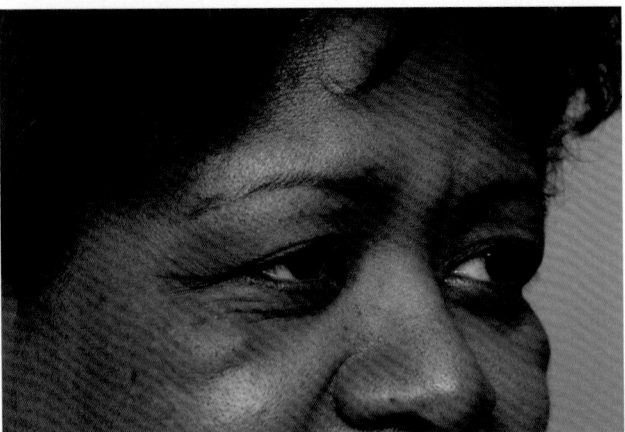

Figure 187.12 Malar mounds. This finding is not easily correctable with standard blepharoplasty approaches.

nature of the ligaments causes a visible disruption in the contour between the eyelid and cheek (Fig. 187.12).

PATIENT SELECTION AND EXAMINATION

The ideal lower eyelid blepharoplasty patient is healthy, has reasonable expectations, and presents with findings easily correctable with a surgical procedure. In order to determine appropriate candidacy, the surgeon must be prepared to look for and elicit for pertinent signs and symptoms.

An evaluation should always begin with an assessment of the patient's motives and expectations. Lower lid blepharoplasty can correct orbital fat pseudoherniation, excess skin and muscle, mild festooning, and tear trough deformities. However, if the patient's main concerns include abnormal skin pigmentation, fine rhytids, or large malar bags, the surgeon must explain that a blepharoplasty is not the appropriate procedure (5) (Fig. 187.13A and B).

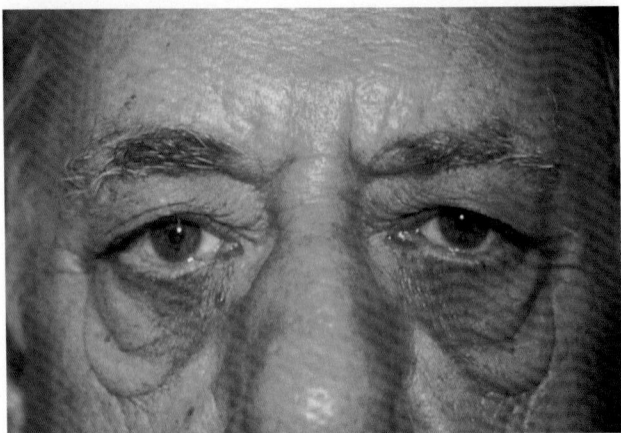

Figure 187.11 Lower eyelid festoons.

When discussing medical history, the surgeon should ask about thyroid eye disease, poorly controlled hypertension, anticoagulant use, blepharitis, facial nerve dysfunction, history of keloid scars or herpes zoster ophthalmicus, and visual field problems (5). Particular attention should be paid to a history of dry eye symptoms or regular use of lubricating drops. The surgeon should inquire about dry eye symptoms in several ways, as some patients may only report "allergic"-type symptoms or watering without emotional stimulation (Fig. 187.14). All patients, and particularly those with symptoms, should be informed that blepharoplasty can cause or exacerbate dry eye symptoms. The surgeon should be aware that a subclinical dry eye condition can worsen to a keratoconjunctivitis sicca with the mechanical alteration that occurs following cosmetic eyelid surgery (6).

A thorough physical examination is critical to selecting the correct procedure and avoiding postoperative complications. The surgeon should look for the following: orbital fat pseudoherniation, orbicularis hypertrophy, dermatochalasis, tear trough deformity, lid laxity, scleral show, negative vector, festooning, malar bags, midface ptosis, and fine rhytids.

Orbital fat pseudoherniation and dermatochalasis are the most common reasons patients seek lower eyelid blepharoplasty. In most cases, fat pseudoherniation is obvious on inspection. This finding can be confirmed by gentle pressure on the globe and examining the patient in upward gaze. Orbicularis hypertrophy can be differentiated from fat pseudoherniation by having the patient smile or squint. While fat pseudoherniation can be treated with either a transconjunctival or transcutaneous approach, skin or muscle excess can only be treated with an incision through the anterior lamella.

The contour of the lower lid should be closely examined. The surgeon should assess for a "tear trough deformity." If a surface depression is noted along the inferomedial aspect of the orbital rim, a fat transposition to efface the "tear trough" should be performed (see procedure section).

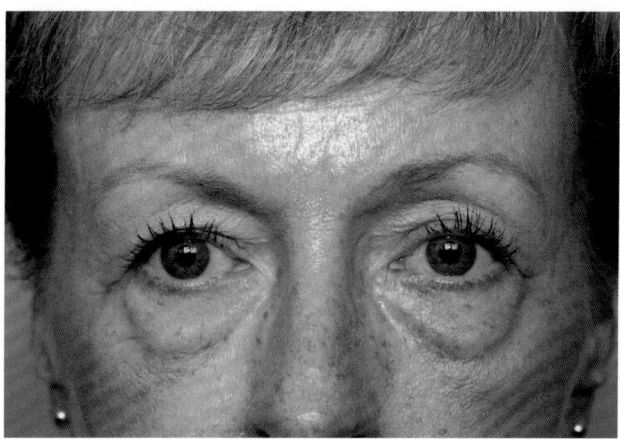 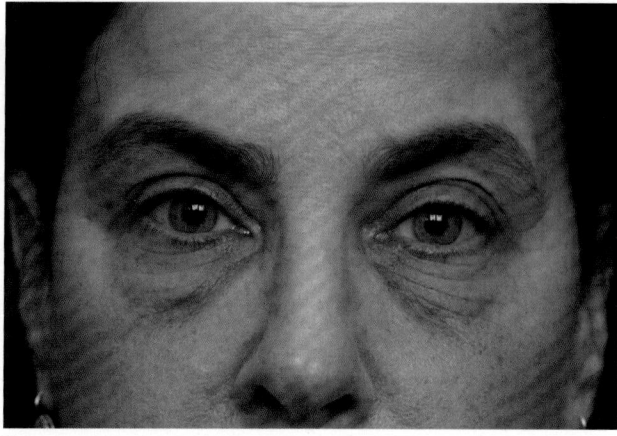

A   **B**

Figure 187.13 A: Excellent candidate for blepharoplasty. This patient has obvious pseudoherniation of orbital fat, tear trough deformity, and some excess skin and muscle. **B:** Poor candidate for blepharoplasty. This patient has hyperpigmentation and fine rhytids of the lower eyelid.

Examination for lid laxity deserves special attention. Failure to note this common sign is a missed opportunity for the surgeon and can result in patient dissatisfaction and an increased risk of postoperative complications. Lower eyelid laxity is evaluated by two common clinical tests: the snap test and distraction test. The snap test assesses canthal stability and orbicularis and tarsal strength (7). The test is performed by gently pulling the lower lid toward the orbital rim and releasing. Obvious scleral show or slow return to the resting position (greater than 1 second) indicates poor lid support. The distraction test is performed by grasping the lower lid and pulling it away from the globe. Distraction of the eyelid greater than 10 mm indicates poor lid support. If the distraction or snap tests are positive, failure to adequately support the lid can lead to ectropion, epiphora, or exposure keratitis (7) (Fig. 187.15A and B).

The position of globe relative to the eyelid and maxilla should also be examined. Assessing for scleral show and negative vector can change the surgical plan and prevent postoperative lid malposition. In a normal-vector orbit, the cornea rests in a vertical plane with the inferior orbital rim. When a negative vector is present, the cornea lies in plane anterior to the inferior orbital rim. In patients with negative vector orbits, transcutaneous approaches with shortening of the anterior lamella can result in significant postoperative lid malposition. If scleral show or negative vector is noted preoperatively, the surgeon can plan procedures to support the lower lid, such as intraoperative canthopexy (see below) or postoperative lid taping. Patients with negative vector orbits should also have conservative fat removal, as they are more prone to developing a "hollowed" appearance.

Festooning and malar bags are signs commonly seen with aging and indicate orbicularis laxity. They can only be corrected with an extended transcutaneous approach to blepharoplasty with undermining in the suborbicularis

plane inferior to the orbital rim. The surgeon should also inspect the lid for horizontal excess, as lid shortening procedures may also be indicated.

Malar edema, midface ptosis, and fine rhytids are not correctable with blepharoplasty. Once noted, the surgeon should educate the patient and discuss adjunctive procedures, such as a midface lift or resurfacing. The surgeon should also discuss the persistent and recurring nature of malar edema, as it may not be corrected with *any* surgical procedure.

PHOTOGRAPHY AND CONSENTS

Although often underestimated as a formality, photography and consents are among the most important aspects of any cosmetic procedure.

Standardized photography for eyelid surgery includes full face and close-up views. Close-up views should extend from just above the eyebrows to the level of the nasal ala. The following close-up views should be obtained: frontal, frontal in upward gaze, frontal with eyes closed, bilateral oblique, and bilateral profile. Full face frontal and bilateral oblique views are also obtained (8) (Fig. 187.16).

A lower eyelid blepharoplasty consent form should include a complete discussion of goals, limitations, alternatives, expected outcomes, risks, and potential for additional surgery. The consent should explicitly state that blepharoplasty will not remove crow feet, malar bags, fine wrinkles, or dark circles. Expected outcomes should include swelling, asymmetric bruising, temporary tearing, need for artificial tears because of dry eye, itching, blurry vision, tightness on eyelid closure, fine scarring of the lower eyelid, slight scleral show, and possible minor asymmetries in eyelid position. Risks outlined should include asymmetry, bleeding, infection, blurriness, double vision, chemosis, ectropion, visual loss, lower lid sagging, rounding of the corner of the eye, and chronic dry eye syndrome.

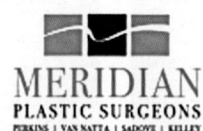

MERIDIAN
PLASTIC SURGEONS
PERKINS | VAN NATTA | SADOVE | KELLEY

Patient Eye Information

Name _____ Date _____

Your Eye Doctor's Name _____

Address _____ Date of last exam _____

Yes No At your last exam, were you told you have any problems with your eyes?
Explain _____
_____

Yes No Do you require glasses or contact lenses?
Yes No Have you had any injuries to the eyes or eyelids?
Explain _____
_____

Yes No Have you had any surgery to the eyes or eyelids? If so, who performed your surgery?
Explain _____
_____

Yes No Do you feel your eyes or eyelids swell excessively?
Yes No Are you bothered by frequent irritations or "allergies" of the eyes or eyelids?
Yes No Do you now take or have you ever taken medications or drops for the eyes?
Explain _____
_____

Yes No Are you bothered by "dry eyes"?
Yes No Do your eyes "water" or tear spontaneously (without emotional stimulation)?
Yes No Do you now have or have you ever had any visual problems with one or both eyes?
Explain _____
_____

Yes No Are there any other problems we have not asked about that you feel we should be aware of?
Explain _____
_____

> ### *Please read the following and carry out the instructions:*

Cover your **Right** eye and read this sentence with your **Left** eye.
Yes No Are you able to read it comfortably _____ without glasses?
_____ with glasses?

Cover your **Left** eye and read this sentence with your **Right** eye.
Yes No Are you able to read it comfortably _____ without glasses?
_____ with glasses?
If there is any difference in your vision, please indicate which eye is stronger. _____ Right eye _____ Left eye

I signify that to the best of my knowledge, the above information is accurate.

Signed _____

Figure 187.14 Typical "dry eye questionnaire." Blepharoplasty surgeons should always inquire about dry eye symptoms prior to embarking on surgery.

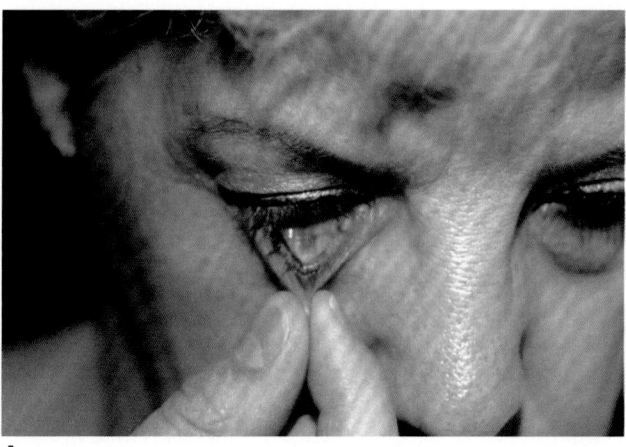 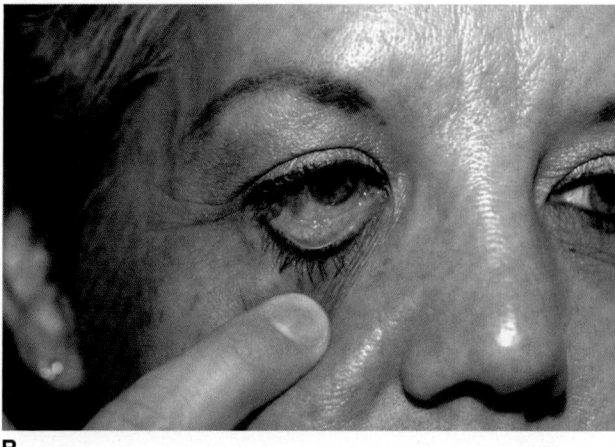

A   **B**

Figure 187.15 **A**: Snap test. The examiner pulls the lower lid toward the orbital rim and releases. Obvious scleral show or slow return to the resting position (greater than 1 second) indicates poor lid support. **B**: Distraction test. The examiner grasps the lower lid and pulls it away from the globe. Distraction of the eyelid greater than 10 mm indicates poor lid support.

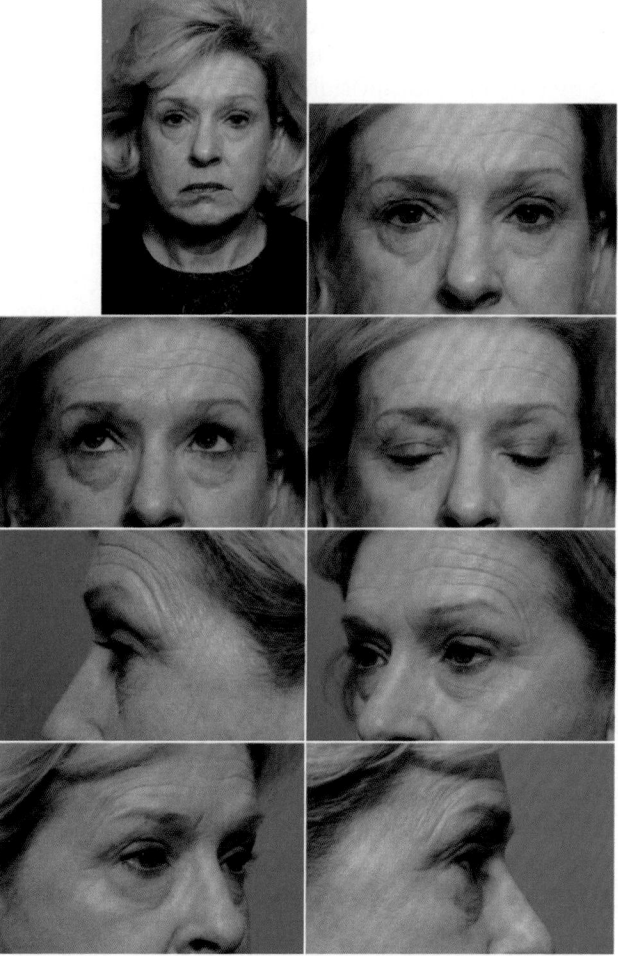

Figure 187.16 Standard views for blepharoplasty photos.

SURGICAL PROCEDURE

The main approaches for lower lid blepharoplasty are transconjunctival and transcutaneous. Both have clear indications and should be part of a surgeon's armamentarium. Once the surgeon has decided on an approach, adjunctive procedures should be considered including canthopexy or canthoplasty and lower lid resurfacing (chemical or laser).

TRANSCONJUNCTIVAL APPROACH

The transconjunctival approach is ideally indicated for younger patients (15 to 35 years old) without anterior lamellar pathology. Otherwise stated, these patients have hereditary pseudoherniation of orbital fat without true excess skin or muscle (Fig. 187.17). Relative indications include patients who do not want an external scar or those with a history of abnormal scarring. The transconjunctival approach can be safely combined with resurfacing procedures or "pinch" skin removal in those with fine rhytids or minimal excess skin of the lower eyelid, respectively (9).

Two transconjunctival approaches are routinely performed: preseptal and postseptal. The preseptal approach involves dissecting inferiorly along the avascular plane between the orbital septum and orbicularis oculi muscle (Fig. 187.18). The postseptal approach is a more direct approach to the orbital fat through the conjunctiva and the lower lid retractors closer to the conjunctival fornix (Fig. 187.19). While the preseptal approach takes slightly longer to perform, it is generally considered to provide better visualization of the individual fat pads and poses less risk to the integrity of the inferior oblique muscle. The

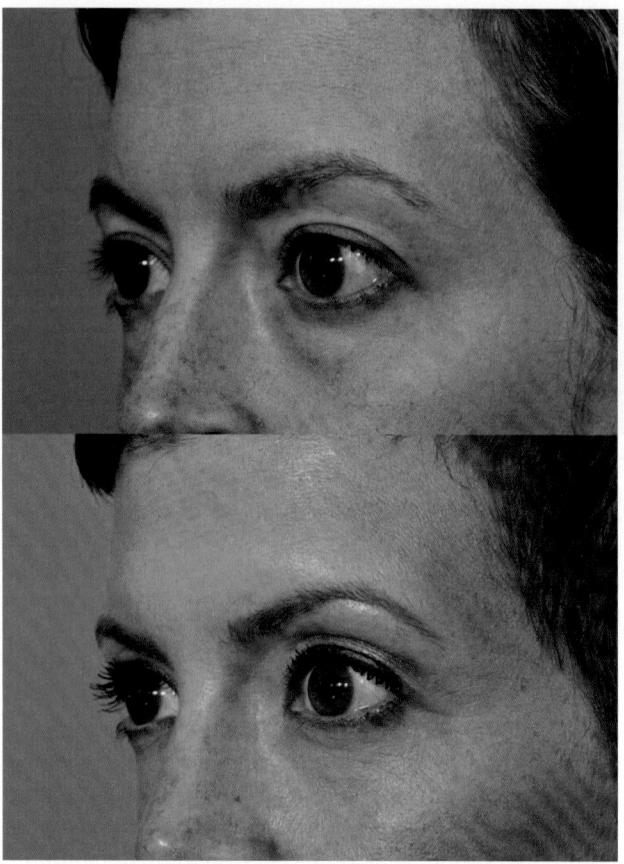

Figure 187.17 Before and after transconjunctival blepharoplasty. Ideal candidates for this approach have pseudoherniation of orbital fat without skin or muscle excess.

preseptal approach also allows the surgeon to approach the individual fat compartments from the same anterior direction as typically seen from the transcutaneous skin–muscle flap approach.

PRESEPTAL TRANSCONJUNCTIVAL TECHNIQUE

Once an appropriate level of sedation is achieved, topical 2% tetracaine is instilled into the inferior fornix of each eye. Local anesthetic (lidocaine with epinephrine) is then injected into the subconjunctival plane of the lower eyelid.

After adequate anesthesia is obtained, a sharp double hook (followed by a Desmarres retractor or double ball hook) is used to retract the lid inferiorly. Light bipolar cautery can be used prior to incision to conservatively cauterize the planned incision site along the central portion of the conjunctiva. An incision is made through the conjunctiva 2 mm inferior to the tarsus. The conjunctiva is then opened laterally and medially; the inferior lid retractors are transected sharply with a small curved scissors. The conjunctiva and inferior retractor muscles are then reflected superiorly over the cornea with a 5-0 silk suture, thus providing corneal protection and countertraction (alternatively, corneal protectors can also be used) (Fig. 187.20A and B).

The orbicularis oculi muscle is then separated from the orbital septum inferiorly to the orbital rim. The surgeon should then closely examine the preoperative pictures and intraoperative findings to determine where to incise the septum and approach the orbital fat pads. Westcott scissors are used to make the incision through the orbital septum. The pseudoherniated fat is very carefully teased out. If fat is not being transposed, it is lightly grasped, cauterized, and excised (Fig. 187.20C). If fat transposition is being performed, a precise pocket is elevated in the suborbicularis plane corresponding to the region of soft tissue depression. The medial fat pad is redraped over the orbital rim and sewn into place using a 6-0 absorbable suture in an interrupted fashion.

After completion of fat resection and/or transposition, the lower eyelid skin is redraped in its anatomic position

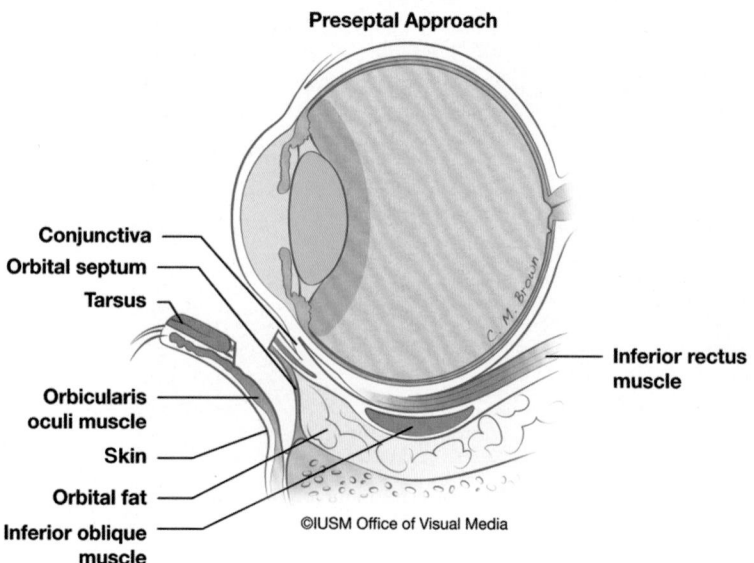

Figure 187.18 Preseptal transconjunctival approach.

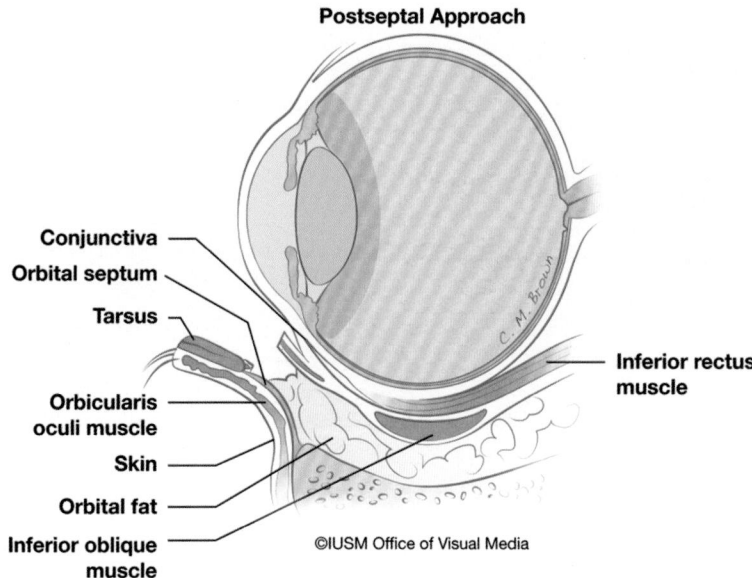

Postseptal Approach

Conjunctiva
Orbital septum
Tarsus
Orbicularis oculi muscle
Skin
Orbital fat
Inferior oblique muscle

Inferior rectus muscle

©IUSM Office of Visual Media

Figure 187.19 Postseptal transconjunctival approach.

A

B

C

D

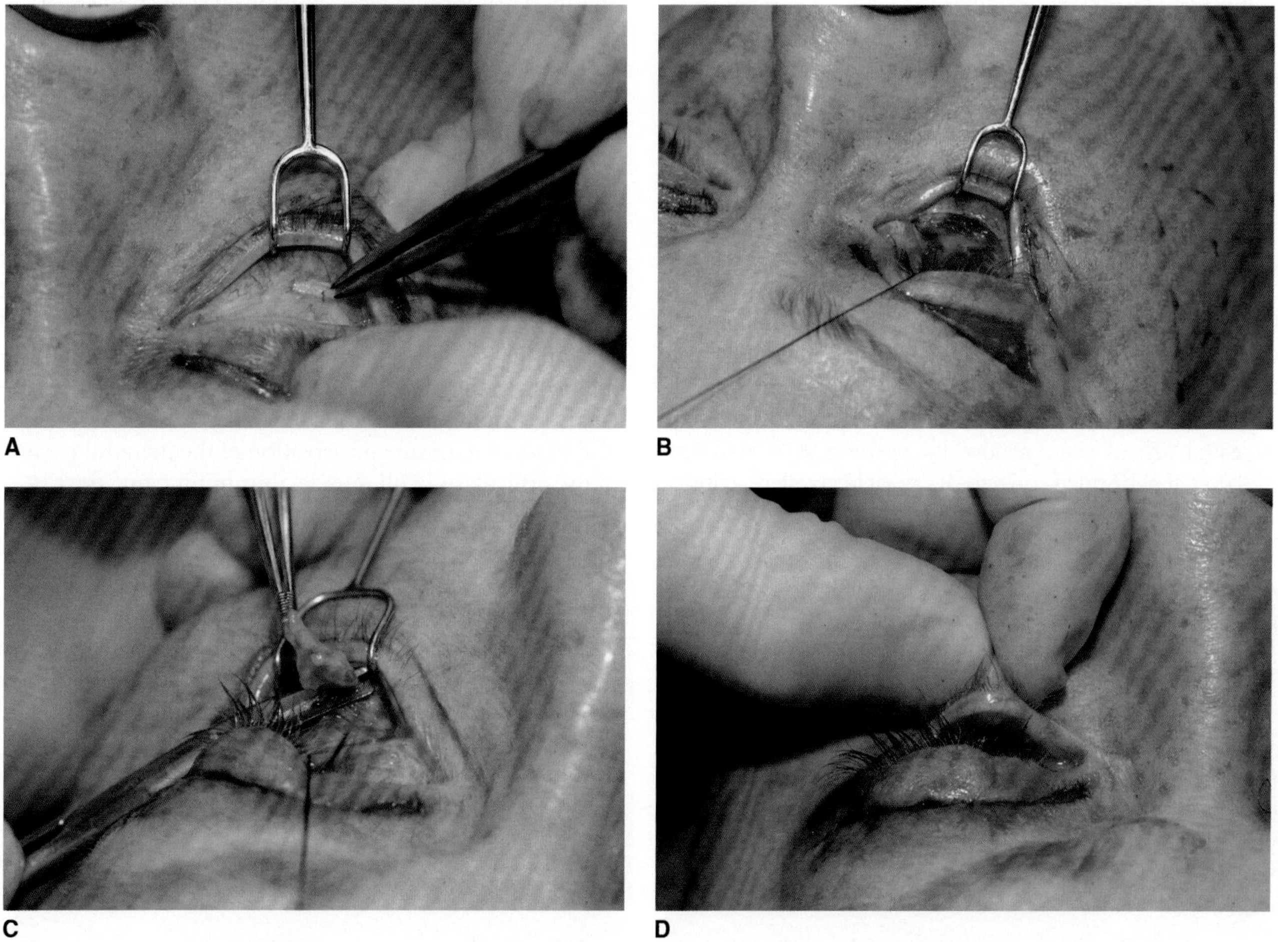

Figure 187.20 Preseptal transconjunctival approach. **A**: Light bipolar cautery is used to conservatively cauterize the planned incision site. **B**: Retraction of the conjunctival flap (comprised of conjunctiva, lower lid retractors, and orbital septum) provides countertraction and corneal protection. **C**: Pseudoherniated fat is gently grasped, cauterized, and excised. **D**: Upon completion of fat resection, the skin is picked up and snapped into place at the inferior limbus. Sutures are not necessary.

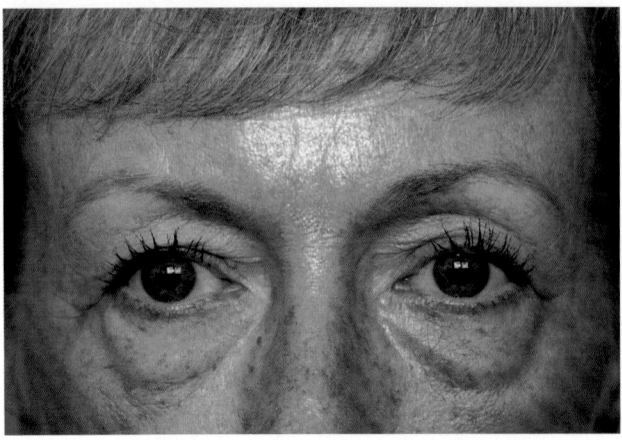 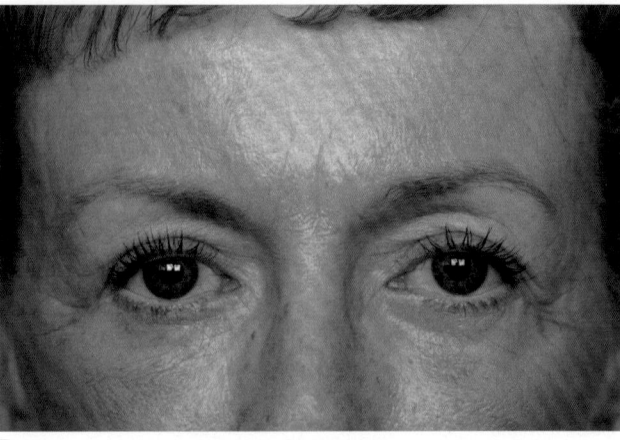

A   B

Figure 187.21 Before and after photos following skin–muscle flap blepharoplasty. **A:** Preoperative. **B:** Postoperative. Note barely perceptible scar.

and evaluated for any residual bulging or irregularity. After acceptable contour is ensured, the silk suture is removed and the skin flap is picked up, raised, and snapped into position over the lower limbus. Sutures are not necessary in this technique (Fig. 187.20D).

If a skin pinch is planned, forceps are used to grasp 2 to 3 mm of redundant skin just inferior to the lash line. Scissors are used to sharply excise the skin. The edges are reapproximated with 6-0 fast absorbing gut sutures or tissue glue (8).

TRANSCUTANEOUS SKIN–MUSCLE FLAP APPROACH

The transcutaneous approach is indicated for patients with anterior lamellar pathology. This is usually an older age group of patients with excess lower eyelid skin, muscle, or both. Some surgeons have avoided this technique due to an increased risk of postoperative lid position abnormalities. However, if performed correctly, it can yield excellent, consistent results with a barely perceptible scar (10) (Fig. 187.21).

SKIN–MUSCLE FLAP TECHNIQUE

Once an appropriate level of anesthesia is achieved, the lower eyelids are infiltrated transcutaneously with local anesthetic (lidocaine with epinephrine) deep to the orbicularis oculi muscle.

The skin incision is performed with a 15 Bard Parker blade 2 mm inferior to the lower lid margin. The incision extends from just lateral to the lower punctum to a position 6 mm lateral to the lateral canthus (Fig. 187.22A and B). Fine curved scissors are then used to dissect through the orbicularis muscle at the lateral aspect of the incision. Blunt scissors are positioned posterior to the muscle at the lateral aspect of the incision, and with spreading motions of the scissors, the skin–muscle flap is elevated off the orbital septum. Dissection proceeds from the inferior orbital rim inferiorly to the incision superiorly (Fig. 187.23). The subciliary incision is then completed using the scissors in a beveled manner to ensure preservation of the pretarsal portion of the orbicularis oculi muscle, thus minimizing the risk of postoperative lower eyelid malposition (Fig. 187.24).

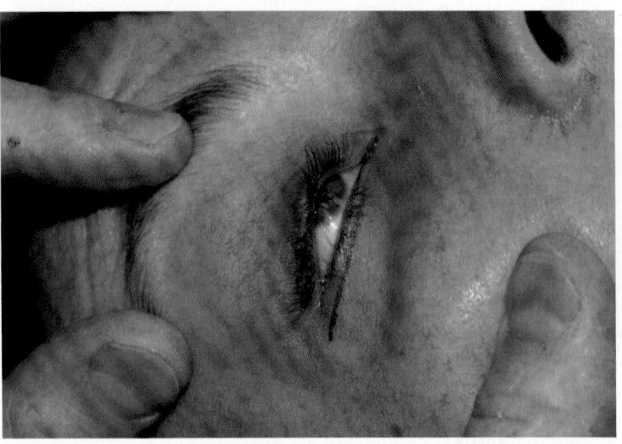 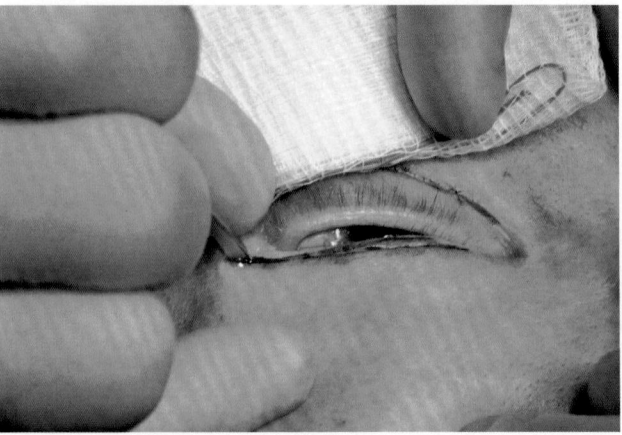

A   B

Figure 187.22 Skin–muscle flap blepharoplasty. **A:** Preoperative marking. **B:** Incision.

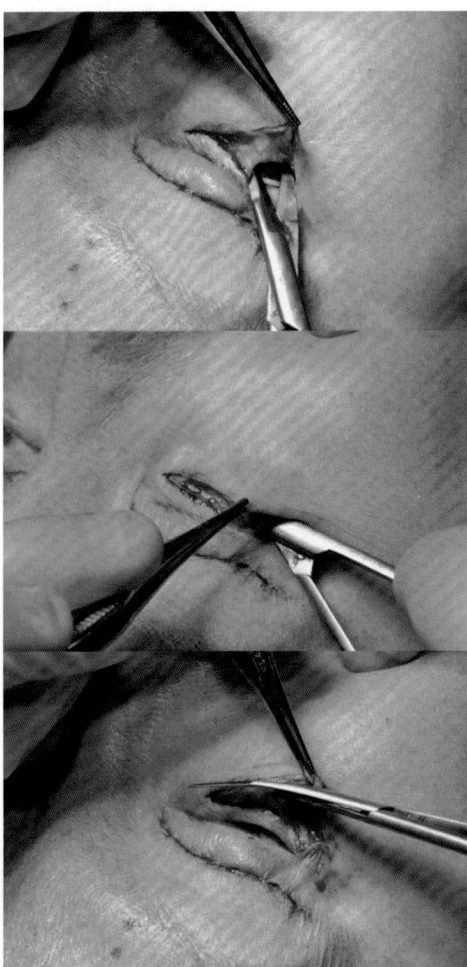

Figure 187.23 Elevation of skin muscle flap during blepharoplasty.

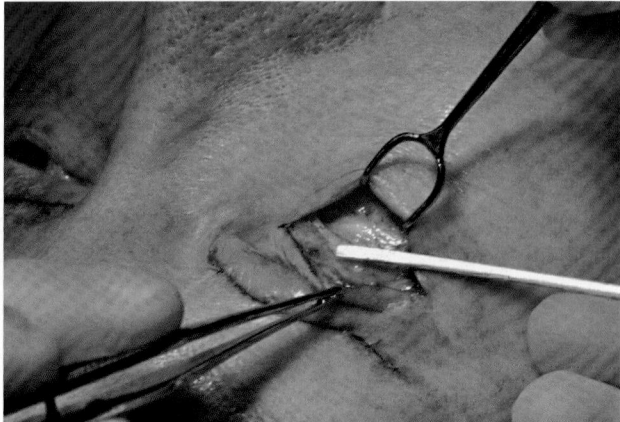

Figure 187.24 Preservation of the pretarsal orbicularis oculi muscle during skin–muscle flap blepharoplasty.

Access to the orbital fat compartments is obtained through small, selected openings of the orbital septum. Gentle palpation of the globe results in herniation of orbital fat through the aforementioned openings of the orbital septum. Bipolar cautery is then used to cauterize the fat pad prior to excision.

This procedure is performed for the lateral, middle, and medial fat compartments, as deemed appropriate. A conservative approach to fat resection is maintained to avoid the creation of a "sunken" or "hollowed" appearance (Fig. 187.25A).

If fat transposition is being performed, dissection inferior to the infraorbital rim is performed and a pocket is created in a supraperiosteal plane in the location of the nasojugal groove. A small opening is made in the orbital septum to gain access to the medial fat pocket. Once the medial fat is isolated, it is transposed over the orbital rim in the suborbicularis plane to efface the corresponding soft tissue depression. The transposed orbital fat is then secured to the periosteum using interrupted 6-0 absorbable suture (Fig. 187.25B).

On completion of fat resection and/or fat transposition, the skin–muscle flap is repositioned. In an anesthetized patient, single-finger pressure is applied at the inferomedial portion of the melolabial mound to create a maximal stretch effect. If the patient is awake, he or she is asked to open his or her mouth and look up. Following this, an inferiorly directed segmental cut is made at the lateral canthus to determine the amount of excess skin to excise. A tacking suture is placed to maintain the position of the skin–muscle flap; overlapping skin is trimmed. A 1- to 2-mm strip of muscle is resected to prevent overlapping of muscle and ridge formation with closure of the subciliary incision. A conservative amount of skin and muscle is resected. The orbicularis oculi muscle is then suspended to the periosteum of the lateral orbital rim with 5-0 poliglecaprone (Monocryl) suture. The deep tissues are then reapproximated at the lateral aspect of the incision using 6-0 absorbable suture (Fig. 187.26A–C).

Following muscle suspension, the subciliary incision is closed with 7-0 blue polypropylene suture at the lateral canthus in a simple interrupted fashion. The remainder of the incision is closed with 6-0 fast absorbing plain gut suture in a running fashion (Fig. 187.26D).

SKIN FLAP TECHNIQUE

The technique of lower lid blepharoplasty using a subciliary incision and "skin-only" flap is rarely used and of historical interest only.

ADJUNCTIVE PROCEDURES

Canthopexy and Canthoplasty

All surgeons performing blepharoplasty should be well versed in procedures to support the lower eyelid. In patients who have weak or lax lower eyelids, the contractile healing forces following blepharoplasty are unopposed, which can lead to retraction and ectropion. To prevent such complications, a canthoplasty or canthopexy should be performed at the time of surgery.

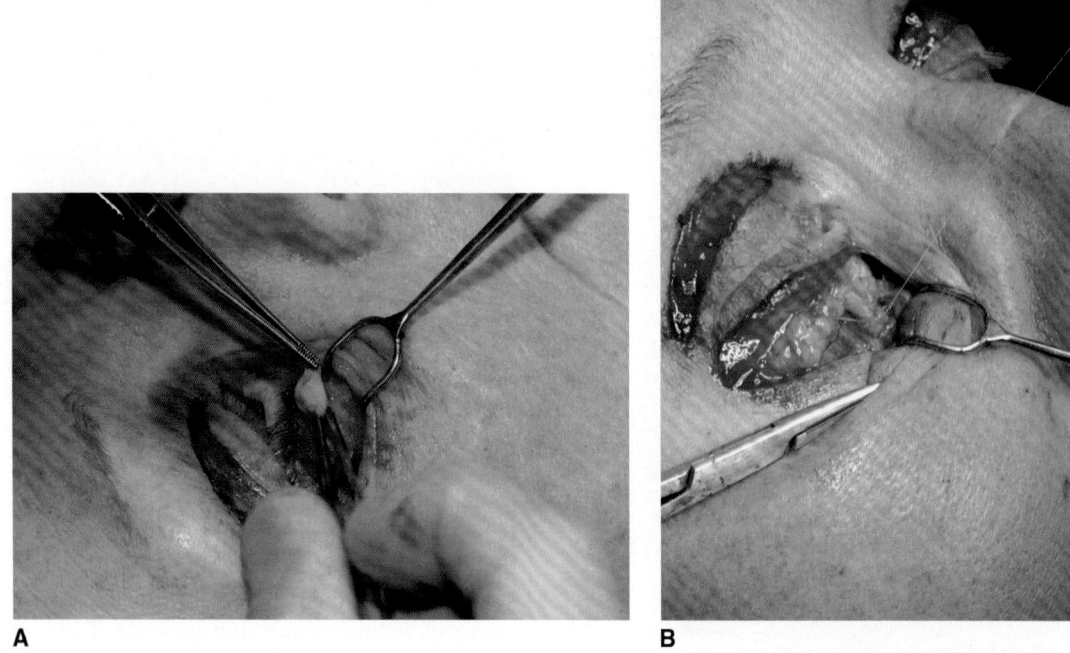

Figure 187.25 Skin–muscle flap blepharoplasty. **A**: Fat resection. **B**: Fat transposition.

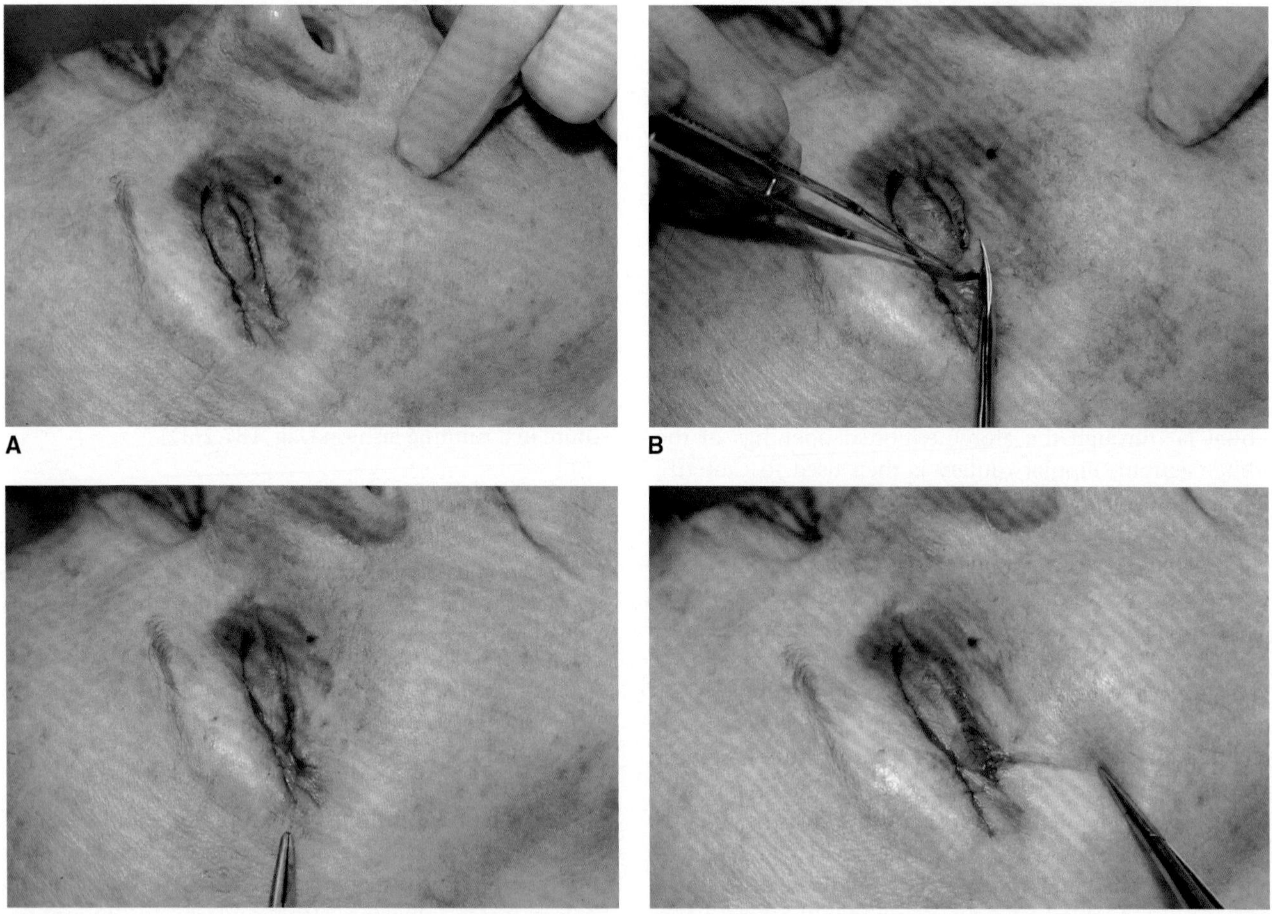

Figure 187.26 Closure of skin–muscle flap approach. **A**: Single finger pressure at the melolabial mound. **B**: Trimming of the skin flap. **C**: Orbicularis suspension suture. **D**: Closure of the external incision.

In cases where temporary support is needed, canthopexy is accomplished before closure of the upper and lower eyelid incisions. A suspension suture of 5-0 poliglecaprone (Monocryl) is placed between the periosteum of the inner aspect of the superolateral orbital rim and the lower lid tarsus, lateral canthal tendon, and pretarsal orbicularis. The suture is tunneled under the bridge of skin between the upper and lower eyelid incisions. If an upper eyelid blepharoplasty is not performed at the time of canthopexy, a separate stab incision can be made at the superolateral orbital rim (Fig. 187.27A–D).

A canthoplasty is performed in cases of significant lid laxity, when horizontal shortening is indicated, or if a more permanent solution is desired. Eyelid scissors are used to perform a lateral canthotomy and inferior cantholysis. Next, the lateral tarsal strip is created by excising conjunctiva from the posterior aspect of the tarsus and excising skin and muscle from the anterior aspect of the tarsus. The tarsal strip is then sutured to the periosteum of the medial aspect of the lateral orbital rim in a posterosuperior position with a 5-0 clear polypropylene suture. The orbicularis is then suspended to the periosteum of the lateral orbital rim at the tubercle with 5-0 poliglecaprone. The lower eyelid incision is then closed in the standard fashion (Fig. 187.28A–D).

LOWER EYELID RESURFACING

Standard blepharoplasty techniques do not treat fine, "crepy" periocular rhytids. While a transcutaneous blepharoplasty can address excess skin, overtightening the skin–muscle flap during surgery to efface fine rhytids can lead to disastrous complications, including rounding, scleral show, or frank ectropion. To safely address crepiness, a resurfacing procedure can be performed at the time of blepharoplasty (Fig. 187.29A and B).

While a complete discussion of lower eyelid resurfacing is beyond the scope of this chapter, it is sufficient to say that resurfacing procedures are characterized as superficial, medium, or deep. Selection of the depth of treatment is based upon degree of preoperative

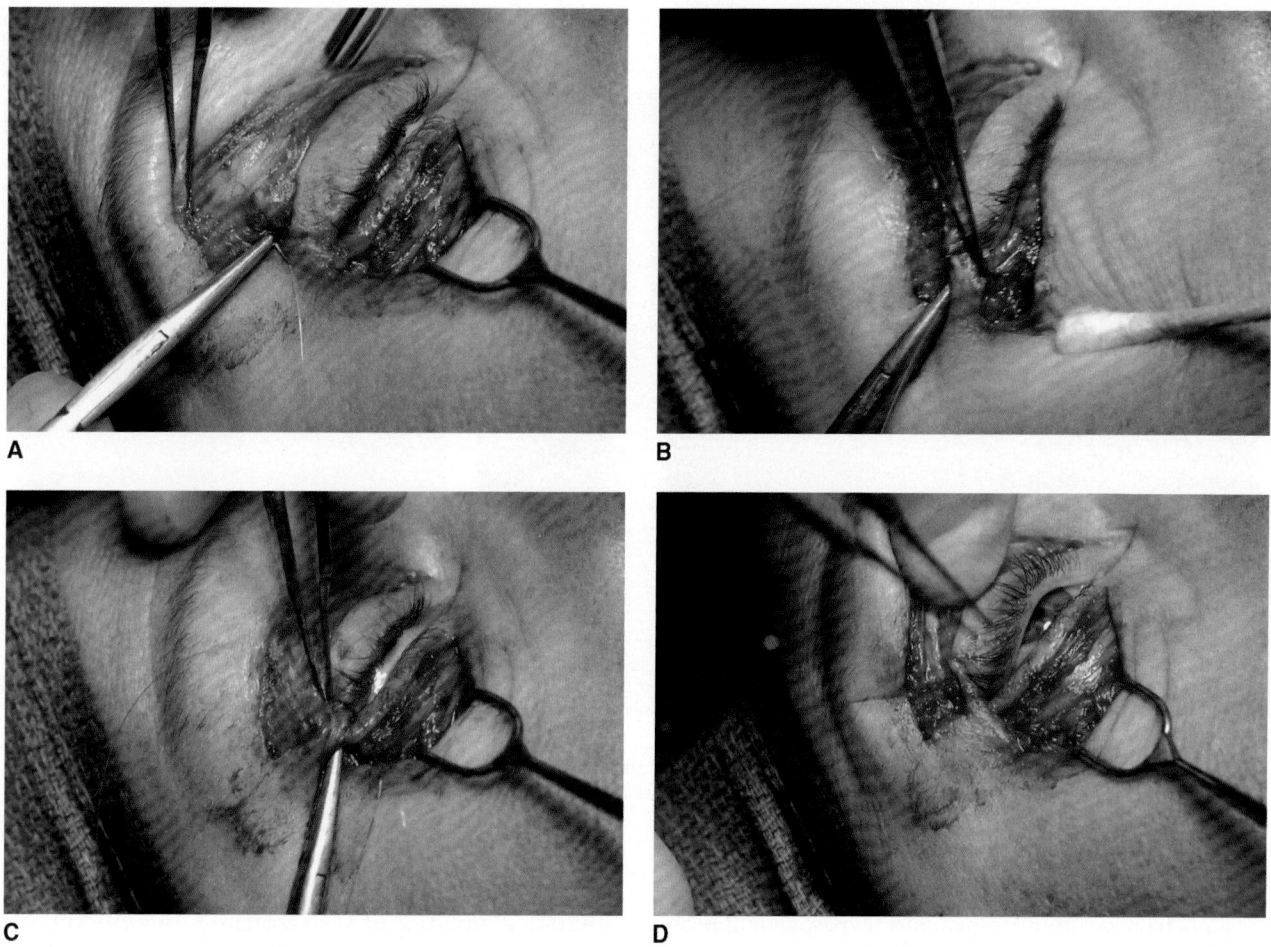

Figure 187.27 Canthopexy. **A:** Suture placed through periosteum of superolateral orbital rim. **B:** Suture placed through the pretarsal orbicularis and tarsus. **C:** Suture tunneled between upper and lower eyelid incisions. **D:** Cinching of suture. Note good support of the lid relative to globe.

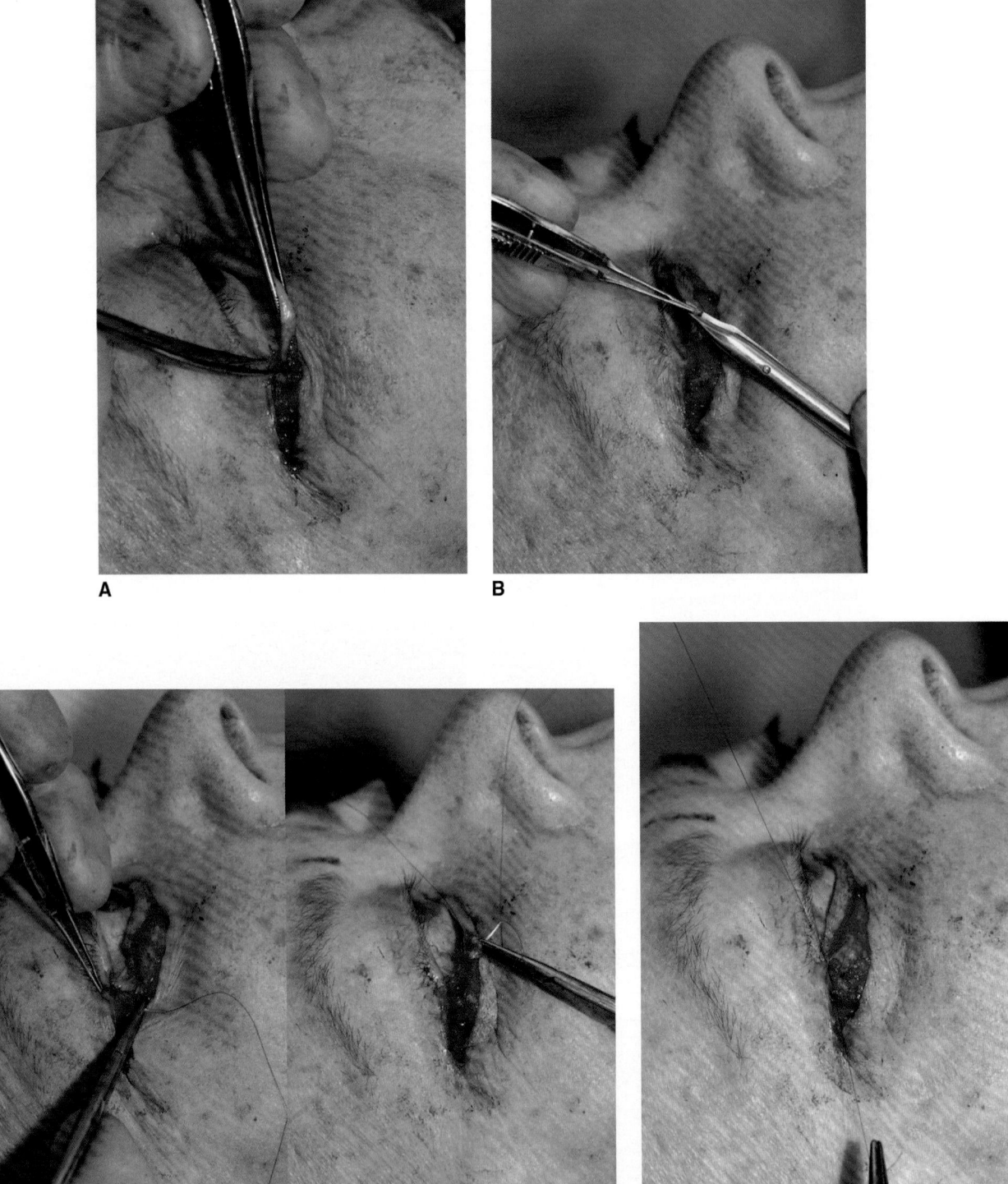

Figure 187.28 Canthoplasty. **A:** Canthotomy and cantholysis. **B:** Creation of lateral tarsal strip. **C:** Suturing of tarsal strip to periosteum of orbital rim. **D:** Cinching of suture. Note good support of the lid relative to the globe.

dermatochalasis, photoaging, and hyperpigmentation. A superficial depth of resurfacing can be achieved with superficial laser treatments. Medium depth modalities include trichloroacetic acid 35% pretreated with Jessner's solution (composed of 14 g resorcinol, 14 g salicylic acid, and 14 mL lactic acid mixed in ethanol) and phenol 88% USP. A deep depth of resurfacing can be achieved with a CO_2 laser or Baker's peel.

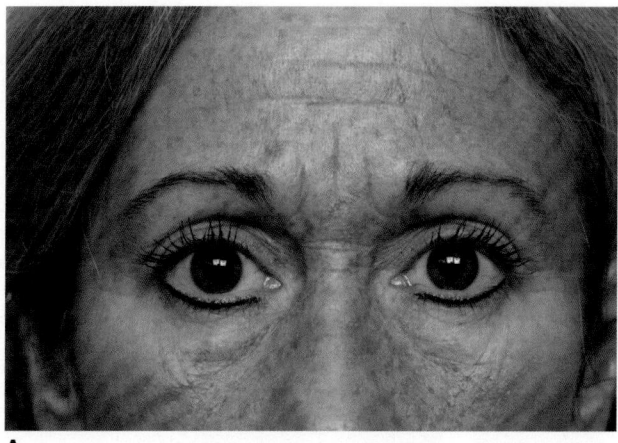
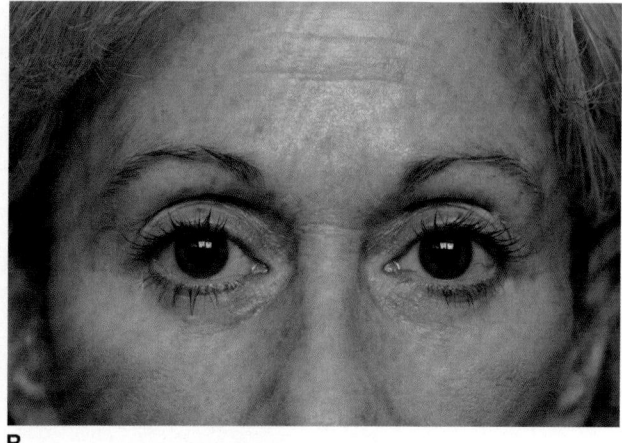

A   B

Figure 187.29 Before and after photos following skin–muscle flap blepharoplasty with lower eyelid chemical peel (phenol 88% USP). **A:** Preoperative. **B:** Postoperative.

FILLERS IN THE LOWER EYELID

Hyaluronic acid fillers can be successfully used as a temporary treatment for the "tear trough" deformity. Selection of filling agent is critical, as overly hydrophilic compounds can lead to an unattractive "puffy" appearance. For this reason, the authors exclusively use Restylane (Medicis Aesthetics Inc., Scottsdale, AZ) in the delicate lower eyelid region. The tear trough region is commonly treated with small incremental aliquots of filler in the supraperiosteal suborbicularis plane with massage following injection to smooth out irregularities (Fig. 187.30A and B).

MIDFACE LIFT

In patients who present with midface ptosis or a double convexity deformity, a midface lift is a useful adjunctive procedure to extended skin–muscle flap blepharoplasty.

While a discussion of midface lift is beyond the scope of this chapter, it is important to note that it does increase recovery time and should only be performed in carefully selected patients (Fig. 187.31A and B).

FAT GRAFTING

Fat grafting has been discussed for decades in the lower eyelid region. It is the senior author's opinion that fat grafting in this region is fraught with complications, such as visible lumps and unevenness, and is not commonly employed as an adjunctive procedure in his practice.

COMPLICATIONS

All blepharoplasty surgeons should expect to encounter and treat complications. Fortunately, sight-threatening complications, such as retroorbital hematoma, are

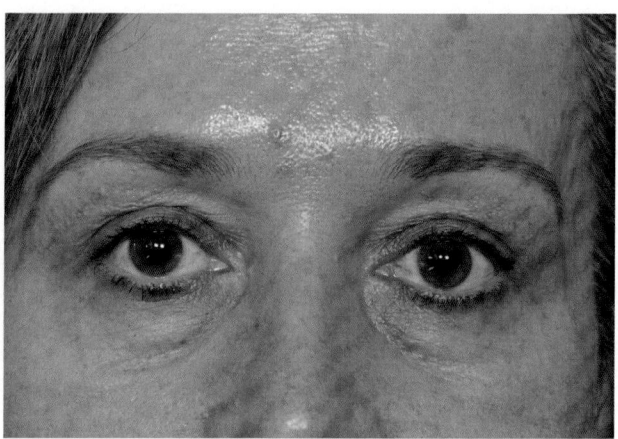
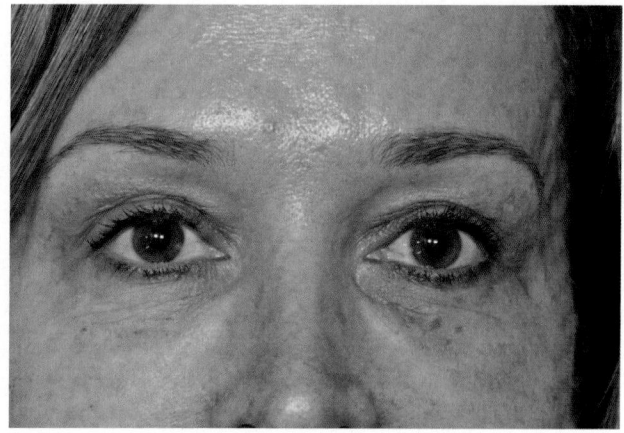

A   B

Figure 187.30 Before and after photos of Restylane filler in the lower eyelid "tear trough" region. **A:** Prefiller. **B:** Postfiller.

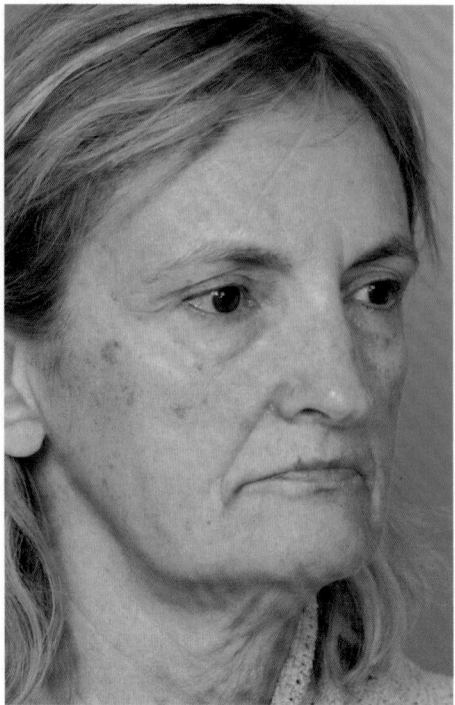 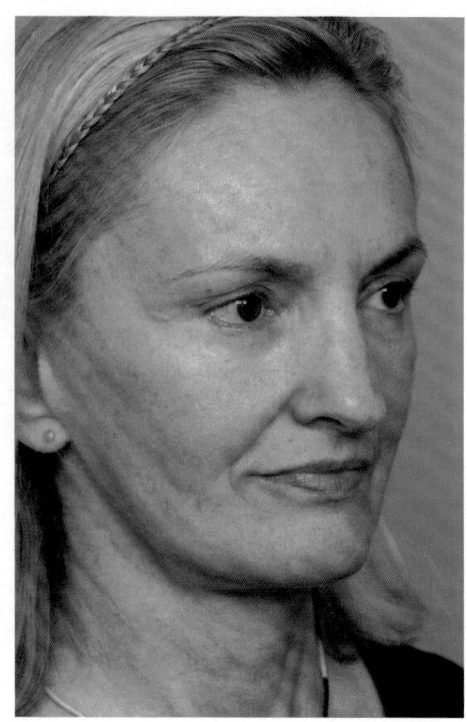

Figure 187.31 Pre and postoperative photos of mid-facelift result with lower lid blepharoplasty. **A:** Preoperative. **B:** Postoperative.   **A**   **B**

extremely rare. The best outcomes are usually achieved with prompt recognition and early treatment.

DRY EYE SYMPTOMS, BLURRY VISION, AND CHEMOSIS

Dry eye symptoms, blurry vision, and chemosis are part of a common spectrum of expected sequelae or complications caused by the mechanical disruption of eyelid function and/or lagophthalmos following surgery.

Prophylaxis for of dry eye symptoms is important following eyelid surgery. All blepharoplasty patients should be placed on an aggressive lubrication regimen consisting of ophthalmic drops and ointment; they should be encouraged to "over-lubricate" in the first 10 days following surgery. Patients should also be told during the preoperative consult that blepharoplasty can lead to "visual downtime," which can last 2 weeks. They should expect to modify their lifestyles (i.e., no driving, contact lenses, or prolonged computer use) during the first several days after surgery. Unfortunately, dry eye symptoms can become chronic, requiring indefinite use of lubrication or adjunctive procedures.

Chemosis is characterized by yellowish conjunctival edema that typically occurs in the first 7 days following blepharoplasty (Fig. 187.32). Large studies have found the incidence to range from less than 1% to 12% (11) of patients following blepharoplasty (12,13). Although the exact cause of chemosis is unknown, disruption of the lower eyelid lymphatics (particularly in the region of the lateral canthus) and conjunctival exposure from

lagophthalmos are thought to be contributing factors. Conservative treatment consists of aggressive lubrication, supportive lid taping, nighttime eye patching, and limiting sodium consumption. Topical steroid drops and rarely surgical procedures, such as drainage conjunctivotomy or temporary tarsorrhaphy, are also occasionally indicated. Most cases resolve within 6 weeks.

LID POSITION ABNORMALITIES

Lid malposition, which includes rounding, retraction, and ectropion, is considered by some to be the most common complication following the transcutaneous approach to blepharoplasty (13) (Fig. 187.33). It has also been

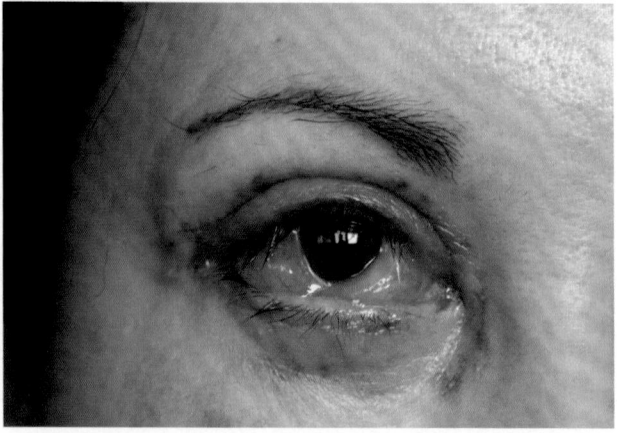

Figure 187.32 Chemosis following skin muscle flap blepharoplasty.

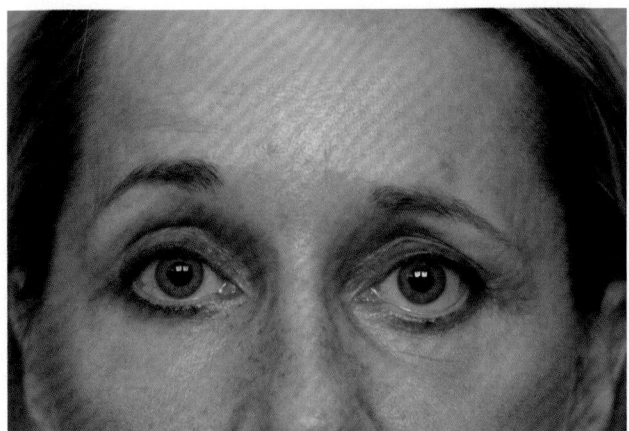

Figure 187.33 Lid malposition following blepharoplasty.

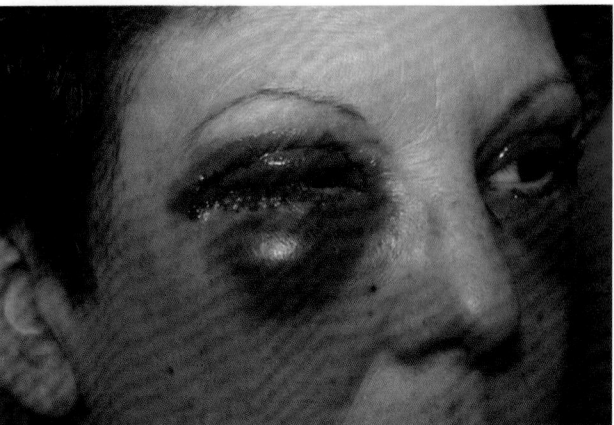

Figure 187.34 Preseptal hematoma immediately following blepharoplasty.

documented following the transconjunctival approach (9). The risk of symptomatic malposition is greater in patients with preexisting lid laxity, leading some to advocate routine canthal support in the form of canthopexy or canthoplasty during blepharoplasty (13).

If mild retraction is noted postoperatively, ocular lubrication, upward massage, and lid taping are recommended. Steroid injections can also be performed to oppose the forces of contracture, particularly if a scar band is palpated. When symptomatic retraction or ectropion develop, surgical management is usually indicated. In cases of horizontal lid excess, a canthoplasty is performed. When scarring of the anterior or posterior lamella is noted, spacer grafts are usually employed.

MILIA

Epithelial remnants can become trapped within the incision, manifesting as small white nodules, or milia. Treatment consists of incision and extraction or marsupialization. This can easily be performed with an 18-gauge needle in the office.

ALLERGIC CONJUNCTIVITIS

Toxoallergic blepharoconjunctivitis can be caused by a variety of topical treatments (prescribed and over the counter) used in the postoperative period. Common causes include preparations containing neomycin or preservatives. Patients will report redness, itching, or increasing swelling and inflammation. Cessation of the offending agent is curative, although topical steroids, cool compresses, and diphenhydramine can be used for symptom relief (5).

INFECTION

The rich vascularity of the eyelids has a protective effect against infection following blepharoplasty. Although extremely rare, infections have been reported, including methicillin-resistant *Staphylococcus aureus*, mycobacterial,

and even necrotizing fasciitis. Clinical suspicion, cultures, and appropriate antibiotics are essential for treatment.

PRESEPTAL HEMATOMA

Although rare, preseptal hematoma can be seen following blepharoplasty (Fig. 187.34). This complication can often be prevented with meticulous intraoperative hemostasis. Treatment consists of opening of incisions, decompression, and cautery of any offending vessels.

RETROORBITAL HEMATOMA

Retroorbital hematoma is considered to be the most feared complication following blepharoplasty. The incidence of orbital hemorrhage has been found to range between 1:2,000 (0.05%) and 1:20,000 (0.005%). The incidence of vision loss due to hematoma has been found to range from 1:10,000 (0.01%) to 1:30,000 (0.003%) (5,14).

Symptoms of retroorbital hematoma usually present within the first 24 hours after surgery. The most commonly reported risk factor is hypertension (14). Patients will complain of pain and pressure. Signs include increased intraocular pressure, eyelid ecchymosis, and a tense orbit. Treatment should consist of immediate decompression by opening all incisions with exploration to identify and cauterize any offending vessel. Medical therapy consists of oxygen, topical beta-blockers, intravenous steroids, mannitol, and acetazolamide. If the wound cannot be adequately explored and decompressed through existing incisions, surgical management consists of lateral canthotomy with inferior cantholysis.

CONCLUSIONS

Lower eyelid blepharoplasty is a detail-oriented procedure. It requires diligence in preoperative planning, intraoperative technique, and postoperative management. Preparation and thoroughness are the keys to success in this rewarding operation.

ACKNOWLEDGMENT

The authors would like to acknowledge Nancy Rothrock for her medical photography and Christopher M. Brown at the Indiana University School of Medicine for his medical illustrations in this chapter.

HIGHLIGHTS

- Thorough knowledge of lower eyelid anatomy is required prior to embarking on blepharoplasty.
- Lower lid blepharoplasty can correct orbital fat pseudoherniation, excess skin and muscle, mild festooning, and tear trough deformities. Blepharoplasty does *not* correct abnormal skin pigmentation, fine rhytids, or large malar bags/edema.
- Physical examination prior to blepharoplasty should always include testing for lower eyelid laxity. Performing blepharoplasty in patients with lid laxity requires lid-supporting adjunctive procedures (canthopexy or canthoplasty). Failure to do this can lead to rounding, scleral show, and frank ectropion.
- The preoperative physical examination should guide the surgeon in selecting the correct approach for blepharoplasty. The transconjunctival and transcutaneous approach each has specific indications.
- Prompt recognition and treatment of complications are essential in avoiding long-term sequelae following blepharoplasty.

REFERENCES

1. Mowlavi A, et al. Lower blepharoplasty using bony anatomical landmarks to identify and avoid injury to the inferior oblique muscle. *Plast Reconstr Surg* 2002;110(5):1318–1322.
2. Lam SM, et al. *Complimentary fat grafting*. Philadelphia, PA: Lippincott Williams & Wilkins, 2007:19.
3. Goldberg RA, et al. Fat repositioning in lower eyelid blepharoplasty. *Semin Ophthalmol* 1998;13(3):103–106.
4. Jacono A. Blepharoplasty, lower lid festoons. http://emedicine.medscape.com/article/1282338-overview. Accessed April, 2008.
5. Klapper SR, Patrinely JR. Management of cosmetic eyelid surgery complications. *Semin Plast Surg* 2007;21(1):80–93.
6. Rees TD, Jelks GW. Blepharoplasty and the dry eye syndrome: guidelines for surgery? *Plast Reconstr Surg* 1981;68(2):249–252.
7. Perkins SW, Latorre R. Blepharoplasty: a facial plastic surgeon's perspective. In: Romo T, ed. *Aesthetic facial plastic surgery*. New York, NY: Thieme, 2000:262–287.
8. Crumley RL, et al. Lower eyelid blepharoplasty. In: Papel I, ed. *Facial plastic and reconstructive surgery*, 3rd ed. New York, NY: Thieme, 2009:271–286.
9. Perkins SW, et al. Transconjunctival approach to lower eyelid blepharoplasty: experience indications, and technique in 300 Patients. *Arch Otolaryngol Head Neck Surg* 1994;120(2): 172–177.
10. Garcia EG, McCollough EG. Transcutaneous lower eyelid blepharoplasty with fat excision: a shift resisting paradigm. *Arch Facial Plast Surg* 2006;8(6):374–380.
11. Honrado CP and Pastorek NJ. Long-term results of lower-lid suspension blepharoplasty: a 30-year experience. *Arch Facial Plast Surg* 2004;6(3):150–154.
12. Weinfeld AB, et al. The comprehensive management of chemosis following cosmetic lower blepharoplasty. *Plast Reconstr Surg* 2008;122(2):579–586.
13. Codner MA, et al. Primary transcutaneous lower blepharoplasty with routine lateral canthal support: a comprehensive 10-year review. *Plast Reconstr Surg* 2008;121(1):241–250.
14. Mejia JD, et al. Visual loss after blepharoplasty: incidence, management, and preventative measures. *Aesthet Surg J* 2011;31(1): 21–29.

Rhytidectomy (Face-Lift) 188

Russell W. H. Kridel   **Zahi Abou Chacra**

The principal role of rhytidectomy is to elevate facial tissues that have descended with the aging process. Although skin excision is performed in a face-lifting procedure, contrary to the once predominant common belief, it is often not the dominant or sole goal one should try to achieve. Most current face-lift techniques rely on resuspension of the superficial musculoaponeurotic system (SMAS), whether through a SMAS or deep plane approach, with redraping and removal of skin without tension. The authors are witness to a steady evolution of technical and anatomical advances producing a new generation of face-lifts. Presently, the authors continue to evaluate these newer techniques in search of the ideal procedure, which will give our patients a long-term, natural correction with rapid recovery and few complications.

GENERAL CONSIDERATIONS AND ADJUNCTIVE PROCEDURES

Aging face patients requesting consultation for a face-lift generally seek a youthful, more rested appearance. These patients have a well-developed self-image and do not want to look different. Rather they desire a natural-appearing result that turns back the hands of time to a more youthful version of themselves. For the surgeon, the goal is to determine what physical characteristics of the face are contributing to the impression of aging, which stigmata are reversible, and by what means. Ideally, the surgeon brings to this consultation a thorough understanding of the processes that lead to an aged appearance and is familiar with a wide variety of medical and surgical interventions appropriate for addressing the clinical problem. As with all elective facial plastic surgery, it is imperative for the surgeon to achieve a balanced, harmonious result. The patient who presents with an interest in face-lift who also has brow ptosis and four-quadrant dermatochalasis can be poorly served if the incongruity is not discussed prior to proceeding with the surgery. Moreover, oftentimes these patients will be left with more stigmata of a lifted appearance should they only address the lower face due to this incongruity. For these reasons, in addition to the face-lift, it is important to discuss the potential benefits of browlift, blepharoplasty, skin resurfacing (laser, chemical peel, and dermabrasion), as well as adjunctive procedures such as soft tissue fillers (like hyaluronic acid and calcium hydroxyapatite), fat injection, alloplastic implants, or muscle-paralyzing agent injections like Botox and newly approved Dysport. These are adjunctive procedures that complement face-lifting surgery and address the general theme of facial rejuvenation, which sometimes face-lifting cannot achieve alone.

A recent paradigm shift among many authors is volume preservation and restoration in the aging face, rather than just resuspension of deep tissues. This paradigm shift is partly demonstrated by the increasing use of biologic and synthetic injectable fillers in facial plastic surgery. Other commonly used volume-augmenting strategies for facial rejuvenation include fat injections and alloplastic implants. Proponents of such techniques argue that fat and tissue atrophy happen along with gravitational changes. Recently, Lambros (1) compared pictures taken up to 50 years apart and studied the effect of aging on the midface and periorbital complex. He concluded that there was little ptosis at the lid–cheek junction and that the aged appearance was partly due to volume loss. In another of his papers, he proposed how the addition of volume may give better results than traditional surgical methods (2). He emphasized that a face that has enough tissue volume is the best predictor of a face-lift outcome. It is our opinion and the one of many other surgeons that volume restoration is an important adjunct but does not replace the need for a surgical lift. The authors do, however, recognize that for some patients with volume loss as well as tissue descent, both problems must be addressed to produce natural, harmonious, and complimentary results.

The term face-lifting is sometimes a misleading term to patients, as it does not spell out which structures will be lifted. It says nothing about the neck, which is a main area of most lifting procedures, and on the other hand, it implies that the upper third of the face will be lifted, which most surgeons consider another procedure that they would address separately, such as with a forehead lift.

Most patients undergoing today's typical face-lift are really getting a lower face- and neck lift. To lift the upper third of the face, for instance, one should rely on a forehead lift. In his recent publication, McCollough stresses that the term face-lift is often inadequately used. He describes five progressive stages of aging and proposes a classification that helps matching the specific aging stage with the appropriate rejuvenation treatment (3). His system describes procedures based on anatomic locations such as temple lift, forehead lift, cheek lift, and neck lift, diminishing confusion around the more generic widely used face-lift term. This chapter focuses only on the anatomy and clinical considerations of the present-day rhytidectomy procedure.

PHYSIOLOGY OF THE AGING FACE

To understand the present-day rhytidectomy procedure, the surgeon must have full knowledge not only of the underlying surgical anatomy but also of the aging physiology of the face, which leads patients to seek rejuvenation

surgery. In general, the aging face presents five landmarks that are points of interest to patients and surgeons alike. These areas include (a) the jowl, (b) the deepened nasolabial folds and lateral perioral jowling, (c) the platysma banding and submental fullness in the neck region, (d) the orbicularis oculi and malar fat pad ptosis, and (e) the aging skin itself (Fig. 188.1A).

In youth, the facial skin is maintained in normal anatomic position by retaining "ligaments" that run from deep facial structures to the dermis itself (4). With aging, attenuation of these "ligamentous" supports then results in malar soft tissue descent. The result of this descent is not only deepening of the melolabial folds but also jowling of the platysma and soft tissue between the masseteric and mandibular ligaments at the jawline. Moreover, this descent of the malar fat pad along with ptosis of the orbicularis oculi also results in hollowing in the infraorbital region. Finally, loss of platysma muscle tone results in anterior banding and the classically pictured "turkey gobbler" neck (5) (Fig. 188.1B).

Separate from the described underlying soft tissue changes, the surgeon must note the cumulative effects of the inherent aging process coupled with the effects of environmental exposure on the skin itself. While a comprehensive review of the changes associated with aging skin is beyond the scope of this chapter, it is important for the surgeon to have a fundamental understanding of

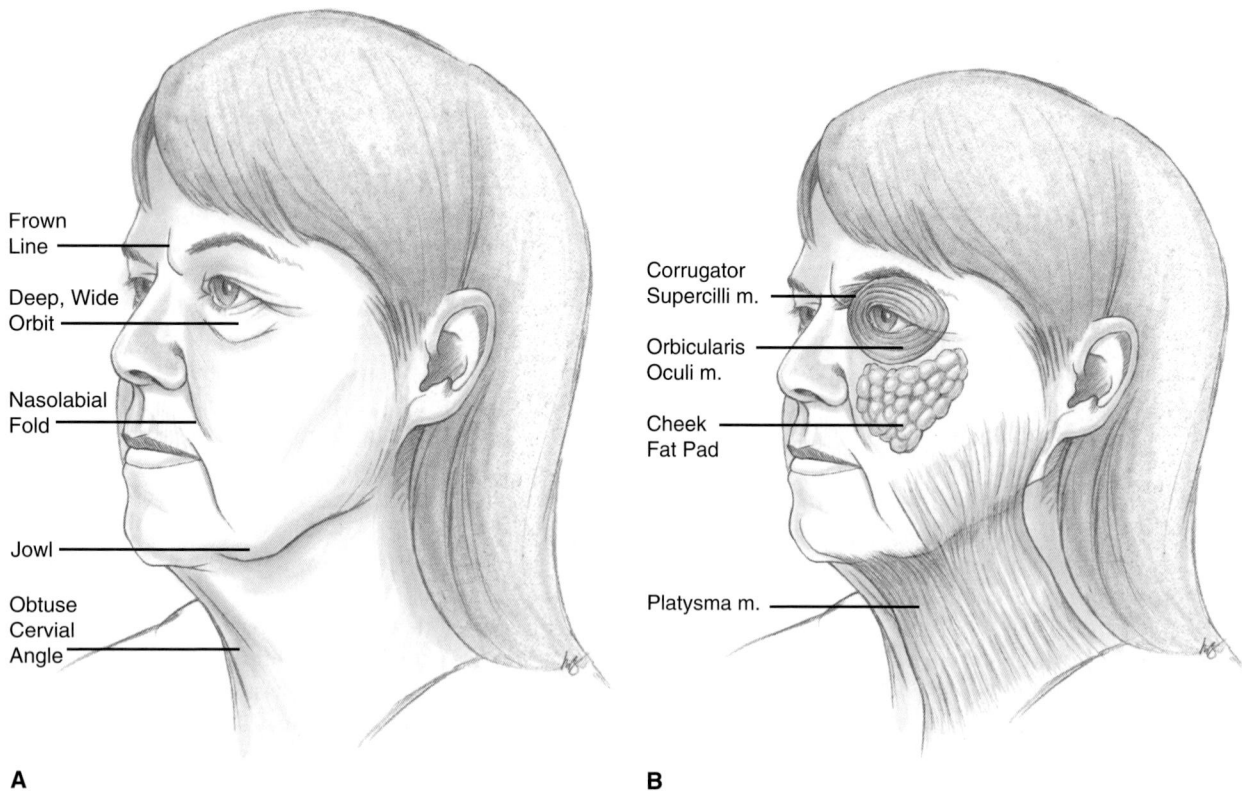

Frown Line

Deep, Wide Orbit

Nasolabial Fold

Jowl

Obtuse Cervial Angle

Corrugator Supercilli m.

Orbicularis Oculi m.

Cheek Fat Pad

Platysma m.

A   **B**

Figure 188.1 A: Topographic changes seen in the face with aging. **B:** Underlying soft tissue and muscular changes seen in the aging face. (Adapted from Zimbler MS, Kokoska MS, Thomas JR. Anatomy and pathophysiology of facial aging. *Facial Plast Surg Clin North Am* 2001;9:179–187.)

these changes. In this regard, it is convenient to think of skin aging in terms of extrinsic and intrinsic factors, affecting both the epidermis and the dermis (6). Extrinsic factors refer to environmental insults such as sun-induced damage (photodamage). Intrinsic aging refers to the natural effects of time and is generally characterized by tissue atrophy and descent and reduction in skin cellular and protein components. In fact, chronologically aged skin has reduced epidermal thickness, flattening of the dermal–epidermal junction, atrophy of the dermis, and a general decline in a variety of cell populations including melanocytes and Langerhans cells (7). This epidermal thinning then makes the skin more susceptible to damage from shearing-type forces (6). Moreover, Yousif and Mendelson (8) showed how habitual facial expressions lead to coarse skin wrinkling and deep folds. However, Kligman et al. (9) noted that in point of fact, there are no histologic features that distinguish the various types of wrinkles from the surrounding skin. He noted that instead there is a configurational change that results from mechanical stress acting on lax, excessive skin, especially in actinically damaged regions.

On the other hand, photoaged epidermis is characterized by striking variability: in its thickness, with alternating areas of atrophy and hyperplasia; in pigmentation, with alternating lentigines and depigmented areas; in the degree of nuclear atypia; and in orderliness of keratinocytes maturation (10). In the past, sun-damaged epidermis was thought to be characterized by a reduction in structural elements, leading to skin wrinkling. In fact, the most striking feature of photodamaged skin is the presence of large quantities of thickened, poorly organized degraded elastic fibers, which degenerate into an amorphous mass, better known as elastosis. This loss of elastin decreases skin elasticity, defined as the loss of the ability of the skin to recoil and redrape once pulled away from the deep tissues (11). The result is aged skin, which does not retain moisture and which loosens and hangs. The ground substance component of the dermal connective tissue matrix is greatly increased. In the dermal cell population, photodamaged skin shows numerous, hyperplastic fibroblasts and abundant, partially degranulated mast cells, which result in a chronic low-grade inflammation termed heliodermatitis. Finally, photodamaged skin shows extensive changes in the microcirculation, which can affect flap viability. Along with skin changes, atrophy of underlying soft tissue and fat have also been described. Skeletal changes pertaining to both bone loss and bone remodeling also occur with aging.

Overall the aging face can be viewed as a coupling of redistributed ptotic underlying soft tissue with overlying skin changes. Together, these changes combine to contribute to the overall impression of the aging face. For most aging face patients, this means that facial rejuvenation will necessitate the surgeon concentrating on five points of interest: (a) the jowl, (b) the deepened melolabial and nasolabial folds, (c) the neck, (d) the malar region, and (e) the skin itself.

SURGICAL ANATOMY

The last 20 years have brought about numerous improvements in the face-lift surgery. These new advances have largely come about through better anatomical understanding as well as an understanding of how the aging process alters these anatomical components throughout the face and neck. Certain salient points of the facial anatomy for rhytidectomy, including vascular supply, details of the SMAS and its relation to the facial nerve, as well as the presence of retaining "ligaments," are described here.

The facial skin is supplied by branches of the external carotid artery. Specifically, the superficial temporal artery, facial artery, transverse facial artery, and infraorbital artery anastomose with one another in the subdermal plexus. The internal carotid artery also contributes to the facial skin centered around the radix and the glabella through branches of the ophthalmic artery. However, this area is not routinely addressed during face-lifting. The elevated subcutaneous flap is based solely on the subdermal plexus, which is supplied by muscular cutaneous arteries arising from branches of the facial and infraorbital arteries. Unfortunately, the standard subcutaneous and SMAS two-layered face-lift effectively divides the skin from its underlying perforating branches. A recent study comparing the vascular anatomy of basic skin flaps in the subcutaneous and SMAS rhytidectomy, the composite rhytidectomy, and the subperiosteal rhytidectomy found, not surprisingly, that the best blood supply was found in subperiosteal dissection while the most tenuous supply was in the subcutaneous flap (12). However, outside of smokers and those patients with small vessel disease, one must consider that each of these techniques has been used for many years with minimal low flap perfusion rate complications (5).

Perhaps the first, and most important, development in the evolution toward the present-day rhytidectomy was the description of the SMAS. In fact, while the precise boundaries of the SMAS continue to be a source of debate, the significance of this fascial layer in relation to present-day rhytidectomy is unquestionable. The SMAS, which is a fibromuscular fascial layer, invests and interlinks the muscles of facial expression. Moreover, in this function it maintains consistent relationships with the facial nerve and major vessels within the facial region. For the operating surgeon, mastery of these relationships and planes of dissection are therefore critical (13).

The regional variations that are found in the relationship between the SMAS and the neurovascular structures are most profound when examining the SMAS and the facial nerve above the zygoma versus below the zygoma (14). Specifically, in the temporal region above the zygoma, the superficial temporal artery and frontal branch *course through the SMAS* (also called temporoparietal fascia). Below the zygoma, the SMAS fans out over the parotid gland and then above the masseter muscle before it surrounds the facial mimetic muscles. Therefore, in the lower face, the facial nerve branches are always *deep to the SMAS* and innervate the facial mimetic muscles on their undersurface (Fig. 188.2).

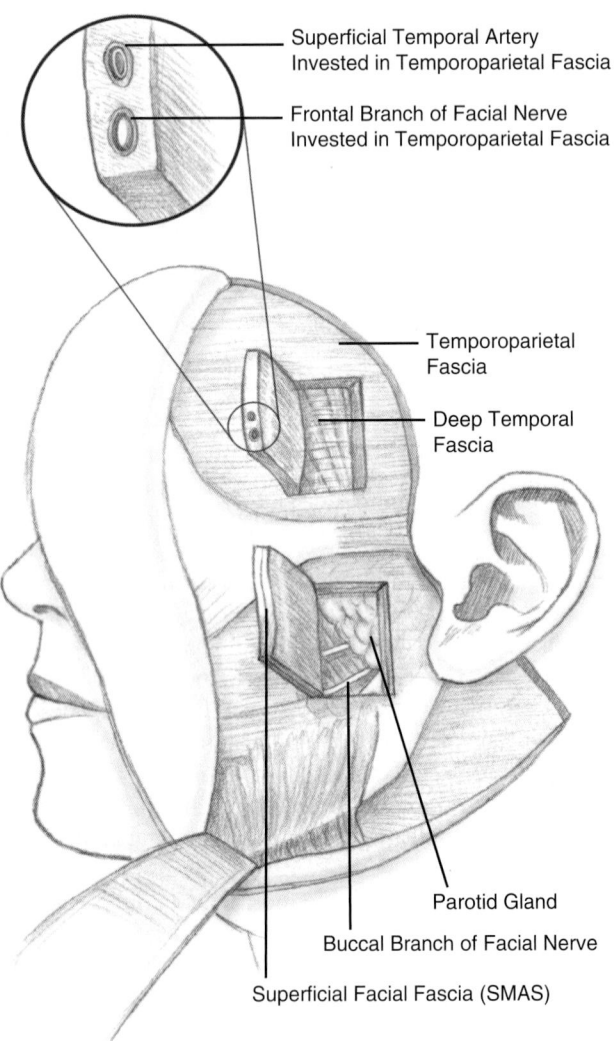

Figure 188.2 In the temporal region, above the zygoma, the frontal branch travels through the SMAS. In the lower face, below the zygoma, the facial nerve branches lie deep to the SMAS and innervate the facial mimetic muscles from their deep surface. (Adapted from Stuzin JM. The relationship of the superficial and deep facial fascias: relevance to rhytidectomy and aging. *Plast Reconstr Surg* 1992;89(3):441–449.)

However, there are three exceptions to that rule. The levator anguli oris, buccinator, and mentalis muscles lie in a somewhat deeper plane making their innervation from the facial nerve from their superficial surface, rather than their undersurface. It should be noted that even in the deep plane and composite lifts, the dissection medial to the zygomaticus major and minor is actually above the SMAS because the SMAS thins out over this region. Moreover, it should be noted that a significant, distinct myofascial layer superficial to the parotid fascia is not always clinically apparent. In fact, Jost and Levet (15) have suggested that the SMAS overlying the parotid includes what the authors have otherwise distinguished as the parotid fascia.

Finally, as previously alluded to, the SMAS has been noted to have a number of "ligamentous" supports, which make it adherent at specific points to the overlying dermis

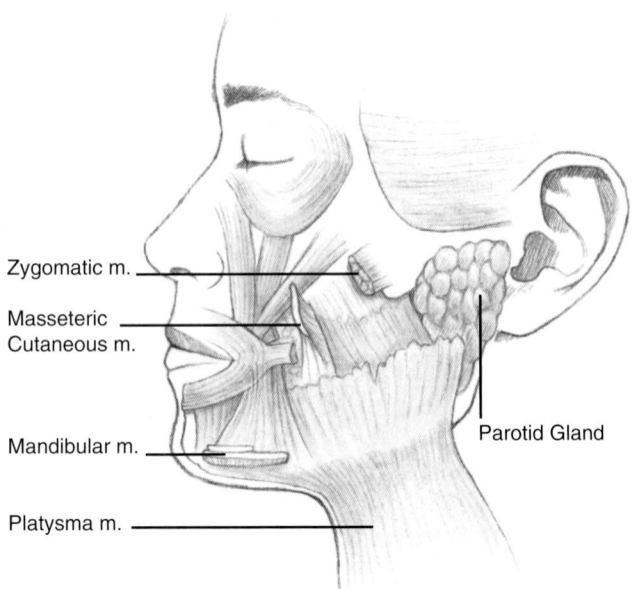

Figure 188.3 The four retaining ligaments of the cheeks.

and underlying muscular/osseous attachments. Specifically, four ligaments support the soft tissues of the cheek: (a) the parotidomasseteric ligament, (b) the platysmal auricular ligament, (c) the zygomatic ligament (McGregor patch), and (d) the mandibular ligament (Fig. 188.3). Although not true ligaments, these fascial condensations are especially important in the deep plane and composite rhytidectomy (16). Release of these ligaments is important and will allow the surgeon to achieve a better pull to redrape the tissue. However, this task must be undertaken with extreme caution as branches of the facial nerve are in close proximity.

SURGICAL EVOLUTION: A HISTORICAL PERSPECTIVE

A steady evolution of anatomically derived technical advances has occurred in the rhytidectomy procedure since the early days of simple skin flap advancement. Reports of face-lifting attempts date back to the very first years of the 20th century and consisted primarily of skin excision and direct closure. This technique was utilized for over 50 years before the first major contribution to advance face-lifting was provided by Skoog. Sometime in the mid-1960s, Skoog began to elevate a "complex morphologic unit" in the cervical region and advance it posteriorly (17). It was observed that this "two-layered shift" of the cervical fascia corrected the anterior banding of the neck and the redundant skin of the cervical region. Skoog subsequently followed this with his description in 1974 of his technique of superficial rhytidectomy of the face and neck based on a subfascial dissection. The new era in face-lift surgery had begun (18–20).

It would take until 1976 before Mitz and Peyronie (21) defined the "complex morphologic unit" referred to by Skoog as the SMAS. The SMAS lift approach, which then became vogue, was a significant step in the evolution of the present-day rhytidectomy. However, some surgeons, in pursuit of the ideal lift, still found the results of the SMAS lift to be short-lived and complicated by perioperative problems. For some surgeons, the SMAS lift did not appear to sufficiently address the ptotic midface and melolabial fold region. In an effort to enhance midface tissue, Faivre (22) described in 1988 the deep temporal face-lift in the sub-SMAS plane. That same year, Psillakis et al. (23) described the subperiosteal midface lift to correct ptotic malar fat pad. In 1990 and 1992, Hamra (24) published his techniques on deep plane face-lift and composite face-lift, respectively (25). In the deep plane face-lift, Hamra innovates on the Skoog technique by adding a superolateral elevation of the malar fat pad. The composite lift added dissection and resuspension of the orbicularis oculi muscle superomedially, thus effacing what the author has termed as the malar crescent, in an effort to rejuvenate the periocular complex and better create harmony with the lower parts of the face.

Recently, many "newly named" face-lift techniques have been heavily marketed: the mini-lift, weekend lift, short flap lift, S lift, and lunchtime lift. Most of these lifts rely on a short skin flap and sometimes a minimal SMAS suspension. These less invasive procedures have the advantages of decreasing associated complications and substantially minimizing patient recovery time. However, in most cases their indications are limited to patients with limited signs of aging, and results from such techniques may be short-lived or less than ideal. Webster had explored short flap face-lifting in 1983, which many later abandoned (26).

To date, it is uncertain what percentage of surgeons are performing the extended sub-SMAS lifts versus the traditional SMAS plication/imbrication techniques. Moreover, questions remain as to the superiority of the results that are achieved in the deep plane versus plication techniques. In fact, while anecdotal reports abound to this effect, it will be very difficult to accomplish the study that can definitively answer this and a whole host of other questions. Proponents of deep plane rhytidectomy claim an improved nasolabial fold in comparison to the traditional SMAS suspension techniques (27). Adamson et al. (28) found a twofold improvement with deep plane measured by the degree of increased volume at the malar eminence and by the amount of effacement of the fold. Becker and Bassichis (29) concluded that results from a deep plane face-lift were not superior to those from SMAS plication in patients that are younger than 70 years old. Baker (30) and Kamer (31) maintain reservations regarding the superiority of the results from the deep plane lifts, especially when these "implied benefits" are weighed in relation to the added risks to the facial nerve. Baker and Conley (32) notes that a review of the world literature in 1979 found an incidence of 0.01% permanent facial nerve injury in deep plane cases. He notes in a later paper (30) that the published articles on the new deep dissection techniques conjure concern as they report a relatively high incidence of facial weakness in the hands of extremely qualified surgeons. He questions what happens when these procedures are attempted by less experienced

surgeons. Time and experience are still needed before the authors will know if the added work and increased potential risk for complication is worth the improved aesthetic results. In a recent systematic review of 39 articles comparing the efficacy and complication rate of different face-lift techniques, Chang concluded there was a lack of quality data to be objectively compared (33). It is also important to note that results will always vary from surgeon to surgeon due to skills and expertise.

ASSESSING CANDIDACY

With an understanding of the physiologic and anatomical changes that present with facial aging, the surgeon is ready to determine whether the patient is a candidate for facial rejuvenation surgery in general and rhytidectomy in particular. This evaluation includes surgical, medical, and psychological components.

The surgical criterion to be addressed is whether rhytidectomy will create physical changes in the patient's face that will contribute meaningfully to a more youthful appearance. In making this determination, it is helpful to divide the stigmata of facial aging into two categories: those that are improved by repositioning of facial tissues and those that require changes in the structure of the tissues themselves. In the first category, one would include ptosis in the jowl, submentum, and anterior neck leading to a disruption of the ideal youthful contours of the jawline, cervicomental angle, and neck, respectively. These are the primary areas improved by rhytidectomy. Malar ptosis will experience modest improvement as well.

On the other hand, intrinsic changes in the tissues themselves are not well addressed by rhytidectomy. As noted earlier, concomitant with the ptosis described above, aging brings about many changes in the skin itself. Fine lines and deeply etched wrinkles in the skin are the grossly visible correlates of crevices in the dermis and subcutaneous tissues formed over time as a result of actinic damage, senescence of connective tissues, and habitual facial expressions. These cosmetic defects will be minimally improved, at best, by rhytidectomy. Instead, they can be addressed more directly by resurfacing techniques, including both chemical and laser exfoliation. In the situation in which such intrinsic properties of the skin comprise a significant portion of the aesthetic problem, the patient should be encouraged to consider skin resurfacing as an adjunct or, in some cases, an alternative to rhytidectomy.

Once the surgeon has determined that a rhytidectomy will address the patient's aesthetic concerns appropriately, it is imperative to assess medical candidacy for the procedure. Most patients who seek cosmetic surgery are in good health, so medical contraindications to the proposed procedure are rarely seen. Vigilance is essential for avoiding disaster. Face-lift candidates—people who feel young inside and want their outward appearance to mirror that vitality—are exactly the same people who tend to minimize medical complaints and even may forget to relate serious medical problems unless questioned directly. Significant bleeding diatheses and American Society of Anesthesiologists (ASA) class IV or V, in which a patient has a dangerously compromising medical condition, should he considered absolute medical contraindications to rhytidectomy. A patient in ASA class III, in which a medical condition impairs the patient's activities to some degree, should be approached with great caution. The severity of the condition and its potential impact on the safe conduct of the operation should be explored in detail. Conditions that may adversely affect healing including uncontrolled diabetes, diseases requiring chronic steroid therapy, or connective tissue abnormalities like the Ehlers-Danlos syndrome should be considered strong relative contraindications to face-lift surgery. Consultation with the primary care physician may be necessary to coordinate prescription medication regimens and facilitate the management of relevant medical conditions.

On the other hand, there are no age limitations for face-lift surgery, and age should not be a reason to deny surgery if the patient is in otherwise good health. A healthy patient in his or her late 70s or early 80s may have 15 or 20 more years of quality life ahead, and the desire to have an improved appearance is indeed valid.

Finally, but not least important, an accurate assessment of the patient's psychological status is central to determining patient candidacy. The surgeon should determine patient motivation and attempt to ascertain whether the patient might fail to view a successful surgical outcome favorably or might react inappropriately to any aspect of the surgery. A thorough discussion of the patient's goals and objectives should provide important clues to his or her psychological profile (34). Although many patients are unaware of exactly what surgery can and cannot accomplish, others have clearly unreasonable expectations, which can include looking exactly as they did 10 or 20 years ago, having surgery without scars, requesting an unnaturally tight lift, or attempting to obtain promises and guarantees. Patients who are excessively occupied with minute flaws also may be poor surgical candidates. Moreover, patients who have recently undergone a major change in their personal status, such as the death of a loved one or divorce, may be subject to depression or psychological unevenness and may require special care.

PREOPERATIVE EVALUATION AND PLANNING

General Considerations

Once a patient is deemed an appropriate candidate for rhytidectomy, they need to be educated clearly before surgery. They must understand that rhytidectomy helps with excessive skin and jowling and provides for redraping of the skin, but it does not change the quality of the skin itself. If fine or deep rhytids are present preoperatively, they will be present postoperatively as soon as the swelling goes down. In severely sun-damaged patients, full-face deep chemical peeling with phenol solution or CO_2 laser resurfacing is often necessary as an adjunct and can be done several weeks after the initial face-lift surgery. If there are significant rhytids limited to the perioral or periorbital areas, these cosmetic units may be safely peeled or removed by laser simultaneously with the rhytidectomy as long as these areas are not undermined during the procedure. Undermined areas are partly devascularized in the immediate postoperative period and further skin insult by laser resurfacing could lead to skin necrosis.

To assess further the overall improvement possible with rhytidectomy, the underlying structure of the face must be critically evaluated. Patients who had a good bony structure of the cheekbones, chin, and jaw during their youth will have the best results, as the redraping of skin will help to highlight these attractive bony structures. Therefore, patients who have a thinner, angular face and good bony definition are generally much better candidates than patients with rounder faces, low cheekbones, or a short mandible (Figs. 188.4 to 188.6).

Adjunctive chin and submalar cheek augmentation may be necessary in conjunction with a face-lift to achieve the desired result. Patients who have a retrusive chin cannot get desired cervicomental definition without a chin implant, even after a face-lift. Also, because the aging process sometimes causes a hollow-cheek deformity due to the atrophy of soft tissue and fat with ptosis of the fat pads, older patients sometimes require submalar augmentation or resupport of the fat pads simultaneously with the face-lift. Redraping the skin alone will not replace soft tissue cheek hollowness.

As the underlying structures of the face dictate the aesthetic results possible above the jawline, those in the neck similarly limit the outcome there. In particular, the position of the hyoid bone relative to the mandible varies from patient to patient. This relationship defines the course of the suprahyoid musculature of the floor of the mouth and limits the maximum improvement possible in the cervicomental angle. A relatively high and posterior hyoid is ideal, allowing maximum elevation of the submental contour and the greatest definition between the submentum and neck in profile. A relatively low and anterior hyoid limits the possible improvement in this area to a predictable degree. It is mandatory, therefore, that hyoid position be assessed and its effects on the possible outcome discussed with the patient in a way that is easily understood. The authors have found the use of diagrams illustrating hyoid position to be very helpful in their practices (Fig. 188.7).

A full evaluation of the facial nerve and muscles should be done preoperatively, particularly noting any asymmetries, especially around the mouth. Sometimes patients have asymmetric smiles or may inadvertently elevate the brow. There may be static asymmetries as well, ranging from minor unilateral cheek or jowl fullness to generalized asymmetry as in hemifacial microsomias. Any asymmetry should be documented, photographed, and discussed with the patient before surgery, or the patient may attribute their asymmetry to the surgery (35). Further, it gives the surgeon the opportunity to

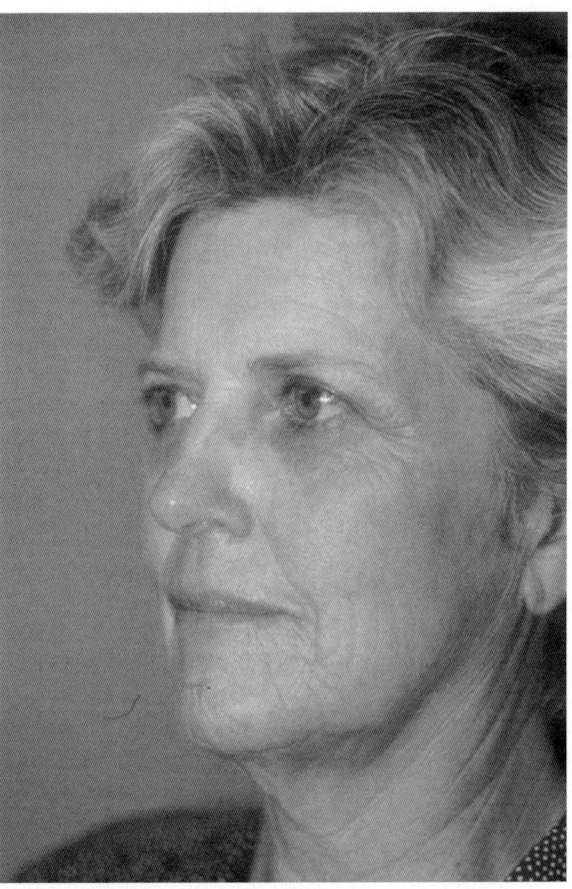

Figure 188.4 Excellent candidate for a face-lift: little fat, good bone structure, and not too much skin.

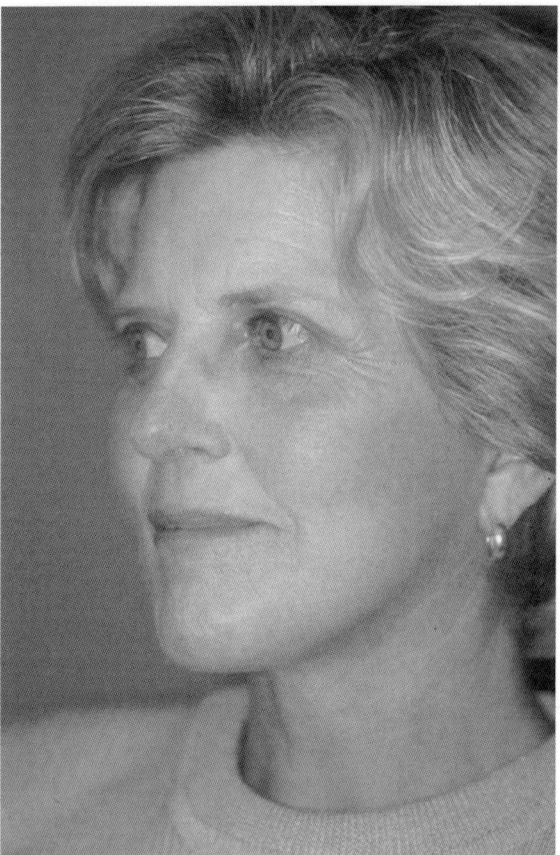

Figure 188.5 Postoperative views of same patient after face-lift and upper eyelid blepharoplasty.

point out that minor asymmetry is normal and that perfect symmetry cannot be a surgical goal. The surgeon also should note any traumatic facial and neck lacerations, sites of previous biopsies, acne scars, facial or neck scars, subcutaneous depressions, surface irregularities, and focal lesions.

Generally, the older patient who presents with voluminous sagging skin or the patient with a fat face and neck would not be as good a candidate as the thinner 40- to 50-year-old patient because postoperative skin re-draping with such excess is less satisfactory, especially if elastosis is present. Such patients should be advised that for a better result, a tuck procedure may be necessary 6 months to 1 year after all the retraction has occurred from the original face-lift (36). If liposis is limited to the submental area, the patient will be a better candidate than one who has a full, rounded face with fat throughout. Liposuction in conjunction with a face-lift exerts its maximal effect in the submental area.

Similarly, if a patient contemplates a weight loss of more than 10 pounds, it may be better to postpone surgery until afterward. The authors discourage patients who have a history of repeated weight gain and loss from considering face-lift surgery because repeated stretching of the facial skin may cause a premature return of skin laxity.

Smoking history is also particularly relevant. Rees and Aston (37) noted that smokers have 12 times greater risk of

skin slough than nonsmokers, possibly secondary to vasoconstriction, and also have a higher incidence of hematoma formation. Postoperative coughing may contribute to this complication. Smoking has long-term effects on the skin that cannot be completely erased by simple cessation perioperatively. If the patient stops smoking for 1 month before and after surgery, many potential complications associated with smoking can be limited. However, even with smoking cessation 1 month prior to surgery, superficial epidermolysis in the preauricular area is not infrequent. Moreover, these patients very likely would be better candidates for a deep plane face-lift in order to limit these possible complications.

Patients with a history of excessive alcohol intake may have characteristic nutritional or liver deficiencies that may lead to poor surgical healing. They also may be uncooperative in the perioperative period, when alcohol consumption is not allowed. Be alert for physical findings associated with excessive alcohol use and hepatic insufficiency.

PREOPERATIVE PREPARATION

Full-disclosure informed consent for surgery and photographs are obtained. The patient is given a packet that includes preoperative and postoperative instructions and a

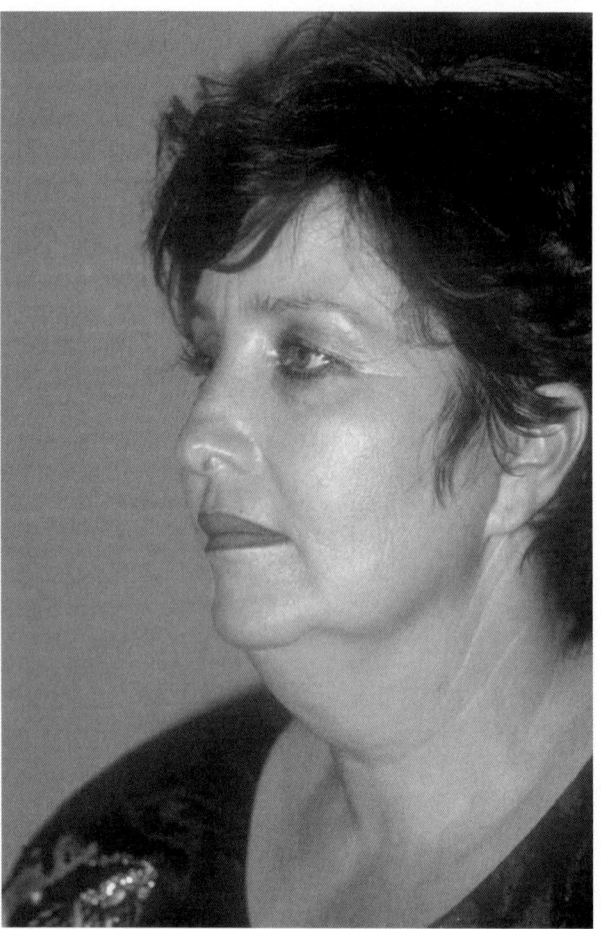

Figure 188.6 A less-than-ideal candidate for a face-lift: excessive skin and fat and rounded bony contours.

description of what to expect during recovery. Having the patient fill all prescriptions in advance serves two purposes: It removes the distraction of a rushed visit to the pharmacy for the patient and caretakers in the early postoperative period when even simple things can be difficult. Also, it allows the patient to take antibiotics the night before surgery to assist in preventing infection and provides the patient with sedatives should sleep be difficult the night before surgery.

The patient is urged to stop smoking 1 month prior to surgery. All medications containing aspirin, steroids, nonsteroidal anti-inflammatory agents, and vitamin E, as well as all herbal medications, should be discontinued at least 2 weeks before surgery. If there is a history consistent with a bleeding diathesis, however tenuous, preoperative bleeding time, platelet count, prothrombin time, and partial thromboplastin time or other coagulation studies should be ordered. The goal is avoidance of hematoma, the most common complication of rhytidectomy.

SURGICAL PLANNING

Successful face-lift surgery is achieved through thoughtful planning and execution of every aspect of the procedure (38). The amount of actual skin excised, the tightness and completeness of the lift in the cheeks, the ability to contour and resuspend the neck, the smoothness of the submental region, and the degree to which the incisions can be camouflaged all are important considerations in achieving a natural, nonoperated appearance. Rhytidectomy is an operation of compromises.

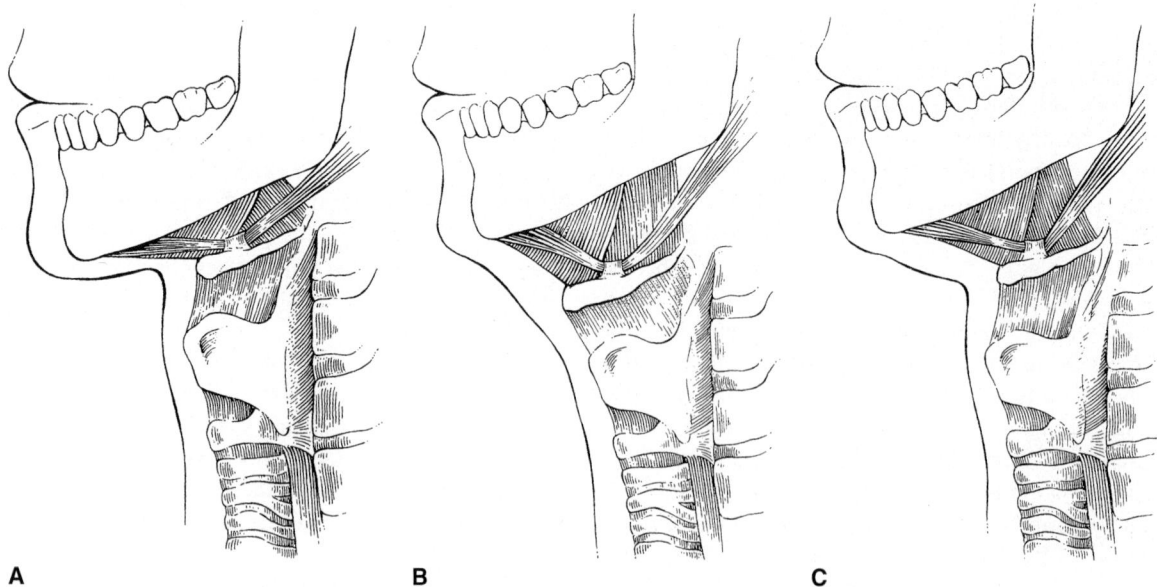

A   **B**   **C**

Figure 188.7 Schematic representation of the limits of improvement in the cervicomental contour imposed by the underlying hyoid bone and suprahyoid musculature. A high posterior hyoid is most favorable for face-lifting (**A**), and a low anterior hyoid is least favorable (**B**); most patients fall somewhere in between (**C**). (Reprinted from Conley J. *Face-lift operation.* Springfield, IL: C. Thomas, 1968:40–41, with permission.)

Anesthesia

The authors prefer to perform face-lifts with the patient under general anesthesia in a hospital ambulatory setting or outpatient surgical center (39). Many patients prefer the idea of complete somnolence and amnesia and are relieved of any anxiety concerning positional discomfort or surgical pain. The presence of an anesthesiologist permits monitoring of the patient's vital signs and status and allows the surgeon to concentrate on the events in the operative field. Communicating any special needs with the anesthesia professionals greatly facilitates the entire operative and postoperative course. The draped endotracheal tube can be moved side to side and does not interfere with the procedure. The anesthesia team strives for rapid, effective anesthesia with a smooth and deep emergence phase coupled with a relatively rapid recovery. Smooth extubation must be guaranteed, as bucking on the endotracheal tube may predispose the patient toward hematoma formation. No long-acting muscle-relaxing agents are permitted, to allow proper intraoperative facial nerve monitoring. Pre-dissection infiltration of local anesthesia with epinephrine is utilized for improved hemostasis. The authors prefer to have the patient emerge from anesthesia after the dressing is in place: this seems to facilitate dressing placement and allows optimal gentle pressure on the skin flaps to decrease the risk of hematoma formation further.

Marking

With the patient in the sitting position, the surgeon better appreciates the descended tissues and the effects of gravitational forces. This helps prevent judgmental errors regarding the amount of fat removal, the degree of laxity, and the amount of SMAS suspension required (40). Markings generally serve two main purposes. On one hand, they help outlining on the skin the areas and the severity of descended tissue, including skin and deeper subcutaneous soft tissue such as SMAS and fat. Attention is precisely drawn to the lower third of the face around the jowl area and the mandibular line. Also the neck is marked for fullness and skin laxity blunting the cervicomental angle as well as for vertical platysmal bands closer to the midline. Weak platysmal bands can be seen best with the patient upright. The patient is asked to jut the lower jaw forward and asked to grimace, and the platysmal bands may be demonstrated more easily. Other important anatomic landmarks to be marked include the anterior borders of the sternocleidomastoid muscles, the submental crease, the region of jowl formation, the angle of the mandible, the inferior mandibular border, and the geniomandibular groove. On the other hand, the authors use markings to delineate our farmost limit of dissection to avoid unnecessary and perhaps dangerous dissection over specific areas. Also it is important to trim hair around the markings before proceeding to the incisions. This will prevent hair from trapping in the incision lines when performing the closure. Hair is pulled away from the incision lines using rubber bands, and clear sticky drapes are placed to maintain hair position out of the surgical field.

Incisions

While much of the recent literature on rhytidectomy describes techniques for improving the quality of the face-lift, far less attention has been devoted on detailing the means of avoiding visible incision lines (41). In fact, while patients present with an interest in facial rejuvenation, rarely would they pursue these goals at the price of visible incision lines.

Several factors can influence incision location, but the authors have found that the most important variable is appreciation for the importance of preserving the temporal hair tuft and the posterior hairline in the female patient. The temporal region is key because a poorly designed and executed incision in this area can lead to temporal alopecia (Fig. 188.8). Descriptions of many of the classic face-lifts include a vertical preauricular incision that enters the temporal scalp posterior to the sideburn hair and then angles forward in a curvilinear fashion. The redraping of the anterior facial skin into the temporal sideburn then creates an area of hair loss. This obvious, unwanted sequela of face-lift surgery results from lifting and removing the natural temporal hair tuft. It is especially apparent in patients requiring a relatively large amount of skin removal from this region, who may already have thin, light-colored hair and a high tuft preoperatively. Unfortunately, no salvage face-lift procedure can improve this complication, which is remedied by hair flaps or follicular unit hair transplantation.

To avoid this problem, the authors use a temporal hair tuft–sparing incision (41) (Fig. 188.9). The incision begins horizontally no higher than the level of the supraauricular crease (segment c to d). As it extends horizontally, the incision has a vertical limb (segment b to c) followed by

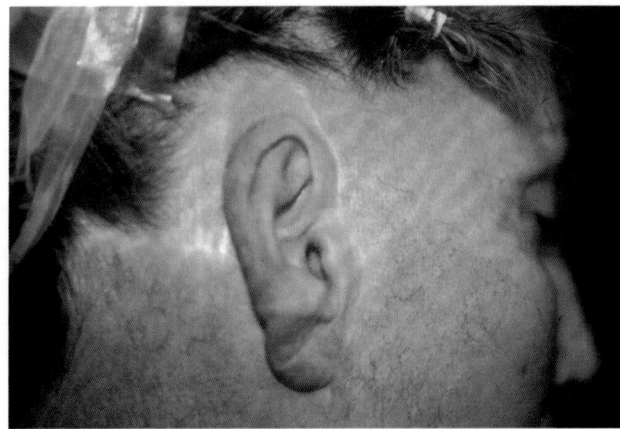

Figure 188.8 This patient had a face-lift performed elsewhere, with improperly placed incisions that caused temporal alopecia, a visible pre-auricular incision, and a post-auricular step-off in the hair line.

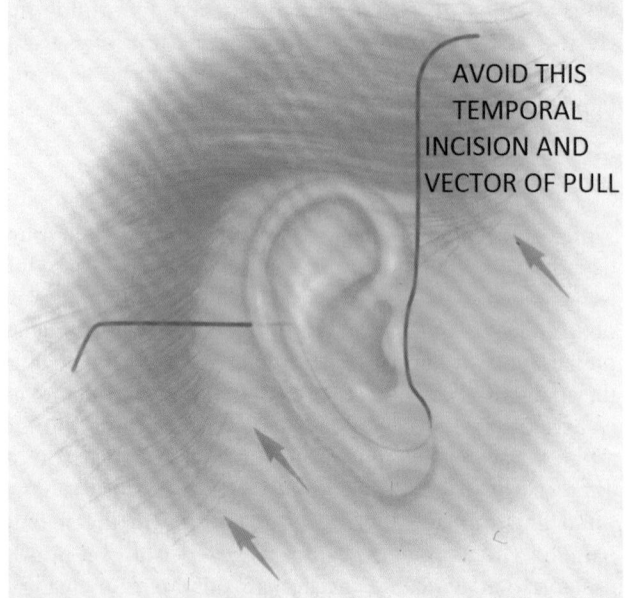

A

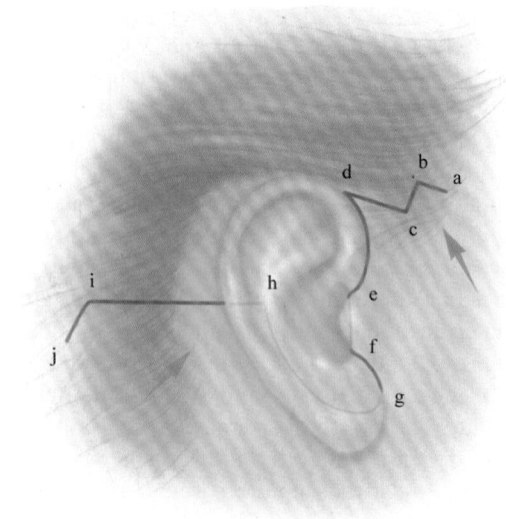

B

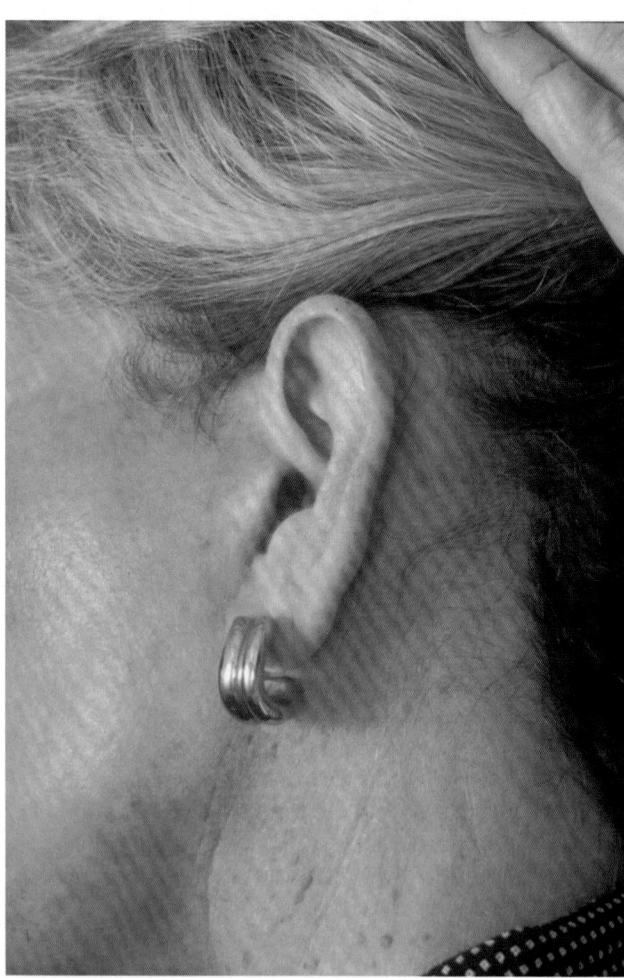

C

Figure 188.9 A: Schema of a poorly planned female face-lift incision performed elsewhere still seen too often; the temporal portion of this incision should be avoided in women because skin excision after a posterosuperior pull leads to loss of the temporal hair tuft and a post-auricular posterior superior pull on the flap causes a hairline step-off. **B:** Schema of our incision with various segments labeled. Note the anterior superior vector for skin re-draping post-auricularly that realigns the hairline. The incision is hidden in the hair, not at its edge. **C:** Postoperative result of a typical patient with our incision showing no temporal hair tuft loss and well-concealed pre- and postauricular incisions. (Reprinted from Kridel RWH. Techniques for inconspicuous face lift scars. *Arch Facial Plast Surg* 2003;5:323–333, with permission.)

an anteroinferior limb (segment a to b) to accommodate any excessive skin reduction and prevent tissue coning. To avoid visibility of this incision, the angle of the first horizontal portion closest to the ear is designed to bevel across the hair follicles; thus, even if there is no hair below this line, the hair follicles above will grow though the advanced lower facial skin flap and hide the scar. The more anterior vertical hair tuft (segment b to c) and then horizontal limb are made parallel to the hair follicles to avoid alopecia (Fig. 188.10). For each segment of this temporal incision, attention must be paid to the direction of beveling.

Several alternatives for the posterior occipital incision must also be carefully considered. Whereas an incision along the inferior edge of the postauricular hairline completely preserves the existing hairline and simplifies redraping, postoperative widening of the scar or potential tissue loss makes this choice less desirable and requires the patient to wear the hair longer to camouflage the scars. Moreover, these patients can no longer wear their hair up because of the conspicuous scars.

Incisions that curve high into the postauricular area are completely hidden; however, potential flap necrosis and derangement of the hairline call for a compromise regarding the placement of the posterior incision. The authors prefer a horizontal incision that extends posteriorly into the hair from slightly below the midconchal region. However, in placement of this incision the authors take into consideration the spacing from the ear to the beginning of the posterior hairline. The incision extends about 5 cm and angles inferiorly at the distal end to reduce the potential cutaneous cone (dog ear) after flap rotation. This incision allows for an anterior vector during redraping maximizing the amount of hairline that is preserved. With experience, these postoperative posterior hairlines look quite full and natural. Respect and consideration for the patient's existing hairline and hair-bearing tissues pay great dividends in terms of patient satisfaction.

Additional factors regarding incision placement involve differences between incision done in men and women, especially in the preauricular limb, but also in the earlobe and postauricular areas (42) (see "Male Face-Lift").

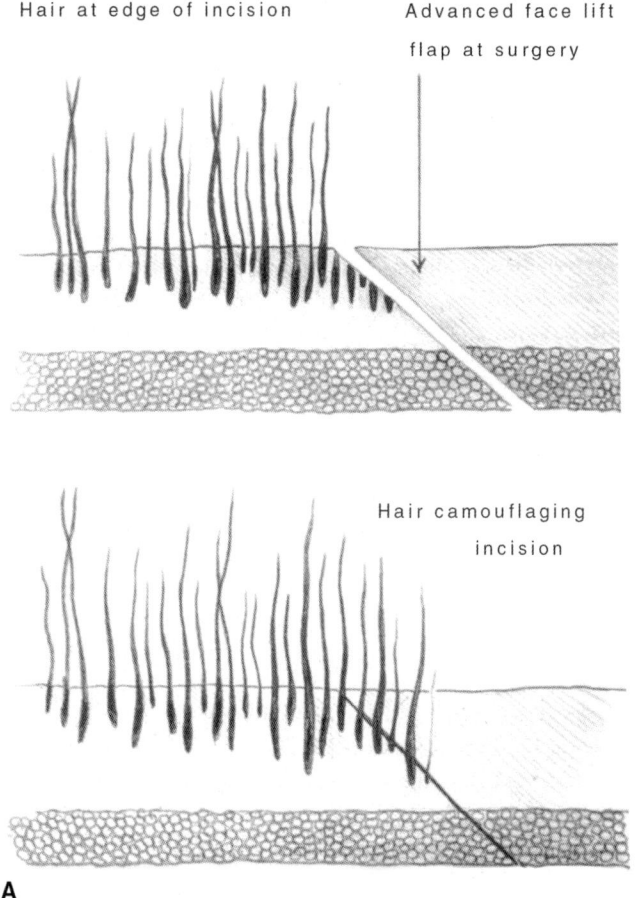

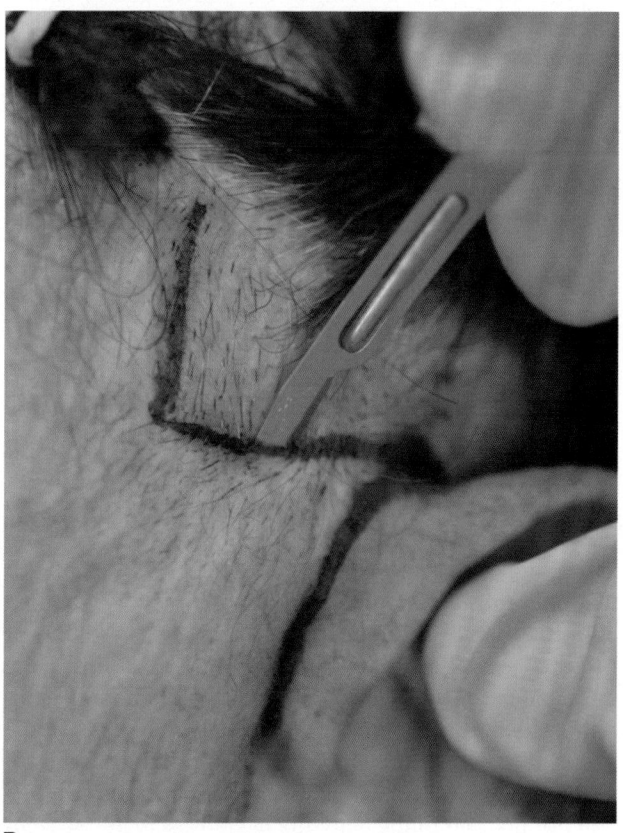

A   **B**

Figure 188.10 A: Beveling of incision *perpendicular* to hair shafts allows hair to grow through the advanced skin flap. **B:** Intraoperative view of incision beveled *perpendicular* to hair follicles. (Reprinted from Kridel RWH. Techniques for inconspicuous face lift scars. *Arch Facial Plast Surg* 2003;5:323–333, with permission.)

OPERATIVE STAGE

The classic, now outdated, face-lift procedure involves only the development of facial skin flaps and the redistribution and excision of excess skin (12). Undermining of the skin in the single-layer skin flap is usually extensive. This older technique is effective; however, the single-layer skin closure often places greater tension on the tissues and results in wider scarring or possible tissue loss. Theoretically, the skin-only, long-flap face-lift may not be as long-lasting and could predispose toward an increased risk of postoperative bleeding.

Contemporary facial plastic surgeons use either the concept of the two-layer cervicofacial rhytidectomy with suspension of the SMAS or the extended sub- SMAS/deep plane rhytidectomy (43). As already discussed, while many surgeons feel that the deep plane lift gives more long-lasting results and decreases the incidence of hematomas, there are as of yet no definitive studies to confirm these findings. In fact, while one study attempted to compare "deep plane versus superficial musculoaponeurotic system plication" face-lifts, Baker noted that many questions remain unanswered (25,44). As such, the authors will proceed with a brief descriptive outline of both procedures.

After appropriate marking of the patient and initiation of general and infiltrative anesthesia, the submentoplasty is performed.

Submentoplasty

The term submentoplasty encompasses submental lipectomy and platysmaplasty, as well as limited skin resection from the submental area on rare occasions. In both the SMAS and sub-SMAS rhytidectomy, surgeons have incorporated the use of suction-assisted lipectomy and platysmaplasty (40,45,46). The two-layer SMAS suspension technique and liposuction has numerous advantages. Open liposuction under direct surgical vision permanently removes fat cells and recontours difficult facial areas, such as the jowl and periparotid region. To gain the maximum improvement in the neck, most patients should undergo platysmaplasty at the time of face-lift. Most patients who are candidates for face-lift also have ptosis of the anterior platysma causing banding. This problem is best handled by low division of the offending bands and resection of the excess muscle under direct vision. Also, unlike the musculature of the face, the platysma of the neck is naturally dehiscent in the midline, with only a tenuous fascial connection between the paired muscles. In the absence of midline platysmal plication, SMAS suspension pulls the anterior margins of the platysma laterally, actually weakening support for the submental fat. Plication of the anterior margins resists this lateral migration and allows suspension to strengthen submental support and enhance recontouring of the neck. Finally, in most patients, a significant proportion of the excess submental fat is actually in the anatomic submental triangle, deep to the platysma, and therefore not accessible by closed liposuction. In these cases, the platysmaplasty approach allows access to this area, with direct open lipectomy. It has been our experience that the addition of routine platysmaplasty to rhytidectomy has both enhanced results in the neck and increased the duration of the aesthetic improvement (Figs. 188.11 and 188.12).

A horizontal incision 1.5 cm long is made in the submental crease. Sharp dissection is used to start a plane just below the dermis. Next, a double-lumen blunt-tipped liposuction cannula is advanced radially to form an even subcutaneous pocket in the submental/cervical region. Then the cannula is advanced, with the lumen toward the deep tissues at all times, in a back-and-forth fashion. Fat is suctioned from the previously delineated areas. Dissection is facilitated by tenting the skin upward and using a rapid motion, which avoids suctioning in the same area for too long. Aggressive suctioning in one position might create dimples and irregularities. Using the "pinch and roll" technique of palpation of the skin between the thumb and forefingers, it must be ensured that no excessive fat deposits are inadvertently omitted during this part of the procedure. Liposuction is carried inferiorly over the hyoid and toward the thyroid notch, then laterally to overlap the anterior borders of the sternocleidomastoid muscles, and then superiorly to the dependent portion of jowl formation and the edge of the mandibular border (Fig. 188.13).

The submental, subcutaneous pocket is inspected with the assistance of a fiberoptic headlight and a modified Converse retractor looking for individual neurovascular septations and controlling any rare bleeding points by using suction cautery. The anterior borders of the platysma are then identified and a small amount of horizontal sectioning is performed of the platysma at the level of the thyroid notch. If fat is found to be excessive between the medial edges of the platysma, one could do a direct lipectomy with the scissors. Staying midline and avoiding undermining the platysmal edges is important. The anterior borders of the platysma are then reapproximated in the midline using a corset platysmaplasty of 2-0 Vicryl suture. At all times, the vector of force is medial and superior. The plication is at least to the level of the hyoid; however, care is taken to avoid excessive tightening, which can strangle the sutured muscle. Also one should perform big enough bites to provide adequate tensile strength without being overaggressive and creating bunching that leads to a nondesirable central band.

The submental incision is left open until the end of the lift to provide access for inspection and further cautery as needed. Only after both flaps have been elevated, trimmed, and sewn into place should the submental incision be closed. This also allows for conservative submental cutaneous resection on rare occasions when excess is substantial

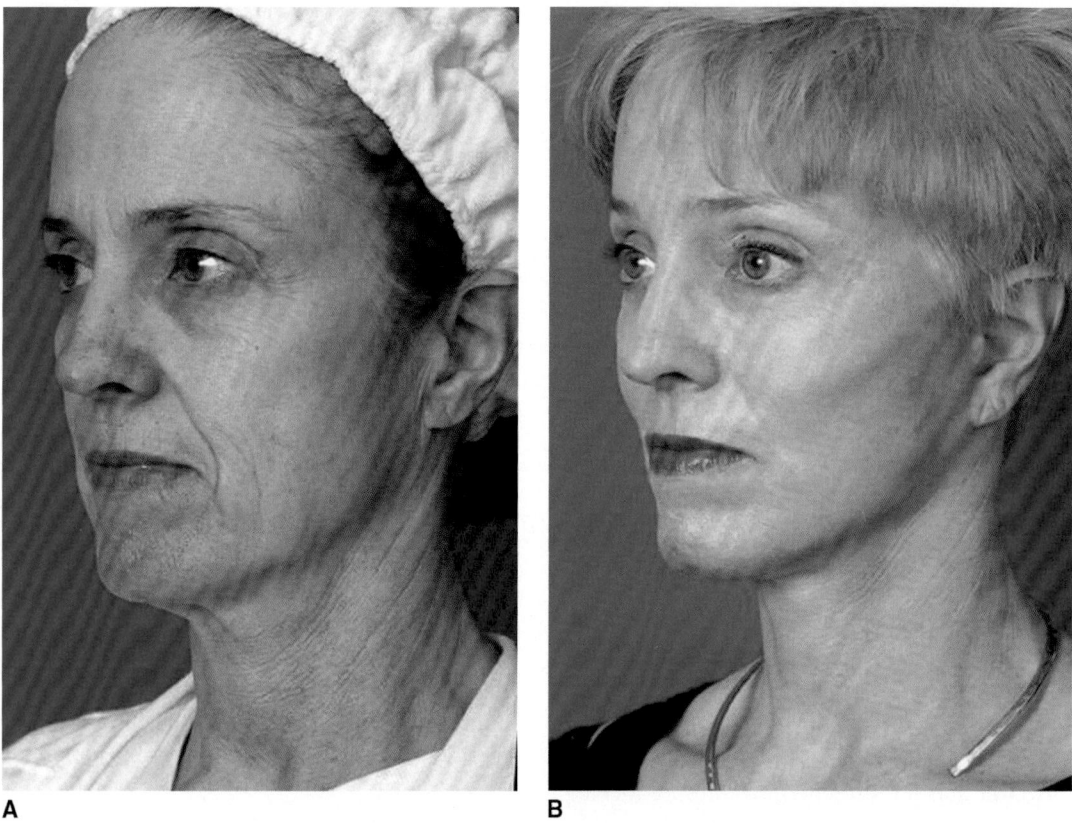

Figure 188.11 A, B: Preoperative and postoperative views after face-lift, submentoplasty, brow-lift, submalar implants, and CO_2 laser resurfacing to the perioral and periorbital regions.

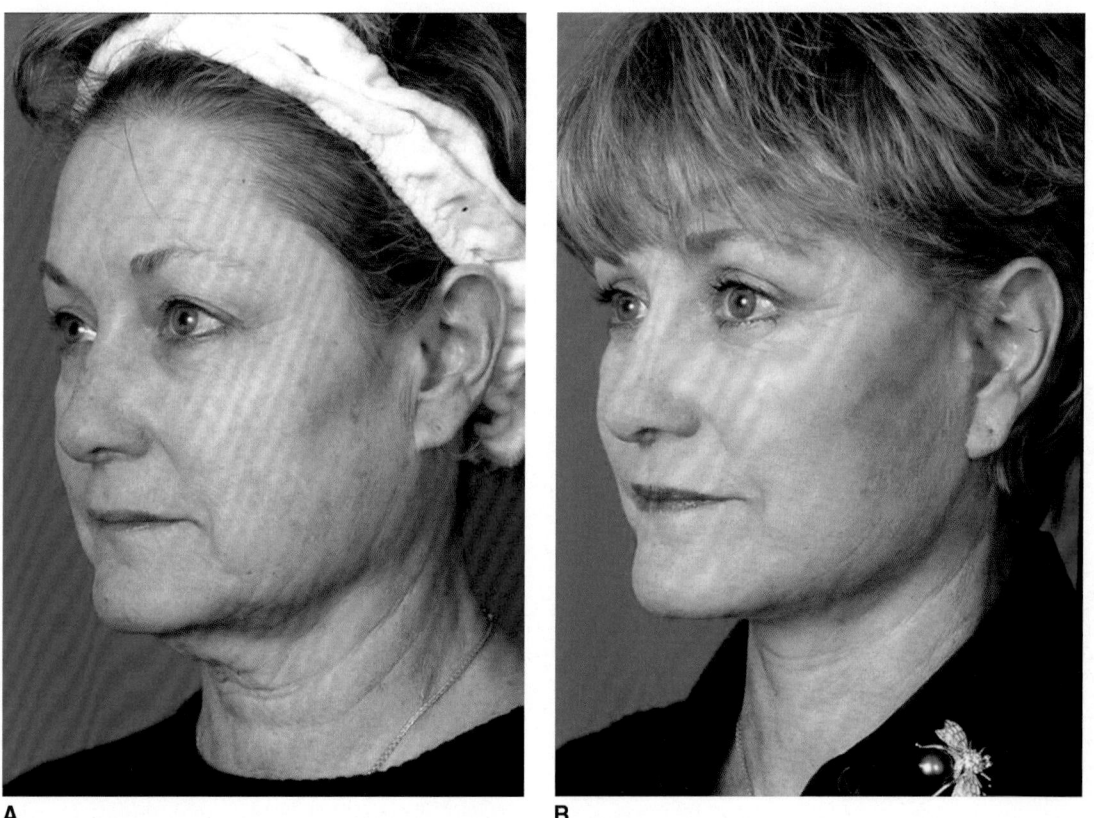

Figure 188.12 A, B: Preoperative and postoperative views after face-lift, submentoplasty, blepharoplasty, and 15% TCA peel to face and neck.

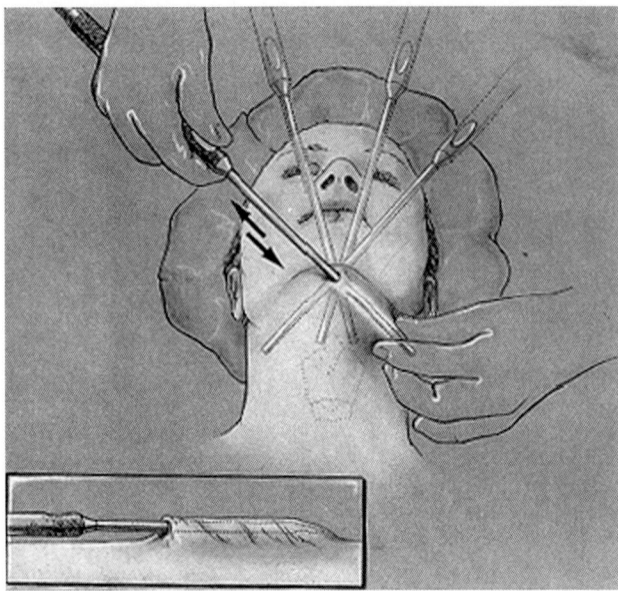

Figure 188.13 The direction of submental liposuction in a fan-like configuration.

even after flap redraping laterally and posteriorly. The authors prefer a layered closure, using 5-0 plain for the subcutaneous layer and 6-0 Prolene in a running locking manner for the skin.

Flap Elevation

Next, beginning on one side, the previously delineated incision is made. Dissection is started occipitally, and the skin flap begun using face-lift scissors. With the scissors tips pointed upward, a gliding motion is used to develop the skin flap (Fig. 188.14). Upward direction of the scissors helps the surgeon better visualize the extent of the dissection. The authors believe that gliding motion rather than spreading prevents stretching trauma to blood vessels and decreases the incidence of telangiectasia encountered in the postoperative period. The skin may be densely adherent to

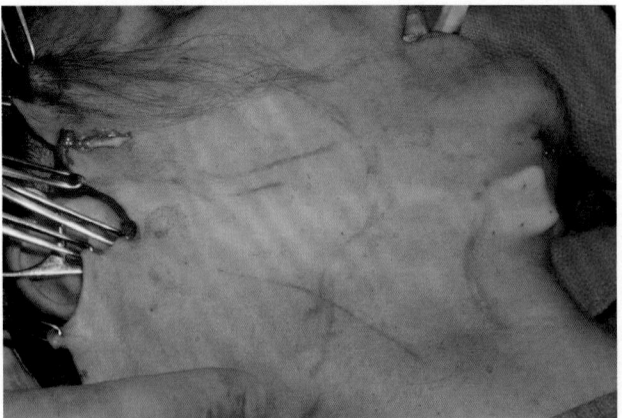

Figure 188.14 Intraoperative use of face-lift scissors, with the skin retracted. Notice the tips of the curved scissors can be seen.

the sternocleidomastoid fascia and the mastoid fascia, and meticulous superficial dissection in this area serves to elevate the flap without injury to the greater auricular nerve. The earlobe is dissected completely free and the skin mobilized over the tragus with small iris or serrated dissecting scissors. Because the temporal incision is placed to preserve the hair tuft, the plane of dissection should not be as deep as the temporalis fascia but rather just under the hair follicles. Superficial flap elevation in this region avoids injury to the frontal branch of the facial nerve, which crosses the zygomatic arch at this point.

The authors usually develop a long flap in the neck and connect broadly with the submental preplatysmal dissection to allow optimal redraping of neck skin. Fat deposits are removed gently under direct visualization, and facial contouring is inspected for uniformity and desired appearance. The area is irrigated with saline to allow an enhanced visualization and better achieve hemostasis. Irrigation also cleans the wound from any free adipose tissue that underwent devascularization during dissection. The authors believe that this tissue would create an increased inflammatory response and prolong the healing phase if it remained in the surgical bed. Bleeding is controlled with bipolar cautery to avoid facial nerve or skin flap injury.

SMAS Suspension

After flap elevation, direct surgical management of the SMAS fascia is performed. SMAS suspension is the foundation on which the longevity, safety, and aesthetically pleasing result is built. SMAS suspension permits tension-free closure of the incision by transferring the strength and support of the face-lift rejuvenation to the deeper structures and tissues. SMAS suspension can be achieved by several different methods (47–50).

Imbrication techniques involve direct incision, resection, or undermining of the SMAS fascia with the reapproximation or overlap of the cut SMAS fascia edges. With imbrication methods, the SMAS is usually identified and incised within the region anterior to the tragus and below the earlobe, overlying the deeper parotid fascia. Many surgeons undermine a separate SMAS fascia layer and resect excess tissue after advancement and redraping. However, one should be careful when elevating two different flaps (cutaneous and SMAS) separately as vascular compromise might ensue if a large area is dissected. Proper suture placement buries each knot to prevent suture spitting or later palpation by the patient. An alternative imbrication technique involves excising a segmental portion of SMAS and resuspending the anterior cut layer without additional undermining. Increased sharp dissection associated with imbrication techniques increases the risks of bleeding, nerve injury, and skin slough. In patients with wide, chubby faces, imbrication and resection tends to flatten the region overlying the parotid gland and therefore may offer some advantages in early surgical definition of this region.

Plication techniques for SMAS suspension avoid direct cutting and undermining of the SMAS layer. The surgeon folds the SMAS fascia on itself and secures the newly folded tissues with permanent buried sutures. Because SMAS plication involves less dissection and surgical time, the potentially decreased risks are thought to offer some significant advantage over imbrication.

With either technique, SMAS suspension lifts and resupports the attached skin layer and reduces the amount of potential cavity space created during flap elevation. The question of which technique is better in terms of long-term results and decreased morbidity is controversial. Webster et al. (51) studied imbrication versus plication by performing each method on opposite sides of the face. By taking exact measurements and confirming the findings on fresh cadaver dissections, they concluded that there was no objective benefit favoring imbrication over plication during the surgical procedure. Subsequent studies failed to demonstrate any long-term advantages either. Because imbrication theoretically involves a greater chance for surgical morbidity, the authors prefer plication for SMAS suspension.

The direction of forces applied to the SMAS layer by sutures is important, and specific vector patterns are used routinely. Plication is done by tugging on the SMAS fascia in a bidirectional vector. Before placing any sutures, the effect of each tug on the face and neck should be noted and the desirable sites secured with 2-0 nonabsorbable sutures. Braided sutures are utilized in order to provide knot security without multiple ties, which can otherwise lead to palpable suture knots. Multiple buried sutures are placed along each vector to avoid relying on only one suture. The first suspension vector generally runs from the angle of the mandible to the fascia near the superior mastoid cortex. Suturing at this point affects the cervicomental angle and the angular bony contour of the mandible, which define a smooth jawline and neck. Attention is then turned to the second vector, which originates in the SMAS of the cheek and mandibular ramus near the anterior border of the parotid. The SMAS here is extended with a more superior than posterior vector toward the preauricular sulcus and tragus. Finally, the third vector extends from the posterior border of the cervical platysma in a predominantly superior direction to the sternocleidomastoid fascia in the region of the mastoid tip. Additional sutures are placed where required for even, firm plication. This is mostly performed around the parotid area to flatten the bumps created by plication sutures, creating a smooth and more natural result over the cheeks.

The overall direction of pull remains superior and only partially posterior (Fig. 188.15). A pull that is too posterior creates a distinctly unattractive and artificial appearance sometimes referred to as the lateral sweep. Posterior lifts tend to widen and flatten the oral commissure, resulting in a disproportionately large mouth. The standard rhytidectomy with SMAS suspension may fail to improve the nasolabial fold to a significant extent unless significant

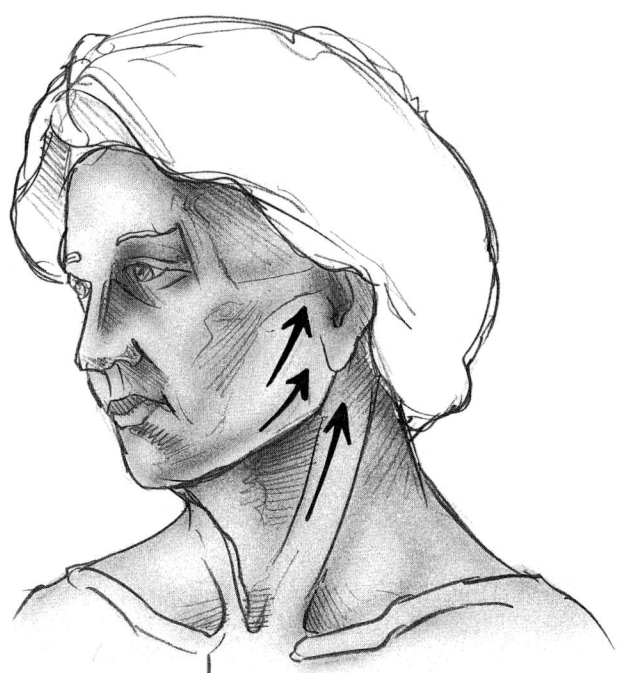

Figure 188.15 *Arrows* indicate the direction of pull for SMAS plication.

subcutaneous dissection is performed. The SMAS inserts on the mimetic muscles of the face (21). In the perioral area, these include the platysma and the same lip retractors and elevators discussed previously. SMAS suspension therefore results in further lateral and superior displacement of the perioral soft tissues, which are densely attached to the mimetic musculature with relatively little effect on the malar soft tissues, which at best are associated only weekly with the muscular plane. In isolation, then, the act of SMAS suspension theoretically could deepen the nasolabial fold even further. That it does not seem to deepen in practice likely results from the excision of excess skin performed after SMAS suspension. The greater the amount of skin excised, the more improvement in the fold. Because of preoperative skin laxity, it is generally possible to excise sufficient skin to result in a small net improvement in the fold without closing under undue skin tension and predisposing to skin slough or scar widening. However, it should be noted that placement of sutures, application of tension, and removal and redraping of skin are so individually variable that different surgeons will find widely disparate results while using the same overall technique.

DEEP PLANE LIFT

The SMAS suspension face-lift is a highly effective operation. With appropriate case selection and planning, both patient and surgeon can expect a technically sound surgery to produce very satisfactory results. However, cosmetic surgeons and their patients are very demanding groups. Therefore, innovative surgeons have continued to attempt to improve the SMAS plication face-lift by doing deep plane/sub-SMAS face-lifts (31,52).

The primary areas of patient and surgeon dissatisfaction with generally accepted face-lift techniques have been the nasolabial fold, the inconsistency in achieving long-term results, and the occurrence of perioperative complications. The family of deep dissection rhytidectomies is aimed primarily at improving the nasolabial fold to a greater extent than is possible using widely accepted SMAS suspension techniques. Of the various techniques that have been reported (22,23,52), the deep plane or, more recently, composite rhytidectomy of Hamra has attracted the most interest. The key distinctions of deep plane rhytidectomy relative to the SMAS plication procedure described in detail already will be discussed and the theoretical advantages and disadvantages noted.

The deep plane rhytidectomy is in fact carried out at three different planes, depending on the area of the face and neck being dissected (31,25) (Fig. 188.16). The dissection of the neck (inferior to the jawline) is preplatysmal

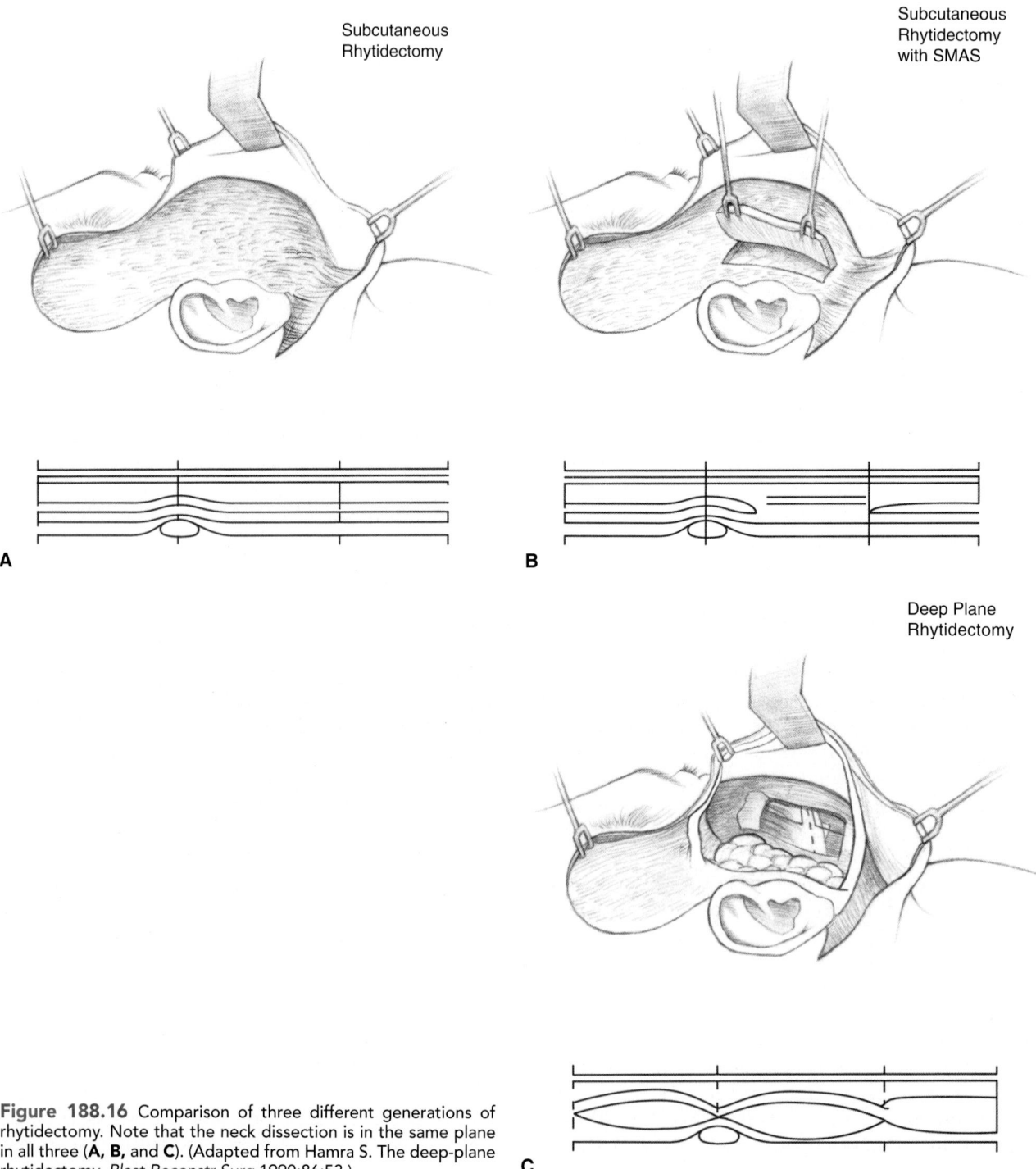

Figure **188.16** Comparison of three different generations of rhytidectomy. Note that the neck dissection is in the same plane in all three (**A, B,** and **C**). (Adapted from Hamra S. The deep-plane rhytidectomy. *Plast Reconstr Surg* 1990;86:53.)

and is connected subcutaneously with the contralateral dissection. A platysmaplasty with submental lipectomy is performed. In this area, the operation is similar to that already described.

Dissection of the lower face is carried out in a sub-SMAS plane, in contradistinction to the subcutaneous plane described previously but similar to most SMAS imbrication techniques. One significant point of difference with established techniques is that the sub-SMAS dissection is carried out anterior to the parotid, where the buccal and marginal branches of the facial nerve may be encountered. A second distinction is that the subcutaneous plane is developed only minimally so that the bulk of the elevated flap contains SMAS along with the skin and subcutaneous fat.

Finally, dissection in the midface is carried out over the malar eminences into the central face. This dissection is much more extensive than in other SMAS suspension techniques. The subcutaneous plane is maintained initially for 2 to 3 cm anterior to the tragus, presumably to avoid injury to the frontal branch of the facial nerve. A thick flap then is developed anteriorly, with dissection immediately superficial to the orbicularis and zygomaticus muscles. No other motor nerve branches should be encountered in this plane, as they enter the muscles from their deep surface (53). The two facial dissection planes are bluntly connected to create a large, thick flap. Excess skin is excised after the flap is resuspended at the SMAS level under tension (25).

The major theoretical advantage of this and similar procedures is that the malar fat and skin can be elevated and resuspended, and the nasolabial fold can be undermined, allowing for its effacement. Additionally, the face-lift flap is maintained as a "myocutaneous" flap (25) consisting of platysma, SMAS, and the superficial tissues, purportedly allowing increased viability and closure under greater tension than is possible with standard procedures. Further possible advantages include a decrease in hematomas because of a more avascular dissection plane and a decrease in skin slough due to the theoretically increased viability. The major theoretical disadvantage of the deep plane dissections is the increased exposure to the facial nerve in the lower face with the concomitant possibility of injury. Moreover, patients with deep rhytids or acne scarring may also find improved results from SMAS suspension with an extended skin flap, which may stretch the skin itself more directly. Because of the widespread interest in this procedure, it is important to evaluate these potential advantages and disadvantages critically.

If ptotic subcutaneous fat in the malar region is a significant contributor to a prominent nasolabial fold, one could predict improvement in the nasolabial fold with infrazygomatic undermining, as described by Hamra and others (24,25,54). This fat is not to be confused with the buccal fat pad (of Bichat), which gives the cheek most of its fullness but lies at a deeper plane, in intimate association with

the facial nerve. On the other hand, anatomic studies of the nasolabial fold demonstrate that it usually consists of little more than skin excess (21,55). In this case, it would seem that only skin resection, and not deep tissue repositioning, is capable of attaining significant improvement in this area. Because the current SMAS suspension procedures usually do not involve undermining medial to the malar eminence, the deep plane procedures as described should obtain some advantage in malar skin redraping and resection.

As for theoretically improved viability with the deeper plane of dissection, this depends on the vascular anatomy of the flap. For the deep plane face-lift flap to be a true fasciocutaneous flap of the SMAS based on the facial artery, as asserted, there must be multiple small perforators from the SMAS to the overlying skin, with only the distal few centimeters immediately anterior to the pinna left random, as this area is undermined subcutaneously. At least one recent study of the vascular anatomy of the face calls this interpretation into question (54). The authors observe vast numbers of small perforators from the facial system in the medial face but only sparse perforators in the transverse facial and posterior auricular distributions. Abundant small perforators from the facial system via the SMAS fascia are not described. Indeed, subcutaneous face-lift dissection results in little bleeding above the jawline and in front of the ear, except for the transection of the transverse facial perforators, which are divided in the deep plane dissection as well. These observations suggest the possibility that both the classic and deep plane face-lift flaps are similarly viable large random flaps. As skin slough is a relatively rare complication, extensive experience with deep plane lifting will be required before reliable empiric judgments can be made.

A much lower incidence of hematoma (about 1%) relative to the classic procedure (8%) is reported for the deep plane procedure (25), providing some indirect evidence that the dissection is more avascular. Given that dissection in the neck for both procedures is in a similar plane, only the facial hematoma incidence is likely to be lower. It may be, however, that neck hematomas can be reduced as well by remaining strictly in the preplatysmal plane as recommended by Hamra (25) rather than hugging the subcutaneous tissues as described above, regardless of whether a deep plane or a more standard SMAS suspension procedure is performed.

In most SMAS suspension procedures practiced today, the facial nerve is well protected. As long as SMAS undermining is not carried forward of the anterior margin of the parotid, the nerve is shielded by the gland parenchyma. Anterior to the gland, the nerve courses within the buccal fat pad deep to the SMAS and therefore is exposed to injury by SMAS undermining in this area. In a similar vein, dissection that remains meticulously superficial to the zygomaticus will protect its innervation; however, the branches to the lower orbicularis are more superficial (the orbicularis lies in a plane superficial to the zygomaticus) and may be vulnerable to injury by dissection over the malar eminence if care is not exercised to remain strictly superficial to the orbicularis as well (53). Both areas are manipulated by the deep plane lifting techniques, which therefore carry theoretically greater risks of nerve injury. A working estimate of the incidence of temporary weakness in deep plane face-lift can be obtained by combining cases from several recent reports (25,56,57). These authors report a total of 23 cases of temporary paralysis in 638 deep plane rhytidectomies, for an estimated incidence of 3.6%. By contrast, a classic review of facial nerve injury in more standard rhytidectomy revealed 50 cases of paralysis in 6,500 rhytidectomies, for an incidence of 0.8%. Seven of these cases were permanent (32). Although no cases of permanent paralysis have yet been reported for deep plane rhytidectomy, it would seem reasonable that the incidence would be correspondingly higher.

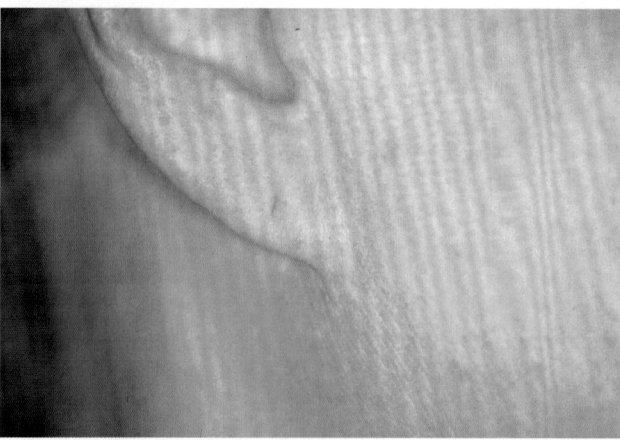

Figure 188.17 Pixie-ear or satyr-ear deformity caused by excessive skin excision or tension at the earlobe.

Flap Closure

Drains

Many surgeons elect not to drain their standard face-lift flaps and reserve drains for excessively long procedures or those in which less-than-perfect hemostasis was achieved (58). A successful argument can be made for omitting drains because the percentage of early seroma and hematoma formation is quite low, and no one has been able to demonstrate that either open or closed suction drainage systems prevent hematoma.

The authors nevertheless favor the use of closed suction drainage in our face-lift patients. The authors have noted great improvement in early skin flap adherence to the deeper layers of dissection because the drains actively remove small amounts of fluid. The authors' patients have reported much less discomfort with suction drains than without them, perhaps because there is no fluid pressure buildup beneath the flap. A Blake perforated drain is placed through a separate posterior stab incision. Aspiration via a bulb suction device continues until the first postoperative day, or longer on rare occasions. A fluffy pressure dressing is still used to support the face and neck and ensure uniform, gentle pressure on the flap.

Earlobe and Tragus

Special attention is given to the flap closure about the earlobe and tragus to prevent postoperative sequelae often associated with these structures. An elongated earlobe directly attached to the facial cheek skin, known as the pixie or satyr earlobe, is a common complication (Fig. 188.17). Other problems include earlobes that are too pendulous and scars visible below the earlobe.

Prevention is by far the best management of these difficulties. During closure, a generous amount of perilobular flap skin needs to be left around the earlobe. Additionally, the skin flap may be fixed to the SMAS or mastoid fascia superiorly. The authors have seen consistently pleasing

earlobes in our face-lift patients by adhering to the following principles. The earlobe complex is dissected completely free from the skin and subcutaneous tissue, rendering it completely mobile. After the initial perilobular flap cut is made before SMAS plication, the authors seldom alter this incision length (Fig. 188.18). Before closure, the earlobe shape is preserved by a horizontal mattress-type suture of 5-0 Prolene, as described by Clyde Litton (personal communication, Washington DC, 1986) (Fig. 188.19). This suture suspends the earlobe superiorly, maintains a normal crease, and prevents the lobe from being pulled downward. The inferior edge of the earlobe is attached to the skin flap by a separate individual Prolene suture.

The tragus shape and projection are similarly affected by flap-closure techniques when a posttragal incision is used. Common postsurgical tragal deformities include blunting, irregularity, and anteriorly dislocated cartilage. Blunting is prevented with a pretragal deep polydioxanone suture (Figs. 188.20 and 188.21). This suture will help recreate the anatomic pretragal sulcus. Moreover, in addition to defatting the skin overlying the tragus, the flap in this area is trimmed to leave a generous portion of extra skin that more than sufficiently covers the tragal cartilage without tension. This segment is sutured to the canal portion of the tragal skin with individual 5-0 plain gut sutures, taking care to avoid needle entry into the cartilaginous tragus.

Wound Closure

The postauricular flap and the temporal region have been trimmed and the incision approximated in these areas by using skin staples. Wound-edge eversion is helpful to fine-line incision healing. The authors oppose the skin edges with a lightly run, locking suture of 5-0 plain gut, even in areas that have been stapled. This hemostatic-type stitch also ensures an airtight flap closure, which allows the suction drain to function more effectively. This extra attention to wound eversion is worth the effort as it seems to improve the appearance of the incisions.

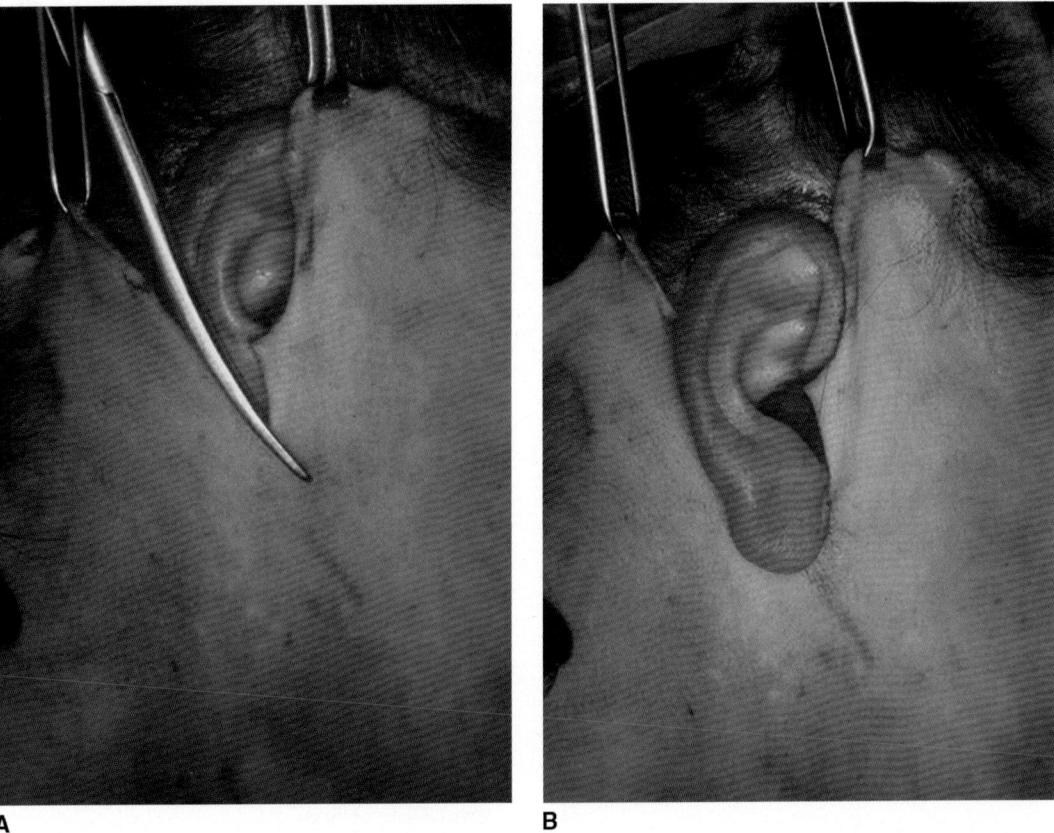

A   B

Figure 188.18 Intraoperative photograph, before plication, showing **A:** the perilobular flap cut to set the lobule and **B:** the flap re-draped around the lobule.

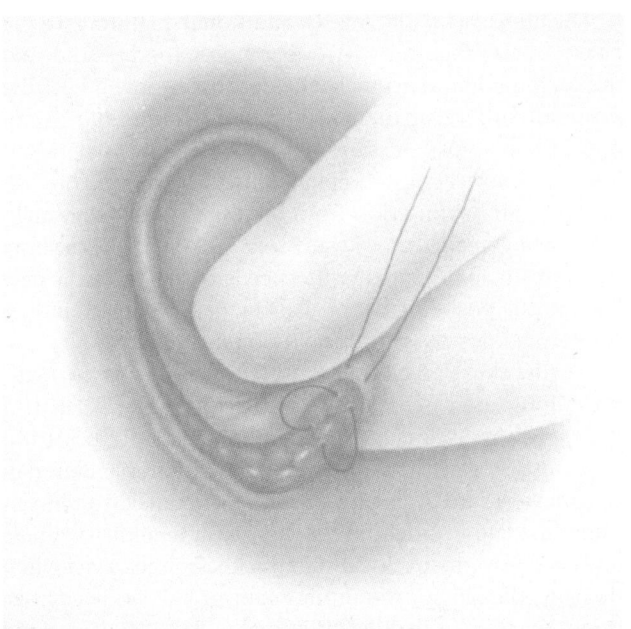

Figure 188.19 To further prevent tethering of the lobule, a mattress stitch with 5-0 polypropylene is placed at the free cut edge of the lobule and secured to the underlying tissues (Clyde Litton, oral communication, 1986). (Reprinted from Kridel RWH. Techniques for inconspicuous face lift scars. *Arch Facial Plast Surg* 2003;5: 323–333, with permission.)

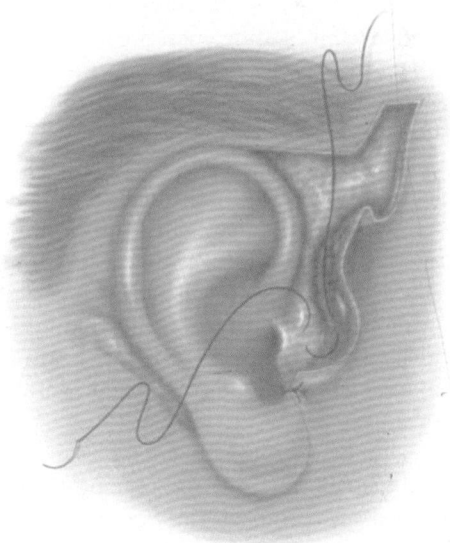

Figure 188.20 Deep suture to recreate the anatomic pretragal sulcus. (Reprinted from Kridel RWH. Techniques for inconspicuous face lift scars. *Arch Facial Plast Surg* 2003;5:323–333, with permission.)

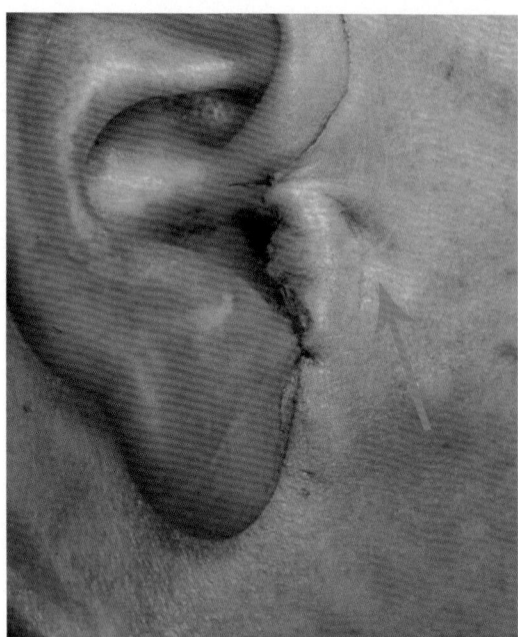

Figure 188.21 Deep suture to recreate the anatomic pretragal sulcus shows as an indentation. (Reprinted from Kridel RWH. Techniques for inconspicuous face lift scars. *Arch Facial Plast Surg* 2003;5:323–333, with permission.)

SPECIAL CONSIDERATIONS

Male Face-Lift

Although men seek facial rejuvenation less commonly than women, the numbers of male face-lifts are increasing. The novice surgeon should be aware of the few differences that exist between male and female face-lifting. Although mostly technical, differences are also on the psychological level. Some authors agree that males seeking rhinoplasty tend to be more detail oriented and demanding than women. However, when it pertains to face-lifting, the authors believe it is quite the opposite phenomenon. Female patients are often very particular about any kind of asymmetry, wrinkle, or bulge that is left or any result that does not return them to the way they were many years ago. Generally, female patients will have better aesthetic results following surgery. This might be due to the fact that men have thicker skin perhaps secondary to beard formation and also have larger parotids that could contribute to a fuller cheek appearance.

From a health perspective, men tend to have more cardiovascular diseases, for instance, making them at an increased surgical risk compared to women of the same age. One should be careful to inquire about past medical and family history to better coordinate patient care with the primary care provider and obtain medical clearance.

The pattern and distribution of facial and temporal hair in a male patient are important preoperative considerations. In a patient with severe temporal recession, in a bald patient or in a patient who shaves his head,

counseling is important as incision placement would be apparent despite the greatest effort in planning. Many factors affect incision placement not only in the preauricular area but also around the earlobe and in the postauricular area. Some surgeons prefer a pretragal rather than a posttragal incision in male, for fear of bringing hair-bearing skin over the tragus (Figs. 188.22 and 188.23). This certainly is a concern, especially in patients with lax skin where the surgeon is planning considerable amount of cutaneous resection. In patients that prefer a retrotragal incision, the authors directly address the hair follicles by cutting them with the scissors flat on the undersurface of the flap. Cautery can often assist in this task as well. This is done when thinning the newly formed tragal skin, remaining careful not to be overaggressive to prevent postoperative epidermolysis over the prominent tragal area. Such planning prevents a scar in the preauricular area, but risks the presence of hair on the tragus, in spite of inactivation of the hair follicles. The authors inform patients that they may need postoperative electrolysis or laser hair removal in this region. Because the male sideburn blends into the beard, loss of the temporal tuft is less problematic than in female patients, as the sideburn could be recreated from growing the beard. Therefore, a curving vertical incision in the posttuft scalp rather than anterior to the tuft is permissible in men.

The incision around the earlobe is generally at the inferior attachment, except in male patients where a margin of non–hair-bearing skin is preserved so hair does not abut the lobe postoperatively, bringing discomfort to the patient and added challenge when shaving in that area.

The third area that needs additional planning is the postauricular incision that extends over the mastoid and the occipital hair. This incision generally is drawn over the posterior surface of the concha before continuing in the hair in female patients. In men, it is preferable to place it lower, at the level of the cephaloauricular groove. This will prevent hair-bearing skin from reaching the concha, making shaving again an awkward task. However, the authors still inform male patients the need to shave over a new zone in the postauricular area as the hair-bearing skin flap is relocated posteriorly and superiorly.

During skin flap elevation over the cheek and the neck, one should be careful not to create too thin of a flap in males. This might inadvertently injure the hair follicles and create areas of permanent patchy beard alopecia. Skin flap thickness should be examined both from outside and from under the flap throughout the dissection to allow evenness and safe movements. Ideal skin thickness is achieved when the surgeon can see the untraumatized hair follicles from under the flap. In that regard in males, the thickness of the flap can vary from patient to patient, and it is often dictated by the depth of the hair follicles.

Last but not least, increased rates of postoperative hematoma have been reported in male patients, perhaps due to the rich subdermal plexus feeding the hair follicles.

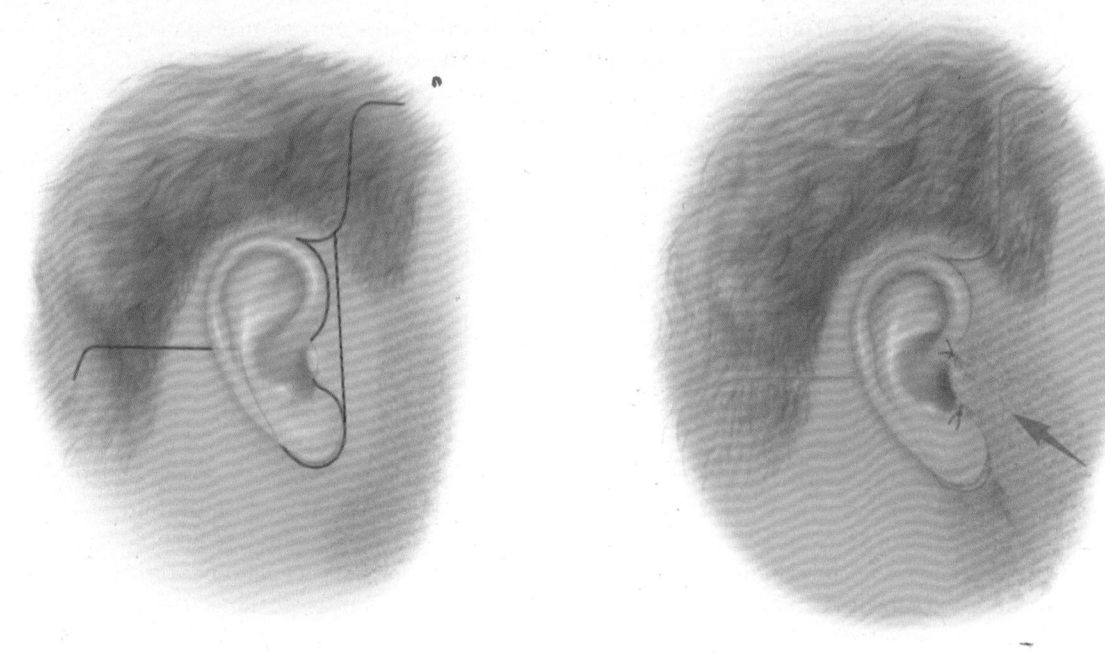

A   **B**

Figure 188.22 A: Schema of two options for male face-lift incision. Note a cuff of non–hair-bearing skin is left around the lobule, and the postauricular incision is placed in the sulcus and not onto the concha, as in women, to prevent men from having to shave in these areas. **B:** Schema of the retrotragal male incision after skin excision and flap redraping. The tragus is now covered with hair-bearing skin. Note also the preserved non–hair-bearing cuff of skin around the lobule. (Reprinted from Kridel RWH. Techniques for inconspicuous face lift scars. *Arch Facial Plast Surg* 2003;5:323–333, with permission.)

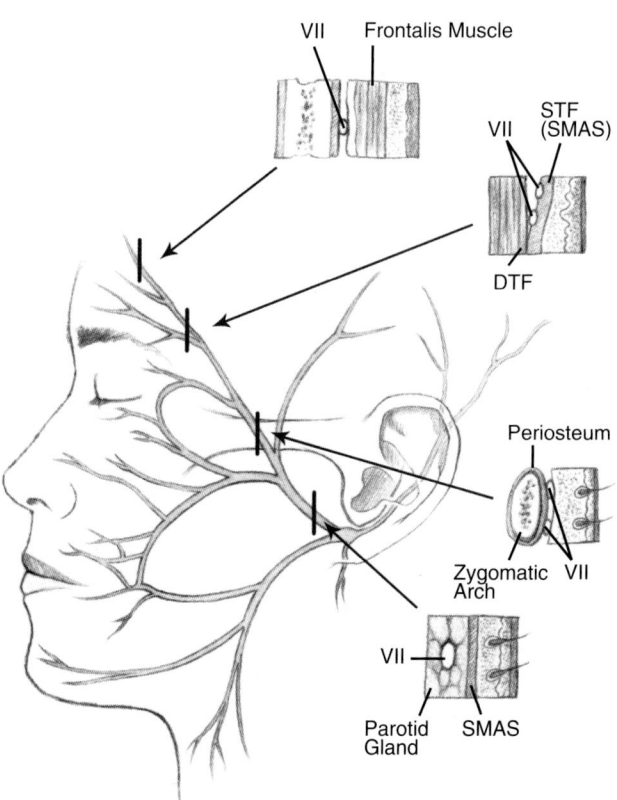

Figure 188.23 The frontal branch of the facial nerve at different locations in its course.

Some surgeons prefer the deep plane lift, advocating a lessened risk of hematoma formation as the ramified subdermal plexus is left intact.

Secondary and Revision Face-Lift

Despite our best intentions, plans, and efforts, some patients may be unhappy because of real or perceived unsatisfactory results. Remember that the patient may not always be as critical of the outcome as the surgeon. The authors consider it inappropriate to impose our desires for near perfection on a patient who otherwise may be perfectly happy with the degree of improvement. On the other hand, mutual concerns over acquired asymmetries, incomplete lifts, persistent facial irregularities, or general unsatisfactory results are best acknowledged openly, with plans made for further correction if possible. Of course, face-lift surgery does not arrest the aging process, and the need for minor tuck-up procedures should not be considered a complication of face-lift surgery. This is especially true in older patients whose skin has lost its elasticity and heavy neck patients who require a lot of fat removal. In fact, some surgeons believe in planned, sequential rhytidectomy and address this issue in the preoperative assessment (36,63). Other than being indicated for recurrence of the signs of aging in the lower two-thirds of the face and neck, a revision or a tuck-up might be indicated when a previous procedure was underdone or overdone or when complications have arisen during the postoperative course. A partial revision could thus be planned to specifically address localized problems. Just as with primary surgery, secondary surgery could be tailored to address one or more specific areas. For instance, a recurrence of platysmal bands in the neck can be corrected with a platysmaplasty alone without having to do a full face-lift. Other indications for secondary surgery include persistent or recurrent jowling, platysmal bands, submental fat, or lax skin.

A prior face-lift or other neck surgery may complicate the proposed procedure. The placement and quality of prior face-lift incisions should be noted and discussed with the patient. Although it may be desirable to revise scars at the time of surgery, the surgeon might not be able to resect the entire width of a scar, specifically when the scar is wider than what could be excised without risking a tension closure after redraping the skin. Closing under tension would risk the same complication one is trying to correct.

Additionally, it may be useful to explore the patient's attitude toward the prior surgery. If the patient was dissatisfied with the result, the surgeon should proceed with caution and further evaluate the patient's motivations. The patient may have been reasonably unhappy with a poor result, but he/she may also be difficult to please, even with a technically sound job.

Dissection might technically be more difficult in a secondary surgery due to previous scarring in the deep tissues. Furthermore, scarring could have incorporated branches of the facial nerve especially if the SMAS has been elevated, rendering dissection more dangerous. If the SMAS was previously addressed with plication, that same technique could be safely utilized again for the revision, as one will not be in a sub-SMAS plane. Nevertheless, plicating the SMAS might still be a challenge as it has possibly been weakened. Sutures might just tear through thinned tissue and desired tension will have to be achieved with the use of an increased number of stitches. Some surgeons have reported that particularly in these revision cases a deep plane lift sometimes allows for better planes of dissection. The surgeon must be honest with himself or herself and with the patient about his or her ability to improve the aesthetic result. Any other prior neck surgery or irradiation might also adversely affect the ease of dissection and progress of healing or, as in the case of neck dissection, might expose deep neck structures to catastrophic injury. Incorporating these considerations into the surgical plan will help avoid a grave outcome.

POSTOPERATIVE CARE

The patient should be given detailed typewritten postoperative instructions before the surgery to allow the patient and his or her family to read the instructions in detail and ask questions before surgery. After surgery, the patient and family are informed again of problems that might arise and instructed to call the physician for any questions.

The authors use a large bulky dressing right after surgery, partly to discourage turning of the head, which can lead to hematoma formation. Patients often complain that their bandage is too tight right after surgery, which usually indicates that they are feeling the tightening of the lift and the bandage. If a compressive dressing is used, the surgeon can make a vertical incision in the midline of the dressing at the inferior border and see if there is any relief, but patients must be ready to accept a feeling of tightness.

Postoperative orders are geared toward keeping the patient calm and as pain-free as possible. Increased pain leads to increased blood pressure, which can increase the likelihood of complications. Likewise, a full bladder after a long procedure can increase blood pressure.

The surgeon should check on the patient the night of surgery. Any unilateral pain that is unrelenting and unresponsive to routine pain medication should alert the physician to possible hematoma formation and must be addressed as soon as possible. The patient also should be seen on the first postoperative day; drains are usually removed at this time, depending on the amount of drainage noted. Before releasing the tension of the bandage and removing the drains, fluffs are held over the area from which the drains are going to be removed, and pressure is applied. Pressure is maintained in those areas until a new bandage can be reapplied. This step helps to keep down the flaps and prevent hematoma or seroma formation. Before placing the new dressing on the first postoperative day, antibiotic ointment or cream is applied on all incisions (we prefer gentamicin cream), making sure to apply some at the external auditory canal to prevent any *Pseudomonas* from the external canal from contaminating the incisions.

Usually by the second or third postoperative day, the large bulky dressing can be totally removed, and an elasticized facial sling can be used. This helps the skin flap to maintain close contact with the subcutaneous tissue and provides faster revascularization and even contraction. It is important to pad the ears because these elasticized bandages can rub the thin skin of the pinna and thus cause irritation.

Usually on the fifth postoperative day, a few of the anterior preauricular stitches are removed, and the patient's hair is washed in a shampoo sink in the office. Patients are cautioned not to use hair dryers in the immediate postoperative period because some numbness of the periauricular and scalp areas will be present, possibly causing patients to burn their skin with the hair dryer due to lack of sensation.

Over ensuing visits, all the sutures are removed and the incisions examined under the microscope, especially in the hair-bearing areas to check for ingrown hairs, which can occur up to several months after surgery. After performing beveled incisions, this step also ensures that the hair will actually grow through the incision for camouflage. Often hairs become trapped and need help to come through the advanced flap.

Almost all patients have significant swelling or bruising postoperatively, and often this is difficult for the patient to accept. Gentle reassurance is key in the first postoperative weeks. As Goin and Goin (59) pointed out, if everything has gone well and the results are good, it is important for the physician to tell the patient so. Patients do not know how they should look and whether things were done well unless the doctor says so. Patients often forget what they looked like before surgery. For that reason, giving them prints of their preoperative photographs at the first or second postoperative visit is extremely helpful. This allows patients to compare their preoperative and postoperative conditions.

COMPLICATIONS

Nerve Injury

Injury to the facial nerve is fortunately a rare complication, with a reported incidence of between 0.4% and 2.6% (35,60–62). The motor nerve branch most vulnerable to direct, technical injury is the frontal branch of the zygomatic–temporal division of the facial nerve. This is because of its superficial location as it traverses the midportion of the zygomatic arch (Fig. 188.23). The authors avoid deep plane dissection entirely in the region superior to the arch and anterior to the temporal hairline to negate the risk of frontal nerve branch injury. Anatomic considerations are important for the marginal mandibular nerve and buccal nerve divisions as well. Marginal nerve injury results in an asymmetrically oriented smile with a higher position of the lower lip on the affected side due to unopposed action of the opposite depressor lip musculature (Fig. 188.24). Platysma transection and excessive SMAS traction in the region near the angle of the mandible and inferior mandibular border can result in marginal nerve paralysis. Buccal motor nerve branches are injured with aggressive dissection medial to the anterior border of the parotid gland. An asymmetric flattening of the midfacial contour may accompany buccal division injury.

Total facial nerve injury is extremely rare. If it is seen postoperatively and complete nerve transection is doubtful, consider a concomitant Bell's palsy (60). Transient paralysis of one or more facial nerve branches often is related to local action imposed by infiltrative anesthesia. Any prolonged paresis merits additional investigation and should not be attributed to the lidocaine effect. Additional causes of facial nerve injury include thermal injury by electrocoagulation; crush or pinch injuries caused by instrumentation or deep suture ligature; excessive SMAS traction; inflammation or infection; pressure from hematoma formation; and distortion, fibrosis, and scarring from previous face-lift surgery (60).

The most commonly injured nerve is the sensory greater auricular nerve because of its intimate association with the firm fascia surrounding the sternocleidomastoid muscle (62,63). Another nerve that is often overlooked both in the literature and clinically is the lesser occipital nerve. Although variable in its innervation pattern, Pantaloni found that in more than half of the cases, it innervated the superior third of the auricle and the mastoid area. And in 21% of patients, it innervated the upper two-thirds of the ear. Also, rarely (in about 5%) it will innervate the majority of the ear (64). Often, the skin flap is adherent in the area of both nerves and sharp dissection or traction can injure the nerve, resulting in permanent sensory deficit of the ear and periauricular skin. Meticulous precautions are paramount in that region.

Hematoma

With a reported incidence as high as 8.5%, hematoma formation remains the most common and feared complication of face-lift surgery (58,60,63). Expanding hematomas require immediate reoperation to control the bleeding source and to evacuate and drain the newly dissected skin flaps. Rapid filling of a suction drain reservoir is a sign of bleeding that must be investigated. Fortunately expanding hematomas are less frequent than small collections. Smaller or delayed hematomas can be managed with serial needle aspiration and pressure dressings. Patient complaints of pain, swelling, or firmness of the buccal region and ecchymosis, especially if unilateral, necessitate immediate inspection of the skin flaps. Intraoral inspection revealing mucosal ecchymosis often signals a hematoma that may be hidden by the external bandage.

Techniques that seem to reduce the incidence of hematoma formation include careful attention to intraoperative hemostasis, closed suction drainage, shorter skin flaps, and two-layer or deep plane face-lift technique. Unrecognized and improperly treated, hematomas result in skin necrosis, infection, prolonged ecchymosis, alopecia, subcutaneous nodules and skin puckering, and scar contracture.

Different factors can help decrease hematoma formation in the postoperative period. Some were already discussed earlier but are reiterated herein and cannot be overemphasized enough. First of all, coordination with the anesthesiologist is crucial for a smooth awakening. Coughing on the endotracheal tube will directly increase the blood pressure and potential bleeding under the flaps. Also, adequate blood pressure control both in the operating room and the postoperative period, especially in patients with a history of increased blood pressure, is paramount. Analgesia and antiemetics help reduce the pain and prevent nausea and vomiting, factors that can otherwise contribute in elevating the blood pressure. Making these medications readily available for the patient in the immediate postoperative period is crucial. Some surgeons have advocated prescribing these medications to be taken regularly rather than on a *pro re nata* regimen, minimizing any potential delays from nursing. Patients are also asked to refrain from exercise as this too can augment the

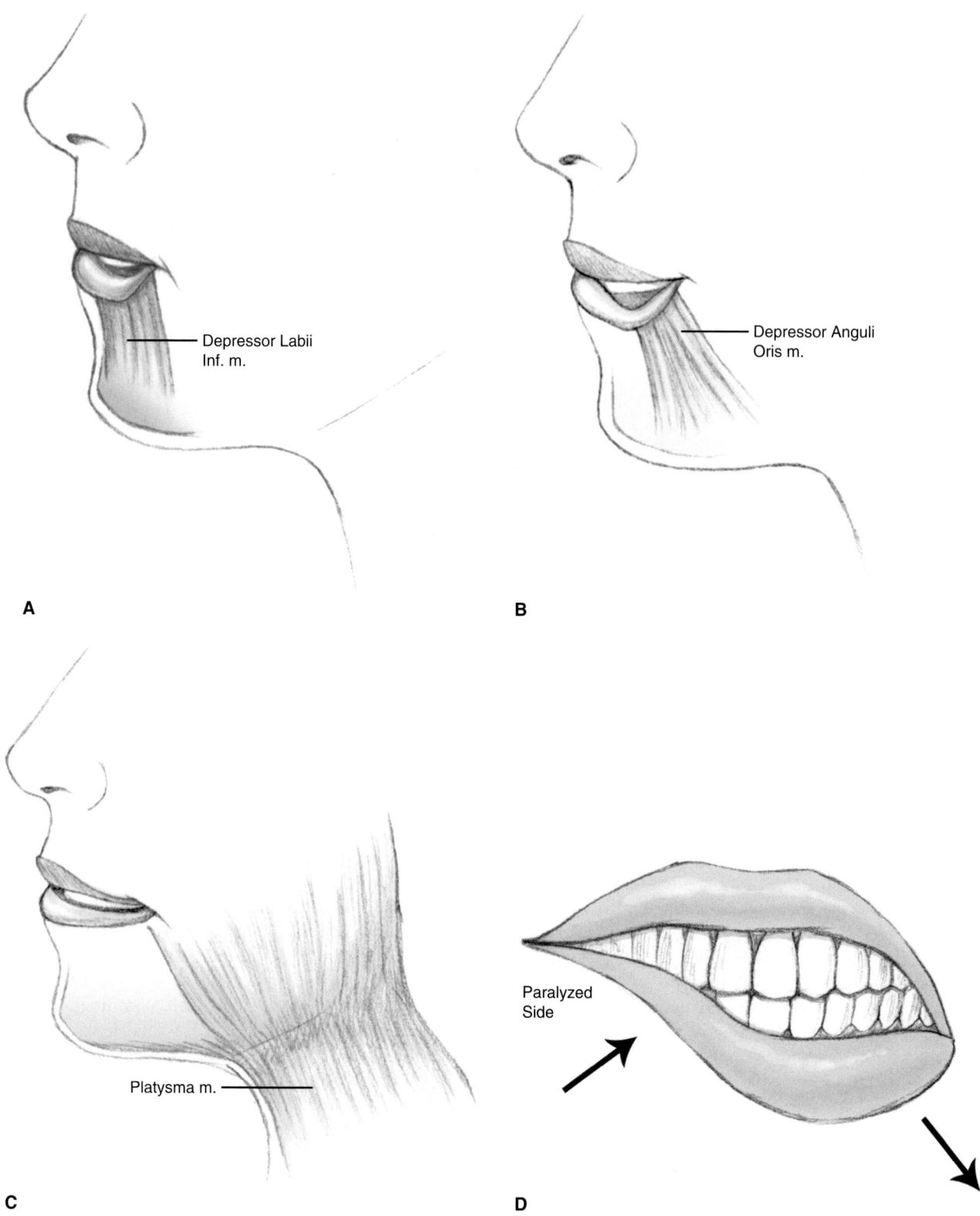

A

Depressor Labii
Inf. m.

B

Depressor Anguli
Oris m.

C

Platysma m.

D

Paralyzed
Side

Figure 188.24 A: The *depressor labii inferioris* everts the vermilion border and also moves the lower lip downward and laterally. **B:** The *depressor anguli oris* moves the lower lip downward and laterally. **C:** The *platysma* also moves the lip downward and laterally. **D:** The deformity caused by marginal mandibular nerve palsy results primarily from the inaction of the two depressor muscles. (Adapted from Baker DC, Conley J. Avoiding facial nerve injuries in rhytidectomy. *Plast Reconstr Surg* 1979;64:784.)

pressure. Compressive dressings, use of drains, and tissue sealants are also advocated by many surgeons.

Incision Problems

Tension on the suture line and skin flaps is the key danger to any face-lift procedure that otherwise may have been executed flawlessly. Careful preparation, incision placement, SMAS suspension, and accurate skin flap redraping without tension minimize incision complications. Preventing tension on skin incisions is the best way to avoid unattractive wide scars, skin slough, and hypertrophic scarring.

Cyanotic changes precede skin necrosis but sometimes can be reversed by increasing the oxygen tension to the skin flap. Often removing a few key sutures is helpful in releasing tension. A skin gap may granulate in if skin slough occurs, spontaneous demarcation with expectant management may limit the extent of tissue loss (65). Superficial debridement and topical antibiotic ointment can clean the wound and begin the process of reepithelialization. Keeping the wound bed moist and avoiding dry and crusted surface have been shown to significantly accelerate reepithelialization.

Active, hypertrophic scars respond to serial injections of triamcinolone at 3- to 4-week intervals. Silastic or silicone sheeting may also prove useful along with scar massaging. Direct excision of residual hypertrophic scars or widened incisions is delayed until after the inflammatory phase, when considerable skin relaxation and healing have occurred. In rare exceptions, one could earlier revise a scar that has obvious and significant deformity with little hope to improvement.

Prevention of structural deformities such as the satyr earlobe or pixie ear, blunted and anteriorly dislocated tragus, elevated temporal hairline, and conspicuous incisions such as suture tracking and posterior hairline step-off has already been thoroughly discussed. Chondritis of the tragus, external auditory canal, and auricle are reported in the literature and may result in structural deformity. Suspected chondritis often responds to ciprofloxacin or other antipseudomonal and antistaphylococcal antibiotics. Undesirable creation of a bloody culture media in the ear canal can be avoided by occluding the canal before surgery with an iodine-soaked cotton ball. Also, no sutures are placed through tragal cartilage, thereby preventing the direct introduction of organisms to the cartilage.

Other incision problems include ingrown hairs, which can establish a nidus of infection and inflammation. During each postoperative visit, ingrown hairs are identified by magnified inspection of the incision and removed. Occasionally, buried permanent sutures used in SMAS suspension find their way to the skin surface. Removing sutures that have extruded after a long follow-up should create no difficulty for the patient. Rarely, persistent hemosiderin deposits are visible beneath the skin and require cosmetic cover.

Alopecia

Other than poorly planned incisions, tension seems to be the main cause of postoperative alopecia. Some loss may be transient and results from temporary surgical stress to the hair follicles during the perioperative period. This phenomenon, better known as telogen effluvium, affects normal hair around the incision sites. These hair follicles do not undergo physical transection from the surgical knife, and hence, patients should be counseled that hair is expected to grow back within 3 months. Many series report an incidence ranging from 0.2% to 1.8% (58).

In contrast, when scars develop, they are usually more noticeable because of the permanent alopecia that accompanies the scar formation. When that is the case, single–follicular unit hair transplantation can be achieved. In males specifically, the donor source should be from an area of the scalp that is not expected to undergo androgenic alopecia with time. This is typically the occipital area. However, if one is planning a revision face-lift with skin resection, follicles from resected scalp in the postauricular area while redraping could be used as a potential transplant source, obviating the need for a separate occipital incision. The small number of follicles harvested from that technique might be a limiting factor if the coverage needed at the recipient site is substantial. It is interesting to note that hair shafts harvested from the lateral occipital regions tend to be thinner. That often is an advantage when reconstructing the temporal hair tuft where shafts are also of a more narrow dimension (Fig. 188.25). Other than hair transplantation, one could rely on excision of the area of alopecia with tissue advancement. Larger areas of alopecia may also require tissue expansion with hair flap rearrangement for aesthetic, full-density hair coverage.

Final Word

The dictum "above all else, do no harm" is of paramount importance in elective aesthetic facial surgery and should be heard loudly in every surgeon's ear while planning and performing facial rejuvenation surgery. Functional, permanent, or disfiguring complications can be particularly devastating to patients who were not ill but simply wanted to look and feel better about themselves. Honesty and integrity must characterize the relationship between the surgeon and patient, and patient education is important to that relationship.

The deep plane techniques have led surgeons to think more rigorously about facial anatomy and the goals of rhytidectomy. Many of these techniques ultimately may be incorporated into standard rhytidectomy practice. Until that time, however, continued critical assessment of the benefits and risks of these procedures is needed, and caution is urged for surgeons contemplating deep dissection in the medial face.

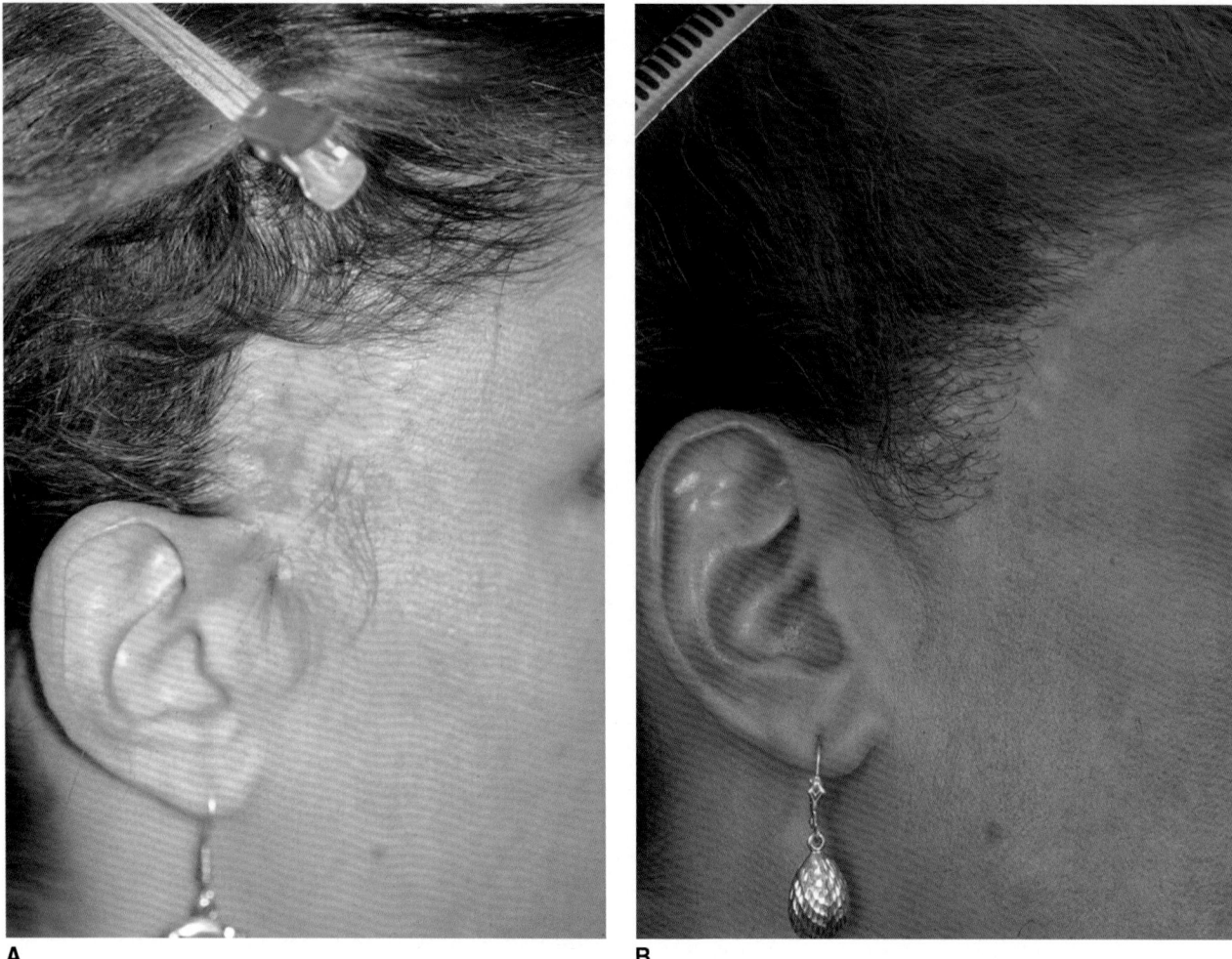

A **B**

Figure 188.25 **A:** Preoperative photograph of a patient with temporal alopecia secondary to scarring. **B:** Postoperative result following tissue expansion, scalp advancement, excision of scars, and two sessions of microfollicular unit hair transplantation. (Reprinted from Kridel RWH. Techniques for inconspicuous face lift scars. *Arch Facial Plast Surg* 2003;5:323–333, with permission.)

HIGHLIGHTS

- The ideal patient for face-lift surgery is aged in the mid-40s to mid-50s and in good general health; has a strong jawline, chin, and cheekbone; and has a high posterior hyoid, a relatively thin neck and face, and minimal photoaging of the skin.
- Rhytidectomy mainly corrects ptosis of the jowl and blunting of the cervicomental angle. If creases and wrinkles of the skin contribute to the aged appearance, one should consider chemexfoliation or laser resurfacing as an adjunct procedure. Periorbital and perioral resurfacing can be done safely at the same sitting as rhytidectomy.
- The "face-lift" is truly only a cheek and neck lift, and often ptosis of other facial regions also contributes

to the aged appearance. Achieving facial harmony between different regions will provide natural non-operated results. Thus, blepharoplasty, forehead lift, and other rejuvenation surgery should be considered at the same sitting as the face-lift. Final face-lift results depend on a good, strong bony framework; augmentation of the cheekbones, submalar areas, and chin also may be necessary.
- To assess whether a patient's expectations are realistic, ensure that improvement and not perfection is the mutual goal, that the patient does not expect to look exactly as she or he did many years ago, and that the patient understands that a face-lift is surgery, with inherent risks and possible complications.
- Thorough preoperative evaluation of the patient's medical condition is mandatory. Because smoking

greatly increases the risk of skin slough, smokers should be operated upon cautiously. Medical conditions that predispose to abnormal bleeding (e.g., coagulopathies, severe hypertension, hepatic or renal disease), if not correctable preoperatively, are contraindications to rhytidectomy. Coordination with the primary care provider is crucial especially in patients with comorbidities that need medical clearance prior to surgery.

- Incisions must be planned differently for men and women. Preserving the anterior hair tuft is key in women. In men, a preauricular incision is preferable, with maintenance of a hair-free border around the ear and under the lobule to prevent beard hair from annoying the patient postoperatively. Furthermore, in males care must be used to preserve the hair follicles during subcutaneous dissection, avoiding beard alopecia.

- In a SMAS suspension rhytidectomy, the pull should be mainly superior, with only a slight posterior vector to counter the chronic effects of gravity. All tension should be carried by this layer with the skin closed under no tension at all. Too much skin tension can lead to skin slough, increased telangiectasias, or a widened scar. Aggressive cutaneous tension can also lead to an unnatural appearance.

- The debate between SMAS suspension rhytidectomy versus deep plane rhytidectomy on routine patients is ongoing. More objective data will be needed to evaluate the effect and longevity of both techniques on different areas of the face.

- Prominent nasolabial folds are a source of concern for patients and surgeons alike, and improvement with standard rhytidectomy is limited. Deep plane rhytidectomy offers some promise as a means of improving this area, but the cosmetic benefit has not yet been clearly established, and the theoretical risk of injury to the facial nerve is greater than with standard techniques. Caution is urged for surgeons contemplating deep plane approaches to the medial face.

- Theories stressing volume loss and tissue atrophy rather than just gravitational changes have shifted some surgeons toward facial fillers, facial implants, and soft tissue augmentation. These techniques are being used alone and in conjunction with traditional lifting procedures. However, surgical lifts will always have a role in resuspending ptotic tissue.

- Submental liposuction and platysmaplasty have enhanced the degree and duration of improvement in submental contour over SMAS plication rhytidectomy alone. These techniques are routinely used along with face-lift and can be tailored to the patient need and age.

- Secondary face-lift surgery is indicated both for recurrence of the signs of aging and for correcting previously obtained results. Planning incision placement is often more challenging in these cases. Dissection can be more tedious and the risk for facial nerve injury higher with SMAS elevation.

- Hematoma is the most common complication of rhytidectomy and is most likely to occur in the first 24 hours after surgery. Vigilance for symptoms and signs of impending problems is mandatory; quality nursing care to prevent postoperative hypertension is essential. Precise postoperative medications and patient adherence to instructions also help to prevent hematoma formation. Meticulous long-term follow-up care will help ensure an optimal result.

REFERENCES

1. Lambros V. Observations on periorbital and midface aging. *Plast Reconstr Surg* 2007;120(5):1367–1376.
2. Lambros V. Models of facial aging and implications for treatment. *Clin Plast Surg* 2008;35(3):319–327.
3. McCollough EG. The McCollough Facial Rejuvenation System: a condition-specific classification algorithm. *Facial Plast Surg* 2011;27(1):112–123.
4. Furnas DW. The retaining ligaments of the cheeks. *Plast Reconstr Surg* 1989;83:11.
5. Sherris DA, Larrabee WF. Anatomic considerations in rhytidectomy. *Facial Plast Surg* 1996;12(3):215.
6. Weiss JS, Swanson NA. Baker S. Anatomy and physiology of aging skin. In: Krause CJ, ed. *Aesthetic facial surgery*. Philadelphia, PA: JB Lippincott, 1991:461.
7. Bhawan J, Andersen W, Lee J, et al. Photoaging versus intrinsic aging: a morphologic assessment of facial skin. *J Cutan Pathol* 1995;22:154.
8. Yousif NJ, Mendelson BC. Anatomy of the midface. *Clin Plast Surg* 1995;22:227.
9. Kligman AM, Zheng P, Lavker RM. The anatomy and pathogenesis of wrinkles. *Br J Dermatol* 1985;113:37.
10. Gilchrest BA. Skin aging and photoaging: an overview. *J Am Acad Dermatol* 1989;21:610.
11. Kligman LH. Photoaging: manifestations, prevention, and treatment. *Dermatol Clin* 1986;4(3):517.
12. Kabaker SS. Kridel RWH, Krugman ME, et al. Tissue expansion in the treatment of alopecia. *Arch Otolaryngol Head Neck Surg* 1986;112:720.
13. Larrabee WF, Henderson JL. Face lift: the anatomic basis for a safe, long-lasting procedure. *Facial Plast Surg* 2000;16(3):239.
14. Stuzin JM, Baker TJ, Gordon HL. The relationship of the superficial and deep facial fascias: relevance to rhytidectomy and aging. *Plast Reconstr Surg* 1992;89(3):441.
15. Jost G, Levet Y. Parotid fascia and face lifting: a critical evaluation of the SMAS concept. *Plast Reconstr Surg* 1984;74:42.
16. Quatela VC, Sabini P. Techniques in deep plane face lifting. *Facial Plast Surg Clin North Am* 2000;8(2):193.
17. Lemmon ML. Superficial fascia rhytidectomy: a restoration of the SMAS with control of the cervicomental angle. *Clin Plast Surg* 1983;10(3):449.
18. Owsley JQ. Platysma- fascia rhytidectomy. *Plast Reconstr Surg* 1977;60:843.
19. Lemmon ML, Hamra ST. Skoog rhytidectomy: a five year experience with 577 patients. *Plast Reconstr Surg* 1980;65:283.

20. Aston SJ. Platysma- SMAS cervicofacial rhytidoplasty. *Clin Plast Surg* 1983;10:507.

21. Mitz V, Peyronie M. The superficial musculoaponeurotic system (SMAS) in the parotid and cheek area. *Plast Reconstr Surg* 1976;58:80.

22. Faivre J. Deep temporal facelift: techniques and indications. *Fr Rev Cosm Surg* 1988;14:53.

23. Psillakis JM, Rumley TO, Camargos A. Subperiosteal approach as an improved concept for correction of the aging face. *Plast Reconstr Surg* 1988;82:383–394.

24. Hamra S. The deep-plane rhytidectomy. *Plast Reconstr Surg* 1990; 86:53.

25. Hamra ST. Composite rhytidectomy. *Plast Reconstr Surg* 1992; 90:1.

26. Webster RC, Smith RC, Smith KF. Facelift, part I: extent of undermining of skin flaps. *Head Neck Surg* 1983;5:525.

27. Becker FF, Bassichis BA. Deep plane facelift vs. superficial musculoaponeurotic system plication face- lift. A comparative study. *Arch Facial Plast Surg* 2004;6:8.

28. Adamson PA, Dahiya R, Litner J. Midface effects of the deep-plane vs superficial musculoaponeurotic system plication face-lift. *Arch Facial Plast Surg* 2007;9:9–11.

29. Becker FF, Bassichis BA. Deep-plane facelift vs superficial musculoaponeurotic system plication face-lift: a comparative study. *Arch Facial Plast Surg* 2004;6:8–13.

30. Baker DC. Deep dissection rhytidectomy: a plea for caution. *Plast Reconstr Surg* 1994;93:1498.

31. Kamer FM. One hundred consecutive deep-plane facelifts. *Arch Otolaryngol Head Neck Surg* 1996;122:17.

32. Baker DC, Conley J. Avoiding facial nerve injuries in rhytidectomy. *Plast Reconstr Surg* 1979;64:781.

33. Chang S, Pusic A, Rohrich RJ. A systematic review of comparison of efficacy and complication rates among facelift techniques. *Plast Reconstr Surg* 2011;127(1):423–433.

34. Tobin HA. Patient motivations and expectations. In: Krause CJ, ed. *Aesthetic facial surgery.* Philadelphia, PA: JB Lippincott, 1991:469.

35. Baker DC. Anatomy and injuries of the facial nerve in cervicofacial rhytidectomy. In: Kaye BI, Gradinger GP, eds. *Symposium on problems and complications in aesthetic plastic surgery of the face.* St. Louis, MO: Mosby, 1984:150.

36. Kamer FM. Sequential rhytidectomy and the two-stage concept. *Otolaryngol Clin North Am* 1980;13:305.

37. Rees TD, Aston SJ. Complications of rhytidectomy. *Clin Plast Surg* 1978;5:109.

38. Webster RC, Davidson TM, White MF, et al. Conservative facelift surgery. *Arch Otolaryngol* 1976;102:657.

39. Colton JJ, Beekhuis GJ. Anesthesia for facial cosmetic surgery. In: Krause CJ, ed. *Aesthetic facial surgery.* Philadelphia, PA: JB Lippincott Co., 1991:503.

40. Kridel RWH, Konior RJ, Buchwach KA. Suction lipectomy. In: Krause CJ, ed. *Aesthetic facial surgery.* Philadelphia, PA: JB Lippincott Co., 1991.

41. Kridel RWH, Liu ES. Techniques for creating inconspicuous facelift scars: avoiding visible incisions and loss of temporal hair. *Arch Facial Plast Surg* 2003;5:325.

42. Webster RC, Fanous N, Smith RC. Male and female facelift incisions. *Arch Otolaryngol* 1982;108:299.

43. McCollough EG, Perkins SW, Langsdon PR. SASMAS suspension rhytidectomy: rationale and long-term experience. *Arch Otolaryngol Head Neck Surg* 1989;115:228.

44. Baker SR. Is deep plane face lift better than superficial musculoaponeurotic system plication facelift? *Arch Facial Plast Surg* 2004;6:8.

45. McCollough EG. Face-lifting in the nineties: selecting the appropriate technique. In: Stuker FJ, ed. *Plastic and reconstructive surgery of the head and neck.* Philadelphia, PA: BC Decker, 1991:165.

46. Feldman JJ. Corset platysmaplasty. *Plast Reconstr Surg* 1990; 85:333.

47. Webster RC, Smith RC, Smith KF. Facelift, part II: etiology of platysma cording and its relationship to treatment. *Head Neck Surg* 1983;6:590.

48. Webster RC, Smith RC, Smith KF. Facelift, part III: plication of the superficial musculoaponeurotic system. *Head Neck Stag* 1983;6:696.

49. Webster RC, Smith RC, Smith KF. Facelift, part IV: use of superficial musculoaponeurotic system suspending sutures. *Head Neck Surg* 1984;6:780.

50. Webster RC, Smith RC, Smith KF. Facelift, part V: suspending sutures for platysma cording. *Head Neck Stag* 1984:6:870.

51. Webster RC, Smith RC, Papsidero MJ, et al. Comparison of SMAS plication with SMAS imbrication in face-lifting. *Laryngoscope* 1982;92:901.

52. Ramirez OM. The subperiosteal rhytidectomy: the third-generation facelift. *Ann Plast Surg* 1992;28:218.

53. Freilinger G, Gruber H, Happak WE, et al. Surgical anatomy of the mimic muscle system and the facial nerve: importance for reconstruction and aesthetic surgery. *Plast Reconstr Surg* 1987;80:686.

54. Whetzel TP. Mathes SJ. Arterial anatomy of the face: analysis of vascular territories and perforating cutaneous vessels. *Plast Reconstr Surg* 1992;89:591.

55. Zutlerey J. Anatomic variations of the nasolabial fold. *Plast Reconstr Surg* 1992;89:225.

56. Barton FE Jr. Rhytidectomy and the nasolabial fold. *Plast Reconstr Surg* 1992;90:601.

57. Mendelson BC. Correction of the nasolabial fold: extended SMAS dissection with periosteal fixation. *Plast Reconstr Surg* 1992;89:822.

58. Kridel RWH, Aguilar EA, Wright WK. Complications of rhytidectomy. *Ear Nose Throat J* 1985;64:44.

59. Goin JM, Goin MK. *Changing the body: psychological effects of plastic surgery.* Baltimore, MD: Williams & Wilkins, 1981.

60. Guerrero-Santos J. Complications of the neck lift. In: Kaye BL, Gradinger GP, eds. *Symposium on problems and complications in aesthetic plastic surgery of the face.* St. Louis, MO: Mosby, 1984:274.

61. Castanares S. Facial nerve paralysis coincident with, or subsequent to, rhytidectomy. *Plast Reconstr Surg* 1974;54:637.

62. Thomas JR. Complications of aesthetic surgery. In: Johns ME, ed. *Complications in otolaryngology-head and neck surgery.* Philadelphia, PA: BC Decker, 1986:281.

63. Anderson JR. The tuck-up operation: a new technique of secondary rhytidectomy. *Arch Otolaryngol* 1975;101:739.

64. Pantaloni M, Sullivan O. Relevance of the lesser occipital nerve in facial rejuvenation surgery. *Plast Reconstr Surg* 1976;1:3.

65. Berman WE. Rhytidectomy. In: Krause CJ, ed. *Aesthetic facial surgery.* Philadelphia, PA: JB Lippincott Co., 1991:513.

The Aging Neck

189

Edwin Francis Williams   **Henry Haipei Chen**

The typical appearance of the aging neck is caused by a constellation of changes associated with both heredity and the aging process. Each patient will demonstrate different anatomic components contributing to the overall appearance of an aging neckline. The anatomic factors that contribute to an ideal cervical contour include a strong chin, a distinct mandibular border, a cervicomental angle of 105 to 120 degrees, a visible subhyoid bone depression, a gentle indentation at the thyroid notch, and visible anterior borders of the sternocleidomastoid muscles (1) (Fig. 189.1). Obtaining these ideal contours should be the goal of any surgical correction of the aging neck. To achieve these goals, however, the surgeon must carefully and systematically analyze each patient to determine the anatomic abnormalities that need to be addressed. An individualized approach ensures that specific deformities are clearly delineated so a youthful and graceful neckline may be restored.

ANATOMY

The aging process exerts an impact on each anatomic element of the cervical region to varying degrees in each patient. Additionally, some patients also display hereditary abnormalities contributing to an unfavorable cervical contour, including a low-positioned hyoid bone, poor chin projection, and a congenital collection of submental fat. Each element of the contributing anatomy should be identified preoperatively and sequentially addressed in the surgical correction to provide an optimal aesthetic outcome. The anatomic areas to be addressed include skin, fat, platysma muscle, chin position, and other unfavorable anatomy (2).

Skin

With time, collagen and elastin fibers degenerate so the overlying skin loses its tone and no longer adheres to the soft tissue contours of the neck. The skin becomes redundant and sags, leading to the development of horizontal cervical rhytids and effacement of the cervicomental angle.

Fat

Fat deposition in the neck can be congenital or acquired. Several anatomic studies have shown that the fat in the submental region is found in discrete compartments (3,4). These areas include (a) a supraplatysmal (subcutaneous) layer diffusely distributed throughout the cervical region, (b) a subplatysmal compartment that overlies the mylohyoid muscle, and (c) facial fat from the cheek and inferior buccal fat pad contributing to a ptotic jowl and loss of the definition of the inferior mandibular border (Fig. 189.2). The subplatysmal layer is further divided into a central compartment between the anterior bellies of the digastric muscles and paired medial and lateral compartments.

Clinically, it is difficult to discern the exact anatomic compartment(s) of submental lipodystrophy, especially in heavy necks. While the use of ultrasonography can be helpful to delineate the areas of excess fat (5), its use is certainly not required as a part of a routine preoperative workup.

Platysma Muscle

The platysma is a paired muscle that is innervated by the cervical branch of the seventh cranial nerve. It originates from the fascia of the pectoralis major and deltoid muscles and ascends in the neck to insert on the inferior border of the mandible (Fig. 189.3). Laterally, the posterior border of the platysma muscle ends in front of the sternocleidomastoid muscle. As the platysma muscle is followed superiorly to the mandible, the medial fibers insert into the periosteum to stabilize one end of the muscle during contraction. The central fibers blend intimately with the risorius muscle. The posterior third of the platysma muscle

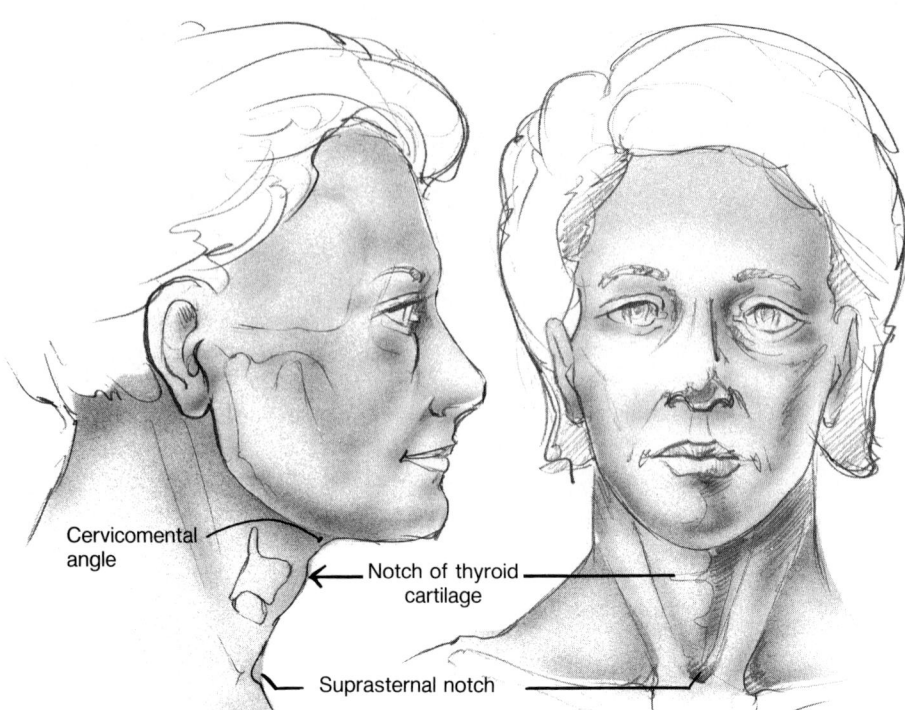

Figure 189.1 The anatomic factors that contribute to an ideal cervical contour include a strong chin, a distinct mandibular border, a cervicomental angle of 90 degrees, a visible subhyoid bone depression, a gentle indentation at the thyroid notch, and visible anterior borders of the sternocleidomastoid muscles.

Cervicomental angle

Notch of thyroid cartilage

Suprasternal notch

sweeps up over the mandible to course anteriorly and fuse with the superficial musculoaponeurotic system (SMAS). The cervical skin receives part of its blood supply from perforating vessels arising from the platysma muscle. These vessels and thick fibrous septa coursing through the subcutaneous fat anchor the dermis to the superficial cervical fascia and platysma muscle.

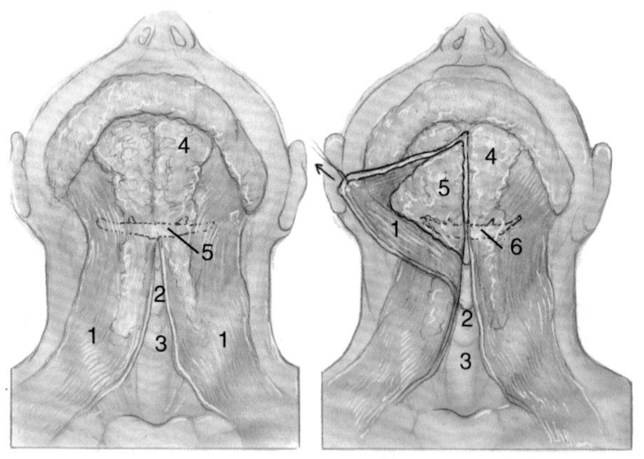

1. Platysma m.
2. Thyroid cartilage
3. Cricoid cartilage
4. Submental fat
5. Outline of hyoid bone

1. Platysma m. reflected laterally
2. Thyroid cartilage
3. Cricoid cartilage
4. Submental fat
5. Fat deep to platysma m. superficial to hyoid and digastric m.
6. Outline of hyoid bone

Figure 189.2 Fat is found both superficial and deep to the platysma.

Different degrees of decussation in the midline of the neck have been documented in anatomic studies, and there is also ethnic variability (6,7). The "turkey gobbler" deformity is caused by a laxity in the platysma muscle that does not decussate in the midline.

The platysma muscle functions to stabilize the chest muscles against the jaw during heavy lifting. It also provides a layer over vital structures of the neck. It is a somewhat vestigial structure in humans, corresponding phylogenetically to the panniculus carnosus muscle that forms a continuous subcutaneous layer in lower mammals (8).

With aging, the platysma muscle becomes atrophic and falls toward the midline. First, convexity occurs in the submental region; then, as the muscle loses tone, it forms the pathognomonic anterior banding of the aged neck. On profile, the apex of the cervicomental angle is blunted by the anterior border of the muscle as it runs diagonally from the mandible to the lower neck. Loss of the platysmal muscle sling also allows ptosis of the underlying cervical contents.

Chin Position

An appropriately projected chin is prerequisite for an optimal aesthetic cervical contour. A poorly projected chin creates an illusion of blunting of the cervicomental angle, and aging contour deformities tend to be worse in patients with smaller mandibles and chins (9,10).

Ideally, in a patient with Angle class I occlusion, the pogonion (the most anterior projecting point of the chin) should touch a line dropped vertically from the vermillion border of the lower lip on profile view. It is aesthetically acceptable in women if the chin is slightly posterior to this

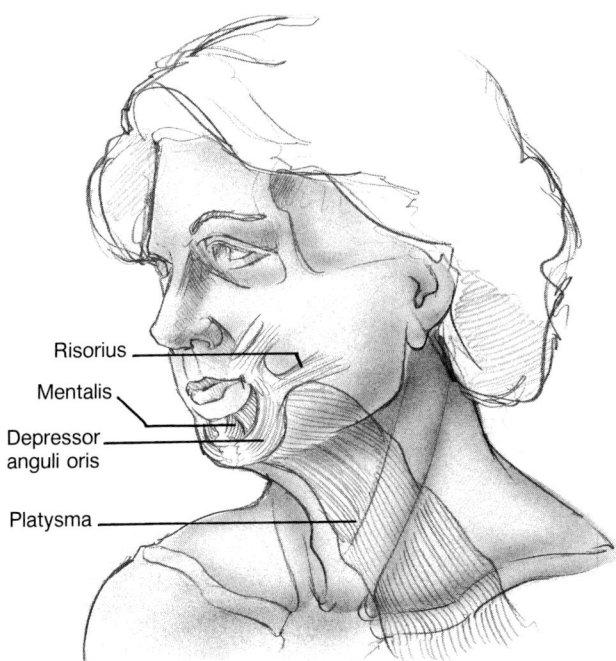

Figure 189.3 The platysma muscle ascends in the neck to blend with the SMAS.

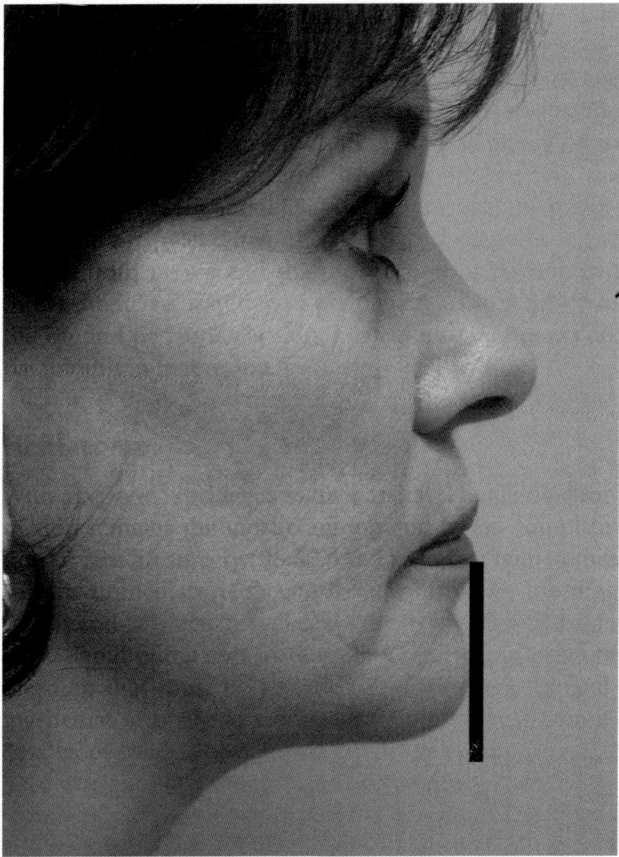

Figure 189.4 The anteriormost projection of the chin (pogonion) should touch a line dropped vertically from the vermillion border of the lower lip on profile view.

line; however, in men, this line should be tangent to the pogonion (11) (Fig. 189.4). The chin contour is determined by the shape and position of the mandible as well as the overlying soft tissues. A weak chin, or microgenia, is most commonly congenital; however, senile absorption of alveolar bone should also be considered in the older patient.

Mandibular hypoplasia is an acquired condition secondary to varying degrees of bony resorption of the mandible. With aging, specific progressive soft tissue atrophy and bone reduction occur in the region between the chin and jowl. This resulting groove has been termed the "prejowl sulcus" (11). Mandibular hypoplasia should not be confused with retrognathia. Patients with retrognathia demonstrate Angle class II occlusion and are optimally treated with a bony advancement technique (e.g., sagittal-split osteotomy), whereas patients with microgenia or mandibular hypoplasia are better treated with alloplastic augmentation.

Unfavorable Anatomy

The hyoid bone supports the floor of the mouth as it is suspended by the digastric, mylohyoid, stylohyoid, and tongue musculature. Ideally, it should be at the level of the third or fourth cervical vertebrae (12). A more posterior and superior hyoid produces a more aesthetic cervical contour. A hyoid bone that is in a relatively inferior position in the neck causes the suprahyoid musculature to course in a more vertical direction, blunting the angle between the chin and neck (13). With advancing age, gravity may favor the drag of the infrahyoid musculature over the suprahyoid

musculature, inducing further descent of the hyoid (12). A low hyoid bone position is a major limiting factor in the optimal rejuvenation of the cervical region.

Submandibular gland ptosis is commonly seen with aging, which is identified as two bulges at the anterior edge of the submandibular triangle. Diagnosis is confirmed by palpation of the gland's cobblestoned surface. The position of the glands should be elucidated preoperatively for both patient counseling and surgical planning.

Overdevelopment of the suprahyoid bone musculature, especially the digastric muscles, can also lead to fullness of the submental region. Identification is facilitated by having the patient flex the neck with the mouth closed (2).

CLASSIFICATION AND EVALUATION

Numerous classification schemes describing the aging neck exist (2,14,15). Dedo's (14) preoperative classification of the neck is the most commonly used. It is a useful tool to help delineate the features contributing to a particular patient's pathology and to help guide targeted surgical intervention (Fig. 189.5).

A patient with a class I neck is typically a younger patient who has minimal, if any, deformity, which may or may not require surgical intervention. A patient with a

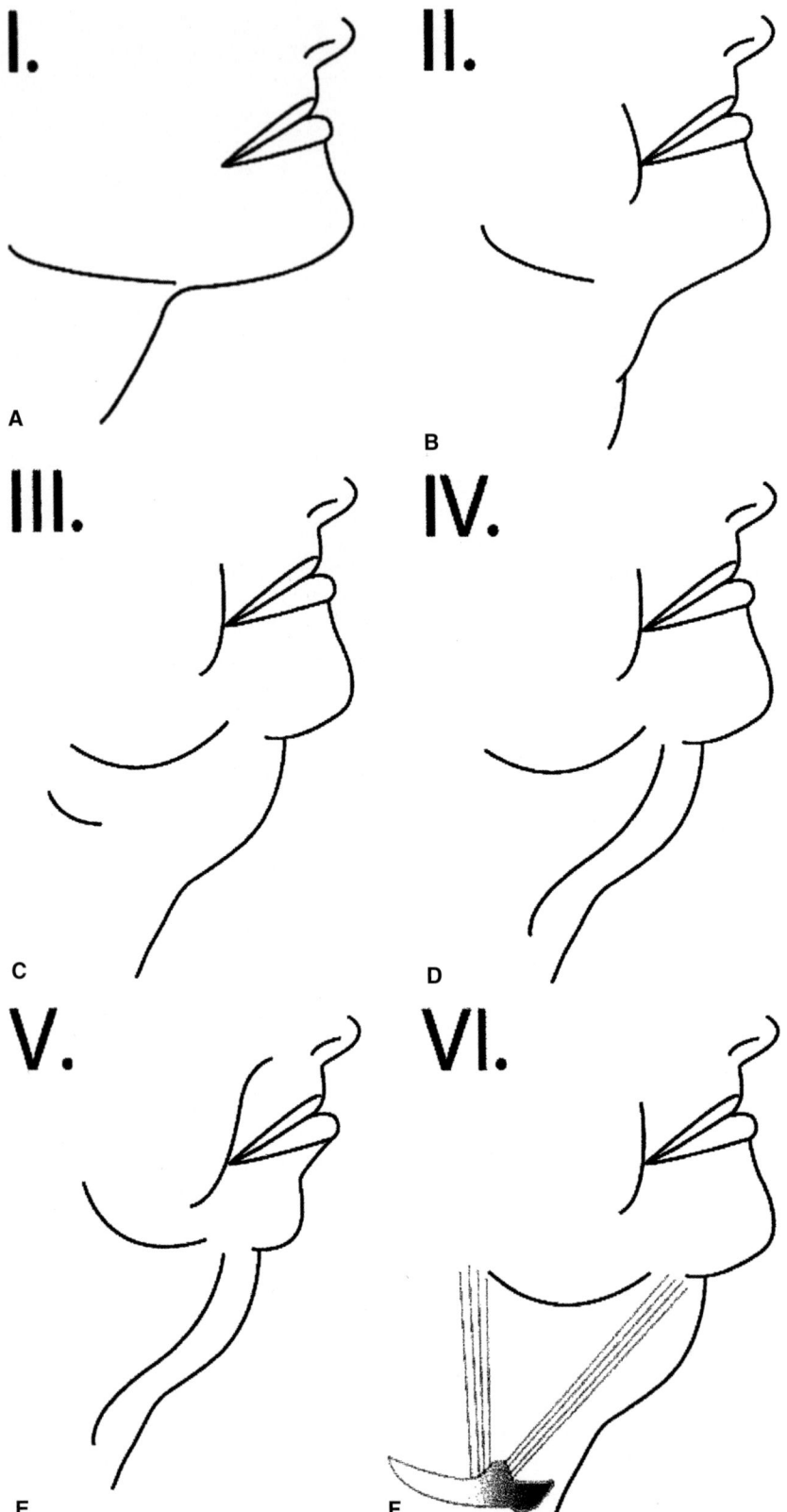

Figure 189.5 Dedo classification of cervical abnormalities: **A:** Class I deformity describes only minimal cosmetic deformity. **B:** Class II deformity describes only skin laxity. **C:** Class III deformity refers to the excessive submandibular and submental adipose. **D:** Class IV deformity refers to anterior banding of the platysma. **E:** Class V deformity describes the condition of microgenia or retrognathia. **F:** Class VI deformity describes a low-positioned hyoid bone.

class I neck should ideally wait until more of an aesthetic problem develops, because any intervention at this time is essentially prophylactic.

The class II patient has skin laxity only, without significant fat or muscle pathology. The class includes the "turkey gobbler" deformity often seen in elderly males.

A class III deformity is caused by excessive cervical liposis. Excess adipose can accumulate in the supra- or subplatysmal layer. Both contribute to jowling.

The class IV patient has a pathologic platysma muscle either in repose or on voluntary contraction. This is usually diagnosed in the thin neck as anterior platysmal banding; however, in patients with submental adiposity or redundant anterior cervical skin, it is often not readily apparent that the platysma muscle is contributing to the deformity. In fact, the full neck does not evidence platysmal banding, even with aging (3). In this case, diagnosis is facilitated by having the patient grimace with the teeth clenched to delineate the medial and lateral borders of the muscle (Fig. 189.6).

The class V patient has a weak mandibular projection from congenital or acquired causes. Although the terms retrognathia and microgenia have been used interchangeably in the scientific literature, each word denotes a different condition. The term microgenia, referring to an underprojected chin, independent of occlusal consideration, is more appropriate to describe most of these patients. Retrognathia, on the other hand, refers to Angle class II occlusion in which the hypoplastic and retruded mandible leads to an overbite and dental malocclusion. It is important to note that prominence of the chin confers strength to the jaw–neck contour and makes the transition between facial and cervical aesthetic units more pronounced, thus giving the illusion of a more acute cervicomental angle (12).

Patients with a class VI neck have an inferiorly positioned hyoid bone that creates an obtuse cervicomental angle. Diagnosis is made by palpating the hyoid bone and evaluating its relationship to the mandible and clavicles. As stated earlier, the hyoid bone should ideally reside at the level of the third or fourth cervical vertebra. A low-positioned hyoid bone is a major limiting factor in optimal aesthetic correction of the aging neck unless more aggressive surgical treatment is undertaken.

TREATMENT

After careful analysis of each anatomic factor contributing to the individual patient's deformity, a targeted surgical treatment plan can be instituted (Table 189.1). It should be noted that a weak chin can be a compounding factor in any of the classification groups. In addition to treating the soft tissue abnormalities, an alloplastic chin implant should be strongly considered in any patient with evidence of microgenia. Again, in patients with significant retrognathia, chin

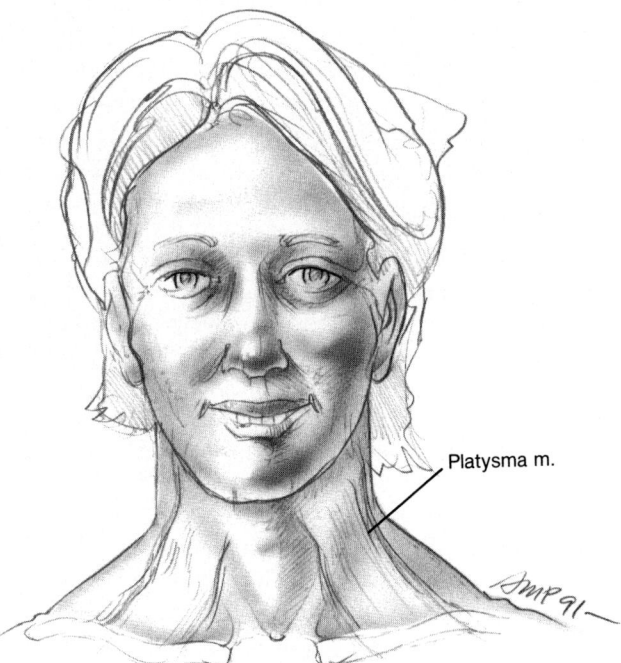

Figure 189.6 The medial and lateral borders of the platysma muscle can be better delineated by having the patient grimace with the teeth clenched.

Platysma m.

TABLE 189.1 ℞	**TARGETED SURGICAL TREATMENT PLAN**
Modified Dedo's Classification	**Treatment Options**
Class I (minimal deformity)	• No surgical intervention • "S lift" • ± Chin augmentation
Class II (laxity of cervical skin)	• Rhytidectomy • ± Chin augmentation
Class III (excess fat)	• Cervical liposuction • ± Anterior platysmaplasty • ± Rhytidectomy (for skin laxity) • ± Chin augmentation
Class IV (platysmal banding)	• Rhytidectomy (with anterior platysmaplasty) • ± Cervical liposuction • ± Chin augmentation
Class V (microgenia or retrognathia)	• Chin augmentation (microgenia) • Bony osteotomy and advancement (retrognathia)
Class VI (low hyoid or other unfavorable anatomy)	• Treat soft tissue abnormalities with standard techniques (with realistic expectations) • ± Division of suprahyoid musculature from mandible • ± Suturing of anterior digastric muscles together • ± Partial excision of anterior digastric muscles • ± Chin augmentation

The "S" Lift

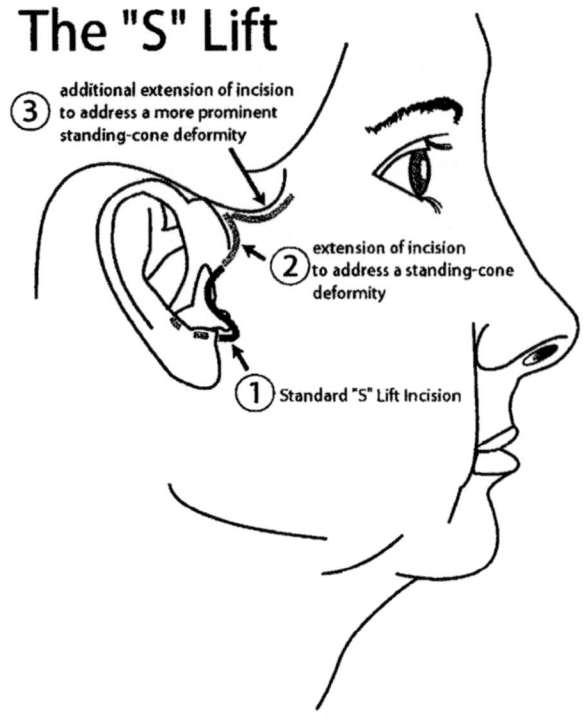

(3) additional extension of incision to address a more prominent standing-cone deformity

(2) extension of incision to address a standing-cone deformity

(1) Standard "S" Lift Incision

Figure 189.7 The configuration of the incision resembles an S shape. The abbreviated length is suitable for younger patients who do not have significant skin redundancy but only some incipient jowling. To address a standing-cone ("dog-ear") deformity that may arise, the anterior skin incision can be extended up to (or all the way around) the temporal tuft, as needed.

augmentation alone may not give optimal aesthetic results, and bony advancement techniques should be considered.

In young patients with minimal deformity (class I), the most prudent course of action would be simply to wait before any surgical intervention is offered. In the patient with good skin and muscle tone, a simple weight loss program could be sufficient (8). The improvement gained by surgical intervention at this time would be minimal; however, intervention may delay soft tissue ptosis from developing as quickly. In the fastidious patient with realistic expectations, a limited rhytidectomy (S lift) can be considered (Fig. 189.7). An incision that extends only under the ear lobule in a lazy-S configuration is made, allowing a limited SMAS suspension and excision of skin without committing the patient to a standard rhytidectomy (16).

In patients with redundant skin of the cervical region (class II), a standard cervicofacial rhytidectomy is generally considered the treatment of choice. To remove excess skin and to efface jowling along the inferior mandibular border, a SMAS imbrication technique is used to provide long-lasting improvement of the contour of the lower one-third of the face and neck. A special note should be made for the "turkey gobbler" deformity, which is commonly seen in men. Multiple techniques have been described to remove the excess skin that often occurs in isolation (12,17). The midline scars that result from these procedures are well hidden in the thick, hair-bearing submental skin of men.

In patients demonstrating isolated fat accumulation (class III), cervical liposuction is the procedure of choice. In the younger patient with good skin elasticity and no platysmal pathology, liposuction can be performed as an isolated procedure. The mild dermal injury inflicted by the liposuction cannula promotes contraction of the overlying skin, thus obviating the need for skin excision in patients with good skin elasticity. Recent reports have suggested that other liposuction techniques (e.g., tumescent, liposhaving, ultrasound assisted) are superior to traditional liposuction. The tumescent technique, which has been applied with success for body liposuction, is less than ideal for the cervicofacial region because the distortion engendered renders assessment difficult, and the persistent edema that arises is an unwarranted drawback. The risk of third space volume shifts further compounds the problem with the tumescent method. Although safety and efficacy of treatment with the liposhaver has been documented in a multi-institutional review (18), the device's ability to cut through muscle and other soft tissue (including blood vessels and nerves) creates the potential for significant complications. The ultrasound method suffers from the attendant risk of increased thermal injury (if internally applied) and neural and cutaneous flap injury. These adverse outcomes are not definitively established because no controlled studies exist, but they remain of concern nevertheless. In essence, these additional technologies have not proved themselves more useful or beneficial than traditional liposuction, even in experienced hands.

The early fourth decade appears to be a transition time when skin elasticity decreases and liposuction alone can result in less than optimal results. Liposuction performed in isolation in a patient with poor skin elasticity and a large accumulation of fat can lead to poor redraping and contraction of the anterior cervical skin, causing postoperative "rippling" and other deformities (13). These patients are typically better candidates for rhytidectomy in conjunction with submental liposuction and anterior platysmaplasty (see "Surgical Technique: Submentoplasty"). The combination of suction lipectomy and rhytidectomy can also predispose the patient to the development of postoperative platysmal banding, even if anterior platysmal banding is not clinically evident preoperatively (3,13). Anterior platysmaplasty, therefore, is suggested when performing liposuction and rhytidectomy concurrently to avoid the untoward sequela of postoperative platysmal banding.

Class IV patients are those with platysmal abnormalities (e.g., muscle ptosis, atrophy, and midline banding). These patients are best served with a rhytidectomy and anterior platysmaplasty. The combination of SMAS suspension rhytidectomy and anterior platysmaplasty creates a "cervical corset" to support the underlying soft tissues. Additionally, if excess fat is also apparent, liposuction can be performed in conjunction with the above procedures.

Class V patients are those with microgenia or retrognathia. As above, a weak chin may be seen in conjunction with other soft tissue abnormalities and should be treated appropriately after determining the occlusal status. Retrognathia is typically corrected with mandibular osteotomies and bony advancement, whereas microgenia is corrected with alloplastic chin augmentation. It should be noted, however, that it is acceptable in certain patients with *mild* retrognathia to perform chin augmentation instead of pursuing the more aggressive treatment with bony advancement. By evaluating the patient's occlusion and distinguishing between true retrognathia and microgenia, the appropriate treatment can be offered to the patient to optimize the aesthetic outcome.

Class VI patients are those with a low-positioned hyoid bone or other unfavorable anatomy such as anterior digastric muscle hypertrophy and submandibular gland ptosis. Preoperatively, these patients should understand the limitations of their particular anatomy so they have a realistic expectation of the outcome. They should be treated appropriately with standard methods; however, more aggressive techniques may be considered to optimize the aesthetic outcome.

Maneuvers to reposition the hyoid include transecting the suprahyoid musculature from the inferior border of the mandible (19) as well as suturing the anterior bellies of the digastric muscles together to create a new vector of pull (9). To treat digastric muscle hypertrophy, tangential shaving of the anterior bellies of the digastric muscles can also be performed (9).

Ptotic submandibular glands, which are commonly seen in elderly patients, represent a limitation to optimal aesthetic outcome. Surgical removal or reduction is certainly beyond the scope of aesthetic surgery; however, by creating a well-supported "cervical corset" with SMAS suspension and anterior platysmaplasty, the ptotic glands will be elevated to a more favorable position.

Surgical Technique: Submentoplasty (Submental Liposuction and Anterior Platysmaplasty)

In the senior author's hands, the submentoplasty (16) is performed at the outset before a rhytidectomy because the medial borders of the platysma muscle are difficult to unite after the lateral pull of the rhytidectomy has been completed. Similarly, submental liposuction precedes platysmaplasty because the removal of adipose and the concomitant undermining permit visualization of the skeletonized platysma. Chin augmentation follows the submentoplasty and precedes the rhytidectomy because the submentoplasty incision is used as a point of entry for chin implantation. Further, vigorous submentoplasty can disturb the position of the implant if done after chin augmentation.

The submentoplasty begins with a straight incision about 1 to 2 mm posterior to the submental crease that extends typically 2 cm in breadth (Fig. 189.8). The incision should fall slightly posterior to the submental crease because placement of the incision directly in the crease will

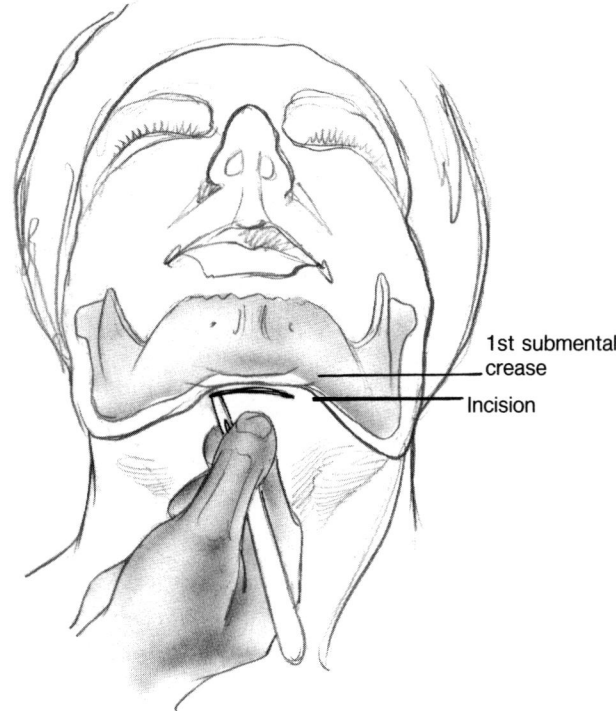

Figure 189.8 The submental incision is placed just behind (1 to 2 mm) the submental crease. If chin augmentation is to be performed, the incision should be placed even further posteriorly (4 to 5 mm behind the crease) to prevent a conspicuous postoperative scar.

deepen over time so that the line may become conspicuous. Additionally, if chin augmentation is to be performed, the incision should be placed even further posteriorly (4 to 5 mm) from the submental crease. This is necessary because following placement of the chin alloplast, the anterior portion of the incision has a tendency to move cephalically, potentially creating a visible incision near the inferior edge of the mandible.

After the initial incision through the skin, wide double-hooked retractors are placed in the superior and inferior aspects of the wound for proper tension and retraction. The assistant retracts the superior flap while the surgeon retracts the inferior flap. The surgeon then performs wide undermining of the flap from just inferior to the jawline (1 to 2 cm below) across the submental region to the contralateral jawline using a pair of Metzenbaum scissors in the subcutaneous plane (Fig. 189.9). Dissection should not pass directly over the jawline to minimize risk of injury to the marginal mandibular nerve. Although the nerve should be protected under the platysma muscle in most cases, an attenuated or dehiscent platysma layer may predispose the nerve to inadvertent harm. The depth of dissection should leave approximately a 3- to 4-mm-thick skin–subcutaneous flap to avoid an uneven contour that may develop after liposuction and to ensure vascularity to the overlying skin flap. The lateral extent of the undermining should be to the anterior borders of the sternocleidomastoid muscle bilaterally.

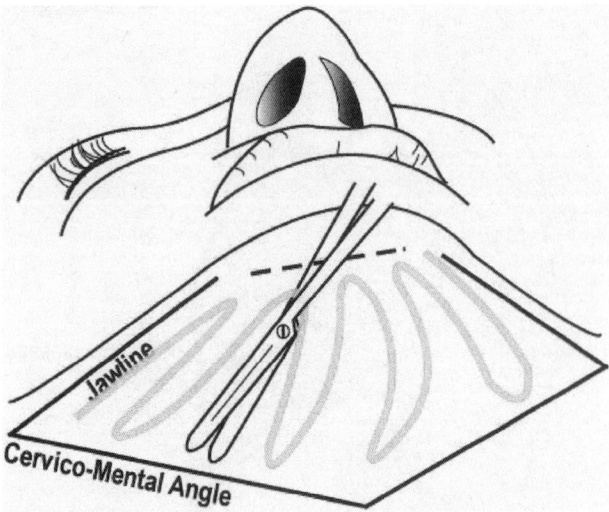

Figure 189.9 Wide undermining of the flap is performed from just inferior to the jaw line (1 to 2 cm below) across the submental region to the contralateral jaw line using a pair of Metzenbaum scissors in the subcutaneous plane.

After the submental region has been widely undermined, a liposuction cannula can be introduced with the aperture *always* facing deep, away from the flap, to avoid the development of an irregular skin contour from suctioning the overlying flap. Furthermore, the vascular supply of the flap emanates from its deep surface, and liposuction under the flap can lead to vascular compromise. The liposuction canister pressure should be set at 29 mm Hg before initiating the procedure. The surgeon should ensure that the instrument is evenly passed over the entire expanse of the undermined submental region, with perhaps additional treatment centrally where a greater adipose deposit may be observed (Fig. 189.10).

Following liposuction, subplatysmal lipectomy and platysmaplasty are performed. With headlight illumination and a Converse retractor, the surgeon should properly visualize the medial terminal fibers of the platysma muscle. If the platysma muscle continues to be obscured by

overlying adipose despite liposuction, a selective lipectomy is performed with scissor dissection. A narrow strip along the medial borders of the platysma is often removed sharply to aid in exposing the subplatysmal fat layer. This step is not performed if the platysma is determined to be minimally redundant and the consequent tension of closure would be too great with additional platysmal resection. If the platysma borders appear widely separated, sufficient undermining is performed to facilitate a relaxed closure. Lipectomy limited to the central subplatysmal compartment is then performed. The anterior digastrics serve as the lateral limit of the dissection. While more aggressive lipectomy may maximize aesthetic outcome, it increases both the likelihood of poorly controlled and visualized hemorrhage and the risk of injury to the marginal mandibular branch of the facial nerve. Additionally, a "cobra deformity" may result from overaggressive fat resection.

Before the platysma muscle can be approximated, the inferior extent of the platysmal closure should be identified (the cervicomental angle, typically located at the thyroid notch). After the platysma borders have been properly exposed and dissected, the anterior free edges are reapproximated with 4-0 polydioxanone, or equivalent, suture in a running, nonlocking fashion (Fig. 189.11). The suture should not be tied very tightly to avoid the complication of a bunched appearance in this area after resolution of edema. To reiterate, the suture should be started at the level of the thyroid notch and proceed in a superior direction. If a chin implant is not planned, then the submental incision is closed with a 6-0 running, locking polypropylene suture (Fig. 189.12).

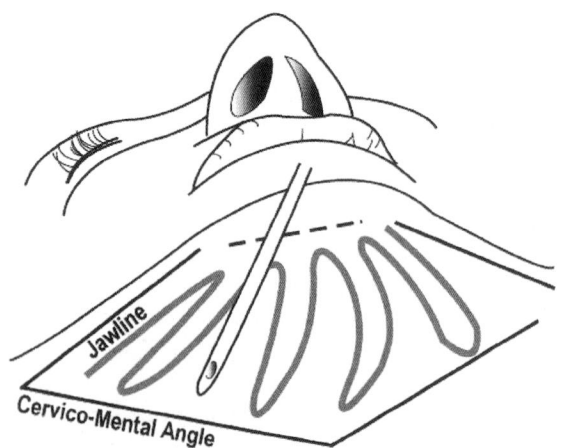

Figure 189.10 The liposuction cannula should be evenly passed over the entire expanse of the undermined submental region.

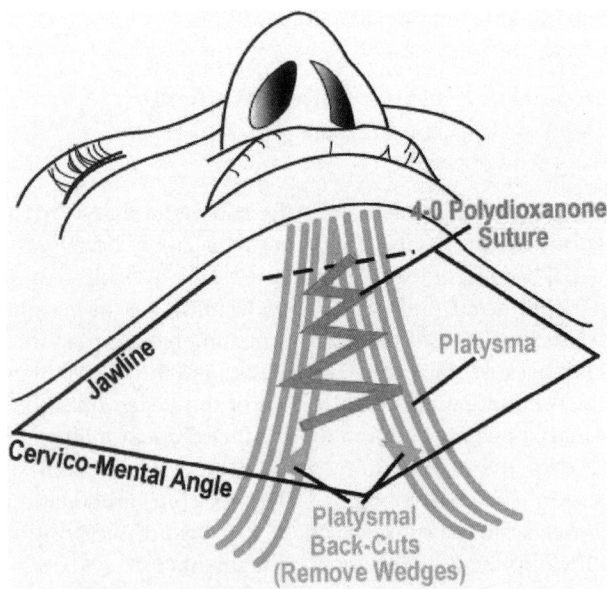

Figure 189.11 After exposure of the anterior platysmal borders, the free edges are approximated with 4-0 polydioxanone suture in a running, nonlocking fashion. The suture should be started approximately at the thyroid notch or cervicomental angle, immediately superior to the platysmal back-cuts.

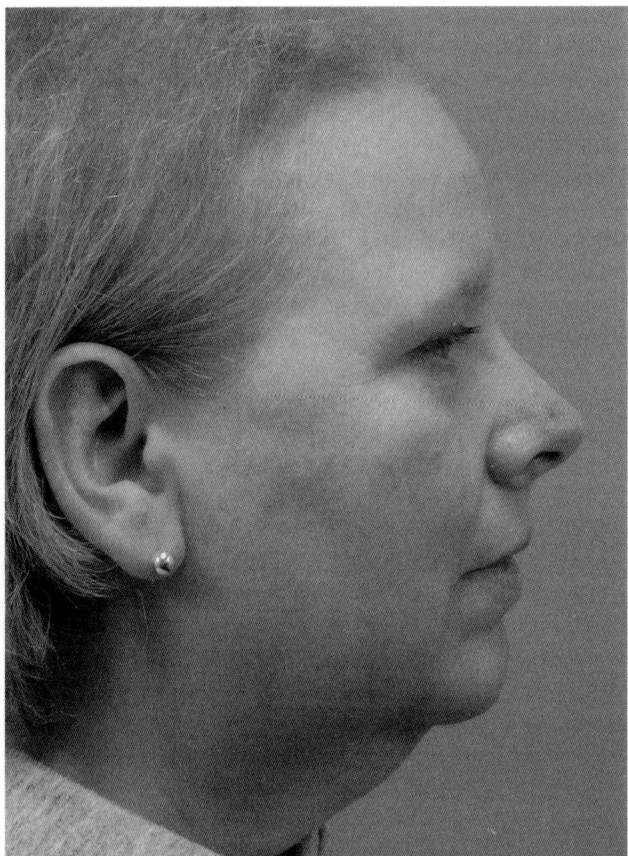
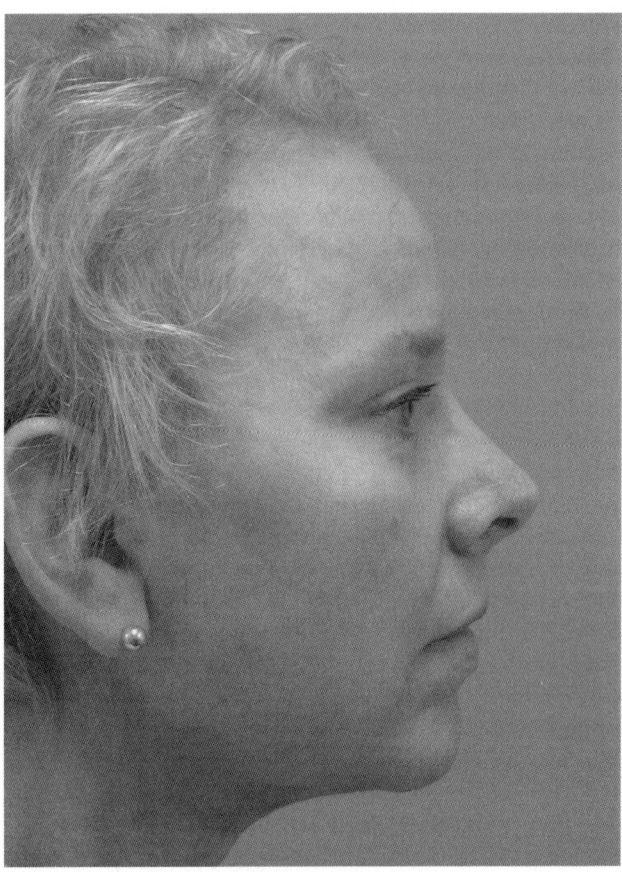

A

B

Figure 189.12 A,B: The pre- and postoperative photographs of a patient who had cervical liposuction–submentoplasty and SMAS imbrication rhytidectomy demonstrate effacement of the jowls and creation of a cervicomental angle of 90 degrees.

COMPLICATIONS AND MANAGEMENT

Early Complications

Early complications following submental liposuction and anterior platysmaplasty include hematoma, seroma, sialocele, infection, contour irregularity, and injury to the marginal mandibular branch of the facial nerve. Hematoma, seroma, or sialocele is seen in less than 1% of patients when liposuction is used as a primary procedure (20). Sialocele is more commonly seen when liposuction is performed over the parotid gland bed in association with a rhytidectomy. Treatment for a sialocele includes pressure dressings, anticholinergics, and repeat aspiration or drainage. A seroma is a collection of serous fluid that occurs in the submental region. They are best treated with needle aspiration and placement of a pressure dressing to prevent reaccumulation.

A large expanding hematoma is an emergency, and the patient should be returned to the operating room for wound exploration, irrigation, and control of all bleeding sites. Smaller hematomas can be managed in the office setting. A limited hematoma discovered on the first postoperative day can be treated by direct aspiration with an 18-gauge needle or by using a gauze sponge to roll out the blood through a small stab incision over the area of concern. A discrete collection discovered somewhat later may require 7 to 10 days to liquefy before it can be aspirated. Persistence of a hematoma predisposes the patient to infection and skin flap necrosis. Because blood is an excellent culture medium, all patients with a hematoma should be placed on prophylactic antibiotics.

Ideally, the best treatment for a hematoma is prevention. In the preoperative phase, the patient's blood pressure should be well controlled. All preoperative medications that could compromise effective coagulation must be ceased for a period of 2 weeks pre- and 2 weeks postoperatively, including prescription medications (e.g., warfarin), over-the-counter medications (e.g., aspirin, ibuprofen), herbal medications (e.g., St. John's wort, ginkgo biloba), supplements (e.g., vitamin E, fish oil, omega-3 fatty acids), and alcohol. In all circumstances, a male patient requires the surgeon to be at an increased level of attention, given the richer vascularity that the hair-bearing skin of the lower face exhibits and the concomitant risk of hematoma formation.

Infections are rare, occurring in less than 1% of patients (20). Most surgeons, however, elect to put their patients on a prophylactic antibiotic regimen despite the lack of scientific evidence to support their use. An alloplastic implant (e.g., chin implant) can be a source for infection. If an abscess develops at the site of implantation, it is almost assured that the implant will require removal. Removal of the implant with reinsertion later when the infection has subsided is the best treatment policy. At the first sign of an infection, a dose of intravenous antibiotics is administered to ensure immediate, proper therapeutic levels, followed by a full regimen of broad-spectrum oral antibiotics until the infection clears.

Early contour irregularities following cervical liposuction are the rule rather than the exception. Most resolve as healing progresses and edema lessens. Patients should be reassured during the first several weeks postoperatively that irregularities generally smooth out over time.

Permanent injury to the marginal mandibular branch of the facial nerve is rare, as long as the surgeon remains superficial to the platysma muscle. Temporary paresis can occur with aggressive liposuction in a patient with an attenuated, thin platysma muscle, which typically resolves within 6 months.

Late Complications

Late complications include scarring, platysmal banding, and irregular neck contour. Hypertrophic or wide scars are rarely seen in the submental incision, but are more commonly seen with rhytidectomy incisions secondary to excessive tension on the skin closure. Additionally, patients with Fitzpatrick V or VI skin types are more susceptible to the development of hypertrophic scars and keloids. Management should include injection of the scars with triamcinolone (10 mg/mL) at 3- to 4-week intervals until improvement is noted. More frequent injections carry the risk of dermal atrophy and hypopigmentation. Additionally, the pulsed dye laser has been shown to be a useful adjunct (16). If the scar persists despite these measures, scar revision may be considered after a 12-month interval.

Platysmal banding, which can occur postoperatively, is most commonly due to unrecognized, and therefore untreated, preoperative platysmal banding. This is most commonly seen in patients with submental obesity and redundant skin (21). To avoid the complication, preoperative recognition is essential. Platysmal banding can be treated primarily, or secondarily, with anterior platysmaplasty.

An irregular neck contour can result from direct, sharp lipectomy, or from an uneven liposuction technique. Especially in the immediate submental region, overzealous excision of fat can produce a central concavity. A "cobra deformity" describes the situation in which a patient has a central submental concavity from overzealous fat removal in combination with prominent platysmal bands, resembling a cobra about to strike. This deformity is even more pronounced when the anterior borders of the platysma muscle are not united following central lipectomy. Irregularities can be prevented by widely undermining the cervical skin with a 3- to 4-mm layer of fat remaining attached to the overlying dermis and by gauging the thickness of this layer with bimanual palpation during liposuction. Additionally, to avoid further irregularities, the surgeon must make sure the aperture of the liposuction cannula is always facing *away* from the dermis.

Even in the best of hands, neck irregularities still occur. If necessary, small localized depressions can be treated with a soft tissue filler (e.g., autologous fat); however, large depressions may require placement of dermal graft materials (e.g., cadaveric acellular dermis) for correction (20). Again, prevention is the best treatment.

HIGHLIGHTS

- The anatomic factors that contribute to an ideal cervical contour include a strong chin, a distinct mandibular border, a cervicomental angle of 105 to 120 degrees, a visible subhyoid bone depression, a gentle indentation at the thyroid notch, and visible anterior borders of the sternocleidomastoid muscles.
- Several anatomic elements contribute to the appearance of an aging neck, including skin, fat, platysma muscle, chin projection, and hyoid bone position.
- Each anatomic element contributing to the deformity should be delineated preoperatively and sequentially addressed to provide an optimal aesthetic outcome.
- A classification system can be used to categorize patients and to target treatment to their specific needs (Table 189.1).
- The rhytidectomy and submentoplasty procedures are the cornerstones of treating the aging neck.
- Early complications of surgery on the aging neck include hematoma, seroma, sialocele, infection, contour irregularity, and injury to the marginal mandibular branch of the facial nerve.
- Late complications include scarring, platysmal banding, and irregular neck contour.

REFERENCES

1. Ellenbogen R, Karlin JV. Visual criteria for success in restoring the youthful neck. *Plast Reconstr Surg* 1980;66:826–837.
2. Dayan SH, Bagal A, Tardy ME Jr. Targeted solutions in submentoplasty. *Facial Plast Surg* 2001;17:141–149.
3. Rohrich RJ, Pessa JE. The subplatysmal supramylohyoid fat. *Plast Reconstr Surg* 2010;126:589–595.
4. Hatef DA, Koshy JC, Sandoval SE, et al. The submental fat compartment of the neck. *Semin Plast Surg* 2009;23:288–291.
5. Mashkevich G, Wang J, Rawnsley J, et al. The utility of ultrasound in the evaluation of submental fullness in aging necks. *Arch Facial Plast Surg* 2009;11:240–245.

6. Cardoso de Castro C. The changing role of platysma in face lifting. *Plast Reconstr Surg* 2000;105:764–775.

7. Kim HJ, Hu KS, Kang MK, et al. Decussation patterns of the platysma in Koreans. *Br J Plast Surg* 2001;54:400–402.

8. Wall SJ, Adamson PA. Surgical options for aesthetic enhancement of the neck. *Facial Plast Surg* 2001;17:109–115.

9. Ramirez OM, Robertson KM. Comprehensive approach to rejuvenation of the neck. *Facial Plast Surg* 2001;17:129–140.

10. Sykes JM. Rejuvenation of the aging neck. *Facial Plast Surg* 2001; 17:99–107.

11. Koch RJ, Hanasono MM. Aesthetic facial analysis. In: Papel ID, ed. *Facial plastic and reconstructive surgery*, 3rd ed. New York: Thieme Medical Publishers, 2009:177–197.

12. Adamson PA, Litner JA. Surgical management of the aging neck. *Facial Plast Surg* 2005;21:11–20.

13. Kamer FM, Pieper PG. Surgical treatment of the aging neck. *Facial Plast Surg* 2001;17:123–128.

14. Dedo DD. "How I do it"—plastic surgery. Practical suggestions on facial plastic surgery. A preoperative classification of the neck for cervicofacial rhytidectomy. *Laryngoscope* 1980;90:1894–1896.

15. Rohrich RJ, Rios JL, Smith PD, et al. Neck rejuvenation revisited. *Plast Reconstr Surg* 2006;118:1251–1263.

16. Lam SM, Williams EF III. Lower facial rejuvenation. In: Williams EF III, Lam SM, eds. *Comprehensive facial rejuvenation: a practical and systematic guide to surgical management of the aging face*. Philadelphia, PA: Lippincott Williams & Wilkins, 2004: 105–151.

17. Bitner JB, Friedman O, Farrior RT, et al. Direct submentoplasty for neck rejuvenation. *Arch Facial Plast Surg* 2007;9:194–200.

18. Becker DG, Cook TA, Wang TD, et al. A 3-year multi-institutional experience with the liposhaver. *Arch Facial Plast Surg* 1999;1: 171–176.

19. Guyuron B. Problem neck, hyoid bone, and submental myotomy. *Plast Reconstr Surg* 1992;90:830–837.

20. Kridel RWH, Kelly PE, Castellano RD. Liposuction of the face and neck: the art of facial sculpture. In: Papel ID, ed. *Facial plastic and reconstructive surgery*, 3rd ed. New York: Thieme Medical Publishers, 2009:286–300.

21. Ahn MS, Kabaker SS. Complications of face lifting. *Facial Plast Surg Clin North Am* 2000;8:211–221.

190

Otoplasty: Anatomy, Embryology, and Technique

Steven Ross Mobley   *Nathan Todd Nelson Schreiber*

In addition to its function in directing sound to the tympanic membrane, the ear plays a complementary role in one's appearance. If abnormal in appearance, however, the ear can command unwanted attention, drawing an observer's eyes away from the rest of the face. Classically, auricular anomalies have resulted in significant social stigma. In a criminology text from 1876, author Cesare Lombroso wrote, "nearly all criminals have jug ears" (1); a number of overtly discriminatory texts from this period contain overtly belittling references to prominent ears as well (2). Although such beliefs are, for the most part, not consciously encouraged today, they persist in more subtle forms. In popular culture, large ears are often exaggerated in jest for cartoons and caricatures. For children especially, prominent or malformed ears may be the subject of ridicule, possibly affecting self-esteem and psychosocial development. It is for this reason that surgical correction of the anomalous ear is often sought.

The goal of otoplasty is to create a more natural appearance and position of the ear. Its origins can be traced back to India in 800 BC, when reconstruction of the lobule using a local cheek flap was first described by Indian surgeon Sushruta (3). Reconstruction of larger ear defects using postauricular scalp flaps was not described until centuries later in textbooks, by Italian surgeon Gaspare Tagliacozzi in 1597, and again by Prussian surgeon Johann Friedrich Dieffenbach in 1845 (4–6). The first truly cosmetic otoplasty, however, was performed in 1881, by American surgeon Edward Ely, on a 12-year-old boy who was ridiculed for having a prominent ear (7,8). In the ensuing years, multiple variations of this operation have been described and provide a number of techniques that may be used to create a more anatomically natural-appearing ear. Given the multitude of techniques, one must understand normal auricular anatomy as well as the goals of surgery in order to successfully perform otoplasty.

ANATOMY AND EMBRYOLOGY

The auricle is essentially an extension of fibroelastic cartilage from the external auditory canal that is covered by perichondrium and a thin layer of skin. The skin is directly adherent to perichondrium anteriorly but is separated from perichondrium by loose areolar tissue posteriorly. Cartilage is deficient at the lobule as well as between the tragus and the beginning of the helix anteriorly. Projections of cartilage from the anterior and inferior ends of the helix are called the spina helicis and the cauda helicis, respectively. Attached to portions of the cartilage itself are six internal auricular muscles: the helicis major, helicis minor, tragicus, and antitragicus along the lateral side of the cartilage and the transversus auriculae and obliquus auriculae along the medial side of the cartilage. Three external auricular muscles, anterior, superior, and posterior, provide additional fixation to the temporal bone and, through the facial nerve, the ability to move one's ear. Auricular sensation is provided by multiple nerves. C2 and C3 through the greater auricular nerve provide sensation posteriorly at the helix, antihelix, and lobule. Cranial nerves IX and X provide sensation to the conchal bowl and posterior external auditory canal. The auriculotemporal branch of the mandibular division of the fifth cranial nerve provides sensation to the tragus, superior helix, and superior and anterior external auditory canal. The superficial temporal, posterior auricular, and occipital branches of the external carotid artery provide the auricle's arterial supply, while the superficial temporal vein, retromandibular vein, external jugular vein, and, in some cases, the mastoid emissary vein provide venous drainage. Lymphatic drainage occurs through the parotid, posterior auricular, and cervical levels 2 and 5 lymph nodes (9). The normal anatomy of the auricle is shown in Figure 190.1.

The external ear develops from six swellings called hillocks of His, which are present at 6 weeks' gestation. The first

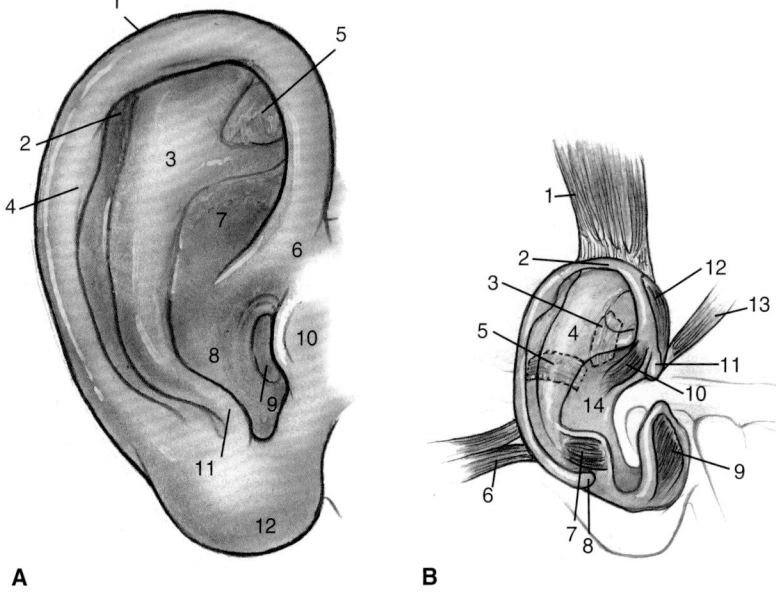

Figure 190.1 A: Normal external auricular anatomy. *1*, Helix; *2*, scaphoid fossa; *3*, antihelix; *4*, auricular (Darwin) tubercle; *5*, triangular fossa; *6*, crus helicis; *7*, cymba concha; *8*, cavum concha; *9*, external auditory meatus; *10*, tragus; *11*, antitragus; *12*, lobule. **B:** Normal external and internal auricular musculature. *1*, Auricularis superior; *2*, helix; *3*, obliquus auriculae; *4*, antihelix; *5*, transversus auriculae; *6*, auricularis posterior; *7*, antitragicus; *8*, cauda helicis; *9*, tragicus; *10*, helicis minor; *11*, spina helicis; *12*, helicis major; *13*, auricularis anterior; *14*, concha.

three hillocks of His develop from the first branchial arch into the tragus, helical crus, and helix, while the second three hillocks of His develop from the second branchial arch into the antihelix, antitragus, and lobule (Fig. 190.2). The hillocks of His are fused by 12 weeks' gestation and reach a final shape around 20 weeks' gestation (9,10).

The ear generally reaches 85% of its ultimate vertical height, 5 cm, by 3 years of age and is nearly full size, 6 cm, by 5 years of age. From this point on, the helix will grow relatively little, while the lobule will grow to a much greater degree, disproportionately lengthening with advancing age (9,11). In general, men have a slightly larger pinna and greater distance from the lateral orbital rim to helical root than do women; these distances are usually equal for each individual and on average measure 6 cm. Ear width, on the other hand, is usually just over half its height. Ear protrusion can be measured by either its distance from or angle to the scalp. The average distance from the helical rim to the scalp is 1.5 to 2 cm while the average auriculocephalic angle is 20 to 35 degrees (Fig. 190.3) (12,13).

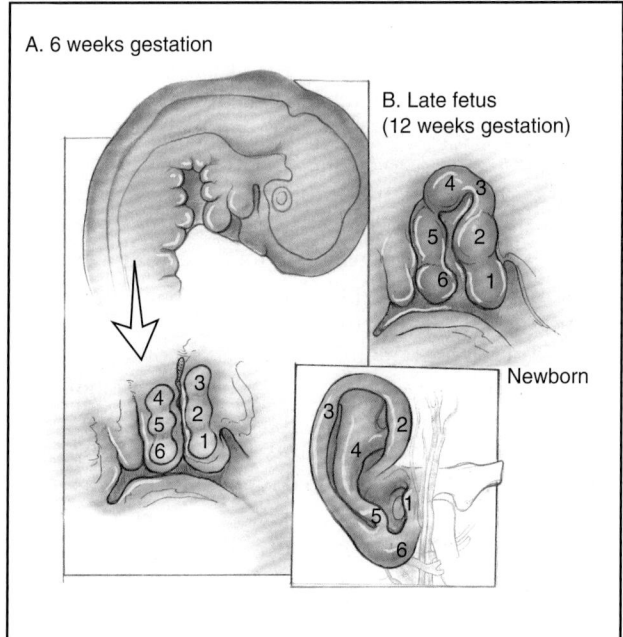

Figure 190.2 Normal ear development from the hillocks of His.

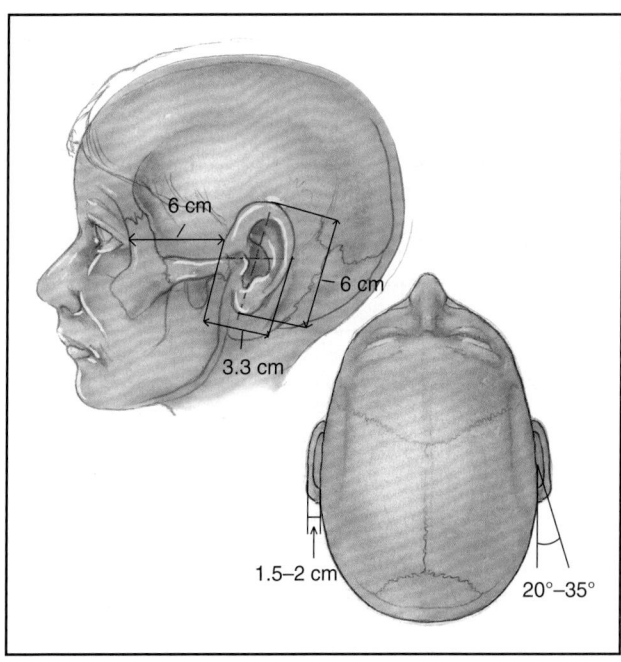

Figure 190.3 Normal ear dimensions.

AURICULAR ANOMALIES

Etiology and Classification

Auricular anomalies occur in approximately 5% of the population, either in isolation or as part of a syndrome (14). Most auricular anomalies are sporadic, but some are hereditary. Their etiologies include genetic mutations, *in utero* insults from exogenous factors, compression from external forces, and abnormal intrinsic ear musculature. There is a wide range of degree to which these anomalies can occur, and there are a number of classification systems, based on extent of anomaly and extent of surgical intervention, that have been devised to group them. Many of the early classification systems were combined by Weerda in 1988, dividing anomalies into first-, second-, and third-degree dysplasia (Table 190.1) (15). In 1997, Tan et al. proposed an even more simplified system that takes ear molding techniques into account and divides anomalies into two groups: deformational auricular anomalies and malformational auricular anomalies. Deformations result from external forces that cause abnormal architecture of tissue that is otherwise normal, while malformations result from abnormal tissue development that leads to abnormal architecture. Deformational auricular anomalies can be manually reduced to create a nearly normal appearance and can be treated early on with ear molding techniques or later with surgery. Malformational auricular anomalies, on the other hand, cannot be manually reduced to a normal appearance. These anomalies require surgery but can, in some cases, be partially treated with ear molding techniques if they also contain deformational components (16,17). In general, these classification systems are useful in clinical evaluation and determining the types of intervention that will be most helpful. However, it is important to keep in mind that auricular anomalies do not always fit cleanly within a single category and a number of treatment options should be considered in every case.

Deformations

Stahl Ear

Stahl ear, alternatively known as Satyr ear, Spock ear, and Vulcan ear, is a first-degree or deformational auricular anomaly characterized by an abnormal transverse crus from the antihelix to the posterior superior helical rim and, often times, an absent superior crus (Fig. 190.4). It may be caused by external forces *in utero* or perhaps an abnormal course of the transversus auriculae, one of the intrinsic muscles of the ear (18). Stahl ear can be treated with molding techniques, suturing techniques, or excision of abnormal cartilage (19,20).

Cryptotia

Cryptotia, a term that means hidden or pocket ear, is a condition in which the superior helical cartilage is buried under the skin (Fig. 190.4). This deformity is thought to be caused by an abnormal attachment of the superior auricular muscle to the scapha rather than to the triangular fossa as well as a shortened transversus auriculae, effectively pulling the superior helix under the skin during development. This condition can be treated with molding or by releasing the superior helix from the scalp with skin grafting, advancing the resulting postauricular defect, performing a Z-plasty, or performing a trefoil flap, a flap consisting of three symmetric triangles based at the superior auricle that is used to cover the posterior cartilage upon release (21,22).

Prominent Ear

The prominent ear is a type of deformational auricular anomaly characterized by an absent antihelical fold and deep conchal bowl (Fig. 190.4). These deformities increase the auriculocephalic angle and the distance from the scalp to the helix. In addition, the prominent ear will often demonstrate a number of secondary findings, including a large helical root, excessive lobule projection, and inadequate helical curl. This condition has been associated with an abnormally distal insertion of the antitragicus muscle that extends along the anterior surface of the ear from the antitragus to the antihelix, pulling the helix laterally during development (23). Ear molding techniques may be successful early in life but, unlike with certain other ear deformities, often fail to adequately treat this condition if older than 3 months (16,24). This failure may be related to resistance created by the antitragicus muscle. In many cases, surgical intervention is required for definitive treatment.

Malformations

Constricted Ear

Constricted ears are characterized by partial absence of cartilage at the upper third of the helical rim and sometimes

TABLE 190.1	AURICULAR DYSPLASIA CLASSIFICATION SYSTEM BY WEERDA	
	Anatomic Definition	Surgical Definition
First-degree dysplasia	Most structures of the normal auricle are recognizable Minor deformities	Reconstruction does not require the use of additional skin or cartilage
Second-degree dysplasia	Some structures of the normal auricle are recognizable Moderate deformities	Partial reconstruction requires the use of additional skin and cartilage
Third-degree dysplasia	None of the structures of the normal ear are recognizable Severe deformities	Total reconstruction requires the use of additional skin and large amounts of cartilage

the concha, resulting in a purse-string effect at the helix (Fig. 190.4). This type of malformation can be classified as either first- or second-degree dysplasia depending on its severity. Constricted ears will demonstrate a combination of helical lidding, protrusion, low position, and decreased size. This category is variably labeled as cup, lop, and cockleshell ear, among other names, in various sources. This malformation can be found in a number of inherited syndromes but is usually sporadic when isolated.

The findings in constricted ears can be divided into three groups based on severity and the treatment that is needed for correction. Mild constriction involves the helix only and can often be corrected with molding techniques as a neonate or later with an otoplasty technique similar to that used for prominent ears. Moderate constriction and severe constriction, however, are defined by hypoplasia of both the helix and scapha and require surgical intervention. Moderate constriction often requires a V-Y helical

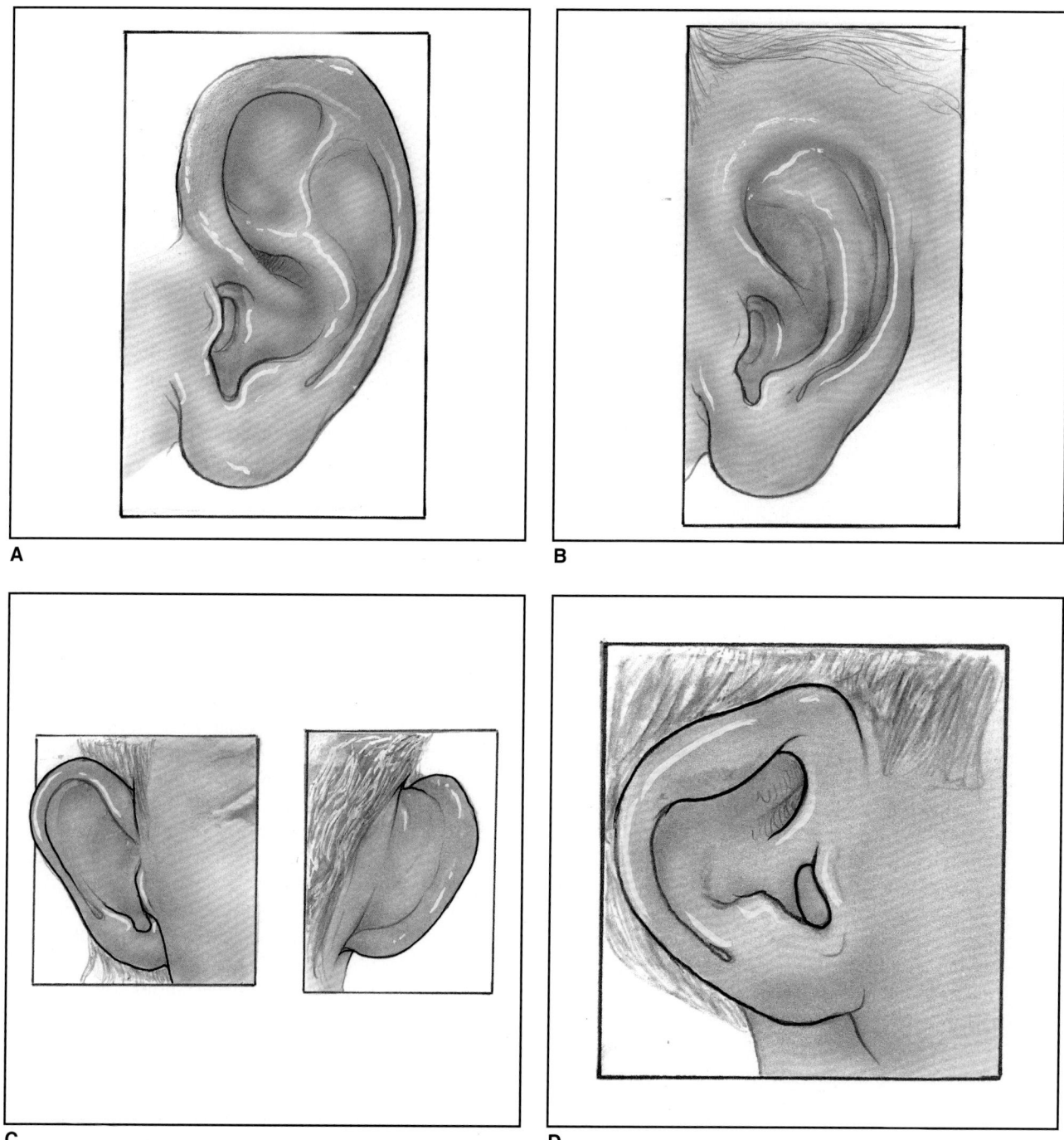

A
B
C
D

Figure 190.4 A: Stahl ear. **B:** Cryptotia. **C:** Prominent ear. **D:** Constricted ear.

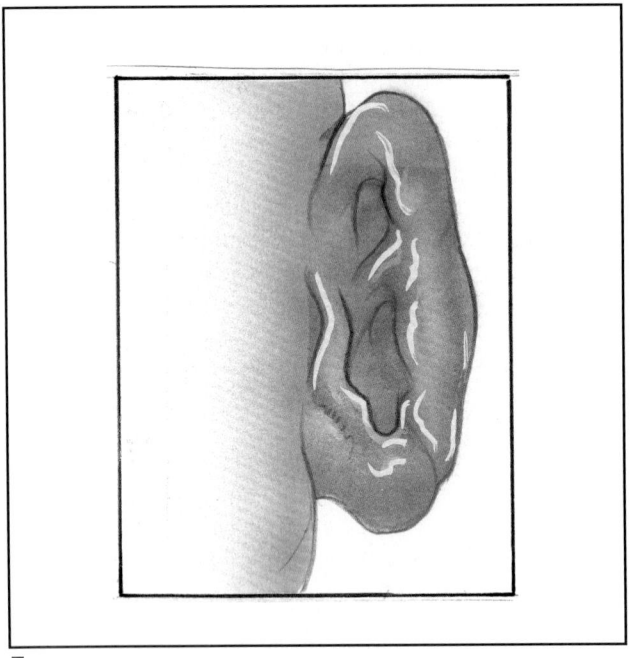

E

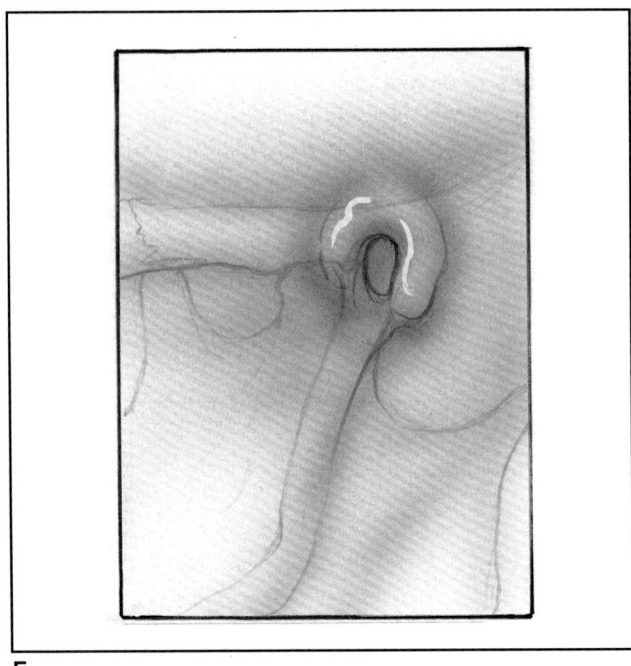

F

Figure 190.4 (*Continued*) **E:** Microtia. **F:** Anotia.

root advancement as well as conchal or sometimes rib cartilage grafting (25). Severe constriction requires subtotal auricular reconstruction with rib cartilage grafting and postauricular skin recruitment (26,27).

Microtia

Microtia is hypoplasia of a majority of the pinna, while anotia is the complete absence of the pinna (Fig. 190.4). These malformations may or may not spare the external auditory canal and are types of third-degree dysplasia. Total auricular reconstruction for microtia and anotia is not addressed in this chapter.

Psychosocial Issues

There have been a handful of studies and anecdotal observations regarding the psychosocial impact of various facial anomalies. The majority of these studies, however, concern children with significant craniofacial malformations. One study that did examine children with isolated ear anomalies noted a 40% incidence of ear anomaly in children who were residents of the Mental Health Center of Norfolk, the majority of which were noted to have had adjustment reactions in childhood or adolescence (12). It is important to note, however, that no evidence of causation could be determined. A more recent study by Sheerin et al. compares children with prominent ears to children with facial port-wine stains and suggests that self-esteem, social, and attention problems may be even more severe in the group with prominent ears. Although the groups were small, the study's authors believe this difference could in part be due to decreased familial support and recognition

of deformity in those with prominent ears, who may be thought of as having an exaggeration of the normal rather than a true deformity. Regardless of the reason for this difference, this study suggests that children who are bothered by their ears are much more likely to have psychosocial problems (28). Further studies may help to determine if otoplasty can help to improve psychosocial adjustment in this population.

PATIENT SELECTION

Initial Evaluation

There are several steps that should be performed when evaluating a patient with auricular dysplasia. The patient's unique ear anatomy should be analyzed, goals and expectations should be addressed, and treatment options should be considered that best meet the agreed-upon goals.

First, the ears should be photographed with full-face and close-up frontal, oblique, lateral, and posterior views. After physical exam, these images are an important adjunct for evaluating the anatomic causes of deformity as well as any differences on one side compared to the other. These images can be viewed with the patient to facilitate a discussion about goals and expectations for treatment, realistic outcomes, and the appropriate techniques that could be employed to achieve this result. In addition, measurements of ear height, width, and distance from the scalp as well as the auriculocephalic angle are useful. Together, these images and measurements can be used to objectively document postoperative and long-term follow-up changes (29).

Nonsurgical Treatment

If a deformational auricular anomaly is identified in a neonate or, according to some, select older individuals, molding techniques should be considered. These techniques usually involve placing a bendable splint along the helical rim, antihelix, and conchal bowl and taping it in place to hold the ear in an appropriate position for 2 to 12 weeks. Molding is able to correct up to 90% of deformational auricular anomalies if started within the first week of life (30,31). Most authors only advocate molding for neonates, but there have been some reports of successful treatment of older children (32). In general, after 3 weeks of age, molding is less successful. Yotsuyanagi noted that improvement declines from 80% if molding is started at 1 to 3 months of age, to 33% if molding is started after 9 years of age. In general, molding failures in this study were most common with moderately and severely constricted ears as well as prominent ears (24,33).

In 2011, Leclere et al. reported a series of 17 patients with prominent ears and an average age of 34.5 years who underwent laser-assisted cartilage reshaping, a new technique in which the ear is treated with an erbium/glass laser to reshape the cartilage without any anesthesia and molded into the desired shape with a silicone splint. The splint is then worn at all times for 2 weeks and then at night only for 4 weeks. At a 30-month follow-up appointment, two patients had incomplete shape correction, which was thought to be related to incorrect splint design and contact dermatitis, and five patients had slight ear asymmetry. Overall, 10 of 17 patients obtained the desired result (34). Although only small series have been published about this technique, it may become a preferred method of treatment in the future.

Ear molding is certainly an attractive option for neonates and perhaps select older children or adults who do not wish to undergo surgery. Importantly, one must gauge a patient's ability to tolerate the discomfort, time, and effort required to wear an ear splint consistently for a period of time. In the future, laser-assisted cartilage reshaping may significantly increase the success rate of molding, although more studies are needed. Surgery can always be performed at a later date for those who do not achieve the desired correction with molding alone.

Surgical Candidates

Prominent ears generally result from a combination of insufficient antihelical fold and excessively large conchal bowl and have been defined in a number of ways. Some define ear prominence as an auriculocephalic angle greater than 40 degrees or a helix to scalp distance greater than 2.5 cm (35). Of the two major components of prominent-ear deformity, unfolding of the antihelical fold has been found to contribute to 73% of ear prominence.

Regardless of published standards, prominent ears, for many people, are primarily a psychological concern, and most will present with their own ideas of how their ears should be. For example, men may present wanting ears very close to the scalp because of balding or a desire to wear their hair short. Women, on the other hand, may tolerate less correction because of longer hair and a greater ability to cover their ears. Alexander et al. (36) found discordance between researcher- and subject-defined ear prominence, with the principal investigator reporting ear prominence in 10% of subjects, but self-reported ear prominence in only 2%, leading the authors to conclude that an ear is prominent when the patient says it is. In a minority of patients, however, prominent ears may interfere with the ability to perform a job or wear safety equipment. Salgado reported a case series of U.S. Army soldiers who underwent otoplasty because of the inability to wear Kevlar helmets without developing skin breakdown along the lateral surfaces of their ears (37). When prominent ears interfere with safety in such a manner, otoplasty is certainly indicated. Constricted ears, however, will often demonstrate more noticeable deformity and are not as subjective of a finding as are prominent ears. Nevertheless, they are apt to produce the same psychological concerns.

Otoplasty has traditionally been delayed until 5 years of age, at which point the ear has nearly reached its adult size, reducing concern for postoperative growth disturbance, and the child has not yet entered grade school, a time before peer ridicule becomes a significant concern. This convention has been challenged, however, and much younger patients, as young as 9 months, have undergone otoplasty without any evidence of altered cartilage growth over a course of several years. The rationale for otoplasty at an earlier age is the observation of excessive caregiver and family focus upon the ears as well as the development of self-image prior to 5 years of age (38,39). Performing otoplasty at an earlier age, however, remains controversial. In a survey of surgeons, psychologists, and parents with children who had undergone otoplasty in the United Kingdom, a majority recommended otoplasty after 6 years of age (40). Regardless, when considering otoplasty in a child, it is imperative to stress to the parents the importance of postoperative care and protective dressings. If it is unlikely that the postoperative care will be tolerated, otoplasty might be best deferred to a later time.

SURGICAL TECHNIQUES

Otoplasty for the Prominent Ear

The main goals of otoplasty for the prominent ear are to create an antihelical fold and reduce the auriculocephalic angle to about 15 to 25 degrees. In addition, a prominent, lateralized helical root and lobule can worsen with otoplasty and often require reduction as well. A wide variety of techniques have been described to achieve these goals and a selection of landmark and novel modifications is presented below, followed by our preferred technique.

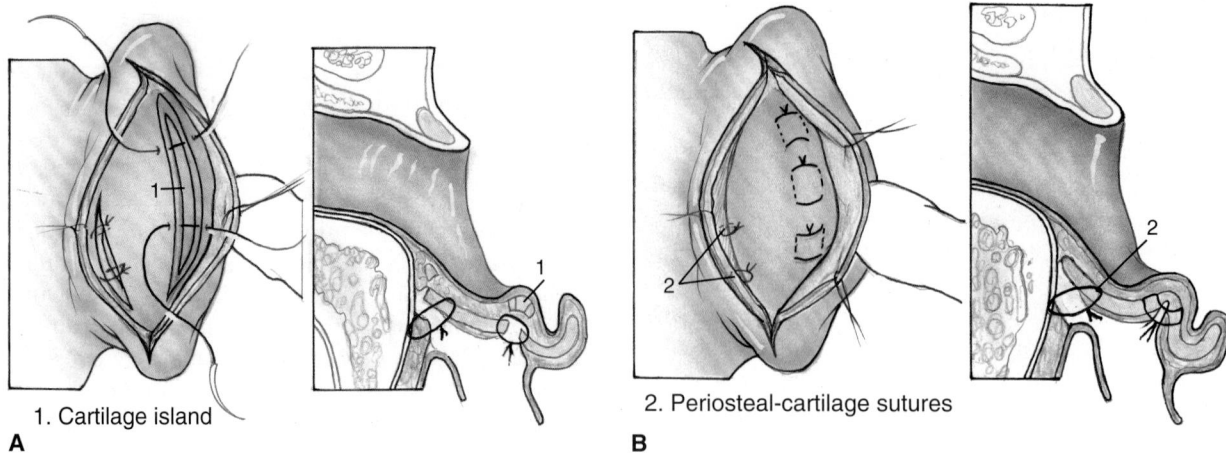

1. Cartilage island

A

2. Periosteal-cartilage sutures

B

Figure 190.5 Comparison of cartilage-cutting (**A**) and cartilage-shaping (**B**) otoplasty techniques.

In 1955, Converse et al. (41) recreated the antihelical fold by making two parallel incisions on either side of the planned antihelix and suturing the edges from either side of the cartilage island together (Fig. 190.5A). In 1959, Farrior (42) described a modification of this technique, excising thin, longitudinal wedges of cartilage posteriorly at the superior crus and antihelical fold; creating a cartilage island at the planned antihelix; and stabilizing the new folds with suture. Hatch (43) noted that the helical root was often displaced laterally in otoplasty and, in 1958, reported securing the helical root to the temporalis fascia to alleviate this problem.

In 1963, Mustarde (44) described a less invasive technique of recreating the antihelical fold, using three permanent horizontal mattress sutures to secure the auricular cartilage to itself without making any cartilage incisions (Fig. 190.5B). In 1967, Kaye (45) described anterior cartilage scoring at the planned antihelical fold with toothed forceps, followed by suture fixation as well as removal of an ellipse of conchal cartilage if needed. In 1968, however, Furnas described a less invasive technique of conchal bowl reduction, simply securing the conchal cartilage to the mastoid periosteum posteriorly. The lobule was reduced by excising a posterior ellipse of skin (46). In 2001, Erol (47) described an anterior approach to otoplasty, placing their incision along the conchal bowl rim, excising a portion of conchal cartilage, scoring the anterior surface of the cartilage to create an antihelical fold, and securing these changes with horizontal mattress sutures.

Incisionless otoplasty was first described by Fritsch in 1994 and involves percutaneously scoring the anterior surface of the cartilage at the planned antihelical fold, creating a small opening at the postauricular sulcus and removing soft tissue for a conchal setback if needed, percutaneously placing horizontal mattress retention sutures from the posterior side of the pinna to create the antihelical fold and pull the concha posteriorly and burying the knots by

pulling skin over them with a single-prong skin hook. The lobule is brought posteriorly by percutaneously dissecting the cauda helicis from the pinna and using the same percutaneous suture technique to secure it to the posterior conchal bowl (48).

In 1999, Epstein et al. (49) described the use of electrocautery to perform partial-thickness ablation of a thin, longitudinal strip of cartilage along its posterior surface at the planned antihelix. The new antihelix was then stabilized with horizontal mattress sutures. Ragab (50) described a modification to this technique in 2010, using the carbon dioxide laser instead of electrocautery in an attempt to curl the cartilage in a controlled fashion.

In general, these techniques fall into one of two categories: cartilage-cutting or cartilage-shaping. Cartilage-cutting techniques involve the incision or scoring of cartilage to create a permanent change to the cartilage shape. These techniques may be best suited for thick, stiff cartilage and often allow greater control over the end result. However, there is greater risk of creating sharp edges and irregularities that are extremely resistant to revision. Cartilage-shaping techniques, on the other hand, involve repositioning the cartilage with sutures to create a more natural shape without the risk of sharp, unnatural-appearing cartilage edges. The end result can easily be adjusted but carries with it the risk of a suture breaking and the ear springing back to its original position.

The surgeon must understand the risks and benefits involved with these techniques. Whenever possible, the senior author (SRM) prefers to use the cartilage-shaping techniques originally described by Mustarde, Furnas, and Hatch. The following is a detailed description of this procedure.

DESIGNING THE INCISION

Prior to injection of local anesthesia, three key landmarks must be identified.

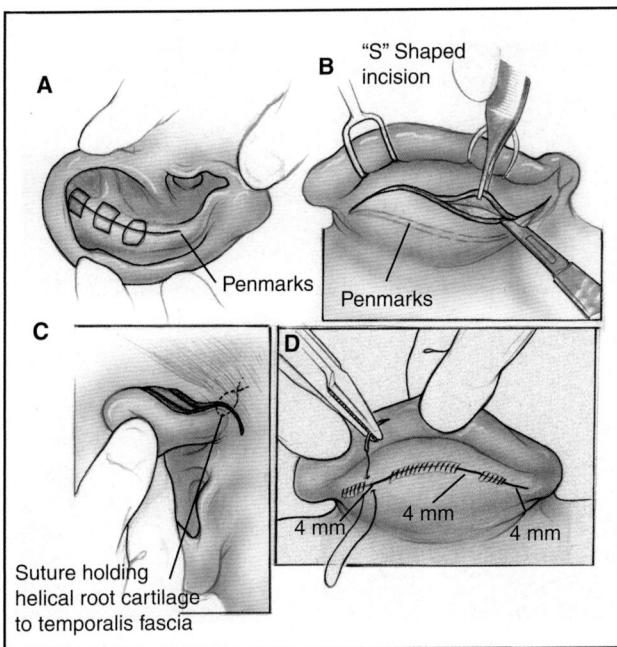

Figure 190.6 Otoplasty incision planning using Mustarde, Furnas, and Hatch techniques. First, the ear is manipulated to create an antihelical fold and Mustarde-type horizontal mattress sutures are planned **(A)**. The ear is then pushed against the scalp and an ellipse of skin that can be excised is marked **(B)**. The planned postauricular incision is extended to the helical root for repositioning to prevent persistent superior ear prominence **(C)**. When closing the postauricular incision, three 4-mm gaps are left (marked by *arrows*) as a controlled drainage pathway to prevent hematoma **(D)**. It is important that these gaps not overlie any stitches.

1. Antihelical fold: The ear should be gently squeezed to identify a naturally appearing antihelical fold (Fig. 190.6A). It is important to mark the central portion of the antihelical fold. This line should not be straight but a gentle anteriorly sloping curve that will create a more natural antihelical fold. We prefer to mark out the future placement of our Mustarde-type horizontal mattress sutures at this time.
2. Conchal setback: A cotton-tipped applicator can be used to press the conchal cartilage against the mastoid to determine where the conchal setback sutures will be placed (Fig. 190.7A and B).
3. Helical root: The placement of the helical root suture should be determined by gently pushing the helical root anteriorly and superiorly against the soft tissue of the scalp in order to determine the location of the relaxed skin tension line in this location (Fig. 190.6C).

With these three landmarks identified, one should design the postauricular incision. With a finger on the area of the future Mustarde-type horizontal mattress sutures, a small dot can be made on the back side of the ear corresponding to the location of each suture. This same technique can be used to identify where the Furnas-type conchal setback sutures will be placed. This will create two lines, which form the basis of the incision (Fig. 190.6B). These

two markings can then be connected with an "S"-shaped line. Now the ear can be pressed back against the scalp and an estimation of how much excess of skin should be removed can be made and the above drawn line can then be converted to a simple ellipse. A dumbbell shape is often advocated for this incision in order to decrease the chances of developing telephone ear deformity, which is discussed later in this chapter. A simple elliptical skin excision, however, can also allow one to address the helical root and lobule and perform a straightforward closure at the end of the procedure.

Injection

Despite the common medical teaching to the contrary, there is no proven contraindication specific to the ear for injecting a local anesthetic containing epinephrine. It is important to keep in mind, however, that epinephrine injection can result in a hypertensive crisis in patients who are taking certain vasoactive medications or have underlying cardiovascular disease, uncontrolled hypertension, hyperthyroidism, or pheochromocytoma (51,52). Patients with cardiovascular disease should be injected with no more than 0.2 mg of epinephrine (20 mL of 1:100,000 epinephrine); some advocate even lower maximum doses of 0.04 mg of epinephrine (4 mL of 1:100,000 epinephrine) up to every 30 minutes in patients with severe cardiovascular disease (53,54). In comparison, doses of 0.3 to 0.5 mg of epinephrine are used for treatment of anaphylaxis.

In the senior author's experience, 1:50,000 concentrations of epinephrine can be used in otoplasty without causing damage to the skin and cartilage. With this technique, the anterior and posterior sides of the ear are each injected with 2 to 3 mL of a custom mixture of 0.25% bupivacaine with 1:50,000 epinephrine. When the procedure is performed under local anesthesia alone, it is helpful to inject 1% lidocaine with 1:50,000 epinephrine followed by 0.25% bupivacaine with 1:50,000 epinephrine after initial anesthesia has been achieved. Firm pressure should be held on the anterior and posterior surfaces of the ear after injection to minimize soft tissue distortion.

Surgical Procedure

The initial skin incision is performed with needlepoint electrocautery, which helps to minimize bleeding, decreases operative time, and results in a very acceptable scar that is well hidden in the postauricular sulcus. Once the incision is complete, the ellipse of skin is excised either sharply or with electrocautery. The converse scissors are then used to undermine the skin in the supraperichondrial plane along the superior half of the ear where the Mustarde-type horizontal mattress sutures will be placed. This dissection should be mostly avascular as long as one remains in this plane. Once this step is complete, a second round of hemostasis is performed with the electrocautery.

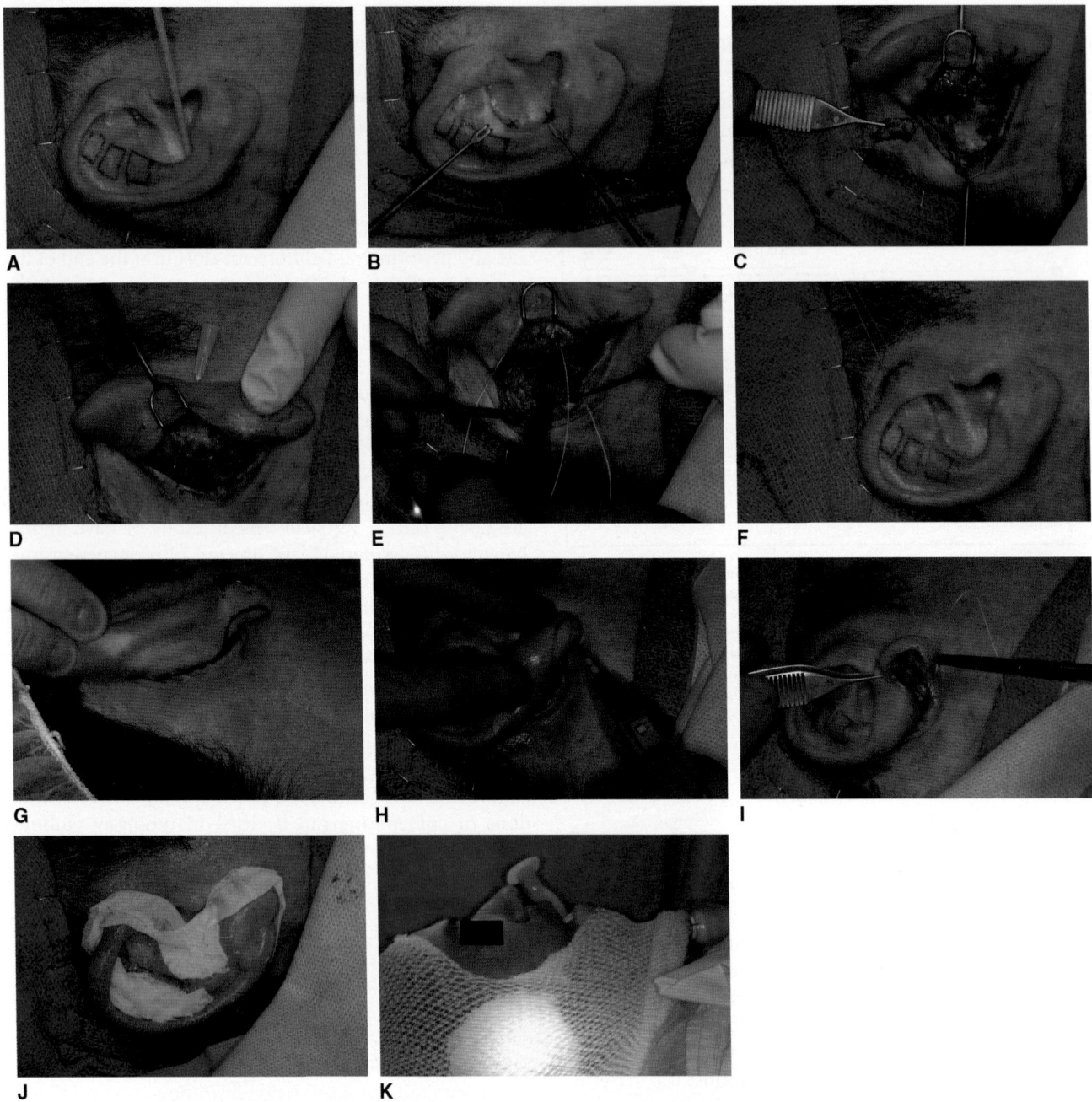

Figure 190.7 Otoplasty technique. Conchal setback sutures are planned by pushing the conchal bowl against the scalp **(A)** and marking the optimal location for suture placement **(B)**. A small amount of soft tissue overlying the mastoid is removed to allow for an appropriate conchal setback, leaving the periosteum for suture placement **(C)**. A 27-gauge needle is placed through the conchal bowl where the suture will be placed and the conchal bowl is secured to the mastoid periosteum **(D,E)**. The helical root can then be secured to temporalis fascia through an incision in a skin fold just anterior to the helical root **(F)**. The lobule can be reduced through an elliptical soft tissue excision **(G–I)**. Once complete, the ear is dressed with petrolatum gauze and wrapped with elastic net bandage **(J,K)**.

In a majority of cases, it may be easier to place Mustarde-type horizontal mattress sutures prior to Furnas-type conchal setback sutures. The reason for this is that once the conchal bowl setback sutures are placed, access to the postauricular cartilage for Mustarde suture placement may be more visually limited. However, in cases where ear prominence mostly results from a large conchal bowl, Furnas-type conchal setback sutures may be placed first without significant visual limitation. It is extremely important to modify one's technique based on each patient's unique anatomy.

Working with the surgical assistant, a repetitive set of maneuvers is then performed: A 27-gauge needle is passed from the anterior to posterior surface in what will be a corner of the Mustarde-type horizontal mattress suture. On the back side of the ear, a cotton-tipped applicator is used to dry the cartilage, and the surgical marker is used to place a very fine dot where the needle will pierce the cartilage. This process is then repeated. In most cases, three Mustarde-type horizontal mattress sutures will be required, but two or four may be appropriate depending on the deformity. The surgeon then places Mustarde-type horizontal mattress sutures (we prefer 4-0 polyester suture), being careful to pass the needle through the full thickness of the cartilage without violating the anterior auricular skin. The initial suture is tightened to ensure that the resulting antihelix is desirable, but is then relaxed and tagged to the surrounding surgical drapes without cutting. The above process is repeated until the desired number of sutures has been placed postauricularly. The Mustarde-type horizontal mattress sutures can be tied from inferior to superior or superior to inferior depending on the case; by gently bending the pinna to create the antihelical fold, it is often evident that bending begins in one direction more naturally. Once the first Mustarde-type horizontal mattress suture is secured with a surgeon's knot, the first assistant gently pinches the edges of the newly formed antihelical fold with a penetrating towel clamp. This will allow the shape to be held in place while the operating surgeon continues to tie the sutures from the posterior side. In order to prevent the postauricular skin from catching as the suture is tied, a side-to-side "windshield wiper" motion can be performed as each knot is tied.

Preparation for Conchal Setback

Before the conchal bowl set back can be performed successfully, there must be a recipient site created into which the conchal bowl can be set. This site is created by using electrocautery to undermine a thin postauricular skin flap and remove a disc of muscle and fascia overlying the mastoid (Fig. 190.7C). It is important to leave a thin layer of tissue over the mastoid periosteum so that the conchal setback suture can be placed securely. The amount of soft tissue that is removed varies based on the amount of setback that is needed, but in general, a region of soft tissue about the diameter of a nickel or quarter and 1 to 4 mm thick should be removed.

Placement of the Furnas Sutures

Furnas-type conchal setback sutures pass through the conchal cartilage and mastoid periosteum. We begin at the conchal cartilage in a backhanded fashion such that the needle can be passed through the mastoid periosteum in a forehanded fashion, allowing better needle control for the second, more technical needle pass (Fig. 190.7D and E). Based on the cartilage rigidity and force that needs to be applied for the conchal bowl setback, the surgeon may use a combination of one or three 4-0 or 3-0 sutures. For example, in a younger patient with more elastic cartilage,

two 4-0 polyester sutures are usually adequate, but in an adult patient with more calcified cartilage, two or three 3-0 polyester sutures may be indicated. It is always best to place the sutures loosely initially and tie them later, just as in creating the antihelical fold. The first assistant can hold the conchal bowl in correct position with a cotton-tipped applicator while the operating surgeon throws surgeon's knots, again with a "windshield wiper" motion.

Helical Root Positioning

An observant surgeon will notice that often after a combination of Mustarde and Furnas sutures, the helical root will almost always protrude laterally. If not corrected, this result will persist postoperatively and is the upper component of the telephone ear deformity. This area of the ear may be overlooked in cosmetic otoplasty but is as important of an area to control as the antihelical fold and the conchal setback. When needed, a helical root incision should be marked prior to the injection of local anesthetics along a natural skin crease (Fig. 190.6C). A small, 6- to 10-mm stab incision is made with a number 11 blade scalpel, and a 4-0 polyester suture is placed deep in the temporalis fascia in a forehanded fashion. The suture should be well seated such that the surgeon should feel that the head could almost be lifted off the table with the suture alone. In a backhanded motion, the suture is now passed through the inferior cartilage of the helical root and tied to bring the antihelical fold into a more natural orientation relative to the newly created antihelical fold and conchal setback (Fig. 190.7F).

Closure

Because the incision at the helical root incision could leave a perceptible scar, it should be closed meticulously with either 6-0 polypropylene or 6-0 fast-absorbing catgut suture. We have achieved good results by everting the skin edges with a few horizontal mattress sutures. As the postauricular incision is closed, three 4-mm gaps are left open to allow for the egress of blood, decreasing the risk of hematoma. The three gaps are placed 5 mm from the apex of the incision, at the midportion of the incision, and at the inferior 4 mm of the incision near the lobule. Closure can be performed in a running fashion between each gap (Fig. 190.6D).

Management of the Lobule

In cosmetic otoplasty, the lobule can sometimes be one of the more challenging structures to shape and position; this is particularly true of large, fleshy lobules that lack rigidity. When the lobule needs to be positioned closer to the scalp, which occurs approximately one-third of the time, a wedge excision can often be the simplest and most direct way to proceed (Fig. 190.7G–I). The amount of tissue that must be excised can be determined by pinching the lobule along its posterior surface. An elliptical wedge of skin should then be marked and excised with needlepoint electrocautery. The resulting defect is closed with a 5-0 fast-absorbing catgut suture, again leaving a purposeful 4-mm gap inferiorly for the postoperative egress of blood.

Dressing

There are many different ways to dress the ear postoperatively that help to support its new shape. In one relatively simple technique, petrolatum gauze (Xeroform) is cut into five 5 mm strips, two of which are packed in the postauricular sulcus, and three of which are packed along the anterior surface of the ear. The petrolatum gauze is pressed into the peaks and valleys of the newly formed antihelix and conchal bowl (Fig. 190.7J). Following placement of the petrolatum gauze, fluffed 4 × 4-inch gauze sponges are placed over each ear and a size 8 elastic net bandage (BandNet) is placed over the face, twisted at the top, and pulled over itself to create a double layer of netting. Younger patients may be better fit with a size 7 elastic net bandage. A gap is cut through the bandage over the eyes, nose, and mouth and the inferior edge of this gap is brought over the anterior mandible like a chin-strap (Fig. 190.7K). The compression created by this dressing is designed to provide three-dimensional support to the skin envelopes overlying cartilage where several sutures have just been placed. It is essential that this pressure dressing be in place prior to extubation, especially in the case of children.

Otoplasty for the Constricted Ear

The goals of otoplasty for patients with constricted ears are to provide adequate, symmetric ear height, projection, and shape. This constellation of deformities is a much more difficult problem to correct and requires the surgeon to be facile in multiple techniques of otoplasty and auricular reconstruction. Several of these techniques for management of the constricted ear will be presented in this section, however, further detail, especially pertaining to rib graft harvest, is beyond the scope of this chapter.

Mild Constricted Ear

Mildly constricted ears, as stated above, can be treated with molding techniques in neonates or even in some older individuals. However, molding is dependent upon cartilage elasticity. Surgically, these patients are often candidates for otoplasty similar to that performed for prominent ears. If standard otoplasty techniques are to be employed, it is critical that the cupped superior helix is able to be manually unfurled into a nearly normal shape. If this manipulation can be performed but requires a significant amount of force, transcutaneous placement of through-and-through 4-0 silk sutures to create the antihelix and reduce helical prominence can be useful in determining if they alone can hold the ear in position for several days to a week preoperatively. If the desired shape can be appropriately retained over this period of time, a standard otoplasty technique

using Mustarde-type horizontal mattress sutures similar to the procedure described above can be used (Fig. 190.8). If sutures are unable to hold the ear in place, however, cartilage-cutting techniques may be required.

Moderate and Severe Constricted Ear

Moderately constricted ears are often difficult to separate from patients who are more appropriately in the mildly or severely constricted categories. Often they will require a V-Y advancement of the helical root to release the helical rim into a more natural position and may require cartilage grafting (Fig. 190.9) (25).

The severely constricted ear, on the other hand, always requires cartilage grafting and often requires an adjacent tissue transfer or skin graft. The most useful cartilage for auricular reconstruction is from the rib. In the constricted ear, partial shaved rib cartilage can be easily harvested with minimal donor-site morbidity. Shaved cartilage will also curl to create a contour very amenable to superior helical reconstruction (Fig. 190.10).

Complications

Fortunately, complications after otoplasty are rare, but they do occur and can in some cases be quite severe. Early complications include infection, chondritis, hematoma, pain, and skin necrosis. Infection and chondritis are the most devastating as they can lead to loss of cartilage and require multiple reconstructive procedures. Generally, a patient developing infection will experience worsening pain around the third or fourth postoperative day, followed by swelling and drainage from the ear. Once infection is suspected, any fluid collections should be drained, a culture should be obtained if possible, and the patient should be treated aggressively with antibiotics. The patient may at first be given oral antibiotics, but if no response is noted within 48 to 72 hours or the infection appears particularly aggressive, broad-spectrum intravenous antibiotics covering skin flora as well as potential pseudomonal infection should be initiated. Hematoma is often a result of either inadequate hemostasis at the time of surgery or postoperative trauma and is suggested by sudden swelling at the surgical site. If detected, a hematoma should be drained expeditiously to prevent infection, calcification, and cartilage loss. Purposeful gaps in closing the postauricular incision can help to prevent this complication if excessive bleeding were to occur. Pain that worsens more than expected in the postoperative period may signal any of the aforementioned complications as well as possible hypersensitivity reactions to the dressing or excessive tightness of the dressing. Skin necrosis is a very rare complication in otoplasty that may be more common in individuals with poor peripheral circulation, such as smokers or diabetics, but may also be caused by excessive dressing tightness (55–58).

Late complications after otoplasty include inadequate correction, telephone ear deformity, abnormal ear

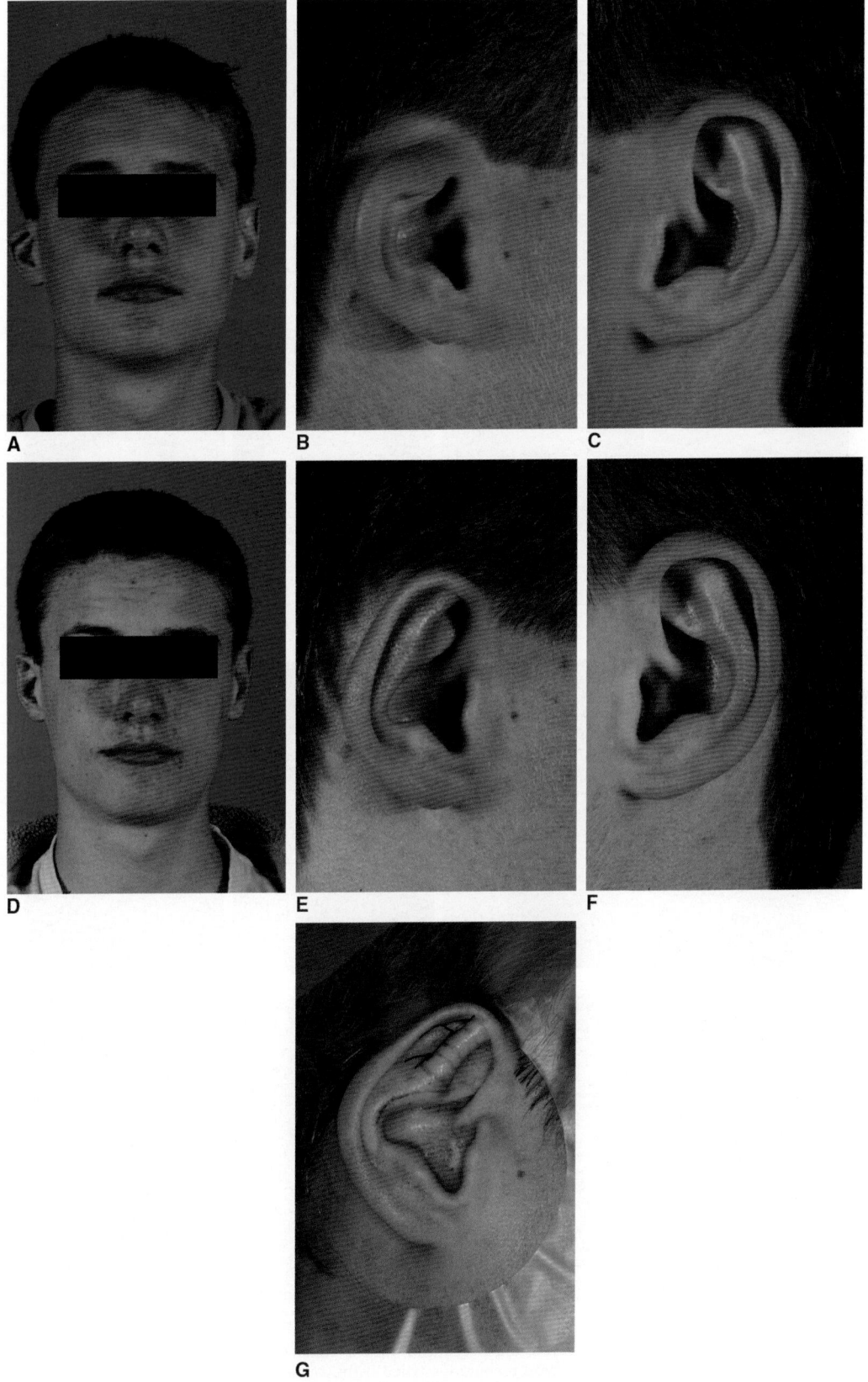

Figure 190.8 Mild to moderately constricted ear. In this 16-year-old with a mild to moderately constricted ear, the ear could be unfurled, but with a significant amount of force (**A–C**). Because the patient was older and able to tolerate an office procedure, through-and-through 4-0 silk sutures were placed transcutaneously to ascertain if they alone would hold the ear in the correct position (**G**). If these sutures had failed, the next treatment option would have been an auricular reconstruction with a partial shaved rib graft. The sutures were placed approximately 1 week preoperatively and held the ear in position. Intraoperatively, a postauricular incision was created, and several, strong Mustarde-type sutures were placed along the superior helix. This patient had a satisfactory result at the 6-week postoperative appointment and ultimately did not require a rib graft as the ear height result was a close enough match to the opposite side that the patient did not feel further surgical intervention was warranted (**D–F**). This suturing technique allowed for better preoperative decision making and demonstrates the difficulty that can be encountered when deciding on a treatment strategy for patients with constricted ears.

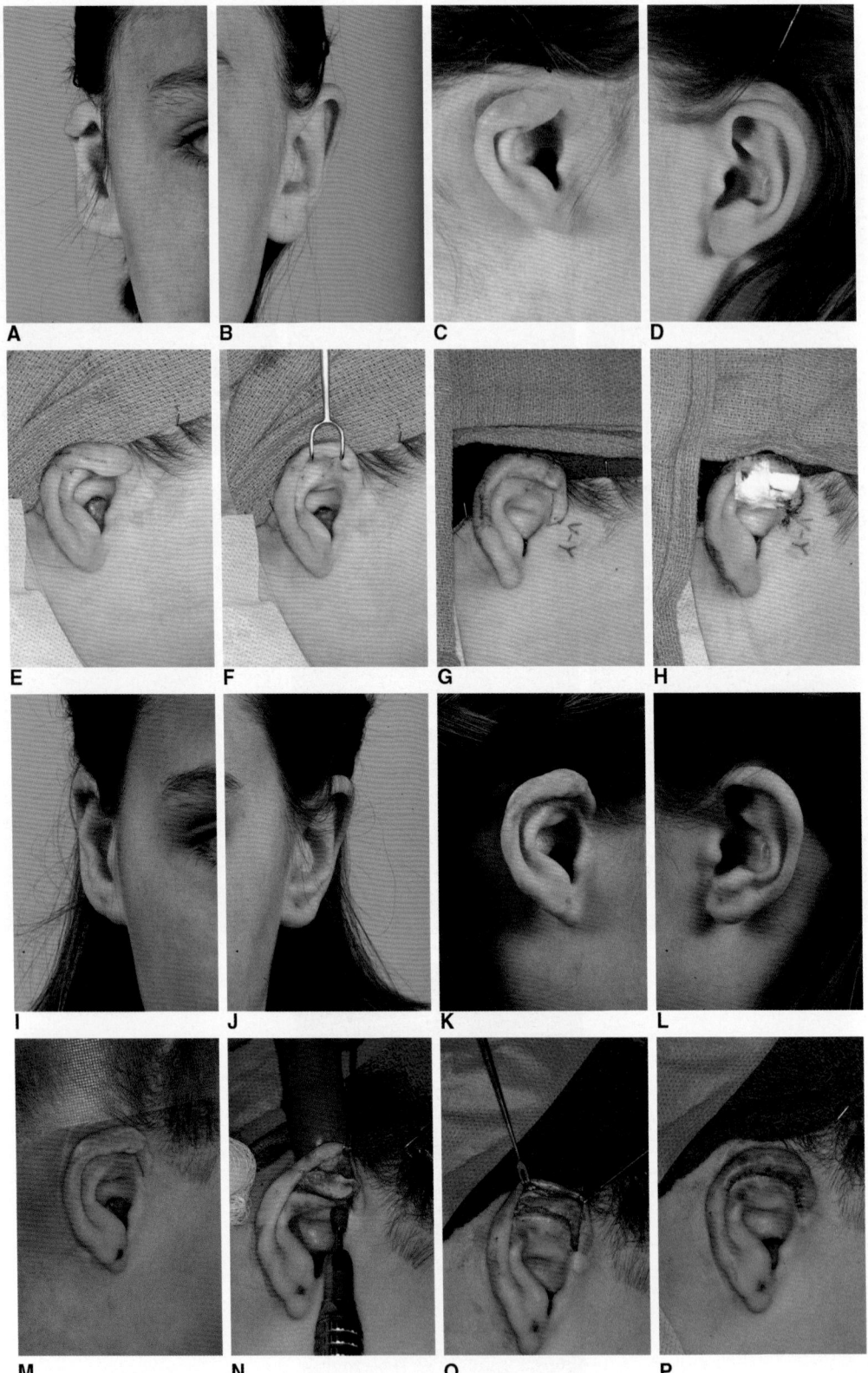

Figure 190.9 Moderately constricted ear. This 7-year-old presented with a constricted upper one-third of the ear that had been attempted to be repaired using standard otoplasty-type techniques twice without success **(A–D)**. The ear was able to be nearly completely unfurled, but was excessively cupped and seemed to be held in place at the helical root **(E,F)**. In addition, the ear had an irregular appearance, and plans were made for a two-stage procedure: the first to correct the height and shape and the second to remove the ear's contour irregularities. In the first stage, an incision was created just posterior to the helical rim along the upper one-third. The cartilage in this region was degloved along its anterior and posterior surfaces, providing broad exposure and allowing the placement of standard Mustarde-type horizontal mattress 4-0 polyester sutures to unfurl the ear. Once unfurled, the skin was brought back over the cartilaginous structure of the ear and a V-Y release of the helical root was performed, allowing the ear to achieve greater vertical height **(G,H)**. A standard bolster dressing was applied because of the wide undermining that was required. About 1 year later, the second-stage surgery was performed to improve the irregular contour of the cartilage. This delay allowed us to ensure that the ear was completely healed and had achieved adequate vertical height correction **(I–L)**. The cartilage was, again, widely degloved, and a diamond-tipped dermabrader was used to correct contour irregularities **(M–O)**. A 1 × 4 cm thick piece of AlloDerm was then evenly spread over the entire upper one-third of cartilage to provide a soft tissue cushion to the overlying skin **(P)**. A bolster dressing was again placed because of wide skin undermining.

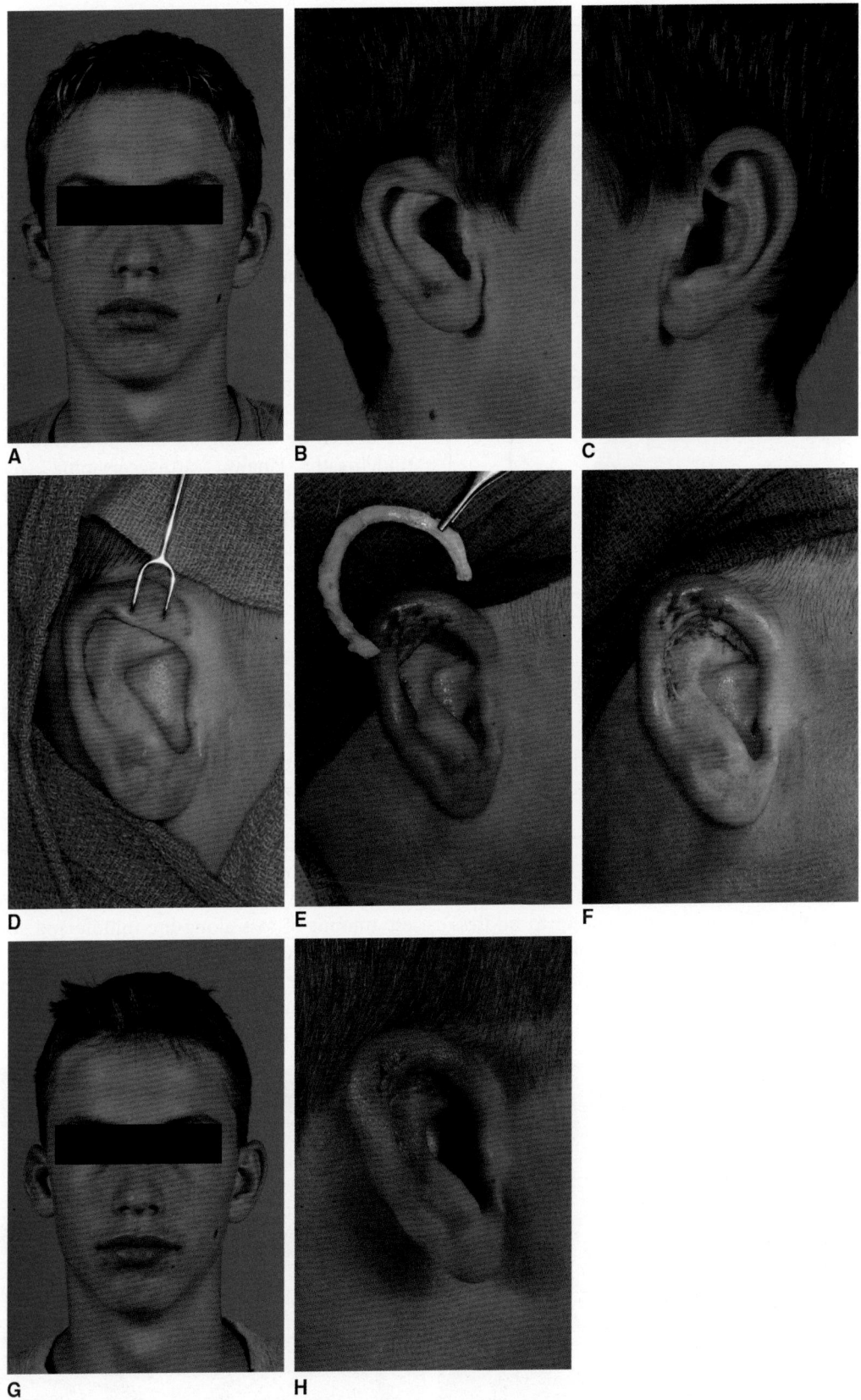

Figure 190.10 Moderate to severely constricted ear. The following 17-year-old had a moderate to severely constricted upper one-third of the ear that would not unfold in the office (**A–C**). The patient was taken to the operating room shortly thereafter for a rib graft to obtain adequate ear height and stability. First, the anterior portion of the helix was incised to allow the ear to release. A template was made of the contralateral ear using sterilized x-ray film, similar to a standard microtia repair, in order to determine the goal for ear height. Next, 5-cm-long, 2- to 3-mm-wide partial-thickness rib graft was harvested, leaving a majority of the rib in the patient's chest, a technique that significantly decreases postoperative pain. The rib was then placed in normal saline while a standard closure of the chest incision was performed and the ear was unfurled. A soft tissue pocket was then created near the root of the helix to the midbody of the helical rim. The rib was then placed in this soft tissue pocket and held in place with through-and-through sutures (**D,E**). Once the ear was completely unfurled and the vertical height of the contralateral ear matched, the anterior auricular skin defect where the ear had been unfurled was measured and a postauricular skin graft harvested for coverage and secured in place (**F**). In the end, a reasonable ear was obtained and the patient was pleased with the result (**G,H**).

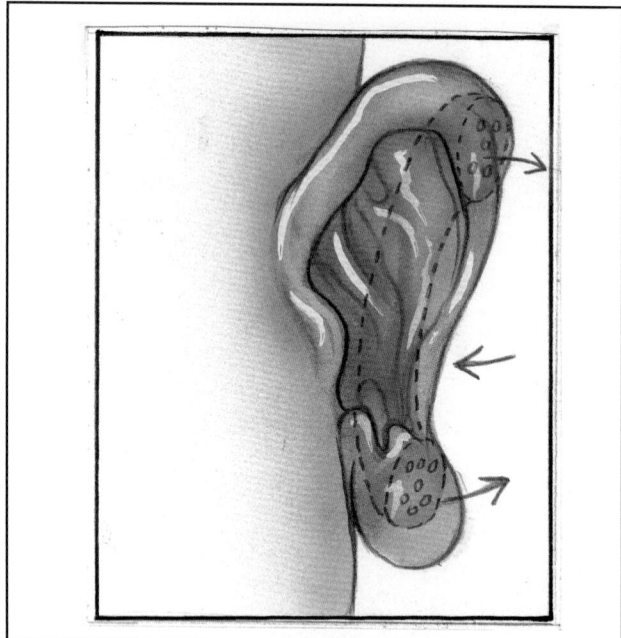

Figure 190.11 Telephone ear deformity is a postoperative result of adequate correction of ear projection in the middle one-third, but inadequate correction of ear projection in the superior and inferior one-third.

contours, keloids, suture granulomas, and extruded or broken sutures. The most common of all complications is inadequate correction of the deformity, often related to the antihelical fold or conchal setback. This problem can be addressed through revision surgery. Telephone ear deformity can be thought of as a type of inadequate correction. This problem is caused by a failure to address a laterally protruding helical root and lobule, both of which are accentuated by the creation of an antihelical fold and conchal setback (Fig. 190.11). This constellation of findings gives the ear a telephone-shaped appearance and can be addressed through revision surgery. Telephone ear deformity can be prevented by the astute surgeon by performing a helical root setback and lobule reduction at the time of initial surgery. Abnormal ear contours may result from cartilage-cutting techniques in which sharp cartilage edges can result. Revision surgery may be required to smoothen these contours. Keloids may form after otoplasty, especially in darker skinned individuals who are prone to them. Keloids can be treated with triamcinolone injection as in any other location. Suture granulomas can occur at any time postoperatively and are often noticed as a subcutaneous lump. These granulomas are treated by incising the skin and removing the suture underneath. Finally, cartilage-shaping techniques are most susceptible to sutures breaking and the ear springing back to its original position (Fig. 190.12). These sutures may also extrude and need to be removed without breaking. Revision surgery may be required in these cases as well (55–58).

LONG-TERM RESULTS

In general, the anatomic results and patient satisfaction for otoplasty are excellent (Figs. 190.13 and 190.14). Some of the immediate postoperative medialization is expected to be lost over time and seems to occur to a greater degree in cartilage-shaping techniques. Messner and Crysdale, using a cartilage-shaping technique similar to the technique described in this chapter, found that 0.9 to 5.8 mm of medialization was lost 1 year after surgery with the greatest amount of loss along the middle and superior thirds of the ear. Overall, 29% of ears returned to their preoperative positions, 28% of ears remained in their immediate postoperative positions, and 43% of ears were found

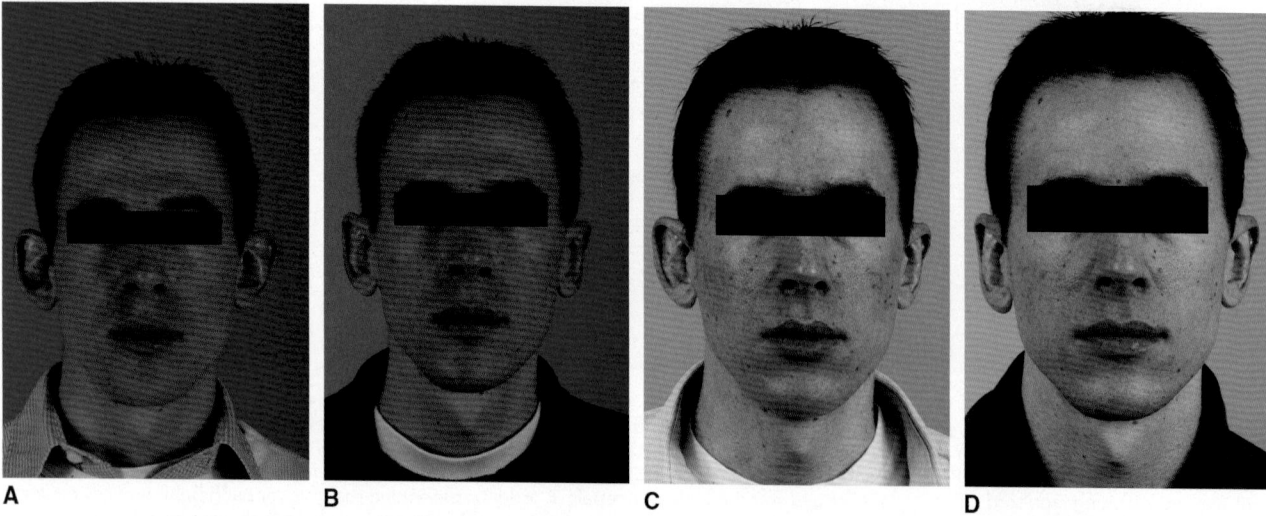

A   B   C   D

Figure 190.12 Example of suture breaking after otoplasty. **A:** Preoperative image of patient with prominent ears. **B:** Initial postoperative ear projection. **C:** Ear projection after Mustarde-type horizontal mattress suture failure at right ear. **D:** Ear projection 1 year after revision surgery for suture failure.

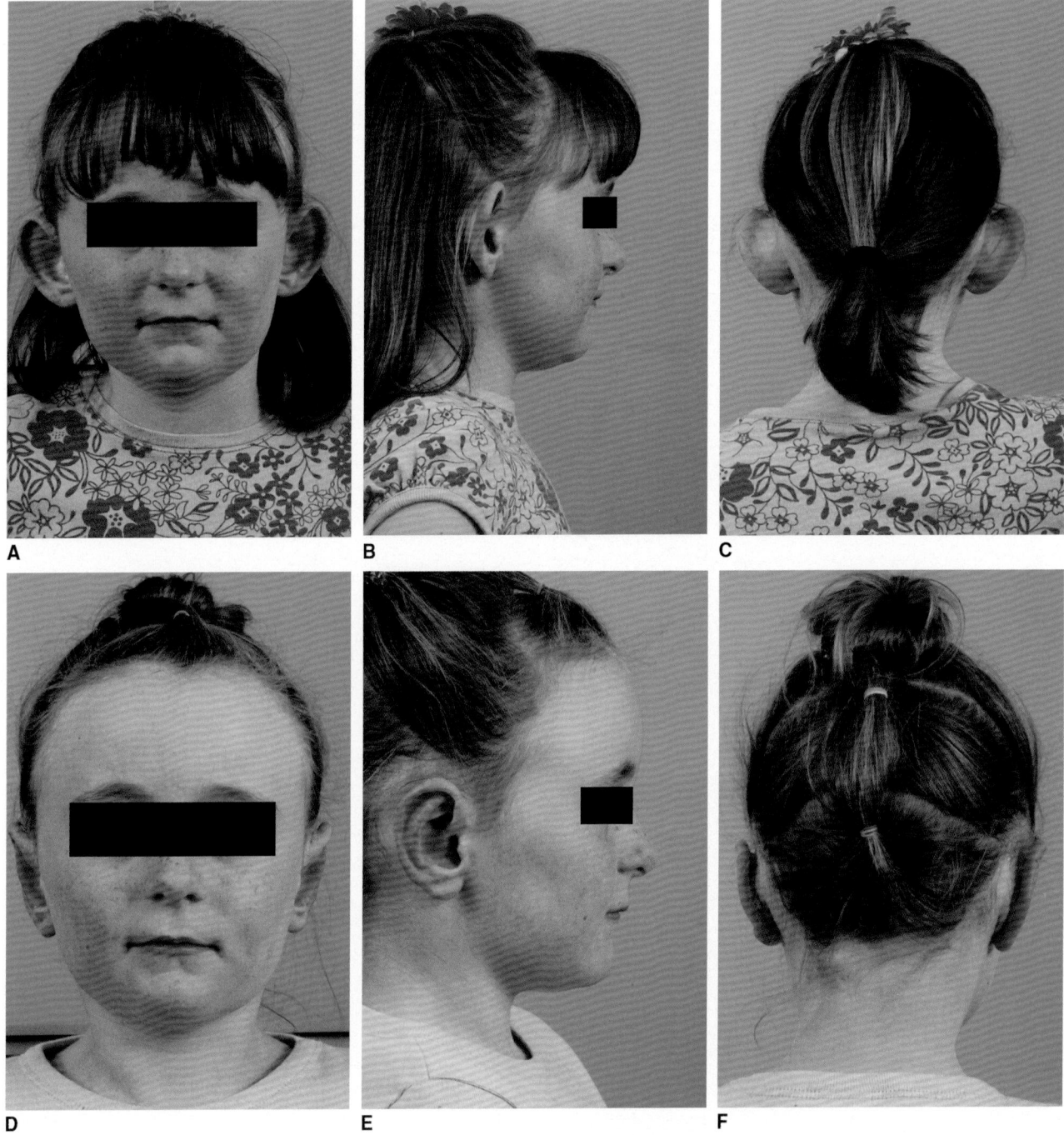

Figure 190.13 Result of otoplasty for prominent ears in a child. Preoperative **(A–C)** and 2-week postoperative results **(D–F)**.

to lie somewhere in between. Despite a 29% return to preoperative position, 85% of patients and their families were happy with the results, but only 73% would choose to undergo otoplasty again (59). Schlegel-Wagner et al., using an anterior cartilage-scoring technique with posterior suture fixation, found that 2 mm of medialization was lost by 6 years postoperatively, with the majority of recurrence along the superior third of the ear. Overall, 90% of patients

and families reported either a "good" or "very good" result (60). Using a cartilage-cutting technique that involves removing a diamond-shaped section of cartilage and suturing it into a tube to create a new antihelix, Lee and Bluestone (61) found that all patients and their families were either "very satisfied" or "extremely satisfied" with the results at 4.6 years postoperatively; however, no measurements were provided.

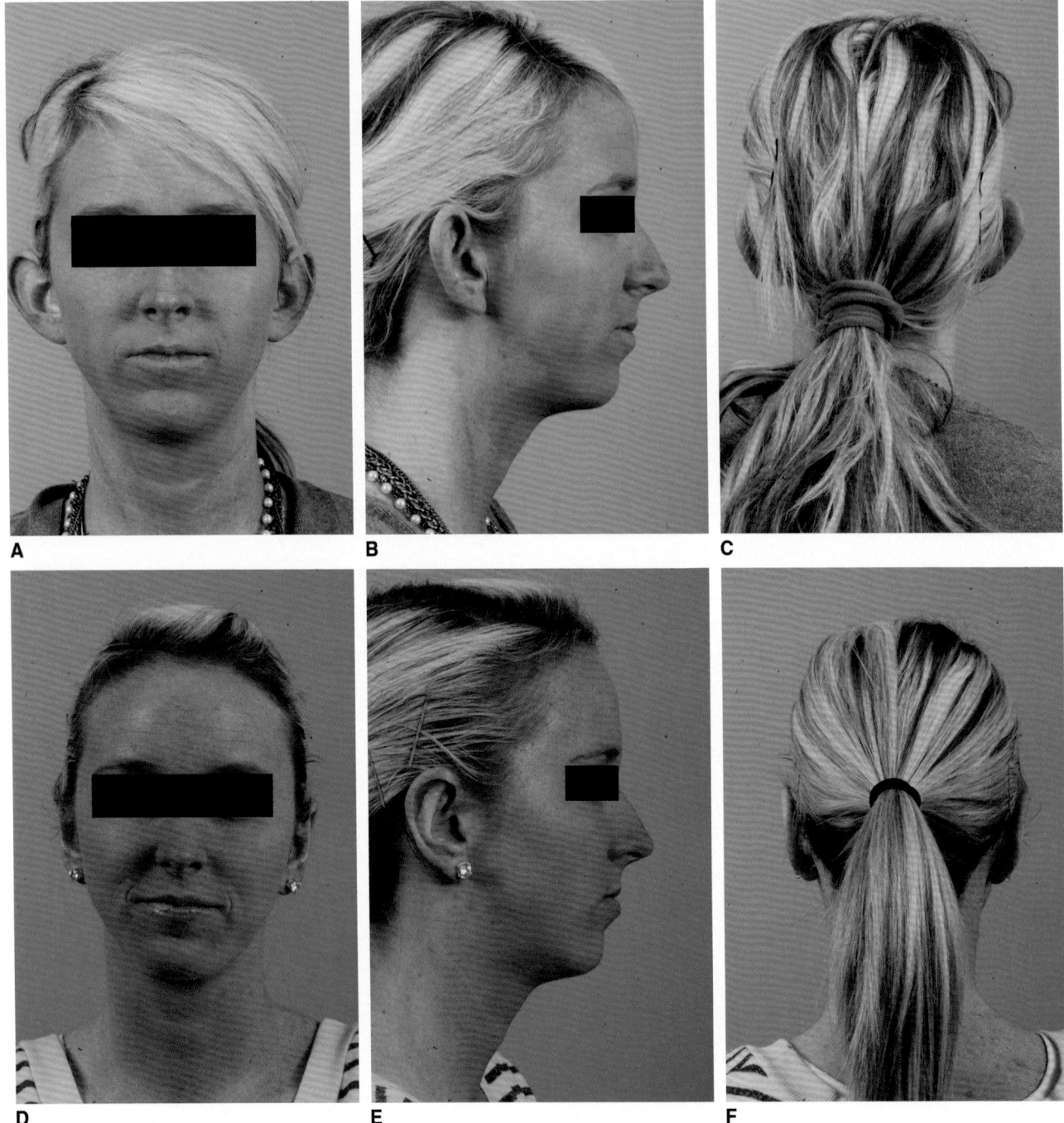

Figure 190.14 Result of otoplasty for prominent ears in an adult. Preoperative **(A–C)** and 6-month postoperative results **(D–F)**.

CONCLUSION

In treating a patient with an anomalous ear, one must consider several factors. Adequate counseling and understanding patient expectations and psychosocial concerns are paramount to patient and family satisfaction. Molding techniques should certainly be considered in newborns with ear deformities but are more controversial in older children. Laser-assisted cartilage reshaping may significantly increase molding success rates, especially in older children and adults, and become a preferred method of treatment in the future. If molding techniques do not adequately correct the deformity or if a child has a mild to moderate malformation, the otoplasty techniques discussed in this chapter may be appropriate. Otoplasty has traditionally been performed after 5 years of age, but this timing has been challenged and otoplasty potentially may be performed at an earlier age. There are a number of otoplasty techniques that have been devised, broadly categorized as cartilage-cutting or cartilage-shaping, and the surgeon should be aware of the pros and cons of these techniques in order to adequately counsel patients preoperatively. Some degree of postoperative lateralization is likely to develop over time, and although the most common complication of otoplasty is inadequate correction, patients and their families can generally expect to be satisfied by the result. Thorough knowledge of auricular anatomy and tailoring surgical technique to each individual ear can help to achieve better, longer-lasting results.

HIGHLIGHTS

- The external ear develops from six hillocks of His that are derived from first and second branchial arch mesoderm.
- The ear reaches 85% of its adult size by 3 years of age and nearly its full adult size by 5 years of age.
- Prominent ears are characterized by an absent antihelical fold and large conchal bowl.
- There is no absolute definition of prominent ear; an ear is prominent when a patient says it is.
- Constricted ears are characterized by a purse-string appearance caused by a lack of cartilage at the upper one-third of the helix and sometimes concha.
- Auricular anomalies may impact psychosocial development.
- Ear molding techniques are most effective in neonates less than 3 weeks old and lose effectiveness with age and increasing cartilage rigidity.
- Most otoplasty surgical techniques can be broadly categorized as either cartilage-cutting or cartilage-shaping.
- Inadequate correction is the most common complication of otoplasty.
- Telephone ear results from failure to address a laterally prominent helical root and lobule.

REFERENCES

1. Lombroso C, Gibson M, Rafter NH. *Criminal man.* Durham, NC: Duke University Press, 2006:53.
2. Gilman SL. *Jewish Frontiers: essays on bodies, histories, and identities.* New York: Palgrave MacMillan, 2003:120–122.
3. Bhishagratna KKL. Piercing and bandaging of the lobules of ears. In: Bhishagratna KKL, ed. *An English translation of the Sushruta Samhita based on the original Sanskrit text, Vol. I—Sutrasthanam.* Calcutta, India: J.N. Bose, 1907:141–154.
4. Tagliacozzi G. Secunda libri, de curtarum aurium chirurgia. In: Tagliacozzi G, ed. *De curtorum chirurgia per Institionem Libri Duo.* Venice, Italy: Reimer Berolini, 1597:91–95.
5. Tagliacozzi G. Praefatio. In: Tagliacozzi G, ed. *De curtorum chirurgia per Institionem Libri Duo.* Venice, Italy: Reimer Berolini, 1597:44–47.
6. Dieffenbach JF. *Die operative chirurgie, erster band.* Leipzig, Germany: F.A. Brockhaus, 1845:395–397.
7. Ely ET. A classic reprint: an operation for prominence of the auricles (with two wood-cuts): by Edward T. Ely, 1881. *Aesthetic Plast Surg* 1987;11(2):73–74.
8. Lam SM. Edward Talbot Ely: father of aesthetic otoplasty. *Arch Facial Plast Surg* 2004;6(1):64.
9. Pham TV, Early SV, Park SS. Surgery of the auricle. *Facial Plast Surg* 2003;19(1):53–74.
10. Rogers BO. Microtic, lop, cup and protruding ears: four directly inheritable deformities? *Plast Reconstr Surg* 1968;41(3):208–231.
11. Brucker MJ, Patel J, Sullivan PK. A morphometric study of the external ear: age- and sex-related differences. *Plast Reconstr Surg* 2003;112:647–652.
12. Adamson JE, Horton CE, Crawford HH. The growth pattern of the external ear. *Plast Reconstr Surg* 1965;36(4):466–470.
13. Farkas LG. Anthropometry of normal and anomalous ears. *Clin Plast Surg* 1978;5:401–412.
14. Ellis DAF, Keohane JD. A simplified approach to otoplasty. *J Otolaryngol* 1992;21(1):66–69.
15. Weerda H. Classification of congenital deformities of the auricle. *Facial Plast Surg* 1988;5(5):385–388.
16. Tan ST, Abramson DL, Macdonald DM, et al. Molding therapy for infants with deformational auricular anomalies. *Ann Plast Surg* 1997;38:263.
17. Porter CJ, Tan ST. Congenital auricular anomalies: topographic anatomy, embryology, classification, and treatment strategies. *Plast Reconstr Surg* 2005;115(6):1701–1712.
18. Yotsuyanagi T, Nihei Y, Shinmyo Y, et al. Stahl's ear caused by an abnormal intrinsic auricular muscle. *Plast Reconstr Surg* 1999;103(1):171–174.
19. Konaklioglu M, Ozmen OA, Unal OF. Stahl syndrome (Satiro's ear). *Otolaryngol Head Neck Surg* 2007;137(4):674–675.
20. Kollali RE. Posterior Z-plasty and J-Y antihelixplasty for correction of Stahl's ear deformity. *J Plast Reconstr Aesthet Surg* 2009;62(11):1418–1423.
21. Yotsuyanagi T, Yamashita K, Shinmyo Y, et al. A new operative method of correcting cryptotia using large Z-plasty. *Br J Plast Surg* 2001;54(1):20–24.
22. Adams MT, Cushing S, Sie K. Cryptotia repair: a modern update to the trefoil flap. *Arch Facial Plast Surg* 2011;13(5):355–358.
23. Bennett SP, Dagash H, McArthur PA. The role of the antitragicus muscle in plical folding of the pinna. *Plast Reconstr Surg* 2005;115(5):1266–1268.
24. Yotsuyanagi T. Nonsurgical correction of congenital auricular deformities in children older than early neonates. *Plast Reconstr Surg* 2004;114(1):190–191.
25. Demir Y. Correction of constricted ear deformity with combined V-Y advancement of the crus helicis and perichondrioplasty technique. *Plast Reconstr Surg* 2005;116(7):2044–2046.
26. Tanzer RC. The constricted (cup and lop) ear. *Plast Reconstr Surg* 1975;55(4):406–415.
27. Janz BA, Cole P, Hollier LH Jr, et al. Treatment of prominent and constricted ear anomalies. *Plast Reconstr Surg* 2009;124 (Suppl 1):27e–37e.
28. Sheerin D, MacLeod M, Kusumakar V. Psychosocial adjustment in children with port-stains and prominent ears. *J Am Acad Child Adolesc Psychiatry* 1995;34(12):1637–1647.
29. Nuara MJ, Mobley SR. Nuances of otoplasty: a comprehensive review of the past 20 years. *Facial Plast Surg Clin North Am* 2006;14(2):89–102, vi.
30. Ullmann Y, Blazer S, Ramon Y, et al. Early nonsurgical correction of congenital auricular deformities. *Plast Reconstr Surg* 2002;109(3):907–913; discussion 914–915.
31. Byrd HS, Langevin CJ, Ghidoni LA. Ear molding in newborn infants with auricular deformities. *Plast Reconstr Surg* 2010;126(4):1191–1200.
32. van Wijk MP, Breugem CC, Kon M. Non-surgical correction of congenital deformities of the auricle: a systematic review of the literature. *J Plast Reconstr Aesthet Surg* 2009;62(6):727–736.
33. Yotsuyanagi T, Yokoi K, Urushidate S, et al. Nonsurgical correction of congenital auricular deformities in children older than early neonates. *Plast Reconstr Surg* 1998;101(4):907–914.
34. Leclère FM, Trelles M, Mordon SR. Cartilage reshaping for protruding ears: a prospective long term follow-up of 32 procedures. *Lasers Surg Med* 2011;43(9):875–880.

35. Adamson PA, McGraw BL, Tropper GJ. Otoplasty: critical review of clinical results. *Laryngoscope* 1991;101(8):883–888.

36. Alexander KS, Stott DJ, Sivakumar B, et al. A morphometric study of the human ear. *J Plast Reconstr Aesthet Surg* 2011;64(1):41–47.

37. Salgado CJ, Mardini S. Corrective otoplasty for symptomatic prominent ears in U.S. soldiers. *Mil Med* 2006;171(2):128–130.

38. Gosain AK, Kumar A, Huang G. Prominent ears in children younger than 4 years of age: what is the appropriate timing for otoplasty? *Plast Reconstr Surg* 2004;114(5):1042–1054.

39. Songu M, Adibelli H. Otoplasty in children younger than 5 years of age. *Int J Pediatr Otorhinolaryngol* 2010;74(3):292–296.

40. Spielmann PM, Harpur RH, Stewart KJ. Timing of otoplasty in children: what age? *Eur Arch Otorhinolaryngol* 2009;266(6): 941–942.

41. Converse JM, Nigro A, Wilson FA, et al. A technique for surgical correction of lop ears. *Plast Reconstr Surg* 1955;15(5):411–418.

42. Farrior RT. A method of otoplasty; normal contour of the antihelix and scaphoid fossa. *Arch Otolaryngol* 1959;69(4):400–408.

43. Hatch MD. Common problems of otoplasty. *J Int Coll Surg* 1958;30(2):171–178.

44. Mustarde JC. The correction of prominent ears using simple mattress sutures. *Br J Plast Surg* 1963;16:170–178.

45. Kaye BL. A simplified method for correcting the prominent ear. *Plast Reconstr Surg* 1967;40(1):44–48.

46. Furnas DW. Correction of prominent ears by conchamastoid sutures. *Plast Reconstr Surg* 1968;42(3):189–193.

47. Erol OO. New modification in otoplasty: anterior approach. *Plast Reconstr Surg* 2001;107(1):193–202; discussion 203–205.

48. Fritsch MH. Incisionless otoplasty. *Otolaryngol Clin N Am* 2009; 49:1199–1208.

49. Epstein JS, Kabaker SS, Swerdloff J. The "electric" otoplasty. *Arch Facial Plast Surg* 1999;1(3):204–207.

50. Ragab A. Carbon dioxide laser-assisted cartilage reshaping otoplasty: a new technique for prominent ears. *Laryngoscope* 2010;120(7):1312–1318.

51. Berbaum MW, Bredle DL, Futamara W. Absence of significant adverse effects from low-dose subcutaneous epinephrine in dermatologic procedures. *Arch Dermatol* 1997;133(10):1318–1319.

52. Rizzi MD, Weil RJ, Lorenz RR. Severe transient hypertension after greater palatine foramen block in a patient taking midodrine. *Am J Otolaryngol* 2010;31(1):67–69.

53. Lowell RJ. The use of epinephrine in local anesthetic solutions for the patient with cardiac and circulatory disturbances. *Newsmonthly* 1957;4(3):13.

54. Becker DE, Reed KL. Essentials of local anesthetic pharmacology. *Anesth Prog* 2006;53(3):98–109.

55. Maniglia AJ, Maniglia JJ, Witten BR. Otoplasty—an eclectic technique. *Laryngoscope* 1977;87(8):1359–1368.

56. Furnas DW. Complications of surgery of the external ear. *Clin Plast Surg* 1990;17(2):305–318.

57. Spira M. Otoplasty: what I do now-a 30-year perspective. *Plast Reconstr Surg* 1999;104(3):834–840.

58. Caouette-Laberge L, Guay N, Bortoluzzi P, et al. Otoplasty: anterior scoring technique and results in 500 cases. *Plast Reconstr Surg* 2000;105(2):504–515.

59. Messner AH, Crysdale WS. Otoplasty. Clinical protocol and long-term results. *Arch Otolaryngol Head Neck Surg* 1996;122(7): 773–777.

60. Schlegel-Wagner C, Pabst G, Müller W, et al. Otoplasty using a modified anterior scoring technique: standardized measurements of long-term results. *Arch Facial Plast Surg* 2010;12(3):143–148.

61. Lee D, Bluestone CD. The Becker technique for otoplasty: modified and revisited with long-term outcomes. *Laryngoscope* 2000;110(6):949–954.

Congenital Auricular Malformation

191

Eugenio A. Aguilar III   *Anthony Echo*

Correction of auricular malformations requires a comprehensive knowledge base of the existing surgical procedures. Surgery, without the knowledge in selecting the proper technique, will cause great harm. As with any surgical operation, successful outcome depends foremost on the surgeon's experience and meticulous attention to detail in both planning and execution. In addition, the plastic surgeon should realize that the care of the patient with an ear deformity may necessitate a team approach that includes an otologist, audiologist, radiologist, and psychiatrist. The family should be an integral part of the surgical planning at the outset. This chapter covers ear deformities ranging from simple protruding ears to major congenital deformities.

ANATOMY AND EMBRYOLOGY

Topographic landmarks in a normal ear are shown in Figure 191.1. Of particular importance are the helix, superior crus, inferior crus, scapha, and antihelix as well as the cymba conchae and the cavum conchae, the two structures that make up the entire conchal bowl.

The development of the auricle is first seen in the 5-week-old embryo. The auricle begins as six mesenchymal proliferations at the dorsal ends of the first and second pharyngeal arches surrounding the first pharyngeal cleft. Initially, the external ear is located in the lower neck. As the mandible develops, the ear ascends to the side of the head at the level of the eyes. The current theory behind auricular development (Fig. 191.2) is that the six hillocks correlate directly with the tragus, helix, cymbum, scapha, antihelix, and antitragus (1).

The ear is made of both intrinsic and extrinsic musculature. The intrinsic muscles are the major and minor helixes, the tragus, the antitragus, the transverse, and the oblique. The extrinsic muscles include the anterior auricularis, superior auricularis, and posterior auricularis.

The auricle receives its blood supply from three arteries: the superficial temporal, the posterior auricular, and the occipital. The venous system involves the posterior auricular, external jugular, superficial temporal, and retromandibular veins. The lymphatic system of the ear drains anteriorly to the parotid lymph nodes and posteriorly to the cervical lymph nodes. Cranial nerve VII supplies the motor innervation of the auricle, with the temporal branch supplying the anterior and superior auricularis muscles and the posterior auricular branch supplying the posterior auricularis muscles. The sensory innervation is supplied primarily by the lesser occipital nerve, the mastoid branch of the lesser occipital nerve, the great auricular nerve (C2, C3), and the auriculotemporal nerve. Arnold nerve, a branch of cranial nerve X, supplies the concha.

A normal auricle and its dimensions are shown in Figure 191.3. The superior aspect of the ear is usually level with the eyebrow (2). The vertical axis of the auricle is typically inclined approximately 20 degrees posteriorly. The vertical height is usually equal to the distance between the lateral orbital rim and the root of the helix at the level of the brow (about 6 cm), and the width is approximately 55% of the length. The helical rim protrudes 1 to 2 cm from the skull at a 21- to 30-degree angle. Traditionally, an ear is considered deformed when the dimensions deviate significantly from these general rules. However, aesthetic appeal is often both subjective and culturally specific. Meticulous preoperative planning with special attention to these factors is essential in achieving normal-appearing and aesthetically pleasing ears.

PROTRUDING EARS

Protruding or prominent ears are a fairly common defect. An extensive array of surgical options is available, and every plastic surgeon should know at least one technique that can be used to achieve reliable results. Optimal

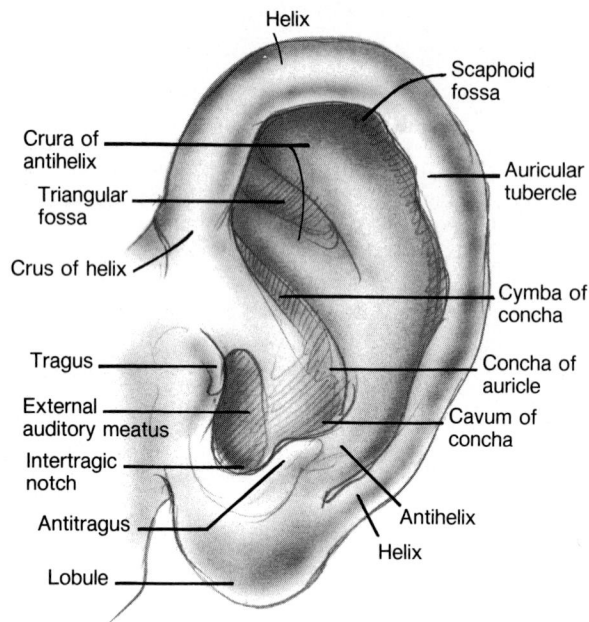

Figure 191.1 Anatomy of the auricle.

surgical outcome depends on a combination of artistic and technical skills. Although the diagnosis of protruding ears is often made by sight, knowing the basic anatomical dimensions will ensure appropriate decisions regarding intervention. The normal angle between the ear and the head should be between 20 and 25 degrees (3). Usually, an angle greater than 30 degrees makes the ears appear overly noticeable. Sometimes the auriculocephalic angle of the ear is less than 30 degrees, but some particular anatomic feature makes the ear offensive to the family or patient; therefore, a thorough preoperative assessment and discussion are necessary.

A prominent ear deformity is usually associated with a poorly formed antihelical fold and an overdeveloped concha. The scapha may be malformed with deficient superior

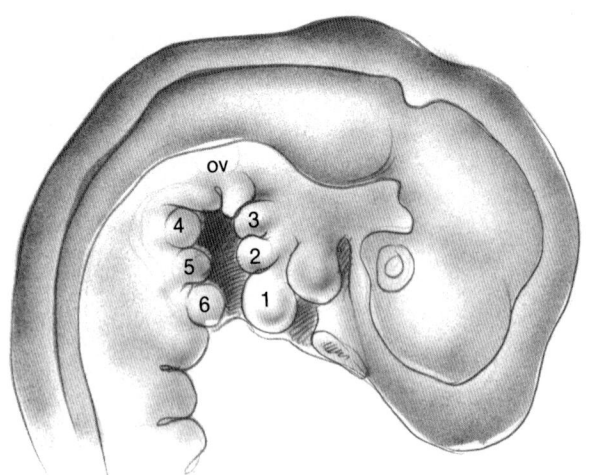

Figure 191.2 Auricle in 5-week human embryo develops from six hillocks.

and inferior crura surrounding the fossa triangularis. In addition, the helix may be abnormal in both definition and curvature.

Preoperative Evaluation

The preoperative evaluation should include good photographs. In addition to the frontal view, adequate documentation should include oblique, lateral, and rear views. Both ears should be compared and evaluated with regard to at least three basic criteria: the thickness and stiffness of the cartilage and the symmetry of one ear compared with the other. Darwinian tubercles should be noted, as should any other preauricular tags that may exist.

A checklist such as that in Table 191.1 will ensure that no important details are missed in the preoperative evaluation. This information should be discussed fully with the patient and family to clarify any points of uncertainty. The more involved the patient is in the planning of the surgical procedure, the more likely the postoperative care will be implemented properly.

Emphasizing the importance of making ear reconstruction a family affair, Eavey (4) counsels parents about the condition as well as techniques to correct the ear. In his study of 92 pediatric patients, Eavey (4) observed that children with microtia and significant auricular malformation require global attention to early family guidance, including expected and unexpected hearing loss, delayed language development, associated medical conditions, and the need for both auricular and otologic reconstruction.

In 1999, Wang (5) advocated that early prosthetic treatment is psychologically beneficial to children with congenital ear deformities. In addition, he described procedures to determine precise locations of craniofacial auricular implants by using computed tomographic (CT) scans. Although CT scan is not typically necessary for the correction of prominent ear deformities, it is a useful tool for more complex congenital deformities.

The usual goal of the operation is to achieve some reduction of the auricle angle to within 15 to 25 degrees while maintaining normal appearance and curvature of the auricular components. The helical curve should remain gentle following surgery, with no unusual breaks or pinching effects. The helical rim should be evaluated after the surgery and its height from the mastoid skin documented. The middle third of the helix should measure 14 to 16 mm and the superior third 16 to 18 mm. Reduction of the overdeveloped conchal bowl may be necessary during the surgery as well.

Otoplasty is best begun before the child starts school, between ages 5 and 6, when the child is old enough to withstand the necessary postoperative manipulations. However, Gosain (6,7) has demonstrated that it is safe to perform otoplasty on children as young as 9 months old without any effect on the development of the ear.

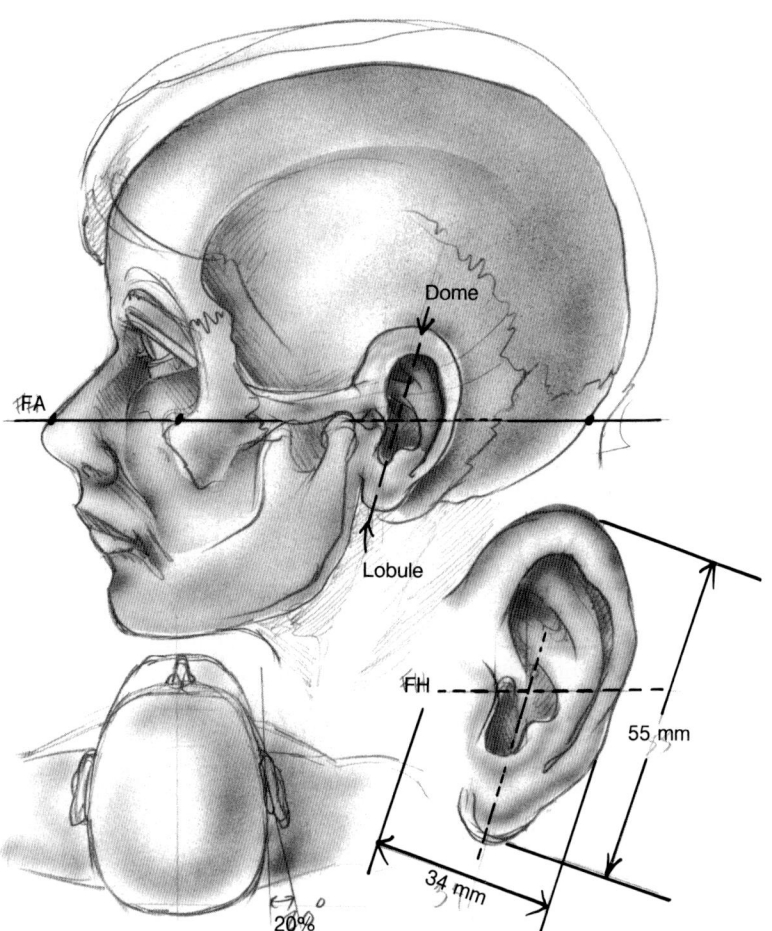

Figure 191.3 Normal ear, with average dimensions for a 6-year-old child.

Surgical Techniques

Mustarde Technique

The Mustardé technique (Fig. 191.4) involves placing several horizontal mattress sutures (usually Ethibon or Ticron) along the scapha in a curved line to create an antihelical sulcus. This technique has several advantages. A normal-appearing antihelical fold can be created, and when placed correctly, the sutures hold indefinitely. Most surgeons tend to forget that a Mustardé suture also can be used to create a more than adequate superior or inferior crus.

Problems can be expected with this technique if the sutures are incorrectly placed since they could become noticeable or erode through the postauricular skin. For this reason, postauricular skin excision is usually not recommended. Furthermore, to improve the placement of the sutures, Brent (8) recently described a hydrodissection technique where normal saline is injected on the antero-lateral surface of the ear to elevate the skin away from the cartilage to allow a full-thickness bite of the perichondrium and cartilage. Should the sutures fail to maintain the proper curve of the antihelical fold, a second operation may be required. Simply using a Mustardé technique is usually not sufficient enough for most otoplasties, because work must be done in the conchal bowl area as well.

Converse Technique

The Converse technique (Fig. 191.5) is more complicated and should be executed only by an experienced surgeon (3). With this technique, an island of cartilage is created that sits anteriorly to the rest of the conchal cartilage. This cartilage produces a normal-appearing fold, with no sharp edges on the corrected antihelix. The advantages of this technique are that it allows more permanent retraction of the auricle and is a potentially more permanent correction of the antihelix. In addition, because the island itself is not sutured, the curvature of the newly created antihelix is gentle.

Farrior Technique

This technique (Fig. 191.6) also requires an experienced surgeon (9). The incisions are made through the cartilage on the conchal rim only; then longitudinal wedges are removed at the level of the superior crus and the future anti-helical fold. An incision then is made through the cartilage at the level of the antihelical fold, creating an island similar to that of the Converse technique. The island widens from the inferior to the superior. This technique produces a more gentle bend of the antihelix. Recent literature has shown that there is approximately a 12% recurrence rate with this technique (10).

TABLE 191.1	D	DIAGNOSIS OTOPLASTY

Deformity criteria
Angle between ear and head 25° to 30° or greater
Dimensions different from normal auricle
Vertical axis—about 20° posteriorly
Vertical height—about 6 cm
Width—about 55% of length
Helical rim—1- to 2-cm protrusion from skull
Angle protrusion—21° to 30°
Superior aspect—usually level with brow
Other anatomy that makes ear offensive to family or patient
One or more significant auricular landmarks of deformity
Very poor antihelical fold
Overdeveloped concha
Abnormally formed scapha
Obvious lack of superior and inferior crus surrounding fossa triangularis
Comparative criteria
Thickness of scaphal cartilage
Stiffness of scaphal cartilage
Symmetry of two ears
Darwinian tubercles
Other preauricular tags
Documentary photographs
Frontal view
Oblique view
Rear view

Pitanguy Technique

The Pitanguy technique (Fig. 191.7) uses a smaller island flap and a conchal setback suture (3). It is appropriate for use with patients who have only a small amount of antihelical cartilage. Again, this technique requires an experienced surgeon and carries a recurrence rate of 4% (11).

Furnas Technique

The Furnas conchalmastoid suture technique (Fig. 191.8) is an important procedure for reducing a conchal bowl, as part of any successful otoplasty procedure. When the conchal bowl is too large, an island can be excised to narrow the dimensions of the bowl and to allow the proximal portion to lie firmly against the mastoid bone. The Furnas technique should always be used in conjunction with a conchal-reducing technique. This technique helps to retract the auricle permanently. If the suture is placed too far anteriorly on the mastoid, it can cause some forward buckling of the conchal bowl at the os of the external canal, leading to partial closure of the canal. To avoid narrowing the external auditory canal, it is important to remember to place the mastoid end of the conchalmastoid suture as far posteriorly as possible. These five otoplasty techniques are summarized in Table 191.2.

Complications and Emergencies

Four major complications can occur following otoplasty (Table 191.3). The most common complication is inadequate correction, and patients and their families should be alerted to this possibility prior to the operation. A secondary operation may be required within a year, even when the initial otoplasty has been performed by a well-trained surgeon.

A hematoma is probably the easiest problem to detect and is often revealed during the first postoperative examination. Simple drainage should treat this complication. Another complication is the "telephone ear" deformity, which is caused by too much flexion of the antihelix at a level equal to the midportion of the ear and inadequate flexion at the superior and inferior poles. This problem can be prevented by repeatedly checking the tension on all sutures during surgery. Reverse telephone ear can occur from overzealous tightening of the superior and inferior third of the ear.

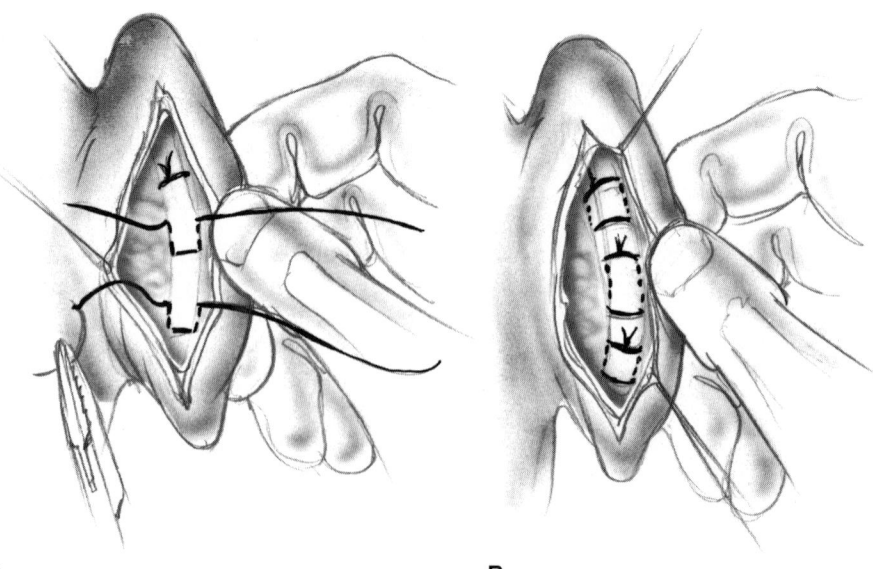

Figure 191.4 Technique of Mustardé. **A:** Marking antihelical fold with methylene blue. **B:** Placing horizontal mattress sutures.

A   B

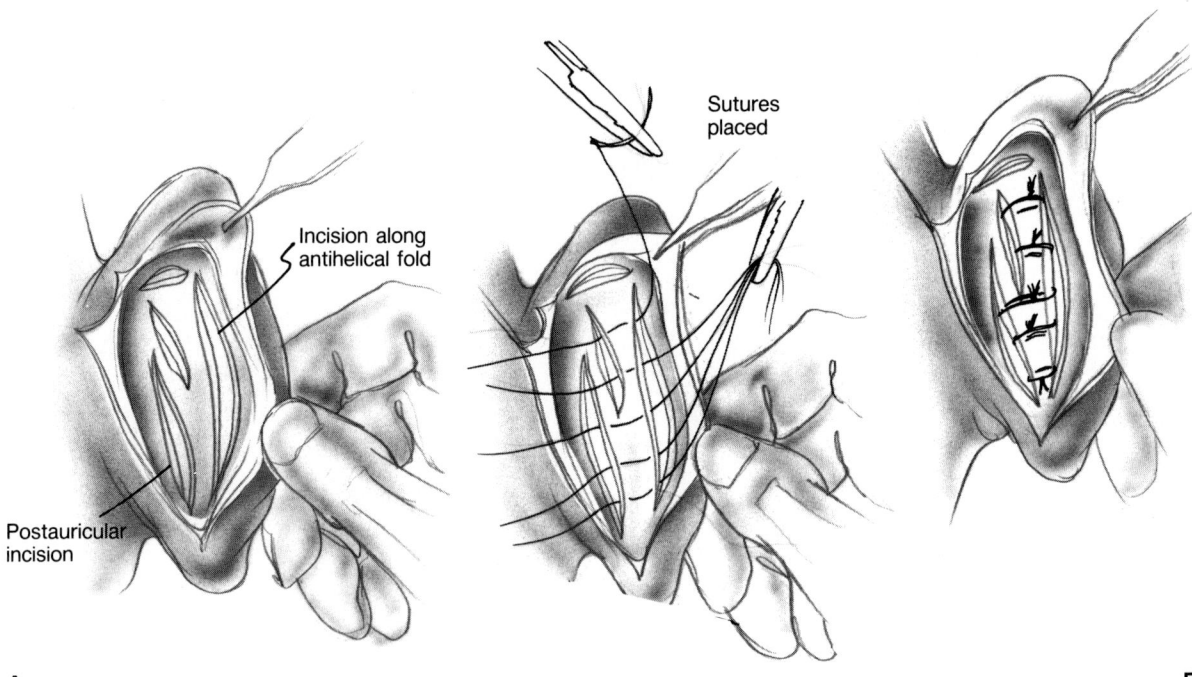

Figure 191.5 Converse technique of otoplasty. **A:** Postauricular incision and incision along antihelical fold. **B:** Sutures along antihelix.

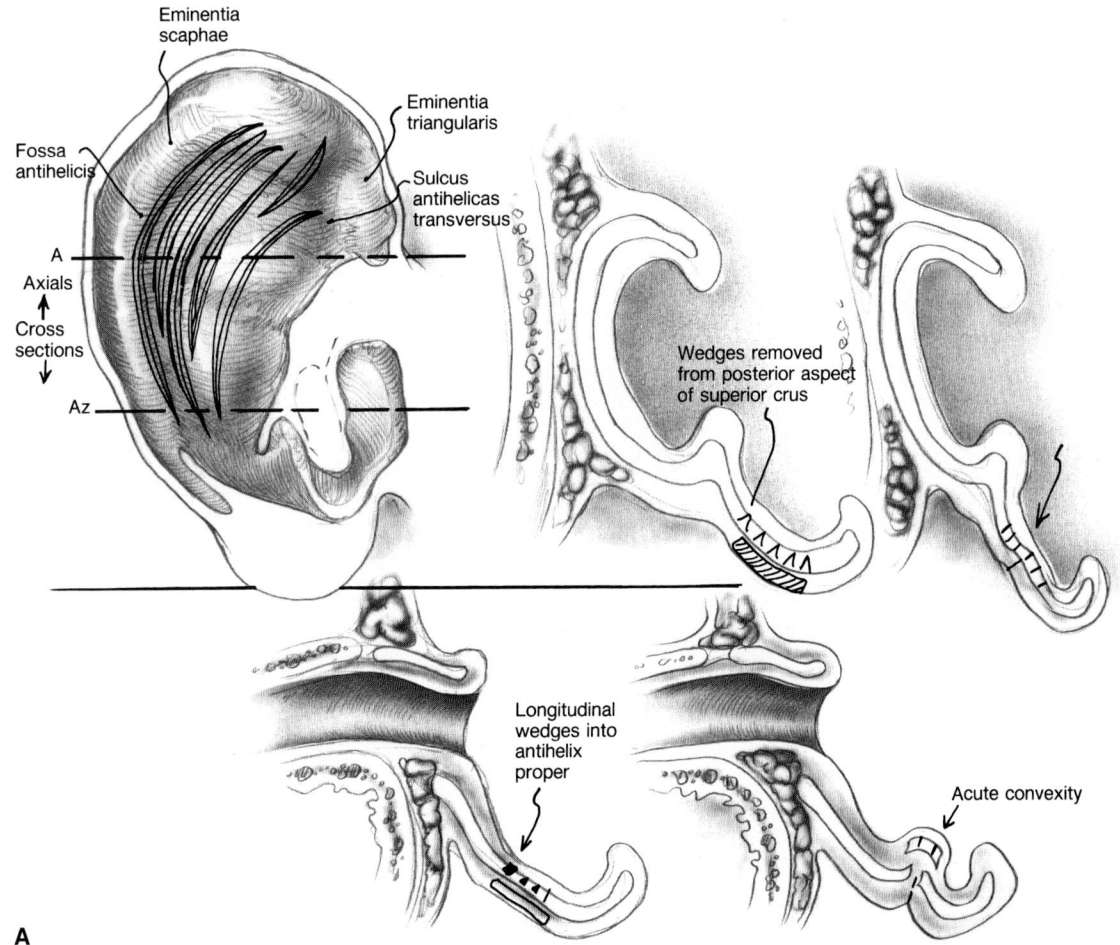

Figure 191.6 Technique of Farrior. **A:** Postauricular incision with incision along antihelical fold, and conchal reduction.

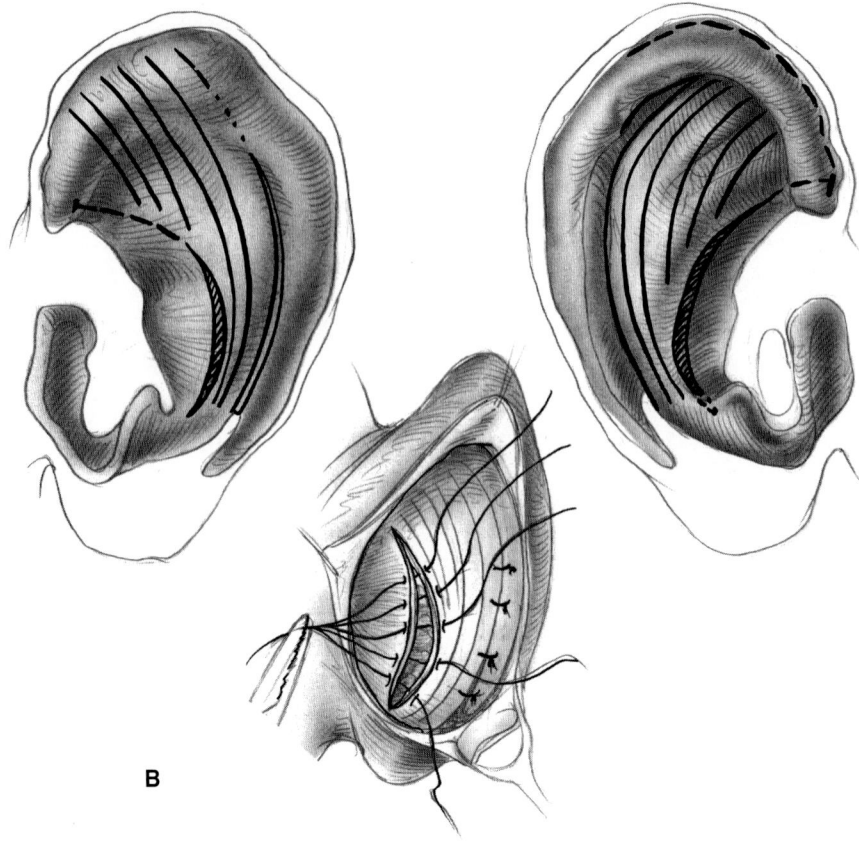

Figure 191.6 *(Continued)*
B: Sutures in place.

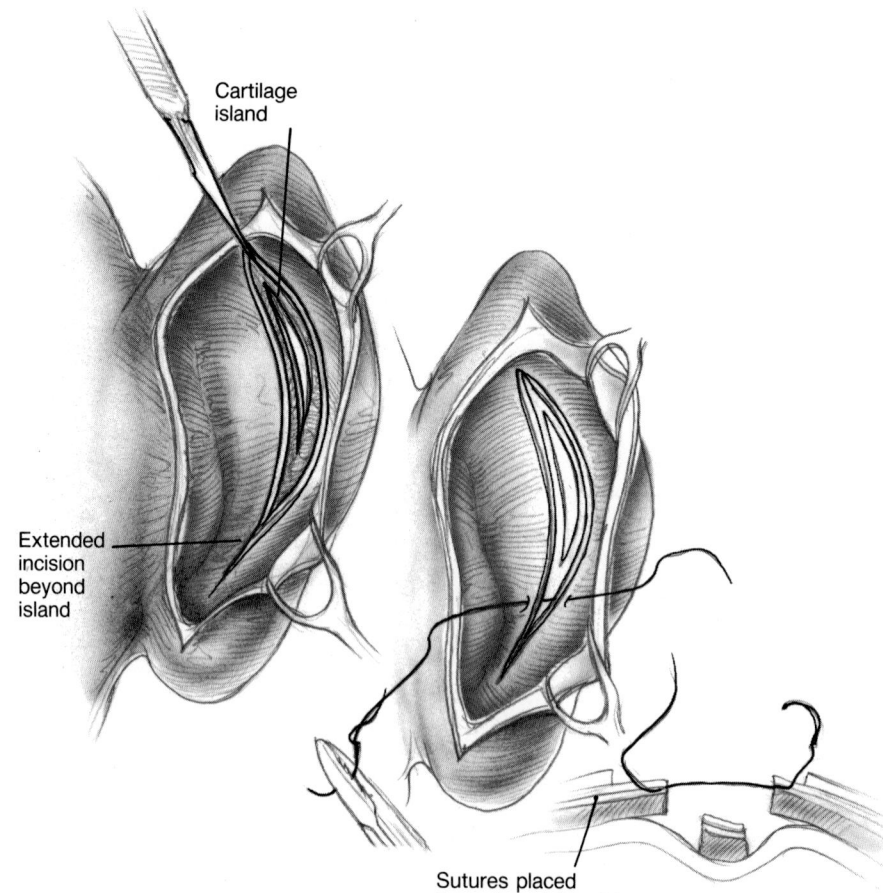

Figure 191.7 Technique of Pitanguy.
A: Postauricular incision and creation of antihelical island flap. **B:** Conchal reduction sutures and sutures around island flap.

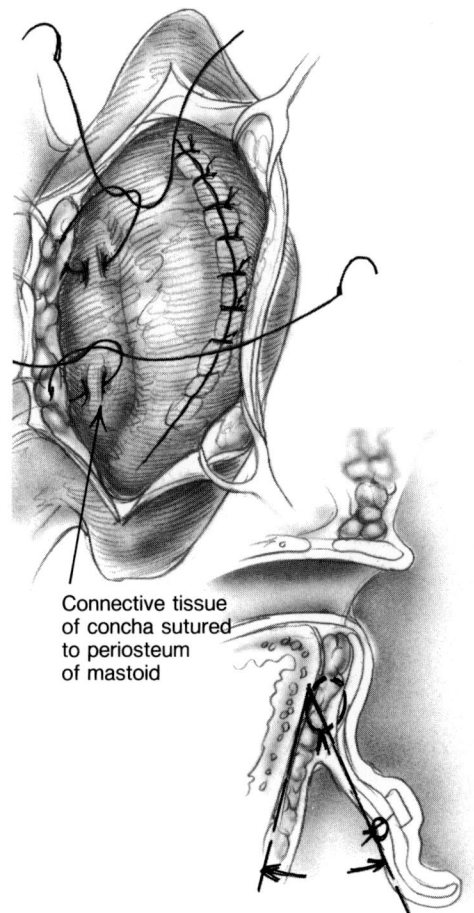

Connective tissue
of concha sutured
to periosteum
of mastoid

Figure 191.8 Conchal mastoid suture of Furnas.

The most feared complication of otoplasty is chondritis. Infection of the cartilage after an otoplasty can cause permanent, devastating changes in the anatomy of the auricle for which no viable solution exists. Therefore, any infection should be treated promptly and aggressively with antibiotics and possible incision and drainage.

Clinical Indicators for Plastic Repair of the External Ear

Strategy
    Indicators (one of the following)
        Congenital or traumatic amputation, defect, or deformity
        Reconstruction following resection of benign or malignant tumor
    Laboratory tests (as indicated)
    Other tests (as indicated)
    Type of anesthesia (as indicated)
    Location of service (as indicated)
Process
    Criteria for discharge
        Recovery from anesthesia
        No bleeding
        Outcome

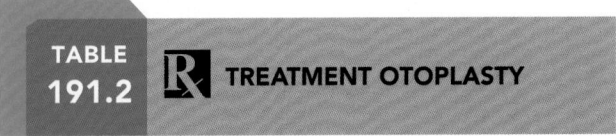

TABLE 191.2 ℞ TREATMENT OTOPLASTY

Mustardé technique
  Advantages
    Very normal-appearing antihelical fold can be created, which sutures can hold indefinitely.
    Sutures also can be used to create good superior or inferior crus.
    Inexperienced surgeons can use this technique successfully.
  Disadvantages
    Incorrectly placed sutures will cause problems.
    Technique is not applicable for work in conchal bowl area.

Converse technique
  Advantages
    Island of cartilage with normal-appearing fold can be created.
    More permanent retraction of auricle is facilitated.
    Gently curved and potentially more permanent correction of antihelix is permitted.
  Disadvantage
    Experienced surgeon must perform.

Farrior technique
  Advantage
    Bend of antihelix is gentle.
  Disadvantage
    Experienced surgeon must perform.

Pitanguy technique
  Advantage
    Patient can have small amount of antihelical cartilage.
  Disadvantage
    Experienced surgeon must perform.

Furna conchal mastoid suture technique
  Advantage
    Permanent retraction of auricle is facilitated.
  Disadvantage
    Partial closure of os of external canal occurs.

Results
    Adequacy of resection margin
    Treatment plan for malignant disease if found
Follow-up
    Wound healing
    Cosmetic result
    Evidence of recurrence
    Counseling of patient regarding disease process

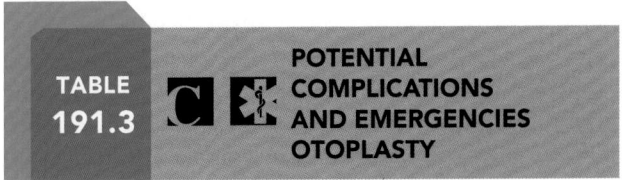

TABLE 191.3 ⚡ POTENTIAL COMPLICATIONS AND EMERGENCIES OTOPLASTY

Complications
  Chondritis (most feared)
  Inadequate correction (most common)
  Hematoma (easiest to detect)
Emergencies
  Acute infection
  Hematoma

The American Academy of Otolaryngology–Head and Neck Surgery and the American Society for Head and Neck Surgery have published clinical indicators for surgical procedures. These clinical indicators are educational statements that have been drafted to assist surgeons in their practice and to promote discussion. These indicators are not practice guidelines nor do they represent standards of practice with which individuals must conform.

CONGENITAL MALFORMATIONS

Congenital malformations of the auricle are present in 1% of births today. Correcting a major congenital malformation of the auricle is a true test of a plastic surgeon's skills.

The definition of microtia has been the subject of numerous publications, as clinicians have attempted to define the different grades that exist. This section focuses on the grades of microtia for which surgeons can initiate surgical reconstruction with a high degree of success.

Tanzer (12,13) published the first article on auricular reconstruction using autogenous rib cartilage in 1959. Shortly after, in 1966, Cronin (14) popularized the use of Silastic as an implant material to reconstruct auricles. Brent (15), who first reported his work in 1974, is considered the world's foremost authority on auricular reconstruction to date.

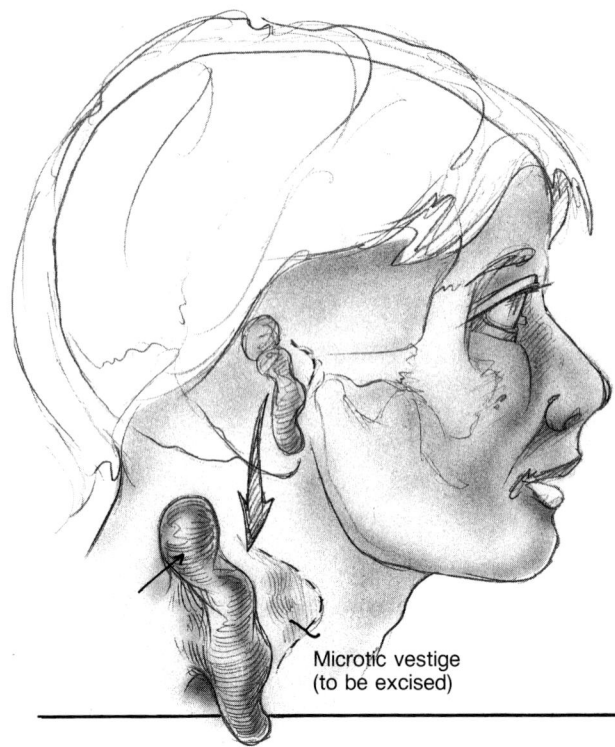

Figure 191.9 Grade III microtia.

Microtic vestige (to be excised)

Classification

In 1988, Aguilar and Jahrsdoerfer (16) amended the 1926 grading system of Marx, and in 1996, Aguilar (17) reaffirmed this concise classification for congenital ear malformations. Grade I is a normal ear. Grade II has some of the auricular framework present, but there are obvious deformities. Grade III is the standard "peanut ear" deformity, which encompasses anotia (Marx's grade IV) (Fig. 191.9).

The concomitant atresia complicates the classification schemes, yet many try to include it as a criterion: Altmann in 1955 (the first schema based on the temporal bone itself, looking at the status of the canal, tympanic bone, drum, and ossicles) and Lapchenko in 1967 and Gill in 1969 (both set up a four-tier scale, examining the degree of middle-ear and external canal development and the presence of ossicular abnormality). Gill also incorporated into his system the degree of pneumatization of the mastoid because this finding seemed to predict the relative success of operative interventions. Ombredonne, Nager, and Colman each sought to establish simplified and clinically practical systems based on Altmann's original classification, but these systems were inconsistent at predicting outcome in those cases of major aplasia or group II anomalies. Fernandez said that Jahrsdoerfer's 1992 system is a grading scale for selecting patients that would most likely benefit from attempts at repair of their atresia. He commended this scale for its "predictive power." Furthermore, the benefit of the Jahrsdoerfer's system is that it is not subject to

interobserver bias and allows for a quantitative analysis of the temporal bone and those structures deemed vital to the success of an operation.

The Jahrsdoerfer scale, based on temporal bone CT findings, assesses nine different parameters that are used in making the determination of candidacy for surgery. Fernandez stated that the stapes and oval window complex account for 3 out of 10 points possible. Other parameters include the middle-ear cleft, facial nerve position, status of the ossicles and round window, and pneumatization of the mastoid. Scores of 6 through 10 range from marginal to excellent candidates for surgery, whereas a score of five or less usually points to a poor outcome.

In 1974, Rogers (18) published a classification system that divided congenital auricular defects into four groups:

1. Macrotia
2. Lop ear
3. Cup ear
4. Prominent ear

In 1977, Tanzer (19) proposed a clinical classification of auricular defects that has been well documented in virtually all articles that have been published since then:

1. Anotia
2. Complete hypoplasia (microtia)
   A. With atresia of the external auditory canal
   B. Without atresia of the external auditory canal

3. Hypoplasia of the middle third of the auricle
4. Hypoplasia of the superior third of the auricle
   A. Constricted (cup and lop) ear
   B. Cryptotia
   C. Hypoplasia of entire superior third
5. Prominent ear

Weerda (20) from Europe in 1988 combined all of the classifications into a concise document. Definitions proposed by Marx and Tanzer and modified by Rogers (21) were presented. This system included surgical guidance for each classification:

1. *First-degree dysplasia.* Average definition: Most structures of a normal auricle are recognizable (minor deformities). Surgical definition: Reconstruction normally does not require the use of additional skin or cartilage.
   A. Macrotia
   B. Protruding ears (synonyms: prominent ears, bat ears)
   C. Cryptotia (synonyms: pocket ear, group IV B [Tanzer])
   D. Absence of upper helix
   E. Small deformities: Absence of the tragus, satyr ear, darwinian tubercle, additional folds (Stahl ear)
   F. Colobomata (synonyms: clefts, transverse coloboma)
   G. Lobule deformities (pixed lobule, macrolobule, absence of lobule, lobule colobomata [bifid lobule])
   H. Cup ear deformities
      i. Type I: Cupped upper portion of the helix, hypertrophic concha, reduced height (synonyms: lidding helix, constricted helix, group IV A [Tanzer], lop ear, minor [mild or moderate] cupping)
      ii. Type II: More severe lopping of the upper pole of the ear; rib cartilage is used as support when a short ear must be expanded or the auricular cartilage is limp.
2. *Second-degree dysplasia.* Average definition: Some structures of a normal auricle are recognizable. Surgical definition: Partial reconstruction requires the use of some additional skin and cartilage (synonym: second-degree microtia [Marx])
   A. Cup ear deformity, type III: The severe cup ear deformity is malformed in all dimensions (synonyms: cockleshell ear, constricted helix, group IV [Tanzer], snail-shell ear)
   B. Mini-ear
3. *Third-degree dysplasia.* Average definition: None of the structures of a normal auricle are recognizable. Surgical definition: Total reconstruction requires the use of skin and large amounts of cartilage (synonyms: complete hypoplasia group II, peanut ear, third-degree microtia [Marx]); normally there is concomitant congenital atresia.
   A. Unilateral: One ear is normal; no middle-ear reconstruction is performed on any child; auricle reconstruction is begun at age 5 or 6 years.

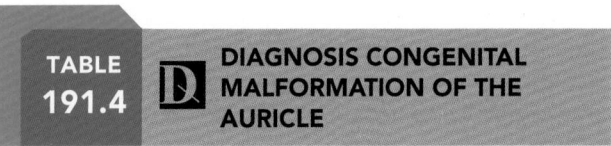

TABLE 191.4	D	DIAGNOSIS CONGENITAL MALFORMATION OF THE AURICLE

Age of patient
Grade of deformity
Size of cartilage
Atresia present
Otologic evaluation
Photographs

   B. Bilateral: Bone-conduction hearing aid before the first birthday; middle-ear surgery at age 4 years without transposition of the vestige; bilateral reconstruction of the auricle at age 5 or 6 years
   C. Anotia

These recommendations can be questioned, however, and there are alternatives. For bilateral microtia, a bone-conduction hearing aid can be placed at birth. In addition, even in bilateral cases, middle-ear surgery can follow the first two stages of auricular reconstruction rather than being the first procedure (22). Guidelines for diagnosis are listed in Table 191.4.

Surgical Reconstruction of Auricular Deformities

In cases of congenital microtia and concomitant atresia, there should be complete coordination between the otologist and the plastic surgeon. Aguilar, in 1996, (17) presented the concept of the Integrated Auricular Reconstruction Protocol. As shown in Table 191.5, microtia repair is accomplished in five stages. The work of the plastic surgeon should be performed first, and the operation should be staged to facilitate total reconstruction of the microtia–atresia complex.

Despite advances made in technique and imaging in recent decades, disagreement remains on several key issues: the prime time for surgery in general, when to operate on cases of unilateral atresia, and the operability of cases with severe craniofacial malformations. Most agree

TABLE 191.5	R	TREATMENT CONGENITAL MALFORMATION OF THE AURICLE

Stage	Treatment
I	Auricular reconstruction (creation of a cartilaginous framework with autogenous rib cartilage)
II	Lobule transposition
III	Atresia repair (by otologist)
IV	Tragal construction
V	Auricular elevation

that the earliest age to proceed is 4 to 5 years, thus allowing time for adequate mastoid and middle-ear pneumatization and increasing patient compliance with postoperative care. Also, most clinicians think that surgery should be instigated earlier in cases of unilateral atresia with evidence of cholesteatoma, infection, or very thin atresia plates. Opinions differ in regard to cases of grade II and III unilateral atresia in patients with normal hearing in the other ear. Jahrsdoerfer believes that the benefit of binaural hearing exceeds the risk of facial nerve injury and other complications. De la Cruz also favors early operations on unilateral atresias if CT findings point to a favorable outcome.

Correction of microtia should begin around the age of 6 years, especially for unilateral cases, and the best material is autogenous costal cartilage. By this age, there is sufficient cartilage to permit surgical reconstruction, and the patient is psychologically able to cooperate with the necessary postoperative care. Bilateral microtia and atresia cases can be started at an earlier age, but only if sufficient costal cartilage exists to form a new ear. Historically, use of other sources for the framework has failed. Neither irradiated cartilage nor Silastic has stood the test of time: irradiated cartilage reabsorbs, and Silastic tends to extrude with time. Furthermore, Silastic implants are notorious for their inability to withstand trauma.

In 1997, Williams et al. (23) reported on the use of polyethylene (Medpor) implants in auricular reconstruction. These implants can be used to support skin grafts when used to reconstruct defects in auricular cartilage. Animal model revealed that these implants are well tolerated as replacements for native cartilage in auricular reconstruction. Polyethylene implants tolerated wound exposure as early as 4 days after implantation and showed the ability to heal these wounds by secondary intention and to support skin grafts. Authors surmised that this is because of the extent of fibrovascular ingrowth from surrounding tissue, which allows the implant material to act more like native tissue and less like a foreign body in this setting.

At the University of Antwerp (Wilrijk) in the year 2000, Somers (24), at a Politzer Society Meeting, described major breakthroughs in reconstructive surgery of the auricle, opening new possibilities in the rehabilitation of patients with an absent auricle. Somers reported on clinicians who had adopted 33 bone-anchored prostheses and performed 22 total auricular reconstructions. These clinicians reported that the surgery for an episthesis, as long as the surgeon takes into consideration the conditions of osseointegration, is easy and has no major risks. Postoperatively, patients were satisfied with their prosthesis and wore it all day without discomfort. For the total auricular repair of major congenital malformations, two techniques were used: the Brent technique followed by the Nagata technique. The Brent technique was found to be safe with good results, but the modification by Nagata had two advantages: two operative stages instead of four and a better definition of the reliefs of structure as the antihelix, crus anterior and posterior, and antitragus tragus. As expected, results of total auricular reconstruction improved with experience.

Surgical Planning and Treatment

Preoperative planning should include photographs of the patient. Most important is the proper preparation of the template. In unilateral cases, the template is based on the patient's contralateral ear; in bilateral cases, the model is made from the mother's ear. The site of implantation of the cartilage framework on the side of the head should be properly measured to avoid malpositioning of the ear.

If radiologic examination has not already been done, it should be ordered before surgery. A high-resolution CT scan of the temporal bones should be obtained. Although a CT scan is unnecessary for the microtia, it does provide important anatomical information to the surgical team. As a team, the plastic surgeon and the otologist should explain and discuss the entire course of the planned reconstruction to the patient and family before any surgical procedure.

The auricular reconstruction (Figs. 191.10 to 191.12) is undertaken during stage I. Note that the dissection of the cartilage is extraperichondrial, and there is no stripping of perichondrium at any point during rib harvesting. Stainless-steel 5-0 wire is used to anchor the eighth rib to the sixth and seventh rib complex. This technique is popularized by Brent (25) and produces reliable results when performed by trained surgeons. The most common complication that can occur from stage I procedure is atelectasis; other complications include pleural tear (which should be appreciated intraoperatively in usual circumstances), pneumothorax, pneumomediastinum, chest wall aberration, hypertrophic scarring, and pneumonia.

Stage II involves lobule transposition and is shown in Figures 191.13 and 191.14 (Fig. 191.14 depicts the peanut ear). To avoid protrusion of the lobule, the incision on the back of the ear should be fairly high. The inferiorly based pedicle flap is quite thin; thus, great care should be taken in its handling.

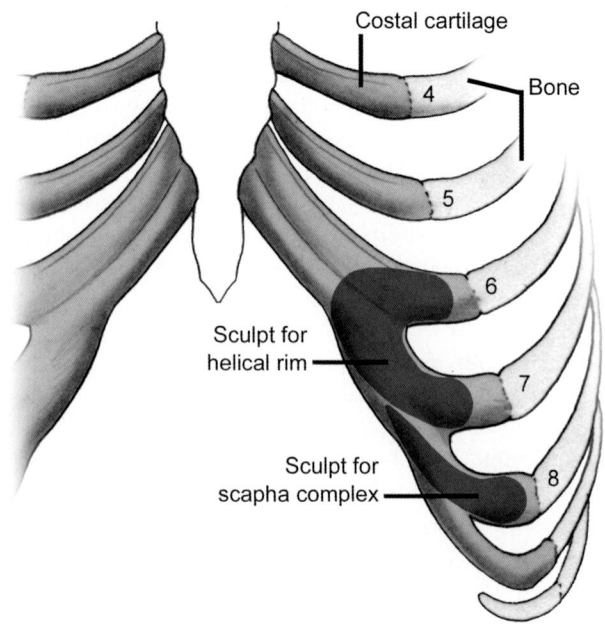

Figure 191.10 Harvesting ribs 6, 7, and 8.

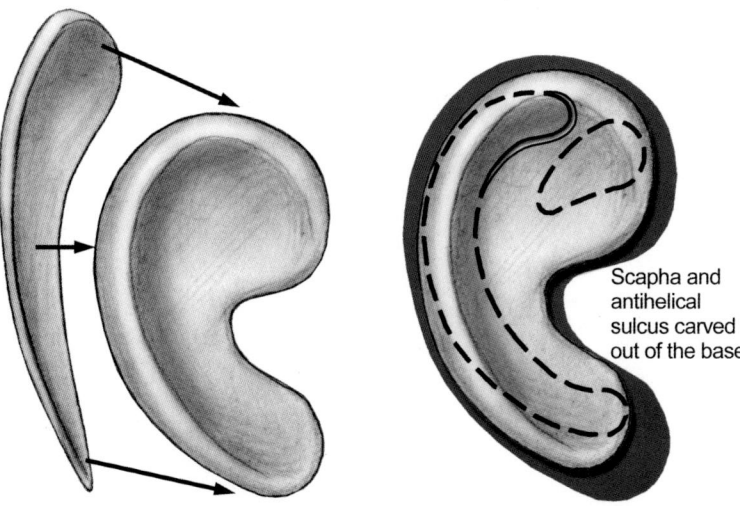

Costal cartilage from 8th rib

Costal cartilage from 6th and 7th ribs

Sculpt 6th and 7th cartilage using template

Scapha and antihelical sulcus carved out of the base

Figure 191.11 Sculpting cartilage to form framework.

Stage III, atresia repair by the otologist, should be undertaken after the first two stages of repair by the plastic surgeon. The temporal bone remnant is in only one location; thus, the opening to that remnant can be made in only one location on the overlying skin. Therefore, it is quite easy to manipulate the framework and line it up where the otologist has drilled the canal. If the otologist drills the canal first, as a stage I procedure, the complication rate is significantly higher, and it is more difficult to place a cartilage framework around an external canal. Moreover, the amount of scarring and the possible compromise to blood flow make complications harder to avoid. The maneuvering of the framework into the proper position on the side of the head is shown in Figures 191.15 and 191.16.

Stage IV, tragal construction, is shown in Figures 191.17 to 191.21. The composite cartilage is taken from the opposite side. Auricular elevation, stage V, is shown in Figures 191.22 and 191.23. The reconstructed ear is shown in Figure 191.24.

Complications

Complications are possible during the surgical reconstruction, as listed in Table 191.6. Placement of the cartilage graft causes severe strain on the overlying skin, which can cause skin necrosis. Skin necrosis of 1 to 2 mm can be treated by the application of ointment and careful observation until skin closure occurs. If the necrosis is greater than 5 mm, the proper course is closure using a pedicled temporal–parietal fascia flap and skin graft. Infection can result in reabsorption of cartilage, and there may be improper placement of the framework. Any grafting procedure always involves the

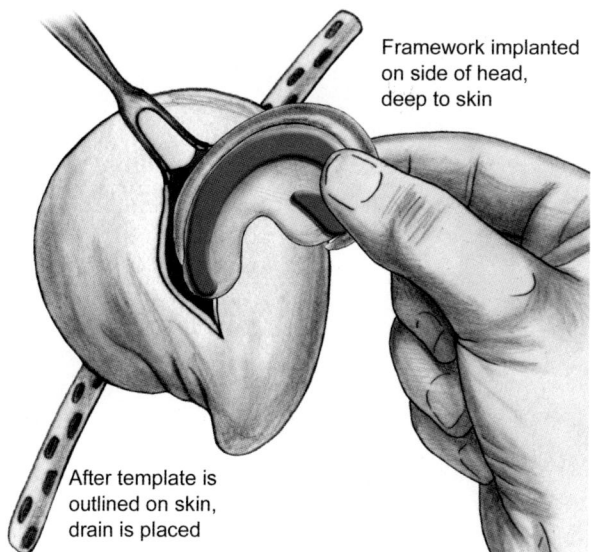

Framework implanted on side of head, deep to skin

After template is outlined on skin, drain is placed

Figure 191.12 Implanting framework on side of head.

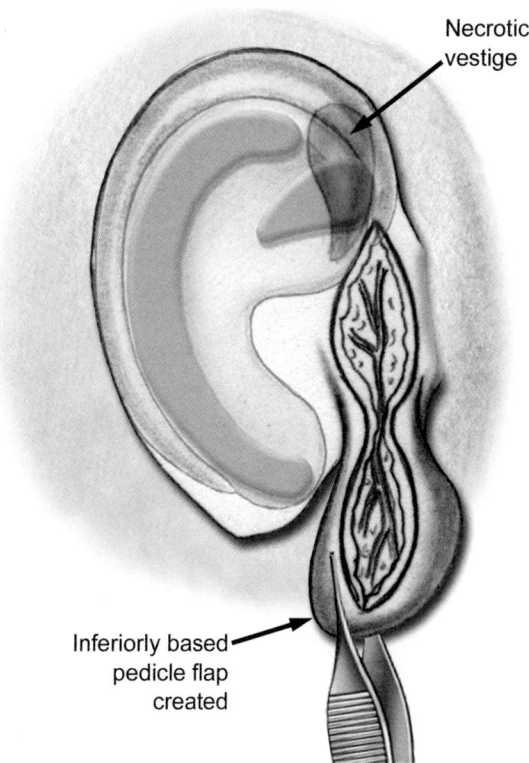

Necrotic vestige

Inferiorly based pedicle flap created

Figure 191.13 Creating inferiorly based pedicle flap.

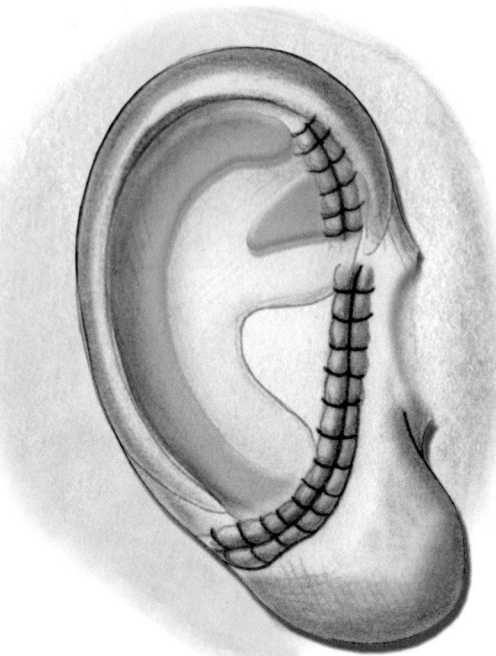

Figure 191.14 Transposing flap into framework.

risk of graft loss. Finally, the possibility of keloid formation is higher when the graft is harvested from the abdomen or the buttocks. Potential emergencies are listed in Table 191.7.

CONCLUSION

The surgery to correct auricular protrusion is more complicated than it appears. Complications can occur with each of the techniques described, even in the hands of experienced surgeons. The surgery always requires postoperative evaluation, and often the surgeon will not be totally

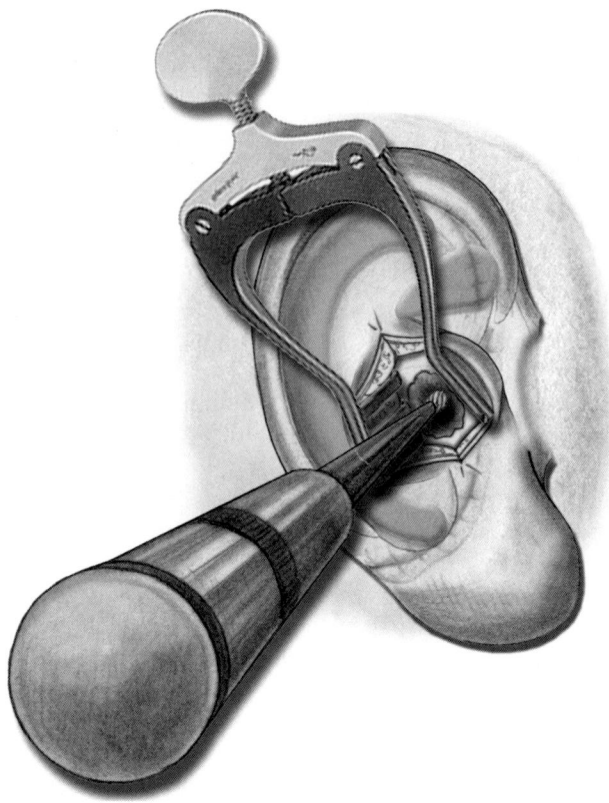

Figure 191.15 Drill-out of temporal bone, creating canal.

satisfied. Therefore, performing this surgery requires a commitment to continuing education and additional experience. Surgical correction of congenital microtia requires commitment by the facial plastic surgeon, who should be performing more than five to ten operations per year to maintain proficiency. The team approach as described in this chapter is invaluable to the families; failure to offer this approach is a significant disservice to the patient.

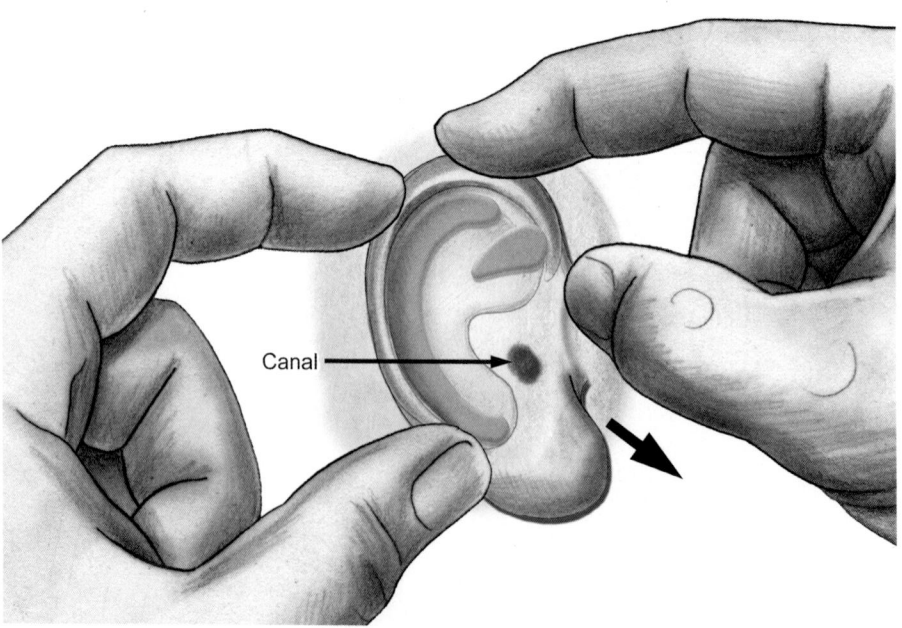

Canal

Figure 191.16 Maneuvering framework into proper position.

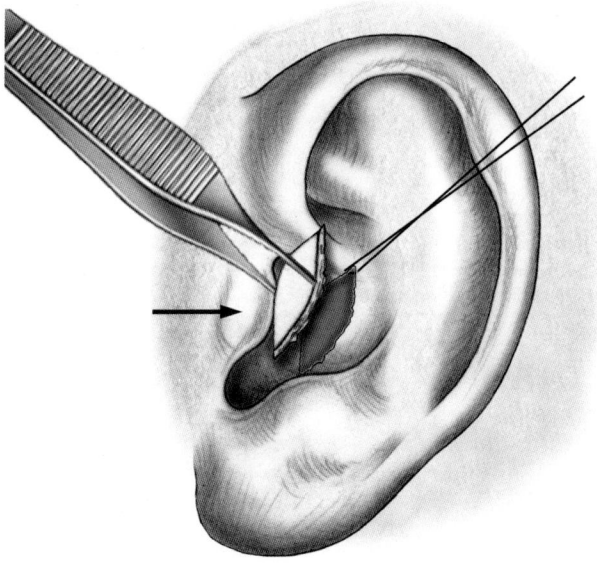

Figure 191.17 Harvesting composite graft.

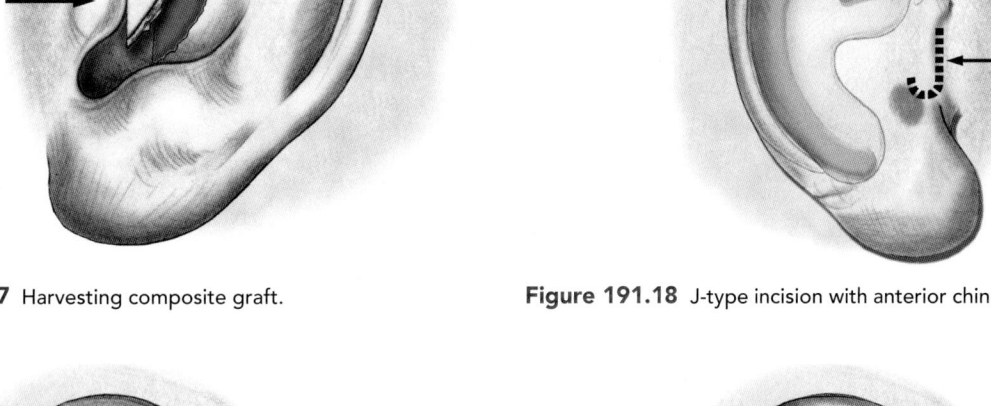

Figure 191.18 J-type incision with anterior chin elevation.

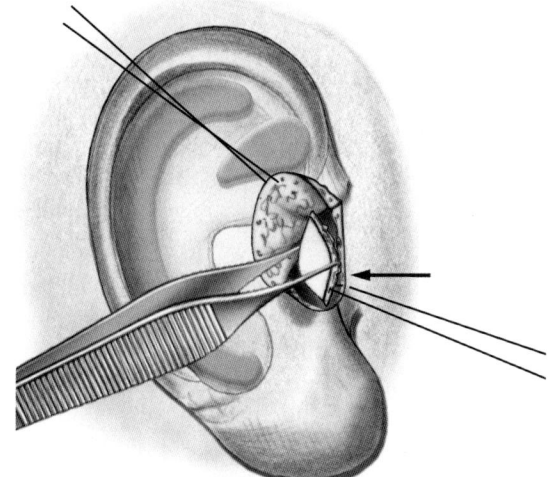

Figure 191.19 Placing composite graft and suturing anterior limb.

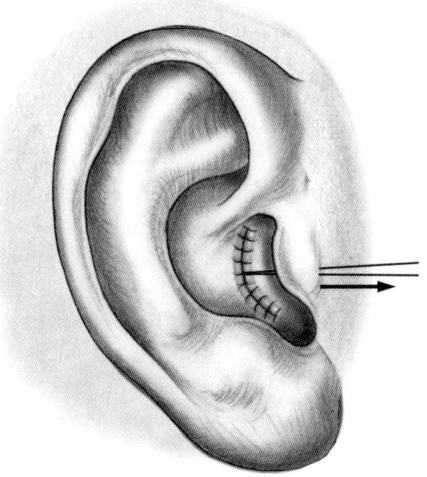

Figure 191.20 Pull-up suture in place with tension.

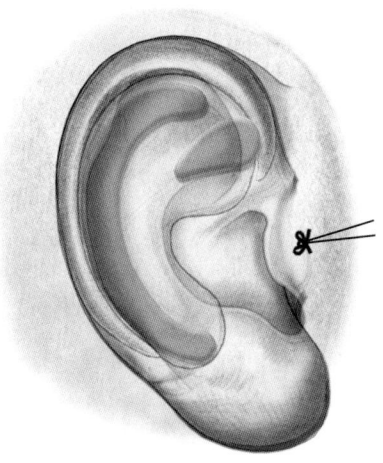

Figure 191.21 Thin graft in place posteriorly.

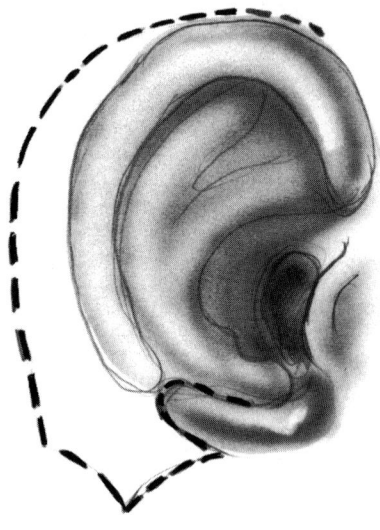

Figure 191.22 Incision in postauricular area.

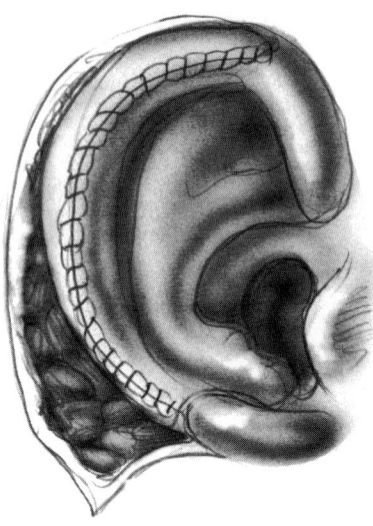

Figure 191.23 Elevating auricle and covering back with split-thickness skin graft.

The future of auricular reconstruction includes the ever-burgeoning field of tissue engineering. The nexus of cell growth biology and cell scaffolding technology is rapidly changing the landscape of surgical options. Many projects are being undertaken to develop biologic ear cartilage framework (26–29) for implantation. However, the technology still has to overcome issues such as tissue rejection and integrity of form. The use of autologous cartilage or synthetic implants will likely be the mainstay options for reconstruction in the foreseeable future. As with other components of the face, the ear is a very specialized structure and once reconstructed will never have the same properties as a native ear even in the best of hands. With the recent advances in composite tissue allotransplantation (30,31), it is possible that patients may receive an ear transplantation in the future for severe defects.

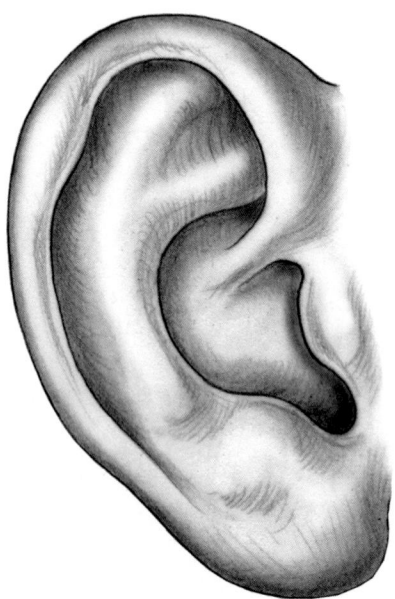

Figure 191.24 Reconstructed ear.

TABLE 191.6	**COMPLICATIONS CONGENITAL MALFORMATION OF THE AURICLE**

Skin necrosis overlying cartilage framework
Chondritis
Reabsorption
Malposition of auricle implant
Tissue breakdown of skin graft or of posterior aspect of ear
Keloiding of donor incision site or skin-graft areas

TABLE 191.7	**EMERGENCIES CONGENITAL MALFORMATION OF THE AURICLE**

Stage	Emergency
I	Pneumothorax, pneumomediastinum, severe skin necrosis
II	Lobule necrosis
III	None
IV and V	Chondritis

HIGHLIGHTS

- The decision to correct protruding ears is based on the angle of the auricle (greater than 30 degrees) and on other specific anatomic defects of the auricle.
- The helical rim should be 14 to 18 mm above the mastoid skin at the middle and superior thirds.
- The vertical axis of the auricle should be inclined approximately 20 degrees posteriorly.
- A detailed checklist is extremely helpful during the preoperative evaluation.
- The best age to perform the otoplasty surgery is 5 or 6 years.
- Mustardé sutures are horizontal mattress sutures used to create an antihelical fold.
- The Furnas technique must be used with caution. The conchal mastoid suture must be directed posteriorly to avoid narrowing the external auditory canal.
- The most feared complication is chondritis, which should be treated promptly with extensive antibiotic therapy.
- Each patient should be seen on the first day postoperatively to allow early intervention for hematoma or infection.
- Every patient and family should be informed of all risks and made aware that a second procedure may be required later (within a year).

- Every surgeon should learn multiple approaches to otoplasty to be able to offer each patient the best chance for success.
- Autogenous cartilage is best because there is no rejection and limited reabsorption.
- Materials such as Silastic and irradiated cartilage are less than satisfactory alternatives to autogenous cartilage.
- Auricular reconstruction should be performed before atresia repair to preserve the integrity of the skin and the blood supply. Atresia repair should be performed after the plastic surgery, because this allows for the movement of the framework to the proper site.
- Age 6 years is appropriate for unilateral microtia correction, both psychologically and anatomically.
- The framework can be maneuvered to align the meatus and the canal.
- The total reconstruction concept is important. A surgical team should be available to handle both the microtia and the atresia.
- For best results, there should be cooperation with the otologist in the staging of the repair.
- Surgeons performing auricular reconstruction should ensure that the cooperating otologist has completed the necessary audiologic evaluations.
- Each surgeon undertaking auricular reconstruction should be committed to this surgery, performing more than 5 to 10 operations per year.

REFERENCES

1. Gulya AJ. Developmental anatomy of the ear. In: Glascock ME III, Shambaugh GE Jr, eds. *Surgery of the ear*, 4th ed. Philadelphia, PA: WB Saunders, 1990.
2. Farkas LG. Anthropometry of normal and anomalous ears. *Clin Plast Surg* 1978;5:401.
3. Pitanguy I, Flemming I. Plastic operations on the auricle. In: Naumann HH, ed. *Head and neck surgery*. Philadelphia, PA: WB Saunders, 1982.
4. Eavey RD. Microtia and significant auricular malformation. Ninety-two pediatric patients. *Arch Otolaryngol Head Neck Surg* 1995;121:57–62.
5. Wang R. Presurgical confirmation of craniofacial implant locations in children requiring implant-retained auricular prosthesis. *J Prosthet Dent* 1999;81:492.
6. Gosain AK, Recinos RF. Otoplasty in children less than four years of age: surgical technique. *J Craniofac Surg* 2002;13(4):505–509.
7. Gosain AK, Kumar A, Huang G. Prominent ears in children younger than 4 years of age: what is the appropriate timing for otoplasty? *Plast Reconstr Surg* 2004;114(5):1042–1054.
8. Brent B. Hydrodissection as key to a natural-appearing otoplasty. *Plast Reconstr Surg* 2008;122(4):1055–1058.
9. Farrior RT. Modified cartilage incisions in otoplasty. *Facial Plast Surg* 1985;2:109.
10. Scharer SA, Farrior EH, Farrior RT. Retrospective analysis of the Farrior technique for otoplasty. *Arch Facial Plast Surg* 2007;9:167–173.
11. Werdin F, Wolter M, Lampe H. Pitanguy's otoplasty: report of 551 operations. *Scand J Plast Reconstr Surg Hand Surg* 2007;41:283–287.
12. Tanzer RC. Total reconstruction of the external ear. *Plast Reconstr Surg* 1959;23:1.
13. Tanzer RC. Correction of microtia with autogenous costal cartilage. In: Tanzer R, Edgerton M, eds. *Symposium on reconstruction of the auricle*. Vol. 10. St. Louis, MO: CV Mosby, 1974.
14. Cronin TD. Use of a Silastic frame for total and subtotal reconstruction of the external ear: preliminary report. *Plast Reconstr Surg* 1966;37:399.
15. Brent B. Ear reconstruction with an expansible framework of autogenous rib cartilage. *Plast Reconstr Surg* 1974;53:619.
16. Aguilar EA III, Jahrsdoerfer RA. The surgical repair of congenital microtia and atresia. *Arch Otolaryngol Head Neck Surg* 1988;98:600.
17. Aguilar EA III. Auricular reconstruction of congenital microtia (grade III). *Laryngoscope* 1996;106(Suppl 82):1–26.
18. Rogers B. Anatomy, embryology and classification of auricular deformities. In: Tanzer R, Edgerton M, eds. *Symposium on reconstruction of the auricle*. Vol. 10. St. Louis, MO: CV Mosby, 1974.
19. Tanzer RC. Congenital deformities. In: Converse JM, ed. *Reconstructive plastic surgery*, 2nd ed. Vol. 3. Philadelphia, PA: WB Saunders, 1977.
20. Weerda H. Classification of congenital deformities of the auricle. *Facial Plast Surg* 1988;5:385.
21. Rogers B. Microtic, lop, cup and protruding ears. *Plast Reconstr Surg* 1968;41:208.
22. Aguilar EA III. Classification of auricular congenital deformities. In: Papel ID, Nachlas NE, eds. *Facial plastic and reconstructive surgery*. St. Louis, MO: Mosby Year Book, 1992.
23. Williams JD, et al. Polyethylene implants in auricular reconstruction. *Arch Otolaryngol Head Neck Surg* 1997;123:578.
24. Somers HT. Politzer Meeting Abstract. St. Augustinus Hospital, University of Antwerp, April 17, 2000.
25. Brent B. Auricular repair with autogenous rib cartilage grafts: two decades of experience with 600 cases. *Plast Reconstr Surg* 1992;90:355–374.
26. Christophel JJ, Chang JS, Park SS. Transplanted tissue-engineering cartilage. *Arch Facial Plast Surg* 2006;8:117–122.
27. Kamil SH, Vacanti MP, Aminuddin BS, et al. Tissue engineering of a human sized and shaped auricle using a mold. *Laryngoscope* 2004;114:867–870.
28. Kamil SH Vacanti MP, Vacanti CA, et al. Microtia chondrocytes as a donor source for tissue-engineered cartilage. *Laryngoscope* 2004;114:2187–2190.
29. Ruszymah BH, Chua KH, Maziyzam AL, et al. Formation of tissue engineered composite construct of cartilage and skin using high density polyethylene as inner scaffold in the shape of human helix. *Int J Pediatr Otorhinolaryngol* 2011;75(6):805–810.
30. Tobin GR, Breidenbach WC III, Pidwell DJ, et al. Transplantation of the hand, face, and composite structures: evolution and current status. *Clin Plast Surg* 2007;34(2)271–278, ix–x.
31. Siemionow MZ, Kulahci Y, Bozkurt M. Composite tissue allotransplantation. *Plast Reconstr Surg* 2009;124(6 Suppl):e327–e339.

192 | Chin Augmentation

Jonathan M. Sykes   *Christina K. Magill*

The chin prominence is not present in any four-legged mammal (1). During evolution, with the adoption of an upright posture and with verticalization of the face, the chin became an important facial feature. The events contributing to the evolutionary development of the chin in humans are open to speculation; however, the importance of the chin in the overall appearance of the face cannot be overstated (2).

Facial beauty arises from symmetry and balanced proportion of all facial features. Although standards of facial beauty are often determined by social media and are time-adjusted, certain elegant features are not affected by time trends. A strong and well-projected chin is one of those features. For this reason, it is not surprising that no United States president has ever had a weak chin. A strong chin helps support the soft tissues of the lower face, and a well-projected chin improves the cervical skin and contributes to a well-defined cervicomental angle (3).

It is important to analyze the chin in three dimensions in order to determine if the deformity is horizontal, vertical, or related to transverse discrepancy or asymmetry (4). Surgical correction of aesthetic deformities of the chin can be performed either by chin augmentation with an implant or by osteotomy and advancement (or reduction) of the bony mentum (5). Simple horizontal deficiencies are often easily corrected with alloplasts. More complex problems of the mentum, such as transverse asymmetry or significant vertical dysmorphia, usually require bony osteotomy of the mentum (genioplasty) with repositioning of the chin into a more ideal three-dimensional position. This chapter outlines the pertinent anatomy and classification of chin deformities and describes an algorithm for correction of these problems.

PATIENT EVALUATION

Careful analysis of the face and chin is important in order to choose and execute the correct procedure. Specifically, the chin should be evaluated as it relates to other skeletal and soft tissue structures, including the lips, teeth, nose, and soft tissues of the neck. A detailed history of past trauma, orthodontic treatment, or prior oral surgery is essential. This is important because many patients with dental malocclusion and underlying facial skeletal abnormalities are treated with orthodontics. Orthodontic therapy may correct the malocclusion, but does not address the underlying facial skeletal deformity (Fig. 192.1). It is also important to identify any past dental extractions, as these can impact future surgical decisions. Lastly, it is important to identify and discuss any temporomandibular joint dysfunction (TMD). Although chin surgery does not directly affect the occlusion, any significant TMD can alter the decision to perform mentoplasty.

Physical examination of the chin should include inspection and palpation of the chin itself and of the adjacent structures such as the lips, teeth, and nose (6). The entire face should be observed at rest and during animation to evaluate the mentalis soft tissue mound and its support. In many patients with either horizontal or vertical microgenia, the mentalis muscle hypertrophies in an effort to create lip competence (7). Overworking of the mentalis muscle causes dimpling of the chin and is referred to as "mentalis strain" (Fig. 192.2). This condition is often associated with open bite deformities and/or microgenia.

Evaluation of patients being considered for chin surgery should include three-dimensional analysis of the chin: (a) vertical (superior–inferior), (b) horizontal (anterior–posterior), and (c) transverse. Analysis should consist of systematic inspection, clinical photographs, and possible radiographic examination (8).

The evaluation of all patients for possible chin surgery should include consistent and reproducible clinical photographs in three views: AP (frontal), lateral (profile), and oblique. These photographs allow analysis of the contour and projection of the chin as it relates to the lips, nose,

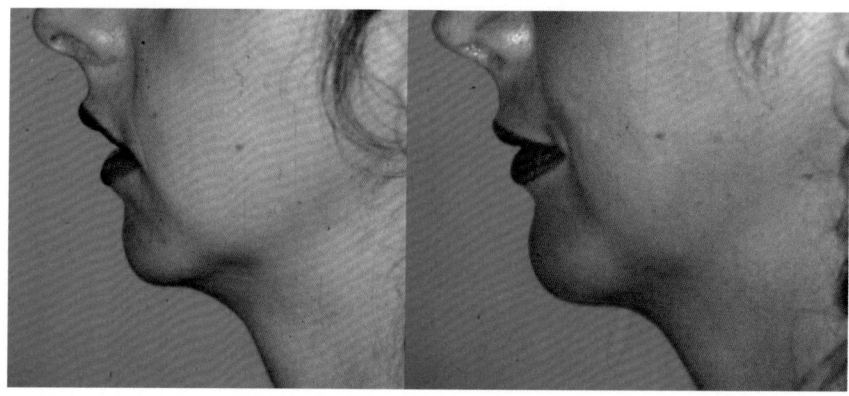

Figure 192.1 **Left:** Lateral photograph of a 23-year-old patient who underwent orthodontic therapy as an adolescent. The patient's occlusion was class I, but the skeletal chin deficiency remained. **Right:** Postoperative image of the patient after chin augmentation with alloplast.

labiomental groove, and soft tissues of the neck. If the physical evaluation and clinical photographs show a minor deformity requiring augmentation with an alloplast, radiographs of the chin are usually not necessary. However, if the deformity is more complex (e.g., vertical chin excess with horizontal deficiency or transverse bony asymmetry), radiographic analysis is essential.

Radiographic evaluation of the chin routinely includes a panoramic radiograph (Panorex) (Fig. 192.3) and cephalometric radiographs in the AP and lateral views (Fig. 192.4A and B). The panoramic radiograph shows the cortical outline of the mandible and the vertical mandibular height. The Panorex also delineates the position of the tooth roots and of the inferior alveolar canals and mental foramina. It is important to know the exact position of the mental foramen and canal preoperatively so intraoperative damage to the mental nerve can be prevented (9). The inferior alveolar nerve, a branch of the third division of the fifth (trigeminal) cranial nerve, travels through the mandibular canal and exits the mental foramen as the mental nerve (10). The mental nerve supplies sensation to the skin and mucous membranes of the lower lip and chin. The mandibular canal is often located 2 to 3 mm below the level

of the mental foramen. Bony osteotomies should therefore be performed at least 5 mm below the mental foramen to avoid injury to the neurovascular bundle.

If orthognathic surgery is considered with bony genioplasty, AP and lateral cephalometric radiographs should be performed. These radiographs allow analysis of skeletal and soft tissue key points, which can be used to predict bony movements after skeletal surgery. The AP cephalometric radiograph allows identification of transverse asymmetries of the chin. Transverse asymmetry of the chin may be associated with more global facial asymmetry (hemifacial microsomia) or with a syndrome such as oculoauricular vertebral (OAV) spectrum, or may be isolated (Fig. 192.5). It is very important to identify chin asymmetries and discuss them with the patient preoperatively. If chin augmentation is performed with an alloplast implant and the asymmetry is not considered, the asymmetry may be magnified.

Lateral cephalometric radiographs provide a soft tissue and skeletal profile upon which key landmarks can be recognized. The radiograph is with the patient's head being stabilized with a headholder in a fixed position at a fixed distance from the radiograph machine (Fig. 192.6).

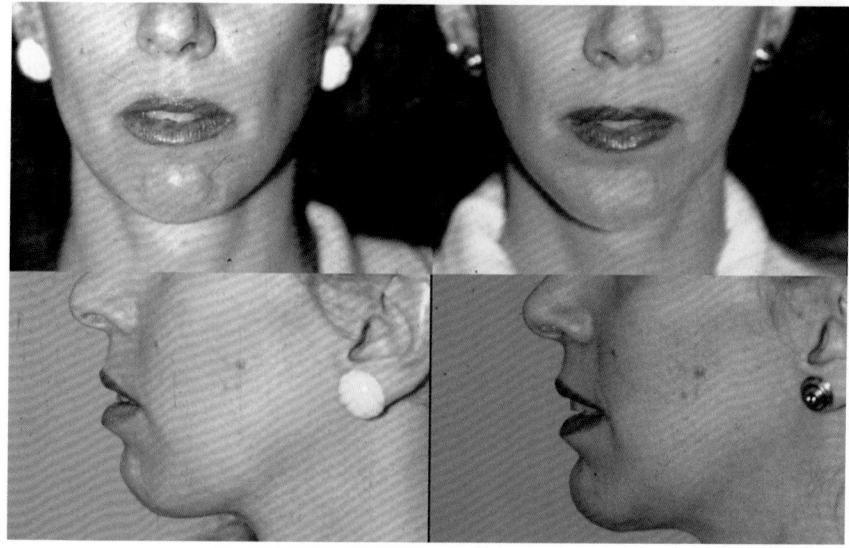

Figure 192.2 **Upper left:** A preoperative frontal photograph of a woman with mentalis muscle strain secondary to microgenia. **Lower left:** A lateral preoperative view is shown. **Upper right:** A frontal postoperative view is shown. The patient has undergone a chin augmentation with an alloplast with resolution of the mentalis strain. **Lower right:** A lateral view of the postoperative result is shown.

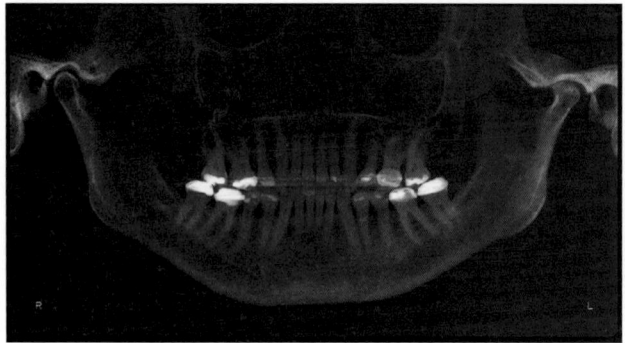

Figure 192.3 A panoramic radiograph is shown.

The head is stabilized with the Frankfort horizontal (from the porion [the superior aspect of the external auditory canal] to the infraorbitale [the inferior orbital rim]) being parallel to the ground. The standardized radiograph produced allows identification of a series of bony and soft tissue landmarks from which various facial analyses can be performed.

The facial analyses created from the lateral cephalometric radiograph produce a two-dimensional prediction of the new postoperative chin position. Various analyses have been described including Ricketts, Burstone, Gonzalez-Ulloa and Stevens, and others. Each of these evaluation methods has positive and negative aspects. The Ricketts analysis, for instance, uses a tangent connecting the soft tissue pogonion (most projecting point) of the chin with the most projecting point of the nasal tip (Fig. 192.7). In this system, the upper lip should lie about 4 mm behind the line, whereas the lower lip is ideally located 2 mm behind the line. While the Ricketts analysis correctly evaluates the lower face in profile, it places great importance on the projection of the nasal tip. The Steiner analysis uses the columellar inflection point ("S") to identify the correct position for the chin point (8). This method places importance on the lip position. The Holdaway "H" angle relates the position of the soft tissue pogonion with important skeletal points on the mid and lower face. No single analysis is ideal, but each method attempts to determine the "ideal" positions for the soft tissues and skeleton of the chin because these structures relate to the remainder of the face.

The aesthetic unit of the chin and upper and lower lips should occupy one-third of the vertical facial height (Fig. 192.8). The lower facial third height can be obtained by measuring the distance between the soft tissue *subnasale* and the soft tissue *gnathion*. If this distance is greater than one-third of the overall facial height, vertical macrogenia exists. If the distance is less than one-third of the facial height, vertical microgenia can be diagnosed. The lower facial third can be further subdivided into subunits that will indicate specifically from where the increase or decrease in vertical height originates. Two methods exist for subdivision of lower facial heights (Fig. 192.9). The first includes a vertical third from *subnasale* to *upper lip stomion* and two thirds from *upper lip stomion* to the *menton*. The second method divides the lower third into two equal parts, from the *subnasale* to the *vermilion border of the lower lip* and from the *lower lip vermilion border* to the *gnathion*. All of these analyses relate the height of the chin and lower face to the total facial height. In complex chin deformities, a vertical discrepancy as well as a horizontal deficiency or excess may often be present (Fig. 192.10).

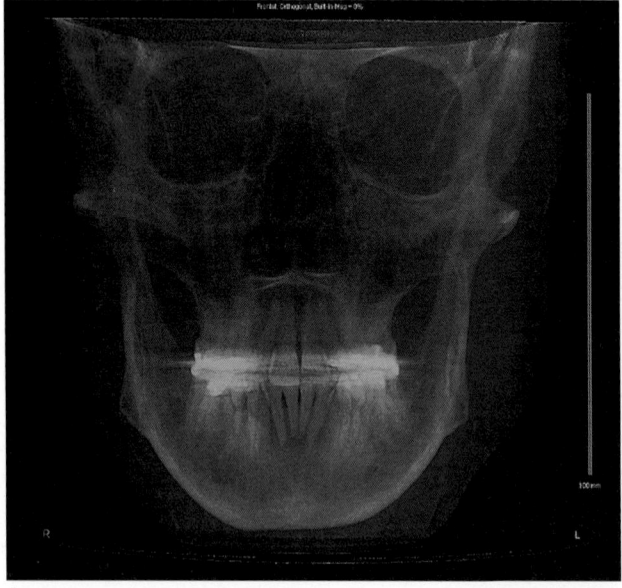

A

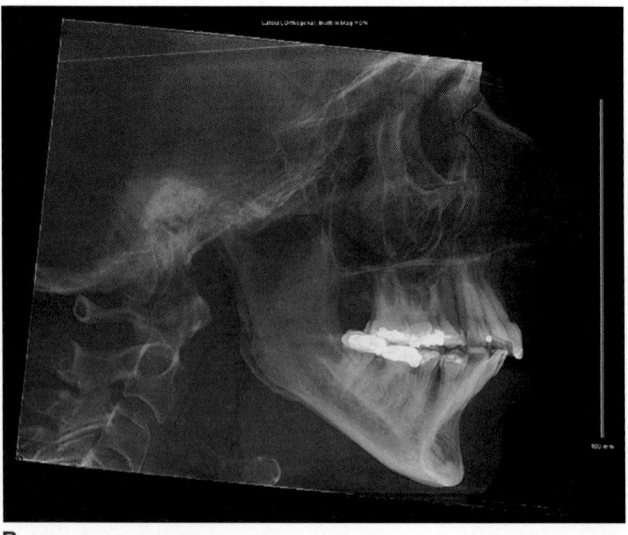

B

Figure 192.4 **A:** A frontal cephalometric radiograph is shown. **B:** A lateral cephalometric radiograph is shown.

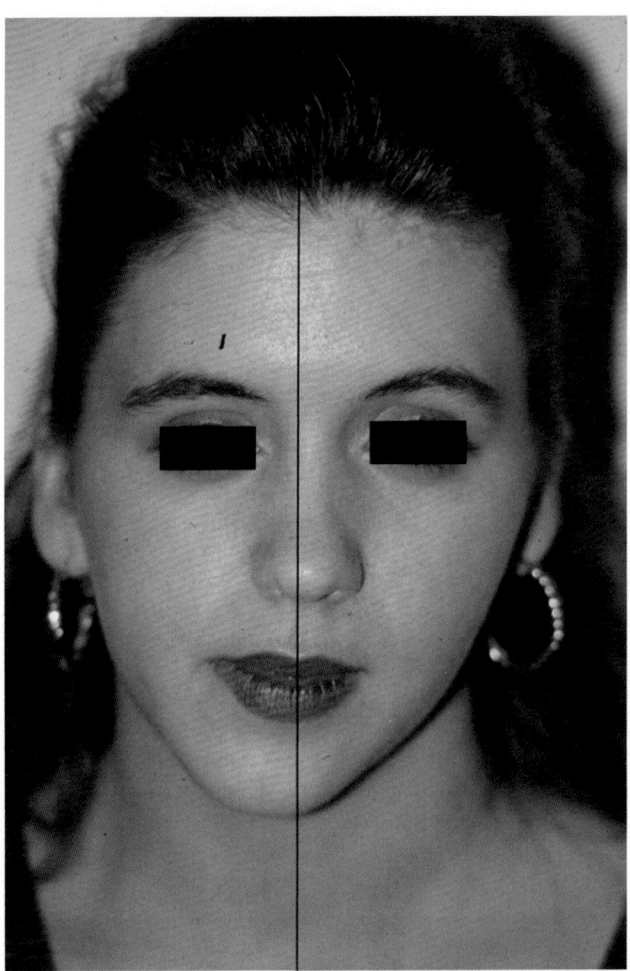

Figure 192.5 Photograph of a 25-year-old female with hemifacial microsomia. A vertical line has been drawn through the center of cupid's bow of the upper lip, demonstrating how the chin deviates to the affected smaller facial side.

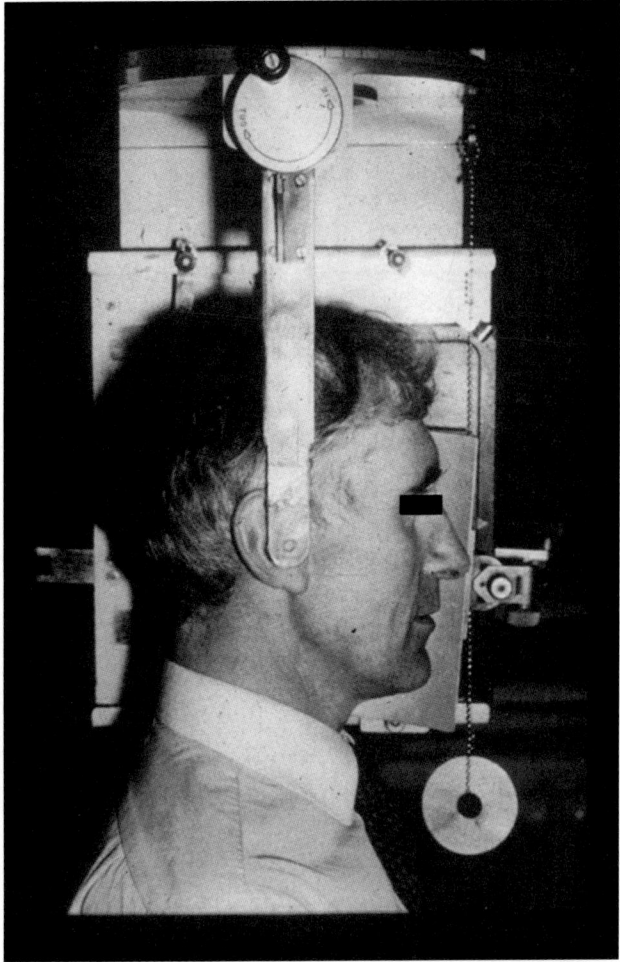

Figure 192.6 A patient in a cephalostat is shown (fixed head holder).

Another parameter that must be analyzed is the transverse dimension of the chin. The transverse dimension can be measured by chin width. The chin can be wide or narrow, and, if asymmetry exists, the midline of the chin may not be aligned with the skeletal midline of the remainder of the face. Transverse asymmetries of the chin exist in many patients with congenital anomalies, such as hemifacial microsomia or OAV spectrum. This congenital malformation is often associated with unequal lengths of the mandibular bodies. In patients with this anomaly, the chin midpoint usually points to the shorter mandibular side (and the smaller side of the face). If a symmetric chin implant is used in a patient with horizontal chin deficiency and transverse asymmetry, the horizontal deficiency may be corrected, but the chin asymmetry may be accentuated. AP cephalometric radiographs allow a comparison of the bony midline of the chin with the dental midlines of the maxilla and the mandible. If the skeletal and soft tissue midline of the chin are not aligned with the dental midlines and with the upper facial skeletal

midline (e.g., nasion), an asymmetric bony genioplasty or chin implant can be performed.

Evaluation of the chin requires careful analysis of both the bony architecture and the soft tissues. Clinical photographs allow evaluation of the soft tissues. Radiographs allow various bony analyses, which enable the surgeon to choose the approach and technique to camouflage, minimize, or correct the deformity. No single analysis precisely identifies every deformity, and no one procedure corrects every chin defect. The surgeon should use a combination of methods to evaluate the chin.

Classification of Chin Deformities

Deformities of the chin and lower face may be related to either bony abnormalities or soft tissue malposition. The chin should be analyzed in all three planes of space: horizontal (AP), vertical (superior–inferior), and transverse. The horizontal and vertical dimensions can each be deficient, normal, or excessive (11). Simple deformities such as

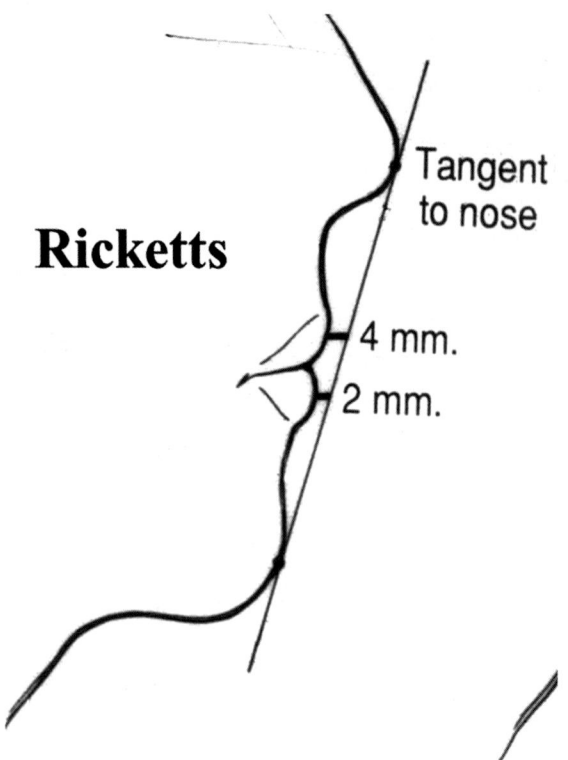

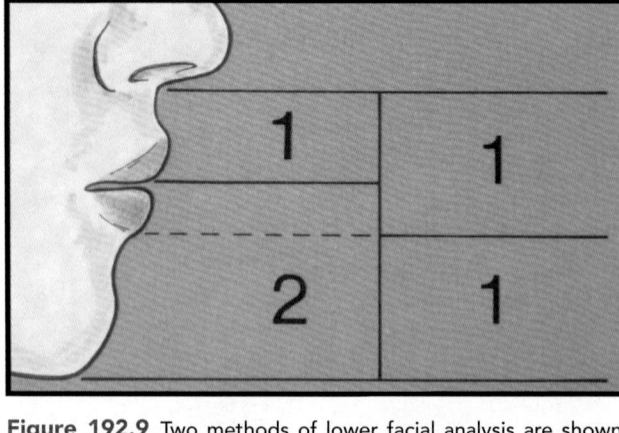

Figure 192.9 Two methods of lower facial analysis are shown: (*1*) The lower face can be divided by a 1/3 ratio from the subnasale to the stomion. The remaining 2/3 of the lower face is drawn from the stomion to the gnathion. (*2*) The lower face is divided into an upper half from the subnasale to the lower lip vermilion cutaneous junction, and a lower half spanning from the vermilion cutaneous junction to the gnathion.

Figure 192.7 Line drawing of the Ricketts analysis showing a tangent between the nasal tip and the most anterior projecting point (pogonion).

mild horizontal chin deficiency (*microgenia*) are easily corrected using either an implant or bony advancement. More complex deformities, such as in a patient with horizontal deficiency and vertical excess, usually require horizontal osteotomy for adequate correction.

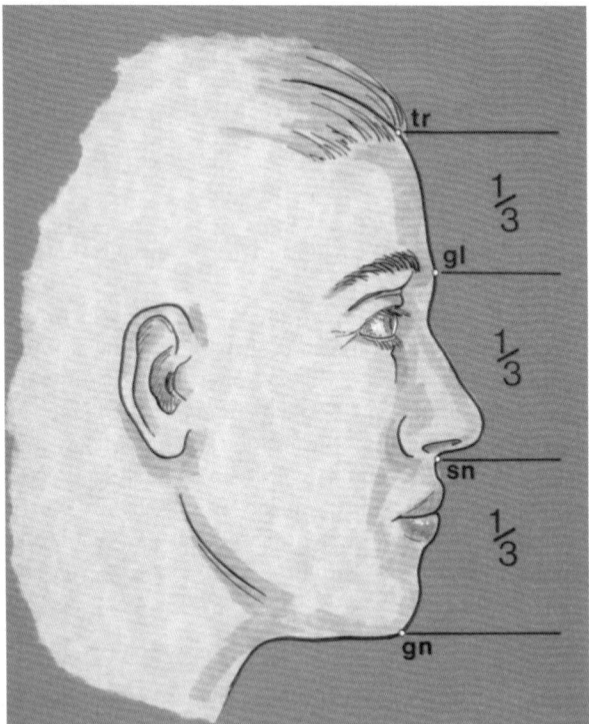

Figure 192.8 A line drawing illustrates the divisions of the face into thirds. The upper third is drawn from the trichion (tr) to the glabella (gl). The middle third is drawn from the glabella to the subnasale (sn). The lower third is drawn from the subnasale to the gnathion (gn).

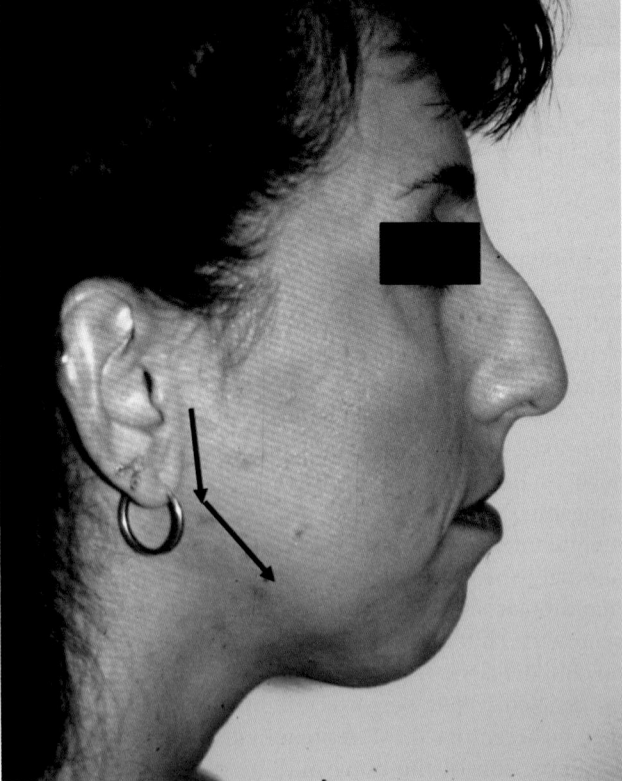

Figure 192.10 A lateral photograph of a patient is shown demonstrating vertical chin height excess and horizontal chin height deficiency.

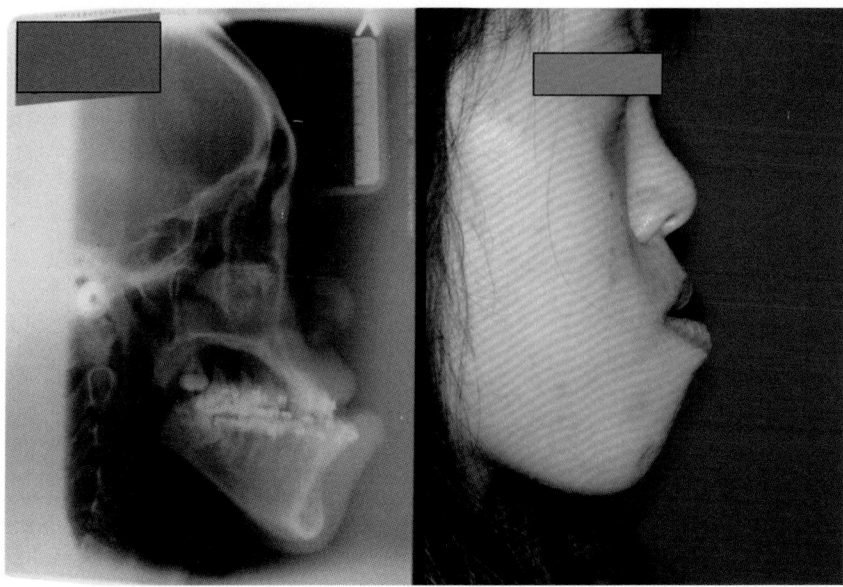

Figure 192.11 Lateral cephalometric radiograph and lateral photograph of a patient with significant vertical macrogenia and mandibular prognathia.

Horizontal chin deficiency is often associated with a small or posteriorly positioned mandible (*retrognathia*) or may involve only a small chin (*microgenia*). Patients with retrognathia often have associated class II malocclusion. Horizontal chin excess is often associated with a large or anteriorly positioned mandible (*prognathia*) or may involve a large mentum only (*macrogenia*) (Fig. 192.11). Patients with mandibular prognathia often have class III malocclusion.

Soft tissue deformities of the chin and submental region also exist. Ptosis of the soft tissues of the chin often accompanies other signs of facial aging. This condition, commonly called witch's chin or senile chin deformity, is caused by a weakening of the muscular attachments of the mentalis and depressor labii inferioris muscles. In this deformity, the soft tissue pad of the chin falls below the mandibular line, and a deep horizontal crease develops in the submental region. Descent of the soft tissue chin pad is accentuated with smiling. This deformity can be inadvertently created or worsened surgically if the mentalis muscles are not reapproximated while inserting a chin implant.

Selection of Procedure

Various procedures exist for correcting aesthetic chin deformities. These include placement of an alloplast, osteotomy and repositioning of the bony mentum (genioplasty), and repositioning of the soft tissues of the chin (12,13). The selection of the best procedure to correct a given deformity of the chin should be based on the type and extent of the deformity.

In patients with horizontal chin deficiency (microgenia), augmentation with an alloplast implant is a simple and effective method to increase chin projection and enhance the profile. In more complex deficiencies, including patients with suboptimal vertical chin height

or transverse asymmetries, alloplasts are less effective and often do not entirely correct the three-dimensional deformity. In cases of horizontal deficiency and vertical excess (patients with a steep mandibular plane), a chin implant may correct the horizontal deficiency, but exacerbate the vertical excess. For these reasons, implant augmentation is an effective method of camouflage for minor chin deformities, but may not be satisfactory for complex deformities.

Osteotomy of the bony mentum (osseous genioplasty) is a versatile and reliable procedure for correcting a variety of skeletal chin deformities. First described by Hofer in 1942, this technique involves horizontal osteotomy and downfracture of the chin, with repositioning and fixation of the distal segment. Osseous genioplasty allows advancement or retrusion in the AP direction as well as lengthening or shortening in the vertical direction. Additionally, the genioplasty procedure provides an approach for correction of transverse asymmetries of the chin. Although customized chin implants can be made to correct chin asymmetries, preformed implants are usually symmetrical.

Correction of soft tissue ptosis has been described. The technique involves the removal of an ellipse of submental skin, creation of a flap of chin soft tissue, and advancement and plication of the soft tissue flap inferiorly. This technique tightens the soft tissue pad and obliterates the horizontal submental crease. However, the soft tissue pogonion is effectively moved posteriorly, and some form of simultaneous augmentation (implant or bony advancement) is usually required.

Surgical Procedures

Chin Augmentation with Alloplast Implant
Placement of a chin implant may be easily performed through either an intraoral or a submental approach. If other

central neck procedures, such as submental liposuction, are being performed simultaneously, a submental incision provides access to both the central neck and the mentum. Additionally, either general anesthesia or local anesthesia with intravenous sedation may be used in placement of an alloplast chin implant.

Prior to anesthetizing the chin, the midline soft tissues of the lip, chin, and thyroid cartilage are marked to ensure midline placement of the implant. Infiltration of the soft tissues of the chin with Xylocaine 1% with 1:100,000 epinephrine is then performed to obtain anesthesia and vasoconstriction. It is important to avoid overinflation and distortion of the soft tissues of the chin with local anesthetic. After anesthetic infiltration, the entire face is prepped and draped.

Placement of a chin implant can be performed through an intraoral or submental approach. A submental approach is often used as this approach allows access to the anterior neck for liposuction and/or platysmaplasty. If a neck procedure is being performed, the neck will be completed prior to definitive placement of the chin implant.

A 2-cm incision is made just inferior to the submental crease (Fig. 192.12). The incision is placed in this area to avoid exposing the scar after the stretching of the soft tissues that naturally occurs after implant placement. Sharp dissection is performed through the inferior chin soft tissues and

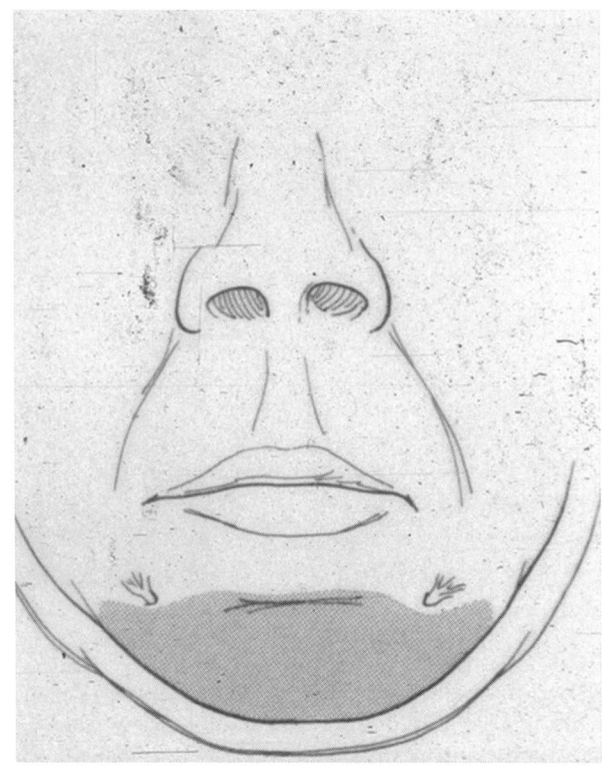

Figure 192.13 The area over the mandible that is shaded illustrates the extent of undermining performed for chin implant placement.

the mentalis muscle (Fig. 192.13). The periosteum is left over the central mentum. Two vertical incisions are made through the periosteum 2 cm lateral to the midline. Bilateral subperiosteal dissections are performed to allow placement of the lateral wings of the implant (Fig. 192.14). The advantage of placing an implant beneath the periosteum is

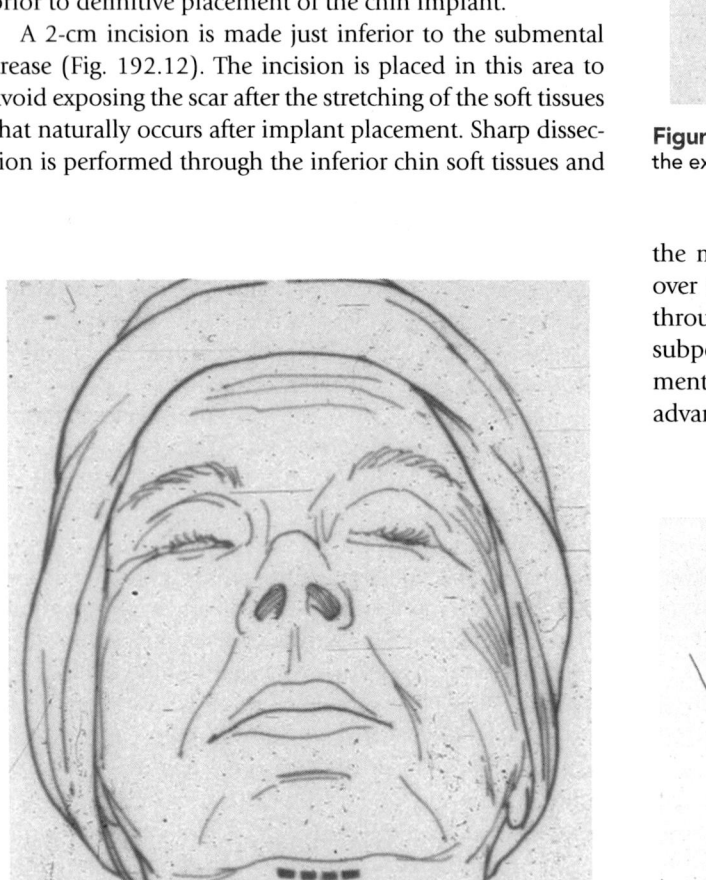

Figure 192.12 Schematic diagram of submental incision.

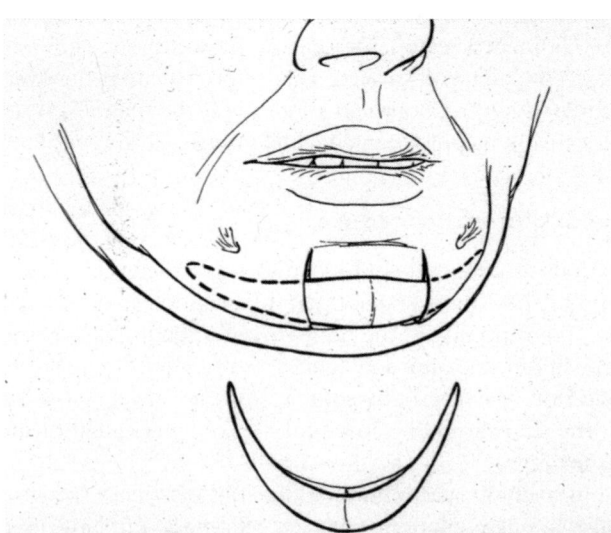

Figure 192.14 Placement of a chin implant is shown with the lateral phalanges lying deep to the periosteum and the middle portion of the implant in the supraperiosteal plane.

improved fixation of the implant. However, subperiosteal placement has been shown to result in some erosion of the anterior mandible. For these reasons, most surgeons advocate dissection in the supraperiosteal plane centrally, with subperiosteal placement laterally. This will theoretically minimize mandibular erosion, while maximally fixing the implant. The subperiosteal dissection is accomplished inferior to the mental foramina to avoid injury to the mental nerves. The size and exact location of the implant pocket created is crucial and often determines the success of the procedure. If the implant pocket is too small, the implant can deform, create irregular contours, or not adhere to the underlying bony mentum. If the pocket is too large, the implant may migrate from the desired midline location and heal in an improper position.

The type, shape, and size of the chin implant used is based on physician preference and individual patient anatomical variation. Common implants used for chin augmentation include expanded polytetrafluoroethylene, silastic (solid silicone), high-density polyethylene (Medpor), and various meshed materials (Mersilene). The implant used should be biocompatible and able to contour well to the underlying mandible curvature. The style of the implants used includes narrow "button" implants and extended or anatomical implants. Extended implants have the advantage of not being as apparent if 1 to 2 mm of displacement occurs. Smaller, central implants are more obvious if slight postoperative displacement of the implant occurs. Additionally, an extended implant is preferred over a narrower, button-style implant, as the wider profile of the extended implant achieves fullness in the pre-jowl region in addition to increasing the projection of the central mentum. A lack of fullness in the pre-jowl region often contributes to an aged or tired look, and augmenting this region helps rejuvenate the lower face.

The size of the implant used is related to the patient's individual chin shape and size. In general, chin augmentation is used to balance the appearance of the lower facial third in relation to the remainder of the face. Prior to placing the actual implant, a "sizer" can be placed into the created pocket and the skin redraped (Fig. 192.15). This maneuver allows the surgeon to determine if the proper size implant has been placed and the appropriate augmentation achieved. Once the proper implant size is chosen, the implant is soaked in antibiotic solution and placed into the prepared pocket.

After placement of the implant, the mentalis muscles should be reapproximated and the soft tissue resuspended meticulously. If the mentalis muscle is not carefully realigned, postoperative ptosis of the soft tissues of the chin may occur. Closure of the mentalis muscle is performed with a No. 4-0 braided absorbable suture. The subcutaneous tissues and dermis are reapproximated with a No. 5-0 chromic suture, followed by skin closure with an interrupted No. 6-0 monofilament nonabsorbable suture (Fig. 192.16A

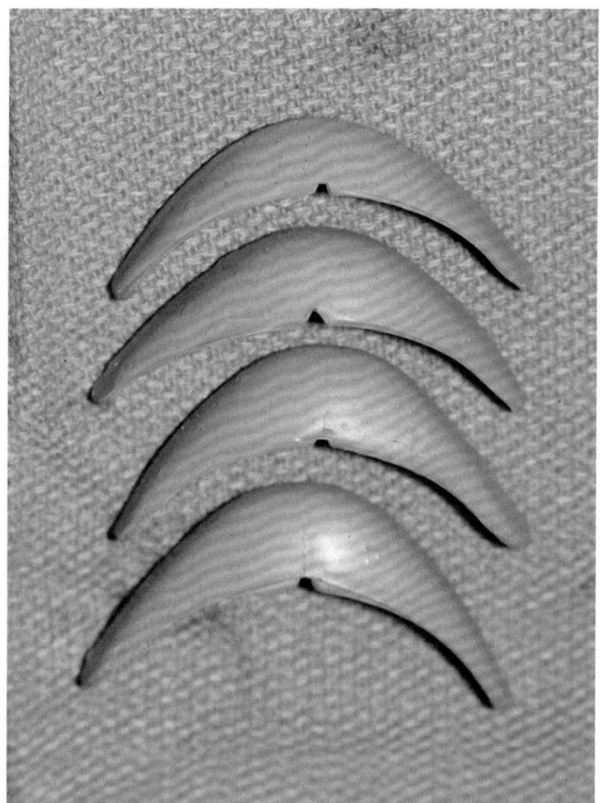

Figure 192.15 Typical size of an extended chin implant with small, medium, large, and extra-large sizes. The photograph shown is of implant sizers (*blue in color*).

and B). A secure chin strap dressing is placed for 3 days to ensure immobility of the implant. Perioperative antibiotics are used for 48 hours.

If an intraoral approach is used, the gingivolabial incision can be either horizontal or vertical. In either case, dissection through the mentalis muscles again occurs with placement of the implant in a supraperiosteal plane centrally and a subperiosteal pocket laterally. Closure is accomplished in two layers with the muscle closure achieving soft tissue resuspension. A chin strap dressing is used for 3 days to secure the position of the implant.

Osseous Genioplasty

First described in 1942 by Hofer, and then popularized by Converse and Wood-Smith in 1964, osseous genioplasty has been developed as a versatile technique in correction of both deficient and excessive chin deformities. Genioplasty can be performed under general anesthesia or intravenous sedation with mentalis nerve block. If general anesthesia is used, nasotracheal intubation is preferred; however, if rhinoplasty is to be performed with the genioplasty, orotracheal intubation should be used.

An intraoral approach is used with a gingivolabial incision from one canine tooth to the other (Fig. 192.17). The incision is made on the labial side of the gingivolabial

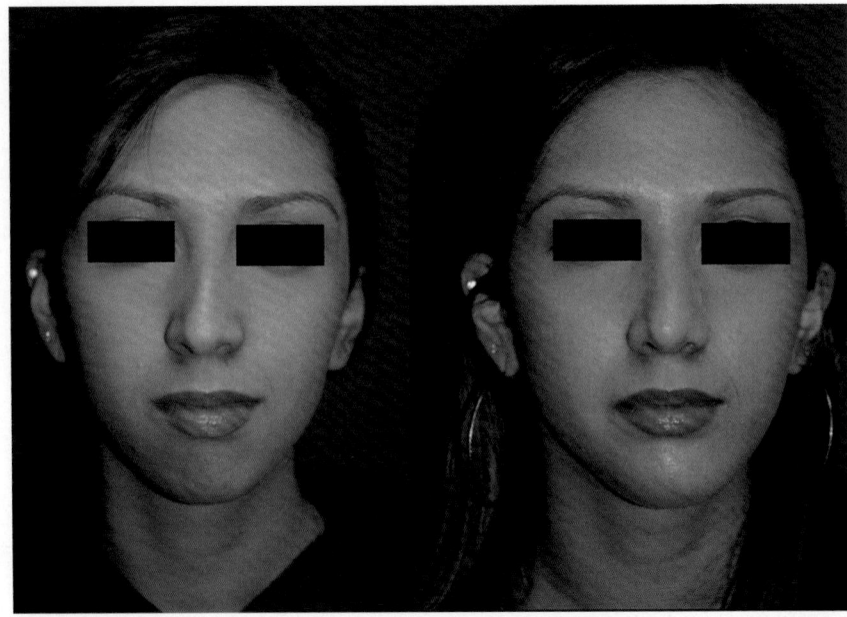

A

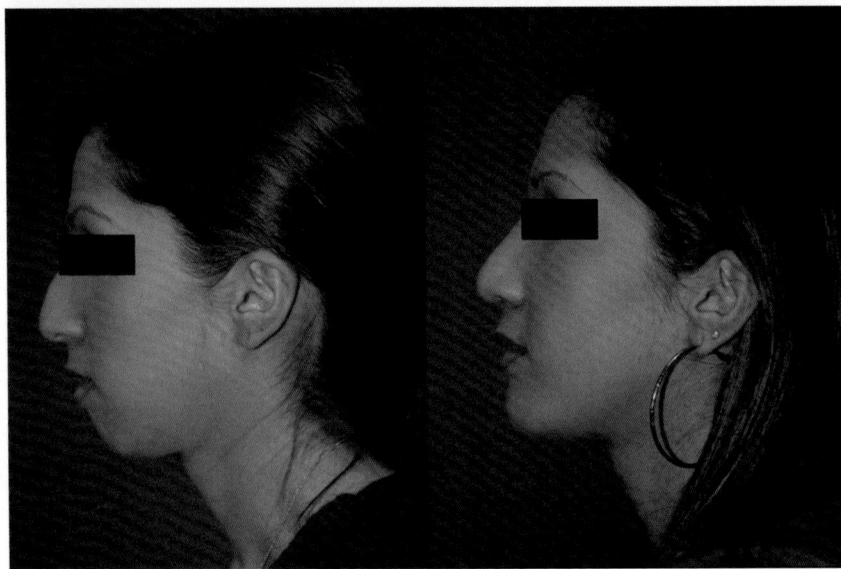

Figure 192.16 A: Frontal photographs of a patient who underwent a chin implant and rhinoplasty. **B:** Lateral preoperative and postoperative photographs of a patient who underwent a chin implant and rhinoplasty.

B

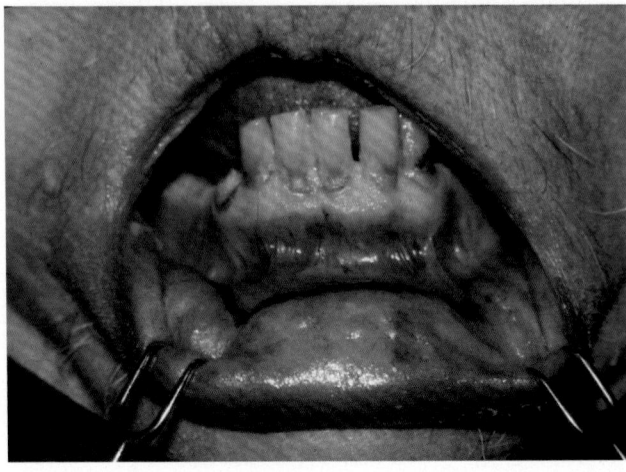

Figure 192.17 An intraoral incision is marked in the gingivolabial mucosa of a cadaver.

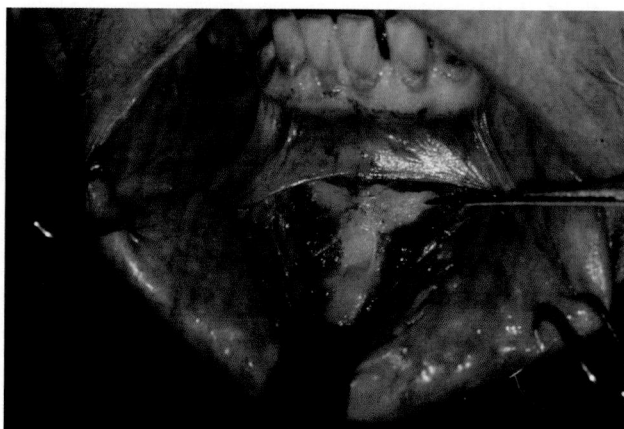

Figure 192.18 A dissection through the mentalis muscle and down to periosteum is shown in preparation for genioplasty.

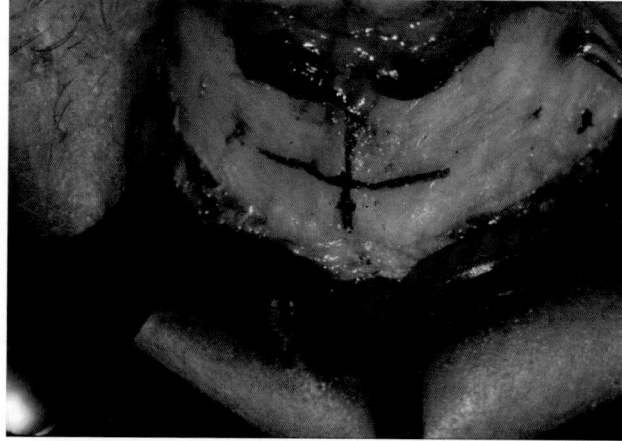

Figure 192.20 Cadaveric dissection showing vertical marking of the midline to facilitate realignment after chin repositioning.

sulcus to allow an adequate mucoperiosteal soft tissue cuff for wound closure. Sharp dissection is performed directly through the mentalis muscle and mandibular periosteum (Fig. 192.18). A subperiosteal dissection is then performed with exposure of both mental nerves (Fig. 192.19). A small inferior segment of soft tissue is preserved over the central segment (bony mentum) of the mandible to provide vascular supply to the distal segment after osteotomy.

After the lateral subperiosteal dissection is completed, the proposed osteotomy is carefully measured and marked. The bony midline is vertically inscribed with a side-cutting burr to allow the proximal and distal segments to be precisely aligned after osteotomy and repositioning (Fig. 192.20). The osteotomy site is then measured and marked with calipers to ensure a symmetrical osteotomy (Fig. 192.21A and B). The horizontal osteotomy should be placed below the level of the tooth roots to prevent dental injury (Fig. 192.22).

The change created by bony osteotomy and repositioning of the chin should be determined by careful preoperative analysis. The chin can be vertically lengthened or shortened, horizontally advanced or retruded, or rotated

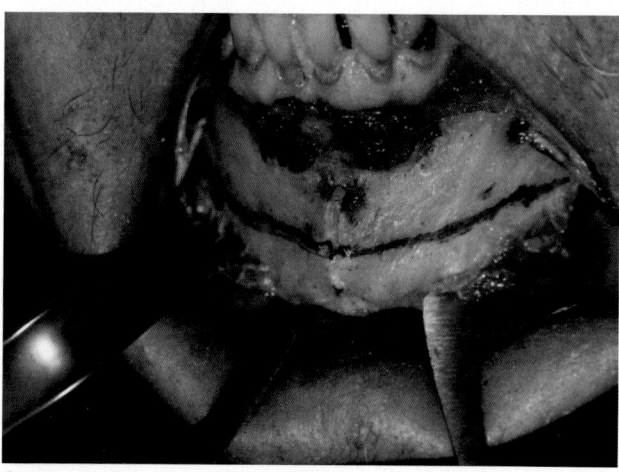

A

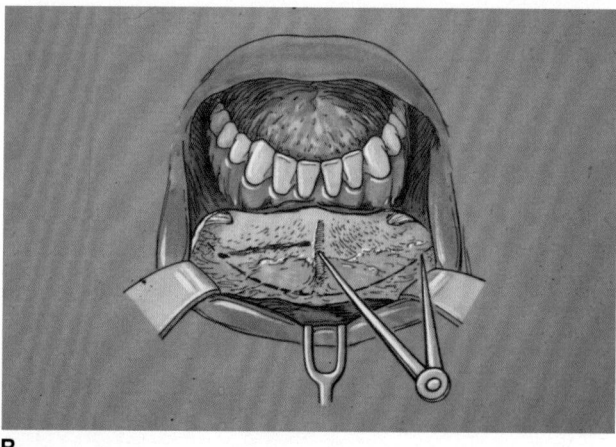

B

Figure 192.21 **A:** Cadaveric dissection showing a horizontal marking at the level of the planned osteotomy. **B:** A schematic illustration is shown using calipers that are used to measure the osteotomy site.

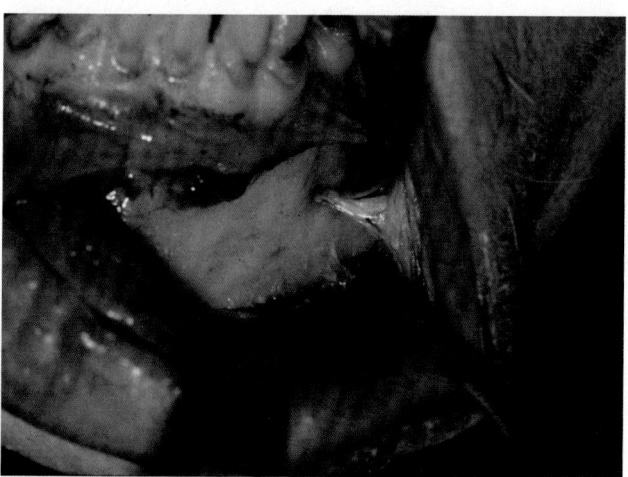

Figure 192.19 Cadaveric dissection of a subperiosteal plane exposing the left mental nerve.

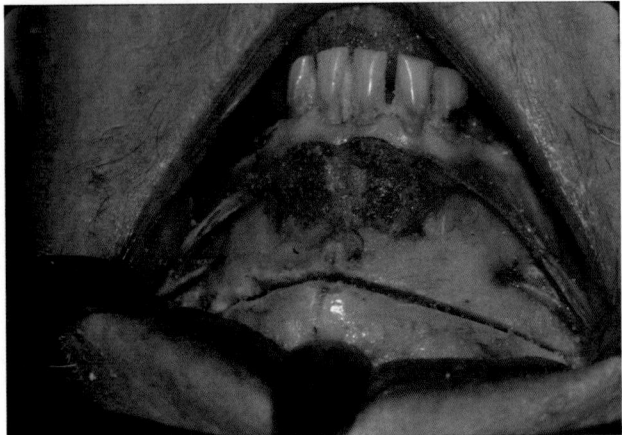

Figure 192.22 A cadaveric dissection is shown in which a horizontal osteotomy has been performed approximately 5 mm inferior to the mental foramen.

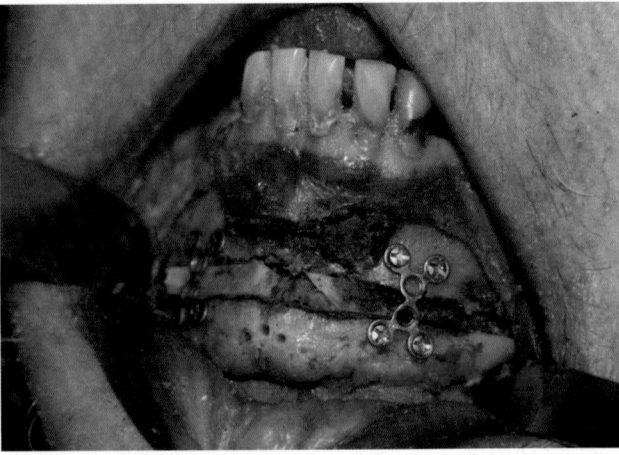

Figure 192.24 Cadaveric rigid fixation of the mentum in a vertically short chin after placement of bone grafts.

to correct transverse asymmetries. This treatment plan will affect the orientation of the osteotomy as well as the actual movement after the osteotomy. If only AP advancement is needed, the osteotomy is made with a horizontal orientation. If vertical movement (shortening) is needed in addition, the osteotomy is made in a more oblique orientation. An oblique osteotomy allows some vertical shortening because the distal segment is advanced. If the chin length is excessive and significant shortening is planned, two oblique osteotomies are made and the intervening bone is removed.

After the osteotomy is marked, the bone cut is created with either a reciprocating or an oscillating saw blade in a lateral-to-medial direction. The lateral extent of the osteotomy should be made at least 5 mm below the mental foramen to avoid injuring the mental nerve. Gentle digital pressure is used to downfracture the bony segment. A small amount of soft tissue must usually be separated from the posterior aspect of the distal segment to facilitate movement.

Repositioning of the distal segment is performed according to the preoperative treatment plan. If vertical

lengthening is required, grafts are placed using autogenous bone or allogenic bone. If vertical shortening is planned, a second parallel osteotomy is made above the first, or the intervening bone is burred away (Fig. 192.23). After the segment is repositioned, it is fixed in position using adaptation plates, positional screws, or interosseous wires (Fig. 192.24). Adaptation plates can be preshaped and provide excellent fixation. The soft tissues of the chin and lips are then replaced, and the new contour is assessed (Fig. 192.25).

The wound is closed in two layers with care taken to resuspend the soft tissues of the chin. Interrupted No. 3-0 catgut is used for the mentalis muscle, and a running locking stitch of No. 3-0 chromic catgut is used for the mucosa.

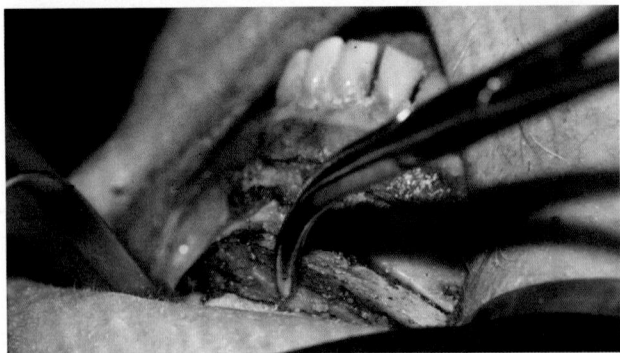

Figure 192.23 A photograph of a cadaveric dissection demonstrating parallel osteotomies and removal of bone (ostectomy) for vertical chin reduction.

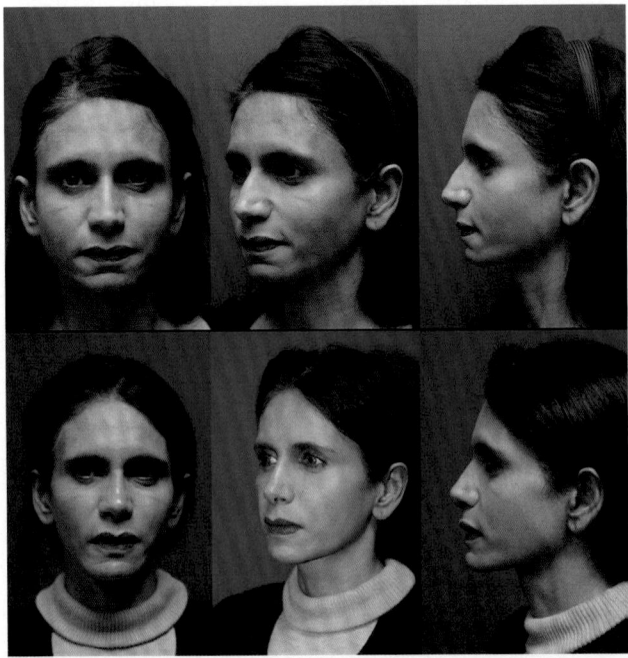

Figure 192.25 AP, oblique, and lateral preoperative (*upper row*) and postoperative (*lower row*) photographs of a woman after septorhinoplasty and bony genioplasty with lengthening and advancement.

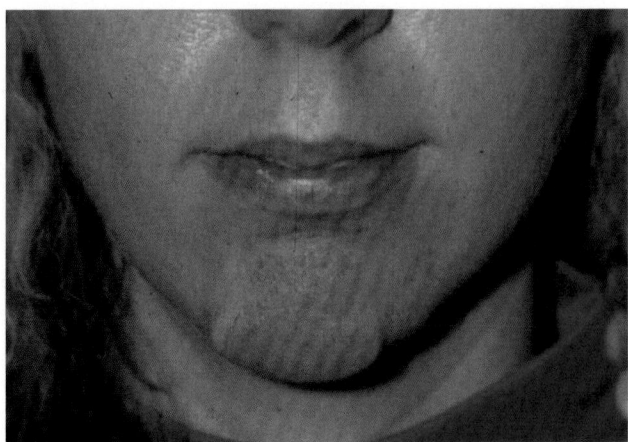

Figure 192.26 Close-up frontal photograph of a patient with a malpositioned chin implant.

A pressure chinstrap dressing is applied for 5 days, and the patient should eat a soft diet for 2 weeks.

Complications

Complications after chin augmentation with an alloplast implant are uncommon. They include hematoma, infection, dysesthesias or anesthesia, and implant malposition. Hematoma and infection are rare and can be avoided with meticulous hemostasis. Sensory nerve disturbances can be minimized with careful anatomic technique. Implant malposition can be avoided by careful creation of an appropriate-sized implant pocket (Fig. 192.26). Chin implants commonly cause mild bony erosion of the anterior mandible (Fig. 192.27). However, this erosion is rarely clinically significant and does not usually cause cosmetic deformity. Finally, mentalis muscle dyskinesis can occur from routine elevation and repositioning of the mentalis muscle. This condition is well treated with 2 to 5 units of botulinum toxin.

Complications after bony genioplasty also are rare and include hematoma and sensory nerve dysesthesias. Additionally, intraoral wound dehiscence can occur. The incidence of dehiscence is low and can be minimized by a careful, layered closure. Plate exposure and infection can also occur. Mentalis muscle dyskinesis also occurs (with an incidence of 5% to 10% post–chin implant or genioplasty) and can be again treated with injection of 2 to 5 units of botulinum toxin.

SUMMARY

The chin plays an important role in the profile and overall facial appearance. In order to evaluate the chin, analysis of the chin as it relates to other facial features should be performed. Three-dimensional evaluation of the chin includes visual inspection, photographic analysis, and radiographs.

Augmentation of the chin can be performed either with placement of an alloplast implant or with osteotomy and movement of the bony mentum. While placement of an implant is a simple procedure and corrects horizontal chin deficiency, bony genioplasty can correct chin deformities in all 3 dimensions. Additionally, bony genioplasty can also correct both horizontal and vertical macrogenia. If carefully performed, chin augmentation with an implant or genioplasty can dramatically improve the appearance of patients with chin deformities.

HIGHLIGHTS

- The chin plays an important role in the facial profile and in overall facial appearance.
- The chin should be evaluated as it relates to other adjacent structures, such as the lips, nose, and teeth.
- It is crucial to evaluate the chin in 3 dimensions: horizontal (AP), vertical, and transverse.
- Horizontal chin deficiency (microgenia) may be associated with class II malocclusion, while chin excess (macrogenia) may be associated with class III malocclusion.
- Horizontal chin deficiency may be camouflaged by an alloplast implant.
- Bony osteotomy of the mentum (genioplasty) can correct vertical and transverse chin deformities.
- Complications of chin surgery include infection, implant malposition, extrusion, and persistent cosmetic deformity.

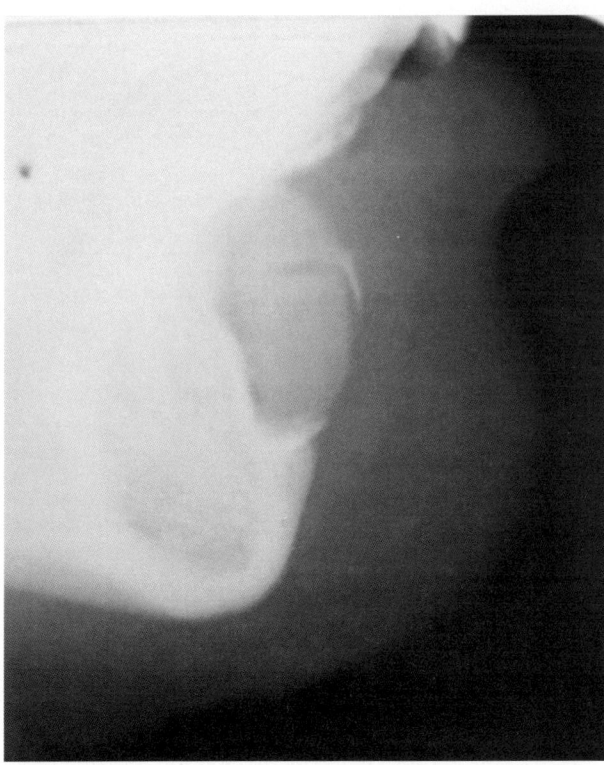

Figure 192.27 Lateral radiograph of a patient with a malpositioned (too superior) chin implant with subsequent bony resorption.

REFERENCES

1. Guyuron BK, Kadi JS. Problems following genioplasty: diagnosis and treatment. *Clin Plast Surg* 1997;24:507–514.
2. Wolfe SA. The chin. In: Wolfe SA, Berkowitz S, eds. *Plastic surgery of facial skeleton*. Boston, MA: Brown, 1989.
3. Rosen HM. Aesthetic guidelines in genioplasty: the role of facial disproportion. *Plast Reconstr Surg* 1995;95:463–472.
4. Sykes J, Donald PJ. Orthognathic surgery. In: Papel I, Nachlas NE, eds. *Facial plastic and reconstructive surgery*. St. Louis, MO: Mosby, 1992.
5. Sykes J, Frodel JL. Genioplasty. *Op Tech Otolaryngol* 1995;6:319.
6. Ricketts RM. Esthetics, environment and the law of lip relation. *Am J Orthod* 1968;54:272.
7. Frodel JL, Sykes JM, Jones JL. Evaluation and treatment of vertical microgenia. *Arch Facial Plast Surg* 2004;6(2):111–119.
8. Steiner CC. Cephalometrics in clinical practice. *Angle Orthod* 1959;29:8.
9. Morris DE, Lo LJ, Margulis A. Pitfalls in orthognathic surgery: avoidance and management of complications. *Clin Plast Surg* 2007;34:17–29.
10. Hwang K, Lee WJ, Song YB, et al. Vulnerability of the inferior alveolar nerve and mental nerve during genioplasty: an anatomic study. *J Craniofac Surg* 2005;16:10–14.
11. Rosen HM. Surgical correction of the vertically deficient chin. *Plast Reconstr Surg* 1988;82:247–256.
12. Chang EW, Lam SM, Karen M, et al. Sliding genioplasty for correction of chin abnormalities. *Arch Fac Plast Surg* 2001;3:8–15.
13. Terino EO. Three-dimensional facial contouring: alloplastic augmentation of the lateral mandible. *Facial Plast Surg Clin North Am* 2002;10:249.

Redefining Skin Resurfacing: The Hetter Chemical Peel

193

Devinder S. Mangat

As medical advancements have increased not only our life span but also our quality of life, it is natural to expect a greater public desire to undo the untoward effects of sunlight, age, and genetics. This has created a myriad of unsubstantiated skin care products, and practitioners of wonder technologies promising unrealistic end results. Chemical peeling has withstood both the harshest critics of safety and of results. Starting with lay peelers in the early 20th century, chemexfoliation has provided not only a stalwart treatment for practitioners of skin rejuvenation but also the standard by which other modalities are judged. Various chemical formulations have provided treatment for rhytids, lentigos, dyschromias, and actinic damage. The goal of this chapter is to address some more recent changes in chemical peel techniques; to uproot some old, outdated tenets; and to discuss the versatility of Hetter chemical peels.

BACKGROUND

The history of chemical peeling did not begin in the hands of physicians but rather in those of the lay peelers. In the 1920s, Hollywood was the fertile ground for these early practitioners as the stars of early motion pictures wished to maintain both a youthful appearance and career longevity. It was not until the 1950s and 1960s when physicians wished not only to learn these practices but also to wrestle them away from prominent lay peelers trained by Jean DeDesly and Antoinette LaGasse. Gregory Hetter, in his four-part series in 2000, eloquently describes a detailed history of the passing of the chemical peeling art from the lay peelers to the plastic surgeons of the 1950s and 1960s.

As chemical peeling transformed to the realm of medical science, much literature was produced regarding the experiences of plastic surgeons. Not all experiences were matched with scientific scrutiny. Instead, in some cases, dogma was written and adhered to for decades. Much of this dogma was born out of the use of the Baker-Gordon phenol–croton oil formulation (Table 193.1), the earliest formula widely used by physician peelers.

PATIENT SELECTION

Defining an individual patient's suitability for chemical peeling is paramount for the cosmetic surgeon. Not only does the patient need to be physically suitable for the peel but also the patient needs to have appropriate expectations of what the peel can accomplish. Rhytids and photodamage must be distinguished from age-related gravitational changes, jowling, and facial fat volume loss.

The ideal chemical peel patient is one with fair skin, blue eyes, and mild, shallow rhytids. However, this only represents a minority of the patients who will present seeking treatment for rhytids and photodamage. In order to help define the patient's skin type, the Fitzpatrick scale (Table 193.2) is most often employed. Patients can also be rated by their skin type, complexion, skin texture, thickness, and photoaging. A useful categorizing scheme is the one described by Glogau (Table 193.3).

The patient's medical history and lifestyle must be thoroughly discussed prior to the planning stages of the peel. Relative contraindications for any resurfacing procedure include cutaneous radiation history, smoking, active or frequent herpes simplex virus (HSV) infections, diabetes mellitus, or a history of hypertrophic scar formation or keloids. Birth control pills, exogenous estrogens (including soaps and cosmetics containing lavender oil), or photosensitizing drugs are to be avoided due to risks of hyperpigmentation. Due to elevated estrogen levels of pregnancy, the patient should not have plans to become pregnant within the first 6 months after the chemical peel (1).

Lifestyle and habitual activities, more specifically, sun exposure and smoking, should be addressed. Due to the

TABLE 193.1	THE "CLASSIC" BAKER AND BAKER-GORDON FORMULATIONS	
Ingredients	Baker-Gordon Solution	Original Baker Formulation
Phenol USP 88%	3 mL	5 mL
Distilled water	2 mL	4 mL
Croton oil (27 guttas = 1 mL)	3 guttas	3 guttas
Septisol	8 guttas	8 guttas

microvascular damage that ensues from nicotine, a chemical peel in the face of chronic smoking can lead to poor tissue healing and poor cosmetic results. Practitioners should be honest and frank regarding the risks of smoking, and a cessation program should be recommended. Smokers should stop smoking 1 month prior to a chemical peel and should avoid smoking for at least 6 months after the peel. Ultraviolet light (UV) exposure can be equally problematic in the postoperative period. A patient's habitual sun exposure should be assessed prior to proceeding with the peel. The patient should be advised that chronic or frequent sun exposure should be avoided after the chemical peel. If this is unacceptable to the patient, the practitioner should consider other options and not perform a peel.

Isotretinoin (Accutane) use is an absolute contraindication to chemical peeling or any other resurfacing procedure. Postpeel reepithelialization relies upon the epidermis within hair follicles and sebaceous glands. Isotretinoin prevents reepithelialization from these locations. Most recommendations include a cessation period of oral isotretinoin for 12 to 24 months prior to the peel.

The patient's expectations should be clarified and agreed upon with the practitioner. The patient's axillary skin can often well represent the final product of a chemical peel, as long as that area has not had excessive UV light exposure over the patient's lifetime (2).

PREPEEL PREPARATION

Proper skin preparation is essential and contributes to optimizing results and minimizing complications. Preoperatively, the use of sunscreens which block UVA and UVB irradiation will decrease melanocyte activity and prevent skin tanning and sunburns. Sunscreen usage should begin 3 months prior to the peel in combination with minimal sun exposure.

Topical tretinoin (Retin-A) is recommended for 6 to 12 weeks prior to the peel. Animal studies have demonstrated clinical and histologic healing benefits of tretinoin prior to dermabrasion. Synergistic qualities of pretreatment topical tretinoin and trichloroacetic acid (TCA) peels have been shown to sustain the effects of the chemical peel (3,4). Tretinoin aids in reepithelialization (5) and leads to increased melanin distribution. After tretinoin treatment, the thickened epidermis displays decreased corneocyte adhesion, decreased stratum corneum thickness, and neocollagen production, all of which are beneficial to the peel and the postoperative result. This thickened and uniform epidermis aids in the uniform application of the peeling agent (6).

The patient should begin nightly treatments with topical tretinoin 6 weeks prior to the peel, and these should be continued after the postpeel reepithelialization is

TABLE 193.2	FITZPATRICK CLASSIFICATION SCALE	
Skin Type	Skin Color	Characteristics
I	White; very fair; red or blond hair; blue eyes; freckles	Always burns, never tans
II	White; fair; red or blond hair; blue; hazel or green eyes	Usually burns, tans with difficulty
III	Cream white; fair with any eye or hair color; very common	Sometimes mild burn, gradually tans
IV	Brown; typical Mediterranean Caucasian skin	Rarely burns, tans with ease
V	Dark brown; mid-eastern skin types	Very rarely burns, tans very easily
VI	Black	Never burns, tans very easily

TABLE 193.3	GLOGAU CLASSIFICATION SCALE

Skin Class	Description

I	"Early Wrinkles"
	   Patient age: 20s–30s
	   Early photoaging
	      Mild pigment changes
	      Minimal wrinkles
	      No "age spots"

II	"Wrinkles in Motion"
	   Patient age: 30s–40s
	   Early to moderate photoaging
	      Appearance of smile lines
	      Early brown "age spots"
	      Skin pores more prominent
	      Early changes in skin texture

III	"Wrinkles at Rest"
	   Patient age: 50s and older
	   Advanced photoaging
	      Prominent brown pigmentation
	      Visible brown "age spots"
	      Prominent, small blood vessels
	      Wrinkles, even at rest

IV	"Only Wrinkles"
	   Patient age: 60s or 70s
	   Severe photoaging
	      Yellow-gray skin color
	      Prior skin cancers
	      Precancerous skin changes (actinic keratosis)

completed. The dose range recommended is between 0.025% and 0.1%. However, there is no literature describing an improved benefit with the higher dosing, suggesting that lower concentrations may be just as effective. Concentration of tretinoin becomes important in those patients who are sensitive to its use. The patient should be warned of the potential side effects including irritation, erythema, and flaking of the skin. When these complications are observed, the dose should be decreased or its use should be discontinued altogether.

Also beneficial in the pretreatment of all peel patients, hydroquinone is most effective in those patients with lentigos, dyschromias, and Fitzpatrick type III, IV, V, and VI skin types, due to the higher risk of postpeel postinflammatory hyperpigmentation (PIH). Hydroquinone blocks the conversion of tyrosine to L-dopa by tyrosinase, thus decreasing melanin production. Hydroquinone, in a concentration of 4% to 8%, should be started 4 to 6 weeks prior to resurfacing. Like tretinoin, hydroquinone should be started after the peel as soon as the patient's skin can tolerate its application.

Even if patients have no recollection of prior herpetic vesicle occurrence, all patients should be warned of the possibility of HSV outbreaks. Patients can have a latent infection even in the setting of a negative history. Common and advisable practice is to start any patient with a negative history on a prophylactic dose of antiviral medication, such as acyclovir 400 mg three times a day, 3 days prior to and continued for at least 7 days after the peel. For those patients with a positive history of active HSV infections, a therapeutic dose of antiviral medication should be employed, such as valacyclovir 1 g three times a day for the aforementioned time period. Postpeel herpetic infections can be unnerving for the practitioner but are devastating for the patient. Therefore, all precautions should be taken to avoid them.

In order to maintain appropriate and uniform depth of penetration of the peeling agent, avoidance of waxing, dermabrasion, and electrolysis should be strictly maintained for 3 to 4 weeks prior to peeling.

BASIC SCIENCE OF HETTER CHEMICAL PEELS

For years, a number of dogmatic suppositions had been purported within the literature regarding the phenol–croton oil peel. These statements date back to the late 1950s and early 1960s when the phenol–croton oil formulas were introduced to the plastic surgery arena. It was from lay peelers from Hollywood in the 1920s and the Miami area in the 1950s that plastic surgeons were able to tease away secret, long-used phenol-based peeling solutions (7). Most formulas contained similar concentrations of croton oil. Litton was the first to present one of these formulas to the American Society of Plastic and Reconstructive Surgery in the late 1950s. However, it is Baker who was credited for the formula he presented in November 1961 and then modified to his classic formula in 1962 (8).

Around the same time that Baker's classic formula was described, Adolph Brown presented three dogmas of phenol peeling. First, that increased concentrations of phenol (80% to 90%) prevented deeper peels by causing an immediate keratocoagulation that prevented further penetration of the phenol solution. Second, Brown believed that by adding a saponin the depth of penetration of phenol increased. Third, he believed that croton oil's role was simply to "buffer" the solution (9). The literature regarding chemexfoliation in the 1960s quickly adopted these assertions and upon them created more dogma. These statements included that phenol was the one and only active ingredient within the Baker formulation and that phenol in lower concentrations penetrated more deeply than in higher concentrations. As a result of these assertions, it was felt that lower concentrations of phenol were more dangerous due to their deeper penetration. As well, it was supposed that septisol caused a deeper penetration and that croton oil had no physiologic role in the peel. Since Brown's assertions in the early 1960s, there have been no scientific studies, animal or human, that lend support to his postulates. That is, until Gregory Hetter, in the late

1990s, questioned these assertions and, more importantly, questioned croton oil's role, or supposed lack thereof, in the standard Baker formula.

Croton oil is pressed from the seeds of *Croton tiglium*, a small shrub found in India and Ceylon. The oil consists mainly of oleic, linoleic, myristic, and arachidonic acids (10). Less than 5% of the oil is made up of a resin, which has been known since 1895 in scientific literature to possess irritant and toxic properties. In 1935, Joseph R. Spies isolated this toxic resin and applied it to the arm of a volunteer, creating severe vesiculations of the skin and a resultant wound taking almost 3 weeks to heal (10). Spies also showed that croton oil was soluble in ethanol and benzene and that it was poorly soluble in a 50:50 phenol to water solution (10). Hetter theorizes that these findings were the basis for using a surfactant, septisol, in the Baker formula.

To refute Brown's postulates and to help elucidate the role of croton oil, Hetter found a patient who was willing to undergo multiple chemical peels of different concentrations of phenol and croton oil. His findings contradicted that which had been previously assumed. At the lowest concentration of 18% phenol, there was minimal postpeel effect. Mild keratolysis occurred with 35% phenol, but there was no clear dermal effect. Hetter noted some desquamation with mild dermal effect after the 50% phenol peel. It was only with 88% phenol that Hetter noted an obvious upper dermal effect, which took 4 to 5 days to heal. With the addition of croton oil, a more profound dermal effect ensued. And, with different croton oil concentrations, there were different healing times. A 0.7% croton oil concentration application required a 7-day healing time, while a 2.1% croton oil concentration, equivalent to that of the classic Baker formula, resulted in an 11-day healing period (10).

From his experience with this one patient, Hetter deduced that phenol peels penetrate more deeply with increased concentrations, that higher concentrations of phenol (88%) without septisol peels penetrate more deeply than lower concentrations (50% and 35%), and that the resultant peel is deeper with increasing concentrations of croton oil.

Hetter used his experience to guide his treatment of five additional patients with varying croton oil concentrations. The results from these five patients allowed him to devise some generalizations of phenol–croton oil peeling. First, the dilution of croton oil, in a constant phenol concentration, shortens the healing time, suggesting a more shallow depth of penetration. Next, he generalized that phenol concentration has little to do with depth of injury. He confirms the observation of Stegman (11) in 1980, which was reiterated by Stone and Lefer (12) in 2001, that multiple coats of peel solution will increase the depth of injury. Obagi (13) first described the need for different depths of peeling for individual subunits of the face. Hetter translated this to his use of varying concentrations of croton oil in different regions of the face. While he found that the lower nose could tolerate croton oil concentrations up to 1.2%, the cheeks and forehead only tolerated concentrations up to 0.8%, and the upper nose, temple, and lateral brow could only withstand concentrations up to 0.4% before the risk of complications rose. Last, Hetter felt 1% croton oil solutions were the upper threshold for safe use to avoid serious risk of hypopigmentation.

Initially, Hetter performed his preliminary work using phenol as a "vehicle" at 33% for the croton oil with one-drop (0.35%), two-drop (0.7%), and three-drop (1.1%) formulations. However, he felt it would be optimal to have a more standardized means of measuring the croton oil concentrations, instead of relying on droppers, which are inherently inconsistent. He converted drops to cubic centimeters by having 25 drops equal 1 mL. Using this conversion, he created a stock solution of 0.04 mL of croton oil per 1 mL of phenol, from which he could make varying croton oil concentrations of 0.4%, 0.8%, 1.2%, and 1.6% in a constant phenol concentration, needing only septisol, phenol, and water. Using his formulations, the practitioner can decide between a phenol concentration of 35% or 48.5%. Table 193.4 depicts the formulas for the varying croton oil concentrations for the Hetter peels using a phenol concentration of 35%.

While Hetter demonstrated that the depth of penetration is partially dictated not only by the components of the peeling solution but also by the concentrations of the components,

TABLE 193.4	**THE HETTER PEEL FORMULA**				
Croton Oil %	0.2%	0.4%	0.8%	1.2%	1.6%
Water	5.5 mL	5.5 mL	5.5 mL	5.5 mL	5.5 mL
Septisol	0.5 mL	0.5 mL	0.5 mL	0.5 mL	0.5 mL
Phenol 88%	3.5 mL	3.0 mL	2.0 mL	1.9 mL	0.0 mL
Stock Solution	0.5 mL	1.0 mL	2.0 mL	3.0 mL	4.0 mL

Adapted from Hetter GP. An examination of the phenol-croton oil peel: part IV. Face peel results with different concentrations of the phenol and croton oil. *Plast Reconstr Surg* 2000;105(3):1061–1083.

Stone emphasized the importance of how application of these varying concentrations must be controlled to create desired results. Stone tested Hetter's posits by performing peels on three case studies using Hetter's varying concentrations, the classic Baker formula with and without croton oil, and varying phenol concentrations without croton oil.

In his first patient, he was able to show on repeat biopsies that the classic Baker formula with and without croton oil would create the same depth of penetration and injury with repeated rubbings and occlusive taping. In the second case, he peeled the patient with alternating concentrations of phenol, 50% and 88%, and alternating concentrations of croton oil, 2.2% and 0.4%, on both thick forehead skin and the thinner nasojugal trough skin. As well, he varied the number of rubs with a wrung-out gauze on the nasojugal trough. On biopsy, he found that all formulas created equal histologic results and similar fibrosis, when applied with 50 rubs. But, by decreasing the number of rubs, he confirmed Hetter's findings that by increasing phenol concentration, the depth of penetration increases. These findings suggest a threshold of injury can be achieved with phenol and croton oil; that threshold can also be achieved by varying concentrations when enough applications are employed. This was confirmed with his third case, in which he used lower phenol concentrations with 2.2%, 0.4%, and 0% croton oil. He found that this aforementioned threshold could be met with all three solutions, but with varying numbers of applications. Stone and Lefer (12) conclude that croton oil serves to lower the threshold number of applications.

Stone's work emphasizes the important point of how the peeling solution is applied to the skin is as important as what active agents are present within the solution. The author feels this is where the experience of the peeler and the "art" of peeling becomes important.

TECHNIQUE

Application of the peeling solution should always be done on sufficiently prepared skin. This preparation begins with vigorous cleaning, with septisol or an acne wash, the evening before and the morning of the procedure.

Preoperative oral sedation, 10 to 15 mg of diazepam and 100 mg of Dramamine, helps relieve the patient's anxiety regarding the intravenous (IV) catheter placement and the upcoming procedure. The antihistamine also reduces oral secretions and helps to protect the patient's airway during periods of deeper sedation. IV fluids should be initiated prior to bringing the patient to the operating room. At this point, additional IV benzodiazepine can be administered if the patient continues to be anxious.

While in a seated position, the patient's submandibular shadow is marked. This step is important to avoid obvious postoperative delineation between peeled and non-peeled areas at the jawline. The patient is then placed in the supine position. After administering a sedating dose of propofol, the nerve blocks (supraorbital, infraorbital,

mental) and field blocks are performed with an equal mixture of 2% lidocaine and 0.5% bupivacaine. The use of epinephrine is avoided, even in the nerve blocks, to allow maximal clearance of phenol. While waiting for maximal anesthesia to occur, the face is thoroughly degreased with an acetone-soaked gauze. Any residual oil on the skin will cause an uneven peel. The acetone cleaning can be repeated throughout the procedure if necessary.

Both Obagi and Hetter recommend using wrung-out cotton, 2-inch by 2-inch gauze, for the application of the peeling agent (10,14). However, the author feels wide cotton-tipped applicators are superior for control of application. As previously mentioned, the depth of the peel is dependent upon the amount of solution on the cotton tip, the uniform application of the solution, as well as the number of strokes applied.

One of the benefits of using a phenol-based solution is that the resultant frost is almost immediate, compared to TCA where the practitioner must safely wait 3 to 4 minutes before assessing a peeled area for needed repeat applications (15). The assessment of peel depth is based on the level of frost observed. In contrast to the TCA peel where the level of frost cannot be determined for 3 or 4 minutes, the phenol-croton oil peel depth can be determined within 20 or 30 seconds. Therefore, areas in need of deeper peeling may be treated again more rapidly. Medium-depth peels create a level II to level III frosting (15) (Table 193.5).

The subunits of the face should be divided by degree of rhytids, lentigos, and photodamage as well as inherent thickness. The author's experience has been to use 0.8% croton oil Hetter solution in areas of deeper rhytids (Glogau III and IV) and thicker skin, such as the perioral, glabellar, and lateral periorbital areas. The intermediate areas (Glogau II and III), such as the inferior periorbital area, are treated with 0.4% croton oil Hetter solution. In order to even the appearance of the face, a simple 88% United States Pharmaceutical (USP) phenol solution is used for all other areas.

An appropriate period, 10 to 15 minutes, must be allowed between each subunit peeled to allow for proper clearance of the phenol solution. The entire face should be peeled over 90 to 120 minutes. In the event that a minor supraventricular arrhythmia occurs, the peel should be stopped, and the practitioner should wait for a return to normal sinus rhythm. The peel should be carried into

TABLE 193.5	CLASSIFICATION OF THE DEGREE OF FROSTING OBTAINED WITH CHEMICAL PEELS

Level I: erythema with stringy or blotchy frosting
Level II: white coat with erythema showing through (should be used for eyelids and areas of bony prominences, i.e., zygomatic arch, malar, chin; higher rate of scarring)
Level III: solid white frost with little or no background erythema

the hairline, as phenol and croton oil will not affect pigment of the hair follicles. The edge of each peeled area will have a margin of reactive hyperemia, which does not represent peeled skin but rather an unpeeled skin reaction. When peeling the adjacent areas, this line of hyperemia (Fig. 193.1) should be included and adequately peeled to avoid obvious lines of demarcation. Similarly, the peel should be carried over the vermilion border. The practitioner can stretch wrinkled skin to allow an even peel over these areas. For deep perioral rhytids, the cotton-tipped applicator can be broken and the wood edge used to apply the peeling agent in the rhytid.

There is no need for neutralization of the peeling solution as the frost represents a completed reaction, which is precipitation of the keratin by the phenol. Great care must be taken around the lower eyelid margin. The peel should be performed to within 3 mm of the ciliary line and stopped. There should be no excess solution on the lower lid. The patient may develop tearing during the procedure. Any tearing should be immediately dried to avoid the tears pooling the peeling solution into the eye. If not adequately anesthetized, the patient will experience an immediate burning sensation for 15 to 20 seconds. However, this sensation will return in 20 minutes and can last 4 to 8 hours later. The longer-lasting effect of the bupivacaine

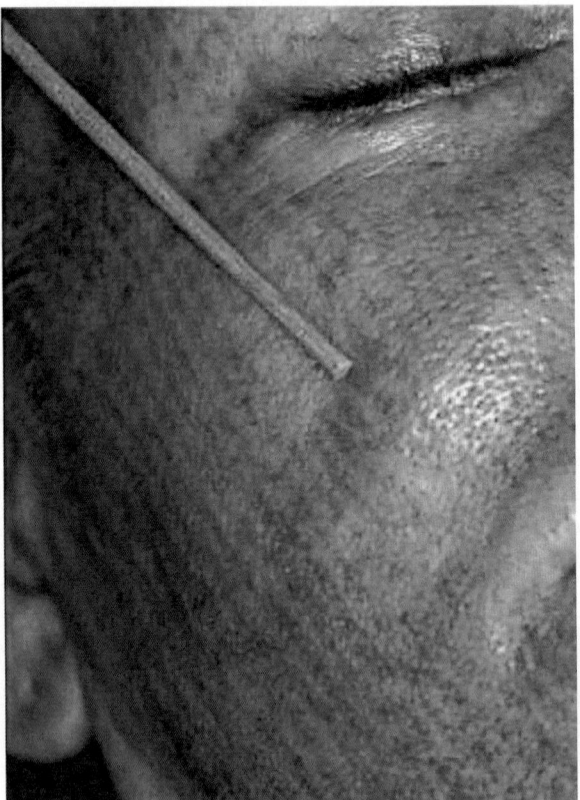

Figure 193.1 This demonstrates the clear line of hyperemia that occurs at the periphery of a peeled area. This hyperemic skin has not been peeled. Care must be taken to peel this area so as to not leave a discrete line of unpeeled skin.

will greatly aid in minimizing the burning sensation in the postoperative period. Therefore, it is essential to perform adequate nerve and field blocks. Even with all precautions in place, accidents may happen. In the case of excess phenol exposure to the patient or the staff, propylene glycol, glycerol, olive oil, castor oil, or cottonseed oil should be poured onto the site to solubilize the phenol. If exposure to the eyes occurs, mineral oil should be immediately applied to the eyes using an eye dropper.

POSTOPERATIVE CARE

Postoperative care begins immediately after the last subunit is peeled.

When the frost subsides and only erythema persists, a thick layer of bland emollient should be applied to all peeled areas, leaving no peeled skin exposed. The senior author prefers Eucerin cream, but Elta or antibiotic ointment may be used. None of these topical agents act as an occlusive dressing, and they will therefore not increase the depth of penetration. Starting with postoperative day 1, the patient will apply the cream three to four times a day to those areas that are exposed. By using the emollient, the peeled skin can be monitored with greater ease on a day-to-day basis.

The patient should have been preoperatively prepared for the expected postoperative edema, erythema, and eventual desquamation. Additionally, patients should also be advised of the burning sensation that may last up to 8 hours following the procedure. The patient's preoprative awareness will aid in the patient's analgesia. The patient should be prescribed an oral narcotic for the postoperative period. The healing process occurs in four stages (15). First, inflammation occurs and increases during the first 12 hours. Next, the epidermis will begin to change in appearance, becoming leathery, and will separate from the dermis. The underlying dermal injury will become necrotic and slough. The emollient will aid in clearing this necrotic tissue from the underlying dermis, which is then recovered with the emollient. Desquamation will occur over 4 to 7 days, exposing the underlying erythematous dermis. The reepithelialization, which typically begins in 48 to 72 hours, will continue through day 7 to 10 (Fig. 193.2), depending on the depth of the peel (15). This reepithelialization will be represented by a conversion of bright red erythema to a lighter shade of pink. The benefit of the peel is born out of the fourth and final stage. This final stage of fibroplasia begins within the first week and continues for 12 to 16 weeks after the peel. This period is marked by neoangiogenesis, new collagen formation, and reorganizing of the collagen.

In the first 12 weeks after the peel, the patient is susceptible to UV light exposure and a resultant hyperpigmentation. Strict avoidance of direct, prolonged sun exposure should be encouraged for that 12-week period. It has been the author's experience that sunscreens should also be avoided for the first 6 weeks. Paraaminobenzoic acid,

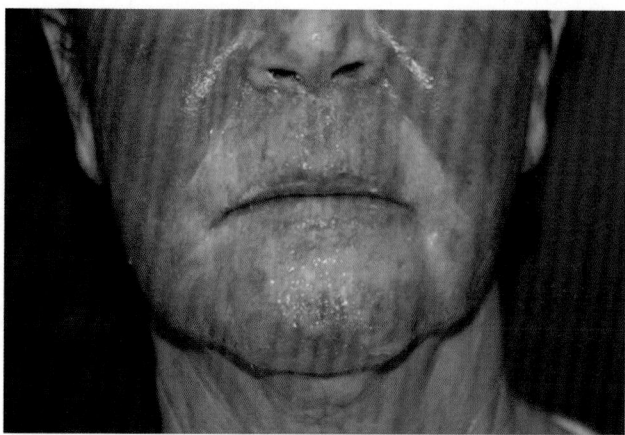

Figure 193.2 Erythematous neoepitheliazation has replaced the sloughed chemoexfoliated skin in this patient who underwent a Hetter chemical peel approximately 7 days ago.

found in many sunscreen preparations, can cause an undesirable reaction, including irritation, increased erythema, and induration. Figures 193.3 to 193.7 demonstrate the exceptional results that are obtained from Hetter peels in the treatment of dyschromia and rhytids.

Women of childbearing age should avoid birth control pills or pregnancy. Increased circulating estrogens can result in hyperpigmentation following chemexfoliation.

COMPLICATIONS

Despite taking all necessary preoperative precautions and measures, the busy practitioner can encounter a litany of postoperative complications. A comprehensive understanding of these complications and their management will serve the peeler well. Proper management of these complications, both minor and major, will make the difference between undesirable and optimal results.

Probably the most feared complication of phenol peels is cardiac arrhythmias. Though no death due to phenol peeling has been described in the literature, the possibility of a potential cardiovascular crisis has led to great fear regarding the use of phenol. Even in patients preoperatively screened and well hydrated, a reversible arrhythmia can occur, especially in patients with undiagnosed myocardial sensitivity. These patients will develop a supraventricular tachycardia within 30 minutes of the onset of the peel, which if exacerbated, can progress into paroxysmal ventricular contractions, paroxysmal atrial tachycardia, ventricular tachycardia, and, possibly, atrial fibrillation. The key is to not allow this progression to occur. Once an irregular rhythm is noted, the peeling should be halted, adequate hydration continued, and the patient's rhythm will return to baseline as the phenol is cleared. At this point, the chemical peeling can proceed, but with vigilant observation of

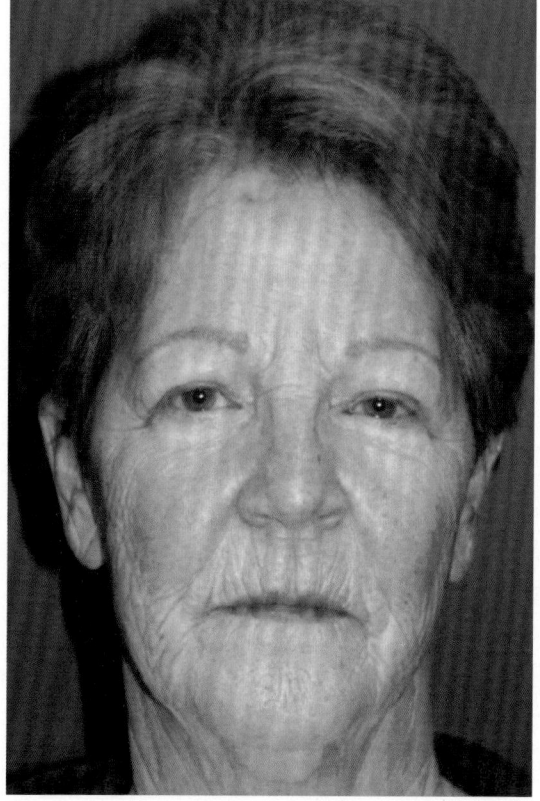
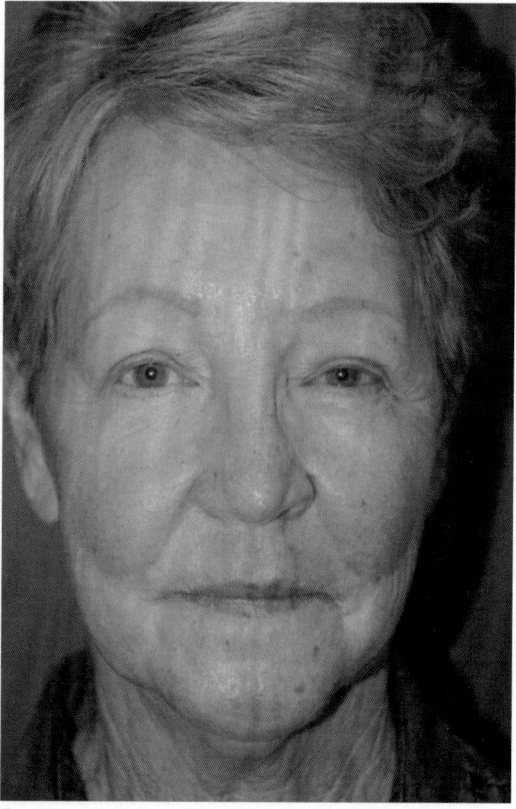

A   B

Figure 193.3 Prepeel **(A)** and postpeel photographs **(B)**. Dramatic improvement in rhytids can be appreciated in this patient who underwent a full-face Hetter chemical peel.

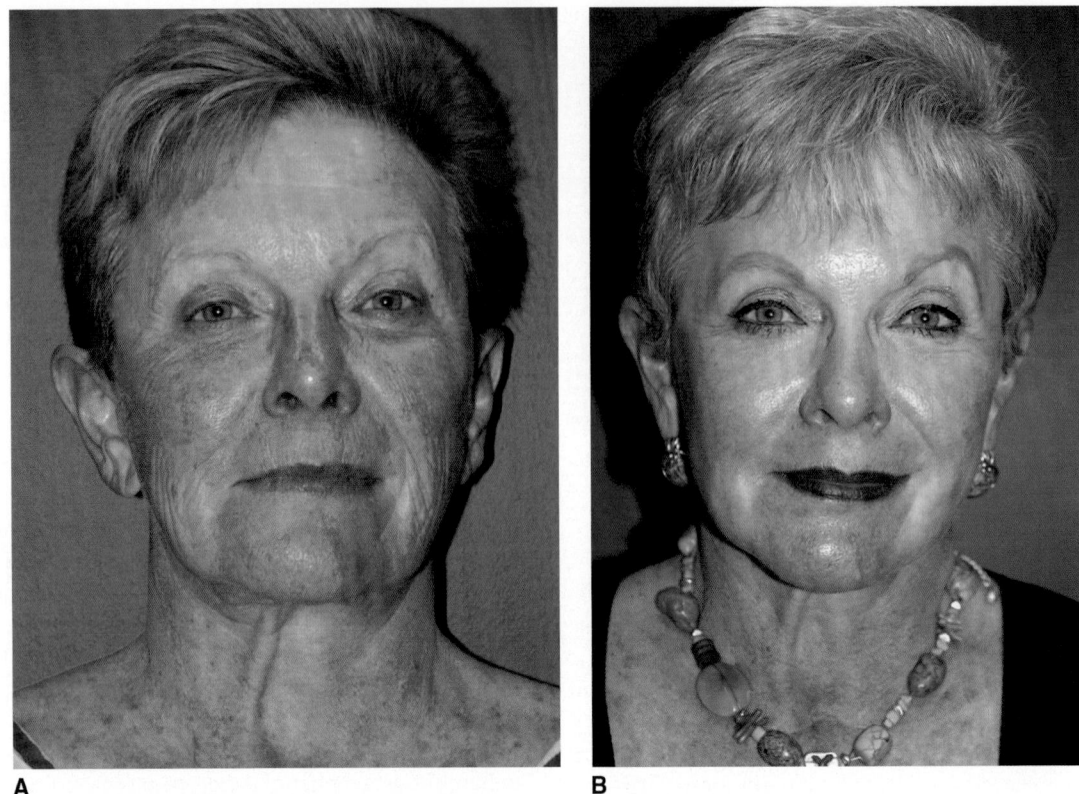

Figure 193.4 Prepeel **(A)** and postpeel photographs **(B)**. Another example of typical expected results in rhytids and dyschromia after a full-face Hetter chemical peel.

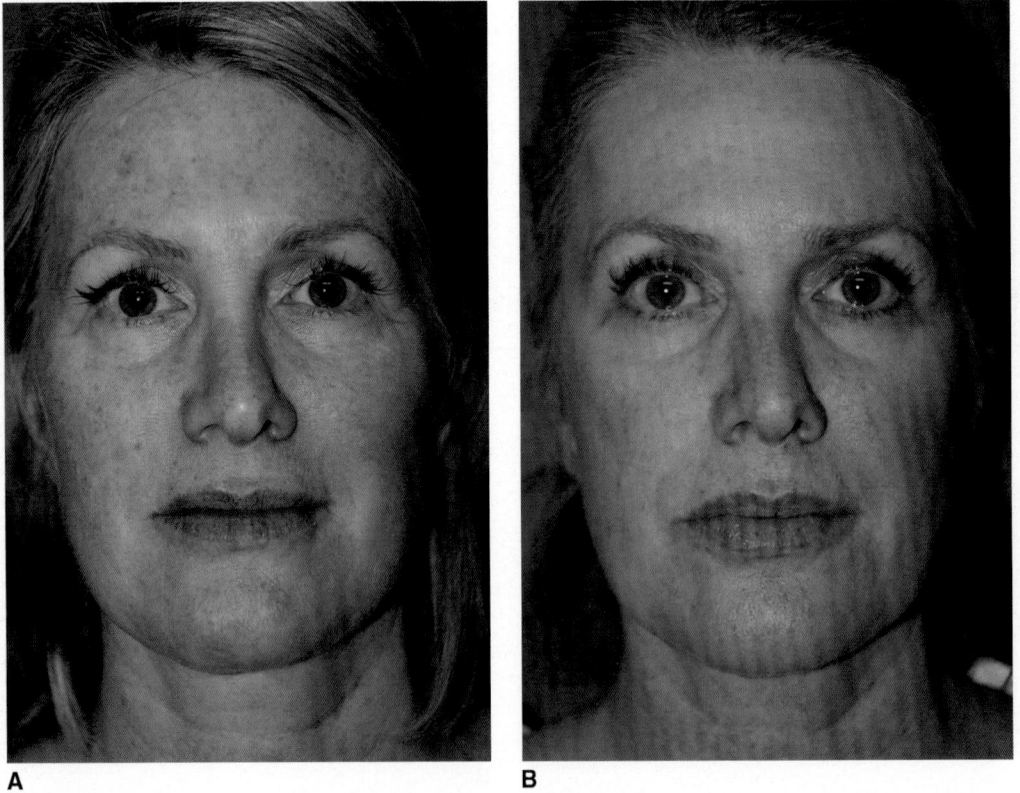

Figure 193.5 Prepeel **(A)** and postpeel photographs **(B)**. A lower croton oil concentration Hetter peel formulation was used here to improve facial dyschromia.

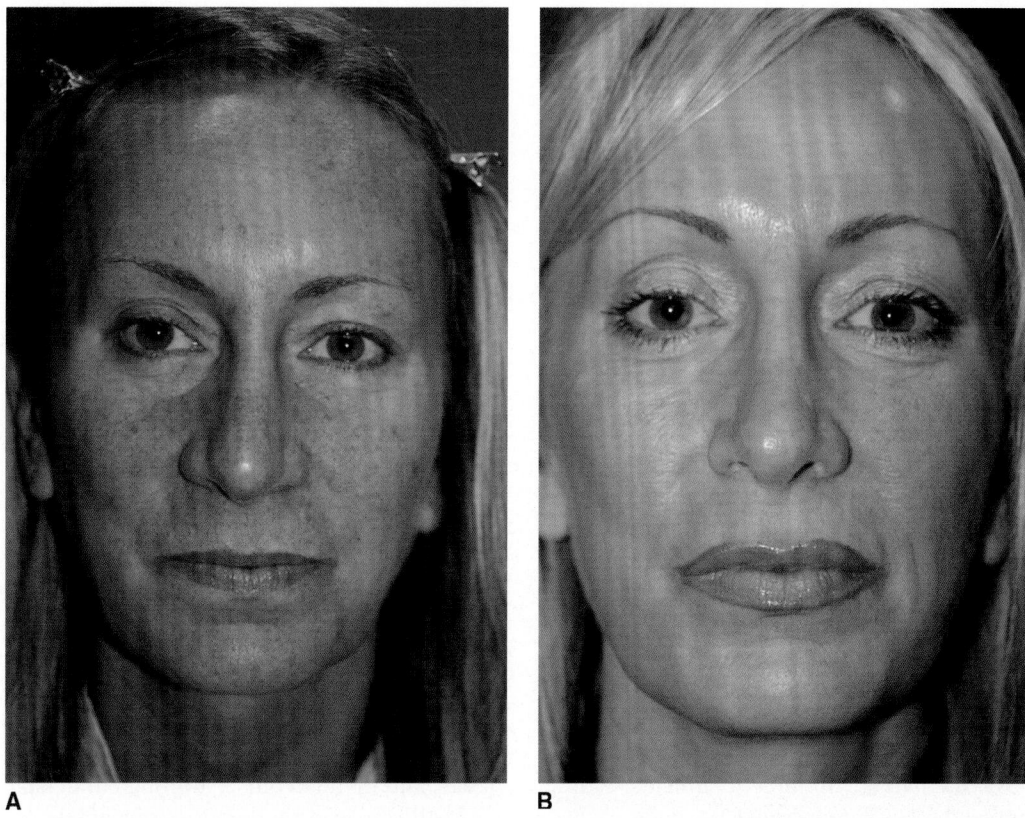

A   B

Figure 193.6 Prepeel **(A)** and postpeel photographs **(B)**. Another example of the use of a lower croton oil concentration Hetter peel formulation to improve facial dyschromia.

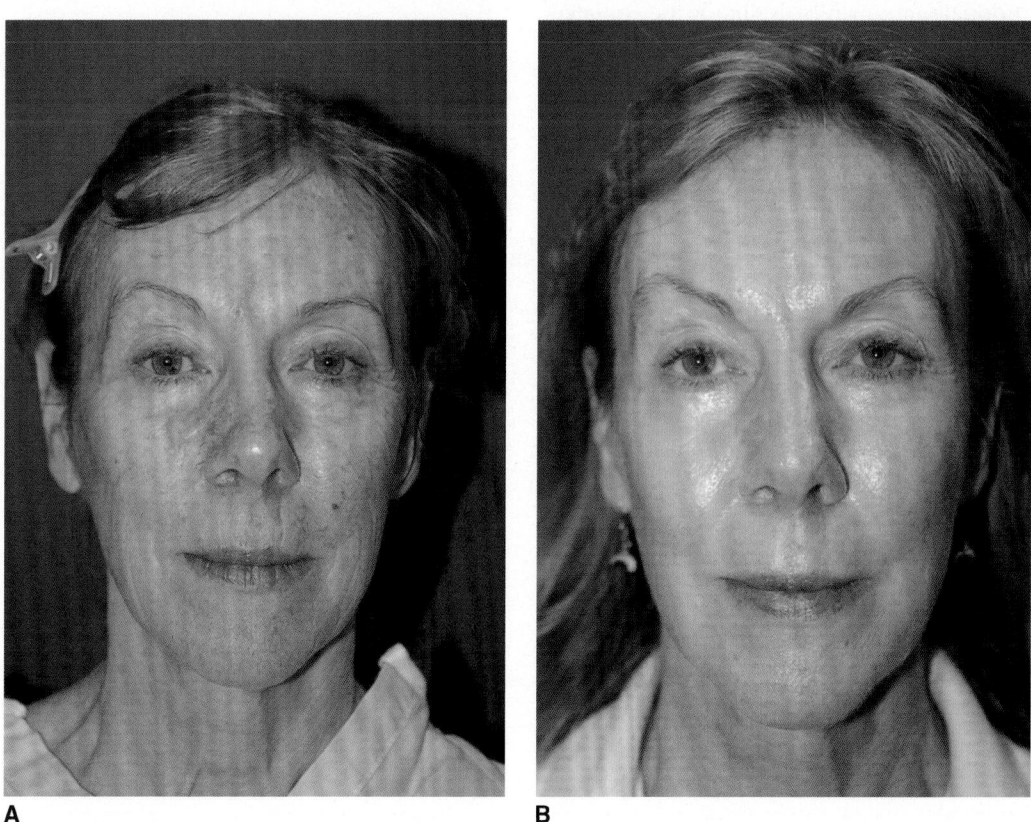

A   B

Figure 193.7 Prepeel **(A)** and postpeel photographs **(B)**. A mid-to-higher croton oil concentration was used here to improve both facial dyschromia and rhytids.

the cardiac rhythm. In the rare cases in which the cardiac rhythm does not return to normal, proper measures should be employed to treat the aberrant rhythm.

Although not as concerning as arrhythmias, prolonged healing times is a nuisance both for the patient and the practitioner. Any area that does not reepithelialize by day 10 should be considered prolonged. Lack of reepithelialization is more common with medium-depth TCA and deeper phenol peels (16). If the wound healing is delayed, daily wound checks should be performed. The practitioner must rule out the presence of infection and treat accordingly. These areas should be treated promptly or they will result in increased risk of scarring.

In the event that scarring occurs, it is going to occur most often in the perioral area, specifically the upper lip. Scarring is most often the result of too deep a peel or from poor postoperative care. The risk of scarring is increased in isotretinoin users. Again, after discontinuing isotretinoin, the practitioner should wait until the patient is clearly developing skin oil. These scars can be treated with Silastic (cross-linked polydimethylsiloxane polymer) sheeting and intralesional steroid injections (Kenalog 20 mg/mL) every 2 to 3 weeks. Overuse of steroids can result in dermal atrophy; therefore, judicious use is recommended. If these scars are erythematous, multiple treatments with a flashlamp-pumped dye laser are helpful (2).

A bacterial pyoderma can aggravate wound healing and lead to scarring. In the rare case of a bacterial or fungal infection, appropriate antimicrobials should be initiated and continued for a 7- to 10-day course.

Similarly, a herpetic infection can be devastatingly uncomfortable for the patient. If, despite prophylaxis, this infection occurs, a maximal antiviral course, valacyclovir 1 g three times a day for 10 days, should be used.

The postoperative erythema that is typical in all peeled patients may last longer than expected. This is more prevalent with patients with sensitive skin or in cases of contact dermatitis. Topical hydrocortisone (2.5%) lotions are helpful for accelerating the resolution of this erythema.

As the erythema is subsiding, some patients, as a result of inadvertent sun exposure or from darker skin type, will develop PIH. This usually occurs weeks after the peel. This is most readily seen in skin overlying bony prominences, such as the lateral malar regions. This is more common in the Fitzpatrick III to VI skin types. A combination of 0.05% retinoic acid, 8% hydroquinone, and hydrocortisone cream is effective at reducing or eliminating this pigmentation. Glycolic acid lotion has been noted to be affective as well (2).

More problematic than hyperpigmentation is hypopigmentation. Classically, this is more common in phenol-based peels. Phenol is thought to eliminate the melanocyte's ability to produce melanin. This can be much more noticeable when single facial subunits are peeled. Hypopigmentation occurred with much greater frequency in the past with the Baker formulation and postoperative occlusive taping or thymol iodide masks. The concentration of the phenol and croton oil, the skin type, and taping are all factors contributing to the risk of hypopigmentation. This complication is irreversible. And patients should be counseled regarding the possible need for makeup use.

CONCLUSION

With the advent of CO_2 laser resurfacing, followed by erbium: YAG laser resurfacing, chemical peeling was marginalized as an outdated practice, supplanted by technologic advances. As well, phenol–croton oil peeling was considered a deep, dangerous peel that had an all-or-none effect at best and a peel riddled with complications at worst. Much like the outdated posits of Adolph Brown and his contemporaries, neither of the aforementioned sentiments is farther from the truth. Chemical peeling should be considered the standard as it is an effective and safe tool for the facial cosmetic surgeon. Furthermore, with our relatively new understanding of the role of croton oil, the modified phenol–croton oil peeling formulations offer a tool that can be tailored for different skin types, skin thicknesses, and rhytid depth. A thorough understanding of this peel will greatly expand the options of what a practitioner can offer his resurfacing patients.

HIGHLIGHTS

- Phenol peels the skin more deeply with increased concentrations, and the resultant peel is deeper with increasing concentrations of croton oil.
- The dilution of croton oil, in a constant phenol concentration, shortens the healing time and suggests a more shallow depth of penetration.
- Hetter peels allow for different depths of peeling for individual subunits of the face by varying concentrations of croton oil for individual facial subunits.
- The depth of the peel is dependent upon the amount of solution on the cotton tip, the uniform application of the solution, as well as the number of applications.
- Experience reveals that 0.8% croton oil Hetter solution works well in areas of deeper rhytids and thicker skin, such as the perioral, glabellar, and lateral periorbital areas.
- Intermediate areas should be treated with 0.4% croton oil Hetter solution such as the inferior periorbital area.
- A simple 88% USP phenol solution is used for all other areas to even the appearance.

REFERENCES

1. Brody HJ. Complications of chemical peeling. *J Dermatol Surg Oncol* 1989;15:1010–1019.
2. Brody HJ. Complications of chemical resurfacing. *Dermatol Clin* 2001;19(3):427–438.
3. Vagotis FL, Brundage SR. Histologic study of dermabrasion and chemical peel in an animal model after pretreatment with retin A. *Aesthetic Plast Surg* 1995;19:243–246.
4. Kim IH, Kim HK, Kye YC. Effects of tretinoin pretreatment on TCA chemical peel in guinea pig skin. *J Korean Med Sci* 1996;11:335–341.
5. Popp C, Kligman AM, Stoudemayer TJ. Pretreatment of photoaged forearm skin with topical tretinoin accelerates healing of full-thickness wounds. Br *J Dermatol* 1995;132:46–53.
6. Hevia O, Nemeth AJ, Taylor JR. Tretinoin accelerates healing after trichloroacetic acid chemical peel. *Arch Dermatol* 1986;15:848.
7. Hetter GP. An examination of the phenol-croton oil peel: part II. The lay peelers and their croton oil formulas. *Plast Reconstr Surg* 2000;105:240–248.
8. Hetter GP. An examination of the phenol-croton oil peel: part III. The plastic surgeon's role. *Plast Reconstr Surg* 2000;105(2):752–763.
9. Brown AM, Kaplan L, Brown ME. Phenol induced histological skin changes: hazards, techniques, and uses. *Br J Plast Surg* 1960;13:158.
10. Hetter GP. An examination of the phenol-croton oil peel: part IV. Face peel results with different concentrations of the phenol and croton oil. *Plast Reconstr Surg* 2000;105(3):1061–1083.
11. Stegman SJ. A comparative histologic study of the effects of three peeling agents and dermabrasion on normal and sundamaged skin. *Aesthetic Plast Surg* 1982;6:123–135.
12. Stone PA, Lefer LG. Modified phenol chemical face peels: recognizing the role of application technique. *Facial Plast Surg Clin North Am* 2001;9(3):351–376.
13. Johnson JB, Ichinose H, Obagi ZE, et al. Obagi's modified trichloroacetic acid (TCA)–controlled variable–depth peel: a study of clinical signs correlating with histological findings. *Ann Plast Surg* 1996;36:225.
14. Hetter GP. An examination of the phenol-croton oil peel: part I. Dissecting the formula. *Plast Reconstr Surg* 2000;105:227–239.
15. Monheit GD. Medium-depth chemical peels. *Dermatol Clin* 2001;19(3):413–425.
16. Szachowicz EH, Wright WK. Delayed healing after full-face chemical peels. *Facial Plast Surg* 1989;6(1):8–13.

194 Lasers in Facial Plastic Surgery

William Russell Ries   *Joseph E. Hall*

"The Quantum Theory of Radiation," published by Einstein in the early 1900s, established laser theory. Maiman built the first laser in 1960, and patient treatment began shortly thereafter (1). The first cutaneous laser treatment with ruby and neodymium pulsed laser systems was performed by Goldman, and Patel subsequently developed the first CO_2 laser in 1964 (2). Lasers have become an integral treatment option for multiple disease processes, and clinical applications for lasers are ever expanding with the concurrent development of imaging systems, computer technology, and robotics (3). Lasers have become increasingly easy to use, and the fundamentals of laser physics are taught to a myriad of health care providers.

In this chapter, laser biophysics, laser–tissue interactions, technical aspects of laser treatment, and complications associated with lasers in facial plastic and reconstructive surgery are discussed. It is the hope of the authors that this chapter will provide a detailed understanding of laser technology, common laser applications, indications and reasons for employment of specific lasers, and practical knowledge related to the technical aspects of laser treatment.

LASER BIOPHYSICS

LASERs (*l*ight *a*mplification by the *s*timulated *e*mission of *r*adiation) produce light energy that travels in a waveform. The distance between two successive peaks of the wave corresponds to the wavelength, while the height of the peak of the wave corresponds to the amplitude. The amplitude is related to the intensity of the light. The period, or the time for the completion of a full wave cycle, is referred to as the frequency (4).

To produce this waveform, lasers follow the fundamentals of quantum mechanics. Specifically, a power source provides energy to a system. Subsequently, photons, units of light energy, present in the system strike atoms in the laser medium and can raise one of its electrons to a higher energy level. Either spontaneous or stimulated emission can occur at this point. Spontaneous emission occurs when the atom in the excited and unstable state reemits a photon and the electron returns to the lower energy level. If an atom in the higher energy state is struck by an additional photon, two photons are emitted. This process is termed stimulated emission (Fig. 194.1). The photons produced will continue to propagate the energy transfer via mirrors within the system. The photons emitted characteristically have the same wavelength, progress in the same direction, and travel in phase (3).

Lasers consist of four main components including a power source, a laser medium, an optical cavity or resonator, and a delivery system (Fig. 194.2). Electrical, light, and high-energy radio frequency waves are examples of possible excitation mechanisms. The optical cavity or resonator contains a medium that may be solid, liquid, gas, or a semiconductive material. Lasers also have a mirror that is 100% reflective and a mirror that is partially transmissive to allow energy to escape the chamber. Delivery systems are variable with most utilizing a fiberoptic delivery system but some using an articulated arm system (CO_2 laser).

The components of the laser together produce light that is of one wavelength (monochromatic), with little divergence (collimated), and in identical temporal and spatial phases (coherent). These properties differentiate laser light from ordinary light.

LASER–TISSUE INTERACTION

Laser energy can have a variety of effects on tissue ranging from activation of biochemical substances or stimulation of biologic tissues at low energy to coagulation or vaporization of biologic tissues at high energy (Fig. 194.3) (3). Most clinically relevant lasers utilize the thermal effects of lasers to coagulate or vaporize. The effect of a laser on a given

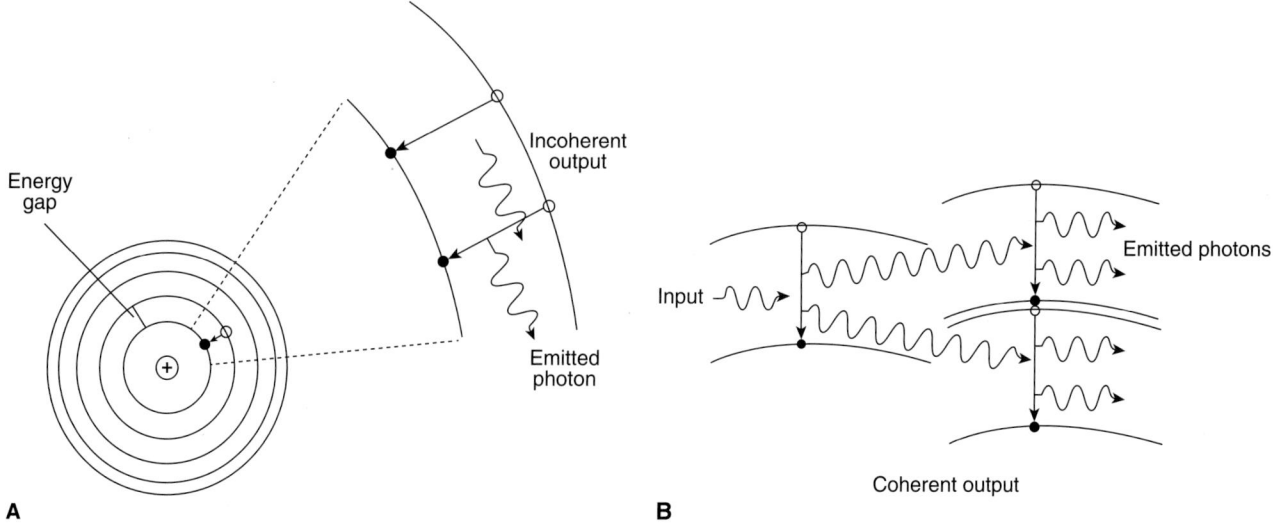

Figure 194.1 The processes of spontaneous and stimulated emission of radiation. (Reprinted from Papel ID, Frodel JL. *Facial plastic and reconstructive surgery*, 3rd ed. New York: Thieme, 2009:100, with permission.)

tissue is a function of the laser wavelength; laser energy density; and the amount of reflection, scatter, absorption, or transmission of energy that occurs (Fig. 194.4) (3).

Chromophores are substances that absorb energy at specific wavelengths. The specific absorption patterns of tissues partly determine the most efficacious laser for a given lesion. The chromophore absorbs light energy, which is then converted to heat. Coagulation of tissues occurs at 60°C to 70°C, and tissue vaporization occurs at 100°C (5). Appropriate laser selection allows for targeted thermal damage in tissues that absorb a specific wavelength of light. This process is termed selective photothermolysis (5). For example, the soft tissues of the body, which consist of mainly of water molecules, absorb CO_2 laser energy efficiently, whereas bone, with little water content, does not. Another important laser property is wavelength, with deeper tissue penetration occurring with longer wavelengths of light (5). The peak absorption wavelength for oxyhemoglobin, which is found in high concentrations in vascular malformations and hemangiomas, is 577 to 585 nm.

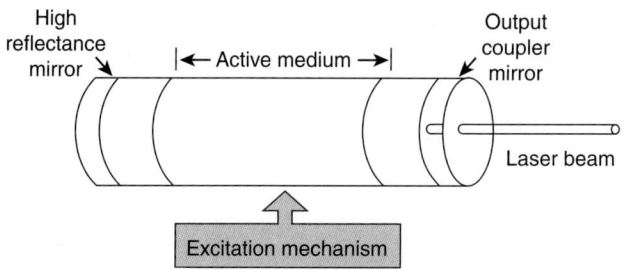

Figure 194.2 Laser apparatus. Lasers use a power source to provide light energy to a system, while photons produce stimulated emission of radiation. (Reprinted from Papel ID, Frodel JL. *Facial plastic and reconstructive surgery*, 3rd ed. New York: Thieme, 2009:100, with permission.)

Two important laser parameters are energy density and power density. Energy density (fluence) is a function of the power density (intensity) of the laser and the time of exposure. Power density is a function of the power divided by the cross-sectional area of the laser beam (spot size). Thus, by altering power density or time of exposure, the amount of energy delivered by a particular laser can be altered. Additionally, by decreasing the laser spot size, power density is increased.

Energy density (fluence) = Power density × Time
Power density = Power (watts)/Cross-sectional area
of laser beam (spot size)

Based on these equations, one can readily deduce that by decreasing the spot size of the laser beam, the power density to the tissue of interest increases. Pulsed energy can also be utilized to alter tissue effects. The pulsed energy mechanism incorporates regular periods of irradiation (on period) with alternating periods of no irradiation (off period). This alternating delivery of laser energy permits heat dissipation during the off period. Thus, thermal heat damage to surrounding tissue is minimized, particularly if the off period is longer than the thermal relaxation time of the tissue of interest. The thermal relaxation time is defined as the amount of time required for an object to dissipate half of its heat. The duty cycle is defined as the ratio of the on interval to the on plus off intervals.

Several pulsed modes have been created for use with lasers. Shuttering can block the delivery of a beam of laser light for specified intervals of time. Superpulse mode refers to a mechanism in which energy is stored during the off period and released during the on period. Q-switched lasers function by storing energy during the off period and releasing high-energy bursts of light for short time intervals using an electro-optical shutter (3). Ultimately, one

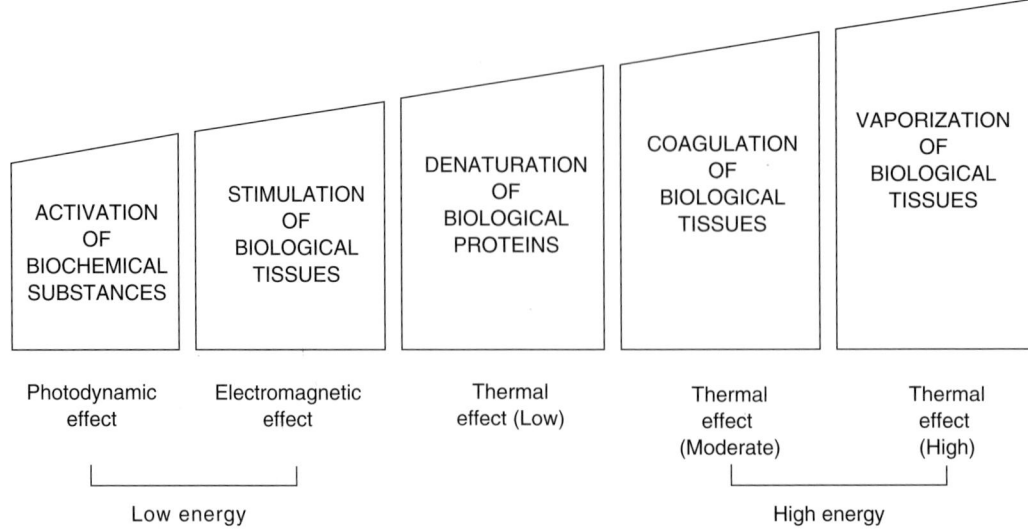

Figure 194.3 High-energy laser treatment causes vaporization and coagulation of tissues, while low-energy causes activation and stimulation of biologic tissues. (Reprinted from Papel ID, Frodel JL. *Facial plastic and reconstructive surgery*, 3rd ed. New York: Thieme, 2009:101, with permission.)

must match the laser wavelength, spot size, energy density, power, and duration of action to the tissue of interest and the desired outcome (5).

LASER CHARACTERISTICS

Flashlamp-Excited Dye Laser

The flashlamp-excited dye laser (FEDL) was designed for the treatment of vascular cutaneous lesions. The laser medium is a rhodamine dye, which is excited optically by a flashlamp. It is delivered by a fiberoptic carrier. This laser produces visible, yellow light (6). The FEDL system is frequently used to treat hemangiomas, port-wine stains, rosacea, and telangiectasias as it emits wavelengths of 585 nm, near the absorption peak of oxyhemoglobin (577 nm) (6,7). The FEDL has a dynamic cooling device that reduces the risk of epidermal injury.

The FEDL has an interchangeable lens system that allows for spot sizes of 3, 5, 7, or 10 mm. The pulse is 450 μs. More recently developed FEDLs can produce longer wavelengths (595 to 600 nm) with spot sizes of 10 to 12 mm and higher peak fluence potentials. These alterations have allowed for more effective treatment of the deeper vessels found in hemangiomas and port-wine stains (6,8). Additionally, longer pulse durations of 1.5 to 40 ms have allowed for telangiectasia treatment without the development of significant purpura (6,8–11). The alterations to the FEDL have provided a treatment that has been shown to reduce erythema, decrease height, and improve texture in scars (12). A decreased rate of recurrence of hypertrophic scars has also been found with the FEDL (13).

Pulsed dye lasers (PDLs) have recently incorporated a unique pulse structure where each macropulse is subdivided into eight micropulses. This technology allows for single-pass treatment with delivery of higher total fluencies with less risk of purpura (14,15). Most patients develop variable erythema and/or purpura following PDL treatments, which may last for 7 to 10 days. Furthermore, patients may develop hyperpigmentation, hypopigmentation, or scarring (6).

Intense Pulsed Light

Intense pulsed light (IPL) uses crystal filters to emit light with wavelengths of 590 to 1,200 nm. The light is noncoherent. The range of wavelengths and pulse durations capable of being produced by this laser are its primary advantages. Cutoff filters produce wavelengths that can be utilized for telangiectasias, skin discoloration, hair removal, or photoaging. Likewise, IPL system filters can eliminate shorter wavelengths to allow for greater dermal penetration with light of longer wavelength (6). IPL systems have also been used to treat port-wine stains and hemangiomas (6). In comparison with the PDL, IPL treatments require more time and have greater associated risks as additive heating occurs with successive passes and longer pulse durations (6).

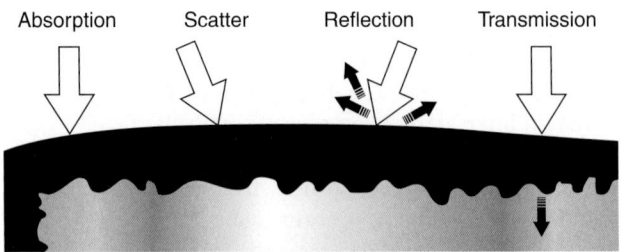

Figure 194.4 The biologic effect of a laser is partially dependent on the amount of absorption, scatter, reflection, or transmission of energy for a given tissue. (Reprinted from Papel ID, Frodel JL. *Facial plastic and reconstructive surgery*, 3rd ed. New York: Thieme, 2009:100, with permission.)

The primary use for IPL systems is treatment of telangiectasias. Selected wavelengths between 470 and 1,400 nm corresponding to absorption peaks of oxyhemoglobin are used to specifically target vessels. The range of wavelengths allows for treatment of vessels at various depths and greater energy penetration into the tissue (6). Newer systems incorporate cooling with chilled sapphire windows.

Potassium Titanyl Phosphate Laser

The potassium titanyl phosphate (KTP) laser is a frequency-doubled (wavelength halved) Nd:YAG laser. This is accomplished by passing the laser energy though a KTP crystal. The resultant light is green with a wavelength of 532 nm, corresponding to a hemoglobin absorption peak. The penetration and scattering of this laser light is intermediate between the CO_2 laser and the Nd:YAG laser. The laser energy is delivered to tissue via a fiber. If the fiber is not in contact with the tissue, vaporization and coagulation occur. Lower settings are typically used for coagulation. If the fiber is in semicontact with the tissue, cutting occurs. The KTP laser has a wide range of pulse durations, from 1 to 100 ms. The KTP laser has a shallow penetration depth. Accordingly, there is low risk of purpura, edema, or crusting (6,16). Atrophic scarring is a concern with the KTP laser.

Red and Infrared Lasers

The alexandrite (755 nm), diode (800 to 940 nm), and Nd:YAG (1,064 nm) lasers are in the red and near-infrared (IR) range. These lasers have been used to treat reticular veins, port-wine stains, and deep vessels in vascular malformations. Red and IR lasers are effective for these lesions as they have wavelengths that target peaks of deoxyhemoglobin in the near-IR range (700 to 1,200 nm), achieve deeper penetration, and allow for higher fluence (6).

The alexandrite laser is a flashlamp-pumped solid-state laser in the red spectrum of light (755 nm) but is not visible. This laser is absorbed by melanin and achieves deep penetration. The alexandrite laser has been used with significant improvement in hypertrophic port-wine stains with settings of 3-mm spot size, fluence range from 30 to 85 J/cm², and dynamic cooling (17). Others use settings of 8-mm spot size for the initial treatment of deep malformations (6). Li et al. (18) also demonstrated the effectiveness of the long-pulse pulsed alexandrite laser for hypertrophic, purple port-wine stains. The authors did note that this laser can cause dyspigmentation but no scarring was noted (18). This wavelength is also absorbed by the blue and black pigments in tattoos and can be used for hair removal.

The diode laser uses superconducting materials that are directly coupled to fiberoptic delivery devices. These lasers result in varying wavelengths depending on the material used. Diode lasers are efficient, converting electrical power to light at efficiencies of 50%, which allows for less heat production and power input (16). The light is fiberoptically delivered.

The Nd:YAG laser emits a wavelength of 1,064 nm, in the near-IR spectrum. The laser medium is neodymium:yttrium aluminum garnet and uses a helium-neon aiming beam. Pigmented tissue is selectively targeted with this laser as it penetrates up to 4 to 6 mm for treatment of deeper vessels (19). The depth of penetration of the Nd:YAG is related to its scatter, which is much greater than with the CO_2 laser. Thus, the Nd:YAG laser can be used for deep vessel coagulation (~3 mm). Yang et al. found the long-pulsed Nd:YAG laser to be equally effective as the PDL for the treatment of port-wine stains in a series of 17 patients (20). The authors found that purpura lasted longer following PDL treatments, but the Nd:YAG caused greater perivascular and epidermal injury with scarring noted in one patient (20).

Depressed scarring and hyperpigmentation are potential complications associated with the Nd:YAG laser (6). Cooling devices assist in minimizing these risks. In comparison with the near-IR diode laser, the Nd:YAG laser has deeper penetration, incurs less surrounding epidermal injury, and may be used more safely in darker pigmented individuals (6).

Carbon Dioxide (CO_2) Laser

The CO_2 laser uses CO_2 gas as a medium and has a wavelength of 10,600 nm. This wavelength is found in the mid-IR range and is absorbed by water. This laser is utilized for tissue with high water content given that it is absorbed well by water molecules. Effects are typically superficial due to minimal scatter and high absorption rates. This laser seals vessels up to 0.5 mm in diameter and nerve fibers.

A helium-neon aiming beam is utilized with this laser system as the laser beam is invisible. Typically, the beam is delivered to tissue through mirrors and lenses in an articulated arm either by a handpiece or attached to an operating microscope (4).

Recently, the fractionated CO_2 laser has gained popularity as it provides several distinct advantages over traditional CO_2 laser treatments. The fractionated CO_2 laser employs the concept of fractionated photothermolysis, which spares the epidermis from significant injury while causing coagulative injury in the dermis (21). Injury to the surrounding tissue is minimized as the fractionated laser delivers microthermal zones that allow for rapid reepithelialization at the periphery. The fractionated CO_2 laser decreases scarring, hypopigmentation, and the recovery time of traditional CO_2 laser treatments (21,22). The fractionated CO_2 laser has been used to treat scars, rhytids, and photodamage (21).

Argon Laser

The argon laser has a range of wavelengths from 488 to 514 nm in the visible spectrum. The resonating chamber and laser medium create a band of wavelengths emitted from this laser. Filters can be used to limit the resultant wavelengths emitted. Hemoglobin absorbs argon laser energy well, thus allowing for use in vascular lesions. A fiberoptic carrier represents the delivery system (4).

Continuous Yellow Dye Laser

The continuous-wave yellow dye laser produces a wavelength of 577 nm in the visible spectrum. The dye is excited by an argon laser. This laser is delivered by a fiberoptic cable. Shutters or a Hexascanner handpiece can pulse the light that is emitted. This laser is well suited for treatment of benign vascular lesions on the face.

Copper Vapor Laser

The copper vapor laser produces two wavelengths of the visible spectrum including a pulsed green light at 511 nm and a pulsed yellow light at 578 nm. A handpiece can deliver the light fiberoptically at spot sizes from 150 to 1,000 μm. This laser also is used to treat benign vascular lesions on the face as well as freckles, nevi, or keratoses.

LASER APPLICATIONS

Treatment Options

Treatment of lesions of the face has been revolutionized with the development and advancements in laser technology. When considering appropriate management for each patient and individual lesions, one must consider all available options. Common nonlaser treatment options consist of observation, ligation, excision, cautery, sclerosant therapy, chemotherapy, radiation, steroid therapy, embolization, systemic medications, or a combination of treatments. However, laser technology remains a mainstay in the treatment of facial lesions as laser selection often allows for targeted and selective photothermolysis. Throughout the discussion below regarding laser applications, treatment options will be further delineated in relation to specific lesions.

Vascular Lesions

Advances in medicine have provided understanding of the biologic basis for many vascular anomalies. Treatment of vascular lesions has evolved at a rapid pace with increasing knowledge of pathophysiology and technical advancements. One of the greatest strides in the treatment of vascular lesions came with the development of the laser.

While the original classification schema for vascular lesions has undergone necessary changes with advancements in the understanding of underlying pathophysiology, vascular lesions continue to be categorized based on structural components and biologic behavior. The general term "vascular lesion" refers to vascular malformations and hemangiomas.

Vascular malformations are differentiated from hemangiomas based upon their presence at birth, increasing size with patient growth, and normal rate of endothelial cell growth. Additionally, capillary vascular malformations have a propensity to become darker in color and develop surface thickening with time. Vascular malformations are often subclassified based on their vessel components: arterial, capillary vascular malformations (port-wine stains), venous, lymphatic, and/or combination lesions. Finally, vascular malformations characteristically have large ectatic vessels and lack endothelial hyperplasia.

In contrast, hemangiomas behave in a similar manner as true neoplasms. Hemangiomas have a proliferative phase with rapid growth and endothelial proliferation, followed by an involution phase. Involution of these lesions is a slow process. Hemangiomas are characteristically absent at birth and demonstrate endothelial hyperplasia in ectatic vessels.

Technical Aspects of Laser Treatment

The ideal laser should have a wavelength that is selectively absorbed by the targeted lesion, minimal epidermal absorption to reduce the incidence of scarring, and a flexible delivery mode capable of pulsed delivery to apply energy consistently based on the thermal relaxation time of the tissue. Multiple lasers have been manufactured and are used for a variety of lesions based on the key laser characteristics discussed above.

Lesion Subtypes

Hemangiomas

Hemangiomas behave in a similar manner as true neoplasms. These lesions typically appear in the few weeks after birth and grow disproportionately with the infant (23). Hemangiomas are more common in Caucasians with a female to male ratio of 3:1. The proportion of all hemangiomas occurring in the head and neck region is 60%. It has been proposed that these lesions result from growth of placental cells transferred to the fetus *in utero* (24). Resolution of these lesions is approximately 50% by age 5 years, 70% by age 7 years, and 90% by age 9 years (25). Following involution of hemangiomas, 40% to 50% of children will have residual telangiectatic cutaneous vessels, fibrous-fatty tissue, or scarring (26). Hemangiomas are classified as superficial (capillary), deep (cavernous), or combined (capillary–cavernous).

Treatment of hemangiomas has recently been modified following numerous reports regarding the success of beta-blocker therapy for these lesions (27–29). Recent studies have demonstrated rapid and consistent therapeutic effects of beta-blockers on infantile hemangiomas (29). Buckmiller et al. treated over 30 patients with propranolol (2 mg/kg/d, t.i.d. dosing), and 97% of lesions displayed improvement in the quality of the hemangioma.

Side effects noted included somnolence (27%) and reflux (10%) (30). While hemangiomas typically undergo spontaneous resolution and have recently been treated with beta-blocker therapy, laser and surgical therapies continue to be utilized for hemangiomas that alter vital functions, demonstrate ulceration, or cause significant cosmetic disfigurement (31). PDLs have been utilized for superficial lesions to lighten the lesion, induce regression, and possibly halt growth (Fig. 194.5) (5,32). Early studies found that PDL treatment possibly prevented enlargement and promoted involution. However, recent studies have called into question the ability of PDL to alter the natural course of hemangiomas. For example, a randomized controlled study by Batta et al. (33) found that PDL treatment versus observation in early hemangiomas resulted in similar clearance or residual signs of hemangioma at 1 year. This study also found that PDL treatment increased the likelihood of skin atrophy ($P = 0.008$) and hypopigmentation ($P = 0.001$) compared with observation (33). Additionally, other studies have noted that early PDL treatment may not decrease deeper hemangioma growth. The KTP and argon lasers can also be used for hemangiomas due to their photocoagulation selectivity.

The 1,064-nm Nd:YAG laser has been used effectively for deeper hemangiomas that failed to respond to other methods of treatment. Clymer et al. (34) treated children with hemangiomas with the 1,064-nm Nd:YAG laser using an interstitial technique and found a reduction in size of lesions and achieved good results without lesion reexpansion (Fig. 194.6).

Combined treatment using both the PDL and the Nd:YAG laser can be utilized for hemangiomas with both superficial and deep components. The Nd:YAG laser is often initially used to treat the deep component percutaneously. Settings typically include a 600-μm bare fiber, 10 to 20 J, and 0.5 to 1.0 pulse width. Ultimately, the settings of each laser type depend on the manufacturer and the specific laser utilized. Lesions are treated in a radial fashion to spare the overlying skin and deeper structures. These treatments may be repeated every 6 to 8 weeks. Once the bulk of the lesion is satisfactorily decreased, the superficial component may be treated with a PDL. Swelling should be expected postoperatively.

Capillary Malformations (Port-Wine Stains)

Port-wine stains (congenital capillary vascular malformations) are benign lesions within the dermis that are usually present at birth. Port-wine stains are present in approximately 0.3% to 0.5% of the population with 5% of these lesions associated with Sturge-Weber syndrome or Klippel-Trenaunay syndrome (3). These lesions are flat and pink to red in color. With age, these lesions can become darker and thicker with increased nodularity. The most common location for port-wine stains is the V_2 distribution of the face. While these lesions are typically not life-threatening, capillary malformations have been found to have significant

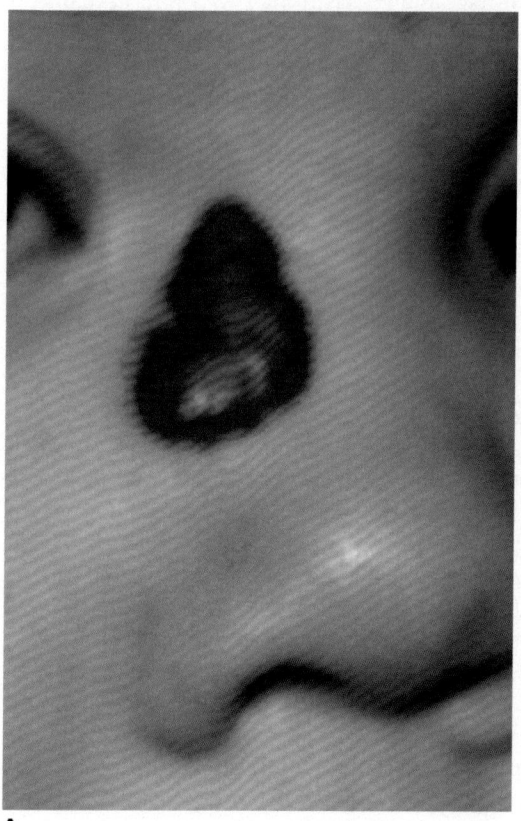
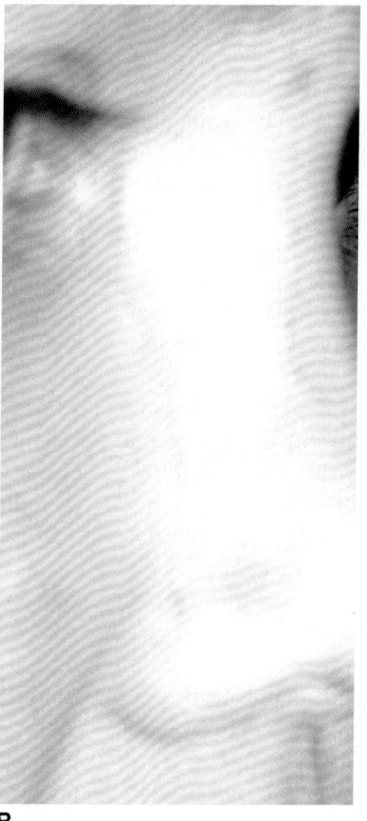

A   **B**

Figure 194.5 A: Right lateral nasal hemangioma, pretreatment. **B:** Appearance following FEDL treatments of hemangioma.

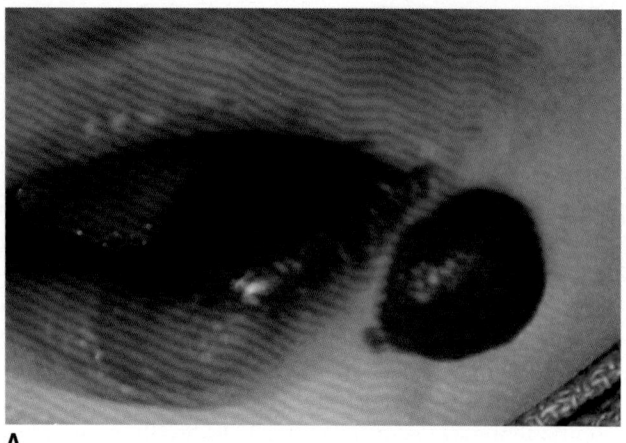
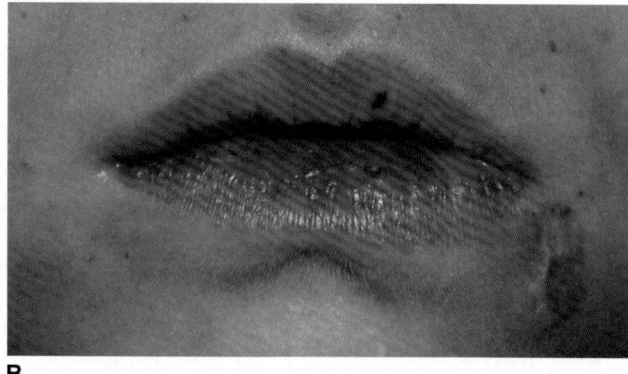

A   **B**

Figure 194.6 A: Left lower lip and buccal hemangioma, pretreatment. **B:** Posttreatment appearance following multiple Nd:YAG laser treatments with serial excisions over 2.5 years.

psychological consequences. Troilius et al. (35) found that port-wine stains negatively affected the lives of 75% of 259 children with these lesions. Additionally, earlier age at treatment has been associated with improved response rates.

The first treatment popularized for port-wine stains was the argon laser (488 to 514 nm). With limited penetration (0.1 mm), significant melanin absorption, and development of blistering and scarring, this treatment has largely been abandoned. Currently, PDLs with wavelengths between 585 and 595 nm are utilized. Treatment response is dependent on location, color, skin type, and age of patient (5). Two types of lesions have been described: type 1 have ectasias of the capillary loops and have a better response to PDL, while type 2 have dilated ectatic vessels in a ring pattern in the superficial horizontal plexus and demonstrate a poor response to PDL treatment. Treatment of port-wine stains with the PDL is effective with two passes per treatment with first pass settings of 5 to 6 J/cm², pulse width of 0.5 ms, and a spot size of 10 mm and second pass settings of 0.5 to 1.0 J/cm², pulse width of 2.0 ms, and a spot size of 10 mm. Cooling devices should be used with all treatments (5). PDL with epidermal cooling has also been used with pulse durations from 0.45 to 3 ms (5,6). Port-wine stains usually require multiple treatments repeated approximately every 2 to 3 months (Fig. 194.7). Ho et al. (36) performed a study with PDL or Nd:YAG treatment of port-wine stains on 107 Chinese patients and noted that 6.1 treatments were necessary for maximal lesional resolution. Additionally, Chan et al. (37) performed a study on port-wine stain treatment with Nd:YAG on 22 Chinese patients and noted that this treatment was only partially effective. The copper vapor laser and continuous dye laser have also been used for the treatment of port-wine stains (38,39). IPL treatment has been used with success in port-wine stains although most believe that patients with port-wine stains respond better to PDL treatment.

Venous Malformations

Venous malformations are treated when causing pain or functional problems (5). Treatment of these lesions typically consists of Nd:YAG laser (1,064 nm) therapy. Previous treatment options consisted of sclerotherapy, compression, or surgical resection. Treatment of these lesions can occur intralesionally or superficially (5). The Nd:YAG laser allows for deep vessel coagulation with penetration up to 4 mm. Superficial cooling is used to limit epidermal damage.

The main goal of treatment is to reduce bulk and improve contour. Settings that have been found to be effective for lesions with traceable vessels from 1 to 3 mm in diameter include a 6-mm spot handpiece, 80 J/cm², 50 ms pulse width, and frequency of 1 Hz (5). For vessels less than 1 mm, settings that have been utilized include a 3-mm spot handpiece, 150 J/cm², and 30 ms pulse width (5). Treatment of these lesions can occur at the earliest 8 weeks following previous treatment. Good results have been noted with Nd:YAG treatment of venous malformations (5,40). Care must be taken with Nd:YAG laser treatment of venous malformations as hypopigmentation, scarring, blistering, or burns can occur. Sclerotherapy for the deep vessels can be combined with laser treatments for the superficial vessels (5).

Telangiectasias

Telangiectasias are dermal lesions characterized by small ectatic vessels. A variety of subtypes have been described including linear, arborizing, punctuate, and spider (nevi or angiomas). The development of telangiectasias is thought to be related to estrogen, nasal trauma, surgery, and genetic susceptibility.

Facial telangiectasia treatment is based on selective thermolysis of oxyhemoglobin. Common lasers used for these lesions include the 595-nm PDL, 532-nm KTP laser, and 520-nm and 1,200-nm IPL (6). Other lasers used include the copper vapor laser and continuous-wave yellow dye laser. Many surgeons use the PDL with pulse stacking and multiple pass technique with good results (41). Common

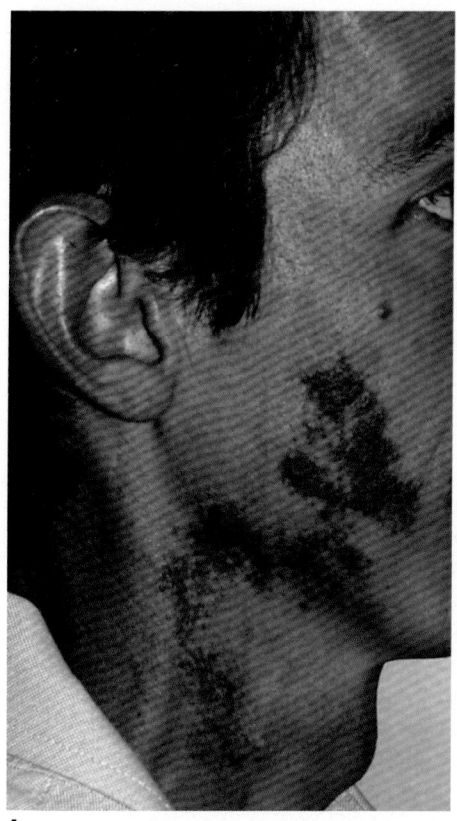
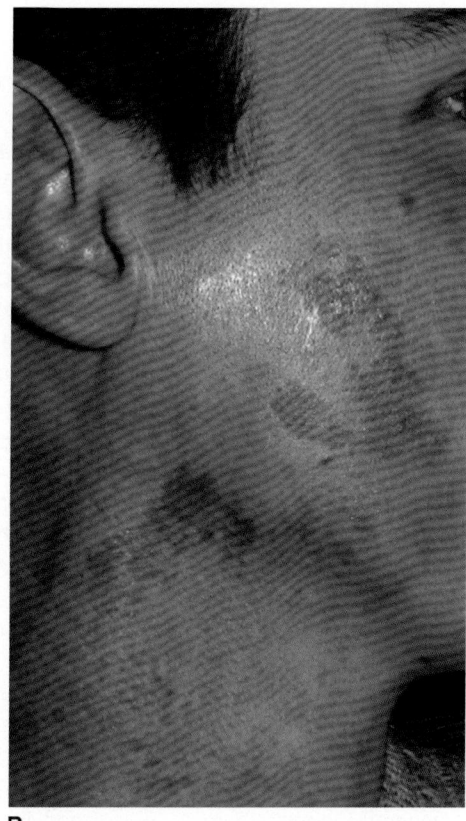

A   **B**

Figure 194.7 A: Pretreatment appearance of a right port-wine stain. **B:** Clinical response of this lesion following multiple FEDL treatments over a 1-year period. Note the decreased size and discoloration.

settings for the PDL for telangiectasias include 10-mm spot size, fluences of 6.5 to 7.5 J/cm^2, and pulse duration of 6 to 10 ms (6). KTP laser treatment has been utilized for telangiectasias with surrounding erythema with single-pass treatments using 10-mm spot size, 20 to 30 ms, and fluences of 7 to 10 J/cm^2 (6). Smaller spot sizes are used for smaller lesions. IPL devices with wavelengths of 520 to 1,200 nm have also been used for telangiectasias. Epidermal cooling and evaluation of skin pigmentation are important for the successful application of this laser. Given the melanin absorption, hypopigmented patches and blistering can be side effects of using this laser on tanned or greater pigmented skin without selective filter utilization (6,42).

Generally, when treating telangiectasias, one should use the smallest spot size and lowest power that will obliterate the dilated vessel. This will avoid nonselective, surrounding tissue damage. Treatment ensues by tracing vessels until the dilated vessel disappears. Spider telangiectasias are treated by obliterating the periphery of the radial vessels and moving toward the center with treatment of the central vessels last (3). Treatment of telangiectasias usually occurs at a lower energy density than that needed for treatment of port-wine stains, and retreatment may occur 6 to 8 weeks following previous treatment.

Hereditary Hemorrhagic Telangiectasia

Hereditary hemorrhagic telangiectasia (HHT, Osler-Weber-Rendu syndrome) is an autosomal dominant disease that causes telangiectatic lesions on the skin and mucous membranes. Patients with HHT often experience epistaxis (~90%) and/or bleeding from lips, gingiva, tongue, buccal mucosa, or hard palate. Patients with this disease may also have arteriovenous malformations in the lungs or brain (43). On histologic examination, ectatic vessels are observed with incomplete surrounding muscular layers.

Septodermoplasty has been utilized, sometimes in combination with lasers, to treat severe epistaxis (44,45). Lasers utilized to treat HHT have included CO_2, argon, Nd:YAG, and KTP. Given its superficial effects and vaporization of the overlying mucous membrane, the CO_2 laser is not the ideal choice for patients with HHT. Argon and KTP lasers provide for vascular selectivity for this disease process. Additionally, the deeper penetration of the Nd:YAG laser allows for effective coagulation of the lesions in HHT (46). Treatment of these lesions is typically performed with a free fiber that is held above the mucosal surface, and the lesion is treated in a rosette fashion by encircling the central portion and subsequently coagulating the central lesion. Nd:YAG treatment generally consists of a power setting of 10 to 25 W with an exposure time of 0.5 seconds. KTP treatment generally consists of a power setting of 6 W with an exposure time of 0.5 seconds with a slightly defocused beam.

Pigmented Lesions

Pigmented lesions can include benign lentigines, freckles, café au lait spots, congenital nevi, melasma, or tattoos. It is unclear how lasers produce pigment destruction but it is believed that photoacoustic damage to the cell by heating and expansion of melanosomes occur causing pigment breakup with phagocytosis and clearing.

Lasers often used to treat pigmented lesions include the pulsed dye (510 nm), copper vapor (511 nm), frequency-doubled Q-switched Nd:YAG (532 nm), KTP (532 nm), Q-switched and long-pulsed ruby (694 nm), Q-switched and long-pulsed alexandrite (755 nm), and Q-switched Nd:YAG (1,064 nm). The PDL is effective for lentigines, freckles, café au lait spots, and bright tattoo pigments such as red, purple, or orange. The ruby laser is preferentially absorbed by melanin and has a deeper level of penetration for effective treatment of the dermis. The Q-switched ruby laser is often used for removal of amateur blue-black tattoos. Red tattoos and other pigmented lesions are often removed with the frequency-doubled Q-switched Nd:YAG laser. The Q-switched alexandrite laser, with deeper penetration, is often used for pigmented lesions, lentigines, café au lait spots, and freckles. This laser can also be used to remove blue and green tattoos. In a previous study, it was shown that lentigines in dark-skinned patients responded better to long-pulsed 532-nm Nd:YAG laser treatment than Q-switched Nd:YAG laser treatment (47). The KTP laser is effective for solar lentigines and photoaging although darker skin types have been shown to have a higher side effect profile (48). Tattoo removal generally requires 5 to 10 treatments, while superficial lentigines and freckles can often be treated once.

Hair Removal

Lasers allow for effective although not permanent hair removal with less pain than electrosurgical techniques. The results of laser hair removal typically outlast traditional techniques including shaving, waxing, plucking, or electrolysis. Laser hair removal is much more effective on hair in the growth or anagen phase. Lasers with wavelengths between 690 and 1,100 nm, to target melanin, are primarily used for hair removal. The lasers often utilized are the red-light, IR, and filtered flashlamp IPL lasers. In removing hair, the pulse width of the laser roughly approximates the thermal relaxation time of the tissue (~10 to 100 ms) to adequately heat the targeted follicles. Cooling systems are used to limit the injury to surrounding areas.

The long-pulsed ruby laser (694 nm), long-pulsed alexandrite laser (755 nm), diode lasers (800 nm), filtered flashlamp IPL, and the Nd:YAG laser (with a carbon suspension) have been used for the process of hair removal. Several of these lasers have been shown to remove hair temporarily and provide long-term hair reduction, although multiple treatments are typically necessary for permanent results to be achieved (49,50). Dark-haired, light-skinned individuals typically have the best results with laser hair removal. Patients with darker skin colors are at a higher risk for hypopigmentation and have been shown to be more safely treated with longer wavelength lasers (51). A new technique that provides skin cooling with longer-pulse width laser treatments has increased the efficiency and decreased the side effects experienced by patients with darker skin colors during hair removal (52,53).

Skin Resurfacing and Rejuvenation

Lasers allow for skin resurfacing and rejuvenation in a controlled and reproducible manner. The water chromophore is targeted by the lasers used for this purpose. Vaporization is typically achieved in skin at approximately 5 J/cm^2 delivered in less than 1 ms. Lasers for skin resurfacing and rejuvenation are typically used for patients with rhytids, photoaging, and scarring.

CO_2 and erbium lasers are typical choices for resurfacing procedures. High-energy, short-pulsed systems with single pulses of 600 ms duration with fluences of 5 to 7 J/cm^2 have been used with the CO_2 laser. These systems minimize thermal damage. Another system utilizes scanning technology. With this system, a continuous laser beam with a microprocessor-controlled scanner moves the beam across the tissue to limit the dwell time at any point. Typical fluences are 5 to 15 J/cm^2 for this system. Erbium lasers rapidly ablate tissue with little thermal effect and cause less tissue shrinkage and faster reepithelialization. The CO_2 laser has also been used effectively for laser-assisted blepharoplasty (54). Rejuvenation of skin is often performed with IPL, PDLs, and Nd:YAG lasers (55–59). Shorter wavelength lasers have been shown to be better for the vascular and pigmentation effects from photoaging, while longer wavelength lasers are more effective for wrinkles (60). More recently, the fractionated CO_2 laser has been employed for laser resurfacing with improved results and less side effects than traditional CO_2 laser treatments (21). To achieve desired results, appropriate perioperative care, skin preparation, herpes prophylaxis, and local anesthesia are important. A pink color occurs following removal of the epidermis, a gray color indicates the papillary dermis, and a chamois yellow color indicates the reticular dermis.

Rhinophyma is a disease characterized by hyperplasia of the sebaceous glands and connective tissue. Most physicians use the CO_2 laser (5 to 10 W, continuous mode) for treatment of this disease. This laser allows the surgeon to sculpt the nose with precise excision and ablation of the tissue. Hemostasis is achieved with this laser and postoperative pain is minimal. The large nodules of rhinophymatous tissue are excised, and a defocused laser is then used to ablate the remainder of the lesion in a paintbrush style (Fig. 194.8).

Cutaneous Malignancies

The CO_2 laser can be used to excise basal and squamous cell carcinomas. This laser allows for sealing of vessels 0.5 mm or larger in diameter in a defocused mode. This laser can also be used for flap elevation or undermining. Postoperative pain is also reduced as nerve endings are sealed during the procedure. Photodynamic therapy is innovative and combines light-sensitive drugs that are

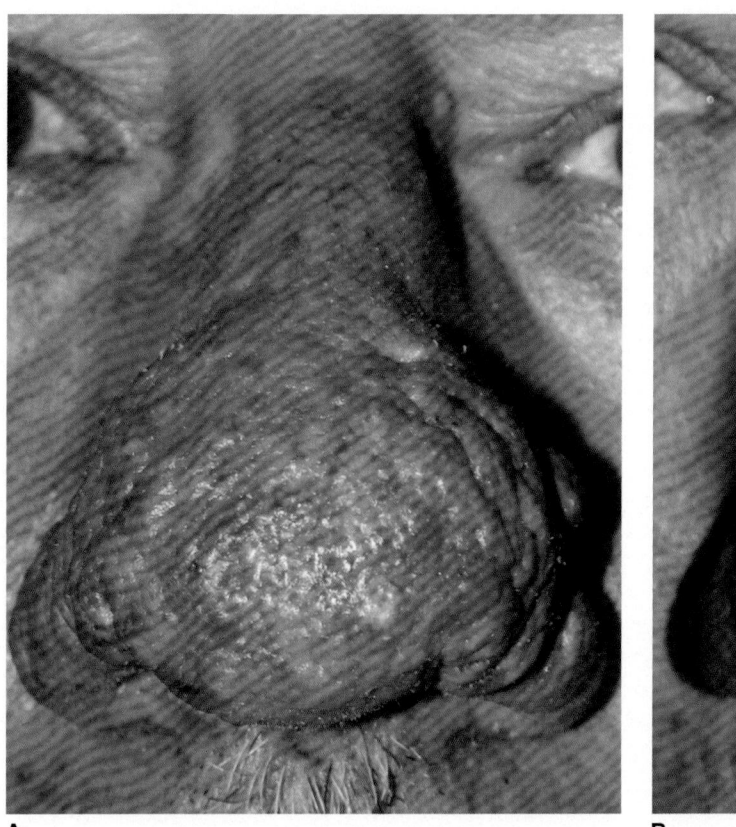 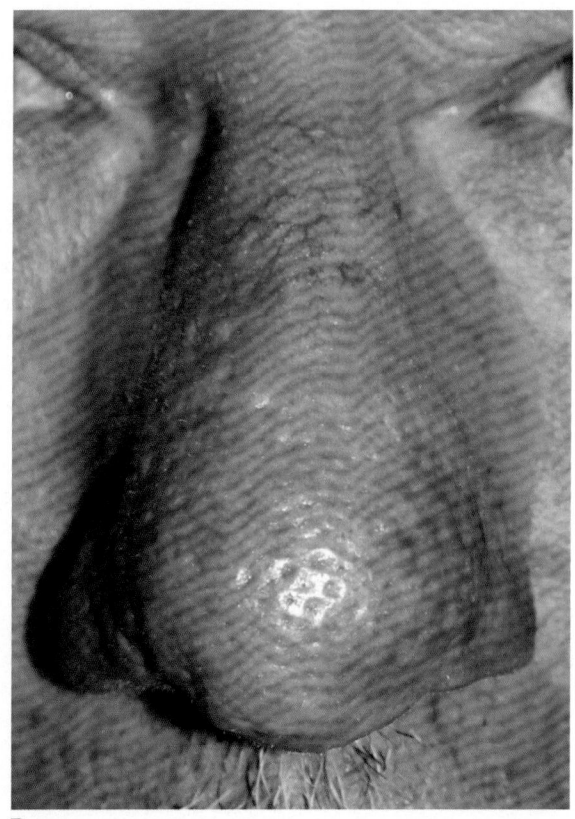

A   B

Figure 194.8 A: Pretreatment appearance of rhinophyma. **B:** Posttreatment appearance of rhinophyma following CO_2 laser ablation and excision.

given intravenously and concentrate in skin and neoplasms with lasers in an attempt to destroy nonmelanoma skin malignancies.

Expected Results

Realistic goals should be outlined with the patient and/or guardian preoperatively. Often, treatment of facial lesions is not designed or even capable of achieving complete resolution, and this should be discussed prior to initiation of any therapy. Risks, benefits, and alternatives should also be discussed in a forthright manner. Outlining the expected goals and demonstrating previous/realistic outcomes with patient photographs can be helpful.

Complications and Management

Complications in laser surgery are primarily avoided by understanding laser physics, laser–tissue interactions, and selecting lasers for appropriate indications. Approved training and safety courses should be attended by all surgeons desiring to perform laser surgery. Additionally, common side effects including hyperpigmentation, hypopigmentation, blistering, crusting, milia, purpura, scarring, infection, and erythema can result from routine laser treatments and should be fully discussed with the patient and family preoperatively.

Radiation hazards can cause injury to the eyes or skin. Eye injury may occur via direct intrabeam viewing or reflected laser light (5,24). Lasers with wavelengths in the 400 to 1,400 nm range of electromagnetic radiation can cause retinal damage as a result of laser beam focusing on the retina (24). Wavelengths of less than 400 nm or greater than 1,400 nm can produce corneal injury (24). Goggles protecting against laser-specific wavelengths should be worn at all times by all individuals in the operating room. Eye protection for the patient is also necessary. The eyes of the patient are often protected by taping the eyelids in the closed position with nonflammable, non-melting tape and covering the eyelids with saline-moistened gauze (5). Aluminum foil is then used to cover the periorbital region (5). Additionally, metallic corneal protectors (instead of plastic) should be used when using lasers in the periorbital region. Furthermore, the patient should have saline-moistened towels draped over all exposed, uninvolved facial skin as misdirected or reflected laser energy can result in burns (5). These inadvertent burns can also be avoided by placing the laser in standby mode or turning off when not utilizing the machine.

Chemical hazards associated with laser are often related to the dyes used for the laser medium. These dyes should only be changed by servicing individuals. Secondary hazards associated with laser usage include fire, noise, and high-voltage irradiation. The risk of fire is reduced by using moistened towels in the operative field and minimizing misdirected laser energy (5). Management of the side effects and complications associated with laser treatment should address the underlying etiology and typically includes symptomatic treatment.

CONCLUSIONS

Laser treatment in facial plastic surgery must be individualized for each patient. Lasers are often important for the targeted treatment of facial lesions. Lasers are selected based on the type of lesion, chromophore content of the tissue, desired biologic effect, and characteristics of the laser including wavelength and energy density. When a surgeon comfortably understands the interplay between lesion or disease pathophysiology and laser characteristics, appropriate treatment and improved patient outcomes can be achieved.

HIGHLIGHTS

- Appropriate treatment of facial lesions requires an understanding of the pathophysiology underlying the etiology of the lesion and knowledge of nonsurgical and surgical options.
- Lasers are important tools in the armamentarium of facial plastic and reconstructive surgeons and are often utilized for the treatment of facial lesions.
- Lasers can allow for targeted treatment of facial lesions and produce light that is monochromatic, collimated, and coherent.
- Lasers are selected based on the type of lesion, chromophore content of the tissue, desired biologic effect, and characteristics of the laser including wavelength and energy density.
- Continued advancements in laser technology have improved results of laser treatment of lesions of the head and neck.

REFERENCES

1. Zweng H, Flocks M, Kapany N, et al. Experimental laser photocoagulation. *Am J Ophthalmol* 1964;58:353–362.
2. Stellar S, Polanyi T. Lasers in neurosurgery: a historical overview. *J Clin Laser Med Surg* 1992;10:399.
3. Ries W, Clymer M. The Appropriate use of lasers in facial plastic surgery. In: Willett J, ed. *Facial plastic surgery*. Stamford, CT: Appleton & Lange, 1997:223–241.
4. Ries W, Wittkopf M. Lasers in facial plastic surgery. In: Papel I, Frodel J, Holt G, et al., eds. *Facial plastic and reconstructive surgery*, 3rd ed. New York: Thieme Medical Publishers, Inc., 2009:99–118.
5. Burns A, Navarro J. Role of laser therapy in pediatric patients. *Plast Reconstr Surg* 2009;124(1 Suppl):82–92.
6. Railan D, Parlette E, Uebelhoer N, et al. Laser treatment of vascular lesions. *Clin Dermatol* 2006;24:8–15.
7. Sommer S, Sheehan-Dave R. Pulsed dye laser treatment of port-wine stains in pigmented skin. *J Am Acad Dermatol* 2000;42:667–671.
8. Lou W, Geronemus R. Treatment of port-wine stains by variable pulsed width pulsed dye laser with cryogen spray: a preliminary study. *Dermatol Surg* 2001;27:963–965.
9. Travelute A, Carniol P, Hruza G. Laser treatment of facial vascular lesions. *Facial Plast Surg* 2001;17(3):193–201.
10. Bernstein E. Treatment of a resistant port wine stain with the 1.5 millisecond pulse duration, tunable, pulsed dye laser. *Dermatol Surg* 2000;26:1007–1009.
11. Kelly K, Nanda V, Nelson J. Treatment of port-wine stain birthmarks using the 1.5-msec pulsed dye laser at high fluences in conjunction with cryogen spray cooling. *Dermatol Surg* 2002;28(4):309–313.
12. Chang C, Ries W. Nonoperative techniques for scar management and revision. *Facial Plast Surg* 2001;17(4):283–288.
13. Bradley D, Park S. Scar revision via resurfacing. *Facial Plast Surg* 2001;17(4):253–262.
14. Ross E, Uebelhoer N, Domankevitz Y. Use of a novel pulse dye laser for rapid single-pass purpura-free treatment of telangiectasias. *Dermatol Surg* 2007;33:1466–1469.
15. Galeckas K. Update on lasers and light devices for the treatment of vascular lesions. *Semin Cutan Med Surg* 2008;27(4):276–284.
16. Ries W, Powitzky E. Lasers in facial plastic surgery. In: Papel I, Frodel J, Holt G, et al., eds. *Facial plastic and reconstructive surgery*, 2nd ed. New York: Thieme Medical Publishers, Inc., 2002:79–95.
17. No D, Dierickx C, McClaren M, et al. Pulsed alexandrite treatment of bulky vascular malformations. *Lasers Surg Med* 2003;15:26.
18. Li L, Kono T, Groff WF, et al. Comparison study of a long-pulse pulsed dye laser and a long-pulse pulsed alexandrite laser in the treatment of port wine stains. *J Cosmet Laser Ther* 2008;10(1):12–15.
19. Rogachefsky A, Silapunt S, Goldberg DJ. Nd:YAG laser (1064 nm) irradiation for lower extremity telangiectases and small reticular veins: efficacy as measured by vessel color and size. *Dermatol Surg* 2002;28(3):220–223.
20. Hunzeker C, Weiss E, Geronemus R. Fractionated CO_2 laser resurfacing: our experience with more than 2000 treatments. *Aesthet Surg J* 2009;29(4):317–322.
21. Tierney E, Hanke C. Treatment of CO_2 laser induced hypopigmentation with ablative fractionated laser resurfacing: case report and review of the literature. *J Drugs Dermatol* 2010;9(11):1420–1426.
22. Yang M, Yaroslavsky A, Farinelli W, et al. Long-pulsed neodymium:yttrium-aluminum-garnet laser treatment for port-wine stains. *J Am Acad Dermatol* 2005;52(3 Pt 1):480–490.
23. Mallucci J. Vascular anomalies must be properly classified. *BMJ* 2000;2:919.
24. North P, Waner M, Mizeracki A, et al. A unique microvascular phenotype shared by juvenile hemangiomas and human placenta. *Arch Dermatol* 2001;137:559–570.
25. Werner J, Dunne A, Folz B, et al. Current concepts in the classification, diagnosis, and treatment of hemangiomas and vascular malformations of the head and neck. *Eur Arch Otorhinolaryngol* 2001;258:141–149.
26. Chang C, Nelson J. Cryogen spray cooling and higher fluence pulsed dye laser treatment improve port-wine stain clearance while minimizing epidermal damage. *Dermatol Surg* 1999;25:767–772.
27. Léauté-Labrèze C, Dumas de la Roque E, Hubiche T, et al. Propranolol for severe hemangiomas of infancy. *N Engl J Med* 2008;358(24):2649–2651.
28. Siegfried E, Keenan W, Al-Jureidini S. More on propranolol for hemangiomas of infancy. *N Engl J Med* 2008;359(26):2846.
29. Sans V, de la Roque E, Berge J, et al. Propranolol for severe infantile hemangiomas: follow-up report. *Pediatrics* 2009;124(3):423–431.
30. Buckmiller L, Richter G, Suen J. Diagnosis and management of hemangiomas and vascular malformations of the head and neck. *Oral Dis* 2010;16:405–418.
31. Vlachakis I, Gardikis S, Michailoudi E, et al. Treatment of hemangiomas in children using a Nd:YAG laser in conjunction with ice cooling of the epidermis: techniques and results. *BMC Pediatr* 2003;3:2.
32. Shafirstein G, Buckmiller L, Waner M, et al. Mathematical modeling of selective photothermolysis to aid the treatment of vascular malformations and hemangioma with pulsed dye laser. *Lasers Med Sci* 2007;22(2):111–118.

33. Batta K, Goodyear H, Moss C, et al. Randomised controlled study of early pulsed dye laser treatment of uncomplicated childhood haemangiomas: results of a 1-year analysis. *Lancet* 2002;360: 521–527.

34. Clymer M, Fortune D, Reinisch L, et al. Interstitial Nd:YAG photocoagulation for vascular malformations and hemangiomas in childhood. *Arch Otolaryngol Head Neck Surg* 1998;124:431–436.

35. Troilius A, Wrangsjö B, Ljunggren B. Potential psychological benefits from early treatment of port-wine stains in children. *Br J Dermatol* 1998;139(1):59–65.

36. Ho W, Chan H, Ying S, et al. Laser treatment of congenital facial port-wine stains: long-term efficacy and complication in Chinese patients. *Lasers Surg Med* 2002;30:44–47.

37. Chan H, Chan E, Kono T, et al. The use of variable width frequency doubled Nd:YAG 532 nm laser in the treatment of port-wine stains in Chinese patients. *Dermatol Surg* 2000;26(7):657–661.

38. Lu Y, Wu J, Yang Y, et al. Photodynamic therapy of port-wine stains. *J Dermatol Treat* 2010;21(4):240–244.

39. Rothfleisch JE, Kosann MK, Levine VJ, et al. Laser treatment of congenital and acquired vascular lesions. A review. *Dermatol Clin* 2002;20(1):1–18.

40. Ulrich H, Gaumler W, Hohenleutner U, et al. Neodymium-YAG laser for hemangiomas and vascular malformations: long term results. *J Dtsch Dermatol Ges* 2005;3:436–440.

41. Iyer S, Fitzpatrick R. Long-pulsed dye laser treatment for facial telangiectasias and erythema: evaluation of a single purpuric pass versus multiple subpurpuric passes. *Dermatol Surg* 2005;31: 898–902.

42. Butler E, McClellan S, Ross E. Split treatment of photodamaged skin with KTP 532 nm laser with 10 mm handpiece versus IPL: a cheek-to-cheek comparison. *Lasers Surg Med* 2006;38(2):124–128.

43. Olitsky S. Hereditary hemorrhagic telangiectasia: diagnosis and management. *Am Fam Physician* 2010;82(7):785–790.

44. Harvey R, Kanagalingam J, Lund V. The impact of septodermoplasty and potassium-titanyl-phosphate (KTP) laser therapy in the treatment of hereditary hemorrhagic telangiectasia-related epistaxis. *Am J Rhinol* 2008;22(2):182–187.

45. Corlett J, Shakespeare P, Wright P, et al. A laser end piece for the treatment of Epistaxis using the Pulsed Dye Laser. *Clin Otolaryngol* 2008;33(1):71–72.

46. Werner A, Bäumler W, Zietz S, et al. Hereditary haemorrhagic telangiectasia treated by pulsed neodymium:yttrium-aluminium-garnet (Nd:YAG) laser (1,064 nm). *Lasers Med Sci* 2008;23(4):385–391.

47. Chan H, Fung W, Ying S, et al. An in vivo trial comparing the use of different types of 532 nm Nd:YAG lasers in the treatment of facial lentigines in Oriental patients. *Dermatol Surg* 2000;26(8):843–849.

48. Bassichis B, Swamy B, Dayan S. Use of the KTP laser in the treatment of rosacea and solar lentigines. *Facial Plast Surg* 2004;20:77–83.

49. Allison K, Kiernan M, Waters R, et al. Evaluation of the ruby 694 chromos for hair removal in various skin sites. *Lasers Med Sci* 2003;18:165–170.

50. Weisberg N, Greenbaum S. Pigmentary changes after alexandrite laser hair removal. *Dermatol Surg* 2003;29:415–419.

51. Hamilton M, Dayan S, Carniol P. Laser hair removal update. *Facial Plast Surg* 2001;17(3):219–222.

52. Nahm W, Tsoukas M, Falanga V, et al. Preliminary study of fine changes in the duration of dynamic cooling during 755-nm laser hair removal on pain and epidermal damage in patients with skin types III-V. *Lasers Surg Med* 2002;31:247–251.

53. Nottingham L, Ries W. Update on lasers in facial plastic surgery. *Curr Opin Otolaryngol Head Neck Surg* 2004;12:323–326.

54. Munker R. Laser blepharoplasty and periorbital laser skin resurfacing. *Facial Plast Surg* 2001;17(3):209–217.

55. Dahiya R, Lam S, Williams E III. A systematic histological analysis of nonablative laser therapy in a porcine model using the pulsed dye laser. *Arch Facial Plast Surg* 2003;5:218–223.

56. Negishi K, Tezuka Y, Kuchikata N, et al. Photorejuvenation for Asian skin by intense pulsed light. *Dermatol Surg* 2001;27:627–632.

57. Bitter P. Noninvasive rejuvenation of photo damaged skin using serial, full face intense pulsed light treatments. *Dermatol Surg* 2000;26:835–883.

58. Goldberg D, Cutler K. Nonablative treatment of rhytids with intense pulsed light. *Lasers Surg Med* 2000;26:196–200.

59. Dayan S, Damrose J, Bhattacharayya T, et al. Histological evaluation following 1064-nm Nd:YAG laser resurfacing. *Lasers Surg Med* 2003;33:126–131.

60. Sadick N. Update on nonablative light therapy for rejuvenation: a review. *Lasers Surg Med* 2003;32:120–128.

195 Management of Benign Facial Lesions

Karen J. Sundby   *John A. Zitelli*

Successful management of facial lesions depends on accurate diagnosis, knowledge of natural history, and use of a specific appropriate treatment. A functional classification scheme, together with history and physical examination, allows narrowing of diagnostic possibilities. Most benign facial lesions are noninflammatory, including various tumors, cysts, and melanocytic lesions (Table 195.1). Important exceptions include specific infectious, degenerative, and metabolic conditions that clinically appear and behave as inflammatory disorders (e.g., verruca, molluscum contagiosum). "Benign" facial lesions can signal serious systemic diseases (Tables 195.2 to 195.4).

HISTORY AND PHYSICAL EXAMINATION

Important questions to ask relate to duration of lesion, family history, fluctuation in size or drainage of any material, rapidity of onset, pain (e.g., leiomyomas are often spontaneously painful), and associated physical findings (e.g., tuberous sclerosis). Inspection and palpation are aided by adequate lighting or side lighting. Diascopy (pressing a clear microscope slide over the lesion to determine whether it is blood-filled—i.e., of vascular origin) also is useful. The lesion is classified by depth (epidermal, dermal, or subcutaneous) and other characteristics (cystic vs. solid; tenderness; color; texture; mobility; surface features, such as smooth or verrucous; presence of a central punctum), distribution and arrangement of lesions, and associated inflammation.

EPIDERMAL LESIONS

Epidermal lesions are most common, including seborrheic keratosis, actinic keratosis, comedones, milia, cutaneous horn, and epidermal cysts (1–5).

Actinic keratosis (or solar or senile keratosis) is composed of small, usually multiple erythematous lesions on sun-exposed areas, such as the face, exposed scalp, and dorsum of the hands. They have a rough, adherent scale and are more easily felt than seen. Actinic keratosis can develop into squamous cell carcinoma (10% to 20%), which usually does not metastasize. The lifetime risk of squamous cell carcinoma in an individual with actinic keratosis has been estimated to be 6% to 10% (6,7).

An analogous lesion to an actinic keratosis, actinic cheilitis (Fig. 195.1), occurs on the lip's vermilion border. It presents with hyperkeratosis, erosions, and a dull opaqueness.

Cutaneous horns (Fig. 195.2) are hyperkeratotic conical lesions whose height is at least half their largest diameter. Various types of lesions may be present at their bases (actinic keratosis, verruca, squamous cell carcinoma, seborrheic keratosis, and rarely trichilemmoma or basal cell carcinoma). Cutaneous horns require adequate removal so their bases can be examined histopathologically (8).

Seborrheic keratoses have brownish-black, verrucous papules or plaques with a "stuck-on" appearance, reflecting their epidermal origin. The sign of Leser-Trélat, the abrupt appearance or explosive expansion in size and number of multiple seborrheic keratoses, especially if accompanied by pruritus, has been implicated as a cutaneous marker of internal malignancy (9,10). In black patients, they may appear on the face as multiple brown to black papules over the cheeks, called dermatosis papulosa nigra.

Epidermal cysts are often compressible and may have visible puncta. If they have been inflamed, they may be fixed to surrounding tissue. It may be difficult to tell epidermal cysts from lipomas or neurofibromas. Lipomas are soft and often lobulated, lack puncta, and are movable against overlying skin. Neurofibromas similarly lack puncta and often display "button-holing" (described later).

Milia are small, yellowish-white, 1- to 2-mm papules. Primary milia develop spontaneously, commonly in newborns and people who are predisposed to them. Secondary

TABLE 195.1 CLASSIFICATION OF BENIGNFACIAL LESIONS

Inflammatory lesions
  Xanthelasma
  Molluscum
  Verruca

Noninflammatory lesions
  Epidermal tumors and cysts
    Seborrheic keratosis
    Epidermal cyst
    Milia
    Dermoid cyst
    Actinic keratosis
    Keratoacanthoma
    Comedones
    Cutaneous horn
  Skin-appendage tumors
    Trichofolliculoma
    Trichoepithelioma
    Pilomatricoma
    Trichilemmoma
    Nevus sebaceous
    Sebaceous hyperplasia/rhinophyma
    Hidrocystoma
    Syringoma

Non–skin-appendage tumors
  Vascular
    Hemangiomas (capillary, cavernous, flammeus)
    Angiomas
    Telangiectasias
    Pyogenic granuloma
    Venous lake
  Fibrous
    Soft fibroma (skin tag)
    Fibrous papule
    Adenoma sebaceum (angiofibroma)
    Hypertrophic scar/keloid
  Neural
    Neurofibroma
  Fatty/muscular/osseous
    Lipoma
    Multiple miliary osteomas
    Leiomyomas
    Melanocytic lesions
    Nevi
    Lentigines
    Ephelides (freckles)
    Nevus of Ota
    Blue nevus
    Spitz nevus

TABLE 195.2 DIFFERENTIAL DIAGNOSIS OF SYNDROMES ASSOCIATED WITH MULTIPLE BENIGNFACIAL LESIONS

Disease	Onset	Cutaneous Features	Systemic Features
Neurofibromatosis	Variable to adulthood, seven types	Neurofibromas Cafe-au-lait macules Axilliary freckling	Multiple skeletal, endocrine, and neurologic abnormalities; increased incidence of malignancy (Wilms, CNS/PNS rhabdomyosarcoma, leukemia)
Tuberous sclerosis	Variable (early childhood to young adult life)	Angiofibromas (adenoma sebaceum, shagreen patches, periungual fibromas, ash leaf white macules)	Mental retardation, epilepsy, multiple organ hamartomas (eye, kidney, heart)
Gardner syndrome	May first appear at age 7–10, 50% display syndrome by age 20	Multiple epidermal cysts	Malignant degeneration (40%), osteomas of facial bones, fibromas, lipomas, leiomyomas of stomach or ileum
Muit-Torre syndrome	Variable	Sebaceous tumors of skin (most are adenomas) with or without keratoacanthomas (often very large)	Visceral neoplasms (often multiple, especially GI, larynx, endometrium)
Cowden disease	Variable	Multiple trichilemmomas, gingival fibromatosis	Greatly increased risk of breast carcinoma, thyroid adenomas, and carcinomas
Multiple endocrine neoplasia (type 2b)	Early childhood	Neuromas of oral and nasal mucosa, upper GI tract, and conjunctiva; lentigines; "blubbery" lips	Increased risk for medullary thyroid carcinoma, pheochromocytoma, marfanoid habitus, kyphoscoliosis

CNS, central nervous system; PNS, peripheral nervous system; GI, gastrointestinal.

| TABLE 195.3 | HEREDITARY TELANGIECTATIC SYNDROMES | | |

Disease	Onset	Cutaneous Features	Systemic Features
Rothmund-Thomson syndrome	3 mo–2 y	Telangiectasias, mottled pigmentation, and atrophy (poikiloderma) of face, arms, legs, buttocks	Moderate dwarfism, sparse hair, cataracts, photosensitivity
Bloom syndrome	Infancy	Erythema and telangiectasias of butterfly area of face, forehead, ears, lids, hands, and forearms	Dwarfism, photosensitivity
Cockayne syndrome	Second year	Erythema and mottled pigmented scarring of butterfly area of face	Physical and mental retardation, loss of subcutaneous fat on face, Mickey Mouse ears
Hereditary hemorrhagic telangiectasia	Childhood	Punctate or linear telangiectasias of face, lips, ears, conjunctiva, upper trunk, arms	Mucosal hemorrhage
Ataxia-telangiectasia	3–5 y	Linear telangiectasias of conjunctiva, eyelids, ears, cheeks	Dwarfism, ataxia

A differential diagnosis also includes the collagen vascular diseases and liver diseases.
Modified from Champion RH, Burton JL, Burns AD, et al., eds. *Rook's textbook of dermatology*, 6th ed. London, UK: Blackwell, 1998, with permission.

| TABLE 195.4 | SYNDROMES WITH MULTIPLE MELANOCYTIC LESIONS | | |

Disease	Onset	Cutaneous Features	Systemic Features
Neurofibromatosis	See Table 195.1	See Table 195.1	See Table 195.1
Albright syndrome	Melanotic macules appear soon after birth.	Melanotic patches (unilateral)	Polyostotic fibrous dysplasia, precocious puberty, endocrine dysfunctions
Peutz-Jeghers	Hyperpigmented macules are usually present at birth or early childhood.	Melanotic macules of lips and oral mucosa	Degeneration (2%–3%) of granulosa cell tumors in females (20%), increased association of duodenal cancer
LEOPARD syndrome	Lentigines appear in infancy and increase in numbers.	Multiple lentigines	Ocular hypertelorism, pulmonary (Moynahan syndrome) stenosis, abnormalities of genitalia, growth restriction, deafness (neural)
Lamb syndrome	—	Facial and genital lentigines, mucocutaneous myxomas, blue nevi	Atrial myxomas
Name syndrome	—	Nevi, myxoid neurofibromata, freckling (ephelides)	Atrial myxoma
Centrofacial lentiginosis	Lentigines appear in first years of life.	Midfacial freckling, sacral hypertrichosis, fusion of eyebrows	High arched palate, missing upper incisors, seizures, mental retardation, scoliosis, spina bifida
Cronkhite-Canada syndrome	—	Melanotic macules on face, extremities, alopecia, onychodystrophy, hyperpigmentation	Gastrointestinal polyposis

LEOPARD, lentigines, electrocardiographic abnormalities, ocular hypertelorism, pulmonary stenosis, abnormal genitalia, retardation of growth, deafness.

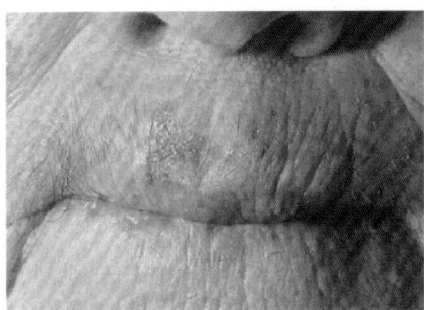

Figure 195.1 Actinic cheilitis. (From Werner R. *Massage therapist's guide to pathology*. Philadelphia, PA: Lippincott Williams & Wilkins, 2012, with permission.)

milia may develop from trauma; from subepidermal blistering diseases, in areas of topical corticosteroid–induced atrophy; or postdermabrasion. In the latter case, the milia are probably a proliferative postinjury epithelial response.

Comedones superficially resemble milia but occur in specific situations. Open comedones (blackheads) are small (1- to 2-mm) papular lesions with a central black plug. They are usually multiple, occurring with acne vulgaris or actinically damaged skin. Closed comedones (whiteheads) are 1- to 2-mm white lesions seen with acne vulgaris. Histologically, comedones are dilated cystic hair follicles filled with keratinous and lipoid material.

SKIN-APPENDAGE TUMORS

Skin-appendage tumors have diverse clinical presentations. They are common on the face and scalp because of the numerous appendageal structures there.

Many facial appendage tumors are small skin-colored papules. Trichofolliculomas occur in adults as solitary facial lesions. They have a central pore with a white wool-like tuft of hair, a diagnostic feature.

Trichoepitheliomas are also small, flesh-colored papules. They are solitary or multiple. Multiple lesions are autosomal dominant, first appearing in childhood, with the number of lesions gradually increasing. Multiple trichoepitheliomas cluster around the central face and can occur with cylindromas, another benign appendage tumor often occurring on the scalp. These can grow together, resembling a turban (turban tumor). At times, trichoepitheliomas can be confused with basal cell carcinomas, both clinically and pathologically.

Trichilemmomas are small, pink to brown facial papules, in solitary and multiple forms. The multiple form can be a feature of the multiple hamartoma syndrome or Cowden disease, an autosomal-dominant genodermatosis associated with a high incidence of neoplasms (both benign and malignant) of the breast and thyroid, which occur in up to two-thirds of patients (11). Multiple trichilemmomas occur in all patients with Cowden disease and precede development of breast cancer, allowing identification of women at risk. These lesions appear nonspecific or can resemble small verrucae. In Cowden disease, oral lesions appear as 1- to 3-mm skin-colored papules that can assume a subtle cobblestone appearance or be so extensive that they involve the entire oral cavity, including the tongue.

Sebaceous hyperplasia is a common papular lesion occurring in older people. It is composed of 2- to 3-mm yellow to orange lobulated papules with a slight central umbilication. They can be solitary or multiple, commonly on the forehead and nose (highest number of sebaceous glands). They are enlargements of normal sebaceous glands. They also can occur with cyclosporine use and can be a feature of acne rosacea (rhinophyma) (Fig. 195.3).

Syringomas are small, flesh-colored to translucent papules that are intraepidermal eccrine duct adenomas. A syringoma may occur at any site on the body but are prone to occur in the periorbital area, especially the eyelids.

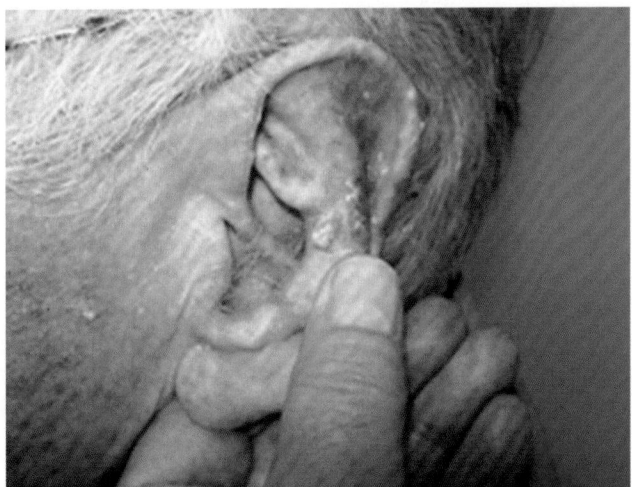

Figure 195.2 Cutaneous horn. (From Goodheart HP. *Goodheart's same-site differential diagnosis: a rapid method of diagnosing and treating common skin disorders*. Philadelphia, PA: Lippincott Williams & Wilkins, 2010, with permission.)

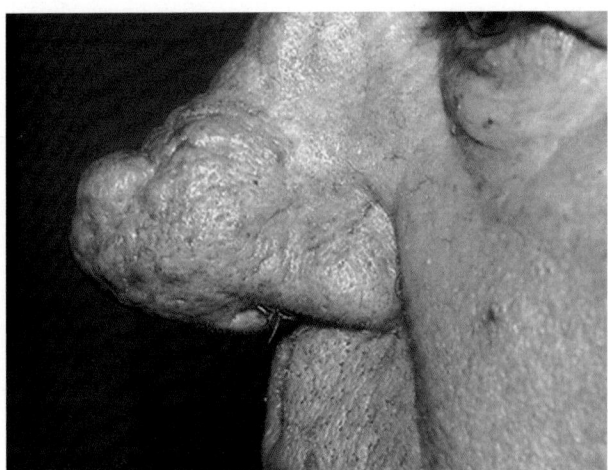

Figure 195.3 Rhinophyma. (From Werner R. *Massage therapist's guide to pathology*. Philadelphia, PA: Lippincott Williams & Wilkins, 2012, with permission.)

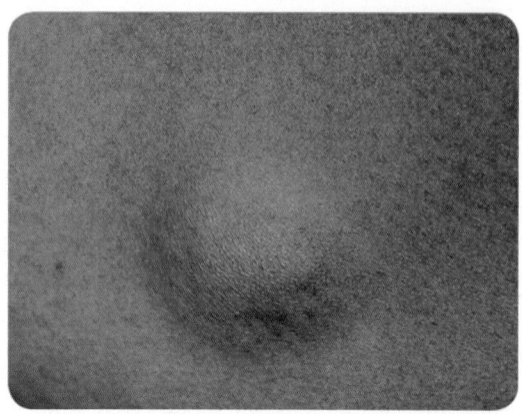

Figure 195.4 Pilomatricoma. (From Lugo-Somolinos A, McKinley-Grant L, Goldsmith LA, et al. *VisualDx: essential dermatology in pigmented skin.* Philadelphia, PA: Lippincott Williams & Wilkins, 2011, with permission.)

Syringomas often have a predilection for apocrine areas (axillae, vulva) or eruptive forms on the trunk or in dermatomal patterns. The lesions are removed from women more commonly than men, although it is not entirely clear that this represents a gender predilection rather than biopsy selection bias resulting from cosmetic or social factors.

Hidrocystomas are small, uncommon cystic periorbital lesions, most commonly seen on the eyelid margin. They are 2 to 15 mm in diameter, with a translucent bluish quality. Apocrine hidrocystomas are larger and solitary, whereas eccrine hidrocystomas are smaller and multiple.

Pilomatricomas (Fig. 195.4) are tumors typified by follicular matrical cornification, usually presenting as a solitary, hard, deep-seated nodule, usually on the face or upper extremities. The nodules may have a faint bluish-red color and are sharply demarcated, ranging in diameter from 0.5 to 3.0 cm. They are common in children and young adults.

Nevus sebaceus (Jadassohn nevus; Fig. 195.5) is a hamartoma that exhibits follicular, sebaceous, and apocrine malformation to varying degrees (12). The lesion is a congenital lesion presenting as a solitary, often linear, slightly raised, orange-yellow hairless plaque on the scalp or face. Its morphologic appearance changes with the activity of underlying sebaceous glands by becoming more verrucous and nodular at puberty. It is well-established that nevus

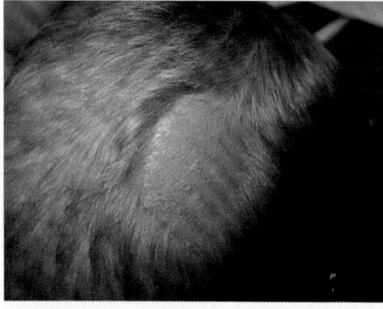

Figure 195.5 Nevus sebaceus. (Image provided by Stedman's.)

sebaceus may develop secondary adnexal neoplasms, most commonly benign but sometimes malignant. Trichoblastoma and syringocystadenoma papilliferum are the most commonly found benign neoplasm, whereas basal cell carcinoma is found in less than 1% of the cases (13–15). Patients rarely have extensive nevus sebaceus plaques with an associated neurocutaneous syndrome (epilepsy, mental retardation, skeletal deformities).

NON–SKIN-APPENDAGE TUMORS

Lesions derived from non–skin-appendage elements include vascular, fibrous, neural, fatty, muscular, and osseous tissues (1–4).

Vascular Tumors

Cherry angiomas are a very common, benign vascular proliferation found on most adults. They are bright-red, dome-shaped papules, 2 to 4 mm in diameter, most commonly found on the trunk and extremities. Patients usually bring these to the attention of the physician when they are chronically traumatized or cosmetically undesirable.

Vascular malformations include capillary malformations (port-wine stain), venous malformations (cavernous hemangioma), lymphatic malformations (lymphangioma, lymphangioma circumscriptum, cystic hygroma), and arteriovenous malformations. It is important therapeutically and prognostically to distinguish among these. Port-wine stains (capillary malformation) are often present at birth as large, flat, pink, well-demarcated patches that demonstrate a growth pattern that parallels the growth of the child. With age, the affected skin develops a more pronounced red color, thickens, and becomes more nodular. Various syndromes are associated with capillary malformations. Sturge-Weber syndrome is a sporadic neurologic disorder in which a facial capillary malformation (usually V1 distribution of the trigeminal nerve) is associated with ipsilateral ocular and leptomeningeal anomalies. When capillary malformations occur on an extremity, a progressive overgrowth of the affected extremity may occur with underlying osteohypertrophy and arteriovenous fistulae, which is known as Klippel-Trenaunay syndrome.

Capillary hemangiomas are more common in females and premature infants. They appear between the third and fifth weeks of life, grow for several months to 1 year, and then regress. Of capillary hemangiomas, 70% regress by age 7 years. Ultimately, only 6% are cosmetically problematic. Histologically, there is vascular endothelial cell proliferation.

The most common acquired hemangioma is a pyogenic granuloma, often found on the face and extremities. It is a rapidly growing, friable, solitary red papule or polyp that frequently ulcerates and easily bleeds. Pyogenic granulomas are often precipitated by minor trauma or pregnancy.

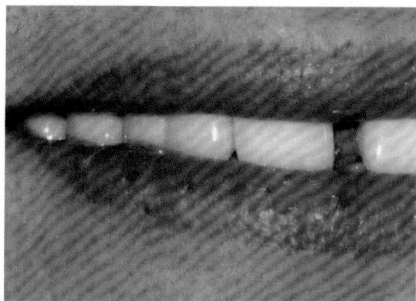

Figure 195.6 Osler-Rendu-Weber disease (hereditary hemorrhagic telangiectasia). (From Schaaf CP, Zschocke J, Potocki L. *Human genetics*. Philadelphia, PA: Lippincott Williams & Wilkins, 2011, with permission.)

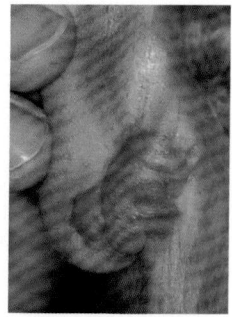

Figure 195.7 Keloid. (From Halperin ECC, Perez CA, Brady LW, et al. *Perez and Brady's principles and practice of radiation oncology*. Philadelphia, PA: Lippincott Williams & Wilkins, 2007, with permission.)

The second major group of vascular lesions of the face are the ectasias, or dilatations of blood vessels (not new vessel growth). These include telangiectasias and venous lakes. Most are acquired or may have syndromal features (Table 195.3).

Facial telangiectasias are extremely common and consist of dilated capillaries that appear as tiny, red, cutaneous vessels that blanch when pressure is applied. Telangiectasias may present in a linear pattern or spider-like with a central feeding vessel and radiating dilated vessels. These lesions occur with conditions such as rosacea, scleroderma, dermatomyositis, radiation dermatitis, chronic alcoholism, liver disease, pregnancy, childhood, Osler-Rendu-Weber disease (Fig. 195.6), carcinoid syndrome, idiopathic telangiectasia (generalized essential telangiectasia), or actinic skin degeneration.

Venous lakes are deep-blue cutaneous nodules usually on the lips, ears, or face. Histologically, they are dilated venules in the dermis that blanch with compression.

Fibrous Tumors

Facial fibrous tissue tumors include skin tags, fibrous papules, adenoma sebaceum, hypertrophic scars, and keloids. A skin tag (soft fibroma) is the most common fibrous lesion. These are small (1 to 2 mm), smooth, filiform, flesh-colored growths commonly located around the eyes or on the neck. They are usually multiple, distinguished from verrucae by their smooth surface. Skin tags occur elsewhere on the body (particularly the inguinal folds and axillae) and can occur as large, solitary, bag-like structures on the lower trunk.

Fibrous papules are solitary, dome-shaped, flesh-colored papules located on the central face of adults, most commonly the nasal ala and alar crease. These can clinically simulate intradermal nevi, adnexal tumors, or basal cell carcinomas. Sampling biopsies are often done to exclude a basal cell carcinoma. Otherwise, these lesions are benign and do not require further treatment unless it is of cosmetic concern to the patient.

Hypertrophic scars can be confused with keloids. Both are red, raised, smooth, and shiny, but hypertrophic scars

remain within the injury area, whereas keloids (Fig. 195.7) extend beyond the original injury site. Hypertrophic scars flatten over time, and keloids proliferate. There is familial and racial predilection (darker skin pigmentation) for keloid formation. Hypertrophic scars develop after wound infection or in certain anatomic locations (deltoid, angle of mandible, sternum). Keloids are uncommon on the face, even in keloid-forming individuals with the exception of the ears.

Adenoma sebaceum (Fig. 195.8) is an uncommon but characteristic feature of tuberous sclerosis. Adenoma sebaceum, mental retardation, and epilepsy form the classic triad of this dominantly inherited neurocutaneous syndrome. Adenoma sebaceum is a misnomer because these growths are not adenomas nor are they sebaceous. These growths are actually angiofibromas. They are numerous small, reddish, smooth papules symmetrically distributed around the nose, cheeks, and chin, sparing the upper lip. They first appear in late childhood, so they are a late sign of tuberous sclerosis.

Fatty/Muscular Tumors

Tumors of fatty, muscular, and osseous tissue occasionally occur on the face (1–5). The most common are lipomas. Clinically, lipomas are single or multiple, soft, rounded,

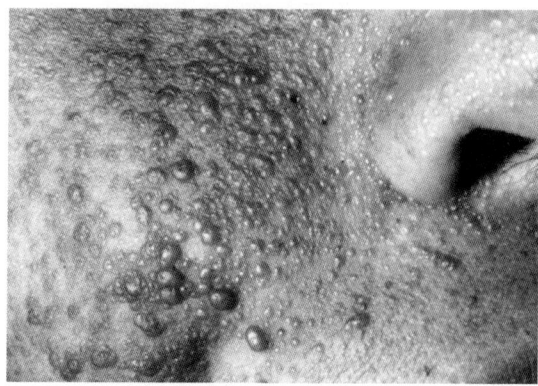

Figure 195.8 Adenoma sebaceum. (From McMillan JA, Feigin RD, DeAngelis C, et al. *Oski solution*. Philadelphia, PA: Lippincott Williams & Wilkins, 2006, with permission.)

lobulated growths that are freely movable against the overlying skin. These collections of mature fat cells with a thin connective tissue capsule must be differentiated from other soft, round growths such as neurofibromas and epidermal cysts.

Leiomyomas occur less commonly on the face. These small, firm, reddish-brown nodules arise from erector pili hair follicle smooth muscle. They are often multiple, arranged in a group or line, and painful.

Neural Tumors

Neurofibromas are benign nerve sheath tumors that can develop as solitary lesions or as multiple lesions as part of neurofibromatosis (NF1) (von Recklinghausen disease). Solitary neurofibromas are soft flesh-colored tumors that resemble normal nevocytic nevi. They may become pedunculated. When pressed, the tumor easily invaginates through a small skin opening (button-hole sign). Subcutaneous neurofibromas are either deep, firm, discrete nodules or, more characteristically, large, flabby, plexiform neuromas that feel like a bag of worms. The plexiform neurofibroma is especially important because it is considered pathognomonic of neurofibromatosis and requires proper patient management (16).

Melanocytic Tumors

Melanocytic nevi contain intraepidermal or dermal collections of nevus cells or both (1–5).

Melanocytic nevi are congenital or acquired and described by their histologic location of the nevus cells within the skin as either junctional, compound, or intradermal. Very few nevi are present at birth; therefore, most nevi are acquired and follow a specific life cycle. Most nevi appear in childhood, adolescence, or early adulthood, with few new nevi developing past middle adulthood. As age increases, the number of nevi progressively decreases. They pass through successive stages of junctional, compound, and intradermal development. Most nevi in children are junctional; in older adults, most nevi are intradermal.

Nevus appearance corresponds with histology. Junctional nevi (Fig. 195.9) are flat and pigmented; dermal

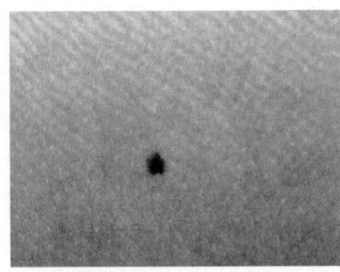

Figure 195.10 Dermal nevi. (From Craft N, Fox, LP. *VisualDx: essential adult dermatology*. Philadelphia, PA: Lippincott Williams & Wilkins, 2010, with permission.)

nevi (Fig. 195.10) are flesh colored and dome shaped or pedunculated; compound nevi (Fig. 195.11) are in between. Congenital nevi are larger than acquired nevi, are pigmented and slightly elevated, and may have increased hair. Compared with acquired nevi, they have deeper nevus cell extension into dermis, distribution of nevus cells near cutaneous appendages, and extension of nevus cells between collagen bundles. Giant congenital nevi have an increased risk for malignant transformation (17,18), whereas small- and medium-sized congenital nevi have little or no increased risk for developing into melanoma.

Spitz nevus (epithelioid and spindle cell nevus) is a rare type of melanocytic nevus (Fig. 195.12). It is a solitary, well-circumscribed, dome-shaped papule or nodule varying in color from pink to tan to brown. Their size varies from about 2 mm to about 2 cm, and they occur on the face and extremities of children and young adults. Although benign, it can resemble malignant melanoma histologically and may require treatment as melanoma unless a definitive distinction of benign versus malignant can be assured by the pathologist.

The principal tumors of epidermal melanocytes are freckles (ephelides) and lentigines. These flat, pigmented lesions are distinct from seborrheic keratoses or junctional nevi, which they resemble. Actinically induced lentigines are lentigo senilis (Fig. 195.13), whereas randomly occurring ones are lentigo simplex. Most facial lesions are lentigo senilis. They are light to dark-brown flat lesions, 5 to 20 mm in diameter or larger. Most are benign, but occasionally on the face they are confused with malignant

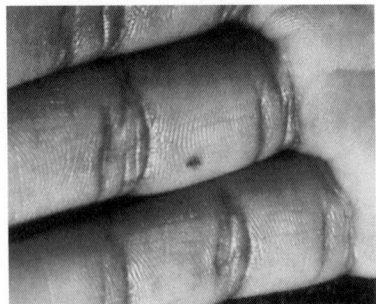

Figure 195.9 Junctional nevus. (From the Institute for Dermatologic Communication and Education, 1976, with permission.)

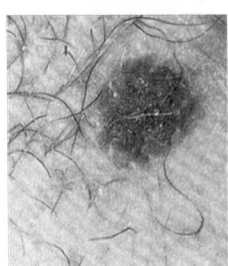

Figure 195.11 Compound nevus. (From Wilkinson EJ. *Wilkinson and Stone atlas of vulvar disease*. Philadelphia, PA: Lippincott Williams & Wilkins, 2013, with permission.)

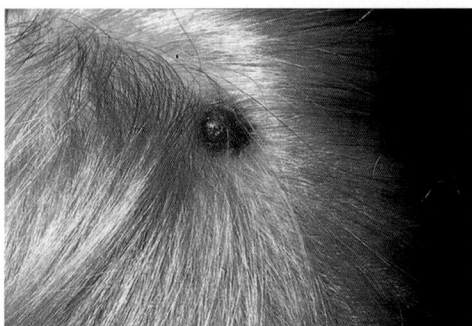

Figure 195.12 Spitz nevus. (From Elder AD, Elenitsas R, Johnson BL, et al. *Synopsis and atlas of Lever's histopathology of the skin.* Philadelphia, PA: Lippincott Williams & Wilkins, 1999, with permission.)

lesions such as lentigo maligna or melanoma *in situ.* Other features distinguishing lentigines from freckles are onset later in life, lack of seasonal variation, and larger size. Psoralen and ultraviolet A photochemotherapy lentigines are lesions precipitated by ultraviolet A phototherapy with psoralen. Freckles, in contrast, are easily recognized as small, brown, scattered macules occurring on sun-exposed areas of fair-skinned people. They have no malignant potential, darken in response to sunlight, and develop in childhood. Multiple facial lentigines are a prominent feature of numerous syndromes (Table 195.4).

The main facial dermal melanocytic lesions are benign intradermal and compound nevi, as described earlier. Other less common lesions include nevus of Ota and common blue nevus. Nevus of Ota is a unilateral blue to brown pigmented patch involving the skin of the periorbital, temple, forehead, or malar areas that occurs predominantly in dark-skinned races. Usually, the ipsilateral sclerae (Fig. 195.14) are involved, and occasionally the conjunctiva, cornea, retina, and oral and nasal mucosa are involved. Nevus of Ota has two times of onset: early childhood before the age of 1 year and around puberty. Malignancies arising in nevi of Ota are rare but when present do not adhere to the typical ABCD rules of melanoma (19). Several cases of primary malignant melanoma of the choroid, orbit, iris, chiasma, and meninges have developed in association with nevus of Ota that exhibited eye involvement (20).

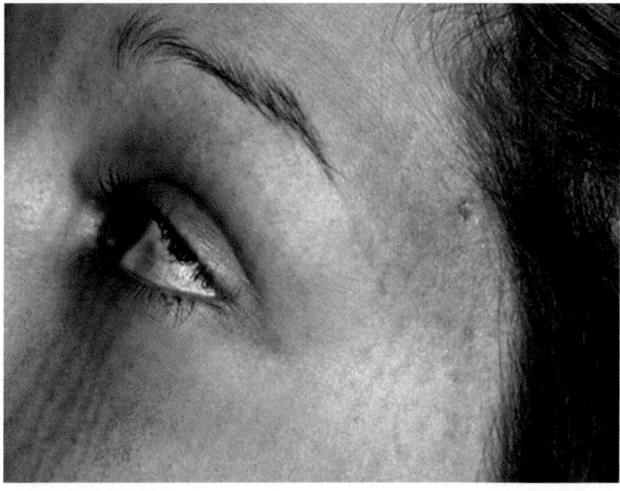

Figure 195.14 Nevus of Ota. (From Craft N, Taylor E, Tumeh PC, et al. *VisualDx: essential adult dermatology.* Philadelphia, PA: Lippincott Williams & Wilkins, 2010, with permission.)

Common blue nevi are small (1 cm), smooth, dome-shaped papules (Fig. 195.15) with a characteristic blue appearance as a result of the presence of deep intradermal melanin pigment that is viewed through intact skin (Tyndall effect). The lesions may appear anywhere, but about 50% of cases are found on the dorsa of the hands and feet.

Infectious Lesions

Warts (verruca vulgaris) are composed of intraepidermal lesions resulting from local infection with the human papilloma virus (1–5). They occur at any age, are spread by local contact or autoinoculation, have an unpredictable course, and are usually asymptomatic. They are more common and resistant to treatment in patients who are immunocompromised.

There are more than 100 genotypes of human papilloma virus, including common, filiform, plantar (including mosaic), flat, and anogenital warts. They have an irregularly corrugated (verrucous) surface, with pinpoint black dots of thrombosed capillaries. On mucosal surfaces, they may be smooth-surfaced papules or on flexible, pedunculated stalks.

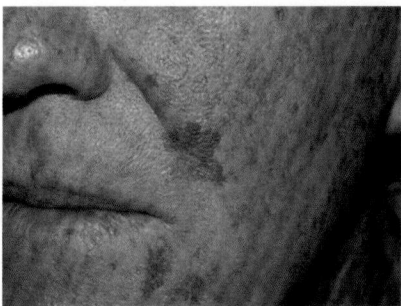

Figure 195.13 Lentigo senilis. (From Werner R. *Massage therapist's guide to pathology.* Philadelphia, PA: Lippincott Williams & Wilkins, 2012, with permission.)

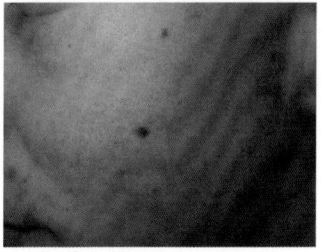

Figure 195.15 Blue nevus.

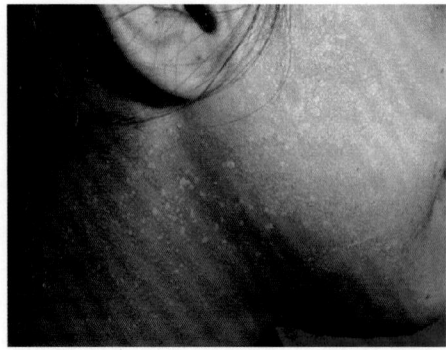

Figure 195.16 Flat warts. (From Burkhart C, Morrell D, Goldsmith LA, et al. *VisualDx: essential pediatric dermatology.* Philadelphia, PA: Lippincott Williams & Wilkins, 2010, with permission.)

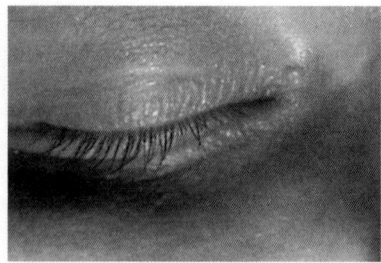

Figure 195.17 Molluscum contagiosum. (From the American Academy of Dermatology, 1977, with permission.)

Common warts are firm, sessile papulonodular growths, uncommon on the face. Filiform warts, common on the face, are tag-like protuberances resembling skin tags. Flat warts (Fig. 195.16) also are common on the face, particularly in young women, and can be missed if not viewed with side lighting. They are slightly elevated, light-brown, 1- to 5-mm grouped discrete lesions.

Molluscum contagiosum (Fig. 195.17) is a cutaneous infection caused by a poxvirus. It produces shiny, flesh-colored to pink, dome-shaped, firm papules with central umbilication. It is spread by local contact or autoinoculation and is common in children, sexually active young adults, and individuals who are immunocompromised. When central umbilication is not apparent, they resemble milia or closed comedones. In patients who are immunocompromised, these lesions can form large crateriform

and plaque-like lesions involving large areas of the face. Molluscum lesions have a central expressible inclusion, which can confirm the diagnosis. In patients who are immunocompromised, disseminated deep fungal infections (e.g., *Cryptococcus)* are also part of the differential diagnosis.

LABORATORY STUDIES

Most dermatologic diagnoses can be made by inspection or skin biopsy (shave, punch, or excision) (2,21,22). A shave biopsy uses a scalpel blade to shave the lesion flush with, or slightly below, the surrounding skin (Fig. 195.18). This biopsy contains epidermis and a small amount of dermis, so it is appropriate for pathology in those layers, such as actinic keratosis, verruca, benign nevi, trichoepithelioma, or trichofolliculoma. A full-thickness skin biopsy (punch or excisional) is used for pathology in the deep dermis (pilomatricoma) or when entire architecture

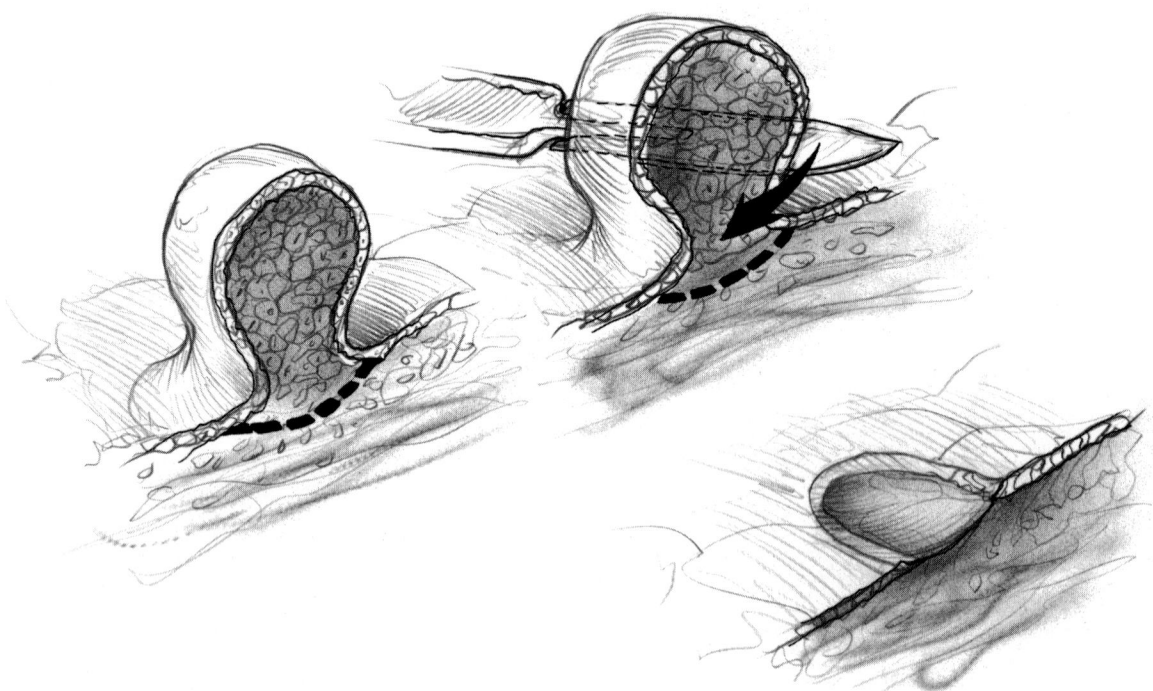

Figure 195.18 Shave biopsy.

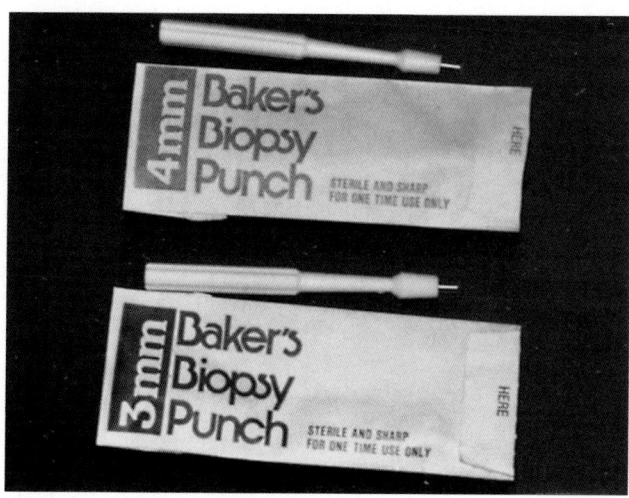

Figure 195.19 Punches (3 and 4 mm).

THERAPEUTIC CONSIDERATIONS: TECHNIQUES AND INSTRUMENTATION

Dermal Curette

The dermal curette is a small instrument with a semisharp round to oval blade of variable size (2 to 10 mm) (Fig. 195.21). This allows the surgeon to distinguish between normal and diseased collagen because the semisharp blade will not normally cut through normal collagen. Dermal curettes also are used to remove superficial epidermal lesions, which may be scraped off the skin's surface (seborrheic keratosis, warts) (Fig. 195.22). The instrument is easy and safe to use, but some experience is needed for the surgeon to distinguish reliably between diseased and normal dermal tissue.

Electrosurgery

In electrosurgery, rapidly oscillating electrical fields destroy tissue thermally and mechanically. A monopolar device (e.g., Hyfrecator) requires no grounding plate and results in superficial tissue destruction; a bipolar device requires a grounding plate and causes deeper tissue destruction. Either can be used for electrodesiccation. For electrosurgery, the needle tip is touched to tissue, destroying a deep sphere of tissue. For electrofulguration, the tip

is required for accurate diagnosis (Spitz nevus). Punch biopsies are performed using a 2- to 8-mm circular sharp blade on a handle (Fig. 195.19). It is pressed firmly against the skin and twisted back and forth to penetrate the full thickness of the skin (Fig. 195.20). These are used to diagnose inflammatory conditions or small tumors. For larger lesions, an excisional biopsy is performed. This is used if carcinoma is suspected or the pathologic process involves the fatty layer.

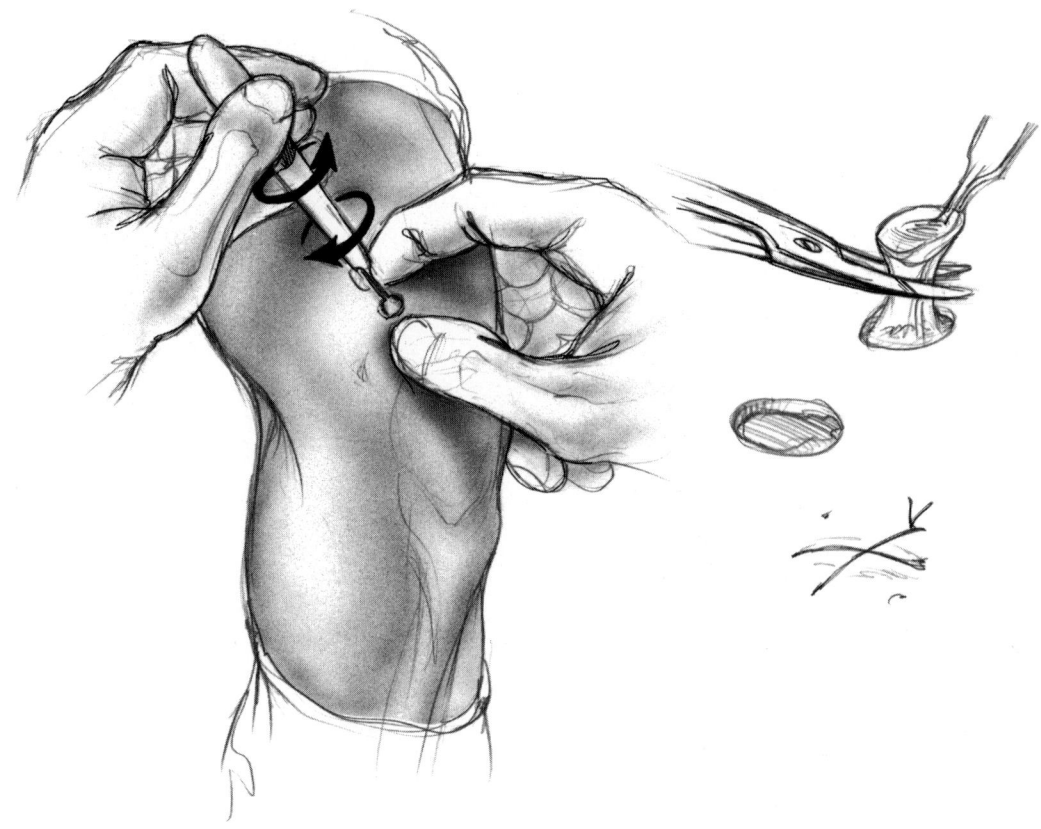

Figure 195.20 Punch biopsy technique.

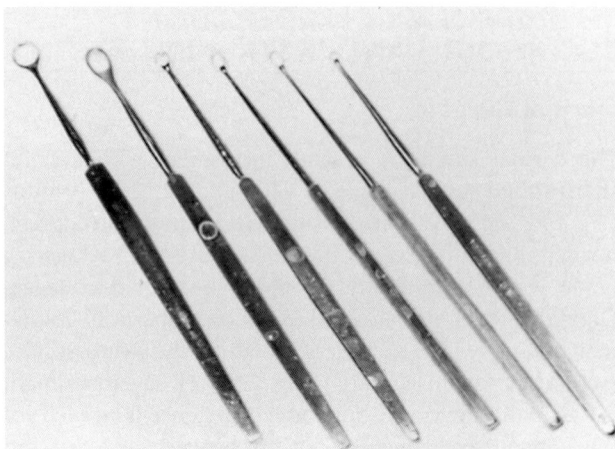

Figure 195.21 Curettes of various sizes.

is held near the lesion, and a spark jumps from needle tip to tissue, destroying a broad superficial arc of tissue. Figure 195.23 shows electrofulguration with curettage to remove a xanthelasma. Electrosurgery is fast with minimal bleeding, but healing by second intent takes 2 to 3 weeks, there is no tissue for histologic examination, and there can be excessive scarring from thermal damage. Electrosurgery is often used with a dermal curette to define lesion margin or to remove tissue as it is destroyed. Complications include combustion of nondry alcohol-treated skin and interruption of certain cardiac pacemakers.

Cryotherapy

In cryotherapy, a cryogen (usually liquid nitrogen) destroys tissue. Freezing causes formation of extracellular and intracellular ice crystals, resulting in cell membrane damage. Most cell damage occurs during thaw, when electrolyte concentrations become abnormal. Rapid freezing followed by slow thawing is most lethal to cells, with melanocytes

being the most susceptible to injury. Tissue destruction is determined by the volume of cryogen applied, the duration of exposure, and the technique used.

A commonly used cryogen is liquid nitrogen, which is the coldest (−196° C) and most versatile agent. Common techniques of application include the cotton-tipped applicator, which is the easiest to learn but evaporates rapidly, necessitating frequent redipping. Spray can also be applied quickly to several lesions but requires skill to direct the cryogen to the specific lesion.

Intralesional Corticosteroid Therapy

Corticosteroid therapy, topical or intralesional, is used to treat inflammatory conditions. Intralesional steroids offer a more concentrated and sustained effect than topical steroids but have more side effects, such as atrophy (usually reversible in 12 months or more) or hypopigmentation (in darker-pigmented skin). Significant systemic absorption can occur when more than 20 mg are injected in a single session or at frequent intervals (Table 195.5).

Intralesional steroids are often used to soften or reduce the size of keloids or hypertrophic scars (10 to 40 mg/mL), repeated every 2 to 3 weeks to minimize systemic toxicity. Intralesional steroid injections also are used after laser or scalpel excision to prevent or reduce recurrence of keloid formation. Intralesional steroids are also used for acne cysts and inflamed epidermal cysts (2.5 to 5.0 mg/mL).

Chemical Peeling

Chemical peeling (chemexfoliation) improves skin quality and texture by applying exfoliants. This causes a variable depth of epidermal and dermal injury that, on healing, has thicker dermal collagen and, in some cases, increased dermal glycosaminoglycans and restoration of elastic fibers in actinically damaged skin. Various peeling agents and

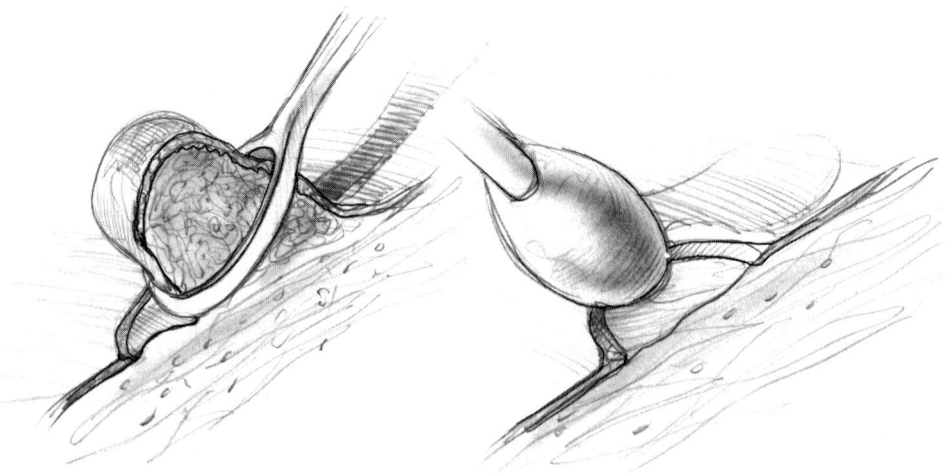

Figure 195.22 Curettage of a seborrheic keratosis.

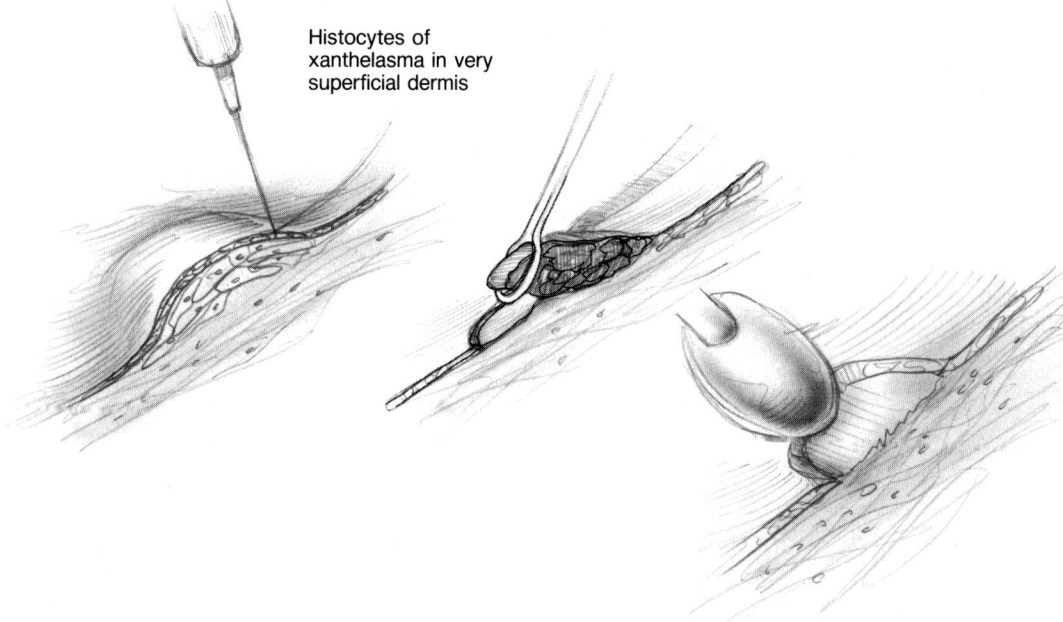

Histocytes of xanthelasma in very superficial dermis

Figure 195.23 Electrofulguration and curettage of a lesion of xanthelasma.

combinations have been used, including trichloroacetic acid, phenol, resorcinol, salicylic acid, and more recently lactic and glycolic acid, each with different properties and depth of penetration. Phenol has a significant risk profile and the potential for systemic toxicity (Table 195.6).

TABLE 195.5	SIDE EFFECTS OF INTRALESIONAL CORTICOSTEROIDS

Local side effects
Atrophy
Striae, stellate pseudoscars
Telangiectasia, purpura, erythema
Hypopigmentation
Impaired wound healing
Exacerbation of cutaneous infections

Systemic side effects
Cardiovascular effects: hypertension
Central nervous system effects: mood alterations, psychosis, pseudotumor cerebri
Endocrine effects: hypothalamic–pituitary–adrenal axis suppression, hirsutism, menstrual irregularities, truncal obesity, moon facies, buffalo hump
Gastrointestinal effects: peptic ulcer, pancreatitis
Hepatic effects: diabetes mellitus
Hematologic effects: lymphopenia, monocytopenia, neutrophilia
Immunologic effects: opportunistic infections
Musculoskeletal effects: osteoporosis, aseptic necrosis of femoral or humeral heads, myopathy
Ophthalmic effects: glaucoma, cataracts (posterior subcapsular)
Renal effects: sodium and fluid retention, hypokalemic alkalosis

Modified from Bondi E, ed. *Dermatology: diagnosis and therapy.* Norwalk, CT: Appleton & Lange, 1991:346, with permission.

Dermabrasion

Dermabrasion is an abrading procedure performed on skin to remove superficial lesions. Initially used to treat acne scars, more recently it has been applied to many cutaneous lesions (Table 195.7). Dermabrasion is performed with a motor-driven instrument with an abrading piece at the end. The abraders (commonly wire brush or diamond fraise) come in various sizes, shapes, and degrees of coarseness.

Competent dermabrasion requires a high level of skill. One must control precisely the depth of the abrasion because prominent scarring occurs if abrasion penetrates reticular dermis. Dermabrasion has similar complications to chemical peeling (Table 195.6). Dermabrasion results can be more predictable than chemical peeling because the extent of wounding can be more precisely controlled.

Laser Surgery

The properties of lasers that make them useful in treating facial lesions (Table 195.8) are precise margination, good

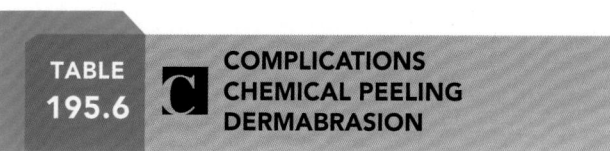

TABLE 195.6	COMPLICATIONS CHEMICAL PEELING DERMABRASION

Pigmentary abnormalities (especially in dark-skinned patients)
Increased sun sensitivity
Hypertrophic scarring (especially over jawline, nasal bridge)
Reactivation or dissemination of herpes simplex
Persistent erythema
Milia

TABLE 195.7	ENTITIES TREATED WITH DERMABRASION

Acne, active
Acne rosacea
Actinically damaged skin
Adenoma sebaceum
Age- and sun-related wrinkle lines
Angiofibromas of tuberous sclerosis
Basal cell carcinoma (superficial type)
Chloasma
Chronic radiation dermatitis
Darier disease
Dermatitis papillaris capillitii
Favre-Racouchot syndrome
Fox-Fordyce
Freckles
Hair transplantation (elevated recipient sites)
Hemangioma
Keratoacanthoma
Leg ulcer
Lentigines
Lichen amyloidosis
Lichenified dermatoses
Molluscum contagiosum
Multiple pigmented nevi
Nevus flammeus
Verrucous
Multiple seborrheic keratoses
Multiple trichoepitheliomas
Neurotic excoriations
Nevi
 • Congenital pigmented nevi
 • Linear epidermal
Porokeratosis of Mibelli
Pseudofolliculitis barbae
Rhinophyma
Scars
 • Early operative
 • Keloids
 • Postacne
 • Traumatic
 • Smallpox or chickenpox
Scleromyxedema
Striae distensae
Syringocystadenoma papilliferum
Syringoma
Systemic lupus erythematosus
Tattoos
 • Amateur (India ink)
 • Blast (gunpowder)
 • Professional
Vitiligo
Telangiectasia
Xanthelasma
Xeroderma pigmentosum

control of destruction depth, good hemostasis, decreased postoperative pain, and target specificity (23). Lasers emit coherent light at specific wavelengths peculiar to the lasing material. This light energy is selectively absorbed by specific skin structures (chromophores) and converted into thermal energy, damaging the tissues. Thermal damage to surrounding tissues can be further reduced by pulsing the laser emission (selective photothermolysis).

Hemostatic Agents

Hemostatic agents are used to control bleeding from removal of superficial cutaneous lesions, which usually results in capillary or venous bleeding.

Monsel solution (ferric subsulfate) is a protein coagulant that is very effective but carries the slight risk of permanent discoloration from iron pigment deposition. Aluminum chloride (20%) is the most commonly used hemostatic agent. It is a colorless but less effective when compared to Monsel solution. Silver nitrate comes conveniently in a stick form or solution but is less effective than Monsel solution or aluminum chloride and can stain skin. It is useful in treating granulation tissue.

All chemical cauterants must be applied to a dry field so there is contact between the bleeding dermal bed and the coagulant. These agents sting when used without local anesthetic.

TREATMENT OF SPECIFIC LESIONS

Seborrheic Keratosis

Seborrheic keratosis lesions are removed by dermal curette or by tangential excision with a scalpel, literally scraped off the skin's surface. If there are numerous lesions, cryotherapy or CO_2 laser can be used. Dermatosis papulosa nigra is treated with light electrodesiccation using fine-tipped cautery needles, then curettage.

Actinic Keratosis

Actinic keratosis lesions usually are treated with cryotherapy. Multiple lesions may require several sessions or alternative therapies, including dermabrasion, chemical peeling, topical 5-fluorouracil (Efudex, Fluoroplex), or topical imiquimod. 5-Fluorouracil comes in concentrations of 1% to 5% and is applied to the face twice daily for 3 weeks. A brisk inflammatory response develops in affected areas. Healing occurs over 6 to 8 weeks and is accelerated by the use of topical corticosteroids. Results are excellent but not permanent, with retreatment often necessary in 2 to 3 years. Imiquimod 5% cream was approved in 2004 for the treatment of actinic keratosis of the face or scalp. Whether administered as monotherapy or adjunctive therapy, topical therapies provide the opportunity to effectively manage actinic keratosis and will likely emerge as an important tool for health care providers (24).

Cutaneous Horns

Cutaneous horns are completely removed (shave or punch technique) so the base can be examined histologically.

TABLE 195.8	LASERS USED IN THE MANAGEMENT OF FACIAL SKIN LESIONS	

Laser	Wavelength	Indications
Argon (continuous)	488, 514 (blue–green)	Telangiectasias, thick PWS in adults, lentigines, and ephelides
Argon-pumped tunable dye (continuous)	504–690 (green–yellow–red)	Telangiectasias, thick PWS in adults, lentigines, and ephelides
Flashlamp-pumped dye (short-pulsed)	510 (green)	Lentigines and ephelides
Copper vapor/bromide (quasicontinuous)	511 (green)	Lentigines and ephelides
Krypton (continuous)	521, 531 (green)	Lentigines and ephelides
KTP (quasicontinuous)	531 (green)	Telangiectasias, thick PWS in adults, lentigines, and ephelides
Frequency-doubled Q-switched Nd:YAG (pulsed)	532 (green)	Lentigines and ephelides
Krypton (continuous)	568 (yellow)	Telangiectasias, thick PWS in adults
Copper vapor/bromide (quasicontinuous)	578 (yellow)	Telangiectasias, thick PWS in adults
Flashlamp-pumped dye (long-pulsed)	585 (yellow)	Flat PWS in children, telangiectasias, hypertrophic scars
Q-switched ruby (pulsed)	694 (red)	Lentigines, ephelides, blue nevus, nevus of Ota
Q-switched alexandrite (pulsed)	755 (near infrared)	Lentigines, ephelides, blue nevus, nevus of Ota
Q-Switched Nd: YAG (pulsed)	1,064 (infrared)	Blue nevus, nevus of Ota
Carbon dioxide (continuous, pulsed, super/ultra-pulsed)	1,060 (infrared)	Rhinophyma, trichoepithelioma, syringoma, angiofibroma, keloids, xanthelasma, scars, and rhytides

PWS, port-wine stain.

Usually an actinic keratosis is found, so it is reasonable to curette and electrodesiccate the base lightly after lesion removal. If a squamous cell or basal cell carcinoma is confirmed by histologic examination, a wider excision is performed.

Epidermal Cysts

Small inflamed cysts occur with acne vulgaris and are treated with intralesional steroids in concentrations of 2 to 5 mg/mL. This results in complete resolution in 3 to 5 days, with a low incidence of recurrence. The injection may cause temporary dermal atrophy, which resolves in 6 to 12 months.

Infected cysts are generally large and of longer duration than small acne-associated cysts. They are tender with surrounding erythema. These are best treated with systemic antibiotics, especially those with additional antiinflammatory effects such as tetracycline and erythromycin. For tense and severely inflamed lesions, incision, drainage, culture, and sensitivity determination should be performed, and the treated lesions should be packed with iodoform gauze. Antibiotics against *Staphylococcus aureus* are empirically started. Surgical therapy is deferred for 4 to 6 weeks after

infection because infection thins the cyst wall and dermal collagen, making the procedure difficult and increasing the chances of infection spreading. Intralesional steroids should not be used on infected cysts.

The treatment of noninfected, noninflamed cysts is surgical, with complete cyst wall removal (to prevent recurrence). Freely mobile cysts have little connection with the overlying epidermis and are easily removed. Injection of local anesthetics between the cyst wall and surrounding tissues (hydrodissection) facilitates surgical removal.

If the cyst is firmly adherent to the surrounding tissues, the entire cyst and surrounding fibrous tissue are excised. The use of a punch biopsy instead of an ellipse may provide an opening large enough to remove the cyst with excellent cosmetic results. Epidermal cysts that are freely or partially mobile may be removed through incisions at distant sites where cosmetic factors are overriding (e.g., a mucosal approach to remove a lip cyst or an incision in the hairline to remove a nearby forehead cyst).

Complications include infection, bleeding, and dehiscence and are usually a result of poor technique. If the cyst wall ruptures with spillage of keratinous material, the area is irrigated with normal saline and all recognizable keratinous debris is removed. Necrosis of overlying skin once a cyst is removed usually occurs when a large cyst has been removed, resulting in large dead space with overlying epidermis. To avoid necrosis, all underlying dead space is removed and tension at the skin edges is minimized. Any redundant skin that may occur in cyst surgery is excised.

Milia

A milia is treated by incising its roof and extracting its keratinous core with a milia comedo extractor. No local anesthetic is required. This technique also may be used for large closed comedones. Smaller closed comedones and open comedones (blackheads) are treated with topical retinoic acid (Retin-A).

Trichofolliculomas

Trichofolliculomas are removed by shaving, punch excision with suturing, or vaporization with a CO_2 laser.

Trichoepitheliomas

Solitary trichoepitheliomas are removed the same way as trichofolliculomas. However, distinction of basal cell carcinoma and solitary trichoepithelioma is difficult both clinically and pathologically. Multiple trichoepitheliomas are removed with dermabrasion and CO_2 laser with excellent results.

Pilomatricomas

Pilomatricomas, deep-seated nodules, require surgical excision in most cases.

Trichilemmomas

Solitary lesions of trichilemmoma are treated as trichofolliculomas. Multiple lesions can be treated with dermabrasion.

Nevus Sebaceus

A nevus sebaceus lesion is sometimes completely excised because it has malignant potential; however, its risk for malignancy is low. It also may be followed for changes of malignancy and treated at a later date if necessary.

Sebaceous Hyperplasia

Sebaceous hyperplasia lesions are treated with cryotherapy or light electrodesiccation with fine-tipped cautery needles.

Rhinophyma

Rhinophyma is treated with electrosurgery, dermabrasion, and argon or CO_2 laser. Excessive sebaceous tissue is excised and the nose is sculpted to its predisease shape. Dermabrasion and CO_2 laser allow the surgeon to sculpt with control and precision, the latter maintaining a relatively bloodless field. Regardless of technique, results are usually excellent. Removing tissue below the pilosebaceous apparatus results in an unattractive, unnaturally smooth, poreless scar.

Hidrocystoma

The hidrocystoma cyst is surgically excised if necessary for cosmetic reasons. Simple incision and drainage result in recurrence.

Syringoma

Syringomas usually present as multiple lesions; therefore, surgical excision is usually not feasible. Dermabrasion and superficial CO_2 laser offer fair results on those selected lesions that are more cosmetically concerning to the patient. Electrodesiccation is sometimes sufficient.

Hemangiomas

Most capillary hemangiomas resolve spontaneously, so treatment is usually not necessary. Exceptions are hemangiomas that ulcerate, encroach on a vital structure (nose, eyes, mouth), or are frequently traumatized (buttock, foot). For these, medical therapy (prednisone and interferon alfa) or intralesional corticosteroids are used. A nevus flammeus (port-wine stain) is treated with tunable dye lasers or, more recently, copper vapor, krypton, or flashlamp-pumped pulsed-dye lasers (Table 195.8). Complications are uncommon with these techniques, with occasional hypopigmentation or skin texture alterations. Scarring and tissue induration are rare. Lesions in dark-skinned patients lighten less than others because epidermal melanin causes some absorption of the laser light.

Pyogenic Granuloma

Pyogenic granulomas are treated aggressively because recurrence is common if excision is incomplete. Shave removal with electrosurgery of the base is simple and effective, as is elliptical excision. Ablation with a CO_2 laser, argon laser, dye laser, or copper vapor laser is also effective.

Telangiectasias

Telangiectasias can be treated simply with electrodesiccation using fine cautery needles (epilating needles). The lowest possible setting on a Hyfrecator or Bovie is used to avoid scarring. Telangiectasias also can be treated with laser therapy (argon, argon-pumped tunable dye, copper vapor, krypton, frequency-doubled Nd:YAG, or flashlamp-pumped pulsed dye). Sclerotherapy (injection of sclerosing agent into the telangiectasia) can be used, but there is the potential of introducing some sclerosant into the cavernous sinus or deep venous drainage of the head and neck, causing potentially grave complications (e.g., blindness, cavernous sinus thrombosis).

Spider Angiomas

Spider angiomas are treated similarly to telangiectasias. In electrosurgery, the needle is placed into the central punctum of the spider angioma. Lesions can recur, so additional treatment may be needed.

Venous Lakes

Small lesions of venous lakes are treated by excision or electrodesiccation. Larger lesions are treated with laser therapy (argon, dye, or copper vapor).

Skin Tags

Skin tags can be snipped off at the base with a sharp curved iris scissors. Local anesthetic is generally not required. Electrodesiccation also can be used.

Fibrous Papule

For a fibrous papule, simple shave excision produces an acceptable cosmetic result and is preferable to superficial destruction methods (CO_2 laser, electrosurgery), which do not permit histologic examination.

Adenoma Sebaceus

Adenoma sebaceus lesions are treated with dermabrasion, CO_2 laser, or argon laser. The argon produces excellent cosmetic results, particularly in patients who have lightly pigmented skin.

Hypertrophic Scars and Keloids

Hypertrophic scars and keloids are managed with intralesional steroids; dermabrasion; pressure; or, most recently, silicone gel matrix. Several treatment strategies often are combined in hopes of better treatment outcomes. Many hypertrophic scars flatten over time. However, long-term results of all treatment options for keloids are poor. Results in the literature are difficult to interpret because most lack long-term follow-up (at least 2 years) and histopathologic criteria to confirm that the lesions are keloids and not hypertrophic scars.

Neurofibromas

Neurofibromas can be excised, CO_2 vaporized, shaved, or removed with electrosurgical cutting current to the base. If the entire lesion is not removed, however, it will regrow slowly. Multiple facial lesions can be dermabraded or excised by CO_2 laser.

Lipomas

Small lipomas can be removed through a small stab incision in the overlying skin. Some lipomas extend insidiously beyond their clinical borders and lie deep to fascia or within muscle. These need to be sharply dissected from surrounding tissue. Giant lipomas may be removed by liposuction. The liposuction cannula is inserted via a small incision. Some lipomas have multiple fibrous septae, requiring careful scissor dissection. Beware of lipomas on the forehead because they often are located beneath the frontalis muscle (subgaleal lipomas). Attempts at excision are frustrating unless the surgeon knows to look in this deeper plane.

Leiomyomas

Leiomyomas are best treated with simple excision.

Melanocytic Nevi

With melanocytic nevi, we are discussing benign nevi, not congenital or dysplastic nevi. Benign nevi can be intradermal, compound, or junctional and can be partly or completely removed. Except for junctional nevi, most nevi are elevated and can be removed by shave technique. This leaves a recurrence risk from residual nevus cells of 10% to 20%. A small hypopigmented area usually results. When a nevus is recurrent, histopathologic interpretation of these often shows atypical or pleomorphic-appearing cells, which can be difficult to distinguish from melanoma (pseudomelanoma).

Two other problems occurring after a shave excision are a depressed scar or peripheral lipping. Depression occurs if local anesthetic infiltration raises the lesion above the skin surface and is avoided by allowing the anesthetic to diffuse out of the lesion before shaving it off. Lipping results if the nevus is not removed flush with surrounding skin because of variable shear forces during shaving. Hemostasis is achieved with aluminum chloride. Monsel solution can hinder histopathologic interpretation of a recurrent nevus because its ferrous subsulfate can be misconstrued as melanin pigment within dermal macrophages.

The second method of removing nevi is complete excision of the lesion. This is necessary for flat nevi. The incision is placed in relaxed skin tension lines. Spot dermabrasion of the scar after 4 to 6 weeks improves the cosmetic result. Complete excision provides a specimen for histologic examination and minimizes recurrence risk.

Spitz Nevi

Spitz nevi are excised for histopathologic examination. This is important because they can resemble malignant melanoma microscopically and the pathologist relies on architectural features lost in a shave biopsy.

Blue Nevi

Simple blue nevi are removed with shave technique or excision. Larger lesions that look like blue nevi are best excised for complete histopathologic examination. Nevi of Ota have been treated successfully with Q-switched Nd:YAG and ruby lasers.

Lentigines and Ephelides

Lentigines and ephelides respond to similar therapy and are similar pathologic processes. For just a few lesions, cryotherapy is probably the easiest treatment. Laser therapy (ruby, alexandrite, pulsed dye, krypton, copper vapor, or frequency-doubled Nd:YAG) is also successful (Table 195.8). For widespread multiple lesions, chemexfoliation is best. A wide variety of agents has been used: retinoic acid, trichloroacetic acid, and alpha hydroxy (glycolic) acids. Retinoic acid carries the fewest risks and is started at low strength (0.025% cream) to minimize irritant effects.

Molluscum Contagiosum

Small numbers of lesions respond well to curettage, cryotherapy, or daily application of topical imiquimod. In patients who are immunocompromised, lesions may number in the thousands and become thick, verrucous, and refractory to treatment. Most recently, chemical peeling with trichloroacetic acid and retinoic acid has been used successfully.

Verrucae

Common and filiform varieties respond well to cryotherapy and electrodesiccation and curettage, although recurrences are common. Flat warts (usually multiple and superficial) respond well to chemexfoliation with retinoic acid or trichloroacetic acid as well as to cryotherapy or topical imiquimod. Harsh keratolytics (e.g., salicylic acid) and blistering agents should not be used in treating facial verrucae because they may lead to scarring.

HIGHLIGHTS

- A classification scheme helps narrow the diagnostic possibilities.
- Seemingly benign facial lesions may be a sign of serious systemic disease.
- Biopsy is the most valuable laboratory aid for diagnosing skin lesions.
- Cosmetic outcomes are important in treating benign facial lesions.
- The risks of all facial surgery should be described to the patient in detail preoperatively.

REFERENCES

1. Freedberg IM, Eisen AZ, Wolff K, et al., eds. *Fitzpatrick's dermatology in general medicine*, 6th ed. New York: McGraw-Hill, 2003.
2. Arndt KA, Leboit PE, Robinson JK, et al., eds. *Cutaneous medicine and surgery.* Philadelphia, PA: WB Saunders, 1996.
3. Champion RH, Burton JL, Burns AD, et al., eds. *Rook's textbook of dermatology*, 6th ed. London, UK: Blackwell Scientific, 1998.
4. Elder DE, Elenitsas R, Jaworsky C, eds. *Lever's histopathology of the skin*, 8th ed. Philadelphia, PA: Lippincott-Raven, 1997.
5. Bolognia JL, Jorizzo JL, Rapini RP. *Dermatology.* London, UK/New York: Mosby, 2003.
6. Salasche SJ. Epidemiology of actinic keratoses and squamous cell carcinoma. *J Am Acad Dermatol* 2000;42:S4–S7.
7. Glogau RG. The risk of progression to invasive disease. *J Am Acad Dermatol* 2000;42:S23–S24.
8. Bondeson J. Everard Home, John Hunter, and cutaneous horns: a historical review. *Am J Dermatopathol* 2001;23:362–369.
9. Vielhauer V, Herzinger T, Korting HC. The sign of Leser-Trélat: a paraneoplastic cutaneous syndrome that facilitates early diagnosis of occult cancer. *Eur J Med Res* 2000;5:512–516.
10. Heaphy MR Jr, Millns JL, Schroeter AL. The sign of Leser-Trélat in a case of adenocarcinoma of the lung. *J Am Acad Dermatol* 2000;43:386–390.
11. Eng C. Will the real Coden syndrome please stand up: revised diagnostic criteria. *J Med Genet* 2000;37:828–830.
12. Prioleau PG, Santa Cruz DJ. Sebaceous gland neoplasia. *J Cutan Pathol* 1984;11:396–414.
13. Jaqueti G, Requena L, Sanchez Yus E. Trichoblastoma is the most common neoplasm developed in nevus sebaceus of Jadassohn: a clinicopathologic study of a series of 155 cases. *Am J Dermatopathol* 2000;22:108–118.
14. Cribier B, Grosshans E. Tumor of the follicular infundibulum: a clinicopathologic study. *J Am Acad Dermatol* 1995;33:979–984.
15. Cribier B, Scrivener Y, Grosshans E. Tumors arising in nevus sebaceus: a study of 596 cases. *J Am Acad Dermatol* 2000;42:263–268.
16. Scheithauer BW, Woodruff JM, Erlandson RA. Tumors of the peripheral nervous system. In: *Atlas of tumor pathology*, Third series, Fascicle 24. Washington, DC: Armed Forces Institute of Pathology, 1999:1–415.
17. DeDavid M, Orlow SJ, Provost N, et al. A study of large congenital melanocytic nevi and associated malignant melanomas: review of cases in the New York University Registry and the world literature. *J Am Acad Dermatol* 1997;36:409–415.
18. Marghoob AA, Schoenbach SP, Kopf AW, et al. Large congenital melanocytic nevi and the risk for the development of malignant melanoma. A prospective study. *Arch Dermatol* 1996;132:170–175.
19. Patel BC, Egan CA, Lucius RW, et al. Cutaneous malignant melanoma in oculodermal melanocytosis (nevus of Ota): report of a case and review of the literature. *J Am Acad Dermatol* 1998;38:862.
20. Teekhasaenee C, Ritch R, Rutnin U, et al. Ocular findings in oculodermal melanocytosis. *Arch Ophthalmol* 1990;108:1114.
21. Roenigk RK, Roenigk HH Jr, eds. *Dermatologic surgery: principles and practice.* New York: Marcel Dekker, 1996.
22. Bennett RG. *Fundamentals of cutaneous surgery.* St. Louis, MO: Mosby, 1988.
23. Wheeland RG. Clinical uses of lasers in dermatology. *Lasers Surg Med* 1995;16:2.
24. Jorizzo JL. Current and novel treatment options for actinic keratosis. *J Cutan Med Surg* 2004;8(Suppl 3):13–21.

Management of Alopecia

196

Raymond J. Konior   Steven Gabel

Burns, traction, infections, autoimmune disease, neoplasms, radiation exposure, psychological disorders, and chemotherapy all can cause hair loss in humans (Table 196.1). The most common type of hair loss in men and women, however, is androgenetic alopecia (AGA), also known as male pattern baldness (MPB). This form of alopecia affects scalp follicles with a genetic potential to androgen inhibition, resulting in the conversion of susceptible terminal hairs to vellus hairs. The hair follicles most likely to demonstrate AGA are in the frontotemporal and the crown regions of the scalp. Several different surgical options are available for restoring hair growth on a balding scalp. The procedure of choice for any given individual will depend on many factors. These include (a) patient's age, (b) degree of baldness, (c) density within the donor region, (d) hair texture, (e) contrast characteristics of the hair and skin, and (f) patient expectations.

A classification system for MPB is essential for planning and comparing the results of different surgical procedures. The Norwood system, the one most often used for men, organizes MPB into seven categories, ranging from class I (minimal frontotemporal recession) to class VII (a very narrow, horseshoe-shaped band of hair in the temporal and low occipital regions) (1). For women, the Ludwig classification system divides hair loss into three grades, ranging from grade I (minimal hair loss) to grade III (severe, generalized thinning) (2). Table 196.2 lists treatment options for MPB.

MEDICAL TREATMENT OF ANDROGENETIC ALOPECIA

Attempts to medically manage MPB are nothing new. Hippocrates, in about 400 BC, prescribed several concoctions composed of animal and plant products to treat baldness.

Ideally, the medical treatment of AGA should be directed against dihydrotestosterone (DHT), the active agent involved in MPB. Finasteride (Propecia), which has been used for years to manage prostate hypertrophy, was approved by the U.S. Food and Drug Administration (FDA) for the treatment of MPB in 1997. Finasteride is a competitive and specific inhibitor of type II 5a-reductase, an intracellular enzyme that converts the androgen testosterone into DHT. Two distinct 5a-reductase isozymes are found in humans. The type II 5a-reductase isozyme is primarily found in the prostate, seminal vesicles, epididymides, and hair follicles. Finasteride has no affinity for androgen receptors but works by blocking the peripheral conversion of testosterone to DHT. Using the recommended dose of 1 mg/d, finasteride produces statistically significant increased hair counts in men with mild-to-moderate degrees of AGA. Systemic therapy that reduces or interferes with androgen levels enough to stop hair loss has the potential to reduce libido and sexual potency, making this form of treatment unacceptable to some men. Drug-related sexual adverse experiences resulting in discontinuation of therapy have been reported in 1.2% of patients on finasteride versus 0.9% of patients on placebo (3,4). Finasteride is not indicated for woman and children.

Minoxidil (Rogaine) was the first drug approved by the FDA for the medical management of MPB. This drug, which traditionally had been used to treat resistant hypertension, was noted to occasionally produce hypertrichosis as a side effect of oral therapy in adults. Minoxidil functions as a potassium channel opener and vasodilator. Currently, the dosages available are 2% and 5% formulations. In men, the 5% minoxidil solution demonstrates a significant advantage over treatment with the 2% solution (5). The mechanism by which minoxidil works to stimulate hair growth remains unclear. In addition, minoxidil does not have any known effect on the production, excretion, or interactions of human androgens. Most, if not all,

TABLE 196.1	ETIOLOGY OF ALOPECIA

Androgenetic alopecia (MPB)
Autoimmune disease (alopecia areata, discoid lupus
    erythematosus)
Thyroid disorders
Burns
Chemotherapy
Dermatologic disorders (e.g., psoriasis, lichen planopilaris,
    bacterial folliculitis)
Neoplasms
Radiation exposure
Traction
Psychological (trichotillomania, stress)

hair transplant surgeons recommend the use of minoxidil and/or finasteride to the majority of their patients (6).

SURGICAL TREATMENT OF ALOPECIA

Patient Evaluation

During the first consultation, the patient's goal of the procedure needs to be discussed. A thorough physical evaluation will need to be performed and an explanation of the surgical options available. The physician must understand the patient's motivations and expectations regarding hair-restoration surgery. Patients who seem emotionally labile may require a psychiatric assessment to evaluate their true motivations, but most patients requesting hair replacement do not have emotional problems; they simply would prefer not to be bald.

Several factors determine what procedure, if any, is appropriate for restoring an alopecic scalp. It is not uncommon for the patient to expect more than can be accomplished with the donor area available. The major reason for rejecting a patient is an inadequate supply of donor hair relative to the patient's final goals.

The ideal patient is one with enough donor hair to completely fill all current or potential areas of alopecia. The

TABLE 196.2	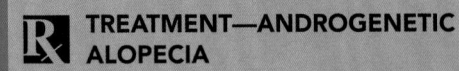 TREATMENT—ANDROGENETIC ALOPECIA

Medications
    Minoxidil (Rogaine)
    Finasteride (Propecia)
Hair-bearing autografts
    Follicular unit grafts
    Micrografts
    Minigrafts
Scalp reduction
Tissue expansion
Scalp flaps

younger the patient, the more conservative the physician must be in estimating the donor hair present and establishing a long-term treatment plan. An accurate assessment of the donor area is required to prevent moving follicles at risk for future alopecia into cosmetically important areas on the scalp, because any future hair loss in those transplanted follicles will result in exposed scars over the scalp. In younger patients whose final hair-loss patterns cannot be determined, the physician should try to delay hair restoration until the physician is secure with the availability of donor hair.

Low-density donor hair may be a contraindication to hair transplantation. Patients with fewer than 40 follicular units/cm² tend to be poor candidates for hair transplantation, unless they are willing to accept very thin hair density from the transplantation procedures. Age is not a contraindication to hair transplantation. Older patients generally have well-established patterns of alopecia that allow a more reliable assessment of the donor area.

Hair color, skin color, and hair texture are important factors in surgical hair restoration. A sharp contrast between the hair and the skin may result in an unnatural-appearing hairline. This is especially true if transplantation is performed with grafts that contain more than one follicle unit. The best hair colors for surgical hair restoration in light-skinned patients are white, salt-and-pepper, and blond. Patients with dark skin and dark hair and those with wiry hair generally are good candidates for hair restoration. Naturally curly hair appears thicker than straight hair, thereby enhancing the results of most hair-replacement procedures.

Hairline Design

The most important goal of hair-replacement surgery is to restore aesthetic balance to the face by recreating a natural, age-appropriate frontal hairline and part (7). The surgically restored hair should be easy to maintain and should not require extraordinary hairstyles for camouflage.

The mature male hairline usually demonstrates distinct triangular regions bilaterally at the junction of the frontal and the temporal hair (Fig. 196.1). These frontotemporal triangles are formed by progressive recession of the frontal hairline superiorly and the temporal hairline posteriorly.

A natural frontal hairline is convex, with the central portion positioned slightly inferior to the frontotemporal triangle region. The most anterior portion of the hairline is placed approximately 7 to 10 cm superior to the glabella. The apex of the frontotemporal triangle marks the lateral aspect of a natural hairline. Regardless of the extent of hairline recession, the apex is designed to fall on a vertical line drawn upward from the lateral canthus of the eye. Because the temporal hairline intersects the lateral extent of the frontal hairline, advanced temporal recessions require a more posterior frontal hairline. Any attempt to fill a large frontotemporal triangle as a means of compensating for

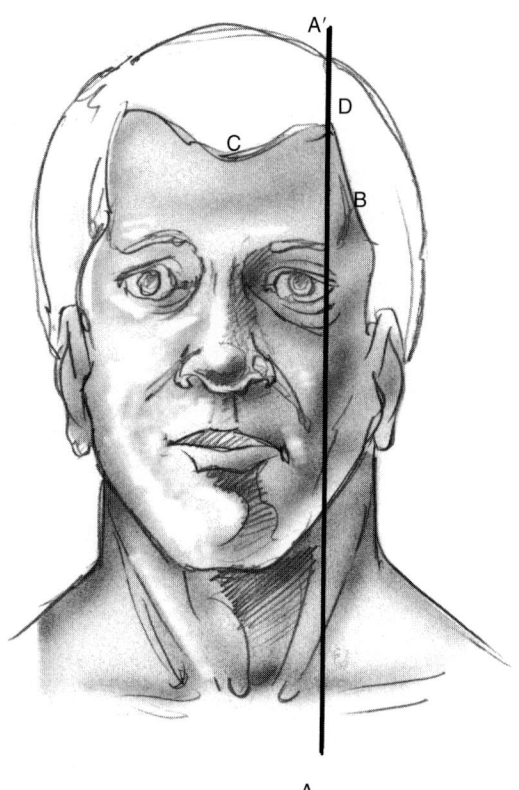

Figure 196.1 The frontotemporal triangle (*BCD*) is defined by the frontal and the temporal hairlines. When planning surgical restoration of the frontal hairline, the apex of the triangle is designed to fall on a vertical line (*AA'*) that intersects the lateral canthus.

advanced temporal recessions will result in an unnatural hairline and part. Modern follicular unit grafting techniques can be used to recreate the temporal hairline in those patients with a low-lying superior temporal fringe.

FEMALE PATTERN HAIR LOSS

In hair restoration, men constitute more than 90% of the patients seeking treatment. As techniques in surgical management continue to improve and public awareness of high patient satisfaction increases, however, there are increasing numbers of women undergoing treatment for hair loss. The approach to female pattern hair loss is much different than MPB, as only 10% of women have an androgenic hair-loss pattern. Therefore, the overwhelming majority of women have hair loss for variety of other reasons, such as hormonal and autoimmune.

The workup involves recognizing the enormous psychological toll hair loss takes on a woman and using appropriate sensitivity when treating women with hair loss. Referral to an endocrinologist is usually part of the workup. Minoxidil 2% solution has been effective in treating female pattern hair loss. Increased dosages of 5% minoxidil have caused unacceptable rates of facial hypertrichosis to occur. Finasteride has not been shown to have benefit in women. Surgical hair restoration remains the only permanent

treatment for hair loss in women. The same principles of adequate donor area and advanced transplantation techniques lead to better outcomes (8).

ANESTHESIA

Because most patients require multiple procedures, an adequate comfort level is essential to maintaining motivation for completion of the entire restoration process. Local anesthesia is sufficient for most hair-restoration procedures, but general anesthesia is occasionally necessary for extensive scalp reductions or flap procedures.

A preoperative sedative is commonly given before the injection of local anesthesia. Regional frontal, occipital, and temporal nerve blocks using 1% lidocaine with 1:100,000 epinephrine are performed before performing a wide-field, circumferential scalp block. This technique anesthetizes the entire hair-bearing scalp.

AUTOGRAFT HAIR TRANSPLANTATION

Okuda (9), a Japanese dermatologist, is generally regarded as the first to describe the successful use of full-thickness hair-bearing autografts for correcting alopecia of the scalp, eyebrow, and mustache areas. Hair transplantation using punch grafts was introduced in the United States in 1959 by Orentreich (10). He coined the term *donor dominance* to describe the fact that autografts maintain characteristics of the donor tissue when transplanted into other regions of the body. Patients followed for more than 30 years continue to demonstrate persistent hair growth following punch-graft hair transplantation (11).

Donor Hair Removal: Elliptical Strip Method

The donor site is that portion of the scalp that contains permanent hair dense enough to permit the harvesting of graft material. This area is usually found on the sides and the back of the head and is limited anteriorly by a vertical line through the external auditory canal. The superior border of the safe donor area in the midoccipital region is generally located beneath a horizontal line that intersects the superior attachment of the auricles to the scalp.

In the past, a multiblade knife was used to harvest the donor hair by simultaneously removing several parallel strips of scalp from the donor region (12). The space between the scalpel blades on this device was adjusted to allow the harvesting of different strip widths. Most often, the donor strips measured 1.5 to 3.0 mm in width; the exact dimensions depended on what size grafts the surgeon required for the recipient site. Because of the increased risk of transection and ultimate follicular loss with the multibladed knife, the preferred method for donor hair removal is with a single 1.0- to 1.5-cm-wide elliptical strip. The width of the strip is determined by several factors, including hair density, hair texture, scalp laxity, and scarring from previous procedures. Using a single scalpel blade to incise the scalp, the donor tissue is obtained with particular care in ensuring the blade is parallel to the angle of follicular growth, thus minimizing damage to the follicles.

Before harvesting grafts, the hair along the donor site is trimmed to about 3 mm. Saline is then infiltrated into the donor site to tense the mobile scalp skin. Donor-site turgidity minimizes the soft tissue distortion that results from pressure generated by the scalpel as it cuts the scalp. Failure to tense the scalp predisposes to irregularly shaped strips and follicular transection. The scalpel blades must parallel the hair follicles to produce an excellent-quality strip. Strip margins are routinely examined during harvesting for evidence of tissue distortion or follicle damage. Poor strip quality may require additional saline infiltration into the surrounding tissues or better alignment of the scalpel blades with the existing hair shafts. The donor strips are removed by incising the subfollicular fat just beneath the base of the follicles. The donor site is reapproximated in the subcutaneous level with a 3-0 Monocryl (poliglecaprone 25) suture, and the cutaneous layer is closed with a running 4-0 nylon suture or staples. A tension-free closure is mandatory to prevent follicular necrosis and a wide scar along the donor-site incision line.

The donor-site strips are examined using magnification, and any transected hair shafts are removed from the edges. Excess subcutaneous fat is trimmed, taking care to leave about 2 mm of fat below the matrix zone of the hair follicles. The strips are then placed flat on a sterile, back-lit cutting surface. Individual grafts (1 to 4 hairs/graft) are made by using a scalpel blade to cut the strips parallel to the path of the embedded follicles. Follicular units used in the hairline should be trimmed to create a teardrop-shaped graft. This method allows for improved density and decreased potential for pitting and graft trauma (13). Different sized grafts can be developed by adjusting the width of the cuts being made along the donor strips. Microscopic dissection techniques are preferred to assure the highest quality, most natural-appearing grafts.

Donor-Site Removal: Follicular Unit Extraction Method

Follicular unit extraction (FUE) is a relatively new technique used for removing individual follicular unit grafts from the donor area using small round punches. In 2002, Rassman et al. (14) developed the FOX system (*follicular unit extraction*), which described the use of 1-mm sharp punches to make a circular incision around the follicles, which are then removed from the scalp. In 2006, Harris (15) described the SAFE method, which uses a two-punch system consisting of a sharp punch to score the epidermis, followed by a dull dissecting punch to separate the follicular unit from the subcutaneous tissue. Recently, powered

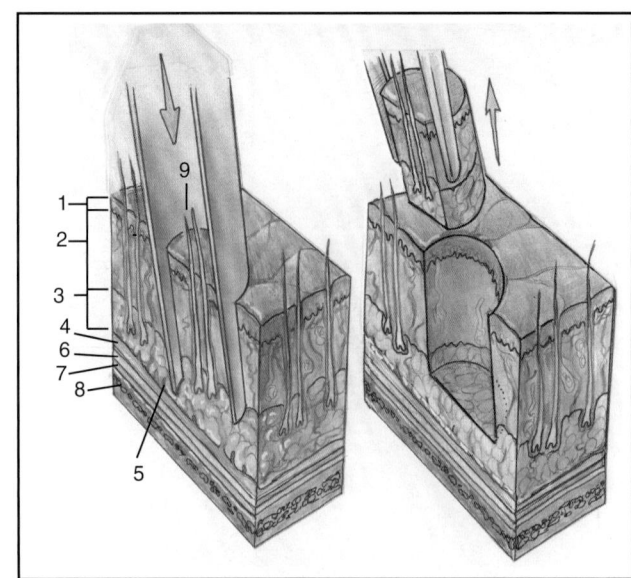

Figure 196.2 FUE is performed using a 1-mm round punch blade to incise the skin down to the subcutaneous tissue. The punch follows the hair(s) in their proper angulation to the base of the follicle. The follicular unit is then gently grasped with an angled forceps and removed. *1*, Epidermis; *2*, dermis; *3*, subcutaneous fat; *4*, galea aponeurotica; *5*, fibrous septum; *6*, subgaleal fascia; *7*, pericranium; *8*, cranium; *9*, 2-hair follicular unit.

instrumentation has replaced handheld instruments to allow the surgeon a more efficient method to extract a greater number of follicular units in a single session with less transection (16).

The donor-area hair is shaved to 2 to 3 mm in length in order to visualize the curvature to the hair. With the patient in a prone position, local anesthesia with 1% lidocaine with 1:100,000 epinephrine is injected to establish a ring block, and saline is sparingly used intradermally to add turgor to the skin. Typically, a 1-mm round punch blade is used to penetrate the epidermis and dermis around the follicular unit to dissect it from the surrounding tissues. Since this is a relatively "blind" procedure, the angle of the hair must be followed accurately to avoid transecting the graft. Once released, the follicular unit is then gently grasped and removed (Fig. 196.2). This procedure is repeated until the desired number of grafts is obtained. The grafts are then examined under the microscope to assure their integrity and remove any excess skin.

The main advantages of FUE include decreased scarring, allowing people to wear their hair very short; decreased pain; and the ability to harvest hairs from other areas of the body. It is also useful to camouflage wide donor-site scars from prior surgery (17).

Recipient Site

Most alopecic areas can be filled with dense-appearing hair using one to three transplant sessions. Grafts are inserted into the recipient sites made by specially designed blades

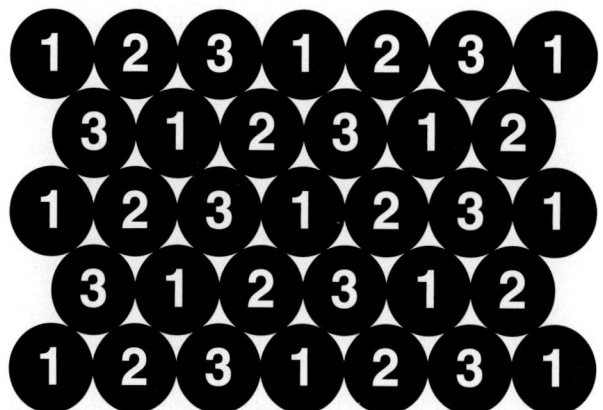

Figure 196.3 Autograft hair transplantation is commonly performed in one to three sessions; a typical grafting sequence is shown. The actual spacing between adjacent grafts during any given session should be sufficient to preserve circulation, but should also maintain a subtle randomness to assure a natural end appearance.

or needles of various sizes. The grafts are spaced evenly apart from each other, taking care to preserve an intact, circumferential bridge of skin between adjacent grafts. This is necessary to maintain adequate circulation around each graft (Fig. 196.3). To maintain a natural hair-growth pattern, the original hair direction and exit angle from the scalp are followed when cutting the recipient site slits or holes. Consistent angling is required throughout all graft sessions to prevent transecting previously transplanted follicles. The hair along the frontal hairline is directed anteriorly at approximately a 10-to-15-degree angle. As the placement of slits extends laterally toward the temple, the hairline is pointed more inferiorly toward the ear and leaves the scalp at a very flat angle.

Modern hair transplantation techniques favor using one of two methods to achieve both density and refinement within the transplanted hairline regions: (a) the exclusive use of follicular unit grafts (18) and (b) combinations of minigrafts and micrografts (19). A follicular unit is a microscopic cluster of closely united follicles. Each cluster of related follicles maintains a microscopically anatomic separation from adjacent follicle unit clusters. A follicle unit usually contains one to four hairs. Follicular unit transplantation requires the use of an operating microscope for optimal graft preparation. The frontal hairline is composed of single hair follicular units, with two to four hair follicular units placed more posteriorly. Microscopic assistance is not used with minigraft and micrograft techniques. Minigrafts contain three to eight hairs, whereas micrografts have only one or two hairs. Micrografts are commonly used to refine the outer perimeter of the transplanted recipient site, especially along the anterior aspect of the frontal hairline. Micrografts soften the transition zone between the bald forehead skin and the transplanted frontal hairline (20). Minigrafts, because of their larger size, are used to create higher density hair, more posteriorly within the recipient site.

Transplantation of the crown requires re-creation of a natural whorl. The center of the whorl usually begins in the middle of the crown's lower quadrant adjacent to the part side. The grafts are angled to mimic a natural whorl, where hair radiates around the predetermined central point.

It is recommended that at least 6 months pass between subsequent transplant sessions. Hair does not grow for an average of 3 months after a transplant session. Therefore, the surgeon should wait 6 months before planning further transplant sessions to evaluate the hair growth from the previous sessions. The surgeon can then examine the quantity and quality of the new hair growth before placing additional grafts. Waiting to see new hair growth also allows the surgeon to precisely and completely fill the spaces left between the previously placed grafts. Crusts form on the grafts soon after surgery and these crusts shed in about 1 to 2 weeks post procedure. The freshly transplanted grafts enter a telogen effluvium phase and lose their preexistent hair over the subsequent 2 to 6 weeks. New hair begins to grow about 10 to 16 weeks after surgery and grows at the normal rate of 1/2 to 1 inch per month. Occasionally, the new hair will appear coarser than the original hair.

Sequelae and Complications

Table 196.3 lists complications of hair-restoration surgery. Most patients experience little discomfort after hair transplantation and require nothing more than acetaminophen with codeine. Severe forehead edema occasionally develops postoperatively; however, this swelling is temporary and may be reduced with postoperative low-dose oral steroids.

Keloidal healing is rare. If any questions regarding a patient's predisposition remain after a thorough preoperative history, a single test graft can be performed at the margin of the fringe. This graft should be observed for 3 to 4 months before scheduling any further transplants. Graft elevation above the surrounding recipient site (cobblestoning) occurs when grafts are not trimmed properly or when there is a size discrepancy between the graft and the recipient opening. Elevated grafts are corrected by shaving the raised epidermal surface parallel to the normal adjacent scalp with a scalpel blade. Cysts can occur when the grafts are placed under the dermis.

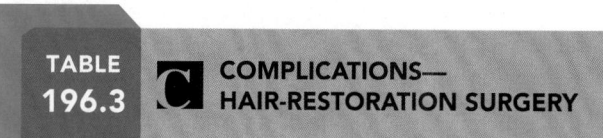

TABLE 196.3	COMPLICATIONS— HAIR-RESTORATION SURGERY

Arteriovenous fistula
Hematoma
Infection
Necrosis
Poor hairline design
Scarring
Telogen
Cysts
Poor preoperative planning (donut deformity)

Tissue necrosis at the donor site is rare and usually results from overaggressive harvesting techniques. Wide scars occur when excessive tension is used to close the donor site. Infections following hair transplants occur in less than 1% of patients. Bleeding is unusual and is usually controlled with firm pressure. Arteriovenous fistulae are rare after transplantation and often resolve spontaneously within 3 to 6 months. Direct steroid injection, suture ligation, or complete excision is required for persistent lesions or progressive enlargement.

Poor preoperative planning can result in an unnatural hairline design, or with regard to future hair loss, a disconnect between a patient's transplanted hair and their natural hair.

SCALP REDUCTION

Scalp reductions, seldom performed today, are used to excise bald skin from the crown and central scalp regions. The hair-bearing scalp is undermined and advanced superiorly to cover the excision site. The inherent flexibility of the scalp determines the success or failure of this technique. Patients with extremely flexible scalps may undergo a tremendous excision of bald scalp in a single operation, whereas patients with very tight scalps realize minimal benefit following a standard scalp reduction. This technique is most useful for reducing crown alopecia in patients with Norwood class IV to VI MPB.

Several scalp reduction patterns have been described (21) (Fig. 196.4). The sagittal midline pattern is the easiest to perform, but it creates a central scar over the vertex of the head and a slot that extends into the midoccipital hair-bearing scalp. Although more time consuming, a Y-pattern reduction can be used in place of the sagittal midline pattern to excise crown alopecia without creating a slot-like deformity at the occipital hairline. A variety of other reduction designs, including C, J, S, and lateral crescent-shaped patterns, use laterally placed scars along the fringe of the bald area to reduce crown alopecia without causing unnatural slot formations in the occipital scalp. Lateral patterns, however, are more difficult to perform than midline patterns, and they produce more central scalp hypesthesia.

Most scalp reductions are performed in a prone position using local anesthesia with intravenous sedation. Skin incisions are carried down through the galea aponeurotica, taking care to bevel the scalpel to avoid transecting adjacent hair follicles. A subgaleal dissection is extended inferiorly to the superior attachment of the auricle and to the nuchal ridge. The surgeon can overlap the undermined scalp to estimate a safe excision margin. This technique prevents overexcising the scalp and reduces the potential for excessive incision line tension. The overlapping bald skin is excised with a scalpel, and the scalp is closed in two layers. A secure galea aponeurotica closure is required to minimize incision line tension.

Few complications occur with standard scalp reductions. Occasionally, a deep suture reaction results in suture extrusion and open wounds along the incision line on the scalp. Suture removal and local wound care remedy this situation. Postoperative bleeding, infection, dehiscence, and permanent hair loss are unusual complications. Graft transplantation is usually required to camouflage the mid-scalp and

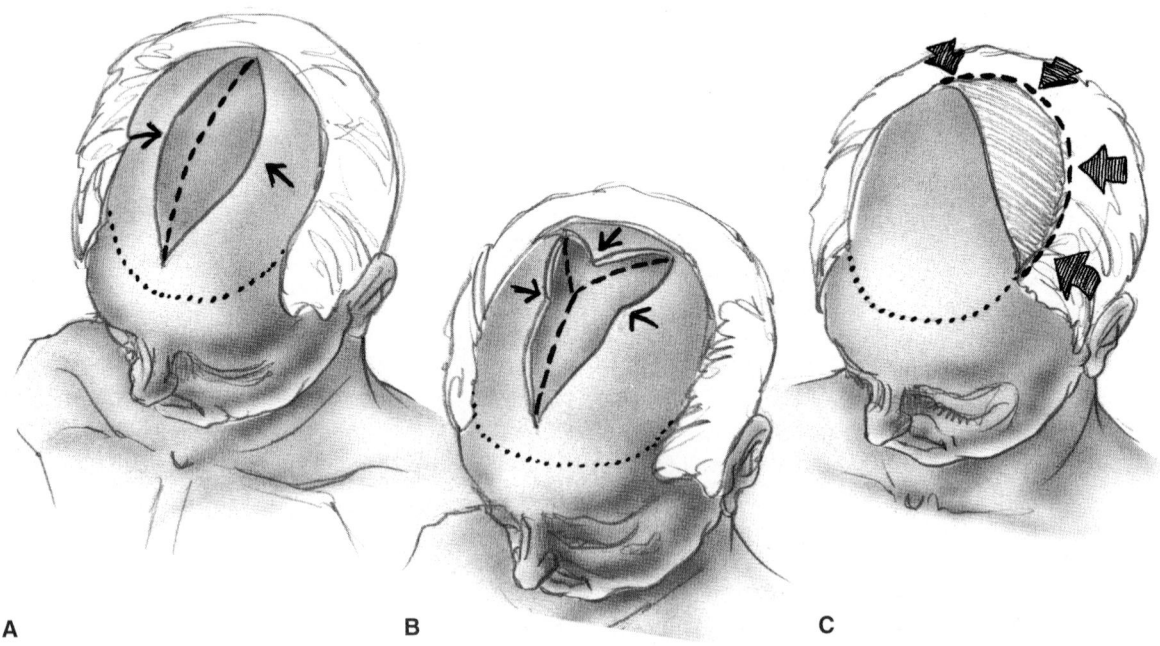

Figure 196.4 Common scalp reduction patterns. **A:** Midline sagittal ellipse. **B:** Y pattern. **C:** Lateral crescent.

crown scars that are produced following a scalp reduction. A poorly executed scalp reduction can produce an unnatural hair direction if the inferiorly directed temporal hairline is pulled too far superiorly to the midline of the scalp.

TISSUE EXPANSION

Scalp tissue expansion redistributes hair follicles in the donor area over a larger surface area on the stretched scalp (22). This technique has been successfully performed in patients with hair loss secondary to trauma, burns, neoplasms, and MPB. Various tissue expanders that allow the surgeon to customize the expansion process for any given area of the scalp are available. This modality is especially useful in patients with MPB who would benefit from a hair-bearing flap or a scalp reduction but are limited by poor scalp flexibility. Tissue expansion enables the surgeon to remove large areas of bald skin without changing the hair color or texture. It is a relatively rapid technique that has few complications when properly performed. The disadvantages include the need for repeated injections to expand the scalp, the pain associated

with the injections, and the temporary cosmetic deformity that results with progressive tissue expansion.

Tissue expansion can be used to provide a relatively rapid restoration of hair-bearing skin over the crown and mid-scalp regions in patients with Norwood class IV to VI MPB and poor scalp flexibility. Scalp expanders are designed to expand the entire temporoparietal and occipital donor regions. This technique does not provide hair coverage in the frontal region, however. In patients with coexistent frontal baldness, standard transplant techniques or a modified transposition flap are used after the expansion procedure is completed.

The expanders are placed through incisions along the temporoparietal and occipital fringe (Fig. 196.5). The hair-bearing scalp is mobilized inferiorly to the superior attachment of the auricle and to the nuchal ridge. Remote injection ports are used to prevent accidental puncture of the tissue expander during the inflation process. The expanders are placed flat against the skull, and the injection ports are placed in a separate pocket under the alopecic mid-scalp region. About 30 mL of sterile saline is

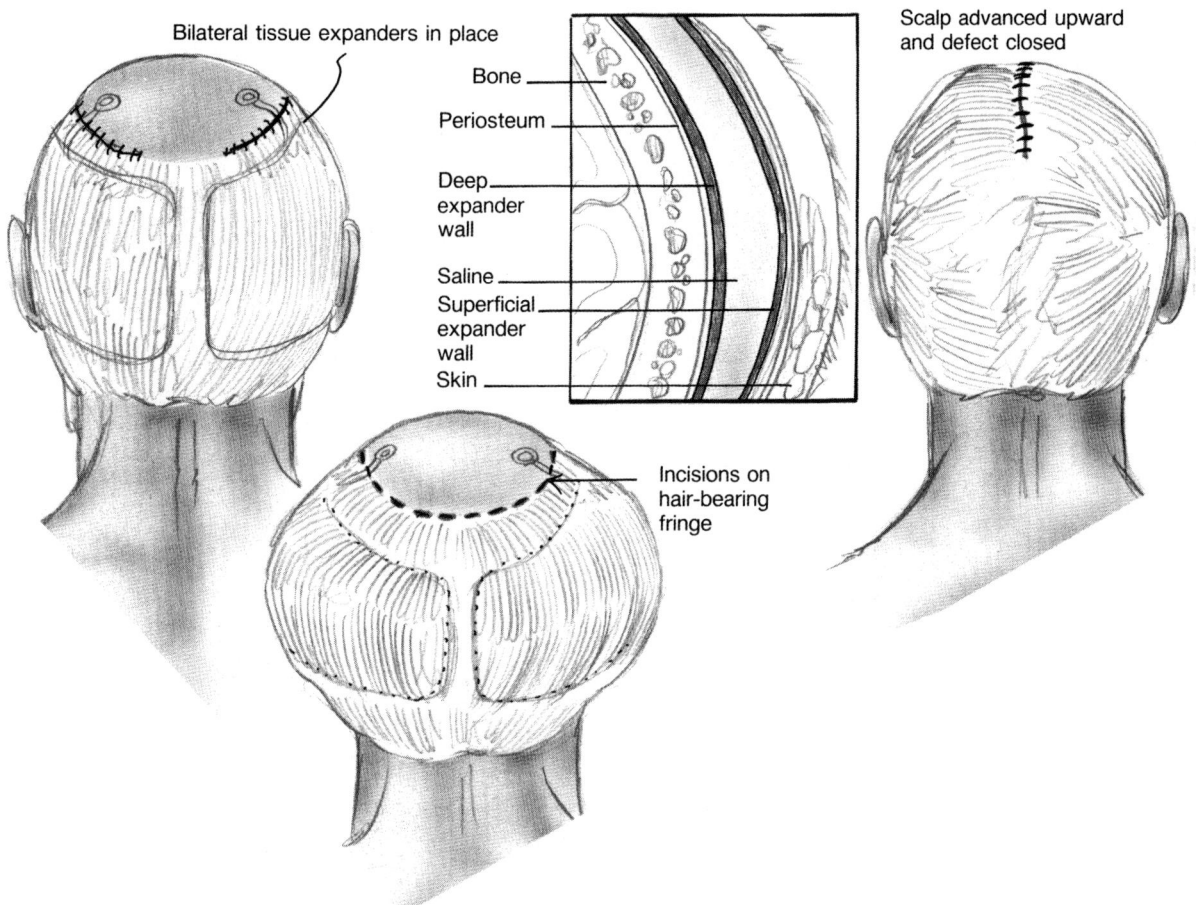

Figure 196.5 Tissue expansion for treating crown and mid-scalp baldness. Tissue expanders are placed bilaterally through incisions (*dashed lines*) along the balding fringe **(left)**. After the expansion process is complete, incisions are made along the hair-bearing fringe, and the bald skin on the crown and mid-scalp is removed **(center)**. The expanded hair-bearing scalp is advanced upward to close the defect **(right)**.

injected into the expanders immediately after skin closure to eliminate dead space.

Tissue expansion begins 2 to 3 weeks postoperatively. The expanders are injected two or three times a week, depending on the patient's pain tolerance during the injection process. Each expander is injected with sterile saline using a 25-gauge needle until the pain threshold is just reached. Each filling session requires about 30 to 60 mL of sterile saline. If pain is a problem, the patient can take a mild analgesic before the injection sessions. The expanders are gradually filled to capacity (500 to 800 mL) over 6 to 8 weeks. Expansion is finished when the cumulative tissue gain across the domes of the expanded tissue exceeds the width of the alopecic defect.

Excision of bald scalp begins by partially deflating the expanders. A horseshoe-shaped incision beginning at the apex of the planned frontotemporal triangle is made superior to the hair-bearing fringe. The expanders are removed, and the expanded scalp is moved superiorly. If additional advancement is required, the capsule is incised inferiorly, and additional undermining is performed. The overlapped

bald skin is excised from the top of the head, and the hair-bearing flaps are brought together in the midline.

Complications of tissue expansion include infection, hematoma, exposure of the implant, and implant failure. Proper technique and the use of preoperative and postoperative antibiotics minimize the potential for these complications.

JURI FLAP

The Juri flap, rarely if ever performed today, is a pedicled transposition flap based on the superficial temporal artery (STA) for surgical restoration of the frontal hairline (23). A single flap is used for frontal hairline restoration in patients with hair loss limited to the frontal region. In suitable candidates with more advanced balding over the top of the head, two flaps and a scalp reduction can be staged to provide about 12 cm of dense hair in the frontal and mid-scalp regions.

The Juri flap requires four stages for completion. The first stage begins with designing a hairline and the flap (Fig. 196.6). The STA is identified by Doppler ultrasonography about 3 cm

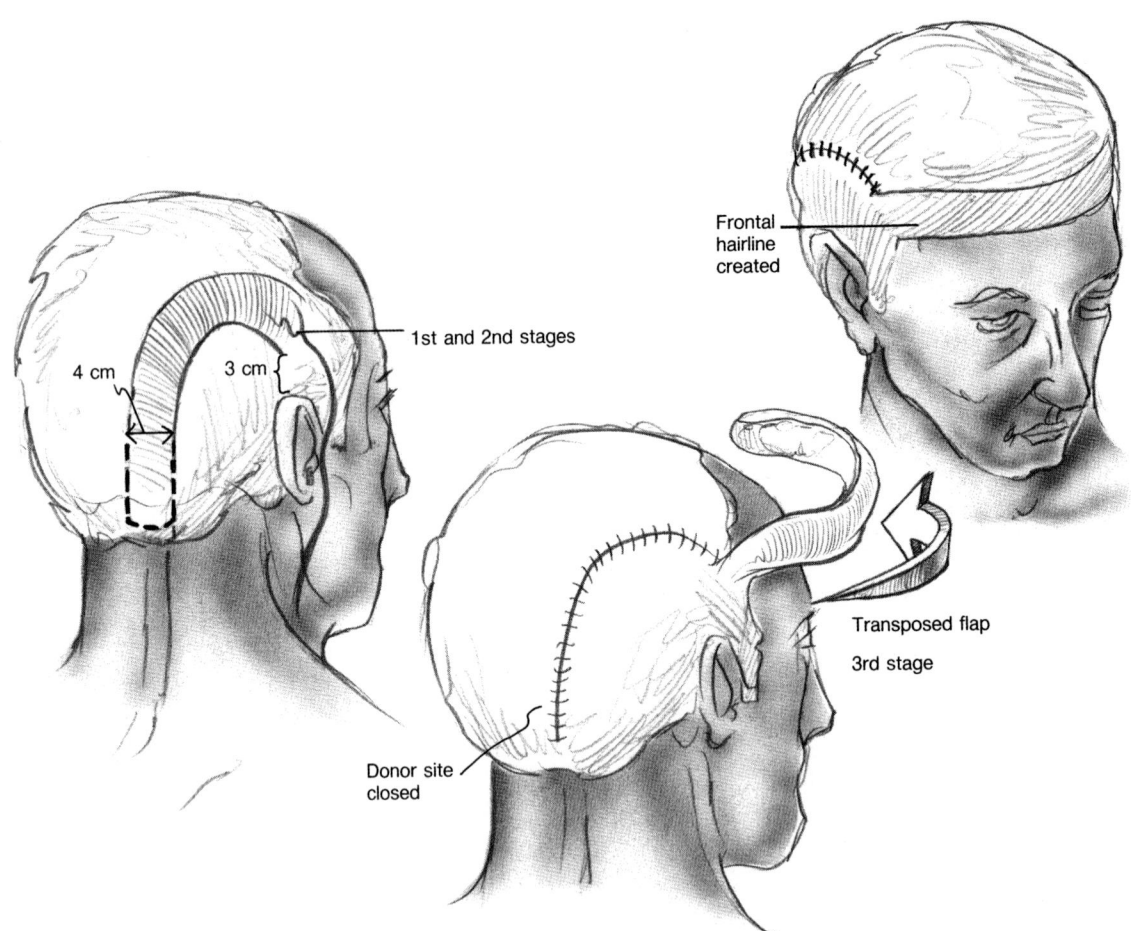

Figure 196.6 The Juri flap. The temporal and parietal portions of the flap are incised during the first stage (*solid lines*). The second stage involves mobilizing the tail of the flap in the occipital region (*dashed lines*) **(left)**. The donor site is closed, and the flap is transposed during the third stage **(center)**. The flap is designed to recreate the frontal hairline **(right)**.

above the root of the helix. The flap is 4 cm wide and has the STA located in the central portion of the base. The base begins posteriorly about 3 cm above the root of the helix and inclines 35 to 45 degrees in an anterior and superior direction. The flap is arched superiorly into the temporal scalp and gently turned posteriorly and inferiorly into the parietal and occipital regions, taking care not to cross the midline or to extend into any areas having the potential for future hair loss. The flap length is determined by measuring the distance from the base of the flap across to the distal end of the frontal hairline. About 4 cm is added to accommodate the "dog ear" that forms when the flap is transposed.

The first two procedures are performed using a local anesthetic. To prevent flap necrosis, epinephrine is never used near the base or the tail of the flap. The first stage consists of incising the proximal three-fourths of the flap through the galea aponeurotica, with attention to maintaining an angle that preserves hair follicles. The flap is not elevated during this stage. One week later, the tail of the flap is incised and elevated to the level of the previous week's incision lines. The occipital vascular plexus is cauterized or ligated and the flap then laid down without entering the region of the prior week's procedure.

The flap is transposed 1 week after the second delay procedure, most often under general anesthesia. The flap is elevated in a subgaleal plane and carefully inspected for adequate circulation at the distal end. A beveled incision is made across the planned anterior hairline, and the scalp is widely undermined in a subgaleal plane superior and inferior to the flap donor site. Homeostasis is checked, and the donor site is closed in layers.

After the donor site is closed, the flap is transposed to lie across the frontal region. A 1-mm strip of epidermis is removed from the frontal edge of the flap with fine forceps and tenotomy scissors. This maneuver allows the surgeon to bury a small strip of dermis along the hairline aspect of the flap below the forehead skin. As hair grows along the deepithelialized strip, it will exit through the overlying forehead skin and incision line, thereby helping to camouflage the frontal scar. The frontal incision line is carefully sutured together. Any overlapping bald skin posterior to the flap is then excised, taking care to avoid tension along the incision line.

Any standing cone deformity that forms at the transposition site is revised 6 weeks after rotating the flap. The flap is cut directly across the dog ear. Limited incisions are made adjacent to this cut along the anterior and posterior margins of the flap. The base of the flap is rotated posteriorly, thus restoring natural hair directionality over the entire temporal scalp. The hairline side of the cut flap is then turned posteriorly to recreate a frontotemporal triangle that is symmetric with the contralateral side. Overlapping bald skin posterior to the flap is excised to accommodate proper flap positioning.

If needed, a second flap is placed 4 cm posterior to the first flap 2 to 3 months after restoration of the frontal hairline. The bald space between the two flaps is excised 2 to 3 months later, resulting in 12 cm of dense hair coverage over the anterior scalp.

One sequela of the Juri flap is the posteriorly oriented frontal hair that results after flap transformation. Severe complications including scalp necrosis and permanent hair loss are more common with flap procedures than with other forms of hair-restoration surgery. These problems are unusual in patients with normal scalp circulation; however, patients with a history of extensive donor graft harvesting over the flap's donor site are especially prone to these complications. Poor hairline design, wide scars, infection, and hematoma are other possible complications of frontal flap hairline restoration (24).

HIGHLIGHTS

- AGA, commonly referred to as MPB, is the most common cause of hair loss in adults.
- Many surgical options are available to manage all but the most severe cases of alopecia.
- Currently, topically applied minoxidil (Rogaine) and oral finasteride (Propecia) are the only medications approved by the FDA for the medical management of hair loss in humans.
- The term *donor dominance* refers to the fact that hair-bearing autografts maintain characteristics of the donor tissue when transplanted into other regions of the body.
- Donor hair is harvested utilizing the elliptical strip method and FUE techniques.
- In the past, standard punch-graft techniques were often criticized for producing unnatural, artificial-appearing hairlines, especially in patients with straight dark hair and light skin color. Technical advances with follicular unit transplants, as well as minigraft and micrograft hair transplants, allow the reconstruction of natural, nonsurgical-appearing frontal hairlines.
- Various scalp reduction techniques are available to reduce crown baldness, offering hope for patients with advanced alopecia who want to attain natural hair restoration over the entire scalp.
- Tissue expansion permits the effective removal and restoration of large alopecic regions in patients with tight, inflexible scalps.

REFERENCES

1. Norwood OT, Shiell RC. *Hair transplant surgery*, 2nd ed. Springfield, IL: Charles C Thomas, 1984.
2. Ludwig E. Classification of the types of androgenetic alopecia (common baldness) occurring in the female sex. *Br J Dermatol* 1977;97(3):247–254.

3. Kaufman KD. Long term (5-year) multinational experience with finasteride 1 mg in the treatment of men with androgenetic alopecia. *Eur J Dermatol* 2002;12:38–49.

4. Whiting DA, Olsen EA, Savin R, et al. Efficacy and tolerability of finasteride 1 mg in men aged 41 to 60 years with male pattern hair loss. *Eur J Dermatol* 2003;12:150–160.

5. Olsen EA, Dunlap MD, Funicella T, et al. A randomized clinical trial of 5% topical minoxidil versus 2% topical minoxidil and placebo in the treatment of androgenetic alopecia in men. *J Am Acad Dermatol* 2002;47:377–385.

6. Avram MR, Cole JP, Gandelman M, et al. The potential role of minoxidil in the hair transplantation setting. *Dermatol Surg* 2002;28:894–900.

7. Shapiro R. Creating a natural hairline in one session using a systematic approach and modern principles of hairline design. *Int J Cosmetic Surg Aesthetic Dermatol* 2001;3(2):89–99.

8. Epstein JS. The treatment of female pattern hair loss and other applications of surgical hair restoration in women. *Facial Plast Surg Clin North Am* 2004;12:241–247.

9. Okuda S. Clinical and experimental studies of transplantation of living hairs. *Jpn J Dermatol Urol* 1939;46:135–138.

10. Orentreich N. Autografts in alopecias and other selected dermatological conditions. *Ann N Y Acad Sci* 1959;83:463.

11. Orentreich D, Orentreich N. Androgenetic alopecia and its treatment. In: Unger W, Nordstrom R, eds. *Hair transplantation.* New York: Marcel Dekker Inc., 1988:1.

12. Buchwach KA. Standard grafts, minigrafts, and micrografts: their use in hair transplantation. *Facial Plast Surg Clin North Am* 1994;2:149.

13. Shapiro R. Principles and techniques used to create a natural hairline in surgical hair restoration. *Facial Plast Surg Clin North Am* 2004;12:201–217.

14. Rassman WR, Bernstein RM, McLellan R, et al. Follicular unit extraction: minimally invasive surgery for hair transplantation. *Dermatol Surg* 2002;28(8):720–728.

15. Harris JA. New methodology and instrumentation for follicular unit extraction: lower follicle transection rates and expanded patient candidacy. *Dermatol Surg* 2006;32(1):56–61.

16. Onda M, Igawa HH, Inoue K, et al. Novel technique of follicular unit extraction hair transplantation with a powered punching device. *Dermatol Surg* 2008;34(12):1683–1688.

17. Bernstein RM, Rassman WR. Follicular unit transplantation: 2005. *Dermatol Clin* 2005;23(3):393–414.

18. Bernstein RM, Rassman WR. The logic of follicular unit transplantation. *Dermatol Clin* 1999;17:277.

19. Konior RJ. Current concepts in hair transplantation. Operative techniques. *Otolaryngol Head Neck Surg* 1995;6:257.

20. Marritt E. Single hair transplantation for hairline refinement: a practical solution. *J Dermatol Surg Oncol* 1984;10:962.

21. Unger MG. Scalp reduction. *Facial Plast Surg Clin North Am* 1994;2:163.

22. Konior RJ. Tissue expansion in scalp surgery. *Facial Plast Surg Clin North Am* 1994;2:203.

23. Juri J. Use of parieto-occipital flaps in the surgical treatment of baldness. *Plast Reconstr Surg* 1975;55:456.

24. Epstein JS, Kabaker SS. Scalp flaps in the treatment of baldness, long-term results. *Dermatol Surg* 1996;22(1):45–50.

Cosmetic Uses of Neurotoxins and Injectable Fillers

197

Grant S. Gillman

Nonsurgical techniques for facial rejuvenation have become the fastest growing area of many cosmetic practices. The use of botulinum toxin and injectable fillers, either alone or in combination, has proven over time to be an effective, minimally invasive and extremely popular treatment option for facial rhytids. Improved safety profiles, lower costs, negligible downtime and increasing duration of effect have led to the veritable explosion of interest in the nonsurgical treatments of facial aging.

One should begin by understanding the basic difference between the neuromodulators and injectable fillers. Whereas botulinum toxin injections are used to eliminate or soften specific *dynamic* facial lines (i.e., wrinkles produced during animation with active contraction of the facial muscles) by selectively weakening the underlying muscles, the fillers as a group are generally used to help efface facial wrinkles or creases that are apparent even *at rest*. In that sense, botulinum toxin can be thought of as *preventing* selected facial wrinkles from developing or deepening, while the injectable fillers on the other hand are used for the treatment of already *established* rhytids. In many cases, the combination of the two might yield a better result than either product alone.

Distinct facial regions are affected by the aging process in different ways. In general, aging of the upper face results more from repetitive action of smaller muscles with the secondary development of dynamic lines—forehead, glabellar and periorbital (crow's feet). Age-related volume loss (aside from the temporal area) contributes less to the aging of the upper face. Accordingly, the use of neuromodulators such as botulinum toxin plays a greater role in the nonsurgical rejuvenation of the upper face than the dermal fillers. On the other hand, gravitational descent, hollowing and volume loss are the primary determinants of aging changes seen in the midface where the approach to volume restoration and nonsurgical rejuvenation focuses primarily more on the use of fillers than neurotoxins. In the lower face, volume loss in the lips and prejowl sulcus as well as deepening of the nasolabial creases are seen with aging in addition to the development of dynamic perioral lines (vertical upper lip rhytids, marionette lines). In the lower face therefore, selective application of either the fillers or neuromodulators can be useful means of addressing the aging changes seen in this region.

While the risk/benefit ratio for these products is extremely favorable, familiarity with the actions, indications, contraindications, treatment expectations and proper patient selection is vital to maximizing patient satisfaction and minimizing complications. Knowledge of the regional anatomy and proper technique are an equally important part of the foundation upon which successful use of these products is built.

REGIONAL ANATOMY

For the most common cosmetic applications of botulinum toxin, one must be intimately familiar with the relevant muscular anatomy of the forehead, glabella, brow, periorbital and perioral regions, and neck (Fig. 197.1).

Horizontal forehead rhytids are caused by repeated contraction of the frontalis muscle—the sole elevator of the brow. In general, there is a midline separation between the two frontalis muscles, and the vertical contraction of those muscles elevates the brow and scalp leading to the formation of transverse lines in the forehead. The frontalis muscle originates from the galea aponeurotica superiorly and interdigitates with the brow depressors inferiorly. From a clinical perspective, it is important to recognize that isolated treatment of the frontalis muscle—the only brow elevator—leaves the action of the brow depressor muscles unopposed. In some patients, this can result in brow ptosis or a heavy, visor-like feeling to the brow.

Brow elevation by the frontalis muscles is opposed by muscles that function as the brow depressors. These

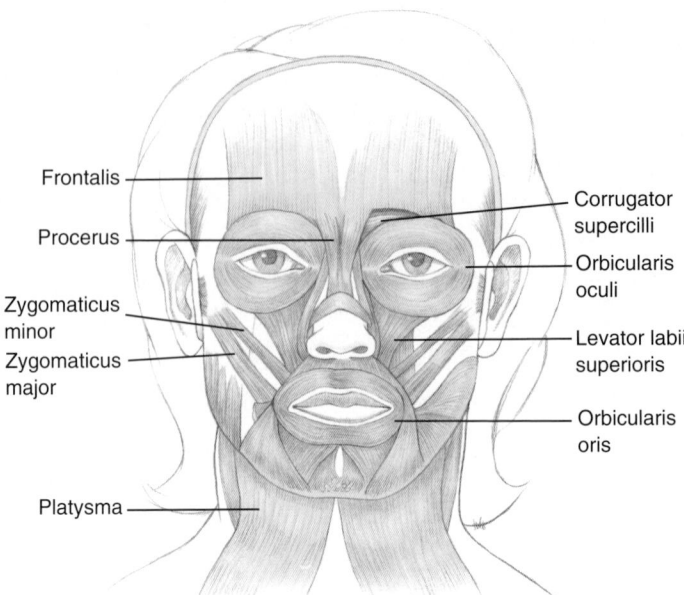

Figure 197.1 Facial musculature.

include the procerus, the corrugator supercilii, the orbicularis oculi and the depressor supercilii (the fibers of the orbicularis below the medial brow).

The procerus muscle originates inferiorly from the lower nasal bones in the midline and runs vertically to blend with the frontalis and insert in the soft tissue between the brows. Contraction of the procerus creates the visible transverse crease at the root of the nose.

The paired corrugator supercilii muscles originate deep to the frontalis and orbicularis muscles near the medial supraorbital ridge where the frontal and nasal bones meet and run superolaterally to insert into the skin and subcutaneous tissue just above the mid-brow. Contraction of the corrugator muscles causes the vertical glabellar lines between the brows (the "frown" lines).

The orbicularis oculi muscle consists of two parts—the orbicular (the outermost portion) and the palpebral, with the latter being divided into preseptal and pretarsal portions. The muscle broadly encircles the orbit, interdigitating with the corrugator muscle medially and superiorly and the frontalis muscle superiorly. Contraction of the orbital portion of the muscle is what produces the lateral orbital rhytids or "crow's feet." Some of the medial fibers of the orbicularis oculi known as the depressor supercilii insert into the skin below the medial eyebrow and also act as medial brow depressors.

The orbicularis oris muscle encircles the mouth and functions both as an oral sphincter and to protrude the lips. Its fibers merge with the depressor anguli oris and the risorius muscles lateral to the oral commissure and the zygomaticus major and minor superiorly. Contraction of the orbicularis oris will result in the fine vertical rhytids that radiate around the upper and lower lips.

The platysma muscle is responsible for horizontal neck creases and vertical bands in the neck. It originates from the fascia overlying the upper chest and clavicle and extends superiorly to insert on the lower mandible and mentum medially and blends with the perioral muscles centrally. More posteriorly and superiorly, the platysma is continuous with the SMAS in the lower two-thirds of the face.

BOTULINUM TOXIN (NEUROTOXINS)

Botulinum toxin injections have become by far the most frequently performed cosmetic procedure over the last decade. In 2008, the use of neurotoxins accounted for almost 25% of all nonsurgical aesthetic procedures (1). Cosmetic applications have expanded, and an increasing number of nonaesthetic applications have been reported as well.

A number of commercially available neuromodulators have been FDA approved for cosmetic applications in the United States. Two of these are formulations of botulinum toxin type A (BoNTA)—onabotulinum toxin A (BoNTA-ONA), which is sold as Botox Cosmetic (Allergan, Inc., Irvine, CA), and abobotulinum toxin A (BoNTA-ABO), which is sold under the trade name Dysport (Medicis Aesthetics, Scottsdale, AZ). Both of these have been approved for the treatment of glabellar lines in addition to their nonaesthetic indications. A third neurotoxin, a formulation of botulinum toxin B, marketed as Myobloc (Solstice Neurosciences, South San Francisco, CA), is FDA approved for nonaesthetic (medical) use and will not be discussed at any length in this chapter. Beyond their FDA-approved medial and aesthetic indications, each of these has been used technically "off-label" in the cosmetic treatment of non-glabellar hyperkinetic facial lines as well.

In addition to differences in the formulation itself, commercial preparations may differ with respect to pH, protein content, purification and manufacturing methods as well as other characteristics (2). It is likely that these differences account somewhat for the variations in clinical characteristics and performance. As a result, there is no single conversion factor that yields *exact* equivalents of efficacy, safety and diffusion between the various preparations, and BoNTA-ABO units are not interchangeable with BoNTA-ONA units (the two main botulinum toxin preparations used clinically). In general, however, BoNTA-ABO (Dysport) is less active on a per unit basis than BoNTA-ONA (Botox Cosmetic), which means that more units are required to achieve a comparable effect. That said, the literature with respect to dose conversions can be confusing, variable in rigor and validity and not free of commercial bias. More recently published literature suggests that one unit of BoNTA-ONA (Botox Cosmetic) is roughly equivalent to 2 to 4 units of BoNTA-ABO (Dysport) for a ratio of 2:1 to 4:1 (3).

Mechanism of Action

Clostridium botulinum is a gram-positive anaerobic bacteria that produces eight antigenically distinct toxins (A, B, C1, C2, D, E, F, and G), seven of which are neuroparalytics. The neurotoxin produces a temporary chemical denervation by inhibiting the release of acetylcholine from the presynaptic neuron at the motor end plates of voluntary muscle. All seven serotypes share the same mechanism of action, inhibiting acetylcholine release at peripheral nerve endings, but differ with respect to molecular complex size, presence or absence of complexing proteins and specific details in their sequence of action (4).

The flaccid paralysis that follows is temporary in nature. Chemodenervation is followed by a two-stage recovery process. Initially, there is growth and sprouting of new axonal collaterals which establish new connections at the motor end plate. At about 3 months, neural transmission through the original (primary) nerve terminal is reestablished and the collateral axons regress (5). This correlates with clinical recovery of function typically in the range of 3 to 4 months postinjection.

Indications and Contraindications

Botox Cosmetic is currently FDA approved for therapeutic use in cervical dystonia, strabismus, blepharospasm and hyperhidrosis and cosmetically for the temporary improvement in vertical glabellar rhytids caused by the action of the corrugator and procerus muscles. Dysport is FDA approved for therapeutic use in the treatment of cervical dystonia in adults and cosmetically for the temporary improvement in glabellar lines. Although technically "off-label," the clinical use of these BoNTA preparations has expanded widely to include the treatment of many other conditions including other facial hyperkinetic lines, migraine headaches, hyperhidrosis, bruxism, Frey syndrome, muscle tension dysphonia, torticollis and bilateral masseteric hypertrophy to name a few.

The use of any botulinum toxin is contraindicated in individuals with preexisting neuromuscular disorders (e.g.,

myasthenia gravis, amyotrophic lateral sclerosis, Eaton-Lambert syndrome) and patients with a sensitivity to any other botulinum toxin product, an albumin allergy, or cow's milk protein allergy (in the case of Dysport; as distinct from patients who are lactose intolerant). Use in pregnant women or lactating mothers is not recommended as there is no safety data regarding use in such circumstances.

Cosmetic Applications of Botulinum Toxin

Commercially available Botox Cosmetic is supplied in a crystalline form as 100 unit vials, whereas Dysport is supplied with 300 units per vial. Both products are diluted with sterile, preservative free normal saline. The volume of dilution depends on the preference of the treating physician. Most prefer dilutions that yield concentrations of 2 to 5 units of Botox Cosmetic per 0.1 mL as this product is typically injected in 2 to 5 unit aliquots (per injection site). Dysport is generally diluted to yield concentrations of either 10 units per 0.1 mL or 10 units per 0.05 mL as this product is typically injected in 10-unit aliquots (per injection site).

The volume of dilution (and hence the concentration) can vary with the clinician's preference, but the underlying principle is that high concentration–low volume injections will help minimize unwanted dispersion of the toxin to surrounding tissues. According to the product information, it is recommended that once reconstituted botulinum toxin should be used within 4 hours, although many clinicians have refrigerated any unused toxin for use up to 30 days (6) and found it to still be clinically effective. In one study of timing of onset and duration of effect in the treatment of forehead rhytids, no difference was found between freshly reconstituted Botox Cosmetic as compared to the same product which was either reconstituted and stored in a refrigerator for 2 weeks or reconstituted and stored in a freezer for 2 weeks prior to use (7).

Following injection, the onset of muscle weakness with BoNTA generally occurs between 2 and 5 days. Botulinum toxin type B (Myobloc) has been shown to have a faster rate of onset than BoNTA formulations—often within 24 hours (8). In general, the duration of response to the BoNTA preparations is similar to one another and should last on average 3 to 4 months before full muscle recovery is noted, though comparative studies looking at physician and patient evaluations of improvement and satisfaction suggest that Botox Cosmetic may have a longer duration of effect than Dysport (9,10). Myobloc on the other hand has a shorter duration of action than either formulation of BoNTA, with efficacy lasting only up to 8 weeks (8).

Although there are many potential applications for the use of botulinum toxin, this chapter will review in general terms only the most common uses for improving facial aesthetics—the treatment of glabellar rhytids ("frown lines"), transverse forehead rhytids, lateral periorbital rhytids ("crow's feet"), the adjustment of brow contour and position (the "chemical" browlift), the treatment of platysmal banding in the neck and vertical upper lip rhytids.

Differences in either injection site specifics or individual adjustments in dose will be apparent from patient to patient and may result from variations in muscle bulk, animation pattern, severity of rhytids, previous results and unique anatomic variations. Keeping detailed treatment records with respect to site, dosage and differences will facilitate reproducibility and improve patient satisfaction. Injection technique is essentially the same regardless of which formulation is used.

Glabellar Rhytids

Glabellar rhytids include the vertical "frown" lines produced by contraction of the corrugator supercilii muscles as well as the transverse crease at the nasion produced by contraction of the procerus. Injection points for glabellar rhytids should target the procerus in the region of the nasion at the intersection of two lines, each of which extends from the medial brow to the opposite medial canthus. Each corrugator muscle is injected medially and laterally into the belly of the muscle above the medial brow roughly in line with the medial canthus and further laterally along the muscle, staying medial to the mid-pupillary line (Fig. 197.2). The latter two injections should always be at or above a transverse line drawn though the mid-eyebrow and above the superior orbital rim to minimize the chance of diffusion into the levator palpebrae of the upper lid which could result in a transient eyelid ptosis (11).

Transverse Forehead Rhytids

As the frontalis muscle is the only elevator of the brow, isolated treatment of horizontal forehead lines must be done with caution. In the patient with heavy glabellar

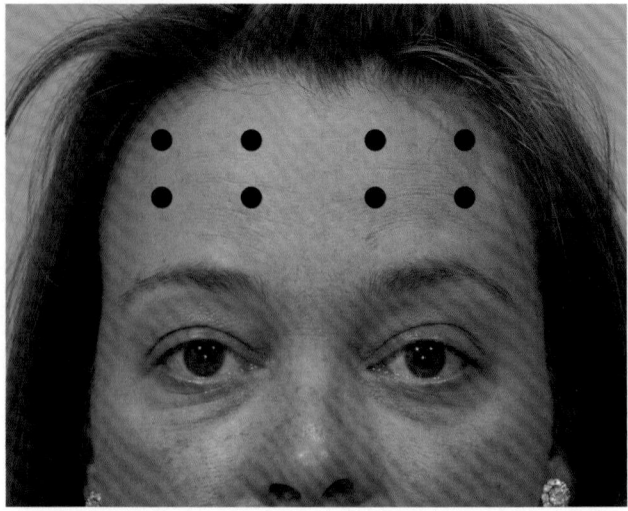

Figure 197.3 Typical grid-like botulinum toxin injection pattern for transverse forehead rhytids.

rhytids or a very low brow one should assume that the brow depressors are quite strong and active, in which case isolated treatment of the frontalis muscle may cause or further aggravate brow ptosis. In such cases, concomitant treatment of the brow depressors (corrugators, procerus) should at the very least be discussed with the patient.

Effective treatment of the transverse forehead rhytids involves subcutaneous or intramuscular injections into the frontalis muscle, either in a relatively uniform grid-like fashion across the forehead (Fig. 197.3) or at four to five equally spaced sites on a horizontal line between the eyebrows and the hairline. Care is taken to stay a minimum of 1 to 1.5 cm above the brow for all injections to minimize the risk of eyebrow ptosis. Simultaneous treatment of brow depressors, if undertaken, can involve the procerus and/or corrugators and/or the lateral orbicularis oculi above the orbital rim and just below the tail of the brow.

Lateral Periorbital Rhytids

Lateral periorbital rhytids ("crow's feet") result from repeated contraction of the lateral portion of the orbicularis oculi muscles. As this muscle is very thin and superficial, intradermal or immediately subdermal injections are sufficiently deep and will help minimize the bruising that can occur commonly in this area. Injections should also be on an arc at least 1.5 cm lateral to the lateral canthus and 1 cm outside the lateral orbital rim to minimize the chance of any diffusion through the lid into the levator palpebrae superioris which could result in upper eyelid ptosis. Treatment of the crow's feet is best avoided in anyone with a preexisting upper eyelid ptosis, lagophthalmos or upper facial palsy.

Having the patient smile or squint will help identify the specific area or lines in need of treatment. Multiple serial injections are then used, typically two to four, perpendicular to the muscle and just outside the orbital

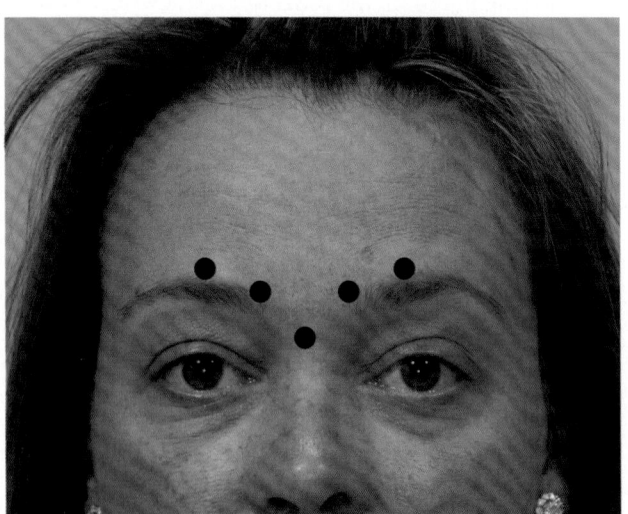

Figure 197.2 Typical botulinum toxin injection pattern for glabellar rhytids/corrugator creases.

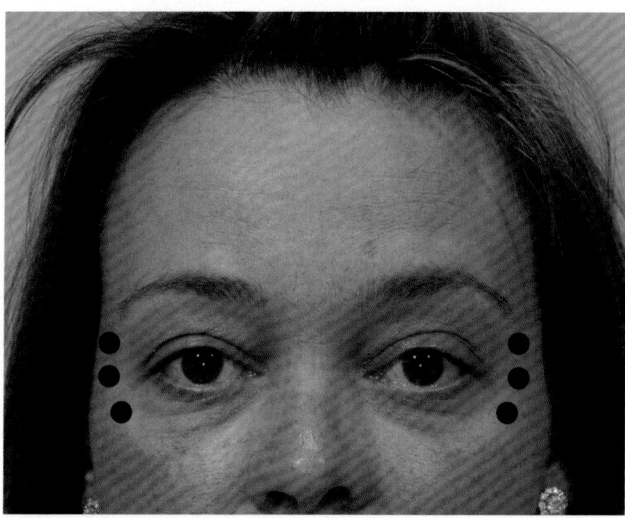

Figure 197.4 Typical botulinum toxin injection pattern for lateral periorbital rhytids.

rim (Fig. 197.4). The amount injected per site will depend on the distribution of the lines and the activity of the underlying orbicularis oculi.

Adjustment of Brow Position and Contour (The "Chemical Browlift")

At least to some degree, brow position is the result of an equilibrium reached between the action of the brow elevator (the frontalis) and the opposing action of the brow depressors (the corrugator, the procerus, the orbicularis oculi and the depressor supercilii) (12,13). As such, selective weakening of the brow depressors with botulinum toxin, either medially or laterally, may result in a modest (several mm) "pharmacologic" brow lift.

Elevation of the entire brow will require attention to both the medial and the lateral brow depressors. Frequently, elevation of only one end of the brow or the other might be desired in which case it suffices to address those muscles only. For elevation of the medial brow, treatment of the corrugators and procerus as well as the depressor supercilii is required. The latter muscle is treated with an injection of a small dose just below and just lateral to the medial head of the brow, taking care to remain outside the orbital rim to avoid unwanted diffusion into adjacent muscles. Elevation of the lateral brow requires a subdermal injection of the orbicularis oculi muscle just below the eyebrow lateral to the high point of the brow, once again remaining outside the orbital rim. One to three injection sites may be required.

Platysmal Banding

Administration of botulinum toxin to platysmal bands can be a useful adjunct in the treatment of the senescent neck (14). Best results are seen with mild to moderate banding

(15), and the changes are most appreciable with dynamic contraction of the platysma than at rest.

Having the patient contract the muscle will best demonstrate the platysmal bands, which are then grasped and injected with botulinum toxin at multiple sites each 1 to 1.5 cm apart, from below the jawline to the lower neck. Typically, each band will receive a total of about 15 units of Botox Cosmetic or 40 to 80 units of Dysport per band. Caution must be exercised to avoid excessive doses and to inject into the muscle but not deep to it. Overly deep injections can increase the risk of dysphagia and/or neck weakness.

Vertical Lip Rhytids

Very low doses of botulinum toxin injected into the orbicularis oris muscle of the upper lip can help efface or soften vertical upper lip lines. This treatment may be an alternative to perioral chemical peels or laser resurfacing and can be used alone or in combination with injectable fillers. In order to avoid problems with oral incompetence the injections are kept very superficial (subdermal), and very small doses are used initially. Nonetheless, professional public speakers and wind instrument musicians may not be ideal candidates for this treatment.

Four evenly spaced injections are given across the upper lip at or immediately above the vermilion border. Starting with lower doses and increasing if necessary is most prudent. In addition to reducing the depth of apparent vertical lip lines, some degree of lip eversion is also frequently noted.

Botulinum Toxin Complications

As noted earlier, the safety profile of neurotoxins when used for cosmetic applications is quite favorable. In fact, the safety, combined with favorable and reproducible outcomes accounts for the popularity of the procedure. Sound knowledge of the regional anatomy, attention to proper doses and technique and the use of high concentration–low volume dilutions all help minimize the incidence of unwanted side effects. Larger volumes can lead to inadvertent and undesirable spread to adjacent nontargeted tissues. Since the effect of any neurotoxin is a temporary one, so too are the complications. There have been no deaths reported or adverse long-term effects from the cosmetic use of neurotoxins (16).

Medications that might potentiate the activity of botulinum toxin include aminoglycosides, cyclosporins, neuromuscular blockers, calcium channel blockers, quinidine, magnesium sulfate and D-penicillamine.

General sequelae of botulinum toxin injections include pain, erythema and bruising at the injection site, headache, flu-like symptoms, malaise and fatigue. Injection pain can be minimized by using small gauge needles as well as slowly inserting the needle and injecting slowly. Aside from

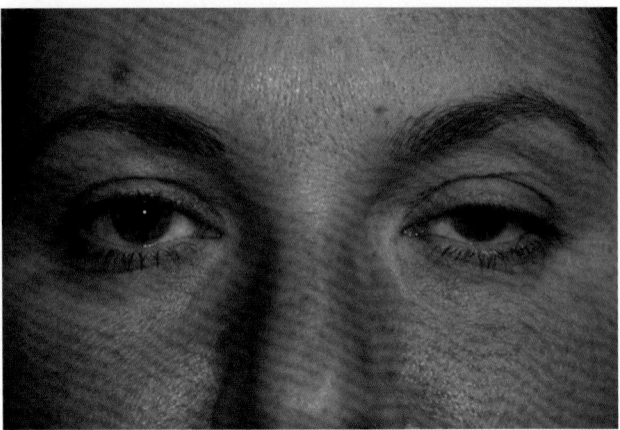

Figure 197.5 Left eyelid ptosis resulting from diffusion of botulinum toxin into levator palpebrae superioris muscle.

injection-related discomfort, erythema and perhaps bruising, the others are much less common. Headaches occur in about 1% of patients, and patients should be informed of this possibility (17).

Site-specific complications should be infrequent if suitable consideration is paid to technical detail. The most significant complication of glabellar or lateral periorbital injections is upper eyelid ptosis (Fig. 197.5). Ptosis results from migration of the injected toxin deep to the orbital septum where it may affect the levator palpebrae superioris of the upper eyelid. Staying outside the orbital rim with all injections (as indicated earlier) should prevent this complication from developing. In addition, one should avoid massaging the area as this may encourage unwanted dispersion of the product. Upper eyelid ptosis can develop up to 1 week after injections and usually resolves within 2 to 6 weeks. Should it develop, ptosis can be treated with alpha-adrenergic ophthalmic drops such as Iopidine 0.5% (Apraclonidine, Alcon Laboratories, Fort Worth, TX) or Mydfrin 2.5% (Phenylephrine 2.5%, Alcon Labs), both of which stimulate Mueller muscle to help elevate the eyelid margin (18). The typical dose is one to two drops three times daily until the ptosis resolves. Injection of the crow's feet can also result in diplopia by affecting the lateral rectus. For this reason, it is important to stay at least 1 cm outside the lateral orbital rim at all times.

Treatment of the frontalis muscle for transverse forehead rhytids can result in brow ptosis, which is best avoided by staying at least 1 to 1.5 cm above the brow. Older patients, those with a low-set brow and those with very active brow depressors are at greatest risk. Should brow ptosis develop, patients can be reassured that the frontalis muscle will return to its baseline activity within 3 to 4 months. Alternatively, brow ptosis can be alleviated, if necessary, by secondary treatment of the brow depressors if this has not already been performed.

Injection of the platysmal bands may also cause unwanted secondary effects. If the injection is too deep it can affect the larynx and hypopharynx, resulting in dysphagia or hoarseness. If the injection is too far lateral weakness of the sternocleidomastoid muscle can occur. Staying superficial and avoiding excessive dosing are critical. Dietary modification (soft foods, liquid diet) and metoclopramide hydrochloride may be necessary for severe dysphagia (18).

Lip weakness or oral incompetence may result from perioral use of botulinum toxin. Prevention is most important and requires use of very low doses initially together with superficial placement.

Resistance to botulinum toxin type A may result from the formation of neutralizing antibodies. This is generally associated with repeated use of high doses (above 300 units) and is relatively uncommon with the lower doses used for cosmetic applications (19). If antibodies to botulinum toxin A develop, the use of botulinum toxin type B may be of benefit (8).

Finally, patient dissatisfaction may result from overtreatment, undertreatment and unmet or unrealistic expectations. Proper patient selection, education and counseling together with consistent procedural skills will help limit the number of unhappy patients.

SOFT TISSUE AUGMENTATION

The use of injectable materials for soft tissue augmentation has a long history dating to Neuber (20) in 1893 when he harvested fat from the arm and injected it into a patient's facial defects. Since that time, many other materials have been developed in the search for a filler substance to correct facial scarring from trauma and acne, static rhytids and malar and lip and melolabial crease augmentation.

In the early part of the 1900s, paraffin injection became popular. This quickly fell out of favor however secondary to repeated granulomatous-type foreign body reactions resulting in paraffinomas. In the 1940 to 1950s, injectable silicone was introduced. Long-term studies with this material however revealed a potential for granulomatous reactions and scarring and so FDA approval was ultimately withdrawn in the 1980s. In the 1970s, Stanford researchers experimented with animal- and human-derived collagen as implantable materials that eventually led to the introduction of bovine collagen (21).

In recent years, research and development in this area has been intense due to the popularity of dermal fillers. Patient demand in this area is high because injectable fillers offer distinct advantages over surgical procedures. The benefits of injectables for soft tissue augmentation include that injections can be performed on an outpatient basis with minimal or no recovery time and they offer immediate results with lower short-term costs than surgical procedures. Additionally, the ease of touch-ups when necessary and consistently improved safety and duration of effect are attractive to patients. Furthermore, certain defects are more easily corrected with contour filling rather than surgical intervention.

However, the *ideal* filler has yet to be found. The ideal filler would be easy to use, biocompatible and without risk of allergic reactions, immunogenic toxicity or carcinogenicity. It would be inexpensive and have an inexhaustible source. The ideal filler material would also be well tolerated and accepted by the host so that long-term correction could be achieved without risk of complication.

In general, most of the currently available materials are made to be injected into the dermis or subdermal. The dermis is the middle layer of the integument composed of viscoelastic tissue lying between the epidermis and the subcutaneous tissue. The predominant cell type in this layer is the fibroblast that secretes the cellular matrix of type I collagen and elastin. Collagen fibers provide tensile strength, while the elastin is responsible for elastic recoil (22). These fibers are embedded in a gel-like ground substance of glycosaminoglycans. The primary polysaccharide of this extracellular matrix is hyaluronic acid (HA), which provides a framework for collagen and elastin to bind and potently binds water maintaining skin turgor. With aging, the concentration of HA in the skin diminishes with a resultant loss of volume, turgor and cellular hydration.

There is no single means of classifying fillers. Currently used dermal fillers can be divided into categories based on the relationship to the donor (xenografts—donor and recipient are different species; autografts—donor and recipient are the same individual; homografts—donor and recipient are same species; and synthetic materials), their duration of effect (temporary vs. permanent) or their chemical makeup (collagens vs. hyaluronic acids vs. biosynthetic polymers). Products available function either as *volumizers* that are relatively neutral and provide bulk (temporarily or permanent) but cause minimal foreign body reaction, or *stimulators* that stimulate tissues by causing a foreign body reaction which then results in new collagen formation.

In general, the deeper the defect the more viscous the filler and the deeper the desired plane of injection. Superficial lines are typically addressed with fillers of smaller particles placed into the upper dermis, whereas fillers of larger particle size (thicker consistency) are injected into the deeper dermis or into the subdermal plane to treat deeper furrows and for larger volume augmentation. Layering techniques, using multiple products, are often used where both volume addition and the effacement of superficial fine lines are desired.

The currently available fillers are approved for the correction of moderate to severe wrinkles and folds and in some cases for the treatment of facial lipoatrophy. The other commonly reported clinical applications such as the correction of soft tissue depressions and volume augmentation (e.g., malar, prejowl sulcus, lips) are off-label uses of these products.

The discussion of dermal fillers that follows is not intended to be exhaustive. There are constantly new products in development that may ultimately prove to be more effective than existing ones, and within little time of any review or publication newer products become available, and others are discontinued. As such, this portion of this chapter is intended to be an overview and should not be regarded as a definitive or comprehensive resource.

Collagen Products

Bovine collagen was the most widely used dermal filler from the time of FDA approval in 1981 until the last decade and has by far the longest track record. Up until the early 21st century, injectable collagen remained the gold standard to which other fillers were compared. As collagen is a major component of the skin's structure, its use as an injectable filler was a logical extension. Owing to widespread development of second- and third-generation dermal and subdermal fillers that are hypoallergenic, safer and longer lasting, distribution of collagen products was halted by the manufacturer in 2010. A brief discussion of collagen is included here for its historical relevance.

Three types of bovine collagen were commercially available. Zyderm I, Zyderm II and Zyplast (Allergan Inc., Irvine, CA) are all derivatives of enzyme-digested bovine collagen—primarily type I—suspended in phosphate buffered saline and lidocaine. During the preparation, antigenicity is reduced by pepsin proteolysis (23). All three of these collagen fillers were made up of 95% type I bovine collagen and 5% type III bovine collagen.

Zyderm I contains 35 mg/mL of collagen and was approved by the FDA in 1981. As the concentration of collagen in Zyderm I was quite low there was significant resorption of this product, and so Zyderm II containing 65 mg/mL of collagen was introduced and approved by the FDA in 1983. It was felt that the higher concentration of collagen translated to longer duration of effect. Zyplast, on the other hand, contains 35 mg/mL of collagen crosslinked with glutaraldehyde in order to make the material less susceptible to enzymatic degradation and resorption, thereby delivering a longer lasting result. All of these products lasted approximately 3 to 5 months—ultimately, a competitive disadvantage.

Zyderm was recommended for superficial mild to moderate wrinkles such as the glabellar creases, periorbital crow's feet and perioral rhytids. The product was injected into the upper dermis. Because of early resorption with this material a slight overcorrection was required. Conversely, Zyplast was injected into the deeper reticular dermis, and since it was more resistant to resorption overcorrection was not needed.

The primary disadvantage of bovine collagen was the risk of a hypersensitivity reaction manifesting as induration, erythema, pruritus and tenderness at the injection site. Skin testing for allergic sensitivity was therefore required prior to definitive use. About 3% to 4% of patients undergoing skin testing developed a hypersensitivity reaction (24,25). Although in the majority of allergic patients a reaction to skin testing was apparent in the first week, about 20% to 30% demonstrated a delayed reaction for which it was necessary to examine the injection site 4 to 6 weeks later. Many considered the need for a second negative skin test to be routine prior to beginning treatments, and even with a negative second skin test the likelihood of an allergic reaction was not entirely eliminated. In addition to a hypersensitivity reaction, bovine collagen injections can result in tissue necrosis (26), foreign body reactions (27) and infrequent systemic reactions such as headache, nausea and arthralgias.

In 2003, the FDA approved release of a bioengineered form of human collagen fillers (Cosmoderm, Cosmoplast—Allergan, Inc, Irvine, CA). The primary advantage of these was a longer duration of effect than bovine collagen, and because these products were derived from bioengineered human fibroblasts no skin pretesting was required. Like the bovine collagen fillers however and for similar reasoning, distribution of these has also been recently discontinued by the manufacturer. A technique for producing autologous collagen was introduced in the mid-1990s—Isolagen (Isolagen Technologies, Houston, TX)—as a way to inject patients with their own fibroblasts that were harvested, cultured, grown *in vitro* and then processed for use. The expense, the time factor in production, the complexity involved in the process and the need for precise coordination between manufacturer, doctor and patient proved to be impractical however, and for that reason the product is no longer available.

Hyaluronic Acid Products

Hyaluronic acid is the main polysaccharide in the extracellular matrix of the human dermis. Because it has the ability to bind 1,000 times its volume in water, HA confers a certain amount of turgor to the skin by affecting dermal volume and compressibility (28). HA is unique in that it is chemically the same in all species, and therefore its derivatives should not be antigenic across species. The injected product is enzymatically degraded locally and then metabolized by the liver into carbon dioxide and water.

HAs are the most widely used of all dermal fillers (29). Commercially available products vary with respect to the source from which they are derived, particle size, degree of cross-linking, viscosity and whether or not lidocaine has been added to the filler. The first HA gels introduced for cosmetic use were derived from rooster combs, whereas most HA products produced today are derived from a non-animal source. Smaller particles used more commonly for finer lines generally last 6 months or more, while larger particles last more in the range of 6 to 12 months. A higher percentage of cross-linking equates with increased resistance to enzymatic biodegradation and therefore a longer duration of effect. HA gels are injected into the mid- to deep dermis to effect a correction of moderate to severe facial wrinkles (Fig. 197.6A and B).

There are two salient advantages to the use of HA gel fillers as compared to collagen. The first is that since HA is identical across species the manufacturers do not recommend or require skin testing prior to injection. Nonetheless, although the current product is highly purified, there are still minute amounts of associated proteins (30). As a result, rare cases of localized hypersensitivity reactions resulting in local erythema and induration resolving in 4 to 20 weeks have been reported (31–33). Overall, the risk of an allergic reaction was less than 1%, and manufacturing processes have evolved to reduce the amount of protein present resulting in fewer reactions. The other notable advantage of the HA products is that in the event of adverse reactions including improper placement (location or

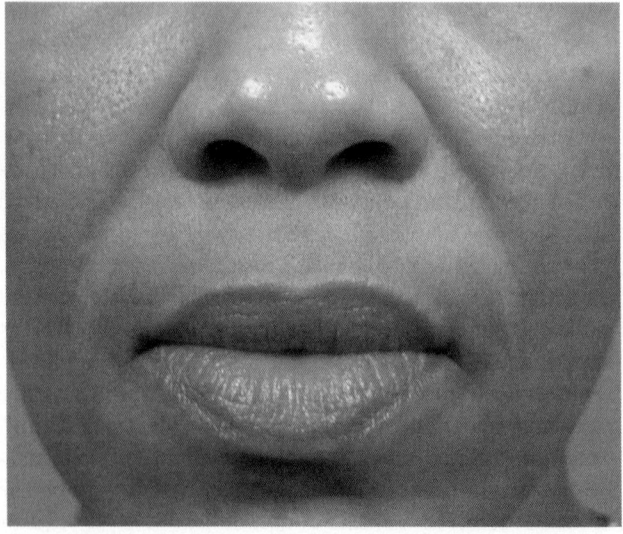
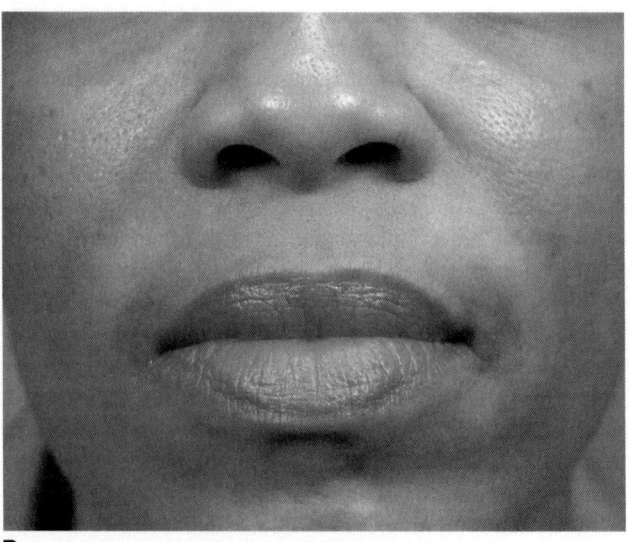

A   **B**

Figure 197.6 Before **(A)** and after **(B)** HA injections to melolabial creases.

volume), the gel can be enzymatically degraded with the use of injectable hyaluronidase giving these products the significant added benefit of being "reversible" (34).

Currently available FDA-approved HA fillers in the United States include Restylane and Perlane products (Medicis, Scottsdale, AZ), Juvederm products (Allergan, Irvine, CA), Prevelle Silk (Mentor, Irving, TX) and Elevess (Anika Therapeutics, Bedford, MA).

Calcium Hydroxylapatite

Radiesse (Bioform Medical, San Mateo, CA) is a biosynthetic polymer composed of 30% calcium hydroxylapatite (CaHA) microspheres (25- to 45-micron diameter particles) suspended in a 70% carrier gel made up of carboxymethylcellulose, water and glycerin. CaHA is naturally occurring component in human bone and teeth, and for that reason skin testing for allergy is not required. Radiesse is the only FDA-approved commercially available CaHA filler.

The FDA-approved cosmetic indications for the use of CaHA are for the correction of moderate to deep facial wrinkles and folds such as the nasolabial folds (Fig. 197.7) and for the treatment of HIV-associated facial lipoatrophy. Off-label facial cosmetic applications have included

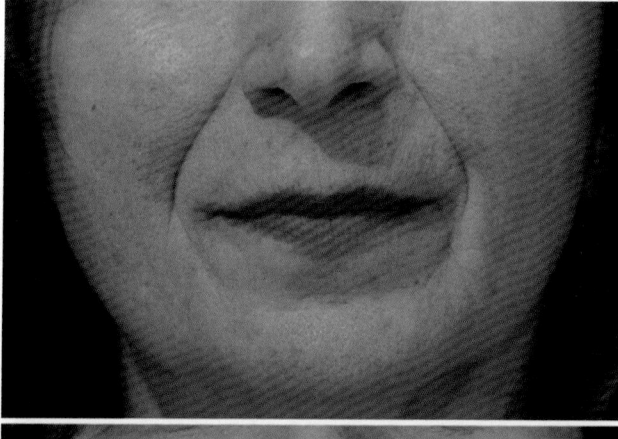
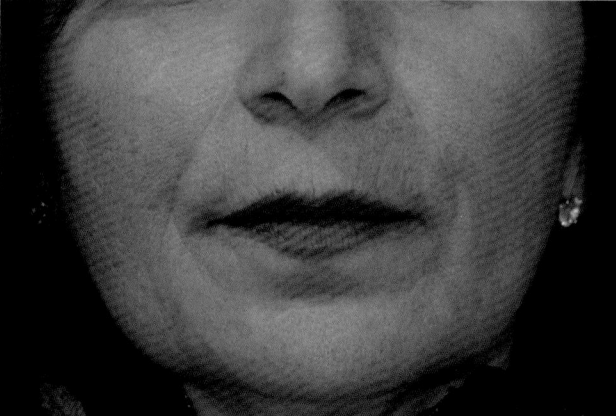

Figure 197.7 Before **(above)** and after **(below)** CaHA (Radiesse) injections to nasolabial creases and marionette lines.

volume augmentation in the malar area, cheek and prejowl sulcus, marionette lines and nasal dorsal irregularities. Deeper folds are augmented with injection into the immediate subdermal plane, whereas volume augmentation (prejowl, malar) is generally done with supraperiosteal deposition of the product. Edema, erythema and ecchymosis are not uncommonly seen with Radiesse injections, but these adverse effects are temporary. Lidocaine can be safely added to the Radiesse syringes without having any deleterious effect on the qualities of the original filler material (35).

When injected, initial volume augmentation results from the displacement of surrounding soft tissue by the carrier gel and CaHA microspheres. Ultimately, the carrier gel undergoes phagocytosis while a process of stimulated neocollagenesis takes place around the CaHA microspheres which serve as a framework or scaffold for the ingrowth of new tissue (36). The duration of effect is typically 12 months or more. The combination of host neocollagenesis and the slow degradation of the CaHA microspheres are thought to account for the more prolonged duration of effect. CaHA is apparent within the soft tissue on CT imaging, but does not generally interfere with interpretation of the images (37).

Poly-L-Lactic Acid

Poly-L-lactic acid (PLLA) is a biodegradable synthetic biopolymer already in use in suture materials and absorbable fixation plates and screws. The commercially available injectable product, Sculptra Aesthetic (Sanofi Aventis, Bridgewater, NJ), is supplied in a vial as a powdered form of PLLA microspheres in a carboxymethylcellulose gel that must be reconstituted with sterile water 2 to 72 hours prior to injection. Skin testing is not necessary.

The product is injected into the subcutaneous plane. The volume that is immediately apparent upon treatment dissipates over the first few days as the water used to reconstitute the powdered PLLA is resorbed. For this reason, the patient must be counseled accordingly so as not to be initially disappointed. Over time, the PLLA microspheres act by stimulating an inflammatory fibrous tissue response in the host that activates collagen neogenesis and deposition around the degrading PLLA particles (38). Several sessions spaced 3 to 4 weeks apart are typically required for complete volume restoration.

As the volume augmentation that occurs results from stimulation of the host to produce new collagen, the effect takes time and the patient should be made to understand that it is not immediate. Strictly speaking, PLLA is not a true filler but rather a collagen growth stimulator.

Sculptra was FDA approved in 2004 for the treatment of facial lipoatrophy in HIV patients, and Sculptra Aesthetic (essentially the same product) was FDA approved in 2009 for the correction of shallow to deep nasolabial fold contour deficiencies (Fig. 197.8). It has been used off-label as

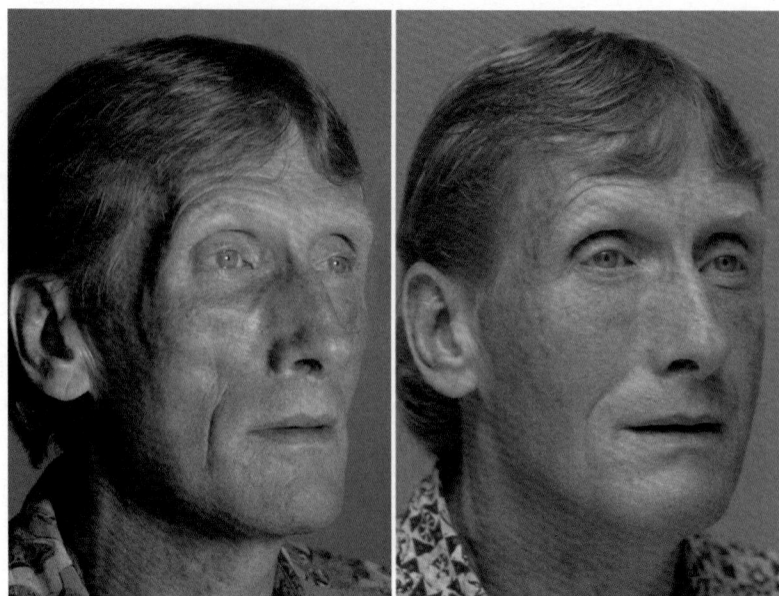

Figure 197.8 Before **(left)** and after **(right)** PLLA (Sculptra) injections to temples, malar eminence and cheeks for the treatment of facial lipoatrophy.

for effective malar, cheek or temple volume augmentation. It is not recommended for use in the periorbital area or lips. The effect may last up to 2 years.

Adverse effects of particular concern with PLLA are the possibility of developing subcutaneous nodules or papules that can develop months after treatment. One can help diminish this risk by insuring an adequate volume of dilution (5 mL or more), preparation of the product at least several hours prior to its use for more complete hydration of the PLLA powder and having the patient massage the treatment area frequently for the first 5 days after each session.

Polymethyl Methacrylate

Injectable polymethyl methacrylate (PMMA), commercially available as Artefill (Suneva Medical, San Diego, CA), is a nonabsorbable permanent filler made up of a suspension of 20% PMMA and 80% bovine collagen. As the collagen carrier is absorbed over 2 to 3 months, the PMMA microspheres stimulate a foreign body reaction and collagen formation. The PMMA acts as a matrix or scaffold for the deposition of the tissue ingrowth, becoming encapsulated by fibrous tissue ensuring a constant augmentation (39).

Skin testing is required because of the presence of the bovine collagen antigens. Artefill was FDA approved in 2006 for the correction of nasolabial folds but has been used off-label for glabellar frown lines, marionette lines and radial lip lines. The material is injected at the junction of the dermal–subdermal junction.

With earlier preparations (used outside the United States), multiple foreign body granulomatous reactions were reported resulting in poor results and increased morbidity and scarring (40). Refinements to the product

were made to lessen that risk and achieve the current FDA-approved preparation. Although the collagen vehicle is resorbed, the PMMA microspheres are non-resorbable and persist in tissue permanently.

Silicone

Injectable silicone is a permanent, non-resorbable filler composed of long chains of polymerized dimethylsiloxane oil. The technique of microdroplet injection was popularized by Webster et al. (41) and Orentreich and Orentreich (42). With this technique, very minute amounts (0.01 mL per injection site) of medical grade liquid silicone are injected into the subdermal plane at 2- to 4-mm intervals. Care is taken not to overcorrect the treatment area as the microdroplets stimulate fibroplasia, and the body thus forms a fibrous collagen capsule around the silicone microdroplets over the ensuing weeks, thereby augmenting the original volume of the liquid silicone microdroplet. Undercorrection is therefore the initial goal, with repeat sessions staged a month or more apart until the desired result is achieved.

Prior to the introduction of injectable collagen, liquid silicone was the filler of choice, although problems arose from products of differing purity, variations in technique and the lack of any standardized FDA-approved product. Webster et al. (41) reported a long-term follow-up with a series of 524 patients with good results and few complications, but others have reported a long list of local and systemic complications some of which may appear even years after injection. These reactions range from chronic inflammation, silicone granulomas, beading, migration, extrusion ulceration and skin necrosis to granulomatous hepatitis, pulmonary embolism and silicone pneumonitis (43–45).

In 1991, the FDA declared the use of injectable silicone illegal. However, with the recent FDA approval of injectable silicone as an intraocular implant in ophthalmology for retinal detachments the off-label use for soft tissue augmentation has been revived. Off-label uses of injectable silicone remain controversial however because of the history of complications with injected silicone, and one must carefully consider the risks versus the benefits (46).

Autologous Fat

Autologous fat has the longest history of use since Neuber (20) first injected it in 1893. The interest in autologous fat transplantation has vacillated over the years due to the variability in results. Some investigators report that between 30% and 60% of the injected fat will be resorbed (47). However, since the advent of liposuction in the 1970s, interest in fat transplantation has increased. Over the last 15 years, techniques and instrumentation for the harvesting, preparation and injection of autologous fat have evolved to improve fat survival and diminish resorption thereby increasing the predictability of the procedure. Some authors such as Coleman (48) recommend injection of small amounts of fat in subcutaneous tunnels to maximize the amount of blood flow to the transplanted fat, thus increasing its viability and the chance of survival. Harvest of fat has to be gently performed with minimal syringe pressure using large-bore cannulas to minimize trauma to the harvested fat cells.

To date, there is no universally accepted method for the harvesting, processing and reinjection of autologous fat, and often results are not reproducible. The advantage of fat transplantation is the large amounts available in the human body, and because it is autologous and natural it negates the concern for allergic reactions and biocompatibility. On the other hand, fat transfer is a surgical procedure, has a more significant recovery period as compared to other injectable fillers and requires a donor site with its own set of potential complications. In addition, fat grafting has the disadvantage of having an unpredictable resorption rate, and touch-ups can be more involved than with off-the-shelf fillers. Over recent years, the surge in interest in commercially supplied dermal fillers has coincided with some decline in the number of fat injection procedures.

Complications of Injectable Fillers

While it is impossible to eliminate complications entirely, most experts will agree that serious complications are rare if the practitioner is committed to accurate facial analysis, proper patient selection and product choice, appropriate training for each filler used and diligent application of technique. Treatment must be individualized and tailored to the needs of the patient, and the limits of what can be accomplished safely must be respected.

While increased product longevity would seem to be a desirable characteristic, one should carefully weigh the risk/benefit of biodegradable, resorbable fillers versus permanent fillers. The fact that visible complications such as bumps, ridges or nodularity will ultimately resolve when a temporary filler has been used may provide some reassurance and comfort to a patient. This comfort level is not available to the patient who has been injected with a permanent filler. At the very least, one should avoid the use of permanent fillers in a given patient until that patient has already used something absorbable with good results.

Complications can be broadly classified into immediate, early, late and permanent. Immediate complications include anaphylaxis, hypersensitivity and pain. Early complications include bruising, edema, overcorrection, infection and vascular compromise. Later complications can include HSV activation, visible irregularities, lumps, granuloma formation and product migration. Permanent complications include scarring (49).

Edema, bruising and injection site pain are not uncommon sequelae and are not truly complications but rather known side effects. Ice packs or cold compresses applied to the treatment area as well as effort directed to avoiding inadvertent puncture of superficial vessels may be helpful in minimizing these.

Allergic or hypersensitivity reactions can theoretically develop with any filler, but are more likely to be an issue with those containing a bovine collagen additive (collagen, Artefill). For these fillers, skin testing is required prior to definitive treatment.

With all fillers, injection technique and proper depth of injection are paramount to success. Superficial injection can result in visible nodularity or lumps. Early-appearing nodules may respond to massage, and in some cases the overlying skin can be nicked and the product extruded (if apparent very early). More delayed appearance or visible nodules may improve by treating the area with small doses of locally injected steroids. HA fillers, if placed too superficially, can result in a bluish discoloration of the skin over the area of injection which is known as a "Tyndall effect." This may be treated with extrusion as noted earlier, or if that fails, the untoward effect HA fillers can be "reversed" with the use of injected hyaluronidase. Naturally, visible irregularities are a much bigger issue if one has used a permanent filler. With permanent fillers, persistent nodules may require surgical removal.

Soft tissue necrosis can occur with vascular compromise resulting from either direct intra-arterial injection or venous obstruction from compression exerted by the filler material. The areas at highest risk are the glabella and the nasal ala in the region of the alar–facial sulcus (medial end of the nasolabial crease). Signs of vascular compromise include blanching of the skin, disproportionate injection pain and discoloration of the surrounding tissue. Management should include immediate cessation of the injection, vigorous massage of the treatment area in an effort to disperse the filler, application of warm compresses and topical nitroglycerine paste for vasodilation and local injection of hyaluronidase (if an HA filler was used).

Conclusion

Although no ideal filler is yet available, very active research and development continues in this area of facial plastic surgery. There are many choices offered on the market that can fulfill patient's needs. It is incumbent upon every practitioner who uses fillers to stay informed on the current materials in order to better inform patients and to make the best possible choices. Often two or more fillers used in combination offer the best results. Likewise, it is not uncommon to combine botulinum toxin in the upper third of the face and fillers in the melolabial folds, marionette lines and perioral region to obtain a refreshed and rejuvenated appearance.

With any permanent synthetic filler, concerns will exist about potential long-term effects or delayed complications. Although permanent complications are uncommon, the wide array of biodegradable, absorbable fillers with favorable safety profiles and relatively predictable results is without doubt a safer alternative, particularly for the inexperienced injector.

As has been stressed throughout this chapter, successful use of both the neurotoxins and injectable fillers begins with familiarity with the strengths and limitations of each product, comfort with the nuances of injection techniques, accurate facial analysis, careful patient selection and realistic management of patient expectations. Properly applied, these minimally invasive nonsurgical techniques can be a valuable and powerful addition to the armamentarium available for the management of facial aging.

HIGHLIGHTS

- Botulinum toxin is used in the treatment of dynamic facial rhytids to prevent them from either developing or deepening.
- Botulinum toxin works by temporarily inhibiting presynaptic release of acetylcholine at the motor end plate. Its use is contraindicated in those with neuromuscular disease and albumin allergy.
- Familiarity with regional facial anatomy, proper technique, and the use of high concentration–low volume dilutions will minimize the risk of adverse outcome with botulinum toxin.
- Injectable fillers are used for soft tissue augmentation to add contour and volume. They are commonly used for camouflage of established facial rhytids and scars and for lip augmentation.
- A great variety of injectable dermal fillers are available. Proper selection will depend on region, patient preference and hypersensitivities.

REFERENCES

1. American Society for Aesthetic Plastic Surgery Web site. Cosmetic Surgery National Data Bank statistics 2008. (Accessed August 2009.)
2. Aoki KR, Ranoux D, Wissel J. Using translational medicine to understand clinical differences between botulinum toxin formulations. *Eur J Neurol* 2006;13(Suppl 4):10–19.
3. Karsai S, Raulin C. Botox and dysport: is there a dose conversion in dermatology and aesthetic medicine? *J Am Acad Dermatol* 2010;62(2):346–347.
4. Dolly JO, Aoki KR. The structure and mode of action of different botulinum toxins. *Eur J Neurol* 2006;13(Suppl 4):1–9.
5. Alderson K, Holds JB, Anderson RL. Botulinum-induced alteration of nerve-muscle interactions in the human orbicularis oculi following treatment for blepharospasm. *Neurology* 1991;41: 1800–1805.
6. Klein AW. Dilution and storage of botulinum toxin. *Dermatol Surg* 1998;24:1179–1180.
7. Yang GC, Chiu RJ, Gillman GS. Questioning the need to use botox within 4 hours of reconstitution: a study of fresh vs. 2-week-old botox. *Arch Facial Plast Surg* 2008;10(4):273–279.
8. Kim EJ, Ramirez AL, Reeck JB, et al. The role of botulinum toxin type B (Myobloc) in the treatment of hyperkinetic facial lines. *Plast Reconstr Surg* 2003;112:88S–93S.
9. Trindade de Almeida AR, Marques E, de Almeida J, et al. Pilot study comparing the diffusion of two formulations of botulinum toxin type A in patients with forehead hyperhidrosis. *Dermatol Surg* 2007;33(1 Spec. No.):S37–S43.
10. Lowe PL, Patnaik R, Lowe NJ. A comparison of two botulinum type A toxin preparations for the treatment of glabellar lines: double-blind, randomized, pilot study. *Dermatol Surg* 2005;31(12):1651–1654.
11. Macdonald MR, Spiegel JH, Raven RB, et al. An anatomical approach to glabellar rhytids. *Arch Otolaryngol Head Neck Surg* 1998;124:1315–1320.
12. Frankel AS, Kamer RM. Chemical browlift. *Arch Otolaryngol Head Neck Surg* 1998;124:321–323.
13. Ahn MS, Catten M, Maas CS. Temporal brow lift using botulinum toxin A. *Plast Reconstr Surg* 2000;105:1129–1135.
14. Brandt FS, Bellman B. Cosmetic use of Botulinum A exotoxin for the aging neck. *Dermatol Surg* 1998;24:1232–1234.
15. Matarasso A, Matarasso SI, Brandt FS, et al. Botulinum A exotoxin for the management of platysmal bands. *Plast Reconstr Surg* 1999;103:645–652.
16. Blitzer A, Binder WJ, Boyd JB, et al. *Management of facial lines and wrinkles.* Philadelphia, PA: Lippincott Williams & Wilkins, 2000.
17. Alam M, Arndt KA, Dover JS. Severe, intractable headache after injection with botulinum toxin A exotoxin: report of 5 cases. *J Am Acad Dermatol* 2002;46:62–65.
18. Klein AW. Complications, adverse reactions, and insights with the use of botulinum toxin. *Dermatol Surg* 2003;29:549–556.
19. Vartanian AJ, Dayan SD. Complications of botulinum toxin A use in facial rejuvenation. *Facial Plast Surg Clin North Am* 2003;11:483–492.
20. Neuber F. Fat transplantation. *Chir Kongr Verhandl Dsch Gesellch Chir* 1890;22:66.
21. Klein A, Elson M. The history of substances for soft tissue augmentation. *Dermatol Surg* 2000;26(12):1096.
22. Parker F. Structure and function of the skin. In: Orkin M, Mailbach HI, Dahl MV, eds. *Dermatology.* San Matteo, CA: Appleton and Lange, 1991:1–14.
23. Wallace DG, McPherson JJ, Ellingsworth LE, et al. Injectable collagen for tissue augmentation. In: Nimni ME, ed. *Collagen,* Vol. 3. Boca Raton, FL: CRC Press, 1988:117–144.
24. Framer FM, Churukium MM. Clinical use of injectable collagen: a three year retrospective review. *Arch Otolaryngol* 1984;110: 93–98.
25. Cooperman LS, Mackinnon V, Bechler G, et al. Injectable collagen: a six year clinical investigation. *Aesthetic Plast Surg* 1985;9:145–151.

26. Hanke CW, Hingley HR, Jolivette DM, et al. Abscess formation and local necrosis after treatment with Zyderm or Zyplast collagen implant. *J Am Acad Dermatol* 1991;25:319–326.

27. Overholt MA, Tschar JA, Font RL. Granulomatous reaction to collagen implant: light and electron microscopic observations. *Cutis* 1993;51:95–98.

28. Haake A, Holbrook K. The structure and development of the skin. In: Freeberg I, Eisen A, Wolff K, et al. eds., *Fitzpatrick's dermatology in general medicine,* 5th ed. New York: McGraw Hill, 1999:89.

29. Beasley KL, Weiss MA, Weiss RA. Hyaluronic acid fillers: a comprehensive review. *Facial Plast Surg* 2009;25:86–94.

30. Duranti F, Salti G, Bovanti B, et al. Injectable hyaluronic acid gel for soft tissue augmentation: a clinical and histologic study. *Dermatol Surg* 1998;24:1317–1325.

31. Lupton JR, Alster TS. Cutaneous hypersensitivity reaction to injectable hyaluronic acid gel. *Dermatol Surg* 2000;26:135–137.

32. Lowe NJ, Maxwell CA, Lowe P, et al. Hyaluronic acid skin fillers: adverse reactions and skin testing. *J Am Acad Dermatol* 2001;45(6):930–933.

33. Friedman PM, Mafong EA, Kauvar AN, et al. Safety data of injectable nonanimal stabilized hyaluronic acid gel for soft tissue augmentation. *Dermatol Surg* 2002;28(6):491–494.

34. Brody HJ. Use of hyaluronidase in the treatment of granulomatous hyaluronic acid reactions or unwanted hyaluronic acid misplacement. *Dermatol Surg* 2005;31(8 Pt 1):893–897.

35. Busso M, Voigts R. An investigation of changes in physical properties of injectable calcium hydroxylapatite in a carrier gel when mixed with lidocaine and with lidocaine/epinephrine. *Dermatol Surg* 2008;34:S16–S23.

36. Coleman KM, Voigts R, DeVore DP, et al. Neocollagenesis after injection of calcium hydoxylapatite composition in a canine model. *Dermatol Surg* 2008;34:S53–S55.

37. Carruthers A, Liebeskind M, Carruthers J, et al. Radiographic and computed tomographic studies of calcium hydroxylapatite for treatment of HIV-associated facial lipoatrophy and correction of nasolabial folds. *Dermatol Surg* 2008;34:S78–S84.

38. Bentkover SH. The biology of facial fillers. *Facial Plast Surg* 2009;25:73–85.

39. Lemperle G, Hazan-Gauthier N, Lemperle M. PMMA microspheres for skin and soft tissue augmentation. Part II: clinical investigations. *Plast Reconstr Surg* 1995;96:627–634.

40. Rudolph CM, Soyer HP, Schuller-Petrovic S, et al. Foreign body granulomas due to injectable aesthetic micro-implants. *Am J Surg Pathol* 1999;23(1):113–117.

41. Webster RC, Fuleihan NS, Gaunt JM, et al. Injectable silicone for small augmentations: twenty year experience in humans. *Am J Cosmet Surg* 1984;1(4):1–10.

42. Orentreich DS, Orentreich N. Injectable fluid silicone. In: Roegnik RK, Roegnik HH, eds. *Dermatologic surgery principles and practice.* New York: Marcel Dekker, 1989:1349–1395.

43. Ellenbogen R, Ellenbogen R, Rubin L. Injectable fluid silicone therapy: human morbidity and mortality. *JAMA* 1975;234:308–309.

44. Ficarra G, Mosqueda-Taylor A, Carlos R. Silicone granuloma of the facial tissues: a report of seven cases. *Oral Surg Oral Med Oral Pathol Oral Radiol Endod* 2002;94(1):65–73.

45. Pearl RM, Laub DR, Kaplan EN. Complications following silicone injections for augmentation of the contours of the face. *Plast Reconstr Surg* 1978;61:888–891.

46. Narins RS, Beer K. Injectable liquid silicone: a review of its' history, immunology, technical considerations, complications and potential. *Plast Reconstr Surg* 2006;118(Suppl 3):77S–84S.

47. Chajchir A, Benzaquen I. Fat grafting injection for soft tissue augmentation. *Plast Reconstr Surg* 1989;84:921–934.

48. Coleman SR. Facial contouring with lipostructure. *Clin Plast Surg* 1997;24(2):347–367.

49. Winslow CP. The management of dermal filler complications. *Facial Plast Surg* 2009;25:124–128.

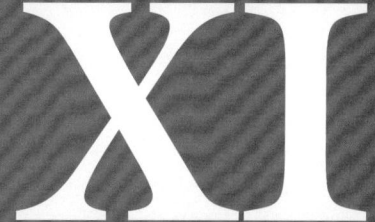

Contemporary Issues in Medical Practice

Shawn D. Newlands   *Karen T. Pitman*

Patient Safety

198

David E. Eibling

"Primum, non nocere" Attributed to Hippocrates (1).

Since the days of Hippocrates, it has generally been assumed that attempts to heal are unpredictable, and those attempts occasionally result in unintentional harm. Injury, and even death, were inevitable for a few unfortunate patients. Health care providers, patients, and the public judged that the natural history of the disease process itself justified these occasional undesired outcomes. When facing imminent surgical or other interventions, patients could only hope that they were protected by their choice of the best doctors and hospitals. Moreover, the statistical odds of themselves or their family members becoming a victim of an iatrogenic injury were small enough to offer some level of comfort. In essence, they relied on hope—hoping it was not "their turn" for something to "go wrong." Physicians likewise were well aware that medical care was imperfect, that diagnoses were sometimes flawed, and that treatment attempts were often poorly conceived, planned, and executed. The occasional medical mistakes were inevitable. Preservation of their own confidence and decision-making ability often relied on the assumption that mistakes were made by other, less able practitioners working in other hospitals and that they were protected by their superior knowledge and skills and superior institution. Many poor outcomes could, (and often were) with minimal effort, be attributed to the patient or their disease process itself.

Of course, not all adverse events that impact patients are due to mistakes. Patients can be harmed by "Acts of God," unforeseen circumstances such as weather or other anomalies that destroy hospitals and infrastructure (tornados, earthquakes, tsunamis, or hurricanes to list just a few from recent years), killing or injuring inpatients along with others in the affected community. Many adverse events, such as infections or falls, long assumed to fall into this "Acts of God" category, are now being shown to be preventable. The growing assumption is that *failing to prevent* potentially

preventable harmful occurrences represents failure and can be interpreted as a mistake. The list of these events continues to increase as investigators demonstrate that interventions can impact the incidence of or harm caused by these occurrences. In recent years, new payment policies in the United States that withhold reimbursement for the treatment of such events add credence to the fact that errors of omission are also mistakes.

Mistakes judged as preventable were interpreted by both society and the medical establishment as indicative of the failings of individual providers who by definition must have been flawed in some way. The assumption that "someone caused this and they have to pay" fed a burgeoning tort claim system whereby the injured patient could seek restitution. The inevitability of human error occurring in the context of ever-increasing complexity and uncertainty led to the flourishing of the medicolegal industry, which grew dramatically in the last half of the 20th century. Accompanying the growth of this industry was wholesale proliferation of armament for the plaintiffs and their legal representation, driven by enormous increases in tort claim awards. Defensive measures were introduced, such as a malpractice insurance industry, often supported by legal mandate, and risk management strategies that sought to protect the health care industry, at the cost of considerable expenditures of resources. As of 2011, efforts to retard the growth of the medical malpractice industry by limiting the amount of financial rewards have been only minimally effective, suggesting that alternative strategies will be required. Shifting the current medical malpractice paradigm to one that improves care, like so many other needed cultural changes, has, by default, been relegated to future generations. The reader is referred to Chapter 199, *Medical Legal Issue*, of this book for a more in-depth discussion of medicolegal implications for otolaryngologic practice.

Contributing to this ongoing impasse is the culture of "name, shame, and blame," an inbred tradition in which most physicians practicing today were trained. The assumption that most mistakes are due to flaws in individual physician performance conveys multiple costs to both the physician and his or her family and colleagues, as well as the organization in which he or she practices. This focus on the individual mandates the identification of the person responsible for the outcome, formal evaluation of his or her performance, and then restriction of his or her practice or enrolling the person in an educational program so that the error does not recur. At times the criminal justice system has been activated, with the result that health care workers who make mistakes are arrested with criminal charges, and even incarceration. Unfortunately, not only does this approach usually fail to identify and rectify the underlying problem, it impairs the objective analysis of human error and assures that the failure will occur again. Examples of misdirected peer review programs are prevalent in 2011 and challenge forward-thinking leaders who are attempting to prevent or mitigate future mistakes. With the exception of a few leaders in patient safety, this paradigm has persisted through the first decade of the current century.

Although these sentiments remain prevalent throughout health care, other industries have long recognized that focusing on individual practitioners is a failed strategy. These industries recognized that human performance is imperfect and highly context dependent, a recognition that drove the adaptation of their corporate structure to this "new" reality. Industries that modified their corporate culture and production systems to adapt to the abilities of their employees, rather than focusing solely on the performance of those employees, excelled in the marketplace due to reduced production costs. Gurus such as Shewforth (2) and Demming (3), initially eschewed by US industries, were embraced by the postwar Japanese, with dramatic results. The effect of this paradigm shift in Japanese industry became evident over the past quarter of a century as automobiles from Japan began to make major inroads into the US automaker's monopoly on the roads and highways of the United States. Medicine was late in accepting the premise that *context* mattered. The recognition that the environment and systems within which human practitioners provided care is a critical factor in outcomes and that it is possible to alter that context through informed system design is only slowly dawning on the industry. As of 2011, medicine was still struggling with the concept that imperfections in complex systems lead to the majority of preventable adverse events, with the focus on error prevention still largely focused on individuals (4,5). Dekker pointed out that this paradigm makes sense to leaders since there are institutional benefits to be had by focusing blame on individuals. Doing so relieves the organization from embarking on often difficult and costly change. *"The judgment that this was human error simply produced too many organizational benefits"* (6). Unfortunately, this strategy simply leads to repeated errors, a lesson learned long ago by other industries. Studying the aviation industry provides insight into the ongoing efforts of the patient safety movement as it attempts to change the entrenched culture of the health care industry (7).

HISTORY OF THE AVIATION SAFETY MOVEMENT

Aviation is generally considered the first industry to position safety as its top priority, a logical choice for the industry since aircraft crashes dramatically impact productivity through loss of not only the aircraft but also often the pilot as well! Following the Second World War (WWII), the United States Air Force (USAF) discovered to their dismay that no amount of pilot training would suffice to prevent crashes if the aircraft could not be safely flown by a human. The advent of jet aviation was met with a rash of accidents due to the increasing mismatch between the capabilities of high-performance aircraft and high-performance pilots. The USAF was instrumental in the development and maturing of the science of *human factors* in order to assess human capabilities during flight and to use this knowledge to inform aircraft design to accommodate to these capabilities. Formal investigation into the limits of human performance drove the development of the science of human factors, a discipline that informs system design to assure that the airplane can be flown by a real human. If the pilot becomes unconscious during a high-G maneuver, it does not matter how well the plane is designed; it will crash and be destroyed along with the pilot. Initial human factors research was directed toward human physiologic capability, such as performance characteristics under high G-forces, or alteration in pressurization and oxygen availability. It became apparent that cognitive resources were also challenged by high-performance flight, and that too little information, too much information, or information provided in a confusing manner would lead to accidents just as well as if the pilot had blacked out. This recognition drove the development of new cockpit information systems, and aviation became the "poster child" for "human-centered design" with reliability and safety as primary goals.

Despite dramatic improvements in aircraft design in the years following WWII, a number of high-visibility aircraft crashes in the 1970s pointed out vividly that even the presence of a highly skilled pilot in the optimally designed cockpit of a technically advanced aircraft could not always avert disaster. The loss of United 193 and Eastern 401 and the improbable crash of two loaded 747s on a fog-shrouded runway in Tenerife in March 1977 (8) were a wake-up call for the industry. Aviation came to the understanding not only that theirs was an imperfect system but that the industry must shoulder the responsibility of improving the system. Inherent in this understanding was the recognition that the established paradigms were untenable and that change was necessary—and the optimism that such change was possible. As a result, multiple innovations were introduced in the 1970s and 1980s, which led to dramatic reductions in the aviation accidents. These include no-fault near-miss reporting, standardized simulator rehearsal, crew resource management (CRM) training (9), and rapid and widespread dissemination of information regarding safety threats (http://www.asrs.arc.nasa.gov. Accessed May, 2011). The most critical change, however, was the fact the industry embraced a "culture of safety" in which all employees are empowered—and expected—to respond immediately and report safety threats (7). Many of these cultural changes are being introduced into health care, but as of 2011, these are best described as "in process." Despite widespread encouragement (10), and although many organizations actively promote the concept of a "safety culture" and survey their employees to assure they are achieving their goals, medicine is still far behind aviation in this regard.

TO ERR IS HUMAN

Medicine was rudely awakened to the extent of the problem of medical error by the publication of the Institute of Medicine report "To Err is Human" published in 1999 (11). This report estimated that somewhere between 44,000 and 98,000 Americans died each year in hospitals as a direct result of medical error. Based on the Harvard Medical Practice study (12) published nearly a decade previously, the figures in the report were initially strongly disputed. It seemed impossible that the same number of deaths occurred each day due to medical errors as would be caused by two 747 crashes *each day*. It has since become apparent that even the 98,000 figure is a gross underestimate of the true magnitude of the number of deaths due to medical error. The numbers are staggering, with the current best estimate is that 1 in 20 Americans will die due to a medical error. Medical mistakes account for the eighth most common cause of death in the United States, more than deaths due to HIV and breast cancer combined! The economic costs are staggering, with a recent estimate that the total societal cost of health care–related adverse events in the United States is now approaching a trillion dollars annually (13)!

Our knowledge of the fundamental science behind medical error is based on the work of psychologists such as James Reason (14) who undertook to determine why humans make mistakes. The research into this area is immense and has recently been recognized by the health care industry as pertinent to an understanding of medical error. Reason classically separates human error into two major types, that of a *mistake*, which is choosing the wrong plan to achieve a specific goal, or a *slip*, which would be defined as failing to execute the plan that one has chosen. Ordering an antibiotic to which the responsible organism is not susceptible might be a mistake, and picking the wrong vial out of the medication drawer might be a slip.

Human error is inevitable as illustrated by the title of the 1999 IOM report "To Err Is Human." Human error is a *by-product* of human attributes, which enable humans to interact with a complex, perceptively rich world. Human error stems from the same cognitive functions that enable the filtering of sensory input, focusing attention on specific goals, pattern recognition, and sequencing of events. Reason quotes Ernest Mach who eloquently stated "accomplishment and error stem from the same source, only the outcome differentiates the two" nearly a century earlier. Other disciplines, particularly those focusing on studying human factors, have adapted these principles through "cognitive engineering" to design strategies whereby the human–technology interface can be improved to reduce the propensity for human error (15).

"PREVENTION" OF HUMAN ERROR

Those who have assimilated the prior paragraphs will quickly recognize that the title of this section is inaccurate. Human error, by its nature, is not preventable. Helmreich (9) pointed out that the goal of error prevention is actually the prevention of injury. He proposed the term "*error troika*" as a fundamental concept useful in designing systems with the goal of injury (or crash) prevention. Errors will happen, but it is possible to design systems to (a) reduce the likelihood of error, (b) "trap" the error before it can progress, or (c) mitigate or prevent the effect of the error once it has occurred. Medication administration strategies often seek to employ all three components of the "troika," with variable success. In a similar vein, the famous "Swiss Cheese" illustration of Reason (14) points out that well-designed systems have multiple layers of protection, or barriers, placed between the error and the "target." These barriers vary in permeability, however, and typically have "holes" that reduce or negate their effectiveness. Whenever the "holes" line up, the effects of the error are experienced by the "target." Keeping this illustration in mind as the reader peruses the examples of safety innovations in this chapter will assist in developing new strategies to protect patients from the unintended actions of well-meaning health care workers.

HISTORY OF THE PATIENT SAFETY MOVEMENT

The seminal article by Lucian Leape published in 1994 (16) was the first to clearly identify medical error as a cause of adverse outcomes in health care. Dr. Leape made a number of pertinent observations, critically by noting that although human error was inevitable, it did not occur randomly. In his paper, he drew heavily on the work of Reason and others, and nearly two decades later, his observations remain critical to our understanding. The concept that error was not random was a particularly crucial observation since it suggests that types and sites of error are *predictable*. Experience in other industries (notably aviation) had demonstrated that prevention of accidents or their sequela was feasible by first investigating accidents that had occurred and using the knowledge gained to inform system redesign. At the time of Leape's report, the Aviation Safety Reporting System (ASRS) (http://www.asrs.arc.nasa.gov) had already been in place for 18 years and had already effected major changes in aviation. Leape pointed out that it was only by studying adverse events in an attempt to identify patterns and discern the causes could future events be prevented or mitigated. Furthermore, Leape emphasized the importance of reporting by frontline staff. Thirty years prior to the publication of "Error in Medicine," Shimmel, chief resident at one of the Yale-New Haven Hospitals, introduced the concept of systematically reporting all adverse events occurring on his inpatient service in an effort to identify and categorize the underlying causes with the ultimate goal of prevention (17).

Anesthesia was the first medical specialty to seek to systematically study medical error. In the late 1970s, faced with mounting public awareness of the risks of anesthesia, the American Society of Anesthesiologists sought to study the problem. The Anesthesia Patient Safety Foundation (APSF) was founded in 1985 and chartered to study anesthesia mishaps and propose interventions, http://www.asahq.org/For-Healthcare-Professionals/Patient-Quality-and-Safety.aspx. The APSF introduced what was at the time a revolutionary approach, the study of "closed claims" in which injured patients or their families had been compensated for an anesthetic adverse event. The story of how a single malpractice insurance company was induced to release this proprietary information (which could have been damaging to its profitability) is one of the intriguing success stories of patient safety and illustrates vividly the effect one or two individuals can make!

The APSF closed claim study (18) revealed that fully one-third of the events that had resulted in a payment to the plaintiff (closed claim) were due to a respiratory cause. This finding prompted the emphasis on the development of new technology (pulse oximetry and capnography) as well as difficult airway algorithms. Astonishingly, within a period of less than 6 years following the report of the APSF and dissemination of its findings, a substantial reduction in the incidence of perioperative respiratory events was reported (19). The success story of the APSF should be viewed as justification to dedicating sufficient resources to identify and study adverse outcomes as the first step in reducing the risk of medical mistakes or the effects of those mistakes.

The National Patient Safety Foundation was established in the 1990s, as a result of a major conference convened in 1996 to address the issues of patient safety (http://www.npsf.org. Accessed May, 2011). This conference brought together members of both the medical community and the human factors communities and was perhaps the first time that the mismatch between the complexity of health care and human capabilities was identified as the fundamental cause of medical error.

Largely unheralded outside of the specialty, it was not until the IOM report in 1999 that the previously unrecognized epidemic of death and injury occurring during medical care reached a level of awareness sufficient to promote action. The IOM report galvanized the nation and prompted the institution of a wide range of investigation and interventions. To quote Robert Wachter (5), "in short, everywhere one looked, one found evidence of major problems with patient safety." The IOM followed with additional reports, new organizations and government agencies (Agency for Healthcare Research and Quality [AHRQ]) were established, and hospitals established patient safety offices to address the issues at the facility level. The Veterans Health Administration (VHA) established the National Center for Patient Safety (NCPS) at Ann Arbor, appointing James Bagian, prior astronaut–physician, as its first director. The NCPS was the first system-wide effort to capture and study adverse events and institutionalized patient safety efforts within the VHA nationwide (http://www.patientsafety.gov. Accessed May, 2011). The state of Pennsylvania established a state level safety agency in 2002 (20) and Congress passed the Patient Safety and Quality Improvement Act in 2005 (available at http://www.govtrack.us/congress/bill.xpd?bill=s109-544. Accessed July, 2011).

Others, such as Peter Pronovost from Johns Hopkins, were unwilling to accept "business as usual" and initiated interventions based on the "basic science" of studying adverse events and near misses. Within a decade, challenges that had been previously assumed to be inevitable and unmanageable, such as hospital-acquired infections such as methicillin-resistant *Staphylococcus aureus* (21) and central line infections (22), were successfully tackled by patient safety investigators. These innovators studied the problems, formulated hypotheses, instituted new practices, and, in these examples, demonstrated remarkable success. It is instructive to note that investigations in patient safety do not follow the classic randomized clinical trial paradigm (RCT) since to do so may be unethical. Rather, most patient safety innovations follow the *"Plan, Do, Study, Act"* paradigm through which innovations are "tested" in actual practice and then studied prior to widespread dissemination and implementation.

The Joint Commission (previously known as the Joint Commission on the Accreditation of Healthcare Organizations) adapted new patient safety goals (JCPSGs) that are updated on a yearly basis and served as criteria for assessing hospital performance in patient safety. Essentially all hospitals in the United States utilize the JCPSGs as a roadmap for improving patient safety in their institutions (http://www.jointcommission.org/assets/1/6/2011_NPSG_Hospital_3_17_11.pdf. Accessed May, 2011). Reviewing these goals is an effective strategy to identify what the organizational targets in patient safety are at any specific time.

Despite these and many other innovations, as of 2011, the epidemic of errors continues to extract an unacceptable toll, both human and financial. In a classic editorial in Health Affairs, "The IOM report: 10 years later" Carolyn Clancy, Director of AHRQ, pointed out that painfully little had occurred, primarily due to an inability to change an intransient culture (23). The rest of this chapter reviews a number of concepts and interventions to guide the otolaryngologist who is beginning his or her "safety journey." The reader will hopefully identify some achievable targets that can be utilized by otolaryngologists, health care teams, and enterprise organizations to reduce the risk of harm to the patients entrusted their care.

SAFETY AND QUALITY

Confusion often exists in defining a perceived boundary between the definitions of *quality* and *safety*. In reality, the boundary is indistinct, although safety can be considered as a prerequisite for quality (5). High-quality care is assumed to be effective care, typically defined by favorable clinical outcomes coupled with cost-effectiveness, usually compliant with established guidelines when such guidelines exist. However, to be high quality, care must, by definition, first be *safe*! Poor quality or ineffective care might be safe, but if the care fails to halt disease progression, one can argue that it is by nature unsafe. A leader in patient safety is reported to have quipped that "*50 years ago healthcare was safe, cheap, … and ineffective, whereas now it is effective, expensive, … and dangerous,*" implying that the complexity required to increase effectiveness of intervention paradoxically increases the risk for injury. Most would assert that the risk is worthwhile. For example, undertreatment of a malignancy to reduce the risk of complications to zero is not desirable since the patient may lose years of valuable life. Regardless of the definition of quality, there are some inherent differences in the strategies employed; quality has the goal of effecting an optimal outcome for the patient, whereas safety seeks to prevent causing harm while doing so.

MEDICAL ERROR AND SYSTEMS SCIENCE

Understanding the causes of medical error requires an in-depth examination of *systems*. Systems consist of people, technology, policies, coordination, and other strategies intended to result in a desired outcome. An aircraft flight occurs due to a closely linked system of the aircraft itself as well as its crew, but also the maintenance and ground personnel and equipment, scheduling, routing, weather, and a plethora of interrelated functions. Systems science has been highly defined in other industries, but only recently has received attention in health care, which by its nature consists of multiple overlapping highly complex systems. Roberson and coauthors emphasized the importance of critically

TABLE 198.1	CHARACTERISTICS OF EFFECTIVE COMPLEX SYSTEMS

Common goal for all system components
Goal-driven system design
Unpredictability expected
Expect and accommodate human error
Feedback loops with short cycle times
Standardization is baseline
Reliant on teams rather than single individuals

From Roberson DW, Kentala E, Healy GB. Quality and safety in a complex world: why systems science matters to otolaryngologists. *Laryngoscope* 2004;114:1810–1814.

examining whole systems when analyzing processes of care and how these processes affect patient outcomes (24). "Systems-based practice" represents one of the six core competencies as defined by the Accreditation Council for Graduate Medical Education and the concepts are familiar to all otolaryngologists who have trained in the past decade. Some of the basic principles of systems are well defined and include the principles enumerated in Table 198.1.

ACCOUNTABILITY AND "JUST CULTURE"

The emphasis on system design as the underlying threat to patient safety shifts the attention from individual performance to system performance. Although this shift is more likely to lead to prevention of adverse events, it has been construed by some to mean that the individual shares less responsibility. This conflict has been addressed at a high level within the aviation industry through the adoption of "*just culture*" (25). A *just culture* recognizes that expert practitioners (i.e., pilots or physicians) typically must accommodate multiple goals, such as keeping on a flight schedule and avoiding stormy weather conditions. In order to perform at high levels, these practitioners must possess some degree of flexibility in order to satisfactorily resolve conflicts and achieve desired outcomes (26). However, within each profession, there exist boundaries within which accomplished practitioners remain. These are often well recognized within the profession, even if not discretely defined by policy or written procedures. Performing outside of these boundaries is not an inadvertent human error but is an intentional act and considered "reckless behavior." In a seminal report published in 2001, David Marx has emphasized that these boundaries must, by nature of their significance, be defined by the profession itself (27). In aviation, an example would be completion of the preflight checklist; examples in surgery include the universal preprocedure pause for "time out" or completion of a postoperative sponge count prior to wound closure. Just as pilots would never consider initiating a flight without completion of the checklist, surgeons would never consider initiating a surgical procedure without first doing a "time out" or closing the wound and leaving the operating room without a reconciled sponge count. In both settings, individuals function within teams that help assure that "forgetting" to do so is extremely unlikely. Refusing to comply with expectations of the profession after being reminded would be considered "outside the norm" and "reckless behavior" and place the practitioner at risk of censure.

Practitioners are also responsible for the systems within which they work. The level of accountability varies by the level of administrative responsibility, but even house staff bear some responsibility and must assume partial "ownership" of the systems in which they work (28). One way in which practitioners can participate in system improvements is by identifying threats to safety, reporting, collecting, collating, and assessing these threats, then develop interventions to reduce them. The challenges are immense, beginning with the task of identification and reporting.

MEASURING PATIENT SAFETY

"Safety shows itself only by the events that do not happen"— Erik Hollnagel

The adage "if you can't measure it, you can't improve it" has been proven correct throughout all of science. Fundamental changes in health care did not begin until pioneer surgeons began assessing their outcomes in an effort to determine whether they were, in fact, effecting positive change for their patients. Over the past several years, a plethora of metrics for quality (although painfully few in otolaryngology) have been introduced, impacting essentially all of health care in the United States (http://www.cms.gov/qualitymeasures. Accessed May 18, 2011). However, few metrics exist to assess patient safety. Attempts to identify differences in outcomes are challenged by the heterogeneous nature of patient selection, institution, treatment and modality, collecting metric, and comorbidity. Nearly 20 years ago, the VHA attempted to measure surgical outcomes to the institution of a risk-adjusted morbidity and mortality (M&M) measure now referred to as Veterans Administration Surgical Quality Improvement Program (VASQIP) (29). An almost identical voluntary program termed National Surgical Quality Improvement Program (NSQIP) (the term originally referred to the VA program well into the first decade of the 21st century) is now managed by the American College of Surgeons. VASQIP and NSQIP measurement systems all involve chart review by trained personnel who attempt to quantify not only outcomes but also comorbidities to assess relative risks. Statistical adjustments are then made utilizing the relative risk to report a "risk-adjusted" outcome in which observed postoperative adverse events are compared with a risk-adjusted "expected" outcome. Although not sufficiently granular to facilitate identification of specific safety threats, use of the data has been demonstrated to drive improvements in quality and safety within the VA (29).

Data entry relies on standardized training of reviewers, who vary nonetheless as they are human. As a result, even with standardized data parameters, variation is introduced into the measurement system. Newer electronic data mining may have the potential to reduce this variability; however, as Pronovost noted in a commentary in 2011 (30), current systems demonstrate substantial variability even when utilized to assess outcomes with an identical patient population. Moreover, although these risk-adjusted measures assume that adverse outcomes are due to suboptimal care or frank medical error (since they assume the risk-adjustment calculations remove patient comorbidities from the result), it is usually impossible to identify the specific events leading to the adverse outcome. For example, a specific episode of postoperative pneumonia might be due to inadequate nursing care with missed opportunity for chest percussion, deep breathing, etc., due to oversedation on the midnight shift, or due to reliance on pain medication technology that was ill suited for the patient for which it was utilized. Or was the occurrence secondary to the primary disease process that the risk-adjusting calculations failed to adequately measure? Quantifying medical error remains an enigma, one that will persist throughout the careers of all currently in practice or in training.

"NEVER EVENTS"

There exists a subset of medical errors that are so egregious, such as amputating the wrong leg, that their identification is straightforward and they are easily identified as errors, even by lay persons. Termed "never events" (as they should "never" occur), these errors, such as retained foreign bodies in surgery, wrong-site surgery, operating on the wrong patient, etc., are unambiguous mistakes. The list of never events, proposed and maintained by the National Quality Forum (http://www.qualityforum.org), currently contains nearly 30 "events." "Never events" are monitored though legally mandated reporting by many states, such as Pennsylvania, which enacted a formal Patient Safety Authority in 2002 (20). An obvious side effect of mandatory reporting is public disclosure, with its attendant institutional public relations challenges. Such mandatory reporting may dramatically impact public opinion, although hospital public relations offices can find comfort in the fact that their competitors are also required to report! However, even in the presence of mandatory reporting, severe adverse events and deaths are often successfully "hidden" from public view, particularly when encountered in a public relations risk–adverse medical environment. The Los Angeles Times reported in November 2010 that 87 hospitals had failed to report a single error in 3 years to the State of California (available at http://articles.latimes.com/2010/nov/27/local/la-me-hospital-errors-20100028. Accessed July 25, 2011). Unfortunately, hiding such information carries with it the risk that if and when the event is discovered the allegation of cover-up (rather than sloppy record keeping) may receive even greater public scrutiny than the error itself.

Implied in the wrong-patient events are patient identification errors, which are considered by many patient safety authorities to be the most common unreported error in health care systems. Some impact of this error can be found in the fact that assuring correct patient identification has been one of the highest priority patient safety goals for the JCPSGs for several years. Although identification errors are common, they only become "never events" when the error results in serious injury to the patient.

Based on the challenges of identifying medical errors (with the exception of "never events"), detection of "surrogate markers" has become the *de facto* strategy utilized to assess patient safety. These include strategies that access electronic health records using data such as bar code medication administration (BCMA) records critical "drug–drug interaction" alert overrides, or rapid switch of prescribed medications. Classen et al. (31) estimated that use of automated triggers will increase the number of detected errors by 10-fold. Although these triggers add sensitivity, they also reduce specificity, so that expert review is often required. An example is identifying patients for whom perioperative antibiotics were not utilized when indicated (part of surgical quality performance measures). The trigger can detect who did and who did not receive perioperative antibiotics but is unable to identify which particular patients require prophylaxis.

ERROR AND NEAR-MISS REPORTING

Voluntary reporting has been consistently demonstrated to be insufficiently sensitive for accurate detection of medical mistakes and adverse events. In a classic study comparing the use of a formal chart review system (the American College of Surgeons National Quality Improvement Program) with standard reporting in M&M conferences, Hutter and colleagues noted that less than one-half of significant complications were reported at the M&M conferences. In a classic quotation, the authors expressed their surprise at their findings: *"we were surprised at our findings as we had always prided ourselves on the veracity of our M&M reporting system"* (32).

Pronovost and Lueford in their recent publication on improving reporting systems made five specific recommendations to improve the current status of reporting (Table 198.2) (20). In the author's opinion, of their recommendations, the most critical, and yet the one least likely to occur, would be the establishment of an independent agency. As noted earlier in this chapter, aviation was able to dramatically improve reporting of near misses by seeking to eliminate the "name, blame, shame" attitudes engendered by most high-performance systems. One critical attribute of the ASRS is that its oversight was assigned to an independent agency within the National Aeronautics and Space Administration (http://www.asrs.arc.nasa.gov.

TABLE 198.2	FIVE RECOMMENDATIONS TO IMPROVE REPORTING SYSTEMS

1. Assure validity and transparency
2. Standardize surveillance systems
3. Trend performance change over time
4. Develop strategies to prioritize measures
5. Create an independent agency

From Pronovost PJ, Lilford R. A road map for improving the performance of performance measures. *Health Aff (Millwood)* 2011;30:569–573.

Accessed July 19, 2011) rather than the licensing agency, the Federal Aviation Administration. It was apparent to those setting up the system that inducing pilots to report their mistakes to FAA would be a doomed strategy since to do so could place the reporter's career in jeopardy.

Studies of medical mistake reporting systems have confirmed that the reporting system itself is often the culprit in reducing the likelihood of reporting by frontline staff (33). Some of the ways in which these systems fail are listed in Table 198.3. One of the more important factors that discourage reporting is the sense of fatalism held by many (most) health care workers: *"why should I bother to report since nothing is going to change?"* Until this assumption is replaced with a "can-do" assumption, it is unlikely that frontline reporting will increase. It can be anticipated that the readers of this chapter will have substantial opportunities to impact this assumption through their interaction with, or even design of, these systems in future years.

As of the second decade of the 21st century, no simple straightforward solution to measuring safety has been identified. The wide range of patient diseases, comorbidities, and treatment algorithms create a complex matrix that defies discrete measurement. As Pronovost and Lueford (30) note, "Let us hope that the efforts in the next decade embrace science instead".

TABLE 198.3	RULES FOR DESIGNING REPORTING SYSTEMS

Improve system usability and reduce inefficiency so that reporting fits easily into workflow

Define purpose of system for potential reporters, and be certain they can access and utilize it within their workplace

Reduce likelihood of adverse consequences by assuring confidentiality

Assure usefulness of reporting by providing feedback and eliminating "black hole" effect

From Holden R, Ben-Tzion K. A review of medical error reporting system design consideration and a proposed cross-level systems research framework. *Hum Factors* 2007;49:257–276.

MEASURING SAFETY IN OTOLARYNGOLOGY

Several investigators have reported on the prevalence of safety issues in otolaryngology. The premier report in this regard was a questionnaire sent to 2,500 otolaryngologists in 2003 with the simple question, "Do you know of a medical error in your practice within the past 6 months?" (34). Four hundred and sixty-six (18%) of surveyed otolaryngologists responded, and of these nearly one-half (210) knew of an error that had occurred. Of these, 78 or 37% had resulted in harm and 9 had led to the death of a patient. Using their findings, the authors estimated that roughly 2,600 patients are injured annually by medical errors in otolaryngology practice in the United States and that these errors lead to 165 deaths. Their estimates were plausible since they were congruent with the order of magnitude of the 1999 IOM report. Based on their findings, the authors proposed a classification system for reporting errors in otolaryngology, which can be summarized as listed on Table 198.4.

Additional studies focusing on specific threats in otolaryngology have addressed a number of threats uniquely encountered within otolaryngology. One of these is *recurrent* angiotensin-converting enzyme inhibitor (ACEI)–induced angioedema. Represcribing an ACEI following a prior episode of ACEI-induced angioedema is an obvious medication error, and despite its improbability, in the review by Roberts and coauthors, had occurred 26 times in a decade in a large academic medical center (35). We revisit this study later in this chapter and review possible strategies to reduce the probability of the event.

Another rare but potentially devastating error is the inadvertent use of concentrated medications. Although the (repeated) inadvertent administration of concentrated heparin to neonates *in lieu* of a lower dose for intravenous flush received the greatest attention (following the accidental overdose of actor Dennis Quaid's twins in 2007), in otolaryngology, the most devastating has been the inadvertent injection of concentrated epinephrine (1:1,000 or 1 mg/mL). The concentrated epinephrine errors are particularly instructive and are discussed in some detail.

In 1995, a 7-year-old boy died after mislabeled concentrated topical epinephrine was inadvertently injected during routine otologic surgery (http://www.ismp.org/newsletters/acutecare/artoc;es/19961204.asp. Accessed July 19, 2011). The sad case received widespread attention throughout North America, and its effect on the providers was featured in the instructional video "Beyond Blame" (available for purchase at http://www.onlinestore.ismp.org). The Joint Commission as well as the Institute for Safe Medication Practices (ISMP) have made specific recommendations intended to reduce the likelihood of similar events occurring, including expressing the concentration of critical medications as milligrams (mg) per milliliter or cubic centimeter (cc) rather than as a ratio (i.e., 1:1,000 epinephrine should be labeled as 1 mg per 1 mL) and requiring clear labeling of all medications, particularly on the "back table" in the operating room (OR) suite. Shah et al. (36) addressed the incidence of erroneous injection of concentrated epinephrine (1 mg per 1 mL rather than the intended 1:100,000 or 1mg per 100 mL concentration) in a survey of otolaryngologists reported in 2008. Of the 126 otolaryngologists who responded the survey, 34, or more than a quarter, had either personally experienced or heard of an epinephrine error *within the past year*, including five deaths. Sixteen, or one in eight, had personally experienced an epinephrine mistake within the past year, and 48, or more than a third, had experienced such an error in their careers (averaging nearly 20 years). Based on their experiences, many otolaryngologists introduced strategies, such as adding a few drops of methylene blue to concentrated topical epinephrine to alert the surgical team. Shah et al. make specific recommendations to prevent or reduce the occurrence (Table 198.5), although anecdotal experience suggests that these errors are still occurring in 2011.

TABLE 198.4	CLASSIFICATION OF ERRORS IN OTOLARYNGOLOGY

History and physical, diagnosis
Testing
Surgical planning or execution (including wrong-site surgery)
Post-op care and medical management
Administrative
Communication

Modified from Shah RK, Kentala E, Healy GB, et al. Classification and consequence of errors in otolaryngology. *Laryngoscope* 2004;114:1322–1335.

TABLE 198.5	RECOMMENDATIONS TO REDUCE LIKELIHOOD OF INADVERTENT INJECTION OF CONCENTRATED (1 mg/mL) EPINEPHRINE

Stock single concentration of epinephrine
Do not stock 1 mg/cc epinephrine in OR suite
Label as dilution by weight rather than ratio, that is, 1 mg/mL rather than 1:1,000
Label all solutions in the surgical field
Draw medications directly from manufacturer's vial directly prior to use
Double-check all solutions with other team members visually and verbally
Review all solutions when changing OR team members
Consider standardization of solution markings

From Shah RK, Hoy E, Roberson DW, et al. Errors with concentrated epinephrine in otolaryngology. *Laryngoscope* 2008;118:1928–1930.

MEDICATION ERRORS

Errors in the administration of concentrated epinephrine or heparin, or ACEIs, are only the tip of the enormous problem of medication error. The pervasiveness of medication errors and the associated costs are staggering. The average hospitalized patient can expect to experience one medication error *each day* they are hospitalized, and the estimated cost of managing medication errors in the elderly is estimated to cost Medicare more than a billion dollars per year. The Institute of Medicine released a report in 2006 as part of the Quality Chasm Series that addressed the extent of the problem and outlined strategies useful for prevention (37). Rosenwasser et al. surveyed otolaryngology residents and attending surgeons operating in a single institution for a 2-month period in 2008 to seek to determine the incidence of perioperative medication errors. Twenty errors were reported occurring in association with a total of 589 surgical procedures. They noted a wide range of error types in their sample, with approximately one-half involving antimicrobials. The authors noted that the fast pace of care seemed to facilitate the mistakes. They made a number of recommendations, many of which relate to information access (38).

AGENCIES AND ORGANIZATIONS

An enormous and ever-growing number of public and private organizations are studying medical mistakes and seeking solutions to the challenge they present. Several organizations have assumed leadership positions in recommending specific interventions. These include the National Quality Forum, the National Safety Foundation, The VA NCPS, as well as AHRQ. The list grows dramatically, and an otolaryngologist could devote her entire waking hours to searching the Internet for information and still access only a small percentage of available information. Some of the sources the author has found useful are listed on Table 198.6.

RESPONDING TO MEDICAL ERROR

Adverse events, many of which are due to medical mistakes, will inevitably occur. Acceptance of this truism leads to the realization that all health care workers, including otolaryngologists, will all experience medical error. It is unlikely that anyone reading this chapter has not encountered medical error in their previous experiences. Poignantly, some have, or will, also experience error from the perspective of the injured patient or family member. Failure to address medical error, regardless of where or how it occurs, or is likely to occur, is unacceptable. Adverse events, in particular those due to error, require a response. Responses may be either productive or counterproductive—and unfortunately the latter often prevails (39). Many in the patient safety arena have addressed the counterproductive responses that are still common in the health care system. The

TABLE 198.6	USEFUL WEB SITES

1. National Patient Safety Foundation. http://www.npsf.org
2. VA National Center for Patient Safety. http://www.patient-safety.gov
3. Institute for Healthcare Improvement. http://www.ihi.org/ihi
4. AHRQ M&M on the web. http://www.webmm.ahrq.gov
5. AHRQ Safety Culture Toolkits. http://www.ahrq.gov/qual/patientsafetyculture/
6. University of Chicago Cognitive Technologies Laboratory. http://www.Ctlab.org
7. Government Usability Web site. http://www.usability.gov
8. Joint Commission National Patient Safety Goals. http://www.jointcommission.org/assets/1/6/2011_NPSG_Hospital_3_17_11.pdf
9. IHI 5 Million Lives Campaign. http://www.ihi.org/IHI/Programs/Campaign/Campaign.htm?Tabid=1ng5.asp
10. WHO Safe Surgery Checklist. http://www.who.int/patient-safety/safesurgery/ss_checklist/en/index.html
11. Pronovost Central Line checklist. http://www.ihi.org/IHI/Programs/Campaign/CentralLineInfection.htm
12. Institute for Safe Medication Practices (ISMP). http://www.ismp.org
13. Aviation Safety Reporting System. http://www.asrs.arc.nasa.gov
14. National Quality Forum (NQF) http://www.qualityforum.org
15. Sorry Works! (disclosure and apology). http://www.sorryworks.net
16. Pennsylvania Patient Safety Authority. http://patientsafetyauthority.org
17. CMS Quality Measures. http://www.cms.gov/qualitymeasures
18. Human Factors and Ergonomics Society. http://www.HFES.org
19. FDA medical device regulations. http://www.fda.gov/MedicalDevices/DeviceRegulationsandGuidance/default.htm

reader is referred to the story of Eric Cropp, an inpatient pharmacist from a children's hospital, who was convicted of manslaughter and sentenced to jail for a medical mistake made by a technician he was supervising (story and commentary available at http://www.ismp.org/Newsletters/acutecare/articles/20091203.asp. Accessed July 22, 2011).

ROOT CAUSE ANALYSIS

Examining errors is the critical first step in effecting substantive changes in health care system functions that threaten safety. A standard technique is to perform a detailed analysis, often termed *"root cause analysis"* or RCA. The term is a misnomer since there is rarely only one cause, nevertheless, when done well, the exercise can inform leadership regarding potential interventions. When done poorly, it gives the illusion of effectiveness without altering risk for future patients. All physicians should be familiar with the strategy, since they will be inevitably involved at some time in their career. The Veterans Administration NCPS has been a leader in this regard (40) and has prepared a number of tools that are available on their Web site (http://www.patientsafety.gov.

TABLE 198.7	ROOT CAUSE ANALYSIS (RCA)

RCA Goals

1. What happened?
2. Why did it happen?
3. What can be done to prevent it from happening again?

RCA Strategies

What?

1. Interview frontline staff
2. Assemble chronology of event, attempting to avoid hindsight bias
3. Outline events and chronology on flow diagram

Why?

4. Consider causation
    a. Information systems
    b. Architecture
    c. Policies or procedures
    d. Equipment
    e. Environment
    f. In-place safety mechanisms
5. Rules of causation
    a. Clear cause–effect
    b. Specific descriptors
    c. Identify preceding cause, not human error
    d. Identify cause of policy/procedure violation
    e. Failure to act only causal if preexisting duty to act

How to prevent?

6. Actions may be strong or weak
    a. Strong actions: architectural, equipment design, forcing functions, interlocks
    b. Weaker actions: double checks, training, new policies
    c. Intermediate actions: workload modification, read-back, documentation, redundancy

From National center for patient safety. http://www.patientsafety.gov.

Accessed July 22, 2011). Some of the key components of an RCA are outlined in Table 198.7. Other resources include the "How to" guide by Sidney Dekker (41), which should be read by all who investigate medical errors. Others have addressed one of the biggest challenges, that is, of so-called "hindsight bias," which must be factored into conclusions reached by all who address human error (42).

OTOLARYNGOLOGIST RESPONSES TO MEDICAL ERROR

In 2006, Landers et al. reported the responses of otolaryngologists from the sample reported earlier by Shah et al. (34). They noted that most otolaryngologists had responded in some manner, and much of the reported data were offered voluntarily by the respondents. One-half had intervened to ameliorate the effect of the error on the patient, in approximately a third the event had resulted in a change in department or hospital practices, and a few (7%) had altered their own individual practice style. Ten percent noted that they had experienced guilt with an associated emotional response, and approximately the same percentage had disclosed the error to the patient (43).

THE SECOND VICTIM, DISCLOSURE, AND APOLOGY

As Lander and others (44,45) have noted, medical error impacts more than the patient and his family. In addition to the obvious medicolegal implications, physicians in particular may be emotionally devastated by medical errors they commit to the point they may become impaired by their response to the error with sleep loss, inability to focus, and secondary effects on their families and coworkers. Wu (46) has famously identified this paradox as the "second victim" and notes that the physicians and other health care workers who commit the error also need assistance in order to return to optimal levels of performance. Wu makes specific recommendations for strategies whereby one can assist coworkers faced with the emotional trauma of committing a medical error.

It is axiomatic that focusing on individual performance, attempting to cover up mistakes, and an institutional priority of protecting the health care team or institution by pulling down a veil of secrecy fails. Not only does this strategy fail to resolve the system design issues that led to the event in the first place, it will most likely exacerbate the negative effects of the error itself. Data exist to suggest that tort claims are often initiated by injured patients and families when they perceive dishonesty or cover-up on the part of the physician, team, or institution. The claim may be initiated "to find out what really happened." When evidence of an error is discovered, the assumption is often that the "doctor must be guilty since (he) tried to cover it up." A considerable body of knowledge exists that supports the benefit of early, honest disclosure to all parties (with the notable exception of tort lawyers). Honest disclosure should be considered integral to ongoing medical care of the patient, as such disclosure will help guide decision-making (47). The effect of disclosure on reducing the risk of tort claims has been well demonstrated, and a number of states have (as of 2011) introduced legislation that offers some degree of protection to health care workers and institutions that disclose errors. The VA has been a leader in this regard, and substantial resources are available online, with the Massachusetts Coalition guideline "When things go wrong: responding to adverse events" particularly useful (available at http://www.macoalition.org/documents/RespondingtoAdverseEvents.pdf). It has been noted that patients expect, and benefit from, an authentic and heartfelt apology as well as full disclosure of the facts. Although difficult to do since doing so is counter to the usual cultural traditions, apology should be considered integral to any response to medical error. Not only does physician acceptance of responsibility and apology assist the patient in "moving past" the error, but it also empowers the physician to engage in actions to improve systems to reduce the likelihood of recurrence of the event. Excellent texts are available to assist the physician faced with the need to disclose (48), and the author has found rehearsal to be valuable in preparation.

SPECIFIC SAFETY INTERVENTIONS

The list of specific patient safety interventions that have been introduced is lengthy and growing at an exponential rate. By the time this chapter has reached publication, much of it will undoubtedly be out-of-date. The following section is not intended to be comprehensive but should be viewed as an overview. The reader is encouraged to seek additional information from the list of Internet sources in Table 198.6.

MEDICAL DEVICE SAFETY

The dramatic increase in the number and complexity of medical devices has added substantial increased risk of medical errors. Although some of these are due to failed automation or function on the part of the equipment itself (particularly noteworthy are the deaths due to programming mistakes in the Therac-25 linear accelerator), most device-related errors occur at the human–device interface. Essentially, instruments that were designed to assisting those seeking to cure may paradoxically occasionally facilitate errors by those same individuals. Among the early investigations into this paradox were the studies by Cook et al. into infusion pumps and other medical devices extending back to the early 1990s (http://www.ctlab.org. Publications accessed July 22, 2011). In the intervening years, the Food and Drug Administration has taken an active role in oversight of devices and recently a greater emphasis on the human–machine interface (http://www.fda.gov/MedicalDevices/DeviceRegulationsandGuidance/default.htm. Accessed July 22, 2011).

ELECTRONIC MEDIAL RECORDS, COMPUTERIZED PHYSICIAN ORDER ENTRY (CPOE), AND BAR CODE MEDICATION ADMINISTRATION

The value of electronic medial record (EMR) systems and particularly CPOE in preventing some types of medical error is obvious and was identified as a critical component of the roadmap for change in essentially all early publications on the topic of patient safety (49,50). As of 2011, there can be no doubt that EMR systems will be universal by the end of the decade. Unfortunately, despite initial promise and high expectations, these systems have also been found to promote new types of error (51–55). Similar to the observations in other medical devices, most threats arise not from the function of the system, but rather are due to insufficient attention paid to the human–system interaction characteristics of the design. Systems that work well in laboratory settings often fail when used in high-stress,

high-stakes settings common in hospitals (55). The opportunity for safety-driven improvement is obvious, and it is the opinion of many that this improvement must be based on formal investigations into cognitive work in complex environments.

One strategy is to study work-arounds, a strategy utilized by Koppel et al. (56) in their study of BCMA implementation published in 2008. Like many other novel technologic advances, postimplementation examination of the technology is frequently associated with surprises. In a classic cognitive engineering text, Woods and Hollnagel (15) emphasize the need to assure that technology is designed to be a team player, with characteristics similar to those of effective human team players, such as transparency and predictability.

COMPUTERIZED DECISION SUPPORT

Decision support for the practitioner is widely considered to be the most valuable potential benefit of EMR systems (57). Human memory is limited, and the design of systems to compensate for human limitations is a critical component of human performance. Don Norman famously quipped that *"the power of the unaided mind is overrated…. (its) real powers come from devising external aids that enhance its cognitive abilities"* (58). The need to design these systems in a way that matches human performance is challenging—and to date most systems fall short of the promise (59,60). The promise is perhaps best illustrated by the title of the definitive text by Robert Greenes *"…the road ahead"* (61). Most EMR systems in use today have some level of decision support integrated into the CPOE component, although none are error-free. The most common form is through view alerts, in which a trigger "pops up" when a potentially unsafe medication (such as ordering an ACEI for a patient with known prior ACEI-related angioedema) is ordered (60). Unfortunately, most systems are "tuned" to eliminate all risk for the institution or EMR vendor, resulting in a plethora of view alerts, most of which are disregarded. Recent studies demonstrate that 90% of view alerts, including a substantial number of critical alerts, are routinely disregarded by physicians (62). It is obvious that much more needs to be done.

SIMULATION IN TRAINING AND ASSESSMENT

Simulation has been an integral component of aviation since WWII. Faced with the need to train thousands of pilots rapidly, the US Army Air Corps realized early that they would quickly run out of airplanes—and pilots—if they did not identify alternative training strategies. One of these was the development of the Link Trainer in which the novice pilot could develop the motor skills that would later function instinctively. The author recently encountered a commercial airline pilot who related the following story confirming the value of simulation training:

"Two weeks ago I lost an engine on take-off. Although the aircraft will fly if it has reached adequate speed for lift-off, there are several procedures which the pilot must do quickly to assure it continues to fly. Losing an engine on take-off is a rare event, and one which most pilots never experience throughout their entire career. However, we practice it—and are tested on it—in every routine training session in the simulator. Two weeks ago was my turn to be tested, this time with a full airplane.

Just as we left the ground I heard the sound, saw the data, and immediately knew what had happened. I and my co-pilot quickly did the correct procedures, just as we had practiced over and over, and the plane responded just as in the simulator. After several minutes when the situation was stable I keyed the intercom to tell the passengers that we had lost an engine and were circling in order to dump fuel (an airplane is too heavy to land with full fuel tanks). As I keyed off the intercom after I had informed them it struck me. My voice wasn't shaking. It was just as I had done in the simulator. Throughout the entire event I had calmly done the correct procedures in the correct order. Our training in the simulator may well have prevented a catastrophe."

Simulation in aviation is now utilized not only for training, and for rehearsal of rare events, but also for certification. In a similar manner, simulation training is becoming ever more utilized as a safety intervention in training health care workers. Many surgical skills such as otologic procedures have been taught in the laboratory for many years, and with the introduction of new simulator technology, it seems inevitable that much learning now done in the OR will occur instead in the simulator laboratory (63,64). In some specialties, "high-stakes" simulation testing is utilized for certification, and there are early investigations into its use in otolaryngology (65). It can be assumed that simulation of all types will represent an ever-increasing role in training and assessment in future years.

PHYSICIAN FATIGUE AND WORK HOURS

The expectation that physicians must work long hours in their training in order to develop the knowledge, skills, and attitudes necessary to provide safe and effective patient care was standard in the United States until early in the 21st century. The death of Libby Zion in 1984 is widely assumed to represent the "beginning of the end" for unlimited work hours for residents. Over the intervening quarter of a century, multiple changes in work regulations have been introduced, many introduced following the 2008 IOM report (available at http://www.IOM.edu/reports/2008/Resident-Duty-Hours-enhancing-sleep-supervision-and-safety.aspx. Accessed July 22, 2011), which reviewed the evidence for fatigue as a patient (and resident) safety issue and made multiple recommendations. The issue is still in flux in 2011 and is likely to be so through the entire life expectancy of this edition. Sexton surveyed surgeons and pilots and noted that although pilots were well aware of the effects of fatigue on their performance, physicians were more likely to believe that

fatigue did not affect their performance (66). One factor limiting the benefit of more rested physicians has been the requirement for more handoffs. The requirement for more structured handoffs (67) is currently generating a number of innovations, of which none have yet been demonstrated to be superior.

CHECKLISTS

Checklists have been part of aviation and other high-stakes industries for years but only recently have become standard in health care. Checklists derive from an understanding of the cognitive limitations of humans—that is, humans have limited memory resources, and these resources degrade even more in periods of stress. Peter Pronovost is well recognized for his work in promoting the use of checklists and has been featured in the lay press for his actions in this regard. His seminal paper in 2006 demonstrating dramatic reductions in the incidence of central line infections after introduction of a simple checklist is viewed as a landmark innovation for patient safety (68). The use of checklists in the OR to assure compliance with Surgical Care Improvement Project (SCIP) standards is now standard in many facilities to assure that perioperative antibiotic and deep venous thrombosis prophylaxis, as well as other interventions, are not inadvertently forgotten. It can be assumed that checklists will become more common in future years.

CREW RESOURCE MANAGEMENT AND MEDICAL TEAMS

Following several high-visibility accidents in the 1970s the aviation industry came to the realization that planes were crashing due to faulty teams rather than faulty aircraft. From this arose the concept of training teams to work as teams, utilizing all the human resources as well as the technologic resources, with set rules and procedures (9). This training was initially termed "cockpit resource management" and later expanded to include the entire crew, hence the term "crew resource management" or CRM. Since its introduction in the late 1970s and early 1980s, there have been few accidents that have occurred due to failure of the cockpit crew to work together. In the intervening period, there has been a substantial effort to introduce CRM into the medical arena, often specifically termed "medical team training." The range of activities and procedures that have been spawned by this paradigm shift has been dramatic, and includes a number of strategies, such as the handoff issue above, with which all physicians are now familiar. The underlying principle is that all members of a team have a stake in team integrity and performance and share the responsibility of the outcomes of its actions. Communication is key to team function, and not only must team members speak up, but effective teams also respond to comments, observations, and recommendations. Effective teams flatten, (but do not eliminate) the hierarchy, by empowering anyone on the team to speak up if necessary. In a manner similar to aviation, standard communication protocols are established, such as the SBAR (situation, background, assessment, recommendation) format for handoffs. "Time out," read-back, CUS words ("I am Concerned," "I am Uncomfortable," "Stop and Step back"), and pre- and post-op briefings are extensions of the concept of teams.

A fundamental requirement of teams is the so-called "basic compact," in which each team member commits to support the ongoing integrity of the team. Teams facilitate coordination among their members. Team members are inter-predicable in that actions of members are predictable by others. Members bear a responsibility to correct faulty knowledge and to be sensitive to factors that degrade the compact. A study of team member perceptions by Makary et al. suggested that considerable disparity exists among team members' opinions of team functioning. Perhaps not surprisingly, surgeons consistently rated team effectiveness at a higher level than either anesthesiologists or nurses (69).

The VA embarked on a formal team training program that sought to train OR teams in all VA hospitals and determine the outcomes of the training. Comparing the VASQIP risk-adjusted mortality in the 74 institutions suggested a dose–response relationship (70). Although it is feasible that the decrease was due to other, possibly unrelated factors, nonetheless the study lends credence to the value of formal team training.

CONCLUSIONS

Patient safety remains a fundamental threat to all who either receive or administer health care. Despite multiple innovations and investment of countless resources, the challenges continue. The otolaryngologist must not become discouraged by the lack of progress but rather must participate in efforts to improve safety for all who are at risk.

HIGHLIGHTS

- Adverse effects of medical care are common, and the personal and fiscal costs impact patients and their families, health care workers, and society. Many adverse effects are due to medical errors, which are estimated to cause the deaths of one in twenty Americans.
- An understanding of human performance and the causes of human error informs us regarding the causes of medical error. Health care workers strive to provide optimal care and do not knowingly put their patients at risk. The roots of most medical errors are due to flawed systems, not flawed individuals; hence fixing systems is a more effective strategy than "fixing" individuals.

- The ultimate goal of patient safety is to protect patients. Since human error cannot be eliminated, strategies to protect the patient from the effects of error are more effective than trying to prevent error. Defenses vary in permeability. Some are more protective than others. "Forcing functions" are more effective strategies than advising health care workers to "be careful."
- Study of the aviation industry can suggest strategies to improve safety within the health care industry, particularly no-fault reporting, simulation and team training, and rapid dissemination of lessons learned.
- Reporting, collating, and studying adverse events and near misses can inform system design to reduce the likelihood of patient injury due to human error.
- Health care workers are not relieved of personal responsibility for patient safety. A just culture seeks to define the balance between system responsibility and individual responsibility.
- Human cognitive performance is affected by fatigue, distraction, and stress. "Time out" and checklists are strategies to compensate for imperfect human performance.
- Most health care today is delivered by teams, not individuals. High-performance teams are safer than high-performance individuals. Teams vary in their effectiveness, and team function is measurable.
- Responding to errors requires attention to the needs of both the patient and health care worker. Honest disclosure and apology are effective in maintaining a healthy ongoing relationship that is healing for both patient and physician.
- Root cause analysis and other tools can be useful in dissecting the causes of adverse events, identifying the causes of error, and informing system design to reduce recurrence of such events.

REFERENCES

1. Smith CM. Origin and uses of primum non nocere—above all, do no harm! *J Clin Pharmacol* 2005;45:371–377. Actual derivation of term unknown. Attributed to Hippocrates Corpus Epidemics Bk. I, Sect. 11, Trans. Adams, but also attributed to Galen.
2. Berwick DM. Controlling variation in health care: a consultation from Walter Shewhart. *Med Care* 1991;29(12):1212–1225.
3. Deming WE. *Out of crisis*. Boston, MA: MIT Press, 1986. Available at http://www.deming.org. Accessed May, 2011.
4. Cook R, Woods D, Miller C. A tale of two stories: contrasting views of patient safety. *Workshop on assembling the scientific basis for progress on patient safety*, 1998. Chicago, IL: National Patient Safety Foundation, 1998. Available at: http://www.npsf.org/rc/tts/front.html. Accessed May, 2011.
5. Wachter RM. *Understanding Patient Safety*. New York: McGraw Hill, 2008.
6. Dekker S. *Patient safety: a human factors approach*. London, UK: CRC Press, 2011.

7. Nance J. *Why hospitals should fly—the ultimate flight plan to patient safety and quality care*. Bozeman, MT: Second River Healthcare Press, 2010.

8. Secretary of Civil Aviation, Spain. Report on Tenerife Crash 1978. Available at http://www.panamair.org/OLDSITE/Accidents/sectererife.htm. Accessed July 20, 2011.

9. Helmreich RL, Merrit AC, Wilhelm JA. The evolution of crew resource management in commercial aviation. *Int J Aviat Psychol* 1997;9:19–32. Available at http://www.mercadodaaviacao.com.br/arquivos/17_04_2010_12_39_57_crm_evolution_-_faa.pdf. Accessed May, 2011.

10. Joint Commission. Leadership committed to safety. Joint Commission Sentinel Event Alert 43. Available at http://www.jointcommission.org/assets/1/18/SEA_43.pdf. Accessed July 20, 2011.

11. Kohn L, Corrigan JM, Donaldson M. *To err is human: building a safer health system*. Washington, DC: National Academy Press, 1999.

12. Brennan T, Leape L, Laird N, et al. Harvard Medical Practice Study I. Incidence of adverse events and negligence in hospitalized patients: results of the Harvard Medical Practice Study I. *N Engl J Med* 1991;324:370–376.

13. Goodman JC, Villarreal P, Jones B. The social cost of adverse medical events, and what we can do about it. *Health Aff (Millwood)* 2011;30:590–595.

14. Reason J. *Human error*. Cambridge, UK: Cambridge University Press, 1990.

15. Woods D, Hollnagel E. *Joint cognitive systems: patterns in cognitive systems engineering*. Boca Raton, FL: Taylor & Francis, 2006.

16. Leape LL. Error in medicine. *JAMA* 1994;272:1851–1857.

17. Schimmel E. The hazards of hospitalization. *Ann Intern Med* 1964;60:1851–1857.

18. Caplan R, Posner K, Ward R, et al. Adverse respiratory events in anesthesia: a closed claims analysis. *Anesthesiology* 1990;72:828–833.

19. Keenan R, Boyan C. Decreasing frequency of anesthetic cardiac arrest. *J Clin Anesth* 1991;3:354–357.

20. Pennsylvania Patient Safety Authority MCARE ACT 13. Available at http://patientsafetyauthority.org/PatientSafetyAuthority?Governance?Documents/act13.pdf. Accessed July 20, 2011.

21. Jain R, Kralovic SM, Evans ME, et al. Veterans affairs initiative to prevent methicillin-resistant *Staphylococcus aureus* infections. *N Engl J Med* 2011;364:1419–1430.

22. Pronovost P, Needham D, Berenholtz S, et al. An intervention to reduce catheter-related bloodstream infections in the ICU. *N Engl J Med* 2006;355:2725–2732.

23. Clancy C. Ten years after to err is human. *Am J Med Qual* 2009;24:525–528.

24. Roberson DW, Kentala E, Healy GB. Quality and safety in a complex world: why systems science matters to otolaryngologists. *Laryngoscope* 2004;114:1810–1814.

25. Global Aviation Information Network Working Group E. *A roadmap to a just culture: enhancing the safety environment* 2004. Available at http://flightsafety.org/files/just_culture.pdf.

26. Dekker S. *Just Culture: balancing safety and accountability*. Aldershot, UK: Ashgate, 2007.

27. Marx D. *Patient safety and the "just culture": a primer for health care executives*. Columbia University, 2001. Available at http://www.mers-tm.org/support/Marx_Primer.pdf.

28. Padmore JS, Jaeger J, Riesenberg LA, et al. "Renters" or "owners"? Residents' perceptions and behaviors regarding error reduction in teaching hospitals: a literature review. *Acad Med* 2009;84:1765–1774.

29. Rowell KS, Turrentine FE, Hutter MM, et al. Use of a national surgical quality improvement data as a catalyst for quality improvement. *J Am Coll Surg* 2007;204:1293–1300.

30. Pronovost PJ, Lilford R. A road map for improving the performance of performance measures. *Health Aff (Millwood)* 2011;30:569–573.

31. Classen DC, Resar R, Griffin F, et al. "Global trigger tool" shows that adverse events in hospitals may be ten times greater than previously measured. *Health Aff (Millwood)* 2011;30:581–589.

32. Hutter MM, et al. Identification of surgical complications of surgical complications and deaths: an assessment of the traditional surgical morbidity and mortality conference compared with the American College of Surgeons-National Surgical Quality Improvement Program. *J Am Coll Surg* 2006;203:618–624.

33. Holden R, Ben-Tzion K. A review of medical error reporting system design consideration and a proposed cross-level systems research framework. *Hum Factors* 2007;49:257–276.

34. Shah RK, Kentala E, Healy GB, et al. Classification and consequence of errors in otolaryngology. *Laryngoscope* 2004;114:1322–1335.

35. Roberts DS, Mahoney EJ, Hutchinson CT, et al. Analysis of recurrent ACE inhibitor–induced angioedema. *Laryngoscope* 2008;118:2115–2120.

36. Shah RK, Hoy E, Roberson DW, et al. Errors with concentrated epinephrine in otolaryngology. *Laryngoscope* 2008;118:1928–1930.

37. Aspden P, Wolcott A, Bootman L, et al. *Preventing medication errors*. Washington, DC: National Academy Press, 2006.

38. Rosenwasser R, Winterstein AG, Rosenberg AF, et al. Perioperative medication errors in otolaryngology. *Laryngoscope* 2010;120:1214–1219.

39. Cook R, Woods D, Miller C. A tale of two stories: contrasting views of patient safety. *Workshop on assembling the scientific basis for progress on patient safety* 1998. Chicago, IL: National Patient Safety Foundation, 1998. Available at http://www.npsf.org/rc/tts/front.html. Accessed May, 2011.

40. Bajian JP, Gosbee JW, Lee CZ, et al. The veterans affairs root cause analysis system in action. *Jt Comm J Qual Improv* 2002;28:531–545.

41. Dekker S. *Field guide to medical error investigation*. Aldershot, UK: Ashgate, 2002.

42. Woods D, Dekker S. *Behind human error*, 2nd ed. Farnham, Surrey England: Ashgate, 2010.

43. Lander LI, Connor JA, Shah RK, et al. Otolaryngologists' responses to errors and adverse events. *Laryngoscope* 2006;116:114–1120.

44. Delbanco T, Bell SK. Guilty, afraid, and alone—struggling with medical error. *N Engl J Med* 2007;357:1682–1683.

45. Wears R, Wu AW. Dealing with failure: the aftermath of errors and adverse events. *Ann Emerg Med* 2002;39(3):344–346.

46. Wu AW. Medical error: the second victim. The doctor who makes the mistake needs help too. *BMJ* 2000;320:726–727.

47. Gallagher TH, Studdert D, Levinson W. Disclosing harmful medical errors to patients. *N Engl J Med* 2007;356:2713–2719.

48. Woods MS, Star JI. *Healing words: the power of apology in medicine*. Chicago, IL: Doctors in Touch, 2004.

49. Bates D, Gawande AA. Patient safety: improving safety with information technology. *N Engl J Med* 2003;348(25):2526–2534.

50. Bates D, Kaushal R. Information technology and medication safety: what is the benefit? (Safer prescribing). *BMJ* 2002;11:261–265.

51. Embi PJ, Yackel TR, Logan JR, et al. Impacts of computerized physician documentation in a teaching hospital: perceptions of faculty and resident physicians. *J Am Med Inform Assoc* 2004;11:300–309.

52. Weiner J, Kfuri T, Chan K, et al. E-Iatrogenesis: an unintended consequence of CPOE and other HIT. *J Am Med Inform Assoc* 2007;14:387–388.

53. Ash J, Berg M, Coiera E. Some unintended consequences of information technology in health care: the nature of patient care information system-related error. *J Am Med Inform Assoc* 2004;11:104–112.

54. Koppel R, Metlay JP, Cohen A, et al. Role of computerized physician order entry systems in facilitating medication errors. *JAMA* 2005;293(10):1197–1203.

55. Han Y, Carcillo J, Venkataraman S, et al. Unexpected increased mortality after implementation of a commercially sold computerized physician order entry system. *Pediatrics* 2005;116(6):1506–1512.

56. Koppel R, Wetterneck T, Telles JL, et al. Work-arounds to barcode medication systems: their occurrences, causes, and threats to patient safety. *J Am Med Inform Assoc* 2008;15:408–409.

57. Teich JM, Osheroff JA, Pifer EA, et al. Clinical decision support in electronic prescribing: recommendations and an action plan. Report of the joint clinical decision support workgroup. *J Am Med Inform Assoc* 2005;12(4):365–376.

58. Norman DA. *Things that make us smart.* Cambridge, MA: Perseus, 1993.
59. Bates D, Kuperman G, Gandhi T, et al. Ten commandments for effective decision support: making the promise of evidence-based medicine a reality. *J Am Med Inform Assoc* 2003;10:523–530.
60. Eibling D. Things that make us smart: why the design of clinical decision support systems is so critical. *Laryngoscope* 2008;118:2121–2124.
61. Greenes RA. *Clinical decision support: the road ahead.* Burlington, MA: Academic Press, Elsevier, 2007.
62. Isaac T, Weissman JS, Davis RB, et al. Overrides of medication alerts in ambulatory care. *Arch Intern Med* 2009;169:305–311.
63. Resnick RK, MacRae H. Teaching surgical skills—changes in the wind. *N Engl J Med* 2006;355:2664–2669.
64. Zirkle M, Blum R, Raemer DB, et al. Teaching emergency airway management using medical simulation: a pilot program. *Laryngoscope* 2005;115:495–500.
65. Zirkle M, Roberson DW, Leuwer R, et al. Using a virtual reality temporal bone simulator to assess otolaryngology trainees. *Laryngoscope* 2007;117:258–263.
66. Sexton JB, Thomas EJ, Helmreich RL. Error, stress, and teamwork in medicine and aviation: cross-sectional surveys. *BMJ* 2000;320:745–749.
67. Horwitz LI, Krumholz HM, Green ML, et al. Transfers of patient care between house staff on internal medicine wards: a national survey. *Arch Intern Med* 2006;166:1173–1177.
68. Pronovost P, Needham D, Berenholtz S. An intervention to decrease catheter-related bloodstream infections. *N Engl J Med* 2006;355:2725–2732.
69. Makary MA, Sexton BJ, Freischlag JA, et al. Operating room teamwork among physicians and nurses: teamwork in the eye of the beholder. *J Am Coll Surg* 2006;202:746–752.
70. Neily J, Mills PD, Young-Xu Y, et al. Association between implementation of a medical team training program and surgical mortality. *JAMA* 2010;304:1693–1700.

BIBLIOGRAPHY

Aspden P, Corrigan JM, Wolcott J, et al. *Patient safety: achieving a new standard for care.* Washington, DC: National Academy Press, 2003.

Casey S. *Set phasers on stun and other true tales of design, technology, and human error.* Santa Barbara, CA: Aegean Publishing Company, 1993.

Cook R, Woods D, Miller C. A tale of two stories: contrasting views of patient safety. *Workshop on assembling the scientific basis for progress on patient safety, 1998.* Chicago, IL: National Patient Safety Foundation, 1998. Available at http://www.npsf.org/rc/tts/front. html. Accessed May, 2011.

Cook R. Two years before the mast: learning how to learn about patient safety. Annenberg Conference 1998. Enhancing patient safety and reducing errors in health care, 1998. Rancho mirage, CA, 1998. Available at http://www.ctlab.org/documents/LearningToLearn. PDF. Accessed May, 2011.

Cooper A, Reimann R, Conin D. *About face 3.0: the essentials of interaction design.* Indianapolis, IN: Wiley, 2007.

Cooper A. *The inmates are running the asylum.* Indianapolis, IN: Sams, 2003.

Dekker S. *Just culture: balancing safety and accountability.* Aldershot, UK: Ashgate, 2007.

Dekker S. *Patient safety: a human factors approach.* London, UK: CRC Press, 2011.

Global Aviation Information Network Working Group E. *A roadmap to a just culture: enhancing the safety environment.* 2004. Available at http://flightsafety.org/files/just_culture.pdf

Kenney C. *The best practice: how the new quality movement is transforming medicine.* New York: Perseus, 2008.

Kohn L, Corrigan JM, Donaldson M. *To err is human: building a safer health system.* Washington, DC: National Academy Press, 1999. Available at http://www.nap.edu/openbook.php?record_id=9728. Accessed May, 2011.

Kumar S, Nash D. *Demand better! Revise our broken healthcare system.* Bozeman, MT: Second River Healthcare Press, 2011.

Kumar S. *Fatal care: survive in the US healthcare system.* Bozeman, MT: Second River Healthcare Press, 2009.

Marx D. *Patient safety and the "just culture": a primer for health care executives.* Columbia University 2001. Available at http://www.merstm.org/support/Marx_Primer.pdf

Massachusetts Coalition. *When things go wrong: responding to adverse events*, 2007. Available at http://www.macoalition.org/documents/RespondingtoAdverseEvents.pdf

Nance J. *Why hospitals should fly—the ultimate flight plan to patient safety and quality care.* Bozeman, MT: Second River Healthcare Press, 2010.

Norman DA. *Design of everyday things.* 2nd ed. New York: Basic Books, 2002.

Norman DA. *Things that make us smart.* Cambridge, MA: Perseus, 1993.

Peters GA, Peters BJ. *Medical error and patient safety: human factors in medicine.* London, UK: CRC Press, 2008.

Shneiderman B, Plaisant C. *Designing the user interface: strategies for effective human-computer interaction*, 4th ed. Reading, MA: Addison–Wesley, 2005.

Tognazzini B. *First principles of interaction design 2004.* Available at: http://www.asktog.com/basics/firstPrinciples.html

Wachter R, Shojania K. *Internal bleeding: the truth behind America's terrifying epidemic of medical mistakes.* New York: Rugged Land, 2004.

Wachter RM. *Understanding patient safety.* New York: McGraw Hill, 2008.

Wickens C, Hollands J. *Engineering psychology and human performance.* New York: Prentice Hall, 2002.

Woods D, Dekker S. *Behind human error*, 2nd ed. Farnham, Surrey England: Ashgate, 2010.

Woods MS, Star JI. *Healing words: the power of apology in medicine.* Chicago, IL: Doctors in Touch, 2004.

Wright A. *Glut: mastering information through the ages.* Washington, DC: National Academies Press, 2005.

Wu AW, Stokes SL. *Removing insult from injury: disclosing adverse events.* [Video]. USA: Johns Hopkins University, 2004. p. 26 Minutes. Available at http://www.jhsph.edu/dept/hpm/research/wu_video. html

199 Business Law and the Practice of Otolaryngology

Robert S. Iwrey   **Stephanie P. Ottenwess**   **Jessica L. Gustafson**
Kathryn Hickner-Cruz   **David M. Ottenwess**   **Reginald Baugh**

With the continuing avalanche of new regulations, the ever-tightening belt of third party payor reimbursement, the increased scrutiny by federal and state enforcement authorities, the increased emphasis on cost-containment and pay-for-performance measures, and the always looming threat of medical malpractice actions, physicians find themselves having to play the role of accountant, attorney, billing consultant, business manager, financial advisor, risk manager, and, if time permits, practicing physician. Long past are the days when a physician could simply devote virtually all of his or her professional time seeing patients and providing high-quality care.

In today's environment, physicians must still focus on providing high-quality care to their patients; however, they may also need to delegate certain aspects of the business side of medicine to the right individuals in order to optimize their success. This may seem counterintuitive to some in that in order to maintain control over their practice as a whole, physicians must learn to let go of some of the pieces.

The most important first step to gaining or regaining control over one's practice is to identify key advisors and specialists. Selecting an experienced health care attorney and an accountant with significant experience in representing physicians and physician practices is crucial as they can help navigate through the often murky waters of the health care regulatory landscape. There are numerous legal and accounting aspects of starting, maintaining, expanding, merging, and even closing a medical practice that require professional advisors to guide physicians so as to avoid the myriad of serious negative consequences that can result from noncompliance with the ever-changing rules of the game. Some of these consequences include, but are not limited to, overpayment demands by third party payors, departicipation or exclusion from third party payors, civil fines, and even criminal sanctions. Experienced, qualified health care attorneys, accountants, and other advisors can mitigate against the risks of facing such consequences as well as assist in crucial administrative matters for example, obtaining

and maintaining the appropriate licenses (such as one's medical license, controlled substance license, drug control license, and Drug Enforcement Administration [DEA] registration), obtaining the best financing for medical and office equipment and supplies, obtaining the appropriate insurance (e.g., professional liability, personal liability, property, workers' compensation, directors and officers liability policies, and even policies now available to insure against fines and defense costs for billing errors and omissions).

Some physicians find it helpful to consult with a business advisor as well to sit down with the other professional advisors and to help develop a business plan based upon the physician's desires and needs. Such plans may include staffing determinations, changes in physical location, adding ancillaries such as imaging and laboratories, marketing, and developing affiliations with other health care providers, entities, and organizations. Prior to implementing such plans, it is a good idea to run them past one's key advisors to assure legal compliance.

Another important step is to make sure that the physician has a good understanding of where his or her practice stands in terms of the billing of professional services rendered. Remember, a physician alone is responsible for the use of his or her provider number. Whether one chooses to do his or her own billing, to employ an in-house biller, to contract with an outside company, or to rely upon his or her employer, ultimately the physician is responsible for the claims submitted under his or her provider number. Thus, if a physician chooses to rely upon others to do his or her billing, the physician should make sure that he or she has the requisite knowledge and experience in his or her specific field of practice. Being proactive, asking the right questions, and researching the prospective biller prior to engagement are time well spent and can save the physician significant headaches in the future. While the enforcement authorities *may* find that the physician did not have the requisite intent for criminal prosecution because his or her biller made the errors and not the physician, the physician will still incur significant costs in both time and money defending the billings, and very often, the physician is subject to significant fines and penalties on top of returning monies to which the physician believed he or she was entitled and upon which he or she relied in the operation of the practice. As such, the physician needs to be familiar with the billing rules as they pertain to his or her specific area of practice. Responsibility for this knowledge and expertise should not be delegated.

Of course, no chapter on the business of medicine would be complete without discussion of medical malpractice and the efforts to reform the system—which to many appears broken and sorely in need of repair but without a viable solution. For the past three decades, medical malpractice tort reform has remained a highly polarizing, heavily contested legal issue, which affects not only physicians and attorneys but also the great many Americans seeking health care each year. But why does this legislation inspire such fervency in those that revile it and in those that champion it? Ask its critics, which typically include much of the plaintiffs' bar, and the answer is simple: medical malpractice tort reform strips individuals of their ability to redress injuries that they have incurred and right the perceived wrongs that have been committed against them. To its advocates, the answer is equally clear: medical malpractice tort reform is the mechanism by which defensive medicine is prevented, doctors' personal and professional livelihoods are protected, and litigious plaintiffs with frivolous lawsuits are deterred from bringing suit. While both sides make frequently valid and often convincing arguments, the reality of medical malpractice tort reform lies somewhere in the middle. It is a legislatively constructed concept, which has made its impact, both positive and negative, on the American legal landscape.

The purpose of this chapter is to provide the physician with a general overview of some, but not all, topics of interest to otolaryngologists regarding the business of medicine. It is by no means an exhaustive list as health care is a broad field and highly regulated with ever-changing laws, regulations, rules, advisory opinions, guidance, and contractual provisions. The goal of this chapter is to provide the physician with a business perspective of medicine and to arm the physician with enough insight and business savvy to recognize certain risk areas so that the physician may timely seek appropriate assistance in compliance with such areas and avoid the negative consequences often associated with a lack of knowledge.

MEDICAL LIABILITY

Medical Liability Claims in the United States

Introduction

Medical malpractice, or negligence law, is just one subset of the legal behemoth that is tort law. A tort is generally defined as a civil wrong that causes an injury, for which a victim may seek damages, typically in the form of money damages, against the alleged wrongdoer (1). Tort law is that body of law that serves as the vehicle by which tort liability can be sought in a court of law against such wrongdoers and generally serves to award damages to a victim sufficient to restore him to the position he would have been in, had the tortious conduct not occurred (1). Tort law typically governs three types of causes of action or, more simply phrased, legal theories of a lawsuit: negligence, strict liability, and intentional torts. A claim for negligence is brought when an injury results from an individual's failure to exercise the standard of care of a reasonably prudent person would have exercised in a similar situation (2). These matters involve unintentional acts that may cause harm. Actions for medical malpractice are classified under the umbrella of negligence claims. Claims for strict liability do not require an intent to harm or the presence of actual negligence but rather are based on the breach of an absolute duty to make something safe (3). Strict liability typically arises in situations that are considered inherently dangerous. For example, an individual who keeps a domesticated Siberian tiger in his home is strictly liable for any injuries that the tiger may cause, no matter the precautions the individual takes in protecting the safety of others. He need not be found to have breached the standard of care to be found strictly liable in such scenarios. Finally, intentional torts are defined as torts committed by a wrongdoer acting with intent (4). Examples of intentional torts include assault and battery, defamation, and false imprisonment.

Historic Analysis of Tort Law and the Evolution of Medical Malpractice Action in the United States

The modern system of American tort law and its district categories are by no means a recent construct. Tort law has existed in some form for hundreds of years, originating from English common law. Common law is defined as law that is issued from judicial decisions and not derived from legislatively enacted laws or statutes. Consequently, centuries-old decisions made by judges in England have greatly affected how the US legal system addresses actions for negligence, strict liability, and intentional tort. Taken one step further, the law that is applied in the most complex medical malpractice case can trace its ancestry to an English judge deciding whether a Welsh farmer's horse was negligently corralled during the 15th century.

The element of damages in tort law is of major significance and is integral to understanding the overall concept of medical malpractice law, mainly because the "runaway juries" have been the subject of great media attention and scrutiny. In tort law, compensatory money damages can be sought by a victim for both economic and noneconomic losses (5). Economic damages seek to compensate an individual for quantifiable economic losses, such as lost income and medical bills, while noneconomic damages are more speculative and seek to compensate an individual for noneconomic losses, such as mental distress and pain and suffering (5). In certain rare scenarios, generally involving egregiously reckless conduct or behavior, a victim may also seek punitive damages against a wrongdoer (6).

Tort law is a function of state law, with each state providing different rules for bringing about a tort claim.[1] Procedurally, various states may approach tort claims differently; however, the basic premise of a tort claim and the elements that a plaintiff must prove in order to bring a successful cause of action remain consistent across all 50 states. This chapter focuses its state-specific discussion of tort law and medical malpractice tort reform on the state of Michigan and utilizes Michigan's experience with medical malpractice tort reform to illustrate how, in recent years, many states have attempted to handle the rising number of suits for medical malpractice.

The modern medical malpractice system in this country dates its origins to the 1840s, when the United States experienced a sudden surge in the number of medical malpractice actions brought in state courts (7). This boom could be attributed to the lack of a national "standard of care" for medical treatment, which often left patients seeking care from unqualified or unskilled medical practitioners (7). As the number of medical malpractice actions spiked, plaintiffs' attorneys also found a new niche in which lucrative careers could be made, primarily due to the availability of contingency fees, wherein a plaintiff's attorney receives as his fee one-third of the plaintiff's overall jury award or settlement. This time frame is typically considered the first medical malpractice "crisis," and the commencement of the long and complicated interplay between the medical community and the legal system.

The second significant medical malpractice crisis in the United States occurred in the 1970s and 1980s (7). During this time period, there was a rapid rise in the number of medical malpractice claims filed, as well as the size of awards made in medical malpractice actions. It has been estimated by the American Medical Association (AMA) that in 1975 as many as 14,000 malpractice suits were filed against physicians. The average jury award in these suits was $171,000 (7). The influx of medical malpractice claims and their subsequent jury awards created a chain reaction that had a far-reaching effect. Many private insurance companies began withdrawing from providing insurance coverage, and the insurers that remained responded by raising malpractice premiums. In 1975, it was documented that malpractice premiums had increased from anywhere from 100% to 750% (7). The sudden increase in insurance premiums, coupled with the loss of many private insurance companies from the market, resulted in some physicians leaving particular practice areas, or retiring from the practice of medicine altogether. It was the culmination of these factors that sparked a call for policy change at both the state and federal levels, and with that, modern medical malpractice tort reform was born.

Before addressing tort "reform" and its impact on the physician's practice, it is important to understand the anatomy of a modern medical malpractice case, as oftentimes the physician is quick to equate "reform" with the altogether elimination of medical malpractice claims from the American legal system. It is not the legal system, however, that is broken. Our civil litigation system has existed for centuries; it is only because it is so interwoven with and dependent on the human element that we see it as controversial. Consequently, a description of a malpractice action is in order that will outline the "theory" of litigation along with the "reality" of being a party defendant in a medical malpractice case.

Medical Malpractice Litigation

Anatomy of a Medical Malpractice Case[2]
General Legal Background

As a practicing physician with a highly advanced degree, years of sophisticated training, and a hard-earned professional license to protect, it is important to gain an understanding of the basic elements of a medical malpractice claim and the procedural aspects of bringing a lawsuit in order to best understand how to limit your exposure to claims of medical negligence. In today's legal environment, physicians often think that a lawsuit is a natural consequence of any "bad result" arising out of care provided to a patient. While a bad result should put the physician on alert that a suit may be on its way, a bad result does not, in and of itself, qualify as a legitimate malpractice claim. To bring, and sustain, an action for medical malpractice, the plaintiff bears the burden of establishing the four basic elements required of any negligence claim, with some variations. Specifically, the plaintiff must establish (a) that a physician or health care provider owed the plaintiff a duty of care, (b) that this duty of care was breached by conduct that was not in accordance with the standard of care that a reasonable physician would have employed under like circumstances, (c) that this breach was a cause of the plaintiff's injury, and (d) that the plaintiff suffered damages as a result of this breach (8).

---

[1] While tort law is primarily a function of state law, there is a Federal Tort Claims Act ("FTCA"), enacted in 1948, that provides that a private individual may sue the United States in a federal district court for most torts committed by persons acting on behalf of the United States. The FTCA imposes some limitations upon actions brought under the Act, specifically that the action must be brought in federal, rather than state court, the matter must be heard in a bench trial, presided over by a judge, and that the United States is not liable for any punitive damages sought by the plaintiff. In a medical malpractice context, claims brought pursuant to the FTCA most typically arise when an individual sues a VA or military hospital for medical negligence.

[2] Most of the authors' medical malpractice work arises out of claims filed in the State of Michigan. Consequently, examples and case law cited here will often involve specific Michigan rules and statutes.

In regard to the third element of causation, a physician's allegedly tortious conduct must be both the cause in fact and the proximate cause of the victim's injury. The cause in fact (or "but-for" cause) of a plaintiff's injury simply means that but for the physician's conduct, the injury would not have occurred. Proximate cause is a complex legal concept, one that is particularly vexing to first-year law students, but essentially, proximate cause can be defined as the initial conduct or act, which sets off a natural and continuous sequence of events that produces an injury.[3] In order for a plaintiff to successfully bring an action for medical malpractice, he or she must establish that the defendant's actions were both the cause in fact and the proximate cause of his or her injuries. Thus, because a bad result may be a natural consequence of treatment, there is no viable claim until a similarly situated physician testifies that the defendant physician breached the standard of care *and* that the breach was a cause of plaintiff's injuries.

Presuit

In a vacuum, a patient who suspects that he or she has been the victim of medical malpractice will retain an attorney who will determine if the plaintiff has a viable claim. If the attorney believes there is evidence of a physician's negligence, the attorney will conduct an investigation, which requires having a qualified physician look at the medical records involved and offer an opinion whether proper treatment was rendered in the case in question. Once the attorney is convinced that the expert will testify adequately about the legal requirements of duty, standard of care, and proximate cause, the attorney may initiate a lawsuit by filing a complaint, almost always in state court. But, in some instances, there may be ways to avoid a lawsuit and circumvent the entire adversarial litigation process.

As a practical matter, a patient who may feel that he or she received inadequate medical treatment due to negligence knows little or nothing about the "burden of proof" or what other legal requirements are necessary to proceed in a court of law. Consequently, a patient who has a negative experience is angry and wishes some redress or, if nothing else, a bit of an explanation as to why *he* fell into that small percentage of patients that his physician quoted as being at risk of a potential complication from the medical treatment in question. As a result, a patient really may only be looking for answers, rather than an attorney.

It is during this period that, in some instances, a physician can head off a lawsuit if her office is receptive to the patient's concerns. Some physicians have gone to great lengths to avoid speaking directly to patients about the "mechanics" of medicine when a less than optimal result has occurred. However, avoidance or vagueness almost always instills suspicion and can, by itself, be the impetus for a patient to head to the nearest attorney's office. One course of action to follow is to be as straightforward and direct with the unhappy patient as possible and to speak with them at length about their complaints if they seek out an explanation. Also, a physician should provide a patient with any requested medical records and may offer to refer a patient to another physician, if the patient so desires. While it is not in the physician's best interest to admit that anything he or she did was inappropriate (unless, of course, what he or she did *was* inappropriate, and then you must let your conscience be your guide), being empathetic to the patient's plight may even go so far as to head off a potential lawsuit.

Suit Filed: Discovery

Assuming that the patient is neither placated nor interested in an informal discussion about the patient's medical care and an attorney is retained who has obtained a positive review from an expert, the formal action is begun in court by filing a pleading known as a complaint.[4] The complaint initiates a civil action and outlines with specificity the basis for the plaintiff's medical malpractice claim and the relief that the plaintiff seeks (9). The complaint is then filed upon the opposing side, who in response must file an answer, which is the defendant's first pleading that addresses the merits of the case and generally denies the plaintiff's allegations and sets forth any of the defendant's defenses and counterclaims (10).

After the complaint and answer have been filed, the pretrial process of gathering evidence to support either party's position, referred to as the discovery stage of the proceedings, begins. During discovery, interrogatories are exchanged between the parties, which are written sets of questions that are required to be answered candidly. Also during the discovery period, depositions of the relevant witnesses are taken. A deposition is a witness' out-of-court testimony, which is taken under oath and recorded for later use at trial or to further additional discovery (11). Depositions are a critical part of the discovery process, as they assist counsel for both parties to focus their discovery requests and identify important issues to be addressed at trial.

The discovery phase of the lawsuit is really the nuts and bolts of the litigation process. The physician learns exactly the nature of the charges being advanced by the patient and what steps will be necessary to defend against the claims. In Michigan, the defendant physician will get some early

---

[3]Proximate cause "normally involves examining the foreseeability of consequences, and whether a defendant should be held legally responsible for such consequences." *Skinner v Square D Co*, 445 Mich 153, 163 (1994).

[4]In some states, such as Michigan, a Notice of Intent to File Claim (NOI) must be served before a formal complaint may be filed with the Court. An NOI puts potential defendants on notice that a case *may* be filed. By law, a claimant must wait approximately 6 months after serving the NOI before proceeding to a court action by filing a legal complaint.

inkling of the specific claims of malpractice being brought, as the plaintiff must file an affidavit of merit with the complaint. This affidavit must be executed by a similarly trained and certified physician who is prepared to testify as an "expert" witness that the defendant physician committed professional negligence. The entire scope of the expert's opinions, however, does not materialize until the witness is actually deposed. It is during the deposition of the expert that the attorneys are given, relatively speaking, free rein to delve into the bases of the expert's opinions and to examine the expert's background and training to verify whether the expert has adequate credentials and/or the adequate background to testify in the case.

Before depositions of experts can be completed, the defendant physician must undergo his or her own deposition. Short of trial, this is typically the most difficult part of the litigation process for a physician. A physician must be very well prepared for his or her deposition testimony, as such testimony usually only can "lose" a case and rarely ever results in one getting dismissed. It is therefore imperative that the pertinent medical records are reviewed in great detail prior to the physician's deposition and that the physician meet with the attorney well in advance of the deposition to ensure a comfort level for both the physician and the attorney. With the expense involved in litigating medical malpractice actions, the defendant physician can fully expect the plaintiff's attorney to be well prepared for the deposition, which makes it crucial that the physician not take the procedure lightly. While the actual process one must undertake to get ready for a deposition could fill another chapter, suffice it to say, the more prepared one is for grueling questioning, the better off the defense of the case will be. Remember, the plaintiff's attorney is not only listening to your every answer; she is also sizing you up to determine just how well you will present before a jury and exactly how you will handle yourself under difficult circumstances.

Having survived the deposition process, it may appear that your case has suddenly disappeared; do not be misled. The lull in the action is only due to the fact that your attorneys are now turning their sights toward taking the discovery of either other defendants or the plaintiff's expert witnesses. This process can usually take several months and only makes it *appear* as if nothing is moving.

Expert Witnesses

In a medical malpractice action in Michigan, as is true in virtually every state, the plaintiff *must* secure medical expert testimony in order to advance the case before a jury.[5] That is to say, before a jury can actually decide the merits of the case, the plaintiff must present expert testimony that the defendant physician breached the standard of care during the treatment of the patient and that that breach was a cause of injury to the plaintiff. This testimony is required because the typical jury does not, as a whole, have the requisite knowledge to decide intricate questions of medical treatment without the assistance of a qualified expert witness. Just what constitutes a qualified expert witness is a matter of discretion for the trial judge and is one of the "human elements" that make litigating a case more difficult. For instance, the judge may have a more liberal interpretation of what the expert needs to be "qualified," which can be frustrating to the defendant.

Because there are no standard rules regarding what is "proper" expert testimony, the use of expert witnesses in medical malpractice cases has become a main source of contention for many advocates of medical malpractice tort reform. As filings of medical malpractice lawsuits have increased throughout the country, the provision of expert witness testimony has become very lucrative for physicians across all medical disciplines. As a result, proponents of tort reform argue that because of the ease at which an expert can be retained to offer expert testimony on a medical malpractice claim, it is increasingly easier for plaintiffs to bring such claims, exacerbating the medical malpractice crisis in the United States. Thus, while theoretically the parties should get well-trained, credible, and reliable experts to testify, this is not always the case.

As a practical matter, proposed expert witnesses are not always bound by their ethical and moral obligations. Because the standard of care is, in most circumstances, neither codified nor objective in nature, there may be wide disagreement as to what really constitutes the "standard of care."[6] For the most part, experts, while genuine in their opinions, will oftentimes confuse their own practice, or what they believe the practice should be, with a national standard of care. For instance, while it is inappropriate for a physician in Michigan to testify about the standard of care in relation to what he or she does or does not do in their practice personally, many experts do just that. Because it is difficult to verify oft-stated, sweeping generalizations made by an expert that their opinions "are common knowledge," "may be heard at any meeting," or "can be readily found in the literature," the defendant physician may risk that a jury will simply accept unsupported statements as true because they do not possess the requisite knowledge of the subject matter. While steps can be taken to hold an expert's feet to the fire on certain medical issues, a liberal judge or

---

[5]In most states, the defendant physician is not necessarily *required* to secure an independent expert to testify on her behalf at trial as the defendant physician is considered an expert in her own right. As a practical matter, however, defense counsel almost always retains an independent, similarly situated physician to assist in the defense of the claim.

[6]In Michigan, the standard of care is defined as what an ordinary board certified physician would do or not do under like or similar circumstances. *Patelczyk v Olson*, 95 Mich App 281, 283; 289 NW2d 910 (1980).

sympathetic jury may be persuaded by an expert who does little else but sit in an office and testify against physicians.

Indeed, there are a few physicians who rely heavily on the income derived from testifying against physicians. It is highly lucrative, and the physician is at little risk for repercussions. Experts on behalf of the plaintiff will typically testify against physicians outside of their state, which gives them a comfort level that they would not ordinarily enjoy if they were testifying against a local colleague.

Progress has been made to limit and correct some of these problems. Various medical organizations have established their own ethical guidelines for expert witness conduct. For example, the American Academy of Otolaryngology–Head and Neck Surgery sets forth that an expert witness to a medical malpractice action should not adopt a position as an advocate or partisan in the legal proceedings; should review all the appropriate medical information in the case and testify to its content fairly, truthfully, and objectively; should review and be thoroughly familiar with the relevant standards of practice and medical literature prevailing at the time of the occurrence and limit their testimony to their areas of expertise; should be prepared to state the basis of the testimony presented and whether it is based on personal experience, specific clinical references, or a generally accepted opinion in the specialty field; should be compensated at a rate that is reasonable and commensurate with the time and effort given in preparation for testifying and should not link their compensation to the outcome of the case; and should be aware that transcripts of their deposition and courtroom testimony are public records, subject to independent peer review (12).

Stringent ethical guidelines, such as the ones imposed by the American Academy of Otolaryngology–Head and Neck Surgery, help ensure that expert witness testimony offered in medical malpractice actions is scientifically truthful and founded in reliable and universally recognized methodologies. These guidelines protect the equitable nature of the civil litigation process and hold accountable expert witnesses who proffer less than truthful medical opinions under oath.

While individual societies are trying to take steps to reign in unreliable testimony, it is not likely to vanish entirely. What constitutes the standard of care is simply too subjective in many instances, and the lines of what constitutes an exercise of judgment and what constitutes medical negligence are often blurred. The important thing to note is that the defendant physician should try to avoid taking any such criticisms personally and should consider the source of those opinions when applicable.

The End Game: Settle or Not to Settle

Once discovery has been completed in a particular case, counsel will begin the process of a cost–benefit analysis of whether a case should, or even can, proceed to trial. This is usually the most difficult part of the case for the defendant physician. The defendant is faced with a Hobson's choice of either grinding it out in trial, with no guarantee of success, or suffer the ignominy of "caving in" to the plaintiff's demands. While those views represent opposite ends of the emotional continuum, the defendant physician experiences these pangs of emotion when deciding what to do.

Before the physician arrives at a decision about settlement versus trial, counsel must first do a complete analysis of the case to determine whether from a factual and legal standpoint, there is a good chance of prevailing at trial. To that end, counsel will analyze all of the opinions of the defendant physicians, the subsequent treating physicians, and the expert witnesses. Counsel will take into account the jurisdiction (where the case is located), the judge involved in the matter, the attorney who is representing the plaintiff, and, perhaps most importantly, the presentation of the client himself. While having excellent experts and a great judge on a case is extraordinarily helpful, those factors may pale in the face of a tentative witness, who also happens to be the defendant. Juries often look to the parties, that is, the plaintiff and the defendant physicians, in order to formulate a decision about the case as, oftentimes, they have heard polar opposite testimony from the experts on the question of whether the defendant breached the standard of care. So, while a case may be extraordinarily "defensible," it may be impossible to move forward with trial because of the personality or fortitude of the defendant physician.

Similarly, many physicians simply cannot afford to be out of the office for several days or several weeks while a trial is being conducted. Trials are typically a session of consecutive days until completion and often take all day to attend. It is easy to "fight to the death" on a case when your physical presence is not needed leading up to trial and your own time and assets are not at risk because your insurance dollars are paying all of the discovery costs and expenses. But when trial is imminent, hard decisions need to be made. It is only when the defendant traverses the "courthouse steps" that either backbones stiffen or knees buckle. Consequently, settlements may be made strictly from a convenience or emotional standpoint, as opposed to on the merits of a case.

Another major reason why cases typically will not proceed to trial is that the defendant physician simply cannot stand the process emotionally. Indeed, it is very difficult to sit through days, if not weeks, watching a parade of witnesses criticizing your every action. Further, the inability to understand the procedural machinations of the court can sometimes make matters extraordinarily frustrating. As a result, it is the rare physician who will take that trip to trial on more than one occasion.

Once it is determined that you want to move forward with trial, new anxieties arise. The question of "How can a jury of lay people possibly understand the medicine and decide in my favor?" is a common concern. Indeed, this fear is often the major reason to settle a case. It is here that counsel must ensure that the issues presented in the case are concise, relevant, and put into language that the jury can understand. For the most part, juries can be trusted to understand the issues presented in a medical malpractice action and with the proper preparation on the part of defense counsel, a jury will typically make an informed decision.

If a defendant physician does in fact decide to go to trial, he must be prepared to enter an entirely different world and face a process that can be potentially grueling and involves going to court on consecutive days until the case is complete. One of the first steps of trial that a physician will witness is jury selection. Initially, a group of individuals, called the veneer, are brought into the courtroom and prospective jurors are selected randomly to hear the case. Before the jury is sworn in, the attorneys and the judge will ask questions to determine whether any of the potential jurors have any biases or prejudices that would render them incapable of arriving at a fair verdict. This process is known as voir dire. Once the jury is impaneled, the parties proceed to opening statements and then evidence is produced, hopefully, in a reasonable fashion. Once all of the evidence has been heard, both sides have rested, and plaintiff has met his burden of proof to present a *prima facie* case of negligence, the jury is charged by the court to decide the case. The jury then deliberates in private and renders a verdict.

This brief overview of the trial process encapsulates what can amount of many weeks worth of events and also is based on the assumption that all the parties involved in the process will be reasonable. More often than not, that is not the case, as in the adversarial setting of a courtroom it is the opponent's job to be unreasonable. Furthermore, some judges, possessing little more than a rudimentary understanding of the medical issues involved, sit and decide important evidentiary issues. Fortunately, the jury decides "guilt" or "innocent"; however, this may provide little comfort to the physician in the hot seat.

As if 2 years of litigation culminating in a long drawn-out trial were not enough, if the physician prevails, the plaintiff has the option to appeal. Depending on the state in which the case sits, the appellate process may take another additional 1 to 4 years. After sweating it out for this period, the appellate court could overturn your hard-fought win and require you to relitigate your case. Thus, given the many unknowns that are associated with trial, physicians and their insurance carriers will look closely at each of the factors involved with a case to determine the best course.

On the other hand, the consequences of settling the case are a bit clearer. First, the case has ended completely with no chance of it hanging over the defendant's head *ad infinitum*. A release and settlement agreement is entered into, which, in some cases, allows for a confidentiality agreement; that is, the terms of the case cannot be discussed by any of the parties. Also, the physician is not admitting negligence by entering into a settlement agreement, only resolving a "disputed" claim. The only real cost with this course of action is a mandatory report to the National Practitioner Data Bank and perhaps a wounded ego. While this is not necessarily desirable, settlement at least allows the physician to move forward without protracted litigation hanging over her head.

Medical Malpractice Insurance

Because of the risks associated with litigation noted above, along with the sheer number of malpractice claims filed annually in the United States, it is not surprising that professional liability insurance has, and should, become a high priority for most practicing physicians and health care professionals. Professional liability insurance can serve a number of goals, the most important of which is the protection of a physician's personal and professional assets and the provision of legal support if a lawsuit is initiated. While most states legally require a physician to purchase a minimum amount of professional liability insurance, there are various other components to consider when deciding what type of coverage best fits a physician's specific needs.

Certain elements affect how much professional liability insurance a physician requires, including the physician's practice area, whether his state requires a minimum level of coverage and whether the physician is willing to jeopardize his personal assets if his level of coverage is insufficient. Once it has been determined exactly what a physician's unique needs are, it is then important to evaluate potential professional liability insurance carriers based upon the levels of protection that they offer against lawsuits, their financial solvency, their process for handling specific medical malpractice claims, and the type of coverage they offer.

Professional liability insurance carriers often offer one of two types of coverage: an occurrence policy or a claims-made policy. An occurrence policy offers protection from losses, which occurred while the policy was in effect, or during the policy term. Furthermore, an occurrence policy will continue to cover those losses any number of years in the future, even if the policy has since expired. For example, if a physician buys an occurrence policy in 1999 and terminates the policy in 2009, he will be covered for any incident of alleged malpractice that occurred in that period of 10 years, even if he is sued for such an incident in 2012, well after the occurrence policy has expired. Essentially, with an occurrence policy, a physician is covered for any incident that occurred during his or her policy term, no matter when he or she is sued. Occurrence policies are especially attractive to physicians because often evidence of alleged medical malpractice is not discovered until many years in the future and occurrence policies allow physicians to remain protected from any potential undetected exposure. Occurrence policies are, however, typically more expensive than a traditional claims-made policy, due to their permanence.

A claims-made policy is also another viable option for professional liability insurance coverage. Claims-made policies differ from occurrence policies in that they offer protection from claims made during a specific time period. A claims-made policy must continually be renewed from the time of the alleged incident to the time the claim is filed, and when a claims-made policy expires, a physician no longer has coverage in the future for alleged incidents of malpractice that occurred in the past. For example, if a physician purchases a claims-made policy in 1999 and renews it until 2009, at which point the physician allows it to expire, the physician will not be covered from a potential claim that is brought in 2011, even if the alleged act of malpractice occurred in 2006, when he or she had claims-made coverage.

In order to reduce their risk of liability exposure, physicians with claims-made policies will often purchase what is called tail coverage. Tail coverage serves to cover losses that occur after a claims-made policy has expired. Functioning much like an occurrence policy, tail coverage protects a physician from claims made after the expiration of the claims-made policy, but which occurred while the policy was effective. For example, a physician purchases a claims-made policy in 2002, which he renews until 2004, at which point he allows it to expire. He then purchases a tail policy in 2004, which protects him from any claims brought against him during the 2002–2004 time frame during which the physician was insured.

The primary difference between tail coverage and an occurrence policy is that when an occurrence policy expires or is terminated, the physician is no longer required to pay premiums on the policy and yet, will continue to have coverage for any losses that occurred during his or her policy term. With tail coverage, the physician must continue to pay premiums until he or she no longer wishes to have protection from incidents that may have occurred during the time the physician's claims-made policy was in effect.

The decision whether to purchase claims-made or tail insurance is a complicated one, which should take into account your particular needs and exposure risks. Claims-made policies offer physicians great flexibility because they are renewed annually, allowing an individual to revise or change his insurance coverage. Furthermore, claims-made policies are portable and may be transferred between insurance carriers, while occurrence policies remain with their original carriers, as they are permanent. Occurrence policies, however, are not without their advantages. An occurrence policy offers protection *ad infinitum*, is not required to be renewed, and does not require the additional purchase of supplemental or tail coverage.

Finally, it is important to consider that in the context of medical malpractice professional liability insurance, a physician's insurance premiums may be covered by the hospital or practice group that employs him. Typically, in such instances, this coverage is made on a claims-made basis. Therefore, if the physician is then to leave the hospital or practice group for other employment, it is critical that he purchases tail coverage to protect against any potential liability that may have occurred while working for his former employer.

No matter the type of insurance coverage a physician chooses to purchase, a physician's protection of his personal assets must be a top priority, particularly in light of the fact that a physician may be personally liable for any portion of a judgment or settlement in excess of his professional liability insurance coverage. After the lengthy and expensive process of obtaining a medical license, a physician must utilize every asset protection strategy available to him to protect his livelihood, including sound tax and estate planning and low-risk financial investments.

Asset protection strategies can be easily implemented by a physician with little expenditure of time or effort. For example, a physician can maximize his contributions to his IRA or other qualified employee benefit plan, which are typically shielded from claims of creditors. Various life insurance arrangements may also be considered, as many jurisdictions exempt all or part of the cash value of a life insurance policy from creditor claims. It is also critical to hire an experienced estate planner, who can suggest trust arrangements that offer significant asset protection and may provide some protection from the claims of creditors, and a knowledgeable accountant or tax expert, who will suggest methods by which to protect assets from various taxing authorities.

While maintaining insurance to protect personal assets is the overreaching goal to the insured, there are other avenues of insurance coverage, which, if appropriately managed, provide security and could ultimately produce income. Offshore captive insurance groups have become very popular with large health systems and large physician groups. Essentially, offshore captives are developed and owned off of the US borders by the insured parties. The captives are subject to the insurance laws of the country of domicile and are not formally required to adhere to US insurance regulations, like a typical domestic or US-domiciled company.

The upside for ownership interest in a captive is a potential return on your premium dollars. Instead of paying a local insurance company tens of thousands of dollars in premiums—money that will never be recouped—these insurance dollars may be placed in a captive, where theoretically, those dollars will grow, ultimately leading to distributions or, at least, a tangible asset. It is important to understand, however, that in order for these entities to become viable and, later, profitable, they must be well capitalized and very well managed—usually with outside underwriters, actuaries, and financial advisers. A well-run offshore captive can turn a liability, insurance premiums, into an asset.

On the other hand, an undercapitalized or poorly managed captive can be a physician's worst nightmare. Poor planning, reckless underwriting, or fraud can spell doom for the captive and could result in zero insurance protection to the participating physician for a period of time. Just to litigate a medical malpractice case up to the time of trial can cost upward of $200,000.00. This figure does not include trial costs, appeals, or a possible verdict, which can be staggeringly expensive. Stated simply, a lack of insurance could result in bankruptcy, humiliation, and a possible legal investigation.

The physician just beginning practice should ask many questions if his or her new group owns its own insurance company and obtain counsel if necessary—as this could make the difference between entering into a practice with a viable, sound captive and entering into a practice with a poorly managed captive destined for failure and economic ruin.

Tort Reform

Theory

In response to the above-mentioned criticisms of medical malpractice litigation and the medical malpractice crisis of the 1970s and 1980s, physicians and malpractice insurance carriers began to lobby heavily for changes to reduce medical malpractice tort liability. Proponents of medical malpractice tort reform argued that as a result of changes to laws governing medical malpractice claims and their associated awards, malpractice insurance premiums would decrease. They further argued that lower insurance premiums for health care providers would increase the number of practicing physicians, lower the costs of health care for consumers, and result in an overall improvement in available medical care. These arguments obviously struck a chord in state legislatures throughout the country because by the mid-1980s, medical malpractice tort reforms had been widely adopted. It is important to note that while medical malpractice reform legislation was introduced at both the state and federal levels, as will be discussed below, attempts to pass real reform have taken hold on the state level, while attempts at passing federal legislation have been unsuccessful.

Typically, medical malpractice tort reform at the state level has focused on legislative reforms to the general doctrines of tort law, such as rules governing punitive damages, noneconomic damages, collateral sources, and joint and several liability (13). These doctrinal reforms have had varying degrees of success throughout the nation, with some reforms being widely adopted across all jurisdictions, and others being less enthusiastically received.

State laws capping noneconomic damages have been just one of the legislatively implicated medical malpractice tort reforms. Advocates of tort reform argue that noneconomic damages are arbitrary and unpredictable and, as such, complicate the settlement process. Further, it is argued that losses for emotional distress and pain and suffering are intangible and exceedingly difficult to assign a dollar value. Currently, over 30 states have caps on noneconomic damages as applied to medical malpractice actions.[7] These limitations on noneconomic damages

vary across jurisdictions: some states employ caps on both economic and noneconomic damages in medical malpractice awards; some states apply noneconomic damage caps only to certain types of malpractice claims, such as obstetrics; and other states allow for increased recovery in particular scenarios, such as where the patient has died or has substantial physical injury (14).[8] Typically, the limit on noneconomic damages varies on a state by state basis, with caps on damages ranging from $250,000 to $500,000 (14).

The tort law concept of joint and several liability has also undergone significant tort reforms in the context of medical malpractice claims. Traditionally, joint and several liability allows a plaintiff, who has been injured by two or more wrongdoers, to recover the full amount of his damages from any one of the defendants that may have been involved in the tortious conduct. This has historically resulted in an injured party seeking damages against the defendant with the most financial resources. A party sued under a theory of joint and several liability may then seek contribution from the additional parties at fault, so that the other defendants have to share in the payment of damages. Oftentimes, however, contribution cannot be achieved because the additional at-fault parties lack the financial means to contribute. As a result, proponents of tort reform argue that joint and several liability is an inequitable concept because one defendant, generally the defendant with the most financial resources, is required to pay damages in an amount considerably more than his share of the total liability. This criticism has caused over 40 states to enact tort reforms to the joint and several liability system, either outright abolishing joint and several liability or requiring an individual defendant to pay an amount of damages proportionate to his share of the overall fault (15).[9]

States Where Tort Reform Has Been Enacted

Michigan serves as an illustrative example of how the specific states have addressed medical malpractice tort reform in an attempt to deal with the modern medical malpractice crisis. In recent years, Michigan has passed sweeping legislation curtailing frivolous litigation in the context of medical malpractice. For example, in 1986 the state passed a rule allowing a court to assess attorneys'

---

[7]States with noneconomic damages caps include Alabama, Alaska, California, Colorado, Florida, Georgia, Hawaii, Idaho, Illinois, Kansas, Maine, Maryland, Massachusetts, Michigan, Minnesota, Mississippi, Missouri, Montana, Nevada, New Hampshire, North Dakota, Ohio, Oklahoma, Oregon, South Carolina, South Dakota, Texas, Utah, Washington, West Virginia, and Wisconsin. American Tort Reform Association, http://atra.org/issues/index.php?issue=7338 (Last visited Dec. 6, 2010).

[8]*Compare* Mont. Code Ann. § 25-9-411 (2005) (cap of $250,000), *with* N.D. Cent. Code § 32-42-02 (1996) (cap of $500,000).

[9]States with such reforms include Alaska, Arizona, Arkansas, California, Colorado, Connecticut, Florida, Georgia, Hawaii, Idaho, Illinois, Indiana, Iowa, Kansas, Kentucky, Louisiana, Massachusetts, Michigan, Minnesota, Mississippi, Missouri, Montana, Nebraska, Nevada, New Hampshire, New Jersey, New Mexico, New York, North Dakota, Ohio, Oklahoma, Oregon, Pennsylvania, Rhode Island, South Carolina, South Dakota, Tennessee, Texas, Utah, Vermont, Virginia, Washington, West Virginia, Wisconsin, and Wyoming. American Tort Reform Association, http://atra.org/issues/index.php?issue=7345 (Last visited Dec. 6, 2010).

fees and costs for filed actions that are perceived as frivolous (16). In 1993, Michigan also enacted noneconomic damages caps in medical malpractice actions, limiting the award of noneconomic damages in medical liability cases to $280,000 for ordinary occurrences and $500,000 in cases where the plaintiff has suffered serious damage to the brain, spinal cord, or reproductive organs (16). In 1995, the state passed a reform to the rule of joint and several liability, barring the application of joint and several liability in the recovery of all damages, except in cases of medical malpractice where the plaintiff is determined to have no allocation of fault (16). The Michigan state legislature additionally passed reforms to the collateral source rule in the context of medical malpractice litigation (16). Prior to passage, the collateral source rule prohibited the presentation of evidence at trial that an injured party has received compensation for his losses from another source, such as an insurance policy. The collateral source rule reform passed by the state of Michigan as part of the overall medical liability reform package now provides that medical malpractice awards be offset by the amount of collateral source payments received by the plaintiff (16).

Through the adoption of comprehensive medical malpractice tort reform, Michigan has done what many other states have wished to achieve: the near-total elimination of all medical malpractice litigation. Indeed, reform began to gain traction in Michigan in the early 2000s following a series of conservative holdings by the State's Supreme Court strictly interpreting the key medical malpractice reform statutory provisions. Reports from the State of Michigan Office of Financial and Insurance Regulation (OFIR) demonstrate that reported claims[10] for the period 2000–2007 show a 77% decrease in court filings (1,142 in 2000 to 263 in 2007). This is a significant drop in cases, which has resulted in a modest drop in insurance premiums. Nonetheless, as will be discussed in the "Compliance and Regulatory Issues" section of this article, health care costs have not declined. Contrary to assertions that less litigation will protect physicians from the constant threat of second-guessing from their patients who have obtained a less than optimal result, health care costs and unnecessary testing has continued to rise.[11]

Despite the adoption of the above-mentioned tort reform measures throughout a variety of US jurisdictions, tort reform has yet to gain momentum on a federal level. Attempts at passing federal legislation restricting medical malpractice liability have failed since the 1970s, when federal tort reform was proposed in response to the first modern medical malpractice crisis. While contemporary presidents and politicians have campaigned for the adoption of far-reaching federal tort reform, all have failed in their efforts. In 2004, President George W. Bush proposed tort reforms affecting the liability exposure of physicians and drug and medical equipment manufacturers; however, opposition in the U.S. Senate prevented the enactment of this federal legislation (17). Additional proposals made in 2005 sought to cap noneconomic damages in medical malpractice actions, restrict the availability of punitive damages, restrict the statute of limitations for medical malpractice suits, and limit contingency fees collected by plaintiffs' attorneys in jury awards (18). Again, this federal legislation failed to get out of Congress.

With efforts at federal tort reform legislation stalled, it is impossible to determine the effect federally implicated restrictions on medical malpractice liability would have on overall national health care costs. It is, therefore, critical to consider whether medical malpractice tort reform at the state level has achieved the movement's stated goal: to reduce health care expenditures.

Relationships between Medical Malpractice Litigation and Health Care Costs

Impact on Rising Health Care Costs

One of the greatest criticisms leveled at the medical malpractice tort system is that the defense of medical malpractice actions needlessly increases the costs of health care in the United States. Medical malpractice tort reform advocates have long argued that the ever-present threat of litigation forces health care providers to charge higher rates to offset the costs of rising malpractice insurance premiums as well as promotes the practice of defensive medicine, which is defined as the overuse of diagnostic testing and health services in order to minimize a physician's liability exposure. The contention that medical malpractice tort reform is the soundest means by which to stabilize malpractice insurance premiums and generally lower health care costs, however, remains a controversial stance among both the legal and medical communities.

Much of the research conducted on the medical liability system suggests that in actuality, costs surrounding medical malpractice litigation are a small fraction of overall health care spending in the United States. Per the National Association of Insurance Commissioners, the overall cost of defending medical malpractice claims and compensating victims of medical malpractice in 2007 was estimated at $7.1 billion, a mere 0.3% of the annual health care costs for that year (19). Even when these figures account for the

---

[10]STATE OF MICHIGAN OFFICE OF FINANCIAL AND INSURANCE REGULATION, EVALUATION OF THE MICHIGAN MEDICAL PROFESSIONAL LIABILITY INSURANCE MARKET (October 2009). Although the OFIR report includes only those entities that filed a "Form A" notice and does not include many filings against self-insured captives insuring many hospitals and physicians in Michigan, the study is still a good indication of the percentage decline throughout the entire state.

[11]Interestingly, although the American Medical Association and other physician organizations wanted substantive medical malpractice reform to avoid "defensive medicine," no such reforms were seriously considered in the recent health reform debate—a debate where rising health care costs was *the* impetus for the resultant enacted legislation.

use of defensive medicine, as well as the expense of defending medical malpractice claims and compensating plaintiffs, the total costs associated with medical malpractice litigation are modest relative to overall health care spending. In 2008, the annual medical malpractice tort system costs, which included the costs of defensive medicine, were estimated to be $55.6 billion, or 2.4% of the total health care costs for the year (20).

If recent statistics appear to reflect that the cost of medical malpractice litigation does not have an overwhelming effect on the overall cost of health care spending, then why have rising health care costs been routinely evoked to demand the adoption of medical malpractice tort reform? The answer may lie with the perception perpetuated by insurance and health care provider lobbyists alike: that the practice of defensive medicine, as well as increased malpractice insurance premiums, is the direct result of increased medical malpractice litigation. Empirical evidence has shown, however, that malpractice insurance premiums are much less affected by medical malpractice litigation than commonly believed and that the costs of defensive medicine are often exaggerated.

Insurance Premiums

During the previously mentioned cycles of medical malpractice crises in the United States, malpractice insurance premiums have generally risen dramatically. Advocates of medical malpractice tort reform point to these premium increases as evidence that medical malpractice claims drive the rising cost of health care. While there is no question that rising insurance premiums place an additional financial burden on physicians seeking malpractice coverage, premium rates are not based solely, or even in large part, upon medical malpractice claim or settlement payouts (21). This is because most insurance companies' profits are not generated from the premiums they receive from their insured physicians (21). Most malpractice insurance carriers face a delay between the time they receive premium payments from their insured physicians and the time they have to pay out medical malpractice claims. Due to this delay, many insurance companies invest the premiums they receive in bonds or other financial securities (21). It is the return on these investments, not malpractice insurance premiums, that generates an insurance company's profits. Therefore, even if the number of malpractice claim payouts an insurance company makes is stable, the company may still be forced to raise premiums if their investments fail to yield adequate returns (21).

In addition, premiums do not only represent a malpractice insurer's indemnification costs. Malpractice insurance premiums represent a variety of costs assumed by an insurance company and passed on to their insured physicians. These costs may include a company's estimated indemnification costs, defense costs, operating fees, reinsurance costs, and profit or surplus building (22). Tort reform opponents argue that even with legislature in place to limit

jury awards or settlements in medical malpractice actions, rising insurance premiums would still be a financial hardship faced by the medical community, as the underwriting cycle and malpractice premiums are affected by much more than the threat of medical malpractice litigation.

Research performed in states that have enacted tort reform in the context of medical malpractice litigation also indicates that rising malpractice premiums are not tied to an influx of medical malpractice filings. In 1986, the state of Florida enacted medical malpractice tort reforms; however, despite this legislation, malpractice premiums in the state have increased on average from 30% to 50% since 2000 (23). In 2003, Florida, after a second bout of tort reform measures, experienced an increase in insurance premium rates by as much as 45% (23).

This empirical evidence challenging the connection between tort reform and malpractice premiums is not just limited to the state of Florida. In 1995, the state of Texas passed legislation limiting the amount of punitive damages available in jury awards (24). Despite this measure, insurance premiums in the state continued to increase. These statistics cast doubts on the claim that tort reform is the most effective way to manage skyrocketing malpractice premium rates and reduce overall health care costs.

Defensive Medicine: Real or Imagined?

Tort reform proponents also typically cite the rise of defensive medicine as the other major negative residual effect of medical malpractice litigation. Those favoring medical malpractice tort reform argue that litigation-weary physicians order unnecessary and exhaustive tests on their patients, which, in turn, drives up the cost of health care. Empirical evidence appears to suggest, however, that both the impact and the prevalence of defensive medicine have been overstated.

Much of the support for the proposition that the practice of defensive medicine is the costly offshoot of medical malpractice litigation comes from a controversial 1996 study conducted by two Stanford University economists, Daniel Kessler and Mark McClellan. In this study, the economists analyzed the costs of care for hospitalized elderly Medicare patients with heart disease in states both with and without medical malpractice tort reforms (25). Based on their findings, Kessler and McClellan concluded that tort reforms resulted in hospital costs savings of 5% to 9% (25). The economists then applied these findings to the entire health care system, hypothesizing that tort reform could lead to a reduction of over $50 billion annually in health care expenditures (25). Tort reform supporters used this study to buttress their claim that without the ever-looming fear of litigation, physicians are freer to order fewer diagnostic tests, which, in fact, reduces their medical spending and lowers overall health care costs.

While Kessler and McClellan's findings became vindication for advocates of medical malpractice tort reform, subsequent research has criticized many of the hypotheses contained within the study. In 2003, the U.S. Government Accountability Office (GAO) issued a statement questioning the applicability of Kessler and McClellan's findings to the entire health care system (26). The GAO's report argued that due to the limited scope of the study and its examination of patient behavior in the specific clinical situation of elderly patients with cardiac issues, "the study results cannot be generalized to estimate the extent and cost of defensive medicine practices across the health care system." (27) The report also concluded that while members of the medical community admitted that defensive medicine exists to some degree, the instance of its actual practice is extremely difficult to measure (27). This difficulty in quantifying the prevalence of defensive medicine in turn makes it more onerous to hypothesize any sort of costs savings for its reduction in practice.

More recent studies performed by the US government also reflect the tenuous connection between tort reform and its impact on the practice of defensive medicine. A 2004 study performed by the Congressional Budget Office (CBO) applied the methods employed by Kessler and McClellan's study to a wider set of medical ailments (26). It was concluded by the agency that there is no evidence linking restrictions on tort liability to reduced medical spending. A second analysis of the link between defensive medicine and health care costs performed by the CBO additionally confirmed no significant statistical difference in medical spending between states with and without medical malpractice tort limits (26).

One of the major reasons that medical malpractice tort reform has not definitively been found to effectively manage the practice of defensive medicine is because defensive medicine has been shown to be motivated by more than just a fear of litigation on physicians' parts. Some behavior that could be characterized as defensive medicine may be motivated more by the increased income additional diagnostic testing can generate for physicians, or the benefits a patient receives from additional testing, and less by fears of liability exposure (26). Additionally, it is unclear exactly how strongly concerns over medical malpractice liability actually affect a physician's treatment decisions. Physicians are highly educated professionals, who have to treat a patient's ailment based on myriad factors and considerations. To assume that all physicians require additional testing merely due to fears of liability exposure is unfounded.

Medical malpractice tort reform may also do little to curtail the practice of defensive medicine because empirical evidence seems to suggest that physicians typically have high levels of malpractice concern, in states both with, and without, tort reform. Research has shown that physicians in states with high malpractice risks have reported nearly the same level of concern over liability exposure as physicians in states with the low malpractice risks due to heightened medical malpractice tort reform (28). These results appear to be further evidence suggesting that tort reform in the context of medical malpractice may do little to assuage physicians' fears of liability or impact their diagnostic behavior in regard to the practice defensive medicine.

Risk Management

Although attempts to curtail medical malpractice litigation have been undertaken by many states with varying degrees of success, it is undisputed that this litigation has decreased over the last two decades. No matter the level of success in your state at instituting tort reform, however, medical malpractice litigation will never disappear entirely. As such, every solo practitioner or ENT practice group must focus its efforts at reducing risk by establishing a comprehensive risk management and compliance program to improve the safety and quality of the care that its physicians and employees provide. A key component of any program is the continuous assessment of quality management processes with a focus on implementing changes where necessary to ensure patient safety and the provision of high-quality and accurate medical care.

While specific areas of risk for otolaryngologists and how such risks can be minimized will be addressed later within this chapter, the structure of any risk management/ quality and performance improvement program will certainly vary depending on the size of your particular practice group. It is widely accepted that with varying degrees of focus, depending on the size and structure of the practice or group, any risk management program must include the implementation of processes to monitor performance, implement change, and meet regulatory requirements in the areas of patient safety, process improvement, quality, and professional staff education and assessment.

Importantly, although voluntarily implementing these quality-related programs in order to reduce exposure to allegations of medical malpractice is necessary for any ENT practice or group to succeed, many of these processes are required by the very organizations that regulate the otolaryngology profession—thus making such implementation of these programs mandatory.

For example, the American Board of Otolaryngology Maintenance of Certification (MOC) program is for diplomats who are working in their ten (10)-year cycle of maintaining their certification. Although the specific requirements of the competencies and components of each MOC program will depend on an ENT's particular practice area, the MOC program generally evaluates four (4) essential competencies on a continuous basis including (a) professional standing, (b) continuing education/ self-assessment, (c) cognitive examination, and (d) performance in practice (29). Evaluation of these competencies seeks to ensure that high standards of health care quality are maintained throughout the ENT practice as a whole, and these exacting quality requirements serve to minimize exposure to individual physicians from the overall risk of medical negligence claims. Other organizations with compliance and regulatory quality requirements include the Joint Commission on Accreditation of Healthcare Organizations and the Accreditation Council for Graduate Medical Education.

Thus, it is clear that every otolaryngology practice, department, or group must focus considerable effort and time in the development and maintenance of a comprehensive quality, risk management, and compliance program to improve patient safety and quality of care not only for the welfare of patients and to maintain a competitive edge but to reduce the ever-present risk of and exposure related to medical malpractice.

COMPLIANCE AND REGULATORY ISSUES

Introduction to Federal Health Care Fraud and Abuse Laws

It is unquestionable that billing and reimbursement have become integral parts of the practice of medicine. It is also unquestionable that few people would devote at least 9 years of their lives to become an otolaryngologist with the intent to cheat the federal government in their billing of medical claims. Various factors, such as greed or carelessness, may contribute to improper behavior by physicians during their careers, but ignorance of the law need not be one of those factors.

Although maintaining proper financial dealings with federal health care programs in the current health care environment is part of being a physician, medical schools and residency programs do not uniformly teach trainees about fraud and abuse. Indeed, in 2010, the Office of the Inspector General (OIG) surveyed all medical school deans and designated officials for institutions that sponsor residency and fellowship programs to determine whether their institutions provide education about fraud, waste, and abuse; to identify knowledge gaps; and to determine how the OIG could best promote education about compliance with the relevant laws. The survey revealed that less than half of the nation's medical schools provide instruction on fraud and abuse (30).

Violating the fraud and abuse laws can result in criminal penalties; civil fines; exclusion from the federal health care programs, which include Medicare and Medicaid; and even loss of your medical license by your State Medical Board. Thus, a good understanding of the five most important federal fraud and abuse laws that apply to physicians is essential.

Enforcement

Three federal government agencies are charged with enforcing the fraud and abuse laws: the Department of Justice, the Department of Health & Human Services Office of the Inspector General (OIG), and the Centers for Medicare & Medicaid Services (CMS). The five laws include the Physician Self-Referral Law (Stark Law), Antikickback Statute (AKS), the False Claims Act, the Exclusion Authorities, and the Civil Monetary Penalties Law.

Physician Self-Referral Law (Stark Law)

The Physician Self-Referral Law,[12] commonly referred to as the Stark Law, (a) prohibits a physician from making referrals of certain designated health services (DHS) payable by Medicare or Medicaid to an entity with which he or she (or an immediate family member) has a financial relationship (ownership or compensation) unless an exception applies[13] and (b) prohibits the entity from filing claims with Medicare or Medicaid (or billing another individual, entity, or third party payor) for those referred services, unless an exception applies. When originally enacted in 1989, the law applied only to physician referrals for clinical laboratory services. In 1993 and 1994, Congress expanded the prohibition to include additional DHS.

DHS now include (a) clinical laboratory services; (b) physical therapy, occupational therapy, and speech–language pathology services; (c) radiology and certain other imaging services; (d) radiation therapy services and supplies; (e) durable medical equipment and supplies; (f) parenteral and enteral nutrients, equipment, and supplies; (g) prosthetics, orthotics, and prosthetic devices and supplies; (h) home health services; (i) outpatient prescription drugs; and (j) inpatient and outpatient hospital services.

Significantly, the Stark Law is a strict liability law, which means that proof of specific intent to violate the law is not required. If Stark is triggered, and an exception is not met, a health care provider will be subject to severe sanctions, including denial of filing claims for those referred services, civil monetary penalties, exclusion from Medicare and Medicaid, and potential False Claims Act liability.

Antikickback Statute

The AKS[14] makes it a criminal offense to knowingly and willfully offer, pay, solicit, or receive any remuneration to induce or reward referrals of items or services reimbursable by a federal health care program. Where remuneration is paid purposefully to induce or reward referrals of items or services payable by a federal health care program, the AKS is violated. By its terms, the statute ascribes criminal liability to parties on both sides of an impermissible "kickback"

---

[12]42 U.S.C. §1395nn.

[13]Stark Law contains approximately 35 exceptions that describe acceptable financial relationships that allow a physician to refer to an entity for the provision of designated health services (42 CFR Part 411, Subpart J). Some commonly applied exceptions to the Stark Law include the exceptions for personal services, bona fide employment relationships, physician recruitment, and physicians practicing in rural areas and locations designated as Health Professional Shortage Areas. Each of the exceptions to the Stark Law has numerous elements that must be met in order to qualify for the exception, and care should be taken to assure compliance with each of these elements.

[14]42 U.S.C. §1320a-7b(b).

transaction. For purposes of the AKS, "remuneration" includes the transfer of anything of value directly or indirectly, overly or covertly, in cash or in kind.

The AKS has been interpreted to cover any arrangement where one purpose of the remuneration was to obtain money for the referral of services or to induce further referrals (31). With the passing of the Patient Protection and Affordable Care Act (PPACA)[15] on March 23, 2010, the AKS "intent" element was revised to remove any specific intent or actual knowledge of an AKS violation. Thus, one does not have to have "knowingly" and "willfully" violated the AKS to make the kickback actionable. Violation of the AKS constitutes a felony punishable by a maximum fine of $25,000, imprisonment up to 5 years, or both. Conviction will also lead to mandatory exclusion from federal health care programs, including Medicare and Medicaid. PPACA[16] also expanded the punishment for violation of the AKS Statute adding that any AKS violation is now a false claim under the False Claims Act, subjecting the provider to civil penalties.

Due to the breadth of the potential application of the AKS, the OIG was required to develop "safe harbor" regulations designed to protect various payment and business practices because such practices would be unlikely to result in fraud or abuse.[17] If an arrangement falls outside of the safe harbor, it is not *per se* illegal, but the facts and circumstances behind the arrangement must be carefully reviewed. The safe harbors set forth specific conditions that, if met, assure entities involved that they will not be prosecuted or sanctioned for the arrangement qualifying for the safe harbor. However, safe harbor protection is afforded only to those arrangements that precisely meet all of the conditions set forth in the safe harbor.

False Claims Act

False Claims Act violations occur when claims are submitted for payment to Medicare or Medicaid that are false or fraudulent. No specific intent to defraud is required. Filing false claims may result in civil penalties of not less than $5,500 and not more than $11,000 for each claim plus three times the programs' loss. Significantly, each instance of an item or a service billed to Medicare or Medicaid counts as a claim; thus, the potential fines can add up quickly. Moreover, a claim that results from a kickback or is made in violation of the Stark Law may also render it false or fraudulent, creating liability under the False Claims Act in addition to the AKS and the Stark Law.

The OIG may initiate administrative proceedings to impose civil monetary penalties and may also initiate administrative proceedings to exclude a party that files a false claim from the federal health care programs. There is also a criminal False Claims Act,[18] which imposes criminal penalties for submitting false claims including imprisonment and criminal fines.

Exclusion Statute[19]

The OIG is required to exclude from participation in all federal health care programs individuals and entities convicted of criminal offenses including (a) Medicare or Medicaid fraud, (b) patient abuse or neglect, and (c) felony convictions for health care–related fraud, theft, financial misconduct, unlawful manufacture, distribution, prescription, or dispensing of controlled substances. The OIG has discretion to exclude individuals and entities on several other grounds. In recent years, the OIG has been exercising its permissive exclusion power with much more frequency in order to combat health care fraud. As of January 2011, more than 5,000 physicians were excluded from participation in the federal health care programs because of these types of violations and cannot treat any of the approximately 100 million Medicare and Medicaid beneficiaries.[20]

Exclusion from participation in the federal health care programs is devastating to any career. The federal programs will not pay the provider for items or services furnished, ordered, or prescribed. As a result, providers may not bill Medicare or Medicaid directly for treating patients nor may their services be billed indirectly through their group practice. Moreover, once excluded from the federal health care programs, it is likely that other third party payors will follow suit, disallowing the excluded provider from submitting claims for reimbursement. As such, an excluded provider will be unemployable as the provider will be unable to receive payment for services rendered from the federal health programs. Unfortunately for such providers, it is impossible to hide from the reality of being excluded as the OIG maintains a List of Excluded Individuals and Entities on its Web site, which can be found at http://oig.hhs.gov/fraud/exclusions.asp.

Civil Monetary Penalties Law[21]

The Civil Monetary Penalties Law grants the OIG the authority to seek civil monetary penalties and, in some instances, exclusion, for a wide variety of conduct. Violations of the law includes violating AKS, presenting claims that the persons knows or should have known is for an item or service that was not provided as claimed or is false or fraudulent or for which payment may not be made. Penalties range from $10,000 to $50,000 per violation and, possibly, exclusion from the federal health programs.

[15]Section 6402(f)(2).
[16]Section 6402(f)(1).
[17]See 42 C.F.R. § 1001.952. Some safe harbors address personal services and rental agreements, investments in ambulatory surgical centers, and payments to *bona fide* employees.

[18]18 U.S.C. §287.
[19]42 U.S.C. §1320a-7.
[20]http://healthpolicyandreform.nejm.org/?p=13576.
[21]42 U.S.C. §1320a-7a.

Application of the Laws

Given that the health care environment has drastically changed over the years, physicians of all experience levels must understand the fraud and abuse laws and how they influence the way medicine is practiced. This is particularly true since physicians must understand that they are personally liable for claims submitted under their national provider identifiers regardless of whether or not they personally code or bill the services. Although a physician can certainly delegate such tasks from a business and administrative perspective, the physician continues to have a significant stake in ensuring compliance. Some physicians are surprised to learn that every CMS 1500 form that is submitted contains a certification statement wherein the physician personally attests that the services were medically necessary and that (absent an exception permitted under the regulations) he or she personally furnished the service.

The key to avoiding violations of the fraud and abuse laws is to have a clear understanding of how they shape and control the three "most common" relationships that physicians encounter in their careers: relationships with payors (like the Medicare and Medicaid programs), relationships with vendors (like drug, biologic, and medical device companies), and relationships with fellow providers (like hospitals, nursing homes, and physician colleagues).

Physician Relationships with Payors

Physicians need to develop and maintain systems in their practice to oversee that they are accurately coding and billing for services rendered to patients and diligently maintaining accurate and complete medical records and documentation to support the fact that the services billed for were necessary and have actually been provided. Physicians must also avoid the misuse of their physician and prescription provider numbers and understand the strict requirements of the Medicare reimbursement rules as a participating or nonparticipating provider. In addition to the fraud and abuse implications resulting from poor documentation practices, physicians should keep in mind that the primary reason for denial in postpayment audit cases (e.g., Medicare audits requesting refunds of alleged overpayments) typically relates to documentation deficiencies. Enhancement of documentation practices in any physician practice should unquestionably be a top priority.

Physician Relationships with Fellow Providers: Physicians, Hospitals, Nursing Homes, Etc.

Within these relationships, physicians must steer clear of any situation in which their decision-making with respect to patient referrals or use of products or services is based on anything other than what is medically necessary and appropriate for the patient. As most physicians have figured out by now, the fraud and abuse laws are complicated; however, physicians are held accountable for ensuring that relationships are structured in a compliant manner. Physicians

can avoid the pitfalls of improper arrangements by making sure that they appropriately consult with experts prior to entering into the relationship. Unfortunately, the fact that a physician was unaware of the implications of the fraud and abuse laws to the relationship is not a legitimate defense.

Physician Relationships with Vendors

A particular area of vulnerability for physicians involves relationships with pharmaceutical and medical device industries. Like physician relationships with fellow providers, physicians must steer clear of allowing the pharmaceutical or medical device industries from buying their loyalty or otherwise inducing them to prescribe or use products based on anything other than what is a medical necessity. The OIG offers some practical questions a physician should self-inquire to test the propriety of any proposed compensation relationship with these entities:

- Does the company really need my particular expertise or input?
- Does the amount of money the company is offering seem fair, appropriate, and commercially reasonable for what it is asking me to do?
- Is it possible the company is paying me for my loyalty so that I will prescribe its drugs or use its devices? (32).

Physicians can also review the OIG's Compliance Program Guidance for Pharmaceutical Manufacturers available at www.oig.hhs.gov/authorities/docs/03/050503FRCPGPharmac. pdf. Moreover, in protecting oneself in these relationships, one must keep in mind that under the PPACA,[22] transparency is coming in the form of requiring drug, device, and biologic companies to publicly report nearly all gifts or payments they make to physicians beginning in 2013.

Compliance Programs

Prior to PPACA, health care providers were encouraged but not required to maintain compliance programs to help ensure their compliance with fraud and abuse laws and federal health program requirements. Under PPACA, if you treat Medicare and Medicaid beneficiaries, you are required to establish a compliance program.[23] Seven

---

[22]Pub. L. 111-148 was signed into law on March 23, 2010.

[23]Section 6401(a). On February 2, 2011, the Centers for Medicare and Medicaid Services ("CMS") published its final rule for establishing new screening requirements for enrollees in Medicare, Medicaid, and the Children's Health Insurance Program ("CHIP") pursuant to Section 6401(a) of PPACA (the "Final Rule") (76 FR 5941). The Final Rule also addressed the compliance program requirement as set forth in Section 6401 of PPACA, which prescribes that, as a condition of enrolling in Medicare, Medicaid, or CHIP, providers and suppliers must establish compliance programs that meet certain "core elements." Notably, however, CMS did not finalize any rules related to mandatory compliance. Instead, CMS noted in the Final Rule that it would continue to do further rule making and would "advance specific proposals at some time in the future."

components to establishing a "solid" compliance program include (a) conducting internal monitoring and auditing, (b) implementing compliance and practice standards, (c) designating a compliance officer or contact, (d) conducting appropriate training and education, (e) responding appropriately to detected offenses and developing corrective action, (f) developing open lines of communication with employees, and (g) enforcing disciplinary standards through well-publicized guidelines.

Notwithstanding the PPACA mandates, in recognition of the increase in enforcement and audit activity, now, more than ever, it is imperative that every physician have in place an effective compliance program that is tailored to his/her particular practice and specialty.

THIRD PARTY PAYOR AUDITS

Third Party Payor Audit(s) Overview

Physicians submitting claims to all third party payors (i.e., Medicare, Medicaid, and private payors) must be cognizant that all claims are under unprecedented payor scrutiny. In an effort to protect the integrity of the Medicare and Medicaid Trust Funds, as well as the bottom line of private insurers, all payors are actively auditing claims. Health care providers must be mindful of this increased claims scrutiny and conduct themselves accordingly.

With respect to claims submitted to Medicare, not only do Medicare Administrative Contractors (MACs) (and/or Medicare Carriers and Intermediaries) conduct their own audits, but also the CMS contracts with various other entities to perform Medicare auditing functions. For example, Medicare's Recovery Audit Contractor (RAC) program is now operational nationwide (and has been expanded to include Part C and Part D claims). RAC auditors are tasked to identify and correct all types of improper Medicare payments and are compensated on a contingency fee basis. In addition, Zone Program Integrity Contractors (ZPICs) (or Program Safeguard Contractors ["PSCs"]) are actively conducting benefit integrity audits nationwide.

With respect to Medicaid claims, in addition to each state conducting their own Medicaid audits, there also exist federal Medicaid auditing programs. Under the Medicaid Integrity Program, Audit Medicaid Integrity Contractors (MICs) are auditing Medicaid claims in every state. The focus of the Audit MICs is on providers with "truly aberrant" claim submissions. In addition, the nationwide RAC program has been expanded to also include Medicaid claims.

Which Physicians Are Likely to Be Audited?

All auditors (Medicare, Medicaid, and private payors) use proprietary "data mining" techniques to determine claims likely to constitute overpayments and to identify providers with utilization patterns that may suggest overpayments

to be occurring. Therefore, physicians providing a high volume of higher-cost procedures, or physicians with a noticeable volume of high-level office visits (e.g., a high volume or level 4 or level 5 office visits), may find themselves under increased claims scrutiny. As noted elsewhere herein, through various guidance documents (e.g., the RAC-approved issues lists), CMS indicates claims likely to be subject to increased scrutiny under the Medicare and Medicaid programs. Physicians submitting these types of claims may see more auditing activity. Moreover, physicians should identify risk areas specific to his or her field of practice. These areas are often identified in specialty publications and can be found in third party payor guidances, local medical review policies, OIG guidances, fraud alerts, and the annual OIG work plan. One such area that has been a significant focus of the enforcement authorities and third party payors is E & M (or Evaluation and Management) services. In addition, physicians can discover their own personal practice risk areas by conducting self-audits focusing on, for example, the ten (10) most-often billed procedures and/or the ten (10) procedures yielding the highest practice revenue, looking at published policies and guidelines for these procedures, meeting with other providers in the physician's office and the billing staff, and discussing the documentation and billing of these procedures.

When conducting such audits, there are a number of significant items to consider. For example, (a) whether the audit should be prospective as opposed to retrospective, (b) whether the audit should be conducted for general educational purposes or for specific reasons (e.g., to quantify a suspected error), (c) whether one should use external auditors or internal auditors, (d) the sample size of the audit, (e) which documents to review, and (f) how often to perform the audit. Importantly, it is highly recommended that any self-audit be done at the direction of legal counsel—not only to help one decide the best manner in which to conduct the audit and to address the aforementioned items, but also to avoid providing a "road map" of any problems revealed by the audit to the enforcement authorities. Self-audits that are not directed by legal counsel are not protected by the attorney work product doctrine and/or attorney–client privilege and thus are discoverable by the enforcement authorities who can use the findings against the physician.

Typical Audit Processes for Medicare

Generally speaking, Medicare audits are conducted to determine whether claims are or were properly submitted to Medicare. When Medicare audits are conducted for medical review purposes, the contractor's focus is to determine whether services are covered, are reasonable and necessary, and are correctly coded. When Medicare audits are conducted for benefit integrity purposes, the focus is different (e.g., looking for possible falsification). Medicare audits may be conducted on either a prepayment or postpayment basis and may be conducted either on-site or via "desk audit."

When initiating either a prepayment review or postpayment audit for medical review purposes, a Medicare contractor is required to issue a written notification to the physician, which includes the following elements:

1. That the physician has been selected for prepayment review or postpayment audit and the reason for the selection. If the reason the physician was selected for audit was comparative data, then the Medicare contractor should provide the comparative data to the physician as part of this notification.
2. Whether the review will be conducted on a prepayment or postpayment basis
3. If postpayment audit, a list of claims requiring medical records to be produced (including the time frames for returning additional documentation—typically 30 to 45 days)

Note: It is essential that physicians adhere to the time frames for submitting requested documentation. If the time frames are not met, the Medicare contractor will deny the subject claims. The contractor thereafter may, but is not required to, reopen the claims upon appeal.

Generally speaking, prepayment review(s) or postpayment audit(s) is conducted within 60 days from receipt of requested medical records.[24] When reviewing claims, the Medicare contractor will use both published Medicare guidance (e.g., National Coverage Decisions (NCDs), Local Coverage Decisions (LCDs), CMS Manuals, CMS Coding Articles, etc.), and internal review guidelines. In a postpayment audit, following the review, the Medicare contractor will prepare a letter to notify the physician regarding the results of the audit, including the rationales for denials and information regarding the statistical extrapolation performed, if applicable. The physician also will receive a demand letter, which triggers relevant appeal deadlines. Prepayment review results will be communicated via Remittance Advice.[25]

The Medicare Appeals Process

Part A and Part B Medicare claim denials arising from Medicare audits are subject to the five-stage appeals process set forth at 42 C.F.R. Part 405, Subpart I. It is essential from a business perspective that physicians understand this appeals process and appeal claim denials as they occur. Denials may be successfully overturned in the Medicare appeals process, resulting in monies returned to the physician. The five-stage appeals process is as follows:

1. *Stage 1: Redetermination.* The first level in the appeals process is redetermination. There is no amount in controversy requirement. Providers must submit redetermination requests in writing within 120 calendar days of receiving notice of initial determination.

   Significantly, federal law prohibits Medicare from recouping an alleged overpayment during the first two stages of the appeals process (i.e., during the redetermination and reconsideration stages of appeal). Although federal regulations grant physicians 120 calendar days to file a request for redetermination, Medicare will begin recouping the alleged overpayment arising from a Medicare audit prior to the expiration of the 120-day appeals time frame if a valid request for redetermination is not first received. Specifically, recoupment will begin on the 41st day from the date of the notice of initial determination, unless a valid request for redetermination is received 30 days following the date of notice of initial determination. If this time frame is not met, Medicare will stop recoupment at whatever point an appeal is received, but it will not refund any amounts withheld prior to that time.

2. *Stage 2: Reconsideration.* Physicians dissatisfied with a redetermination decision may file a request for reconsideration to be conducted by a Qualified Independent Contractor (QIC). A QIC is a Medicare contractor tasked to complete this second level of appeal (reconsideration level of appeal). There is no amount in controversy requirement. This second level of appeal must be filed within 180 calendar days of receiving notice of the redetermination decision.

   Although federal regulations grant physicians 180 calendar days to file a request for reconsideration, Medicare will again begin recouping its alleged overpayment following the redetermination stage prior to the expiration of the 180-day appeals time frame if a valid request for reconsideration is not first received. Specifically, recoupment may begin on the 61st day from the date of redetermination decision, unless a valid request for reconsideration is received. If this time frame is not met, Medicare will stop recoupment at whatever point an appeal is received.

   Significantly, physicians must submit a "full and early presentation of evidence" in the reconsideration stage. When filing a reconsideration request, a physician must present evidence and allegations related to the dispute and explain the reasons for the disagreement with the initial determination and redetermination. Absent good cause, failure of a physician to submit evidence prior to the issuance of the notice of reconsideration precludes subsequent consideration of the evidence. Accordingly, physicians may be prohibited from introducing evidence in later stages of the appeals process if such evidence is not presented at the reconsideration stage.

---

[24]This 60-day time period does not apply to reviews for benefit integrity purposes (PSC or ZPIC audits).
[25]*See generally*, Medicare Program Integrity Manual (CMS Pub. 100-08), Chapter 3, Section 30.4 *et seq.*

3. *Stage 3: Administrative Law Judge (ALJ) Hearing.* A provider dissatisfied with a reconsideration decision may request an ALJ hearing. The request must be filed within 60 days following receipt of the QIC's decision and must meet an amount in controversy requirement. ALJ hearings can be conducted by video teleconference (VTC), in person, or by telephone. The regulations require the hearing to be conducted by VTC if the technology is available; however, if VTC is unavailable or in other extraordinary circumstances, the ALJ may hold an in-person hearing. Additionally, the ALJ may offer a telephone hearing.

4. *Stage 4: Medicare Appeals Council (MAC) Review.* The fourth level of appeal is the Medicare Appeals Council (MAC) Review. The MAC is within the Departmental Appeals Board of HHS. A MAC Review request must be filed within 60 days following receipt of the ALJ's decision. Among other requirements, a request for MAC Review must identify and explain the parts of the ALJ action with which the party disagrees. Unless the request is from an unrepresented beneficiary, the MAC will limit its review to the issues raised in the written request for review.

5. *Stage 5: Federal District Court.* The final step in the appeals process is judicial review in federal district court. A request for review in district court must be filed within 60 days of receipt of the MAC's decision and meet an amount in controversy requirement.

Audit Defenses

In preparing a Medicare appeal, physicians should both challenge the merits of the claim denials and employ applicable legal defenses. In arguing the merits, physicians should prepare a position paper and/or a summary of the documentation relevant to the claims at issue, setting forth the justification for the services as billed. Attached to the position paper should be all records supporting the claims at issue, organized in a user-friendly manner. Note that this likely will involve more records than just the records for the specific dates of service denied. For example, if a procedure is denied, the submitted documentation should include any office visit preceding the procedure supporting the medical necessity for the procedure. In arguing the merits of the claim, physicians should engage the services of a qualified medical/coding/statistical expert, as applicable. In addition to arguing the merits, physicians may choose to employ the following legal defenses, as applicable:

1. *Provider without Fault:* As a general rule, a provider will be considered without fault if it exercised reasonable care in billing for and accepting payment (i.e., it complied with all pertinent regulations, made full disclosure of material facts, and, on the basis of the information available, had a reasonable basis for assuming

that the payment was correct). A provider or supplier will be presumed to be without fault if an overpayment is discovered subsequent to the third year following initial determination.[26]

2. *Waiver of Liability:* In the event a Medicare contractor denies a service as not medically reasonable and/or necessary, the denial constitutes a denial under Section 1862 (a) of the Social Security Act, subjecting the claims to waiver of liability consideration. The statutory authority for the application of Waiver of Liability is set forth in Section 1879 (a) of the Social Security Act. Generally speaking, once waiver of liability applies, the relevant inquiry focuses on whether the provider or supplier knew or could have reasonably been expected to know that payment would not have been made for the services.

3. *Treating Physician's Rule:* The legal theory of the Treating Physician's Rule provides that the treating physician's determination that a service is medically necessary and appropriate should predominate over a reviewer's determination.

4. *Challenges to Statistics:* Providers may also legally challenge the statistics in connection with extrapolated audits. This will involve the retention of a qualified statistical expert to review the statistical sample and extrapolation performed for compliance with Medicare guidelines. Challenging the statistical extrapolation performed (which, if successful, would bring the overpayment demand to the "actual" overpayment, rather than the projected overpayment) should be a key focus of any appeal where a statistical extrapolation is performed.[27]

Compliance Tips

Although physicians may not be able to prevent a Medicare audit from occurring, physicians should prepare for increased claims scrutiny and audit activity by dedicating resources to the following:

1. Regularly *monitoring* guidance documents educating physicians regarding the types of claims subject to increased Medicare claims scrutiny, including historical audit data (such as the review results arising from the RAC Demonstration Program), the RACs' Web sites identifying approved audit issues (links available from www.cms.hhs.gov/RAC), the OIG Work Plan, etc.

   Note that the RAC demonstration program did not focus on ENT physicians specifically; thus, a review of the RAC demonstration results is not particularly helpful for ENT physicians with the exception of vestibular

---

[26]Section 1870 of the Social Security Act. *See also* Medicare Financial Management Manual, CMS 100-06, Chapter 3, Section 70 *et seq.*
[27]*See* Section 1893 of the Social Security Act and Medicare Program Integrity Manual, CMS Pub. 100-08, Chapter 3, Section 3.10 *et seq.*

function testing.[28] As of the date of publication of this chapter, the RACs' Web sites did include certain ENT physician-specific issues presently under RAC review (e.g., the RACs are presently reviewing certain E & M issues). These Web sites should be continuously monitored as Medicare approves additional areas for RAC review. A review of other guidance documents, such as the OIG Work Plan, will be helpful to identify areas that may be subject to scrutiny. For example, the 2011 OIG Work Plan states that payments for E & M services will be subject to scrutiny in 2011.

2. *Reviewing* and educating physicians regarding any Medicare NCDs and LCDs applicable to claims submitted by the physicians

3. *Designating* an audit "point person" responsible to monitor communications from Medicare and its contractors, which will include monitoring records requests and ensuring that such requests are responded to within the requisite time frames

4. *Implementing* compliance efforts, including but not limited to (a) educating staff members regarding the potential business impact of Medicare audits and the corresponding importance of compliance and appropriate response to records requests and claim determinations and (b) performing documentation and coding education. Documentation and coding education may entail engaging a qualified health care legal professional and coding professional to conduct a formal compliance audit of high-risk claims.

5. *Tracking* claim denials, monitoring and abiding by appeal deadlines, and properly working up appeals to challenge denials in the appeals process

PHYSICIAN LICENSING ACTIONS AND THEIR COLLATERAL EFFECTS

Introduction

Whether an otolaryngologist is a medical doctor or an osteopath, his or her ability to practice in any given state within the United States (other than at a federal institution such as a VA hospital) is governed by the laws of that state. While some states allow a physician who is not licensed in their particular state, but who is licensed in another state in good standing, to practice in their state under certain special circumstances (e.g., in an educational setting or in emergency circumstances), the far majority of the time a physician must be compliant with the laws, rules, and regulations of each state in which the physician practices.

Physicians will be deemed to have constructive knowledge of such laws, rules, and regulations regardless of whether he or she has actual knowledge thereof. As such, it is imperative for a physician seeking licensure in a given state to become familiar with that state's governing laws, rules, and regulations, especially since there are some significant differences (e.g., in some states there are express prohibitions against prescribing medication to family members regardless of the circumstances, whereas in other states, such prescribing is allowed as long as the physician determines that he or she can maintain objectivity when treating the patient). Typically, states have boards of medicine that promulgate administrative rules and guidance to which physicians should adhere, in addition to public health codes and other statutory and case law, in order to avoid disciplinary action taken against a physician's license. Some states have one board of medicine that governs both medical doctors and osteopaths while other states have separate boards for each—although the rules and guidance for medical doctors often mirror those for osteopaths. These medical boards are administrative agencies often composed of not just physicians but other health care providers and members of the public appointed by state executive officials (such as the governor) and serve to govern the medical profession and help to protect the health, safety, and welfare of the public.

The bases for disciplinary action are often codified by statutory law in each state and are enforced by the state's medical board. Some bases may be very specific (e.g., violation of a particular state statute regarding prescribing a medication for an illegitimate, nontherapeutic purpose), while other bases are rather broad (e.g., acting outside the applicable standard of practice). An important distinction for physicians to keep in mind is the difference between a licensing action and a medical malpractice action. In a medical malpractice action, the physician's actions or omissions must cause damages for liability to arise. In a licensing action, causing damages is not a requisite element. As such, a physician may find himself/herself subject to a licensing action for failing to document information where the applicable standard of practice requires such documentation in the medical record even though the lack of documentation did not result in any harm to a patient.

How Licensure Actions Arise

An action against a physician's license typically arises from a complaint filed with the state medical board by a person or entity with firsthand knowledge of alleged wrongdoing by the physician (e.g., a patient, employee, or employer of the physician). Some states allow for completely anonymous complaints while others require the complainant to identify himself or herself in order to commence an investigation. In some scenarios, the complainant is the court clerk who under legal authority is required to report to the medical board when a physician is convicted of a crime

---

[28]The majority of physician claim denials made during the RAC demonstration program involved pharmaceutical injectables, Neulasta (incorrect coding), Vestibular function testing, and duplicate claims. See "The Medicare Recovery Audit Contractor (RAC) Program: An Evaluation of the 3-Year Demonstration," *available at* http://www.cms.gov/RAC/Downloads/RACEvaluationReport.pdf.

or an alcohol- or drug-related offense. In some states, the complainant may be the physician's medical malpractice defense attorney who is required to report to the medical board a verdict or settlement against the physician in a medical malpractice action. The complainant may be a hospital where the physician had his or her medical staff privileges reduced, limited, suspended, or revoked or employment terminated. The physician himself or herself may even be the complainant as, in nearly every state, the physician has a duty to self-report a disciplinary action or criminal conviction against the physician in another state within a certain prescribed time frame (e.g., 30 days from the date of the final order or conviction).

Typical allegations asserted against a physician are for quality of care concerns, a scope-of-practice concern issue or the conduct of the physician—which may include potential criminal conduct (e.g., a patient who is billed for services that he or she never received may submit a written allegation against the physician to the applicable state medical board). After receiving an allegation, the medical board typically reviews it and determines whether the alleged facts, if true, could be deemed a violation of the state's public health code or other statutory laws or case law and thereby warrant an investigation.

An investigation into an allegation usually involves interviewing the person filing the allegation, interviewing the physician, identifying and interviewing other persons such as coworkers or employers who may provide relevant information, and collecting other evidence.

Administrative Complaint and Hearing

If the medical board determines that there is sufficient evidence to demonstrate a violation of the applicable public health code or law, a formal administrative complaint is typically filed by the state against the physician (often called the "licensee" in such matters) charging the physician with specific statutory violations or other violations of the law.

Nearly every state also provides the medical board with grounds for the issuance of an administrative complaint for numerous preceding criminal violations. For example, a conviction of any criminal sexual conduct; reckless or intentional inappropriate destruction or alteration of medical records; a misdemeanor or felony involving fraud to obtain professional fees; a misdemeanor related to the ability to practice safely/competently; and practicing under the influence of alcohol or drugs in many states provides a basis for a licensing action against the convicted physician.

Since the state medical board is charged with protecting the health, safety, and welfare of its citizens, if the medical board believes that there could be an immediate risk to the public health, safety, or welfare, it may order a summary suspension of the physician's license until an administrative hearing is held. Under such circumstances, the physician must immediately cease practicing medicine even before he or she is given an opportunity to defend his or her actions and cannot practice medicine until otherwise authorized to do so by the medical board. Summary suspension typically occurs where the physician is convicted of a felony or a misdemeanor involving the illegal delivery, possession, or use of a controlled substance.

The procedures to be followed after the issuance of an administrative complaint differ from state to state; however, they typically require the physician to file an answer to the administrative complaint and provide the licensee an opportunity to meet with members of the medical board to attempt to reach a resolution of the administrative complaint short of attending a formal administrative hearing. These procedures usually have specific deadlines associated with answering the administrative complaints, requesting and attending settlement conferences and other procedures for which failure to comply can have severe adverse consequence for the physician (e.g., failing to timely answer an administrative complaint in some states results in all of the allegations being deemed admitted and the matter goes straight to the medical board for imposition of sanctions against the physician). Proposed settlements usually require formal approval by the medical board and are typically available to the public.

If a settlement cannot be reached, the matter proceeds to an administrative hearing to be conducted in accordance with established state administrative procedures and rules governing the conduct of the hearing, introduction of evidence, and the examination of witnesses. The purpose of the hearing is to determine the facts of the case and the laws and rules that should be applied to the case. Should the physician be found to have violated the applicable state laws, sanctions will be imposed upon the physician and/or his or her license, which can include a monetary fine, probation, reprimand, restriction on the license, additional medical education beyond the standard requirements for continuing medical education, community service, and/or suspension or revocation of the license.

Licensing Actions May Lead to Criminal Prosecution

While state public health codes have numerous grounds upon which the medical boards may rely for the issuance of an administrative complaint, some provisions are more apt to lead to criminal prosecution, for example, allegations of an inappropriate sexual relationship with a patient, a pattern of providing controlled substances without medical necessity, a pattern of fraudulent billing, and a pattern of performing medically unnecessary procedures for personal financial gain. All of these offenses typically fall within express provisions of state public health codes giving rise to a licensing action and also fall within the ambit of numerous state and federal criminal statutes, thereby leaving the physician exposed to potential criminal prosecution.

Furthermore, it is important to understand that some actions by physicians subsequent to being served with an Administrative Complaint may also lead to criminal prosecution. One common allegation contained within an administrative complaint is that the physician violated his or her general duty due to inadequate, insufficient and/or missing documentation. Such an allegation can lead a concerned physician to attempt to "correct" the situation by creating records where none existed or supplementing the records to address the alleged inadequacy or insufficiency without including sufficient information to make it clear when these new records were added. Such action by a physician is typically a felony under state statutory law.

When defending a health care licensing matter, it is important to always consider the possibility of criminal exposure for the subject physician. Such consideration is integral to the decision of whether to have the physician testify at an administrative hearing. Physicians have to weigh the risk of asserting their Fifth Amendment rights against self-incrimination in order to avoid having admissions made during administrative proceedings that could be used against them in a criminal matter.

A physician facing a health care investigation or an administrative action by a state medical board cannot afford to take a myopic view of his or her predicament. Due to the criminal implications and the domino effect that often accompanies the imposition of state-imposed sanctions, such physician are well advised to obtain experienced health care counsel as early as possible in the process who will take an expansive view of the matter in order to assess the collateral damage that could result from a proposed settlement of a state action. Although most attorneys are knowledgeable enough to inform their clients of their Fifth Amendment rights against self-incrimination in order to avoid having their clients make any admissions during the administrative proceedings, which could lead to criminal charges, many attorneys are unaware of the effects that collateral sanctions may have on their clients. Any settlement strategy should take into consideration all of the collateral sanctions and enforcement actions that could arise as a result of a settlement.

Collateral Effects of a Licensing Action Other Than Criminal Prosecution

In addition to the aforementioned potential for criminal prosecution, there are numerous consequences and collateral effects that a licensing action may have on a physician. Any sanctions imposed upon the physician are typically published online and in the state's disciplinary action report, and notice of the sanctions is sent to numerous state and federal authorities (which, for physicians, may include the National Practitioner Data Bank), along with applicable professional associations, and various national and local news associations (e.g., the Associated Press and the United Press International). The severity of the sanction imposed by the state medical board will determine the extent of the collateral damage to the physician. The following is a list of some, but not all, of the repercussions that a sanctioned physician may encounter: loss of hospital privileges, loss of participation and enrollment with state professional associations, loss of participation in preferred provider organizations (PPOs), loss of enrollment with third party payors, loss of DEA registration, loss of board certification, and exclusion from participation with Medicare, Medicaid, and other federal and state government programs.

As noted above, nearly every state requires a physician who is disciplined in another state to report such discipline to their state. Thereafter, such state has the right to file its own disciplinary action against the physician even though all of the facts and circumstances that gave rise to the original disciplinary action took place in the other state. As a result, the derivative state may impose even a harsher sanction against the physician than the sanction imposed by the originating state depending upon the laws, policies, politics, and mind-set of the derivative state.

Conclusion

Unfortunately, some physicians fail to appreciate the serious magnitude of an allegation filed against them with their state licensing body. Whether a physician is contacted directly by an investigator or whether he or she hears from a patient or an employee that an investigator has been asking questions regarding the professional behavior/conduct of the physician, the physician should immediately contact an experienced and knowledgeable health care attorney to provide assistance and guidance at the earliest possible stage. All too often, physicians believe that they can explain away or justify the alleged inappropriate behavior/conduct only to learn later on that such admissions are used as direct evidence against them to support a sanction against his or her health care license. Moreover, depending on the severity of the sanction imposed, there are numerous collateral effects that a state licensing action may have on the physician, including, but not limited to

1. Loss of hospital privileges and/or employment
2. Loss of enrollment with state professional associations and their associated benefits (e.g., health, disability, and life insurance)
3. Loss of participation in PPOs and other third party payors
4. Loss of DEA registration, state-controlled substance licenses, and other health care licenses/registrations
5. Loss of board certification
6. Exclusion from participation with Medicare, Medicaid, and other federal and state governmental programs
7. Commencement of other judicial or administrative proceedings (e.g., criminal proceedings, civil monetary proceedings, malpractice actions, and other state licensing actions)
8. Permanent reports to the National Practitioner Data Bank and state licensing data banks

Prior to the commencement of a formal hearing, there is often a window of opportunity in which an experienced and knowledgeable health care attorney can help the physician to develop and implement prophylactic measures and to take certain actions that may convince the licensing authorities not to proceed with disciplinary action or to accept a sanction less severe than originally recommended. Due to this relatively small time frame, it is imperative that the physician contact an attorney at the earliest recognizable stage of a potential licensing matter. As Benjamin Franklin once said: "an ounce of prevention is worth a pound of cure"—a physician that retains an experienced and knowledgeable health care attorney early in the process can often avoid the increased time and financial resources involved in trying to win a licensure case at an administrative hearing, when compared to resources needed to implement reasonable measures to rectify the alleged inappropriate behavior/conduct.

SETTING UP A PHYSICIAN PRACTICE

Introduction

Physicians very rarely graduate from medical school knowing how to successfully run a business. And a physician practice is just that: a business. Fortunately, physicians are often successful in organizing and operating their own medical practices, especially when they rely upon a team of qualified and experienced professionals, such as accountants, financial advisors, attorneys, billing companies, and third party payor enrollment consultants.

As discussed further below, from a corporate perspective, organization of a new business generally involves several steps, including each of the following:

a. Establishing the business entity (typically through a state-level filing of Articles of Incorporation, Certificates of Incorporation, Articles of Organization, or other equivalent document, as appropriate)
b. Applying to the Internal Revenue Service (IRS) for a federal tax identification number (EIN)
c. Protecting the name and other intellectual property of the practice, as appropriate
d. Negotiating and adopting governing documents (Bylaws, Shareholders' Agreement, Operating Agreement, Buy-Sell Agreement, etc.)
e. Adopting initial corporate resolutions to ratify the organization of the entity; adopting the governing documents; electing directors, managers, and officers, as the case may be; authorizing the establishment of a bank account; etc.
f. Enrolling in Medicare and other third party payors
g. Opening bank accounts and obtaining necessary insurance

Physicians who refrain from obtaining the valuable guidance of legal, financial, and reimbursement professionals in order to limit the associated costs often eventually incur unnecessary (and sometimes substantial) expenses to correct problems that would have been avoidable had the practice adopted a more conscientious approach to its organization. Examples of the unfortunate circumstances that sometimes face practices that have acted in an uninformed and/or careless manner include the following:

a. Failure to officially organize the business entity or provision of incorrect information when applying for an EIN, resulting in delay in receiving Medicare billing numbers and lost revenue
b. Disregard for corporate practice of medicine doctrines, if applicable, eventually requiring the practice to restructure
c. Misunderstanding of the nature of, and the benefits offered by, the form of business entity resulting in the physician entering agreements with hospitals and others in the physician's individual capacity instead of through the business, which can lead to unanticipated adverse tax consequences
d. Lack of appreciation for the importance of maintaining corporate formalities (such as holding annual meetings, adopting corporate resolutions, maintaining corporate records and minutes, etc.), which makes it more likely that creditors will attempt to impose personal liability upon the owners of an entity who otherwise have the protection of limited liability (often referred to as "piercing the corporate veil")

The purpose of this section is to provide a broad overview of certain considerations with respect to the organization of a new physician practice. As discussed above, it is highly advisable for physicians to engage professional advisors who are able to position the new practice for success. Nothing set forth below is a substitute for such guidance.

Choice and Formation of Business Entity

The form of a business entity, the relationship of such business entity to its owner(s) and creditors, and its operations are governed, at least in part, by the state in which the business is organized and the states in which the business operates.

Each state has its own specific statutes, regulations, and other guidance with respect to the various corporate forms recognized by such state. Most states publish an abundance of helpful information on their Web sites that explain the pros and cons of choosing one form of entity over another and the process for organizing such entity. State publications on these topics are often geared toward small businesses and include references to other related legal requirements, including those pertaining to taxes, licenses, and securities requirements. Although it is common for business entities to organize themselves in states other than those in which they operate (e.g., in the State of Delaware because of the favorable and well-developed corporate laws in such jurisdiction), physician practices are generally organized in the same state in which they operate due to their relatively limited size and their heavily regulated nature.

A brief overview of certain common forms of business entities follow below. Although such descriptions are generally true, each state has its own unique requirements, and physicians should work with their legal and financial advisors with state-specific knowledge when making a final determination regarding choice of entity.

Sole Proprietorship

A sole proprietorship is a form of entity that is owned by one person who generally owns all of the assets of the business and is personally liable for the debts of the business. Because a sole proprietorship is not a business entity that is distinct from its owner, a sole proprietorship cannot continue beyond the life of the owner. Sole proprietorships generally do not need to file documents at the state level to form their business; however, they sometimes need to file their name and other information in the counties in which they operate. For the reasons just stated and others, it is rarely advisable for a physician to form a physician practice as a sole proprietorship.

Partnerships

Many states recognize at least two types of partnerships: (a) general partnerships and (b) limited partnerships.

General Partnerships

A general partnership is a form of entity that is owned by at least two people. All of the owners are personally liable for the debts of the business. All profits and losses of a partnership generally flow through to the partners for tax purposes. Partners often enter into a written partnership agreement to govern their relations. Typically no state-level filing is required to form a partnership, but partnerships sometimes need to file their name and other information in the counties in which they operate. Similar to sole proprietorships, it is typically inadvisable for a physician to form a physician practice as a partnership.

Limited Partnerships

A limited partnership is a form of entity that is owned by at least two people, at least one of which is a general partner who has personal liability for partnership debts and has the majority of management rights. Limited partnerships are typically distinct from general partnerships in that limited partnerships are generally created by filing documents at the state level and offer limited liability to some of its investors. Today, it is not common for physician practices to be formed as limited partnerships because of the lack of flexibility offered by most state limited partnership laws.

Nonprofit Corporation

Although rare, physician practices can be formed as nonprofit corporations, which are formed through state-level filings typically referred to as Articles of Incorporation. Depending upon the specific state law, nonprofit corporations may be formed on a stock, membership, or directorship basis for any lawful purpose not involving pecuniary gain or profit for its officers, directors, shareholders, or members. It is important to note that not all nonprofit corporations are federally tax-exempt organizations. Although many health care organizations are exempt from federal income tax under 501(a) of the Internal Revenue Code, such tax-exempt status is generally only available when all applicable requirements are satisfied and the entity submits an Application for Recognition of Exemption to the IRS.

Corporations

Profit corporations are generally formed by submitting a state-level filing for the purpose of generating profit for their owners, who are referred to as shareholders. The internal affairs of a corporation and the relationships among the shareholders are often governed by the corporation's Bylaws, Shareholders' Agreement, and Buy–Sell Agreement, as applicable. Such document filed with the state is usually referred to as the corporation's Articles of Incorporation or Certificate of Incorporation. Most corporations are governed by three layers of management: shareholders, directors, and officers. Shareholders, directors, and officers are generally not liable for the corporation's obligations unless they sign a personal guarantee or enter a contract in their individual capacity on behalf of the corporation. A corporation can exist indefinitely and its existence is not affected by the death of a shareholder. Except in the case of an S Corporation as described below, a corporation is taxed separate from its owners.

S Corporation

An S Corporation is a profit corporation that elects "S Corporation" status for federal tax purposes by filing Form 2553 (Election by a Small Business Corporation) with the IRS. S Corporations are distinct from other general profit corporations in that the profits and losses of the S Corporation flow through to the shareholders, who report the S Corporation's income and losses on their personal tax returns. There are several requirements that a corporation must satisfy in order to be eligible for S Corporation status, including, without limitation, the following: (a) be organized as a domestic corporation, (b) have only allowable shareholders (i.e., no partnerships, corporations, or nonresident alien shareholders as shareholders), (c) have no more than one hundred shareholders, and (d) have only one class of stock.

Limited Liability Company

Limited liability companies (LLCs) are created through state-level filings, which are generally referred to as an LLC's Articles of Organization. LLCs are sometimes managed by their owners, referred to as members. In other cases, LLCs are managed by a manager or group of managers (i.e., a Board of Managers), but the members continue to have ultimate authority over certain major decisions pertaining to the LLC. In addition to the Articles of Organization or equivalent document, the internal affairs of a company and the relationships among the members are often governed by the company's Operating Agreement, as applicable. Members are generally not liable for the obligations of their LLC unless they sign a personal guarantee or enter a contract in their individual capacity on behalf of the company. For purposes of federal income tax, LLCs are taxed as sole proprietorships, partnerships, corporations, or S Corporations depending upon the number of members and the elections made by the LLC. An LLC can exist indefinitely and its existence is not affected by the death of a member.

Professional Service Entities

Many states either require or permit business entities that provide professional services such as medicine to be organized as a professional corporation, professional limited liability company, or other professional entity and be owned exclusively by licensed professionals who are legally authorized to provide such professional service. These requirements are typically set forth in the corporate statutory laws of such states.

Corporate Practice of Medicine

Many states prohibit a business entity from practicing medicine or employing a physician to provide medical services (often referred to as the "corporate practice of medicine") unless an exception applies. The state corporate practice of medicine prohibitions and exceptions is set forth in state statutes, regulations, case law, and attorney general opinions. Such prohibitions are intended to protect physician decision making and prevent a physician's loyalty from being divided between the needs of a corporation and the needs of the patient. States generally limit application of the corporate practice of medicine doctrine through certain exceptions, including those created for hospitals and other licensed health care facilities and also professional business entities such as professional corporations and professional LLCs. States often adopt these exceptions because the entities covered by the exception are either licensed themselves or owned by licensed physicians, and therefore, applying the corporate practice of medicine to such businesses is not necessary to advance the underlying purpose of the doctrine.

Name Protection

Physician practices, like most businesses, have an interest in protecting their identity and reputation. For those business entities that are formed through state-level filings, the applicable state will generally only accept the filing if the name of the business entity is distinguishable from other active names on the business records of the state. For many small physician practices, the level of protection offered by state corporate laws with respect to a corporate name is sufficient. However, business entity's that are more concerned about protecting their corporate names can register their name as a trade mark or service mark. Additional information regarding this process can be found at http://www.uspto.gov/smallbusiness/trademarks/.

Securing a Business Loan

Newly formed physician practices require capital to procure the resources required to commence operations (e.g., office space, office and medical equipment, IT/EHR software and hardware, furnishings, supplies, payroll, insurance premiums, legal and other professional expenses, etc.), and such capital may be obtained in several different ways. First, practice owners (usually referred to as the partners, members, or shareholders depending upon the form of business entity selected) often contribute capital or loan money to the business. Yet most physicians are unable to independently provide all of the necessary financing. Second, the initial financial burden of commencing the practice operations can be mitigated if the practice leases the items, or obtains financing from the vendor, instead of purchasing the items immediately in cash. Third, it is also important to note that federal law, including the federal Stark Law and Antikickback Law, permits hospitals to provide certain financial support and income guarantees to physicians that relocate and establish a practice within the geographic area served by a hospital when certain requirements are satisfied. Such support is most prevalent in underserved areas. Fourth, in the event that the options just described are insufficient, traditional third party financing is an attractive option. The legal and financial advisors to the practice often have strong relationships with banks and finance companies and can therefore recommend those that provide competitive interest rates on fair terms. However, it is important to understand that most lenders will require personal guarantees or other security interests necessary to sufficiently protect them if the practice defaults on the loan.

Securing Insurance

It is highly advisable for physician practices to acquire insurance coverage that is appropriate for the size and nature of the practice's business. Such insurance policies may include, without limitation, the following:

a. Commercial liability
b. Auto
c. Employment practices
d. Professional liability
e. Errors and omissions
f. Directors and officers
g. Premises liability
h. Personal property
i. Workers' compensation
j. Key-Man life
k. Health, disability, long-term care, etc.

Before contacting insurance agents to obtain information and quotes for coverage, physician practices should understand their insurance needs. For example, the practice should consider the following terms: coverage limits, naming additional insureds, whether the insurance should be on a claims-made or occurrence basis, who needs to be covered (i.e., employees, volunteers, etc.), etc. Practices also need to be cognizant of those insurance requirements imposed upon the practice by applicable state law (e.g., pertaining to workers' compensation insurance and often professional liability insurance) and those insurance requirements imposed upon the practice by contract (e.g., office space and equipment leases, employment and independent contractor agreements, agreements with hospitals, third party payors, etc.).

Obtaining a Federal Tax Identification Number

After a new business entity is officially organized (through the filing of Articles of Incorporation, Certificate of Incorporation, Articles of Organization, or otherwise), the next priority is generally to file for a federal employer identification number (often referred to as a TIN or an EIN). Additional information regarding federal tax identification numbers and the process for applying for such number can be found at http://www.irs.gov/businesses/small/. Irrespective of whether the application is submitted online, by telephone, by fax, or by mail, applicants must be very careful to complete the forms in a diligent manner to ensure that all information provided is complete and correct to avoid subsequent problems from arising. Physician practices should maintain a copy of the application and all related documentation, including IRS Form CP575 (which provides verification of the EIN), as it will often be required to open a bank account and apply for a Medicare provider number. Further, it is advisable for physician practices to work closely with their financial advisors in this regard to ensure that the S election, if applicable, and other related filings are timely filed.

Enrolling with Third Party Payors

In order for a physician practice to operate and thrive, it will be necessary for the practice to effectively and efficiently obtain reimbursement for its services. Therefore, enrollment with Medicare and other third party payors is an important part of organizing a physician practice. Today, Medicare enrollment can be accomplished electronically through CMS' Internet-based Provider Enrollment, Chain, and Ownership System established by the CMS, which is the branch of the U.S. Department of Health & Human Services (HHS) that administers the Medicare program. CMS Form 855B is the enrollment application used by clinics and group practices, and CMS Form 855I is the enrollment application used by physicians. Such applications require the submission of an abundance of information and documentation in a complete and accurate manner. Additional information pertaining to Medicare provider enrollment is available at http://www.cms.gov/MedicareProviderSupEnroll/. Each third party payor also has its own unique provider enrollment policies and procedures although many such payors utilize a universal credentialing application called Universal Provider Datasource, which is described at http://www.caqh.org/ucd.php.

IMPLEMENTING HIPAA PRIVACY AND SECURITY IN A PHYSICIAN'S OFFICE

Introduction

HIPAA, the Health Insurance Portability and Accountability Act,[29] was passed by Congress in 1996 and was designed to improve the efficiency and effectiveness of the health care system. Although the primary purpose of HIPAA is to protect health care coverage for individuals who lose or change their jobs, it also includes Title II, better known as the Administrative Simplification Act. Title II requires the U.S. Department of HHS to adopt national standards for electronic health care transactions in order for the health care industry to become more efficient. Congress also recognized, however, that advances in electronic technology could erode the privacy and security of health information. Consequently, Congress incorporated into HIPAA provisions that mandate the adoption of federal privacy and security protections for individually identifiable health information.

HIPAA Privacy Rule

The HIPAA Privacy Rule pertains to three categories of "covered entities"—health care providers, health plans,[30] and health care clearinghouses.[31] Health care providers are covered if they transmit health information electronically. Even a doctor in a small practice who keeps only paper records will almost certainly use a billing service that transmits information electronically. In short, it is nearly impossible to provide health care today without using electronic means in some way and therefore fall under the purview of the HIPAA Privacy Rule.

---

[29]Pub. L. 104–191.

[30]Health plan means almost anyone that pays for the cost of medical care. This includes health insurance companies, HMOs (health maintenance organizations), group health plans sponsored by an employer, Medicare and Medicaid, and virtually any other company or arrangement that pays for your health care.

[31]Health care clearinghouses can be any number of organizations that work as a go-between for health care providers and health plans. An example of this would be a billing service that takes information from a doctor and puts it into a standard coded format. Patients rarely deal directly with clearinghouses.

The HIPAA Privacy Rule generally safeguards the confidentiality of protected health information (PHI), which is defined as "individually identifiable health information" that is transmitted electronically, maintained electronically, or transmitted or maintained in any other form or medium.[32] It includes not only paper and electronic records but oral statements as well. Common documents that would be considered to contain PHI would include (a) all components of the medical record, (b) information contained on billing cards or superbills, (c) information contained on hospital face sheets, and (d) information contained on other forms such as the financial consent, informed consent, and patient information sheets.

The HIPAA Privacy Rule places restrictions on how a physician group can use PHI within the practice and how and when PHI can be disclosed to entities outside the practice. In general (with exceptions for emergencies), the privacy rule prohibits health care providers from using or disclosing PHI without first obtaining the patient's HIPAA consent. The HIPAA consent is different from informed and financial consents in that the HIPAA consent is for "use" and "disclosure" of PHI. However, HIPAA consent is not required to use and disclose PHI for treatment, payment, and operations.[33] If the physician group uses or discloses information for other purposes such as for certain research or marketing activities, a HIPAA authorization would have to be signed by the patient.

Another important document that must be provided to the patient at the time of the HIPAA consent is the group's HIPAA Notice of Privacy Practices.[34] This document is separate and apart from the HIPAA consent and must be posted in a conspicuous place in the physician's office. The HIPAA notice is a document that must set forth a number of items including, but not limited to, (a) all of the different uses and disclosures of PHI that the physician group is permitted to make under the privacy rule, (b) how the patients can get access to their information, (c) the manner in which patients can complain to the group with regard to potential breaches of privacy, (d) a statement that the patient has the right under HIPAA to request certain restrictions on their PHI (note that the group is not required to agree to all restrictions), and (e) an explanation of the privacy policies and procedures that the practice has put in place.

In addition to the HIPAA consent and notice requirements, physician groups are also required under the privacy rule to implement privacy policies, establish formal safeguards, and train the practice's staff to ensure the privacy of PHI. In order to meet these administrative requirements,

organizations must first formally designate an individual within the organization as the "Privacy Officer." The Privacy Officer will be responsible for the "development and implementation" of the policies and procedures necessary for compliance under the HIPAA privacy rule.[35] These administrative requirements impose a focus on privacy that may have previously taken a back seat in the hectic, business-like atmosphere that often characterizes modern-day health care.

In order to effectuate the required training, physician practices should have compliance programs in place, which should include HIPAA education as part of an annual compliance education in service. The education should focus on providing employees with a general understanding of HIPAA as well as explaining the policies and forms that will be put in place. Education should also include practical tips to make certain that a patient's privacy is not breached, such as the following:

1. Following phone protocols. A medical office must have specific guidelines for what information is given over the phone. Certain individuals like health insurance representatives or family members might have clearance to be told patient information, but other callers should be given only basic information that does not violate HIPAA.
2. Protect workstations. A computer that has access to PHI, should always be locked when the person who uses it is away from the desk to prevent unauthorized use.
3. Protect papers. Documents like medical claims and bills should be turned face down when the person who is responsible for them is away from the desk. The files must be kept in secure containers where they cannot be read by someone passing by.
4. Use HIPAA-compliant waste baskets and shredders. Some offices have color-coded trash bins, one set for regular trash like apple cores and gum wrappers and another covered set of bins for documents. The documents that go in the secure bins get shredded every day. The other trash bins get emptied by cleaning people at night.

In addition to training its employees, practice groups must enter into agreements with each of their business associates (BAs) wherein the BAs agree to safeguard PHI provided by the group or PHI that the BAs access via permission of the group.[36] In general, BAs are independent entities that provide services on behalf of the group that involve PHI. A list of common BAs for a practice may include the following:

1. Billing companies
2. Practice management companies
3. Collection agencies
4. CPA firms and law firms

---

[32] 45 C.F.R. §160.103.
[33] The privacy rule incorporates what it calls a "minimum necessary" standard when it comes to how much information should be disclosed. Covered entities are required to limit the amount of information disclosed to others to the minimum necessary to accomplish the intended purpose. 45 CFR §§164.502(b), 164.514(d).
[34] 45 CFR §164.520(a) and (b).

[35] 45 CFR §164.530(a)(1).
[36] 45 CFR §§164.502€ & 164.504(e).

5. Independent compliance auditors
6. Record storage companies
7. Software vendors
8. Cleaning services

The HIPAA Security Rule

Privacy and data security go hand in hand. The security rule, like the privacy rule, creates a national standard. This means that all health care providers, health plans, and health care clearinghouses that transmit information electronically must adopt a data security plan.

Only PHI maintained or transmitted in electronic format (EPHI) is covered by the security rule.[37] For example, EPHI would include billing information contained on a computer system, electronic medical records, and computerized patient scheduling systems in an ENT practice. Although nonelectronic PHI (e.g., hardcopy medical charts) is not covered by the HIPAA security rules, this information is still protected by the HIPAA privacy rules.

The security rule, according to the HHS, was designed to be flexible, establishing a security framework for small practices as well as large institutions. All covered entities must have a written security plan.[38]

The general requirements of the HIPAA Security Rule mandate that covered entities do all of the following:

1. Ensure the confidentiality, integrity, and availability of all EPHI that the entity creates, receives, maintains, or transmits
2. Protect against any reasonably anticipated threats or hazards to the security or integrity of such information
3. Protect against any reasonably anticipated uses or disclosures of such information that are not permitted or required by the HIPAA Privacy Rule
4. Ensure workforce compliance[39]

To achieve compliance with the general HIPAA Security Rule requirements set forth above, covered entities are required to meet 18 standards. In order to meet each of these standards, the HIPAA Security Rule sets forth implementation specifications that serve as the instructions for compliance with each standard. There are two types of implementation specifications, "required" and "addressable."

Required implementation specifications must be implemented as set forth in the HIPAA Security Rule. Addressable implementation specifications allow covered entities to implement alternative specifications instead of, or in combination with, the implementation specification set forth in the HIPAA Security Rule. If an alternative approach is taken, the entity must document its decision

not to implement the HIPAA Security Rule's implementation specification, the rationale behind its decision, and the alternative approach that it has chosen. The standards and their related implementation specifications are broken down into three broad categories: (a) administrative safeguards,[40] (b) physical safeguards,[41] and (c) technical safeguards.[42] The administrative safeguard standards require entities to analyze the risks of unauthorized disclosure of EPHI within the entity, implement a number of required policies and procedures, and maintain certain documentation to manage and minimize risk. Physical safeguard standards deal with the security measures taken to protect buildings and equipment, which house EPHI, from natural and environmental hazards and unauthorized intrusion. The policies and procedures required under this standard include policies to protect the physical locations that house electronic equipment, as well as to protect the equipment itself. Technical safeguard standards deal with the technologic measures to safeguard and control access to EPHI as well as the development and implementation of policies and procedures dealing with the use of technology.

To address HIPAA security, the following action plan should be implemented:

1. Appoint a Security Officer (this is required under the rule[43]) who must review and understand the requirements of the rule. The Security Officer may need to seek outside assistance from attorneys or consultants versed in the HIPAA Security Rule.
2. Identify BAs that are creating, receiving, or transmitting EPHI for the practice and include HIPAA security language in the BA agreement.
3. Inventory EPHI and electronic systems within the practice and begin working on the required policies and procedures.
4. Conduct required security training with all workforce members.

Why Physician Offices Must Be HIPAA Compliant

HIPAA sets a national standard for accessing and handling medical information. Before HIPAA, the right to privacy of health information varied from state to state. Now, health care providers, health plans, and other health care services that operate in all states have to abide by the minimum standards set by HIPAA. Any state is free to adopt laws that give patients more privacy, but it cannot take away the basic rights given by HIPAA.[44] Compliance with HIPAA's privacy and security requirements is mandatory, and failure to

---

[37]45 CFR §160.103.
[38]45 CFR §§164.306(b)(2) and (e).
[39]45 CFR §164.306(a).

[40]45 CFR §164.308(a).
[41]45 CFR §164.301(a) to (d).
[42]45 CFR §164.312(a), (b), (c), and (e).
[43]45 CFR §164.308(a)(2).
[44]45 CFR §§164.202, 164.203.

comply could lead to civil and criminal penalties. In 2009, the Health Information Technology for Economic and Clinical Health (HITECH) Act was passed, which, in part, strengthens HIPAA's privacy and security protections and, notably, increases its enforcement rules.

The HHS Office of Civil Rights (OCR), which in addition to its responsibility for enforcing the HIPAA Privacy Rule was given responsibility in July 2010 for security rule enforcement too, has implemented a stronger enforcement program in the form of HIPAA privacy and security audits. The OCR's implementation of proactive HIPAA compliance audits, required under the provisions of the HITECH Act, marked a shift from the largely reactive approach to compliance and enforcement seen since the HIPAA Privacy and Security Rules went into effect in 2003 and 2005, respectively. The audits will focus on how covered entities are meeting specific HIPAA requirements such as implementation of appropriate safeguards and seek evidence that risk analysis, contingency planning, and other key activities are in fact being carried out. In concert with stronger procedural methods for enforcement, the HITECH Act also increased the civil and criminal penalties for noncompliance, gave state attorneys general the right to sue covered entities for violations on behalf of state residents, and mandated formal investigations for any cases of HIPAA violations involving willful neglect. Collectively, all of these measures must make compliance a bigger priority for HIPAA-covered entities (and BAs too, since HITECH extended most HIPAA requirements to apply directly to them as well).

OPERATIONAL ISSUES

Office Electronic Medical Records

Electronic medical records lie at the center of any computerized health information system. However, there is no law that requires medical practices to adopt electronic records. Nonetheless, the HITECH stimulus act does threaten non-adopters with cuts in their Medicare reimbursements. The cuts begin in 2015 and increase to a maximum of 5% of the reimbursements. As such, while not a mandate or law requiring the adoption of electronic medical records, the HITECH Act strongly encourages physicians to do so.

One of the primary purposes of the HITECH Act and the regulations promulgated under HITECH is to promote use of electronic health records (EHRs) in a manner that advances quality, safety, and efficiency of patient care. To that end, the HITECH Act not only includes provisions to protect the privacy and security of patient health information contained within EHRs but also provides for significant financial incentives under Medicare and Medicaid to eligible health providers who demonstrate meaningful use of EHRs. HITECH specifically authorizes the CMS to provide reimbursement incentives for eligible professionals and eligible hospitals who are successful in becoming "meaningful users" of EHRs.

On July 13, 2010, CMS issued the Final Rule[45] titled "Medicare and Medicaid Programs; Electronic Health Record Incentive Program" (the "Final Rule"), which sets forth the criteria that eligible health providers must satisfy to demonstrate meaningful use of EHRs sufficient to receive incentive payments from the federal government.

Meaningful Use Criteria

Under the Final Rule, achieving meaningful use requires using certified EHR technology to achieve improvements in quality, safety, and efficiency in health care (i.e., physicians will not be able to achieve meaningful use through the adoption of EHRs alone). The Final Rule divides the meaningful use criteria into a "core" group of required objectives and a "menu set" of procedures from which providers can choose. This "two-track" approach ensures that the most basic elements of meaningful EHR use will be met by all providers qualifying for incentive payments while also allowing latitude in other areas to reflect the varying needs of providers pursuing full EHR use.

This Final Rule (Stage 1 of 3) will apply only to the first two (2) years of the federal meaningful use incentive programs. Stages 2 and 3 will include more stringent requirements for achieving meaningful use of EHRs in the future.[46]

Physician Eligibility

Eligible physicians, who for purposes of Medicare generally include doctors of medicine or osteopathy, dentists or dental surgeons, podiatrists, optometrists, and chiropractors, began registering for the EHR meaningful use Medicare/Medicaid incentive program in January 2011. Payments under the incentive program began in May 2011. Importantly, hospital-based physicians are not eligible for the Medicare incentive payments and, subject to certain limited exceptions, are also not eligible for the Medicaid incentive payments. Under the Final Rule, CMS defines hospital-based physicians as those who furnish at least 90% of their professional services within an inpatient hospital or an emergency room hospital. Typical examples of hospital-based physicians include pathologists, anesthesiologists, hospitalists, or emergency physicians. CMS will determine noneligibility based upon site of service codes. In other words, physicians providing services in outpatient settings, including ambulatory clinics, are eligible for incentives.

Some physicians believe that being exempt from eligibility for the Medicare/Medicaid EHR incentives is a desirable result. This is due to the fact that hospital-based physicians who are exempt from otherwise available incentives

---

[45]75 FR 44590.

[46]The requirements contained within each of the three stages have been hotly debated, most notably by the physician specialists. These specialists have repeatedly complained that the requirements are only realistically attainable by the primary care physicians, and as a result, they will face financial sanctions for being unable to meet unattainable goals in the meaningful use of EHR.

will also be exempt from the penalties that will begin in 2015 if a provider fails to meet the meaningful use requirements. According to many specialty groups, this is particularly significant since they will find it difficult to meet the meaningful use requirements because the measures either do not apply to their specialty or they are not reportable through their specific practice's information management systems.

Understanding Your Electronic Medical Record

As noted earlier in this chapter, physicians are facing unprecedented scrutiny in the submission of claims. For example, with respect to Medicare claims, not only do Medicare Affiliated Contractors (MACs), Medicare Carriers, and Intermediaries conduct their own audits, but also Medicare's RAC program is operational nationwide and has been expanded to include Part C and Part D claims, and Zone Program Integrity Auditors (ZPICs) and PSCs are conducting nationwide benefit integrity audits. With respect to Medicaid claims, MICs are actively auditing claims, and the RAC program is expanding to Medicaid claims as well. Physicians must be cognizant of this increased claims scrutiny and conduct themselves accordingly, with an increased focus on compliance.

Certain compliance issues are heightened with the use of electronic medical records. Auditors and medical reviewers routinely deny claims because an item or service is found not to be medically necessary. As such, it is essential that when a physician documents a service performed, such documentation must establish for the reviewer the medical necessity of the service rendered. There are special compliance issues that arise with respect to the use of electronic medical records, particularly with respect to issues of medical necessity. For example, many electronic medical records have built in "time savers," such as self-populating fields that insert a patient's medical history or procedural history into each record. These time-saving devices ultimately may hurt a provider if not used correctly, should the provider be subject to an audit. Auditors and claim reviewers may deny claims for medical necessity if it appears that the documentation is not tailored to the service performed but is merely a template. Each record should be distinct from the next. Additionally, auditors and claim reviewers may deny claims if they find that the medical records associated with the service or procedure are internally inconsistent. For example, claims have been denied because the medical record states in one area: "patient has no complaints of pain," but in another area states: "patient presents with severe pain." Providers using electronic medical records must ensure that they understand the capabilities of the software, have knowledge regarding which fields self-populate, and tailor each record to the patient's condition at the time of assessment.

With the coming of quality assessment programs from the government or commercial payers, the need exists for the inexpensive collection of quality data through a limited series of questions, typically less than 10. Independent of any externally mandated data collection effort you need to understand your practice and how you can better serve your patients. Several kinds of systems are available for use including the manual review of paper or electronic medical records, paper forms completed by the patient or staff, interactive voice response systems, local electronic data capture systems, or central web-based systems. The advantages and disadvantages of each system are beyond the scope of this chapter. Your chosen system should permit you to capture information easily into a readily accessible format (usually electronic) easily manipulated by you or your staff. Careful consideration should be given to the capacity of a practice through its EMR or other systems to acquire information in a cost-effective timely manner.

Use of the Shewhart cycle or PDCA (Plan, Do, Check, Act—repeat) has proven to be a useful tool for process improvement. Focus on the correction of issues preventable by process improvement. Identify the root cause (people, processes, tools, materials) of issues. The purpose of data acquisition is not to improve the outcome by measuring it, but to improve its production process. However, if the outcome is unknown or variable in its outcome, document the processes that produce the desired outcome. If the process is variable, the process must first be stabilized, and then measured against stakeholder expectations. As long as the process is unstable, it will be impossible to make systematic changes to the process and get uniform results. A stable production process will prevent errors and assure ongoing consistent quality outcomes. Often true medical outcomes are often too costly in time, effort, or money to measure, and interim process measures must be utilized. Picking an interim process step or outcome that has face validity maybe acceptable alternative. Whenever possible, identify and use standardized data definitions to facilitate comparisons with surrogate data.

Social Media and E-mail Communication

As with all businesses, medical practices face competition from other offices in their area and must differentiate themselves by portraying value and quality to their prospective clients. The use of social media outlets like Facebook, or collaboration tools like blogs or wikis, has provided a place for patients to learn about a physician's practice and decide on the value and quality of the practice before they become a patient. As a result, health care providers are more frequently utilizing social media to market their practices and to dispense health information. In doing so, however, it is critical for any provider or practice to ensure that their use of social media outlets does not inappropriately invade the physician–patient relationship or erode a continued positive Internet presence for health care providers.

With these goals in mind, the AMA adopted recommendations for physician use of social media.[47] The guidelines recommend that physicians utilize privacy settings on social media Web sites and develop appropriate mechanisms to monitor their Internet presence for accuracy and appropriateness. The AMA also suggests that health care providers maintain proper boundaries when interacting with patients on the Internet and exercise good faith efforts to protect their clients' privacy and confidentiality. Finally, the AMA cautions physicians to be mindful of the potential negative implications arising from the use of social media on their reputations and professional careers.

E-mail communication between physicians and patients within a professional relationship, in which the physician has taken responsibility for the patient's care, is also on the rise. Although the use of e-mail communication within this professional relationship can certainly be useful and effective, caution must be exercised when used for urgent matters or when relaying confidential information in that privacy and security measures are in place. Those patients who a provider communicates with via e-mail must have an understanding of the need to call the provider's office directly if the matter is urgent (requiring a response on the same day) and have a clear understanding of the expected response time on nonurgent e-mails. This can best be accomplished by written statements on all e-mail communications with patients that clearly states the relevant expectations and understandings.

The AMA has also issued guidelines governing the use of e-mail within the physician–patient relationship.[48] Within these guidelines, the AMA urges against the use of e-mail communications as replacing "the crucial interpersonal contacts that are the very basis of the patient-physician relationship" but that it only be used to enhance such contacts.

Hospital Call

A physician's duty to undertake hospital emergency department call and whether or not the hospital is required to pay for such call coverage (and if so, how much) is a complicated and evolving matter with vast ethical, legal, and medical implications. Typically, hospitals require physicians within certain specialties to share in some minimal amount of emergency department call coverage in order for the hospitals to meet certain federal and state quality of care requirements (e.g., EMTALA) and therefore mandate that these physicians provide some minimal call coverage in order to obtain and maintain medical staff privileges at the hospitals. However, over the years, in certain geographic areas, there has been a

reduction in the willingness of physicians to provide such coverage, in part, due to an increase in the number of uninsured patients receiving their only care in emergency rooms, a shortage of certain specialty physicians, falling reimbursement for certain specialty physician services, and a perceived increase in the risk of lawsuits to the physician if the physician provides such coverage. In August 1992, the OIG published a report on Specialty Coverage in Hospital Emergency Departments, which found that "sixty-seven percent of hospitals report that they encounter difficulty ensuring coverage for at least one specialty service they offer in their emergency departments." The report also indicated that only about 10% of the hospitals encouraged specialty physicians to provide emergency care by offering them direct compensation for being on the on-call list. At the time, the OIG strongly encouraged physicians, hospital administrators and boards, consumers and advocacy groups, health insurers, and government officials to get together and address the issue immediately. Unfortunately, approximately 20 years later, we are still faced with the same issues.

When physicians request compensation for providing the additional emergency department call coverage requested by the hospital in order to offset the physicians' aforementioned financial concerns, legal issues arise. Such compensation may run afoul of numerous federal and state laws governing hospital–physician relationships including, but not limited to, the federal AKS and Stark regulations. Moreover, nonprofit hospitals also need to be aware of IRS regulations pertaining to private inurement and benefit issues to maintain their nonprofit status. The remainder of this article focuses on how such compensation may run afoul of the federal AKS.

The OIG has expressed concern that payments by hospitals for ER call coverage could be easily misused to entice physicians to join or remain on the hospital's staff or to generate additional business for the hospital in violation of the AKS. While the AKS bars the parties from making unlawful kickback payments in any form, it does not compel physicians to provide on-call services for free. As with any compensation relationship between a hospital and a physician, compensation for ER call coverage must be at fair market value for actual and necessary services rendered based upon an arm's length transaction and cannot take into account, directly or indirectly, the value or volume of any past or future referrals or other business between the parties. On-call compensation will be scrutinized to ensure that it is not a vehicle to disguise improper payments for referrals. Although the OIG does not opine on whether a certain dollar amount is or is not at fair market value *per se*, it has published two instructive advisory opinions that should guide physicians and hospitals when deciding an appropriate on-call compensation arrangement.

On September 20, 2007, the OIG issued Advisory Opinion 07-10, which provides some guidance as to how

---

[47]AMA Policy: Professionalism in the Use of Social Media. www.ama-assn.org/ama/pub/meeting/professionalism-social-media_print.html
[48]AMA H-478.997 Guidelines for Patient-Physician Electronic Mail

to structure such compensation arrangements to avoid AKS violations. Included in the Advisory Opinion were statements by the OIG that warned against on-call compensation arrangements: (a) based upon lost opportunity (i.e., payments that do not reflect bona fide/actual lost income to the physician), (b) where physicians are compensated and there are no identifiable services provided, (c) involving aggregate payments that are disproportionately high compared to the physician's regular practice income, and (d) wherein the physician receives separate reimbursement from insurers or patients in addition to the hospital's on-call payment resulting in the physician being paid twice for the same services. The OIG approved the per diem payment arrangement to physicians who were willing to (a) participate in an equal prorate share of on-call coverage, (b) provide follow-up inpatient care, (c) timely respond to calls, (d) appropriately document the services provided, (e) participate in quality programs, and (f) provide 1.5 days of uncompensated on-call coverage per month. The per diem rate was based upon (a) the physician's specialty, (b) the severity of the illness typically seen by that specialty, (c) the likelihood of having to respond to call or provide follow-up care, and (d) whether the coverage was on a weekday or weekend (which resulted in a slightly higher fee).

On May 14, 2009, the OIG issued Advisory Opinion 09-05, which provided some additional guidance on how to structure an AKS-compliant on-call compensation arrangement. The OIG approved an alleged FMV flat fee-for-service arrangement where, in order to be reimbursed for claims provided to indigent and uninsured patients treated at the hospital's ER, the physicians were required to (a) participate in an on-call rotation, (b) provide follow-up inpatient care, (c) timely respond to calls, and (d) evaluate the patient in person. The flat fee schedule was determined based upon patient acuity levels, average length of stay, physician time commitment for each kind of service, and consideration of the fees paid by public, private, and self-payors for such services.

On October 23, 2012, the OIG issued Advisory Opinion 12-15, to address an inquiry regarding a hospital's payment of per diem fees to physicians for providing on-call coverage for unassigned patients presenting to the hospital's ER. The hospital's arrangement involved 130 specialist physicians who provide unrestricted call coverage for the ER per written agreement whereby they agree to respond within a required time frame, provide inpatient care and follow-up care in their office practices for ER patients whom they admit, timely prepare medical records, and participate in medical staff committee appointments—all regardless of an ER patient's insurance status or ability to pay. The hospital created an uniform per diem fee to be paid to the physicians providing such call in each specialty based upon numerous factors associated with each specialty's call burden including the number of days per month that a specialist would likely be called, the number

of patients likely to be seen per call day, and the number of patients likely to require inpatient and follow-up care. The hospital retained an independent consultant who opined that the per diem rate was consistent with fair market value without regard to the volume or value of referrals or any individual physician's referral pattern. The OIG warned against arrangements that pay for "lost opportunity" (as opposed to true lost income), which pay more than FMV, or which pay physicians for services for which they already receive separate reimbursement. Nonetheless, the OIG approved the arrangement based upon similar factors set forth within Advisory Opinions 07-10 and 09-05 including that the per diem payments: (a) were consistent with fair market value and tailored to reflect the call coverage burden applicable to each specialty; (b) were calculated and allocated in advance each year without regard to physician referral patterns; (c) were the only payment available to the physicians for a significant amount of care provided; (d) were offered to all specialists in staff required to provide unrestricted call coverage under the hospital's bylaws; and (e) did not result in any additional costs to the federal health healthcare programs.

With the increasing desire to have specialists on call at hospitals, there will likely be more guidance issued in the future to address such matters.

HIGHLIGHTS

- The business of medicine is complex. Obtain key advisors and specialists to assist you in the management of your practice.
- Ultimately, you, the physician, are responsible for your provider number. You need to be familiar with the billing rules.
- Bad results do not in and of themselves result in a potential malpractice risk. Communication breakdowns are often at the heart of many malpractice actions.
- Malpractice claims require four basic elements: establishing the medical provider had a duty of care, that the duty was breached by conduct not in accordance with a standard of care, that the breech was the cause of the injury, and the plaintiff suffered damages.
- The discovery phase is the nuts and bolts of the litigation process. In it the physician learns the exact nature of the charges being advanced and the steps necessary to defend the claim. Preparation is paramount as few cases are won during the discovery but many more are lost.
- Settlement of a malpractice action may be the best course of action based upon the jurisdiction, judge, attorney, physician factors, convenience, merit, or an emotional standpoint.

- Two professional liability insurance policies are available: occurrence and claims made. The former offers protection from losses that occur while the policy is in effect. Claims-made policies offer protection from claims made during a specific time period. Upon termination, tail coverage is often necessary with a claims-made policy.

- Protection of your personal assets is a top priority. Professional liability insurance, the use of IRAs or employee benefit plans, life insurance, and the services of an experienced estate planner, accountant, or tax expert may be a few of the strategies used to protect personal assets.

- Empiric evidence tying malpractice and tort reform to medical malpractice litigation is limited and provides little support for the contention that it is the most effective means of managing skyrocketing malpractice premium rates or reducing health care costs. Further defensive medicine is motivated by more than fear of litigation.

- The Physician Self-Referral Law, commonly referred to as the Stark Law, prohibits a physician (or immediate family member) from making referrals of DHS such as laboratory services, DME, home health, hospital services, radiology and other imaging services, PT, OT and speech services, and radiation therapy for Medicaid or Medicare patients to an entity they have a financial relationship with without an exception. Proof of specific intent to violate the law is not required.

- The Antikickback Statute makes it a crime to knowingly and willfully offer, pay, solicit, or receive any remuneration (anything of value) for referral of items or services reimbursable by a federal health care program.

- Physicians need to develop and maintain systems in their practice to oversee coding, billing, and documentation for services rendered. Physicians should steer clear of any situation in which their decision making with respect of patient referrals or use of products is based upon anything other than what is medically necessary and appropriate.

- The seven components of a compliance program include conducting internal monitoring and auditing, implementing compliance standards, having a compliance officer or designate, conducting education and training, responding in a timely and appropriate fashion to detached offenses and developing corrective action plans, keeping communication avenues open with patients and staff, and enforcing disciplinary standards.

- Licensure actions arise out of complaints and should prompt appropriate counsel and response at the earliest possible stage.

- Organizing a practice has seven basic steps: establishing the business entity, obtaining an IRS federal tax identification number, protecting the name and any intellectual property, developing the governing documents of the business, adopting the necessary corporate resolutions to ratify the business entity, enrolling in third party insurance plans, and opening business accounts and obtaining the necessary insurance.

- The HIPAA safeguards the confidentiality of PHI that is transmitted electronically. Virtually every practice is covered by this act even if you chose not to use an electronic medical record.

- Compliance issues related to medical necessity are highlighted when documentation in the electronic medical records is not tailored to the service performed but is merely a template.

REFERENCES

1. F. Patrick Hubbard. *The Nature and Impact of the "Tort Reform" Movement*, 35 HOFSTRA L. REV. 438, 439 (2006).
2. Black's Law Dictionary 470 (Second Pocket ed. 2001).
3. F. Patrick Hubbard. *The Nature and Impact of the "Tort Reform" Movement*, 35 HOFSTRA L. REV. 417 (2006).
4. Black's Law Dictionary 713 (Second Pocket ed. 2001).
5. F. Patrick Hubbard. *The Nature and Impact of the "Tort Reform" Movement*, 35 HOFSTRA L. REV. 439 (2006).
6. F. Patrick Hubbard. *The Nature and Impact of the "Tort Reform" Movement*, 35 HOFSTRA L. REV. 441 (2006).
7. Cecilia Loh. An Overview of Medical Malpractice and the Tort Reform Debate, April 23, 2003, at http://www.case.edu/med/epidbio/mphp439/Malpractice.htm
8. Black's Law Dictionary 470 (Second Pocket ed. 2001).
9. Black's Law Dictionary 119 (Second Pocket ed. 2001).
10. Black's Law Dictionary 37 (Second Pocket ed. 2001).
11. Black's Law Dictionary 156 (Second Pocket ed. 2001).
12. http://www.entnet.org/aboutus/Ethics.cfm (Last accessed April 28, 2011).
13. F. Patrick Hubbard. *The Nature and Impact of the "Tort Reform" Movement*, 35 HOFSTRA L. REV. 475 (2006).
14. F. Patrick Hubbard. *The Nature and Impact of the "Tort Reform" Movement*, 35 HOFSTRA L. REV. 498–499 (2006).
15. Joanna M. Shepherd. *Tort Reforms' Winners and Losers: The Competing Effects of Care and Activity Levels*, 55 UCLA L. REV. 905, 920 (2008).
16. American Tort Reform Association, http://www.atra.org/states/MI (Last visited Dec. 6, 2010).
17. Douglas A. Kysar et al. *Medical Malpractice Myths and Realities: Why an Insurance Crisis is Not a Lawsuit Crisis*, 39 Loy. L.A. L. Rev. 785, 789 (2006).
18. Douglas A. Kysar et al. *Medical Malpractice Myths and Realities: Why an Insurance Crisis is Not a Lawsuit Crisis*, 39 Loy. L.A. L. Rev. 790 (2006).
19. National Association of Insurance Commissioners. *Countrywide Summary of Medical Malpractice Insurance Calendar Years 1991-2008* (2009).
20. Michelle Mello et al. *National Costs of the Medical Liability System*, Health Affairs, Sept. 2010, at 1569.
21. Douglas A. Kysar et al. *Medical Malpractice Myths and Realities: Why an Insurance Crisis is Not a Lawsuit Crisis*, 39 Loy. L.A. L. Rev. 798 (2006).
22. Michelle Mello et al. *National Costs of the Medical Liability System*, Health Affairs, Sept. 2010, at 1570.
23. Douglas A. Kysar et al. *Medical Malpractice Myths and Realities: Why an Insurance Crisis is Not a Lawsuit Crisis*, 39 Loy. L.A. L. Rev. 803 (2006).

24. Douglas A. Kysar et al. *Medical Malpractice Myths and Realities: Why an Insurance Crisis is Not a Lawsuit Crisis*, 39 Loy. L.A. L. Rev. 795 (2006).

25. Douglas A. Kysar et al. *Medical Malpractice Myths and Realities: Why an Insurance Crisis is Not a Lawsuit Crisis*, 39 Loy. L.A. L. Rev. 808 (2006).

26. Douglas A. Kysar et al. *Medical Malpractice Myths and Realities: Why an Insurance Crisis is Not a Lawsuit Crisis*, 39 Loy. L.A. L. Rev. 809 (2006).

27. *Medical Malpractice: Implications of Rising Premiums on Access to Health Care*, Government Accountability Office, August 29, 2003.

28. Emily Carrier et al. *Physicians' Fears of Malpractice Lawsuits Are Not Assuaged by Tort Reforms*, Health Affairs, Sept. 2010, at 1585.

29. http://www.aboto.org/Resident%20Handbook.pdf. Last accessed April 27, 2011.

30. http://oig.hhs.gov/oei/reports/OEI-01-10-00140.pdf

31. *United States v. Kats*, 871 F.2d 105 (9th Cir. 1989); *United States v. Greber*, 760 F.2d 68 (3d Cir.), cert. denied, 474 U.S. 988 (1985).

32. http://oig.hhs.gov/fraud/PhysicianEducation/roadmap_web_version.pdf

Compliant Documentation, Coding, and Billing in the Practice of Otolaryngology— Head and Neck Surgery

200

Stephen R. Levinson

How many physicians look forward to learning about documentation and coding? Probably as few as the number of businessmen who want to learn the details of the tax code. Yet documentation and coding are as integral to the practice of medicine as accurate bookkeeping and correctly filing taxes are to anyone operating a business. From their earliest exposure to performing history and physical examinations, medical students who have great teachers are admonished that their documented medical record for each patient encounter should be an accurate and understandable reflection of the medical care they provided and the thought process they followed. (As summarized by the great medical record innovator Dr. Lawrence Weed, "It's not sufficient to just know what was done. It's a very incomplete record if we don't know why it was done" (1). What is, however, seldom appreciated and rarely taught is that the use of creatively designed medical record documentation tools can improve quality, compliance, and efficiency for recording diagnostic and surgical procedures and especially for documenting and coding evaluation and management (E/M) care. When used for documenting E/M services, effective medical record tools also increase workflow efficiency and promote physicians' diagnostic patient care process. The benefits of effective documentation further extend to include audit compliance, medicolegal protection, communication with other physicians, and, most importantly, helping to ensure optimal patient care for both current and future visits.

While physicians almost universally understand the role that coding plays in filing claims for insurance, they must also appreciate its role in data retrieval and information processing. In the office setting, diagnostic and procedure codes are the gateway to accessing the records of patients who have undergone specific procedures or who have been diagnosed with particular illnesses. Accurate coding facilitates chart review and analysis of the success of various treatment options, as well as initiating patient recalls under appropriate circumstances. These individual practice benefits are magnified by combining related data from large numbers of physician practices, facilitating "comparative effectiveness research" (CER), which is one of the promised benefits of widespread use of electronic health records (EHRs). The requirement for coding correctly has been underscored by the proliferation of coding and health information management (HIM) professionals, who in various settings may be employed to review, assist, or even replace coding by physicians. However, even if their hospital or practice employs coding professionals, physicians need to understand coding fundamentals to achieve correct codification of patient care and to ensure receiving proper payments for their services.

SURVEYING THE CURRENT ENVIRONMENT AND SEARCHING FOR SOLUTIONS

Why do physicians so frequently complain that the tasks of creating consistently compliant (2) documentation and coding are confusing, challenging, and/or unrelated to their goals for medical practice? It is far easier to learn how to identify the precise procedure and diagnostic codes for excision of a benign neoplasm of the lateral lobe of a parotid gland with dissection and preservation of the facial nerve (CPT code 42145 and ICD-9 code 201.2) than it is to master the surgical technique required to perform that challenging operation safely and well. Similarly, with a relatively small amount of training combined with compliantly designed (and physician-friendly) medical record forms, it is far easier to perform and document the medically indicated level of care for a new patient with probable Meniere's disease (CPT code 99204 and ICD-9 code 386.01) than it is to master the optimal evaluation and management pathways for each patient who presents with significant vertigo.

This author believes there are three factors creating barriers to logically and naturally incorporating precise documentation and accurate coding into optimal medical workflow and patient care excellence:

- Lack of early training in coding principles and their integration into medical care
- Lack of efficient and compliant documentation tools that can enable physicians to create documentation at the level and precision that is taught and required
- Lack of teaching physician and practicing physician role models who excel in compliant documentation and coding

All three of these deficiencies could, and should, be remedied by introducing effective curricula and documentation tools at the appropriate junctures during medical education. For example, effective *documentation* of a comprehensive history and physical examination (the "H&P") is traditionally taught as the first medical school course in clinical medicine, and this meaningful clinical documentation almost exactly parallels the compliant H&P required for evaluation and management (E/M) documentation and coding. This would be an optimal time to introduce sophisticated documentation tools to help young physicians provide and document the desired level of care compliantly. Use of such tools would also allow students to achieve good care far more efficiently than the "time-honored" approach of documenting with only a blank sheet of paper and a pen. As almost all physicians have experienced, performing and documenting a comprehensive H&P with such primitive technology requires between 45 and 90 minutes per patient encounter; this is the medical record equivalent of training students to examine the tympanic membrane using nothing more advanced than direct vision with an open ear speculum or to auscultate the heart by placing their ear directly against the patient's chest.

The demands of our current medical environment require practicing physicians, academic physicians, residents, and even medical students to complete patient encounters within 10 to 20 minutes. Unfortunately, failure to provide sophisticated documentation tools that facilitate performing and documenting extensive care within this time frame has forced student physicians (and now their professional supervisors and role models) to abandon the high-quality history taking and physical examination they were taught to perform. As a consequence, most physicians currently provide and record only "problem-focused" patient care, which creates compliance problems for their evaluation and management services. The current transformation to EHRs offers a welcome window of opportunity to provide such tools, but unfortunately most current EHR data entry designs have failed to facilitate the recording of *individualized* (patient-specific and visit-specific) documentation that "meet all of the optimal standards that physicians should apply to introduction of any medical record technology... usability, efficiency, E/M compliance, promotion of individualized quality care, and data integrity" (3).

Linking the Quality History and Physical Examination with E/M Documentation and Coding

Since the mid-1970s, probably the most commonly used reference text for teaching medical students the principles of obtaining and documenting a high-quality history and physical examination is the Bates' "Guide to Physical Examination and History Taking" (4). Revealingly, comparing both the E/M section of the AMA publication "Current Procedural Terminology" (5) (CPT) and the American Medical Association (AMA)/Centers for Medicare and Medicaid Services (CMS) publication "Documentation Guidelines" (6) with the Bates' Guide text of clinical practice makes it apparent that "this reference book is unquestionably the source of the E/M coding system. The descriptions of medical history and physical examination match concept for concept, paragraph for paragraph, and often almost word-for-word among the three documents. This includes not only the broad concepts, but also the details such as the various organ systems listed in the review of systems and physical examination and the specific definitions for chief complaint (CC) and history of present illness. It also includes a similar overview of formulating and documenting clinical assessments and treatment plans. Most impressively, the Bates' Guide also presents the concept of the 'nature of the patient's problem.' This component of patient assessment parallels CPT's similarly named E/M component 'nature of the presenting problem' (NPP), which plays a pivotal role ... in helping physicians understand how an effective E/M system promotes excellence in patient care.

In summary, the E/M coding system is actually a codification of the medical diagnostic process that all physicians learn in their training as being the most effective method for providing high-quality patient care. Making physicians aware of this relationship allows them to view compliance-based records from a fresh perspective: rather than being an added chore at the conclusion of patient care, carefully designed IMR *(Intelligent Medical Record)* tools can help physicians comfortably provide optimal care within a time frame that meets the limitations of the current health care environment" (7).

In the optimal documentation and coding model presented here, medical students would receive medical record tools and instruction that together facilitate their ability to provide the comprehensive (and compliant) H&P taught during their early clinical training. This monitoring and mentoring of patient care and *documentation* should continue throughout residency training as well. In addition, it appears reasonable and logical that, at the onset of residency training, effective and compliant *documentation* templates should be introduced for recording diagnostic and therapeutic procedures, helping residents develop, practice, and thereby maintain effective procedure documentation techniques from the outset.

Finally, the beginning of residency training would also be an optimal time to introduce the fundamental concepts of *coding* for procedures (CPT coding) and diagnoses (ICD-9 coding, soon-to-be replaced by ICD-10 coding). These alphanumeric codes provide a shorthand "language" for recording and reporting the care physicians provide. Just as early childhood is the most successful learning time frame for introducing an individual to a new language, incorporating coding as a parallel language early in residency will enable young physicians to speak this language fluently.

Unfortunately, our medical training programs do not currently provide this idealized approach to incorporating effective documentation and coding skills and tools as an integral component of learning medical care excellence. Instead, upon completing residency training, most physicians are plunged unprepared into the chilling waters of creating documentation that must meet regulatory demands for coding and billing, performance measures, medicolegal protection, and compliance reviews. This current reality calls for an explanation of documentation and coding that can make these principles understandable and workable for practicing and academic physicians, for residents, and even for medical students.

The remainder of this chapter is devoted to presenting the basic principles of each component of coding and documentation and examining their interplay with the current payment system in the United States. This includes examples of structured documentation tools capable of incorporating these principles into the normal workflow of quality patient care, and it underscores the basic tenet that proper coding and documentation must accurately *report* the care provided, not *distort* that care to meet external regulatory demands.

DOCUMENTATION FUNDAMENTALS

Hippocrates probably documented his patient care by writing freehand on parchment with a quill pen. As his patient volume increased with his widening fame, he probably began to experience the time limitations of creating accurate records using such limited technology. Yet over the next several thousand years, the only significant technologic advances for improving medical documentation were the introduction of milled paper and the ballpoint pen. With mounting time pressures, many physicians increased their writing speed by becoming less and less legible, some even attaining a level of illegibility that left them unable to read their own notes. A significant alternative for recording care finally appeared in the 20th century in the form of dictation. This offered physicians an option that was definitely legible and could also be faster than writing an entire record in longhand. In addition, however, it added the often-significant cost of transcribing the dictated records into paper documents.

Whether created by handwriting or dictation, the final medical records were stored as paper documents, which have inherent limitations in ease of access and costs of storing, retrieving, and sharing the records, as well as mining them for data. The heralded introduction of EHRs offers solutions to these information storage and retrieval problems, but it has also introduced a broad spectrum of challenges to effective data entry. Early on, physicians adopting EHRs were required to type their medical observations into the software programs, a process that is not only usually slower than either dictation or writing but also creates barriers to good patient–physician interaction (or alternatively leads to the double effort of physicians writing notes to themselves on paper, which they then use to type their notes at the end of the day, long after seeing their patients; this is a suboptimal and perhaps noncompliant solution to the data entry challenge). Eventually, some electronic records introduced full or partial dictation alternatives, but many have also introduced a variety of automated data entry shortcuts by copying and pasting blocks of text from previous records and/or from preloaded generic descriptions. While speeding the process of documenting a patient encounter, these shortcuts severely curtail *individualized* documentation, introducing significant problems with compliance (8–10) and challenges in understanding what was actually performed (and why it was performed) during each encounter. Fortunately, effective data entry solutions are achievable, and these are also able to provide documentation that is accurate, individualized, and efficient. Physicians should therefore establish criteria that the data entry features of EHR systems must meet to ensure usability, efficiency, compliance, data integrity, and promoting quality care.

Toolkit for Designing Medical Records to Meet Physicians' Needs

There are several medical record documentation tools that can help physicians create records that surpass the standard written or dictated format. These include

1. **Choice of interface** (graphic and narrative): Traditional medical record documentation required that all information be entered as free text. This approach necessitates a time commitment that is unreasonably excessive to meet today's medical care demands.
   a. **Narrative interface**: There remains a critical requirement for free-text narrative descriptions for those portions of a medical procedure or visit that call for analog (expository) documentation (e.g., an individualized history of the patient's present illness during a visit for evaluation and management care).
   b. **Graphic interface**: A preprinted list of questions or descriptions from which to select appropriate responses using check boxes or similar indicators (e.g., a survey of possible medical illnesses in the past

medical history section of the H&P screen or form). A more sophisticated variation expands this option by also allowing the entry of brief written details along with positive responses to the preentered questions.

2. **Use of preloaded information** (templates and macros): Criteria for proper medical record design for documentation of procedures and, particularly, of evaluation and management services must carefully distinguish between *template* designs that facilitate efficiently recording *individualized* care and *macro* designs that automatically enter identical clinical information in visit after visit and case after case (a process that is labeled "cloned documentation"). While these features have become pervasive in many EHRs, some physicians have incorporated templates or macros into their written or dictated paper records, where they have similar advantages and potential dangers.

a. **Template**: A preloaded graphic interface section that provides detailed structure but no substance until active documentation is entered

   i. An effective office template should list all the elements of a comprehensive ENT physical examination with blank check boxes after each element to indicate either "normal" or "abnormal" findings. The physician checks the appropriate finding for each area examined and leaves blank those boxes for exam elements not performed during a particular patient encounter (all abnormal findings are further described with supplemental narrative detail).

   ii. In other words, until a physician *documents* his or her actual findings, the paper form or electronic screen shows only a blank template of information. There is NO preloaded documentation that anything has yet been performed.

   iii. Well-designed templates provide similar advantages for documentation of PFSH (past history, family history, social history) and Review of Systems obtained during initial E/M visits.

b. **Macro**: A preloaded graphic interface section that provides detailed structure plus standardized substance, because all of the check boxes have been prefilled to indicate normal findings (alternatively, in EHRs, a template form may be converted to a macro when a single electronic "click" *automatically* checks all of the normal boxes). In its narrative form, a macro's preloaded information presents as one or more completed descriptive paragraphs that appear identical to a dictated normal head and neck examination (or a completely negative background history and review of systems).

   i. In other words, before the physician even meets the patient, the macro-loaded paper form or electronic screen attest that he or she has performed a comprehensive head and neck examination and the findings were 100% normal.

   ii. Hypothetically, such macros require "documentation by exception"; that is, the physician is supposed to undocument all exam elements that were not performed and to re-document all exam elements that were found to be abnormal. If done correctly, this undocumentation and re-documentation process, though compliant, actually requires more time and effort than individually checking the blank boxes of a template. It is also subject to multiple oversights that can result in erroneous documentation. In practice, few physicians expend the effort to re-document their macros. As a result, even when physicians using macros perform a limited or focused examination, their records commonly report a comprehensive examination for every visit, almost always with all normal findings except for the one or two areas related to the patient's presenting problem.

   iii. Unless a physician meticulously reviews each item of a macro and undocuments and re-documents each element that was not normal (or negative), the use of macros inevitably results in "cloned documentation." (A recent analysis from the Department of Biomedical Informatics at Columbia University reported that EHRs using macros created medical records where 54% of the wording was identical on progress notes and 78% was identical on discharge notes (11).)

   iv. The use of macros in creating medical documentation will usually fail to support a physician under the scrutiny of a compliance audit, as noted below, or a medicolegal inquiry. Clinically, unless extensively modified line-by-line, macros also fail to convey meaningful patient-specific and visit-specific information needed to assist the physician in the ongoing care of his or her patients.

The Compliance Verdict on "Cloned" Medical Record Documentation

Over many years, CMS and various Medicare Carriers have released a series of critiques of "cloned" medical records, that is, records created by various macro techniques such as "copy forward" (of information from a patient's previous visits), "copy/paste" (of preloaded generic history or examination descriptions), and/or documentation by exception. In 2007, First Coast Service Options, the Florida Medicare carrier, issued a persuasive condemnation of these documentation techniques:

"Cloned documentation does not meet medical necessity requirements for coverage of services rendered due to the lack of specific, individual information. All documentation in the medical record must be specific to the patient and her/his situation at the time of the encounter. Cloning of documentation is considered a misrepresentation of the medical necessity requirement for coverage of services. Identification of this type of documentation will lead to denial of services for lack of medical necessity and recoupment of all overpayments made" (12).

The compliance (and potential financial) danger of improperly employing these data entry techniques was further underscored in a white paper issued in 2007 by the Department of Health and Human Services (HHS) and the Office of the National Coordinator for Health Information Technology (ONCHIT). Their assessment uses the term "templates" to indicate the characteristics of "macros" as described above:

"These tools include the use of defaults, templates (i.e., *macros*), copying, and others. These are legitimate benefits of using an automated system and can be extremely helpful if used correctly; however, the tools can also open the EHR-S up to fraud or abuse" (13).

   v. For E/M services, it is clear that macros should not be used for documenting any portions of the medical history or physical examination. On the other hand, the "correct use" cited above would permit macros to be used effectively and compliantly in portions of the medical decision-making E/M component, to import standard lists of diagnostic tests and/or treatment programs for specific diagnoses. However, such use still requires review for appropriateness and individualized customization during each encounter, prior to incorporating a macro into the medical record.

   vi. Similarly, it appears that macros should have only carefully controlled use in operative reports, permissible only for standard manipulations and only if there is additional individualized narrative information describing the key portions of the diagnostic or therapeutic procedures.

3. **Optimal use of *data entry personnel*:** Although all documentation of the medical history and physical examination has traditionally been entered by the physician (as instructed in medical school), the 1995 and 1997 editions of the *Documentation Guidelines* provide two far less time-consuming alternatives for obtaining and documenting multiple subcomponents of the medical history. They instruct, "The ROS (*Review of Systems*) and/or PFSH (*Past History, Family History, and Social History*) may be recorded by ancillary staff or on a form completed by the patient" (14). This guidance is highly logical, because each physician employs his or her own standard set of questions for each of these medical history elements. Permitting patients to review and respond to these inquiries is extraordinarily efficient. It allows physicians to elicit and record a *comprehensive* medical history without significant time expenditure. Further, the information obtained promotes quality care by providing full background information, identifying both contributory and unrelated medical issues. These insights allow physicians to accurately determine a preliminary differential diagnosis and a preliminary assessment of the nature of the patient's problem ("NPP"—the E/M coding system's measure of *medical necessity*).

Of course, medically it is insufficient just to obtain and document this medical history information; the physician must also review the responses and further investigate all positive findings (i.e., it is not sufficient to simply record that a patient has chest pain—the physician must inquire about the details to determine whether this symptom may be medically significant, potentially health endangering, and/or require assessment). The *Documentation Guidelines* reflects this quality care mandate by requiring "to document that the physician reviewed the information, there must be a notation supplementing or confirming the information recorded by others" (14) (note: clearly the advice to "supplement" refers to all positive responses, while "confirm"—with an attestation by signature—is appropriate to indicate review of all the negative responses).

4. **Optimal use of appropriate *data entry modalities*:** Effective documentation requires the use of data entry tools that facilitate the efficient entry of individualized and accurate medical information. In the traditional paper environment, physicians elect to write or dictate their documentation. Prior to the introduction of EHRs, few, if any, physicians chose to record the H&P by typing, either during the care process or as an additional step following each encounter. The process would be too time-consuming and/or too intrusive into the physician–patient interaction.

Considering these drawbacks, it is remarkable that numerous EHR software systems have chosen to require the use of keyboard and mouse as the primary or only technology available for physicians to document their care. Therefore, to meet the usability, efficiency, and patient interaction requirements of all physicians, it should be required that EHRs provide at least one alternative for each data entry option

a. For physicians who prefer direct computer entry, use of keyboard and mouse
b. For physicians who prefer to dictate some or all of their records, use of (i) voice recognition software or (ii) dictation with transcription
c. For physicians who prefer to write (legibly) some or all of their records, use of (i) a tablet PC or (ii) a digital pen with digital paper

In addition to physicians' personal preferences, each of these technologies offers its own particular advantages and limitations (15). Often overlooked is the potential added efficiency and usability of combining two or more of these modalities, each being employed where it is most comfortable for the physician. For example, a physician with poor handwriting might elect to use a tablet PC or mouse entry with clicks to rapidly place Xs in the check boxes of the graphic interface section of the physical examination (see Fig. 200.7) while dictating the free-text narrative required to precisely describe the details of each of the abnormal findings.

CODING AND BILLING FUNDAMENTALS

Whereas the principles and practice of physicians accurately *documenting* their patient care have been evolving since Hippocrates saw his first patient, the concept of "codifying" that patient care is a relatively recent phenomenon. It was not until the 1980s that Medicare and most insurers began requiring that physicians submit their claims for payment using CPT procedure codes and ICD diagnostic codes. Prior to that time, physicians submitted most insurance forms with a free-text description of the procedure performed (e.g., "tonsillectomy and adenoidectomy") and the accompanying diagnosis (e.g., "chronic tonsillitis"). Following the transition to payments based on coding, the purpose of which "is to provide a uniform language that will accurately describe medical, surgical, and diagnostic services" (16), practices have been required to select the most appropriate CPT procedure code (e.g., 42820, for tonsillectomy and adenoidectomy, younger than age 12) and the most appropriate ICD diagnosis code (e.g., 474.02, for chronic tonsillitis and adenoiditis).

Resources for Compliant Coding and Documentation (publications are available through various medical and compliance organizations)

1. CPT: Current Procedural Terminology" (*procedure codes, including E/M codes*)
2. "CPT Assistant" (*periodical, which publishes explanations and clarifications of CPT codes and instructions*)
3. "International Classification of Diseases, ICD-9-CM" (*diagnosis codes*)
4. "HCPCS Level 2" (*additional procedure codes*)
5. "Documentation Guidelines for Evaluation and Management Services," 1995 and 1997 editions (*Evaluation and Management Documentation principles*)
6. "Medicare RBRVS: The Physicians' Guide" (*Medicare RVUs and payments, global periods, assistant at surgery restrictions, cosurgeon adjustments*)
7. "CPT Reference of Clinical Examples" (AMA scenarios for correct coding of procedures and E/M services)
8. "National Correct Coding Initiative (NCCI) Edits" (Medicare scenarios for correct coding of procedures)

Resources for Compliance in Otolaryngology—Head and Neck Surgery (Available through the American Academy of Otolaryngology—Head and Neck Surgery)

1. AAO-HNS Clinical Indicators Compendium: http://www.entnet.org/Practice/clinicalIndicators.cfm
2. AAO-HNS Policy Statements: http://www.entnet.org/Practice/policystatements.cfm
3. AAO-HNS Clinical Practice Guidelines and Clinical Consensus Statements: http://www.entnet.org/Practice/clinicalPracticeguidelines.cfm

---

Although physician practices and hospitals view procedure and diagnosis coding almost exclusively through the lens of its role in reporting claims for proper payment, these codes also play additional roles in improving health care. CPT advises that its procedure code functions extend to "the development of guidelines for medical care review... to medical education and outcomes, health services, and quality research by providing a useful basis for local, regional, and national utilization comparisons" (16). ICD-9-CM codes are a United States "clinical modification" of the World Health Organization's International Classification of Disease. Its published intent is "to serve as a useful tool to classify morbidity data for indexing medical records, medical care review, and ambulatory and other medical care programs, as well as for basic health statistics" (17). These functions provide the foundation for some of the goals for system-wide use of EHRs, which are intended to facilitate the collection of coded information about symptoms and diseases, including the relative success of various procedures used to diagnose and treat them.

While these coding benefits promise to advance medical science and improve population health, the primary impact of coding on practicing U.S. physicians is accurate submission of claims to obtain correct payment in a timely manner. Reliable coding for payment depends on accurate documentation, and these demands will increase with the greater coding specificity being introduced in 2014 with the transition to ICD-10 diagnostic codes.

Integrating Coding and Billing Principles into Documentation and Patient Care

Commonly underemphasized or even overlooked in discussions of coding and billing practices, the critical factors in achieving compliant coding and documentation are *specificity* and *medical necessity*.

Specificity

Specificity is a central feature in identification of correct *procedure codes*, E/M codes, and diagnosis codes. CPT, the guide for procedure codes, instructs physicians to

"Select the name of the procedure or service that *accurately identifies* the service performed. Do not select a CPT code that merely approximates the service provided. If no such specific code exists, then report the service using the appropriate unlisted procedure or service code. In surgery, it may be an operation; in medicine, a diagnostic or therapeutic procedure; in radiology, a radiograph... Any service or procedure should be *adequately documented* in the medical record" (18).

These instructions not only underscore the need for specificity in identifying correct codes, they highlight the direct compliance link between coding and documentation. Physicians must have an appreciation and understanding of procedure codes in order to ensure that their *documentation* supports (i.e., verifies) that the procedure being coded was, in fact, performed. The potential hazards of nonspecific documentation and noncompliant coding are emphasized below.

Specificity is similarly a central feature in identification of correct *diagnosis codes*. ICD-9, the current guide for *diagnosis* codes, instructs physicians to

"Describe the patient's condition using terminology that uses **specific** diagnoses as well as symptoms, problems or reasons for the encounter. If symptoms are present but a definitive diagnosis has not been determined, code the symptoms... Determine whether the code is at the highest level of *specificity*. Assign three digit codes (category codes) if there are no four-digit codes within the code category. Assign four-digit codes (subcategory codes) if there are no five-digit codes for that category. Assign five-digit codes (fifth digit subclassification codes) for those categories where they are available" (19).

Medical Necessity

Medical necessity introduces the concepts of "standards of care" and, more recently, "evidence-based medicine" (EBM) into correct billing practices. Physicians are comfortable considering the *medical indications* for ordering tests, diagnostic procedures, medical treatments, and therapeutic procedures. *Medical necessity* is the parallel terminology used as a prime determinant for appropriate payment in insurance reviews. (This concept may also carry considerable weight in evaluations of quality care or professional liability.) Physicians commonly assume that their personal decision to provide various levels of office care, perform diagnostic or therapeutic procedures, or order certain diagnostic tests automatically qualify as a certification of medical necessity. In response to concerns about some of these decisions, Medicare and private insurers elected to establish and apply their own standards of medical necessity, at times using them as a basis for denying payment for correctly coded services. The resultant conflicts, appeals, and failure to have a common understanding of

this concept between physicians and insurers became one of the pivotal issues in the national class action lawsuits filed by physician organizations against health insurers in the first decade of the 21st century (20). The negotiations on this issue prompted the AMA and its affiliated specialty organizations to promulgate a definition of medical necessity that, with modifications during the negotiations, has become an established standard applied by physicians and insurers alike:

"'Medically Necessary' or 'Medical Necessity' shall mean health care services that a physician, exercising prudent clinical judgment, would provide to a patient for the purpose of preventing, evaluating, diagnosing or treating an illness, injury, disease or its symptoms, and that are: (a) in accordance with generally accepted standards of medical practice; (b) clinically appropriate, in terms of type, frequency, extent, site and duration, and considered effective for the patient's illness, injury or disease; and (c) not primarily for the convenience of the patient, physician, or other health care provider, and not more costly than an alternative service or sequence of services at least as likely to produce equivalent therapeutic or diagnostic results as to the diagnosis or treatment of that patient's illness, injury or disease. For these purposes, "generally accepted standards of medical practice" means standards that are based on credible scientific evidence published in peer-reviewed medical literature generally recognized by the *relevant* medical community, Physician Specialty Society recommendations and the views of physicians practicing in *relevant* clinical areas, and any other *relevant* factors" (21).

The introduction of the word "relevant" in multiple portions of this definition addressed concerns in broad language commonly found in insurer contracts that gave carriers wide latitude to consider any factors they chose. (Note: This definition's compromise language concerning *relative cost* of alternative services raises concerns about patients' rights to choose their care, even if more costly, under the doctrine of informed consent. While this notion could raise issues between patients and their insurers, physicians must be aware of the potential for insurers to deny payment for more costly service options; under such circumstances, it is advisable that they seek approval for payment prior to initiating such care.)

Fundamental Precepts of Billing, Coding, and Documentation

Three fundamental principles of medical record auditing provide the insight physicians need to understand correct billing and coding and to conceptualize their requirements for properly designed documentation tools needed to facilitate compliant coding while promoting optimal patient care:

1. Medicare stipulates, "*Medical necessity* of a service is the overarching criterion for payment in addition to the individual requirements of a CPT code" (22).
   a. This statement reflects criteria in section 1862 of Social Security Law that stipulate, "no payment may be made under (*Medicare*) part A or part B for any expenses incurred for items or services which… are not *reasonable and necessary* for the diagnosis or treatment of illness or injury or to improve the functioning of a malformed body member" (23).
   b. Finally, in its section reviewing payment for E/M services, the Trailblazer MAC's website further clarifies, "Federal law requires that *all expenses* paid by Medicare, including expenses for Evaluation and Management (E/M) services, are '*medically reasonable and necessary*'… Medicare's *determination of medical necessity is separate* from its determination that the E/M service was rendered as billed… At audit, Medicare will deny or downcode E/M services that, in its judgment, *exceed the patient's documented needs*" (24).
2. "If medical care is not documented in the medical record, it is treated as if it had not been performed." (25)
   a. Although this statement is no longer found in the current CMS Carriers' Manual, it was obtained from section 7103.1(i) of an older version. Related language also appears on the Trailblazer MAC website, reporting that an error in coding occurs when "Documentation is incomplete/insufficient: (*i.e.,*) documentation does not support the level of service billed" (26).
3. "Automation is not documentation" (27).
   a. Preloaded generic clinical information that is copied and inserted from previous encounters (copy forward), from preloaded macros (copy/paste) or created by filling in multiple check boxes with a single click (documentation by exception) fail to record individualized clinical information related to each patient and each encounter. Although the use of automated data entry is most frequently found in suboptimal designs for EHRs, similar functionality has found its way into dictated operative reports and E/M records with distressingly increasing frequency.
   b. Reviewing records created with automated documentation reveals that physicians using this approach almost always undocument and redocument only the clinical information that is relevant to their patient's presenting illness. Because of the automated defaults to "normal findings," all other aspects of the patient's health almost always appear in the completed H&P as normal—a circumstance that is not compatible with the reality of most patients' health status. In other words, such "cloned records" attempt to give the impression that the physician performed *comprehensive care*, when in fact the repetitive "normal" findings in history and examination related to other organ systems attest to the fact that the physician performed and accurately documented only *problem-focused care*.
   c. As noted above in the box reporting a "final verdict" on cloned documentation, automated documentation consistently fails to provide both of the critical factors needed for compliant coding and documentation: it is insufficient to record the *specificity* required for individualized clinical information, and it is therefore "considered a misrepresentation of the *medical necessity* requirement for coverage of services" (28).

Fortunately, these three auditing principles can be transformed into three powerful core documentation principles that physicians can employ to ensure compliant documentation, coding, and billing:

1. When (patient-specific and visit-specific) care is documented, it was done.
2. When care is medically necessary, and that necessity is *documented* in the medical record, payment must be made.
3. Nonautomated (i.e., individually documented) records promote compliance and can also enhance quality of care.

DESIGNING MEDICAL RECORDS TO MEET PHYSICIANS' NEEDS

These three documentation principles can be used as cornerstones for medical record designs that meet all of physicians' requirements for effective documentation and coding tools:

- Usability: Ease of data entry with options to use multiple data entry modalities—dictation, legible handwriting, and/or keyboard and mouse
- Efficiency: Completing care and individualized documentation in a reasonable time frame without sacrificing compliance or data integrity
- Compliance: For both procedure and E/M records, the documentation should verify specific details of what was performed and the medical necessity of performing that care.
- Data integrity: The documented record should clearly and easily convey all the care performed and the reasons why it was performed (to another physician, to a reviewer, and most importantly to the physician himself/herself during subsequent visits).
- Promoting quality patient care: During E/M services, compliance-based documentation tools follow the diagnostic paradigm taught to physicians from the Bates' Guide; this facilitates providing levels of care warranted by the NPPs during each encounter.
- Appropriate productivity: Care, documentation, coding, and billing are all achieved at medically indicated levels, which the physician determines and sets based on his or her assessment of medical necessity.

Compliant Designs for Documenting Operative Procedures

While surgeons have been dictating operative reports for many years, the traditional approach commonly includes only demographic information, preoperative and postoperative diagnoses, the name(s) of the operation(s) performed, and a free-text narrative of the procedure. However, the operative note frequently fails to provide an explanation of the medical indications (i.e., the *medical necessity*) for performing the procedure. More recently, some physicians have also sought to save time in creating their operative reports by instructing their transcriptionists to insert generic macros to describe the procedure performed, in lieu of individualized dictation. This effort to save dictation time and costs illustrates the danger of replacing documentation with automation: every operation for every patient reads almost exactly the same, thereby sacrificing *specificity*.

These deficits can be remedied. *Medical necessity* should be documented by adding a section for "indications" near the beginning of the report. Here the physician dictates a narrative description of the clinical rationale warranting the performance of the surgical procedure. *Specificity* for the significant observations made during the course of the operation should be documented by dictating individualized narrative descriptions of the steps in the procedure and insertion of an additional section labeled "Operative Findings." This section conveys the nuances of the operation and significant anatomic findings and challenges. For example, when dictating a tonsillectomy, the surgeon can document whether significant scar tissue or aberrant blood vessels were found in the dissection plane of each of the two tonsils, as well as the approximate amount of bleeding and how readily it was controlled. Figure 200.1 illustrates a sample template for operative procedures, including sections to document indications and operative findings.

Can macros ever be used compliantly in an operative report? Only under stringent guidelines. Most surgeons employ a reasonably standard technique when performing the straightforward procedures of tonsillectomy and adenoidectomy (T&A) or myringotomy with tube insertion. A physician could employ a detailed macro that reports this standardized procedure, providing that the physician adds specificity by dictating individualized narrative sections for "Indications" and "Operative Findings." In addition, if a particular procedure presents unusual challenges, difficulties, and/or complications, the procedure section should be documented individually instead of attempting to modify the macro. For more extensive operations that have greater complexity and/or variation in anatomic and pathologic findings, it is preferable for specificity that physicians avoid macros and dictate the procedures as free text.

Similar principles apply to creating compliant templates for minor diagnostic procedures performed in the office setting, such as fiberoptic laryngoscopy, fiberoptic nasal endoscopy, and fiberoptic nasopharyngoscopy. Because examination of the larynx, pharynx, and nasal passages are included elements of the physical examination portion of E/M visits in the practice of Otolaryngology—Head and Neck Surgery, there must be appropriate medical indications documented to warrant billing for these services in addition to the usual direct and indirect (mirror) examinations of the internal nose, pharynx, and larynx.

```
Patient Name:       _____

Date of Operation: _____/_____/_____

Operation(s) Performed: _____
                        _____

Surgeon: _____

Pre-Operative Diagnoses: _____

Post-Operative Diagnoses: _____

Indications:


Operative Findings:


Procedure:
```

Figure 200.1 Sample operative report for operating room procedures.

A user-friendly, efficient, and compliant operative report template, as illustrated below, can include

- A graphic interface for rapid documentation of the appropriate medical indication(s)
- A brief macro describing the standard topical anesthesia, passage of the endoscope, and areas examined
- A section for documenting specific operative findings that combines graphic elements to record normal findings plus narrative sections (indicated by blank lines) to record details of all significant or abnormal findings

For physicians who prefer to dictate (or whose handwriting is illegible), the same template can be used with only the free-text sections being dictated instead of writing on the blank lines. When the operative report thereby becomes a hybrid of written template plus dictation, it is preferable to check the box labeled "see attached dictation" to ensure that the record is not misinterpreted in the case of an audit or medicolegal review.

Below are sample templates of operative reports for fiberoptic laryngoscopy and diagnostic nasal endoscopy (Fig. 200.2).

Patient: _____   Account #: _____

Date of Operation: _____ / _____ / _____   ☐ **With Video Review**

Surgeon: ☐ Dr. A   ☐ Dr. B
                ☐ Dr. C   ☐ Dr. D

Procedure: **Flexible Fiberoptic Flexible Pharyngo-Laryngoscopy**

Pre-operative Diagnosis: _____

Post-operative Diagnosis: _____

Indications for use of fiberoptic examination: Need for improved visualization due to:

☐ Hyperactive gag reflex   ☐ Posterior epiglottis position

☐ Obstructive base of tongue   ☐ Inability to visualize anterior commissure

☐ Detailed evaluation of lesion   ☐ History of treated neoplasm

☐ Enhanced mucosal visualization (to evaluate inflammation and edema)

☐ Evaluation of documented obstructive sleep apnea, with Mueller maneuver

☐ Other: _____

Procedure: The patient's nose was prepared with topical anesthesia, using cotton pledgets moistened with a solution of 4% lidocaine combined with 0.5% neosynephrine. Five minutes was allowed for anesthetic and vasoconstrictive effect, and the pledgets were removed. A flexible fiberoptic laryngoscope was advanced through the nostril to sequentially examine the nasopharynx, palate, oropharynx, base of tongue, epiglottis, larynx, hypopharynx, and piriform sinuses.

Findings:
  Nasopharynx:
    ☐ Normal mucosa   ☐ Diffuse inflammation: mild moderate severe
    _____

  Larynx and hypopharynx:
  Vocal cords: ☐ normal   ☐ abnormal   Arytenoids: ☐ normal   ☐ abnormal
  Retrocricoid: ☐ normal   ☐ abnormal   Post commiss: ☐ normal   ☐ abnormal
  _____

  Palate and oropharynx/Other:
  _____
  _____

                                              ☐ See attached dictation
_____
Signature

Figure 200.2 Sample procedure reports for diagnostic nasopharyngolaryngoscopy and nasal endoscopy.

Patient: _____   Account #: _____

Date of Operation: _____ / _____ / _____   ☐ **With Video Review**

Surgeon: ☐ Dr. A   ☐ Dr. B
                        ☐ Dr. C   ☐ Dr. D

Procedure: **Diagnostic Fiberoptic Nasal Endoscopy**

Pre-operative Diagnosis: _____

Post-operative Diagnosis: _____

Indications for use of fiberoptic examination: Need for improved visualization of intranasal anatomy, due to:

☐ Assess chronic sinusitis (post Rx)   ☐ Need to visualize ostiomeatal complex

☐ Assess nasal polyp(s) (post Rx)   ☐ Need to visualize posterior nasal space

☐ Chronic headache/facial pain   ☐ Need to evaluate compression points

☐ Uncontrolled posterior epistaxis   ☐ Need to visualize nasopharynx

☐ Pre-operative planning for endoscopic sinus surgery

☐ Other: _____

Procedure: The patient's nose was prepared with topical anesthesia, using cotton pledgets moistened with a solution of 4% lidocaine combined with 0.5% neosynephrine. Five minutes was allowed for anesthetic and vasoconstrictive effect, and the pledgets were removed. The rigid fiberoptic nasal endoscope was advanced through each nostril in turn to sequentially examine the septum, turbinates, ostiomeatal complex, and nasopharynx.

Findings:
  Right nostril:
    Mucosa: ☐ normal ☐ inflamed ☐ edematous   Mucus: ☐ normal ☐ abnormal
    Septum: ☐ normal ☐ abnormal   Turbinates: ☐ normal ☐ abnormal
    Ostiomeatal complex: ☐ normal ☐ abnormal   Nasopharynx: ☐ normal ☐ abnormal
    _____
    _____

  Left nostril:
    Mucosa: ☐ normal ☐ inflamed ☐ edematous   Mucus: ☐ normal ☐ abnormal
    Septum: ☐ normal ☐ abnormal   Turbinates: ☐ normal ☐ abnormal
    Ostiomeatal complex: ☐ normal ☐ abnormal   Nasopharynx: ☐ normal ☐ abnormal
    _____
    _____

                                                 ☐ See attached dictation
_____
Signature

Figure 200.2 *(Continued)*

Compliant Designs for Documenting Evaluation and Management (E/M) Services

The E/M documentation and coding system first appeared in the 1992 edition of the AMA's publications of CPT. It is built on the economic principles of the resource-based relative value system (RBRVS), also introduced in 1992, which for each service provided (and coded) seeks to quantify the relative values of physicians' individual work, practice expense, and liability insurance costs. Early E/M training focused almost exclusively on the system's three "key components": medical history, physical examination, and medical decision-making. These are the E/M elements used to report the *specificity* of care provided. However, as E/M training evolved, compliance experts recognized the importance of placing equal emphasis on NPPs, which is one of the E/M system's four contributory factors. "[A] critical insight to coordinating coding and documentation with *medical necessity* and appropriate quality care is to include NPP as a mandatory fourth factor" (29).

Performing and documenting effective evaluation and management services has received steadily increasing emphasis over the last several years through recent initiatives for (a) implementation of quality measures; (b) MS-DRG requirements for sophisticated reporting of hospital inpatient E/M services; (c) adoption of EHRs; (d) increasing oversight through audits by Medicare Administrative Contractors (MACs), the Office of the Inspector General (OIG), Recovery Audit Contractors (RACs), and the new Zone Program Integrity Contractors (ZPICs); and (e) continued economic constriction (relative to practice costs) in the Medicare and insurer payment systems.

"As physicians and administrators confront the challenges created by these and other changes in the health care environment, they consistently discover that meaningful solutions depend upon effective, compliant, and efficient medical record documentation. Meeting this goal begins with documentation of a meaningful history and physical examination (H&P), which helps physicians ensure that their patients receive levels of clinical care that are appropriately matched to the severity of their illnesses (i.e., matched to the nature of the presenting problems)" (30). Although a comprehensive analysis and presentation of complete solutions to the E/M compliance challenge are beyond the scope of a single chapter, reviewing a set of core principles can provide the basis for incorporating reliable and compliant E/M documentation and coding into patient care. In addition to the three core documentation principles cited previously, effective E/M methodology and documentation tools can be built on a foundation of five basic postulates:

1. *Quality care must be the principle measure for effective medical records.* This principle puts documentation and coding into proper perspective; patient care comes first, and rules and guidelines must conform to this framework to be considered credible.
2. *The E/M process must "work" for clinicians.* That is, the protocol for evaluating patients must be compatible with physicians' optimal diagnostic process and patient care workflow. Since the E/M system is a codification of the workflow presented in the *Bates' Guide to Physical Examination and History Taking*, incorporating E/M guidelines into the structure of a medical record form results in a document that is familiar to physicians (the comprehensive H&P learned in medical school) and intuitive for them to learn and use.
3. *Medical record forms must incorporate consideration and documentation of the NPPs.* This inclusion provides documentation of medical necessity, based on the physician's case-specific assessment. It also allows the forms to include compliant documentation prompts, which

can guide physicians to perform, document, and code for medically indicated levels of care that are warranted by the severity of patients' illnesses.

4. *Appropriate documentation and coding must be integrated into the process of providing care,* not added on as an additional challenging task at the end of a patient visit.
5. *Use of tools, not rules.* Successful medical record designs incorporate all E/M requirements and guidelines into sophisticated documentation *tools,* instead of demanding physicians to memorize long lists of complex compliance rules.

Effective *E/M methodology* reflects the ideal care process and workflow that physicians are taught during their training. Unfortunately, the demand for completing this care in a limited time frame prevents physicians from implementing this optimal workflow due to lack of appropriate documentation tools. Providing effective and efficient tools, as described below, gives physicians the ability to reapply the optimal diagnostic process. This process begins with a comprehensive medical history (complete PFSH and review of systems plus an extended history of present illness) during every patient visit. This global review of each patient's status not only facilitates developing an accurate and inclusive differential diagnosis; it also provides the perspective physicians need to determine the relative severity of illness (i.e., the NPPs). Armed with this insight, plus helpful documentation prompts on their H&P templates, physicians can then perform and document the appropriate level of physical examination and medical decision making that are medically indicated by the severity of the NPP. Of course, while history-based severity assessments are frequently accurate, they are confirmed or modified on the basis of findings during the physical examination and review of available diagnostic tests.

Precise documentation of *all* E/M elements is critical to ensuring E/M compliance, particularly in the event of an external audit. This includes documentation of the traditional H&P components: (a) complete medical history, (b) normal and abnormal examination findings, (c) data reviewed, (d) assessment (differential diagnosis), and (e) plans (treatments and data ordered). However, two critical elements required for E/M compliance should be added to this standard approach: (f) documentation of the physician's assessment of the three levels of risk and (g) documentation of the physician's final assessment of the NPPs. The three levels of risk are described in CPT and the Documentation Guidelines Table of Risk (31) as

"The risk of significant complications, morbidity, and/ or mortality, as well as comorbidities, associated with (1) the patient's presenting problem(s), (2) the diagnostic procedure(s), and/or (3) the possible management options" (32).

The additional documentation of a physician's assessment of levels of risk and the NPP can be accomplished efficiently through the use of check boxes on the H&P form, and this supplemental documentation provides irrefutable support for the *medical necessity* of the level of care provided.

Effective *H&P forms* should be designed for usability and efficiency, with inclusion of E/M compliance rules to ensure appropriate care and documentation. Figures 200.3 to 200.9 illustrate portions of E/M forms for outpatient services (appropriately modified forms can be designed for inpatient care or other E/M services as well). These templates are compatible with the specialty of Otolaryngology—Head and Neck Surgery, including the single organ system ENT examination from the 1997 Documentation Guidelines.

Physicians at Teaching Hospits and "Physician Presence"

On December 13, 1995, The New York Times published a report that sent a compliance shock wave through the community of academic physicians. It reported that the "University of Pennsylvania's Health System has agreed to pay thirty million dollars to settle government complaints that it filed improper Medicare bills for doctors' services.... This substantial settlement followed a Government audit of one hundred patients treated in 1993" (45). The government had extrapolated the outcome of this limited audit over all of the comparable records for multiple years, calculating a fine that was significantly higher than the final settlement amount.

The audit identified two significant issues. One concerned submission of claims for E/M services at levels significantly exceeding the level of care documented in the medical record by residents and physicians (the same E/M issues discussed above). The second issue highlighted a new concept that subsequently became known as "physician presence." Charges had been submitted by attending physicians for E/M services that were clearly provided and documented by residents. Although physicians had placed their signature on the residents' charts, there was no documented evidence of the attending physicians being present during the residents' care of the patients or of independently performing any of the billed patient care. Instead, the audits determined that the teaching physicians' signatures on the charts indicated only they had reviewed the resident's notes, not that they had provided actual E/M services. The audit concluded that this practice was evidence of billing twice for the same service, since Medicare pays an additional fee to teaching hospitals for the residents' care of covered patients, and that was the only care documented as having been performed.

In establishing requirements for teaching physician to submit E/M claims when caring for patients in conjunction with residents, Medicare and the OIG referred to established rules published by the Health Care Financing Administration (HCFA; now CMS) in Intermediary Letter 372 (IL-372). HCFA subsequently clarified these guidelines in 1996 in a new "Final Rule for Teaching Physicians," presented in section 15016 of the Medicare Carriers Manual. In 2002s Transmittal 1780, CMS augmented section 15016 with several clarifications and examples for writing attestations of care, though without substantially altering the established principles and documentation requirements for teaching physicians to submit E/M claims. It is noteworthy that adhering to these more recent shortcut suggestions frequently leads once again to imprecise documentation of the actual care that teaching physicians perform. It can therefore be advised that incorporating the actual details of IL-372 and section 15016 into templates to document physician presence provides superior guidance and increased probability of compliance.

Teaching physicians are cautioned that if they elect to simply sign residents' notes, they should not submit claims for these services. However, following such an approach would not only be inadequate to meet payment requirements, it would also fail to reflect care provided, fulfillment of resident teaching responsibilities, and protection in the event of a professional liability claim.

On the positive side, the IL-372 and section 15016 guidelines provide three scenarios that permit attending physicians to submit claims for E/M services when they share care with residents. In the first scenario, the teaching physician would personally perform, document, and code only for the elements of an E/M service that he or she completed independent of the resident (46); this approach requires more time for comprehensive care and documentation than optimal in the teaching situation. In the second option, the resident performs the elements required for an E/M service in the presence of, or jointly with, the teaching physician, and the resident documents the service (47); except under unusual circumstances, this approach also requires excess teaching physician time and creates awkward scheduling challenges.

The final compliant option fortunately matches up extremely well with appropriate patient care workflow for teaching physicians. In this approach, the resident provides and documents the level of care medically indicated for the patient, and "the teaching physician independently performs the critical or key portion(s) of the service with or without the resident present and, as appropriate, discusses the case with the resident. In this instance, the teaching physician must document that he or she personally saw the patient, personally performed critical or key portions of the service, and participated in the management of the patient. The teaching physician's note should reference the resident's note. For payment, the composite of the teaching physician's entry and the resident's entry together

Patient Name:_____   Account No._____   DOB:____/____/____

Initial Visit Medical History Form (p. 1): Please provide the following medical information to the best of your ability:

Date:	Age:	List any **ALLERGIES TO MEDICATIONS:**
What problems are you here for today?		

Past Medical History:

1) Please check the "Yes" or "No" box to indicate if you have any of the following illnesses; for "Yes" answers, please explain

	Yes	No			Yes	No	
Diabetes (Circle: type I / type II)	☐	☐	_____	Stomach or Intestinal problems	☐	☐	_____
Hypertension (high blood press)	☐	☐	_____	Allergy problems/therapy	☐	☐	_____
Thyroid problems	☐	☐	_____	Kidney problems	☐	☐	_____
Heart Disease/cholesterol probs	☐	☐	_____	Neurological problems	☐	☐	_____
Respiratory problems	☐	☐	_____	Cancer	☐	☐	_____
Bleeding disorder	☐	☐		Other Medical Diagnosis	☐	☐	_____

2) **Please list any operations (and dates) you have ever had** *(including tonsils & adenoids)*:

3) **Please list any current medications (and amounts, times per day);**
(include aspirin, antacids, vitamins, hormone replacement, birth control, herbal supplements, OTC meds including sinus/allergy/weight loss meds):

Social History:

	Yes	No	Please list details below:	
Do you use tobacco?	☐	☐	List type and how much:_____	
If no, did you use it previously?	☐	☐	List type and how much:_____	**When did you quit?**
Do you drink alcohol?	☐	☐	List type and how much:_____	
Do you use recrational drugs?	☐	☐	List type and how much:_____	
What is your occupation?			_____	

Family History:

Please check the "Yes" or "No" box to indicate whether any relatives have any of the following illnesses:
If yes, please indicate which relative(s) have the problem

	Yes	No	
Heart problems / murmurs	☐	☐	_____
Allergy	☐	☐	_____
Diabetes	☐	☐	_____
Cancer	☐	☐	_____
Bleeding disorder	☐	☐	_____
Anesthesia problems	☐	☐	_____

☐ See attached dictation   Reviewed by:

Figure 200.3 Initial outpatient visit—CC and PFSH (33). This section is presented in questionnaire format, as encouraged by the Documentation Guidelines, for patients to complete and for physicians to review, confirm, and supplement positive responses (34) (by writing on the blank lines or by supplemental dictation).

Date____/____/____

Patient Name:_____   Account No._____   DOB:____/____/____

Patient Medical History Form (p. 2): Please provide the following medical information to the best of your ability:

Review of Systems:

1) Please check the "Yes" or "No" box to indicate whether you presently have any of the following symptoms:

2) For any "yes" responses, please check the "current" box if this symptom relates to the reason for your visit today

		Yes	No	Current		Yes	No	Current
GENERAL	chills	☐	☐	☐	weight loss or gain	☐	☐	☐
	fatigue	☐	☐	☐	daytime sleepiness	☐	☐	☐
ALLERGY	environmental allergy	☐	☐	☐	sneezing fits	☐	☐	☐
NEURO	headache	☐	☐	☐	weakness	☐	☐	☐
	passing out	☐	☐	☐	numbness, tingling	☐	☐	☐
EYES	eye pain / pressure	☐	☐	☐	vision changes	☐	☐	☐
	watery or itchy eyes	☐	☐	☐				
ENT	hearing loss	☐	☐	☐	ear noises	☐	☐	☐
	dizziness	☐	☐	☐	lightheadedness	☐	☐	☐
	nasal congestion	☐	☐	☐	sinus pressure or pain	☐	☐	☐
	hoarseness	☐	☐	☐	problem snoring, apnea	☐	☐	☐
	throat clearing	☐	☐	☐	throat pain	☐	☐	☐
RESPIR.	cough	☐	☐	☐	coughing blood	☐	☐	☐
	wheezing	☐	☐	☐	shortness of breath	☐	☐	☐
CARDIAC	chest pain	☐	☐	☐	palpitations	☐	☐	☐
	wake short of breath	☐	☐	☐	ankle swelling	☐	☐	☐
GI	difficulty swallowing	☐	☐	☐	heartburn	☐	☐	☐
	abdominal pain	☐	☐	☐	nausea/vomiting	☐	☐	☐
	bowel irregularity	☐	☐	☐	rectal bleeding	☐	☐	☐
GU	frequent urination	☐	☐	☐	painful urination	☐	☐	☐
	blood in urine	☐	☐	☐	prostate problems	☐	☐	☐
HEME/LYM	swollen glands	☐	☐	☐	sweating at night	☐	☐	☐
	bleeding problems	☐	☐	☐	easy bruising	☐	☐	☐
ENDO	feel warmer than others	☐	☐	☐	feel cooler than others	☐	☐	☐
MSK	joint aches	☐	☐	☐	muscle aches	☐	☐	☐
SKIN	rash	☐	☐	☐	hives	☐	☐	☐
	itching	☐	☐	☐	skin or hair changes	☐	☐	☐
PSYCH	depression	☐	☐	☐	anxiety or panic	☐	☐	☐

PLEASE STOP HERE   ☐ See attached dictation

Reviewed by:

Figure 200.4 Initial outpatient visit—ROS (review of systems) (35). This section is presented in questionnaire format, as encouraged by the Documentation Guidelines, for patients to complete and for physicians to review, confirm, and supplement positive responses (36) (by writing on the blank lines or by supplemental dictation).

Established Patient Visit Form

| Patient Name:_____ | | Account No._____ | DOB:____/____/____ |

Date: ____/____/____   **PMH/SH/FH**   no change since last visit date: _____

   Except: _____

_____

New Allergies: _____   **Existing allergies:** _____

Current Medications: _____

Reviewed by:

ROS   no change since last visit date: _____

   Except: _____

Reviewed by:

Figure 200.5 Established outpatient visit—update of PFSH and ROS (37). This use of an "update" to obtain and document the equivalent of a complete PFSH and ROS is indicated by the Documentation Guidelines (38). If obtained by a nurse or medical assistant, physicians must review, confirm, and supplement positive responses (by writing on the blank lines or by supplemental dictation).

must support the medical necessity of the billed service and the level of the service billed by the teaching physician" (47). This third scenario allows teaching physicians to see their patients independently, where they can review their residents' "comprehensive" medical notes and then perform and document care that is "problem focused" on the patients' major medical issues. This also allows for the common practice where attending physicians regularly communicate with and teach their residents about these issues during normal teaching rounds. There are two requirements for effective documentation tools for teaching physicians to achieve compliant documentation and coding in this setting. First, the resident requires compliant documentation tools such as those described above (appropriate forms for inpatient care are available (48)) to ensure that his or her care and medical record documentation support the appropriate level of service. The resident's

H&P record should also report the name of the attending physician. Second, the teaching physician will benefit from a compliant medical record template built on the principles and vocabulary of IL-372 and CMS section 15016 guidelines. A sample form is shown in Figure 200.10.

CODING COMPLEXITIES, RBRVS, AND USE OF MODIFIERS

Excellent documentation and correct coding of each procedure or E/M service are essential for compliance and for billing, but they are only the first steps towards successful submission of claims for payment to MACs and private insurers. These fiscal organizations use sophisticated software systems with complex paradigms of coding relationships to determine the circumstances under which they will authorize payments for your claims.

Established Patient Visit Form

PRESENT ILLNESS	Chronology with:	1. one to three elements [level 2 or 3] 2. four to eight elements; OR status of 3 chronic or inactive conditions [level 4 or 5]
	(1) duration (2) timing (3) severity; (4) location (5) quality (6) context (7) modifying factors (8) assoc. signs & symptoms	
Chief Complaint:		☐ See attached dictation

Figure 200.6 Established outpatient visit—CC and history of present illness (39). This section requires free-text narrative for quality care and compliance. This may be documented by writing on the blank lines or by dictation. Note the documentation prompt, based on medically indicated level of care. In addition to listing the eight elements of the HPI, this prompt stresses obtaining and documenting a "chronological description of the development of the patient's present illness from the first sign and/or symptom [for initial visits] or from the previous encounter [for established patient visits] to the present" (40).

Date ____/____/____   Patient States Consultation Requested By_____

PHYSICAL EXAMINATION:		Ear Nose & Throat						

GENERAL   (at least 3 measurements of vital signs)

BP sitting-standing ____/____mm Hg

PULSE ____/min   regular - irregular

HT___ft____in   WT_____lbs

BP supine____/____mm Hg

RESP ____/min   TEMP _____o (F-C)

			Normal/AB				Normal/AB
	GENERAL APPEARANCE	Stature, nutrition	☐ ☐	NECK	MASSES & TRACHEA	Symmetry, masses	☐ ☐
	COMMUNICATION & VOICE	Pitch, clarity	☐ ☐		THYROID	Size, nodules	☐ ☐
HEAD/	INSPECTION	Lesions, masses	☐ ☐	EYES	OCULAR MOTILITY & GAZE	EOMs, nystagmus	☐ ☐
FACE	PALPATION / PERCUSSION	Skeleton, sinuses	☐ ☐	RESP.	RESPIRATORY EFFORT	Inspiratory-expiratory	☐ ☐
	SALIVARY GLANDS	Masses, tenderness	☐ ☐		AUSCULTATION	Lung sounds	☐ ☐
	FACIAL STRENGTH	Symmetry	☐ ☐	CVS	HEART AUSCULTATION	rhythm, heart sounds	☐ ☐
ENT	PNEUMO-OTOSCOPY	EACs; TMs mobile	☐ ☐		PERIPH VASC SYSTEM	Edema, color	☐ ☐
	HEARING ASSESSMENT	Gross; Weber/Rinne	☐ ☐	LYMPH.	NECK/AXILLAE/GROIN/ETC.	Adenopathy	☐ ☐
	EXTERNAL EAR & NOSE	Appearance	☐ ☐	NEURO/	CRANIAL NERVES	II - XII	☐ ☐
	INTERNAL NOSE	Mucosa, turbinates	☐ ☐	PSYCH.	ORIENTATION	Person, place, time	☐ ☐
	*AFTER DECONGESTANT	Septum, OMCs	☐ ☐		MOOD & AFFECT	Comments	☐ ☐
	LIPS,TEETH & GUMS	Mucosa, dentition	☐ ☐		*ROMBERG		☐ ☐
	ORAL CAVITY, OROPHARYNX	Mucosa, tonsils, palate	☐ ☐		*TANDEM ROMBERG		☐ ☐
	HYPOPHARYNX	Mucosa, pyriforms	☐ ☐		*PAST POINTING		☐ ☐
	LARYNX (mirror: adults)	Anatomy, vocal cord mobility	☐ ☐				
	NASOPHAR. (mirror: adults)	Mucosa, choanae	☐ ☐		☐ See attached dictation		

1. problem focused = 1-5 elements [level 1]   2. expanded = 6-11 elements [level 2]   3. detailed = 12 or more elements [level 3]
4. comprehensive = document every element in basic areas AND at least 1 element in each optional area [level 4 or 5]   *optional

Figure 200.7 Initial outpatient visit—physical examination (41). This section is based on the single organ system examination for "ear, nose, mouth, and throat" presented in the 1997 Documentation Guidelines. Physicians must document findings for all elements examined as normal or abnormal. Pertinent normal descriptions are preloaded, and physicians must provide detailed descriptions for all abnormal findings (42) (by writing on the blank lines or by supplemental dictation). Note the documentation prompt, based on medically indicated level of care, located at the bottom of the section.

Claims for Individual Services Only

The most straightforward of these paradigms certify that procedures are age and gender appropriate and cross-check databases to ensure that charges are not made for surgery on body parts that had previously been removed. For example, a claim for CPT code 99385 (initial preventive medicine evaluation, age 18 to 39 years) will be rejected if the insurer's records indicate the patient is only 13 years old. Similarly, claims will be rejected for a prostate biopsy on a female patient or for gallbladder surgery on a patient whose records document previous performance of a cholecystectomy.

On a more sophisticated level, payers' claims processing software compares for appropriateness each procedure code with the associated diagnosis code(s). It will automatically reject procedure code 31575 (fiberoptic laryngoscopy) if it is submitted with diagnosis code 470 (deviated nasal septum); the diagnosis does not support medical necessity for performing this type of procedure. Most of these software programs also assign an assumed level of illness severity to various diagnosis codes as well as medical necessity indicators for many pairings of procedure and diagnosis codes. As a result, for example, the programs will generally deny claims for E/M code 99214 (moderate to high NPP) when submitted with the sole diagnosis code of 460 (acute nasopharyngitis or common cold) or 461.2 (acute ethmoid sinusitis); these diagnoses are not usually associated with sufficient illness severity to warrant high-level E/M services. They will also reject claims for CPT code 31231 (diagnostic nasal endoscopy) if submitted with either code 460 or

MEDICAL DECISION MAKING	2 of the 3 sections (a vs a', b vs b vs b''', c vs c' vs c'') must meet or exceed indicated level of care	
DATA REVIEWED (c):	1. Minimal (level 2) 2. Limited (level 3) 3. Moderate (level 4) 4. Extensive (level 5)	

☐ Audiology   ☐ See attached dictation

☐ X-ray / CT scan

☐ Lab/ blood work

IMPRESSIONS / DIFFERENTIAL DIAGNOSES (a):   **PLANS / MANAGEMENT OPTIONS (a')**

1. Minimal (level 2)   2. Limited (level 3)   3. Multiple (level 4)   4. Extensive (level 5)

1) _____   1) _____   ☐ See attached dictation

2) _____   2) _____

3) _____   3) _____

4) _____   4) _____

5) _____   5) _____

DATA ORDERED (c'):   1. Minimal or none (level 2)   2. Limited (level 3)   3. Moderate (level 4)   4. Extensive (level 5)

☐ Audiology   ☐ Sinus CT scan   ☐ MRI of IACs w gad.   ☐ Allergy testing

                                                                                      ☐ See attached dictation

---

COMPLEXITY OF DATA REVIEWED OR ORDERED (c'')

1. Minimal (level 2)   2. Limited (level 3)   3. Moderate (level 4)   4. Extensive (level 5)

1. min   2. limited   3. mod   4. extensive

RISK OF COMPLICATIONS &/OR MORBIDITY OR MORTALITY (see examples in Table of Risk)

1. Minimal (level 2)   2. Low (level 3)   3. Moderate (level 4)   4. High (level 5)

risk of presenting problem(s) (b):   1. min   2. low   3. mod   4. high

risk of diagnostic procedure(s) ordered or reviewed (b'):   1. min   2. low   3. mod   4. high

risk of management option(s) selected (b''):   1. min   2. low   3. mod   4. high

Figure 200.8 Initial or established outpatient visit—medical decision-making (MDM) (43). This section includes all three subcomponents of MDM, separated into their related elements and organized to be compatible with physicians' diagnostic process. Note particularly the inclusion of a section for documentation of the three levels of risk. Also note the documentation prompts, based on medically indicated level of care, located in each subsection.

461.2 because of lack of medical necessity (medical indications) for performing this procedure under these circumstances. It is therefore essential for physicians and/or their staff (billing specialists or certified coders) to match each CPT code with one or more appropriate diagnosis codes. In addition, many accounts receivable systems for medical practices are equipped with "claims scrubbers," software programs that review the coding and identify potential coding discrepancies for review and possible correction prior to claim submission.

Claims for Multiple Procedures on Same Date of Service

The magnitude of coding and billing challenges increases significantly when claims are submitted for two or more procedures, or for a procedure and an E/M service, performed on the same date of service. Addressing the complexity of claims for multiple CPT services requires an appreciation of a number of fundamental coding and billing principles.

Principle #1: The claims processing software of Medicare Carriers and essentially all private insurers are programmed to authorize payment for only one service per day. (The exceptions to this policy are codes labeled as "add-on codes" and codes with an "XXX" designation, indicating they are exempt from being combined under a surgical package or global concept.) Achieving payment for more than one appropriately coded service on the same day requires the use of appropriate *modifiers* to alert payers' software that the claims should be paid. Modifiers are described in detail in Appendix A of CPT (49) and summarized below.

NATURE OF PRESENTING PROBLEM(S)

☐ minor   (level 1)   Problem runs definite and prescribed course, is transient in nature, and is not likely to permanently alter health status; OR, has a good prognosis with management and compliance.

☐ low   (level 1)   Problem where the risk of morbidity without treatment is low; there is little to no risk of mortality
      (level 2 for consult)   without treatment; full recovery without functional impairment is expected.

☐ low - mod   (level 2)   Problem where the risk of morbidity without treatment is low to moderate; there is low to moderate risk of mortality without treatment; full recovery without functional impairment is expected in most cases, with low probability of prolonged functional impairment

☐ moderate   (level 3)   Problem where the risk of morbidity without treatment is moderate; there is moderate risk of mortality without treatment; prognosis is uncertain, or there is an increased probability of prolonged functional impairment.

☐ mod - high   (level 4,5)   Problem where the risk of morbidity without treatment is moderate to high; there is moderate risk of mortality without treatment; uncertain prognosis or increased probability of prolonged functional impairment

☐ high   (level 4,5)   Problem where the risk of morbidity without treatment is high to extreme; there is moderate to high risk of mortality without treatment, or high probability of severe prolonged functional impairment.

Figure 200.9 Initial Outpatient Visit - Nature of the Presenting Problem(s) (NPP) (44). This section provides CPT descriptions of illness severity associated with various levels of NPP; these are supplemented by associated levels of care presented in the CPT descriptors. Appropriate templates for NPP of established outpatient visits and other types of service are also available (44). Clinical examples, approved by various specialty societies including AAO-HNS, are provided in Appendix C of CPT.

Principle #2: Most surgical procedures include a "surgical package" of additional care services (50). The surgical package also includes expected E/M services related to the procedure for a particular time span. Additionally, the appropriate time span for each procedure is specified by CMS as the "global period," which may be zero days or 10 days for "minor procedures" and is 90 days for "major procedures." Certain other minor procedures (e.g., audiology codes) have an "XXX" designation, which indicates, "the global concept does not apply to the code" (51).

Principle #3: Many procedures include performance of other less complex procedures as "components."

Principle #4: The relative value units (RVUs) assigned to each procedure are determined on the basis of vignettes that take into consideration the procedure itself, the surgical package, and all less complex component procedures. These vignettes are developed by an AMA committee that includes representatives of most major specialty societies, including Otolaryngology—Head and Neck Surgery. They are available in the AMA publication "CPT Reference of Clinical Examples."

Principle #5: CPT principles for correct coding of multiple procedures all seem to reinforce a unifying basic premise: "Every medical service performed should be compensated once, but only once. For example, the physician should not submit a code for E/M services if another service (such as a procedure with a global period, as described below) also includes the value of that same E/M service" (52).

Principle #6: Medicare provides an NCCI that indicates procedures it considers should not be billed (i.e., should not be coded) in combination with other procedures. There are currently more than 600,000 edits in the NCCI (53). Fortunately, most of these are "category 1/category 2" combining (i.e., "bundling") edits that are compliant with CPT's vignettes. However, Medicare also includes "mutually exclusive edits" and defined payment policies that may differ from CPT's assignment of RVUs.

Principle #7: Most private insurers use claims processing software from a common vendor. While these systems also include combining or bundling edits, the number of edits is several magnitudes greater than in NCCI (54); most of the extra edits are necessarily inconsistent with CPT and with NCCI edits, and they are therefore noncompliant. When the explanation of benefits (EOBs) from private insurers deny claims based on these noncompliant edits, the justification is usually conveyed either as one procedure being "incidental to" another or the two procedures being "mutually exclusive." Neither these two terms nor the explanations of what they mean are found in CPT or in NCCI; they are noncompliant with CPT principles and practices.

Unfortunately, even though insurers require medical practices to use the CPT coding system to submit claims, and they pay on the basis of CPT codes, they are not legally required to follow CPT coding compliance principles. Despite this, it remains important for physicians to understand and adhere to proper coding and compliant use of modifiers so that they can identify and challenge noncompliant payment practices they encounter when dealing with payers.

Patient Name: _____   Record # _____   Date: ___/___/____

Physician Presence - <u>Attending Physician should indicate either presence and participation in, or repeat and confirmation of,</u>
<u>   key elements of each component below and, in either event, enter summary comments on review of</u>
<u>   resident's documentation and confirmation or revision of findings.</u>

A. 3/3 elements required for initial visit and consultation	*B. 2/3 elements required for subsequent care visit*

☐ <u>Please refer to resident medical record note by Dr.</u> _____ dated ___/___/____

HISTORY: ☐ Physically Present   ☐ Personally Repeated (history of present illness and prior tests)
☐ Review of history confirms the resident's documentation, with the following modifications and/or summary comments:

_____
_____
_____
_____
_____

EXAMINATION: ☐ Physically Present   ☐ Personally Repeated (major exam findings)
☐ Review of physical exam confirms the resident's documentation, with the following modifications &/or summary comments:

_____
_____
_____
_____

MED DECISION MAKING: ☐ Physically Present   ☐ Personally Repeated: assessment, diagnosis, plan of care
☐ Review of decision making confirms the resident's documentation, with the following modifications and/or summary comments:

_____
_____
_____
_____
_____
_____
_____
_____

Complete this section only if documented below >50% of visit time involved counseling and/or coordinating care.

TIME: _____ minutes   ☐ > 50% of visit time involved counseling and/or coordination of care

Attending physician's signature:

Figure 200.10 Sample form for teaching physicians to document care provided under *the rules of physician presence.*

Commonly Used Modifiers for Multiple Procedures

When submitting claims for two or more independent surgical procedures on the same date of service, the modifiers that are most commonly added to all procedure codes other than the principle code are .50, .51, and .59. *The .50 modifier* should be applied whenever the physician performs a *bilateral procedure* at the same session. Examples of correct use of this modifier are

- 69436.50 to report bilateral tympanostomy with insertion of tubes (under general anesthesia)
- 31255.50 to report bilateral endoscopic total ethmoidectomy (surgery on anterior and posterior ethmoid cells)
- 30901.50 to report bilateral control of anterior nasal hemorrhage (simple)

These example codes show procedures that are also frequently performed unilaterally, so the RVU values assigned to them incorporate the value of a single procedure. For services that are most often performed as bilateral procedures or whose CPT descriptions specify that the procedure is designated as bilateral, it is not necessary or appropriate to add the .50 modifier. Examples of intrinsically bilateral codes include

- 42826: Tonsillectomy, age 12 or over (*this is an example of an intrinsically bilateral procedure*)
- 30801: Ablation, soft tissue of inferior turbinates, *unilateral or bilateral*, any method

The .51 modifier is appropriate when two procedures are performed, and one is not a component of the other. This modifier signals to the payer's software that the procedures are independent, and they should both be paid. The highest valued code should always be listed first, without the .51 modifier, because (as noted below) this procedure will be paid at full value while the others are each paid at 50% of their value. A common example of correct use of this modifier is

- 31254 (endoscopic anterior ethmoidectomy), 31256.51 (endoscopic maxillary antrostomy)

CPT describes that the .59 modifier is to be used to indicate a "distinct procedural service." This meaning is further clarified by stating that it "is used to identify procedures/services, other than E/M services, that are not normally reported together, but are appropriate under the circumstances. Documentation must support a different session, different procedure or surgery, different site or organ system, separate incision/excision, separate lesion, or separate injury" (55). CPT further cautions, "When another already established modifier is appropriate, it should be used rather than modifier 59" (55). An example of correct use of this modifier is

- 31255 (endoscopic total ethmoidectomy), 31254.59 (endoscopic anterior ethmoidectomy)
  - When performed on the same nasal passage, 31254 is a component of 31255 and should not be billed separately. However, if the procedures are performed on opposite sides of the nose, the .59 modifier is required to indicate that the procedures were not performed in the same location.
  - The .51 modifier could not be appropriately used, because software programs would assume the coding was for both procedures on the same side and would disallow the 31254 completely.

The .59 modifier is effective in indicating that payment is appropriate for otherwise non-billable code combinations. However, it must only be used judiciously and correctly, as excessive use will likely trigger an audit and significant financial penalties if improper utilization is found.

From the perspective of insurer payments, unfortunately Medicare long ago made a decision that it would reduce payments by 50% for all secondary procedures (those submitted with a .50, .51, or .59 modifier). This decision

came in 1992 with the introduction of the RBRVS system and a unilateral determination that the absence of distinct pre- and postoperative care for the secondary procedures justified the reduction. Almost all surgeons would dispute the validity of such a severe reduction, and its magnitude is even self-contradicted by Medicare's use of only a 20% reduction when a surgeon delegates pre- and postoperative care to another clinician (indicated by use of modifier .54). However, this is a long-standing policy for Medicare, and it is duplicated by almost all private insurers (although some implement even greater reductions for third and fourth procedures).

Commonly Used Modifiers for E/M Services Related to Procedures

All diagnostic and surgical procedures that have an associated global period are subject to the guidelines of the surgical package definition, and the RVUs designated for these services *include* all E/M services provided under two particular circumstances:

- "Subsequent to the decision for surgery, one related Evaluation and Management (E/M) encounter on the date immediately prior to or on the date of the procedure (including history and physical)."
- "Typical postoperative follow-up care" (56)

These guidelines advise that *under normal circumstances an E/M code should not be submitted when a procedure is performed on the same day* (because the value for this service is already included in the value assigned to the procedure). However, there are several defined circumstances in which the E/M service is more extensive than normally anticipated. When these conditions arise, physicians are advised to submit a code for the E/M service with an appropriate modifier. The three modifiers that may apply are .24, .25, and .57.

Compliant use of the .25 modifier, "significant, separately identifiable evaluation and management service by the same physician on the same day of the procedure or other service": Although E/M services on the day of a procedure are included in the "surgical package," certain well-defined circumstances warrant submission of an E/M code with a .25 or .57 modifier attached. The .25 modifier is applied only for minor procedures, that is, procedures with a zero-day or 10-day global period. The two situations that should justify this coding are

- If "the patient's condition required a significant, separately identifiable E/M service above and beyond the other service provided or beyond the usual preoperative and postoperative care associated with the procedure that was performed" (57). This situation is most commonly appropriate when the procedure is performed for one diagnosis (e.g., nasal endoscopy performed for evaluation of chronic sinusitis), and the E/M service is performed for a separate problem (e.g., acute otitis externa). With two *unrelated* diagnosis codes, a payer's claims processing software should readily identify that the E/M service was for a significant and separately identifiable condition.

- If the E/M care resulted in the decision to perform a minor or diagnostic procedure, because CPT coding guidelines specify that the surgical package includes (only) E/M care that is performed "subsequent to the decision for surgery"

However, the case of E/M as the basis of the decision for a minor procedure still requires a significant and separately identifiable E/M service, not simply problem-focused care. This interpretation is clarified in the Medicare RBRVS Physician's Guide section describing minor surgeries and endoscopies: "Payment for a visit would be allowed in addition to payment for suturing a scalp wound if, in addition, a full neurologic exam is made for a patient with head trauma. If the physician only identified the need for sutures and confirmed allergy and immunization status, billing for a visit would not be appropriate" (58).

An excellent example of *appropriate* use of the .25 modifier with decision for surgery would be an initial visit for a patient who is a smoker, has three months of persistent hoarseness, and has a hyperactive gag reflex that precludes an adequate mirror examination of the larynx. Since this is an initial visit, it is logical and obvious that the E/M service was the basis for making a decision to perform a medically indicated fiberoptic laryngoscopy (CPT code 31575). Therefore, the appropriate E/M code should be submitted with a .25 modifier (assuming the physician performs and documents an appropriately high level of E/M service that is warranted for this patient). Unfortunately, there is a significant billing/payment challenge under the same circumstances if the patient is an established patient in the practice and presents with a new problem. When the same (or a related) diagnosis code is submitted for both the procedure and the E/M service, the payer's software has no means of confirming that the E/M service was truly the basis for the decision to perform the procedure. "The result is frequently denial or delay of claims processing, necessitating appeals for payment and causing significant administrative burden for the physician's staff" (59).

Compliant use of the .57 modifier, "decision for surgery": The CPT codebook specifies only that this modifier is used with an E/M service that results in the initial decision to perform surgery. However, Medicare provides clarification that specifically differentiates correct use of the .57 modifier from modifier 25, by stating, "use of modifier .57 is limited to operations with 90-day global periods" (60). A hypothetical example for use of this modifier would be evaluation in the emergency department of an adult patient found to have a large parapharyngeal space abscess. The E/M evaluation would be billed (e.g., 99284.57) as the basis for the decision to take the patient to the operating

room and perform an open draining of the abscess (CPT code 21501, which has a 90-day global period).

Compliant use of the .24 modifier, "unrelated evaluation and management service by the same physician during a postoperative period." Most diagnostic procedures, such as fiberoptic laryngoscopy and fiberoptic nasal endoscopy, are assigned a zero-day global period. Therapeutic surgical procedures may have global periods of 0, 10, or 90 days. Normally, no E/M codes should be submitted during the designated postoperative time frame. There are, however, two circumstances under which an E/M code should be submitted with an attached .24 modifier:

- Provision of an E/M service for a problem unrelated to the original procedure. For example, if a patient who has undergone a superficial parotidectomy develops acute ethmoid sinusitis during the 90-day global period, the evaluation and management of this episode should be coded (e.g., CPT code 99213.24 with a diagnosis code of 461.2).
- Treatment of a postoperative complication. CPT's surgical package description of "typical" follow-up care encompasses the E/M services normally provided during the assigned global periods (0, 10, or 90 days). CPT further specifies. "Complications, exacerbations, recurrence, or the presence of other diseases or injuries requiring additional services should be separately reported" (61). Therefore, if the patient who is postoperative from a superficial parotidectomy develops a fistula, the E/M care of this complication should be coded and submitted (e.g., 99213.24 with a diagnosis code of 527.4 [salivary gland fistula]).

The Medicare Conundrum for Billing Postoperative Complications

Although in most instances Medicare's national policy for use of modifiers is compliant with CPT conventions, it has unilaterally adopted a number of "payment rules and policies" that contradict certain principles of the CPT coding system. One such policy concerns reimbursement for complications that occur during the global period of an operation. Instead of recognizing that the RBRVS values for surgical procedures do not include any RVUs for potential care of postoperative complications, Medicare will not provide payment for any medical or surgical care that does not require a trip to the operating room. Its policy states, "Medicare will include these services (*for complications*) in the approved amount for the global surgery with no separate payment made" (62). Medicare therefore instructs that physicians should not submit any claims for E/M services provided for care of complications during the postoperative global period.

CODING AND BILLING RISKS AND CHALLENGES IN OTOLARYNGOLOGY—HEAD AND NECK SURGERY

Precise descriptive documentation of procedures and E/M services is the foundation for accurate coding. When applied to the billing process, documentation and coding are subject to review by Medicare and insurance carriers, which can lead to two potential issues for medical practices.

The first issue is that practices must be alert to the potential for insurers' noncompliant payment practices through improper "bundling" of payments and/or denial of services. For example, insurers have at times programmed their claims processing software to improperly deny payment for performance of a nasal septal reconstruction (CPT code 30520) by "bundling" it into endoscopic sinus surgery procedures (e.g., CPT code 31254), using the improper and nonspecific rationale that the septum operation is "incidental to" the performance of the sinus surgery. This noncompliant payment practice was another of the critical issues in the national class action lawsuits filed by physician organizations against health insurers in the first decade of the 21st century (63). Practices must rise to the challenge of meticulous scrutiny of each line item of the EOBs they receive from payers, with follow-up inquiries and appeals to attempt to receive correct payment. This important concern is covered in the chapter on billing and accounts receivable.

The second issue is that practices must be alert to compliance risks and potentially severe financial penalties in the event of audits of their coding and documentation practices by Medicare and/or private insurers. Although Medicare in particular does perform "random reviews," the use of "targeted audits" is more prevalent, from Medicare-related organizations and private insurers alike. Targeted reviews are initiated when an automated (by computer) analysis of a physician's coding and billing patterns reveals statistically significant disparities in frequency and/or intensity of services when compared with the patterns of fellow practitioners. This finding then triggers a request for medical records, which are evaluated by trained reviewers for appropriateness of care and coding.

In the event of an audit by a MAC, other government agency (64), or private insurer, payment will be denied if the physician's medical documentation is inadequate to support performance of the services claimed, if the coding is inaccurate (i.e., inadequate *specificity*), or if the documentation fails to support *medical necessity* for performing the care. If the audit reveals only occasional problems, the medical practice may be provided educational materials and re-reviewed within a reasonable time frame. On the other hand, consequences escalate dramatically if a review reveals a high frequency of improper coding practices:

- At a minimum, the practice will be required to refund the improper payments identified in the audits. (It is noteworthy that under the requirements of the recently passed Affordable Health Care for America Act, practices must promptly self-report any overpayments they identify, or they face additional financial penalties for non-reporting.)

- If medical record documentation consistently fails to support the specificity or medical necessity of claims submitted, the MAC or insurer may extrapolate the discovered errors to include all claims for those identified services filed over a period of multiple years. Extrapolation can result in economically devastating repayments.

- Practices may be placed under a "corporate integrity agreement" (CIA), requiring strict independent oversight of a formal compliance plan and prepayment review of all claims.

- Under more egregious circumstances, a MAC auditor (or an auditor from the OIG or other government agencies) may conclude that such unsupported bills were "false claims," resulting in additional fines of up to $11,000 per claim. This determination may even lead to criminal prosecution.

- Practices may be prohibited from participation in the Medicare or Medicaid programs.

Recognized Risk Areas

While some recognized risk areas for disparities in coding and billing practices relate to lack of specificity or misunderstanding of component procedures, the most prevalent risk category is failure of the documentation to support *medical necessity*. This vulnerability includes risks related to levels of E/M care, decisions for surgery, timing of surgery, and extent of surgery. As noted above in the definition of medical necessity agreed upon in the national class action lawsuit settlements, medical necessity includes care that is "in accordance with generally accepted standards of medical practice" (65), and those accepted standards include "standards that are based on credible scientific evidence published in peer-reviewed medical literature generally recognized by the *relevant* medical community, Physician Specialty Society recommendations..." (66). In the specialty of Otolaryngology—Head and Neck Surgery, the Quality Improvement Committee and appropriate specialty committees of the AAO-HNS have adhered to the practices of "EBM" in evaluating applicable peer-reviewed medical literature to compile its Clinical Indicators Compendium, Policy Statements, and Clinical Practice Guidelines and Clinical Consensus Statements (cited previously as resources for compliance). As noted below, the tenets of EBM advocate using best evidence and guidelines as a starting point for care; that is, they should be considered a platform and not a box. However, *it is incumbent upon physicians to **document** the basis for care decisions that significantly vary from these standards*, particularly if they are to withstand reviews for compliance and quality of care.

As one perplexed physician reviewer observed in evaluating coding for the performance of endoscopic sinus surgeries, "the decisions for timing and extent of surgery relate to physician preferences rather than to patients' medical indications."

Fundamentals of Evidence Based Medicine (EBM)

Dr. David Sackett, commonly recognized as the "father of evidence-based medicine," describes the principles and practice of EBM as the integration of best clinical evidence with individual clinical expertise and patient's individual values and expectations: "EBM is the conscientious, explicit and judicious use of current best evidence in making decisions about the care of individual patients. The practice of EBM means integrating individual clinical expertise with the best available external clinical evidence from systematic research… Good doctors use both individual clinical expertise and the best available external evidence, and neither alone is enough. Without clinical expertise, practice risks becoming tyrannized by external evidence, for even excellent external evidence may be inapplicable to or inappropriate for an individual patient. Without current best external evidence, practice risks becoming rapidly out of date, to the detriment of patients" (67).

Specific Coding and Billing Risks

Following is an overview of some of the most significant risk areas in Otolaryngology—Head and Neck Surgery, selected by frequency and intensity of service, including a brief summary of critical compliance concerns.

Evaluation and Management Coding (E/M)

1. **Indicators for potential risk**: Frequent use of high-level E/M codes (i.e., level 4 and level 5), particularly in association with diagnosis codes not usually associated with relatively high severity illness (i.e., moderate to high NPP)
   a. See Appendix C of CPT for Clinical Examples of patients whose severity of illness (NPP) is deemed sufficient to warrant various levels of care.
2. **Documentation dangers**: E/M documentation frequently fails to comply with principles presented in CPT and the Documentation Guidelines. This particularly includes failure to document qualitative features of E/M, the three levels of risk, and an assessment of the NPPs.
   a. Risk levels may be significantly increased in many EHRs that use noncompliant screen designs and noncompliant data entry shortcuts (resulting in "cloned" documentation).

b. Reports of Medicare/OIG audits of physicians using such noncompliant EHRs have documented repayment penalties in excess of $175,000 per physician (68). Noncompliant E/M coding in EHRs is near the top of the OIG's list of items to audit in its 2011 - 2013 work plans.

Ear Procedures

1. **Removal of ventilation tube(s) in the operating room (CPT code 69424)** (performed for prolonged retention).
   a. **Indicators for potential risk**: Codes submitted for performing a tympanic membrane repair (CPT code 69610), myringoplasty [69620], or tympanoplasty without mastoidectomy [69631] instead of, or in addition to, code 69424 (particularly if performed routinely)
   b. **Compliance risk**: Standard practice followed by most physicians is removal of the retained tube allowing spontaneous closure without the *medical necessity* of a repair procedure; there is no *evidence* for a significant failure rate of this less complex treatment.
      i. If there are conditions in a specific case warranting such a repair (e.g., a widened perforation or a monomeric membrane around the retained tube), these should be well-documented in the medical record and in the "indications" section of the operative report; additional diagnosis code(s) might also be indicated.
   c. Note: If tube removal is performed in office setting, no procedure code is applicable; the procedure is a component of the E/M service.

Nose and Sinus Procedures

Review of the coding and billing practices related to most of the procedures in this section reveals significant physician disparities in frequency of performing the procedures, timing of performing the procedures, and/or extent of procedures performed. Detailed review of documentation frequently reveals additional disparities among physicians in clinical indications for performing the procedures. These variations occur despite the existence of evidence-based standards for care and the absence of clinical evidence of significant differences in outcomes with more extensive techniques.

1. **Diagnostic nasal endoscopy (CPT code 31231)**
   a. **Indicators for potential risk**: Codes submitted with high frequency, especially when associated with diagnostic codes not commonly associated with *medical necessity* for performing this procedure and particularly when employed during an initial evaluation of a new medical problem
   b. **Compliance risk**: The appropriate ear, nose, and throat physical examination (under both 1995

and 1997 Documentation Guidelines protocols) includes an intranasal examination using anterior rhinoscopy, with or without utilization of a topical decongestant spray. Routine use of a nasal endoscope to perform all or part of this standard intranasal examination, instead of or in addition to use of anterior rhinoscopy, is considered to be "primarily for the convenience of the physician," and it therefore fails to meet the criteria for "*medical necessity*." Figure 200.2's documentation form for nasal endoscopy includes a number of clinical indications that support the medical necessity of performing this procedure to supplement anterior rhinoscopy.

2. **Nasopharyngoscopy with (fiberoptic) endoscope** (CPT code 92511)

   a. **Indicators for potential risk**: Codes submitted with high frequency, especially when associated with diagnostic codes not commonly associated with *medical necessity* for performing this procedure

   b. **Compliance risk**: The appropriate ear, nose, and throat physical examination (under both 1995 and 1997 Documentation Guidelines protocols) includes a mirror examination of the nasopharynx. Routine use of a fiberoptic endoscope to perform this standard examination instead of or in addition to use of a mirror, while clinically acceptable, is considered to be "primarily for the convenience of the physician," and it therefore fails to meet the criteria for "*medical necessity*." Documentation of medical necessity should include two components: (a) the medical indication for examining the nasopharynx and (b) a reason why mirror examination provides inadequate visualization.

3. **Turbinate surgery**: Mucosal cauterization (CPT codes 30801 and 30802), partial or complete resection inferior turbinate (CPT code 30130), submucous resection inferior turbinate (CPT code 30140), and therapeutic fracture of inferior turbinate (CPT code 30930)

   a. **Indicators for potential risk**: Codes submitted with high frequency, particularly as a *routine* component of most sinus operations and/or nasal septal reconstructive surgery

   b. **Compliance risk**: The AAO-HNS "Clinical Indicators Compendium" emphasizes that one of the *required* indications for performing surgery of the inferior turbinate is "chronic nasal obstruction, *management inadequate*" (69). Standard management for unilateral compensatory turbinate hypertrophy associated with a deviated nasal septum is correction of the septal deformity, with physiologic return to normal mucosal thickness and airway patency over a relatively short period of several weeks. Similarly, standard management for reactive turbinate hypertrophy associated with chronic unilateral or bilateral sinusitis is medical or surgical correction of the sinus pathology, with physiologic return to normal

mucosal thickness and airway patency over a relatively short period of several weeks. These guidelines reserve turbinate intervention solely for those unusual cases that demonstrate continued turbinate pathology with airway obstruction after this primary surgical management. Therefore, the routine use of turbinate surgery, prior to evaluating the outcome of corrective surgery, appears to be "primarily for the convenience of the physician," and it therefore fails to meet the criteria for *medical necessity*.

4. **Endoscopic sinus surgery**: Anterior ethmoidectomy (CPT code 31254), total ethmoidectomy (CPT code 31255), maxillary sinusotomy (CPT codes 31256 and 31257), frontal sinus exploration (CPT code 31276), and sphenoidotomy (CPT codes 31287 and 31288)

   a. **Indicators for potential risk**: Two high-risk issues stand out in reviewing coding and billing patterns for endoscopic sinus surgery. The first is frequent or consistent performance of surgery in close proximity to the initial evaluation for nasal and sinus symptoms, which suggests significant variance from *medical necessity* guidelines. The second risk factor is high frequency of multiple procedures during each surgical episode; that is, many or most surgeries including total ethmoidectomy, frontal sinus surgery, and/or sphenoid sinus surgery. This finding suggests the possibility of significant variance from both *specificity* and *medical necessity* guidelines.

   b. **Compliance risk**: The AAO-HNS "Clinical Indicators Compendium" provides comprehensive guidelines on appropriate indications for performing endoscopic surgery as well as specifications that affect timing and extent of surgery. These include "failure of medical management for chronic sinus pathology ... *(including)* optimal medical therapy prior to obtaining sinus CT scan, prior to nasal endoscopy, and prior to surgery ... *(this therapy includes)* antibiotic therapy consisting of four to six consecutive weeks of appropriate antibiotic drugs" (70). The timing required for adequate medical therapy raises significant concerns when claims consistently reveal performance of surgery in less than 6 weeks after initial consultation. Another of these guidelines relates medical necessity for each component of surgery to specificity of diagnostic findings: "Surgical procedure and findings must be compatible with clinical status, CT findings, and nasal endoscopic findings *(all determined after optimal medical therapy)*. That is, only patients with significant persistent sinus symptoms and pathology should undergo surgery" (71). High frequency of multiple extensive surgeries, particularly after optimal medical evaluation and therapy, is also inconsistent with the practices of many physicians who experience excellent outcomes with endoscopic surgery that in the majority of cases is confined to the anterior ethmoid sinus and the maxillary ostium.

c. Sinus care and documentation should reflect the standards presented in the Clinical Indicators Compendium. In the event of variance from these standards, documentation should clearly support the medical indications for discrepancies.

5. **Debridement** (CPT code 31237)

   a. **Indicators for potential risk**: Codes submitted for a significant majority of cases of endoscopic sinus surgery, particularly with multiple and frequent debridements. Claims reviews commonly reveal that physicians who submit for multiple debridements do so in essentially every case. Particular concern relates to both *medical necessity* for performing the procedures and whether the procedures performed meet the *specificity* required to qualify as a true debridement (rather than just cleaning debris).

   b. **Compliance risks**

      i. In the postoperative management of primary and noncomplex endoscopic sinus surgery patients, there is no *evidence* of more favorable outcomes in patients undergoing multiple debridement procedures. In its Policy Statement on Debridement of the Sinus Cavity after FESS, while the AAO-HNS affirms, "The frequency with which the above mentioned procedure should be performed is a clinical judgment best made by the surgeon," it also advises that this frequency should be *"determined on a case by case basis"* (72). However, for surgeons whose use of debridement following noncomplicated procedures is *routine* rather than individually determined, it appears to be "primarily for the convenience of the physician" and therefore fails to meet the criteria for *medical necessity*.

      ii. Of greater concern is a potential *specificity* issue related to submission of claims for nasal cleaning treatments whose intensity of service fails to qualify as a true debridement. The AAO-HNS Policy Statement on debridement also specifies that debridement "involves transnasal insertion of the endoscope for visualization and parallel insertion of various instruments for the purpose of removal of postsurgical crusting, devitalized mucosa or other contaminated tissue. *It is performed under local or general anesthesia* in an office suitably equipped or operating room, depending on the clinical circumstances of the case" (72). However, documentation of debridement procedures frequently reports only use of suction and forceps to remove loose crusts, rather than more demanding procedures requiring injected local anesthesia or general anesthesia. Such documentation fails to support the *specificity* required to code for a true debridement procedure.

Oral Cavity

1. **Coding for uvulopalatopharyngoplasty (UPPP) and tonsillectomy** (CPT codes 42145 and 42826):

   a. **Indicators for potential risk**: Most surgeons express the opinion that the combination of these two procedures involves greater skill, effort, and time than performing a UPPP alone. However, Medicare's NCCI edits designate tonsillectomy to be a component service of the UPPP procedure. Therefore, submitting claims for performing both services during the same operation is an example of "unbundling." In other words, the value of a tonsillectomy is included in the RVUs assigned to the more complex UPPP procedure, so it should not also be coded and billed separately.

Larynx

1. **Flexible fiberoptic laryngoscopy** (CPT code 31575):

   a. **Indicators for potential risk**: Codes submitted with high frequency, especially when associated with diagnostic codes not commonly associated with *medical necessity* for performing this procedure

   b. **Compliance risk**: The appropriate ear, nose, and throat physical examination (under both 1995 and 1997 Documentation Guidelines protocols) includes a mirror examination of the larynx. Routine use of a fiberoptic endoscope to perform this standard examination instead of, or in addition to, use of a mirror, while clinically acceptable, is considered to be "primarily for the convenience of the physician," and it therefore fails to meet the criteria for *"medical necessity."* Documentation of medical necessity should include two components: (a) the medical indication for examining the larynx and (b) a reason that mirror examination provides inadequate visualization. The documentation form for fiberoptic laryngoscopy shown in Figure 200.2 includes a number of clinical indications that support the medical necessity of performing this procedure.

SUMMARY

High-quality documentation accurately reflects the procedures and cognitive services physicians provide for their patients. In addition, the introduction of effective documentation templates that integrate compliance principles and enable efficient data entry can facilitate accurate coding and actually promote quality patient care. Even when working in practices that include certified professional coders, physicians need to understand and practice the basic concepts of compliant documentation and coding. Not only does their knowledge assist coders by providing the specificity they require for accurate identification of services, but it is also addresses the critical area of medical necessity, which only physicians can provide. For the practice of Otolaryngology—Head and Neck Surgery, the "generally accepted standards of medical practice" that are the foundation of medical necessity include the evidence-based recommendations found in the AAO-HNS's Clinical Indicators, Policy Statements, and Practice Guidelines.

HIGHLIGHTS

- The E/M coding system is actually derived from the recognized medical student text "Bates' Guide to Physical Examination and History Taking."
  - The E/M system is therefore a codification of the medical diagnostic process that all physicians learn in their training as being the most effective method for providing high-quality patient care.
  - Therefore, compliantly designed medical record tools can actually help physicians provide optimal care within a time frame that meets the limitations of the current health care environment.
- Physicians require a toolkit of usable, efficient, and compliant data entry options for efficient and compliant documentation, including
  - Proper application of graphic and narrative interface designs
  - Proper application of templates, with limited and cautious use of macros
  - Optimal use of appropriate data entry personnel, including staff and/or patients
  - Optimal use of appropriate data entry modalities for dictation, legible handwriting, and/or keyboard and mouse (with electronic health records)
- Coding principles rely on reporting the most appropriate procedure codes using CPT designations and the most appropriate diagnosis codes using ICD-9 designations:
  - Codification has multiple uses, including reporting for CER, population studies for public health, and (in the United States) submission of claims for payment.
- The critical factors in achieving compliant coding and documentation are specificity and medical necessity.
  - Specificity is required for selection of correct procedure and diagnosis codes.
  - Medical necessity is a central factor in appropriateness of claims, including consideration of standards of care and application of evidence-based medicine.
- The three central concepts to compliant coding and billing are:
  - "Medical necessity of a service is the overarching criterion for payment in addition to the individual requirements of a CPT code."

- "If medical care is not documented in the medical record, it is treated as if it had not been performed."
- "Automation is not documentation."
- Physicians' requirements for effective medical record documentation and coding tools include usability, efficiency, compliance, data integrity, promoting quality patient care, and appropriate productivity.
  - Appropriate template designs for procedures and for evaluation and management services (E/M) incorporate specificity and medical necessity to fulfill these goals.
- Physicians at teaching hospitals can and should incorporate the concepts of Medicare's compliance requirements (IL-372 and section 15016 of the Carriers Manual) to integrate personal problem-focused care and documentation plus teaching responsibilities with the comprehensive care and documentation provided by their resident physicians. This requires compliant E/M documentation tools for the residents and compliant "physician presence" documentation tools for the teaching physicians.
- To ensure proper billing and payment, physicians need to understand the basic concepts related to the RBRVS and appropriate use of modifiers.
- Physicians should be aware of noncompliant payment practices employed by Medicare and private insurers to improperly "bundle" services and deny appropriate payments.
- Physicians should be aware of possible compliance risks and potentially severe financial penalties in the event of audits of their coding and documentation practices by Medicare and/or private insurers:
  - A number of recognized risk areas are reviewed for both E/M services and specific procedures.
  - Physicians should be aware of and familiar with standards of care compiled by the AAO-HNS in its "Clinical Indicators," "Policy Statements," and "Clinical Practice Guidelines and Clinical Consensus Statements."

REFERENCES

1. Versel N. Dr. Weed's Software Cure, Digital HealthCare & Productivity. com, http:///www.health-itworld.com/emag/070104/289.html?page:int=-1, accessed June 7, 2007.
2. "Compliance" may be defined as "conformity in fulfilling official requirements." Merriam Webster Dictionary, http://www.merriam-webster.com/dictionary/compliance, accessed March 11, 2011.
3. Levinson SR. *Practical EHR: Electronic record solutions for compliance and quality care.* AMA Press, 2008:26, Chapter 2.
4. Bickley LS, Szilagyi PG. *Bates guide to physical examination and history taking,* 10th ed. Lippincott Williams & Wilkins, 2008.
5. American Medical Association. *Current Procedural Terminology (CPT) 2011,* Professional Edition. AMA Press, 2010.

6. American Medical Association and Health Care Financing Administration. 1997 Documentation Guidelines for Evaluation and Management Services, https://www.cms.gov/MLNProducts/Downloads/MASTER1.pdf, accessed April 21, 2011.

7. Levinson SR. *Practical E/M: documentation and coding solutions for quality patient care*, 2nd ed. AMA Press, 2008:6–7.

8. Hartzband P, Groopman J. Avoiding the pitfalls of going electronic. *N Engl J Med* 2008;358:1656–1657.

9. Dimick C. *Documentation bad habits: shortcuts in electronic records pose risk. J AHIMA* 2008;79(6):40–43.

10. Cuvo JB, Dinh AK, Fahrenholz CG. Quality data and documentation for EHRs in physician practice. Practice Brief appearing in *Journal of AHIMA* 2008;79(8):43–48.

11. Wrenn J, Stein D, Bakken S, et al. Quantifying clinical narrative redundancy in an electronic health record. *JAMIA* 2010;17:49–53, http://jamia.bmj.com/content/17/1/49.short

12. Winter E. *Requirements for the payment of medicare claims—a selection of some important criteria*, http://www.cbhc.org/news/wp-content/uploads/2010/07/Session-2002-2.pdf, accessed April 21, 2011.

13. ONCHIT and HHS. *Recommended requirements for enhancing data quality in electronic health record systems*, 2007, p. 46, http://www.rti.org/pubs/enhancing_data_quality_in_ehrs.pdf, accessed April 21, 2011.

14. American Medical Association and Health Care Financing Administration. 1997 Documentation Guidelines for Evaluation and Management Services, p. 6, https://www.cms.gov/MLNProducts/Downloads/MASTER1.pdf, accessed April 21, 2011.

15. Levinson SR. *Practical EHR: electronic record solutions for compliance and quality care*. AMA Press, 2008:177–184, Chapter 11.

16. American Medical Association. *Current Procedural Terminology (CPT) 2011*, Professional Edition. AMA Press, 2010:v.

17. "ICD-9-CM 2009, Physician, Volumes 1 and 2, 9th Revision—Clinical Modification," Ingenix, 2008, p. 1.

18. American Medical Association. *Current Procedural Terminology (CPT) 2011*, Professional Edition. AMA Press, 2010:X (Instructions for Use of the CPT Codebook).

19. "ICD-9-CM 2009, Physician, Volumes 1 and 2, 9th Revision—Clinical Modification," Ingenix, 2008, p. 3.

20. For detailed information about the lawsuit and settlements with various carriers, please review the information at http://www.hmosettlements.com/pages/about.html, accessed April 21, 2011.

21. Practice Management Center, American Medical Association, http://www.ama-assn.org/ama1/pub/upload/mm/368/bcbsflyer.pdf, accessed April 21, 2011.

22. Medicare Claims Processing Manual, Chapter 12, section 30.6.1, https://www.cms.gov/manuals/downloads/clm104c12.pdf, p. 38, accessed April 21, 2011.

23. Social Security Act, section 1862, http://www.ssa.gov/OP_Home/ssact/title18/1862.htm, accessed April 21, 2011.

24. Trailblazer MAC web site, http://www.trailblazerhealth.com/Publications/Job%20Aid/medical%20necessity.pdf, accessed April 21, 2011.

25. Levinson SR. *Practical E/M: documentation and coding solutions for quality patient care*. AMA Press, 2008:49, Chapter 6.

26. Trailblazer MAC web site, http://www.trailblazerhealth.com/Tools/Notices.aspx?ID=13039&DomainID=1, accessed April 21, 2011.

27. Levinson SR. *Practical EHR: electronic record solutions for compliance and quality care*. AMA Press, 2008:99, Chapter 7.

28. Winter E. *Requirements for the payment of medicare claims—a selection of some important criteria*, http://www.cbhc.org/news/wp-content/uploads/2010/07/Session-2002-2.pdf, accessed April 21, 2011.

29. Levinson SR. *Practical E/M: documentation and coding solutions for quality patient care*, 2nd ed. AMA Press, 2008:39, Chapter 5.

30. Levinson SR. *Practical E/M: documentation and coding solutions for quality patient care*, 2nd ed. AMA Press, 2008: ix, Prologue.

31. 1997 Documentation Guidelines for Evaluation and Management Services, Table of Risk, p. 50, https://www.cms.gov/MLNProducts/Downloads/MASTER1.pdf, accessed April 21, 2011.

32. American Medical Association. *Current Procedural Terminology (CPT) 2011*, Professional Edition. AMA Press, 2010:9.

33. Levinson SR. *Practical E/M: documentation and coding solutions for quality patient care*, 2nd ed. (enclosed CD ROM), Copyright 2008, American Medical Association, 2008. All Rights Reserved.

34. 1997 Documentation Guidelines for Evaluation and Management Services, p. 6, https://www.cms.gov/MLNProducts/Downloads/MASTER1.pdf, accessed April 21, 2011.

35. Levinson SR. *Practical E/M: documentation and coding solutions for quality patient care*, 2nd ed. (enclosed CD ROM), Copyright 2008, American Medical Association, 2008. All Rights Reserved.

36. 1997 Documentation Guidelines for Evaluation and Management Services, p. 6 https://www.cms.gov/MLNProducts/Downloads/MASTER1.pdf, accessed April 21, 2011.

37. Levinson SR. *Practical E/M: documentation and coding solutions for quality patient care*, 2nd ed. (enclosed CD ROM), Copyright 2008, American Medical Association, 2008. All Rights Reserved.

38. 1997 Documentation Guidelines for Evaluation and Management Services, p. 6 https://www.cms.gov/MLNProducts/Downloads/MASTER1.pdf, accessed April 21, 2011.

39. Levinson SR. *Practical E/M: documentation and coding solutions for quality patient care*, 2nd ed. (enclosed CD ROM), Copyright 2008, American Medical Association, 2008. All Rights Reserved.

40. 1997 Documentation Guidelines for Evaluation and Management Services, p. 7 https://www.cms.gov/MLNProducts/Downloads/MASTER1.pdf, accessed April 21, 2011.

41. Levinson SR. *Practical E/M: documentation and coding solutions for quality patient care*, 2nd ed. (enclosed CD ROM), Copyright 2008, American Medical Association, 2008. All Rights Reserved.

42. 1997 Documentation Guidelines for Evaluation and Management Services, p. 11, https://www.cms.gov/MLNProducts/Downloads/MASTER1.pdf, accessed April 21, 2011.

43. Levinson SR. *Practical E/M: documentation and coding solutions for quality patient care*, 2nd ed. (enclosed CD ROM), Copyright 2008, American Medical Association, 2008. All Rights Reserved.

44. Levinson SR. *Practical E/M: documentation and coding solutions for quality patient care*, 2nd ed. (enclosed CD ROM), Copyright 2008, American Medical Association, 2008. All Rights Reserved.

45. Johnston D. University agrees to pay in settlement on Medicare, New York Times, December 13, 1995:A18.

46. Medicare Carriers Manual Part 3 Claims Process, Transmittal 1780, November 22, 2002:3, https://www.cms.gov/Transmittals/Downloads/R1780B3.pdf, accessed April 21, 2011.

47. Medicare Carriers Manual Part 3 Claims Process, Transmittal 1780, November 22, 2002:4, https://www.cms.gov/Transmittals/Downloads/R1780B3.pdf, accessed April 21, 2011.

48. Levinson SR. *Practical E/M: documentation and coding solutions for quality patient care*, 2nd ed. (enclosed CD ROM). AMA Press, 2008:173–178, Chapter 19.

49. American Medical Association. *Current Procedural Terminology (CPT) 2011*, Professional Edition. AMA Press, 2010:549–551.

50. American Medical Association. *Current Procedural Terminology (CPT) 2011*, Professional Edition. AMA Press, 2010:52.

51. Smith S. ed. *Medicare RBRVS: the physicians' guide*. Chicago, IL: AMA Press, 2008:155.

52. Levinson SR. *Practical E/M: documentation and coding solutions for quality patient care*, 2nd ed. AMA Press, 2008:294.

53. Interesting Trend in NCCI Edits, Wolters Kluwer MediBlog, 2009, http://www.mediregs.com/blog/2009/06/interesting-trend-ncci-edits.htm, accessed April 21, 2011.

54. Personal communication with insurer compliance expert.

55. American Medical Association. *Current Procedural Terminology (CPT) 2011*, Professional Edition. AMA Press, 2010:550.

56. American Medical Association. *Current Procedural Terminology (CPT) 2011*, Professional Edition. AMA Press, 2010:52.

57. American Medical Association. *Current Procedural Terminology (CPT) 2011*, Professional Edition. AMA Press, 2010:549.

58. Smith S. ed. *Medicare RBRVS: the physicians' guide*. Chicago, IL: AMA Press, 2008:93.

59. Levinson SR. *Practical E/M: documentation and coding solutions for quality patient care*, 2nd ed. AMA Press, 2008:299.

60. Smith S. ed. *Medicare RBRVS: the physicians' guide*. Chicago, IL: AMA Press, 2008:96.

61. Smith S. ed. *Medicare RBRVS: the physicians' guide*. Chicago, IL: AMA Press, 2008:52.

62. Smith S. ed. *Medicare RBRVS: the physicians' guide*. Chicago, IL: AMA Press, 2008:91.

63. For detailed information about the lawsuit and settlements with various carriers, please review the information at http://www.hmosettlements.com/pages/about.html, accessed April 21, 2011.

64. Other agencies that may perform review of Medicare or Medicaid payments include the Office of the Inspector General ("OIG") and Zone Program Integrity Contractors ("ZPIC"—an organization that focuses on the potential of fraudulent billing).

65. Practice Management Center, American Medical Association, Definition of "Medical Necessity," http://www.ama-assn.org/ama1/pub/upload/mm/368/bcbsflyer.pdf, accessed April 21, 2011.

66. Practice Management Center, American Medical Association, Definition of "Medical Necessity," http://www.ama-assn.org/ama1/pub/upload/mm/368/bcbsflyer.pdf, accessed April 21, 2011.

67. Sackett DL. Evidence Based Medicine, Seminars in Perinatology, Feb 21, 1997, Vol. 1, pp. 3–5, http://www.ncbi.nlm.nih.gov/pubmed/9190027, accessed April 21, 2011.

68. Levinson S, Grider D, Linker R, et al. The perfect storm. *Med Econ* April 3, 2009:18–27, http://www.practicalem.com/perfectstorm.htm, accessed April 21, 2011.

69. AAO-HNS Clinical Indicators Compendium. Inferior turbinectomy, http://www.entnet.org/Practice/clinicalIndicators.cfm, p. 27, accessed April 21, 2011.

70. AAO-HNS Clinical Indicators Compendium. "Endoscopic Sinus Surgery, Adult" and "Endoscopic Sinus Surgery, Pediatric," http://www.entnet.org/Practice/clinicalIndicators.cfm, pp. 22–25, accessed April 21, 2011.

71. AAO-HNS Clinical Indicators Compendium. "Endoscopic Sinus Surgery, Adult" and "Endoscopic Sinus Surgery, Pediatric," http://www.entnet.org/Practice/clinicalIndicators.cfm, pp. 23, 25, accessed April 21, 2011.

72. AAO-HNS Policy Statements. Debridement of the sinus cavity after FESS, http://www.entnet.org/Practice/policystatements.cfm, accessed April 21, 2011.

BIBLIOGRAPHY

AAO-HNS. Clinical Indicators Compendium, http://www.entnet.org/Practice/clinicalIndicators.cfm

AAO-HNS. Policy Statements: Debridement of the Sinus Cavity after FESS, http://www.entnet.org/Practice/policystatements.cfm

American Medical Association, *Current Procedural Terminology (CPT) 2011*, Professional Edition, Chicago: AMA Press, 2010.

American Medical Association and Health Care Financing Administration, 1995 Documentation Guidelines for Evaluation and Management Services, https://www.cms.gov/MLNProducts/Downloads/1995dg.pdf

American Medical Association and Health Care Financing Administration, 1997 Documentation Guidelines for Evaluation and Management Services, https://www.cms.gov/MLNProducts/Downloads/MASTER1.pdf

Bickley LS, Szilagyi PG. *Bates guide to physical examination and history taking*, 10th ed. Philadelphia, PA: Lippincott Williams & Wilkins, 2008.

Class Action Lawsuit Settlements, http://www.hmosettlements.com/pages/about.html

Cuvo JB, Dinh AK, Fahrenholz CG. Quality data and documentation for EHRs in physician practice. Practice Brief appearing in *Journal of AHIMA* 2008;79(8):43–48.

Dimick C. Documentation bad habits: shortcuts in electronic records pose risk. *J AHIMA* 2008;79(6):40–43.

Hartzband P, Groopman J. Avoiding the pitfalls of going electronic. *N Engl J Med* 2008;358:1656–1657.

ICD-9-CM 2009, Physician, Volumes 1 and 2, 9th Revision—Clinical Modification, Salt Lake City: Ingenix, 2008.

Interesting Trend in NCCI Edits, Wolters Kluwer MediBlog, 2009, http://www.mediregs.com/blog/2009/06/interesting-trend-ncci-edits.htm

Johnston D, University agrees to pay in settlement on Medicare. *New York Times*, December 13, 1995:A18.

Levinson SR. *Practical EHR: electronic record solutions for compliance and quality care*. Chicago: AMA Press, 2008.

Levinson SR. *Practical E/M: documentation and coding solutions for quality patient care*, 2nd ed., Chicago: AMA Press, 2008.

Levinson S, Grider D, Linker R, et al. The perfect storm. *Med Econ* April 3, 2009:18–27, http://www.practicalem.com/perfectstorm.htm

Medicare Carriers Manual Part 3 Claims Process, Transmittal 1780, November 22, 2002:3, https://www.cms.gov/Transmittals/Downloads/R1780B3.pdf

Medicare Claims Processing Manual, Chapter 12, section 30.6.1, https://www.cms.gov/manuals/downloads/clm104c12.pdf

ONCHIT and HHS, Recommended requirements for enhancing data quality in electronic health record systems, 2007, p. 46, http://www.rti.org/pubs/enhancing_data_quality_in_ehrs.pdf

Practice Management Center, American Medical Association, http://www.ama-assn.org/ama1/pub/upload/mm/368/bcbsflyer.pdf

Sackett DL. Evidence Based Medicine. *Semin Perinatol* Feb 21, 1997;1:3–5, http://www.ncbi.nlm.nih.gov/pubmed/9190027

Smith S, ed., *Medicare RBRVS: the physicians' guide*. Chicago, IL: AMA Press, 2008.

Social Security Act, section 1862, http://www.ssa.gov/OP_Home/ssact/title18/1862.htm

Trailblazer MAC web site, http://www.trailblazerhealth.com/Publications/Job%20Aid/medical%20necessity.pdf

Trailblazer MAC web site, http://www.trailblazerhealth.com/Tools/Notices.aspx?ID=13039&DomainID=1

Versel N, Dr. Weed's Software Cure, Digital HealthCare & Productivity.com, June 7, 2007; http:///www.health-itworld.com/emag/070104/289.html?page:int=-1

Winter E. Requirements for the payment of medicare claims—a selection of some important criteria, http://www.cbhc.org/news/wp-content/uploads/2010/07/Session-2002-2.pdf

Wrenn J, Stein D, Bakken S, et al. Quantifying clinical narrative redundancy in an electronic health record. *JAMIA* 2010;17:49–53, http://jamia.bmj.com/content/17/1/49.short

201 Clinic Management

Dana E. Habers   *Scott P. Stringer*

ABSTRACT

This chapter works in concert with others in this book to provide residents, medical students, and physicians with a high-level overview of the core skills required to successfully manage a clinical practice. It is meant to build a practical awareness of ambulatory (outpatient) clinic operations, not as an exhaustive manual. The core elements of establishing a practice, promoting access for patients to your services, retaining patients and referral sources, and sustaining financial viability are discussed. The core elements of a clinical practice include

- Human Resources
- Access Management
- Clinic Efficiency
- Managed Care Contracting and Financial Management
- Critical Communication and Protecting Patient Privacy
- Information Technology
- Marketing

Beyond the operating and exam room, there are fundamental skills critical to a physician's success in the medical business. Too many medical students and residents graduate with high honors and a list of academic achievements, but fail in their careers because of a lack of basic business savvy. A full business education is simply too vast to include in the educational journey of a medical school and residency, and this chapter outlines the core skills required to successfully manage a clinical practice and a practical understanding of ambulatory (outpatient) operations. Throughout the text, *Key Resource* inserts are included that lead to more extensive sources of information on each subject.

HUMAN RESOURCES

Above all else, personnel and the human element of any clinical practice will drive its success. Management is one area where the art to medical science comes into play; it requires a significant time investment and is the area most likely to provide a return on investment than any other aspect of clinic management. People make the business. From the provider and their staff to the patients and their families, having the right people on the team will make all the difference.

Whether a physician is in private practice or joins the faculty of a large academic medical center, their role in clinic is inherently that of a leader. The physician sets the tone for a practice, and support staff will revere and respect a physician who is a good leader. What good news for the ego, but the responsibility that comes with this role cannot be underestimated. Leadership is refined with experience and does not come naturally to every medical school graduate. It is worth the time and energy for physicians to hone their leadership skills and work towards greatness in this regard. Top leaders are "differentiated from other levels of leaders in that they have a wonderful blend of personal humility combined with extraordinary professional will. Understand that they are very ambitious; but their ambition, first and foremost, is for the company's success. They realize that the most important step they must make to become a Level 5 leader is to subjugate their ego to the company's performance. When asked for interviews, these leaders will agree only if it's about the company and not about them" (1).

Beyond the physician, the people supporting their provision of care carry tone and culture throughout the practice. Relationships between the physician and patient are pivotal, but the amount of time patients spend interacting with the clinic staff far outweighs time spent with their physician. A positive patient care experience hinges on whether each team member they interact with consistently demonstrates helpfulness and kindness and promotes an environment of safety, security, and confidentiality. Hiring staff who subscribe to common philosophies on customer service and priorities in the workplace forms the foundational stability for a thriving, oftentimes unpredictably busy clinical practice.

In addition to hiring the right people for the right roles, it is important to rightsize the number of employees. There are several organizations in the market that offer benchmarking data for staffing levels. It is important to gauge, but difficult to compare unequivocally to other practices, as support needs vary widely from practice to practice and will depend on several factors.

Key Resource: Health Care Management Networking

Several health care management organizations exist for benchmarking and idea sharing: to name a few, the Medical Group Managers Association, Healthcare Financial Management Association, Healthcare Information and Management Systems Society, American College of Healthcare Executives, and many more that dive deeper into specialties or delineate between academic medicine and private practices.

Patient volumes, socioeconomic characteristics of the patient population, mix of services provided, and even the physician's personal style of practice all factor into determining the right number of support staff per physician. Key operational roles include registered nurses (RNs); licensed practical nurses (LPNs); medical assistants (MAs); and nonmedical administrative support including management, schedulers, patient accounting, housekeeping, information technology, and medical receptionists.

Retention of excellent employees saves a practice both time and money and improves the quality of care. National studies have estimated the average cost of replacing an RN to be anywhere from about $22,000 to over $64,000 (2). Turnover costs are estimated to range between 0.75 and 2.0 times the salary of the departing individual (3), while nurse turnover costs have been estimated at 1.3 times the salary of a departing nurse (4). Patient care can suffer when the nursing and administrative staff members are inexperienced or unfamiliar with the clinic operations.

Beyond just being a great leader and setting a productive cultural tone, there are tactical strategies to retain good people. Making the financial investment in your staff is the most obvious. Paying market-competitive salaries that keep pace with inflation and offering a competitive benefits package to supplement take-home pay are strategies. People are also motivated by nonmonetary rewards and recognition that can be as simple as a note of appreciation when they've done a good job or getting recognition for making a positive impression on a patient. Retention is not a mystery—consider what drives each individual on your team and ensure that his or her intrinsic needs to be a happy and productive employee are met. Support

the sharing of ideas, get to know staff, and listen to their concerns. Provide opportunities for their personal and professional growth. These are valuable investments in the core of the clinical practice, the people.

ACCESS MANAGEMENT

Access to health care has sparked ongoing debate and political division in the United States for years. Physicians are inherently committed to treating patients who come to them in need of care. However, health care professionals are not immune to economic realities. In the current system, the cost of health care often exceeds individual affordability. While many Americans have insurance coverage, there are a vast number of individuals and families who do not. There are also people with high deductible insurance plans who, while covered by an insurance plan, will struggle with affordability. Health care providers must balance both missions: to provide care to those in need, while remaining viable as a business and able to sustain continued services over the course of time. Increasingly, ethical pressure builds on the physician to walk this fine line.

One method used to promote sustainability is to divide a portion of patient appointment slots between various payer classes. This mechanism builds in both the accommodation of patients with a variety of payment sources as well as the funding from enough insured patients to sustain the practice.

Logistical access points are another component of access to health care. Requests for physician services come from a variety of constituents: referring primary care doctors, referring specialists, their office staff, and patients themselves. To accommodate all requests, it is advisable to develop policies and consistent protocols around both who is authorized to refer a patient to the clinic and what process they must follow to do so. For example, if a referring physician calls to request an appointment for one of his or her patients, copies of applicable clinical information from the patient's chart will need to be sent prior to the appointment. Labs or other ancillary test results from outside sources will avoid ordering duplicate studies or tests and achieve a continuum of care for the patient. Such policies must be built in advance and adhered to consistently in order to ensure equity in access. Another consideration in access points is how requests are received—whether by inbound phone, fax, e-mail, or other mechanisms, a quick turnaround and bidirectional communication with the requester is important to promote access and survive in a competitive market. Acquiring a reputation of being difficult to access or slow to respond to appointment requests will quickly drive referring physicians to send their patients elsewhere.

Scheduling template design is also critical. It impacts not only revenue but also clinic throughput, efficiency, staff morale, and patient satisfaction. Length of appointment will naturally vary by provider, but a good rule of thumb for a new physician starting to build the practice is to allot 15-minute increments for every standard patient visit. The template can be adjusted accordingly to properly account for a typical new or established patient visit with each provider.

There are several examples of template design techniques that can be used to promote access, the most common include

- Stream scheduling: Patients are each given a unique appointment time and arrive in a steady stream throughout clinic. Setting realistic appointment times is critical for smooth patient flow. This is the most common model.
- Open access: No appointment is required. Patients are seen during specified hours on a first-come, first-serve basis. This technique works well for brief visit types and when clinic staffing levels are flexible to accommodate variations in demand.
- Double booking: Two or more patients are given the same appointment time. This works best for patients whose needs can be met simultaneously, for example, patient A requires lab work and will have a wait time while results are processed, during which the physician can see patient B for suture removal. Double booking is also used where patient populations have a high rate of no shows or last-minute cancellations, in order to ensure a full schedule despite last-minute decline in patient demand.
- Clustering: Patients with similar problems or who require an assembly line procedure are seen consecutively. This is useful if the patient care involves a particular piece of equipment and efficiencies are gained by seeing patients back to back.
- Wave or modified wave scheduling: Two or three patients who have complex or time-consuming problems are scheduled at the beginning of each hour, followed by single appointments every 10 to 20 minutes the rest of the hour devoted to patients with minor problems or for same day walk-ins. In wave or modified wave, the appropriate triage of patient needs when scheduling the appointments is critical to success.

Once an appointment is scheduled, the process to obtain approval for any procedures should begin immediately. The difficulty for physicians in this system is that each insurance company typically develops a unique set of rules around which procedures require an authorization, the process physicians must follow to obtain pre-approval, and even the level of detail or data sets required to obtaining an authorization. The best approach is to have dedicated office personnel for this function who can become familiar with each of the rule sets, keep abreast as they change, and allow as much time as possible to follow their protocols before a service is rendered.

The patients' arrival to the clinic presents a prime opportunity to validate their demographic and insurance information. This information must be accurately captured to process medical claims or advance their account through the collections cycles for payments due after the date of service. Many insurance companies provide eligibility verification tools on their Web sites, or there are clearinghouse vendors whose technology will automatically validate discreet data fields against various insurance company databases to guide correction of inaccuracies.

CLINIC EFFICIENCY

Physicians in training are often criticized for the time it takes to do many of the things they have been taught to do well. For example, documentation that is thorough and detailed takes time, as does visiting with a patient during a routine evaluation and management visit. However, in order to stay afloat, a clinical practice will survive off volume. As long as the reimbursement environment is based on a fee-for-service infrastructure, the more services a physician can provide in a day, the more financially viable the physician's practice will be. The challenge for physicians is to find balance and work towards efficiency, trimming any wasted time from the day. Clinic layout and flow is one way to save steps for physicians, nurses, and other support staff. It is important to have the right number of support staff, but each one must have the ability to do his or her job efficiently and without, or at least with minimal, waste.

Bottlenecks can arise in the physical layout of the clinic space, the stocking and flow of medical supplies and equipment, or even in the logistical characteristics of the support staff. For example, to run two exam rooms in parallel, the vitals station must be set up to filter patients through from the waiting area to exam room in a timely manner. Having a vitals space that is in an awkward location or having too few staff to support patient movement through the hallways can result in exam rooms sitting vacant for periods of time or worse sitting idle with waiting patients inside. Flow diagrams, Pareto charts, spaghetti diagrams, and process time studies are all excellent continuous quality improvement tools available to help troubleshoot clinic flow issues.

It will be obvious that there is a problem; the difficulty comes with identifying the root cause and implementing and monitoring the fix. Successful improvement initiatives begin with a clear goal and an understanding of the information needed to identify and monitor measures of resolution. According to Raymond Carey, "The goal of data collection is to gain an objective view of the process under investigation and to understand how it is performing over time. The healthcare field is replete with data. Few industries collect as much data as we do in healthcare. The problem we face, therefore, is not a data problem, it is an information problem" (5).

OPERATIONAL ADAPTABILITY

Health care is an amorphous industry, one in which the physician and their support team must continuously evolve to meet the needs of their customer. Clinic operations management is complex in that it requires standardization and structure, while remaining flexible enough to adapt as the regulatory, technologic, financial, and medical environments change. Leading change is a critical skill for physicians in light of this challenge.

"Change is a physical event so it's not surprising that many people have strong reactions to it…. To get any idea rolling, it is important to build understanding and enthusiasm. When the idea is supported by a sufficient number of key people, it takes off under its own steam, building its own sense of momentum" (6). When planning change, there are key steps that will ensure adoption by even the most reluctant support staff.

First, communicate about what is driving the change—what is the catalyst? Context helps people understand and often empathize with the change leader. Second, gain critical mass in the organization. Identify key opinion leaders who will more readily shift from neutral to supportive and allow their influence to drive peers who are resistant from their state of resistance to one of neutrality. Third, actively listen to concerns and address them consistently and persistently, allowing emotional reactions to change to subside under the limelight of good information.

Even with extensive planning and communication, there will remain those who simply will not accept change. As a change leader, be mindful that late adopters can easily drain time and resources. Identify late adopters early on and have a plan in place to address their resistance without sacrificing support for the adoptive group. Change is never easy, but will always be a part of what physicians must embrace.

A CLIMATE OF SAFETY AND QUALITY

The term *culture of safety* is typically associated with production industries like automotive manufacturing or nuclear power. "Accident-free" signs hang near construction sites, and certifications such as ISO-9000 indicate the success of assembly line industries in meeting measurable quality standards. The application of safety-oriented research is incredibly important to health care, despite its differences from a factory. Health care poses a challenge most other industries do not have: each patient is unique, so standardized processes must also adapt in consideration of each patient's needs. There is no one size fits all or mechanical assembly line. However, the benefits of standardization where applicable ensure quality and serve to reduce medical errors.

Clinic support staff must feel comfortable bringing forward matters they believe to be potential quality or safety issues. They need an open, safe forum for passing this information up to the management or physician team to proactively address. Many organizations provide an anonymous mechanism to promote honest, open feedback and solicit input from those who are on the front lines and therefore more likely to notice potential safety land mines.

The response when a medical error or safety breach does occur is also a key indicator of the culture. Health care involves many potential points of failure, and delivery of health services is a complex web of people, resources, and systems. "Errors are not synonymous with negligence. Medicine's ethos of infallibility leads, wrongly, to a culture that sees mistakes as individual problems or weaknesses and remedies them with blame and punishment. Instead people should be looking for the multiple contributing factors, which can be resolved only by improving systems" (7).

MANAGED CARE CONTRACTING

Contracting to become an in-network provider with a managed care company promotes business for the population of patients who are covered by that insurance plan. In the process of contracting, one key negotiation is the amount agreed to accept as payment in full, also called the *allowable*. Universal billing codes called Current Procedural Terminology (CPT) codes are used to both negotiate rates by procedure, as well as in the submission of claims for payment. Reimbursement for each CPT code will depend on the up front negotiation, typically phrased as a percent of Medicare reimbursement. Other contract terms include termination clauses, processes for claims submission and payment remittances, methods used to recoup overpayments or address underpayments, and length of the agreement. Small private practices are advised to seek legal counsel on all contract negotiations from an attorney experienced in health care reimbursement, and larger group practices typically employ their own contracting and legal departments to facilitate discussions with the insurance carriers and advocate for fair reimbursement for physicians work.

Overview of Negotiation Goals

Provider goals in a negotiation:	Insurance company goals in a negotiation:
Maximize payment per service provided	Minimize payment per service provided
Minimize authorization requirements for procedures, autonomy in decision-making for medical necessity	Utilization review—control procedure volumes, limit to medical necessity only
Minimize administrative burden in claims adjudication (file claims and receive payments electronically, etc.)	
Promote access to physicians for insured patients/members	

There is a delicately balanced trade-off between rates and volumes. Once the contract is signed, your role in the relationship must remain proactive and continuous. Each payer requires ongoing maintenance. Specifically, close monitoring of claims payments over time to assess whether payers are complying with the terms and agreed upon rates. Several tools in the marketplace have the capacity to electronically scrub or analyze claims payment data and identify under- and overpayments. These tools provide the data, but reacting to it in a timely fashion is critical to your relationships and ultimately the bottom line. If payers are overpaying, they will likely request a recoupment down the road and oftentimes not at opportune moments given clinic cash flow. If they are underpaying, you must connect with your representative to identify the issue, fix it, and ensure proper payment for your services according to the agreed upon terms both retroactively and going forward. It is likely there will be errors in payment as systems on both the insurer and provider side are complicated and interwoven. Expecting payment terms to be met without constant monitoring is overly optimistic.

Key Resource: Medicare Reimbursement

Medicare allowables are public information. Rates by CPT code are published on the Centers for Medicare and Medicaid Services at https://www.cms.gov. This Web site contains up-to-date information for physicians on repayment for care of Medicare beneficiaries.

The current formula used to calculate rate of reimbursement is founded on a measure of physician productivity called a relative value unit (RVU) and on a geographic cost of living/practice adjustment called a geographic practice cost index (GPCI), as follows:

2010 Non-Facility Pricing Amount

$$= ([\text{Work RVU} \times \text{Work GPCI}]$$
$$+ [\text{Transitioned Non-Facility PE RVU} \times \text{PE GPCI}]$$
$$+ [\text{MP RVU} \times \text{MP GPCI}]) \times \text{Conversion Factor (CF)}$$

2010 Facility Pricing Amount

$$= ([\text{Work RVU} \times \text{Work GPCI}]$$
$$+ [\text{Transitioned Facility PE RVU} \times \text{PE GPCI}]$$
$$+ [\text{MP RVU} \times \text{MP GPCI}]) \times \text{CF}$$

The conversion factor for CY 2010 is $36.0846.

Specific reimbursement rates and detail on each code is available in a lookup reference on Medicare's Web site at: https://www.cms.gov/apps/physician-fee-schedule/overview.aspx.

FINANCIAL MANAGEMENT

As health care becomes increasingly complex, so too do the financial mechanisms layered beneath the practitioner in support of their clinical practice. Despite national recognition of the need to revolutionize how much our nation is spending on health care, as of 2011, the payment methodology used to reimburse physicians for their time and expertise is based on the volume of services provided. A standard value unit is applied to each procedural code available to a physician for billing (CPT Coding), and further, a dollar value is assigned to that work. As such, payment models intrinsically motivate physicians to generate the greatest volume possible. Pay for performance and value-based purchasing are new buzz words to the reimbursement scene in the early 2000s and are each an attempt to tie in quality of care in addition to volume. The idea being, rather than paying providers simply for a specific service, payers would reimburse providers based on their clinical outcomes or on measurable indicators of *effective* health care services. These systems are imperfect and exist in a variety of pilot modes across the country, but they are driving providers to pay attention to quality measures and patient population management strategies in addition to daily clinic operations. Whether or not our industry adopts these models, it is generally agreed across political platforms that the current model in the United States is unsustainable. Health care financing is convoluted and has evolved over time into a difficult to understand stratosphere of funds flows.

Where consumers (patients) are accustomed in most industries to paying for goods or services at the time they are rendered, in health care there are third-party fiscal guarantors who may be responsible for payment on the patient's behalf and most often payment from patients is not due or due several weeks after a service has been provided. The process to determine financial responsibility and pursue payment takes time, introducing days of lag between the point when a service is rendered and when it is fully paid for by either the insurance agent or patient.

Reducing this lag is a goal of any financially savvy clinic manager. There are several methods to do so, but most effective is to attempt to collect the patient portion of payment on the day of their office visit. This point of service opportunity allows the provider to make decisions about their willingness to see patients who are in debt for prior services or unwilling to resolve those balances in a timely manner. It is also a key time to educate patients about their expected out-of-pocket expense, and patients may need to make decisions about the services they receive when care is optional. Estimating the actual out-of-pocket expense for any visit is a challenge since information around the full complement of services that will be provided to a specific patient are often undefined until after a patient needs assessment is complete. Estimating as accurately as possible and practicing consistent policies for services rendered before, after, or regardless of payment is critical to establish. Typically, offices collect at a minimum the co-pay amount for their visits up front, and it is common to balance bill the coinsurance, deductible, or other cash outlay by patient statement on the back end post-adjudication of any insurance claims.

Another method to expedite payment for health care services is to file claims to the payer sources electronically. A standard, Health Insurance Portability and Accountability Act (HIPAA)-compliant file format exists to promote this mode of claims processing. It is beneficial for both the provider and insurance agent because it reduces manual intervention and labor associated with the claims adjudication process.

Patient responsibility for health care costs ebbs and flows over time. Insurance companies are shifting more out-of-pocket responsibility to patients as health care costs rise and threaten to shrink their margins. This trend has made it increasingly difficult for physicians and hospitals to accurately collect payment for their services. "The economic recession and rising unemployment—plus changing demographics and baby boomers aging into Medicare—are among the factors expected to influence health spending during 2009 to 2019. In 2009 the health share of gross domestic product is expected to have increased 1.1% points to 17.3%—the largest single-year increase since 1960. Average public spending growth rates for hospital, physician and clinical services, and prescription drugs are expected to exceed private spending growth in the first 4 years of the projections. As a result, public spending is projected to account for more than half of all US health care spending by 2012" (8). What this means to the average physician is the expectation of increased productivity, despite the inevitability that reimbursements will hit a plateau.

Enrollment in private health insurance plans is also changing the composition of guarantors responsible to pay for physician services. "Private health insurance premiums grew 1.3% in 2009, a deceleration from 3.5% growth in 2008. Benefit payment growth also slowed, from 4.4% in 2008 to 2.8% in 2009. These trends were heavily influenced by the recession as private health insurance enrollment declined. In 2009, spending for benefits increased faster than premiums, and as a result, the net cost of private health insurance (or the difference between premiums and benefits) fell to an 11.1% share of total private health insurance spending from 12.4% in 2008—a continuation of its recent decline" (9).

Given these climate changes, it is critical that physicians and health care managers work towards efficiency and contain overhead costs to the degree feasible. Again, there is a delicate balance in this task—one must continue to provide excellence in health care and promote a positive patient experience, while capturing enough revenue to sustain the practice over the long term.

CRITICAL PATIENT COMMUNICATION

Established and dependable communication pathways between providers and their patients are a requirement of any ambulatory clinic. Nurses often manage most of the triage and alleviate the provider from having to be involved in every patient care call. The key to building an effective system of triage is to empower clinic staff at the lowest common denominator to address patient needs. For example, calls from patients requesting appointments or seeking driving directions should be managed by an administrative support staff member, where a prescription refill request requires the medical expertise of a nurse to respond. Physicians may receive an escalated call if, for example, another physician is requesting a consult or advice on patient care. There must be systematic accountability built into the flow for prompt response times and follow through in meeting the caller's needs. Physicians face great competing interests for the time in their day, so building a strong team of dependable, capable staff to manage the patient care needs expands the breadth and impact of the physician's clinic day.

Patients will inevitably need to consult their physician after business hours, and a process must be in place for ensuring patient needs continue to be met during those times. Rotating a provider on call is the most common method used to promote work–life balance for physicians; having some resource available will prevent patients from defaulting to the emergency room when faced with an after-hours need.

Technology has promoted communication through electronic mail. Health care is still relatively uncharted, and physicians face liabilities on medical advice or treatment offered via e-mail. It is not yet sophisticated enough as a technology to fully assess patient status, but can be an effective tool of working with established patients to refill prescriptions or schedule follow-up appointments. While much of this is physician preference, availability of a provider by e-mail can be a major point of satisfaction for patients who are accustomed to this mode of communication for other aspects of their lives. There are CPT codes available for consults provided over e-mail; however, many insurance companies refuse to reimburse for this service. Undoubtedly, as technologies change, the potential for varying modes of communication between patients and their providers will continue to expand and evolve.

A useful tool for gauging whether a patient population is satisfied with their provider relationship and care experience is by conducting randomized patient satisfaction surveys. There are several vendors on the market that will conduct a survey by phone, e-mail, or mail; collate the responses; and provide statistical data and comment data back to their provider clients. Feedback on the physician and the patient's experience in the clinic is useful to gauge likelihood of practice growth, identify weaknesses or opportunities for improved bedside manner, and supplement face to face impressions with measurable, ongoing evaluation of care. Patients who feel confident in the abilities of their provider often demonstrate higher likelihood of compliance with treatment plans, and ultimately a solid relationship with their caregiver can mean a healthier lifestyle through medication compliance and motivated lifestyle choices. In the end, making patients healthy is not enough—making patients happy in addition is important to a physician's success.

PATIENT PRIVACY

Clinics must be physically and operationally designed to protect patient privacy. The Health Insurance Portability and Accountability Act of 1996, or HIPAA sets national standards for the security of individual identity and health information. These guidelines are enforced by the Office of Civil Rights, and failure of a practice to comply or breach can result in serious penalties.

Key Resource: Patient Privacy Rule

Visit the U.S. Department of Health and Human Services Web site for detail on who is covered by the Privacy Rule, what information is protected, and permitted uses and disclosures (http://www.hhs.gov/ocr/privacy/).

Promote privacy in the clinic setting by following simple but often overlooked behaviors:

- Do not discuss patient cases in the hallways. Conversations can easily be overheard.
- Do not discuss patient cases with anyone other than those who need to know in order to care for the patient.
- Secure all medical records, paper and electronic. No exceptions.
- Restrict access to information systems at the appropriate levels, and track individual activity in any system containing protected health information.
- Design work spaces to promote privacy. Shade visible computer monitors, ensure patients are offered a space to carry on private or sensitive conversations with staff at registration desks and vitals stations, and insulate exam room walls to prevent noise pollution.
- Properly disclose breaches, and immediately address the security weakness in order to prevent it from impacting additional patients.

INFORMATION TECHNOLOGY

Information technology has drastically changed the way clinicians function. From the medical technologies and connectivity between them, to electronic visits and telemedicine, technologic advancement has set the stage for physicians to reach further distances to apply their skills. At the same time, technology has complicated the clinical setting by introducing a nonhuman element to patient care.

Providers often document medical record information electronically throughout a patient encounter, which can distract the physician's attention from the actual patient encounter. Balancing bedside manner with the need to efficiently and thoroughly document their treatment will be a growing challenge for physicians as technology continues to become an integral part of the health care experience.

Electronic medical records come in as many varieties as patients—there are systems designed specifically for subspecialists or generic ambulatory models that can cross multiple specialties. There are also varying degrees of connectivity. Some systems allow a community of providers to connect seamlessly to one another's medical records, with patient permission, and promote the sharing of information at the click of a button. However they are designed, their role in health care and clinic day-to-day operations is growing and critical. When implemented and used properly, the benefits of an electronic health record far outweigh the burdens. Medicare has begun tying reimbursement amounts to the use of this technology by providers through a program called Meaningful Use. The choice between paper and electronic medical charting is becoming obsolete, and drivers point towards a very near future where all medical doctors function on some degree of electronic medical records, often interconnected across practice lines.

Key Resource: Meaningful Use

Medicare is introducing financial penalties, which follow closely behind a brief period of financial incentives, for providers based on their ability to demonstrate Meaningful Use. For a full review of the program, refer to https://www.cms.gov/EHRIncentivePrograms/30_Meaningful_Use.asp.

Information technology is opening doors, not only for patient care and quality but also for management of physician practices as business entities. Making informed decisions is critical to survival in the health care industry. Regulatory and financial environments dictate constant change and require frequent reevaluation of practice viability. It is important to invest in a technology infrastructure that will allow decisions to be driven by data. There is a vast array of performance metrics, and within each metric there can also be multiple means of calculating the metric. Trending performance against both industry competitors and collaborators must be done with caution due to this variability. It is also highly recommended that trending be done against internal benchmarks, for example, reviewing the visit volumes of a practice in the current month compared to the same month prior year. This allows you to monitor both the health and viability of the practice as well as its likelihood to compete in a given market.

Below is a list of some basic key performance indicators typical of a clinical practice dashboard.

Key Measures of Practice Performance

Metric	Importance to Clinic Management
Charges	Total dollar value of services provided in a given time period. Charges are an indicator of volume of work completed by a clinician. In managed care contracts, recall that the final reimbursement amount will be the contractual allowable, not the actual charge. Always charge equal to or greater than the contractual allowable to maximize collections. Charge amounts have a greater impact on self-pay patients, unless your practice has a discount policy. Tracking charges month to month can be skewed by changes in the fee schedule.
Collection rates	Calculations for collection rates vary greatly, but the most common are Gross Collection Rate (GCR) and Net Collection Rate (NCR). GCR = Total Amount Collected/Total Amount Billed, does not account for differences in contractual allowances, subject to fluctuation with fee schedule changes which may not have corresponding impact on actual reimbursement. NCR = Total Amount Collected/Total Amount Billed—Contractual Allowances + Refunds and Overpayments. Most accurate measure of collections performance by calculating effectiveness of collecting total potential revenue.
Patient revenue	Total dollars received for services provided in a given time period. The primary source of income for most practices is fee-for-service patient care revenue; although some have other inputs such as contractual arrangements to provide consultative work or inpatient hospital coverage.
Payer mix	Patient population broken out into payer classifications. Percentages are commonly broken down into the main five to six payer classes with the remainder defined as Other. Practices often measure Medicare, Medicaid, Insured, Uninsured, and break Insured down into the top three to four coverage plans. Knowing the percent of your patient population in each category will gauge whether reimbursement rates will suffice to cover overhead.
Resource utilization	How many patients are seen per exam room per hour, or how many of the allotted clinic hours are spent providing patient care gives some measure of productivity and also use of fixed overhead on space.
Physician work relative value units (wRVU)	The relative level of time, skill, training, and intensity required to render a service. The resource-based relative value scale, developed for the Center for Medicare and Medicaid Services, assigns a relative value to each CPT code relative to all of the other CPT codes. RVUs are determined by committees of the American Medical Association. The committees' members come from all medical specialties and include representatives from other health professions, including nursing. The committees assign a relative value after hearing testimony from specialty groups on how many hours or minutes it takes to perform a procedure, the level of skill required, the level of education/training required, and the practice expense associated with a procedure. Measuring wRVU totals over time gauge the level of complexity and volume of services being provided, and are commonly used in productivity-based compensation plans for physicians.
Visit volumes	Basic count of visits attended or billed by a physician can be a gauge of patient demand for services, supply or availability of the physician, or both.

MARKETING

There will always be a need for doctors, nurses, and clinical care teams to serve patient health needs. However, success in the health care market is not a given. While demand continues to grow, in some markets supply of health care providers exceeds the community need. Marketing and attention to the public perception and understanding of your practice remain important survival tactics in the field. An investment in a marketing firm for guidance on practice name, and most effective mediums in your market will pay off. Typical mediums include

- Yellow and white pages, update both print and online directories
- Web sites—invest in both an owned and operated Web site as well as update your information found on go-to resources for the general public such as Health Grades, WebMD, and Angie's List.
- Social media networks like Facebook or Twitter
- Becoming involved in your local community through chamber of commerce memberships, local charity and volunteer work, guest speaking at conferences, and other networking business opportunities
- Outreach to referring doctor's offices through regular visits

- Direct mail campaigns or newsletters to patients and their families
- Provide opportunities for members of your local community to become engaged in your practice by offering community educational seminars or free screening days.

Any of the above incrementally or in combination will reach key audiences and promote growth. Above all, word of mouth prevails, and patients who have come to see you and had a stellar experience will be the most powerful marketing tool you have to grow your practice.

SUMMARY

This chapter introduced several fundamental skills critical to a physician's success in the medical business. While not meant to be an exhaustive manual on how practitioners can become business savvy, we have introduced the core considerations for physicians whether running a small private practice setting or becoming a member of a large physician practice plan. Business acumen comes in time and with experience, but the highlights on clinic management include

- Human resources—people are at the core of health care, and it is the most important investment of time and money you can make to develop a dependable, talented, aligned support staff. Physicians set the tone, and the attitude and citizenship of the provider will permeate all others in a clinic setting.
- Access management—making it easy for patients to get appointments will improve their satisfaction and promote relationships with the referring community.
- Clinic efficiency, remaining adaptable, and promoting a climate of safety and quality care will improve the likelihood that patients will return or recommend their physician to others.
- Financial viability of the practice hinges on managed care contracting, financial management, and accurately capturing any reimbursement for all services provided.
- Remaining available to patients for critical communication and protecting patient privacy are both a responsibility of the physician and a right of the patient.
- Information technology continues to shape health care, and it is inevitable and something that when embraced can enhance both the life of a physician and the quality of care given to patients.
- Marketing and setting oneself apart from competitors will be key in establishing an identity not as an individual physician but as a leader in the field of medicine.

REFERENCES

1. Collins J. *Good to great: why some companies make the leap... and others don't!* New York: HarperBusiness, 2001.
2. Advisory Board Company. A misplaced focus: reexamining the recruiting/retention trade-off. *Nursing Watch* 1999;11:114.
3. McConnell CR. Staff turnover: occasional friend, frequent foe, and continuing frustration. *Health Care Manag* 1999;8:1–13.
4. Jones CB. The costs of nursing turnover, part 2: application of the nursing turnover cost calculation methodology. *J Nurs Admin* 2005;35(1):41–49.
5. Carey RG. *Measuring quality improvement in healthcare: a guide to statistical process control applications.* New York: American Society for Quality, 2001.
6. Scholtes PR. *The team handbook,* 3rd ed. 2003.
7. Nelson EC. *Quality by design: a clinical microsystems approach.* 2007.
8. Truffer CJ, Keehan S, Smith S, et al. Health spending projections through 2019: the recession's impact continues. *Health Aff* 2010;29(3):522–529.
9. Centers for Medicare & Medicaid Services. Highlights, National Health Expenditures, 2009. https://www.cms.gov/NationalHealthExpendData/downloads/highlights.pdf. Accessed on March, 2011.

RECOMMENDED READING

- Medical Group Managers Association—www.mgma.com
- Healthcare Financial Management Association—www.hfma.org
- Healthcare Information and Management Systems Society—www.himss.org
- American College of Healthcare Executives—www.ache.org
- Centers for Medical Services—www.cms.gov
- Department of Health and Human Services—www.dhhs.gov
- Certification Commission for Health Information Technology—www.cchit.org
- Huss J, Coleman M. *Start your own medical practice: a guide to all the things they don't teach you in medical school about starting your own practice.* 2006.
- Stanley K, Daigrepont J. *Starting a medical practice: the physician's handbook for successful practice start up.* 2003.

Comparative Medical Systems

202

William Anthony Wood

OVERVIEW

Every year in the United States, over 40,000 people die because of lack of health insurance (1). Among industrialized democracies, only the United States fails to provide universal health coverage. According to the U.S. Census Bureau, in 2010, 49.9 million Americans—over 16% of the population—lack health insurance (2). This is an increase in the uninsured, from 2008, of several million individuals, and an increase of over one percentage point of the nation's total population. About 10% of American children under 18 were uninsured in 2009.

Among those *with* coverage, the number of people with employment-based insurance is falling. Due to recent job losses in the current economic downturn, another 2010 study by the independent Commonwealth Fund estimates that "nine million working-age adults—57 percent of people who had health insurance through a job that was lost—became uninsured in the last two years" (3). The study further notes that "an estimated 44 million people were paying off medical debt in 2010, up from 37 million in 2005," and that "4 million declared bankruptcy because of medical bills."

Most physicians are not experts on the topic of comparative medical systems. This chapter serves as an introduction, from one doctor's perspective. The topic is huge and covered in detail by peer-reviewed journals such as *Health Affairs,* along with regular commentaries in *The New England Journal of Medicine,* frequently updated books and Web sites, and in-depth reports by national and international expert organizations such as the Institute of Medicine (IOM) and the World Health Organization (WHO).

Although we do not cover everyone in the United States, we spend far more per capita than other similar countries and yet have significantly worse outcomes. Figures from 2009 from the Organisation for Economic Co-operation and Development (OECD), whose 34 countries include most of the world's wealthy industrial democracies, show total health expenditure per capita in the United States at currently nearly $8,000. This compares to an estimated $5,350 in Norway, the next highest spender, and $4,363 in neighboring Canada (4). In fact, the OECD notes that although US *government* spending on health care is less than half of *total* health care expenditures, at 47.7%,

> ...the level of health spending in the United States is so high that public (i.e., government) spending on health per capita is *greater (emphasis in original)* than in all other OECD countries, except Norway and the Netherlands. For this amount of public expenditure in the United States, government provided in 2009 insurance coverage only for the elderly and disabled people (through Medicare) and some of the poor (through Medicaid and the State Children's Health Insurance Program [SCHIP]), whereas in most other OECD countries this was enough for government to provide universal health insurance (4).

In effect, one could say that we pay enough in taxes to achieve universal coverage, but do not receive it. Other analyses point to a significantly higher percentage of total US health care spending from taxes—as much as 60%—without universal coverage (5).

Despite our outlier expenditures, our results are significantly below average, compared to similarly wealthy nations. Our average life expectancy is 78 years, compared to 80.7 years in Canada, for example (putting Canada more than 1 year higher than the OECD average, of 79.5 years, in 2009) (6). Similarly, our infant mortality is 6.5 (in 2008, latest available), which is much higher than the average in other OECD countries, of 4.4 in 2009. Our infant mortality rate is much higher than Canada's, which was 5.1 in 2007. The OECD notes that "... while life expectancy in the United States used to be 1½ year *above* the OECD average in 1960, it is now... almost 1½ year *below* the average of 79.5 years" (7) (*emphasis in original*).

There are numerous ways, aside from the standard overall statistics of life expectancy and infant mortality, to compare different countries' medical systems and outcomes. One approach looks at "deaths from treatable conditions," termed "amenable mortality." A study comparing the United States with 18 other industrialized countries, evaluating "trends in deaths considered amenable to health care before age seventy-five between 1997–98 and 2002–3," found a decline in all countries in amenable mortality over this period, averaging 17%. However, "the United States was an outlier, with a decline of only 4 percent" (8).

While our higher per capita health expenditures buy us more MRI and CT machines, on average, than other OECD countries, we have fewer doctors and hospital beds. The 2011 OECD comparison report notes that "in 2009, the United States had 2.4 practising physicians per 1,000 population, below the OECD average of 3.1." The report notes that we have 2.7 hospital beds per 1,000 population in 2007 (latest year available), lower than the OECD average of 3.5 beds in 2009. We have 34.3 CT scanners per million population in 2007 (latest year available), much higher than the OECD average of 22.1, and 25.9 MRIs per million population, "more than twice the OECD average of 12.0" (9). But more machines, and fewer doctors and hospital beds, do not equate to longer life expectancy nor lower infant mortality.

Among other participants in the field, thousands of physicians, including this author, are active in Physicians for a National Health Program (PNHP.org), a nonprofit advocacy group working for single-payer national health insurance in the United States, also termed Medicare for All. My personal perspective, based on my reading of relevant research, is that such a system would provide the most rational and cost-effective solution to the problem of the uninsured. You will make your living as an otolaryngologist via compensation from our medical system (or fragmented parts of it, as detailed below), throughout your career. If your doors are open to them, self-pay patients—a euphemism for the uninsured—will likely present themselves in your clinic every week.

THE PROBLEM: LACK OF UNIVERSAL COVERAGE IN THE UNITED STATES

Through diverse approaches, the citizens of every industrialized democracy but ours have passed universal health coverage for their populations. We are also alone in having a predominantly for-profit health insurance industry, in which insurers are private corporations that (must) generate dividends for stockholders and multimillion-dollar incomes for top executives. Here, of course, any patient "can always go to the ER," but this inadequate "safety net" approach does not constitute universal coverage.

Most otolaryngology residents see patients in the ER who have delayed seeking medical attention due to lack of health insurance. Of course, this delay often worsens

their prognoses and outcomes. A study of over 60,000 laryngeal cancer patients in the National Cancer Database from 1996 to 2003 found that "individuals lacking insurance or having Medicaid are at greatest risk for presenting with advanced laryngeal cancer" (10). (The study's authors further note that "results for the Medicaid group may be influenced by the postdiagnosis enrollment of uninsured patients." Medicaid is the public insurance program for the poor, jointly funded by federal and state governments.) They comment that "in multivariate analysis, the type of health insurance remained the strongest predictor of stage at diagnosis and tumor size."

The authors of the laryngeal cancer study also looked at over 40,000 oropharyngeal cancer patients in the same national database. They found that, "after controlling for other sociodemographic characteristics, patients with advanced oropharyngeal cancer at diagnosis were more likely to be uninsured (odds ratio 1.37; 95% confidence interval 1.21–1.55)" (11). They noted that, after "controlling for covariates [patient sex, age, race, treatment facility type, zip code–based education and income categories, and U.S. Census region]," this association reached a very high statistical significance, with a value of $P < 0.0001$.

From my own residency, I remember more than one patient with laryngeal cancer who waited until experiencing acute airway compromise, after having been hoarse with odynophagia for weeks or months, before coming to the ER. These patients then usually needed a total laryngectomy for their T4 tumor. An earlier diagnosis would likely have required a less extirpative treatment. In a long-standing free annual community head and neck screening clinic conducted by the University of Michigan Department of Otolaryngology, "lack of insurance ($P = 0.05$) was a significant predictor of a lesion suspicious for malignancy" (12).

The IOM, the health arm of our National Academies, has noted for a number of years that, "for adults *without* health insurance [emphasis in original], the evidence shows: … adults are more likely to be diagnosed with later-stage cancers that are detectable by screening or by contact with a clinician who can assess worrisome symptoms" (13). The IOM physician representative who testified before Congress on its most recent report on the uninsured, Dr. John Ayanian of Harvard Medical School, noted in his testimony that "Uninsured adults are 25 percent more likely to die prematurely than insured adults overall, and with serious conditions such as heart disease, diabetes or cancer, their risk of premature death can be 40 to 50 percent higher" (14).

Lack of insurance, of course, is not the *only* factor contributing to the delay of diagnosis and treatment in seriously ill patients, including head and neck cancer patients. There are what have been termed "patient delay" factors, including vague or nonurgent-appearing symptoms. There are also "professional delay" factors, attributable to clinicians initially evaluating head and neck malignancies, in diagnosis and/or referral. These delays have been identified for over two decades as a contributing factor in the advanced stage at which oral and oropharyngeal carcinomas are often diagnosed (15), for example.

THE SOLUTION(S)—WHAT OTHER RICH COUNTRIES DO

There are numerous different classification schema for comparing countries' medical systems. With his permission, I borrow a classification system published by the journalist and author T.R. Reid, a longtime correspondent for *The Washington Post*. He served as chief of the *Post's* Tokyo and London bureaus, and hence lived in those countries, and utilized their health systems, for extended periods of time. He recently spent over a year surveying other rich countries' health care systems, using his own stiff and painful shoulder as an entrée for a personal evaluation of these other systems. He also interviewed many physicians and policymakers, in many industrialized democracies.

He detailed his experiences and conclusions in a television documentary and a best-selling book. The documentary aired on the PBS program *Frontline*, entitled "Sick Around the World—Can the United States learn anything from the rest of the world about how to run a health care system?" (16). The countries' systems differ quite significantly, from one to the other, but they each provide universal coverage. One section of the program's website is entitled "Five Capitalist Democracies & How They Do It." His subsequent book is entitled *The Healing of Democracy: A Global Quest for Better, Cheaper, and Fairer Health Care* (17) and provides an entertaining and very readable introduction to comparative medical systems. Michael Moore's 2007 popular movie *Sicko* (18) also compared our system to other countries and includes numerous personal vignettes of American uninsured individuals.

Reid writes at length about his conversations with the Harvard economist William Hsiao, who has been involved in setting up health care systems in over a dozen countries. Hsiao (19) has coauthored a prominent textbook, *Getting Health Reform Right*, and his "team of health system analysts was commissioned by the Vermont Legislature to develop and evaluate three options for health system reform and determine which option would best achieve the stated goals" (20). His team "found that the system capable of producing the greatest potential savings and achieving universal coverage was a single-payer system." Hsiao was very involved in setting up Taiwan's relatively new single-payer system. Reid reports that his conversations with Hsiao focused on first principles:

> "Before you can set up a health care system for any country," Hsiao told me, "you have to know that country's basic ethical values. The first question is: Do people in your country have a right to health care? If the people believe that medical care is a basic right, you design a system that means anybody who is sick can see a doctor.

> If a society considers medical care to be an economic commodity, then you set up a system that distributes health care based on the ability to pay. And then the poor, pretty much, are left out" (17).

As Reid notes, "all the developed countries except the United States have decided that every human has a basic right to health care." He divides health care systems into four basic models:

- The "Beveridge" model (the United Kingdom, Spain, and others)
- The "Bismarck" model (Germany, Japan, Switzerland, and others)
- The National Health Insurance model (Canada, Taiwan, and others)
- The Out-of-Pocket model

While most wealthy democracies have adopted one of the first three models exclusively, our "system" in the United States comprises parts of all four of these models, including the last, which is neither "coverage" nor a "system."

One important distinction among medical systems is often initially difficult for some Americans, including many American physicians, to grasp, in part because of imprecise rhetorical attacks on "socialized" medicine: There is a significant difference between national health *insurance*, with doctors in private practice, and a national health *system*, with doctors sometimes employed by the government. Additionally, in a universal coverage approach with *insurance*, health insurance can be single-payer, or multi-payer. The United States has a hodgepodge of different approaches, but its multi-payer (usually for-profit) *insurance* system does *not* provide universal coverage and access.

Our Medicare program is single-payer national health *insurance* program for seniors. Medicare reimburses physicians in private (or academic) practice who care for these seniors. Medicare is a "third-party payer," separate from the patient (first party) and the provider (second party). Physicians compete against one another, in the marketplace, for these senior patients, although all physicians get paid by the same government *insurance* system. In contrast, the Veterans Administration (VA) is a pure national health *system*, where the physicians are *employed* directly by the government and receive a salary for providing care to patients in that system. VA physicians do not compete among one another for patients, for example.

THE "BEVERIDGE" MODEL

The United Kingdom and a number of other industrialized democracies have health care systems in which the government is the owner of hospitals and heavily involved in doctors' compensation. Patients do not pay for care at the point of service (doctors' offices or the hospital). General taxation provides the revenues to pay physicians' and other providers' salaries. In Britain, hospital-affiliated specialists, like surgeons, are government employees, while "general practitioners" (GPs) have their own businesses. T.R. Reid names this model after Lord William Beveridge, the aristocratic reformer who was one of the prime architects of Britain's National Health Service (NHS), which was conceived and implemented during World War II. As Reid notes, the system has "minimal paperwork and no billing." The NHS

> "cares for roughly one-fifth the population of the United States but spends only one-fifteenth of the U.S. health care bill. And yet the results are good: Britain has lower child mortality, longer healthy life spans, and better recovery rates from most major diseases than does the United States" (21).

Just as there are downsides to the lack of universal coverage in the United States, including avoidable deaths, the Beveridge model has downsides. The NHS limits medications and procedures which are covered, just as American private insurers do. Patients often have to wait for nonurgent, elective procedures. The NHS decides on these limits through an open, public process, via its National Institute for Health and Clinical Excellence, or NICE (22). Following NICE guidelines also insulates British physicians from malpractice suits. In the case of T.R. Reid's shoulder, for which an American orthopod had recommended a total arthroplasty, his GP told him that the NHS would most likely *not* pay for surgery, because he did not have a serious disability from the condition.

The NHS doesn't directly *employ* GPs in Britain, but it does provide their only source of payment. A doctor receives a capitation fee for each patient in her practice, whether the patient needs the doctor's care regularly or not. This incentivizes the doctor to provide preventative care, to reduce the number of patients with long-term sequelae from diabetes, hypertension, etc., for whom she must care. The more patients a doctor has in her practice, the higher her income. Reid notes that Britain has far more GPs than specialists, about 60%, because "the GPs in Britain generally make more money than the specialists—on average, about twice as much" (23).

THE "BISMARCK" MODEL

Before the latter part of the 19th century, "Germany" was a collection of separate principalities. Otto von Bismarck unified these fiefdoms into one empire. He also pushed Germany's parliament, the Reichstag, in 1883 to pass what is now termed "statutory health insurance (SHI)"(24). A detailed history of the evolution of the Bismarck model in Germany is available from The European Observatory on Health Systems and Policies. This institution is a collaboration of the WHO and many European governments and other institutions and publishes "health system profiles (HiTs)" on most countries in Europe and some

additional countries outside of Europe, as well (e.g., Australia, Israel).

In the German system, a fixed percentage of an employee's paycheck, about 15%, goes toward membership in one of many competing, but *nonprofit*, health insurance plans, termed "sickness funds" (*Krankenkassen*), which the employee chooses. Employers and employees divide this expense, and joining a sickness fund is mandatory, except for the highest earners. Unlike American insurers, though, the sickness funds must accept anyone and pay any legitimate claims by providers. Elected representatives of employers and employees control the sickness funds (25), and local hospitals and doctors' organizations negotiate reimbursement fees with the funds. The sickness funds compete against one another for patients. The wealthy can "opt out" and buy private coverage from for-profit companies, which about 7% of the population chooses to do (17). The government pays the employers' share for unemployed and retired enrollees.

In 1994, with a largely private for-profit health insurance system and rising numbers of uninsured, like the current US situation, Switzerland adopted a Bismarck-type system of private nonprofit health insurance plans. The plan was approved by national referendum and took effect in 1996. Reid also details his experiences in other Bismarck-type systems, in France and Japan.

THE NATIONAL HEALTH INSURANCE MODEL

A single-payer insurance system eliminates many unnecessary expenses. First of all, the insurance system does not have to generate profits, above and beyond providing care for enrollees. Because there is no reason to exclude sick patients, the system does not have to expend resources "cherry-picking" healthy individuals. Nor does the insurance system need to spend money on marketing. Physicians and other providers do not have to employ staff to sort through different payers, claims processes, denials of coverage for appropriate services, and other similar administrative headaches.

A study of the administrative costs of health care in the United States and Canada in fiscal 1999 found total administrative costs in the United States of $1,059 per capita, compared to $307 per capita in Canada. For practitioners (e.g., readers of this chapter), administrative costs were $324 per capita in the United States versus $107 in Canada. The authors note that "Canadian physicians send virtually all bills to a single insurer" (26).

Though both Canada and Taiwan have a single-payer system, there is a notable "policy" difference between them. When Taiwan adopted a single-payer system in 1994, one of its authors, Harvard economist William Hsiao, made sure that employee and employer contributions to fund the system were termed a health insurance "premium," rather than a "tax." Canada's single-payer system is funded through general taxation, although three provinces do charge premiums (27). Taiwan's program led to coverage for 11 million previously uninsured, and this led to a "sudden explosion of new suppliers," Hsiao notes in Reid's (28) book, with intense competition among providers, who are independent businesspeople.

WHAT WE DO—INCLUDING "OUT OF POCKET" FOR UNINSURED AND UNDERINSURED

In the United States, we have different "systems" for different classes of patients. If you are 65 or older (disabled or have end-stage renal disease), you are in a single-payer government-*financed* insurance system, and you can see your choice of any participating, competing private provider, through Medicare. If you are poor enough (criteria vary by state), you may qualify for government-financed Medicaid, though generally fewer private providers accept that third-party payer for their services, because of low reimbursement. If you are a veteran or Native American, you may qualify for a Beveridge-style government-*run* system, through the VA or the Indian Health Service.

If you have a job with good benefits, you may be able to choose from one of a number of competing Bismarck-style insurers—with the significant difference that the insurers are for-profit and hence financially interested in limiting their coverage of your claims. If, however, you are *not* poor enough to qualify for Medicaid, and your employer does *not* offer an affordable health insurance option, you will pay "out of pocket" for your health expenses. The out-of-pocket "model," or "self-pay," is of course predominant in poor countries without the resources to provide universal coverage, also.

RECENT AND ONGOING DEVELOPMENTS IN THE UNITED STATES—THE "PATIENT PROTECTION AND AFFORDABLE CARE ACT" (PPACA OR ACA) OF 2010 AND MEDICARE "REFORM"

In the spring of 2010, President Obama signed a massive new health care bill into law, attacked by critics as "Obamacare," and known more neutrally by its acronym PPACA or simply the "Affordable Care Act" (ACA). On the last day of its 2011–2012 term, a majority of the Supreme Court upheld the constitutionality of the ACA (29). The ruling is complex and incorporates several separate decisions, specifically about the mandate on individuals to purchase health insurance, and state Medicaid expansion.

The ACA's individual mandate, requiring most people and their dependents to have health insurance coverage,

begins in 2014. The ACA includes a range of acceptable plans ("silver level," etc.), varying by an individual's income, subsidized for individuals through tax credits, and a tax-like penalty for noncompliance. (More details are available at the Kaiser Family Fund[KFF] website and document cited in reference 29.) The KFF analysis notes that "almost 9 in 10 non-elderly people would either satisfy the mandate automatically because they already are insured or be exempt from it."

In February 2013, Florida Republican Governor Rick Scott, who had sued to block ACA on the day of its signing by the President (one of the lawsuits that led, in conjunction with other states' actions, to the Supreme Court case), reversed his opposition to expanding Medicaid in his state (30). Numerous other Republican Governors have taken similar steps in their states. In a contrasting state-level development, in the spring of 2011 the Governor of Vermont "signed a bill… that sets Vermont on a path to creating the nation's first publicly financed health care system." (31)

The Congressional Budget Office, as of February 2013, predicts that by 2023 ACA will result in insurance coverage for an additional 27 million currently uninsured Americans, who would not otherwise have had insurance (32). Unfortunately, it also predicts that 30 million other nonelderly people will continue to remain uninsured in 2023. Legislators continue to introduce bills for a single-payer, Medicare-for-all system (33).

Prominent specialist observers of our health care system, like Jonathan Oberlander (34), a political scientist on the faculty of the School of Medicine, at the University of North Carolina at Chapel Hill, note that "there is broad agreement that the United States must slow rising health care costs." But he notes also that

> …the predominance of fiscal issues also distorts health policy by producing "reforms" that are exercises in cost shifting, not cost saving. For example, raising Medicare's eligibility age would actually increase total health care spending while shifting federal costs to employers, private health insurance, and seniors…
>
> The United States needs systemwide cost control, not budget gimmicks (34).

Canada's road to a single-payer health insurance system began with passage in one province, Saskatchewan, and perhaps a similar evolution will occur in the United States. The state legislature of our largest state, California, passed single-payer legislation in 2006 and again in 2008, which Governor Schwarzenegger subsequently vetoed (35). The father of Canada's Medicare system, Tommy Douglas, was premier of Saskatchewan when he overcame a doctors' strike in 1962 to implement the plan there. Mr. Douglas (who coincidentally is actor Kiefer Sutherland's grandfather) was chosen as "The Greatest Canadian," in a 2004 nationwide poll conducted by the Canadian Broadcasting Corporation (36).

OBSTACLES TO UNIVERSAL COVERAGE IN THE UNITED STATES

Of course, the biggest obstacle to changing the current fragmented, inadequate health care system in the United States is the political power of the for-profit health insurance industry. Aside from the dependency of federally elected officials on private campaign contributions, the US Supreme Court has ruled in January 2010 that "No sufficient governmental interest justifies limits on the political speech of nonprofit or for-profit corporations" (37). The private insurers' trade group, "America's Health Insurance Plans" (AHIP) made up of companies "providing health benefits for over 200 million Americans," is essentially silent with respect to the issue of the uninsured (38).

Wendell Potter was the head of corporate communications at the multibillion dollar health insurance giant CIGNA, before becoming a whistle-blower about the industry's dumping of sick patients to boost profits. His book, *Deadly Spin: An Insurance Company Insider Speaks Out on How Corporate PR is Killing Health Care and Deceiving Americans* (39), details the mechanics and tactics of AHIP in Washington. He testified before House and Senate committees in the run-up to the passage of ACA. He notes in his book that he warned legislators that if

> ...the so-called solutions insurers were "bringing to the table"... did not include a public insurance option to

compete with private insurers, it might as well be called the "Health Insurance Industry Profit Protection and Enhancement Act."

Although he somewhat reluctantly supports the law, given that some of the millions of uninsured patients will get coverage, he notes that

> ...insurers will get billions of dollars in new revenues from people required by law to buy their products and billions more from the government to subsidize premiums for people who can't afford them (40).

His book is a detailed primer on how the insurance industry has used vast public relations (PR) efforts, like the focus-group tested phrase, "government takeover," successfully, in "every campaign the industry has conducted in recent decades to defeat reform efforts" (41). In his ongoing on-line coverage, he notes how the health insurance industry pursues "clear obscurity" to obfuscate the waste and expense of our for-profit, private system (42).

PHYSICIAN SUPPORT FOR NATIONAL HEALTH INSURANCE IN THE UNITED STATES

In a recent survey of over 2,000 US physicians, a majority support national health insurance (43). Only 42% support the federal government as the sole payer, in

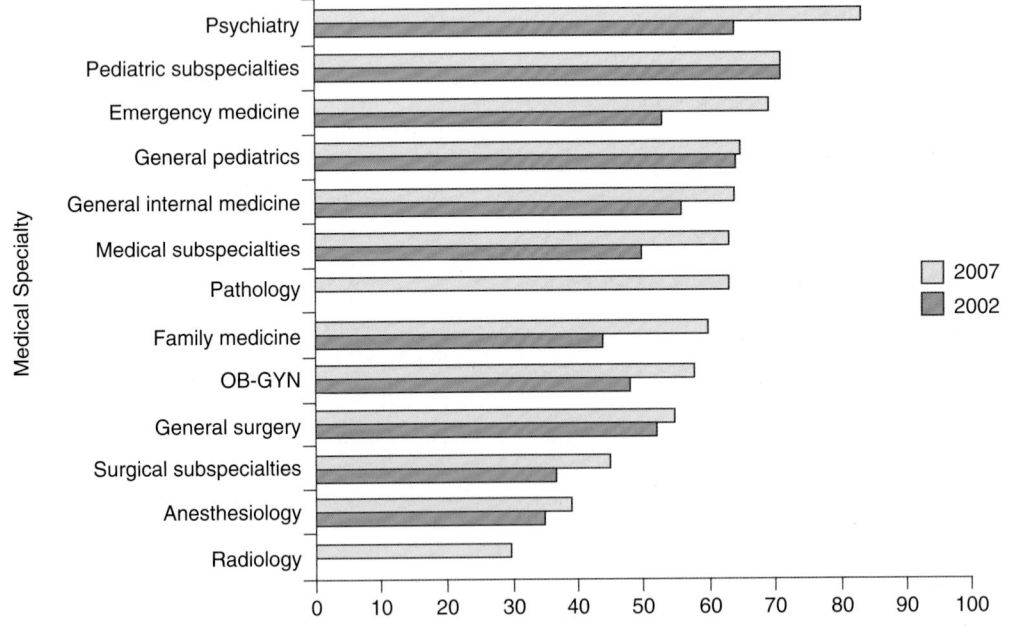

Support for government legislation to establish National Health Insurance in 2007 and 2002, by specialty

2002 data are not available for pathology and radiology because of lack of response in those categories. OB-GYN = obstetrics and gynecology.

From Carroll AE, Ackerman RT. Support for national health insurance among U.S. physicians: 5 years later. *Ann Intern Med* 2008;148(7):566.

another survey of over 1,500 physicians from 2009, however (44). The authors of the first survey note that "more than one half of the respondents from every medical specialty supported national health insurance legislation, with the exception of respondents in surgical subspecialties, anesthesiologists, and radiologists." With respect to physician satisfaction in countries that do have universal coverage, T.R. Reid (17) notes in his medical travels that "almost every doctor in almost every country…complains that he isn't paid enough for his hard work."

ALL HEALTH CARE SYSTEMS "RATION" CARE

All medical care exists in a framework of virtually unlimited demand from patients, constrained by a limited supply by providers and institutions. Any such phenomenon requires "rationing," though countries use different methods to distribute this limited resource. In the United States, we ration by economic status: If you have a good job with benefits, or fall into one of the patchwork government systems, you have coverage. A former British health minister, John Reid, describes rationing in the UK's Beveridge system with the phrase, "We cover everybody, but we don't cover everything" (45). Canada has waiting lists for many elective surgeries, but has better overall health outcomes than the United States. No other country, though, arranges its health system to provide a profit to investors and disproportionate salaries to insurance company executives, and squeezes patients to generate those funds, as we do.

The prominent health care economist Uwe Reinhardt (46), Professor of Political Economy at Princeton, notes that "The price system constitutes just one of many ways to ration scarce resources." He details one vignette of price rationing, which leads to many physicians not treating patients on Medicaid:

> Consider the legislators of my home state, New Jersey, who apparently think nothing of limiting compensation to a pediatrician to $30 for a Medicaid office visit, while bestowing upon themselves insurance that pays that same pediatrician $90 or more for treating their children.

He later notes that

> It is not clear to me on what ethical or scientific basis one could judge this (US) approach to rationing health care to be more "efficient" than rationing by queue….
>
> As already suggested, few Canadians would consider it ethically acceptable to pay a pediatrician much less for treating a poor child than for treating a rich child (46).

I urge readers, particularly residents, to become more than lay people, when it comes to the system by which you will make your living.

HIGHLIGHTS

- The United States is the only industrialized democracy without a system of universal health care.
- The United States spends far more per capita on health care than other rich countries, with worse health outcomes—for example, higher infant mortality and shorter average life expectancy. This results in large part from far higher administrative costs, generated by private, for-profit health insurance.
- Lack of health insurance in the United States leads to avoidable deaths and advanced disease at presentation. For example, laryngeal and oropharyngeal tumor stage is more likely to be advanced at time of diagnosis, in patients without health insurance.
- Other industrialized democracies have a variety of universal health care systems, including the "Beveridge" model of a National Health Service (e.g., the NHS in the United Kingdom), the "Bismarck" model of nonprofit cooperative insurance funds with physicians in private practice (e.g., Germany), and single-payer National Health Insurance (e.g., Canada's Medicare system), also with physicians in private practice.
- The United States has different systems for different populations: National Health Insurance for seniors (our Medicare), a Beveridge system for veterans and Native Americans (the VA and Indian Health Service), for-profit private insurance for some employees, and "self-pay" (no insurance) for many other individuals.
- The United States is the only industrialized democracy with a predominantly private, for-profit insurance industry. These companies must generate a return for stockholders and high salaries for executives, leading to necessary rationing of patient care on the basis of expanding company profit.
- The ACA of 2010 will insure tens of millions of currently uninsured Americans, but will still leave tens of millions of others uninsured.
- The primary obstacle to universal coverage is the stranglehold on reform exercised by the for-profit private insurance industry, through deceptive public relations strategies, multimillion-dollar lobbying campaigns, and privately financed elections of Congress.

REFERENCES

1. Wilper AP, Woolhandler S, Lasser KE, et al. Health insurance and mortality in US adults. *Am J Public Health* 2009;99:2289–2295.
2. "Income, poverty and health insurance coverage in the United States. 2010," press release dated September 13, 2011, available at: http://www.census.gov/newsroom/releases/archives/income_wealth/cb11-157.html; accessed October 5, 2011.

3. "New health insurance survey: 9 million adults joined ranks of uninsured due to job loss in 2010; few viable health insurance options exist for unemployed," press release dated March 16, 2011, The Commonwealth Fund, available at: http://www.commonwealthfund.org/Content/Surveys/2011/Mar/2010-Biennial-Health-Insurance-Survey.aspx; accessed May 22, 2011.

4. "OECD Health Data 2011—How Does the United States Compare," http://www.oecd.org/dataoecd/46/2/38980580.pdf, accessed October 5, 2011.

5. Woolhandler S, Himmelstein DU. Paying for national health insurance—and not getting it. *Health Aff* 2002:88–98. Available at: http://www.pnhp.org/publications/payingnotgetting.pdf, accessed October 5, 2011.

6. "OECD Health Data 2011—How Does Canada Compare," available at: http://www.oecd.org/dataoecd/46/33/38979719.pdf, accessed October 5, 2011.

7. "OECD Health Data 2011—How Does the United States Compare."

8. Nolte E, McKee CM. Measuring the health of nations: updating an earlier analysis. *Health Aff* 2008;(1):58–71.

9. "OECD Health Data 2011—How Does the United States Compare," accessed October 5, 2011.

10. Chen AY, Schrag NM, Halpern M, et al. Health insurance and state at diagnosis of laryngeal cancer: does insurance type predict stage at diagnosis? *Arch Otolaryngol Head Neck Surg* 2007;133(8):784–790.

11. Chen AY, Schrag NM, Halpern M, et al. The impact of health insurance status on stage at diagnosis of oropharyngeal cancer. *Cancer* 2007;110(2):395–402.

12. Shuman AG, Entezami P, Chernin AS, et al. Demographics and efficacy of head and neck cancer screening. *Otolaryngol Head Neck Surg* 2010;143(3):353–360.

13. "America's uninsured crisis: Consequences for health and health care—report brief," February 2009. Available online at www.iom.edu/americasuninsuredcrisis.

14. "America's uninsured crisis: Congressional testimony," March 11, 2009, available at IoM website.

15. Guggenheimer J, Verbin RS, Johnson JT, et al. Factors delaying the diagnosis of oral and oropharyngeal carcinomas. *Cancer* 1989;64:932–935 [full text available on-line].

16. Full program available online at http://www.pbs.org/wgbh/pages/frontline/sickaroundtheworld/.

17. Reid TR. *The healing of America*. New York: Penguin Books, 2009 & 2010, 215, 76–77, 140.

18. http://sickothemovie.com/index.html, Accessed on May 22, 2011.

19. Roberts M, Hsiao W, Berman P, et al. *Getting health reform right*. Oxford: Oxford University Press, 2008.

20. Hsiao WC. State-based single payer health care—a solution for the United States? *N Engl J Med* 2011;364:1188–1190.

21. Reid TR. *The healing of America*. New York: Penguin Books, 2009 & 2010:105.

22. http://www.nice.org.uk/.

23. http://www.nice.org.uk/.123.

24. Busse R, Riesberg A. "Health systems in transition: Germany," 2004, published by the European Observatory on Health Systems and Policies, available online at http://www.euro.who.int/__data/assets/pdf_file/0018/80703/E85472.pdf

25. Busse R, Riesberg A. "Health systems in transition: Germany," 2004, published by the European Observatory on Health Systems and Policies, p. 35; available online at http://www.euro.who.int/__data/assets/pdf_file/0018/80703/E85472.pdf.

26. Woolhandler S, Campbell T, Himmelstein DU. Costs of health care administration in the United States and Canada. *N Engl J Med* 2003;349:768–775.

27. "Canada's Health Care System," Health Canada/Santé Canada, C. 2005, accessible via http://www.hc-sc.gc.ca/hcs-sss/alt_formats/hpb-dgps/pdf/pubs/2005-hcs-sss/2005-hcs-sss-eng.pdf, p. 5; accessed May 22, 2011.

28. Reid TR. *The healing of America*. New York: Penguin Books, 2009 & 2010. pp. 172–173.

29. A thorough and readable review of the court's decision is available at The Kaiser Family Fund's site, at http://www.kff.org/healthreform/upload/8332.pdf; accessed on April 1, 2013.

30. See for example, http://www.nytimes.com/2013/02/21/us/in-reversal-florida-says-it-will-expand-medicaid-program.html?_r=0; accessed on April 1, 2013.

31. http://www.nytimes.com/2011/05/27/us/27brfs-Vermont.html?scp=1&sq=Vermont%20health&st=cse

32. "CBO's February 2013 Estimate of the Effects of the Affordable Care Act on Health Insurance Coverage," http://www.cbo.gov/sites/default/files/cbofiles/attachments/43900_ACAInsuranceCoverageEffects.pdf, accessed on April 1, 2013.

33. H.R. 676, "Expanded and Improved Medicare for All Act," Rep. John Conyers' (D-MI), 41 cosponsors as of April 1, 2013; accessed via http://thomas.loc.gov/; also http://conyers.house.gov/index.cfm/healthcare.

34. Oberlander J. "Health care policy in an age of austerity." *N Engl J Med* 2011;365:12; accessible for free online at http://www.nejm.org/doi/pdf/10.1056/NEJMp1109352.

35. see, for example, http://www.scrippsnews.com/node/12361.

36. video clip at http://archives.cbc.ca/politics/parties_leaders/clips/11120/.

37. *Citizens United v. Federal Election Commission*, Supreme Court opinion, January 21, 2010, p. 50, accessed via http://www.supremecourt.gov/opinions/09pdf/08-205.pdf on May 22, 2011.

38. A search on the organization's website using the term "uninsured," on May 22, 2011, found 127 documents, but no document published after the passage of ACA appeared to address this topic with any proposal for coverage; http://www.ahip.org/.

39. Potter W. *Deadly Spin*, New York: Bloomsbury Press, C. 2010.

40. Potter W. *Deadly Spin*, New York: Bloomsbury Press, C. 2010:6–7.

41. Potter W. *Deadly Spin*, New York: Bloomsbury Press, C. 2010:39.

42. http://wendellpotter.com/2011/05/the-clear-obscurity-of-the-health-insurance-industry/.

43. Carroll AE, Ackermann RT. Support for national health insurance among U.S. physicians: 5 years later. *Ann Intern Med* 2008;148:566.

44. McCormick D, Woolhandler S, Bose-Kolanu A. et al. U.S. physicians' views on financing options to expand health insurance coverage: a national survey. *J Gen Intern Med* 2009;24(4):526–531.

45. Reid TR. *The healing of America*. New York: Penguin Books, 2009 & 2010:224.

46. Reinhardt UE. "Keeping Health Care Afloat," The Milken Institute Review, Sec. Quar. 2007, pp. 36-43. http://www.princeton.edu/~reinhard/pdfs/MILKEN%20REVIEW%20CANADA%20vs%20US.pdf.

Effective Education in Medical Practice

203

John M. Schweinfurth

Graduation from a residency training program and entry into surgical practice represents an abrupt and often permanent change in learning styles. Professors are fond of telling the graduate, "This is just the beginning of your education, not the end." The divide is dramatic. Nothing in didactic form approaches the learning experience of the real world, where there is no textbook, no lesson plan, and no instructor to fall back on. Indeed, many early decisions are based on the teacher's transplanted wisdom. Often the transition is abrupt; the educational process up to graduation is based on a teacher-directed model of learning for which there is no direct continuity in practice. Currently, there are multiple, instructor-led resources for long-term learning including opportunities for continuing medical education (CME) from annual national and regional professional meetings, home study courses, audio digests, and online reviews.

This chapter, however, is not about formal, teacher-directed learning activities such as lectures and CME. The reality is that instructor-led CME activity, while valuable, represents not only an artificial learning environment but a relatively ineffective one at that (1). Active engagement in self-planned learning activities tends to be more effective than the passive learning, which commonly characterizes formal CME. The vast majority of postgraduate, or lifetime, learning is problem specific and occurs in the context of real experience: the clinic, on an Internet search engine at night, or over the phone with a colleague; those conversations that invariably begin, "I have this patient...."

Lifetime learning involves finding and implementing solutions to everyday problems encountered in the clinic, in the emergency room, in the operating room, and on the wards. The process by which much of this education occurs is via *self-directed learning* (SDL). According to Gibbons, a paradigm shift in instruction is "teaching students to challenge themselves to pursue activities that arise from their own experiences, employing their own emerging styles to find patterns of meaning and processes of productivity that lead them to a high level of achievement and fulfillment. The prime imperative... is not to enhance teacher-directed learning, but to develop a more student-directed model" (2).

WHAT IS SELF-DIRECTED LEARNING?

Initially described by Malcolm Knowles, in its broadest meaning "self-directed learning" is a process

"... in which individuals take the initiative... in diagnosing their learning needs, formulating learning goals, identifying human and material resources for learning, choosing and implementing appropriate learning strategies, and evaluating learning outcomes" (3).

Knowles argues that proactive learners learn more things better than do passive, or "reactive," learners. They enter into learning purposefully with greater motivation and better long-term retention. Finally, because of rapid changes in our understanding of the world, it is no longer realistic to define education as the transmission of static knowledge but to develop instead skills of inquiry.

Hammond and Collins (4) describe SDL as "a process in which learners take the initiative, with the support and collaboration of others. For increasing self- and social awareness; critically analyzing and reflecting on their situations; diagnosing their learning needs with specific reference to competencies they have helped identify; formulating socially and personally relevant learning goals; identifying human and material resources for learning; choosing and implementing appropriate learning strategies; and reflecting on and evaluating their learning." This humanistic characterization of SDL implies a sense of social awareness, self-actualization, and the acceptance of personal responsibility for one's own learning.

TABLE 203.1	SKILLS AND COMPETENCIES OF THE LIFELONG LEARNER

The lifelong learner would:
- Be methodical and disciplined
- Be logical and analytical
- Be reflective and self-aware
- Demonstrate curiosity, openness, and motivation
- Be flexible
- Be interdependent and interpersonally competent
- Be persistent and responsible
- Be venturesome and creative
- Show confidence and have a positive self-concept
- Be independent and self-sufficient
- Have developed information-seeking and retrieval skills
- Have developed knowledge about, and skill at, learning generally
- Develop and use defensible criteria for evaluating learning

The acquisition of SDL is a complex process, involving numerous skills and competencies relied upon to complete challenges such as medical school and residency. Unlike the classroom setting, where the emphasis is on mastery of content, SDL emphasizes *personal* action taken to become more productive. Testing is no longer an issue, but performance certainly is. Many authors have identified SDL as essential to continuing education efforts in adults (5,6).

Not everyone is ready to accomplish SDL, however; this is because certain traits are essential for becoming a successful, productive individual. Candy (7) synthesized an essential character list from over 100 such traits (Table 203.1).

Barrows called for the application of SDL in medical education because "the curricula of many medical schools put too heavy an emphasis on memorization of facts and little stress on problem solving or self-directed study skills necessary for the practice of medicine. Problem-based SDL is a teaching–learning method specifically designed to emphasize these skills and to increase the retention of facts and their recall in the clinical situation" (8). Generally, SDL is not limited to specific settings but can occur as a part of any process and include formal learning activities as well. Among Tough's factors are three common patterns in independent study: a specified learning need, curiosity, and a general desire to learn (9). Houle (10) described three groups of adult learners: goal oriented, activity oriented, and learning oriented based on their immediate educational needs, not necessarily on individual learning styles. Of these, most practicing physicians clearly fall into the first category, as they embark on a learning project to acquire new procedural skills, to become familiar with new medications, or updates in coding and reimbursement schedules, for example. Activity-oriented learners participate for social interaction and learning-oriented for the sake of knowledge itself.

THE CHALLENGE MODEL OF SELF-DIRECTED LEARNING

Possibly the most influential essay on SDL is *The Walkabout* by Maurice Gibbons published in the 1974 edition of the Phi Delta Kappan. At the heart of the essay is the movie of two children lost in the desert wilderness of the Australian outback. Facing certain death, the two are found and cared for by a young aborigine on his walkabout, a 6-month long endurance test during which he must survive alone in the wilderness and return to his tribe an adult. Gibbons surveys the ramifications of the story from a societal standpoint:

"The movie is a haunting comment on education. What I find most provocative is the stark contrast between the aborigine's walkabout experience and the test of adolescent's readiness for adulthood in our own society. The young native faces a severe but extremely appropriate trial, one in which he must demonstrate the knowledge and skills necessary to make him a contributor to the tribe rather than a drain on its meager resources. By contrast, the young North American is faced with written examinations that test skills very far removed from the actual experience he will have in real life. He solves familiar theoretical problems; he does not apply what he knows in strange but real situations…. His preparation is primarily for the mastery of content and skills in the disciplines and has little to do with reaching maturity, achieving adulthood, or developing fully as a person."

The walkabout model is quite applicable to the learning required by the practicing physician. First of all, it should be experiential and the experience should be "hands-on." Second, it should be a challenge that extends the capacities of the learner. Third, it should be a challenge specific to or, better, designed by the learner. A productive learning experience depends on the learner's ability to make appropriate choices, but in most teacher-directed situations the student is not called upon to make any meaningful choices. "The test of the walkabout, and of life, is not what (the learner) can do under a teacher's direction, but what the teacher has enabled him to decide and to do on his own" (Gibbons, 1974). Most importantly, the trial should be an important learning experience in itself and should involve not only the demonstration of the student's knowledge and skill but also his or her self-awareness, flexibility, and nature as a person.

THE "CHANGE" MODEL

Fox et al. (11) developed a model of learning and change based on 700 incidents in over 300 physicians. The authors found that the most common forces for change were professional: a general desire for competence or the perception of a changing clinical environment. Once a need for change is identified, the physician develops an image of how the practice would appear following the change.

Information is gathered to help analyze the gap between existing skills and those necessary to complete the change. It is the process of analyzing and describing the gap that provides the jumping-off point for planning, development, implementation, and assessing learning activities. The process of change involves three stages: preparing to change, making the change, and sustaining the change (12).

LEARNING THROUGH EXPERIENCE

The process of learning through experience has been described in Kolb's (13) experiential learning cycle.

1. *Concrete experience*: In the first stage, a physician may encounter an unexpected situation that differs from expected practice, for example, a complaint of hoarseness with a normal-appearing larynx.
2. *Reflective observation*: Following the encounter, the physician reflects on the experience, performs an Internet search, consults with a colleague, or perhaps takes no further action.
3. *Abstract conceptualization*: The physician combines the results of reflection with any new knowledge gained to conceive of a possible new approach, which would theoretically encompass the problem, in this case a neurologic disorder such as spasmodic dysphonia or vocal scarring.
4. *Active experimentation*: A new approach may be taken. In the present example, a videostroboscopy might be performed or a new diagnosis considered and tested. The experience with the new approach, for example, findings on videostroboscopy, immediately lead to a new concrete experience and the cycle begins anew.

Kolb's cycle provides an excellent model for conceptualizing the learning process a practitioner might undergo as a result of clinical challenges encountered on a regular basis. There is an abundance of adult learning research that supports the role of experience and reflection in continuing education (14–18). In reality, the process is likely to be more dynamic, complex, and interrupted with fits and starts, dead ends, misinterpreted experiences, and incorrect conclusions. An awareness of the process will assist the learner and educator in designing and promoting educational experiences, which allow for each stage to occur and mature.

PROMOTING SELF-DIRECTED LEARNING

Although an internal motivation for learning is more powerful and enduring than external forces, near-term goals such as recertification and renewal of medical licenses and hospital privileges will be the order of the day when time is limited, as is always the case. Factors that may both facilitate and combine these processes will ultimately be more productive and satisfying to the learners and to professional boards and licensing bodies. Specialty literature, national and regional conferences, and other CME activities may help learners identify gaps between needed skills and current capabilities as well as help learners to visualize an image of change to see how it might look to do something differently.

Computerized learning modules and portfolio projects may potentially bridge these knowledge gaps. Similar to a teacher-directed learning experience, computer modules may serve to drive Kolb's learning cycle by providing prompts and asking questions that require reflection or application of new knowledge. Online searches offer access to very specific sources of knowledge not readily available in texts. Portfolio projects can serve to document the SDL process, both for refinement and potentially for CME credit or recertification. A portfolio is a purposeful collection of work that chronicles learning needs, goals, efforts, progress, and achievements. These can take the shape of a collection of loose papers or a sophisticated interactive computer-based module. Presented to a professional or licensing board, they represent the comprehensive learning efforts of the individual as opposed to strict learning outcomes as obtained through exams. Portfolios, consequently, provide both instruction and assessment simultaneously. Unlike standardized tests, portfolios are as unique as their creators and can be used to discover the needs of individual learners and their evolution over time, as opposed to legislating knowledge from a central authority.

Identifying Needs

Once a strong professional identity has formed, usually after the first year of training, resident learning may be described in a manner similar to that of practicing physicians by the "change model" of Fox et al. (11). In interviews with over 300 practicing physicians, the authors found that the desire to learn and change can come from professional, personal, and social reasons. In their experience, the most common reasons for change included a desire for general competence or the recognition of a changing practice environment (such as competition, improved patient self-education, and access to the Internet). Physicians respond to areas of deficient knowledge by referring complex patients, discussions with colleagues, and consultation of the literature (14). These behaviors are typically stimulated by perceived deficiencies from caring for a particular patient, discussion, or reading. However, these deficiencies are often subjective and may not accurately reflect actual needs. Objective needs assessment is therefore needed in order to provide a more realistic image of knowledge gaps. Systematic assessments, such as performance audits and outcomes measures; patient care benchmarks; billing; and documentation audits are examples of measures that provide objective measures. Other examples include independently reviewed portfolio projects and written or computerized tests and problem-based scenarios. Regardless of the assessment strategy used, it is important to allow the physician to develop a self-monitoring strategy rather than to merely respond to external events.

Computerized Self-directed Learning Modules

Adult learning theory, including Kolb's cycle and the principles of SDL, depends on the developments of practical tools that help individuals take charge of their learning and apply the theory to their own practice. As the personal computer and the Internet have enjoyed growing widespread use among physicians as an essential resource, the potential for their application in CME has also expanded. Although the full potential of computerized SDL has not yet been reached, several models are available in fields other than otolaryngology, which serve as examples of potential structured programs.

The Maintenance of Competence (MOCOMP) program is designed to encourage specialists to take charge of their own CME efforts (19). The program has three components: (a) a credit system to promote production of high-quality, practice-based, educational programs; (b) a self-directed CME plan designed to motivate individual specialists to record and critically appraise their CME activities; and (c) an annual, personalized CME profile. There are many ways that physicians obtain information, that is, reading, consultations, rounds, research, etc., but these activities are too numerous to record on a regular basis and rarely lead to a change in practice. This information screening is defined as "General Professional Activity" in the revised MOCOMP program and consists of scanning the professional environment for new ideas. Occasionally information does capture the interest of the specialist who might then explore the area in more detail, known as "In-Depth Review." These activities are focused and goal oriented and should lead to one of the following outcomes after completion (20):

1. I will modify my practice.
2. I will wait for further information before I modify my practice.
3. I see no need to modify my practice.

The Computerized Evaluative Learning Tool (CELT) is based on the adult learning principles that learning should acknowledge prior experience, allow reflection, be participative, provide ownership, and be self-directed (21). The users enter data under four menus depending on whether they have a specific learning need, wish to apply new knowledge, or learn from an event to reduce future risk and/or to analyze and learn from the emotions the event caused. The four menus are as follows:

1. *Educational need*: The user starts with a learning need and the program takes them through meeting the need and then applying the learning in practice.
2. *Educational event*: The user recollects a specific learning point and is guided to apply it in practice.

3. *Emotional response*: This allows learning from an emotional experience to take place and enables a change in future behavior.
4. *Significant event analysis*: This allows learning to take place following a significant event in the workplace and enables the user to make changes to minimize the risk of a subsequent event.

CELT provides a learning structure to enable physicians to recognize and document that learning has taken place, to be specific about what has been learned through reflection, and then, if appropriate, to act on the learning and apply it in practice.

Portfolio Projects as a Model for Future Recertification

The computer models described above provide not only a framework for SDL but documentation of the process, which becomes an individual portfolio. Indeed, this process and the accompanying documentation could potentially be used not only for CME credits but for recertification itself as discussed previously. The Royal College of Physicians and Surgeons of Canada and several of the specialty societies, including the Canadian Anesthetists' Society, have developed the MOCOMP project as part of the recertification process. The philosophy of MOCOMP is to develop a comprehensive CME strategy, which will motivate specialists to continuously update their clinical practice.

Whether through the use of a software-based SDL computer module or simply documentation on the computer, the use of portfolio projects as part of the recertification process benefits physicians in several ways. First, it encourages and formalizes the process of SDL. It is likely that the documentation will encourage both an increase in quality of the process and product as well as the learning experience. Second, it encourages familiarity and therefore skill with the process so that each time SDL is initiated with less reservation. Finally, and most importantly, the physician can be rewarded with specialty CME hours or potentially with partial recertification credit depending on acceptance from accreditation bodies.

INTRODUCTION OF SDL IN THE UNDERGRADUATE CURRICULUM

The origins of Kolb's work may be traced back to a famous dictum of Confucius circa 450 BC: "Tell me, and I will forget. Show me, and I may remember. Involve me, and I will understand." As discussed at the beginning of the chapter, the transition from teacher-led to learner-directed activity is unnecessarily abrupt. Given the rapid changes in medical knowledge and practice, the need to keep abreast of the field is the one constant. But are graduates really ready for SDL? Seemingly not, as residency prepares them for learning passively from lectures and actively only from studying textbooks, board preparation materials, and journals. These activities are directed toward mastery of a body of knowledge. As described previously, real-world learning is typically problem based, not comprehensive. So, it seems intuitive that incorporation of problem-based learning in residency is more preparatory for SDL than simply memorizing a body of knowledge.

The goals of teaching as described by Isaacs (22) are (a) to arouse and keep students' interest, (b) to give facts and details, (c) to make students think critically about the subject, and (d) to prepare students for independent studies by demonstration of problem solving and professional reasoning. Isaacs notes, however, that only two of these purposes are well suited to didactic lectures. The problem then is how to organize lecture material so that individual student's learning needs are better addressed. Gibbs (23) suggests that lecture sessions contain a variety of activities designed to stimulate individual students to think including small group discussion, working problems during lecture time, questions included in the lecture, and quizzes at the end of lecture, among others. Possibilities considered include standard interactive lecturing, facilitated discussion, brainstorming, small group activities, problem solving, competitive large group exercises, and the use of illustrative cliff hanger and incident cases. Kell and Van Deursen (24) identified a preference toward teacher-directed learning in average age learners and student-directed in mature learners. The differences in learning preference persisted 6 months after graduation. The results suggest that mature students enter the course with skills that equip them to be more flexible in their learning, less dependent on instructor direction, and more self-reliant. Although further research is needed to identify which life skills are practiced by mature students and those that would promote SDL if encouraged in younger students, activities that promote involvement and active learning would be expected to promote SDL in later life (25).

CONCLUSION

This chapter is intended as a primer and not a comprehensive discourse on SDL and its application in CME. It is every teacher's responsibility to realize the impact of their teaching on their learners so that the learners' natural tendency for self-direction, displayed in their personal lives, can be transferred to their educational and working environments (26). Similarly, national specialty boards and associations, licensing boards, and governing bodies should recognize the importance of continuous SDL motivated by an internal desire to improve rather than as merely a reaction to external mandates.

REFERENCES

1. Wentz DK. Continuous medical education at a crossroads. *JAMA* 1990;264:2425–2426.
2. Gibbons M. Pardon me, didn't I just hear a paradigm shift? *Phi Delta Kappa* 2004;85(6):461–467.
3. Knowles MS. *Self-directed learning. A guide for learners and teachers.* Englewood Cliffs, NJ: Prentice Hall/Cambridge, 1975:135.
4. Hammond M, Collins R. *SDL: critical practice.* New York: Nichols/GP Publishing, 1991.
5. Fox RD, Bennett NL. Continuing medical education: learning and change: implications for continuing medical education. *BMJ* 1998;316:466–468.
6. Towle A. Continuing medical education: changes in health care and continuing medical education for the 21st century. *BMJ* 1998;316:301–304.
7. Candy PC. *Self-direction in life-long learning.* San Francisco, CA: Jossey-Bass Publishers, 1991.
8. Barrows HS. Problem-based, self-directed learning. *JAMA* 1983;250(22):3077–3080.
9. Tough A. *Why adults learn: a study of the major reasons for beginning and continuing a learning project. Monographs in adult education,* vol 3. Toronto, ON: Ontario Institute for Studies in Education, 1968.
10. Houle CO. *The inquiring mind.* Madison, WI: University of Wisconsin Press, 1961.
11. Fox RD, Mazmanian PE, Putnam RW. *Changing and learning in the lives of physicians.* New York: Praeger Publishers, 1989.
12. Putnam RW, Campbell MC. Competence. In: Fox RD, Mazmanian PE, Putnam RW, eds. *Changing and learning in the lives of physicians.* New York: Praeger Publishers, 1989.
13. Kolb DA. *Experiential learning: experience as a source of learning and development.* Englewood Cliffs, NJ: Prentice-Hall, 1984.
14. Slotnick HB. How doctors learn: the role of clinical problems across the medical school-to-practice continuum. *Acad Med* 1996;71(1):28–34.
15. Smith F, Singleton A, Hilton S. General practitioners' continuing education: a review of policies, strategies and effectiveness, and their implications for the future. *Br J Gen Pract* 1998;48(435):1689–1695.
16. Boud D, Keogh R, Walker D, eds. *Reflection: turning experience into learning.* London, UK: Kogan Page, 1985.
17. Brigley S, Young Y, Littlejohns P, et al. Continuing education for medical professionals: a reflective model. *Postgrad Med J* 1997;73(855):23–26.
18. Sobral DT. An appraisal of medical students' reflection-in-learning. *Med Educ* 2000;34(3):182–187.
19. Parboosingh J. Learning portfolios: potential to assist health professionals with self-directed learning. *J Contin Educ Health Prof* 1996;16:75–81.
20. Clark AJ, Doig GA. The maintenance of competence programme (MOCOMP). *Can J Anaesth* 1993;40(6):477–479.
21. Kelly DR, MacKay L. CELT: a computerised evaluative learning tool for continuing professional development. *Med Educ* 2003;37:358–367.
22. Isaacs G. Lecturing practices and note-taking purposes. *Studies in Higher Education* 1994;19(2):203–217.
23. Gibbs G. *Lecturing to more students.* Oxford, UK: Polytechnics and Colleges Funding Council, 1992.
24. Kell C, Van Deursen R. The fight against professional obsolescence should begin in the undergraduate curriculum. *Med Teach* 2000;22(2):160–163.
25. Schweinfurth JM. Interactive instruction in otolaryngology resident education. *Otolaryngol Clin North Am* 2007;40(6):1203–1214.
26. Turner P, Whitfield T. Physiotherapists' use of evidence based practice: a cross-national study. *Physiother Res Int* 1997;2(1):17–29.

204 Medical Informatics and Databases

John C. Sok   *Richard K. McHugh*

Our ability to obtain medical information has increased exponentially with public access to the Internet (1). As more hospitals and health care systems transition to the use of electronic health records (EHRs), the potential for machine-searchable clinical data significantly increases. EHRs store various forms of data including clinical diagnosis, drug prescriptions, treatment interventions, testing, and other associated medical records. We have more clinical data available to us now than at any other time in history, and the volume only continues to increase. This chapter describes the emerging field of medical informatics in otolaryngology and serves as an introduction to data mining and searchable clinical databases.

Collections of clinical data comprise various forms of databases. Smaller studies are amenable to researcher-performed manual searches through primary data. However, given the increasing volume and complexity of the data, medical informatics will become even more essential when performing clinical studies. Data mining of clinical databases also has the potential to find associations that would not otherwise be uncovered by traditional manual search and analyses. Furthermore, genomics and other translational forms of data are adding more complexity to clinical databases. This volume and variety of data is likely to continue to increase and become more complex as we shift from analysis of static targets (e.g., DNA, RNA, protein sequences) to dynamic targets (e.g., transcription, expression, metabolism, and genomics). Although daunting, such data present us with unparalleled opportunities. The medical informatics required to perform successful analyses of large clinical databases entails the combination of biostatistics and computational biology, among many other disciplines. Here we provide a framework to understand and apply medical informatics to clinical and translational studies in otolaryngology.

INTRODUCTION TO CLINICAL DATABASES

A database represents any organized collection of information, usually in digital form. There are several types of databases utilized in clinical medicine as reviewed by Harrison and Aller in 2008 (2). Larger regional and national data may be obtained from insurance or care provider claims data, single or cooperative provider repositories, or public health and government databases. Unfortunately, insurance databases and most government databases are not designed to record complete clinical records. Furthermore, such databases may be greatly impacted by selection, analysis, and interpretation biases (3). For instance, billing codes may be used to identify a study group. However, such codes may have been submitted as "rule out" diagnoses and may not represent the actual diagnosis. Moreover, the choice of codes utilized may be influenced by financial incentives. Further, only billed interventions may be listed such that the study lacks a complete clinical record of observations due to nonbillable interventions being excluded. Therefore, databases comprised of insurance claims data or similarly compiled data may be used to draw broad population-based associations but are not suitable for higher complexity clinical questions.

An individual clinician or clinical service often creates clinical databases composed of a series of patients with a common disease process, symptom, or treatment paradigm. Although this type of data is more precise and prone to fewer selection errors than insurance claims data, the population study size and size of the geographic area are generally small. The creation of such databases is usually under the auspices of a single Institutional Review Board (IRB) approval and designed to study a focused set of questions. These databases are usually small enough to facilitate manual analyses performed by one or more researchers.

Unfortunately, databases created in this format are not broadly applicable to other clinical data mining queries.

Although there still remains some resistance by physicians to adopt EHR systems, EHRs are becoming more prevalent (4). In February 2009, US Congress enacted into law the Health Information Technology for Economic and Clinical Health (HITECH) Act, which implemented new policies to induce adoption and "meaningful use" of EHRs by hospitals and physicians. Therefore, the American Academy of Otolaryngology—Head and Neck Surgery Medical Informatics Committee recently published formal recommendations and guidelines to encourage the adoption of EHRs (5). EHRs yield a wealth of clinical data. When planning a study that uses EHRs, the specific types of data and analyses should be predetermined prior to beginning the study. For instance, the population under study should be definable such that conclusions have wide applicability. Other factors to consider include age, gender, interventions, follow-up, and others. These factors produce many types of data. All of the temporal data and some laboratory results may be represented by numerical data. Binary coding may be used for gender, qualitative laboratory results, and status changes such as recurrence of a disease. Staging systems, ICD-9, and CPT numbers yield commonly accepted codes. However, a significant proportion of clinical data is textual and is in analog form derived from various health practitioner notes including clinic and operative notes, or descriptive reports from imaging studies.

Outcome measures, narrative text, and other textual data are most cumbersome to evaluate. It requires a researcher to manually evaluate each case individually in order to ascertain the data and often presents additional challenges related to the analysis of such data. Furthermore, text-based data sets are generally not conducive to data mining analyses for several reasons (6). First, EHRs record a significant portion of data in nonsearchable textual form. Nonsearchable text-based data need to either be transferred to a data warehouse as coded and searchable data, or a text-based search engine capable of utilizing the EHR directly must be in place. Second, there are a multitude of incompatible EHR systems. The differences in these systems limit one's ability to merge the data for collaborative efforts. Natural language processing presents a possible solution for recording and analyzing textual data, and it has been proven to have had at least limited success for data mining in the field of Allergy (7).

The Veterans Administration (VA) manages a nationwide system of EHRs. This is perhaps the best documentation of EHR models, and it has been noted to have significant advantages and disadvantages (8). The VA EHR system is known as the Veterans Health Information Systems and Technology Architecture, or VistA. The greatest advantage of the VA EHR database is the immense volume of available clinical data. However, at this time, its data searches are not perfect and can produce duplicative results, requiring manual review and thereby creating inefficiencies. There are plans to update VistA to improve its data mining capabilities and to support evidence-based medicine studies.

Since EHR databases are difficult to utilize due to textual data and inefficient search strategies that were not designed to facilitate clinical studies, researchers have created data warehouses (6). Data warehouses are comprised of EHR data that is coded, structured, and inclusive of all personal patient information deidentified for Health Insurance Portability and Accountability Act (HIPAA) of 1996 compliance. The software for such a warehouse is designed to support clinical databases studies and data mining. As such, data warehouses represent a powerful source for associative clinical studies. However, the cost to create and maintain a data warehouse is substantial. Usage of such clinical data framework for research on a population at a national level has been examined for the United States (9).

Regardless of the source, data must be accurate and standardized in order to be useful in any study. Therefore, the first step to answering a research question that proposes to query a database should be to ensure that the data is of acceptable quality for such analysis. Likewise, the first step in creating a database should be to set universal standards for how data are recorded to maintain or increase relevance for studies.

BASICS OF CLINICAL DATABASE ANALYSES

As clinical databases grow to provide increased statistical power and become representative of the overall population, the methods to perform clinical analysis of these databases grow beyond the limit of manual search strategies. Medical informatics seeks to create and utilize robust computational methods in database studies. The basic principles of clinical trial design and statistical analyses are the foundation for medical informatics. Although the details of these principles are beyond the scope of this chapter, many reviews on this topics have been published (3,10–12). It should be noted that nonrandomized or noncontrolled data are not able to establish causality. However, population-based correlative studies may be extremely powerful at revealing associations and limiting bias and may be applicable to situations in which a randomized, controlled trial could not otherwise be performed.

Unfortunately, studies that are not randomized and controlled are more likely to be predisposed to bias. Bias entails random, systematic, or intentional disagreement between the results and the true occurrence. Bias may influence any part of a clinical study including population accrual, data collection, analysis, or interpretation. Formulation of any clinical study should include efforts to understand and limit potential biases (3).

Data mining involves "extraction of implicit, previously unknown, and potentially useful information" through mathematical analysis (13). Therefore, through pattern discovery, clustering, and other methods, it may reveal clinically significant associations. By definition, data mining is different from the standard statistical analyses used in clinical studies. Brown and Harrison provide encompassing reviews of data mining and the complex analyses possible (14,15). As with any database study, data mining requires complete, accurate, structured, and coded data to perform adequate calculations. Unfortunately, medical data are perhaps the most difficult on which to perform data mining due to multiple factors including high dimensionality, heterogeneity, imprecision, and temporal patterns (15). A number of premade tools for data mining exist. "Open-source" tools created in a collaborative, nonprofit, and expandable manner have distinct advantages over commercial data mining software packages (16). Specific usage of data mining tools is beyond the scope of this introduction, and collaboration with a statistician familiar with these methods is recommended.

CLINICAL DATABASE APPLICATIONS

Clinical databases may take many forms based on the type of data, structure, and other features (see Table 204.1). Here we describe the steps to complete three types of clinical study based on specific databases. First, we describe the meta-analysis study using the PubMed and other literature databases, which is a commonly employed study for clinical research. Second, we describe the Surveillance Epidemiology and End Results (SEER) database for cancer population studies. Lastly, we describe the utility of the VA EHR VistA. A published study relating to laryngeal cancer is utilized for each database study example. Each example study may be obtained for in-depth information and assist extrapolation to similar types of studies and databases.

Although software-based search and analysis has become more commonplace, these studies required manual review by a researcher to some degree.

PubMed and Literature Databases (e.g., Meta-Analyses)

The PubMed database is a free resource that was developed and is maintained by the National Center for Biotechnology Information (NCBI). It is one of the most commonly accessed literature databases in clinical medicine and basic science research. The PubMed database from the National Institute for Health (NIH) and National Library of Medicine (NLM) comprises almost 21 million citations for biomedical literature. It includes all citations from MEDLINE, life science journals, NLM, as well as older citations from the print version of Index Medicus going back to1951. It also includes some new citations prior to publication and indexing in MEDLINE. For most clinical researchers, PubMed provides the majority of the data to perform meta-analyses and practice evidence-based medicine. Searching on PubMed is facilitated through several key concepts. Searches are best performed for concepts while being as specific as possible. By using several conceptual words, a search may be narrowed. Searching for English language only or review articles may further narrow a search. Combining searches may be useful to understanding the volume of literature available for topics. For instance, a search for "chemotherapy" returns over 2 million citations. A second search for "laryngeal cancer" returns just over 25,000 citations. Next, combining these searches (e.g., searching for both "chemotherapy" *and* "laryngeal cancer") returns just over 2,300 citations.

TABLE 204.1	COMMON DATABASES		
Database	**Type of Data**	**Type of Studies**	**References**
Cochrane Collaboration	In-depth clinical reviews	Systematic review Meta-analysis RevMan statistical analysis software	www.cochrane.org
ENSEMBL	Genomic sequences	Sequence comparison	www.ensembl.org
NCCN	Cancer registries Medical records		
Nucleotide/BLAST (NCBI)	DNA sequences Protein sequences	Sequence comparison	www.ncbi.nlm.nih.gov/ nuccore
PubMed (NCBI)	Compilation of biomedical citations from MEDLINE, life science journals, and online books		www.ncbi.nlm.nih.gov/ pubmed/
Research Portfolio Online Reporting Tools (RePORT)	Reports, data, and analysis of NIH research activities	Ongoing NIH research activities	www.report.nih.gov/
Surveillance Epidemiology and End Results (SEER)	US cancer statistics	Population trends	www.seer.cancer.gov/
VA	EMR Million Veteran Program		www.research.va.gov/

Although not exact, this combination gives the impression that approximately 10% of the literature on laryngeal cancer involves chemotherapeutic treatments. Or approximately 0.1% of the literature concerning chemotherapy is also concerned with laryngeal cancer. Finally, by registering and opening an individual account with NCBI, a researcher may save the searches for future study. There are also other methods used to manipulate searches, and an online training tutorial can be found on PubMed (http://www.nlm.nih.gov/bsd/disted/pubmed.html).

The Cochrane Collaboration is a nonprofit international organization established in 1993 and designed to support best evidence-based comprehensive reviews of treatment modalities (www.cochrane.org) (17). Submission of a review begins with registering your topic in order to prevent duplication and to judge the appropriateness of the topic. The process of developing a Cochrane review topic is undertaken by a team with expertise that covers both the topic and the statistics required for analysis. Such reviews require data mining literature, most commonly utilizing PubMed. Most Cochrane reviews analyze randomized control studies and study interventions or diagnostic tests. Therefore, a Cochrane Review represents both a powerful resource for data mining results and a database of evidence-based reviews. It is perhaps the pinnacle of evidence-based medicine studies utilizing other literature databases to perform systematic reviews.

A meta-analysis involves statistical analysis from a compilation of multiple related studies. Features extracted from each study must include similarities in the type of data and population such that the data may be grouped and reanalyzed. By employing multiple studies, power may be increased in the analysis of a potential clinical result. The use of multiple studies seeks to reduce the effect of systematic error in most cases. However, publication bias may occur due to the increased probability that research with statistically significant results will be published, while studies without significant results are less likely to be published. Therefore, a meta-analysis involving multiple published studies may be more affected by publication bias. A funnel plot may demonstrate that publication bias is minimized.

Performing a meta-analysis requires a stepwise approach (see Table 204.2) and, often, the assistance of a biostatistician. Resources required for performing a comprehensive meta-analysis is detailed in literature (17,18). A meta-analysis begins with a research question or a clearly stated hypothesis. Often, both published and unpublished studies are incorporated into the meta-analysis. "Gray literature" includes studies that are not available in the standard search engines, such as unpublished results, abstracts, conference proceedings, graduate theses, and book chapters (18). In some instances, the incorporation of gray literature improves the quality of the meta-analysis as it may serve to reduce publication bias (19). However, gray literature is often not peer reviewed and tends to be smaller studies of generally lower statistical power. To obtain homogenous data between studies, definable criteria such as age, sex, tumor site, stage, performance status, treatment allocated, date of randomization, date and site of first recurrence, date of second primary cancer, and cause of death are collected. Survival status and latest follow-up data are also collected. Often, each study is statistically analyzed independently for internal consistency.

TABLE 204.2	STEPS IN COMPLETING A META-ANALYSIS	

Step No.	Action	Further Information
1	Formulate a hypothesis.	This is the basic research question(s).
2	Define the search parameters (database).	Type(s) of studies to review? What years? Follow-up? What database(s) will be searched? Will gray literature be included?
3	Define the inclusion criteria (study).	Create a grading system for literature based on inclusion criteria.
4	Perform the search.	This will identify specific literature that fits the criteria and provide a quality grade for each. If fewer than expected studies are included, consider modifying the hypothesis to fit available literature.
5	Analyze the included literature.	Calculate effect sizes. Code moderating variables. Summary estimate of effect (with 95% confidence interval) Test of homogeneity Provide a descriptive analysis.
6	Interpret the results.	Relate the results to the hypothesis Consider possible mechanism(s) Consider limitations (appropriateness of data to hypothesis, type and quality of studies, power)
7	Future directions	Consider future directions for further research.

The analyzed data then undergo interpretation and discussion. It is common to compare the result to that of other prominent literature in terms of proposed mechanism, study design, results, and study limitations.

Population Databases and Data Warehouses (e.g., SEER Database)

The SEER database collects cancer data including incidence, prevalence, and survival and represents 26% of the US population. The SEER database is an example of a clinical data warehouse based on collections of data from defined populations. It comprises 17 population-based cancer registries from the Alaskan Native Tumor Registry, Arizona Indians, greater California, Connecticut, Detroit, Atlanta, greater and rural Georgia, Hawaii, Iowa, Kentucky, Los Angeles, Louisiana, New Jersey, New Mexico, San Francisco–Oakland, San Jose–Monterey, Seattle–Puget Sound, and Utah. SEER also contains data on cancer mortality for the entire United States. This database is primarily employed for comparative cancer statistics based on age, geographic region, socioeconomic class, and race. Among the many possible comparisons, this broad data set also allows analyses related to health disparities. The SEER system includes both a database of cancer registry patients and software to perform statistical analyses. Population databases such as the SEER database provide access to high-quality clinical data and a relatively easy interface to perform studies for retrospective association.

Institutional Database Studies (e.g., Veterans Administration)

The VA employs EHRs of all veterans who undergo medical evaluation and treatment at their facilities. Not only does this wealth of clinical data provide the ability to perform powerful retrospective studies, the VA also enrolls veterans into prospective studies including random controlled trials. IRB approval is required to perform human research utilizing VA materials.

The VA has completely transitioned to the use of EHRs ahead of national mandate. This created a very comprehensive database in terms of clinical details; however, the issue here is that most of the data are textual (8). Coding variables that include ICD-9 and CPT codes are available but have not been universally applied given the VA's status as a single-payer system. Furthermore, the software systems available for searching and extracting patient data from VistA are limited with respect to data mining and clinical studies.

BASIC SCIENCE ADJUNCTS TO TRANSLATIONAL MEDICINE

The complete sequencing of the human genome in 2001 opened the door to a new world of analyses (20,21). Knowledge of genomic, proteomic, and related resources is often essential in transitioning clinical data into translational data. Here we present just a few of the possible resources that assist in bridging basic science and clinical data. Most of these resources are available to the public and represent open-source data.

ENSEMBL is a database comprising multiple vertebrate and eukaryotic genomes that is freely available (www.ensembl.org). Multiple search methods and types of analysis are possible. Searches can also be based on disease names or physiologic functions. Therefore, one may quickly search for genes involved in disease or other processes.

The NCBI provides a multitude of searchable resources including PubMed (see Clinical Database Applications), OMIM, SNP, and others. A review of their functions and tutorials can be readily obtained by going directly to the NCBI home page (www.ncbi.nlm.nih.gov).

The Research Portfolio Online Reporting Tool (RePORT) provides information on all funded research grants from the NIH including areas of research, funded organizations, success rates, and budgets. In addition, the RePORT Expenditures and Results (RePORTER) supports queries of all current and historical funded grants. Most importantly, this allows for searches of funded grants by terms related to the research topic. Therefore, a researcher can identify funded studies in the RePORTER database in order to prevent redundancy in their research grant application (www.report.nih.gov/).

Bioinformatics supports the analysis of a multitude of areas in basic science research. In genomics, gene identification and genome assembly may be predicted. Protein structure predictions and protein interactions may also be predicted. These can lead to rational drug design and discovery. If a potential candidate protein or genetic sequence is isolated as a target molecule during pathogenesis, these resources may assist in identifying additional mechanisms or pathways, providing new directions in translational research and interceptive therapeutics.

Translational Research Databases

As advances in molecular biology and refinements in techniques such as gene therapy develop, translational research databases are steadily emerging. However, they are perhaps the most difficult kind of database to populate and analyze. Currently there are a small number of standard genetic tests reported in EHRs. In the future, genetic screening tests, such as a disease-specific cDNA microarray test, may become readily available and incorporated into EHRs. Textual data are common in genomics, proteomics, PubMed literature, and EHRs (22). Multiple text associations are possible per entity, such as abbreviations, syntax, semantics, and specific sequences. Effective search methods utilizing text-based data sets require either exhaustive manual effort if the database is limited or search engines for larger databases.

Obtaining sufficient power in databases requires larger populations. To effectively populate translational databases, collaboration between collection centers is necessary. Collaborative efforts may include private hospital systems, state and federal systems, and academic hospitals. Data themselves may present a problem, particularly in collaborative databases. If data are to be compared across multiple sources, then standardized coding must be presented such that data are presented in an equivalent manner. This may require manual coding and incorporation of translational data into translational databases.

Private and public databases of genetic information from human tissue samples are another source of translational databases (Reviewed in 26). These either record a limited set of clinical data along with the genetic information or link to the genetic information such that associated clinical data may be acquired from EHR.

Ethical Issues in Translational Research

Translational databases create ethical challenges due to the inclusion of genetic and other personal data. Discrimination based on genetic data may occur at a variety of levels or influence insurance coverage. In response to this evolving concern, Congress passed the Genetic Information Nondiscriminating Act (GINA) in 2008 (23). Title I of GINA seeks protection for alteration of health insurance coverage based on genetic information. Title II provides individuals with protection related to genetic information from employer and workplace discrimination. GINA also amends genetic information to be part of the clinical information protected under HIPAA. Some researchers have fought against the stringent restrictions in GINA, believing that they will create a bureaucracy of increased costs and compliance to perform studies involving genetic information. This has been deemed akin to the effect of HIPAA on human research. Finally, genetic information about a patient opens doors to similar information about related family members, against whom similar discrimination may ensue. These issues have undergone philosophical debate for many years and will create a greater impact as advances in genetic testing further develop.

Translational Database Studies

Small-scale translational databases can be readily formed from patient cohorts at a single institution. Such collections may be prospective, randomized, and controlled. Given the generally limited numbers of patients, textual clinical data coding and the security overseen by an IRB may be managed by a few researchers. Although powerful in answering a limited number of questions related to specific accrual criteria, small translational studies cannot compare to the statistical power of a large-scale database.

The electronic MEdical Records and GEnomics (eMERGE) network is a consortium of five institutions collaborating to merge DNA repositories and EHRs (24,25). Currently, genome-wide association studies to provide genotyping have been performed for a small number of specific primary disease phenotypes. Each of the five sites has created a biobank combining genomic data and EHR-based clinical correlative data. Challenges in synthesis of data between the sites have been addressed. Unfortunately, the cohorts may not be comparable for some conditions. However, the eMERGE system provides a valuable example for the feasibility of collaborative translational research.

As part of EHRs, comprehensive medication histories are recorded, which may provide important translational associations. Both clinical utility and technical difficulties in synthesizing these data into multi-institutional data warehouses, also referred to as biobanks, have been reviewed (26). Collaborative efforts of Johnson and Johnson, the Cancer Institute of New Jersey, and St. Jude Children's Research Hospital has created a translational database combining biomarker data (e.g., gene expression profiles, genotypes, serum protein panels, and others) with clinical correlations from internal clinical trials (27). Open-source tools were used to analyze the data. This database has been mined for multiple drug discovery functions including indication selection and trial design. The related intuitive graphical interface allows for quick validation of hypotheses such that the effect of small changes may be evaluated. One problem with such systems is the propensity to create analysis and interpretation biases by tailoring search parameters to find significant effects.

Crowley et al. (28) furthered a research-based translational database of deidentified clinical and tissue specimen data by integration with the Cancer Biomedical Informatics Grid (caBIG). This created standardized architectural grouping and vocabulary with graphical interfaces and text-based search mechanisms. Although the caBIG database was successfully generated, no multi-institutional collaborative data mining studies have yet been produced. This also exemplifies the multidisciplinary and costly nature of creating a multi-institutional translational data warehouse.

Currently, translational databases represent a promising and novel technology that is under continuous development. Given that the establishment of translational data warehouses requires significant financial commitments, for smaller groups we recommend seeking opportunities to be included in existing and emerging institutional and multi-institutional studies.

CONCLUSION

Clinical information from patient records and medical research has been stored in paper-based form for centuries. Over time, this paper-based system has consumed increasing space, created inefficiencies in storage and acquisitions, and most notably, delayed access to medical care. In contrast, the ability to store clinical information digitally into a computer database allows for instant and more efficient access to patient records and research data, and has revolutionized all aspects of medical care and research. To this end, the field of medical informatics is an emerging discipline that relates computer applications and algorithms in the delivery of medical care to ultimately improve human health.

HIGHLIGHTS

- In 2009, US Congress enacted into law the HITECH Act, which implemented new policies to induce adoption and "meaningful use" of EHRs by hospitals and physicians. Therefore, the American Academy of Otolaryngology—Head and Neck Surgery Medical Informatics Committee recently published formal recommendations and guidelines to encourage the adoption of EHRs.

- Most EHR databases currently available are stored as narrative text and other textual data, presenting research challenges for data mining and other clinical research.

- There are many clinical databases available for the researcher; examples include PubMed, SEER database for cancer population studies, VA EHR, or VistA.

- The complete sequencing of the human genome in 2001 is uncovering the molecular basis of human pathologies. Basic Science database includes ENSEMBL, which is a database comprising multiple vertebrate and eukaryotic genomes and the NCBI.

- Translational Research databases are emerging; however, they are the most difficult kind of database to populate and analyze due to limits in technology and small population size.

REFERENCES

1. Balatsouras DG, Kaberos A, Korres SG, et al. Internet resources available to otolaryngologists. *Ann Otol Rhinol Laryngol* 2002;1 11:1139–1143.
2. Harrison JH, Aller RD. Regional and national health care data repositories. *Clin Lab Med* 2008;28:101–117.
3. Hartman JM, Forsen JW, Wallace MS, et al. Tutorials in clinical research: Part IV: recognizing and controlling bias. *Laryngoscope* 2002;112:23–31.
4. Castillo VH, Martinez-Garcia AI, Pulido JRG. A knowledge-based taxonomy of critical factors for adopting electronic health record systems by physicians: a systematic literature review. *BMC Med Inform Decis mak* 2010;10:60–76.
5. Das S, Eisenberg LD, House JW, et al. Meaningful use of electronic health records in otolaryngology: recommendations from the American Academy of Otolaryngology—Head and Neck

6. Surgery Medical Informatics Committee. *Otolaryngol Head Neck Surg* 2011;144(2):135–141.
6. Lyman JA, Scully K, Harrison JH. The development of health care data warehouses to support data mining. *Clin Lab Med* 2008;28:55–71.
7. Dalan D. Clinical data mining and research in the allergy office. *Curr Opin Allergy Clin Immun* 2010;10(3):171–177.
8. Millard WB. Electronic health records: promises and realities. Part II: some early voyages in partially charted waters. *Ann Emerg Med* 2010;56(3):A17–A21.
9. Safran C, Bloomrosen M, Hammond WE, et al. Toward a national framework for the secondary use of health data: an american medical informatics association white paper. *J Am Med Inform Assoc* 2007;14(1):1–9.
10. Neely JG, Hartman JM, Forsen JW, et al. Tutorials in clinical research. Part VII: understanding comparative statistics (contrast)—Part A: general concepts of statistical significance. *Laryngoscope* 2003;113:1534–1540.
11. Neely JG, Hartman JM, Forsen JW, et al. Tutorials in clinical research: VII. Understanding comparative statistics (contrast)—Part B: application of T-Test, Mann-Whitney U, and Chi-Square. *Laryngoscope* 2003;113:1719–1724.
12. Stewart MG, Neely JG, Hartman JM, et al. Tutorials in clinical research: Part V: outcomes research. *Laryngoscope* 2002;112: 248–254.
13. Lee S, Siau K. A review of data mining techniques. *Ind Manage Data Syst* 2001;100(1):41–46.
14. Brown DE. Introduction to data mining for medical informatics. *Clin Lab Med* 2008;28(1):9–35.
15. Harrison JH. Introduction to the mining of clinical data. *Clin Lab Med* 2008;28:1–7.
16. Zupan B, Demsar J. Open-source tools for data mining. *Clin Lab Med* 2008;28:37–54.
17. Henderson LK, Craig JC, Willis NS, et al. How to write a Cochrane systematic review. *Nephro* 2010;15:617–624.
18. Khoshdel A, Attia J, Carney SL. Basic concepts in a meta-analysis: a primer for clinicians. *J Clin Pract* 2006;60(10):1287–1294.
19. Song, F, Parekh S, Hooper L, et al. Dissemination and publication of research findings: an updated review of related biases. *Health Technol Assess* 2010;14(8):iii, ix–xi,1–193.
20. Venter JC, Adams MD, Myers EW, et al. The sequence of the human genome. *Science* 2001;291(5507):1304–1351.
21. Lander ES, Linton LM, Birren B, et al. Initial sequencing and analysis of the human genome. *Nature* 2001;409(6822):860–921.
22. Krallinger M, Valencia A, Hirschman L. Linking genes to literature: text mining, information extraction, and retrieval applications for biology. *Genome Biol* 2008;9(Suppl 2):S8.1–S8.14.
23. Sethi P, Theodos K. Translational bioinformatics and healthcare informatics: computational and ethical challenges. *Perspect Health Inf Manag* 2009;6:1–13.
24. McCarty CA, Chisholm RL, Chute CG, et al. The eMERGE Network: a consortium of biorepositories linked to electronic medical records data for conducting genomics studies. *BMC Med Genomics* 2011;4:13–23.
25. McGuire AL, Basford M, Dressler LG, et al. Ethical and practical challenges of sharing data from genome-wide association studies: The eMERGE consortium experience. *Genome Res* 2011;21(7):1001–1007. [Epub Jun 1, 2011.]
26. Wilke RA, Xu H, Denny JC, et al. The emerging role of electronic medical records in pharmacogenomics. *Clin Pharmacol Ther* 2011;89(3):379–386.
27. Szalma S, Koka V, Knasanova T, et al. Effective knowledge management in translational medicine. *J Transl Med* 2010;8:68–76.
28. Crowley RS, Castine M, Mitchell K, et al. caTIES: a grid based system for coding and retrieval of surgical pathology reports and tissue specimens in support of translational research. *J Am Med Inform Assoc* 2010;17:253–264.

Telemedicine for Otolaryngology

205

John Kokesh   Chris Patricoski   A. Stewart Ferguson

Telemedicine utilizes technology to enhance communication and provide services over a distance. In this way, "telemedicine" represents an evolution in health care that has adopted the technologies and communication infrastructure now available in society. The telephone and fax machine were the earliest telecommunication tools used in clinical practice, and are now so ubiquitous that we can hardly imagine medicine without them.

With the rapid advances in technology and telecommunications, and perhaps more importantly, widespread societal acceptance of technology, a new generation will redefine how medicine is practiced in the future. "Telemedicine" will likely become an antiquated term requiring redefinition, no longer describing a niche area in certain medical specialties but rather a methodology by which modern information transfer is used to improve the practice of medicine.

This chapter examines the current telemedicine technologies and present applications of telemedicine in otolaryngology. While telemedicine has grown significantly in the last 10 years, there is a need for further adoption throughout the United States. The realization that improvements are needed in access for care, costs of care delivery, and availability of medical specialists will likely help remove some of the barriers that have thus far thwarted widespread innovation and adoption of telemedicine in otolaryngology. The nature of the specialty, with well-developed and extensive use of endoscopy, microscopy, photographic imaging, and physiologic data, makes otolaryngology a potential beneficiary of an expanded role for telemedicine in the future practice of medicine.

DEFINITIONS

The American Telemedicine Association (ATA) defines telemedicine as "the use of medical information exchanged from one site to another via electronic communications to improve patients' health status" (1). Telemedicine has been traditionally divided into three areas: Interactive Video Teleconferencing (VTC), Asynchronous Store-and-Forward (S&F), and Remote Patient Monitoring (RPM). While the distinction between these categories has begun to blur with advances in device technology and means of information transfer, it is worthwhile to review each as well their current usage in medicine.

The term "VTC" telemedicine applies to a medical encounter performed over a live teleconference link with video and audio and, in some instances, a live display of data from remote medical devices. As commonly practiced, a "presenting provider" is physically present with the patient to assist with the interview, conduct aspects of the examination, and operate devices to obtain parts of the examination to be transmitted. The presenting provider, for example, may operate an endoscope to provide live video of the examined body system. The "consulting provider" is located at a distance and receives the live video feed. There is synchronous communication between the providers and the patient; questions can be asked and immediately answered. The consulting provider may direct certain parts of the examination. The encounter may be recorded for future reference. Some of the advantages of VTC are that it is interactive, patient movement and affect can be assessed, and a "human" connection between the involved parties can be established. The consulting provider has the ability to conduct an interview similar to an in-person exam and can help direct the encounter. The disadvantages of VTC are that all involved parties must be available simultaneously for the encounter, technical and network support is needed to ensure full function at the time of the scheduled encounter, and sufficient bandwidth is required for adequate video quality. VTC has generally been most successful when used as part of an integrated health system where coordinated scheduling, technical support, training, and funding are provided (2). Examples of medical specialties where VTC has been successfully used include psychiatry and mental health services, cardiology, and intensive care unit consultation (Tele–ICU) (3,4). VTC has also been used in the recent development of "telestroke" networks, where a remotely located neurologist assesses patients with evolving strokes and decides whether thrombolytic therapy should be administered (5).

"S&F" telemedicine involves the capture, storage, and transmission of data between providers for the purpose of obtaining medical advice and opinion. As commonly practiced, the "creator" is physically present when interviewing the patient, conducting an examination, capturing data, and documenting the encounter in a telemedicine case. The "consultant" at a remote location would then review the transmitted data after it was sent in its entirety. S&F is asynchronous; the providers need not be available at the same time, and the created "case" may be viewed minutes, hours, or days after it was created and transmitted. Typical data that are captured and utilized in S&F include clinical histories, vital signs, digital photos, radiology images, endoscopic images, scanned documents, audiograms, tympanograms, and heart and lung sounds. The advantages of

S&F are that it does not require simultaneous availability of providers, thereby avoiding scheduling and logistic problems. It can be extremely time efficient for the consultant as complete data collection and organization of information have occurred during creation of the case, often along predetermined guidelines (Fig. 205.1). S&F can be used with low or interrupted bandwidth, enabling its use in very remote or infrastructure-deprived locations. Finally, once set up with the appropriate software, security, and operational standards, S&F "works like e-mail" requiring much less ongoing maintenance and support than VTC. Disadvantages of S&F are that real-time interaction between providers is not possible; the consulting provider cannot direct the exam (though they can asynchronously request additional information), and sustained movement, voice, and affect of the patient cannot be assessed (though short video files are now easily transferrable). S&F has long been successfully used in those specialties where the assessment or "read" of the consultant regarding static clinical data is the valued service. Well-established examples are teleradiology (6), teledermatology (7), and telepathology (8).

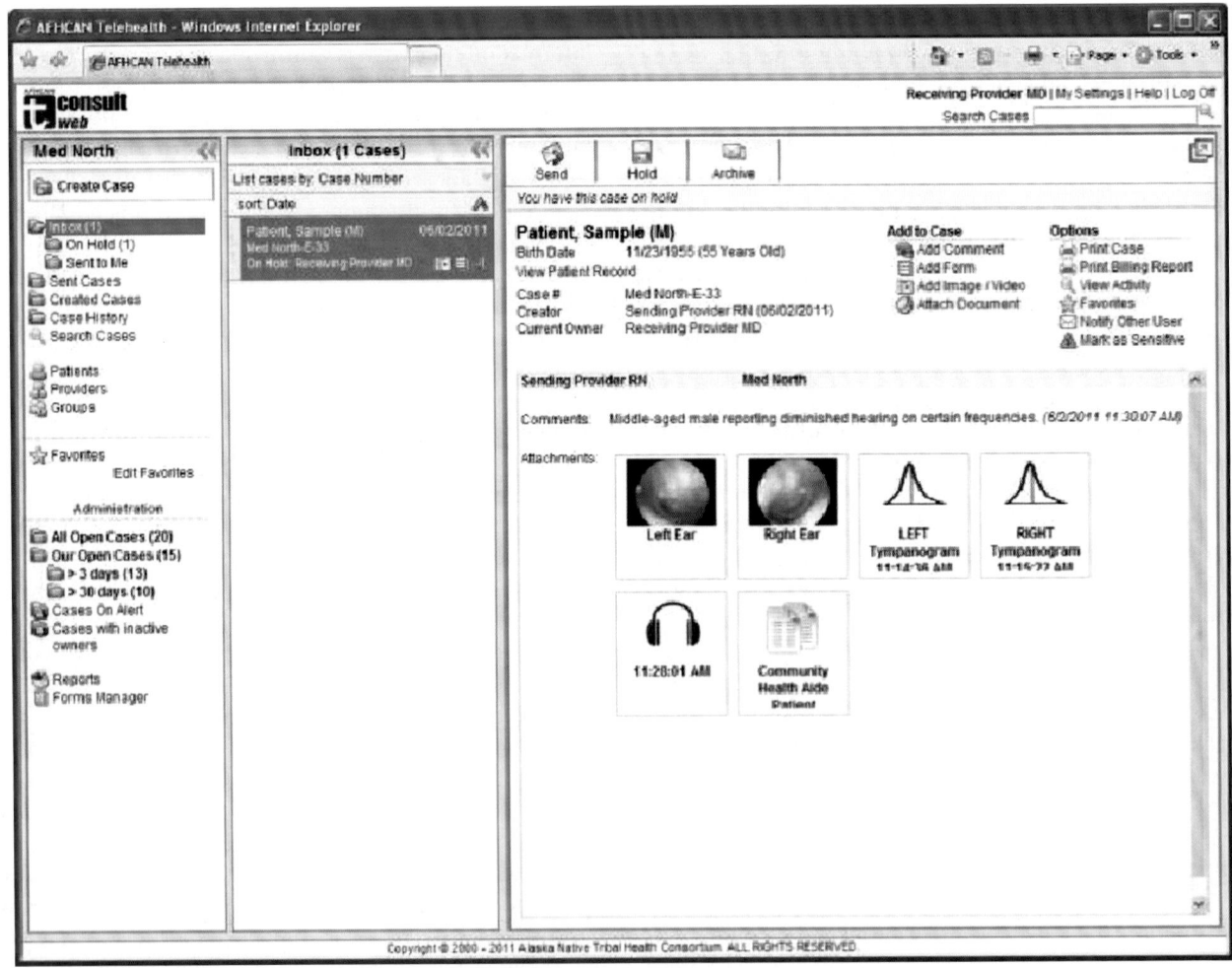

Figure 205.1 Alaska Federal Health Care Access Network (AFHCAN) tConsult software. Clinical information and data have been organized for review by the consultant.

RMP technology enables the monitoring of patient health data originated from the patient's home, nursing facility, place of employment, school, and other locations. It is most often employed in the patient's home and, as such, is often called "home telehealth." RPM almost always involves capture of data similar to S&F and sometimes includes video. To date, RPM has proven useful for the management of chronic disease states such as diabetes, congestive heart failure, and chronic pulmonary disease (9,10). Used appropriately, RPM facilitates access to care, patient and family involvement and education, and early identification and intervention for acute illness or health status decompensations. RPM holds tremendous promise for cost savings through improved chronic disease management, especially for integrated health systems (11). From a commercial standpoint, RPM represents a large potential market, and device manufacturers are rapidly adding new products to the field. For these reasons, this is the most rapidly growing field in telemedicine, and clinicians will likely have increasing opportunities to use home monitoring in the future.

A final category of telemedicine deserving mention relates to the use of telemedicine technologies in the performance of surgical procedures. In telementoring and teleproctoring, a distantly located "expert" surgeon monitors and assists a surgeon at a distant location performing a surgery. A typical current application would involve using a live VTC link used to mentor an endoscopic procedure (12). Telesurgery, the performance of a surgical procedure by a remotely located surgeon using robotic devices, is currently the subject of feasibility studies and demonstration projects (13).

SECURITY AND HIPAA

Telemedicine is no different from other forms of clinical care in regard to the applicability of regulations governing privacy and security. The use and disclosure of an individuals' health information (protected health information [PHI]) by providers and organizations are subject to national standards and regulations—regardless of the care delivery model. Most notable among these are the so-called HIPAA Privacy and Security Rules and the more recent HITECH Act:

■ The Standards for Privacy of Individually Identifiable Health Information (Privacy Rule) was issued by the US Department of Health and Human Services in 2000 to implement the requirements of the Health Insurance Portability and Accountability Act of 1996 (HIPAA). The Privacy Rule standards address the use and disclosure of individuals' health information called "protected health information" by organizations subject to the Privacy Rule (covered entities) as well as standards for individuals' privacy rights to understand and control how their health information is used.

■ HIPAA also mandated the creation of national standards for the security of electronic health care information, which were then released in the final "HIPAA Security Rule" in 2003. This final rule specified a range of administrative, technical, and physical security procedures for covered entities to use to for electronic protected health information (ePHI); the standards were delineated into either required or addressable (optional) implementation specifications.

■ More recently, the Health Information Technology for Economic and Clinical Health Act (HITECH Act) was passed as part of the American Recovery and Reinvestment Act of 2009 (ARRA). Because HITECH contains incentives designed to accelerate the adoption of electronic health record (EHR) systems and potentially generate a massive growth in the exchange of ePHI, the HITECH Act further broadened the scope of privacy and security protections established under HIPAA.

A good "rule of thumb" is to recognize that a telehealth system should be treated no different than an EHR system in regard to privacy and security. Telehealth systems are designed to capture, transmit, store, and display ePHI—as are EHR systems. Many telehealth systems interface to EHRs and share information in a back-and-forth manner to provide a more complete view of the patient record. Telehealth systems sometimes contain information that is potentially "more identifiable" of the patient as they may contain images of the patients face or other body parts.

It is not possible to provide a thorough review of the HIPAA and HITECH regulations as they apply to telehealth systems, but the following features are recommended in any telehealth system to maximize the ability to comply with HIPPA and HITECH. While the general concepts apply to VTC, S&F, and RPM, the remainder of this section uses S&F telehealth as an example for how these standards and regulations may apply.

■ All data should be encrypted "at rest" and during "transport." Data flow (i.e., "transport") in a telehealth system from a computer (or system) in the patient exam room to other systems where remote providers (or specialists) can view the data. Data may stay on a server (at rest) or a desktop PC for hours or days until a provider can view that data. Data that are encrypted are not "readable" or "viewable" without the right key to "decrypt" the data. This prevents unauthorized users from accessing the data and provides a significant level of privacy and security protection. While some organizations elect to not encrypt data flowing within their private network, telehealth services are becoming much more common between organizations with data flowing outside of organizational networks and potentially across Internet links, further accentuating the need to encrypt the data.

■ Access to data through a browser—such as Internet Explorer or Safari—should rely on an encrypted connection (e.g., "https" instead of "http"). When this access occurs across the Internet or outside of an organization's trusted network, the Web site should provide "https" connectivity using a security certificate from a trusted organization—thereby allowing users to have greater trust in the web server's authenticity.

- Systems that require data to move between organizations or across nonsecure networks should include a mechanism to make sure the data do not change (data validation) and a mechanism to verify the site or provider that originated the data (nonrepudiation). This is usually accomplished through electronic signatures and "hash" algorithms.

- The telehealth system should integrate with the user authentication mechanism used by the organization, so the user account can be managed through a central mechanism and password policies can be enforced (e.g., regular changes, minimum password length, and complexity).

- All major user activities should be tracked within the telehealth system through an audit mechanism. As a minimum, all successful and unsuccessful log-in attempts should be logged as well as any changes that impact patient data.

- Users should have sufficient access for their needs, but no more. Role-based security is an excellent mechanism whereby users are assigned to various roles (e.g., consultant, trainer, clinical administrator) that define their access to telehealth data and functionality. Time-outs should be employed to limit access to data should a provider leave a workstation prior to logging out.

- Recognizing that not all telehealth cases are necessarily equal, the telehealth system should provide a mechanism to indicate when a case is "sensitive" or requires tighter security than other cases. Such cases might include abuse cases, mental health cases, or HIV/AIDS cases.

- Similar to EHR systems, telehealth equipment (workstations, servers, medical devices) can all contain ePHI and as such need to be physically secured to prevent loss of data due to theft or unauthorized access.

- The telehealth system needs to be managed and protected similar to an EHR system. This would include, for example, accepting updates only when tested and provided by a reputable source, backing up data and providing for disaster recovery efforts, active defenses against viruses and other malware, and protecting equipment against loss of power or intermittent power surges.

It is not uncommon to find providers that rely on e-mail as a simple telehealth solution—allowing for the exchange of images and basic textual information about a patient. This should raise significant concern based on the proceeding information, as an e-mail system is often not considered a secure system by most organizations and will limit or impede and organization's ability to achieve HIPAA compliance.

USES OF TELEMEDICINE IN OTOLARYNGOLOGY

Telemedicine has been used in the field of otolaryngology since the early 1990s. Use has occurred primarily in those situations where there was a remote, isolated population to serve; a shortage or lack of availability of otolaryngologist; or, more recently, backlogs of patients needing otolaryngology care inadequately addressed by the existing delivery system. Applications have been partially driven by available technologies and their cost, and the spectrum of clinical services that can be delivered at a distance has increased with advances in technology and communication infrastructure. Finally, most of the usage and research in the use of telemedicine in otolaryngology has occurred in those settings where the financial and regulatory barriers that have limited the widespread use of telemedicine in the United States are less formidable and where telemedicine programs have been designed to meet a specific clinical or population need. Examples include programs run through the United States Department of Defense and the United States Public Health Service as well as programs in countries with national health plans.

Otology and Neurotology

The ability to obtain and transmit diagnostic quality images of the tympanic membrane and middle ear has been well established. Pedersen, in pioneering work done in Norway, showed that a video otoscope coupled to a VTC network could be used to allow a remotely located otolaryngologist to direct patient examinations and establish diagnoses and treatment plans. This resulted in improved access for otolaryngology care as well as reduced cost for care delivery to isolated populations (14). Additional work using this methodology has verified that high-quality images can be routinely obtained with the video endoscope, even in pediatric populations (15). Still images of tympanic membrane obtained by a video otoscope and accompanied by audiologic and tympanometric data and transmitted using S&F technology were used to deliver otology consultations to patients in remote areas of Western Australia (16). Exam findings and diagnoses based on S&F examination using digital images from a video otoscope for children with previously placed tympanostomy tubes were found to correlate highly with those established by in-person encounters with otolaryngologists using binocular operating microscopes (17). S&F telemedicine using tympanic membrane images, clinical histories, and audiologic data has been shown to allow for accurate planning for chronic ear surgery (18).

This work has demonstrated that telemedicine, whether VTC or S&F, is a useful tool for delivering otology care. As diagnosis depends to a great degree on the physical characteristics of the tympanic membrane, image quality is critically important. Images must be in focus, adequately

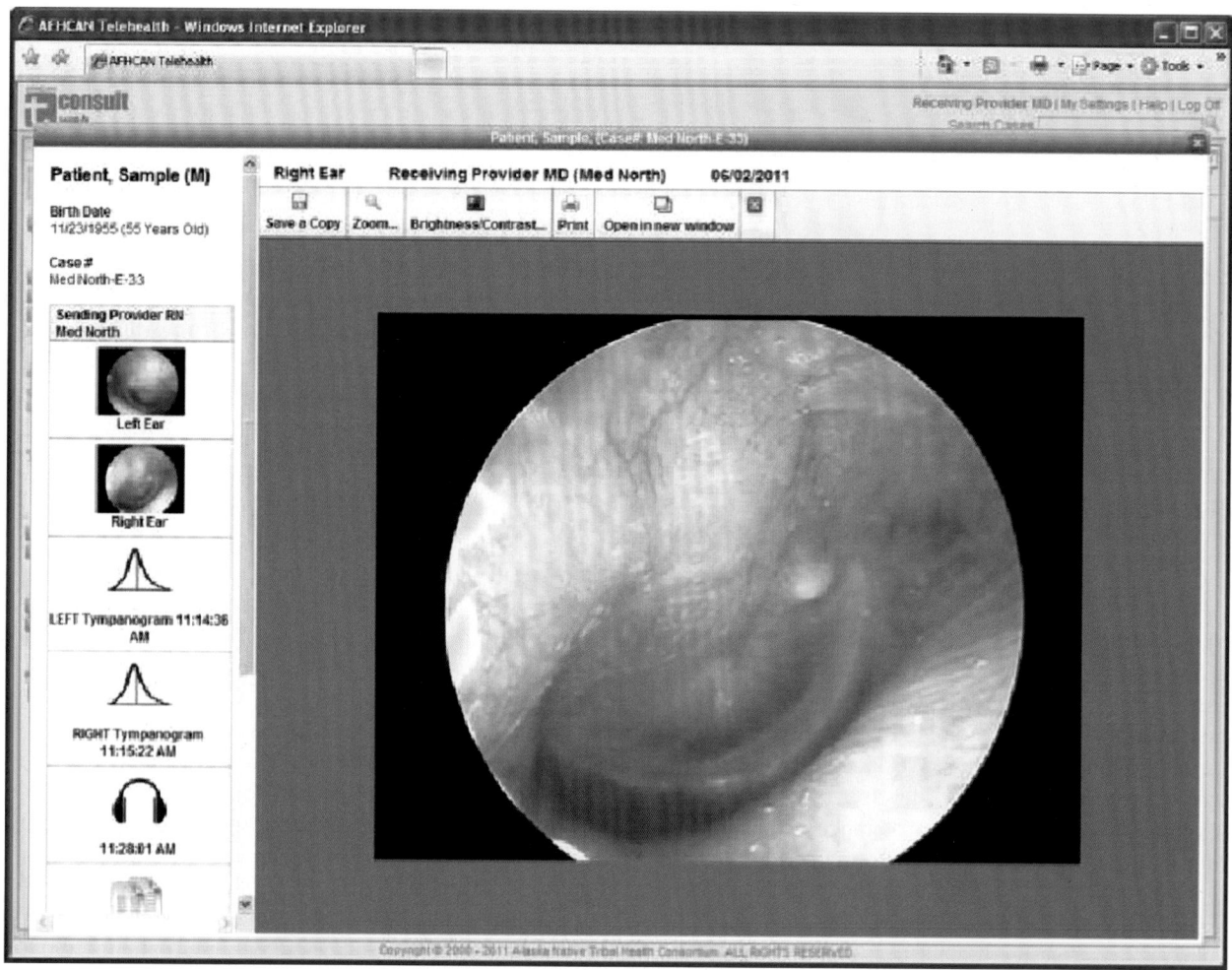

Figure 205.2 Typical otology case in AFHCAN tConsult software. Case includes images, audiogram, tympanogram, and clinical history.

illuminated, and free of obstruction. A high-performing video otoscope proves to be a worthwhile investment, and training must be provided to those acquiring the images to ensure consistent high quality. While most video otoscopes do allow for insufflation, and tympanic membrane mobility can be assessed if VTC is used, the addition of tympanometric data has generally found to be a useful adjunct to images. When "packaged" with digitized clinical histories and audiograms, an otology "case" can be created that can be reviewed by the otolaryngologist and in most cases lead to an accurate diagnosis and treatment plan (Fig. 205.2). When used over an S&F platform and coupled with clinical guidelines and standards for the information required by the consultant, telemedicine can become an extraordinarily efficient way to diagnosis, triage, and offer treatment advice for otologic disease.

Recent experiences have demonstrated the utility of telemedicine in delivering otologic and neurotologic care. S&F telemedicine has been used in rural Alaska to deliver otology care with dramatic effects on access and reduced waiting times. Alaska Natives have a high burden of middle ear disease, and many are remotely located with difficult access

to specialty care (19). To address these issues, a statewide telemedicine system, the Alaska Federal Health Care Access Network (AFHCAN), was created (20). To manage otologic disease, primary care physicians and midlevel providers have been trained in the use of otoscopes, tympanometers, and screening audiometers and use S&F telemedicine to obtain consultation from otolaryngologists at an urban referral center (21). Populations receiving this care model realized markedly reduced waiting times for care and overall improved access to the opinion of an otolaryngologist (Fig. 205.3) (22). Audiologists trained in video otoscope image acquisition and the use of S&F telemedicine have partnered with consulting otolaryngologists to deliver care to extremely remote populations in Alaska, making use of mobile devices and equipment (Fig. 205.4). Effective triage, cost savings from avoided travel, and identification of undiagnosed, serious disease states were demonstrated (23). In post hurricane Katrina in southeast Louisiana, clinical protocols were combined with a blend of S&F and VTC telemedicine to allow a distantly located consulting neurootologist to assist local providers in providing neurotologic care. With appropriate planning, this model was

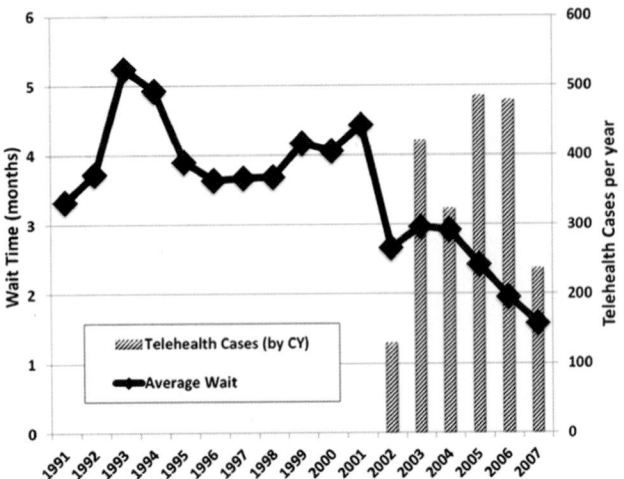

Figure 205.3 Average wait times for otolaryngology appointments. Nome, Alaska, 1991 to 2007. Wait times for in-person clinic appointments steadily decrease as telemedicine usage increases.

found to be very effective for service delivery in this area of need (24).

An effective and gratifying use of S&F telemedicine in rural Alaska has been for the identification and treatment of sensorineural hearing loss. Working closely with audiologists, protocols have been developed to allow for an audiologist to obtain medical clearance for hearing aid fitting without requiring an in-person encounter with the otolaryngologist. This has resulted in savings of travel costs and inconvenience for the patient and has meant for many patients access to a hearing aid that they would not have otherwise had. This model has also greatly strengthened the working relationship between audiologist and otolaryngologist. In the future, S&F telemedicine may assist otolaryngologists and audiologists in maintaining a collaborative approach to the management of patients with hearing impairment, an area of some recent controversy (25).

In summary, telemedicine is an effective *tool* that can be used to *assist* the otolaryngologist in delivering care for otologic disease. Pathologies can be diagnosed, advice can be given to primary care providers, and patients can be triaged to their most appropriate level for care—all by the specialist with the most expertise in the disease process. However, as with all telemedicine, there must be a means to deliver traditional, in-person medical or surgical care for those identified to need such.

Pediatric Otolaryngology

Isolated pediatric populations with limited access to the care of an otolaryngologist have been the subject of studies evaluating telemedicine as a care delivery model. VTC was used to evaluate children with problems such as sleep disorder breathing, otitis media, and sinusitis. Otoscopes were used for ear imaging, and a modified, diffuse light source coupled to an otoscope was used to image the oral cavity and pharynx. Diagnoses and treatment plans given by remotely located otolaryngologist were found to correlate highly with those made during a traditional in-person encounter with an otolaryngologist (26). This same methodology was used to do a cost minimization analysis for a telepediatric otolaryngology screening program in Western Australia. By avoiding travel costs for patients and their families, telemedicine-based services were found to be less

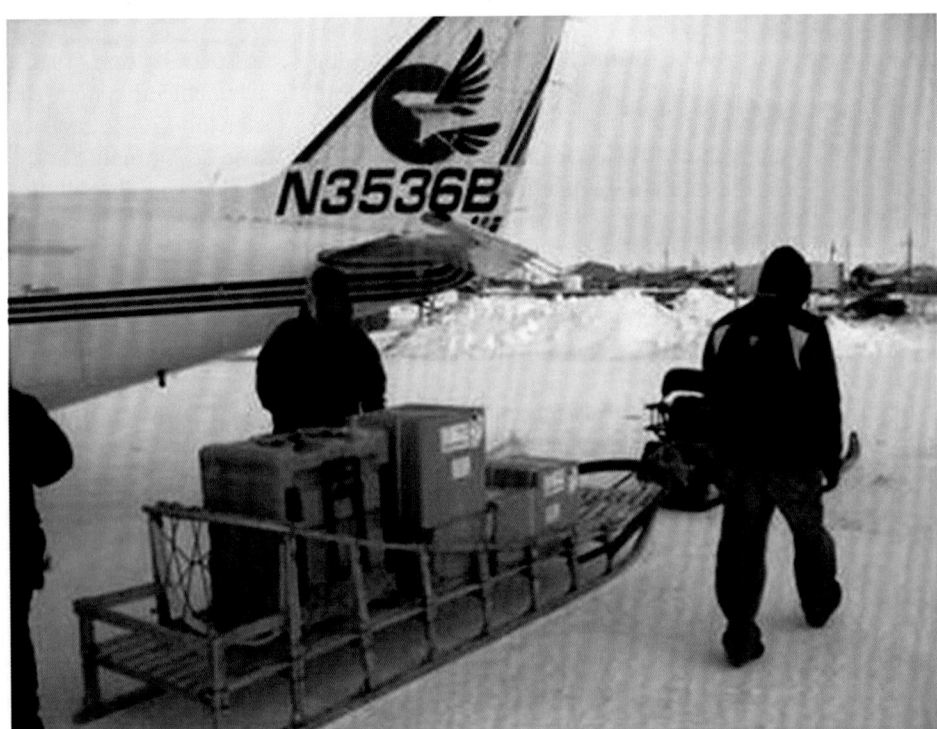

Figure 205.4 Mobile audiology and telemedicine equipment transported to a highly remote Arctic area. Specialty care is provided by a midlevel provider telecommuting store-and-forward cases to specialist in an urban center.

expensive than those delivered through a traditional outpatient clinic, once adequate telemedicine volume was achieved (27). A similar screening service directed at ear disease using a medical van with wireless connectivity served children in remote Australia, with high satisfaction levels for those patients served (28). Telemedicine appears to offer one solution for delivering basic otolaryngology diagnostic services to otherwise underserved pediatric populations.

Head and Neck Oncology

An interesting use of VTC has been for extending the availability of multidisciplinary teams (MDTs) for the diagnosis and management of patients with head and neck cancer. MDTs are used to establish diagnosis, staging, and treatment plans. In addition, they ideally involve specialties such as nutrition and speech pathology to develop comprehensive plans tailored to the patients needs. It can be a challenge to bring together all the participants for MDTs, and there are costs associated with travel and time away from work. Also, MDTs function best when all the necessary information has been prepared and distributed prior to the meeting. VTC has been used to address these issues allowing providers and, at times, patients to participate remotely and share information. Provider satisfaction and cost savings have been demonstrated (29,30).

As MDTs function best when they manage a large number of cases per year, they tend to be offered primarily in major centers. VTCs have allowed for both patients and their local providers from remote areas to fully participate and benefit from fully resourced, more centrally located MDTs (31). In this way, telemedicine again allows for widespread access to concentrated medical expertise.

Home monitoring may become a more important adjunct in the care of head and neck cancer patients as devices and services become more widely available. Pain control, nutrition, and respiratory status can all be monitored remotely, allowing for earlier management at home in the perioperative period. Patients with chronic needs could benefit from regular virtual nursing "visits" addressing concerns and identifying and intervening on problems early. Patient education and family involvement can also be promoted using videoconferencing made available through home devices.

Excellent images of the nasopharynx, nasal cavity, oral cavity, pharynx, and larynx can be obtained and transmitted using standard rigid endoscopes and cameras. Formal studies examining the diagnostic accuracy of transmitted images for head and neck tumors have not been done.

Laryngology and Speech Disorders

With advances in endoscopes and imaging technology, it has become a relatively routine matter to visualize and image the larynx. Most family practitioners and emergency room physicians are trained in the use of flexible scopes, though recognition of pathology is often a difficult task for the occasional examiner of the larynx. A means by which to easily obtain the opinion of an otolaryngologist would be useful. There has been some work showing that asynchronous examination of either still laryngeal images or short video clips correlates well with in-person examination (32,33). Flexible laryngoscope images transmitted by VTC to a consulting otolaryngologist have been used to establish diagnosis and treatment plans for US military personnel (34). It is now possible to capture and transmit short video clips of a dynamic laryngeal exam using an S&F platform, which creates interesting possibilities for asynchronous expert consultation. Technologic advances, such as high-resolution distal chip camera endoscopes that allow for improved digital images of the larynx, may lead to more interest in developing telemedicine applications for laryngology.

For speech disorders, telemedicine applications are being investigated for both diagnosis and treatment. Early work indicates that it may be feasible to identify some voice disorders by analyzing remotely transmitted voice, using either standard telephone networks or voice over the Internet (35,36). Automated systems could be set up to facilitate screening for new diagnoses or monitoring of existing voice disorders. VTC has been used to deliver speech pathology services to remote patient populations. In small studies, efficacy has been shown to be comparable to standard in-person speech therapy, and patient acceptance has been good (37). Given that speech pathology can be very difficult to make available to isolated or underserved populations, telemedicine holds great promise to address this problem (38).

Facial Plastics and Trauma

Images have long been used in facial plastics for the purposes of documentation, planning, and follow-up, though a role for remote diagnosis and consultation is still being developed. Telemedicine has established utility in the field of dermatology, and high-quality images transmitted to a consultant dermatologist have been shown to have comparable diagnostic accuracy to an in-person evaluation for conditions such as skin malignancy (39). In remote Alaska, transmittal of store-and-forward images to consultants at a regional trauma center has been used to remotely give advice on wound closure for traumatic soft tissue facial injuries. For more severe injuries and for patients with facial fractures, a combination of photographic and radiologic images "packaged" with clinical histories is used to make triage decisions and to assist in preoperative planning (40). With the widespread availability of "smartphones," patients can take and send their own images for review. Interesting early work is being done with this model, and patient-generated telemedicine may play an increasing role in the future, especially in the area of facial plastics (41).

Telemedicine in the Operating Room

Telemedicine can be used to bring remotely located expertise into the operating room, allowing a more experienced or specialized surgeon to advise and mentor another surgeon both before and during an operation. Telementoring may involve the use of image review and even computer simulation prior to an operation to plan a procedure and receive input from a remotely located surgeon (42). During an operation, VTC can be employed so that the remotely located surgeon may counsel the surgeon performing the operation. This method of remote consultation has successful applications for endoscopic sinus surgery where the video from the endoscope is fed simultaneously to both surgeons (43) and a VTC connection has been used to supply intraoperative consultations for other complicated procedures to surgeons in remote Pacific islands (44). Remote monitoring and intraoperative testing for cochlear implantation surgery have been shown to be cost-effective and to maximize the availability of audiologists skilled in this area (45). The advent of robotic surgery presents the possibility that telesurgery, where a remotely located surgeon controls the robotic device, may someday become clinically applicable.

BARRIERS TO ADOPTION

Cost of technology, immature telecommunications infrastructure, and lack of evidence of clinical utility were often reasons that initial interest in telemedicine did not progress to actual clinical use. In the past, the barriers to entry were simply too high for most physicians, practices, and health care systems. For example, the costs of a dedicated VTC system were close to being prohibitive. Many of these previous problems have been resolved. The situation is different today with other challenges that need to be addressed.

One key barrier to adoption of telemedicine is the learning curve and hesitation associated with a new technology and confidence that the technology is a solution to the user's problem (46–48). The adoption of technology by the typical American consumer is making this less of an issue, as comfort using software, smartphones, and tablet PCs has disseminated into the workplace.

There are additional economic, organizational, and behavioral knowledge barriers that inhibit the diffusion of telemedicine (49). Further barriers to setting up a telemedicine program are related to organizational communication and structure (50).

The most perplexing issues facing telemedicine are more sociopolitical. They have been identified during the early growth of telemedicine and include (a) interstate licensing and institutional credentialing of physicians, (b) legal liability and litigation, (c) individual client or patient autonomy and right to privacy, (d) reimbursement, (e) knowledge about telemedicine, and (f) system design and infrastructure (51).

Licensure and Credentialing

A telemedicine encounter by its nature may create a licensure and credentialing quandary; the patient may reside in a different state where the consulting physician may not hold a license and may be receiving care at a facility at which the consulting provider may not be credentialed. In general, the consulting provider must have a license to practice medicine in the state from which the patient is presented. The state-based licensure model makes it more difficult to easily expand telemedicine across state lines. Some states have addressed this issue with consultation exceptions, reciprocity agreements, or special telemedicine licenses. There is some interest in a joint state–federal approach to designate a national telemedicine license (52). More likely, the state model will be retained, but efficiencies in multi-licensure will grow with entities such as the federal credentialing verification service. The federal health care system requires physicians to have only one state medical license. The Veteran's Administration, Department of Defense, and Indian Health Service have been able to take advantage of this to grow cross-state telemedicine.

The consulting provider also needs to be credentialed at the originating facility. Again, advocacy groups are proposing less onerous "credentialing by proxy" rules that would allow facilities to enter agreements whereby for the purposes of providing telemedicine, the consulting provider need only apply and obtain full credentials at one facility. At the time of this writing, clarification on credentialing for telemedicine is forthcoming from CMS (Center for Medicaid and Medicare Services.)

Professional Liability

Providers interested in offering care through telemedicine would be best advised to discuss their coverage with their carrier. The authors are unaware of instances where coverage was denied specifically for medical care within the provider's scope of practice delivered through telemedicine.

The experience delivering neurotology care by means of telemedicine to patients in post-Katrina New Orleans gives an excellent recounting of how the barriers described above were addressed to allow for this program to carry forward, giving a sense of what difficulties the current environment presents (24).

Reimbursement

Past Medicare rules allowed reimbursement only for VTC in rural areas. A professional fee was paid to the consulting provider, and a small facility fee was paid to the origination site. Reimbursement for VTC was extremely low considering the technology and network costs and the time commitment required of the providers for a typical VTC session. This made VTC impractical in the fee for service environment. This situation essentially persists today, and a strong economic case for VTC can be made only in a systems context where savings such as avoided patient travel costs offset the costs of VTC and provider time commitment. Adoption of VTC for the provision of otolaryngology services outside of systems such as the US military will require a different economic model. The cost of VTC has dropped significantly with the advent of excellent, low-cost web cameras and the ability to do VTC over the Internet rather than on more expensive dedicated point to point networks. This coupled with changes in the reimbursement model could lead to a wider array of economically feasible clinical applications.

The reimbursement environment for S&F telemedicine is variable by state and payer and therefore complex and confusing. At least 21 states currently offer Medicaid reimbursement for telemedicine services, some of which include S&F: Alaska, Arkansas, California, Georgia, Hawaii, Illinois, Iowa, Kansas, Kentucky, Louisiana, Minnesota, Montana, Nebraska, North Carolina, North Dakota, Oklahoma, South Dakota, Texas, Utah, Virginia, and West Virginia, and each state has its own guidelines for dealing with reimbursement (53,54).

Reimbursement for two forms of S&F telemedicine—teleradiology and telepathology—has long been allowed, and successful business plans for both exist. In Alaska, Medicaid began to offer reimbursement for telehealth for both "store-and-forward" and live videoconferencing in 2002. Alaska Medicaid established a practice of reimbursing S&F encounters using the evaluation and management coding system, stipulating that a GQ modifier be used to designate S&F telemedicine. Private insurers eventually adopted this practice, and now most in Alaska reimburse for S&F telemedicine at rates equivalent to a face-to-face encounter coded at a similar level.

In both Arizona and New Mexico, a flat fee structure has been designed for this purpose. The ATA has been active in lobbying for a comprehensive national policy for S&F telemedicine reimbursement. Until that is achieved, providers should check with payers in their state for their current policy. Until there is more clarity and predictability about reimbursement for S&F otolaryngology, it will be difficult to develop the business case for it in the fee for service environment.

Program Building and the Problem of Scale

The benefits of telemedicine are best seen in the context of a program or a health care system, where a coordinated network of providers delivers care using telemedicine to a population of patients, matching clinical need with the capacity to meet that need. A successful telemedicine program depends on a well thought-out and executed plan that addresses the many aspects that underlie a telemedicine effort. Technology must be assessed and selected to best suit clinical needs, and it must be assessed on an ongoing basis, as devices in particular evolve rapidly. Workflows need to be planned to deliver consistent service

and to ensure that telemedicine is never a "step-down" from traditional face-to-face medicine. Transitions to traditional medicine need to be smooth and efficient when the patient's needs can no longer be met by telemedicine. Providers, both initiating and consulting, must be trained initially and recurrently to maintain high-quality standards and to accommodate for new technologies. Organizational and administrative support in the form of business planning and operations, legal assistance, contracting, and marketing are important. Since telemedicine by its nature occurs between a patient and at least two providers and often in a very immediate fashion, the building and maintaining of relationships between providers is essential. Finally, telemedicine is a new and rapidly changing area of health care delivery for which there is no true "gold standard" or established "right way" to emulate. Those entering the world of telemedicine need to be flexible and creative and understand that constant troubleshooting and adjustment to changing situations are to be expected.

The problem of scale is unique to S&F telemedicine and is essentially the problem of matching capacity to demand. While a consultant can only physically see one patient at a time in their clinic or only be involved in one VTC at time, there is virtually no limit to how many S&F cases can be sent to a consultant in any period of time. When serving a large population of patients or a large number of referring providers, this can become a difficult workload problem. The potential answer to this problem lies in "scaling up" by creating a network of consultants, possibly geographically distant or time zone disparate, who can be recruiting in to handle heavy workload as needed. This is possible since telemedicine holds the possibility of routing workload to available providers without restriction by location or time zone. This model has been effectively applied by commercial teleradiology reading services.

Future Directions

The future in telemedicine is exciting. New technologies are rapidly emerging and will undoubtedly change the telemedicine space radically. High-definition technologies have already substantially upgraded the quality of VTC and will soon lead to enhanced ability to capture still images of extraordinary high quality. A new generation of home monitoring devices will result in telemedicine extending into the home of many patients and will change how care is delivered for chronic conditions and for preventive care. Improvements in broadband infrastructure should make telemedicine available to larger segments of the population and should improve its quality and speed. The ability to perform VTC over the Internet rather than over dedicated networks has already made VTC more available and has drastically dropped its cost. Finally, Accountable Care Organizations will have very strong financial incentives to reduce costs through the improved management of chronic disease, early diagnosis of conditions, and enhanced provider efficiency. It is expected that telemedicine will be an important tool in the integrated care delivery plans for these organizations.

With the adoption of EHRs and emerging health information exchange networks, health care data will be made available for physicians located distances from the patients. Compilation of the information and remote access will indeed have an impact on telemedicine as practice workflows adopt and change.

Probably the most exciting future area of telemedicine is that of mobile health or mHealth. The use of mobile phones worldwide has undergone exponential growth in recent years. As networks become more available, faster, and able to accommodate more data, and as "smartphones" become more capable, their use for personal health care will undoubtedly explode in ways that most of us cannot imagine. This is already occurring with a large number of health-related "apps" coming on the market on a daily basis. Innovative health care systems are experimenting ways to leverage mobile phones to improve efficiency, outcomes, and customer satisfaction. The future consumers and providers of health care are technology savvy and will expect health care to be delivered in a way commensurate with their use and understanding of personal, mobile technology. The evolution of personal health records will further involve the patient in record collection, documentation, and care. It is possible that some day in the near future, "telemedicine" may become an archaic term referring to a past era when health care delivery and telecommunications and technology were somehow distinct and separate.

HIGHLIGHTS

- The three main areas of telemedicine are Interactive VTC, Asynchronous Store-and-Forward (S&F), and RPM.
- With regard to privacy and security standards, telemedicine should be treated no differently than an electronic health record.
- Telemedicine thus far has proven to be most useful in situations where there are remote populations to be served or a shortage of providers.
- Both S&F and VTC have been shown to have useful clinical applications in otology and neurotology.
- Reimbursement, credentialing, and professional liability related to telemedicine currently lack national standardization.

REFERENCES

1. ATA Defining Telemedicine. *http://www.americantelemed.org/learn*
2. Moehr JR, Anglin CR, Schaafsma JP, et al. Video conferencing-based telehealth—its implications for health promotion and health care. *Methods Inf Med* 2005;44(2):334–341.
3. Norman S. The use of telemedicine in psychiatry. *J Psychiatr Ment Health Nurs* 2006;13(6):771–777.
4. Franzini L, Sail KR, Thomas EJ, et al. Costs and cost-effectiveness of a telemedicine intensive care unit program in 6 intensive care units in a large health care system. *J Crit Care* 2011;26(3):329.e1–6.
5. Meyer BC, Raman R, Chacon MR, et al. Reliability of site-independent telemedicine when assessed by telemedicine-naive stroke practitioners. *J Stroke Cerebrovasc Dis* 2008;17(4):181–186.
6. Barneveld Binkhuysen FH, Ranschaert ER. Teleradiology: Evolution and concepts. *Eur J Radiol* 2011;78(2):205–209.
7. Warshaw EM, Hillman YJ, Greer NL, et al. Teledermatology for diagnosis and management of skin conditions: a systematic review. *J Am Acad Dermatol* 2011;64(4):759–772.e21. [Epub Oct 30, 2010.]
8. Weinstein RS, Graham AR, Richter LC, et al. Overview of telepathology, virtual microscopy, and whole slide imaging: prospects for the future. *Hum Pathol* 2009;40(8):1057–1069. [Epub Jun 24, 2009.]
9. Dang S, Dimmick S, Kelkar G. Evaluating the evidence base for the use of home telehealth remote monitoring in elderly with heart failure. *Telemed J E Health* 2009;15(8):783–796.
10. Chumbler NR, Neugaard B, Ryan P, et al. An observational study of veterans with diabetes receiving weekly or daily home telehealth monitoring. *J Telemed Telecare* 2005;11(3):150–156.
11. Finkelstein SM, Speedie SM, Potthoff S. Home telehealth improves clinical outcomes at lower cost for home healthcare. *Telemed J E Health* 2006;12(2):128–136.
12. Latifi R, Peck K, Satava R, et al. Telepresence and telementoring in surgery. *Stud Health Technol Inform* 2004;104:200–206.
13. Whitten P, Mair F. Telesurgery versus telemedicine in surgery—an overview. *Surg Technol Int* 2004;12:68–72.
14. Pedersen S, Hartviksen G, Haga D. Teleconsultation of patients with otorhinolaryngologic conditions. A telendoscopic pilot study. *Arch Otolaryngol Head Neck Surg* 1994;120(2):133–136.
15. Lundberg T, Westman G, Hellstrom S, et al. Digital imaging and telemedicine as a tool for studying inflammatory conditions in the middle ear—evaluation of image quality and agreement between examiners. *Int J Pediatr Otorhinolaryngol* 2008;72(1):73–79. [Epub Nov 5, 2007.]
16. Eikelboom RH, Mbao MN, Coates HL, et al. Validation of tele-otology to diagnose ear disease in children. *Int J Pediatr Otorhinolaryngol* 2005;69(6):739–744. [Epub Feb 16, 2005.]
17. Patricoski C, Kokesh J, Ferguson AS, et al. A comparison of in-person examination and video otoscope imaging for tympanostomy tube follow-up. *Telemed J E Health* 2003;9(4):331–344.
18. Kokesh J, Ferguson AS, Patricoski C. Preoperative planning for ear surgery using store-and-forward telemedicine. *Otolaryngol Head Neck Surg* 2010;143(2):253–257.
19. Singleton RJ, Holman RC, Plant R, et al. Trends in otitis media and myringotomy with tube placement among American Indian/Alaska native children and the US general population of children. *Pediatr Infect Dis J* 2009;28(2):102–107.
20. Patricoski C. Alaska telemedicine: growth through collaboration. *Int J Circumpolar Health* 2004;63(4):365–386.
21. Kokesh J, Ferguson AS, Patricoski C, et al. Digital images for postsurgical follow-up of tympanostomy tubes in remote Alaska. *Otolaryngol Head Neck Surg* 2008;139(1):87–93.
22. Hofstetter PJ, Kokesh J, Ferguson AS, et al. The impact of telehealth on wait time for ENT specialty care. *Telemed J E Health* 2010;16(5):551–556.
23. Kokesh J, Ferguson AS, Patricoski C, et al. Traveling an audiologist to provide otolaryngology care using store-and-forward telemedicine. *Telemed J E Health* 2009;15(8):758–763.
24. Arriaga MA, Nuss D, Scrantz K, et al. Telemedicine-assisted neurotology in post-Katrina Southeast Louisiana. *Otol Neurotol* 2010;31(3):524–527.
25. Zapala DA, Stamper GC, Shelfer JS, et al. Safety of audiology direct access for medicare patients complaining of impaired hearing. *J Am Acad Audiol* 2010;21(6):365–379.
26. Smith AC, Dowthwaite S, Agnew J, et al. Concordance between real-time telemedicine assessments and face-to-face consultations in paediatric otolaryngology. *Med J Aust* 2008;188(8):457–460.
27. Xu CQ, Smith AC, Scuffham PA, et al. A cost minimisation analysis of a telepaediatric otolaryngology service. *BMC Health Serv Res* 2008;8:30.

28. Elliott G, Smith AC, Bensink ME, et al. The feasibility of a community-based mobile telehealth screening service for Aboriginal and Torres Strait Islander children in Australia. *Telemed J E Health* 2010;16(9):950–956. [Epub Oct 29, 2010.]

29. Savage SA, Nixon I, MacKenzie K. Teleconferencing in the management of head and neck cancer. *Clin Otolaryngol* 2007;32(2):130–132.

30. Stalfors J, Björholt I, Westin T. A cost analysis of participation via personal attendance versus telemedicine at a head and neck oncology multidisciplinary team meeting. *J Telemed Telecare* 2005;11(4):205–210.

31. Stalfors J, Lundberg C, Westin T. Quality assessment of a multidisciplinary tumour meeting for patients with head and neck cancer. *Acta Otolaryngol* 2007;127(1):82–87.

32. Furukawa M, Furukawa MK, Mizojiri G, et al. Telemedicine in laryngology. *Telemed J* 1998;4(4):329–333.

33. Lemonnier LA, Treadway CK, Ho-Sheng L, et al. The feasibility of telemedicine in fiberoptic laryngology. *Laryngoscope* 2010;120:S10.

34. Haegen TW, Cupp CC, Hunsaker DH. Teleotolaryngology: a retrospective review at a military tertiary treatment facility. *Otolaryngol Head Neck Surg* 2004;130(5):511–518.

35. Wormald RN, Moran RJ, Reilly RB, et al. Performance of an automated, remote system to detect vocal fold paralysis. *Ann Otol Rhinol Laryngol* 2008;117(11):834–838.

36. Zhu Y, Witt RE, MacCallum JK, et al. Effects of the Voice over Internet Protocol on perturbation analysis of normal and pathological phonation. *Folia Phoniatr Logop* 2010;62(6):288–296. [Epub Jun 28, 2010.]

37. Grogan-Johnson S, Alvares R, Rowan L, et al. A pilot study comparing the effectiveness of speech language therapy provided by telemedicine with conventional on-site therapy. *J Telemed Telecare* 2010;16(3):134–139. [Epub Mar 2, 2010.]

38. Mashima PA, Doarn CR. Overview of telehealth activities in speech-language pathology. *Telemed J E Health* 2008;14(10):1101–1117.

39. Tadros A, Murdoch R, Stevenson JH. Digital image referral for suspected skin malignancy—a pilot study of 300 patients. *J Plast Reconstr Aesthet Surg* 2009;62(8):1048–1053. [Epub Oct 10, 2008.]

40. Kokesh J, Ferguson AS, Patricoski C. Telehealth in Alaska: delivery of health care services from a specialist's perspective. *Int J Circumpolar Health* 2004;63(4):387–400.

41. Moumoulidis I, Mani N, Patel H, et al. A novel use of photo messaging in the assessment of nasal fractures. *J Telemed Telecare* 2007;13(8):387–390.

42. Klapan I, Vranjes Z, Risavi R, et al. Computer-assisted surgery and computer-assisted telesurgery in otorhinolaryngology. *Ear Nose Throat J* 2006;85(5):318–321. [Review.]

43. Burgess LP, Syms MJ, Holtel MR, et al. Telemedicine: teleproctored endoscopic sinus surgery. *Laryngoscope* 2002;112(2):216–219.

44. Holtel MR, Burgess LP. Telemedicine in otolaryngology. *Otolaryngol Clin North Am* 2002;35(6):1263–1281.

45. Shapiro WH, Huang T, Shaw T, et al. Remote intraoperative monitoring during cochlear implant surgery is feasible and efficient. *Otol Neurotol* 2008;29(4):495–498.

46. Attewell P. Technology diffusion and organizational learning: the case of business computing. *Org Sci* 1992;3:1–19.

47. Fichman RG, Kemerer CF. The assimilation of software process innovations: an organizational learning perspective. *Manage Sci* 1997;43:1345–1363.

48. Bashshur RL. Critical issues in telemedicine. *Telemed J* 1997;3(2):113–126.

49. Tanriverdi H, Iacono CS. Diffusion of telemedicine: a knowledge barrier perspective. *Telemed J* 1999;5(3):223–244.

50. Whitten PS, Allen A. Analysis of telemedicine from an organizational perspective. *Telemed J* 1995;1(3):203–213.

51. Sanders JH, Bashshur RL. Challenges to the implementation of telemedicine. *Telemed J* 1995;1(2):115–123.

52. Jacobsen PD, Selvin E. Licensing telemedicine: the need for a national system. *Telemed J eHealth* 2000;6(4):429–439.

53. Naditz A. Medicare's and Medicaid's new reimbursement policies for telemedicine. *Telemed eHealth* 2008;14(1):21–24.

54. Palsbo SE. Medicaid payment for telerehabilitation. *Arch Phys Med Rehabil* 2004;85(7):1188–1191.

206 Quality Improvement in Otolaryngology

Rahul K. Shah   Jean Brereton   David W. Roberson

The otolaryngologist may sometimes feel that the word "quality" is used by everyone, in every situation, to address every issue and to mean whatever the speaker or writer wishes it to mean. The busy physician may be pardoned if he/she concludes that the term has no fixed meaning and that it is safe to tune out of any conversation where it comes up.

This chapter starts by trying not to define quality in medicine but to at least characterize it. We then make the case that, while the term is overused, there is a core set of principles and behaviors that can substantially improve the life of the otolaryngologist and his/her patients.

Quality in medicine refers to two very different, but complementary, things:

1. The rigorous measurement of actual outcomes and the use of that data to drive improvement
2. A set of principles and behaviors that have been shown to bring about improvements in a wide variety of diverse complex systems, including medicine and surgery

There is a large body of literature and practical experience about each of these domains. Much is known about how to measure real-world outcomes of complex processes, including medical and surgical care. Much is also known about how one can successfully bring about improvement in a complex organization (such as a physician practice, a hospital, or an operating room) (1).

Although the skills and practices needed for each domain are very different, it should be obvious that the two processes are complementary. If one sets out to improve a complex organization, it will be helpful to know whether the resulting outcomes are better, worse, or the same. Similarly, there is little if any value to measuring outcomes rigorously unless one has tools with which to improve low-performing organizations.

In order to provide a context for the quality improvement (QI) efforts within medicine, this chapter reviews the historical background for quality in surgery and medicine and the specific data in otolaryngology. Next, we describe the role of measurement for QI and discuss the organizations that are trying to create valid measures in medicine today and some of the current and future external standards for quality. We then discuss the performance of complex systems and how some organizations achieve high performance in complex systems and conclude with a very basic primer on how to engage in local QI.

HISTORICAL BACKGROUND

The concept of QI in medicine is not novel; some of our current-day practices were espoused by surgeons decades ago (2,3). Dr. Ernest Avery Codman (1869 to 1940) conceived of what he called "The End Result Idea" in Boston in the first decade of the 20th century (2,3). By rigorously following outcomes, he demonstrated that some surgeons far outperformed others and justified the need for specialization and extra training in specific surgical domains (2,3). He was essentially forced out of organized medicine and converted his home to a surgical hospital (2,3). It is impossible to know to what extent he was forced out because his ideas were threatening and to what extent his undiplomatic approach contributed. One high point of his not-so-subtle approach was distributing, at a meeting of the Boston county surgical society, a caricature of the Boston medical system that included (among other things) a caricature of the president of Harvard, musing "Could my clinical professors make a living without humbug?" (2,3).

Codman's work was later validated in many venues. He was one of the first surgeons to advocate for a surgical morbidity and mortality conference, now almost universal. He later chaired the committee for Standardization of Hospital for the American College of Surgeons—which ultimately morphed into the Joint Commission. Dr. Codman might be impressed with our surgical virtuosity and the technical advances within our hospitals, but he would surely be extremely disappointed that most of us still do not follow the "End Result System" (2,3).

Much as the Flexner report in 1910 revolutionized and codified the medical education process, the Institute of Medicine's (IOM) 2000 report, To Err is Human, is seen by many as a watershed moment in our awareness of patient safety and quality (4). This report did not present any new data, but it did organize and synthesize the vast body of existing data on medical error and called it out publically and prominently. While some argued that the estimate of over 100,000 preventable deaths annually from extrapolated data from one state was unfair, subsequent research has generally indicated that the IOM report did "size" the problem reasonably accurately (4). The result has been a decade of tremendous contributions in the literature and actual improvement in outcomes for patients and hospitals. The initiatives have been broad based—from pediatrics to geriatrics and from private practices toward health systems.

QUALITY IN OTOLARYNGOLOGY: THE EVIDENCE IN OUR SPECIALTY

As noted above, some have doubted the conclusion of the IOM report, To Err is Human, about the number of errors and adverse events in American medicine. Specialty-specific data within otolaryngology have been generally confirmatory (5,6). A study of self-reports in a survey methodology revealed that approximately 2,500 preventable deaths occur annually in otolaryngology! (5). Aside from the mortalities, the study highlighted zones of risk for surgery. Specific areas where errors could be potentially ameliorated include zones of high risk, such as sinus surgery, surgery around major cranial nerves, use of concentrated epinephrine, and the immediate perioperative period (5). Targeted research has been performed to specifically address each of these areas and have further supported these areas as zones of risk.

Definitions

An *adverse event* is defined as a negative consequence resulting from medical treatment (4,7,8), and a *medical error* has multiple definitions, but the most broadly termed is an incorrect plan or failure to execute a correct plan (4,7,8). Some errors cause adverse events and some do not. Likewise, some adverse events are due to errors and some are not. For example, a patient with culture-positive streptococcal pharyngitis who is treated with amoxicillin and has anaphylaxis to the amoxicillin has experienced an adverse event, although there was no error. An error would be prescribing amoxicillin to a patient with a documented allergy to amoxicillin. This error might or might not lead to a reaction (an adverse event).

Currently, a great deal of effort is being put into reducing medical error. The goal is to reduce preventable adverse events (broadly defined as those adverse events which are due to errors). Adverse events not due to errors (e.g., mucositis from a correct dose of chemotherapy) might be considered unpreventable. However, this has not always proven to be true. When the senior author of this chapter (DWR) was a resident, ventilator-associated pneumonia affected about 10% of patients on ventilators, and was considered an unavoidable adverse event. With the advent of ventilator management bundles, ventilator-associated pneumonia has become quite rare in the United States. Thus the line between what is "preventable" and what is "unpreventable" may be at times unclear, and innovative thinking can allow us to prevent complications once thought unavoidable.

THE ROLE OF MEASUREMENT IN QI

There are two fundamental differences in the way that measurement is performed for QI purposes, compared to the measurement that is done for basic or clinical research (Tables 206.1 and 206.2):

1. For local improvement efforts, the overriding concern is that measurement should be inexpensive. Perfect accuracy and statistical significance are secondary considerations.
2. To compare physicians, hospitals, or health care systems, one needs not just measures but *metrics*—defined by Webster as "standards for measurement." All players need to measure something the same way in order for comparisons to be fair.

Most of us are trained to perform basic and/or clinical research. Extremely rigorous measurement, and an insistence on statistical validity, is the norm. In local clinical QI processes, the best measures are the cheapest ones—because you can afford to make them and afford to repeat them. When your practice introduces a new "check-in" form, you do not have the time, personnel, or money to study its effect with scientific rigor. Instead, you will use some type of "quick and dirty" measure of success. Often the measure will be as simple as asking your receptionist if it is working well. If it's not obvious there has been a change, you might go so far as to track check-in times for a couple of weeks. It would be foolish and wasteful to try to prove that the new form is better or worse with statistical significance. For ongoing improvement efforts, the major measurement consideration is opportunity cost, and one should strive for the simplest, roughest measure that will provide useful (even if imperfect) information. *One of the biggest obstacles to local improvement is the insistence on "scientific quality" data when "quick and dirty" measures should be used.*

TABLE 206.1	KEY DIFFERENCES IN MEASUREMENT IN RESEARCH VERSUS QUALITY: LOCAL QI EFFORTS

	Measurement for Local QI	
	Research	**Quality**
Measurement accuracy	*"Get it right"* Goal is perfect accuracy.	*"Spend wisely"* The resources for quality measurement are finite, and there are many important things to measure. Measuring something perfectly will usually take resources away from measurement of other important things. We should spend the least amount of money and human resources possible to get reasonably accurate information.
Data-based decision-making	*"Is P < 0.05?"* Clinical practice will not typically alter unless convincing statistical evidence builds up that a new treatment/process is better.	*"What do we think is the best decision?"* Quality is more like clinical medicine. Just as we must often make a clinical decision for a patient without perfect data, in quality, we often have to make decisions about our department and our processes without perfect data. If data are suggestive but not statistically significant that, for example, there is a problem or an area for improvement, the important question is not "Is $P < 0.05$?" but "Do we believe that this is concerning and we should do something about it?"
Follow-up	*"Next case"* There is no universal standard for performing follow-up research studies. Large studies are often elaborate, expensive, and only possible as "one-offs."	*"Never stop checking"* Important domains should be monitored forever since change can sneak in anytime. Ongoing monitoring provides a way of checking in case decisions made with imperfect data (see above) turn out to be wrong.

On the other hand, if your results are to be compared with your peers' results in public (e.g., on a government Web site), you would wish to insist on very rigorous measurement using fair, risk-adjusted data. When measures are used for comparison purposes, once again there is an important difference between the sorts of measures that most physicians are familiar with and the *metrics* that must be used for quality purposes. To compare different physicians or institutions, one must use rigorously defined metrics, in which every player uses the same definitions of (a) which patients are to be included, (b) what a "success" or "failure" is, and (c) exactly how the measurement will be performed. In addition, most metrics also require risk adjustment, since different physicians or hospitals may treat very different patient populations—and risk adjustment for many types of medical and surgical care is very difficult. But the point is that, under quality metrics, we are not free to define "success" or failure as we wish—everyone must work

TABLE 206.2	KEY DIFFERENCES IN MEASUREMENT IN RESEARCH VERSUS QUALITY: METRIC DEVELOPMENT

	Metric Development for "High Stakes" or Public Reporting and Comparison	
	Research	**Quality**
"Measurement" versus "Metric"	*"My way or the highway"* Each researcher must define for himself/herself how to measure clinical "success" or "failure." Rarely possible to compare fairly across institutions/settings.	*"Get on the bus"* Metric = "Standard for measurement" A metric is a rigorous definition of how to conduct a particular measurement. Only when different institutions agree on metrics can meaningful benchmarking take place. It is important to use accepted metrics, even if we do not feel they are the "ideal" definition.

with the same definitions. Naturally, it is rare that everyone agrees on what the correct metric is. Physicians, independent by nature, would often prefer to publish their personal definition of success in stapedectomy or cancer surgery. In clinical research this is normal, but in quality comparison metrics it completely defeats the purpose.

It is extraordinarily difficult to create good metrics for most clinical medicine and surgery. It is instructive to consider cases where metric development has succeeded and has indeed driven improvement.

One resounding success has been The Society of Thoracic Surgeons' surgical data registry, which now captures almost all cardiac cases done in the United States (9). This database has demonstrated significant variability between different hospitals and systems and served as a major impetus for improvement and reduction in postoperative mortality (9). The reasons that this database has been successful are that (a) cardiac surgeons repeatedly perform hundreds or thousands of very similar operations, (b) the vast majority of cardiac surgical complications are in just a few categories (death, cardiac arrest, stroke, venous thrombosis, and pulmonary embolus), and (c) cardiac surgery has a significant, measurable frequency of "nongameable" adverse events. It is easy to determine even from hospital administrative data if patients survived to discharge. Thus the measurement challenge, while very large, could be overcome with persistence.

Another huge success has been the sharing and distribution of data on cystic fibrosis (CF) outcomes. There is no question that this has spurred underperforming centers to improve and higher-performing centers to strive to "stay ahead," with the result that overall outcomes have improved considerably over the last decades (10). The reasons for this success are also similar. CF patients are almost all treated in CF centers; they usually spend most or all of their lives under the care of one center; there is an appreciable mortality (a non-gameable outcome) and an intermediate clinical outcome (FEV1) that is extraordinarily tightly linked to ultimate outcome (risk of death) (10). Therefore, CF centers can compare themselves to each other by looking at fairly simple measures of mortality and FEV1, with reasonable accuracy.

Consider how much more difficult it will be to compare two different otolaryngologists' performances at treating sinus disease. Major complications are extremely rare. Minor complications are highly "gameable"—it is difficult or impossible to determine with certainty whether or not every patient has a postoperative infection or transient bleeding. Few of us collect validated outcome data on our patients' results. There is no good risk-stratification system to indicate which patients are likely to be refractory to all treatment. Finally, the true measure of our success with sinus disease would measure how we do with all our patients—not just the ones who require surgery. The need to measure our performance at the medical aspect of management will be confounded by the fact that in some locations, the medical management is primarily done by allergists, internists, pediatricians, and family practitioners, while in other settings, the otolaryngologist may do much of the nonsurgical management. A measure that focused only on surgical outcomes, for example, would "reward" an otolaryngologist who performed unnecessary surgery on patients with mild, self-limited sinus disease. It is fallacious to argue, as some have done (footnote Porter and Teisberg, Redefining Health Care), that because measurement has improved care in relatively straightforward situations such as CF and cardiac surgery, it will be easy to extend this strategy to all conditions. Many national organizations, including the American Academy of Otolaryngology-Head and Neck Surgery (AAO-HNS), are working hard to develop valid metrics for many medical and surgical conditions, but the task is extremely difficult.

ORGANIZATIONS ENDORSING QUALITY MEASURES OR MEASURING QUALITY

There are myriad organizations, both public and private, that constitute the health care quality landscape. As many of these are involved in measuring, assessing, and reporting on physicians and the clinical care that they provide, we have included a brief description of some of the major entities tied to physician quality; however, this is not an exhaustive list, and, with the implementation of health care reform, the list will most certainly continue to expand. As of this writing (2011), it is fair to say that the national landscape of quality measurement organizations is cluttered. Some of these organizations will certainly survive; some may collapse or become superfluous; new ones may also be founded. An alphabetical listing of some of the important quality organizations on the national landscape, and a brief description of each, follows here.

Agency for Health Care Quality and Research

The Agency for Health Care Quality and Research (AHRQ) is a government agency within the Department of Health and Human Services that evaluates quality and safety in the delivery of health care, helps translate what works in health care, provides funding for health services research, and partners with both the public and private sectors in how to improve the health care delivery models.

Ambulatory Quality Alliance

The Ambulatory Quality Alliance (AQA) is a multi-stakeholder group (i.e., clinicians, health plans, consumer groups, employer groups) that is focused on improving quality and patient safety of health care in the outpatient setting. The group looks at the effectiveness of health care delivery by determining best practice in performance measurement, data integrity, and public reporting. The AQA is unique in that in attempts to have multi-stakeholders convene, they can potentially align the stakeholders and secure broader-based support (11).

Centers for Medicare/Medicaid Services

As the government sponsored (Department of Health and Human Services) provider of Medicare and the oversight organization to State Medicaid programs, Centers for Medicare/Medicaid Services (CMS), the nation's largest insurer, was one of the earliest organizations to develop programs to assess quality in the provision of care and to evaluate the relationship between quality and cost (12). Beginning in the 1980s with the introduction of peer review organizations focused on inappropriate admissions and retrospective review of hospital length of stay, continuing with the adoption of QI organizations in the 1990s that focused on utilization of hospital services as a way to control costs, and most recently with the introduction of Pay for Performance, Compare Web sites, and the Physician Quality Reporting System, the government has been at the forefront of this movement toward the provision of high-quality, effective care with efficient use of resources.

Institute for Healthcare Improvement

The Institute for Healthcare Improvement (IHI) is a non-profit Massachusetts-based institute that strives to optimize patient safety and outcomes. They are known for the tools and education they provide to health care professionals and the crucial role they play in assisting the prioritization of the myriad initiatives which exist. Indeed, they were so successful that Dr. Berwick, whom was president and chief executive officer of IHI, was recently appointed the head of the Centers for Medicare and Medicaid Services.

Institute of Medicine

The IOM is a nonprofit, nongovernmental organization dedicated to the improvement of health and health care. It is the organization within the National Academy of Sciences that responds to inquiries from governmental and private organizations on health policy issues. In 1999, the IOM produced the landmark report To Err is Human, a report that outlines how medical errors can be prevented and set a mandate to reduce errors by 50% over 5 years (4).

Joint Commission

As noted in this chapter, the Joint Commission can trace its root back to Dr. Codman, whom was always advocating for rigorous study of one's outcomes. At present, the Joint Commission serves many roles, the most prominent being a regulatory accrediting agency. In such a role, they have been pivotal in helping to advocate and push for real gains in transparency of outcomes, benchmarking, and tangible patient safety and QI metrics and results.

National Quality Forum

The National Quality Forum (NQF) is a private, non-profit membership organization concentrated on establishing national patient safety priorities and performance improvement goals. NQF evaluates and endorses measures across a wide spectrum of specialties. NQF is contracted with the US Department of Health and Human Services to develop a process to evaluate and encourage measured development for the nation's top medical conditions, that is, those conditions that account for 95% of Medicare spending (13,14).

Physician Consortium for Performance Improvement

The American Medical Association formed the Physician Consortium for Performance Improvement (PCPI) in 2000 as the first physician-led initiative for the development of evidence-based measures, measure implementation, and outcomes reporting tools. PCPI membership includes representation from over 100 national medical societies and state medical societies as well as the AHRQ, the Council for Medical Specialty Societies, and the American Board of Medical Specialties (ABMS). To date, the PCPI has developed over 30 measure sets and close to 200 individual measures. PCPI measures represent the majority of measures contained with the Center for Medicare and Medicaid Services Physician Quality Reporting System.

Surgical Quality Alliance

The American College of Surgeons convened the Surgical Quality Alliance in 2005 to bring together over 20 surgical specialties (including Otolaryngology—Head and Neck Surgery) and anesthesia to address quality performance in surgery. The group ensures collaboration on quality measures across surgery and provides feedback to federal and private payer policy on issues addressing surgical quality of care (15).

EXTERNAL REQUIREMENTS FOR QUALITY

The ABMS sets the standards for 24 member boards for certification and maintenance of certification including for Otolaryngology—Head and Neck Surgery. In recognition that the boards play a major role in ensuring that physicians are continuously engaged in performance improvement over the course of their careers, they have developed a four-part framework for accessing physician competency (16). The four areas for physician assessment are *Part I* Licensure and professional standing, *Part II* Lifelong learning and periodic self-assessment, *Part III* Cognitive expertise as demonstrated through exam, and *Part IV* Performance in practice. By 2014 physicians must demonstrate assessment of performance in practice and QI (every 2 to 5 years), the use of an approved survey tool that measures physician communication skills, and skill assessment through utilization of peer survey (17). Most medical boards now require physicians to demonstrate quality in their practice. There has been demonstrated value in such as improved outcomes have been associated with board certification/maintenance of certification (18).

QUALITY WITHIN HEALTH CARE INSTITUTIONS

Health System Programs

In response to market-driven competition and financial pressures from employers and payers, and most importantly, in the desire to provide, safe, high-quality care, hospital systems have been at the forefront of the QI movement. Hospitals develop QI programs that assess and measure physician performance across a multitude of clinical quality indicators. Much of this has been driven in response to external forces such as meeting Joint Commission standards, the public reporting of hospital-specific performance measures (CMS' Hospital Compare Web site and similarly from the Leapfrog Group), and pressures from government and private payers. Increasingly health systems executives and their respective boards are placing as much focus on clinical quality as has historically been placed on financial and operational data when assessing hospital performance. It has become clear that such importance to patient safety and quality also drives the financial metrics of the institutions. Hospital departments are being asked to provide specialty-specific measures as their hospitals embark on organization-wide QI programs, and performance on these measures is being taken into account in the development of physician compensation programs as well as for regulatory compliance with Ongoing Professional Practice Evaluation (OPPE) from the Joint Commission. Fortunately with the convergence of a robust information technology infrastructure in health care, much of these efforts and analysis have been made easier with continued implementation of electronic health records at the system level (19).

Department-Specific Initiatives

Starting in 2008, every health system was required to assess physician performance with regard to the six core competencies defined by the Joint Commission, the ABMS, and the American Council for Graduate Medical Education. Previously, these six areas of assessment were utilized solely in the assessment of house officers, but the Joint Commission has now extended these requirements to every physician on a hospital's medical staff. Called the OPPE, the core areas measured are Medical/Clinical Knowledge, Patient Care, Interpersonal Skills and Communication, Practice-Based Learning, Professionalism, and System-Based

Practice. If there are issues identified with individual physician performance or if a physician is new to the hospital or is seeking privileges for a procedure, the physician may be assessed utilizing a Focused Professional Performance Evaluation (FPPE), a time-limited period during which an organization evaluates and determines a practitioner's performance in practice. This can be done through chart review, monitoring practice, simulation, or peer review. As these tools, the OPPE and FPPE, are relatively new introductions for physicians to assess quality, there will certainly be iterations to such as the specific measurement tools are developed and trialed (20).

QUALITY AND REIMBURSEMENT

While there have been many gains in quality particularly in the prior couple of decades, improvements have mainly been focused within individual hospitals and health systems and related to specific conditions. For instance, the Joint Commission reported that scores on meeting quality parameters for heart attack, pneumonia, surgery, and childhood asthma rose from 81.8% to 95.4% between 2002 and 2009 (21). However, there has not been consistent, widespread improvement over many health conditions in inpatient and ambulatory health settings (22). To speed the journey and increase the consistency over time of health QI, many hospitals and insurers, including Medicare, have tied improvement in quality metrics to financial incentives associated with compensation (salary incentives) or through enhancements to reimbursement for services rendered (e.g., Pay for Performance programs and CMS' Physician Quality Reporting System). Most of these programs focus on evaluating physician performance across a broad set of measures including those derived from medical records, billing and administrative data, electronic health records, and patient and provider surveys. It is not yet clear to what extent financial incentives can drive fundamental, long-term changes in behavior and health systems, and other physician organizations are looking at a number of approaches (i.e., peer review, public reporting, financial incentives), which taken together may potentially drive lasting change (23).

QUALITY AND HEALTH CARE REFORM

When discussing reform of any nature, it is with caution that the three issues below are highlighted as it maybe, a decade from now, these entities may not even exist or may have been substantially changed by legislation in their scope, etc. In 2010, the Patient Protection and Healthcare Affordable Care Act was signed into law. The act is designed to make significant changes to the delivery and financing of health care in the United States. The goal of health care reform is to eliminate the fragmentation of the current health delivery system and improve health care effectiveness and quality while slowing spending. Two of the major tenets of the legislation were the creation of accountable care organizations (ACOs) and creation of the CMS Innovation Center. The act sets forth the Medicare Shared Savings Program for ACO. What is envisioned is an organization (physician led or hospital) that takes accountability for a set group of Medicare patients and, based on delivering high-quality care and reducing the cost of that care below expected levels, can share in the realized savings. It is anticipated that ACOs could aid in reducing the fragmentary nature of the current health care delivery model and provide vertical integration of care rather than the more traditional horizontal integration of care. The concept is different from shared risk arrangements of the past in that there are built in safeguards against downside risk at least for the initial years of the arrangement. Many of the details of how ACOs would be structured and who will fund the necessary upfront costs have yet to be fully addressed (24). The act also stipulated the creation of the CMS Innovation Center that will create new payment and health services delivery models designed to reduce cost while maintaining and enhancing quality of care. The initial focus of the Innovation Center will be the Partnership for Patients that has the dual purpose of (a) reducing health care–acquired conditions 40% from 2010 to 2013 and (b) reducing hospital readmissions 20% during this time period. It is estimated that in meeting these two measures alone, 60,000 lives could be saved and many complications of care eliminated. The financial impact is purported to be as much as $50 billion in savings over ten years (25).

COMPLEX SYSTEMS AND HIGH PERFORMANCE WITHIN SYSTEMS

Dr. Avedis Donabedian (1919 to 2000) laid the foundation for an understanding of systems science applications to health care QI. His significant contribution was the concept of the framework for QI that included structure, process, and outcome. Much of the organizational QI processes in health care come from his prescient teachings. Systems science is the fundamental concept that in health care, the delivery of care is made up of overlapping systems. These systems interact to ensure the patient is cared for. For example, a critically injured child in a motor vehicle accident is triaged by an emergency medicine team (system) that brings the child to the hospital (system), where the child is managed by the trauma team (system) that decides the patient needs to have surgery (system) and the patient is whisked to the operating room and managed by a cadre of health care professionals (system) that successfully operates on her, and she recuperates on the ward (system) to be discharged without issue back to her home (system).

The myriad systems that one encounters mandate that we consider health care organizations to be amenable to application of concepts of systems science. A spectrum exists as there are, of course, those systems that are exemplars and others that barely function. The later are easy to conjure; the most successful systems include the nuclear industry, airline industry, and chemical manufacturing. Unfortunately, health care lies in the middle of such spectrum. In an effort to imbue health care, specifically, otolaryngology, which such characteristics, it is imperative to identify such so that we can learn from other industries. Systems that function at a very high level with consistent reliability are called high-reliability organizations or high-performance systems. Characteristics of such systems include many variables, the most pertinent to otolaryngology include (1) an understanding that (a) common aims are essential, (b) outstanding systems are created from outstanding elements, (c) complex systems are inherently unpredictable, (d) feedback loops improve performance, (e) standardization improves function for repetitive processes, (f) standardization is the only baseline, (g) shortened cycle time improves function, (h) system features should be driven by system goal, (i) human error is ubiquitous, (j) respect for persons improves systems performance, and (k) strong constructive leadership is essential. A failure by physicians, especially otolaryngologists, to embrace and understand the nuances of high-performance systems will result in inefficiencies and frustrations. An excellent cognitive process is to choose one of the identified characteristics of high-reliability organizations above and apply it to your realm and see the outcomes. For example, try dictating and signing charts immediately—the downstream effects in terms of improved communication, improved patient care, and ultimately outcomes will be eye-opening.

A PRIMER ON LOCAL QI INITIATIVES

It is imperative for surgeons to lead QI initiatives as we are presumably the experts of our patients. However we are not experts on QI projects, as such, in large or academic health systems, you may be able to partner with your patient safety and QI offices. In smaller hospitals or practices, you may have to design your own initiatives. With any QI project, it is important to start small and periodically measure the effect of the intervention. A basic and classic model for a QI initiative is the PDSA cycle. This involves the steps of (P)lanning an intervention, (D)oing the intervention, (S)tudying the impact of the intervention, and (A)cting to improve the outcomes further. This iterative cycle is one of the most basic QI tools.

Nationally, with regard to otolaryngology, there are several anecdotal best practices that have been implemented as QI initiatives. Some of the standout projects include calling posttonsillectomy patients back instead of having them come back to the office for follow-up (26). An example that is not in the peer-reviewed literature was a practice in which, after misadministration of allergy sera to the wrong patient with an untoward outcome, the practice implemented a check where the patient corroborates with the technician that he or she is going to receive the intended allergy sera.

CONCLUSION

"Quality," properly understood, refers to two different but complementary sets of activities:

1. The use of basic, well-known principles to improve processes locally
2. The rigorous measurement of outcomes and the use of that data to drive improvement

The two processes require very different actions and skill sets, but are highly complementary. Every physician should understand the basics of local QI, and every physician should understand what distinguishes local improvement measures from rigorous national metrics. Not every physician can or should be expert in national outcome metrics; it is critical that physicians as groups (e.g., through national specialty societies) are engaged in the process of developing, validating, and deploying national metrics.

HIGHLIGHTS

- There is potential for significant benefit from implementation of QI initiatives in otolaryngology.
- There are fundamental differences in the way that measurement is performed for QI purposes, compared to the measurement that is done for basic or clinical research.
- Nationally, there are several quality organizations that are driving the initiatives on a broad level.
- Quality in medicine can be achieved by application of systems science principles to move organizations toward high-reliability organizations.
- Local QI efforts are easily implemented and can be done successfully by following the (p)lan, (d)o, (s)tudy, and (a)ct cycle.

REFERENCES

1. Roberson DW, Kentala E, Healy GB. Quality and safety in a complex world: why systems science matters to otolaryngologists. *Laryngoscope* 2004;114(10):1810–1814.
2. Rodkey GV, Itani KMF. Evaluation of healthcare quality: a tale of three giants. *Am J Surg* 2009;198(Suppl 5):S3–S8.
3. Brand RA. Ernest Avery Codman, MD, 1869–1940. *Clin Orthop Relat Res* 2009;(467):2763–2765.
4. Kohn L, Corrigan J, Donaldson M. *To Err Is Human: building a safer health system*. Washington, DC: National Academy Press, 2000.
5. Shah RK, Kentala E, Healy GB, et al. Classification and consequences of errors in otolaryngology. *Laryngoscope* 2004;114: 1322–1335.
6. Shah RK, Lander L, Forbes P, et al. Safety on an inpatient pediatric otolaryngology service: many small errors, few adverse events. *Laryngoscope* 2009;119(5):871–879.
7. Rothschild JM, Landrigan CP, Cronin JW. The critical care safety study: the incidence and nature of adverse events and serious medical errors in intensive care. *Crit Care Med* 2005;33:1694–1700.
8. Brennan TA, Leape LL, Laird NM, et al. Incidence of adverse events and negligence in hospitalized patients: results of the Harvard medical practice quality improvement initiative I. *N Engl J Med* 1991;324:370–376.
9. New Initiatives. http://www.sts.org/national-database. Accessed July 16, 2011.
10. Annals of Medicine. The Bell Curve: What happens when patients find out how good their doctors really are. http://newyorker.com/archive/2004/12/06/041206fa_fact. Accessed July 16, 2011.
11. AQA Background: improving clinical quality and consumer decision-making (revised Oct 2010). http://www.aqalliance.org. Accessed May 15, 2011.
12. Chassin MR, Loeb JM. The ongoing quality improvement journey. Next stop, high reliability. *Health Aff (Millwood)* 2011;30(4): 559–568.
13. Corrigan JM, Burstin H. Measuring quality of performance: where is it headed and who is making the decisions? *Curr Clin Pract* 2007;1(1):4–7.
14. http://www.qualityforum.org/. Accessed May 15, 2011.
15. Surgical Quality Alliance. http://www.facs.org/ahp/sqa/index.html. Accessed March 2, 2013.
16. Weiss KB. ABMS maintenance of certification: raising the bar in measuring physician competency. NAMSS *Synergy* Jan-Feb 2009:20–22.
17. ABMS updates: standards for quality, safety. http//www.internalmedicinenews.Ault A.5/15/09 Accessed March 2, 2013
18. Brennan TA, Horwitz RI, Duffy FD, et al. The role of physician specialty board certification status in the quality movement. *JAMA* 2004;292(9):1038–1043.
19. Pham HH, Bernabeo EC, Chesluk BJ, et al. The roles of practice systems and individual effort in quality performance. *BMJ Qual Saf* 2011;20:704–710. DOI:10.1136/bmjqs.2010.048991.
20. Catalano EW, Ruby SG, Talbert ML, et al. College of American Pathologists considerations for the delineation of pathology clinical privileges. *Arch Pathol Lab Med* 2009;133:613–618.
21. Joint Commission reports gains in hospital quality care. http://www.ahanews.com/ahanews_app/jsp/display.jsp?dcrpath=AHANEWS/AHANewsNowArticle/data/ann_092210_TJC&domain=AHANEWS. Accessed June 5, 2011.
22. Chassin MR, Loeb JM. The ongoing quality improvement journey: next stop, high reliability. *Health Aff (Millwood)* 2011;30(4): 559–568.
23. Gosfield AG. Compensation for quality: the next inevitable step medical groups respond to provider payment reform. *Group Pract J* 2008:10–15.
24. Fisher ES, McClellan MB, Bertko J, et al. Fostering accountable health care: moving forward in medicare. *Health Aff (Millwood)* 2009;28:219–231.
25. An Innovative "Menu" of Options for Partnership. http://www.innovations.cms.gov/files/reports/Innovations-Center-Year-One-Summary-document.pdf. Accessed March 2, 2013.
26. Jones DT, Yoon MJ, Licameli G. Effectiveness of postoperative follow-up telephone interviews for patients who underwent adenotonsillectomy: a retrospective study. *Arch Otolaryngol Head Neck Surg* 2007;133(11):1091–1095.

207 | Conflict of Interest

Andrew H. Murr   *Susan J. Murr*

The views expressed in this chapter are the personal views of the authors and do not represent the views of their respective employers.

Conflicts of interest between physicians and industry have received much attention in the headlines lately, perhaps driven by the increasing complexity of potential relationships. Relationships between the physician community and industry are important in helping patients through the development of new medicines and technologies that enable patients to live longer and healthier lives. In short, these relationships are essential to medical innovation. At the same time, these relationships must be managed in a transparent, ethical manner to insure that first and foremost, the best interests of the patient are kept in the forefront. This chapter explores the definition of a conflict using examples from the news, the types of relationships that may pose conflicts, some of the rules governing conflicts, and best practices in the management of conflicts.

DEFINITION OF CONFLICT OF INTEREST

The definition of conflict of interest is variable, but according to Merriam-Webster's online dictionary a conflict of interest is "a conflict between the private interests and the official responsibilities of a person in a position of trust" (1). This conflict may commonly be based upon financial rewards, but it can also be based upon a set of circumstances that achieves a specific outcome. An example of an outcome as a component of a conflict of interest is when a judge must excuse himself or herself because of a type of knowledge or relationship that is possessed that may then skew or give the appearance of skewing the outcome of a legal case. Another term, duality of interest, is used when a person has two roles, which may lead to an influence on judgment. An example of duality of interest is when a board member of a foundation that gives research grants is also part of a team that has applied for one of the foundation's grants.

Several examples of possible perceived conflicts of interest have been prominent in news reports over the past several years, and these examples can be instructive. In 2009, Liz Kowalczyk of the Boston Globe wrote an article about a potential conflict of interest at Massachusetts General Hospital involving Dr. Joseph Biederman who oversaw a study involving risperidone in treating psychosis in children under age 10 between 2002 and 2005. Johnson and Johnson, the company that manufactured the drug via Janssen Pharmaceuticals, had given $700,000 to support the research center at Massachusetts General, and it was reported that Dr. Biederman appeared to have received $1.5 million in consulting and speaking fees from them. This income was allegedly not reported in a timely fashion to Harvard University. Although Dr. Biederman did not own stock in J&J, J&J was alleged to be intimately involved in the research center that Dr. Biederman oversaw. As Dr. Marcia Angell summarized in a comment for the Boston Globe on March 20, 2009, "Even if you have the best intentions, it's hard to remain objective about people who've been so good to you" (2). Whether or not the income and support from J&J influenced the outcome of ongoing research work is unknown. However, large amounts of monetary support for studies in the form of research center support and income and consulting fees can have the appearance of influencing the accumulation of objective results.

Another story depicting a possible conflict of interest involved the development and marketing of an orthopedic hip implant manufactured by DePuy. The implant was developed by several physicians including Dr. Thomas Schmalzried and Dr. Thomas Vail and was known as the ASR Implant. The implant was released in the United States in 2005 without undergoing FDA trials after being used abroad, but by 2008 there were over 200 problems reported with the implant, and by 2009 over 300 problems were reported. A high percentage of reported problems resulted in a need to replace the implant. DePuy was reportedly slow to react to information about problems with the product and continued to market the device. The developers of the device were also reported to be supportive of it even in the face of mounting failure data. Dr. Schmalzried was reported as receiving $3.4 million in payments over a 2-year period for work and royalties related to the device. The company and the physicians were accused of continuing to support the device after data showed it to be failing at a high rate. Finally, DePuy pulled the device from the market (3). Taking this information at face value, news reports speculated that it appeared that financial incentives and profit may have interfered with timely decision making in light of accumulating negative clinical information concerning the clinical performance and failure rate of the device in which the doctors had a financial interest (4).

The main tool used to combat the appearance of conflict of interest is disclosure. Disclosure allows a person with a potential conflict to report the issue prior to beginning work on a study or publication or presentation. In this way, any judgmental body such as an editorial review board or an audience at a lecture can be apprised of the relationship of an individual to a technology or drug or research question. Disclosure also allows the possibility of screening slides or other presentation material by a disinterested third party to make sure that biased information is not being disseminated in a scientific or educational setting that awards educational credits to people who are in the audience. Obviously, one way to control conflict of interest in presented material would be to have a zero tolerance approach whereby any person who has any financial or other interest in a project or outcome would not be welcome to participate in publically speaking or writing about the subject. This extreme position, however, would essentially be a prohibition upon allowing some of the most creative and expert scientists and investigators from being involved in the education process. It would also deter experts from becoming involved in promising investigations that could have translational and commercial applications. Certainly, translational science should be encouraged and not discouraged as the benefit to society as a whole is an overriding principle. As a result, conflict of interest can be managed through a process of transparency rather than being prohibited outright.

CONFLICT OF INTEREST IN PUBLISHING

Because of variability in defining conflict of interest, each journal or publication theoretically can define its own individual set of standards for its authors and readers. Standardization, however, certainly has some advantages. The International Committee of Medical Journal Editors (ICMJE) has recently adopted a standard form for disclosure formally referred to as "ICMJE Form for Disclosure of Potential Conflicts of Interest" (5) (Fig. 207.1). This form has been embraced by many journals including JAMA (6,7). The form is a fairly simple PDF document that has four sections. Section 1 is identifying information. Section 2 elicits information about personal or institutional payment from

a third party to support any aspect of the submitted work. This includes grants, consulting fees, travel support, fees for data monitoring or statistical analysis, fees for writing or reviewing the work, writing assistance or administrative support, or others. Section 3 probes financial activities outside of the submitted work, including relationships present during the 36 months prior to the actual submission. This includes board memberships, consultancies, employment, expert testimony, grants, payment for lectures, payment for manuscript preparation, patents, royalties, payment for developing educational presentations, stock options, travel accommodations and meeting expenses, or other. Finally, Section 4 asks for any other relevant information that the author can think of that may have influenced the work. Section 4 was added after a period of review and comment elicited feedback that itemizing every conceivable conflict, such as conflicts involving spouses or children, is impractical. To resolve this challenge, Section 4 was added as an open-ended section to allow the author to submit any other potential category of conflict that had been missed in the above sections (6). Not every otolaryngology—head and neck surgery–based journal has adopted this ICMJE form, but the thoroughness and thoughtfulness of this form is a relatively concise guide to what would be expected in disclosing all aspects of potential bias when submitting an article for publication consideration.

CONFLICT OF INTEREST IN RESEARCH

Recently, the National Institutes of Health (NIH) proposed the first major overhaul of conflict of interest guidelines in over a decade. Old standards triggered financial reporting at $10,000. The new guidelines require disclosure of support that exceeds $5,000. This includes reporting stock ownership, speaking fees, consulting arrangements, and other financial relationships with foundations or industry. Disclosure of these potential conflicts is to be made to the parent institution, and so the parent institution is therefore tasked with monitoring compliance with ethical standards. The parent institution is also responsible for allowing public scrutiny of any reported disclosure items. As a dual check on reporting, the Patient Protection and Affordable Care Act, commonly known as the Obama Health Care Plan, also included a "sunshine provision" that mandated that industry report to a government database any payment or gift to a physician greater than $10 (8,9).

INSTITUTIONAL CONFLICT OF INTEREST

Individuals are not the only people who can benefit from financial arrangements with industry. Very often, entire institutions have a stake in a certain technology or drug. A case in point involved a situation at the Cleveland Clinic. According to news reports, Delos M. Cosgrove, M.D., was the head of the Cleveland Clinic Foundation and had received royalties from a company called AtriCure.

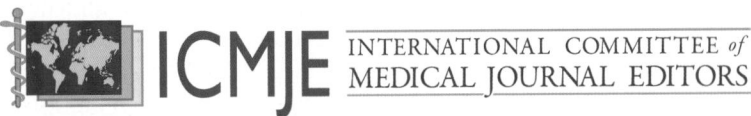

ICMJE Form for Disclosure of Potential Con⊠icts of Interest

The purpose of this form is to provide readers of your manuscript with information about your other interests that could in⊠uence how they receive and understand your work. The form is designed to be completed electronically and stored electronically. It contains programming that allows appropriate data display. Each author should submit a separate form and is responsible for the accuracy and completeness of the submitted information. The form is in four parts.

1. Identifying information.

Enter your full name. If you are NOT the corresponding author please check the box "no" and a space to enter the name of the corresponding author in the space that appears. Provide the requested manuscript information. Double-check the manuscript number and enter it.

2. The work under consideration for publication.

This section asks for information about the work that you have submitted for publication. The time frame for this reporting is that of the work itself, from the initial conception and planning to the present. The requested information is about resources that you received, either directly or indirectly (via your institution), to enable you to complete the work. Checking "No" means that you did the work without receiving any ⊠nancial support from any third party -- that is, the work was supported by funds from the same institution that pays your salary and that institution did not receive third-party funds with which to pay you. If you or your institution received funds from a third party to support the work, such as a government granting agency, charitable foundation or commercial sponsor, check "Yes". Then complete the appropriate boxes to indicate the type of support and whether the payment went to you, or to your institution, or both.

3. Relevant ⊠nancial activities outside the submitted work.

This section asks about your ⊠nancial relationships with entities in the bio-medical arena that could be perceived to in⊠uence, or that give the appearance of potentially in⊠uencing, what you wrote in the submitted work. You should disclose interactions with ANY entity that could be considered broadly relevant to the work. For example, if your article is about testing an epidermal growth factor receptor (EGFR) antagonist in lung cancer, you should report all associations with entities pursuing diagnostic or therapeutic strategies in cancer in general, not just in the area of EGFR or lung cancer.

Report all sources of revenue paid (or promised to be paid) directly to you or your institution on your behalf over the 36 months prior to submission of the work. This should include all monies from sources with relevance to the submitted work, not just monies from the entity that sponsored the research. Please note that your interactions with the work's sponsor that are outside the submitted work should also be listed here. If there is any question, it is usually better to disclose a relationship than not to do so.

For grants you have received for work outside the submitted work, you should disclose support ONLY from entities that could be perceived to be a⊠ected ⊠nancially by the published work, such as drug companies, or foundations supported by entities that could be perceived to have a ⊠nancial stake in the outcome. Public funding sources, such as government agencies, charitable foundations or academic institutions, need not be disclosed. For example, if a government agency sponsored a study in which you have been involved and drugs were provided by a pharmaceutical company, you need only list the pharmaceutical company.

4. Other relationships.

Use this section to report other relationships or activities that readers could perceive to have in⊠uenced, or that give the appearance of potentially in⊠uencing, what you wrote in the submitted work.

1

Figure 207.1 ICMJE disclosure form. This ICMJE disclosure form is designed to provide transparency with regard to any conflicts an author might have in developing material for publication. It succinctly covers most issues likely to be encountered when considering conflict of interest.

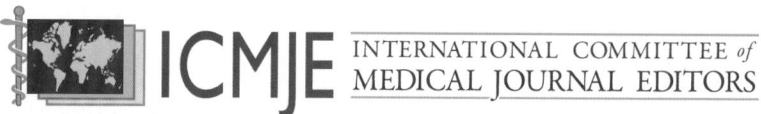

ICMJE Form for Disclosure of Potential Conflicts of Interest

Section 1.   **Identifying Information**

1. Given Name (First Name)

2. Surname (Last Name)

3. Effective Date (07-August-2008)

4. Are you the corresponding author?   ☐ Yes   ☐ No

5. Manuscript Title

6. Manuscript Identifying Number (if you know it)

Section 2.   **The Work Under Consideration for Publication**

Did you or your institution at any time receive payment or services from a third party for any aspect of the submitted work (including but not limited to grants, data monitoring board, study design, manuscript preparation, statistical analysis, etc...)?

Complete each row by checking "No" or providing the requested information. If you have more than one relationship click the "Add" button to add a row. Excess rows can be removed by clicking the "X" button.

The Work Under Consideration for Publication						
Type	No	Money Paid to You	Money to Your Institution*	Name of Entity	Comments**	
1. Grant	☐	☐	☐			✕ / ADD
2. Consulting fee or honorarium	☐	☐	☐			✕ / ADD
3. Support for travel to meetings for the study or other purposes	☐	☐	☐			✕ / ADD
4. Fees for participation in review activities such as data monitoring boards, statistical analysis, end point committees, and the like	☐	☐	☐			✕ / ADD
5. Payment for writing or reviewing the manuscript	☐	☐	☐			✕ / ADD
6. Provision of writing assistance, medicines, equipment, or administrative support	☐	☐	☐			✕

2

Figure 207.1 *(Continued)*

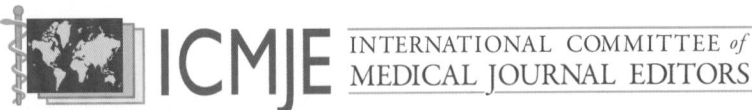

ICMJE Form for Disclosure of Potential Conflicts of Interest

The Work Under Consideration for Publication						
Type	No	Money Paid to You	Money to Your Institution*	Name of Entity	Comments**	ADD
7. Other	☐	☐	☐			✕
						ADD

* This means money that your institution received for your efforts on this study.
** Use this section to provide any needed explanation.

Section 3. Relevant financial activities outside the submitted work.

Place a check in the appropriate boxes in the table to indicate whether you have financial relationships (regardless of amount of compensation) with entities as described in the instructions. Use one line for each entity; add as many lines as you need by clicking the "Add +" box. You should report relationships that were present during the 36 months prior to submission.

Complete each row by checking "No" or providing the requested information. If you have more than one relationship click the "Add" button to add a row. Excess rows can be removed by clicking the "X" button.

Relevant financial activities outside the submitted work						
Type of Relationship (in alphabetical order)	No	Money Paid to You	Money to Your Institution*	Entity	Comments	
1. Board membership	☐	☐	☐			✕
						ADD
2. Consultancy	☐	☐	☐			✕
						ADD
3. Employment	☐	☐	☐			✕
						ADD
4. Expert testimony	☐	☐	☐			✕
						ADD
5. Grants/grants pending	☐	☐	☐			✕
						ADD
6. Payment for lectures including service on speakers bureaus	☐	☐	☐			✕
						ADD
7. Payment for manuscript preparation	☐	☐	☐			✕

3

Figure 207.1 *(Continued)*

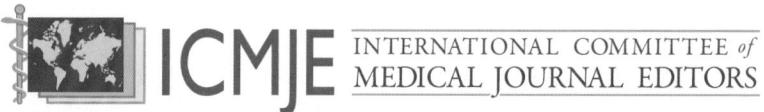

ICMJE Form for Disclosure of Potential Conflicts of Interest

Relevant financial activities outside the submitted work						
Type of Relationship (in alphabetical order)	**No**	**Money Paid to You**	**Money to Your Institution***	**Entity**	**Comments**	
						ADD
8. Patents (planned, pending or issued)	☐	☐	☐			✕
						ADD
9. Royalties	☐	☐	☐			✕
						ADD
10. Payment for development of educational presentations	☐	☐	☐			✕
						ADD
11. Stock/stock options	☐	☐	☐			✕
						ADD
12. Travel/accommodations/ meeting expenses unrelated to activities listed**	☐	☐	☐			✕
						ADD
13. Other (err on the side of full disclosure)	☐	☐	☐			✕
						ADD

* This means money that your institution received for your efforts.
** For example, if you report a consultancy above there is no need to report travel related to that consultancy on this line.

Section 4. Other relationships

Are there other relationships or activities that readers could perceive to have influenced, or that give the appearance of potentially influencing, what you wrote in the submitted work?

☐ No other relationships/conditions/circumstances that present a potential conflict of interest

☐ Yes, the following relationships/conditions/circumstances are present (explain below):

At the time of manuscript acceptance, journals will ask authors to confirm and, if necessary, update their disclosure statements. On occasion, journals may ask authors to disclose further information about reported relationships.

Hide All Table Rows Checked 'No'   **SAVE**

4

Figure 207.1 *(Continued)*

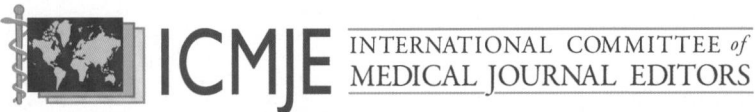

ICMJE Form for Disclosure of Potential Conflicts of Interest

Evaluation and Feedback

Please visit http://www.icmje.org/cgi-bin/feedback to provide feedback on your experience with completing this form.

Figure 207.1 *(Continued)*

AtriCure produced a surgical tool that was not specifically FDA approved for heart surgery in 2005, but the Cleveland Clinic had been conducting research on using the tool to ablate atrial fibrillation. The Cleveland Clinic itself apparently also had an investment interest in the company. Yet, in conducting the research, patients were not initially made aware of the institution's financial interest and the foundation director's financial relationship to the technology. Eventually, Dr. Cosgrove removed himself from overseeing the Cleveland Clinic Foundation's investment section, and the institution created the Cleveland Clinic's Innovation Management and Conflict of Interest Committee to vet promising technologies and their relationship to the organization (10). Thus, Cleveland Clinic developed an individual approach to managing the institution's expertise, creativity in translational research, and economic investments in a presumably ethical fashion. Other organizations such as the American Association of Medical Colleges and the Institute of Medicine (IOM) have constructed guidelines and recommendations to allow institutions to ethically manage conflict of interest while still benefiting from expertise in translational research and industry partnerships (11). Uniformity in adopting these guidelines has been relatively unsuccessful as recently shown in a report published by Ehringhaus in Journal of the American Medical Association, which showed that only 38% of institutions had policies which oversaw the institution's own investment portfolio (12).

CONFLICT OF INTEREST IN MEDICAL PRACTICE

Conflicts of interest can be encountered in the direct delivery of health care. The federal government has identified this potential conflict and has through the legislature weighed in by developing laws that concern direct medical practice.

Although beyond the scope of this chapter to discuss in detail, the prohibition on collective bargaining by physicians by the federal government certainly has its roots in a valuation judgment concerning conflict of interest. The idea that physicians would "price fix" is deemed to be in direct conflict with societal well-being, presumably. More directly, the federal Stark legislation has developed rules to prevent physicians and practices from directly referring business to entities in which they have a financial interest. The Stark legislation was passed in three parts: Part I in 1989, Part II in 1993, and Part III became effective in 2007. Obviously legislation of this sort is complex and subject to interpretation and opinion and judgment. In general, Part I addressed the issue of physicians referring laboratory work to laboratories in which they had a financial interest. Part II addressed other medical practice venues and also set aside exceptions or "safe harbors." One particular exception was in the development of outpatient surgicenters. Finally, Part III was signed into law by President Clinton as part of

Medicare legislation and contained an "antikickback" provision so that referrals to a center of care could not result in a financial bonus to the physician who made the referral. Also, these laws are designed to govern Medicare and Medicaid billing issues (13–16). Another area of conflict of interest in direct medical practice has to do with complicated rules governing the submission of bills to the government Medicare program. The federal government has often claimed that fraudulent billing in the Medicare system is a source of financial waste and ill-gotten gains. In the 1990s under the Clinton administration, PATH audits were accomplished. PATH stands for "Physicians At Teaching Hospitals." The government's position was that Medicare Part A dollars paid for resident salaries. Because the resident salaries were supported partly by these Part A dollars, any further billing for services provided by residents were considered to be duplicative. Therefore, overseeing faculty could not bill for resident services under Part B of Medicare unless they were actively taking part in direct teaching or supervision of the work. In general, direct patient care services are billed through Medicare Part B in all practices that participate in this government program.

Financial conflicts of interest in the government system became apparent in three general categories during PATH audits. One category was when a physician billed for a service that was not at the correct level of complexity. Billing levels were generally divided into five categories of complexity on the outpatient side of medicine, and reimbursements were made by higher amounts or remuneration as the complexity of the patient encounter, time spent, and decision making increased. Audits were directed to determine if the amount billed was consistent with the documentation that described the visit. If the documentation did not match the billing level, fines and penalties could be assessed. A conflict of interest was therefore inherent between the physician's desire to be maximally reimbursed at the discounted Medicare rate and the documentation that the physician could provide to support the level of service claimed. A second category of investigation pertained to procedural billing. A system was developed to valuate the relative complexity and worth of various surgical and other procedures. The concept of a Relative Value Unit, or RVU, was invented to provide a basis for creating a differential financial value scale that could be applied to various interventions in surgery and medicine. A conflict of interest would exist if a surgeon billed for a certain procedure that was more complex and more highly valued while a less complex or valued procedure was actually performed. The third category of conflict of interest addressed the problem of a supervising physician billing for a service that was accomplished by a resident while the attending physician was not properly present to supervise or accomplish the procedure in person.

An example of the power inherent in the federal government's ability to conduct an audit is reflected in the experience of H. Richard Winn, the former Chief of

Neurosurgery at University of Washington. As he reports in the *Journal of Neurosurgery*, Dr. Winn was the subject of a detailed investigation by the federal government. He was accused of improperly billing Medicare for services rendered by residents who were not properly supervised as well as several other charges. The final outcome was that Dr. Winn pleaded guilty to "one count of obstructing 'communication of information to a criminal investigator'" after a 3-year federal investigation. A $500,000 fine was also levied, which "represented 0.5% and 1.3% of billings and revenues, respectively." The institution itself was also the subject of controversy for not properly educating its faculty on the nuances of proper billing procedures. Dr. Winn left the University of Washington and was required to write an account of the audit, which revealed errors in compliance with federal rules which was published in the *Journal of Neurosurgery* (17). The stakes for maintaining an appropriate compliance with federal regulations governing conflict of interest and economic practices are quite high.

CONFLICT OF INTEREST IN CONTINUING MEDICAL EDUCATION

Continuing medical education (CME) programs are designed to deliver credits to learners who participate in enhancing their knowledge and competency to practice medicine. CME credits are typically required to renew medical licensure. The Accreditation Council for Continuing Medical Education (ACCME) is the governing body that accredits institutions to oversee and run CME programs. Conflict of interest can be part of this process in two general categories. First, individuals invited to speak at a program may have worked on a technology in which they have a financial interest, which can impact the objective presentation of information. Second, companies often support programs through contribution of funds, which help to underwrite the event. This may come in the form of direct support for the program activity or in the form of paying to be able to set up a marketing display at the event. Marketing displays must be physically separated from the presentation of educational material.

Each organization that runs an event for credit must have a policy that governs these conflicts in accordance with oversight of the ACCME. The ACCME requires that all individuals in a position to oversee the educational content of a CME event disclose any "relevant financial relationships." The financial conflicts of interest may be in any amount occurring within the last 12 months. To be pertinent, relevant conflicts of interest must also affect the content of the presentation. Relevant conflicts also include financial or other interests held by a spouse or partner. Individual institutions must develop a specific policy on faculty disclosure and an oversight process to vet disclosures. Valid disclosure typically pertains to salary, royalties, intellectual property rights, consulting fees, honoraria, ownership interest, employment or management

positions, speaking fees, consulting fees, or advisory panel, review panel, or board memberships. If such a relationship is identified, it is still valid for a speaker to deliver content at a CME meeting as long as the presentation and/or slides are reviewed in advance by a person who is impartial. The validation process generally includes review of literature cited to make sure it is objective, surveying the presented information to assure balance, and assessing the presentation to assure that it is nonpromotional (18).

SPECIFIC RULES GOVERNING CONFLICTS IN INDUSTRY

The topic of rules governing conflicts of interest between industry and the medical profession is complex, as requirements can take many forms. In this emerging area, requirements can come from many different sources. This section provides an overview of some of these requirements. The intention is not to be all-inclusive, which in this rapidly developing area is not possible, but instead to help raise awareness of the potential sources for and common types of these varying requirements.

At the federal level, the antikickback statutes require that industry not provide unlawful inducements to health care professionals for the purchase of products. The antikickback statutes prohibit for the health care industry some practices which may be common in other industries. These statutes contain criminal prohibitions against payment (or the solicitation of payment) in any form, whether direct or indirect, for the referral or purchase of any item or service that is reimbursable under a federal health care program. As such, their scope is broad (19).

These requirements are further illuminated in the Office of Inspector General for the U.S. Department of Health and Human Services (OIG) Compliance Program Guide for Pharmaceutical Manufacturers. This guide provides practical examples in many areas of activity, including discounts, product support services, educational grants, research funding, business courtesies (entertainment, travel, meals, gifts, etc.), and samples. As such, the guide provides a road map to industry and the physician community of the types of activities that may be risky or prohibited as applied to the vast array of different types of health care professionals' relationships with industry (20).

The pharmaceutical and medical device industries have also been self-policing, with trade associations and their members adopting the Code on Interactions with Healthcare Professionals (PhRMA Code) and Code of Ethics on Interactions with Health Care Professionals (AdvaMed Code), respectively (21,22). These codes are meant to provide a practical framework by which industry can maintain compliance with the complex requirements of the federal antikickback statutes, among others. These codes not only require industry to maintain a compliance program but provide practical guidance in the areas of product training and education, educational conference support, sales, promotional and business meetings, consulting arrangements, royalty payments, prohibitions on entertainment and recreation, guidelines for modest meals, educational items and prohibitions on gifts, provision of coverage, reimbursement and health economics information, research and educational grants and charitable donations, and evaluation and demonstration products. The two industry codes cover industry behavior and differ slightly in content, taking into account the differences between the two industries, which is why medical device sales representatives and pharmaceutical sales representatives may interact with health care professionals in slightly different ways.

States have increasingly begun to promulgate legislation in the area as well, with requirements aimed at industry behavior. These requirements typically take one of two forms: (a) conduct requirements that regulate manufacturer's interactions with health care professionals and (b) disclosure requirements that require manufacturers to report the amount of certain spending, such as consulting agreements, provision of educational items, meals, and product training, among other things, to certain recipients including physicians. Some states require both conduct and disclosure requirements and in several instances those conduct requirements in effect codify, or make into law, the existing industry codes. There are currently 10 jurisdictions that have laws in this area. California, Connecticut, Massachusetts, Minnesota, Nevada, and Vermont have conduct requirements, while Colorado, Maine, Massachusetts, Minnesota, Vermont, Washington DC, and West Virginia have public disclosure requirements (23).

In addition to state law, a relatively unpublicized provision of the Obama administration's health care reform, the Patient Protection and Affordable Care Act, commonly referred to as the "Sunshine Act," extends disclosure requirements at the federal level to physicians and teaching hospitals while including some conduct requirements as well. Effective January 1, 2012, pharmaceutical and medical device companies will need to collect and report payments to physicians and teaching hospitals for consulting fees, compensation for services, honoraria, gifts, entertainment, food, travel, education, research, charitable contributions, royalty or license fees, ownership or investment interest, speaker fees, grants, and anything else defined in the regulations. These requirements are sweeping and reports will be done at the individual recipient level to provide greater transparency of these relationships, which will be published by the federal government on a publically available and searchable database (24).

Conflict of interest rules are not confined to industry. CME has long been overseen by ACCME, which provides strict requirements to help insure that CME programs are fair, balanced, and independent of commercial bias and influence, while still allowing industry support (25). ACCME requires that commercial support associated with

any CME activity be given with full knowledge of the educational provider. Social events associated with CME activities must be subordinate to the educational component of the meeting. Product promotion is prohibited during the CME activity and any promotional activity or product advertisement must occur in a space separate from the educational event space. In this manner, CME events can provide objective information that can be used by physicians to independently evaluate practices and procedures without the shadow of any actual or perceived conflicts with industry, while allowing industry to continue to provide valuable support of educational events.

Medical societies have also gotten into the act. For example, the Council of Medical Specialty Societies in April 2010 developed a Code for Interactions with Companies (26). These guidelines apply to the individual specialty societies that belong to the council and establish core principles to help minimize actual or perceived conflicts of interest. The principles for interaction with industry include independence, transparency, accepting charitable contributions, accepting corporate sponsorships, society meetings, research grants, clinical practice guidelines, journals, advertising, and licensing. In this manner, by setting standards which medical specialty societies can adapt and adopt, the council helps to ensure that society members' interactions with companies remain focused on the benefit of patients and members and the improvement of patient care.

Likewise, the American Academy of Orthopedic Surgeons (AAOS) has recently developed some new disclosure rules, which are notable in requiring public disclosure and providing a publically available searchable online database. In announcing the new database in December 2009, AAOS acknowledged that it is responding to increasing public and government scrutiny of the relationship between orthopedic surgeons and industry. The enhanced policy requires each participant in an AAOS CME program, or author, and members of AAOS governance groups to disclose all potential conflicts of interests. Using a uniform format, these participants are responsible for recording their relationships with commercial entities relating to orthopedics and must review and update this information at least semiannually. Information to be provided includes royalties, speakers bureaus, industry employment, consulting (paid or unpaid), stock options, research support, and other financial support. Failure to participate can result in the physician being asked to not participate in the program or governance group. The information in the AAOS Orthopaedic Disclosure Program is available both to members and to the public, and individual disclosures are included in meeting materials (27).

The American Academy of Otolaryngology—Head and Neck Surgery has promulgated a Statement of Principles and Code of Ethics (Code) that succinctly addresses industry relations:

"This Code of Ethics does not seek to restrict legal trade practices. However, a physician's commercial or financial interests should never be placed ahead of the interests and welfare of patients. Conflicts of interest undermine the trust that patients place in their physician. For this reason, physicians should endeavor to avoid any venture that creates a conflict of interest between personal financial interests and the best interests of the patient. Conflicts that develop between a physician's financial interests and the physician's responsibilities to the patient should be resolved to the benefit of the patient."

The Code also covers inventions and fee-setting, among other topics (28).

Institutions are also developing conflict of interest and disclosure requirements—and are making headlines as they do so. In late 2008 the Cleveland Clinic led the way by becoming the first major medical center to announce that they would be making a complete disclosure of doctors' and researchers' financial ties to industry on their Web site (29). In 2009 Harvard University–affiliated hospitals adopted new conflict of interest guidelines, which forbid industry gifts and ban meals and doctors' participation in speaker programs (30). Harvard Medical School has followed suit, banning faculty members from giving promotional talks or accepting personal gifts, travel, or meals from industry and placing strict limits on the income faculty can earn from consulting, joining boards, and other work with industry while publically disclosing payments of more than $5,000. Johns Hopkins has addressed this issue by prohibiting gifts, entertainment, and food; barring sales representatives from patient care areas; only allowing invited sales representatives into their facility; and requiring donations to be made to the institution rather than individual doctors (31). Stanford University School of Medicine has made public its faculty members' income from consulting with outside groups and royalty payments for inventions (32).

Institutions that address institutional as well as individual conflicts may well be ahead of the curve. In January 2011, the OIG reviewed the NIH grant process and concluded that there are currently no federal requirements that grantee institutions identify, report, or manage actual or potential institutional conflicts (33). Since 1995, there have been federal regulations regarding investigators' and researchers' conflicts of interest and requiring that those conflicts be managed, but the report found a dearth of guidance—and written policies and procedures at the grantee institution level—to address institutional conflicts. The report concluded that the NIH lacks information on institutional conflicts and their impact on NIH-sponsored research and recommended new regulations to address these issues. Additional activity in this area can be anticipated as members of congress, particularly Senators Grassley and Baucus, continue to advocate for aggressive oversight.

Given the number and types of entities, ranging from industry associations to medical societies to health care institutions and even state and federal government that are involved in crafting rules regarding conflicts of interest, physicians need to stay constantly on top of these requirements. As this area has become increasingly complex, the best advice may be to remain cognizant of the changing landscape and seek appropriate guidance when necessary.

BEST PRACTICES

Advancing health care goals and improving patient care depends in part on close collaboration between health care professionals and industry. As these relationships become increasingly complex, it is more important than ever to insure that actual or perceived conflicts of interest are appropriately addressed. The integrity of the relationship between patient and physician must always be preserved. At the same time, avoiding even the appearance of a conflict and abiding by the increase in transparency requirements helps maintain public—and patient—trust.

The first step is awareness. Be vigilant about activities that, by their nature, may lead to a perceived conflict. In so doing, retain common sense and put yourself in the shoes of the public. A good test for any activity is "what would this look like as a headline in tomorrow's newspaper?"

Be educated about these emerging requirements. There are many sources for information. Begin with your local or national medical society. Both AdvaMed and PhRMA maintain public Web sites full of accessible information about their respective code requirements (21,22). The health care institutions with which you are affiliated may maintain policies that directly or indirectly govern conduct with or disclosure of the industry affiliations of staff, so make sure that applicable policy manuals are checked. Finally, read the fine print of any grant that you may be involved with to make sure you are knowledgeable about any conflict or disclosure requirements.

Another consideration is transparency. To meet this requirement, think about what a typical patient would want to know. Transparency helps provide information to make informed decisions, maintain trust, and minimize conflicts. Expect to see increasing activity in this regard. Transparency is here, so carefully consider industry relationships and funding through the lens of public disclosure.

Finally, keeping up with developments and emerging requirements is important. To avoid making any missteps, stay up to date on what your industry partners and the institutions that you work for require. Don't be blindsided by the specter of public disclosure but instead embrace it as a way to increase the information available to members of the public as they make that all-important decision of who they chose to provide their health care. Ultimately, all of us—the public, the medical community, and industry—will benefit.

HIGHLIGHTS

- Conflict of interest is present when a responsible individual has private circumstances that influence the normal progression of their professional tasks or trust. These conflicts may include financial interests but may also relate to other benefits or outcomes.
- Continuing collaboration between health care professionals and industry is essential to the advancement of health care through innovation, so it is essential to manage conflicts appropriately.
- Disclosure of conflict is the key element to maintaining trust and objectivity.
- Conflict of interest can occur in publishing, in research, in CME, and in the practice of medicine. Various organizations have created guidelines to help manage conflict of interest including the ICMJE, NIH, IOM, ACCME, and the federal government.
- Institutions, through their investments and business interests, can also be subject to conflict of interest problems.
- Medically related industry including medical device manufacturers and the pharmaceutical industry should have internal policies in place to meet legal and ethical guidelines designed to minimize and manage conflict of interest. These policies should encourage the creation of intellectual property and should strive to separate marketing efforts from educational and developmental endeavors.
- Specialty societies including the American Academy of Otolaryngology—Head and Neck Surgery have created guidelines to help maintain the highest standards of professionalism with regard to conflict of interest.

REFERENCES

1. Conflict of interest. http://www.merriam-webster.com. Accessed May 20, 2011.
2. Kowalczyk L. Senator broadens inquiry into psychiatrist. *Boston Globe* March 21, 2009:B1.
3. Meier B. With warning, a hip device is withdrawn. *The New York Times* March 10, 2010:B1.
4. Voreacos D, Nussbaum A, Farrel G. "Johnson & Johnson Reaches for a Band Aid", Bloomberg Business Week, April 3, 2011. http://www.msnbc.msn.com/id/42383262/ns/business-vs_business/t/johnson-johnson-reaches-band-aid/ Accessed online June 23, 2011.
5. International Committee of Medical Journal Editors. ICMJE form for disclosure of potential conflicts of interest. http://www.icmje.org/coi_disclosure.pdf. Accessed May 20, 2011.
6. Drazen JM, de Leeuw PW, Laine C, et al. Toward more uniform conflict disclosures: the updated ICMJE conflict of interest reporting form. *JAMA* 2010;304(2):212–213. PMID: 20595375. [Epub Jul 1, 2010.]
7. Fontanarosa PB, Flanagin A, DeAngelis CD. Implementation of the ICMJE Form for reporting potential conflicts of interest. *JAMA* 2010;304(13):1496. PMID: 20924020.
8. Goozner M. NIH proposes new conflict-of-interest rules for investigators. *J Natl Cancer Inst* 2010;102(14):1006–1007. PMID: 20616352. [Epub Jul 8, 2010.]
9. Kaiser J, National Institutes of Health. Lowering the boom on financial conflicts. *Science* 2010;328(5982):1091. PMID: 20508102.
10. Armstrong D. How a famed hospital invests in device it uses and promotes. *The Wall Street* December 12, 2005. online.wsj.com/article/SB113435097142119825-search.html. Accessed online February 26, 2013.
11. Kaiser J. Conflicts of interest. IOM panel backs public disclosure of drug company payments. *Science* 2009;324(5927):579. PMID: 19407172.
12. Ehringhaus SH, Weissman JS, Sears JL, et al. Responses of medical schools to institutional conflicts of interest. *JAMA* 2008;299(6):665–671. PMID: 18270355.
13. Kolber MJ. Stark regulation: a historical and current review of the self-referral laws. *HEC Forum* 2006;18(1):61–84. PMID: 17076130.
14. Glaser DM. Legal issues affecting ancillaries and orthopedic practice. *Orthop Clin North Am* 2008;39(1):89–102, vii. PMID: 18061773.
15. Satiani B. Exceptions to the stark law: practical considerations for surgeons. *Plast Reconstr Surg* 2006;117(3):1012–1022; discussion 1023. PMID: 16525301.
16. Pacella SJ. Exceptions to the stark law: the ambulatory surgery center exemption. *Plast Reconstr Surg* 2006;118(3):822–823; author reply 823. PMID: 16932222.
17. Winn HR. Errors in compliance with federal rules and regulations relating to healthcare benefits programs: the University of Washington Department of Neurological Surgery experience. *J Neurosurg* 2004;100(1):47–55. PMID: 14743911.
18. ACCME standards for commercial support. http://www.accme.org/dir_docs/doc_upload/68b2902a-fb73-44d1-8725-80a1504e520c_uploaddocument.pdf. Accessed May 20, 2011.
19. 42 U.S.C. § 1320a-7b.
20. Office of Inspector General, U.S. Department of Health and Human Services. Compliance program guide for pharmaceutical manufacturers. April 23, 2003. Federal Register, Vol. 68, No. 86, Monday, May 5, 2003, p. 23731–23742. https://oig.hhs.gov/authorities/docs/03/050503FRCPGPharmac.pdf. Accessed online February 26, 2013.
21. http://www.advamed.org, accessed February 26, 2013, pdf pp. 1–23, http://advamed.org/res/112/advamed-code-of-ethics-on-interactions-with-health-care-professionals
22. http://www.phrma.org, Code on Interactions with Healthcare Professionals, accessed February 26, 2013, pp. 1–36, http://www.phrma.org/sites/default/files/108/phrma_marketing_code_2008.pdf
23. Health Industry Distributors Association 2011 Gift Disclosure Report. http://www.hida.org. Updated January 2011. http://www.hida.org/App_Themes/Member/docs/Healthcare%20reform/2011%20Gift%20Disclosure%20Rpt.pdf. Accessed February 26, 2013.
24. P.L. 111-148, Section 6002: transparency reports and reporting of physician ownership of investment interest. Accessed online February 26, 2013, 124 stat. 689–124 stat. 696. http://www.gpo.gov/fdsys/pkg/PLAW-111publ148/pdf/PLAW-111publ148.pdf
25. ACCME Standards for commercial support, http://www.accme.org/dir_docs/doc_upload/68b2902a-fb73-44d1-8725-80a1504e520c_uploaddocument.pdf. Accessed April 25, 2011.
26. CMSS code for interactions with companies. http://www.cmss.org/codeforinteractions.aspx. Accessed May 26, 2011.
27. AAOS orthopedic disclosure program. http://www3.aaos.org/education/disclosure/disclosure_intro.cfm. Accessed May 26, 2011.
28. American Academy of Otolaryngology—Head and Neck Surgeons statement of principles and code of ethics. http://www.entnet.org/aboutus/Ethics.cfm. Accessed May 26, 2011.
29. Abelson R. Cleveland clinic discloses doctors' industry ties. *The New York Times* December 2, 2008. http://www.nytimes.com/2008/12/03/business/03clinic.html?pagewanted=all. Accessed online February 26, 2013.
30. Kowalczyk L. Harvard puts tighter limits on medical faculty. *Boston Globe* July 21, 2010. http://www.boston.com/news/education/higher/articles/2010/07/21/harvard_puts_tighter_limits_on_medical_faculty/ Accessed online February 26, 2013.

31. TheWallStreetJournalHealthBlog.http://blogs.wsj.com/health.April 8, 2009. http://blogs.wsj.com/health/2009/04/08/johns-hopkins-bans-free-drug-samples-gifts-from-industry/ Accessed February 26, 2013.

32. Stanford University School of Medicine News, September 15, 2009. http://med.stanford.edu/ism/2009/september/coi.html.   Accessed May 26, 2011.

33. King & Spalding, Client Alert, Government Advocacy and Public Policy Practice Group. HHS OIG recommends new federal regulations to govern NIH grantee institutions. January 31, 2011. http://www.kslaw.com/imageserver/KSPublic/library/publication/ca013111.pdf. Accessed February 26, 2013.

INDEX

(Note: Page numbers followed by *f* indicate figures; those followed by *t* indicate tables.)

A

Aarskog syndrome, 1635–1636
Abbe flap, in lip reconstruction, 1797, 1798, 1799*f*
Abdominal injuries, secondary survey of trauma, 1103–1104
Abductor spasmodic dysphonia, 1032–1033
Ablative resurfacing lasers, 2866–2867
Ablative therapy, 2622
Abrasions, soft tissue injuries, 1109
Abscess(es)
  cerebellar/temporal lobe, 2444
  epidural, 580–581, 581*f*
  odontogenic infection
    buccal space, 773, 773*f*
    dentoalveolar, 771, 772*t*
    submandibular space, 773, 774*f*
  orbital, 576
  periosteal, 2444
  retropharyngeal, 169, 169*f*
  subdural, 581, 581*f*
  subperiosteal, 575, 576*f*
Absorbable suture material, 22
Accent method, voice therapy, 1050
Acetaminophen, 45–46
Achalasia, 854–855, 855*f*
Achondroplasia, 1636
Acinic cell carcinoma, salivary gland, 1765–1766, 1765*f*
Acne rosacea, 3215, 3215*f*
Acoustic neuroma, 213, 213*f*
Acoustic rhinometry, 366, 455–456
Acoustic stapedial reflex measurement, 2279–2280
Acoustic transformer theory, 2466
Acoustic voice analysis, 1072, 1072*f*
Acquired immunodeficiency syndrome. *See also* Human immunodeficiency virus infection
  hairy cell leukoplakia, 743
  lymphoma, 2039
  otologic manifestations, 2520
  Sjögren syndrome, 705
Acral lentiginous melanoma, 1741. *See also* Malignant melanoma
Acrocephalosyndactyly, type I, 1622–1623, 1623*f*
Actinic cheilitis, 3212, 3215*f*
Actinic keratoses, 1726–1727, 1727*f*, 3212
  treatment of, 3224
Actinomycosis, 287–288, 287*f*
Adaptive immune system, 382–383

Adductor spasmodic dysphonia, 1032–1033
Adenocarcinoma, 2047
  ceruminous, 2369
  salivary gland, 1766
    polymorphous low-grade, 1766
Adenoid(s). *See also* Adenotonsillar disease, in children
  enlargement of, 1460*f*
Adenoid cystic carcinoma, 192*f*, 1992*f*, 2047, 2369
  MRI, 154, 155*f*–156*f*
  salivary gland, 1765, 1765*f*
  tracheal tumors, 1996
Adenoidectomy, 2225
  adenotonsillar disease, in children, 1437–1438
  pediatric rhinosinusitis, 1459–1460, 1460*f*
Adenoma
  ceruminous, 2368
  pleomorphic, 2369
  salivary
    basal cell adenoma, 1764
    malignant, 1766–1767, 1766*f*
    pleomorphic adenoma, 1760–1762, 1762*f*
    warthin tumor, 186*f*
  thyroid, 2120
Adenoma sebaceum, 3217, 3217*f*
  treatment of, 3227
Adenomatoid odontogenic tumor, 2104–2105
Adenomatous tumors, of middle ear, 2370–2372
Adenotonsillar disease, in children
  clinical practice guidelines, 1440–1441, 1441*t*
  clinical presentation
    adenoids, 1434
    hypertrophy, 1433–1434
    infections, 1433
    tonsils, 1434–1435, 1435*f*
  complications, 1439
  contraindications, 1438–1439
  controversy, 1440
  embryology
    components and properties, 1431, 1432*t*
    ICA, 1432
    palatoglossus muscle, 1431
    palatopharyngeus muscle, 1431
    pharyngeal pouch, 1430

  structure of, 1430
    Waldeyer ring, 1431, 1431*f*
  epidemiology, 1430
  immunophysiology, 1432
  management
    infection/inflammation, 1435–1436, 1436*t*
    sleep disorders/breathing, 1436–1437
  neoplasia, 1433*t*, 1442
  outcomes, 1436*t*, 1438
  peritonsillar abscess, 1439–1440
  surgical techniques
    adenoidectomy, 1437–1438
    tonsillectomy, 1437
Adenotonsillar surgery
  pediatric otolaryngology, 1300–1301
Adenotonsillectomy, 2225, 2225*f*
Adenovirus, 1433
Adrenal glands
  adrenal insufficiency, 259
  Cushing's syndrome, 259–260
  pheochromocytoma, 260
  primary aldosteronism, 258–259
  secondary aldosteronism, 259
Adrenal insufficiency, 259
  preoperative management of, 33–34, 34*t*
Adrenocorticotropic hormone, 258–259
Adson forceps, 22
Advanced trauma life support, 1212
Adverse event, 3373
Adynamic ileus, 40
Aerodigestive tract
  congenital anomalies of
    pathophysiology
      hypopharyngeal/laryngeal, 1308
      nasopharyngeal obstruction, 1306, 1308*f*
      oral, 1306–1307
      oropharyngeal, 1307, 1308*f*
      tracheobronchial and esophageal, 1308–1309
    postnatal diagnosis
      CT scanning, 1311
      flexible endoscopic evaluation of swallowing, 1310–1311, 1311*f*
      functions of, 1310
      hypopharyngeal/laryngeal, 1313–1314, 1313*f*, 1315*f*
      nasopharyngeal obstruction, 1311–1312, 1312*f*
      oral, 1312–1313, 1312*f*
      oropharyngeal, 1313
      physical examination, 1309–1311

Aerodigestive tract (*Continued*)
   tracheobronchial and esophageal, 1314–1316, 1315*f*
   ventilating bronchoscope, 1311, 1312*f*
  prenatal diagnosis, 1309, 1309*f*–1310*f*
  treatment
   hypopharyngeal/laryngeal, 1320–1321, 1320*f*–1321*f*
   nasopharyngeal obstruction, 1316–1318, 1316*f*–1318*f*
   oral, 1318–1319, 1319*f*
   oropharyngeal, 1319–1320, 1320*f*
   principles of, 1316
   tracheobronchial and esophageal, 1322–1324, 1322*f*–1324*f*
  ingestion injury
   chest radiograph, 1405, 1405*f*
   clinical presentation, 1400
   complications, 1401–1402, 1402*f*
   diagnosis and treatment, 1400–1401, 1401*t*
   disc battery, 1406, 1406*f*
   foreign-body aspiration, 1402–1403
   mass effect, 1405
   mechanism of, 1399–1400
   treatment, 1404
   upper esophageal sphincter, 1405, 1405*f*–1406*f*
   workup, 1403–1404, 1403*f*–1404*f*
  Munchausen syndrome, 1407
Afferent pupillary defect, midface fracture, 1213
Agency for Health Care Quality and Research, 3375
Aging. *See also* Elderly patients
  ablative therapy, 2622
  auditory system
   dysfunction, 2615–2616, 2616*t*
   presbycusis, 2616–2618, 2617*f*, 2617*t*
   rehabilitation, 2618
  definitions, 298
  demographics and disability, 298–299
  diagnostic evaluation, 2621
  disease and disability, 299–300
  dizziness
   definition, 2615
   differential diagnosis, 2615, 2616*t*
   etiology of, 2616*t*
   evaluation of, 2620*t*
   types of, 2618*t*
  face, anatomy of, 3104–3105, 3104*f*
  health care, 302
  management of, 2621–2622
  patient history, 2619, 2619*t*, 2620*t*
  physical examination, 2619, 2619*t*, 2620*t*
  physiology of, 3055, 3056*f*
  vestibular dysfunction, 2620–2621
  vestibular systems, 2618–2619, 2618*t*
Air embolism
  as complication of mastoid surgery, 2463
Airtraq optical laryngoscope, 901, 901*f*
Airway
  larynx and protection of, 951
  stenotic lesions, larynx, 963–964

trauma to, primary survey of, 1094–1096, 1095*f*, 1096*f*
Airway endoscopy
  recurrent respiratory papillomatosis, 1415
Airway management, 246–248
  in lip cancer, 1804, 1804*t*
Airway obstruction, 1571–1572
  cleft lip/palate, 1571
  intubation, 917
Airway pressure release ventilation, 60
Airway stents, upper airway obstruction, 890–891
Alar rim grafts, nasal tip surgery, 2973, 2975*f*
Alaryngeal speech, 1978
Alaska Federal Health Care Access Network, 3362, 3362*f*
Alcohol use/abuse
  fetal alcohol syndrome and, 1635, 1635*f*
  surgery in, 46
Alcohol withdrawal syndrome
  atrial fibrillation, 71–72, 72*t*
  benzodiazepines, 68
  Clostridium difficile colitis, 70–71, 71*t*
  contrast-induced nephropathy, 69–70, 69*t*, 70*f*
  gastric acid suppression, 68–69, 69*t*
  incidence of, 68
  symptoms, 68, 68*t*
Aldosteronism
  primary, 258–259
  secondary, 259
Alexander syndrome, 1536
Alexander's law, 2685
Alfentanil, 241
Allergan, for soft tissue augmentation, 3246
Allergic fungal rhinosinusitis
  allergic bronchopulmonary aspergillosis, 567, 569
  clinical presentation, 567
  diagnosis, 567–568
  eosinophilic mucin rhinosinusitis, 569
  fungal cultures, 569
  pathology, 568, 570*f*
  radiology, 568, 568*t*, 569*f*
  treatment approach
   antifungal agents, 571
   endoscopic sinus surgery, 570
   immunomodulation, 570–571
Allergic rhinitis
  allergen exposure, 551
  antigen processing, 551
  asthma, 379–380, 551
  clinical characteristics, 550–551
  definition, 460
  development of
   allergic response, 398–399, 398*f*, 399*f*
   early response, 399
   environmental changes, 396, 397*f*
   family history, 396
   genetics, 396, 396*t*
   hygiene hypothesis, 397–398
   late response, 399–400, 400*f*
   lifestyle changes, 396–397
  diagnosis, 401–402
   allergy testing, 463
   history, 461–462, 462*t*
   physical findings, 462, 463*f*

economic impact of, 379
epidemiology, 461
genetics, 460
immunology of, 460–461
immunotherapy
  adverse reactions, 404
  allergen tolerance, 404
  allergen-specific immunotherapy, 402–403
  clinical recommendations for, 404*t*
  grass pollen immunotherapy, 404
  immune mechanisms, 403–404
  sublingual immunotherapy, 404
  symptoms, 405*t*
management
  allergens avoidance, 402
  pharmacotherapy, 402, 403*f*
  pregnant patients, 402
nasal and nonnasal symptoms, 551*t*
neural component
  nasal cycle, 400
  nasal-ocular reflex, 401
  nasonasal reflex, 400–401
  neuropeptides and neurogenic inflammation, 401
prevalence of, 379
and rhinosinusitis, 538
symptoms, 379
treatment of
  environmental control, 463–464
  immunotherapy, 465–466
  pharmacologic therapy, 464, 465*t*
  surgery, 464–465
Allergy testing
  allergen extract variability, 413
  allergen selection
   abundance, 413
   arthropod allergy, 414
   cross-reactivity, 413
   inhalant mold allergy, 414
   pollen allergens, 413–414
   potency, 413
   proteins, animal dander, 414
  antigen screens, 414
  interpretion, 419–420, 420*f*
  negative allergy test, 412
  positive allergy test, 412
  sensitivity and tolerance, 413
  skin testing
   blended techniques, 417–418, 418*f*
   intradermal, 416–417, 416*f*
   positive and negative controls, 415
   sIgE testing, 418–419, 419*f*
   skin prick tests, 415–416, 415*f*
   total IgE, 419
Alloderm, 53
Alloplast implantion, 3181–3183, 3182*f*, 3183*f*
Alopecia
  following forehead lift, 3071
  medical treatment of, 3229–3230
  rhytidectomy, 3127, 3128*f*
  surgical treatment of
   anesthesia, 3231
   autograft hair transplantation, 3231–3234
   female pattern hair loss, 3231

hair-replacement surgery, 3230–3231
juri flap, 3236–3237
patient evaluation, 3230
scalp reduction, 3234–3235
tissue expansion, 3235–3236
Alport syndrome, 125, 1636
hearing loss in, 1543t, 1551
Alternative medicine. See Complementary
and alternative medicine
Alveolar bone grafting, 1562, 1568
Alveolar nerve, inferior, nerve blocks
of, 237
Alveolar rhabdomyosarcoma, 2373
Amblyopia, 230
Ambulatory quality alliance,
3375–3376
Ameloblastic fibroma, 2106, 2106f
Ameloblastoma, 2102–2104, 2103f
American college of chest physicians,
1348
Aminoglycosides, 133, 2542, 2545
Amiodarone, 37
Amphotericin B
acute invasive fungal rhinosinusitis, 561
Amplification, subjective nonpulsatile tinnitus, 2602
Amyloidosis, 294–295, 981, 981f
Amyotrophic lateral sclerosis, 208–209,
209t, 1037
Anaerobes, 134
Anaplastic carcinoma, 2120–2121
Anesthesia
airway management, 246–248
anesthesia monitoring
anesthesia machine, 244–245
depth of anesthesia, 246
emergencies, 244t
hemodynamic, 245–246
intraoperative, 245
temperature control, 246
antiemetics, 244
endoscopic procedures, 248
general. See General anesthetic agents
and intraoperative monitoring of facial
nerve, 2326
intravenous sedative agents, 241
local, 1110–1111
local anesthesia. See Local anesthesia
narcotic agonists and antagonists
alfentanil, 241
fentanyl, 241–242
morphine, 241
naloxone, 242
remifentanil, 242
sufentanil, 241
neuromuscular blocking agents, 242t
categories, 243
cisatracurium, 243
edrophonium, 243
pancuronium, 243
succinylcholine, 243
sugammadex, 244
tubocurarine, 243
preoperative preparation, 248
regional, 1111, 1111f
Aneuploidy, 122
Angelman syndrome, 121

Angiofibroma
juvenile
diagnosis of, 2025, 2026f
endoscopic and endoscopic-assisted
approaches, 2028
epidemiology and pathogenesis, 2023
growth patterns, 2024–2025, 2024f,
2025f
open surgery, 2027–2028, 2027t
radiation therapy, 2028
staging, 2025–2026, 2027t
surgical approaches, 2026–2027
nasopharyngeal, 440, 441f
Angiogenesis, wound healing, 79
Angiography, paraganglioma, 2006–2008,
2008f, 2009f
Angiolytic lasers, 52
Angiomas
cherry, 3216
spider treatment of, 3227
Angiosarcoma
epidemiology, 2019–2020
etiologic factors, 2020, 2020t
molecular analysis, 2020–2021
pathology, 2020
staging, 2021, 2021t
treatment, 2021–2023, 2022f
Angle, of mandible
fracture
management, 1196f, 1202–1203,
1203f
transoral approach, 1189, 1190f
Angular cheilitis, 740, 740f
Angular vestibuloocular reflex
Ménière syndrome, 2703
Animal-scratch disease, salivary glands,
704–705
Ankyloglossia, 1318
Ann Arbor staging system, 2035, 2035t
Anosmia, 373–374
Anotia, otoplasty, 3146, 3146f
Anterior airway, larynx, 870f
Anterior glottic stenosis, 884, 884f
Anterior neck dissection, 1820
Anterior saccular cyst, 986f
Antibiotic sore mouth, 740
Antibiotics
in acute rhinosinusitis, 543–544
chronic rhinosinusitis, 588–589
diarrhea, 40
odontogenic infection, 779, 780t
preoperative, 22–23, 23t
wounds, 1111–1112
Anticholinergics, chronic rhinosinusitis,
591
Anticoagulants
preoperative management in use of,
29–30
in thromboembolic disease, 31
Antidepressants
subjective nonpulsatile tinnitus, 2603
tobacco cessation, 335
Antidiuretic hormone, 252–253
syndrome of inappropriate secretion
of, 34

Antiemetics, 244
Antifungals, 133–134
Antihistamines, 464, 590
Anti-inflammatory agent, sudden sensorineural hearing loss, 2592
Antimicrobial agents, 131–138
aminoglycosides, 133
antifungals, 133–134
antiviral agents, 134
cephalosporins, 131, 132t
clindamycin, 132
croup, 138
fluoroquinolones, 133
macrolide, 134
otitis externa, 136–137
otitis media, 135–136
penicillins, 131, 132t
peritonsillar abscess, 138
pharyngitis, 138
salivary gland infections, 138
sinusitis, 137, 138f
supraglottitis, 138
trimethoprim-sulfamethoxazole, 133
upper respiratory infections, 134–135
vancomycin, 133
Antiviral agents, sudden sensorineural
hearing loss, 2592
Antley-Bixler syndrome, 1636
Antral lavage, pediatric rhinosinusitis,
1460
Antrostomy
inferior meatal, complications of, 1460
pediatric rhinosinusitis, 1460
Aortopulmonary window metastatic
lymphadenopathy, 146f
Apert syndrome, 1622–1623, 1623f
Aphakia, 221
Aphthous stomatitis, recurrent, 749–751,
749f–751f, 750t
Apligraf, 53
Apnea, after neck dissection, 1832
Appendicular coordination, 2722
Arachnoid cyst, 2577
Arcanobacterium haemolyticum infection,
765
Arnold-Chiari malformation, 1034, 1035f,
1320, 2729
Arterial supply
facial nerve, 2505
to nose, 2924–2925
Arteriosclerosis, 232
Arteriovenous fistula, 2608, 2608f
Arteriovenous malformations, 1586–1587,
1586f
Arthritis, rheumatoid. See Rheumatoid
arthritis
Arthrocentesis, temporomandibular joint,
789
Arthropod allergy, 414
Arthroscopy, temporomandibular joint,
789–790
Arytenoidectomy, 885, 885f
Arytenoids
abduction of, for bilateral vocal fold
immobility, 1022
larynx and, 945–947
Aspergillosis, 134

Aspiration, 859–866
  diagnosis
    endoscopy, 1345
    laryngeal clefts, 1345–1346
    radiology, 1345
    tracheoesophageal fistula, 1346
  diagnosis of, 860t
  etiology of, 859–860
  evaluation of, 861, 861f
  identification of, 859, 860t
  laryngeal closure procedures, 864–866,
    865f, 866f
  management, 1346, 1347t
  management of
    decision making in, 861–862
    initial, 862t
  sensory loss, 861
  sialorrhea, control of, 1346–1347
  swallowing, 860–861, 860f
  therapeutic options
    esophageal run-off, 863
    esophageal strictures, 863–864
    glottic closure, 862–863
    nonoral feedings and airway manage-
      ment, 862, 862t, 863f, 863t
  tracheostomy, 861
  upper esophageal sphincter, 864
  Zenker diverticulum, 864
Aspiration biopsy. See Biopsy
Aspirin, 28, 33
Aspirin exacerbated respiratory disease,
  531–532
Assistive listening devices. See Hearing aids
  and assistive listening devices
Ataxia, 1034, 2722
Atelectasis, 2476–2477
  postoperative management, 38–39
  preoperative management of, 38
Atelectatic sinus, 428, 429f–430f
Atenolol, 35
Atherosclerotic carotid artery disease, 2608
Atresia
  aural. See Aural atresia, congenital
  choanal. See Choanal atresia
  esophageal, 1322
Atrophic rhinitis
  clinical findings, 482
  diagnosis, 483
  inferior turbinate hypertrophy, 619
  K. ozaenae, 483
  pathophysiology, 482
  primary form, 482
  secondary form, 482
  treatment, 483–484
Atropine, 37
Audiogram, in otosclerosis, 2490, 2491f,
  2492f
Audiologic test battery, 2274–2280
Audiometry. See also Hearing evaluation
  otitis media, 1480–1481
  pure-tone, 2274–2277, 2275f
  speech, 2277–2278
Auditory brainstem audiometry, 1481
Auditory brainstem implant
  complications, 2649
  indications, 2648
  outcomes, 2650

overview of, 2647
  patient history, 2647–2648
  principles of, 2648, 2648f
  surgery, 2648–2649, 2649f, 2650f
Auditory brainstem response, 1524,
  2280–2282, 2281f, 2282f,
  2315–2317, 2316f–2319f
  testing, 1510–1512
    auditory neuropathy spectrum disor-
      der, 1511
    auditory steady-state response,
      1511–1512
    measurement, 1510–1511
    used for, 1510
Auditory canal
  external
    development of, 2241
    embryology of, 2384
    and pinna, neoplasms of, 2365–2370
  internal
    neoplasms of, 2376–2381
Auditory evoked potentials
  recording options, 2317
Auditory evoked responses, 2280–2284,
  2281f–2283f
  cortical, 2283–2284
Auditory function, peripheral and central,
  assessment of, 2274–2289
Auditory nerve, physiology of, 2263, 2264f
Auditory neuropathy, 1545
Auditory neuropathy spectrum disorder, 1533
Auditory processing disorders
  assessment of, 2285–2286
  central auditory nervous system
    dysfunction, 2285
  test battery, 2285–2286
Auditory steady-state response, 1511–1512,
  2270–2271
Auditory system, aging
  dysfunction, 2615–2616, 2616t
  presbycusis, 2616–2618, 2617f, 2617t
  rehabilitation, 2618
Aural atresia, congenital
  audiometric evaluation of, 2386–2387
  classification of, 2386
  computed tomography, 2387
  grading system for, 2389t
  medical management, 2387
  patient evaluation in, 2386
  physical examination in, 2386–2387
  surgery for, 2387–2390
    facial nerve monitoring during, 2328,
      2328t
    patient selection, 2388–2389, 2389t
    timing of, 2389
    unilateral and bilateral, repair of,
      2387–2388
  technique of, 2390–2394
    drilling canal in, 2390–2391, 2391f
    incision, 2390
Aural immittance (impedance)
  measurement, 2278
Auricle(s)
  acid burn, 2347
  anatomy and embryology, 3161, 3162f,
    3163f
  anatomy of, 2333, 2334f

congenital malformations
  classification, 3168–3169, 3168f
  complications, 3171–3172, 3174t
  emergencies, 3174t
  surgical reconstruction
    atresia repair, 3171, 3172f
    auricular elevation, 3171, 3173f, 3174f
    auricular reconstruction, 3170,
      3170f, 3171f
    Brent and Nagata technique, 3170
    lobule transposition, 3170, 3171f,
      3172f
    microtia, 3169–3170
    polyethylene implants, 3170
    preoperative planning, 3171
    radiologic examination, 3170
    reconstructed ear, 3174f
    tragal construction, 3170, 3173f
  development of, 2239–2240
    anomalies, 2240–2241
    major malformation, 2386
    minor malformation, 2386
    sharp trauma, 2346–2347
Auricular cartilage graft, 2470
Auricular injury, 1123–1126, 1123f–1125f
Auriculotemporal nerve, 695
Autografts
  hair transplantation
    donor hair removal, 3231–3232
    donor-site removal, 3232
    recipient site, 3232–3233
    sequelae and complication, 3233–3234
  for soft tissue augmentation, 3245
Autoimmune inner ear disease, 2591
  clinical presentation, 2524
  corticosteroid therapy
    cyclophosphamide, 2526
    etanercept, 2525
    intratympanic steroid therapy, 2526
    limitations, 2525
    low-dose methotrexate, 2525
    patterns of response, 2525
    prednisone, 2525
  diagnosis, 2524–2525
  differential diagnosis, 2524
  epidemiology, 2523
  pathophysiology, 2523–2524
Autoimmune neurologic diseases
  myasthenia gravis, 211–212
  Susac syndrome, 212–213, 213f
Autonomic rhinitis, 482
Autosomal dominant inheritance, 1618f
Autosomal recessive inheritance, 1618f, 1619
Aviation safety movement, 3256–3257
Aviation safety reporting system, 3258
Avitene, 52
Avulsion, soft tissue injuries, 1109
Ayurveda, 319
Azelastine, 471

B
Bacillary angiomatosis, 283–284
Bacterial infections
  acute bacterial sialadenitis, 1467
  pharyngitis due to, 758–761, 760f, 765
  tuberculosis, stomatitis, 743–744
Bacterial laryngitis, 978–979, 979f

Bacterial meningitis, 1530
Bacterial pyoderma, 3198
Balloon catheter dilation procedures
    complications, 649
Balloon sinuplasty, 600–601
Barbiturates, 42, 42t, 46, 240
Bard-Parker handle, 22
Barium swallow, 165, 166f
    to demonstrate aspiration, 861, 861f
    modified, of upper aerodigestive tract, 165
Basal cell nevus syndrome, 2102
Basal-bolus insulin treatment, 31, 32t
Basaloid squamous cell carcinoma, 191f
Basic surgical principles
    antibiotic selection, 22–23, 23t
    informed consent, 20
    patient positioning and exposure, 22
    postoperative care, 23
    preoperative assessment and evaluation
        anticoagulation and antiplatelet
            therapy, 20
        beta-blockade, 18, 20
        cardiac evaluation and care algorithm,
            18, 19f
        clinical risk factors, 18
        energy requirements, 18, 19t
        functional capacity, 18
        pulmonary evaluation, 20
        renal and hepatic function, 20
        suture material, 22
    sterile technique, 21
    surgical instruments
        forceps, 22
        scalpels, 21–22
        scissors, 22
    universal precautions, 20–21
    venous thromboembolism prophylaxis
        complications, 23–24
        incidence, 24
        risk profiles, 24, 24t
Basilar migraine, 2727–2728
Beals syndrome, 1636
Beaver handle, 22
Beckwith-Wiedemann syndrome, 120–121,
    1636
Bedside swallow evaluation
    acute stroke, 828
    examination and observation, 827
    feeding history, 825–826
    flexible endoscopic evaluation of
            swallowing
        epiglottis tip, 828, 828f
        equipment requirement, 828
        FEESST versus fluoroscopy, 830t
        laryngeal adductor reflex, 828–829
        patient position, 828
        penetration aspiration scale, 830, 830t
        pharyngeal squeeze maneuver,
            828–829, 829f
        premature spillage, 830
        rising tide sign, 830
        videofluoroscopic swallow study, 831
    oral cavity and oropharynx, 827
    silent aspiration, 827–828
    used for, 825
Behavior observation audiometry, 1513
Behavioral audiometry, 1481

Behçet disease, 278, 748
Behind-the-ear hearing aids, 2660, 2660f,
    2661f, 2667, 2667f
Bell palsy, 2510–2512
Benedikt syndrome, 202
Benign esophageal neoplasms, 857
Benign mixed tumor
    of salivary gland, 1760, 1766, 1766f
Benign necrotizing otitis externa, 137
Benign nonepithelial tumors, 2048
Benign paroxysmal positional vertigo,
    2708–2710
Benign salivary neoplasia, 984
Benign vocal fold lesions, professional
    voice, 1067–1068
Benjamin-Inglis classification, 1321
Benzodiazepines, 42, 42t, 65, 65t, 241
Bernard cheiloplasty, Webster modification
    of, 1800, 1801f
β-blockade therapy, preoperative, in car-
    diac abnormalities, 35
Betahistine
    Ménière syndrome, 2704
Bethesda system, thyroid cytopathology,
    2118t
Bicoronal flap incision, 2059f–2060f
Bifrontal craniotomy, 2087
Bilateral vestibular hypofunction, 2712
Bilateral vocal fold immobility
    clinical presentation and evaluation, 1017
        fiberoptic laryngoscopy, 1018, 1018f
        history, 1018–1019
        imaging, 1019
        laryngeal electromyography, 1019
        laryngoscopy and palpation,
            1019–1020, 1020f
        physical examination, 1019
        serology, 1019
    etiology of, 1017, 1017t, 1018t
    management
        airway, 1020
        long-term surgical solutions,
            1021–1022, 1021f
        temporizing (reversible) treatments,
            1020–1021
Bilevel positive pressure (BIPAP), 2175
Bilobed flaps
    in cutaneous nasal defects, 2877,
        2879–2880, 2882f
Binder syndrome, 1636
Bing-Siebenmann malformation, 1536
Biofilms, 1486–1487
Biologic and mechanical creeps, 2850, 2851t
Biologic materials, as implants, 2785t,
    2787
Biopsy
    cutaneous lesion, 178–179
    of lip, 1790, 1791, 1791t, 1793
    of lymph nodes, 1813, 1814
        sentinel node, 1814–1815
    mucosal sites, 179
    neoplasms, 2049
    of salivary gland
        fine-needle aspiration, 1769, 1769t
        surgical, 1770
    subcutaneous masses, 179–180
Bishop-Harmon forceps, 22

Bisoprolol, 35
Bites, soft tissue injuries, 1127–1128
Bivalirudin, 29
Blastomycosis, 290
Bleeding. See also Hemorrhage
    as complication of mastoid surgery,
        2463
    intraoperative and postoperative,
        testing/management in, 30
    percutaneous dilatational tracheotomy,
        942
Blepharitis, 224
Blepharochalasis, 3076
Blepharoplasty
    lower eyelid
        canthopexy and canthoplasty, 3095,
            3096f, 3097
        complications of, 3099–3100
        dermatochalasis, 3086, 3086f
        double convexity deformity, 3086,
            3088f
        dy eye symptoms, blurry vision and
            chemosis, 3100, 3100f
        ectropion and entropion, 3086,
            3087f
        fat grafting, 3099
        festoons, 3086, 3088f
        hyaluronic acid fillers, 3099, 3099f
        infection of, 3101
        laxity, 3086, 3087f
        lid position abnormalities, 3100–3101,
            3101f
        malar mounds, 3086, 3088, 3088f
        midface lift, 3099, 3100f
        milia, 3101
        negative vector, 3086, 3087f
        orbicularis hypertrophy, 3086, 3087f
        orbital fat pseudoherniation/palpebral
            bags, 3085–3086, 3086f
        patient selection and examination,
            3088–3089, 3089f–3091f
        photography, 3089, 3091f
        preseptal hematoma, 3101, 3101f
        preseptal transconjunctival technique,
            3092, 3093f, 3094, 3094f
        resurfacing, 3097–3098, 3099f
        retroorbital hematoma, 3101
        scleral show, 3086, 3087f
        skin flap technique, 3095
        skin-muscle flap
            technique for, 3094–3095, 3094f,
                3095f
            transcutaneous approach, 3094,
                3094f
        surgical procedure for, 3091
        tear trough deformity, 3086, 3087f
        toxoallergic blepharoconjunctivitis,
            3101
        transconjunctival approach, 3091–
            3092, 3092f, 3093f
    upper eyelid
        complications of, 3084
        patients history, 3077–3078
        periocular rejuvenation, 3081, 3081f
        photography, 3081
        physical examination, 3078–3081,
            3080f

Blepharoplasty (*Continued*)
  surgical anatomy of
    levator muscle and Müller muscle,
      3076–3077
    orbicularis oculi muscle hyperfunc-
      tion, 3074–3075, 3075*f*
    periorbital musculature, 3075, 3076*f*
    postseptal orbital compartment,
      3076, 3076*f*
    tarsal plate level, 3077, 3078*f*
    upper eyelid-brow complex, 3074,
      3075*f*
  surgical technique, 3081–3083, 3082*f*,
    3083*f*
Blindness. *See* Vision loss
Blood components
  preoperative transfusion of, 27–28, 27*t*
Blood dyscrasia, ocular manifestations
  of, 227
Blood supply, eyelids, 4–5
Blood vessels
  of forehead, 3053, 3054*f*
  sinus surgery complications, 658
Blow-out fracture
  demographics and etiology, 1227–1228,
    1228*f*
  surgical indications, 1231
Blowout, jugular vein, after neck dissection, 1834
Blue nevus, 3219, 3220*f*
  treatment of, 3228
Blunt injuries, traumatic disorders,
  external ear, 2346
Body dysmorphic disorder, 2759
Body, of mandible fracture, 1196*f*, 1202
Bone(s)
  anchored hearing system
    complications, 2641
    conductive or mixed hearing losses,
      2640
    single-sided deafness, 2640
    surgery, 2640–2641, 2641*f*
  contour, forehead, 3057
  lesions
    fibrous dysplasia, 292–293, 293*f*
    ossifying fibroma, 293
    Paget disease, 293–294
  vaults, nasal dorsum
    anatomy, 2953
    defects of, 2956, 2956*t*
    grafts, 2961–2962
    hump reduction, 2959–2960, 2960*f*
    iatrogenic deformities, 2956*t*, 2959
    osteotomies, 2960–2961, 2961*f*, 2962*f*
Bone healing, 1153–1154
BOR syndrome, 124
Borderline personality disorder, 2759
Botox
  for brow adjustment, 3243
  complications associated with,
    3243–3244
  contraindications, 3241
  cosmetic applications of, 3241–3242
  in glabellar rhytids, 3242
  indications, 3241
  and injectable fillers, cosmetic uses of,
    3239–3250

in lateral periorbital rhytids, 3242–3243,
    3243*f*
  mechanism of action, 3241
  for platysmal banding, 3243
  in transverse forehead rhytids, 3242,
    3242*f*
  in vertical lip rhytids, 3243
Botryoid tumors, 2373
Botulism, 1041–1042
Bovine collagen, for soft tissue augmenta-
  tion, 3245
Bowen disease, 1727
Boxcar sign, 222
Brachytherapy. *See also* Radiation therapy
  in recurrent nasopharyngeal cancer,
    1886, 1888–1893, 1889*f*
Braided suture, 22
Brain, 305–306, 306*f*. *See also* Central
    nervous system
Brain abscess, 2405–2406
Brain herniation
  in cholesteatoma, 2444
Brainstem, vestibular, 2299–2300
Branchial cleft anomalies
  anatomic pathways, 1608, 1608*t*
  branchial cleft lesions, 1608–1609, 1609*f*
  CT scan, 1609, 1609*f*
  pyriform sinus, 1609, 1609*f*
  seventh nerve dissection, 1608, 1608*f*
  surgical exposure of, 1607, 1608*f*
Branchiootorenal syndrome, 1533–1534,
    1543*t*, 1548, 1611–1612, 1611*t*,
    1623–1624, 1624*f*
Breathing. *See also* Respiration
  sleep-disordered. *See* Sleep-disordered
    breathing
  trauma and, primary survey of, 1097,
    1097*f*, 1098*f*
Bronchiectasis, in Kartagener syndrome,
    1629
Bronchoscope, 1311, 1312*f*
Brow(s)
  adjustment of, Botox for, 3243
  asymmetries of, forehead lift and, 3057
Brow lift
  browpexy, 3067
  chemical, 3243
  direct, 3065, 3065*f*, 3066*f*
  indirect, 3066–3067
  surgical procedure for, 3067
  technique for, 3066, 3066*f*
  and upper blepharoplasty, surgical pro-
    cedure for, 3061
Browpexy, 3067
Brucellosis, 284
Brun nystagmus, 2685
Buccal space, odontogenic infection, 773,
    773*f*, 774*f*
Bulbar palsy, 1037
Bullard laryngoscope, 900, 900*f*
Bullous pemphigoid, 745, 745*f*
Bupivacaine, 46, 236
Burning mouth syndrome, 753, 753*t*
Burns
  ocular trauma, 229
  oral cavity cancer, 1869–1870
  soft tissue injuries, 1128

Business law, 3270–3301
  compliance and regulatory issues
    compliance programs, 3284–3285
    enforcement, 3282–3283
    federal health care fraud and abuse
      laws, 3282
    law applications, 3284
  medical liability
    claims in the United States, 3271–3272
    health care costs, 3280–3282
    medical malpractice insurance,
      3276–3278
    medical malpractice litigation
      expert witnesses, 3274–3275
      general legal background,
        3272–3273
      Hobson's choice, 3275
      presuit, 3273
      settlement *versus* trial, 3275
      suit filed, 3273–3274
      trials, 3275–3276
    tort reform, 3278–3279
  medical malpractice, 3271
  operational issues
    hospital call, 3299–3300
    office electronic medical records
      meaningful use criteria, 3297
      Medicare Affiliated Contractors, 3298
      physician eligibility, 3297–3298
      Zone Program Integrity Auditors,
        3298
    social media and e-mail communica-
      tion, 3298–3299
  physician licensing actions
    administrative complaint and hearing,
      3289
    criminal prosecution, 3289–3290
    licensure actions, 3288–3289
  physician practice setting
    business entity, 3292–3293
    business loan, 3293
    corporate perspective, 3291
    federal tax identification number,
      3294
    Hipaa privacy and security,
      3294–3296
    securing insurance, 3293–3294
    third party payors enrolling, 3294
  professional services billing, 3270–3271
  third party payor audits
    audit defenses, 3287
    audit processes for medicare,
      3285–3286
    compliance tips, 3287–3288
    Medicare appeals process, 3286–3287
    overview of, 3285
Butanol threshold test, 454
Buttress graft, nasal tip surgery, 2975
Butyl-2-cyanoacrylate
  implant, 2795

C
Calcifying epithelial odontogenic tumor,
    2105
Calcitonin, 254
Calcium
  excess of, 255

in thyroid surgery, 33
Calcium carbonate, 33
Calcium gluconate, 33
Calcium homeostasis, hyperparathyroidism, 2131–2132, 2132f
Calcium hydroxyapatite-based injectable implant, 2793
Calculi, salivary. See Sialolithiasis
Caldwell-Luc operation
    complications, 644–645
    maxillary sinus, 604
Caloric and head impulse testing
    Ménière syndrome, 2703
Caloric requirements, daily, 26
Calvaria, anatomy of, 3, 4f
Canalicular injury, 1119f
Canalplasty, 2465
Candidiasis
    acute atrophic, 740
    esophagitis, 852, 853f
    pharyngeal, 766
    stomatitis, 740–741, 740f, 740t, 741f
Canine space, odontogenic infection, 773
Capillary hemangiomas, 2066, 3216
Capillary malformations, 3205–3207, 3207f
Capsaicin, nonallergic rhinitis, 472
Carbon dioxide laser. See also Laser(s)
    for skin cancer, 1732–1734, 1733f, 1733t, 1734t
Carbunculosis, 2344
Carcinoid tumors, 264–265
Carcinoma
    anaplastic, 2120–2121
    follicular, 2120
    papillary, 2120
Carcinoma ex-pleomorphic adenoma, salivary gland, 1766–1767, 1766f
Cardiogenic shock, 1099–1100, 1100f
Cardiovascular disorders
    ACC/AHA guidelines, 35
    β-blockade therapy, 35
    dysrhythmia, 37
    hypertension, 35–36, 36t
    hypotension, 36–37, 36t
    postoperative, risk factors for, 35
Cardioversion, 37
Carotid artery dissection, 313, 1807, 1809–1811, 1814, 1824–1826, 1832–1834
Carotid artery rupture, after neck dissection, 1832
Carotid body tumors, 2003–2005, 2004f, 2004t, 2005t, 2011–2012, 2012f, 2013f
Carotid space, deep neck, 797, 799
Carotid-cavernous fistula, 2608–2609
Carotidynia, 313
Cartilage, nasal, for nasal reconstruction, 2872
Cartilage-shaping technique, otoplasty, 3156–3157, 3157f, 3158f
Cartilaginous vaults
    anatomy, 2953
    defects of, 2956–2957
    management of, 2957–2958, 2958f, 2959f
Castleman disease, 1599

Cataract formation, 221–222
Catch-up saccades, 2687
Catecholamine-secreting tumors, 263–264
Catenary lever effect, 2466
Cathelicidin, 382
Cathode ray tubes, 2782
Cat-scratch disease, 283–284, 704–705, 1595–1596
Caudal excess nasal deformity, 3017
Caustic ingestions
    esophageal disorders, 857
    laryngeal stenosis, 1361
Cavernous hemangioma, 2066, 2067f
Cavernous sinus thrombophlebitis, 576–577
Cefazolin, 44
Celecoxib (celebrex), 1423
Cell cycle
    cell proliferation, 1652–1654
    epidermal growth factor, 1648–1650
    inhibitors, 1654–1655
    p53, 1655–1656
    transforming growth factor beta, 1651–1652
Cell population, radiation therapy, 1682, 1683f
Cellulitis
    lip swelling, 771, 772f
    orbital, 575–576, 576f
Centenarians, 298
Centers for Disease Control, 20–21
Central compartment dissection, 1820, 1823
Central nervous system
    auditory, 2263, 2269–2271
    neurologic disorder
        ataxic disorders, 1034
        hyperkinetic disorders, 1032–1034
        hypokinetic disorders, 1030–1032, 1031f, 1032t
        mixed disorders, 1034–1037
        spastic disorder, 1030
Central vestibular disorders, 2738–2739
    eye movement examination
        gaze-evoked nystagmus, 2721
        head-shaking nystagmus, 2720
        ocular tilt reaction, 2720
        positional nystagmus, 2720
        rebound nystagmus, 2721
        saccades, 2720
        smooth pursuit, 2719–2720
        spontaneous downbeat nystagmus, 2720–2721
        vibration-induced nystagmus, 2720
    focal neurologic examination findings, 2721–2722
    migraine-associated vertigo
        basilar migraine, 2727–2728, 2727t
        definite migrainous vertigo, 2727, 2727t
        diagnostic criteria, 2726, 2726t
        motion sickness, 2728
        probable migrainous vertigo, 2727, 2727t
        treatment, 2728
        vestibulopathy and hearing loss, 2728
    multiple sclerosis, 2728–2730

versus peripheral cause of vertigo, 2719t
    dizziness, 2718
    spontaneous nystagmus, 2718–2719
symptoms, 2722–2723, 2723t
vertebrobasilar TIAs
    AICA stroke and hearing loss, 2725, 2725t
    cerebellar infarction, 2726
    isolated vertigo, 2724, 2724t
    labyrinthine infarct, 2724–2725
    vascular risk factors, 2723–2724
    vertebrobasilar ischemia and imaging, 2726
    Wallenberg syndrome, 2725–2726
Central vestibular system, 2717–2718
Cephalic trim technique, 3004
Cephalometrics, in facial analysis, 2768
Cephalosporins, 131, 132t
Ceramic implants, 2786
Cerebellar hemorrhage, 204
Cerebellar infarction, 203, 204f, 2726
Cerebellar/temporal lobe abscesses, 2444
Cerebellopontine angle
    anatomy, 2556–2558, 2557f, 2558f
    neoplasms of, 2376–2381
    tumors of
        arachnoid cyst, 2577
        epidermoid and dermoid cyst, 2577, 2578f
        facial nerve monitoring during, 2327
        intraaxial lesions, 2580
        lipoma, 2577, 2579f
        meningioma, 2575–2577, 2576f
        miscellaneous extraaxial lesions, 2578–2580, 2579f
        nonvestibular cranial nerve schwannomas, 2574, 2574f
        patient history, 2556
        radiology, 2584t
        skull base lesions, 2580–2583, 2581f–2583f
        vestibular schwannoma. See Vestibular schwannoma
Cerebral edema, after neck dissection, 1832
Cerebrospinal fluid, 1273, 1282
    fistula, 655–656
    leakage of, 662–673
        as complication of mastoid surgery, 2462–2463
        etiology, 662–663
            accidental trauma, 663, 663f
            congenital CSF leaks, 665
            spontaneous CSF leaks, 664–665
            surgical trauma, 663–664, 664f
            tumors, 665
        history of surgery for, 662
        long-term management, 672
        patient workup
            imaging studies, 666–667, 667f
            laboratory testing, 665–666
            patient history, 665
            physical examination, 665, 666f
        perioperative issues
            antibiotics, 668
            intrathecal fluorescein, 667–668, 668f
            lumbar drain, 668

Cerebrospinal fluid (*Continued*)
  postoperative care, 672
  reconstructive techniques, 671
  site-specific repair strategy
    anterior skull base, 670–671, 671*f*
    cribriform plate/ethmoid roof, 669
    frontal sinus CSF leaks, 670
    outcomes, 672
    pedicled flaps, 671
    sella and clivus, 671
    sphenoid sinus, 669–670, 670*f*
  surgical management
    principles, 669
    rationale for repair, 668–669
  physiology and intracranial pressure
    basics, 662
Cerebrovascular disease
  cerebellar hemorrhage, 204
  cerebellar infarction, 203, 204*f*
  clinical evaluation and management
    acute spontaneous vertigo, 204
    CT, 205
    magnetic resonance angiogram,
      205, 206*f*
    MRI, 205*f*
  lateral medullary syndrome, 200, 203*f*
  lateral pontomedullary syndrome, 200,
    203*f*
  midbrain syndromes, 202–203, 204*f*
  stroke, 199
  subarachnoid hemorrhage, 204
  vertebrobasilar insufficiency, 199–200
Ceruminous adenocarcinoma, 2369
Cervical esophageal carcinoma
  complications, 1936, 1936*t*
  diagnosis
    imaging, 1920–1921
    nutritional evaluation, 1921
    patient evaluation, 1919–1920, 1920*t*
    physical examination, 1920
  epidemiology, 1918–1919
  esophagus reconstruction, 1932–1933,
    1933*f*, 1934*f*
  etiology, 1919
  functional rehabilitation, 1936
  neck management, 1932
  nonsurgical therapy, 1933, 1935
  organ preservation protocol, 1936
  pathology
    molecular staging, 1923
    patterns of spread, 1921–1922, 1921*t*,
      1922*f*
    TNM staging, 1922–1923
  prognosis, 1923–1924, 1923*t*, 1924*t*
  salvage surgery, 1935–1936
  surgery of
    advanced-stage pyriform sinus cancer,
      1925, 1927
    cervical esophagus, 1932
    early-stage pyriform sinus cancer,
      1924–1925, 1925*f*, 1926*f*
    postcricoid cancer, 1929
    posterior hypopharyngeal wall cancer,
      1927–1928, 1928*f*–1931*f*
    preoperative considerations, 1924
    transoral laser and robotic surgery,
      1929

Cervical fascia, deep neck, 796
Cervical metastasis, 2057–2058
Cervical necrotizing fasciitis, 779
Cervical plexus, nerve block of, 238
Cervical spine injury, 917
Cervical subcutaneous emphysema, 1142
Cervical tracheal tumors, 1996
Cervicogenic headache, 314
Chalazion, 224
CHARGE association, 1625
Charged coupled devices, 2779
Cheek, soft tissue injuries, 1120–1121,
  1121*f*, 1122*f*
Cheilitis, actinic, 3212, 3215*f*
Cheilitis glandularis, 713
Cheilitis granulomatosa, 1629–1630,
  1629*f*
Cheiloplasty. *See* Lip(s), cancer of, surgery
  for
Chemical hazards, lasers, 3209–3210
Chemical peeling
  in benign lesions, 3222–3223, 3223*t*
  Hetter
    basic science of, 3191–3193, 3192*t*
    complications, 3195, 3198
    historical background of, 3189, 3190*t*
    patient selection, 3189–3190, 3190*t*,
      3191*t*
    postoperative care, 3194–3195,
      3195*f*–3197*f*
    prepeel preparation, 3190–3191
    technique of, 3193–3194, 3193*t*, 3194*f*
Chemokines, 389
  receptor families, 395*t*
  receptor involvement, human disease,
    396*t*
Chemosis, following blepharoplasty, 3100,
  3100*f*
Chemotherapy, 341–342
  administration schedules, 1694
  biologic therapy, 1701–1702
  clinical trials
    phase I trials, 1694
    phase II trials, 1694
    phase III trials, 1694
  drugs used
    biologic modifier, 1693–1694
    5-fluorouracil, 1693
    methotrexate, 1693
    platinum-based agents, 1693
    taxanes, 1693
  free tissue transfer
    hypopharynx, 1715–1717, 1716*f*
    larynx, 1715
    nasopharynx/skull base/paranasal
      sinuses, 1712–1713
    oral cavity, 1713, 1714*f*
    oropharynx, 1713–1715
    radial forearm free flaps, 1711–1712
    skin flap necrosis, 1711, 1711*f*
    in wound healing, 1711
  head and neck cancer, 1694
    carotids, CT angio, 1709, 1709*f*
    chondroradionecrosis, 1710
    osteoradionecrosis, 1709, 1709*f*
    radiation therapy, 1709
    role of, 1708

laryngeal cancer
  induction chemotherapy, 1968–1969
  radiation therapy, 1967–1968
locally advanced unresectable disease
  cisplatin and 5-fluorouracil,
    1700–1701
  concurrent chemoradiation, 1700
in nasopharyngeal carcinoma,
  1887–1888, 1893
neoplasms, 2051, 2053, 2057*t*
oral cavity cancer, 1864
organ preservation
  hypopharyngeal cancer, 1696–1697
  larynx cancer, 1695–1696
  nasopharyngeal cancer, 1698–1699
  oral cavity cancer, 1699–1700
  oropharyngeal cancer, 1697–1698
overview of, 1692
postoperative management, high-risk
  disease, 1701
recurrent or distant metastatic disease,
  1702–1703
for salivary gland tumors, 1781, 1781*t*
tracheal tumors, 1996
Cherry angiomas, 3216
Chiari malformations, 214, 214*f*
Chicago classification, high-resolution
  manometry, 834, 834*t*
Children. *See* Pediatric patients
Chin
  augmentation
    aesthetics of, 3178, 3180*f*
    alloplast implant, 3181–3183, 3182*f*,
      3183*f*
    cephalostat, 3177–3178, 3179*f*
    chin deformities, 3178–3181, 3180*f*,
      3181*f*
    congenital malformation, 3179
    contour and projection of, 3176–3177
    facial skeletal deformity, 3176, 3177*f*
    hemifacial microsomia, 3177, 3179*f*
    lower facial analysis, 3178, 3180*f*
    mentalis strain, 3176, 3177*f*
    orthognathic surgery, 3177
    osseous genioplasty. *See* Osseous
      genioplasty
    physical examination, 3176
    radiography, 3177, 3178*f*, 3179*f*
    Ricketts analysis, 3178, 3180*f*
    surgical procedure selection, 3181
  facial features, 3176
  and neck, assessment of, for plastic sur-
    gery of face, 2767
  soft tissue injuries, 1126, 1126*f*
Chin tuck posture, 839
Chinese medicine, traditional, acupunc-
  ture and, 319–320
Chiropractic medicine, 318–319
Chlamydia pneumoniae, 1433
Chlorhexidine gluconate, 21
Choanal atresia
  in nasal obstruction, 1330–1331,
    1330*f*–1331*f*
Cholesteatoma, 2362–2364, 2433–2445
  acquired, 2434–2436
  complications and emergency,
    2442–2445, 2443*f*, 2444*f*

congenital, 2363, 2434–2435, 2434f
diagnosis of, 2363–2364
extratemporal, 2444, 2444f
infections of, 2444
morphologic appearance, 2363
otitis media, 1499
pathogenesis of, 2434–2436, 2434t, 2435f, 2436f
preoperative evaluation, 2438–2440, 2440t
prevention of, 2437, 2439f
surgical anatomy of, 2436–2437, 2437f–2439f
surgical goals for, 2440t
surgical management of, 2389–2390, 2440–2442, 2441t
treatment of, 2364
Cholesterol granuloma
causes of, 2375–2376
cerebellopontine angle, 2581, 2581f, 2582f
diagnosis of, 2376
of petrous apex, 2376
Choline transporter-like-2, 2707
Chondritis, 2344
Chondrodermatitis nodularis chronica helicis, 2370
Chondroma, 983
Chondromatous lesions
cerebellopontine angle, 2581, 2582f
Chondroradionecrosis, 1720
Chondrosarcoma, 2049
MRI, 152, 153f
of skull base, 2373–2374
Chordoma
cerebellopontine angle, 2583, 2583f
of skull base, 2374
Choristoma, in middle ear, 2375
Chromosomes, 1541
Chronic daily headache, 309–310, 310t
Chronic sialadenitis, 706–707, 707f
Chronic sinusitis, 1456t
Chronic suppurative otitis media, 136, 2400
Chronic ulcerative stomatitis, 747
Chronic vocal fold scar, voice therapy, 1054
Chronically inadequate vestibular function, 2712
Churg-Strauss syndrome, 276, 495–496, 496f
Chylous fistula
after neck dissection, 1831–1832
Ciaglia Blue Rhino Introducer Kit, 938f
Ciliary dyskinesia
primary, 367, 539
secondary, 367–368
Circulation, in trauma patients, primary survey of, 1097–1100, 1110f
Cisatracurium, 243
Cisplatin
in metastasis of nasopharyngeal cancer, 1888, 1893
ototoxicity, 2545–2546
Cleft lip/palate, 1561, 1565
anatomical classification systems
LAHSHAL system, 1560

Veau classification system, 1560, 1561f
anatomy
bilateral cleft lip, 1559
palatal anatomy, 1559–1560, 1560f
unilateral cleft lip, 1559
embryology
facial development, 1557, 1558f
palatal anatomy, 1557
sonic hedgehog, 1557
epidemiology, 1556–1557
oral feeding, 1559
otolaryngologic considerations
airway obstruction, 1571
eustachian tube dysfunction, 1570–1571
hoarseness, 1572
obstructive sleep apnea, 1571–1572
prenatal diagnosis and counseling, 1557–1558, 1558t
in Robin sequence, 1631
surgical management
alveolar bone grafting, 1562, 1568
bilateral cleft lip and nose repair, 1564–1565, 1564f
cleft lip and nose repair, 1561
cleft palate repair, 1561, 1565
cleft rhinoplasty, 1562, 1570
furlow double opposing Z-plasty, 1565–1566, 1566f
intravelar veloplasty, 1566–1568, 1567f
lip adhesion, 1562–1563
nasoalveolar molding, 1562
orthognathic surgery, 1562, 1568–1570
presurgical infant orthopedics, 1560–1561
pulsed-dye laser therapy, 1562
speech surgery, 1561–1562, 1568
unilateral cleft lip and nose repair, 1563–1564, 1563f
Cleft rhinoplasty, 1562, 1570
Clindamycin, 132
Clinic management
access management, 3333–3334
clinic efficiency, 3334
critical patient communication, 3337–3338
financial management, 3336–3337
human resources, 3332–3333
information technology, 3338, 3339t
managed care contracting
negotiation goals, 3335–3336
marketing, 3339–3340
operational adaptability, 3334–3335
patient privacy, 3338
safety and quality, 3335
Clinical data
causality of
analysis of, measurement scales for, 90, 90t
assessment of, 90
interpretation of
numerical, descriptive statistics and, 91t
questions for, 87–100
study design for, 87, 88t, 89
sampling population for, 97–98, 97t

statistical significance of, versus clinical importance of, 94
understanding of, 86–100
Clinical databases
applications
institutional database studies, 3358
population databases and data warehouses, 3358
PubMed and literature databases, 3356–3358
basics of, 3355–3356
billing codes, 3354
EHR systems, 3355
institutional review board, 3354
insurance database, 3354
translational medicine
ethical issues in, 3359
translational database studies, 3359
translational research databases, 3358–3359
types of, 3354
Veterans Administration, 3355
Clinical guidelines
AGREE instrument principles, 1674, 1674t
flawed guideline, 1673
goals of, 1673
resources for, 1674, 1674t
Clinical pathways
laryngectomy, 1675
lengths of stay, 1674
for unilateral neck dissection, 1674
unknown primary tumor, 1675, 1675f
Clinical status, 1673
Clinical studies
results of, validity of, 94–95
types of, 102–103, 103t
Clinical-severity index, creation of, 103–104
Clonidine, in smoking cessation therapy, 335
Clonidine-withdrawal syndrome, 35
Clostridium difficile colitis, 70–71, 71t
Cluster headache, 309, 310t
Coagulation phase, of wound healing, 77–78, 78f
Coalescent mastoiditis, 801f
Cocaine, 236
Coccidioidomycosis, 290
Cochlea
anatomy of, 2256–2262, 2257f–2262f
clinical and histopathologic changes, 2617–2618, 2617t
gross extracellular potentials, 2262–2263
transduction and, 2258, 2261f, 2262f
Cochlear aplasia, inner ear anomaly, 1535
Cochlear hypoplasia, 1535
Cochlear implants
auditory system, 2626–2627
clinical evaluation, 2637–2638, 2638t
coding strategies, 2627
complications, 2636, 2636t
current device technology, 2628, 2628t
meningitis, 2636–2637

Cochlear implants (*Continued*)
  outcomes of, 2625
  overview of, 2625
  patient history, 2625–2626
  patient selection, 2628–2629, 2629*t*
  surgery
    cochleostomy, 2633, 2634*f*
    electrode insertion, 2633
    inner ear malformation, 2630*f*–2631*f*,
      2633–2634, 2635*f*
    inner ear obstruction, 2634–2635,
      2635*f*
    otitis media, 2635–2636
    patient preparation, 2632, 2632*f*
    patient setup, 2631–2632
    receiver-stimulator placement and
      fixation, 2632–2633
    standard mastoidectomy, 2633
    telemetry, 2633
    temporal bone imaging, 2629–2631,
      2630*f*–2632*f*
    trauma and bone dust, 2627–2628
Cochlear modifier, 2258
Cochlear nucleus, 2269, 2270*f*
Cochleostomy, 2633, 2634*f*
Cochrane, 1354
Codeine, 45
Coding and billing
  fundamentals
    auditing principles, 3310
    documentation and patient care
      medical necessity, 3309
      specificity, 3308–3309
    medicare, 3310
    preloaded generic clinical informa-
      tion, 3310
    records review, 3310
  ICD-9, 3305
  modifiers use
    E/M services related to procedures,
      3323–3324
    individual services claims, 3319–3320
    multiple procedures, 3322–3323
    multiple procedures, date of service,
      3320–3321
  in otolaryngology
    ear procedures, 3326
    evaluation and management coding,
      3326
    larynx, 3328
    nose and sinus procedures,
      3326–3328
    oral cavity, 3328
    recognized risk areas, 3325–3326
    specific coding and billing risks, 3326
Coffin-Lowry syndrome, 1636
Cogan syndrome, 278–279, 2522
Cognitive impairment, 43
Cohen syndrome, 1637
Cold dry air provocation test, 471
Collagen
  bovine, for soft tissue augmentation,
    3245
  metabolism of, and wound healing, 82
Collagen vascular disease, 267, 268*f*
Colony-stimulation factor leak, neo-
    plasms, 19

Comedones, 3215
Comorbid conditions
  definition of, 104
  identification of, 104
Comparative medical systems
  amenable mortality, 3342
  Bismarck-style insurers, 3345
  government-financed insurance system,
    3345
  lack of universal coverage
    beveridge model, 3343–3344
    Medicaid, 3342
    national health insurance model,
      3344–3345
    for oropharyngeal cancer patients,
      3342
    patient delay factors, 3342–3343
    solution(s) for, 3343
  national health insurance, 3346–3347
  obstacles to, 3346
  Organisation for Economic Co-operation
    and Development, 3341
  Patient Protection And Affordable Care
    Act, 3345
  Physicians for a National Health
    Program, 3342
  ration care, 3347
  universal health coverage, 3341
Compensatory treatment techniques, 838
  bolus consistency, 840
  feeding, 840
  intraoral prosthetics, 840–841
  postures, 839–840, 839*t*
  sensory enhancement technique, 840
Complementary and alternative medicine,
    316–326
  allergic rhinitis and rhinosinusitis, 325
  head and neck oncology, 324–325
  manipulative and body-based tech-
    niques
    chiropractic medicine, 318–319
    massage, 319
    osteopathic medicine, 318
  mind-body medicine, 317–318
  natural products, 317
  otitis media, 323–324
  in otolaryngology patients
    drug-herb interactions, 321–322
    perioperative management, 322–323
  tinnitus, 323
  vertigo, 323
  whole medical systems
    ayurveda, 319
    homeopathy, 320
    naturopathic medicine, 320–321
    traditional chinese medicine, 319–320
Complete glottic stenosis, 885
Completion rhinoplasty, 2991
Compliant documentation
  comparative effectiveness research, 3303
  comprehensive history and physical
    examination, 3304
  electronic health records, 3303
  evaluation and management documen-
    tation, 3304
  factors, 3304
  toolkit for, 3305–3308

Composite grafts, in cutaneous nasal
    defects, 2877
Composite perichondrium-cartilage island
    graft, 2472–2473, 2473*f*
Compound nevi, 3218, 3219*f*
Compression of morbidity, 299
Computed tomography
  atrophic rhinitis, 483, 483*f*
  central skull base, 142–143, 143*f*
  fungus ball, 423*f*
  granulomatous sinusitis, 437, 437*f*
  indications, 422, 423*t*
  invasive fungal rhinosinusitis, 559
  invasive fungal sinusitis, 435–437, 436*f*
  maxillofacial structures and sinonasal
    cavities, 144, 144*f*
  midface fracture, 1210*f*, 1213–1214,
    1214*t*
  of nasopharyngeal cancer, 1878, 1879,
    1879*f*, 1883, 1883*f*, 1884*f*, 1885,
    1888, 1892*f*
  neonatal respiratory distress
    nasal obstruction, 1330, 1331*f*
    oral cavity/oropharynx/hypopharynx,
      1331
    trachea/bronchi, 1334
    vocal fold paralysis, 1333
  noninvasive fungal sinusitis, 435,
    435*f*–436*f*
  orbit, 144–145, 145*f*
  paraganglioma, 2005–2006, 2006*f*–2007*f*
  principles, 141, 142*f*
  rhinosinusitis
    acute, 425–426, 425*f*
    atelectatic sinus, 428, 429*f*–430*f*
    bony destruction, sinonasal sarcoma,
      430, 431*f*
    chronic, 541–542, 542*f*
    chronic sinusitis, 426, 426*f*
    encephalocele, 432, 433*f*
    endoscopic sinus surgery, 432–435
    frontal sinus mucocele with proptosis,
      428, 429*f*
    intracerebral abscess and epidural
      abscess, 581*f*
    normal paranasal sinus anatomy, 426,
      427*f*
    odontogenic maxillary sinusitis, 426,
      426*f*
    orbital cellulitis, 576*f*
    orbital subperiosteal abscess, 430, 430*f*
    pott puffy tumor, 583*f*
    pott puffy tumor with epidural empy-
      ema, 430, 431*f*
    preseptal abscess, 576*f*
    retention cysts, 428, 430
    sinonasal polyposis, 426, 428*f*
    subdural empyema, 430, 431*f*
    subperiosteal orbital abscess, 576*f*
  sinonasal neoplasm
    arrested skull base pneumatization,
      440, 442*f*
    breast carcinoma metastasis, 437, 439*f*
    intracranial and orbital invasion, 438*f*
    inverted papilloma, 440, 441*f*
    juvenile nasopharyngeal angiofi-
      broma, 440, 441*f*

mass/inflammation prediction, 437
soft tissues, 145
temporal bone, 141–142, 142f
terminology, 422
tumor staging, 440–441, 443
Computed tomography angiography, 145,
147–148
Concha bullosa, nasal obstruction in, 364
Conditioned play audiometry, 1514
Conductive hearing loss, 2640. *See also*
Hearing loss
Condyle, mandibular fracture, 1279, 1279f
management, 1196f, 1203–1204, 1204t
Confidential voice therapy, 1050–1051
Configuration, 2276–2277
Conflicts of interest
best practices, 3390
continuing medical education, 3388
definition of
disclosure, 3381
duality of interest, 3380
institutional, 3381, 3387
in medical practice, 3387–3388
in publishing, 3381
in research, 3381
rules governing, 3388–3390
Confocal microscopy, 51
Congenital carotid anomalies, 2608
Congenital CSF leaks, 665
Congenital high-airway obstruction syndrome, 1321
Congenital malformations
airway, 1296–1297
auricular, 1295
definition of, 1620
formes frustes of, 1620
inheritance of, 1619, 1619f
midline, 1296
nares, 1295–1296
neck, 1297
oral cavity, 1296
otolaryngologic, 1621–1622
Congenital nasal pyriform aperture stenosis, 1316–1317, 1317f
Congenital nystagmus, 2685
Congenital stapes disorders, 1533
Congenital tracheal stenosis, 1322–1324,
1322f–1324f
Congenital upper airway obstruction,
1328–1329, 1331
Conjunctivitis, 224
Conjunctivodacryocystorhinostomy, 629–630
Consensual light reflex, 218
Constricted ear, otoplasty, 3144–3146,
3145f, 3152, 3153f–3155f
Continuing medical education
learning through experience
abstract conceptualization, 3351
active experimentation, 3351
concrete experience, 3351
reflective observation, 3351
self-directed learning. *See* Self-directed
learning
Continuous positive airway pressure, 2192,
2224
autotitrating, 2175
inspiration and expiration, 2174–2175

Contralateral routing of signal, 2656–2657
Contrast agents, 167
Contusions, soft tissue injuries, 1109
Conus elasticus, larynx, 946
Conventional audiometry, 1481
Conventional behavioral audiometry, 1514
Conventional long-term tissue expansion,
2852–2853, 2853f–2856f
Cook Airway Exchange Catheter, 902, 902f
Core biopsies, 180
Cornea
ulceration of, due to forehead lift, 3071
Corneal abrasion, 228, 228f
Coronavirus, 1433
Cortical auditory evoked responses,
2283–2284
Corticosteroids, 2593
for adrenal suppression, 34t
for benign lesions, 3222, 3223t
intralesional, side effects, 3222, 3223t
for management of scars and keloids,
2866
Corynebacterium diphtheriae infection, 762,
1433
Cosmetics, for scar camouflage, 2868
Cosmoderm, for soft tissue augmentation,
3246
Cosmoplast, for soft tissue augmentation,
3246
Cough
and airway lesions, 1351–1352
antibiotics, 1353–1354
antihistamines, 1353–1354
chronic nocturnal cough, 1352
decongestants, 1353–1354
environmental toxicants, 1352
etiology, 1351
foreign body, 1352
gastroesophageal reflux disease,
1352–1353
otolaryngologist
ACCP, 1348
causes, 1350
clinical significance, 1349
commission crimes, 1351
cystic fibrosis, 1351
diagnosis, 1350
etiology, 1349–1350
evaluation, 1348
expiratory phase, 1351
false focal folds, 1351
immunodeficiency, 1351
pathology, 1349
physical examination, 1350
primary ciliary dyskinesia, 1351
red herrings, 1349
post-infectious, 1352
sinonasal causes of, 1351
treatment, 1353
Cowden syndrome, 125
COX-2 inhibitors, platelet dysfunction
and, 28
Coxsackie virus infection, 760–761, 1433
Cranial anatomy, 3, 4f
Cranial base
anterior
craniofacial resection, 2087–2088

endoscopic endonasal resection, 2088,
2089f–2090f
ethmoid bone, 2083
intracranial surface of, 2082
sphenoid sinus, 2083
middle, 2083–2084
endoscopic endonasal approach,
2090, 2092f
lateral infratemporal skull base
approach, 2090, 2091f
pathology, 2085, 2085t
physical examination of, 2085–2086
posterior cranial fossa, 2084–2085
Cranial base surgery
craniofacial resection, 2087–2088, 2087t
endoscopic endonasal resection, 2088,
2089f–2090f
history, 2081–2082
imaging in
balloon occlusion test, 2086, 2086t
computed tomography, 2086
positron emission tomography, 2086
operative management, 2086–2087
Cranial fossae, anatomy of, 3
Craniofacial dysostosis, 1625–1626, 1625f
Craniofacial resection, 2087–2088, 2087t
Craniofacial surgery, 2233
Craniotomy, 1454
C-reactive protein, 2707
Creep, 2850
Crescent-shaped ostium, 707f
Crew resource management, 3257
Cribriform plate, 360
Cricoarytenoid joint, 947
Cricoid cartilage, 945
Cricothyrotomy, 1096, 1096f
Cri-du-chat syndrome, 1637
Critical care
alcohol withdrawal syndrome. *See*
Alcohol withdrawal syndrome
anaerobic metabolism, 56
analgesia, 64
blood transfusions, ICU, 56–57
mechanical ventilation. *See* Mechanical
ventilation
nasogastric tube, 62–63, 62f
oliguria, postoperative period, 63–64,
63t, 64t
oxygen delivery, 55
oxygen extraction, 55–56
perioperative beta blockade, 66, 66t, 67t
sedatives, 64–66
shock, 57
tissue oxygenation and organ perfusion,
55
vasoactive agents. *See* Vasoactive agents
Critical patient communication, Clinic
management, 3337–3338
Crohn disease, 747–748
pharyngitis in, 767
Cromolyn sodium, allergic rhinitis, 464
Crooked nose
camouflage grafts, 2987
etiology, 2977
patient history and physical examination
asymmetries and deviations,
2977–2978, 2978f

Crooked nose (*Continued*)
  division and permutation of, 2978, 2978f
  endonasal examination, 2978–2979
  radiographic assessment, 2979
  three-quarter base and bird's-eye view, 2979, 2979f
  treatment
    lower third, 2987, 2987f
    middle third, 2981, 2981f–2986f, 2987
    septum, 2979–2980
    upper third, 2980–2981, 2980f
Crosseal (Ethicon), 52
Cross-lip flaps, 1797, 1800
Croup, 138
Crouzon syndrome, 124, 1625–1627, 1625f, 1626t, 1627f
Crush injuries, wounds, 1109–1110
Cryotherapy, 2868, 3222
Cryptotia, otoplasty, 3144, 3145f
C-spine injury
  midface fracture, 1213
Cupid's bow, cleft lip/palate, 1563
Curettage, 3221
  with electrodesiccation, for skin, 1730
Curettes, dermal, 3221
Cushing's syndrome, 259–260
Cutaneous horns, 3212, 3215f
  treatment of, 3224–3225
Cutaneous malignancy, lasers, 3208–3209
Cutaneous malignant melanoma
  clinical presentation and diagnosis
    childhood history, 1740
    fine-needle aspiration, 1740
    melanin lack, 1739–1740
    physical examination, 1740
    pigmented lesions, 1739
  epidemiology, 1739
  initial management of, 1743, 1744f
  lymphadenectomy, 1749–1750, 1750f
  mucosal, 1742
  occult lymph node disease detection
    elective lymph node dissection, 1745
    sentinel lymph node identification, 1745–1748
  radiotherapy, 1750–1751
  risk factors for, 1739
  staging system
    metastatic workup, 1744
    primary tumor, 1742
    regional nodal staging, 1742–1744
  subtypes
    acral lentiginous, 1741
    desmoplastic melanoma, 1741
    lentigo maligna, 1740
    nodular melanoma, 1741
    superficial spreading melanoma, 1741
  surveillance in, 1754–1755, 1754f
  systemic therapy
    biochemotherapy, 1753–1754
    chemotherapeutic agents, 1753
    interferon, 1751–1752
    interleukin-2, 1752
    ipilimumab, 1752–1753
    tumor vaccines, 1752
  TNM staging, 1742, 1743t
  treatment of, 1748–1749

Cutaneous manifestations, 745f
Cyanoacrylate adhesives, 52–53
Cyclic adenosine monophosphate, 372
Cyclic hematopoiesis, 749
Cyst(s)
  arachnoid, 2577
  dentigerous, 2098–2099, 2098f
  epidermal, 3212
    treatment of, 3225–3226
  epidermoid and dermoid, 2577, 2578f
  Epstein-Barr virus infection, 1470
  Gorlin, 2099
  incisive canal, 2100
  nasopalatine duct, 2100
  odontogenic, 2097–2113. *See also* Odontogenic cysts
  orbital tumors, 2071–2072
  periapical, 2097–2098, 2098f
  radicular, 2097–2098
  sialo-odontogenic, 2099–2100, 2100f
  voice therapy, 1054–1055
Cystic fibrosis, 126, 489–490, 490t, 538, 1300
Cystic fibrosis transmembrane conductance regulator dysfunction, 450
Cytokines
  characteristics of, 390t–394t
  production, lymphocytes, 389, 389t
Cytomegalovirus infection, 1433, 1527–1528
  pharyngitis due to, 764
  recurrent respiratory papillomatosis, 1421

D
Dacryocystitis, 225
Dacryocystorhinostomy
  background, 624–625
  complications
    conjunctivodacryocystorhinostomy, 629–630
    perioperative, 628
    revisions, 629
    surgical failures, 628–629
  evaluation, 625–626
  technique options, 629–630
Danger spaces, deep neck infection, 797, 806–807, 808f
Data. *See* Clinical data
Deafness dystonia optic atrophy syndrome, 1551
Debakey forceps, 22
Decongestants
  chronic rhinosinusitis, 590
  nonallergic rhinitis, 472
Deformations, 1620. *See also* Otolaryngologic syndromes
  glottic closure, 860, 860f
  physiology of, 860–861, 860f
  upper esophageal sphincter relaxation, 860–861
Deformity, 2757
Deglutition
  aspiration, 860
  peripheral sensory and motor components, 818t
  phases of, 1899–1900
  physiology, 807, 1899–1900

Delirium tremens, 46
Demeclocycline, 34
Dendritic cells, 387
Dental infections. *See* Odontogenic infections
Dental numbering system, universal, 1195, 1197f
Dental occlusion, 2165, 2166f
Dentigerous cysts, 2098–2099
Dentoalveolar abscess, odontogenic infection, 771, 772t
Dentoalveolar fracture, 1280
Denture-related stomatitis, 741–742, 741f
Depression, 2758
Dermabrasion
  complications, 3223, 3223t
  conditions treated with, 3223, 3224t
  for scar camouflage, 2867, 2867f, 2868f
Dermal augmentation, collagen injection, 2795
Dermal curettes, 3221
Dermal nevi, 3218, 3218f
Dermatitis, infectious eczematoid, 2344, 2344f
Dermatochalasis, lower eyelid blepharoplasty, 3086, 3086f
Dermatography, 2868
Dermatomyositis, 1042
  associated disorders, 274
  diagnostic criteria for, 273, 274t
  head and neck manifestations, 274
  incidence, 273
  treatment, 274
Dermatoses, 2345–2346
Dermoid cysts, 1614–1615, 1614f, 1615f, 2375, 2577, 2578f
  orbital tumor, 2072
  of temporal bone, 2375
Desmoplastic melanoma, 1741
Desmopressin, 29
Desquamative gingivitis, 744f, 746f
Dexmetomidine, 66
Dextrocardia, in Kartagener syndrome, 1629
DFNB gene, in hearing loss, 1543t, 1544, 1544f
Diabetes insipidus, 34, 253
Diabetes mellitus
  basal-bolus insulin treatment, 31, 32t
  diabetic ketoacidosis, 32
  hyperglycemia, 31
  hyperosmolar nonketotic syndrome, 32
  POC glucose testing, 31
  regular insulin, 32
Diabetic ketoacidosis, 32, 261–262
Diagnostic tests, statistical terms associated with, 92t
Dialysis, preoperative, in chronic renal failure, 40
Diarrhea, antibiotic-associated, 40
Diazepam, 42, 42t, 65, 65t
Diced cartilage-fascia graft, 3008, 3024, 3024f, 3025
Differentiated thyroid cancer
  long-term management
    follow-up methods, 2126
    locoregional recurrent/persistent disease, 2126

reoperation for
 distant metastatic disease, 2127
 preoperative evaluation, 2126
surgical management
 hypocalcemia, 2124
 midline cervical fascia dissection, 2122
 MIVAT, 2123
 parathyroid glands, autotransplanatation, 2123
 postoperative hematoma, 2124
 preoperative laryngoscopy, 2121–2122
 recurrent laryngeal nerve, 2122–2124, 2122f, 2123f
 regional lymphatics management, 2123–2124
 special patient populations, 2124
 superior laryngeal nerve injury, 2124
 total thyroidectomy, 2123
 tracheal /esophageal invasion, 2124
Difficult airway management
 algorithm, 896, 897f
 cricothyroidotomy
  indications, 905
  needle cricothyroidotom, 906
  procedure, 906
 ex utero intrapartum treatment procedure, 898, 898f
 flexible fiberoptic bronchoscopy
  advantages, 899–890
  endotracheal tube, 900
  modified nasal trumpet, 890, 890f
  positioning for, 890
  sedated, 898
 indirect rigid fiberoptic-enhanced laryngoscope, 900, 900f
 intubating or lighted stylets, 901–903, 902f
 laryngeal mask airway guided intubation, 904–905, 905f
 laryngoscope blade placement, 889, 899f
 retromolar technique, 889, 899f
 rigid fiberoptic bronchoscopy, 901, 901f
 rigid fiberoptic stylets, 901, 901f
 ventilation, 905, 905f
 video laryngoscopy, 903–904
DiGeorge sequence, 1637
Digestive tract, upper, anatomy and physiology of, 817–823
Digital light projectors, 2782
Digital photography, for pictorial documentation
 archiving, 2782
 compression, 2781
 editing and morphing, 2781–2782
 input devices
  cameras, 2780–2781, 2780f
  scanners, 2781
 output devices
  printers, 2782
  projectors, 2782–2783
 storage, 2782
Dihydroergotamine, 306
Diltiazem, 37
Dimethylbenzanthracene, 1647

Diphtheroid infection, pharyngitis due to, 760–761
Diplopia, 223
 orbital fracture, 1238
 orbital tumors, 2064
Direct light reflex, 218
Discoid lupus erythematosus, 747
Disease-modifying antirheumatic drug, 271
Disease-specific HRQOL, 721, 724t–725t
Disruptions, 1620
Distal esophageal spasm, 854, 854f
Diuretics
 ototoxicity of, 2544
 sudden sensorineural hearing loss, 2592
Dix-Hallpike test, dizziness, 2692, 2692f
Dizziness, 2733, 2734
 definition, 2615
 differential diagnosis, 2615
 etiology of, 2616t, 2674
 evaluation of, 2618, 2618t
 multifactorial nature of, 2673–2674, 2674f
 neurotologic examination
  dynamic visual acuity, 2691
  equipments for, 2683–2684, 2684f
  gait and posture test, 2695–2696, 2696f
  gaze-evoked nystagmus, 2685
  head heave test, 2689–2690
  head impulse test, 2687–2689, 2688f, 2689f
  hyperventilation-induced nystagmus, 2698
  limb coordination test, 2694–2695, 2694t
  malleolar sign, 2697
  mastoid vibration, 2697
  positional versus positioning testing, 2691–2693, 2692f, 2693t
  postheadshake nystagmus test, 2690–2691, 2690f
  rotation-induced nystagmus, 2687
  sensory evaluation, 2674
  skew deviation and ocular torsion reaction test, 2690
  smooth pursuit, 2686–2687
  sound-evoked or pressure-evoked eye movements, 2697–2698, 2697f
  spontaneous nystagmus, 2684–2685
  structure of, 2682, 2682t–2683t
 patient evaluation, 2302
 patient history
  accompanying symptoms, 2680
  discovery of, 2674
  exacerbating factors, 2679t, 2680
  medications and comorbidity, 2680–2682, 2681t
  posttraumatic vertigo, 2679–2680
  questionnaire and direct questioning, 2674–2678
  time duration, 2679
  vertigo, disequilibrium and light-headedness, 2678–2679, 2679t
 population problem, 2673
 sensory evaluation, 2674
 simulation battery of, 2620t
 types of, 2618t

DNA, 1542
DNA repair pathway, HNSCC
 base excision repair, 1658
 double-strand break repair, 1658–1659
 interstrand cross-link repair, 1656–1658
 nucleotide excision repair, 1656–1658
 single-strand break repair, 1658
Dobutamine, 36t, 39, 59
Dominant traits, 1541
Dopamine, 36t, 41, 59
Dorsolateral medullary syndrome, 2725–2726
Double convexity deformity, lower eyelid blepharoplasty, 3086, 3088f
Down syndrome
 in hearing loss, 1552
 hearing loss in, 1626
Drug-induced sleep endoscopy, 2227
 epiglottic prolapse, 2208, 2209f
 oropharyngeal lateral wall collapse, 2208, 2208f
 tongue base prolapse, 2208, 2209f
Dry-eye syndrome, 233
Dual-mode acoustic rhinometry, 456
Duckbill voice prosthesis, 1985f
Duction, 220
Duragen, 53
Duraguard, 53
Dural arteriovenous fistula, 2608, 2608f
Dural defect, 2088
Dural substitutes, 53
Durarepair, 53
Dynamic visual acuity, 2691
Dysarthria, 2722
Dysdiadochokinesis, 2722
Dysgeusia
 as complication of mastoid surgery, 2462
Dysmetria, 2686, 2694
Dysmorphology. See Congenital malformations
Dysosmia, 376
Dysphagia, 825, 826t
 upper digestive tract, 817
Dysplasia
 orbital and ethmoid fibrous, 2072–2073, 2073f
 squamous
  mild, 187f
  moderate, 188f
  mucosa, 194
  severe, 188f
Dysrhythmias, preoperative management of, 37
Dysthyroid orbitopathy, 630
Dystonia, 1032

E
Eagle syndrome, 312
Ear
 congenital malformation, 2384–2397
 development of, 2239–2250, 2240t
  auricular, 2239–2240
  control of, 2249–2250
  external and middle ear, 2241–2243
  inner ear, 2245–2246
  ossicles, 2242, 2243f

Ear (*Continued*)
  evaluation of, for plastic surgery of face, 2764
  external
    anatomy and physiology of, 2253–2272, 2254f, 2333–2335, 2334f, 2335f
    development of, 2241–2243
    noninflammatory lesions
      aural polyp, 2353
      bacterial perichondritis, 2349
      cerumen impaction, 2351–2352
      chondrodermatitis nodularis chronica, 2349
      cutaneous cysts, 2348
      dermatologic conditions, 2353–2356
      external auditory canal cholesteatoma, 2351
      foreign body, 2353
      furuncle, 2353
      gouty tophi, 2349
      hypertrophic scars and keloids, 2349–2350
      keratoacanthoma, 2349
      keratosis obturans, 2350–2351
      microtia/congenital auricular atresia, 2348
      preauricular pits and skin tags, 2348
      sebaceous cysts, 2349
    sound pressure and, 2253, 2254f
    traumatic disorders, 2346–2348
  implants for, 2790. *See also* Cochlear implants
  inner
    autoimmune disease, 2591
    development of, 2245–2246
    malformation of, cochlear implants, 2630f–2631f, 2633–2634, 2635f
    obstruction of, cochlear implants, 2634–2635, 2635f
    and lateral skull base, neoplams of, 2359t, 2360f
  middle
    anatomy, 2255
    embryology of, 2242, 2384–2385
    function of, 2255, 2255f
    maldevelopment, 2242–2243
    maldevelopment of, 2242–2243
    neoplasms of, 2370–2376
    temporal bone trauma, 2410–2430
    nonlinear properties of, 2266–2269, 2267f, 2268f
  surgery of, facial nerve monitoring during, 2328
Eastlander flap, in lip reconstruction, 1797, 1798, 1800, 1800f
Eating Assessment Tool, 825, 826t
Ectopic thyroid, 1613–1614
Ectrodactyly-ectodermal dysplasia clefting syndrome, 1637
Ectropion, lower eyelid blepharoplasty, 3086, 3087f
Edema
  cerebral, 1832
  facial, after neck dissection, 1832
  pulmonary, 39

Reinke, 996, 996f
Edentulous mandible fractures, 1204, 1205f
Edrophonium, 243
Ehlers-Danlos syndrome, 3108
Eighth nerve monitoring, direct, 2315, 2315f, 2319–2321
Elasticity, suture material selection, 22
Elder dependency ratio, 299
Elderly patients
  clinical care, 300
  clinical management
    communication and collaboration, 302
    delirium, 301
    falls and fall-related injuries, 301–302
    geriatric social workers, 302
    patient satisfaction, 302
    physical and occupational therapists, 302
    polypharmacy, 301
Elective lymph node dissection, 1745
Electrocochleography, 2282–2283, 2283f, 2317–2319, 2320f
  evoked, for facial nerve monitoring, 2324–2326
  Ménière syndrome, 2703
Electrodesiccation, with curettage, for skin, 1730
Electromyography
  laryngeal
    bilateral vocal fold immobility, 1019
    unilateral vocal fold paralysis, 1011, 1012f, 1013f
  neurologic disorder
    applications, 1044–1045, 1045f
    needle electromyography, 1043–1044
    technique of, 1043–1044, 1043f, 1044f
Electronystagmography
  caloric irrigation testing, 2306–2307
  electrodes, 2303
  hallpike and roll tests, 2306
  headshake test, 2305–2306
  hyperventilation testing, 2305
  oculomotor evaluations
    gaze stability testing, 2303–2304
    optokinetic nystagmus, 2305
    saccade evaluation, 2304–2305
    smooth pursuit tracking, 2305
  spontaneous nystagmus, 2305
  static positional testing, 2306
Electro-olfactogram, 455
Electrophysiologic testing, facial paralysis, 2508–2510, 2509t, 2510f
Electrosurgery, 3221–3222, 3223f
Embolism
  air, 2463
  pulmonary, 31
Empty nose syndrome, 618–619
Encephalocele
  as complication of mastoid surgery, 2462–2463
  embryology, 1447, 1448f
  nasal, congenital development of, 1451
Endochondral pseudocysts, auricular, 2370

Endocrine abnormalities, perioperative management
  adrenal glucocorticoids, 33–34, 34t
  diabetes mellitus, 31–32, 32t
  pituitary, 34–35
  thyroid and parathyroid disorders, 32–33, 33t
Endocrine system
  adrenal glands
    adrenal insufficiency, 259
    Cushing's syndrome, 259–260
    pheochromocytoma, 260
    primary aldosteronism, 258–259
    secondary aldosteronism, 259
  pancreas
    diabetes mellitus, 261
    diabetic ketoacidosis, 261–262
    glucagon, 260–261
    glucose metabolism, 260
    hyperglycemic hyperosmolar state, 262
    hypoglycemia, 262
    insulin, 261
    multiple endocrine neoplasia syndromes, 262–263, 263t
  parathyroid glands. *See* Parathyroid gland(s)
  pituitary gland. *See* Pituitary
  thyroid gland
    myxedema coma, 258
    synthesis, 256–257
    thyroid storm, 257–258
    triiodothyronine and thyroxine, 256, 257
Endocrinology, 250–266
Endo-extralaryngeal suture lateralization, bilateral vocal fold immobility, 1020
End-of-life care, head and neck cancer, 350–353
Endolaryngeal stenosis, 1145
Endolaryngeal stent, 1148–1149, 1148f
Endolymphatic hydrops, 2702
Endolymphatic sac tumors, 2371
  bony invasion, 2371
  cerebellopontine angle, 2583
  clinical manifestations of, 2371
  diagnosis of, 2372
  extension of, 2371–2372
Endolymphatic shunt, in surgery of mastoid, 2456–2458
Endoscopes, for nasal endoscopy, 541, 541f
Endoscopic forehead lift
  advantages of, 3068, 3070
  flap suspension and fixation, 3069–3070
  incisions for, 3068–3069, 3069f
  moderate brow ptosis, 3067–3068, 3068f
  supraorbital dissection, 3069, 3069f
Endoscopic laser partial arytenoidectomy, bilateral vocal fold immobility, 1021–1022
Endoscopic sinus surgery
  allergic fungal rhinosinusitis, 570
  balloon sinuplasty, 600–601
  clinical outcomes, 602
  concha bullosa, 599

ethmoid sinus
   anatomical landmarks, 598, 598f
   anterior ethmoidectomy, 598–599, 598f
   posterior ethmoidectomy, 599, 599f
  history and physical exam, 595
  image guidance, 601
  imaging, 595
  maxillary sinus
   antrostomy, 598
   middle turbinate, 596
   minimally invasive maxillary technique, 597f
   uncinate process, 596, 596f
  nasal cavity injection sites, 595, 596f
  preparation, 595
  revision surgery
   anterior arch of the middle turbinate, 601
   lamina papyracea, 601
   maxillary sinus antrostomy, 601
   posterior choanal arch, 602
   sphenoid sinus roof, 601f, 602
   sphenoid sinus, 600, 600f
Endoscopic skull base surgery, 2077
Endoscopic total laser arytenoidectomy, bilateral vocal fold immobility, 1021, 1021f
Endoscopic transoral laser microsurgery, 1969, 1970f
Endoscopic voice restoration, 1981f
Endoscopic-assisted nasal cautery, 504
Endoscopy
  culture equipment for, 542
  fiberoptic, 2207–2208
  in mastoid surgery, 2456
  nasal, 541, 541f
  in nasopharyngeal cancer, 1878, 1883–1884, 1884f–1886f, 1888, 1890f, 1891, 1891f
  pediatric voice, 1373, 1373f–1374f
Endotracheal intubation, 1384–1386, 1385t
End-point nystagmus, 2685
Enlarged vestibular aqueduct syndrome, 1546, 1546f
Eosinophilic esophagitis, 852, 853f
  pediatric voice, 1374, 1375f
Eosinophilic granuloma, 2372–2373
Eosinophilic mucin rhinosinusitis, 569
Ephelides, 3218
  treatment of, 3228
Epidermal cyst(s), 2577, 2578f, 3212
  treatment of, 3225–3226
Epidermolysis bullosa
  acquisita, 745
  pharyngitis due to, 762–763
Epidural abscess, 580–581, 581f
Epigenetics, 299
Epiglottis
  larynx, 946
  upper digestive tract, inverted, 821, 821f
Epinephrine, 59
Episcleritis, 224
Episodic ataxias, 2729
Epistaxis, 501–507
  clinical management

absorbable nasal packing, 504–505, 505f
  comorbid systemic factors, 505–506
  endoscopic-assisted nasal cautery, 504
  nonabsorbable nasal packing, 505, 505f
  patient assessment, 504
  endovascular embolization, 507
  epidemiology, 501–503
  etiology
   bleeding, 501
   hereditary hemorrhagic telangiectasia, 501–502, 502t
   hypertension, 503
   inherited bleeding diatheses, 503
   secondary epistaxis, 501, 502f, 502t
   systemic causes, 502–503
  incidence, 501
  surgical management
   ethmoidal artery ligation, 506, 506f
   intranasal bleeding, 506–507
   septodermoplasty, 507
   sphenopalatine artery ligation, 506, 506f
Epithelial inclusion cysts, 2072
Epithelialization, wound healing, 79
Epithelial-myoepithelial carcinoma, 192f
Epithelium
  neoplasm
   benign tumors, 1473–1474
   diagnosis, 1472
   malignant tumors, 1474–1475
   parotid gland, 1472
  vocal fold lesions
   keratotic lesions, 989–990
   pathophysiology, 989
Epstein-Barr virus, 1433
  pharyngitis due to, 763–764
  sialadenitis, 1469
Epworth Sleepiness Score, 2183
Ergotamine, 306
Erythema migrans, 753–754
Erythrocyte abnormalities, preoperative management of, 28
Erythroplakia, 1646
Esophageal achalasia, 854–855, 855f
Esophageal atresia, 1322
Esophageal disorders
  caustic ingestion, 857
  diverticula, 856
  emergencies associated with, 856–857
  esophageal motility, 853–855, 854f, 855f
  esophageal rings, 855–856
  esophageal strictures, 855
  esophageal webs, 855
  esophagitis
   infectious, 852, 853f
   noninfectious, 852, 853f
  gastroesophageal reflux disease, 853
  neoplasms, 857
  progressive systemic sclerosis, 855
Esophageal diverticula, 856
Esophageal foreign body, 857
Esophageal motility drugs, 844–845, 845t
Esophageal perforation, 856
Esophageal sphincter, upper, 864
Esophageal strictures, 863–864

Esophagoscopy
  transnasal, 832–834
   complications, 834
   endoscope placement, 832–833, 833f
   flexible endoscopic evaluation of swallowing, 834
   fluoroscopic video-esophagram, 832
   indications, 831–832
   patient position, 832, 832f
Esophagram, 165, 166f
Esophagus
  cervical
   carcinoma. See Cervical esophageal carcinoma
   surgery of, 1932
  neck injury, 1139
  nutcracker, 854
  reconstruction, 1932–1933, 1933f, 1934f
Esotropia, 229
Essential tremor, voice therapy, 1055
Esthesioneuroblastoma, 440f
Ethmoid sinuses, 359–360, 360f, 361f, 362. See also Sinus(es)
  anatomy of, 8, 8f
  complications, 607t, 610
  endoscopic sinus surgery
   anatomical landmarks, 598, 598f
   anterior ethmoidectomy, 598–599, 598f
   posterior ethmoidectomy, 599, 599f
   operative technique, 609–610
Ethmoidectomy, pediatric rhinosinusitis, 1460–1461, 1461f, 1462f
Ethyl-2-cyanoacrylate implant, 2795
Etomidate, 240
Eustachian tube
  dysfunction, 1570–1571
  function, 1485–1486, 1485f
Evidence-based medicine, 102–110
  appraisal of quality of evidence in, 107–108, 108t
  asking answerable question in, 107
  evidence levels for studies in, 108t
  evidence-based guidelines, 109–110, 109t
  grading of, 108t
  integration of evidence with clinical experience, 108
  results and recommendations in, 108, 108t
  search for best available evidence in, 107
Evoked otoacoustic emission screening, 1524
Ewing sarcoma, 2374
Ex utero intrapartum treatment, 898, 898f, 1336
Exophytic Schneiderian papilloma, 186f
Exotropia, 230
Extensibility, 2849–2850
External auditory canal atresia, 1533
External beam radiation therapy, 2126
Extracorporeal membrane oxygenation, 1526
Extradural (epidural) granulation tissue/abscess, 2405
Extraesophageal reflux, 484
  connection of, 962–963
  middle ear, 962
  nose and paranasal sinuses, 963
  stenotic lesions, 963–964

Extratemporal cholesteatoma, 2444, 2444f
Extremity injuries, secondary survey of trauma, 1104
Extrinsic laryngeal musculature, professional voice, 1059, 1060f
Eye
    anatomy of, 5–6, 6f
    assessment of, for plastic surgery of, 2763–2764, 2764f
    care of, in facial paralysis, 2517
    midface fracture, 1221
    red. See Red eye
Eye examination
    external inspection and pupil examination, 218–219
    indications, 217
    intraocular pressure, 220
    motility, 220, 220f
    ophthalmoscopy, 220–221
    Schirmer test, 221
    visual acuity, 217–218, 219f, 219t
Eyebrow. See Brow(s)
Eyelid
    anatomy of, 4–6, 5f
    lower
        anatomy of, 3085, 3086f
        blepharoplasty. See Blepharoplasty
    soft tissue injuries, 1117–1119, 1117f–1119f
    upper blepharoplasty, 3074–3084
    upper eyelid-brow complex, 3074, 3075f

F
Face
    anatomy of, 8–9, 9f
    benign lesions of
        classification of, 3212, 3213t
        epidermal, 3212–3215
        history taking and physical examination of, 3212
        laboratory studies in, 3220–3221, 3220f, 3221f
        management of, 3212–3228
        syndromes associated with, differential diagnosis of, 3212, 3213t
        therapeutic considerations, 3221–3224
    fatty/muscular tumors, 3217–3218, 3218f
    fibrous tumors, 3217, 3217f
    infectious lesions of, 3219–3220, 3220f
    melanocytic tumors of, 3218–3219, 3218f–3220f
    muscles of, 3239, 3240f
    neural tumors, 3218
    non-skin-appendage tumors, 3216–3220
    plastic surgery of
        anatomic landmarks in, 2760t, 2762t
        general, 2760–2768
        methods of, 2768–2769
    and preoperative evaluation, 2757–2758
    regional anatomy of, 3239–3240, 3240f
    rhytidectomy. See Rhytidectomy
    skin-appendage tumors, 3215–3216, 3216f
    temporal region, 1116f
    vascular tumors, 3216–3217, 3217f

Facial analysis
    anatomic landmarks in, 2760t, 2762t
    cephalometrics, 2768
    chin, 2767
    "divine" proportions, 2759, 2759f
    ears, 2764
    eyebrows, 2763, 2763f
    eyes/eyelids, 2763–2764, 2764f
    forehead
        nasofrontal angle, 2762, 2763f
        shape, 2761–2762
    general facial assessment
        facial height, 2760–2761, 2761f
        frontal symmetry and proportion, 2760, 2760f
        lateral view assessment, 2761, 2762t
        lower facial symmetry, 2761
        zero meridian and Frankfort horizontal line, 2761, 2761f
    history, 2759, 2759f
    lip, 2767
    midface, 2766–2767
    nasal angles, 2765
    nasal tip projection
        Goode's method, 2765–2766, 2765f
        Powell and Humphries method, 2765, 2765f
        Simons's method, 2765
        versus tip rotation, 2765, 2765f
    nasal width, 2766, 2766f
    neck, 2767–2768, 2767f
    nose, 2764–2765
    pathologic conditions
        body dysmorphic disorder, 2759
        depression, 2758
        personality disorder, 2759
    photometrics, 2768
    profile planes and angles, 2762t
    standard reference points, 2760, 2760f, 2760t
    three-dimensional photography, 2768–2769, 2768f
Facial edema, after neck dissection, 1832
Facial fracture
    in children
        condyle, 1279, 1279f
        craniofacial growth and trauma, 1274–1275, 1275f
        dentoalveolar, 1280
        epidemiology, 1272–1273
        etiology/injury mechanism, 1274
        frontal bone, 1281–1282
        frontal sinus, 1282
        management, 1273–1274, 1273t–1274t
        mandible, 1278–1279, 1278f
        mandible arch, 1279–1280, 1280f
        medial orbital wall, 1281
        midface, 1280
        nasal fracture, 1277
        nasoorbitoethmoid complex, 1277, 1281–1282, 1282f
        newborn nasal deformity, 1277
        orbit, 1281
        orbital floor and roof, 1281–1282
        orbital rim, 1277
        radiographic examination, 1274

        supraorbital rim, 1282
        transcaruncular incision, 1277
        zygomaticomaxillary complex, 1280–1281
    panfacial, 1163–1167, 1164t, 1165f, 1166f
    panfacial, approach to
    rigid fixation, 1275–1277, 1276t
Facial injury
    bone fracture, 1134
    complications, 1134, 1135t
    Gant and Epstein system, 1132, 1132f
    gunshot wounds, 1133–1134, 1134f
    management algorithm, 1133, 1133f
    nerve injury, 1134
    parotid duct, 1134
    shotgun injury, 1133
    stab wounds, 1133
Facial muscles, 8, 9f
Facial nerve, 9
    abnormalities
        in aural atresia, 2385
    abnormalities of, 2505
    anatomy of, 2503–2504, 2504f
    anesthesia and, 2326
    arterial supply to, 2505
    development of, 2243–2245, 2244f
    embryology of, 2385
    injury to
        facial paralysis. See Facial paralysis
        during otologic surgery management of, 2461
        soft tissue, 1121–1123
    intraoperative monitoring, 2323
        benefits and applications, 2327
        direct, 2326
        history of, 2323–2324
        indications for, 2326–2327, 2326t
        monitoring systems, 2324, 2324t
        objectives of, 2324t
        types of, 2323, 2323t
    maldevelopment, 2244–2245, 2244f
    in parotid surgery, 1770
    parotidectomy
        complications, 1781, 1781t
        identification of, 1176, 1778t
        injury of, 1782
        monitoring of, 1782
    pathophysiology of, 2508–2510
    schwannomas, 2377
    surgical, 2504–2505, 2504f, 2505f
    topographical organization of, 2505
    tumors of skull base and, 2515–2516
Facial pain
    acute sinusitis, 311, 311t
    central, 305
    peripheral, 305
    primary headache. See Primary headache
    secondary headache. See Secondary headache
Facial palsy, 1533
Facial paralysis, 2443–2444
    acute, 2503–2518
        differential diagnosis of, 2508
        assessment of, 2506
        due to trauma, 2513–2515, 2515f, 2516f
        history taking in, 2505–2506

laboratory studies in, 2507–2508
management of injuries in, 2514t
in newborn, 2516–2517
in otitis media, 2513
physical examination in, 2506–2507
Facial reanimation
  hypoglossal facial nerve transfer, 2907, 2908f
  nerve injury classification, 2905
  neural discontinuity, 2905–2907, 2906f, 2907f
  surgical technique
    split XII-VII transfer, 2907, 2908f, 2909
    VII-VII cross-face grafting, 2909
  zonal approach
    middle facial zone. See Middle facial zone
    upper facial zone, 2909–2910
Facial sensory loss, 2721
Facial skeletal trauma
  computed tomography scanning, 1171
  coronal approach
    complications, 1176–1177, 1177f
    coronal flaps, 1171
    curvilinear coronal incision, 1171, 1172f, 1173f
    pericranial flap elevation, 1173, 1174f
    Raney clips, 1172–1173
    sawtooth design, 1172, 1173f
    straight-line incision, 1171, 1172f
    supraorbital structures, 1174, 1175f
    zygomatic arches, 1173–1174, 1177f
  hemicoronal incision, 1171
  lower midface and maxilla
    mandibular fracture. See Mandibular fractures
    upper labial sulcus approach, 1187, 1187f, 1188f
  midfacial skeleton
    orbit, 1177, 1177f, 1178f
    orbital rim, floor and wall. See Lower eyelid
Facial weakness, 2721
Facioauriculovertebral sequence, 1627–1629
Familial hypocalciuric hypercalcemia, 2133
Family Assessment of Treatment at the End of Life, 352
Fat
  autologous, for soft tissue augmentation, 3249
  orbital decompression, 632
Fatty/muscular tumors, 3217–3218, 3218f
Fenestral otosclerosis, computed tomography, 141, 142f
Fentanyl, 64, 241
Festoons, lower eyelid blepharoplasty, 3086, 3088f
Fetal alcohol syndrome
  Aarskog syndrome, 1635–1636
  achondroplasia, 1636
  Alport syndrome, 1636
  Antley-Bixler syndrome, 1636
  Beals syndrome, 1636
  Beckwith-Wiedemann syndrome, 1636

Binder syndrome, 1636
Coffin-Lowry syndrome, 1636
Cohen syndrome, 1637
Cri-du-chat syndrome, 1637
DiGeorge sequence, 1637
ectrodactyly-ectodermal dysplasia cleft-ing syndrome, 1637
fetal rubella syndrome, 1637
fragile X syndrome, 1637
Fraser syndrome, 1637
Gardner syndrome, 1637–1638
Gorlin syndrome, 1638
Klippel-Feil anomaly, 1638
Larsen syndrome, 1638
LEOPARD syndrome, 1638
Marfan syndrome, 1638
Miller syndrome, 1638
Möbius syndrome, 1638–1639
multiple mucosal melanoma syndrome, 1639
Nager acrofacial dysostosis syndrome, 1639
Noonan syndrome, 1639
Opitz (BBB/G syndrome), 1639
orofaciodigital syndrome type I and II, 1639
osteogenesis imperfecta, 1639–1640
otopalatodigital syndrome type I and II, 1640
Smith-Lemli-Opitz syndrome, 1640
Stickler syndrome, 1640
Sturge-Weber syndrome, 1640
Turner syndrome, 1640
van der Woude syndrome, 1640–1641
whistling face syndrome, 1641
Williams syndrome, 1641
Fetal rubella syndrome, 1637
Fever, postoperative
  causes of, 43, 44t
  evaluation of, 43–44
  nosocomial infection, 44
  treatment of, 44
Fiberoptic endoscopy, 2207–2208
Fiberoptic laryngoscopy
  bilateral vocal fold immobility, 1018, 1018f
  unilateral vocal fold paralysis, 1015, 1016f
Fibrin sealants, 52
Fibroelastic membranes of larynx, 873f
Fibroma, 984–985
  ameloblastic, 2106, 2106f
  ossifying, 293
Fibromatosis colli, 1600–1601
Fibromyalgia, 2160
Fibronectin
  wound healing, 80
Fibrosarcoma, 2048, 2374
Fibrous dysplasia, 2527
  in bone, 292–293, 293f
  in jaw, 2109, 2110f
  orbital tumor, 2072–2073, 2073f
  in skull base, 143, 143f
Fibrous histiocytoma, 281
Fibrous masses, voice therapy, 1054–1055
Fibrous papules, 3217, 3227
Fibrous tumors, facial, 3217, 3217f

Fibular osteocutaneous flap, 2835–2836, 2837f, 2838
Financial planning, medical practice, 3336–3337
Fine needle aspiration
  biopsy
    cell blocks, 179
    Diff-Quik staining, 179
    25-gauge needle, 179
    specimen adequacy, 179–180
    ultrasound-guided, 180
  molecular markers, 2118–2119, 2118t
Fistula
  cerebrospinal fluid, 655–656
  chylous, after neck dissection, 1831–1832
  dural arteriovenous, 2608, 2608f
  salivary, postoperative, 1782
Flail chest, trauma, 1102f
Flaps
  in lip reconstruction, 1794, 1795f, 1796–1798, 1800, 1801, 1802f, 1803f, 1804
  microvascular free
    composite, 2835–2842
    fascial and fasciocutaneous, 2824–2831
    muscle and musculocutaneous, 2831–2835
    visceral, 2842–2844
Flap-type tracheostomy, bilateral vocal fold immobility, 1022
Flashlamp-excited dye laser, 3202
Flexible endoscopic evaluation of swallow-ing, 1310–1311, 1311f, 1332–1333
  epiglottis tip, 828, 828f
  equipment requirement, 828
  versus fluoroscopy, 830t
  laryngeal adductor reflex, 828–829
  patient position, 828
  penetration aspiration scale, 830, 830t
  pharyngeal squeeze maneuver, 828–829, 829f
  premature spillage, 830
  rising tide sign, 830
  videofluoroscopic swallow study, 831
Flexible fiber delivery, 52
Floseal (Baxter), 52
Flow phonation, voice therapy, 1052–1053
Fluoroquinolones, 133
Fluoroscopy, 165, 166f
Focal length multiplier, 2779
Follicle-stimulating hormone, 252
Follicular carcinoma, 2120
Foramen cecum, congenital anomalies, nose, 1445, 1447f
Forceps, 22
Forehead
  aging, 3053–3072
  analysis of, for plastic surgery of face, 2761–2762, 2763f
  anatomy of, 3053–3055, 3054f, 3055f
  assessment of, 3056–3057
  brow aesthetics, 3056
  patient history, 3053
  preoperative counseling, 3057
  transverse rhytids of, Botox injections in, 3242, 3242f

Forehead flaps, for nasal restoration, 2885–2886, 2885t, 2886f–2892f, 2888–2889

Forehead lift
    browpexy, 3067
    complications of, 3070–3071
    coronal
        advantages and disadvantages of, 3059, 3059f
        contraindications to, 3059
        incision for, 3058, 3058f, 3059f
        technique for, 3059–3061, 3060f, 3061f
    direct brow, 3065, 3065f, 3066f
    endoscopic. See Endoscopic forehead lift
    indirect brow, 3066–3067
    midforehead, 3058f, 3064–3065
    pretrichial, 3058f, 3062–3063, 3062f
    surgical management, 3057–3058
    trichophytic, 3058f, 3063–3064, 3063f, 3064f

Foreign bodies
    cough, 1352
    esophageal, 857

Formant frequencies, professional voice, 1062–1063, 1062f

Forme fruste, 1620

Fosphenytoin, 42

Fraceschetti-Zwahlen-Klein syndrome, 1632–1633, 1633f

Fragile X syndrome, 1637

Frailty, 299–300

Fraser syndrome, 1637

Freckles, 3218

Freidman staging system, 2196, 2196f

Frey syndrome, 698, 1770, 1782–1783, 1782f

Friable tumors, neoplasms, 2061, 2061t

Friedreich ataxia, 1034, 2729

Frontal bone fracture, 1281–1282

Frontal bulla cell, 679f

Frontal drillout procedure, 683

Frontal sinus
    anatomy of, 362
    complications, 607t, 609
    CSF leaks, 670
    fractures of, 1282
        anatomic parameter, 1257, 1258f
        anatomy, 1255, 1256f
        anterior table, 1259, 1259f
        diagnosis, 1255–1256, 1256f–1257f
        frontal recess, 1257–1258, 1258t, 1259f
        pathophysiology, 1255, 1256f
        posterior table, 1258t, 1259–1260, 1260f
        surgical technique. See Sinus surgery
    indications, 605–606, 605t
    operative techniques
        bicoronal incision, 608–609
        eyebrow incision, 607–608, 608f
        lynch incision, 606–607, 607f
        mid-forehead incision, 608
        trephination, 606
    surgery
        complications of, 647, 649, 682
        controversies in, 686
        cranialization, 1269–1270, 1269f–1270f
        draf III/EMLP/drillout procedure
            bilateral Draf IIB, 684, 685f
            bur passage, 684, 685f
            efficacy, 683
            frontal process, 684, 684f
            frontal T and olfactory neuron, 684–685, 685f
            oval-shaped neo-ostium, 685, 686f
            septal window, 684, 684f
            unilateral drillout, 684, 685f
        endoscopic anterior table repair, 1261–1262, 1261f–1263f
        mini-trephination, 683
        obliteration
            autologous material, 1268
            bipolar forceps, 1267, 1267f
            coronal incision, 1266
            intracranial penetration, 1267, 1268f
            osteotomy, 1267, 1267f
            parietal region, 1268, 1269f
            scalloped area, 1268, 1269f
            side-cutting burr, 1267, 1268f
        open reduction and internal fixation
            bone fragment, 1265–1266, 1266f
            incision line, 1263, 1263f
            pericranial flap, 1265, 1265f
            risk of, 1262–1263
            supraorbital neurovascular pedicle, 1264–1265, 1265f
            temporoparietal fascia, 1264, 1264f, 1266f
            "zig-zag" incision, 1263, 1264f
        operative technique
            axillary flap technique, 682–683
            in chronic rhinosinusitis, 680, 682
            3D reconstruction, 681f
            draf IIB approach, 680
            mucosal thickening, 676, 680
            preoperative planning and assessment, 682
        postoperative care, 685–686
        surgical anatomy
            agger nasi cell, 676, 677f
            anterior and medial drainage pathway, 676, 677f
            frontal bulla cell, 679f
            frontal recess and sinus cells, 675, 676f
            frontal sinus development, 675
            fronto-ethmoidal cells, 677f
            intersinus septal cell, 680f
            suprabullar cell, 679f
            trephination, 1260, 1260f–1261f

Frontolateral vertical hemilaryngectomy, 1953

Frontoorbitotemporal craniotomy, 2076, 2076f

Frostbite, 1128

Full transfixion incisions, 2945

Functional status, 1673

Fungal ball
    clinical presentation, 565
    pathology, 566–567, 566f
    radiology, 565–566, 566f
    treatment, 567

Fungal infections
    pharyngitis in, 766
    stomatitis
        candidiasis, 740–741, 740f, 740t, 741f
        denture-related, 741–742, 741f

Fungal laryngitis, 979, 979f

Fungal rhinosinusitis
    classification of, 557, 558t
    invasive fungal sinusitis. See Invasive fungal sinusitis
    noninvasive fungal sinus infections
        allergic fungal rhinosinusitis. See Allergic fungal rhinosinusitis
        fungal ball. See Fungal ball
        localized fungal colonization, 565
    spores, 557
    yeast and molds, 557

Furlow double opposing Z-plasty
    Dingman retractor, 1565, 1565f
    velar nasal flaps, 1566, 1566f
    velum infiltration, 1565

Furosemide, 39, 41

Furunculosis, 2344

G

Gabapentin, 208

Gadopentetate dimeglumine, 167

Gardner syndrome, 125, 1637–1638

Gastric acid
    biological role of, 959
    nature of, 958–959
    neutralization, 959
    pharmacology, 959
    secretion and regulation, 959

Gastric pull-up with pharyngogastric anastomosis, 1934f

Gastroesophageal reflux disease, 845, 961
    esophageal disorder, 853, 853f
    neonatal respiratory distress
        evaluation and treatment of, 1328–1330, 1329f
        laryngomalacia, 1332
        laryngospasm, 1333

Gastrointestinal disorders, preoperative management of, 39–40

Gastroomentum, microvascular flaps of, 2843–2844, 2843f

Gaze stabilization test, 2303–2304, 2309

Gaze-evoked nystagmus, 2685

Gelatin-based products, 52

Gelfoam (Baxter), 52

Gene therapy
    Atoh1, 2749
    translational research, 3358

General anesthetic agents
    inhalational anesthetic agents
        characteristics, 238t
        halothane, 239
        malignant hyperthermia, 239–240
        minimum alveolar concentration, 238
        nitrous oxide, 239
        sevoflurane and desflurane, 239
    intravenous anesthetic agents, 240t
        barbiturates, 240
        etomidate, 240
        ketamine, 241
        propofol, 240–241

Generic HRQOL instruments, 720–721, 720t
Genetic disorders
    diagnosis and treatment of, 126–127
    in head and neck cancer, 125–126
    in laryngology, 126
    in otology and neurotology, 123–124
    in rhinology, 126
Genetic therapy, 127–128
Genetics, 111–128. *See also* Inheritance
    Mendelian genetics
        autosomal dominant inheritance, 115, 116f
        autosomal recessive inheritance, 115–117, 117f
        basic terminology, 115t
        penetrance and expressivity, 119
        sex-linked inheritance, 117–118, 118f
        molecular therapy in, 127–128
    non-mendelian genetics
        additional epigenetic influences, 121
        chromosomal anomalies, 122–123
        complex genetics, 122
        digenic inheritance, 121–122
        genomic imprinting, 119–121
        mitochondrial inheritance and mutations, 119
    principles of, 1541–1542
Genioglossus advancement, 2211, 2212f
Genioplasty. *See* Osseous genioplasty
Genomic imprinting, 119–121
Gentamicin, 2704
Geometric broken-line closure, for scar camouflage, 2863, 2865f, 2866f
Geriatrics. *See* Elderly patients
Giant cell (temporal) arteritis, 277–278
Gingivostomatitis, herpetic, 764
GJB genes, in hearing loss, 1544–1545
Glabellar rhytids, Botox injections in, 3242
Glandular hypertrophy, 713
Glandular tumors
    of external auditory canal, 2368–2369
    of external ears
        diagnosis of, 2369
        treatment of, 2369
Glasgow coma scale, 1101t
Glioma, 1447
Glomus tympanicum tumors, 2359–2360
Glossopexy, 1332
Glossopharyngeal nerve, 695
Glossopharyngeal neuralgia, 312
Glossoptosis, 2231
Glottal leukoplakia, 1088
Glottic cancer, early
    carcinoma in situ, 1950
    endoscopic surgical procedure, 1951–1953, 1951f, 1952f
    laryngofissure and cordectomy, 1953, 1953f
    outcomes of, 1954
    photodynamic therapy, 1955
    radiotherapy, 1955
    stages and diagnosis, 1943t, 1950
    surgical pathology, 1949–1950
    treatment, 1945t, 1950
    vertical partial laryngectomy, 1953, 1953f

Glottic closure, swallowing, 860, 860f
Glucagon, 260–261
Glucose-6-phosphate dehydrogenase deficiency, 28
Goiter, 1627–1629, 1627f, 1628f
Goldenhar syndrome, 124
Gonadotropin-releasing hormone, 252
Gonorrhea, pharyngitis due to, 765
Gorlin cyst, 2099
Gorlin syndrome, 125, 1638
Gout, 283
Gouty tophi, noninflammatory lesions, 2349
G-protein-coupled receptor-mediated signal, 730
Gracilis flap, 2835, 2836f
Gradle scissors, 22
Gradual loss of vision, 221–222
Grafts, in facial, head, and neck surgery, 2784–2796
Graft-*versus*-host disease, 738–739, 739f
Granular cell tumor, 985
Granuloma
    cholesterol. *See* Cholesterol granuloma
    eosinophilic, 2372–2373
    pyogenic, 3216, 3226
Granulomatous disease
    bacterial infections
        actinomycosis and nocardia, 287–288, 287f
        brucellosis, 284
        cat-scratch disease and bacillary angiomatosis, 283–284
        leprosy, 286–287, 287t
        nontuberculous mycobacteria, 286
        rhinoscleroma, 284
        syphilis, 288–289, 289f
        tuberculosis, 284–286, 285f
        tularemia, 289
    fungal infections
        blastomycosis, 290
        coccidioidomycosis, 290
        histoplasmosis, 289–290
    gout, 283
    neoplastic disorders
        fibrous histiocytoma, 281
        langerhans cell histiocytosis, 280–281
        necrotizing sialometaplasia, 281
        pyogenic granuloma, 281
        reparative granuloma, 281
    parasitic infections
        leishmaniasis, 290–291
        myiasis, 291
        rhinosporidiosis, 291–292
        toxoplasmosis, 291
    pharyngitis in, 767
    physical examination, 280
    sarcoidosis, 281–283, 282f
Granulomatous invasive fungal rhinosinusitis
    axial and coronal CT scans, 564, 564f
    pathology, 564–565, 565f
    treatment and prognosis, 565
Granulomatous lesions, 1470
Great auricular nerve, 694–695
Group A beta-hemolytic streptococci, 1433
Growth and development

abnormal. *See* Otolaryngologic syndromes
    patterns of, 1288–1295, 1288f–1294f, 1291t
Growth hormone, 251
Guillain-Barré syndrome, 210, 1039–1040, 1040f
Gustatory sweating, 1770, 1782–1783, 1782f

H
Haemophilus influenzae, 1383
    rhinosinusitis due to, 1458, 1458t
    tonsillar hypertrophy, 1433
    type B, 1298
Hair cell regeneration
    Atoh1 gene therapy, 2749
    cell cycle inhibition, 2749–2750
    embryonic stem cells, 2750–2751
    nonmammalian vertebrates *versus* mammals, 2747–2748
    notch signaling pathway, 2749
    somatic stem cells, 2750
    stem cell transplantation, 2751, 2751f
Hair cell stimulators, 2624
Hair loss. *See* Alopecia
Hair removal, lasers, 3208
Hair transplantation, autograft
    donor hair removal, 3231–3232
    donor-site removal, 3232
    recipient site, 3232–3233
    sequelae and complication, 3233–3234
Hairline patterns, forehead lift and, 3057
Hairy cell leukoplakia
    in AIDS, 743
Hallgren syndrome, 1633
Hallpike and roll tests, 2306
Halmagyi maneuver, 2721–2722
Halothane, 239
Hamartoma, 983
Hand-Schüller-Christian disease, 2373
Hard failure, 2636
Hard palate. *See* Palate
Harmonic sound source, professional voice, 1061–1062, 1062t
Hashimoto thyroiditis, 2071
Head and neck
    surgery
        anatomy of, 3–17
        pictorial documentation for. *See* Photodocumentation
    vascular tumor. *See* Vascular tumor
Head and neck cancer
    NO neck in, 1839–1846
    orbital. *See* Orbital tumors
    pain
        acute pain, 345
        cancer pain, 345
        end-of-life care, 350–353
        head and neck pain, 345
        methadone, 348
        neuropathic pain, 348, 350
        opioid analgesic drugs, 348, 349t
        pain management principles, 346–347, 346t
        percutaneous gastrostomy, 348
        pharmacologic approach, 347–348

Head and neck cancer (*Continued*)
  shoulder and arm pain, 345
  treatment regimens, 345
radiation therapy for. *See* Radiation
    therapy
salivary gland, 1760. *See also* Salivary
    gland disease
treatment of
  chemotherapy in. *See* Chemotherapy
  multidisciplinary team approach,
    1676–1677
Head and neck masses
  history of
    branchio-oto-renal syndrome,
      1590–1591
    cervical lymphadenitis, 1590
    periodic fever, 1590
  imaging
    computerized tomography, 1592
    magnetic resonance imaging, 1593
    plain radiographs, 1592
    ultrasound, 1592
  inflammatory masses
    characterization of infection, anatomi-
      cal location, 1596–1598
    congenital masses, 1596
    infectious etiologies for, 1595–1596
    noninfectious etiologies, 1598–1599
  laboratory testing, 1591
  neoplastic masses
    fibromatosis colli, 1600–1601
    lipomas, 1600
    lymphoma, 1601
    nasopharyngeal carcinoma, 1603
    neural tumors, 1600
    neuroblastoma, 1602–1603
    pilomatrixoma, 1600
    posttransplant lymphoproliferative
      disease, 1601–1602
    rhabdomyosarcoma, 1602
    sarcomas, 1602
    teratomas, 1600
    thyroid malignancies, 1603
  physical examination, 1591
  tissue diagnosis
    fine-needle aspiration biopsy, 1593
    incisional/excisional biopsy,
      1593–1594
Head and neck squamous cell carcinoma
  angiogenesis and vasculogenesis,
    1664–1665
  apoptosis counterbalances proliferation,
    1659–1662
  cell cycle
    cell cycle inhibitors, 1654–1655
    cell proliferation, 1652–1654
    epidermal growth factor, 1648–1650
    p53, 1655–1656
    transforming growth factor beta,
      1651–1652
  chemotherapy
    carotids, 1709, 1709f
    chondroradionecrosis, 1710
    osteoradionecrosis, 1709, 1709f
    role of, 1708
  DNA repair pathway
    base excision repair, 1658

double-strand break repair,
  1658–1659
interstrand cross-link repair,
  1656–1658
nucleotide excision repair, 1656–1658
single-strand break repair, 1658
free tissue transfer
  hypopharynx, 1715–1717, 1716f
  larynx, 1715
  nasopharynx/skull base/paranasal
    sinuses, 1712–1713
  oral cavity, 1713, 1714f
  oropharynx, 1713–1715
  radial forearm free flaps, 1711–1712
  skin flap necrosis, 1711, 1711f
  in wound healing, 1711
microvascular surgery
  chondroradionecrosis, 1720
  osteoradionecrosis, 1718–1720
pathogenesis and field cancerization
  dimethylbenzanthracene, 1647
  loss of heterozygosity, 1647–1648
  oral leukoplakia and erythroplakia,
    1646
  proto-oncogenes, 1647
  tumor induction and promotion,
    1647
  tumor progression, 1647, 1648f
  tumor suppressor, 1647, 1647t
recurrent, 1710–1711
subtypes of
  based on risk factors, 1645–1646
  genetic backgrounds, 1646
tumor heterogeneity, 1662–1664
unresectable, 1717–1718
Head heave test, 2689–2690
Head impulse test, 2308, 2687–2689,
  2688f, 2689f
Head injuries, secondary survey of trauma,
  1100–1101, 1100f, 1101t
Head thrust test, 2721–2722
Head trauma, 373, 1531–1532
Headaches, 2444
  primary. *See* Primary headache
  secondary. *See* Secondary headache
Health technology assessments, 719
Health-related quality of life
  assessment instruments selection
    relevance, 722
    reliability, 723
    responsiveness, 723
    validity, 723
  effectiveness, 726–727
  feedback, 726–727
  functional health status
    handicap and disability, 719, 719f
    impairment, 719, 719f
  head and neck surgery, 723–726
  measurement of
    health technology assessments, 719
    humanistic issues, 718
    NIH demonstration project, 719
    outcomes-adjusted reimbursement, 718
    patient-reported outcome measures,
      718–719
    quality-adjusted life years, 719
  quality of practice, 726–727

types of
  disease-specific scales, 721, 724t–725t
  generic HRQOL instruments,
    720–721, 720t
  symptom-specific instruments, 721
Hearing
  anatomy and physiology of, 2253–2272
Hearing aids and assistive listening devices
  amplification system, 2654–2655, 2655f
  assistive technology, 2669–2670, 2670t
  batteries, 2663
  coupling choices, 2662, 2663f
  digital noise reduction, 2666–2667
  directional microphones, 2665–2666,
    2666f
  earmolds, 2660–2661
  evaluation of, 2655–2656, 2657t
  fitting, 2655, 2663–2665, 2664f, 2667
  hearing loss and candidacy, 2655
  in noise, 2665
  orientation of, 2669, 2669t
  outcome assessment of, 2669
  population, 2654
  preselection decisions, 2656
  presetting and verification, 2667–2669,
    2667f–2669f
  remote control, 2662–2663
  routing of signal, 2656–2658
  sound sources, 2662
  styles in, 2658, 2658f–2661f, 2660
  telephone access, 2661–2662, 2662t
Hearing devices, implantable. *See also*
    Cochlear implants
  auditory brainstem response testing
    ASSR, 1511–1512
    auditory neuropathy spectrum disor-
      der, 1511
    measurement, 1510–1511
    used for, 1510
  congenital hearing loss, 1507
  development of auditory behavior, 1509
  hearing loss
    classification, 1515, 1515t
    evaluation, 1515
    management of, 1515
  immittance testing, 1513
  otoacoustic emission testing, 1512–1513
  otolaryngologist's role in
    bone-anchored hearing appliances,
      1519, 1519f
    hearing aid fitting, 1515–1517
    implantation, 1517–1518, 1517t
    meningitis vaccination, 1518–1519
    otitis media, 1518
  pure-tone testing, 1513–1514, 1514f
  screening
    joint committee on infant hearing,
      1507–1508, 1508t
    neonatal intensive care unit, 1508
    newborn period, 1509
    risk factor, 1507
  test battery, 1509–1510
  universal newborn hearing screening,
    1507
Hearing evaluation
  audiologic testing in, 2490, 2491f, 2492f
  in children, 1553

epidemiology of, 2489
history taking in, 2489–2490
indications for, 2286
in infants, 1545
in otosclerosis, 2490, 2491f, 2492f
physical examination in, 2489–2490
Hearing handicap
evaluation of, 2277, 2277t
permanent, definition of, 2277
Hearing impairment, permanent definition of, 2277
Hearing loss
after mastoid surgery, 2461
in Alport syndrome, 1543t, 1551
assistive listening devices. See Hearing aids and assistive listening devices
auditory neuropathy, 1545
in branchiootorenal syndrome, 1543t, 1548, 1623–1624, 1624f
causes of
etiology of, 1525–1526
extra-corporeal membrane oxygenation, 1526
infectious causes, 1526–1530
in CHARGE association, 1625
cholesteatoma and, 2442
in Crouzon syndrome, 1626
in deafness dystonia syndrome, 1551
in Down syndrome, 1552, 1626
enlarged vestibular aqueduct syndrome, 1546, 1546f
genetics
in autosomal dominant disorders, 1547
in autosomal recessive disorders, 1542–1551
in chromosomal disorders, 1552
diagnosis of, 1544
genetic counseling for, 1553
genetic principles and, 1541–1542
in mitochondrial disorders, 1543t, 1551–1552
in multifactorial disorders, 1552
in otolaryngologic syndromes, 1621–1622
X-linked disorders, 1543t
in Goldenhar syndrome, 1552, 1628
hearing devices, implantable
classification, 1515, 1515t
evaluation, 1515
management of, 1515
in Jervell and Lange-Nielsen syndrome, 1543t, 1546
in Kartagener syndrome, 1629
in Kearns-Sayre syndrome, 1552
in Klippel-Feil syndrome, 1550–1551
in MELAS syndrome, 1551–1552
in Melnick-Fraser syndrome, 1623
in MIDD syndrome, 1552
in neurofibromatosis, 1548–1549
newborn hearing screening
auditory brainstem response, 1524
Crib-O-Gram, 1524
electrodermal response audiometry, 1524
evoked otoacoustic emission, 1524

goals for, 1525
Joint Committee on Infant Hearing recommendations, 1523
otoacoustic emission, 1524
otolaryngologist, role of, 1525
in school-aged children, 1523
statewide infant hearing screening programs, 1524
tests used for, 1525
transient evoked otoacoustic emission, 1524
in Norrie disease, 1543t, 1550
in otopalatodigital syndrome, 1550
in Pendred syndrome, 1543t, 1546
permanent, definition of, 2277
sensorineural hearing loss. See Sensorineural hearing loss
in Stickler syndrome, 1543t, 1549
trauma
head trauma, 1531–1532
noise-related hearing loss, 1530–1531
ototoxicity, 1531
in Treacher Collins syndrome, 1543t, 1549
treatment of, 2364
in Turner syndrome, 1552
in Usher syndrome, 1543t, 1547
in Waardenburg syndrome, 1543t, 1549, 1634
Heerfordt disease, 282
Hemangiomas, 984, 985f, 2610
in beard distribution, 1578
capillary, 3216
classification of, 2364
congenital, 1575
facial nerve, 2364
geniculate, 2364
head and neck, morphologic variations, 1575, 1577f
infantile
cosmetic outcome, 1574
diagnostic evaluation, 1579–1582
GLUT1, 1575
growth phase, 1575
natural regression, 1574, 1576f
lasers, 3204–3205, 3205f, 3206f
nose, 1578
periocular, 1578, 1578f
phaces, 1577–1578
subglottic, 1578, 1579f
Hemangiopericytoma, 2048–2049, 2364–2365
architectural pattern of, 2017
chemotherapy, 2019
clinical presentation, 2018–2019
diagnosis of, 2018
radiation therapy, 2019
treatment, 2019
Hematologic abnormalities, preoperative management of, 27–30
Hematoma, 2124
following forehead lift, 3071
rhytidectomy, 3125, 3127
soft tissue injuries, 1109
Hematopoietic tumors, 2067–2068
Hemifacial microsomia, 1627

Hemitransfixion incisions, 2945, 2946f
Hemoglobinopathies, preoperative management of, 28
Hemolytic streptococci, pediatric rhinosinusitis, 1458, 1458t
Hemophilia A and B, 498–499
Hemorrhage. See also Bleeding
as complication of forehead surgery, 3070
sinus surgery complications, 656–657
Hemostatic agents, 52–53
in benign facial lesions, 3224
Hemostatic disorders
preoperative management of, 29–30, 29t
Heparin, 29
Hereditary telangiectasia
hemorrhagic, 497–498, 3207, 3212, 3214t, 3217f
Herpes simplex virus infection, 743f, 1433, 1528
of external auditory canal, 2345
pharyngeal, 764
stomatitis, 742–743, 742f
Herpes ulceration, 742–743, 742f
Herpes zoster oticus, 2345, 2512–2513
Heterogeneity, 1542
Heterotropia, 220, 220f
Heterozygosity, 1542
Hidrocystomas, 3216, 3226
High frequency oscillation, 60
High-resolution manometry
Chicago classification, 834, 834t
pressure topography, 834, 835f
High-resolution microendoscopy, 51
Histamine receptor blockers (H$_2$ blockers), 68–69
Histiocytoma, fibrous, 281
Histiocytosis X, 2068. See also Langerhans cell histiocytosis
Histoplasmosis, 289–290
Hoarseness, 953, 1572
Hodgkin lymphoma, 2036
Hogan technique, 1568
Hollinger telescope, 905f
Homeopathy, 320
Homografts, for soft-tissue augmentation, 3245
Hordeolum, 223
Hormone-induced rhinitis, 480–481, 481t
Horner syndrome, 2361, 2721, 3077
Human acellular dermis matrix, 2787
Human immunodeficiency virus infection, 1529. See also Acquired immunodeficiency syndrome
external ear disease in, 2346
otologic manifestations, 2520
pharyngitis in, 764
viral sialadenitis, 704
Human papillomavirus. See also Recurrent respiratory papillomatosis
pharyngitis in, 764–765
recurrent respiratory papillomatosis, 1409–1410
skin cancer and, 1724
squamous cell carcinoma, 196

Human resources, 3332–3333
Hurthle cell carcinoma, 2120
Hyaluronic acid products, for soft tissue augmentation, 3246–3247, 3246f
Hydration, voice therapy, 1049
Hydrocortisone, for adrenal suppression, 34t
Hydromorphone, 64
Hydroxyapatite, 2786, 2790
Hygiene hypothesis, 397–398
Hyoid bone
    anatomy of, 11–12, 11f
    deep neck space
        anterior visceral space, 800
        masticator space, 800
        parapharyngeal space, 799, 799f
        parotid space, 800
        peritonsillar space, 800
        submandibular and sublingual spaces, 799–800
        suprasternal space, 800
        temporal space, 800
Hyoid suspension procedure, 2211, 2212f
Hyperbaric oxygen therapy, 2592
Hyperbilirubinemia, 1533
Hypercalcemia
    calcium level, 255
    pathogenesis, 255
    treatment
        bisphosphonates, 255
        calcitonin, 255
        glucocorticoids, 256
        hydration and diuretics, 255
Hypercapnia, trauma, 1094
Hyperemia, 3194, 3194f
Hyperfractionation, 1684
Hyperglycemia, 31
Hyperglycemic hyperosmolar state, 262
Hyperkinetic disorders
    dystonia, 1032
    essential tremor, 1033–1034
    lower esophageal sphincter, 854
    oculopalatolaryngopharyngeal myoclonus, 1034
    spasmodic dysphonia, 1032–1033
    tic disorders, 1034
Hyperkinetic esophageal motility disorders
    distal esophageal spasm, 854, 854f
    nutcracker esophagus, 854
Hypermetria, 2686
Hyperopia, 221
Hyperosmolar nonketotic syndrome, 32
Hyperparathyroidism
    calcium homeostasis, 2131–2132, 2132f
    clinical manifestations of, 2133
    embryology and anatomical considerations, 2131
    evaluation
        CT with contrast, 2135, 2136f
        family history of, 2133
        plasma calcium and parathyroid levels, 2133–2134
        Sestamibi parathyroid scan, 2134, 2135f
        ultrasound of, 2134, 2134f
        vitamin D level measurements, 2134
    familial hypocalciuric hypercalcemia, 2133

mediastinal adenoma, 2141, 2142f
parathyroid carcinoma, 2132, 2141–2142, 2142f
parathyroid gland histology, 2132, 2132f
parathyroidectomy
    anterior approach, 2140, 2140f
    bilateral exploration, 2136–2138, 2137f, 2138f
    indications for, 2135, 2136t
    intraoperative rapid parathyroid hormone, 2138–2139
    lateral approach, 2140, 2141f, 2142f
    minimally invasive, 2138, 2139
    patient outcome, 2140
    postoperative care, 2142–2143
    primary, 2132
    secondary and tertiary, 2132
Hypersalivation, 699
Hypersensitivity. See Allergy
Hypertension
    cardiovascular disorders, 35–36, 36t
    epistaxis, 503
    perioperative pharmacologic control, 36t
    preoperative management of, 35–36
Hypertonic lower facial paralysis, 2917
Hypertrophic scars, 3217, 3217f
    treatment of, 3227
Hypertrophy, inferior turbinate. See Turbinate(s), hypertrophy of
Hyperventilation-induced nystagmus, 2698
Hyphema, 228
Hypocalcemia, 33, 256, 2124
Hypofractionation, 1684
Hypoglycemia, 262
Hypokinetic disorders
    esophageal motility
        achalasia, 854–855, 855f
        ineffective esophageal motility, 854
    multiple systems atrophy, 1031–1032
    Parkinson disease, 1030–1031, 1031f, 1032t
    parkinsonism, 1030
Hypomobility disorder, 785
Hypopharyngeal cancer
    chemotherapy, 1696–1697
    complications, 1936, 1936t
    diagnosis
        imaging, 1920–1921
        nutritional evaluation, 1921
        patient evaluation, 1919–1920, 1920t
        physical examination, 1920
    epidemiology, 1918–1919
    esophagus reconstruction, 1932–1933, 1933f, 1934f
    etiology, 1919
    functional rehabilitation, 1936
    neck management, 1932
    nonsurgical therapy, 1933, 1935
    organ preservation protocol, 1936
    pathology
        molecular staging, 1923
        patterns of spread, 1921–1922, 1921t, 1922f
        TNM staging, 1922–1923
    prognosis, 1923–1924, 1923t, 1924t

salvage surgery, 1935–1936
surgery of
    advanced-stage pyriform sinus cancer, 1925, 1927
    cervical esophagus, 1932
    early-stage pyriform sinus cancer, 1924–1925, 1925f, 1926f
    postcricoid cancer, 1929
    posterior hypopharyngeal wall cancer, 1927–1928, 1928f–1931f
    preoperative considerations, 1924
    transoral laser and robotic surgery, 1929
Hypopharyngeal/laryngeal obstruction
    postnatal diagnosis, 1313–1314, 1313f, 1315f
    prenatal diagnosis, 1309, 1309f–1310f
    treatment
        Arnold-Chiari malformation, 1320
        laryngeal cleft, 1320–1321, 1321f
        laryngeal web, 1321
        propranolol, 1320
        supraglottoplasty, 1320
Hypopharynx, 12f, 13, 1917–1918, 1918f, 1919f
Hypopigmentation, 2868
Hypotension
    perioperative, pharmacologic control, 36t
    postoperative, prevention of, 36–37
Hypotheses, testing of, analytic statistics and, 93t
Hypothyroidism, 32
Hypotonia, 2722
Hypovolemic shock, 1098–1099
Hypoxia, 1093, 1094

I
Idiopathic intracranial hypertension, 313–314, 2610
Idiopathic orbital inflammation, 226, 2071
Idiopathic stenosis, 881
Idiopathic ulcerative laryngitis, 980
Ileus, adynamic, postoperative management of, 40
Iliac crest flaps, osteocutaneous and osteomusculocutaneous, 2838–2839
Image guidance
    for biopsy, 180
    revision sinus surgery, 52
    rhinology and allergy, 601
Image-guided endoscopic sinus surgery, 650
Image-guided navigation, 52
Imagined ugliness syndrome, 2996
Imipenem, 288
Immune complex-mediated vasculitides, 276
Immune response
    B lymphocytes, 386–387
    basophils, 384
    dendritic cells, 387
    eosinophils, 384
    monocytes, 384–385
    neutrophils, 383–384
    T lymphocytes, 385–386
Immune-mediated inner ear disease
    Behcet disease, 2707

Cogan syndrome, 2707
histopathologic patterns, 2706
relapsing polychondritis, 2707
sarcoidosis, 2707
serologic tests, 2707
systemic immune disease, 2706–2707
treatment, 2708
Immunization
for melanoma, 1751–1752
for otitis media, 1487–1488
for *Streptococcus pneumoniae*, in infants
and children, 2520
Immunodeficiency, otitis media and,
1487–1488
Immunoglobulins
IgA, 388
IgD, 388
IgE, 388–389
IgG, 387–388
IgM, 388
Immunotherapy
active, 404
allergen-specific, 402–404
in allergy, 386, 402–404
chronic rhinosinusitis, 591
rhinitis, 325
Impacted tooth, dentigerous cysts, 2098,
2098f
Implants
biocompatibility of, 2784–2785
biologic materials as, 2785t, 2787
ceramic, 2786
in face, head, and neck, 2784–2796
characteristics of, 2785–2787
complications and emergencies associated with, 2795–2796, 2796t
indications for, 2787–2788
patient evaluation for
preoperative counseling for, 2788
qualities needed for, 2787–2788
surgical management for, 2788–2795
metallic, 2785–2786
patient-specific, 2787
polymers as, 2786–2787
In vitro testing, in rhinitis, 453
Incisions. *See also* specific procedures and
approaches
bicoronal flap, 2059f–2060f
endoscopic forehead lift, 3068–3069,
3069f
facial skeletal trauma, 117, 1172f, 1173f
rhinoplasty
hemitransfixion, 2945, 2946f
Killian incision, 2945, 2946f
nasal-tip, 2943, 2945f
transcolumellar and intercartilaginous, 2944, 2945f
septoplasty, 615, 615f
Incisive canal cyst, 2100
Inclusion body myositis, 1042
Indirect rigid fiberoptic-enhanced laryngoscope, 900, 900f
Ineffective esophageal motility disorder,
854
Infantile hemangioma
cosmetic outcome, 1574
diagnostic evaluation

corticosteroids, 1580–1581
history and physical examination,
1579
indications for, 1582, 1582t
magnetic resonance imaging, 1580,
1580t
multimodal therapy, 1580
periorbital hemangiomas, 1582
propranolol, 1581–1582, 1581t
pulse dye laser, 1582
ulceration, 1580
ulcerative scalp hemangiomas, 1582,
1582f
ultrasound, 1579, 1579f
GLUT1, 1575
growth phase, 1575
natural regression, 1574, 1576f
Infectable fillers, Botox and, cosmetic uses
of, 3239–3250
Infections
anaerobes, 134
antimicrobial agents. *See* Antimicrobial
agents
Aspergillus, 134
bacteria
acute bacterial sialadenitis, 1467
*methicillin-resistant Staphylococcus
aureus,* 134
pharyngitis due to, 758–761, 760f,
765
Pseudomonas aeruginosa, 134
tuberculosis, stomatitis, 743–744
facial, 3219–3220, 3220f
hygiene hypothesis, 397–398
implant, 2795
otologic manifestations, 2519–2521
percutaneous dilatational tracheotomy,
942
Infectious disease
otitis media, 1299–1300
rhinosinusitis, 1300
Streptococcus pneumoniae, 1300
Infectious mononucleosis, Epstein-Barr-
associated
clinical course of, 763
complications of, 763–764
diagnosis of, 763
pharyngitis in, 763–764
symptoms of, 763
Inferior alveolar nerve block, 237
Inferior meatal antrostomy
complications, 644, 644t
Inferior turbinate hypertrophy. *See*
Turbinate(s), hypertrophy of
Inflammatory bowel disease, 747–748
Inflammatory masses, head and neck
masses
characterization of infection, anatomical
location
buccal space, 1598
mandibular space, 1597
masticator space, 1597–1598
parapharyngeal space, 1597
parotid space/parotitis, 1598
peritonsillar space, 1596
prevertebral space/danger space, 1597
retropharyngeal space, 1596–1597

submandibular space/submandibular
sialadenitis, 1597
infectious etiologies for
acute bacterial lymphadenitis, 1595
acute viral lymphadenitis, 1595
cat-scratch disease, 1595–1596
fungal infections, 1596
mycobacterial lymphadenitis, 1595
opportunistic infections, 1596
parasitic infections, 1596
noninfectious etiologies
Castleman disease, 1599
Kawasaki disease, 1598
Kikuchi-Fujimoto disease, 1598
Rosai-Dorfman disease, 1598–1599
sarcoidosis, 1598
Inflammatory muscle disease, 273–274
Inflammatory myopathies, 1042
associated disorders, 274
diagnostic criteria for, 273, 274t
head and neck manifestations, 274
incidence, 273
treatment, 274
Inflammatory tumors, orbital, 2071
Informed consent, 20
Infrahyoid epiglottis, 1945–1946, 1945f
Infratemporal fossa, 2058, 2059f–2060f
Ingestion injury, aerodigestive tract
chest radiograph, 1405, 1405f
clinical presentation, 1400
complications, 1401–1402, 1402f
diagnosis and treatment, 1400–1401,
1401t
disc battery, 1406, 1406f
foreign-body aspiration, 1402–1403
mass effect, 1405
mechanism of, 1399–1400
treatment, 1404
upper esophageal sphincter, 1405,
1405f–1406f
workup, 1403–1404, 1403f–1404f
Inhalant mold allergy, 414
Inhalation injuries, secondary survey of
trauma, 1104–1105
Inheritance. *See also* Genetics
autosomal dominant, 115, 116f, 1617,
1618f
autosomal recessive, 115–117, 117f,
1617, 1618f
digenic, 121–122
expressivity, 119, 1620
heterogeneity, 1620
molecular basis of
DNA and chromosomes, 111–113,
112f, 113f
RNA and proteins, 113–115,
113f, 114f
penetrance in, 119, 1620
pleiotropy and, 1620
polygenic, 122
sex-linked, 117–118, 118f
X-linked, 1617, 1619f
Injection augmentation laryngoplasty, 994,
1014–1015, 1014t, 1015f
Injury
auricular, 1123–1126, 1123f–1125f
canalicular, 1119f

Injury (*Continued*)
  eyelid, full-thickness, 1118, 1118*f*
  facial nerve, 1121–1123
  trauma
    abdominal, 1103–1104
    extremity, 1104
    head and spine, 1100–1101, 1100*f*,
      1101*t*
    inhalation, 1104–1105
    neck, 1101–1102, 1101*f*
    thoracic, 1102–1103, 1102*f*
Innate immune system
  allergic sensitization, 383
  antimicrobial peptides, 382
  complement system, 381–382
  defensins, 382
  nasal glandular products, 380
  natural killer cells, 381
  pattern recognition receptors, 380
  physical barriers, 380
Inner ear. *See* Ear, inner
Institute for healthcare improvement,
  3376
Institute of medicine, 3376
Insulin, preoperative, in diabetes mellitus,
  32, 261
Insulin-like growth factor 2 gene, 121
Integrins, wound healing, 79
Intense pulsed light, 3202–3203
Intensity-modulated radiation therapy
  advantages of, 1687–1688
  versus 3D plan, 1687, 1687*f*
  multiple radiation beams, 1687
  tongue cancer, 1688, 1688*f*
Intention tremor, 2722
Intercartilaginous incisions, 2944, 2945*f*
Interferon(s)
  malignant melanoma, 1751–1752
  recurrent respiratory papillomatosis,
    1423–1424
  for skin cancer, 1731
Interleukins, 737
  cutaneous malignant melanoma, 1752
  recurrent respiratory papillomatosis,
    1410
Internal carotid artery, 1432
Internuclear ophthalmoplegia, 2686
Intersinus septal cell, 680*f*
Intracerebral abscess, 581–582
Intracochlear membrane rupture
  sudden sensorineural hearing loss,
    2590–2591
Intraconal orbital tumor, 2077, 2078*f*
Intracranial abscess and orbital phlegmon
  computed tomography, 144, 144*f*
Intracranial and extracranial aneurysms,
  2609, 2609*f*
Intradermal dilutional testing, 417, 417*t*
Intradermal skin testing, 416, 416*f*
  dilutional testing, 417, 417*t*
  positive response and negative control,
    416, 416*f*
  single intradermal testing, 416–417
Intralesional fillers, 2868
Intranasal antihistamines, 464
Intranasal corticosteroids, 464
Intranasal ethmoidectomy, 645

Intraoperative monitoring, neurophysiologic, 2314–2330
  auditory system monitoring, 2315, 2315*f*
  of facial nerve, 2323
Intraoperative photography, 2776–2777
Intrathecal fluorescein, 667–668, 668*f*
Intravelar veloplasty, 1566–1568, 1567*f*
Intravenous sedative agents, 241
Intrinsic laryngeal muscles
  larynx, 948*f*
  professional voice, 1059–1061, 1060*f*,
    1061*f*
Intubation
  airway assessment
    patient history, 909, 909*t*
    physical examination, 909, 909*t*
  complications
    airway obstruction and barotrauma, 917
    bronchial and esophageal intubation,
      917
    cervical spine injury, 917
    corneal abrasions, 917
    dental injuries, 916
    intracranial intubation, 917
    laryngeal trauma, 916
    macroglossia, 916
    mucosal injury, 916
    nasal and lip trauma, 916
    nerve injuries, 916
    pulmonary edema, 917
    tracheal trauma, 916–917
  difficult airway
    GlideScope, 913–914, 913*f*
    MacIntosh laryngoscope, 912, 913*f*
    Miller laryngoscope blade, 913, 913*f*
  endotracheal tube selection, 4*t*, 910
  factors affecting, 909–910
  history of, 908
  Hunsaker Mon-Jet tube
    advantages of, 914, 914*t*
    complications, 915, 915*t*
    subglottic ventilation, 914
  indications, 908–909, 909*t*
  laryngeal mask airway, 915–916, 915*f*,
    915*t*
  Mallampati classification, 909, 909*f*
  nasotracheal intubation, 911–912, 911*f*
  noninvasive ventilation, 916, 916*f*
  orotracheal intubation, 910–911, 911*f*
  versus tracheotomy, 910, 910*t*
Invasive fungal sinusitis, 375–376
  acute invasive fungal rhinosinusitis. *See*
    Rhinosinusitis
  chronic invasive fungal rhinosinusitis,
    562–564
  clinical features of, 376*t*
  diagnosis, 376
  granulomatous invasive fungal rhinosi-
    nusitis
    axial and coronal CT scans, 564, 564*f*
    pathology, 564–565, 564*f*
    treatment and prognosis, 565
Inverted Schneiderian papilloma, 187*f*
Inverted-V deformity, 2991, 2993*f*, 3023
Invisible in canal hearing aid, 2658, 2658*f*
Ipratropium bromide
  nonallergic rhinitis, 472

Iridocyclitis, 225
Iris scissors, 22
Iritis, 225
Isolagen, for soft tissue augmentation,
  3246

J
Jadassohn nevus, 3216, 3216*f*
Jaundice, neonatal, hearing loss and, 1526
Jaw. *See also* Mandible; Maxilla
  aneurysmal bone cyst, 2111
  central giant cell lesion, 2109, 2111, 2112*f*
  cysts of, 2097–2113
  fibrous dysplasia, 2109, 2110*f*
  ossifying fibroma, 2108–2109, 2109*f*
  osteochondroma of, 2107–2108, 2108*f*
  osteoma of, 2107
  torus of, 2106–2107
  vascular malformations, 2111–2112
Jejunum, microvascular flaps of,
  2842–2843, 2842*f*
Jerk nystagmus, 2684
Jervell Lange-Nielsen syndrome, 124
Joint Committee on Infant Hearing, 1507,
  1508, 1508*t*
Journal articles
  grandeur in, signs of, 87*t*
  interpretation of, 86–100
  worth reading, identification of, 86–87,
    87*t*
Jugular bulb anomalies, 2605, 2607, 2607*f*
Jugular thrombophlebitis, internal, 805*f*
Jugular vein thrombosis, 1832
Jugulotympanic paragangliomas
  clinical presentation and classification,
    2003–2005, 2004*f*, 2004*t*, 2005*t*
  embolization, 2012–2014, 2014*f*
Junctional nevus, 3218, 3218*f*
Juvenile nasopharyngeal angiofibroma,
  440, 441*f*
  diagnosis of, 2025, 2026*f*
  endoscopic and endoscopic-assisted
    approaches, 2028
  epidemiology and pathogenesis, 2023
  growth patterns, 2024–2025, 2024*f*,
    2025*f*
  open surgery, 2027–2028, 2027*t*
  radiation therapy, 2028
  staging, 2025–2026, 2027*t*
  surgical approaches, 2026–2027
Juvenile recurrent parotitis, 707–708, 708*f*,
  1469

K
Kallmann syndrome, 117, 118*f*
Kanamycin, 2542, 2681
Kaposi sarcoma, 2021, 2039, 2346
Kaposiform hemangioendothelioma,
  1575*f*, 1579
Karapandzic labioplasty, 1797, 1798*f*
Kartagener syndrome, 126, 1629
Kasabach-Merritt phenomenon, 1579
Kawasaki disease, 279, 762, 1598
Kearns-Sayre syndrome, 1552
Keipert syndrome, 124–125
Keloids, 3217, 3217*f*, 3227
Keratitis, 224

Keratoacanthoma, 1727
    of lip, 1791
    noninflammatory lesions, 2349
Keratocysts, odontogenic tumor, 2101–2102
Keratoses
    actinic, 3212
        treatment of, 3224
    seborrheic
        treatment of, 3224
    senile, 1726
Keratosis obturans, 2350–2351
Ketamine, 241
Kidney injury, acute, 63–64, 63t
Kikuchi-Fujimoto disease, 279, 1598
Killian incision, 2945, 2946f
Klack's solution, 269
Klebsiella rhinoscleromatis, 284
Klinefelter syndrome, 122
Klippel-Feil syndrome, 1550–1551, 1638
Koplik spots, 2520
Kussmaul disease, 713

L
Labial arteries, 1788, 1794, 1798
Labyrinth
    ethmoid, 522, 643
    membranous
        development of, 2245–2246
        innervation of, development of,
            2246–2247
    osseous, development of, 2247–2249
    vestibular, 2673
Labyrinthectomy
    Ménière syndrome, 2704
    translabyrinthine tumor, 2571f
Labyrinthine fistula, as complications of
            cholesteatoma, 2442–2443
Labyrinthitis, 2404
    bacterial infection, 1530, 2520
    otitis media, 2400t
    otogenic suppurative, 2404
    serous/toxic, 2404
    vestibular injury, 2462
Lacerations
    repair
        drains, 1114
        postoperative care, 1113–1114
        suture techniques, 1112–1113, 1112f,
            1113f
    soft tissue injuries, 1109
Lacrimal system, 5–6, 5f, 1117–1119,
        1117f–1119f
Lacrimal tumors, orbital, 2074
Lag screw application, 1157, 1158f
Lagophthalmos, 3070–3071, 3078
Lambert-Eaton myasthenic syndrome, 1041
Lamina papyracea, 360
Lamina propria, 949–950
    development of, 1068
    granuloma, 995
    midmembranous vocal fold lesions
        cysts, 990–991, 991f–992f
        fibrous mass, 991, 992f
        nodules, 990, 990f
        nonspecific vocal fold lesion,
            991–992, 993f
        polyps, 990, 991f

pseudoscyt, 992–993, 993f
        reactive vocal fold lesion, 991, 993f
        striking zone, 990
    rheumatologic lesions, 994–995
    vocal fold scar and sulcus vocalis,
            993–994, 994f
Langerhans cell histiocytosis, 280–281,
        2068, 2521–2522
Laparoscopic Nissen fundoplication,
        972–973
Large agger cell, 677f
Large left skull base chondrosarcoma, 152,
        153f
Larsen syndrome, 1638
Laryngeal adductor reflex, 828–829
Laryngeal atresia, 1333, 1333f
Laryngeal cancer
    advanced
        differential diagnosis of, 1967, 1967f
        emergencies in, 1975
        evaluation and diagnosis of,
            1964–1967, 1965f, 1966f
        history and physical examination,
            1964–1965, 1965f
        imaging, 1965–1966, 1965f
        laboratory tests and consultations,
            1966
        nonsurgical treatment, 1967–1969
        patterns of spread, 1962–1963, 1963f
        posttreatment quality of, 1974–1975
        staging of, 1963, 1964t
        surgical evaluation, 1966–1967, 1966f
        surgical treatment, 1969–1974, 1970f,
            1971f, 1974f, 1974t
    chemoradiation, 1695–1696
    clinical database, 3356, 3357
    early
        epidemiology, 1940
        glottic cancer
            carcinoma in situ, 1950
            endoscopic surgerical procedure,
                1951–1953, 1951f, 1952f
            laryngofissure and cordectomy,
                1953, 1953f
            outcomes of, 1954
            photodynamic therapy, 1955
            radiotherapy, 1955
            stages and diagnosis, 1943t, 1950
            surgical pathology, 1949–1950
            treatment, 1945t, 1950
            vertical partial laryngectomy, 1953,
                1953f
        risk factor, 1940
        subglottic cancer
            surgical pathology, 1955–1956
            treatment, 1956
        supraglottic cancer
            diagnosis, 1942, 1943t
            horizontal supraglottic laryngec-
                tomy, 1947
            neck management, 1948–1949
            outcomes of, 1949
            radiotherapy, 1949
            supracricoid laryngectomy,
                1947–1948
            supraglottic laryngectomy, 1943,
                1944f

surgical pathology, 1942
        transoral laser microsurgery. See
            Transoral laser microsurgery
        transoral robotic surgery,
            1946–1947
        treatment, 1942–1943
    tumor biology
        genetics, 1940–1941
        pathology, 1941
    epidemiology of, 1961–1962, 1962f,
        1962t
    external beam radiation, 982
Laryngeal disease, 961–962
Laryngeal dysfunction, neurologic disor-
        der, 1037
Laryngeal electromyography, 1377
    bilateral vocal fold immobility, 1019
    unilateral vocal fold paralysis, 1011,
        1012f, 1013f
Laryngeal framework surgery, 1015–1017
Laryngeal lymphomas, 2039
Laryngeal pacing, bilateral vocal fold
        immobility, 1022
Laryngeal palpation, 1071, 1071f
Laryngeal pemphigus, 982, 982f
Laryngeal skeleton, 871f
Laryngeal stenosis
    anatomy, 1356–1357
    atresia, 1359
    caustic ingestions, 1361
    complications, 1369
    decision making, 1368
    differential diagnosis of, 1362, 1362t
    gastric acid reflux disease and eosino-
        philic esophagitis, 1361
    granulomatous disease, 1360
    management
        anterior cartilage graft, 1364, 1366,
            1366f
        cricotracheal resection, 1366, 1367f
        endoscopic evaluation, 1363
        extubation, 1364, 1365t
        history, 1362
        medical therapy, 1362
        posterior cartilage graft, 1364–1366
        preoperative assessment, 1362–1363
        slide and cervical slide tracheoplasty,
            1366, 1368
        stenting option, 1368, 1369f
        surgical, 1363–1364, 1363t–1364t
    postintubation stenosis, 1359–1360
    postreconstruction restenosis, 1360
    posttracheotomy, 1360
    radiation effects, 1361
    signs and symptoms, 1357, 1357t
    subglottic stenosis, 1357–1358, 1358t
    supraglottic webs, 1358–1359, 1359t
    systemic diseases, 1360–1361
    thermal injuries, 1361
    tracheal stenosis, 1361
    trauma, 1360
Laryngeal trauma
    complications, 1149–1150, 1149t–1150t
    diagnosis and evaluation
        history, 1142, 1142t
        physical examination of, 1142–1143
        radiologic evaluation, 1143–1144, 1143f

Laryngeal trauma (*Continued*)
  management
    algorithm for, 1144, 1144*f*
    cricotracheal separation, 1149
    emergency care, 1144–1145, 1145*t*
    grafting, 1147
    medical treatment, 1145–1146
    severed recurrent laryngeal nerve, 1149
    stents, 1148–1149, 1148*f*
    surgical treatment, 1146–1147,
      1147*f*–1148*f*
    treatment decision making, 1145,
      1145*t*
  pathophysiology of, 1141–1142
Laryngeal vibration, professional voice,
  1068, 1068*f*
Laryngectomy, 1969–1970
  near-total, 1972
  postlaryngectomy, 1972–1973
  supracricoid partial, 1971, 1971*f*
  supraglottic, 1970–1971
  total, 1972
  vertical hemilaryngectomy, 1970
Laryngitis, 881–882, 979*f*
  infectious
    bacterial, 978–979, 979*f*
    fungal, 979, 979*f*
    idiopathic ulcerative, 980
    viral, 978, 979*f*
  peripheral nervous system, 1042
  upper airway stenosis, 881–882
Laryngoceles, 985–986, 986*f*
Laryngomalacia, 1339–1340, 1340*f*
  neonatal respiratory distress, 1332,
    1332*f*
  stridor, 1339–1340, 1340*f*
Laryngopharyngeal reflux
  diagnosis
    esophagoscopy, 965, 967
    laryngopharyngoscopy, 964–965,
      965*f*–967*f*, 965*t*
    pepsin detection, 968–969
    quality of life, 964, 964*t*
    radiologic imaging, 968
    reflux detection, 967–968
  extraesophageal reflux
    connection of, 962–963
    middle ear, 963
    nose and paranasal sinuses, 963
    stenotic lesions, 963–964
  gastric reflux
    bile, 960–961
    gastric acid, 958–959
    pepsin, 959–960
    pharmacology, 959
    trypsin, 961
  pathophysiology
    versus gastroesophageal reflux disease,
      961
    nonacid and weakly acid reflux,
      961–962
  pediatric voice, 1373, 1373*f*–1374*f*
  symptoms of, 958
  treatment
    alcohol, 970
    alginate, 971
    assessment and management of, 970*f*

bicarbonate gum, 971
dietary factors, 969
elevation of head, bed, 971
H$_{959}$ receptor antagonists, 971
medications, 969
prokinetic agents, 971
proton pump inhibitors, 971–972
recommended lifestyle modifications,
  969*t*
smoking, 969–970
sucralfate, 971
surgical management of, 972–973
tight-fitting clothes, 970
weight loss, 969
  voice therapy, 1049
Laryngotracheobronchitis, 1342
Laryngovideostroboscopy, 1010*f*
Larynx
  anatomy, 13, 14*f*, 1941, 1962, 1962*f*
    age-related changes in, 950–951, 950*f*
    anterior airway, 870*f*
    cricoarytenoid joint, 947
    cricoid cartilage, 945
    endoscopic appearence, 870*f*
    epiglottis, 946
    fibroblastic membranes, 946, 946*f*
    membranous vocal fold, 949–950,
      949*f*
    mucosal cover, 873–874, 874*f*
    muscles and nerves, 871–872, 872*f*,
      947–949, 948*f*
    nerve supply, 873
    posterolateral projection, 945–946
    skeleton, 870–871, 871*f*–873*f*
    supporting framework of, 945, 946*f*
    vertical section, 870*f*, 946*f*
  benign neoplasia
    benign salivary neoplasia, 984
    chondroma, 983
    fibroma, 984–985
    granular cell tumor, 985
    hamartoma, 983
    hemangioma, 984, 985*f*
    respiratory papillomatosis, 983–984,
      984*f*
    rhabdomyoma, 983
    schwannomas, 985
  cancer, chemotherapy, 1695–1696
  infection
    bacterial laryngitis, 978–979, 979*f*
    fungal laryngitis, 979, 979*f*
    idiopathic ulcerative laryngitis, 980
    mycobacterial infection, 979–980
    syphilis, 980
    viral laryngitis, 978, 979*f*
  infiltration
    amyloidosis, 981, 981*f*
    external beam radiation, 982–983, 983*f*
    pemphigus and pemphigoid,
      981–982, 982*f*
    relapsing polychondritis, 981
    rheumatoid arthritis, 980–981
    sarcoidosis, 982, 982*f*
    systemic lupus erythematous, 981
    Wegener granulomatosis, 980
  laryngoceles and saccular cysts,
    985–986, 986*f*

membranous vocal fold, 949, 949*f*
neonatal respiratory distress
  flexible endoscopic evaluation of
    swallowing, 1332–1333
  laryngeal atresia, 1333, 1333*f*
  laryngomalacia, 1332, 1332*f*
  subglottic hemangioma, 1334, 1334*f*
neuroanatomy
  cerebellum and extrapyramidal sys-
    tems, 1027–1028
  cerebral cortex, 1026–1027
  lesions of, 1028–1029
  motor neurons, 1028
  vagus pathway, 1026, 1028*f*
neurologic disorder
  central nervous system
    ataxic disorders, 1034
    dystonia, 1032
    essential tremor, 1033–1034
    laryngeal dysfunction, 1037
    mixed disorders, 1034–1037
    multiple sclerosis, 1036–1037, 1036*f*
    multiple systems atrophy,
      1031–1032
    oculopalatolaryngopharyngeal
      myoclonus, 1034
    Parkinson disease, 1030–1031,
      1031*f*, 1032*t*
    parkinsonism, 1030
    spasmodic dysphonia, 1032–1033
    spastic disorder, 1030
    stroke, 1034–1036
    tic disorders, 1034
  diagnosis and treatment, 1029–1030,
    1029*t*
  electromyography, 1043–1045, 1043*f*,
    1044*f*
  hoarseness, 1026
  human vocal process, 1026, 1027*f*
  laryngeal presentation, 1045*t*
  peripheral nervous system
    amyotrophic lateral sclerosis, 1037
    botulism, 1041–1042
    bulbar palsy, 1037
    Guillain-Barré syndrome,
      1039–1040, 1040*f*
    inflammatory myopathies, 1042
    Lambert-Eaton myasthenic
      syndrome, 1041
    mononeuropathy, 1038
    muscular dystrophies, 1042
    myasthenia gravis, 1040–1041
    myelinopathy, 1038
    myopathies, 1042
    poliomyelitis, 1038
    postpolio syndrome, 1038
    progressive bulbar palsy, 1037–1038
    spinal muscular atrophy, 1038
    superior laryngeal nerve paresis,
      1039, 1040*f*
    vocal fold paralysis, 1038–1039,
      1039*f*
  physiology
    airflow regulation, 874–875
    airway protection, 951
    cough, 874
    respiration, 951–952

sensory receptors, 875
valsalva maneuver, 874, 952
voice, 952–953, 952f
stenotic lesions, airway, 963–964
Laser(s), 52
for benign facial lesions, 3223–3224
biophysics of
coagulation/vaporization, 3200, 3202f
components of, 3200, 3201f
characteristics of
argon laser, 3203–3204
CO$_2$ laser, 3203
continuous-wave yellow dye laser, 3204
copper vapor laser, 3204
flashlamp-excited dye laser, 3202
intense pulsed light, 3202–3203
potassium titanyl phosphate laser, 3203
red and infrared lasers, 3203
complications, 3209–3210
expected results, 3209
laser-tissue interaction
chromophores, 3201
coagulation/vaporization, 3200, 3202f
energy density, 3201
power density, 3201
spontaneous and stimulated emission, 3200, 3201f
thermal relaxation time, 3201
lesion subtypes
capillary malformations, 3205–3206, 3207f
cutaneous malignancy, 3208–3209
hair removal, 3208
hemangiomas, 3204–3205, 3205f, 3206f
hereditary hemorrhagic telangiectasia, 3207
pigmented lesions, 3207–3208
rejuvenation, 3208, 3209f
skin resurfacing, 3208, 3209f
telangiectasias, 3206–3207
venous malformations, 3206
patient management, 3209–3210
for skin cancer, 1731
skin resurfacing
for scar camouflage, 2866–2867
technical aspects of, 3204
treatment options, 3204
vascular lesions, 3204
Lateral arm flap, 2827, 2828f
Lateral crural strut grafts, 2973, 2973f, 2976f, 3019–3021, 3020f
Lateral lamella of the cribriform plate, 664
Lateral medullary syndrome, 200, 203f
Lateral neck dissection, 1819, 1820f, 1823, 1832
Lateral orbital decompression, 631, 632f
Lateral osteotomy, nasal dorsum, 2960, 2961f
Lateral pharyngotomy, 1907–1908, 1908f
Lateral pontomedullary syndrome, 200, 203f
Lateral sinus thrombosis, 2444
Lateral thigh flap, 2828
Latissimus dorsi flap, 2833–2835, 2834f
Laxity, lower eyelid blepharoplasty, 3086, 3087f

Lee Silverman voice therapy, 1031, 1032t, 1051
Left buccal carcinoma, 170, 170f
Left faucial tonsil carcinoma, 147f
Left hepatocellular carcinoma metastasis, 170, 171f
Leiomyomas
multiple, 3218, 3218f
treatment of, 3227
Leishmaniasis, 290–291
Lemierre syndrome, 804–805, 805f
Lentigines, 3218
treatment of, 3228
Lentigo maligna, 1740
Lentigo senilis, 3218, 3219f
LEOPARD syndrome, 1638
Leprosy, 286–287, 287t
Leptomeningeal carcinomatosis, 2578
Lesion subtypes
capillary malformations, 3205–3206, 3207f
cutaneous malignancy, 3208–3209
hair removal, 3208
hemangiomas, 3204–3205, 3205f, 3206f
pigmented lesions, 3207–3208
rejuvenation, 3208, 3209f
skin resurfacing, 3208, 3209f
telangiectasias, 3206–3207
venous malformations, 3206
Letterer-Siwe disease, 2373
Leukemia
orbital tumor, 2068
temporal bone involvement in, 2365
Leukotriene
inhibitors, 591
modifiers, 464
Levator palpebrae superioris muscle, 3076, 3077f
Lidocaine, 37, 235–236
subjective nonpulsatile tinnitus, 2603
Lingual choristomas, 1318–1319, 1319f
Lingual thyroid, 1613–1614
Lingual tonsil surgery, 2213, 2215f, 2231
Lip(s)
adhesion, 1562–1563
anatomy and physiology of, 1788–1790, 1789f
biopsy of, 1790, 1791, 1791t, 1793
cancer of
airway management, 1804, 1804t
biologic behavior of, 1788, 1790, 1804
clinical evaluation of, 1790–1791, 1791t
diagnosis of, 1790, 1791, 1791t, 1793
etiology of, 1790
nodal metastases in, 1793
nutrition in, 1804
cellulitis, 771, 772f
evaluation of, for plastic surgery of face, 2767, 2767f
keratoacanthoma, 1791, 1791t
nodal metastases in, 1793
premalignant lesions of, 1792
radiation therapy for
complications of, 1792, 1792t, 1804
risk factors for, 1792, 1793

soft tissue injuries, 1126, 1126f
staging of, 1790, 1791f
surgery for, 1792–1794
reconstructive, 1792, 1794–1804
swelling of, in Melkersson-Rosenthal syndrome, 1630
ulcers of, differential diagnosis of, 1790
Lipomas, 1600
cerebellopontine angle, 2380, 2577, 2579f
imaging of, 2381
of internal auditory canal, 2381
treatment of, 3227
Liquid crystal displays, 2782
Literature. See also Journal articles
interpretation of, 86–100
Local anesthesia, 236t
cationic form, 235
cocaine, 236
lidocaine, 235–236
lipophilic and hydrophilic end, 235
local anesthetic systemic toxicity, 236–237
metabolism, 235
nerve blocks
cervical plexus, 238
inferior alveolar nerve, 237
infraorbital nerve, 237
sensory innervation, 237
superior laryngeal nerve, 238
supraorbital and supratrochlear nerves, 237
trigeminal nerve, 237
Lorazepam, 65, 65t
Loss of heterozygosity, 1647–1648
Lower eyelid
transconjunctival approach
caruncular approach, 1182–1183, 1184f
conjunctiva and lower lid retractors flap, 1179, 1180f
corneal shield, 1178–1179
lateral canthotomy and cantholysis, 1179, 1181, 1182f
medial extension, 1181–1182, 1183f
orbital retractors, 1182
preseptal/post septal dissection, 1179, 1181f
transcutaneous approach
inferior rim incision, 1184, 1184f
malposition, 1185, 1187, 1187f
plane of dissection, 1184, 1185f
postoperative view, 1186f
skin-muscle flap, 1184, 1185f
subciliary incision, 1184, 1184f
Lower lid malposition, 1238
Ludwig angina
deep neck infection, 807–809, 808f, 809f
odontogenic infection, 777–778
Lumbar puncture, 2405
Lund-Kennedy endoscopic scores, 587
Lund-Mackay staging system, 587, 587t
Lupus cheilitis, 747

Lyme disease, 1529, 2521
Lymph node
    biopsy, 1814–1815
    metastases
        in lip cancer, 1793
        in skin cancer, 1735
Lymphadenitis, 1595
Lymphangioma, orbital tumor, 2066–2067
Lymphatic drainage
    of lips, 1789f, 1790
Lymphatic vessels, of neck, 17
Lymphoepithelial carcinoma, 190f
Lymphoepithelial cysts, 704
Lymphomas, 490–491, 1601, 2032–2040,
    2121
    AIDS-related, 2039
    diagnosis
        imaging, 2033–2034, 2034f
        tissue, 2034–2035
    epidemiology of, 2032–2033, 2033f
    Hodgkin, 2036
    laryngeal, 2039
    non-Hodgkin, 2036–2037
    posttransplant lymphoproliferative dis-
        order, 2039–2040
    salivary gland, 1768, 2037–2039, 2038f
    sinonasal, 2037
    staging of, 2035–2036, 2035t
    of temporal bone, 2365
    thyroid, 2039
    Waldeyer ring, 2037, 2038f
Lymphoproliferative lesions, 2067–2068
Lyric hearing aid, 2658, 2658f

M
Macrogenia, chin augmentation, 3181,
    3181f
Macroglossia, 2231
Macrolides, 134
    in chronic hypertrophic rhinosinusitis,
        591
    ototoxicity, 2544
Magnetic resonance imaging
    brachial plexus, 154, 156, 159f
    esthesioneuroblastoma, 440f
    indications, 422, 423t
    of nasopharyngeal cancer, 1878, 1879,
        1880f–1883f, 1882, 1883, 1885,
        1888, 1893f
    nasopharynx and skull base, 152–153,
        153f, 155f
    neonatal respiratory distress
        congenital subglottic stenosis, 1334
        evaluation and treatment of,
            1328–1330, 1329f
        fetal assessment, 1335–1336, 1335f
        nasal obstruction, 1330–1331, 1331f
        oral cavity/oropharynx/hypopharynx,
            1331–1332
        trachea/bronchi, 1334
        vocal fold paralysis, 1333
    orbits, 154
    paraganglioma, 2006, 2007f, 2008f
    paranasal sinuses, 153–154
    principles, 148
    salivary glands, 154
    sinonasal carcinoma, 424f

soft tissue neck, aerodigestive tract and
    larynx, 149–150, 151f
technical considerations, 148–149, 149f,
    150f
temporal bone, 150, 152, 152f
temporomandibular joint, 154, 787, 787f
terminology, 422, 425
tumor staging, 443
Malar augmentation, 2776t
Malar fat pad, 3104, 3104f, 3107
Malar mounds, lower eyelid blepharo-
    plasty, 3086, 3088, 3088f
Malignant esophageal neoplasms, 857
Malignant fibrous histiocytoma, 1602,
    1791, 1991t
Malignant hyperthermia, 44–45, 45t
Malignant melanoma
    clinical presentation and diagnosis
        childhood history, 1740
        excisional biopsy, 1740
        fine-needle aspiration, 1740
        melanin lack, 1739–1740
        physical examination, 1740
        pigmented lesions, 1739
    epidemiology, 1739
    of external ear
        diagnosis of, 2368
        growth phase, 2367
        incidence of, 2367
        treatment of, 2368
    lymphadenectomy, 1749–1750, 1750f
    metastases from, 1762
    mucosal, 1742
    occult lymph node disease detection
        elective lymph node dissection, 1745
        sentinel lymph node identification,
            1745–1748
    radiotherapy, 1750–1751
    staging system
        metastatic workup, 1744
        primary tumor, 1742
        regional nodal staging, 1742–1744
    subtypes
        acral lentiginous, 1741
        desmoplastic melanoma, 1741
        lentigo maligna, 1740
        nodular melanoma, 1741
        superficial spreading melanoma, 1741
    surveillance in, 1754–1755, 1754f
    systemic therapy
        biochemotherapy, 1753–1754
        chemotherapeutic agents, 1753
        interferon, 1751–1752
        interleukin-2, 1752
        ipilimumab, 1752–1753
        tumor vaccines, 1752
    treatment of, 1748–1749
Malignant necrotizing otitis externa, 136
Malignant tumors
    epithelial, 2046–2048, 2047t, 2048t
    nonepithelial, 2048–2049
Malleoincudal lever effect, 2466
Malnutrition
    preoperative, 26–27
    protein-calorie, 26
Mandible. See also Jaw
    anatomy, 10–11

arch fracture, 1279–1280, 1280f
implants for, 2793–2794, 2794f
reconstruction of, following oropharyn-
    geal surgery, 1913
tori, 2106
Mandibular fractures, 1278–1279, 1278f
    anatomy, 1195, 1196f–1197f
    bone morphogenetic protein, 1206
    complications, 1206, 1206t
    edentulous fracture, 1204, 1205f
    emergencies, 1206, 1206t
    evaluation and diagnosis
        history, 1196, 1198t
        physical examination, 1196,
            1198–1199f
        radiographic evaluation, 1198, 1199f
    external fixation, 1204, 1205f
    hardware removal, 1205–1206
    management
        angle, 1196f, 1202–1203, 1203f
        body, 1196f, 1202
        closed reduction, 1200
        condyle, 1196f, 1203–1204, 1204t
        goals of, 1198
        hardware selection, 1201–1202, 1201f
        open reduction, 1200–1201, 1200t,
            1201f
        ramus, 1196f, 1204
        symphysis/parasymphysis, 1196f,
            1202, 1202f
    mandible, biomechanics, 1195–1196,
        1197f
    medical modeling, 1206
    pediatric fracture, 1204–1205
    resorbable fixation system, 1206
    stereotactic image guidance, 1206
    teeth management, fracture line, 1204
    transcutaneous approach
        blunt dissection, 1191
        laceration, 1190
        marginal mandibular nerve, 1190, 1190f
        passive drain, 1191
        retromandibular or preauricular
            approach, 1191, 1192f, 1193
        submandibular approach, 1191, 1191f
        symphysis, 1190
    transoral approach
        disadvantage, 1188
        labial sulcus approach, 1188, 1189f
        mandibular angle fracture, 1189, 1190f
Mandibular hypoplasia, 3133
Mandibular lingual release, 1906–1907,
    1906f
Mandibular space, odontogenic infection
    mylohyoid, 774, 775f
    sublingual space, 774, 776, 776f
    submandibular space, 776, 776f
    submental space, 776–777
Mandibular swing approach, osteotomy,
    1908–1909, 1910f
Mandibulectomy, 1909–1910, 1911f
Mandibulofacial dysostosis, 1632–1633,
    1633f
    in hearing loss, 1543t
Maneuvers, 842–844, 842t, 843f
Manipulative and body-based techniques
    chiropractic medicine, 318–319

massage, 319
osteopathic medicine, 318
Manual circumlaryngeal techniques, voice therapy, 1051–1052
Marfan syndrome, 1638
Marketing, clinic management, 3339–3340
Marshall syndrome, 754
Mask interface, 2179
Massage therapy, 319
Mast cells, allergic rhinitis, 399
Mastoid
embryology of, 2384–2385
history, 2447, 2448t
neoplasms of, 2370–2376
obliteration of, 2455–2456
surgery of, 2447–2463
complication of, 2461–2463, 2461t
facial nerve monitoring during, 2328
Mastoidectomy
complete, 2451–2453, 2451f–2453f
incisions of, 2447–2450, 2448f, 2449f
indications for, 2448t
intact canal (open) versus canal-wall-down (closed), 2453–2454, 2454t
radical, 2454
Bondy procedure for, 2455
modified, 2454–2455, 2455f
simple, 2450–2451, 2451f
surface landmarks for, 2450, 2450f, 2451f
technique of, 2447–2455
Mastoiditis, 2401
Maternally inherited diabetes and deafness syndrome, hearing loss in, 1552
Maxilla, 9, 10f. See also Jaw
Maxillary sinus. See also Sinus(es)
anatomy of, 8, 8f, 362
Caldwell-Luc procedure, 604
complications, 605, 607t
endoscopic sinus surgery
antrostomy, 598
middle turbinate, 596
minimally invasive maxillary technique, 597f
uncinate process, 596, 596f
indications, 604, 605t
operative technique, 604–605, 606f
Maxillectomy
inferior, 2056f
medial, 2046, 2051f
total, 2050, 2054f–2055f
Maxillofacial trauma, temporomandibular joint, 785
Maxillomandibular advancement, 2214, 2215f, 2216
Maximal interincisal opening, 1196
Maximal voluntary ventilation test, 38
Mayo scissors, 22
Measles, 1529
Meatoplasty, 2456, 2457f, 2465
Mechanical ventilation
discontinuation of, 60–61, 61f
modes of
airway pressure release ventilation, 60
high frequency oscillation, 60
pressure control ventilation, 60
pressure regulated volume control, 60
pressure support ventilation, 60

proportional assist ventilation, 60
synchronized intermittent mechanical ventilation, 59–60
volume control, 59
tracheostomy
percutaneous versus open tracheostomy, 62
timing of, 61–62
ventilator dysynchrony, 59
Mederma, scar camouflage, 2869
Medial orbital decompression, 631, 631f
Median rhomboid glossitis, 740–741, 740t, 741f
Mediastinal adenoma, hyperparathyroidism, 2141, 2142f
Mediastinitis, 779–780, 805
Medical error
agencies and organizations, 3263
drug-drug interaction, 3261
history of
accountability, 3260
anesthesia, 3258
anesthesia patient safety foundation, 3258
aviation safety reporting system, 3258
institute of medicine report, 3258
just culture, 3259–3260
measurement of, 3260
safety and quality, 3259
systems science, 3259, 3259t
in otolaryngology
classification of, 3262, 3262t
concentrated medications, 3262
epinephrine injections, 3262, 3262t
otolaryngologist responses, 3264
patient identification errors, 3261
public disclosure, 3260
reporting systems
recommendations to, 3261, 3261t
rules for, 3261, 3261t
sense of fatalism, 3261
voluntary reporting, 3261
responding to, 3263
Medical errors, 1678
Medical liability
claims in the United States, 3271–3272
health care costs
defensive medicine, 3280–3281
insurance premiums, 3280
risk management, 3281–3282
medical malpractice litigation
expert witnesses, 3274–3275
general legal background, 3272–3273
Hobson's choice, 3275
presuit, 3273
settlement versus trial, 3275
suit filed, 3273–3274
trials, 3275–3276
tort reform, 3278–3279
Medical records
physician's needs
appropriate productivity, 3310
compliance, 3310
data integrity, 3310
efficiency, 3310
evaluation and management services, 3313–3315

established outpatient visit, 3315, 3318f
initial outpatient visit, 3315, 3316f, 3317f
nature of presenting problems, 3314
quality care, effective medical records, 3314
resource-based relative value system, 3313
work for clinicians, 3314
operative procedures
fiberoptic laryngoscopy and diagnostic nasal endoscopy, 3312, 3312f, 3313f
sample operative report, 3311, 3311f
promoting quality patient care, 3310
teaching hospitals, 3315, 3318
usability, 3310
toolkit for
choice of interface, 3305–3306
data entry, 3307–3308
preloaded information, 3306–3307
Medicare/medicaid services, 3376
Medication overuse headache, 309–310
Medullary thyroid carcinoma
extent of surgery, 2128
genetics of, 2127
postoperative follow-up, 2128
preoperative workup, 2127
Melanocytic lesions, multiple syndromes with, 3212, 3214t
Melanocytic nevi, 3218, 3227
MELAS syndrome, in hearing loss, 1551–1552
Melkersson-Rosenthal syndrome, 1629–1630, 1629f
Melnick-Fraser syndrome, 124, 1611–1612, 1611t, 1623–1624, 1624f
Melolabial flap, in cutaneous nasal defects, 2881, 2883f, 2884
Memory, suture material selection, 22
Mendelian genetics
autosomal dominant inheritance, 115, 116f
autosomal recessive inheritance, 115–117, 117f
basic terminology, 115t
penetrance and expressivity, 119
sex-linked inheritance, 117–118, 118f
Mendelsohn maneuver, 842, 843f
Ménière syndrome
clinical features, 2702, 2702t
endolymphatic hydrops, 2702
physiologic tests, 2703–2704
prevalence, 2702
signs and symptoms, 2701–2702
treatment, 2704
Meningioma
clinical presentation, 2575
diagnosis, 2379
diagnostic evaluation, 2575–2576, 2576f
epidemiology, 2575
etiology of, 2379
histopathology, 2575
incidence of, 2378–2379
molecular biology, 2575

Meningioma (*Continued*)
orbital, 2069, 2070*f*
temporal bone, 2380
treatment of, 2380, 2576–2577
Meningitis, 582–583
clinician evaluation, 2404–2405
cochlear implants, 2636–2637
treatment of
dexamethasone, 2405
direct disease extension, 2405
myringotomy, 2405
Mentalis strain, chin augmentation, 3176, 3177*f*
Mentocervical angle
assessment of, for plastic surgery of face, 2767–2768
Mentoplasty implants, 2793–2794
Meperidine, 44, 45, 64
Mepivacaine, 236
Merkel cell carcinoma, 2370
American Joint Committee on Cancer classification, 1736, 1737*t*
H & E staining of, 1736, 1736*f*
incidence of, 1735
MeroGel (bioresorbable nasal dressing), 1461, 1461*f*
Mesenchymal tumors
diagnosis and management, 1472*t*, 1473*t*
epithelial neoplasms, 1472–1475
hemangiomas, 1470–1471
lymphatic vascular malformations, 1471
orbital tumor, 2072–2074, 2073*f*
rhabdomyosarcoma, 1471–1472
Metabolic disorders
otologic manifestations, 2527
Metabolic imbalances, 42
Metallic implants, 2785–2786
Metastases
cerebellopontine angle, 2578–2579, 2579*f*
from lip cancer, 1790, 1793
occult, 1839–1840, 1840*t*
from salivary gland tumors, 1762
Metastatic melanoma, 173, 173*f*
Metastatic tumors, 1997
neoplasms, 2049
orbital, 2075
Methicillin-resistant *Staphylococcus aureus*, 134
Methimazole, 32
Methylprednisolone, 33
Metoprolol, 35
Metronidazole, 40
Metzenbaum scissors, 22
Microdebrider-assisted inferior turbinate reduction, 618, 618*f*
Microfibrillar collagen products, 52
Microflap surgery, 1076
Microgenia, chin augmentation, 3177*f*, 3181
Micromotion, implant, 2795–2796
Microscopic polyangiitis, 277
Microsomia, hemifacial, 1627
Microsurgery, vestibular schwannoma, 2563–2565, 2564*f*, 2565*f*
Microtia, otoplasty, 3146, 3146*f*

Microvascular decompression
subjective nonpulsatile tinnitus, 2603–2604
Microvascular free tissue harvest, 50
Microvascular reconstruction approaches, midface, 2845–2846
Midazolam, 65, 65*t*, 241
Midbrain syndromes, 202–203, 204*f*
Middle ear implants
biological aspect of, 2644
complications of, 2647
current device technology, 2643*f*, 2644–2645, 2644*f*
direct cochlear fluid stimulation, 2643–2644, 2644*f*
direct ossicular or cochlear stimulation, 2642–2643
indications, 2645–2646, 2645*f*
ossicular attachment, 2643, 2643*f*
outcomes of, 2647
overview of, 2641–2642
patients history, 2642
postimplantation and fitting, 2646–2647
surgery, 2646
Middle ear myoclonus, 2611
Middle facial zone
functional and aesthetic issues, 2910
reanimation
first-stage cross-face nerve grafting, 2914
free muscle transfer, 2913, 2914, 2916–2917
lower facial zone, 2917
nasolabial fold, 2911
nose, 2911, 2914*f*
oral commissure and smile, 2911–2912, 2915*f*
temporalis transfer, 2912–2913
Midface
assessment of, for plastic surgery of face, 2766–2767
augmentation of, implants for, 2792–2793, 2792*f*
defects of, microvascular reconstructive approaches to, 2845–2846
fracture, 1280
anatomy
buttresses, 1209, 1210*f*
maxilla, 1209
zygoma, 1209–1210, 1210*f*
complications
eye/eyelid/orbital, 1221
implant, 1221–1222
lip distortion, 1221
malocclusion, 1222
sensory disturbance, 1222
temporal hollowing, 1222
computed tomography, 1210*f*, 1213–1214, 1214*t*
management
extended access approach, 1215
immediate reconstruction, 1214, 1214*t*
maxillomandibular fixation, 1214–1215
stable internal fixation, 1215

zygomaticomaxillary complex. *See* Zygomaticomaxillary complex
pathophysiology
maxilla, 1210–1211, 1211*f*, 1219*f*
zygoma, 1211–1212, 1211*f*–1212*f*
patient evaluation
facial assessment, 1213
ophthalmologic exam, 1213
physical exam, 1212–1213
technical adjuvant
computer-aided surgery, 1222
intraoperative CT scanning, 1222–1223
Midfacial degloving approach, 2088
Midforehead lift, 3058*f*, 3064–3065
Midline labiomandibular glossotomy, 1908, 1909*f*
Midline osteotomy genioglossus advancement, 2231–2232, 2232*f*
Midline posterior glossectomy, 2232, 2232*f*
Migraine
auditory symptoms, 207
clinical symptoms, 205
diagnosis and classification, 205, 206*t*
etiology, 207
management, 207–208, 208*f*
neurologic symptoms, 207
vertigo manifestations, 205–206
vestibular symptoms, 206–207
Migraine disorders, vestibular and balance laboratory study, 2302
Migraine-associated vestibulopathy, 2728
Migrainous vertigo
clinical features, 2704
pathophysiologic mechanisms, 2704–2705
treatment, 2705
Milia, 3212, 3215
lower eyelid blepharoplasty, 3101
treatment of, 3226
Miller Fisher syndrome, 1040
Miller syndrome, 1638
Mind-body medicine, 317–318
Mini split-thickness skin graft, 2473
Minimally invasive endoscopic resection, 670
Minimally invasive video-assisted thyroidectomy, 2123
Mini-trephination, 683
Minor intrinsic laryngeal cartilages, professional voice, 1061
Mitochondrial genomic deletions, 125
Mitomycin C, 1150
Mixed connective tissue disease, 275
Mixed hearing loss, 2640. *See also* Hearing loss
Möbius syndrome, 1638–1639
Modified barium swallow, 165
Mohs surgery
for lip cancer, 1793, 1795*f*
for skin cancer, 1731
Molluscum contagiosum, 3220, 3220*f*
treatment of, 3228
Mondini malformation, 1534
Monofilament suture, 22
Mononeuropathy, 1038

Moraxella catarrhalis, 1354
   pediatric rhinosinusitis and, 1458, 1458*t*
Morphine, 45, 45*t*, 64, 241
Mosaic cartilage tympanoplasty, 2480, 2482*f*
Motion sickness, 206
Motor nerve, injury to, during forehead lift, 3070
Motor neuron disorders
   amyotrophic lateral sclerosis, 1037
   poliomyelitis, 1038
   progressive bulbar palsy, 1037–1038
   spinal muscular atrophy, 1038
Mucoepidermoid carcinoma, 193*f*
   salivary gland, 1764–1765, 1764*f*, 1782
Mucolytics, chronic rhinosinusitis, 591–592
Mucopolysaccharidoses
   otologic manifestations, 2527
Mucosal edema, 2401
Mucous membrane pemphigoid, 744–745, 744*f*
Mulliken method, single-stage bilateral nasolabial cleft repair, 1564, 1564*f*
Multidisciplinary team approach
   components of, 1676, 1676*t*
   efficacy of, 1676–1677
   presentations, 1676, 1677*f*
Multiple endocrine neoplasia syndromes, 262–263, 263*t*
Multiple mucosal melanoma syndrome, 1639
Multiple sclerosis
   Arnold-Chiari syndrome, 2729
   ataxia syndromes, 2729
   examination findings, 2728–2729
   neurologic disorder, 1036–1037, 1036*f*
   neurotologic signs and symptoms, 2728
   thiamine deficiency, 2729–2730
Multiple systems atrophy, 1031–1032
Mumps, 703–704, 1529
   otologic manifestations, 2520
   sialadenitis, 1468
Munchausen syndrome
   aerodigestive tract, 1407
Muscle(s)
   face, 3239, 3240*f*
   of forehead, 3054, 3055*f*
   of nose, 2924, 2924*t*
Muscle tension dysphonia, voice therapy, 1055
Muscular dystrophies, 1042
Myasthenia gravis, 211–212, 1040–1041
   perioperative management, 42–43
Myasthenic syndrome, 1041
Mycobacterial infection, 979–980
Mycobacterial lymphadenitis, 1595
Mycoses, pharyngitis in, 766
Myelinopathy, 1038
Myeloid differentiation primary response (MyD88)-dependent signaling, 380, 380*f*
Myiasis, 291
Myopathic disorders, 1042
Myopathies, 1042
Myopia, 221

Myotonic dystrophy, 1042
Myringotomy, 2405
Myxedema coma, 258

N
Nager acrofacial dysostosis syndrome, 1639
Naloxone, 242
Naltrexone, tobacco cessation, 335
Narcotic agonists and antagonists, 241–242
Nasal airway resistance, 365
Nasal and palatal surgery. *See* Sleep apnea
Nasal and paranasal sinuses
   autoimmune disease
      Churg-Strauss syndrome, 495–496, 496*f*
      relapsing polychondritis, 494–495, 495*f*
      Sjogren syndrome, 496, 497*f*
      Wegener granulomatosis, 493–494, 494*t*
   congenital/genetic disorder
      cystic fibrosis, 489–490, 490*t*
      lymphoma, 490–491
   granulomatous. *See* Sarcoidosis
   hematologic disorders
      coagulation disorders, 498–499
      hereditary hemorrhagic telangiectasia, 497–498
      thrombocytopenia, 498
Nasal base
   stabilizing of, in nasal tip surgery, 2965*f*, 2969–2971, 2969*f*, 2970*f*
   structures of, 2932–2933
Nasal cavity, anatomy of, 7–8, 7*f*
Nasal dorsum
   anatomy
      aesthetic subunits, 2952, 2953*f*
      nasal bones and upper lateral cartilages, 2952–2953, 2954*f*
      nasion, alar groove, 2952, 2953*f*
      skin and subcutaneous tissue, 2952
   bony vaults
      anatomy, 2953
      defects of, 2956, 2956*t*
      management of, 2956*t*, 2959–2962, 2959*f*–2962*f*
   cartilaginous vaults
      anatomy, 2953
      defects of, 2956–2957
      management of, 2957–2958, 2958*f*, 2959*f*
   nasal analysis
      aesthetic angles, 2954
      brow-tip aesthetic line, 2955, 2956*f*
      chin-down view, 2954, 2955*f*
      dorsal projection, 2955–2956, 2956*f*
      nasal length, 2954, 2955*f*
Nasal fracture, 1277
   anatomy, 1241–1242, 1242*f*
   in children, 1250–1251
   complications, 1252–1253, 1252*t*
   diagnosis
      history, 1245–1246
      imaging, 1247
      physical examination, 1246, 1246*f*

   management of
      classification, 1248–1249, 1249*f*
      closed reduction, 1248–1249
      general anesthesia, 1247
      goal of, 1247–1248
      ice pack, 1247
      open reduction, 1248, 1250, 1250*f*
      primary septal repair, 1250
      septum, 1248
   pathophysiology
      bilateral displaced fracture, 1242, 1243*f*
      bony nasal cap, 1243, 1244*f*
      curvature illusion, 1242, 1243*f*
      impact force, 1242
      nasal pyramid and obstruction, 1242, 1244*f*
      naso-orbital-ethmoid complex, 1243
      septum fracture, 1244, 1245*f*
      unilateral depressed fracture, 1242–1243, 1243*f*
   technique, 1251–1252, 1251*f*–1252*f*
Nasal obstruction, 2193
   anatomic causes of, 363–365
   clinical history, 612
   clinical investigations, 613
   Cottle maneuver, 619, 619*f*
   differential diagnosis, 613, 613*t*
   external and internal nasal valves, 619, 619*f*
   imaging, 613
   nasolacrimal duct cyst, 1330, 1330*f*
   operative procedures
      cartilaginous grafts, 619–620
      Park suture placement, 620, 620*f*
      spreader grafts, 619, 620*f*
   physical examination, 612–613
   septoplasty. *See* Septoplasty
   treatment options, 613–614, 614*t*
   turbinate reduction. *See* Inferior turbinate hypertrophy
Nasal polyps
   allergy, 530–531
   aspirin exacerbated respiratory disease, 531–532
   asthma, 531
   clinical presentation
      anterior rhinoscopy, 526–527, 526*f*–527*f*
      histopathologic examination, 526
      imaging studies, 527–528, 528*f*
      nasal endoscopy, 527, 527*f*
      sinonasal symptoms, 526
   cystic fibrosis, 532
   differential diagnosis, 526*t*
   epidemiology
      age, 526
      autopsy study report, 525
      ethnic and geographic differences, 525–526
      genetic predisposition, 526
      questionnaire and survey studies, 525
   etiology, 530
   fungi, 531
   histopathology, 529–530, 529*f*
   natural history of, 529
   severity classification in, 528

Nasal septum
    anatomy of, 363, 363f, 2933
    deviated
        causes, 614
        septoplasty. See Septoplasty
        submucous resection, 614
    role of, 2934
Nasal surgery
    breathing and impact on sleep
        airflow, 2193
        nasal obstruction, 2193
        polysomnogram, 2194, 2194t
        sleep disturbance, 2194
        Starling resistor, 2193–2194
    nasal resistance, 2192–2193
    nasal turbinates, 2194–2195
    patients evaluation, 2193
    symptoms of, 2192–2193
Nasal tip
    anatomy of, 2964–2969, 2965f–2968f
    devastated
        central tip support
            alter tip location, 3014, 3014f
            case studies, 3018
            caudal excess nasal deformity, 3017
            collapsed/displaced alar cartilages,
                3016, 3017f–3018f
            overresected nose, 3014–3015
            septal extension graft. See septal
                extension graft
            sidewall tensioning, 3017f–3018f,
                3018–3019
        lateral tip support
            alar rim graft, 3020–3021, 3020f
            alter tip location, 3016f, 3019
            composite graft, 3020
            lateral crural strut graft, 3019–3021,
                3020f
            severe scar contracture, 2992f,
                3019–3020
            sidewall tensioning, 3021
            structural grafting, 3019
    ideal contour of, 2964, 2966f
    position of, 2923f
    projection, assessment of, for plastic sur-
            gery of face
        Goode's method, 2765–2766, 2765f
        Powell and Humphries method, 2765,
            2765f
        Simons's method, 2765
        versus tip rotation, 2765, 2765f
    support of, 2935–2936
        Tardy classification of, 2935
        tripod concept of, 2935
    surgery of, 2964–2976
        analysis and diagnosis for,
            2964–2969, 2965f–2968f
        modification of tip in, 2971–2976,
            2971f–2976f
        preoperative planning for, 2969
        stabilizing nasal base in, 2965f,
            2969–2971, 2969f, 2970f
        techniques for, 2969–2976
Nasal valve
    anatomy of, 363, 363f
    collapse of, nasal obstruction in, 364
Nasal wall, lateral, anatomy of, 359–360

Nasal-tip incisions, 2943, 2945f
Nasoalveolar molding, 1562
Nasofacial angle, 2765
Nasofrontal angle, 2762, 2763f
Nasogastric tube, 62–63, 62f
Nasolabial angle, 2765
Nasolacrimal duct cyst, nasal obstruction,
        1330, 1330f
Nasoorbitoethmoid fracture, 1277,
        1281–1282, 1282f
Nasopalatine duct cyst, 2100
Nasopharyngeal anatomy, 12f, 13
Nasopharyngeal carcinoma, 191f, 1603
    chemotherapy, 1698–1699
    clinical presentations of, 1876–1878
    computed tomography, 141, 142f
    diagnosis of, 1878, 1883, 1888
        imaging studies in, 1878–1883, 1888
    histologic classification of, 1876
    histopathology of, 1875–1876
    nonkeratinizing, 1876, 1876f
    oncogenic factors, 1875
    persistent or recurrent, management of,
        1888–1893
    recurrent management of, 1888–1893,
        1891f, 1892f, 1893f
    squamous cell, 1875
    staging of, 1878, 1883–1886, 1887t
    treatment in
        chemotherapy, 1887–1888, 1893
        radiotherapy, 1876, 1879, 1886–1887,
            1889, 1893
    undifferentiated, 1875, 1876, 1876f,
        1887t
Nasopharyngeal obstruction
    pathophysiology, 1306, 1308f
    postnatal diagnosis, 1311–1312, 1312f
    prenatal diagnosis, 1309, 1309f–1310f
    treatment, 1316–1318, 1317f–1318f
Nasopharyngectomy, in recurrent naso-
        pharyngeal cancer, 1889–1893,
        1893f
National Comprehensive Cancer Network
        guidelines, malignant melanoma,
        1744
National quality forum, 3376
Natural products, 317
Naturopathic medicine, 320–321
Naugle exophthalmometer, 1230
Near-total laryngectomy, 1972
Neck
    aging
        anatomy, 3131–3133, 3132f, 3133f
        classification and evaluation, 3133,
            3134f, 3135, 3135f
        complications and management,
            3139–3140
        treatment
            ptotic submandibular glands, 3137
            retrognathia, 3137
            rhytidectomy, 3136
            submental liposuction and ante-
                rior platysmaplasty, 3137–3138,
                3138f, 3139f
            targeted surgical treatment plan,
                3135, 3135t
            tumescent technique, 3136

anatomy of
    arterial supply, 15, 15f
    cervical triangles, 13–14, 14f
    inferior portion, 14, 15f
    lateral portion, 15
    lymphatic system, 16
    venous supply, 16, 16f
    visceral structures, 16–17, 16f
assessment of, for plastic surgery of face,
        2767–2768
deep spaces of
    classification, 796–797, 797t
    entire neck, 797–799, 797f, 798f
    fascial organization
        classification, 794, 795t
        deep cervical fascia, 796
        midsagittal visualization, 794, 795f
        superficial cervical fascia, 795
    hyoid bone
        anterior visceral space, 800
        masticator space, 800
        parapharyngeal space, 799, 799f
        parotid space, 800
        peritonsillar space, 800
        submandibular and sublingual
            spaces, 799–800
        suprasternal space, 800
        temporal space, 800
    infections of
        bacteriology of, 800–801
        complications, 804–805, 805f
        danger spaces, 806–807, 808f
        diagnosis, 801–803, 801f
        etiology, 794
        management, 803–804, 804f
        masticator space, 810
        mediastinitis, 805
        necrotizing cervical fasciitis,
            805–806
        parapharyngeal space, 809–810,
            809f
        parotid space, 810
        prevertebral spaces, 806–807
        retropharyngeal spaces, 806–807,
            807f
        submandibular space and ludwig
            angina, 807–809, 808f, 809f
implants for, 2794–2795
injury
    penetrating
        anatomy, 1135, 1135f
        clinical signs and symptoms, 1136,
            1136t
        complications, 1139
        laryngotracheal, 1139
        management algorithm, 1136, 1137f
        pharynx and esophagus, 1139
        vascular evaluation, 1138–1139
        zone I, 1137–1138
        zone II, 1138
        zone III, 1138
    secondary survey of trauma,
        1101–1102, 1101f
larynx cancer treatment, 1973, 1974t
Neck dissection
    adjuvant therapy with, 1827
    air leaks after, 1830–1831

anatomy of
  anterior, 1807–1811
  fascial compartment, 1810
  lymphatics, 1810–1812, 1811f
  marginal mandibular branch of facial nerve, 1807–1808
  nerve to levator scapulae, 1809
  platysma muscle, 1807
  spinal accessory nerve, 1808–1809
  thoracic duct, 1809–1810
  vasculature, 1807, 1808f
apnea after, 1832
biopsy for
  fine-needle aspiration, 1813, 1814
  sentinel node, 1814–1815
bleeding in, 1831, 1833, 1834
blindness after, 1832
carotid artery rupture after, 1832–1834
central compartment, 1820, 1823
chylous fistula after, 1831–1832
classification of, 1810, 1815–1826, 1816t
complications of, 1807, 1814, 1830–1834
current controversies in, 1827–1830
diagnostic evaluation for, 1812–1815, 1826
extended supraomohyoid, 1819, 1822
extent of, 1807, 1815, 1817, 1820, 1826, 1827, 1829, 1830, 1832
facial/cerebral edema after, 1832
imaging studies for, 1811–1813, 1824, 1833
incisions in, 1807, 1809, 1832
indications for
  rationale for, 1820–1822
infection after, 1830, 1831
jugular vein
  blow-out after, 1834
  thrombosis after, 1832
lateral, 120, 1807–1812, 1816, 1817, 1819, 1820f, 1823–1825, 1830, 1832
paratracheal, 1811, 1812, 1820, 1824, 1825
physiology of, 1812
planned, after organ-preservation surgery, 1828–1830
posterolateral, 1807, 1820, 1821f
radiation therapy after, 1812, 1822–1824, 1827–1829, 1832, 1833
radical, 1809, 1815–1817, 1816f, 1816t, 1818–1820, 1822, 1829
retropharyngeal, 1811, 1812, 1814, 1824–1825
selective
  extended, 1815, 1816t, 1819, 1822, 1824
  indications for, 1822, 1823, 1829
  rationale for, 1820–1822
  sequelae of, 1830, 1834
  types of, 1819, 1822, 1823, 1829
staging and, 1814, 1815, 1822
upper mediastinal, 1814, 1824, 1825
Necrotizing cervical fasciitis, 805–806, 806f
Necrotizing sialometaplasia, 281, 713
  versus minor salivary gland tumor, 1770
Needle thoracentesis, 1098f

Neisseria gonorrhea infection, 1433
  pharyngitis in, 765
Neonatal intensive care unit, 1508
Neonatal respiratory distress
  anatomy and physiology, 1328
  evaluation and treatment of, 1328–1330, 1329f
  fetal assessment, 1335–1336, 1335f
  larynx
    flexible endoscopic evaluation of swallowing, 1332–1333
    laryngeal atresia, 1333, 1333f
    laryngomalacia, 1332, 1332f
    subglottic hemangioma, 1334, 1334f
  nasal obstruction, 1330–1331, 1330f–1331f
  oral cavity/oropharynx/hypopharynx, 1331–1332
  trachea/bronchi, 1334–1335, 1335f
Neoplasms
  of cell-specific origin, 2358–2365
  ear and lateral skull base, 2358–2382, 2359t, 2360f
  head and neck masses
    benign neoplasms, 1600–1601
    malignant neoplasm, 1601–1603
  of the internal auditory canal and cerebellopontine angle, 2376–2381
  of nose and paranasal sinuses, 2044–2062
  of pinna and external auditory canal, 2365–2370
Neural discontinuity
  auricular nerve, 2906, 2906f
  donor nerves, 2906, 2906f
  sural nerve, 2906, 2906f
Neural stimulators, 2624
Neural tumors, 1600
  orbital, 2068–2069, 2070f
Neurilemmoma, 2069
Neuroblastoma, 1602–1603
Neurodegenerative diseases, 374
Neurofibromas
  facial, 3218
  treatment of, 3227
Neurofibromatosis
  in hearing loss, 1548–1549
  type-1, 1630, 1631f
  type 2, 1630
Neurogenic sarcomas, 2048
Neurogenic shock, 1099
Neurohypophysis, 257
Neurologic disorder
  larynx
    ataxic disorders, 1034
    bulbar palsy, 1037
    diagnosis and treatment, 1029–1030, 1029t
    electromyography
      applications, 1044–1045, 1045f
      needle electromyography, 1043–1044
      technique of, 1043–1044, 1043f, 1044f
    hoarseness, 1026
    human vocal process, 1026, 1027f
    hyperkinetic disorders, 1032–1034

    hypokinetic disorders, 1030–1032, 1031f, 1032t
    laryngeal presentation, 1045t
    mixed disorders, 1034–1037
    motor neuron disorders, 1037–1038
    myopathic disorders, 1042
    neuromuscular junction, 1040–1042
    peripheral neuropathies, 1038–1040, 1039f, 1040f
    postpolio syndrome, 1038
    spastic disorder, 1030
  midface fracture, 1213
Neurology
  autoimmune neurologic diseases
    myasthenia gravis, 211–212
    Susac syndrome, 212–213, 213f
  cerebrovascular disease. See Cerebrovascular disease
  Chiari malformations, 214, 214f
  cranial nerve anatomy and function, 199, 200f, 201f, 202t
  and internal medicine workup, bilateral vocal fold immobility, 1019
  migraine
    auditory symptoms, 207
    clinical symptoms, 205
    diagnosis and classification, 205, 206t
    etiology, 207
    management, 207–208, 208f
    neurologic symptoms, 207
    vertigo manifestations, 205–206
    vestibular symptoms, 206–207
  neoplasms
    brainstem, 213–214
    cerebellar, 214
    vestibular schwannomas, 213, 213f
  neuromuscular disorders
    amyotrophic lateral sclerosis, 208–209, 209t
    Guillain-Barré syndrome, 210
    multiple sclerosis, 210–211
    pseudobulbar palsy, 209–210
  normal-pressure hydrocephalus, 214
Neuromonics, 2603
Neuromuscular blocking agents, 242–244, 242t
Neuropathic pain, 312, 348, 350
Neurophysiologic monitor, ideal, characteristics of, 2315t
Neuropsychiatric problems, postoperative management of, 41–43
Nevoid basal cell carcinoma syndrome, 2102
Nevus
  basal cell, 2102
  blue, 3219, 3220f
    treatment of, 3228
  compound, 3218, 3219f
  dermal, 3218, 3218f
  Jadassohn, 3216, 3216f
  junctional, 3218, 3218f
  melanocytic, 3218, 3227
    treatment of, 3227
  of Ota, 3219, 3219f
    treatment of, 3226
Nevus sebaceus, 3216, 3216f
  treatment of, 3226

Newborn nasal deformity, 1277
Nicardipine, 35
Nicotine replacement therapy, 333
Nitroprusside, 35, 36t, 39
NO neck
  management of
    biopsy in
      sentinel lymph node biopsy,
        1844–1845
      ultrasound-guided fine needle aspiration, 1841
    controversies in, 1843–1844
    elective neck dissection, 1842–1843
    elective neck irradiation, 1843
    future directions in, 1844–1845
    lateral and anterior-posterior lymphoscintigraphy, 1845, 1845f
    occult metastases, 1839–1840, 1840t
      impact of, 1840
      incidence of, 1839–1840, 1840t
      risk factors for, 1842, 1842t
    overview of, 1839–1846
    pathologic predictors of, 1846
    radiographic imaging
      computed tomography,
        1840–1841
      magnetic resonance imaging,
        1840–1841
      positron emission tomography,
        1841
    oral cavity cancer
      lip cancer, 1866
      mandibular involvement, 1866
    pathologic predictors of, 1846
Nocardia infection, 287f, 288
Nodular melanoma, 1741
Noise-induced hearing loss
  acoustic trauma, 2532
  compensation and, 2537
  diagnosis of, 2536, 2536t
  epidemiology of
    damage risk criteria, 2534–2535,
      2535f
    industrial noise exposure, 2534,
      2534t
    nonoccupational exposures,
      2535–2536
  management of
    clinical presentation, 2538–2539
    hearing conservation, 2537–2538,
      2538t
  nonauditory effects of, 2539
  pathogenesis of
    age-related hearing changes, 2531f,
      2532–2533
    drugs and chemicals, 2533–2534
    otoacoustic emissions, 2534
    pathology, 2532, 2532f, 2533f
    pathophysiology, 2534
    pure-tone threshold shifts,
      2530–2531, 2531f
    vibration interaction, 2532
  prevention of, 2539
Noise-induced permanent threshold shift,
  2530–2532, 2534–2536
Nonablative resurfacing lasers, 2867
Nonabsorbable suture material, 22

Nonallergic rhinitis
  aging, 485
  atrophic rhinitis, 482–484
  autonomic rhinitis, 482
  classification, 470
  drug-induced rhinitis
    aspirin exacerbated respiratory disease,
      477–479
    rhinitis medicamentosa, 477t,
      479–480, 479f
    systemic anti-hypertensive medications, 475, 476t, 477
  eosinophilia syndrome, 473
  epidemiology and social impact,
    469–470
  hormone-induced rhinitis, 480–481,
    481t
  idiopathic rhinitis
    anterior rhinoscopy and endoscopy,
      471
    cold dry air provocation test, 471
    CT scan, 471
    etiology, 470
    nasal symptoms, 471, 471t
    pharmacologic therapy, 471–472
    smoking history, 471
    surgical options, 472–473
  occupational rhinitis
    causes of, 474
    diagnosis of, 475
    immunologic testing, 475
    nasal provocation, 475
    prevalence of, 474, 474t
    risk factors, 474–475
    treatment, 475
  physiology, 470
  systemic causes of, 484, 484t
Nonarteritic ischemic optic neuropathy, 233
Non-HIV-related lymphoepithelial
  cysts, 704
Non-Hodgkin lymphomas
  aggressive, 2036–2037
  indolent, 2036
Non-mendelian genetics
  additional epigenetic influences, 121
  chromosomal anomalies, 122–123
  complex genetics, 122
  digenic inheritance, 121–122
  genomic imprinting, 119–121
  mitochondrial inheritance and mutations, 119
Nonsurgical organ preservation therapy,
  160–161, 161f
Nontuberculous mycobacterial infections,
  286, 704
Noonan syndrome, 1639
Norepinephrine, 59
Normal-pressure hydrocephalus, 214
Norrie disease, in hearing loss, 1543t, 1550
Nose, 2919–2939
  acquired immune response in, 368–369
  aesthetic subunits of, 2874, 2874f
  alar lobule and nasal sidewall of, 2873
  anatomy
    surface, 2919, 2920f, 2921, 2921f
    subunits of, 2919, 2921

  topography and, 2921–2924
  surgical, 2919–2939
  valvular, 2937–2938
  anatomy of, 2872–2873
  areas of structural void, 2936–2937
  assessment of, for plastic surgery of face,
    2764–2765
  blood supply to, 2872–2873, 2924–2925
  bony piriform platform surrounding,
    2873
  cantilever concept of, 2934
  congenital anomalies
    clinical and pathologic features
      congenital nasal mass, 1451, 1452t
      nasoethmoidal, 1449, 1450
      nasofrontal, 1449, 1451f
      nasoorbital, 1449, 1450f
      occipital encephaloceles, 1451
      sinus tract, 1447, 1449f
    embryology
      dermoid, 1446–1447, 1447f
      encephalocele, 1447, 1448f
      fonticulus nasofrontalis, 1445,
        1447f
      foramen cecum, 1445, 1447f
      glioma, 1447
      nasal capsule, 1445, 1447f
      neural tube formation, 1445,
        1446f
      prenasal space, 1445, 1447f
    evaluation, 1451, 1452f
    surgical treatment
      craniotomy, 1454
      CSF rhinorrhea, 1454
      rhinoplasty incision, 1452, 1453f
      vertical midline incision, 1452, 1453f
  defects of
    analysis of, 2873–2875, 2874f, 2874t
    etiology of, 2872
    large
      forehead flap in, 2885–2886, 2885t,
        2886f–2892f, 2888–2889
      preoperative considerations in,
        2884
    small
      bilobed flap in, 2877, 2879–2880,
        2882f
      grafts and flaps for, 2875–2876,
        2876t
      melolabial flap in, 2881,
        2883f–2884f, 2884
      primary closure of, 2877, 2879f,
        2880f, 2881f
      reconstructive options for, 2876t
      Reiger flap in, 2880
      rhomboid flap in, 2877
      second intention healing in, 2876
      skin and composite grafts in, 2877,
        2877t, 2878f
  dorsal, reconstruction of, with composite septal flap, 2895
  ethnic variations in, 2938–2939
  external, anatomy of, 7, 7f
  external nasal skin, 2872
  function of, maintenance of, following
    nasal restoration with flaps and
    grafts, 2991

grafting of
for form, 2891, 2894f, 2984
techniques of, 2894–2895, 2896f, 2897f
inner lining of, 2925
intermediate crus of, 2930–2931, 2931f
internal lining defects of, repair of
cutaneous epithelium for, 2898, 2900, 2901f
full-thickness skin grafts for, 2895, 2898, 2899f
intranasal tissue for, 2900, 2902–2903
pericranial flap for, 2903
intranasal mucosa, 2873
lateral crus of, 2931–2932, 2931f
ligamentous attachments of, 2934–2935
lower cartilaginous vault of, 2929–2930
mechanics and stability of, 2933–2937
medial crus of, 2930
musculature of, 2872
nasal tip surgery. See Nasal tip
neoplasms, 2044–2062
nerve supply to, 2925
osseous vault of, 2927–2928
physiology of, 365–369
protection of, 367–369
reconstruction of
with flaps and grafts, 2871–2903
history of, 2871–2872
rhinoplasty. See Rhinoplasty
sensory nerve supply of, 2873
skeletal framework of, 2925–2932
skin-soft tissue envelope of, 2924–2925
soft tissue injuries, 1119–1120
soft tissue of, 2872
structural framework of, 2873
structural support and grafting for, 2889, 2891, 2893f, 2894–2895
upper cartilaginous vault of, 2928–2929
vascular anatomy, 503f
external carotid arterial system, 503
internal carotid arterial system, 503, 503f
vascular anastomoses, 504
venous drainage, 503–504
Nosocomial acute bacterial rhinosinusitis, 512
Nosocomial infection, 44
Nuclear medicine, 158
Nuclear scintigraphy, 161
Nutcracker esophagus, 854
Nutrition
lip cancer, 1804
preoperative, 26
Nystagmus
gaze-evoked nystagmus, 2685
hyperventilation-induced, 2698
rotation-induced, 2687
spontaneous, 2684–2685, 2719

O

Obesity, obstructive sleep apnea and, 2206–2207
Obstructive adenoid hyperplasia, 1434

Obstructive sleep apnea. See Sleep apnea, obstructive
Occipital encephaloceles, congenital anomalies, nose, 1451
Occipital neuralgia, 312
Occlusal appliance therapy, temporomandibular joint, 788–789, 789f
Occlusion, dental. See Dental occlusion
Occult lymph node disease detection
elective lymph node dissection, 1745
sentinel lymph node identification, 1745–1748
Occult metastases
impact of, 1840
incidence of, 1839–1840, 1840t
Ocular torsion reaction test, dizziness, 2690
Ocular trauma
blunt trauma, 228
burns, 229
cornea and conjunctiva
blood dyscrasia, 227
contact lens misplacement, 228
corneal abrasion, 228
foreign bodies, 228
subconjunctival hemorrhage, 227–228
eyelid laceration, 227
history and examination, 226–227
orbital trauma, 227
penetrating injuries, 228–229
Oculoauriculovertebral dysplasia, 1552, 1627–1629, 1627f
Oculopalatolaryngopharyngeal myoclonus, 1034
Oculopharyngeal muscular dystrophy, 1042
Odontogenic cysts, 2097–2113
adenomatoid tumor, 2104–2105
calcifying (Gorlin), 2099
dentigerous, 2098–2099, 2098f
glandular, 2099–2100, 2100f
keratocysts, 2101–2102
in nevoid basal cell carcinoma, 2102
periapical, 2097–2098, 2098f
radicular, 2097–2098
Odontogenic infections
buccal space, 773, 773f, 774f
canine space, 773
complications of
cervical necrotizing fasciitis, 779
deep neck space, 779
mediastinitis, 779–780
demographics of, 770
localized, 771, 771f–773f, 772t
ludwig angina, 777–778
mandibular space, 774, 775f, 776–777, 776f
masticator space, 774, 775f
microbiology of, 770
treatment
antibiotics, 779, 780t
dental management, 778
diagnostic imaging of, 778–779
surgical approaches, 778

Odontogenic tumors, 2100–2106
adenomatoid cysts, 2104–2105
ameloblastoma, 2102–2104, 2103f
calcifying epithelial, 2105
myxoma, 2105–2106, 2105f
Pindborg, 2105
Odontomas, 2101
Odors identification of, 371. See also Olfaction
Office-based laryngeal procedure
advantages, 1078
airway and esophageal dilation, 1089
airway evaluation and assessment
anesthesia, 1080–1081
cricoarytenoid joint fixation, 1081
posterior glottic stenosis, 1081
subglottic and tracheal stenosis, 1081
anesthesia
equipment and medications, 1079f
superior laryngeal nerve block, 1080
topical application, 1079, 1080
biopsy, 1081–1082, 1081f, 1082f
laryngeal visualization, 1078
laser procedures
clinical indications, 1088
CO2 laser, 1087–1088
patient and surgeon positioning, 1086–1087, 1087f
potassium titanyl phosphate laser, 1088
pulse dye laser, 1088
thulium laser, 1088
monitoring, 1080
patient selection and preparation, 1078–1079, 1080f
secondary tracheoesophageal puncture, 1089
transnasal esophagoscopy, 1089
vocal fold injection
advantages, 1082
complications, 1086
general anesthesia, 1082
indications, 1082
injection materials, 1086
location and amount, 1083
peroral approach, 1083, 1083f
postprocedure care, 1086
thyrohyoid approach, 1083–1085, 1084f
transcricothyroid membrane approach, 1085–1086, 1085f
treatment, 1082
OK-432, for lymphatic malformations, 1471
Olfaction
anatomy
craniofacial resections, 374
olfactory epithelium, 371
olfactory mucosa, 372, 372f
olfactory neurons, 372
olfactory loss
chronic rhinosinusitis, 373
congenital anosmia, 373–374
dysosmia, 376
electrophysiologic tests, 375
evaluation, 374

Olfaction (*Continued*)
head trauma, 373
imaging studies, 375–376
neurodegenerative diseases, 374
phantosmia, 376
psychophysical tests, 375, 375*f*
sinus surgery complications, 658
treatment, 376–377
upper respiratory infection, 373
physiology of, 366–367, 372–373
Olfactory neuroblastoma, 2047, 2047*t*,
2048*t*
Olfactory-event related potentials, 455
Omentum, microvascular flaps of,
2843–2844, 2843*f*
Oncocytic Schneiderian papilloma, 187*f*
Oncocytoma, salivary gland, 1763–1764,
1763*f*
Ondine curse, 918
Open conservation laryngeal surgery,
1969–1970
near-total laryngectomy, 1972
postlaryngectomy, 1972–1973
supracricoid partial laryngectomy, 1971,
1971*f*
supraglottic laryngectomy, 1970–1971
total laryngectomy, 1972
vertical hemilaryngectomy, 1970
Open mastoid cavity, 2477
Open surgery, temporomandibular joint,
790, 790*f*
Operational adaptability, clinic management, 3334–3335
Operative technologies
dissection/hemostasis, 49–50
operative field visualization, 50–51
robotic resection oro/ hypopharyngeal
lesion, 51–53
Ophthalmologic evaluation
imaging in, 232–233
ocular trauma. *See* Ocular trauma
pediatric ophthalmology, 229–230
red eye. *See* Red eye
in systemic disease
arteriosclerosis, 232
blood dyscrasia, 231
collagen vascular disease, 231
diabetes, 231–232
hypertension, 232
metastatic cancer, 231
neurologic disease, 230–231
ocular side effects, medications, 231
systemic infection, 231
thyroid-associated orbitopathy, 231,
231*f*
vision loss
gradual, 221–222
sudden, 222–223
transient, 223
Ophthalmoscopy, 220–221
Opiates, 64, 65*t*
Opitz (BBB/G syndrome), 1639
Opitz-Frias syndrome, 126
Opitz-G syndrome, 1320
Optic canal meningioma, 2070*f*
Optic nerve
decompression, 635
glioma, 2068–2069

technique, 635–636
Optic neuritis, 223, 223*f*
Optic neuropathy, midface fracture, 1213
Optokinetic nystagmus, 2305
Oral appliances, obstructive sleep apnea,
2182–2183
Oral cancer
alveolar ridge
floor of mouth, 1867–1868
hard palate, 1868–1869
oral tongue, 1868
chemotherapy, 1699–1700
clinical presentation
bleeding, 1857–1858
erythroplakia, 1856*f*, 1857
leukoplakia, 1856–1857, 1856*f*
ulcerative lesion, 1857
complication
acute airway obstruction, 1870
bleeding/hematoma formation, 1870
osteoradionecrosis, 1870
superficial burns, 1869–1870
tooth decay, 1870
diagnosis and evaluation of
alcohol use, 1858
dysarthria, 1858
evaluation under anesthesia, 1861
imaging use, 1858–1860
lymphadenopathy, 1861
physical examination, 1858
pulmonary metastasis, 1860
risk factors for, 1858
staging of, 1860–1861
trismus, 1858
epidemiology, 1854–1855, 1855*t*
etiology of, 1855–1856
future directions in, 1871
management of, N0 neck, 1865–1866
retromolar trigone, 1869
staging and prognosis of, 1862–1863
treatment
chemotherapy, 1864
radiation, 1863–1864
surgery of, 1864
Oral cavity
anatomy
AJCC staging manual, 1849, 1851*f*
atomic structures, 1849, 1850*f*
buccal mucosa, 1854
floor of mouth, 1852, 1853*f*
hard palate, 1853
intrinsic muscles, tongue, 1852,
1854*f*
lower alveolar ridge, 1849
musculature of, 1849, 1851*f*
oral tongue, 1852, 1853*f*
retromolar trigone, 1854
superficial anatomic landmark, 1849,
1850*f*
upper alveolar ridge, 1852–1853
microvascular reconstruction
approaches, 2845
odontogenic, 2097
structures of, anatomy of, 9–12
Oral decongestants, nonallergic rhinitis,
472
Oral dysphagia, 819
Oral leukoplakia, 1646

Oral lichen planus, 751–752, 752*f*
Oral obstruction
pathophysiology, 1306–1307
postnatal diagnosis, 1312–1313, 1312*f*
prenatal diagnosis, 1309, 1309*f*–1310*f*
treatment
ankyloglossia, 1318
lingual choristomas, 1318–1319,
1319*f*
Orbicularis hypertrophy, lower eyelid
blepharoplasty, 3086, 3087*f*
Orbicularis oculi muscle hyperfunction,
3074–3075, 3075*f*
Orbicularis oris muscle, 1788, 1789*f*,
1794, 1798, 1798*f*
Orbit
anatomy, 2065–2066, 2065*f*
bones, 638
extraconal space, 638–639, 639*f*
intraconal space, 638
lamina papyracea, 639
opticocarotid recess, 639, 640*f*
computed tomography, 144–145, 145*f*
implants for, 2790–2791, 2791*f*
sinus surgery complications
bindness, 653–655
diplopia, 655
epiphora, 655
hematoma, 650–653
Orbit floor fracture, 1281
Orbital abscess, 576
Orbital cellulitis, 575–576, 576*f*, 630
Orbital decompression
background, 630
endoscopic access
endoscopic orbital decompression,
633
endoscopic transnasal, 632
maxillary trephination, 633
surgical risks, 633–634
transcaruncular, 633
fat, 632
floor, 631–632, 632*f*
indications, 630, 630*f*
lateral, 631, 632*f*
medial, 631, 631*f*
superior, 632
Orbital exenteration, 442
Orbital fractures
biomechanics, 1229
clinical evaluation
color perception, 1230
CT scans, 1229–1230
extraocular movements, 1230
Naugle exophthalmometer, 1230
ocular injury, 1230
periorbital edema, 1229
physical examination, 1230
demographics and etiology
blow-out fracture, 1227–1228, 1228*f*
orbital roof fractures, 1229
zygomaticomaxillary complex fractures, 1228, 1228*f*
floor
transantral endoscopic approach,
1234–1235, 1234*f*, 1235*f*
transconjunctival approach, 1233,
1233*f*

transcutaneous approach, 1232–1233, 1232f
lateral orbit and orbital roof
  coronal approach, 1237
  lateral brow approach, 1236–1237
  upper blepharoplasty approach, 1237, 1237f
medial orbit
  transcaruncular incision, 1235–1236, 1236f
  transcutaneous approach, 1235
  transnasal approaches, 1236
pathophysiology, 1229
postoperative care, 1237–1238
postoperative complications, 1238
surgical indications
  blow-out fracture, 1231
  orbital roof fractures, 1231–1232, 1231f
  zygomaticomaxillary complex fractures, 1231
Orbital pseudotumor, 226
Orbital roof fractures, 1281–1282
demographics and etiology, 1229
surgical indications, 1231–1232, 1231f
Orbital tumors
classification, 2063–2064, 2064t
clinical presentation, 2064–2065
cystic lesions, 2071–2072
hematopoietic, 2067–2068
inflammatory, 2071
lacrimal, 2074
mesenchymal, 2072–2074, 2073f
metastatic, 2075
neural, 2068–2069, 2070f
orbital anatomy, 2065–2066, 2065f
postoperative care, 2077
secondary lesions, 2074–2075
surgical approaches to, 2075–2077, 2076f, 2078f
vascular, 2066–2067, 2067f
Orbital varices, 2067
Orbitozygomatic craniotomy, 2076, 2076f
Organ of Corti, 2257–2258, 2259f, 2260f, 2260t, 2747, 2748f
Orofacial clefting, 1556
Orofacial granulomatosis, 753
Orofaciodigital syndrome, 1639
Oropharyngeal cancer
chemotherapy, 1697–1698
diagnosis of
  endoscopic staging in, 1903, 1903t
  evaluation, 1902–1903, 1902t, 1903t
  history taking in, 1902
  physical examination in, 1902
emergencies in, 1913, 1913t
etiology of, 1900
histopathology of, 1900–1901
natural history of, 1901–1902, 1901t
prognosis in, 1914, 1914t
surgery in, complications of, 1900
treatment of
  complications of, 1913, 1913t
  follow-up after, 1913–1914, 1913t
  mandibular lingual release in, 1906–1907, 1906f
  new and developing, 1914
  nonsurgical, 1905
  organ preservation, 1903

primary tumor, 1905
reconstruction of defects following, 1910–1913, 1912f
for squamous cell carcinoma, 1903–1905, 1904t
transmandibular, 1908–1910, 1909f–1911f
transoral approach, 1905
transoral robotic surgery, 1905–1906
transpharyngeal approaches, 1907–1908, 1907f, 1908f
Oropharyngeal defects, microvascular reconstructive approaches to, 2845
Oropharyngeal obstruction
pathophysiology, 1307, 1308f
postnatal diagnosis, 1313
prenatal diagnosis, 1309, 1309f–1310f
treatment, 1319–1320, 1320f
Oropharynx
anatomy of, 12f, 13, 1898–1899, 1899f
physiology of, 1899–1900
surgery for, 2845
Orotracheal intubation, 512
Orthognathic surgery, 1562, 1568–1570
Osler-Weber-Rendu syndrome, 126, 3217, 3217f
Osseointegrated devices
biological aspect of, 2639
bone anchored hearing system
  complications, 2641
  conductive or mixed hearing losses, 2640
  single-sided deafness, 2640
  surgery, 2640–2641, 2641f
bone conduction, 2638–2639, 2639f
current device technology, 2639, 2639f
new device development, 2641
outcome of, 2641
overview of, 2638
pediatric population, 2640
Osseous genioplasty
complications, 3187, 3187f
gingivolabial incision, 3183, 3184f, 3185
osteotomy, 3185–3186, 3185f, 3186f
soft tissue replacement, 3186, 3186f
subperiosteal dissection, 3185, 3185f
vertical chin reduction, 3186, 3186f
wound care, 3186–3187
Ossicles
in aural atresia, 2348
development of, 2242, 2243f
Ossiculoplasty
applied middle ear mechanics, 2478
fixed ossicular chain, 2484
gain mechanisms, 2466–2467, 2468t
incus and stapes, 2481–2482, 2483f
incus erosion
  applebaum prosthesis, 2479
  contour of prosthesis, 2480, 2481f
  incudostapedial joint reconstruction, 2478
  incus interposition, 2479, 2480f
  middle ear anatomy, 2479, 2479f
  mosaic cartilage tympanoplasty, 2480, 2482f
  partial ossicular replacement prosthesis, 2480

malleus, 2482–2484, 2483f
principles, 2477–2478
synthetic materials, 2478
tympanoplasty. See Tympanoplasty
Ossifying fibroma, 293
Osteogenesis imperfecta, 1639–1640, 2492
otologic manifestations, 2526–2527
Osteogenic sarcoma, 2049, 2374
Osteoma
of external ear, 2369–2370
of jaw, 2107
orbital tumor, 2074
Osteopathic medicine, 318
Osteopetrosis
otologic manifestations, 2527
Osteoradionecrosis
causes of, 1718
fibular free flap, 1719, 1719f
pathogenesis of, 1718
reconstructive option, 1718–1719
scapular/iliac crest free flaps, 1719
treatment for, 1718
Ostiomeatal complex, 538
Otic capsule, development of, 2247–2249, 2248f
Otitic hydrocephalus, 2407
Otitis externa, 136–137, 2335
acute, 2335
bacteriology, 2336
bullous, 2343
chronic stage, 2335, 2339
complications of, 2340t
conditions related to, 2343
dermatoses, 2345–2346
diagnosis, 2336, 2338t
differential diagnosis, 2336–2337
furunculosis and carbunculosis, 2344
granular, 2343
herpes zoster and herpes simplex virus, 2345
history taking in, 2336
hypertrophic, surgical management of, 2340, 2340t
infectious eczematoid dermatitis, 2344, 2344f
medical treatment of, 2337–2338
moderate stage, 2338–2339
natural history of, 2337
necrotizing (malignant), 2340
  clinical and radiographic findings, 2341–2342
  diagnosis, 2340–2341
  medical treatment, 2345–2356
  surgical treatment of, 2343–2344
otomycosis, 2345
perichondritis and chondritis, 2344
physical examination in, 2336
radiation-induced, 2343
relapsing polychondritis, 2344
severe stage, 2339
staging of, 2336, 2337f, 2338f, 2338t
Otitis media, 135–136
antibiotic prophylaxis, 1493
bacteriology of, 2399, 2400t
clinical guidelines for, 1494t, 1497
cochlear implants, 2635–2636
complementary and alternative medicine, 323–324

Otitis media (*Continued*)
  complications of, 1500–1501, 2399,
    2400*t*
    bezold abscess, 2403
    chronic suppurative otitis media, 2400
    differential diagnosis of, 2403
    eustachian tube function, 2401
    intracranial complications,
      2404–2407
    labyrinthine fistula, 2401, 2403
    labyrinthitis, 2404
    malodorous discharge, 2400
    masked mastoiditis, 2403
    mastoiditis, 2401
    meningitis, 2401
    mucosal edema, 2401
    patterns of presentation, 2401, 2401*t*
    petrositis, 2401, 2403
    retrograde thrombophlebitis, 2401
    signs and symptoms, 2401, 2401*t*
    tissue edema production, 2400
    uncomplicated chronic otorrhea,
      2400
  diagnosis
    audiometry, 1480–1481
    immittance testing (tympanometry),
      1480
    pneumatic otoscopy, 1479
    symptoms and signs, 1479, 1480*f*
  environmental factor
    day careand siblings, 1483–1484
    feeding, 1484
    obesity, 1484–1485
    pacifier use, 1484
    socioeconomic status, 1484
    tobacco smoke exposure, 1484
    upper respiratory infection, 1483
  epidemiology, 1481
  facial paralysis in, 2513
  hearing devices, implantable, 1518
  host response factors, 1482–1483, 2399
  incidence of, 1481, 1481*f*
  leukotriene inhibitors, 1495
  local anatomy, 2399
  medications and substances, 1493
  pathogens exposure, 2399
  pathophysiology and pathogenesis,
    1485*f*, 2399
    allergy and immunology, 1487–1488
    bacterial infection, 1486
    biofilms, 1486–1487
    eustachian tube function, 1485–1486,
      1485*f*
    gastroesophageal reflux, 1488
    viral infection, 1487
  persistent perforation, 1499
  prevention
    bacterial vaccines, 1488–1489
    environmental factors management,
      1488
    viral vaccines, 1489–1490
  surgical treatment
    adenoidectomy, 1493–1494, 1496–1497
    myringotomy, 1493, 1495–1496
    otitis media with effusion. *See* Otitis
      media with effusion
    tympanocentesis, 1493

  treatment, 1490–1492, 1491*t*
    antibiotic prophylaxis, 1493
    decongestants/antihistamines, 1492
    steroids, 1492–1493
  tympanostomy tube
    audiologic examination, 1497–1498
    complications, 1498
    displacement of, 1499
    indications for, 1499
    ototopical drops, 1497
    selection of, 1497
    tympanosclerosis and atrophy, 1498
    water precautions, 1499–1500
Otitis media with effusion, 136
  clinical guidelines for, 1494*t*, 1497
  incidence of, 1482
  risk factors, 1482
  treatment, 1494–1495, 1494*t*
Otoacoustic emissions, 1512–1513, 1524,
    2258, 2266–2267, 2268*f*, 2269,
    2534
  clinical applications of, 2285, 2285*t*
  measurement of, 2284–2285, 2284*f*
    equipment of, 2284, 2284*f*
OTOF gene, in hearing loss, 1545
Otolaryngologic syndromes
  Apert syndrome, 1622–1623, 1623*f*
  associations in, 1621
  branchiootorenal syndrome,
    1623–1624, 1624*f*
  CHARGE association, 1625
  classification of, 1621–1622
  Crouzon syndrome, 1625–1627, 1625*f*,
    1626*t*, 1627*f*
  deformations, 1620
  disruptions, 1620
  Down syndrome, 1626–1627, 1626*t*
  fetal alcohol syndrome, 1635–1641,
    1635*f*
  forme fruste, 1620
  genetic counseling for, 1617, 1621
  Goldenhar syndrome, 1552,
    1627–1629, 1627*f*
  heterogeneity of, 1620
  history in, 1621
  inheritance of, 1617, 1618*f*, 1619, 1619*f*
  Kartagener syndrome, 1629
  malformations in, 1620
  Melkersson-Rosenthal syndrome,
    1629–1630, 1629*f*
  Melnick-Fraser syndrome, 1623–1624,
    1624*f*
  neurofibromatosis, 1630, 1631*f*
  physical examination in, 1621
  practical approach to, 1621–1622
  in Robin sequence, 1631, 1631*f*
  sequences in, 1620
  Shprintzen syndrome, 1631–1632,
    1631*f*
  Treacher Collins syndrome, 1632–1633,
    1633*f*
  Usher syndrome, 1633–1634
  Waardenburg syndrome, 1634, 1634*f*
Otolaryngologist, in cough
  ACCP, 1348
  causes, 1350
  clinical significance, 1349

  commission crimes, 1351
  cystic fibrosis, 1351
  diagnosis, 1350
  etiology, 1349–1350
  evaluation, 1348
  expiratory phase, 1351
  false focal folds, 1351
  immunodeficiency, 1351
  pathology, 1349
  physical examination, 1350
  primary ciliary dyskinesia, 1351
  red herrings, 1349
Otolaryngology
  geriatric, 298–302
  outcomes research in, 105
Otologic manifestations
  autoimmune disease
    autoimmune inner ear disease,
      2523–2526
    Cogan syndrome, 2522
    polyarteritis nodosa, 2522–2523
    relapsing polychondritis, 2523
    rheumatoid arthritis, 2523
  bone disease
    osteogenesis imperfecta, 2526–2527
    Paget disease, 2526
  granulomatous disease
    langerhans histiocytosis, 2521–2522
    sarcoidosis, 2522
    Wegener granulomatosis, 2522
  infectious diseases
    bacterial infections, 2520
    cytomegalovirus, 2519
    HIV infection, 2520
    lyme disease, 2521
    mumps and measles viruses, 2520
    rubella, 2519
    syphilis, 2520–2521
    varicella-zoster virus, 2520
Otomycosis, 2345
Otopalatodigital syndrome, 125, 1550, 1640
Otoplasty
  anatomy and embryology, 3142–3143,
    3143*f*
  auricular anomalies
    deformations, 3144, 3145*f*–3146*f*
    etiology and classification, 3144
    psychosocial issues, 3146
  cartilage-shaping technique, 3156–3157,
    3157*f*, 3158*f*
  incision design
    antihelical fold, 3149, 3150*f*
    closure, 3151
    complications, 3152, 3156, 3156*f*
    conchal setback preparation, 3149,
      3150*f*, 3151
    constricted ear, 3152, 3153*f*–3155*f*
    dressing, 3152
    Furnas sutures placement, 3151
    helical root, 3149, 3149*f*, 3151
    injection, 3149
    lobule management, 3151–3152
    surgical procedure, 3149–3151
  malformations, 3144–3146, 3145*f*–3146*f*
  origins, 3142
  patient selection
    initial evaluation, 3146

nonsurgical treatment, 3147
surgical candidates, 3147
surgical techniques, 3147–3148, 3148f
Otorrhea, 1498
Otosclerosis, 2487–2501, 2611
amplification in, 2492
bone remodeling, 2488
differential diagnosis, 2490–2492, 2492t
embryology of, 2487
etiology of, 2488
histology of, 2487–2488
management of, 2492
medical management of, 2492–2493, 2493t
pathophysiology of, 2488–2489, 2488f
surgery
anesthesia, 2494–2495
anterior crurotomy, 2495–2496
complications of, 2493t, 2500–2501
contraindications to, 2493–2494
indication, 2500, 2500t
laser treatment, 2496
management of, 2493
notched bucket-handle prosthesis, 2499
numerous stapes prosthesis, 2498
patient counseling for, 2494
patient selection for, 2493–2494
perilymph gusher, 2499
perioperative steroids, 2498
pitfalls of, 2500–2501
postoperative care, 2498–2499
prosthesis placement, 2497, 2498f
rosette pattern, 2497, 2498f
stapedial superstructure, 2496–2497, 2497f
technique for, 2494–2500, 2495f–2498f, 2500t
tissue graft, 2497, 2498f
Otospongiosis, computed tomography, 141, 142f
Ototoxicity
clinical monitoring of, 2547
genetics of
aminoglycoside, 2545
cisplatin, 2545–2546
hearing loss, 1531
otoprotective strategies, 2546–2547
systemic ototoxicity, 2543t
aminoglycosides, 2542
heavy metals, 2544
iron-chelating agent, 2544
loop diuretics, 2544
macrolides, 2544
platinum compounds, 2542–2543
salicylates, nsaids and quinine, 2544
vancomycin, 2544
vinca alkaloids, 2543–2544
topical ototoxicity, 2545
Outcomes research
definition of, 102
and evidence-based medicine, 106–109
history, 102
in otolaryngology, results from, 105
outcomes to be measured in, 104–105
quality of life measurements and, 104
steps in performing, 103–105

types of, 102, 103t, 105–106
validity and, 104
Outer ear. See Ear, external
Overlay tympanoplasty, 2474, 2475f, 2476
Overresected nose
augmentation graft, 3003–3004
postsurgical deformities, 2991, 2992f
Oxidized cellulose, 52
Oxygen delivery, 55
Oxygen extraction, 55–56
Oxytocin, 253

P
Paget disease, 2491–2492
bone(s), 293–294
otologic manifestations, 2526
Pain
definition, 344
facial. See Facial pain
in head and neck cancer. See Head and neck cancer
headache. See Headaches
postoperative, pharmacologic management of, 45–46, 45t
Palatal augmentation, 840
Palatal myoclonus, 2610–2611
Palatal obdurator, 840
Palate
adult tonsillectomy, 2197–2198
anatomy of, 10, 11f
diagnosis and evaluation, 2196, 2196f
expansion sphincter pharyngoplasty, 2199–2200, 2200f
failure of, 2199
palatopharyngoplasty, 2197
tori, 2106
transpalatal advancement pharyngoplasty, 2198–2199, 2198f, 2199f
upper pharynx anatomy, 2195–2196
uvulopalatopharyngoplasty, 2197
Palate surgery, in obstructive sleep apnea, 2210, 2211t
Palifermin, 738
Palliative care
antineoplastic therapies
chemotherapy, 341–342
radiation therapy, 342
surgery, 342
clinical practice guidelines
care structure and process, 343
cultural aspects, 344
ethical and legal aspects, 344
imminently dying patient care, 344
physical aspects, 343
psychosocial and psychiatric aspects, 343
social aspects, 343
spiritual, religious, and existential aspects, 343–344
versus hospice care, 340
pain in head and neck cancer. See Pain
quality of life, 340
Pallister-Hall syndrome, 126, 1320
Pancreas
diabetes mellitus, 261
diabetic ketoacidosis, 261–262
dysfunction of, 489

glucagon, 260–261
glucose metabolism, 260
hyperglycemic hyperosmolar state, 262
hypoglycemia, 262
insulin, 261
multiple endocrine neoplasia syndromes, 262–263, 263t
Pancuronium, 243
Panfacial fracture
anatomic reduction, 1165
dimensions, 1165, 1166f
emergency, 1163, 1164t
fracture fixation, 1165, 1166f
history and physical examination, 1163
nasoethmoid complex, 1167
orbital floor continuity, 1166–1167
orbital/periorbital fracture, 1164
radiologic evaluation, 1164
skull base, 1165, 1165f
subcranial approach, 1164–1165
zygomatic arch fracture, 1166
Papillary carcinoma, 2120
Papillary thyroid carcinoma, 2116
Papilloma
laser procedures, 1088
sinonasal tract, 2046t
squamous cell, 2370
voice therapy, 1054
Paracoccidioidomycosis, 742, 742t
Paraganglioma(s), 2609–2610
anatomy and physiology, 1999–2000, 2000f–2002f
angiographic evaluation, 2010–2011, 2011f
cerebellopontine angle, 2580–2581, 2581f
clinical presentation and classification, 2003–2005, 2004f, 2004t, 2005t
complications
baroreflex failure, 2015
carotid body tumors, 2013f, 2017, 2018f
cranial nerve injury, 2015–2016, 2016f
external beam radiation, 2016
radiation, 2016–2017
salvage therapy, 2017, 2018f
vascular injury, 2014–2015
diagnosis
angiography, 2006–2008, 2008f, 2009f
computed tomography, 2005–2006, 2006f–2007f
magnetic resonance imaging, 2006, 2007f, 2008f
radionuclide, 2008
embolization
carotid body tumors, 2012–2014, 2014f
inflammatory response, 2011, 2012f
jugulotympanic paragangliomas, 2012–2014, 2014f
vagal paragangliomas, 2014
epidemiology and pathophysiology
annual incidence of, 2000
catecholamines, 2001
genetics, 2002–2003
malignancy, 2001

Paraganglioma(s) (*Continued*)
  surgery, 2010
  of temporal bone, 2358–2362
    diagnosis of, 2358
    growth patterns of, 2358
    incidence of, 2359
    treatment of, 2362
  treatment, 2010, 2012*f*
Parainfluenza virus, 761, 1433
Paralysis
  bilateral vocal fold
    clinical presentation and evaluation,
      1017–1020, 1018*f*, 1020*f*
    etiology, 1017, 1017*t*, 1018*t*
    fiberoptic laryngoscopy, 1018, 1018*f*
    history, 1018–1019
    imaging, 1019
    laryngeal electromyography, 1019
    laryngoscopy and palpation,
      1019–1020, 1020*f*
    management, 1020–1022, 1021*f*
    physical examination, 1019
    serology, 1019
  unilateral vocal fold
    classical teaching, 1012–1013
    early surgical intervention, 1014
    etiology, 1004–1007, 1005*f*, 1006*t*
    history, 1007–1008
    imaging, 1011
    injection augmentation, 1014–1015,
      1014*t*, 1015*f*
    laryngeal electromyography, 1011,
      1012*f*, 1013*f*
    laryngeal framework surgery, 1015–1017
    laryngeal reinnervation, 1017
    management, 1011–1012
    nimodipine, 1017
    patient factors, 1012, 1013*t*
    physical examination, 1008–1010,
      1008*f*–1010*f*
    serology, 1010–1011
Paramedian midbrain syndrome, 202
Paranasal sinuses. *See* Sinus(es)
Parapharyngeal space, deep neck infection,
  809–810, 809*f*
Parathyroid carcinoma, 2132, 2141–2142,
  2142*f*
Parathyroid gland(s)
  anatomy of, 16–17, 16*f*
  blood supply, 253
  calcium metabolism
    calcitonin, 254
    hyocalcemia, 256
    hypercalcemia, 255–256
    vitamin D, 254–255
  disorders of, preoperative management
    of, 32–33
  ectopic locations, 253
  histology of, 2132, 2132*f*
  parathyroid hormone
    primary hyperparathyroidism, 254
    secretion, 254
    structure and metabolism, 253
Parathyroid hormone
  primary hyperparathyroidism, 254
  secretion, 254
  structure and metabolism, 253

Parathyroidectomy
  anterior approach, 2140, 2140*f*
  bilateral exploration, 2136–2138, 2137*f*,
    2138*f*
  indications for, 2135, 2136*t*
  lateral approach, 2140, 2141*f*, 2142*f*
  minimally invasive, 2138, 2139
  patient outcome, 2140
  pitfalls of IOPTH, 2138–2139
Paratracheal neck dissection, 1811, 1812,
  1820, 1824, 1825
Parenteral nutrition, preoperative, 26
Paresthesia and hypesthesia, sinus surgery
  complications, 658
Parinaud syndrome, 203
Parkinson disease, 1030–1031, 1031*f*, 1032*t*
Parkinsonism, 1030
Parodoxic vocal fold motion disorder,
  1301
Parotid duct(s), soft tissue injuries,
  1120–1121, 1121*f*, 1122*f*
Parotid gland
  accessory, 692, 693*f*
  anatomy of, 9, 9*f*
  arterial blood supply, 692
  facial nerve
    auriculotemporal nerve, 695
    branches, 693–694
    great auricular nerve, 694–695
    parotidectomy, 694, 694*f*
  histology, 691
  lymphatic system, 695
  parasympathetic stimulation, 695
  parotid fascia, 692
  parotid space, 691
  Stensen duct, 692, 693*f*
  superficial and deep layer, 692, 693*f*
  superficial compartment, 692
  surgery of
    facial nerve identification/monitoring,
      1176, 1778*t*
    technique of, 1770
    tumors of, 1760
  sympathetic stimulation, 695
  venous drainage, 692
Parotid space, deep neck infection, 810
Parotidectomy, 51, 694, 694*f*
Partial ossicular replacement prosthesis,
  2466, 2480–2482, 2481*f*
Pathogen-associated molecular patterns,
  380
Patient care
  clinical guidelines, 1673–1674, 1674*t*
  clinical pathways, 1674–1675
  cost of care, 1679–1680
  health care disparity, 1678–1679
  medical errors, 1678
  multidisciplinary team approach
    components of, 1676, 1676*t*
    efficacy of, 1676–1677
    presentations, 1676, 1677*f*
  quality care. *See* Quality care
  surgical safety checklist, 1678, 1679*f*
Patient privacy, clinic management, 3338
Patient reported outcome measurement
    information system, 718–719
Patient safety

agencies and organizations, 3263
aviation safety movement, 3256–3257
human error
  prevention of, 3257
medical error. *See* Medical error
medication errors, 3263
in otolaryngology, 3262
root cause analysis. *See* Root cause
  analysis
Patient satisfaction, 1673
Patient-controlled analgesia, 45
Patient-specific implants, 2787
Pattern recognition receptors, 380
Patulous eustachian tube, 2611
Pediatric patients
  audiology and hearing devices. *See*
    Hearing devices, implantable
  congenital malformations in
  diagnostic audiologic assessment in,
    2286
  facial fracture
    condyle, 1279, 1279*f*
    craniofacial growth and trauma,
      1274–1275, 1275*f*
    dentoalveolar, 1280
    epidemiology, 1272–1273
    etiology/injury mechanism, 1274
    frontal bone, 1281–1282
    frontal sinus, 1282
    management, 1273–1274,
      1273*t*–1274*t*
    mandible arch, 1278–1280, 1278*f*,
      1280*f*
    medial orbital wall, 1281
    midface, 1280
    nasal fracture, 1277
    nasoorbitoethmoid complex, 1277,
      1281–1282, 1282*f*
    newborn nasal deformity, 1277
    orbit, 1281
    orbital floor and roof, 1281–1282
    orbital rim, 1277
    radiographic examination, 1274
    rigid fixation, 1275–1277, 1276*t*
    supraorbital rim, 1282
    transcaruncular incision, 1277
    zygomaticomaxillary complex,
      1280–1281
  head and neck masses. *See* head and
    neck masses
  ophthalmology
    congenital abnormalities
      amblyopia, 230
      esotropia, 229
      exotropia, 230
      pseudostrabismus, 230
      strabismus, 229
  otolaryngology
    adenotonsillar surgery, 1300–1301
    application, 1288
    congenital malformation
      airway, 1296–1297
      auricular, 1295
      midline, 1296
      nares, 1295–1296
      neck, 1297
      oral cavity, 1296

cystic fibrosis, 1300
growth and development, patterns of
  in boys, 1288, 1288f
  cervical lymph node, 1295
  craniofacial skeletal comparison,
    1289, 1290f
  endoscopic view, 1294, 1294f
  eustachian tube, 1292, 1292f
  facial configuration, 1289, 1290f
  in girls, 1288, 1289f
  larynx, 1293, 1293f
  paranasal sinus, 1291–1292, 1291f,
    1291t
  postnatal growth, 1288, 1289f
  temporal bone development, 1293,
    1293f
infectious disease
  otitis media, 1299–1300
  rhinosinusitis, 1300
  Streptococcus pneumoniae, 1300
issues, 1301–1302
polysomnography study, 1287–1288
sensory impairment
  facial paralysis, 1299
  haemophilus influenzae type B,
    1298
  multichannel cochlear implanta-
    tion, 1298
  otolaryngologist, 1297, 1298t
  pediatric otolaryngologists, 1299
  vertiginous disorder, 1299
  vocal fold paralysis, 1299
speech and voice, 1301
otologic procedures in, facial nerve
  monitoring during, 2328
rhinosinusitis
  adenoidectomy, 1459–1460, 1460f
  antral lavage, 1460
  bacteriology, 1458, 1458t
  chronic pediatric sinusitis, 1459t
  differential diagnosis, 1455, 1456t
  ethmoidectomy, 1460–1461, 1461f,
    1462f
  etiology, 1456–1457
  facial growth, 1461
  guided imaging in, 1462f
  inferior meatal antrostomy, 1460
  intracranial complications, 1464
  medical management, 1458–1459,
    1459t
  middle meatal antrostomy, 1460
  nasal antral windows, 1460
  orbital complications, 1461–1463,
    1463f, 1464f
  other diagnostic aids, 1456–1457,
    1456t, 1457f
  persistent sinus disease, 1461, 1463t
  physical examination, 1455–1456
  signs and symptoms, 1455, 1456t
salivary gland disease
  autoimmune conditions, Sjögren syn-
    drome, 1475
  inflammatory conditions, 1467–1470,
    1468t
  mesenchymal tumors. See
    Mesenchymal tumors
  sialorrhea, 1475–1477

trauma, 1477
salivary gland tumors in, 1760, 1762t
sleep disordered breathing, 2220–2233
tracheotomy
  communication, 1396
  complications of
    accidental decannulation, 1392
    cartilaginous collapse, 1393
    esophageal injury, 1392
    granulomas, 1392–1393
    intraoperative, 1391–1392
    obstruction/plugging, 1392
    stomal stenosis, 1392, 1393f
    stoma/wound breakdown, 1392
    suprastomal airway obstruction,
      1392, 1393f
    tracheoesophageal fistula forma-
      tion, 1392
    tracheo-innominate artery fistula,
      1393
    tracheostomy-related mortality rate,
      1394
    tube occlusion, 1392
  decannulation of, 1395–1396
  versus endotracheal intubation,
    1384–1386, 1385t
  history of, 1382–1383
  indications for, 1383–1384, 1384t
  postoperative care, 1390–1391
  swallowing, 1396
  technique
    anatomy of, 1386, 1386f
    excess subcutaneous fat deep, 1386,
      1387f
    operating table, 1386, 1386f
    pretracheal fascia, 1387, 1388f
    skin incision, 1387, 1387f
    strap muscles, 1386, 1387f–1388f
    thyroid isthmus, 1386, 1388f
    tracheal cartilage, 1389, 1390f
    tracheal stenosis, 1387
    tracheostomy stoma tract, 1387,
      1388f
    tracheostomy tube, 1389, 1389f
    Z-plasty principles, 1390
  tracheostomy tube, 1394–1395,
    1394f–1395f
Pediatric voice
  acoustic and aerodynamic evaluation,
    1373
  airway reconstruction, dysphonia, 1379,
    1379f
  bilateral vocal cord paralysis, 1378
  congenital laryngeal webs, 1378
  endoscopy and videostroboscopy, 1373,
    1373f–1374f
  evaluation, 1374
  functional disorders, 1378–1379
  history, 1373
  laryngopharyngeal reflux and eosino-
    philic esophagitis, 1374, 1375f
  recurrent respiratory papillomatosis,
    1377
  unilateral vocal fold paralysis,
    1377–1378
vocal fold
  microstructure of, 1372

nodules, cysts, and polyps
  endoscopic examination, 1375,
    1376f
  hourglass closure configuration,
    1375, 1375f
  nonoperative management, 1376
  operative management, 1376–1377
  phono-traumatic event, 1375
vocal process granulomas, 1379
voice-related quality-of-life/handicap-
  ping assessment, 1374
Pedicled flaps, 671
Pemphigoid, pharyngitis due to,
  762–763
Pemphigus vulgaris, 745–747, 745f, 746f,
  747t
Pendred syndrome, 1535, 1543t
Pendular nystagmus, 2684, 2685
Penetrance, 1541
  of gene/trait, 1620
Penetrating injuries
  cavitation effects, 1131, 1132f
  emergency, 1136, 1136t
  principles of, 1131–1132
  rotational ballistics, 1131, 1132f
Penicillin(s)
  antimicrobial agents, 131, 132t
  in streptococcal pharyngitis, 759
Peptococci/peptostreptococci, pediatric
  rhinosinusitis and, 1458, 1458t
Percutaneous dilatational tracheotomy, 62
  anesthesia, 938–939
  complications
    accidental decannulation, 943
    accidental extubation, 942
    bleeding, 942
    desaturation, 942
    infection, 942
    posterior wall injury, 942–943
    subcutaneous emphysema, 943
    technical misadventures, 943
  cost analyses, 936
  critically ill patients, 936
  instruments, 937–938, 938f, 939f
  patient selection, 937, 937t
  personnel, 937
  postoperative considerations, 941
  preoperative planning, 937
  technique, 939–941, 639f–641f
Percutaneous gastrostomy, 348
Periapical cysts, 2097–2098, 2098f
Pericardiocentesis, 1099, 1100f
Perichondritis, 2344
Perilymphatic fistula, 1534, 2705–2706
Periocular hemangiomas, 1578, 1578f
Periodic acid-Schiff staining, 741f
Periodic alternating nystagmus, 2685
Periodic fevers with aphthous,
  761–762
Perioperative management issues
  cardiovascular disorders
    American College of Cardiology/
      American Heart Association
      guidelines, 35
    β-blockade therapy, 35
    dysrhythmia, 37
    hypertension, 35–36, 36t

Perioperative management issues
(*Continued*)
hypotension, 36–37, 36*t*
postoperative, risk factors for, 35
endocrine abnormalities
adrenal glucocorticoids, 33–34, 34*t*
diabetes mellitus, 31–32, 32*t*
pituitary, 34–35
thyroid and parathyroid disorders, 32–33, 33*t*
fever, 43–44, 44*f*
gastrointestinal disorders
adynamic ileus, 40
diarrhea, 40
stress ulcers, 39
hematologic abnormalities
blood components and transfusion, 27–28, 27*t*
erythrocyte abnormalities, 28
hemostatic disorders, 29–30, 29*t*
intraoperative and postoperative bleeding, 30
platelet abnormalities, 28–29
malignant hyperthermia, 44–45, 45*t*
neuropsychiatric problems, 41–43
postoperative pain, 45–46, 45*t*
preoperative malnutrition, 26–27
pulmonary disorders, 37–39
renal disease, 40–41
thromboembolic diseases
diagnosis, 31
management, 31
preventive measures, 30–31
pulmonary embolism, 31
Perioral region, implants for, 2793
Periorbital hemangiomas, 1582
Periorbital musculature, upper eyelid blepharoplasty, 3075, 3076*f*
Periorbital rhytids, lateral Botox injections in, 3242–3243, 3243*f*
Periosteal abscess, 2444
Peripheral neuropathy
Guillain-Barré syndrome, 1039–1040, 1040*f*
mononeuropathy, 1038
myelinopathy, 1038
superior laryngeal nerve paresis, 1039, 1040*f*
vocal fold paresis and paralysis, 1038–1039, 1039*f*
Peripheral vestibular disorders
benign paroxysmal positional vertigo, 2736–2737
bilateral vestibular hypofunction, 2738
medications, 2734
Meniere disease, 2738
vestibular neuritis, 2738
Peripheral vestibular system, 2717
Peritonsillar abscess, 138
Personality disorder, 2759
Pertinent orbital anatomy
bony anatomy, 622, 623*f*
lacrimal anatomy, 624, 625*f*
neuromuscular anatomy, 623, 624*f*
vascular anatomy, 622–623, 623*f*
Petrosa, surgery of, 2447–2463
Petrositis, 2401

Petrous apex, surgical access to, 2458–2460, 2459*f*, 2460*f*
Petrous apicectomy, 2458–2460, 2459*f*, 2460*f*
Phaces, 1577–1578
Phacoemulsification, 222
Phantosmia, 376
Pharmacotherapy
subjective nonpulsatile tinnitus, 2603
temporomandibular joint, 789
tobacco cessation
antidepressants, 335
clonidine, 335
combination therapy, 335
effectiveness and abstinence rates, 336*t*
naltrexone, 335
nicotine replacement therapy, 333
varenicline, 333, 335
Pharyngeal constrictor
myotomy, 1983, 1983*f*
spasm, 1984, 1984*f*
Pharyngeal squeeze maneuver, 828–829, 829*f*, 841
Pharyngitis, 138, 757–767
in adult
due to bacterial infections, 765
due to fungal infections, 766
due to inflammatory infections
due to viral infections, 763–765
in child
due to bacterial infections, 758–761, 760*f*
due to inflammatory infections, 761–763
due to viral infections, 760*f*, 761
differential diagnosis, 757, 758*t*
Pharyngoesophageal defects, microvascular reconstructive approaches to, 2844–2845
Pharynx
airway physiology, 869
anatomy of, 12–13, 12*f*, 757–758
functions of, 365
Phenobarbital, 42, 42*t*
Phenol peels. *See* Chemical peeling
Phenotypic expressivity, 1620
Phenylephrine, 59
Phenytoin, 42, 42*t*
Pheochromocytoma, 260
Phonation, myoelastic-aerodynamic theory of, 952
Phonatory glottic cycle, 952–953, 952*f*
Phonomicrosurgery
complications, 1002, 1002*f*
equipments for
laryngoscope, 997–998
long Hopkins rod telescope, 998
microscope and laser, 998
patient evaluation, 997
preoperative measures, 997
preoperative stroboscopy examination, 997
procedure and technique
anesthesia, 998
microflap approach, 999–1001, 1000*f*, 1001*f*

microscope and laryngoscope position, 999
patient positioning, 998–999
ventilation options, 998
Phonotrauma, 953
Photoaged epidermis, 3105
Photodocumentation
digital, 2780–2783, 2780*f*
informed consent, 2772
intraoperative, 2776–2777
principles of, 2772–2777
standardization of, 2773–2776
distracting elements removal, 2775
equipment, 2773
lighting and background, 2775–2776, 2777*f*
patient positioning, 2773, 2774*f*, 2775, 2775*f*
traditional, 2777–2780
camera, 2778
data back, 2779
film, 2779–2780
lenses, 2779
tripod, 2779
viewfinder grid, 2779
Photodynamic therapy, 52, 1730–1731
Photometrics, in facial analysis, 2768
Physician consortium for performance improvement, 3376
Physician practice setting
business entity
corporate practice of medicine, 3293
corporations, 3292
limited liability company, 3292–3293
name protection, 3293
nonprofit corporation, 3292
partnership, 3292
professional service entities, 3293
sole proprietorship, 3292
business loan, 3293
corporate perspective, 3291
federal tax identification number, 3294
Health Insurance Portability and Accountability Act[29] privacy and security, 3294–3296
securing insurance, 3293–3294
third party payors enrolling, 3294
Physician self-referral law, 3282
Pictorial documentation. *See* Photodocumentation
Pigmented lesions, lasers, 3207–3208
Pill-induced esophagitis, 852, 853*f*
Pilomatricomas, 3216, 3216*f*
treatment of, 3226
Pilomatrixoma, 1600, 2370
Pindborg tumors, 2105
Pinna, and external auditory canal, neoplasms of, 2365–2370
Piriform aperture, nasal dorsum, 2952
Piriform apex, 1918*f*
Piriform fossa cancer, 1922*f*
Pitressin, 34
Pituitary
anatomy and embryology, 250
anterior pituitary
adrenocorticotropic hormone, 251–252

follicle-stimulating hormone, 252
gonadotrophs, 252
growth hormone, 251
luteinizing hormone, 252
prolactin, 251
thyroid-stimulating hormone, 252
posterior pituitary
antidiuretic hormone, 252–253
oxytocin, 253
Pituitary adenoma, preoperative management in, 34
Plasmacytoma
extramedullary, temporal bone, 2365
of temporal bone, 2365
Plate application, skeletal facial trauma, rigid fixation, 1157–1158, 1158t
Platelet abnormalities, preoperative management of, 28–29
Platelet derived growth factor, wound healing, 80
Platysma muscle, 3131–3132, 3133f
Platysmal banding, Botox for, 3243
Platysmaplasty, 3118–3119, 3118f
Platysmectomy, 2918
Play audiometry, 1481
Pleiotropy, 1620
Pleomorphic adenoma, 171–172, 171f–172f, 186f
malignant variations of
recurrence of, 1781
of salivary glands, 1760–1762, 1762f
Plummer-Vinson syndrome, 125
Plunging ranula, 170, 170f
Pneumomediastinum, percutaneous dilatational tracheotomy, 943
Pneumoparotitis, 713
Pneumothorax
management in trauma patients, 1097
percutaneous dilatational tracheotomy, 943
Poliomyelitis, 1038
Pollen allergens, 413–414
Polyarteritis nodosa, 275–276
otologic manifestations, 2522–2523
Polycythemia vera, 28
Polydioxanone, 2787
Polyetheretherketone, 2787
Polyglactin 910, 2790
Polyhydramnios, 1322
Polymers, as implants, 2786–2787
Polymethyl methacrylate, 2787
Polymorphous low-grade adenocarcinoma, 193f, 1766
Polymyositis, 1042
associated disorders, 274
diagnostic criteria for, 273, 274t
head and neck manifestations, 274
incidence, 273
treatment, 274
Polypharmacy, 301
Polyps, voice therapy, 1054–1055
Polysomnogram, 2194t
Port-wine stains, 1583, 1583f
Posaconazole, acute invasive fungal rhinosinusitis, 562
Positional nystagmus, 2719
Positional vertigo, 2719

Positive airway pressure therapy, 2228
Positron emission tomography
applications of, 160–161
in nasopharyngeal cancer, 1882, 1883, 1883f, 1884f, 1888
principles, 158–160
Postcricoid cancer, 1922f, 1929
Posterior commissure hypertrophy, 967f
Posterior glottic chink, professional voice, 1061f
Posterior glottic stenosis, 884, 884f, 885t
larygoscopy, 1019f
Posterior inferior cerebellar artery syndrome, 2725–2726, 2726t
Posterior triangle lipoma, 173, 173f
Posterior wall injury
percutaneous dilatational tracheotomy, 942–943
Posterolateral neck dissection, 1807, 1820, 1821f
Postheadshake nystagmus test, dizziness, 2690–2691, 2690f
Postintubation stenosis
laryngeal, 1359–1360
Postlaryngectomy, 1972–1973
Postnasal drip, pharyngitis due to, 766–767
Postpolio syndrome, 1038
Postreconstruction restenosis
laryngeal stenosis, 1360
Posttracheotomy, laryngeal stenosis, 1360
Posttransplant lymphoproliferative disorder
in children, 1601–1602
lymphoma, 2039–2040
pharyngitis in, 762
Postural control assessment
positioning, 2309, 2309f
principle protocols, 2310
sensory organization test, 2309, 2310f
Postures, 839–840, 839t
Potassium titanyl phosphate laser, 52, 1088, 3203
recurrent respiratory papillomatosis, 1416–1417
Pott puffy tumor, 520
frontal sinusitis, 583, 583f
Povidone-iodine scrub, 21
Prader-Willi syndrome, 121
Preauricular cysts and sinuses, 1610–1611, 1610f, 1611f
Prednisone, 33
Pregnancy, alcohol abuse in, fetal alcohol syndrome and, 1637
Presbycusis, aging, 2616–2618, 2617f, 2617t
Presbyopia, 221
Pressure dressings, scar camouflage, 2869
Pressure regulated volume control, 60
Presurgical infant orthopedics, 1560–1561
Pretrichial lift, 3058f, 3062–3063, 3062f
Prevertebral spaces, deep neck infection, 797, 799, 806–807
Primary ciliary dyskinesia, 367, 456
ciliary motility analysis, 457
ciliary ultrastructure analysis, 457
genetic analysis, 457

nasal nitric oxide, 456
saccharin test, 456
Primary headache
chronic daily headaches, 309–310, 310t
cluster headache, 309, 310t
medication overuse, 309–310
migraine
clinical symptoms, 306
diagnosis of, 306
diagnostic criteria, 307t
treatment, 306–308
prevalence, 306
tension-type headache, 308–309, 308t
Primary lateral sclerosis, 1030
Primary squamous cell carcinoma, 2121
Professional voice
anatomy and physiology for voice production
extrinsic laryngeal musculature, 1059, 1060f
intrinsic laryngeal musculature, 1059–1061, 1060f, 1061f
minor intrinsic laryngeal cartilages, 1061
care of, 1074–1075
management
laryngeal hygiene measures, 1073, 1073t
multidisciplinary evaluation, 1073
schedule and style performance, 1073
voice therapy, 1073–1074
pathophysiology
benign vocal fold lesions, 1067–1068
laryngeal vibration, 1068, 1068f
loss of pliability, 1067, 1067f
pediatric patient, 1068
performance styles, 1066–1067
reflux, 1072–1073
sound production principles
formant frequencies, 1062–1063, 1062f
harmonic sound source, 1061–1062, 1062t
human communication, 1061
vocal tract, 1061, 1061f
surgical management
indications, 1075
microflap surgery, 1076
telangiectatic vessel and vibratory asymmetry, 1067f
vocal difficulties
acoustic analysis, 1072, 1072f
complaints, 1069
finding discussion, 1072
history, 1069, 1069t, 1070f–1071f, 1071
laryngeal examination, 1071
physical examination, 1071, 1071f
stroboscopy, 1071–1072
vocal performance styles, 1065–1066, 1065f, 1066t
voice production mechanism
subglottic pressure, 1063–1064, 1063f
vibratory source, 1063, 1063t
vocal fold approximation, 1064
vocal fold tension, 1064–1065, 1064f
Prognathia, chin augmentation, 3181
Progressive bulbar palsy, 1037–1038

Progressive systemic sclerosis, 855
Proliferative retinopathy, 232
Prominent ear, otoplasty, 3144, 3145f
Propofol, 66, 240–241
Proportional assist ventilation, 60
Propranolol, 207, 1320
Proptosis, 226
Propylthiouracil, 32–33
Protein-calorie malnutrition, 26
Proton pump inhibitors, 68–69,
        971–972
Protruding ears
    otoplasty
        complications and emergencies, 3164,
            3167, 3167t
        converse technique, 3163, 3165f
        diagnosis, 3164t
        farrior technique, 3163, 3165f–3166f
        Furnas technique, 3164, 3167f
        Mustardé technique, 3163, 3164f
        Pitanguy technique, 3164, 3166f
        preoperative evaluation, 3162
Pseudobulbar palsy, 209–210, 1030
Pseudomonas aeruginosa, 134, 1149, 1363,
        1458, 1458t
Pseudostrabismus, 230
Pseudosulcus vocalis versus sulcus vocalis,
        965f
Pterygium, 224
Pterygopalatine fossa, neoplasms, 2058
Ptosis, forehead lift and, 3056–3057
Ptyalism, 699
Pull-down maneuver, 1051–1052
Pulmonary complications
    of anesthesia and surgery, 37
    predisposing factors for, 38
Pulmonary disorders
    postoperative pulmonary insufficiency
        in, 38–39
    preoperative management of
        anesthesia choice, 38
        arterial blood gases, 38
        chest radiograph, 37
        lung function tests, 37–38
        physical examination, 37
Pulmonary edema
    acute, endotracheal intubation, 270
    postoperative management, 39
Pulmonary embolism, 31
Pulmonary insufficiency, postoperative,
        38–39
Pulp necrosis, 771, 771f
Pulsatile tinnitus
    diagnostic evaluation
        algorithm, 2605, 2605f
        imaging techniques, 2604–2605,
            2606f, 2607f
    etiology, 2604, 2604t
    nonvascular etiologies
        idiopathic intracranial hypertension,
            2610
        middle ear myoclonus, 2611
        otosclerosis, 2611
        palatal myoclonus, 2610–2611
        patulous eustachian tube, 2611
        semicircular canal dehiscence,
            2610

    vascular anomalies
        atherosclerotic carotid artery disease,
            2608
        carotid-cavernous fistula, 2608–2609
        congenital carotid anomalies, 2608
        dural arteriovenous fistula, 2608,
            2608f
        intracranial and extracranial aneu-
            rysms, 2609, 2609f
        jugular bulb anomalies, 2605, 2607,
            2607f
        sigmoid sinus diverticula, 2607
    vascular neoplasms
        hemangioma, 2610
        paragangliomas, 2609–2610
Pulse dye laser, 1088, 1416, 1562, 3202
Punch biopsy, 3221f
Punch biopsy, technique of, 3221f
Puncture, soft tissue injuries, 1109
Push-back maneuver, 1051–1052
Pyogenic granuloma, 281, 3216, 3226
    treatment of, 3226

Q
Qinine, ototoxicity of, 2544
Quality care
    definition of, 1672–1673
    historical background, 1672
    organizations for, 1673
    outcomes of care, 1673
    purpose of, 1672
Quality improvement
    complex systems and high performance,
        3378
    external requirements for, 3376–3377
    health care institutions
        department-specific initiatives, 3377
        health system programs, 3377
    health care reform, 3377–3378
    historical background, 3372–3373
    organizations endorsing
        Agency for Healthcare Research and
            Quality, 3375
        ambulatory quality alliance,
            3375–3376
        institute for healthcare improvement,
            3376
        institute of medicine, 3376
        joint commission, 3376
        medicare/medicaid services, 3376
        national quality forum, 3376
        physician consortium for performance
            improvement, 3376
        surgical quality alliance, 3376
    in otolaryngology, 3373
    primer, 3378
    reimbursement, 3377
    role of measurement, 3373–3375,
        3374t
Quality-adjusted life years, 719

R
Radial forearm flap, 2824–2826, 2825f
Radial forearm-palmaris longus flap, in lip
        reconstruction, 1801
Radiation hazards, lasers, 3209
Radiation pharyngitis, 767

Radiation therapy, 342
    dose and delivery
        fractions, 1683–1684
        linear accelerator, 1683, 1683f
        thermoplastic head mask, 1683, 1683f
    fractionation and treatment time, 1684
    hemangiopericytoma
        radiation therapy, 2019
    hypopharyngeal and cervical esophageal
        carcinoma, 1924
    innovations in, 1689–1690
    juvenile nasopharyngeal angiofibroma,
        2028
    laryngeal cancer, 1967–1968
    for lip cancer, 1792–1794, 1803f,
        1804
        complications of, 1792, 1792t,
            1804
    nasopharyngeal carcinoma, 1876, 1879,
        1886–1887, 1889, 1893
    neoplasms, 2050–2051, 2058, 2060t
    oral cavity cancer, 1863–1864
    planning
        computed tomography, 1684–1685
        dose volume histogram, 1685, 1686f
        normal structure dose tolerance, 1685,
            1685t
        oncologist consultation, 1684
        oradiation terms, 1685, 1685t
        plastic mask, 1684–1685
        target doses, 1685, 1685t
        treatment time, 1686
    radiation delivery, 1686–1689
    radiation toxicity, 1689
    radiobiology, 1682–1683, 1683f
    for salivary gland tumors, 1779, 1781
    for skin cancer, 1730
    tracheal tumors, 1995–1996
Radicular cysts, 2097–2098
Radiesse, for soft tissue augmentation,
        3247
Radioactive iodine treatment, 2125
Radiography, 165–166
Radiology, in cerebellopontine angle,
        2584t
Radionuclide scanning
    paraganglioma, 2008
    of thyroid gland, 2118
Radiosurgery, 1690
Radiotherapy. See Chemotherapy
Rapid intraoperative tissue expansion,
        2853–2854, 2857t
Rathke pouch, 257
Real-ear to coupler difference, 1515–1517
Rebound nystagmus, 2685
Receiver in the ear, 2660, 2661f
Reckless behavior, 3259–3260
Reconstructive ladder, 2849, 2850f
Rectus abdominis flap, 2831–2833,
        2832f
Recurrent aphthous stomatitis, 749–751,
        749f–751f, 750t
Recurrent laryngeal nerve, 873,
        1377–1378
    injury, 2124
    unilateral vocal fold paralysis, 1004,
        1005f, 1007

Recurrent respiratory papillomatosis, 1377
  adjuvant medical therapy
    antireflux, 1424
    avastin, 1425
    celecoxib (celebrex), 1423
    cidofovir use, 1423
    cytomegalovirus retinitis, 1421
    Derkay severity score, 1422
    indole-3-carbinol, 1424
    interferon, 1423–1424
    low-risk HPV (type 6)-related disease, 1423
    Mycobacterium bovis, 1424
    quadrivalent HPV vaccine, 1425–1426, 1426f, 1426t
  clinical feature, 1413–1414
  epidemiology
    clinical practice, 1411
    pilot study, 1412
    population rate, 1411
    transmission, 1412–1413, 1413f
  etiology
    connective tissue stroma, 1410, 1411f
    human papillomavirus, 1409–1410
    papilloma lesions, 1410–1411, 1411f
  laser-safe endotracheal tube, 1417
  medical management, 1421, 1423t
  operative technique
    CO_2 laser, 1419–1420
    endoscopic microdebrider, 1418–1419
  patient assessment, 1414–1415, 1414t
  postoperative care, 1420
  preoperative planning, 1417–1418
  repeat flexible fiberoptic laryngoscopy, 1415
  staging, 1420–1421, 1421f–1422f
  surgical management
    distal-chip scopes, 1416
    goals of, 1415
    microdebrider, 1416
    potassium-titanyl-phosphate laser, 1416–1417
    potential surgical modality, 1416, 1416t
    pulse dye lasers, 1416
Red and infrared lasers, 3203
Red cell abnormalities, preoperative management of, 28
Red eye
  conjunctivitis, 224
  episcleritis, 224
  eyelid abnormalities
    blepharitis, 224
    chalazion, 224
    sty, 223–224
  iritis and iridocyclitis, 225
  keratitis, 224
  scleritis, 224
  signs and symptoms, 225t, 226t
  treatment guidelines, 226
Reed-Sternberg cell lymphoma, 2032, 2033f
Reflux finding score, 965, 965t
Reflux pharyngitis, 766
Reflux symptom index, 825, 827t, 964, 964t
Refractive error, 221

Refsum disease, 123–124
Regional nodal staging, malignant melanoma, 1742–1744
Reinke edema, 996, 996f
Rejuvenation, lasers, 3208, 3209f
Relapsing polychondritis, 274–275, 494–495, 495f, 881, 981
  diagnosis, 274
  head and neck manifestations, 274–275
  otologic manifestations, 2523
  treatment, 275
Relaxed open-throat breathing, 1052
Relaxed skin tension lines, 1112, 1112f
Remifentanil, 242
Remote patient monitoring, 3361, 3363
Renal disease
  chronic, 733
  perioperative management of, 40–41
Renal failure
  acute, 41
  chronic
    perioperative management, 40–41
    perioperative management of, 40–41
    postoperative management in, 41
Reparative granuloma, 281
Repose genioglossus tongue suspension, 2231, 2232f
Respiration
  larynx, 951–952
  nose, 365–366
Respiratory distress syndrome, adult, 39
Respiratory papillomatosis, 983–984, 984f
Restylane, for soft tissue augmentation, 3247
Retinal detachment, 222–223
Retinal infarcts, 232
Retinitis pigmentosa, in Usher syndrome, 1543t, 1547, 1633
Retinitis proliferans, 232
Retrognathia
  aging neck, 3137
  chin augmentation, 3181
Retromolar trigone
  oral cavity cancer, 1869
Retropharyngeal abscess, 169, 169f
Retropharyngeal neck dissection, 1811, 1812, 1814, 1824–1825
Retropharyngeal spaces, deep neck infection, 797, 797f, 798f, 806–807, 807f
Revision rhinoplasty
  augmentation graft, 3003–3004
  case presentation
    central tip support restoration, 3033, 3033f–3036f, 3036
    completion rhinoplasty, 3029, 3029f–3032f, 3033
    narrow nose revision, 3039, 3040f–3042f, 3042
    overresected tip and dorsum, 3036, 3037f–3039f, 3039
    severely collapsed nose revision, 3043, 3043f–3049f, 3049
  computer imaging, 3000–3001
  contemporary techniques, 2989–2990
  cosmetic nasal surgery, 2989

  devastated nasal dorsum
    dorsal augmentation, 3023–3025, 3024f
    middle vault, 3021–3022
    osteotomies, 2993f, 3022–3023, 3022f, 3023f
    postsurgical collapse, 3021, 3022f
    spreader graft, 3025–3026
  devastated nasal tip. *See* Nasal tip
  external rhinoplasty approach, 3010–3011
  patient evaluation, 2993
  physical assessment, 2999–3000
  post operative care
    dressing, 3026–3027
    ice, cooling, 3027, 3027f
    postsurgical care and monitoring, 3026
    soft tissue edema, 3026
    steroid injection, 3028
    swelling, 3027–3028
  postsurgical deformities of
    coexisting nasal airway dysfunction, 2991, 2993
    inverted-V deformity, 2991, 2993f
    overresected and overgrafted nose, 2991, 2992f
    patients history, 2991
    physical examination, 2990
    skeletal tissue deficiency, 2990–2991
    tissue limitations, 2990, 2990f
  prognostic indicators, 2997–2999
  psychological aspects
    botched nose job, 2995
    complications, 2994–2995
    internet, treatment advice, 2995
    patient care, 2994
    patient history, 2993
    somatoform and personality disorders, 2996–2997
  skeletal tissue replacement
    autologous tissue graft, 3004
    complications, 3004–3005
    conchal cartilage graft, 3007, 3007f
    costal cartilage graft, 3007–3008, 3008f
    nasal morphology, 3005
    septal cartilage graft, 3005–3006, 3006f
    soft tissue graft, 3008–3010, 3009f
  soft tissue surgical technique, 3011
  surgical deconstruction
    alar retraction, 3012
    en bloc excision, 3013, 3014f
    histology, 3013
    nasal size reduction, 3013–3014
    revision surgeon, 3013
    severe tip cartilage distortion, 3011, 3011f
    skeletal distortion, 3012
    skeletal remnant, 3011
    structural cartilage graft, 3012
  surgical reconstruction, 3002–3003
  treatment for
    finalization, 3001–3002
    planning, 2993

Rhabdomyoma, 983
Rhabdomyosarcoma, 1602
  alveolar, 2373
  orbit, 2072
  pleomorphic, 2373
  sinonasal tract, 2048
Rheologic agents
  sudden sensorineural hearing loss,
    2592
Rheumatic fever, 760
Rheumatoid arthritis, 980–981
  head and neck manifestations, 270
  nonarticular manifestations, 269, 270t
  otologic manifestations, 2523
  physical findings, 269
Rheumatologic diseases
  inflammatory muscle disease,
    273–274
  mixed connective tissue disease, 275
  relapsing polychondritis, 274–275
  rheumatoid arthritis, 269–271
  Sjögren syndrome, 271–272
  systemic lupus erythematosus,
    267–269
  systemic sclerosis, 272–273
  vasculitides. See Vasculitides
Rhinion, nasal dorsum, 2953
Rhinitis, 2179
  allergic. See Allergic rhinitis
  atrophic, 482
  capsaicin, nonallergic, 472
  decongestants, 472
  definition, 509
  hormone-induced, 480–481, 481t
  ipratropium bromide, 472
  mast cells, 399
Rhinitis medicamentosa, 477t, 479–480,
    479f
Rhinitis sicca, inferior turbinate hypertro-
    phy, 618
Rhinomanometry, 364, 366, 456, 456t
Rhinometry, acoustic, 366
Rhinophyma, 3208, 3209f, 3215, 3215f
  treatment of, 3226
Rhinoplasty
  anatomy, 2941, 2942f
  nasal analysis, 2946
    base view, 2950
    facial proportion, 2947, 2947f
    frontal view, 2948, 2948f
    oblique view, 2948–2950, 2949f,
      2950f
    patient evaluation, 2947
  nasal and facial angle, 2942–2943,
    2942f, 2943f
  revision rhinoplasty. See Revision rhino-
    plasty
  surgical approaches
    disadvantages of, 2946
    external/endonasal, 2943, 2944f,
      2946
    guidelines for, 2943, 2944t
    retrograde and transcartilaginous,
      2946
  surgical incisions
    full transfixion, 2945
    hemitransfixion, 2945, 2946f

    Killian incision, 2945, 2946f
    nasal-tip, 2943, 2945f
    transcolumellar and intercartilagi-
      nous, 2944, 2945f
Rhinoscleroma, 284
Rhinosinusitis
  acute, 509–522, 794
    bacterial
      bacterial infection, 512
      medical management of, 517–519
      microbiology, 512
    clinical courses, 519
    clinical presentation, 513
    complications
      acute bacterial rhinosinusitis,
        519–520
      extracranial, 520–521
      intracranial, 520, 520f
    definition, 509
    economic burden of, 510
    endoscopic evaluation, 515, 515t
    epidemiology
      incidence and prevalence,
        509–510
      predisposing factors and contribu-
        tors, 510t
    imaging modalities, 515t
      computed tomography, 516
      magnetic resonance imaging, 516
      ultrasound, 515
      X-ray, 516
    pathophysiology and microbiology
      acute bacterial rhinosinusitis, 512
      acute fulminant invasive fungal
        sinusitis, 512–513, 513f
      acute viral rhinosinusitis, 511–512,
        511t
      infection, 511
      inflammation, 511
      nosocomial acute bacterial rhinosi-
        nusitis, 512
    pathophysiology of, 535–536
    patient history, 513–514, 514t
    pediatric patients, 521–522
    physical examination, 514–515
    temporal classification, 510t
    treatment, 516–519
    treatment of, 543–544
    viral
      etiology, 511, 511t
      history, 511–512
      medical management of, 517–518
      pathogenesis, 511
  bony complications, 583, 583f
  chronic
    and allergic rhinitis, 538
    asthma, 551
    computed tomography in, 541–542,
      542f
    costs of, 353
    diagnosis, 586
    diagnostic correlates of, 543
    diagnostic criteria, 540, 540t
    endoscopic sinus surgery. See
      Endoscopic sinus surgery
    environmental factors in, 537–538
    genetic factors, 538

    medical management
      antibiotics, 588–589
      anticholinergics, 591
      antihistamines, 590
      decongestants, 590
      immunotherapy, 591
      leukotriene inhibitors, 591
      macrolide antibiotics, 591
      mucolytics, 591–592
      steroids, 587–588
      surfactants, 592
    with nasal polyposis
      classification and features, 526t
      histopathology, 525
      pathophysiology of, 525
    olfactory loss, 373
    pathophysiology of, 536–539, 537f
    physiologic factors in, 539
    prevalence, 586
    signs and symptoms, 551t
    sinonasal methicillin-resistant
      Staphylococcus aureus
      antibiotics, 589–590
      prevalence, 589
      saline irrigation, 590
    staging systems, 586–587
    staging systems for, 542–543, 543t
    structural factors in, 538, 538f
    symptoms and clinical signs, 586
    treatment of
      anti-inflammatory therapy, 546–547
      antimicrobial therapy, 544–546, 545t
  complementary and alternative medi-
    cine, 325
  incidence of, 535
  intracranial complications
    anatomic considerations, 580
    diagnosis and classification, 580, 580f
    epidural abscess, 580–581, 581f
    intracerebral abscess, 581–582
    meningitis, 582–583
    prevention, 584
    risk factors, 579
    subdural abscess, 581, 581f
    symptoms, 579–580
    venous sinus thrombosis, 582
  invasive fungal
    chronic, 562–563
      clinical presentation, 563
      diagnosis, 563
      imaging, 563
      pathology, 563
      prognosis, 564
      treatment, 563
    clinical presentation and diagnosis
      biopsy and frozen section studies,
        559–560
      computed tomography, 559
      fungal culture, 560
      immune function, 558–559
      nasal endoscopy, 559
      signs and symptoms, 559, 559f
    pathology, 560–561
    prognosis, 562
    radiology, 560, 560f
    treatment, 561–562
  nonpolypoid, 535–547

orbital complications
  anatomic considerations, 573
  cavernous sinus thrombophlebitis, 576–577
  Chandler classification, 573, 574f
  microbiology, 577–578, 578t
  orbital abscess, 576
  orbital cellulitis, 575–576, 576f
  preseptal infections, 573, 575, 576f
  radiography, 577
  subperiosteal abscess, 575, 576f
  treatment, 578–579, 579f
pediatric
  adenoidectomy, 1459–1460, 1460f
  antral lavage, 1460
  bacteriology, 1458, 1458t
  chronic pediatric sinusitis, 1459t
  differential diagnosis, 1455, 1456t
  ethmoidectomy, 1460–1461, 1461f, 1462f
  etiology, 1456–1457
  facial growth, 1461
  guided imaging in, 1462f
  inferior meatal antrostomy, 1460
  intracranial complications, 1464
  medical management, 1458–1459, 1459t
  middle meatal antrostomy, 1460
  nasal antral windows, 1460
  orbital complications, 1461–1463, 1463f, 1464f
  other diagnostic aids, 1456–1457, 1456t, 1457f
  persistent sinus disease, 1461, 1463t
  physical examination, 1455–1456
  signs and symptoms, 1455, 1456t
signs and symptoms of, 540t
Rhinosporidiosis, 291–292
Rhinotomy, 2087–2088
Rhinovirus, 1433
Rhombic flaps
  in cutaneous nasal defects, 2877
Rhytidectomy, 3136
  adjunctive procedures to, 3103–3104
  anatomy of aging face, 3104–3105, 3104f
  assessing candidacy, 3107–3108
  complications
    alopecia, 3127, 3128f
    hematoma, 3125, 3127
    incision problems, 3127
    nerve injury, 3125, 3126f
  deep plane lift
    advantage of, 3118
    dissection, 3119
    earlobe and tragus, 3120, 3120f–3122f
    flap closure, 3120
    platysmaplasty, 3118–3119, 3118f
    ptotic subcutaneous fat, 3119
  general considerations in, 3103–3104
  operative stage
    flap elevation, 3116, 3116f
    submentoplasty, 3114, 3115f, 3116, 3116f
    superficial musculo-aponeurotic system suspension, 3116–3117, 3117f
  postoperative care, 3124–3125
  preoperative planning and evaluation

face structure, 3108, 3109f, 3110f
facial nerve and muscle, 3108–3109, 3110f
hyoid bone and suprahyoid musculature, 3108, 3110f
patient preparation, 3109
smoking history, 3109
special considerations
  male face-lift, 3122–3123, 3123f
  secondary and revision face-lift, 3123–3124
surgery
  anatomy of, 3105–3106, 3106f
  anesthesia, 3111
  incision for, 3111–3113, 3111f–3113f
  marking for, 3111
  patient history, 3106–3107
Rhytids
  forehead lift and, 3057
  glabellar, Botox injections in, 3242
  lateral periorbital, Botox injections in, 3242–3243, 3243f
  in transverse forehead, Botox injections in, 3242, 3242f
  in vertical lip, Botox injections in, 3243
Rieger flap, in cutaneous nasal defects, 2880
Riga-Fede disease, 754
Right glomus vagale, 172, 172f
Right internal carotid artery pseudoaneurysm
  computed tomography, 147–148, 148f
Right vestibular schwannoma, 150, 152, 152f
Robin sequence, 1631, 1631f
Robot master hand controller, 50, 50f
Robot stereo viewer, 50, 50f
Rocker deformity, nasal dorsum, 2960
Romberg position, 2722
Romberg test, 2695, 2696f
Root cause analysis, 3263–3264, 3264t
Rosai-Dorfman disease, 1598–1599
Rotation-induced nystagmus, 2687
Rubella, 5

S
Saccade, 2304–2305, 2686
Saccharin test, 367, 456
Saddle-nose deformity, 2960
Saline spray
  nonallergic rhinitis, 472
Saliva
  functions
    antibacterial activity, 697
    buffering action, 697–698
    lubrication and protection, 698
    taste and digestion, 698
    tooth integrity maintenance, 698
  secretion of, 698
Salivary fistula, 1782
Salivary gland(s)
  adenoma
    pleomorphic adenoma, 186f
    warthin tumor, 186f
  anatomy of, 762t, 1760, 1761t
  biopsy of
    fine-needle aspiration, 1769, 1769t
    surgical, 1770

carcinoma
  acinic cell, 192f
  adenoid cystic, 192f
  epithelial-myoepithelial, 192f
  mucoepidermoid, 193f
  polymorphous low-grade adenocarcinoma, 193f
embryology
  embryogenesis, 691, 692f
  lymphatic system, 691
  minor salivary glands, 697
  parotid gland. See Parotid gland
  sublingual gland, 696–697
  submandibular gland, 695–696, 696f
imaging, 699, 699f
infections, 138
lymphoma of, 1768, 2037–2039, 2038f
major, 762t, 1760, 1761t
minor, 762t, 1760, 1761t
nonneoplastic diseases of, 702–714
physiology
  functions, 697–698
  microstructure, 697
  salivary flow rates, 698–699
  secretion, 698
physiology of, 762t, 1760, 1761t
sialendoscopy, 700
Salivary gland disease
  aberrant salivary gland tissue, 713
  acute suppurative sialadenitis
    bimanual palpation, 703
    causative microbes, 703
    incidence, 702
    salivary stasis, 702
    treatment, 703
  autoimmune conditions, Sjögren syndrome, 1475
  benign
    basal cell adenoma, 1764
    oncocytoma, 1763–1764, 1763f
    pleomorphic adenoma, 1760–1762, 1762f
    Warthin Tumor, 1762, 1763f
  cheilitis glandularis, 713
  chemotherapy, 1781, 1781t
  classification of, 1760, 1761t
  complications of, 713–714
  diagnosis and management, 714t
  differential diagnosis of, 1770
  etiology of, 1678
  glandular hypertrophy, 713
  granulomatous infections
    Cat-scratch disease, 704–705
    chronic sialadenitis, 706–707, 707f
    cystic lesions, 710–711
    juvenile recurrent parotitis, 707–708, 708f
    sarcoidosis, 705
    sialendoscopy, 709–710, 709f, 710f
    sialolithiasis, 708–709, 708f
    Sjögren syndrome, 705–706, 705f, 706f
    tuberculosis, 704
  history in, 1768–1769, 1768f
  imaging, 1769–1770, 1769f, 1770f
  incidence of, 1762t
  inflammatory conditions

Salivary gland disease (*Continued*)
  acute sialadenitis, 1467–1469
  chronic inflammation, 1469–1470
  diagnosis and management, 1468*t*
 of lip, 1791, 1794
 location of, 1784
 malignant
   acinic cell carcinoma, 1765–1766,
     1765*f*
   adenocarcinoma, 1766
   adenoid cystic carcinoma, 1765, 1765*f*
   carcinoma ex pleomorphic adenoma,
     1766–1767, 1766*f*
   lymphoma, 1768
   mucoepidermoid carcinoma,
     1764–1765, 1764*f*
   polymorphous low-grade adenocar-
     cinoma
   primary squamous cell carcinoma,
     1767
   salivary duct carcinoma, 1767–1768,
     1767*f*
   sarcoma, 1768
   undifferentiated carcinoma, 1767
 mesenchymal tumors. *See* Mesenchymal
   tumors
 metastases, 1784
 necrotizing sialometaplasia, 713
 pediatric, 1760
 physical examination, 1769
 pneumoparotitis, 713
 prognosis of, 1767, 1784
 radiation injury
   radioactive iodine-induced sialadeni-
     tis, 711
   sialadenosis, 712–713
   trauma, 711–712, 712*f*
 radiation therapy, 1779, 1781
 risk factor for, 1762, 1768, 1782
 sialorrhea, 1475–1477
 surgery for
   minor salivary gland, 1779
   for parotid tumors, 1770
   for submandibular gland tumors,
     1778–1779
 trauma, 1477
 viral sialadenitis
   HIV, 704
   mumps, 703–704
Sampling population, for clinical data,
  97–98, 97*t*
Sarcoidosis, 281–283, 282*f*, 539, 705,
  748–749, 982, 982*f*, 1598
 cerebellopontine angle, 2580
 childhood
   Marshall syndrome, 754
   traumatic eosinophilic granuloma,
     754
 differential diagnosis, 492, 492*f*
 erythema multiforme, 754
 otologic manifestations, 2522
 physical examination, 491–492, 492*f*
 sinonasal manifestations, 491, 492
 treatment, 493
Sarcoma, 1602, 2074
 salivary gland, 1768
 of temporal bone, 2374

Scalp, 2084–2085
 anatomy of, 3, 4*f*
 implants for, 2789–2790
Scalpels, 21–22
Scapular and parascapular flaps, fasciocutaneous and osteofasciocutaneous, 2839–2842
Scar(s)
 camouflage, 2859–2869
   adjunctive nonsurgical interventions
     direct camouflage, 2868
     intralesional injections, 2866
     resurfacing techniques, 2866–2868
     topical agents, 2868–2869
   dermabrasion for, 2867, 2867*f*, 2868*f*
   excisional techniques for, 2863–2864
   laser resurfacing for, 2866–2867
   scar irregularization for, 2861–2863,
     2862*f*–2866*f*
   scar types, 2860
   soft tissue fillers for, 2868
   surgical techniques
     flaps, 2861–2863
     grafts, 2864
     prevention, 2865–2866
     serial excision, 2863–2864
     surgical planning and scar reloca-
       tion, 2860–2861, 2861*f*
     tissue expansion, 2864
   wound healing process
     inflammatory phase, 2859
     proliferative phase, 2859
     remodeling phase, 2860
 depressed, management of, 2860
 hypertrophic, 3217, 3217*f*
   treatment of, 3227
 techniques of, 2860–2861
 widening of, following forehead lift, 3071
Scarlet fever, 759
Scheibe malformation, 1536
Schirmer test, 221
Schneiderian papilloma
 exophytic, 186*f*
 inverted, 187*f*
 oncocytic, 187*f*
Schwannoma, 985, 2069
 facial nerve, 2377
 jugular foramen, 2377
 of temporal bone
   categories of, 2377
   diagnosis of, 2377–2378
 trigeminal, 2377
 vestibular, 2377
Scintigraphy
 99mTc pertechnetate, 163
 nuclear scintigraphy, 161
 parathyroid, 162–163
 somatostatin, 163
 thyroid, 161–162, 162*f*, 162*t*
Scleritis, 224
Screw application
 skeletal facial trauma, rigid fixation,
   1156–1157, 1157*f*
Sebaceous hyperplasia, 3215
 treatment of, 3226
Seborrheic keratoses, 3212
 treatment of, 3224

Secondary ciliary dyskinesia, 367–368
Secondary headache
 carotidynia and carotid artery dissection,
   313
 craniofacial or cervical disorders, 314
 neuropathic pain
   glossopharyngeal neuralgia, 312
   occipital neuralgia, 312
   trigeminal neuralgia, 312, 312*t*
 nonvascular intracranial disorders,
   313–314
 signs and symptoms, 310*t*, 311*t*
 sinogenic pain, 310–312
 Sluder syndrome, 313
 subdural hematoma, 313
 temporal arteritis, 313
 temporomandibular joint syndrome,
   314
 vascular disorders, 313, 313*t*
Secondary intention healing, of cutaneous
   nasal defects, 2876
Sedatives
 benzodiazepines, 65, 65*t*
 dexmetomidine, 66
 propofol, 66
 ventilator days and ICU length of stay,
   64–65
Selective serotonin reuptake inhibitors,
  208
Self-directed learning
 activity oriented, 3350
 analyzing process, 3351
 goal oriented, 3350
 learning oriented, 3350
 personal action, 3350
 promoting
   computerized learning modules,
     3351
   computerized self-directed learning
     modules, 3352
   identifying needs, 3351–3352
   portfolio projects, 3351, 3352
   skills and competencies, 3350*t*
   undergraduate curriculum,
     3352–3353
 walkabout model, 3350
Sella turcica, 257
Semicircular canal dehiscence, 2610
Semioccluded vocal tract, voice therapy,
  1053
Senescence, 298
Senile chin deformity, 3181
Senile keratosis, 1726
Senile macular degeneration, 222
Sensitization, aesthetic self-assessment,
   peer Group comparison and
   avoidance behaviors, 2758
Sensorineural hearing loss
 causes of, 1532
 definition of, 1532
 diagnostic evaluation of, 1536–1537
 inner ear anomaly
   cochlear aplasia, 1535
   cochlear hypoplasia, 1535
   intracochlear partition type I and
     type II, 1534
   labyrinthine malformations, 1534

large vestibular aqueduct, 1535
Mondini malformation, 1534
Pendred syndrome, 1535
membranous anomalies
Alexander malformation, 1536
Bing-Siebenmann malformation, 1536
Scheibe malformation, 1536
middle and inner ear structural anomaly
branchio-oto-renal syndromes, 1533–1534
CHARGE, 1533
congenital stapes disorders, 1533
external auditory canal atresia, 1533
facial palsy, 1533
perilymphatic fistula, 1534
very low birth weight, NICU infants
auditory neuropathy spectrum disorder, 1533
hyperbilirubinemia, 1533
incidence of, 1532
vestibular anomaly, 1536
Sensory impairment
facial paralysis, 1299
haemophilus influenzae type B, 1298
multichannel cochlear implantation, 1298
otolaryngologist, 1297, 1298t
pediatric otolaryngologists, 1299
vertiginous disorder, 1299
vocal fold paralysis, 1299
Sensory loss, aspiration in, 861
Sensory nerve, injury to, during forehead lift, 3070
Sensory organization test, 2309, 2310f
Sentinel lymph node biopsy, 1814–1815
pathologic analysis of, 1748
potential therapeutic benefit, 1748
surgical management of, 1745, 1746f
technical considerations
handheld gamma probe, 1748
localization and mapping of, 1746
lymphazurin, 1746
radioactivity use, 1746
SPECT-CT, 1746, 1747f
Septal deviation, nasal obstruction in, 363–364
Septal extension graft
caudal excess nasal deformity, 3017
caudal septum placement, 3015–3016, 3015f, 3016f
overresected nasal tip, 3016, 3016f
rigid stability, 3018
uses of, 3015
Septodermoplasty, 507
Septoplasty, 2979–2980
cartilaginous septum, 615
clinical indications for, 614t
complications, 616–617
endoscopic, 615, 616f
extracorporeal, 616, 616f
Freer's hemitransfixion incision, 615, 615f
hemostatic agent, 615
Killian incision, 615
mucoperichondrial flap elevation, 615, 615f
outcomes, 616

septal anatomy, 614, 614f
Severe reinke edema, voice therapy, 1054
Shave biopsy, 3220f
Shield grafts, nasal tip surgery, 2974–2975, 2975f
Shikani optical stylet, 901, 901f
Shock, in trauma patients, 1097–1098
cardiogenic, 1099–1100, 1100f
hypovolemic, 1098–1099
neurogenic, 1099
Shprintzen syndrome, 1631–1632, 1631f
Sialadenitis
acute
bacterial, 1467
neonatal, 1467–1468
viral, 1468–1469
acute suppurative
bimanual palpation, 703
causative microbes, 703
incidence, 702
salivary stasis, 702
treatment, 703
chronic, 706–707, 707f
radioactive iodine-induced, 711
Sialadenosis, 712–713
Sialectasis, in children, 1469
Sialendoscopy, 700
Sialography, 164–165, 165f
Sialolithiasis, 1469–1470
Sialometaplasia, necrotizing
versus minor salivary gland tumor, 1770
Sialo-odontogenic cyst, 2099–2100, 2100f
Sialorrhea
salivary gland disease, 1475–1477
Sickle cell disease, 28
Side-lying posture, 839–840
sIgE testing, 418–419, 419f
Sigmoid sinus
diverticula, 2607
thrombophlebitis, 2406–2407
Silicone
for management of scars, 2868
for soft tissue augmentation, 3248–3249
Silver-Russell syndrome, 121
Single lens reflex photography, 2777, 2778
Single-nucleotide polymorphisms, 460
Single-sided deafness, 2640. See also Hearing loss
Sinogenic pain
causes of, 310, 311
rhinosinusitis, 311, 311t
treatment, 312
Sinonasal disease
allergy testing
in vitro skin testing, 453–454
in vivo skin testing, 452–453, 452t
ciliary testing
ciliary motility analysis, 457
ciliary ultrastructure analysis, 457
genetic analysis, 457
nasal nitric oxide, 456
primary ciliary dyskinesia, 456
saccharin test, 456
in-office CT scanning
advantages, 458
disadvantages, 458, 458t

versus traditional sinus CT scans, 457–458
types, 457, 458t
laboratory investigations
cystic fibrosis testing, 450–451
infectious testing, 451
primary immunodeficiency testing, 451
systemic inflammatory disease testing, 451–452, 452t
nasal airway patency evaluation
acoustic rhinometry, 455–456
rhinomanometry, 456, 456t
olfactory testing
electrophysiologic olfactory tests, 455
psychological olfactory tests, 454–455
radiographic imaging, 446–447
computed tomography, 449, 449t
magnetic resonance imaging, 449–450, 450t
plain films (Roentgenographs), 447, 449
rigid sinonasal endoscopy, 446, 447t
Sinonasal lymphoma, 2037
Sinonasal papilloma
exophytic Schneiderian papilloma, 186f
inverted Schneiderian papilloma, 187f
oncocytic Schneiderian papilloma, 187f
Sinonasal tract
anatomy of, 361f
embryology of, 359
and external environment, 369
Sinonasal undifferentiated carcinoma, 194f, 2048
Sinus(es)
anatomy of, 8, 8f
neoplasms
benign epithelial tumors, 2045–2046, 2046t, 2047t
benign nonepithelial tumors, 2048
biopsy, 2049
chemotherapy, 2051, 2053, 2057t
diagnosis, 2044–2045, 2045t
emergencies in, 2061–2062, 2061t
ethmoid sinus, 2055
frontal sinus, 2057
malignant epithelial tumors, 2046–2048, 2047t, 2048t
malignant nonepithelial tumors, 2048–2049
maxillary antrum, 2063
metastatic tumors, 2049
nasal cavity, 2063
pathology, 2045, 2045t
postsurgical rehabilitation, 2050
radiation therapy, 2050–2051
sphenoid sinus, 2055, 2057
squamous cell carcinoma, 2053
staging, 2049, 2050t
surgical resection, 2050, 2051f–2056f
tumors management, 2056f, 2057–2058, 2057t
Sinus obstruction, causes of, 538
Sinus surgery, 50, 644t
anterior skull base
choanal bridge, 642, 643f

Sinus surgery (*Continued*)
 cribriform plate, 640–641
 fovea ethmoidalis, 641–642
 Keros catagorization, 642, 642*f*
 maxillary and ethmoid sinuses,
  642–643, 643*f*
 middle turbinate, 642
 planum sphenoidale, 640
 sphenoid sinus, 641
brain and blood vessel injury, 658
cerebrospinal fluid fistula, 655–656
endoscopic surgical procedures
 balloon catheter dilation procedures,
  649
 frontal sinus surgery, 649
 image-guided endoscopic sinus surgery, 650
 middle meatal antrostomy, 647–648,
  648*f*
 powered endoscopic sinus surgery,
  649–650, 650*f*
 sphenoidotomy, 648–649, 648*f*, 649*f*
external approaches, 604–611
growth and sinus development abnormality, 658, 660
hemorrhage, 656–657
olfactory loss, 658
open surgical procedures
 Caldwell-Luc operation, 644–645
 frontal sinus trephination, 646
 inferior meatal antrostomy,
  644, 644*t*
 intranasal ethmoidectomy, 645
 open frontal sinus surgery, 647
 sphenoidotomy, 646, 646*f*
 transantral and external ethmoidectomy, 645–646
orbital complications
 bindness, 653–655
 diplopia, 655
 epiphora, 655
 hematoma, 650–653
paresthesia and hypesthesia, 658
subcutaneous emphysema, 655
synechia, 657–658
Sinusitis, 137, 1456
 chronic
  pediatric rhinosinusitis, 1459*t*
  definition, 509
 in Kartagener syndrome, 1629
Sistrunk procedure, 1612, 1612*f*
Sjögren syndrome, 164, 165*f*, 271–272,
  496, 497*f*, 1475
 acquired immunodeficiency syndrome-
  related complex, 705
 clinical manifestations of, 271
 diagnostic criteria, 705
 early lymphocytic infiltrate pattern, 272
 head and neck manifestations, 272
 imaging, 705, 706*f*
 pathophysiology, 705
 primary and secondary form, 271
 treatment, 272, 705–706
Skeletal facial trauma, rigid fixation
 bone healing, 1153–1154
 complications, 1167–1169, 1169*t*
 fracture reduction, 1159–1160, 1160*f*

incisions and exposure, 1162–1163,
  1162*f*–1163*f*
instrumentation, 1158–1159
lag screw, 1157, 1158*f*
occlusion, 1161, 1161*f*
panfacial fracture
 anatomic reduction, 1165
 dimensions, 1165, 1166*f*
 emergency, 1163, 1164*t*
 fracture fixation, 1165, 1166*f*
 history and physical examination, 1163
 nasoethmoid complex, 1167
 orbital floor continuity, 1166–1167
 orbital/periorbital fracture, 1164
 radiologic evaluation, 1164
 skull base, 1165, 1165*f*
 subcranial approach, 1164–1165
 zygomatic arch fracture, 1166
pathophysiology and classification,
  1154, 1154*f*
plate application, 1157–1158, 1158*t*
principles of, 1155, 1155*f*–1156*f*
rationale, 1154–1155
screw application, 1156–1157, 1157*f*
soft tissue loss, 1167, 1168*f*
terminology, 1155–1156
Skew deviation, dizziness, 2690
Skin
 of forehead, 3054, 3054*f*
 nasal, 2924
 premalignant lesions, 1726–1727, 1727*f*
Skin cancer, 1723–1737
 anatomic location of, 1727, 1728*t*
 cryosurgery in, 1730
  curettage with electrodesiccation, for
   skin, 1730
  laser therapy, 1731
  Mohs surgery, 1731
  photodynamic therapy, 1730–1731
  radiation therapy, 1730
  reconstructive surgery in, 1733–1734
 epidemiology of, 1723
 etiology of, 1723–1724
 evaluation of, 1723
 excisional surgery in, 1731
 human papillomavirus and, 1724
 merkel cell carcinoma, 1735–1736
 metastases from
  nodal, 1735
 premalignant lesions, 1726–1727, 1727*f*
 prognosis of, 1728
 recurrent, 1729–1730
 risk factors for, 1723–1724
 squamous cell
  evaluation, 1725
  histopathology of, 1725–1726
 TNM classification of, 1727
 treatment of, 1730–1735
 tumor behavior in, 1727–1728
Skin grafts, in cutaneous nasal defects,
  2877, 2877*t*
Skin prick tests, 415–416, 415*f*
Skin resurfacing
 Hetter chemical peel
  basic science of, 3191–3193, 3192*t*
  complications, 3195, 3198
  historical background of, 3189, 3190*t*

 patient selection, 3189–3190, 3190*t*,
  3191*t*
 postoperative care, 3194–3195,
  3195*f*–3197*f*
 prepeel preparation, 3190–3191
 technique of, 3193–3194, 3193*t*,
  3194*f*
lasers, facial plastic surgery, 3208, 3209*f*
Skin substitutes, 53
Skin tags, treatment of, 3227
Skin-appendage tumors, 3215–3216,
  3216*f*
Skull
 bony lesions of, 292–295
 implants for, 2790
Skull base
 defects of, microvascular reconstructive
  approaches to, 2846–2847
 endoscopic surgery, 2077
 fibrous dysplasia, 143, 143*f*
 lateral
  and ear, neoplasms of, 2358–2382
  metastatic disease, 2381
 neoplasms, 2058, 2059*f*–2060*f*, 2061
 surgery of, facial nerve monitoring during, 2327–2328
 tumors of, facial nerve and, 2515–2516
Sleep apnea
 obstructive
  anesthetic complications, 2226
  behavioral modifications, 2185–2186
  conditions causing, 2221*t*
  consequences of, 2220–2221
  continuous positive airway pressure,
   2224
  hypersomnia, 2186
  hypopharyngeal procedures
   direct tissue excision, 2213
   epiglottis posterior displacement/
    retroflexion, 2213–2214
   genioglossus advancement, 2211,
    2212*f*
   hyoid suspension procedure, 2211,
    2212*f*
   lingual tonsillectomy, 2213, 2215*f*
   palate surgery, 2210, 2211*t*
   submucosal tongue radiofrequency,
    2213, 2214*f*
   tongue advancement, 2211
   tongue reduction procedures, 2213
   tongue stabilization, 2213
  hypoxemia, 2186
  insomnia, 2186
  medical therapy, 2183
  medical treatment, 2224, 2224*f*
  nasal obstruction treatment, 2183
  nasal surgery
   impact on sleep, 2193–2194, 2194*t*
   nasal resistance, 2192–2193
   patients evaluation, 2193
   symptoms of, 2192–2193
  oral appliances
   adherence, 2182–2183
   effectiveness, 2181–2182, 2182*f*
   mandibular repositioning appli-
    ance, 2180, 2181*f*
   side effects and complications, 2183

thermoplastic splints, 2180–2181
tongue retaining device, 2180, 2181*f*
oropharyngeal airway, obstruction
　cine magnetic resonance imaging,
　　2227–2228, 2228*f*, 2229*f*, 2230*t*
　drug-induced sleep endoscopy,
　　2227
　Mueller maneuver grading system,
　　2226–2227
　persistent nasal airway obstruction,
　　2227
　radiographic study, 2227
oropharyngeal exercises, 2185
outcome assessment
　clinical outcomes, 2209, 2209*t*
　sleep testing outcomes, 2209–2210
oxygen therapy, 2185
palate surgery
　adult tonsillectomy, 2197–2198
　diagnosis and evaluation, 2196,
　　2196*f*
　expansion sphincter pharyngo-
　　plasty, 2199–2200, 2200*f*
　failure of, 2199
　palatopharyngoplasty, 2197
　transpalatal advancement pharyngo-
　　plasty, 2198–2199, 2198*f*, 2199*f*
　upper pharynx anatomy, 2195–2196
　uvulopalatopharyngoplasty, 2197
positional therapy, 2184–2185
positive airway pressure
　adherence, 2178–2179
　effectiveness, 2176–2178
　interfaces, 2176
　modality, 2174–2175
　pathophysiology of, 2174, 2175*f*
　side effects and complications, 2179
　titration methods, 2175–2176
postoperative evaluation, 2226
preoperative evaluation, 2225–2226
skeletal surgery
　maxillomandibular advancement,
　　2214, 2215*f*, 2216
snoring
　minimally invasive techniques and
　　procedures, 2200–2203
Stanford protocol, 2192
surgical evaluation
　airway evaluation techniques, 2206,
　　2207*t*
　axial T2-weighted MRI, 2208, 2208*f*
　drug-induced sleep endoscopy,
　　2208, 2208*f*, 2209*f*
　fiberoptic endoscopy, 2207–2208
　history and physical examination,
　　2206
　lateral cephalometry, 2207
　mandible and dentition, positions
　　and dimensions, 2207
　modified Mallampati position, 2207
　obesity and weight gain, 2206–2207
surgical treatment
　adenoidectomy, 2225
　adenotonsillectomy, 2225, 2225*f*
treatment of
　anatomic locations, upper airway
　　obstruction, 2230, 2231*f*

medical therapy, 2230
　nasal surgery, 2230–2233
　oral appliances, 2229
　oropharyngeal scarring and stenosis,
　　2230
　positional therapy, 2230, 2230*f*
　positive airway pressure therapy,
　　2228
　weight loss, 2229
　weight loss, 2184, 2184*f*
Sleep disorders
　airway, radiologic evaluation
　　computed tomography, 2167, 2167*f*
　　fluoroscopy, 2167
　　magnetic resonance imaging, 2167,
　　　2168*f*
　　somnofluoroscopy, 2167
　　X-ray cephalometry, 2166–2167, 2167*f*
　circadian rhythm disorders
　　delayed sleep phase type, 2153
　　jet lag type, 2153
　　shift work type, 2153
　diagnosis of, 2168–2170, 2168*f*, 2169*t*
　inadequate sleep, 2152–2153
　insomnia, 2153
　international classification of, 2149,
　　2151*t*
　narcolepsy, 2153–2154
　patient evaluation
　　abdominal obesity, 2166
　　age and gender, 2160
　　body mass index, 2164, 2164*t*
　　dental occlusion, 2165, 2166*f*
　　drug-induced sleep endoscopy, 2166
　　ESS questionnaire, 2155, 2156*t*
　　Friedman clinical staging system, 2165
　　head and neck examination, 2165
　　height and weight, 2160
　　history, 2154
　　Mallampati rating, oral cavity, 2165,
　　　2165*f*
　　nasopharyngeal endoscopy, 2166
　　nocturnal awakening, 2155
　　patient's daily schedule, 2155
　　review of systems, 2159–2160
　　sleep diary, 2155, 2156*f*
　　sleep hygiene and quality, 2154, 2155*t*
　　snoring, 2154–2155
　　standardized history and physical
　　　form, 2157, 2157*f*, 2158*f*
　　tonsil size, 2165, 2165*f*
　　waist-hip ratio, 2166
　rapid eye movement, 2154
　restless legs syndrome, 2154
　sleep-disordered breathing
　　central sleep apnea/complex sleep
　　　apnea, 2152
　　obesity-hypoventilation syndrome,
　　　2152
　　obstructive sleep apnea, 2150–2152,
　　　2152*t*
　treatment of, 2170–2171
Sleep-disordered breathing
　adenotonsillar disease, in children, 1438
　conditions causing, 2221*t*
　diagnosis
　　flexible laryngoscopy, 2223

history, 2221, 2221*t*
　nasopharyngoscopy, 2223
　physical examination, 2221–2223,
　　2222*f*, 2222*t*
　polysomnography, 2223–2224, 2223*t*
　epidemiology, 2220, 2221*t*
Sluder syndrome, 313
Small agger cel, 677*f*
Smell identification test, 375, 454–455,
　455*f*
Smith-Lemli-Opitz syndrome, 1640
Smoking
　nicotine, 329
　prevalence, 329
　secondhand smoke, 330
　socioeconomic status, 329
　tobacco. *See* Tobacco use
Smooth pursuit, dizziness, 2686–2687
Sniffing sticks testing, 454–455
Snoring
　obstructive sleep apnea, 2191–2192
　minimally invasive techniques and pro-
　　cedures
　　anterior palatoplasty, 2202–2203
　　coblation techniques, 2201–2202
　　factors influencing, 2201
　　injection snoreplasty, 2202
　　mortality of, 2201
　　pillar soft palate implants, 2202
　　prevalence of, 2201
　　radiofrequency tissue ablation,
　　　2201–2202
Soft tissue
　augmentation, 3244–3250
　　autografts, 3245
　　autologous fat, 3249
　　calcium hydroxylapatite, 3247, 3247*f*
　　homografts, 3245
　　hyaluronic acid products, 3245*f*,
　　　3246–3247
　　poly-L-lactic acid, 3247–3248, 3248*f*
　　polymethyl methacrylate, 3248
　　silicone, 3248–3249
　　xenographs, 3245
　reconstruction of, following oropharyn-
　　geal surgery, 1912–1913, 1912*f*
　subcutaneous, nasal, 2924
　xenografts, 3245
Soft-tissue defects, external, microvascular
　reconstructive approaches to,
　2847
Soft tissue fillers, 2868
Soft tissue injuries
　anatomical location
　　auricle, 1123–1126, 1123*f*–1125*f*
　　cheek and parotid, 1120–1121, 1121*f*,
　　　1122*f*
　　eyelids and lacrimal system,
　　　1117–1119, 1117*f*–1119*f*
　　facial nerve injury, 1121–1123
　　forehead, temple and brow,
　　　1115–1117, 1116*f*
　　lips and chin, 1126, 1126*f*
　　nose, 1119–1120
　　scalp, 1114–1115, 1114*f*
　etiology, 1108
　evaluation, 1108–1109

Soft tissue injuries (*Continued*)
laceration repair
drains, 1114
postoperative care, 1113–1114
suture techniques, 1112–1113, 1112*f*,
1113*f*
mechanism of, 1108
pediatric, 1128–1129
special considerations for
bites, 1127–1128
burns, 1128
wounds
classification, 1109–1110
management, 1110–1112, 1111*f*, 1112*t*
Solar keratosis, 1726
Solitary fibrous tumor, 2073–2074
Solitary median maxillary central incisor,
1316
Space-based approach, image interpretation
buccal space, 170, 170*f*
carotid sheath, 172–173
differential diagnoses, 168*t*
masticator space, 170, 171*f*
parapharyngeal space, 170–172, 171*f*,
172*f*
parotid space, 173
pharyngeal mucosal space, 168
posterior triangle space, 173, 173*f*
prevertebral space, 173, 173*f*
retropharyngeal space, 168–169, 169*f*
sublingual space, 169, 169*f*
submandibular space, 169–170, 170*f*
visceral space, 173
Spasmodic dysphonia, 1032–1033, 1055
Spectrogram, professional voice, 1062*f*
Speech surgery, 1561–1562, 1568
Speech threshold, 2278
Sphenoid sinus, 607*t*, 610. *See also* Sinus(es)
Sphenoidotomy, complications
endoscopic surgical procedures,
648–649, 648*f*, 649*f*
open surgery, 646, 646*f*
Sphenopalatine artery ligation, 506, 506*f*
Sphincter pharyngoplasty, 1568
Spider angiomas, treatment of, 3227
Spinal muscular atrophy, 1038
Spine injuries, secondary survey of trauma,
1100–1101, 1100*f*, 1101*t*
Spitz nevus, 3218, 3219*f*
treatment of, 3227
Splint therapy
temporomandibular joint, 788–789, 789*f*
Spondee words, 2277–2278
Spontaneous central nystagmus, 2719
Spontaneous cerebro spina fluid leaks,
664–665
Spontaneous nystagmus, 2305
dizziness, 2684–2685
Spontaneous peripheral nystagmus,
2718–2719
Squamous cell carcinoma, 2046–2048,
2047*t*, 2048*t*
adverse pathologic features in, 196
benign neoplasms
salivary gland type adenomas, 186*f*
sinonasal papillomas, 186*f*–187*f*
squamous precursor lesions,
187*f*–188*f*

ear and lateral skull base, 2367
histologic variants of, 194–195
HPV-related, 196
malignant neoplasms
basaloid SCC, 191*f*
dysplasia, 194
invasive and in situ SCC, 188*f*
lymphoepithelial carcinoma, 190*f*
nasopharyngeal carcinoma, 191*f*
perineural invasion, 190*f*
poorly differentiated SCC, 189*f*
salivary gland type carcinoma,
192*f*–193*f*
verrucous carcinoma, 191*f*
well and moderately differentiated
SCC, 189*f*
oropharyngeal, treatment of,
1903–1905, 1904*t*
of pinna, 2367
salivary gland, 1767
tracheal tumors, 1996
treatment of, 2367
Squamous cell papilloma, 2370
Squamous dysplasia
mild, 187*f*
moderate, 188*f*
severe, 188*f*
Staging system
creation of, 103–104
malignant melanoma
National Comprehensive Cancer
Network guidelines, 1744
primary tumor, 1742
regional nodal staging, 1742–1744
Stahl ear, otoplasty, 3144, 3145*f*
Standard mastoidectomy, 2633
Stapedectomy
complications of, 2493*t*, 2500–2501
facial nerve monitoring during, 2328
indication, 2500, 2500*t*
patient counseling for, 2494
patient selection for, 2493–2494
pitfalls of, 2500–2501
technique for, 2494–2500, 2495*f*–2498*f*,
2500*t*
Stapedial reflex measurement, acoustic,
2279–2280
Staphylococcus aureus, 1149, 1363, 1433,
1458, 1458*t*
Static positional testing, 2306
Statistical tests
for related samples, 95
results of, strength and consistency of,
99–100
for valid analysis, 94–95
Status epilepticus
pharmacologic management of, 42, 42*t*
Stem cell factor, 399
Stenosis
laryngeal trauma, 1146, 1149, 1150
Stenotic lesions, larynx and airway,
963–964
Stents
upper airway stenosis, tracheal
autografts, 891
placement, 890
tracheotomy tube, 891, 891*f*
used for, 890

Stereotactic radiotherapy
in recurrent nasopharyngeal cancer,
1889
Sterile technique, 21
Steroids
chronic rhinosinusitis, 587–588
scar camouflage, 2866
subjective nonpulsatile tinnitus, 2603
Stevens-Johnson syndrome, pharyngitis
due, 762–763
Stickler syndrome, 124, 1640
in hearing loss, 1543*t*, 1549
Robin sequence, 1620
Stomatitis
clinical assessment of, 736–737
etiology, 737
fungal infection
candidiasis, 740–741, 740*f*, 740*t*, 741*f*
denture-related, 741–742, 741*f*
paracoccidioidomycosis, 742, 742*t*
idiopathic
burning mouth syndrome, 753, 753*t*
erythema migrans, 753–754
oral lichen planus, 751–752, 752*f*
orofacial granulomatosis, 753
recurrent aphthous stomatitis,
749–751, 749*f*–751*f*, 750*t*
malnutrition and deficiency, 749
systemic condition
Behcet disease, 748
Crohn disease, 747–748
cyclic hematopoiesis, 749
lupus, 747
pregnancy, 748
sarcoidosis, 748–749
ulcerative colitis, 748
Wegener granulomatosis, 747
treatment-related
drugs administration, 737–738
lichenoid reaction, 739–740,
739*f*, 739*t*
medications, 738
mucositis, 737, 737*f*, 738
tuberculosis, 743–744
vesiculobullous lesions
bullous pemphigoid, 745, 745*f*
epidermolysis bullosa acquisita, 745
mucous membrane pemphigoid,
744–745, 744*f*
pemphigus vulgaris, 745–747, 745*f*,
746*f*, 747*t*
viral infection
herpes simplex virus, 742–743, 742*f*
HIV-associated stomatitis, 742–743
Strabismus, 229
Streptococcal infections
complications of, 760
pharyngitis due to, 758–760, 760*f*, 765
Streptococcus pneumoniae, 1300
pediatric rhinosinusitis and, 1458, 1458*t*
Stress relaxation, 2850
Stress ulcers
preventive management of, 39
prophylaxis, indications, 69*t*
treatment of, 39
Stridor
diagnosis for
laryngomalacia, 1339–1340, 1340*f*

laryngotracheobronchitis, 1342
subglottic stenosis, 1343–1344, 1343f
vascular anomalies, 1340–1342, 1341f
vocal cord immobility, 1342–1343
endoscopy, 1339
management of, 1344
perinatal history, 1338–1339
physical examination, 1339
radiology, 1339
Stroboscopy,
vocal difficulties, 1071–1072
voice examination, 955
Stroke, 199
after carotid artery dissection, 1826
neurologic deficitsdisorder, 1034–1036
Sturge-Weber syndrome, 1584, 1640
Sty, 223–224
Subacute necrotizing sialadenitis, 713
Subarachnoid hemorrhage, 204
Subcutaneous emphysema
percutaneous dilatational tracheotomy, 943
sinus surgery complications, 655
Subcutaneous immunotherapy, 591
allergic rhinitis, 465
Subdural abscess, 581, 581f
Subdural empyema, 2406
Subdural hematoma, 313
Subglottic cancer, early
surgical pathology, 1955–1956
treatment, 1956
Subglottic carcinoma, 1973
Subglottic hemangioma, 1578, 1579f
Subglottic pressure, professional voice, 1063–1064, 1063f
Subglottic stenosis, 1149
Sublingual gland
anatomy, 696
arterial blood supply, 696–697
ducts, 696
sympathetic and parasympathetic innervation, 697
tumors of, 1768
Sublingual immunotherapy, 404, 591
allergic rhinitis, 466
Submandibular gland(s)
anatomy, 12, 12f, 695, 695f
arterial blood supply, 696
capsule, 696
complications of, 1783t
technique, 1779, 1780f
ptosis, 3133
superficial and deep lobes, 695, 696f
surgery of, 1778–1779
sympathetic innervation, 696
tumors of, 1760, 1778
Submandibular space, deep neck infection, 807–809, 808f, 809f
Submucosal minimally invasive lingual excision procedure, 2232–2233
Subperiosteal abscess, 575, 576f
Succinylcholine, 243
Sudden loss of vision, 222–223, 223f
Sudden sensorineural hearing loss
autoimmune inner ear disease, 2591
corticosteroid therapy, 2593
definition of, 2589

differential diagnosis, 2589–2590, 2590t
epidemiology of, 2589
intracochlear membrane rupture, 2590–2591
patient evaluation, 2591, 2591t
spontaneous recovery rate, 2592–2593
therapeutic regimens, 2593
transtympanic steroid application, 2593
treatment, 2592
vascular compromise, 2590
viral infection, 2590, 2593–2594
Sugammadex, 244
Sulcus vocalis, 993–994, 994f
Sumatriptan (Imitrex), 207
Sun exposure
lip cancer and, 1790
skin cancer, 1723
Supercentenarians, 298
Superficial cervical fascia, deep neck space, 795
Superficial spreading melanoma, 1741
Superior canal dehiscence syndrome
chronically inadequate vestibular function, 2712
clinical features, 2710
diagnostic tests, 2710–2711
treatment, 2711–2712
Superior laryngeal nerve, 873
block, 238
injury, 2124
paresis, 1039, 1040f
Superior orbital decompression, 632
Superior semicircular canal dehiscence
computed tomography, 141, 142f
Suprabullar cell, 679f
Supracricoid laryngectomy
early laryngeal cancer, 1947–1948
partial, 1971, 1971f
Supraglottic cancer, early
diagnosis, 1942, 1943t
horizontal supraglottic laryngectomy, 1947
neck management, 1948–1949
outcomes of, 1949
radiotherapy, 1949
supracricoid laryngectomy, 1947–1948
surgical pathology, 1942
transoral laser microsurgery. See Transoral laser microsurgery
transoral robotic surgery, 1946–1947
treatment, 1942–1943
Supraglottic laryngectomy, 1970–1971
early laryngeal cancer, 1943, 1944f
Supraglottic quadrangular membrane, larynx, 946
Supraglottic stenosis, 1150
Supraglottic swallow, 842
Supraglottitis, 138
Suprahyoid epiglottis, 1944
Suprahyoid pharyngotomy, 1907, 1907f
Supraomohyoid neck dissection, 1819, 1819f, 1822–1824
Surfactants
chronic rhinosinusitis, 592
Surgery
versus chemoradiation, 1973
preoperative evaluation for, 26

Surgical Care Improvement Project, 21
Surgical pathology
biopsy
cutaneous lesion, 178–179
mucosal sites, 179
subcutaneous masses, 179–180
frozen section
cervical lymph node specimens, 183–184
medical cost containment, 183
patterns of, 183
surgical margins, 183
time-consuming fixation/dehydration, 182
histopathology
hematoxylin and eosin stain, 185
squamous cell carcinoma. See Squamous cell carcinoma
pathology laboratory
reporting standards, 185
specimen handoff and processing, 184–185
surgical margins
adequacy, 180–181
orientation, 181–182
shrinkage, 182
surgical instruments choice, 182
Surgical site infection, 44
Surgical tattooing, 2868
Surgicel (Ethicon), 52
Susac syndrome, 212–213
Suture material, 22
Suture-guided transhyoid pharyngotomy, 1613
Swallowing
functional assessment, 825–836
bedside swallow evaluation. See Bedside swallow evaluation
dysphagia, 825, 826t
high-resolution manometry, 834, 835f, 835t
transnasal esophagoscopy. See Transnasal esophagoscopy
glottic closure, 860, 860f
nonsurgical management of, 838–847
compensatory treatment techniques, 838–841, 839t
direct therapy, 841
immunocompromised host, 847
maneuvers, 842–844, 842t, 843f
medical management, 844
motility drugs, 844–845, 845t
motion, resistance and control exercises, 841
nutrition, 846
oral care, 847
pulmonary status, 846
radiographic examination, 838
reflux disease control, 845–846
sensory-motor integration procedures, 841–842
upper esophageal sphincter relaxation, 860–861
Sweating, gustatory, 1782, 1782f
Symptom-specific instruments, 721
Syndactyly, in Apert syndrome, 1622–1623, 1623f

Syndrome of inappropriate antidiuretic hormone secretion
  preoperative management in, 34
Syndromes
  definitions of, 1620
  otolaryngologic, 1621–1622
Synechia, sinus surgery complications, 657–658
Syphilis, 288–289, 289f, 1528–1529
  larynx, 980
  pharyngitis in, 765
  tertiary, 765
Syringomas, 3215–3216
  treatment of, 3226
Systemic lupus erythematosus, 267–269, 747, 981
  diagnosis, 267–268, 268t
  head and neck manifestations
    discoid lesions, 268
    discoid lupus erythematosus, 269
    localized telangiectasia, 268–269
    neuropathy, 269
    ulcerative lesions, 269
  incidence, 267
  treatment, 270–271
Systemic sclerosis, 272–273
  American College of Rheumatology criteria for, 272
  diffuse cutaneous disease, 272
  head and neck manifestations, 272–273, 273f
  incidence, 272
  limited cutaneous disease, 272
  treatment, 273
  visceral and fatal manifestations, 272
Systemic steroids
  allergic rhinitis, 464

T
T1 cell, 677f
T2 cell, 677f, 678f
T3 cell, 678f
Tachydysrhythmias, preoperative management of, 37
Tandem walk, 2722
Tantalum implant, 2786
Tarsorrhaphy, 2912f
Tarsus, anatomy of, 4, 5f
Taste
  anatomy of, 729–730, 730f
  development of, 729
  innervation of tongue
    central pathways, 731
    genetic variations, 731
    glossopharyngeal (IX cranial) nerve, 730
    trigeminal and superior laryngeal nerve, 731
  taste altering conditions
    aging, 732–733
    nerve damage, 733
    radiation and chemotherapy, 733–734
    systemic diseases, 733
  taste loss
    effects of, 734
    therapy for, 734

testing
  electrogustometry, 732
  regional taste test, 732
  taste detection and recognition, 731
  threshold or intensity testing, 732
  videomicroscopy, 732, 732f, 733f
  whole-mouth taste, 731–732
transduction, 730
T-box transcription factor, 389
Tear trough deformity, lower eyelid blepharoplasty, 3086, 3087f
Technical misadventures
  percutaneous dilatational tracheotomy, 943
Teeth
  impacted, dentigerous cysts and, 2098, 2098f
Telangiectasia, 3206–3207
  hereditary, 3213, 3214t
  treatment, 3226–3227
Telemedicine
  barriers to adoption
    future directions in, 3369–3370
    licensure and credentialing, 3368
    problem of scale, 3369
    professional liability, 3368
    program building, 3369
    reimbursement, 3368–3369
  definitions
    Alaska Federal Health Care Access Network, 3362, 3362f
    asynchronous store-and-forward, 3362
    remote patient monitoring, 3361, 3363
    video teleconferencing, 3361–3362
  in otolaryngology
    facial plastics and trauma, 3367
    head and neck oncology, 3367
    laryngology and speech disorders, 3367
    neurotology, 3364–3366
    in operating room, 3368
    pediatric otolaryngology, 3366–3367
  security and HIPAA, 3363–3364
Temple lift, bilateral, surgical procedure for, 3058f, 3061–3062
Temporal arteritis, 223, 313
Temporal bone
  classification of, 2411–2413
  epidemiology of, 2410
  evaluation
    clinical evaluation, 2413–2414
    radiographic evaluation, 2414–2416
  implants for, 2790
  management
    cholesteatoma and external auditory stenosis, 2429
    CSF fistulae, 2423–2426
    facial nerve injury, 2416–2423
    hearing loss, 2426–2429
    vascular injuries, 2429–2430
  otosclerosis, 2488, 2488f
  paraganglioma, 2358
  pathophysiology, 2410–2411
Temporal region, 1116f
Temporomandibular joint, 782–791, 1195

anatomy of, 782–783, 783f
differential diagnosis, 787
magnetic resonance imaging, 787, 787f
management
  excessive over jet, 788
  occlusal appliance therapy, 788–789, 789f
  pharmacotherapy, 789
  physical therapy, 789
  surgery, 788
pathophysiology
  hypomobility disorder, 785
  intracapsular disorder, 783–784
  molecular biologic mechanism, 784–785
  muscle-related pain, 783
  posttraumatic, 785–786, 786f
  psychosocial comorbidity, 784
  Wilkes classification, 3f
physical examination, 786
physiology of, 782–783, 783f
surgery-closed
  arthrocentesis, 789
  arthroscopy, 789–790
  open surgery, 790, 790f
  reconstruction, 790
Temporomandibular joint syndrome, 314
Temporoparietal fascial flap, 2830, 2831f
Tension, 2849
Tension-type headache
  diagnostic criteria, 308–309, 308t
  epidemiology, 308
  pathogenesis, 308
  treatment, 309
Teratomas, 1600, 2375
Tetanus, wounds, 1111, 1112t
Thermal injuries, external ear, 2347
Thermoplastic splints, 2180–2181
Thiamine deficiency, 2729–2730
Thoracic injuries, secondary survey of trauma, 1102–1103, 1102f
Thoracostomy, tube, in trauma patients, 1097, 1097f
Thornton adjustable positioner, 2180, 2181f
Three-dimensional photography, 2768–2769, 2768f
Thrombocytopenia, 28, 498
Thromboembolic disease
  diagnosis of, 31
  management of, 31
  prevention of, 30–31
  pulmonary embolism in, 31
  preoperative, 31
  risk factors for, 30
Thrombosis
  jugular vein, 1832
  lateral sinus, 2444
  venous sinus, 582
Thulium laser, 1088
Thyroglossal duct cysts, 2115
  antimicrobials, 1613
  dermoid cysts, 1614–1615, 1615f
  ectopic thyroid, 1613–1614
  lingual thyroid, 1613–1614

in midline of neck, 1612, 1612*f*
postsurgical recurrence of, 1612–1613
Sistrunk procedure, 1612, 1612*f*, 1613*f*
suture-guided transhyoid pharyngotomy, 1613
Thyroid
adenoma, 2120
anatomy of, 16, 16*f*
disorders of, preoperative management of, 32–33
myxedema coma, 258
neoplasms. *See* Thyroid cancer
orbitopathy, 144, 145*f*
and parathyroid surgery, 50–51, 50*f*
scintigraphy, 161–162, 162*f*, 162*t*
synthesis, 256–257
thyroid storm, 257–258
triiodothyronine and thyroxine, 256, 257
Thyroid cancer, 125, 1603
anaplastic carcinoma, 2120–2121
differentiated. *See* Differentiated thyroid cancer
EBRT, 2126
follicular carcinoma, 2120
Hurthle cell carcinoma, 2120
lymphoma, 2121, 2039
medullary thyroid carcinoma, 2127–2128
molecular basis of, 2116–2117, 2117*f*
nodules, evaluation
clinical assessment, 2117
CT, MRI, and PET/CT, 2118
fine-needle aspiration and molecular markers, 2118–2119, 2118*t*
laboratory studies, 2117–2118
radionuclide thyroid scan, 2118
ultrasound, 2118
workup, 2119–2120, 2119*f*
papillary carcinoma, 2120
postoperative risk stratification, 2125, 2125*t*
postoperative staging system, 2125
primary squamous cell carcinoma, 2121
radioactive iodine treatment, 2125
risk factors of, 2116
stage groupings, 2121, 2122*t*
surgical anatomy and embryology
ectopic thyroid tissue, 2115
parafollicular C cells, 2115
thyroglossal duct cyst, 2115
systemic therapy, 2126
thyroid adenoma, 2120
TNM staging for, 2121, 2121*t*
total thyroidectomy, 2123
TSH suppression, 2125
Thyroid cartilage fracture
blunt cervical trauma, 1141
diagnosis, 1142
surgical treatment, 1146–1147, 1147*f*
thyrotomy, 1147, 1148*f*
treatment decision making, 1145, 1145*t*
Thyroid isthmus
pediatric tracheotomy, 1386, 1388*f*
Thyroid storm, 257–258
medical control of, 33, 33*t*

Thyroid-associated orbitopathy, 231, 231*f*, 2071
Thyroidectomy, 49
Thyroid-stimulating hormone, 252
Thyrotoxic crisis, preoperative management of, 33, 33*t*
Tic disorders, 1034
Tinnitus
classification, 2597
complementary and alternative medicine, 323
diagnostic evaluation, 2598
history, 2597–2598
physical examination, 2598
pulsatile tinnitus. *See* Pulsatile tinnitus
subjective nonpulsatile tinnitus
diagnostic evaluation, 2601–2602, 2601*f*
etiology, 2598–2600, 2599*t*, 2600*t*
hyperacusis, 2601
retraining therapy, 2602–2603, 2602*f*
risk factors, 2600–2601, 2600*t*
treatment, 2602–2604
Tisseel (Baxter), 52
Tissue expansion
advantages and disadvantages, 2849, 2850*t*
alopecia
applications, 2851–2852
complications, 2854
conventional long-term, 2852–2853, 2852*f*–2856*f*
physiology, 2851
rapid intraoperative, 2853–2854
skin biomechanics, 2849–2850
tissue expanders, 2852, 2852*f*
types, 2850–2851, 2851*t*
Tissue reactivity, suture material selection, 22
Tissue substitutes, 53
Titanium implant, 2786
Tobacco use
clinical intervention, 330*t*
advise, 331
arrange, 332
ask, 330
assess, 331
assist, 331–332, 332*t*
multimodality treatment
intensive counseling, 332
pharmacotherapy, 333–336, 334*t*
perioperative considerations, 336–337
programs and resources, 336
Toll-like receptors, 380
expression of, 380, 381*t*
signaling, cell biology, 380*f*
Tongue
anatomy of, 11–12, 11*f*
retaining device, 2180, 2181*f*
squamous cell carcinoma, 146*f*
Tongue-hold maneuver, 842, 843*f*
Tonsillectomy, 49
adenotonsillar disease, in children, 1437
Topical decongestants
nonallergic rhinitis, 472

Topical hemostatic agents, 52
Tori, 2106
Tort reform, 3278–3279
Total laryngectomy, 1972
Total ossicular replacement prosthesis, 2466, 2481–2485, 2483*f*
Total parenteral nutrition, preoperative, 26, 27
Total thyroidectomy, 2123
Toxoplasmosis, 291, 1526–1527
Trachea
pediatric tracheotomy, 1389, 1390*f*
stenosis, 1361
transplantation
allograft, 891–892
bioengineered tissue, 892
tumors
clinical presentation
history, 1990, 1991*t*
imaging, 1990, 1992*f*
definitive surgical management
cricotracheal resection, 1994
extended resection, 1995
laryngeal-tracheal resections, 1995
lymphadenectomy, 1995
tracheal resection, 1992–1994, 1994*t*
endoscopic and nonoperative management, 1995–1996
initial airway management, 1991–1992
pathology of, 1990, 1991*t*, 1996–1997
adenoid cystic carcinoma, 1996
cervical trachea, 1996
metastatic tumors, 1997
squamous cell carcinoma, 1996
Tracheitis, 881–882
Tracheobronchial and esophageal obstruction
pathophysiology, 1308–1309
postnatal diagnosis, 1314–1316, 1315*f*
prenatal diagnosis, 1309, 1309*f*–1310*f*
treatment
congenital tracheal stenosis, 1322–1324, 1322*f*–1324*f*
tracheoesophageal fistula, 1322, 1322*f*–1323*f*
Tracheoesophageal fistula, 1322, 1322*f*–1323*f*, 1346
Tracheoesophageal puncture
for voice restoration during laryngectomy, 1979–1981, 1981*f*, 1982*f*
Tracheo-innominate artery fistula
pediatric tracheotomy, 1393
Tracheostoma construction, 1982
Tracheostomy
and aspiration, 861
bilateral vocal fold immobility, 1020
Tracheotomy, 2233. *See also* Pediatric patients
cricothyrotomy, 919–920, 920*f*, 921*f*
emergency tracheotomy, 920–924
history of, 917–918

Tracheotomy (*Continued*)
  indications for, 918–919
  intraoperative complications, 933t
    fire, 934
    hemorrhage, 933
    pneumomediastinum, 933
    pneumothorax, 933
    tracheoesophageal fistula, 933
  modifications
    Bjork flap, 927
    complications, 929
    cuffed tracheostomy tube, 928–929
    inferior skin flap, 928, 932f
    omega skin incision, 928, 930f
    superiorly based flap, 928, 931f
  open surgical tracheotomy
    adults, 926, 928f
    children, 926, 928f
    electrocautery, 927
    neck tapes, 926
    patient position, 925
    preoperative planning, 924–925, 925t
    thyroid isthmus, 926, 927f
    thyroid isthmus retraction, 926, 927f
    trachea, 927
    traction sutures, 926, 928f
    transverse incision, 925–926, 926f
    Trousseau dilator insertion, 926, 929f
  percutaneous dilatational tracheotomy
    anesthesia, 938–939
    complications, 941–942
    cost analyses, 936
    critically ill patients, 936
    instruments, 937–938, 938f, 939f
    patient selection, 937, 937t
    personnel, 937
    postoperative considerations, 941
    preoperative planning, 937
    technique, 939–941, 639f–641f
  postoperative care
    accidental decannulation, 931, 932f
    decannulation, 932–933
    humidification, 931
    meticulous local wound care, 931
    patient positioning, 930
    preoperative teaching, 929–930
    speaking valve, 932
    tracheal suctioning, 930–931
    tracheostomy tube exchanger, 931–932
  postoperative complications
    depressed scar, 936
    displaced tracheostomy tube, 934
    granulation tissue, 935, 935t
    hemorrhage, 934
    subcutaneous emphysema, 935
    tracheal stenosis and tracheomalacia, 936
    tracheocutaneous fistula, 936
    tracheoesophageal fistula, 935
    tracheoinnominate artery rupture, 935–936
    tube obstruction, 934
    wound infection, 934
Traditional chinese medicine, 319–320
Transcolumellar incisions, 2944, 2945f
Transfusion Requirement in Critical Care trial, 57

Transfusions
  complications of, 27
  preoperative, 27–28
Transient evoked otoacoustic emissions, 1524
Transient loss of vision, 223
Transient receptor potential vanilloid type receptor, 472
Transitory otoacoustic emission, 1481
Transnasal esophagoscopy
  complications, 834
  endoscope placement, 832–833, 833f
  flexible endoscopic evaluation of swallowing, 834
  fluoroscopic video-esophagram, 832
  indications, 831–832
  patient position, 832, 832f
Transoral laser microsurgery
  glottic cancer, 1951, 1951f, 1952f
  supraglottic cancer, 1944f, 1945f
    aryepiglottic fold, 1946
    complications, 1946
    contraindications, 1943–1944
    endoscopic surgery classification, 1943, 1945t
    false cord, 1946
    frozen section analysis, 1946
    hemostasis, 1946
    infrahyoid epiglottis, 1944–1946, 1944f
    postoperative care, 1946
    suprahyoid epiglottis, 1944
    surgical procedure, 1944
Transoral robotic surgery, 1905–1906
Transorbital neuroendoscopic surgery, 2077
Transverse cordotomy
  bilateral vocal fold immobility, 1021, 1021f
Trauma, 711–712, 712f
  acoustic, 2532
  blunt, 1141–1142
  hearing loss
    head trauma, 1531–1532
    noise-related hearing loss, 1530–1531
    ototoxicity, 1531
  management, 1105
  metabolic response, 1094
  neuroendocrine response, 1093–194
  penetrating, 1142
  primary survey
    airway, 1094–1096, 1095f, 1096f
    breathing, 1097, 1097f, 1098f
    circulation and shock, 1097–1100, 1110f
  role of otolaryngologist, 1105
  salivary gland disease, 1477
  secondary survey
    abdominal injuries, 1103–1104
    extremity injuries, 1104
    head and spine injuries, 1100–1101, 1100f, 1101t
    inhalation injuries, 1104–1105
    neck injuries, 1101–1102, 1101f
    thoracic injuries, 1102–1103, 1102f
Traumatic displacement, implant, 2795
Traumatic eosinophilic granuloma, 754

Treacher Collins syndrome, 124
  in hearing loss, 1543t, 1549
  hearing loss in, 1632–1633, 1633f
Trichilemmomas, 3215
  treatment of, 3226
Trichoepitheliomas, 3215
  treatment of, 3226
Trichofolliculomas, treatment of, 3226
Trichophytic forehead lift, 3058f, 3063–3064, 3063f, 3064f
Tricyclic antidepressants, 207–208
Trigeminal nerve block, 237
Trigeminal neuralgia, 312, 312t
Triiodobenzoic acid derivatives
  sudden sensorineural hearing loss, 2592
Trimethoprim-sulfamethoxazole, 133
Trisomy, 122
Trisomy 21
  hearing loss in, 1552, 1626
Tube feeding, preoperative, 27
Tube thoracostomy, 1097, 1097f
Tuberculosis, 284–286, 285f, 704
  cerebellopontine angle, 2580
  stomatitis, 743–744
Tuberculous
  adenitis, 804f
Tubocurarine, 243
Tubular necrosis
  acute, 63–64, 64t
Tularemia, 289
Tumor
  debulking, 1995
  hypoxia imaging, 166
  perfusion imaging, 166–167
Turbinate(s)
  hypertrophy of
    complications
      atrophic rhinitis, 619
      empty nose syndrome, 618–619
      rhinitis sicca, 618
    reduction in
      carbon dioxide laser, 617–618
      cryosurgery, 618
      electrocautery, 617
      inferior turbinate outfracture, 617, 617f
      microdebrider-assisted inferior turbinate reduction, 618, 618f
      radiofrequency-assisted, 617
      submucosal resection, 618, 618f
      submucous diathermy, 617
  inferior
    anatomy and function of, 362
    hypertrophy of, nasal obstruction, 364
Turner syndrome, 122, 1640
  in hearing loss, 1552
Tylosis, 125
Tympanic membrane, 1479, 1480, 1480f
  development of, 2241
Tympanomeatal flap
  design of, 2495, 2495f
  elevation technique, 2495, 2495f, 2496f
Tympanometry, 1480, 2278–2279, 2279f
Tympano-ossicular reconstruction, 2482, 2483f

Tympanoplasty
   applied tympanic membrane mechanics, 2469
   atelectasis, 2476–2477
   auricular cartilage graft, 2470
   canal incisions, 2469, 2470f–2472f
   composite perichondrium-cartilage island graft, 2472–2473, 2473f
   definition, 2465
   drumhead preparation, 2469–2470
   lateralized tympanic membrane, 2477
   mini split-thickness skin graft, 2473
   open mastoid cavity, 2477
   overlay repair, 2474, 2475f, 2476
   preoperative evaluation, 2467, 2469
   principles, 2469
   surgical exposure of, 2469, 2470t
   types of, 2465–2466
   underlay repair, 2473, 2474f
Tympanostomy tube
   audiologic examination, 1497–1498
   complications, 1498
   displacement of, 1499
   indications for, 1499
   ototopical drops, 1497
   selection of, 1497
   tympanosclerosis and atrophy, 1498
   water precautions, 1499–1500

U

Ulcerative colitis, 748
Ulcerative hemangiomas, 1582, 1582f
Ulcerative laryngitis, idiopathic, 980
Ulcerative scalp hemangiomas, 1582, 1582f
Ulcers
   of lip, differential diagnosis of, 1790
   stress
      preventive management of, 39
      treatment of, 39
Ultrasound
   advantages of, 157
   fine needle aspiration, 160f
   indications and technique, 157–158
   principles, 156
Ultrasound-guided biopsy, 180
Uncomplicated chronic otorrhea, 2400
Underlay tympanoplasty, 2473, 2474f
Unified airway
   allergic rhinitis
      allergic march, 553
      pathophysiology and inflammation, 553–554
      treatment, 554
   chronic otitis media with effusion, 553
   chronic rhinosinusitis and asthma
      cystic fibrosis, 555
      inflammation, 554
      medical and surgical treatment, 554
      Samter triad, 554–555
   loss of nasal protection, 553
   nasobronchial reflex, 553
   upper and lower airways, 550
Unilateral vestibular function
   episodic excitation
      benign paroxysmal positional vertigo, 2708–2710, 2709f

bilateral vestibular hypofunction, 2712
      superior canal dehiscence syndrome, 2710–2712
      immune-mediated inner ear disease, 2706–2707
      Ménière syndrome, 2701–2704
      migrainous vertigo, 2704–2705
      perilymph fistula, 2705–2706
Unilateral vocal fold paralysis
   etiology
      bilateral innervation of interarytenoid, 1005f
      causes of, 1004, 1006t
      idiopathic and miscellaneous, 1007
      medications, 1007
      neurological disease, 1006–1007
      nonlaryngeal malignancies, 1006t
      recurrent laryngeal nerve, 1004, 1005f, 1007
      surgical or iatrogenic of, 1006, 1006t
      systemic diseases, 1007
   history
      airway, 1008
      vocal inventory, 1008
      vocal quality and swallowing, 1007
   pediatric voice, 1377–1378
   physical examination
      laryngeal, 1008–1010, 1008f–1010f
      neck, 1008
   treatment
      classical teaching, 1012–1013
      early surgical intervention, 1014
      injection augmentation, 1014–1015, 1014t, 1015f
      laryngeal framework surgery, 1015–1017
      laryngeal reinnervation, 1017
      management, 1011–1012
      nimodipine, 1017
      patient factors, 1012, 1013t
   workup
      imaging, 1011
      laryngeal electromyography, 1011, 1012f, 1013f
      serology, 1010–1011
Universal newborn hearing screening, 1507
Unsteadiness, 2302
   vestibular and balance laboratory study, 2302
Unterberger (Fukuda) stepping test, 2695
Upper airway anatomy and function
   circulatory reflexes, 875–876
   larynx
      anatomy, 870–874
      physiology, 874–875
   in nonhuman mammals, 868
   pharyngeal
      anatomy, 868, 869f
      physiology, 869
   sagittal view of, 869f
   speech regulation
      articulation, 877
      phonation, 876
      resonance, 876–877
      voice control, 877

Upper airway stenosis
   etiology, 880t
      idiopathic stenosis, 881
      laryngitis and tracheitis, 881–882
      laryngopharyngeal reflux, 881
      origin of, 879
      relapsing polychondritis, 881
      trauma, 879–880
      Wegener granulomatosis, 880–881
   evaluation
      imaging, 882–883
      operating room-based direct laryngoscopy, 883
      physical examination and office endoscopy, 882
      pulmonary physiologic testing, 883
      reflux testing, 883
   glottic stenosis, 884–885, 884f, 885f, 885t
   nonoperative management, 883
   subglottic and tracheal stenosis
      corkscrew subtype, 886, 886f
      Cotton-Meyer staging system, 885–886, 885t
      cricotracheal resection, 887–889, 888f
      endoscopic management, 886–887
      inflammatory tissue and cartilaginous collapse, 886, 886f
      laryngeal releasing procedures, 890
      mitomycin-C, 887
      simple thin fibrous, 886, 886f
      tracheal resection, 889–890, 889f
   supraglottic stenosis, 883–884, 884f
   tracheal stents
      autografts, 891
      placement, 890
      tracheotomy tube, 891, 891f
      used for, 890
   tracheal transplantation/tissue engineering
      allograft, 891–892
      bioengineered tissue, 892
Upper digestive tract
   anticipatory phase, 817–818
   breathing and swallowing, 823
   dysphagia, 817
   esophageal phase, 822, 822f
   oral preparatory phase, 818–819, 818t
   oral transfer phase, 819, 820f
   pharyngeal phase
      hyolaryngeal complex elevation, 821, 821f
      inverted epiglottis, 821, 821f
      relaxed upper esophageal sphincter, 821, 822f
      velum elevation, 820, 820f
Upper mediastinal lymph node dissection, 1825
Upper respiratory infection, 134–135, 373
Usher syndrome, 123, 1543t, 1547, 1633–1634
Uvulopalatopharyngoplasty, 2230–2231

V

Vaccines
   meningitis, 1518–1519
   for otitis media, 1488–1490
   P. multocida, 483
   for Streptococcus Pneumoniae, 1300

7-Valent pneumococcal conjugate vaccine, 135
Valsalva maneuver
    larynx, 952
van der Woude syndrome, 1557, 1640–1641
Vanadium implant, 2786
Vancomycin, 40, 133
Varenicline
    tobacco cessation, 333, 335
Vascular cell adhesion molecule 1, 400
Vascular ectasias, laser procedures, 1088
Vascular tumor(s)
    angiosarcoma
        epidemiology, 2019–2020
        etiologic factors, 2020, 2020t
        molecular analysis, 2020–2021
        pathology, 2020
        staging, 2021, 2021t
        treatment, 2021–2023, 2022f
    cerebellopontine angle, 2579–2580
    classification of, 1999, 2000t
    facial, 3216–3217, 3217f
    hemangioma. See Hemangiomas
    hemangiopericytoma
        architectural pattern of, 2017
        chemotherapy, 2019
        clinical presentation, 2018–2019
        diagnosis of, 2018
        radiation therapy, 2019
        treatment, 2019
    juvenile nasopharyngeal angiofibroma
        diagnosis of, 2025, 2026f
        endoscopic and endoscopic-assisted
            approaches, 2028
        epidemiology and pathogenesis, 2023
        growth patterns, 2024–2025, 2024f, 2025f
        open surgery, 2027–2028, 2027t
        radiation therapy, 2028
        staging, 2025–2026, 2027t
        surgical approaches, 2026–2027
    Kasabach-Merritt phenomenon, 1579
    lymphatic malformations
        cystic hygromas, 1585
        microcystic and macrocystic malfor-
            mations, 1585, 1585f
        microcystic malformations, 1585
        respiratory obstruction, 1586
        sclerotherapy, 1586
        Turner syndrome, 1586
    neoplasms, 2061, 2061t
    orbital
        capillary hemangioma, 2066
        cavernous hemangioma, 2066, 2067f
        lymphangioma, 2066–2067
    paraganglioma. See Paraganglioma
    vascular malformations
        capillary malformations, 1583–1584, 1583f
        diagnostic modalities, 1583
        venous malformations, 1584, 1584f
Vasculitides
    Behçet disease, 278
    Churg-Strauss syndrome, 276
    Cogan syndrome, 278–279

    giant cell (temporal) arteritis, 277–278
    immune complex-mediated, 276
    Kawasaki disease, 279
    Kikuchi-Fujimoto disease, 279
    microscopic polyangiitis, 277
    polyarteritis nodosa, 275–276
    Wegener granulomatosis, 276–277
Vasculitis, orbital, 2071
Vasoactive agents
    cardiovascular effects of, 58t
    pitfalls
        cardiac valvular disease, 58
        diastolic dysfunction, 57–58
        systolic left ventricular failure, 57
        tachycardia, 58
    relative receptor activity of, 58t
    vasopressor requirements, 58–59
Vasodilators
    sudden sensorineural hearing loss, 2592
Vasopressin, 59
Velocardiofacial syndrome, 1632, 1632f
Velopharyngeal incompetence, in
        Shprintzen syndrome, 1631–1632, 1632f
Velopharyngeal insufficiency, 1561–1562, 1568
Venous lakes, 3217
    treatment, 3227
Venous malformations, 1584, 1584f, 3206
Venous sinus thrombosis, 582
Venous thromboembolism prophylaxis
    surgery
        complications, 23–24
        incidence, 24
        risk profiles, 24, 24t
Ventricular obliteration, 966f
Vermilionectomy, for cancer
    reconstruction after, 1794
Verrucae, 3228
    treatment of, 3228
Verrucous carcinoma, 191f
Vertebrobasilar insufficiency, 199–200
Vertebrobasilar ischemia, 2726
Vertical hemilaryngectomy, 1970
Vertical partial laryngectomy, 1953
Vertigo, 323, 2302. See Dizziness
Vestibular and balance laboratory study
    case examples, 2310–2312
    dizziness, 2302
    dynamic visual acuity, 2309
    electronystagmography/videonystag-
        mography, 2303–2307
    gaze stabilization test, 2309
    head-impulse test, 2308
    migraine disorders, 2302
    off-axis total body rotation, 2307, 2308f
    on-axis total body rotation, 2307, 2308f
    unsteadiness, 2302
    VEMP threshold response curves, 2308, 2309f
    vertigo, 2302
    vestibular-evoked myogenic potential, 2307
    video oculography, 2310
    visual acuity problems, 2310
    in young child, 2302

Vestibular brainstem
    reciprocal inhibition, 2300
    vestibular nuclei, 2299–2300
    vestibuloocular reflexes, 2300
Vestibular disorders
    peripheral, 2701–2713
        clinical presentation, 2702t
        in unilateral lesions
            benign paroxysmal positional ver-
                tigo, 2708–2710, 2709f
            bilateral vestibular hypofunction, 2712
            immune-mediated inner ear disease, 2706–2707
            Ménière syndrome, 2701–2704
            migrainous vertigo, 2704–2705
            perilymph fistula, 2705–2706
            superior canal dehiscence syn-
                drome, 2710–2712
Vestibular dysfunction, aging, 2620–2621
Vestibular hair cells
    cupula, 2293–2294
    mechanoelectrical transduction chan-
        nels, 2294
    polarization of, 2295f
    polarization vector, 2294
    sensory neuroepithelium, anatomy and
        physiology of, 2293, 2294f
Vestibular injury, as complication of tym-
        panomastoid surgery, 2462
Vestibular labyrinth
    ampulla, 2292
    head rotation, 2292
    innervation, 2291, 2292f
    otolith organs, 2291
    vertical canals orientation, 2291, 2292f
Vestibular neuritis, 2706
Vestibular rehabilitation, 2733–2742
    factors affecting recovery, 2736
    innovations in, 2739–2742, 2740f, 2741f
    outcome measures
        Activities-specific Balance Confidence
            scale, 2735
        clinical test of sensory integration and
            balance, 2736
        five times sit to stand test, 2736
        gait and balance measurement, 2735
        Timed Up and Go test, 2736
        Verbal and visual analog scales, 2735
Vestibular schwannoma, 213, 213f
    clinical presentation, 2559
    diagnosis
        audiologic behavioral evaluation, 2559–2560
        computed tomography, 2561
        electrophysiologic evaluation, 2559–2560
        magnetic resonance imaging, 2560–2561, 2560f, 2561f
        vestibular assessment, 2560
    epidemiology, 2558
    histopathology, 2558–2559
    microsurgery, 2563–2565, 2564f, 2565f
    molecular biology, 2559
    surgery for
        emergencies after tumor removal, 2573–2574, 2573t

middle cranial fossa approach, 2565, 2566f–2567f, 2567–2568
retrosigmoid-suboccipital approach, 2568, 2569f–2570f
stereotactic radiosurgery as, 2562–2563, 2562f
translabyrinthine approach, 2568, 2570, 2571f–2572f, 2572–2573
treatment, 2561–2562
Vestibular system
aging, 2618–2619, 2618t
cellular anatomy of
supporting cells, 2295
vestibular afferent neurons, 2295–2296
vestibular efferent neurons, 2296
vestibular hair cells, 2293–2295, 2294f, 2295f
function and anatomy of, 2291–2301
gross anatomy of, 2291–2293
mechanotransduction
basic physics of, 2296–2297
in otolith organs, 2298–2299
in semicircular canals, 2297–2298
vestibular brainstem, 2299–2300
Vestibular-evoked myogenic potential
Ménière syndrome, 2703–2704
vestibular and balance laboratory study, 2307
Vestibuloocular reflexes, 2300
Vibratory source, professional voice, 1063, 1063t
Video oculography, 2310
Video teleconferencing, 3361–3362
Videoendoscopy, middle ear states, 1480f
Videonystagmography
caloric irrigation testing, 2306–2307
electrodes, 2303
hallpike and roll tests, 2306
headshake test, 2305–2306
hyperventilation testing, 2305
monocular recordings, 2303, 2304f
oculomotor evaluations
gaze stability testing, 2303–2304
optokinetic nystagmus, 2305
saccade evaluation, 2304–2305
smooth pursuit tracking, 2305
spontaneous nystagmus, 2305
static positional testing, 2306
Videostroboscopy
pediatric voice, 1373, 1373f–1374f
Vidian neurectomy, 472–473
Villaret syndrome, 2361
Viral infection(s)
pharyngitis in, 758t, 760, 761, 763–765
stomatitis
herpes simplex virus, 742–743, 742f
HIV-associated stomatitis, 742–743
sudden sensorineural hearing loss, 2590, 2593–2594
viral sialadenitis, 1468–1469
Viral laryngitis, 978, 979f
Viral lymphadenitis
acute, 1595
Viscoelasticity, 2850
Vision loss
gradual, 221–222

orbital fracture, 1238
sudden, 222–223
transient, 223
Visual acuity problems, 2310
Visual reinforcement audiometry, 1481, 1513–1514, 1514f
Vitamin D, 254–255
Vitamin E
scar camouflage, 2868–2869
Vinca alkaloids, ototoxicity, 2543–2544
Vincomycin, ototoxicity, 2544
Vocal difficulties
acoustic analysis, 1072, 1072f
complaints, 1069
finding discussion, 1072
history, 1069, 1069t, 1070f–1071f, 1071
laryngeal examination, 1071
physical examination, 1071, 1071f
stroboscopy, 1071–1072
Vocal fold(s)
atrophy, voice therapy, 1055
bilateral paralysis of
clinical presentation and evaluation, 1017–1020, 1018f, 1020f
etiology, 1017, 1017t, 1018t
fiberoptic laryngoscopy, 1018, 1018f
history, 1018–1019
imaging, 1019
laryngeal electromyography, 1019
laryngoscopy and palpation, 1019–1020, 1020f
management, 1020–1022, 1021f
physical examination, 1019
serology, 1019
edema, 966f
laceration, repair of, 1146, 1147f
larynx, 949, 949f
lesions
epithelial abnormalities
keratotic lesions, 989–990
pathophysiology, 989
lamina propria. See Lamina propria; Lamina propria, vocal fold
phonomicrosurgery. See Phonomicrosurgery
Reinke edema, 996, 996f
vascular lesions, 996
mucosa, larynx, 874f
nodules, cysts, and polyps
pediatric voice
endoscopic examination, 1375, 1376f
hourglass closure configuration, 1375, 1375f
nonoperative management, 1376
operative management, 1376–1377
phono-traumatic event, 1375
paralysis, voice therapy, 1055
professional voice
approximation, 1064
tension, 1064–1065, 1064f
unilateral paralysis of
classical teaching, 1012–1013
early surgical intervention, 1014
etiology, 1004–1007, 1005f, 1006t
history, 1007–1008
imaging, 1011

injection augmentation, 1014–1015, 1014t, 1015f
laryngeal electromyography, 1011, 1012f, 1013f
laryngeal framework surgery, 1015–1017
laryngeal reinnervation, 1017
management, 1011–1012
nimodipine, 1017
patient factors, 1012, 1013t
physical examination, 1008–1010, 1008f–1010f
serology, 1010–1011
Vocal function exercises, voice therapy, 1053
Vocal performance styles, professional voice, 1065–1066, 1065f, 1066t
Vocal registers, 1066, 1066t
Vocal tract, professional voice, 1061, 1061f
Voice. See also Larynx
abuse of
vocal therapy and reduction of, 1049
anatomy
age-related changes in, 950–951, 950f
cricoarytenoid joint, 947
cricoid cartilage, 945
epiglottis, 946
fibroblastic membranes, 946, 946f
membranous vocal fold, 949–950, 949f
muscles and nerves, 947–949, 948f
posterolateral projection, 945–946
supporting framework of, 945, 946f
vertical section, 946f
classification, 1065–1066, 1065f
clinical evaluation
examination, 954–955
history, 953–954
physiology
airway protection, 951
phonatory glottic cycle, 952–953, 952f
respiration, 951–952
valsalva maneuver, 952
Voice Handicap Index, 825, 826t, 953, 1070f–1071f
Voice rehabilitation following laryngectomy, 1978–1987
alaryngeal speech, 1978
complications of, 1984–1985, 1985t
emergencies in, 1987
operative procedure, 1978
pharyngeal constrictor
separation, 1978, 1979f
spasm, 1984, 1984f
postoperative rehabilitation, 1985–1986, 1985f, 1986f
primary voice restoration
selection criteria, 1981–1982
surgical technique, 1982–1983, 1982f, 1983f
shunts and valves, 1979
tracheoesophageal puncture
surgical procedure, 1980–1981, 1981f
timing and patient selection, 1979–1980
tracheoesophageal speech, 1986–1987
voice quality, 1987

Voice therapy
    approaches
        accent method, 1050
        confidential, 1050–1051
        flow phonation, 1052–1053
        Lee Silverman voice treatment,
            1051
        manual circumlaryngeal techniques,
            1051–1052
        resonant voice, 1052
        respiratory retraining, 1052
        semioccluded vocal tract, 1053
        vocal function exercises, 1053
    appropriate referrals for, 1054–1055,
        1054t
    limitation to success, 1055
    phonotrauma reduction, 1049–1050,
        1050f
    professional voice, 1073–1074
    reasons for success or failure, 1056t
    success, connotations of, 1056
    venn diagram, 1048, 1049f
    vocal hygiene, 1048–1049
Von Recklinghausen disease, 1630
    hearing loss, 1548–1549
von Willebrand disease, 27, 28, 498

W
Waardenburg syndrome, 124, 1543t,
    1549–1550, 1634, 1634f
Waldeyer ring lymphomas, 2037,
    2038f
Wallenberg syndrome, 2721, 2725–2726
Warfarin, 29
Warthin tumor, 186f, 1762, 1763f
Warts, 3219–3220, 3220f
    treatment of, 3228
Weber syndrome, 202
Webster-modified Bernard cheiloplasty,
    1800, 1801f
Wedge excision technique, 2232
Wegener granulomatosis, 276–277, 539,
    747, 880–881, 980
    clinical diagnosis, 493
    clinical presentation, 494
    diagnostic criteria of, 493, 494t
    etiology, 493

immunosuppressive therapy, 494
    otologic manifestations, 2522
    respiratory symptoms, 494
    signs and symptoms, 493
    surgical treatment, 494
Well-differentiated thyroid cancer, 2116
Whistling face syndrome, 1641
Wildervanck syndrome, 125
Wilkes classification, temporomandibular
    joint, 3f
Williams syndrome, 1641
Winkler disease, 2370
Witch's chin deformity, 3181
Wolff-Chaikoff phenomenon, 257
Work-related rhinitis, 474–475
Wound(s)
    adhesive, 52–53
    classification, 23t
    neoplasms, 2059–2060, 2061t
    soft tissue injuries
        classification, 1109–1110
        management, 1110–1112, 1111f, 1112t
Wound healing
    acute wounds, 75
    antimicrobial peptides, 84
    calreticulin, 84
    chronic wounds, 75
    coagulation and hemostasis phase,
        77–78, 78f
    cytokines in, 77t
    derangements of, 83
    factors affecting
        alcohol, 82
        arginine, 82–83
        collagen, 82
        diabetics, 81–82
        estrogen, age-related impairment, 81
        infections, 80–81
        inflammation, 81
        ischemia and tissue hypoxia, 80
        local edema, 80
        neuropathy, 82
        NSAIDs and glucocorticoids, 82
        obesity, 82
        protein, 82
        radiotherapy, 83
        smoking, 82

stress, 81
        vitamin C and A deficiency, 83
        zinc deficiency, 83
    gene transfer, 84
    history, 75
    hyperbaric oxygen treatment, 83–84
    inflammatory phase, 76, 76f
        early inflammatory phase, 78
        late inflammatory phase, 78–79
    pH changes, 84
    proliferative phase, 79
    remodeling phase, 79–80, 80t
    tissue injury, 76, 76f
W-plasty, for scar camouflage, 2862–2863,
    2863f

X
Xenographs, for soft tissue augmentation,
    3245
Xeroderma pigmentosa, 125
X-linked inheritance, 1629

Z
Zafirluka, 532
Zenker diverticula, 166f, 864
Zidovudine, 739t
Zileuton, 532, 546
Zithromax (Azithromycin), 1459t
Z-line, assessment of, 834
Z-plasty, for scar camouflage, 2861–2862,
    2862f
Zygomaticomaxillary complex fractures,
    1280–1281
    articulation, 1215–1216, 1216t
    demographics and etiology, 1228,
        1228f
    goals of, 1215
    hardware, 1217, 1217f
    incisions, 1215–1216, 1216f
    issue, 1215
    maxilla, 1220–1221, 1220f
    orbital floor management, 1217–1218
    palate, 1219–1220, 1219f
    reduction method, 1217
    surgical indications, 1231
    zygomatic arch, 1218–1219,
        1218f–1219f